THIRD EDITION

CLINICAL VIROLOGY

THIRD EDITION

CLINICAL VIROLOGY

EDITORS

DOUGLAS D. RICHMAN

Departments of Pathology and Medicine, University of California, San Diego School of Medicine, La Jolla, California, and Veterans Affairs San Diego Healthcare System, San Diego, California

RICHARD J. WHITLEY

Division of Infectious Diseases, Department of Pediatrics, School of Medicine, University of Alabama at Birmingham, Birmingham, Alabama

FREDERICK G. HAYDEN

Departments of Medicine and Pathology, University of Virginia School of Medicine, University of Virginia Health Sciences Center, Charlottesville, Virginia

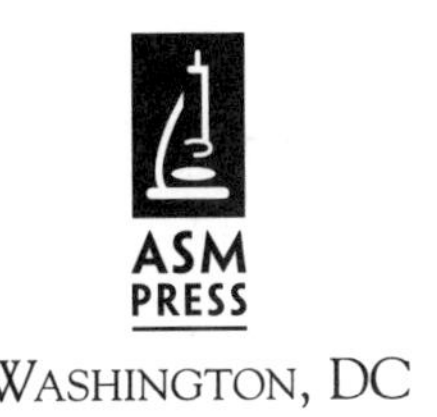

WASHINGTON, DC

Address editorial correspondence to ASM Press, 1752 N St. NW,
Washington, DC 20036-2904, USA

Send orders to ASM Press, P.O. Box 605, Herndon, VA 20172, USA
Phone: 800-546-2416; 703-661-1593
Fax: 703-661-1501
E-mail: books@asmusa.org
Online: estore.asm.org

Library of Congress Cataloging-in-Publication Data

Clinical virology / editors, Douglas D. Richman, Richard J. Whitley, Frederick G. Hayden.—3rd ed.
p. ; cm.
Includes bibliographical references and index.
ISBN 978-1-55581-425-0
1. Virus diseases. 2. Diagnostic virology. I. Richman, Douglas D. II. Whitley, Richard J. III. Hayden, Frederick G.
[DNLM: 1. Virus Diseases—diagnosis. 2. Virus Diseases—therapy. 3. Antiviral Agents—therapeutic use. 4. Viruses—pathogenicity. WC 500 C639 2009]
RC114.5.C56 2009
616.9′1—dc22

2008019983

10 9 8 7 6 5 4 3 2 1

To our families—Eva, Sara, Matthew, Adam, and Isabella; Kevin, Christopher, Jennifer, and Katherine; Melissa, Dan, Gabriella, Gretta, and Geoffrey—and to our many colleagues and friends, who have inspired and supported us throughout the years.

Contents

SECTION II
The Agents / 385

PART A DNA VIRUSES

PART B RNA VIRUSES

Contributors

ADRIANO AGUZZI
University Hospital Zürich, Institute of Neuropathology, CH-8091 Zürich, Switzerland

GÖRAN AKUSJÄRVI
Department of Medical Biochemistry and Microbiology, BMC, 751 23 Uppsala, Sweden

DAVID A. ANDERSON
Macfarlane Burnet Institute for Medical Research and Public Health, Alfred Medical Research and Education Precinct, Melbourne 3004, Victoria, Australia

LARRY J. ANDERSON
Division of Viral Diseases, National Center for Immunization and Respiratory Diseases, Centers for Disease Control and Prevention, Atlanta, GA 30333

CARLOS F. ARIAS
Departamento de Genética del Desarrollo y Fisiología Molecular, Instituto de Biotecnología, Universidad Nacional Autónoma de México, Cuernavaca, Morelos 62210, Mexico

ROBERT L. ATMAR
Departments of Medicine and of Molecular Virology and Microbiology, Baylor College of Medicine, Houston, TX 77030

ALAN D. T. BARRETT
Department of Pathology, Center for Biodefense and Emerging Infectious Diseases, Sealy Center for Vaccine Development and Institute for Human Infections and Immunity, University of Texas Medical Branch, Galveston, TX 77555

BRENDA L. BARTLETT
Center for Clinical Studies, Houston, TX 77030

SALLY J. BELL
Department of Gastroenterology, St. Vincent's Hospital, Melbourne, Fitzroy, Victoria, Australia 3065

WILLIAM J. BELLINI
Measles, Mumps, Rubella, and Herpesvirus Laboratory Branch, Division of Viral Diseases, National Center for Immunization and Respiratory Diseases, Centers for Disease Control and Prevention, Atlanta, GA 30333

JACK R. BENNINK
Laboratory of Viral Diseases, National Institute of Allergy and Infectious Diseases, Bethesda, MD 20892

WILLIAM A. BLATTNER
Institute of Human Virology, University of Maryland School of Medicine, Baltimore, MD 21201

THOMAS P. BLECK
Department of Neurology, Evanston Northwestern Healthcare, Evanston, IL 60201

GUY BOIVIN
CHUQ-CHUL, Quebec City, Quebec, Canada G1V 4G2

WILLIAM BONNEZ
University of Rochester School of Medicine and Dentistry, Rochester, NY 14642

MIKE BRAY
Division of Clinical Research, National Institute of Allergy and Infectious Diseases, National Institutes of Health, Bethesda, MD 20892

JAMES C. M. BRUST
Division of Infectious Diseases, Columbia University Medical Center, New York, NY 10032

R. MARK BULLER
Department of Molecular Microbiology and Immunology, Saint Louis University, St. Louis, MO 63104

BARRIE J. CARTER
Targeted Genetics Corporation, Seattle, WA 98109

KEVIN A. CASSADY
Department of Pediatrics, University of Alabama at Birmingham, Birmingham, AL 35233

YUAN CHANG
Molecular Virology Program, University of Pittsburgh Cancer Institute, Pittsburgh, PA 15213

MANHATTAN E. CHARURAT
Institute of Human Virology, University of Maryland School of Medicine, Baltimore, MD 21201

ALESSIA CIANCIO
Division of Gastroenterology and Hepatology, Torino University Medical School, Torino 10126, Italy

MICHEL COUILLARD
Laboratoire de Santé Publique du Québec, Institut National de Santé Publique de Québec, Sainte-Anne-de-Bellevue, Quebec, Canada H9X 3R5

JULES L. DIENSTAG
Gastrointestinal Unit, Massachusetts General Hospital, Boston, MA 02114

DAVID EASTY
Department of Ophthalmology, Bristol Eye Hospital, Bristol BS1 2LX, United Kingdom

VINCENT CLIVE EMERY
Centre for Virology, Hampstead Campus, Royal Free and University College Medical School, London NW3 2PF, United Kingdom

JANET A. ENGLUND
Department of Pediatrics, Children's Hospital and Regional Medical Center, University of Washington, and Fred Hutchinson Cancer Research Center, Seattle, WA 98105

DEAN D. ERDMAN
Division of Viral Diseases, National Center for Immunization and Respiratory Diseases, Centers for Disease Control and Prevention, Atlanta, GA 30333

MARY K. ESTES
Departments of Molecular Virology and Microbiology and of Medicine, Baylor College of Medicine, Houston, TX 77030

STEPHEN M. FEINSTONE
Laboratory of Hepatitis Viruses, Division of Viral Products, Center for Biologics Evaluation and Research, FDA, Bethesda, MD 20892

FRANK FENNER
The John Curtin School of Medical Research, The Australian National University, Canberra 2601, Australia

MANUEL A. FRANCO
Instituto de Genética Humana, Pontificia Universidad Javeriana, Bogotá, Colombia

ANNE A. GERSHON
Departments of Pediatrics and Microbiology, Columbia University College of Physicians & Surgeons, New York, NY 10032

ROGER I. GLASS
Fogarty International Center, National Institutes of Health, Bethesda, MD 20892

JOSEPH C. GLORIOSO
Department of Molecular Genetics and Biochemistry, University of Pittsburgh School of Medicine, Pittsburgh, PA 15261

JOHN W. GNANN, JR.
Department of Medicine, Division of Infectious Diseases, University of Alabama at Birmingham, Birmingham, AL 35294, and Veterans Affairs Medical Center, Birmingham, AL 35233

BARNEY S. GRAHAM
Vaccine Research Center, National Institute of Allergy and Infectious Diseases, National Institutes of Health, Bethesda, MD 20892

PAOLO GRANDI
Department of Neurological Surgery, University of Pittsburgh School of Medicine, Pittsburgh, PA 15261

HARRY B. GREENBERG
Departments of Medicine, Microbiology, and Immunology, Stanford University School of Medicine and Veterans Affairs Palo Alto Health Care System, Palo Alto, CA 94305

JOHN E. GREENLEE
Neurology Service, VA Salt Lake City Healthcare System, and Department of Neurology, University of Utah School of Medicine, Salt Lake City, UT 84132

DIANE E. GRIFFIN
Department of Molecular Microbiology and Immunology, Johns Hopkins Bloomberg School of Public Health, Baltimore, MD 21205

PAUL DAVID GRIFFITHS
Centre for Virology, Hampstead Campus, Royal Free and University College Medical School, London NW3 2PF, United Kingdom

JOHN C. GUATELLI
Department of Medicine, University of California San Diego, La Jolla, CA 92093

SCOTT M. HAMMER
Division of Infectious Diseases, Columbia University Medical Center, New York, NY 10032

FREDERICK G. HAYDEN
Departments of Medicine and Pathology, University of Virginia Health Sciences Center, Charlottesville, VA 22908

IAN HICKIE
Brain and Mind Research Institute, University of New South Wales, Sydney 2052, Australia

KARL M. JOHNSON
Special Pathogens Branch, Centers for Disease Control and Prevention, Atlanta (retired), 10 Calle Final, Placitas, NM 87043

DAVID W. KIMBERLIN
Division of Pediatric Infectious Diseases, The University of Alabama at Birmingham, Birmingham, AL 35233

DONALD B. KOHN
Departments of Pediatrics and Molecular Microbiology & Immunology, University of Southern California Keck School of Medicine, Division of Research Immunology/Bone Marrow Transplantation, Childrens Hospital Los Angeles, Los Angeles, CA 90027

THOMAS G. KSIAZEK
Special Pathogens Branch, Division of Viral and Rickettsial Diseases, National Center for Zoonotic, Vector-Borne, and Enteric Diseases, Centers for Disease Control and Prevention, Atlanta, GA 30333

DANIEL R. KURITZKES
Section of Retroviral Therapeutics, Brigham and Women's Hospital, Division of AIDS, Harvard Medical School, Cambridge, MA 02139

WAI-MING LEE
Department of Pediatrics, University of Wisconsin Clinical Sciences Center, Madison, WI 53706

T. JAKE LIANG
Liver Diseases Branch, National Institute of Diabetes and Digestive and Kidney Diseases, National Institutes of Health, Bethesda, MD 20892

ANDREW R. LLOYD
The Inflammatory Diseases Research Unit, School of Medical Sciences, University of New South Wales, Sydney 2052, Australia

STEPHEN A. LOCARNINI
Department of Molecular Research and Development, Victorian Infectious Diseases Reference Laboratory, North Melbourne, Victoria, Australia 3051

KATHERINE LUZURIAGA
Department of Pediatrics and Program in Molecular Medicine, University of Massachusetts Medical School, Worcester, MA 01605

JOHN S. MACKENZIE
Australian Biosecurity CRC, Curtin University of Technology, Perth, Western Australia 6845, Australia

ANNETTE MARTIN
Department of Virology, Laboratory of Molecular Genetics of Respiratory Viruses, CNRS URA 3015, Institut Pasteur, 75724 Paris, France

JULIE E. MARTIN
Vaccine Research Center, National Institute of Allergy and Infectious Diseases, National Institutes of Health, Bethesda, MD 20892

TONY MAZZULLI
Department of Microbiology, Mount Sinai Hospital, Toronto, Ontario, Canada M5G 1X5

KENNETH McINTOSH
Division of Infectious Diseases, Children's Hospital, Boston, MA 02115

ERNESTO MÉNDEZ
Departamento de Genética del Desarrollo y Fisiología Molecular, Instituto de Biotecnología, Universidad Nacional Autónoma de México, Cuernavaca, Morelos 62210, Mexico

GREGORY J. MERTZ
Department of Internal Medicine, University of New Mexico Health Sciences Center, Albuquerque, NM 87131

JORDAN P. METCALF
Pulmonary and Critical Care Medicine, Department of Medicine, University of Oklahoma Health Sciences Center, Oklahoma City, OK 73104

OLLI MEURMAN
Department of Microbiology, Turku University Hospital, PL 52, 20521 Turku, Finland

RICHARD MILNE
Centre for Virology, Hampstead Campus, Royal Free and University College Medical School, London NW3 2PF, United Kingdom

PATRICK S. MOORE
Molecular Virology Program, University of Pittsburgh Cancer Institute, Pittsburgh, PA 15213

YASUKO MORI
National Institute of Biomedical Innovation, Ibaraki, Osaka 567-0085, Japan

WILLIAM J. MOSS
Departments of Epidemiology, International Health, and Molecular Microbiology and Immunology, Johns Hopkins Bloomberg School of Public Health, Baltimore, MD 21205

FRANK J. O'NEILL
VA Salt Lake City Healthcare System and Department of Oncological Sciences, Division of Molecular Biology and Genetics, University of Utah School of Medicine, Salt Lake City, UT 84148

PETER PALESE
Departments of Microbiology and of Medicine, Mount Sinai School of Medicine, New York, NY 10029

MANISH PATEL
Division of Viral Diseases, National Center for Immunization and Respiratory Diseases, Centers for Disease Control and Prevention, Atlanta, GA 30333

J. S. M. PEIRIS
Department of Microbiology, The University of Hong Kong, Queen Mary Hospital, Pokfulam, Hong Kong SAR

C. J. PETERS
University of Texas Medical Branch, Galveston, TX 77555

LYLE R. PETERSEN
Division of Vector-Borne Infectious Diseases, Centers for Disease Control and Prevention, Fort Collins, CO 80522

MARTIN PETRIC
British Columbia Centre for Disease Control, Vancouver, British Columbia, Canada V5Z 4R4

PEDRO A. PIEDRA
Departments of Molecular Virology and Microbiology and of Pediatrics, Baylor College of Medicine, Houston, TX 77030

THEODORE C. PIERSON
Laboratory of Viral Diseases, National Institute of Allergy and Infectious Diseases, Bethesda, MD 20892

DOUGLAS D. RICHMAN
Departments of Pathology and Medicine, University of California San Diego, La Jolla, CA 92093

MARIO RIZZETTO
Division of Gastroenterology and Hepatology, Torino University Medical School, Torino 10126, Italy

BERNARD ROIZMAN
The Marjorie B. Kovler Viral Oncology Laboratories, The University of Chicago, Chicago, IL 60637

JOSÉ R. ROMERO
Division of Pediatric Infectious Diseases, Arkansas Children's Hospital and University of Arkansas for Medical Sciences, Little Rock, AR 72202

PAUL A. ROTA
Measles, Mumps, Rubella, and Herpesvirus Laboratory Branch, Division of Viral Diseases, National Center for Immunization and Respiratory Diseases, Centers for Disease Control and Prevention, Atlanta, GA 30333

YARON ROTMAN
Liver Diseases Branch, National Institute of Diabetes and Digestive and Kidney Diseases, National Institutes of Health, Bethesda, MD 20892

CHARLES E. RUPPRECHT
Poxvirus and Rabies Branch, Division of Viral and Rickettsial Diseases, Centers for Disease Control and Prevention, Atlanta, GA 30333

OLLI RUUSKANEN
Department of Pediatrics, Turku University Hospital, PL 52, 20521 Turku, Finland

ISWAR L. SHRESTHA
Siddhi Polyclinic, Dilli Bazar, Kathmandu, Nepal

GARRY SHUTTLEWORTH
Department of Ophthalmology, Singleton Hospital, Swansea SA2 8QA, United Kingdom

ROBERT F. SILICIANO
Department of Medicine, Johns Hopkins University School of Medicine, Baltimore, MD 21205

SAUL J. SILVERSTEIN
Departments of Pediatrics and Microbiology, Columbia University College of Physicians & Surgeons, New York, NY 10032

PETER SIMMONDS
Centre for Infectious Diseases, University of Edinburgh, Summerhall, Edinburgh EH9 1QH, United Kingdom

ANTONINA SMEDILE
Division of Gastroenterology and Hepatology, Torino University Medical School, Torino 10126, Italy

DAVID W. SMITH
Division of Microbiology and Infectious Diseases, PathWest Laboratory Medicine WA, Nedlands, Western Australia 6009, Australia

MAGDALENA E. SOBIESZCZYK
Division of Infectious Diseases, Columbia University Medical Center, New York, NY 10032

PHILIP R. SPRADLING
Surveillance and Epidemiology Branch, Division of Viral Hepatitis, Centers for Disease Control and Prevention, Atlanta, GA 30333

JOHN L. SULLIVAN
Department of Pediatrics and Program in Molecular Medicine, Office of Research, University of Massachusetts Medical School, Worcester, MA 01655

ANDREW W. TAI
Gastrointestinal Unit, Massachusetts General Hospital, Boston, MA 02114

BARBARA S. TAYLOR
Division of Infectious Diseases, Columbia University Medical Center, New York, NY 10032

ALEXANDER J. V. THOMPSON
Department of Gastroenterology, St. Vincent's Hospital, Melbourne, Fitzroy, Victoria, Australia 3065

HONG VAN TIEU
Division of Infectious Diseases, Columbia University Medical Center, New York, NY 10032

JEFFREY A. TOWBIN
Texas Children's Hospital, Baylor College of Medicine, Houston, TX 77030

JOHN J. TREANOR
Infectious Diseases Unit, University of Rochester School of Medicine, Rochester, NY 14642

RONALD B. TURNER
Department of Pediatrics, University of Virginia School of Medicine, Charlottesville, VA 22908

STEPHEN K. TYRING
Department of Dermatology, University of Texas Health Science Center, Houston, TX 77030

DENIS WAKEFIELD
The Inflammatory Diseases Research Unit, School of Medical Sciences, University of New South Wales, Sydney 2052, Australia

SCOTT C. WEAVER
Department of Pathology, University of Texas Medical Branch, Galveston, TX 77555

RICHARD J. WHITLEY
Departments of Pediatrics, Microbiology, and Medicine, University of Alabama at Birmingham, Birmingham, AL 35233

JOHN V. WILLIAMS
Departments of Pediatrics and of Microbiology and Immunology, Vanderbilt University School of Medicine, Nashville, TN 37232

JOSEPH K. WONG
Department of Medicine, Veterans Affairs Medical Center and University of California San Francisco, San Francisco, CA 94121

KOICHI YAMANISHI
National Institute of Biomedical Innovation, Ibaraki, Osaka 567-0085, Japan

JONATHAN W. YEWDELL
Laboratory of Viral Diseases, National Institute of Allergy and Infectious Diseases, Bethesda, MD 20892

MICHAEL T. YIN
Division of Infectious Diseases, Columbia University Medical Center, New York, NY 10032

STEVEN YUKL
Department of Medicine, Veterans Affairs Medical Center and University of California San Francisco, San Francisco, CA 94121

JOHN A. ZAIA
Division of Virology, Beckman Research Institute City of Hope, Duarte, CA 91010

Preface

Virology is currently one of the most dynamic areas of clinical medicine. Challenges related to novel viruses, changing epidemiologic patterns, new syndromes, unmet vaccine needs, antiviral drug resistance, and threats of bioterrorism are balanced against improved insights into viral pathogenesis, better diagnostic tools, novel immunization strategies, and an expanding array of antiviral agents. The demands on clinicians, public health workers, and laboratorians will continue to increase as will the opportunities for effective intervention. This text, now in its third edition, is designed to inform scientists and health care professionals about the medically relevant aspects of this rapidly evolving field.

Clinical Virology has two major sections. The first addresses infections and syndromes related to particular organ systems, as well as the fundamentals of modern medical virology, including immune responses and vaccinology, diagnostics, antivirals, and the nascent field of gene therapy. The second provides agent-specific chapters that detail the virology, epidemiology, pathogenesis, clinical manifestations, laboratory diagnosis, and prevention and treatment of important viral pathogens. In a multiauthored text like *Clinical Virology*, the selection of authors is key. The senior authors for individual chapters were chosen because of their internationally recognized expertise and active involvement in their respective fields. In addition, common templates for the syndrome-specific and separately for the agent-specific chapters allow the reader to readily access material. Since publication of the second edition in 2002, all of the chapters have been extensively revised to incorporate new information and relevant citations. In addition, the rapidly expanding field of antiviral drugs demanded dividing the subject into two chapters.

We have been particularly fortunate in receiving invaluable help from our administrative assistants, Bryna Block, Stephanie McKinney, Dunia Ritchey, and Diane Ramm. In addition, we express our appreciation for the enthusiastic professional support provided by Jeff Holtmeier, Jennifer Adelman, and Susan Birch of ASM Press.

DOUGLAS D. RICHMAN
RICHARD J. WHITLEY
FREDERICK G. HAYDEN

Important Notice (Please Read)

This book is intended for qualified medical professionals who are aware that medical knowledge is constantly changing. As new information becomes available, changes in treatment, diagnostic procedures, equipment, and the use of drugs and biologicals become necessary. The editors, authors, and publisher have, as far as it is possible, taken care to ensure that the information given in this text is accurate and up-to-date but cannot guarantee that it is. Consequently, readers are strongly advised to confirm that the information, especially with regard to drug usage, complies with the latest legislation and standards of practice. The authors, editors, and publisher make no warranty, expressed or implied, that the information in this book is accurate or appropriate or represents the standard of care for any particular facility or environment or any individual's personal situation.

Introduction

DOUGLAS D. RICHMAN, RICHARD J. WHITLEY, AND FREDERICK G. HAYDEN

1

Clinical virology incorporates a spectrum of disciplines and information ranging from the X-ray crystallographic structure of viruses and viral proteins to the global socioeconomic impact of disease. Clinical virology is the domain of molecular biologists, geneticists, pharmacologists, microbiologists, vaccinologists, immunologists, practitioners of public health, epidemiologists, and clinicians, both pediatric and adult. It encompasses events that include accounts ranging from epidemics impacting history and Jennerian vaccination to the identification of new agents and mechanisms of disease. For example, since the previous edition of this text, multiple new viral pathogens have emerged or been recognized, including coronaviruses (NL63, HKU1, and severe acute respiratory syndrome), parvoviruses (bocavirus and PARV4), polyomaviruses, the recently reported arenavirus following transplantation (4), mimivirus (5), adenovirus 14 as a lethal pneumonia agent, and the reemergence of influenza A (H5N1) as a global threat. Previously recognized agents, like metapneumoviruses and rhinoviruses, have been appreciated to cause more disease than originally thought (2), and previously recognized agents, like Chikungunya virus, responsible for endemic local disease have reemerged in epidemic proportions (1). Morbidity and mortality due to chronic viral infections, especially human immunodeficiency virus and chronic hepatitis B and C viruses, are being increasingly documented. We hope that the fascinating breadth and importance of the subject of clinical virology will be conveyed by this text. In this edition, we have attempted to update and improve upon the information in the previous edition.

A few facts about nomenclature should be noted. Students (among others) are bewildered by virus classification. Historically, classification reflected the information available from general descriptive biology. Viruses were thus classified by host (e.g., plant, insect, mouse, or bird), by disease or target organ (e.g., respiratory, hepatitis, or enteric), or by vector (e.g., arboviruses). These classifications were often overlapping and inconsistent. Molecular biology now permits us to classify by genomic and biophysical structure, which can be quantitative and evolutionarily meaningful. Table 1 is derived from the comprehensive *Virus Taxonomy: Eighth Report of the International Committee on Taxonomy of Viruses* (3).

The list in Table 1 represents viruses known to infect humans. Many of the agents are primarily animal viruses that incidentally infect humans, e.g., herpesvirus B, rabies virus, the *Arenoviridae*, the *Filoviridae*, the *Bunyaviridae*, and many arthropod-borne viruses. The role of intraspecies transmission of viruses is becoming increasingly appreciated. Although its contribution to zoonotic infections like H5N1 and antigenic shift of influenza A virus is well documented, the role of intraspecies transmission is a major consideration in the emerging diseases caused by Sin Nombre virus and related hantaviruses, Nipah virus, Ebola virus, arenavirus, hemorrhagic fever viruses, the agent of variant bovine spongiform encephalopathy, and, most importantly, the human immunodeficiency viruses. Although not a documented risk, the theoretical threats of organ transplants from primates and pigs prompted a section on xenotransplantation in the chapter on transplantation. There are, in addition, a number of human viruses that have not been recognized to cause human disease, including spumaretroviruses, reoviruses, and the adeno-associated parvoviruses. The text does not elaborate on these viruses in detail, but we did elect to include a chapter on TT virus (TTV) and the circoviruses, despite any proven disease association, because of their remarkably high prevalence in human populations globally and the remarkably high titers achieved in the blood. We elected not to cover other viruses that are uncertain pathogens in humans but recognized causes of disease in animals, such as bornaviruses.

In order to provide a comprehensive yet concise treatment of the diverse agents and diseases associated with human viral infections, we have chosen to organize this book into two major sections. The first provides information regarding broad topics in virology, including immune responses, vaccinology, laboratory diagnosis, principles of antiviral therapy, and detailed considerations of important organ system manifestations and syndromes caused by viral infections. The second section provides overviews of specific etiologic agents and discusses their biology, epidemiology, pathogenesis of disease causation, clinical manifestations, laboratory diagnosis, and management. We have attempted to ensure that the basic elements are covered for each of the viruses of interest, but it is the authors of each of these chapters who have done the real work and to whom we owe our gratitude.

TABLE 1 Taxonomy of human viruses

Family[a]	Subfamily or genus	Type species or example[b]	Morphology	Envelope	Chapter
DNA viruses					
dsDNA viruses					
Poxviridae			Brick shaped or ovoid	+	18
	Chordopoxvirinae				
	Orthopoxvirus	Vaccinia virus, variola virus			
	Parapoxvirus	Orf virus			
	Molluscipoxvirus	Molluscum contagiosum virus			
	Yatapoxvirus	Yaba monkey tumor virus			
Herpesviridae			Icosahedral	+	
	Alphaherpesvirinae				
	Simplexvirus	Human herpesviruses (HSV) 1 and 2			19
		Cercopithecine herpesvirus 1 (herpesvirus B)			20
	Varicellovirus	Human herpesvirus 3 (VZV)			21
	Betaherpesvirinae				
	Cytomegalovirus	Human herpesvirus 5 (CMV)			22
	Roseolovirus	Human herpesviruses 6 and 7			23
	Gammaherpesvirinae				
	Lymphocryptovirus	Human herpesvirus 4 (EBV)			24
	Rhadinovirus	Human herpesvirus 8 (KSHV)			25
Adenoviridae	*Mastadenovirus*	Human adenoviruses	Icosahedral	–	26
Polyomaviridae	*Polyomavirus*	JC virus	Icosahedral	–	27
Papillomaviridae	*Papillomavirus*	Human papillomaviruses	Icosahedral	–	28
ssDNA viruses					
Parvoviridae	*Parvovirinae*		Icosahedral	–	
	Erythrovirus	B19 virus			29
	Dependovirus	Adeno-associated virus 2[c]			
	Bocavirus	Human bocavirus			
Circoviridae	*Circovirus*	TTV	Icosahedral	–	30
DNA and RNA reverse-transcribing viruses					
Hepadnaviridae	*Orthohepadnavirus*	Hepatitis B virus	Icosahedral	+	31
Retroviridae			Spherical	+	
	Deltaretrovirus	HTLV-1 and -2			32
	Lentivirus	Human immunodeficiency viruses 1 and 2			33
	Spumavirus	Spumavirus (foamy virus)[c]			

(Continued on next page)

TABLE 1 *(Continued)*

Family[a]	Subfamily or genus	Type species or example[b]	Morphology	Envelope	Chapter
RNA viruses					
dsRNA viruses					
Reoviridae			Icosahedral	–	
	Orthoreovirus	Reovirus 3[c]			
	Orbivirus	Kemerovo virus			34
	Rotavirus	Human rotaviruses			35
	Coltivirus	Colorado tick fever virus			34
	Seadornavirus	Banna virus			34
Negative-stranded ssRNA viruses					
Paramyxoviridae			Spherical	+	
	Paramyxovirinae				
	Respirovirus	Human parainfluenza viruses			36
	Morbillivirus	Measles virus			37
	Rubulavirus	Mumps virus			38
	Henipavirus	Nipah virus			39
	Pneumovirinae				
	Pneumovirus	Human respiratory syncytial virus			36
	Metapneumovirus	Human metapneumovirus			36
Rhabdoviridae			Bacilliform	+	40
	Vesiculovirus	Vesicular stomatitis virus			
	Lyssavirus	Rabies virus			
Filoviridae	*Filovirus*	Ebola virus	Bacilliform	+	41
Orthomyxoviridae			Spherical	+	42
	Influenzavirus A	Influenza A virus			
	Influenzavirus B	Influenza B virus			
	Influenzavirus C	Influenza C virus			
Bunyaviridae	*Orthobunyavirus*	Bunyamwera virus, La Crosse virus	Amorphic	+	43
	Hantavirus	Hantaan virus, Sin Nombre virus			
	Nairovirus	Crimean-Congo hemorrhagic fever virus			
	Phlebovirus	Rift Valley fever virus			
Arenaviridae	*Arenavirus*	Lymphocytic choriomeningitis virus	Spherical	+	44
Positive-stranded ssRNA viruses					
Picornaviridae	*Enterovirus*	Polioviruses	Icosahedral	–	45
	Rhinovirus	Human rhinoviruses			46
	Hepatovirus	Hepatitis A virus			47
Caliciviridae	*Calicivirus*	Norwalk virus	Icosahedral	–	48
Hepeviridae	*Hepevirus*	Hepatitis E virus	Icosahedral	–	49
Astroviridae	*Mamastrovirus*	Human astrovirus 1	Icosahedral	–	50

(Continued on next page)

TABLE 1 Taxonomy of human viruses *(Continued)*

Family[a]	Subfamily or genus	Type species or example[b]	Morphology	Envelope	Chapter
Coronaviridae	*Coronavirus*	Human coronavirus	Pleomorphic	+	51
Flaviviridae			Spherical	+	
	Flavivirus	Yellow fever virus			52
	Hepacivirus	Hepatitis C virus			53
Togaviridae			Spherical	+	
	Alphavirus	Western equine encephalitis virus			54
	Rubivirus	Rubella virus			55
Subviral agents: satellites, viroids, and agents of spongiform encephalopathies					
Satellites (ssRNA)	*Deltavirus*	Hepatitis delta virus	Spherical	+	56
Prion protein agents		Creutzfeldt-Jakob agent	?	–	57

[a] ds, double stranded; ss, single stranded.
[b] HSV, herpes simplex virus; VZV, varicella-zoster virus; CMV, cytomegalovirus; EBV, Epstein-Barr virus; KSHV, Kaposi's sarcoma-associated herpesvirus; HTLV-1, human T-cell lymphotropic virus type 1; TTV, TT virus.
[c] Human virus with no recognized human disease.

REFERENCES

1. **Charrel, R. N., X. de Lamballerie, and D. Raoult.** 2007. Chikungunya outbreaks—the globalization of vectorborne diseases. *N. Engl. J. Med.* **356:**769–771.
2. **Deffrasnes, C., M. E. Hamelin, and G. Boivin.** 2007. Human metapneumovirus. *Semin. Respir. Crit. Care Med.* **28:** 213–221.
3. **Fauquet, C. M., M. A. Mayo, J. Maniloff, U. Desselberger, and L. A. Ball (ed.).** 2005. *Virus Taxonomy: Eighth Report of the International Committee on Taxonomy of Viruses.* Elsevier Academic Press, San Diego, CA.
4. **Palacios, G., J. Druce, L. Du, T. Tran, C. Birch, T. Briese, S. Conlan, P.-L. Quan, J. Hui, J. Marshall, J. F. Simons, M. Egholm, C. D. Paddock, W.-J. Shieh, C. S. Goldsmith, S. R. Zaki, M. Catton, and W. I. Lipkin.** 2008. A new arenavirus in a cluster of fatal transplant-associated diseases. *N. Engl. J. Med.* **358:**991–998.
5. **Raoult, D., B. La Scola, and R. Birtles.** 2007. The discovery and characterization of mimivirus, the largest known virus and putative pneumonia agent. *Clin. Infect. Dis.* **45:**95–102.

Viral Syndromes and General Principles

SECTION I

Respiratory Infections

JOHN J. TREANOR

2

Respiratory viral infections have a major impact on health. Acute respiratory illnesses, largely caused by viruses, are the most common illnesses experienced by otherwise healthy adults and children. In the United States, the 1992 National Health Interview Survey data suggest that such illnesses are experienced at a rate of 85.6 illnesses per 100 persons per year and account for 54% of all acute conditions exclusive of injuries (26). A total of 44% of these illnesses require medical attention and result in 287 days of restricted activity, 94.4 days lost from work, and 182 days lost from school per 100 persons per year. The morbidity of acute respiratory disease in the family setting is significant. The Tecumseh study, a family-based surveillance study of respiratory illness, estimated that respiratory viral infections result in 2.4 illnesses per person per year; approximately one-quarter of these illnesses result in consultation with a physician (103). Illness rates for all acute respiratory conditions are highest in young children; children below the age of 9 years are estimated to experience between five and nine respiratory illnesses per year (85), while adults experience between three and five such illnesses (103).

Mortality due to acute viral respiratory infection in otherwise healthy individuals is rare in economically developed countries, with the exception of epidemic influenza and possibly respiratory syncytial virus (RSV) or adenovirus infection. However, acute respiratory infection is a major cause of childhood mortality in developing countries (11), and it is estimated that 4.5 million children under 5 years of age die annually from acute respiratory illness. Viruses are identified in about 3 to 40% of cases of respiratory disease in this setting and are estimated to play a contributing role in approximately 20 to 30% of deaths (11). Measles alone accounts for 6 to 21% of the morbidity and from 8 to 93% of the mortality due to acute lower respiratory infection in developing countries (96).

Both RNA and DNA viruses are responsible for these infections, producing clinical syndromes ranging in severity from merely uncomfortable to life-threatening. Each of these viruses may be responsible for different clinical syndromes depending on the age and immune status of the host. Furthermore, each of the respiratory syndromes associated with viral infection may be caused by a variety of specific viral pathogens (Table 1). This chapter describes the clinical syndromes of respiratory virus infection, the spectrum of viruses associated with these syndromes, and the pathophysiology of these illnesses. Specific features of the virology and pathophysiology of disease induced by individual viral agents are described in greater detail in each of the virus-specific chapters.

SEASONAL PATTERNS OF RESPIRATORY VIRUS INFECTION

Many of the viruses associated with acute respiratory disease display a significant seasonal variation in incidence, especially in temperate climates (Fig. 1). Although the exact seasonal arrival of each virus in the community cannot be predicted with precision, certain generalizations are useful diagnostically and in planning control strategies. For example, both influenza virus and RSV epidemics occur predominantly in the winter months, with a peak prevalence in January to March in the northern hemisphere. Parainfluenza virus type 3 (PIV-3) infections show a predominance in the spring, while PIV-1 and PIV-2 cause outbreaks in the fall to early winter. Rhinoviruses may be isolated throughout the year, with increases in frequency in the spring and fall. The peak prevalence of enteroviral isolations is in late summer and early fall, while adenoviruses are isolated at roughly equal rates throughout the year. The herpesviruses do not show significant seasonal variation in incidence, except for varicella-zoster virus infection, which occurs throughout the year but more commonly in late winter and early spring.

COMMON COLDS

Clinical Features and Syndrome Definition

The term "cold" really does not constitute a single viral entity, but rather a syndrome with a variety of causes. Most observers consider colds to include symptoms of rhinitis with variable degrees of pharyngitis; the predominant associated symptoms include nasal stuffiness, sneezing, runny nose, and sore throat. Patients often report chills, but significant fever is unusual in adults. Cough and hoarseness are variably present and may be more frequent in the elderly (39). Headache and mild malaise may occur. Although a multitude of viruses may be associated with this syndrome, the pattern of symptoms associated with colds

TABLE 1 Estimated frequency with which individual viral respiratory syndromes are caused by specific viral pathogens

Virus	Frequency[a] of syndrome							
	Colds	Pharyngitis	Tracheobronchitis	Croup	Bronchiolitis	Pneumonia		
						Children[b]	Adults	Immunocompromised individuals
RNA viruses								
Influenza virus								
Type A	+	++	+++	++	+	++	++++	+
Type B	+	++	++	+	+	+	++	+
PIV								
Type 1	+	++	+	++++	+			
Type 2	+	++	+	++	+			
Type 3	+	++	+	+++	++	+++	+	+
RSV	++	+		++	++++	++++	+	++
hMPV	+				++	++		±
Measles virus			+	+		++	+	+
Rhinovirus	++++	++	+	+	+	+		±
Enterovirus	++	++			+	+		
Coronavirus	++	+		++				±
SARS coronavirus							+[c]	
DNA viruses								
Adenovirus		++	+	++	++	++	++	++
Herpes simplex virus		+			+	+		++
Varicella-zoster virus						+	+	+
EBV		++						
CMV		+				++		++++

[a] The relative frequency of causation is graded semiquantitatively as follows: +, causes some cases (1 to 5% of cases); ++, fairly common cause (5 to 15% of cases); +++, common cause (15 to 25% of cases); ++++, major cause (>25% of cases); ±, rarely reported, occasional case reports.

[b] Individuals under the age of 5 years.

[c] Only during the outbreak of SARS.

does not appear to vary significantly between agents. Physical findings are nonspecific and most commonly include nasal discharge and pharyngeal inflammation. More severe disease, with higher fever, may be seen in children.

Overall, colds are one of the most common of disease experiences. Adults average six to eight colds per 1,000 person-days during the peak cold season and from two to four colds per person per year (56). Rates of colds are higher in children, who average six to eight colds per year. Adults with children at home have a higher frequency of colds, and women are generally affected more often than men.

Colds are self-limited, with a median duration of illness of approximately 9 to 10 days in adults (7). Recognized complications of colds include secondary bacterial infections of the paranasal sinuses and middle ear and exacerbations of asthma, chronic bronchitis, and emphysema. Involvement of the middle ear is common, and changes in middle-ear pressures have been documented following both experimentally induced and naturally occurring rhinovirus (32) and influenza virus (16) infections. These abnormalities are likely due to eustachian tube dysfunction and probably account for the frequency with which otitis media complicates colds. Colds are associated with symptomatic otitis media in approximately 2% of cases in adults (28) and in a higher proportion in young children (69). Rhinoviruses and other common-cold viruses have been detected in middle-ear fluids in approximately 20 to 40% of cases of otitis media with effusion in children (113). Infections with RSV, influenza virus, and adenoviruses are often also associated with otitis media (69).

Colds are also associated with abnormalities of the paranasal sinuses which may or may not be evident clinically. Mucosal thickening and/or sinus exudates have been observed acutely in as many as 77% of subjects with colds (57, 129). However, clinically manifest acute sinusitis is seen only in a small (0.5 to 5%) proportion of adults with naturally occurring colds.

Clinical colds in atopic individuals may be more severe or more likely to result in wheezing than in nonatopic individuals, and rhinoviruses have been identified as major causes of asthma exacerbations in children and adults (42). The mechanism of this increased susceptibility is unclear but may be related to an altered immune response to infection. Rhinovirus colds may increase asthma by augmenting airway allergic responses such as histamine release

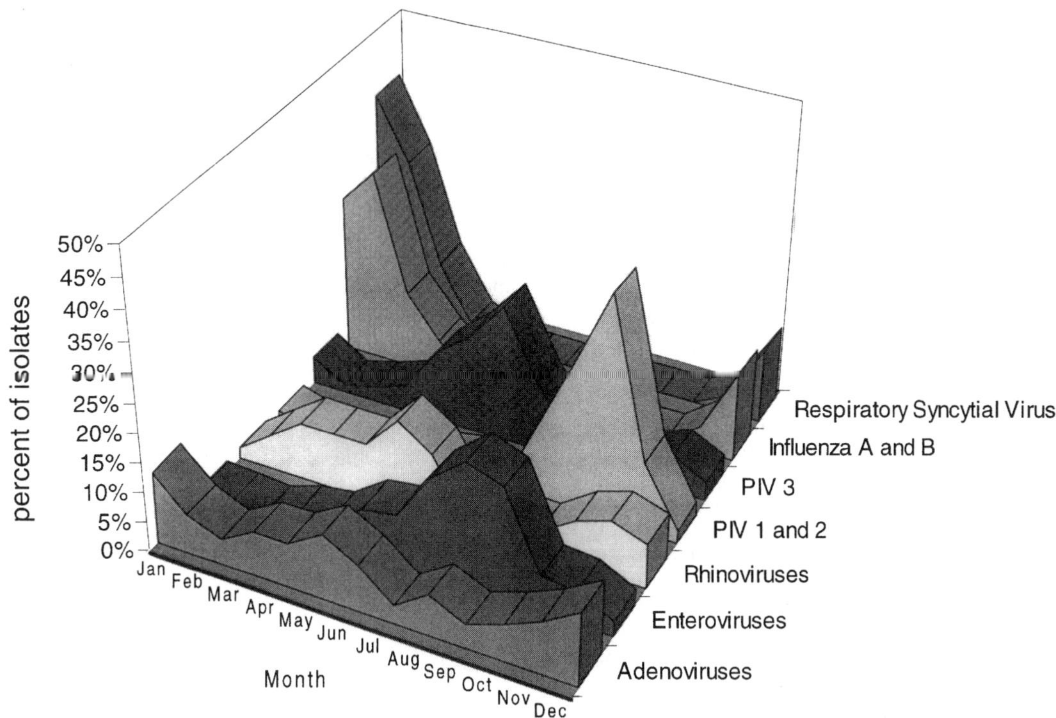

FIGURE 1 Many of the viruses which affect the respiratory tract exhibit a seasonal variation in prevalence. In this figure, numbers of virus isolates from children seen in private pediatric practices in Rochester, NY, are plotted by month of isolation. Data represent the 6-year average from 1990 to 1995 and are expressed as the percentage of all isolates of each virus which occurred in the given month.

and eosinophil influx after antigen challenge. Rhinoviruses have also been identified as important causes of exacerbations of chronic obstructive pulmonary disease (95, 139).

Etiology and Differential Diagnostic Features

The majority of common colds are associated with infection with rhinoviruses or other picornaviruses, particularly when very sensitive techniques, such as PCR, are used for diagnosis (7, 73). Other agents frequently associated with common colds include coronaviruses and, in nonprimary infections, PIV and RSV, with a variety of other agents implicated occasionally (Table 1).

The differential diagnosis of individuals presenting with typical signs and symptoms is limited. However, in the presence of additional signs or symptoms which are not part of this clinical description, such as high, persistent fever, signs of respiratory distress, or lower respiratory tract disease, alternative diagnoses should be sought. Allergic causes should be considered in individuals who present with recurrent symptoms restricted to the upper respiratory tract.

Pathogenesis

Studies of the pathogenesis of the common cold have largely focused on rhinoviruses, the most commonly implicated viral etiology. Transmission of most of the viruses responsible for the common cold is by direct contact or large droplets, with inoculation of virus into the upper respiratory tract. In situ hybridization studies of nasal biopsy specimens from rhinovirus-infected subjects demonstrate that infection is largely confined to relatively small numbers of ciliated nasal mucosal epithelial cells (6), although occasional nonciliated cells are also infected (6). Sloughing of these epithelial cells is seen in naturally occurring colds, but the epithelial lining remains intact, with structurally normal cell borders. Infection is not associated with significant increases in the numbers of lymphocytes in the nasal mucosa, but increases in the numbers of polymorphonuclear leukocytes have been detected in nasal mucosa and secretions, probably due to elaboration of interleukin 8 (IL-8) by infected cells (131). Although rhinoviruses are not able to grow efficiently at body temperature, virus can be detected within cells of the lower airway even in uncomplicated colds in healthy subjects (104).

In general, the number of infected cells appears to be quite limited, even in fairly symptomatic individuals (7). Such findings suggest that virus-induced cellular injury is not the direct cause of symptoms in rhinovirus colds and that inflammatory mediators play an important role. The nasal secretions during the initial response to rhinovirus infection are predominantly the result of increased vascular permeability, as demonstrated by elevated levels of plasma proteins in nasal secretions (74). Glandular secretions (lactoferrin, lysozyme, and secretory immunoglobulin A) predominate later in colds (74). Similar observations have been made in allergic rhinitis. However, in contrast to the situation in allergic rhinitis, histamine does not appear to play a role in the induction of symptoms in colds, as nasal histamine levels do not increase, and therapy with selective H1 antihistamines is not effective (114). Nasal secretion kinin, IL-1, IL-6, and IL-8 levels increase during colds, and kinin and IL-8 concentrations correlate with symptoms (106). In addition, intranasal administration of bradykinin mimics the induction of signs and symptoms in the common cold, including increased nasal vascular permeability, rhinitis, and sore throat (118). Enhanced synthesis of proinflammatory cytokines and cell adhesion molecules in the middle ear may also contribute to the pathogenesis of otitis media associated with colds (108).

Treatment and Prevention

Treatment of colds is directed toward alleviation of symptoms. Nasal irrigation with isotonic saline effectively reduces sore throat, cough, nasal congestion, and nasal secretion in children (124). Symptoms of sneezing and rhinorrhea can be alleviated with nonselective antihistamines such as brompheniramine, chlorpheniramine, or clemastine fumarate, at the cost of some sedation (58, 130). The effect is probably due to the anticholinergic properties of these drugs because, as mentioned earlier, treatment with selective H1 inhibitors is not effective. Topical application of vasoconstrictors such as phenylephrine or ephedrine provides relief of nasal obstruction but may be associated with a rebound of symptoms upon discontinuation if used for more than a few days. Studies of pseudoephedrine have demonstrated measurable improvements in nasal airflow consistent with a decongestant effect (77, 128). Topical application of ipratropium, a quaternary anticholinergic agent that is minimally absorbed across biological membranes, reduces rhinorrhea significantly in naturally occurring colds (27). This agent probably exerts its major effect on the parasympathetic regulation of mucous and seromucous glands. Nonsteroidal anti-inflammatory drugs such as naproxen moderate the systemic symptoms of rhinovirus infection (125). Symptomatic therapy with systemic anticholinergic drugs or anticholinergic-sympathomimetic combinations has not been shown to confer any benefit and has been shown to be associated with significant side effects (29). In particular, the use of the decongestant phenylpropanolamine has recently been shown to be associated with an increased risk of hemorrhagic stroke (145), and this drug has been removed from over-the-counter cold remedies. In fact, most over-the-counter cough and cold remedies have not been studied at all in pediatric populations, in which they may be associated with significant side effects and generally should not be used (122). As expected, there is also no benefit in treatment of colds with antibacterial agents, although they are frequently prescribed for colds, particularly in children.

Development of a vaccine to prevent the common cold would be a difficult undertaking because more than 100 serotypes of rhinovirus have been characterized, and many noncultivatable rhinoviruses appear to exist (88). In addition, with the exception of influenza viruses, vaccines for the other viruses responsible for colds have yet to become available. Since colds due to PIV and RSV represent reinfection of individuals who already have been exposed multiple times, it may be difficult to effectively prevent them by vaccination. Although many agents with potent in vitro activity against rhinoviruses have been evaluated in clinical trials, only intranasal interferon for prophylaxis of rhinovirus colds and oral pleconaril for their treatment have some evidence of clinical benefit (67). No antivirals are currently available for therapy of common colds.

PHARYNGITIS

Clinical Features and Syndrome Definition

Pharyngitis is a common complaint of both adults and children and is one of the more common reasons for seeking outpatient medical care. In general, this term refers to individuals who present with the primary complaint of sore throat, and the term should probably be reserved for those individuals who manifest some objective evidence of pharyngeal inflammation as well. The clinical manifestations of pharyngitis are dominated by the specific causative agent. However, generally the syndrome can be divided into those cases in which nasal symptoms accompany pharyngitis, which are predominantly viral in nature, and those cases without nasal symptoms, which have a somewhat more diverse spectrum of etiologic considerations, including both group A and non-group A streptococci, *Chlamydia* (strain TWAR), *Mycoplasma*, and other agents (72).

Etiology and Differential Diagnostic Features

Viral pathogens associated with acute pharyngitis are summarized in Table 1. Rhinovirus colds are frequently accompanied by pharyngitis, although objective signs of pharyngeal inflammation are uncommon. Adenovirus infections are frequently associated with pharyngitis, and a specific syndrome of pharyngoconjunctival fever, consisting of fever, pharyngitis, and bilateral conjunctivitis, is associated with adenovirus types 3 and 7. A variety of enteroviral serotypes are associated with febrile pharyngitis. Herpangina is a specific coxsackievirus-induced pharyngitis in which small (1- to 2-mm) vesicular lesions of the soft palate rupture to become small white ulcers. Pharyngitis is a typical component of acute influenza in which individuals experience the sudden onset of systemic symptoms of fever, myalgias, and malaise accompanied by upper respiratory signs and symptoms, including pharyngitis. Primary oral infection with herpes simplex virus may present with pharyngitis, typically with vesicles and shallow ulcers of the palate, tongue, and pharyngeal mucosa and cervical lymphadenopathy.

Pharyngitis may be the presenting or predominating symptom in more generalized viral infections. Pharyngitis is a significant complaint in approximately one-half of cases of the acute mononucleosis syndrome due to Epstein-Barr virus (EBV). Pharyngitis in this syndrome is generally exudative and is accompanied by cervical and generalized lymphadenopathy, as well as fever, hepatosplenomegaly, and other systemic symptoms. The heterophile antibody test is typically positive in the second week of illness. Cytomegalovirus (CMV) can cause an identical syndrome which is monospot negative and may be associated with pharyngitis more commonly in children than adults. An acute mononucleosis-like syndrome with pharyngitis may also be the presenting manifestation of primary human immunodeficiency virus infection.

The differential diagnosis of acute pharyngitis generally centers upon the differentiation of streptococcal from viral etiologies. Features suggestive of streptococcal pharyngitis include tonsillar swelling, moderate to severe tenderness on palpation, enlargement of lymph nodes, presence of scarlatiniform rash, and absence of coryza (8). The presence of nasal symptoms or of conjunctivitis favors a viral etiology, and as described above, some viral syndromes may present with distinguishing characteristics which help in their identification. Generally, acute pharyngitis in children less than 3 years of age is predominantly viral in origin. The presence of exudate is suggestive of bacterial etiology, but exudates may also be seen with adenovirus or EBV. Rapid diagnostic tests for the office identification of group A streptococci are widely available and are indicated in most cases where the etiology is uncertain. When highly sensitive tests are used, backup cultures are generally not necessary (46). Routine studies for other bacterial and nonbacterial pathogens are usually not obtained.

Pathogenesis

As described above, pharyngitis in the common cold is probably the result of chemical mediators of inflammation, which are potent stimulators of pain nerve endings. Potentially similar mechanisms may account for pharyngitis in other viral syndromes as well. Direct viral damage and other host inflammatory responses may also contribute.

Treatment and Prevention

The treatment of most cases of viral pharyngitis is symptomatic. Patients suspected of having influenzal pharyngitis who are seen within the first 2 days of illness can be treated with antiviral therapy (see chapter 42). In immunosuppressed patients with chronic herpetic pharyngitis or healthy hosts with primary gingivostomatitis, acyclovir therapy is recommended (see chapter 19).

Treatment of group A streptococcal infections with antimicrobial agents is generally initiated to prevent rheumatologic complications of this infection, and because treatment of acute streptococcal pharyngitis is associated with more rapid resolution of symptoms, although the absolute benefits are rather modest (24). Guideline recommendations for the selective use of throat cultures and antibiotic treatment can reduce unnecessary use of antibiotics for treatment of pharyngitis (99).

CROUP (ACUTE LARYNGOTRACHEOBRONCHITIS)

Clinical Features and Syndrome Definition

Croup, or viral laryngotracheobronchitis, is a clinically distinct illness that predominantly affects children under the age of 3 years (19). The illness typically begins with upper respiratory tract symptoms of rhinorrhea and sore throat, often with a mild cough. After 2 or 3 days, the cough deepens and develops a characteristic brassy, barking quality, which is similar to a seal's bark. Fever is usually present, generally between 38 and 40°C, although those with croup due to RSV may have normal temperatures. The child may appear to be apprehensive and most comfortable sitting forward in bed. The respiratory rate is elevated, but usually not over 50; this contrasts with bronchiolitis, where more severe tachypnea is often seen. Chest wall retractions, particularly in the supraclavicular and suprasternal areas, may be observed. Children with this finding on presentation have a higher risk of hospitalization or of requiring ventilatory support.

The characteristic physical finding of croup is inspiratory stridor. Inspiration is prolonged, and in very severe cases, some degree of expiratory obstruction may also be seen. Rales, rhonchi, and wheezing, which reflect the characteristic involvement of the lower respiratory tract, may be heard on physical examination. A fluctuating course is typical, and the child may appear to worsen or improve within an hour. Hypoxemia occurs in 80% of children with croup severe enough to require hospitalization. The degree of hypoxia is generally difficult to ascertain clinically, but pulse oximetry provides a reliable and noninvasive means to monitor the state of oxygenation. Children who develop respiratory insufficiency as a result of increasing fatigue also may have elevations in partial pressure of CO_2 in arterial blood ($PaCO_2$). Other routine laboratory assays are generally unremarkable. Children with croup characteristically exhibit subglottic narrowing of the tracheal air shadow on posteroanterior films of the neck, the so-called "steeple" sign (Fig. 2). This finding may be useful in differentiating croup from epiglottitis. Chest X rays may reveal parenchymal infiltrates, which are part of the characteristic involvement of the lower respiratory tract in this syndrome.

Croup is predominantly a disease of young children, with a peak age incidence in the second year of life. In the Seattle virus watch family study, the annual incidence of croup was 5.2 per 1,000 in the first 6 months of life, 11.0 per 1,000 in the second 6 months, 14.9 per 1,000 in the second year of life, and 7.5 per 1,000 in those 2 to 3 years of age, with a marked drop after that age (41).

Etiology and Differential Diagnostic Features

An estimate of the relative importance of individual infectious agents in croup is shown in Table 1. The PIVs are the most common viruses responsible for croup, accounting for about 75% of cases (25). Of the PIVs, PIV-1 and -2 are most commonly associated with croup (25), and the seasonal incidence of croup reflects the seasonal variations in PIV incidence (Fig. 1). Less common causes of croup include RSV, influenza A or B viruses, rhinoviruses, coronaviruses, CMV, adenoviruses, and *Mycoplasma pneumoniae*. Measles virus is a relatively less common cause of croup but is associated with especially severe disease (119). My-

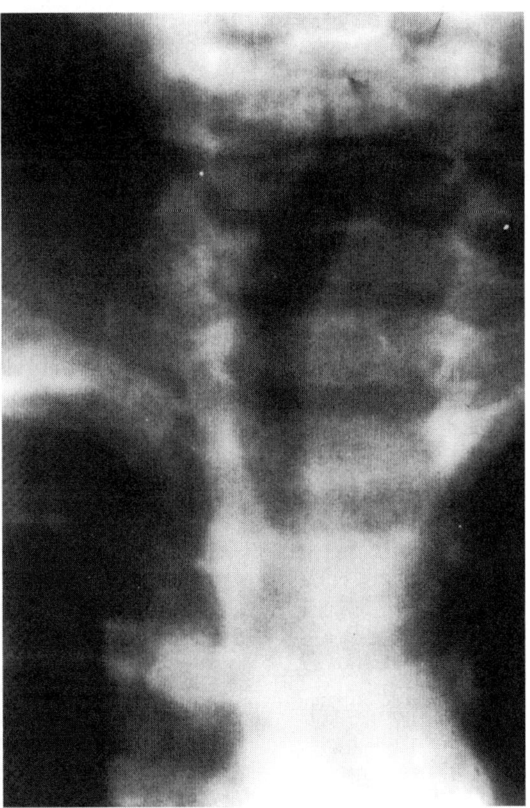

FIGURE 2 Posteroanterior roentgenogram of the neck of a child with viral croup that shows the characteristic narrowing of the air shadow of the trachea in the subglottic area. (Courtesy of Carolyn B. Hall, University of Rochester.)

coplasma pneumoniae and influenza viruses tend to be isolated more commonly from older children with croup (25). PIV-2 and influenza A viruses are associated with more severe disease (82), but generally the clinical manifestations of the croup syndrome due to individual agents are similar. Specific viral diagnosis is not routinely attempted since the clinical syndrome is sufficient for diagnosis, and management generally does not depend on identification of the specific agent.

The majority of cases of inspiratory stridor in children are caused by viral croup. However, it is critical to distinguish these syndromes from other, potentially more serious causes of airway obstruction such as bacterial epiglottitis and tracheitis. Epiglottitis is an acute cellulitis of the epiglottis and surrounding structures. Patients present with acute respiratory distress and drooling, but the barking cough of croup is absent. Epiglottitis in children was usually caused by *Haemophilus influenzae* type b, but this infection has virtually vanished in the United States since the introduction of polysaccharide conjugate vaccines, and the incidence of epiglottitis in children has also declined considerably (98). In adults, and rarely in children, epiglottitis may be caused by a variety of other bacterial agents such as *Haemophilus parainfluenzae* or beta-hemolytic streptococci, which may spread from a contiguous focus of infection. Bacterial tracheitis is a relatively rare syndrome that mimics croup. Abundant purulent sputum is often present. Bacterial tracheitis is usually caused by *Staphylococcus aureus* or *H. influenzae* type b; other bacteria such as beta-hemolytic streptococci and *Streptococcus pneumoniae* have also been associated with this syndrome. Other infectious causes of stridor, including peritonsillar or retropharyngeal abscess or diphtheria, and noninfectious causes of stridor, such as trauma or aspiration of a foreign body, should be considered.

Direct visualization of the epiglottis may be necessary to exclude bacterial etiologies, and facilities and personnel for this procedure and for emergency airway management should be available. Lateral neck radiographs may show edema of the epiglottis (Fig. 3) or thickening of the retropharyngeal space in individuals with retropharyngeal abscess. However, radiographs are limited in accuracy and should be performed with caution for individuals with respiratory distress. It may be useful to administer racemic epinephrine, as a rapid response is suggestive of croup.

Pathogenesis

The severity of clinical symptoms in PIV croup appears to be directly related to the level of virus replication (61). The viral infection in croup produces inflammation in both the upper respiratory tract and the lung parenchyma. The classic signs of croup, including the barking cough and inspiratory stridor, arise mostly from inflammation occurring in the larynx and trachea. Inflammatory changes are seen by histology in the epithelial mucosa and submucosa of the larynx and trachea. The cellular infiltrate includes histiocytes, lymphocytes, plasma cells, and polymorphonuclear leukocytes. The inflammation and obstruction are greatest at the subglottic level, which is the least distensible part of the airway because it is encircled by the cricoid cartilage. Consequently, localized inflammation and edema lead to obstruction to airflow. The impeded flow of air through this narrowed area produces the classic high-pitched vibration. Obstruction is greater during inspiration because the narrowing occurs in the extrathoracic portion of the airway and is enhanced in small children because the walls of the airways in these individuals are relatively compliant and can collapse to a greater extent. Obstruction of airflow results in an initial decline in tidal volume, which is compensated by an increase in respiratory rate to maintain

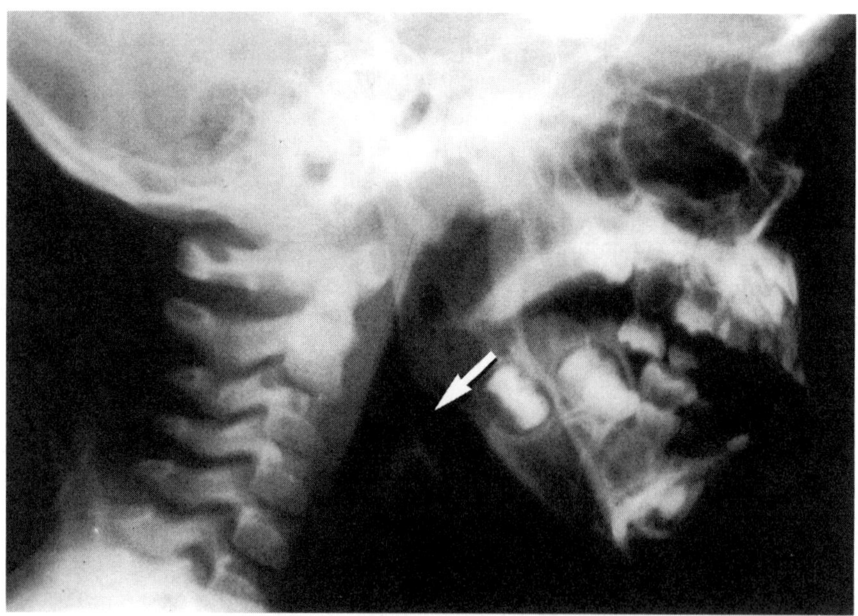

FIGURE 3 Lateral neck radiograph of the neck of a child with epiglottitis demonstrates the characteristic thickening of the epiglottis in this disease and may be helpful in distinguishing this illness from croup or retropharyngeal abscess. (Courtesy of Carolyn B. Hall, University of Rochester.)

adequate alveolar ventilation. However, if the obstruction increases, the work of breathing may increase until the child tires, and as the respiratory rate declines, the child develops hypercarbia and respiratory failure.

Involvement of the lower respiratory tract is integral to the pathophysiology of croup (Fig. 4) (63). Inflammatory changes are noted throughout the respiratory tract, including the linings of the bronchi, bronchioles, and even the alveoli. Consistent with these findings, hypoxemia is detected in about 80% of children hospitalized with croup. Although some degree of hypoxia can be explained on the basis of hypercarbia, the major pathophysiological mechanism is ventilation-perfusion mismatching. Pulmonary edema may complicate severe croup and upper airway obstruction (86). The onset of pulmonary edema often is immediately following intubation. Pulmonary edema in these cases appears to be due not to pulmonary artery hypertension but to local hypoxia and increased alveolar capillary transmural pressure.

Treatment and Prevention

Because the majority of hospitalized children are hypoxic, oxygen is important for severe disease and should be given to all hypoxemic patients. Humidified air, or mist, therapy is commonly used and has several potential roles. Desiccation of the inflamed epithelial surfaces is decreased, and the viscosity of the exudate is reduced. However, the value of mist therapy has not been proven, and removal of the child from the parents and placement in a mist tent can be more distressing to the child than beneficial.

Steroids have been shown to confer significant benefits in the management of mild, moderate, and severe croup, including more rapid improvement in symptoms, reduced length of hospital stay, and reduced rates of intubation. Administrations of a single dose of dexamethazone intramuscularly or orally and of budesonide by nebulizer are all effective, and comparative trials have shown all three strategies to be equally effective (78, 83). Administration of single-dose steroid therapy in this setting has not been associated with significant side effects and should probably be used in most patients with significant illness (12).

Administration of nebulized racemic epinephrine generally gives rapid, symptomatic relief in croup. It is believed that α-adrenergic stimulation by this drug causes mucosal vasoconstriction, leading to decreased subglottic edema. The onset of action is rapid, often within minutes, but the duration of relief is also limited, 2 h or less. Therefore, treated subjects should be observed closely for clinical deterioration. While symptomatic relief is considerable, use of epinephrine is not associated with improvements in oxy-

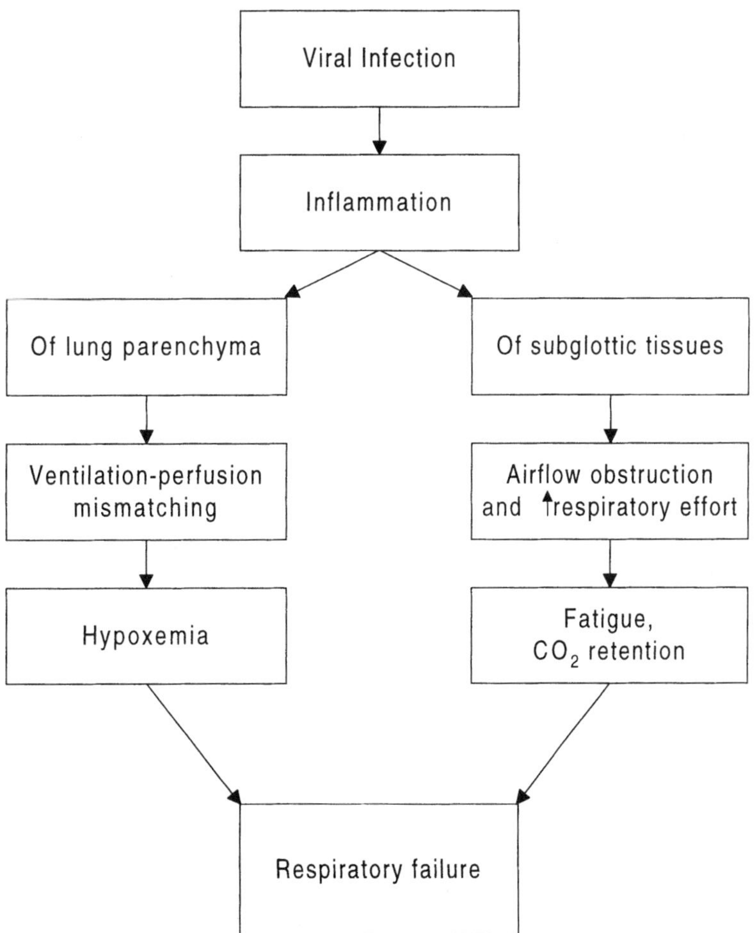

FIGURE 4 Pathophysiology of croup. Both mechanical obstruction of airflow and ventilation-perfusion mismatching due to parenchymal infection of the lung are responsible for the hypoxia and respiratory distress of croup. (Modified from reference 60 with permission.)

genation, probably because the defect in oxygen is associated with ventilation-perfusion mismatching due to lower respiratory tract involvement. In addition, tachycardia may occur. Thus, inhaled epinephrine is generally reserved for children who fail to respond to more conservative management.

Antiviral agents effective against some of the viruses responsible for croup are available but have not been tested for clinical efficacy. However, the potential benefit of the use of antiviral agents in the typical self-limited course of croup would likely be limited. Since croup is a viral illness, antibiotic therapy is of no benefit. Effective prevention of croup will largely depend on development of vaccines for the individual viral agents responsible for this syndrome. Vaccines are currently available for both measles and influenza viruses. There are currently no vaccines available for PIV, although live vaccines are in clinical development (51).

TRACHEITIS AND TRACHEOBRONCHITIS

Clinical Features and Syndrome Definition

In addition to causing croup and bronchiolitis, viral infection of the trachea and bronchi may cause tracheitis or tracheobronchitis. Tracheitis is characterized by tracheal tenderness, which can be elicited by gentle pressure on the anterior trachea just below the cricoid cartilage. Substernal discomfort on inhalation and nonproductive paroxysmal cough are noted. Nonproductive paroxysmal cough is also characteristic of tracheobronchitis and is usually much more severe at night. Later in the course of illness, small amounts of clear or whitish sputum may be produced. Accompanying symptoms may include fever, headache, myalgias, malaise, and anorexia. After several days of coughing, chest wall or abdominal discomfort which is muscular in nature may be noted. Physical findings are generally nonspecific; examination of the chest commonly reveals scattered rhonchi and occasional wheezing. Egophony, pleural friction rubs, or areas of dullness to percussion are not present.

Etiology and Differential Diagnostic Features

Tracheobronchitis is most typically caused by influenza A or B virus (Table 1). Herpes simplex has been associated with necrotizing tracheobronchitis in nonimmunocompromised hosts (123), and this syndrome is often accompanied by refractory bronchospasm.

The differential diagnosis of acute bronchitis includes nonviral infections and noninfectious etiologies such as cough-variant asthma. *Mycoplasma pneumoniae* and *Chlamydia pneumoniae* infections cause prolonged cough. *Bordetella pertussis* infection should also be considered in the differential diagnosis of prolonged cough illness. In otherwise healthy persons, workup of acute cough should be directed toward determining the presence of pneumonia.

Treatment and Prevention

Treatment in adults is best effected by prescribing rest, aspirin for headache and fever, cold-water vapor inhalation, and a cough suppressant such as guaifenesin with dextromethorphan. If coughing is particularly bothersome at night and interferes with sleep, a sedative together with one or two doses of cough syrup often is effective. For children, a recent trial has demonstrated that a single nocturnal dose of honey is as effective as dextromethorphan for suppressing cough due to upper respiratory tract infections (111). Herpetic disease has been treated successfully with acyclovir. In the absence of signs of pneumonia, treatment of prolonged cough with antibacterial agents is of no benefit (49, 136).

BRONCHIOLITIS

Clinical Features and Syndrome Definition

Bronchiolitis is a fairly characteristic syndrome of infants and young children whose presenting symptoms are dominated by the major pathophysiological defect, obstruction to expiratory airflow (141). The onset of lower respiratory symptoms is usually preceded by rhinitis, often with nasal congestion and discharge. More severe symptoms characteristically occur 2 to 3 days later, but in some cases they are concurrent with the onset of upper respiratory symptoms. In many instances, there may be a history of exposure to an adult or sibling with a cold or other minor respiratory illness or a history of exposure to other cases of bronchiolitis in the day care setting.

The hallmark of disease is wheezing, which can be quite marked, with flaring of the nostrils and use of accessory muscles of respiration. Cough may or may not be prominent initially, and when cough is present, it may be paroxysmal in nature. Slight cyanosis is often observed, but the presence or absence of cyanosis is not a reliable indicator of the degree of oxygenation or of the severity of disease. Physical findings are generally confined to the chest, with development of rales, which are usually musical in the beginning and then become more moist. Hyperresonance of the chest may be observed, and the liver may be displaced downward due to hyperinflation. The respiratory rate is elevated, with rates of 50 to 80 breaths per minute. Fever is frequently present at the beginning of the illness but may no longer be present at the time lower respiratory tract involvement develops. Among hospitalized infants, one-third or more are afebrile, despite marked lower respiratory tract disease. Thus, the presence or absence of fever does not indicate the severity of the child's illness. Mild conjunctivitis is noted in about a third of cases, with pharyngitis of varied severity in about half and otitis media in 5 to 10%. The hospital course is variable, but most infants will show improvement in 3 to 4 days (62).

Radiological findings are generally nonspecific, with reported findings including air trapping, consolidation, and collapse (80). Air trapping is particularly indicative of RSV bronchiolitis and may be the only radiological finding (Fig. 5). However, there is no correlation between the radiographic findings and the clinical course (43). Chest radiographs should be obtained to rule out alveolar filling defects suggestive of bacterial pneumonia and for those infants with severe disease, sudden deterioration, or underlying disorders (23). Results of routine laboratory tests are generally unremarkable, and the peripheral leukocyte count is usually not elevated. Abnormal water, electrolyte, and endocrine homeostasis may be seen during acute illness, including elevated antidiuretic hormone secretion and low fractional excretion of sodium (50). Electrolyte disturbances, most notably hyponatremia, may be seen with severe disease, particularly if excessive amounts of hypotonic fluid are administered (126). Acute disease may be associated with elevations in pulmonary artery pressure,

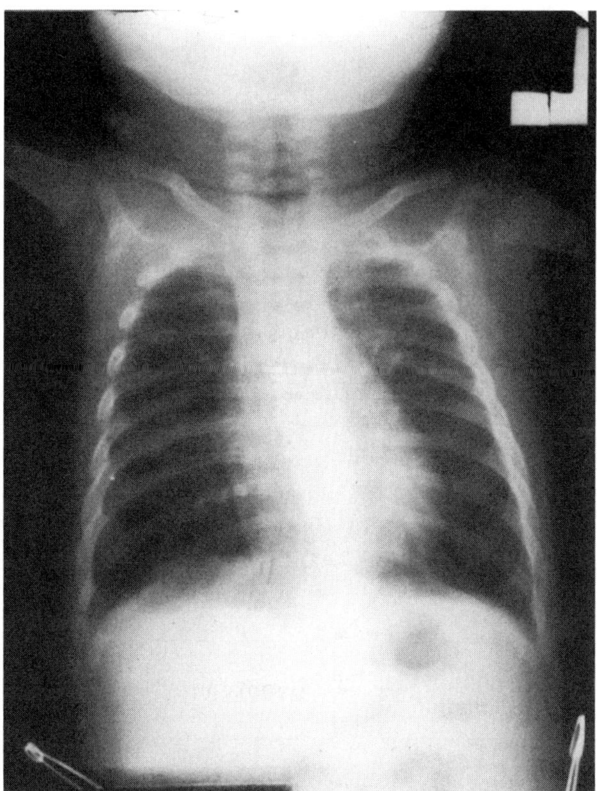

FIGURE 5 The chest radiograph in bronchiolitis characteristically shows hyperinflation due to obstruction of airflow. A variety of other findings may be present, including interstitial infiltrates or lobar consolidation. (Courtesy of Carolyn B. Hall, University of Rochester.)

but echocardiographic studies are usually unremarkable in infants with structurally normal hearts (109).

Bronchiolitis is a disease predominantly of infancy, and the epidemiology of this disease closely parallels that of the major infectious cause, RSV. The peak age incidence is between 2 and 6 months of age, with over 80% of cases occurring in the first year of life (110). The rate of hospitalization of infants during the first 12 months of life for bronchiolitis is estimated to be approximately 10 per 1,000 population (81), with the peak age of hospitalization between 1 and 3 months. Hospitalization rates are highest in children who reside in industrialized urban settings. In North Carolina, the rates of hospitalization for bronchiolitis in children less than 5 years of age were 1/714, 1/588, and 1/227 in rural, urban, and heavily industrialized areas, respectively (68). Among groups of a lower socioeconomic status, hospitalization rates of 0.5 to 1% of the entire population of infants in the first year of life are not uncommon (48).

The risk of hospitalization and severe bronchiolitis is particularly high in infants with congenital heart or lung disease or with immunodeficiency (64). In addition, infants born prematurely and those who are less than 6 weeks of age at the time of presentation are also at risk (89). More severe disease has also been documented to occur in children with a family history of asthma and those exposed to cigarette smoke in the family setting.

Etiology and Differential Diagnostic Features

RSV causes the majority of cases of bronchiolitis, and during the RSV epidemic season, essentially all cases are due to this virus (142). Overall, RSV is recovered from about three-fourths of all infants admitted to the hospital with bronchiolitis (141). Other respiratory viruses causing bronchiolitis include PIV, influenza virus, mumps virus, and rhinoviruses (Table 1). Adenovirus types 3, 7, and 21 are relatively uncommon causes but may be associated with more severe disease, including bronchiolitis obliterans (10). Rhinoviruses represent a small but significant proportion of cases of bronchiolitis (100). Rhinoviruses can also mimic RSV infection in infants with bronchopulmonary dysplasia (20).

Human metapneumovirus (hMPV) is also a significant cause of bronchiolitis (132, 140). The clinical picture most closely resembles that of RSV, and bronchiolitis is the major manifestation in children. Clinical features include wheezing and hypoxia. There are no clinical features that can distinguish between disease caused by hMPV and RSV, although generally that due to RSV may be more severe. Novel human coronaviruses, such as NL-63, have also been associated with lower respiratory tract disease in infants (36). An additional recently described human parvovirus, the human bocavirus, has been found in as many as 20% of cases of acute wheezing in young children (2). This virus is often detected in the presence of other viruses, and the exact role it plays in this syndrome has not been determined completely (4).

The differential diagnosis of diseases characterized by expiratory airflow obstruction in infants is relatively small. Pertussis can occasionally be confused with bronchiolitis, but more frequent vomiting, more paroxysmal cough, and lymphocytosis would be clues to the diagnosis of pertussis. Differentiation of acute infectious bronchiolitis from the initial presentation of allergic asthma is difficult, and this contributes to the difficulty in assessing therapeutic interventions in this disease. Anatomic defects such as vascular rings can cause obstruction of the airway. Foreign bodies should be considered, especially in young infants. Gastroesophageal reflux is an additional consideration.

RSV and some of the other viral agents responsible for bronchiolitis can be isolated from nasopharyngeal secretions in cell culture, but nucleic acid detection techniques are more sensitive and detect a wider range of viruses (135). Rapid antigen detection techniques are widely used, and the sensitivity of such techniques is dependent on the quality of the nasopharyngeal specimen, with nasopharyngeal aspirates superior to brushings or swabs (9). Their utility in routine management is unclear, although they may be useful for infection control purposes.

Pathogenesis

The pathophysiology of infectious bronchiolitis has been described most completely in the case of infection with RSV. The basic pathophysiological changes in bronchiolitis are summarized in Fig. 6 (141). Viral infection of epithelial cells of the bronchioles leads to destruction and necrosis of the ciliated epithelium. Leukocytes, predominantly lymphocytes, can be seen in increased numbers in the peribronchial tissues (1). The submucosa becomes edematous, and there is increased production of mucus. Ultimately, dense plugs of alveolar debris and strands of fibrin form within small bronchi and bronchioles, which may partially or completely obstruct airflow. The patho-

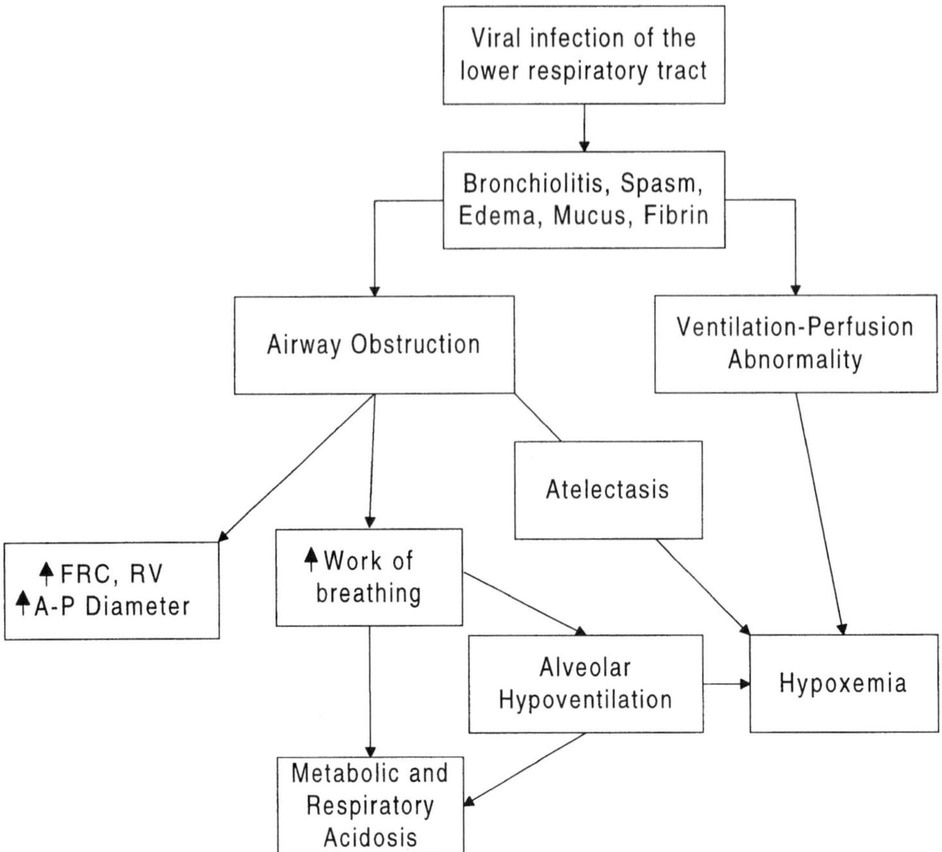

FIGURE 6 Pathophysiology of bronchiolitis. Viral infection of the lower respiratory tract results in inflammation and increased mucus production. Both airway obstruction and ventilation-perfusion mismatching are responsible for the clinical findings of hypoxia, hyperinflation, and hypoventilation. If uncorrected, these defects can lead to apnea or sudden death. FRC, functional residual capacity; RV, residual volume; A-P, anterior-posterior. (Modified from reference 141 with permission.)

genic basis for respiratory difficulty in bronchiolitis is related to obstruction of these small airways (141). Hypoxemia is the major abnormality of gas exchange, with ventilation-perfusion imbalance the major cause of the hypoxemia. In addition to hypoxia, hypercarbia and respiratory acidosis have been observed in some severely ill infants.

Infants appear to be particularly susceptible to the consequences of viral infection for several reasons. The peripheral airways are disproportionately narrow in the early years of life. In addition, collateral channels of ventilation, such as the pores of Kohn, are deficient in both number and size in the infant lung. Finally, the airways of infants are intrinsically more reactive to bronchospastic stimuli than are the airways of older children (91). However, it is not clear how RSV infection results in the observed histologic damage, and the reasons why some children experience relatively mild disease while others go on to respiratory failure are unknown.

The possibility that immune responses are involved in the pathogenesis of RSV bronchiolitis has received considerable attention. The presence of preexisting infection-induced antibody does not appear to play a role in enhancing the severity of disease because maternal antibody, or passively transferred antibody, is protective. Factors identified as potentially playing a role include overproduction of immunoglobulin E in response to infection, alteration in the cytokine phenotype of responding T cells, and release of leukotrienes in the airways (133).

Following recovery from acute bronchiolitis, some children experience continued episodes of wheezing, especially during apparently viral upper respiratory infections. Estimates are that the risk of either infrequent or frequent wheezing following recovery from documented RSV lower respiratory tract infection is increased about three- to fourfold (127). The mechanisms underlying this increased risk are unknown.

Treatment and Prevention

Recommendations regarding the treatment and prophylaxis of bronchiolitis have been summarized recently (3). Correction of hypoxemia is the most important aspect of managing RSV lower respiratory tract disease. Oxygenation should be monitored by pulse oximetry, and oxygen should be administered to infants whose oxygen saturation consistently falls below 90%. Since bronchiolitis is a viral disease which is infrequently complicated by bacterial superinfection, routine treatment with antibiotics is not warranted. Because of the dehydrating effect of tachypnea and reduced oral intake in some hospitalized infants, parenteral rehydration is often needed, but care must be taken to avoid inducing hyponatremia. Fluid intake and electrolyte concentrations should be carefully monitored in all infants with severe bronchiolitis, as hyponatremia and syndrome of inappropriate secretion of antidiuretic hormone may occur.

Data concerning the potential benefits of bronchodilator therapy are somewhat conflicting. Generally, bronchodilators produce modest short-term improvements in clinical scores but do not improve oxygenation, rates of hospitalization, or duration of hospital stay (134). The majority of studies of systemic corticosteroids have also failed to demonstrate a beneficial effect in acute bronchiolitis, and oral corticosteroids do not appear to have beneficial effects (21).

Antiviral therapy is available for some of the viruses responsible for bronchiolitis, but the use of such therapy for the most common etiology, RSV, remains controversial. Initial randomized placebo-controlled trials of ribavirin small-particle aerosol showed benefit in treatment of bronchiolitis in healthy infants, infants with high-risk underlying disease, and infants requiring mechanical ventilation. However, subsequent experience with use of the drug in clinical practice did not confirm this clinical benefit. In addition, when randomized trials were performed using normal saline instead of distilled water as a placebo, ribavirin did not appear to have clinical efficacy (55, 101). These findings, and the expense of this drug, suggest that ribavirin should be considered primarily in selected infants and young children with severe illness or at high risk of serious RSV disease.

A humanized neutralizing monoclonal antibody to the RSV F protein, palivizumab (Synagis), has had significant protective efficacy in a population of infants with prematurity or bronchopulmonary dysplasia, as well as in children with hemodynamically significant congenital heart disease. Administration of palivizumab intramuscularly at a dose of 0.15 mg/kg of body weight once per month resulted in a 55% reduction in RSV-related hospitalizations and a lower incidence of intensive care unit admissions in this population (75). Current recommendations for the use of passive antibody prophylaxis in the United States are to consider use in infants and children less than 2 years of age with chronic lung disease or congenital heart disease and in infants born at 32 weeks of gestation or earlier (who would be expected to receive little placental transfer of maternal antibody). Palivizumab may be considered for infants born between 32 and 35 weeks of gestation who have at least two additional risk factors, such as exposure to secondhand smoke or attendance at day care (3). Palivizumab is not effective for therapy of RSV disease.

Interruption of nosocomial transmission may be facilitated by thorough hand washing, decontamination of surfaces and inanimate objects, and isolation or cohorting of infected infants. Use of disposable eye-nose goggles by pediatric staff reduces the risk of nosocomial RSV infection in both staff and patients. Regular use of gowns, gloves, and possibly masks by hospital staff caring for infected children may also reduce the risk of nosocomial RSV spread. Protective isolation of high-risk infants or deferring their elective admission during institutional outbreaks of RSV has been recommended.

Vaccines are available to prevent bronchiolitis due to influenza virus and mumps virus, but there is no vaccine currently available for prevention of bronchiolitis due to RSV or PIV. There are multiple significant hurdles to the development of such vaccines, including the very young age at which the disease manifests, the suppressive effect of maternal antibody on vaccine responses, and, in the case of RSV, the potential for enhanced disease in vaccine recipients (44). However, several promising live vaccine candidates are in clinical development, and it has been demonstrated that it is possible to prevent RSV lower respiratory tract disease with such a vaccine (143).

VIRAL PNEUMONIA

Clinical Features and Syndrome Definition

Viral infections of the lower respiratory tract represent a wide spectrum of clinical entities, including croup and bronchiolitis, tracheobronchitis, and reactive airway changes. The development of pneumonia is defined by the development of abnormalities of alveolar gas exchange accompanied by inflammation of the lung parenchyma, often associated with visible changes on chest radiographs or abnormalities of other radiological studies such as computerized tomography or gallium scanning. Considerable variety exists in the presentation of viral pneumonia depending on the age and immunologic competence of the host and the specific viral pathogen, but there are certain general features which are described below.

The clinical features of primary viral pneumonia in immunocompetent adults have been best described for influenza viruses (chapter 42). Cough is generally nonproductive initially, although scant mucoid sputum develops commonly and production of frothy, pink-tinged sputum is seen in some severely ill individuals. Almost all reported cases have emphasized the predominant cyanosis and hypoxemia which are typical of severe primary viral pneumonia. Physical findings are often nonspecific; the patient generally appears to be acutely ill, conjunctivitis and rhinitis may be noted, and the trachea may be somewhat tender. Chest exam reveals increased respiratory rate and diffuse rales and wheezes. A variety of chest X-ray patterns have been described, but most typically diffuse, bilateral interstitial infiltrates are present. However, there are really no radiographic patterns that reliably differentiate between bacterial and viral pneumonia. The sputum is relatively scant and generally shows few polymorphonuclear leukocytes, and Gram's stain reveals minimal numbers of bacteria. In the original reports of influenza pneumonia, before the availability of mechanical ventilation, the clinical course was often progressively downhill, with a high mortality rate. However, there is a spectrum of disease severity, and the mortality rate in healthy adults in the nonpandemic era is low.

The basic presentation of viral pneumonia in children is similar but usually somewhat milder. The clinical presentation typically includes fever and lower respiratory tract signs and symptoms, such as difficulty breathing, nonproductive cough, and physical findings of wheezing or increased breath sounds. Young infants may present with apneic episodes with minimal fever. The clinical presentation may be dominated by the associated croup or bronchiolitis, both of which are frequently present.

Underlying cardiopulmonary diseases, such as valvular heart disease or chronic obstructive pulmonary disease, are well-recognized risk factors for viral pneumonia in adults and children. Pregnancy has mainly been recognized as a risk factor for pneumonia during pandemic influenza, but pregnancy has also been recognized as a risk factor for cardiopulmonary hospitalizations in the interpandemic period (107).

Bacterial superinfection is a common complication of viral lower respiratory tract infection, particularly in adults. The classic presentation is that of a typical episode of viral illness with more or less complete recovery, followed 2 to 14 days later by a recurrence of fever and development of cough and dyspnea (94). Chest X ray reveals lobar infiltrates, and the clinical course is typical of bacterial pneumonia. In addition, combined bacterial and viral pneumonia, with clinical features of each, is common in adults and with certain viruses in children. Bacterial superinfection of the lung in cases of viral pneumonia can occur with many bacteria, but the most common bacterium responsible for bacterial pneumonia complicating influenza is *Streptococcus pneumoniae*. There are also increases in the relative frequency of *Staphylococcus aureus*, including community-acquired methicillin-resistant organisms, and *Haemophilus influenzae* (121).

Etiology and Differential Diagnostic Features

Evaluation of the specific cause of acute pneumonia, and, in particular, attribution of pneumonia to a particular viral etiology, is complicated by difficulty in obtaining appropriate samples for culture, difficulty in detecting certain pathogens, and the frequent asymptomatic shedding of some viruses, such as herpesviruses or adenoviruses. Serologic diagnosis essentially establishes a temporal, but not causal, relationship between viral infection and a clinical syndrome and may be misleading during times of high prevalence of a particular viral agent. With these qualifications in mind, it is reasonable to make several broad generalizations regarding the role of viruses in acute pneumonia. The impact of viral pneumonia and the spectrum of associated viral agents are highly dependent on the age group and immune status of the host. While viruses are clearly important and frequent causes of pneumonia in young children, their role is less apparent in older children. In healthy adults, pure viral pneumonia is rare and is predominantly due to influenza or adenovirus. Elderly adults may experience more significant lower respiratory tract signs and symptoms following infection with agents which normally cause upper respiratory tract illness in younger adults, like RSV. Finally, viral pneumonia is an important cause of morbidity and mortality in individuals with compromised immune systems, with a broader spectrum of viral agents than seen in immunologically intact individuals.

Healthy Adults

The use of PCR and other sensitive diagnostic techniques has led to a greater appreciation of the role of viruses in community-acquired pneumonia in both adults (5) and the elderly (37). The majority of cases are associated with influenza viruses (Table 1), with a variety of other viruses also playing important roles, including RSV, hMPV, coronavirus, PIV, and rhinoviruses. Adenoviruses have been described as causes of significant outbreaks of atypical pneumonia in military recruits and, less often, in civilians. Illness is typically mild and clinically resembles that due to M. *pneumoniae*, but more severe disseminated infections and deaths have been reported (84). Multiple X-ray patterns are noted; there may be large pleural effusions. Prodromal symptoms of upper respiratory infection are reported by most patients, and pharyngitis is often found on presentation. Bacterial superinfection, particularly with *Neisseria meningitidis*, may occur. Adenovirus serotypes 4 and 7 are most often implicated, but recent reports have emphasized the emergence of a relatively rare adenovirus, serotype 14, responsible for severe community-acquired pneumonia in adults and children (93).

Varicella also occasionally causes pneumonia in adults (102). Chest radiographs taken in adults with varicella will reveal infiltrates in 10 to 20%, most frequently with a nodular infiltrate with peribronchial distribution involving both lungs; however, the majority of these individuals are asymptomatic. More severe illness is seen occasionally, and fatal varicella pneumonia has been reported to occur in pregnancy. The severity of the pulmonary lesions in varicella generally correlates better with the extent of the rash than with findings on pulmonary exam. Following recovery from chickenpox, the development of diffuse pulmonary calcifications has been documented.

RSV frequently causes detectably altered airway reactivity in adults (65), and on occasion, lower respiratory tract involvement becomes clinically manifest as pneumonia in otherwise healthy adults (147). RSV is being increasingly recognized as a cause of significant lower respiratory tract disease in the elderly (38). It has been estimated that 2 to 4% of pneumonia deaths among the elderly in the United States may be due to RSV (66). PIVs have also been reported as occasional causes of pneumonia in adults and in the elderly (97). Measles can be complicated by clinically severe pneumonitis in a small percentage of healthy adults, and bacterial superinfection is common. Diffuse pneumonitis and respiratory failure have been described in association with EBV acute mononucleosis in otherwise healthy adults.

Hantaviruses are associated with hantavirus cardiopulmonary syndrome (HCPS), characterized by the onset of severe pulmonary dysfunction after a 2- to 3-day prodrome of nonspecific influenza-like symptoms of fever, myalgias, cough, gastrointestinal symptoms, and headache (30). Coryza or upper respiratory tract symptoms suggest an alternative diagnosis. Laboratory abnormalities include leukocytosis, increased hematocrit due to hemoconcentration, and thrombocytopenia with coagulopathy. However, clinical bleeding is unusual, in contrast to the case with other systemic hantavirus syndromes (30). Moderately elevated levels of serum lactate dehydrogenase and aspartate aminotransferase are typically seen. A variety of radiographic abnormalities have been described. Radiographic findings which may help to distinguish hantavirus pulmonary syndrome from adult respiratory distress syndrome include early, prominent interstitial edema and nonperipheral distribution of initial airspace disease (17).

The novel human coronavirus causing severe acute respiratory syndrome (SARS) was associated with epidemics of severe respiratory disease initially in southern China and subsequently in multiple locations in Asia and elsewhere in the early spring of 2003 (112). After an intense epidemic associated with 8,096 cases and 774 deaths, the disease disappeared, largely due to aggressive infection control practices. The human SARS coronavirus was probably introduced into human populations from an animal species, likely the palm civet or a related animal, and subsequent transmission took place largely in the health care setting.

The most common symptoms on presentation were fever, chills and/or rigors, and myalgias (13, 90). Cough and dyspnea were the predominant respiratory symptoms but were not always present initially, while upper respiratory symptoms, such as rhinorrhea or sore throat, were infrequent. In addition, about a third of patients had diarrhea at some point in the clinical course. Respiratory disease was progressive and became more severe over 4 to 7 days, leading to significant hypoxemia. About 20% of patients required respiratory support, and the overall case fatality rate was about 10%. Laboratory abnormalities on presentation included elevations in lactate dehydrogenase, transaminases, and creatine kinase and hematologic abnormalities, particularly lymphopenia, as well as thrombocytopenia. The lymphopenia included depletion of both CD4 and CD8 cells (22). Radiological abnormalities included unilateral or bilateral ground-glass opacities or focal unilateral or bilateral areas of consolidation (52, 105). This syndrome is described in more detail in chapter 51.

Children

Overall, viruses are relatively more common causes of pneumonia in children than in adults. In most series, RSV has been associated with the largest proportion of viral pneumonia in young children, particularly when accompanied by bronchiolitis (142) (Table 1). It should be noted in this regard that bronchiolitis and pneumonia represent a spectrum of lower respiratory tract involvement with RSV, frequently coexist, and are not clearly distinguishable. The most typical radiographic finding is diffuse interstitial pneumonitis, although lobar or segmental consolidation is evident in about one-fourth of children with RSV lower respiratory tract disease, often involving the right upper or middle lobe.

The PIVs are second only to RSV as causes of pneumonia in this age group. As described earlier, lower respiratory tract involvement is integral to the pathophysiology of croup, but pneumonia with pulmonary infiltrates is most commonly associated with PIV-3. Influenza A and B viruses are both significant causes of pneumonia in children during epidemics. In infants and children, the most frequent manifestation of influenza pneumonia is an interstitial pneumonitis similar in appearance and course to the pneumonias caused by the other predominant viral agents of pneumonia in this age group, except that a secondary bacterial pneumonia may occur more frequently than with RSV or PIV.

Adenoviruses are frequently isolated from children with respiratory disease and are implicated in about 10% of childhood pneumonias. However, the true impact of adenoviruses as causes of pneumonia in this age group is difficult to assess because of the long and intermittent asymptomatic respiratory shedding of these viruses in children. Hilar adenopathy on chest X ray is somewhat more common with this form of pneumonia than with other types (138). Pneumonia is the most frequent serious complication of measles. Rhinoviruses have also been associated with a significant proportion of community-acquired pneumonias in children. Other viruses which may occasionally cause viral pneumonia in children include enteroviruses, rubella virus, and herpes simplex virus.

Differentiation between viral and bacterial forms of pneumonia on clinical grounds can be difficult in this age group, and radiological criteria do not always distinguish these entities well. Mixed viral and bacterial pneumonia may be present. However, in healthy infants and children with RSV or PIV pneumonia, bacteria do not appear to play an important role, and routine addition of antibacterial agents is not useful. The exception to this observation is in developing countries, where mixed viral and bacterial pneumonias in children are frequent and severe.

Immunocompromised Hosts

Individuals with diminished immunity, particularly diminished cellular immunity, may develop severe, life-threatening pulmonary infections with the entire spectrum of RNA and DNA viruses, including both viruses that are typical causes of lower respiratory tract disease in healthy hosts and other, more opportunistic viral pathogens (Table 1). DNA viruses have received the most recognition in this regard.

CMV is a frequent cause of severe pneumonitis in immunosuppressed individuals, particularly transplant recipients (76). The highest risk in the transplant population is 1 to 3 months posttransplantation, with the peak incidence at 8 weeks posttransplantation. Diffuse interstitial pneumonitis is the most frequent manifestation, but multiple other radiographic presentations have been reported, including nodular infiltrates resembling nocardiae. Multiple associated findings are present in severe infection and reflect the disseminated nature of the infection; the presence of neutropenia, abnormalities of liver function tests, and mucosal ulcerations may be clinical clues to the diagnosis.

Herpes simplex pneumonia has been reported to occur largely in immunocompromised or debilitated individuals. These cases are variably preceded by clinically evident mucocutaneous disease. The majority of cases present as a focal pneumonia as a result of contiguous spread from the upper respiratory tract; diffuse interstitial disease resulting from hematogenous spread occurs in up to 40% of cases (115). Risk groups include neonates, transplant recipients, and burn patients, particularly with inhalation injury, prolonged mechanical ventilation, cardiothoracic surgery, and trauma.

Varicella-zoster virus is an important problem in individuals with hematologic malignancies and others with iatrogenic immunosuppression, with the greatest risk seen in organ transplantation. Prolonged fever and/or recurrent crops of lesions are predictors of visceral dissemination, and pneumonia is generally seen in this setting. Pulmonary manifestations may include pleuritic chest pain due to vesicular lesions of the pleura, and, as also true for healthy hosts, the chest radiographs may demonstrate diffuse nodular lesions.

Adenoviruses are significant causes of morbidity and mortality in immunocompromised patients, particularly after transplantation. In contrast to infection in healthy hosts, infection in immunocompromised subjects tends to be disseminated, with isolation of virus from multiple body sites, including the lungs, liver, gastrointestinal tract, and urine (87). In addition, the spectrum of serotypes includes both those found in immunocompetent individuals and a markedly increased frequency of isolation of higher-numbered serotypes found rarely in immunologically normal subjects (71).

RNA viruses have also received increasing recognition as potential causes of significant morbidity and mortality in this population (120). RSV has been well recognized as a cause of pneumonia in recipients of bone marrow (70) and solid-organ (34) transplants. Nosocomial transmission of RSV in this setting has been well documented and may be the source of many infections in this susceptible population. The illness typically begins with nondescript upper respiratory symptoms that progress over several days to severe, life-threatening lower respiratory tract involvement. Mortality rates of 50% or higher are typical if pneumonia supervenes, particularly if disease occurs in the preengraftment period (47). PIVs have also been reported as infrequent lower respiratory tract pathogens in both solid-organ and bone marrow transplantation. Type 3 has been the most common serotype isolated, but all four serotypes have been implicated (120). Influenza virus may also cause severe disease in transplant recipients (137) and leukemic subjects. Rhinovirus and coronavirus infections have also been detected in this population (14).

Measles giant cell pneumonia is a severe, usually fatal form of pneumonia in immunosuppressed individuals. Most cases have occurred in those with hematologic or other malignancies or in individuals with AIDS (79). Recent outbreaks of measles worldwide, coupled with the increasing incidence of human immunodeficiency virus infection, have increased the frequency and impact of measles giant cell pneumonia. Giant cell pneumonia also occurs in significantly malnourished individuals. Multinucleated giant cells with intranuclear inclusions are seen and may be demonstrable in fluid obtained by bronchoalveolar lavage. An important feature of measles pneumonia in immunocompromised hosts is that many patients present without rash or other typical manifestations of measles, and a high index of suspicion must be maintained (79). Such hosts may not mount the cellular immune responses involved in the pathogenesis of rash in immunologically intact individuals.

Diagnosis

Epidemiological or clinical features of viral pneumonia, like season, exposure history, and systemic signs or symptoms, such as rash, may be very useful in establishing the potential viral etiologies in specific cases of viral pneumonia. However, the clinical presentation is rarely distinctive enough to permit a specific viral diagnosis to be made on clinical grounds alone, which instead generally depends on detection of the viral agent in appropriate respiratory specimens. Many of these viruses can be isolated from upper respiratory tract samples, but lower respiratory tract samples often have higher yield, particularly for adults or immunocompromised hosts. Assessment of the lower respiratory tract may require bronchoalveolar lavage with supporting histopathology or immunohistochemistry. Rapid antigen detection tests are available for detection of RSV and influenza viruses in respiratory secretions but lack sensitivity. Reverse transcription-PCR assays are more sensitive, and several multiplex ones are commercially available. Definitive attribution of pneumonia to viruses which are typically shed asymptomatically in the upper respiratory tract, such as herpes simplex virus, is more difficult and requires detection of virus in the lower respiratory tract, usually in association with pathological evidence of invasive disease.

Pathogenesis

The pathogenesis of viral infections of the lower respiratory tract can conveniently be categorized as (i) infections initiated in and primarily confined to the respiratory tract, such as with influenza virus or RSV; (ii) processes in which infection is initiated in the respiratory tract with subsequent systemic manifestations, such as in measles or varicella; and (iii) processes in which respiratory tract involvement is secondary to a systemic infection, such as with CMV. Each of these situations may lead to what is recognized clinically as a viral pneumonia. The general features of primary viral pneumonia are discussed below using influenza as a model, and pathogenesis of other forms of viral pneumonia is discussed briefly in comparison.

In primary pneumonia in the first category, virus infection reaches the lungs either by contiguous spread from the upper respiratory tract or by inhalation of small-particle aerosols. Infection initially occurs in ciliated respiratory mucosal epithelial cells of the trachea, bronchi, and lower respiratory tract and leads to widespread destruction of these cells. The mucosa is hyperemic, and the trachea and bronchi contain bloody fluid. Tracheitis, bronchitis, and bronchiolitis are seen, with loss of normal ciliated epithelial cells. Submucosal hyperemia, focal hemorrhage, edema, and cellular infiltrate are present. The alveolar spaces contain various numbers of neutrophils and mononuclear cells admixed with fibrin and edema fluid. The alveolar capillaries may be markedly hyperemic, with intra-alveolar hemorrhage. Acellular, hyaline membranes line many of the alveolar ducts and alveoli. Pathological findings seen by biopsy of lung in nonfatal cases during nonpandemic situations are similar to those described for fatal cases (144).

The pathological changes in the lower respiratory tract in children with viral pneumonia due to RSV and PIV are nonspecific and include epithelial necrosis with bronchiolar mucus plugging and widespread inflammation and necrosis of lung parenchyma, and severe lesions of the bronchial and bronchiolar mucosa as well (1). In fatal cases of RSV pneumonia in children, hemorrhagic pneumonia with peribronchial mononuclear infiltration and cytoplasmic inclusion bodies in epithelial cells are seen. Giant cell pneumonia with virally induced multinucleated syncytial cells may be seen in RSV, PIV, or measles virus infections in immunocompromised hosts.

Bacterial superinfection is a well-recognized complication of viral pneumonia and accounts for a large proportion of the morbidity and mortality of viral lower respiratory tract disease, especially in adults. Consequently, the spectrum of disease and pathophysiology of bacterial superinfection have been studied intensively, and a number of factors in viral respiratory disease which could play a role in increasing the risk of bacterial infection have been identified. The disruption of the normal epithelial cell barrier to infection and the loss of mucociliary clearance undoubtedly contribute to the enhancement of bacterial pathogenesis (92). In addition, increased adherence of bacteria to virus-infected epithelial cells has been demonstrated. Polymorphonuclear leukocytes and mononuclear cells are susceptible to abortive infection by some respiratory viruses, with resulting decreased function, which may also contribute to enhanced bacterial infection.

Infection with influenza virus, RSV, PIV, and adenoviruses is usually limited to the respiratory tract by mechanisms which are not completely clear. In contrast, respiratory tract infection with measles or varicella-zoster virus leads to dissemination and systemic manifestations. In more severe cases of varicella, vesicles may be found within the tracheobronchial tree and on pleural surfaces. Microscopic examination demonstrates interstitial pneumonitis with edema, intranuclear inclusion bodies within septal cells, and peribronchiolar inflammation.

HCPS represents an additional example of a viral infection which involves the lungs as part of a systemic infection. The pathogenesis of HCPS involves extensive infection of endothelial cells throughout the body, which is particularly intensive within the vascular endothelial cells of the lung (146). Abundant viral antigen and nucleic acid can be detected within these cells. Microscopic examination of the lung reveals mild to moderate interstitial pneumonitis with variable degrees of congestion, edema, and mononuclear cell infiltration. The cellular infiltrate is composed of a mixture of small and large mononuclear cells, which consist predominantly of T lymphocytes and monocytes/macrophages. The picture is one of immune mediated capillary leak and not of cell necrosis or inflammatory pneumonitis. High levels of cytokines have been detected in the blood and likely mediate the endothelial damage.

There are several features of CMV pneumonitis in the transplant setting that suggest that host and viral factors interact in pathogenesis (53). CMV pathogenicity is enhanced in transplant recipients and frequently occurs at the site of the transplanted organ. The risk of CMV pneumonitis is highest in individuals at the highest risk of graft-versus-host disease (35). Finally, treatment with antivirals alone is ineffective (116), while treatment with antivirals and immune globulin, which serve to mitigate the graft-versus-host component, is effective (33, 117).

Treatment and Prevention

Therapy of viral pneumonia is dependent on the severity of disease, the age and immune status of the host, and the specific causative viral agent. General supportive measures, particularly the management of hypoxia, are critical, and some patients have required high-frequency ventilation or extracorporeal membrane oxygenation. Since mixed viral-bacterial infections and bacterial superinfections are common, antibacterial agents may be required as indicated by appropriate microbiological studies.

Antiviral therapy should be guided by the results of diagnostic tests (Table 2). The neuraminidase inhibitors oseltamivir (Tamiflu) and zanamivir (Relenza) are active against both influenza A and B viruses (54). It should be noted that these agents have mostly been studied in uncomplicated influenza in healthy adults, in whom the main effect is reduction of the duration of illness. There are no controlled data on which to base recommendations regarding treatment of pneumonia, but it seems reasonable to use antiviral agents if the patient is still virus positive at the time of presentation. Although the M2 inhibitors amantadine and rimantadine are effective against sensitive viruses, the great majority of influenza A (H3N2) viruses worldwide, as well as most clade 1 H5N1 viruses, are completely resistant to M2 inhibitors (15). Therefore, M2 inhibitors are no longer recommended for use as antiviral agents against influenza.

The only option available for the other RNA viruses is ribavirin, but there is little evidence of efficacy of this agent for treating established viral pneumonia (see "Bronchiolitis" above). In immunocompromised hosts, treatment of RSV pulmonary infection associated with respiratory failure has not been successful. One approach that appears to be promising is treatment with ribavirin, possibly in combination with immune globulin, early in the illness, when upper respiratory symptoms predominate (120). Controlled trials in PIV infection are not available, although anecdotal reports suggest potential efficacy (45). Limited controlled trials have suggested that aerosolized ribavirin may reduce the severity of symptoms in children with measles, and some immunocompromised patients with measles pneumonia have done well following treatment with aerosolized (79) or intravenous (40) forms of the drug. Intravenous ribavirin is effective in the treatment of hemorrhagic fever with renal syndrome but does not appear to be useful for treatment of hantavirus pulmonary syndrome (18).

Acyclovir is active in vitro against herpes simplex virus types 1 and 2 and against varicella-zoster virus but does not have clinically useful activity for treatment of CMV or EBV disease. Although controlled clinical trials of this drug in herpes simplex pneumonia have not been conducted, the drug has proven clinical efficacy in other herpesvirus infections and would be indicated in any serious herpes simplex virus lower respiratory tract infection. Acyclovir is also effective in the therapy of varicella, and intravenous acyclovir has been effective when initiated early in the course of varicella pneumonia (59). The related drugs famciclovir and penciclovir are similar to acyclovir in their spectrum of activity against herpesviruses. Viruses resistant to the activity of these drugs have been isolated from treated immunocompromised patients and may be susceptible to the antiherpes drug phosphonoformic acid (foscarnet).

Once CMV pneumonitis is established, particularly in allogeneic bone marrow transplant patients, it is very difficult to treat. Ganciclovir is highly active against CMV in vitro, but monotherapy is not effective against pneumonitis in bone marrow transplant recipients. The combination of ganciclovir therapy and intravenous CMV immune globulin can reduce the mortality rate from approximately 90 to 50% or lower in these patients. The effect of the immune globulin in this situation may mostly be to ameliorate graft-versus-host disease. Whether combination therapy is required in solid-organ transplant recipients with CMV pneumonia is uncertain. Cidofovir and foscarnet are other antiviral drugs with activity against CMV. Both have been used to successfully treat CMV retinitis, but their effectiveness for treating CMV pneumonia has not been established. All of the available CMV antivirals have serious side effects that limit their usefulness.

Guidelines for reducing the risk of CMV disease in stem cell transplant recipients have been published (31). Transplant candidates should be screened for evidence of CMV immunity, and CMV-seronegative recipients of allogeneic stem cell transplants from CMV-seronegative donors should receive only leukocyte-reduced or CMV-seronegative erythrocytes and/or leukocyte-reduced platelets. In mismatched solid-organ transplant recipients (donor positive/recipient negative), posttransplantation prophylaxis with oral ganciclovir or its prodrug valganciclovir significantly reduces the risk of CMV disease, although late-onset disease still occurs. Another strategy is preemptive therapy with ganciclovir or another anti-CMV agent when screening detects infection, but before disease develops. This strategy requires the use of sensitive and specific laboratory tests for diagnosis.

Antiviral treatment of proven value for adenovirus infection is not available. Both ganciclovir and cidofovir are active in vitro, and there are anecdotal reports of clinical use in immunocompromised patients.

TABLE 2 Therapies of potential benefit in viral pneumonia

Viral etiology	Potential therapy[a]	Comments
RSV	Ribavirin	Controlled studies show some efficacy in RSV bronchiolitis; not recommended for routine use but may be considered for use in high-risk or severely ill children
	Palivizumab (Synagis)	Prevention of RSV in high-risk children; not useful for therapy
PIV	Ribavirin	Case reports of efficacy in PIV infection; no controlled studies are available
Influenza A virus	M2 inhibitors (amantadine, rimantadine)	Widespread resistance limits usefulness of these agents; generally not recommended
	Neuraminidase inhibitors (zanamivir [inhaled], oseltamivir [oral])	Effective in uncomplicated influenza in adults, children, and the elderly when administered within 48 h of illness; reductions in complications; efficacy unproven in complicated disease or pneumonia; frequency of resistance appears to be less than with M2 inhibitors
Influenza B virus	Neuraminidase inhibitors (zanamivir [inhaled], oseltamivir [oral])	Active in vitro but less than for influenza A; clinical data suggest that efficacy may also be lower
Measles virus	Ribavirin	Ribavirin may shorten the duration of illness in children with measles; use in measles pneumonia is unproven
	IVIG[b]	IVIG may decrease risk of measles when administered to susceptible individuals and may decrease symptoms in those infected
Herpes simplex virus	Acyclovir (famciclovir, penciclovir)	Controlled trials have demonstrated efficacy of acyclovir in a variety of herpes simplex diseases; cross-resistance between agents
	Foscarnet	May be useful for treatment of herpesviruses resistant to acyclovir
Varicella-zoster virus	Acyclovir (famciclovir, penciclovir)	Demonstrated efficacy in varicella and in varicella pneumonia; must use relatively high doses
	Foscarnet	May be useful for management of acyclovir-resistant cases
CMV	Ganciclovir	Clinical efficacy in CMV pneumonitis in AIDS and solid-organ transplantation; in bone marrow transplant patients, efficacious when combined with IVIG
	Foscarnet	Predominant use in ganciclovir resistance or in individuals who cannot tolerate ganciclovir due to hematologic toxicity

[a] Note that this is a listing of potential therapies only and is not to be considered a recommendation for use.
[b] IVIG, intravenous immune globulin.

Although recent years have witnessed a significant increase in the spectrum and potency of available antiviral agents, drug therapy for viral pneumonia remains burdened by the toxicity of drugs, the development of antiviral resistance, and the complex pathogenesis of many viral syndromes in which viral replication is only part of the disease process. Vaccines of variable effectiveness currently exist for influenza, measles, and varicella-zoster viruses. Development of additional effective vaccines for the viral pathogens causing pneumonia will contribute to the control of this important problem.

REFERENCES

1. **Aherne, W., T. Bird, S. D. M. Court, P. S. Gardner, and J. McQuillin.** 1970. Pathologic changes in virus infections of the lower respiratory tract in children. *J. Clin. Pathol.* **23:**7–18.
2. **Allander, T., T. Jartti, S. Gupta, H. G. M. Niesters, P. Lehtinen, R. Osterback, T. Vuorinen, M. Waris, A. Bjerkner, A. Tiveljung-Lindell, B. G. van den Hoogen, T. Hyypia, and O. Ruuskanen.** 2007. Human bocavirus and acute wheezing in children. *Clin. Infect. Dis.* **44:**904–910.
3. **American Academy of Pediatrics Subcommittee on Diagnosis and Management of Bronchiolitis.** 2006. Diagnosis and management of bronchiolitis. *Pediatrics* **118:**1774–1793.
4. **Anderson, L. J.** 2007. Human bocavirus: a new viral pathogen. *Clin. Infect. Dis.* **44:**911–912.
5. **Angeles-Marcos, M., M. Camps, T. Pumarola, J. Antonio-Martinez, E. Martinez, J. Mensa, E. Garcia, G. Penarroja, P. Dambrava, I. Casas, M. T. Jimenez de Anta, and A. Torres.** 2006. The role of viruses in the aetiology of community-acquired pneumonia in adults. *Antivir. Ther.* **11:**351–359.
6. **Arruda, E., T. R. Boyle, B. Winther, D. C. Pevear, J. M. Gwaltney, Jr., and F. G. Hayden.** 1995. Localization of human rhinovirus replication in the upper respiratory tract by in situ hybridization. *J. Infect. Dis.* **171:**1329–1333.
7. **Arruda, E., A. Pitkaranta, T. J. J. Witek, C. A. Doyle, and F. G. Hayden.** 1997. Frequency and natural history of rhinovirus infections during autumn. *J. Clin. Microbiol.* **35:**2684–2688.
8. **Attia, M., T. Zaoutis, S. Eppes, J. O. Klein, and F. Meier.** 1999. Multivariate predictive models for group A beta-hemolytic streptococcal pharyngitis in children. *Acad. Emerg. Med.* **6:**8–13.
9. **Barnes, S. D., J. M. Leclair, M. S. Forman, T. R. Townsend, G. M. Laughlin, and P. Charache.** 1989. Comparison of nasal brush and nasopharyngeal aspirate

techniques in obtaining specimens for detection of respiratory syncytial viral antigen by immunofluorescence. *Pediatr. Infect. Dis. J.* **8:**598–601.

10. **Becroft, D. M. O.** 1971. Brochiolitis obliterans, bronchiolitis, and other sequelae of adenovirus type 21 infection in young children. *J. Clin. Pathol.* **24:**72–81.
11. **Berman, S.** 1991. Epidemiology of acute respiratory infections in children of developing countries. *Rev. Infect. Dis.* **13:**S454–S462.
12. **Bjornson, C. L., T. P. Klassen, J. Williamson, R. Brant, C. Mitton, A. Plint, B. Bulloch, L. Evered, and D. W. Johnson.** 2004. A randomized trial of a single dose of oral dexamethasone for mild croup. *N. Engl. J. Med.* **351:**1306–1313.
13. **Booth, C. M., L. M. Matukas, G. A. Tomlinson, A. R. Rachlis, D. B. Rose, H. A. Dwosh, S. L. Walmsley, T. Mazzulli, M. Avendano, P. Derkach, I. E. Ephtimios, I. Kitai, B. D. Mederski, S. B. Shadowitz, W. L. Gold, L. A. Hawryluck, E. Rea, J. S. Chenkin, D. W. Cescon, S. M. Poutanen, and A. S. Detsky.** 2003. Clinical features and short-term outcomes of 144 patients with SARS in the greater Toronto area. *JAMA* **289:**2801–2809.
14. **Bowden, R. A.** 1997. Respiratory virus infections after marrow transplant: the Fred Hutchinson Cancer Research Center experience. *Am. J. Med.* **102(3A):**27–30.
15. **Bright, R. A., D. K. Shay, B. Shu, N. J. Cox, and A. I. Klimov.** 2006. Adamantane resistance among influenza A viruses isolated early during the 2005–2006 influenza season in the United States. *JAMA* **295:**891–894.
16. **Buchman, C. A., W. J. Doyle, D. P. Skoner, J. C. Post, C. M. Alper, J. T. Seroky, K. Anderson, R. A. Preston, F. G. Hayden, P. Fireman, and G. D. Ehrlich.** 1995. Influenza A virus-induced acute otitis media. *J. Infect. Dis.* **172:**1348–1351.
17. **Butler, J. C., and C. J. Peters.** 1994. Hantaviruses and hantavirus pulmonary syndrome. *Clin. Infect. Dis.* **19:**387–395.
18. **Chapman, L. E., G. J. Mertz, C. J. Peters, H. M. Jolson, A. S. Khan, T. G. Ksiazek, F. T. Koster, K. F. Baum, P. E. Rollin, A. T. Pavia, R. C. Holman, J. C. Christenson, P. J. Rubin, R. E. Behrman, L. J. Bell, G. L. Simpson, and R. F. Sadek for the Ribavirin Study Group.** 1999. Intravenous ribavirin for hantavirus pulmonary syndrome: safety and tolerance during 1 year of open-label experience. *Antivir. Res.* **4:**211–219.
19. **Cherry, J. D.** 2008. Croup. *N. Engl. J. Med.* **358:**384–391.
20. **Chidekel, A. S., A. R. Bazzy, and C. L. Rosen.** 1994. Rhinovirus infection associated with severe lower respiratory tract illness and worsening lung disease in infants with bronchopulmonary dysplasia. *Pediatr. Pulmonol.* **18:**261–263.
21. **Corneli, H. M., J. J. Zorc, P. Mahajan, K. N. Shaw, R. Holubkov, S. D. Reeves, R. M. Ruddy, B. Malik, K. A. Nelson, J. S. Bregstein, K. M. Brown, M. N. Denenberg, K. A. Lillis, L. B. Cimpello, J. W. Tsung, D. A. Borgialli, M. N. Baskin, G. Teshome, M. A. Goldstein, D. Monroe, J. M. Dean, N. Kuppermann, and the Bronchiolitis Study Group of the Pediatric Emergency Care Applied Research Network (PECARN).** 2007. A multicenter, randomized, controlled trial of dexamethasone for bronchiolitis. *N. Engl. J. Med.* **357:**331–339.
22. **Cui, W., Y. Fan, W. Wu, F. Zhang, J. Y. Wang, and A. P. Ni.** 2003. Expression of lymphocytes and lymphocyte subsets in patients with severe acute respiratory syndrome. *Clin. Infect. Dis.* **37:**857–859.
23. **Dawson, K. P., A. Long, J. Kennedy, and N. Mogridge.** 1990. The chest radiograph in acute bronchiolitis. *J. Paediatr. Child Health* **26:**209–211.
24. **Del Mar, C. B., P. P. Glasziou, and A. B. Spinks.** 2000. Antibiotics for sore throat. *Cochrane Database of Systemic Reviews* CD000023.
25. **Denny, F. W., T. F. Murphy, W. A. J. Clyde, A. M. Collier, and F. W. Henderson.** 1983. Croup: an 11-year study in a pediatric practice. *Pediatrics* **71:**871–876.
26. **Department of Health and Human Services.** 1994. Current estimates from the National Health Interview survey, 1992. DHHS publication no. (PHS) 94-1517. Department of Health and Human Services, Hyattsville, MD.
27. **Diamond, L., R. J. Dockhorn, J. Grossman, J. C. Kisicki, M. Posner, M. A. Zinny, P. Koker, D. Korts, and M. T. Wecker.** 1995. A dose-response study of the efficacy and safety of ipratropium bromide nasal spray in the treatment of the common cold. *J. Allergy Clin. Immunol.* **95:**1139–1146.
28. **Dingle, J. H., G. F. Badger, and W. S. Jordan, Jr.** 1964. Illness in the home: study of 25,000 illnesses in a group of Cleveland families. Press of Case Western University, Cleveland, OH.
29. **Doyle, W. J., D. K. Riker, T. P. McBride, F. G. Hayden, J. O. Hendley, J. D. Swarts, and J. M. Gwaltney, Jr.** 1993. Therapeutic effects of an anticholinergic-sympathomimetic combination in induced rhinovirus colds. *Ann. Otol. Rhinol. Laryngol.* **102:**521–527.
30. **Duchin, J. S., F. T. Koster, C. J. Peters, G. L. Simpson, B. Tempest, S. R. Zaki, T. G. Ksiazer, P. E. Rollin, S. Nichohl, E. T. Umland, R. L. Moolenaar, S. E. Reef, K. B. Nolte, M. M. Gallaher, J. C. Butler, and R. F. Breiman.** 1994. Hantavirus pulmonary syndrome: a clinical description of 17 patients with a newly recognized disease. *N. Engl. J. Med.* **330:**949–955.
31. **Dykewicz, C.** 2001. Summary of the guidelines for preventing opportunistic infections among hematopoietic stem cell transplant recipients. *Clin. Infect. Dis.* **33:**139–144.
32. **Elkhatieb, A., G. Hipskind, D. Woerner, and F. G. Hayden.** 1993. Middle ear abnormalities during natural rhinovirus colds in adults. *J. Infect. Dis.* **168:**618–621.
33. **Emanuel, D., I. Cunningham, K. Jules-Elysee, J. A. Brochstein, N. A. Kernan, J. Laver, D. Stover, D. A. White, A. Fels, B. Polsky, H. Castro-Malaspina, J. R. Peppard, B. P. U. Hammerling, and R. J. O'Reilly.** 1988. Cytomegalovirus pneumonia after bone marrow transplantation successfully treated with the combination of ganciclovir and high-dose intravenous immune globulin. *Ann. Intern. Med.* **109:**777–782.
34. **Englund, J. A., C. J. Sullivan, and M. C. Jordan.** 1988. Respiratory syncytial virus infection in immunocompromised adults. *Ann. Intern. Med.* **109:**203–208.
35. **Enright, H., R. Haake, D. Weisdorf, N. Ramsay, P. McGlave, J. Kersey, W. Thomas, D. McKenzie, and W. Miller.** 1993. Cytomegalovirus pneumonia after bone marrow transplantation: risk factors and response to therapy. *Transplantation* **55:**1339–1346.
36. **Esper, F., C. Weibel, D. Ferguson, M. L. Landry, and J. S. Kahn.** 2005. Evidence of a novel human coronavirus that is associated with respiratory tract disease in infants and young children. *J. Infect. Dis.* **191:**492–498.
37. **Falsey, A., and E. E. Walsh.** 2006. Viral pneumonia in older adults. *Clin. Infect. Dis.* **42:**518–524.
38. **Falsey, A. R.** 1998. Respiratory syncytial virus infection in older persons. *Vaccine* **16:**1775–1778.
39. **Falsey, A. R., R. M. McCann, W. J. Hall, M. M. Criddle, M. A. Formica, D. Wycoff, and J. E. Kolassa.** 1997. The "common cold" in frail older persons: impact of rhinovirus and coronavirus in a senior daycare center. *J. Am. Geriatr. Soc.* **45:**706–711.

40. **Forni, A. L., N. W. Schluger, and R. B. Roberts.** 1994. Severe measles pneumonitis in adults: evaluation of clinical characteristics and therapy with intravenous ribavirin. *Clin. Infect. Dis.* **19:**454–462.
41. **Foy, H. M., M. K. Cooney, A. J. Maletzky, and J. T. Grayston.** 1973. Incidence and etiology of pneumonia, croup, and bronchiolitis in preschool children belonging to a prepaid medical care group over a four-year period. *Am. J. Epidemiol.* **97:**80–92.
42. **Friedlander, S. L., and W. W. Busse.** 2005. The role of rhinovirus in asthma exacerbations. *J. Allergy Clin. Immunol.* **116:**267–273.
43. **Friis, B., M. Eiken, A. Hornsleth, and A. Jensen.** 1990. Chest X-ray appearances in pneumonia and bronchiolitis. Correlation to virological diagnosis and secretory bacterial findings. *Acta Paediatr. Scand.* **79:**219–225.
44. **Fulginiti, V. A., J. J. Eller, O. F. Sieber, J. W. Joyner, M. Minamitani, and G. Meiklejohn.** 1969. Respiratory virus immunization. I. A field trial of two inactivated respiratory virus vaccines: an aqueous trivalent parainfluenza virus vaccine and an alum-precipitated respiratory syncytial virus vaccine. *Am. J. Epidemiol.* **89:**435–448.
45. **Gelfand, E. W., D. McCurdy, and D. P. Rao.** 1983. Ribavirin treatment of viral pneumonitis in severe combined immunodeficiency disease. *Lancet* **ii:**732–783.
46. **Gerber, M. A., R. R. Tanz, W. Kabat, E. Dennis, G. L. Bell, E. L. Kaplan, and S. T. Shulman.** 1997. Optical immunoassay for group A beta-hemolytic streptococcal pharyngitis. An office-based, multicenter investigation. *JAMA* **277:**899–903.
47. **Ghosh, S., R. E. Champlin, J. Englund, S. A. Giralt, K. Rolston, I. Raad, K. Jacobson, J. Neumann, C. Ippoliti, S. Mallik, and E. Whimbey.** 2000. Respiratory syncytial virus upper respiratory tract illnesses in adult blood and marrow transplant recipients: combination therapy with aerosolized ribavirin and intravenous immunoglobulin. *Bone Marrow Transplant.* **25:**751–755.
48. **Glezen, W. P., L. H. Taber, A. L. Frank, and J. A. Kasel.** 1986. Risk of primary infection and re-infection with respiratory syncytial virus. *Am. J. Dis. Child.* **140:**543–546.
49. **Gonzales, R., and M. A. Sande.** 2000. Uncomplicated acute bronchitis. *Ann. Intern. Med.* **133:**981–991.
50. **Gozal, D., A. A. Colin, M. Jaffe, and Z. Hochberg.** 1990. Water, electrolyte, and endocrine homeostasis in infants with bronchiolitis. *Pediatr. Res.* **27:**204–209.
51. **Greenberg, D., R. Walker, M. S. Lee, K. Reisinger, J. Ward, R. Yogev, M. Blatter, S. Yeh, R. Karron, C. Sangli, L. Eubank, K. Coelingh, J. Cordova, M. August, and H. Mehta.** 2005. A bovine parainfluenza virus type 3 vaccine is safe and immunogenic in early infancy. *J. Infect. Dis.* **191:**1116–1122.
52. **Grinblat, L., H. Shulman, A. Glickman, L. Matukas, and N. Paul.** 2003. Severe acute respiratory syndrome: radiographic review of 40 probable cases in Toronto, Canada. *Radiology* **228:**802–809.
53. **Grundy, J. E.** 1990. Virologic and pathogenetic aspects of cytomegalovirus infection. *Rev. Infect. Dis.* **12:**S711–S719.
54. **Gubareva, L. V., L. Kaiser, and F. G. Hayden.** 2000. Influenza virus neuraminidase inhibitors. *Lancet* **355:**827–835.
55. **Guerguerian, A. M., M. Gauthier, M. H. Lebel, C. A. Farrell, and J. Lacroix.** 1999. Ribavirin in ventilated respiratory syncytial virus bronchiolitis. A randomized, placebo-controlled trial. *Am. J. Resp. Crit. Care Med.* **160:**829–834.
56. **Gwaltney, J. M., Jr., J. O. Hendley, G. Simon, and W. S. Jordan, Jr.** 1966. Rhinovirus infections in an industrial population. I. The occurrence of illness. *N. Engl. J. Med.* **275:**1261–1268.
57. **Gwaltney, J. M., Jr., C. D. Phillips, R. D. Miller, and D. K. Riker.** 1994. Computed tomographic study of the common cold. *N. Engl. J. Med.* **330:**25–30.
58. **Gwaltney, J. M., Jr., and H. M. Druce.** 1997. Efficacy of brompheniramine maleate for the treatment of rhinovirus colds. *Clin. Infect. Dis.* **25:**1188–1194.
59. **Haake, D. A., P. C. Zakowski, D. L. Haake, and Y. J. Bryson.** 1990. Early treatment with acyclovir for varicella pneumonia in otherwise healthy adults: retrospective controlled study and review. *Rev. Infect. Dis.* **12:**788–798.
60. **Hall, C. B.** 1995. Acute laryngotracheobronchitis (croup), p. 573–579. *In* G. L. Mandell, J. E. Bennett, and R. Dolin (ed.), *Principles and Practice of Infectious Diseases*, 4th ed. Churchill Livingstone, New York, NY.
61. **Hall, C. B., J. M. Geiman, B. B. Breese, and R. G. Douglas, Jr.** 1977. Parainfluenza viral infections in children: correlation of shedding with clinical manifestations. *J. Pediatr.* **91:**194–198.
62. **Hall, C. B., W. J. Hall, and D. M. Speers.** 1979. Clinical and physiological manifestations of bronchiolitis and pneumonia: outcome of respiratory syncytial virus. *Am. J. Dis. Child.* **133:**798–802.
63. **Hall, C. B., and J. T. McBride.** 2000. Acute laryngotracheobronchitis, p. 663–669. *In* G. L. Mandell, J. E. Bennett, and R. Dolin (ed.), *Principles and Practice of Infectious Diseases*, 5th ed. Churchill Livingstone, Philadelphia, PA.
64. **Hall, C. B., K. R. Powell, N. E. MacDonald, C. L. Gala, M. E. Menegus, S. C. Suffin, and H. J. Cohen.** 1986. Respiratory syncytial viral infection in children with compromised immune function. *N. Engl. J. Med.* **315:**77–81.
65. **Hall, W. J., C. B. Hall, and D. M. Speers.** 1978. Respiratory syncytial virus infection in adults: clinical, virologic, and serial pulmonary function studies. *Ann. Intern. Med.* **88:**203–205.
66. **Han, L. L., J. P. Alexander, and L. J. Anderson.** 1999. Respiratory syncytial virus pneumonia among the elderly: an assessment of disease burden. *J. Infect. Dis.* **179:**25–30.
67. **Hayden, F., D. Herrington, T. Coats, K. Kim, E. Cooper, S. Villano, S. Liu, S. Hudson, D. Pevear, M. Collett, and M. McKinlay.** 2003. Efficacy and safety of oral pleconaril for treatment of colds due to picornaviruses in adults: results of 2 double-blind, randomized, placebo-controlled trials. *Clin. Infect. Dis.* **36:**1523–1532.
68. **Henderson, F. W., W. A. Clyde, Jr., A. M. Collier, F. W. Denny, R. J. Senior, C. I. Sheaffer, W. G. Conley, and R. M. Christian.** 1979. The etiologic and epidemiologic spectrum of bronchiolitis in pediatric practice. *J. Pediatr.* **95:**183–190.
69. **Henderson, F. W., A. M. Collier, M. A. Sanyal, J. M. Watkins, D. L. Fairclough, W. A. Clyde, Jr., and F. W. Denny.** 1982. A longitudinal study of respiratory viruses and bacteria in the etiology of acute otitis media with effusion. *N. Engl. J. Med.* **306:**1377–1383.
70. **Hertz, M. I., J. A. Englund, D. Snover, P. B. Bitterman, and P. B. McGlave.** 1989. Respiratory syncytial virus-induced acute lung injury in adult patients with bone marrow transplants: a clinical approach and review of the literature. *Medicine* **68:**269–281.
71. **Hierholzer, J. C., R. Wigand, L. J. Anderson, T. Adrian, and J. W. M. Gold.** 1988. Adenoviruses from patients with AIDS: a plethora of serotypes and a description of five new serotypes of subgenus D (types 43–47). *J. Infect. Dis.* **158:**804–813.
72. **Huovinen, P., R. Lahtonen, T. Ziegler, O. Meurman, K. Hakkarainen, A. Miettinen, P. Arstila, J. Eskola, and P.**

Saikku. 1989. Pharyngitis in adults: the presence and coexistence of viruses and bacterial organisms. *Ann. Intern. Med.* **110:**612–616.

73. **Hyypia, T., T. Puhakka, O. Ruuskanen, M. Makela, A. Arola, and P. Arstila.** 1998. Molecular diagnosis of human rhinovirus infection: comparison with virus isolation. *J. Clin. Microbiol.* **36:**2081–2083.
74. **Igarashi, Y., D. P. Skoner, W. J. Doyle, M. V. White, P. Fireman, and M. A. Kaliner.** 1993. Analysis of nasal secretions during experimental rhinovirus upper respiratory infections. *J. Allergy Clin. Immunol.* **92:**722–731.
75. **Impact-RSV Study Group.** 1998. Palivizumab, a humanized respiratory syncytial virus monoclonal antibody, reduces hospitalization from respiratory syncytial virus infection in high-risk infants. *Pediatrics* **102:**531–537.
76. **Ison, M. G., and J. A. Fishman.** 2005. Cytomegalovirus pneumonia in transplant recipients. *Clin. Chest Med.* **26:** 691–705.
77. **Jawad, S. S., and R. Eccles.** 1998. Effect of pseudoephedrine on nasal airflow in patients with nasal congestion associated with common cold. *Rhinology* **36:**73–76.
78. **Johnson, D. W., S. Jacobson, P. C. Edney, P. Hadfield, M. E. Mundy, and S. Schuh.** 1998. A comparison of nebulized budesonide, intramuscular dexamethasone, and placebo for moderately severe croup. *N. Engl. J. Med.* **339:** 498–503.
79. **Kaplan, L. J., R. S. Daum, M. Smaron, and C. A. McCarthy.** 1992. Severe measles in immunocompromised patients. *JAMA* **267:**1237–1241.
80. **Khamapirad, T., and W. P. Gelzen.** 1987. Clinical and radiographic assessment of acute lower respiratory tract disease in infants and children. *Semin. Respir. Infect.* **2:** 130–144.
81. **Kim, H. W., J. O. Arrobio, C. D. Brandt, B. C. Jeffries, G. Pyles, J. L. Reid, R. M. Chanock, and R. H. Parrott.** 1973. Epidemiology of respiratory syncytial virus infection in Washington, D.C. I. Importance of the virus in different respiratory tract disease syndromes and temporal distribution of infection. *Am. J. Epidemiol.* **98:**216–225.
82. **Kim, H. W., C. D. Brandt, J. O. Arrobio, B. Murphy, R. M. Chanock, and R. H. Parrott.** 1979. Influenza A and B virus infection in infants and young children during the years 1957–1976. *Am. J. Epidemiol.* **109:**464–479.
83. **Klassen, T. P., M. E. Feldman, L. K. Watters, T. Sutcliffe, and P. C. Rowe.** 1994. Nebulized budesonide for children with mild-to-moderate croup. *N. Engl. J. Med.* **331:**285–289.
84. **Klinger, J. R., M. P. Sanchez, L. A. Curtin, M. Durkin, and B. Matyas.** 1998. Multiple cases of life-threatening adenovirus pneumonia in a mental health care center. *Am. J. Respir. Crit. Care Med.* **157:**645–649.
85. **Lambert, S. B., K. M. Allen, J. D. Druce, C. J. Birch, I. M. Mackay, J. B. Carlin, J. R. Carapetis, T. P. Sloots, M. D. Nissen, and T. M. Nolan.** 2007. Community epidemiology of human metapneumovirus, human coronavirus NL63, and other respiratory viruses in healthy preschool-aged children using parent-collected specimens. *Pediatrics* **120:**e929–e937.
86. **Lang, S. A., P. G. Duncan, D. A. Shephard, and H. C. Ha.** 1990. Pulmonary edema associated with airway obstruction. *Can. J. Anesth.* **37:**210–218.
87. **La Rosa, A. M., R. E. Champlin, N. B. Mirza, J. Gajewski, S. Giralt, K. V. Rolston, I. Raad, K. Jacobson, D. Kontoyiannis, L. Elting, and E. Whimbey.** 2001. Adenovirus infections in adult recipients of blood and marrow transplants. *Clin. Infect. Dis.* **32:**871–875.
88. **Lau, S. K. P., C. C. Y. Yip, H.-W. Tsoi, R. A. Lee, L.-Y. So, Y.-L. Lau, K.-H. Chan, P. C. Y. Woo, and K.-Y. Yuen.** 2007. Clinical features and complete genome characterization of a distinct human rhinovirus (HRV) genetic cluster, probably representing a previously undetected HRV species, HRV-C, associated with acute respiratory illness in children. *J. Clin. Microbiol.* **45:**3655–3664.
89. **Lebel, M. H., M. Gauthier, J. Lacroix, E. Rousseau, and M. Buithieu.** 1989. Respiratory failure and mechanical ventilation in severe bronchiolitis. *Arch. Dis. Child.* **64:**1431–1437.
90. **Lee, N., D. Hui, A. Wu, P. Chan, P. Cameron, G. M. Joynt, A. Ahuja, M. Y. Yung, C. B. Leung, K. F. To, S. F. Lui, C. C. Szeto, S. Chung, and J. J. Sung.** 2003. A major outbreak of severe acute respiratory syndrome in Hong Kong. *N. Engl. J. Med.* **348:**1986–1994.
91. **Lesouef, P. N., G. C. Geelhoed, D. J. Turner, S. E. Morgan, and L. I. Landau.** 1989. Response of normal infants to inhaled histamine. *Am. Rev. Respir. Dis.* **139:** 62–66.
92. **Levandowski, R. A., T. R. Gerrity, and C. S. Garrard.** 1985. Modifications of lung clearance mechanisms by acute influenza A infection. *J. Lab. Clin. Med.* **106:**428–432.
93. **Louie, J., A. Kajon, M. Holodniy, L. Guardia-LaBar, B. Lee, A. Petru, J. Hacker, and D. Schnurr.** 2008. Severe pneumonia due to adenovirus serotype 14: a new respiratory threat? *Clin. Infect. Dis.* **46:**421–425.
94. **Louria, D. B., H. L. Blumenfeld, J. T. Ellis, E. D. Kilbourne, and D. E. Rogers.** 1959. Studies on influenza in the pandemic of 1957–1958. II. Pulmonary complications of influenza. *J. Clin. Investig.* **38:**213–265.
95. **Mallia, P., and S. L. Johnston.** 2006. How viral infections cause exacerbation of airway diseases. *Chest* **130:** 1203–1210.
96. **Markowitz, L. E., and P. Neiburg.** 1991. The burden of acute respiratory infection due to measles in developing countries and the potential impact of measles vaccine. *Rev. Infect. Dis.* **13:**S555–S561.
97. **Marx, A., H. E. Gary, Jr., B. J. Marston, D. D. Erdman, R. F. Breiman, T. J. Torok, J. F. Plouffe, T. M. File, Jr., and L. J. Anderson.** 1999. Parainfluenza virus infection among adults hospitalized for lower respiratory tract infection. *Clin. Infect. Dis.* **29:**134–140.
98. **Mayo-Smith, M. F., J. W. Spinale, C. J. Donskey, M. Yukawa, R. H. Li, and F. J. Schiffman.** 1995. Acute epiglottitis: an 18-year experience in Rhode Island. *Chest* **108:**1640–1647.
99. **McIsaac, W. J., J. D. Kellner, P. Aufricht, A. Vanjaka, and D. E. Low.** 2004. Empirical validation of guidelines for the management of pharyngitis in children and adults. *JAMA* **291:**1587–1595. (Erratum, **294:**2700, 2005.)
100. **McMillan, J. A., L. B. Weiner, A. M. Higgins, and K. MacKnight.** 1993. Rhinovirus infection associated with serious illness among pediatric patients. *Pediatr. Infect. Dis. J.* **12:**321–325.
101. **Meert, K. L., A. P. Sarnaik, M. J. Gelmini, and M. W. Lich-Lai.** 1994. Aerosolized ribavirin in mechanically ventilated children with respiratory syncytial virus lower respiratory tract disease: a prospective, double-blind, randomized trial. *Crit. Care Med.* **22:**566–572.
102. **Mohsen, A. H., and M. McKendrick.** 2003. Varicella pneumonia in adults. *Eur. Respir. J.* **21:**886–891.
103. **Monto, A. S., and K. M. Sullivan.** 1993. Acute respiratory illness in the community: frequency of illness and the agents involved. *Epidemiol. Infect.* **110:**145–160.
104. **Mosser, A. G., R. Vrtis, L. Burchell, W. M. Lee, C. R. Dick, E. Weisshaar, D. Bock, C. A. Swenson, R. D. Cornwell, K. C. Meyer, N. N. Jarjour, W. W. Busse, and J. E. Gern.** 2005. Quantitative and qualitative anal-

ysis of rhinovirus infection in bronchial tissues. *Am. J. Respir. Crit. Care Med.* **171:**645–651.

105. **Müller, N. L., G. C. Ooi, P. L. Khong, and S. Nicolaou.** 2003. Severe acute respiratory syndrome: radiographic and CT findings. *Am. J. Roentgenol.* **181:**3–8.
106. **Naclerio, R. M., D. Proud, A. Kagey-Sobotka, L. M. Lichtenstein, J. O. Hendley, and J. M. Gwaltney, Jr.** 1988. Kinins are generated during experimental rhinovirus colds. *J. Infect. Dis.* **157:**133–142.
107. **Neuzil, K. M., G. W. Reed, E. F. Mitchel, L. Simonsen, and M. R. Griffin.** 1998. The impact of influenza on acute cardiopulmonary hospitalizations in pregnant women. *Am. J. Epidemiol.* **148:**1094–1102.
108. **Okamoto, Y., K. Kudo, K. Ishikawa, E. Ito, K. Togawa, I. Saito, I. Moro, J. A. Patel, and P. L. Ogra.** 1993. Presence of respiratory syncytial virus genomic sequences in middle ear fluid and its relationship to expression of cytokines and cell adhesion molecules. *J. Infect. Dis.* **168:**1277–1281.
109. **Pahl, E., and S. S. Gidding.** 1988. Echocardiographic assessment of cardiac function during respiratory syncytial virus infection. *Pediatrics* **81:**830–834.
110. **Parrott, R. H., H. W. Kim, and J. O. Arrobio.** 1973. Epidemiology of respiratory syncytial virus infection in Washington, D.C. *Am. J. Epidemiol.* **98:**289–300.
111. **Paul, I. M., J. Beiler, A. McMonagle, M. L. Shaffer, L. Duda, and C. M. Berlin, Jr.** 2007. Effect of honey, dextromethorphan, and no treatment on nocturnal cough and sleep quality for coughing children and their parents. *Arch. Pediatr. Adolesc. Med.* **161:**1140–1146.
112. **Peiris, J. S., S. T. Lai, L. L. M. Poon, Y. Guan, L. Y. C. Yam, W. Lim, J. Nicholls, W. K. S. Yee, W. W. Yan, M. T. Cheung, V. C. C. Cheng, K. H. Chan, D. N. C. Tsang, R. W. H. Yung, T. K. Ng, K. Y. Yuen, and Members of the SARS Study Group.** 2003. Coronavirus as a possible cause of severe acute respiratory syndrome. *Lancet* **361:**1319–1325.
113. **Pitkaranta, A., A. Virolainen, J. Jero, E. Arruda, and F. G. Hayden.** 1998. Detection of rhinovirus, respiratory syncytial virus, and coronavirus infections in acute otitis media by reverse transcriptase polymerase chain reaction. *Pediatrics* **102:**291–295.
114. **Proud, D., C. J. Reynolds, S. Lacapra, A. Kagey-Sobotka, L. M. Lichtenstein, and R. M. Naclerio.** 1988. Nasal provocation with bradykinin induces symptoms of rhinitis and sore throat. *Am. Rev. Respir. Dis.* **137:**613–616.
115. **Ramsey, P. G., K. H. Fife, R. C. Hackman, J. D. Meyers, and L. Corey.** 1982. Herpes simplex virus pneumonia: clinical, virologic, and pathologic features in 20 patients. *Ann. Intern. Med.* **97:**813–820.
116. **Reed, E. C., R. A. Bowden, P. S. Dandliker, C. A. Gleaves, and J. D. Meyers.** 1986. Treatment of cytomegalovirus pneumonia with 9-[2-hydroxy-1-(hydroxymethyl) ethoxymethyl] guanine and high-dose corticosteroids. *Ann. Intern. Med.* **105:**214–215.
117. **Reed, E. C., R. A. Bowden, P. S. Dandliker, K. E. Lilleby, and J. D. Meyers.** 1988. Treatment of cytomegalovirus pneumonia with ganciclovir and intravenous cytomegalovirus immunoglobulin in patients with bone marrow transplants. *Ann. Intern. Med.* **109:**783–788.
118. **Rees, G. L., and R. Eccles.** 1994. Sore throat following nasal and orophayrngeal bradykinin challenge. *Acta Oto-Laryngol.* **114:**311–314.
119. **Ross, L. A., W. H. Mason, J. Lanson, T. W. Deakers, and C. J. L. Newth.** 1992. Laryngotracheobronchitis as a complication of measles during an urban epidemic. *J. Pediatr.* **121:**511–515.
120. **Sable, C. A., and F. G. Hayden.** 1995. Orthomyxoviral and paramyxoviral infections in transplant patients. *Infect. Dis. Clin. N. Am.* **9:**987–1003.
121. **Schwarzmann, S. W., J. L. Adler, R. F. J. Sullivan, and W. M. Marine.** 1971. Bacterial pneumonia during the Hong Kong influenza epidemic of 1968–1969. *Arch. Intern. Med.* **127:**1037–1041.
122. **Sharfstein, J. M., M. North, and J. R. Serwint.** 2007. Over the counter but no longer under the radar—pediatric cough and cold medications. *N. Engl. J. Med.* **357:**2321–2324.
123. **Sherry, M. K., A. S. Klainer, M. Wolff, and H. Gerhard.** 1988. Herpetic tracheobronchitis. *Ann. Intern. Med.* **109:**229–233.
124. **Slapak, I., J. Skoupa, P. Strnad, and P. Hornik.** 2008. Efficacy of isotonic nasal wash (seawater) in the treatment and prevention of rhinitis in children. *Arch. Otolaryngol. Head Neck Surg.* **134:**67–74.
125. **Sperber, S. J., J. O. Hendley, F. G. Hayden, D. K. Riker, J. V. Sorrentino, and J. M. Gwaltney, Jr.** 1992. Effects of naproxen on experimental rhinovirus colds. A randomized, double-blind, controlled trial. *Ann. Intern. Med.* **117:**37–41.
126. **Steensel-Moll, H. A., J. A. Hazelzet, E. V. D. Voort, H. J. Neijens, and W. H. L. Hackeng.** 1990. Excessive secretion of antidiuretic hormone in infections with respiratory syncytial virus. *Arch. Dis. Child.* **65:**1237–1239.
127. **Stein, R. T., D. Sherrill, W. J. Morgan, C. J. Holberg, M. Halonen, L. M. Taussig, A. L. Wright, and F. D. Martinez.** 1999. Respiratory syncytial virus in early life and risk of wheeze and allergy by age 13 years. *Lancet* **354:**541–545.
128. **Taverner, D., C. Danz, and D. Econimos.** 1999. The effects of oral pseudoephedrine on nasal patency in the common cold: a double-blind single-dose placebo-controlled trial. *Clin. Otolaryngol. Allied Sci.* **24:**47–51.
129. **Turner, B. W., W. S. Cail, J. O. Hendley, F. G. Hayden, W. J. Doyle, J. V. Sorrention, and J. M. Gwaltney, Jr.** 1992. Physiologic abnormalities in the paranasal sinuses during experimental rhinovirus colds. *J. Allergy Clin. Immunol.* **90:**474–478.
130. **Turner, R. B., S. J. Sperber, J. V. Sorrentino, R. R. O'Connor, J. Rogers, A. R. Batouli, and J. M. Gwaltney, Jr.** 1997. Effectiveness of clemastine fumarate for treatment of rhinorrhea and sneezing associated with the common cold. *Clin. Infect. Dis.* **25:**824–830.
131. **Turner, R. B., M. T. Wecker, G. Pohl, T. J. Witek, E. McNally, R. St. George, B. Winther, and F. G. Hayden.** 1999. Efficacy of tremacamra, a soluble intercellular adhesion molecule 1, for experimental rhinovirus infection: a randomized clinical trial. *JAMA* **281:**1797–1804.
132. **van den Hoogen, B. G., J. C. de Jong, J. Groen, T. Kuiken, R. de Groot, R. A. Fouchier, and A. D. Osterhaus.** 2001. A newly discovered human pneumovirus isolated from young children with respiratory tract disease. *Nat. Med.* **7:**719–724.
133. **van Schaik, S. M., R. C. Welliver, and J. L. L. Kimpen.** 2000. Novel pathways in the pathogenesis of respiratory syncytial virus disease. *Pediatr. Pulmonol.* **30:**131–138.
134. **Wainwright, C., L. Altamirano, M. Cheney, J. Cheney, S. Barber, D. Price, S. Moloney, A. Kimberley, N. Woolfield, S. Cadzow, F. Fiumara, P. Wilson, S. Mego, D. VandeVelde, S. Sanders, P. O'Rourke, and P. Francis.** 2003. A multicenter, randomized, double-blind, controlled trial of nebulized epinephrine in infants with acute bronchiolitis. *N. Engl. J. Med.* **349:**27–35.
135. **Waner, J. L., N. J. Whitehurst, S. J. Todd, H. Shalaby, and L. V. Wall.** 1990. Comparison of Directigen RSV with viral isolation and direct immunofluorescence for

the identification of respiratory syncytial virus. *J. Clin. Microbiol.* **28:**480–483.

136. **Wenzel, R. P., and A. A. Fowler.** 2006. Acute bronchitis. *N. Engl. J. Med.* **355:**2125–2130.
137. **Whimbey, E., L. S. Eling, R. B. Couch, W. Lo, L. Williams, R. E. Champlin, and G. P. Bodey.** 1994. Influenza A virus infection among hospitalized adult bone marrow transplant recipients. *Bone Marrow Transplant.* **13:**437–440.
138. **Wildin, S. R., T. Chonmaitree, and L. E. Swischuk.** 1988. Roentgenographic features of common pediatric viral respiratory tract infections. *Am. J. Dis. Child.* **142:** 43–46.
139. **Wilkinson, T. M., J. R. Hurst, W. R. Perera, M. Wilks, G. C. Donaldson, and J. A. Wedzicha.** 2006. Effect of interactions between lower airway bacterial and rhinoviral infection in exacerbations of COPD. *Chest* **129:** 317–324.
140. **Williams, J. V., P. A. Harris, S. J. Tollefson, L. L. Halburnt-Rush, J. M. Pingsterhaus, K. M. Edwards, P. F. Wright, and J. E. Crowe, Jr.** 2004. Human metapneumovirus and lower respiratory tract disease in otherwise healthy infants and children. *N. Engl. J. Med.* **350:**443–450.
141. **Wohl, M. E. B., and V. Chernick.** 1978. Bronchiolitis. *Am. Rev. Respir. Dis.* **118:**759–781.
142. **Wright, A. L., L. M. Taussig, C. G. Ray, H. R. Harrison, and C. J. Holberg.** 1989. The Tucson Children's Respiratory Study. II. Lower respiratory tract illness in the first year of life. *Am. J. Epidemiol.* **129:**1232–1246.
143. **Wright, P. F., R. A. Karron, R. B. Belshe, J. Thompson, J. E. J. Crowe, T. G. Boyce, L. L. Halburnt, G. W. Reed, S. S. Whitehead, E. L. Anderson, A. E. Wittek, R. C. Casey, M. Eichelberger, B. Thumar, V. B. Randolph, S. A. Udem, R. M. Chanock, and B. R. Murphy.** 2000. Evaluation of a live, cold-passaged, temperature-sensitive, respiratory syncytial virus vaccine candidate in infancy. *J. Infect. Dis.* **182:**1331–1342.
144. **Yelandi, A. V., and T. V. Colby.** 1994. Pathologic features of lung biopsy specimens from influenza pneumonia cases. *Hum. Pathol.* **25:**47–53.
145. **Yoon, B. W., H. J. Bae, K. S. Hong, S. M. Lee, B. J. Park, K. H. Yu, M. K. Han, Y. S. Lee, D. K. Chung, J. M. Park, S. W. Jeong, B. C. Lee, K. H. Cho, J. S. Kim, S. H. Lee, K. M. Yoo, and Acute Brain Bleeding Analysis (ABBA) Study Investigators.** 2007. Phenylpropanolamine contained in cold remedies and risk of hemorrhagic stroke. *Neurology* **68:**146–149.
146. **Zaki, S. R., P. W. Greer, L. M. Coffield, C. S. Goldsmith, K. B. Nolte, K. Foucar, R. M. Feddersen, R. E. Zumwalt, G. L. Miller, A. S. Khan, P. E. Rollin, T. G. Ksiazek, S. T. Nichol, B. W. J. Mahy, and C. J. Peters.** 1995. Hantavirus pulmonary syndrome: pathogenesis of an emerging infectious disease. *Am. J. Pathol.* **146:**552–579.
147. **Zaroukian, M. H., and I. Leader.** 1988. Community-acquired pneumonia and infection with respiratory syncytial virus. *Ann. Intern. Med.* **109:**515–516.

Viral Central Nervous System Infections

KEVIN A. CASSADY AND RICHARD J. WHITLEY

3

Central nervous system (CNS) symptoms (headache, lethargy, and impaired psychomotor performance) are frequent components of viral infections; however, viral infections of the CNS occur infrequently and most often result in relatively benign, self-limited disease. Nevertheless, these infections have tremendous importance because of the potential for death and neurologic damage. Neural tissues are exquisitely sensitive to metabolic derangements, and injured brain tissue recovers slowly and often incompletely (7, 49). Clinical presentation and patient history, while frequently suggestive of a diagnosis, remain unreliable methods for determining the specific etiology of CNS disease (7, 84). Tumors, infections, and autoimmune processes in the CNS often produce similar signs and symptoms (84). Different diseases may share a common pathogenic mechanism and therefore result in similar clinical presentations. Furthermore, understanding the pathogenic mechanism of a disease provides a rational basis for the development of antiviral medications and strategies for the prevention of viral CNS infections.

The definitions of viral CNS disease are often based on both virus tropism and disease duration. Inflammation occurs at multiple sites within the CNS and accounts for the myriad of clinical descriptors of viral neurologic disease. Inflammation of the spinal cord, leptomeninges, dorsal nerve roots, or nerves results in myelitis, meningitis, radiculitis, or neuritis, respectively. Aseptic meningitis is a misnomer frequently used to refer to a benign, self-limited viral infection causing inflammation of the leptomeninges (69). The term hinders epidemiological studies, as the definition fails to differentiate between infectious (fungal, tuberculous, viral, or other infectious etiologies) and noninfectious causes of meningitis. Encephalitis refers to inflammation of parenchymal brain tissue and is usually accompanied by a depressed level of consciousness, altered cognition, and frequently focal neurologic signs. Acute encephalitis occurs over a relatively short period (days), while chronic encephalitis presents over weeks to months. The temporal course of slow infections of the CNS (kuru, visna, and variant Creutzfeldt-Jakob disease [vCJD]) overlaps with the chronic encephalitides. Slow infections of the CNS are distinguished by their long incubation period combined with a slow replication rate, eventually resulting in death or extreme neurologic disability over months to years (86).

Viral disease in the CNS can also be classified by pathogenesis. Neurologic disease is frequently categorized as either primary or postinfectious. Primary encephalitis results from direct viral entry into the CNS that produces clinically evident cortical or brain stem dysfunction (69). Subsequent damage results from a combination of virus-induced cytopathic effects and the host immune response. Viral invasion, however, remains the initiating event (69). The parenchyma exhibits neuronophagia and the presence of viral antigens or nucleic acids (48). A postinfectious or parainfectious encephalitis produces signs and symptoms of encephalitis temporally associated with a systemic viral infection, without evidence of direct viral invasion in the CNS. Pathological specimens demonstrate demyelination and perivascular aggregation of immune cells, without evidence of virus or viral antigen, leading some to hypothesize an autoimmune etiology (69).

Meningitis and encephalitis represent separate clinical entities; however, a continuum exists between these distinct forms of disease. A change in a patient's clinical condition can reflect disease progression with involvement of different regions of the brain. Therefore, in many cases it is difficult to accurately and prospectively predict the etiology and extent of CNS infection. Epidemiological data in many cases provide clues to the etiology of the illness. An overview is difficult, as each pathogen fills a different ecological niche with unique seasonal, host, and vector properties (Tables 1 and 2)(69). Instead, it is useful to analyze the prototypes of viral CNS infection, meningitis and encephalitis, and the approach to patients with presumed viral infections of the CNS.

VIRAL MENINGITIS

Epidemiology

Acute viral meningitis and meningoencephalitis represent the majority of viral CNS infections and frequently occur in epidemics or in seasonal distribution (55, 69). While there have been changes in the epidemiology of viral meningitis in North America through the recent introduction of West Nile virus, enteroviruses cause the majority of viral meningitis cases. Arboviruses constitute the second most common cause of viral meningitis in the United States (7, 43, 56, 62). Mumps virus remains an important cause of

TABLE 1 DNA viruses: type of disease, epidemiological data, and pathogenesis of viral infections of the CNS

Viral agent	CNS disease	Temporal course	Transmission	Pathway to CNS	Relative frequency[a]	Laboratory confirmation
Herpesviridae						
HSV-1	Encephalitis	Acute (congenital), sporadic (latent)	Human	Neuronal, blood	+++	PCR of CSF; cell culture of brain biopsy sample
HSV-2	Meningitis Encephalitis	Primary, recurrent Acute (congenital)	Human	Neuronal, blood Blood, neuronal	++	Cell culture of genital, rectal, and skin samples; PCR of CSF
CMV	Encephalitis (neonate and immunosuppressed)	Acute, subacute	Human	Blood	++	PCR; cell culture of brain biopsy sample or CSF
EBV	Encephalitis, meningitis, myelitis, Guillain-Barré syndrome	Acute	Human	Blood	+	PCR
VZV	Cerebellitis, encephalitis, meningitis, myelitis	Postinfectious (acute), latent reactivation (zoster)	Human	Blood, neuronal	++	PCR, clinical findings, cell culture from a lesion, brain biopsy sample, or necroscopy (rarely)
Human herpesvirus 6	Encephalitis, febrile seizures, latent form?	Acute	Human	Blood	++	PCR
B virus (cercopithecine herpesvirus 1)	Encephalitis	Acute	Animal bite and human	Blood	+	Culture, PCR (high frequency of detection; unknown significance)
Adenoviridae						
Adenovirus	Meningitis, encephalitis	Acute	Human	Blood	+	Cell culture of CSF or brain
Poxviridae						
Vaccinia virus	Encephalomyelitis	Postinfectious	Vaccine	Blood	Presumed extinct	Recent vaccination

[a] +++, frequent; ++, infrequent; +, rare; ?, unknown.

viral CNS disease in countries that do not immunize against this virus. Recent data indicate that the risk of meningitis from natural mumps virus infection outweighs the risk of aseptic meningitis associated with the vaccine; nonetheless, not all countries vaccinate against mumps (7, 44, 52). There are greater than 74,000 cases of viral meningitis a year in the United States (68). Most cases occur from the late spring to autumn months, reflecting increased enteroviral and arboviral infections during these seasons (7, 68). A retrospective survey performed in the 1980s found that the annual incidence of "aseptic meningitis" was approximately 10.9/100,000 persons, or at least four times the incidence passively reported to the CDC during the period (55). Virus was identified in only 11% of patients in this study. With the advent of improved nucleic acid-based diagnostic methods these data have changed, and isolation rates now approach 50 to 86% (7, 41, 42).

Pathogenesis

The pathogenesis of viral meningitis is incompletely understood. Inferences regarding the pathogenesis of viral meningitis are largely derived from data on encephalitis, experimental animal models of meningitis, and clinical observations (69). Viruses use two basic pathways to gain access to the CNS: hematogenous and neuronal spread. Most cases of viral meningitis occur following a high-titer secondary viremia. Host and viral factors combined with seasonal, geographic, and epidemiological probabilities influence the proclivity to develop viral CNS infection. For example, arboviral infections occur more frequently in epidemics and show a seasonal variation, reflecting the prevalence of the transmitting vector (7, 48). Enteroviral meningitis occurs with greater frequency during the summer and early autumn months, reflecting the seasonal increase in enteroviral infections. Enteroviral infections also exemplify the difference host physiology makes in determining the extent of viral disease. In children less than 2 weeks of age, enterovirus infections can produce a severe systemic infection, including meningitis or meningoencephalitis (68). Ten percent of neonates with systemic enteroviral infections die, while as many as 76% are left with permanent sequelae. In children over 2 weeks of age, however, enteroviral infections are rarely associated with severe disease or significant morbidity (68).

The sequence of viral hematogenous spread to the CNS is illustrated in Fig. 1 (69). A virus must first bypass or attach to and enter host epithelial cells to produce infection. Virus then spreads and initially replicates in the regional lymph nodes (e.g., measles and influenza viruses) or enters the circulatory system, where it seeds other tissues (e.g., arboviruses, enteroviruses, and varicella-zoster virus [VZV]) (69). Primary viremia allows virus to seed distant locations of the body and frequently marks the onset of clinical illness. In rare circumstances such as disseminated neonatal herpes simplex virus (HSV) infection, viruses infect the CNS during primary viremia (37, 75); however, most viral infections involve an intermediate organ prior to reaching the CNS. The liver and spleen provide ideal locations for secondary viral replication due to their highly vascular structure and reticuloendothelial network. Secondary viremia results in high titers of virus in the bloodstream for prolonged periods, facilitating viral CNS spread. The pathophysiology of viral transport from blood to the brain and viral endothelial cell tropism is poorly understood. Virus infects endothelial cells, leaks across the damaged endothelium, passively channels through the endothelium (pinocytosis or colloidal transport), or bridges the endothelium within migrating leukocytes (69). This transendothelial passage occurs in vessels of the choroid plexus, meninges, or cerebrum, as depicted in Fig. 2.

Numerous barriers and host defenses limit viral dissemination to the CNS. The skin and mucosal surfaces possess mechanical, chemical, and cellular defenses that protect the cells from viral infection (69). Leukocytes and secretory factors (interleukins, interferons, and antibodies) further augment these defenses and help eliminate viruses that bridge the epithelial layer. Local immune responses are crucial in limiting systemic viral infection. A swift inflammatory response can limit viremia and symptoms of infection. In the liver and spleen, the high degree of parenchymal contact and large number of fixed mononuclear macrophages provide an excellent opportunity for host eradication of viremia (69). The blood-brain or blood-cerebrospinal fluid (blood-CSF) barrier, a network of tight endothelial junctions sheathed by glial cells that regulate molecular access to the CNS, further limits viral access to the CNS (21, 53).

Viral meningitis is a relatively benign self-limited illness, and pathological specimens are rarely available for study (68). The CSF, however, is frequently sampled and demonstrates a mononuclear immune cell response to most viral infections. Certain viral infections, most notably mumps virus and some enterovirus infections, elicit a polymorphonuclear cell infiltrate in the CSF early during disease. The initial CSF formula mimics bacterial meningitis and later shifts to a mononuclear predominance. Viral antigen presentation by mononuclear histiocytes stimulates the influx of immune cells. Recruited immune cells release soluble factors (interleukins and vasoactive amines) that mobilize other cells and change the permeability of the blood-brain barrier (5, 7). The viral etiology and type of CNS disease (meningitis versus encephalitis) can produce differences in CSF gamma interferon, interleukin 2 (IL-2), IL-6, and IL-12 levels (31, 51, 83). While research data suggest that these may be used to differentiate CNS disease, CSF cytokine measurements are not a routine commercial diagnostic method and are limited to research institutions. Furthermore, these cytokines are also elevated in autoimmune CNS disease (23). Physical and chemical changes in the blood-brain barrier allow the entry of serum proteins like immunoglobulins and interleukins, further augmenting the antiviral process. The cell-mediated immune response is important for eliminating virus from the CNS; however, immunoglobulin also has a role in protecting the host in some viral infections. This is best illustrated by the devastating clinical course of enteroviral meningitis in agammaglobulinemic patients as well as X-linked hyper-immunoglobulin M syndrome (13, 68, 70). Patients with impaired cell-mediated immunity have a higher incidence of CNS infections with certain viruses (VZV, measles virus, and cytomegalovirus [CMV])(69).

Clinical Manifestations

Age, immune status, and viral etiology influence the clinical manifestations of viral meningitis. Patients with enteroviral meningitis often present with nonspecific symptoms such as fever (38 to 40°C) of 3 to 5 days' duration, malaise, and headache (7, 68). Approximately 50% of patients have nausea or vomiting (7). While nuchal rigidity and photophobia are the hallmark sign and symp-

TABLE 2 RNA viruses: type of disease, epidemiological data, and pathogenesis of viral infections of the CNS[a]

Viral taxonomy	CNS disease	Case fatality rate (%)	Vector	Geographic distribution	Disease pattern	Pathway to CNS	Frequency[e]	Laboratory confirmation[f]
Togaviridae, *Alphavirus* (arbovirus)								
Western equine encephalitis virus	Meningitis, encephalitis	3–10	Mosquitoes, birds	United States, west of the Mississippi River	Epidemic	Blood	++	Serologic titer (HI, CF, N, IFA); viral antigen detection in brain; rarely culture
Eastern equine encephalitis virus		>30		United States, Atlantic and Gulf Coast states	Sporadic		+	Viral culture or antigen detection in brain; serologic titer (HI, CF, N, IFA); CSF IgM ELISA
Venezuelan equine encephalitis virus		<1	Mosquitoes, horses	Central and South America, southwestern United States, and Florida	Sporadic, epidemic		+	Serologic titer (HI, CF, N, IFA); CSF IgM ELISA
Flaviviridae, *Flavivirus* (arbovirus)								
Japanese encephalitis virus	Meningitis, encephalitis	25	Mosquitoes, swine, or birds	Japan, China, Korea, Taiwan, Southeast Asia, India, Nepal	Epidemic, endemic	Blood	+++	Peripheral blood ELISA; serologic titer (HI, CF, N, IFA); CSF antigen tests or PCR
St. Louis encephalitis virus		7		United States			+++	CSF IgM ELISA, serologic titer (HI, CF, N, IFA); PCR; rarely culture
West Nile virus		Higher attack rate in elderly (11–33)		Africa, Middle East, India, Eastern Europe; recently imported into the United States and spreading rapidly			+++	Culture (rare), serologic titer (HI, IFA), PCR
Murray Valley virus	Encephalitis	20–60		Australia			++	Viral culture, serologic titer (HI, CF, N)
Tick-borne encephalitis virus complex		20	Ticks, unpasteurized milk	Eastern Russia and Central Europe	Epidemic, sporadic		++	Serologic titer (HI, CF, N), IgM ELISA PCR
Bunyaviridae (arbovirus)								
California (La Crosse) encephalitis virus	Meningitis, encephalitis	<1	Mosquitoes, rodents	Northern Midwest and northeastern United States	Endemic	Blood	+++ (LCV) + (CEV)	Viral culture. CSF IgM ELISA; serologic titer (HI, CF, N, IFA); CIE; PCR

Reoviridae, *Coltivirus* (arbovirus)								
Colorado tick fever virus	Meningitis, encephalitis	<1	Ticks, rodents	Rocky Mountains, Pacific Coast states of the United States	Endemic	Blood	+	Antigen detection on erythrocyte membrane; viral culture; serologic titer (HI, CF, N, IFA)
Picornaviridae (enterovirus)								
Poliovirus	Meningitis, myelitis	4.5–50[b]	Fecal-oral	Worldwide	Endemic	Blood and neuronal	++	Viral culture from CSF or brain; viral culture from another site; serologic testing for some serotypes; PCR
Coxsackievirus	Meningitis, meningoencephalitis, myelitis	Rarely[c]				Blood	+++	
Echovirus							+++	
Paramyxoviridae (exanthematous virus)								
Measles virus	Encephalitis, SSPE[d]	15	Postinfectious, blood	Worldwide	Sporadic	Blood	++	Serology, ELISA, clinically
Mumps virus	Meningitis, encephalitis, myelitis	<1	Blood				+++	CSF viral culture
Orthomyxoviridae (upper respiratory virus)								
Influenza viruses	Encephalitis	<1	Postinfectious	Worldwide	Sporadic	Blood	+	Viral culture from another site
Rhabdoviridae								
Rabies virus	Encephalitis, encephalomyelitis	~100	Mammals	Worldwide	Sporadic	Neuronal	+++	Antigen detection in brain; serologic tests (IFA, CF, HA, CIE); viral culture
Retroviridae								
HIV type 1	Encephalopathy, encephalitis, leukoencephalopathy	Majority	Humans	Worldwide	Progressive	Blood	++	PCR of CSF or autopsy samples; MRI findings; isolation; in situ antigen detection
Arenaviridae								
Lymphocytic choriomeningitis virus	Meningitis, encephalitis	<2.5	Rodents	Worldwide	Sporadic	Blood	+	CSF, blood culture; urine culture; serology

[a] Data from reference 7.

[b] The case fatality rate from poliomyelitis is increased in sporadic cases. With vaccination, the epidemic forms of polio have decreased, as has morbidity. In turn, the calculated case fatality rate in the United States has increased as sporadic and vaccine-associated disease has increased relative to the number of cases of disease.

[c] Rarely fatal except in nenonate and agammaglobulinemic patient where fatality rates can approach 50% even with treatment.

[d] SSPE, subacute sclerosing parencephalitis.

[e] +++, frequent; ++, infrequent; +, rare; ?, unknown.

[f] HI, hemagglutination inhibition; CF, complement fixation; NA, neutralizing antibody titer; CIE, counterimmunoelectrophoresis; IFA, immunofluorescent antibody; ELISA, enzyme-linked immunosorbent assay.

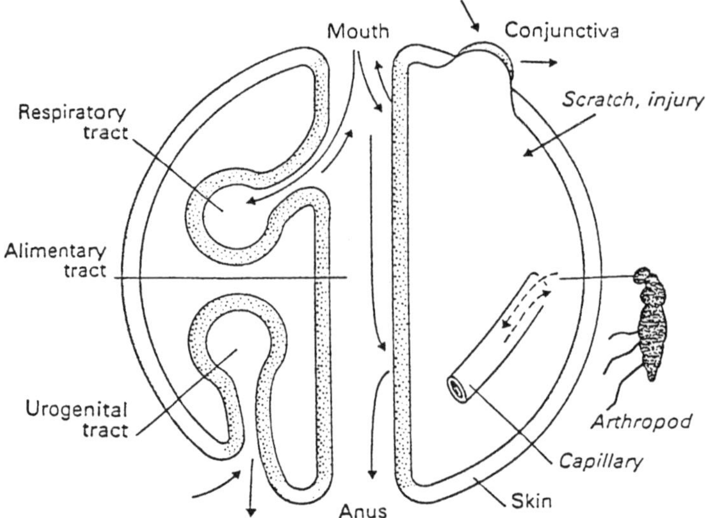

FIGURE 1 Body surfaces as sites of virus infection and shedding.

tom for meningitis, 33% of patients with viral meningitis have no evidence of meningismus (7). Less than 10% of children younger than 2 years of age develop signs of meningeal irritation. The majority of these children with meningitis present with fever and irritability (64). Children may also present with seizures secondary to fever, electrolyte disturbances, or the infection itself. The clinician must have a high index of suspicion for meningitis, especially in younger patients. In the immunocompromised host, enteroviral infection is both a diagnostic quandary and a potentially life-threatening disease. Immunocompromised patients frequently do not mount a brisk immune cell response; therefore, CSF analysis does not reflect evidence of disease (namely, CNS involvement).

Symptoms of meningitis (stiff neck, headache, and photophobia) occur in approximately 11% of men and 36% of women with primary HSV type 2 (HSV-2) genital infection. In one study, 5% of patients with primary HSV genital infection had severe enough meningitis to require hospitalization. All of the hospitalized patients had evidence of a lymphocytic pleocytosis on CSF analysis (7). In another study, HSV-2 was cultured from the CSF of 78% of patients with meningitis symptoms during primary genital infection. These patients also exhibited a CSF leukocytosis and increases in CSF antibody titers (6). Examples exist of recurrent HSV-2 meningitis (with or without genital lesions), although cases associated with primary infection are more common (33). HSV meningitis may spread to the CSF by neuronal spread along the sacral nerves.

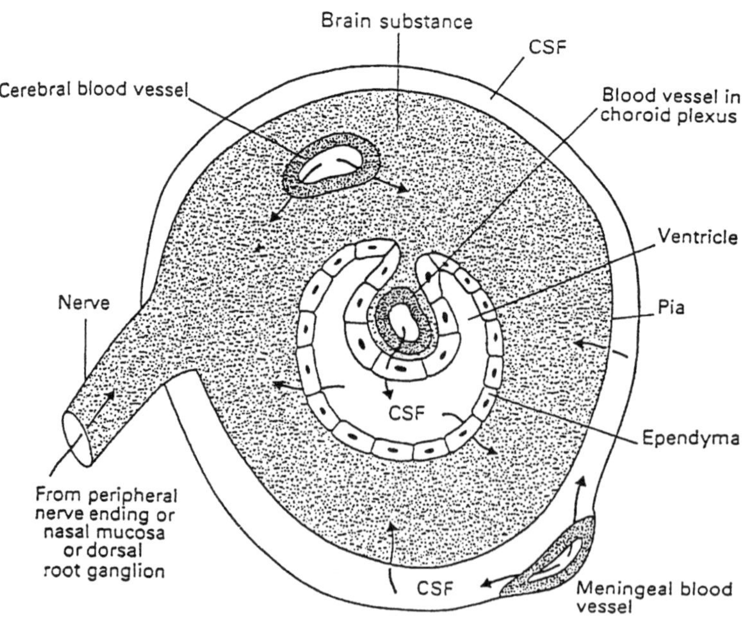

FIGURE 2 Routes of viral invasion of the CNS.

Alternatively, the virus may reach the CSF by hematogenous spread, as the virus has been cultured from the blood buffy coat layer (7). VZV, CMV, Epstein-Barr virus (EBV), and parainfluenza virus have all been cultured or detected by PCR from the CSF of patients with meningitis (7, 30, 41). The three herpesvirus infections occur more frequently in immunocompromised patients and rarely produce isolated meningitis. Instead, these infections usually progress and involve the parenchyma.

Laboratory Findings

Initial CSF samples, while frequently suggestive of a diagnosis, are not sensitive or specific enough predictors to differentiate viral from bacterial meningitis (54). Instead, epidemiological trends, patient history, and accompanying laboratory information are important adjuncts in predicting the etiology of meningitis. CSF in patients with viral meningitis typically exhibits a pleocytosis with 10 to 500 leukocytes, as well as a slightly elevated protein level (<100 mg/dl). The glucose level in the CSF is typically greater than 40% of the level in a simultaneously drawn serum sample. Tremendous variation in CSF formulas exists, with significant overlap between viral and bacterial CSF laboratory findings (54). In a retrospective review of more than 400 patients with acute viral or bacterial meningitis performed before the *Haemophilus influenzae* type b conjugate vaccine was made available, investigators found that approximately 20% of the CSF samples that grew bacteria exhibited a CSF pleocytosis of less than 250 leukocytes/mm^3 (7). Fifteen percent of the patients with bacterial meningitis had a CSF lymphocytosis, while 40% of the patients with viral meningitis had a predominance of polymorphonuclear cells. Some investigators recommend repeating the lumbar puncture 6 to 12 h later, as the CSF profile of patients with viral meningitis will shift from a polymorphonuclear to a lymphocytic pleocytosis over this period (7). However, in one study performed during an echovirus epidemic, 8 of 9 children with presumed enteroviral meningitis failed to develop CSF lymphocyte predominance when a lumbar puncture was repeated 5 to 8 h later (54). A recent retrospective study found that during an enterovirus outbreak, 51% of patients demonstrated polymorphonuclear leukocyte predominance in their CSF profile despite a symptom duration of >24 h. Of note, the investigators in this study were unable to confirm the etiology of meningitis in most cases, as this was a retrospective study (54). Other investigators have confirmed that the change to a lymphocytic CSF profile occurs 18 to 36 h into the illness (82). A multifactorial method examining the CSF profile, peripheral blood profile, and history of seizures resulting in a bacterial meningitis score has also been investigated to differentiate bacterial from viral meningitis. This provides improved sensitivity but still failed to detect all cases of bacterial meningitis, including some cases in infants (57). With the increasing use of highly sensitive and specific nucleic acid-based diagnostic techniques, a viral etiology for the meningitis can often be established within 24 to 36 h, limiting the duration of hospitalization, antibiotic use, and additional diagnostic procedures (42, 43, 62).

Etiologic Diagnosis

Historically, the techniques for identifying viral meningitis were insensitive and often impractical. Depending upon the study cited and diagnostic methods used, investigators identified an agent in only 25 to 67% of presumed CNS infections (7, 32, 41). The diagnosis of viral meningitis relied on viral culture, and CSF viral culture rates differ based on etiology (7).

A synopsis of viral detection techniques for different viruses is presented in Tables 1 and 2 (69). The rapidity and sensitivity of enterovirus diagnosis have improved with the advent of molecular diagnostic techniques such as reverse transcriptase PCR (RT-PCR). Demonstration of viral nucleic acid in the CSF of patients with symptoms of meningitis has replaced viral culture and serologic diagnosis. One of the advantageous features of viral culture is the ability to identify virus serotypes for epidemiological studies; however, for clinical purposes, nucleic acid-based assays have largely replaced viral culture because of their speed and sensitivity (62, 68). As with any PCR-based technique, nucleic acid contamination of the laboratory area is a concern, and results must always be interpreted within the clinical context.

In the past, serologic testing confirmed the clinical suspicion of an arboviral infection. While virus can be cultured from CSF during the early stages of the infection, this has little utility in the acute management of a patient with CNS disease. Recently, the use of RT-PCR for diagnosis of arbovirus infections in the CNS has met with mixed results. Because of the diverse viral etiologies of arboviral infections, the development of specific primers that can hybridize across multiple viral families (*Togaviridae*, *Flaviviridae*, and *Bunyaviridae*) has been difficult. Currently there is an emphasis on the development of improved "universal group primers" to perform an initial group screening, followed by RT-PCR using higher-specificity primers as a second viral diagnostic test (40). Many laboratories have chosen instead to concentrate efforts on establishing diagnostic studies for the more common viral etiologies regionally as a more cost-effective method for diagnosis and patient management (43).

Differential Diagnosis

Unusual but treatable infections should always be considered and investigated in patients with a CSF pleocytosis and negative conventional bacterial cultures. Spirochetes (*Treponema*, *Borrelia*, and *Leptospira*), mycoplasmas, bartonellae, and mycobacteria can produce a pleocytosis with both negative Gram stain and bacterial cultures. Fastidious bacteria (*Listeria*) may fail to grow in culture and occasionally produce a mononuclear pleocytosis similar to viral meningitis. This is of particular concern in infants and elderly and immunocompromised patients. Some bacteria, while not directly infecting the CNS, can release toxins that create a change in the level of consciousness, specifically *Staphylococcus aureus* and *Streptococcus pyogenes* exotoxin-mediated toxic shock syndrome. Frequently, children with streptococcal throat infections present with "neck stiffness" secondary to localized pharyngeal inflammation and tender anterior cervical lymphadenopathy. Parameningeal infections, especially from infected sinuses, produce CNS symptoms and pleocytosis presenting with nuchal rigidity, focal neurologic changes, and altered mental status. Similarly, partially treated bacterial infections can have CSF findings resembling viral meningitis. Questions regarding history of self-medication with leftover antibiotics should be included in a review of systems.

Fungal and parasitic infections can produce CNS infections, although they uncommonly produce only meningitis. The exceptions to this rule are *Coccidioides* and *Cryptococ-*

cus. These pathogens characteristically produce meningitis rather than any focal CNS disease. *Cryptococcus*, for example, produces meningitis primarily in immunosuppressed patients and remains the leading cause of fungal meningitis (7). Many of these infections are treatable and need to be investigated with a thorough history for possible exposures. Fungi such as *Candida, Aspergillus, Histoplasma*, and *Blastomyces* most frequently cause focal parenchymal disease when infecting the CNS. These fungi, while frequently in the differential for an immunocompromised host, can also cause disease in the healthy host. Parasites like *Naegleria fowleri* or *Balamuthia mandrillaris* produce meningoencephalitis with purulent CSF (36, 71). A history of recent summertime swimming in a stagnant pond or recent travel in Central or South America should raise suspicion for these infections.

Noninfectious processes that can produce true aseptic meningitis include hematologic malignancies, medications (especially immunomodulatory, nonsteroidal anti-inflammatory, and trimethoprim-sulfa medications), autoimmune diseases, and foreign material and proteins. Leukemia produces a CSF pleocytosis with cancerous cells; this occurs most frequently with acute lymphocytic leukemia, although subarachnoid involvement can also occur in acute myelogenous leukemia. Immunomodulatory drugs such as intravenous immunoglobulin or antilymphocyte globulin (OKT-3) also cause aseptic meningitis. Of the medications associated with meningitis, nonsteroidal anti-inflammatory agents, sulfa-containing drugs, and cytosine arabinoside are the most common offenders. Drug-induced aseptic meningitis frequently occurs in patients with underlying connective tissue or rheumatologic diseases. A patient with drug-induced aseptic meningitis warrants investigation for a possible underlying autoimmune disease (63). Epithelial or endothelial cysts can rupture and spill their contents (keratin and protein), producing a brisk inflammatory response mimicking acute viral meningitis.

Treatment and Prognosis

The fundamental principle of therapy for viral meningitis lies in the identification of potentially treatable diseases. Until recently, no therapy existed for most cases of viral meningitis. Efforts instead focused on preventive strategies (largely through vaccination) as well as identification of treatable nonviral etiologies of meningitis. Despite these advances, patients with meningitis warrant careful assessment for treatable nonviral etiologies. The clinician must also anticipate and treat the complications of viral CNS disease (seizures, syndrome of inappropriate secretion of antidiuretic hormone, hydrocephalus, and raised intracranial pressure). Supportive therapy includes hydration and antipyretics and analgesics.

In the healthy host, viral meningitis is a relatively benign self-limited disease. A prospective study of children less than 2 years of age, for example, found that even for the 9% of children who develop evidence of acute neurologic disease (complex seizures, increased intracerebral pressure, or coma), the long-term prognosis is excellent. During long-term follow-up (42 months of age), children with acute CNS complications performed neurodevelopmental tasks and achieved developmental milestones as well as children with an uncomplicated course (64). An overview of the approach to a patient with suspected viral CNS disease is presented in a later section.

Antibody preparations and an antiviral agent, pleconaril, have shown activity against enterovirus in small series (2, 81) and animal studies (4, 58, 66). However, randomized controlled trials have not supported their routine use in enterovirus meningitis (1, 17). Case reports exist in the literature of immunoglobulin preparations improving outcome in agammaglobulinemic patients with enteroviral meningitis. Despite the administration of immunoglobulin, these patients did not eliminate the virus from the CSF and developed chronic enteroviral meningitis (7). Enteroviral infections in neonates frequently produce overwhelming viremia and CNS disease. Ten percent of neonates with systemic enteroviral infections die, while as many as 76% are left with permanent sequelae. A blinded randomized control trial did not demonstrate clinical benefit for neonates with severe life-threatening enteroviral infection who received intravenous immunoglobulin (2). While the role of antibody in immunocompromised patients with life-threatening infections remains unproven but debatable, there are currently no data supporting the use of immunoglobulin preparations for non-life-threatening infections in the healthy host.

Specific antiviral agents are available for several other viral etiologies of meningitis. Although no definitive clinical trials have been conducted, most authors recommend the use of intravenous acyclovir for HSV meningitis, as it decreases the duration of primary herpes disease and may limit meningeal involvement (85). Recurrent HSV-2 meningitis occurs rarely, and recently a single case of meningitis associated with HSV-1 reactivation was reported. At this time there are no data on the benefit of antiviral treatment or on suppressive therapy for recurrent HSV CNS disease (7, 12). VZV, CMV, EBV, and parainfluenza virus have all been cultured from the CSF of patients with meningitis. The three herpesvirus infections occur more frequently in immunocompromised patients and can progress to more serious disease such as encephalitis or myelitis. Effective antiviral therapy exists for VZV infections of the CNS and should be instituted in these patients (15, 24). The issue of therapy for CMV CNS infection in the immunocompromised host is more problematic, and therapy should be tailored to the clinical likelihood of infection.

VIRAL ENCEPHALITIS

Epidemiology and Prevalence

Similar to the case with viral meningitis, passive reporting systems underestimate the incidence of viral encephalitis (7). An estimated 20,000 cases of encephalitis occur each year in the United States; however, the CDC received only 740 (0.3/100,000) to 1,340 (0.54/100,000) annual reports of persons with encephalitis from 1990 to 1994 (7). A review of the cases in Olmsted County, MN, from 1950 to 1980 found that the incidence of viral encephalitis was at least twice as frequent as the incidence reported by the CDC (55). A prospective multicenter study in Finland demonstrated results similar to those of the Olmsted study and demonstrated an incidence of encephalitis of 10.5/100,000 (38). Although the introduction of nucleic acid-based diagnostic testing has enhanced the detection of many viruses, a viral etiology is never found in the majority (83%) of cases of encephalitis (41). While the etiology of encephalitis has changed with alterations in the viral reservoirs in North America, the overall death rates from encephalitis have not changed since the late 1970s to 1980s

(35). HSV CNS infections occur without seasonal variation, affect all ages, and constitute the majority of fatal cases of endemic encephalitis in the United States (7). Arboviruses, a group of over 500 arthropod-transmitted RNA viruses, are the leading cause of encephalitis worldwide and in the United States (69). Arboviral infections occur in epidemics and show a seasonal predilection, reflecting the prevalence of the transmitting vector (7). Asymptomatic infections vastly outnumber symptomatic infections. Patients with disease may develop a mild systemic febrile illness or viral meningitis (7). Encephalitis occurs in a minority of persons with arboviral infections, but the case fatality rate varies extremely, from 5 to 70%, depending upon viral etiology and age of the patient. Based upon passive reporting to the CDC, neuroinvasive West Nile virus infections now far outnumber other arboviral causes of encephalitis in the United States (47). It is unknown if this is a function of improved testing and more active surveillance for this disease. Historically, La Crosse virus encephalitis has been the most commonly reported arboviral disease in the United States, while St. Louis virus encephalitis is the most frequent cause of epidemic encephalitis (7, 72). Characteristically, eastern equine encephalitis virus and most arboviral infections occur in the late summer following amplification of the virus and peak mosquito activity (7). This case report demonstrates that in warm climates, the clinician must have a high index of suspicion for insect-borne diseases.

Japanese B virus encephalitis and rabies constitute the majority of cases of encephalitis outside of North America. Japanese encephalitis virus, a member of the *Flavivirus* genus, occurs throughout Asia and causes epidemics in China despite routine immunization (3, 7). In warmer locations, the virus occurs endemically (7, 26). The disease typically affects children, although adults with no history of exposure to the virus are also susceptible (7). As with the other arboviral infections, asymptomatic infections occur more frequently than symptomatic infections. However, the disease has a high case fatality rate and leaves half of the survivors with a significant degree of neurologic morbidity (7). Rabies virus remains endemic around much of the world. Human infections in the United States decreased over the last decades to one to three cases per year due to the immunization of domesticated animals. Bat exposure is increasingly recognized as the source of infection. Fifteen percent (685 of 4,470) of bats tested carried the rabies virus in one study analyzing risk of bat exposure and rabies (60). Bat-associated variants of the virus accounted for 24 of the 32 cases occurring since 1990. In most cases (22 of 24) there was no evidence of bite; however, in half of the cases, direct contact (handling of bats) was documented (9). In areas outside the United States, human cases of rabies virus encephalitis number in the thousands and are caused by unvaccinated domestic animals following contact with infected wild animals.

Postinfectious encephalitis, an acute demyelinating process, has also been referred to as acute disseminated encephalomyelitis (ADEM) or autoimmune encephalitis and accounts for approximately 100 to 200 additional cases of encephalitis annually (7, 77). The disease historically produced approximately one-third of the encephalitis cases in the United States and was associated with measles, mumps, and other exanthematous viral infections (7, 77). Postinfectious encephalitis is now associated with antecedent upper respiratory virus (notably influenza virus) and VZV infections in the United States (7). Autoimmune encephalitis complicates 1 of every 1,000 measles infections, making measles virus the leading cause of postinfectious encephalitis worldwide (7).

The slow infections of the CNS known as transmissible spongiform encephalopathies (TSEs) occur sporadically worldwide. The prototypical TSE is CJD; it occurs at high rates within families and has an estimated incidence of 0.5 to 1.5 cases per million population (86). In 1986, cases of a TSE in cattle, bovine spongiform encephalopathy (BSE), were reported in the United Kingdom. In addition to affecting other livestock throughout Europe that were fed supplements containing meat and bonemeal, cross-species transmission of BSE has been documented, leading to a ban in the use of bovine offal in fertilizers, pet food, and other animal feed (86). A decrease in the recognized cases of BSE has occurred since the institution of these restrictions. Concomitant with the increased cases of BSE in Europe, an increase in cases of an atypical CJD also occurred, suggesting animal-to-human transmission. The report of atypical CJD (unique clinical and histopathological findings) affecting young adults (CJD rarely has been diagnosed in young adults) and a characteristic methionine at the polymorphic codon 129 led to the designation of a new disease, vCJD. As of 2006, a total of 160 cases of vCJD were diagnosed in the United Kingdom and 28 cases were diagnosed outside of the United Kingdom (11).

Pathogenesis

The pathogenesis of encephalitis requires that viruses reach the CNS by hematogenous or neuronal spread. As in meningitis, viruses most frequently access the CNS after a high-titer secondary viremia and cell-free or cell-associated CNS entry (69). Other than direct entry via cerebral vessels, virus can initially infect the meninges and CSF and then enter the parenchyma across either ependymal cells or the pial linings. Viruses exhibit differences in neurotropism and neurovirulence. For example, reovirus types 1 and 3 produce different CNS diseases in mice based on differences in receptor affinities. Hemagglutinin receptors on reovirus type 3 bind to neuronal receptors, enabling fatal encephalitis. Reovirus type 1 has a distinct hemagglutinin antigen and binds to ependymal cells and produces a hydrocephalus and an ependymitis (7). Receptor difference is only one determinant of viral neurotropism. For example, enteroviruses with similar receptors produce very different diseases. Five coxsackie B viruses (B1 to B5) readily produce CNS infections, while type B6 rarely produces neurologic infection (65, 69). Viral genes have been discovered that influence the neurovirulence of HSV-1 (10). HSV-1 mutants with either $\gamma_1 34.5$ gene deletions or stop codons inserted into the gene have a decreased ability to cause encephalitis and death following intracerebral inoculation in mice compared to wild-type virus (10, 44).

In addition to viral factors, host physiology is also important in determining the extent and location of viral CNS disease. Age, sex, and genetic differences between hosts influence viral infections and clinical course (25, 68). Host age influences the clinical manifestations and sequelae of a viral infection. For example, Sindbis virus infection produces lethal encephalitis in newborn mice, while weanling mice experience persistent but nonfatal encephalitis. The reason for the difference in outcome is twofold. Mature neurons resist virus-induced apoptosis, and older mice have an improved antibody response, thus limiting viral replication (25). Variations in macrophage function between individuals can result in clinically distinct infections and disease. Moreover, macrophage antigen response can change with age and is important in limiting spread of infection within a patient (7). In addition to age, physical activity may be another important host factor that determines the severity of infection. Exercise has been associated with increased risk for paralytic poliomyelitis and may result in an increased incidence of enteroviral myocarditis and aseptic meningitis (7). Increasingly, host differences are recognized as equally important determinants of disease at the cellular and molecular levels.

Historically, the peripheral neural pathway was considered the only pathway of viral neurologic infection. Contemporary data, however, demonstrate that the circulatory system provides the principal pathway for most CNS infections in humans (7). HSV and rabies virus are examples of viruses that infect the CNS by neuronal spread. Sensory and motor neurons contain transport systems that carry materials along the axon to (retrograde) and from (anterograde) the nucleus. Peripheral or cranial nerves provide access to the CNS and shield the virus from immunoregulation.

Rabies virus classically infects by the myoneural route and provides a prototype for peripheral neuronal spread (9, 69). Rabies virus replicates locally in the soft tissue following a bite from a rabid animal. After primary replication, the virus enters the peripheral nerve by acetylcholine receptor binding. Once in the muscle, the virus buds from the plasma membrane and crosses myoneural spindles or enters across the motor end plate (69). The virus travels by anterograde and retrograde axonal transport to infect neurons in the brain stem and limbic system. Eventually the virus spreads from the diencephalic and hippocampal structures to the remainder of the brain, killing the animal (69).

Virus also infects the CNS through cranial nerves. Animal studies have shown that HSV can infect the brain through the olfactory system as well as the trigeminal nerve (69). Early HSV encephalitis damages the inferomedial temporal lobe and contains direct connections with the olfactory bulb (7). The route of human HSV infections, however, is less clear. Despite data supporting olfactory and trigeminal spread of virus to the CNS, definitive proof in humans is lacking. The association of viral latency in the trigeminal ganglia, the relative infrequency of HSV encephalitis, and the confusing data regarding encephalitis from HSV reactivation suggest that the pathogenesis is more complex than described above (85).

In patients with acute encephalitis, the parenchyma exhibits neuronophagia and cells containing viral nucleic acids or antigens. The pathological findings are unique for different viruses and reflect differences in pathogenesis and virulence. In the case of typical HSV encephalitis, a hemorrhagic necrosis occurs in the inferomedial temporal lobe, with evidence of perivascular cuffing, lymphocytic infiltration, and neuronophagia (69). Pathological specimens from animals with rabies virus encephalitis demonstrate microglial proliferation, perivascular infiltrates, and neuronal destruction. The location of the pathological findings can be limited to the brain stem areas (dumb rabies) or the diencephalic, hippocampal, and hypothalamic areas (furious rabies) based on the immune response mounted against the infection (69). Pathological findings relate to the viral etiology and are discussed in subsequent sections.

Some viruses do not directly infect the CNS but produce immune system changes that result in parenchymal damage. Patients with postinfectious encephalitis (ADEM) exhibit focal neurologic deficits and altered consciousness associated temporally with a recent (1- to 2-week) viral infection or immunization (77). Pathological specimens, while showing evidence of demyelination by histologic or radiographic analysis, do not demonstrate evidence of viral infection in the CNS by culture or antigen tests. Patients with postinfectious encephalitis have subtle differences in their immune systems, and some authors have proposed an autoimmune reaction as the pathogenic mechanism of disease (7). Postinfectious encephalitis occurs most commonly following VZV and measles, mumps, influenza, and parainfluenza virus infections. With immunization, the incidence of postinfectious encephalitis has decreased in the United States; however, measles continues to be the leading cause of postinfectious encephalitis worldwide (7).

The TSEs are noninflammatory CNS diseases involving the accumulation of an abnormal form of a normal glycoprotein, the prion protein (PrP) (7). These encephalopathies differ in mode of transmission. While most of the TSEs are experimentally transmissible by direct inoculation in the CNS, this mode rarely occurs except for iatrogenic transmissions (79). The scrapie agent spreads by contact and lateral transmission. There is no evidence for lateral transmission in the case of BSE or vCJD, and all cases appear to have occurred following parenteral intake or ingestion of affected materials. The transmissible agents remain infectious after treatments that would normally inactivate viruses or nucleic acids (detergent formalin, ionizing radiation, and nucleases) (7). Most of the experimental work on TSEs has involved analysis of the scrapie agent. The current working model is that posttranslational alteration of the normally α-helical form of PrP results in a protease-resistant β-pleated sheet structure that accumulates in neurons, leading to progressive dysfunction, cell death, and subsequent astrocytosis. In studies on the scrapie agent and recently with vCJD, gastrointestinal tract involvement with infection of abdominal lymph nodes was found to occur first, followed by hematogenous spread through the reticuloendothelial system and brain involvement a year or more later (7, 28). Experimental subcutaneous inoculation in mice and goats also leads to local lymph node involvement followed by splenic spread and then CNS involvement. Cases of vCJD by blood transfusion have also occurred (27). Based upon animal studies, there is an equal distribution of the agent associated with leukocytes and free in the plasma, with negligible levels associated with the erythrocytes and platelets (18).

Clinical Manifestations

Clinical symptoms have a pathophysiological basis. Patients with encephalitis have clinical and laboratory evidence of parenchymal disease; however, infection rarely involves only the brain parenchyma. Some viruses (rabies virus and B virus) produce encephalitis without significant meningeal involvement. However, most patients with encephalitis have concomitant meningitis. Most patients also have a prodromal illness with myalgias, fever, and anorexia reflecting the systemic viremia. Neurologic symptoms can range from fever, headache, and subtle neurologic deficits or change in level of consciousness to severe disease with seizures, behavioral changes, focal neurologic deficits, and coma (69). Clinical manifestations reflect the location and degree of parenchymal involvement, and they differ based on viral etiology. For example, HSV encephalitis affects the inferomedial frontal area of the cortex, resulting in focal seizures, personality changes, and aphasia. These symptoms reflect the neuroanatomic location of infection with inflammation near the internal capsule, limbic, and Broca regions (69). Parethesias near the location of the animal bite and change in behavior correlate temporally with the axoplasmic transport of rabies virus and the viral infection of the brain stem and hippocampal region (7, 78). Rabies has a predilection for the limbic system, producing personality changes. The damage spares cortical regions during this phase, allowing humans to vacillate between periods of calm, normal activity and short episodes of rage and disorientation (69). Alternatively, Japanese encephalitis virus initially produces a systemic illness with fever, malaise, and anorexia, followed by photophobia, vomiting, headache, and changes in brain stem function. Most children die from respiratory failure and frequently have evidence of cardiac and respiratory instability, reflecting viremic spread via the vertebral vessels and infection of brain stem nuclei (69). Other patients have evidence of multifocal CNS disease involving the basal ganglia, thalamus, and lower cortex and develop tremors, dystonia, and parkinsonian symptoms (69).

Encephalitis, unlike meningitis, has high mortality and complication rates. Case fatality rates differ based on the viral etiology and host factors (7, 73). For example, within the arthropod-borne viral encephalitides, St. Louis encephalitis virus infection has an overall case mortality rate of 10%. The mortality rate is only 2% in children but increases to 20% in the elderly (29). Other viruses, like western equine and eastern equine encephalitis viruses, produce higher mortality and morbidity in children than in adults (29).

The TSEs are slowly progressing diseases with long incubation periods. Sporadic CJD occurs between the ages of 50 and 70 years and is characterized by dementia, tremors, and, more rarely, abnormal movements and ataxia. Unlike sporadic CJD, vCJD disease affects young adults and adolescents and produces cerebellar ataxia and sensory involvement (dysesthesias), with florid amyloid plaques detected in the brain on autopsy. Neurologic deterioration progresses relentlessly, and most patients die less than a year after onset of their neurologic manifestations.

Laboratory Findings and Diagnosis

Establishing a diagnosis requires a meticulous history, knowledge of epidemiological factors, and a systematic evaluation of possible treatable diseases. In the past, investigators failed 50 to 75% of the time to identify an etiology for encephalitis, depending on the study and diagnostic tests used (7). Encephalitis can occur as a separate clinical entity, although meningitis usually coexists. A CSF pleocytosis usually occurs in encephalitis but is not necessary for the diagnosis. Leukocyte counts typically number in the 10s to 100s in viral encephalitis, although higher counts occur (7). CSF glucose levels are usually normal, although some viral etiologies (eastern equine encephalitis) produce CSF studies consistent with acute bacterial meningitis (7). Some viruses (HSV) produce a hemorrhagic necrosis, and the CSF exhibits this with moderately high protein levels and evidence of erythrocytes. Supratentorial and cerebellar tumors can produce increased intracranial pressure and can mimic encephalitis. A careful fundoscopic exam and appropriate radiographic imaging should be performed to rule out any evidence of papilledema and increased intracranial pressure prior to obtaining CSF.

Unlike meningitis, encephalitis often requires additional laboratory and radiologic tests to establish the diagnosis. The clinical circumstances of the patient and the likely etiologies dictate specific laboratory and radiologic evaluations. Historically, the standard for diagnosis has been brain biopsy and viral culture. For many viruses (HSV, enterovirus, EBV, VZV, JC virus, human herpesvirus 6, and TBE), detection of viral nucleic acids by PCR or RT-PCR from the CSF has replaced culture and brain biopsy as the standard for diagnosing encephalitis (7, 14, 76). Radiographic studies that support the diagnosis of focal encephalitis are computerized tomography (CT scan) and magnetic resonance imaging (MRI). The increased sensitivity of MRI to alterations in brain water content and the lack of bone artifacts make this the neuroradiologic modality of choice for CNS infections (16, 22). MRI and, especially, diffusion-weighted imaging detect parenchymal changes earlier than CT scan and better define the extent of a lesion (46). Furthermore, MRI is more sensitive for detecting evidence of demyelinating lesions in the periventricular and deep white matter, thus allowing the differentiation of parainfectious from acute viral encephalitis. Patients with viral encephalitis frequently have diffuse or focal epileptiform discharges with background slowing (69). These electroencephalogram (EEG) changes precede CT scan evidence of encephalitis and provide a sensitive, although nonspecific, diagnostic test. EEG changes in the temporal lobe area strongly support the diagnosis of HSV encephalitis; however, the absence of these changes does not rule out HSV encephalitis.

Historically, patients with viral encephalitis required a battery of different diagnostic tests. HSV encephalitis, for example, could be diagnosed acutely by brain biopsy and viral culture or retrospectively by CSF antibody and convalescent-phase serologic tests (69). The diagnosis of enterovirus meningitis previously required virus isolation from the throat or rectum acutely or serologic studies retrospectively. The advent of PCR has simplified and improved the diagnosis of many viral CNS infections. Molecular techniques are not routinely used for the diagnosis of most viral CNS infections (34, 69). Primers also exist for the detection of certain arboviral encephalitides (California encephalitis group viruses, Japanese encephalitis virus, West Nile virus, St. Louis encephalitis virus, dengue fever viruses 1 to 4, and yellow fever virus); however, the development of universal arboviral primers has been more difficult (7, 40, 48). The successful detection of viral nucleic acids in the CSF is influenced by the duration, extent, and etiology of disease. The laboratory test is relatively rapid, has high sensitivity, and provides a less invasive means to diagnose encephalitis. For example, only 4% of CSF cultures are positive for patients with sporadic HSV encephalitis; however, 53 of 54 patients with biopsy-proven HSV encephalitis had evidence of HSV DNA in the CSF by PCR. CSF PCR has a sensitivity of >95% and a specificity approaching 100% for patients with HSV encephalitis (19). Interestingly, in the three cases in which the CSF PCR was positive but the brain biopsy was negative, biopsy samples had been improperly prepared prior to viral culture or the biopsy site was suboptimal (7). Recent efforts have focused on correlating viral nucleic acid copy number as a reflection of virus quantity to predict clinical outcome (67).

The clinical diagnosis of a TSE is supported by detection of characteristic EEG changes (periodic sharp and slow wave complexes), the presence of 14-3-3 protein in the CSF, and characteristic MRI findings (increased signal in the basal ganglia in sporadic CJD or evidence of increased signal in the pulvinar in vCJD) (39). Most laboratory tests are of little value in the diagnosis in humans. CSF examination shows normal values or slightly elevated protein levels. The EEG in classic CJD reveals generalized slowing early in the disease, punctuated by biphasic or triphasic peaks late in the disease with the onset of myoclonus. MRI changes late in the illness reveal global atrophy with hyperintense signal from the basal ganglia (86). Diffusion weighted imaging and fluid attenuation inversion recovery remain the most reliable and sensitive imaging techniques for CJD (39, 80). Histopathological examination of the brain using a specific antibody to the PrP-res protein confirms the disease. In addition, evidence of gliosis, neuronal loss, and spongiform changes supports the diagnosis. In cases of vCJD, characteristic amyloid plaques (so-called florid plaques) microscopically define the disease. The florid plaques are not seen in other TSEs and consist of flower-like amyloid deposits surrounded by vacuolor halos. The detection of PrP-res in the tonsillar tissue by immunohistochemical staining is also strongly supportive of vCJD diagnosis (86).

Differential Diagnosis

Identifying treatable disease expeditiously is a priority in patients presenting with neurologic changes. In patients with suspected HSV encephalitis undergoing brain biopsy for confirmation of disease, alternate diagnoses are frequently found. Of 432 patients, only 45% had biopsy-confirmed HSV encephalitis and 22% had another etiology established by brain biopsy. Of these, 40% had a treatable disease (9% of the biopsy group), including bacterial abscess, tuberculosis, fungal infection, tumor, subdural hematoma, or autoimmune disease. The majority of the remaining 60% identifiable but untreatable causes of encephalitis were of viral etiology. A third group of 142 patients (33%) went undiagnosed even after brain biopsy and the conventional diagnostic tests (84).

Pathological processes in the CNS have limited clinical expressions and thus often produce similar signs and symptoms (69). Other causes of encephalitis are presented in Table 3. Mass lesions in the CNS (tumor, abscess, or blood) can cause focal neurologic changes, fever, and seizures, similar to encephalitis. Metabolic (hypoglycemia, uremia, and inborn errors of metabolism) and toxin-mediated disorders (ingestions, tick paralysis, or Reye syndrome) can cause decreased consciousness, seizures, and evidence of background slowing on EEG. Limbic encephalitis can produce protracted encephalitis and is caused by paraneoplastic phenomena. Furthermore, treatable infectious causes of encephalitis must be vigorously investigated. Mycoplasmas produce demyelinating brain stem encephalitis in approximately 0.1% of infections.

Prevention

Prevention of viral infection remains the mainstay of therapy. Historically the most frequent cause of viral CNS disease, mumps, has largely been eliminated through vaccination. Live attenuated vaccines against measles, mumps, and rubella have resulted in a dramatic decrease in the incidence of encephalitis in industrialized countries. Measles continues to be the leading cause of postinfectious encephalitis in developing countries, however, and complicates 1 of every 1,000 measles virus infections (7). Vaccination has also changed the character of previously common viral CNS disease. In 1952, poliomyelitis affected 57,879 Americans. Widespread vaccination has eradicated the disease currently from the western hemisphere. Vaccines exist for some arboviral infections. Vaccination against Japanese encephalitis virus has reduced the incidence of encephalitis in Asia; however, cases still occur annually even with vaccination (3, 61, 74).

Vaccination is not cost-effective for preventing all viral infections. For example, vector avoidance, the use of mosquito deterrents, and mosquito abatement programs provide less costly strategies for preventing arboviral encephalitides in the United States (7, 59). Ideally, chemoprophylaxis taken during outbreaks would provide the least costly and most effective prevention; however, at this time no drug exists. Preexposure prophylaxis and immediate postexposure prophylaxis are the only ways known to prevent death in rabies-exposed individuals (50). Case reports exist of patients surviving symptomatic rabies, but all of these patients had some prior immunity or received postexposure prophylaxis prior to developing symptoms. Individuals exposed to rabies require vigorous cleansing of the wound, postexposure vaccination, and direct administration of rabies virus hyperimmunoglobulin at the site of the animal bite. Individuals with frequent contact with potentially rabid animals (veterinarians, animal control staff, workers in rabies laboratories, and travelers to areas where rabies is endemic) should receive preexposure vaccination. The U.S. Food and Drug Administration (FDA), to reduce the potential exposure to TSE agents in the blood supply, has implemented guidelines eliminating whole blood or blood components prepared from individuals who later developed CJD or vCJD. While four cases of transfusion-associated vCJD have been reported, the risk associated with packed red blood cell and platelet transfusion is less than that for patients receiving large amounts of whole blood (18). Changes in the agricultural practices in Europe, testing for infected cattle, and bans on infected cattle have been associated with a decline in the number of cases of vCJD. In North America no cases of vCJD have been reported and the U.S. Department of Agriculture has programs in place to monitor for TSEs in livestock (8).

Treatment

Patients with encephalitis, depending on the etiology and extent of CNS involvement, require treatment tailored to their clinical situation. Currently few antiviral medications are available to treat CNS infections. Antiviral therapy exists for HSV-1, HSV-2, VZV, CMV, and human immunodeficiency virus (HIV). The introduction of acyclovir and vidarabine has resulted in a sharp decline in mortality and morbidity from herpesvirus infections. Neonatal mortality from disseminated HSV disease and HSV encephalitis has declined from 70 to 40% since the development of acyclovir and vidarabine (7). Antiviral treatment of disseminated HSV encephalitis decreases the morbidity from 90 to 50% of survivors and reduces the severity of their neurologic impairment (7). VZV immunoglobulin and acyclovir have reduced the complications from primary VZV infection and zoster in neonates and immunocompromised patients, respectively. Although controlled trials have not evaluated the efficacy of acyclovir in VZV encephalitis, the

TABLE 3 Nonviral etiologies for encephalitis and meningitis

- Infectious
  - Bacteria
    - Common organisms (*Streptococcus pneumoniae*, *Streptococcus agalactiae*, *Neisseria meningititis*, *Haemophilus influenzae*)
    - Complex bacteria (*Mycobacterium*, *Actinomyces*, *Nocardia*)
    - Spirochetes (*Treponema*, *Borrelia*, *Leptospira*)
    - Cell associated (*Rickettsia*, *Ehrlichia*, *Mycoplasma*)
    - *Brucella*, *Listeria*, *Bartonella*
    - Partially treated bacterial infection
    - Abscess (brain, parameningeal)
    - Bacterially produced toxin
  - Fungi
    - *Blastomyces*, *Candida*, *Histoplasma*, *Coccidioides*, *Aspergillus*, *Sporothrix*, *Zygomyces*, others
  - Parasites and protozoa
    - *Toxoplasma*, *Taenia solium*, *Echinococcus*, *Strongyloides*, *Schistosoma*, *Acanthamoeba*, *Naegleria fowleri*, *Balamuthia mandrillaris*, *Trypanosoma*, *Plasmodium*
- Postinfectious
  - Guillain-Barré syndrome
  - Brain stem encephalitis
  - Miller-Fisher syndrome
  - ADEM postviral (VZV; RSV; measles, parainfluenza, and influenza viruses)
- Unknown
  - Limbic encephalitis
  - Paraneoplastic syndrome

medication is routinely used to treat this complication (7, 20). With the increase in the rate of HIV infection, diseases previously limited to the neonatal and postnatal period now occur with increasing frequency in the adult population. Ganciclovir and foscarnet are used for the treatment of CMV encephalitis, although controlled clinical trials have not confirmed the efficacy of treatment. Data also suggest that antiretroviral therapy decreases the frequency and severity of HIV CNS disease. Studies have not determined if this is because of a direct reduction in HIV activity in the CNS or a secondary effect due to improved immune function and decreased opportunistic infections affecting the CNS (45). In cases of postinfectious encephalitis (ADEM), no randomized controlled trial has confirmed the benefit of immunomodulatory drugs. In practice, clinicians often treat ADEM with different immunomodulators in an attempt to limit T-cell-mediated destruction of the CNS (77). It must be emphasized, however, that no placebo-controlled studies have been performed and immunomodulatory therapy is based simply on isolated case reports. As with most case reports, clinical failures and iatrogenic morbidity from a therapeutic modality are rarely ever reported.

APPROACH TO PATIENTS WITH VIRAL CNS DISEASE

The approach to a patient with a presumed CNS viral infection must be tailored to the severity and distribution of neurologic involvement. The degree of diagnostic as well as therapeutic intervention differs based on the type of CNS disease. For example, a patient with photophobia and nuchal rigidity but a nonfocal neurologic exam does not require invasive intracranial pressure monitoring like a patient with encephalitis and evidence of increased intracranial pressure. After establishing the degree of CNS disease by history and physical exam, and stabilizing the patient (airway, breathing, and circulation), the clinician next must ascertain a diagnosis. The first step of any intervention hinges on establishing the correct diagnosis. A history and physical exam are logical first steps. The thoroughness of the initial history and physical exam is tailored to the stability of the patient. A comatose individual with apneustic respirations requires immediate intervention, whereas the individual with nuchal rigidity and photophobia can afford a more detailed investigation for the etiology of the patient's symptoms prior to instituting any therapy.

Treatable causes of CNS dysfunction require rapid evaluation and intervention in an effort to prevent permanent or further CNS damage. Potentially treatable diseases (fungal CNS infections, partially treated bacterial meningitis, tuberculous meningitis, parameningeal infection, mycoplasma infection, and fastidious bacterial infections) can mimic viral CNS disease and should be vigorously investigated before the illness is attributed to an untreatable viral etiology. The same logic applies to treatable viral infections and noninfectious etiologies. The radiographic and laboratory studies available for establishing a diagnosis must be prioritized based on the likely etiology and the stability of the patient.

After establishing a presumptive diagnosis and instituting therapy, the clinician must also vigilantly anticipate and treat complications associated with the viral CNS disease or the therapeutic interventions. Seizures secondary to direct viral CNS damage, inflammatory vasculitis, and electrolyte changes require anticonvulsant therapy with benzodiazepams, phenytoin, and barbiturates (7). Patients with cerebral edema may require intracranial pressure monitoring and hyperventilation, osmotic therapy, and CSF removal in an attempt to maintain cerebral pressures (7). The ultimate goal of intracranial pressure monitoring is to maintain adequate cerebral perfusion. While a physician struggles to maintain an adequate intravascular blood volume, intracranial pressures can rise to dangerous levels as capillary leakage complicates the patient's course. The risks of increased intracranial pressure from aggressive fluid resuscitation or the syndrome of inappropriate antidiuretic hormone release necessitates fastidious fluid management and frequent electrolyte monitoring. Cardiac arrhythmias can also develop in patients with encephalitis secondary to electrolyte changes or brain stem damage. Cardiac and respiratory arrest can occur early in disease; therefore, equipment for intubation and cardioversion should be readily available for a patient with encephalitis. In addition to the direct damage the virus can cause in the CNS, certain viruses can also produce systemic damage and complicate the management of the CNS disease. Patients can develop overwhelming hepatitis, pneumonitis, disseminated intravascular coagulation, and shock. Patients in a coma from encephalitis can recover after long periods of unconsciousness. The physician should limit the amount of iatrogenic damage and vigorously support the patient during the acute phase of the illness.

CONCLUSION

Numerous factors influence the clinical manifestations of viral CNS infections. An individual's age, immune history, cultural practices, and genetic makeup can influence the clinical expression of viral infection as readily as the viral serotype, receptor preference, viral load, and cell tropism (7). Changes in behavior or in cultural beliefs, increased travel, and modification of the environment alter disease patterns and expose individuals to new infectious agents. CNS infections therefore must be examined in a geographic, cultural, and environmental context as well as at the cellular, molecular, and genetic levels. Improvements in our ability to diagnose CNS infections will produce a better understanding of the pathogenesis and true extent of CNS viral disease.

These studies were supported by awards from the NIAID (N01-1-I-15113), NCI (CA RO-1-13148), and Division of Research Resources (DRR) (RR-032) and a grant from the State of Alabama.

REFERENCES

1. **Abzug, M. J., G. Cloud, J. Bradley, P. J. Sanchez, J. Romero, D. Powell, M. Lepow, C. Mani, E. V. Capparelli, S. Blount, F. Lakeman, R. J. Whitley, and D. W. Kimberlin.** 2003. Double blind placebo-controlled trial of pleconaril in infants with enterovirus meningitis. *Pediatr. Infect. Dis. J.* **22:**335–341.
2. **Abzug, M. J., H. L. Keyserling, M. L. Lee, M. J. Levin, and H. A. Rotbart.** 1995. Neonatal enterovirus infection: virology, serology, and effects of intravenous immune globulin. *Clin. Infect. Dis.* **20:**1201–1206.
3. **Ayukawa, R., H. Fujimoto, M. Ayabe, H. Shoji, R. Matsui, Y. Iwata, H. Fukuda, K. Ochi, K. Noda, Y. Ono, K. Sakai, Y. Takehisa, and K. Yasui.** 2004. An unexpected outbreak of Japanese encephalitis in the Chugoku District of Japan, 2002. *Jpn. J. Infect. Dis.* **57:**63–66.
4. **Bauer, S., G. Gottesman, L. Sirota, I. Litmanovitz, S. Ashkenazi, and I. Levi.** 2002. Severe coxsackie virus b infection in preterm newborns treated with pleconaril. *Eur. J. Pediatr.* **161:**491–493.
5. **Becher, B., A. Prat, and J. P. Antel.** 2000. Brain-immune connection: immuno-regulatory properties of CNS-resident cells. *Glia* **29:**293–304.
6. **Bergstrom, T., A. Vahlne, K. Alestig, S. Jeansson, M. Forsgren, and E. Lycke.** 1990. Primary and recurrent herpes simplex virus type 2-induced meningitis. *J. Infect. Dis.* **162:**322–330.
7. **Cassady, K. A., and R. J. Whitley.** 2002. Viral central nervous system infections, p. 27–44. *In* D. D. Richman, R. J. Whitley, and F. G. Hayden (ed.), *Clinical Virology*, 2nd ed. ASM Press, Washington, DC.
8. **Centers for Disease Control and Prevention.** 2004. Bovine spongiform encephalopathy in a dairy cow—Washington State, 2003. *Morb. Mortal. Wkly. Rep.* **52:**1280–1285.
9. **Centers for Disease Control and Prevention.** 2000. Human rabies—California, Georgia, Minnesota, New York, and Wisconsin, 2000. *Morb. Mortal. Wkly. Rep.* **49:**1111–1115.
10. **Chou, J., E. R. Kern, R. J. Whitley, and B. Roizman.** 1990. Mapping of herpes simplex virus-1 neurovirulence to gamma 134.5, a gene nonessential for growth in culture. *Science* **250:**1262–1266.
11. **Collee, J. G., R. Bradley, and P. P. Liberski.** 2006. Variant CJD (vCJD) and bovine spongiform encephalopathy (BSE): 10 and 20 years on: part 2. *Folia Neuropathol.* **44:**102–110.
12. **Conway, J. H., A. Weinberg, R. L. Ashley, J. Amer, and M. J. Levin.** 1997. Viral meningitis in a preadolescent child caused by reactivation of latent herpes simplex (type 1). *Pediatr. Infect. Dis. J.* **16:**627–629.
13. **Cunningham, C. K., C. A. Bonville, H. D. Ochs, K. Seyama, P. A. John, H. A. Rotbart, and L. B. Weiner.** 1999. Enteroviral meningoencephalitis as a complication of X-linked hyper IgM syndrome. *J. Pediatr.* **134:**584–588.
14. **Debiasi, R. L., and K. L. Tyler.** 2004. Molecular methods for diagnosis of viral encephalitis. *Clin. Microbiol. Rev.* **17:**903–925, table of contents.
15. **De La Blanchardiere, A., F. Rozenberg, E. Caumes, O. Picard, F. Lionnet, J. Livartowski, J. Coste, D. Sicard, P. Lebon, and D. Salmon-Ceron.** 2000. Neurological complications of varicella-zoster virus infection in adults with human immunodeficiency virus infection. *Scand. J. Infect. Dis.* **32:**263–269.
16. **Deresiewicz, R. L., S. J. Thaler, L. Hsu, and A. A. Zamani. 1997.** Clinical and neuroradiographic manifestations of eastern equine encephalitis. *N. Engl. J. Med.* **336:**1867–1874.
17. **Desmond, R. A., N. A. Accortt, L. Talley, S. A. Villano, S. J. Soong, and R. J. Whitley.** 2006. Enteroviral meningitis: natural history and outcome of pleconaril therapy. *Antimicrob. Agents Chemother.* **50:**2409–2414.
18. **Dobra, S. A., and P. G. Bennett.** 2006. vCJD and blood transfusion: risk assessment in the United Kingdom. *Transfus. Clin. Biol.* **13:**307–311.
19. **Domingues, R. B., F. D. Lakeman, M. S. Mayo, and R. J. Whitley.** 1998. Application of competitive PCR to cerebrospinal fluid samples from patients with herpes simplex encephalitis. *J. Clin. Microbiol.* **36:**2229–2234.
20. **Echevarria, J. M., I. Casas, and P. Martinez-Martin.** 1997. Infections of the nervous system caused by varicella-zoster virus: a review. *Intervirology* **40:**72–84.
21. **Edens, H. A., and C. A. Parkos.** 2000. Modulation of epithelial and endothelial paracellular permeability by leukocytes. *Adv. Drug Delivery Rev.* **41:**315–328.

22. **Fonseca-Aten, M., A. F. Messina, H. S. Jafri, and P. J. Sanchez.** 2005. Herpes simplex virus encephalitis during suppressive therapy with acyclovir in a premature infant. *Pediatrics* **115:**804–809.
23. **Fragoso-Loyo, H., Y. Richaud-Patin, A. Orozco-Narvaez, L. Davila-Maldonado, Y. Atisha-Fregoso, L. Llorente, and J. Sanchez-Guerrero.** 2007. Interleukin-6 and chemokines in the neuropsychiatric manifestations of systemic lupus erythematosus. *Arthritis Rheum.* **56:**1242–1250.
24. **Gilden, D. H., B. K. Kleinschmidt-DeMasters, J. J. LaGuardia, R. Mahalingam, and R. J. Cohrs.** 2001. Neurologic complications of the reactivation of varicella-zoster virus. *N. Engl. J. Med.* **342:**635–645.
25. **Griffin, D. E.** 1998. A review of alphavirus replication in neurons. *Neurosci. Biobehav. Rev.* **22:**721–723.
26. **Handy, R., and S. Lang.** 2004. Flavivirus encephalitis. *N. Engl. J. Med.* **351:**1803–1804. (Author's reply, **351:** 1803–1804.)
27. **Hewitt, P.** 2006. vCJD and blood transfusion in the United Kingdom. *Transfus. Clin. Biol.* **13:**312–316.
28. **Hilton, D. A.** 2006. Pathogenesis and prevalence of variant Creutzfeldt-Jakob disease. *J. Pathol.* **208:**134–141.
29. **Ho, D. D., and M. S. Hirsch.** 1985. Acute viral encephalitis. *Med. Clin. N. Am.* **69:**415–429.
30. **Hosoya, M., K. Honzumi, M. Sato, M. Katayose, K. Kato, and H. Suzuki.** 1998. Application of PCR for various neurotropic viruses on the diagnosis of viral meningitis. *J. Clin. Virol.* **11:**117–124.
31. **Ichiyama, T., S. Maeba, N. Suenaga, K. Saito, T. Matsubara, and S. Furukawa.** 2005. Analysis of cytokine levels in cerebrospinal fluid in mumps meningitis: comparison with echovirus type 30 meningitis. *Cytokine* **30:** 243–247.
32. **Jeffery, K. J., S. J. Read, T. E. Peto, R. T. Mayon-White, and C. R. Bangham.** 1997. Diagnosis of viral infections of the central nervous system: clinical interpretation of PCR results. *Lancet* **349:**313–317.
33. **Jensenius, M., B. Myrvang, G. Storvold, A. Bucher, K. B. Hellum, and A. L. Bruu.** 1998. Herpes simplex virus type 2 DNA detected in cerebrospinal fluid of 9 patients with Mollaret's meningitis. *Acta Neurol. Scand.* **98:**209–212.
34. **Kennedy, P. G.** 2005. Viral encephalitis. *J. Neurol.* **252:** 268–272.
35. **Khetsuriani, N., R. C. Holman, A. C. Lamonte-Fowlkes, R. M. Selik, and L. J. Anderson.** 2007. Trends in encephalitis-associated deaths in the United States. *Epidemiol. Infect.* **135:**583–591.
36. **Kiderlen, A. F., and U. Laube.** 2004. Balamuthia mandrillaris, an opportunistic agent of granulomatous amebic encephalitis, infects the brain via the olfactory nerve pathway. *Parasitol. Res.* **94:**49–52.
37. **Kimura, H., M. Futamura, H. Kito, T. Ando, M. Goto, K. Kuzushima, M. Shibata, and T. Morishima.** 1991. Detection of viral DNA in neonatal herpes simplex virus infections: frequent and prolonged presence in serum and cerebrospinal fluid. *J. Infect. Dis.* **164:**289–293.
38. **Koskiniemi, M., M. Korppi, K. Mustonen, H. Rantala, M. Muttilainen, E. Herrgard, P. Ukkonen, and A. Vaheri.** 1997. Epidemiology of encephalitis in children. A prospective multicentre study. *Eur. J. Pediatr.* **156:**541–545.
39. **Krasnianski, A., B. Meissner, U. Heinemann, and I. Zerr.** 2004. Clinical findings and diagnostic tests in Creutzfeldt-Jakob disease and variant Creutzfeldt-Jakob disease. *Folia Neuropathol.* **42**(Suppl. B):24–38.
40. **Kuno, G.** 1998. Universal diagnostic RT-PCR protocol for arboviruses. *J. Virol. Methods* **72:**27–41.
41. **Kupila, L., T. Vuorinen, R. Vainionpaa, V. Hukkanen, R. J. Marttila, and P. Kotilainen.** 2006. Etiology of aseptic meningitis and encephalitis in an adult population. *Neurology* **66:**75–80.
42. **Kupila, L., T. Vuorinen, R. Vainionpaa, R. J. Marttila, and P. Kotilainen.** 2005. Diagnosis of enteroviral meningitis by use of polymerase chain reaction of cerebrospinal fluid, stool, and serum specimens. *Clin. Infect. Dis.* **40:**982–987.
43. **Lee, B. E., and H. D. Davies.** 2007. Aseptic meningitis. *Curr. Opin. Infect. Dis.* **20:**272–277.
44. **Markovitz, N. S., D. Baunoch, and B. Roizman.** 1997. The range and distribution of murine central nervous system cells infected with the $\gamma_1 34.5^-$ mutant of herpes simplex virus 1. *J. Virol.* **71:**5560–5569.
45. **Maschke, M., O. Kastrup, S. Esser, B. Ross, U. Hengge, and A. Hufnagel.** 2000. Incidence and prevalence of neurological disorders associated with HIV since the introduction of highly active antiretroviral therapy (HAART). *J. Neurol. Neurosurg. Psychiatry* **69:**376–380.
46. **Maschke, M., O. Kastrup, M. Forsting, and H. C. Diener.** 2004. Update on neuroimaging in infectious central nervous system disease. *Curr. Opin. Neurol.* **17:**475–480.
47. **McNabb, S. J., R. A. Jajosky, P. A. Hall-Baker, D. A. Adams, P. Sharp, W. J. Anderson, A. J. Javier, G. J. Jones, D. A. Nitschke, C. A. Worshams, and R. A. Richard, Jr.** 2007. Summary of notifiable diseases—United States, 2005. *Morb. Mortal. Wkly. Rep.* **54:**1–92.
48. **Meece, J. K., J. S. Henkel, L. Glaser, and K. D. Reed.** 2003. Mosquito surveillance for West Nile virus in southeastern Wisconsin—2002. *Clin. Med. Res.* **1:**37–42.
49. **Moorthi, S., W. N. Schneider, and M. L. Dombovy.** 1999. Rehabilitation outcomes in encephalitis—a retrospective study 1990–1997. *Brain Inj.* **13:**139–146.
50. **Moran, G. J., D. A. Talan, W. Mower, M. Newdow, S. Ong, J. Y. Nakase, R. W. Pinner, and J. E. Childs for the Emergency ID Net Study Group.** 2000. Appropriateness of rabies postexposure prophylaxis treatment for animal exposures. *JAMA* **284:**1001–1007.
51. **Nagafuchi, M., Y. Nagafuchi, R. Sato, T. Imaizumi, M. Ayabe, H. Shoji, and T. Ichiyama.** 2006. Adult meningism and viral meningitis, 1997–2004: clinical data and cerebrospinal fluid cytokines. *Intern. Med.* **45:**1209–1212.
52. **Nagai, T., T. Okafuji, C. Miyazaki, Y. Ito, M. Kamada, T. Kumagai, K. Yuri, H. Sakiyama, A. Miyata, T. Ihara, H. Ochiai, K. Shimomura, E. Suzuki, S. Torigoe, M. Igarashi, T. Kase, Y. Okuno, and T. Nakayama.** 2007. A comparative study of the incidence of aseptic meningitis in symptomatic natural mumps patients and monovalent mumps vaccine recipients in Japan. *Vaccine* **25:** 2742–2747.
53. **Nagy, Z., and K. Martinez.** 1991. Astrocytic induction of endothelial tight junctions. *Ann. N. Y. Acad. Sci.* **633:** 395–404.
54. **Negrini, B., K. J. Kelleher, and E. R. Wald.** 2000. Cerebrospinal fluid findings in aseptic versus bacterial meningitis. *Pediatrics* **105:**316–319.
55. **Nicolosi, A., W. A. Hauser, E. Beghi, and L. T. Kurland.** 1986. Epidemiology of central nervous system infections in Olmsted County, Minnesota, 1950–1981. *J. Infect. Dis.* **154:**399–408.
56. **Nigrovic, L. E., and V. W. Chiang.** 2000. Cost analysis of enteroviral polymerase chain reaction in infants with fever and cerebrospinal fluid pleocytosis. *Arch. Pediatr. Adolesc. Med.* **154:**817–821.
57. **Nigrovic, L. E., N. Kuppermann, C. G. Macias, C. R. Cannavino, D. M. Moro-Sutherland, R. D. Schremmer, S. H. Schwab, D. Agrawal, K. M. Mansour, J. E. Bennett, Y. L. Katsogridakis, M. M. Mohseni, B. Bulloch,

D. W. Steele, R. L. Kaplan, M. I. Herman, S. Bandyopadhyay, P. Dayan, U. T. Truong, V. J. Wang, B. K. Bonsu, J. L. Chapman, J. T. Kanegaye, and R. Malley. 2007. Clinical prediction rule for identifying children with cerebrospinal fluid pleocytosis at very low risk of bacterial meningitis. *JAMA* **297:**52–60.

58. **Nowak-Wegrzyn, A., W. Phipatanakul, J. A. Winkelstein, M. S. Forman, and H. M. Lederman.** 2001. Successful treatment of enterovirus infection with the use of pleconaril in 2 infants with severe combined immunodeficiency. *Clin. Infect. Dis.* **32:**E13–E14.
59. **Palmisano, C. T., V. Taylor, K. Caillouet, B. Byrd, and D. M. Wesson.** 2005. Impact of West Nile virus outbreak upon St. Tammany Parish Mosquito Abatement District. *J. Am. Mosq. Control Assoc.* **21:**33–38.
60. **Pape, W. J., T. D. Fitzsimmons, and R. E. Hoffman.** 1999. Risk for rabies transmission from encounters with bats, Colorado, 1977–1996. *Emerg. Infect. Dis.* **5:**433–437.
61. **Parida, M., P. K. Dash, N. K. Tripathi, S. Ambuj, S. Sannarangaiah, P. Saxena, S. Agarwal, A. K. Sahni, S. P. Singh, A. K. Rathi, R. Bhargava, A. Abhyankar, S. K. Verma, P. V. Rao, and K. Sekhar.** 2006. Japanese encephalitis outbreak, India, 2005. *Emerg. Infect. Dis.* **12:**1427–1430.
62. **Ramers, C., G. Billman, M. Hartin, S. Ho, and M. H. Sawyer.** 2000. Impact of a diagnostic cerebrospinal fluid enterovirus polymerase chain reaction test on patient management. *JAMA* **283:**2680–2685.
63. **Rodriguez, S. C., A. M. Olguin, C. P. Miralles, and P. F. Viladrich.** 2006. Characteristics of meningitis caused by ibuprofen: report of 2 cases with recurrent episodes and review of the literature. *Medicine* (Baltimore) **85:**214–220.
64. **Rorabaugh, M. L., L. E. Berlin, F. Heldrich, K. Roberts, L. A. Rosenberg, T. Doran, and J. F. Modlin.** 1993. Aseptic meningitis in infants younger than 2 years of age: acute illness and neurologic complications. *Pediatrics* **92:**206–211.
65. **Rotbart, H. A., P. J. Brennan, K. H. Fife, J. R. Romero, J. A. Griffin, M. A. McKinlay, and F. G. Hayden.** 1998. Enterovirus meningitis in adults. *Clin. Infect. Dis.* **27:**896–898.
66. **Rotbart, H. A., and A. D. Webster.** 2001. Treatment of potentially life-threatening enterovirus infections with pleconaril. *Clin. Infect. Dis.* **32:**228–235.
67. **Santhosh, S. R., M. M. Parida, P. K. Dash, A. Pateriya, B. Pattnaik, H. K. Pradhan, N. K. Tripathi, S. Ambuj, N. Gupta, P. Saxena, and P. V. Lakshmana Rao.** 2007. Development and evaluation of SYBR Green I-based one-step real-time RT-PCR assay for detection and quantitation of Japanese encephalitis virus. *J. Virol. Methods* **143:**73–80.
68. **Sawyer, M. H. 1999.** Enterovirus infections: diagnosis and treatment. *Pediatr. Infect. Dis. J.* **18:**1033–1039.
69. **Scheld, W. M., R. J. Whitley, and C. M. Marra (ed.).** 2004. *Infections of the Central Nervous System*, 3rd ed. Lippincott Williams & Wilkins, Philadelphia, Pa.
70. **Schmugge, M., R. Lauener, R. A. Seger, T. Gungor, and W. Bossart.** 1999. Chronic enteroviral meningoencephalitis in X-linked agammaglobulinaemia: favourable response to anti-enteroviral treatment. *Eur. J. Pediatr.* **158:**1010–1011. (Letter.)
71. **Schuster, F. L., C. Glaser, S. Honarmand, J. H. Maguire, and G. S. Visvesvara.** 2004. Balamuthia amebic encephalitis risk, Hispanic Americans. *Emerg. Infect. Dis.* **10:**1510–1512.
72. **Sejvar, J. J.** 2006. The evolving epidemiology of viral encephalitis. *Curr. Opin. Neurol.* **19:**350–357.
73. **Sejvar, J. J.** 2007. The long-term outcomes of human West Nile virus infection. *Clin. Infect. Dis.* **44:**1617–1624.
74. **Solomon, T.** 2006. Control of Japanese encephalitis—within our grasp? *N. Engl. J. Med.* **355:**869–871.
75. **Stanberry, L. R., S. A. Floyd-Reising, B. L. Connelly, S. J. Alter, M. J. Gilchrist, C. Rubio, and M. G. Myers.** 1994. Herpes simplex viremia: report of eight pediatric cases and review of the literature. *Clin. Infect. Dis.* **18:**401–407.
76. **Steiner, I., H. Budka, A. Chaudhuri, M. Koskiniemi, K. Sainio, O. Salonen, and P. G. Kennedy.** 2005. Viral encephalitis: a review of diagnostic methods and guidelines for management. *Eur. J. Neurol.* **12:**331–343.
77. **Stuve, O., and S. S. Zamvil.** 1999. Pathogenesis, diagnosis, and treatment of acute disseminated encephalomyelitis. *Curr. Opin. Neurol.* **12:**395–401.
78. **Suja, M. S., A. Mahadevan, C. Sundaram, J. Mani, B. C. Sagar, T. Hemachudha, S. Wacharapluesadee, S. N. Madhusudana, and S. K. Shankar.** 2004. Rabies encephalitis following fox bite—histological and immunohistochemical evaluation of lesions caused by virus. *Clin. Neuropathol.* **23:**271–276.
79. **Sutton, J. M., J. Dickinson, J. T. Walker, and N. D. Raven.** 2006. Methods to minimize the risks of Creutzfeldt-Jakob disease transmission by surgical procedures: where to set the standard? *Clin. Infect. Dis.* **43:**757–764.
80. **Tschampa, H. J., K. Kallenberg, H. Urbach, B. Meissner, C. Nicolay, H. A. Kretzschmar, M. Knauth, and I. Zerr.** 2005. MRI in the diagnosis of sporadic Creutzfeldt-Jakob disease: a study on inter-observer agreement. *Brain* **128:**2026–2033.
81. **Valduss, D., D. L. Murray, P. Karna, K. Lapour, and J. Dyke.** 1993. Use of intravenous immunoglobulin in twin neonates with disseminated coxsackie b1 infection. *Clin. Pediatr.* **32:**561–563.
82. **Varki, A. P., and P. Puthuran.** 1979. Value of second lumbar puncture in confirming a diagnosis of aseptic meningitis. A prospective study. *Arch. Neurol.* **36:**581–582.
83. **Wang, S. M., H. Y. Lei, L. Y. Su, J. M. Wu, C. K. Yu, J. R. Wang, and C. C. Liu.** 2007. Cerebrospinal fluid cytokines in enterovirus 71 brain stem encephalitis and echovirus meningitis infections of varying severity. *Clin. Microbiol. Infect.* **13:**677–682.
84. **Whitley, R. J., C. G. Cobbs, C. A. Alford, Jr., S. J. Soong, M. S. Hirsch, J. D. Connor, L. Corey, D. F. Hanley, M. Levin, and D. A. Powell for the NIAID Collaborative Antiviral Study Group.** 1989. Diseases that mimic herpes simplex encephalitis. Diagnosis, presentation, and outcome. *JAMA* **262:**234–239.
85. **Whitley, R. J., and J. W. J. Gnann.** 1992. Acyclovir: a decade later. *N. Engl. J. Med.* **327:**782–793.
86. **Whitley, R. J., N. Macdonald, D. M. Ascher, and the Committee on Infectious Diseases.** 2000. Technical report: transmissible spongiform encephalopathies: a review for pediatricians. *Pediatrics* **106:**1160–1165.

Gastrointestinal Syndromes

MANISH PATEL AND ROGER I. GLASS

4

Gastroenteritis is one of the most common illnesses affecting infants, children, and adults and accounts for more than 2.5 million deaths annually in children under 5 years of age worldwide (87). The term gastroenteritis implies an inflammation of the stomach and intestine, but depending on the specific etiology, the pathophysiology of illness can be quite diverse. In fact, gastroenteritis can be caused by multiple different pathogens—viruses, bacteria, and parasites—many of which produce no inflammation and some of which are increasingly being recognized as causes of potentially vaccine-preventable diseases. The clinical presentation can vary widely from purely upper gastrointestinal symptoms of vomiting (e.g., winter vomiting disease) to acute diarrhea without any upper gastrointestinal complaints (10, 54). Although gastroenteritis most often presents as mild diarrhea, it is a frequent cause of severe disease leading to hospitalizations and deaths among infants, children, and the elderly, particularly among infants and children in developing countries. These episodes are characterized by a variety of symptoms, including abdominal cramping, malaise, anorexia, headache, myalgia, nausea, vomiting, and diarrhea. These symptoms can appear alone or together and can mimic illness caused by toxins, drugs, or other medical conditions. In this chapter, we use the terms gastroenteritis and diarrhea interchangeably and concentrate on those illnesses caused specifically by viruses.

HISTORICAL BACKGROUND

Our understanding of the role played by gastrointestinal viruses has been determined entirely by our ability to detect these agents through direct observation, through measurement of an immune response to infection, or through more recently developed genetic analysis of clinical specimens collected from patients (Table 1). Historically, viruses have been implicated as agents of acute gastroenteritis when no other pathogens could be identified in fecal specimens (33). Moreover, as recently as 1970, infectious agents could be identified in such a small percentage of patients with diarrhea that explanations such as the diarrhea of malnutrition, weaning, or physiological constitution were invoked as the underlying cause of these disease episodes.

The ability to detect viral agents of gastroenteritis has followed the major historical advances in virology (Table 1). Early investigators demonstrated that "transmissible agents" present in fecal filtrates were able to transmit gastroenteritis to animals and humans (21, 33). With the refinement of cell culture techniques for growing viruses from the 1950s through 1970s, a new generation of advances allowed a number of viruses—echoviruses, adenoviruses, and coxsackie A and B viruses—to be isolated from fecal specimens of patients with diarrhea (25, 90, 94, 103). Although these viruses were identified from patients with symptoms of gastroenteritis, establishing these agents as causes of disease has been challenging because these viruses have also been isolated from patients who had other syndromes or were asymptomatic.

In 1972, the Norwalk agent became the first virus discovered that was determined to be a causative agent of gastroenteritis (55). Using immunoelectron microscopy, Kapikian et al. visualized grape-like clusters of small round structured viruses (SRSVs) in fecal specimens of patients in an outbreak of diarrhea, but not in controls, and applied the same technique to document the patients' immune responses. Since then, electron microscopy has been critical to identifying or confirming all new viral agents of gastroenteritis, including rotaviruses (8), adenovirus (114), astroviruses (74), and the "classic human" caliciviruses (75). Human caliciviruses have recently been placed in their own genus, *Norovirus* (previously called "Norwalk-like viruses"), along with *Sapovirus* (previously called "Sapporo-like viruses") (36).

While many viruses have been identified in fecal specimens, the etiologic association of these viruses with disease requires further investigation and must meet certain criteria for causality. In order to document an infection causing disease, the patient should exhibit a measurable immune response to the specific agent. The virus should also be present more often in patients with gastroenteritis than in persons without gastroenteritis. The onset of clinical signs and symptoms should correspond in time with the onset of virus detection, and the termination of disease should in some way correspond with the end of detection. Some viruses from fecal filtrates have been given to animals to demonstrate the biological plausibility of illness and to human volunteers to fulfill Koch's postulates of disease causation. Consequently, while many viruses have

TABLE 1 Historical advances in the identification of viral agents of gastroenteritis

Yr	Agent	Advance and comment
1940–1950	"Transmissable" agents	Fecal filtrates transmit gastroenteritis in animals and humans
1950–1970	Echoviruses, adenoviruses, coxsackie A and B viruses	Viruses cultivated from stools of patients with diarrhea; causal relationship to disease unclear
1972	Norwalk virus	First virus clearly associated with diarrhea (55)
	Rotavirus group A	Virus discovered by Bishop et al. (8) in duodenal mucosa and now recognized as the most common cause of severe diarrhea in children
1975	Enteric adenovirus serotypes 40 and 41, group F	Unique serotypes and group of fastidious adenoviruses associated with diarrhea
	Astrovirus	Virus rarely identified in fecal specimens now recognized to be a more common cause of disease in children
1979	Calicivirus	"Classic" human calicivirus associated with disease in children, genetically related to the Norwalk family of viruses
1980s	Rotavirus groups B and C	Pathogens recognized in animals found to cause disease in humans; animal and human strains distinct
1970s–1980s	Norwalk-like viruses or SRSVs now recognized to be human caliciviruses, e.g., Snow Mountain agent, Hawaii agent, Toronto agent, minireovirus, Parramatta agent, Taunton agent, Montgomery County agent, and Desert Storm virus	Each virus morphologically identical but antigenically and genetically distinct; variant in the family *Caliciviridae*
1980s–1990s	Novel agents, e.g., torovirus, picobirnavirus, and enterovirus 22	Found in fecal specimens of patients with diarrhea more often than controls, but full association with disease is unclear

been found in fecal specimens, some, like torovirus (59), coronavirus (95), picobirnavirus (98), enterovirus (16), the Aichi agent (123), and pestivirus (124), have yet to fulfill these strict criteria and be accepted as pathogens of the gastrointestinal tract in humans. These agents require further laboratory, clinical, and epidemiological investigations in order to confirm their association with gastrointestinal disease. We now suspect that—at least in the United States—most gastrointestinal illnesses in children are due to viruses. However, our understanding of the full spectrum of disease associated with these viruses, except rotavirus, remains incomplete.

VIRAL AGENTS

The viral agents that are proven causes of gastroenteritis fall into four distinct families—rotaviruses *(Reoviridae)*, human caliciviruses *(Caliciviridae)*, enteric adenoviruses *(Adenoviridae)*, and astroviruses *(Astroviridae)* (Table 2; Fig. 1). The diversity in viral genomic structures among these agents ranges from those containing single-stranded RNA (astroviruses and caliciviruses) to those with double-stranded RNA (rotaviruses) and to those with double-stranded DNA (adenoviruses). Despite the diversity of these agents and their epidemiological characteristics, the clinical presentations of disease caused by these agents are indistinguishable. Moreover, while viruses in the same families also cause disease in animals, the amount of transmission between animals and humans is likely to be limited, if present at all. All of these viruses can be detected using electron microscopy, but the amount of virus shed in fecal specimens ranges from 10^{12} particles per gram (rotavirus) to subdetectable levels ($<10^6$ in calicivirus infections). Our knowledge of the epidemiology of these agents is a direct function of both this level of shedding and the quality of techniques available to detect the virus present in fecal specimens.

EPIDEMIOLOGY

Viral gastroenteritis occurs in two distinct epidemiological settings: childhood diarrhea (i.e., endemic disease) and outbreaks (i.e., epidemic disease) (Table 3). In developed countries, a majority of the diarrheal illnesses in children aged less than 5 years is due to a variety of viral agents—rotavirus (46), adenovirus (13, 114), caliciviruses (85), and astrovirus (67). Infants may be infected in the first few months of life, and the prevalence of antibody to these agents approaches 100% by 5 years of age (18). Globally, rotavirus is the most common cause of severe gastroenter-

TABLE 2 Microbiological and epidemiological characteristics of viral agents that cause gastroenteritis[a]

Virus	Microbiological characteristics		Epidemiological characteristics	
	Morphology	Detection method	Setting	Comment
Rotavirus				
Group A	70-nm double-capsid wheel-shaped ("rota") virus with 11 segments of dsRNA	EIA, EM, PAGE, RT-PCR, culture	Endemic in children	Most common cause of severe diarrhea in children; accounts for ca. 1/3 hospitalizations for diarrhea in U.S. children; mode of transmission unknown; may be preventable by vaccines under development
			Outbreaks in high-risk groups in adults	Affects travelers, immunocompromised patients, parents of infected children, and caretakers in day care centers
Group B	Same as group A	EM, PAGE, EIA, RT-PCR	Epidemic	Found only in China; associated with cholera-like disease in adults; transmitted by water
Group C	Same as group A	EM, PAGE, EIA, RT-PCR	Epidemic	Worldwide distribution; outbreaks in children (newborns to school-age); sporadic cases in Japan, the United States, and the United Kingdom; mode of transmission and prevalence of outbreaks unknown
Noroviruses (human calicivirus)	27- to 32-nm SRSV with ssRNA	EM (IEM), RT-PCR/Southern blot hybridization; seroconversion using expressed antigens	Epidemic and endemic in all age groups	All age groups affected; most common cause of outbreaks of nonbacterial gastroenteritis; may be a common pathogen of children; transmission via contaminated water, food, and shellfish
Sapoviruses (human calicivirus)	Distinguishable by EM from Norwalk by calices and Star-of-David morphology; otherwise identical	Expressed antigens not available; otherwise identical	Endemic in children	Mode of transmission unknown
Adenovirus, enteric	70-nm icosahedral virus with dsDNA; serotypes 31, 40, and 41 associated with diarrhea	EM, EIA for hexon and serotypes 40 and 41	Endemic in children	Disease may be more severe than rotavirus-induced diarrhea
Astrovirus	27- to 32-nm, ssRNA small round virus (star configuration)	EM, EIA, RT-PCR	Endemic in children; may cause outbreaks	All children infected in first 3 yr of life; less severe than rotavirus; mode of transmission unknown; outbreaks reported in day care centers, schools, and nursing homes; winter seasonality

[a] EIA, enzyme immunoassay; EM, electron microscopy; PAGE, polyacrylamide gel electrophoresis; IEM, immunoelectron microscopy; dsRNA, double-stranded RNA; ssRNA, single-stranded RNA.

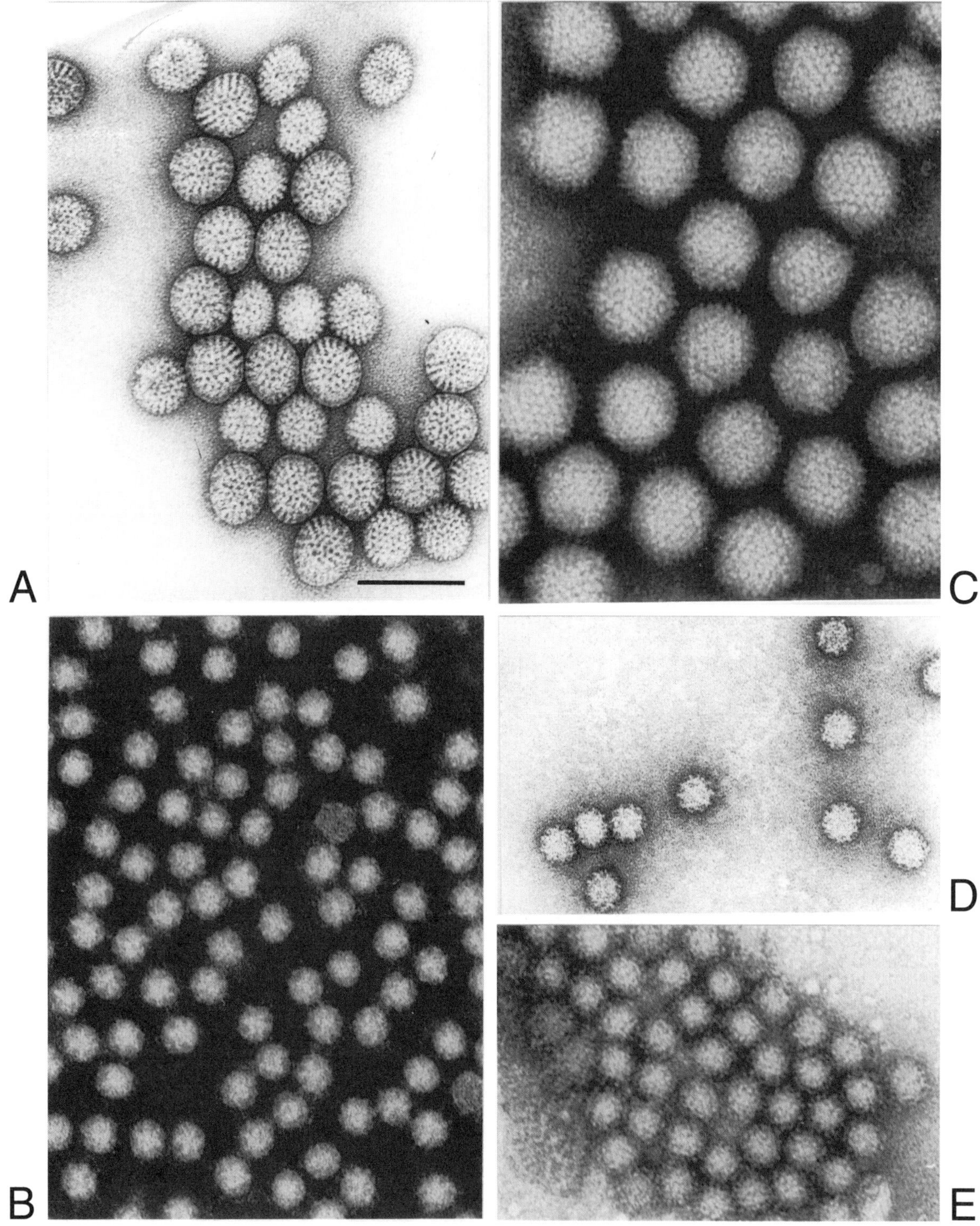

FIGURE 1 Electron micrographs showing agents of viral gastroenteritis. (A) Rotavirus; (B) astrovirus; (C) adenovirus; (D and E) Norwalk-like viruses of the family *Caliciviridae*.

itis in children <5 years of age, accounting for an estimated 2.4 million hospital admissions and 600,000 deaths each year (87). Hospital-based surveillance systems for childhood diarrhea have demonstrated that nearly 40 to 50% of diarrheal hospitalizations year-round are caused by rotavirus, a proportion that is much higher than previously estimated (14). Despite documenting the major role of rotavirus as a cause of severe childhood diarrhea, an "etiologic gap" continues to exist for 30 to 40% of all cases of diarrhea. Recent advances in diagnostics are likely to demonstrate that other viruses (e.g., noroviruses and sapoviruses) are likely to fill in this etiologic gap (32, 88).

TABLE 3 Contrasting epidemiological patterns of viral gastroenteritis

Characteristic	Pattern in:	
	Childhood diarrhea (endemic)	Outbreaks (epidemic)
Viruses	Rotavirus group A, adenovirus, astrovirus, human caliciviruses	Human caliciviruses, rotavirus groups B and C ± astrovirus or rotavirus (special settings)
Age	<5 yr	All ages
Antibody interpretation	Seroprevalence is 100% by age 5	Seroprevalence high or low but seroconversions in affected cases
Mode(s) of transmission	?, droplets, contact	Food (shellfish), water, person-to-person contact
Prevention and control	Effective vaccines for rotavirus licensed and in use	Public health measures to stop transmission by removing contaminated food or water

Precise modes of transmission for most of these agents are unknown, and their incidence rates, where documented, are similar among children in developed and developing countries. Epidemiological studies suggest that transmission within families, communities, and special settings may occur despite the availability of sanitary food and water. Because interrupting the transmission of these agents may be impossible when the mode of transmission remains elusive, no primary prevention is available. For this reason, secondary prevention is aimed at stopping dehydration caused by prolonged vomiting and/or diarrhea using oral or parenteral rehydration therapy (23).

Outbreaks of viral gastroenteritis occur in all age groups and in many different settings (56). Since viral gastroenteritis is often mild, we know much more about large outbreaks that occur in identifiable settings (e.g., weddings, cruise ships, long-term care facilities, and hospital wards) than about small outbreaks or sporadic cases, where the source of infection cannot easily be traced (10). Caliciviruses are the most common cause of epidemic gastroenteritis, accounting for more than 50% of all-cause gastroenteritis and 90% of viral gastroenteritis outbreaks worldwide (71, 122). Outbreaks of calicivirus infections are also frequently reported in institutional settings, such as nursing homes and day care centers (116). Large outbreaks of group B rotavirus have also been well documented in China (48), and smaller outbreaks of group C rotavirus have been identified among children and adults in a global distribution (15, 92). Outbreaks of astrovirus (83) and rotavirus (97), two viruses endemic to children, have also been documented among people who should already be immune following their first infections as children. Rotavirus outbreaks among attendants in day care centers (3, 4), mothers of children with rotavirus (4), travelers (109), and patients in long-term care facilities (42) may be due to alternate modes of transmission in which direct contact with a large fecal inoculum overwhelms an individual's preexisting immunity.

In epidemics of viral gastroenteritis, particularly those caused by caliciviruses, a mode of transmission can often be documented (5). Fecally contaminated food (43), especially raw shellfish (22, 57), and water (6, 63) are among the most commonly identified vehicles for transmission, perhaps because the spread of viruses by airborne droplets (105), vomitus (45), or direct person-to-person contact (5, 105) is more difficult to prove. Even produce, such as raspberries, contaminated before retail distribution may be a source of infection (26). Contamination of environmental surfaces with caliciviruses has occurred during outbreaks in institutional settings and may serve as a reservoir that sustains an outbreak (51). Inapparent contamination of restrooms may be a source of infection in many settings (45, 122). Primary prevention efforts can be directed at interrupting transmission by removing the contaminated vehicle of infection.

While rotaviruses and caliciviruses occur in distinct epidemiological patterns, there is considerable crossover in presentation. Winter seasonal epidemics among infants and children are the most common presentation of rotaviruses, but these agents do cause disease in adults and the elderly, suggesting that these groups may be exposed to unusually large inocula in the context of special settings or that immunity to rotaviruses wanes over time. Epidemics of caliciviruses are common in older children and adults despite the fact that most children possess antibody to both genera of the family *Caliciviridae*—noroviruses and the sapoviruses (37). This suggests that infection with caliciviruses is common in children, although confirmation of infection is difficult due to the limited duration of viral shedding and other diagnostic limitations (32). Consequently, caliciviruses may be an important cause of endemic diarrhea in children, second only to rotaviruses as an important cause of severe gastroenteritis among children worldwide (85, 88). Although a rapid and accurate diagnostic assay is not available for diagnosing calicivirus infections, epidemiological features are useful in confirming calicivirus as a cause of outbreaks (56). Recently, these criteria were validated to be highly specific in discriminating calicivirus outbreaks from other etiologies and could continue to be used until diagnostic assays become widely available (112).

Risk factors for fatal disease include social-system and health care system characteristics, such as access to proper rehydration therapy, and biological factors, such as the nutritional status and immunocompetence of the child (7, 46). Diarrheal deaths are not uncommon in the elderly (65) and have been identified among patients who became ill in outbreaks of gastroenteritis associated with caliciviruses. Electrolyte disturbances in those patients in this group with preexisting health problems have appeared to place these individuals at particular risk.

CLINICAL MANIFESTATIONS AND PATHOGENESIS

Despite the variety of viral agents that cause gastroenteritis, a number of key features in their epidemiology and clinical presentation can be explained by the pathophysiology of infection and disease. For those agents studied, the inoculum size is small: fewer than 100 viral particles properly buffered can cause disease (35). The small inoculum size would permit transmission by airborne droplet spread or direct contact, although the importance of these modes of spread has been difficult to document (5, 45, 105). Following ingestion but prior to the onset of clinical manifestations, the virus replicates in the epithelial cells of the small intestine during an incubation process that can range from 15 to 48 h, depending upon the inoculum size (21, 106). The incubation period of 12 to 36 h for food poisoning due to a virus (e.g., noroviruses) helps in distinguishing these agents from organisms that produce a preformed bacterial toxin (e.g., *Staphylococcus aureus* or *Bacillus cereus*) and typically have a shorter incubation period (<12 h).

Viral replication may be associated with low-grade fever, myalgia, and malaise. Disease is generally of short duration and lasts from 3 to 5 days, perhaps representing the period required for the small intestine to replace cells damaged by infection and to mount an immune response necessary to clear the infection. Shedding of virus at low levels can be confirmed for days to weeks after the clinical illness, depending upon the sensitivity of the assays used for detection (80, 93).

Acute episodes of viral gastroenteritis are distinguished by the presence of watery diarrhea and vomiting. A majority of patients with diarrhea experience vomiting as an associated symptom, but some patients may present with vomiting alone (e.g., winter vomiting disease) (113). The mechanism of emesis during viral gastroenteritis is poorly understood, but it is likely different from the mechanism of the associated secretory diarrhea. In animal models, different gastrointestinal viruses exhibit tropism for different locations in the intestine and for different target cells within the intestine (41). For humans, much less is known about the pathogenesis of viral gastroenteritis. While diarrhea was traditionally believed to result from cellular damage in the intestine, newer data for rotavirus indicate that tissue invasion may not be necessary to cause disease (72), as inactivated rotavirus can cause a secretory diarrhea in animal models. A nonstructural viral antigen has recently been identified that may act as a cellular toxin mediating watery diarrhea after viral infection. The enteric nervous system in the wall of the intestine is likely to be stimulated by rotavirus, leading to intestinal water and electrolyte secretion (72). Receptor blockade at these neurotransmitter sites could be a potential target for treatment of rotavirus and possibly other viral causes of diarrhea (61). Although bloody diarrhea has been occasionally described in the context of rotavirus infections, classic dysentery associated with tissue invasion and an intense cellular infiltration of the intestinal mucosa has not been described with viral gastroenteritis. Indeed, the lack of blood in the stool distinguishes viral diarrheas from the bacterial or amoebic dysenteries.

Chronic, prolonged diarrhea may be associated with coronaviruses and picobirnaviruses. Although investigators identified coronaviruses in patients with tropical sprue almost 20 years ago, this observation has not been replicated in other patient cohorts (2). Picobirnaviruses have been identified in patients infected with human immunodeficiency virus (HIV) who have chronic diarrhea. However, in one recent study these viruses were not found in HIV-infected children (70). Proof of pathogenicity has not been established (38).

Viral infections of the intestinal tract cause clinical syndromes that can range from asymptomatic infections to severe, complicated, dehydrating diarrhea and death. In infants and young children, the rates of mortality due to rotavirus are particularly high in developing countries (87). The key clinical features determining disease severity of viral gastroenteritis are the degree and rate at which fluids and electrolytes are lost and the rapidity with which these losses can be replaced by oral and/or parenteral rehydration therapy.

HIGH-RISK GROUPS

Hospital wards, day care centers, and extended care facilities for the elderly provide special settings where outbreaks of viral gastroenteritis commonly occur (28, 30, 71). Similarly, infections with viral agents are common in American travelers to developing countries (12). Even childhood pathogens such as rotavirus can cause gastroenteritis in immune travelers, suggesting that the inoculum to which they are exposed may be large enough to overwhelm preexisting immunity and involve alternate routes of transmission, such as the respiratory tract. Viral gastroenteritis remains an important cause of illness among U.S. military personnel and was found to be the main cause of lost work time among U.S. personnel serving in the Gulf during Operation Desert Shield (50). Large outbreaks of gastroenteritis due to caliciviruses have also been documented among naval personnel deployed on aircraft carriers (78) and among tourists aboard cruise ships (122) and commercial airplane flights (121), where viral gastroenteritis can spread rapidly, disable passengers and crew, and pose challenging problems for control (45).

Some populations are at particularly high risk of viral gastroenteritis due to either their increased exposure to the viruses or their increased susceptibility to infection (Table 4). The predisposition of young children and the elderly to viral gastroenteritis probably reflects a lack of immunity or waning immunity with age plus a concentrated exposure to the agents in settings like day care centers or long-term care facilities, where hygienic precautions can be easily breached (30). In the early studies with volunteers challenged with noroviruses, approximately 13 to 40% of vol-

TABLE 4 Groups at high risk for viral gastroenteritis

Increased exposure to viruses
Children and the elderly
Parents and caretakers of children
Hospital wards, day care centers, nursing homes
Travelers in developing countries
Increased susceptibility
Children and the elderly
Immunodeficient
Congenital, e.g., SCID
Acquired, e.g., HIV infection
Chemotherapy, e.g., bone marrow transplant

unteers never became infected and only 50% developed illness. Genetic susceptibility to norovirus infection is a prominent factor in the development of norovirus infection; specifically, norovirus infection depends on the presence of histocompatibility blood group antigen (HBGA) receptors in the gut of susceptible hosts (49, 69). The genetic polymorphism of HBGAs results in a highly variable phenotypic expression of these receptors in humans, with various patterns of binding of norovirus strains to these different HBGA receptors (47). The combination of the strain-specific binding and the variable expression of the HBGA receptors explains the various host susceptibilities that are observed in norovirus outbreaks and studies (47, 49, 89). The host specificity may also explain why persons with higher levels of preexisting antibody to noroviruses were more likely to develop illness on rechallenge with noroviruses (89). Those without antibodies to noroviruses may not get infected because they lack genetic susceptibility to infection and thus never mount an immune response to a particular strain.

Children as well as adults with congenital or acquired immunodeficiencies are easily infected with viral agents of gastroenteritis and often experience prolonged shedding of these viruses (38, 104, 126). Children undergoing ablative chemotherapy preceding bone marrow transplantation or children with severe combined immunodeficiency (SCID) are at particular risk for viral gastroenteritis with prolonged shedding of virus (104, 126). Children as well as adults with HIV infections commonly experience viral gastroenteritis as an opportunistic infection as their illness progresses (62). Several studies in adults but not in children have identified viruses to be the most common pathogens in general, although parasites and HIV may themselves cause gastrointestinal symptoms (38). In HIV-infected patients in whom viruses have been intensively sought, both common viruses (rotaviruses and enteric adenoviruses) and the less common agents (astroviruses and caliciviruses) have been identified. However, in a large study in Malawi, the severity and duration of clinical symptoms from rotavirus disease were no different in children with and without HIV infection (19).

OTHER VIRAL AGENTS OF GASTROENTERITIS

In addition to detection of picobirnaviruses in immunocompromised patients, other viruses have been identified in humans in association with gastroenteritis. Toroviruses (enveloped, positive-stranded RNA viruses in the family *Coronaviridae*) have been shown to cause infection and diarrhea in animals, but their role as a cause of gastroenteritis in humans remains unclear (52, 60). Toroviruses have been identified by electron microscopy in human stool, with confirmation by enzyme immunoassay using reagents specific to bovine toroviruses. A survey of specimens found torovirus to be present in 8% of 2,800 specimens screened (60). One study reported torovirus detection among 35% of 206 hospitalized children with nosocomial gastroenteritis, compared with 14% of 206 controls without gastroenteritis (52). Patients infected with torovirus were more often immunocompromised and infected in the hospital than were patients infected with rotavirus or astrovirus. Clinically, patients with torovirus exhibited bloody diarrhea more often but vomiting less often than patients infected with rotavirus or astrovirus. Improved molecular assays will help evaluate the relative importance of toroviruses as an etiology of gastroenteritis in humans.

Coronaviruses are important causes of respiratory infections in humans and other species and have been identified as a cause of gastroenteritis in several animal species. Earlier studies with humans found coronavirus in association with diarrhea and tropical sprue (16, 76). Coronaviruses have been observed by electron microscopy in 0 to 6% of stool specimens examined (66, 91). In 2002, coronavirus was identified as the cause of the newly emerging severe acute respiratory syndrome (SARS), which initially began in China but soon spread across the globe. Interestingly, over a third of the SARS patients had diarrhea, and in some, diarrhea was the presenting symptom (64). Fecal-oral transmission was documented, and fecal shedding occurred in one patient for 73 days after onset of illness (17). Gastrointestinal coronavirus infection during the global SARS outbreak demonstrates the public health and clinical importance of heeding this finding with regard to interruption of fecal-oral transmission and use of stool samples to diagnose illness, since stool samples have the highest yield for coronavirus and pose less risk for transmitting illness to health care workers collecting the samples. In the future, use of molecular diagnostic tests may help clarify the role of coronaviruses as a cause of both sporadic and epidemic gastroenteritis in humans.

ASSOCIATED DISEASES

The group of viruses that cause gastroenteritis in humans also cause a variety of other illnesses in other animal species. Rotavirus and astrovirus can cause fatal hepatitis in SCID mice and normal ducks, respectively, and a calicivirus (hepatitis E virus) causes hepatitis, while other caliciviruses cause a variety of bullous lesions in many animal species (34, 96, 108). Nonenteric adenoviruses have a wide diversity of clinical presentations in humans. Yet despite these biological similarities, it has been difficult to document important extraintestinal manifestations of this group of human gastrointestinal viruses in humans. Increasingly, rotavirus has been found in extraintestinal sites such as hepatic tissue of children who died with SCID (31) and in the cerebrospinal fluid of children with rotavirus diarrhea who had convulsions (11, 73, 115). These systemic complications have been unusual findings, but antigenemia and viremia after rotavirus infection may be more common than previously suspected (11). While rotavirus has been reported for children with a wide variety of clinical problems—including gastrointestinal bleeding (20), sudden infant death syndrome (125), ulcerative colitis (29), Reye syndrome (102), Kawasaki disease (77), intussusception (58), and necrotizing enterocolitis (99)—the association with disease has not been confirmed and rotavirus is probably not the causal agent of disease for most of these conditions. For the other viruses, the availability of simple diagnostic tests has not permitted the more in-depth search for other nongastrointestinal manifestations of disease in humans.

DETECTION METHODS

The greatest impediment to our understanding of the viral agents of gastroenteritis has been the lack of simple and sensitive diagnostic tests that would permit physicians to make a rapid diagnosis and epidemiologists to study the burden and spread of disease. A diagnosis of viral gastroenteritis rests on finding the virus or one of its components in a fecal specimen or detecting a rise in significant antibody titer in the sera of an infected patient. Shortly after the first identification of rotavirus as a cause of infant gastroenteritis, simple enzyme immunoassays were developed that were sensitive, specific, inexpensive, and easy to use in the field (127). Currently, commercial diagnostic tests based on immunoassays are available only to detect rotavirus and adenovirus in fecal specimens, although reliable diagnostic methods for caliciviruses may also be on the horizon (86).

These and the other viruses can sometimes be visualized by electron microscopy in fecal specimens if the concentration of virus exceeds 10^6 to 10^7, the threshold for detection (79). It is not surprising that we know the most about rotavirus, since this virus is shed in huge numbers (up to 10^{12}/g of feces) during the acute illness. Unfortunately, some viruses (e.g., astrovirus and calicivirus) often cannot be visualized by electron microscopy even during acute diarrheal episodes, indicating that their concentration in stool is below the level of detection. Virus is shed in greatest concentrations during the period of acute diarrhea. Thus, fecal samples collected within 48 h of disease onset are most likely to yield a positive diagnosis. Virus can be shed in smaller quantities for several hours before the onset of disease and for days to weeks after the illness is resolved, but special research techniques (e.g., nucleic acid detection and cultivation) are needed for detection (93).

The arrival of molecular diagnostic methods in the last 15 years has helped to close this diagnostic gap in the etiology of gastroenteritis, and human caliciviruses are emerging as one of the leading causes of diarrhea worldwide (86, 88). For example, the known epidemiology of astrovirus has been altered with each new advance in diagnosis. When electron microscopy was the only method available, astrovirus was thought to be a rare pathogen of children found occasionally in small outbreaks and sporadic cases. With the development of an enzyme immunoassay and molecular methods, the reported incidence in hospitalized patients jumped from <1% to 8 to 10% (40, 44, 83). The full understanding of the epidemiology of this and other novel viral agents will necessarily await further use of more sensitive PCR-based assays (40). Real-time quantitative reverse transcriptase PCR (RT-PCR), which is faster and more sensitive than conventional RT-PCR, has recently been developed for calicivirus detection. It should be useful for rapidly detecting caliciviruses, as well as simultaneously identifying multiple other enteric pathogens (e.g., astrovirus, enterovirus, and adenovirus) in large numbers of stool samples during epidemic and endemic gastroenteritis (86). RT-PCR followed by nucleotide sequencing has been particularly useful in molecular epidemiology studies to identify the point source of infection as well as to differentiate outbreaks that were mistakenly assumed to be connected (51).

For epidemiological research, serosurveys can provide additional understanding of the extent of infection. While current methods may not detect virus in fecal specimens, documentation of a rise in the titer of antibody to a specific agent can help confirm that the patient was infected, even though the patient's illness has usually passed. For norovirus, serology has long been the diagnostic test of choice for outbreaks, since it is often easier to collect and test paired sera from many patients than it is to detect virus in stool (81). Seroprevalence studies have also increased appreciation of caliciviruses as a common infection in young children, and the virus can now be detected in their stool samples (37, 86, 88). The discrepancy between a high seroprevalence of antibodies to the virus but low rates of detection noted in the past can now be explained because past assays of virus in stool specimens were quite insensitive (32). Serologic assays have been developed for the other viral agents of gastroenteritis (e.g., astrovirus and group B and C rotaviruses) but are available only in reference laboratories.

TREATMENT AND PREVENTION

Therapeutic interventions and recommended therapy for acute viral gastroenteritis have remained essentially unchanged since approximately 1985, when the American Academy of Pediatrics recommended oral rehydration solution as first-line therapy for uncomplicated diarrheal illness (23). These oral solutions provide essential electrolyte replacement plus sugar (glucose or sucrose) and may be administered as outpatient therapy. As tolerated, patients should begin taking food early in the illness, since adequate caloric intake has been found to enhance patient recovery. Oral rehydration therapy may be used for traveler's diarrhea of either viral or bacterial origin (23, 24). Additionally, bismuth subsalicylate has been found to reduce stool output requirements and duration of hospitalization among children with acute watery diarrhea (27). There is no role for antibiotic therapy in the treatment of uncomplicated viral gastroenteritis. While such agents as diphenoxylate or loperamide may reduce symptoms such as abdominal cramping or stool frequency, they have not been demonstrated to reduce intestinal fluid losses, have no practical value, and should be avoided since they may be harmful in some cases, particularly in children younger than 3 years of age (68, 84).

The volume of fluid to be replaced may be assessed clinically by determining the severity of dehydration. When severe dehydration is present, more rapid fluid replacement using intravenous fluids may be necessary (23). Great attention must be paid to infants and younger children presenting with diarrhea, vomiting, and clinically significant dehydration (i.e., moderate to severe dehydration). Such patients require early oral or parenteral fluid plus electrolyte replacement. In the case of rotavirus-induced diarrhea, vomiting, and diarrhea may occur together, but diarrhea and subsequent dehydration often persist from 4 to 8 days after onset, necessitating persistent and regular fluid replacement (23).

Those patients in special populations discussed above with persistent or chronic diarrhea may need additional nutritional support in conjunction with fluid and electrolyte replacement. Clinical investigations suggest that micronutrient replacement—especially zinc—may shorten the duration of diarrheal episodes (9). Such findings are particularly important for rapidly growing infants and children and for those who may already be undernourished from prior illness or social factors. Selected children who are immunodeficient and develop chronic rotavirus illness may be treated with oral feedings of human milk containing antirotavirus antibody (39). At present, no specific antiviral agents have been recommended to treat gastroenteritis due to viral agents, although several agents, including protease inhibitors, have been studied (118).

In some settings, elderly patients may develop acute vomiting and diarrhea. Such illnesses in high-risk elderly patients who may be immunocompromised or undernourished or who have underlying diabetes or heart disease must be recognized as potentially life threatening (119). Given these risk factors for gastroenteritis in the elderly, prompt attention and treatment of dehydration and electrolyte imbalances during acute gastroenteritis may be critical to patient survival. Routine infection control procedures during care of ill residents, including hand washing and barrier precautions (e.g., gloves), should help reduce transmission of viral gastroenteritis in long-term care facilities for the elderly.

While no chemoprophylaxis for agents of viral gastroenteritis is currently available, many investigators feel that breast milk protects against the development of clinically severe rotavirus-induced diarrhea with dehydration in feeding infants (82, 107, 120). In premature infants, oral human serum globulin that contains antirotavirus antibody has been administered prophylactically and shown to protect against rotavirus gastroenteritis. Also, bovine colostrum containing antirotavirus antibodies has been administered to infants and young children as a form of passive immunization, and this was found to prevent rotavirus-induced diarrhea (107). *Lactobacillus* spp. have been used as an adjunct to fluid and electrolyte replacement as a method to enhance recovery of normal gut flora that is disrupted during the course of acute gastroenteritis episodes (110). Finally, newer methods under investigation include the use, in the gut, of commensal bacteria such as *Bifidobacterium*, which may prevent clinically significant rotavirus-induced diarrhea by inhibiting or reducing viral attachment and replication in the intestinal mucosa (101).

Prevention of viral gastroenteritis depends upon the epidemiological setting. For childhood disease, prevention strategies may be of limited value. Recommendations include proper diaper handling and disposal of feces by caregivers, double diapering of infants, routine hand washing, and use of barrier precautions to reduce transmission in hospital and day care settings. For outbreaks associated with calicivirus, identification of the mode of transmission can lead to specific public health interventions to remove contaminated foods or water.

In 2006, two live oral rotavirus vaccines—RotaTeq (Merck Vaccines, Whitehouse Station, NJ) and Rotarix (GlaxoSmithKline Biologicals, Rixensart, Belgium)—were licensed for use in many countries. Large prelicensure clinical trials of each of these vaccines have demonstrated high efficacy (85 to 98%) against severe group A rotavirus (i.e., the most common cause of endemic diarrhea in children <5 years of age) disease and a good safety profile (100, 117). Hopefully, the global use of these vaccines and other new candidate vaccines in development will reduce rotavirus disease burden and the overall impact of diarrhea among children worldwide. The observation that adults are repeatedly at risk of infections with the caliciviruses suggests either that immunity is short-lived (53) or that the antigenic diversity of strains is too great to permit natural immunity to all the virus strains most often responsible for human disease (1). However, vaccination, possibly with an antigen load that is several logs higher than that which causes natural disease, might provide longer-term protection than natural immunity (111). Vaccines against other viruses may be warranted when the full disease burden of these infections can be fully assessed.

SUMMARY

Gastroenteritis is a major cause of morbidity and mortality in humans, and viruses represent an important cause of this disease. While many viruses have been discovered that are associated with diarrhea in humans, we know the most about rotavirus because the methods to detect it are the best developed. Rotavirus remains the most important cause of severe diarrhea in children worldwide, and the recent licensure of effective vaccines will likely have a major impact on the reduction of this global disease. The gastroenteritis viruses fall into two distinct epidemiological groups: those that cause common childhood diarrhea in children in the first few years of life—rotavirus, adenovirus, calicivirus, and astrovirus—and those responsible for epidemic disease, primarily calicivirus but also astrovirus and group B rotavirus. All of these viruses cause clinical syndromes of diarrhea and vomiting that are generally similar, extraintestinal manifestations of disease are rare, and other disease syndromes associated with these viruses in humans have not been well documented. Some groups of people are at particularly high risk for disease with these agents by virtue of their age (the young and the old), their extent of exposure, or their host susceptibility, and special precautions for these groups are needed. The primary treatment of all these diseases is replacement of fluids and electrolytes. Prevention of the main childhood disease, rotavirus-induced diarrhea, rests with the recently introduced vaccines. Prevention of viral gastroenteritis epidemics will rest with the identification of the vehicle of infection, interruption of the mode of transmission, and the potential development of vaccines.

REFERENCES

1. **Ando, T., J. S. Noel, and R. L. Fankhauser.** 2000. Genetic classification of "Norwalk-like viruses." *J. Infect. Dis.* **181** (Suppl. 2):S336–S348.
2. **Baker, S. J., M. Mathan, V. I. Mathan, S. Jesudoss, and S. P. Swaminathan.** 1982. Chronic enterocyte infection with coronavirus. One possible cause of the syndrome of tropical sprue? *Dig. Dis. Sci.* **27:**1039–1043.
3. **Bartlett, A. V., M. Moore, G. W. Gary, K. M. Starko, J. J. Erben, and B. A. Meredith.** 1985. Diarrheal illness among infants and toddlers in day care centers. I. Epidemiology and pathogens. *J. Pediatr.* **107:**495–502.
4. **Bartlett, A. V., M. Moore, G. W. Gary, K. M. Starko, J. J. Erben, and B. A. Meredith.** 1985. Diarrheal illness among infants and toddlers in day care centers. II. Comparison with day care homes and households. *J. Pediatr.* **107:**503–509.
5. **Becker, K. M., C. L. Moe, K. L. Southwick, and J. N. MacCormack.** 2000. Transmission of Norwalk virus during football game. *N. Engl. J. Med.* **343:**1223–1227.
6. **Beller, M., A. Ellis, S. H. Lee, M. A. Drebot, S. A. Jenkerson, E. Funk, M. D. Sobsey, O. D. Simmons III, S. S. Monroe, T. Ando, J. Noel, M. Petric, J. P. Middaugh, and J. S. Spika.** 1997. Outbreak of viral gastroenteritis due to a contaminated well. International consequences. *JAMA* **278:**563–568.
7. **Bern, C., J. Lew, P. McFeeley, D. Ing, R. T. Ing, and R. I. Glass.** 1993. Diarrheal deaths in children living in New Mexico: toward a strategy of preventive interventions. *J. Pediatr.* **122:**920–922.

8. **Bishop, R. F., G. P. Davidson, I. H. Holmes, and B. J. Ruck.** 1973. Virus particles in epithelial cells of duodenal mucosa from children with acute nonbacterial gastroenteritis. *Lancet* **ii:**1281–1283.
9. **Black, R. E.** 1993. Persistent diarrhea in children of developing countries. *Pediatr. Infect. Dis. J.* **12:**751–761.
10. **Blacklow, N. R., and H. B. Greenberg.** 1991. Viral gastroenteritis. *N. Engl. J. Med.* **325:**252–264.
11. **Blutt, S. E., C. D. Kirkwood, V. Parreno, K. L. Warfield, M. Ciarlet, M. K. Estes, K. Bok, R. F. Bishop, and M. E. Conner.** 2003. Rotavirus antigenaemia and viraemia: a common event? *Lancet* **362:**1445–1449.
12. **Bolivar, R., R. H. Conklin, J. J. Vollet, L. K. Pickering, H. L. DuPont, D. L. Walters, and S. Kohl.** 1978. Rotavirus in travelers' diarrhea: study of an adult student population in Mexico. *J. Infect. Dis.* **137:**324–327.
13. **Brandt, C. D., H. W. Kim, W. J. Rodriguez, J. O. Arrobio, B. C. Jeffries, E. P. Stallings, C. Lewis, A. J. Miles, M. K. Gardner, and R. H. Parrott.** 1985. Adenoviruses and pediatric gastroenteritis. *J. Infect. Dis.* **151:** 437–443.
14. **Bresee, J. S., E. Hummelman, E. A. Nelson, and R. I. Glass.** 2005. Rotavirus in Asia: the value of surveillance for informing decisions about the introduction of new vaccines. *J. Infect. Dis.* **192**(Suppl. 1)**:**S1–S5.
15. **Brown, D. W., L. Campbell, D. S. Tomkins, and M. H. Hambling.** 1989. School outbreak of gastroenteritis due to atypical rotavirus. *Lancet* **ii:**737–738.
16. **Caul, E. O., and S. I. Egglestone.** 1977. Further studies on human enteric coronaviruses. *Arch. Virol.* **54:**107–117.
17. **Cheng, P. K., D. A. Wong, L. K. Tong, S. M. Ip, A. C. Lo, C. S. Lau, E. Y. Yeung, and W. W. Lim.** 2004. Viral shedding patterns of coronavirus in patients with probable severe acute respiratory syndrome. *Lancet* **363:**1699–1700.
18. **Cubitt, W. D., and D. A. McSwiggan.** 1987. Seroepidemiological survey of the prevalence of antibodies to a strain of human calicivirus. *J. Med. Virol.* **21:**361–368.
19. **Cunliffe, N. A., J. S. Gondwe, C. D. Kirkwood, S. M. Graham, N. M. Nhlane, B. D. Thindwa, W. Dove, R. L. Broadhead, M. E. Molyneux, and C. A. Hart.** 2001. Effect of concomitant HIV infection on presentation and outcome of rotavirus gastroenteritis in Malawian children. *Lancet* **358:**550–555.
20. **Delage, G., B. McLaughlin, and L. Berthiaume.** 1978. A clinical study of rotavirus gastroenteritis. *J. Pediatr.* **93:** 455–457.
21. **Dolin, R., N. R. Blacklow, H. DuPont, S. Formal, R. F. Buscho, J. A. Kasel, R. P. Chames, R. Hornick, and R. M. Chanock.** 1971. Transmission of acute infectious nonbacterial gastroenteritis to volunteers by oral administration of stool filtrates. *J. Infect. Dis.* **123:**307–312.
22. **Dowell, S. F., C. Groves, K. B. Kirkland, H. G. Cicirello, T. Ando, Q. Jin, J. R. Gentsch, S. S. Monroe, C. D. Humphrey, C. Slemp, D. M. Dwyer, R. A. Meriwether, and R. I. Glass.** 1995. A multistate outbreak of oyster-associated gastroenteritis: implications for interstate tracing of contaminated shellfish. *J. Infect. Dis.* **171:** 1497–1503.
23. **Duggan, C., M. Santosham, and R. I. Glass** for the Centers for Disease Control and Prevention. 1992. The management of acute diarrhea in children: oral rehydration, maintenance, and nutritional therapy. *Morb. Mortal. Wkly. Rep. Recomm. Rep.* **41:**1–20.
24. **DuPont, H. L., and C. D. Ericsson.** 1993. Prevention and treatment of traveler's diarrhea. *N. Engl. J. Med.* **328:** 1821–1827.
25. **Eichenwald, H. F., A. Ababio, A. M. Arky, and A. P. Hartman.** 1958. Epidemic diarrhea in premature and older infants caused by ECHO virus type 18. *JAMA* **166:** 1563–1566.
26. **Falkenhorst, G., L. Krusell, M. Lisby, S. B. Madsen, B. Böttiger, and K. Mølbak.** 2005. Imported frozen raspberries cause a series of norovirus outbreaks in Denmark, 2005. *Euro. Surveill.* **10:**E050922.2.
27. **Figueroa-Quintanilla, D., E. Salazar-Lindo, R. B. Sack, R. Leon-Barua, S. Sarabia-Arce, M. Campos-Sanchez, and E. Eyzaguirre-Maccan.** 1993. A controlled trial of bismuth subsalicylate in infants with acute watery diarrheal disease. *N. Engl. J. Med.* **328:**1653–1658.
28. **Gaggero, A., L. F. Avendano, J. Fernandez, and E. Spencer.** 1992. Nosocomial transmission of rotavirus from patients admitted with diarrhea. *J. Clin. Microbiol.* **30:**3294–3297.
29. **Gebhard, R. L., H. B. Greenberg, N. Singh, P. Henry, H. L. Sharp, L. Kaplan, and A. Z. Kapikian.** 1982. Acute viral enteritis and exacerbations of inflammatory bowel disease. *Gastroenterology* **83:**1207–1209.
30. **Gellert, G. A., S. H. Waterman, D. Ewert, L. Oshiro, M. P. Giles, S. S. Monroe, L. Gorelkin, and R. I. Glass.** 1990. An outbreak of acute gastroenteritis caused by a small round structured virus in a geriatric convalescent facility. *Infect. Control Hosp. Epidemiol.* **11:**459–464.
31. **Gilger, M. A., D. O. Matson, M. E. Conner, H. M. Rosenblatt, M. J. Finegold, and M. K. Estes.** 1992. Extraintestinal rotavirus infections in children with immunodeficiency. *J. Pediatr.* **120:**912–917.
32. **Glass, R. I., J. Noel, T. Ando, R. Fankhauser, G. Belliot, A. Mounts, U. D. Parashar, J. S. Bresee, and S. S. Monroe.** 2000. The epidemiology of enteric caliciviruses from humans: a reassessment using new diagnostics. *J. Infect. Dis.* **181**(Suppl. 2)**:**S254–S261.
33. **Gordon, I., H. S. Ingraham, and R. F. Korns.** 1947. Transmission of epidemic gastroenteritis to human volunteers by oral administration of fecal filtrates. *J. Exp. Med.* **86:**409–422.
34. **Gough, R. E., M. S. Collins, E. Borland, and L. F. Keymer.** 1984. Astrovirus-like particles associated with hepatitis in ducklings. *Vet. Rec.* **114:**279.
35. **Graham, D. Y., X. Jiang, T. Tanaka, A. R. Opekun, H. P. Madore, and M. K. Estes.** 1994. Norwalk virus infection of volunteers: new insights based on improved assays. *J. Infect. Dis.* **170:**34–43.
36. **Green, K. Y., T. Ando, M. S. Balayan, T. Berke, I. N. Clarke, M. K. Estes, D. O. Matson, S. Nakata, J. D. Neill, M. J. Studdert, and H. J. Thiel.** 2000. Taxonomy of the caliciviruses. *J. Infect. Dis.* **181**(Suppl. 2)**:**S322–S330.
37. **Greenberg, H. B., J. Valdesuso, A. Z. Kapikian, R. M. Chanock, R. G. Wyatt, W. Szmuness, J. Larrick, J. Kaplan, R. H. Gilman, and D. A. Sack.** 1979. Prevalence of antibody to the Norwalk virus in various countries. *Infect. Immun.* **26:**270–273.
38. **Grohmann, G. S., R. I. Glass, H. G. Pereira, S. S. Monroe, A. W. Hightower, R. Weber, and R. T. Bryan** for The Enteric Opportunistic Infections Working Group. 1993. Enteric viruses and diarrhea in HIV-infected patients. *N. Engl. J. Med.* **329:**14–20.
39. **Guarino, A., R. B. Canani, S. Russo, F. Albano, M. B. Canani, F. M. Ruggeri, G. Donelli, and A. Rubino.** 1994. Oral immunoglobulins for treatment of acute rotaviral gastroenteritis. *Pediatrics* **93:**12–16.
40. **Guix, S., A. Bosch, and R. M. Pinto.** 2005. Human astrovirus diagnosis and typing: current and future prospects. *Lett. Appl. Microbiol.* **41:**103–105.

41. **Hall, G. A.** 1987. Comparative pathology of infection by novel diarrhoea viruses. *Ciba Found. Symp.* **128:**192–217.
42. **Halvorsrud, J., and I. Orstavik.** 1980. An epidemic of rotavirus-associated gastroenteritis in a nursing home for the elderly. *Scand. J. Infect. Dis.* **12:**161–164.
43. **Hedberg, C. W., and M. T. Osterholm.** 1993. Outbreaks of food-borne and waterborne viral gastroenteritis. *Clin. Microbiol. Rev.* **6:**199–210.
44. **Herrmann, J. E., D. N. Taylor, P. Echeverria, and N. R. Blacklow.** 1991. Astroviruses as a cause of gastroenteritis in children. *N. Engl. J. Med.* **324:**1757–1760.
45. **Ho, M. S., R. I. Glass, S. S. Monroe, H. P. Madore, S. Stine, P. F. Pinsky, D. Cubitt, C. Ashley, and E. O. Caul.** 1989. Viral gastroenteritis aboard a cruise ship. *Lancet* **ii:**961–965.
46. **Ho, M. S., R. I. Glass, P. F. Pinsky, N. C. Young-Okoh, W. M. Sappenfield, J. W. Buehler, N. Gunter, and L. J. Anderson.** 1988. Diarrheal deaths in American children. Are they preventable? *JAMA* **260:**3281–3285.
47. **Huang, P., T. Farkas, W. Zhong, M. Tan, S. Thornton, A. L. Morrow, and X. Jiang.** 2005. Norovirus and histo-blood group antigens: demonstration of a wide spectrum of strain specificities and classification of two major binding groups among multiple binding patterns. *J. Virol.* **79:**6714–6722.
48. **Hung, T., G. M. Chen, C. G. Wang, H. L. Yao, Z. Y. Fang, T. X. Chao, Z. Y. Chou, W. Ye, X. J. Chang, and S. S. Den.** 1984. Waterborne outbreak of rotavirus diarrhoea in adults in China caused by a novel rotavirus. *Lancet* **i:**1139–1142.
49. **Hutson, A. M., R. L. Atmar, D. Y. Graham, and M. K. Estes.** 2002. Norwalk virus infection and disease is associated with ABO histo-blood group type. *J. Infect. Dis.* **185:**1335–1337.
50. **Hyams, K. C., A. L. Bourgeois, B. R. Merrell, P. Rozmajzl, J. Escamilla, S. A. Thornton, G. M. Wasserman, A. Burke, P. Echeverria, K. Y. Green, A. Z. Kapikian, and J. N. Woody.** 1991. Diarrheal disease during Operation Desert Shield. *N. Engl. J. Med.* **325:**1423–1428.
51. **Isakbaeva, E. T., M. A. Widdowson, R. S. Beard, S. N. Bulens, J. Mullins, S. S. Monroe, J. Bresee, P. Sassano, E. H. Cramer, and R. I. Glass.** 2005. Norovirus transmission on cruise ship. *Emerg. Infect. Dis.* **11:**154–158.
52. **Jamieson, F. B., E. E. Wang, C. Bain, J. Good, L. Duckmanton, and M. Petric.** 1998. Human torovirus: a new nosocomial gastrointestinal pathogen. *J. Infect. Dis.* **178:**1263–1269.
53. **Johnson, P. C., J. J. Mathewson, H. L. DuPont, and H. B. Greenberg.** 1990. Multiple-challenge study of host susceptibility to Norwalk gastroenteritis in US adults. *J. Infect. Dis.* **161:**18–21.
54. **Kapikian, A. Z., H. W. Kim, R. G. Wyatt, W. L. Cline, J. O. Arrobio, C. D. Brandt, W. J. Rodriguez, D. A. Sack, R. M. Chanock, and R. H. Parrott.** 1976. Human reovirus-like agent as the major pathogen associated with "winter" gastroenteritis in hospitalized infants and young children. *N. Engl. J. Med.* **294:**965–972.
55. **Kapikian, A. Z., R. G. Wyatt, R. Dolin, T. S. Thornhill, A. R. Kalica, and R. M. Chanock.** 1972. Visualization by immune electron microscopy of a 27-nm particle associated with acute infectious nonbacterial gastroenteritis. *J. Virol.* **10:**1075–1081.
56. **Kaplan, J. E., G. W. Gary, R. C. Baron, N. Singh, L. B. Schonberger, R. Feldman, and H. B. Greenberg.** 1982. Epidemiology of Norwalk gastroenteritis and the role of Norwalk virus in outbreaks of acute nonbacterial gastroenteritis. *Ann. Intern. Med.* **96:**756–761.
57. **Kohn, M. A., T. A. Farley, T. Ando, M. Curtis, S. A. Wilson, Q. Jin, S. S. Monroe, R. C. Baron, L. M. McFarland, and R. I. Glass.** 1995. An outbreak of Norwalk virus gastroenteritis associated with eating raw oysters. Implications for maintaining safe oyster beds. *JAMA* **273:**466–471.
58. **Konno, T., H. Suzuki, T. Kutsuzawa, A. Imai, N. Katsushima, M. Sakamoto, and S. Kitaoka.** 1977. Human rotavirus and intussusception. *N. Engl. J. Med.* **297:**945.
59. **Koopmans, M., and M. C. Horzinek.** 1994. Toroviruses of animals and humans: a review. *Adv. Virus Res.* **43:**233–273.
60. **Koopmans, M., M. Petric, R. I. Glass, and S. S. Monroe.** 1993. Enzyme-linked immunosorbent assay reactivity of torovirus-like particles in fecal specimens from humans with diarrhea. *J. Clin. Microbiol.* **31:**2738–2744.
61. **Kordasti, S., H. Sjovall, O. Lundgren, and L. Svensson.** 2004. Serotonin and vasoactive intestinal peptide antagonists attenuate rotavirus diarrhoea. *Gut* **53:**952–957.
62. **Kotler, D. P., H. P. Gaetz, M. Lange, E. B. Klein, and P. R. Holt.** 1984. Enteropathy associated with the acquired immunodeficiency syndrome. *Ann. Intern. Med.* **101:**421–428.
63. **Lawson, H. W., M. M. Braun, R. I. Glass, S. E. Stine, S. S. Monroe, H. K. Atrash, L. E. Lee, and S. J. Englender.** 1991. Waterborne outbreak of Norwalk virus gastroenteritis at a southwest US resort: role of geological formations in contamination of well water. *Lancet* **337:**1200–1204.
64. **Leung, W. K., K. F. To, P. K. Chan, H. L. Chan, A. K. Wu, N. Lee, K. Y. Yuen, and J. J. Sung.** 2003. Enteric involvement of severe acute respiratory syndrome-associated coronavirus infection. *Gastroenterology* **125:**1011–1017.
65. **Lew, J. F., R. I. Glass, R. E. Gangarosa, I. P. Cohen, C. Bern, and C. L. Moe.** 1991. Diarrheal deaths in the United States, 1979 through 1987. A special problem for the elderly. *JAMA* **265:**3280–3284.
66. **Lew, J. F., R. I. Glass, M. Petric, C. W. Lebaron, G. W. Hammond, S. E. Miller, C. Robinson, J. Boutilier, M. Riepenhoff-Talty, C. M. Payne, R. Franklin, L. Oshiro, and M. Jaqua.** 1990. Six-year retrospective surveillance of gastroenteritis viruses identified at ten electron microscopy centers in the United States and Canada. *Pediatr. Infect. Dis. J.* **9:**709–714.
67. **Lew, J. F., C. L. Moe, S. S. Monroe, J. R. Allen, B. M. Harrison, B. D. Forrester, S. E. Stine, P. A. Woods, J. C. Hierholzer, J. E. Herrmann, N. R. Blacklow, A. V. Bartlett, and R. I. Glass.** 1991. Astrovirus and adenovirus associated with diarrhea in children in day care settings. *J. Infect. Dis.* **164:**673–678.
68. **Li, S. T., D. C. Grossman, and P. Cummings.** 2007. Loperamide therapy for acute diarrhea in children: systematic review and meta-analysis. *PLoS Med.* **4:**e98.
69. **Lindesmith, L., C. Moe, S. Marionneau, N. Ruvoen, X. Jiang, L. Lindblad, P. Stewart, J. LePendu, and R. Baric.** 2003. Human susceptibility and resistance to Norwalk virus infection. *Nat. Med.* **9:**548–553.
70. **Liste, M. B., I. Natera, J. A. Suarez, F. H. Pujol, F. Liprandi, and J. E. Ludert.** 2000. Enteric virus infections and diarrhea in healthy and human immunodeficiency virus-infected children. *J. Clin. Microbiol.* **38:**2873–2877.
71. **Lopman, B., H. Vennema, E. Kohli, P. Pothier, A. Sanchez, A. Negredo, J. Buesa, E. Schreier, M. Reacher, D. Brown, J. Gray, M. Iturriza, C. Gallimore, B. Bottiger, K. O. Hedlund, M. Torven, C. H. von Bonsdorff, L. Maunula, M. Poljsak-Prijatelj, J. Zimsek, G. Reuter, G. Szucs, B. Melegh, L. Svennson, Y. van Duijnhoven, and M. Koopmans.** 2004. Increase in viral gastroenteritis outbreaks in Europe and epidemic spread of new norovirus variant. *Lancet* **363:**682–688.

72. **Lundgren, O., A. T. Peregrin, K. Persson, S. Kordasti, I. Uhnoo, and L. Svensson.** 2000. Role of the enteric nervous system in the fluid and electrolyte secretion of rotavirus diarrhea. *Science* **287:**491–495.
73. **Lynch, M., B. Lee, P. Azimi, J. Gentsch, C. Glaser, S. Gilliam, H. G. Chang, R. Ward, and R. I. Glass.** 2001. Rotavirus and central nervous system symptoms: cause or contaminant? Case reports and review. *Clin. Infect. Dis.* **33:**932–938.
74. **Madeley, C. R., and B. P. Cosgrove.** 1975. Letter: 28 nm particles in faeces in infantile gastroenteritis. *Lancet* **ii:** 451–452.
75. **Madeley, C. R., and B. P. Cosgrove.** 1976. Letter: caliciviruses in man. *Lancet* **i:**199–200.
76. **Mathan, M., V. I. Mathan, S. P. Swaminathan, and S. Yesudoss.** 1975. Pleomorphic virus-like particles in human faeces. *Lancet* **i:**1068–1069.
77. **Matsuno, S., E. Utagawa, and A. Sugiura.** 1983. Association of rotavirus infection with Kawasaki syndrome. *J. Infect. Dis.* **148:**177.
78. **McCarthy, M., M. K. Estes, and K. C. Hyams.** 2000. Norwalk-like virus infection in military forces: epidemic potential, sporadic disease, and the future direction of prevention and control efforts. *J. Infect. Dis.* **181**(Suppl. 2)**:** S387–S391.
79. **Miller, S. E.** 1986. Detection and identification of viruses by electron microscopy. *J. Electron Microsc.* **4:**265–301.
80. **Mitchell, D. K., R. Van, A. L. Morrow, S. S. Monroe, R. I. Glass, and L. K. Pickering.** 1993. Outbreaks of astrovirus gastroenteritis in day care centers. *J. Pediatr.* **123:**725–732.
81. **Monroe, S. S., R. I. Glass, N. Noah, T. H. Flewett, E. O. Caul, C. I. Ashton, A. Curry, A. M. Field, R. Madeley, and P. J. Pead.** 1991. Electron microscopic reporting of gastrointestinal viruses in the United Kingdom, 1985–1987. *J. Med. Virol.* **33:**193–198.
82. **Newburg, D. S., J. A. Peterson, G. M. Ruiz-Palacios, D. O. Matson, A. L. Morrow, J. Shults, M. L. Guerrero, P. Chaturvedi, S. O. Newburg, C. D. Scallan, M. R. Taylor, R. L. Ceriani, and L. K. Pickering.** 1998. Role of human-milk lactadherin in protection against symptomatic rotavirus infection. *Lancet* **351:**1160–1164.
83. **Oishi, I., K. Yamazaki, T. Kimoto, Y. Minekawa, E. Utagawa, S. Yamazaki, S. Inouye, G. S. Grohmann, S. S. Monroe, S. E. Stine, C. Carcamo, T. Ando, and R. I. Glass.** 1994. A large outbreak of acute gastroenteritis associated with astrovirus among students and teachers in Osaka, Japan. *J. Infect. Dis.* **170:**439–443.
84. **Owens, J. R., R. Broadhead, R. G. Hendrickse, O. P. Jaswal, and R. N. Gangal.** 1981. Loperamide in the treatment of acute gastroenteritis in early childhood. Report of a two centre, double-blind, controlled clinical trial. *Ann. Trop. Paediatr.* **1:**135–141.
85. **Pang, X. L., S. Honma, S. Nakata, and T. Vesikari.** 2000. Human caliciviruses in acute gastroenteritis of young children in the community. *J. Infect. Dis.* **181**(Suppl. 2)**:**S288–S294.
86. **Pang, X. L., J. K. Preiksaitis, and B. Lee.** 2005. Multiplex real time RT-PCR for the detection and quantitation of norovirus genogroups I and II in patients with acute gastroenteritis. *J. Clin. Virol.* **33:**168–171.
87. **Parashar, U. D., E. G. Hummelman, J. S. Bresee, M. A. Miller, and R. I. Glass.** 2003. Global illness and deaths caused by rotavirus disease in children. *Emerg. Infect. Dis.* **9:**565–572.
88. **Parashar, U. D., J. F. Li, R. Cama, M. DeZalia, S. S. Monroe, D. N. Taylor, D. Figueroa, R. H. Gilman, and R. I. Glass.** 2004. Human caliciviruses as a cause of severe gastroenteritis in Peruvian children. *J. Infect. Dis.* **190:** 1088–1092.
89. **Parrino, T. A., D. S. Schreiber, J. S. Trier, A. Z. Kapikian, and N. R. Blacklow.** 1977. Clinical immunity in acute gastroenteritis caused by Norwalk agent. *N. Engl. J. Med.* **297:**86–89.
90. **Parrott, R. H.** 1957. The clinical importance of group A Coxsackie viruses. *Ann. N. Y. Acad. Sci.* **67:**230–240.
91. **Payne, C. M., C. G. Ray, V. Borduin, L. L. Minnich, and M. D. Lebowitz.** 1986. An eight-year study of the viral agents of acute gastroenteritis in humans: ultrastructural observations and seasonal distribution with a major emphasis on coronavirus-like particles. *Diagn. Microbiol. Infect. Dis.* **5:**39–54.
92. **Penaranda, M. E., W. D. Cubitt, P. Sinarachatanant, D. N. Taylor, S. Likanonsakul, L. Saif, and R. I. Glass.** 1989. Group C rotavirus infections in patients with diarrhea in Thailand, Nepal, and England. *J. Infect. Dis.* **160:**392–397.
93. **Pickering, L. K., A. V. Bartlett III, R. R. Reves, and A. Morrow.** 1988. Asymptomatic excretion of rotavirus before and after rotavirus diarrhea in children in day care centers. *J. Pediatr.* **112:**361–365.
94. **Ramos-Alvarez, M., and A. B. Sabin.** 1958. Enteropathogenic viruses and bacteria; role in summer diarrheal diseases of infancy and early childhood. *JAMA* **167:** 147–156.
95. **Resta, S., J. P. Luby, C. R. Rosenfeld, and J. D. Siegel.** 1985. Isolation and propagation of a human enteric coronavirus. *Science* **229:**978–981.
96. **Riepenhoff-Talty, M., K. Schaekel, H. F. Clark, W. Mueller, I. Uhnoo, T. Rossi, J. Fisher, and P. L. Ogra.** 1993. Group A rotaviruses produce extrahepatic biliary obstruction in orally inoculated newborn mice. *Pediatr. Res.* **33:**394–399.
97. **Rodriguez, W. J., H. W. Kim, C. D. Brandt, R. H. Schwartz, M. K. Gardner, B. Jeffries, R. H. Parrott, R. A. Kaslow, J. I. Smith, and A. Z. Kapikian.** 1987. Longitudinal study of rotavirus infection and gastroenteritis in families served by a pediatric medical practice: clinical and epidemiologic observations. *Pediatr. Infect. Dis. J.* **6:**170–176.
98. **Rosen, B. I., Z. Y. Fang, R. I. Glass, and S. S. Monroe.** 2000. Cloning of human picobirnavirus genomic segments and development of an RT-PCR detection assay. *Virology* **277:**316–329.
99. **Rotbart, H. A., W. L. Nelson, M. P. Glode, T. C. Triffon, S. J. Kogut, R. H. Yolken, J. A. Hernandez, and M. J. Levin.** 1988. Neonatal rotavirus-associated necrotizing enterocolitis: case control study and prospective surveillance during an outbreak. *J. Pediatr.* **112:**87–93.
100. **Ruiz-Palacios, G. M., I. Perez-Schael, F. R. Velazquez, H. Abate, T. Breuer, S. C. Clemens, B. Cheuvart, F. Espinoza, P. Gillard, B. L. Innis, Y. Cervantes, A. C. Linhares, P. Lopez, M. Macias-Parra, E. Ortega-Barria, V. Richardson, D. M. Rivera-Medina, L. Rivera, B. Salinas, N. Pavia-Ruz, J. Salmeron, R. Ruttimann, J. C. Tinoco, P. Rubio, E. Nunez, M. L. Guerrero, J. P. Yarzabal, S. Damaso, N. Tornieporth, X. Saez-Llorens, R. F. Vergara, T. Vesikari, A. Bouckenooghe, R. Clemens, B. De Vos, and M. O'Ryan.** 2006. Safety and efficacy of an attenuated vaccine against severe rotavirus gastroenteritis. *N. Engl. J. Med.* **354:**11–22.
101. **Saavedra, J. M., N. A. Bauman, I. Oung, J. A. Perman, and R. H. Yolken.** 1994. Feeding of Bifidobacterium bifidum and Streptococcus thermophilus to infants in hospital for prevention of diarrhoea and shedding of rotavirus. *Lancet* **344:**1046–1049.

102. **Salmi, T. T., P. Arstila, and A. Koivikko.** 1978. Central nervous system involvement in patients with rotavirus gastroenteritis. *Scand. J. Infect. Dis.* **10:**29–31.
103. **Sanford, J. P., and S. E. Sulkin.** 1959. The clinical spectrum of ECHO-virus infection. *N. Engl. J. Med.* **261:**1113–1122.
104. **Saulsbury, F. T., J. A. Winkelstein, and R. H. Yolken.** 1980. Chronic rotavirus infection in immunodeficiency. *J. Pediatr.* **97:**61–65.
105. **Sawyer, L. A., J. J. Murphy, J. E. Kaplan, P. F. Pinsky, D. Chacon, S. Walmsley, L. B. Schonberger, A. Phillips, K. Forward, C. Goldman, J. Brunton, R. A. Fralick, A. O. Carter, G. W. Gary, R. I. Glass, and D. E. Low.** 1988. 25- to 30-nm virus particle associated with a hospital outbreak of acute gastroenteritis with evidence for airborne transmission. *Am. J. Epidemiol.* **127:**1261–1271.
106. **Schreiber, D. S., N. R. Blacklow, and J. S. Trier.** 1973. The mucosal lesion of the proximal small intestine in acute infectious nonbacterial gastroenteritis. *N. Engl. J. Med.* **288:**1318–1323.
107. **Simhon, A., and L. Mata.** 1978. Anti-rotavirus antibody in human colostrum. *Lancet* **i:**39–40.
108. **Smith, A. W., D. E. Skilling, and S. Ridgway.** 1983. Calicivirus-induced vesicular disease in cetaceans and probable interspecies transmission. *J. Am. Vet. Med. Assoc.* **183:**1223–1225.
109. **Steffen, R., F. Collard, N. Tornieporth, S. Campbell-Forrester, D. Ashley, S. Thompson, J. J. Mathewson, E. Maes, B. Stephenson, H. L. DuPont, and F. von Sonnenburg.** 1999. Epidemiology, etiology, and impact of traveler's diarrhea in Jamaica. *JAMA* **281:**811–817.
110. **Szajewska, H., M. Kotowska, J. Z. Mrukowicz, M. Armanska, and W. Mikolajczyk.** 2001. Efficacy of Lactobacillus GG in prevention of nosocomial diarrhea in infants. *J. Pediatr.* **138:**361–365.
111. **Tacket, C. O., M. B. Sztein, G. A. Losonsky, S. S. Wasserman, and M. K. Estes.** 2003. Humoral, mucosal, and cellular immune responses to oral Norwalk virus-like particles in volunteers. *Clin. Immunol.* **108:**241–247.
112. **Turcios, R. M., M. A. Widdowson, A. C. Sulka, P. S. Mead, and R. I. Glass.** 2006. Reevaluation of epidemiological criteria for identifying outbreaks of acute gastroenteritis due to norovirus: United States, 1998–2000. *Clin. Infect. Dis.* **42:**964–969.
113. **Uhnoo, I., E. Olding-Stenkvist, and A. Kreuger.** 1986. Clinical features of acute gastroenteritis associated with rotavirus, enteric adenoviruses, and bacteria. *Arch. Dis. Child.* **61:**732–738.
114. **Uhnoo, I., G. Wadell, L. Svensson, and M. E. Johansson.** 1984. Importance of enteric adenoviruses 40 and 41 in acute gastroenteritis in infants and young children. *J. Clin. Microbiol.* **20:**365–372.
115. **Ushijima, H., K. Q. Xin, S. Nishimura, S. Morikawa, and T. Abe.** 1994. Detection and sequencing of rotavirus VP7 gene from human materials (stools, sera, cerebrospinal fluids, and throat swabs) by reverse transcription and PCR. *J. Clin. Microbiol.* **32:**2893–2897.
116. **van Duynhoven, Y. T., C. M. de Jager, L. M. Kortbeek, H. Vennema, M. P. Koopmans, F. van Leusden, W. H. van der Poel, and M. J. van den Broek.** 2005. A one-year intensified study of outbreaks of gastroenteritis in The Netherlands. *Epidemiol. Infect.* **133:**9–21.
117. **Vesikari, T., D. O. Matson, P. Dennehy, P. Van Damme, M. Santosham, Z. Rodriguez, M. J. Dallas, J. F. Heyse, M. G. Goveia, S. B. Black, H. R. Shinefield, C. D. Christie, S. Ylitalo, R. F. Itzler, M. L. Coia, M. T. Onorato, B. A. Adeyi, G. S. Marshall, L. Gothefors, D. Campens, A. Karvonen, J. P. Watt, K. L. O'Brien, M. J. DiNubile, H. F. Clark, J. W. Boslego, P. A. Offit, and P. M. Heaton.** 2006. Safety and efficacy of a pentavalent human-bovine (WC3) reassortant rotavirus vaccine. *N. Engl. J. Med.* **354:**23–33.
118. **Vonderfecht, S. L., R. L. Miskuff, S. B. Wee, S. Sato, R. R. Tidwell, J. D. Geratz, and R. H. Yolken.** 1988. Protease inhibitors suppress the in vitro and in vivo replication of rotavirus. *J. Clin. Investig.* **82:**2011–2016.
119. **Weinberg, A. D., and K. L. Minaker for the Council on Scientific Affairs, American Medical Association.** 1995. Dehydration. Evaluation and management in older adults. *JAMA* **274:**1552–1556.
120. **Welsh, J. K., and J. T. May.** 1979. Anti-infective properties of breast milk. *J. Pediatr.* **94:**1–9.
121. **Widdowson, M. A., R. Glass, S. Monroe, R. S. Beard, J. W. Bateman, P. Lurie, and C. Johnson.** 2005. Probable transmission of norovirus on an airplane. *JAMA* **293:**1859–1860.
122. **Widdowson, M. A., A. Sulka, S. N. Bulens, R. S. Beard, S. S. Chaves, R. Hammond, E. D. Salehi, E. Swanson, J. Totaro, R. Woron, P. S. Mead, J. S. Bresee, S. S. Monroe, and R. I. Glass.** 2005. Norovirus and foodborne disease, United States, 1991–2000. *Emerg. Infect. Dis.* **11:**95–102.
123. **Yamashita, T.** 1999. Biological and epidemiological characteristics of Aichi virus, as a new member of Picornaviridae. *Virus* (Nagoya) **49:**183–191. (In Japanese.)
124. **Yolken, R., E. Dubovi, F. Leister, R. Reid, J. Almeido-Hill, and M. Santosham.** 1989. Infantile gastroenteritis associated with excretion of pestivirus antigens. *Lancet* **i:**517–520.
125. **Yolken, R., and M. Murphy.** 1982. Sudden infant death syndrome associated with rotavirus infection. *J. Med. Virol.* **10:**291–296.
126. **Yolken, R. H., C. A. Bishop, T. R. Townsend, E. A. Bolyard, J. Bartlett, G. W. Santos, and R. Saral.** 1982. Infectious gastroenteritis in bone-marrow-transplant recipients. *N. Engl. J. Med.* **306:**1010–1012.
127. **Yolken, R. H., H. W. Kim, T. Clem, R. G. Wyatt, A. R. Kalica, R. M. Chanock, and A. Z. Kapikian.** 1977. Enzyme-linked immunosorbent assay (ELISA) for detection of human reovirus-like agent of infantile gastroenteritis. *Lancet* **ii:**263–267.

Viral Hepatitis

ANDREW W. TAI AND JULES L. DIENSTAG

5

Viral hepatitis is a systemic infection primarily affecting the liver. Five different human hepatitis viruses have been recognized and characterized in detail. The five established agents are hepatitis A virus (HAV), hepatitis B virus (HBV), hepatitis C virus (HCV), hepatitis D virus (HDV), and hepatitis E virus (HEV), all RNA viruses, except for HBV, a DNA virus. The hepatitis viruses differ widely not only in their phylogeny but also in their modes of transmission and clinical features. However, common themes exist among human hepatitis viruses: all are hepatotropic and cause a characteristic necroinflammatory process that is recognized clinically and pathologically as "hepatitis." While all of them can cause acute hepatitis, only HBV, HCV, and HDV cause chronic hepatitis and long-term infections.

In this chapter, we discuss the typical clinical and pathological features of viral hepatitis as well as the suggested initial evaluation of a patient presenting with suspected viral hepatitis.

HISTORICAL PERSPECTIVES

The understanding of viral hepatitis has evolved more rapidly in the last 40 years than at any other time in history. Although epidemics of jaundice were recognized as early as the Middle Ages, the notion that such outbreaks were the result of infectious agents was not secured until the Second World War. Two observations established that epidemics of jaundice were caused by a filterable infectious agent, i.e., a virus. First, outbreaks of hepatitis in military personnel immunized with yellow fever vaccine were shown to have resulted from contamination of the vaccine by an agent in the serum used to supplement viral culture media. Second, viral hepatitis was transmissible to volunteers with filtered inocula (75).

Subsequent studies demonstrated definitively the existence of more than one hepatitis virus. Foremost among these was the elegant work performed by Krugman and his colleagues in the 1950s and 1960s at the Willowbrook State School in Staten Island, NY. These investigations led to the identification of two immunologically distinct hepatitis viruses, HAV and HBV, with different incubation periods and different primary modes of transmission (65). By demonstrating the protective effects of inoculating susceptible individuals with boiled hepatitis B serum, Krugman and colleagues laid the foundation for the first-generation, plasma-derived hepatitis B vaccine developed in the 1970s (63, 64).

Perhaps the most seminal observation ushering in the modern era of viral hepatitis research was the discovery in 1965 by Blumberg and colleagues of Australia antigen, the HBV surface antigen (14). Independently, Prince found an identical antigen in the serum of patients with transfusion-associated hepatitis (89).

Further characterization of HBV followed close on the heels of the discovery of the Australia antigen. The application of immunologic, electron microscopic, immunohistochemical, and biophysical techniques led to the identification in 1970 of the 42-nm hepatitis B virion (31) with its hepatitis B surface antigen (HBsAg) envelope and its internal 27-nm nucleocapsid core expressing hepatitis B core antigen. HBV was found to be a DNA virus of the family *Hepadnaviridae* with an endogenous DNA-dependent DNA polymerase. The entire HBV genome was cloned and characterized by 1979 (18, 21, 104, 114). The availability of precise serologic tools for the study and diagnosis of hepatitis B provided new clinical insights about the disease and its pathogenesis. Several studies documented a link between HBV infection and immune complex disorders, including a prodromal dermatitis-arthritis syndrome, glomerulonephritis, and generalized vasculitis (48). The availability of serologic markers and molecular probes for HBV DNA also established an undeniable link between HBV infection and hepatocellular carcinoma (9). Molecular studies of hepatitis B subsequently identified several HBV genotypes, some of which are associated with more rapidly progressive liver injury refractory to therapy and others with hepatocellular carcinoma (57).

As mentioned previously, Krugman and colleagues found that boiling serum containing HBV could inactivate the virus without destroying its antigenicity and that such material injected into susceptible hosts could protect them from infection with live virus. This discovery led to the development of an unconventional but highly effective plasma-derived vaccine against HBV (105) that was deployed for clinical use in 1981. Development of an effective hepatitis B vaccine within approximately 15 years of the discovery of Australia antigen and without the benefit of in vitro cultivation of the virus was hailed as one of the major medical breakthroughs of the time. No sooner had the first-generation, plasma-derived vaccine been released than a second-generation, recombinant HBsAg vaccine was developed, supplanting the plasma-derived one. Initially, hepatitis B vaccination was targeted at high-risk groups; however, this approach failed to have an impact on reducing the frequency of new cases in the general population. Instead, adoption of neonatal and universal childhood vaccination programs was required to reduce the prevalence of chronic HBV infection, fulminant hepatitis, and hepatocellular carcinoma, especially in areas of high HBV endemicity (20). Epidemiological projections suggest that universal childhood vaccination has the potential to reduce or even eliminate hepatitis B as a public health problem within two generations (56).

Following the discovery of HBV came recognition of the existence of other hepatitis viruses, and advances in understanding these other agents paralleled progress in our understanding of HBV. HAV transmission was characterized by Krugman and colleagues, but this type of hepatitis had been described earlier in 1912 by Cockayne and in 1923 by Blumer (15) as an epidemic hepatitis that they termed "infectious hepatitis." Most of the infections occurred in children or young adults, developed 7 to 10 days after exposure to a jaundiced person, peaked in frequency in the fall and winter, and were transmitted largely by person-to-person contact. In 1947, MacCallum introduced the terms hepatitis A and hepatitis B to distinguish "infectious hepatitis" (hepatitis A) from "serum hepatitis" (hepatitis B). In the late 1960s, convincing evidence of transmission of HAV to nonhuman primates (marmosets) was published by Holmes et al. (53), but further progress in HAV research was limited until 1973, when Feinstone et al. visualized 27-nm viral particles by immune electron microscopy of filtrates of feces obtained from persons with hepatitis A (44). Subsequent serologic and virologic advances provided the basis for laboratory tests to detect and characterize HAV; the virus was cultivated in vitro; the biochemical properties, molecular structure, and seroepidemiology of HAV were defined; and the virus genome was cloned and sequenced (5, 27). Twenty-two years after the 1973 detection of HAV, a highly effective, inactivated hepatitis A vaccine became available (25).

The next hepatitis agent to be discovered was the delta hepatitis virus, or HDV, a defective RNA virus that requires the helper function of HBV for its replication and expression. HDV was discovered in 1977 by Rizzetto and colleagues (93), who detected a new nuclear antigen—distinct from known HBV antigens—by immunofluorescence microscopy in the livers of patients with chronic HBV infection. Delta antigen was purified from the liver of an Italian patient, following which a sensitive radioimmunoassay was developed for delta antigen and antibody. An elegant series of biochemical characterization studies, clinical correlations, and chimpanzee transmission studies demonstrated that HDV was unlike any virus that had been described for animals but instead resembled certain plant satellite viruses or viroids (94). Delta hepatitis can occur at the time of primary HBV infection (coinfection) or at any time during chronic HBV infection (superinfection). Because HDV relies on HBV for its replication and expression, delta hepatitis infection cannot persist following HBV clearance, and persons immune to HBV as a result of either previous HBV infection and recovery or vaccination are also immune to HDV.

Until the early 1970s, conventional wisdom held that only two hepatitis viruses, HAV and HBV, existed. Development of diagnostic serologic tests for these two viruses during the 1970s and the application of these serologic tests to stored serum samples from prospectively studied patients with transfusion-associated hepatitis revealed that most of these cases were, in fact, caused by neither HAV nor HBV (43). In fact, "non-A, non-B" cases accounted for most instances of transfusion-associated hepatitis even after the introduction of HBsAg screening to exclude blood donors with HBV infection. Identification of a specific viral agent associated with non-A, non-B hepatitis proved to be a long, difficult quest, even after the presumptive agent was transmitted experimentally in chimpanzees in 1978 (106). The virus was finally identified more than a decade later, as reported in 1989 by Choo et al. (23), who identified a virus-specific clone from a cDNA expression library constructed from the plasma of a chimpanzee with experimental non-A, non-B hepatitis. This advance allowed the entire genome to be cloned, and analysis of the genome revealed that this new agent, designated HCV, was a single-stranded RNA virus belonging to the *Flaviviridae* family, with substantial genotypic diversity. The availability of serologic tests for HCV infection provided tools for defining its seroepidemiology, demonstrated a nearly 3% worldwide prevalence of chronic HCV infection (13), and defined HCV as the leading cause of chronic viral hepatitis, cirrhosis, and hepatocellular carcinoma in Western countries.

At a time when only two hepatitis viruses were recognized, HAV was believed to cause all cases of hepatitis attributed to fecal-oral transmission. Several waterborne epidemics of viral hepatitis occurred in underdeveloped countries in the mid-20th century, including a massive epidemic in Delhi, India, in 1955. These were initially attributed to infection with HAV and explained by the hypothesis that overwhelming water contamination by HAV overcame immunity to HAV, which was almost universal among Indian adults. Such epidemics and sporadic cases were caused by fecal-oral transmission, struck young to middle-aged adults, and, like HAV, were not associated with chronic liver disease. However, the age distribution was older than was typical for hepatitis A, the incubation period was longer, and secondary cases in households were rare (16). Cholestasis was a prominent histologic feature of this epidemic hepatitis, and acute liver failure (ALF) occurred in approximately 10% of cases, primarily in pregnant women, which is also highly unusual for hepatitis A (82). In 1980, serologic tests applied to stored clinical samples collected during these waterborne epidemics failed to implicate HAV (or HBV) (120). In 1983, HAV-like 27- to 30-nm viral particles were detected in stool, and antibodies to these particles appeared during convalescence (4). This virus, HEV, was transmissible experimentally to nonhuman primates. Because HEV could not be grown in cell culture and the amount of virus recoverable from naturally infected humans and experimentally infected primates was so limited, progress in understanding HEV was slow until HEV was finally cloned in 1990 (92). HEV is a nonenveloped single-stranded positive-sense RNA virus and is the only member of the genus *Hepevirus*.

HAV through HEV account for most cases of acute and chronic viral hepatitis, but a small proportion of cases (up to 5% of transfusion-associated cases and approximately 3% of all reported community-acquired cases) remains for which the specific viral cause is not known. Research to identify novel viruses that cause hepatitis has been disappointing. During the 1980s and 1990s, several candidate viruses were identified, including GB virus A, GB virus B, GB virus C/hepatitis G, TT virus, and SEN virus (35, 67, 71, 72, 85, 95, 102). No convincing evidence, however, implicates any of these agents as a cause of acute or chronic liver disease. Therefore, to date, no hepatitis agents besides the five known hepatitis viruses have been identified.

EPIDEMIOLOGY

A summary of clinical and epidemiological features of hepatitis A to hepatitis E is included in Table 1.

Enterically Transmitted Agents

Of the known hepatitis viruses, HAV and HEV are transmitted almost exclusively by the fecal-oral route. HAV has a worldwide distribution and is typically an infection of childhood, facilitated by poor sanitation, crowding, and lack of access to clean water. Large outbreaks as well as sporadic cases have been traced to contaminated food (including fruits and vegetables imported from developing countries, where infection is endemic, to developed countries), water, milk, and shellfish. In countries that have enjoyed a steady improvement in environmental hygiene and sanitation over recent decades, the frequency of HAV infection has declined, and the mean age of exposure has increased correspondingly. Whereas hepatitis A in children is usually subclinical and anicteric, adults tend to have clinically apparent, often severe acute hepatitis A. Therefore, as the frequency of childhood infection decreases in developed countries, and as a susceptible cohort of adults emerges, more cases of severe acute hepatitis A in adults occur. The paradox, then, is that as HAV infection becomes less frequent in a population, the age of infection and severity of hepatitis A increase in the few cases that do occur.

Outbreaks and sporadic cases of hepatitis E, the other recognized enterically transmitted type of viral hepatitis, have been reported and confirmed serologically in Asia, Africa, India, and North and Central America. Most cases can be traced to exposure to contaminated water, and secondary cases within households are rare. Infections arise in populations and age groups that are immune to HAV; young to middle-aged adults between 15 and 40 years of age are the most common targets.

The application of serologic tests has demonstrated the presence of antibodies to HEV (anti-HEV) worldwide, including developed countries where the incidence is believed to be very low. In the United States, where up to 2% of blood donors have been found to be anti-HEV reactive (34), most reported cases of HEV have been in travelers returning from areas of endemicity; however, autochthonous cases of HEV infection have been reported in developed countries such as the United Kingdom and France. The mode of transmission in these cases remains uncertain, but reports of HEV isolation from swine, rodents, and deer suggest that HEV may be a zoonosis (109), and animal reservoirs of HEV may account for autochthonous HEV infection. A substantial increase in disease severity (10 to 20% mortality) among pregnant women is a recognized but unexplained phenomenon.

TABLE 1 Clinical and epidemiological features of viral hepatitis

Feature	HAV	HBV	HCV	HDV	HEV
Incubation period (days)	15–45; mean, 30	30–180; mean, 60–90	15–160; mean, 50	30–180; mean, 60–90	14–60; mean, 40
Onset	Acute	Acute or subclinical	Subclinical, uncommonly acute	Acute or subclinical	Acute
Age preference	Children, young adults	Young adults, infants, toddlers	Any age; more common in adults	Same as HBV	Young adults (20–40 yrs)
Transmission					
Enteric	+++	–	–	–	+++
Percutaneous	–	+++	+++	+++	–
Perinatal	–	+++	+	+	–
Sexual	–	++	++	++	–
Development of chronic infection (%)	0	1–10 (90% of neonates)	70–85	Common (invariable in HDV superinfection)	0
Development of ALF (%)	0.1	0.1–1	Rare	5–20	1–2 (10–20% in pregnant women)
Prognosis	Excellent	Worse with age, debility	Variable	Acute, good; chronic, poor	Good except in pregnancy

Percutaneously Transmitted Agents

HBV, HCV, and HDV are blood-borne agents transmitted primarily by percutaneous routes. Chronically infected human hosts, rather than environmental reservoirs such as water or food, sustain these viral agents within populations.

Transmission of HBV occurs principally by exposure to blood, blood products, blood-contaminated instruments, and sexual contact. Globally, perinatal transmission from mother to baby is the most common route of HBV infection. Currently, in the United States, sexual contact (both heterosexual and homosexual) is the most commonly recognized risk factor, accounting for at least half of new cases per year. In volunteer blood donors, the prevalence of antibody to hepatitis B surface antigen (anti-HBs), a reflection of previous HBV infection, ranges from 5 to 10%, but the prevalence is higher in persons with certain risk factors, such as injection drug use, chronic hemodialysis, multiple sexual partners, and birth in an area of endemicity.

Perinatal transmission from HBsAg-positive mothers is uncommon in North America and Western Europe but is the most important mode of HBV transmission in East Asia, sub-Saharan Africa, and developing countries. The risk is substantially greater for infants born to mothers with high levels of HBV replication, e.g., those who have circulating hepatitis B e antigen (HBeAg), of whom 90% become infected, than for infants born to mothers with antibodies to HBeAg (anti-HBe), of whom only 10% become infected. In most cases, acute infection in the neonate is clinically silent, but the child is very likely to remain infected chronically.

Prevalence of infection, modes of transmission, and human behavior result in geographically different epidemiological patterns of HBV infection. In East Asia and Africa, HBV infection is a disease of newborn and young children and is perpetuated by a cycle of maternal-neonatal spread. In North America and Western Europe, HBV infection is primarily a disease of adolescence and early adulthood, when intimate sexual contact as well as recreational and occupational percutaneous exposures tend to occur. Because infection in early life is associated with a high likelihood of chronic infection, most of the HBV infections in East Asia and Africa become chronic and can be complicated decades later by cirrhosis and hepatocellular carcinoma. In contrast, in North America and Western Europe, where most infections are acquired in adulthood, the likelihood of clinically apparent hepatitis is high but that of chronic infection is low. Therefore, in such "western" populations, chronic hepatitis is a relatively rare complication of acute hepatitis B and progression to end-stage cirrhosis and hepatocellular carcinoma is infrequent.

Modes of HDV transmission are similar to those for HBV, with percutaneous exposures the most efficient. Sexual transmission of HDV is less efficient than for HBV, and perinatal transmission of HDV is uncommon (77). Although infection with HDV is distributed worldwide, only about 5% of the world's HBV-infected persons are also infected with HDV (38). Generally, three different epidemiological patterns of HDV infection exist. (i) In countries with a low prevalence of chronic HBV infection, HDV prevalence is generally low among both inactive HBV carriers and patients with chronic HBV-related liver disease. In such countries, HDV infection occurs most commonly among injection drug users and hemophiliacs (i.e., populations with substantial exposure to blood products). (ii) In Mediterranean countries, HDV infection is endemic, and HDV is transmitted predominantly by close personal and sexual contact. (iii) In most of East Asia, where the prevalence of chronic HBV is very high, HDV infection is uncommon. Hepatitis D can be introduced into a population through injection drug users or by migration of persons from areas of endemicity to areas of nonendemicity. Disease related to HDV outbreaks has been very severe, often progressing to fulminant hepatitis, with case fatality rates of up to 20% for outbreaks of superinfection (51) and 5% for coinfection. These sustained outbreaks tend to blur the distinctions between geographic areas of endemicity and nonendemicity.

The worldwide prevalence of HCV infection, based on serologic testing for anti-HCV, is approximately 2 to 3%; however, geographic variability exists (117). Prevalence rates of 0.5 to 1.8% have been documented in the United States, southern Europe, and Japan. Rates are as high as 10% in parts of Africa and even higher, >20%, in parts of Egypt. Transmission of HCV appears to occur primarily via percutaneous routes. HCV has been incriminated as the culpable agent in more than 90 to 95% of cases of transfusion-associated hepatitis prior to the introduction of HCV screening tests. Since the introduction of blood donor screening for anti-HCV (and, more recently, HCV RNA), transfusion-associated hepatitis has been reduced dramatically and now is very rare (1, 97).

Nonpercutaneous transmission of HCV does occur but appears to be much less efficient than percutaneous routes. Although sexual transmission of HCV does occur (83, 108, 110, 119), most studies fail to identify a substantial risk of sexual transmission to stable sexual partners of patients with chronic HCV. The annual risk of transmission has been estimated to be 0.6% or less in mismatched heterosexual monogamous couples. Based on this estimate, an expert panel concluded that sexual transmission is sufficiently rare that a change in sexual practice is not advocated for monogamous couples in long-term relationships, although they should be advised that the potential for transmission exists and that barrier protection may reduce the risk of transmission (84). Nonsexual household contacts appear to be at very low risk for HCV infection.

The route of transmission is undefined in 30 to 40% of all known cases of HCV infection (55). Low socioeconomic level and other high-risk attributes such as use of noninjection illegal drugs, contact with a sexual partner who has used injection drugs, or history of sexually transmitted diseases have been identified frequently in this population, as has almost-forgotten, limited injection drug use in the remote past. HCV infection in volunteer blood donors (0.5 to 1.8%), who have been screened to exclude risk factors for exposure to blood-borne viruses, is also attributable to long-forgotten percutaneous exposure. Indeed, studies in recent decades of the age-specific prevalence of HCV infection implicate an epidemic of injection drug use in the 1960s and 1970s as the primary risk factor in the cohort of persons infected currently.

In contrast to the high efficiency of perinatal transmission of HBV, perinatal transmission of HCV is rare and then likely only in babies born to highly viremic women. Prospective studies of perinatal transmission of HCV have yielded an average rate of 5% in women with HCV alone and up to 15% in mothers coinfected with human immunodeficiency virus (HIV) and HCV (111).

PATHOPHYSIOLOGY OF VIRAL HEPATITIS

The mechanisms by which the hepatotropic viruses cause liver injury have not been determined definitively but most likely involve a combination of immune-mediated injury to infected hepatocytes, induction of hepatocyte apoptosis, and, in unusual circumstances, from a direct viral cytopathic effect. Both innate and adaptive immune responses are likely to be involved in viral clearance as well as hepatocyte injury.

For example, cytotoxic T lymphocytes (CTLs) are generated against infected hepatocytes in both HBV and HCV. In hepatitis B, CTLs appear to be directed at nucleocapsid proteins, HBcAg and HBeAg, on the liver cell surface (11). The presence of HCV-specific CTL activity in hepatitis C has been documented as well (62), and in both HBV and HCV infections, viral epitopes that represent CTL targets have been identified. Cytotoxic-T-cell activity has also been identified in patients with hepatitis A, and in all likelihood, similar CTL-derived responses to the other hepatitis viruses occur.

There is also evidence that the hepatitis viruses can be directly cytopathic. In situations in which the immune response is compromised, the accumulation of large amounts of HBsAg in hepatocytes may result in direct liver cell injury. This phenomenon has been postulated to explain the severe hepatitis (fibrosing cholestatic hepatitis; see below) that occurs in patients with recurrent disease after liver transplantation for end-stage liver disease associated with hepatitis B, and a comparable process has been observed in severe recurrent hepatitis C following liver transplantation. This hypothesis is supported by a transgenic-mouse model in which HBsAg accumulates in mouse liver cells and results in hepatocyte injury (22). The degree to which HBsAg contributes to hepatocyte injury in immunocompetent humans, however, is unknown.

The host and viral factors that distinguish reliably between infected patients who will recover and those who develop chronicity remain to be elucidated. Certain viral factors may play a role in the pathogenicity of viral hepatitis. Coinfection with two hepatitis viruses (e.g., HBV plus HDV, HCV plus HBV, or HAV plus HCV) can increase the severity of liver disease, and several genotypes of HCV and HBV are thought to be associated with more severe liver disease than others. Precore/core promoter variants of HBV are associated with more severe liver disease (severe chronic hepatitis and fulminant hepatitis) than wild-type HBV. For hepatitis C, patients with the most robust and viral epitope-broad CTL responses appear to be more likely to recover from acute infection.

The extrahepatic manifestations of HBV infection appear to result from immune-complex-mediated injury. Deposition in affected tissue vessels of HBV antigens, antibodies, and complement components has been implicated in the prodromal serum sickness-like syndrome of arthritis and dermatitis in acute infection and in glomerulonephritis and generalized vasculitis (polyarteritis nodosa) in chronic infection. In chronic hepatitis C, HCV-containing immune complexes have been implicated in the pathogenesis of essential mixed cryoglobulinemia. The B-cell proliferation associated with chronic HCV infection may increase the risk of developing B-cell non-Hodgkin's lymphomas, though this association displays strong geographic variation (47).

CLINICAL FEATURES

Acute Viral Hepatitis

The clinical features and course of uncomplicated acute viral hepatitis are similar among the several types of viral hepatitis. The prodromal symptoms are typically nonspecific and quite variable and occur after an incubation period that varies with the viral agent. Constitutional symptoms, if present, usually precede the onset of jaundice by 1 to 2 weeks and may include headache, myalgia, arthralgia, fatigue, weakness, anorexia, nausea, vomiting, cough, pharyngitis, photophobia, and coryza. Low-grade fever, right upper quadrant or epigastric discomfort, and alteration in taste and smell occur often. These symptoms typically last 1 to 2 weeks and are coincident with elevations in aminotransferase levels. Dark urine may precede the onset of clinical jaundice by several days, and acholic stools can be seen for a proportion of patients with hepatitis A and especially with hepatitis E. In HCV infection, the symptoms are usually milder—often clinically inapparent—than in HBV, HAV, or HEV infection.

Acute viral hepatitis may be icteric or anicteric. Over 75% of acute HCV infections are anicteric, as are the vast majority of HAV and HBV infections in children. With the onset of clinical jaundice, constitutional prodromal symptoms usually diminish. The liver becomes swollen and tender and may be associated with right upper quadrant pain. Infrequently, patients present with a cholestatic picture that can be confused with extrahepatic biliary obstruction; such a cholestatic presentation has been observed in a subset of HAV and especially in HEV infections. During the recovery phase, constitutional symptoms disappear, but liver enlargement and abnormalities in liver biochemical tests persist. Complete clinical and biochemical recovery is to be expected 1 to 2 months after the onset of acute HAV and HEV infections and 3 to 6 months after onset in 95 to 99% of uncomplicated cases of acute hepatitis B in immunocompetent adults. In hepatitis B, the likelihood of viral clearance and recovery is higher after clinically apparent than after inapparent acute infection. For hepatitis C, however, this pattern is less obvious. Earlier observations suggested no difference in outcome between symptomatic and asymptomatic or between severe and mild acute hepatitis C among prospectively monitored (unselected) persons with transfusion-associated (2) or reported (selected) cases of community-acquired hepatitis C (30). More recently, among patients selected for referral to research centers in Germany (45), clearance of acute HCV infection was observed in 52% of 46 patients with symptomatic illness but in none of 9 patients with asymptomatic illness. In contrast, in a cohort of 214 consecutive patients with acute hepatitis C enrolled in an epidemiological study in Italy over a 5-year period, although the frequency of spontaneous recovery was relatively high, 36%, the likelihood of chronicity was the same for patients with symptomatic and asymptomatic acute infection (96). Patients who fail to recover within 6 months of the onset of acute hepatitis are considered to have chronic hepatitis (see "Chronic Viral Hepatitis" below).

Each of the acute viral hepatitides has a number of unusual or distinguishing clinical features. A small proportion of patients with HAV infection experience relapsing or polyphasic hepatitis—aminotransferase elevation, fecal excretion of HAV, and, sometimes, symptoms—weeks to months after apparent recovery from acute hepatitis. An equally small proportion of patients experience a cholestatic variant of HAV infection, characterized by prolonged jaundice (>12 weeks) with symptoms of pruritus and fatigue. Even among patients with relapsing hepatitis or cholestatic hepatitis, HAV remains a self-limited infection.

Except for the very small proportion of patients with fulminant hepatitis A (see below), virtually all previously healthy patients with acute HAV infection recover completely. Cholestatic features are especially common in patients with acute hepatitis E, which, like hepatitis A, does not lead to chronic infection.

Acute HBV infection can be associated with extrahepatic manifestations, HDV coinfection, and, rarely, ALF (see below). The extrahepatic manifestations of acute HBV infection result from the deposition of viral antigen-antibody immune complexes. Several clinical syndromes are now recognized. In approximately 10 to 20% of patients with acute HBV infection, a serum sickness-like "arthritis-dermatitis" prodrome occurs during the incubation period or early acute phase. This syndrome consists of an urticarial rash, angioedema, fever, or symmetrical polyarthritis or polyarthralgias; activation of the classical and alternative complement pathways is associated with hypocomplementemia (116). This serum sickness-like syndrome is self-limited and resolves as acute illness develops and is not associated with chronic joint disease or irreversible joint damage. Other syndromes include mixed cryoglobulinemia and papular acrodermatitis of childhood (Gianotti-Crosti syndrome), which consists of a papular rash that typically spares the trunk, with associated lymphadenopathy.

Acute HDV infection can occur simultaneously with acute HBV infection or can be superimposed upon chronic HBV infection. When acute HDV and HBV infections occur simultaneously, clinical and biochemical features may be indistinguishable from those of HBV infection alone; however, simultaneous HBV and HDV infections may be associated with more severe or fulminant hepatitis. When HDV superinfection occurs in a patient with chronic hepatitis B, clinical worsening is likely.

The case-fatality rate for acute viral hepatitis is, overall, very low (approximately 0.1%) but is higher in older patients with acute HAV infection (see above), patients with acute HBV and HDV coinfection (5%), and pregnant women with acute hepatitis E (10 to 20%).

Non-Virus-Specific Biochemical and Serologic Changes

Characteristic biochemistry test abnormalities occur among all forms of acute viral hepatitis. Elevations of the serum alanine aminotransferase (ALT) and aspartate aminotransferase (AST) levels represent the earliest indicators of hepatocellular injury during acute viral hepatitis. These changes begin during the prodromal phase and precede a rise in serum bilirubin. In typical acute viral hepatitis, ALT levels exceed AST levels, and peak aminotransferase levels above 1,000 U/liter are not uncommon. Aminotransferase levels diminish progressively during recovery. Total serum bilirubin usually increases for 1 to 2 weeks to 5 to 20 mg/dl and may continue to rise despite falling serum aminotransferase levels before falling gradually thereafter over several weeks. Jaundice is usually visible in the sclera or skin when the serum bilirubin concentration exceeds 2.5 to 3 mg/dl. Serum alkaline phosphatase may be normal or mildly elevated. Other recognized laboratory abnormalities include mild neutropenia, relative lymphocytosis, atypical lymphocytosis, and the presence of low titers of nonspecific autoantibodies such as rheumatoid factor, smooth muscle, and nuclear antibodies. Serum globulins, especially gamma globulin, are either normal or slightly elevated, and acute hepatitis A is accompanied often by a nonspecific increase in serum immunoglobulin M (IgM) levels. Although the serum aminotransferases and bilirubin can reach substantial levels, their magnitude is not generally predictive of disease severity or prognosis. In contrast, severe cases of acute viral hepatitis are evidenced by impairment of hepatic synthetic function, reflected in prolongation of the prothrombin time and, when sustained, reduction in serum albumin levels.

Virus-Specific Serologic Features

A summary of serologic markers of hepatitis A to hepatitis E appears in Table 2.

HAV

Fecal excretion of HAV begins during the late incubation period, peaks just before jaundice becomes apparent

TABLE 2 Common serologic patterns and their interpretations

Virus	Serologic pattern	Interpretation
HAV	IgM anti-HAV$^+$	Acute infection
	IgG anti-HAV$^+$	Remote infection
HBV	HBsAg$^+$, IgM anti-HBc$^+$	Acute infection
	HBsAg$^+$, IgG anti-HBc$^+$, HBeAg$^+$, HBV DNA$^+$	Chronic, replicative infection
	HBsAg$^+$, IgG anti-HBc$^+$, HBeAg$^-$, anti-HBe$^+$, HBV DNA $> 10^4$ copies/ml	Chronic, replicative infection with a precore or core promoter mutant
	HBsAg$^+$, IgG anti-HBc$^+$, HBeAg$^-$, anti-HBe$^+$, HBV DNA $< 10^3$–10^4 copies/ml	Chronic, minimally replicative infection
	HBsAg$^-$, anti-HBs$^+$, IgG anti-HBc$^+$	"Resolved" infection
	HBsAg$^-$, anti-HBs$^+$, IgG anti-HBc$^-$	Vaccinated
HDV	Anti-HDV$^+$, HBsAg$^+$	HDV infection
	IgM anti-HBc$^+$	Coinfection
	IgG anti-HBc$^+$	Superinfection
HCV	Anti-HCV$^+$, HCV RNA$^+$	HCV infection
	Anti-HCV$^+$, HCV RNA$^-$	Resolved infection or false-positive antibody
HEV	IgM anti-HEV$^+$	Acute infection
	IgG anti-HEV$^+$	Remote infection

(in icteric cases), and falls to barely detectable levels as the clinical illness evolves. Serologic markers are more convenient and reliable in establishing a diagnosis of acute infection. The primary humoral immune response to HAV infection is IgM antibody to HAV (anti-HAV), and its serologic detection is the basis for the diagnosis of acute hepatitis A. IgM anti-HAV becomes detectable during the prodrome and persists at high levels for approximately 3 months. Low-level IgM anti-HAV may persist in some patients for 6 to 12 months. As the clinical illness resolves, and beyond the first 3 months, IgG anti-HAV replaces IgM anti-HAV as the predominant antibody and persists indefinitely thereafter, correlating with immunity to reinfection.

HBV

In acute HBV infection, HBsAg is the first serologic marker to appear, usually preceding biochemical and clinical evidence of hepatitis by several weeks. Within 1 to 2 weeks of the appearance of HBsAg in serum, antibody to hepatitis B core antigen (anti-HBc) can be detected in serum; initially, and for approximately the first 6 months of HBV infection, the predominant anti-HBc is of the IgM class. Therefore, in the small proportion of patients (<5%) in whom circulating levels of HBsAg do not exceed the detection threshold, a diagnosis of acute HBV infection can be established by demonstrating the presence of IgM anti-HBc. Typically, in acute HBV infection, IgM anti-HBc declines to undetectable levels approximately 6 months after the onset of infection. As IgM anti-HBc declines, IgG anti-HBc becomes the predominant class of anti-HBc and persists indefinitely.

As HBsAg levels decline after acute hepatitis B, usually within 4 to 6 months after the onset of infection, anti-HBs, present heretofore but obscured by excess HBsAg, becomes detectable. Patients with circulating anti-HBs resulting from prior HBV infection or HBV vaccination are felt to be immune to HBV infection. In some cases, persons with apparent clinical recovery following HBV infection, as evidenced by the presence of anti-HBs and/or IgG anti-HBc, can experience reactivation of HBV infection following myeloablative therapy or certain types of immunosuppression (59).

Some individuals have detectable IgG anti-HBc but no detectable anti-HBs or HBsAg. The frequency of "isolated anti-HBc" ranges from 0.5 to 2% in blood donors in areas of nonendemicity to ~10% in regions of endemicity. Within areas of nonendemicity, subpopulations with high HBV prevalence (injection drug users and persons with HIV or HCV infection) also have higher rates of isolated anti-HBc. Some cases of isolated anti-HBc represent remote HBV infection with waning titers of anti-HBs, as shown by a prompt, anamnestic rise in anti-HBs titers after single-dose HBV vaccination. A false-positive anti-HBc test is another possibility, particularly for people without risk factors for HBV infection and with normal aminotransferase levels. Occult HBV infection (i.e., detectable HBV DNA) in this setting is uncommon (100) but should be considered in patients from high-prevalence populations or in patients with abnormal aminotransferase levels or chronic liver disease.

Another serologic marker of HBV infection is HBeAg, which appears during periods of active HBV replication. HBeAg is almost invariably present during acute HBV infection and is replaced by anti-HBe once peak replication ceases and biochemical and clinical recovery begin. The exception is acute infection by precore or core promoter HBV mutants, which block transcription or translation of the precore gene and therefore do not express HBeAg. Consequently, little is to be gained by HBeAg testing during acute hepatitis B. When acute hepatitis B is slow to resolve based on persistently high serum aminotransferase levels, persistence of HBeAg (beyond 3 months) tends to predict progression to chronicity. Markers of HBV replication, such as HBeAg and HBV DNA, are rarely of help in the management of patients with acute hepatitis B, but they assume importance in the evaluation, management, and monitoring of patients with chronic hepatitis B (see below).

HCV

Current third-generation enzyme immunoassays are 97% sensitive for detection of current or resolved HCV infection. Furthermore, reactivity in third-generation immunoassays develops significantly earlier (during acute illness) than with older assays (often delayed until several months after acute illness) (7). Over half of patients with acute HCV hepatitis are anti-HCV positive at the time of presentation, and about 95% are antibody positive 1 month later (6). Despite the high specificity of third-generation enzyme immunoassays (99.7%), false-positive anti-HCV tests do occur for populations with a low prevalence of HCV exposure (e.g., asymptomatic blood donors) and for persons with autoimmune disease and hyperglobulinemia. Specificity of serologic assays for anti-HCV is assessed nowadays by demonstrating the presence of circulating HCV RNA.

The earliest and most sensitive serum marker of HCV infection is the presence of HCV RNA based on sensitive amplification techniques such as reverse transcriptase PCR (RT-PCR). False-negative anti-HCV tests may occur in the setting of immunosuppression (including HIV infection) and for patients undergoing chronic hemodialysis. HCV RNA should be assayed in seronegative immunocompromised individuals if clinical suspicion of HCV infection is high. On the other hand, a positive HCV RNA result for seronegative healthy blood donors lacking anti-HCV is more likely to be the result of a false-positive RT-PCR than of true infection (90). In such cases, retesting for HCV RNA in a different laboratory or with a different assay may be useful.

HDV

During HDV infection, HDV antigen can be detected in hepatocyte nuclei by immunohistochemical techniques, but in most cases, liver tissue is unavailable. The most reliable serologic marker of HDV infection is antibody to HDV antigen (anti-HDV), which can be detected by routinely available immunoassays. Although IgM anti-HDV responses occur, they do not distinguish reliably between acute and chronic HDV infection; a serologic diagnosis of hepatitis D relies on testing for total anti-HDV. During simultaneous acute HDV-HBV coinfection, levels of anti-HDV are usually low, time to initial appearance of anti-HDV is variable, and anti-HDV may persist for only a short time beyond the resolution of acute infection, leaving no evidence of previous infection. In contrast, when hepatitis D causes acute superinfection of a patient with preexisting chronic hepatitis B, anti-HDV appears early, increases to very high levels, and persists indefinitely. In this setting, serologic diagnosis of HDV infection is quite reliable. Although HDV antigen can also be detected in serum, its appearance tends to be transient. PCR for HDV RNA is specific and sensitive, provides information about HDV replication, but is not commercially available. When a patient presents with acute hepatitis and has HBsAg and anti-HDV in serum, determination of the class of anti-HBc is helpful in establishing the relationship between HBV and HDV infection. In simultaneous acute HBV and HDV infections, IgM anti-HBc will be detectable, while in acute HDV infection superimposed upon chronic HBV infection, IgG anti-HBc will be identified.

HEV

The serologic and virologic events accompanying acute hepatitis E mirror those observed in acute hepatitis A. As in acute HAV infection, acute HEV infection can be diagnosed by detection of IgM antibodies to HEV. As with hepatitis A, IgG anti-HEV persists for many years, perhaps indefinitely, following exposure. Enzyme immunoassays for both IgG and IgM anti-HEV as well as RT-PCR for HEV RNA in serum or stool can also be performed in selected research and reference laboratories.

Fulminant Viral Hepatitis

The most severe form of acute hepatitis is known as fulminant hepatitis, which is one cause of ALF. ALF is defined by the occurrence of hepatic encephalopathy (ranging from drowsiness, confusion, and disorientation to stupor and deep coma) and hepatic synthetic dysfunction (based usually on a prolonged prothrombin time) within 8 weeks of onset in individuals without preexisting liver disease. ALF can also be caused by drugs or toxins, various metabolic liver disorders, autoimmune hepatitis, and vascular disorders.

Acute viral hepatitis used to account for the majority of cases of ALF in the United States, France, and Great Britain (58) but more recently has been surpassed by acetaminophen overdose and idiosyncratic drug reactions. Only 12% of the cases of ALF treated in 17 referral centers in the United States between 1998 and 2001 were attributed to HAV or HBV (107). Hepatitis B accounts for the majority of cases of fulminant viral hepatitis. Depending on the population studied, a sizable proportion of these HBV-associated cases may be associated with HDV infection (50). In addition, infection with precore/core promoter mutant HBV strains has been linked to instances of ALF in Israel and Japan (69), but not in cases of fulminant hepatitis elsewhere. Fulminant HAV infection is uncommon, and its frequency in ALF appears to be falling, accounting for 5% of all cases of ALF in persons enrolled in the ALF Study Group in the United States in 1998 but only 0.8% in 2005 (107). Among those with fulminant hepatitis A, adults 60 years of age and older had a case fatality rate of 1.8%, compared to a rate of 0.5% in the 15- to 39-year-old age group and 0% in those under the age of 15 (118). Fulminant hepatitis has been associated with acute hepatitis E in areas of endemicity, primarily in pregnant women (81); however, recent studies suggest that HEV is not an identifiable cause of presumed non-A, non-B fulminant hepatitis in the United States (70). HCV causes fulminant hepatitis only extremely rarely, if ever.

Although in most cases of ALF a cause can be established, clinicians are faced occasionally with patients who have ALF and whose clinical presentation suggests a viral cause but without evidence of infection by conventional hepatitis viruses. Covert viral infection has been observed classically in fulminant hepatitis B infection during which an overwhelming host immune response results in severe liver injury. With a rapid and overwhelming destruction of hepatocytes, patients who have fulminant hepatitis B may lose all viable substrate for HBV synthesis by the time they present clinically; in such instances HBsAg, HbeAg, and HBV DNA may be undetectable (121). Another infectious cause of ALF is herpes simplex virus (HSV; see "Diagnostic Considerations" below). Other possible causes of unexplained ALF include occult acetaminophen or other toxin-mediated injury (32) or novel viruses (41).

Patients with ALF have signs and symptoms of encephalopathy that may begin subtly with sleep-wake cycle disturbances and mood lability or irritability, which may then progress to drowsiness, asterixis, confusion, and then coma. Altered hepatic synthetic function with coagulopathy is often accompanied by multisystem organ failure. These patients invariably have a hemorrhagic diathesis, with thrombocytopenia as well as prolonged prothrombin time and partial thromboplastin time. Low-grade disseminated intravascular coagulation may also be present, and renal dysfunction is common. The mortality rate is extremely high, exceeding 80% among patients in deep coma who do not undergo liver transplantation. On the other hand, patients who survive may have complete biochemical and histologic recovery. Death results typically from cerebral edema causing brain stem herniation, sepsis, bleeding, or multisystem organ failure.

Chronic Viral Hepatitis

The clinical features of chronic HBV, chronic HBV plus HDV, and chronic HCV infections are similar and run the entire clinical spectrum from asymptomatic infection to end-stage liver failure. Fatigue, malaise, and anorexia are common symptoms and can accompany all types of chronic viral hepatitis. Jaundice may be seen in advanced chronic hepatitis with cirrhosis or may be seen in acute exacerbations of chronic hepatitis B with or without concomitant HDV infection. Such flares of chronic hepatitis B may lead to progressive liver injury and clinical decompensation of previously compensated cirrhosis. Chronic HDV infection is associated with more severe hepatitis than chronic hepatitis B alone; moderate to severe chronic hepatitis, with or without cirrhosis, is the rule rather than the exception. Cirrhosis may develop in either chronic HBV (with or without HDV) or HCV infection.

In chronic hepatitis B, progression to more severe histopathological lesions and cirrhosis tends to be confined primarily to patients with ongoing HBV replication, as evidenced by detectable HBeAg and high titers of HBV DNA or, in patients with precore/core promoter mutant HBV, by the presence of high levels of HBV DNA. Coinfection with HDV further increases the risk of cirrhosis. Among patients with chronic HCV infection, cirrhosis develops in approximately 20% over the course of two decades. Complications of cirrhosis, including ascites, gastrointestinal bleeding, hepatic encephalopathy, and hepatocellular carcinoma, are common in end-stage disease.

The rate at which liver injury progresses to cirrhosis is determined by both viral and host factors. Viral factors such as genotype and level of viremia have been discussed previously. Recognized host factors include the presence of coexisting liver disease, alcohol intake, and the integrity of the host immune response. The influence of the host immune system has been studied in the context of cohorts with coexisting viral liver disease and immunodeficiencies, including those with HIV infection, recipients of organ allografts, and persons with hypogammaglobulinemia and HCV.

Among persons with HIV infection (see below), 10% are estimated to have chronic HBV infection and, depending on the population studied, 10 to 90% are coinfected with HCV. HIV coinfection is associated with increased HBV replication and an increased risk for the development of cirrhosis (28). Similarly, the risk of progression to cirrhosis is higher in HIV-HCV coinfection (37). Much of the data collected on these coinfected populations predates the widespread use of highly active antiretroviral therapy (HAART); however, in HIV infection, the potential benefit of therapy-associated immune reconstitution on slowing viral liver disease may be offset by a higher proportion of patients with clinically apparent liver disease as a result of their extended longevity.

Extrahepatic disease may complicate chronic HBV, HCV, or HDV infection. Polyarthralgia and, less commonly, polyarthritis are occasionally observed in patients with chronic hepatitis B. While generalized vasculitis (polyarteritis nodosa [PAN]) develops in considerably less than 1% of patients with chronic HBV infection, 30 to 40% of patients with PAN have HBsAg in serum and deposition of HBV antigen-containing immune complexes in small and medium-sized arteriolar walls. The clinical characteristics of patients with HBsAg-positive PAN are similar to those of patients who have PAN without HBsAg antigenemia. Similarly, immune-complex glomerulonephritis has been documented in association with chronic HBV infection.

Extrahepatic complications of chronic hepatitis C are less common than in chronic hepatitis B, with the exception of essential mixed cryoglobulinemia (74, 80). This disease is characterized by the production of a polyclonal IgG and monoclonal IgM with rheumatoid factor activity, forming an immune complex that precipitates upon cooling. Clinically, this phenomenon presents with arthralgias/arthritis, cutaneous vasculitis, and, occasionally, membranoproliferative glomerulonephritis resulting from immune-complex deposition. Over 90% of patients with essential mixed cryoglobulinemia have chronic HCV infection. In both HBV and HCV infections, the institution of antiviral therapy can be an effective treatment of these extrahepatic manifestations. HCV has also been associated with porphyria cutanea tarda and sicca syndrome, among other extrahepatic features.

The most devastating clinical complication of chronic viral hepatitis is hepatocellular carcinoma (HCC). Although almost all patients with HCC and hepatitis B are cirrhotic, chronic HBV infection can cause HCC in the absence of cirrhosis and is seen primarily in persons infected early in life or in immunocompromised patients (9). In a retrospective study, the presence of anti-HDV was found to be associated with a threefold-increased risk of HCC compared to the risk in HDV-seronegative patients with chronic HBV infection (42). HCC can also complicate HCV infection but, unlike HBV, occurs almost exclusively in patients with cirrhosis (36, 101).

Laboratory features of chronic viral hepatitis do not distinguish adequately between histologically mild and severe hepatitis. Aminotransferase elevations may fluctuate in the range of 100 to 1,000 U, and ALT (serum glutamic pyruvic transaminase) activity tends to be more elevated than AST (serum glutamic oxalacetic transaminase) activity; however, once cirrhosis is established, AST usually exceeds ALT. Alkaline phosphatase activity tends to be normal or mildly elevated. Hyperbilirubinemia may be quite pronounced in advanced cases of chronic viral hepatitis with cirrhosis but is rare or very mild during earlier phases of chronic hepatitis. Hypoalbuminemia, thrombocytopenia, and prolongation of the prothrombin time are associated with advanced chronic viral hepatitis with cirrhosis.

Virus-Specific Features

HBV

The likelihood of chronicity after acute HBV infection varies as a function of age and is most common at the extremes of life. Chronicity of HBV infection occurs in 90% of infants born to mothers with HBeAg-positive chronic HBV infection and is also more likely in the elderly. Immunocompromised persons and patients with comorbid conditions also have an increased risk of chronic HBV infection.

Once the diagnosis of chronic HBV infection has been established by detection of circulating HBsAg, testing for HBeAg, anti-HBe, and HBV DNA should be done as markers of viral replication and for monitoring responses to antiviral therapy.

Patients with chronic hepatitis B can be subdivided into those with detectable HBeAg and those without. In chronic HBV infection, serologic detection of HBeAg identifies patients with highly replicative chronic infection. Such HBeAg-positive patients are highly infectious and tend to have histologic evidence of substantial liver injury. Studies of the natural history of chronic HBV infection have shown that, annually, approximately 10% of patients with HBeAg-positive chronic HBV infection seroconvert spontaneously to a relatively nonreplicative state in which HBeAg is lost, anti-HBe is acquired, and circulating HBV DNA falls below a threshold of $<10^3$ to 10^4 copies/ml. Those in the replicative state tend to have more severe chronic hepatitis than those in the nonreplicative state. In the nonreplicative state, infectivity and liver injury (as reflected by biochemical tests and liver histology) are limited; these patients tend to be inactive HBV carriers.

HBeAg-negative chronic hepatitis B falls into two categories. One group, as described above, is composed of "inactive carriers." Approximately 4 to 20% of these individuals can revert to HBeAg positivity in the future, however, and should be monitored with periodic testing to confirm maintenance of the inactive state. The other group is characterized by persistent HBV replication as indicated by elevated HBV DNA levels (typically $>10^4$ copies/ml) and histologic evidence of ongoing hepatic inflammation. These individuals are most often infected with precore/core promoter variants of HBV (17). Precore/core promoter mutations block transcription or translation of the precore gene, which encodes HBeAg. In HBeAg-negative chronic hepatitis B, the level of liver injury correlates with levels of HBV DNA; while some patients have persistently elevated aminotransferase levels and HBV DNA, in others, HBV DNA and ALT levels fluctuate widely. Not uncommonly, in the latter patients, periods of undetectable HBV DNA and normal ALT activity may alternate with periods of high HBV DNA levels and substantial elevations of ALT. Generally, patients with HBeAg-negative chronic hepatitis B have lower HBV

DNA levels (10^5 to 10^6 virions/ml) than patients with HBeAg-positive chronic hepatitis B ($\geq 10^6$ virions/ml).

HDV

Although coinfection with HBV and HDV is associated with a higher mortality rate than acute HBV infection alone, simultaneous acute infections with these agents does not increase the frequency of chronicity. Superinfection by HDV of a patient with chronic HBV infection almost always results in chronic HDV infection. In this setting, the likelihood of fulminant hepatitis is increased (103). Outbreaks of severe HDV superinfection in isolated populations with a high hepatitis B carrier rate have been described in which the mortality rate exceeded 20%. The laboratory features of chronic HDV infection are similar to those of chronic HBV infection alone.

HCV

Although acute HCV infection is usually anicteric and subclinical, chronicity follows in about 85% of cases, and progression to cirrhosis occurs in at least 20% of patients with chronic HCV infection within 20 years (98). Progression of chronic HCV infection, which occurs even in patients with mild histologic lesions, may be influenced by HCV genotype, level of viremia, coexisting other hepatitis viral infection, age of acquisition, immunosuppression, coexisting alcohol abuse, the presence of fatty liver infiltration, and the presence of other comorbid illnesses.

Most patients with hypogammaglobulinemia and HCV infection acquired their viral hepatitis as a result of contaminated human immunoglobulin preparations. This class of patients includes those with selective immunoglobulin deficiencies and common variable immunodeficiency. Progression to cirrhosis is particularly high in this subgroup, the members of which have rates of cirrhosis as high as 30% in as little as 5 to 10 years (12). Identification of HCV infection may be delayed in these patients, who fail frequently to produce anti-HCV. Accelerated liver injury, including the development of fibrosing cholestatic hepatitis (see below), may also be seen in recipients of organ allografts.

Chronic HCV infection is associated with more episodic fluctuations in aminotransferase levels, which tend to be elevated to a lesser degree than in chronic HBV infection. A high prevalence of autoantibodies occurs in patients with chronic HCV infection, most notably, nuclear antibodies, smooth muscle antibodies, and rheumatoid factor (26). Autoantibodies to liver-kidney microsomes, commonly seen in patients with type 2 autoimmune hepatitis, are found in approximately 5% of patients with chronic hepatitis C (68). Patients with chronic HCV infection and autoantibodies do not appear to be more prone to the development of autoimmune complications of interferon therapy than those without autoantibodies.

Pathology

In acute viral hepatitis, both spotty and panlobular hepatocyte injury and necrosis occur in a characteristic pattern. Typical histologic findings include panlobular infiltration with mononuclear cells, hepatocyte necrosis, Kupffer cell hyperplasia, and variable degrees of cholestasis. Hepatocellular steatosis can be present but is usually mild and macrovesicular in nature. The mononuclear cell infiltrate is predominately lymphocytic but may include plasma cells, eosinophils, and neutrophils. Hepatocyte damage occurs in the form of ballooning degeneration as well as acidophilic bodies (also known as Councilman bodies); the latter are the result of apoptosis (Fig. 1). In uncomplicated acute viral hepatitis, the reticulin framework is typically preserved. Large hepatocytes with a ground-glass cytoplasmic appearance may be seen in chronic HBV infection; these cells contain HBsAg and can be identified by immunohistochemical staining for HBsAg.

In HCV infection, prominent eosinophilic degeneration may be seen, and the degree of inflammatory lymphocytic infiltration is relatively sparse relative to the degree of liver cell necrosis (49). HCV infection is also remarkable for a marked increase in activation of sinusoidal lining cells, the presence of steatosis, and, occasionally, bile duct lesions in which biliary epithelial cells appear to be piled up without interruption of the basement membrane. Lymphoid aggregates are also a recognized histologic feature of HCV infection.

In HEV infection, cholestasis is a common histologic feature, characterized by bile stasis in canaliculi and gland-like transformation of parenchymal cells. The remaining hepatocytes may be swollen, with a foamy appearance. Portal vein and central vein branches may show signs of phlebitis, with edema and an inflammatory infiltrate.

A more severe histologic lesion, bridging hepatic necrosis (Fig. 2), is occasionally observed in some patients with acute hepatitis. This is characterized by loss of all the liver cells in multiple acini, producing the appearance of massive or submassive hepatic necrosis. Bridging necrosis between lobules results from large areas of hepatic cell dropout, with collapse of the reticulin framework. The bridge consists of condensed reticulin, inflammatory debris, and degenerating liver cells that span adjacent portal areas, portal to central veins, or central vein to central vein. Bridging necrosis occurs in approximately 1 to 5% of cases in uncomplicated acute viral hepatitis and is not a poor prognostic finding.

As mentioned previously, the most severe form of viral hepatitis is fulminant hepatitis. Small, shrunken livers of patients with fulminant hepatitis demonstrate massive necrosis and dropout of liver cells in most, if not all, lobules, with extensive collapse and condensation of the reticulin framework.

In chronic viral hepatitis, a spectrum of histologic activity occurs, and the histologic "grade" of necroinflammatory activity can be categorized from minimal to severe. Minimal inflammation confined to portal tracts represents the mildest histologic form of chronic viral hepatitis. When the inflammatory infiltrate spills out beyond the confines of the portal tract and disrupts the integrity of the limiting plate of periportal hepatocytes (so-called "piecemeal necrosis" or "interface hepatitis"), the chronic hepatitis is categorized as mild to moderate, and an even more advanced degree of severity (that may fall into a moderate or a severe grade) is characterized by necrosis that spans or bridges portal tracts or portal to central areas of the lobule ("bridging necrosis"), as defined above for acute hepatitis (Fig. 2). In the most severe form of chronic hepatitis, multilobular collapse, the necroinflammatory process is very extensive.

In addition to the severity of inflammation, chronic hepatitis is also categorized by relative "stage," defined by the presence and extent of fibrosis. When fibrosis is sufficiently severe to alter the normal architecture of the liver

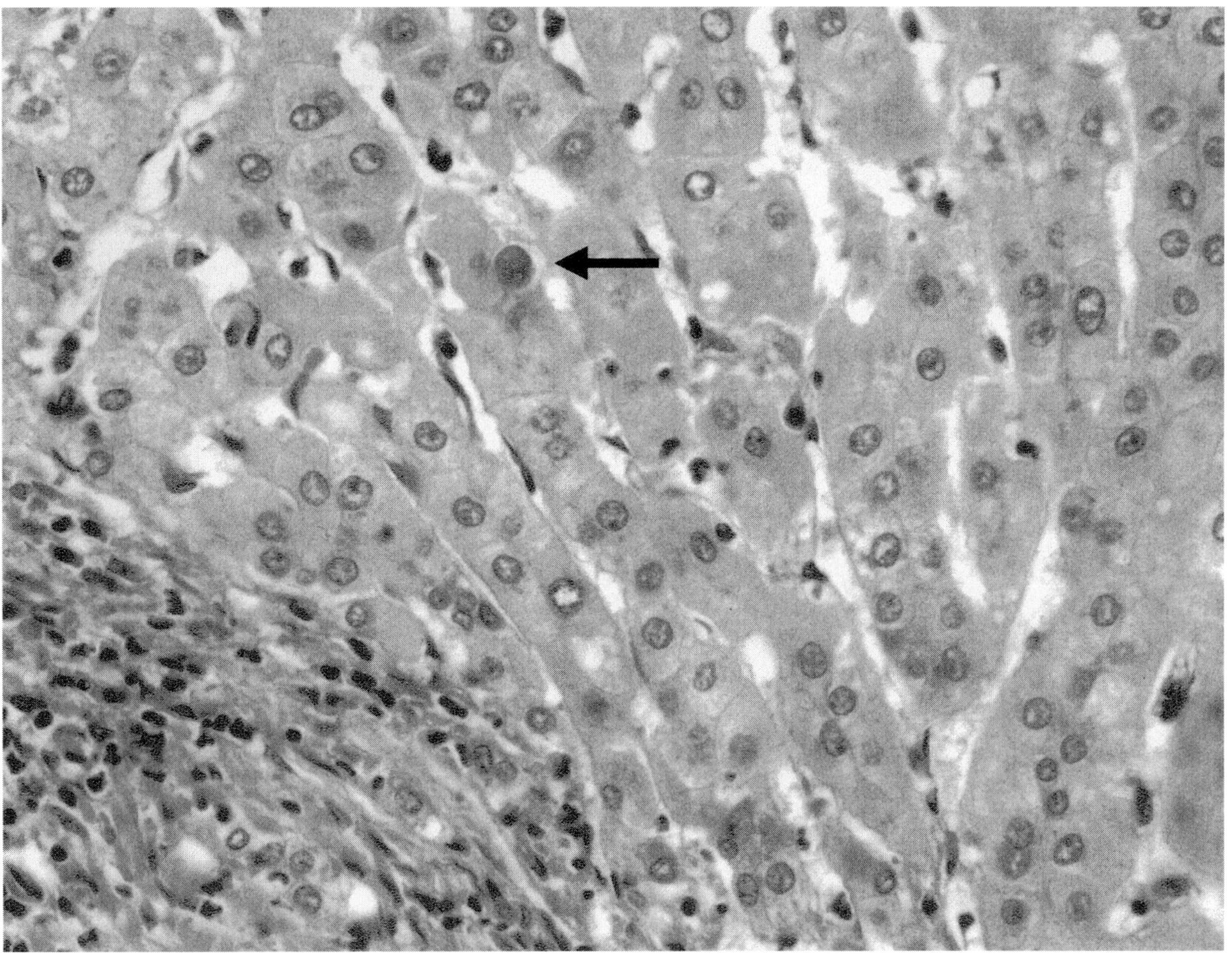

FIGURE 1 Round, eosinophilic Councilman bodies (arrow) signifying apoptosis of hepatocytes. (Courtesy of G. Y. Lauwers.)

and the relationship of architectural landmarks with each other, the process is defined as cirrhosis (Fig. 3). Characterization of histologic stage and grade has supplanted the abandoned terminology of "chronic persistent hepatitis," "chronic lobular hepatitis," and "chronic active hepatitis." Semiquantitative systems to grade the degree of inflammation and stage the extent of fibrosis have been developed to allow comparison of specimens from different patients and comparison of specimens from the same patient over time (54, 60).

Fibrosing cholestatic hepatitis is a pathological variation that deserves special mention. This entity was described originally in 1991 for HBV-infected recipients of liver allografts (33). Since its original description, fibrosing cholestatic hepatitis has also been seen in HBV-infected and HCV-infected recipients of heart, kidney, and liver allografts. Pathological features include marked periportal fibrosis and cholestasis with ballooning degeneration of hepatocytes out of proportion to the degree of inflammatory infiltrate. Rapid progression to clinically decompensated cirrhosis occurs without treatment. The imbalance between hepatocyte injury and inflammatory infiltrate, the clinical association with an immunosuppressed population, and the high levels of viremia typically found in these patients have led to speculation that this process may represent a viral cytopathic effect.

Immunohistochemical studies of HBV-infected livers have demonstrated HBsAg in the cytoplasm and on the plasma membrane of infected liver cells. In contrast, HBcAg predominates in the nucleus, but scant amounts are also seen in the cytoplasm and on the cell membrane. Electron microscopic studies of liver biopsy material have demonstrated the presence of HBsAg particles in the cytoplasm and HBcAg particles in the nucleus of liver cells during HBV infection. These morphological observations suggest that DNA is synthesized and packaged within core particles in the nucleus, while the surface coat is assembled in the cytoplasm, resulting in the formation of intact hepatitis B virions. Delta virus antigen, like HBcAg, is localized to the hepatocyte nucleus, while HAV, HCV, and HEV antigens are localized to the cytoplasm.

Diagnostic Considerations

Acute viral hepatitis is suspected most often by the clinician in a patient presenting with new elevations in serum aminotransferase levels and/or other liver biochemical tests in the setting of typical constitutional symptoms, with or without icterus. In such settings, however, the clinician

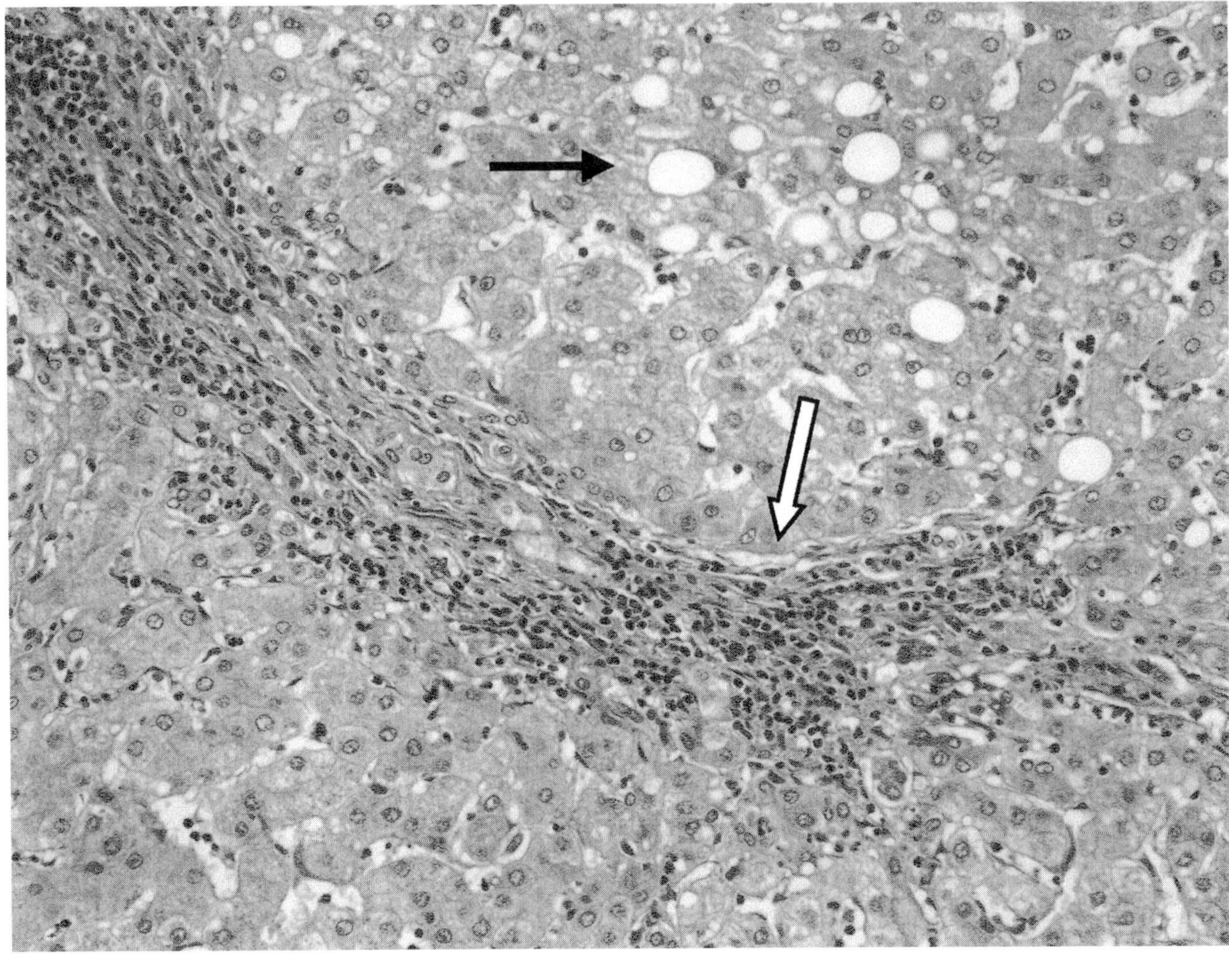

FIGURE 2 Bridging necrosis (also known as interface hepatitis or piecemeal necrosis). An inflammatory infiltrate is visible within the portal tracts, spilling out into the hepatic lobule and resulting in piecemeal necrosis or interface hepatitis (white arrow). The hepatic lobule contains fat (black arrow) within hepatocytes, a common finding in viral hepatitis. (Courtesy of G. Y. Lauwers.)

should be careful to consider noninfectious causes in the differential diagnosis of suspected acute viral hepatitis.

Drug- or toxin-induced hepatitis may cause a clinical picture indistinguishable from that of viral hepatitis. A careful medication and alcohol history should be obtained in all cases, and the clinician should ask explicitly about herbal medications, vitamins, and other nutritional supplements, which often will not be volunteered by the patient. Marked aminotransferase elevation (over 1,000 IU/ml) can be seen in acute viral hepatitis and toxin- or drug-induced hepatitis but also in hepatic ischemia (typically resulting from systemic hypotension) and in autoimmune hepatitis. Acute biliary obstruction or acute cholecystitis may present occasionally with aminotransferase elevation but is typically accompanied by epigastric or right upper quadrant pain; ultrasonography is helpful if either of these is suspected. Other possible causes to be considered include passive congestion of the liver resulting from elevated right-sided venous pressures or Budd-Chiari syndrome, a variety of genetic or metabolic liver disorders (e.g., Wilson's disease, alpha-1 antitrypsin deficiency, and acute fatty liver of pregnancy), and, very rarely, multiple liver metastases.

Acute viral hepatitis may also result from infections other than HAV to HEV. Several of the herpesviruses can cause an acute hepatitis in certain circumstances. HSV can cause a severe or even fulminant hepatitis in primary infection of neonates or pregnant women. Primary infection with or reactivation of HSV can also cause severe hepatitis in immunocompromised persons and occasionally in immunocompetent individuals. The presence of associated oral, genital, or skin lesions should be carefully sought out if this diagnosis is suspected, but only about half of patients with HSV hepatitis will have mucocutaneous lesions. Classic features of HSV hepatitis include very high aminotransferase levels and fever with normal or only slightly elevated serum bilirubin levels. Infectious mononucleosis, caused by Epstein-Barr virus, may present with hepatitis in addition to a myriad of other symptoms, including sore throat, fever, lymphadenopathy, and constitutional symptoms. In some cases, hepatitis may be both severe and the predominant clinical feature. Cytomegalovirus can cause acute hepatitis in all age groups and in both immunocompetent and immunocompromised hosts. Varicella-zoster virus infection commonly causes mild or subclinical hepatitis in primary

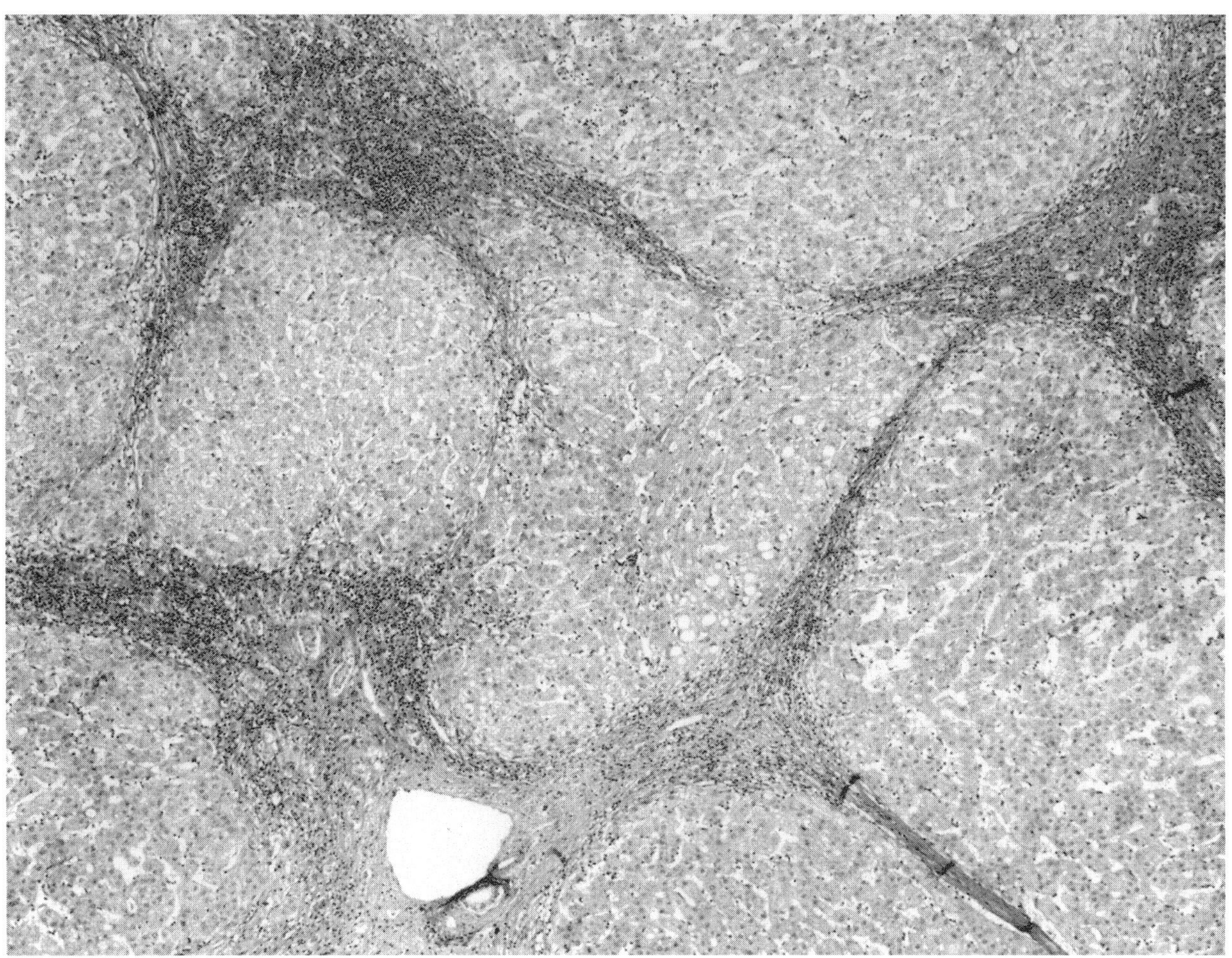

FIGURE 3 Cirrhosis resulting from chronic hepatitis C. The portal tracts contain numerous chronic inflammatory cells, which occasionally disrupt the limiting plate and spill out into the hepatocyte lobules (interface hepatitis). The lobules are separated from one another by fibrous septa to create nodules. (Courtesy of G. Y. Lauwers.)

childhood infection but may cause severe or fulminant hepatitis in immunocompromised persons with disseminated varicella-zoster virus infection. There are case reports of human herpesvirus 6-associated ALF in immunocompetent individuals (19).

Rubella (German measles) has been associated with hepatitis in both congenital and acquired disease. The hemorrhagic fever viruses (Rift Valley Fever, Congo-Crimean hemorrhagic fever, Lassa, Marburg, and Ebola viruses) can all cause hepatitis during the course of their severe, generalized infection. Yellow fever, caused by a group B arbovirus, causes hepatitis in severe disease. Adenoviruses and several enteroviruses, including coxsackievirus group B and echoviruses, have been associated with hepatitis. Parasitic infestations such as toxoplasmosis can, in rare instances, cause hepatitis in neonates and immunocompromised adults.

When confronted with a patient with suspected acute viral hepatitis, a clinician should be able to establish the absence or presence of HAV, HBV, and HCV infection by testing for four serologic markers (Fig. 4): IgM anti-HAV, HBsAg, IgM anti-HBc, and anti-HCV. The presence of HBsAg, with or without IgM anti-HBc, indicates HBV infection. If IgM anti-HBc is also identified, then most likely the patient has acute or recent HBV infection. Less commonly, IgM anti-HBc may be detected during reactivation of chronic HBV infection. If the patient is HBsAg$^+$ IgM anti-HBc$^-$, the HBV infection was acquired in the remote past and is now chronic. A diagnosis of acute HBV infection can be made as well in the presence of IgM anti-HBc alone, as the patient may be in the window period of acute HBV infection during which HBs antigenemia has resolved but anti-HBs have not yet appeared (the window period is rarely, if ever, seen currently due to increasing sensitivity of HBsAg and anti-HBs assays). A negative test for IgM anti-HBc for a patient with detectable serum HBsAg and a clinical picture consistent with acute hepatitis should raise several possibilities. These include superinfection with another virus (e.g., HDV, HAV, or HCV) as well as the flare in aminotransferase activity seen when a patient with highly replicative HBeAg-positive chronic HBV infection spontaneously seroconverts to anti-HBe reactivity and clears HBeAg. Other possibilities include reactivation of chronic hepatitis B (but in some cases IgM anti-HBc becomes detectable during reactivation) or a nonviral

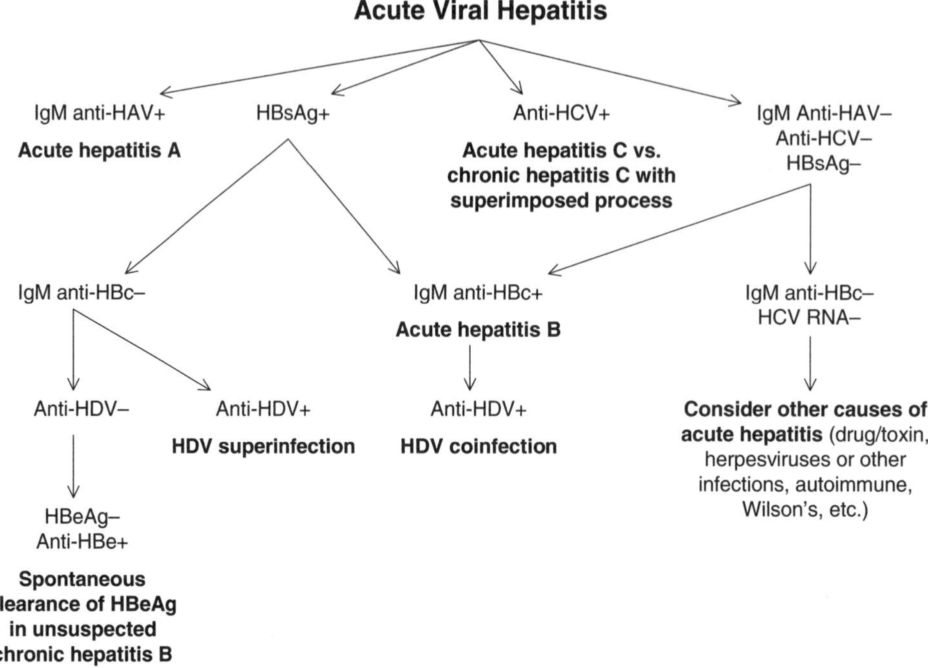

FIGURE 4 Diagnostic approach to a patient with acute viral hepatitis.

cause of liver injury, such as drug-induced hepatitis superimposed upon chronic hepatitis B.

A diagnosis of acute HAV infection relies on the identification of IgM anti-HAV. If IgM anti-HAV coexists with HBsAg, a diagnosis of acute HAV in the setting of either acute or chronic HBV infection can be made. If IgM anti-HBc coexists with IgM anti-HAV, a diagnosis of simultaneous acute HAV and acute HBV infection can be made, and if IgM anti-HBc is undetectable, the patient likely has acute HAV infection superimposed upon chronic HBV infection.

The presence of anti-HCV in a patient with acute hepatitis suggests a diagnosis of acute HCV infection, particularly if the patient is known to have been seronegative in the past; however, the relative infrequency of symptomatic acute HCV infection should alert the clinician to the possibility that the acute hepatitis is in fact caused by another viral agent or a nonviral process superimposed upon chronic HCV infection. Testing for HCV RNA may be considered if the clinical picture is consistent with acute viral hepatitis but all of the above serologic markers are negative.

Serologic testing for anti-HDV is reserved for patients with acute HBV infection who have risk factors for hepatitis D (injection drug use, frequent exposure to blood and blood products, or origin from an area where HDV is endemic) or who have very severe acute hepatitis. When all four serologic markers are absent, a diagnosis of acute HEV infection should be entertained if the epidemiological setting is appropriate. Alternatively, a nonviral process or another infection (as discussed above) may be responsible. Immunoassays for anti-HEV are available through reference laboratories.

For patients with chronic hepatitis, a virologic diagnosis can be achieved by testing for HBsAg, anti-HBc, anti-HCV, and, when appropriate, anti-HDV (Fig. 5). The presence of HBsAg and IgG anti-HBc establishes a diagnosis of chronic HBV infection. If a serologic diagnosis of chronic HBV infection is made, HBeAg, anti-HBe, and HBV DNA should then be tested as markers of viral replication and to subcategorize further the type of chronic HBV infection, as discussed above.

The presence of anti-HCV suggests chronic HCV infection; in this case, HCV RNA testing should then be performed, because up to 15% of patients have spontaneously cleared HCV infection and are persistently HCV RNA negative. HCV RNA testing may also be useful if chronic viral hepatitis is suspected but other serologic markers (including anti-HCV) are negative, particularly in immunocompromised individuals or those on chronic hemodialysis.

The presence of anti-HDV in a patient with HBsAg and IgG anti-HBc establishes a diagnosis of chronic HDV and HBV infection. Testing for anti-HDV in the setting of chronic HBV infection is indicated for patients with very severe chronic hepatitis, when a dramatic flare in biochemical activity occurs, and when epidemiological risk factors support a potential diagnosis of concurrent HDV infection.

Special Clinical Situations

Transmission in Health Care Workers

Health care workers exposed to blood and body fluids are at risk for infection with all three blood-borne hepatitis viruses. Transmission of infection is most commonly the result of accidental needlestick injuries with instruments contaminated by infected blood, although infections resulting from other types of exposure, such as blood exposures to abraded skin or mucosa, have been documented as well.

The risk of seroconversion following percutaneous exposure to HBV-infected blood averages 26%, and such seroconversion is most likely to occur when the source is

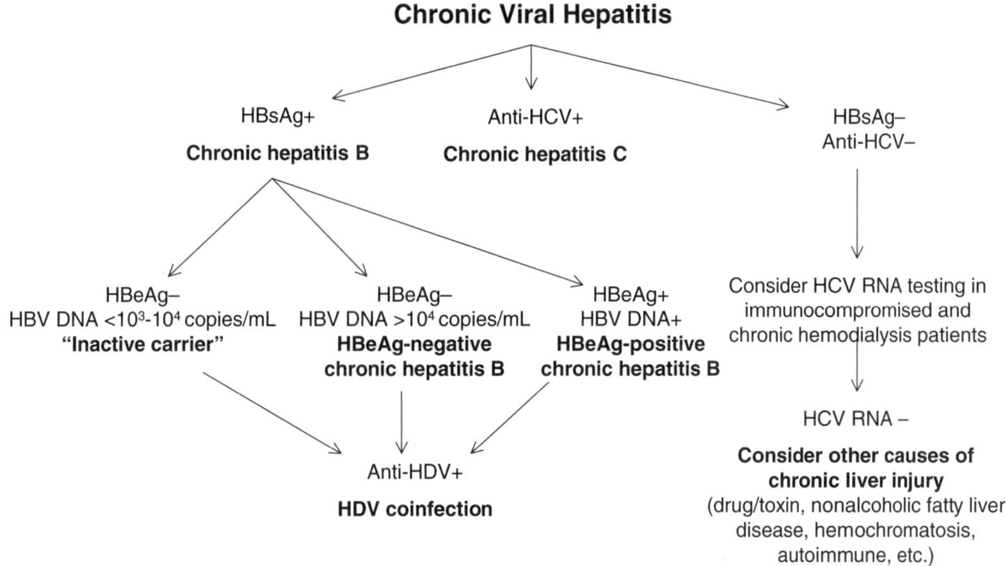

FIGURE 5 Diagnostic approach to a patient with chronic viral hepatitis.

HBeAg positive (3); the risk of HBV infection after an HBeAg-negative needlestick exposure is as low as 0.1%. A fundamental strategy to prevent workplace transmission of hepatitis B has been the vaccination of all nonimmune health care workers. In the United States, federal rules mandate that employers make available and pay for vaccination of all health care workers at risk. Vaccination, which is given as a series of three intramuscular injections at 0, 1, and 6 months, elicits neutralizing antibodies in >95% of vaccinees. Postexposure prophylaxis (PEP) is necessitated only after exposure to the blood or body fluids of HBsAg-positive persons. Exposed health care workers who have been previously immunized should have their antibody titers measured, and if they are adequate, no further intervention is required. Health care workers with suboptimal antibody titers, vaccine nonresponders, and the unvaccinated should all receive hepatitis B immunoglobulin (HBIG) after an HBsAg-positive needlestick. HBIG is prepared from pooled plasma containing a high titer of anti-HBs and is highly effective in preventing infection if given within 72 h of an exposure (99). Vaccine recipients with suboptimal antibody titers should also receive a booster vaccination; nonresponders and the unvaccinated should receive a complete course of vaccination. HBIG and hepatitis B vaccine can be given simultaneously provided they are injected at separate sites. All exposed health care workers should have HBsAg and anti-HBs assayed upon exposure and then at 1 to 2 months following exposure. Because of the unique dependence of hepatitis D on hepatitis B for infection, the above strategy for PEP of hepatitis B applies as well to the prevention of HDV transmission.

The risk of seroconversion following exposure to a needlestick from an HCV-infected person averages 2 to 3%, with a range of 0 to 7% (52). Baseline testing for anti-HCV and serum aminotransferase levels should be performed for all exposed individuals and at 3 to 6 months after exposure. Neither the immediate administration of interferon nor hyperimmunoglobulin has an established role in PEP for hepatitis C, and the delayed introduction of antiviral therapy until after confirmation of infection does not seem to alter its effectiveness (113); antiviral therapy introduced a mean of ~90 days after exposure, once HCV infection is established, prevents progression to chronicity in >95% of cases.

Strict adherence to universal precautions is the cornerstone of all strategies designed to eliminate occupational exposures. All exposures in health care workers should be promptly reported to local occupational health authorities to facilitate implementation of the most current recommendations for PEP.

Viral Hepatitis in Pregnancy

Abnormalities in liver biochemistry tests are not uncommonly encountered in pregnancy. Acute hepatitis or elevations in liver biochemistry tests in pregnancy can be caused by any of the viral hepatitides described above, by nonviral disorders such as gallstone disease, and by conditions unique to pregnancy. Although beyond the scope of this chapter, acute fatty liver of pregnancy and HELLP syndrome (hemolysis, elevated liver function tests, and low platelets) occur late in pregnancy and are associated with a high rate of maternal and fetal morbidity and mortality unless promptly recognized and treated. Both of these entities should be considered in any patient in her third trimester of pregnancy with a significant elevation in liver biochemistry tests. HELLP syndrome can develop in the second trimester or even in the first week postpartum.

Acute HAV infection in pregnancy is associated with an increased risk of preterm labor but no apparent increase in fetal or maternal mortality (39). The clinical course of HAV infection in the mother does not appear to be altered by pregnancy. HAV is not teratogenic, and the risk of fetal transmission in utero is thought to be negligible.

In contrast to the relatively benign course of HAV infection in pregnancy, the severity of acute HEV infection is greatly increased in pregnancy. In areas where HEV is endemic, HEV accounts for about 60% of clinically apparent cases of jaundice and acute viral hepatitis in pregnancy (86). Fulminant hepatic failure develops in a substantial fraction (22 to 55%) of women with acute HEV infection; the maternal case fatality rate may be as high as 40%, and the risk in HEV-infected mothers of preterm labor and fetal mortality is increased substantially. As determined by testing of cord blood for HEV RNA, the risk of perinatal transmission of HEV infection has been recorded to be as high as 33% (66). The reason for the greatly increased severity of HEV infection in pregnancy is not understood.

The course of acute or chronic maternal HBV infection does not appear to be altered by pregnancy or to increase the risk of fetal complications; however, the risk of perinatal HBV transmission approaches 90% in mothers who are HBeAg positive, and chronic HBV infection will develop in 85 to 90% of those infected. Fortunately, administration of HBIG and hepatitis B vaccine to neonates born to HBV-infected mothers is 85 to 95% effective at preventing chronic HBV infection (8). Because of this highly effective intervention, the U.S. Public Health Service recommends that all pregnant women be screened routinely for HBsAg early in pregnancy and that the infants of all HBsAg-positive mothers be treated with HBIG and hepatitis B vaccine at birth.

As observed in a small nonrandomized study, lamivudine given in the last month of pregnancy to highly viremic mothers (HBV DNA $\geq 1.2 \times 10^9$ copies/ml), when combined with neonatal HBIG and vaccination, appeared to reduce the risk of perinatal transmission compared to that in historical controls given HBIG and vaccine alone (115); however, the efficacy of lamivudine treatment during pregnancy in reducing the frequency of HBV infection in newborns has not been tested in a randomized controlled trial.

The effect of pregnancy on chronic hepatitis C is minimal; liver biochemical tests tend to improve during the third trimester and then revert to prepregnancy levels following delivery (29). In contrast to the high efficiency of perinatal transmission of HBV, perinatal transmission of HCV is relatively infrequent. Prospective studies of perinatal transmission of HCV have yielded an average rate of 5% in women with HCV alone and up to 15% in mothers coinfected with HIV and HCV (111). The risk of perinatal HCV transmission is increased in highly viremic mothers. Unfortunately, no effective interventions to reduce the risk of perinatal HCV transmission are available. Alpha interferon and, especially, ribavirin are teratogenic (U.S. Food and Drug Administration class X) and should not be given in pregnancy.

Cesarean section delivery has not been found to reduce the frequency of perinatal transmission of hepatitis B or hepatitis C. In a Cochrane review published in 2006, the evidence for and against the value of elective cesarean section over vaginal delivery in reducing the risk of HCV transmission was compiled, but the conclusion reached was that insufficient data existed to justify cesarean section delivery in this setting (78).

Viral Hepatitis in HIV Infection

Chronic viral hepatitis is becoming an increasingly important clinical problem in HIV-infected people. As mortality from traditional AIDS-related complications declines in areas where HAART is available, the morbidity and mortality resulting from chronic viral hepatitis are increasing (73). Approximately 10% of HIV-infected patients have chronic HBV coinfection. In the Western world, about 25% of HIV-infected patients are coinfected with HCV, and this rate may be as high as 90% in HIV-infected injection drug users. Therefore, all HIV-infected patients should be screened for HBV and HCV. Up to 6% of HIV-HCV-coinfected patients fail to produce detectable anti-HCV; if clinical suspicion of HCV coinfection is sufficiently high, HCV RNA testing should be done. All HIV-infected patients who are not immune to HBV and/or HAV should be vaccinated.

HIV is highly detrimental to the course of HCV infection; HIV accelerates the progression of liver fibrosis, increases the risk of cirrhosis and end-stage liver disease, and shortens the survival of patients with decompensated HCV-associated cirrhosis (10, 87). Therefore, all HIV-HCV-coinfected patients should be evaluated as candidates for HCV antiviral therapy. Unfortunately, the rates of response to treatment with pegylated interferon and ribavirin for hepatitis C are significantly lower in patients with HIV-HCV coinfection, particularly in those with HCV genotype 1 infection (24, 112).

Whether HCV infection alters the clinical course of HIV infection is controversial. Although HCV infection does not appear to accelerate the progression of HIV infection to AIDS, in some studies (but not others), HCV infection has been shown to lower the degree of immune reconstitution (as measured by CD4 cell count) after the initiation of HAART (79).

Less is known about the effect of HIV on chronic HBV infection. HIV infection appears to alter the natural course of HBV infection, although the effect of HIV infection on hepatitis B is not as profound as that of HIV infection on hepatitis C. HIV-infected patients have an increased risk of progression to chronic HBV infection following acute infection, and the rates of spontaneous HBeAg clearance and seroconversion are lower (46, 88). Chronic HBV infection does not alter the course of HIV infection. The decision to treat hepatitis B in patients with HIV-HBV coinfection should be based on whether HIV treatment is ongoing or planned. Nucleoside/nucleotide analogs with activity against both HBV and HIV (lamivudine, emtricitabine, tenofovir, and, on a more limited basis, entecavir) should never be used as monotherapy to treat hepatitis B in HIV-HBV-coinfected patients who are not receiving HAART; in this setting, the risk of selecting for resistant HIV quasispecies is prohibitively high. Conversely, HAART regimens in HIV-HBV-coinfected patients should include an agent that is active against HBV.

The risk of serious HAART-related hepatotoxicity, which is increased in patients with HIV-HBV or HIV-HCV coinfection, can be difficult to distinguish from a flare of viral hepatitis resulting from HAART-related immune reconstitution. This clinical dilemma is rendered even more challenging by other potentially confounding causes of liver injury in patients with HIV/AIDS, e.g., fatty liver infiltration, mycobacterial or fungal infection, infiltrative malignancy, etc.

Viral Hepatitis in Solid-Organ Transplantation

Antiviral therapy of chronic hepatitis B and C, both in immunocompetent and in immunosuppressed patients, is addressed in the chapters elsewhere in this volume on these agents. Therefore, the reader should refer to these respective agent-specific chapters for a discussion of the management of HBV and HCV infection prior to and following liver transplantation.

Viral hepatitis can be a complicating issue in patients with chronic renal failure, many of whom become candidates for renal transplantation. Although the prevalence of chronic HBV and HCV infection in hemodialysis patients declined following the adoption of stringent measures in dialysis centers to prevent transmission of blood-borne agents, a substantial number of patients being evaluated for renal transplantation have chronic HBV (3 to 15%) and/or HCV infection (10 to 45%).

Mortality may be higher following renal transplantation in patients with chronic HBV infection than in patients without HBV infection (40). In addition, clinically severe HBV reactivation and fibrosing cholestatic hepatitis have both been reported following renal transplantation. The literature contains conflicting reports about the effect of chronic HBV infection on the rate of renal allograft failure, and the optimal strategy for managing chronic hepatitis B prior to, during, and after renal transplantation has not been defined. In some transplantation centers, "prophylactic" therapy is given pretransplantation to patients with HBsAg positivity regardless of HBV DNA level, while, in other centers, "preemptive" antiviral therapy is initiated for rising serial HBV DNA levels, even if liver biochemistry tests remain normal. Although randomized controlled trials to compare these two approaches have not been done, the results of small studies suggest that either the prophylactic or preemptive approach is superior to a "reactive" approach in which antiviral therapy is not started until clinically evident HBV-related liver injury has occurred. Viral resistance to nucleoside analogs is likely to become an increasing problem in patients receiving long-term antiviral therapy posttransplantation; therefore, strategies to limit such resistance, e.g., limiting the duration of pretransplantation therapy, delaying the onset of posttransplantation therapy, or relying on combination-drug therapy, should be considered for patients with chronic HBV undergoing solid-organ transplantation.

Chronic hepatitis C infection may increase the risk of mortality and allograft failure in renal allograft recipients. Unfortunately, treatment of hepatitis C in this population is challenging. Because interferon has been associated with an increased risk of acute allograft rejection, interferon is avoided, generally, following renal transplantation (76) but may be considered in patients with substantial liver injury associated with chronic HCV infection or in patients with HCV-related glomerulonephropathy. Therefore, in light of the difficulty in treating hepatitis C after renal transplantation, patients with renal failure and hepatitis C should be considered as candidates for antiviral therapy prior to renal transplantation. Ribavirin, however, is cleared renally and should be avoided in patients with end-stage renal disease because of the high risk of severe, ribavirin-related hemolytic anemia. The use of low-dose ribavirin combined with pegylated interferon has been studied in small populations of hemodialyzed patients with chronic hepatitis C (91), but larger studies need to be performed before this approach can be recommended routinely. Prior to renal transplantation, if antiviral therapy for hepatitis C is required, patients are more likely to be treated with pegylated interferon monotherapy, which, however, is associated with a lower sustained virologic response rate.

Limited data exist to inform approaches to transplantation of solid organs other than the liver and kidney in patients with chronic hepatitis B or C, and in many transplantation centers, patients with chronic viral hepatitis are excluded as candidates for heart or lung transplantation.

Hepatitis in Patients Undergoing Myeloablative Chemotherapy

Myeloablative chemotherapy can lead to HBV reactivation in patients with chronic HBV infection, usually as chemotherapy is withdrawn and treatment-blunted cytolytic immune activity is restored. Such episodes of reactivation can range from mild, asymptomatic increases in serum aminotransferase levels to fulminant hepatic failure or fibrosing cholestatic hepatitis. In one study of patients undergoing cytotoxic chemotherapy, 26% of HBsAg-positive patients experienced HBV reactivation (122). The risk increases with more myelosuppressive regimens, such as those used for hematopoietic stem cell transplantation or for hematologic malignancies. Rituximab, a monoclonal antibody targeting CD20 on B cells, has also been associated with severe HBV reactivation. The risk of HBV reactivation is also higher in those with high baseline HBV DNA levels; on the other hand, HBV reactivation can occur in those with low or undetectable HBV DNA, and rare cases of HBV reactivation have been described even for patients with serologic markers at baseline consistent with recovery from HBV infection, i.e., HbsAg negative and anti-HBs positive.

Prophylactic antiviral therapy (as opposed to reactive antiviral therapy after HBV reactivation has begun) with lamivudine has been shown consistently to minimize the risk of, and prevent the serious consequences of, HBV reactivation in high-risk patients undergoing cytotoxic chemotherapy (reviewed in reference 61). Therefore, all patients who are being considered for cytotoxic chemotherapy, particularly those with hematologic malignancies, should be screened for HBV infection by testing for HBsAg, anti-HBs, and anti-HBc. All HBsAg-positive patients should start prophylactic antiviral therapy (most of the published experience in the literature involved lamivudine therapy, but the more potent, less resistance-prone newer agents [see chapter 31] may be preferable) at least 1 week prior to the initiation of chemotherapy; although the optimal duration of such antiviral therapy is not known, and although some patients cannot be weaned from antiviral therapy, most authorities would recommend continuing antiviral therapy for at least 12 months after completion of chemotherapy; serial monitoring for HBV DNA and aminotransferase levels should be done during antiviral therapy.

The management of patients with isolated anti-HBc (HBsAg and anti-HBs negative) is not well defined; however, the risk of HBV reactivation is also increased in this population. One approach is to test for HBV DNA and to start antiviral prophylaxis in those with detectable HBV DNA. Those with undetectable HBV DNA as well as patients who are HbsAg negative, anti-HBc positive, and anti-HBs positive are at low risk for reactivation but should be monitored with serial HBV DNA measurements during and after chemotherapy. Because, in these patients, a rise in HBV DNA usually precedes clinically overt HBV reactivation by weeks to months, HBV DNA monitoring should provide sufficient warning to implement timely initiation of preemptive antiviral therapy.

Typically, patients with chronic HCV infection tolerate myeloablative chemotherapy well from the standpoint of their HCV. Although HCV RNA and ALT may rise during or after a course of myeloablative chemotherapy, significant hepatic dysfunction as a result of an HCV flare is extremely uncommon (123). Therefore, prophylactic antiviral therapy and HCV RNA monitoring are not indicated in patients with hepatitis C who are undergoing chemotherapy.

Other potential causes of liver inflammation and/or dysfunction should always be considered in patients in whom abnormalities in liver biochemistry tests develop during the course of cytotoxic chemotherapy and/or stem cell transplantation. As already described above, other infections such as cytomegalovirus and other herpesviruses may cause serious hepatitis in immunocompromised patients. A cholestatic pattern of liver biochemistry tests may suggest other infections such as hepatosplenic candidiasis or disseminated mycobacterial infection, or noninfectious processes such as cholestasis associated with total parenteral nutrition. In addition, chemotherapeutic agents and other drugs may themselves cause hepatotoxicity. Finally, venoocclusive disease and graft-versus-host disease are two important and frequently encountered causes of liver dysfunction in patients undergoing stem cell transplantation.

REFERENCES

1. **Aach, R. D., C. E. Stevens, F. B. Hollinger, J. W. Mosley, D. A. Peterson, P. E. Taylor, R. G. Johnson, L. H. Barbosa, and G. J. Nemo.** 1991. Hepatitis C virus infection in post-transfusion hepatitis. An analysis with first- and second-generation assays. *N. Engl. J. Med.* **325:** 1325–1329.
2. **Alter, H. J., P. V. Holland, A. G. Morrow, R. H. Purcell, S. M. Feinstone, and Y. Moritsugu.** 1975. Clinical and serological analysis of transfusion-associated hepatitis. *Lancet* **ii:**838–841.
3. **Alter, H. J., L. B. Seef, P. M. Kaplan, V. J. McAuliffe, E. C. Wright, J. L. Gerin, R. H. Purcell, P. V. Holland, and H. J. Zimmerman.** 1976. Type B hepatitis: the infectivity of blood positive for e antigen and DNA polymerase after accidental needlestick exposure. *N. Engl. J. Med.* **295:**909–913.
4. **Balayan, M. S., A. G. Andjaparidze, S. S. Savinskaya, E. S. Ketiladze, D. M. Braginsky, A. P. Savinov, and V. F. Poleschuk.** 1983. Evidence for a virus in non-A, non-B hepatitis transmitted via the fecal-oral route. *Intervirology* **20:**23–31.
5. **Baroudy, B. M., J. R. Ticehurst, T. A. Miele, J. V. Maizel, Jr., R. H. Purcell, and S. M. Feinstone.** 1985. Sequence analysis of hepatitis A virus cDNA coding for capsid proteins and RNA polymerase. *Proc. Natl. Acad. Sci. USA* **82:**2143–2147.
6. **Barrera, J. M., M. Bruguera, M. G. Ercilla, C. Gil, R. Celis, M. P. Gil, M. del Valle Onorato, J. Rodes, and A. Ordinas.** 1995. Persistent hepatitis C viremia after acute self-limiting posttransfusion hepatitis C. *Hepatology* **21:** 639–644.
7. **Barrera, J. M., B. Francis, G. Ercilla, M. Nelles, D. Achord, J. Darner, and S. R. Lee.** 1995. Improved detection of anti-HCV in post-transfusion hepatitis by a third-generation ELISA. *Vox Sang.* **68:**15–18.
8. **Beasley, R. P., L. Y. Hwang, G. C. Lee, C. C. Lan, C. H. Roan, F. Y. Huang, and C. L. Chen.** 1983. Prevention of perinatally transmitted hepatitis B virus infections with hepatitis B immune globulin and hepatitis B vaccine. *Lancet* **ii:**1099–1102.
9. **Beasley, R. P., L. Y. Hwang, C. C. Lin, and C. S. Chien.** 1981. Hepatocellular carcinoma and hepatitis B virus: a prospective study of 22707 men in Taiwan. *Lancet* **ii:** 1129–1132.
10. **Benhamou, Y., M. Bochet, V. Di Martino, F. Charlotte, F. Azria, A. Coutellier, M. Vidaud, F. Bricaire, P. Opolon, C. Katlama, and T. Poynard for the MULTIVIRC Group.** 1999. Liver fibrosis progression in human immunodeficiency virus and hepatitis C virus coinfected patients. *Hepatology* **30:**1054–1058.
11. **Bertoletti, A., C. Ferrari, F. Fiaccodori, A. Penna, R. Margolskee, H. Schlicht, P. Fowler, S. Guilhot, and F. V. Chisari.** 1991. HLA class 1-restricted cytotoxic T cells recognize endogenously synthesized hepatitis B virus nucleocapsid antigen. *Proc. Natl. Acad. Sci. USA* **88:**10445–10449.
12. **Bjoro, K., S. S. Froland, Z. Yun, H. H. Samdal, and T. Haaland.** 1994. Hepatitis C infection in patients with primary hypogammaglobulinemia after treatment with contaminated immune globulin. *N. Engl. J. Med.* **331:**1607–1611.
13. **Blackwell Publishing.** 1999. Global surveillance and control of hepatitis C. Report of a WHO Consultation organized in collaboration with the Viral Hepatitis Prevention Board, Antwerp, Belgium. *J. Viral Hepat.* **6:**35–47.
14. **Blumberg, B. S., H. J. Alter, and S. Visnich.** 1965. A "new" antigen in leukemia sera. *JAMA* **191:**541–546.
15. **Blumer, G.** 1923. Infectious jaundice in the United States. *JAMA* **81:**353–358.
16. **Bradley, D. W.** 1992. Hepatitis E: epidemiology, aetiology and molecular biology. *Rev. Med. Virol.* **2:**19–28.
17. **Brunetto, M. R., M. Stemler, and F. Schodel.** 1989. Identification of HBV variant which cannot produce precore derived HBeAg and may be responsible for severe hepatitis. *Ital. J. Gastroenterol.* **21:**151–154.
18. **Burrell, C. J., P. Mackay, P. J. Grennaway, P. H. Hofschneider, and K. Murray.** 1979. Expression in Escherichia coli of hepatitis B virus sequences cloned in plasmid pBR-322. *Nature* **279:**43–47.
19. **Cacheux, W., N. Carbonell, O. Rosmorduc, D. Wendum, F. Paye, R. Poupon, O. Chazouillères, and J. Gozlan.** 2005. HHV-6-related acute liver failure in two immunocompetent adults: favourable outcome after liver transplantation and/or ganciclovir therapy. *J. Intern. Med.* **258:**573–578.
20. **Chang, M. H., C. J. Chen, M. S. Lai, H. M. Hsu, T. C. Wu, M. S. Kong, D. C. Liang, W. Y. Shau, and D. S. Chen for the Taiwan Childhood Hepatoma Study Group.** 1997. Universal hepatitis B vaccination in Taiwan and the incidence of hepatocellular carcinoma in children. *N. Engl. J. Med.* **336:**1855–1859.
21. **Charnay, P., C. Pourcel, A. Louise, A. Fritsch, and P. Tiollais.** 1979. Cloning in Escherichia coli and physical structure of hepatitis B virion DNA. *Proc. Natl. Acad. Sci. USA* **76:**2222–2226.
22. **Chisari, F. W., K. Hopchin, T. Moriyama, C. Pasquinelli, H. A. Dunsford, S. Sells, and C. A. Pinkert.** 1989. Molecular pathogenesis of hepatocellular carcinoma in hepatitis B virus transgenic mice. *Cell* **59:**1145–1156.
23. **Choo, Q. L., G. Kuo, A. J. Weiner, L. R. Overby, D. W. Bradley, and M. Houghton.** 1989. Isolation of a cDNA clone derived from a blood borne non-A, non-B viral hepatitis genome. *Science* **244:**359–362.
24. **Chung, R. T., J. Andersen, P. Volberding, G. K. Robbins, T. Liu, K. E. Sherman, M. G. Peters, M. J. Koziel, A. K. Bhan, B. Alston, D. Colquhoun, T. Nevin, G. Harb, C. van der Horst, and AIDS Clinical Trials Group A5071 Study Team.** 2004. Peginterferon alfa-2a plus ribavirin versus interferon alfa-2a plus ribavirin for chronic hepatitis C in HIV-coinfected persons. *N. Engl. J. Med.* **351:**451–459.

25. **Clemens, R., A. Safary, A. Hepburn, C. Roche, W. J. Stanbury, and F. E. André.** 1995. Clinical experience with an inactivated hepatitis A vaccine. *J. Infect. Dis.* **171:**S44–S49.
26. **Clifford, B. D., D. Donahue, L. Smith, E. Cable, B. Luttig, M. Manns, and H. L. Bonkovsky.** 1995. High prevalence of serological markers of autoimmunity in patients with chronic hepatitis C. *Hepatology* **21:**613–619.
27. **Cohen, J. I., J. R. Ticehurst, R. H. Purcell, A. Buckler-White, and B. M. Baroudy.** 1987. Complete nucleotide sequence of wild-type hepatitis A virus: comparison with different strains of hepatitis A virus and other picornaviruses. *J. Virol.* **61:**50–59.
28. **Colin, J. F., D. Cazals-Hatem, M. A. Loriot, M. Martinot-Peignoux, B. N. Pham, A. Auperin, C. Degott, J. P. Benhamou, S. Erlinger, D. Valla, and P. Marcellin.** 1999. Influence of human immunodeficiency virus infection on chronic hepatitis B in homosexual men. *Hepatology* **29:**1306–1310.
29. **Conte, D., M. Fraquelli, D. Prati, A. Colucci, and E. Minola.** 2000. Prevalence and clinical course in chronic hepatitis C virus (HCV) infection and rate of HCV vertical transmission in a cohort of 15,250 pregnant women. *Hepatology* **31:**751–755.
30. **Czaja, A. J.** 1992. Chronic hepatitis C virus infection—a disease in waiting? *N. Engl. J. Med.* **327:**1949–1950.
31. **Dane, D. S., C. H. Cameron, and M. Briggs.** 1970. Virus-like particles in serum of patients with Australia antigen associated hepatitis. *Lancet* **ii:**695–698.
32. **Davern, T. J., L. P. James, J. A. Hinson, J. Polson, A. M. Larson, R. J. Fontana, E. Lalani, S. Munoz, A. O. Shakil, W. M. Lee, and Acute Liver Failure Study Group.** 2006. Measurement of serum acetaminophen-protein adducts in patients with acute liver failure. *Gastroenterology* **130:**687–694.
33. **Davies, S. E., B. C. Portmann, J. G. O'Grady, P. M. Aldis, K. Chaggar, G. J. Alexander, and R. Williams.** 1991. Hepatic histological findings after transplantation for chronic hepatitis B virus infection, including a unique pattern of fibrosing cholestatic hepatitis. *Hepatology* **13:**150–157.
34. **Dawson, G. J., K. H. Chau, C. M. Cabal, P. O. Yarbough, G. R. Reyes, and I. K. Mushahwar.** 1992. Solid-phase enzyme-linked immunosorbent assay for hepatitis E virus IgG and IgM antibodies utilizing recombinant antigens and synthetic peptides. *J. Virol. Methods* **38:**175–186.
35. **Deinhardt, F., A. W. Holmes, R. B. Capps, and H. Popper.** 1967. Studies on the transmission of viral hepatitis to marmoset monkeys. I. Transmission of disease, serial passage, and descriptions of liver lesions. *J. Exp. Med.* **125:**673–688.
36. **DiBisceglie, A. M., S. E. Order, J. L. Klein, J. G. Waggoner, M. H. Sjogren, G. Kuo, M. Houghton, Q. L. Choo, and J. H. Hoofnagle.** 1991. The role of chronic viral hepatitis in hepatocellular carcinoma in the United States. *Am. J. Gastroenterol.* **86:**335–338.
37. **Di Martino, V., P. Rufat, N. Boyer, P. Renard, F. Degos, M. Martinot-Peignoux, S. Matheron, V. Le Moing, F. Vachon, C. Degott, D. Valla, and P. Marcellin.** 2001. The influence of human immunodeficiency virus coinfection on chronic hepatitis C in injection drug users: a long-term retrospective cohort study. *Hepatology* **34:**1193–1199.
38. **Dusheiko, G. M.** 1994. Rolling review—the pathogenesis, diagnosis and management of viral hepatitis. *Aliment. Pharmacol. Ther.* **8:**229–253.
39. **Elinav, E., I. Z. Ben-Dov, Y. Shapira, N. Daudi, R. Adler, D. Shouval, and Z. Ackerman.** 2006. Acute hepatitis A infection in pregnancy is associated with high rates of gestational complications and preterm labor. *Gastroenterology* **130:**1129–1134.
40. **Fabrizi, F., P. Martin, V. Dixit, F. Kanwal, and G. Dulai.** 2005. HBsAg seropositive status and survival after renal transplantation: meta-analysis of observational studies. *Am. J. Transplant.* **5:**2913–2921.
41. **Fagan, E. A.** 1994. Acute liver failure of unknown pathogenesis: the hidden agenda. *Hepatology* **19:**1307–1312.
42. **Fattovich, G., G. Giustina, E. Christensen, M. Pantalena, I. Zagni, G. Realdi, S. W. Schalm, and The European Concerted Action on Viral Hepatitis (Eurohep).** 2000. Influence of hepatitis delta virus infection on morbidity and mortality in compensated cirrhosis type B. *Gut* **46:**420–426.
43. **Feinstone, S., A. Kapikian, R. Purcell, H. Alter, and P. Holland.** 1975. Transfusion-associated hepatitis not due to viral hepatitis type A or B. *N. Engl. J. Med.* **292:**767–770.
44. **Feinstone, S. M., A. Z. Kapikian, and R. H. Purcell.** 1973. Hepatitis A: detection by immune electron microscopy of a virus-like antigen associated with acute illness. *Science* **182:**1026–1028.
45. **Gerlach, J. T., H. M. Diepolder, R. Zachoval, N. H. Gruener, M. C. Jung, A. Ulsenheimer, W. W. Schraut, C. A. Schirren, M. Waechtler, M. Backmund, and G. R. Pape.** 2003. Acute hepatitis C: high rate of both spontaneous and treatment-induced viral clearance. *Gastroenterology* **125:**80–88.
46. **Gilson, R. J., A. E. Hawkins, M. R. Beecham, E. Ross, J. Waite, M. Briggs, T. McNally, G. E. Kelly, R. S. Tedder, and I. V. Weller.** 1997. Interactions between HIV and hepatitis B virus in homosexual men: effects on the natural history of infection. *AIDS* **11:**597–606.
47. **Gisbert, J. P., L. García-Buey, J. M. Pajares, and R. Moreno-Otero.** 2003. Prevalence of hepatitis C virus infection in B-cell non-Hodgkin's lymphoma: systematic review and meta-analysis. *Gastroenterology* **125:**1723–1732.
48. **Gocke, D. J.** 1978. Immune complex phenomena associated with hepatitis, p. 277–283. *In* G. N. Vyas, S. N. Cohen, and R. Schmid (ed.), *Viral Hepatitis: a Contemporary Assessment of Etiology, Epidemiology, Pathogenesis and Prevention*. The Franklin Institute Press, Philadelphia, PA.
49. **Goodman, Z. D., and K. G. Ishak.** 1995. Histopathology of hepatitis C virus infection. *Semin. Liver Dis.* **15:**70–81.
50. **Govindarajan, S., K. P. Chin, A. G. Redeker, and R. L. Peters.** 1984. Fulminant B viral hepatitis: role of delta agent. *Gastroenterology* **86:**1417–1420.
51. **Hadler, S. C., M. De Monzon, A. Ponzetto, E. Anzola, D. Rivero, A. Mondolfi, A. Bracho, D. P. Francis, M. A. Gerber, S. Thung, J. Gerin, J. E. Maynard, H. Popper, and R. H. Purcell.** 1984. Delta virus infection and severe hepatitis: an epidemic in Yupca Indians of Venezuela. *Ann. Intern. Med.* **100:**339–344.
52. **Hernandez, M. E., M. Bruguera, T. Puyuelo, J. M. Barrera, J. M. Sanchez Tapias, and J. Rodes.** 1992. Risk of needlestick injuries in the transmission of hepatitis C virus in hospital personnel. *J. Hepatol.* **16:**56–58.
53. **Holmes, A., L. Wolfe, H. Rosenblate, and F. Deinhardt.** 1969. Hepatitis in marmosets: induction of disease and coded specimens. *Science* **165:**816–817.
54. **Ishak, K., A. Baptista, L. Bianchi, F. Callea, J. De Groote, F. Gudat, H. Denk, V. Desmet, G. Korb, R. N. M. MacSween, M. J. Phillips, B. G. Portmann, H. Poulsen, P. J. Scheuer, M. Schmid, and H. Thaler.** 1995. Histological grading and staging of chronic hepatitis. *J. Hepatol.* **22:**696–699.

55. **Iwarson, S., G. Norkrans, and R. Wejstal.** 1995. Hepatitis C: natural history of a unique infection. *Clin. Infect. Dis.* **20:**1361–1370.
56. **Kao, J. H., and D. S. Chen.** 2002. Global control of hepatitis B virus infection. *Lancet Infect. Dis.* **2:**395–403.
57. **Kao, J. H., P. J. Chen, M. Y. Lai, and D. S. Chen.** 2000. Hepatitis B genotypes correlate with clinical outcomes in patients with chronic hepatitis B. *Gastroenterology* **118:** 554–559.
58. **Katelaris, P. H., and D. B. Jones.** 1989. Fulminant hepatic failure. *Med. Clin. N. Am.* **73:**955–970.
59. **Kempinska, A., E. J. Kwak, and J. B. Angel.** 2005. Reactivation of hepatitis B infection following allogeneic bone marrow transplantation in a hepatitis B-immune patient: case report and review of the literature. *Clin. Infect. Dis.* **41:**1277–1282.
60. **Knodell, K. G., K. G. Ishak, W. C. Black, T. S. Chen, N. Kaplowitz, T. W. Kiernan, and J. Wollman.** 1981. Formulation and application of a numerical scoring system for assessing histological activity in asymptomatic chronic active hepatitis. *Hepatology* **1:**432–435.
61. **Kohrt, H. E., D. L. Ouyang, and E. B. Keeffe.** 2006. Systematic review: lamivudine prophylaxis for chemotherapy-induced reactivation of chronic hepatitis B virus infection. *Aliment. Pharmacol. Ther.* **24:**1003–1016.
62. **Koziel, M. J., D. Dudley, N. Afdhal, Q. L. Choo, M. Houghton, R. Ralston, and B. D. Walker.** 1993. Hepatitis C virus (HCV)-specific cytotoxic T lymphocytes recognize epitopes in the core and envelope proteins of HCV. *J. Virol.* **67:**7522–7532.
63. **Krugman, S., J. Giles, and J. Hammond.** 1970. Hepatitis virus: effect of heat on the infectivity and antigenicity of the MS-a and MS-2 strains. *J. Infect. Dis.* **122:**432.
64. **Krugman, S., J. Giles, and J. Hammond.** 1971. Viral hepatitis type B (MS-2 strain): studies on active immunization. *JAMA* **217:**41.
65. **Krugman, S., J. P. Giles, and J. Hammond.** 1967. Infectious hepatitis: evidence for two distinctive clinical, epidemiological and immunological types of infection. *JAMA* **200:**365–373.
66. **Kumar, A., M. Beniwal, P. Kar, J. B. Sharma, and N. S. Murthy.** 2004. Hepatitis E in pregnancy. *Int. J. Gynecol. Obstet.* **85:**240–244.
67. **Leary, T. P., A. S. Muerhoff, J. N. Simons, T. J. Pilot-Matias, J. C. Erker, M. L. Chalmers, G. G. Schlauder, G. J. Dawson, S. M. Desai, and I. K. Mushahwar.** 1996. Sequence and genomic organization of GBV-C: a novel member of the flaviviridae associated with human non-A-E hepatitis. *J. Med. Virol.* **48:**60–67.
68. **Lenzi, M., G. Ballardini, M. Fusconi, F. Cassani, L. Selleri, U. Volta, D. Zauli, and F. B. Bianchi.** 1990. Type 2 autoimmune hepatitis and hepatitis C virus infection. *Lancet* **335:**258–259.
69. **Liang, T. J., K. Hasegawa, N. Rimon, J. R. Wands, and E. Ben-Porath.** 1991. A hepatitis B virus mutant associated with an epidemic of fulminant hepatitis. *N. Engl. J. Med.* **324:**1705–1709.
70. **Liang, T. J., L. Jeffers, R. K. Reddy, M. O. Silva, H. Cheinquer, A. Findor, M. De Medina, P. O. Yarbough, G. R. Reyes, and E. R. Schiff.** 1993. Fulminant or subfulminant non-A, non-B viral hepatitis: the role of hepatitis C and E viruses. *Gastroenterology* **104:**556–562.
71. **Linnen, J., J. Wages, Z. Y. Zhang-Keck, K. E. Fry, K. Z. Krawczynski, H. Alter, E. Koonin, M. Gallagher, M. Alter, S. Hadziyannis, P. Karayiannis, K. Fung, Y. Nakatsuji, J. W. Shih, L. Young, M. Piatak, C. Hoover, J. Fernandez, S. Chen, J. C. Zou, T. Morris, K. C. Hyams, S. Ismay, J. D. Lifson, G. Hess, S. K. Foung, H. Thomas, D. Bradley, H. Margolis, and J. P. Kim.** 1996. Molecular cloning and disease association of hepatitis G virus: a transfusion-transmissible agent. *Science* **271:**505–508.
72. **Lou, S., X. Qiu, G. Tegtmeier, S. Leitza, J. Brackett, K. Cousineau, A. Varma, H. Seballos, S. Kundu, S. Kuemmerle, and J. Hunt.** 1997. Immunoassays to study prevalence of antibody against GB virus C in blood donors. *J. Virol. Methods* **68:**45–55.
73. **Louie, J. K., L. C. Hsu, D. H. Osmond, M. H. Katz, and S. K. Schwarcz.** 2002. Trends in causes of death among persons with acquired immunodeficiency syndrome in the era of highly active antiretroviral therapy, San Francisco, 1994–1998. *J. Infect. Dis.* **186:**1023–1027.
74. **Lunel, F., L. Musset, P. Cacoub, L. Frangeul, P. Cresta, M. Perrin, P. Grippon, C. Hoang, J. C. Piette, J. M. Huraux, and P. Opolon.** 1994. Cryoglobulinemia in chronic liver diseases: role of hepatitis C virus and liver damage. *Gastroenterology* **106:**1291–1300.
75. **MacCallum, F. O., and D. J. Bauer.** 1944. Homologous serum jaundice: transmission experiments with human volunteers. *Lancet* **i:**622–627.
76. **Magnone, M., J. L. Holley, R. Shapiro, V. Scantlebury, J. McCauley, M. Jordan, C. Vivas, T. Starzl, and J. P. Johnson.** 1995. Interferon-alpha-induced acute renal allograft rejection. *Transplantation* **59:**1068–1070.
77. **Mast, E. E., and M. J. Alter.** 1993. Epidemiology of viral hepatitis: an overview. *Semin. Virol.* **4:**273–283.
78. **McIntyre, P. G., K. Tosh, and W. McGuire.** 2006. Caesarean section versus vaginal delivery for preventing mother to infant hepatitis C virus transmission. *Cochrane Database of Systematic Reviews* CD005546.
79. **Miller, M. F., C. Haley, M. J. Koziel, and C. F. Rowley.** 2005. Impact of hepatitis C virus on immune restoration in HIV-infected patients who start highly active antiretroviral therapy: a meta-analysis. *Clin. Infect. Dis.* **41:** 713–720.
80. **Misiani, R., P. Bellavita, D. Fenili, G. Borelli, D. Marchesi, M. Massazza, G. Vendramin, B. Comotti, E. Tanzi, G. Scudeller, and A. Zanetti.** 1992. Hepatitis C virus infection in patients with essential mixed cryoglobulinemia. *Ann. Intern. Med.* **117:**573–577.
81. **Munoz, S. J., D. W. Bradley, P. Martin, K. Krawczynski, M. A. Purdy, and S. Westerberg.** 1992. Hepatitis E virus found in patients with apparent fulminant non-A, non-B hepatitis. *Hepatology* **16:**76A.
82. **Naidu, S., and R. Viewanath.** 1957. Infectious hepatitis in Delhi 1955–1956: a critical study; observations in pregnant women. *Indian J. Med. Res.* **45:**71–76.
83. **Nakashima, K., S. Kashiwagi, J. Hayashi, A. Noguchi, M. Hirata, W. Kajiyama, K. Urabe, K. Minami, and Y. Maeda.** 1992. Sexual transmission of hepatitis C virus among female prostitutes and patients with sexually transmitted diseases in Fukuoka, Kyushu, Japan. *Am. J. Epidemiol.* **136:**1132–1137.
84. **National Institutes of Health.** 2002. Management of hepatitis C: 2002. *NIH Consens. State Sci. Statements* **19:** 1–46.
85. **Nishizawa, T., H. Okamoto, K. Konishi, H. Yoshizawa, Y. Miyakawa, and M. Mayumi.** 1997. A novel DNA virus (TTV) associated with elevated transaminase levels in posttransfusion hepatitis of unknown etiology. *Biochem. Biophys. Res. Commun.* **14:**92–97.
86. **Patra, S., A. Kumar, S. S. Trivedi, M. Puri, and S. K. Sarin.** 2007. Maternal and fetal outcomes in pregnant women with acute hepatitis E virus infection. *Ann. Intern. Med.* **147:**28–33.
87. **Pineda, J. A., M. Romero-Goméz, F. Díaz-García, J. A. Girón-González, J. L. Montero, J. Torre-Cisneros, R. J. Andrade, M. González-Serrano, J. Aguilar, M. Aguilar-**

Guisado, J. M. Navarro, J. Salmerón, F. J. Caballero-Granado, J. A. García-García, Grupo Andaluz para el Estudio de las Enfermedades Infecciosas, and Grupo Analuz para el Estudio del Hígado. 2005. HIV coinfection shortens the survival of patients with hepatitis C virus-related decompensated cirrhosis. *Hepatology* **41:** 779–789.

88. **Piroth, L., D. Sène, S. Pol, I. Goderel, K. Lacombe, B. Martha, D. Rey, V. Loustau-Ratti, J. F. Bergmann, G. Pialoux, A. Gervais, C. Lascoux-Combe, F. Carrat, and P. Cacoub.** 2007. Epidemiology, diagnosis and treatment of chronic hepatitis B in HIV-infected patients (EPIB 2005 STUDY). *AIDS* **21:**1323–1331.
89. **Prince, A. M.** 1968. An antigen detected in the blood during the incubation period of serum hepatitis. *Proc. Natl. Acad. Sci. USA* **60:**814–821.
90. **Prince, A. M., J. W. Scheffel, and B. Moore.** 1997. A search for hepatitis C virus polymerase chain reaction-positive but seronegative subjects among blood donors with elevated alanine aminotransferase. *Transfusion* (Paris) **37:**211–214.
91. **Rendina, M., A. Schena, N. M. Castellaneta, F. Losito, A. C. Amoruso, G. Stallone, F. P. Schena, A. Di Leo, and A. Francavilla.** 2007. The treatment of chronic hepatitis C with peginterferon alfa-2a (40 kDa) plus ribavirin in haemodialysed patients awaiting renal transplant. *J. Hepatol.* **46:**768–774.
92. **Reyes, G. R., M. A. Purdy, J. P. Kim, K. C. Luk, L. M. Young, K. E. Fry, and D. W. Bradley.** 1990. Isolation of a cDNA from the virus responsible for enterically transmitted non-A, non-B hepatitis. *Science* **247:**1335–1339.
93. **Rizzetto, M., M. G. Canese, S. Arico, O. Crivelli, F. Bonino, C. G. Trepo, and G. Verme.** 1977. Immunofluorescence detection of a new antigen-antibody system (δ/anti-δ) associated with the hepatitis B virus in the liver and in the serum of HBsAg carriers. *Gut* **18:**997–1003.
94. **Rizzetto, M., J. W. Shih, and J. L. Gerin.** 1980. The hepatitis B virus-associated delta antigen: isolation from liver, development of solid-phase radioimmunoassays for delta antigen and anti-delta and partial characterization of delta antigen. *J. Immunol.* **125:**318–324.
95. **Roth, W. K., D. Waschk, S. Marx, S. Tschauder, S. Zeuzem, H. Bialleck, H. Weber, and E. Seifried.** 1997. Prevalence of hepatitis G virus and its strain variant, the GB agent, in blood donations and their transmission to recipients. *Transfusion* (Paris) **37:**651–656.
96. **Santantonio, T., E. Medda, C. Ferrari, P. Fabris, G. Cariti, M. Massari, S. Babudieri, M. Toti, R. Francavilla, F. Ancarani, G. Antonucci, G. Scotto, V. Di Marco, G. Pastore, and T. Stroffolini.** 2006. Risk factors and outcome among a large patient cohort with community-acquired acute hepatitis C in Italy. *Clin. Infect. Dis.* **43:** 1154–1159.
97. **Schreiber, G. B., M. P. Busch, S. H. Kleinman, and J. J. Korelitz.** 1996. The risk of transfusion transmitted viral infection. *N. Engl. J. Med.* **334:**1685–1690.
98. **Seeff, L. B.** 2002. Natural history of chronic hepatitis C. *Hepatology* **36:**S35–S46.
99. **Seeff, L. B., E. C. Wright, H. J. Zimmerman, H. J. Alter, A. A. Dietz, B. F. Felsher, J. D. Finkelstein, P. Garcia-Pont, J. L. Gerin, H. B. Greenlee, J. Hamilton, P. V. Holland, P. M. Kaplan, T. Kiernan, R. S. Koff, C. M. Leevy, V. J. McAuliffe, N. Nath, R. H. Purcell, E. R. Schiff, C. C. Schwartz, C. H. Tamburro, Z. Vlahcevic, R. Zemel, and D. S. Zimmon.** 1978. Type B hepatitis after needle-stick exposure: prevention with hepatitis B immune globulin. Final report of the Veterans Administration Cooperative Study. *Ann. Intern. Med.* **88:**285–293.
100. **Silva, A. E., B. J. McMahon, A. J. Parkinson, M. H. Sjogren, J. H. Hoofnagle, and A. M. Di Bisceglie.** 1998. Hepatitis B virus DNA in persons with isolated antibody to hepatitis B core antigen who subsequently received hepatitis B vaccine. *Clin. Infect. Dis.* **26:**895–897.
101. **Simonetti, R. G., C. Camma, F. Fiorello, M. Cottone, M. Rapicetta, L. Marino, G. Fiorentino, A. Craxi, A. Ciccaglione, R. Giuseppetti, T. Stroffolini, and L. Pagliaro.** 1992. Hepatitis C virus infection as a risk factor for hepatocellular carcinoma in patients with cirrhosis. *Ann. Intern. Med.* **116:**97–102.
102. **Simons, J. N., T. J. Pilot-Matias, T. P. Leary, G. J. Dawson, and S. M. Desai.** 1995. Identification of two flavivirus-like genomes in the GB hepatitis agent. *Proc. Natl. Acad. Sci. USA* **92:**3401–3405.
103. **Smedile, A., G. Verme, A. Cargnel, P. Dentico, P. Opolon, D. Vergani, P. Farci, F. Caredda, N. Caporaso, C. Trepo, A. Gimson, R. Williams, and M. Rizzetto.** 1982. Influence of delta infection on severity of hepatitis B. *Lancet* **ii:**945–947.
104. **Sninsky, J. J., A. Siddiqui, W. S. Robinson, and S. N. Cohen.** 1979. Cloning and endonuclease mapping of the hepatitis B viral genome. *Nature* **279:**346–348.
105. **Szmuness, W., C. E. Stevens, E. J. Harley, E. A. Zang, W. R. Oleszko, D. C. William, R. Sadovsky, J. M. Morrison, and A. Kellner.** 1980. Hepatitis B vaccine: demonstration of efficacy in a controlled clinical trial in a high-risk population in the United States. *N. Engl. J. Med.* **303:**833–841.
106. **Tabor, E., R. J. Gerety, J. A. Drucker, L. B. Seeff, J. H. Hoofnagle, D. R. Jackson, M. April, L. F. Barker, and G. Pineda-Tamondong.** 1978. Transmission of non-A, non-B hepatitis from man to chimpanzee. *Lancet* **ii:** 463–466.
107. **Taylor, R. M., T. Davern, S. Munoz, S. H. Han, B. McGuire, A. M. Larson, L. Hynan, W. M. Lee, R. J. Fontana, and U.S. Acute Liver Failure Study Group.** 2006. Fulminant hepatitis A virus infection in the United States: incidence, prognosis, and outcomes. *Hepatology* **44:**1589–1597.
108. **Tedder, R. S., R. J. Gilson, M. Briggs, C. Loveday, C. H. Cameron, J. A. Garson, G. E. Kelly, and I. V. Weller.** 1991. Hepatitis C virus: evidence for sexual transmission. *Br. Med. J.* **302:**1299–1302.
109. **Tei, S., N. Kitajima, K. Takahashi, and S. Mishiro.** 2003. Zoonotic transmission of hepatitis E virus from deer to human beings. *Lancet* **362:**371–373.
110. **Thomas, D. L., J. M. Zenilman, H. J. Alter, J. W. Shih, N. Galai, A. V. Carella, and T. C. Quinn.** 1995. Sexual transmission of hepatitis C virus among patients attending sexually transmitted diseases clinics in Baltimore—an analysis of 309 sex partnerships. *J. Infect. Dis.* **171:** 768–775.
111. **Thomas, S. L., M. L. Newell, C. S. Peckham, A. E. Ades, and A. J. Hall.** 1998. A review of hepatitis c virus (HCV) vertical transmission: risks of transmission to infants born to mothers with and without HCV viraemia or human immunodeficiency virus infection. *Int. J. Epidemiol.* **27:**108–117.
112. **Torriani, F. J., M. Rodriguez-Torres, J. K. Rockstroh, E. Lissen, J. Gonzalez-García, A. Lazzarin, G. Carosi, J. Sasadeusz, C. Katlama, J. Montaner, H. Sette, Jr., S. Passe, J. De Pamphilis, F. Duff, U. M. Schrenk, and D. T. Dieterich for the APRICOT Study Group.** 2004. Peginterferon alfa-2a plus ribavirin for chronic hepatitis

C virus infection in HIV-infected patients. *N. Engl. J. Med.* **351:**438–450.

113. **U.S. Public Health Service.** 2001. Updated U.S. Public Health Service Guidelines for the management of occupational exposures to HBV, HCV, and HIV and recommendations for postexposure prophylaxis. *Morb. Mortal. Wkly. Rep. Recomm. Rep.* **50:**1–52.
114. **Valenzuela, P., P. Gray, M. Quiroga, J. Zaldivar, H. M. Goodman, and W. J. Rutter.** 1979. Nucleotide sequence of the gene coding for the major protein of hepatitis B virus surface antigen. *Nature* **280:**815–819.
115. **van Zonneveld, M., A. B. van Nunen, H. G. Niesters, R. A. de Man, S. W. Schalm, and H. L. Janssen.** 2003. Lamivudine treatment during pregnancy to prevent perinatal transmission of hepatitis B virus infection. *J. Viral Hepat.* **10:**294–297.
116. **Wands, J. R., E. Mann, E. Alpert, and K. J. Isselbacher.** 1975. The pathogenesis of arthritis associated with acute hepatitis-B surface antigen-positive hepatitis: complement activation and characterization of circulating immune complexes. *J. Clin. Investig.* **55:**930–936.
117. **Wasley, A., and M. J. Alter.** 2000. Epidemiology of hepatitis C: geographic differences and temporal trends. *Semin. Liver Dis.* **21:**1–16.
118. **Wasley, A., J. T. Miller, L. Finelli, and Centers for Disease Control and Prevention (CDC).** 2007. Surveillance for acute viral hepatitis—United States, 2005. *Morb. Mortal. Wkly. Rep. CDC Surveill. Summ.* **16:**1–24.
119. **Weinstock, H. S., G. Bolan, A. L. Reingold, and L. B. Polish.** 1993. Hepatitis C virus infection among patients attending a clinic for sexually transmitted diseases. *JAMA* **269:**392–394.
120. **Wong, D. C., R. H. Purcell, M. A. Sreenivasan, S. R. Prasad, and K. M. Pavri.** 1980. Epidemic and endemic hepatitis in India: evidence for a non-A, non-B hepatitis aetiology. *Lancet* **ii:**876–879.
121. **Wright, T. L., D. Mamish, C. Combs, M. Kim, E. Donegan, L. Ferrell, J. Lake, J. Roberts, and N. L. Ascher.** 1992. Hepatitis B virus and apparent fulminant non-A and non-B hepatitis. *Lancet* **339:**952–955.
122. **Yeo, W., B. Zee, S. Zhong, P. K. Chan, W. L. Wong, W. M. Ho, K. C. Lam, and P. J. Johnson.** 2004. Comprehensive analysis of risk factors associating with hepatitis B virus (HBV) reactivation in cancer patients undergoing cytotoxic chemotherapy. *Br. J. Cancer* **90:** 1306–1311.
123. **Zuckerman, E., T. Zuckerman, D. Douer, D. Qian, and A. M. Levine.** 1998. Liver dysfunction in patients infected with hepatitis C virus undergoing chemotherapy for hematologic malignancies. *Cancer* **83:**1224–1230.

Infections in Organ Transplant Recipients

JOHN A. ZAIA

6

Organ transplantation represents a continually expanding field of medicine, and with each innovative method for subverting the natural process of host immunity, new and unusual presentations for virus infections have occurred. For example, in the mid-1960s, with the introduction of cytotoxic drugs such as azathioprine and cyclophosphamide for renal transplantation, pneumonitis associated with human cytomegalovirus (CMV) infection was first observed (65). It was soon noted that transplant recipients who acquired Epstein-Barr virus (EBV) infection developed a previously unrecognized clinical syndrome, posttransplantation lymphoproliferative disease (PTLD) (112). There are many other viruses, for example, respiratory viruses, herpes simplex virus (HSV), and varicella-zoster virus (VZV), for which infection in organ recipients can lead to serious complications. The time of onset of these viral infections after transplantation is fairly predictable (Fig. 1). The herpesviruses HSV, EBV, CMV, and human herpesvirus 6 (HHV-6) reactivate during the first 1 to 3 months. Problems with hepatitis and polyomaviruses (e.g., BK virus) occur in later months. With the increasing use of xenotransplantation, the concern about introducing viral zoonoses increases, as is discussed below. But from a management standpoint, CMV, EBV, adenovirus (AV), and hepatitis virus infections consume a major focus of attention. However, certain unusual infections such as rabies, West Nile virus, and Creutzfeldt-Jakob disease (CJD) can be a concern after transplantation and are discussed here. A variety of respiratory virus infections cause more severe illnesses with higher rates of pneumonitis and solid-organ graft rejection episodes in transplant patients (59); specific agents are discussed elsewhere in this volume.

CMV INFECTION

Background

Despite the fact that CMV was initially noticed and, in fact, was named because of its effect on the fetus (143), its major clinical significance, perhaps until the AIDS era, has been in the organ transplant recipient (54). CMV produces disease principally in the immunologically impaired individual and, in doing so, demonstrates considerable variability in the types of clinical syndromes that are seen in different at-risk groups. In the fetus and in the person with advanced AIDS, in whom the level of immunodeficiency is relatively constant, CMV produces predominantly retinal, central nervous system (CNS), and gut diseases (61, 147). In transplant populations, in which immunodeficiency is iatrogenic and can vary, it produces mononucleosis-like syndromes, involvement of the transplanted organ (e.g., liver, heart, or lung), and pneumonitis (119). With the introduction of preventive antiviral strategies over the past 15 years, there have been significant changes in the occurrence of life-threatening CMV infection and in the management of transplant patients. In the 1980s, the rate of CMV-related mortality was 10 to 30% for recipients of allogeneic marrow transplantation (91), but with the use of ganciclovir, it has dropped to 2 to 5% (146). The use of antiviral chemotherapy has also altered the natural course of posttransplantation CMV. In the preantiviral era, the onset of disease was 2 to 3 months posttransplantation, but with the use of antiviral suppression, CMV reactivation and disease onset are delayed and occur 4 to 12 months posttransplantation, and there can be toxic effects of the antiviral intervention. With a shift in disease onset to later times after transplantation and with the side effects of antiviral treatment, the strategies for management of the transplant recipient have become more complicated. Treatment plans must weigh these risks, including costs, against the anticipated benefits and develop a rational approach. Thus, the person with responsibility for the care of transplant recipients requires familiarity with the changing aspects of CMV infection and prevention.

Pathogenesis of CMV Infection and Its Effect in the Transplant Recipient

CMV-associated diseases in transplant populations are acquired by transmission of infection from the transplanted organ or from reactivation of endogenous infection in the recipient (24, 54). As with other herpesviruses, CMV can reactivate from a latent infection in the absence of functional CMV-specific cell-mediated immunity and lead to persistent infection which can progress to organ-specific disease or to systemic infection. With regard to the requirement for progressive infection to produce disease, the recovery of CMV at sites like urine or the throat does not correlate with disease, while CMV viremia and asymptomatic pulmonary infection strongly correlate with subse-

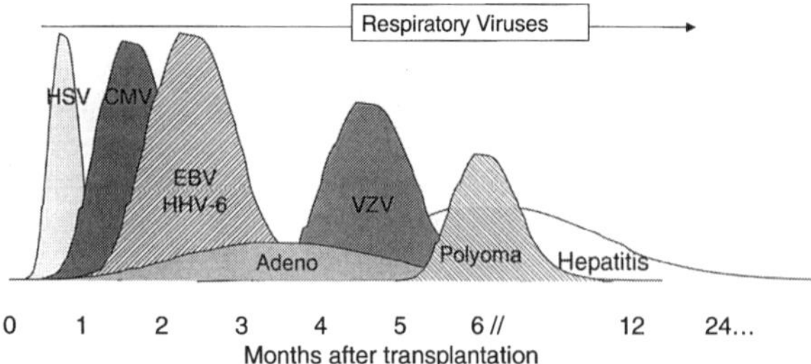

FIGURE 1 Occurrence of the most frequent virus infections after transplantation. Shown are the times after both SOT and marrow transplantation that recipients present with characteristic types of virus infections, ranging from HSV at the earliest time to CMV, EBV, and HHV-6 at 1 to 3 months after transplantation and AV, VZV, polyomavirus, and hepatitis viruses at later times.

quent disease (93, 123). Progression of CMV infection from regional to disseminated infection is necessary prior to the onset of serious CMV disease in this setting.

The pathogenesis of CMV-associated diseases is poorly understood, but it is possible to surmise important features of the disease process from its clinical presentations. In the non-hematopoietic cell transplantation (non-HCT) setting, this variation in the types of symptom complex that occur in association with CMV infection ranges from the extreme of severe organ dysfunction (e.g., encephalitis, retinitis, adrenalitis, enteritis, and hepatitis) seen in association with profound immunologic impairment, as in patients with AIDS or in neonates (61, 147), to mononucleosis syndromes, with malaise and fatigue, as occur in adolescents and in young adults (70). The usual asymptomatic course of CMV infection of immunocompetent persons is also seen with CMV infection after HCT or solid-organ transplantation (SOT) (53, 93). When renal, heart and/or lung, and marrow transplant populations are compared, it can be seen that the rates of infection with CMV and the incubation periods are similar, but the types of disease vary. For example, CMV-associated interstitial pneumonia (CMV-IP) is a more frequent problem for marrow allograft recipients (54, 91, 118). In AIDS patients and in fetuses, CMV infection is progressive and unchecked, and in these settings the virus demonstrates a neurotropism, with direct tissue damage in the CNS. The neurotropic aspect of CMV infection is rarely seen in transplant recipients (53, 91, 118). The principal differences in presentation of CMV disease between these groups are the predominance of mononucleosis-like symptoms in the transplantation patients and direct involvement of the transplanted organ in the case of SOT (118).

In addition to direct effects of viral infection on organ function, CMV infection after transplantation is associated with events such as graft rejection, atherosclerosis, and increased rates of bacterial and fungal infections (99, 103). Because these effects have been associated with immunologic abnormalities specific for transplantation populations, like graft-versus-host disease (GVHD), the symptom complex associated with CMV appears to be due not only to a direct toxic effect of infection on cell or organ function but also to a secondary or indirect effect on host responses to infection. Understanding the pathogenesis of CMV disease in the transplant recipient, therefore, involves elements related both to the onset and progression of virus infection and to the effect of this infection on general cellular function and on specific immune function.

Risk Factors for CMV Complications

To better understand the biological aspects of CMV infection and to minimize CMV complications after transplantation, the risk factors for CMV disease must be recognized (Table 1). The most significant risk factor is the development of CMV infection itself, and for that reason, a patient age of >20 years, a prior infection of the donor with CMV, and a prior infection of the recipient with CMV are most important factors. Seroepidemiological (54) and molecular (24) evidence indicates that the donated organ is the source of CMV reinfection in most instances. Primary CMV infection occurs in mismatched donations (infected donor and previously uninfected recipient), but more frequently, reinfection occurs in the recipient who has had prior CMV infection and acquires a new CMV strain from the donor (24). In SOT patients, CMV disease is much more likely after primary than secondary infection, whereas this is not necessarily true for HCT patients (92, 118). In addition, liver and heart transplant patients have a greater incidence of CMV disease than do renal transplant patients (36). Cadaver organ transplants are associated with more CMV infections than are transplants of organs from living donors (14).

Immunosuppression is of primary importance in considering risk factors of CMV disease after transplantation. Patients with detectable cytotoxic T-lymphocyte (CTL) activity targeted to CMV have significantly less disease than those without CTLs (113, 117, 135). The absence of CMV-specific $CD4^+$ T-cell function is a marker for CMV disease (72, 82). The frequency of CMV-specific CD4 and $CD8^+$ T cells can be assessed and evaluated quantitatively (74), and studies have linked the absolute numbers of CMV-reactive T cells to protection from disease (46). In addition, donor immunity contributes to the CMV-specific cellular immune status of HCT recipients (29). The post-transplantation reacquisition of CMV-specific cellular immunity following marrow ablation is improved when the donor has prior immunity to CMV (78). Similarly, in SOT, the influence of cellular immune modification by the use of anti-T-cell antibody or of other agents which can influence CTLs will significantly increase the risk of progressive CMV infection (14, 118).

In HCT, the presence of GVHD is considered the most important additional factor for the development of CMV

TABLE 1 Risk factors for CMV complications in the transplant recipient

CMV infection
Seropositive donor and seronegative recipient
Graft as source of reinfection
Age
Mismatch status of solid-organ donor
Mismatch number
HLA type: DR7, DRw6, B7
Organ type
Liver, heart > renal transplant
Cadaver > living donor solid-organ transplant
Allogeneic > autologous marrow transplant
Immune status
Anti-T-cell antibody therapy
CMV-specific lymphocyte immunity

disease (92). Marrow transplant recipients with minimal risk for GVHD, like autologous and syngeneic transplant recipients, have nearly the same prevalence of CMV infection but have almost no CMV disease (144). Patients over 20 years of age are also at increased risk either because of increased rates of prior CMV infection or because GVHD occurs with a greater frequency in this group (92).

Clinical Course of CMV Diseases in Transplant Recipients

In SOT recipients, the early descriptions of infection continue to be true, and SOT recipients with CMV-associated complications present with fever, malaise, and, variably, neutropenia and thrombocytopenia (53, 118). These can be associated with subsequent fungal and bacterial complications. HCT recipients with CMV-associated complications present with fever with or without gastroenteritis or CMV-IP (91). CMV enterocolitis and hepatitis occur in both transplant populations but are less frequently observed in HCT recipients. Although CMV disease can manifest in a variety of ways, certain serious syndromes are associated with specific transplant patient groups. For example, with heart and lung transplantation, bronchiolitis obliterans can occur following CMV infection and following acute rejection. Bronchiolitis obliterans is defined as a decline in forced expiratory volume in one second <80% posttransplantation baseline and the histologic presence of obliterative brochiolitis (128). Acute rejection is associated with CMV in all solid-organ transplants, including heart (48), lung (6), kidney (133), and liver (40) transplants. Within the subgroups of solid-organ recipients, those with liver and pancreas transplants have significantly more CMV disease than those with kidney transplants (36). Gastrointestinal (GI) CMV infection occurs in any area of the GI tract and manifests similarly in HCT and SOT recipients, producing diarrhea, abdominal pain, cramping, nausea, and vomiting (37).

For HCT, the most life-threatening CMV-associated syndrome is CMV-IP, which manifests with dyspnea and oxygen desaturation and progresses to respiratory failure in a majority of cases (91). In the 1990s, the use of antiviral prophylaxis produced a marked reduction in serious CMV-IP, but this complication remains a problem long after allogeneic transplantation (11).

Treatment and Prevention of CMV Infection in Transplant Recipients

Prevention of CMV Infection in the Seronegative Transplant Recipient

For the CMV-seronegative marrow transplant recipient for whom there is a CMV-seronegative organ donor, the risk of infection is determined by the exposure to posttransplantation blood products. Virtually all primary CMV infections can be prevented by careful preparation or processing of the blood components (15). Thus, in HCT, 90% of all disease occurs in the CMV-seropositive recipient. In SOT, the option to use CMV-seronegative organ donors is usually not available, and the risk of CMV disease is associated with the CMV antibody-positive (+) or -negative (−) serostatus of donor (D) and recipient (R), such that $D^+ R^-$ transplants are at highest risk for CMV disease (56). A significant amount of disease occurs because of endogenous CMV reactivation either from the recipient or from the donor organ, but improved antiviral chemotherapy can modify this virus reactivation or, if reactivation does occur, influence the progression of CMV infection.

Role of Acyclovir in CMV Prophylaxis

Initial attempts to suppress the reactivation of CMV infection in HCT and SOT recipients used either oral or intravenous (i.v.) acyclovir (5, 94). The mean 50% inhibitory dose of acyclovir for CMV strains (63.1 ± 30.2 μM) (27) is similar to the peak acyclovir levels in plasma with these regimens (ranging from 25 to 100 μM), and acyclovir significantly reduced CMV reactivation and disease. Long-term use of high-dose oral acyclovir (800 mg four times daily for 6 months) had no effect on CMV disease but led to a significant improvement in the survival rate after marrow transplantation (110). These early observations indicated that antivirals could influence CMV reactivation rates after transplantation and that this could perturb the natural course of CMV infection and the associated clinical disease.

Valacyclovir, a prodrug of acyclovir that provides levels in blood comparable to those obtained with i.v. acyclovir (58), with an oral dosage of 2 g four times daily for >900 days after renal transplantation, was effective in significantly reducing CMV disease in high-risk, mismatched ($D^+ R^-$) patients (45%, versus 16%) and in lowering the rate of acute rejection episodes (52%, versus 26%) (88). Similar inhibition of CMV reactivation has been reported to occur in allogeneic HCT recipients (137). Valacyclovir is not currently approved for CMV prophylaxis, and because other agents with high antiviral potency exist, its use in the transplant setting is reserved for low-risk patients.

Role of Ganciclovir in CMV Prophylaxis

The prevention of CMV disease with i.v. ganciclovir was first shown in studies after marrow transplantation (44, 123). With ganciclovir, two strategies have been used: either all at-risk patients are treated for a defined period or only transplant recipients with documented CMV infection are treated. The first approach is termed general prophylaxis, and the second strategy is termed preemptive or early antiviral therapy. There is no best strategy for use of ganciclovir, and the clinical situation determines the appropriate approach. For example, in HCT, ganciclovir preemptive treatment has been shown to be associated with improved survival rates, whereas general prophylaxis has no survival advantage (44, 45). The pretransplantation use of ganciclovir is no longer recommended.

Ganciclovir is associated with marrow toxicity, and drug-related neutropenia occurs in approximately 30% of transplant recipients receiving ganciclovir (121). The median time of onset of neutropenia is 36 days (range, 6 to 74 days) after starting treatment, and the neutropenia persists for a median of 12 days (range, 4 to 20 days) (44, 45). The use of prophylactic ganciclovir has also been associated with the failure of development of CMV-specific cell-mediated immunity and an increase in late CMV-associated disease (11, 78).

Prevention of CMV Disease Using Ganciclovir after SOT

In SOT recipients, ganciclovir prophylaxis prevents disease associated with CMV reactivation or reinfection, but it has been less effective in modifying the clinical course of primary CMV infection (126). Considerable controversy remains about whether preemptive (based on detecting virus antigen or DNA) or prophylactic ganciclovir should be used in SOT recipients (64, 67, 126). The goal is to protect the highest-risk patients with antiviral therapy aimed at reduction of reactivated infection and prevention of reinfection and early disease. In high-risk groups such as D^+ R^- SOT recipients, CMV-associated disease occurs significantly less in the ganciclovir-treated patients who initiate preemptive therapy for CMV-positive culture than in those receiving acyclovir prophylaxis (126). Thus, it is current practice in many solid-organ transplant centers to use ganciclovir i.v. for a short period (1 to 2 weeks posttransplantation) and then treat the patient preemptively thereafter. When oral ganciclovir was compared to placebo in liver transplant recipients for the first 3 months after transplantation, there was found to be a significant reduction in the CMV disease rate for all patients (19%, versus 5%), for primary infection (44%, versus 15%), and for those receiving antilymphocyte antibody treatment (33%, versus 5%) (42). There have been few comparative studies of preemptive treatment versus prophylactic ganciclovir in SOT, but one such study in renal transplant recipients showed more CMV viremia as measured by DNA in the preemptive group and more late CMV disease in the prophylactic group (67). A meta-analysis evaluating these strategies in SOT recipients concluded that both strategies for ganciclovir use, as well as prophylactic acyclovir, reduced CMV organ disease, but only prophylactic ganciclovir reduced the associated bacterial and fungal infections and death (64).

Prevention of CMV Disease Using Ganciclovir after Marrow Transplantation

The use of the preemptive strategy was established in HCT when ganciclovir, given to asymptomatic transplant recipients at the time of laboratory evidence of active pulmonary CMV infection, significantly reduced progression to CMV disease (123). Of HCT patients with initially asymptomatic CMV pulmonary infection, approximately 60 to 70% will subsequently develop CMV-IP (123). Ganciclovir is given at a dosage of 5 mg/kg of body weight i.v. twice daily for 7 days and then maintained at 5 mg/kg once daily for 5 to 6 days per week for 2 to 6 weeks based on the clearance of CMV DNA from blood (Table 2). The use of preemptive ganciclovir is effective in preventing the morbidity of CMV infection while sparing the toxicity of ganciclovir in those who are at a lower risk of disease. However, the need to identify those with significant CMV infection places a requirement for continued monitoring, and it is limited by the sensitivity of the assays used to detect CMV.

Use of Other Antiviral Agents for Prevention of CMV Disease in Transplant Patients

Foscarnet

The optimal method for prevention of CMV disease after HCT and SOT usually relies on a preemptive strategy that uses ganciclovir. However, with evidence of drug-related marrow toxicity or clinical suspicion of ganciclovir resistance, based on failure to clear virus, foscarnet should be used instead of ganciclovir. Also, during ganciclovir treatment, it is not unusual to observe breakthrough CMV viremia, which is usually associated with increased immunosuppressive therapy and not with drug-resistant virus (100). Resistance to ganciclovir does occur, however, especially in SOT recipients (79). In this situation, foscarnet can be used alone or in combination with ganciclovir for CMV suppression. Although renal toxicity can be limiting, foscarnet can be safely used in this population by following recommendations regarding pretreatment hydration (85).

TABLE 2 CMV prophylaxis in transplant recipients[a]

General prophylaxis using ganciclovir[b]
Treat all CMV-seropositive recipients
Dosage: 5 mg/kg b.i.d. for 7 days and then q.d. 5–6 days/wk
Start when ANC is 750 × 10^{-9} liter
Stop when immunosuppression is significantly reduced or when the ANC is <750 × 10^{-9} liter for 2 consecutive days
Preemptive therapy[c]
Treat all recipients with CMV infection of blood or when concomitant use of immunosuppressive therapy suggests high risk of CMV reactivation
Ganciclovir dosage: 5 mg/kg b.i.d. for 7–14 days and then q.d. 5 days/wk
Foscarnet[d] dosage: 60 mg/kg t.i.d. or 90 mg/kg with fluid diuresis
Stop after 4–6 wks, when CMV DNA is undetectable in blood, or when immunosuppression is significantly reduced

[a] b.i.d., twice a day; q.d., once a day; t.i.d., three times a day.
[b] General prophylaxis is used in all CMV-seropositive transplants.
[c] Preemptive therapy is used when CMV is detected in blood.
[d] Substituted for ganciclovir when there is marrow toxicity or drug resistance.

Oral Ganciclovir and Valganciclovir

Oral ganciclovir is poorly absorbed, although its use has been approved in the United States for CMV prophylaxis after SOT. Oral valganciclovir is well absorbed and can be substituted for i.v. drug during maintenance therapy for control of CMV reactivation. Valganciclovir is approved for use in adult AIDS patients and adult kidney, heart, and kidney-pancreas transplant patients with CMV infection. The dosage of oral ganciclovir for adults is 1 g three times daily. The dosage of valganciclovir is 900 mg once daily in adults. The toxicity of these drugs is similar to that of the i.v. formulation.

Cidofovir

Cidofovir has been used in transplant patients as second-line therapy for patients with CMV disease unresponsive to ganciclovir or foscarnet (83), but its renal toxicity severely limits its use.

Cellular Immunotherapy for Prevention of CMV Disease

Older observations indicated that patients who were able to develop CMV-specific CTL function after allogeneic HCT survived serious CMV infection, and those who failed to develop a positive response to CMV infection often succumbed with CMV-IP (113). The posttransplantation cellular immune response appears to develop from memory cells present in the donor graft for patients receiving non-T-cell depleted transplants (75). Although controversial, when the HCT involves a seropositive donor and a seropositive recipient, there is less CMV disease than when there is a CMV-seronegative donor for such a recipient. Several approaches for augmenting this donor-derived viral immunity with adoptive immunotherapy have been suggested. An initial study found that a high-risk group of HCT recipients receiving adoptive immunotherapy had both an absence of CMV disease and CMV infection in blood (139). Subsequently the feasibility of adoptive cellular therapy by various methods (25, 38, 76) suggested the potency of the immune system in protection against CMV infection. Use of this currently investigative method or other methods involving boosting donor immunity using vaccines may eventually become standard therapy for CMV prevention.

EBV INFECTION

Background

In the general population, EBV infection is the cause of infectious mononucleosis and is associated with important neoplastic diseases such as nasopharyngeal carcinoma (114), African Burkitt's lymphoma (52, 69), non-Hodgkin's lymphoma in AIDS (26), and Hodgkin's disease (142). In the transplant population, all aspects of these clinical manifestations of EBV infection can be seen, and for this reason, EBV is among the most important infectious problems after either HCT or SOT. The seminal observation that linked EBV to certain lymphoproliferative syndromes in SOT recipients was the description of the X-linked lymphoproliferative (XLP) syndrome in 1975 (see the review in reference 112). The chronic immunosuppression necessary to maintain the viability of the solid-organ graft or the suppression of GVHD can mimic XLP syndrome with resulting prolonged and extensive EBV infection, leading to lymphoid and other malignancies (see chapter 24 for a general description of the pathogenesis of EBV infection).

The occurrence of lymphomas in renal transplant recipients was first documented in 1969 (107). The direct link to immunosuppressive agents was established with the development of a lymphoid malignancy at the actual site of injection of antilymphocyte globulin (34). Shortly thereafter, both the association of lymphoid malignancies with immunodeficiency and the observation that the neoplasms associated with organ transplantation can regress with cessation of immunosuppressive therapy were made. With the description of XLP syndrome, EBV was linked to malignant lymphoproliferation after infectious mononucleosis, organ transplantation, and other immunodeficiency conditions (112). The most significant clinical syndrome associated with EBV infection in SOT and HCT recipients is PTLD. PTLD is defined as an abnormal proliferation of lymphoid cells in a transplant recipient. PTLD is not necessarily a malignant neoplastic change, although this is an important aspect in the spectrum of PTLD (112, 120). The prevalence of PTLD varies with the type of organ transplant, with rare occurrence after T-cell-replete HCT and increasing occurrence after renal, liver, and heart-lung, and kidney-pancreas SOT and after HCT with T-cell-depleted organs (8). The reported incidence rates per 100 person-years during the first 2 years posttransplantation are 1.4 for liver, 2.0 for heart, 6.2 for lung, and 5.2 for kidney-pancreas transplants (138). In allogeneic HCT, the risk of PTLD is increased 30-fold by the use of T-cell depletion and 12-fold by the use of anti-T-cell therapy for GVHD (95).

Pathogenesis of EBV-Related Diseases after Transplantation

Primary EBV infection is a major risk factor in PTLD in renal transplant recipients (55), and use of PCR methods has confirmed that quantitative assessment of EBV infection can identify those at risk for PTLD (80). The total immunopathological response to EBV infection results in enlarged lymph nodes, painful cervical lymphadenitis, tonsillitis, and splenomegaly, which characterize the clinical syndrome called "infectious mononucleosis." In the absence of an immunologic control on B-cell infection, progressive EBV infection occurs and results in B-cell lymphoproliferative disorders (20). It is the iatrogenic immunosuppression used in organ transplant recipients that impairs the anti-EBV CTL response and allows continued EBV replication, B-cell proliferation, and consequent PTLD. EBV-induced proliferation of lymphoid cells is the first of two stages of cancer induction; the second stage involves the development of a fixed genetic change by means of chromosomal or other mutational alterations (68, 69). Although there are polymorphic cellular changes during the proliferative stage that can be detected by use of either cellular or viral markers, there are only a few fixed genetic changes. These result in the convergent cytogenetic abnormalities observed (69), usually involving chromosome 14 translocations, c-*myc* or N-Ras proto-oncogene mutations, or T-cell receptor alterations (68).

Risk Factors for PTLD

Certain risk factors that determine which transplant patients are more likely to develop PTLD are well recognized. The development of EBV infection, especially primary infection, is the most important factor (55), and the amount of detectable EBV in the blood is directly related to occurrence of PTLD (109). Sequential analysis of the EBV DNA levels from subjects with PTLD and SOT controls without PTLD have shown that EBV DNA levels increase in both groups with the induction of immunosuppression, but markedly elevated levels of EBV DNA are seen in the majority of patients before or at the onset of PTLD (66). PCR assays for EBV DNA in blood can detect elevated levels of EBV DNA for up to 3 weeks before onset of PTLD, and prospective quantitative PCR assays for EBV DNA can be used for early detection of PTLD (130). Of the immunosuppressive regimens that influence the ability to control EBV infection, the antibodies that directly target T lymphocytes, like polyclonal antilymphocyte globulins and OKT3, are important risk factors for PTLD. In addition, cyclosporine and tacrolimus (FK506), which are used prophylactically to suppress graft rejection or GVHD, are also significant risk factors, although this might not be a simple direct relationship. Some studies, for example, have shown that cyclosporine is a risk factor only in relation to the total amount of immunosuppression (97). As noted before, the type of organ transplanted will also affect the risk of PTLD, with heart and/or lung having the highest risk and non-T-cell-depleted HCT associated with the lowest (8, 138). However, in HCT, it has been observed that certain subgroups, such as those with T-cell-depleted transplants, especially with higher numbers of stem cells (136) and matched unrelated marrow recipients (124), have a higher incidence of PTLD than allogeneic related transplant recipients.

Source of EBV in the Transplant Patient with PTLD

Similar to the case with CMV, the source of the EBV in persons with PTLD appears to be the donor organ, and the risk of PTLD is higher in children experiencing primary EBV infection after SOT. In one case cluster, analysis of the EBV strains from a single donor and two recipients showed that the virus associated with PTLD in both recipients was identical to that detected in the donor (21). Using a DNA minisatellite probe to distinguish the DNA from lymphoblastic cell lines (LCLs) isolated from PTLD specimens and from the donor spleen, it was found that all LCLs were distinct, indicating that the lymphoid proliferation in the individuals with PTLD was of B cells from the recipients. With some exceptions, the cell of origin for PTLD is from the recipient after SOT, but in HCT PTLD usually derives from the donor lymphoid cells, presumably because the recipient marrow is ablated (21, 47). The exceptions to this rule are important to note because of their importance to our understanding of the full spectrum of pathogenesis. In this regard, some studies have shown both recipient and donor cells in PTLD after marrow transplantation (148) and PTLD of donor origin after renal transplantation (115).

Clinical Manifestations of EBV Infection after Transplantation

Mononucleosis-Like Syndrome

Mononucleosis can occur after EBV infection in transplant recipients as it does in immunocompetent persons. The clinical triad of sore throat with exudative pharyngitis, fever, and lymphoadenopathy appears and can include other signs and symptoms such as malaise, headache, anorexia, myalgias, and hepatosplenomegaly. CNS complications, including aseptic meningitis, encephalitis, and Guillain-Barré syndrome, can occur. Unlike infection in immunologically normal persons, in which the T-lymphocyte response contributes the "mononuclear" element to the hematologic findings, in the transplant recipient one does not expect to see a true hematologic mononucleosis. The symptom complex of pharyngitis, fever, and lymphoadenopathy should suggest EBV infection in this population. The serologic findings normally utilized for diagnostic purposes are not reliable in the immunosuppressed population, and direct EBV-specific PCR-based detection methods should be used for assessing infection (109).

PTLD

Although nonspecific signs of fever and malaise can be a hallmark of PTLD, especially persisting nonspecific signs and symptoms in the patient who has been treated for CMV infection, this disease ultimately manifests as a focal or multifocal occurrence of lymphoid proliferation (51). The most common areas for disease are the CNS, the gut, and the allograft itself. The involvement of the allograft is particularly frequent in heart and/or lung recipients, for whom the differential diagnosis will include pneumonitis, graft rejection, and PTLD. Aggressive immunoblastic lymphoma can occasionally be seen, and this usually occurs in the first 100 days posttransplantation.

Other Cancers

After HCT, non-Hodgkin's lymphomas are the predominant malignancy associated with EBV, occurring in 90% of instances of this lymphoproliferative complication. In other transplant patient groups, the association of EBV with non-Hodgkin's lymphoma occurs in >70% of PTLD cases (8, 112). In addition to B-cell neoplasms, EBV has been found in association with approximately 25% of T-cell lymphomas occurring in transplant recipients. EBV is recognized to be associated with Hodgkin's disease (141), but Hodgkin's disease remains a relatively rare observation after transplantation. Unlike PTLD, which usually occurs during the first year after transplantation, Hodgkin's disease occurs later, at a mean time of 49 months posttransplantation. In addition to lymphoid neoplasms, secondary malignancies of the stomach and colon may have EBV markers in renal transplant recipients (132).

Oral Hairy Leukoplakia

As in AIDS, chronic EBV infection of the transplant recipient can cause oral hairy leukoplakia (26). Oral hairy leukoplakia is a lesion on the tongue or oral mucosa due to epithelial hyperplasia. EBV and human papillomavirus have been associated with this syndrome. When EBV is present, it can be detected in the epithelial cells in these lesions, and it is known to replicate in linear form, with high copy number of infectious virus. The lesion rarely undergoes malignant transformation.

Treatment of EBV Infection

General Approach

PTLD is a life-threatening complication of transplantation and is associated with a mortality rate of more than 50%. Reduction in immunosuppression can result in regression of PTLD, and therefore monitoring for EBV infection using PCR analysis and preemptive reduction in immunosuppression is the first aspect of patient management. Local surgical control of disease is often necessary, particularly if the disease is associated with GI bleeding, and in general, surgical excision of the PTLD lesion is performed when possible. The role of antiviral therapy is unknown, but antiviral therapy has appeared to improve PTLD according to some anecdotal reports. However, since no single aspect of treatment is performed alone, it is not possible to know what role any of these treatments has played. The treatment of PTLD was changed dramatically with the observations that adoptive humoral and cellular immunotherapy could positively impact disease progression (104). At present, then, treatment includes reduction in immunosuppression, surgical control of local disease, anti-B-cell therapy, introduction of donor T cells, and use of antiviral chemotherapy.

Antiviral Therapy

EBV is inhibited in vitro by several antiviral agents, including acyclovir, ganciclovir, foscarnet, penciclovir, and interferon. However, except for oral hairy leukoplakia, in which acyclovir is effective therapy (116), there is little clinical benefit from antiviral agents during infectious mononucleosis (2), chronic mononucleosis (131), and even fulminant infection associated with X-linked immunoproliferative syndrome (102). As noted above, these agents inhibit only the replication of linear EBV DNA, in which the EBV-encoded DNA polymerase is active, as in hairy leukoplakia, and have no influence on the episomal form of virus found in latently infected cells, which replicates using cellular enzymes. Thus, EBV-seropositive persons treated with acyclovir continue to have cultivable EBV in circulating lymphocytes (145). Despite this, however, acyclovir and ganciclovir have been used in PTLD, with occasional reports of success, and some experts recommend the use of acyclovir based on their early experience (51). Ganciclovir is more active than acyclovir against EBV in vitro and can effectively reduce the nasopharygeal excretion of EBV after SOT (109). Others have reported anecdotal experiences with acyclovir or ganciclovir for EBV infection after transplantation, and even interferon has also been used for treatment of PTLD, but the results are inconclusive. No formal evaluation of prophylactic ganciclovir or foscarnet for prevention of PTLD has been performed, but retrospective analysis found a lower incidence of PTLD in high-risk solid-organ transplant recipients who were administered i.v. ganciclovir followed by high-dose oral acyclovir (31). Because of the general use of ganciclovir for prevention of CMV disease in this population, it will be difficult to design an adequate controlled study of antiviral prevention of PTLD.

Cellular Immunotherapy

Because remissions of both polyclonal and monoclonal tumors can occur after reduction or withdrawal of immunosuppressive therapy, adoptive cellular immunotherapy directed toward improvement of immune function has been attempted, with remarkable results. Infusion of unirradiated donor leukocytes (approximately 10^6 $CD3^+$ T cells/kg) into recipients of T-cell-depleted marrow transplants who developed PTLD resulted in clinical responses within 8 to 21 days after infusion, including sustained remissions in three long-term survivors (104). Methods for preparing and genetically marking EBV-specific CTLs of donor origin have been developed, and these cells have been safely infused into marrow transplant recipients (76). This type of approach illustrates the potential for cellular therapy to eliminate EBV complications after transplantation.

Humoral Immunotherapy for PTLD of B-Cell Origin

The availability of monoclonal antibody therapy for B-cell lymphoid malignancy has greatly improved the management of PTLD. Rituximab, a mouse-human chimeric monoclonal antibody with specificity for CD20, a B-cell antigen, has been approved for treatment of B-cell lymphomas (77), and this agent has become useful in both prevention and treatment of PTLD. Rituximab at a dose of 375 mg/m^2, in four infusions over 1 month, resulted in an overall response rate of 69% in 32 PTLD patients, with 20 complete responses. The initial approach to PTLD is reduction in immunosuppression, then rituximab therapy, and, for resistant disease, conventional lymphoma chemoradiotherapy (39, 134). Current recommendations are for rituximab to be used preemptively when EBV PCR assays indicate increasing virus replication (98). Treatment with rituximab is given as 375 mg/m^2 i.v. in a single infusion and repeated weekly for up to 4 weeks if there is no decrease in EBV levels as determined by PCR. When administered early in the course of EBV infection, a single treatment can be sufficient. Adverse effects of rituximab include infusional reactions, and the agent should be given after antihistamine treatment.

OTHER HERPESVIRUSES

HSV and VZV

HSV and VZV infections are described in chapters 19 and 21, respectively. They manifest clinically after transplantation with the same type of infection and severity as seen in other immunosuppressed populations. Infection usually derives from reactivation of latent virus, with HSV manifesting as oral or genital skin infection, with the potential for visceral infection in the GI system or brain. VZV usually manifests as herpes zoster, with dissemination of infection in a proportion of patients depending on the level of immunosuppression. HSV reactivation occurs in approximately 70% of HSV-seropositive transplant recipients and can be suppressed with acyclovir (250 mg/m^2 i.v. twice daily for 1 month after transplantation). VZV reactivation occurs in up to 50% of allogeneic transplant recipients, and this can be prevented by long-term use of acyclovir (800 mg orally twice daily), although this is not an approved indication (10). For acyclovir-resistant HSV or VZV infection, foscarnet is substituted for treatment.

HHV-6 and -8

The epidemiology of HHV-6 and its important disease syndromes are described in chapter 23. Following bone marrow transplantation, HHV-6 reactivates in 36 to 46% of bone marrow transplant recipients during the first 2 to 3 months after transplantation (62). HHV-6 is neurotropic in other populations, and an evaluation of encephalitis after allogeneic bone marrow transplantation has suggested a correlation with HHV-6 infection. HHV-6 DNA has been identified in cerebrospinal fluid specimens from up to one-quarter of marrow transplant patients with CNS symptoms (140). HHV-6 encephalitis is associated with seizures and with abnormal electroencephalogram, but not with cerebrospinal fluid pleocytosis or pathognomonic findings from imaging studies. HHV-6 has also been associated with pneumonitis and with marrow failure. HHV-6 is susceptible to ganciclovir and foscarnet and only relatively susceptible to acyclovir (33). Foscarnet is generally used for treatment of this infection.

HHV-8 infection is associated with Kaposi's sarcoma, multicentric Castleman's disease, and primary effusion lymphoma, as discussed in more detail in chapter 25. Although rare, these syndromes have been observed in HHV-8-infected HCT and SOT recipients (3, 19), as have pancytopenia and other hematopoietic abnormalities (89). With the increase in organ transplantation in AIDS patients, complications of HHV-8 infection will undoubtedly be seen more frequently. Reduction in immunosuppression is the first approach to management of transplant recipients with symptomatic HHV-8 infection. Although there is no antiviral drug approved for HHV-8 infection, both ganciclovir and foscarnet are active against HHV-8 (33) and have been used in this setting.

HBV AND HCV

Pathogenesis of Viral Hepatitis after Transplantation

The pathogenesis of disease due to hepatitis B virus (HBV) and HCV is described elsewhere (see chapters 31 and 53, respectively). In the transplant population, HBV infection is influenced by genetic variants of these viruses. For example, the mutated precore region of HBV results in a stop codon that prevents cleavage and secretion of HBV e antigen (HbeAg) during virus replication (41). The presence of the HBV precore strain mutation appears to increase the risk of complications of HBV following liver transplantation. Those who are HBV DNA negative pretransplantation have no recurrence of HBV infection. Of those with wild-type virus detected pretransplantation, ~70%

become reinfected with HBV. Of those with precore mutant HBV strains noted pretransplantation, all become reinfected, and most of these will develop HBV-related graft loss or fibrosing cholestatic hepatitis.

HCV infection recurs in virtually all patients after liver transplantation. This can lead to chronic hepatitis of variable severity. HCV quasispecies complexity and diversity are greatest in those with the least severe hepatitis, and the level of viremia is predictive of the histologic severity of disease (122). This suggests that the potency of the immune response, which provides strong pressure for virus quasispecies dynamics, protects the recipient from progressive HCV hepatitis. It is likely that the main determinant of HCV disease in the transplant recipient will be shown to be the posttransplantation development of HCV-specific immune function.

Hepatitis Virus Infection in SOT

Much clinical information regarding HBV and HCV has come from the solid-organ transplant setting (30). As with marrow transplantation (see below), there are situations that are acceptable for both the donor and recipient to be hepatitis virus infected, although the outcome clearly is affected by the activity of virus infection. The risk of transmission of HBV is increased from donors who are HBV core antibody (HBcAb) positive but HBV surface antigen (HbsAg) negative. Some experts recommend not accepting livers from any donors with past HBV infection but accepting kidneys from donors who are both HBcAb positive and HBsAg negative.

Among 235 kidney transplant recipients infected with HBV, HCV, or both, chronic hepatitis developed in 50% of those who were HCV positive and HBV negative and in 64% of those who were both HCV and HBV positive (108). Liver failure occurred in 7% of the HCV-positive, HBV-negative patients and in 17% of the HCV-positive, HBV-positive patients. In renal transplant recipients who were either HBV or HCV infected, no difference in the prevalence of chronic hepatitis was noted. However, among those with chronic hepatitis in the HBV group, there was more frequent progression to end-stage liver disease or carcinoma. The 10-year follow-up of graft and patient survival following liver transplantation is not influenced by the HCV serostatus of the recipient (13). However, 90% of liver allografts show histologic evidence of hepatitis and 20% have cirrhosis at 5 years after transplantation (43).

Not only is the course of chronic hepatitis after renal transplantation more severe with HBV infection, but also the rate of acute rejection episodes appears to be increased (49). Graft survival rates were similar between groups with and without HBV infection after 1 year, but the rate was significantly lower in the HBV group 5 years after transplantation. The critical issue, of course, is the long-term survival of persons transplanted with HBV or HCV infection. Virtually all patients with severe chronic active hepatitis and the majority of those with even mild chronic active hepatitis will progress to cirrhosis following transplantation. The morbidity usually is not observed for 5 to 10 years posttransplantation, and no reliable markers for predicting outcome have been identified.

Hepatitis Virus Infection in HCT

The clinical course of HCT in persons receiving marrow from HBsAg-positive donors has been described previously (87). HBsAg positivity occurred transiently posttransplantation in approximately 25% of patients, and <10% became chronic HBsAg carriers. Antigenemia developed more frequently in those with no antibody to HBV surface antigen (HBsAb), but this pretransplantation antibody did not prevent antigenemia posttransplantation. Liver failure with death occurred in 20% of recipients, and those with anti-HBe-positive donors had a higher frequency of liver failure (28%, versus 0%). No liver failure occurred in recipients who were anti-HBsAb positive pretransplantation. The occurrence of veno-occlusive disease after HBV infection has not been confirmed, but fibrosing cholestatic hepatitis can be a serious complication of HBV infection in this setting.

Almost all HCV RNA-positive patients undergoing HCT show transaminase elevations between days 40 and 50 after HCT and again after day 100, when immunosuppression is reduced (90). Deaths due to hepatic failure may occur, although one long-term follow-up study of marrow recipients having HCV infection found no difference in the frequency or degree of liver dysfunction between patients who were HCV RNA positive and those who were negative prior to marrow transplantation (84). Subjects did develop severe liver dysfunction after transplantation, and this occurred in association with tapering of the immunosuppression. No patient developed liver failure, but serum transaminase levels were abnormal in 68% without evidence of liver cirrhosis.

Of 96 HCV-seropositive thalassemia patients undergoing allogeneic HCT, 4 had transient and 5 had persistent HCV seronegativity after transplantation. Again, the long-term survival was not influenced by the presence of HCV hepatitis in this group. No liver failure occurred in patients with anti-HCV antibody undergoing marrow transplantation, but it did occur in approximately 10% of those without pretransplantation HCV antibody who subsequently developed HCV infection (41).

Are marrow donors who are HCV antibody positive but HCV RNA negative able to transmit virus to the recipient? All patients undergoing HCT from HCV-seropositive donors can be expected to develop plasma HCV RNA after cell infusion from those with positive serum HCV RNA (125). However, the recipients of cells from donors who are only HCV antibody positive remain free of plasma HCV RNA.

In summary, HBV and HCV infection in a donor or recipient is not a contraindication for HCT. Experience suggests that HCV RNA levels in the serum of donors are predictive for transmission of infection to the recipient. The presence of anti-HCV antibody in the donor appears to predict a favorable outcome. Before transplantation, patients with hepatitis must be screened for status of liver dysfunction and might require a liver biopsy to rule out cirrhosis before proceeding with the transplantation.

Antiviral Management of HBV and HCV

Interferons were once the only treatment modality for HBV and HCV infection, but nucleoside analogs are now the preferred treatment for HBV infection (see chapters 12 and 31 for detailed discussions of the nucleoside analogs and their use for HBV infection). Ribavirin in combination with interferon is the approved treatment for HCV, but large-scale studies with transplant patients are not available (24) (see chapters 12 and 53 for treatment of HCV infection).

Hepatitis B Immunoglobulin

Whether HBV infection will recur after liver transplantation performed for chronic HBV with cirrhosis is determined by both host and viral factors, and the role of HBsAb in supporting the immunologic status of the recipient has been controversial (111). Early studies failed to prove convincingly the effectiveness of passive immunotherapy with hepatitis B immunoglobulin (HBIG), but HBIG may influence outcome. With the use of HBIG, most remain HBsAg negative during the course of HBIG therapy, but ultimately HBV reinfection occurs. Nevertheless, the long-term survival rate can be improved in chronic HBV-positive recipients, and HBIG is approved in the United States for prophylaxis in liver transplant recipients.

The duration of HBIG administration appears to be important, as one would expect in this chronic virus infection. Patients receiving only 1 week of prophylaxis developed HBV infection in nearly 90% of cases, and one-half of the patients lost their graft because of fulminant hepatitis. Among those who received long-term immunoprophylaxis, 43% developed HBV reinfection. The preoperative level of HBV DNA was predictive for virologic outcome irrespective of the use of the immunoprophylaxis. The dosing is undoubtedly important, and it has been recommended to keep the anti-HBsA levels above 400 IU/ml during the posttransplantation period.

HBIG in combination with lamivudine has shown promise for control of infection of the allograft, but the optimal timing, patient selection, and duration of therapy remain issues to be resolved (35). The cost-effectiveness of using lamivudine plus HBIG has been evaluated, and combination therapy was a significant cost-effective strategy in a setting of liver transplantation in the presence of HBV infection (50).

AV INFECTION IN TRANSPLANT PATIENTS

AV infection can be isolated by tissue culture from approximately 5 to 20% of HCT recipients, but when surveillance includes PCR and electron microscopy of stool, infection can be documented in a high proportion of patients, with incidence rates of 60 to 90% in the first 3 months in pediatric populations (23, 96). Infection occurs in the respiratory tract, eyes, GI tract, and bladder, and the most frequent site of infection is the GI tract. AV-associated hemorrhagic cystitis can be a particular problem in this population (18, 96). Approximately two-thirds of PCR-based infections are asymptomatic, and disease risk is related to the level of immunodeficiency (96). HCT recipients of T-cell-depleted or nonrelated donor grafts and those with severe GVHD are at highest risk (22). Blood infection, as monitored with PCR, is associated with a high risk of disease (18), and disseminated AV can result in fulminant hepatitis, nephritis, and other life-threatening organ involvement. In a cohort of 5,000 HCT recipients, for example, AV infection occurred in 8 to 12% of allogeneic HCT recipients and 6% of autologous HCT recipients (18).

Treatment is based on a preemptive management strategy for those at highest risk, with monitoring of stool and blood by PCR. Reduction in immunosuppressant therapy is the first line of treatment, since there is no agent currently approved for treatment of AV in the United States. Of note, preemptive ganciclovir use has been associated with a significantly lower risk of AV infection (18). Cidofovir has been used for AV infection in uncontrolled studies, and there is no single recommended dosing regimen. Low-dose cidofovir (1 mg/kg i.v. three times weekly for 2 weeks with probenicid) (57) and 3- to 5-mg/kg doses (86) have been used in the treatment of AV infection. In these uncontrolled studies, cidofovir has been used with or without ribavirin (127). Adoptive T-cell immunotherapy has also been proposed as a treatment for AV infection in high-risk patients (76).

POLYOMAVIRUS INFECTIONS IN TRANSPLANT RECIPIENTS

Of the polyomaviruses of humans, BK virus and JC virus produce disease in transplant recipients. Polyomaviruses are ubiquitous in humans, and infection is acquired at an early age (see chapter 27). Excretion of both BK and JC viruses in the urine is common in the transplant population (4), as is polyomavirus DNA in blood after transplantation (12). These viruses share common gene sequences, and there is cross-reactive T-cell immunity to both BK and JC viruses (73).

BK Virus Infection

BK virus infection is common in SOT (7) but is a particular problem in renal transplant recipients (32). BK virus infection of the kidney produces an interstitial nephritis that mimics acute rejection, but this can be differentiated from rejection effects by the presence of viral antigen or DNA and by an increase in B cells (1). In addition to interstitial nephritis, BK virus has been linked to ureteric stenosis and hemorrhagic cystitis. BK virus can be detected in urine from approximately 50% of HCT recipients, and in this population it is not clear whether the hemorrhagic cystis is due to prior chemotherapy, to BK virus, or to other viruses such as AV (9). Although frequently associated with cystitis, BK virus excretion has been observed in up to 30% of HCT recipients without hemorrhagic cystitis. Nevertheless, when the BK virus infection is characterized by quantitative BK virus DNA measurement in urine, there is a correlation between disease and virus load (81). Although unapproved for this indication, low-dose cidofovir (1 mg/kg three times weekly) has been used for treatment of symptomatic BK virus infection (63).

JC Virus Infection

Progressive multifocal leukoencephalopathy (PML) is a rare but serious occurrence in SOT and marrow transplantation (16). JC virus infects oligodendrocytes of the CNS, leading to a fatal demyelinization disease characterized by hemiparesis, seizures, deteriorating mental status, and death. JC virus infection, although thought of as a CNS problem, has been observed in 37% of cases of interstitial nephritis after renal transplantation (4). Regarding therapy, reduction in immunosuppression is most important. The largest experience with antiviral treatment of PML, using cidofovir, is in AIDS, and it is not clear whether cidofovir treatment with adequate antiretroviral therapy is any more effective than use of antiretroviral therapy alone (71). Cidofovir has been used in SOT and HCT recipients with PML without the success observed in AIDS.

RESPIRATORY VIRAL INFECTIONS IN TRANSPLANT RECIPIENTS

The common respiratory virus infections, i.e., with respiratory syncytial virus, parainfluenza virus, influenza virus, and human metapneumovirus, occur in transplant patients, and except for the potential for serious pulmonary complications, the infections are not qualitatively different from those seen in otherwise healthy populations. The description and management of these infections are presented elsewhere in this volume (see chapters 36 and 42).

UNUSUAL INFECTIONS ASSOCIATED WITH TRANSPLANT GRAFTS

The time between donor death and organ procurement does not allow for testing for rare infections within the policies of the National Organ Procurement and Transplantation Network (see http://www.optn.org/policiesAndBylaws/charterAndBylaws.asp). For this reason, SOT recipients will continue to be at risk for certain infections such as rabies, West Nile virus, and CJD. Rabies was first transmitted from human to human via a corneal transplant more than 30 years ago, and since then rabies has been transmitted with SOT grafts (129). Rabies should be part of the differential diagnosis of any transplant patient who develops encephalitis within the first 30 days after SOT or HCT. Similarly, West Nile virus infection can be transmitted by means of organ transplantation (60).

The transmissible spongiform encephalopathies can be transmitted from person to person by direct inoculation of prions, and the acquired or iatrogenic form of CJD is rare, accounting for less than 1% of CJD cases (28). Organ grafts, especially cadaveric cornea and dura, have been associated with transmission of CJD (101), but posttransplantation CJD has been waning in incidence since the peak in the 1990s and is now extremely rare (17). The incubation period for disease is a function of inoculum exposure, with onset of cornea-related CJD at 16 to 28 months and of dura-transmitted disease at 18 months to 18 years (28). Disease presentation also differs with exposure, with cornea-related CJD manifesting as dementia and dura-related disease manifesting as ataxic gait and relatively slow progression (28, 101). A variant of CJD is transmitted from animals with bovine spongiform encephalopathy (mad cow disease) to humans and has been associated with blood transfusions, but it has not yet been observed after SOT (28). There is no treatment for CJD, and prevention of transmission by SOT is done by rigorous screening of the medical history of potential tissue donors.

VIRUS INFECTIONS OF XENOTRANSPLANTATION

Xenotransplantation is defined as any procedure that involves the transplantation, implantation, or infusion into a human recipient of either (i) "live cells," tissues, or organs from a nonhuman animal source or (ii) human body fluids, cells, tissues, or organs that have had ex vivo contact with live nonhuman animal cells, tissues, or organs. Because of the increasing clinical need for life-saving organ transplantation to replace diseased organs and the current use of vascular and valvular tissues from nonhuman animal sources in clinical medicine, there is a concern about development of infections in this setting. A U.S. Public Health Service Guideline discussing infectious-disease issues in xenotransplantation was published in 2001 (22). This guideline emphasizes that transplantation clinicians and infectious-disease specialists have a responsibility to participate in the oversight, education, and implementation of xenotransplantation protocols. Thus, it is important to understand the infectious-disease risks and the methods of reducing these risks for both the recipients and their close contacts. The guideline further emphasizes that the education and counseling process for the recipients and their close contacts, including associated health care professionals, is the responsibility of the transplant team, including the infectious-disease consultants. Infectious-disease public health concerns about xenotransplantation focus not just on transmission of potential zoonoses but also on transmission of infectious agents as yet unrecognized (106).

Under current guidelines, nonhuman primate tissues are restricted from xenotransplantation in the United States because of concern about cross-species transmission of infections which might be more common or more serious when derived from a closely related species (22). To date, the largest experience in xenotransplantation is with use of swine-derived cell products or tissues. Swine have been shown to have at least three types of viruses of significance to humans, namely, pig endogenous retrovirus (PERV), swine hepatitis E virus (HEV), and a porcine gammaherpesvirus capable of producing PTLD (22). Viruses such as swine HEV are very closely related to human HEV, and source herds can be screened to eliminate this as a problem. However, PERVs are present in germ line tissue, and since there are three classes of PERV known to infect human cells, considerable attention has been directed at the issue of PERV-related disease in humans (22). To date, long-term studies of pig-to-human xenotransplantation have failed to demonstrate evidence of PERV infection in humans exposed to pig tissue (105).

REFERENCES

1. **Ahuja, M., E. P. Cohen, A. M. Dayer, B. Kampalath, C. C. Chang, B. A. Bresnahan, and S. Hariharan.** 2001. Polyoma virus infection after renal transplantation. Use of immunostaining as a guide to diagnosis. *Transplantation* **71:**896–899.
2. **Andersson, J., B. Skoldenberg, W. Henle, G. Giesecke, A. Ortqvist, and I. Julander.** 1986. Effect of acyclovir on infectious mononucleosis: a double-blind, placebo-controlled study. *J. Infect. Dis.* **153:**283–290.
3. **Andreoni, M., D. Goletti, P. Pezzotti, A. Pozzetto, P. Monini, L. Sarmati, F. Farchi, G. Tisone, A. Piazza, F. Pisani, M. Angelico, P. Leone, F. Citterio, B. Ensoli, and G. Rezza.** 2001. Prevalence, incidence and correlates of HHV-8/KSHV infection and Kaposi's sarcoma in renal and liver transplant recipients. *J. Infect.* **43:**195–199.
4. **Baksh, F. K., S. D. Finkelstein, P. A. Swalsky, G. L. Stoner, C. F. Ryschkewitsch, and P. Randhawa.** 2001. Molecular genotyping of BK and JC viruses in human polyomavirus-associated interstitial nephritis after renal transplantation. *Am. J. Kidney Dis.* **38:**354–365.
5. **Balfour, H. H., Jr., B. A. Chace, J. T. Stapleton, R. L. Simmons, and D. S. Fryd.** 1989. A randomized, placebo-controlled trial of oral acyclovir for the prevention of cytomegalovirus disease in recipients of renal allografts. *N. Engl. J. Med.* **320:**1381–1387.
6. **Bando, K., I. L. Paradis, S. Similo, H. Konishi, K. Komatsu, T. G. Zullo, S. A. Yousem, J. M. Close, A. Zeevi, and R. J. Duquesnoy.** 1995. Obliterative bronchiolitis af-

ter lung and heart-lung transplantation. An analysis of risk factors and management. *J. Thorac. Cardiovasc. Surg.* **110:**4–13.

7. **Barton, T. D., E. A. Blumberg, A. Doyle, V. N. Ahya, J. M. Ferrenberg, S. C. Brozena, and A. P. Limaye.** 2006. A prospective cross-sectional study of BK virus infection in non-renal solid organ transplant recipients with chronic renal dysfunction. *Transplant Infect. Dis.* **8:**102–107.
8. **Basgoz, N., and J. K. Preiksaitis.** 1995. Post-transplant lymphoproliferative disorder. *Infect. Dis. Clin. N. Am.* **9:** 901–923.
9. **Bedi, A., C. B. Miller, J. L. Hanson, S. Goodman, R. F. Ambinder, P. Charache, R. R. Arthur, and R. J. Jones.** 1995. Association of BK virus with failure of prophylaxis against hemorrhagic cystitis following bone marrow transplantation. *J. Clin. Oncol.* **13:**1103–1109.
10. **Boeckh, M., H. W. Kim, M. E. Flowers, J. D. Meyers, and R. A. Bowden.** 2006. Long-term acyclovir for prevention of varicella zoster virus disease after allogeneic hematopoietic cell transplantation—a randomized double-blind placebo-controlled study. *Blood* **107:**1800–1805.
11. **Boeckh, M., W. Leisenring, S. R. Riddell, R. A. Bowden, M. L. Huang, D. Myerson, T. Stevens-Ayers, M. E. Flowers, T. Cunningham, and L. Corey.** 2003. Late cytomegalovirus disease and mortality in recipients of allogeneic hematopoietic stem cell transplants: importance of viral load and T-cell immunity. *Blood* **101:**407–414.
12. **Bogdanovic, G., P. Ljungman, F. Wang, and T. Dalianis.** 1996. Presence of human polyomavirus DNA in the peripheral circulation of bone marrow transplant patients with and without hemorrhagic cystitis. *Bone Marrow Transplant.* **17:**573–576.
13. **Boker, K., G. Dalley, and M. Bahr.** 1997. Long-term outcome of hepatitis C virus infection after liver transplantation. *Hepatology* **25:**203–210.
14. **Boland, G. J., R. J. Hene, C. Ververs, M. A. M. DeHaan, and G. C. DeGast.** 1993. Factors influencing the occurrence of active cytomegalovirus (CMV) infections after organ transplantation. *Clin. Exp. Immunol.* **94:** 306–312.
15. **Bowden, R. A., S. J. Slichter, M. H. Sayers, M. Mori, M. J. Cays, and J. D. Meyers.** 1991. Use of leukocyte-depleted platelets and cytomegalovirus-seronegative red blood cells for prevention of primary cytomegalovirus infection after marrow transplant. *Blood* **78:**246–250.
16. **Bronster, D. J., M. W. Lidov, D. Wolfe, M. E. Schwartz, and C. M. Miller.** 1995. Progressive multifocal leukoencephalopathy after orthotopic liver transplantation. *Liver Transplant. Surg.* **1:**371–372.
17. **Brown, P., J. P. Brandel, M. Preece, and T. Sato.** 2006. Iatrogenic Creutzfeldt-Jakob disease: the waning of an era. *Neurology* **67:**389–393.
18. **Bruno, B., T. Gooley, R. C. Hackman, C. Davis, L. Corey, and M. Boeckh.** 2003. Adenovirus infection in hematopoietic stem cell transplantation: effect of ganciclovir and impact on survival. *Biol. Blood Marrow Transplant.* **9:**341–352.
19. **Bruno, B., R. Sorasio, P. Barozzi, J. Vieira, P. Omede, F. Giaretta, M. Rotta, L. Giaccone, M. Massaia, M. Luppi, and M. Boccadoro.** 2006. Kaposi's sarcoma triggered by endogenous HHV-8 reactivation after non-myeloablative allogeneic haematopoietic transplantation. *Eur. J. Haematol.* **76:**342–347.
20. **Buchsbaum, R. J., J. A. Fabry, and J. Lieberman.** 1996. EBV-specific cytotoxic T lymphocytes protect against human EBV-associated lymphoma in scid mice. *Immunol. Lett.* **52:**145–150.
21. **Cen, H., M. C. Breinig, R. W. Atchison, M. Ho, and J. L. McKnight.** 1991. Epstein-Barr virus transmission via the donor organs in solid organ transplantation: polymerase chain reaction and restriction fragment length polymorphism analysis of IR2, IR3, and IR4. *J. Virol.* **65:**976–980.
22. **Centers for Disease Control and Prevention.** 2001. U.S. Public Health Service guideline on infectious disease issues in xenotransplantation. *Morb. Mortal. Wkly. Rep. Recomm. Rep.* **50:**1–46.
23. **Chakrabarti, S.** 2007. Adenovirus infections after hematopoietic stem cell transplantation: still unravelling the story. *Clin. Infect. Dis.* **45:**966–968.
24. **Chou, S. W.** 1986. Acquisition of donor strains of cytomegalovirus by renal-transplant recipients. *N. Engl. J. Med.* **314:**1418–1423.
25. **Cobbold, M., N. Khan, B. Pourgheysari, S. Tauro, D. McDonald, H. Osman, M. Assenmacher, L. Billingham, C. Steward, C. Crawley, E. Olavarria, J. Goldman, R. Chakraverty, P. Mahendra, C. Craddock, and P. A. Moss.** 2005. Adoptive transfer of cytomegalovirus-specific CTL to stem cell transplant patients after selection by HLA-peptide tetramers. *J. Exp. Med.* **202:**379–386.
26. **Cohen, J. I.** 1991. Epstein-Barr virus lymphoproliferative disease associated with acquired immunodeficiency. *Medicine* (Baltimore) **70:**17–60.
27. **Cole, N. L., and H. H. Balfour, Jr.** 1987. In vitro susceptibility of cytomegalovirus isolates from immunocompromised patients to acyclovir and ganciclovir. *Diagn. Microbiol. Infect. Dis.* **6:**255–261.
28. **Collins, S. J., V. A. Lawson, and C. L. Masters.** 2004. Transmissible spongiform encephalopathies. *Lancet* **363:** 51–61.
29. **Cwynarski, K., J. Ainsworth, M. Cobbold, S. Wagner, P. Mahendra, J. Apperley, J. Goldman, C. Craddock, and P. A. Moss.** 2001. Direct visualization of cytomegalovirus-specific T-cell reconstitution after allogeneic stem cell transplantation. *Blood* **97:**1232–1240.
30. **Davis, C. L., D. R. Gretch, and R. L. Carithers, Jr.** 1995. Hepatitis B and transplantation. *Infect. Dis. Clin. N. Am.* **9:**925–941.
31. **Davis, C. L., K. L. Harrison, J. P. McVicar, P. J. Forg, M. P. Bronner, and C. L. Marsh.** 1995. Antiviral prophylaxis and the Epstein-Barr virus-related post-transplant lymphoproliferative disorder. *Clin. Transplant.* **9:**53–59.
32. **de Bruyn, G., and A. P. Limaye.** 2004. BK virus-associated nephropathy in kidney transplant recipients. *Rev. Med. Virol.* **14:**193–205.
33. **De Clercq, E., L. Naesens, L. De Bolle, D. Schols, Y. Zhang, and J. Neyts.** 2001. Antiviral agents active against human herpesviruses HHV-6, HHV-7 and HHV-8. *Rev. Med. Virol.* **11:**381–395.
34. **Deodhar, S. D., A. G. Kuklinca, D. Vidt, A. L. Robertson, and J. B. Hazard.** 1969. Development of reticulum-cell sarcoma at the site of antilymphocyte globulin injection in a patient with renal transplant. *N. Engl. J. Med.* **280:**1104–1106.
35. **Dodson, S. F., M. E. de Vera, C. A. Bonham, D. A. Geller, J. Rakela, and J. J. Fung.** 2000. Lamivudine after hepatitis B immune globulin is effective in preventing hepatitis B recurrence after liver transplantation. *Liver Transplant.* **6:**434–439.
36. **Dunn, D. L., K. J. Gillingham, M. A. Kramer, W. J. Schmidt, A. Erice, H. H. Balfour, Jr., P. F. Gores, R. W. B. Gruessner, A. J. Matas, W. D. Payne, D. E. R. Sutherland, and J. S. Najarian.** 1994. A prospective randomized study of acyclovir versus ganciclovir plus human immune globulin prophylaxis for cytomegalovirus in-

fection after solid organ transplantation. *Transplantation* **57:**876–884.

37. **Einsele, H., G. Ehninger, H. Hebart, P. Weber, S. Dette, H. Link, H. P. Horny, V. Meuter, S. Wagner, H. D. Waller, et al.** 1994. Incidence of local CMV infection and acute intestinal GVHD in marrow transplant recipients with severe diarrhoea. *Bone Marrow Transplant.* **14:**955–963.
38. **Einsele, H., E. Roosnek, N. Rufer, C. Sinzger, S. Riegler, J. Loffler, U. Grigoleit, A. Moris, H. G. Rammensee, L. Kanz, A. Kleihauer, F. Frank, G. Jahn, and H. Hebart.** 2002. Infusion of cytomegalovirus (CMV)-specific T cells for the treatment of CMV infection not responding to antiviral chemotherapy. *Blood* **99:**3916–3922.
39. **Elstrom, R. L., C. Andreadis, N. A. Aqui, V. N. Ahya, R. D. Bloom, S. C. Brozena, K. M. Olthoff, S. J. Schuster, S. D. Nasta, E. A. Stadtmauer, and D. E. Tsai.** 2006. Treatment of PTLD with rituximab or chemotherapy. *Am. J. Transplant.* **6:**569–576.
40. **Evans, P. C., A. Soin, T. G. Wreghitt, C. J. Taylor, D. G. Wight, and G. J. Alexander.** 2000. An association between cytomegalovirus infection and chronic rejection after liver transplantation. *Transplantation* **69:**30–35.
41. **Fujii, Y., K. Kaku, M. Tanaka, and T. Kaneko.** 1994. Hepatitis C virus infection and liver disease after allogeneic bone marrow transplantation. *Bone Marrow Transplant.* **13:**523–526.
42. **Gane, E., F. Saliba, G. J. C. Valdecasas, J. O'Grady, M. D. Pescovitz, S. Lyman, and C. A. Robinson for The Oral Ganciclovir International Transplantation Study Group.** 1997. Randomised trial of efficacy and safety of oral ganciclovir in the prevention of cytomegalovirus disease in liver-transplant recipients. *Lancet* **350:**1729–1733.
43. **Gane, E. J., B. C. Portmann, and N. V. Naoumouv.** 1996. Long-term outcome of hepatitis C infection after liver transplantation. *N. Engl. J. Med.* **334:**821–827.
44. **Goodrich, J. M., R. A. Bowden, L. Fisher, C. Keller, G. Schoch, and J. D. Meyers.** 1993. Ganciclovir prophylaxis to prevent cytomegalovirus disease after allogeneic marrow transplant. *Ann. Intern. Med.* **118:**173–178.
45. **Goodrich, J. M., M. Mori, C. A. Gleaves, C. Du Mond, M. Cays, D. F. Ebeling, W. C. Buhles, B. DeArmond, and J. D. Meyers.** 1991. Early treatment with ganciclovir to prevent cytomegalovirus disease after allogeneic bone marrow transplantation. *N. Engl. J. Med.* **325:**1601–1607.
46. **Gratama, J. W., and J. J. Cornelissen.** 2003. Diagnostic potential of tetramer-based monitoring of cytomegalovirus-specific CD8$^+$ T lymphocytes in allogeneic stem cell transplantation. *Clin. Immunol.* **106:**29–35.
47. **Gratama, J. W., J. A. P. Oosterveer, J. M. M. Lepoutre, J. J. van Rood, F. E. Zwaan, J. M. J. J. Vossen, J. G. Kapsenberg, D. Richel, G. Klein, and I. Ernberg.** 1990. Serological and molecular studies of Epstein-Barr virus infection in allogeneic marrow graft recipients. *Transplantation* **49:**725–730.
48. **Grattan, M. T., C. E. Moreno-Cabral, V. A. Starnes, P. E. Oyer, E. B. Stinson, and N. E. Shumway.** 1989. Cytomegalovirus infection is associated with cardiac allograft rejection and atherosclerosis. *JAMA* **261:**3561–3566.
49. **Grekas, D., C. Dioudis, K. Mandraveli, and P. Alivanis.** 1995. Renal transplantation in asymptomatic carriers of hepatitis B surface antigen. *Nephron* **69:**267–272.
50. **Han, S. H., J. Ofman, C. Holt, K. King, G. Kunder, P. Chen, S. Dawson, L. Goldstein, H. Yersiz, D. G. Farmer, R. M. Ghobrial, R. W. Busuttil, and P. Martin.** 2000. An efficacy and cost-effectiveness analysis of combination hepatitis B immune globulin and lamivudine to prevent recurrent hepatitis B after orthotopic liver transplantation compared with hepatitis B immune globulin monotherapy. *Liver Transplant.* **6:**741–748.
51. **Hanto, D. W., G. Fizzera, and K. J. Gajl-Peczalska.** 1982. Epstein-Barr virus (EBV)-induced B cells lymphoma after renal transplantation: acyclovir therapy and transition from polyclonal to monoclonal B-cell proliferation. *N. Engl. J. Med.* **306:**913–918.
52. **Henle, G., W. Henle, and R. Dielh.** 1968. Relation of Burkitt's tumor-associated herpes-type virus to infectious mononucleosis. *Proc. Natl. Acad. Sci. USA* **59:**94–101.
53. **Hibberd, P. L., and D. R. Snydman.** 1995. Cytomegalovirus infection in organ transplant recipients. *Infect. Dis. Clin. N. Am.* **9:**863–877.
54. **Ho, M.** 1991. *Cytomegalovirus, Biology and Infection*, 2nd ed. Plenum Publishing, New York, NY.
55. **Ho, M., G. Miller, and R. W. Atchinson.** 1985. Epstein-Barr virus infections and DNA hybridization studies in post-transplantation lymphoma and lymphoproliferative lesions: the role of primary infection. *J. Infect. Dis.* **152:** 876–886.
56. **Ho, M., S. Suwansirikul, J. N. Dowling, L. A. Youngblood, and J. A. Armstrong.** 1975. The transplanted kidney as a source of cytomegalovirus infections. *N. Engl. J. Med.* **293:**1109–1112.
57. **Hoffman, J. A., A. J. Shah, L. A. Ross, and N. Kapoor.** 2001. Adenoviral infections and a prospective trial of cidofovir in pediatric hematopoietic stem cell transplantation. *Biol. Blood Marrow Transplant.* **7:**388–394.
58. **Höglund, M., P. Ljungman, and S. Weller.** 2001. Comparable aciclovir exposures produced by oral valaciclovir and intravenous aciclovir in immunocompromised cancer patients. *J. Antimicrob. Chemother.* **47:**855–861.
59. **Ison, M. G.** 2007. Respiratory viral infections in transplant recipients. *Antivir. Ther.* **12:**627–638.
60. **Iwamoto, M., D. B. Jernigan, A. Guasch, M. J. Trepka, C. G. Blackmore, W. C. Hellinger, S. M. Pham, S. Zaki, R. S. Lanciotti, S. E. Lance-Parker, C. A. Diaz-Granados, A. G. Winquist, C. A. Perlino, S. Wiersma, K. L. Hillyer, J. L. Goodman, A. A. Marfin, M. E. Chamberland, and L. R. Petersen.** 2003. Transmission of West Nile virus from an organ donor to four transplant recipients. *N. Engl. J. Med.* **348:**2196–2203.
61. **Jacobson, M. A., and J. Mills.** 1988. Serious cytomegalovirus disease in the acquired immunodeficiency syndrome (AIDS). Clinical findings, diagnosis, and treatment. *Ann. Intern. Med.* **108:**585–594.
62. **Kadakia, M. P., W. B. Rybka, and J. A. Stewart.** 1996. Human herpesvirus-6 infection in bone marrow transplantation. *Blood* **87:**5341–5354.
63. **Kadambi, P. V., M. A. Josephson, J. Williams, L. Corey, K. R. Jerome, S. M. Meehan, and A. P. Limaye.** 2003. Treatment of refractory BK virus-associated nephropathy with cidofovir. *Am. J. Transplant.* **3:**186–191.
64. **Kalil, A. C., J. Levitsky, E. Lyden, J. Stoner, and A. G. Freifeld.** 2005. Meta-analysis: the efficacy of strategies to prevent organ disease by cytomegalovirus in solid organ transplant recipients. *Ann. Intern. Med.* **143:**870–880.
65. **Kanich, R. E.** 1966. Human cytomegalovirus and cytomegalovirus disease in renal homotransplant recipients. *Am. J. Med.* **40:**8874–8882.
66. **Kenagy, D. N., Y. Schlesinger, K. Weck, J. H. Ritter, M. M. Gaudreault-Keener, and G. A. Storch.** 1995. Epstein-Barr virus DNA in peripheral blood leukocytes of patients with posttransplant lymphoproliferative disease. *Transplantation* **60:**547.

67. **Khoury, J. A., G. A. Storch, D. L. Bohl, R. M. Schuessler, S. M. Torrence, M. Lockwood, M. Gaudreault-Keener, M. J. Koch, B. W. Miller, K. L. Hardinger, M. A. Schnitzler, and D. C. Brennan.** 2006. Prophylactic versus preemptive oral valganciclovir for the management of cytomegalovirus infection in adult renal transplant recipients. *Am. J. Transplant.* **6:**2134–2143.
68. **Klein, G.** 1994. Epstein-Barr virus strategy in normal and neoplastic B cells. *Cell* **77:**791–793.
69. **Klein, G.** 1979. Lymphoma development in mice and human: diversity of initiation is followed by convergent cytogenetic evolution. *Proc. Natl. Acad. Sci. USA* **76:**2442–2446.
70. **Klemola, E.** 1973. Cytomegalovirus infection in previously healthy adults. *Ann. Intern. Med.* **79:**267–268.
71. **Kraemer, C., S. Evers, T. Nolting, G. Arendt, and I. W. Husstedt.** 18 January 2008. Cidofovir in combination with HAART and survival in AIDS-associated progressive multifocal leukoencephalopathy. *J. Neurol.* doi: 10.1007/s00415-008-0731-z.
72. **Krause, H., H. Hebart, G. Jahn, C. A. Muller, and H. Einsele.** 1997. Screening for CMV-specific T cell proliferation to identify patients at risk of developing late onset CMV disease. *Bone Marrow Transplant.* **19:**1111–1116.
73. **Krymskaya, L., M. C. Sharma, J. Martinez, W. Haq, E. C. Huang, A. P. Limaye, D. J. Diamond, and S. F. Lacey.** 2005. Cross-reactivity of T lymphocytes recognizing a human cytotoxic T-lymphocyte epitope within BK and JC virus VP1 polypeptides. *J. Virol.* **79:**11170–11178.
74. **Lacey, S. F., D. J. Diamond, and J. A. Zaia.** 2004. Assessment of cellular immunity to human cytomegalovirus in recipients of allogeneic stem cell transplants. *Biol. Blood Marrow Transplant.* **10:**433–447.
75. **Lacey, S. F., G. Gallez-Hawkins, M. Crooks, J. Martinez, D. Senitzer, S. J. Forman, R. Spielberger, J. A. Zaia, and D. J. Diamond.** 2002. Characterization of cytotoxic function of CMV-pp65-specific $CD8^+$ T-lymphocytes identified by HLA tetramers in recipients and donors of stem-cell transplants. *Transplantation* **74:**722–732.
76. **Leen, A. M., G. D. Myers, U. Sili, M. H. Huls, H. Weiss, K. S. Leung, G. Carrum, R. A. Krance, C. C. Chang, J. J. Molldrem, A. P. Gee, M. K. Brenner, H. E. Heslop, C. M. Rooney, and C. M. Bollard.** 2006. Monoculture-derived T lymphocytes specific for multiple viruses expand and produce clinically relevant effects in immunocompromised individuals. *Nat. Med.* **12:**1160–1166.
77. **Leget, G. A., and M. S. Czuczman.** 1998. Use of rituximab, the new FDA-approved antibody. *Curr. Opin. Oncol.* **10:**548–551.
78. **Li, C. R., P. D. Greenberg, M. J. Gilbert, J. M. Goodrich, and S. R. Riddell.** 1994. Recovery of HLA-restricted cytomegalovirus (CMV)-specific T-cell responses after allogeneic bone marrow transplant: correlation with CMV disease and effect of ganciclovir prophylaxis. *Blood* **83:**1971–1979.
79. **Limaye, A. P., L. Corey, D. M. Koelle, C. L. Davis, and M. Boeckh.** 2000. Emergence of ganciclovir-resistant cytomegalovirus disease among recipients of solid-organ transplants. *Lancet* **356:**645–649.
80. **Limaye, A. P., M. L. Huang, E. E. Atienza, J. M. Ferrenberg, and L. Corey.** 1999. Detection of Epstein-Barr virus DNA in sera from transplant recipients with lymphoproliferative disorders. *J. Clin. Microbiol.* **37:**1113–1116.
81. **Limaye, A. P., K. R. Jerome, C. S. Kuhr, J. Ferrenberg, M. L. Huang, C. L. Davis, L. Corey, and C. L. Marsh.** 2001. Quantitation of BK virus load in serum for the diagnosis of BK virus-associated nephropathy in renal transplant recipients. *J. Infect. Dis.* **183:**1669–1672.
82. **Ljungman, P., J. Aschan, J. N. Azinge, L. Brandt, A. Ehrnst, V. Hammarström, S. Klaesson, A. Linde, B. Lönnqvist, O. Ringdén, et al.** 1993. Cytomegalovirus viraemia and specific T-helper cell responses as predictors of disease after allogeneic marrow transplantation. *Br. J. Haematol.* **83:**118–124.
83. **Ljungman, P., G. L. Deliliers, U. Platzbecker, S. Matthes-Martin, A. Bacigalupo, H. Einsele, J. Ullmann, M. Musso, R. Trenschel, P. Ribaud, M. Bornhäuser, S. Cesaro, B. Crooks, A. Dekker, N. Gratecos, T. Klingebiel, E. Tagliaferri, A. J. Ullmann, P. Wacker, and C. Cordonnier for the Infectious Diseases Working Party of the European Group for Blood and Marrow Transplantation.** 2001. Cidofovir for cytomegalovirus infection and disease in allogeneic stem cell transplant recipients. *Blood* **97:**388–392.
84. **Ljungman, P., N. Johansson, J. Aschan, and H. Glaumann.** 1995. Long-term effects of hepatitis C virus infection in allogeneic bone marrow transplant recipients. *Blood* **86:**1614–1618.
85. **Ljungman, P., G. Oberg, J. Aschan, A. Ehrnst, B. Lonnqvist, K. Pauksen, and P. Sulila.** 1996. Foscarnet for pre-emptive therapy of CMV infection detected by a leukocyte-based nested PCR in allogeneic bone marrow transplant patients. *Bone Marrow Transplant.* **18:**565–568.
86. **Ljungman, P., P. Ribaud, M. Eyrich, S. Matthes-Martin, H. Einsele, M. Bleakley, M. Machaczka, M. Bierings, A. Bosi, N. Gratecos, and C. Cordonnier.** 2003. Cidofovir for adenovirus infections after allogeneic hematopoietic stem cell transplantation: a survey by the Infectious Diseases Working Party of the European Group for Blood and Marrow Transplantation. *Bone Marrow Transplant.* **31:**481–486.
87. **Locasciulli, A., A. Alberti, G. Bandini, and P. Polchi.** 1995. Allogeneic bone marrow transplantation from HBsAg+ donors: a multicenter study from the Gruppo Italiano Trapianto di Midollo Osseo (GITMO). *Blood* **86:**3236–3240.
88. **Lowance, D., H.-H. Neumayer, C. M. Legendre, J.-P. Squifflet, J. Kovarik, P. J. Brennan, D. Norman, R. Mendez, M. R. Keating, G. L. Coggon, A. Crisp, and I. C. Lee for The International Valacyclovir Cytomegalovirus Prophylaxis Transplantation Study Group.** 1999. Valacyclovir for the prevention of cytomegalovirus disease after renal transplantation. *N. Engl. J. Med.* **340:**1462–1470.
89. **Luppi, M., P. Barozzi, V. Rasini, G. Riva, A. Re, G. Rossi, G. Setti, S. Sandrini, F. Facchetti, and G. Torelli.** 2002. Severe pancytopenia and hemophagocytosis after HHV-8 primary infection in a renal transplant patient successfully treated with foscarnet. *Transplantation* **74:**131–132.
90. **Maruta, A., H. Kanamori, H. Fukawa, and H. Harano.** 1994. Liver function tests of recipients with hepatitis C virus infection after bone marrow transplantation. *Bone Marrow Transplant.* **13:**417–422.
91. **Meyers, J. D., N. Flournoy, and E. D. Thomas.** 1982. Nonbacterial pneumonia after allogeneic marrow transplantation: a review of ten years' experience. *Rev. Infect. Dis.* **4:**1119–1132.
92. **Meyers, J. D., N. Flournoy, and E. D. Thomas.** 1986. Risk factors for cytomegalovirus infection after human marrow transplantation. *J. Infect. Dis.* **153:**478–488.
93. **Meyers, J. D., P. Ljungman, and L. D. Fisher.** 1990. Cytomegalovirus excretion as a predictor of cytomegalovirus disease after marrow transplantation: importance of cytomegalovirus viremia. *J. Infect. Dis.* **162:**373–380.

94. **Meyers, J. D., E. C. Reed, D. H. Shepp, M. Thornquist, P. S. Dandliker, C. A. Vicary, N. Flournoy, L. E. Kirk, J. H. Kersey, E. D. Thomas, et al.** 1988. Acyclovir for prevention of cytomegalovirus infection and disease after allogeneic marrow transplantation. *N. Engl. J. Med.* **318:**70–75.

95. **Micallef, I. N., M. Chhanabhai, R. D. Gascoyne, J. D. Shepherd, H. C. Fung, S. H. Nantel, C. L. Toze, H. G. Klingemann, H. J. Sutherland, D. E. Hogge, T. J. Nevill, A. Le, and M. J. Barnett.** 1998. Lymphoproliferative disorders following allogeneic bone marrow transplantation: the Vancouver experience. *Bone Marrow Transplant.* **22:**981–987.

96. **Myers, G. D., C. M. Bollard, M. F. Wu, H. Weiss, C. M. Rooney, H. E. Heslop, and A. M. Leen.** 2007. Reconstitution of adenovirus-specific cell-mediated immunity in pediatric patients after hematopoietic stem cell transplantation. *Bone Marrow Transplant.* **39:**677–686.

97. **Nalesnik, M. A., R. Jaffe, and T. E. Starzl.** 1988. The pathology of post-transplant lymphoproliferative disorders occurring in the setting of cyclosporine-A prednisone immunosuppression. *Am. J. Pathol.* **133:**173–192.

98. **Nephrology Dialysis Transplantation.** 2002. European best practice guidelines for renal transplantation. Section IV: long-term management of the transplant recipient. IV.6.1. Cancer risk after renal transplantation. Post-transplant lymphoproliferative disease (PTLD): prevention and treatment. *Nephrol. Dial. Transplant.* **17**(Suppl. 4)**:**31–33, 35–36.

99. **Nichols, W. G., L. Corey, T. Gooley, C. Davis, and M. Boeckh.** 2002. High risk of death due to bacterial and fungal infection among cytomegalovirus (CMV)-seronegative recipients of stem cell transplants from seropositive donors: evidence for indirect effects of primary CMV infection. *J. Infect. Dis.* **185:**273–282.

100. **Nichols, W. G., L. Corey, T. Gooley, W. L. Drew, R. Miner, M. Huang, C. Davis, and M. Boeckh.** 2001. Rising pp65 antigenemia during preemptive anticytomegalovirus therapy after allogeneic hematopoietic stem cell transplantation: risk factors, correlation with DNA load, and outcomes. *Blood* **97:**867–874.

101. **Noguchi-Shinohara, M., T. Hamaguchi, T. Kitamoto, T. Sato, Y. Nakamura, H. Mizusawa, and M. Yamada.** 2007. Clinical features and diagnosis of dura mater graft associated Creutzfeldt Jakob disease. *Neurology* **69:**360–367.

102. **Okano, M., G. M. Thiele, and J. R. Davis.** 1988. Epstein-Barr virus and human diseases: recent advances in diagnosis. *Clin. Microbiol. Rev.* **1:**300–312.

103. **Ozdemir, F. N., A. Akgul, A. Altunoglu, A. Bilgic, Z. Arat, and M. Haberal.** 2007. The association between cytomegalovirus infection and atherosclerotic events in renal transplant recipients. *Transplant. Proc.* **39:**990–992.

104. **Papadopoulos, E. B., M. Ladanyi, D. Emanuel, and S. Mackinnon.** 1994. Infusions of donor leukocytes to treat Epstein-Barr virus-associated lymphoproliferative disorders after allogeneic bone marrow transplantation. *N. Engl. J. Med.* **330:**1185–1191.

105. **Paradis, K., G. Langford, Z. Long, W. Heneine, P. Sandstrom, W. M. Switzer, L. E. Chapman, C. Lockey, D. Onions, and E. Otto for The XEN 111 Study Group.** 1999. Search for cross-species transmission of porcine endogenous retrovirus in patients treated with living pig tissue. *Science* **285:**1236–1241.

106. **Patience, C., Y. Takeuchi, and R. A. Weiss.** 1998. Zoonosis in xenotransplantation. *Curr. Opin. Immunol.* **10:** 539–542.

107. **Penn, I., W. Hammond, L. Brettschneider, and T. E. Starzl.** 1969. Malignant lymphomas in transplantation patients. *Transplant. Proc.* **1:**106–112.

108. **Pouteil-Noble, C., J. C. Tardy, P. Chossegros, F. Mion, M. Chevallier, F. Gérard, P. Chevallier, F. Megas, N. Lefrançois, and J. L. Touraine.** 1995. Co-infection by hepatitis B virus and hepatitis C virus in renal transplantation: morbidity and mortality in 1098 patients. *Nephrol. Dial. Transplant.* **10**(Suppl. 6)**:**122–124.

109. **Preiksaitis, J., F. Diaz-Mitoma, and F. Mirzayans.** 1992. Quantitative oropharyngeal Epstein-Barr virus shedding in renal and cardiac transplant recipients: relationship to immunosuppressive therapy, serological responses and the risk of post-transplant lymphoproliferative disorder. *J. Infect. Dis.* **166:**986–994.

110. **Prentice, H. G., E. Gluckman, R. L. Powles, P. Ljungman, N. J. Milpied, R. Camara, F. Mandelli, P. Kho, L. Kennedy, and A. R. Bell for the European Acyclovir for CMV Prophylaxis Study Group.** 1997. Long-term survival in allogeneic bone marrow transplant recipients following acyclovir prophylaxis for CMV infection. *Bone Marrow Transplant.* **19:**129–133.

111. **Pruett, T. L., and R. McGory.** 2000. Hepatitis B immune globulin: the US experience. *Clin. Transplant.* **14:** 7–13.

112. **Purtilo, D. R., R. S. Strobach, M. Okano, and J. R. Davis.** 1992. Biology of disease: Epstein-Barr virus-associated lymphoproliferative disorders. *Lab. Investig.* **67:**5–23.

113. **Quinnan, G. V., Jr., N. Kirmani, A. H. Rook, J. F. Manischewitz, L. Jackson, G. Moreschi, G. W. Santos, R. Saral, and W. H. Burns.** 1982. Cytotoxic T cells in cytomegalovirus infection: HLA-restricted T-lymphocyte and non-T-lymphocyte cytotoxic responses correlate with recovery from cytomegalovirus infection in bone-marrow-transplant recipients. *N. Engl. J. Med.* **307:**7–13.

114. **Raab-Traub, N., K. Flynn, C. Klein, G. Pizza, C. De Vinci, L. Occhiuzzi, G. Farneti, U. Caliceti, and E. Pirodda.** 1987. EBV associated malignancies. *J. Exp. Pathol.* **3:**449–456.

115. **Renoult, E., B. Aymard, M. J. Gregoire, and A. Bellow.** 1995. Epstein-Barr virus lymphoproliferative disease of donor origin after kidney transplantation: a case report. *Am. J. Kidney Dis.* **26:**84–87.

116. **Resnick, L., J. S. Herbst, D. V. Ablashi, S. Atherton, B. Frank, and L. Rosen.** 1988. Regression of oral hairy leukoplakia after orally administered acyclovir therapy. *JAMA* **259:**384–388.

117. **Reusser, P., S. R. Riddell, J. D. Meyers, and P. D. Greenberg.** 1991. Cytotoxic T-lymphocyte response to cytomegalovirus after human allogeneic bone marrow transplantation: pattern of recovery and correlation with cytomegalovirus infection and disease. *Blood* **78:**1373–1380.

118. **Rubin, R. H., A. B. Cosimi, N. E. Tolkoff-Rubin, P. S. Russell, and M. S. Hirsch.** 1977. Infectious disease syndromes attributable to cytomegalovirus and their significance among renal transplant recipients. *Transplantation* **24:**458–464.

119. **Rubin, R. H.** 1990. Impact of cytomegalovirus infection on organ transplant recipients. *Rev. Infect. Dis.* **12**(Suppl. 7)**:**S754–S766.

120. **Saemundsen, A. K., D. T. Purtilo, K. Sakamoto, J. L. Sullivan, A. C. Synnerholm, D. Hanto, R. Simmons, M. Anvret, R. Collins, and G. Klein.** 1981. Documentation of Epstein-Barr virus infection in immunodeficient patients with life-threatening lymphoproliferative diseases by Epstein-Barr virus complementary RNA/

DNA and viral DNA/DNA hybridization. *Cancer Res.* **41:**4237–4242.

121. **Salzberger, B., R. A. Bowden, R. C. Hackman, C. Davis, and M. Boeckh.** 1997. Neutropenia in allogeneic marrow transplant recipients receiving ganciclovir for prevention of cytomegalovirus disease: risk factors and outcome. *Blood* **90:**2502–2508.
122. **Sanchez-Fueyo, A., M. Gimenez-Barcons, F. Puig-Basagoiti, A. Rimola, J. M. Sanchez-Tapias, J. C. Saiz, and J. Rodes.** 2001. Influence of the dynamics of the hypervariable region 1 of hepatitis C virus (HCV) on the histological severity of HCV recurrence after liver transplantation. *J. Med. Virol.* **65:**266–275.
123. **Schmidt, G. M., D. A. Horak, J. C. Niland, S. R. Duncan, S. J. Forman, and J. A. Zaia for The City of Hope-Stanford-Syntex CMV Study Group.** 1991. A randomized, controlled trial of prophylactic ganciclovir for cytomegalovirus pulmonary infection in recipients of allogeneic bone marrow transplants. *N. Engl. J. Med.* **324:**1005–1011.
124. **Shapiro, R. S., K. McClain, and G. Frizzera.** 1988. Epstein-Barr virus associated B cell lymphoproliferative disorders following bone marrow transplantation. *Blood* **71:**1234–1243.
125. **Shuahart, M. C., D. Myerson, B. H. Childs, and J. D. Fingeroth.** 1994. Marrow transplantation from hepatitis C virus seropositive donors: transmission rate and clinical course. *Blood* **85:**3229–3235.
126. **Singh, N.** 2006. Antiviral drugs for cytomegalovirus in transplant recipients: advantages of preemptive therapy. *Rev. Med. Virol.* **16:**281–287.
127. **Sivaprakasam, P., T. F. Carr, M. Coussons, T. Khalid, A. S. Bailey, M. Guiver, K. J. Mutton, A. J. Turner, J. D. Grainger, and R. F. Wynn.** 2007. Improved outcome from invasive adenovirus infection in pediatric patients after hemopoietic stem cell transplantation using intensive clinical surveillance and early intervention. *J. Pediatr. Hematol. Oncol.* **29:**81–85.
128. **Smith, M. A., S. Sundaresan, T. Mohanakumar, E. P. Trulock, J. P. Lynch, D. L. Phelan, J. D. Cooper, and G. A. Patterson.** 1998. Effect of development of antibodies to HLA and cytomegalovirus mismatch on lung transplantation survival and development of bronchiolitis obliterans syndrome. *J. Thorac. Cardiovasc. Surg.* **116:**812–820.
129. **Srinivasan, A., E. C. Burton, M. J. Kuehnert, C. Rupprecht, W. L. Sutker, T. G. Ksiazek, C. D. Paddock, J. Guarner, W. J. Shieh, C. Goldsmith, C. A. Hanlon, J. Zoretic, B. Fischbach, M. Niezgoda, W. H. El-Feky, L. Orciari, E. Q. Sanchez, A. Likos, G. B. Klintmalm, D. Cardo, J. LeDuc, M. E. Chamberland, D. B. Jernigan, and S. R. Zaki.** 2005. Transmission of rabies virus from an organ donor to four transplant recipients. *N. Engl. J. Med.* **352:**1103–1111.
130. **Stevens, S. J. C., E. A. M. Verschuuren, I. Pronk, W. van der Big, M. C. Harmsen, T. H. The, C. J. L. M. Meijer, A. J. C. van den Brule, and J. M. Middeldorp.** 2001. Frequent monitoring of Epstein-Barr virus DNA load in unfractionated whole blood is essential for early detection of posttransplant lymphoproliferative disease in high-risk patients. *Blood* **97:**1165–1171.
131. **Sullivan, J. L., K. S. Byron, F. E. Brewster, K. Sakamoto, J. E. Show, and J. S. Pagano.** 1982. Treatment of life-threatening Epstein-Barr virus infection with acyclovir. *Am. J. Med.* **73:**262–266.
132. **Suzuki, T., Y. Takano, K. Yamashita, and K. Sato.** 1993. A possible role for Epstein-Barr virus in tumorigenesis after immunosuppression in cases of renal transplantation. *J. Cancer Res. Clin. Oncol.* **119:**627–629.
133. **Toupance, O., M. C. Bouedjoro-Camus, J. Carquin, J. L. Novella, S. Lavaud, A. Wynckel, D. Jolly, and J. Chanard.** 2000. Cytomegalovirus-related disease and risk of acute rejection in renal transplant recipients: a cohort study with case-control analyses. *Transplant Int.* **13:**413–419.
134. **Trappe, R., H. Riess, N. Babel, M. Hummel, H. Lehmkuhl, S. Jonas, I. Anagnostopoulos, M. Papp-Vary, P. Reinke, R. Hetzer, B. Dorken, and S. Oertel.** 2007. Salvage chemotherapy for refractory and relapsed posttransplant lymphoproliferative disorders (PTLD) after treatment with single-agent rituximab. *Transplantation* **83:**912–918.
135. **Tu, W., L. Potena, P. Stepick-Biek, L. Liu, K. Y. Dionis, H. Luikart, W. F. Fearon, T. H. Holmes, C. Chin, J. P. Cooke, H. A. Valantine, E. S. Mocarski, and D. B. Lewis.** 2006. T-cell immunity to subclinical cytomegalovirus infection reduces cardiac allograft disease. *Circulation* **114:**1608–1615.
136. **van Esser, J. W. J., B. van der Holt, E. Meijer, H. G. M. Niesters, R. Trenschel, S. F. T. Thijsen, A. M. van Loon, F. Frassoni, A. Bacigalupo, U. W. Schaefer, A. D. M. E. Osterhaus, J. W. Gratama, B. Lowenberg, L. F. Verdonck, and J. J. Cornelissen.** 2001. Epstein-Barr virus (EBV) reactivation is a frequent event after allogeneic stem cell transplantation (SCT) and quantitatively predicts EBV-lymphoproliferative disease following T-cell-depleted SCT. *Blood* **98:**972–978.
137. **Vusirikala, M., S. N. Wolff, R. S. Stein, S. J. Brandt, D. S. Morgan, J. P. Greer, F. G. Schuening, J. S. Dummer, and S. A. Goodman.** 2001. Valacyclovir for the prevention of cytomegalovirus infection after allogeneic stem cell transplantation: a single institution retrospective cohort analysis. *Bone Marrow Transplant.* **28:**265–270.
138. **Walker, R. C., C. C. V. Paya, W. F. Marshall, J. G. Strickler, R. H. Wiesner, J. A. Veloza, T. M. Habermann, R. C. Daly, and C. G. McGregor.** 1995. Pretransplantation seronegative Epstein-Barr virus status is the primary risk factor for posttransplant lymphoproliferative disorder in adult heart, lung, and other solid organ transplantations. *J. Heart Lung Transplant.* **14:**214–221.
139. **Walter, E. A., P. D. Greenberg, M. J. Gilbert, R. J. Finch, K. S. Watanabe, E. D. Thomas, and S. R. Riddell.** 1995. Reconstitution of cellular immunity against cytomegalovirus in recipients of allogeneic bone marrow by transfer of T-cell clones from the donor. *N. Engl. J. Med.* **333:**1038–1044.
140. **Wang, F. Z., A. Linde, H. Hagglund, M. Testa, A. Locasciulli, and P. Ljungman.** 1999. Human herpesvirus 6 DNA in cerebrospinal fluid specimens from allogeneic bone marrow transplant patients: does it have clinical significance? *Clin. Infect. Dis.* **28:**562–568.
141. **Weiss, L. M., and K. L. Chang.** 1992. Molecular biologic studies of Hodgkin's disease. *Semin. Diagn. Pathol.* **9:**272–278.
142. **Weiss, L. M., L. A. Movahed, R. A. Warnke, and J. Sklar.** 1989. Detection of Epstein-Barr viral genomes in Reed-Stemberg cells of Hodgkin's disease. *N. Engl. J. Med.* **320:**502–506.
143. **Weller, T. H., J. C. Macauley, J. M. Craig, and P. Wirth.** 1957. Isolation of intranuclear inclusion producing agents from infants with illnesses resembling cytomegalic inclusion disease. *Proc. Soc. Exp. Biol. Med.* **94:**4–12.
144. **Wingard, J. R., D. Y. Chen, W. H. Burns, D. J. Fuller, H. G. Braine, A. M. Yeager, H. Kaiser, P. J. Burke, M. L. Graham, and G. W. Santos.** 1988. Cytomegalo-

virus infection after autologous bone marrow transplantation with comparison to infection after allogeneic bone marrow transplantation. *Blood* **71:**1432–1437.

145. **Yao, Q. Y., P. Ogan, M. Rowe, M. Wood, and A. B. Rickinson.** 1989. Epstein-Barr virus-infected B cells persist in the circulation of acyclovir-treated virus carriers. *Int. J. Cancer* **43:**67–71.
146. **Zaia, J. A.** 2004. Cytomegalovirus infection, p. 701–726. *In* K. G. Blume, S. J. Forman, and F. R. Appelbaum (ed.), *Thomas' Hematopoietic Cell Transplantation*. Blackwell Publications, Boston, MA.
147. **Zaia, J. A., and D. J. Lang.** 1984. Cytomegalovirus infection of the fetus and neonate. *Neurol. Clin.* **2:**387–410.
148. **Zutter, M. M., P. J. Martin, G. E. Sale, H. M. Shulman, L. Fisher, E. D. Thomas, and D. M. Durnam.** 1988. Epstein-Barr virus lymphoproliferation after bone marrow transplantation. *Blood* **72:**520–529.

Viral Myocarditis

JEFFREY A. TOWBIN

7

Myocarditis is a process characterized pathologically by an inflammatory infiltrate of the myocardium with necrosis and/or degeneration of adjacent myocytes not typical of the ischemic damage associated with coronary artery disease. It has been defined as an inflammatory process affecting the heart and causing ventricular dysfunction. The inflammation may involve myocytes, interstitium, vascular elements, and/or pericardium and may be an acute or chronic process. This definition does not take into account the underlying etiology (132). Clinically, myocarditis most commonly manifests with signs of congestive heart failure, which include breathlessness, exercise intolerance, and fatigue, and may be associated with abdominal pain, chest pain, palpitations, syncope, and sudden death. In childhood, myocarditis is usually an acute process with left ventricular (LV) systolic dysfunction with or without dilation of the LV, while adult presentation is most typically chronic and mimics dilated cardiomyopathy (DCM) with LV dilation and systolic dysfunction or LV dysfunction without dilation.

ETIOLOGY

Most cases of myocarditis in the United States and Western Europe result from viral infections (11, 18, 30). In the 1970s and 1980s, coxsackieviruses, including coxsackievirus A (CVA) and CVB, as well as echoviruses were the most commonly identified viral etiologies, but in the 1990s and early 21st century, other viral causes, including adenoviruses, especially serotypes 2 and 5 (15, 78), and enteroviruses (CVA and CVB, echovirus, and poliovirus), particularly CVB (5, 51, 131), were recognized (Table 1). Most recently, parvovirus B19 has become a commonly identified virus in patients with suspected myocarditis, supplanting adenovirus as the most commonly identified etiologic agent (36, 73, 95, 110, 127). However, a wide variety of other viral causes of myocarditis (17, 98) in children have been described, including influenza virus (102), cytomegalovirus (CMV) (108), herpes simplex virus (HSV) (71), hepatitis C virus (83, 84, 93), rubella virus (1), varicella virus (70), mumps virus (25), Epstein-Barr virus (EBV) (39), human immunodeficiency virus (HIV) (104a), and respiratory syncytial virus (103), among others.

PCR evaluation of cardiac samples from subjects suspected of having myocarditis has demonstrated that a variety of viral genomes can be identified. In addition to the enteroviruses and adenovirus genomes, CMV, parvovirus B19, respiratory syncytial virus, EBV, HSV, and influenza A virus have been reported (17, 18, 61, 75). Mumps virus was responsible for endocardial fibroelastosis (EFE), a previously important cause of heart failure in children that has disappeared over the past 20 years (89). Since 2000, parvovirus B19 has become the predominant viral genome identified in the heart, but a cause-and-effect relationship has not been proven (17, 36, 73, 95, 110, 127). In Japan, hepatitis C virus has been shown to be a common etiologic agent, with the other viral genomes typically seen in North America and Europe playing a lesser role. (83, 84, 93). Other viruses, such as human herpesviruses 6 and 7, have been occasionally reported as well. More recently, outbreaks of chikungunya virus have been reported, especially in countries in the Indian subcontinent. The acute stage of infection with chikungunya virus is characterized by fever, polyarthritis, and occasional rash and can be complicated by myocarditis and pericarditis (64, 114). This virus was previously identified in the 1960s to 1970s as a cause of myocarditis in Asia and Africa, along with other arboviruses such as dengue virus (90). Other viral causes of myocarditis are likely to develop and be identified during the following decade(s).

EPIDEMIOLOGY

Myocarditis is a disorder that is underdiagnosed (18, 132). The incidence of the usual lymphocytic form of myocarditis reportedly ranges from 4 to 5% from reports of young men dying of trauma (42) to as high as 16 to 21% in autopsy series of children dying suddenly. In adults with unexplained DCM, the incidence ranges from 3 to 63% (55, 132), although the large multicenter Myocarditis Treatment Trial, which was strictly based on specific diagnostic criteria (the so-called Dallas criteria; see below) reported a 9% incidence (80).

Usually sporadic, viral myocarditis can also occur as an epidemic (42). Epidemics usually are seen in newborns, most commonly in association with CVB. Intrauterine myocarditis occurs during community epidemics as well as sporadically (125). Postnatal spread of coxsackievirus is via the fecal-oral or respiratory route (6, 38). The World Health Organization (WHO) reports that this ubiquitous

TABLE 1 Viral causes of myocarditis

Enteroviruses
CVA
CVB
Echovirus
Poliovirus
Adenovirus
Parvovirus B19
CMV
Herpesvirus
Influenza A virus
Varicella-zoster virus
Mumps virus
Measles virus
Rabies virus
Hepatitis B and C viruses
Rubella virus
Rubeola virus
Respiratory syncytial virus
HIV
EBV
Chikungunya virus

family of viruses results in cardiovascular sequelae in less than 1% of infections, although this increases to 4% when CVB alone is considered (42). Other important viral causes, like adenovirus (2, 87) and influenza A virus, are transmitted primarily via the respiratory route.

PATHOPHYSIOLOGY

Viral infection triggers interstitial inflammation or myocardial injury, resulting in cardiac enlargement and an increase in the ventricular end-diastolic volume (38, 56, 87, 132). Normally, this increase in volume results in an increased force of contraction, improved ejection fraction, and improved cardiac output as described by the Starling mechanism. The myocardium is unable to respond to these stimuli, resulting in reduced cardiac output. A domino effect of changes occurs, and this results in the pathophysiological response in patients with myocarditis.

1. Interactions with the sympathetic nervous system may preserve systemic blood flow via vasoconstriction and elevated afterload. This sympathetic nervous system input results in tachycardia and diaphoresis.
2. Congestive heart failure ensues with disease progression. A progressive increase in ventricular end-diastolic volume and pressure results in increased left atrial pressure. This is transmitted to the pulmonary venous system, causing increasing hydrostatic forces that overcome the colloid osmotic pressure that normally prevents fluid transudation across capillary membranes. This results in pulmonary edema.
3. Concomitantly, all cardiac chambers dilate, particularly the LV. This dilation, in addition to poor ventricular function, creates worsening pulmonary edema and worsening cardiac function. The ventricular dilation also results in stretching of the mitral annulus and resultant mitral regurgitation, further increasing left atrial volume and pressure.
4. During the healing stages of myocarditis, fibroblasts replace normal myofibers and result in scar formation. Reduced elasticity and ventricular performance can result in persistent heart failure. In addition, ventricular arrhythmias commonly accompany this fibrosis.

PATHOLOGY

Gross and Microscopic Findings

Pathological findings are nonspecific, with similar gross and microscopic changes noted irrespective of the causative agent (30, 38, 132). The heart weight is increased. and all four chambers are affected. The muscle is flabby and pale, with petechial hemorrhages often seen on the epicardial surfaces, especially in cases of CVB infection. A bloody pericardial effusion also may be seen relating to the often-combined finding of pericarditis. The ventricular wall is frequently thin, although hypertrophy may be found as well. The valves and endocardium are not involved.

In cases of chronic myocarditis, the valves may be glistening white, suggesting that EFE may be the result of an in utero viral myocarditis (56). Children with myocarditis typically have symptoms for less than 2 weeks, whereas those with EFE have symptoms for more than 4 months. Mumps virus and CVB3 have been identified in the myocardium of infants with EFE (89).

Mural thrombi occur in the LV, and small emboli are often found in the coronary and cerebral vessels (106). Coronary emboli, although rare, may produce areas of ischemia or injury with resultant production of the cardiac arrhythmias that sometimes occur during the acute disease.

An interstitial collection of mononuclear cells, including lymphocytes, plasma cells, and eosinophils (Fig. 1), is typical of early myocarditis (131). Polymorphonuclear cells are rare, as are viral particles. Extensive necrosis of the myocardium, with loss of cross-striation in the muscle fibers and edema, is seen in severe infections, but especially with coxsackievirus. Perivascular accumulation of lymphocytes and plasma cells has been described with CVB myocarditis but is usually a minor finding. In disease due to rickettsiae, varicella virus, and trypanosomes or other parasites, and in reactions to sulfonamides, this is a much more prominent finding (12, 19, 67, 77, 101, 126).

Diphtheria myocarditis is frequently complicated by arrhythmias and complete atrioventricular block (22). Diphtheria exotoxin attaches to conductive tissue and interferes with protein synthesis by inhibiting a translocating enzyme

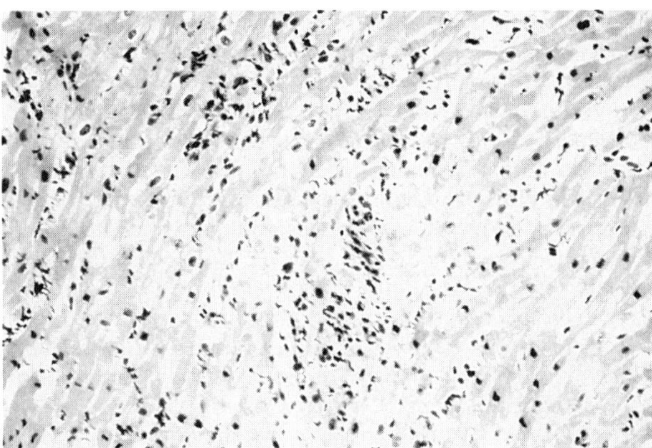

FIGURE 1 Endomyocardial biopsy histology demonstrates lymphocytic infiltrates, myocardial edema, and necrosis.

in the delivery of amino acids (44). Triglyceride accumulates, producing fatty changes of the myofibers.

Bacterial myocarditis produces microabscesses and patchy focal suppurative changes. A combined perimyocarditis is also frequently encountered. Parasitic myocarditis caused by *Trichinella* has a focal infiltrate with lymphocytes and eosinophils, but larvae are usually not identified (12).

A severe myocarditis caused by *Trypanosoma cruzi* (77, 101) results in Chagas' disease. Rare in North America, Chagas' disease is endemic in South America, affecting up to 50% of some populations. Microscopic examination reveals the organism as well as neutrophils, lymphocytes, macrophages, and eosinophils.

Sudden death in infancy may result from myocardial inflammation. James (57) described a resorptive, degenerative process in the His bundle and left margin of the atrioventricular node with the absence of inflammatory cells in cases he studied of infants who died in Northern Ireland.

Giant cell myocarditis (27, 29, 94, 105, 116) occurs with tuberculosis, syphilis, rheumatoid arthritis, rheumatic heart disease, sarcoidosis, and fungal or parasitic infections. Giant cells also occur in idiopathic (Fiedler's) myocarditis. There are two types of giant cells: cells originating from the myocardium and cells derived from interstitial histiocytes.

CLINICAL MANIFESTATIONS

Presentation depends on the age of the affected individual, the immune status, the specific viral trigger, genetic factors, and the environment (17, 30, 38). Nonspecific flu-like illness or episodes of gastroenteritis may precede symptoms of congestive heart failure.

Newborns and Infants

Newborns or infants present with poor appetite, fever, irritability or listlessness, periodic episodes of pallor, and diaphoresis. Sudden death may occur in this subgroup of children (17, 38, 111). On physical examination, pallor and mild cyanosis in addition to classic symptoms of congestive heart failure are commonly noted. It is important to keep in mind that the younger the child, the more likely that the disease was triggered as an intrauterine event and, therefore, this form of myocarditis is expressed as a chronic disease that mimicks chronic DCM (17, 89).

Children, Adolescents, and Adults

Older children, adolescents, and adults commonly have a recent history of nonspecific illness, typically presenting as upper respiratory or gastrointestinal symptoms (with or without fever) 10 to 14 days prior to presentation (38). Initial symptoms include lethargy, low-grade fever, and pallor; the child usually has decreased appetite and may complain of abdominal pain. Diaphoresis, palpitations, rashes, exercise intolerance, and general malaise are common signs and symptoms. Later in the course of illness, respiratory symptoms such as breathlessness and cough become predominant; syncope or sudden death may occur due to cardiac collapse. Findings on physical examination are consistent with congestive heart failure (15, 38), as described above. Unlike with newborns, jugular venous distention and pulmonary rales may be observed, and resting tachycardia may be prominent. Arrhythmias, including atrial fibrillation, supraventricular tachycardia, or ventricular tachycardia, as well as atrioventricular block, may occur (37, 38).

The prognosis of acute myocarditis in newborns is poor (43). In one study, a 75% mortality rate was observed in 25 infants with suspected CVB myocarditis (43). Most deaths occurred in the first week of the illness. Older infants and children have a better prognosis, with a mortality rate between 10 and 25% in clinically recognizable cases; however, a subgroup of patients present to the emergency center dead. In other cases, the children present with signs and symptoms of very common childhood disorders such as a viral respiratory illness, gastroenteritis, or dehydration and therefore are treated for these disorders initially. However, over hours or days, these children may very rapidly deteriorate and succumb, usually after a cardiac or respiratory arrest. On autopsy, myocarditis is diagnosed. These patients are extremely difficult to diagnose and, even if identified, have limited therapeutic options.

Complete recovery occurs in about 50% of patients (33, 81). Twenty-five percent of the patients continued to have an abnormal electrocardiogram or chest radiograph even though they were clinically asymptomatic. Abnormalities in the resting electrocardiogram may not be seen, but they may be brought out with exercise. Adult patients who recover may be asymptomatic at rest or with light exertion but may demonstrate a reduced working capacity with exercise stress testing.

DIAGNOSTIC EVALUATION

The diagnosis of myocarditis is often difficult to establish but should be suspected in any patient who presents with unexplained congestive heart failure or ventricular tachycardia in the absence of predisposing cardiac conditions. Appropriate diagnostic studies include the following (46).

Chest Radiography

Cardiomegaly with pulmonary edema is classically demonstrable radiographically.

Electrocardiography

Sinus tachycardia with low-voltage QRS complexes with or without low-voltage or inverted T waves are classically described. A pattern of myocardial infarction with wide Q waves and ST-segment changes also may be seen (119) (Fig. 2). Ventricular tachycardia, supraventricular tachycardia, atrial fibrillation, or atrioventricular block occurs in some children (37).

Echocardiography

A dilated and dysfunctional LV consistent with DCM is seen on two-dimensional and M-mode echocardiography (Color Plate 1). Segmental wall motion abnormalities are relatively common, but global hypokinesis is predominant. Pericardial effusion frequently occurs. Doppler and color Doppler commonly demonstrate mitral regurgitation. Dilation of other chambers also may be seen.

Endomyocardial Biopsy

Cardiac catherization shows low cardiac output and elevated end-diastolic pressures. Right ventricular endomyocardial biopsy (Fig. 3) is used to examine for inflammatory infiltrate (Fig. 1), which is usually patchy and scattered in the ventricular myocardium. A mononuclear cell infiltrate is diagnostic of myocarditis, although this does not delineate etiology. Myocardial biopsy is diagnostically sensitive

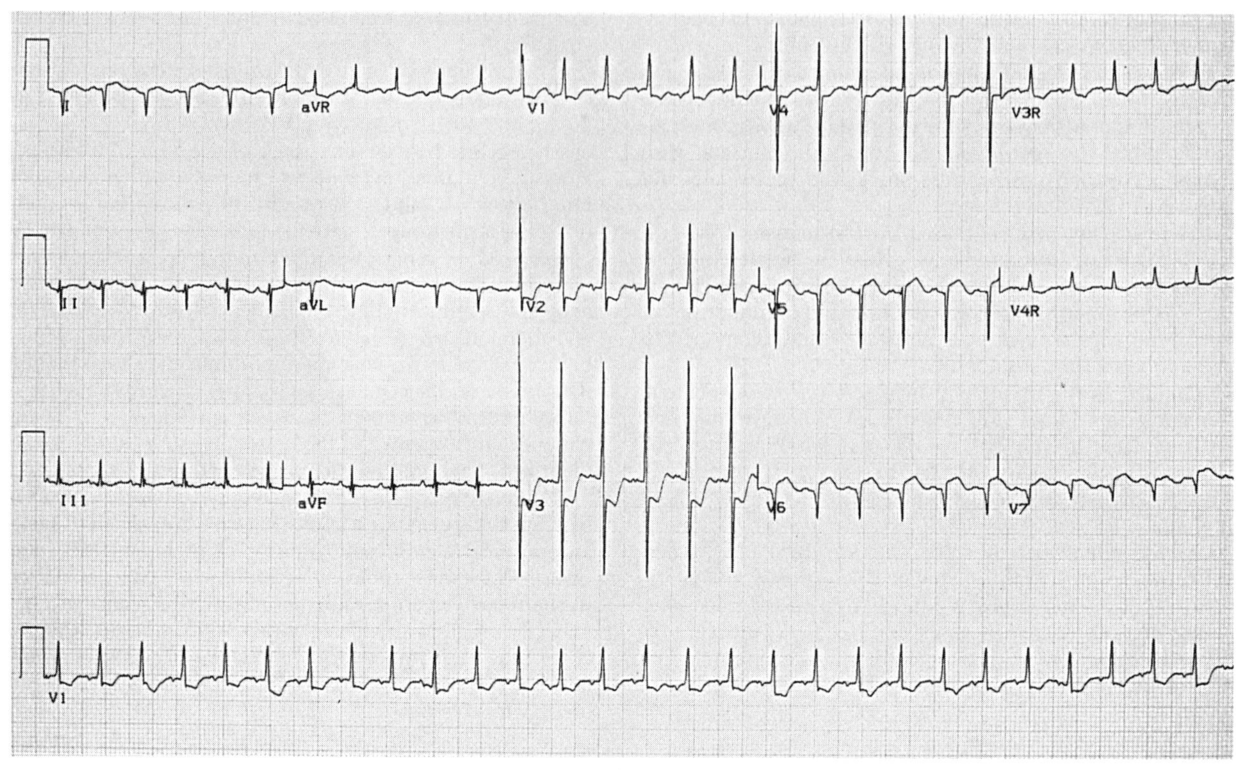

FIGURE 2 Electrocardiogram from a child with myocarditis. Sinus tachycardia and low-voltage QRS complexes with inverted T waves and a pattern of myocardial infarction with wide Q waves in leads I and aVL, and ST-segment changes consistent with ischemia, are noted throughout.

in 3 to 63% of cases (4, 26, 38, 47, 112). Because there is a risk associated with biopsy, particularly in young children or those with severe ventricular dilation, some centers have abandoned this procedure, particularly on young and small children (<10 kg) and those with severe dilation.

The Dallas Criteria

The Dallas criteria define myocarditis as "a process characterized by an inflammatory infiltrate of the myocardium with necrosis and/or degeneration of adjacent myocytes not typical of ischemic damage" due to coronary artery or other disease (4). At the time of initial biopsy, a specimen may be classified as active myocarditis, borderline myocarditis, or no myocarditis, depending on whether an inflammatory infiltrate occurs in association with myocyte degeneration or necrosis (active) or too sparse of an infiltrate or no myocyte degeneration occurs (borderline) (14, 80). Repeat endomyocardial biopsy may be appropriate in cases where strong suspicion of myocarditis exists clinically; on repeat endomyocardial biopsy, histology may be classified as ongoing myocarditis, resolving myocarditis, or resolved myocarditis.

Viral Studies

A positive viral culture from myocardium has been considered the diagnostic standard in the past. Viral culture of peripheral specimens, such as blood, stool, or urine, is commonly performed but is unreliable at identifying the causative infection. A fourfold increase in antibody titer correlates with infection (99, 115). However, these studies are nonspecific, because prior infection with the causative virus is commonplace.

First reported in 1986, in situ hybridization was performed on myocardial tissue using probes for coxsackievirus (13, 14). This technique is difficult to use in a hospital setting and therefore lost favor and never gained widespread use. PCR (15, 18, 78) amplifies viral sequences from cardiac tissue samples, is extremely sensitive, and is typically specific (15, 18, 78). In 25 to 50% of cases, the enterovirus genome was initially identified by PCR (3, 5, 6, 17, 18, 53, 73, 78, 79, 97, 128); however, no other viral genomes were sought in these early studies (3, 28, 58). Subsequently, PCR was used to screen for other viral genomes within cardiac tissue specimens, and adenovirus (Fig. 4) was identified as commonly as enterovirus in heart tissue specimens of patients with myocarditis or DCM (Table 2) (15, 17, 18, 78). PCR analysis usually does not identify the viral genome in peripheral blood of patients with myocarditis, but the viral genome can be identified in tracheal aspirates of intubated children with myocarditis, potentially reducing the need for endomyocardial biopsy (2).

DIFFERENTIAL DIAGNOSIS

Any cause of acute circulatory failure may mimic myocarditis. Other nonviral etiologies include other infectious agents such as rickettsiae, bacteria, protozoa and other parasites, fungi, and yeasts (12, 22, 53, 55, 59, 67, 69, 76, 77, 85, 101, 106, 126); various drugs, including antimicrobial medications (132); hypersensitivity, autoimmune, or collagen-vascular diseases, such as systemic lupus erythematosus, mixed connective tissue disease, rheumatic fever, rheumatoid arthritis, and scleroderma; toxic reactions to

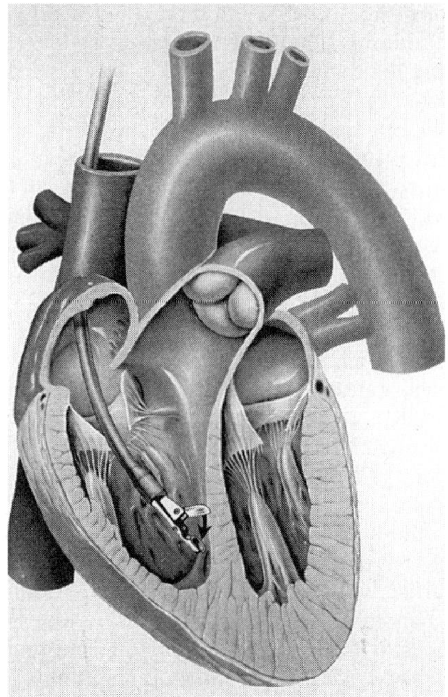

FIGURE 3 Endomyocardial biopsy technique. The bioptome is advanced via the superior vena cava into the right atrium, across the tricuspid valve into the right ventricle, and finally situated against the interventricular septum, where the biopsy is performed. The bioptome can also be advanced via the inferior vena cava with similar results. (Reprinted from reference 120 with permission of Elsevier.)

infectious agents (25, 35, 39, 60, 66, 72, 89, 94) (e.g., mumps or diphtheria); or other disorders such as Kawasaki disease and sarcoidosis (94, 133). In most cases, however, the cause goes unrecognized and idiopathic myocarditis is diagnosed.

Immunology

The immunopathogenesis of CVB and encephalomyocarditis has been studied in mice. CMV, HIV, and adenovirus

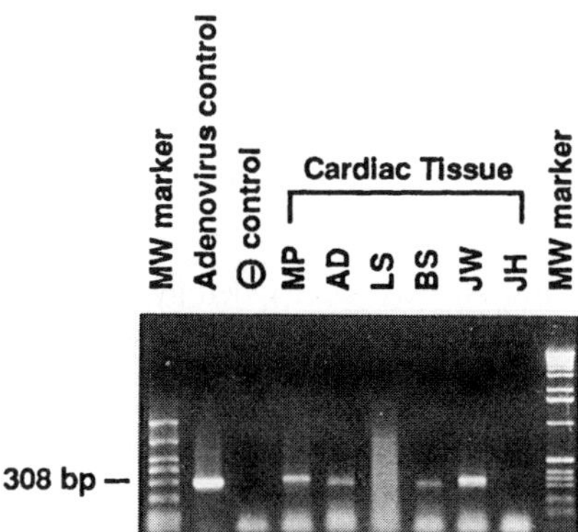

FIGURE 4 Nested PCR for the adenovirus genome. The agarose gel demonstrates a 308-bp PCR-positive band in the adenovirus-positive control lane, as well as in lanes designated MP, AD, BS, and JW, in which DNA was extracted from myocardial tissue samples obtained from patients with myocarditis. Patients designated LS and JH are PCR negative, as is the negative (−) control lane. MW, molecular weight.

TABLE 2 Myocarditis etiologies in children by PCR analysis

Diagnosis	No. of samples	No. of PCR$^+$ samples	PCR amplimer (#)
Myocarditis	624	239 (38%)	Adenovirus 142 (23%)
			Enterovirus 85 (14%)
			CMV 18 (3%)
			Parvovirus 6 (<1%)
			Influenza A5 virus (<1%)
			HSV 5 (<1%)
			EBV 3 (<1%)
			RSV[a] 1 (<1%)
DCM	149	30 (20%)	Adenovirus 18 (12%)
			Enterovirus 12 (8%)
Controls	215	3 (1.4%)	Enterovirus 1 (<1%)
			CMV 2 (<1%)

[a]RSV, respiratory syncytial virus.

models also have been described (21, 41, 48, 50, 52, 62, 65, 68). In mice, CVB viremia occurs 24 to 72 h after infection, and maximum tissue viral loads develop at 72 to 96 h (131). Virus titers subsequently decline, with no infectivity detectable 7 to 10 days after inoculation. Antibody concentrations decline as virus titers increase, implying an active role for antibody in viral clearance. Macrophages appear 5 to 10 days after infection in the murine CVB model of myocarditis (131). Risk factors for severe myocarditis include age, mouse strain, viral variant, exercise, and gender (131). Pathogenetic mechanisms include direct viral myofiber destruction and T-lymphocyte cytolysis (41, 48, 50, 54, 72, 130). Animals with absent or blocked T-cell function have less myocardial injury. In BALB/c mice, the greatest susceptibility is between 16 and 18 weeks; males have a more rapid and severe course of myocarditis than females. Estradiol has been shown to decrease severity, and testosterone increases cytolytic activity in males. Either a preferential stimulation of T-helper cells or an inadequate stimulation of T-cytolytic/suppressor cells could explain why antibody responses to various antigens may be enhanced and cellular immune responses depressed in females.

The natural killer (NK) cell is important in the pathogenesis of myocarditis. Animals depleted of NK cells prior to infection with coxsackievirus develop more severe myocarditis (41). NK cells are activated by interferon, an indirect modulator of myocardial injury. Murine skin fibroblasts serve as target cells for CVB-sensitized cytotoxic T cells. The NK cells specifically limit the nonenveloped virus infection by killing the virally infected cells. Male mice are less efficient in activating NK cells. Presumably, the more efficiently viral clearance occurs, the less virally induced neoantigen production occurs, reducing recognition by cytotoxic T lymphocytes. T cells can affect injury by accumulation of activated macrophages, production of antibody and antibody-dependent cell-mediated cytotoxicity, direct lysis by antibody and complement, and direct action of cytotoxic T cells (130).

Host genetic factors have been shown to affect the severity of disease, as well as the pathogenic mechanisms that participate in disease development (21, 62, 68, 82). Cytolytic T cells mediate myocarditis in the BALB/c mouse, and two distinct cytolytic T-cell populations are formed in the BALB/c mouse: one recognizing virus-infected cells and producing direct myocytolysis and another that destroys uninfected myocytes and is believed to be an autoreactive lymphocyte. Complement depletion increases the amount of inflammation in this species, and no reactive immunoglobulin G antibody is found in the myocytes. In the DBA/2 mouse, the T-helper cells indirectly mediate the course of disease, and complement depletion reduces inflammation. Cytolytic T cells are produced but apparently are not pathogenic; immunoglobulin G antibody is found in the myocytes.

In humans, antibody-mediated cytolysis is found among 30% of patients with suspected myocarditis, as well as in almost all patients with proven infections with CVB, influenza A virus, or mumps virus (72). A muscle-specific antimyolemmal antibody has been found in these patients and correlated with the degree of in vitro-induced cytolysis of rat cardiocytes. A CVB-specific complementary DNA hybridization probe detected virus nucleic acid sequences in patients diagnosed as having active or healed myocarditis or DCM (13, 14). Patients with unrelated disorders had no virus-specific sequences (13), suggesting that viral genomic material persists in patients with congestive cardiomyopathy or healing myocarditis. Although viral cultures are usually negative, continued viral replication may occur at a low level or abortively. The latter may conceal viral antigens by a process that prevents correct posttranslational processing of capsid proteins. Another study found that adult patients with myocarditis more often have neutralizing antibody responses to CVB1 to CVB6 (30). One hypothesis is that sequential infection and immune responses against several types of CVB are essential in the development of myocarditis; however, some cases of myocarditis clearly involve exposure to only one type of CVB.

Defective cell-mediated immunity compared with that in healthy controls occurs in patients with myocarditis and DCM. The pathogenesis of adenoviral myocarditis differs from that of CVB (48, 54, 117), and the inflammatory infiltrate is substantially less in adenoviral infection (18, 78, 97), specifically the numbers of CD2, CD3, and CD45RO T lymphocytes seen in the adenovirus-infected patients compared to those with myocarditis not due to adenovirus (97). Adenoviruses have a number of strategies for modulating the immune response that could affect the number of activated lymphocytes in the adenovirus-infected myocardium (48). Adenovirus E3 protein can protect cells from tumor necrosis factor-mediated lysis, as well as down-regulate major histocompatibility complex class I antigen expression. The E1A proteins can promote the induction of apoptosis (88) and inhibit interleukin 6 (IL-6) expression, as well as interfere with IL-6 signal transduction pathways. These functions of E1A may be pertinent to the development of the myocardial pathology seen in DCM. IL-6 promotes lymphocyte activation, which is reduced in adenovirus-infected patients. Apoptotic cells are also observed in the myocardium of patients with DCM. Taken together, these events are likely to result in DCM.

LONG-TERM SEQUELAE

In those cases in which resolution of cardiac dysfunction does not occur, a chronic DCM results, which is characterized by a dilated LV and LV systolic function, with or without diastolic dysfunction and/or right ventricular dilation and dysfunction (6, 9, 34, 43, 79, 86). The underlying etiology of DCM is uncertain, but viral persistence and autoimmunity have been widely speculated. In addition, cytoskeletal protein disruption has also been demonstrated (121). Enteroviral protease 2A directly cleaves the cytoskeletal protein dystrophin, resulting in dysfunction of this protein (7). Because mutations in dystrophin are known to cause an inherited form of DCM (as well as the DCM associated with the neuromuscular diseases Duchenne muscular dystrophy and Becker muscular dystrophy), it is possible that this contributes to the chronic DCM seen in enteroviral myocarditis (122, 123). Adenoviruses also have enzymes that cleave membrane structural proteins or result in activation or inactivation of transcription factors, cytokines, or adhesion molecules to cause chronic DCM (23, 45, 48). Therefore, it appears as if a complex interaction between the viral genome and the heart occurs and results in the long-term outcome of affected patients.

As in mice, myocarditis in humans may have a genetic basis (92). Support for this includes the frequent finding of myocardial lymphocytic infiltrates in patients with familial and sporadic DCM (91), as well as the few reports of families in which two or more related individuals have been diagnosed with myocarditis on endomyocardial biopsy. Of note, the common receptor for the four most common viral causes of myocarditis (CVB3 and CVB4 and adenoviruses 2 and 5) is the human coxsackievirus and adenovirus receptor (10, 118). Mutations in this receptor might result in host differences leading to myocarditis, although this hypothesis requires study.

SUPPORT FOR VIRAL CAUSE-AND-EFFECT RELATIONSHIP WITH MYOCARDITIS

Despite the increasingly common association of the viral genome within the myocardium in patients with myocarditis, limited definitive data exist to prove that the virus causes ventricular disturbance directly leading to the clinical phenotype. Myocarditis is defined as a primary inflammatory disorder; however, definitive data to support this concept are limited. In many cases of myocarditis, frank, fulminant inflammation with lymphocytic or other infiltrate, edema, and cell necrosis with or without fibrosis is seen. In other circumstances, little infiltrate, necrosis, or edema is seen in subjects with acute-onset heart failure and ventricular dysfunction. In both situations, the viral genome can be identified in up to 30 to 40% of those studied by PCR. In addition, PCR analysis of "controls," specimens from subjects not thought to have clinical symptoms consistent with myocarditis and not having recent infectious or febrile illness, very rarely identify the viral genome. However, since a relatively low percentage of biopsies are currently performed in children suspected of having myocarditis and, of those, a limited number have PCR performed on the myocardium, definitive cause-and-effect data are lacking.

An excellent human model exists, however, and has been used to study this issue. Cardiac transplant recipients undergo routine surveillance biopsies for rejection at most institutions, and in all cases, histopathology is performed. At Texas Children's Hospital, all subjects also undergo myocardial PCR analysis with screening for adenovirus, enterovirus (including coxsackievirus), parvovirus B19, CMV, and EBV (16, 100). Detection of the viral genome in these samples has been shown to correlate with outcome. Shirali et al. demonstrated that those subjects not having any PCR-positive studies during a 5-year follow-up period had a 96% 5-year survival rate, while those with at least a single PCR-positive result have a 5-year survival rate of 67% (109, 113, 123). Survival did not closely correlate with the level of inflammatory infiltrate seen on histopathology, and the specific virus identified in the myocardium appeared to be an important variable regarding both the outcome and the inflammatory response. For instance, adenovirus was shown by Pauschinger et al. (97) and Shirali et al. (113) to cause a lower level of inflammatory infiltrate than enteroviruses or parvovirus B19. Similar findings have been obtained for lung transplant recipients (20).

MANAGEMENT

Care of a patient presenting with a clinical picture and history strongly suggestive of myocarditis depends on the severity of myocardial involvement (96). Many patients present with relatively mild disease, with minimal or no respiratory compromise and only mild signs of congestive heart failure. These patients require close monitoring to assess whether the disease will progress to worsening heart failure and the need for intensive medical care. Experimental animal studies suggest that bed rest may prevent an increase in intramyocardial viral replication in the acute stage. Thus, it appears to be prudent to place patients under this restriction at the time of diagnosis. Normal arterial blood oxygen levels should be maintained for any patient with compromised hemodynamics resulting in hypoxemia.

Positive Inotropic Agents Support Cardiac Output

The current strategy for therapy includes supporting the blood pressure to achieve end-organ perfusion and urine output without "driving" the myocardium with inotropic agents. Phosphodiesterase inhibitors such as intravenous milrinone have been used to provide both inotropy and afterload reduction and in typical cases are used in association with diuretics. More recently, nesiritide has been used either along with one or both of these agents or in place of this combination. For blood pressure support, calcium and/or vasopressin infusions may be used. The use of intravenous agents such as high-dose dopamine, dobutamine, norepinephrine, and epinephrine may improve blood pressure but may have the associated cost of increasing heart rate and increasing mechanical stress on the heart, as well as increasing the possibility for arrhythmias. Therefore, these agents should be used cautiously, if at all, perhaps only as a bridge to the placement of a mechanical assist device. When chronic oral therapy is possible and hypotension is not present, an afterload-reducing drug such as captopril or enalapril (104) may be used with beta-blockers such as carvedilol or metoprolol with or without diuretics.

Arrhythmias should be vigorously treated (37). Supraventricular tachyarrhythmias respond to digitalis. Ventricular arrhythmias respond to lidocaine or intravenous amiodarone. Despite aggressive treatment of these arrhythmias, rapid deterioration to ventricular fibrillation, especially in the very young, may occur and should be treated immediately by direct-current cardioversion. In some cases an internal cardioverter defibrillator is necessary. Complete atrioventricular block requires a temporary transvenous pacemaker. Chronic arrhythmias may persist long after the acute disease has passed (37). Thus, children who recover from myocarditis, regardless of etiology, should be monitored indefinitely.

The use of immunosuppressive agents in suspected or proven viral myocarditis is controversial (24, 40, 129). Some animal studies have suggested an exacerbation of virus-induced cytotoxicity in the presence of immunosuppressive drugs, possibly due to reduced interferon production. The Myocarditis Treatment Trial analyzed the use of immunosuppressive and steroid therapy (81). Although the study was performed with adult patients, the results are potentially applicable to children. There was no difference among patients treated with azathioprine and prednisone, cyclosporine and prednisone, or conventional therapy. Immunosuppressive therapy was not beneficial in most patients with histologically confirmed myocarditis.

Another important therapeutic option is the use of intravenous gamma globulin in children with myocarditis. One study (32) used this agent in 21 of 46 children with myocarditis; patients who received this drug had better LV function at follow-up and a trend toward a higher survival rate at 1 year. Whether this proves to be beneficial or whether these early results mirror the early published experience with corticosteroids remains to be seen (63, 74).

One study (63) reported efficacy of beta interferon treatment in myocarditis, with viral clearance and prevention of progressive deterioration of LV function. In this phase II study, 22 consecutive patients with chronic LV dysfunction and PCR-proven enteroviral or adenoviral infection were given subcutaneous beta interferon three times weekly for approximately 6 months; all 22 patients demonstrated viral clearance, reduced LV dilation, and improved systolic function. Another uncontrolled study reported similar success with alpha interferon in patients with enterovirus-induced myocarditis (28).

LV assist devices and aortic balloon pumps have been used to support the cardiovascular system in some cases, whereas extracorporeal membrane oxygenator therapy has been used in others (31, 49, 107, 124). When they are necessary, the devices may be lifesaving and should be considered an option in children large enough to allow placement of the device successfully. In some circumstances, transplantation becomes necessary (92, 123).

Vaccination

Vaccination is not currently available for the principal viral agents causing myocarditis. The efficacy of the polio vaccine has led to the suggestion that a broadly reactive enteroviral vaccine, if possible, or at least a CVB-specific vaccine, could be beneficial for reducing the incidence of myocarditis or DCM. Immunization is protective in mice (134). The possibility of success in this regard is supported by the study of EFE. This form of DCM was the most common form identified in children until the late 1960s, with an incidence of 1 in 5,000 live births in the United States. Since that time, the incidence has declined significantly. Mumps virus genomic RNA sequences were found in 90% of myocardial samples from EFE patients analyzed (89) (Fig. 5). Thus, EFE may result from persistent in utero mumps virus infection of the myocardium. The mumps virus vaccine has all but eliminated this form of DCM.

I am funded by the Abby Glaser Children's Heart Fund, TexGen, the Pediatric Cardiomyopathy Registry grant (NIH 2 R01 HL53392-11), the Pediatric Cardiomyopathy Specimen Repository grant (NIH

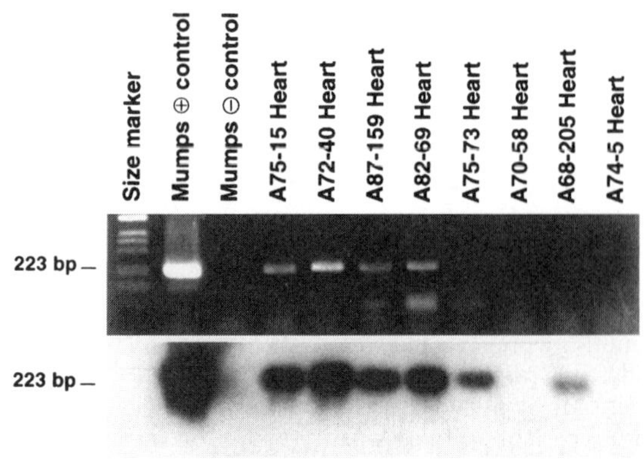

FIGURE 5 PCR analysis of fixed heart samples obtained from infants with EFE. Note the PCR-positive bands at 223 bp indicative of mumps virus. Sequence analysis confirmed the viral genome as that consistent with mumps.

1 R01 HL087000-01A1), the Children's Cardiomyopathy Foundation, and the John Patrick Albright Foundation.

REFERENCES

1. **Ainger, L. E., N. G. Lawyer, and C. W. Fitch.** 1966. Neonatal rubella myocarditis. *Br. Heart J.* **28:**691–697.
2. **Akhtar, N., J. Ni, C. Langston, G. J. Demmler, and J. A. Towbin.** 1996. PCR diagnosis of viral pneumonitis from fixed-lung tissue in children. *Biochem. Mol. Med.* **58:** 66–76.
3. **Archard, L. C., M. A. Khan, B. A. Soteriou, H. Zhang, H. J. Why, N. M. Robinson, and P. J. Richardson.** 1998. Characterization of coxsackie B virus RNA in myocardium from patients with dilated cardiomyopathy by nucleotide sequencing of reverse transcription-nested polymerase chain reaction products. *Hum. Pathol.* **29:** 578–584.
4. **Aretz, H. T.** 1987. Myocarditis: the Dallas criteria. *Hum. Pathol.* **18:**619–624.
5. **Baboonian, C., M. J. Davies, J. C. Booth, and W. J. McKenna.** 1997. Coxsackie B viruses and human heart disease. *Curr. Top. Microbiol. Immunol.* **223:**31–52.
6. **Baboonian, C., and T. Treasure.** 1997. Meta-analysis of the association of enteroviruses with human heart disease. *Heart* **78:**539–543.
7. **Badorff, C., G.-H. Lee, B. J. Lamphear, M. E. Martone, K. P. Campbell, R. E. Rhoads, and K. U. Knowlton.** 1999. Enteroviral protease 2A cleaves dystrophin: evidence of cytoskeletal disruption in an acquired cardiomyopathy. *Nat. Med.* **5:**320–326.
8. Reference deleted.
9. **Bengtssen, E., and B. Lamberger.** 1966. Five year follow-up study of cases suggestive of acute myocarditis. *Am. Heart J.* **72:**751–763.
10. **Bergelson, J. M., J. A. Cunningham, G. Drouguett, E. A. Kurt-Jones, A. Krithivas, J. S. Hong, M. S. Horwitz, R. L. Crowell, and R. W. Finberg.** 1997. Isolation of a common receptor for coxsackie B viruses and adenoviruses 2 and 5. *Science* **275:**1320–1323.
11. **Berkovich, S., R. Rodriguez-Torres, and J. S. Lin.** 1968. Virologic studies in children with acute myocarditis. *Am. J. Dis. Child.* **115:**207–221.
12. **Bessoudo, R., T. J. Marrie, and E. R. Smith.** 1981. Cardiac involvement in trichinosis. *Chest* **79:**698–699.
13. **Bowles, N. E., P. J. Richardson, E. G. J. Olsen, and L. C. Archard.** 1986. Detection of coxsackie-B virus specific RNA sequences in myocardial biopsy samples from patients with myocarditis and dilated cardiomyopathy. *Lancet* **1:**1120–1123.
14. **Bowles, N. E., M. L. Rose, P. Taylor, N. R. Banner, P. Morgan-Capner, L. Cunningham, L. C. Archard, and M. H. Yacoub.** 1989. End-stage dilated cardiomyopathy. Persistence of enterovirus RNA in myocardium at cardiac transplantation and lack of immune response. *Circulation* **80:**1128–1136.
15. **Bowles, N. E., and J. A. Towbin.** 1998. Molecular aspects of myocarditis. *Curr. Opin. Cardiol.* **13:**179–184.
16. **Bowles, N. E., F. Javier Fuentes-Garcia, K. A. Makar, H. Li, J. Gibson, F. Soto, P. L. Schwimmbeck, H. P. Schultheiss, and M. Pauschinger.** 2002. Analysis of the coxsackievirus or dilated cardiomyopathy. *Mol. Genet. Metab.* **77:**257–259.
17. **Bowles, N. E., J. Ni, D. L. Kearney, M. Pauschinger, H. P. Schultheiss, R. McCarthy, J. Hare, J. T. Bricker, K. R. Bowles, and J. A. Towbin.** 2003. Detection of viruses in myocardial tissues by polymerase chain reaction: evidence of adenovirus as a common cause of myocarditis in children and adults. *J. Am. Coll. Cardiol.* **42:**466–472.
18. **Bowles, N. E., K. R. Bowles, and J. A. Towbin.** 2005. Viral genome detection and outcome in myocarditis. *Heart Failure Clin.* **1:**407–417.
19. **Braiser, A. R., J. D. Macklis, D. Vaughan, L. Warner, and J. M. Kirshenbaum.** 1987. Myopericarditis as an initial presentation of meningococcemia. *Am. J. Med.* **82:** 641–644.
20. **Bridges, N. D., T. L. Spray, M. H. Collins, N. E. Bowles, and J. A. Towbin.** 1998. Adenovirus infection in the lung results in graft failure after lung transplantation. *J. Thorac. Cardiovasc. Surg.* **116:**617–623.
21. **Brownstein, D. G.** 1998. Comparative genetics of resistance to viruses. *Am. J. Hum. Genet.* **62:**211–214.
22. **Burch, G. E., S.-C. Sun, R. S. Sohal, K. C. Chu, and H. L. Colcolough.** 1968. Diphtheritic myocarditis. *Am. J. Cardiol.* **21:**261–268.
23. **Calabrese, F., and G. Thiene.** 2003. Myocarditis and inflammatory cardiomyopathy: microbiological and molecular aspects. *Cardiovasc. Res.* **60:**11–25.
24. **Chan, K. Y., M. Iwahara, L. N. Benson, G. J. Wilson, and R. M. Freedom.** 1991. Immunosuppressive therapy in the management of acute myocarditis in children: a clinical trial. *J. Am. Coll. Cardiol.* **17:**458–460.
25. **Chaudary, S., and B. E. Jaski.** 1989. Fulminant mumps myocarditis. *Ann. Intern. Med.* **110:**569–570.
26. **Chow, L. H., S. J. Radio, T. D. Sears, and B. M. McManus.** 1989. Insensitivity of right ventricular biopsy in the diagnosis of myocarditis. *J. Am. Coll. Cardiol.* **14:** 915–920.
27. **Cooper, L. T., Jr.** 2003. Idiopathic giant cell myocarditis, p. 405–420. *In* L. T. Cooper, Jr. (ed.), *Myocarditis: from Bench to Bedside*. Humana Press, Totowa, NJ.
28. **Daliento, L., F. Calabrese, F. Tona, A. L. Caforio, G. Tarsia, A. Angelini, and G. Thiene.** 2003. Successful treatment of enterovirus-induced myocarditis with interferon alpha. *J. Heart Lung Transplant.* **22:**214–217.
29. **Davidoff, R., I. Palacios, J. Southern, J. T. Fallon, J. Newell, and G. W. Dec.** 1991. Giant cell versus lymphocytic myocarditis. A comparison of their clinical features and long-term outcomes. *Circulation* **83:**953–961.
30. **Dec, G. W., I. F. Palacios, J. T. Fallon, H. T. Aretz, J. Mills, D. C. Lee, and R. A. Johnson.** 1985. Active myocarditis in the spectrum of acute dilated cardiomyopathies: clinical features, histologic correlates, and clinical outcome. *N. Engl. J. Med.* **312:**885–890.
31. **Deiwick, M., A. Hoffmeier, T. D. Tjan, T. Krasemann, C. Schmid, and H. H. Scheld.** 2005. Heart failure in

children—mechanical assistance. *Thorac. Cardiovasc. Surg.* **53**(Suppl. 2):S135–S140.
32. **Drucker, N. A., S. D. Colan, A. B. Lewis, A. S. Beiser, D. L. Wessel, M. Takahashi, A. L. Baker, A. R. Perez-Atayde, and J. W. Newburger.** 1994. Gamma-globulin treatment of acute myocarditis in the pediatric population. *Circulation* **89:**252–257.
33. **English, R. F., J. E. Janosky, J. A. Ettedgui, and S. A. Webber.** 2004. Outcomes for children with acute myocarditis. *Cardiol. Young* **14:**488–493.
34. **Felker, G. M., C. J. Jaeger, E. Klodas, D. R. Thiemann, J. M. Hare, R. H. Hruban, E. K. Kasper, and K. L. Baughman.** 2000. Myocarditis and long-term survival in peripartum cardiomyopathy. *Am. Heart J.* **140:**785–791.
35. **Ferrans, V. J., and E. R. Rodriguez.** 1985. Cardiovascular lesions in collagen-vascular diseases. *Heart Vessels* **1:**256–261.
36. **Francalanci, P., J. L. Chance, M. Vatta, S. Jimenez, H. Li, J. A. Towbin, and N. E. Bowles.** 2004. Cardiotropic viruses in the myocardium of children with end-stage heart disease. *J. Heart Lung Transplant* **23:**1046–1052.
37. **Friedman, R. A., D. L. Kearney, J. P. Moak, A. L. Fenrich, and J. C. Perry.** 1994. Persistence of ventricular arrhythmia after resolution of occult myocarditis in children and young adults. *J. Am. Coll. Cardiol.* **24:**780–783.
38. **Friedman, R. A., J. A. Schowengerdt, and J. A. Towbin.** 1998. Myocarditis, p. 1777–1794. *In* J. T. Bricker, A. Garson, Jr., D. J. Fisher, and S. R. Neish (ed.), *The Science and Practice of Pediatric Cardiology*, 2nd ed. Williams & Wilkins, Baltimore, MD.
39. **Frishman, W., M. E. Kraus, J. Zabkar, V. Brooks, D. Alonso, and L. M. Dixon.** 1977. Infectious mononucleosis and fatal myocarditis. *Chest* **72:**535–538.
40. **Frustaci, A., C. Chimenti, F. Calabrese, M. Pieroni, G. Thiene, and A. Maseri.** 2003. Immunosuppressive therapy for active lymphocytic myocarditis: virological and immunologic profile of responders versus nonresponders. *Circulation* **107:**857–863.
41. **Godeny, E. K., and C. J. Gauntt.** 1987. Murine natural killer cells limit coxsackievirus B3 replication. *J. Immunol.* **139:**913–918.
42. **Grist, N. R., and D. Reid.** 1988. General pathogenicity and epidemiology, p. 241–252. *In* M. Bendinelli and H. Friedman (ed.), *Coxsackieviruses: a General Update*. Plenum, New York, NY.
43. **Grogan, M., M. M. Redfield, K. R. Bailey, G. S. Reeder, B. J. Gersh, W. D. Edwards, and R. J. Rodeheffer.** 1995. Long-term outcome of patients with biopsy-proven myocarditis: comparison with idiopathic dilated cardiomyopathy. *J. Am. Coll. Cardiol.* **26:**80–84.
44. **Gross, D., H. Willens, and S. M. Zeldis.** 1981. Myocarditis in Legionnaires' disease. *Chest* **79:**232–234.
45. **Grumbach, I. M., A. Heim, P. Pring-Akerblom, S. Vonhof, W. J. Hein, V. Muller, and H. R. Figulla.** 1999. Adenoviruses and enteroviruses as pathogens in myocarditis and dilated cardiomyopathy. *Acta Cardiol.* **54:**83–88.
46. **Hastreiter, A. R., and R. A. Miller.** 1964. Diagnosis and treatment of myocarditis and other myocardial diseases. *Adv. Cardiopulm. Dis.* **22:**250–258.
47. **Hauck, A. J., D. L. Kearney, and W. D. Edwards.** 1989. Evaluation of postmortem endomyocardial biopsy specimens from 38 patients with lymphocytic myocarditis: implications for role of sampling error. *Mayo Clin. Proc.* **64:** 1235–1245.
48. **Hayder, H., and A. Mullbacher.** 1996. Molecular basis of immune evasion strategies by adenoviruses. *Immunol. Cell Biol.* **74:**504–512.
49. **Helman, D. N., L. J. Addonizio, D. L. Morales, K. A. Catanese, M. A. Flannery, J. M. Quagebeur, N. M. Edwards, M. E. Galantowicz, and M. C. Oz.** 2000. Implantable left ventricular assist devices can successfully bridge adolescent patients to transplant. *J. Heart Lung Transplant.* **19:**121–126.
50. **Henke, A., S. Huber, A. Stelzner, and J. L. Whitton.** 1995. The role of $CD8^+$ T lymphocytes in coxsackievirus B3-induced myocarditis. *J. Virol.* **69:**6720–6728.
51. **Hirschman, Z. S., and S. G. Hammer.** 1974. Coxsackie virus myopericarditis: a microbiological and clinical review. *Am. J. Cardiol.* **34:**224–232.
52. **Hori, H., T. Matoba, M. Shingu, and H. Toshima.** 1981. The role of cell mediated immunity in coxsackie B viral myocarditis. *Jpn. Circ. J.* **45:**1409–1414.
53. **Horn, H., and O. Saphir.** 1935. The involvement of the myocardium in tuberculosis. *Ann. Rev. Tuberc.* **32:**492–506.
54. **Huber, S. A.** 1997. Coxsackievirus-induced myocarditis is dependent on distinct immunopathogenic responses in different strains of mice. *Lab. Investig.* **76:**691–701.
55. **Hudson, R. E. B.** 1965. Myocardial involvement (myocarditis) in infections, infestation and drug therapy. *Cardiovasc. Pathol.* **1:**782–854.
56. **Hutchins, G. M., and S. A. Vie.** 1972. The progression of interstitial myocarditis to idiopathic endocardial fibroelastosis. *Am. J. Pathol.* **66:**483–496.
57. **James, T. N.** 1968. Sudden death in babies: new observations on the heart. *Am. J. Cardiol.* **22:**479–506.
58. **Jin, O., M. J. Sole, J. W. Butany, W. K. Chia, P. R. McLaughlin, P. Liu, and C. C. Liew.** 1990. Detection of enterovirus RNA in myocardial biopsies from patients with myocarditis and cardiomyopathy using gene amplification by polymerase chain reaction. *Circulation* **82:**8–16.
59. **Karjalainen, J.** 1989. Streptococcal tonsillitis and acute nonrheumatic myopericarditis. *Chest* **95:**359–363.
60. **Kerr, L. D., and H. Spiera.** 1993. Myocarditis as a complication in scleroderma patients with myositis. *Clin. Cardiol.* **16:**895–899.
61. **Klingel, K., M. Sauter, C. T. Bock, G. Szalay, J. J. Schnorr, and R. Kandolf.** 2004. Molecular pathology of inflammatory cardiomyopathy. *Med. Microbiol. Immunol.* **193:**101–107.
62. **Knowlton, K. U., E. S. Jeon, N. Berkley, R. Wessely, and S. Huber.** 1996. A mutation in the puff region of VP2 attenuates the myocarditic phenotype of an infectious cDNA of the Woodruff variant of coxsackievirus B3. *J. Virol.* **70:**7811–7818.
63. **Kuhl, U., M. Pauschinger, P. L. Schwimmbeck, B. Seeberg, C. Lober, M. Noutsias, W. Poller, and H. P. Schulheiss.** 2003. Interferon-β treatment eliminates cardiotropic viruses and improves left ventricular function in patients with myocardial persistence of viral genomes and left ventricular dysfunction. *Circulation* **107:**2793–2798.
64. **Lahariya, C., and S. K. Pradhan.** 2006. Emergence of chikungunya virus in Indian subcontinent after 32 years: a review. *J. Vector Borne Dis.* **43**(4)**:**151–160.
65. **Langley, R. J., G. A. Prince, and H. S. Ginsberg.** 1998. HIV type-1 infection of the cotton rat (Sigmodon fulviventer and S. hispidus). *Proc. Natl. Acad. Sci. USA* **95:** 14355–14360.
66. **Lash, A. D., A. L. Wittman, and F. P. Quismorio, Jr.** 1986. Myocarditis in mixed connective tissue disease: clinical and pathologic study of three cases and review of the literature. *Semin. Arthritis Rheum.* **15:**288–296.
67. **Leak, D., and M. Meghji.** 1979. Toxoplasmic infection in cardiac disease. *Am. J. Cardiol.* **43:**841–849.
68. **Lee, C., E. Maull, N. Chapman, S. Tacy, and C. Gauntt.** 1997. Genomic regions of coxsackievirus B3 associated with cardiovirulence. *J. Med. Virol.* **52:**341–347.

69. **Lewes, D., D. J. Rainford, and W. F. Lane.** 1974. Symptomless myocarditis and myalgia in viral and Mycoplasma pneumoniae infections. *Br. Heart J.* **36:**924–932.
70. **Lorber, A., A. Zonis, E. Maisuls, L. Dembo, A. Palant, and T. C. Iancu.** 1988. The scale of myocardial involvement in varicella myocarditis. *Int. J. Cardiol.* **20:**257–262.
71. **Lowry, P. J., R. A. Thompson, and W. A. Little.** 1983. Humoral immunity in cardiomyopathy. *Br. Heart J.* **50:** 390–394.
72. **Maisch, B., R. Trostel-Soeder, E. Strechemesser, P. A. Berg, and K. Kochsiek.** 1982. Diagnostic relevance of humoral and cell-mediated immune reactions in patients with acute viral myocarditis. *Clin. Exp. Immunol.* **48:**533–545.
73. **Maisch, B., A. D. Ristic, I. Portig, and S. Pankuweit.** 2003. Human viral cardiomyopathy. *Front. Biosci.* **8:**s39–s67.
74. **Maisch, B., G. Hufnagel, S. Kölsch, R. Funck, A. Richter, H. Rupp, M. Herzum, and S. Pankuweit.** 2004. Treatment of inflammatory dilated cardiomyopathy and (peri)myocarditis with immunosuppression and i.v. immunoglobulins. *Herz* **29:**624–636.
75. **Mantke, O. D., R. Meyer, S. Prosch, A. Nitsche, K. Leitmeyer, R. Kallies, and M. Niedrig.** 2005. High prevalence of cardiotropic viruses in myocardial tissue from explanted hearts of heart transplant recipients and heart donors: a 3-year retrospective study from a German patients' pool. *J. Heart Lung Transplant.* **24:**1632–1638.
76. **Marin-Garcia, J., and F. F. Barrett.** 1983. Myocardial function in Rocky Mountain spotted fever: echocardiographic assessment. *Am. J. Cardiol.* **51:**341–343.
77. **Marsden, P. D.** 1971. South American trypanosomiasis (Chagas' disease). *Int. Rev. Trop. Med.* **4:**97–121.
78. **Martin, A. B., S. Webber, F. J. Fricker, R. Jaffe, G. Demmler, D. Kearney, Y.-H. Zhang, B. Gelb, J. Ni, J. T. Bricker, and J. A. Towbin.** 1994. Acute myocarditis: rapid diagnosis by PCR in children. *Circulation* **90:**330–333.
79. **Martino, T. A., P. Liu, and M. J. Sole.** 1994. Viral infection and the pathogenesis of dilated cardiomyopathy. *Circ. Res.* **74:**182–188.
80. **Mason, J. W.** 1991. Distinct forms of myocarditis. *Circulation* **83:**1110–1111.
81. **Mason, J. W., J. B. O'Connell, A. Herskowitz, N. R. Rose, B. M. McManus, M. E. Billingham, and T. E. Moon.** 1995. A clinical trial of immunosuppressive therapy for myocarditis. *N. Engl. J. Med.* **333:**269–275.
82. **Matsumori, A.** 1997. Molecular and immune mechanisms in the pathogenesis of cardiomyopathy: role of viruses, cytokines and nitric oxide. *Jpn. Circ. J.* **61:**275–291.
83. **Matsumori, A.** 2005. Hepatitis C virus infection and cardiomyopathies. *Circ. Res.* **96:**144–147.
84. **Matsumori, A.** 2006. Role of hepatitis C virus in cardiomyopathies. *Ernst Schering Res. Found. Workshop* **55:** 99–120.
85. **McAlister, H. F., P. T. Klemontowicz, C. Andrews, J. D. Fisher, M. Feld, and S. Furman.** 1989. Lyme carditis: an important cause of reversible heart block. *Ann. Intern. Med.* **110:**339–345.
86. **McCarthy, R. E., J. P. Boehmer, R. H. Hruban, G. M. Hutchins, E. K. Kasper, J. M. Hare, and K. L. Baughman.** 2000. Long-term outcome of fulminant myocarditis as compared with acute (nonfulminant) myocarditis. *N. Engl. J. Med.* **342:**690–695.
87. **McManus, B. M., and R. Kandolf.** 1991. Evolving concepts of cause, consequence and control in myocarditis. *Curr. Opin. Cardiol.* **6:**418–427.
88. **Narula, J., N. Haider, R. Virmani, T. G. DiSalvo, F. D. Kolodgie, R. J. Hajjar, U. Schmidt, M. J. Semigran, G. W. Dec, and B. A. Khaw.** 1996. Apoptosis in myocytes in end-stage heart disease. *N. Engl. J. Med.* **335:** 1182–1189.
89. **Ni, J., N. E. Bowles, Y.-H. Kim, G. J. Demmler, D. L. Kearney, J. T. Bricker, and J. A. Towbin.** 1997. Viral infection of the myocardium in endocardial fibroelastosis: molecular evidence for the role of mumps virus as an etiological agent. *Circulation* **95:**133–139.
90. **Obeyesekere, I., and Y. Hermon.** 1972. Myocarditis and cardiomyopathy after arbovirus infections (dengue and chikungunya fever). *Br. Heart J.* **34:**821–827.
91. **O'Connell, J. B., R. E. Fowles, J. A. Robinson, R. Subramanian, R. E. Henkin, and R. M. Gunnar.** 1984. Clinical and pathologic findings of myocarditis in two families with dilated cardiomyopathy. *Am. Heart J.* **167:** 127–135.
92. **O'Connell, J. B., G. W. Dec, I. F. Goldenberg, R. C. Starling, G. H. Mudge, S. M. Augustine, M. R. Costanzo-Nordin, M. L. Hess, J. D. Hosenpud, and T. B. Icengl.** 1990. Results of heart transplantation for active lymphocytic myocarditis. *J. Heart Transplant.* **9:** 351–356.
93. **Okabe, M., K. Fukuda, K. Arakawa, and M. Kikuchi.** 1997. Chronic variant myocarditis associated with hepatitis C virus infection. *Circulation* **96:**22–24.
94. **Okura, Y., G. W. Dec, J. M. Hare, M. Kodama, G. J. Berry, H. D. Tazelaar, K. R. Bailey, and L. T. Cooper.** 2003. A clinical and histopathologic comparison of cardiac sarcoidosis and idiopathic giant cell myocarditis. *J. Am. Coll. Cardiol.* **41:**322–329.
95. **Pankuweit, S., S. Lamparter, M. Schoppet, and B. Maisch.** 2004. Parvovirus B19 genome in endomyocardial biopsy specimen. *Circulation* **109:**e179.
96. **Parrillo, J. E.** 1998. Myocarditis: how should we treat in 1998? *J. Heart Lung Transplant.* **17:**941–944.
97. **Pauschinger, M., N. E. Bowles, F. J. Fuentes-Garcia, V. Pham, U. Kuhl, P. L. Schwimmbeck, H. P. Schultheiss, and J. A. Towbin.** 1999. Detection of adenoviral genome in the myocardium of adult patients with idiopathic left ventricular dysfunction. *Circulation* **99:**1348–1354.
98. **Perez Pulido, S.** 1984. Acute and subacute myocarditis. *Cardiovasc. Rev. Rep.* **5:**912–926.
99. **Piedra, P. A., G. A. Poveda, B. Ramsey, K. McKoy, and P. W. Hiatt.** 1998. Incidence and prevalence of neutralizing antibodies to the common adenoviruses in children with cystic fibrosis: implication for gene therapy with adenovirus vectors. *Pediatrics* **101:**1013–1019.
100. **Poller, W., H. Fechner, M. Noutsias, C. Tschoepe, and H. P. Schultheiss.** 2002. Highly variable expression of virus receptors in the human cardiovascular system. Implications for cardiotropic viral infections and gene therapy. *Z. Kardiol.* **91:**978–991.
101. **Poltera, A. A., J. N. Cox, and R. Owor.** 1976. Pancarditis affecting the conducting system and all valves in human African trypanosomiasis. *Br. Heart J.* **38:**827–837.
102. **Proby, C. M., D. Hackett, S. Gupta, and T. M. Cox.** 1986. Acute myopericarditis in influenza A infection. *Q. J. Med.* **60:**887–892.
103. **Puchkov, G. F., and B. M. Minkovich.** 1972. A case of respiratory syncytial infection in a child by interstitial myocarditis with lethal outcome. *Arkh. Patol.* **34:**70–73.
104. **Rezkalla, S., R. A. Kloner, G. Khatib, and R. Khatib.** 1990. Beneficial effects of captopril in acute coxsackievirus B3 murine myocarditis. *Circulation* **81:**1039–1046.
104a. **Rodriguez, E. R., S. Nasim, J. Hsia, R. L. Sandin, A. Ferreira, B. A. Hilliard, A. M. Ross, and C. T. Garrett.** 1991. Cardiac myocytes and dendritic cells harbor hu-

man immunodeficiency virus in infected patients with and without cardiac dysfunction: detection by multiplex, nested, polymerase chain reaction in individually microdissected cells from right ventricular endomyocardial biopsy tissue. *Am. J. Cardiol.* **68:**1511–1520.

105. **Rosenstein, E. D., M. J. Zucker, and N. Kramer.** 2000. Giant cell myocarditis: most fatal of autoimmune diseases. *Semin. Arthritis Rheum.* **30:**1–16.
106. **Saphir, O., and M. Field.** 1954. Complications of myocarditis in children. *J. Pediatr.* **45:**457–463.
107. **Schindler, E., M. Muller, M. Kwapisz, H. Akinturk, K. Valeske, J. Thul, and G. Hempelmann.** 2003. Ventricular cardiac-assist devices in infants and children: anesthetic considerations. *J. Cardiothorac. Vasc. Anesth.* **17:**617–621.
108. **Schonian, U., M. Crombach, S. Maser, and B. Maisch.** 1995. Cytomegalovirus associated heart muscle disease. *Eur. Heart J.* **16**(Suppl. 10)**:**46–49.
109. **Schowengerdt, K. O., J. Ni, S. W. Denfield, R. J. Gajarski, B. Radovancevic, O. H. Frazier, G. J. Demmler, D. L. Kearney, J. T. Bricker, and J. A. Towbin.** 1996. Diagnosis, surveillance, and epidemiologic evaluation of viral infections in pediatric cardiac transplant recipients with the use of polymerase chain reaction. *J. Heart Lung Transplant.* **15:**111–123.
110. **Schowengerdt, K. O., J. Ni, S. W. Denfield, R. J. Gajarski, N. E. Bowles, G. Rosenthal, D. L. Kearney, J. K. Price, B. B. Rogers, G. M. Schauer, R. E. Chinnock, and J. A. Towbin.** 1997. Association of parvovirus B19 genome in children with myocarditis and cardiac allograft rejection: diagnosis using the polymerase chain reaction. *Circulation* **96:**3549–3554.
111. **Shimizu, C., C. Rambaud, G. Cheron, C. Rouzioux, G. M. Lozinski, A. Rao, G. Stanway, H. F. Krous, and J. C. Burns.** 1995. Molecular identification of viruses in sudden infant death associated with myocarditis and pericarditis. *Pediatr. Infect. Dis. J.* **14:**584–588.
112. **Shingu, M.** 1989. Laboratory diagnosis of viral myocarditis: a review. *Jpn. Circ. J.* **53:**87–93.
113. **Shirali, G. S., J. Ni, R. E. Chinnock, J. K. Johnston, G. L. Rosenthal, N. E. Bowles, and J. A. Towbin.** 2001. Association of viral genome with graft loss in children after cardiac transplantation. *N. Engl. J. Med.* **344:**1498–1503.
114. **Simon, F., P. Paule, and M. Oliver.** 2008. Chikungunya virus-induced myopericarditis: toward an increase of dilated cardiomyopathy in countries with epidemics? *Am. J. Trop. Med. Hyg.* **78:**212–213.
115. **Sole, M. J., and P. Liu.** 1993. Viral myocarditis: a paradigm for understanding the pathogenesis and treatment of dilated cardiomyopathy. *J. Am. Coll. Cardiol.* **22:**99A–105A.
116. **Stoica, S. C., M. Goddard, S. Tsuiu, J. Dunning, K. McNeil, J. Parameshwar, amd S. R. Large.** 2003. Ventricular assist surprise: giant cell myocarditis or sarcoidosis? *J. Thorac. Cardiovasc. Surg.* **126:**2072–2074.
117. **Strand, S., W. J. Hofmann, H. Hug, M. Muller, G. Otto, D. Strand, S. M. Mariani, W. Stremmel, P. H. Krammer, and P. R. Galle.** 1996. Lymphocyte apoptosis induced by CD95 (APO-1/Fas) ligand-expressing tumor cells—a mechanism of immune evasion? *Nat. Med.* **2:**1361–1366.
118. **Tomko, R. P., R. Xu, and L. Philipson.** 1997. HCAR and MCAR: the human and mouse cellular receptors for subgroup C adenoviruses and group B coxsackieviruses. *Proc. Natl. Acad. Sci. USA* **94:**3352–3356.
119. **Towbin, J. A., J. T. Bricker, and A. Garson, Jr.** 1992. Electrocardiographic criteria for diagnosis of acute myocardial infarction in childhood. *Am. J. Cardiol.* **69:**1545–1548.
120. **Towbin, J. A.** 1993. Molecular genetic aspects of cardiomyopathy. *Biochem. Med. Metab. Biol.* **49:**285–320.
121. **Towbin, J. A.** 1998. The role of cytoskeletal proteins in cardiomyopathies. *Curr. Opin. Cell Biol.* **10:**131–139.
122. **Towbin, J. A., and N. E. Bowles.** 2002. The failing heart. *Nature* **415:**227–233.
123. **Towbin, J. A.** 2002. Cardiomyopathy and heart transplantation in children. *Curr. Opin. Cardiol.* **17:**274–279.
124. **Undar, A., E. D. McKenzie, M. C. McGarry, W. R. Owens, D. L. Surprise, V. D. Kilpack, M. W. Mueller, S. A. Stayer, D. B. Andropoulos, J. A. Towbin, and C. D. Fraser, Jr.** 2004. Outcomes of congenital heart surgery patients after extracorporeal life support at Texas Children's Hospital. *Artif. Organs* **28:**963–966.
125. **Van den Veyver, I. B., J. Ni, N. Bowles, R. J. Carpenter, Jr., C. P. Weiner, J. Yankowitz, K. J. Moise, Jr., J. Henderson, and J. A. Towbin.** 1998. Detection of intrauterine viral infection using the polymerase chain reaction (PCR). *Mol. Genet. Metab.* **63:**85–95.
126. **Vargo, T. A., D. B. Singer, P. C. Gillette, and D. J. Fernbach.** 1977. Myocarditis due to visceral larva migrans. *J. Pediatr.* **90:**322–323.
127. **Wang, X., G. Zhang, F. Liu, M. Han, D. Xu, and Y. Zang.** 2004. Prevalence of human parvovirus B19 DNA in cardiac tissues of patients with congenital heart diseases indicated by nested PCR and in situ hybridization. *J. Clin. Virol.* **31:**20–24.
128. **Weiss, L. M., X. F. Liu, K. L. Chang, and M. E. Billingham.** 1992. Detection of enteroviral RNA in idiopathic dilated cardiomyopathy and other human cardiac tissues. *J. Clin. Investig.* **90:**156–159.
129. **Weller, A. H., M. Hall, and S. A. Huber.** 1992. Polyclonal immunoglobulin therapy protects against cardiac damage in experimental coxsackievirus-induced myocarditis. *Eur. Heart J.* **13:**115–119.
130. **Wong, C. Y., J. J. Woodruff, and J. F. Woodruff.** 1997. Generation of cytotoxic T lymphocytes during coxsackie B-3 infection. II. Characterization of effector cells and demonstration of cytotoxicity against viral infected fibers. *J. Immunol.* **118:**165–169.
131. **Woodruff, J. F.** 1980. Viral myocarditis: a review. *Am. J. Pathol.* **101:**427–484.
132. **Wynn, J., and E. Braunwald.** 1997. The cardiomyopathies and myocarditides, p. 1404–1463. *In* E. Braunwald (ed.), *Heart Disease: a Textbook of Cardiovascular Medicine*. W. B. Saunders, Philadelphia, PA.
133. **Yamamoto, L. G.** 2003. Kawasaki disease. *Pediatr. Emerg. Care* **19:**422–424.
134. **Zhang, H. Y., P. Morgan-Capner, N. Latif, Y. A. Pandolfino, W. Fan, M. J. Dunn, and L. C. Archard.** 1997. Coxsackievirus B3-induced myocarditis: characterization of stable attenuated variants that protect against infection with the cardiovirulent wild-type strain. *Am. J. Pathol.* **150:**2197–2207.

Viral Infections of the Skin

BRENDA L. BARTLETT AND STEPHEN K. TYRING

8

Viral infections produce a variety of cutaneous manifestations. Skin and mucosal findings either are the result of primary viral replication within the epidermis or are a secondary effect of viral replication elsewhere in the body. Three groups of viruses represent most primary epidermal viral replications: human papillomaviruses (HPV), herpesviruses, and poxviruses. Several virus families, such as retroviruses, paramyxoviruses, togaviruses, parvoviruses, and picornaviruses, produce skin lesions secondarily. Other viruses, such as rhabdoviruses, orthomyxoviruses, and reoviruses, rarely induce skin lesions.

CLINICAL MANIFESTATIONS

A wide spectrum of skin lesions can result from viral infections. For example, while infection with HPV is most known for causing verrucous papules, other manifestations of this viral infection include erythematous macules in epidermodysplasia verruciformis (EV), smooth papules in bowenoid papulosis, and fungating Buschke-Lowenstein tumors. Vesicles are considered the primary lesion in herpes simplex virus (HSV), varicella-zoster virus (VZV), and many coxsackievirus infections. However, the vesicles are often preceded by erythema and papules and followed by pustules, crusts, or shallow ulcers. Ulcers without other stages can be seen with cytomegalovirus (CMV) infections of the skin and mucous membranes as well as with HSV, VZV, or coxsackievirus infections of mucous membranes. Both macules and papules are seen with measles and rubella. Macules coalescing into larger erythematous patches are seen in Epstein-Barr virus (EBV), human herpesvirus 6 (HHV-6), and parvovirus B19 infections.

Some viruses induce skin changes that are highly suggestive of the diagnosis, such as the verrucous papules seen with papillomavirus infection or the smooth umbilicated papules resulting from poxvirus infection. However, other viruses produce nonspecific skin lesions, including urticaria, erythema multiforme, and petechiae. In these cases, a differential including viral and nonviral etiologies must be considered. Depending on the clinical picture, vesicles induced by HSV type 1 (HSV-1), HSV-2, or VZV may be diagnostic or may necessitate a broad differential. Other herpesviruses, such as EBV, CMV, and HHV-6, less frequently produce skin manifestations and are most accurately diagnosed when the systemic manifestations of the viral infection are also considered. Cutaneous manifestations of viral diseases can range from very specific (e.g., dermatomal vesicles of herpes zoster) to very general (e.g., urticaria), and the differential diagnosis must take the total clinical presentation of the patient into consideration.

PATHOPHYSIOLOGY

Viruses infect the skin via three different routes: direct inoculation, local spread from an internal focus, and systemic infection. Viruses that infect the skin by direct inoculation include primary HSV, papillomaviruses, and most poxviruses (except smallpox). Primary VZV produces systemic infection with viremia and dissemination to the skin and mucous membranes. Recurrent VZV (shingles) or recurrent HSV reaches the skin from an internal focus, the sensory ganglia.

The effect of viral replication on infected cells may directly produce skin lesions, or the skin lesions may result from the host response to the virus. Alternatively, the lesions may be the result of the interaction between the viral replication and the host response. In general, viruses that replicate in the epidermis directly produce skin lesions. On the other hand, viruses that replicate elsewhere in the body typically produce skin manifestations via the host's response to viral replication. For example, the host's cell-mediated immune response to rubella and measles viruses is thought to be at least partly responsible for the skin manifestations associated with these viruses, and rashless measles can manifest as pneumonitis or central nervous system (CNS) disease in highly immunocompromised hosts.

DIAGNOSIS

Laboratory Diagnosis

Five general methods of laboratory diagnosis are available to confirm suspected viral diseases: viral culture, microscopic examination of infected tissue, detection of viral antigens, detection of viral DNA or RNA, and serology. Viral culture is the preferred method of diagnosis when a good culture system is available. If HSV-1 or HSV-2 is responsible for the lesion, a positive culture can be obtained within 1 to 2 days. Viral cultures are most likely to be positive if the sample is taken from the vesicular stage, while later stages of healing are less likely to be positive. Positive cultures are more difficult to obtain from VZV, even when fresh vesicular fluid is used to inoculate the cell culture.

A second method of diagnosis is microscopic evaluation of the involved skin. Such examination can reveal histologic changes consistent with a particular viral family but is usually not helpful in identifying the specific virus responsible. For example, benign warts caused by different HPV types have a similar histologic appearance under the microscope. Histologic changes induced by HSV-1 and HSV-2, as well as by VZV, are similar to each other but distinctive from changes associated with other herpesviruses. A more rapid procedure in suspected HSV-1, HSV-2, and VZV infection is the Tzanck smear. After scraping cells from the base of a vesicle, a smear is prepared on a glass slide and stained with Wright or Giemsa stain. The presence of multinucleated giant cells confirms that one of the three viruses is responsible for the vesicle, though it cannot specify which virus. Another viral infection that can be diagnosed directly from smears from a skin lesion is molluscum contagiosum (MC). The presence of intracytoplasmic inclusion bodies will help to distinguish papules associated with MC virus from skin lesions of *Cryptococcus neoformans*, which can appear very similar in human immunodeficiency virus (HIV)-infected patients.

Among rapid diagnostic tests, perhaps the most frequently used for detection of viral infections of the skin is fluorescent-antibody detection of HSV-1, HSV-2, and VZV. This technique distinguishes among these three viruses, in contrast to the Tzanck smear. Immunoperoxidase techniques are sometimes used to detect HPV capsid antigens. However, these techniques can lead to false-negative results in oncogenic types of HPV, as the viral DNA may not have associated capsid antigens. Labor-intensive techniques such as electron microscopy or immunoelectron microscopy can be used to detect viral particles or viral antigens.

Assays to detect viral nucleic acid are becoming more widely used, especially when no effective culture or serologic assay is available. In situ hybridization allows not only detection of the viral nucleic acid but also histologic localization of the virus to specific cells. PCR primers can be designed to detect a range of viruses within a particular family (i.e., consensus primers) or may be specific for a particular virus (i.e., type-specific primers). Further information can be gained from in situ PCR, which combines the sensitivity of PCR with localization of the virus on histology.

A hybrid capture assay is now routinely used to detect HPV DNA from Papanicolaou (Pap) smears. This is a non-radioactive, relatively rapid, liquid hybridization assay designed to detect 18 HPV types divided into high- and low-risk groups; it has the advantage of being able to provide qualitative estimates of viral load, which may correlate with the grade and the natural history of cervical pathology. This assay uses specific RNA probes which hybridize with the target HPV DNA obtained from Pap smears. The hybrids are then captured onto a solid phase with antibodies specific for RNA-DNA hybrids. The captured hybrids are detected with antibodies conjugated to alkaline phosphatase. The resulting signal is then amplified. This additional process augments the sensitivity of the Pap smear alone. Hybrid capture assay may be particularly useful when the Pap smear is read as ASCUS (atypical squamous cells of undetermined significance) (23).

Differential Diagnosis

The differential diagnosis of various types of viral exanthemata requires the consideration of a spectrum of both viral and nonviral conditions. Vesicles may be due to HSV-1, HSV-2, VZV, poxviruses, hand-foot-and-mouth disease viruses, and other coxsackieviruses. Most vesicles develop into pustules during the process of healing. Therefore, the differential diagnosis of vesiculopustules must include nonviral entities such as bullous impetigo, insect bite reactions, drug eruptions, contact dermatitis, and gonococcemia. Macules may be observed in rubella, EBV infection (infectious mononucleosis), and HHV-6 infection (roseola), as well as a variety of coxsackievirus A and B and echovirus infections. Nonviral etiologies of macules may include drug eruptions and bacterial infections (scarlet fever, Rocky Mountain spotted fever, and erysipelas). Macules may manifest with papules in measles, echovirus infections, and human parvovirus B19 infections (erythema infectiosum). Maculopapular lesions may also be seen in erythema multiforme, which is commonly of viral etiology (HSV) or may be associated with nonviral infections or drug eruptions. Papules are seen in a variety of poxviruses and HPV infections, as well as in Gianotti-Crosti syndrome, which may be a manifestation of hepatitis B or another viral infection. Papules may also be seen with bacterial infection (*Bartonella* and *Mycobacterium*), fungal infections (*Cryptococcus*), and noninfectious conditions (seborrheic keratoses and basal cell carcinomas). Nodules may be observed in poxvirus infections (orf and milker's nodules), HPV (squamous cell carcinomas associated with HPV-16), or HHV-8 (Kaposi's sarcoma), as well as in mycobacterial and *Bartonella* infections (bacillary angiomatosis) and noninfectious tumors (basal cell carcinomas, squamous cell carcinoma, melanoma, and pyogenic granuloma). Urticaria is usually associated with allergic reactions, including drug eruptions, but may be due to hepatitis B virus or coxsackievirus infections. Petechiae are seen in dengue fever and other hemorrhagic fevers (Lassa fever) but may occur in nonviral conditions producing thrombocytopenia. Ulcerations of the mucous membranes commonly occur with HSV-1, HSV-2, VZV, CMV, and hand-foot-and-mouth disease (HFMD) viral infections. Anogenital ulcers in immunocompromised persons are sometimes due to CMV or may involve a coinfection of CMV and HSV. Oral ulcers of viral etiology must be distinguished from nonviral ulcers such as aphthous ulcers. Cutaneous ulcers may be related to stasis dermatitis or to other causes of decreased circulation.

LOCAL IMMUNITY TO VIRAL INFECTIONS

Not only does the epidermis serve as a primary line of defense against infections, but because of its anatomic structure, it also contains the basic elements needed for the immune response against infection. Therefore, the concept of skin-associated lymphoid tissue (SALT) has been proposed (140). SALT is made up of the following: (i) keratinocytes, which phagocytize foreign particles, release cytokines, and express major histocompatibility complex (MHC) class II antigens upon incubation with gamma interferon (IFN-γ); (ii) epidermal Langerhans cells, which have surface expression of MHC class II, CD1, C3biR, and CD4 molecules and are the predominant scavenger antigen-presenting cell of the epidermis; (iii) skin-trophic T cells, which in the epidermis include mainly "inactive" memory T cells of predominantly $CD8^+$ phenotype, although $CD4^+$ and $CD4^-$ $CD8^-$ $\gamma\delta^+$ T cells are also present; and (iv) skin endothelial cells, which direct cellular traffic in and out of the skin (Fig. 1).

DNA VIRUSES

Human Papillomaviruses

Virology

HPV, which belong to the *Papovaviridae* family, are nonenveloped, double-stranded, circular DNA viruses with approximately 8,000 bp. The HPV genome encodes early proteins (E1 to E7) and late proteins (L1 and L2). Most early proteins direct DNA replication and RNA transcription. The late proteins are viral capsids that are assembled into virions. Proteins E6 and E7 are involved in oncogenesis. E6 binds to and inactivates the tumor suppressor protein p53 and thereby blocks cell apoptosis. E7 inactivates Rb family proteins and thereby interferes with transforming growth factor beta and induces cell proliferation. E5 has recently also been found to affect host cell tumoral transformations by modulating growth factor receptors (22).

Epidemiology

Anogenital HPV infection is extremely common, with an annual incidence of 5.5 million cases in the United States (115). Approximately 75% of sexually active adults will have had an HPV infection by age 50. Of these, approximately 60% have had a prior infection, 14% have subclinical infection, and 1% have clinically evident lesions (74). Peak prevalence of anogenital HPV is in women younger than 25 years old; there is a second peak in women over age 55 (12).

Condyloma acuminata, or genital (venereal) warts, are the most frequently diagnosed sexually transmitted disease, with an annual incidence of approximately 1 million new cases in the United States (Fig. 2; Color Plate 2). Over 90% of cases of condyloma acuminatum are due to HPV-6 or -11 and are clinically benign. Genital warts are most often spread by sexual contact, with a 60% transmission rate during sexual contact with an infected partner. The mean incubation period of HPV is 2 to 3 months but ranges from 3 weeks to beyond 8 months (124).

The prevalence of anogenital infection, particularly that caused by HPV-16, varies geographically. For example, the prevalence of HPV-16 among HPV-positive women is higher in North America and Europe than in sub-Saharan Africa. There is a relatively low proportion of HPV-16 among HPV-infected women in Africa and a relatively high rate of HPV-35, -45, and -58. Asian populations dis-

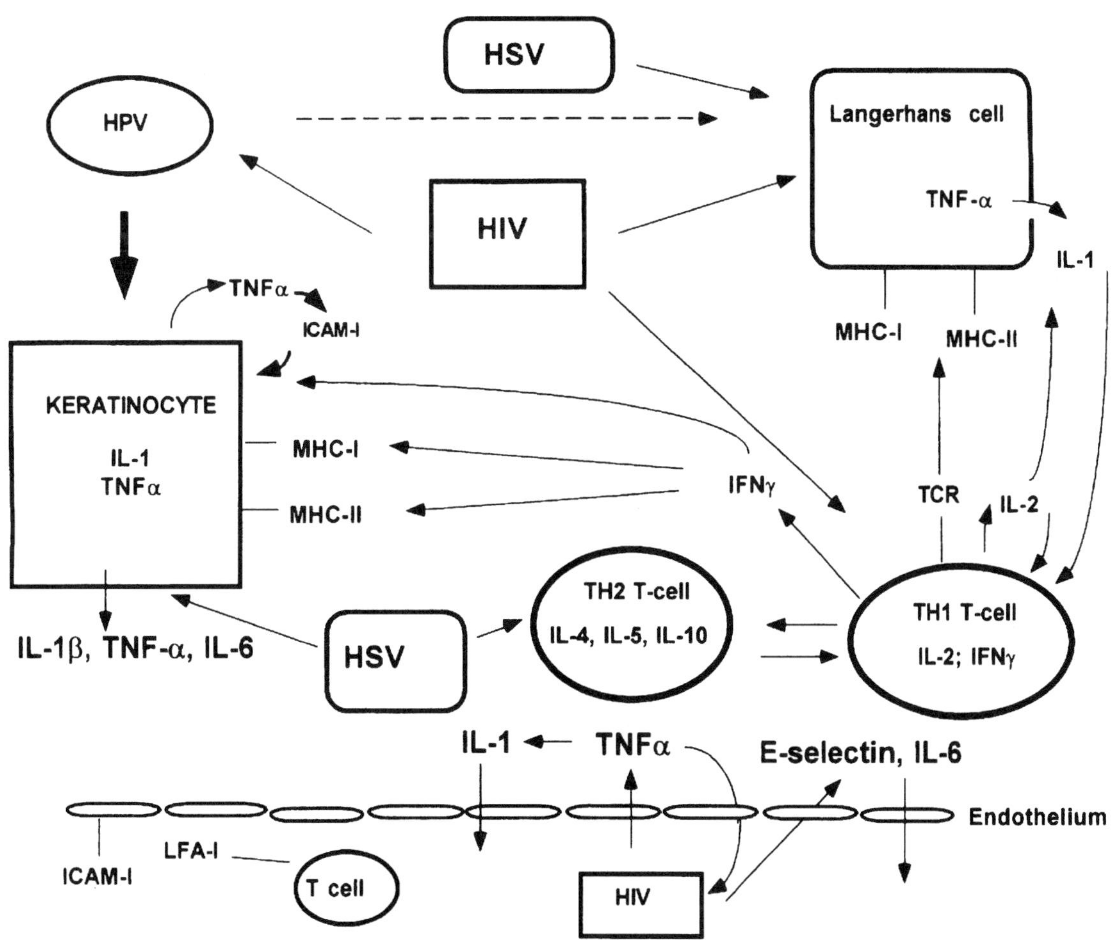

FIGURE 1 Pathways of the cutaneous immune response to infection with HPV, HSV, and HIV.

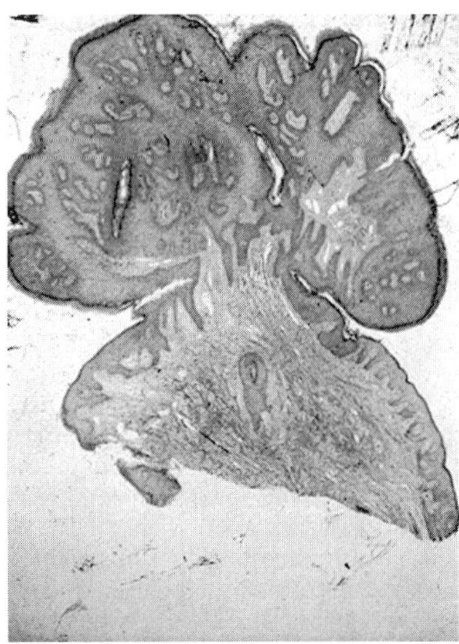

FIGURE 2 Photomicrograph of condyloma acuminatum showing acanthosis, papillomatosis, and parakeratosis.

play heterogeneous HPV types. The proportions of women infected with HPV-18 are relatively similar across regions (32). HPV infection also appears to be very common in men but is less well studied. Most studies report prevalence in men comparable to that in women. However, men have lower seropositivity of HPV-6, -11, -16, and -18 (44).

The most significant risk factor for anogenital infection in both men and women is a high number of sexual partners. HPV has also been positively correlated with smoking. A possible association with oral contraceptive use has been suggested (12). Circumcision has been postulated as helpful in preventing HPV, but the role of circumcision remains unclear (44). One 15-year study from 2002 (International Agency for Research) concluded that male circumcision is associated with a decreased risk of penile HPV infection. In the case of men with a history of multiple sexual partners, a decreased risk of cervical cancer in their current female partners was seen. The mechanism by which circumcision helps protect against HPV infection is unclear but is thought to go beyond increased probability of good penile hygiene. The keratinized stratified squamous epithelium of the penile shaft is likely less vulnerable to infection than the nonkeratinized mucosal lining of the prepuce (24).

Nongenital cutaneous HPV infections occur in 10% of children, with a peak incidence between the ages of 12 and 16 (4). Adults are also affected by cutaneous HPV but less commonly than children. Close personal contact is the main risk factor for transmission, as these lesions spread by direct skin-to-skin or skin-to-mucosa contact. However, transmission of both anogenital and nongenital cutaneous HPV infections depends on lesion location, HPV quantity in the lesion, type of contact, and immune status of the exposed individual.

Clinical Features

HPV can be categorized based on regional tropism—that is, whether they cause genitomucosal lesions, nongenital cutaneous lesions, or lesions associated with epidermodysplasia verruciformis (EV). The most prevalent clinical form of genitomucosal lesions is condyloma acuminata. These warts are exophytic, cauliflower-like lesions typically located near moist surfaces. Papular warts and flat lesions occur less commonly. These lesions are smaller and less obvious on exam than condyloma acuminata. Examination under a colposcope or other type of magnification may be necessary for identification (134). Anogenital HPV infection is commonly associated with cancer, as described in more detail below (see chapter 28).

An uncommon manifestation of genital HPV infection is the Buschke-Lowenstein tumor, or "giant condyloma." This lesion typically manifests as a slow-growing, large, malodorous, cauliflower-like mass. These lesions resemble condyloma acuminata histologically but exhibit both downward and upward growth, thus appearing locally invasive. Recurrences of Buschke-Lowenstein tumors are common (134).

Bowenoid papulosis is an anogenital neoplasia that manifests as multiple, verrucous, brown-red papules that may coalesce. Lesions are more common in females, in whom they occur around the labia minora and majora, inguinal folds, and perianal areas. In men, lesions occur on the glans or shaft of the penis (134).

Nonanogenital mucosal disease can occur in the nares, mouth, larynx, and conjunctiva. HPV from genital lesions can be transmitted to distant mucous membranes via orogenital sex (causing oral condyloma acuminatum) or nonsexually, as in cases of vertical transmission during vaginal delivery (142). In the latter case, HPV from vaginal warts may be transmitted to the oral or respiratory tract of the infant and manifest as respiratory (laryngeal) papillomas (86); alternatively, anogenital warts may develop in infants within a few months of birth as a result of acquisition during vaginal delivery. Children may also develop anogenital warts due to incidental spread from cutaneous warts or from sexual abuse (94).

Cutaneous HPV lesions are common and can manifest as verruca vulgaris (HPV-2), plantar warts (HPV-1), or verruca plana (HPV-3). These common warts can manifest on any skin surface but are most commonly seen on the hands and fingers. They manifest as flesh-colored exophytic papules and nodules that are usually benign and self-limited; however, they can be annoying and difficult to eradicate.

Cutaneous warts in EV, on the other hand, can lead to major morbidity and mortality (62). EV is a rare autosomal recessive genodermatosis and was the first model of cutaneous viral oncogenesis in humans. EV patients develop disseminated warty papules and erythematous macules during childhood. These lesions progress to cutaneous carcinomas in adulthood in approximately one-half of these patients (Color Plate 3). At least 19 HPV types are associated with EV. Several of these genotypes have oncogenic potential, most notably HPV-5 and -8 (96). Nonsense mutations in adjacent novel genes, *EVER1* and *EVER2*, are associated with EV. These genes encode integral membrane proteins in the endoplasmic reticulum (109). Oncogenic HPV genotypes in EV appear to be necessary but not sufficient for malignant transformation. The most important cofactor, in the case of EV, is UV irradiation, which is illustrated by the fact that the highest incidence of carcinomas in EV patients is in areas of greatest sunlight exposure (61).

Diagnosis

Often no laboratory tests are carried out if, by clinical appearance, the lesion is presumed to be HPV related and benign. When biopsies of verrucae are carried out, the following general patterns may be observed in tissues: acanthosis, papillomatosis, hyperkeratosis, parakeratosis, and prominent and often thrombosed dermal capillary vessels. Koilocytes, large keratinocytes with an eccentric, pyknotic nucleus surrounded by a perinuclear halo, are often observed. Frequently, a biopsy is conducted to determine if the lesion is dysplastic or neoplastic. In the general population, such biopsies would most likely be taken in the anogenital region. In this population, dysplastic or neoplastic lesions are most frequent on the cervix and therefore would be detectable via cytopathology taken with the Pap smear.

Immunohistochemical staining for HPV capsid antigens provides more specific detection of HPV. Since dysplastic or neoplastic lesions contain few, if any, capsid antigens, this method may give false-negative results with such lesions. Since HPV cannot be readily grown in tissue culture and serology is not routinely useful, the only specific method of diagnosing HPV is via DNA or RNA detection methods. The hybrid capture assay II, which detects hybrids formed between HPV DNA and an RNA probe, and PCR are by far the most sensitive methods of detecting HPV DNA (106).

Whereas verrucae are usually clinically evident, they may resemble seborrheic keratoses, nevi, or acrochordons. Verrucae planae may mimic papules of lichen planus. Condyloma acuminatum must be differentiated from condyloma latum, the skin lesion associated with secondary syphilis. Bowenoid papulosis can be confused with lichen planus, psoriasis, seborrheic keratoses, or condyloma acuminata (134). Benign verrucae also must be differentiated from dysplastic and neoplastic lesions.

Treatment

Treatment for most benign verrucae consists of surgery, cryotherapy, or topical chemotherapy. In each case, the objective is to eradicate the lesion and allow the immune system to hold latent HPV in surrounding (normal-appearing) tissue in check so as to prevent recurrences. Surgical therapy includes simple excision, electrodesiccation, and removal with a CO_2 laser. Cryotherapy involves application of liquid nitrogen, which induces dermal and epidermal cellular necrosis. Topical chemotherapy options include podophyllin resin, purified podophyllotoxin, 5-fluorouracil, retinoic acid, cantharidin, salicylic acid, lactic acid, bichloroacetic acid, and trichloroacetic acid (124). Selection of the most appropriate therapy depends on the size and location of the wart, as well as on the history of previous therapies.

IFN-α is also approved for treatment of condyloma acuminatum. Combinations of interferon and other treatments do not appear to be more effective than other treatments used alone. Interferon is costly and inconsistently effective and should not be considered a primary treatment (124). Therapy of HPV-related malignant lesions includes surgery; if metastases are present, chemotherapy is usually included. Imiquimod is an immunomodulatory agent demonstrated to be very effective for condyloma acuminatum (148). It is applied topically by the patient and produces minimal local inflammation and no systemic side effects. Its mode of action is via induction of endogenous IFN-α as well as a host of other cytokines. In contrast to therapies without antiviral or immunomodulatory mechanisms of action, a very low rate of recurrence is observed following clearance of condyloma acumination with imiquimod. Use of imiquimod in conjunction with surgical treatment may be even more effective. One retrospective study found that the rate of recurrent anogenital warts was much lower in patients treated with a 16-week course of imiquimod (5% cream) monotherapy and surgical excision of residual warts than in those treated with surgical excision alone.

Prophylactic vaccines for HPV have recently been developed. Gardasil is a quadrivalent vaccine targeting HPV-6, -11, -16, and -18 that was approved by the Food and Drug Administration (FDA) in June 2006 for prevention of genital warts, cervical cancer, and certain precancerous lesions in women 9 to 26 years old. Cervarix, a bivalent vaccine targeting HPV-16 and -18, was approved in Australia in May 2007 for women 10 to 45 years old. Both vaccines appear to be nearly 100% effective in preventing cervical lesions. The quadrivalent vaccine also effectively prevents vaginal and vulvar neoplasia (125).

Poxviruses

Virology

Poxviruses are large enveloped double-stranded linear DNA viruses that belong to the family *Poxviridae*. Poxviruses of clinical significance include those causing smallpox, vaccinia, monkeypox, MC, orf, and milker's nodules. Although smallpox was declared eradicated worldwide by the World Health Organization in 1980, it remains a clinical issue because of its potential use as a biological weapon (19). Variola virus (the causative agent of smallpox), vaccinia virus (the virus used to vaccinate against smallpox), and monkeypox virus belong to the genus *Orthopoxvirus*. The genomes of variola virus and vaccinia virus are closely related. MC virus belongs to a distinct genus, *Molluscipoxvirus*. Orf and milker's nodules are both caused by parapoxviruses.

Epidemiology

Smallpox was endemic throughout the world but has been eradicated by a worldwide vaccination program. Vaccination against smallpox has not been routine in the United States for over 30 years. Virtually all citizens are currently susceptible to variola because vaccination is believed to be protective for only 5 to 10 years (54). Currently, smallpox virus is known to exist in only two laboratories: the Centers for Disease Control and Prevention in Atlanta, GA, and a laboratory in Novosibirsk, Russia. However, there is concern that the virus exists elsewhere and could be used in biological warfare. Viral transmission is primarily via respiratory droplets. Historically, the incidence of infection was highest in the winter and early spring because aerosolized variola virus survives better at lower temperatures and low humidity levels (21).

Monkeypox has historically been significant only in sub-Saharan Africa, where it was recognized as a distinct disease in 1970 despite its presumable existence for thousands of years. Early studies suggested that most cases occurred in children under age 10 and were associated with animal contact, although secondary human-to-human transmission did occur. The first documentation of monkeypox in the western hemisphere was a cluster of cases in the U.S. Midwest in 2003. This outbreak was spread by prairie dogs that apparently acquired the virus from Gambian rats when housed with them at a distribution center in Illinois. Person-to-person spread of monkeypox through close contact with infected individuals appears to occur inefficiently. Vaccination with vaccinia virus is protective against monkeypox (90).

MC is the most prevalent poxvirus infection and commonly occurs on the trunk in children and as a sexually transmitted disease in the genital area of adults. Most children with MC are healthy and younger than 8 years of age. Fewer than 5% of children in the United States have clinical evidence of MC virus infection (42). MC virus most commonly infects individuals 15 to 29 years old (42, 147). Infection with MC virus occurs at increased rates among immunocompromised individuals, and the prevalence of MC among HIV-positive patients is 5 to 18% (147). The occurrence of MC virus infection in HIV-positive patients has decreased significantly since the introduction of highly active antiretroviral therapy (HAART). Other immunodeficient states, such as that occurring with corticosteroid use, and perhaps atopic dermatitis can also predispose to MC virus infection. MC spreads primarily by direct skin-to-skin contact, including autoinoculation; spread via fomites can also occur.

Clinical Features

Smallpox

Smallpox replicates in the epidermis and is spread not only via direct skin contact and fomites but also by respiratory transmission. Preceding the development of skin lesions, patients experience 3 days of apprehension, sudden prostrating fever, severe headache, back pain, and vomiting. Erythematous macules then develop and progress to tense, deep-seated papules and vesicles (Fig. 3). The vesicles are followed by pustules, then crusts, and finally scar formation. The rash appears in a centrifugal distribution with all lesions in the same stage of development. Overall, the mortality rate with smallpox is approximately 30%, but the hemorrhagic form results in almost 100% mortality even before development of skin lesions. Variola minor is caused by a less virulent strain of variola virus. The clinical manifestations are similar to those of variola major, or classical smallpox, as described above, but the severity and mortality rate (<1%) are lower (19).

Vaccinia

Vaccination with vaccinia virus is no longer routine but is still used in certain target populations. The live virus vaccine occasionally leads to serious complications, including bacterial superinfections, vaccinia necrosum, generalized vaccinia, eczema vaccinatum, erythema multiforme, accidental inoculation, and encephalitis (54). These are discussed in chapter 18.

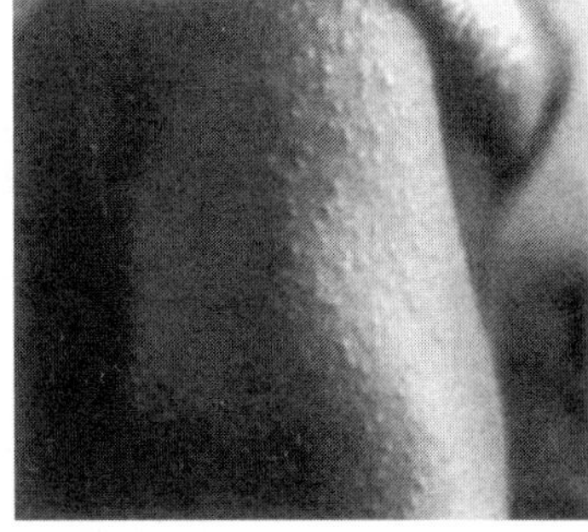

FIGURE 3 Variola major (smallpox).

Monkeypox

The clinical picture of human monkeypox virus infection resembles that of smallpox. There is a 10- to 14-day incubation period followed by a prodromal illness consisting of fever, malaise, and lymphadenopathy. After 1 to 3 days, patients break out in a maculopapular rash that usually begins on the trunk and spreads peripherally. Lesions can occur on the palms and soles and on mucous membranes. The mortality rate is 10%, and death usually occurs during the second week of the illness (90).

Monkeypox and smallpox have very similar clinical manifestations. One distinguishing feature clinically is lymphadenopathy, which is common in the prodromal phase of monkeypox virus infection but not smallpox (90). However, poxviruses cannot be readily identified from one another except by PCR assay (19).

MC

The incubation period of MC is 2 to 7 weeks. It manifests as 3- to 6-mm skin-colored papules with a central umbilication. Although four different strains of MC virus (I through IV) have been identified (based on restriction endonuclease digestion patterns), all strains produce similar clinical pictures. MCV I is responsible for the vast majority of infections in immunocompetent hosts in the United States. Clinical presentations of MC often follow one of two patterns in immunocompetent individuals: widespread papules on the trunk and face of children, transmitted by direct skin-to-skin (nonsexual) contact, or genital papules in adults, spread by sexual contact. In either case it is unusual to see more than 15 lesions in an individual patient. In immunocompromised persons, especially those who are HIV positive, MC can manifest with thousands of papules and be a major source of morbidity (Fig. 4; Color Plate 4); HIV-positive patients also commonly have facial involvement as well as increased likelihood of bacterial superinfection and treatment resistance (42).

Orf

Orf, contagious ecthyma, is a less common poxvirus infection that is transmitted from sheep, goats, and other animals to the hands of humans (Color Plate 5). Orf man-

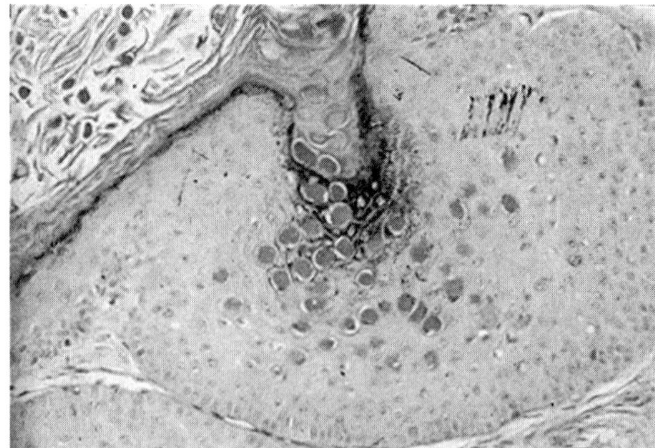

FIGURE 4 Photomicrograph of MC demonstrating central umbilication and epidermal hyperplasia containing intracytoplasmic inclusions (Henderson-Paterson bodies) compressing nuclei.

ifests as cutaneous nodules averaging 1.6 cm in diameter associated with regional lymphadenopathy, lymphangitis, and fever. Lesions spontaneously progress through six stages, resulting in healing in about 35 days (76).

Milker's Nodules

Milker's nodules are caused by paravaccinia virus. Clinically similar to orf, the lesions result from manual contact with teats of infected cows and have an incubation period of 4 to 7 days. Also similar to orf, the nodules heal in 4 to 6 weeks after progressing through six clinical stages (50).

When smallpox was epidemic, it was occasionally confused with chickenpox, dengue fever, or enterovirus infections. An important distinguishing feature between smallpox and chickenpox is that the crops of lesions are in the same stage of development in smallpox infection, whereas lesions occur in different stages of development in chickenpox. The hemorrhagic form of smallpox had to be distinguished from other viral hemorrhagic exanthems, coagulation disorders, typhus, and meningococcal septicemia.

A number of entities can mimic MC in the healthy host, such as warts, basal cell carcinomas, and lichen planus. In HIV-positive patients, MC must be distinguished from cutaneous cryptococcal infection (116). Orf and milker's nodules can mimic one another or can be confused with pyogenic granulomas, sporotrichosis, or atypical mycobacterial infection.

Treatment

For patients with smallpox or disseminated vaccinia, management of symptoms and prevention of bacterial superinfection were paramount. The effectiveness of thiosemicarbezone and antivariola or antivaccinia sera was limited. Similarly, there is no proven effective treatment for monkeypox, but the vaccination virus is highly protective. However, eradication of monkeypox is not possible due to the existence of an animal reservoir (90).

MC is a self-limited condition, but resolution may take 6 months to 5 years. Therefore, most physicians recommend treatment, particularly for genital lesions, to reduce the risk of spread and patient discomfort. Treatment options include local excision by electrocautery, curettage, or cryotherapy and chemical ablation via application of trichloroacetic acid or podophyllin. Patients may opt to treat their lesions at home by self-administering topical treatments such as podophyllotoxin, retinoic acid, or imiquimod cream (147). Recurrences are common in immunocompromised persons. Lesions of orf or milker's nodules can be removed via excision and cautery, but this is usually not necessary since spontaneous resolution can be expected in approximately 6 weeks.

Human Herpesviruses

HSV-1 and HSV-2

Epidemiology and Clinical Manifestations

HSV-1 is most known for causing oral herpes, or herpes labialis. The virus is typically transmitted via direct inoculation of the skin and mucous membranes. Herpes labialis is extremely common, with up to 90% of adults having serologic evidence of HSV-1 infection (10). While the majority of primary infections with HSV-1 are asymptomatic, the virus remains dormant in the host's neuronal ganglia and can reactivate to produce recurrent symptomatic disease. Recurrent episodes occur in up to one-third of infected individuals and can be induced by stress, trauma, menstruation, fever, colds, and UV light. Upon reactivation, the virus travels down the sensory nerve, producing prodromal sensations of pruritus or tingling. When the virus reaches the skin, grouped vesicles with surrounding erythema form on or near the vermillion border of the lip. There is often regional lymphadenopathy and occasionally fever, headache, and malaise. Vesicles ulcerate, crust, and resolve in 2 to 4 weeks, frequently with postinflammatory hypo- or hyperpigmentation.

At least 45 million individuals in the United States, or one in four adults, are estimated to be seropositive for HSV-2 (49). HSV-2 is most known for causing genital herpes or herpes genitalis. As with HSV-1, most primary infections with HSV-2 are asymptomatic, with only 10 to 25% of seropositive individuals indicating a history of genital ulcers (49). Primary HSV-2 infection classically manifests with widespread genital vesicles and ulcers with surrounding erythema (Color Plate 6). There may be associated edema, pain, inguinal lymphadenopathy, discharge, dysuria, malaise, fever, and photophobia. These signs and symptoms typically occur within 3 to 14 days of sexual contact with an infected individual. Viral shedding from active lesions lasts up to 14 days in women and approximately 10 days in men (34); however, HSV-2-seropositive individuals can still shed the virus and infect others when no lesions are present. Symptoms are typically more severe in women than in men, and skin lesions often require 3 to 4 weeks for complete healing.

Similar to HSV-1, recurrences of HSV-2 may be triggered by a variety of factors, such as emotional or physical stress or mild trauma. Recurrent episodes of HSV are usually less severe than initial outbreaks and often heal in 7 to 10 days without therapy. Men suffer 20% more recurrences than women, which may contribute to the higher rate of herpes transmission from men to women. In immunocompromised individuals, HSV recurrences may be chronic and result in significant morbidity if untreated.

It is estimated that up to 30% of first-episode genital herpes is due to HSV-1, which is often attributable to orogenital contact. Genital herpes due to HSV-1 is usually less severe than disease due to HSV-2. In addition, genital herpes due to HSV-1 recurs less frequently than HSV-2-associated disease.

In addition to herpes labialis and genitalis (Color Plate 7), HSV-1 and HSV-2 can also cause gingivostomatitis, herpetic whitlow (Color Plate 8), HSV gladiatorum, neonatal herpes, herpetic keratoconjunctivitis, aseptic meningitis, and herpes encephalitis. Complications of HSV infection include erythema multiforme (Fig. 5; Color Plate 9) and eczema herpeticum due to autoinoculation of the virus onto areas of atopic dermatitis. With immunocompromise, infection with HSV-1 or HSV-2 can lead to widespread local infection, as well as disseminated cutaneous and visceral infection.

Neonatal herpes is caused by HSV-1 or HSV-2 transmitted in utero, intrapartum, or postnatally. The details of newborn HSV infection are described in chapter 19.

Diagnosis

Diagnosis of HSV-1 and HSV-2 infection is often made clinically but can be confirmed by viral culture, Tzanck smear, PCR, serology, and antigen detection. HSV-1 and HSV-2 typically grow readily within 1 to 2 days in cell culture (130). Using fluid from an intact vesicle, the

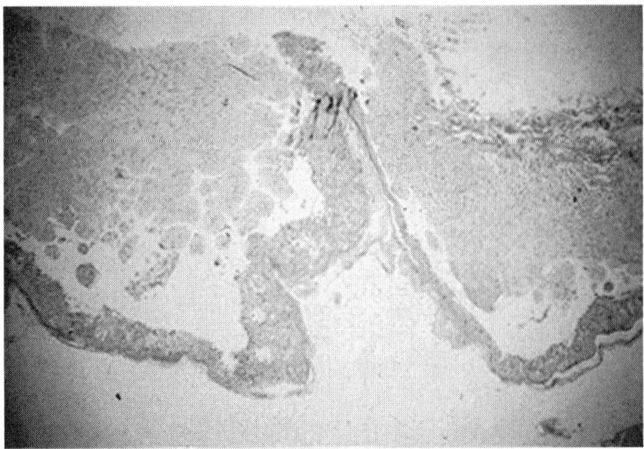

FIGURE 5 Photomicrograph of erythema multiforme associated with HSV-1, showing subepidermal vesicles, necrotic keratinocytes, and balloon cell degeneration.

Tzanck smear is positive if acantholytic keratinocytes or multinucleated giant acantholytic keratinocytes are detected (Fig. 6). As the prognosis is different for herpes genitalis caused by HSV-1 versus HSV-2, differentiating between the two is important for patient counseling. Antigen detection using antibodies specific for HSV-1 and HSV-2 can be helpful. Serology not only can differentiate between HSV-1 and HSV-2 but also can be helpful in distinguishing primary genital herpes with a predominance of immunoglobulin M (IgM) antibodies from nonprimary genital herpes with a high proportion of IgG.

The differential diagnosis for vesicular lesions associated with HSV infection includes contact dermatitis, bullous impetigo, and insect bites. For lesions that are located specifically in the orolabial region, aphthous stomatitis, HFMD, and herpangina should be considered. In addition, erythema multiforme should be considered, as HSV is the most common identifiable etiologic agent (35, 37). The differential for lesions in the genital region includes urethritis, urinary tract infections, tinea cruris, and vaginitis.

Treatment and Prevention

HSV-1 and HSV-2 are commonly treated with nucleoside analogs that block viral DNA polymerase, such as acyclovir. Topical, oral, and intravenous acyclovir are available, though the topical formulation is rarely used due to its limited penetration of the stratum corneum. Oral acyclovir, especially if started early, accelerates the rate of lesion crusting in oral and genital herpes (135). In patients with severe or frequent recurrences or with ocular HSV, suppressive therapy with acyclovir has been shown to decrease the recurrence rate by 50% (135). Acyclovir has also been shown to reduce asymptomatic viral shedding of HSV-2 by 95% (154).

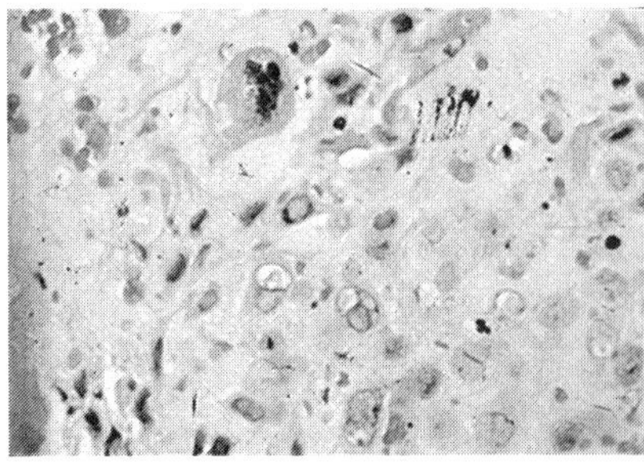

FIGURE 6 Photomicrograph of an ulcer resulting from HSV-2, in which multinucleated giant cells with eosinophilic intranuclear inclusions can be seen.

The efficacy of oral acyclovir is limited by frequent dosing and low bioavailability. Therefore, in immunocompromised patients with mucocutaneous HSV, especially in disseminated disease, the intravenous preparation is favored. Intravenous acyclovir is also used for infection in neonates, eczema herpeticum, and herpes encephalitis (157). Foscarnet is approved for the treatment of acyclovir-resistant HSV infections.

Currently, valacyclovir and famciclovir along with acyclovir are the mainstay drugs for treating as well as suppressing genital herpes. One study demonstrated a 50% decrease in HSV-2 transmission with once-daily valacyclovir (34). Famciclovir has also been shown to be an effective, well-tolerated option for the suppression of genital herpes among individuals with multiple recurrences (149). Topical cidofovir has been shown to be another effective agent for treatment of genital herpes but is not approved for this purpose (122).

The development of an effective vaccine against HSV-1 and HSV-2 has proven challenging, though recent advances allow for cautious optimism. Two recent studies of a prophylactic glycoprotein D2 alum/MPL vaccine demonstrated prevention of genital herpes disease in 73 and 74% of seronegative women whose regular sexual partner had a history of genital herpes (137). A second prophylactic vaccine (ICP10ΔPK, AuRx) was shown to prevent recurrent disease in 44% of immunized subjects and to reduce the frequency and severity of recurrences in subjects that were not fully protected (9).

Varicella-Zoster Virus

Epidemiology and Clinical Manifestations

VZV, or HHV-3, is a highly prevalent member of the *Herpesviridae* family, with 98% of the adult population in the United States having serologic evidence of previous infection. Primary infection with VZV nearly always manifests symptomatically as varicella (chickenpox). Before the introduction of a vaccine in 1995, 3 million to 4 million cases of varicella leading to approximately 10,000 hospitalizations and 100 deaths were reported each year (158). Transmission occurs via direct contact or airborne droplets. Primary varicella typically manifests in younger children as low-grade fever, malaise, and disseminated pruritic vesicles classically described as "dewdrops on a rose petal." Skin lesions first appear on the face and trunk as erythematous macules and rapidly progress over 12 to 14 h to papules, vesicles, pustules, and crusts (Color Plate 10). Most of the lesions are seen centrally and on the proximal extremities. Vesicles also appear on mucous membranes but rapidly erode to form shallow, painful ulcers. Due to the rapid evolution of successive crops of lesions, varicella is characterized by the simultaneous presence of lesions in all stages of development within the same anatomic region. In older children and adults, the exanthem is often preceded by up to 3 days of prodromal symptoms, including headache, myalgias, anorexia, nausea, and vomiting.

The most common cutaneous complication of varicella in young, immunocompetent individuals is scarring, which is often secondary to bacterial superinfection with *Staphy-*

lococcus aureus or *Streptococcus pyogenes*. In adults and immunocompromised individuals, significant morbidity and occasional mortality can result from complications of VZV infection, including myelitis, large vessel granulomatous arteritis, encephalitis, varicella pneumonia, and varicella hepatitis (27). Maternal infection with VZV in the first trimester is associated with a 2% risk of congenital malformations, such as intrauterine growth retardation, limb hypoplasia, cataracts, chorioretinitis, microcephaly, cortical atrophy, and skin lesions. The skin lesions typically consist of areas of hypertrophic scarring with induration and erythema located especially on the extremities.

In 20% of immunocompetent individuals and in up to 50% of immunocompromised individuals, VZV reactivates years or even decades later to produce herpes zoster. Though in most cases the exact trigger for reactivation is unknown, advancing age appears to be an important factor, with 66% of cases reported to occur in individuals over 50. Upon reactivation, the virus spreads down the sensory nerve, and transient virema occurs with associated prodromal symptoms of pain, fever, regional lymphadenopathy, and malaise (35). After a few days to weeks of pain, vesicles appear along the distribution of the sensory nerve (Color Plate 11). Although vesicles generally occur only along one dermatome, it is not unusual for a few lesions to appear in neighboring dermatomes. The predilection for zoster to appear in certain anatomic regions (face and trunk) usually corresponds to the areas most affected by primary varicella. After a few days the vesicles become pustules, and within 1 to 2 weeks the pustules become crusts. The skin lesions found in herpes zoster can shed VZV and cause primary varicella in seronegative individuals. Currently, more than 1,000,000 cases of herpes zoster occur each year in the United States; however, the utilization of the VZV vaccine may significantly alter the epidemiology of herpes zoster.

Although scarring can occur, particularly in darker-skinned individuals, cutaneous complications of herpes zoster are rare. The most prevalent complication is postherpetic neuralgia, which is defined as persistent pain for more than 8 to 12 weeks after initial rash appearance (27). The pain, which may be extremely severe, can last for months to years and be highly resistant to treatment. Other complications of herpes zoster include vision impairment or blindness with involvement of the ophthalmic branch of the trigeminal nerve and painful facial paralysis (Ramsay Hunt syndrome) with involvement of the facial and auditory nerves (57). Rarely, sensory defects, motor paralysis, and encephalomyelitis can occur (66, 119). Dissemination of herpes zoster, defined as more than 20 vesicles outside the primary and adjacent dermatomes, is rare in healthy hosts but can occur in up to 40% of severely immunocompromised individuals. Cutaneous dissemination may be a marker of visceral involvement (liver, lungs, and the CNS) and therefore can herald significant morbidity and mortality.

Diagnosis

Varicella and herpes zoster are usually diagnosed clinically, though viral cultures, Tzanck smear, and serology can confirm the diagnosis. Antigen and viral DNA detection are the most useful techniques for rapid virologic diagnosis. Samples for culture should be taken from the vesicular stage, and growth requires at least 7 to 10 days. Herpes zoster can be retrospectively diagnosed by a ≥4-fold increase in the titer of antibody to VZV between the acute and convalescent phases.

The differential diagnosis for primary varicella includes disseminated HSV, eczema herpeticum, eczema vaccinatum, disseminated vaccinia in immunosuppressed patients, enterovirus, and the bullous form of impetigo (158). The differential diagnosis for herpes zoster includes poison ivy, poison oak, contact dermatitis, zosteriform HSV infection, erysipelas, bullous impetigo, and necrotizing fasciitis (158). In immunocompromised patients with pulmonary involvement, the differential diagnosis should include both varicella pneumonia and *Pneumocystis carinii* pneumonia, which also commonly affects this patient population.

Treatment

For most individuals, primary varicella is a benign, self-limited disease and treatment is largely supportive. However, pregnant women and neonates are at considerable risk for morbidity and mortality and are treated with antivirals such as intravenous acyclovir (51, 131). Treatment for herpes zoster includes antivirals and analgesics for pain control. Acyclovir, valacyclovir, and famciclovir are FDA approved for the management of acute herpes zoster, though they may not decrease the rate of development of postherpetic neuralgia (51). Antiviral therapy is imperative in patients with herpes zoster that involves the ophthalmic branch of the trigeminal nerve, to prevent vision loss (51). Pain management is especially difficult with conventional analgesics in herpes zoster patients who develop postherpetic neuralgia. Tricyclic antidepressants, notably doxepin and amitriptyline, have been shown to reduce the pain associated with postherpetic neuralgia (83). In addition, two controlled trials have shown the benefit of the anticonvulsants gabapentin and pregabalin for postherpetic neuralgia (136).

Prevention

Vaccines are currently available for prophylaxis of varicella and herpes zoster. The live attenuated viral vaccine (Oka strain) was approved in 1995 and produces a 95% seroconversion rate (155). Significant adverse events with the vaccine are rare, with fewer than 5% experiencing a mild varicella-like disease. There has been a significant decrease in varicella since the vaccine was instituted, and vaccination will likely alter the epidemiology of herpes zoster as well (128). Children should get the first dose of the vaccine at 12 to 15 months and the second dose at 4 to 6 years. Children over 13 years of age who have never had varicella or the vaccine should get two doses at least 28 days apart. The VZV vaccine is contraindicated in immunocompromised individuals, in persons with a history of anaphylactic or anaphylactoid reactions to gelatin or neomycin, and in pregnant women (71). Varicella-zoster immunoglobulin is recommended for postexposure prophylaxis in immunocompromised persons, pregnant women, and neonates born to mothers who acquired varicella a week before or up to 2 days after delivery.

A second vaccine for herpes zoster prevention has a higher titer of the same live attenuated virus. One study found that the incidence of herpes zoster was 51% lower in the vaccinated group than in the placebo-treated group and the incidence of postherpetic neuralgia was 67% lower with the vaccine (97). In 2006, the Advisory Committee on Immunization Practices recommended a single dose of zoster vaccine for adults 60 years of age or older, whether or not they have had a previous episode of herpes zoster (25).

EBV

Epidemiology and Clinical Manifestations

EBV, or HHV-4, causes infectious mononucleosis, also known as "the kissing disease," as the virus is typically transmitted through oral secretions (25). Infectious mononucleosis first manifests as prodromal symptoms of malaise, headache, and fatigue, followed by fever, sore throat, and cervical adenopathy. Hepatomegaly and splenomegaly can also occur. Cutaneous manifestations of infectious mononucleosis include macules, papules, and, less commonly, erythema, vesicles, and purpura. These lesions are the result of viral replication and manifest during the first week of illness. In approximately one-third of patients, small petechiae are observed at the border of the hard and soft palates. If infectious mononucleosis is inappropriately treated with ampicillin or certain other penicillins, a high percentage of patients develop erythematous macules and papules over the trunk and extremities (100). These lesions persist for about 1 week, followed by desquamation.

EBV has a pathogenic role in the development of many cancers, especially in immunocompromised individuals; these cancers include Burkitt's lymphoma, Hodgkin's disease, nasopharyngeal carcinoma, and posttransplantation B-cell lymphoma (27). EBV expression has also been detected in cutaneous T-cell lymphomas, including mycosis fungoides, though its role is yet to be determined (129). Mycosis fungoides initially manifests as annular pink scaly patches that over time develop into patches and plaques that may resemble psoriasis. Finally, large irregular tumors form that may ulcerate. EBV DNA has also been detected in epithelial cells of oral hairy leukoplakia, an oral lesion closely associated with HIV infection (53) (Color Plate 12). Finally, Gianotti-Crosti syndrome, manifested as symmetric, nonpruritic, lichenoid papules of the face, limbs, and buttocks, has also been associated with primary EBV infection (80) (Color Plate 13).

Diagnosis

Diagnosis is usually made through the detection of antibodies to EBV. In particular, the monospot test, which detects heterophile antibodies, is used to diagnose infectious mononucleosis. This test is not commonly used for children due to its high false-negativity rate. Peripheral smears can support the diagnosis if greater than 10% atypical lymphocytes are noted. Specific EBV antibody assays are available, as well as PCR (27).

The differential diagnosis for the classic symptoms of sore throat, malaise, and lymphadenopathy associated with infectious mononucleosis includes streptococcal pharyngitis and other viral causes of pharyngitis. Acute HIV syndrome can also manifest as malaise, lymphadenopathy, and nonspecific mucocutaneous manifestations. Acute CMV infection can cause infectious mononucleosis similar to EBV mononucleosis, with hepatomegaly and atypical lymphocytosis. The cutaneous manifestations of infectious mononucleosis may resemble a number of nonspecific viral exanthems. However, if the findings are preceded by the recent administration of ampicillin, the probability of EBV infection is high.

Treatment

Treatment for infectious mononucleosis due to EBV is largely supportive. Antivirals, such as acyclovir, and corticosteroids have not been shown to be effective (120, 150). The development of anti-B-cell antibodies such as rituximab has greatly enhanced the therapeutic options for EBV-associated cancers (33, 52).

Cytomegalovirus

Epidemiology and Clinical Manifestations

CMV is a ubiquitous virus that is transmitted through infectious secretions. In developing countries, close to 100% of the adult population are seropositive, while in developed countries only about 50% of adults have evidence of infection. Primary infection is usually subclinical in immunocompetent individuals, although CMV mononucleosis syndrome occurs. Symptoms include fever, fatigue, and, less commonly, lymphadenopathy, sore throat, and organomegaly. Up to one-third of patients with CMV mononucleosis develop a maculopapular generalized rash.

Primary CMV infection in pregnant women poses a serious threat to the fetus. Maternal CMV infection is considered a leading viral cause of congenital malformations, CNS injury, and hearing loss in the neonate. If primary maternal infection occurs during pregnancy, especially during the first trimester, the rate of transmission is about 40% (3). Many of these infants have clinical manifestations at birth, including intrauterine growth retardation, microcephaly, cerebral atrophy, periventricular calcifications, chorioretinitis, sensorineural hearing loss, thrombocytopenia, and hepatosplenomegaly. Cutaneous manifestations include jaundice and purpuric macules and papules, secondary to persistent dermal hematopoiesis, resulting in the clinical picture of the "blueberry muffin baby." With recurrent maternal infection during pregnancy, the risk of transmission is only about 1%, and most of these infants have clinically silent disease at birth (3).

In immunocompromised patients, in whom CMV is associated with a variety of clinical entities, including retinitis, hepatitis, and colitis, infection may be associated with a variety of skin lesions, from vesicles to verrucous plaques. The most prevalent cutaneous manifestation is ulceration, especially in the perianal area (60). These cutaneous ulcerations are the result of CMV infection of the vascular endothelium and subsequent destruction of blood vessels.

Diagnosis

CMV DNA levels in acute CMV infection can provide prognostic information for immunocompromised patients. Histology can also be beneficial in diagnosis. CMV-infected cells have characteristic intranuclear inclusions surrounded by clear halos resembling "owl's eyes."

In the neonate with congenital CMV infection, the differential diagnosis includes other congenital infections, including toxoplasmosis, rubella, HSV, syphilis, and lymphocytic choriomeningitis virus. For older patients, the differential diagnosis for CMV infectious mononucleosis includes EBV mononucleosis. The monospot test is generally negative in CMV mononucleosis.

Treatment

Ganciclovir, a nucleoside analog of guanosine, has been shown to be effective in the treatment and prophylaxis of CMV infections (36, 82). Valganciclovir, a prodrug of ganciclovir, is available orally and has significantly increased bioavailability compared to ganciclovir, with similar safety and efficacy profiles (82). Valganciclovir has been approved for the treatment of CMV retinitis in adult patients with AIDS, as well as for prophylaxis of CMV disease in organ transplant recipients (1). For ganciclovir- and valganciclovir-resistant CMV infections, intravenous foscarnet is the drug of choice. For further discussion, see also chapters 12 and 22.

HHV-6 and HHV-7

Epidemiology and Clinical Manifestations

HHV-6 and HHV-7 are highly prevalent members of the *Herpesviridae* family; 90% of children have serologic evidence of HHV-6 infection by 2 years of age (162). HHV-7 infection usually occurs later, with most children seropositive by 5 to 6 years of age (159). Transmission is through oropharyngeal secretions. Primary infection with HHV-6 is a common cause of fever, irritability, and rhinorrhea in children. One study found that primary HHV-6 infection accounted for 20% of fevers in children between 6 and 12 months of age (56). HHV-6, as well as HHV-7, is also associated with the common childhood exanthem roseola infantum (exanthem subitum or sixth disease). Roseola infantum manifests as a high fever lasting 3 to 5 days followed by the development of a nonpruritic, blanchable, pink, maculopapular rash on the neck and trunk. Other cutaneous manifestations include palpebral edema and lesions on the soft palate. Roseola infantum is usually self-limited but can, rarely, cause seizures and encephalitis (8).

HHV-7 is also suspected to play a role in the pathogenesis of pityriasis rosea, another acute, self-limited exanthem. Pityriasis rosea begins with the development of a herald patch, a single plaque that is salmon colored to red with fine scale at the periphery. The herald patch is followed by the development of pink papules and plaques in a "Christmas tree" distribution on the trunk.

Diagnosis

Diagnosis is usually made clinically but can be confirmed via serology, peripheral blood mononuclear cell culture, or PCR (56). The clinical presentation of roseola infantum and its rapid resolution distinguish it from other entities on the differential diagnosis, including drug eruptions, scarlet fever, rubella, measles, erythema infectiosum, and other viral exanthems. The differential diagnosis for pityriasis rosea includes drug eruptions, secondary syphilis, guttate psoriasis, erythema multiforme, and tinea corporis. The presence of a herald patch and the resolution of pityriasis rosea without treatment can aid in diagnosis.

Treatment

There have been no controlled trials of antiviral therapy or specific recommendations for the management of HHV-6 and HHV-7 (38). Treatment is largely supportive.

HHV-8

Epidemiology

The prevalence of HHV-8 varies significantly in the population worldwide. In the United States, less than 5% of the adult population has serologic evidence of HHV-8, whereas in areas of high endemicity, such as Africa, more than 50% are seropositive (101). HHV-8 is predominantly shed in the saliva and to a lesser degree in semen and other body fluids. The source of transmission of HHV-8 also varies. In low-prevalence areas, transmission is mainly through sexual contact, while in areas of high endemicity, transmission is typically from mother to child and between siblings (101). HHV-8 is associated with the development of Kaposi's sarcoma. It was initially described to occur in HIV-infected persons who developed Kaposi's sarcoma, but it was later detected in HIV-negative Kaposi's sarcoma as well (28, 107).

Clinical Manifestations

Kaposi's sarcomas are vascular neoplasias that initially present as deep red-purple macules (Color Plate 14). The macules evolve into papules, plaques, and tumors that can be pink, red, purple, or brown. Classically, the lesions begin on the feet and hands and spread proximally. There is often associated lymphedema, especially of the lower extremities. Kaposi's sarcomas can present with oral lesions as well and involve almost any internal organ. It is the most common AIDS-associated malignancy in the developed world and one of the most common cancers in developing nations.

HHV-8 is also associated with primary effusion lymphoma and multicentric Castleman's disease. Castleman's disease is caused by the hyperproliferation of B cells forming tumors in lymph nodes throughout the body. In addition, HHV-8 DNA has also been detected in squamous cell carcinomas and other epithelial lesions in organ transplant recipients (107). The role of HHV-8 in the pathogenesis of these epithelial tumors is still unclear.

Diagnosis and Differential Diagnosis

The differential for Kaposi's sarcoma includes dermatofibroma, pyogenic granuloma, hemangioma, bacillary (epithelioid) angiomatosis, melanocytic nevus, ecchymosis, granuloma annulare, stasis dermatitis, and insect bites (158). Both PCR and serologic markers can aid in diagnosis, although skin biopsy is usually necessary for confirmation (37, 117) (Fig. 7).

Treatment

HHV-8 found in Kaposi's sarcomas is usually in the latent stage, rendering these lesions resistant to typical antiherpes medications that block viral replication. However, HHV-8 in multicentric Castleman's disease is typically in the lytic stage, allowing antiherpes drugs to be effective in

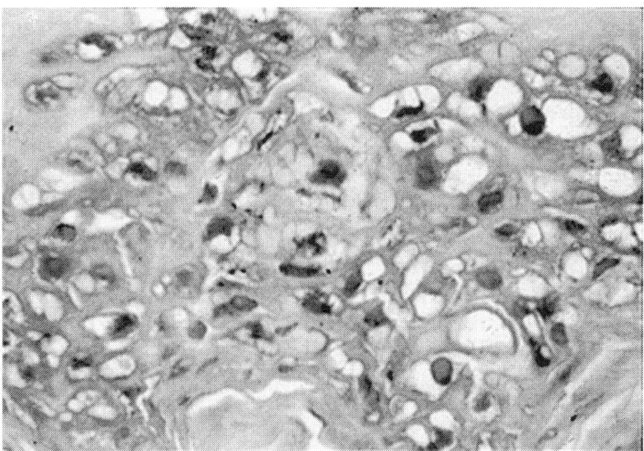

FIGURE 7 Photomicrograph of Kaposi's sarcoma associated with HHV-8, demonstrating neovascularization, endothelial proliferation, and plump hyperchromatic atypical nuclei lining vascular spaces.

this disease (72). For progressive and disseminated Kaposi's sarcomas, chemotherapy and IFN-α can be used (41). Local disease can be treated with radiotherapy, intralesional chemotherapy, cryotherapy, and alitretinoin gel (20, 45). The prognosis of HHV-8-associated Kaposi's sarcomas in AIDS patients has benefited greatly from the development of HAART. HAART has led to a significant decrease in the prevalence of AIDS-related Kaposi's sarcomas and has lowered morbidity and mortality rates in patients when they do develop (46).

B Virus (Herpesvirus Simiae)

An animal herpesvirus, B virus (herpesvirus simiae), can also rarely cause human disease, most significantly a fatal encephalomyelitis. This virus usually infects humans following a bite or scratch from a macaque monkey. Erythema, induration, and vesicles develop at the inoculation site and are followed by fever, lymphangitis, lymphadenopathy, gastrointestinal symptoms, and myalgias. These symptoms are followed by rapid progression to the neurologic signs and symptoms of encephalomyelitis (16). Although many nonhuman herpesviruses exist, B virus is of particular importance due to the high mortality rate in infected humans (156). Diagnosis is typically made through viral culture. The virus can be recovered from vesicular skin lesions at the point of inoculation, as well as from vesicles following reactivation of the latent B virus.

Parvovirus B19

Virology

Parvoviruses are nonenveloped, icosahedral viruses, about 25 nm in diameter, containing a single-stranded, nonenveloped DNA (151). Parvovirus B19 is a member of the *Erythrovirus* genus within the *Parvoviridae* family. It is among the smallest of the DNA animal viruses and has an approximate genome size of 5,000 bp. The only known natural host cell of parvovirus B19 is the human erythroid progenitor (84). After experimental inoculation of parvovirus B19, the number of erythroid progenitors in the bone marrow declines within a few days (104). A distinctive cytopathic effect and assembled parvovirus particles can be seen in erythroid progenitors in cultures of bone marrow (98), peripheral blood (126), and fetal liver (160).

Epidemiology

Parvovirus B19 infection is common worldwide and occurs both sporadically and as epidemics. Parvovirus B19 has been recognized since the 1980s as the cause of erythema infectiosum (fifth disease) (6). This syndrome presents most commonly in children 4 to 10 years of age and often in epidemics in late winter and early spring (144). Viremia appears 6 to 14 days after a susceptible patient contracts parvovirus B19 via the respiratory route, but the rash appears 17 to 18 days following infection. Approximately 60 to 70% of adults are parvovirus B19 IgG seropositive, with prevalence rates increasing with age (69). The rate of primary parvovirus B19 infection in adults is much higher in those who are immunocompromised. Parvovirus B19 typically affects 1 to 5% of pregnant women, but higher attack rates (up to 20%) occur during an epidemic. Infection of a pregnant woman, particularly during the first or second trimester, can lead to nonimmune hydrops fetalis and fetal death (47). The virus is spread by respiratory droplets, but nosocomial infections have been described (14). Parvovirus B19 has also been transmitted by blood products, especially pooled factor VIII and factor IX concentrates. Since January 2002, producers of plasma derivatives have voluntarily instituted quantitative measurements of B19 DNA to reduce the risk of iatrogenic transmission. Iatrogenic transmission of parvovirus B19 via blood products continues to occur in part because the virus' small size, heat resistance, and high viral load make it difficult to eradicate from blood and plasma derivatives (18).

Clinical Features

Erythema infectiosum begins with nonspecific symptoms approximately 4 to 14 days after exposure to parvovirus B19 but can begin as late as 21 days after exposure (5). Confluent erythematous, edematous plaques appear on the cheeks with circumoral pallor after about 2 days of low-grade fever, headache, and coryza. The rash gives the cheeks a "slapped" appearance (Color Plate 15) and is accompanied by continuation of the above-mentioned symptoms and the appearance of cough, conjunctivitis, pharyngitis, malaise, myalgias, nausea, diarrhea, and occasional arthralgias. After 1 to 4 days, the facial rash fades coinciding with the appearance of erythematous macules and papules with a reticulated pattern on the extensor surfaces of the extremities, neck, and trunk. The rash can be pruritic and usually lasts for 1 to 2 weeks but can persist for months. The rash may be evanescent, and recurrences can be provoked by exposure to sunlight, heat, emotional stress, or exercise. Patients with erythema infectiosum appear to be infectious only before the appearance of the rash, since parvovirus B19 is usually not found in respiratory secretions or in the serum after the appearance of cutaneous manifestations. Parvovirus myocarditis (13) and heart failure (92) have followed fifth disease in a small number of cases. Parvovirus infection has been associated with severe but self-limited hepatitis in a few children (133).

The gloves-and-socks syndrome, an exanthem localized to the hands and feet, with edema, erythema, paresthesia, and pruritus, has also been linked to parvovirus B19 (132). Chronic fatigue syndrome may follow infection with parvovirus B19 (68). Meningitis, encephalitis, and a variety of neurologic complications may occur with fifth disease and parvovirus infection (67). In adults, primary parvovirus B19 infection is often associated with an acute arthropathy without rash. Other clinical presentations of parvovirus B19 infection, potentially much more serious than erythema infectiosum but uncommonly accompanied by rash, include transient aplastic crisis in patients with chronic hemolytic anemia, parvovirus-related chronic anemia in immunocompromised patients, and nonimmune fetal hydrops (65).

Diagnosis

Nonspecific laboratory tests such as complete blood count and serum chemistries are usually normal in erythema infectiosum, although elevated levels of hepatic aminotransferases can accompany fifth disease. Detection of serum IgM directed to parvovirus B19 indicates recent infection. The serum IgM levels start to decline after 1 month, but IgM is still detectable for 6 months after infection. Parvovirus B19-specific IgG can be detected 1 week following infection and persists for years. Tests such as radioimmunoassay, counterimmunoelectrophoresis, enzyme-linked immunosorbent assay (ELISA), dot blot hybridization, and PCR exist for detection of the virus. The virus may be cultured in human erythroid progenitors.

The macular and papular stages of erythema infectiosum must be differentiated from drug eruptions, bacterial infections (such as scarlet fever and erysipelas), and other viral infections (such as those due to enteroviruses and rubella, measles, and roseola viruses).

Treatment

Since erythema infectiosum is a self-limited and mild illness, no treatment is usually indicated. No specific antiviral therapy exists for parvovirus B19. Nonsteroidal anti-inflammatory drugs are often used to relieve arthralgias and arthritis.

Pure red cell aplasia and the underlying persistent parvovirus B19 infection may be terminated rapidly by discontinuing immunosuppressive therapy or by instituting antiretroviral drug therapy in patients with HIV. Commercial immune globulins are a good source of antibodies against parvovirus; a persistent B19 infection responds to a 5- or 10-day course of immune globulin at a dose of 0.4 g per kg of body weight, with a prompt decline in serum viral DNA, accompanied by reticulocytosis and increased hemoglobin levels (75).

Prevention of infection can best be achieved via good infection control practices, including frequent hand washing and not sharing food or drinks. One infection with parvovirus B19 produces lifelong immunity. No vaccine against parvovirus B19 is currently available, but a recombinant human parvovirus B19 vaccine composed of viral capsid proteins is currently in clinical trials (11).

RNA VIRUSES

Enteroviruses

Virology

The enterovirus genus belongs to the *Picornaviridae* family, all of the members of which contain a small, positive-sense, single-stranded RNA genome. Enteroviruses are nonenveloped and contain four specific structural proteins (VP1, VP2, VP3, and VP4) that compose the icosahededral capsid. Traditionally, the taxonomy of the enterovirus genus was subdivided into groups based on the associated disease in humans and animal models. These subgroups included polioviruses, coxsackievirus group A (CVA), coxsackievirus group B (CVB), echoviruses, and the other nongrouped enteroviruses. However, a new classification system (Table 1) combines and separates some of the old subgroups into four groups (human enterovirus A, B, C, and D) based on molecular and biological characteristics (139). Although there is a new classification system, the names of the individual serotypes of the old system are still commonly used.

Epidemiology

Enteroviruses are highly contagious and are typically transmitted by human oral-oral and fecal-oral mechanisms. Direct contact with fluid from cutaneous and ocular lesions, fomites, and contaminated water sources may also be mechanisms of transmission, but more evidence is needed. After infection via the buccal mucosa, pharynx, or gastrointestinal tract, the virus travels to regional lymph nodes and a later viremia carries the virus to secondary locations, including mucocutaneous sites, resulting in intraepidermal vesicles containing neutrophils, mononuclear cells, and proteinaceous eosinophilic material. The subvesicular dermis is edematous and contains a perivascular polymorphous infiltrate composed of lymphocytes and neutrophils. The lower gastrointestinal tract may remain infected, thereby releasing virus into the feces for days, weeks, or even months after initial infection, thus allowing the potential for spread (30).

Enterovirus infections occur worldwide. It has been estimated that each year there are approximately 10 million to 15 million symptomatic enterovirus infections in the United States (141). These infections tend to have a seasonal preference for summer and fall, and a higher incidence in children younger than 10 years of age has been reported (70).

Enterovirus 71 (EV71) has received widespread attention since it caused epidemics in Malaysia and Taiwan in 1997 and 1998, respectively. Among an estimated 1.3 million infections in Taiwan, 405 reported severe cases needed hospitalization and 78 deaths occurred (59). Since then, there have been outbreaks all over the Asian-Pacific region. EV71 not only has mucocutaneous manifestions but also is associated with severe neurologic and cardiopulmonary complications.

Clinical Features

Enteroviruses can cause a variety of clinical manifestations. Although the majority of infections are benign and usually only manifest as a fever, common mucocutaneous presentations (Table 2) and less common manifestions (Table 3) are recognized.

While a variety of enteroviruses, particularly coxsackieviruses, cause mucocutaneous manifestations, the two most distinctive clinical syndromes are HFMD and herpangina.

HFMD

HFMD is a mucocutaneous manifestation that usually affects persons in their preteen and teenage years (143). The associated viruses that cause HFMD are transmitted via the oral-oral or fecal-oral route. Serotypes CVA16 and EV71 are responsible for most epidemic cases of HFMD, but occasionally HFMD may be associated with CVA4 to CVA7, CVA9, CVA10, CVB1 to CVB3, and CVB5. In one study, echovirus 4, which is commonly associated with aseptic meningitis and the cause of outbreaks in Cuba, Cape Town, South Africa, Spain, and India, was also found to be associated with HFMD (121). After an incubation period of 3 to 6 days, a prodrome characterized by low fever, malaise, and abdominal or respiratory symptoms precedes the mucocutaneous lesions by 12 to 24 h.

Oral lesions typically appear first and are most common on the hard palate, tongue, and buccal mucosa. The lesions can vary in number from 1 to 10 and typically begin as macules that rapidly progress to 2- to 3-mm vesicles and then to shallow, yellow-gray painful ulcers with an erythematous halo.

Cutaneous vesicles appear concomitantly with or soon after the oral lesions and are most prevalent on the hands and feet, including the palms and soles, but can appear on the face, legs, and buttocks. These lesions can vary in number from a few to over 100. Cutaneous lesions also begin as erythematous macules but are larger (3 to 7 mm) and develop into cloudy, white oval vesicles with a red halo (55). Both oral and cutaneous lesions are usually tender or painful and resolve in 5 to 10 days without treatment or scarring.

TABLE 1 Taxonomy of enteroviruses

Traditional taxonomy	Current taxonomy
Polioviruses PV1–PV3[a]	Human enterovirus A CVA2–CVA8, CVA10, CVA12, CVA14, CVA16, EV71, EV76, EV89, EV90, EV91
Coxsackie A viruses CVA1–CVA22, CVA24	Human enterovirus B CVA9, CVB1–CVB6, E1–E7, E9, E11–E21, E24–E27, E29–E33, EV69, EV73–EV75, EV77–EV88, EV100–EV101
Coxsackie B viruses CVB1–CVB6	Human enterovirus C CVA1, CVA11, CVA13, CVA17, CVA19–CVA22, CVA24, PV1–PV3
Echoviruses E1–E7, E9, E11–E21, E24–E27, E29–E33	Human enterovirus D EV68, EV70
Numbered enteroviruses EV68–EV71	

[a] PV, poliovirus.

Herpangina

Herpangina is a self-limiting, acute illness that characteristically affects the posterior oropharyngeal structures. Viruses causing herpangina are spread via routes similar to those causing HFMD. Herpangina is usually caused by CVA2, CVA4, CVA5, CVA6, CVA8, or CVA10; however, less commonly, the syndrome can be caused by various group B coxsackieviruses, echoviruses, and nonspecific enteroviruses. Herpangina usually affects children from 1 to 7 years of age and begins abruptly with a high fever, sore throat, dysphagia, anorexia, and malaise (89). Small, gray-white vesicles (less than 5 mm) surrounded by erythema appear on the posterior palate, uvula, and tonsils; the vesicles usually ulcerate. Systemic symptoms usually resolve within 4 to 5 days, and the ulcers heal spontaneously within 1 week.

Diagnosis

Exanthematous enteroviral infections are usually diagnosed based on clinical presentation. In both HFMD and herpangina, a mild leukocytosis (i.e., 10,000 to 15,000/mm^3) may be seen. If a specific diagnosis must be made, virus isolation, type-specific serology, or reverse transcriptase PCR may be used to identify the responsible virus type. PCR-based assays used to detect enterovirus serotypes are superior to viral culture for diagnosis of severe enterovirus infections, such as aseptic meningitis and encephalitis (111, 118). When a patient presents with vesicles, it is best to take samples from both throat swabs and vesicle swabs in attempts to isolate the virus. For those patients who do not have vesicles, it is best to take throat and rectal swabs (95).

Oral lesions of HFMD and herpangina can be distinguished from each other based on the total clinical presentation (e.g., cutaneous and anterior oral lesions in HFMD) as well as serology. Oral lesions can sometimes be confused with aphthous stomatitis, which are larger and less uniform than the oral erosions in HFMD. More importantly, the mucous membrane ulcers should be differentiated from those associated with HSV and VZV. Both HSV and VZV yield multinucleated, giant cells on a characteristic Tzanck smear, while HFMD and herpangina do not. Cutaneous vesicles of HFMD should also be differentiated from HSV and VZV infections as well as from erythema multiforme, rubella, drug eruptions, and gonococcemia.

Therapy

There is no specific antiviral therapy or vaccine for HFMD or herpangina; management is symptomatic. Fluid replacement and limited physical activity are strongly encouraged. Proper hygiene and avoiding contaminated food can help prevent viral infection. Breast-feeding has also been found to reduce the number of enterovirus infections in infants and provides an overall protective effect (123).

Measles Virus

Virology and Epidemiology

Measles, also known as rubeola, is a highly contagious childhood infection caused by an enveloped, single-stranded RNA virus from the *Paramyxoviridae* family. Since the development of the measles vaccine in 1963, the incidence of measles has decreased by 98% in the United States (158). In many developing nations, however, mea-

TABLE 2 Common mucocutaneous manifestations of enteroviruses

HFMD
Herpangina
Macular rash
Maculopapular rash
Urticarial rash
Roseola-like lesions
Boston exanthem disease
Eruptive pseudoangiomatosis

TABLE 3 Associated manifestations of enteroviruses

Mild	Serious
Exanthem	Encephalitis
Enanthem	Meningitis
Fever	Neonatal sepsis
Pleurodynia	Myocarditis
Pharyngitis	Pericarditis
Croup	Hepatitis
	Acute paralysis

sles is still highly prevalent; mortality rates range from 1 to 5% and can reach 30% in malnourished children and in refugee areas (48). Approximately 800,000 people worldwide still die from measles virus infection every year, with over half of these deaths in Africa (39).

Clinical Features

Measles outbreaks typically occur in the late winter to early spring. Transmission is through respiratory droplets from sneezing and coughing. Infected persons are contagious for several days before signs and symptoms develop. Infection is characterized by a prodromal phase of fever, coryza, cough, and conjunctivitis for 3 to 4 days. Splenomegaly and lymphadenopathy may also be noted. Cutaneous manifestations include pathognomonic Koplik's spots and a maculopapular morbilliform eruption. Koplik's spots, which appear several days before the onset of the rash, are characterized by clusters of blue-white spots on an erythematous base located on the buccal mucosa. The rash first appears on the forehead and behind the ears and then spreads inferiorly to the face, then the trunk and extremities, and finally to the palms and soles (Color Plate 16). The macules and papules may coalesce, especially on the face. As the exanthema progresses, the systemic symptoms typically subside. The rash gradually fades to a yellow-tan color with faint desquamation, resolving entirely in 4 to 6 days. Although the rash may be partly due to viral damage to epithelial and vascular endothelial cells, the appearance of skin lesions simultaneously with detectable serum antibody suggests that virus-antibody complexes may initiate the damage.

Complications of measles virus infection include otitis media, pneumonia, diarrhea, purpura, and thrombocytopenia. In immunocompromised patients, pneumonitis and encephalitis can occur. In one prospective study, HIV-infected children were documented to have a higher rate of hospitalization from measles, a younger age of presentation, and a higher fatality rate (85). The complications of encephalitis and thrombocytopenic purpura may be due to the formation of immune complexes. Atypical measles can occur in individuals previously given the killed measles virus vaccine who are subsequently exposed to wild-type measles or to live attenuated measles virus vaccine (31). Coryza, conjunctivitis, and Koplik's spots are absent in atypical measles. Unlike in typical measles, the eruption spreads centripetally, usually beginning on the hands and feet. Initially the exanthema consists of erythematous macules and papules which may progress to vesicular and petechial lesions (125).

Diagnosis

Diagnosis is usually made clinically, but serology using ELISA, complement fixation, neutralization, or hemagglutination inhibition tests can be used for confirmation. In addition, cultures, antigen detection, and PCR can be used. On cytological examination of secretions, multinucleated giant cells can be seen. Biopsy of the measles exanthem reveals hyaline necrosis of epithelial cells, formation of a serum exudate around superficial dermal vessels, proliferation of endothelial cells followed by a leukocytic infiltrate of the dermis, and lymphocytic cuffing of vessels.

The differential diagnosis for measles includes other viral exanthems such as rubella, roseola, and enterovirus, as well as drug eruptions, scarlet fever, Kawasaki disease, infectious mononucleosis, toxoplasmosis, and *Mycoplasma pneumoniae* infection (158).

Treatment

Immunization against measles has been available since 1963. Worldwide, the mortality rate from measles fell by 60% between 1999 and 2005 (48). The WHO, the CDC, and the Pan-American Health Organization have established a goal of global measles eradication by 2010 (26). The first dose of the vaccine is typically given between 12 and 15 months, and a second dose is given at 4 to 6 years. It is commonly given as part of the measles-mumps-rubella (MMR) combination vaccine or, more recently, the measles-mumps-rubella-varicella (MMRV) vaccine. Fever is the most common side effect of the vaccine, occurring in 5 to 15% of recipients. Another 5% of individuals develop a mild rash.

Measles is a self-limited disease in most patients, and treatment is largely supportive. Vitamin A deficiency is considered a risk factor for measles virus infection, and the WHO recommends vitamin A supplementation for all hospitalized patients in areas of high endemicity (43). There are currently no antiviral drugs specifically approved for the treatment of measles. Passive immunity via serum immunoglobulins may modify or prevent measles if administered within 6 days of exposure to the virus. Ribavirin may be beneficial in patients with severe complications of measles (145).

Rubella Virus

Virology and Epidemiology

Rubella, also known as German measles, is caused by rubella virus, from the *Togaviridae* family. Before the development of a vaccine in 1969, rubella was a worldwide disease with epidemics every 6 to 9 years, typically in the spring. Since the implementation of the vaccine, the incidence of rubella has decreased by 99% in the United States (158). However, with inadequate immunization programs in developing countries, rubella virus infection continues to be a significant health concern.

Clinical Features

Rubella is an acute viral illness typically seen in children, although all age groups are susceptible. Transmission is through airborne droplets and can occur up to 7 days before and after the onset of symptoms. Fifty percent of rubella virus infections are asymptomatic. When symptoms do occur, they usually begin with prodromal symptoms starting 14 to 21 days after infection. Prodromal symptoms are more prominent with increasing age and consist of low-grade fever, headache, conjunctivitis, upper respiratory tract symptoms, and sore throat. Lymphadenopathy is common, especially in the posterior auricular, suboccipital, and posterior cervical lymph nodes. Arthritis and splenomegaly can also occur, especially in adults. From 1 to 4 days after the initiation of the prodrome, an erythematous macular to papular rash appears. It begins on the face and spreads to the neck, trunk, and extremities within 24 h. Lesions often coalesce to form a scarlatiniform eruption. The cutaneous manifestations typically resolve completely within 3 days without residual pigment changes. The rash appears simultaneously with a rise in antibody titers, suggesting that the exanthem may be due to the inflammatory effects of antibody-virus complexes rather than direct viral infection.

Rubella virus infection is typically a benign illness, though complications such as encephalitis, neuritis, orchitis, and thrombocytopenia can occur (40). Infection during pregnancy, especially in the first trimester, can lead to congenital malformations in approximately 50% of infected neonates. Neonates with congenital rubella can present with cataracts, deafness, congenital heart defects, intrauterine growth retardation, microcephaly, mental retardation, thrombocytopenia, hepatosplenomegaly, and encephalitis. Infection of the bone marrow produces the characteristic cutaneous findings of petechiae and ecchymoses (17).

Diagnosis

Diagnosis is typically made clinically, although it can be difficult to differentiate rubella from other viral exanthems. Serology is commonly used to confirm the diagnosis. Viral culture and PCR can also be employed. Recently, samples of saliva have been used to detect rubella-specific RNA, IgM, and IgG (15, 153). Increased numbers of atypical lymphocytes and plasma cells may be found in peripheral blood but are not diagnostic.

Diagnosis of congenital rubella can be made through viral culture, PCR, or serology using samples from amniocentesis, cordocentesis, and chorionic villous sampling (40). During the first trimester, PCR of a sample of amniotic fluid can provide a diagnosis of prenatal infection with rubella virus within 48 h (114). After delivery, the detection of rubella-specific IgM antibodies can make the diagnosis of congenital rubella, as the maternally derived antibody is IgG.

The differential diagnosis for rubella includes other infectious exanthems, adverse drug eruptions, scarlet fever, and enterovirus infection (158). If arthritis is present, the differential diagnosis also includes acute rheumatic fever, rheumatoid arthritis, and erythema infectiosum (158). Congenital rubella syndrome may resemble other congenital infections due to toxoplasmosis and CMV.

Treatment

Rubella is typically a benign, self-limited illness, and treatment is symptomatic. There are currently no antiviral medications specifically approved for rubella virus infection. Prevention is carried out with a live attenuated vaccine that is often administered as part of the MMR vaccine or the recently developed MMRV vaccine. The first dose is typically given at 12 to 15 months, and the second is given at 4 to 6 years. Since the implementation of the vaccine, rubella is no longer considered endemic in the United States (112). As with the measles vaccine, the rubella vaccine is contraindicated in pregnant women and in severely immunocompromised individuals.

Human Immunodeficiency Virus

Virology

HIV is a member of the genus *Lentivirus* within the family *Retroviridae*. Like other retroviruses, HIV carries an RNA-dependent DNA polymerase (i.e., reverse transcriptase), which allows viral RNA to be converted into a proviral DNA sequence.

Epidemiology

Although other retroviruses, such as human T-cell leukemia virus type 1 (HTLV-1) and HTLV-2, can have cutaneous manifestations, particularly due to the association of HTLV-1 with adult T-cell lymphoma/leukemia (93), the most important retrovirus medically and in terms of cutaneous manifestations is HIV type 1. Mucocutaneous manifestations of HIV infection are often responsible for the signs and symptoms that lead to suspicion and serologic testing for HIV (78). Similarly, a variety of mucocutaneous manifestations may serve as clinical markers of progression from asymptomatic HIV infection to full-blown AIDS (16).

Transmission of HIV is primarily via sexual contact with an infected person, significant exposure to infected blood or blood products, or perinatally from an infected mother to her child. After sufficient contact with HIV, the virus infects $CD4^+$ T lymphocytes by attachment to the CD4 molecule and coreceptors (CCR5 or CXCR4). Other $CD4^+$ cells such as monocytes and macrophages are also infected by HIV and help to spread the virus to susceptible cells in the brain, lymph nodes, skin, lungs, and gastrointestinal tract. HIV produces disease by killing $CD4^+$ cells, by syncytium formation, and by induction of certain cytokines that may play a direct role in induction of malignancy, neurologic disease, and other clinical manifestations.

Clinical Features

Upon initial infection with HIV, many patients are asymptomatic. Patients who develop an acute primary HIV infection 3 to 6 weeks after exposure manifest fever, mononucleosis-like symptoms, and a characteristic erythematous, maculopapular exanthem appearing on the trunk and extremities. The exanthem and symptoms of the acute illness generally resolve spontaneously within 2 weeks (64). Biopsy material from the exanthem associated with primary HIV infection usually demonstrates nonspecific changes, such as a superficial perivascular and perifollicular mononuclear cell infiltrate predominately composed of $CD4^+$ cells. Detectable formation of antibody to HIV usually requires several weeks after infection and in some cases may follow infection by more than 1 year.

As the $CD4^+$ T cells decline and the disease progresses from asymptomatic HIV infection through advanced AIDS, over 90% of patients will develop secondary mucocutaneous manifestations of their infection (161). Such signs may be infectious, neoplastic, or noninfectious and nonneoplastic. A summary of the dermatologic findings of opportunistic HIV/AIDS-related pathogens is presented in Table 4. These include viral, bacterial, fungal, and parasitic infections, as well as neoplastic malignancies associated with HIV infection. Nonneoplastic and noninfectious mucocutaneous findings include inflammatory diseases (e.g., psoriasis and Reiter's disease); vascular diseases; hypersensitivities to drugs, insect bites, and UV light; pruritus; xerosis; ichthyosis; and seborrheic dermatitis.

Laboratory Findings

ELISA is used to screen for HIV infection, and the Western blot assay is used to confirm the diagnosis. Although seroconversion does not occur until approximately 6 weeks after the acute illness, viremia can be detected approximately 10 days after infection (103). The presence of HIV may be detected by PCR or isolation of virus from the blood or demonstration of HIV p24 antigenemia. Semiquantification of HIV RNA in the serum, which is useful in assessing the response to antiretroviral therapy, can also be done using PCR. Disease progression is also accompa-

TABLE 4 Dermatologic findings of opportunistic diseases in HIV-infected patients

Organism(s)	Dermatologic findings
Viruses	
MC virus	Dome-shaped, flesh-colored papules with a central umbilication; larger, coalescent, and persistent lesions occur in HIV-infected patients; lesions may be widespread and atypical; observed in unusual sites such as the face, neck, and scalp; unusual forms include solitary, endophytic, aggregated, inflamed, and giant MCs (73)
HSV	Clusters of vesicles that may rupture, crust, and form multiple small or large confluent painful ulcers; recurrent oral and anogenital HSV may lead to chronic ulcerations in HIV-infected patients (127)
Herpes zoster virus (shingles)	Dermatomal eruption of vesicles that arise in clusters from a red base that either umbilicate or rupture before forming crusts; in HIV-infected patients, the eruption may also be multidermatomal, recurrent, ulcerative, and widely disseminated with systemic involvement (29)
VZV (chickenpox)	HIV-infected patients often have chronic infections that begin as vesicles and progress to necrotic, nonhealing ulcers (77)
HPV (warts)	Flesh-colored papules that evolve into dome-shaped, gray to brown, hyperkeratotic discrete and rough papules, often with black dots on the surface; HIV-infected patients can have severe, widespread, and chronic warts, which may arise on mucosal surfaces, the face, perianal region, and the female genital tract; HPV is associated with cervical cancer in women (81) and anal cancer in both sexes
EBV (oral hairy leukoplakia)	White plaques with hair-like projections localized on the lateral aspect of the tongue (113)
CMV	Persistent perineal ulcers are the most common presentation; ulcers may be coinfected with HSV; also associated with nonspecific cutaneous lesions such as verrucous or purpuric papules, vesicles, morbilliform eruptions, and hyperpigmented indurated plaques (29, 81, 91)
Bacteria	
Staphylococcus aureus	Primary infections include impetigo, folliculitis, furuncles, carbuncles, abscesses, and necrotizing fasciitis; recurrent infections are common due to increased prevalence of nasal and perineal colonization in HIV-infected patients (63, 105)
Pseudomonas aeruginosa	Ecthyma gangrenosum, infection of catheter sites, and secondary infection of underlying disorders such as Kaposi's sarcoma in advanced HIV disease (81)
Bartonella spp. (bacillary angiomatosis)	Bacillary angiomatosis is characterized by red to purple papules, nodules, or plaques resembling Kaposi's sarcoma (Color Plate 17); any site except the palms, soles, and oral cavity may be involved; hematogenous or lymphatic dissemination to bone marrow and other lymphoid organs may occur (102)
Mycobacterium tuberculosis	Cutaneous tuberculosis is rare; multifocal lupus vulgaris, tuberculous gummata, orofacial tuberculosis, scrofuloderma, and miliary abscesses may be seen (81)
Mycobacterium avium-intracellulare complex	Cutaneous manifestations are extremely rare, and some reports describe scaling plaques, crusted ulcers, ecthyma-like lesions, verrucous ulcers, inflammatory nodules, pustular lesions, and draining sinuses (81)
Treponema pallidum (syphilis)	Although the classic papulosquamous secondary lesions are often seen, unusual presentations may be observed in HIV-infected patients including rapidly progressing noduloulcerative forms, papular eruptions that mimic MC, and lues maligna (110)
Fungus or infection	
Candida (candidiasis)	Generally causes mucosal disease: cutaneous, oropharyngeal, vulvovaginal, and esophageal; recurrent and persistent mucocutaneous candidiasis is common in HIV-infected patients; manifests as whitish, curd-like exudates on the dorsal or buccal mucosa that are easily scraped away; recurrent vulvovaginal candidiasis presents with creamy-white vaginal discharge, with itching and burning pain; the vaginal mucosa is inflamed, and pseudomembranous plaques are often seen (63, 105)
Tinea versicolor (dermatophytosis)	Numerous small, circular, white, scaling papules on the upper trunk; may involve the upper arms, neck, and abdomen; in HIV-infected patients, cutaneous involvement is often more atypical in appearance, widespread, and resistant to therapy (58)

(Continued on next page)

TABLE 4 Dermatologic findings of opportunistic diseases in HIV-infected patients *(Continued)*

Organism(s)	Dermatologic findings
Cryptococcus neoformans (cutaneous cryptococcosis)	Translucent, dome-shaped, umbilicated lesions resembling MC on the head, face, and neck; cellulitis, ulcers, papules, plaques, and pustules are other presentations (81)
Histoplasma capsulatum (cutaneous histoplasmosis)	Mucocutaneous erosions, oral ulcerations, disseminated and erythematous macules and papules, cellulitis-like eruptions, MC-like lesions (108)
Coccidioides immitis (coccidioidomycosis)	Begin as papules and evolving to pustules, plaques, or nodules with minimal surrounding erythema; hemorrhagic papules or nodules; lesions may resemble MC (81)
Sporothrix schenckii (sporotrichosis)	Hematogenous dissemination to the skin may manifest as papules to nodules that become eroded, ulcerated, crusted, or hyperkeratotic, usually sparing the palms, soles, and oral mucosa (79)
Penicillium marneffei (penicilliosis)	Most common skin lesions are umbilicated papules resembling MC, occurring most frequently on the face, ears, upper trunk, and arms (81)
Aspergillus spp.	Necrotic papulonodules; subcutaneous nodules (138)
Parasites	
Leishmania donovani (leishmaniasis)	Papular, maculopapular or nodular lesions; typically ulcerated nodules on the extremities; in atypical presentations, the lesions are disseminated (99)
Acanthamoeba castellani (acanthamebiasis)	Dissemination to the skin is common in AIDS; necrotic nodules and painful ulcerations of the trunk and extremities develop in HIV-infected patients (29, 146)
Toxoplasma gondii (toxoplasmosis)	Cutaneous involvement is rare; manifests as an eruption of macules, papules, or vesicles involving the trunk and extremities (81)
Pneumocystis carinii	Disseminated infection may appear as MC-like papules, bluish cellulitic plaques, and deeply seated abscesses in the external ear or nares (81)
Malignancies	
Kaposi's sarcoma	Purple patches on the distal lower extremities that progress proximally and become multifocal; individual lesions darken and thicken, eventually becoming brown and verrucous; lesions in HIV-infected patients have a predilection for the face, torso, and oral mucosa (7)
Non-Hodgkin's lymphoma	Non-Hodgkin's lymphoma tends to be more progressive and aggressive (88); pink to purple papules are usually seen when the skin is affected; the lesions often ulcerate and sometimes stimulate panniculitis (103); younger age of onset, more advanced stages, and extranodal site involvement at presentation, in particular the CNS, intestine, and skin, are found in HIV-infected patients (87)
Squamous and basal cell carcinomas	In HIV infection, these tumors appear earlier and more often on unexposed sites such as the trunk and extremities; metastases of basal cell carcinoma have been recorded (103, 152)
Malignant melanoma	Appears to be more aggressive, with shorter disease-free periods and lower overall survival rates in patients with melanoma and HIV than in patients with melanoma without HIV (2)

nied by a marked decline in $CD4^+$ cells, an increase in $CD8^+$ cells, and an inverted CD4/CD8 cell ratio.

Cutaneous manifestations of acute HIV infection are nonspecific and can resemble those of a variety of benign viral diseases, including enterovirus infection, infectious mononucleosis, secondary syphilis, acute infection with hepatitis A or B virus, roseola, and toxoplasmosis (64). The papulosquamous eruption of HIV most closely mirrors that of secondary syphilis, but drug eruptions are also included in the differential diagnosis. Because a wide variety of skin problems develop in persons with advanced HIV disease, the differential diagnosis usually expands into a myriad of possibilities that often can be differentiated one from another only via a skin biopsy.

Treatment

There are currently more than 22 drugs which have been approved for treatment of HIV infection (see chapters 11 and 33).

We are indebted to the following contributors for their help in the preparation of the manuscript: Melissa Diamantis, Joanna Harp, Emily Moglovkin, Brandon Christianson, Jeff Drucker, Natalia Mendoza, Aron Gewirtzman, and Anne Marie Tremaine.

REFERENCES

1. **Abdel-Haq, N., P. Chearskul, H. Al-Tatari, and B. Asmar.** 2006. New antiviral agents. *Indian J. Pediatr.* **73:** 313–321.
2. **Aboulafia, D. M.** 1998. Malignant melanoma in an HIV-infected man: a case report and literature review. *Cancer Investig.* **16:**217–224.
3. **Alford, C. A., S. Stagno, R. F. Pass, and W. J. Britt.** 1990. Congenital and perinatal cytomegalovirus infections. *Rev. Infect. Dis.* **12**(Suppl. 7)**:**S745–S753.
4. **Allen, A. L., and E. C. Siegfried.** 2000. What's new in human papillomavirus infection. *Curr. Opin. Pediatr.* **12:** 365–369.

5. **American Academy of Pediatrics.** 2007. Parvovirus B19 (erythema infectiosum, fifth disease). *Red Book 2006: Report of the Committee on Infectious Diseases*, 26th ed. 2006. American Academy of Pediatrics, Elk Grove Village, IL.
6. **Anderson, M. J., E. Lewis, I. M. Kidd, S. M. Hall, and B. J. Cohen.** 1984. An outbreak of erythema infectiosum associated with human parvovirus infection. *J. Hyg.* **93:** 85–93.
7. **Antman, K., and Y. Chang.** 2000. Kaposi's sarcoma. *N. Engl. J. Med.* **342:**1027–1038.
8. **Asano, Y., T. Yoshikawa, S. Suga, I. Kobayashi, T. Nakashima, T. Yazaki, Y. Kajita, and T. Ozaki.** 1994. Clinical features of infants with primary human herpesvirus 6 infection (exanthem subitum, roseola infantum). *Pediatrics* **93:**104–108.
9. **Aurelian, L.** 2004. Herpes simplex virus type 2 vaccines: new ground for optimism? *Clin. Diagn. Lab. Immunol.* **11:** 437–445.
10. **Bader, C., C. S. Crumpacker, L. E. Schnipper, B. Ransil, J. E. Clark, K. Arndt, and I. M. Freedberg.** 1978. The natural history of recurrent facial-oral infection with herpes simplex virus. *J. Infect. Dis.* **138:**897–905.
11. **Ballou, W. R., J. L. Reed, W. Noble, N. S. Young, and S. Koenig.** 2003. Safety and immunogenicity of a recombinant parvovirus B19 vaccine formulated with MF59C.1. *J. Infect. Dis.* **187:**675–678.
12. **Baseman, J. G., and L. A. Koutsky.** 2005. The epidemiology of human papillomavirus infections. *J. Clin. Virol.* **32**(Suppl. 1)**:**S16–S24.
13. **Beghetti, M., A. Gervaix, C. A. Haenggeli, M. Berner, and P. C. Rimensberger.** 2000. Myocarditis associated with parvovirus B19 infection in two siblings with merosin-deficient congenital muscular dystrophy. *Eur. J. Pediatr.* **159:**135–136.
14. **Bell, L. M., S. J. Naides, P. Stoffman, R. L. Hodinka, and S. A. Plotkin.** 1989. Human parvovirus B19 infection among hospital staff members after contact with infected patients. *N. Engl. J. Med.* **321:**485–491.
15. **Ben Salah, A., A. Zaâtour, L. Pomery, B. J. Cohen, D. W. Brown, and N. Andrews.** 2003. Validation of a modified commercial assay for the detection of rubella-specific IgG in oral fluid for use in population studies. *J. Virol. Methods* **114:**151–158.
16. **Benson, P. M., S. L. Malane, R. Banks, C. B. Hicks, and J. Hilliard.** 1989. B virus (herpesvirus simiae) and human infection. *Arch. Dermatol.* **125:**1247–1248.
17. **Bialecki, C., H. M. Feder, Jr., and J. M. Grant-Kels.** 1989. The six classic childhood exanthems: a review and update. *J. Am. Acad. Dermatol.* **21:**891–903.
18. **Bonvicini, F., G. Gallinella, G. A. Gentilomi, S. Ambretti, M. Musiani, and M. Zerbini.** 2006. Prevention of iatrogenic transmission of B19 infection: different approaches to detect, remove or inactivate virus contamination. *Clin. Lab.* **52:**263–268.
19. **Bossi, P., A. Tegnell, A. Baka, F. Van Loock, J. Hendriks, A. Werner, H. Maidhof, and G. Gouvras.** 2004. Bichat guidelines for the clinical management of smallpox and bioterrorism-related smallpox. *Euro. Surveill.* **9:**E7–E8.
20. **Boudreaux, A. A., L. L. Smith, C. D. Cosby, M. M. Bason, J. W. Tappero, and T. G. Berger.** 1993. Intralesional vinblastine for cutaneous Kaposi's sarcoma associated with acquired immunodeficiency syndrome. A clinical trial to evaluate efficacy and discomfort associated with infection. *J. Am. Acad. Dermatol.* **28:**61–65.
21. **Breman, J. G., and D. A. Henderson.** 2002. Diagnosis and management of smallpox. *N. Engl. J. Med.* **346:** 1300–1308.
22. **Campisi, G., V. Panzarella, M. Giuliani, C. Lajolo, O. Di Fede, S. Falaschini, C. Di Liberto, C. Scully, and L. Lo Muzio.** 2007. Human papillomavirus: its identity and controversial role in oral oncogenesis, premalignant and malignant lesions. *Int. J. Oncol.* **30:**813–823.
23. **Carvalho, M. O., R. W. Almeida, F. M. Leite, I. B. Fellows, M. H. Teixeira, L. H. Oliveira, and S. M. Cavalcanti.** 2003. Detection of human papillomavirus DNA by the hybrid capture assay. *Braz. J. Infect. Dis.* **7:**121–125.
24. **Castellsague, X., F. X. Bosch, N. Munoz, C. J. Meijer, K. V. Shah, S. de Sanjose, J. Eluf-Neto, C. A. Ngelangel, S. Chichareon, J. S. Smith, R. Herrero, V. Moreno, and S. Franceschi.** 2002. Male circumcision, penile human papillomavirus infection, and cervical cancer in female partners. *N. Engl. J. Med.* **346:**1105–1112.
25. **Centers for Disease Control and Prevention.** 2008, posting date. Prevention of herpes zoster. Recommendations of the Advisory Committee on Immunization Practices (ACIP). Centers for Disease Control and Prevention, Atlanta, GA. [Online.] http://www.cdc.gov/mmwr/preview/mmwrhtml/rr57e0515a1.htm.
26. **Centers for Disease Control and Prevention.** 1997. Measles eradication: recommendations from a meeting cosponsored by the World Health Organization, the Pan American Health Organization, and CDC. *Morb. Mortal. Wkly. Rep. Recomm. Rep.* **46**(RR-11)**:**1–20.
27. **Chakrabarty, A., and K. Beutner.** 2004. Therapy of other viral infections: herpes to hepatitis. *Dermatol. Ther.* **17:** 465–490.
28. **Chang, Y., E. Cesarman, M. S. Pessin, F. Lee, J. Culpepper, D. M. Knowles, and P. S. Moore.** 1994. Identification of herpesvirus-like DNA sequences in AIDS-associated Kaposi's sarcoma. *Science* **266:**1865–1869.
29. **Chen, M., and C. Cockerell.** 2003. Cutaneous manifestations of HIV infection and HIV-related disorders, p. 1199–1215. *In* J. Bolognia and J. Jorizzo (ed.), *Dermatology*. Elsevier, London, England.
30. **Cherry, J.** 1998. Enteroviruses: coxsackieviruses, echoviruses, and polioviruses, p. 1787–1839. *In* R. Feigen and J. Cherry (ed.), *Textbook of Pediatric Infectious Disease*, 4th ed. W. B. Saunders, Philadelphia, PA.
31. **Cherry, J. D.** 1993. Contemporary infectious exanthems. *Clin. Infect. Dis.* **16:**199–205.
32. **Clifford, G. M., S. Gallus, R. Herrero, N. Munoz, P. J. Snijders, S. Vaccarella, P. T. Anh, C. Ferreccio, N. T. Hieu, E. Matos, M. Molano, R. Rajkumar, G. Ronco, S. de Sanjose, H. R. Shin, S. Sukvirach, J. O. Thomas, S. Tunsakul, C. J. Meijer, and S. Franceschi.** 2005. Worldwide distribution of human papillomavirus types in cytologically normal women in the international agency for research on cancer HPV prevalence surveys: a pooled analysis. *Lancet* **366:**991–998.
33. **Collins-Burow, B., and E. S. Santos.** 2007. Rituximab and its role as maintenance therapy in non-Hodgkin lymphoma. *Expert Rev. Anticancer Ther.* **7:**257–273.
34. **Corey, L., A. Wald, R. Patel, S. L. Sacks, S. K. Tyring, T. Warren, J. M. Douglas, Jr., J. Paavonen, R. A. Morrow, K. R. Beutner, L. S. Stratchounsky, G. Mertz, O. N. Keene, H. A. Watson, D. Tait, and M. Vargas-Cortes.** 2004. Once-daily valacyclovir to reduce the risk of transmission of genital herpes. *N. Engl. J. Med.* **350:** 11–20.
35. **Croen, K. D., and S. E. Straus.** 1991. Varicella-zoster virus latency. *Annu. Rev. Microbiol.* **45:**265–282.
36. **Crumpacker, C. S.** 1996. Ganciclovir. *N. Engl. J. Med.* **335:**721–729.
37. **Curreli, F., M. A. Robles, A. E. Friedman-Kien, and O. Flore.** 2003. Detection and quantitation of Kaposi's

sarcoma-associated herpesvirus (KSHV) by a single competitive-quantitative polymerase chain reaction. *J. Virol. Methods* **107:**261–267.
38. **De Bolle, L., L. Naesens, and E. De Clercq.** 2005. Update on human herpesvirus 6 biology, clinical features, and therapy. *Clin. Microbiol. Rev.* **18:**217–245.
39. **de Quadros, C. A.** 2006. Is global measles eradication feasible? *Curr. Top. Microbiol. Immunol.* **304:**153–163.
40. **De Santis, M., A. F. Cavaliere, G. Straface, and A. Caruso.** 2006. Rubella infection in pregnancy. *Reprod. Toxicol.* **21:**390–398.
41. **de Wit, R., J. K. Schattenkerk, C. A. Boucher, P. J. Bakker, K. H. Veenhof, and S. A. Danner.** 1988. Clinical and virological effects of high-dose recombinant interferon-alpha in disseminated AIDS-related Kaposi's sarcoma. *Lancet* **ii:**1214–1217.
42. **Dohil, M. A., P. Lin, J. Lee, A. W. Lucky, A. S. Paller, and L. F. Eichenfield.** 2006. The epidemiology of molluscum contagiosum in children. *J. Am. Acad. Dermatol.* **54:**47–54.
43. **D'Souza, R. M., and R. D'Souza.** 2002. Vitamin A for the treatment of children with measles—a systematic review. *J. Trop. Pediatr.* **48:**323–327.
44. **Dunne, E. F., C. M. Nielson, K. M. Stone, L. E. Markowitz, and A. R. Giuliano.** 2006. Prevalence of HPV infection among men: a systematic review of the literature. *J. Infect. Dis.* **194:**1044–1057.
45. **Duvic, M., A. E. Friedman-Kien, D. J. Looney, S. A. Miles, P. L. Myskowski, D. T. Scadden, J. Von Roenn, J. E. Galpin, J. Groopman, G. Loewen, V. Stevens, J. A. Truglia, and R. C. Yocum.** 2000. Topical treatment of cutaneous lesions of acquired immunodeficiency syndrome-related Kaposi sarcoma using alitretinoin gel: results of phase 1 and 2 trials. *Arch. Dermatol.* **136:**1461–1469.
46. **Engels, E. A., R. M. Pfeiffer, J. J. Goedert, P. Virgo, T. S. McNeel, S. M. Scoppa, and R. J. Biggar.** 2006. Trends in cancer risk among people with AIDS in the United States 1980–2002. *AIDS* **20:**1645–1654.
47. **Ergaz, Z., and A. Ornoy.** 2006. Parvovirus B19 in pregnancy. *Reprod. Toxicol.* **21:**421–435.
48. **Eurosurveillance.** 2007. Measles deaths fall by 60 percent worldwide. *Euro Surveill.* **12:**E070125.1.
49. **Fleming, D. T., G. M. McQuillan, R. E. Johnson, A. J. Nahmias, S. O. Aral, F. K. Lee, and M. E. St. Louis.** 1997. Herpes simplex virus type 2 in the United States, 1976 to 1994. *N. Engl. J. Med.* **337:**1105–1111.
50. **Friedman-Kien, A. E., W. P. Rowe, and W. G. Banfield.** 1963. Milker's nodules: isolation of a poxvirus from a human case. *Science* **140:**1335–1336.
51. **Gnann, J. W., Jr., and R. J. Whitley.** 2002. Clinical practice. Herpes zoster. *N. Engl. J. Med.* **347:**340–346.
52. **Gökbuget, N., and D. Hoelzer.** 2006. Novel antibody-based therapy for acute lymphoblastic leukaemia. *Best Pract. Res. Clin. Haematol.* **19:**701–713.
53. **Greenspan, D., J. S. Greenspan, M. Conant, V. Petersen, S. Silverman, Jr., and Y. de Souza.** 1984. Oral "hairy" leucoplakia in male homosexuals: evidence of association with both papillomavirus and a herpes-group virus. *Lancet* **ii:**831–834.
54. **Guharoy, R., R. Panzik, J. A. Noviasky, E. P. Krenzelok, and D. C. Blair.** 2004. Smallpox: clinical features, prevention, and management. *Ann. Pharmacother.* **38:**440–447.
55. **Habif, T.** 2004. Exanthems and drug eruptions, p. 462–464. *In* T. Habif (ed.), *Clinical Dermatology: a Color Guide to Diagnosis and Therapy*. Mosby, Philadelphia, PA.
56. **Hall, C. B., C. E. Long, K. C. Schnabel, M. T. Caserta, K. M. McIntyre, M. A. Costanzo, A. Knott, S. Dewhurst, R. A. Insel, and L. G. Epstein.** 1994. Human herpesvirus-6 infection in children. A prospective study of complications and reactivation. *N. Engl. J. Med.* **331:**432–438.
57. **Harding, S. P., J. R. Lipton, and J. C. Wells.** 1987. Natural history of herpes zoster ophthalmicus: predictors of postherpetic neuralgia and ocular involvement. *Br. J. Ophthalmol.* **71:**353–358.
58. **Helton, J. L.** 1997. Genital dermatology in the HIV-infected patient. *AIDS Patient Care STDS* **11:**237–243.
59. **Ho, M., E.-R. Chen, K.-H. Hsu, S.-J. Twu, K.-T. Chen, S.-F. Tsai, J.-R. Wang, and S.-R. Shih for the Taiwan Enterovirus Epidemic Working Group.** 1999. An epidemic of enterovirus 71 infection in Taiwan. *N. Engl. J. Med.* **341:**929–935.
60. **Horn, T. D., and A. F. Hood.** 1990. Cytomegalovirus is predictably present in perineal ulcers from immunosuppressed patients. *Arch. Dermatol.* **126:**642–644.
61. **Jablonska, S., J. Dabrowski, and K. Jakubowicz.** 1972. Epidermodysplasia verruciformis as a model in studies on the role of papovaviruses in oncogenesis. *Cancer Res.* **32:**583–589.
62. **Jablonska, S., and G. Orth.** 1985. Epidermodysplasia verruciformis. *Clin. Dermatol.* **3:**83–96.
63. **Johnson, R.** 2003. Cutaneous manifestations of human immunodeficiency virus disease, p. 2138–2150. *In* T. Fitzpatrick, A. Eisen, and K. Wolff (ed.), *Dermatology in Internal Medicine*, 6th ed. McGraw Hill, New York, NY.
64. **Kahn, J. O., and B. D. Walker.** 1998. Acute human immunodeficiency virus type 1 infection. *N. Engl. J. Med.* **339:**33–39.
65. **Keeler, M. L.** 1992. Human parvovirus B-19: not just a pediatric problem. *J. Emerg. Med.* **10:**39–44.
66. **Kendall, D.** 1957. Motor complications of herpes zoster. *Br. Med. J.* **2:**616–618.
67. **Kerr, J. R., F. Barah, M. L. Chiswick, G. V. McDonnell, J. Smith, M. D. Chapman, J. B. Bingham, P. Kelleher, and M. N. Sheppard.** 2002. Evidence for the role of demyelination, HLA-DR alleles, and cytokines in the pathogenesis of parvovirus B19 meningoencephalitis and its sequelae. *J. Neurol. Neurosurg. Psychiatry* **73:**739–746.
68. **Kerr, J. R., J. Bracewell, I. Laing, D. L. Mattey, R. M. Bernstein, I. N. Bruce, and D. A. Tyrrell.** 2002. Chronic fatigue syndrome and arthralgia following parvovirus B19 infection. *J. Rheumatol.* **29:**595–602.
69. **Kerr, S., G. O'Keeffe, C. Kilty, and S. Doyle.** 1999. Undenatured parvovirus B19 antigens are essential for the accurate detection of parvovirus B19 IgG. *J. Med. Virol.* **57:**179–185.
70. **Khetsuriani, N., A. Lamonte-Fowlkes, S. Oberst, and M. A. Pallansch for the Centers for Disease Control and Prevention.** 2006. Enterovirus surveillance—United States, 1970–2005. *Morb. Mortal. Wkly. Rep. Surveill. Summ.* **55:**1–20.
71. **Kimberlin, D. W., C. Y. Lin, P. J. Sanchez, G. J. Demmler, W. Dankner, M. Shelton, R. F. Jacobs, W. Vaudry, R. F. Pass, J. M. Kiell, S. J. Soong, and R. J. Whitley.** 2003. Effect of ganciclovir therapy on hearing in symptomatic congenital cytomegalovirus disease involving the central nervous system: a randomized, controlled trial. *J. Pediatr.* **143:**16–25.
72. **Klass, C. M., and M. K. Offermann.** 2005. Targeting human herpesvirus-8 for treatment of Kaposi's sarcoma and primary effusion lymphoma. *Curr. Opin. Oncol.* **17:**447–455.
73. **Kolokotronis, A., D. Antoniades, E. Katsoulidis, and V. Kioses.** 2000. Facial and perioral molluscum contagiosum as a manifestation of HIV infection. *Aust. Dent. J.* **45:**49–52.

74. **Koutsky, L.** 1997. Epidemiology of genital human papillomavirus infection. *Am. J. Med.* **102:**3–8.
75. **Kurtzman, G., N. Frickhofen, J. Kimball, D. W. Jenkins, A. W. Nienhuis, and N. S. Young.** 1989. Pure red-cell aplasia of 10 years' duration due to persistent parvovirus B19 infection and its cure with immunoglobulin therapy. *N. Engl. J. Med.* **321:**519–523.
76. **Leavell, U. W., Jr., M. J. McNamara, R. Muelling, W. M. Talbert, R. C. Rucker, and A. J. Dalton.** 1968. Orf. Report of 19 human cases with clinical and pathological observations. *JAMA* **204:**657–664.
77. **Leibovitz, E., A. Kaul, M. Rigaud, D. Bebenroth, K. Krasinski, and W. Borkowsky.** 1992. Chronic varicella zoster in a child infected with human immunodeficiency virus: case report and review of the literature. *Cutis* **49:** 27–31.
78. **Libman, H., and R. A. Witzburg.** 1993. *HIV Infection: a Clinical Manual,* 2nd ed., Little, Brown, Boston, MA.
79. **Lipstein-Kresch, E., H. D. Isenberg, C. Singer, O. Cooke, and R. A. Greenwald.** 1985. Disseminated Sporothrix schenckii infection with arthritis in a patient with acquired immunodeficiency syndrome. *J. Rheumatol.* **12:** 805–808.
80. **Lowe, L., A. A. Hebert, and M. Duvic.** 1989. Gianotti-Crosti syndrome associated with Epstein-Barr virus infection. *J. Am. Acad. Dermatol.* **20:**336–338.
81. **Maniar, J., and R. Kamath.** 2006. HIV and HIV-associated disorders, p. 93–124. *In* S. Tyring, O. Lupi, and U. Hengge (ed.), *Tropical Dermatology.* Elsevier, Philadelphia, PA.
82. **Martin, D. F., J. Sierra-Madero, S. Walmsley, R. A. Wolitz, K. Macey, P. Georgiou, C. A. Robinson, and M. J. Stempien.** 2002. A controlled trial of valganciclovir as induction therapy for cytomegalovirus retinitis. *N. Engl. J. Med.* **346:**1119–1126.
83. **Max, M. B., S. C. Schafer, M. Culnane, B. Smoller, R. Dubner, and R. H. Gracely.** 1988. Amitriptyline, but not lorazepam, relieves postherpetic neuralgia. *Neurology* **38:** 1427–1432.
84. **Mortimer, P. P., R. K. Humphries, J. G. Moore, R. H. Purcell, and N. S. Young.** 1983. A human parvovirus-like virus inhibits haematopoietic colony formation in vitro. *Nature* **302:**426–429.
85. **Moss, W. J., M. Monze, J. J. Ryon, T. C. Quinn, D. E. Griffin, and F. Cutts.** 2002. Prospective study of measles in hospitalized, human immunodeficiency virus (HIV)-infected and HIV-uninfected children in Zambia. *Clin. Infect. Dis.* **35:**189–196.
86. **Mounts, P., and K. V. Shah.** 1984. Respiratory papillomatosis: etiological relation to genital tract papillomaviruses. *Prog. Med. Virol.* **29:**90–114.
87. **Myskowski, P. L., and R. Ahkami.** 1996. Dermatologic complications of HIV infection. *Med. Clin. N. Am.* **80:** 1415–1435.
88. **Myskowski, P. L., D. J. Straus, and B. Safai.** 1990. Lymphoma and other HIV-associated malignancies. *J. Am. Acad. Dermatol.* **22:**1253–1260.
89. **Nakayama, T., T. Urano, M. Osano, Y. Hayashi, S. Sekine, T. Ando, and S. Makinom.** 1989. Outbreak of herpangina associated with coxsackievirus B3 infection. *Pediatr. Infect. Dis. J.* **8:**495–498.
90. **Nalca, A., A. W. Rimoin, S. Bavari, and C. A. Whitehouse.** 2005. Reemergence of monkeypox: prevalence, diagnostics, and countermeasures. *Clin. Infect. Dis.* **41:** 1765–1771.
91. **Nico, M. M., N. C. Cymbalista, Y. C. Hurtado, and L. H. Borges.** 2000. Perianal cytomegalovirus ulcer in an HIV infected patient: case report and review of literature. *J. Dermatol.* **27:**99–105.
92. **Nigro, G., V. Bastianon, V. Colloridi, F. Ventriglia, P. Gallo, G. D'Amati, W. C. Koch, and S. P. Adler.** 2000. Human parvovirus B19 infection in infancy associated with acute and chronic lymphocytic myocarditis and high cytokine levels: report of 3 cases and review. *Clin. Infect. Dis.* **31:**65–69.
93. **Nobre, V., A. C. Guedes, M. L. Martins, E. F. Barbosa-Stancioli, J. C. Serufo, F. A. Proietti, J. G. Ribas, C. E. Ferreira, and J. R. Lambertucci.** 2006. Dermatological findings in 3 generations of a family with a high prevalence of human T cell lymphotropic virus type 1 infection in Brazil. *Clin. Infect. Dis.* **43:**1257–1263.
94. **Obalek, S., S. Jablonska, M. Favre, L. Walczak, and G. Orth.** 1990. Condylomata acuminata in children: frequent association with human papillomaviruses responsible for cutaneous warts. *J. Am. Acad. Dermatol.* **23:** 205–213.
95. **Ooi, M. H., T. Solomon, Y. Podin, A. Mohan, W. Akin, M. A. Yusuf, S. del Sel, K. M. Kontol, B. F. Lai, D. Clear, C. H. Chieng, E. Blake, D. Perera, S. C. Wong, and J. Cardosa.** 2007. Evaluation of different clinical sample types in diagnosis of human enterovirus 71-associated hand-foot-and-mouth disease. *J. Clin. Microbiol.* **45:**1858–1866.
96. **Orth, G.** 2006. Genetics of epidermodysplasia verruciformis: insights into host defense against papillomaviruses. *Semin. Immunol.* **18:**362–374.
97. **Oxman, M. N., M. J. Levin, G. R. Johnson, K. E. Schmader, S. E. Straus, L. D. Gelb, R. D. Arbeit, M. S. Simberkoff, A. A. Gershon, L. E. Davis, A. Weinberg, K. D. Boardman, H. M. Williams, J. H. Zhang, P. N. Peduzzi, C. E. Beisel, V. A. Morrison, J. C. Guatelli, P. A. Brooks, C. A. Kauffman, C. T. Pachucki, K. M. Neuzil, R. F. Betts, P. F. Wright, M. R. Griffin, P. Brunell, N. E. Soto, A. R. Marques, S. K. Keay, R. P. Goodman, D. J. Cotton, J. W. Gnann, Jr., J. Loutit, M. Holodniy, W. A. Keitel, G. E. Crawford, S. S. Yeh, Z. Lobo, J. F. Toney, R. N. Greenberg, P. M. Keller, R. Harbecke, A. R. Hayward, M. R. Irwin, T. C. Kyriakides, C. Y. Chan, I. S. Chan, W. W. Wang, P. W. Annunziato, and J. L. Silber.** 2005. A vaccine to prevent herpes zoster and postherpetic neuralgia in older adults. *N. Engl. J. Med.* **352:**2271–2284.
98. **Ozawa, K., G. Kurtzman, and N. Young.** 1986. Replication of the B19 parvovirus in human bone marrow cell cultures. *Science* **233:**883–886.
99. **Paredes, R., J. Munoz, I. Diaz, P. Domingo, M. Gurgui, and B. Clotet.** 2003. Leishmaniasis in HIV infection. *J. Postgrad. Med.* **49:**39–49.
100. **Patel, B. M.** 1967. Skin rash with infectious mononucleosis and ampicillin. *Pediatrics* **40:**910–911.
101. **Plancoulaine, S., and A. Gessain.** 2005. Epidemiological aspects of human herpesvirus 8 infection and of Kaposi's sarcoma. *Med. Mal. Infect.* **35:**314–321. (In French.)
102. **Plettenberg, A., U. van Dyk, A. Stoehr, H. Albrecht, H. J. Stellbrink, J. Berger, and W. Meigel.** 1997. Increased risk for opportunistic infections during chemotherapy in HIV-infected patients with Kaposi's sarcoma. *Dermatology* **194:**234–237.
103. **Porras, B., M. Costner, A. E. Friedman-Kien, and C. J. Cockerell.** 1998. Update on cutaneous manifestations of HIV infection. *Med. Clin. N. Am.* **82:**1033–1080, v.
104. **Potter, C. G., A. C. Potter, C. S. Hatton, H. M. Chapel, M. J. Anderson, J. R. Pattison, D. A. Tyrrell, P. G. Higgins, J. S. Willman, and H. F. Parry.** 1987. Variation of erythroid and myeloid precursors in the marrow and peripheral blood of volunteer subjects in-

fected with human parvovirus (B19). *J. Clin. Investig.* **79:**1486–1492.

105. **Powderley, W.** 2001. Dermatological manifestations of human immunodeficiency virus infection, p. 107–112. *In* W. Powderley (ed.), *Manual of HIV Therapeutics*, 2nd ed. Lippincott/Williams and Wilkins, Philadelphia, PA.
106. **Rady, P. L., R. Chin, I. Arany, T. K. Hughes, and S. K. Tyring.** 1993. Direct sequencing of consensus primer generated PCR fragments of human papillomaviruses. *J. Virol. Methods* **43:**335–350.
107. **Rady, P. L., A. Yen, J. L. Rollefson, I. Orengo, S. Bruce, T. K. Hughes, and S. K. Tyring.** 1995. Herpesvirus-like DNA sequences in non-Kaposi's sarcoma skin lesions of transplant patients. *Lancet* **345:** 1339–1340.
108. **Ramdial, P. K., A. Mosam, N. C. Dlova, B. N. Satar, J. Aboobaker, and S. M. Singh.** 2002. Disseminated cutaneous histoplasmosis in patients infected with human immunodeficiency virus. *J. Cutan. Pathol.* **29:**215–225.
109. **Ramoz, N., L. A. Rueda, B. Bouadjar, L. S. Montoya, G. Orth, and M. Favre.** 2002. Mutations in two adjacent novel genes are associated with epidermodysplasia verruciformis. *Nat. Genet.* **32:**579–581.
110. **Ray, M. C., and L. E. Gately III.** 1994. Dermatologic manifestations of HIV infection and AIDS. *Infect. Dis. Clin. N. Am.* **8:**583–605.
111. **Read, S. J., K. J. Jeffery, and C. R. Bangham.** 1997. Aseptic meningitis and encephalitis: the role of PCR in the diagnostic laboratory. *J. Clin. Microbiol.* **35:**691–696.
112. **Reef, S. E., T. K. Frey, K. Theall, E. Abernathy, C. L. Burnett, J. Icenogle, M. M. McCauley, and M. Wharton.** 2002. The changing epidemiology of rubella in the 1990s: on the verge of elimination and new challenges for control and prevention. *JAMA* **287:**464–472.
113. **Resnick, L., J. S. Herbst, and N. Raab-Traub.** 1990. Oral hairy leukoplakia. *J. Am. Acad. Dermatol.* **22:** 1278–1282.
114. **Revello, M. G., F. Baldanti, A. Sarasini, M. Zavattoni, M. Torsellini, and G. Gerna.** 1997. Prenatal diagnosis of rubella virus infection by direct detection and semiquantitation of viral RNA in clinical samples by reverse transcription-PCR. *J. Clin. Microbiol.* **35:**708–713.
115. **Revzina, N. V., and R. J. Diclemente.** 2005. Prevalence and incidence of human papillomavirus infection in women in the USA: a systematic review. *Int. J. STD AIDS* **16:**528–537.
116. **Rico, M. J., and N. S. Penneys.** 1985. Cutaneous cryptococcosis resembling molluscum contagiosum in a patient with AIDS. *Arch. Dermatol.* **121:**901–902.
117. **Robin, Y. M., L. Guillou, J. J. Michels, and J. M. Coindre.** 2004. Human herpesvirus 8 immunostaining: a sensitive and specific method for diagnosing Kaposi sarcoma in paraffin-embedded sections. *Am. J. Clin. Pathol.* **121:** 330–334.
118. **Romero, J. R.** 1999. Reverse-transcription polymerase chain reaction detection of the enteroviruses. *Arch. Pathol. Lab. Med.* **123:**1161–1169.
119. **Rose, F. C., E. M. Brett, and J. Burston.** 1964. Zoster encephalomyelitis. *Arch. Neurol.* **11:**155–172.
120. **Roy, M., B. Bailey, D. K. Amre, J. B. Girodias, J. F. Bussieres, and P. Gaudreault.** 2004. Dexamethasone for the treatment of sore throat in children with suspected infectious mononucleosis: a randomized, double-blind, placebo-controlled, clinical trial. *Arch. Pediatr. Adolesc. Med.* **158:**250–254.
121. **Russo, D. H., A. Luchs, B. C. Machado, C. Carmona Rde, and C. Timenetsky Mdo.** 2006. Echovirus 4 associated to hand, foot and mouth disease. *Rev. Inst. Med. Trop. São Paulo* **48:**197–199.
122. **Sacks, S. L., S. D. Shafran, F. Diaz-Mitoma, S. Trottier, R. G. Sibbald, A. Hughes, S. Safrin, J. Rudy, B. McGuire, and H. S. Jaffe.** 1998. A multicenter phase I/II dose escalation study of single-dose cidofovir gel for treatment of recurrent genital herpes. *Antimicrob. Agents Chemother.* **42:**2996–2999.
123. **Sadeharju, K., M. Knip, S. M. Virtanen, E. Savilahti, S. Tauriainen, P. Koskela, H. K. Akerblom, and H. Hyoty.** 2007. Maternal antibodies in breast milk protect the child from enterovirus infections. *Pediatrics* **119:** 941–946.
124. **Scheinfeld, N., and D. S. Lehman.** 2006. An evidence-based review of medical and surgical treatments of genital warts. *Dermatol. Online J.* **12:**5.
125. **Schmiedeskamp, M. R., and D. R. Kockler.** 2006. Human papillomavirus vaccines. *Ann. Pharmacother.* **40:** 1344–1352.
126. **Serke, S., T. F. Schwarz, H. Baurmann, A. Kirsch, B. Hottentrager, A. Von Brunn, M. Roggendorf, D. Huhn, and F. Deinhardt.** 1991. Productive infection of in vitro generated haemopoietic progenitor cells from normal human adult peripheral blood with parvovirus B19: studies by morphology, immunocytochemistry, flow-cytometry and DNA-hybridization. *Br. J. Haematol.* **79:** 6–13.
127. **Severson, J. L., and S. K. Tyring.** 1999. Relation between herpes simplex viruses and human immunodeficiency virus infections. *Arch. Dermatol.* **135:**1393–1397.
128. **Seward, J. F., B. M. Watson, C. L. Peterson, L. Mascola, J. W. Pelosi, J. X. Zhang, T. J. Maupin, G. S. Goldman, L. J. Tabony, K. G. Brodovicz, A. O. Jumaan, and M. Wharton.** 2002. Varicella disease after introduction of varicella vaccine in the United States, 1995–2000. *JAMA* **287:**606–611.
129. **Shimakage, M., T. Sasagawa, K. Kawahara, M. Yutsudo, H. Kusuoka, and T. Kozuka.** 2001. Expression of Epstein-Barr virus in cutaneous T-cell lymphoma including mycosis fungoides. *Int. J. Cancer* **92:**226–231.
130. **Slomka, M. J.** 2000. Current diagnostic techniques in genital herpes: their role in controlling the epidemic. *Clin. Lab.* **46:**591–607.
131. **Smego, R. A., Jr., and M. O. Asperilla.** 1991. Use of acyclovir for varicella pneumonia during pregnancy. *Obstet. Gynecol.* **78:**1112–1116.
132. **Smith, S. B., L. F. Libow, D. M. Elston, R. A. Bernert, and K. E. Warschaw.** 2002. Gloves and socks syndrome: early and late histopathologic features. *J. Am. Acad. Dermatol.* **47:**749–754.
133. **Sokal, E. M., M. Melchior, C. Cornu, A. T. Vandenbroucke, J. P. Buts, B. J. Cohen, and G. Burtonboy.** 1998. Acute parvovirus B19 infection associated with fulminant hepatitis of favourable prognosis in young children. *Lancet* **352:**1739–1741.
134. **Sonnex, C.** 1998. Human papillomavirus infection with particular reference to genital disease. *J. Clin. Pathol.* **51:** 643–648.
135. **Spruance, S. L., J. C. Stewart, N. H. Rowe, M. B. McKeough, G. Wenerstrom, and D. J. Freeman.** 1990. Treatment of recurrent herpes simplex labialis with oral acyclovir. *J. Infect. Dis.* **161:**185–190.
136. **Stacey, B. R., and R. L. Glanzman.** 2003. Use of gabapentin for postherpetic neuralgia: results of two randomized, placebo-controlled studies. *Clin. Ther.* **25:** 2597–2608.
137. **Stanberry, L. R., S. L. Spruance, A. L. Cunningham, D. I. Bernstein, A. Mindel, S. Sacks, S. Tyring, F. Y. Aoki, M. Slaoui, M. Denis, P. Vandepapeliere, and G. Dubin for the GlaxoSmithKline Herpes Vaccine Efficacy Study Group.** 2002. Glycoprotein-D–adjuvant vac-

cine to prevent genital herpes. *N. Engl. J. Med.* **347:** 1652–1661.

138. **Stanford, D., M. Boyle, and R. Gillespie.** 2000. Human immunodeficiency virus-related primary cutaneous aspergillosis. *Australas. J. Dermatol.* **41:**112–116.

139. **Stanway, G., F. Brown, and P. Christian.** 2005. *Picornaviridae*, p. 757–778. *In* C. Fauquet, M. Mayo, J. Maniloff, U. Desselberger, and L. Ball (ed.), *Virus Taxonomy: Classification and Nomenclature of Viruses. Eighth Report of the International Committee on Taxonomy of Viruses.* Elsevier Academic Press, San Deigo, CA.

140. **Streilein, J.** 1990. Skin-associated tissues (salt): the next generation, p. 25. *In* J. Bos (ed.), *Skin Immune System (SIS).* CRC Press, Boca Raton, FL.

141. **Strikas, R. A., L. J. Anderson, and R. A. Parker.** 1986. Temporal and geographic patterns of isolates of nonpolio enterovirus in the United States, 1970–1983. *J. Infect. Dis.* **153:**346–351.

142. **Syrjanen, S.** 1987. Human papillomavirus infections in the oral cavity, p. 104. *In* K. Syrjanen, L. Grissman, and L. G. Koss (ed.), *Papillomaviruses and Human Disease.* Springer-Verlag KG, Berlin, Germany.

143. **Thomas, I., and C. K. Janniger.** 1993. Hand, foot, and mouth disease. *Cutis* **52:**265–266.

144. **Thurn, J.** 1988. Human parvovirus B19: historical and clinical review. *Rev. Infect. Dis.* **10:**1005–1011.

145. **Tomoda, A., K. Nomura, S. Shiraishi, A. Hamada, T. Ohmura, M. Hosoya, T. Miike, Y. Sawaishi, H. Kimura, H. Takashima, Y. Tohda, K. Mori, Z. Kato, A. Fukushima, H. Nishio, A. Nezu, and K. Nihei.** 2003. Trial of intraventricular ribavirin therapy for subacute sclerosing panencephalitis in Japan. *Brain Dev.* **25:**514–517.

146. **Torno, M. S., Jr., R. Babapour, A. Gurevitch, and M. D. Witt.** 2000. Cutaneous acanthamoebiasis in AIDS. *J. Am. Acad. Dermatol.* **42:**351–354.

147. **Tyring, S. K.** 2003. Molluscum contagiosum: the importance of early diagnosis and treatment. *Am. J. Obstet. Gynecol.* **189:**S12–S16.

148. **Tyring, S. K., I. Arany, M. A. Stanley, M. A. Tomai, R. L. Miller, M. H. Smith, D. J. McDermott, and H. B. Slade.** 1998. A randomized, controlled, molecular study of condylomata acuminata clearance during treatment with imiquimod. *J. Infect. Dis.* **178:**551–555.

149. **Tyring, S. K., F. Diaz-Mitoma, S. D. Shafran, L. A. Locke, S. L. Sacks, and C. L. Young.** 2003. Oral famciclovir for the suppression of recurrent genital herpes: the combined data from two randomized controlled trials. *J. Cutan. Med. Surg.* **7:**449–454.

150. **van der Horst, C., J. Joncas, G. Ahronheim, N. Gustafson, G. Stein, M. Gurwith, G. Fleisher, J. Sullivan, J. Sixbey, S. Roland, et al.** 1991. Lack of effect of peroral acyclovir for the treatment of acute infectious mononucleosis. *J. Infect. Dis.* **164:**788–792.

151. **van Regenmortel, M. H. V., C. M. Fauquet, and D. H. L. Bishop.** 2001. *Virus Taxonomy Deluxe: Classification and Nomenclature of Viruses. Seventh Report of the International Committee on Taxonomy of Viruses + Online Database.* Academic Press, San Diego, CA.

152. **Volm, M. D., and J. H. Von Roenn.** 1996. Non-AIDS-defining malignancies in patients with HIV infection. *Curr. Opin. Oncol.* **8:**386–391.

153. **Vyse, A. J., and L. Jin.** 2002. An RT-PCR assay using oral fluid samples to detect rubella virus genome for epidemiological surveillance. *Mol. Cell. Probes* **16:**93–97.

154. **Wald, A., J. Zeh, G. Barnum, L. G. Davis, and L. Corey.** 1996. Suppression of subclinical shedding of herpes simplex virus type 2 with acyclovir. *Ann. Intern. Med.* **124:**8–15.

155. **Watson, B., R. Gupta, T. Randall, and S. Starr.** 1994. Persistence of cell-mediated and humoral immune responses in healthy children immunized with live attenuated varicella vaccine. *J. Infect. Dis.* **169:**197–199.

156. **Whitley, R. J.** 1993. The biology of B virus (cercopithecine virus), p. 317. *In* B. Roizman, R. J. Whitley, and C. Lopez (ed.), *The Human Herpesviruses.* Lippincott-Raven, New York, NY.

157. **Whitley, R. J., C. A. Alford, M. S. Hirsch, R. T. Schooley, J. P. Luby, F. Y. Aoki, D. Hanley, A. J. Nahmias, and S. J. Soong.** 1986. Vidarabine versus acyclovir therapy in herpes simplex encephalitis. *N. Engl. J. Med.* **314:**144–149.

158. **Wolff, K., R. Johnson, and D. Suurmond.** 2005. *Fitzpatrick's Color Atlas and Synopsis of Clinical Dermatology,* 5th ed. McGraw-Hill Publishing, New York, NY.

159. **Wyatt, L. S., W. J. Rodriguez, N. Balachandran, and N. Frenkel.** 1991. Human herpesvirus 7: antigenic properties and prevalence in children and adults. *J. Virol.* **65:** 6260–6265.

160. **Yaegashi, N., H. Shiraishi, T. Takeshita, M. Nakamura, A. Yajima, and K. Sugamura.** 1989. Propagation of human parvovirus B19 in primary culture of erythroid lineage cells derived from fetal liver. *J. Virol.* **63:**2422–2426.

161. **Zalla, M. J., W. P. Su, and A. F. Fransway.** 1992. Dermatologic manifestations of human immunodeficiency virus infection. *Mayo Clin. Proc.* **67:**1089–1108.

162. **Zerr, D. M., A. S. Meier, S. S. Selke, L. M. Frenkel, M. L. Huang, A. Wald, M. P. Rhoads, L. Nguy, R. Bornemann, R. A. Morrow, and L. Corey.** 2005. A population-based study of primary human herpesvirus 6 infection. *N. Engl. J. Med.* **352:**768–776.

Viral Hemorrhagic Fevers: a Comparative Appraisal

MIKE BRAY AND KARL M. JOHNSON

9

The term viral hemorrhagic fever (VHF) designates a group of similar diseases caused by some 15 different RNA viruses from four different taxonomic families (Table 1). Although they differ in certain features, all types of VHF are characterized by fever and malaise, a fall in blood pressure that can lead to shock, and the development of coagulation defects that can result in bleeding. With the exception of dengue virus, which is maintained among human populations by mosquito transmission, all of the HF agents persist in nature through cycles of infection in animals. The geographic range of each disease therefore reflects that of the reservoir species. Human illness is an accidental event resulting from contact with an infected animal or its excretions or the bite of an infected arthropod. Its pathogenesis only indirectly reflects the mechanisms by which the causative agent replicates in its reservoir host.

In contrast to diseases such as viral hepatitis or encephalitis, VHF is not localized to one organ of the body. Instead, HF viruses replicate primarily in monocytes, macrophages, and dendritic cells, which are present in all tissues. The fact that these cells, which normally serve as the first line of defense against microbial invaders, are the principal sites of viral replication goes far to explain the ability of these pathogens to cause rapidly overwhelming infection. In some types of VHF, virus also infects parenchymal cells in the liver and other tissues, causing various degrees of damage. The HF agents also differ in their interactions with the immune system: the most severe diseases, such as Ebola and Marburg HF, are characterized by a failure of adaptive immunity, while hantavirus pulmonary syndrome (HPS) and Rift Valley fever (RVF) proceed either despite or because of the host immune response. Despite the syndrome's name, hemorrhage is generally a minor feature of VHF. Instead, as in other severe inflammatory syndromes, such as septic shock, the major pathophysiological lesion is an increase in vascular permeability ("capillary leak") brought about by mediators released from infected cells. Careful physiological management to maintain sufficient blood flow to critical organs is therefore the hallmark of patient care.

Because most of types of VHF occur in regions remote from modern medical facilities, few clinical data have been obtained from patients, and most information on their pathogenesis comes from studies of infected animals in high-containment laboratories. The fact that these diseases are generally found in rural areas of developing countries that lack the resources to pay for advanced medical care also helps to explain why only a single antiviral drug, ribavirin, is available to treat just a few of these diseases, and why only a handful of vaccines are in use. The development of new types of prophylaxis and therapy is benefiting from current efforts to defend against the possible threat of bioterrorism and the real and present danger of emerging infectious diseases. This chapter provides a general survey of VHF, comparing individual diseases to each other and to other types of human illness. Additional information on individual viruses and the diseases they cause can be found in the appropriate chapters of this book.

CAUSATIVE AGENTS

The HF viruses belong to four different families, the *Arenaviridae*, *Bunyaviridae*, *Filoviridae*, and *Flaviviridae*. All are enveloped viruses with single-stranded RNA genomes. The flavivirus genome consists of one strand of positive-sense RNA. Viruses in the other three families have negative-sense genomes, which consist of a single strand in the case of the filoviruses, two separate segments for the arenaviruses, and three for the bunyaviruses.

HISTORICAL PERSPECTIVE

The various types of VHF have presumably occurred for millennia, whenever humans have come into contact with reservoir animals or been bitten by infected arthropods. The first to be recognized by the European medical community was yellow fever (YF), which was encountered by early travelers to sub-Saharan Africa and was transferred to the New World through the slave trade. Its frequently fatal outcome was long attributed to the severe hepatic damage and jaundice that gave the disease its name, but it was eventually realized that gastrointestinal hemorrhage and compromised renal function resulting from hypovolemic shock were more common causes of death. A correct appreciation of the role of diminished intravascular volume in this disease did not emerge until clinical tools for blood pressure measurement were developed in the 1920s, when urban YF had been largely suppressed by mosquito control efforts. Recent studies have in fact shown that host inflam-

TABLE 1 Some epidemiological features of the principal types of VHF

Virus family	Disease	Virus	Geographic distribution	Reservoir host	Patients[a] and areas affected; seasonal pattern
Arenaviridae	Argentine HF	Junin virus	North-central Argentina	Mouse (*Calomys musculinus*)	M; corn harvest; March–June
	Bolivian HF	Machupo virus	Northeastern Bolivia	Mouse (*Calomys callosus*)	All ages, both sexes; villages; February–July
	Venezuelan HF	Guanarito virus	Central Venezuela	Mouse (*Zygodontomys brevicauda*)	All ages, M = F; houses, gardens; no seasonality
	Lassa fever	Lassa virus	West Africa	Mouse (*Mastomys natalensis*)	All ages, both sexes; villages; no seasonality
Bunyaviridae	CCHF	CCHF virus	Africa, Middle East to west China	Livestock, crows, hares, *Hyalomma* ticks	Adults, M > F; cattle, pasture contact; summer
	RVF	RVF virus	Africa	Livestock, several mosquito genera	All ages, M > F; late summer; arthropods
	HFRS	Hantaan, Seoul, and Puumula viruses	Northern Asia and Europe, including the Balkans and Scandinavia	Mice and rats (*Apodemus*, *Rattus*, *Clethrionomys*)	Mostly adults, M > F; rodent excreta; fall-winter
	Hantavirus cardiopulmonary syndrome	Sin Nombre, Andes, many others	North, Central, and South America	Mice (*Peromyscus* sp., *Sigmodon hispidus*, ?others)	Adults, M = F; rodent excreta; late spring-summer peak
Flaviviridae	YF	YF virus	Tropical Africa, Amazon basin	Primates, including humans; tree hole mosquitoes	M > F, all ages; arthropod contact; dry season
	Dengue HF/shock syndrome	Dengue virus types 1–4	Southeast Asia, Caribbean, coastal South and Central America	*Aedes aegypti* > *Aedes albopictus*	Children <12 yr; peak in late rainy, early dry seasons
	Kyasanur Forest disease	Kyasanur Forest virus	Karnatake State (India)	Monkeys, birds, livestock, ixodid ticks	Adults, M > F; tick contact; summer-fall, dry season
	Omsk HF	Omsk virus	Western Siberia	Vole (*Arvicola terrestris*), ixodid ticks	Adult males; muskrat hunt; winter
Filoviridae	Marburg and Ebola HF	Marburg and Ebola viruses	Sub-Saharan Africa	Reservoir and vector unknown	Mainly adults, M = F; sporadic; late summer

[a] M, male; F, female.

matory responses are as important in the pathogenesis of severe YF as in other types of VHF (30, 35).

Other types of VHF began to be identified in the early 1900s, when the severe hantaviral infection that is now termed HF with renal syndrome (HFRS) was described in Siberia, and a milder form, nephropathia epidemica, was recognized in Scandinavia (8, 12, 31). However, it was not until several thousands of cases of HFRS occurred among United Nations troops in the Korean War that VHF was brought forcefully to the attention of Western medicine. Over the ensuing five decades, a number of "new" types of VHF have been described and their causative agents have been isolated. The Old World arenavirus Lassa fever virus and the New World agent Machupo virus were both characterized during investigations of disease outbreaks in the 1960s. Marburg virus was discovered in 1967 as a result of the inadvertent importation of infected monkeys from Uganda to Europe, while the other filovirus genus, Ebola virus, came to attention when its Zaire and Sudan species caused large epidemics in Africa in 1976. RVF, first recognized in the 1930s, caused a massive mosquito-borne outbreak in Egypt in 1977. The spectrum of disease continued to expand in the 1990s, with the discovery of a previously unrecognized condition, HPS, which shares features of VHF and an acute respiratory distress syndrome (23). New World hantavirus strains, their rodent hosts, and cases of human illness have been identified throughout North and South America. The list of arenaviruses has also continued to grow with the recognition of fatal human infections caused by Whitewater Arroyo virus in California. There is no reason to believe that the list of HF viruses is now complete.

EPIDEMIOLOGY

The occurrence of VHF reflects the fact that humans are often exposed to viruses that are maintained in animals. In the vast majority of cases, such cross-species transfer does not result in disease. For a foreign virus to cause illness, appropriate cell surface receptors and intracellular cofactors must be present to permit its replication in human cells, and innate defenses must fail sufficiently to permit its cell-to-cell spread. VHF represents the extreme end of the spectrum of possible outcomes of cross-species virus transfer, in which an agent replicates so well and disseminates so quickly that it causes a severe inflammatory syndrome.

Maintenance hosts have been identified for nearly all of the HF agents (Table 1). In most cases, the natural reservoir is a species of rodent, probably because these animals' large numbers and high population density favor the continuous circulation of viruses. Old and New World primates are reservoirs for sylvatic YF, and a variety of species are involved in the circulation of Crimean-Congo HF (CCHF) virus. Only in the case of the filoviruses has a host animal not been identified, but various species of bats are the prime suspects (see chapter 41).

The transmission of a virus from animals to humans can occur through direct physical contact, exposure to virus-containing excretions, or the bite of an infected mosquito or tick. The identity of the host and the mode of transmission strongly influence the pattern of human disease. For example, HPS, which results from contact with the aerosolized excretions of infected rodents, and CCHF, which is transmitted by tick bite, tend to occur as sporadic single cases. By contrast, mosquito-borne agents such as YF virus and dengue virus can be carried from person to person to cause explosive epidemics.

The arenaviruses and hantaviruses provide interesting examples of coevolution, in which each agent has a single rodent species as its primary host (3). Animals that harbor arenaviruses display partial immune "tolerance," permitting chronic viremia and viruria; the latter probably represents the major source of environmental exposure. The epidemiological pattern of arenaviral HF is determined by the intersection of rodent ecology and human activities. In Argentina and Venezuela, animal reservoirs are found in or adjacent to cultivars, placing adult males who harvest corn in the fall at greatest risk of infection. In contrast, because the reservoir rodents invade dwellings and gardens, Bolivian HF and Lassa fever are largely acquired in or near houses, and persons of both sexes and all ages are at risk. Lassa fever is a truly endemic disease, because the *Mastomys* reservoir breeds year-round, and a nearly constant fraction of animals are chronically infected. Hantaviruses also cause chronic infection in their rodent hosts, which excrete virus in saliva and feces for short periods and in urine for many months. Human infection is most often associated with agriculture, mining, or military activity. Nephropathia epidemica has a well-marked cyclic activity, in which rodent population density and prevalence of infection correlate with transmission to humans.

The epidemiology of arthropod-borne VHF reflects the biology of viral infection in the mosquito or tick. Both vectors acquire the virus through blood feeding, indicating that viremia occurs in the animal reservoir. Mosquitoes competent to transmit flaviviruses are chronically infected, but their vector competence is reduced by their relatively short lifetimes. Multiple human infections are often the result of interrupted blood feeding and movement to a second host. Among the various types of VHF, only CCHF and Kyasanur Forest disease are transmitted by ticks. "Vertical" (transstadial and transovarial) transmission is an important feature of their natural history. Ticks use the blood of birds and mammals primarily as an energy source for the next stage of their life cycle. Because far less than 100% of eggs from an adult female are infected, vertebrate viremia is also important for tick-borne transmission of virus to humans.

Dengue fever is the exception to the rule that the HF viruses are maintained in animals. The disease may at one time have been confined to a small region of the tropics and maintained through infection of wild primates, in a manner similar to YF. However, the successful adaptation of the virus to person-to-person transmission by mosquitoes, combined with a vast increase in the human population in tropical regions and a failure of mosquito control efforts, has permitted the agent to disperse widely and evolve into four distinct serotypes (18). As discussed below, the circulation of more than one serotype in the same geographic region sets the stage for the occurrence of secondary infections, in which nonneutralizing antibodies can enhance virus uptake into cells, causing intense inflammation and increased vascular permeability (dengue HF/shock syndrome). Even though only a small fraction of secondary cases result in HF, because of its global distribution, dengue virus is the most important cause of VHF.

Once an individual becomes ill with VHF, there is great variation in the potential for further human-to-human transmission. A number of diseases, including RVF and dengue HF, rarely or never spread directly from person to person and thus pose little or no threat to medical personnel. However, some of the most virulent agents, including Ebola, Marburg, Lassa, and CCHF viruses, cause prolonged high viremia and can therefore be spread through direct contact with blood and other body fluids. Hospital-based outbreaks have occurred when proper infection control measures were not practiced (11).

Although normally confined to the geographic range of its reservoir host, any type of VHF can potentially be carried to other parts of the world through the movement of infected humans or animals. The likelihood that one of these "exotic" diseases will appear in an unexpected location has increased markedly with the growth of worldwide air travel. The most spectacular event of this type is still the 1967 Marburg outbreak. Although patients with Lassa fever have traveled from Africa to Europe and North America on a number of occasions, no further transmission of disease occurred during their medical care. Perhaps the most effective dissemination of an HF virus has been the worldwide spread of the Seoul hantavirus, carried by Asian rats that have stowed away on ships.

CLINICAL MANIFESTATIONS

Most of the signs and symptoms of VHF reflect the release of proinflammatory mediators from virus-infected cells and their effects on temperature regulation, cardiac function, gastrointestinal tract motility, control of vascular tone and endothelial permeability, and the blood clotting system. Fever, malaise, myalgia, and headache are typical early manifestations that tend to evolve insidiously in the case of Lassa fever but can begin so abruptly in YF, CCHF, and the filovirus diseases that patients can report the hour of onset. Fever is usually high and unremitting. Bradycardia may be notable, particularly in arenavirus and filovirus diseases and in YF. Vomiting and diarrhea frequently occur. Abdominal pain can be sufficiently prominent to lead to surgical intervention; hospital-based outbreaks of CCHF and Ebola HF have begun in this fashion.

Vasodilatation and increased permeability of the endothelial linings of blood vessels are manifested in a number of physical signs. Capillary dilatation is often signaled by diffuse erythema of the skin of the upper trunk and face that blanches on pressure. Conjunctival injection with petechial hemorrhages is common. An erythematous rash is characteristic in Marburg and Ebola HF but may be difficult to see in dark-skinned persons. Edema of the face and sometimes of the extremities is another manifestation of a capillary leak syndrome, but it may only become evident when a severely ill, dehydrated patient is treated with intravenous fluids. The development of coagulation defects leads to easy bruising, failure of venipuncture sites to clot, hemorrhage from the gastrointestinal and urinary tracts, and menorrhagia. Large ecchymoses are a characteristic sign of CCHF but are rare in the other diseases. Although massive bleeding can occur in severely ill or moribund patients, it is much less common than popular descriptions of these diseases would suggest.

Other clinical manifestations reflect the involvement of specific organ systems. Some degree of hepatic infection is seen in most types of VHF, but it varies markedly in severity among the different diseases. Levels of liver enzymes (aspartate and alanine aminotransferase) in serum are markedly elevated in filoviral HF, YF, and RVF, but clinical jaundice is commonly observed only in the latter two conditions. Other than the acute pulmonary edema seen in HPS, VHF rarely produces specific changes in the lungs. As regards kidney function, the renal compromise phase of HFRS is characterized by severe oliguria with increased blood urea nitrogen and creatinine levels; a diuretic phase typically follows. New World hantavirus infections are characterized by a low cardiac index and high systemic vascular resistance, resulting in severe lactic acidosis and an oxygen perfusion deficit, in recognition of which these diseases have been designated hantavirus cardiopulmonary syndrome. Encephalitis and ophthalmic inflammation are late complications of RVF whose etiology remains undetermined.

The systemic inflammation of VHF leads to numerous changes in clinical laboratory tests, none of which are specific to these diseases. Blood leukocyte patterns vary widely. Leukopenia is frequently observed, but patients with dengue HF usually have normal white blood cell counts. Leukopenia is minimal in Lassa fever, and fatal disease may be heralded by a frank polymorphonuclear leukocytosis. An increase in white blood cells with atypical lymphocytes is characteristic of hantavirus infections. With the exception of Lassa fever, thrombocytopenia is a universal finding, but it is usually not severe enough in itself to account for hemorrhagic manifestations. Signs of hemoconcentration include a rise in the hemoglobin, hematocrit, and plasma protein levels. Monitored sequentially, these can provide an index of the loss of plasma volume resulting from the capillary leak syndrome and the efficacy of therapeutic countermeasures. Proteinuria is a hallmark of VHF and may be severe in Lassa, Marburg, and Ebola fevers as well as in HFRS. Coagulation factors are variously reduced, but major increases in prothrombin and partial prothrombin times are common only in YF, CCHF, RVF, and the filoviral diseases. Limited testing during outbreaks has shown that fibrin split products and D-dimers, indicative of disseminated intravascular coagulation, are present in Ebola HF and CCHF; they would probably be found in many of the other diseases if testing capability were available.

Those who survive VHF generally suffer few long-term sequelae. Patients with filoviral HF show sloughing of skin and hair loss during convalescence, probably reflecting diffuse viral infection and necrosis of cutaneous structures. Arthralgia may persist for months. The retinal vasculitis of RVF can result in permanent loss of central vision. About 3% of Lassa fever survivors have permanent eighth-nerve damage, making it the most common cause of deafness in young people in its region of endemicity.

PATHOGENESIS

The transmission of HF viruses from animals to humans is unidirectional: infected patients do not serve as a source of infection for the reservoir host. Because human infections are "dead-end" events from the point of view of virus evolution, the pathogenesis of VHF does not represent the outcome of any sort of adaptation or viral "survival strategy" but simply reflects the fortuitous ability of an animal virus to replicate efficiently in human cells.

At present, the best-understood form of VHF is the fulminant illness caused by Ebola Zaire virus, which displays all the classic features of the HF syndrome (see chapter 41). Although only limited data have been obtained during epidemics in Africa, careful time course experiments with mice, guinea pigs, and nonhuman primates have provided a detailed day-by-day picture of the course of illness. These studies have identified several basic pathophysiological mechanisms that are responsible for the lethal course of Ebola HF and probably contribute to some degree to all types of VHF (5, 27). First, Ebola virus replicates quickly in monocytes and macrophages, with the release of large numbers of new virions and the secretion of large quantities of proinflammatory cytokines, chemokines, and other mediators (6). The principal stimulus for macrophage activation is probably the presence of double-stranded RNA, which triggers signaling cascades that result in the production of interleukin 1β (IL-1β), IL-6, tumor necrosis factor alpha (TNF-α), and nitric oxide, a potent stimulant of vasodilatation. Activated macrophages synthesize and display tissue factor on their surfaces, triggering the extrinsic coagulation pathway (16).

Although early discussions of the pathogenesis of VHF attributed vascular leak and hemorrhage to viral infection or injury of the endothelial lining of blood vessels, and designations for the diseases included expressions such as "capillary toxicosis," it now appears more likely that alterations in vascular function and the development of coagulopathy represent physiological responses to circulating proinflammatory mediators, in the same way that changes in blood flow occur about an infected wound. In VHF, however, the release of large amounts of these substances into the plasma causes vascular dilatation and increased permeability to take place "everywhere at once," with catastrophic effects on intravascular volume and blood pressure. That, of course, does not mean that viral infection of blood vessel linings cannot also occur. Infected endothelial cells have been observed, for example, in tissues from persons with fatal cases of CCHF (7). However, the studies of Ebola virus-infected macaques noted above found infected endothelial cells only on the last 1 to 2 days of illness, suggesting that the vascular lining is initially resistant to infection but becomes susceptible under the influence of inflammatory mediators (17).

A second major factor that has been shown to play an important role in filoviral HF, and presumably contributes to all types of VHF, is viral suppression of type I interferon responses. Ebola virus, for example, encodes two different interferon antagonists, one that suppresses the initial production of interferon by the infected cell and another that prevents the cell from responding to exogenous type I and type II interferons (2). A number of other HF agents, including RVF virus, dengue virus, and some arenaviruses, have also been shown to block interferon responses through a variety of mechanisms (1). The importance of the interferon system to the control of viral dissemination helps to explain why all of the HF agents are RNA viruses. Because the double-stranded RNA molecules that are generated in the course of their transcription and genome duplication are a strong stimulus for type I interferon responses, each RNA virus must evolve ways of evading or suppressing interferon responses in its host, to the extent needed to ensure its own continued survival. The outcome of human infection with a novel virus will therefore depend in part on the extent to which the agent blocks human interferon responses. The HF viruses may constitute that small subset of RNA viruses that suppress human interferon responses so effectively that they cause rapidly overwhelming disease.

The third factor that helps to explain the very high case fatality rate of filoviral HF is the ability of these viruses to infect and kill a wide variety of parenchymal cells, resulting in extensive tissue damage. All HF viruses can replicate in human monocytes and macrophages, but they differ in their abilities to infect other types of cells. At one end of the spectrum, dengue virus principally infects only those two cell types, without causing their death. At the other extreme, Ebola and Marburg viruses are apparently capable of infecting and killing almost every type of cell in the body except for lymphocytes and neurons. Their lack of host cell specificity appears to reflect the ability of the filoviral surface glycoprotein to bind to widely distributed cell surface lectins. Material released from dying cells is itself a stimulus for inflammation, contributing further to the fulminant systemic illness. Most HF viruses produce a degree of tissue damage intermediate between the minimal injury of dengue fever and the massive destruction caused by the filoviruses, with the liver as the principal target. Hepatic involvement probably begins with the spread of virus through the bloodstream to fixed macrophages (Kupffer cells) in sinusoids, from which infection then extends to parenchymal cells, giving rise to increased levels of "liver-associated" enzymes in the plasma. As noted, hepatic injury is a prominent feature of YF, causing the jaundice that gave the disease its name, and is seen in some cases of RVF. It also occurs in CCHF and some other infections, but without producing the high levels of bilirubin that lead to jaundice.

Although similar in the above respects, the various types of VHF appear to differ in the relationship between viral infection and host immune responses. At one end of the spectrum, patients dying from filoviral HF show no sign of an antibody response despite the presence of high levels of virus in the bloodstream, indicating that the immune system is unable to detect and respond to the infection (25). Because dendritic cells play a critical role in initiating adaptive responses by presenting microbial antigens to $CD4^+$ and $CD8^+$ T cells, this suggests that infection interferes with dendritic cell function. These cells are in fact a major site of filoviral replication, but instead of undergoing normal maturation, infected cells do not up-regulate stimulatory cofactors, are unable to present antigens, and do not stimulate naïve lymphocytes to proliferate (28). Lassa virus produces a similar effect on dendritic cells, and Lassa fever is also characterized by uncontrolled viral replication, in which the circulating viral titer correlates with the likelihood of death.

Failure of adaptive immunity is made even worse in filoviral infections, and probably in other types of severe HF, by a massive loss of lymphocytes resulting from programmed cell death (14). Lymphocyte apoptosis leading to "immune paralysis" is now recognized to contribute to mortality from septic shock resulting from infections with gram-negative bacteria (32). Destruction of these cells does not result from their infection by Ebola virus but is driven indirectly by the binding of TNF-α, Fas ligand, and other inflammatory mediators to cell surface receptors and perhaps by changes in cellular metabolism that affect mitochondrial membrane function. Although recent experimental evidence indicates that virus-specific T cells begin to proliferate during the course of filoviral HF, the cells do not arrive in time to prevent death (4).

In contrast to the failure of immune responses in filoviral HF, virtually all patients with hantavirus infections have circulating virus-specific immunoglobulin M, immunoglobulin G, or both at the time of diagnosis. In the case of HPS, titers at hospital admission vary inversely with the severity of illness, suggesting that antibodies have a protective role. Viral antigens are detectable on the surfaces of capillary endothelial cells, most intensely in the lungs in HPS and in the kidneys in HFRS (37). In HPS, the capillary leak often ceases abruptly, suggesting that immune-mediated cytokine release is the primary mechanism of illness. The development of HFRS and its resolution take much longer, indicating that tissue damage is greater, needs more time for repair, and may be partly the result of viral destruction of cells or the effects of immune viral complexes. Proposed explanations for the reversal of the capillary leak include the maturation of high-affinity antibodies that block sites for immune cell targets, a change in the ratio of circulating antigens and antibodies that inhibits the formation and deposition of complexes, or a cytokine feedback loop that calms the chemical storm. The answer to this question may have important therapeutic implications.

RVF also provides an example of how human immune responses influence the course of illness. Most cases are acute, self-limited febrile episodes. Viremia may be very high at onset but disappears within 3 to 5 days, by which time virus-specific antibodies are detectable. However, about 1 to 2% of patients continue to have virus in the blood, respiratory secretions, and spinal fluid, even in the presence of antibodies, and progress to fulminant VHF with hepatitis, jaundice, and hemorrhage. Large amounts of virus are present in the liver and other organs at death. Uncontrolled viral replication in these RVF patients therefore resembles that seen in filoviral HF, but it appears to result from a defective immune response in certain patients rather than the increased virulence of a viral strain. In another disease variant, some RVF patients appear to be stable or improving after 5 to 15 days of illness and then develop an apparently immune-mediated meningoencephalitis or retinal vasculitis. The neurologic disease has been temporally associated with the greatest production of antiviral antibodies seen in any of the forms of RVF.

Dengue HF has a unique pathogenesis that is a consequence of the virus's evolution into four different serotypes. Primary dengue is an unpleasant, but rarely fatal, flu-like illness that results from the transient release of proinflammatory cytokines from virus-infected monocytes and macrophages. Viremia is already ending by the time of symptom onset, and the illness resolves uneventfully. The recovered individual is thenceforth resistant to reinfection by that serotype. In a small percentage of cases, however, reinfection by a second serotype results in severe disease in which viremia persists and high levels of IL-6, TNF-α, and other mediators in plasma induce vascular leak and shock (26). Two immune mechanisms appear to be responsible for the occurrence of dengue HF. First, nonneutralizing antibodies remaining from a previous infection can enhance viral replication by linking virions to Fc receptors on the surfaces of target cells, which then take them up into the cytoplasm. This antibody-mediated "virus delivery system" causes severe illness by increasing the number of infected cells, the number of viral particles that enter each cell, and the release of cytokines and other vasoactive mediators. Second, cross-reactive memory $CD8^+$ T cells can attack monocytes and macrophages expressing viral epitopes on their surfaces, triggering an explosive inflammatory response. Because tissue damage is minimal and adaptive immune responses remain intact, patients who are treated promptly with intravenous fluids can recover within a matter of days.

DIAGNOSIS

The signs and symptoms of VHF resemble those of a wide range of infectious diseases, so a specific diagnosis can be made only by means of specialized laboratory tests that directly identify the pathogen. Such assays are generally not performed by hospital laboratories but require the participation of a containment facility able to conduct live-virus research. Only in rare circumstances will the clinician evaluating an acutely ill patient proceed directly to such tests. VHF would be high on the list of possible diagnoses only when a patient reports having been exposed to a sick person or a disease vector during an identified VHF outbreak, but more often the patient's recent travel history will only suggest a range of possibilities, rather than a specific diagnosis. Thus, although someone who develops fever and malaise soon after returning from central Africa could be infected with Ebola or Marburg virus, it is much more likely that he or she has a more common (and treatable) disease, such as malaria or typhoid fever. An appropriate diagnostic strategy for the clinician faced with a possible case of VHF would therefore be to collect blood and other samples needed to diagnose the most likely diseases, based on the physical examination and history, while determining how specific assays could be carried out if initial tests prove negative.

A variety of diagnostic tests have been developed for VHF. Viral antigens and antibodies are now detected most commonly by enzyme-linked immunosorbent assay, often employing recombinant antigens and monoclonal antibodies as defined reagents. PCR is being utilized with great success to identify virus-specific nucleotide sequences. Because many types of VHF are characterized by prolonged viremia, blood is generally the best sample for testing. Information on diagnostic assays for various types of VHF can be found in the appropriate chapters of this book and on a number of infectious-disease websites. In the United States, further information can also be obtained by contacting the local section of the Laboratory Response Network or the Special Pathogens Branch at the Centers for Disease Control and Prevention in Atlanta, GA.

MANAGEMENT

The first priority in treating a patient with VHF is to prevent the further spread of infection. The risk of person-to-person transmission varies greatly for the different diseases. Although respiratory spread appears to be rare for most types of VHF, it was documented in a hospital outbreak of Lassa fever in Nigeria in which a patient in an open ward had a persistent cough. The Andes strain of hantavirus has also been transmitted from patients to medical personnel or family members. Several diseases characterized by prolonged high viremia, including Lassa, Ebola, and Marburg fevers and CCHF, can be spread through direct contact with body fluids. In the case of the filoviruses, this has been shown to include blood, saliva, vomitus, feces, and even sweat. The risk of transmission is obviously highest when a specific diagnosis has not yet been made and family members and medical personnel are not taking precautions to avoid contamination.

Whatever type of VHF is being treated, medical personnel must observe universal precautions in handling diagnostic specimens and take special care to avoid exposure to aerosolized material, whether during patient care procedures or in the laboratory. Gloves, gowns, and other standard protective measures against blood-borne or enteric diseases should be supplemented with face or eye shields and HEPA-filtered masks or portable air-purifying respirators to protect against aerosols. The patient's room should be under negative directional air pressure, if possible. Up-to-date advice on the collection, processing, and disposal of diagnostic specimens and other aspects of biohazard management during patient care is available from the Centers for Disease Control and Prevention. Emergency consultation regarding these guidelines and for diagnostic assistance can be obtained by calling (404) 639-1511 during the day and (404) 639-2888 at night.

Therapeutic interventions for VHF can be divided into nonspecific and specific measures. General supportive management should, whenever possible, be based on careful monitoring of circulating blood volume and correction of electrolyte abnormalities (21, 33). The hematocrit should be measured frequently, and a Swan-Ganz catheter should be used when available. Human albumin has formed an important part of treatment of dengue HF in children, but its use in other types of VHF should be undertaken with caution because of the risk of precipitating pulmonary edema. In HPS, in which massive amounts of plasma may be lost into pulmonary airways, tissue edema can be greater than is clinically evident, so the judicious use of diuretics may be helpful. Inotropic agents and vasopressors may also be indicated. Because of the low cardiac index and high peripheral resistance that appear to characterize hantaviral infections, the administration of such drugs should be started early, before the advent of clinical shock. Extracorporeal membrane oxygenation has been used to rescue HPS patients with otherwise invariably fatal physiological abnormalities (23). Although corticosteroids in various doses have been administered to patients with many types of VHF, there is no evidence that they are of benefit for any of these conditions.

Specific therapeutic measures are available for only a few of these diseases. Intravenous administration of the guanosine analog ribavirin was shown to improve the survival rate in severe Lassa fever in a clinical trial in Sierra Leone in the 1980s (29), and treatment has also reduced the rate of mortality from HFRS (20). Anecdotal reports indicate that it is beneficial in CCHF, though proof of efficacy suffers from the lack of an animal model of the disease (10). Purified immunoglobulin from survivors of Argentine HF has been proven effective in the treatment of that disease if begun before day 8 of illness (9).

A number of experimental therapies have shown efficacy in laboratory animal models of various types of VHF, as described in the corresponding chapters of this book. The most effort has gone into the treatment of Ebola HF. Although no small-molecule drug has been found to inhibit filovirus replication, antisense and small interfering RNA molecules targeting specific genomic sequences have proven effective as pre- and postexposure prophylaxis in rodents and nonhuman primates (34). Interventions aimed at modifying host responses to infection have also been surprisingly successful. Recombinant nematode anticoagulant protein c2, which blocks the interaction of tissue factor with factor VIIa, provided significant protection to Ebola virus-infected macaques when initiated soon after exposure (15), and activated protein C, which has shown benefit in human septic shock, was also protective (19).

Perhaps the most exciting advance in postexposure therapy has been the discovery that a single injection of a live, recombinant vesicular stomatitis virus vaccine encoding a filovirus surface glycoprotein, given 30 min after exposure to the corresponding pathogen, completely protected rhesus macaques against otherwise lethal challenge with Marburg or Ebola Sudan virus and gave a 50% survival rate for Ebola Zaire infection (13, 22). No cross-protection was observed, indicating that protection was based on the rapid induction of a specific immune response. This success in preventing an otherwise lethal illness with a single vaccination supports the hypothesis that the virulence of the filoviruses is based in part on the failure of the human immune system to respond to their presence. Delivering appropriate viral antigens to dendritic cells soon after pathogen exposure triggers the antigen-specific response that is needed to prevent disease.

Success in developing experimental treatments for VHF in animal models has so far been limited to interventions that begin early in the incubation period, before the development of symptoms. If the same approaches prove to be safe and effective in humans, they could be lifesaving for a laboratory worker accidentally exposed to a pathogen and could have many applications in the setting of a disease outbreak. In contrast, developing an effective treatment for full-blown VHF, with its combination of vascular insufficiency, disseminated intravasular coagulation, tissue damage, and impaired immune function, is likely to remain a challenging medical problem for the foreseeable future.

PREVENTION

Only a few vaccines are in use for the prevention of VHF. The live attenuated 17D YF vaccine, first introduced in the 1930s, remains one of the finest ever developed, but its use in tropical countries, where sylvatic infection is endemic, is unfortunately insufficient to prevent recurrent epidemics.The attenuated Candid-1 vaccine for Argentine HF has also proven to be highly effective and has played an important role in reducing the incidence of disease in its zone of endemicity.

Considerable progress has been made in developing experimental vaccines for a number of types of VHF, based on a variety of platforms. Several approaches to a Lassa fever vaccine have proven protective in laboratory animals, but none has yet gone forward to a clinical trial. Recent progress in restoring research capacity at the Kenema Lassa fever ward in Sierra Leone suggests that such testing should soon be feasible (24). Given the extreme virulence of the filoviruses, progress in developing vaccines that protect nonhuman primates against Marburg and Ebola viruses has been remarkable. Successful approaches now include a DNA-adenovirus prime-boost strategy, noninfectious virus-like particles, and the vesicular stomatitis virus vaccine described above (see chapter 41).

The most problematic disease from the point of view of vaccine development is dengue fever. As discussed above, the immunity that follows infection by one of the four dengue virus serotypes can predispose an individual to severe disease (dengue HF/shock syndrome) if he or she is later exposed to a second serotype. So as not to place vaccinees at risk of severe illness, it is now generally accepted that a dengue vaccine must protect against all four serotypes at once (36). The current status of this effort is described in chapter 52.

REFERENCES

1. **Basler, C. F.** 2005. Interferon antagonists encoded by emerging RNA viruses, p. 197–220. *In* P. Palese (ed.), *Modulation of Host Gene Expression and Innate Immunity by Viruses*. Springer, Dordrecht, The Netherlands.
2. **Basler, C. F., A. Mikulasova, L. Martinez-Sobrido, J. Paragas, E. Muhlberger, M. Bray, H. D. Klenk, P. Palese, and A. Garcia-Sastre.** 2003. The Ebola virus VP35 protein inhibits activation of interferon regulatory factor 3. *J. Virol.* **77:**7945–7956.
3. **Bowen, M., C. J. Peters, and S. T. Nichol.** 1997. Phylogenetic analysis of the Arenaviridae: patterns of virus evolution and evidence for cospeciation among arenaviruses and their rodent hosts. *Mol. Phylogenet. Evol.* **8:**301–316.
4. **Bradfute, S. B., K. L. Warfield, and S. Bavari.** 2008. Functional CD8+ T cell responses in lethal Ebola virus infection. *J. Immunol.* **180:**4058–4066.
5. **Bray, M.** 2005. Pathogenesis of viral hemorrhagic fever. *Curr. Opin. Immunol.* **17:**399–403.
6. **Bray, M., and T. W. Geisbert.** 2005. Ebola virus: the role of macrophages and dendritic cells in the pathogenesis of Ebola hemorrhagic fever. *Int. J. Biochem. Cell Biol.* **37:** 1560–1566.
7. **Burt, F. J., R. Swanepoel, W. J. Shieh, J. F. Smith, P. A. Leman, P. W. Greer, L. M. Coffield, P. E. Rollin, T. G. Ksiazek, C. J. Peters, and S. R. Zaki.** 1997. Immunohistochemical and in situ localization of Crimean-Congo hemorrhagic fever (CCHF) virus in human tissues and implications for CCHF pathogenesis. *Arch. Pathol. Lab. Med.* **121:**839–846.
8. **Casals, J., H. Hoogstraal, K. M. Johnson, A. Shelokov, N. H. Wiebenga, and T. H. Work.** 1966. A current appraisal of hemorrhagic fevers in the U.S.S.R. *Am. J. Trop. Med. Hyg.* **15:**751–764.
9. **Enria, D. A., A. M. Briggiler, and Z. Sanchez.** 2008. Treatment of Argentine hemorrhagic fever. *Antiviral. Res.* **78:**132–139.
10. **Ergonul, O.** 2006. Crimean-Congo haemorrhagic fever. *Lancet Infect. Dis.* **6:**203–214.
11. **Fisher-Hoch, S. P.** 2005. Lessons from nosocomial viral haemorrhagic fever outbreaks. *Br. Med. Bull.* **73–74:**123–137.
12. **Gajdusek, D. C.** 1962. Virus hemorrhagic fevers. Special reference to hemorrhagic fever with renal syndrome (epidemic hemorrhagic fever). *J. Pediatr.* **60:**841–857.
13. **Geisbert, T. W., K. M. Daddario-DiCaprio, K. J. Williams, J. B. Geisbert, A. Leung, F. Feldmann, L. E. Hensley, H. Feldmann, and S. M. Jones.** 2008. Recombinant vesicular stomatitis virus vector mediates postexposure protection against Sudan Ebola hemorrhagic fever in nonhuman primates. *J. Virol.* **82:**5664–5668.
14. **Geisbert, T. W., L. E. Hensley, T. R. Gibb, K. E. Steele, N. K. Jaax, and P. B. Jahrling.** 2000. Apoptosis induced in vitro and in vivo during infection by Ebola and Marburg viruses. *Lab. Investig.* **80:**171–186.
15. **Geisbert, T. W., L. E. Hensley, P. B. Jahrling, T. Larsen, J. B. Geisbert, J. Paragas, H. A. Young, T. M. Fredeking, W. E. Rote, and G. P. Vlasuk.** 2003. Treatment of Ebola virus infection with a recombinant inhibitor of factor VIIa/tissue factor: a study in rhesus monkeys. *Lancet* **362:**1953–1958.
16. **Geisbert, T. W., H. A. Young, P. B. Jahrling, K. J. Davis, E. Kagan, and L. E. Hensley.** 2003. Mechanisms underlying coagulation abnormalities in Ebola hemorrhagic fever: overexpression of tissue factor in primate monocytes/macrophages is a key event. *J. Infect. Dis.* **188:**1618–1629.
17. **Geisbert, T. W., H. A. Young, P. B. Jahrling, K. J. Davis, T. Larsen, E. Kagan, and L. E. Hensley.** 2003. Pathogenesis of Ebola hemorrhagic fever in primate models: evidence that hemorrhage is not a direct effect of virus-induced cytolysis of endothelial cells. *Am. J. Pathol.* **163:** 2371–2382.
18. **Gubler, D. J.** 2006. Dengue/dengue haemorrhagic fever: history and current status. *Novartis Found. Symp.* **277:**3–16; discussion, 16–22, 71–73, 251–253.
19. **Hensley, L. E., E. L. Stevens, S. B. Yan, J. B. Geisbert, W. L. Macias, T. Larsen, K. M. Daddario-DiCaprio, G. H. Cassell, P. B. Jahrling, and T. W. Geisbert.** 2007. Recombinant human activated protein C for the postexposure treatment of Ebola hemorrhagic fever. *J. Infect. Dis.* **196**(Suppl. 2):S390–S399.
20. **Huggins, J. W.** 1989. Prospects for treatment of viral hemorrhagic fevers with ribavirin, a broad-spectrum antiviral drug. *Rev. Infect. Dis.* **11**(Suppl. 4):S750–S761.
21. **Jeffs, B.** 2006. A clinical guide to viral haemorrhagic fevers: Ebola, Marburg and Lassa. *Trop. Dr.* **36:**1–4.
22. **Jones, S. M., H. Feldmann, U. Stroher, J. B. Geisbert, L. Fernando, A. Grolla, H. D. Klenk, N. J. Sullivan, V. E. Volchkov, E. A. Fritz, K. M. Daddario, L. E. Hensley, P. B. Jahrling, and T. W. Geisbert.** 2005. Live attenuated recombinant vaccine protects nonhuman primates against Ebola and Marburg viruses. *Nat. Med.* 11:786–790.
23. **Jonsson, C. B., J. Hooper, and G. Mertz.** 2008. Treatment of hantavirus pulmonary syndrome. *Antivir. Res.* **78:** 162–169.
24. **Khan, S. H., A. Goba, M. Chu, C. Roth, T. Healing, A. Marx, J. Fair, M. C. Guttieri, P. Ferro, T. Imes, C. Monagin, R. F. Garry, and D. G. Bausch.** 2008. New opportunities for field research on the pathogenesis and treatment of Lassa fever. *Antivir. Res.* **78:**103–115.
25. **Ksiazek, T. G., P. E. Rollin, A. J. Williams, D. S. Bressler, M. L. Martin, R. Swanepoel, F. J. Burt, P. A. Leman, A. S. Khan, A. K. Rowe, R. Mukunu, A. Sanchez, and C. J. Peters.** 1999. Clinical virology of Ebola hemorrhagic fever (EHF): virus, virus antigen, and IgG and IgM antibody findings among EHF patients in Kikwit, Democratic Republic of the Congo, 1995. *J. Infect. Dis.* **179**(Suppl. 1):S177–S187.
26. **Kurane, I.** 2007. Dengue hemorrhagic fever with special emphasis on immunopathogenesis. *Comp. Immunol. Microbiol. Infect. Dis.* **30:**329–340.
27. **Mahanty, S., and M. Bray.** 2004. Pathogenesis of filoviral haemorrhagic fevers. *Lancet Infect. Dis.* **4:**487–498.
28. **Mahanty, S., K. Hutchinson, S. Agarwal, M. McRae, P. E. Rollin, and B. Pulendran.** 2003. Cutting edge: impairment of dendritic cells and adaptive immunity by Ebola and Lassa viruses. *J. Immunol.* **170:**2797–2801.
29. **McCormick, J. B., I. J. King, P. A. Webb, C. L. Scribner, R. B. Craven, K. M. Johnson, L. H. Elliott, and R. Belmont-Williams.** 1986. Lassa fever. Effective therapy with ribavirin. *N. Engl. J. Med.* **314:**20–26.
30. **Monath, T. P.** 2008. Treatment of yellow fever. *Antivir. Res.* **78:**116–124.
31. **Myhrman, G.** 1951. Nephropathia epidemica: a new infectious disease in northern Scandinavia. *Acta Med. Scand.* 140:52–56.
32. **Parrino, J., R. S. Hotchkiss, and M. Bray.** 2007. Prevention of immune cell apoptosis as potential therapeutic

strategy for severe infections. *Emerg. Infect. Dis.* **13:**191–198.

33. **Pigott, D. C.** 2005. Hemorrhagic fever viruses. *Crit. Care Clin.* **21:**765–783.
34. **Spurgers, K. B., C. M. Sharkey, K. L. Warfield, and S. Bavari.** 2008. Oligonucleotide antiviral therapeutics: antisense and RNA interference for highly pathogenic RNA viruses. *Antivir. Res.* **78:**26–36.
35. **ter Meulen, J., M. Sakho, K. Koulemou, N. Magassouba, A. Bah, W. Preiser, S. Daffis, C. Klewitz, H. G. Bae, M. Niedrig, H. Zeller, M. Heinzel-Gutenbrunner, L. Koivogui, and A. Kaufmann.** 2004. Activation of the cytokine network and unfavorable outcome in patients with yellow fever. *J. Infect. Dis.* **190:**1821–1827.
36. **Whitehead, S. S., J. E. Blaney, A. P. Durbin, and B. R. Murphy.** 2007. Prospects for a dengue virus vaccine. *Nat. Rev. Microbiol.* **5:**518–528.
37. **Zaki, S. R., P. W. Greer, L. M. Coffield, C. S. Goldsmith, K. B. Nolte, K. Foucar, R. M. Feddersen, R. E. Zumwalt, G. L. Miller, A. S. Khan, P. E. Rollin, T. G. Ksiazek, S. T. Nichol, B. W. J. Mahy, and C. J. Peters.** 1995. Hantavirus pulmonary syndrome. Pathogenesis of an emerging infectious disease. *Am. J. Pathol.* **146:**552–579.

Viral Disease of the Eye

GARRY SHUTTLEWORTH AND DAVID EASTY

10

The eye and its adnexal structures are subject to a number of viral diseases. The initial part of this chapter discusses anatomic and physiological considerations of the eye and its principal clinical syndromes. Ocular disorders are classified according to the affected anatomic structures, for the most part, for example, keratitis, uveitis, cataract, and retinitis. The latter part of this chapter discusses its major viral diseases and highlights selected risk groups (infants and persons infected with human immunodeficiency virus [HIV]). The development of and advances in antiviral therapies have made many of the viral diseases of the eye amenable to treatment.

ANATOMY AND PHYSIOLOGY

The eye is unique in that it has structures with a high blood flow per unit mass (retina and choroids) directly adjacent to structures that, crucial to their optical functions, are avascular (vitreous cavity, anterior chamber, crystalline lens, and cornea) (Fig. 1). Specialized cellular barriers and pumps maintain the internal milieu of the eye. These control delivery of nutrients and removal of waste products from the avascular structures. By the very nature of the high degree of specialization and organization of its component structures, viral damage results in at least transient impairment of visual functions (visual acuity, visual field, color perception, or depth perception). Although the less specialized structures of the eye can effect adequate functional repair, provided damage is limited (e.g., corneal and conjunctival epithelium), the inability of certain ocular components to regenerate (e.g., retina, crystalline lens, and vitreous) or remodel (e.g., cornea) sufficiently to regain normal function often results in permanent visual impairment.

In the eyelids and conjunctival sac, immune cells guard the sites at which ocular exposure to antigens occurs. Lymphocytes and antigen-presenting cells of the conjunctiva-associated lymphatic tissue (CALT) form a distinct layer in the substantia propria and in places cluster to form follicles. The CALT is considered part of the mucosa-associated lymphatic tissues, which also include the gastrointestinal, tracheobronchial, and urogenital mucosae. These tissues are protected primarily by immunoglobulin A (IgA) antibodies and T-cell-mediated immunity. Antigen-presenting cells in the CALT process antigenic material and migrate to the periocular lymphatics in the eyelids that drain forward, down the face to the superficial lymph nodes around the base of the skull, and hence to the bloodstream and spleen, the primary recipient of eye-derived antigens. Following proliferation (clonal expansion), activated effector cells travel in the bloodstream to the eye, where they migrate to the site of infection to coordinate the specific immunologic response.

Visual function is critically dependent upon normal structural integrity, as reparative processes are incapable of remodelling all ocular components where tissues are damaged. Consequently, host immune responses to combat infection, viral or otherwise, may permanently damage ocular structures. In order to reduce this likelihood, the eye has evolved mechanisms whereby intraocular antigen-presenting cells, influenced by intraocular cytokines and acting in conjunction with the spleen, evoke specific immunologic adaptations. These adaptations have been termed anterior chamber-associated immune deviation and consist of suppression of relatively nonspecific, delayed-type hypersensitivity responses, with preservation of specific non-complement-fixing humoral immunity and up-regulation of suppressor T-cell responses. In addition, blood ocular barriers in the retina and anterior segment (tight cellular junctions of the capillary endothelial cells and retinal pigment epithelium) limit the ocular immune responses by restriction of cellular and macromolecular traffic, and programmed intraocular apoptosis of inflammatory cells may occur. These immune modulations and adaptations modify the severity and extent of nonspecific intraocular inflammation and serve to reduce collateral ocular damage. In a similar manner, the immune system is prevented from mounting autoimmune responses to tissue-restricted antigens, e.g., interphotoreceptor retinal binding protein and retinal S antigen.

MAJOR CLINICAL SYNDROMES

Conjunctivitis

Conjunctivitis may occur in isolation or in association with keratitis; combined inflammation is known as keratoconjunctivitis. The most common viral cause is adenovirus (Table 1). Typically conjunctivitis is associated with conjunctival hyperemia that is most marked in the con-

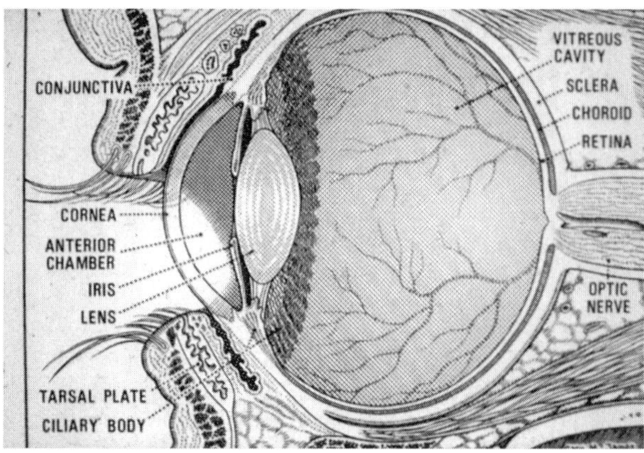

FIGURE 1 Diagram depicting a cross-section of the eyelids and globe. (Courtesy of Lloyd-Luke Ltd.)

junctival fornices, a discharge that in uncomplicated viral disease is usually watery but which may contain mucus, mild ocular irritation, and lid mattering. Visual function usually remains normal.

Conjunctival inflammatory responses, which can be examined in the everted upper and lower eyelids, are divided into nonspecific papillary responses, which under magnification have a velvety red appearance and are a consequence of tissue edema (Color Plate 18), and follicular responses, which have the appearance of grains of rice due to the formation of aggregates of activated lymphocytes. Occasionally, conjunctival inflammation is so severe that transudates rich in proteins and fibrin coagulate to form membranes or pseudomembranes on the conjunctival surfaces.

Keratitis

Keratitis is the result of inflammation affecting the cornea. It may occur in isolation or be associated with conjunctivitis or blepharitis. There are a plethora of clinical syndromes associated with keratitis; some are highly specific, but many share common features (Table 2).

Significant inflammation affecting the cornea results in limbal vascular dilatation with erythema most marked at the corneoscleral limbus. While pain can be variable, it is usually moderate to severe. Photophobia is almost always present and is thought to be due to reflex inflammation and spasm of the iris in response to light. A watery discharge is the result of reflex lacrimation and mucous-buildup corneal surface compromise. Visual compromise may occur as a consequence of reactive blepharospasm or, more significantly, inflammatory cell infitration and structural damage or perforation.

Appropriate investigation, accurate diagnosis, and effective treatment of keratitis are mandatory if damage to visual function is to be avoided.

Scleritis and Episcleritis (Table 3)

Scleritis manifests as either a localized or diffuse inflammation of the sclera and its overlying tissues. The lesions have a dusky red or violaceous appearance, although this may vary according to severity and ambient lighting. Typically, scleritis produces a relatively severe, chronic, deep, gnawing pain. Vision may be affected, particularly if there is corneal or uveal involvement, as in sclero-uveo-keratitis, or if the inflammation is posterior (posterior scleritis). Episodes of scleritis may be prolonged and can be sight threatening.

Initial treatment usually consists of systemic anti-inflammatory agents, including nonsteroidal anti-inflammatory drugs (NSIADs) and corticosteroids. However, cytotoxic agents are sometimes required to control the inflammation or to allow steroid sparing.

Episcleritis refers to inflammation of the episclera and overlying tissues. Lesions may superficially resemble scleritis, but closer examination will reveal a lack of scleral involvement and a brighter red coloration. Symptoms vary from cosmetic erythema only to mild ocular irritation. Episcleritis is not sight threatening, episodes are usually self-limited, and treatment is usually not indicated.

TABLE 1 Viral causes of conjunctivitis

Virus	Type of conjunctival inflammation
Adenovirus	Follicular conjunctivitis, pseudomembranous/membranous conjunctivitis
Picornavirus	Enterovirus 70, coxsackievirus A24, acute hemorrhagic conjunctivitis (tropical disease)
HSV	Primary infection—follicular conjunctivitis, neonatal ophthalmia
VZV	Lid margin lesions cause a mucopurulent conjunctivitis
EBV	Follicular conjunctivitis, membranous conjunctivitis
Measles virus	Mucopurulent keratoconjunctivitis with conjunctival (Koplik's) spots
Mumps virus	Follicular or papillary conjunctivitis
Echovirus	Keratoconjunctivitis
Influenza virus	Papillary conjunctivitis
Molluscum contagiosum virus	Toxic follicular conjunctivitis—reaction to shedding of molluscum bodies into tear film
NDV	Follicular conjunctivitis
Vaccinia virus	Papillary conjunctivitis, pseudomembranous/membranous conjunctivitis

TABLE 2 Viral causes of keratitis

Virus	Type of corneal inflammation
HSV	Epithelial disease (dendritic/geographic), stromal disease (disciform/interstitial)
VZV (zoster)	Epithelial disease (occasional atypical dendritic/neurotrophic/mucous plaque), stromal disease (nummular/disciform)
VZV (varicella)	Small transient dendritic figures, punctate epithelial keratitis, disciform keratitis
Adenovirus	Fine keratitis/subepithelial punctate opacities
Measles virus	Epithelial keratitis/ulceration and perforation in malnourished or immunocompromised populations, complicated by secondary HSV and bacterial infection
Mumps virus	Punctate epithelial keratitis, disciform keratitis
Rubella virus	Punctate epithelial keratitis, stromal keratitis
Vaccinia virus	Punctate epithelial keratitis, interstitial keratitis, disciform keratitis, necrotizing stromal keratitis

Uveitis

The term uveitis covers an enormous range of ocular inflammatory diseases, includes inflammation of any part of the uvea (iris, ciliary body, and choroid), and may be associated with several viral infections (Table 4). In practical terms, uveitis additionally includes vitritis, chorioretinitis, retinochoroiditis, retinitis, endophthalmitis, and panuveitis, as viruses do not usually produce isolated uveal inflammation.

Typically, anterior uveal inflammation is associated with limbal hyperemia, moderate to severe pain, photophobia, and reflex lacrimation. During acute attacks, visual function may be compromised by corneal edema, the accumulation of endothelial debris, turbidity of the aqueous humor, elevation of the intraocular pressure, or cystoid macular edema.

Incompetence of the endothelial vascular barrier of the iris capillaries allows leakage of plasma proteins and migration of cells into the aqueous humor. These proteins may be visualized as flare, light scattered from the slit lamp beam known as the Tyndall effect, while the cellular infiltration is seen as bright dust-like specks. If significant amounts of fibrinogen gain access to the aqueous humor, polymerization may result in adherence between the iris, lens, and cornea. Small clusters of cells that collect on the posterior surface of the corneal endothelium are known as keratic precipitates and are usually visible only with the slit lamp. Complications of anterior uveitis include cataract formation, corneal endothelial damage, and glaucoma. Treatment is directed toward reducing the ocular inflammatory responses with topical and sometimes systemic corticosteroid or NSAIDs, with treatment of any underlying etiology when possible.

TABLE 3 Viral causes of scleritis and episcleritis

Virus	Feature(s)
HSV	Scleritis, episcleritis
VZV	Scleritis, episcleritis
Mumps virus	Scleritis, episcleritis
Influenza virus	Episcleritis
EBV	Scleritis, episcleritis

Viral uveitis occurs most commonly following a previous epithelial infection due to herpes simplex virus (HSV) and may occur without simultaneous corneal involvement. Classically, there is an acute inflammatory reaction with large keratic precipitates ("mutton fat") that are rarely seen with other causes of uveitis. In addition to the marked anterior chamber flare and cellular infiltration, there may be involvement of the iris with sectorial iris atrophy that probably results from virus proliferation in the pigmentary epithelium (Fig. 2).

Retinitis

Viral causes of retinal disease have become prominent since the onset of HIV infection (Table 5). In the normal eye, the blood retinal barriers, which consist of the zonulae occludens of the retinal pigment epithelium (the pigmented monolayer of cells upon which the retina rests) and the vascular endothelia of the retinal arterioles and capillaries, limit the passage of both cellular and macromolecular traffic into the retina. Blood retinal barrier incompetence may produce retinal edema (which may be cystoid in appearance when located at the macula), bleeding, and exudation. Damage to the retinal barriers may result from retinal inflammatory cellular infiltrates and retinal ischemia, severe forms of which may result in retinal necrosis. Once the retinal barriers are breached, inflammatory cells may enter the vitreous cavity, cluster together, producing opacities, and give rise to symptoms of visual floaters. All of these processes may, depending upon location, affect visual function.

TABLE 4 Viral causes of uveitis

Virus	Feature(s)
VZV	Anterior uveitis, sectorial iris infarction and atrophy
HSV	Anterior uveitis and sectorial atrophy
EBV	Anterior uveitis, choroiditis
Adenovirus	Anterior uveitis (rare)
Vaccinia virus	Anterior uveitis, choroiditis
Influenza virus	Anterior uveitis
Mumps virus	Anterior uveitis

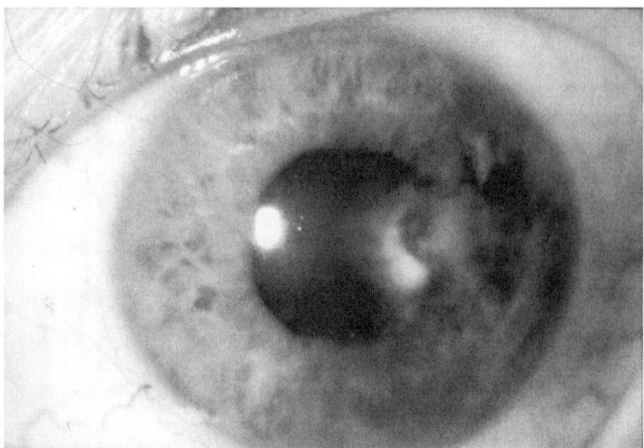

FIGURE 2 Sectorial atrophy of the iris and localized cataract secondary to HSV uveitis.

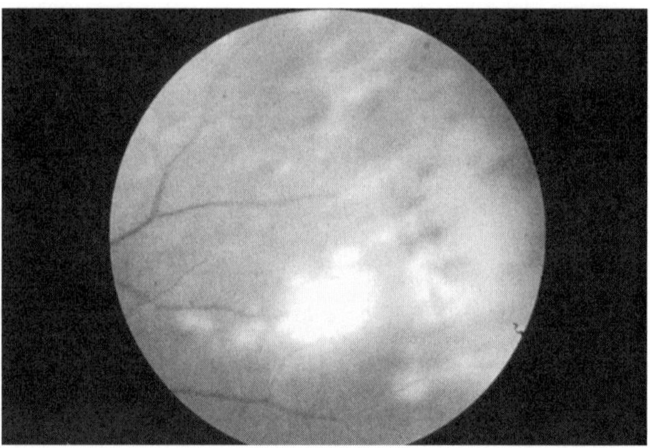

FIGURE 3 ARN syndrome demonstrating peripheral necrotic retinal lesions, the view of which is impeded to some extent by vitreous inflammation. (Courtesy of S. Lightman.)

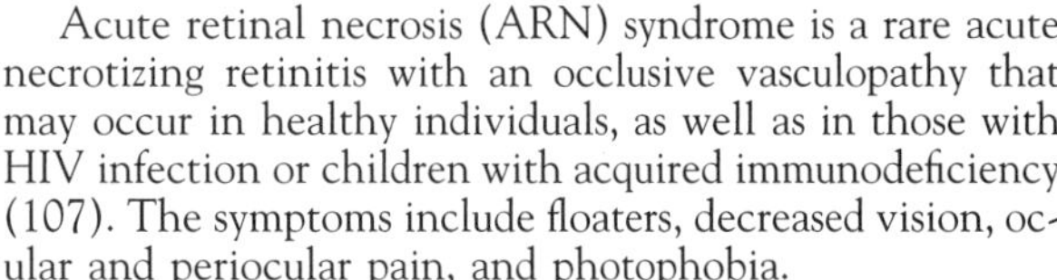

Acute retinal necrosis (ARN) syndrome is a rare acute necrotizing retinitis with an occlusive vasculopathy that may occur in healthy individuals, as well as in those with HIV infection or children with acquired immunodeficiency (107). The symptoms include floaters, decreased vision, ocular and periocular pain, and photophobia.

ARN is most commonly caused by varicella-zoster virus (VZV) infection (18) but it may also be caused by HSV (88, 101), cytomegalovirus (CMV), or Epstein-Barr virus (EBV) (10) infection. The development of ARN may be related to an impairment of cell-mediated immunity. Both VZV and HSV are neurotropic viruses and are thought to reach the retina via the optic nerve from the brain. The typical fundal picture shows areas of focal peripheral necrotic retinitis (Fig. 3) which rapidly spread to form large confluent circumferential geographic lesions. Other findings include moderate to severe vitritis, optic disk edema, retinal arteritis, retinal detachment (1), vascular occlusion, and a granulomatous anterior uveitis. Involvement of the central nervous system (CNS) can also occur. Progression to involve the optic nerve causes a profound deterioration of vision. The retinitis usually spares the posterior pole of the eye, and in those without optic nerve involvement or retinal detachment, central vision may be retained. ARN is differentiated from CMV retinitis by its moderate to marked vitritis and rapid progression. A posterior retinal form of ARN can also occur (83, 94).

Bilateral involvement occurs in 30 to 60% of individuals, usually within the first 3 months. The risk of bilateral involvement may be reduced by the systemic administration of acyclovir. Retinal breaks, which occur at the edges of the necrotic retina, lead to retinal detachment in up to 75% of cases. Without treatment, ARN can destroy the entire retina within 6 weeks.

Intravenous acyclovir has been used successfully in otherwise healthy adults to treat ARN resulting from HSV. Although evidence regarding the potential benefits of such treatment is controversial, where the clinical appearance suggests a high probability of HSV or VZV retinitis, high-dose intravenous acyclovir should be instituted (133) and subsequent oral antiviral therapy (acyclovir, valacyclovir, or famciclovir) should be continued for 3 to 4 months or indefinitely in ARN associated with HIV infection. Other forms of antiviral treatment have included systemic ganciclovir and intravitreal acyclovir. Systemic steroids have been used in an attempt to suppress the intraocular inflammation, and anticoagulants have been used to combat the occlusive vasculopathy. However, the benefits of such treatments remain uncertain. Laser photocoagulation may be employed to "wall off" spreading areas of necrosis, and vitreoretinal surgery may be indicated in those at risk of developing, or who have developed, retinal detachments.

However, the results of treatment and the visual prognosis are poor, especially in those with extensive disease or AIDS and in the elderly. Only 60% of those affected will retain a visual acuity of 20/200 or better. Recently, the use of valacyclovir, famciclovir, or valganciclovir, alone or in combination with adjunctive intravitreal foscarnet or ganciclovir injections, has been reported to have therapeutic effect (2, 3, 38).

Progressive outer retinal necrosis (PORN) is a severe form of VZV or HSV type 1 (HSV-1) retinitis that occurs in AIDS patients and sometimes in other immunocompromised patients (65, 87). PORN typically manifests following a previous episode of cutaneous zoster and in association with severe immunodeficiency (CD4 cell count of $<50/\mu l$), and it is thought that it may represent a dis-

TABLE 5 Viral causes of retinal disease

Virus or syndrome	Feature(s)
CMV	Necrotizing retinitis, most common in patients with AIDS but may also occur in neonates and immunosuppressed patients
HIV	Asymptomatic microangiopathy
ARN syndrome	Acute necrotizing retinitis, panuveitis due to HSV or VZV

tinct form of ARN occurring in the severely immunocompromised.

The condition usually manifests with painless, unilateral visual loss. Fundus examination reveals a fulminant, multifocal outer retinal necrosis. While lesions typically appear in the peripheral retina, lesions at the posterior pole are also frequent. The initial lesions progress rapidly to confluence, resulting in complete retinal atrophy and frequently retinal detachment (36). Vitritis and retinal vasculitis are not usually features of PORN. Identification of VZV as the etiologic agent has resulted from viral cultures, antigen detection, and identification of VZV DNA by PCR in vitreous (102) and retinal (36) biopsy specimens. However, HSV-1 has also been implicated (94).

Ocular Adnexal Disease

The ocular adnexa comprise those tissues that are anatomically or functionally related to the eye. These include the eyelids, the periocular skin and associated structures, the lacrimal and accessory glands, and the lacrimal drainage apparatus. The features of disease depend upon the structures involved and are beyond a general description. There are a significant number of inflammatory conditions of the adnexa that are caused by viruses (Table 6).

MAJOR OCULAR VIRAL PATHOGENS

Adenoviruses

Forty-seven adenovirus serotypes have been described, and a large number of these have been reported as causing ocular disease (see chapter 26). Some serotypes have gained particular notoriety for the clinical manifestations that they induce, their infectivity, and their mode of infection. However, ocular manifestations are not strain specific (147). The prevalence of the milder forms of ocular disease is unclear, but local epidemics of the more severe infections occur episodically, including in modern ophthalmic units (139), where water or instrument contamination can be responsible for disease transmission (62).

Traditionally, the clinical manifestations of ocular adenoviral disease have been divided into epidemic keratoconjunctivitis (types 8, 19, and 37), a highly infective condition with marked corneal involvement (13, 14) usually occurring in adults and with clustering of cases around ophthalmic units, and pharyngoconjunctival fever (types 3, 4, and 7) exhibiting a triad of infectious follicular conjunctivitis, upper respiratory tract illness, and pyrexia, which is most commonly seen in children. The mode of virus transmission relates to the features of the illness. In the case of type 8 infection, which usually lacks any respiratory or gastrointestinal component, spread is by direct contact and via fomites. In disease due to types 3, 4, 7, 19, and 37, which may have respiratory or gastrointestinal components, transmission includes droplet spread.

Clinical Manifestations

Ocular adenoviral infection results in an acute, self-limited disease that varies considerably in severity and typically affects children and young adults. In temperate regions, peaks of infection occur in the winter and summer. The incubation period ranges between 2 and 14 days, and the virus is shed in ocular secretions for 10 to 14 days following onset. Symptoms include pain, lacrimation, and foreign-body sensations in more severe cases. Corneal involvement and anterior uveitis may produce considerable discomfort and photophobia. Vision may be reduced in the acute stages by corneal epithelial and stromal inflammation and later by scarring. Typically, the other eye also becomes involved but is not usually as severely affected as the first eye due to immune activation and the appearance of neutralizing antibodies.

Follicular conjunctivitis is the most common finding in patients with ocular adenoviral infection and may be difficult to differentiate from the rare follicular conjunctivitis caused by HSV-1 (143). The follicular response is variable but is usually most marked in the lower recesses of the conjunctival sac. A papillary response may be most marked under the upper lid in those patients with severe ocular disease and foreign-body sensations. Conjunctival hemorrhages may occur, particularly in infection due to serotypes 3, 7, 8, 10, and 19, and range from petechiae to frank subconjunctival hemorrhage. Exudation and membrane or pseudomembrane formation may occur in the more severe forms of involvement and may lead to conjunctival scarring and symblepharon formation. Chemosis, periorbital and lid edema, sufficient to close the palpebral aperture, may also occur. Less common ocular features include anterior uveitis and disciform keratitis.

Subepithelial punctate opacities (Fig. 4) are the hallmark of corneal disease and result from cellular infiltration in response to the subepithelial viral antigen deposition that may occur during an initial diffuse punctate epithelial keratitis. These opacities vary considerably in number and when located centrally may interfere with visual function.

Although the acute disease process is self-limited, the subepithelial punctate opacities may persist from weeks to years, giving symptoms of mild ocular irritation and visual disturbance. Those infiltrates that resolve rapidly do so without sequelae, but those that persist may result in various degrees of scarring. Membranous or pseudomembranous cicatrizing conjunctivitis and involvement of the cornea are the most important features in determining both the short- and longer-term ocular morbidity.

TABLE 6 Viral causes of ocular adnexal disease

Virus	Feature(s)
VZV	Herpes zoster ophthalmicus, lid cicatrization
HSV	Primary infection—vesicular blepharoconjunctivitis, canaliculitis
Mumps virus	Dacryoadenitis
Measles virus	Dacryoadenitis, dacryocystitis
Molluscum contagiosum virus	Molluscum nodules
Papillomavirus	Papillomas of the lid, conjunctiva
HHV-8 (KSHV)[a]	Kaposi's sarcoma in AIDS

[a] HHV-8, human herpesvirus 8; KSHV, Kaposi's sarcoma-associated herpesvirus.

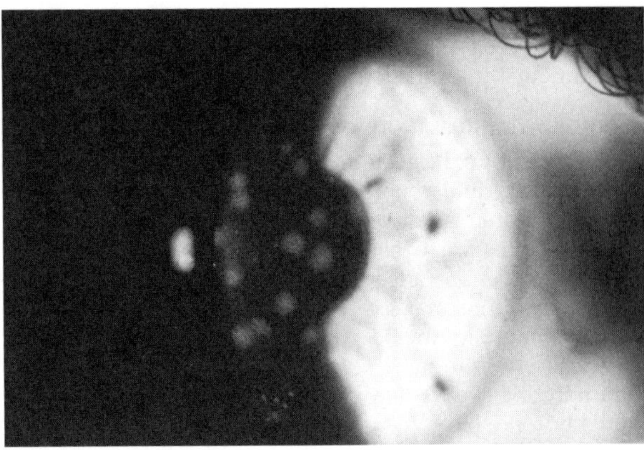

FIGURE 4 Subepithelial punctate infiltrates of established adenoviral keratitis.

Diagnosis

Diagnosis depends upon not only the ocular manifestations but also associated systemic features and history of infectious contacts. Definitive diagnosis of adenoviral disease can be made by virus isolation in cell culture; however, results take 1 to 3 weeks to obtain. PCR (20, 24, 98, 130) and modified cell cultures combined with immunofluorescent techniques (75) facilitate rapid diagnosis.

Treatment

Despite the existence of an animal model for ocular adenoviral disease and some varied results from the use of nucleoside analogs like cidofovir in both animals and humans (43, 44, 54, 112, 142), there is still no specific antiviral agent available for ocular adenovirus. Treatment is currently directed at the prevention of serious sequelae, the alleviation of distressing symptoms, and the prevention of transmission by promoting hygiene. In the acute stage, antibiotic drops are often administered to prevent secondary infections and cycloplegic agents may be offered for pain relief. The use of topical corticosteroid drops remains controversial. Although associated with a resolution of the corneal infiltrates and opacities, this benefit is often at the expense of recurrence of the lesions on withdrawal of therapy. Treatment with topical corticosteroids may provide general comfort but also enhances viral replication in the early stage of infection (113). As most infections with adenovirus are self-limited and resolve without sequelae, the only indications for corticosteroid use are cicatrizing conjunctival disease or visual compromise resulting from corneal cellular infiltrates or scarring. Phototherapeutic keratectomy has been successfully employed to treat persistent adenoviral subepithelial infiltrates.

Picornaviruses

The best-described ocular disorder that results from picornavirus infections is acute hemorrhagic conjunctivitis. During the last quarter century, picornaviruses have been recognized to cause epidemics of conjunctivitis in the tropics and smaller outbreaks in temperate zones. The first recognized outbreaks occurred in Africa and Asia in the late 1960s, and a subsequent epidemic swept around the globe involving many millions of people in overcrowded and underprivileged conditions. Continued activity occurred in the 1980s and 1990s in India, Singapore, Taiwan, Japan, South America, South Africa, China, and several states in the United States. More recent outbreaks have been recorded to occur in infants in Russia (82) and in the Caribbean (29) and Nepal (77).

Acute hemorrhagic conjunctivitis is caused by one of two picornaviruses, one a prime variant of coxsackievirus A24 and the other enterovirus 70. These viruses produce indistinguishable clinical manifestations. Epidemics of mixed virus infection have also been reported. Viral infection occurs either by direct contact with infected secretions or via fecal-oral contamination and follows a short incubation period ranging from 12 to 48 h.

Clinical Manifestations

Ocular infection is typically bilateral, and symptoms include local pain, foreign-body sensations, and lacrimation. Clinical features include eyelid edema, follicular conjunctivitis with serous discharge, chemosis, and subconjunctival hemorrhages (Color Plate 19). Occasionally, hemorrhages occur in the skin of the eyelids. Although subconjunctival hemorrhages were widely present in the early epidemics in the tropics, they have been less evident subsequently and have also been reported to occur in other viral infections, including infection with adenovirus serotype 11. Corneal involvement is limited to a superficial epithelial keratitis, although bacterial superinfection has been reported to occur, particularly in patients treated with topical corticosteroids (146). Variable findings include preauricular lymphadenopathy, respiratory tract illness, and constitutional upset. Cataract and uveitis were recorded in a Russian outbreak (81).

Diagnosis

Diagnosis may be made by viral isolation from ocular secretions within the first 2 days of infection before neutralizing antibodies appear, or from serologic evidence of infection. Virus has also been isolated from the pharynx and feces of affected persons. More recently, a reverse transcription-PCR has been developed to detect enterovirus 70 (145).

Treatment

The condition usually resolves without sequelae within 2 weeks. Although in the vast majority of cases the condition is entirely benign, very rarely, neurologic complications have been reported with enterovirus 70 infections (62). Radiculomyelitis may occur up to 2 months following the ocular disease (61), producing a motor paralysis, not unlike poliomyelitis, which tends to involve the proximal muscles of the lower limbs. Recovery is typically incomplete. Single or multiple cranial nerve palsies which follow the ocular disease more closely are also reported.

While there is no specific treatment for acute hemorrhagic conjunctivitis, antibiotic drops may be administered to prevent secondary infections and cold compresses may be used to relieve discomfort. The use of topical corticosteroids may predispose to the development of microbial keratitis and should be discouraged (146). Greatest attention should be paid to measures to prevent the spread of infection, including education and improvements in hygiene and sanitation.

Epstein-Barr Virus

Direct involvement of the eye or its adnexa may precede or follow generalized disease due to EBV. The most common ocular manifestation of infection is a follicular conjunctivitis (34). This response may be associated with white spots, which probably represent collections of inflammatory cells, and may occasionally be associated with a membranous conjunctivitis (127). Keratitis is uncommon, but punctate epithelial keratitis, dendritic keratitis, and stromal keratitis are reported. The stromal lesions have been described as discrete, sharply demarcated, multifocal, pleomorphic, or ring shaped and distinct from adenoviral or HSV stromal keratitis (115). Nummular keratitis with anterior subepithelial coin-shaped infiltrates may be associated with infectious mononucleosis.

Less commonly, dacryoadenitis with periorbital edema, periocular masses, Sjögren syndrome (135) (although recent evidence implies that this is unlikely [156]), episcleritis, uveitis (17, 99), optic neuritis, retinal vasculitis, extraocular muscle palsies, and nystagmus have been reported in association with EBV. However, the evidence for involvement of EBV in uveitis must be held as conjectural until better diagnostic tools become available.

The diagnosis of EBV infection may be made clinically but often requires detection of atypical lymphocytes, heterophile antibody or EBV-specific antibody to viral capsid antigen, or nuclear antigen or early antigen (see chapter 24). Despite in vitro inhibition of viral replication by acyclovir, bromovinyl-deoxyuridine, and ganciclovir, there is little clinical evidence to recommend the use of such agents currently. Ocular management is therefore aimed at local control of inflammation, prevention of secondary infection, and relief of discomfort.

Measles Virus

The ocular manifestations of measles first appear during the prodromal stage of the infection and include a subepithelial conjunctivitis with elevated papules (Koplik's spots). This develops into an epithelial keratoconjunctivitis that first appears on the exposed parts of the conjunctiva and progresses toward the center of the cornea. Lesions may coalesce to form large epithelial erosions, but corneal ulceration and perforation are rare in well-nourished populations. Involvement of the cornea gives rise to the photophobia that is characteristic of measles virus infection.

Other ocular manifestations include membranous conjunctivitis, optic neuritis, neuroretinitis resulting in a "salt and pepper" fundus, stellate macular lesions, uveitis, neuro-ophthalmic features, and a delayed peripheral lipid keratopathy sometimes seen in an adult patient with a history of severe measles in childhood. Intrauterine infection with measles virus has also been implicated in congenital dacryostenosis and a pigmentary retinopathy.

In underdeveloped countries where there is poor sanitation and malnutrition, particularly vitamin A deficiency, measles virus infections may result in severe corneal disease with ulceration, keratomalacia, secondary bacterial or HSV infections (Color Plate 20), and corneal perforation (134), so blindness is a common sequela of measles. Ultimately, preventive measures in the form of worldwide nutritional programs (for example, 200,000 IU of vitamin A on two occasions) and vaccination programs will serve to significantly reduce both the morbidity and fatalities that result from measles virus infection.

A very rare complication of measles, subacute sclerosing panencephalopathy (SSPE), may occur some years following the infection. SSPE may manifest as visual system involvement, including optic neuritis, cortical blindness, nystagmus, papilledema, macular pigmentary changes, chorioretinitis, and optic atrophy. The condition is untreatable and invariably fatal (25, 117).

Newcastle Disease Virus

Newcastle disease virus (NDV) primarily affects fowl, causing pneumoencephalitic infections. Human infection occurs uncommonly as a result of contact with infected poultry or from laboratory accidents and manifests as mild fever and malaise. The disease is self-limited and runs a course of 7 to 10 days. Ocular involvement consists of a follicular conjunctivitis associated with preauricular lympadenopathy that is usually unilateral. Rarely, a fine punctate keratitis may develop which may persist for some months (47). No specific therapy exists, and treatment is directed at symptom relief and prevention of secondary infection.

Herpes Simplex Virus

Among the viral causes of keratitis (Table 2), HSV infection ranks highly as a serious clinical condition that leads to significant morbidity and occasionally to loss of sight. The resultant corneal scarring may necessitate corneal transplantation to restore clarity to the visual axis and requires prolonged treatment and intensive follow-up.

HSV infection is one of the more common causes of ocular infection in Western communities. One 7-year study of 157 patients with at least one episode estimated that 500 patients with dendritic ulceration of the cornea were seen per year per million population. The maximum incidence occurred in persons between 40 and 50 years of age, with a greater number of males than females affected. Associated recurrent herpes labialis was reported for 50%. Recurrence was reported for 61%, and the average number of attacks was 3.4. Primary HSV infections account for 5% of new presentations.

Pathogenesis

HSV-1 infection of the eye may cause blepharitis, keratitis, conjunctivitis, uveitis, and retinitis. The most common manifestation, however, is keratitis. This may manifest as corneal edema due to endothelial dysfunction, as epithelial ulceration, or as white stromal inflammatory infiltrates. Persistent inflammation may result in either superficial or deep vascularization. As a result of the inability of the repair process to remodel precisely the orthogonal collagen fibers of the original corneal structure, inflammatory processes produce permanent scarring, loss of transparency, and visual handicap. While removal of corneal opacities by corneal transplantation can be attempted, results are unpredictable and latent virus may reactivate, resulting in recurrent disease and corneal graft rejection.

Experimental evidence in mice suggests two major routes of primary eye infection: direct infection by droplet spread or contact with infected secretions and initial infection at a nonocular site (120), with neuronal spread of virus along nerves supplying the cornea. Autoinoculation appears to be an unlikely source of eye infection (138). Virus may enter the cornea and the sensory nervous system via nontraumatic mechanisms (67).

In mice, primary ocular disease is accompanied by rapid invasion of the nervous system by the virus, and HSV can be detected in the ophthalmic part of the trigeminal ganglion 2 days after corneal inoculation (140). Subsequently, virus spreads to the nonophthalmic parts of this ganglion and then to sites within the same dermatome but separate from the inoculation site. Thus, other ocular sites such as the eyelids and iris can become infected by zosteriform spread via ocular sensory nerves rather than by direct intercellular spread via the cells of the skin.

Following corneal inoculation, HSV-1 can establish a latent infection in the sensory neurons of all three parts of the trigeminal ganglion, and studies with replication-defective virus mutants have shown that latency is established very rapidly and without prior synthesis of viral proteins, making intervention difficult.

Recurrent murine ocular HSV disease induced by UV irradiation of the cornea results in virus shedding in the tear film and production of recurrent corneal disease with a spectrum similar to that seen in humans (89, 121, 123). While we should be cautious in extrapolation of experimental findings to human pathology, animal studies continue to yield information about the immunopathology (69, 78, 119, 125, 128) and virology (8, 148) of disease, to guide improvements in treatment, and to develop effective vaccines.

Pathology

Epithelial disease in the form of dendritic keratitis is associated with formation of multinucleated giant cells and intranuclear inclusion bodies, as well as necrosis of the cells alongside the area of ulceration and infiltration with neutrophils in the underlying stroma. In stromal keratitis, in addition to the influx of neutrophils, lymphocytes are present and are critical in the cascade of events that predispose to chronic inflammatory sequelae. The mechanism by which HSV reaches the stroma is not clear. However, it seems likely that virus introduced into the epithelium via the sensory neuron escapes into the superficial stromal layers from the subepithelial nerve plexus, then enters keratocytes, and subsequently disseminates into the stroma by intercellular spread. Such spread would be enhanced where inhibitory immunologic responses are reduced by local corticosteroid use (30).

Granulomatous reactions can be seen at the level of Descemet's membrane, midstroma, and Bowman's layer. HSV antigens can be detected in keratocytes, endothelial cells, and epithelioid histiocytes together with multinucleated giant cells in necrotizing stromal keratitis, in contrast to inactive disease, in which viral antigens are not apparent. Endotheleitis has been described, associated with HSV DNA in the aqueous humor demonstrated by PCR. The pathogenesis of stromal disease is complex and has yet to be fully understood (66).

Possible latent virus has been identified in corneal tissue taken from patients who have undergone transplantation for stromal keratitis, in whom the tissue had apparently been in a quiescent state without any evidence of active inflammatory disease (124). Isolations have been made at a frequency of 12 to 29% of corneas sampled. Virus could be isolated from the areas with clinical disease in the form of scarring but not from relatively transparent regions. One study of patients with inactive stromal disease reported antigen detection in 82% of corneas of patients with herpetic keratitis and in 22% of corneas from patients with no history of keratitis. Latency-associated transcripts were not detected in this study, although HSV-1 was isolated by culture from 2% of patients. However, in spite of these studies and others, the verdict on corneal latency remains uncertain (162).

Clinical Manifestations

HSV may cause epithelial ulcerative keratitis, which is generally self-limited but responds rapidly to treatment with antiviral therapy. Stromal keratitis results in temporary or permanent loss of corneal transparency. A useful clinical sign that can be assessed by clinicians is loss of corneal sensation, seen most characteristically in areas of stromal scarring following an attack of stromal inflammation.

Primary or recurrent disease can occur, usually affecting the cornea or the anterior uvea. Primary disease (Fig. 5) is rare and involves the lid margins as small vesicles, the tarsal conjunctiva as a follicular inflammatory response, and the cornea as a single, often large dendritic ulcer. Occasionally, there may be multiple small ulcers extending on to the conjunctiva. Involvement of the deeper stroma does not generally occur.

In recurrent disease, in addition to dendritic ulceration of the epithelium, the corneal stroma can also become involved, producing a severe stromal keratitis. The anterior part of the uvea can also be involved, manifesting as iritis. In this there is a flare visible in the anterior chamber along with inflammatory cells (easily seen with the slit lamp microscope). On rare occasions the posterior segment of the eye can become involved, resulting in ARN syndrome.

Epithelial disease causes moderate to severe pain, watering, and photophobia. The infection is generally unilateral, and recurrences are associated with the classical trigger factors, including pyrexia, trauma (26), and exposure to sunlight. Dendritic ulcers are the common feature of ulcerative disease and are associated with conjunctival hyperemia. The ulcers are narrow and branching and are best seen after instilling dilute fluorescein drops and illuminating with a cobalt blue light (Color Plate 21). The surrounding epithelium becomes loose and can be easily debrided using a cotton-wool applicator, sometimes used for treatment. The ulcer has an irregular zig zag configuration with side branchings presenting a complicated arborescent pattern. The ulcer margin is vertical where the cells are opaque and are laden with virus. Ulcers usually heal in 5 to 12 days in the untreated state. However, epithelial defects or ulcers may persist for longer and probably represent poor epithelial regeneration rather than viral persistence. Dendritic ulcers occurring in malnourished children with simultaneous measles virus infection are extensive and are

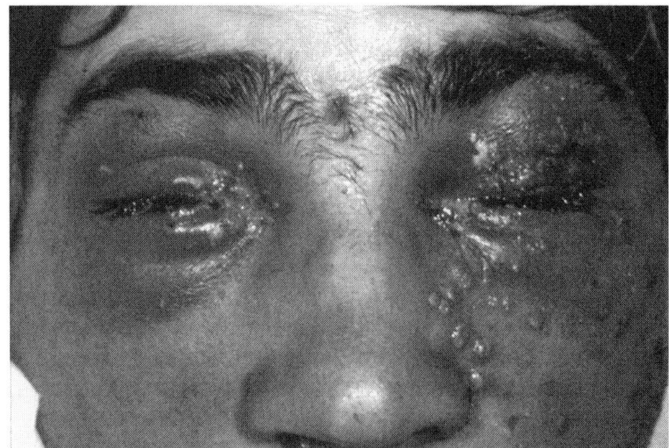

FIGURE 5 Primary HSV infection affecting the face and eyes bilaterally in an atopic individual.

known as amoeboid ulcers (Color Plate 20). Likewise, when a dendritic ulcer is treated erroneously with topical corticosteroid, immune responses are curtailed, and an extensive amoeboid ulcer results (Color Plate 22).

Stromal keratitis by definition is the inflammatory reaction that occurs in the presence of, or following, a dendritic figure and is the most common sight-threatening manifestation of HSV (90). The basement membrane of the epithelium and Bowman's layer (the anterior-most part of the corneal stroma) act as relative barriers to prevent the spread of viral particles from the epithelium, where the sensory nerve endings are clustered, into the deep stroma. However, in approximately 30% of patients with ulcerative disease, virus or its antigens penetrate into the corneal stroma (68, 162). The clinical appearances are summarized in Table 7.

Permanent stromal scarring generally follows which may not be sufficient to cause permanent visual handicap but when marked and involving the visual axis results in significant visual compromise for which a corneal transplant may be required (28). Corneal thinning or perforation may be seen in neglected cases of stromal keratitis and may require urgent corneal grafting. The vascularization induced by stromal keratitis increases the risk of graft rejection, and studies are under way to investigate the vascular inhibitory effects of anti-vascular endothelial cell growth factor antibodies (Avastin) (57).

Diagnosis

Diagnosis of ulcerative keratitis is made by viral culture or by immunofluorescent techniques. Enzyme-linked immunosorbent assays have proved to be useful and remain positive for viral antigen following treatment when culture has become negative. Such tests are rapid and correlate with culture results.

Occasionally, "trophic ulcers," which are quite different from dendritic ulcers, are seen, and they are thought to be the result of the corneal anesthesia that is caused by the herpetic infection. They can be perpetuated by the prolonged use of topical antivirals that in the past have been quite toxic. Since topical acyclovir ointment has become available, they are seen less frequently.

Treatment

The objective of treatment is to inhibit viral replication and concurrently to reduce the inflammatory and immune reaction in the stroma that can lead to lasting damage to the collagen fibrils (153, 154). Topical corticosteroid should never be used in isolation for treatment of dendritic ulcers, because the virus can replicate freely in the presence of local steroid-induced immunosuppression. Such ulcers are known as amoeboid or geographic because of their appearance, which is due to diffuse viral spread both within the epithelium and to the stroma (Color Plate 22).

Before antiviral agents became available, dendritic ulcers were treated by cautery using carbolic acid, ether, or iodine. Although this resulted in resolution of the ulceration, these treatments were associated with stromal scarring (20a) and even recurrent epithelial erosions. Debridement employing a sterile cotton-tipped applicator to gently remove the loose epithelium is reasonably successful, as inferred from clinical trials where debridement has been compared with idoxuridine (149), and may be reasonably employed as treatment where antiviral therapy is unavailable.

Antivirals

Treatment of HSV keratouveitis requires antiviral agents with good intraocular penetration, such as trifluorothymidine or acyclovir employed in conjunction with topical corticosteroids. Although the results of the multicenter Herpetic Eye Disease Study (51, 52) were not conclusive, a trend emerged showing the potential beneficial effect of oral acyclovir. Acyclovir is more active than idoxuridine, trifluorothymidine, vidarabine, or phosphonoacetic acid against HSV in vitro. Clinical studies have confirmed the in vitro findings and shown that tolerability is superior to that of the first-generation antivirals. A number of uncontrolled studies have reported a therapeutic effect of systemic acyclovir with topical corticosteroid in treatment of stromal keratouveitis (106).

Toxicity was a problem with the early antiviral agents (e.g., idoxuridine), particularly after prolonged use, but was rarely a problem after short-term use such as in the treatment of recurrent ulcerative disease. Toxic effects include follicular conjunctivitis, bulbar conjunctival chemosis and hyperemia, constriction of the lacrimal puncta, punctate epithelial keratopathy, chronic epithelial deficits, reduction of tear secretion, and keratinization of tarsal plates. Toxic changes are not seen with acyclovir, although after prolonged use, punctate epithelial keratopathy may occur.

TABLE 7 Stromal manifestations of HSV

Stromal manifestation	Feature(s)
Ghosting of dendritic figures	Occurs in the stroma underlying the previous ulcer, initially as a branched area of stromal edema and then persisting as a scar that may slowly disappear over many months or years
Superficial punctate keratitis	Opacities distributed mainly in the superficial stroma, variable in position, size, and shape; may persist for many months
Disciform keratitis	Represents an immunologic reaction to persisting viral antigen; inflammatory-cell infiltration and diffuse stromal edema cause folds in the deep layers of the cornea (Descemet's membrane)
Immune ring (Wessely ring) formation	Due to antibody-antigen complex formation within the stromal compartment, attracting inflammatory cells
Necrotic stromal keratitis	A persistent form of keratitis that is associated with foci of cellular infiltration, white or yellowish; does not respond to anti-inflammatory treatment

Systemic acyclovir or other antivirals must be used in the treatment of primary HSV keratitis in association with topical acyclovir when there are significant mucocutaneous or facial lesions (Fig. 5). In addition, topical antibiotic therapy may be required, as a dendritic ulcer may act as a portal of entry for bacteria and the development of microbial keratitis. Where full-strength or dilutions of topical corticosteroid are used for treatment of stromal herpes simplex keratitis, an antiviral "umbrella" should be simultaneously employed.

Long-term systemic acyclovir effectively reduces recurrences of stromal keratitis (6, 9, 12, 80). In addition, where corneal grafts have been performed for stromal scarring due to HSV keratitis, it is judicious to use both topical steroids and a nontoxic topical antiviral in an effort to prevent recurrences during the postoperative period. Many physicians employ systemic acyclovir as additional prophylaxis. Long-term prophylaxis with oral acyclovir appears to reduce the rate of recurrence of epithelial and stromal herpes simplex keratitis (51, 52, 104) and corneal graft failure in patients with a history of recurrent HSV keratitis (80, 126, 129, 161).

Resistance to antiviral therapy in HSV keratitis has been reported, although the evidence for this is not very convincing. One series of stromal isolates from 12 patients undergoing keratoplasty were found to be sensitive to a battery of antivirals, notwithstanding the long-term antiviral treatment which had been administered (97, 124). However, chronic infection due to HSV that fails to respond to high-dose acyclovir therapy has been reported to occur in patients with AIDS, and isolates have been shown to be thymidine kinase negative (15).

Corticosteroids

Topical corticosteroids are employed to reduce the stromal infiltration and consequent damage to the collagenous structure of the cornea in stromal keratitis. Likewise, they must be used in HSV uveitis to reduce the characteristic severe inflammatory reaction. Because of the risk of promoting virus recurrence in the epithelium or increasing viral proliferation, the concomitant use of an antiviral (e.g., acyclovir) with good stromal and anterior chamber penetration is essential (51).

The objective is to employ the minimal concentration of topical steroid that will achieve a therapeutic effect. A low concentration should be used in the first instance, and where no therapeutic effect is obtained, a higher concentration should be considered. High-dose corticosteroids should be tapered in stages over several days or even weeks to avoid the risk of a severe rebound inflammatory response (31). More recently the use of topical cyclosporine has been shown to be beneficial in herpetic stromal keratitis, although larger studies are awaited (48, 109).

Prevention

Vaccination may protect animals against ocular HSV, but no vaccines are available for human use at present. However, local periocular vaccination in rabbits with HSV-1 KOS or gB2/gD2 in MF59 emulsion provided significant protection against conjunctivitis or iritis to a greater extent than systemic injection (100). Research using laboratory models of recurrence shows that vaccination with HSV-1 glycoproteins with adjuvant can reduce spread of virus in the ocular model (110, 122). Vaccination with heat shock-inactivated HSV seems to reduce the number and duration of recurrences in keratitis or keratouveitis in humans, although this is not very convincing, and further studies will be necessary to confirm such data (105).

Varicella-Zoster Virus

Varicella

Varicella occasionally causes small papular lesions on the margins of the eyelids, conjunctiva, or limbus. Those on the lids can develop into excavated ulcers that cause considerable inflammation. Rarely, varicella can induce severe scleritis (46, 92). The cornea may show a superficial punctate keratitis and marginal keratitis in the presence of limbal pustules. Corneal involvement may also occur late in the disease, weeks or months after resolution of the exanthema. Small bleb-like lesions in the presence of corneal edema have been described, and, rarely, disciform keratitis and dendritic figures have been recorded. The disciform keratitis appears identical to herpes simplex keratitis, but unlike the latter, the disciform keratitis responds to topical corticosteroid without the need for simultaneous topical antiviral cover.

Herpes Zoster

Many ocular tissues can be affected by herpes zoster ophthalmicus, including the skin of the forehead and eyelids, cornea, uveal tract, retina, and optic and cranial nerves. As with nonophthalmic zoster, the severity of an attack is increased in immunocompromised patients.

Typically, an erythematous, pustular rash within the distribution of the first division of the trigeminal nerve is present (Fig. 6). The rash may extend from the nose and the eye to the skull vertex but does not cross the midline. Involvement of the nasociliary nerve occurs in about 30% of patients and correlates closely with ocular involvement, which occurs in approximately 50% of patients. The eye may be damaged by a number of processes, including viral replication, vasculitis, corneal anesthesia and neurotrophic damage, tear film abnormalities, conjunctival scarring and eyelid abnormalities, and the inflammatory responses to the virus. Postherpetic neuralgia is one of the most serious effects of herpes zoster ophthalmicus and may be associated with the extent and severity of the eruption, advanced age, and the inability of the immune system to control the

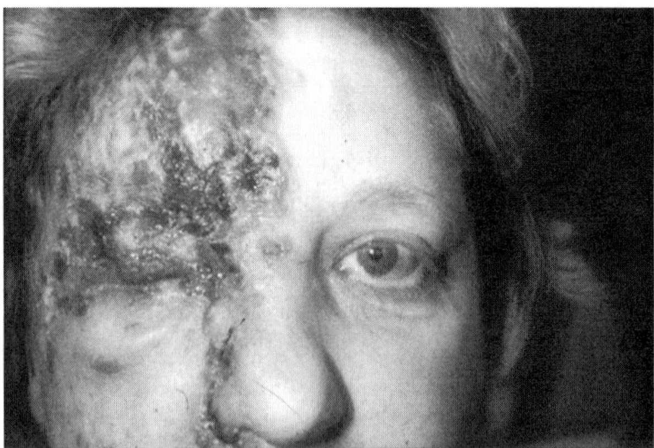

FIGURE 6 Herpes zoster affecting the first ophthalmic division of the trigeminal nerve. Note the periocular edema, vesicles, and crusts.

spread of virus (160). Postherpetic neuralgia is not prevented by early systemic antivirals or corticosteroids.

Clinical Manifestations

An attack of herpes zoster is usually preceded by neuralgic pain and associated with the appearance of a vesicular cutaneous eruption within the same dermatome. Ocular involvement does not correlate with the severity of the cutaneous eruption; mild cutaneous features occasionally precede a severe ocular disease.

Eyelid vesicles resolve with pitting, pigmentation, and scarring, sometimes resulting in eyelid retraction, malposition, and corneal exposure. The lash follicles and meibomian glands may also be damaged.

Nodular or diffuse scleritis (Color Plate 23) and keratitis may occur, sometimes months later. The keratitis may be epithelial with an atypical dendriform ulceration, a pseudodendritic ulceration due to persistent erosions or mucous plaque formation. Stromal disease may be punctate, focal, or diffuse and lead to persistent scarring (Fig. 7 and 8), often associated with lipid deposition (Fig. 9). Damage to the corneal nerves may result in profound corneal anesthesia. Vasculitis may occur in the iris, where it causes sectoral atrophy, or in the retina as part of ARN syndrome. Cranial nerve palsies and CNS involvement are also occasionally seen. Long-term sequelae include postherpetic neuralgia, permanent scarring of the eyelids, entropion, keratoconjunctivitis sicca, and neurotrophic keratopathy.

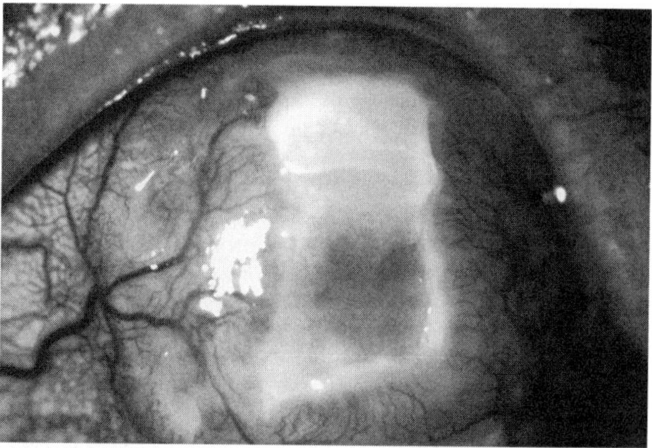

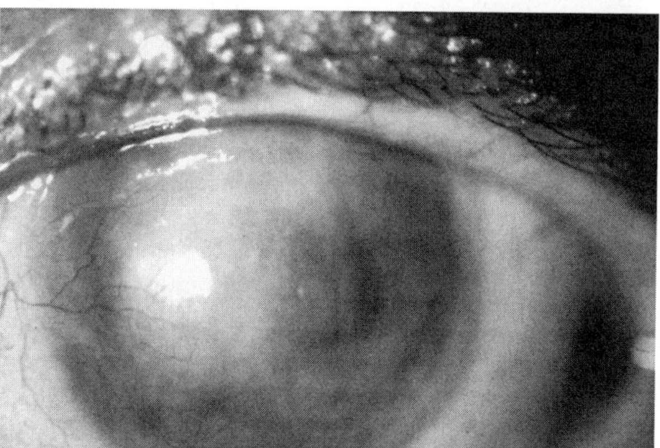

FIGURE 7 (Top) Persisting epithelial ulceration secondary to unsatisfactory herpes zoster pretreatment. (Bottom) Resolution of the ulceration with inactive corneal scarring following treatment with ocular lubricants and steroids 2 years later.

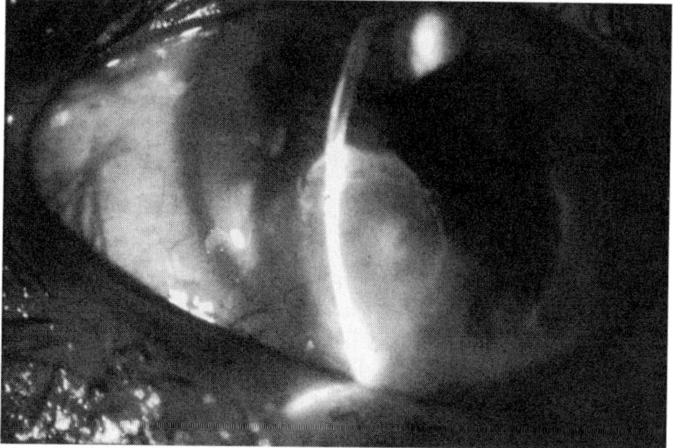

FIGURE 8 Inactive corneal scarring secondary to VZV infection.

In the congenital varicella syndrome, in which a mother suffers VZV infection in the first two trimesters of pregnancy, skin lesions in a dermatomal distribution and eye lesions can be identified in about 2% of births.

Treatment

The puzzle in treatment of herpes zoster ophthalmicus is the lack of clear insight into the pathology induced by the virus. Since many of the inflammatory sequelae occur after the acute attack has resolved, it is not known whether they are due to the persistence of the virus within the ocular tissue or whether the reactions are immunologic. However, VZV DNA can be identified in the cornea up to 8 years after an attack, suggesting that viral persistence may play a role (150).

In the acute stages (within 72 h of onset), systemic treatment with oral acyclovir hastens the resolution of skin lesions, reduces the acute pain and viral shedding, and reduces the incidence of episcleritis, keratitis, and iritis. Other antiviral agents, specifically valacyclovir and famciclovir, are at least as effective in preventing ocular complications and have simpler dosing schedules because of their high oral bioavailability (19, 141). In addition, topical treatment with acyclovir has been shown to hasten

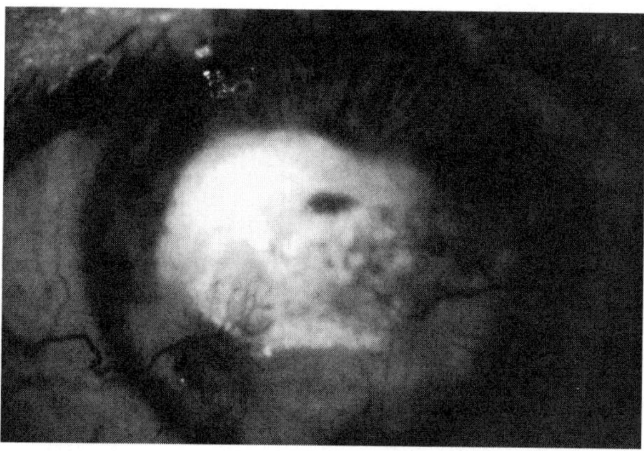

FIGURE 9 Lipid keratopathy resulting from scarring and vascularization of the cornea as a result of VZV.

the resolution of corneal epithelial disease and to reduce the incidence of recurrent disease. Interferon has also been used with some success in herpes zoster, but adverse effects are frequent and postherpetic neuralgia remains unaffected. Evidence relating to the role of systemic corticosteroids in the prevention of postherpetic neuralgia remains controversial (91).

Vaccinia Virus

Ocular disease due to vaccinia virus may occur following autoinoculation or infection from the vaccination site of another individual. The clinical manifestations are more severe in nonimmune individuals and include ulcerating eyelid pustules, blepharoconjunctivitis, eyelid edema, and an occasionally membranous purulent papillary conjunctivitis. Corneal involvement occurs in about 30% of individuals with eye disease and ranges from a mild superficial punctate keratitis to a necrotizing stromal keratitis, which may occur up to 3 months following the original infection and which can result in perforation. Small dendrites, geographic ulceration, and chronic disciform keratitis are also described in association with vaccinia, as are uveitis, choroiditis, extraocular muscle palsy, and optic neuritis.

With the eradication of smallpox and discontinuance of vaccination programs in the early 1970s, ocular disease due to vaccinia is rare. However, with a recent resurgence of vaccinations, 16 cases of ocular vaccinia were reported from in excess of 450,000 smallpox vaccinations (35). While the majority of ocular complications of smallpox vaccination in immunocompetent patients are self-limited, some cases may require treatment with trifluridine drops, topical corticosteroids, and vaccinia immune globulin. Vaccinia virus does not appear to be sensitive to acyclovir.

Cytomegalovirus

CMV retinitis is the most common of the severe ocular infections that occur in patients with HIV and was first noted in the early 1980s shortly after the original descriptions of AIDS. It occurs in around one-third of AIDS patients (59, 103), typically when the $CD4^+$ lymphocyte count falls to below 50 cells/mm^3 (16), and is commonly associated with systemic CMV infection (colitis, encephalitis, pneumonitis, adrenalitis, and radiculopathy), which may be subclinical. It is an AIDS-associated illness, accounting for about 5% of AIDS diagnoses. Interestingly, CMV retinitis is less common in African patients and children with AIDS. Although CMV retinitis may occur in patients who are immunosuppressed and occasionally in neonates, it is most commonly seen in the latter stages of HIV infection. However, the use of highly active antiretroviral therapy has led to a very significant decline in the incidence of HIV-related CMV retinitis (22, 111).

Pathogenesis

CMV retinitis occurs following chronic CMV viremia. The virus is thought to reach the retina either via infected monocytes or, more rarely, by direct extension from the CNS via the optic nerve. The processes that give rise to HIV microangiopathy possibly facilitate the passage of CMV-infected cells into the retina and may explain the higher incidence of CMV retinitis in patients with HIV infection than in immunosuppressed transplant patients. Simultaneous infections in the retina occur with HIV and CMV and with CMV and HSV. Once within the retina, the virus rapidly spreads in antero- and retrograde directions along the nerve fiber layer before spreading cell to cell into the adjacent retina.

Pathology

Histologic examination reveals areas of extensive retinal necrosis but little inflammatory response. Cells containing viral intranuclear and intracytoplasmic inclusions may be found in all layers of the retina, some of which are large, with a characteristic perinuclear halo (owl eye cells). Occasionally, multinucleate giant cells may be seen. Immunohistochemistry, in situ hydridization, and electron microscopy have revealed the presence of CMV antigens, DNA, and virions in both the nuclei and cytoplasm of infected cells. Gliosis or calcium deposition marks areas of burned-out disease where retinal vessels show perivascular fibrosis and narrowing.

Clinical Manifestations

Typically, CMV retinitis is painless or associated with mild or vague ocular discomfort. Visual symptomatology depends upon the part of the retina involved and upon complications, for example, retinal detachment (70). Vitreous involvement produces floaters, which are usually best seen against a uniformly illuminated background (e.g., a blue sky), or a reduction in vision. Additional symptoms may include those due to associated systemic CMV disease.

Ocular involvement is bilateral in about half of those affected, with a significant proportion of patients losing vision before death. Approximately 80% of those with unilateral disease will develop bilateral disease without treatment (86).

Visual function may be markedly affected as a result of involvement of the optic nerve head (Color Plate 24) or the macula; however, many cases are asymptomatic and regular fundoscopic screening for the disease is required, particularly in those with $CD4^+$ lymphocyte counts below 100 cells/mm^3. Those who are symptomatic may complain of the gradual onset of floaters, photopsia (flashing lights), blurred vision, and visual field defects. Pain and photophobia are not usual features of CMV retinitis and suggest an alternative HIV-associated diagnosis, e.g., VZV, HSV, syphilis, or toxoplasma retinitis.

Fundus examination may reveal an appearance which has been termed the "cottage cheese and ketchup fundus" or "pizza fundus." This consists of large unifocal, but sometimes multifocal, areas of cheesy, yellow-white, full-thickness retinal necrosis often centered upon blood vessels, with associated intraretinal hemorrhages and perivenous and, less commonly, arteriolar sheathing (Fig. 10).

The necrotic process usually starts in the periphery (49) and is slowly but relentlessly progressive, spreading through the fundus with a mean doubling time of around 3 weeks. Untreated, the entire retina may be destroyed within 6 months. The necrotic area is surrounded by an active yellow-white leading edge, in front of which small granular satellite lesions may be seen. Progression of the necrotic process is likened to the spread of a bushfire. In patients treated with antiviral agents, the active edge of a lesion may be narrow and easily missed. More peripheral lesions are less hemorrhagic, have a more granular appearance, and tend to be oval or circular. Areas of burned-out disease appear gliotic, with fine granulations of the retinal pigment epithelium. Macular exudative retinal detachments are also

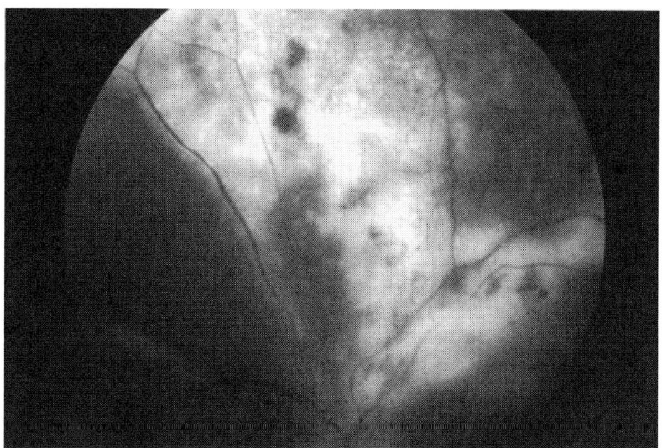

FIGURE 10 CMV retinitis with a large superior sector of necrosis and perivenous sheathing. (Courtesy of R. Markham.)

reported and may resolve with antiviral therapy (39). Vitreous hemorrhages suggest a retinal tear occurring at the active edge of a lesion or herald a retinal detachment (37).

Typically the vitreous cavity, choroid, and anterior segment show little or no inflammatory reaction, although fine scattered deposits are commonly observed on the corneal endothelium (118). Involvement of the optic nerve head (45), whether as a result of a primary optic nerve head infection or as a result of spread from intracranial or adjacent retinal disease, produces similar yellow-white necrosis and associated hemorrhage.

Diagnosis

The differential diagnosis of hemorrhagic retinal necrosis in an HIV-positive individual includes ARN, PORN, toxoplasma retinochoroiditis (27), fungal infection, syphilitic retinitis, intraocular lymphoma, and HIV microangiopathy. Typically, the slow progression, unifocality, characteristic appearance, and absence of intraocular inflammation help to establish the diagnosis of CMV retinitis. However, in atypical cases the diagnosis may be aided by electron microscopy or PCR amplification of viral DNA obtained from an endoretinal, choroidal, or vitreous biopsy (74). Virus isolation from blood or urine may help to confirm the diagnosis.

Treatment

While spontaneous regression may occur, possibly as a result of improved immunocompetence, the prognosis for visual recovery is poor. Without treatment the disease will progress relentlessly, leaving an atrophic, gliotic retina with retinal vascular attenuation, optic atrophy, and little or no visual function. Immune reconstitution as a result of potent antiretroviral drug therapies has produced CMV immune-reconstitution diseases, which include a benign transient vitritis and retinitis and a delayed-onset uveitis with a poor visual prognosis.

In the small proportion (1.3 to 5%) of therapeutically immunosuppressed transplant patients with CMV retinitis, withdrawal or modification of immunosuppressive therapy may be all that is required to arrest the disease process. Antiviral therapy may be indicated if immune recovery is slow or withdrawal of immunosuppressive therapy is unwise (137). Therapeutic agents with activity against CMV include foscarnet (86), ganciclovir (5, 55, 158), cidofovir (40, 56), and valganciclovir. Although therapeutic effects are usually clinically apparent within 3 to 4 weeks, inhibition of viral activity is not absolute (104) and recurrence occurs following cessation of therapy. Eventually recurrence occurs in many on maintenance therapies as a result of acquired antiviral resistance.

Systemic administration of valganciclovir, ganciclovir, foscarnet, or cidofovir (79) leads to suppression of the retinitis and delay in the progression of the disease. However, all are associated with serious systemic side effects, which has prompted the search for local therapies. Systemic treatments, however, have the advantage of treating associated disseminated disease and protecting the other eye (see chapters 12 and 22). Treatment is typically administered through an indwelling catheter in the form of a high induction dose followed by a lower maintenance dose. However, valganciclovir, a prodrug of ganciclovir with excellent oral bioavailability, offers the benefits of an oral drug with pharmacokinetics comparable to those of ganciclovir (23).

Reactivation of the disease or the development of antiviral resistance requires a change of antiviral agent or combination therapy. The occurrence of CMV retinitis at such an advanced stage of HIV infection and the associated systemic infection mean that even with systemic treatment, survival may be limited.

Local treatments take the form of repeated ganciclovir or foscarnet intravitreal injections (4, 50, 159) or implantation, via the pars plana, of an intraocular sustained-release device 5. Intravitreal injections of cidofovir (72, 73, 108) are also efficacious but may be associated with inflammation and hypotony (132). Although systemic toxicity is avoided, complications associated with repeated intraocular injections and intraocular procedures include hemorrhage, endophthalmitis (155), and retinal detachment. The incidence of retinal detachment is lower following intravitreal therapy than after systemic therapy (158). An antisense oligonucleotide (fomivirsen) has been approved for intravitreal therapy for the local treatment of CMV retinitis in patients with AIDS for whom other therapy is ineffective or unsuitable.

Although the visual prognosis with treatment is good (90% retain 40/20 vision at 6 months), retinal detachment occurs in between 10 and 30% (38, 42, 116) of cases. Retinal detachments result from large ragged retinal tears that occur at the active leading edges of areas of necrosis or in the resultant atrophic retina. Both the presence of active disease and the extent of retinal involvement are independent risk factors for the development of retinal detachment. Although laser retinal photocoagulation has not been proven to contain the spread of retinal infection, it may be of use in treating retinal breaks and localized peripheral detachments. Treatment of full-blown retinal detachments is best performed by pars plana vitrectomy, internal silicone oil tamponade, and endolaser (38).

Following the introduction of potent antiretroviral therapy, improvements in immune function have led to a very significant decline in the incidence of HIV-related CMV retinitis (32) and a dramatic improvement in the prognosis. Some of those who respond may no longer require maintenance anti-CMV therapy (41, 56, 58, 93, 151, 152). The incidence of visual impairment during follow-up is high but is substantially lower among patients who receive potent antiretroviral therapy, especially those observed to have immune recovery (101). However, potent antiretroviral therapy itself has been associated with severe lymphocytic intraocular inflammatory response, possibly the result of improved immunocompetence leading to an exaggerated response to existing intraocular antigen (42, 60, 63, 101). These CMV immune-reconstitution diseases include a benign transient vitritis and retinitis and a delayed-onset uveitis. The last requires early recognition and treatment with systemic corticosteroids, as cystoid macular oedema and epiretinal membrane formation often lead to visual impairment (71). How best to identify, screen, and treat those at risk is currently uncertain.

Mumps

The most common form of ocular involvement in mumps is dacryoadenitis, although a papillary or follicular conjunctivitis, which may be associated with subconjunctival hemorrhage, is not unusual. Episcleritis, scleritis, anterior uveitis, stromal keratitis, and optic neuritis may also occur and usually resolve without complications. In addition, neuroretinitis and a possible association with acute posterior multifocal placoid pigment epitheliopathy (11) have also been reported. The diagnosis is usually made clinically without recourse to serology or virus isolation.

Treatment of the acute infection is both supportive and symptomatic. Vaccination is effective in preventing the complications of mumps. A live attenuated vaccine, which is usually administered to children in combination with measles and rubella vaccination, produces immunity in over 90% of subjects.

Molluscum Contagiosum

Molluscum contagiosum is a relatively common viral disease with a prevalence of around 1% in healthy subjects, rising to 10 to 15% in those with HIV, in whom the infection may be atypical and extensive (85). Molluscum nodules are most common in the axilla or on the trunk but can occur on most parts of the body, including the periocular skin and, rarely, conjunctiva. An intraocular molluscum lesion has even been reported following traumatic implantation of infected epithelial cells. Transmission occurs through contact of abraded skin with infectious virus particles, with an incubation period of between 2 and 6 weeks. The typical lesions are pale, painless nodules between 2 and 5 mm in diameter which may appear in groups. Classically, lesions are said to be umbilicated, but this is not an invariable feature.

Ocular disease may occur as a result of eyelid lesions, particularly those occurring on the lid margins (Fig. 11), which may be difficult to detect among the eyelashes and which frequently lack the classical umbilicated appearance. A uniocular chronic follicular conjunctivitis is typical and represents a reaction to virus particles shed from molluscum bodies into the tear film. However, conjunctivitis is less common in those with HIV-associated disease. A punctate epithelial keratitis may also occur, as may a filamentary keratopathy and a superior corneal vascular pannus.

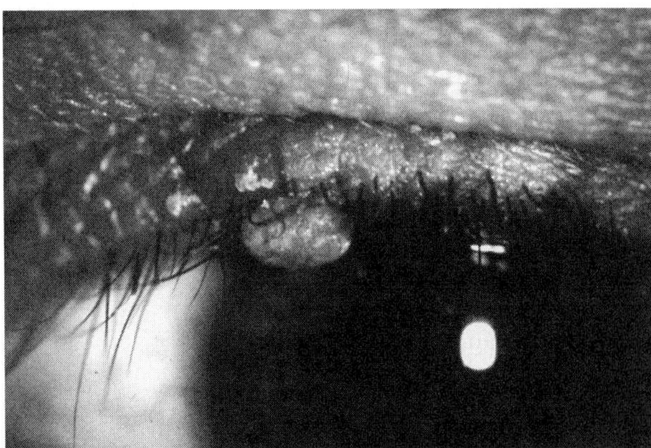

FIGURE 11 Molluscum lesion of the upper eyelid margin. Note the lack of umbilication.

Molluscum nodules resolve spontaneously over several weeks but may, rarely, lead to a trachoma-like picture of conjunctival scarring with visual loss. However, molluscum nodules associated with HIV do not resolve spontaneously. Should treatment be required, excision, incision, curettage, or merely expression of the contents is effective in eradicating the lesions, after which ocular features clear rapidly. Cidofovir may contribute to clearance of advanced lesions in HIV-associated disease (96).

Papillomavirus

Papillomaviruses can cause a variety of ocular epithelial disorders ranging from the common wart on the eyelid to multiple conjunctival papillomas in the fornices or at the limbus. Lesions occurring on the eyelids may be sessile or pedunculated and share the same general histologic features as lesions occurring on other keratinizing epithelia, with epithelial proliferation overlying a fibrovascular core derived from the underlying connective tissue. Eyelid papillomas may be disfiguring or cause a ptosis, while those on the eyelid margin may cause a mild chronic papillary conjunctivitis or a punctate epithelial keratitis.

Papillomavirus types 6, 11, 16, and 18 have been associated with conjunctival disease. Types 6 and 11 have been associated with benign-type papillomas, while types 16 and 18 have been associated with conjunctival dysplasia and carcinoma (95) but may also be detectable in non-neoplastic lesions and healthy conjunctiva (64, 84).

Conjunctival papillomas are more common in younger patients (<10 years) and can arise anywhere within the conjunctival sac, appearing either as pedunculated growths with finger-like processes emanating from the fornices or as sessile lesions at the limbus. Less commonly, inverted lesions may also occur, particularly in the lacrimal gland. Conjunctival papillomas may be multiple and have a propensity to recur following excision. Recurrent conjunctival papillomas can sometimes be so severe as to involve the entire conjunctival surface.

Conjunctival dysplasia and carcinomas are not common but may occur in elderly subjects and are slightly more common in men. Lesions vary considerably in appearance and location but are usually solitary, vascular, sessile epithelial thickenings that arise in the region of the limbus (where there is high mitotic activity). Multiple and pedunculated lesions are, however, reported, and recurrence following excision is not uncommon.

Treatment of these conjunctival lesions is usually by surgical excision, taking a suitable margin of healthy tissue. Adjunctive therapies include cryotherapy and cautery to the base of the lesion and courses of topical antimetabolite drops (e.g., mitomycin C). Incomplete excision or bleeding from the lesion may result in multiple seeding and recurrence of the lesions. Recurrent or severe disease may be treated with systemic interferon or topical cytotoxic agents.

Neurologic Disorders

Many viruses are capable of producing neuro-ophthalmological disease (Table 8). The spectrum of disease is broad, ranging from isolated extraocular muscle palsy to sinister CNS disease. However, in the majority of such disorders, neurologic involvement represents only an occasional feature or complication and nonneurologic features predominate.

Ocular Manifestations of HIV Infection

The ocular manifestations of HIV type 1 (HIV-1) and HIV-2 take a variety of forms, but opportunistic infections are the most important and commonly encountered. Such infections are often associated with disseminated involvement of other body systems, necessitating a thorough clinical assessment in all cases. The response of the ocular tissues is modified by the profound immunocompromise associated with AIDS, with the result that inflammatory responses are less marked than in immunocompetent individuals. In addition, infections tend to be more severe and are more commonly multicentric and bilateral.

The diagnosis of opportunistic infection in HIV is usually made clinically, but laboratory investigation may be of value in atypical cases. However, serology may be difficult to interpret, and invasive investigations such as tissue biopsy are dangerous and difficult. Therapeutic interventions tend to be less effective and are often capable only of disease suppression, necessitating the use of secondary prophylactic or maintenance regimens to prevent disease recurrence (131).

Keratoconjunctivitis sicca, HIV microangiopathy, retinal vasculitis, Reiter's syndrome, and orbital inflammatory syndrome may occur early in the course of HIV infection. In late HIV infection (AIDS), CMV retinitis, Kaposi's sarcoma, and other neoplastic and opportunistic lesions may arise.

HIV has been detected in the conjunctiva, cornea, iris, and retina. It has also been recovered from tears, the aqueous humor, the vitreous body, and the ciliary body. However, no case of HIV transmission as a result of corneal transplantation has been reported to date.

The anterior-segment manifestations of HIV infection are varied (Table 9). HSV-1, HSV-2, and occasionally both simultaneously may cause HSV keratitis. Typical dendritic ulcers may occur, but atypical peripheral corneal lesions are not uncommon. Stromal disease is, however, unusual in HIV infection. Involvement is more likely to be bilateral, multifocal, less responsive to treatment, of longer duration, and more likely to recur than disease in immunocompetent individuals. Recurrent disease may require lifelong maintenance therapy, and resistance to acyclovir may necessitate the use of foscarnet.

Ophthalmic zoster is probably the most common external ocular infection to occur in AIDS. In a young patient with immunodeficiency, a diagnosis of ophthalmic zoster necessitates the exclusion of HIV. Clinically, infections may be similar to those occurring in immunocompetent hosts but tend to be more severe (Fig. 12) and less responsive to treatment with high-dose systemic acyclovir. Ocular complications, including keratitis, uveitis, and retinitis (see below), occur more frequently in HIV-associated disease. Resistance to acyclovir may require treatment with parenteral foscarnet.

HIV-positive patients may also demonstrate asymptomatic abnormalities of the conjunctival vessels. These include microaneurysms, irregular vessel caliber, curved or comma-shaped vascular segments, and a granular appearance of the blood column. Similar appearances are sometimes encountered in sickle cell disease and diabetes. The abnormalities may represent the extraocular equivalent of HIV retinal microangiopathy (see below) and are thought to be associated with elevated levels of blood fibrinogen, which result in vascular sludging, occlusion, and ischemia.

Several disorders associated with HIV infection may manifest in the posterior segment of the eye (Table 10). HIV microangiopathy is the most common form of posterior-segment involvement in AIDS, occurring in 60 to 70% of patients (87). It is usually asymptomatic, although some patients report photopsia and a subjective dimming of vision. HIV microangiopathy can occur in any stage of HIV infection but is more usual in advanced HIV disease. The pathogenesis of HIV microangiopathy is controversial, with direct vascular endothelial infection by HIV, HIV-associated immune-complex deposition (103), opportunistic infectious agents, elevated levels of blood fibrinogen, abnormal polymorphonuclear leukocyte rigidity

TABLE 8 Viral causes of neurologic ocular disease

Virus	Feature(s)
VZV	Optic neuritis, extraocular muscle palsy, internal ophthalmoplegia
Influenza virus	Optic neuritis, extraocular muscle palsy, accommodative abnormalities, mydriasis, papilledema
Measles virus	Optic neuritis, VI nerve palsy, mydriasis, accommodative abnormalities, strabismus, SSPE
Mumps virus	Optic neuritis, extraocular muscle palsy
EBV	Optic neuritis, ophthalmoplegia, nystagmus, accommodative abnormalities
Poliomyelitis virus	Optic neuritis, extraocular muscle palsy
Rabies virus	Extraocular muscle palsy, facial nerve palsy
Polyomaviruses	Progressive multifocal leukoencephalopathy, a diffuse progressive leukoencephalopathy most commonly seen in patients with AIDS. Ocular manifestations of the condition include multiple visual deficits, ocular motility disturbances, nystagmus, and optic neuropathies secondary to CNS disease. There is no effective treatment.
Vaccinia virus	Optic neuritis

TABLE 9 Anterior-segment manifestations of HIV infection

Clinical entity	Comment(s)
Blepharitis	Seborrheic or staphylococcal
Sicca syndrome	Tear deficiency/primary Sjögren's syndrome (lymphocytic infiltration of the lacrimal gland) occurs with increased frequency in HIV
Molluscum contagiosum	Common infection in HIV-positive individuals—atypical/large lesions, widely disseminated. The lesions do not resolve spontaneously, and they often recur and spread.
External ocular infections	Bacterial conjunctivitis, cryptococcal conjunctivitis, chlamydial inclusion disease
Conjunctival microvascular abnormalities	May represent the external counterpart of retinal HIV microangiopathy
Herpes zoster ophthalmicus	Tends to be severe and difficult to treat
Herpes simplex keratitis	Often manifest as peripheral corneal ulcers that may be difficult to treat and recur
Bacterial and fungal keratitis	Although these infections are not common in the HIV-positive community, once established they tend to be particularly severe.
Microsporidiosis	Intracellular parasite may cause a chronic bilateral superficial keratitis and follicular conjunctivitis. Topical treatment with fumigillin may need to be prolonged.
Uveitis	May occur in association with ARN, toxoplasma retinitis, syphilis, fungal infection, or microsporidiosis. CMV may also cause primary infection involving the ciliary body, and HIV itself has been implicated as causing irideocyclitis. Immune dysregulation in early HIV infection may lead to anterior uveitis or Reiter's syndrome, and rifabutin can cause an anterior uveitis/vitritis.
Kaposi's sarcoma	The most common tumor in AIDS patients. May occur on the skin of the eyelids, the conjunctiva, and, rarely, in the orbit. HHV-8[a] is implicated in the pathogenesis. Treatment is by cryotherapy or radiotherapy when symptomatically indicated.
Conjunctival carcinoma	Prevalence increased and more aggressive when associated with HIV
Lymphoma	Malignant large-cell lymphoma occurring in the ocular tissues is usually associated with systemic lymphoma but may occasionally occur as a primary malignancy within the eyelid and orbit and intraocularly.

[a] HHV-8, human herpersvirus 8.

(136), or a combination of these factors cited as possible causes.

Clinical features of HIV microangiopathy fluctuate and consist of peripapillary cotton-wool spots (nerve fiber layer infarcts), microaneurysms and hemorrhages in the posterior pole and periphery (Fig. 13). The capillary damage that results from HIV microangiopathy may provide CMV-infected monocytes direct access to the retina from the bloodstream and may explain both the higher frequency of CMV retinitis in AIDS patients than in immunosuppressed transplant patients and the paravascular location of most areas of CMV retinitis.

Treatment neither exists nor is indicated for HIV microangiopathy, as visual function remains unaffected. Whether antiretroviral therapy has any effect on the appearance of HIV microangiopathy is unclear.

PORN is the most serious of the HIV-related retinal infections. Despite the use of aggressive high-dose therapeutic combinations of systemic and intravitreal antiviral agents, including ganciclovir, foscarnet, and acyclovir (114), the prognosis is poor, with two-thirds of patients losing all vision within 1 month (33). The prognosis is better with intravitreal therapy directed at VZV, together with potent antiretroviral therapy (157), but reactivation after initial control is common (18).

Neuro-ophthalmic manifestations associated with HIV infection are listed in Table 11.

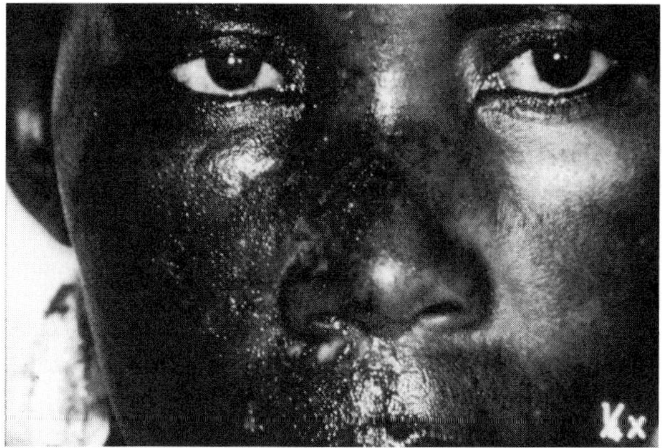

FIGURE 12 Herpes zoster ophthalmicus occurring in a young African patient with HIV infection. (Courtesy of I. Mohammed.)

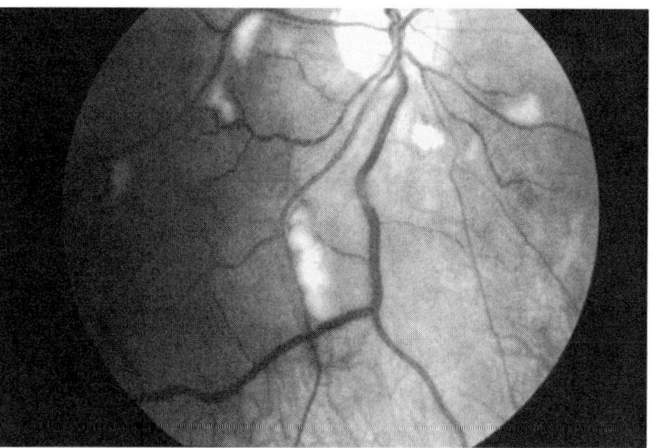

FIGURE 13 HIV microangiopathy showing retinal nerve fiber infarcts.

Viruses Associated with Congenital Ocular Disease (Table 12)

Congenital Rubella

The three most common ocular abnormalities that result from congenital rubella are cataract, infantile glaucoma, and retinopathy. Congenital cataracts or cataracts appearing shortly after birth usually result from infection acquired within the first trimester of pregnancy. They are often associated with other ocular and systemic abnormalities, including microphthalmia, corneal abnormalities, glaucoma, retinopathy, and iris hypoplasia. Cataracts may be bilateral, nuclear (affecting the center of the lens), lamellar (affecting a lamellar shell of lens fibers), or total (throughout all layers of the lens) and may progress to complete opacity. Cataract has also been reported to appear after birth in previously clear lenses, and this together with progression

TABLE 10 Posterior-segment manifestations of HIV infection

Clinical entity	Features
HIV microangiopathy	Cotton-wool spots, retinal hemorrhage (flame or blot), retinal microaneurysms
CMV retinitis	Necrotizing retinitis, "cottage cheese and ketchup fundus" or "pizza fundus"—cheesy necrosis and retinal hemorrhage
ARN	Acute necrotizing retinitis, panuveitis due to HSV or VZV
Progressive outer retinal necrosis	Fulminant outer retinal necrosis; most severe posterior-segment manifestation of HIV
Toxoplasma retinochorioditis	Associated with disseminated disease or CNS disease (50%). Focal retinitis, moderate vitritis, or granulomatous anterior uveitis may be multifocal and bilateral. Not self-limited and requires treatment. Newly acquired or dissemination of latent infection.
Pneumocystis carinii choroidopathy	More common in patients using inhaled PCP[a] prophylaxis. Asymptomatic, multifocal choroidal infiltrates at posterior pole. Implies disseminated infection which requires treatment.
Syphilitic retinitis	Often associated with neurosyphilis. Panuveitis, retinitis, mild to severe vitritis which is often bilateral. Optic disk edema may indicate syphilitic meningitis.
Mycobacterial choroidopathy	Granulomatous uveitis, vitritis, and multifocal choroidal granulomas

[a] PCP, *Pneumocystis carinii* pneumonia.

TABLE 11 Neuro-ophthalmic manifestations associated with HIV infection

Manifestation	Comment(s)
Enhancing cranial-space-occupying lesions[a]	
Opportunistic infections	*Toxoplasma gondii* encephalitis CMV encephalitis Syphilis Mycobacterial encephalitis Cryptococcal meningitis
Malignancy	High-grade B-cell lymphoma—primary tumors manifest as vitritis, while secondary tumors manifest as choroidal lesions.
Progressive multifocal leukoencephalopathy	Diffuse progressive leukoencephalopathy most commonly seen in patients with AIDS. Ocular manifestations of the condition include multiple visual deficits, ocular motility disturbances, nystagmus, and optic neuropathies secondary to CNS disease. There is no effective treatment.
Other neuro-ophthalmic manifestations	Optic neuritis, cranial nerve palsies, and myositis

[a] Lesions apparent upon cranial imaging; may be associated with raised intracranial pressure and optic nerve head swelling or papilledema.

of congenital lenticular opacities probably results from the persistence of live virus within the lens after birth (53). Indeed, rubella virus has been isolated from cataracts and infected brain (21) 12 years after birth. Surgical treatment of the cataract may be required if vision is impaired and is best performed early, particularly in cases of bilateral disease, in an attempt to facilitate visual development.

Infantile glaucoma associated with the congenital rubella syndrome is probably the result of anomalous development of the anterior chamber angle although chronic uveitis and an enlarged cataractous lens may also contribute. Raised intraocular pressure in a child may result not only in damage to the optic nerve but also in enlargement of the entire globe (buphthalmos) (Fig. 14). Surgical intervention to facilitate aqueous egress is often required.

Rubella retinopathy is usually bilateral but can be unilateral and even sectoral. The retinopathy affects the retinal pigment epithelium in isolation, resulting in a fundal appearance described as "salt and pepper," with widespread irregular pigment deposits of variable size most numerous at the macula. Other features include a loss of the foveal reflex and a dust-like stippling of the peripheral retina. Optic atrophy without vascular attenuation has also been reported.

Visual functions, including visual acuity, visual field, and electrophysiology, remain normal or near normal, and fluorescein angiographic appearances are consistent with the pathological changes noted in the retinal pigment epithelium (76). Similar retinal appearances have also been described to result from in utero infection with measles virus, VZV, and influenza virus. Although rubella retinopathy is not usually a cause of poor vision, other rubella-associated ocular abnormalities (cataract, glaucoma, and microphthalmos) may lead to significant visual impairment.

In order to prevent intrauterine infection with rubella virus, the mother must be prevented from acquiring the disease while pregnant. This is best achieved by ensuring that the mother has acquired either natural (previous infection) or artificial (vaccine) active immunity by the time she reaches childbearing age. Immunization programs which achieve long-term protection using strains of live attenuated virus have been implemented throughout the world for this purpose, with a significant reduction in the number of rubella virus-infected children being born.

Congenital CMV

Ocular abnormalities associated with intrauterine CMV infection include chorioretinitis which may be associated

TABLE 12 Viruses associated with congenital ocular disease

Virus	Type of congenital abnormality
CMV	Necrotizing retinitis, cataract, optic atrophy, optic disk and anterior-segment abnormalities
Rubella virus	Pigmentary retinopathy, congenital cataract, congenital glaucoma
VZV	Optic atrophy, chorioretinopathy, congenital cataract, neurologic abnormalities
Measles virus	Pigmentary retinopathy, cataract, macular lesion, dacryostenosis
HSV	Ophthalmia neonatorum, keratitis, chorioretinitis, optic neuritis, cataract, uveitis, microphthalmia
Mumps virus	Cataract, corneal opacity, posterior uveitis, microphthalmos
Influenza virus	Cataract, pigmentary retinopathy

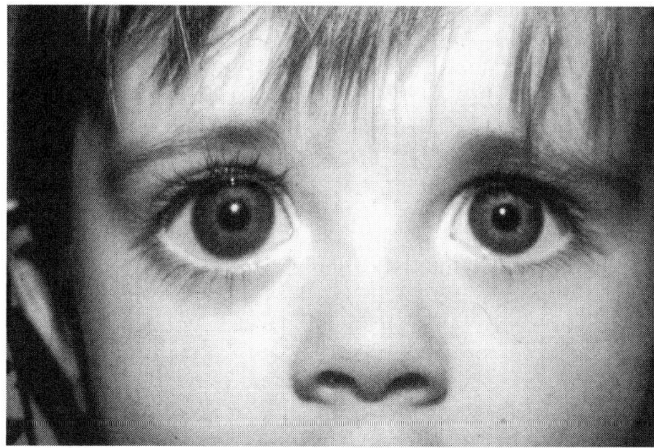

FIGURE 14 Buphthalmos associated with congenital glaucoma with obvious enlargement of both the right and left corneas.

with CMV encephalitis, cataract, retinal necrosis with calcification, optic atrophy, optic-disk and anterior-chamber abnormalities, uveitis, and strabismus.

VZV Infection

The effects of VZV infection occurring during the course of pregnancy were first reported in 1947. Congenital infection has been associated with a wide spectrum of multisystem abnormalities, including optic atrophy, pigmentary retinopathy, nystagmus, abnormal pupillary responses, and cataract.

REFERENCES

1. **Abegg, M., M. Kurz-Levin, and H. Helbig.** 2007. Retinal detachment in patients with acute retinal necrosis: a case series. *Klin. Monatsbl. Augenheilkd.* **224:**360–363.
2. **Aizman, A.** 2006. Treatment of acute retinal necrosis syndrome. *Drugs Today* **42:**545–551.
3. **Aizman, A., M. W. Johnson, and S. G. Elmer.** 2007. Treatment of acute retinal necrosis syndrome with oral antiviral medications. *Ophthalmology* **114:**307–312.
4. **Akula, S. K., P. E. Ma, G. A. Peyman, M. H. Rahimy, N. E. Hyslop, Jr., A. Janney, and P. Ashton.** 1994. Treatment of cytomegalovirus retinitis with intravitreal injection of liposome encapsulated ganciclovir in a patient with AIDS. *Br. J. Ophthalmol.* **78:**677–680.
5. **Anand, R., S. D. Nightingale, R. H Fish, T. J. Smith, and P. Ashton.** 1993. Control of cytomegalovirus retinitis using sustained release of intraocular ganciclovir. *Arch. Ophthalmol.* **111:**223–227.
6. **Beck, R. W., P. A. Asbell, E. J. Cohen, C. R. Dawson, R. A. Hyndiuk, D. B. Jones, H. E. Kaufman, K. E. Kip, N. Kurinij, P. S. Moke, R. D. Stulting, J. Sugar, and K. R. Wilhelimus.** 2000. Oral acyclovir for herpes simplex virus eye disease: effect on prevention of epithelial keratitis and stromal keratitis. *Arch. Ophthalmol.* **118:** 1030–1036.
7. Reference deleted.
8. **Biswas, P. S., and B. T. Rouse.** 2005. Early events in HSV keratitis—setting the stage for a blinding disease. *Microbes Infect.* **7:**799–810.
9. **Blatt, A. N., K. A. Laycock, R. H. Brady, P. Traynor, D. J. Krogstad, and J. S. Pepose.** 1993. Prophylactic acyclovir effectively reduces herpes simplex virus type 1 reactivation after exposure of latently infected mice to ultraviolet B. *Investig. Ophthalmol. Vis. Sci.* **34:**3459–3465.
10. **Bonfioli, A. A., and A. W. Eller.** 2005. Acute retinal necrosis. *Semin. Ophthalmol.* **20:**155–160.
11. **Borruat, F. X., B. Piguet, and C. P. Herbort.** 1998. Acute posterior multifocal placoid pigment epitheliopathy following mumps. *Ocul. Immunol. Inflamm.* **6:**189–193.
12. **Brigden, D., A. Gowle, and A. Rosling.** 1985. Acyclovir, a new antiherpetic drug; early experience in man with systemically administered drug, p. 53. *In* L. H. Collier and J. Oxford (ed.), *Developments in Antiviral Therapy.* Academic Press, London, United Kingdom.
13. **Chaberny, I. E., P. Schnitzler, H. K. Geiss, and C. Wendt.** 2003. An outbreak of epidemic keratoconjunctivitis in a pediatric unit due to adenovirus type 8. *Infect. Control Hosp. Epidemiol* **24:**514–519.
14. **Chang, C. H., M. M. Sheu, K. H. Lin, and C. W. Chen.** 2001. Hemorrhagic viral keratoconjunctivitis in Taiwan caused by adenovirus types 19 and 37: applicability of polymerase chain reaction-restriction fragment length polymorphism in detecting adenovirus genotypes. *Cornea* **20:**295–300.
15. **Chatis, P. A., and C. S. Crumpacker.** 1992. Resistance of herpesviruses to antiviral drugs. *Antimicrob. Agents Chemother.* **36:**1589–1595.
16. **Cheong, I., P. J. Flegg, R. P. Brettle, P. D. Welsby, S. M. Burns, B. Dhillon, C. L. Leen, and J. A. Gray.** 1992. Cytomegalovirus disease in AIDS: the Edinburgh experience. *Int. J. STD AIDS* **3:**324–328.
17. **Cigni, A., G. Soro, R. Faedda, F. Caucci, F. Amadori, A. Manca, F. Tanda, and A. E. Satta.** 2003. A case of adult-onset tubulointerstitial nephritis and uveitis ("TINU syndrome") associated with sacroileitis and Epstein-Barr virus infection with good spontaneous outcome. *Am. J. Kidney Dis.* **42:**E4–E10.
18. **Ciulla, T. A., B. K. Rutledge, M. G. Morley, and J. S. Duker.** 1998. The progressive outer retinal necrosis syndrome: successful treatment with combination antiviral therapy. *Ophthalmic Surg. Lasers* **29:**198–206.
19. **Colin, J., O. Prisant, B. Cochener, O. Lescale, B. Rolland, and T. Hoang-Xuan.** 2000. Comparison of the efficacy and safety of valaciclovir and acyclovir for the treatment of herpes zoster ophthalmicus. *Ophthalmology* **107:**1507–1511.
20. **Cooper, R. J., A. C. Yeo, A. S. Bailey, and A. B. Tullo.** 1999. Adenovirus polymerase chain reaction assay for rapid diagnosis of conjunctivitis. *Investig. Ophthalmol. Vis. Sci.* **40:**90–95.

20a. **Coster, D. L., J. R. McKinnon, and M. C. Falcon.** 1977. Role of debridement in the treatment of herpetic keratitis. *Trans. Ophthalmol. Soc. U.K.* **97:**314–317.

21. **Cremer, N. E., L. S. Oshiro, M. L. Weil, E. H. Lennette, H. H. Itabashi, and L. Carnay.** 1975. Isolation of rubella virus from the brain in chronic progressive panencephalitis. *J. Gen. Virol.* **29:**143–153.
22. **Culbertson, W. W., M. S. Blumenkranz, J. S. Pepose, and V. T. Curtis.** 1986. Varicella zoster virus is a cause of acute retinal necrosis syndrome. *Ophthalmology* **93:** 559–569.
23. **Cvetkovic, R. S., and K. Wellington.** 2005. Valganciclovir: a review of its use in the management of CMV infection and disease in immunocompromised patients. *Drugs* **65:**859–878.
24. **Dalapathy, S., T. K. Lily, and H. N. Madhaven.** 1998. Development and use of nested polymerase chain reaction for detection of adenovirus from conjunctivitis. *J. Clin. Virol.* **11:**77–84.
25. **De Laey, J. J., M. Hanssens, P. Colette, L. Geerts, and H. Priem.** 1983. Subacute sclerosing panencephalitis:

fundus changes and histopathologic correlations. *Doc. Ophthalmol.* **56**(1–2):11–21.
26. **Dhaliwal, D. K., E. G. Romanowski, K. A. Yates, D. Hu, M. Goldstein, and Y. J. Gordon.** 2001. Experimental laser-assisted in situ keratomileusis induces the reactivation of latent herpes simplex virus. *Am. J. Ophthalmol.* **131**:506–507.
27. **Doft, B. H., and J. D. M. Gass.** 1985. Punctate outer retinal toxoplasmosis. *Arch. Ophthalmol.* **103**:1332–1336.
28. **Dong, X., W. Shi, and L. Xie.** 2001. Penetrating keratoplasty in active herpes simplex stromal keratitis. *Zhonghua Yan Ke Za Zhi* **37**:118–120 (In Chinese.)
29. **Dussart, P., G. Cartet, P. Huguet, N. Leveque, C. Hajjar, J. Morvan, J. Vanderkerckhove, K. Ferret, B. Lina, J. J. Chomel, and H Norder.** 2005. Outbreak of acute hemorrhagic conjunctivitis in French Guiana and West Indies caused by coxsackievirus A24 variant: phylogenetic analysis reveals Asian import. *J. Med. Virol.* **75**:559–565.
30. **Easty, D. L., C. Shimeld, C. M. P. Claoué, and M. Menage.** 1987. Herpes simplex virus isolation in chronic stromal keratitis: human and laboratory studies. *Curr. Eye Res.* **6**:69–74.
31. **Easty, D. L.** 1985. The management of herpes simplex keratitis, p. 179–227. *In* D. L. Easty (ed.), *Virus Disease of the Eye.* Lloyd-Luke (Medical Books) Ltd., London, United Kingdom.
32. **Eong, K. G., S. Beatty, and S. J. Charles.** 2000. The changing pattern of cytomegalovirus retinitis in human immunodeficiency virus disease. *Singap. Med. J.* **41**:298–300.
33. **Ergstrom, R. E., Jr., G. N. Holland, T. P. Margolis, C. Muccioli, J. I. Lindley, R. Belfort, Jr., S. P. Holland, W. H. Johnston, R. A. Wolitz, and A. E. Kreiger.** 1994. The progressive outer retinal necrosis syndrome. A variant of necrotising herpetic retinopathy in patients with AIDS. *Ophthalmology* **101**:1488–1502.
34. **Feinberg, A. S., C. W. Spraul, J. T. Holden, and H. E. Grossniklaus.** 2000. Conjunctival lymphocytic infiltrates associated with Epstein-Barr virus. *Ophthalmology* **107**: 159–163.
35. **Fillmore, G. L., T. P. Ward, K. S. Bower, E. J. Dudenhoefer, J. D. Grabenstein, G. K. Berry, and W. P. Madigan, Jr.** 2004. Ocular complications in the Department of Defense Smallpox Vaccination Program. *Ophthalmology* **111**:2086–2093.
36. **Forster, D. J., P. U. Dugel, G. T. Frangieh, P. E. Liggett, and N. A. Rao.** 1990. Rapidly progressive outer retinal necrosis in the acquired immune deficiency syndrome. *Am. J. Ophthalmol.* **110**:341–348.
37. **Freeman, W. R., D. N. Friedberg, C. Berry, J. I. Quiceno, M. Behette, S. C. Fullerton, and D. Munguia.** 1993. Risk factors for development of rhegmatogenous retinal detachment in patients with cytomegalovirus retinitis. *Am. J. Ophthalmol.* **116**:713–720.
38. **Freeman, W. R., D. E. Henderly, W. L. Wan, D. Causey, M. Trousdale, R. L. Green, and N. A. Rao.** 1987. Prevalence, pathophysiology and treatment of retinal detachment in treated cytomegalovirus retinitis. *Am. J. Ophthalmol.* **103**:527–536.
39. **Gangan, P. A., G. Besen, D. Munguia, and W. R. Freeman.** 1994. Macular serous exudation in patients with acquired immune deficiency syndrome and cytomegalovirus retinitis. *Am. J. Ophthalmol.* **118**:212–219.
40. **Garcia, C. R., F. J. Torriani, and W. R. Freeman.** 1998. Cidofovir in the treatment of cytomegalovirus (CMV) retinitis. *Ocul. Immunol. Inflamm.* **6**:195–203.
41. **Goldberg, D. E., L. M. Smithen, A. Angelilli, and W. R. Freeman.** 2005. HIV-associated retinopathy in the HAART era. *Retina* **25**:633–649; quiz, 682–683.
42. **Goldberg, D. E., H. Wang, S. P. Azen, and W. R. Freeman.** 2003. Long term visual outcome of patients with cytomegalovirus retinitis treated with highly active antiretroviral therapy. *Br. J. Ophthalmol.* **87**:853–855.
43. **Gordon, Y. J., E. G. Romanowski, and T. Araullo-Cruz.** 1994 Topical HPMPC inhibits adenovirus type 5 in the New Zealand rabbit ocular replication model. *Investig. Ophthalmol. Vis. Sci.* **35**:4135–4143.
44. **Gordon, Y. J., E. Romanowski, T. Araullo-Cruz, L. Seaberg, S. Erzurum, R. Tolman, and E. De Clercq.** 1991. Inhibitory effect of (S)-HPMPC, (S)-HPMPA, and 2′-nor-cyclic GMP on clinical ocular adenoviral isolates is serotype-dependent in vitro. *Antivir. Res.* **16**:11–16.
45. **Grossniklaus, H. E., K. E. Frank, and R. L. Tomsak.** 1987. Cytomegalovirus retinitis and optic neuritis in aquired immune deficiency syndrome. *Ophthalmology* **94**: 1601–1604.
46. **Gungor, I. U., N. Ariturk, U. Beden, and O. Darka.** 2006. Necrotizing scleritis due to varicella zoster infection: a case report. *Ocul. Immunol. Inflamm.* **14**:317–319.
47. **Hales, R. H., and H. B. Ostler.** 1973. Newcastle disease conjunctivitis with subepithelial infiltrates. *Br. J. Ophthalmol.* **57**:694–697.
48. **Heiligenhaus, A., and K. P. Steuhl.** 1999. Treatment of HSV-1 stromal keratitis with topical cyclosporin A: a pilot study. *Graefe's Arch. Clin. Exp. Ophthalmol.* **237**:435–438.
49. **Henderly, D. E., W. R. Freeman, D. M. Causey, and N. A. Rao.** 1987. Cytomegalovirus retinitis and response to therapy with ganciclovir. *Ophthalmology* **94**:425–434.
50. **Henry, A., H. Cantrill, C. Fletcher, B. J. Chinnock, and H. H. Balfour.** 1987. Use of intravitreal ganciclovir for cytomegalovirus retinitis in a patient with AIDS. *Am. J. Ophthalmol.* **103**:17–23.
51. **Herpetic Eye Disease Study Group.** 1998. Acyclovir for the prevention of recurrent herpes simplex virus eye disease. *N. Engl. J. Med.* **339**:300–306.
52. **Herpetic Eye Disease Study Group.** 2000. Oral acyclovir for herpes simplex virus eye disease: effect on prevention of epithelial keratitis and stromal keratitis. *Arch. Ophthalmol.* **118**:1030–1036.
53. **Hertzberg, R.** 1968. Twenty-five year follow-up of ocular defects in congenital rubella. *Am. J. Ophthalmol.* **66**:269–271.
54. **Hillenkamp, J., T. Reinhard, R. S. Ross, D. Böhringer, O. Cartsburg, M. Roggendorf, E. De Clercq, E. Godehardt, and R. Sundmacher.** 2001. Topical treatment of acute adenoviral keratoconjunctivitis with 0.2% cidofovir and 1% cyclosporine: a controlled clinical pilot study. *Arch. Ophthalmol.* **119**:1487–1491.
55. **Holland, G. N., Y. Sidikaro, A. E. Krieger, D. Hardy, M. J. Sakamoto, L. M. Frenkel, D. J. Winston, M. S. Gottlieb, Y. J. Bryson, and R. E. Champlin.** 1987. Treatment of cytomegalovirus retinopathy with ganciclovir. *Ophthalmology* **94**:815–823.
56. **Holland, G. N.** 2000. New issues in the management of patients with AIDS-related cytomegalovirus retinitis. *Arch. Ophthalmol.* **118**:704–706.
57. **Hosseini, H., and M. R. Khalili.** 2007. Therapeutic potential of bevacizumab (Avastin) in herpetic stromal keratitis (HSK). *Med. Hypotheses* **69**:568–570.
58. **Jabs, D. A., S. G. Bolton, J. P. Dunn, and A. G. Palestine.** 1998. Discontinuing anticytomegalovirus therapy in patients with immune reconstitution after combination antiretroviral therapy. *Am. J. Ophthalmol.* **126**:817–822.
59. **Jabs, D. A., W. R. Green, R. Fox, B. F. Polk, and J. G. Bartlett.** 1989. Ocular manifestations of acquired immune deficiency syndrome. *Ophthalmology* **96**:1092–1099.

60. **Jackson, T. L., W. Meacock, M. Youle, and E. M. Graham.** 2000. Severe intraocular inflammation after a change of potent antiretroviral therapy. *Br. J. Ophthalmol.* **84:**933–934.
61. **Jiang, S. C.** 2006. Human adenoviruses in water: occurrence and health implications: a critical review. *Environ. Sci. Technol.* **40:**7132–7140.
62. **John, J. J., S. Christopher, and J. Abraham.** 1981. Neurological manifestations of acute haemorrhagic conjunctivitis due to enterovirus 70. *Lancet* **ii:**1283–1284.
63. **Karavellas, M. P., C. Y. Lowder, C. Macdonald, C. P. Avila, Jr., and W. R. Freeman.** 1998. Immune recovery vitritis associated with inactive cytomegalovirus retinitis: a new syndrome. *Arch. Ophthalmol.* **116:**169–175.
64. **Karcioglu, Z. A., and T. M. Issa.** 1997. Human papilloma virus in neoplastic and non-neoplastic conditions of the external eye. *Br. J. Ophthalmol.* **81:**595–598.
65. **Kashiwase, M., T. Sata, Y. Yamauchi, H. Minoda, N. Usui, T. Iwasaki, T. Kurata, and M. Usui.** 2000. Progressive outer retinal necrosis caused by herpes simplex virus type 1 in a patient with acquired immunodeficiency syndrome. *Ophthalmology* **107:**790–794.
66. **Kaye, S., and A. Choudhary.** 2006. Herpes simplex keratitis. *Prog. Retin. Eye Res.* **25:**355–380.
67. **Kaye, S., C. Shimeld, E. Grinfeld, N. J. Maitland, T. J. Hill, and D. L. Easty.** 1992. Non-traumatic acquisition of herpes simplex virus infection through the eye. *Br. J. Ophthalmol.* **76:**412–418.
68. **Kaye, S. B., K. Bakere, R. Bonshek, H. Maseruka, E. Grinfeld, A. Tullo, D. L. Easty, and C. A Hart.** 2000. Human herpesviruses in the cornea. *Br. J. Ophthalmol.* **84:**563–571.
69. **Keadle, T. L., N. Usui, K. A. Laycock, J. K. Miller, J. S. Pepose, and P. M. Stuart.** 2000. IL-1 and TNF-α are important factors in the pathogenesis of murine recurrent herpetic stromal keratitis. *Investig. Ophthalmol. Vis. Sci.* **41:**96–102.
70. **Kempen, J. H., D. A. Jabs, L. A. Wilson, J. P. Dunn, S. K. West, and J. A. Tonascia.** 2003. Risk of vision loss in patients with cytomegalovirus retinitis and the acquired immunodeficiency syndrome. *Arch. Ophthalmol.* **121:**466–476.
71. **Kempen, J. H., Y. I. Min, W. R. Freeman, G. N. Holland, D. N. Friedberg, D. T. Dieterich, and D. A. Jabs.** 2006. Risk of immune recovery uveitis in patients with AIDS and cytomegalovirus retinitis. *Ophthalmology* **113:**684–694.
72. **Kirsch, L. S., J. F. Arevalo, E. Chavez de la Paz, D. Munguia, E. De Clercq, and W. R. Freeman.** 1995. Intravitreal cidofovir (HPMPC) treatment of cytomegalovirus retinitis in patients with acquired immunodeficiency syndrome. *Ophthalmology* **102:**533–542.
73. **Kirsch, L. S., J. F. Arevalo, E. De Clercq, E. Chavez de la Paz, D. Munguia, R. Garcia, and W. R. Freeman.** 1995. Phase III study of intravitreal cidofovir for the treatment of cytomegalovirus retinitis in patients with the acquired immune deficiency syndrome. *Am. J. Ophthalmol.* **119:**466–476.
74. **Knox, C. M., D. Chandler, G. A. Short, and T. P. Margolis.** 1998. Polymerase chain reaction-based assays of vitreous samples for the diagnosis of viral retinitis. Use in diagnostic dilemmas. *Ophthalmology* **105:**37–44.
75. **Kowalski, R. P., L. M. Karenchak, E. G. Romanowski, and Y. J. Gordon.** 1999. Evaluation of the shell vial technique for detection of ocular adenovirus. Community Ophthalmologists of Pittsburgh, Pennsylvania. *Ophthalmology* **106:**1324–1327.
76. **Krill, A. E.** 1972. Retinopathy secondary to rubella. *Int. Ophthalmol. Clin.* **12:**89.
77. **Kurokawa, M., S. K. Rai, K. Ono, R. Gurung, and S. Ruit.** 2006. Viral investigation of acute hemorrhagic conjunctivitis outbreak (2003) in Nepal using molecular methods. *Southeast Asian J. Trop. Med. Public Health* **37:**904–910.
78. **Lairson, D. R., C. E. Begley, T. F. Reynolds, and K. R. Wilhelmus.** 2003. Prevention of herpes simplex virus eye disease: a cost-effectiveness analysis. *Arch. Ophthalmol.* **121:**108–112.
79. **Lalezari, J. P., R. J. Stagg, B. D. Kuppermann, G. N. Holland, F. Kramer, D. V. Ives, M. Youle, M. R. Robinson, W. L. Drew, and H. S. Jaffe.** 1997. Intravenous cidofovir for peripheral cytomegalovirus retinitis in patients with AIDS. A randomized, controlled trial. *Ann. Intern. Med.* **126:**257–263.
80. **Langston, D. P.** 1999. Oral acyclovir suppresses recurrent epithelial and stromal herpes simplex. *Arch. Ophthalmol.* **117:**391–392.
81. **Lashkevich, V. A., G. A. Koroleva, A. N. Lukashev, E. V. Denisova, and L. A Katargina.** 2004. Enterovirus uveitis. *Rev. Med. Virol.* **14:**241–254.
82. **Lashkevich, V. A., G. A. Koroleva, A. N. Lukashev, E. V. Denisova, L. A. Katargina, and I. P. Khoroshilova-Maslova.** 2005. Acute enterovirus uveitis in infants. *Vopr. Virusol.* **50:**36–45. (In Russian.)
83. **Lau, C. H., T. Missotten, J. Salzmann, and S. L. Lightman.** 2007. Acute retinal necrosis features, management, and outcomes. *Ophthalmology* **114:**756–762.
84. **Lauer, S. A., J. S. Malter, and J. R. Meier.** 1990. Human papillomavirus type 18 in conjunctival intraepithelial neoplasia. *Am. J. Ophthalmol.* **110:**23–27.
85. **Leahey, A. B., J. J. Shane, A. Listhaus, and M. Trachtman.** 1997. Molluscum contagiosum eyelid lesions as the initial manifestation of acquired immunodeficiency syndrome. *Am. J. Ophthalmol.* **124:**240–241.
86. **LeHoang, P., B. Girard, M. Robinet, P. Marcel, L. Zazoun, S. Matheron, W. Rozenbaum, C. Katlama, I. Morer, and J. O. Lernestedt.** 1989. Foscarnet in the treatment of cytomegalovirus retinitis in acquired immune deficiency syndrome. *Ophthalmology* **96:**865–873; discussion, 873–874.
87. **Lewis, J. M., Y. Nagae, and Y. Tano.** 1996. Progressive outer retinal necrosis after bone marrow transplantation. *Am. J. Ophthalmol.* **122:**892–895.
88. **Lewis, M. L., W. W. Culbertson, J. D. Post, D. Miller, G. T. Kokame, and R. D. Dix.** 1989. Herpes simplex virus type 1. A cause of acute retinal necrosis syndrome. *Ophthalmology* **96:**875–878.
89. **Liesegang, T. J.** 1989. Epidemiology of ocular herpes simplex. Natural history in Rochester, Minn., 1950 through 1982. *Arch. Ophthalmol.* **107:**1160–1165.
90. **Liesegang, T. J.** 1999. Classification of herpes simplex virus keratitis and anterior uveitis. *Cornea* **18:**127–143.
91. **Liesegang, T. J.** 2004. Herpes zoster virus infection. *Curr. Opin. Ophthalmol.* **15:**531–536.
92. **Livir-Rallatos, C., Y. El-Shabrawi, P. Zatirakis, P. E. Pellett, F. R. Stamey, and C. S. Foster.** 1998. Recurrent nodular scleritis associated with varicella zoster virus. *Am. J. Ophthalmol.* **126:**594–597.
93. **MacDonald, J. C., M. P. Karavellas, F. J. Torriani, L. S. Morse, I. L. Smith, J. B. Reed, and W. R. Freeman.** 2000. Highly active antiretroviral therapy-related immune recovery in AIDS patients with cytomegalovirus retinitis. *Ophthalmology* **107:**877–881.
94. **Margolis, R., O. F. Brasil, C. Y. Lowder, S. D. Smith, D. M. Moshfeghi, J. E. Sears, and P. K. Kaiser.** 2007. Multifocal posterior necrotizing retinitis. *Am. J. Ophthalmol.* **143:**1003–1008.

95. **McDonnell, J. M., P. J. McDonnell, and Y. Y. Sunn.** 1992. Human papillomavirus DNA in tissues and ocular surface swabs of patients with conjunctival epithelial neoplasia. *Investig. Ophthalmol. Vis. Sci.* **33:**184–189.

96. **Meadows, K. P., S. K. Tyring, A. T. Pavia, and T. M. Rallis.** 1997. Resolution of recalcitrant molluscum contagiosum virus lesions in human immunodeficiency virus-infected patients treated with cidofovir. *Arch. Dermatol.* **133:**987–990.

97. **Menage, M. J., E. De Clerq, A. van Lierde, V. S. Easty, J. M. Darville, S. D. Cook, and D. L. Easty.** 1990. Antiviral drug sensitivity in ocular herpes simplex virus infection. *Br. J. Ophthalmol.* **74:**532–535.

98. **Mielke, J., M. Grub, N. Freudenthaler, C. M. Deuter, R. Beck, and M. Zierhut.** 2005. Epidemic keratoconjunctivitis. Detecting adenoviruses. *Ophthalmologe* **102:** 968–970. (In German.)

99. **Morishima, N., S. Miyakawa, Y. Akazawa, and S. Takagi.** 1996. A case of uveitis associated with chronic active Epstein-Barr virus infection. *Ophthalmologica* **210:** 186–188.

100. **Nesburn, A. B., S. Slanina, R. L. Burke, H. Ghiasi, S. Bahri, and S. L. Wechsler.** 1998. Local periocular vaccination protects against eye disease more effectively than systemic vaccination following primary ocular herpes simplex virus infection in rabbits. *J. Virol.* **72:**7715–7721.

101. **Nguyen, Q. D., J. H. Kempen, S. G. Bolton, J. P. Dunn, and D. A. Jabs.** 2000. Immune recovery uveitis in patients with AIDS and cytomegalovirus retinitis after highly active antiretroviral therapy. *Am. J. Ophthalmol.* **129:**634–639.

102. **Pavesio, C. E., S. M. Mitchell, K. Barton, S. D. Schwartz, H. M. Towler, and S. Lightman.** 1995. Progressive outer retinal necrosis (PORN) in AIDS patients: a different appearance of varicella-zoster retinitis. *Eye* **9:**271–276.

103. **Pepose, J. S., G. N. Holland, M. S. Nestor, A. J. Cochran, and R. Y. Foos.** 1985. Acquired immune deficiency syndrome. Pathogenic mechanisms of ocular disease. *Ophthalmology* **92:**472–484.

104. **Pepose, J. S., C. Newman, M. C. Bach, T. C. Quinn, R. F. Ambinder, G. N. Holland, P. S. Hodstrom, H. M. Frey, and R. Y. Foos.** 1987. Pathological features of cytomegalovirus retinopathy after treatment with the antiviral agent ganciclovir. *Ophthalmology* **94:**414–424.

105. **Pivetti-Pezzi, P., M. Accorinti, R. A. Colabelli-Gisoldi, M. P. Pirraglia, and M. C. Sirianni.** 1999. Herpes simplex virus vaccine in recurrent herpetic ocular infection. *Cornea* **18:**47–51.

106. **Porter, S. M., A. Patterson, and P. Kho.** 1990. A comparison of local and systemic acyclovir in the management of herpetic disciform keratitis. *Br. J. Ophthalmol.* **74:**283–285.

107. **Purdy, K. W., J. R. Heckenlively, J. A. Church, and M. A. Keller.** 2003. Progressive outer retinal necrosis caused by varicella-zoster virus in children with acquired immunodeficiency syndrome. *Pediatr. Infect. Dis. J.* **22:** 384–386.

108. **Rahhal, F. M., J. F. Arevalo, D. Munguia, I. Taskintuna, E. Chavez de la Paz, S. P. Azen, and W. R. Freeman.** 1996. Intravitreal cidofovir for the maintenance treatment of cytomegalovirus retinitis. *Ophthalmology* **103:**1078–1083.

109. **Rao, S. N.** 2006. Treatment of herpes simplex virus stromal keratitis unresponsive to topical prednisolone 1% with topical cyclosporine 0.05%. *Am. J. Ophthalmol.* **141:**771–772.

110. **Richards, C. M., R. Case, T. R. Hirst, T. J. Hill, and N. A. Williams.** 2003. Protection against recurrent ocular herpes simplex virus type 1 disease after therapeutic vaccination of latently infected mice. *J. Virol.* **77:**6692–6699.

111. **Rodrigues, M. M., A. Palestine, R. Nussenblatt, H. Masur, and A. M. Macher.** 1983. Unilateral cytomegalovirus retinochoroiditis and bilateral cytoid bodies in a bisexual man with the acquired immune deficiency syndrome. *Ophthalmology* **90:**1577–1582.

112. **Romanowski, E. G., and Y. J. Gordon.** 2000. Efficacy of topical cidofovir on multiple adenoviral serotypes in the New Zealand rabbit ocular model. *Investig. Ophthalmol. Vis. Sci.* **41:**460–463.

113. **Romanowski, E. G., K. A. Yates, and Y. J. Gordon.** 2002. Topical corticosteroids of limited potency promote adenovirus replication in the Ad5/NZW rabbit ocular model. *Cornea* **21:**289–291.

114. **Rosenthal, G., K. U. Bartz-Schmidt, P. Walter, B. Kirchhof, and K. Heimann.** 1998. Failure of sorivudine therapy in progressive outer retinal necrosis caused by varicella zoster virus. *Aust. N. Z. J. Ophthalmol.* **26:**327–328.

115. **Sajjadi, H., and M. Parvin.** 1994. A case of severe symptomatic superficial keratitis associated with Epstein-Barr virus. *Eye* **8:**362–364.

116. **Sandy, C. J., P. A. Bloom, E. M. Graham, J. D. Ferris, S. M. Shah, W. E. Schulenburg, and C. S. Migdal.** 1995. Retinal detachment in AIDS related cytomegalovirus retinitis. *Eye* **9:**277–281.

117. **Serdaroglu, A., K. Gucuyener, I. Dursun, K. Aydin, C. Okuyaz, M. Subasi, M. Or, and B. Ozkan.** 2005. Macular retinitis as a first sign of subacute sclerosing panencephalitis: the importance of early diagnosis. *Ocul. Immunol. Inflamm.* **13:**405–410.

118. **Severin, M., and C. Hartmann.** 1988. Endothelial alteration in AIDS with cytomegalovirus infection. *Ophthalmologica* **196:**7–10.

119. **Shimeld, C., D. L. Easty, and T. J. Hill.** 1999. Reactivation of herpes simplex virus type 1 in the mouse trigeminal ganglion: an in vivo study of virus antigen and cytokines. *J. Virol.* **73:**1767–1773.

120. **Shimeld, C., A. B. Tullo, T. J. Hill, and W. A. Blyth.** 1984. Spread of herpes simplex virus to the eye following cutaneous inoculation in the skin of the snout of the mouse, p. 39. *In* P. C. Maudgal and L. Misotten (ed.), *Herpetic Eye Diseases*. Dr. W. Junk, Dordrecht, The Netherlands.

121. **Shimeld, C., T. J. Hill, W. A. Blyth, and D. L. Easty.** 1989. An improved model of recurrent herpetic eye disease in mice. *Curr. Eye Res.* **8:**1193–1205.

122. **Shimeld, C., T. J. Hill, W. A. Blyth, and D. L. Easty.** 1990. Passive immunization protects the mouse eye from damage after herpes simplex virus infection by limiting spread of virus in the nervous system. *J. Gen. Virol.* **71**(Pt. 3):681–687.

123. **Shimeld, C., T. J. Hill, W. A. Blyth, and D. L. Easty.** 1990. Reactivation of latent infection and induction of recurrent herpetic eye disease in mice. *J. Gen. Virol.* **71**(Pt. 2):397–404.

124. **Shimeld, C., A. B. Tullo, D. L. Easty, and J. Thomsitt.** 1981. Isolation of herpes simplex virus from the cornea in chronic stromal keratitis. *Br. J. Ophthalmol.* **66:**643–647.

125. **Shimeld, C., J. L. Whiteland, N. A. Williams, D. L. Easty, and T. J. Hill.** 1996. Reactivation of herpes simplex virus type 1 in the mouse trigeminal ganglion: an in vivo study of virus antigen and immune cell infiltration. *J. Gen. Virol.* **77:**2583–2590.

126. **Simon, A. L., and D. Pavan-Langston.** 1996. Long-term oral acyclovir therapy. Effect on recurrent infectious herpes simplex keratitis in patients with and without grafts. *Ophthalmology* **103:**1399–1404.
127. **Slobod, K. S., J. T. Sandlund, P. H. Spiegel, B. Haik, J. L. Hurwitz, M. E. Conley, L. C. Bowman, E. Benaim, J. J. Jenkins, R. M Stocks, Y. Gan, and J. W. Sixbey.** 2000. Molecular evidence of ocular Epstein-Barr virus infection. *Clin. Infect. Dis.* **31:**184–188.
128. **Stumpf, T. H., C. Shimeld, D. L. Easty, and T. J. Hill.** 2001. Cytokine production in a murine model of recurrent herpetic stromal keratitis. *Investig. Ophthalmol. Vis. Sci.* **42:**372–378.
129. **Sudesh, S., and P. R. Laibson.** 1999. The impact of the herpetic eye disease studies on the management of herpes simplex virus ocular infections. *Curr. Opin. Ophthalmol.* **10:**230–233.
130. **Takeuchi, S., N. Itoh, E. Uchio, K. Aoki, and S. Ohno.** 1999. Serotyping of adenoviruses on conjunctival scrapings by PCR and sequence analysis. *J. Clin. Microbiol.* **37:**1839–1845.
131. **Tantisiriwat, W., and W. G. Powderly.** 2000. Prophylaxis of opportunistic infections. *Infect. Dis. Clin. N. Am.* **14:**929–944.
132. **Taskintuna, I., F. M. Rahhal, N. A. Rao, C. A. Wiley, A. J. Mueller, A. S. Banker, E. De Clercq, J. F. Arevalo, and W. R. Freeman.** 1997. Adverse events and autopsy findings after intravitreous cidofovir (HPMPC) therapy in patients with acquired immune deficiency syndrome (AIDS). *Ophthalmology* **104:**1827–1836.
133. **Teich, S. A., T. W. Cheung, and A. H. Friedman.** 1992. Systemic antiviral drugs used in ophthalmology. *Surv. Ophthalmol.* **37:**19–53.
134. **Titiyal, J. S., N. Pal, G. V. Murthy, S. K. Gupta, R. Tandon, R. B. Vajpayee, and C. Gilbert.** 2003. Causes and temporal trends of blindness and severe visual impairment in children in schools for the blind in North India. *Br. J. Ophthalmol.* **87:**941–945.
135. **Tsubota, K., S. Nishimura, I. Kudo, I. Saito, and I. Moro.** 1991. Detection of Epstein-Barr virus in dry eyes with Sjogren syndrome. *Jpn. J. Clin. Ophthalmol.* **45:** 1611–1613.
136. **Tufail, A., G. N. Holland, T. C. Fisher, W. G. Cumberland, and H. J. Meiselman.** 2000. Increased polymorphonuclear leucocyte rigidity in HIV infected individuals. *Br. J. Ophthalmol.* **84:**727–731.
137. **Tugal-Tutkun, I., N. Kir, A. Gul, M. Konice, and M. Urgancioglu.** 2000. Cytomegalovirus retinitis in a patient with Wegener's granulomatosis. *Ophthalmologica* **214:**149–152.
138. **Tullo, A. B., D. L. Easty, T. J. Hill, and W. A. Blyth.** 1982. Ocular herpes simplex and the establishment of latent infection. *Trans. Ophthalmol. Soc. U.K.* **102**(Pt. 1)**:**15–18.
139. **Tullo, A. B., and P. G. Higgins.** 1980. An outbreak of adenovirus type 4 conjunctivitis. *Br. J. Ophthalmol.* **64:** 489–493.
140. **Tullo, A. B., C. Shimeld, W. A. Blyth, T. J. Hill, and D. L. Easty.** 1982. Spread of virus and distribution of latent infection following ocular herpes simplex in the non-immune and immune mouse. *J. Gen. Virol.* **63**(Pt. 1)**:**95–101.
141. **Tyring, S., R. A. Barbarash, J. E. Nahlik, A. Cunningham, J. Marley, M. Heng, T. Jones, T. Rea, R. Boon, and R. Saltzman.** 1995. Famciclovir for the treatment of acute herpes zoster: effects on acute disease and postherpetic neuralgia. *Ann. Intern. Med.* **123:**89–96.
142. **Uchio, E.** 2005. New medical treatment for viral conjunctivitis. *Nippon Ganka Gakkai Zasshi* **109:**962–984; discussion, 985. (In Japanese.)
143. **Uchio, E., S. Takeuchi, N. Itoh, N. Matsuura, S. Ohno, and K. Aoki.** 2000. Clinical and epidemiological features of acute follicular conjunctivitis with special reference to that caused by herpes simplex virus type 1. *Br. J. Ophthalmol.* **84:**968–972.
144. Reference deleted.
145. **Uchio, E., K. Yamazaki, K. Aoki, and S. Ohno.** 1996. Detection of enterovirus 70 by polymerase chain reaction in acute hemorrhagic conjunctivitis. *Am. J. Ophthalmol.* **122:**273–275.
146. **Vajpayee, R. B., N. Sharma, M. Chand, G. C. Tabin, M. Vajpayee, and J. R. Anand.** 1998. Corneal superinfection in acute hemorrhagic conjunctivitis. *Cornea* **17:**614–617.
147. **Viswalingam, N. D.** 1993. Adenovirus keratoconjunctivitis: an enigma. *Eye Suppl.* **7**(Suppl. 3)**:**5–7.
148. **Wander, A. H., Y. M. Centifanto, and H. E. Kaufman.** 1980. Strain specificity of clinical isolates of herpes simplex virus. *Arch. Ophthalmol.* **98:**1458–1461.
149. **Wellings, C., P. N. Awdry, F. H. Bors, B. R. Jones, D. C. Brown, and H. E. Kaufman.** 1972. Clinical evaluation of trifluorothymidine in the treatment of herpes simplex corneal ulcers. *Am. J. Ophthalmol.* **73:**932–942.
150. **Wenkel, H., C. Rummelt, B. Fleckenstein, and G. O. Naumann.** 1993. Detection of varicella zoster virus DNA and viral antigen in human cornea after herpes zoster ophthalmicus. *Cornea* **12:**131–137.
151. **Whitcup, S. M., E. Fortin, A. S. Lindblad, P. Griffiths, J. A. Metcalf, M. R. Robinson, J. Manischewitz, B. Baird, C. Perry, I. M. Kidd, T. Vrabec, R. T. Davey, Jr., J. Falloon, R. E. Walker, J. A. Kovacs, H. C. Lane, R. B. Nussenblatt, J. Smith, H. Masur, and M. A. Polis.** 1999. Discontinuation of anticytomegalovirus therapy in patients with HIV infection and cytomegalovirus retinitis. *JAMA* **282:**1633–1637.
152. **Whitcup, S. M.** 2000. Cytomegalovirus retinitis in the era of highly active antiretroviral therapy. *JAMA* **283:** 653–657.
153. **Wilhelmus, K.** 2007. Therapeutic interventions for herpes simplex virus epithelial keratitis. *Cochrane Database Systematic Reviews* CD002898.
154. **Wilhelmus, K. R.** 2000. The treatment of herpes simplex virus epithelial keratitis. *Trans. Am. Ophthalmol. Soc.* **98:**505–532.
155. **Williamson, J. C., S. R. Virata, R. H. Raasch, and J. A. Kylstra.** 2000. Oxacillin-resistant Staphylococcus aureus endophthalmitis after ganciclovir intraocular implant. *Am. J. Ophthalmol.* **129:**554–555.
156. **Willoughby, C. E., K. Baker, S. B. Kaye, P. Carey, N. O'Donnell, A. Field, L. Longman, R. Bucknall, and C. A. Hart.** 2002. Epstein-Barr virus (types 1 and 2) in the tear film in Sjogren's syndrome and HIV infection. *J. Med. Virol.* **68:**378–383.
157. **Yin, P. D., S. K. Kurup, S. H. Fischer, H. H. Rhee, G. A. Byrnes, G. A. Levy-Clarke, R. R. Buggage, R. B. Nussenblatt, J. M. Mican, and M. E. Wright.** 2007. Progressive outer retinal necrosis in the era of highly active antiretroviral therapy: successful management with intravitreal injections and monitoring with quantitative PCR. *J. Clin. Virol.* **38:**254–259.
158. **Young, S., P. McCluskey, D. C. Minassian, P. Joblin, C. Jones, M. T. Coroneo, and S. Lightman.** 2003. Retinal detachment in cytomegalovirus retinitis: intravenous versus intravitreal therapy. *Clin. Exp. Ophthalmol.* **31:**96–102.
159. **Young, S., N. Morlet, G. Besen, C. A. Wiley, P. Jones, J. Gold, Y. Li, W. R. Freeman, and M. T. Coroneo.** 1998. High-dose (2000-microgram) intravitreous ganci-

clovir in the treatment of cytomegalovirus retinitis. *Ophthalmology* **105:**1404–1410.

160. **Zaal, M. J., H. J. Völker-Dieben, and J. D'Amaro.** 2000. Risk and prognostic factors of postherpetic neuralgia and focal sensory denervation: a prospective evaluation in acute herpes zoster ophthalmicus. *Clin. J. Pain* **16:**345–351.

161. **Zhang, W., T. Suzuki, A. Shiraishi, I. Shimamura, Y. Inoue, and Y. Ohashi.** 2007. Dendritic keratitis caused by an acyclovir-resistant herpes simplex virus with frameshift mutation. *Cornea* **26:**105–106.

162. **Zheng, X.** 2002. Reactivation and donor-host transmission of herpes simplex virus after corneal transplantation. *Cornea* **21**(7 Suppl.)**:**S90–S93.

Antiretroviral Agents

MAGDALENA E. SOBIESZCZYK, BARBARA S. TAYLOR, AND SCOTT M. HAMMER

11

In 1987, zidovudine became the first approved agent in the United States for the treatment of human immunodeficiency virus type 1 (HIV-1) infection. Two decades later, 24 additional agents in six drug classes had been approved. These include nucleoside analog reverse transcriptase inhibitors (NRTIs), a nucleotide analog reverse transcriptase inhibitor, nonnucleoside reverse transcriptase inhibitors (NNRTIs), protease inhibitors (PIs), entry inhibitors, and an integrase inhibitor (Table 1). This success is the result of a prodigious effort to dissect the virus' life cycle and the virion's interaction with its major target cell, the $CD4^+$ T lymphocyte, to identify promising drug targets. It also illustrates the interdependency of the drug development process, knowledge of disease pathogenesis, and use of sensitive monitoring tools available like plasma HIV-1 RNA and drug resistance testing. This chapter describes the major characteristics of antiretroviral agents that are currently approved, or at a promising stage of development, and is organized according to the virus' replication cycle (Fig. 1). This chapter complements chapter 33, which discusses the virologic and clinical aspects of HIV disease and in which the principles of antiretroviral treatment and the prevention of resistance are discussed.

HIV-1 ENTRY INHIBITORS

HIV cell entry is characterized by a series of complex virus-host cell interactions that are each a potential site for inhibition. HIV entry into the CD4 cell requires nonspecific interactions with the cell surface heparin sulfates, followed by highly specific binding to the CD4 receptor and CXCR4/CCR5 coreceptor, leading to conformational change in the envelope transmembrane subunit, and, finally, virus-host cell membrane fusion (43, 158, 243). Currently, two approved drugs, and several others in clinical development, target either the viral attachment or subsequent fusion (Fig. 1). Selected investigational agents are summarized in Table 2.

Enfuvirtide

Enfuvirtide (Fuzeon, T-20; formerly DP-178, pentafuside) is a membrane fusion inhibitor that interferes with HIV gp41 protein-mediated virus-cell fusion (Fig. 1 and 2). The agent is a 36-amino-acid synthetic peptide that is derived from the second heptad repeat (HR2) of HIV-1 gp41. This molecule interacts with sequences within the first heptad repeat (HR1) of the prehairpin intermediate, thereby perturbing the transition of gp41 into an active state (49, 158).

Spectrum of Activity

Enfuvirtide 50% inhibitory concentrations (IC_{50}s) were initially reported to vary with the coreceptor specificity of an HIV-1 isolate. The IC_{50}s for R5 clinical isolates are 0.2 to 0.8 $\log_{10}$ unit higher than those for a corresponding X4 virus (49); the median IC_{50} is 1.7 ng/ml for wild-type strains. Enfuvirtide inhibits a broad range of non-clade B viruses and strains resistant to other classes of antiretroviral agents but has no activity against HIV-2. It exhibits additive to synergistic activity when combined with members of other antiretroviral drug classes. Although enfuvirtide is a gp41 derivative, its pharmacokinetics and antiviral effects are not affected by preexisting anti-gp41 antibodies.

Pharmacology

The low oral bioavailability of enfuvirtide necessitates parenteral administration of this agent. It is available in powder form and must be reconstituted with sterile water prior to administration by subcutaneous injection. The bioavailability of the 90-mg dose is about 84%. The current dosage in adults is 90 mg twice daily (b.i.d.). The median steady-state trough level with a 100-mg dose was 1.02 μg/ml. Following a single 90-mg subcutaneous dose of the drug, the mean elimination half-life ($t_{1/2}$) is 3.8 h (1.8 h after intravenous dosing). The drug is approximately 92% protein bound. No dose adjustments are required in hepatic or renal impairment.

Drug Interactions

Enfuvirtide is not an inhibitor of cytochrome P450 (CYP450) enzymes. No clinically significant interactions with other antiretroviral agents have been identified to date.

Adverse Effects

Adverse effects include local inflammation around the infusion or injection site, which may be related to its ability to function as a phagocyte chemoattractant and a chemotactic agonist via the phagocyte *N*-formylpeptide receptor (89). Painful, erythematous, indurated nodules have

TABLE 1 Antiviral agents: indications and dosing regimens

Antiretroviral agent (year approved)	Indication	Standard dosing[a]
Entry inhibitors		
Enfuvirtide (2003)	HIV-1 and HIV-2 infections	90 mg (1 ml) s.c. b.i.d.
Maraviroc (2007)	HIV-1 and HIV-2 infections	Dose depends on whether interacting medications are taken concurrently: 150 mg p.o. b.i.d. with CYP3A inhibitors; 600 mg p.o. b.i.d. with CYP3A inducers; 300 mg p.o. b.i.d. with all NRTIs, nevirapine, tipranavir, and enfuvirtide
NRTIs		
Zidovudine (1987)	HIV-1 and HIV-2 infections	200 mg p.o. t.i.d. *or* 300 mg p.o. b.i.d.
Didanosine (1991)	HIV-1 and HIV-2 infections	Tablet formulation ≥60 kg, 200 mg p.o. b.i.d. or 400 mg p.o. q.d. <60 kg, 125 mg p.o. b.i.d. or 250 mg p.o. q.d. Powder formulation ≥60 kg, 250 mg p.o. b.i.d. <60 kg, 167 mg p.o. b.i.d. Delayed-release capsule (enteric coated) ≥60 kg, 400 mg p.o. q.d. <60 kg, 250 mg p.o. q.d. Dosing adjustment with tenofovir: ≥60 kg, 250 mg p.o. q.d. <60 kg, appropriate dose not established, probably <250 mg/day
Zalcitabine (1992) (discontinued by manufacturer in 2006)	HIV-1 and HIV-2 infections	0.75 mg p.o. t.i.d.
Stavudine (1994)	HIV-1 and HIV-2 infections	≥60 kg, 40 mg p.o. b.i.d. <60 kg, 30 mg p.o. b.i.d.
Lamivudine (1995)	HIV-1 and HIV-2 infections (also used for treatment of chronic HBV infections; see chapter 12, Table 1)	150 mg p.o. b.i.d. or 300 mg q.d.
Abacavir (1998)	HIV-1 and HIV-2 infections	300 mg p.o. b.i.d. or 600 mg q.d.
Emtricitabine (2003)	HIV-1 and HIV-2 infections	200 mg p.o. q.d. or 240 mg (24 ml) of oral solution q.d.
Nucleotide analog reverse transcriptase inhibitor		
Tenofovir (2001)		300 mg p.o. q.d.
NRTIs		
Nevirapine (1996)	HIV-1 infections	200 mg p.o. q.d. for 2 wks, then 200 mg p.o. b.i.d.
Efavirenz (1998)	HIV-1 infections	600 mg q.h.s. on an empty stomach
Delavirdine (1997)	HIV-1 infections	400 mg p.o. t.i.d.; separate administration of didanosine or antacids by 1 h
Etravirine (2008)	HIV-1 infections	200 mg p.o. b.i.d.
Integrase inhibitor		
Raltegravir (2007)	HIV-1 and HIV-2 infections	400 mg p.o. b.i.d.
HIV PIs		
Saquinavir, hard-gelatin capsule (1996)	HIV-1 and HIV-2 infections	600 mg p.o. t.i.d.
Saquinavir, soft-gelatin capsule (discontinued distribution in 2006)	HIV-1 and HIV-2 infections	1,200 mg p.o. t.i.d.; with ritonavir at 1,000 mg b.i.d.
Indinavir (1996)	HIV-1 and HIV-2 infections	800 mg p.o. t.i.d.; with ritonavir at 800 mg b.i.d.
Ritonavir (1996)	HIV-1 and HIV-2 infections	600 mg p.o. b.i.d.; 100–400 mg/day as a pharmacokinetic booster for other PIs
Nelfinavir (1997)	HIV-1 and HIV-2 infections	750 mg p.o. t.i.d. or 1,250 mg b.i.d.

(Continued on next page)

TABLE 1 *(Continued)*

Antiretroviral agent (year approved)	Indication	Standard dosing[a]
Amprenavir (1999) (discontinued by manufacturer in 2007)	HIV-1 and HIV-2 infections	See Fosamprenavir
Fosamprenavir (2003)	HIV-1 and HIV-2 infections	1,400 mg p.o. b.i.d. *or* 1,400 mg p.o. q.d. + ritonavir at 200 mg p.o. q.d. *or* 1,400 mg p.o. q.d. + ritonavir at 100 mg p.o. q.d. *or* 700 mg p.o. b.i.d. + ritonavir at 100 mg p.o. b.i.d.
Lopinavir-ritonavir (2000)	HIV-1 and HIV-2 infections	400 mg/100 mg p.o. b.i.d.
Tipranavir (2005)	HIV-1 and HIV-2 infections	500 mg p.o. b.i.d.
Atazanavir (2003)	HIV-1 and HIV-2 infections	400 mg p.o. q.d.
Darunavir (2006)	HIV-1 and HIV-2 infections	600 mg p.o. b.i.d.

[a] s.c., subcutaneously; p.o., per os; t.i.d., three times a day; q.d., once a day; q.h.s., every night.

been reported to occur in up to 98% of individuals participating in clinical studies, but this uncommonly (7% of subjects) led to drug discontinuation or local infection (1.7%). The majority of individuals experience their first injection site reaction during the first week of treatment. Bacterial pneumonia occurs with greater frequency among patients on enfuvirtide. Risk factors for pneumonia included low initial $CD4^+$ cell count, high initial viral load, intravenous drug use, smoking, and a history of lung disease (229). Laboratory abnormalities include development of eosinophilia.

Resistance

Resistance to enfuvirtide in vitro is associated primarily with amino acid substitutions in positions 36 to 43 within the HR1 target domain of gp41 (110). These changes confer alterations in HR1 binding affinities and corresponding changes, up to 34-fold, in the IC_{50} (224). Enfuvirtide has a low genetic barrier to resistance, and resistant variants appear within 2 to 4 weeks during monotherapy. In patients with early treatment failure, the most common mutations are G36E/D/S and V38A/G/M; mutations at codons 40 (Q40H) and 43 (N43D) seem to emerge more slowly than mutations at codons 36 and 38 (142). These findings highlight the importance of combining enfuvirtide with other active agents to ensure the probability of virologic suppression. In growth competition assays, enfuvirtide-resistant isolates containing I37T, V38M, or G36S/V38M HR1 domain mutations appear to be less fit. The N43D single mutation confers decreased fitness for which the E137K mutation can compensate.

These mutations in the envelope gene do not appear to diminish the susceptibility of HIV-1 to other classes of viral entry inhibitors, including coreceptor (CCR5 and

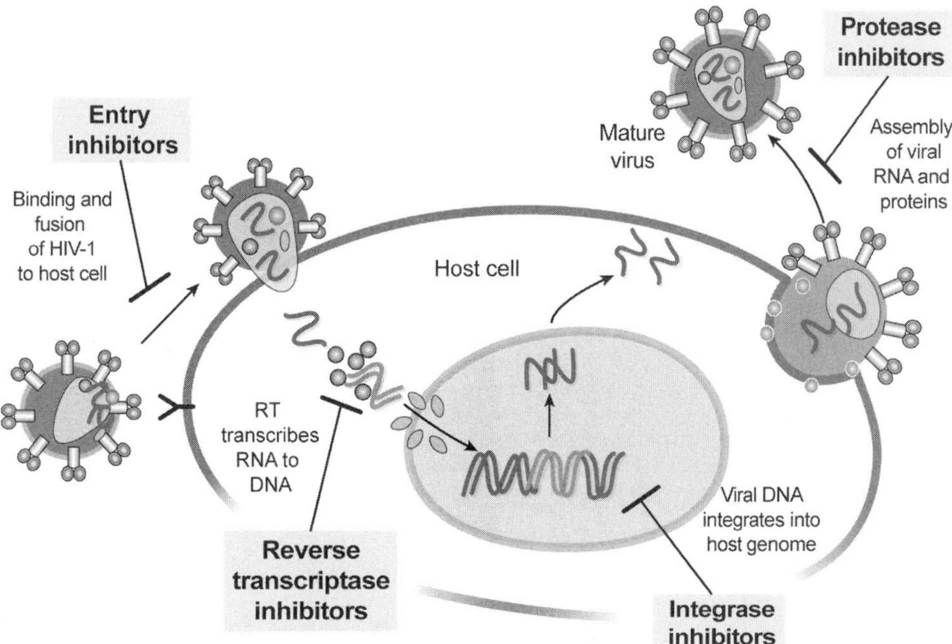

FIGURE 1 Replication cycle of HIV-1 with current targets for antiretroviral therapy. (Adapted from reference 50a with permission [http://clinicaloptions.com/hiventry].)

TABLE 2 Selected investigational agents

Agent	Mechanism of action	Study phase	Comments
TNX-355	Entry inhibitor; anti-CD4 monoclonal Ab[a]	II	IC_{50} of 0.0004–0.152 mg/ml for HIV-1. In a phase II trial of treatment-experienced HIV-1 patients failing therapy, TNX-355 in combination with an optimized background resulted in 48-wk viral load reductions of 0.96 and 0.7 log at 10 and 15 mg/kg intravenously every 2 wks (vs 0.14 log for placebo). A viral load reduction of >1 log was achieved in 39% at a lower dose, vs 11% in the placebo arm.
HGS004	Entry inhibitor; monoclonal Ab to CCR5 blocker	I	In a phase I trial, dose escalation resulted in a viral load reduction of ≥1 log with concurrent increases in CD4 cell counts. Two events of moderately severe transient infusion-related rash occurred at a dose of 2 mg/kg. At >8 mg/kg, there was a CCR5 receptor occupancy of >80% from days 14–28.
PRO 140	Fusion inhibitor	II	Acts synergistically with enfuvirtide. In a dose escalation phase I trial, well tolerated at doses of 0.1–5.0 mg/kg. At 60 days after administration, binding of PRO 140 to CCR5-expressing cells was detected for the highest dose. Ongoing phase Ib trial in HIV patients.
SPO1A	Entry inhibitor	II	
TAK 652	Entry inhibitor; CCR5 blocker	I	
Apricitabine (AVX-754, formerly SPD754)	Reverse transcriptase inhibitor	II	Active against M184V-, L74V-, and K103N-harboring viruses; dose-dependent median plasma HIV-1 RNA reduction of 1.18 to 1.58 log_{10}; compared to lamivudine in treatment-experienced patients with M184V mutation, demonstrated greater reductions in plasma HIV-1 RNA levels; lamivudine or emtricitabine may cause reduced intracellular phosphorylation of apricitabine and diminished antiviral activity
Racivir	Reverse transcriptase inhibitor	II	50:50 racemic mixture of the (−)-β-enantiomers and (+)-β-enantiomers of emtricitabine; pharmacokinetic profile supports once-daily dosing; well tolerated; in treatment-naïve patients, racivir in combination with stavudine and efavirenz results in mean HIV-1 RNA reduction of up to 2.43 log_{10}
Elvucitabine (ACH-126,443)	Reverse transcriptase inhibitor	II	Excellent oral bioavailability and a $t_{1/2}$ of >100 h; at doses of 5–10 mg once daily or 20 mg b.i.d. in combination with lopinavir-ritonavir, decreased HIV-1 RNA levels up to 2.0 log_{10}; doses of >50 mg resulted in reversible bone marrow suppression and decline in CD4 cell counts in several patients
MIV-210	Reverse transcriptase inhibitor	I	Oral bioavailability, >80%
Stampidine	Reverse transcriptase inhibitor	Preclinical	
4′E-d2-FA	Reverse transcriptase inhibitor	Preclinical	

IDX12899 IDX12989	Reverse transcriptase inhibitor	II	Animal data support once-daily dosing; longer time for development of resistance to both compounds than to efavirenz in serial-passage studies
RDEA427	Reverse transcriptase inhibitor	Preclinical	
RDEA806	Reverse transcriptase inhibitor	II	
BILR 355 BS	Reverse transcriptase inhibitor	IIa	50% effective concentrations of 0.25 nM (wild-type virus) to 13 nM; requires ritonavir boosting
R1206	Reverse transcriptase inhibitor	Preclinical	
UK-453,061	Reverse transcriptase inhibitor	II	IC_{90} averages 12 nM; binds both wild-type and K103N reverse transcriptase mutants by inducing conformational changes in tyrosine residues 181 and 188 that are different from those observed with other NNRTIs. After 7 days of monotherapy, viral load was reduced by up to 2 $\log_{10}$ at the highest doses (750 mg once daily or 500 mg b.i.d.) compared to placebo; no evidence of CNS side effects emerged during the first week of treatment.
GSK364735	Integrase inhibitor	I	IC_{50} of 1.2 nM in vitro; well absorbed after oral dose; C_{max} reached 0.75 to 5.0 h after dose
MK-2048	Integrase inhibitor	Preclinical	IC_{95} of 41 nM in 50% normal human serum
GSK364735 (GRZ105655)	Integrase inhibitor	II	Protein-adjusted IC_{50} of 42 nM. The compound was safe and well tolerated in healthy subjects; the most common adverse effects were dizziness and headache.
Elvitegravir (GS-9137, JTK-303)	Integrase inhibitor	II	IC_{50} of 16 nM for HIV-1; ≥1.0 $\log_{10}$ reduction of HIV-1 RNA in a 10-day monotherapy study
GS-8374	PI	Preclinical	Mean IC_{50} change of 6.2-fold
PPL-100	PI	I	Prodrug is phosphorylated to active drug, PL-100; long $t_{1/2}$ supports development as a once-a-day drug. Demonstrated high genetic barrier to resistance.
Bevirimat (PA457)	Maturation inhibitor	IIb	Well absorbed; long $t_{1/2}$ (60–80 h); hepatic clearance; phase I/IIa clinical trials demonstrate reductions of up to 0.72 $\log_{10}$ HIV RNA copy/ml after a single dose of 75, 150, or 250 mg; the greatest mean reduction in viral load occurred at higher doses of the drug. Preliminary results of a 14-day monotherapy study demonstrate that 34% of individuals achieved a viral load reduction of 1.42 $\log_{10}$ HIV-1 RNA.

Enfuvirtide

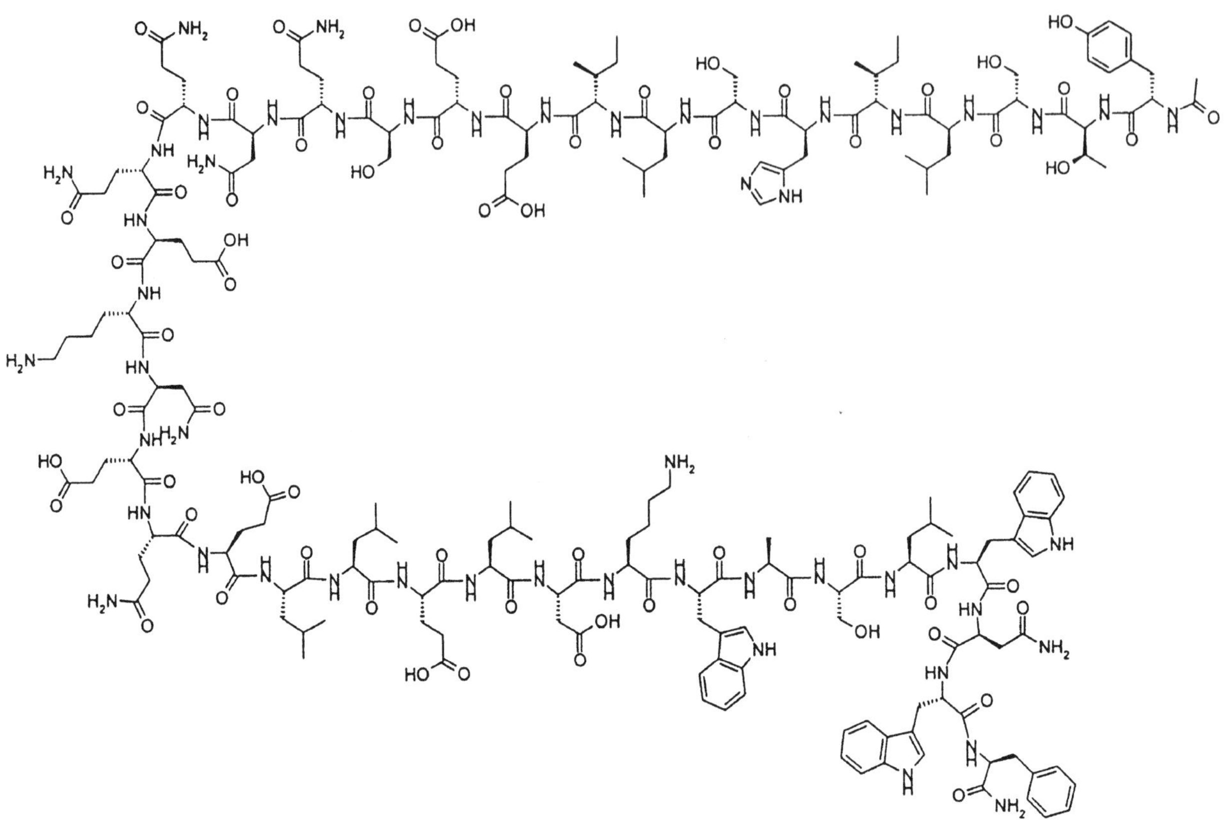

Maraviroc

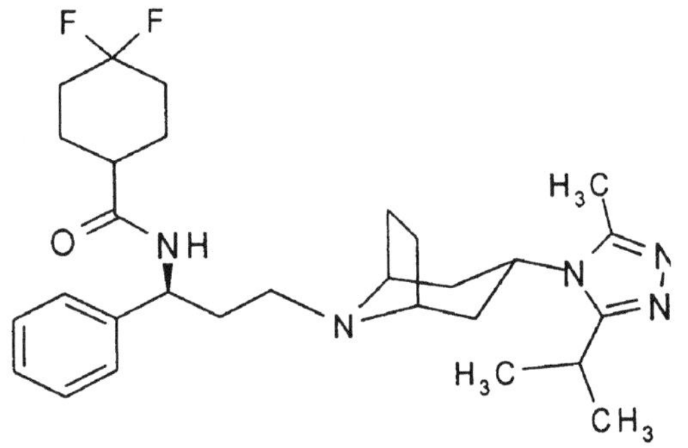

FIGURE 2 Chemical structures of entry inhibitors.

CXCR4) antagonists (192). In patients with virologic failure, changes other than those described for the HR1 region may contribute to the poor response (193), like mutations or polymorphisms in the HR2 region, as well as CCR5 coreceptor usage and density (246).

Clinical Applications

Enfuvirtide, when utilized in a potent combination regimen, has proven beneficial in highly treatment-experienced patients. The week 12 virologic and immunologic responses to enfuvirtide are highly predictive of subsequent response (190). There are no data on the use of enfuvirtide in treatment-naïve individuals. Studies of highly treatment experienced patients with preexisting 3 class resistance have established that (i) addition of enfuvirtide to an optimized background significantly improves rates of viral suppression to <400 copies/ml and results in greater CD4 cell increases in the enfuvirtide group (TORO-1 and TORO-2 trials) (131, 177); (ii) enfuvirtide-naïve patients who add enfuvirtide to the PIs darunavir-ritonavir or tipranavir-ritonavir and with raltegravir and maraviroc achieve better rates of virologic suppression to

<50 copies of HIV-1 RNA/ml than patients whose optimized background did not include enfuvirtide (34, 98). The greatest benefit of enfuvirtide has been seen in patients with CD4 cell counts of >100 cells/mm^3, HIV-1 RNA levels of <100,000 copies/ml, and at least two active drugs in the background regimen (169).

CCR5 Antagonists

The rationale for development of CCR5 antagonists in the treatment of HIV-1 infection is based on the observations that (i) HIV-1 uses the CCR5 chemokine receptor for entry into human cells and (ii) a 32-bp deletion in the CCR5 coding region confers natural resistance to infection with R5 virus in individuals failing to express the receptor on the host cell (2, 52, 139, 170). The current therapeutic niche of CCR5 inhibitors is as one component of combination regimens for patients with multidrug-resistant R5 virus. These agents are not active against HIV-1 strains that use CXCR4 (245).

Maraviroc

Maraviroc {4,4-difluoro-*N*-((1*S*)-3-[exo-3-(3-isopropyl-5-methyl-4*H*-1,2,4-triazol-4-yl)-8-azabicyclo[3.2.1]oct-8-yl]-1-phenylpropyl)cyclohexanecarboxamide; Selzentry, UK-427,857} (Fig. 1 and 2) is a selective, slowly reversible antagonist that blocks the interaction between HIV-1 gp120 and the chemokine receptor CCR5 on host cells (51), thereby preventing gp41 from inserting the fusion peptide into the host membrane. Maraviroc is only active against CCR5-tropic virus, and patients should be screened for their virus coreceptor tropism prior to commencing treatment.

Spectrum of Activity

Maraviroc is the first drug of its class to be approved for use in treatment-experienced patients infected with CCR5-tropic HIV-1. In vitro, maraviroc demonstrates no antagonism with existing antiretroviral agents and additive or synergistic activity in combination with enfuvirtide.

Pharmacology

Formulations of maraviroc include 150- and 300-mg film-coated tablets. The recommended dosage is 150, 300, or 600 mg b.i.d. depending on concomitant therapy.

The bioavailability of the 100-mg dose is 23%, and that of the 300-mg dose is predicted to be 33%. Coadministration of this agent with a high-fat meal reduced its area under the concentration-time curve (AUC) by 33%, although in clinical trials the antiviral effects of maraviroc were not affected by food. It can therefore be administered without food restrictions. Approximately 76% of the drug is protein bound, and it has a volume of distribution of approximately 194 liters. The plasma elimination $t_{1/2}$ of the 300-mg-b.i.d. dosage averages 22.9 h. It is primarily excreted via feces, with only a limited amount of renal excretion (25%). Drug concentrations may be increased in patients with renal impairment and when CYP3A inhibitors are coadministered.

Drug Interactions

Maraviroc is metabolized by CYP3A, so inhibitors of CYP3A (e.g., ketoconazole, lopinavir-ritonavir, and atazanavir) increase the concentrations of maraviroc in plasma, while CYP3A inducers (efavirenz, rifampin, and St. John's wort) decrease the AUC of maraviroc.

Adverse Effects

Hepatotoxicity has been reported with maraviroc's use. Evidence of a systemic allergic reaction (e.g., pruritic rash, eosinophilia, or elevated immunoglobulin E) may occur before the development of hepatotoxicity. The safety of this agent has not been studied in patients with significant underlying liver disease, and caution is advised for such patients. In large efficacy trials, the most common adverse events reported with dosages of up to 300 mg b.i.d. were paresthesias, upper respiratory tract infections, rash, abdominal pain, and dizziness. Drug discontinuations were infrequent. The effect of maraviroc on serum lipids appears to be minimal.

The consequences of targeting a CCR5 coreceptor on host defenses, particularly in the setting of underlying immunodeficiency, remain to be seen (139). The possibility that pharmacological blockade might increase the risk of opportunistic events, including malignancies, has not been substantiated in clinical trials to date. An increased rate of malignancies, particularly lymphomas, has been suggested with another CCR5 antagonist, vicriviroc, but this still remains an open question (84) (see below). An increase in susceptibility to severe West Nile virus infection and tick-borne encephalitis in European populations is a concern with pharmacological blockade of CCR5, given the reports of this complication in individuals who do not express an intact CCR5 coreceptor (123, 140).

Resistance

Several potential mechanisms of resistance to maraviroc have been described. R5 virus can acquire mutations that allow it to utilize the CCR5 coreceptor in the presence of bound drug (242). Two or three amino acid residue substitutions in the V3 loop region of the envelope allow the protein to interact with CCR5 in the drug-bound conformation and are the most likely cause of the resistance phenotype. Shifts in IC_{50}s may not be predictive of maraviroc resistance; rather, there is a flattening of the susceptibility curve representing the virus' acquired ability to utilize maraviroc-bound receptor for entry into the cell (242). CXCR4- or dually tropic virus may emerge from a preexisting reservoir of X4-tropic virus not detected before the initiation of treatment (241). Individuals with X4-tropic virus at baseline demonstrate a reduced virologic response to maraviroc (95).

Clinical Applications

Maraviroc has been approved for treatment of CCR5-tropic virus in patients with evidence of ongoing viral replication and at least 3 drug class experience. Two large efficacy trials of treatment-experienced patients (MOTIVATE 1 and 2) demonstrated significantly higher rates of virologic suppression to HIV-1 RNA levels of <50 copies/ml and higher mean increases in CD4 cell counts in the maraviroc group than in the placebo group. Among patients who experienced virologic failure on maraviroc, the majority harbored X4 virus.

CXCR4-tropic or dually tropic virus emerges more frequently in patients with disease progression and with antiretroviral treatment experience (100). Patients infected with an X4-tropic or dually tropic virus do not derive the same benefit from addition of maraviroc to their regimen as those with pure R5 virus. Of note, 44% of screened patients in the major efficacy trials harbored X4-tropic or dually/mixed-tropic virus, and among treatment-experienced patients or those with first-line regimen failure, the prevalence of dually tropic virus is even higher (162, 244).

The role of maraviroc in treatment-naïve patients with CCR5-tropic virus has not been established yet. Maraviroc in combination with zidovudine-lamivudine compared to efavirenz-zidovudine-lamivudine did not meet the criterion for noninferiority, although greatest virologic benefit was seen in individuals with baseline HIV-1 plasma RNA levels of >100,000 copies/ml.

Vicriviroc

Vicriviroc is an investigational CCR5 antagonist that acts similarly to maraviroc.

Spectrum of Activity

Vicriviroc is a potent inhibitor of most R5 viruses in vitro, with an IC_{50} in the range of 20 nM. It demonstrates additive or synergistic activity in combination with other approved antiretroviral agents (223).

Pharmacology

Vicriviroc is rapidly absorbed, achieving maximum concentration (C_{max}) within 1 to 1.5 h of administration; the elimination $t_{1/2}$ in plasma ranges from 28 to 34 h. The AUC is not affected by a high-fat meal, and the drug may be administered with no food restrictions.

Drug Interactions

Vicriviroc is a substrate of the CYP450 isoenzyme system, and its AUC may be increased by ritonavir and other CYP3A inhibitors. However, the combination of vicriviroc with different ritonavir-boosted PIs does not appear to significantly change plasma vicriviroc levels, and thus dose adjustment may not be required.

Adverse Effects

The most commonly reported adverse effects include fatigue, headache, nausea, and extremity pain. Eight cases of malignancies were reported in a number of patients in the first 48 weeks of vicriviroc therapy. No new malignancies, however, were noted during a median of 2.3 years of follow-up in the ACTG A5211 trial or in blinded follow-up on 20- or 30-mg vicriviroc treatment (249). Phase III trials of 30-mg dose of vicriviroc are currently underway.

Resistance

Resistance to vicriviroc is associated with accumulation of mutations in the V3 loop of gp120 protein allowing the virus to recognize the inhibitor-bound form of the CCR5 receptor (187, 230).

Clinical Applications

Vicriviroc results in reductions of HIV RNA of 1 to 1.5 $\log_{10}$ copies/ml at dosages of 25 and 50 mg b.i.d. during 14 days of monotherapy (209, 223). In treatment-experienced patients with R5 virus, those given 10 and 15 mg of vicriviroc in an optimized background maintained plasma viral loads 2.1 to 2.4 $\log_{10}$ copies/ml below baseline levels at 48 weeks (84). A dose of 30 mg resulted in higher minimum concentrations (C_{min}s) than did the 20-mg dose and was associated with a trend toward better virologic control and increased CD4 cell counts over 48 weeks. However, in treatment-naïve patients, one study comparing vicriviroc to efavirenz, both in combination with fixed-dose zidovudine-lamivudine, was discontinued early due to poor virologic responses in the vicriviroc arms.

INVESTIGATIONAL HIV-1 ENTRY INHIBITORS

A number of investigational agents were in various stages of clinical and preclinical testing in 2008 (Table 2). They include (i) a humanized anti-CD4 monoclonal antibody (TNX-355) which, when administered intravenously to treatment-experienced patients in combination with optimized background therapy, resulted in up to a 0.96 $\log_{10}$ reduction in the HIV-1 RNA level at 48 weeks; (ii) a soluble attachment inhibitor (PRO 542) that binds to gp120 to block attachment and entry of the virus and demonstrated good antiviral activity in individuals with advanced disease; and (iii) CXCR4 antagonists (AMD11070) which have proven challenging to develop but could be used in patients with dually/mixed-tropic virus.

NUCLEOSIDE ANALOG REVERSE TRANSCRIPTASE INHIBITORS

Reverse transcriptase catalyzes the conversion of single-stranded genomic viral RNA into double-stranded DNA with duplicated long terminal repeats, which is subsequently integrated into cellular DNA by the viral integrase enzyme. The mature p66/p51 heterodimeric reverse transcriptase is generated by the viral protease from a homodimer by cleavage of the C-terminal RNase H domain during maturation of the viral particle. The polymerase and RNase H catalytic sites are located on p66, while p51 plays a structural role. Nucleoside analogs require intracellular triphosphorylation by host cell enzymes before incorporation by reverse transcriptase into the growing chain of viral DNA. All the currently approved nucleoside analogs target the polymerase activity of the reverse transcriptase. As with the other nucleoside analogs, the HIV-1-inhibitory concentrations of NRTIs in vitro depend on a number of factors, including the assay system, cell type, and virus isolate used. The cell types account for differences in activity obtained in vivo. The pharmacology and adverse effects of these agents are summarized in Table 3.

Zidovudine

Zidovudine (3′-azido-2′,3′-dideoxythymidine; azidothymidine, Retrovir) (Fig. 1 and 3; Tables 1 and 4) is a synthetic thymidine analog with an azido group substituting for the 3′-hydroxyl group on the ribose ring.

Spectrum of Activity

In peripheral blood lymphocytes, zidovudine has an IC_{50} for HIV-1 between 0.003 and 0.013 μg/ml. It has in vitro activity against other retroviruses, including HIV-2 and human T lymphotropic virus type 1 (HTLV-1).

Mechanism of Action

The antiviral activity of zidovudine is mediated by its intracellular 5′-triphosphate derivative. The mono- and diphosphate forms of zidovudine are generated by cellular thymidine and thymidylate kinases, respectively. The formation of zidovudine diphosphate appears to be a rate-limiting step, as reflected by higher intracellular zidovudine monophosphate levels due to inhibition of thymidylate kinase. The final phosphorylation is completed by a cellular

TABLE 3 Reverse transcriptase inhibitors: pharmacokinetic, major toxicity, and drug interaction characteristics

Agent	Oral bioavailability	Effect of food on AUC	$t_{1/2}$ (intracellular $t_{1/2}$), h	Major route of elimination	Adjustment for renal insufficiency	Major toxicities	Major drug interactions
Zidovudine	65%	Modest decrease	1 (3)	Major inactive metabolite, G-zidovudine is renally excreted	Yes	Neutropenia, anemia, myopathy, nausea, headache, lactic acidosis, and hepatic steatosis (rare)	Myelosuppressive agents (e.g., ganciclovir): increased risk of neutropenia, anemia Rifampin, rifabutin: decreased zidovudine levels Probenecid, valproic acid, atovaquone, fluconazole, phenytoin, methadone: increased zidovudine levels
Didanosine	36% for standard formulations; 42% for enteric formulation	Decrease	1.6 (8–24)	Metabolized to hypoxanthine; ≤55% of didanosine is renally excreted unchanged	Yes	Peripheral neuropathy, pancreatitis, diarrhea, lactic acidosis	Neurotoxic agents (e.g., vinca alkaloids): increased risk of didanosine neurotoxic effects Pancreatitis-associated agents (e.g., pentamidine): increased risk of didanosine pancreatitis. Didanosine's associated buffer decreases the absorption of agents requiring an acidic pH. Ranitidine may increase oral absorption by blocking acid secretion. Stavudine: increases didanosine toxicity (peripheral neuropathy, hyperlactemia) Tenofovir: increases levels of didanosine in serum
Stavudine	86%	No	1.4 (3–4)	Metabolized to thymidine; 40% of stavudine is renally excreted unchanged.	Yes	Peripheral neuropathy, pancreatitis, lipodystrophy and hyperlipidemia, lactic acidosis with hepatic steatosis (higher incidence than with other NRTIs)	Neurotoxic agents: increased risk of stavudine neurotoxicity; do not coadminister with zidovudine; methadone decreases levels
Lamivudine	86%	No	3–4 (10.5–15.5)	Mainly renally excreted unchanged	Yes	Peripheral neuropathy and pancreatitis in pediatric patients	No clinically relevant interactions reported

(*Continued on next page*)

TABLE 3 Reverse transcriptase inhibitors: pharmacokinetic, major toxicity, and drug interaction characteristics *(Continued)*

Agent	Oral bioavailability	Effect of food on AUC	$t_{1/2}$ (intracellular $t_{1/2}$), h	Major route of elimination	Adjustment for renal insufficiency	Major toxicities	Major drug interactions
Abacavir	96%	No	1.2 (20.9)	Metabolized by alcohol dehydrogenase and glucuronyl transferase to inactive forms which are then mainly renally excreted.	No	Potentially fatal hypersensitivity reaction in 3% of cases. Asthenia, abdominal pain, headache, diarrhea, dyspepsia, and transaminitis are also reported.	Methadone: increased clearance by 22%
Emtricitabine	93%	No	10 (>20)	Renally excreted	Yes	Headache, nausea, insomnia; lactic acidosis and hepatomegaly with steatosis (rare), hyperpigmentation of palms and soles	No known significant interactions
Tenofovir	>40%	Increase	>12	Mainly renally excreted unchanged	Yes	Neutropenia, headache, fatigue	May decrease levels of atazanavir; administer 300 mg of atazanavir with 100 mg of ritonavir when used as part of a tenofovir-containing regimen Didanosine: increased levels Raltegravir, saquinavir, cidofovir, ganciclovir: increased levels
Nevirapine	64%	Not available	>24 (?)	Hepatic (CYP450 system)	No	Rash, including Stevens-Johnson syndrome; fever; myalgias; hepatic toxicity, including acute hepatic failure	Etravirine: decreased levels Fluconazole: increased nevirapine AUC by 100% Rifampin and rifabutin: decreased nevirapine levels

Efavirenz	Not reported for humans; 42% in animal studies	A high-fat meal increases the oral bioavailability in humans by 50%.	40–55	Hepatic enzymes PDP and CYP450 CYP2D6	No	Rash, CNS symptoms (e.g., dizziness, abnormal dreams), hepatotoxicity	Amprenavir, nelfinavir, saquinavir, lopinavir-ritonavir, atorvastatin, simvastatin: decreased levels Methadone, rifabutin, clarithromycin: decreased levels Efavirenz decreases fosamprenavir levels by 36%; the recommended dosage increase is either 1,400 mg of fosamprenavir with 300 mg of ritonavir q.d. or standard doses along with 200 mg of ritonavir b.i.d.
Delavirdine	85%	Decrease	1.4 (?)	Hepatic (CYP450 system)	No	Rash; nausea; fatigue; diarrhea	CYP450 system inducers (e.g., rifampin, rifabutin, phenytoin): decreased delavirdine levels CYP450 system inhibitors (e.g., clarithromycin, ketoconazole): increased delavirdine levels CYP450 enzyme substrates (e.g., terfenadine, astemizole, warfarin, cyclosporine): increased levels
Etravirine	Unknown	Food increases oral bioavailability; should be taken following a meal	41 (?)	Hepatic (CYP450 system)	Renal: no Hepatic: no	Nausea, rash	Efavirenz, nevirapine: decreased etravirine levels Lopinavir-ritonavir: increased etravirine AUC by 85% CYP3A4, CYP2C9, and/or CYP2C19 inducers: may decrease level of etravirine in serum Voriconazole: increased levels of both drugs Ritonavir and tipranavir-ritonavir: decreased levels of etravirine

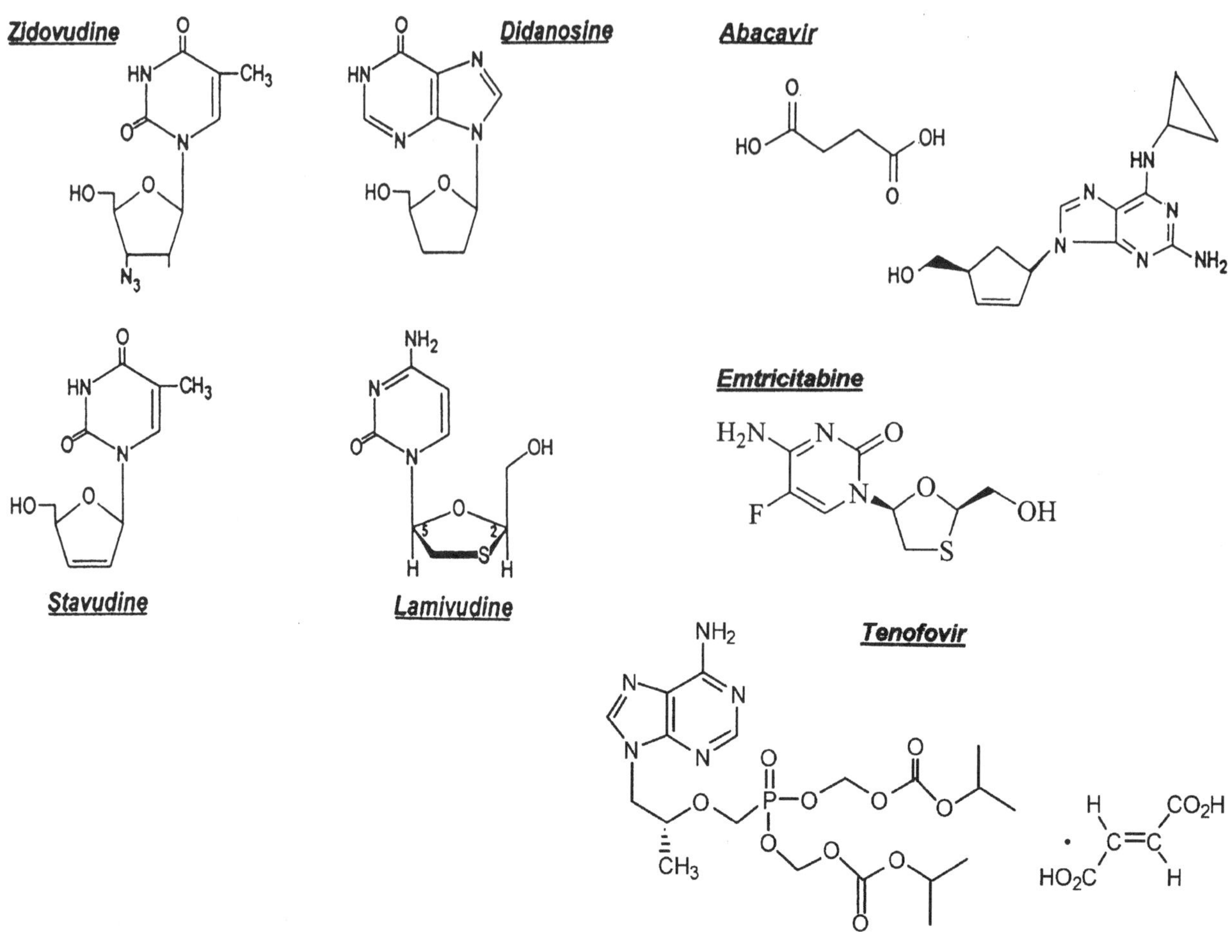

FIGURE 3 Chemical structures of NRTIs.

nucleoside diphosphate kinase. Zidovudine triphosphate then acts as a competitive substrate for the HIV reverse transcriptase and is incorporated into the elongating 3′ end of the yet-unintegrated proviral DNA. This results in the premature termination of chain elongation due to the inability of the nucleoside analog to form a normal 3′-5′ phosphodiester linkage.

Zidovudine and the other nucleoside analogs may vary in their antiviral activities within different primary cell types in vitro. Zidovudine is more potent in activated cells than nonactivated cells. The thymidine kinase required for zidovudine phosphorylation is an S-phase-specific enzyme and thus has increased activity in stimulated cells and lowered activity in resting cells.

Pharmacology

Zidovudine is available in capsule, syrup, and intravenous formulations. Based on its intracellular $t_{1/2}$ (11), the current dosage in adults is 300 mg b.i.d. It is available in a fixed-dose formulation with lamivudine (Combivir) and in combination with abacavir and lamivudine (Trizivir), with no differences in bioavailability or side effects compared to those of the drugs taken separately. The oral forms of zidovudine are rapidly absorbed and undergo extensive first-pass metabolism. The resulting overall bioavailability is ~64%. Zidovudine reaches C_{max}s of 2.35 to 5.5 μM in plasma at 0.5 to 1.5 h after a 200-mg dose. The mean $t_{1/2}$ of zidovudine in serum is approximately 1 h after oral dosing, but the intracellular $t_{1/2}$ of zidovudine 5′-triphosphate is approximately 3 h. Zidovudine C_{max}s in plasma are decreased by >50% when the drug is taken with food; however, the AUC remains unchanged.

Zidovudine has limited plasma protein binding (about 34 to 38%). Cerebrospinal fluid (CSF)-to-plasma ratios vary widely (15 to 135%) but average 50% 2 to 4 h after dosing. The mean CSF drug concentrations in adults range from 0.05 to 1.06 μmol/liter over a dose range of 200 to 1,250 mg. Drug appearance in semen correlates with clearance of HIV-1 from semen. The ratios of the concentrations of zidovudine, amprenavir, and lamivudine in semen and blood were found to be 12.9, <1, and 5.3, respectively (182). Zidovudine levels in breast milk and serum are comparable after a single dose. Zidovudine rapidly crosses the placenta by passive diffusion, and therefore fetal and maternal concentrations are proportional. Pregnancy does not appear to alter the maternal metabolism of zidovudine.

Zidovudine is predominantly metabolized hepatically by a uridine diphosphoglucuronosyl transferase (UGT) to its major active metabolite, zidovudine glucuronide, which undergoes renal elimination with a $t_{1/2}$ of 0.61 to 1.73 h. Urinary recoveries of zidovudine and the glucuronide are 14 and 74%, respectively. Patients with hepatic dysfunction have two- to threefold increases in the peak plasma zidovudine level and elimination $t_{1/2}$ (55). The metabolism

TABLE 4 PIs: pharmacokinetic, major toxicity, and drug interaction characteristics

Agent	Oral bioavailability	Effect of food on AUC	$t_{1/2}$ (h)	Route of metabolism	Adjustment for hepatic and renal insufficiency	Major toxicities	Major drug interactions
Saquinavir	4%; erratic for tablets and hard-gel capsules when taken as the only PI	Increase for soft-gel capsule; take tablet and hard-gel capsule within 2 h of a meal when taken with ritonavir	1–2	CYP450 CYP3A4 inhibitor and substrate	Hepatic: no	Nausea, diarrhea, abdominal pain, headache, hyperlipidemia, elevated transaminases, fat redistribution, potential for increased bleeding in patients with hemophilia, oral ulceration	Clarithromycin and saquinavir: increased levels Ketoconazole, grapefruit juice: increased saquinavir levels Efavirenz and rifampin (CYP450 inducers): decreased saquinavir levels
Indinavir	65%	Decrease by 77%	1.5–2	CYP450 CYP3A4 inhibitor and substrate	Hepatic: yes Renal: no	Nephrolithiasis, renal colic, indirect hyperbilirubinemia, nausea, hyperglycemia, fat redistribution, headache, asthenia, blurred vision, insomnia, alopecia, dry skin, ingrown nails, metallic taste, thrombocytopenia, hemolytic anemia	Coadministration with atorvastatin may increase risk of myopathy and rhabdomyolysis Itraconazole and ketoconazole: increased indinavir levels Rifampin: decreased indinavir AUC by >80%; use adjusted dose of rifabutin as an alternative
Ritonavir	Not determined	Increase	3–5	CYP450 system (CYP3A4 > CYP2D6; potent CYP3A4 inhibitor)	Hepatic: no[a] Renal: no	Nausea, vomiting, diarrhea, abdominal pain, paresthesias (circumoral and peripheral), asthenia, taste perversion, fat redistribution, hyperlipidemia, hypertriglyceridemia, hyperglycemia, elevated transaminases, pancreatitis, potential for increased bleeding in patients with hemophilia	Antihistamines (astemizole, terfenadine), hypnotics (alprazolam, diazepam, triazolam), antiarrhythmics (amidarone), or lipid-lowering agents (simvastatin, lovastatin): levels increased Rifampin: decreased ritonavir AUC by 35% Voriconazole: decreased AUC up to 80% Warfarin, phenytoin, atovaquone: decreased levels
Nelfinavir	20–80%	Increase	3.5–5	CYP50 CYP3A4 inhibitor and substrate	Hepatic: no Renal: no	Diarrhea, elevated transaminases, hyperglycemia, fat redistribution, fatigue, potential for increased bleeding in patients with hemophilia	Lovastatin, simvastatin: levels increased Methadone: levels increased Anticonvulsants (carbamazepine, phenobarbital): decreased nelfinavir levels

(*Continued on next page*)

TABLE 4 PIs: pharmacokinetic, major toxicity, and drug interaction characteristics *(Continued)*

Agent	Oral bioavailability	Effect of food on AUC	$t_{1/2}$ (h)	Route of metabolism	Adjustment for hepatic and renal insufficiency	Major toxicities	Major drug interactions
Fosamprenavir	Not determined	No	7.7	CYP450 CYP3A4 inhibitor, substrate, and inducer	Hepatic: yes Renal: no	Skin rash (particularly in patients sensitive to sulfonamides), diarrhea, nausea, vomiting, headache, elevated transaminase, hyperglycemia, hyperlipidemia and fat redistribution, potential for increased bleeding in patients with hemophilia	Etravirine: increased fosamprenavir levels Antifungals (voriconazole, itraconazole): may result in bidirectional inhibition Sildenafil, tadalafil, vardenafil: increased levels
Lopinavir-ritonavir	Not determined	Increase	5–6	CYP50 CYP3A4 inhibitor and substrate	Hepatic: no	Diarrhea, nausea, vomiting, elevated transaminases, hyperlipidemia, hypertriglyceridemia, fat redistribution, metallic taste, asthenia, potential for increased bleeding in patients with hemophilia	Decrease methadone levels
Tipranavir	Increased by high-fat meal	Not determined	6	CYP450 CYP3A4 inducer and substrate; combined with ritonavir CYP3A4 inhibitor and CYP2D6 inhibitor; potent inducer of P-glycoprotein	Hepatic: use with caution in moderate to severe impairment Renal: no	Rash (especially patients with sulfonamide allergy); nausea; vomiting; diarrhea; hepatotoxicity, including hepatic decompensation (especially with underlying liver disease); hyperlipidemia; hypertriglyceridemia; fat redistribution; case reports of intracranial hemorrhage; potential for increased bleeding in patients with hemophilia	Clarithromycin, azole antifungals, erectile dysfunction agents: increased levels Lipid-lowering agents (lovastatin, simvastatin): increased potential for myopathy or rhabdomyolysis Amiodarone: increased potential for serious or life-threatening cardiac arrhythmias Rifampin and St. John's wort: decreased tipranavir levels Etravirine, zidovudine: decreased levels

Atazanavir	Not determined	Increase	6.5–7.9	CYP450 CYP3A4 inhibitor and substrate	Hepatic: yes Renal: no	Prolonged PR interval and first-degree AV block (asymptomatic), indirect hyperbilirubinemia, abnormal liver enzymes, hyperglycemia, fat redistribution, potential for increased bleeding in patients with hemophilia	Proton pump inhibitors decrease atazanavir absorption, and concurrent administration is contraindicated; other antacids and H2 blockers should be used with caution Efavirenz decreases concentrations in plasma; addition of ritonavir may compensate for the interaction. Coadminstration with indinavir is not recommended due to increased risk of hyperbilirubinemia.
Darunavir	37%; 82% with ritonavir	Increase	7	CYP450 CYP3A4 inhibitor and substrate	Hepatic: yes Renal: no	Rash; diarrhea; nausea; headache; cold-like symptoms, including runny nose or sore throat; elevated transaminases; hyperlipidemia; hypertriglyceridemia	Lipid-lowering agents, calcium channel blockers, antiarrhythmics, erectile dysfunction agents, clarithromycin, tenofovir: increased concentrations Rifampin: decreased darunavir levels; increased rifabutin effect, requires reduced rifabutin dose; use with caution with lopinavir-ritonavir or efavirenz (decreased darunavir and increased coadministered drug levels) Maraviroc: increased levels; adjust dose to 150 mg b.i.d.

[a] No dosage adjustment in mild hepatic impairment; no data for moderate to severe impairment; use with caution.

of zidovudine also leads to the formation of a minor but cytotoxic compound, 3′-amino-3′-deoxythymidine, which may be partially responsible for the adverse effects of zidovudine (55). This metabolite has a $t_{1/2}$ of approximately 2.7 h. Renal dysfunction (mean creatinine clearance, 18 ml/min) increases the elimination $t_{1/2}$ of zidovudine to 1.4 h and doubles its AUC; total daily dosages of 300 to 400 mg are therefore recommended for patients with severe renal impairment. Although zidovudine glucuronide is effectively removed by dialysis, negligible amounts of zidovudine are cleared by either hemodialysis or peritoneal dialysis.

Adverse Effects

The most prominent zidovudine toxicities are neutropenia and anemia, which occur in 16 and 24% of patients at higher doses. In zidovudine-induced anemia, the reticulocyte count is usually depressed and the erythropoietin level is elevated, suggesting inhibition of erythroid stem cell lines. Myelosuppression has been associated with increased doses and duration of zidovudine, as well as with lower baseline hematologic parameters (e.g., CD4 cell count, neutrophil count, hemoglobin concentration, and vitamin B_{12} levels).

Anemia occurs as early as 4 to 6 weeks after initiation of therapy and in nearly 7% of patients with advanced HIV disease, compared to 1% in those with early asymptomatic infection. Although macrocytosis occurs in more than 90% of zidovudine recipients, it does not correlate with the development of anemia. Neutropenia is also seen more frequently in advanced HIV infection (37%) than in the early stages (8%) and is usually detected within 12 to 24 weeks after initiation of therapy. In addition to zidovudine dose reduction or discontinuation, management options for zidovudine-related hematologic toxicity include the use of hematopoietic growth factors (erythropoietin or granulocyte colony-stimulating factors).

Zidovudine is also associated with both skeletal and cardiac muscle toxicities. Zidovudine-related polymyositis occurs in approximately 6 to 18% of patients who have been treated for more than 6 months. Clinically, this myopathy is manifested by the insidious onset of myalgias, muscle tenderness, and proximal-muscle weakness, mainly in the lower extremities. Diagnostic features include elevated creatine phosphokinase levels and a myopathic pattern on electromyography. Muscle biopsy reveals minimal to moderate inflammation and myonecrosis with an excess of abnormal mitochondria and a decrease in mitochondrial DNA, probably secondary to the inhibition of DNA polymerase Y. The cessation of zidovudine treatment usually results in a gradual resolution over the ensuing 6 to 8 weeks.

Nausea, abdominal discomfort, headache, insomnia, malaise, and fatigue are relatively common side effects. These are early symptoms in a substantial number of patients but often resolve despite continued drug administration. Gastrointestinal effects such as bloating, dyspepsia, hepatitis, and esophageal ulceration have also been described. Zidovudine can cause nail and skin hyperpigmentation. Zidovudine-related seizures and macular edema have been reported, as have cases of lactic acidosis characterized by elevated liver transaminase levels and hepatomegaly due to steatosis, which can be fatal.

Zidovudine has been associated with abnormalities of body fat distribution and lipid metabolism (173). In the Gilead 934 study comparing zidovudine-lamivudine with tenofovir-emtricitabine, each with efavirenz in treatment-naïve patients, more patients taking zidovudine experienced loss of limb fat as assessed by dual-energy X-ray absorptiometry scans than in the tenofovir arm. No teratogenicity in human studies has been reported thus far; zidovudine is mutagenic and carcinogenic in rodents.

Drug Interactions

Agents that interfere with the hepatic metabolism or renal excretion of zidovudine can accentuate zidovudine-associated toxicities. Probenecid increases zidovudine levels by inhibiting renal excretion or glucuronidation. Valproic acid, atovaquone, fluconazole, indomethacin, naproxen, cimetidine, phenytoin, testosterone, ethinyl estradiol, chloramphenicol, methadone, and codeine have all been associated with increased zidovudine levels. Rifampin and rifabutin can lower zidovudine concentrations. Although concomitant use of trimethoprim-sulfamethoxazole could affect zidovudine elimination, in theory due to use of the same glucuronidation pathway, no pharmacokinetic or clinically relevant effects have been noted. Other drugs which also have myelosuppressive effects, such as ganciclovir, dapsone, flucytosine, and oncological chemotherapeutic agents, may add to the hematologic adverse effects of zidovudine. Ribavirin inhibits phosphorylation of zidovudine; therefore, this combination should be avoided if possible.

Resistance

The reverse transcriptase coding region from high-level zidovudine-resistant HIV-1 isolates reveals amino acid substitutions at one or more of six positions (M41L, D67N, K70R, L210W, T215F or Y, and K219Q) (110, 135).

Two distinct mechanisms of resistance to zidovudine and other nucleotide and nucleoside analogs have been elucidated: (i) impairment of the incorporation of the analog into DNA and (ii) removal of the analog from the prematurely terminated DNA chain (33, 129). Reverse transcriptase mutations like thymidine analog mutations (TAMs) at positions 41, 67, 210, 215, and 219 promote ATP-mediated and pyrophosphate-mediated excision of the incorporated terminator (28), whereas M184V or Q151M complex mutations impair the ability of reverse transcriptase to incorporate nucleoside analogs. The M184V mutation severely compromises pyrophosphorolysis, an in vitro finding which is consistent with clinical data indicating an increase in zidovudine sensitivity in the presence of the M184V mutation (75).

The degree of zidovudine resistance is proportional to the number of mutations in the reverse transcriptase coding region. Moreover, the mutations appear and accumulate in a serial manner and confer a degree of cross-resistance to all NRTIs. Subspecies demonstrating differential genotypic and phenotypic resistance patterns can coexist, and these may differ among tissue compartments. TAMs evolve in one of two distinct pathways: (i) T215Y alone or with M41L, L210W (TAM1) and (ii) T215F, which commonly occurs with D67N, K70R, and K219Q (TAM2) (87, 99).

In addition to TAMs, two multinucleoside resistance mutational pathways have been described that confer zidovudine resistance. The Q151M complex includes A62V, V75I, F116Y, and Q151M, with the Q151M mutation being the critical mutation for multidrug resistance. The second pathway is a 2-amino-acid insertion at reverse transcriptase position 69. Most resistance assays evaluate the polymerase domain and do not look for resistance mutations in the connection and RNase H domains of the HIV-1 reverse transcriptase. Mutations in these domains may be clinically significant. RNase H cleaves the RNA template as the DNA reverse transcript elongates. Mutations in the RNase H domain increase NRTI resistance, probably by decreasing RNase H activity, allowing more time for excision of zidovudine (178). In vivo evaluation of mutations outside of the catalytic domain identified the A371V mutation in the connection domain and Q509L in the RNase H domain; these mutations were 1.7 times more resistant to zidovudine than wild-type virus, in combination with TAMs (17). The N348I mutation in the connection domain inhibits movement of the thumb region of the polymerase domain, thereby allowing more time for zidovudine excision. It occurs more frequently in treatment-experienced patients and, in combination with TAMs, confers a fourfold decrease in susceptibility to zidovudine.

Clinical Applications

Zidovudine was the first approved antiretroviral agent and consequently has been the agent most widely used in clinical trials and practice. Zidovudine in combination with another nucleoside analog and either a PI (with or without ritonavir enhancement) or an NNRTI became one of the standard-of-care regimens in the era of potent antiretroviral therapy beginning in 1996. As part of initial therapy, the combination of zidovudine and lamivudine has been a key dual-NRTI component in multiple clinical trials and has demonstrated considerable durability, tolerability, and clinical benefit (198, 219, 234).

Comparison of zidovudine with abacavir, in combination with lamivudine and efavirenz, showed similar virologic responses in both arms; however, the CD4 cell count rise was greater in the abacavir-lamivudine-treated patients than in the zidovudine-lamivudine-treated patients (45). A comparison of zidovudine-lamivudine with tenofovir-emtricitabine as part of an efavirenz-based regimen in treatment-naïve patients demonstrated lower rates of virologic suppression to <50 copies/ml and higher rates of anemia with the zidovudine regimen (69). Zidovudine-lamivudine has been supplanted by tenofovir-emtricitabine and abacavir-lamivudine as recommended dual-nucleoside components of either NNRTI- or ritonavir-boosted PI-based initial therapeutic regimens (in persons with susceptible virus strains).

Zidovudine was the first antiretroviral agent evaluated as a prophylactic agent in HIV-infected pregnant women and accidentally exposed health care workers. In a landmark study (ACTG 076), zidovudine reduced the risk of mother-to-child transmission of HIV-1 by two-thirds compared to placebo (38). For accidentally exposed health care workers, a retrospective case control study found that zidovudine reduced the hazard of HIV transmission by 81% (22). Combination therapy is now, of course, recommended when HIV-1 prophylaxis is indicated.

Zidovudine in combination with alpha interferon may have some efficacy in the treatment of adult T-cell leukemia-lymphoma caused by HTLV-1.

Didanosine

Didanosine (2′,3′-dideoxyinosine; Videx) is a nucleoside analog (Fig. 1 and 3; Tables 1 and 3) and was the second antiretroviral agent approved by the Food and Drug Administration (FDA).

Spectrum of Activity

Didanosine has similar inhibitory activities against HIV-1 and HIV-2. The inhibitory concentration of didanosine for HIV-1 varies depending upon a number of factors, including the assay system, cell type, and virus isolate used. The IC_{50}s range from 0.6 to 2.4 μg/ml in lymphocyte cell lines and 0.0024 to 0.024 μg/ml in monocyte/macrophage cell cultures. Didanosine also has in vitro activity against simian immunodeficiency virus and HTLV-1.

Mechanism of Action

As with the other dideoxynucleosides, didanosine requires intracellular phosphorylation to achieve antiviral activity. However, didanosine also requires additional cellular metabolism, first to 2′,3′-dideoxy-IMP by a 5′-nucleotidase and then to 2′,3′-dideoxy-AMP by amination by adenylosuccinate synthetase and adenylosuccinate lyase. Two subsequent phosphorylations then lead to its final active form, 2′,3′-dideoxy-ATP (ddATP), which competes with the physiological nucleoside, 2′-dideoxy-ATP (dATP). ddATP functions as a competitive inhibitor of HIV reverse transcriptase by chain termination due to lack of the 5′-hydroxyl group required for continued reverse transcription. Didanosine acts synergistically with other antiretroviral agents.

Pharmacology

The N-glycosidic bond of didanosine is hydrolyzed at low pH (pK_a = 9.13), which limits the oral delivery of the drug. To overcome this challenge, didanosine has undergone serial formulation changes since its introduction. Eating can lower didanosine bioavailability by stimulating gastric acid secretion. Consequently, dosing is recommended at least 30 min to 1 h before or 2 h after eating. In 2001, a new encapsulated formulation of enteric beadlets (ddI-EC, Videx EC) was introduced and has shown better tolerability than the previously buffered didanosine chewable tablet.

Although the elimination $t_{1/2}$ in plasma averages 1.6 h after oral administration, the intracellular $t_{1/2}$ of ddATP ranges from 8 to 24 h, justifying once-daily dosing. Protein binding is less than 5%. Unlike other purine analogs, didanosine enters erythrocyte membranes via facilitated diffusion. The concentrations in CSF approach 20% of those in plasma (range, 12 to 85%). Pregnancy does not appear to alter the pharmacokinetics of didanosine, and 20 to 50% of maternal levels of didanosine are found in the placental and fetal circulation (239). Didanosine is metabolized to hypoxanthine and then to uric acid by xanthine oxidase. Approximately 40% of didanosine is excreted unchanged via glomerular filtration and tubular secretion. Uremia decreases didanosine clearance at least threefold. Dose adjustments for renal dysfunction may be indicated due to the magnesium and aluminum contents of the buffered tablets. Didanosine is partially dialyzable, with an extraction ratio of 53%.

Adverse Effects

The most clinically significant toxicities are dose-related painful peripheral neuropathy and pancreatitis. The risk of pancreatitis during therapy increases in patients with a history of pancreatitis (30%, versus 5%), a history of alcohol or drug use, hypertriglyceridemia, or the concurrent use of hydroxyurea. Salivary gland toxicity also occurs, and some patients develop sialadenitis and even sicca syndrome.

Didanosine-related peripheral neuropathy presents as symmetrical foot pain and paresthesias, which typically resolve slowly after didanosine withdrawal. Symptoms may continue to increase in the first few weeks after its discontinuation. Mechanistically, it may be related to the inhibition of neuron DNA polymerase γ (mitochondrial DNA polymerase). Didanosine-related peripheral neuropathy is more frequent in patients with advanced HIV disease and preexisting neuropathy.

Myelosuppression is rarely seen with didanosine. Other adverse effects include headache, rash, nausea, vomiting, hepatotoxicity, xerostomia, and pediatric retinal depigmentation. The combination of didanosine with stavudine may potentiate the risk of pancreatitis, peripheral neuropathy, and lactic acidosis and should not be used (14, 36, 198). No evidence of mutagenicity is seen on Ames testing, and there is no evidence of teratogenicity in human or animal studies.

Drug Interactions

Coadministration of ganciclovir increases the maximum didanosine concentrations in plasma by 59%, and dosage reduction of didanosine should be considered in this situation if side effects consistent with didanosine toxicity occur. Coadministration of other drugs with didanosine may potentiate peripheral neuropathy (e.g., metronidazole, isoniazid, ethambutol, pentamidine, and vinca alkaloids) and pancreatitis (e.g., azathioprine, pentamidine, and vinca alkaloids). Itraconazole and ketoconazole should be administered at least 2 h before or 2 to 6 h after didanosine because of decreased absorption from the buffer content of didanosine. Absorption of tetracycline and ciprofloxacin is reduced by the divalent-cation content of buffer-containing didanosine formulations. Methadone treatment drecreases serum didanosine levels (mean decrease in AUC of 57%) via decreased bioavailability and possibly increased first-pass metabolism. Coadministration of tenofovir increases the AUC of didanosine and may potentiate didanosine-associated toxicities. This combination is associated with a high rate of early virology failure, CD4 cell count decline, and development of resistance (also see section on tenofovir below).

Concomitant use of hydroxyurea (27, 172) or ribavirin (130) increases the ratio of intracellular triphosphorylated didanosine to physiological nucleoside triphosphates and increases the risk of mitochondrial toxicity (lactic acidosis, pancreatitis, and hepatic steatosis).

Resistance

The L74V and M184V mutations have been associated with a 3- to 10-fold decrease in didanosine sensitivity in vitro. The K65R mutation confers a 3- to 5-fold decrease in sensitivity, the Q151M and K65R mutations confer >10-fold changes in susceptibility, and isolates with L74V and T215F have a median change of approximately a factor of 5 (134). The 69-insert multinucleoside resistance mutation confers resistance to didanosine as well. The presence of three or more TAMs (41L, 210W, 215Y/F, 219Q/E, 44D, 67N, 70R, and 118I) confers intermediate or high-level resistance to didanosine in vitro.

The L74V mutation has been associated with increased levels of viremia in vivo. HIV-1 isolates from patients whose antiviral regimen has been changed to didanosine after prior zidovudine monotherapy reveal L74V and M184V mutations. Combination therapy with didanosine and zidovudine has resulted in A62V, F77L, F116Y, and Q151M mutations and in vitro conferred at least partial cross-resistance to lamivudine, stavudine, and zalcitabine. Although L74V is the most common mutation selected in vivo by didanosine, the zidovudine-associated resistance mutations are probably responsible for most of the reduced susceptibility to this agent. When L74V is present with M184V, it may lead to further losses of susceptibility to abacavir and didanosine. The presence of zidovudine-associated mutations at the start of therapy predicts more rapid virologic failure of didanosine-containing regimens.

Clinical Applications

Because of limited clinical experience with didanosine in combination with emtricitabine or lamivudine as part of a dual-nucleoside component, current guidelines recommend that didanosine be considered an alternative nucleoside backbone for use in combination therapy. Didanosine's current use is largely restricted to an adjunctive role in regimens designed for treatment-experienced patients with virologic failure.

Stavudine

Stavudine (2′,3′-didehydro-2′,3′-deoxythymidine; Zerit), like zidovudine, is a thymidine analog (Fig. 1 and 3; Tables 1 and 3). Stavudine is available in capsule strengths of 15, 20, 30, and 40 mg and in an oral solution.

Spectrum of Activity

Stavudine has activity against HIV-1, with 50% effective concentrations of 0.04 μM in peripheral blood mononuclear cells (PBMCs) and 0.3 μM in monocyte/macrophage cell lines. Stavudine has similar activity against HIV-2 and has demonstrated activity against other animal retroviruses. Additive or synergistic in vitro inhibition has been reported with double or triple combinations of numerous antiretroviral agents, except for zidovudine-stavudine, which is an antagonistic combination.

Mechanism of Action

Stavudine has a mechanism of action similar to that of zidovudine. Following passive diffusion into cells, stavudine is activated by a series of thymidine kinases to the active triphosphorylated form. The initial phosphorylation of stavudine monophosphate by thymidylate kinase is the rate-limiting step. Triphosphorylated stavudine competes with the natural substrate of HIV reverse transcriptase, 2′-deoxythymidine-5′-triphosphate, and its lack of a 3′-OH prevents formation of the 3′-5′ phosphodiester bond essential for nucleotide elongation. Stavudine is more active against HIV in mitogen-stimulated peripheral blood lymphocytes and less active in quiescent cells due to decreased phosphorylation by the cell cycle-dependent thymidine kinase.

Pharmacology

Stavudine has high oral bioavailability due in part to its acid stability and the lack of significant first-pass metabolism. Ingestion with a meal reduces the C_{max} but not the overall absorption (AUC) compared to those in the fasting state. A C_{max} in plasma of approximately 1.2 μg/ml is reached in less than 1 h after a dose of 0.67 mg/kg of body weight. The CSF-to-plasma ratio is estimated at 0.40. Placental concentrations of stavudine are about half those of zidovudine.

The mean elimination $t_{1/2}$ is 1.4 h. Renal excretion of unchanged drug, in part by renal tubular secretion, accounts for about 40% of stavudine elimination. Stavudine is also converted to thymine, which then enters the pyrimidine pool. Alternatively, it is metabolized further to β-aminoisobutyric acid. A small proportion may also be excreted in the form of other miscellaneous metabolites. Due to the contribution of renal clearance to stavudine elimination, the $t_{1/2}$s after a 40-mg dose increase to 3.5 and 4.8 h in patients with creatinine clearances of 25 to 50 and 9 to 25 ml/min, respectively. Stavudine therefore requires dose adjustments in the setting of renal impairment and hemodialysis. No dose adjustments are necessary in patients with hepatic impairment.

Adverse Effects

Dose-related peripheral neuropathy is the principal limiting toxicity of stavudine. The risk of neuropathy is related to higher dosages (≥2 mg/kg/day), longer duration of treatment, and the presence of more advanced disease. Other potential predictors of neuropathy are a lower baseline CD4 cell count, past or current neuropathy, concomitant excessive alcohol use, and renal impairment. Neuropathy is infrequent during the initial 12 weeks of stavudine treatment. After the withdrawal of stavudine, the neuropathy frequently resolves, but the median time to resolution varies from about 1 week with a 0.1-mg/kg/day dosage to 3 weeks with a 2.0-mg/kg/day regimen.

Thymidine nucleoside analogs (stavudine and zidovudine) contribute to development of lipodystrophy and lipid metabolism abnormalities (71, 92, 111). Switching these agents with nonthymidine nucleoside analogs decreases the frequency and progression of lipodystrophy (92). Of all NRTIs, stavudine has been most frequently implicated in lipodystrophy and mitochondrial toxicity, including fatal lactic acidosis. The combination of stavudine and didanosine should not be used because of enhanced risk of peripheral neuropathy, hyperlactatemia, and clinical lactic acidosis (14, 36).

Myelosuppression with stavudine is uncommon. Stavudine incorporation into nuclear DNA is 50 to 100 times lower than that of zidovudine. Although the K_m of stavudine triphosphate is lower than that of zidovudine triphosphate, the 3′-5′ exonuclease-mediated excision of zidovudine from nuclear DNA is inhibited by zidovudine monophosphate but not by stavudine monophosphate (217). Additionally, cytotoxicity is limited by cellular enzymes in hematopoietic stem cells, which readily metabolize stavudine to thymidine and thymidine 5′-triphosphate. Other adverse effects associated with stavudine include elevation of hepatic enzyme levels, nausea, vomiting, headache, rash, fever, and diarrhea.

Drug Interactions

Stavudine enjoys relatively few drug-drug interactions compared to other antiretroviral agents. Drugs with neurotoxic side effects may increase the risk of peripheral neuropathy when combined with stavudine. Because stavudine and zidovudine compete for thymidine kinase in the cell, these two agents are antagonistic and should not be prescribed together. Clinical antagonism of stavudine and zidovudine results from the inhibition of stavudine phosphorylation by zidovudine.

Resistance

Although the V75T mutation selected in vitro confers a sevenfold decrease in stavudine susceptibility, decreased virologic responses to stavudine usually result from the TAMs associated with zidovudine resistance. There is a high degree of cross-resistance between zidovudine and stavudine. TAMs M41L, D67N, K70R, L210W, T215Y/F, and K219Q/E are selected by both thymidine analogs, zidovudine and stavudine, and are associated with cross-resistance to all currently approved NRTIs (109). The Q151M mutation can also be seen in patients receiving zidovudine with didanosine.

Clinical Applications

Stavudine as a component of standard triple therapy with two NRTIs and one PI has largely shown equivalence to other NRTIs (60, 220). Studies of stavudine in combination with other reverse transcriptase inhibitors and efavirenz in antiretroviral-naïve patients indicate the following: (i) comparison of stavudine with tenofovir demonstrated equivalent rates of suppression to plasma HIV-1 RNA levels of <50 copies/ml but increased rates of lipodystrophy in the stavudine arm (71), and (ii) stavudine compared with emtricitabine, combined with didanosine, proved to be virologically inferior (59% of stavudine versus 78% of emtricitabine patients achieved HIV-1 RNA levels of <50 copies/ml) (203). Consequently, stavudine is no longer a first-line NRTI because of its toxicity profile, and its use is discouraged.

Lamivudine

Lamivudine [(−)-2′,3′-dideoxy-3′-thiacytidine; Epivir] (Fig. 1 and 3; Tables 1 and 3) is the (−) enantiomer of a cytidine analog with a sulfur substituted for the 3′ carbon atom in the furanose ring. To streamline the dosing of the nucleoside analog component of combination therapy, fixed-dose formulations of lamivudine-zidovudine (Combivir), lamivudine-zidovudine-abacavir (Trizivir), and lamivudine-abacavir (Epzicom) in single capsules have been approved. The standard dosage of lamivudine is 150 mg b.i.d. or 300 mg once daily.

Spectrum of Activity

Lamivudine displays activity against HIV-1 and -2, as well as hepatitis B virus (HBV). Inhibitory concentrations range from 2 nM to 15 μM in in vitro susceptibility assays. Synergy has been noted in combination with the thymidine analogs and tenofovir.

Mechanism of Action

Although both lamivudine enantiomers have in vitro antiviral activity, the (−) enantiomer form is more potent, possibly on the basis of its resistance to 3′-5′ exonuclease excision, and less cytotoxic because (−) enantiomers of nucleosides are poorly recognized by mammalian polymerases. Lamivudine requires phosphorylation to the triphosphate metabolite for antiviral activity; the triphosphate competitively inhibits the viral reverse transcriptase and interrupts proviral DNA chain elongation.

Pharmacology

Oral lamivudine is rapidly absorbed, and bioavailability in adults is approximately 86% for doses between 0.25 and

8.0 mg/kg. Although absorption of lamivudine is slowed in the postprandial state, there is no significant decrease in the AUC with food. Lamivudine has low protein binding (<36%). A C_{max} in serum of 1.5 μg/ml is attained in 1 to 1.5 h. The mean elimination $t_{1/2}$ in plasma is approximately 2 to 4 h, but the intracellular $t_{1/2}$ varies between 10.5 and 15.5 h. As a consequence of predominant renal elimination in an unchanged form via glomerular filtration and active tubular excretion, lamivudine dose adjustments are required in individuals with severe renal functional impairment.

Adverse Effects

Lamivudine has a very favorable toxicity profile and is well tolerated at dosages ranging from 0.5 to 20.0 mg/kg/day (184). A trend toward neutropenia is seen only with the highest doses. Insomnia, headache, diarrhea, abdominal pain, and pruritus have been reported but are infrequent (184). Reports of rash, arthralgias, myalgias, pancreatitis, hepatitis, and peripheral neuropathy have an unclear association with lamivudine in adults. In children, rare associations of pancreatitis or hepatitis with lamivudine have been noted.

Drug Interactions

Trimethoprim-sulfamethoxazole decreases the renal clearance of lamivudine and consequently increases systemic exposure to the drugs (171). Coadministration of lamivudine with zidovudine results in a rise in peak plasma zidovudine concentrations, but this is not thought to be clinically significant. Lamivudine and emtricitabine have nearly identical resistance profiles, have minimal additive antiviral activity, and should not be used together.

Resistance

Resistance to lamivudine develops rapidly and uniformly in treated patients who are not on a fully suppressive antiretroviral regimen or who are poorly compliant. Mutations at codon 184 that lead to either an isoleucine or a valine substitution for methionine occur rapidly and confer 100- to 1,000-fold decreases in susceptibility (15). While zidovudine resistance mutations allow for increased DNA synthetic rescue of zidovudine triphosphate termination through pyrophosphorolysis, the M184V mutation generates lamivudine resistance by decreasing the efficiency of incorporation of lamivudine monophosphate 20- to 100-fold relative to those of the wild-type reverse transcriptase HIV strains (75).

Plasma HIV-1 RNA levels show a decline of approximately 95% below baseline within 2 weeks of initiation of therapy, but this is followed by a rebound in viral load with the appearance of the M184V mutation in nonsuppressive regimens (118). Low-level resistance to didanosine is also conferred by this substitution. M184V has been reported to increase reverse transcriptase fidelity 2.4-fold, likely the consequence of reduced processivity (62, 137). The observed persistent antiviral effects in the presence of the M184V mutation may be the result of impaired fitness.

Although low-level cross-resistance (two- to fourfold) has been noted with M184V for didanosine and abacavir, the presence of the M184V mutation in isolation does not appear to compromise subsequent treatment with didanosine- or abacavir-containing regimens (88, 167). The M184V mutation reverses reduced susceptibility to the thymidine analogs and tenofovir conferred by the TAMs. Lamivudine also delays the emergence of zidovudine resistance mutations. These effects may, in part, underlie the efficacy of combination therapy of lamivudine and emtricitabine with thymidine analogs and tenofovir. The molecular basis for this effect relates to the fact that the M184V mutation, although decreasing the rate of incorporation of lamivudine monophosphate and conferring lamivudine resistance, also reduces pyrophosphorolytic rescue of DNA synthesis chain-terminating zidovudine triphosphate and therefore blocks the key zidovudine resistance mechanism (75).

Multidrug resistance mutations and mutation clusters may also confer various degrees of cross-resistance with lamivudine. The Q151M resistance complex (V75I, F77L, F116Y, and Q151M) is associated with a modest (4- to 10-fold) decrease in lamivudine susceptibility (101). A variety of substitution, deletion, and insertion mutations around codon 69, corresponding to the β3-β4 hairpin loop of the finger domain of the reverse transcriptase, diminish nucleoside susceptibilities, including that to lamivudine, more than 10-fold.

Clinical Applications

Lamivudine (or emtricitabine; see below) is a key component of current initial regimens in treatment-naïve persons with drug-susceptible virus because of its potency and excellent tolerability. It is typically combined with abacavir or zidovudine to form the dual-nucleoside component of NNRTI- or ritonavir-boosted PI-based regimens. Several studies examining three-nucleoside analog combinations have demonstrated high rates of virologic failure in treatment-naïve individuals. These regimens should be avoided (83, 121). In patients with viruses containing M184V, there may be benefit in continuing lamivudine to maintain this mutation because viruses with M184V replicate less well than wild-type viruses when a fully suppressive new regimen cannot be constructed.

Lamivudine and emtricitabine are essentially clinically interchangeable; the choice depends on which nucleoside or nucleotide analog is chosen to pair it with given the availability of fixed-dose combinations.

Abacavir

Abacavir sulfate {(−)-(1*S*,4*R*)-4-[2-amino-6-(cyclopropylamino)-9*H*-purin-9-yl]-2-cyclopentene-1-methanol; 1592U89, Ziagen} is a carbocyclic guanine analog (Fig. 1 and 3; Tables 1 and 3). It is available as both a 300-mg tablet and a 20-mg/ml solution, as well as in a fixed-dose formulation with lamivudine (Epzicom) and in combination with zidovudine and lamivudine (Trizivir).

Spectrum of Activity

Abacavir has an IC_{50} of 0.26 μM in human peripheral blood lymphocytes for HIV-1 strains. It is additive with NNRTIs, PIs, and other nucleoside analogs.

Mechanism of Action

Abacavir undergoes intracellular metabolism to its active triphosphate form, which interrupts HIV proviral DNA chain elongation. However, abacavir is also a prodrug that, prior to triphosphorylation, requires a modification to carbovir. Thus, abacavir activation is characterized by an initial phosphorylation by adenosine phosphotransferase to a monophosphate form, which is then further processed by a cytosolic 5′-nucleotidase to produce carbovir monophosphate; the latter is subsequently converted to di- and triphosphates of carbovir by cellular kinases.

Pharmacology

Abacavir sulfate is well absorbed, with an oral bioavailability of 83% and no important food effect. Similar pharmacokinetic profiles are seen with the abacavir-zidovudine-lamivudine fixed-dose formulation and with the three drugs given separately. C_{max}s in serum of 2.87 and 4.73 μg/ml are attained in less than 2 h after dosages of 300-mg b.i.d. and 600 mg, respectively. As the most lipophilic of the nucleoside analogs, abacavir exhibits good central nervous system (CNS) distribution, with mean levels in CSF that are twice the IC_{50} for wild-type HIV-1 and CSF-to-plasma AUC ratios ranging from 27 to 33% (128). Despite an elimination $t_{1/2}$ in plasma of 1.2 h for abacavir, the intracellular $t_{1/2}$ of carbovir triphosphate at an abacavir dosage of 300 mg/day is 20.6 h. Thus, the prolonged intracellular $t_{1/2}$ of the active carbovir triphosphate supports the approved b.i.d. or once-daily dosing.

Adverse Effects

Because abacavir is a relatively selective inhibitor of the HIV reverse transcriptase relative to cellular DNA polymerases, myelotoxicity is infrequent (114). Abacavir is generally well tolerated, with asthenia, abdominal pain, headache, diarrhea, and dyspepsia being the most commonly reported side effects. Laboratory abnormalities include elevations in liver enzyme levels.

The most significant adverse effect associated with abacavir is the idiosyncratic hypersensitivity reaction. This syndrome has an incidence of approximately 8% and is characterized by the appearance over several days of fever (80%), rash (70%), gastrointestinal symptoms (50%), malaise (40%), and respiratory symptoms. Fever or rash occurs in 98% of cases. Hypersensitivity cases typically occur within 6 weeks of the initiation of abacavir therapy (94%), with a median onset of 11 days. Accompanying laboratory abnormalities can include lymphopenia, thrombocytopenia, and elevated transaminase or creatine phosphokinase levels. This syndrome usually improves within days after the discontinuation of abacavir therapy. Rechallenge in individuals suspected of having this condition is contraindicated because severe allergic reactions, including fatalities, may occur within hours. Individuals who have tolerated abacavir in the past are unlikely to experience hypersensitivity reactions after reinitiating treatment; several severe or fatal exceptions, however, have been reported among these individuals (10, 141). HLA B*5701 predicts abacavir hypersensitivity (149), and screening for HLA B*5701 before initiating the drug is recommended, as it has been shown to significantly reduce the rate of hypersensitivity reactions in white populations; this feature may be generalizable to other groups (150, 191).

In a direct comparison between abacavir-lamivudine and tenofovir-emtricitabine, the former combination contributed to a greater increase in mean total cholesterol (increase of 12 mg/dl, versus 0), and triglyceride levels. In the ACTG A5202 study (see "Clinical applications" below), patients in the abacavir-lamivudine group with a baseline HIV RNA level of ≥100,000 copies/ml developed cholesterol and triglyceride abnormalities more rapidly than those in the tenofovir-emtricitabine group. Whether this translates into an increased risk of cardiovascular complications remains to be seen. A large prospective cohort study of over 333,000 patients suggested that recent use of abacavir may be associated with increased risk of myocardial infarction, particularly in patients with underlying risk of coronary artery disease (205). The significance of these findings is as yet unclear.

Drug Interactions

No significant drug interactions have been noted with abacavir.

Resistance

Selection for resistance to abacavir in vitro is characterized by the accumulation of multiple mutations within the HIV-1 reverse transcriptase. An initial M184V mutation, conferring a two- to fivefold increase in resistance, is followed by the appearance of either L74V/K65R or L74V/Y115F. While individually these mutations are associated with a low-level (2- to 4-fold) loss of susceptibility, M184V-containing double mutants have increased (7- to 11-fold) resistance. Abacavir-resistant isolates containing permutations of these mutations have various degrees of cross-resistance to lamivudine and didanosine.

Isolates obtained after abacavir monotherapy revealed substitutions at codons 65, 74, and 184. The addition of zidovudine appeared to delay the selection of the M184V mutation. In vivo studies identified the following mutations: K65R, L74V, Y115F, and M184V, as well as TAMs M41L, D67N, K70R, L210W, T215F/Y, and K219E/Q; the Q151M complex, usually in combination with V75I, F77L, F116Y; and T69 insertion mutations (110).

Failure to respond to abacavir combined with zidovudine-lamivudine generally is associated with the selection of the M184V mutation followed by the gradual accumulation of TAMs. Increasing numbers of TAMs (>4) result in a loss of virologic response to abacavir (133). Multinucleoside analog resistance-associated insertions at position 68 or 69 and the Q151M resistance complex (with codon 62, 68, 75, 77, and 116 changes) also confer cross-resistance to abacavir (110).

Clinical Applications

Abacavir has demonstrated durable efficacy in combination with lamivudine and either a PI or an NNRTI in treatment-naïve patients (45, 59, 72, 174, 199, 204). Abacavir may be administered either as a separate pill or in a more convenient fixed-dose combination, single-pill formulation that might favorably impact drug adherence. As noted above, triple-nucleoside-only regimens containing abacavir have higher rates of virologic failure than do efavirenz-containing combinations (83, 121) and should be avoided as initial regimens.

Studies evaluating the efficacies of combinations of nucleoside or nucleotide analogs indicate that (i) abacavir-lamivudine and zidovudine-lamivudine, each combined with efavirenz in treatment-naïve individuals, show comparable rates of virologic suppression to <50 copies/ml, but there is a greater increase in CD4 cell counts in the abacavir-lamivudine group (209 cells/mm^3, versus 155 cells/mm^3) (45); (ii) abacavir-lamivudine is comparable to tenofovir-emtricitabine, both regimens combined with lopinavir-ritonavir, but abacavir-lamivudine demonstrates a greater median increase in CD4 cell count than does tenofovir-emtricitabine (216). However, in the BICOMBO trial, noninferiority of abacavir-lamivudine relative to tenofovir-emtricitabine could not be demonstrated. Preliminary data from ACTG A5202, a study comparing abacavir-lamivudine with tenofovir-emtricitabine in combination with either efavirenz or atazanavir-ritonavir in treatment-naïve patients, suggested that individuals with higher baseline HIV-1 RNA levels were more likely to experience virologic failure in the abacavir-lamivudine arm than in the tenofovir-emtricitabine arm. Until further data are obtained, a degree of caution should be exercised when initiating therapy in patients with viral loads of >100,000 RNA copies/ml. For the treatment of antiretroviral-experienced patients, the use of abacavir-containing regimens has demonstrated limited clinical utility (35, 179).

Emtricitabine

Emtricitabine {5-fluoro-1-(2*R*,5*S*)-[2-(hydroxymethyl)-1,3-oxathiolan-5-yl]cytosine; Emtriva} is a cytidine analog that is the (−) enantiomer of a thio analog of cytidine; it differs from other cytidine analogs in that it has a fluorine in the 5 position (Fig. 1 and 3; Tables 1 and 3). It is available as both a 200-mg tablet and a 10-mg/ml solution, as well as in fixed-dose formulations with tenofovir (Truvada) and tenofovir and efavirenz (Atripla). Emtricitabine is administered in a once-daily dosage of 200 mg (48).

Spectrum of Activity

Relative to other cytidine analogs like lamivudine, emtricitabine is 4- to 10-fold more potent; for a laboratory-adapted strain, it has an IC_{50} of 0.009 to 0.5 μM in human cell lines (196, 207). This heightened potency may be the result of a greater efficiency of incorporation of emtricitabine triphosphate than of lamivudine triphosphate by the HIV-1 reverse transcriptase (62). It has activity against HIV-1, HIV-2, and HBV. The role of emtricitabine as an anti-HBV agent is discussed in chapter 12. Emtricitabine has demonstrated synergistic or additive activity with other nucleoside analogs, PIs, and NNRTIs.

Mechanism of Action

Emtricitabine undergoes serial intracellular phosphorylations to an active triphosphate form. Emtricitabine 5′-triphosphate inhibits the activity of the HIV-1 reverse transcriptase by competing with the natural substrate deoxycytidine 5′-triphosphate. Because it lacks a hydroxyl group at the 3′ position of the oxothiolane moiety (41, 196), incorporation of emtricitabine 5′-triphosphate interrupts HIV proviral DNA chain elongation in susceptible strains (62).

Pharmacology

Emtricitabine is rapidly absorbed, and the C_{max} in plasma is reached in 1 to 2 h. The AUC of emtricitabine is not affected by coadministration of food. The drug has low protein binding (<4%). The elimination $t_{1/2}$ in plasma averages approximately 10 h, and the intracellular $t_{1/2}$ of emtricitabine triphosphate is longer than 20 h.

Emtricitabine is predominantly renally eliminated by both glomerular filtration and active tubular secretion; thus, dosing interval adjustments are required in individuals with creatinine clearances of <50 ml/min. Hemodialysis removes approximately 30% of the emtricitabine dose.

Adverse Effects

Emtricitabine, like lamivudine, is well tolerated. Adverse effects attributed to emtricitabine have been mild to moderate CNS and gastrointestinal symptoms (Table 3). For HBV-coinfected individuals, exacerbations of hepatitis B have been reported after discontinuation of emtricitabine.

Drug Interactions

There are no clinically significant drug interactions.

Resistance

As with lamivudine, high-level resistance to emtricitabine is associated with M184I/V reverse transcriptase mutations. In clinical studies, the combination of tenofovir with emtricitabine was less likely to select for the M184V mutation than the zidovudine-lamivudine combination. The emtricitabine-containing regimen was also less likely to select for the K65R mutation than lamivudine in the presence of tenofovir.

Clinical Applications

Emtricitabine or lamivudine in combination with stavudine and a nonnucleoside inhibitor (nevirapine or efavirenz) results in equivalent antiviral effects after 48 weeks of therapy (16% probability of virologic failure for emtricitabine, versus 11% for lamivudine). Once-daily combination of emtricitabine compared to b.i.d. stavudine with a background regimen of didanosine and efavirenz results in higher rates of virologic suppression (<50 copies/ml with 76% with emtricitabine, versus 54% with stavudine) (203). Emtricitabine has also shown efficacy in treatment-experienced patients with plasma HIV-1 RNA levels of <400 copies/ml who switch from lamivudine- or PI-containing regimens to emtricitabine-containing ones. The simplification to once-daily emtricitabine does not affect the proportion of patients with plasma HIV-1 RNA level suppression to <400 or <50 copies/ml. Emtricitabine in combination with tenofovir has demonstrated considerable potency and durability of virologic control as part of PI- or NNRTI-based regimens (5).

SELECTED INVESTIGATIONAL NRTIs

Numerous nucleoside analogs have been and will continue to be evaluated as antiretrovirals. A few have progressed through early stages of clinical evaluation and are listed in Table 2.

NUCLEOTIDE ANALOG REVERSE TRANSCRIPTASE INHIBITORS

Tenofovir Disoproxil Fumarate

Tenofovir [bis(isopropyloxymethylcarbonyl)PMPA; Viread] (Fig. 1 and 3; Tables 1 and 3) is a prodrug of the cyclic nucleoside phosphonate 9-*R*-(2-phosphonomethoxypropyl)adenine (PMPA). This agent is available in 300-mg tablets approved for once-daily dosing. It is available in combination with emtricitabine (Truvada) and emtricitabine and efavirenz (Atripla) in fixed-dose combination tablets.

Spectrum of Activity

Tenofovir is an inhibitor of retroviruses, including HIV-1, simian immunodeficiency virus, and feline leukemia virus, as well as hepadnaviruses.

Mechanism of Action

Tenofovir disoproxil fumarate is converted to tenofovir by diester hydrolysis and subsequently undergoes phosphorylation to form tenofovir diphosphate. The antiviral activity of this agent is due to the inhibition of viral DNA polymerases. With respect to HIV-1, this class of agents inhibits HIV-1 reverse transcriptase more potently than it inhibits cellular DNA polymerases, which may be the basis for the excellent tolerability of tenofovir.

Pharmacology

Because of the drug's hydrophilic properties, tenofovir demonstrates a permeability-limited oral absorption (bioavailability of 25 to 40%). To overcome this, tenofovir is formulated as the *bis*-ester prodrug, tenofovir disoproxil fumarate (232). Administration of tenofovir with a high-fat meal increases its bioavailability from 25 to 39%; bioavailability is not appreciably affected by lower-fat meals, so it is dosed without regard to food. Tenofovir disoproxil fumarate has a $t_{1/2}$ of approximately 17.1 h, with intracellular $t_{1/2}$s of the diphosphate form of 12 to 15 h in activated PBMCs and 33 to 50 h in resting PBMCs, thus permitting once-daily dosing. The drug is excreted renally by both glomerular filtration and active tubular secretion.

Adverse Effects

A small proportion of patients taking tenofovir experience increases in serum creatinine, glycosuria, hypophosphatemia, and acute tubular necrosis. However, renal impairment was not common in patients with normal renal function at baseline (248). Patients with more advanced HIV disease, greater treatment experience, concomitant PI use, and preexisting renal impairment may be at an increased risk of this complication (70). The mechanism of tenofovir's infrequent renal dysfunction remains an active area of investigation. The agent should be used with caution in individuals with preexisting renal disease, and alternative nucleoside analogs should be considered. In individuals coinfected with HBV, discontinuation of tenofovir may cause flares of viral replication and hepatitis; close monitoring of such patients is advised.

Fat maldistribution is not commonly seen with tenofovir-based regimens (71), and switching from zidovudine- or stavudine-containing regimens to tenofovir or abacavir may slow or halt the progression of this syndrome. Tenofovir may have a more pronounced effect on bone loss than other agents (79). The safety of tenofovir in pregnancy has not yet been established, but animal studies indicate impaired fetal growth and decreased fetal bone porosity within 2 months of starting maternal therapy. Human teratogenicity has not yet been reported.

Drug Interactions

Tenofovir has exhibited strong antiviral activity in combination with other antiretroviral agents. Tenofovir decreases the AUC of atazanavir by 25%; therefore, patients who receive concomitant therapy with tenofovir should use ritonavir-boosted atazanavir.

In clinical studies, the combination of tenofovir and didanosine has been associated with increased didanosine toxicity and a high rate of early virologic failure as well as CD4 cell decline in treated individuals, although conflicting data on this point exist (148, 185). Coadministration of darunavir with tenofovir has resulted in an increased tenofovir AUC, but the clinical significance of this interaction has not been established.

Resistance

Tenofovir retains activity against a range of nucleoside-resistant HIV strains. In vitro, the K65R mutation of HIV-1 confers a ninefold decrease in sensitivity to tenofovir, and the M184V mutation partially reverses this resistance. Insertions at codon 69 also confer decreased susceptibility to tenofovir. The effect of this mutation is potentiated in the presence of the M184V mutation. Nonresponse to tenofovir is more likely to occur when the drug is added to a failing regimen in heavily pretreated patients, as opposed to its use as a part of a new regimen with other active medications. Clinical data suggest that the presence of >2 TAMs, particularly M41L or L210W, is associated with decreased susceptibility to tenofovir. The activity of tenofovir is retained in the presence of the Q151M complex mutations (153, 164).

Clinical Applications

Potent and durable virologic suppression is seen in treatment-naïve individuals with tenofovir and lamivudine or emtricitabine in combination with efavirenz (68, 71; J. R. Arribas, A. Pozniak, J. Gallant, E. DeJesus, R. Campo, S. S. Chen, D. McColl, A. Cheng, and J. Enejosa, poster exhibition at the 4th IAS Conference on HIV Pathogenesis, Treatment, and Prevention, Sydney, Australia). In direct comparison with lamivudine-zidovudine, tenofovir-emtricitabine demonstrates a greater increase in CD4 cell counts and a higher rate of virologic suppression to <50 copies/ml sustained over 144 weeks (5). Importantly, the tenofovir-emtricitabine fixed-dose combination has been better tolerated than the fixed-dose zidovudine-lamivudine. Experience with tenofovir-emtricitabine compared to abacavir-lamivudine in combination with either efavirenz or atazanavir-ritonavir is described in the section on abacavir above. Higher rates of virologic failure occur with the combination of tenofovir, abacavir, and lamivudine in treatment-naïve individuals (121, 132). These combinations should not be used.

In treatment-experienced individuals with incomplete virologic suppression and baseline nucleoside resistance mutations, the addition of tenofovir to stable regimens usually results in reductions in plasma HIV-1 RNA levels (208). In patients with suppressed viral loads at baseline, switching the nucleoside component to tenofivir-emtricitabine results in fewer treatment failures and drug discontinuations than switching to abacavir-lamivudine. Discontinuations have been higher with abacavir-lamivudine, possibly due to abacavir hypersensitivity when patients given abacavir have not been screened at baseline for the presence of HLA-B*5701.

The potency, convenience, and favorable safety profile make tenofovir, when paired with emtricitabine in a fixed-dose combination, an important component of an initial three-drug regimen that includes a PI or NNRTI (86).

NONNUCLEOSIDE REVERSE TRANSCRIPTASE INHIBITORS

Although structurally diverse, the nonnucleoside inhibitors share similar HIV-1 reverse transcriptase binding sites and function by noncompetitive allosteric binding to a hydrophobic pocket created by the p66 palm-and-thumb subdomains of the reverse transcriptase (214). This alters the structure and function of the HIV-1 reverse transcriptase (181). When the NNRTI is bound to this site, it interacts with multiple amino acid residues within the pocket. Mutations in the codons of these key amino acids alter inhibitor binding properties and form the mechanistic basis for NNRTI resistance. The binding of an NNRTI to the enzyme-DNA complex is proposed to slow reverse transcriptase-mediated catalysis by causing a distortion of the normal spatial configuration of the carboxyl groups and associated Mg^{2+} ions of three aspartic acid residues in the adjacent polymerase active site (218). As a consequence, nucleotide triphosphate molecules destined to be added to the elongating proviral DNA chain are bound but inefficiently utilized. The narrow spectrum of antiviral activity is conferred by a tyrosine at amino acid position 181 in HIV-1 but not present in HIV-2 or the HIV-1 O clade, against which these compounds are inactive (122).

Nevirapine

Nevirapine (11-cyclopropyl-5,11-dihydro-4-methyl-6*H*-dipyrido[3,2-b:2′,3′-e][1,4]diazepin-6-one; Viramune) (Fig. 1 and 4; Tables 1 and 3) formulations include 200-mg tablets and a 50-mg/ml oral suspension. Nevirapine antiviral activity is limited to HIV-1, with an IC_{50} of 10 to 100 nM, while 50% cytotoxicity requires 321,000 nM concentrations.

Pharmacology

Nevirapine is rapidly absorbed, with an oral bioavailability of >90%. An initial C_{max} in serum of 2.0 ng/ml is reached approximately 4 h after a 200-mg oral dose. Steady-state trough concentrations average 4.5 ng/ml (~16 μM) at a nevirapine dosage of 400 mg/day. Concentrations in plasma do not appear to be altered by food or antacids. Secondary peak levels are seen, which may reflect enterohepatic recirculation. Plasma protein binding is approximately 60%. Although in one study, the concentrations in CSF ranged from 336 to 2,781 μg/liter (above the IC_{50} for laboratory and clinical isolates, 2.66 to 26.7 μg/liter), these concentrations are below that predicted by plasma protein binding (117). Nevirapine crosses the placenta and is present in breast milk and semen.

The clearance of nevirapine increases through the first 2 to 4 weeks of dosing, such that the elimination $t_{1/2}$ of nevirapine in plasma decreases from 45 h after single doses to 25 to 30 h with multiple ones. Detectable levels of nevirapine have been found in chronically treated children and adults for up to 7 days after nevirapine cessation (40). Detectable levels may persist longer in treatment-naïve

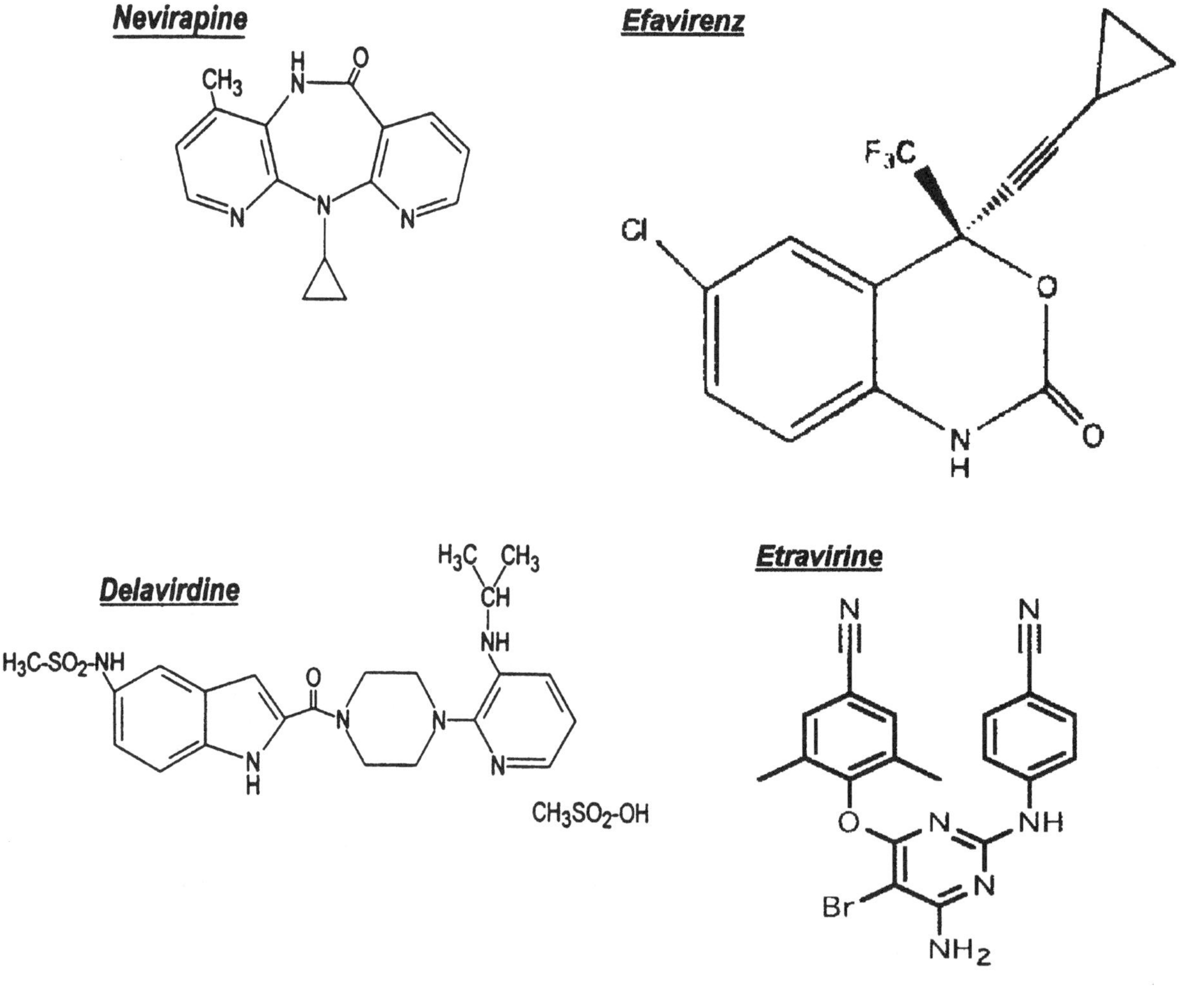

FIGURE 4 Chemical structures of NNRTIs.

women who receive single-dose nevirapine for prophylaxis of mother-to-child transmission of HIV-1. Nevirapine is metabolized to hydroxymethylnevirapine in liver microsomes and also dose dependently induces the CYP450 family CYP3A and CYP2B1 isozymes.

Adverse Effects

The most common adverse reaction associated with nevirapine is a nonpruritic macular rash distributed on the face, trunk, and extremities, excluding the palms and soles; the rash usually occurs within the first 6 weeks of therapy. Rash has occurred in 48% of nevirapine recipients who received 400 mg/day. Severe rash may be more common in women. Stevens-Johnson syndrome has been reported. The incidence of rash does not appear to be related to plasma drug levels, stage of HIV disease, history of rash with other agents, gender, or race. The risk may be attenuated by administering a lower initial dosage of 200 mg/day for 2 weeks and then increasing the dosage to 200 mg b.i.d. The rash may be accompanied by hepatotoxicity, fever, and myalgias.

Liver toxicity occurs in about 4% of patients. The risk of hepatotoxicity is higher in women and in patients with higher CD4 cell counts (>250 cells/μl in women and >400 cells/μl in men), and thus nevirapine should not be initiated in these populations. Coinfection with HBV or HCV increases the risk of liver toxicity. Life-threatening and fatal cases of hepatotoxicity as well as severe, even fatal, skin reactions, including Stevens-Johnson syndrome, toxic epidermal necrolysis, and hypersensitivity reactions, have been reported and can occur duirng the first 18 weeks of therapy. The overall rate of hypersensitivity reaction has been about 6%; increased risk has been associated with high pretreatment plasma HIV-1 RNA levels, high CD4 cell counts, and female gender.

Drug Interactions

Nevirapine has no pharmacokinetic interactions with nucleosides, but it does decrease the AUCs of the PIs. Given the involvement of the CYP450 system in its metabolism, nevirapine would be expected to have effects on coadministered drugs which also utilize the CYP3A4 metabolic pathway, such as rifampin and rifabutin. Coadministration of rifampin and nevirapine or efavirenz is associated with lower nevirapine concentrations and greater variability in plasma drug levels. Some data suggest that combining efavirenz or nevirapine at standard doses in combination with rifampin results in comparable virologic and clinical outcomes (6, 64). Nevirapine-induced methadone withdrawal has been reported, and the methadone dose should be increased before commencing nevirapine (31).

Resistance

The nevirapine binding site is created mainly by amino acid residues 100 to 110 and 180 to 190, comprising the 2β sheets that form the binding pocket in the HIV-1 reverse transcriptase. Consequently, mutations associated with resistance generally fall within these regions. In vitro and clinical isolate data indicate several mutations which are responsible for conferring nevirapine resistance. These include L100I, K103N, V106A, V108I, Y181C/I, Y188C/L/H, and G190A (109). Several of these mutations engender variable cross-resistance to other NNRTIs.

In vivo, nevirapine-resistant isolates are genotypically mixed, and the most common ones in patients with virologic failure occur at positions 103, 181, 190, 188, and 106. Each mutation reduces nevirapine susceptibility at least 50-fold (110). The in vitro introduction of the nevirapine-associated Y181C substitution in zidovudine-resistant HIV strains causes an increase in zidovudine susceptibility. Mutations at positions 138 and 227 selected by etravirine appear to reduce susceptibility to nevirapine and efavirenz, and V179F in combination with Y181C causes high-level resistance to nevirapine and etravirine.

Clinical Applications

In a direct comparison with efavirenz and nevirapine, both given in combination with stavudine and lamivudine, nevirapine b.i.d. demonstrated a similar rate of virologic suppression to a plasma HIV-1 RNA level of <50 copies/ml, and there were no significant differences in treatment failure between regimens (233). Despite these data, nevirapine's b.i.d. dosing and risk of heptatotoxicity make it a less attractive option as initial therapy than efavirenz in nonpregnant women or those seeking to become pregnant. Its major use in the developed world is as an alternative to efavirenz in patients intolerant to the latter agent's CNS side effects. In the developing world, nevirapine is a key component of initial regimens because of its low cost and availability in fixed-dose generic combinations.

Nevirapine is safe in pregnant women with CD4 cell counts of <250 cells/μl. Administering single-dose nevirapine to both the mother and infant in the peripartum period significantly reduces vertical transmission of HIV-1 but is associated with a substantial incidence of resistance in women (up to 40 to 60%) and infants (33 to 87%), especially if techniques for low-frequency mutant detection are employed (61, 212). Addition of a short course of nucleoside analogs (zidovudine-lamivudine or tenofovir-emtricitabine) decreases the development of maternal and pediatric resistance after single dose nevirapine (30, 161).

Efavirenz

Efavirenz {[(S)-6-chloro-4-(cyclopropylethyn)-1,4-dihydro-4-(trifluoromethyl)-2*H*-3,1-benzoxazin-2-one]; L-743,726, DMP 266, Sustiva} is available in tablet and capsule formulations (Fig. 1 and 4; Tables 1 and 3). It is also available in combination with emtricitabine and tenofovir as a single tablet (Atripla). It has IC_{90}s ranging from 0.003 to 0.009 μM for wild-type clinical and laboratory HIV-1 isolates.

Pharmacology

The bioavailability of efavirenz in humans has not been reported; a meal high in fat content increases the bioavailability of efavirenz by 50%. The C_{max} averages 4.0 μM and the C_{min} averages 1.6 μM at a 600-mg daily dosage. Variability in plasma drug levels may be in part explained by the allelic pattern of two genes responsible for the metabolism and transport of efavirenz, the genes for P-glycoprotein and CYP450 isozyme CYP2D6. The levels of efavirenz in CSF reflect only 1% of the concentration of the drug in plasma due to almost complete protein binding. Efavirenz achieves therapeutic concentrations in semen throughout the dosing interval and can suppress HIV-1 levels in the seminal compartment.

Hepatic metabolism of efavirenz is the major mechanism of drug clearance via the CYP3A4 and CYP2D6 systems; therefore, liver disease decreases the C_{max} of efavirenz compared with that in healthy subjects. The hepatic cytochrome system metabolizes efavirenz to hydroxylated metabolites, with subsequent glucuronidation, and these metabolites are excreted in the urine.

Adverse Effects

Efavirenz toxicities include maculopapular rash, dizziness (27%, versus 9% in the control group), impaired concentration (11%, versus 4%), depression (9%, versus 5%), abnormal dreaming (6%, versus 1%), and euphoria (5%, versus 2%). CNS adverse events occur more often in subjects taking efavirenz (54%, versus 27%), although these symptoms tend to resolve over the course of a few weeks probably due to self-induction of hepatic metabolism and increased clearance of the drug. The incidence of adverse events does not differ with the timing of the dose, splitting of the dose, or age of the subject, although when efavirenz is taken at night, the CNS side effects may be more tolerable. The incidence and severity of rash are not related to dose. Efavirenz administration can generally be continued despite the occurrence of a rash, with resolution over 3 to 4 weeks. As with other NNRTIs, metabolic abnormalities such as lipoatrophy and elevations in high-density lipoprotein cholesterol and total cholesterol have also been observed in subjects taking efavirenz (46, 92). Efavirenz has been associated with an increased risk of lipoatrophy compared to lopinavir-ritonavir, whereas derangements in lipid profiles (triglycerides in particular) were similar in the two groups (92).

Efavirenz is assigned an FDA pregnancy category C status. In pregnant cynomolgus monkeys treated throughout pregnancy with doses of efavirenz which resulted in plasma drug levels similar to those in humans dosed with 600 mg/day, craniofacial malformations (anencephaly, unilateral anopthalmia, microophthalmia, and cleft palate) occurred. Several cases of neural tube defects have been reported after early human gestational exposure to efavirenz (67). Pregnancy should be avoided in women receiving efavirenz, and women should undergo pregnancy testing prior to starting this agent. Women taking a regimen that includes efavirenz should receive counseling regarding contraceptive practices.

Drug Interactions

Efavirenz is a substrate of CYP450 and thus affects the hepatic metabolism of many coadministered drugs. It lowers the concentrations of maraviroc and etravirine. Atazanavir levels are decreased by 74%; therefore, it has to be administered with ritonavir and the response has to be monitored (180). Dosage adjustment is indicated for rifabutin and methadone (32), and an alternative to clarithromycin is recommended when efavirenz is used.

Resistance

Efavirenz selects for the Y181C/I, V106M, L100I, K103N, G190S/A, P225H, V108I, K103N, Y188L, G190S/A, and P225H mutations (109). The K103N mutation confers cross-resistance to nevirapine and delavirdine but not to etravirine. Patients failing efavirenz combination therapy have shown 19- to 36-fold resistance to efavirenz in isolates containing the K103N reverse transcriptase mutation and 280-fold resistance in isolates with the G190S mutation. Resistance to efavirenz increases to 100-fold with the development of additional mutations at codons 106, 188, 190, and 106 (194). Several nucleoside analog mutations (e.g., 118I, 298Y, and 215Y) can result in phenotypic hypersusceptibility to efavirenz in patients with extensive NRTI experience (213). The underlying mechanism may include increased reverse transcriptase enzyme susceptibility to the NNRTI (e.g., with 118I/215Y) or decreased virion-associated levels of reverse transcriptase (with 208Y/215Y and 118I/208Y/215Y).

Clinical Applications

Efavirenz-containing regimens compare favorably to PI-based therapy, including atazanavir and lopinavir/ritonavir-based regimens (198, 219, 221), and to triple-nucleoside-based regimens (83). In combination with the dual-nucleoside backbone of tenofovir-emtricitabine, zidovudine-lamivudine, or abacavir-lamivudine, efavirenz has achieved high rates of virologic suppression (45, 71, 82). Efavirenz compared with nevirapine, each in combination with lamivudine-stavudine, showed no significant differences in rates of virologic suppression or increases in CD4 cell counts (233). Efavirenz has shown an efficacy comparable to that of PI-based regimens in two retrospective and one open-label study of treatment-naïve patients with advanced HIV-1 disease (165, 188).

Delavirdine

Delavirdine {1-(5-methanesulfonamido-1*H*-indol-2-yl-carbonyl)-4-[3-(1-methylethylamino)pyridinyl] piperazine; Rescriptor} (Fig. 1 and 4; Tables 1 and 3) has a recommended dosage in adults of 400 mg three times daily when combined with agents that do not affect its metabolism.

Pharmacology

Delavirdine is rapidly absorbed, with an oral bioavailability of more than 60%. Antacids or a high gastric pH decreases the AUC of delavirdine. A large proportion of delavirdine is protein bound (98%), and the median CSF-to-plasma ratio is approximately 0.39. Delavirdine is metabolized through human liver microsomal CYP450 and can partially inhibit CYP2C9, -2C19, -2D6, and -3A4.

Adverse Effects

The most common adverse effect is a pruritic maculopapular rash that characteristically presents during the first 2 weeks of therapy and can usually be managed without discontinuation of the drug. Stevens-Johnson syndrome and erythema multiforme can occur.

Drug Interactions

By inhibiting the CYP450 CYP3A4 isozyme, delavirdine enhances the pharmacokinetic profile of the PIs indinavir, saquinavir, and fosamprenavir, whereas nelfinavir decreases delavirdine levels by approximately 50% (13, 180).

Resistance

In patients experiencing virologic failure on delavirdine therapy, isolates manifest the K103N and Y181C mutations and the P236L substitution; each individual mutation reduces the susceptibility to delavirdine approximately 50-fold (26, 195). Mutations G190A/S and P225H, which confer resistance to nevirapine and efavirenz, have been shown to produce hypersensitivity to delavirdine.

Clinical Applications

Early studies of delavirdine in combination with one or two NRTIs showed modest potency and durability (65, 112). Given the limited efficacy of delavirdine in treatment-naïve and -experienced individuals (80, 81), the agent's high pill burden, and the availability of more potent agents in this class, delavirdine is rarely prescribed.

Etravirine

Etravirine {4-[[6-amino-5-bromo-2-[(4-cyanophenyl)-amino]-4-pyrimidinyl]oxy]-3,5-dimethylbenzonitrile; Intelence, TMC 125} is a diaryl-pyrimidine derivative that binds to HIV reverse transcriptase with mutations within the hydrophobic pocket (Fig. 1 and 4; Tables 1 and 3). It is approved for use in individuals who have experienced virologic failure with other NNRTIs and harbor a multi-drug-resistant virus (235). Formulations of this agent include 100-mg tablets. Etravirine exhibits activity against laboratory as well as wild-type strains of HIV-1, with median IC_{50}s ranging from 0.9 to 5.5 nM (0.4 to 2.4 ng/ml).

Pharmacology

The oral bioavailability of etravine has not been determined. The AUC of the drug under fasting conditions is diminished by 50%; therefore, etravirine should be taken with food. The C_{max} averages 390 ng/ml at 4 h after dosing. It is highly protein bound, and its distribution in other compartments (CSF and genital tract secretions) has not been evaluated to date. Although the elimination $t_{1/2}$ of etravirine in plasma (41 h) is long enough to support once-daily dosing, such dosing has not been tested in controlled trials to date. It is primarily excreted via feces, with only a limited amount of renal excretion (1.2%).

Drug Interactions

Like nevirapine and efavirenz, etravirine is hepatically metabolized by the CYP450 system. It is both a substrate and an inducer of CYP3A4, as well as an inhibitor of CYP2C9 and CYP2C19. As a result, coadministration of etravirine with inhibitors or inducers of these CYP450 enzymes may alter levels of etravirine in serum, and coadministration of etravine with drugs that are substrates of these enzymes may alter their levels in serum. Certain antiretrovirals should not be coadministered with etravirine, including other NNRTIs, all unboosted PIs, and ritonavir-boosted tipranavir or fosamprenavir. Combining etravirine with lopinavir-ritonavir is possible but should be done with caution. Darunavir-ritonavir reduces the AUC of etravirine by about 37%; etravirine has been safe and effective with darunavir-ritonavir as part of the background regimen without dosage adjustments. The maraviroc AUC is decreased by 53%, and the dosage of maraviroc needs be adjusted to 600 mg b.i.d. if it is coadministered with etravirine. If maraviroc is being dosed with a ritonavir-boosted PI as well as etravirine, the dosage of maraviroc should be 150 mg b.i.d. Etravirine can be combined with the integrase inhibitor, raltegravir.

Adverse Effects

The most commonly reported adverse events are nausea and rash (91, 107). The rash is mild to moderate in severity, occurs most frequently in the second week of therapy, and generally resolves within 1 to 2 weeks on continued therapy. It is a rare cause of drug discontinuation (91, 107, 138, 146). There are no observable effects on lipids or liver function enzymes.

Rare cases of serious skin reactions, like Stevens-Johnson syndrome and erythema multiforme, were reported during clinical development, but the risk appears to be low (no cases among over 500 treated patients in phase III studies). Patients with a history of NNRTI-related rash did not appear to be at an increased risk for the development of rash while taking etravirine.

Resistance

Mutations at the following codons present at baseline appear to affect the response to etravirine: V90I, A98G, L100I, K101E/P, V106I, V179D/F, Y181C/I/V, and G190A/S (109, 116). In in vitro studies, the highest levels of resistance to etravirine were observed for HIV-1 harboring a combination of substitutions: V179F plus Y181C (187-fold change), V179F plus Y181I (123-fold change), or V179F plus Y181C plus F227C (888-fold change). The K103N mutation does not confer resistance to etravirine.

The presence of at least three of these mutations at baseline (particularly V179D, V179F, Y181V, and G190S) has been associated with a diminished response to the drug (19, 138, 146). The development of cross-resistance to other NNRTIs in patients failing etravirine-based regimens is expected but remains to be elucidated.

Clinical Applications

Etravirine monotherapy demonstrated considerable potency and tolerability over 7 days in treatment-naïve individuals (78). Subsequent short-term studies in treatment-experienced individuals failing initial NNRTI regimens demonstrated that etravirine had virologic activity against NNRTI-resistant virus (73). Etravirine's niche lies in combination with at least one other active agent in highly treatment-experienced individuals; the addition of etravirine results in an increased proportion of individuals achieving sustained virologic suppression to <50 copies/ml and greater increases in CD4 cell counts than with placebo (138, 145). Among patients with a moderate loss of susceptibility to darunavir (darunavir change, <40-fold), the presence of at least two active drugs in the background regimen correlates with a better virologic response in the etravirine arm. The additive benefit of etravirine, however, is least pronounced in individuals with ≥2 active agents in the background regimen (91, 107).

INVESTIGATIONAL NNRTIs

A number of investigational NNRTI compounds continue through preclinical and clinical development. These agents are typically characterized by activity against HIV-1 strains that are resistant to efavirenz or nevirapine. Selected agents are described below; other promising drugs in phase I or preclinical testing are listed in Table 2.

Rilpivirine

Rilpivirine [4-((4-5(4-((1E)-2-cyanoethyl)-2,6-dimethylphenyl)amino)-2-pyrimydinyl)amino)benzonitrile; TMC 278], is a diaryl-pyrimidine analog that demonstrates conformational "flexibility" enabling it to bind to the hydrophobic pocket of the reverse transcriptase enzyme in both wild-type and drug-resistant variants (42). It has an IC_{50} of <1 nM and both good oral bioavailability and a prolonged elimination $t_{1/2}$, >30 h, in humans, allowing for once-daily dosing (74). The agent is a substrate of the CYP3A4 isoenzyme, and therefore exposure to rilpivirine is increased during coadministration with ritonavir and decreased during coadministration of rifabutin.

Rilpivirine has demonstrated activity in antiretroviral-naïve and -experienced patients. In treatment-naïve patients, no significant differences occurred in plasma HIV-1 RNA changes from baseline between the rilpivirine and efavirenz arms: at 48 weeks, 77 to 81% of subjects in the rilpivirine arm achieved the primary endpoint of <50 HIV-1 RNA copies/ml, compared to 81% in the efavirenz arm. Changes in the CD4 cell counts were also similar between the two arms. Rilpivirine has been well tolerated and less likely than efavirenz to cause a rash and CNS adverse effects. The most common side effects are dizziness and headache. Compared to efavirenz, rilpivirine appears to have a minimal effect on total cholesterol and virtually no effect on low-density lipoprotein cholesterol or triglyceride levels. Drug discontinuations are more common with the 150-mg dose. The 75-mg once-daily dosage was selected for further testing in phase III trials that will compare the drug to efavirenz in treatment-naïve patients.

The agent appears to have a relatively high genetic barrier to resistance. Mutations selected by rilpivirine in vitro include Y181C alone or in combination with other mutations such as E40K, K101E/I, V108I, V179F, M230I, H221Y, F227C, and T386A. It remains to be seen what this drug's role might be in individuals with resistance to first-generation NNRTIs.

INTEGRASE INHIBITORS

HIV integrase is a virally encoded enzyme that is responsible for integrating the viral DNA into the genome of the host cell (186). Integration of the viral genome is essential for stable maintenance of the genome and for viral gene expression and replication. Integration is a multistep event that involves processing of the viral DNA by removing the terminal dinucleotide from each end, formation of the preintegration complex, and integration of the DNA strand into the cellular DNA. The enzyme incorporates viral DNA strands into the host chromosome through strand transfer. Integrase inhibitors belong to a new class of antiretroviral agents that selectively inhibit the strand transfer function of the HIV integrase enzyme, thereby preventing integration and inhibiting HIV replication (93, 94).

Raltegravir

Raltegravir {*N*-(4-fluorobenzyl)5-hydroxy-1-methyl-2-(1-methyl-1-([(5-methyl-1,3,4-oxadiazol-2-yl)carbonyl]amino)-ethyl)-6-oxo-1,6-dihydropyrimidine-4-carboxamide; MK-0518, Isentress} was approved by the FDA in October 2007 at a dosage of 400 mg orally b.i.d. for use in treatment-experienced patients with resistance to other antiretroviral drug classes.

Spectrum of Activity

Raltegravir is active against viruses resistant to all other classes of antiretrovirals, with IC_{95}s of 31 ± 20 nM against the H9IIIB variant of HIV-1 in human cell lines.

Pharmacology

The C_{max} in plasma averages 4.94 μM 1 h after a single dose of 200 mg of raltegravir in healthy volunteers (115), and levels in plasma decline below the limits of detection by 24 h. In single and multiple dose-ranging studies in healthy and infected subjects, concentrations in serum declined in a biphasic manner, with an initial-phase elimination $t_{1/2}$ of approximately 1 h and a terminal-phase elimination $t_{1/2}$ of 7 to 12 h. Steady-state concentrations are achieved within 2 days. The major mechanism of clearance of raltegravir in humans is by hepatic UGT-1A1. Glucuronidated raltegravir is excreted primarily in feces (51% of the dose) and urine (32% of the dose) (115). No dose adjustment appears to be necessary in patients with severe renal insufficiency. In clinical trials using combination antiretroviral therapy, raltegravir pharmacokinetic parameter values (AUC from 0 to 12 h, C_{max}, and C_{max} at 12 h) were increased 1.33- to 1.42-fold compared with monotherapy (156).

Adverse Effects

Raltegravir is well tolerated and does not seem to be associated with lipid abnormalities. Possible side effects include nausea and elevated liver enzymes. To date, the risk of developing a malignancy has not been increased in individuals receiving raltegravir (77, 155).

Drug Interactions

Raltegravir is eliminated primarily by the UGT1A1-mediated glucuronidation pathway; therefore, it may be subject to drug interactions when coadministered with UGT1A1 inducers or inhibitors (e.g., atazanavir). The addition of atazanavir-ritonavir to a regimen of raltegravir at 400 mg every 12 h increases the raltegravir AUC by 41% and the C_{max} by 24% (103). Levels of raltegravir in plasma may be mildly increased during concomitant use of tenofovir, but this does not require dose adjustment. Levels in plasma were moderately reduced when raltegravir was coadministered with efavirenz and rifampin (the C_{max} decreased by 38% with the latter), but the clinical significance of this interaction remains to be determined (104). Levels of raltegravir in plasma were not affected by coadministration with ritonavir or tipranavir.

Resistance

HIV-1 develops resistance to raltegravir with mutations in the active site of the integrase gene. In the phase III clinical studies of raltegravir in treatment-experienced individuals, virologic failure was associated with mutations Q148H/K/R and N155H, which represent signature mutations that define two pathways of resistance. Each of these mutations is typically accompanied by one or more additional mutations in isolates derived from patients exhibiting virologic failure on raltegravir.

Clinical Applications

Raltegravir has been evaluated as part of initial therapy in treatment-naïve individuals and as salvage therapy in individuals harboring a multidrug-resistant HIV strain.

In a 10-day monotherapy study, raltegravir monotherapy (100, 200, 400, and 600 mg) resulted in mean HIV-1 RNA decreases of 1.99 $\log_{10}$ copies/ml at the 600-mg dose (154). Compared to efavirenz, in combination with tenofovir and lamivudine, raltegravir demonstrates higher rates of early virologic suppression to <50 copies/ml; at 48 weeks, however, comparable rates of virologic suppression and mean changes in $CD4^+$ cell counts (144 to 221 cells/μl) are seen in both groups (156).

When used in combination with optimized background therapy in treatment-experienced individuals with evidence of resistance to at least one drug in each of the three classes, raltegravir has resulted in up to a 2-$\log_{10}$ decrease in week 24 HIV-1 RNA levels compared to optimized background therapy alone. Significantly greater proportions of patients in the raltegravir treatment arm achieve HIV-1 RNA levels of <50 copies/ml. Higher doses of the drug resulted in greater CD4 cell recovery (77). Favorable responses have been sustained at 48 weeks (77), thus leading to the selection of raltegravir at 400 mg orally b.i.d. as the dosage to take forward in clinical development.

In two pivotal studies, week 48 data confirmed the superior potency and durability of raltegravir compared to placebo, each in combination with an optimized background, in individuals with triple-class resistant virus: 64% in the raltegravir arm achieved viral suppression to <50 copies/ml, compared to 34% in the placebo arm (39, 222). The availability of raltegravir has contributed substantially to being able to achieve the therapeutic target of full virologic suppression (i.e., plasma HIV-1 RNA level of <50 copies/ml) in highly treatment-experienced patients with multidrug-resistant virus.

INVESTIGATIONAL INTEGRASE INHIBITORS

Elvitegravir

Elvitegravir (GS-9137, JTK-303) is a modified quinolone antibiotic that inhibits HIV-1 integrase. It is under investigation in phase II and III clinical trials at a dosage of 150 mg orally b.i.d. in combination with ritonavir at 100 mg orally b.i.d. Elvitegravir is metabolized by CYP450-mediated oxidation and glucuronidation (UGTs 1A1 and -1A3). In vitro passaging studies revealed a primary mutation, E92Q, which conferred 36-fold resistance to elvitegravir. During a 24-week phase II dose-ranging study of elvitegravir plus optimized background therapy in highly treatment-experienced patients, the most common integrase mutations were E92Q, E138K, Q148R/K/H, and N155H (each observed in 39%); S147G (32%); and T66I/A/K (18%). Mutations at integrase codons E92, E138, Q148, and N155 have been reported to be selected by raltegravir in vivo, and thus cross-resistance exists between these two integrase inhibitors (160).

In a 10-day dose-finding monotherapy study in treatment-naïve and -experienced patients with HIV-1 RNA levels between 10,000 and 300,000 copies/ml, elvitegravir resulted in a $\geq$1.0 $\log_{10}$ reduction of HIV-1 RNA (44).

HIV PROTEASE INHIBITORS

Retrovirus replication requires virus-mediated proteolytic cleavage of *gag* and *gag-pol* polypeptide precursors mediated by the viral dimeric aspartyl protease. There are currently 10 approved HIV-1 PIs that share several characteristics: (i) they are all peptidomimetics; (ii) they bind to the active site with a noncleavable scissile bond; (iii) they have potent in vivo activity against HIV-1 when used in combination regimens; (iv) they have in vitro activity against both HIV-1 and HIV-2; (v) they have various degrees of cross-resistance that can be extensive and treatment limiting; and (vi) they have pharmacological profiles that confer a significant potential for drug interactions with other antiviral and nonantiviral agents. For a number of agents in this class, this characteristic can be exploited to improve pharmacological profiles with "ritonavir boosting." The unique resistance characteristics (e.g., large number of mutations required to confer resistance) and antiviral efficacy of ritonavir-boosted PIs make them attractive choices for initial as well as salvage therapy (211, 236). Second-generation PIs such as tipranavir and darunavir present additional options for patients who are highly treatment experienced and have HIV-1 strains resistant to other PIs.

Potential interactions with PIs may result from the coadministration of drugs that affect the CYP3A4 isozyme. Major drug interactions for PIs are listed in Table 4. Specific drugs and/or drug classes of this kind (e.g., astemizole and terfenadine, midazolam, triazolam, simvastatin, lovastatin, cisapride, and ergot alkaloids) may lead to severe toxicity and are therefore contraindicated in combination with CYP3A4-metabolized PIs. Conversely, inducers of the CYP3A4 isozyme (e.g., rifabutin and rifampin) can enhance PI clearance and lead to subtherapeutic levels.

Caution is required in administering PIs along with nonprescription herbal remedies. Since the currently available PIs are P-glycoprotein substrates and since constituents of St. John's wort are P-glycoprotein inducers, their coadministration should be avoided because therapeutic failure could result from reduced PI bioavailability.

Metabolic disorders have been increasingly recognized in the era of more potent antiretroviral therapy. Beginning in the late 1990s, case reports and studies began implicating PIs in causing abnormal glycemic control, insulin resistance, and increased triglyceride and cholesterol levels as soon as 14 days after treatment initiation. Accompanying body morphology changes have been described (23–25). These include fat distribution changes like truncal obesity, dorsocervical fat ("buffalo hump"), lipomatosis, and gynecomastia, as well as lipoatrophy from the buttocks, face, and extremities. The lipoatrophic changes have also been attributed to nucleoside analog therapy, and attempts to dissect the causality of the morphological changes continue. Lipodystrophic changes may be accompanied by insulin resistance and hypertriglyceridemia.

Saquinavir

Saquinavir {*cis-N-tert*-butyl-decahydro-2[2(*R*)-hydroxy-4-[iw-1]phenyl-3-(S)-[[N-(2-quinolylcarbonyl)-L-asparginyl]amino][ol0]butyl]-(4aS,8aS)-isoquinoline-3(S)-carboxyamide methanesufonate; Invirase} (Fig. 1 and 5; Tables 1 and 4) is a hydroxyethylamine-derived peptidomimetic HIV PI that is available in hard-gelatin capsule and tablet formulations. It should be used at a dosage of 1,000 mg b.i.d. or 2,000 mg daily with 100 mg of ritonavir to improve the agent's pharmacokinetics and enhance its efficacy.

Spectrum of Activity

The IC_{50} of saquinavir ranges from 1 to 30 nM for both HIV-1 and -2 assessed in peripheral blood lymphocytes. Saquinavir is inhibitory for human cell proteases at 50,000-fold-higher concentrations. It demonstrates additive interactions when combined with nucleoside analogs like zidovudine, didanosine, and lamivudine and with other PIs like amprenavir and ritonavir (163).

Pharmacology

The poor bioavailability of the saquinavir hard-gelatin capsule results from both modest absorption (30%) and extensive first-pass hepatic metabolism, precluding its appropriate use without ritonavir boosting. A high proportion of saquinavir in plasma is protein bound (>98%), predominantly to α_1-acid glycoprotein. CSF-to-plasma ratios and penetration into the male genital tract are low, if

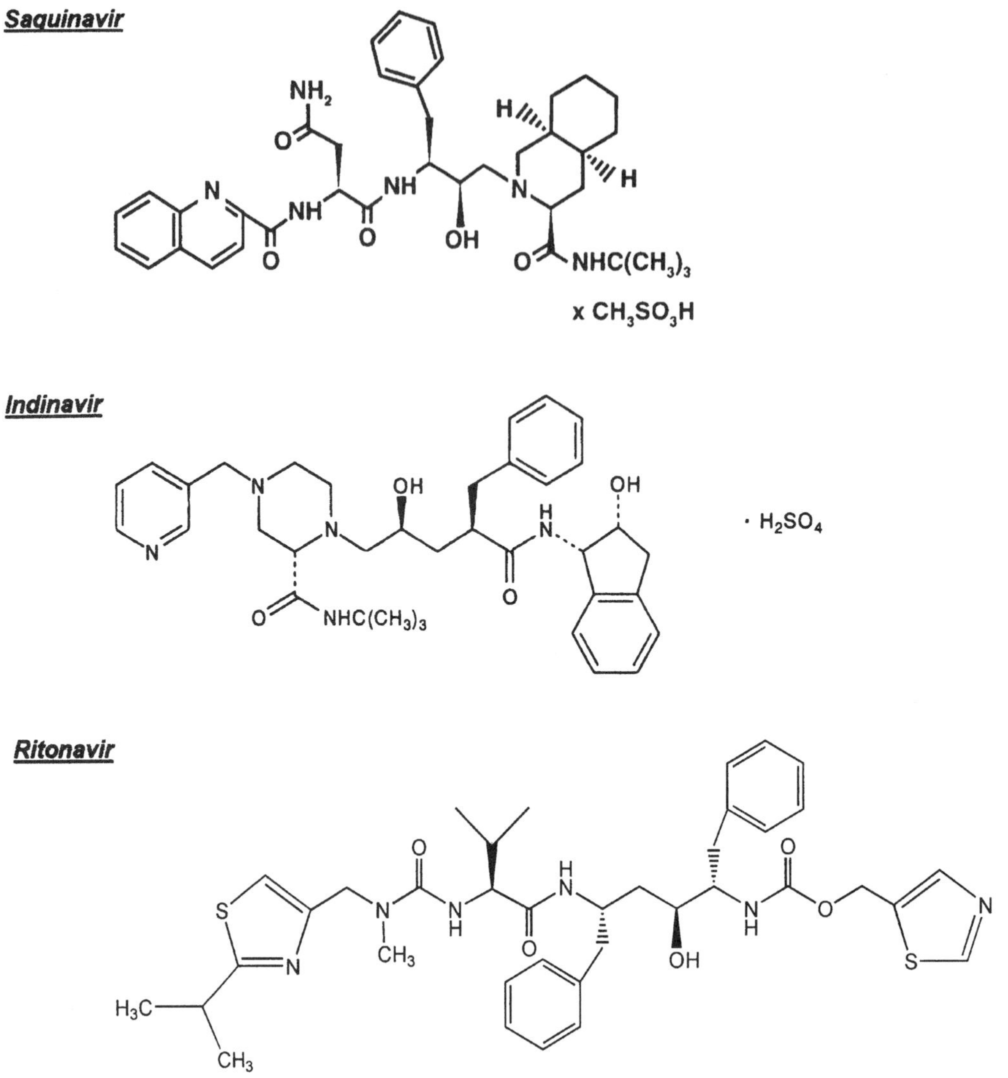

Saquinavir

$\times\ CH_3SO_3H$

Indinavir

$\cdot\ H_2SO_4$

Ritonavir

FIGURE 5 Chemical structures of PIs.

not unmeasurable, even with ritonavir boosting (227). Saquinavir is metabolized primarily by the CYP3A4 isozyme into various inactive mono- and dihydroxylated forms. Saquinavir is also a P-glycoprotein substrate and inhibitor, which may account for its poor oral bioavailability and its efflux from body compartments like the CNS and male genital tract.

Adverse Effects

Diarrhea, abdominal discomfort, and nausea are the most commonly reported adverse effects (126). A greater number of episodes of spontaneous bleeding have occurred in HIV-infected hemophiliacs taking PIs than in those taking nucleoside analogs, but a mechanism has not been defined (189).

Drug Interactions

Saquinavir is metabolized by the CYP450 CYP3A4 isoenzyme and may alter the concentration of drugs metabolized by this enzyme, for example, antiarrhythmic agents and lipid-lowering agents. Specific interactions with other PIs are notable for saquinavir AUC changes (ritonavir, +20-fold; indinavir, +6.2-fold; nelfinavir, +3.9-fold; atazanavir, +5.4- to +7.1-fold; and amprenavir, +0.19-fold). Because nevirapine and efavirenz decrease the saquinavir AUC by 24 and 62%, respectively, these combinations are not recommended without ritonavir boosting. Tipranavir decreases the saquinavir AUC by 76% and should not be coadministered. Rifampin, an inducer of the CYP450 enzyme, decreases saquinavir levels by up to 84%. Marked elevations of transaminases have been reported with coadministration, and thus this combination should be avoided.

Resistance

Selection for saquinavir-resistant mutants in vitro yields characteristic amino acid changes L90M and G48V, which result in a 3- to 40-fold decrease in saquinavir susceptibility (105, 152). These mutations confer a lower affinity of the protease for saquinavir and a diminished catalytic efficiency relative to the wild-type enzyme.

As predicted by in vitro studies, substitutions at codons 90 and 48, principally the L90M mutation, were identified in early saquinavir clinical trials (102). The L90M mutation is found in approximately 18% of resistant isolates

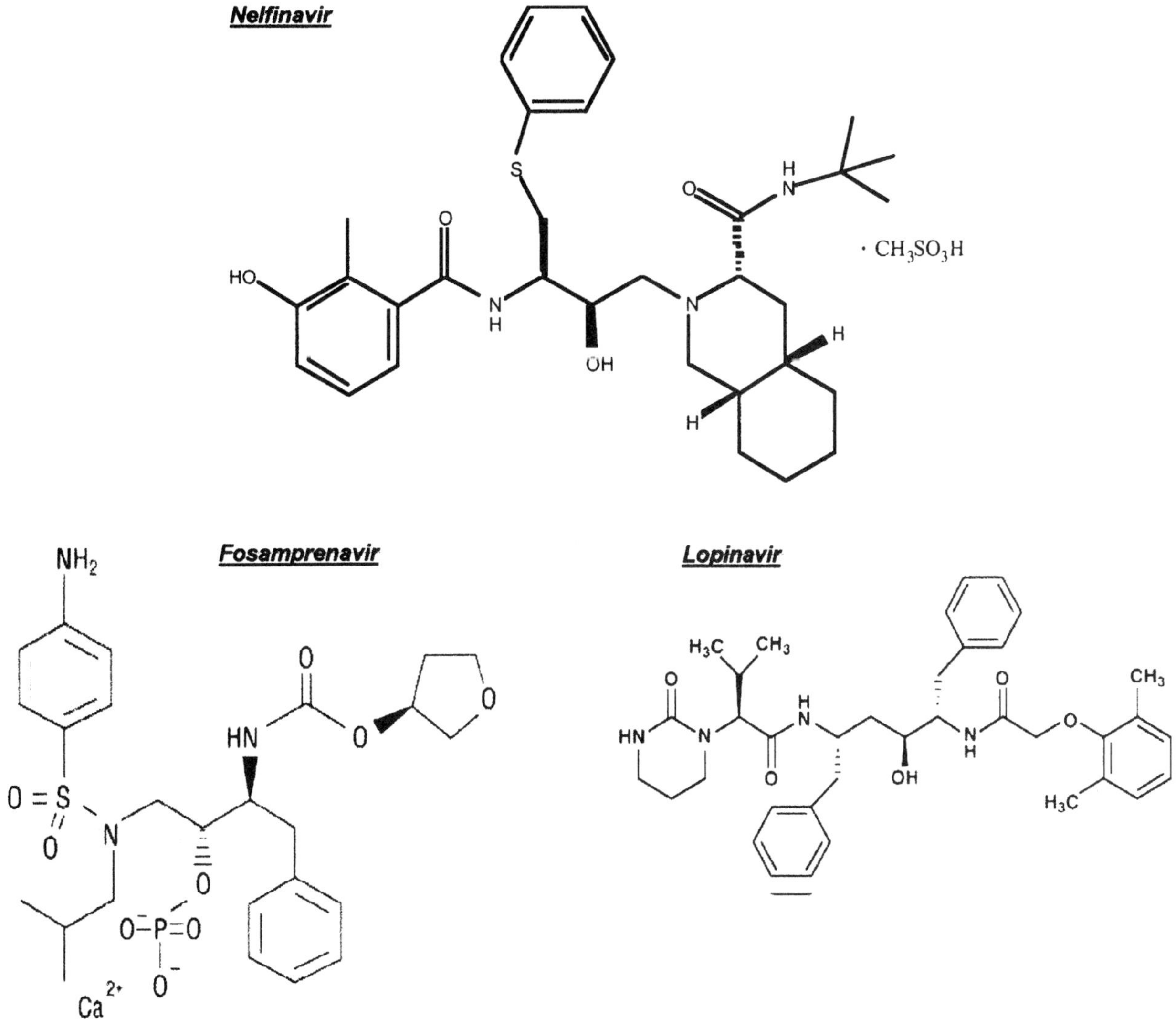

Nelfinavir

$\cdot CH_3SO_3H$

Fosamprenavir

Lopinavir

FIGURE 5 *(Continued)*

obtained after 7 to 12 months of therapy, particularly in patients receiving unboosted saquinavir. In contrast, the G48V mutation has occurred in only 2% of isolates, and the L90M G48V double mutation was even less common. Other substitutions seen in combination with L90M include mutations at codons 10, 36, 46, 63, 71, and 84. The accumulation of A71V/T or I54V/T with the V82A/F, L10I/V pattern resulted in high-level, >100-fold, saquinavir resistance in clinical samples (210). Mutations conferring cross-resistance occur at codons 46, 54, and 82. The prevalence of this cross-resistance ranges from 60 to 90% and correlates with increasing numbers of mutations in protease. The L90M mutation correlates with a lower likelihood of response to other PIs like nelfinavir (54).

Clinical Applications

When combined with low-dose ritonavir and two NRTIs, saquinavir provides potent and durable anti-HIV-1 activity (1, 53, 125). Saquinavir-ritonavir has been shown to be noninferior to lopinavir-ritonavir, each in combination with tenofovir-emtricitabine. Saquinavir-ritonavir can be used as part of initial regimens but is mostly viewed as an alternative to lopinavir-ritonavir or atazanavir-ritonavir in this circumstance. In patients with PI resistance, darunavir-ritonavir or tipranavir-ritonavir predictably will have greater activity.

Indinavir

Indinavir {*N*-[2(*R*)-hydroxy-1(*S*)-indanyl]-5-((2(*S*)-(1,1-dimethylethylaminocarbonyl)-4-[pyridin-3-yl)methyl]piperazin-1-yl)-4(*S*)-hydroxy-2(2)-phenylmethylpentanamide; Crixivan} (Fig. 1 and 5; Tables 1 and 4) is a peptidomimetic HIV-1 and HIV-2 PI. The original dosing scheme for indinavir was 800 mg every 8 h. However, in combination with ritonavir boosting, b.i.d. dosing schedules of indinavir became standard.

Spectrum of Activity

Indinavir has an IC_{50} for HIV-1 isolates ranging from 0.025 to 0.1 μmol/liter for clinical isolates tested in peripheral blood lymphocytes. It demonstrates synergy with other antiretroviral agents, including NRTIs.

Tipranavir

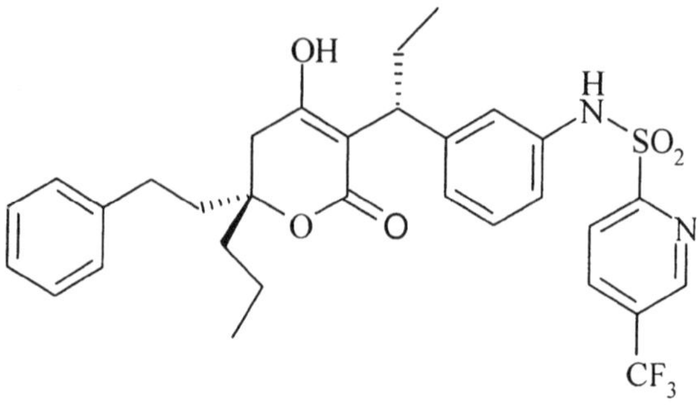

Atazanavir

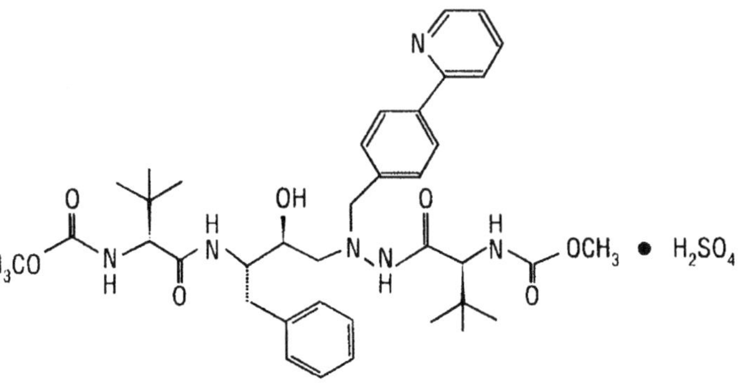

Darunavir

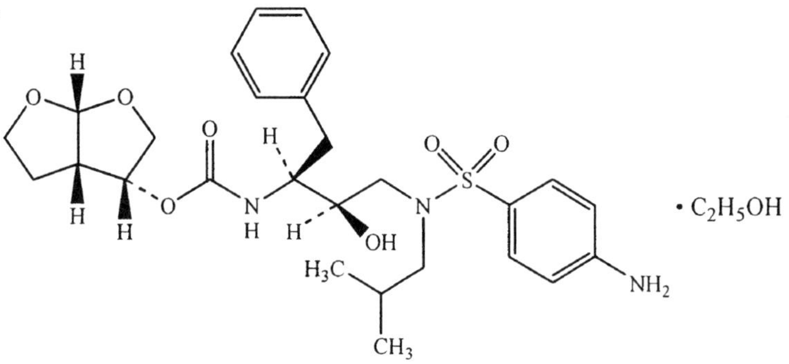

FIGURE 5 *(Continued)*

Pharmacology

Indinavir, as a capsule formulation, is rapidly absorbed, with a bioavailability of 60%, and reaches a C_{max} in plasma of 12 μM at 0.8 h after an 800-mg oral dose. Absorption is diminished by the coadministration of high-fat, high-protein foods. Plasma protein binding is approximately 60%, and the elimination $t_{1/2}$ in plasma is 1.8 h. The mean concentration of indinavir in CSF is only 1.7% of the concentration in plasma. The indinavir semen-to-blood ratio varies between 0.6 and 1.4 depending on the measurement time after administration, but it generally is better than that of saquinavir or ritonavir. Semen and CSF indinavir levels are enhanced 7.5- and 3-fold, respectively, with the addition of ritonavir at a dosage of 100 mg b.i.d. (85). The hepatic CYP3A4 isozyme plays a major role in the metabolism of indinavir, and a modest dose reduction is recommended for patients with significant hepatic dysfunction. Less than 20% of the drug is excreted in the urine, but the urine is supersaturated in the early postdose period.

Adverse Effects

The most commonly encountered adverse effect of indinavir is an asymptomatic and reversible indirect hyperbilirubinemia, seen in at least 10 to 15% of patients, presumed to be secondary to direct inhibition of UGT1A1-mediated bilirubin glucuronidation. This effect is dose related and is typically independent of elevations in hepatic enzyme levels. Patients with Gilbert and Crigler-Najjar syndromes harbor polymorphisms in the UGT1A1 gene and demonstrate higher levels of indirect bilirubin after treatment with either indinavir or atazanavir than do untreated patients (247).

Nephrolithiasis and acute interstitial nephritis have also been associated with indinavir use. The renal stones consist of indinavir precipitated from supersaturated urine. In a 3-year follow-up study, this complication occurred in up to 36% of subjects; the frequency decreases with adequate hydration (2 to 3%). Nephrolithiasis was significantly reduced with ritonavir boosting of indinavir (3, 16, 63).

Drug Interactions

Since indinavir is metabolized in hepatic microsomes, interactions with agents that affect the CYP450 metabolic pathway can be expected. Indinavir is a P-glycoprotein substrate. Therefore, as with other PIs, its bioavailability and compartmental distribution may be altered by compounds that affect this efflux pump.

Resistance

Reduction in indinavir susceptibility is associated with substitutions at 11 amino acid residues: L10I/V/R, K20M/R, L24I, V32I, M36I, M46I/L, I54V, A71V/T, G73SA, L76V, V77I, V82A/F/T, I84V, L90M, L63P/A/C/H/Q/S/T, and I64V (37, 47, 109). V82A/T/F/S and, less frequently, L90M and I84V, substitutions are found in individuals experiencing virologic failure on an indinavir-containing regimen. The degree of reduced susceptibility is proportional to the number of amino acid substitutions encoded in the HIV protease gene. The accumulation of at least three mutations is necessary before phenotypic resistance (>4- to 10-fold) can be demonstrated. Despite a wide range of accumulated mutational permutations that could impart resistance, V82A/F/T, M46I/L, I54V/T/A, I84V, and L90M are the key mutations most frequently present in indinavir-resistant isolates (50). V82A/F/T, L90M, and I84V in combination with substitution at codon 46 or 54 are associated with 10-fold reductions in susceptibility (195).

Clinical Applications

Indinavir holds an important place in the history of antiretroviral therapy development, as it helped usher in the period of potent antiretroviral therapy, when controlled clinical trials of indinavir plus two NRTIs demonstrated clear superiority of this combination over dual-nucleoside therapy alone. However, in the developed world, indinavir usage is now very limited. When administered, it should be combined with low-dose ritonavir to improve its pharmacokinetic profile. Its relatively low cost has permitted the drug to be useful in second-line therapies in the developing world.

Ritonavir

Ritonavir {10-hydroxy-2-methyl-5-(1-methylethyl)-1-[2-(1-methylethyl)-4-thiazolyl]-3,6-dioxo-8,11-bis(phenylmethyl)-2,4,7,12-tetraazatridecan-13-oicacid, 5-thiazolylmethyl ester [5*S*-(5*R**,8*R**,10*R**11*R**)], Norvir} (Fig. 1 and 5; Tables 1 and 4) is a C2-symmetric HIV PI that is more commonly used as a pharmacoenhancer of coadministered PIs. Ritonavir is available in tablet and oral solution formulations.

Spectrum of Activity

Synergy with ritonavir is seen in combination with nucleoside analogs and with other HIV PIs. As a symmetric inhibitor, ritonavir was specifically designed to correspond to the C2 symmetric active site of the HIV protease homodimer. In peripheral blood lymphocytes, the IC_{50} of the drug for HIV-1 ranges from 3.8 to 153 nM.

Pharmacology

Ritonavir has an oral bioavailability of 78%. A C_{max} in plasma of approximately 1.8 μM is attained 3.4 h after oral dosing. The elimination $t_{1/2}$ in plasma after oral dosing is about 3 h. Despite high plasma protein binding (in the range of 99%), ICs are achieved by oral doses of at least 400 mg every 12 h. Furthermore, the distribution of ritonavir is likely to be affected by P-glycoprotein since it is both a substrate and an inhibitor of this efflux pump. The distribution of ritonavir into CSF is relatively limited, and levels of ritonavir in semen are likewise low.

Ritonavir is metabolized in hepatic microsomes, predominantly by the CYP450 CYP3A4 and -3A5 isozymes and to a lesser extent by CYP2D6. A ritonavir isopropylthiazole metabolite retains antiviral activity but has low concentrations in plasma. In addition to being a hepatic microsomal substrate, ritonavir exhibits inhibitory activity against CYP3A4, CYP2D6, CYP2C9, CYP2D19, CYP2A6, CYP1A2, and CYP2E1. Consequently, significant drug interactions are to be expected, and in the case of its interaction with other HIV-1 PIs, this can be exploited to boost their drug levels.

Adverse Effects

The most common adverse effects observed in clinical trials include gastrointestinal symptoms and altered taste sensation. Laboratory abnormalities observed with ritonavir at dosages of 400 mg b.i.d. or higher include hypercholesterolemia, hypertriglyceridemia, and elevated liver enzyme levels (20, 231). Ritonavir used in combination with other PIs is also associated with abnormalities in glucose metabolism and body fat distribution (18, 23, 56, 175).

Drug Interactions

Ritonavir reversibly but potently inhibits the metabolism of drugs that are substrates of multiple P450 isozymes (above), including other PIs such as saquinavir, indinavir, amprenavir, lopinavir, tipranavir, and darunavir. It is a much stronger inhibitor of CYP3A4 than are other HIV PIs, and therefore the drug interactions are more complex with ritonavir (Table 4). Ritonavir is also a substrate for the CYP450 CYP3A4 isozyme and, to a lesser extent, CYP2D6.

Resistance

Resistance to ritonavir is similar to that to indinavir. The initial mutation is characteristically V82A/F, followed by the appearance of V82T (168). In vivo changes at residue 82 correlate with increases in plasma HIV-1 RNA levels during ritonavir treatment (168). Subsequent resistance-associated mutations include I54V, M36I, A71V, K20R, I84V, and M46I and, in contrast to indinavir, appear to accumulate in a patterned fashion. At the low dose employed for boosting of other PIs, ritonavir is thought to exert limited anti-HIV-1 activity in vivo and therefore contributes to the emergence of PI-associated resistance mutations indirectly (i.e., through the selective pressure exerted by the paired PI which is boosted).

Clinical Applications

Ritonavir pharmacoenhancement of other PIs may lead to improved antiretroviral regimens by (i) enhancing antiviral activity by elevating the trough levels of the coadministered PI well above the IC_{50} or IC_{90} associated with certain drug-resistant isolates and (ii) improving the ease of administration by diminished frequency of dosing and elimination of food effects. Intolerance to, or side effects from, ritonavir, even when used at a low dose, may be limiting.

Nelfinavir

Nelfinavir {[3S-(3R*,4aR*,8aR*,22′S*,3′S*)]-2-[2′-hydroxy-3′-phenylthiomethyl-4′-aza-5′-oxo-5′-(2″-methyl-3′-hydroxyphenyl)pentyl]decahydroiso-quinoline-3-N-t-butylcarboxamide methanesulfonic acid salt; AG1343, Viracept} (Fig. 1 and 5; Tables 1 and 4) is available in tablet and oral powder formulations at standard dosing of 750 mg three times daily or 1,250 mg b.i.d. The drug was recalled temporarily from the European market in July 2007 because of high levels of ethyl methanesulfonate (EMS), a carcinogen and teratogen in animals. Nelfinavir manufactured in the United States has lower levels of EMS.

Spectrum of Activity

Nelfinavir exhibits activity against HIV-1, with IC_{50}s ranging from 23 to 28 μM for susceptible HIV-1 clinical and laboratory strains in monocytes and peripheral blood lymphocytes.

Pharmacology

Oral bioavailability ranges from 20 to 80%, and C_{max}s of 2 to 3 μg/ml in plasma are achieved at 3.4 h; concentrations in plasma exceed the in vitro IC_{95} for HIV-1 isolates for up to 24 h after a single 800-mg dose. The oral bioavailability of nelfinavir increases two- to threefold when the drug is administered with food. Nelfinavir is 99% protein bound, predominantly to α_1-acid glycoprotein; however, antiviral activity is not appreciably affected. Its presence in CSF and the male genital tract is minimal.

The elimination $t_{1/2}$ of nelfinavir is approximately 3.5 to 5 h. Nelfinavir is metabolized in hepatic microsomes, predominantly by CYP3A isozymes (52%), followed by CYP2C19, CYP2D6, and possibly CYP2C9, into a number of oxidative metabolites. Produced by the CYP2C19 isoenzyme, the major metabolite, M8 (previously designated AG-1402), retains antiretroviral activity comparable to that of nelfinavir. Because less than 2% of nelfinavir is excreted in urine, renal impairment has modest effects on nelfinavir clearance, but nelfinavir is removed by hemodialysis and should be redosed after dialysis. In patients with severe hepatic function impairment, a nelfinavir dosing change may not be necessary because the nelfinavir AUC is increased 49 to 75% while there is concurrently decreased M8 production.

Adverse Effects

The adverse effects most commonly associated with nelfinavir include diarrhea (69%), headache (23%), and weakness (15%). Diarrhea was significantly more common in the three-times-daily than in the b.i.d. dosing arm, but in some cases it could be symptomatically relieved with antidiarrheal agents.

Drug Interactions

Since nelfinavir is both a substrate and inducer/inhibitor of CYP450 CYP3A4 isozyme and P-glycoprotein, there are multiple interactions that could potentially result from the coadministration of nelfinavir with other drugs. However, nelfinavir is not boosted by ritonavir to a clinically useful extent. In addition, nelfinavir inhibits the CYP2B6 isoenzyme and therefore has the potential to affect the metabolism of drugs such as bupropion.

Resistance

The D30N mutation is the most commonly seen initial mutation in subtype B virus, although the L90M pathway, which confers nelfinavir resistance almost exclusively on non-subtype B strains, is also noted in a significant minority of subtype B strains. Subsequently, an M46I/I84V double mutant is selected, with a 30-fold reduction in susceptibility relative to the wild type. Other mutations observed in vitro and in vivo include L10F/I, M36I, M46I, A71T/V, V82A/F/T, I84V, N88D/S, and L90M. Isolates with nelfinavir resistance on the basis of the D30N mutation retain susceptibility to other PIs.

In a survey of more than 6,000 HIV-1 isolates obtained from specimens submitted for clinical testing, the frequency of the D30N mutation was low (1%) (96). While this unique resistance pattern may be prominent when nelfinavir is administered as the first PI, high-level resistance to nelfinavir and cross-resistance to other PIs can occur in the absence of the D30N mutation. For example, dual mutations at 10I and 90M conferred broad PI cross-resistance, which was enhanced by the addition of other substitutions at codons 54, 71, 77, 82, and 84.

Clinical Applications

Compared to those of nonnucleoside analog-based regimens (198) and other PI-based regimens such as lopinavir-ritonavir or fosamprenavir-ritonavir in previously untreated individuals, the overall potency, spectrum of activity, and durability of nelfinavir are lower (72, 238). At present, nelfinavir is no longer recommended for treatment-naïve patients. Moreover, given the low genetic barrier to resistance of this drug and cross-resistance with other PIs in highly antiretroviral-experienced individuals, the efficacy of nelfinavir as part of a salvage regimen is poor. Nelfinavir has been used in pregnancy, but concerns about its potency and about contamination with EMS, a by-product of manufacturing, make it less desirable for pregnant women or women planning to become pregnant.

Amprenavir

Amprenavir {(3S)-tetrahydro-3-furyl-N-(1S,2R)-3-(4-[iw-1]amino-N-isobutylbenzenesulfonamido)-1-benzyl-2-hydroxypropyl carbamate; Agenerase} (Fig. 1; Table 1) is a structure-based designed hydroxyethylamine sulfonamide peptidomimetic isostere. Formulations of this agent include 50- and 150-mg capsules and a 15-mg/ml solution. In 2007, the manufacturer discontinued production and sale of amprenavir in the United States, as it has been supplanted by the prodrug, fosamprenavir. The dosing, pharmacokinetic, major toxicity, and drug interaction characteristics of amprenavir are similar to those of fosamprenavir, for which it is the parent drug (see below).

Fosamprenavir

Fosamprenavir {N-[3-[N-(4-aminophenylsulfenylsulfonyl)-N-sobutylamino]-1(S)-benzyl-2-(R)-(phosphonoxy)propyl] carbamic acid tetrahydrofuran-3(S)-yl ester calcium salt; Lexiva} (Fig. 1 and 5; Tables 1 and 4) is a prodrug that is rapidly hydrolyzed to amprenavir and inorganic phosphate by cellular phophatases in the gut epithelium. Fosamprenavir allows for lower pill burden and improved bioavailability compared to the parent drug. Fosamprenavir formulations include 700-mg tablets and a 50-mg/ml oral suspension. Pharmacokinetic data support a 700-mg-b.i.d. dosing schedule with 100 mg of ritonavir b.i.d. or 1,400-

mg-once-daily dosing with either 100 or 200 mg of ritonavir (202).

Spectrum of Activity

Fosamprenavir has little or no antiviral activity in vitro. It is rapidly metabolized to amprenavir, which exhibits activity against both HIV-1 and HIV-2, with an IC_{50} of 0.054 μM for the HIV-1_{IIIB} laboratory clone in MT-4 cells. Amprenavir is additive with a number of other antiretroviral agents (zidovudine, didanosine, abacavir, saquinavir, indinavir, and ritonavir).

Pharmacology

Fosamprenavir displays good oral bioavailability, reaches peak levels 1.5 to 2 h after dosing, and has an elimination $t_{1/2}$ in plasma of approximately 8 h. There is secondary absorption, with a second peak occurring 10 to 12 h after dosing. Its absorption is not affected by food when the drug is coadministered with low-dose ritonavir. Fosamprenavir is 90% plasma protein bound and has a large volume of distribution. It is metabolized hepatically through CYP450 CYP3A4 and is a potent inducer of the same enzyme. Only <1% of each dose is excreted through the urine.

Drug Interactions

Once fosamprenavir is desphosphorylated to amprenavir, it is metabolized by the CYP450 CYP3A4 isoenzyme system. It also inhibits the CYP450 pathway. The effect of ritonavir on fosamprenavir pharmacokinetics has been exploited to enhance amprenavir trough levels (202).

Adverse Effects

The most common toxicities are rash (up to 19%), gastrointestinal symptoms (diarrhea, nausea, and vomiting), and abnormal fat redistribution. Common laboratory abnormalities include liver enzyme abnormalities, hyperglycemia, and hyperlipidemia. A higher incidence of gastrointestinal side effects occurs with once-daily, compared to b.i.d., dosing of unboosted fosamprenavir. Data suggest more favorable tolerability and virologic efficacy of once-daily fosamprenavir combined with the 100-mg dose of ritonavir than with the 200-mg dose (97).

Resistance

The L10F/I/R/V,V32I, M46I/L, I47V, I50V, I54M/L, G73S, V82A/F/S/T, I84V, L76V, and L90M mutations are selected in vitro. Most of the in vitro and in vivo data are based on studies of amprenavir, which is the drug used for susceptibility testing.

A triple mutant with the codon 50, 46, and 47 changes displays higher levels of resistance (14- to 20-fold). Further analysis of in vitro-selected isolates have shown that p1/p6 Gag-Pol cleavage site mutations appear early and concurrently with the L10F and I84V protease mutations in the selection process.

Amprenavir resistance patterns generated in vivo are more complex. The most common mutations to develop in patients with virologic failure on fosamprenavir and amprenavir include V32I, M46I/L, I47V, I50V, I54M/L, and I84V (110, 147). The I50V mutation appears to have the greatest effect on amprenavir susceptibility, in some studies reducing it about eightfold (195).

Clinical Applications

Compared to lopinavir-ritonavir, each in combination with abacavir-lamivudine, b.i.d. boosted fosamprenavir demonstrates comparable virologic efficacy (65% in the lopinavir-ritonavir arm vs. 66% in the fosamprenavir-ritonavir arm, with plasma HIV-1 RNA at <50 copies/ml) over 96 weeks (59). Compared to nelfinavir, fosamprenavir-ritonavir, either b.i.d. or once daily, demonstrates lower rates of virologic failure (72, 199). The efficacy of once-daily fosamprenavir with 100 mg of ritonavir is comparable to the efficacy of atazanavir-ritonavir (215).

Lopinavir (Coformulated with Ritonavir)

Lopinavir {*N*-[(1*S*,3*S*,4*S*)-4-[[(2,6-dimethylphenoxy)acetyl]amino]-3-hydroxy-5-phenyl-1-(phenylmethyl)pentyl] tetrahydro-a-(1-methylethyl)-2-oxo-1(2*H*)-pyrimidineacetamide; Kaletra} is structurally related to ritonavir (Fig. 1 and 5; Tables 1 and 4). For pharmacological enhancement, it is formulated in a fixed-dose combination with ritonavir in a tablet containing 200 mg of lopinavir and 50 mg of ritonavir. The liquid formulation contains 80 mg of lopinavir and 20 mg of ritonavir per ml; the capsule formulation has been discontinued. The new formulation offers lower pill burden, less drug level variability, enhanced tolerability, and heat stability. Ritonavir-boosted lopinavir has been approved for once-daily dosing in treatment-naïve individuals.

Spectrum of Activity

Lopinavir was designed primarily to reduce the dependence of PI activity on the drug molecule interacting with the isopropyl side chain of the V82 amino acid of the target HIV-1 protease. As a result, lopinavir exhibits more potent activity against both wild-type and mutant HIV-1 strains than does ritonavir. The IC_{50} of lopinavir is approximately 10-fold lower than that of ritonavir. The mean IC_{50} of lopinavir ranged from 4 to 11 nM for HIV-1 subtype B clinical isolates.

Pharmacology

In healthy volunteers, a 400-mg dose of lopinavir alone only transiently produces plasma drug levels of >0.1 μg/ml. To compensate for this low oral bioavailability, lopinavir was developed with pharmacokinetic enhancement by ritonavir. The resulting lopinavir has an AUC from 0 to 24 h that is 77-fold greater than that of lopinavir alone, and it has an elimination $t_{1/2}$ in plasma of 10.0 ± 3.7 h. Lopinavir is over 98% protein bound, but lopinavir-ritonavir's penetration into the CSF results in levels which exceed the IC_{50} for wild-type HIV-1. Lopinavir is metabolized in hepatic microsomes via NADPH- and CYP3A4/5-dependent pathways. Lopinavir metabolism results in the formation of at least 12 compounds, most notably, M-1 (4-oxo), M-3, and M-4 (two 4-hydroxy epimers).

Drug Interactions

Efavirenz reduces the levels of lopinavir-ritonavir due to its CYP450-inducing activity; therefore, the dose of lopinavir-ritonavir should be increased when used in combination with efavirenz. Other PIs, including fosamprenavir and tipranavir, decrease lopinavir levels significantly and should not be coadministered. Lopinavir-ritonavir has been shown to significantly reduce methadone levels, resulting in opiate withdrawal symptoms; this interaction is due to the lopinavir, not ritonavir, component.

Adverse Effects

Gastrointestinal adverse effects (diarrhea and nausea) are the most commonly reported symptoms associated with a regimen that includes lopinavir-ritonavir plus stavudine and lamivudine. These symptoms typically occur in the initial 2 months of therapy and subsequently diminish in frequency. Lopinavir-ritonavir has a greater impact on cholesterol, particularly on triglycerides, than do atazanavir-ritonavir and saquinavir-ritonavir (106); some of these abnormalities may be reversible upon switching to another PI, like atazanavir or a nonnucleoside inhibitor. Like other PIs, lopinavir-ritonavir may contribute to abnormalities of body fat redistribution.

Diarrhea was reported with a greater frequency at the 800-mg/200-mg once-daily dosing schedule approved for antiretroviral-naïve patients than with conventional dosing (17%, vs. 5%) (166). The most frequently seen laboratory abnormalities with lopinavir-ritonavir use are changes in the lipid profile, with most of the changes occurring in the first month of treatment (238).

Resistance

The characterization of in vitro-selected lopinavir-resistant HIV-1 strains reveals a sequential accumulation of mutations in the protease gene that include L10F/I/R/V, K20M/R, L24I, V32I, L33F, M46I/L, I47V/A, I50V, F53L, I54V, I63P, A71V/T, G73S, L76V, V82A, I84V, and L90M (110). Accompanying p1/p6 and p7/p1 cleavage site mutations are seen. The genotypic correlates of reduced lopinavir susceptibility have been characterized through an analysis of in vitro lopinavir susceptibility to HIV-1 isolates derived from patients failing to respond to single- or multiple-PI regimens. Isolates with reduced in vitro lopinavir susceptibility require the accumulation of six or more protease mutations. These mutations have occurred at 11 protease residues: positions 10, 20, 24, 46, 53, 54, 63, 71, 82, 84, and 90 (120, 157). Resistance significantly correlates with the number of these mutations, and the cumulative effect of multiple mutations leads to virologic failure; however, the combination of lopinavir with ritonavir has a higher genetic barrier to resistance (12, 119, 124). At least 10-fold reductions in susceptibility are needed before a change in virologic response is observed, and ≥60-fold reductions in susceptibility are required before the activity of a standard dose of the drug is no longer sufficient to reduce plasma HIV-1 RNA levels by half a log. Mutations at positions 46, 54, and 82, together with accessory mutations at positions 10 and 20, reduce lopinavir susceptibility >50-fold and have been shown to reduce virologic responses to lopinavir-ritonavir therapy of treatment-experienced patients (195). The mutations at positions 84 and 90 modestly reduce lopinavir/ritonavir susceptibility but contribute to reduced susceptibility to other PIs (195). In lopinavir-ritonavir-naïve patients with wild-type virus who experience virologic failure, emergence of resistance mutations is rare (66, 113).

Clinical Applications

For initial treatment in antiretroviral-naïve patients, once-daily dosing has an efficacy similar to that of b.i.d. lopinavir-ritonavir (106), with the possible exception of individuals with more advanced disease and plasma HIV-1 RNA levels of >100,000 copies/ml.

The efficacy of lopinavir-ritonavir compares favorably to those of other PIs or NNRTIs. A direct comparison with fosamprenavir in treatment-naïve individuals demonstrated comparable potencies for lopinavir-ritonavir and ritonavir-boosted fosamprenavir regimens (59). Better virologic responses were seen with an efavirenz-based regimen than with a lopinavir-ritonavir-based regimen, but better CD4 cell responses and less resistance were seen following virologic failure with lopinavir-ritonavir plus two nucleoside analogs (197). Atazanavir-ritonavir and b.i.d. lopinavir-ritonavir, each in combination with tenofovir-emtricitabine, show similar efficacies, although atazanavir-ritonavir confers better lipid profiles and fewer gastrointestinal side effects.

Lopinavir-ritonavir also plays an important role in salvage therapy. In combination with NNRTIs and NRTIs, lopinavir-ritonavir has resulted in virologic suppression to <400 copies of HIV RNA/ml in patients failing to respond to their initial or multiple PI regimens (9). In patients with prior failure on a PI-based regimen, lopinavir-ritonavir demonstrates an efficacy comparable to that of ritonavir-boosted atazanavir for suppression of plasma HIV-1 RNA levels to <50 copies/ml (108). The greatest benefit has been seen in patients with ≥4 major protease mutations at baseline (176). Addition of lopinavir-ritonavir to the fusion inhibitor enfuvirtide in patients naïve to lopinavir-ritonavir results in enhanced virologic and immunologic responses relative to those with no concurrent use of the agent (177). In lopinavir-naïve, treatment-experienced patients, the newer PIs like darunavir-ritonavir or tipranavir-ritonavir proved noninferior to lopinavir-ritonavir treatment (145). Once-daily dosing is not recommended in PI-experienced patients.

While there has been some interest in exploring the role of lopinavir-ritonavir in novel treatment strategies, including the use of lopinavir-ritonavir monotherapy (i.e., simplification regimens) following a fully suppressive regimen, its role as a component of simplification therapy remains to be determined. Two studies (MONARK and M03-613) found that large proportions of patients on lopinavir/ritonavir monotherapy after initial virologic suppression experienced suboptimal virologic responses compared to those who continued use of combinations. The monotherapy intervention may have been associated with an increased risk of development of resistance (21). Therefore, this strategy is not one that should be routinely employed.

Tipranavir

Tipranavir {(6*R*)-3-{(1*R*)-1-[3-{{[5-(trifluoromethyl)(2-pyridyl)]sulfonyl}amino}phenyl]propyl}-4-hydroxy-6-(2-phenylethyl)-6-propyl-5,6-dihydro-2*H*-pyran-2-one; Aptivus} is a nonpeptidic PI of HIV belonging to the class of 4-hydroxy-5,6-dihydro-2-pyrone sulfonamides (Fig. 1 and 5; Tables 1 and 4). It is available as a 250-mg soft-gelatin capsule coadministered with ritonavir to achieve effective concentrations in plasma. Ritonavir increases tipranavir concentrations 24- to 70-fold; thus, to achieve adequate concentrations in plasma, 500 mg of the drug must be coadministered with 200 mg of ritonavir.

Spectrum of Activity

Tipranavir is active against a wide range of drug-resistant isolates and demonstrated a mean IC_{50} of 0.23 mM for highly multidrug-resistant clinical isolates (136). Potential mechanisms of its enhanced potency against PI-resistant virus include ability to bind to the active site of the protease enzyme with fewer hydrogen bonds, thereby creating greater flexibility at the active site (136) or strong hydrogen bonding interaction with the amide backbone of the protease active-site Asp30 (206, 228). The drug demonstrates additive interactions with other PIs, NNRTIs, and nucleoside analogs and synergistic interaction with the HIV fusion inhibitor, enfuvirtide.

Pharmacology

Maximum tipranavir concentrations of 61 to 115 μmol/liter were achieved in healthy volunteers 3 h postdosing, and the 12-h AUC ranged from 503 to 1,160 μmol/liter/h. Oral absorption is increased twofold by administration with a high-fat meal or light snack, and the elimination $t_{1/2}$ in plasma is 5.5 to 6 h. As tipranavir is a substrate for CYP450 CYP3A4, boosting with ritonavir is necessary for appropriate pharmacodynamics. To achieve adequate concentrations, tipranavir must be coadministered with 200 mg of ritonavir daily. The higher dose is required because tipranavir is both a substrate and potent inducer of P-glycoprotein and may initially induce its own metabolism (144, 159). Tipranavir is over 99.9% protein bound.

There are no data regarding the CSF penetration by tipranavir. Tipranavir use is contraindicated in patients with moderate to severe hepatic impairment. Though mild hepatic impairment increases tipranavir-ritonavir concentrations, dose adjustment is not indicated.

Drug Interactions

Tipranavir both inhibits and induces the CYP450 enzyme system, and when tipranavir is used in combination with ritonavir, the net effect is inhibition of the CYP3A4 enzyme. Tipranavir is also an inducer of the P-glycoprotein transporter. Thus, tipranavir may alter the concentrations of many other drugs metabolized by these pathways (Table 4). Tipranavir decreases the concentrations of amprenavir, indinavir, lopinavir-ritonavir, and saquinavir and nucleoside analogs like abacavir, zidovudine, and didanosine. It also appears that coadminstration of tipranavir-ritonavir with enfuvirtide may affect the volume of distribution and elimination $t_{1/2}$ of tipranavir, thereby resuting in an increased C_{min} of this agent, although this interaction does not appear to result in an increased risk of hepatotoxicity.

Adverse Effects

The most common adverse effects associated with tipranavir are predominantly gastrointestinal and include diarrhea, dyspepsia, abdominal distention, and pancreatitis. In two large clinical trials (RESIST 1 and RESIST 2) of more than 1,400 patients which included patients coinfected with HBV or HCV but with stable liver enzymes at baseline, hepatic and lipid-related adverse effects occurred with greater frequency in the tipranavir-ritonavir arm but were rarely a cause for drug discontinuation. Hepatitis virus coinfection and a baseline CD4 cell count of >200 cells/mm^3 were predictors of liver function abnormalities (225). However, only 1.9% of patients who developed grade 3/4 liver enzyme abnormalities discontinued therapy. Cases of clinical hepatitis and hepatic decompensation in patients with chronic HBV or HCV infection who received tipranavir-ritonavir have been reported.

Ritonavir-boosted tipranavir was linked to 14 cases of fatal or nonfatal intracranial hemorrhage in clinical trials of 6,840 HIV-1-infected patients, but a direct causative effect has not been proven. Many of the patients had other contributing risk factors, like CNS lesions, head trauma, coagulopathy, recent neurosurgery, hypertension, or concurrent use of antiplatelet and anticoagulant agents. In vitro and in vivo data suggest that tipranavir can inhibit platelet aggregation and thus should be used with caution in patients receiving antiplatelet agents or anticoagulants or who are at risk of increased bleeding after trauma or surgery (76).

Resistance

A pivotal characteristic of tipranavir's efficacy is its activity against many HIV-1 isolates with resistance to previously approved PIs (136). Ninety percent of highly resistant clinical isolates (>10-fold resistance to three or more PIs) remain susceptible to tipranavir, and only 2% have >10-fold resistance to tipranavir (136); however, in order for tipranavir to be effective, <3- to 4-fold resistance is required. Critical mutations include codons 33, 82, 84, and 90, and accumulation of two or more of them has been associated with decreased susceptibility to the drug. A total of 21 mutations at 16 protease codons have been shown to correlate with a decreased response to tipranavir-ritonavir therapy in treatment-experienced patients: L10V, I13V, K20M/R/V, L33F, E35G, M36I, K43T, M46L, I47V, I54A/M/V, Q58E, H69K, T74P, V82L/T, N83D, and I84V. A tipranavir mutation score developed based on these mutations predicted that the presence of ≥8 of these mutations resulted in a loss of the week 24 virologic response to tipranavir; the week 24 virologic response decreased from 1.3 logs with three mutations to 0.64 log when four mutations were present (8). Mutation I50V has been associated with increased tipranavir susceptibility (57).

Clinical Applications

Given the activity of tipranavir against a broad spectrum of PI-resistant clinical isolates, the optimal use of tipranavir is as a component of combination regimens designed for treatment-experienced patients experiencing treatment failure with PI-resistant virus (98). In such patients, tipranavir-ritonavir has been superior in achieving virologic suppression to HIV RNA levels of <50 copies/ml to a comparator ritonavir-boosted PI (indinavir, amprenavir, lopinavir, or saquinavir). The tipranavir-ritonavir regimen also has demonstrated greater increases in CD4 cell counts than the comparator PIs. To ensure the magnitude and durability of response, a successful regimen should contain other active agents in the optimized background.

Atazanavir

Atazanavir {(3S,8S,9S,12S)-3,12-*bis*(1,1-dimethylethyl)-8-hydroxy-4,11-dioxo-9-(phenylmethyl)-6-[[4-(2-pyridinyl)phenyl]methyl]-2,5,6,10,13-pentaazatetradecanedioic acid dimethyl ester, sulfate (1:1); BMS-232632, Zrivada, Reyetaz} (Fig. 1 and 5; Tables 1 and 4) is an azapeptide aspartyl PI. It is available in capsule formulations of 100, 150, 200, and 300 mg.

Spectrum of Activity

Atazanavir has activity against laboratory and clinical HIV-1 isolates grown in peripheral mononuclear cells and macrophages (IC_{50}, 2 to 5 nM) and variable activity against HIV-2 isolates (1.9 to 32 nM). Clinical isolates that are resistant to one or two of the currently approved PIs typically remain susceptible to this compound. However, isolates with high-level resistance and hence a larger number of protease gene mutations are more likely to be associated with resistance to atazanavir.

Pharmacology

Atazanavir has rapid absorption that requires food and gastric acid; coadministration of a single dose with a light meal leads to a 70% increase in the AUC. A 400-mg once-daily dosage attains mean steady-state levels above the protein-binding-adjusted IC_{90}. Atazanavir alone has an elimination $t_{1/2}$ in plasma of approximately 7 h. It is 86% protein bound and is metabolized by hepatic CYP450 isoenzyme CYP3A4. Only 13% of unmetabolized drug is excreted in the urine, and there is no recommendation for dose adjustment with renal insufficiency. It is contraindicated in those with a Child-Pugh score over 9, and the dosage is decreased to 300 mg daily in those with a score between 7 and 9. The CSF-to-plasma ratio is 0.002 to 0.02, comparable to that of indinavir.

Adverse Effects

A prominent adverse effect has been a dose-dependent, reversible indirect hyperbilirubinemia, typically occurring in the first 60 days of treatment (Table 4). It is more frequent in persons with the UGT1A1-28 genotype or the CC genotype of the 3435C → T polymorphism in the multidrug resistance (MDR1) gene (86, 183, 200, 201). Patients with Gilbert and Crigler-Najjar syndromes harbor polymorphisms in the UGT1A1 gene and demonstrate higher levels of indirect bilirubin after treatment with either indinavir or atazanavir than do untreated patients. Prolongation of the PR and QTc intervals, usually asymptomatic, has also been noted with high doses of atazanavir. A case of torsade de pointes has been reported (143). Caution is advised when coadministering atazanavir with other drugs that cause PR interval prolongation.

Nephrolithiasis has been reported with use of ritonavir-boosted or unboosted atazanavir (29), and lipid abnormalities have been slightly more pronounced in patients receiving ritonavir-boosted atazanavir than in those receiving atazanavir.

Drug Interactions

Atazanavir is a substrate and inhibitor of CYP3A as well as an inhibitor of CYP2C8 isoenzymes. Therefore, atazanavir should not be coadministered with agents with narrow therapeutic windows that are substrates of these isoenzymes (Table 4). Atazanavir, however, does not appear to induce its own metabolism. Drugs that induce or inhibit CYP3A activity may decrease or increase, respectively, concentrations of atazanavir in plasma. Coadministration with tenofovir decreases serum atazanavir concentrations and increases concentrations of tenofovir (226); addition of low-dose ritonavir may compensate for this interaction. Atazanavir requires acidic gastric pH for dissolution; therefore, administration with proton pump inhibitors, which raise the gastric pH, significantly interferes with the absorption of atazanavir and can cause subtherapeutic serum atazanavir levels. H2 receptor antagonists may be an alternative if atazanavir is administered at least 2 h before and ≥10 h after the H2 receptor antagonist.

Resistance

In vitro, accumulation of the mutations I50L, N88S, I84V, A71V, and M46I decreases susceptibility to atazanavir 93- to 183-fold. Changes are also observed at the protease cleavage sites following drug selection. In PI-naïve patients failing unboosted atazanavir, I50L is the most commonly observed mutation (240), but it appears less frequently in patients receiving ritonavir-boosted atazanavir (110). Recombinant viruses containing the I50L mutation displayed increased in vitro susceptibility to other PIs (amprenavir, indinavir, lopinavir, nelfinavir, ritonavir, and saquinavir). In patients failing an atazanavir-ritonavir-based regimen, accumulations of L10F/I/V, G16E, L33F/I/V, M46I/L, I54L/V/M/T, D60E, I62V, A71I/T/L, V82A/T, I84V, I85V, L90M, and I93L are seen in various combinations (110). A genotypic resistance score composed of 8 mutations (10F/I/V, G16E, L33I/F/V, M46I/L, D60E, I84V, I85V and L90M) predicted that the occurrence of >3 of these mutations correlated with a reduced virologic response at 3 months, particularly when L90M was present (237). The presence of a mutation at positions 46, 73, 84, or 90 at baseline was associated with a poorer virologic response (176).

For unboosted atazanavir, the presence of 0, 1 to 2, 3, or ≥4 of the following mutations has been associated with 83, 67, 6, and 0% response rates: G16E, V32I, K20I/M/R/T/V, L33F/I/V, F53L/Y, I64L/M/V, A71I/T/V, I85V, and I93L/M.

Clinical Applications

Atazanavir as a once-daily administered PI with a favorable lipid profile offers an attractive option for both antiretroviral-naïve and -experienced individuals. In previously untreated patients, ritonavir-boosted atazanavir shows an efficacy similar to that of unboosted atazanavir but is associated with fewer virologic failures and a higher barrier to development of resistance. Unboosted atazanavir demonstrates a potency comparable to that of efavirenz, each in combination with two nucleoside analogs (219). Atazanavir-ritonavir and fosamprenavir-ritonavir, each in combination with tenofovir-emtricitabine, show comparable potencies (215). Atazanavir-ritonavir has been used successfully in treatment-experienced patients (106), but it has not performed as well as the newer PIs tipranavir-ritonavir and darunavir-ritonavir in patients failing to respond to multiple PI regimens (34).

Darunavir

Darunavir {[(1S,2*R*)-3-[[(4-aminophenyl)sulfonyl](2-methylpropyl)amino]-2-hydroxy-1-(phenylmethyl)propyl]-carbamic acid (3*R*,3aS,6a*R*)-hexahydrofuro[2,3-*b*]furan-3-yl ester monoethanolate; Prezista, TMC-114}, is approved for use as part of combination therapy against HIV-1 strains that are resistant to other PIs (Fig. 1 and 5; Tables 1 and 4). It is available as a film-coated tablet for oral administration in a 300-mg dose. When darunavir is given orally in combination with 100 mg of ritonavir b.i.d., the systemic exposure of darunavir increases approximately 14-fold; therefore, the agent should only be administered with 100 mg of ritonavir to achieve sufficient concentrations in plasma.

Spectrum of Activity

Darunavir exhibits activity against HIV-1 and HIV-2, with median IC_{50}s ranging from 1.2 to 8.5 nM (0.7 to 5.0 ng/ml) in PBMCs (7).

Pharmacology

Darunavir is rapidly absorbed and reaches the C_{max} in plasma after 2.5 to 4 h. Systemic absorption of darunavir is increased by 30% when it is taken with a meal, though the content of the meal does not appear to matter. In the presence of ritonavir at 100 mg, darunavir has a rapid distribution and elimination phase followed by a slower elimination phase, yielding a terminal elimination $t_{1/2}$ of 15 h. Darunavir is approximately 95% protein bound.

Like other PIs, darunavir is metabolized by hepatic CYP450 CYP3A4, and coadministration with ritonavir leads to an increase in darunavir bioavailability from 37 to 82%. Only 14% of darunavir is excreted in feces. There are no current dose adjustment recommendations for either renal or hepatic insufficiency. Considering darunavir's metabolism, caution is recommended in its administration to individuals with hepatic insufficiency.

Adverse Effects

The most common adverse effects occurring in >10% of patients have been diarrhea, nausea, and headache. Mild to moderate skin rash, typically self-limited maculopapular skin eruptions, is uncommon (<10%), and severe skin rash, including erythema multiforme and Stevens-Johnson syndrome, is rare. Darunavir contains a sulfonamide moiety and should be used with caution in patients with a known sulfonamide allergy. Cases of new-onset diabetes mellitus, exacerbation of preexisting diabetes mellitus, and hyperglycemia have been reported. There are reports of severe hepatitis occurring in approximately 0.5% of patients, particularly those with preexisting liver disease or viral hepatitis.

Drug Interactions

Darunavir is both a substrate and an inhibitor of the CYP450 enzyme system (CYP3A). As with other PIs, coadministration with drugs primarily metabolized by CYP3A may alter concentrations of darunavir and the other drug in plasma (Table 4). For example, carbamazepine, phenobarbital, and phenytoin are inducers of CYP450 enzymes, and darunavir should not be used in combination with these agents, as coadministration may cause significant decreases in plasma darunavir concentrations. Darunavir interacts with other antiretroviral agents: coadministration with efavirenz decreases the concentration of darunavir while increasing that of the coadministered antiretroviral; therefore, caution is recommended when administering darunavir with efavirenz. Coadministration with etravirine decreases its levels (AUC by 37% and C_{min} by 49%) without affecting the darunavir concentration.

Resistance

Mutations associated with a diminished response to darunavir include V11I, V32I, L33F, I47V, I50V, I54L or M, G73S, L76V, I84V, and L89V. In treatment-experienced patients, the presence of three or more of these mutations at baseline is correlated with a diminished virologic response to darunavir-ritonavir (34). In a clinical trial of darunavir-ritonavir as salvage therapy, the mutations V32I and I54L or M were present in more than 30 and 20% of virologic failure isolates, respectively, and the median darunavir phenotype (change from the reference virus strain) of the virologic failure isolates was 21-fold at baseline and 94-fold at failure. I50V, I54M, L76V, and I84V result in the greatest degree of reduced susceptibility. A higher probability of virologic response to darunavir-ritonavir occurs if the baseline darunavir change in the IC_{50} (compared with reference darunavir susceptibility) is less than 10-fold (34); 10- to 40-fold or >40-fold changes in phenotypic susceptibility to darunavir are a commonly used cutoff to differentiate between an intermediate or low likelihood of response to darunavir-ritonavir, respectively.

The specifics of cross-resistance of darunavir to other PIs like atazanavir and tipranavir need to be further defined (58, 127, 151). To date, data from the largest studies evaluating tipranavir and darunavir suggest that the overlap in mutations is limited to codons 33, 47, 54, and 84. In one study, the majority of viral strains from patients remained susceptible to tipranavir after the patients experienced treatment failure on a darunavir-containing regimen; another analysis revealed no correlations between tipranavir-ritonavir and darunavir-ritonavir resistance profiles, and isolates remained susceptible to darunavir even after tipranavir failure (58).

Clinical Applications

In treatment-experienced patients with evidence of resistance to PIs, darunavir-ritonavir in combination with nucleoside analogs, with or without enfuvirtide, provides higher rates of viral suppression to <50 copies/ml and immunologic recovery than in patients in the ritonavir-boosted PI comparator group (34, 90). The addition of enfuvirtide to the regimen among enfuvirtide-naïve individuals significantly improves the rates of virologic suppression to <50 copies/ml (58 and 44% for patients with and without enfuvirtide, respectively) (34). Darunavir-ritonavir in patients with limited treatment experience (82% were susceptible to >4 PIs, all lopinavir-ritonavir naïve) demonstrates noninferiority to lopinavir-ritonavir with respect to virologic suppression. Individuals with virologic failure on darunavir-ritonavir are more likely to maintain susceptibility to other PIs than individuals failing lopinavir-ritonavir regimens. Darunavir-ritonavir in combination with tenofovir-emtricitabine in treatment-naïve patients appears to be noninferior to lopinavir-ritonavir with respect to virologic suppression to HIV RNA levels of <50 copies/ml at week 48 (ARTEMIS study). In patients with plasma HIV-1 RNA levels of >100,000 copies/ml, darunavir-ritonavir achieves higher rates of virologic suppression (79%, versus 67% in the lopinavir/ritonavir arm).

INVESTIGATIONAL HIV-1 PROTEASE INHIBITORS

While PIs exhibit potent in vitro activity and the recent addition of second-generation PIs has marked a major advance in antiretroviral therapy, patients continue to experience virologic failure on these regimens. The search for newer agents with improved efficacy and toxicity profiles continues. Examples of investigational PIs are described in Table 2.

MATURATION INHIBITORS

Agents targeting later stages of the life cycle of the virus, such as bevirimat, represent a new class of antiretroviral drugs, the maturation inhibitors (Table 2). The drug disrupts a late step in the processing of HIV-1 Gag that involves the conversion of the capsid precursor p25 to mature capsid protein p24, thereby resulting in production of noninfectious virions with abnormal capsid morphology. Mutations for resistance to the drug have been found at the p25-to-p24 cleavage site. The drug has been well tolerated in healthy volunteers, and its long $t_{1/2}$ may allow b.i.d. dosing. A subset of wild-type viruses, however, carries amino acid substitutions in the CA-SP1 cleavage site conferring resistance to bevirimat and thereby reducing its ability to associate with the HIV-1 Gag protein.

REFERENCES

1. **Ananworanich, J., A. Hill, U. Siangphoe, K. Ruxrungtham, W. Prasithsirikul, P. Chetchotisakd, S. Kiertiburanakul, W. Munsakul, P. Raksakulkarn, S. Tansuphasawadikul, R. Nuesch, D. A. Cooper, and B. Hirschel.** 2005. A prospective study of efficacy and safety of once-daily saquinavir/ritonavir plus two nucleoside reverse transcriptase inhibitors in treatment-naive Thai patients. *Antivir. Ther.* **10:**761–767.
2. **Arenzana-Seisdedos, F., J. L. Virelizier, D. Rousset, I. Clark-Lewis, P. Loetscher, B. Moser, and M. Baggiolini.** 1996. HIV blocked by chemokine antagonist. *Nature* **383:**400.
3. **Arnaiz, J. A., J. Mallolas, D. Podzamczer, J. Gerstoft, J. D. Lundgren, P. Cahn, G. Fatkenheuer, A. D'Arminio-Monforte, A. Casiro, P. Reiss, D. M. Burger, M. Stek, and J. M. Gatell.** 2003. Continued indinavir versus switching to indinavir/ritonavir in HIV-infected patients with suppressed viral load. *AIDS* **17:**831–840.
4. Reference deleted.
5. **Arribas, J. R., A. L. Pozniak, J. E. Gallant, E. Dejesus, B. Gazzard, R. E. Campo, S. S. Chen, D. McColl, C. B. Holmes, J. Enejosa, J. J. Toole, and A. K. Cheng.** 2008. Tenofovir disoproxil fumarate, emtricitabine, and efavirenz compared with zidovudine/lamivudine and efavirenz in treatment-naive patients: 144-week analysis. *J. Acquir. Immune Defic. Syndr.* **47:**74–78.
6. **Avinhingsanon, A., W. Monsuthi, P. Kantipong, C. Chuchotaworn, S. Moolphate, N. Yamada, H. Yanai, P. Phanuphak, D. Burger, and K. Ruxrungtham.** 2007. Pharmacokinetics and 12 weeks efficacy of nevirapine 600 mg per day in HIV infected patients with active TB receiving rifampicin: a multicenter study, abstr. 576. *14th Conf. Retrovir. Opportunistic Infect., Los Angeles, CA.*
7. **Back, D., V. Sekar, and R. M. Hoetelmans.** 2008. Darunavir: pharmacokinetics and drug interactions. *Antivir. Ther.* **13:**1–13.
8. **Baxter, J. D., J. M. Schapiro, C. A. Boucher, V. M. Kohlbrenner, D. B. Hall, J. R. Scherer, and D. L. Mayers.** 2006. Genotypic changes in human immunodeficiency virus type 1 protease associated with reduced susceptibility and virologic response to the protease inhibitor tipranavir. *J. Virol.* **80:**10794–10801.
9. **Benson, C. A., S. G. Deeks, S. C. Brun, R. M. Gulick, J. J. Eron, H. A. Kessler, R. L. Murphy, C. Hicks, M. King, D. Wheeler, J. Feinberg, R. Stryker, P. E. Sax, S. Riddler, M. Thompson, K. Real, A. Hsu, D. Kempf, A. J. Japour, and E. Sun.** 2002. Safety and antiviral activity at 48 weeks of lopinavir/ritonavir plus nevirapine and 2 nucleoside reverse-transcriptase inhibitors in human immunodeficiency virus type 1-infected protease inhibitor-experienced patients. *J. Infect. Dis.* **185:**599–607.
10. **Berenguer, J., B. Padilla, V. Estrada, C. Martin, P. Domingo, J. M. Kindelán, and J. M. Ruiz-Guiardin.** 2002. Safety of abacavir therapy after temporary interruptions in patients without hypersensitivity reactions to the drug. *AIDS* **16:**1299–1301.
11. **Blum, M. R., S. H. Liao, S. S. Good, and P. de Miranda.** 1988. Pharmacokinetics and bioavailability of zidovudine in humans. *Am. J. Med.* **85:**189–194.
12. **Bongiovanni, M., T. Bini, F. Adorni, P. Meraviglia, A. Capetti, F. Tordato, P. Cicconi, E. Chiesa, L. Cordier, A. Cargnel, S. Landonio, S. Rusconi, and A. d'Arminio Monforte.** 2003. Virological success of lopinavir/ritonavir salvage regimen is affected by an increasing number of lopinavir/ritonavir-related mutations. *Antivir. Ther.* **8:**209–214.
13. **Borin, M. T., J. H. Chambers, B. J. Carel, W. W. Freimuth, S. Aksentijevich, and A. A. Piergies.** 1997. Pharmacokinetic study of the interaction between rifabutin and delavirdine mesylate in HIV-1 infected patients. *Antivir. Res.* **35:**53–63.
14. **Boubaker, K., M. Flepp, P. Sudre, H. Furrer, A. Haensel, B. Hirschel, K. Boggian, J. P. Chave, E. Bernasconi, M. Egger, M. Opravil, M. Rickenbach, P. Francioli, and A. Telenti.** 2001. Hyperlactatemia and antiretroviral therapy: the Swiss HIV Cohort Study. *Clin. Infect. Dis.* **33:**1931–1937.
15. **Boucher, C. A., N. Cammack, P. Schipper, R. Schuurman, P. Rouse, M. A. Wainberg, and J. M. Cameron.** 1993. High-level resistance to (−) enantiomeric 2′-deoxy-3′-thiacytidine in vitro is due to one amino acid substitution in the catalytic site of human immunodeficiency virus type 1 reverse transcriptase. *Antimicrob. Agents Chemother.* **37:**2231–2234.
16. **Boyd, M., C. Duncombe, K. Ruxrungthram, M. Khongphattanayothin, E. Hassink, P. Srasuebkul, J. Sangkote, P. Reiss, M. Stek, J. Lange, D. A. Cooper, and P. Phanuphak.** 2002. Indinavir TID vs indinavir/ritonavir BID in combination with AZT/3TC for HIV infection in nucleoside pretreated patients: HIV-NAT 005 76-week follow up, abstr. 422-W. *9th Conf. Retrovir. Opportunistic Infect., Seattle, WA.*
17. **Brehm, J., D. Koontz, S. Zelina, N. Sluis-Cremer, and J. Mellors.** 2007. 3′-Azido-3′-dideoxythymidine selects mutations in the connection (A371V) and RNase H (Q509L) domains of reverse transcriptase that increase AZT resistance in combination with thymidine analog mutations without affecting the rate of AZT excision on a DNA/DNA template/primer, abstr. 90. *14th Conf. Retrovir. Opportunistic Infect., Los Angeles, CA.*
18. **Brown, T. T., S. R. Cole, X. Li, L. A. Kingsley, F. J. Palella, S. A. Riddler, B. R. Visscher, J. B. Margolick, and A. S. Dobs.** 2005. Antiretroviral therapy and the prevalence and incidence of diabetes mellitus in the multicenter AIDS cohort study. *Arch. Intern. Med.* **165:**1179–1184.
19. **Cahn, P., R. Haubrich, J. Leider, G. Pialoux, M. Schechter, S. Walmsley, J. Vingerhoets, M. Peeters, G. De Smedt, M. P. de Béthune, and B. Woodfall.** 2007. Pooled 24-week results of DUET-1 and -2: TMC125 (etravirine; ETR) vs placebo in 1203 treatment-experienced HIV-1-infected patients, abstr. H-717. *Abstr. 47th Intersci. Conf. Antimicrob. Agents Chemother.*
20. **Calza, L., R. Manfredi, B. Farneti, and F. Chiodo.** 2003. Incidence of hyperlipidaemia in a cohort of 212 HIV-infected patients receiving a protease inhibitor-based antiretroviral therapy. *Int. J. Antimicrob. Agents* **22:**54–59.
21. **Campo, R., B. da Silva, L. Cotte, J Gathe, B. Gazzard, C. Hicks, M. Dehaan, K. Wikstrom, M. King, and G. Hanna.** 2007. Predictors of loss of virologic response in subjects who deintensified to lopinavir/ritonavir monotherapy after achieving plasma HIV-1 RNA <50 copies/mL on LPV/r plus zidovudine/lamivudine, abstr. 514. *14th Conf. Retrovir. Opportunistic Infect., Los Angeles, CA.*
22. **Cardo, D. M., D. H. Culver, C. A. Ciesielski, P. U. Srivastava, R. Marcus, D. Abiteboul, J. Heptonstall, G. Ippolito, F. Lot, P. S. McKibben, and D. M. Bell for The Centers for Disease Control and Prevention Needlestick**

Surveillance Group. 1997. A case-control study of HIV seroconversion in health care workers after percutaneous exposure. *N. Engl. J. Med.* **337:**1485–1490.

23. **Carr, A.** 2003. HIV lipodystrophy: risk factors, pathogenesis, diagnosis and management. *AIDS* **17**(Suppl. 1)**:** S141–S148.

24. **Carr, A.** 2000. HIV protease inhibitor-related lipodystrophy syndrome. *Clin. Infect. Dis.* **30**(Suppl. 2)**:**S135–S142.

25. **Carr, A., and D. A. Cooper.** 2000. Adverse effects of antiretroviral therapy. *Lancet* **356:**1423–1430.

26. **Ceccherini-Silberstein, F., V. Svicher, T. Sing, A. Artese, M. M. Santoro, F. Forbici, A. Bertoli, S. Alcaro, G. Palamara, A. d'Arminio Monforte, J. Balzarini, A. Antinori, T. Lengauer, and C. F. Perno.** 2007. Characterization and structural analysis of novel mutations in human immunodeficiency virus type 1 reverse transcriptase involved in the regulation of resistance to nonnucleoside inhibitors. *J. Virol.* **81:**11507–11519.

27. **Cepeda, J. A., and D. Wilks.** 2000. Excess peripheral neuropathy in patients treated with hydroxyurea plus didanosine and stavudine for HIV infection. *AIDS* **14:**332–333.

28. **Chamberlain, P. P., J. Ren, C. E. Nichols, L. Douglas, J. Lennerstrand, B. A. Larder, D. I. Stuart, and D. K. Stammers.** 2002. Crystal structures of zidovudine- or lamivudine-resistant human immunodeficiency virus type 1 reverse transcriptases containing mutations at codons 41, 184, and 215. *J. Virol.* **76:**10015–10019.

29. **Chan-Tack, K. M., M. M. Truffa, K. A. Struble, and D. B. Birnkrant.** 2007. Atazanavir-associated nephrolithiasis: cases from the US Food and Drug Administration's Adverse Event Reporting System. *AIDS* **21:**1215–1218.

30. **Chi, B. H., M. Sinkala, F. Mbewe, R. A. Cantrell, G. Kruse, N. Chintu, G. M. Aldrovandi, E. M. Stringer, C. Kankasa, J. T. Safrit, and J. S. Stringer.** 2007. Single-dose tenofovir and emtricitabine for reduction of viral resistance to non-nucleoside reverse transcriptase inhibitor drugs in women given intrapartum nevirapine for perinatal HIV prevention: an open-label randomised trial. *Lancet* **370:**1698–1705.

31. **Clarke, S. M., F. M. Mulcahy, J. Tjia, H. E. Reynolds, S. E. Gibbons, M. G. Barry, and D. J. Back.** 2001. Pharmacokinetic interactions of nevirapine and methadone and guidelines for use of nevirapine to treat injection drug users. *Clin. Infect. Dis.* **33:**1595–1597.

32. **Clarke, S. M., F. M. Mulcahy, J. Tjia, H. E. Reynolds, S. E. Gibbons, M. G. Barry, and D. J. Back.** 2001. The pharmacokinetics of methadone in HIV-positive patients receiving the non-nucleoside reverse transcriptase inhibitor efavirenz. *Br. J. Clin. Pharmacol.* **51:**213–217.

33. **Clavel, F., and A. J. Hance.** 2004. HIV drug resistance. *N. Engl. J. Med.* **350:**1023–1035.

34. **Clotet, B., N. Bellos, J. M. Molina, D. Cooper, J. C. Goffard, A. Lazzarin, A. Wohrmann, C. Katlama, T. Wilkin, R. Haubrich, C. Cohen, C. Farthing, D. Jayaweera, M. Markowitz, P. Ruane, S. Spinosa-Guzman, and E. Lefebvre.** 2007. Efficacy and safety of darunavir-ritonavir at week 48 in treatment-experienced patients with HIV-1 infection in POWER 1 and 2: a pooled subgroup analysis of data from two randomised trials. *Lancet* **369:**1169–1178.

35. **Clumeck, N., F. Goebel, W. Rozenbaum, J. Gerstoft, S. Staszewski, J. Montaner, M. Johnson, B. Gazzard, C. Stone, R. Athisegaran, and S. Moore.** 2001. Simplification with abacavir-based triple nucleoside therapy versus continued protease inhibitor-based highly active antiretroviral therapy in HIV-1-infected patients with undetectable plasma HIV-1 RNA. *AIDS* **15:**1517–1526.

36. **Coghlan, M. E., J. P. Sommadossi, N. C. Jhala, W. J. Many, M. S. Saag, and V. A. Johnson.** 2001. Symptomatic lactic acidosis in hospitalized antiretroviral-treated patients with human immunodeficiency virus infection: a report of 12 cases. *Clin. Infect. Dis.* **33:**1914–1921.

37. **Condra, J. H., W. A. Schleif, O. M. Blahy, L. J. Gabryelski, D. J. Graham, J. C. Quintero, A. Rhodes, H. L. Robbins, E. Roth, M. Shivaprakash, D. Titus, T. Yang, H. Tepplert, K. E. Squires, P. J. Deutsch, and E. A. Emini.** 1995. *In vivo* emergence of HIV-1 variants resistant to multiple protease inhibitors. *Nature* **374:**569–571.

38. **Connor, E. M., R. S. Sperling, R. Gelber, P. Kiselev, G. Scott, M. J. O'Sullivan, R. VanDyke, M. Bey, W. Shearer, R. L. Jacobson, E. Jimenez, E. O'Neill, B. Bazin, J.-F. Delfraissy, M. Culnane, R. Coombs, M. Elkins, J. Moye, P. Stratton, and J. Balsley for The Pediatric AIDS Clinical Trials Group Protocol 076 Study Group.** 1994. Reduction of maternal-infant transmission of human immunodeficiency virus type 1 with zidovudine treatment. *N. Engl. J. Med.* **331:**1173–1180.

39. **Cooper, D., J. G., J. Rockstroh, C. Katlama, P. Yeni, A. Lazzarin, X. Xu, R. Isaacs, H. Teppler, and B. Y. Nguyen.** 2008. 48-Week results from BENCHMRK-1, a phase III study of raltegravir in patients failing ART with triple-class resistant HIV-1, abstr. 788. *15th Conf. Retrovir. Opportunistic Infect., Boston, MA.*

40. **Cressey, T. R., H. Green, S. Khoo, J. M. Treluyer, A. Compagnucci, Y. Saidi, M. Lallemant, D. M. Gibb, and D. M. Burger.** 2008. Plasma drug concentrations and virologic evaluations after stopping treatment with nonnucleoside reverse-transcriptase inhibitors in HIV type 1-infected children. *Clin. Infect. Dis.* **46:**1601–1608.

41. **Cui, L., R. F. Schinazi, G. Gosselin, J. L. Imbach, C. K. Chu, R. F. Rando, G. R. Revankar, and J. P. Sommadossi.** 1996. Effect of beta-enantiomeric and racemic nucleoside analogues on mitochondrial functions in HepG2 cells. Implications for predicting drug hepatotoxicity. *Biochem. Pharmacol.* **52:**1577–1584.

42. **Das, K., A. D. Clark, Jr., P. J. Lewi, J. Heeres, M. R. De Jonge, L. M. Koymans, H. M. Vinkers, F. Daeyaert, D. W. Ludovici, M. J. Kukla, B. De Corte, R. W. Kavash, C. Y. Ho, H. Ye, M. A. Lichtenstein, K. Andries, R. Pauwels, M. P. De Bethune, P. L. Boyer, P. Clark, S. H. Hughes, P. A. Janssen, and E. Arnold.** 2004. Roles of conformational and positional adaptability in structure-based design of TMC125-R165335 (etravirine) and related non-nucleoside reverse transcriptase inhibitors that are highly potent and effective against wild-type and drug-resistant HIV-1 variants. *J. Med. Chem.* **47:**2550–2560.

43. **De Clercq, E.** 2007. The design of drugs for HIV and HCV. *Nat. Rev. Drug Discov.* **6:**1001–1018.

44. **DeJesus, E., D. Berger, M. Markowitz, C. Cohen, T. Hawkins, P. Ruane, R. Elion, C. Farthing, L. Zhong, A. K. Cheng, D. McColl, and B. P. Kearney.** 2006. Antiviral activity, pharmacokinetics, and dose response of the HIV-1 integrase inhibitor GS-9137 (JTK-303) in treatment-naive and treatment-experienced patients. *J. Acquir. Immune Defic. Syndr.* **43:**1–5.

45. **DeJesus, E., G. Herrera, E. Teofilo, J. Gerstoft, C. B. Buendia, J. D. Brand, C. H. Brothers, J. Hernandez, S. A. Castillo, T. Bonny, E. R. Lanier, and T. R. Scott.** 2004. Abacavir versus zidovudine combined with lamivudine and efavirenz, for the treatment of antiretroviral-naive HIV-infected adults. *Clin. Infect. Dis.* **39:**1038–1046.

46. **DeJesus, E., S. Walmsley, C. Cohen, D. Cooper, B. Hirschel, J. Goodrich, H. Valdez, J. Heera, N. Rajicic, and N. Maye.** 2008. Fasted lipid changes after administration

of maraviroc or efavirenz in combination with zidovudine and lamivudine for 48 weeks to treatment-naïve HIV-infected patients, abstr. 929. *15th Conf. Retrovir. Opportunistic Infect., Boston, MA.*

47. **Delaunay, C., F. Brun-Vezinet, R. Landman, G. Collin, G. Peytavin, A. Trylesinski, P. Flandre, M. Miller, and D. Descamps.** 2005. Comparative selection of the K65R and M184V/I mutations in human immunodeficiency virus type 1-infected patients enrolled in a trial of first-line triple-nucleoside analog therapy (Tonus IMEA 021). *J. Virol.* **79:**9572–9578.
48. **Delehanty, J., C. Wakeford, L. Hulett, J. Quinn, B. McCreedy, M. Almond, D. Miralles, F. Rousseau.** 1999. A phase I/II randomized, controlled study of FTC versus 3TC in HIV-infected patients, abstr. 16. *6th Conf. Retrovir. Opportunistic Infect., Chicago, IL.*
49. **Derdeyn, C. A., J. M. Decker, J. N. Sfakianos, X. Wu, W. A. O'Brien, L. Ratner, J. C. Kappes, G. M. Shaw, and E. Hunter.** 2000. Sensitivity of human immunodeficiency virus type 1 to the fusion inhibitor T-20 is modulated by coreceptor specificity defined by the V3 loop of gp120. *J. Virol.* **74:**8358–8367.
50. **Descamps, D., V. Joly, P. Flandre, G. Peytavin, V. Meiffredy, S. Delarue, S. Lastere, J. P. Aboulker, P. Yeni, and F. Brun-Vezinet.** 2005. Genotypic resistance analyses in nucleoside-pretreated patients failing an indinavir containing regimen: results from a randomized comparative trial (Novavir ANRS 073). *J. Clin. Virol.* **33:**99–103.

50a. **Doms, R. W.** 5 October 2007, posting date. Understanding HIV entry and targets for therapy. *Clinical Care Options HIV.* Clinical Care Options, Reston, VA. http://clinicaloptions.com/hiventry.

51. **Dorr, P., M. Westby, S. Dobbs, P. Griffin, B. Irvine, M. Macartney, J. Mori, G. Rickett, C. Smith-Burchnell, C. Napier, R. Webster, D. Armour, D. Price, B. Stammen, A. Wood, and M. Perros.** 2005. Maraviroc (UK-427,857), a potent, orally bioavailable, and selective small-molecule inhibitor of chemokine receptor CCR5 with broad-spectrum anti-human immunodeficiency virus type 1 activity. *Antimicrob. Agents Chemother.* **49:**4721–4732.
52. **Dragic, T., V. Litwin, G. P. Allaway, S. R. Martin, Y. Huang, K. A. Nagashima, C. Cayanan, P. J. Maddon, R. A. Koup, J. P. Moore, and W. A. Paxton.** 1996. HIV-1 entry into CD4+ cells is mediated by the chemokine receptor CC-CKR-5. *Nature* **381:**667–673.
53. **Dragsted, U. B., J. Gerstoft, C. Pedersen, B. Peters, A. Duran, N. Obel, A. Castagna, P. Cahn, N. Clumeck, J. N. Bruun, J. Benetucci, A. Hill, I. Cassetti, P. Vernazza, M. Youle, Z. Fox, and J. D. Lundgren.** 2003. Randomized trial to evaluate indinavir/ritonavir versus saquinavir/ritonavir in human immunodeficiency virus type 1-infected patients: the MaxCmin1 Trial. *J. Infect. Dis.* **188:**635–642.
54. **Dronda, F., J. L. Casado, S. Moreno, K. Hertogs, I. Garcia-Arata, A. Antela, M. J. Perez-Elias, L. Ruiz, and B. Larder.** 2001. Phenotypic cross-resistance to nelfinavir: the role of prior antiretroviral therapy and the number of mutations in the protease gene. *AIDS Res. Hum. Retrovir.* **17:**211–215.
55. **Dudley, M. N.** 1995. Clinical pharmacokinetics of nucleoside antiretroviral agents. *J. Infect. Dis.* **171**(Suppl. 2)**:**S99–S112.
56. **Dufer, M., Y. Neye, P. Krippeit-Drews, and G. Drews.** 2004. Direct interference of HIV protease inhibitors with pancreatic beta-cell function. *Naunyn-Schmiedeberg's Arch. Pharmacol.* **369:**583–590.
57. **Elston, R., J. Scherer, D. Hall, J. Schapiro, R. Bethell, V. Kohlbrenner, and D. Mayers.** 2006. De-selection of the I50V mutation occurs in clinical isolates during aptivus/r (tipranavir/ritonavir)-based therapy, abstr. 92. 15th Int. HIV Drug Resistance Workshop, Sitges, Spain.
58. **Elston, R. C., D. R. Kuritzkes, and R. Bethell.** 2007. An investigation into the influence of the tipranavir-associated V82L/T mutations on the susceptibility to darunavir and brecanavir, abstr. 602. *14th Conf. Retrovir. Opportunistic Infect., Los Angeles, CA.*
59. **Eron, J., Jr., P. Yeni, J. Gathe, Jr., V. Estrada, E. DeJesus, S. Staszewski, P. Lackey, C. Katlama, B. Young, L. Yau, D. Sutherland-Phillips, P. Wannamaker, C. Vavro, L. Patel, J. Yeo, and M. Shaefer.** 2006. The KLEAN study of fosamprenavir-ritonavir versus lopinavir-ritonavir, each in combination with abacavir-lamivudine, for initial treatment of HIV infection over 48 weeks: a randomised non-inferiority trial. *Lancet* **368:**476–482.
60. **Eron, J. J., Jr., R. L. Murphy, D. Peterson, J. Pottage, D. M. Parenti, J. Jemsek, S. Swindells, G. Sepulveda, N. Bellos, B. C. Rashbaum, J. Esinhart, N. Schoellkopf, R. Grosso, and M. Stevens.** 2000. A comparison of stavudine, didanosine and indinavir with zidovudine, lamivudine and indinavir for the initial treatment of HIV-1 infected individuals: selection of thymidine analog regimen therapy (START II). *AIDS* **14:**1601–1610.
61. **Eshleman, S. H., D. R. Hoover, S. Chen, S. E. Hudelson, L. A. Guay, A. Mwatha, S. A. Fiscus, F. Mmiro, P. Musoke, J. B. Jackson, N. Kumwenda, and T. Taha.** 2005. Resistance after single-dose nevirapine prophylaxis emerges in a high proportion of Malawian newborns. *AIDS* **19:**2167–2169.
62. **Feng, J. Y., J. Shi, R. F. Schinazi, and K. S. Anderson.** 1999. Mechanistic studies show that (−)-FTC-TP is a better inhibitor of HIV-1 reverse transcriptase than 3TC-TP. *FASEB J.* **13:**1511–1517.
63. **Fischl, M., B. Young, M. Watkins, R. Arduino, E. Jensen, H. Wilson, C. Carey, A. Desai, and J. Schranz.** 2001. Direct study: a multicenter, open-label, 24-wk pilot study with a 24-wk extension to evaluate the safety, tolerability and efficacy of indinavir (IDV)-ritonavir (RTV) 800/100 bid in combination with D4T plus 3TC in HIV-infected individuals (Merck Protocol 094), abstr. I-1923. *41st Intersci. Conf. Antimicrob. Agents Chemother.*
64. **Friedland, G., S. Khoo, C. Jack, and U. Lalloo.** 2006. Administration of efavirenz (600 mg/day) with rifampicin results in highly variable levels but excellent clinical outcomes in patients treated for tuberculosis and HIV. *J. Antimicrob. Chemother.* **58:**1299–1302.
65. **Friedland, G. H., R. Pollard, B. Griffith, M. Hughes, G. Morse, R. Bassett, W. Freimuth, L. Demeter, E. Connick, T. Nevin, M. Hirsch, and M. Fischl for the ACTG 261 Team.** 1999. Efficacy and safety of delavirdine mesylate with zidovudine and didanosine compared with two-drug combinations of these agents in persons with HIV disease with CD4 counts of 100 to 500 cells/mm^3 (ACTG 261). *J. Acquir. Immune Defic. Syndr.* **21:**281–292.
66. **Friend, J., N. Parkin, T. Liegler, J. N. Martin, and S. G. Deeks.** 2004. Isolated lopinavir resistance after virological rebound of a ritonavir/lopinavir-based regimen. *AIDS* **18:**1965–1966.
67. **Fundaro, C., O. Genovese, C. Rendeli, E. Tamburrini, and E. Salvaggio.** 2002. Myelomeningocele in a child with intrauterine exposure to efavirenz. *AIDS* **16:**299–300.
68. **Gallant, J., A. Pozniak, E. DeJesus, J. Arribas, R. Campo, S.-S. Chen, D. McColl, J. Enejosa, and A. Cheng.** 2006. Efficacy and safety of tenofovir DF (TDF), emtricitabine (FTC) and efavirenz (EFV) compared to fixed dose zidovudine/lamivudine (CBV) and EFV

through 96 weeks in antiretroviral treatment-naïve patients, abstr. TUPE0064. *XVI Int. AIDS Conf., Toronto, Canada.*

69. **Gallant, J. E., E. DeJesus, J. R. Arribas, A. L. Pozniak, B. Gazzard, R. E. Campo, B. Lu, D. McColl, S. Chuck, J. Enejosa, J. J. Toole, and A. K. Cheng.** 2006. Tenofovir DF, emtricitabine, and efavirenz vs. zidovudine, lamivudine, and efavirenz for HIV. *N. Engl. J. Med.* **354:**251–260.
70. **Gallant, J. E., M. A. Parish, J. C. Keruly, and R. D. Moore.** 2005. Changes in renal function associated with tenofovir disoproxil fumarate treatment, compared with nucleoside reverse-transcriptase inhibitor treatment. *Clin. Infect. Dis.* **40:**1194–1198.
71. **Gallant, J. E., S. Staszewski, A. L. Pozniak, E. DeJesus, J. M. Suleiman, M. D. Miller, D. F. Coakley, B. Lu, J. J. Toole, and A. K. Cheng.** 2004. Efficacy and safety of tenofovir DF vs stavudine in combination therapy in antiretroviral-naive patients: a 3-year randomized trial. *JAMA* **292:**191–201.
72. **Gathe, J. C., Jr., P. Ive, R. Wood, D. Schurmann, N. C. Bellos, E. DeJesus, A. Gladysz, C. Garris, and J. Yeo.** 2004. SOLO: 48-week efficacy and safety comparison of once-daily fosamprenavir/ritonavir versus twice-daily nelfinavir in naive HIV-1-infected patients. *AIDS* **18:**1529–1537.
73. **Gazzard, B. G., A. L. Pozniak, W. Rosenbaum, G. P. Yeni, S. Staszewski, K. Arasteh, K. De Dier, M. Peeters, B. Woodfall, J. Stebbing, and G. A. vant' Klooster.** 2003. An open-label assessment of TMC 125—a new, next-generation NNRTI, for 7 days in HIV-1 infected individuals with NNRTI resistance. *AIDS* **17:**F49–F54.
74. **Goebel, F., A. Yakovlev, A. L. Pozniak, E. Vinogradova, G. Boogaerts, R. Hoetelmans, M. P. de Bethune, M. Peeters, and B. Woodfall.** 2006. Short-term antiviral activity of TMC278—a novel NNRTI—in treatment-naive HIV-1-infected subjects. *AIDS* **20:**1721–1726.
75. **Gotte, M., D. Arion, M. A. Parniak, and M. A. Wainberg.** 2000. The M184V mutation in the reverse transcriptase of human immunodeficiency virus type 1 impairs rescue of chain-terminated DNA synthesis. *J. Virol.* **74:**3579–3585.
76. **Graff, J., N. von Hentig, K. Kuczka, C. Angioni, P. Gute, S. Klauke, E. Babacan, and S. Harder.** 2008. Significant effects of tipranavir on platelet aggregation and thromboxane B2 formation in vitro and in vivo. *J. Antimicrob. Chemother.* **61:**394–399.
77. **Grinsztejn, B., B. Y. Nguyen, C. Katlama, J. M. Gatell, A. Lazzarin, D. Vittecoq, C. J. Gonzalez, J. Chen, C. M. Harvey, and R. D. Isaacs.** 2007. Safety and efficacy of the HIV-1 integrase inhibitor raltegravir (MK-0518) in treatment-experienced patients with multidrug-resistant virus: a phase II randomised controlled trial. *Lancet* **369:**1261–1269.
78. **Gruzdev, B., A. Rakhmanova, E. Doubovskaya, A. Yakovlev, M. Peeters, A. Rinehart, K. de Dier, P. Baede-Van Dijk, W. Parys, and G. van't Klooster.** 2003. A randomized, double-blind, placebo-controlled trial of TMC125 as 7-day monotherapy in antiretroviral naive, HIV-1 infected subjects. *AIDS* **17:**2487–2494.
79. **Guillemi, S., F. Ng, W. Zhang, V. Lima, C. Rocha, M. Harris, G. Bondy, A. Belzberg, and J. Montaner.** 2008. Risk factors for reduced bone mineral density in HIV-infected individuals in the modern HAART era, abstr. 969. *15th Conf. Retrovir. Opportunistic Infect., Boston, MA.*
80. **Gulick, R. M., X. J. Hu, S. A. Fiscus, C. V. Fletcher, R. Haubrich, H. Cheng, E. Acosta, S. W. Lagakos, R. Swanstrom, W. Freimuth, S. Snyder, C. Mills, M. Fischl, C. Pettinelli, and D. Katzenstein.** 2002. Durability of response to treatment among antiretroviral-experienced subjects: 48-week results from AIDS Clinical Trials Group Protocol 359. *J. Infect. Dis.* **186:**626–633.
81. **Gulick, R. M., X. J. Hu, S. A. Fiscus, C. V. Fletcher, R. Haubrich, H. Cheng, E. Acosta, S. W. Lagakos, R. Swanstrom, W. Freimuth, S. Snyder, C. Mills, M. Fischl, C. Pettinelli, and D. Katzenstein.** 2000. Randomized study of saquinavir with ritonavir or nelfinavir together with delavirdine, adefovir, or both in human immunodeficiency virus-infected adults with virologic failure on indinavir: AIDS Clinical Trials Group Study 359. *J. Infect. Dis.* **182:**1375–1384.
82. **Gulick, R. M., H. J. Ribaudo, C. M. Shikuma, C. Lalama, B. R. Schackman, W. A. Meyer III, E. P. Acosta, J. Schouten, K. E. Squires, C. D. Pilcher, R. L. Murphy, S. L. Koletar, M. Carlson, R. C. Reichman, B. Bastow, K. L. Klingman, and D. R. Kuritzkes.** 2006. Three- vs four-drug antiretroviral regimens for the initial treatment of HIV-1 infection: a randomized controlled trial. *JAMA* **296:**769–781.
83. **Gulick, R. M., H. J. Ribaudo, C. M. Shikuma, S. Lustgarten, K. E. Squires, W. A. Meyer III, E. P. Acosta, B. R. Schackman, C. D. Pilcher, R. L. Murphy, W. E. Maher, M. D. Witt, R. C. Reichman, S. Snyder, K. L. Klingman, and D. R. Kuritzkes.** 2004. Triple-nucleoside regimens versus efavirenz-containing regimens for the initial treatment of HIV-1 infection. *N. Engl. J. Med.* **350:**1850–1861.
84. **Gulick, R. M., Z. Su, C. Flexner, M. D. Hughes, P. R. Skolnik, T. J. Wilkin, R. Gross, A. Krambrink, E. Coakley, W. L. Greaves, A. Zolopa, R. Reichman, C. Godfrey, M. Hirsch, and D. R. Kuritzkes for the AIDS Clinical Trials Group 5211 Team.** 2007. Phase 2 study of the safety and efficacy of vicriviroc, a CCR5 inhibitor, in HIV-1-infected, treatment-experienced patients: AIDS Clinical Trials Group 5211. *J. Infect. Dis.* **196:**304–312.
85. **Haas, D. W., B. Johnson, J. Nicotera, V. L. Bailey, V. L. Harris, F. B. Bowles, S. Raffanti, J. Schranz, T. S. Finn, A. J. Saah, and J. Stone.** 2003. Effects of ritonavir on indinavir pharmacokinetics in cerebrospinal fluid and plasma. *Antimicrob. Agents Chemother.* **47:**2131–2137.
86. **Hammer, S. M., M. S. Saag, M. Schechter, J. S. Montaner, R. T. Schooley, D. M. Jacobsen, M. A. Thompson, C. C. Carpenter, M. A. Fischl, B. G. Gazzard, J. M. Gatell, M. S. Hirsch, D. A. Katzenstein, D. D. Richman, S. Vella, P. G. Yeni, and P. A. Volberding.** 2006. Treatment for adult HIV infection: 2006 recommendations of the International AIDS Society—USA panel. *Top. HIV Med* **14:**827–843.
87. **Hanna, G. J., V. A. Johnson, D. R. Kuritzkes, D. D. Richman, A. J. Brown, A. V. Savara, J. D. Hazelwood, and R. T. D'Aquila.** 2000. Patterns of resistance mutations selected by treatment of human immunodeficiency virus type 1 infection with zidovudine, didanosine, and nevirapine. *J. Infect. Dis.* **181:**904–911.
88. **Harrigan, P. R., C. Stone, P. Griffin, I. Nájera, S. Bloor, S. Kemp, M. Tisdale, B. Larder, and the CNA2001 Investigative Group.** 2000. Resistance profile of the human immunodeficiency virus type 1 reverse transcriptase inhibitor abacavir (1592U89) after monotherapy and combination therapy. *J. Infect. Dis.* **181:**912–920.
89. **Hartt, J. K., T. Liang, A. Sahagun-Ruiz, J. M. Wang, J. L. Gao, and P. M. Murphy.** 2000. The HIV-1 cell entry inhibitor T-20 potently chemoattracts neutrophils by specifically activating the N-formylpeptide receptor. *Biochem. Biophys. Res. Commun.* **272:**699–704.
90. **Haubrich, R., D. Berger, P. Chiliade, A. Colson, M. Conant, J. Gallant, T. Wilkin, J. Nadler, G. Pierone, M.**

Saag, B. van Baelen, and E. Lefebvre. 2007. Week 24 efficacy and safety of TMC114/ritonavir in treatment-experienced HIV patients. *AIDS* **21:**F11–F18.

91. **Haubrich, R., P. Cahn, B. Grinsztejn, J. Lalezari, J. Madruga, A. Mills, M. Peeters, J. Vingerhoets, K. Iveson, and G. De Smedt.** 2008. DUET-1: week 48 results of a phase III randomized double-blind trial to evaluate the efficacy and safety of TMC125 vs placebo in 612 treatment-experienced HIV-1-infected patients, abstr. 790. *15th Conf. Retrovir. Opportunistic Infect., Boston, MA.*
92. **Haubrich, R. H., S. Riddler, G. DiRienzo, L. Komarow, W. Powderly, K. Garren, T. George, J. Rooney, J. Mellors, and D. Havlir.** 2007. Metabolic outcomes of ACTG 5142: a prospective, randomized, phase III trial of NRTI-, PI-, and NNRTI-sparing regimens for initial treatment of HIV-1 infection, abstr. 38. *14th Conf. Retrovir. Opportunistic Infect., Los Angeles, CA.*
93. **Hazuda, D. J., P. Felock, M. Witmer, A. Wolfe, K. Stillmock, J. A. Grobler, A. Espeseth, L. Gabryelski, W. Schleif, C. Blau, and M. D. Miller.** 2000. Inhibitors of strand transfer that prevent integration and inhibit HIV-1 replication in cells. *Science* **287:**646–650.
94. **Hazuda, D. J., S. D. Young, J. P. Guare, N. J. Anthony, R. P. Gomez, J. S. Wai, J. P. Vacca, L. Handt, S. L. Motzel, H. J. Klein, G. Dornadula, R. M. Danovich, M. V. Witmer, K. A. Wilson, L. Tussey, W. A. Schleif, L. S. Gabryelski, L. Jin, M. D. Miller, D. R. Casimiro, E. A. Emini, and J. W. Shiver.** 2004. Integrase inhibitors and cellular immunity suppress retroviral replication in rhesus macaques. *Science* **305:**528–532.
95. **Heera, J., M. Saag, P. Ive, J. Whitcomb, M. Lewis, L. McFadyen, J. Goodrich, H. Mayer, E. van der Ryst, and M. Westby.** 2008. Virological correlates associated with treatment failure at week 48 in the phase 3 study of maraviroc in treatment-naive patients, abstr. 40LB. *15th Conf. Retrovir. Opportunistic Infect., Boston, MA.*
96. **Hertogs, K., S. Bloor, S. D. Kemp, C. Van den Eynde, T. M. Alcorn, R. Pauwels, M. Van Houtte, S. Staszewski, V. Miller, and B. A. Larder.** 2000. Phenotypic and genotypic analysis of clinical HIV-1 isolates reveals extensive protease inhibitor cross-resistance: a survey of over 6000 samples. *AIDS* **14:**1203–1210.
97. **Hicks, C., E. DeJesus, D. Wohl, Q. Liao, K. Pappa, and T. Lancaster.** 2007. Once-daily fosamprenavir (FPV) boosted with either 100mg or 200mg of ritonavir (r) along with abacavir (ABC)/lamivudine (3TC): 48 week safety and efficacy results from COL100758. *11th Eur. AIDS Conf., Madrid, Spain.*
98. **Hicks, C. B., P. Cahn, D. A. Cooper, S. L. Walmsley, C. Katlama, B. Clotet, A. Lazzarin, M. A. Johnson, D. Neubacher, D. Mayers, and H. Valdez.** 2006. Durable efficacy of tipranavir-ritonavir in combination with an optimised background regimen of antiretroviral drugs for treatment-experienced HIV-1-infected patients at 48 weeks in the Randomized Evaluation of Strategic Intervention in multi-drug reSistant patients with Tipranavir (RESIST) studies: an analysis of combined data from two randomised open-label trials. *Lancet* **368:**466–475.
99. **Hu, Z., F. Giguel, H. Hatano, P. Reid, J. Lu, and D. R. Kuritzkes.** 2006. Fitness comparison of thymidine analog resistance pathways in human immunodeficiency virus type 1. *J. Virol.* **80:**7020–7027.
100. **Hunt, P. W., P. R. Harrigan, W. Huang, M. Bates, D. W. Williamson, J. M. McCune, R. W. Price, S. S. Spudich, H. Lampiris, R. Hoh, T. Leigler, J. N. Martin, and S. G. Deeks.** 2006. Prevalence of CXCR4 tropism among antiretroviral-treated HIV-1-infected patients with detectable viremia. *J. Infect. Dis.* **194:**926–930.
101. **Iversen, A. K., R. W. Shafer, K. Wehrly, M. A. Winters, J. I. Mullins, B. Chesebro, and T. C. Merigan.** 1996. Multidrug-resistant human immunodeficiency virus type 1 strains resulting from combination antiretroviral therapy. *J. Virol.* **70:**1086–1090.
102. **Ives, K. J., H. Jacobsen, S. A. Galpin, M. M. Garaev, L. Dorrell, J. Mous, K. Bragman, and J. N. Weber.** 1997. Emergence of resistant variants of HIV in vivo during monotherapy with the proteinase inhibitor saquinavir. *J. Antimicrob. Chemother.* **39:**771–779.
103. **Iwamoto, M., L. A. Wenning, G. C. Mistry, A. S. Petry, S. Y. Liou, K. Ghosh, S. Breidinger, N. Azrolan, M. J. Gutierrez, W. E. Bridson, J. A. Stone, K. M. Gottesdiener, and J. A. Wagner.** 2008. Atazanavir modestly increases plasma levels of raltegravir in healthy subjects. *Clin. Infect. Dis.* **47:**137–140.
104. **Iwamoto, M., L. A. Wenning, A. S. Petry, T. Laethem, M. Desmet, J. T. Kost, S. Merschman, E. Mangin, N. Azrolan, H. E. Greenberg, W. Haazen, J. A. Stone, K. M. Gottesdiener, and J. A. Wagner.** 2006. Minimal effect of ritonavir (RTV) and efavirenz (EFV) on the pharmacokinetics (PK) of Mk-0518, abstr. A-373. *46th Intersci. Conf. Antimicrob. Agents Chemother.*
105. **Jacobsen, H., K. Yasargil, D. L. Winslow, J. C. Craig, A. Krohn, I. B. Duncan, and J. Mous.** 1995. Characterization of human immunodeficiency virus type 1 mutants with decreased sensitivity to proteinase inhibitor Ro 31-8959. *Virology* **206:**527–534.
106. **Johnson, M., B. Grinsztejn, C. Rodriguez, J. Coco, E. DeJesus, A. Lazzarin, K. Lichtenstein, V. Wirtz, A. Rightmire, L. Odeshoo, and C. McLaren.** 2006. 96-week comparison of once-daily atazanavir/ritonavir and twice-daily lopinavir/ritonavir in patients with multiple virologic failures. *AIDS* **20:**711–718.
107. **Johnson, M., T. Campbell, B. Clotet, C. Katlama, A. Lazzarin, W. Towner, M. Peeters, J. Vingerhoets, S. Bollen, and G. De Smedt.** 2008. DUET-2: week-48 results of a phase III randomized double-blind trial to evaluate the efficacy and safety of TMC125 vs placebo in 591 treatment-experienced HIV-1-infected patients, abstr. 791. *15th Conf. Retrovir. Opportunistic Infect., Boston, MA.*
108. **Johnson, M. A., J. C. Gathe, Jr., D. Podzamczer, J. M. Molina, C. T. Naylor, Y. L. Chiu, M. S. King, T. J. Podsadecki, G. J. Hanna, and S. C. Brun.** 2006. A once-daily lopinavir/ritonavir-based regimen provides noninferior antiviral activity compared with a twice-daily regimen. *J. Acquir. Immune Defic. Syndr.* **43:**153–160.
109. **Johnson, V. A., F. Brun-Vezinet, B. Clotet, H. F. Gunthard, D. R. Kuritzkes, D. Pillay, J. M. Schapiro, and D. D. Richman.** 2007. Update of the drug resistance mutations in HIV-1: 2007. *Top. HIV Med.* **15:**119–125.
110. **Johnson, V. A., F. Brun-Vezinet, B. Clotet, H. F. Gunthard, D. R. Kuritzkes, D. Pillay, J. M. Schapiro, and D. D. Richman.** 2008. Update of the drug resistance mutations in HIV-1: spring 2008. *Top. HIV Med.* **16:**62–68.
111. **Joly, V., P. Flandre, V. Meiffredy, N. Leturque, M. Harel, J. P. Aboulker, and P. Yeni.** 2002. Increased risk of lipoatrophy under stavudine in HIV-1-infected patients: results of a substudy from a comparative trial. *AIDS* **16:**2447–2454.
112. **Joly, V., M. Moroni, E. Concia, A. Lazzarin, B. Hirschel, J. Jost, F. Chiodo, Z. Bentwich, W. C. Love, D. A. Hawkins, E. G. L. Wilkins, A. J. Gatell, N. Vetter, C. Greenwald, W. W. Freimuth, W. de Cian,**

and The M/3331/0013B Study Group. 2000. Delavirdine in combination with zidovudine in treatment of human immunodeficiency virus type 1-infected patients: evaluation of efficacy and emergence of viral resistance in a randomized, comparative phase III trial. *Antimicrob. Agents Chemother.* **44:**3155–3157.

113. **Kagan, R. M., M. D. Shenderovich, P. N. Heseltine, and K. Ramnarayan.** 2005. Structural analysis of an HIV-1 protease I47A mutant resistant to the protease inhibitor lopinavir. *Protein Sci.* **14:**1870–1878.
114. **Kakuda, T.** 2000. Pharmacology of nucleoside and nucleotide reverse transcriptase inhibitor-induced mitochondrial toxicity. *Clin. Ther.* **22:**685–708.
115. **Kassahun, K., I. McIntosh, D. Cui, D. Hreniuk, S. Merschman, K. Lasseter, N. Azrolan, M. Iwamoto, J. A. Wagner, and L. A. Wenning.** 2007. Metabolism and disposition in humans of raltegravir (MK-0518), an anti-AIDS drug targeting the human immunodeficiency virus 1 integrase enzyme. *Drug Metab. Dispos.* **35:**1657–1663.
116. **Katlama, C., T. Campbell, B. Clotet, M. Johnson, A. Lazzarin, K. Arasteh, W. Towner, B. Trottier, M. Peeters, J. Vingerhoets, G. De Smedt, B. Baeten, G. Beets, R. Sinha, and B. Woodfall.** 2007. DUET-2: 24-week results of a phase III randomised double-blind trial to evaluate the efficacy and safety of TMC125 vs placebo in 591 treatment-experienced HIV-1 infected patients, abstr. WESS204-2. *4th IAS Conf. HIV Pathog. Treatment Prev., Sydney, Australia.*
117. **Kearney, B., R. Price, L. Sheiner, E. Bellibas, S. Staprans, L. Thevanayagam, and F. Aweeka.** 1999. Estimation of nevirapine exposure within the cerebrospinal fluid using CSF: plasma area under the curve ratios, abstr. 406. *Program Abstr. 6th Conf. Retrovir. Opportunistic Infect., Chicago, IL.*
118. **Kellam, P., C. A. Boucher, and B. A. Larder.** 1992. Fifth mutation in human immunodeficiency virus type 1 reverse transcriptase contributes to the development of high-level resistance to zidovudine. *Proc. Natl. Acad. Sci. USA* **89:**1934–1938.
119. **Kempf, D. J., J. D. Isaacson, M. S. King, S. C. Brun, J. Sylte, B. Richards, B. Bernstein, R. Rode, and E. Sun.** 2002. Analysis of the virological response with respect to baseline viral phenotype and genotype in protease inhibitor-experienced HIV-1-infected patients receiving lopinavir/ritonavir therapy. *Antivir. Ther.* **7:**165–174.
120. **Kempf, D. J., J. D. Isaacson, M. S. King, S. C. Brun, Y. Xu, K. Real, B. M. Bernstein, A. J. Japour, E. Sun, and R. A. Rode.** 2001. Identification of genotypic changes in human immunodeficiency virus protease that correlate with reduced susceptibility to the protease inhibitor lopinavir among viral isolates from protease inhibitor-experienced patients. *J. Virol.* **75:**7462–7469.
121. **Khanlou, H., V. Yeh, B. Guyer, and C. Farthing.** 2005. Early virologic failure in a pilot study evaluating the efficacy of therapy containing once-daily abacavir, lamivudine, and tenofovir DF in treatment-naive HIV-infected patients. *AIDS Patient Care STDS* **19:**135–140.
122. **Kim, E. Y., L. Vrang, B. Oberg, and T. C. Merigan.** 2001. Anti-HIV type 1 activity of 3′-fluoro-3′-deoxythymidine for several different multidrug-resistant mutants. *AIDS Res. Hum. Retrovir.* **17:**401–407.
123. **Kindberg, E., A. Mickiene, C. Ax, B. Akerlind, S. Vene, L. Lindquist, A. Lundkvist, and L. Svensson.** 2008. A deletion in the chemokine receptor 5 (CCR5) gene is associated with tickborne encephalitis. *J. Infect. Dis.* **197:**266–269.
124. **King, M. S., R. Rode, I. Cohen-Codar, V. Calvez, A. G. Marcelin, G. J. Hanna, and D. J. Kempf.** 2007. Predictive genotypic algorithm for virologic response to lopinavir-ritonavir in protease inhibitor-experienced patients. *Antimicrob. Agents Chemother.* **51:**3067–3074.
125. **Kirk, O., T. L. Katzenstein, J. Gerstoft, L. Mathiesen, H. Nielsen, C. Pedersen, and J. D. Lundgren.** 1999. Combination therapy containing ritonavir plus saquinavir has superior short-term antiretroviral efficacy: a randomized trial. *AIDS* **13:**F9–F16.
126. **Kitchen, V. S., C. Skinner, K. Ariyoshi, E. A. Lane, I. B. Duncan, J. Burckhardt, H. U. Burger, K. Bragman, A. J. Pinching, and J. N. Weber.** 1995. Safety and activity of saquinavir in HIV infection. *Lancet* **345:**952–955.
127. **Koh, Y., T. Towata, A. Ghosh, and H. Mitsuya.** 2007. Selection in vitro of HIV-1 variants highly resistant to darunavir using a mixture of HIV-1 isolates resistant to multiple PI, abstr. 606. *14th Conf. Retrovir. Opportunistic Infect., Los Angeles, CA.*
128. **Kumar, P. N., D. E. Sweet, J. A. McDowell, W. Symonds, Y. Lou, S. Hetherington, and S. LaFon.** 1999. Safety and pharmacokinetics of abacavir (1592U89) following oral administration of escalating single doses in human immunodeficiency virus type 1-infected adults. *Antimicrob. Agents Chemother.* **43:**603–608.
129. **Kuritzkes, D. R., R. L. Bassett, J. D. Hazelwood, H. Barrett, R. A. Rhodes, R. K. Young, and V. A. Johnson.** 2004. Rate of thymidine analogue resistance mutation accumulation with zidovudine- or stavudine-based regimens. *J. Acquir. Immune Defic. Syndr.* **36:**600–603.
130. **Lafeuillade, A., G. Hittinger, and S. Chadapaud.** 2001. Increased mitochondrial toxicity with ribavirin in HIV/HCV coinfection. *Lancet* **357:**280–281.
131. **Lalezari, J. P., K. Henry, M. O'Hearn, J. S. Montaner, P. J. Piliero, B. Trottier, S. Walmsley, C. Cohen, D. R. Kuritzkes, J. J. Eron, Jr., J. Chung, R. DeMasi, L. Donatacci, C. Drobnes, J. Delehanty, and M. Salgo.** 2003. Enfuvirtide, an HIV-1 fusion inhibitor, for drug-resistant HIV infection in North and South America. *N. Engl. J. Med.* **348:**2175–2185.
132. **Landman, R., D. Descamps, G. Peytavin, A. Trylesinski, C. Katlama, P. M. Girard, B. Bonnet, P. Yeni, M. Bentata, C. Michelet, A. Benalycherif, F. Brun Vezinet, M. D. Miller, and P. Flandre.** 2005. Early virologic failure and rescue therapy of tenofovir, abacavir, and lamivudine for initial treatment of HIV-1 infection: TONUS study. *HIV Clin. Trials* **6:**291–301.
133. **Lanier, E. R., M. Ait-Khaled, J. Scott, C. Stone, T. Melby, G. Sturge, M. St. Clair, H. Steel, S. Hetherington, G. Pearce, W. Spreen, and S. Lafon.** 2004. Antiviral efficacy of abacavir in antiretroviral therapy-experienced adults harbouring HIV-1 with specific patterns of resistance to nucleoside reverse transcriptase inhibitors. *Antivir. Ther.* **9:**37–45.
134. **Larder, B. A., and S. Boor.** 2001. Analysis of clinical isolates and site directed mutants reveals the genetic determinants of didanosine resistance, abstr. 47. *5th Int. Workshop on HIV Drug Resistance and Treatment Strategies, Scottsdale, AZ.*
135. **Larder, B. A., G. Darby, and D. D. Richman.** 1989. HIV with reduced sensitivity to zidovudine (AZT) isolated during prolonged therapy. *Science* **243:**1731–1734.
136. **Larder, B. A., K. Hertogs, S. Bloor, C. H. van den Eynde, W. DeCian, Y. Wang, W. W. Freimuth, and G. Tarpley.** 2000. Tipranavir inhibits broadly protease inhibitor-resistant HIV-1 clinical samples. *AIDS* **14:**1943–1948.
137. **Larder, B. A., S. D. Kemp, and P. R. Harrigan.** 1995. Potential mechanism for sustained antiretroviral efficacy

of AZT-3TC combination therapy. *Science* **269:**696–699.

138. **Lazzarin, A., T. Campbell, B. Clotet, M. Johnson, C. Katlama, A. Moll, W. Towner, B. Trottier, M. Peeters, J. Vingerhoets, G. de Smedt, B. Baeten, G. Beets, R. Sinha, and B. Woodfall.** 2007. Efficacy and safety of TMC125 (etravirine) in treatment-experienced HIV-1-infected patients in DUET-2: 24-week results from a randomised, double-blind, placebo-controlled trial. *Lancet* **370:**39–48.
139. **Lederman, M. M., A. Penn-Nicholson, M. Cho, and D. Mosier.** 2006. Biology of CCR5 and its role in HIV infection and treatment. *JAMA* **296:**815–826.
140. **Lim, J. K., C. Y. Louie, C. Glaser, C. Jean, B. Johnson, H. Johnson, D. H. McDermott, and P. M. Murphy.** 2008. Genetic deficiency of chemokine receptor CCR5 is a strong risk factor for symptomatic West Nile virus infection: a meta-analysis of 4 cohorts in the US epidemic. *J. Infect. Dis.* **197:**262–265.
141. **Loeliger, A. E., H. Steel, S. McGuirk, W. S. Powell, and S. V. Hetherington.** 2001. The abacavir hypersensitivity reaction and interruptions in therapy. *AIDS* **15:** 1325–1326.
142. **Lu, J., S. G. Deeks, R. Hoh, G. Beatty, B. A. Kuritzkes, J. N. Martin, and D. R. Kuritzkes.** 2006. Rapid emergence of enfuvirtide resistance in HIV-1-infected patients: results of a clonal analysis. *J. Acquir. Immune Defic. Syndr.* **43:**60–64.
143. **Ly, T., and M. E. Ruiz.** 2007. Prolonged QT interval and torsades de pointes associated with atazanavir therapy. *Clin. Infect. Dis.* **44:**e67–e68.
144. **MacGregor, T. R., J. P. Sabo, S. H. Norris, P. Johnson, L. Galitz, and S. McCallister.** 2004. Pharmacokinetic characterization of different dose combinations of coadministered tipranavir and ritonavir in healthy volunteers. *HIV Clin. Trials* **5:**371–382.
145. **Madruga, J. V., D. Berger, M. McMurchie, F. Suter, D. Banhegyi, K. Ruxrungtham, D. Norris, E. Lefebvre, M. P. de Bethune, F. Tomaka, M. De Pauw, T. Vangeneugden, and S. Spinosa-Guzman.** 2007. Efficacy and safety of darunavir-ritonavir compared with that of lopinavir-ritonavir at 48 weeks in treatment-experienced, HIV-infected patients in TITAN: a randomised controlled phase III trial. *Lancet* **370:**49–58.
146. **Madruga, J. V., P. Cahn, B. Grinsztejn, R. Haubrich, J. Lalezari, A. Mills, G. Pialoux, T. Wilkin, M. Peeters, J. Vingerhoets, G. de Smedt, L. Leopold, R. Trefiglio, and B. Woodfall.** 2007. Efficacy and safety of TMC125 (etravirine) in treatment-experienced HIV-1-infected patients in DUET-1: 24-week results from a randomised, double-blind, placebo-controlled trial. *Lancet* **370:**29–38.
147. **Maguire, M., D. Shortino, A. Klein, W. Harris, V. Manohitharajah, M. Tisdale, R. Elston, J. Yeo, S. Randall, F. Xu, H. Parker, J. May, and W. Snowden.** 2002. Emergence of resistance to protease inhibitor amprenavir in human immunodeficiency virus type 1-infected patients: selection of four alternative viral protease genotypes and influence of viral susceptibility to coadministered reverse transcriptase nucleoside inhibitors. *Antimicrob. Agents Chemother.* **46:**731–738.
148. **Maitland, D., G. Moyle, J. Hand, S. Mandalia, M. Boffito, M. Nelson, and B. Gazzard.** 2005. Early virologic failure in HIV-1 infected subjects on didanosine/tenofovir/efavirenz: 12-week results from a randomized trial. *AIDS* **19:**1183–1188.
149. **Mallal, S., D. Nolan, C. Witt, G. Masel, A. M. Martin, C. Moore, D. Sayer, A. Castley, C. Mamotte, D. Maxwell, I. James, and F. T. Christiansen.** 2002. Association between presence of HLA-B*5701, HLA-DR7, and HLA-DQ3 and hypersensitivity to HIV-1 reverse-transcriptase inhibitor abacavir. *Lancet* **359:**727–732.
150. **Mallal, S., E. Phillips, G. Carosi, J. M. Molina, C. Workman, J. Tomazic, E. Jagel-Guedes, S. Rugina, O. Kozyrev, J. F. Cid, P. Hay, D. Nolan, S. Hughes, A. Hughes, S. Ryan, N. Fitch, D. Thorborn, and A. Benbow.** 2008. HLA-B*5701 screening for hypersensitivity to abacavir. *N. Engl. J. Med.* **358:**568–579.
151. **Marcelin, A. G., B. Masquelier, D. Descamps, J. Izopet, C. Charpentier, C. Alloui, G. Peytavin, M. Lavignon, P. Flandre, and C. Vincent.** 2007. Mutations associated with response to boosted tipranavir in HIV-1-infected PI-experienced patients, abstr. 612. *14th Conf. Retrovir. Opportunistic Infect., Los Angeles, CA.*
152. **Marcelin, A. G., C. Dalban, G. Peytavin, C. Lamotte, R. Agher, C. Delaugerre, M. Wirden, F. Conan, S. Dantin, C. Katlama, D. Costagliola, and V. Calvez.** 2004. Clinically relevant interpretation of genotype and relationship to plasma drug concentrations for resistance to saquinavir-ritonavir in human immunodeficiency virus type 1 protease inhibitor-experienced patients. *Antimicrob. Agents Chemother.* **48:**4687–4692.
153. **Margot, N. A., E. Isaacson, I. McGowan, A. Cheng, and M. D. Miller.** 2003. Extended treatment with tenofovir disoproxil fumarate in treatment-experienced HIV-1-infected patients: genotypic, phenotypic, and rebound analyses. *J. Acquir. Immune Defic. Syndr.* **33:**15–21.
154. **Markowitz, M., J. O. Morales-Ramirez, B. Y. Nguyen, C. M. Kovacs, R. T. Steigbigel, D. A. Cooper, R. Liporace, R. Schwartz, R. Isaacs, L. R. Gilde, L. Wenning, J. Zhao, and H. Teppler.** 2006. Antiretroviral activity, pharmacokinetics, and tolerability of MK-0518, a novel inhibitor of HIV-1 integrase, dosed as monotherapy for 10 days in treatment-naive HIV-1-infected individuals. *J. Acquir. Immune Defic. Syndr.* **43:**509–515.
155. **Markowitz, M., B. Y. Nguyen, E. Gotuzzo, F. Mendo, W. Ratanasuwan, C. Kovacs, G. Prada, J. O. Morales-Ramirez, C. S. Crumpacker, R. D. Isaacs, L. R. Gilde, H. Wan, M. D. Miller, L. A. Wenning, and H. Teppler.** 2007. Rapid and durable antiretroviral effect of the HIV-1 integrase inhibitor raltegravir as part of combination therapy in treatment-naive patients with HIV-1 infection: results of a 48-week controlled study. *J. Acquir. Immune Defic. Syndr.* **46:**125–133.
156. **Markowitz, M., L. N. Slater, R. Schwartz, P. H. Kazanjian, B. Hathaway, D. Wheeler, M. Goldman, D. Neubacher, D. Mayers, H. Valdez, and S. McCallister.** 2007. Long-term efficacy and safety of tipranavir boosted with ritonavir in HIV-1-infected patients failing multiple protease inhibitor regimens: 80-week data from a phase 2 study. *J. Acquir. Immune Defic. Syndr.* **45:**401–410.
157. **Masquelier, B., D. Breilh, D. Neau, S. Lawson-Ayayi, V. Lavignolle, J. M. Ragnaud, M. Dupon, P. Morlat, F. Dabis, and H. Fleury.** 2002. Human immunodeficiency virus type 1 genotypic and pharmacokinetic determinants of the virological response to lopinavir-ritonavir-containing therapy in protease inhibitor-experienced patients. *Antimicrob. Agents Chemother.* **46:**2926–2932.
158. **Matthews, T., M. Salgo, M. Greenberg, J. Chung, R. DeMasi, and D. Bolognesi.** 2004. Enfuvirtide: the first therapy to inhibit the entry of HIV-1 into host CD4 lymphocytes. *Nat. Rev. Drug Discov.* **3:**215–225.
159. **McCallister, S., H. Valdez, K. Curry, T. MacGregor, M. Borin, W. Freimuth, Y. Wang, and D. L. Mayers.** 2004. A 14-day dose-response study of the efficacy, safety, and pharmacokinetics of the nonpeptidic protease

inhibitor tipranavir in treatment-naive HIV-1-infected patients. *J. Acquir. Immune Defic. Syndr.* **35:**376–382.

160. **McColl, D. J., S. Fransen, S. Gupta, N. Parkin, N. Margot, S. Chuck, A. K. Cheng, and M. D. Miller.** 2007. Resistance and cross-resistance to first generation integrase inhibitors: insights from a phase II study of elvitegravir (GS-9137), abstr. 9. *16th Int. HIV Drug Resistance Workshop, Barbados, West Indies.*
161. **McIntyre, J. A., N. Martinson, G. E. Gray, M. Hopley, T. Kimura, P. Robinson, and D. Mayers.** 2005. Addition of short course Combivir to single dose Viramune for the prevention of mother to child transmission of HIV-1 can significantly decrease the subsequent development of maternal and paediatric NNRTI-resistant virus, abstr. TuFo0204. *3rd Int. AIDS Soc. Conf. HIV Pathog. Treatment, Rio de Janeiro, Brazil.*
162. **Melby, T., M. Despirito, R. Demasi, G. Heilek-Snyder, M. L. Greenberg, and N. Graham.** 2006. HIV-1 coreceptor use in triple-class treatment-experienced patients: baseline prevalence, correlates, and relationship to enfuvirtide response. *J. Infect. Dis.* **194:**238–246.
163. **Merrill, D. P., M. Moonis, T. C. Chou, and M. S. Hirsch.** 1996. Lamivudine or stavudine in two- and three-drug combinations against human immunodeficiency virus type 1 replication in vitro. *J. Infect. Dis.* **173:**355–364.
164. **Miller, M. D., N. Margot, B. Lu, L. Zhong, S. S. Chen, A. Cheng, and M. Wulfsohn.** 2004. Genotypic and phenotypic predictors of the magnitude of response to tenofovir disoproxil fumarate treatment in antiretroviral-experienced patients. *J. Infect. Dis.* **189:**837–846.
165. **Miro, J. M., J. Pich, P. Domingo, D. Podzamczer, J. R. Arribas, E. Ribera, J. Arrizabalaga, M. Lonca, E. De Lazzari, and M. Plana.** 2007. Immunological reconstitution in severely immunosuppressed antiretroviral-naive patients (<100 CD4þ T cells/mm^3) using a nonnucleoside reverse transcriptase inhibitor (NNRTI)- or a boosted protease inhibitor (PI)-based antiretroviral therapy regimen: 3 year results (the ADVANZ trial), abstr. P-1915. *17th Eur. Congr. Clin. Microbiol. Infect. Dis. (ECCMID) Int. Cong. Chemother., Munich, Germany.*
166. **Molina, J. M., A. Wilkin, P. Domingo, R. Myers, J. Hairrell, C. Naylor, T. Podsadecki, M. King, and G. Hanna.** 2005. Once daily vs twice daily lopinavir/ritonavir in antiretroviral-naive patients: 96-week results, abstr. WePe12.3C12. *3rd Int. AIDS Soc. Conf. HIV Pathog. Treatment, Rio de Janeiro, Brazil.*
167. **Molina, J. M., A. G. Marcelin, J. Pavie, L. Heripret, C. M. De Boever, M. Troccaz, G. Leleu, and V. Calvez.** 2005. Didanosine in HIV-1-infected patients experiencing failure of antiretroviral therapy: a randomized placebo-controlled trial. *J. Infect. Dis.* **191:**840–847.
168. **Molla, A., M. Korneyeva, Q. Gao, S. Vasavanonda, P. J. Schipper, H. M. Mo, M. Markowitz, T. Chernyavskiy, P. Niu, N. Lyons, A. Hsu, G. R. Granneman, D. D. Ho, C. A. Boucher, J. M. Leonard, D. W. Norbeck, and D. J. Kempf.** 1996. Ordered accumulation of mutations in HIV protease confers resistance to ritonavir. *Nat. Med.* **2:**760–766.
169. **Montaner, J., R. D. Masi, J. Delehanty, J. Chung, Z. Gafoor, and M. Salgo.** 2003. Optimizing T-20 treatment: analysis of factors leading to therapeutic success from the registration trials TORO 1 and TORO 2, abstr. 116. *2nd Int. AIDS Soc. Conf. on HIV Pathogenesis and Treatment, Paris, France.*
170. **Moore, J. P., S. G. Kitchen, P. Pugach, and J. A. Zack.** 2004. The CCR5 and CXCR4 coreceptors—central to understanding the transmission and pathogenesis of human immunodeficiency virus type 1 infection. *AIDS Res. Hum. Retrovir.* **20:**111–126.
171. **Moore, K. H., G. J. Yuen, R. H. Raasch, J. J. Eron, D. Martin, P. K. Mydlow, and E. K. Hussey.** 1996. Pharmacokinetics of lamivudine administered alone and with trimethoprim-sulfamethoxazole. *Clin. Pharmacol. Ther.* **59:**550–558.
172. **Moore, R. D., W. M. Wong, J. C. Keruly, and J. C. McArthur.** 2000. Incidence of neuropathy in HIV-infected patients on monotherapy versus those on combination therapy with didanosine, stavudine and hydroxyurea. *AIDS* **14:**273–278.
173. **Moyle, G.** 2000. Clinical manifestations and management of antiretroviral nucleoside analog-related mitochondrial toxicity. *Clin. Ther.* **22:**911–936; discussion, 898.
174. **Moyle, G. J., E. DeJesus, P. Cahn, S. A. Castillo, H. Zhao, D. N. Gordon, C. Craig, and T. R. Scott.** 2005. Abacavir once or twice daily combined with once-daily lamivudine and efavirenz for the treatment of antiretroviral-naive HIV-infected adults: results of the Ziagen Once Daily in Antiretroviral Combination Study. *J. Acquir. Immune Defic. Syndr.* **38:**417–425.
175. **Murata, H., P. W. Hruz, and M. Mueckler.** 2000. The mechanism of insulin resistance caused by HIV protease inhibitor therapy. *J. Biol. Chem.* **275:**20251–20254.
176. **Naeger, L. K., and K. A. Struble.** 2006. Effect of baseline protease genotype and phenotype on HIV response to atazanavir/ritonavir in treatment-experienced patients. *AIDS* **20:**847–853.
177. **Nelson, M., K. Arasteh, B. Clotet, D. A. Cooper, K. Henry, C. Katlama, J. P. Lalezari, A. Lazzarin, J. S. Montaner, M. O'Hearn, P. J. Piliero, J. Reynes, B. Trottier, S. L. Walmsley, C. Cohen, J. J. Eron, Jr., D. R. Kuritzkes, J. Lange, H. J. Stellbrink, J. F. Delfraissy, N. E. Buss, L. Donatacci, C. Wat, L. Smiley, M. Wilkinson, A. Valentine, D. Guimaraes, R. Demasi, J. Chung, and M. P. Salgo.** 2005. Durable efficacy of enfuvirtide over 48 weeks in heavily treatment-experienced HIV-1-infected patients in the T-20 versus optimized background regimen only 1 and 2 clinical trials. *J. Acquir. Immune Defic. Syndr.* **40:**404–412.
178. **Nikolenko, G. N., S. Palmer, F. Maldarelli, J. W. Mellors, J. M. Coffin, and V. K. Pathak.** 2005. Mechanism for nucleoside analog-mediated abrogation of HIV-1 replication: balance between RNase H activity and nucleotide excision. *Proc. Natl. Acad. Sci. USA* **102:**2093–2098.
179. **Opravil, M., B. Hirschel, A. Lazzarin, H. Furrer, J. P. Chave, S. Yerly, L. R. Bisset, M. Fischer, P. Vernazza, E. Bernasconi, M. Battegay, B. Ledergerber, H. Gunthard, C. Howe, R. Weber, and L. Perrin.** 2002. A randomized trial of simplified maintenance therapy with abacavir, lamivudine, and zidovudine in human immunodeficiency virus infection. *J. Infect. Dis.* **185:**1251–1260.
180. **Panel on Antiretroviral Guidelines for Adults and Adolescents.** 29 January 2008. Guidelines for the use of antiretroviral agents in HIV-1-infected adults and adolescents—January 29, 2008. Department of Health and Human Services, Washington, DC. www.aidsinfo.nih.gov/ContentFiles/AdultAdolescentGL.pdf.
181. **Pata, J. D., W. G. Stirtan, S. W. Goldstein, and T. A. Steitz.** 2004. Structure of HIV-1 reverse transcriptase bound to an inhibitor active against mutant reverse transcriptases resistant to other nonnucleoside inhibitors. *Proc. Natl. Acad. Sci. USA* **101:**10548–10553.

182. **Pereira, A. S., L. M. Smeaton, J. G. Gerber, E. P. Acosta, S. Snyder, S. A. Fiscus, R. R. Tidwell, R. M. Gulick, R. L. Murphy, and J. J. Eron, Jr.** 2002. The pharmacokinetics of amprenavir, zidovudine, and lamivudine in the genital tracts of men infected with human immunodeficiency virus type 1 (AIDS clinical trials group study 850). *J. Infect. Dis.* **186:**198–204.
183. **Persico, M., E. Persico, C. T. Bakker, I. Rigato, A. Amoroso, R. Torella, P. J. Bosma, C. Tiribelli, and J. D. Ostrow.** 2001. Hepatic uptake of organic anions affects the plasma bilirubin level in subjects with Gilbert's syndrome mutations in UGT1A1. *Hepatology* **33:** 627–632.
184. **Pluda, J. M., T. P. Cooley, J. S. Montaner, L. E. Shay, N. E. Reinhalter, S. N. Warthan, J. Ruedy, H. M. Hirst, C. A. Vicary, J. B. Quinn, et al.** 1995. A phase I/II study of 2′-deoxy-3′-thiacytidine (lamivudine) in patients with advanced human immunodeficiency virus infection. *J. Infect. Dis.* **171:**1438–1447.
185. **Podzamczer, D., E. Ferrer, J. M. Gatell, J. Niubo, D. Dalmau, A. Leon, H. Knobel, C. Polo, D. Iniguez, and I. Ruiz.** 2005. Early virological failure with a combination of tenofovir, didanosine and efavirenz. *Antivir. Ther.* **10:**171–177.
186. **Pommier, Y., A. A. Johnson, and C. Marchand.** 2005. Integrase inhibitors to treat HIV/AIDS. *Nat. Rev. Drug Discov.* **4:**236–248.
187. **Pugach, P., A. J. Marozsan, T. J. Ketas, E. L. Landes, J. P. Moore, and S. E. Kuhmann.** 2007. HIV-1 clones resistant to a small molecule CCR5 inhibitor use the inhibitor-bound form of CCR5 for entry. *Virology* **361:** 212–228.
188. **Pulido, F., J. R. Arribas, J. M. Miro, M. A. Costa, J. Gonzalez, R. Rubio, J. M. Pena, M. Torralba, M. Lonca, A. Lorenzo, C. Cepeda, J. J. Vazquez, and J. M. Gatell.** 2004. Clinical, virologic, and immunologic response to efavirenz or protease inhibitor-based highly active antiretroviral therapy in a cohort of antiretroviral-naive patients with advanced HIV infection (EfaVIP 2 study). *J. Acquir. Immune Defic. Syndr.* **35:**343–350.
189. **Racoosin, J. A., and C. M. Kessler.** 1999. Bleeding episodes in HIV-positive patients taking HIV protease inhibitors: a case series. *Haemophilia* **5:**266–269.
190. **Raffi, F., C. Katlama, M. Saag, M. Wilkinson, J. Chung, L. Smiley, and M. Salgo.** 2006. Week-12 response to therapy as a predictor of week 24, 48, and 96 outcome in patients receiving the HIV fusion inhibitor enfuvirtide in the T-20 versus Optimized Regimen Only (TORO) trials. *Clin. Infect. Dis.* **42:**870–877.
191. **Rauch, A., D. Nolan, A. Martin, E. McKinnon, C. Almeida, and S. Mallal.** 2006. Prospective genetic screening decreases the incidence of abacavir hypersensitivity reactions in the Western Australian HIV cohort study. *Clin. Infect. Dis.* **43:**99–102.
192. **Ray, N., J. E. Harrison, L. A. Blackburn, J. N. Martin, S. G. Deeks, and R. W. Doms.** 2007. Clinical resistance to enfuvirtide does not affect susceptibility of human immunodeficiency virus type 1 to other classes of entry inhibitors. *J. Virol.* **81:**3240–3250.
193. **Reeves, J. D., S. A. Gallo, N. Ahmad, J. L. Miamidian, P. E. Harvey, M. Sharron, S. Pohlmann, J. N. Sfakianos, C. A. Derdeyn, R. Blumenthal, E. Hunter, and R. W. Doms.** 2002. Sensitivity of HIV-1 to entry inhibitors correlates with envelope/coreceptor affinity, receptor density, and fusion kinetics. *Proc. Natl. Acad. Sci. USA* **99:**16249–16254.
194. **Rhee, S. Y., M. J. Gonzales, R. Kantor, B. J. Betts, J. Ravela, and R. W. Shafer.** 2003. Human immunodeficiency virus reverse transcriptase and protease sequence database. *Nucleic Acids Res.* **31:**298–303.
195. **Rhee, S. Y., J. Taylor, G. Wadhera, A. Ben-Hur, D. L. Brutlag, and R. W. Shafer.** 2006. Genotypic predictors of human immunodeficiency virus type 1 drug resistance. *Proc. Natl. Acad. Sci. USA* **103:**17355–17360.
196. **Richman, D. D.** 2001. Antiretroviral activity of emtricitabine, a potent nucleoside reverse transcriptase inhibitor. *Antivir. Ther.* **6:**83–88.
197. **Riddler, S. A., R. Haubrich, A. G. DiRienzo, L. Peeples, W. G. Powderly, K. L. Klingman, K. W. Garren, T. George, J. F. Rooney, B. Brizz, U. G. Lalloo, R. L. Murphy, S. Swindells, D. Havlir, and J. W. Mellors.** 2008. Class-sparing regimens for initial treatment of HIV-1 infection. *N. Engl. J. Med.* **358:**2095–2106.
198. **Robbins, G. K., V. De Gruttola, R. W. Shafer, L. M. Smeaton, S. W. Snyder, C. Pettinelli, M. P. Dube, M. A. Fischl, R. B. Pollard, R. Delapenha, L. Gedeon, C. van der Horst, R. L. Murphy, M. I. Becker, R. T. D'Aquila, S. Vella, T. C. Merigan, and M. S. Hirsch.** 2003. Comparison of sequential three-drug regimens as initial therapy for HIV-1 infection. *N. Engl. J. Med.* **349:**2293–2303.
199. **Rodriguez-French, A., J. Boghossian, G. E. Gray, J. P. Nadler, A. R. Quinones, G. E. Sepulveda, J. M. Millard, and P. G. Wannamaker.** 2004. The NEAT study: a 48-week open-label study to compare the antiviral efficacy and safety of GW433908 versus nelfinavir in antiretroviral therapy-naive HIV-1-infected patients. *J. Acquir. Immune Defic. Syndr.* **35:**22–32.
200. **Rodriguez Novoa, S., P. Barreiro, A. Rendon, A. Barrios, A. Corral, I. Jimenez-Nacher, J. Gonzalez-Lahoz, and V. Soriano.** 2006. Plasma levels of atazanavir and the risk of hyperbilirubinemia are predicted by the 3435C→T polymorphism at the multidrug resistance gene 1. *Clin. Infect. Dis.* **42:**291–295.
201. **Rotger, M., P. Taffe, G. Bleiber, H. F. Gunthard, H. Furrer, P. Vernazza, H. Drechsler, E. Bernasconi, M. Rickenbach, and A. Telenti.** 2005. Gilbert syndrome and the development of antiretroviral therapy-associated hyperbilirubinemia. *J. Infect. Dis.* **192:**1381–1386.
202. **Ruane, P. J., A. D. Luber, M. B. Wire, Y. Lou, M. J. Shelton, C. T. Lancaster, and K. A. Pappa.** 2007. Plasma amprenavir pharmacokinetics and tolerability following administration of 1,400 milligrams of fosamprenavir once daily in combination with either 100 or 200 milligrams of ritonavir in healthy volunteers. *Antimicrob. Agents Chemother.* **51:**560–565.
203. **Saag, M. S., P. Cahn, F. Raffi, M. Wolff, D. Pearce, J. M. Molina, W. Powderly, A. L. Shaw, E. Mondou, J. Hinkle, K. Borroto-Esoda, J. B. Quinn, D. W. Barry, and F. Rousseau.** 2004. Efficacy and safety of emtricitabine vs stavudine in combination therapy in antiretroviral-naive patients: a randomized trial. *JAMA* **292:**180–189.
204. **Saag, M. S., A. Sonnerborg, R. A. Torres, D. Lancaster, B. G. Gazzard, R. T. Schooley, C. Romero, D. Kelleher, W. Spreen, S. LaFon, and the Abacavir Phase 2 Clinical Team.** 1998. Antiretroviral effect and safety of abacavir alone and in combination with zidovudine in HIV-infected adults. *AIDS* **12:**F203–F209.
205. **Sabin, C., S. Worm, R. Weber, W. El-Sadr, P. Reiss, R. Thiebaut, S. DeWit, M. Law, A. Phillips, and J. Lundgren.** 2008. Do thymidine analogues, abacavir, didanosine and lamivudine contribute to the risk of myocardial infarction? The D:A:D Study, abstr. 957c. *15th Conf. Retrovir. Opportunistic Infect., Boston,* MA.
206. **Schake, D.** 2004. How flexible is tipranavir in complex with the HIV-1 protease active site? *AIDS* **18:**579–580.

207. **Schinazi, R. F., A. McMillan, D. Cannon, R. Mathis, R. M. Lloyd, A. Peck, J. P. Sommadossi, M. St. Clair, J. Wilson, and P. A. Furman.** 1992. Selective inhibition of human immunodeficiency viruses by racemates and enantiomers of *cis*-5-fluoro-1-[2-(hydroxymethyl)-1,3-oxathiolan-5-yl]cytosine. *Antimicrob. Agents Chemother.* **36:**2423–2431.
208. **Schooley, R. T., P. Ruane, R. A. Myers, G. Beall, H. Lampiris, D. Berger, S. S. Chen, M. D. Miller, E. Isaacson, and A. K. Cheng.** 2002. Tenofovir DF in antiretroviral-experienced patients: results from a 48-week, randomized, double-blind study. *AIDS* **16:**1257–1263.
209. **Schurmann, D., G. Fatkenheuer, J. Reynes, C. Michelet, F. Raffi, J. van Lier, M. Caceres, A. Keung, A. Sansone-Parsons, L. M. Dunkle, and C. Hoffmann.** 2007. Antiviral activity, pharmacokinetics and safety of vicriviroc, an oral CCR5 antagonist, during 14-day monotherapy in HIV-infected adults. *AIDS* **21:**1293–1299.
210. **Servais, J., J. M. Plesséria, C. Lambert, E. Fontaine, I. Robert, V. Arendt, T. Staub, F. Schneide, R. Hemme, and J. C. Schmit.** 2001. Genotypic correlates of resistance to HIV-1 protease inhibitors on longitudinal data: the role of secondary mutations. *Antivir. Ther.* **6:**239–248.
211. **Shafer, R. W., and J. M. Schapiro.** 2005. Drug resistance and antiretroviral drug development. *J. Antimicrob. Chemother.* **55:**817–820.
212. **Shapiro, R. L., I. Thior, P. B. Gilbert, S. Lockman, C. Wester, L. M. Smeaton, L. Stevens, S. J. Heymann, T. Ndung'u, S. Gaseitsiwe, V. Novitsky, J. Makhema, S. Lagakos, and M. Essex.** 2006. Maternal single-dose nevirapine versus placebo as part of an antiretroviral strategy to prevent mother-to-child HIV transmission in Botswana. *AIDS* **20:**1281–1288.
213. **Shulman, N. S., R. J. Bosch, J. W. Mellors, M. A. Albrecht, and D. A. Katzenstein.** 2004. Genetic correlates of efavirenz hypersusceptibility. *AIDS* **18:**1781–1785.
214. **Smerdon, S. J., J. Jager, J. Wang, L. A. Kohlstaedt, A. J. Chirino, J. M. Friedman, P. A. Rice, and T. A. Steitz.** 1994. Structure of the binding site for nonnucleoside inhibitors of the reverse transcriptase of human immunodeficiency virus type 1. *Proc. Natl. Acad. Sci. USA* **91:**3911–3915.
215. **Smith, K. Y., W. G. Weinberg, E. Dejesus, M. A. Fischl, Q. Liao, L. L. Ross, G. E. Pakes, K. A. Pappa, and C. T. Lancaster.** 2008. Fosamprenavir or atazanavir once daily boosted with ritonavir 100 mg, plus tenofovir/emtricitabine, for the initial treatment of HIV infection: 48-week results of ALERT. *AIDS Res. Ther.* **5:**5.
216. **Smith, K. Y., D. Fine, P. Patel, N. Bellos, L. Sloan, P. Lackey, D. Sutherland-Phillips, C. Vavro, Q. Liao, and M. Shaefe.** 2008. Efficacy and safety of abacavir/lamivudine combined to tenofovir/emtricitabine in combination with once-daily lopinavir/ritonavir through 48 weeks in the HEAT study, abstr. 774. *15th Conf. Retrovir. Opportunistic Infect., Boston, MA.*
217. **Sommadossi, J. P.** 1995. Comparison of metabolism and in vitro antiviral activity of stavudine versus other 2′,3′-dideoxynucleoside analogues. *J. Infect. Dis.* **171**(Suppl. 2):S88–S92.
218. **Spence, R. A., W. M. Kati, K. S. Anderson, and K. A. Johnson.** 1995. Mechanism of inhibition of HIV-1 reverse transcriptase by nonnucleoside inhibitors. *Science* **267:**988–993.
219. **Squires, K., A. Lazzarin, J. M. Gatell, W. G. Powderly, V. Pokrovskiy, J. F. Delfraissy, J. Jemsek, A. Rivero, W. Rozenbaum, S. Schrader, M. Sension, A. Vibhagool, A. Thiry, and M. Giordano.** 2004. Comparison of once-daily atazanavir with efavirenz, each in combination with fixed-dose zidovudine and lamivudine, as initial therapy for patients infected with HIV. *J. Acquir. Immune Defic. Syndr.* **36:**1011–1019.
220. **Squires, K. E., R. Gulick, P. Tebas, J. Santana, V. Mulanovich, R. Clark, B. Yangco, S. I. Marlowe, D. Wright, C. Cohen, T. Cooley, J. Mauney, K. Uffelman, N. Schoellkopf, R. Grosso, and M. Stevens.** 2000. A comparison of stavudine plus lamivudine versus zidovudine plus lamivudine in combination with indinavir in antiretroviral naive individuals with HIV infection: selection of thymidine analog regimen therapy (START I). *AIDS* **14:**1591–1600.
221. **Staszewski, S., J. Morales-Ramirez, K. T. Tashima, A. Rachlis, D. Skiest, J. Stanford, R. Stryker, P. Johnson, D. F. Labriola, D. Farina, D. J. Manion, and N. M. Ruiz for The Study 006 Team.** 1999. Efavirenz plus zidovudine and lamivudine, efavirenz plus indinavir, and indinavir plus zidovudine and lamivudine in the treatment of HIV-1 infection in adults. *N. Engl. J. Med.* **341:** 1865–1873.
222. **Steigbigel, R., P. Kumar, J. Eron, M. Schechter, M. Markowitz, M. Loutfy, J. Zhao, R. Isaacs, B. Y. Nguyen, and H. Teppler.** 2008. 48-Week results from BENCHMRK-2, a phase III study of raltegravir in patients failing ART with triple-class resistant HIV, abstr. 789. *15th Conf. Retrovir. Opportunistic Infect., Boston, MA.*
223. **Strizki, J. M., C. Tremblay, S. Xu, L. Wojcik, N. Wagner, W. Gonsiorek, R. W. Hipkin, C.-C. Chou, C. Pugliese-Sivo, Y. Xiao, J. R. Tagat, K. Cox, T. Priestley, S. Sorota, W. Huang, M. Hirsch, G. R. Reyes, and B. M. Baroudy.** 2005. Discovery and characterization of vicriviroc (SCH 417690), a CCR5 antagonist with potent activity against human immunodeficiency virus type 1. *Antimicrob. Agents Chemother.* **49:**4911–4919.
224. **Su, C., T. Melby, R. DeMasi, P. Ravindran, and G. Heilek-Snyder.** 2006. Genotypic changes in human immunodeficiency virus type 1 envelope glycoproteins on treatment with the fusion inhibitor enfuvirtide and their influence on changes in drug susceptibility in vitro. *J. Clin. Virol.* **36:**249–257.
225. **Sulkowski, M., J. Rockstroh, V. Soriano, J. O. Stern, and J. Miki.** 2006. Clinical course of increased LFTs and hepatic events associated with ritonavir (RTV) boosted tipranavir (TPV/r) based therapy in the RESIST studies, abstr. H-1899. *46th Intersci. Conf. Antimicrob. Agents Chemother.* American Society for Microbiology, Washington, DC.
226. **Taburet, A. M., C. Piketty, C. Chazallon, I. Vincent, L. Gerard, V. Calvez, F. Clavel, J. P. Aboulker, and P. M. Girard.** 2004. Interactions between atazanavir-ritonavir and tenofovir in heavily pretreated human immunodeficiency virus-infected patients. *Antimicrob. Agents Chemother.* **48:**2091–2096.
227. **Taylor, S., D. J. Back, J. Workman, S. M. Drake, D. J. White, B. Choudhury, P. A. Cane, G. M. Beards, K. Halifax, and D. Pillay.** 1999. Poor penetration of the male genital tract by HIV-1 protease inhibitors. *AIDS* **13:**859–860.
228. **Temesgen, Z., and J. Feinberg.** 2007. Tipranavir: a new option for the treatment of drug-resistant HIV infection. *Clin. Infect. Dis.* **45:**761–769.
229. **Trottier, B., S. Walmsley, J. Reynes, P. Piliero, M. O'Hearn, M. Nelson, J. Montaner, A. Lazzarin, J. Lalezari, C. Katlama, K. Henry, D. Cooper, B. Clotet, K. Arasteh, J. F. Delfraissy, H. J. Stellbrink, J. Lange, D. Kuritzkes, J. J. Eron, Jr., C. Cohen, T. Kinchelow, A.

Bertasso, E. Labriola-Tompkins, A. Shikhman, B. Atkins, L. Bourdeau, C. Natale, F. Hughes, J. Chung, D. Guimaraes, C. Drobnes, S. Bader-Weder, R. Demasi, L. Smiley, and M. P. Salgo. 2005. Safety of enfuvirtide in combination with an optimized background of antiretrovirals in treatment-experienced HIV-1-infected adults over 48 weeks. *J. Acquir. Immune Defic. Syndr.* **40:**413–421.

230. **Tsibris, M. N., M Sagar, Z. Su, C. Flexner, W. Greaves, P. Skolnik, E. Coakley, M. Subramanian, R. Gulick, and D. Kuritzkes.** 2008. Emergence in vivo of vicriviroc resistance in HIV-1 subtype C: role of V3 loop and susceptibility to other CCR5 antagonists, abstr. 870. *15th Conf. Retrovir. Opportunistic Infect., Boston, MA.*

231. **Tsiodras, S., C. Mantzoros, S. Hammer, and M. Samore.** 2000. Effects of protease inhibitors on hyperglycemia, hyperlipidemia, and lipodystrophy: a 5-year cohort study. *Arch. Intern. Med.* **160:**2050–2056.

232. **van Gelder, J., S. Deferme, L. Naesens, E. De Clercq, G. van den Mooter, R. Kinget, and P. Augustijns.** 2002. Intestinal absorption enhancement of the ester prodrug tenofovir disoproxil fumarate through modulation of the biochemical barrier by defined ester mixtures. *Drug Metab. Dispos.* **30:**924–930.

233. **van Leth, F., P. Phanuphak, K. Ruxrungtham, E. Baraldi, S. Miller, B. Gazzard, P. Cahn, U. G. Lalloo, I. P. van der Westhuizen, D. R. Malan, M. A. Johnson, B. R. Santos, F. Mulcahy, R. Wood, G. C. Levi, G. Reboredo, K. Squires, I. Cassetti, D. Petit, F. Raffi, C. Katlama, R. L. Murphy, A. Horban, J. P. Dam, E. Hassink, R. van Leeuwen, P. Robinson, F. W. Wit, and J. M. A. Lange for the 2NN Study Team.** 2004. Comparison of first-line antiretroviral therapy with regimens including nevirapine, efavirenz, or both drugs, plus stavudine and lamivudine: a randomised open-label trial, the 2NN Study. *Lancet* **363:**1253–1263.

234. **Vibhagool, A., P. Cahn, M. Schechter, F. Smaill, L. Soto-Ramirez, G. Carosi, M. Montroni, C. E. Pharo, J. C. Jordan, N. E. Thomas, and G. Pearce.** 2004. Triple nucleoside treatment with abacavir plus the lamivudine/zidovudine combination tablet (COM) compared to indinavir/COM in antiretroviral therapy-naive adults: results of a 48-week open-label, equivalence trial (CNA3014). *Curr. Med. Res. Opin.* **20:**1103–1114.

235. **Vingerhoets, J., H. Azijn, E. Fransen, I. De Baere, L. Smeulders, D. Jochmans, K. Andries, R. Pauwels, and M. P. de Bethune.** 2005. TMC125 displays a high genetic barrier to the development of resistance: evidence from in vitro selection experiments. *J. Virol.* **79:**12773–12782.

236. **von Wyl, V., S. Yerly, J. Boni, P. Burgisser, T. Klimkait, M. Battegay, H. Furrer, A. Telenti, B. Hirschel, P. L. Vernazza, E. Bernasconi, M. Rickenbach, L. Perrin, B. Ledergerber, and H. F. Gunthard.** 2007. Emergence of HIV-1 drug resistance in previously untreated patients initiating combination antiretroviral treatment: a comparison of different regimen types. *Arch. Intern. Med.* **167:**1782–1790.

237. **Vora, S., A. G. Marcelin, H. F. Gunthard, P. Flandre, H. H. Hirsch, B. Masquelier, A. Zinkernagel, G. Peytavin, V. Calvez, L. Perrin, and S. Yerly.** 2006. Clinical validation of atazanavir/ritonavir genotypic resistance score in protease inhibitor-experienced patients. *AIDS* **20:**35–40.

238. **Walmsley, S., B. Bernstein, M. King, J. Arribas, G. Beall, P. Ruane, M. Johnson, D. Johnson, R. Lalonde, A. Japour, S. Brun, and E. Sun.** 2002. Lopinavir-ritonavir versus nelfinavir for the initial treatment of HIV infection. *N. Engl. J. Med.* **346:**2039–2046.

239. **Wang, Y., E. Livingston, S. Patil, R. E. McKinney, A. D. Bardeguez, J. Gandia, M. J. O'Sullivan, P. Clax, S. Huang, and J. D. Unadkat.** 1999. Pharmacokinetics of didanosine in antepartum and postpartum human immunodeficiency virus-infected pregnant women and their neonates: an AIDS clinical trials group study. *J. Infect. Dis.* **180:**1536–1541.

240. **Weinheimer, S., L. Discotto, J. Friborg, H. Yang, and R. Colonno.** 2005. Atazanavir signature I50L resistance substitution accounts for unique phenotype of increased susceptibility to other protease inhibitors in a variety of human immunodeficiency virus type 1 genetic backbones. *Antimicrob. Agents Chemother.* **49:**3816–3824.

241. **Westby, M., M. Lewis, J. Whitcomb, M. Youle, A. L. Pozniak, I. T. James, T. M. Jenkins, M. Perros, and E. van der Ryst.** 2006. Emergence of CXCR4-using human immunodeficiency virus type 1 (HIV-1) variants in a minority of HIV-1-infected patients following treatment with the CCR5 antagonist maraviroc is from a pretreatment CXCR4-using virus reservoir. *J. Virol.* **80:**4909–4920.

242. **Westby, M., C. Smith-Burchnell, J. Mori, M. Lewis, M. Mosley, M. Stockdale, P. Dorr, G. Ciaramella, and M. Perros.** 2007. Reduced maximal inhibition in phenotypic susceptibility assays indicates that viral strains resistant to the CCR5 antagonist maraviroc utilize inhibitor-bound receptor for entry. *J. Virol.* **81:**2359–2371.

243. **Westby, M., and E. van der Ryst.** 2005. CCR5 antagonists: host-targeted antivirals for the treatment of HIV infection. *Antivir. Chem. Chemother.* **16:**339–354.

244. **Wilkin, T. J., Z. Su, D. R. Kuritzkes, M. Hughes, C. Flexner, R. Gross, E. Coakley, W. Greaves, C. Godfrey, P. R. Skolnik, J. Timpone, B. Rodriguez, and R. M. Gulick.** 2007. HIV type 1 chemokine coreceptor use among antiretroviral-experienced patients screened for a clinical trial of a CCR5 inhibitor: AIDS Clinical Trial Group A5211. *Clin. Infect. Dis.* **44:**591–595.

245. **Wolinsky, S. M., R. S. Veazey, K. J. Kunstman, P. J. Klasse, J. Dufour, A. J. Marozsan, M. S. Springer, and J. P. Moore.** 2004. Effect of a CCR5 inhibitor on viral loads in macaques dual-infected with R5 and X4 primate immunodeficiency viruses. *Virology* **328:**19–29.

246. **Xu, L., A. Pozniak, A. Wildfire, S. A. Stanfield-Oakley, S. M. Mosier, D. Ratcliffe, J. Workman, A. Joall, R. Myers, E. Smit, P. A. Cane, M. L. Greenberg, and D. Pillay.** 2005. Emergence and evolution of enfuvirtide resistance following long-term therapy involves heptad repeat 2 mutations within gp41. *Antimicrob. Agents Chemother.* **49:**1113–1119.

247. **Zhang, D., T. J. Chando, D. W. Everett, C. J. Patten, S. S. Dehal, and W. G. Humphreys.** 2005. In vitro inhibition of UDP glucuronosyltransferases by atazanavir and other HIV protease inhibitors and the relationship of this property to in vivo bilirubin glucuronidation. *Drug Metab. Dispos.* **33:**1729–1739.

248. **Zimmermann, A. E., T. Pizzoferrato, J. Bedford, A. Morris, R. Hoffman, and G. Braden.** 2006. Tenofovir-associated acute and chronic kidney disease: a case of multiple drug interactions. *Clin. Infect. Dis.* **42:**283–290.

249. **Zingman, B., J. Suleiman, E. DeJesus, J. Slim, M. McCarthy, M. Lee, N. Case, C. Mak, and L. Dunkle.** 2008. Vicriviroc, a next generation CCR5 antagonist, exhibits potent, sustained suppression of viral replication in treatment-experienced adults: VICTOR-E1 48-week results, abstr. 39LB. *15th Conf. Retrovir. Opportunistic Infect., Boston, MA.*

Antiherpesvirus, Anti-Hepatitis Virus, and Anti-Respiratory Virus Agents

MICHAEL T. YIN, JAMES C. M. BRUST, HONG VAN TIEU, AND SCOTT M. HAMMER

12

This chapter reviews agents which have been, or are being, developed to treat herpesvirus, hepatitis virus, and respiratory virus infections. Detailed information is provided for approved agents and those in more advanced stages of clinical development. Agents in phase I human studies or promising approaches which are still in preclinical development are described briefly. The reader is referred to the respective disease-specific chapters for full discussions of the viral agents and the diseases they cause. Agents like imiquimod and interferon (IFN) for papillomavirus infections are discussed in chapter 28 on papillomavirus.

ANTIHERPESVIRUS AGENTS

See chapter 19 on herpes simplex virus (HSV), chapter 21 on varicella-zoster virus (VZV), and chapter 22 on cytomegalovirus (CMV) for additional information.

Acyclovir

Acyclovir {9-[(2-hydroxyethoxy)methyl]guanine; Zovirax} (Fig. 1; Tables 1 and 2) represents a landmark in the history of antiviral agent development. The anti-HSV activity of acyclovir demonstrated that analogs of guanosine were active and that acyclic side chains could substitute for the ribose moiety, conferring specificity by the selective uptake and activation of acyclovir in HSV-infected cells.

Spectrum of Activity

Acyclovir's greatest and clinically most important activity is against HSV type 1 (HSV-1), HSV-2, and VZV. The inhibitory concentrations for susceptible isolates of HSV-1 average 0.04 μg/ml. HSV-2 is approximately twofold less susceptible and VZV is approximately eightfold less susceptible than HSV-1. Acyclovir also has activity against Epstein-Barr virus (EBV), but CMV susceptibilities are quite variable and a substantial proportion of isolates are resistant (197). Human herpesvirus 6 (HHV-6) is only modestly susceptible to acyclovir.

Mechanism of Action

Acyclovir is a poor substrate for cellular enzymes. Intracellular phosphorylation of acyclovir monophosphate is facilitated by HSV thymidine kinase. The di- and triphosphorylation of acyclovir occurs by cellular kinases to generate the active form of the drug, acyclovir triphosphate. Selectivity for HSV is conferred because cellular kinases are far more active in virus-infected cells (67). Acyclovir triphosphate is both a competitive inhibitor of the viral DNA polymerase and a chain terminator. Because it lacks the 3′-hydroxy group necessary to form 3′-5′ phosphodiester bonds, incorporation of acyclovir triphosphate into the growing viral DNA chain leads to chain termination. Cellular DNA polymerases are much less susceptible to inhibition by acyclovir triphosphate (10- to 30-fold), which is another component of the selectivity of this agent.

Adverse Effects

Given the widespread use of acyclovir in both healthy and immunocompromised hosts for more than 25 years, acyclovir has been remarkably well tolerated. Following intravenous administration, local reactions at the injection site have been reported, and headache and nausea may occur. Neurotoxicity, albeit relatively rare, may manifest as tremors, myoclonus, confusion, lethargy, agitation, and hallucination, as well as dysarthria, ataxia, hemiparesthesias, and seizures. Symptoms of neurotoxicity usually appear within the first 24 to 72 h of administration and are more likely to occur when levels in plasma are elevated, as with intravenous administration or in the setting of renal insufficiency. Acyclovir is relatively insoluble in urine, with a maximum solubility of 2.5 mg/ml at physiological pH. As a result of the low urine solubility, acyclovir crystallization may occur in kidney tubules, especially in the setting of elevated plasma acyclovir levels and dehydration. Prevention of acyclovir crystal deposition can be accomplished by volume repletion prior to drug administration and avoidance of rapid infusions. Acute tubular toxicity leading to renal failure has also been reported with acyclovir, especially for patients with underlying renal disease or receiving concomitant nephrotoxic drugs. Topical acyclovir is usually well tolerated, but there have been reports of local burning, stinging, and erythema.

In vitro, acyclovir is neither immunosuppressive nor toxic to bone marrow precursor cells. Although mutagenic in some preclincial assays, acyclovir lacks carcinogenicity and teratogenicity in animal studies. In healthy subjects receiving chronic prophylaxis for genital HSV infection for over a decade, no chronic toxicities, including abnormal-

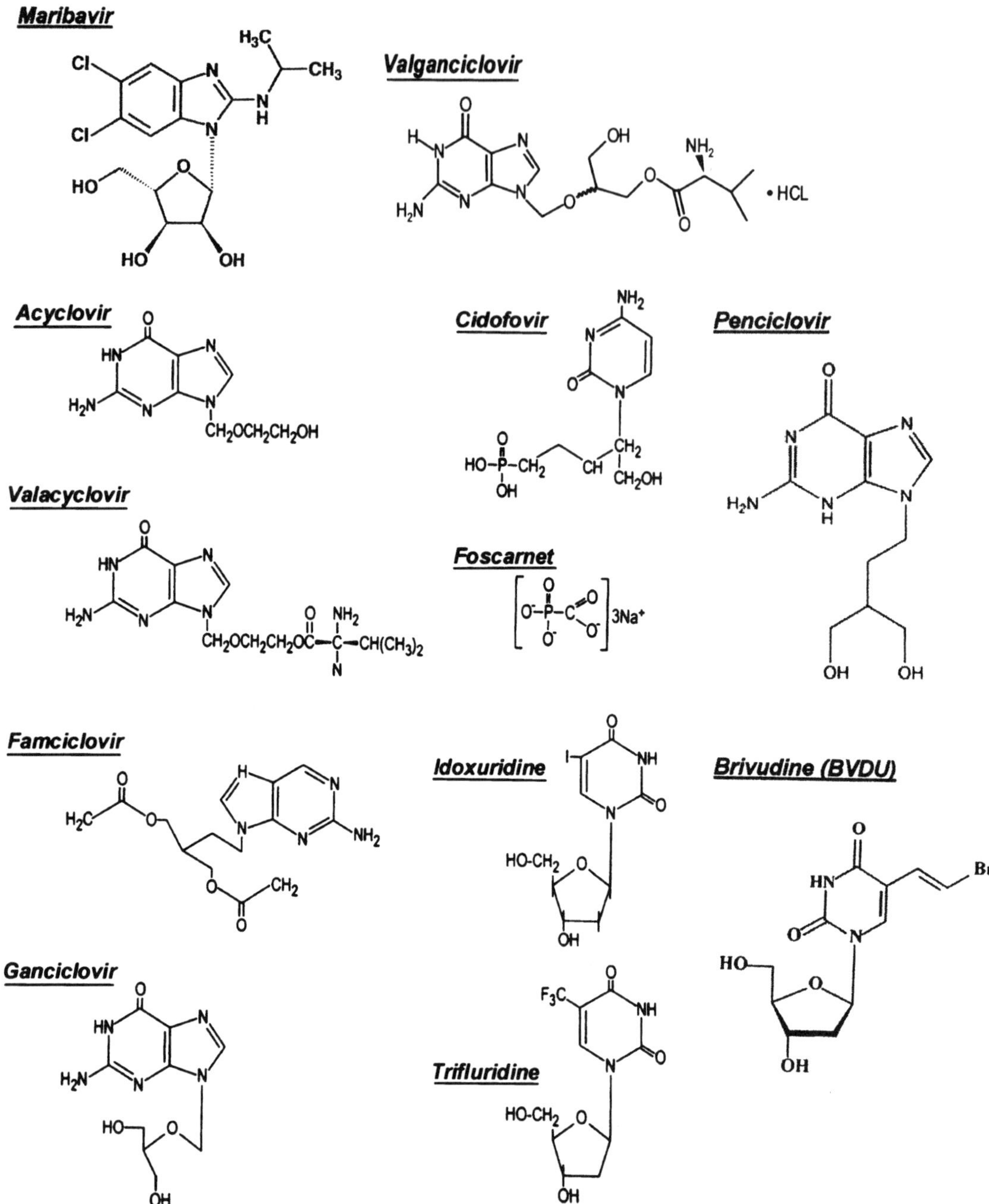

FIGURE 1 Chemical structures of antiherpesvirus agents.

ities of spermatogenesis, have been reported. HSV-specific immune responses can be diminished by acyclovir treatment of primary infection, which may be related to diminution of antigen expression (9).

Pharmacokinetics

Oral, intravenous, and topical preparations of acyclovir are available. Ophthalmic formulations are available outside the United States. The maximum concentrations (C_{max}s) in plasma average approximately 10 μg/ml after an intravenous infusion of 5 mg/kg of body weight and 0.6 μg/ml following a 200-mg oral dose; the levels in plasma proportionately increase with increasing doses. Oral bioavailability is 15 to 30% and may be lower, on average, in immunocompromised hosts. Minimal, if any, drug is absorbed after topical administration. The elimination half-life ($t_{1/2}$) in plasma averages 3 h in subjects with normal renal function. The primary mode of excretion is renal and occurs through both glomerular filtration and tubular secretion. Approximately 85% of administered drug is excreted unchanged in the urine; the remainder is metabolized to 9-carboxymethoxymethylguanine before excretion. Dose adjustments for renal insufficiency are necessary.

TABLE 1 Antiviral agents: approved and potential indications and dosing regimens

Agent	Formulation	Indication	Standard adult dosing[a]
Antiherpesvirus agents			
Acyclovir	Oral Intravenous Topical	Immunocompetent host	
		Genital HSV infection	
		Primary	400 mg p.o. t.i.d. for 7–10 days *or* 200 mg p.o. 5×/day for 7–10 days or apply topically 6×/day for 7 days. For more severe cases (e.g., accompanied by aseptic meningitis, etc.), 5–10 mg/kg i.v. q8h initially, followed by p.o. to complete at least 10 days of total therapy
		Recurrent	400 mg p.o. t.i.d. for 5 days *or* 800 mg p.o. b.i.d. for 5 days *or* 800 mg p.o. t.i.d. for 2 days *or* 200 mg p.o. q4h, 5×/day for 5 days, initiated at earliest sign or symptom of recurrence
		Suppression	400 mg p.o. b.i.d.
		Herpes labialis	Apply 5×/day for 4 days 400 mg p.o. 5×/day for 5 days
		Herpes simplex encephalitis or other invasive syndromes	10 mg/kg i.v. q8h for 10 days
		Varicella, chickenpox	800 mg p.o. 5×/day for 5 days *or* 10 mg/kg i.v. q8h for 7 days if invasive (e.g., encephalomyelitis)
		Herpes zoster, shingles	800 mg p.o. 5×/day for 7–10 days
		Immunosuppressed host	
		Mucocutaneous HSV	400 mg p.o. 5×/day for 7–10 days *or* 5 mg/kg i.v. q8h in more severe cases for 7 days
		Herpes labialis	Apply 6×/day for 7 days
		Suppression	400–800 mg p.o. b.i.d. or t.i.d.
		HSV encephalitis	10 mg/kg i.v. q8h for 10 days
		Herpes zoster, shingles	10 mg/kg i.v. q8h for 7 days
		Varicella, chickenpox	800 mg p.o. 5×/day for 7 days *or* 10 mg/kg i.v. q8h for 7–10 days if invasive (e.g., encephalomyelitis)
Valacyclovir	Oral	Immunocompetent host	
		Genital HSV infection	
		Primary	1 g p.o. b.i.d. for 7–10 days
		Recurrent	500 mg p.o. b.i.d. for 3 days *or* 1 g p.o. daily for 5 days
		Suppression	1 g p.o. daily or 500 mg p.o. daily
		Herpes labialis	2 g p.o. b.i.d. for 1 day
		Herpes zoster, shingles	1 g p.o. t.i.d. for 7 days
		HIV-infected host	
		Genital HSV	
		Recurrent	1 g p.o. b.i.d. for 5–10 days
		Suppression	500 mg p.o. b.i.d.
Famciclovir	Oral	Immunocompetent host	
		Genital HSV infection	
		Primary	250 mg p.o. t.i.d. for 7–10 days
		Recurrent	1 g p.o. b.i.d. for 1 day
		Suppression	250 mg p.o. b.i.d.
		Herpes labialis	1,500 mg p.o. in one dose, initiated at earliest sign
		Herpes zoster, shingles	500 mg p.o. t.i.d. for 7 days
		HIV-infected host	
		Genital HSV	
		Recurrent	500 mg p.o. b.i.d. for 5–10 days
		Suppression	500 mg p.o. b.i.d.
Penciclovir	Topical	Herpes labialis	Apply q2h for 4 days
Brivudine	Oral	Herpes zoster, shingles	125 mg p.o. daily for 7 days in immunocompetent host
	Ophthalmic	Herpes simplex keratitis	Apply to conjunctiva 5×/day
Trifluridine	Ophthalmic	Herpes simplex keratitis	1 drop of 1% solution q2h (maximum, 9 drops/day) for 10 days
Idoxuridine	Ophthalmic	Herpes simplex keratitis	1 drop q4h

(Continued on next page)

TABLE 1 Antiviral agents: approved and potential indications and dosing regimens *(Continued)*

Agent	Formulation	Indication	Standard adult dosing[a]
Ganciclovir	Oral Intravenous Intraocular implant	HIV-infected host	
		CMV retinitis	5 mg/kg i.v. q12h for 14–21 days for induction treatment, followed by maintenance therapy (5 mg/kg i.v. daily for 7 days/wk *or* 6 mg/kg i.v. daily for 5 days/wk *or* 1 g p.o. t.i.d. or 500 mg 6×/day) *or* ocular implant every 6–9 mo with or without ganciclovir at 1–1.5 g p.o. t.i.d.
		CMV, gastrointestinal	5 mg/kg i.v. q12h for 21–28 days (need for maintenance not proven, but advisable)
		Other immunosuppressed host	
		CMV infection	5 mg/kg i.v. q12h for 14–21 days (maintenance therapy not generally necessary)
		Prophylaxis or preemptive therapy of CMV in transplant recipients	5 mg/kg i.v. q12h for 7–14 days and then 5 mg/kg i.v. daily 7 days/wk *or* 6 mg/kg i.v. daily 5 days/wk during "risk" period for transplant patients *or* 1 g p.o. t.i.d. in solid-organ transplant patients
		CMV pneumonia in bone marrow transplant recipients	5 mg/kg i.v. q12h for 10–14 days combined with i.v. immune (or CMV hyperimmune) globulin
Valganciclovir	Oral	HIV-infected host	
		CMV retinitis	900 mg p.o. b.i.d. for 21 days for induction therapy, followed by 900 mg p.o. daily for maintenance
		CMV prophylaxis in high-risk kidney, heart, and kidney-pancreas transplant patients	900 mg p.o. daily
Foscarnet	Intravenous	HIV-infected host	
		CMV retinitis	60 mg/kg i.v. q8h *or* 90 mg/kg i.v. q12h for 14–21 days for induction treatment, followed by maintenance therapy (90–120 mg/kg i.v. daily)
		CMV, gastrointestinal or CNS disease	60 mg/kg i.v. q8h *or* 90 mg/kg i.v. q12h for 14–21 days (need for maintenance therapy not proven, but advisable)
		Other immunosuppressed host	
		CMV disease	60 mg/kg i.v. q8h *or* 90 mg/kg i.v. q12h for 14–21 days
		HIV- or non-HIV-infected immunosuppressed host	
		Acyclovir-resistant HSV or VZV infection	40 mg/kg i.v. q8h *or* 60 mg/kg i.v. q12h for 14 days
		Invasive HHV-6 disease	60 mg/kg i.v. q8h *or* 90 mg/kg i.v. q12h for 14–21 days
Cidofovir	Intravenous	CMV retinitis	5 mg/kg i.v. every wk for 2 wks and then 5 mg/kg i.v. every other wk (combined with probenecid and hydration for nephroprotection)
Fomivirsen	Intravitreal	CMV retinitis	330 μg intravitreally every other wk for two doses and then once every 4 wks for maintenance
Docosanol	Topical	Recurrent herpes labialis	Apply topically 5×/day
Anti-hepatitis virus agents			
Lamivudine	Oral	Chronic hepatitis B	100 mg p.o. daily
Adefovir	Oral	Chronic hepatitis B	10 mg p.o. daily
Entecavir	Oral	Chronic hepatitis B	0.5 mg p.o. daily for nucleoside-naïve hepatitis B, 1 mg p.o. daily for lamivudine-resistant hepatitis B
Telbivudine	Oral	Chronic hepatitis B	600 mg p.o. daily
Emtricitabine	Oral	Hepatitis B activity; not FDA approved for chronic hepatitis B	200 mg p.o. daily (capsule), 240 mg p.o. daily (solution)
Tenofovir	Oral	Hepatitis B activity; not FDA approved for chronic hepatitis B	300 mg p.o. daily

(Continued on next page)

TABLE 1 *(Continued)*

Agent	Formulation	Indication	Standard adult dosing[a]
Ribavirin	Oral	Chronic hepatitis C	In combination with peg-IFN-α2a Monoinfection, genotypes 1 and 4: <75 kg, 1,000 mg p.o. daily in two divided doses for 48 wks; ≥75 kg, 1,200 mg p.o. daily in two divided doses for 48 wks Monoinfection, genotypes 2 and 3: 800 mg p.o. daily in two divided doses for 24 wks Coinfection with HIV: 800 mg p.o. daily in two divided doses for 48 wks In combination with peg-IFN-α2b 400 mg p.o. b.i.d. for 1 yr; after 24 wks of treatment, if serum HCV RNA is not below the limit of detection of assay, consider discontinuation In combination with IFN-α2b ≤75 kg, 400 mg p.o. q.a.m., 600 mg p.o. q.p.m. >75 kg, 600 mg p.o. b.i.d. If HCV RNA is undetectable at 24 wks, duration of therapy is 48 wks
Anti-respiratory virus agents			
Amantadine	Oral	Influenza A virus	
		Prophylaxis	100 mg p.o. b.i.d. during risk period
		Treatment	100 mg p.o. b.i.d.; discontinue within 3–5 days or within 24–48 h after symptoms disappear
Rimantadine	Oral	Influenza A virus	
		Prophylaxis	100 mg p.o. b.i.d. during risk period
		Treatment	100 mg p.o. b.i.d. for 5 days
Oseltamivir	Oral	Influenza A and B viruses	
		Prophylaxis	75 mg p.o. daily for 10 days (up to 6 wks)
		Treatment	75 mg p.o. b.i.d. for 5 days
Zanamivir	Inhalational	Influenza A and B viruses	
		Prophylaxis (household)	Two oral inhalations (10 mg) daily for 10 days
		Prophylaxis (community)	Two oral inhalations (10 mg) daily for 28 days
		Treatment	Two oral inhalations (10 mg) b.i.d. for 5 days
Ribavirin	Inhalational	RSV	6 g (20 mg/ml) administered via aerosol over 12–18 h/day for 3–7 days

[a] Abbreviations: p.o., per as; i.v., intravenously; 5×, five times; q.a.m., every morning; q.p.m., every evening.

Drug Interactions

Few potentially important drug interactions have been noted. Caution should be exercised when other potentially nephrotoxic or neurotoxic agents are being used concurrently, but whether there is additive toxicity with specific agents is unclear. In vitro, mycophenolate mofetil potentiates the anti-HSV activity of acyclovir through depletion of dGTP pools, but the clinical significance of this observation is unclear.

Resistance

The descriptions of persistent or progressive clinical disease with acyclovir-resistant HSV or VZV isolates in immunocompromised hosts, particularly patients with human immunodeficiency virus (HIV) infection, helped to establish the clear-cut clinical significance of antiviral resistance. HSV resistance may be based on mutations in the viral thymidine kinase or DNA polymerase genes. Thymidine kinase-based resistance may be the result of absent or low-level enzyme production or the elaboration of a thymidine kinase with altered substrate specificity. Thymidine kinase deficiency is more often due to production of a truncated protein than to production of a functional but altered enzyme. Acyclovir-resistant subpopulations exist among clinical isolates of HSV in the absence of drug exposure, but the clinical expression of resistance only occurs in the face of drug treatment. Such isolates may be the result of the selection of a preexistent drug-resistant subpopulation or a new mutational event. DNA polymerase mutants due to mutations in HSV genome regions I, II, III, V, VII, and A have been described to occur rarely in clinical isolates of HSV (45).

Although acyclovir-resistant HSV strains are less pathogenic in animal models, they can cause serious clinical disease in immunocompromised hosts. In such hosts, HSV resistance is usually manifested by chronic mucocutaneous ulceration, but invasive visceral and central nervous system (CNS) disease, which may be fatal, occurs with either HSV-1 or HSV-2 (191). Following resolution of mucocutaneous lesions due to resistant HSV, subsequent recurrences are usually acyclovir susceptible (in the absence of acyclovir exposure), implying that latent ganglionic virus is not altered. Recurrent disease due to thymidine kinase-altered virus in an immunocompetent host has been reported. Thymidine kinase-deficient or -altered HSV or VZV isolates resistant to acyclovir remain susceptible in vitro to foscarnet, cidofovir, and brivudine but are fully cross-resistant to ganciclovir and famciclovir. When re-

TABLE 2 Antiherpesvirus agents: pharmacokinetics, major toxicity, and drug interaction characteristics

Agent	Oral bioavailability (%)	Effect of food on AUC	$t_{1/2}$ (h) in adults	Major route of elimination	Adjustment for renal insufficiency	Major toxicities	Major drug interactions
Acyclovir	15–30	No	3	85% renally excreted unchanged, catabolite also renally excreted	Yes	Headache, nausea, nephrotoxicity, neurotoxicity	Possible additive effects with other nephrotoxic or neurotoxic agents
Valacyclovir	55 (of acyclovir)	No	3	Renal	Yes	Same as acyclovir; possible association with HUS/TTP[b] when used in immunocompromised persons at high dosages	Same as acyclovir; cimetidine and probenecid decrease the rate but not the degree of valacyclovir-to-acyclovir conversion
Famciclovir	77	No	2	Penciclovir catabolite is renally excreted	Yes	Headache, nausea	Probenecid, theophylline: increased plasma famciclovir levels Digoxin levels increased
Brivudine	30	No	16	Metabolized by liver to inactive metabolite	No	Nausea, headaches	Potentiates toxicity of 5-FU or other fluoropyrimidines
Trifluridine	NA[a]	NA	NA	Negligible systemic absorption and metabolism	No	Local eye irritation; mutagenic, carcinogenic, and teratogenic potential	None reported
Idoxuridine	NA	NA	NA	Negligible systemic absorption and metabolism	No	Local eye irritation; mutagenic, carcinogenic, and teratogenic potential. DMSO preparation can be associated with headache, lightheadedness, and nausea.	None reported

Ganciclovir	5	Increases by 8–9%	3–4	Mainly renally excreted unchanged	Yes	Neutropenia, thrombocytopenia	Bone marrow-suppressive agents: increased risk of myelosuppression
Valganciclovir	61	Increases by 14–30%	3–4	Mainly renally excreted unchanged	Yes	Neutropenia, thrombocytopenia	Bone marrow-suppressive agents: increased risk of myelosuppression
Foscarnet	NA	NA	4.5–8.2	Renal	Yes	Nephrotoxicity, electrolyte disturbances, neurotoxicity, anemia, neutropenia	Nephrotoxic agents: increased risk of foscarnet nephrotoxic adverse effects Pentamidine: increased risk of hypocalcemia
Cidofovir	NA	NA	2.6	Renal	Yes	Nephrotoxicity, cardiomyopathy, rash, iritis (with intravitreal administration)	Probenecid: nephroprotective at cidofovir doses of >3 mg/kg
Fomivirsen	NA	NA	78 (retinal $t_{1/2}$)	Exonucleases	No	Increased intraocular pressure, intraocular inflammation, cataracts, retinal toxicity	Potential for additive ocular toxicity with coadministered cidofovir
Docosanol	NA	NA	NA	NA	No	Rash, pruritus, dry skin, burning and stinging at application site	None reported

[a]NA, not applicable.
[b]HUS/TTP, hemolytic-uremic syndrome/thrombotic thrombocytopenic purpura.

sistance is due to a DNA polymerase mutation, cross-resistance to foscarnet may exist, but susceptibility to cidofovir and brivudine is usually maintained (15).

Clinical Applications

Acyclovir has been extensively studied for the prophylaxis and treatment of herpesvirus infections in both immunocompetent and immunocompromised hosts. The intravenous formulation was shown to be superior to vidarabine in treating HSV encephalitis in healthy hosts and VZV infections in immunosuppressed subjects and to be equivalent to vidarabine in treating neonatal HSV infection in early landmark studies. For serious mucocutaneous, visceral, or CNS disease due to HSV or VZV, parenteral acyclovir is the agent of choice, unless acyclovir resistance is suspected. For subjects with normal renal function, a dosage of 5 mg/kg every 8 h (q8h) is appropriate for mucocutaneous disease. A dosage of 10 mg/kg q8h should be used for VZV infections and for invasive HSV disease. For neonatal HSV disease, a dosage as high as 20 mg/kg q8h has been recommended. Acyclovir at 10 mg/kg q8h is indicated for VZV disease because of the generally lower susceptibility of VZV isolates.

Acyclovir does not appear to be beneficial for patients with acute infectious mononucleosis despite the demonstration of a decrease in EBV shedding, or for patients with chronic fatigue syndrome. Oral hairy leukoplakia regresses with acyclovir treatment. Acyclovir has been reported anecdotally to induce regression in some patients with polyclonal B-cell posttransplantation lymphoproliferative disorders (PTLD). Antiviral therapy is often used in conjunction with reduced immunosuppression and other therapies in PTLD despite clear evidence of acyclovir efficacy. Most EBV-infected cells within PTLD lesions are transformed B cells that are not undergoing lytic replication and therefore will not be inhibited by acyclovir or ganciclovir. Prophylactic use of acyclovir or ganciclovir after transplantation may reduce the risk of PTLD, especially during the first posttransplantation year (79).

In healthy hosts, the intravenous and oral forms of acyclovir decrease the period of virus shedding and speed healing in patients with primary genital HSV infection (238). Topical acyclovir ointment demonstrates some efficacy for primary genital HSV infection (47), but it is inferior to systemic therapy. For recurrent genital HSV infection, oral acyclovir for 5 days reduces the duration of pain and virus shedding, but topical acyclovir is clinically ineffective. Short-course acyclovir therapy, consisting of 2 days of 800 mg three times daily (t.i.d.) started within 12 h of symptom onset, decreased time to healing and episode duration by 2 days compared to placebo (228). For recurrent orolabial HSV, a 5% acyclovir cream preparation has been FDA approved (121), and oral acyclovir at 400 mg five times per day has been demonstrated to be effective. Oral acyclovir is also beneficial for the treatment of herpes zoster in adults and varicella in children. The acute pain of herpes zoster is consistently diminished by acyclovir, and a meta-analysis suggested that it reduces postherpetic neuralgia (243). Oral acyclovir alone or in combination with prednisolone does not improve the likelihood of complete recovery from Bell's palsy beyond the benefit of prednisolone alone (212).

Acyclovir is also effective for prophylaxis of HSV infections in immunosuppressed patients undergoing solid-organ or bone marrow transplantation and in patients receiving cancer chemotherapy (202). Although therapeutically ineffective for established CMV infections, acyclovir does have efficacy for the prophylaxis of CMV infection in renal, liver, and bone marrow transplant recipients (148); however, this role has been largely supplanted by valganciclovir.

In healthy hosts, oral acyclovir is very effective for the suppression of recurrent genital herpes, reducing recurrences by approximately 90% (189). Safety, efficacy, and lack of emergence of resistance for periods up to 10 years have been demonstrated (221). Subclinical shedding of HSV-2 from the genital tract in women can also be successfully suppressed by twice-daily (b.i.d.) oral acyclovir (229). Prevention of herpetic whitlow and recurrent erythema multiforme associated with recurrent HSV infection is also possible. Short-term prophylaxis of recurrent oral HSV infection can be effective when initiated prior to a known stimulus for reactivation, such as occurs with exposure to UV light (e.g., such as that experienced by skiers).

Valacyclovir

Valacyclovir (2-[2-amino-1,6-dihydro-6-oxo-9*H*-purin-9-yl-methoxy]ethyl-L-valinate hydrochloride; Valtrex) (Fig. 1; Tables 1 and 2) is the L-valyl ester of acyclovir. It was designed to enhance the oral bioavailability of the parent compound and is one of a series of such compounds that has been investigated. Valacyclovir is converted to acyclovir prior to anabolic phosphorylation, thus avoiding unwanted toxicity. The antiviral spectrum of activity of valacyclovir is identical to that of acyclovir.

Mechanism of Action and Pharmacokinetics

The L-valyl esterification of acyclovir increases the bioavailability of acyclovir and does not alter the mechanism of action of the drug. Absorption of valacyclovir in the gastrointestinal tract is facilitated by a stereospecific transporter system; first-pass intestinal and hepatic hydrolysis by valacyclovir hydrolase yields complete conversion of valacyclovir to acyclovir, resulting in a three- to fivefold increase in acyclovir bioavailability. Once the drug is converted to acyclovir, the elimination $t_{1/2}$, excretion, and metabolism are the same as those noted for acyclovir. In healthy volunteers given doses of 500 and 1,000 mg of valacyclovir, C_{max}s are reached in 1.5 to 1.75 h and average 3.3 and 5.7 μg/ml, respectively. Pharmacokinetic parameters in patients with advanced HIV infection are similar to those in healthy volunteers.

Drug Interactions and Adverse Effects

The drug interaction and side effect profiles are similar to those of acyclovir. In patients with advanced HIV infection, gastrointestinal complaints and neutropenia were seen in 31 and 19% of subjects, respectively (111). Cases resembling thrombotic microangiopathy have been reported for subjects with advanced HIV infection and for recipients of allogeneic bone marrow transplants treated with high dosages of valacyclovir (8,000 mg/day) for prolonged periods for CMV prophylaxis (18), but such events have not been reported for immunocompetent or HIV-infected subjects receiving valacyclovir for suppression of genital herpes. Although a causal association with valacyclovir has not been elucidated, the implication is that the occurrence of thrombotic microangiopathy is restricted to severely immunocompromised individuals receiving high dosages of valacyclovir or sometimes other drugs.

Resistance

Acyclovir-resistant HSV or VZV may emerge during valacyclovir therapy, and the mechanisms are similar to those reported for acyclovir.

Clinical Applications

Valacyclovir has demonstrated efficacy in the treatment of herpes zoster and genital HSV infections. Valacyclovir at 1,000 mg b.i.d. was found to be comparable to acyclovir at 200 mg five times daily in terms of efficacy and safety for the treatment of initial genital herpes infection (73). Valacyclovir at 1,000 or 500 mg b.i.d. for 5 days has an efficacy comparable to that of acyclovir at 200 mg five times daily for 5 days in immunocompetent individuals with recurrent genital herpes (223). Short-course therapy with valacyclovir at 500 mg b.i.d. for 3 days was equivalent to the 5-day course of valacyclovir (143). Suppressive therapy for recurrent genital herpes is also successful with valacyclovir, and once-daily dosing with 500 or 1,000 mg appears to be as effective as acyclovir at 400 mg b.i.d. (172). Valacyclovir at 1,000 mg t.i.d. is an effective therapy for herpes zoster and is superior to acyclovir but equivalent to famciclovir (222) in reducing the likelihood of prolonged pain.

Oral valacyclovir at a dosage of 2,000 mg four times daily is effective in the prophylaxis of CMV (and HSV) infections in renal transplant recipients. In HIV-infected persons, valacyclovir appeared to be superior to acyclovir in preventing CMV disease, but the study was terminated early because of a higher mortality rate in the valacyclovir arm, a finding which is unexplained (85). Valganciclovir has largely replaced valacyclovir for prophylaxis of CMV disease.

Famciclovir and Penciclovir

Famciclovir [9-(4-hydroxy-3-hydroxymethylbut-1-yl)guanine; Famvir] (Fig. 1; Tables 1 and 2) is the inactive diacetyl 6-deoxy prodrug ester of penciclovir [9-(4-hydroxy-3-hydroxy-3-hydroxymethylbut-1-yl)guanine], an acyclic nucleoside analog of guanosine.

Spectrum of Activity

Famciclovir is a prodrug lacking intrinsic antiviral activity and must be converted to penciclovir triphosphate, which is its active form. HSV-1, HSV-2, and VZV are susceptible to penciclovir; the average inhibitory concentrations are 0.4, 1.5, and 5.0 μg/ml, respectively, in MRC-5 cells (64). EBV and hepatitis B virus (HBV) are also susceptible in vitro. Famciclovir also shows antiviral activity in animal models of hepadnavirus infection but is not a clinically useful anti-HBV agent.

Mechanism of Action

Penciclovir is selectively monophosphorylated by the HSV or VZV thymidine kinase; formation of penciclovir di- and triphosphate is catalyzed by cellular kinases. Penciclovir triphosphate competitively inhibits the viral DNA polymerase and can also be incorporated into the growing viral DNA chain. Because of the presence of the hydroxyl group on the acyclic side chain, viral DNA chain extension may occur to a limited extent after incorporation (64). This aspect of its mechanism of action contrasts with that of acyclovir triphosphate, which is an obligate chain terminator. Penciclovir triphosphate is a less potent inhibitor of HSV DNA polymerase than acyclovir triphosphate, but this is balanced by much higher intracellular levels of penciclovir triphosphate and by its much longer intracellular $t_{1/2}$. The intracellular $t_{1/2}$s of penciclovir are 10 to 20 h in HSV-infected cells and 9 h in VZV-infected cells (64).

Pharmacokinetics

Famciclovir is rapidly converted to penciclovir by deacetylation and oxidation. Famciclovir undergoes extensive first-pass metabolism, with aldehyde oxidase probably responsible for the oxidation at the 6 position. Following an oral dose of 500 mg of famciclovir, a C_{max} of 3.3 μg/ml is achieved by 1 h (74). Sixty to seventy percent of the drug is excreted as penciclovir in the urine by both glomerular filtration and tubular secretion, and the remainder is excreted in the feces or as 6-deoxy-penciclovir and other minor metabolites in the urine or feces (74). In subjects with hepatic disease, the time to peak plasma drug level and the concentration achieved are decreased relative to those in healthy volunteers, but overall exposure is not reduced.

Adverse Effects

Famciclovir is generally very well tolerated. Headache and nausea are the most common side effects. Famciclovir and penciclovir have yielded positive results in some preclinical carcinogenesis models, including rodent tumor induction and mutagenesis assays, although not in tests of teratogenicity.

Drug Interactions

Probenecid would predictably increase plasma penciclovir concentrations because of the inhibition of renal tubular secretion of the drug, but formal interaction studies have not been performed. Theophylline can increase penciclovir levels moderately, but dose adjustments are not necessary. Allopurinol has no effect on penciclovir pharmacokinetics. Penciclovir, on the other hand, can increase digoxin levels modestly (mean increase, 19%) but does not alter the digoxin area under the concentration-time curve (AUC).

Resistance

The prevalences of penciclovir-resistant HSV isolates among subjects participating in clinical trials involving penciclovir (topical and intravenous) or famciclovir were 0.22 and 2.1% of immunocompetent and immunocompromised subjects, respectively, similar to the prevalence of acyclovir resistance (193). Most HSV and VZV isolates resistant to acyclovir on the basis of thymidine kinase deficiency are cross-resistant to famciclovir and penciclovir. Interestingly, mutations associated with penciclovir resistance in the thymidine kinase gene are distributed throughout the gene, in contrast to those associated with acyclovir, which are preferentially localized to the homopolymeric hot spots (193). Some acyclovir-resistant isolates with altered thymidine kinase substrate specificity may still retain their ability to phosphorylate penciclovir and remain susceptible.

Clinical Applications

Famciclovir is approved in the United States for the treatment of genital herpes, herpes labialis, and herpes zoster. For recurrent genital herpes, famciclovir at 125 mg was similar to acyclovir at 200 mg in 5-day treatment courses (40). Recent studies have led to the approval of short courses of famciclovir for treatment of recurrent genital herpes (1,000 mg b.i.d. for 1 day) and herpes labialis

(1,500-mg single dose) (8, 210). Topical 1% penciclovir cream has moderate efficacy in treatment of orolabial herpes, decreasing the time to healing in comparison to that with placebo by a median of 1 day (27). In the treatment of herpes zoster, famciclovir at 500 mg t.i.d. decreases the time of lesion healing and shortens the duration of postherpetic neuralgia (219). In a controlled trial comparing famciclovir dosages of 250, 500, and 750 mg t.i.d. with acyclovir at 800 mg five times per day in immunocompetent adults, acute measures of healing and pain were equivalent (28). Famciclovir at 500 mg t.i.d. has efficacy and tolerability similar to those of acyclovir at 800 mg five times daily in immunocompetent persons with ophthalmic zoster (220) and similar to those of valacyclovir at 1,000 mg t.i.d. in immunocompetent persons over 50 years of age with herpes zoster (222). The more convenient dosing schedule of famciclovir and the potentially shorter duration of postherpetic neuralgia argue in favor of employing famciclovir or valacyclovir for herpes zoster, particularly in older individuals, in whom the complication of postherpetic neuralgia is more frequent.

Brivudine

Brivudine [(*E*)-5-(2-bromovinyl)-2′-deoxyuridine, Zostex, Zerpex, Brivirac, Helpin] is a selective nucleoside analog (Fig. 1; Tables 1 and 2) utilized for treatment of herpes keratitis and herpes zoster in immunocompetent patients in Europe.

Spectrum of Activity

Brivudine is a potent and selective inhibitor of HSV-1 and VZV replication. EBV is also sensitive to brivudine, but CMV and HSV-2 are relatively resistant to its antiviral action. In vitro, the 50% effective concentration (EC_{50}) of brivudine is 0.0024 μg/ml for VZV, compared to 4.64 g/ml for acyclovir (208).

Mechanism of Action and Pharmacokinetics

Brivudine activation depends upon a specific phosphorylation by the HSV-1 or VZV thymidine kinase that converts brivudine to its 5′-monophosphate and 5′-diphosphate. HSV-2-encoded thymidine kinase is unable to phosphorylate brivudine 5′-monophosphate to 5′-diphosphate (81). After further phosphorylation by cellular kinases, brivudine 5′-triphosphate interacts with viral DNA polymerase either as a competitive inhibitor or as an alternative substrate allowing incorporation into the growing DNA chain. Incorporation may affect both the stability and function of viral DNA during the replication and transcription processes (54).

Brivudine has a low bioavailability (30%) and is highly protein bound (>95%) to plasma protein. The C_{max} at steady state (1.7 μg/ml) is achieved 1 h after administration of once-daily oral brivudine at 125 mg and is 1,700-fold greater than the in vitro 50% inhibitory concentration (IC_{50}) for VZV. Brivudine is rapidly metabolized by thymidine phosphorylase into inactive compounds, BVU [(*E*)-5-(2-bromovinyl)uracil] and 2-deoxyribose-1-phosphate. However, BVU can be reconverted in vitro and in vivo to brivudine through a pentosyl transfer reaction which restores the antiviral potential of the compound (55).

Adverse Effects

Oral brivudine is generally well tolerated, and the incidences of potentially treatment-related adverse events were similar for brivudine (8%) and acyclovir (10%), with nausea as the most commonly reported adverse event (232).

Drug Interactions

The main metabolite of brivudine, BVU, irreversibly inhibits dihydropyrimidine dehydrogenase, the enzyme that regulates the metabolism of natural nucleosides like thymidine and of pyrimidine derivatives, including the fluoropyrimidine 5-fluorouracil (5-FU). Coadministration of brivudine and 5-FU increases the systemic exposure to 5-FU and increases its toxicity. When a congener analog, bromovinyl arabinosyl uracil (BVaraU), was administered to patients in Japan receiving 5-FU, several deaths occurred. In healthy adults who received brivudine at 125 mg once daily for 7 days, dihydropyrimidine dehydrogenase activity was fully restored by 18 days after the final dose of brivudine. Therefore, coadministration of brivudine and fluoropyrimidine derivatives, or administration of these agents within 4 weeks of each other, is contraindicated (119).

Resistance

There are no reports of clinical isolates with brivudine resistance that developed during therapy. A broad variety of HSV-1 clones were selected under a single round of high-dose brivudine, including acyclovir-susceptible and brivudine-resistant phenotypes, and mutations associated with brivudine resistance occurred in the homopolymer stretches of G's and C's of the thymidine kinase gene (2). Serial passage of VZV under the pressure of acyclovir, brivudine, and BVaraU was cross-resistant to all drugs that depend on the viral thymidine kinase for activation (3). In contrast, virus strains selected under pressure of penciclovir were resistant to acyclovir, but not brivudine.

Clinical Applications

Brivudine is available in Europe for topical treatment of herpetic keratitis as 0.1% eyedrops and orally for treatment of VZV and HSV-1. The efficacy of brivudine at 125 mg orally once daily for 1 week for treatment of herpes zoster in immunocompetent subjects >50 years of age is generally comparable to that of acyclovir (232) or famciclovir (231). Incidence of postherpetic neuralgia was less with brivudine than with acyclovir (33%, versus 44%) (232) but similar to that with famciclovir (231). Brivudine appears to be effective for treatment of herpes zoster in immunocompromised patients (218). Topical brivudine has also been utilized to treat herpetic keratitis that is clinically resistant to other antiviral agents.

Trifluridine

Trifluridine (5-trifluoromethyl-2′-deoxyuridine; Viroptic) is a halogenated nucleoside analog (Fig. 1; Tables 1 and 2) that is approved in the United States for the treatment of herpetic keratitis.

Spectrum of Activity

Trifluridine has activity against the DNA viruses HSV-1 and -2, CMV, and vaccinia virus; there is inconsistent activity against adenovirus. Inhibitory concentrations for strains of HSV average 10 μg/ml, and, importantly, acyclovir-resistant strains of HSV remain sensitive to trifluridine.

Mechanism of Action

Trifluridine is anabolically phosphorylated by cellular kinases to the triphosphate form, which is a competitive inhibitor of the HSV DNA polymerase. Trifluridine is available only as a 1% ophthalmic solution in the United States. There is no significant systemic absorption.

Adverse Effects

The most frequent adverse reactions reported during clinical trials were mild, transient burning or stinging upon instillation (5%) and palpebral edema (3%). Other, less common adverse reactions were superficial punctate keratopathy, epithelial keratopathy, hypersensitivity reaction, stromal edema, keratitis sicca, hyperemia, and increased intraocular pressure. The potential for corneal epithelial keratopathy is lower with trifluridine than with topical idoxuridine. Trifluridine has shown carcinogenic, mutagenic, and potentially teratogenic activities in preclinical assays.

Drug Interactions

No adverse drug interactions have been reported with the simultaneous treatment of the eye with topical antibacterial, steroid, or atropine preparations.

Resistance

No reports of clinical isolates of HSV resistant to trifluridine have appeared, although there is one report of laboratory selection of trifluridine resistance (69).

Clinical Applications

The primary and approved indication for topical trifluridine is for primary and recurrent HSV infections of the cornea and conjunctiva. Its efficacy is comparable to those of other topical antiherpetic agents, but trifluridine is generally better tolerated and thus is considered the agent of choice. Topical trifluridine has also demonstrated clinical utility in the treatment of persistent cutaneous ulcers due to acyclovir-resistant HSV infections in patients with AIDS and can be considered when faced with HSV ulcers that are due to acyclovir- and foscarnet-resistant strains. However, systemic or topical treatment with cidofovir is a preferable alternative.

Idoxuridine

Idoxuridine (5-iodo-2′-deoxyuridine; Stoxil) is a pyrimidine nucleoside analog (Fig. 1; Tables 1 and 2) available for topical administration. Idoxuridine is approved only for topical ophthalmic use in the United States, although a topical preparation in dimethyl sulfoxide (DMSO) is available in Europe. Although idoxuridine was originally developed in the 1960s as a parenteral agent, the first placebo-controlled trial in herpesvirus infections showed its toxicity and lack of efficacy and led to the cessation of its development by this route.

Spectrum of Activity

Idoxuridine is active against HSV-1 and -2, other herpesviruses, and poxviruses. Inhibitory concentrations for strains of HSV average ≤10 μg/ml.

Mechanism of Action

Idoxuridine is anabolically phosphorylated by cellular kinases to its active form. Idoxuridine triphosphate is a competitive inhibitor of HSV DNA polymerase and can also be incorporated into the growing DNA chain and act as a chain terminator. There is negligible systemic absorption of idoxuridine after ocular application. Topical idoxuridine in DMSO is absorbed to a modest extent.

Adverse Effects

Topical application in the eye can result in local irritation and inflammatory reactions, including punctate keratopathy. The DMSO preparations can result in local irritation and mild systemic symptoms of headache, lightheadedness, and nausea. Intravenous idoxuridine causes severe bone marrow toxicity as its major side effect. The drug has mutagenic, carcinogenic, and teratogenic potential.

Drug Interactions

No significant drug interactions with other topically applied ophthalmic medications have been reported.

Resistance

HSV strains resistant to idoxuridine can be selected in vitro and have been isolated from treated patients (69). Mutations in viral DNA polymerase mediate this resistance.

Clinical Applications

In the United States, the only role for idoxuridine is in the topical treatment of HSV keratitis. Topical idoxuridine in DMSO, which is still available in a few countries in Europe and Asia, has marginal utility for the treatment of HSV labialis, HSV genitalis, and localized herpes zoster and cannot be recommended.

Ganciclovir

Ganciclovir [9-(1,3-dihydroxy-propoxymethyl)guanine; Cytovene] (Fig. 1; Tables 1 and 2) is an acyclic nucleoside analog of guanosine that is structurally similar to acyclovir, differing only by the presence of a hydroxymethyl group. This difference confers markedly improved activity against CMV but also a different toxicity profile.

Spectrum of Activity

The clinical usefulness of ganciclovir derives from its improved anti-CMV activity; inhibitory concentrations are 0.2 to 3.0 μg/ml for susceptible clinical isolates (72). Ganciclovir also has activity against HSV-1 and -2, VZV, and EBV, with in vitro inhibitory concentrations in the range of 1 to 3, 1 to 2, and 1 to 5 μg/ml, respectively (72). It is inhibitory for HHV-6. Activity against HBV has also been demonstrated but is not clinically useful.

Mechanism of Action

As for other nucleoside analog antiherpesviral agents, ganciclovir requires intracellular phosphorylation to its active form. Monophosphorylation in HSV- and VZV-infected cells is accomplished by the virus-encoded thymidine kinase that phosphorylates acyclovir (72). In CMV-infected cells, ganciclovir is monophosphorylated by the product of the UL97 gene. Ganciclovir monophosphate is converted to the di- and triphosphorylated derivatives by cellular kinases. Ganciclovir triphosphate is a competitive inhibitor of herpesviral DNA polymerases and is incorporated into the growing viral DNA chain, where it slows chain elongation (72). The intracellular $t_{1/2}$ of ganciclovir triphosphate in CMV-infected cells is >18 h; the prolonged intracellular $t_{1/2}$ of ganciclovir triphosphate compared to that of acyclovir triphosphate may be partially responsible for the improved anti-CMV activity of ganciclovir.

Pharmacokinetics

Ganciclovir is available in both intravenous and oral formulations and can be administered by direct intravitreal injection and through an implantable intraocular device. Following an intravenous dose of 5 mg/kg, the C_{max} is 8 μg/ml; dose-independent kinetics have been observed at intravenous doses of $\leq$5 mg/kg (249). Intravitreal levels averaging 1.2 μg/ml have been reported for patients on induction doses of intravenous ganciclovir (130). Despite poor oral absorption, peak levels in plasma of 1 μg/ml can be achieved with an oral dose of 1,000 mg taken with food. However, the availability of oral valganciclovir, which results in plasma ganciclovir levels comparable to that seen with parenteral administration, has supplanted the use of oral ganciclovir (see below). CNS penetration occurs, with ratios of drug concentrations in cerebrospinal fluid (CSF) to those in plasma ranging from 0.24 to 0.70.

Adverse Effects

Hematologic toxicity is the most important adverse reaction noted following intravenous ganciclovir administration (153). Absolute neutrophil counts below 1,000/mm^3 have been noted in approximately 40% of patients with HIV infection and in 7 and 40% of heart and bone marrow transplant recipients, respectively. Thrombocytopenia (platelet counts of <50,000/mm^3) occurs with a reported frequency of 13% in HIV-infected subjects and 8 to 57% in transplant recipients. The incidence of neutropenia after oral administration of ganciclovir is lower (14 to 24%) in patients with HIV infection, presumably due to the lower overall drug exposure. Granulocyte and granulocyte-macrophage colony-stimulating factors are effective in reversing the neutropenia associated with ganciclovir and permit its continued use at efficacious doses (92).

Other adverse effects noted in patients receiving ganciclovir include headache, neurotoxic reactions, fever, rash, gastrointestinal complaints (including diarrhea) in subjects taking the oral capsule formulation, anemia, and abnormal liver enzymes (153).

Retinal detachment may occur during the course of treatment of CMV retinitis (113). Detachment, which is probably not due to a direct toxic effect of the drug, results from scarring and retraction as the infection is controlled or as the disease progresses. Detachments are also seen in untreated patients, especially newborns with congenital CMV infection. In patients treated locally with ganciclovir via an implanted device, local inflammatory reactions, scleral thinning, and retinal detachments have been described to occur. Ganciclovir is mutagenic, carcinogenic, and teratogenic in preclinical assays and inhibits the growth of bone marrow progenitor cells in vitro.

Drug Interactions

In HIV-infected subjects, the use of zidovudine in combination with induction doses of ganciclovir results in a high incidence of neutropenia that often precludes their simultaneous use, unless granulocyte or granulocyte-macrophage colony-stimulating factor support is employed. Similarly, caution must be exercised when administering potentially marrow-suppressive agents to any individual receiving ganciclovir.

Resistance

HSV and VZV isolates that are resistant to acyclovir on the basis of thymidine kinase deficiency exhibit cross-resistance to ganciclovir. HSV isolates resistant to acyclovir on the basis of mutations in the viral DNA polymerase may remain susceptible to ganciclovir. Given their relative infrequency in comparison to thymidine kinase-deficient mutants, ganciclovir should not be used empirically in cases in which acyclovir resistance is suspected or proven.

Two basic mechanisms cause resistance to ganciclovir in CMV clinical isolates. The first and more common is due to mutations in the UL97 phosphotransferase gene, which encodes a protein kinase responsible for the monophosphorylation of ganciclovir. Almost all mutations of the UL97 gene have been found within two clusters of codons, codons 460 to 520 and 590 to 607, spanning the proposed ATP-binding and substrate recognition sites, respectively (82). Mutations at codons 460, 594, and 595 in the UL97 gene appear to be the most frequently encountered, but other codon site mutations or deletions have also been implicated. Isolates resistant to ganciclovir on the basis of UL97 gene mutations remain susceptible to foscarnet and cidofovir. The second, and less common, mechanism of ganciclovir resistance in clinical CMV isolates consists of mutations in the conserved subdomains of the UL54 DNA polymerase gene (68). In such instances, cross-resistance to cidofovir or foscarnet may be present. Further, mutations in both the UL97 and UL54 genes may coexist and lead to high-level ganciclovir resistance.

Before the advent of the era of potent antiretroviral therapy, the level and degree of immunosuppression in individuals with AIDS, combined with the need to continue maintenance therapy in subjects with retinitis, provided an appropriate milieu for viral resistance to emerge (62). In one series of CMV retinitis patients, 7.6% excreted resistant virus following 3 or more months of therapy (62). Resistant isolates have been isolated from organ transplant recipients and patients with hematologic malignancies, but the incidence of phenotypic CMV resistance is relatively low. In a study of 240 solid-organ transplant recipients who received oral ganciclovir prophylaxis, the overall incidence of ganciclovir-resistant CMV disease as determined by the plaque reduction assay performed on blood isolates was 2.1% (145). All of the subjects with resistant CMV disease were CMV-seronegative recipients of organs from CMV-positive donors.

Clinical Applications

Ganciclovir is useful for the treatment and prophylaxis of CMV infections in immunocompromised hosts. In HIV-infected patients with CMV retinitis, rates of initial response to intravenous ganciclovir are generally 75 to 85% (61). Induction courses of 5 mg/kg b.i.d. for 14 to 21 days must be followed by maintenance therapy; otherwise, predictable recurrence and progression of CMV retinitis will occur in the absence of immune restoration by potent antiretroviral therapy. Foscarnet is comparable to ganciclovir as primary therapy of CMV retinitis and has been reported to confer a median 4-month survival advantage (4). Ganciclovir delivered locally by ocular implants is effective in controlling CMV retinitis in patients intolerant of systemic ganciclovir. The combination of ganciclovir implants and oral ganciclovir provides both systemic and local drug activity and decreases progression of existing disease and incidence of new CMV disease (154). Use of implants has decreased dramatically in the era of potent antiretroviral therapy.

Ganciclovir also appears to be effective for gastrointestinal disease due to CMV in HIV-infected subjects, although the need for maintenance therapy is still debated. CNS disease and CMV polyradiculopathy have more variable response rates. Combination regimens with foscarnet suggest that these two agents can be used safely when administered concurrently or in alternating regimens (112). In severe or immediately life-threatening circumstances such as CMV encephalitis, combined initial treatment with ganciclovir and foscarnet is a consideration. In vitro data suggest that a combination of ganciclovir and foscarnet is synergistic against ganciclovir-susceptible or weakly resistant CMV isolates; however, there are insufficient clinical data to determine whether combination antiviral therapy is superior to monotherapy.

In other immunocompromised hosts, such as solid-organ transplant recipients, ganciclovir appears to be effective for treating invasive CMV disease, but responses in bone marrow transplant recipients are variable. Ganciclovir monotherapy is ineffective in treating CMV pneumonia in this population, and ganciclovir was not better than placebo for CMV gastrointestinal disease (185). However, ganciclovir combined with immunoglobulin appears to have some efficacy for the treatment of CMV pneumonia in marrow transplant recipients.

Ganciclovir has been studied extensively for prevention of CMV disease in organ transplant recipients. Effective regimens include prophylaxis, targeted prophylaxis, and preemptive therapy. Prophylaxis refers to the treatment of all patients prior to detection of CMV viremia during the highest-risk period, usually for a predetermined time after transplantation. Targeted prophylaxis refers to treatment during a defined period of increased immunosuppression such as OKT3 or antilymphocyte globulin treatment for rejection, prior to detection of CMV viremia. Preemptive therapy refers to initiation of treatment following the detection of CMV viremia or a positive CMV antigen test in the absence of clinically evident CMV disease.

Valganciclovir

Valganciclovir {L-valine, 2-[(2-amino-1,6-dihydro-6-oxo-9*H*-purin-9-yl)methoxy]-3-hydroxypropyl ester, monohydrochloride; Valcyte} is the L-valyl ester of ganciclovir and was designed, in a manner similar to that for valacyclovir, as a prodrug to enhance the oral bioavailability of the parent compound (Fig. 1; Tables 1 and 2). It has been approved for induction and maintenance therapy of CMV retinitis in patients with HIV infection and for posttransplantation prophylaxis in high-risk kidney, heart, and kidney-pancreas transplant patients.

Spectrum of Activity

Since valganciclovir is completely converted to ganciclovir, their spectra of activity are identical. Following oral administration, valganciclovir is recognized by the PEPT1 intestinal peptide transporter, which facilitates its absorption. After transport into intestinal cells, the drug is converted to ganciclovir by intracellular esterases. Ganciclovir levels were detected in serum within 15 min of valganciclovir administration, with a C_{max} of 2.98 μg/ml. The C_{max} and the time to attaining the peak were greater and shorter, respectively, than those achieved with oral ganciclovir. A dose of 900 mg of valganciclovir produces the same drug exposure as a 5-mg/kg intravenous dose of ganciclovir in liver transplant recipients (176).

Adverse Effects

In the pharmacokinetic studies to date, headache, nausea, and diarrhea have been most frequently noted, with neutropenia also seen with longer-term dosing.

Drug Interactions

No formal drug interaction studies with valganciclovir have been reported, but the profile would be expected to be similar to that for ganciclovir.

Resistance

New UL97 and polymerase mutations have been reported to occur in allogeneic stem cell transplant recipients who received prolonged valganciclovir as preemptive therapy for CMV disease (152). The UL97 mutation (deletion of codons 601 to 603) conferred a 15-fold-increased ganciclovir resistance, and the DNA polymerase mutation (D413A) conferred cross-resistance to cidofovir. Initial studies in solid-organ transplant patients receiving valganciclovir prophylaxis suggest that genotypic resistance is rare (25). However, among 225 CMV donor-seropositive, recipient-seronegative kidney, pancreas, liver, and heart recipients, 9 of 65 (15%) of patients who developed CMV disease had clinically suspected drug-resistant virus, 4 of whom had confirmed UL97 or UL54 mutations (65). Allograft loss and mortality occurred in two of four patients with proven drug-resistant CMV disease and in three of five patients with clinically suspected drug-resistant CMV disease.

Clinical Applications

In HIV-infected subjects, oral valganciclovir (900 mg b.i.d. for 3 weeks and then 900 mg once daily for 1 week) has been shown to be comparable to intravenous ganciclovir (5 mg/kg b.i.d. for 3 weeks and then 5 mg/kg once daily for 1 week) in the induction phase of treatment for CMV retinitis (49). At week 4, 86% of ganciclovir recipients and 88% of valganciclovir recipients showed no evidence of disease progression by fundoscopic photography, and the percentage of subjects with CMV viremia declined comparably in both groups. The approved dosage of valganciclovir is 900 mg orally b.i.d. for induction therapy of CMV disease and 900 mg once daily for maintenance and prophylaxis after transplantation. The benefit of valganciclovir therapy to prevent CMV disease after solid-organ transplantation has been established, but the best strategy (preemptive or prophylactic), treatment regimen (full-dose or low-dose valganciclovir), and duration have not yet been fully delineated (209).

Foscarnet

Foscarnet (trisodium phosphonoformate, Foscavir) (Fig. 1; Tables 1 and 2) is a pyrophosphate analog that differs from the other major antiherpesviral agents in that it is not a nucleoside or nucleotide analog.

Spectrum of Activity

Foscarnet has in vitro activity against HSV-1 and -2, VZV, CMV, EBV, HHV-6, HIV, and HBV. Inhibitory concentrations of foscarnet for viral DNA polymerases are 0.4 to 3.5 μM for HSV-1, 0.6 to 22 μM for HSV-2, 0.4 μM for VZV, 0.3 μM for CMV, 0.5 to 3.0 μM for EBV, and 0.1 to 0.5

μM for HIV. Inhibitory concentrations for viral replication vary considerably. For example, IC_{50}s of foscarnet for isolates of HSV, CMV, and HIV are 10 to 130, 100 to 300, and 10 to 25 μM, respectively (227). The different concentrations needed for enzyme inhibition and inhibition of virus replication are due to inefficient transport of this highly charged molecule across cell membranes. Isolates of HSV, VZV, and CMV that are resistant to acyclovir and ganciclovir on the basis of diminished ability to phosphorylate these agents remain susceptible to foscarnet.

Mechanism of Action

Foscarnet differs from nucleoside analog inhibitors in a number of important respects: it does not require intracellular metabolism for activation, is a noncompetitive inhibitor of viral DNA polymerases, and is not incorporated into the growing viral DNA chain. It blocks the pyrophosphate-binding site on the viral DNA polymerase, thereby interfering with pyrophosphate exchange from deoxynucleotide triphosphate moieties.

Foscarnet is available as an intravenous formulation and can be administered as a continuous or intermittent infusion. Following intravenous administration of doses of 60 and 90 mg/kg, the C_{max}s are 509 and 766 μM, respectively (10). The initial $t_{1/2}$ in plasma is 4.5 to 8.2 h in subjects with normal renal function, but there is a more prolonged terminal $t_{1/2}$ that may extend as long as 88 h. This relates to the deposition of the drug in bone, which can account for 20% of an administered dose (10). The CSF-to-plasma ratio of foscarnet averages 0.66, but a wide interpatient variability exists (100).

Adverse Effects

Foscarnet has a number of important potential side effects. Most frequent is nephrotoxicity, with elevations of creatinine noted in the majority of treated subjects. Saline hydration can reduce the risk of nephrotoxicity. Metabolic abnormalities include hypo- and hypercalcemia, hypomagnesemia, hypokalemia, and hypo- and hyperphosphatemia. Direct complexing of ionized calcium by foscarnet in the plasma may be responsible for hypocalcemia, and inhibition of the tubular reabsorption of phosphate may be responsible for the hypophosphatemia. Decreases in ionized calcium may not be reflected by the total serum calcium, and thus close observation for manifestations of hypocalcemia, such as paresthesias and tetany, is important. Neurologic toxicities include tremor, altered sensorium, and seizures; the last is potentiated by the tendency for foscarnet to cause hypocalcemia. Anemia and neutropenia occur in up to 33 and 17% of patients, respectively. Other side effects include headache, nausea, vomiting, and genital ulcerations, the last probably the result of local toxicity from the high concentrations of foscarnet excreted in the urine. In some test systems, foscarnet has demonstrated mutagenic and teratogenic effects, and its safety in pregnancy has not been evaluated. Its poor solubility requires administration of large fluid volumes; slow infusion is needed to minimize the risks of seizures and other manifestations of hypocalcemia.

Drug Interactions

Foscarnet should be used with particular caution in patients receiving pentamidine, as hypocalcemia can be potentiated by their concomitant use. Zidovudine and foscarnet exhibit no pharmacokinetic interactions, but together they may increase the risk for anemia (12). Any potentially nephrotoxic agent should be used with caution in patients receiving foscarnet. Ganciclovir exhibits no pharmacokinetic interactions with foscarnet, but dose adjustments of both drugs are necessary if a decrease in creatinine clearance occurs.

Resistance

Since foscarnet does not require intracellular activation, resistance to this agent occurs exclusively at the level of the viral DNA polymerase. Clinical isolates of HSV, CMV, and VZV resistant to foscarnet have been described, and the in vitro susceptibility of HSV strains derived from HIV patients correlates with foscarnet treatment success or failure (124). For resistant isolates of HSV, CMV, and VZV, there are three- to eightfold increases in inhibitory concentrations, and progressive CNS disease has been associated with foscarnet-resistant HSV strains (183). Foscarnet-resistant HSV and CMV strains may remain susceptible to acyclovir and ganciclovir, respectively, although dually resistant clinical isolates have been described (124). For such isolates, cidofovir remains a therapeutic option. Resistance of HIV to foscarnet has been linked to mutations in reverse transcriptase.

Clinical Applications

Foscarnet is effective treatment for CMV retinitis, either as primary therapy or when there is suspicion or proof of ganciclovir resistance. It is also useful for acyclovir-resistant mucocutaneous HSV or VZV infection in patients with HIV infection. One comparative trial of foscarnet and ganciclovir found that the two drugs were equivalent with respect to CMV outcome, but the foscarnet group exhibited an improved survival rate, with foscarnet extending life by an average of 4 months (4). When used as maintenance therapy for established CMV retinitis, the time to recurrence is inversely proportional to the foscarnet dosage employed. Therefore, a maintenance dosage of 120 mg/kg/day results in a delayed time to progression compared to that obtained with 90 mg/kg/day (102). Uncontrolled studies suggest a benefit for foscarnet in visceral disease due to CMV, except for CMV pneumonitis in bone marrow transplant recipients. Foscarnet can be used safely in conjunction with ganciclovir given either concomitantly in full doses for severe syndromes such as CMV ventriculoencephalitis in patients with AIDS or in alternating maintenance regimens (11). Intravitreal foscarnet has been employed in CMV retinitis.

Foscarnet may have a particular role in the prophylaxis of CMV infections in marrow transplant recipients. In patients with allogeneic hematopoietic stem cell transplantation and CMV antigenemia or viremia, preemptive foscarnet therapy demonstrated an efficacy similar to that of ganciclovir but was associated with a lower rate of neutropenia and treatment-limiting hematotoxicity (188). Although foscarnet exhibits in vitro and in vivo anti-HIV activities, its toxicity profile and requirement for parenteral administration preclude its use. It has been ineffective for HBV.

Cidofovir

Cidofovir {(S)-1-[3-hydroxy-2-(phosphonylmethoxy)propyl]cytosine; Vistide} (Fig. 1; Tables 1 and 2) is an acyclic phosphonate nucleotide analog which belongs to a family of phosphonylmethoxyalkyl derivatives of purines and pyrimidines.

Spectrum of Activity

Cidofovir has been primarily developed as an anti-CMV agent but has broad antiherpesvirus activity. The in vitro IC_{50}s for clinical CMV isolates are in the range of 0.1 μg/ml (165). In general, ganciclovir- and foscarnet-resistant strains of CMV and HSV remain susceptible to cidofovir. Cidofovir also has in vitro activity against human papillomaviruses, adenoviruses, poxviruses, and JC virus.

Mechanism of Action

Cidofovir is taken up by both virally infected and uninfected cells and does not require the action of a virus-induced kinase to be converted to its active moiety (101). The structure of cidofovir represents a monophosphorylated nucleotide. Cellular enzymes convert cidofovir to its diphosphate form, which, as an analog of a nucleotide triphosphate, is a competitive inhibitor of the viral DNA polymerase and causes premature chain termination. Cidofovir diphosphate has an intracellular $t_{1/2}$ of >48 h, an important factor that permits intermittent dosing schemes not previously possible for other anti-CMV agents. There is a 25- to 50-fold selectivity of cidofovir diphosphate for the viral compared to the cellular DNA polymerase (101).

Pharmacology

Cidofovir can be administered intravenously, topically, and by ocular implant. C_{max}s of 3.1 to 23.6 μg/ml are achieved with intravenous doses of 1.0 to 10.0 mg/kg, respectively. Cidofovir has poor CSF penetration, and ocular penetration has not been well characterized. The elimination $t_{1/2}$ in plasma is 2.6 h, and 90% of the drug is excreted in the urine, with renal tubular secretion contributing substantially to clearance (138). Dose reduction is necessary in the setting of renal insufficiency if the benefit of the drug is thought to outweigh the risk of worsening renal function.

Adverse Effects

The major adverse effect of cidofovir is nephrotoxicity, which appears to result from renal tubular damage (179). At a dosage of 5 mg/kg twice weekly without concomitant probenecid, renal toxicity is common and manifested by proteinuria and glycosuria (179). Concomitant use of high-dose probenecid appears to permit dosages of cidofovir of 5 mg/kg weekly or biweekly to be tolerated. Cardiomyopathy has been reported to occur in one HIV-infected subject treated simultaneously with stavudine, and erythematous cutaneous eruptions have been described to occur in subjects treated with cidofovir and probenecid (179). Iritis and hypotony (decreased intraocular pressure) are notable complications of both systemically and intravitreally administered cidofovir (53). Topical corticosteroids are effective in controlling the iritis associated with cidofovir if it is deemed in the patient's best interest to continue the drug. Neutropenia occurs in approximately 20% and requires monitoring. When cidofovir is administered with probenecid, hypersensitivity reactions, nausea, vomiting, and diarrhea occur commonly. Preclinical studies indicate that cidofovir has mutagenic, gonadotoxic, embryotoxic, and teratogenic effects. Cidofovir is associated with tumors in rats.

Drug Interactions

Probenecid has a nephroprotective effect in animal models and likely in humans. At cidofovir doses of 3 mg/kg, probenecid does not affect the clearance of cidofovir. However, at higher doses of cidofovir, probenecid given pre- and postinfusion reduces renal clearance (48). This differential effect of probenecid, dependent on the cidofovir dose, is not fully explained but has been hypothesized to reflect the presence of multiple tubular secretion pathways (48). The first may be high affinity, probenecid insensitive, and saturable. Once saturated, a probenecid-sensitive secretory mechanism may then be operative. Coadministration with other nephrotoxic drugs such as foscarnet or aminoglycosides should be avoided.

Resistance

CMV resistance to cidofovir may emerge during chronic use. After 3 months of cidofovir therapy for CMV retinitis, 29% of subjects had CMV isolates with reduced susceptibility to cidofovir (109). However, reduced susceptibility to cidofovir in vitro may not predict clinical progression (38). Most of the known mutations that confer cross-resistance between ganciclovir and cidofovir map in the exonuclease domains located between amino acids 300 and 545 of UL54 (156).

Clinical Applications

Cidofovir is effective in some HIV-infected patients with CMV retinitis and failure to respond or intolerance to ganciclovir and foscarnet. An induction course of cidofovir of 5 mg/kg weekly for 2 weeks is followed by dose frequency reduction to every other week. In patients with relapsed CMV retinitis, the 5-mg/kg-every-other-week maintenance regimen was more effective in delaying recurrence but was associated with a higher incidence of nephrotoxicity than the lower-dose regimen (3 mg/kg) (139). Combining cidofovir with oral ganciclovir might be an alternative treatment approach that avoids placement of a central venous catheter (114), but the toxicity of this regimen and the approval of valganciclovir make this a less attractive approach. Intravitreal cidofovir given as 20-μg injections may be an alternative maintenance regimen for patients with CMV retinitis, although the risk of ocular inflammation and hypotony is high (122).

Cidofovir can also be considered for the treatment of acyclovir-resistant HSV infections, either by the intravenous route or topically as a gel, which is not available as a commercial formulation (136). Cidofovir has also been studied as an investigational drug for the topical treatment of human papillomavirus infections in immunosuppressed patients, for the systemic treatment of progressive multifocal leukoencephalopathy in HIV-infected patients receiving potent antiretroviral therapy, and for respiratory papillomatosis.

Cidofovir interferes with poxviral DNA replication at concentrations well below those that are toxic for human cells and has a remarkably long intracellular $t_{1/2}$, making it an attractive agent for prophylaxis against smallpox were it to be utilized in a bioterrorism attack. Aerosolized doses of cidofovir prevented lethal intranasal or aerosol cowpox virus infection in murine models (29). Alkoxyalkyl esters of cidofovir have been developed that show improved uptake and absorption without the renal toxicity. Two esters, hexadecyloxypropyl-cidofovir (HDP-CDV) and octadecyloxyethyl-cidofovir, have been shown to be more active than cidofovir against CMV and other herpesviruses. HDP-CDV (CMX001) is currently under development as an oral drug for the treatment of CMV and smallpox infection, and phase I clinical studies are in progress (171).

Fomivirsen

Fomivirsen (ISIS 2922, Vitravene) is a phosphorothioate antisense oligonucleotide (5′-GCG TTT GCT CTT CTT CTT GCG-3′) that is 21 nucleotides in length (Tables 1 and 2). Fomivirsen is approved for the intravitreal treatment of CMV retinitis, and is also the first antisense compound approved as an antiviral agent.

Spectrum of Activity

Fomivirsen is active only against CMV. The IC_{50} for the AD169 laboratory strain of CMV is 0.37 μM. It is substantially more potent than ganciclovir and is active against ganciclovir-resistant strains of CMV.

Mechanism of Action

Fomivirsen, as an antisense compound, binds to the mRNA of the immediate-early 2 gene of CMV and presumably blocks the expression of immediate-early 2 protein, resulting in the inhibition of CMV replication. Additional antiviral activity may be conferred by the inhibition of virus adsorption to target cells.

Pharmacokinetics

Fomivirsen is administered only by intravitreal injection. The elimination $t_{1/2}$s from the vitreous humor and retina in rabbits are 62 and 79 h, respectively, with gradual breakdown of the oligonucleotide chain. The concentration of the drug in the retina follows a slower time course than in the vitreous humor; C_{max}s in the retinas of rabbits are seen 5 days after injection, and levels are maintained at 10 times those in the vitreous humor at the 10-day mark (142). In cynomolgus monkeys, vitreal concentrations peak at 2 days after administration and are undetectable at 14 days. Accumulation in the monkey retina occurs with multiple doses; the estimated elimination $t_{1/2}$ from the monkey retina is 78 h.

Adverse Effects

Intraocular inflammation (anterior chamber inflammation, uveitis, and vitritis) and increased intraocular pressure are the major adverse effects of fomivirsen. Incidence rates for ocular adverse events are dose and schedule dependent. Approximately 10% of eyes will experience an ocular adverse event with each injection (110). Anterior chamber inflammation and increased intraocular pressure can be controlled medically. Retinal pigment epitheliopathy and retinal detachments also occur more commonly with more intensive regimens, but it is unclear whether these result from an unanticipated drug toxicity or the presence of more severe CMV disease in patients receiving the more intensive regimens.

Drug Interactions

There is a potential for additive ocular toxicity of treatment with fomivirsen if it overlaps temporally with the administration of cidofovir. It is thus recommended that fomivirsen not be given to patients who have received cidofovir in the previous 2 to 4 weeks.

Resistance

A mutant resistant to fomivirsen has been isolated following serial laboratory passage in the presence of the drug. However, analysis of the target sequence in the mutant virus revealed no changes in the region complementary to fomivirsen; therefore, the mechanism of resistance is unclear (163). Clinical isolates that have developed resistance to fomivirsen on therapy have not been reported.

Clinical Applications

In a small study of newly diagnosed peripheral CMV retinitis in AIDS patients, fomivirsen (165 μg once weekly for 3 weeks as induction and then 165 μg every 2 weeks as maintenance) significantly delayed progression of the disease (71 versus 13 days) (5). A dose comparison study in AIDS patients with refractory CMV retinitis comparing more (330 μg weekly for 3 weeks followed by 330 μg every other week) and less (330 μg on days 1 and 15 and then 330 μg monthly) intense schedules found no significant difference between regimens in median time to progression (6). The approved dosage is 330 μg injected intravitreally once every other week as induction therapy and 330 μg intravitreally once every 4 weeks for maintenance.

Maribavir

Maribavir [5,6-dichloro-2-(isopropylamino)-1-β-L-ribofuranosyl-1*H*-benzimidazole; GW1263W94] belongs to a new class of drugs, the benzimidazole ribosides, and has a mechanism of action that differs from those of available CMV drugs that target the viral DNA polymerase.

Spectrum of Activity

Maribavir has activity against only two of the human herpesviruses: CMV and EBV. Maribavir inhibits CMV replication in vitro, with a mean IC_{50} of 0.12 μM as measured by multicycle DNA hybridization (22).

Mechanism of Action

Maribavir does not require intracellular activation, and its phosphorylated forms do not directly inhibit the viral DNA polymerase. Instead, maribavir inhibits the viral protein kinase, UL97, which severely impairs viral replication through mechanisms that are not fully understood (22). Maribavir also has been shown to interfere with viral nucleocapsid egress from the nucleus (128).

Pharmacology

Maribavir is rapidly absorbed after oral administration, with the C_{max} in plasma occurring 1 to 3 h after dosing and with an elimination $t_{1/2}$ of 3 to 5 h (230). Maribavir is extensively metabolized by the hepatic cytochrome P450 3A4 isozyme to an inactive metabolite (449W94) which is excreted in the urine (230). More than 98% of maribavir in the plasma is bound to protein, and less than 2% of the administered dose is eliminated unchanged in the urine; therefore, no dose adjustments are necessary with renal impairment (213). CNS and ocular penetration has not been studied.

Adverse Effects

Maribavir shows minimal cytotoxicity against bone marrow progenitors and human leukemic cell lines in vitro and limited toxicity in rats and monkeys. In healthy and HIV-infected subjects, the major adverse effects were mild to moderate taste disturbance in 80% of subjects, presumably resulting from secretion of the drug into the saliva after systemic absorption, and headache in 53% of subjects (230).

Drug Interactions

Maribavir, which is a UL97 kinase inhibitor, may inhibit the phosphorylation of ganciclovir, thereby antagonizing its antiviral effect. Checkerboard assays of maribavir paired with ganciclovir suggest that maribavir antagonizes the anti-CMV effect of ganciclovir, increasing the IC_{50} for a sensitive strain up to 13-fold, whereas it had no effect on the activities of foscarnet and cidofovir (41).

Resistance

CMV strains containing UL97 or UL54 DNA polymerase mutations, which are resistant to ganciclovir, foscarnet, or cidofovir, are sensitive to maribavir (63). Two clinical CMV isolates serially passaged in cell culture with maribavir developed UL97 mutations V353A and T409M, which conferred 15- and 80-fold increases in resistance, respectively, without significantly affecting ganciclovir susceptibility (42). CMV strains resistant to maribavir remain susceptible to current CMV antivirals (63).

Clinical Applications

In a 28-day dosing study in HIV-infected men with asymptomatic CMV shedding, maribavir demonstrated activity at all tested dosage regimens (100, 200, and 400 mg t.i.d. and 600 mg b.i.d.), with mean reductions in semen CMV titers of 2.9 to 3.9 log_{10} PFU/ml (137). A randomized, double-blind, dose-ranging study of maribavir prophylaxis (100 mg b.i.d., 400 mg once daily, and 400 mg b.i.d.) for prevention of CMV infection in allogeneic stem cell transplant patients demonstrated that the incidence of CMV infection, based on CMV DNA, was lower in each of the respective maribavir groups (7, 11, and 19%) than in the placebo group (46%) (241). Anti-CMV therapy was also used less often in the maribavir group, and maribavir had no adverse effect on neutrophil or platelet count.

Other Antiherpesvirus Agents

Docosanol

Docosanol ($C_{22}H_{46}OC$; Abreva) is a 22-carbon saturated alcohol that inhibits replication of HSV-1 and -2. Topical docosanol was approved by the FDA in July 2000 for the treatment of recurrent herpes labialis in adults and children aged 12 years and over. It is the only nonprescription drug available for this indication.

A highly lipophilic compound, docosanol inhibits entry of lipid-enveloped viruses into target cells by fusion with the cell plasma membrane. As a result, the virus remains on the cell surface and is blocked from entering the nucleus for viral replication. Docosanol lacks direct virucidal activity (150), and cellular metabolism may be required for its antiviral activity. Although it is active in vitro against VZV, CMV, HHV-6, and respiratory syncytial virus (RSV), the most important clinical activity of docosanol is against HSV-1 and -2 (150). In one clinical trial, persons with herpes labialis who received early docosanol treatment had a significant decrease in healing time of lesions, by a median difference of 18 h. Significant reductions in the duration of the ulcer or soft-crust stage of lesions and of associated symptoms, such as pain, burning, and pruritus, were also observed (190). Mild side effects, including headache and application site reactions, have been reported with docosanol.

Docosanol has activity against acyclovir-resistant HSV strains, since it does not interact with viral thymidine kinase or DNA polymerase. Anti-HSV activities of acyclovir and docosanol were synergistically additive in vitro. The emergence of acyclovir-resistant herpesvirus strains was decreased with the combination therapy, highlighting the potential role of docosanol in combination therapy with antiviral nucleoside analogs to treat mucocutaneous herpes infections (150). Off-label use of the drug to treat Kaposi's sarcoma in HIV-infected patients has shown partial reduction in lesion size.

Imiquimod

Imiquimod {1-(2-methylpropyl)-1*H*-imidazo[4,5-c]quinolin-4-amine; Aldara} is an agonist for Toll-like receptor 7 (TLR-7). Binding promotes maturation of dendritic cells as well as production of IFN-α, IFN-γ (indirectly), interleukin 12 (IL-12), IL-6, IL-8, and/or tumor necrosis factor from dendritic and other innate immune cells.

Imiquimod is available in a 5% topical cream. Following application to affected skin, some systemic absorption is seen, with levels in serum ranging from 0.1 to 3.5 ng/ml, depending on the dose applied. Urinary recoveries of up to 0.15% are seen following thrice-weekly treatment with 75 mg for 16 weeks. Use of imiquimod is often limited by local toxicity, which, although usually mild or moderate, can be severe. Common adverse events include erythema, burning, pain, erosion, induration, and edema.

Imiquimod is approved for the treatment of actinic keratosis, superficial basal cell carcinoma, and external genital or perianal warts. Because of its immunomodulatory and consequent antiviral effects, it has been studied for treatment of both oral and genital HSV infection. Several case reports have noted more rapid healing of primary HSV-2 lesions and decreased viral shedding in patients with acyclovir-resistant HSV lesions. In an open-label, controlled study for treatment of herpes labialis, subjects receiving imiquimod had a longer time to recurrence, but the trial was stopped early due to severe local toxicity in the imiquimod group (20). A controlled dose-ranging study for herpes genitalis found no effect of imiquimod on time to recurrence (196).

Investigational Antiherpesvirus Agents

There are several novel and potentially effective compounds under preclinical and early clinical investigation, some of which are listed in Table 3. New antiherpesvirus drugs include inhibitors of immediate early gene expression, nonnucleoside DNA polymerase inhibitors, helicase-primase inhibitors, inhibitors of protein-protein interactions among DNA replication proteins, and inhibitors of assembly, encapsidation, and nuclear egress (46, 156).

ANTI-HEPATITIS VIRUS AGENTS

This section describes agents that are primarily or exclusively directed at treatment of hepatitis virus infection (also see chapter 5 on viral hepatitis, chapter 31 on HBV, and chapter 53 on HCV). For ribavirin, which has other applications, its other antiviral activities are described in "Antiviral Agents for Respiratory Viruses" below.

TABLE 3 Investigational antiherpesvirus drugs

Agent	Chemical backbone	Spectrum	Mechanism(s) of action	Stage of development
HDP-CDV (CMX001)	Alkoxyalkyl ester of cidofovir	CMV, smallpox virus	Inhibition of DNA synthesis	Phase I
ODE-CDV[a]	Alkoxyalkyl ester of cidofovir	CMV, smallpox virus	Inhibition of DNA synthesis	Preclinical
PNU-183792	4-Oxo-dihydro-quinoline	Multiple herpesviruses	Inhibition of UL54	Preclinical
BAY 57-1293	Thiazole urea derivative	HSV-1, HSV-2	Helicase-primase inhibitor	Preclinical
BILS 179 BS	Thioazolylphenyl compound	HSV-1, HSV-2	Helicase-primase inhibitor	Preclinical
T-902611	Nitro-imidazolyl-pyrimidine	CMV	Helicase-primase inhibitor; inhibition of UL70	Phase II clinical, abandoned

[a]ODE-CDV, octadecyloxyethyl-cidofovir.

Antiviral Agents for HCV

IFNs

IFNs are part of the repertoire of human cytokines that have important multifunctional capabilities, including antiviral, immunomodulatory, and antiproliferative effects. There are currently nine approved IFN preparations for clinical use, of which five are approved for the treatment of chronic HCV (Table 4). The nomenclature for this group of cytokines has evolved over the past four decades, although the term interferon stems from the original discovery of these compounds, which produce viral interference. There are two major types of human IFNs that have been studied clinically: IFN-α/β (leukocyte/fibroblast) and IFN-γ. IFN-α and -β are encoded by genes on human chromosome 9; IFN-γ is encoded by a gene on human chromosome 12. There are over 12 subtypes of IFN-α but only 1 IFN-β subtype and 1 IFN-γ subtype. IFN-α and -β have 45% DNA homology and 30% amino acid homology. It is not clear why an array of closely related IFN-α subtypes exist, but one postulate is that the redundancy ensures that this natural defense system remains operative.

Spectrum of Activity

IFNs possess inhibitory activity against a broad array of DNA and RNA viruses. IFN-α and -β typically have greater antiviral activity than does IFN-γ, and the subspecies of IFN-α may express differential activities against a particular viral agent.

Mechanisms of Action

IFNs are not constitutively produced but are synthesized in response to a wide variety of infections and stimuli of the innate immune system and are an integral component of the complex cytokine network (see chapter 14). Nearly all cell types can produce IFN-α and -β, while IFN-γ is produced largely by T and natural killer (NK) cells. Once produced, IFNs possess no inherent antiviral activity but act by inducing an antiviral state within target cells. IFNs bind to specific receptors on the cell surface: IFN-α and -β have the same receptor, coded for by a gene on chromosome 21; IFN-γ binds to a receptor coded for by a gene on chromosome 6. These receptors are composed of at least two subunits which must be present to ensure that full IFN action is induced (70). Following receptor binding, receptor-associated tyrosine kinases (Tyk2 and JAK1 for IFN-α and -β and JAK1 and JAK2 for IFN-γ) are activated and, in turn, phosphorylate specific cytoplasmic proteins (termed STAT proteins). These proteins move to the nucleus, where they bind to specific *cis*-acting elements in the promoter regions of IFN-inducible genes (51). Transcription of these genes occurs within minutes of IFNs' binding to the cell receptors.

Depending upon the viral agent and cell type, IFNs can inhibit viral replication at nearly all steps from penetration to particle release. For some viral agents, inhibition occurs at more than one step, and for others the mechanism(s) of inhibition remains undefined. Several mechanisms of IFN-induced antiviral activity have been described: (i)

TABLE 4 IFNs used in the management of viral hepatitis[a]

IFN type	Brand name	Indication(s)	$t_{1/2}$ (h)	Usual dose
IFN-α2a	Roferon	Chronic HCV	3.7–8.5 (i.v.)	Chronic HCV: 3 million IU i.m. or s.c. t.i.w. for 12 mo
IFN-α2b	Intron A	Chronic HCV, chronic HBV	2 (i.v.) 2–3 (s.c.)	Chronic HCV: 3 million units i.m. or s.c. t.i.w. Chronic HBV: 5 million units/day or 10 million units t.i.w. i.m. or s.c.
peg-IFN-α2a	Pegasys	Chronic HCV, chronic active HBV	50–140 (s.c.)	Chronic HCV and HBV: 180 μg s.c. weekly
peg-IFN-α2b	PegIntron	Chronic HCV	40 (s.c.)	1–1.5 mg/kg/wk
IFN alphacon-1	Infergen	Chronic HCV	NA	9 μg s.c. t.i.w.

[a]i.v., intravenous; i.m., intramuscular; s.c., subcutaneous; t.i.w., thrice per week; NA, not available.

2′-5′ oligoadenylate synthetases are activated by double-stranded (viral) RNA and are responsible for the conversion of ATP into a series of oligonucleotides designated 2′,5′-oligo(A)s. The 2′,5′-oligo(A)s then activate an RNase, RNase L, which can cleave single-stranded mRNAs (205). (ii) A double-stranded RNA-dependent protein kinase termed PKR (P68 kinase, P1, DAI, dsl, and eukaryotic initiation factor 2 [eIF2] kinase) is activated by double-stranded (viral) RNA and autophosphorylated, which, in turn, phosphorylates the alpha subunit of eIF2. This prevents the recycling of eIF2 with inhibition of protein synthesis (157). (iii) The induction of a phosphodiesterase inhibits peptide chain elongation (226). (iv) MxA protein, which binds to cytoskeletal proteins and inhibits viral transcriptases, is synthesized (173). (v) Nitric oxide synthetase is induced by IFN-γ in macrophages (117).

Although some of the IFN-inducible functions have been linked to the inhibition of replication of individual viruses, for the most part there is uncertainty in trying to dissect out single activities of IFNs in this process, since more than one mechanism may be operative simultaneously. In addition, some antiviral effects of IFNs result indirectly from stimulation of antiviral immune functions. For example, the immunomodulatory activities of IFN, such as induction of cytotoxic T-cell and NK cell activity and the induction of major histocompatibility complex proteins, may also help control viral infections.

Pharmacology

IFNs have no in vivo activity when administered orally. For systemic effects, they must be administered intravenously, intramuscularly, or subcutaneously. The elimination $t_{1/2}$ of IFN-α in plasma following intravenous administration is 2 to 3 h; this is extended to 4 to 6 h following intramuscular or subcutaneous administration, with 80% of an administered dose absorbed following injection by the latter routes. The levels achieved in plasma are dose proportional. The relevance of classic pharmacokinetic parameters of IFNs in relation to their antiviral activity is questionable, since systemic effects are measurable in the absence of detectable IFN levels in plasma. Two long-acting, slow-release formulations of IFN combined with polyethylene glycol are currently available (PegIntron and Pegasys). These products can be administered subcutaneously once per week and achieve sustained levels in blood equivalent to those of standard IFN given three times a week. Penetration into CSF and respiratory secretions is minimal.

Adverse Effects

IFNs cause a broad range of side effects, most commonly systemic and hematologic. Dose-related influenza-like symptoms are common with initiation of treatment and generally include fever, chills, headache, nausea, myalgias, and arthralgias. Gradual dose escalation may be helpful; tolerance to these side effects can develop with time, but this is not uniform. The most common hematologic side effects are leukopenia and thrombocytopenia, and thus treatment of immunocompromised hosts or patients taking other myelotoxic agents can be difficult. Other important side effects include neurotoxicity (including somnolence, confusion, electroencephalographic changes, behavioral changes, and seizures), psychiatric disturbances (especially depression), hepatotoxicity, nephrotoxicity, thyroiditis, and alopecia. Topical intranasal administration of IFN-α has been associated with local irritation and mucosal friability. Intralesional injection of condylomata can have both local and systemic side effects, such as flu-like symptoms, fatigue, anorexia, and local pain.

Drug Interactions

Few formal drug interaction studies with the approved preparations of IFNs have been performed. Care must be exercised when coadministering other potentially myelosuppressive or neurotoxic drugs. Pegylated IFN-α2a and -α2b (collectively referred to hereafter as "peg-IFN" unless specified otherwise) inhibit cytochrome P450 (CYP) 1A2 enzymes but do not affect the pharmacokinetics of drugs metabolized by CYP2C9, CYP2C19, CYP2D6, or CYP3A4 hepatic microsomal enzymes. No studies of drug interactions have been performed with IFN-β.

Resistance

Many viruses have developed strategies to evade or inhibit IFN-mediated antiviral effects (see chapter 14 on immunity to viral infections). However, acquired resistance to the actions of IFNs through specific mutations during therapeutic administration has not been well documented. Variability in the response of HCV to IFN therapy has been associated in vitro with amino acid substitutions in the NS5A protein, although the significance of this association remains unclear. Specifically, heterogeneity between codons 2209 and 2248 may affect the ability of IFN to bind to double-stranded-RNA-dependent protein kinase, thereby reducing the host antiviral response (50). In HCV replicon cells, IFN-resistant HCV strains have decreased expression and activity of Tyk2 and JAK1, two proteins in the JAK-STAT pathway which are intermediates in IFN-mediated intracellular signaling (98).

Clinical Applications

IFN-α preparations are beneficial in the treatment of chronic HBV (see below) and HCV infections, although responses are not uniform and relapse rates after discontinuation of treatment are substantial. The response to IFN therapy in patients with chronic hepatitis C is higher than in patients with hepatitis B and depends on host factors such as a younger age, less advanced disease state, ethnicity, and a lower degree of hepatocyte HLA antigen expression. Virologic factors, including a lower degree of viremia and HCV genotype, also affect IFN responsiveness, with genotypes 2 and 3 having better rates of response to IFN than genotypes 1 and 4 (78, 217). peg-IFN in combination with ribavirin achieves rates of viral response superior to those of standard IFN-ribavirin therapy and peg-IFN alone and is now the standard of care for chronic hepatitis C (78, 149). Though the efficacy is lower in patients coinfected with HIV and HCV, peg-IFN and ribavirin are superior to standard IFN-ribavirin in this patient population as well (217).

A new form of IFN-α consisting of recombinant human IFN-α2b genetically fused to recombinant human serum albumin is currently under investigation for the treatment of chronic hepatitis C. Albumin–IFN-α has a prolonged elimination $t_{1/2}$ and provides greater drug exposure than does standard IFN-α, so this fusion protein will probably be dosed every 2 weeks (14). A phase II study in treatment-naïve genotype 1 HCV-infected subjects demonstrated reductions in HCV RNA of $>3 \log_{10}$ IU/mol after 4 weeks of therapy. Two large phase III studies comparing albumin–IFN-α plus ribavirin to peg-IFN plus ribavirin are currently underway.

Intralesional and systemic administration of IFN-α can lead to regression of condyloma acuminata (187), although its efficacy in HIV-infected individuals is lower than in other populations and other modalities of treatment may be equally effective and/or less toxic. IFNs have demonstrated activity in the prophylaxis and treatment of herpesvirus infections, but the degree of activity and the toxicity profile limit the usefulness of this approach. IFN in combination with an antiviral agent may be effective in refractory herpes simplex keratitis (239). IFNs have in vitro and in vivo activities against HIV, but the toxicity profile makes administration difficult. IFN-α is approved for the treatment of Kaposi's sarcoma and exhibits the greatest activity in subjects with CD4 cell counts of >200/mm^3 (129). In the prophylaxis of respiratory virus infections, IFNs have demonstrated efficacy against rhinovirus, but the local toxicity of intranasal administration has greatly limited this approach. IFN-γ can reduce the risk of recurrent infections in patients with chronic granulomatous disease.

Ribavirin

Ribavirin (1-β-D-ribofuranosyl-1,2,4-triazole-3-carboxamide; Rebetol, Copegys, Ribapak, Ribasphere, Virazole) (Fig. 2; Tables 1 and 5) is a synthetic nucleoside analog of guanosine approved in the United States for the treatment of RSV infection and in combination with IFN-α for the treatment of HCV.

Spectrum of Activity

Ribavirin has in vitro activity against a broad range of both RNA and DNA viruses, including flaviviruses, paramyxoviruses, bunyaviruses, arenaviruses, retroviruses, herpesviruses, adenoviruses, and poxviruses. In structure-activity studies, both the ribose moiety and the base are essential for maintenance of antiviral activity.

Mechanism of Action

The mechanism of action of ribavirin is incompletely understood and likely multifactorial. Ribavirin is phosphorylated by host cell enzymes to ribavirin triphosphate. In influenza virus, ribavirin triphosphate interferes with capping and elongation of mRNA and may directly inhibit viral RNA polymerase activity. Some studies have suggested a direct antiviral effect of ribavirin on HCV, although the data are not consistent and this effect, if present, is probably small. Ribavirin inhibits HCV RNA polymerase, but only at concentrations exceeding those achieved clinically. Inhibition of inosine-5′-monophosphate dehydrogenase by ribavirin monophosphate depletes the intracellular pools of GTP required for RNA synthesis. Ribavirin may also act indirectly by immunomodulatory effects, causing a change in the host T-cell response from a T-helper 2 (Th2) to a Th1 response. For hepatitis C, the shift to a Th1 profile with production of Th1 cytokines, especially IFN-γ, is believed to halt virion production, increase lysis of infected hepatocytes, stop transformation to neoplastic cells, and limit fibrogenesis (83). Finally, ribavirin may act as a mutagen, increasing the error rate in replicating RNA strands and pushing the virus over the threshold of error catastrophe. There is evidence to support this theory from HCV replicon studies, but human data remain inconclusive.

Pharmacology

Aerosol, oral, and intravenous formulations of ribavirin exist, but the aerosol and oral preparations are the only ones approved in the United States. Concentration of ribavirin in plasma after a single oral dose has three phases: rapid absorption, rapid distribution, and a long elimination phase. Following a 600-mg dose, the C_{max} was 782 ng/ml, the elimination $t_{1/2}$ was 79 h, and the AUC was 13,394 ng · h/ml. Administration with food enhances absorption and results in a 70% increase in the concentration in plasma. Following intravenous doses of 1,000 and 500 mg, the concentrations in plasma were approximately 2,400 and 1,700 ng/ml, respectively. The plasma-to-CSF ratio is approximately 0.7. Aerosol ribavirin must be delivered through a small-particle aerosol generator (designated SPAG-2). When ribavirin is given at a 20-mg/ml concentration via aerosol, the concentrations in respiratory secretions may reach 1,000 μg/ml, with levels of 2 to 3 μg/ml in plasma. The $t_{1/2}$ in respiratory secretions is approximately 2 h. The drug is generally delivered to children in a tent, but a mask can also be used. For intubated patients, caution must be exercised in delivering ribavirin via the endotracheal tube because precipitation of the drug may raise airway pressures.

Adverse Effects

Oral and intravenous administration is associated with anemia, which is related to intravascular hemolysis and bone marrow-suppressive effects. Depression, pruritus, rash, nausea, and cough have been reported. When the drug is given as an aerosol preparation, bronchospastic reactions can occur, and ocular irritation has been reported. Ribavirin also has immunosuppressive effects. In vitro, antigen- and mitogen-driven lymphocyte proliferative responses are suppressed by ribavirin, and release of mast cell mediators may be inhibited.

Ribavirin has teratogenic, carcinogenic, and mutagenic properties in preclinical assays, and therefore its use in pregnant women is contraindicated. Potential occupational exposure to aerosolized ribavirin has caused considerable concern, and appropriate precautions should be taken to protect health care workers. Guidelines for the drug's aerosol administration have been published (71).

Drug Interactions

In vitro studies suggest that ribavirin can antagonize the activity of zidovudine by inhibiting its phosphorylation, although such an effect has not been observed in vivo (13). Conversely, ribavirin can potentiate the anti-HIV activity of didanosine by facilitating its phosphorylation, but there have been reports of severe mitochondrial toxicity resulting in fatal and nonfatal lactic acidosis in patients receiving didanosine and ribavirin concurrently (31). Guidelines for management of patients coinfected with HIV and HCV advise against the use of didanosine and ribavirin together.

Resistance

Diminished susceptibility of Sindbis virus to ribavirin has been reported (198). It is caused by resistance to nsP1, which is believed to mediate mRNA capping and is encoded by the virus. Replicon studies with HCV Huh7

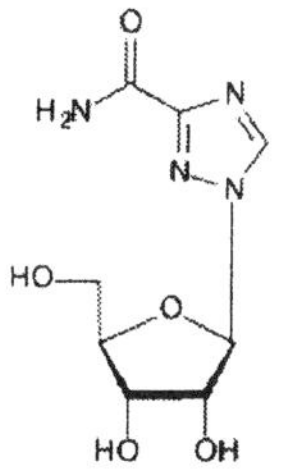

Ribavirin

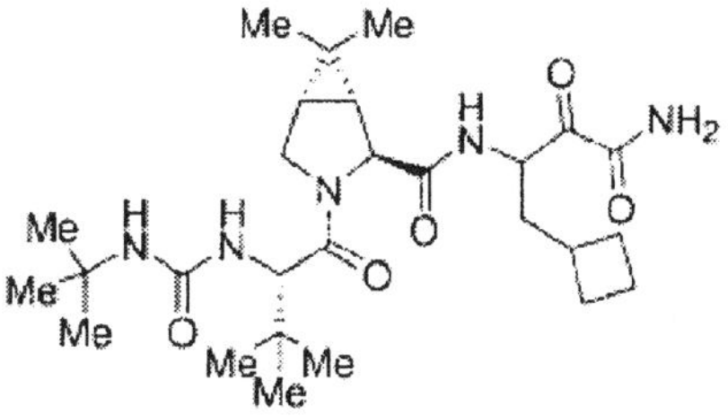

Boceprevir

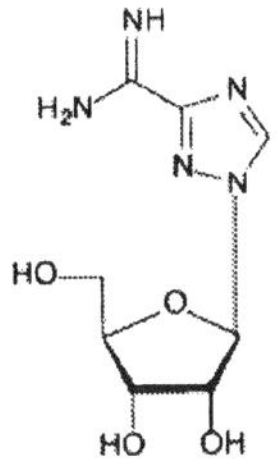

Viramidine (ribavirin prodrug)

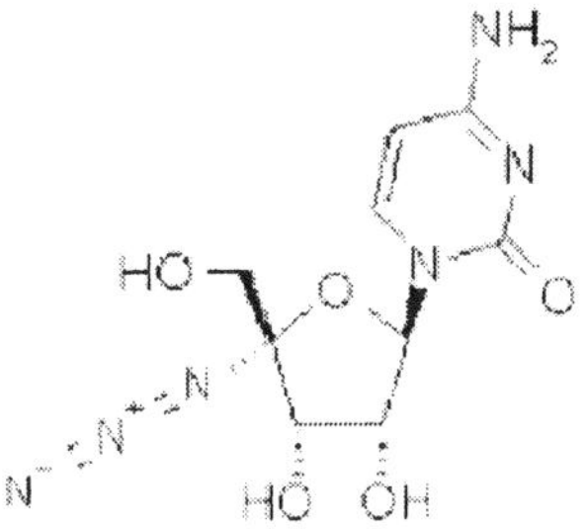

R1479 (R1626 is prodrug of R1479)

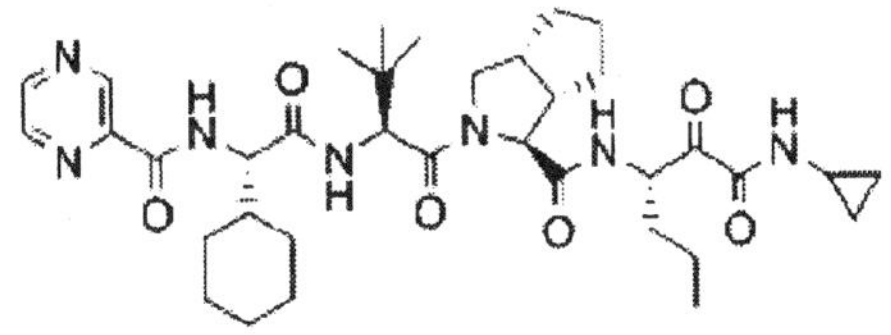

Telaprevir

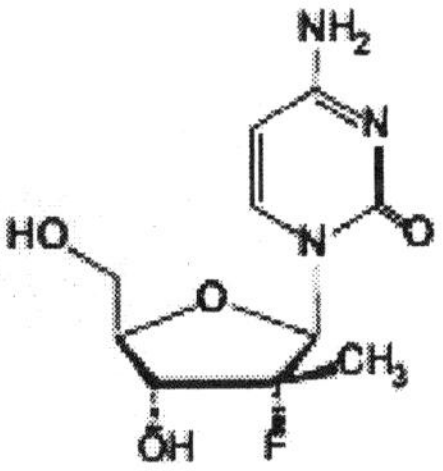

PSI-6130

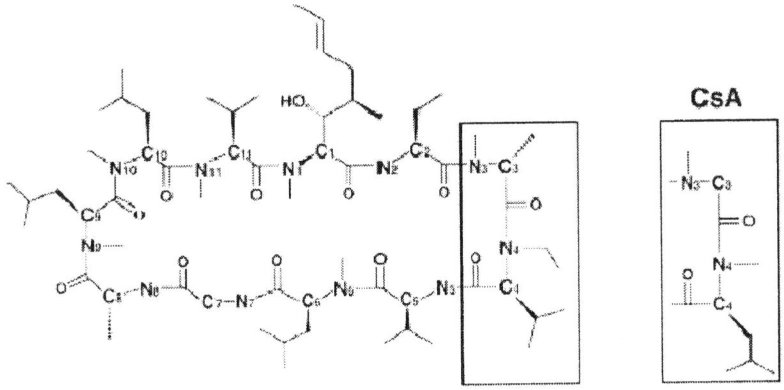

CsA

FIGURE 2 Chemical structures of anti-HCV agents.

TABLE 5 HBV and HCV agents: pharmacokinetics, major toxicities, and drug interaction characteristics

Agent	Oral bioavailability (%)	Effect of food on AUC	$t_{1/2}$ (h) in adults	Major route of elimination	Adjustment for renal insufficiency	Major toxicities	Major drug interactions
Lamivudine	80–88	No	3–7	Mainly renally excreted unchanged	Yes	Abdominal pain, nausea, vomiting	Probable interaction with ribavirin (lactic acidosis); IFN-α (hepatic decompensation)
Adefovir	59	No	7.5	Renally excreted (45%)	Yes	Rash, pruritus, abdominal pain, nausea, diarrhea, renal impairment	Nephrotoxic agents may increase renal toxicity; ribavirin may increase risk of hepatic decompensation and other mitochondrial toxicity
Entecavir	100	Decreases by 18–20%	128–149	Mainly renally excreted, 60–70% unchanged	Yes	Hepatitis, headache, dizziness, hematuria	None
Telbivudine	100	No	40–49	Renally excreted, 42% unchanged	Yes	Abdominal pain, elevated creatine kinase, headache, nasopharyngitis, upper respiratory infection, malaise/fatigue, lactic acidosis, hepatitis	None
Emtricitabine	93 (capsule), 75 (solution)	No	10	Renally excreted, 86% unchanged and 13% as metabolites	Yes	Dizziness, headache, diarrhea, rash, weakness, cough, rhinitis, anemia, neutropenia	Ganciclovir and valganciclovir may increase hematologic toxicity; ribavirin may increase risk of hepatotoxicity and other mitochondrial toxicity
Tenofovir	25–40	Increases by 40% with high-fat meal; no with light meal	17	Renally excreted, 70–80%, primarily unchanged	Yes	Diarrhea, nausea, renal impairment, weakness	May increase didanosine levels. May decrease serum atazanavir levels; serum tenofovir levels may increase with acyclovir and ganciclovir
Ribavirin	45	Increases by 42% with high-fat meal	21–36 (plasma); 40 days (erythrocyte compartment)	Renal and hepatic	Yes	Anemia, neurotoxicity, gastrointestinal effects; teratogenic, carcinogenic, and mutagenic potential	Mitochondrial toxicity with didanosine; ? antagonize zidovudine

strains have demonstrated the appearance of the B415F-to-Y mutation in the NS5B RNA polymerase when exposed to ribavirin. Strains with the 415Y mutation have a replicative advantage over the 415F strains in the presence of ribavirin, but when ribavirin is removed, all strains revert to the 415F variant and demonstrate improved replicative capacity over the 415Y mutant (248). In another study, the G404S and E442G mutations in the NS5A protein were both associated with low-level ribavirin resistance (178). There have been no reports of RSV, influenza virus, or HIV isolates resistant to ribavirin.

Clinical Applications

Ribavirin in combination with peg-IFN (IFN-α2a or -α2b) is currently the standard therapy for chronic HCV infection and is approved for this indication. These agents, when given together for 6 months (genotypes 2 and 3) or 12 months (genotypes 1 and 4), significantly improve sustained response rates compared to the use of peg-IFN alone or the combination of ribavirin with standard (thrice-weekly) IFN-α for initial treatment of chronic HCV infection (78). In retreatment of relapses and nonresponders to prior IFN-based therapy with ribavirin and peg-IFN, combination therapy has yielded increased rates of sustained viral response. Maximal response rates, however, remain lower than 20% in previous nonresponders (127). peg-IFN and ribavirin are also used in combination for the treatment of chronic HCV infection in HIV-coinfected patients, although response rates appear to be lower than in patients with HCV monoinfection (217).

Investigational HCV Agents

Taribavirin (Viramidine)

Taribavirin (1-β-D-ribofuranosyl-1*H*-1,2,4-triazole-3-carboxamidine; Virazole) (Fig. 2) is a guanosine analog and a prodrug of ribavirin.

Mechanism of action and pharmacology. Taribavirin is an oral formulation that is rapidly absorbed and extensively converted to ribavirin by hepatic adenosine deaminase. The C_{max} is obtained after approximately 1.5 h, and at a dosage of 1,200 mg daily, the C_{max} averages 437 ng/ml. The plasma AUC of ribavirin is two to four times higher than that of taribavirin. In monkeys, taribavirin resulted in liver drug levels that were three times that achieved with ribavirin, whereas intraerythrocyte drug levels were half of that achieved with ribavirin (147). Intracellular levels of ribavirin have been shown to correlate with degree of hemolytic and resultant anemia.

Clinical applications. One study comparing peg-IFN with either ribavirin (weight based) or taribavirin (800 to 1,600 mg) found that severe anemia (defined as a hemoglobin of <10 g/dl) occurred more often in the ribavirin group than in the taribavirin group (27%, versus 0 to 2%) but that the proportion of patients with undetectable HCV RNA did not differ between any of the taribavirin groups and the ribavirin group (84). Two phase III studies, however, examining the combination of peg-IFN with either taribavirin or ribavirin demonstrated that, despite lower rates of anemia, taribavirin therapy was not comparable with ribavirin in sustained virologic responses (SVR) (38 to 40%, versus 52 to 55%). In post hoc analyses, subjects receiving greater than 18 mg of taribavirin per kg were more likely to have an SVR than those receiving a lower relative dose, suggesting that higher doses of taribavirin should be utilized in future studies. Dosing of taribavirin prior to initiation of combination therapy with peg-IFN is also being explored.

HCV Protease Inhibitors

The HCV NS3 serine protease is an attractive target for antiviral development. The HCV genome is translated to a polypeptide which undergoes posttranslational processing to produce 10 different peptides. The NS3 serine protease is one of the proteases responsible for such processing and also functions in the evasion of the host immune response and the establishment of chronic infection (195) (Fig. 3). NS3 interferes with RIG-1, a cellular helicase which binds HCV RNA and activates factors that result in IFN-β production. NS3 also cleaves Cardiff, an additional factor downstream of RIG-1, to further decrease IFN-β production (158), and blocks Toll-IL-1 receptor domain-containing adaptor (TRIF), which normally serves as another activator for interferon regulatory factor 3 and NF-κB (144). HCV protease inhibitors that are in clinical trials are summarized below; preclinical and early-phase agents are listed in Table 6.

Telaprevir (VX-950). Telaprevir {2-(2-[2-cyclohexyl-2-[(pyrazine-2-carbonyl)-amino]-acetylamino]-3,3-dimethyl-butyryl)-octahydro-cyclopenta[c]pyrrole-1-carboxylic acid; 1-cyclopropylaminooxalyl-butyl)-amide; VX-950) (Fig. 2) is a peptidomimetic inhibitor of the HCV NS3-4A protease.

SPECTRUM OF ACTIVITY. Telaprevir appears to bind variably to the NS3-4A proteases of different HCV genotypes. One study found that the inhibition constants for genotypes 2a and 3a are approximately 7- and 40-fold higher than for genotype 1a, respectively (174), but another reported that the activity of telaprevir against genotypes 2a, 2b, 3a, and 4a are within 10-fold that for genotype 1a or 1b (C. Lin, B. L. Hanzelka, U. Muh, L. Kovari, D. J. Bartels, A. M. Tigges, J. Miller, B. G. Rao, and A. D. Kwong, presented at the 42nd Annual Meeting of the European Association for the Study of Liver Disease, Barcelona, Spain).

MECHANISM OF ACTION. Telaprevir's interaction with the NS3-4A protease is thought to follow a biphasic process marked initially by weak binding and subsequently by rearranging to form a tightly bound, long-lived complex that inhibits the enzyme. The inhibitory constant for this reaction at equilibrium is approximately 7 nM (174).

PHARMACOLOGY. In humans, telaprevir accumulates with multiple dosing and appears to be associated with trough concentration (C_{trough})-dependent inhibiton of HCV. Subjects receiving 750 mg q8h had a mean C_{trough} of 1,054 ng/ml and a $\geq$4-$\log_{10}$ decline in HCV RNA, while those receiving 450 mg q8h had a C_{trough} of 781 and a $\geq$3-$\log_{10}$ decline in HCV RNA (186).

DRUG INTERACTIONS. Coadministration of telaprevir with the CYP3A inhibitor, ritonavir, results in >15-fold increases in drug exposure and >50-fold increases in concentrations in plasma 8 h after dosing (120).

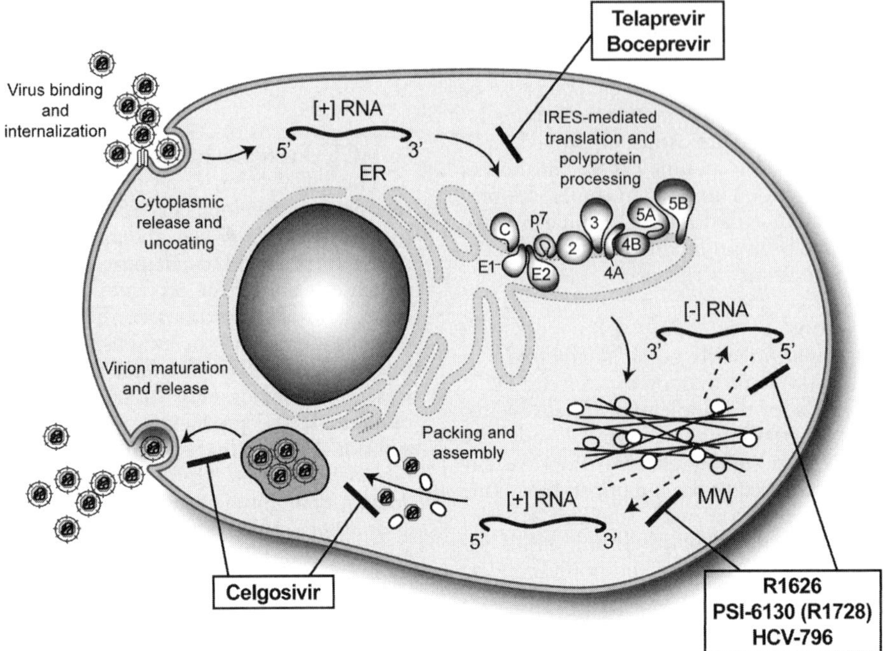

FIGURE 3 Inhibition of HCV replication cycle by antiviral agents. After surface-bound HCV is internalized via receptor-mediated endocytosis, fusion of the viral envelope and cellular endosomal membrane occurs and the HCV RNA is passaged to the endoplasmic reticulum (ER). The internal ribosome entry site (IRES) directs the binding of the viral RNA to cytoplasmic ribosomal subunits and initiates translation. The large polyprotein precursor is processed by cellular and viral proteases into structural and nonstructural proteins. The viral NS3/NS4A protease is the target of HCV protease inhibitors. The viral NS5B enzyme, RNA polymerase, is responsible for the initial synthesis of a complementary negative-strand RNA template and the subsequent synthesis of positive-strand RNA [(+)RNA] and is the target of the HCV polymerase inhibitors. The final step of HCV replication consists of viral assembly and release. α-Glucosidase I is a host enzyme that is essential for the proper glycosylation of viral envelope proteins, and is the target of α-glucosidase inhibitors. MW, membranous web. (Adapted from reference 205a with permission [http://clinicaloptions.com/hiventry].)

RESISTANCE. Subjects receiving lower dosages of telaprevir (450 mg q8h or 1,250 mg b.i.d.) have decreases in HCV RNA within the first 3 days, followed by either no further decline or an increase in viral load from days 7 to 14. Mutations in the NS4-4A protease domain develop by day 14 and confer various levels of decreased sensitivity to telaprevir (186). Several mutations in NS3-4A confer resistance to telaprevir in vitro, including A156V/T (>50-fold resistance), V36A/M and R155K/T (both <25-fold resistance), and T54S/A. The double mutations confer high-level resistance. Variants with these resistance mutations have decreased replication capacity both in vitro and in vivo, perhaps related to impaired cleavage of the HCV substrates. Wild-type virus reappears in patients by 7 months after discontinuation of telaprevir and more rapidly in patients with highly resistant, less fit virus (194). It

TABLE 6 HCV investigational drugs in early-phase studies

Agent	Mechanism of action	Stage of development
GS-9190	HCV polymerase inhibitor	Phase I
GSK625433	HCV polymerase inhibitor	Phase I
VCH-759	HCV polymerase inhibitor	Phase I
RO-0622	HCV polymerase inhibitor	Preclinical
ANA598	HCV polymerase inhibitor	Preclinical
HCV-796	HCV polymerase inhibitor	Phase II (development on hold because of possible hepatotoxicity)
TMC435350	HCV protease inhibitor	Phase I
ITMN-191 (R-7227)	HCV protease inhibitor	Phase I
GI-5005	Yeast-based immunotherapy	Phase I
CPG10101	TLR-9 agonist	Phase II (on hold)

is not yet known if resistant HCV prospecies will reappear after reintroduction of drug pressure, as no long-lived reservoir for HCV has yet been demonstrated.

ADVERSE EFFECTS. Initial studies have found no serious adverse effects. Diarrhea, nausea, fatigue, and dry skin occur at a higher incidence with telaprevir than with placebo (186), and during combination therapy with peg-IFN and ribavirin, drug discontinuations appear to be more frequent in telaprevir than placebo recipients (9%, versus 3%). The most commonly reported adverse effects have been rash and gastrointestinal events.

CLINICAL APPLICATIONS. In initial studies, HCV genotype 1-infected patients receiving telaprevir achieved HCV RNA reductions of $\geq 2 \log_{10}$ (median reduction of 4.4 $\log_{10}$ at a dosage of 750 mg q8h after a 14-day course) and decreases in median alanine aminotransferase (ALT) from baseline (186), as well as significant decreases in the size of perihepatic lymph nodes, compared with those of patients receiving placebo, suggesting that by suppressing viral replication, telaprevir may indirectly decrease inflammatory activity in the liver. Preliminary results from two ongoing phase II studies indicate that a greater proportion of subjects receiving telaprevir at 750 mg orally q8h in combination with peg-IFN and ribavirin achieved an undetectable HCV RNA level at 12 weeks than those receiving peg-IFN and ribavirin alone (88%, versus 52%). Seven percent of subjects in the telaprevir arms of PROVE-1 experienced viral rebound with detection of resistance to telaprevir.

Boceprevir (SCH-503034)

SPECTRUM OF ACTIVITY. Boceprevir {(1*R*,5*S*)-*N*-[3-amino-1-(cyclobutylmethyl)-2,3-dioxopropyl]-3-[2(*S*)-[[[(1,1-dimethyl)amino]carbonyl]amino]-3,3-dimethyl-1-oxobutyl]-6,6-dimethyl-3-azabicyclo[3.1.0]hexan-2(*S*)-carboxamide} (Fig. 2) is an HCV NS3-4A protease inhibitor.

MECHANISM OF ACTION. Boceprevir is a potent inhibitor of the NS3-4A HCV protease, with an inhibitory constant of 14 nM (180).

PHARMACOLOGY. Boceprevir dosages of 200 and 400 mg t.i.d. provide C_{max}s of 351 and 523 ng/ml, respectively, when administered in combination with peg-IFN-α2b. C_{max} was achieved in 1 h, and the elimination $t_{1/2}$ in healthy controls is approximately 7 h.

ADVERSE EFFECTS. Boceprevir has been generally well tolerated. The most commonly reported side effects are headache, myalgias, rigor, and fever, which occur more frequently with combination therapy with peg-IFN. No significant laboratory or electrocardiographic abnormalities have been observed.

DRUG INTERACTIONS. Minimal changes in AUC were detected with the 200-mg t.i.d. dosage but not the 400-mg-t.i.d. dosage of boceprevir when administered with peg-IFN (195). There are no published studies of interactions with other medications, but because boceprevir is not an inhibitor of the CYP enzymes, it should not affect the levels of drugs metabolized via this pathway.

RESISTANCE. Three mutations in the NS3 protease, T54A, V170A, and A156S, can confer resistance to boceprevir. A156S results in the greatest change (>100-fold) but is also associated with a significant loss of viral fitness. By contrast, the V170A mutation does not affect replicon fitness and has consistently appeared as the dominant mutation following prolonged exposure to boceprevir (216). Viral variants resistant to either boceprevir or the HCV polymerase inhibitor HCV-796 do not show cross-resistance, which suggests that the two classes of drugs could be used together in combination therapy and potentially forestall the development of resistance.

CLINICAL APPLICATIONS. In small numbers of chronically HCV genotype 1-infected nonresponders to prior peg-IFN therapy, 1 week of boceprevir monotherapy was associated with a mean decrease in HCV RNA of 1.61 $\log_{10}$ at the 400-mg-t.i.d. dosage. When given in combination with peg-IFN, mean decreases in HCV RNA were 2.48 $\log_{10}$ after 1 week and 2.88 $\log_{10}$ after 2 weeks (195). A phase II study examining the combination of boceprevir with peg-IFN and ribavirin for prior nonresponders is underway.

HCV Polymerase Inhibitors

The HCV NS5B RNA-dependent RNA polymerase synthesizes the initial complementary negative-strand RNA template, as well as the subsequent positive-strand genomic RNA. Nucleoside and nonnucleoside inhibitors of this enzyme that are currently undergoing clinical trials are summarized below; preclinical-phase and early-phase agents are listed in Table 6.

R1626. R1626, a prodrug of R1479 (4′-azidocytidine) (Fig. 2), is a nucleoside HCV polymerase inhibitor. The triphosphorylated form, R1479-TP, inhibits NS5B-dependent RNA polymerase by competing with CTP (123). In replicon cells, R1479 inhibited HCV genotype 1b replication, with an IC_{50} of 1.28 μM. No changes in cell viability were seen in doses of R1479 up to 2 mM. The S282T mutation in the NS5B polymerase, which confers resistance to other inhibitors (e.g., valopicitabine), does not affect R1479's ability to inhibit NS5B in replicon models, raising the possibility of future combination therapy within the nucleoside polymerase inhibitor class (123).

An initial study in HCV genotype 1-infected subjects showed that R1626 was generally well tolerated, was efficiently converted to R1479, and reversibly inhibited HCV in a dose-dependent manner. After 15 days of therapy with R1626, eight of nine subjects receiving 4,500 mg b.i.d. had normalization of ALT, and their mean reduction in HCV viral load in the 4,500-mg arm was 3.7 $\log_{10}$. After 4 weeks, R1626 in combination with peg-IFN and ribavirin resulted in an undetectable viral load in 81% of subjects, compared with 5% of those receiving peg-IFN and ribavirin together. Severe neutropenia and thrombocytopenia occurred in R1626 recipients, but these resolved after discontinuation of drug. Several mutations are associated with decreased sensitivity to R1626, including S96T and N142T, but neither mutation was found at baseline or after 4 weeks of therapy in one study.

PSI-6130 (R7128). PSI-6130 (β-D-2′-deoxy-2′fluoro-2′C-methylcytidine; R7128) (Fig. 2) is a pyrimidine nucleoside analog and a potent inhibitor of the HCV NS5B polymerase that acts as a chain terminator. It must be phosphorylated to the 5′-triphosphate form through the activities of deoxycytidine kinase, UMP-CMP kinase, and nucleoside diphosphate kinase. In a replicon model, PSI-6130 inhibited HCV genotypes 1a and 1b with similar activities. It has an EC_{90} of 5.4 μM in Huh 7 replicon cells, with no cytotoxicity or cytostasis (43).

A preliminary study of R7128, an oral prodrug of PSI-6130, in genotype 1-infected subjects who had failed to respond to prior peg-IFN and ribavirin therapy found that those receiving at least 750 mg b.i.d. achieved a >2-$\log_{10}$ drop in viral load after 14 days of monotherapy (183a). Of those with baseline ALT abnormalities, 78% had normalization of ALT after 14 days of R7128. The most common side effect was headache. After oral dosing of R7128, the $t_{1/2}$ of PSI-6130 in plasma was found to be approximately 5 h, but the active metabolite, PSI-6206, had a $t_{1/2}$ in plasma of approximately 20 h.

Immunomodulators

CsA. Discovered more than 30 years ago, the cyclic octapeptide cyclosporine (formerly called cyclosporin A) (CsA) is now widely used as an immunosuppressant. By binding cyclophilin, it forms a complex which inhibits calcineurin, thereby decreasing transcription of IL-2 and other lymphokines. CsA inhibits HCV in a replicon culture system (233) in a concentration-dependent manner, with an IC_{50} of approximately 0.5 μg/ml. The mechanism of action against HCV is not yet well understood but is likely mediated by its blockade of cyclophilins and appears to be independent of the IFN pathway and its immunosuppressive effects. The combination of CsA and IFN-α2b for 24 weeks was associated with a greater likelihood of SVR than IFN alone (55%, versus 32%), especially in those with genotype 1 and high baseline viral loads (SVR of 42%, versus 5%). CsA does not appear to exacerbate the many side effects of IFN, and the nephrotoxicity risk is low at the reduced CsA dose utilized (105). The anti-HCV activity of CsA has prompted research into the development of related molecules which might have similar activity but without the same immunosuppressive effects. Such development has led to the discovery of DEBIO-025.

DEBIO-025. DEBIO-025 is a synthetic, nonimmunosuppressive cyclosporine (Fig. 2). It differs from CsA in three ways: sarcosine is replaced by methylalanine at position 3, leucine is replaced by valine at position 4, and the nitrogen is ethylated instead of methylated (170).

SPECTRUM OF ACTIVITY. In Huh 5-2 replicon systems, both CsA and DEBIO-025 inhibit HCV replication, with a mean EC_{50} for DEBIO-025 of 0.27 μg/ml, which is 10-fold lower than that for CsA (2.8 μg/ml). In an HCV culture model in Huh 7-Lunet or Huh 7.5 cells, DEBIO-025 is also 10 times more potent than CsA and is able to completely clear cells of their HCV replicon, whereas CsA could not at similar concentrations. This raises the promising possibility of sustained viral eradication with use of DEBIO-025 (170). In HCV genotype 1b-infected chimeric mice transplanted with functional human hepatocytes, DEBIO-025 does not inhibit HCV replication, but when combined with peg-IFN it results in a 100-fold reduction, suggesting that these two agents may be synergistic against HCV genotype 1b. In contrast, when genotype 1a-infected chimeric mice were treated with CsA and peg-IFN, all mice died within 4 days (106).

MECHANISM OF ACTION. Because DEBIO-025 has been shown to inhibit HCV in subgenomic replicon models, it must have a mechanism of action which is independent of the structural proteins. One theory is that both CsA and DEBIO-025 inhibit the peptidyl-propyl *cis/trans* isomerase (PPIase) activity of cyclophilins (170). Cyclophilin B regulates HCV RNA-dependent RNA polymerase, and CsA was recently reported to inhibit this activity.

Both CsA and DEBIO-025 have activity against HIV type 1 (HIV-1) and prevent binding of cyclophilin A to the capsid of HIV-1. By binding to the viral capsid, cyclophilin A normally saturates the binding sites for TRIM5α/Ref1 host cell restriction factor and prevents it from inhibiting the viral Gag protein (94). Because of two modifications in the presumed calcineurin-binding domain, DEBIO-025 has very low affinity for calcineurin and thus lacks the immunosuppressive effects of CsA (170). The immunosuppressive effect of DEBIO-025 appears to be 7,000-fold lower than that of CsA in vitro.

PHARMACOLOGY. A 10-day course of DEBIO-025 at daily doses up to 1,200 mg appears to be safe and well tolerated. The drug has linear pharmacokinetics, and levels in plasma are 10 to 50 times higher than the replicon EC_{50} for HCV, with excellent tissue penetration. At doses of 1,200 mg given orally b.i.d., levels in plasma peak after approximately 2 h; accumulate over several weeks of dosing, with 5-fold increases in C_{max} and 10-fold increases in AUC; and show a multiphase decline, with a mean terminal $t_{1/2}$ of 100 h.

ADVERSE EFFECTS. At dosages of 1,200 mg b.i.d., 21% of those receiving DEBIO-025 discontinued therapy for hyperbilirubinemia. Bilirubin levels returned to normal following discontinuation of the study drug. High doses of DEBIO-025 may saturate biliary canalicular transporters, resulting in elevations of total bilirubin. Subjects receiving DEBIO-025 also show greater decreases in platelet counts than those treated with placebo; these also rapidly returned to normal levels following treatment completion. No data on adverse drug interactions are currently available.

RESISTANCE. Using replicon models, exposure of cells to increasing doses of DEBIO-025 can result in the generation of resistant strains which, although cross-resistant to CsA, remain sensitive to IFN and various protease and polymerase inhibitors (L. Coelmont, J. Paeshuyse, S. Kaptein, I. Vliegen, A. Kaul, E. de Clercq, B. Rosenwirth, P. Scalfaro, R. Crabbé, R. Bartenschlager, J. Dumont, and J. Neyts, presented at the International Conference on Antiviral Research, Palm Springs, CA, 2007).

CLINICAL APPLICATIONS. One recent controlled trial of DEBIO-025 (14 days at 1,200 mg b.i.d.) in human subjects coinfected with HIV and HCV found that the mean HCV viral load decreased by 3.6 $\log_{10}$, compared with 0.7 $\log_{10}$ in the placebo group (76). Recent data showing inhibition of HIV by DEBIO-025 have raised the possibility that the drug could be useful in the management of patients coinfected with HIV and HCV (181). Phase II studies examining the combination of DEBIO-025 with peg-IFN therapy in HCV-monoinfected subjects are currently underway.

TLR Agonists

TLRs are pattern recognition receptors which recognize diverse epitopes from a broad range of pathogens and stimulate an innate immune system response. There has been recent interest in the therapeutic potential of synthetic agonists against TLR-7 or TLR-9, with the hope that they could induce expression and release of endogenous IFN-α, eliminating the need for exogenous IFN injections (200). Several pharmaceutical companies have been developing such agents for the treatment of hepatitis C, although studies to date have been disappointing.

Miscellaneous

Celgosivir. Celgosivir is an investigational inhibitor of α-glucosidase I, a host enzyme required for HCV viral assembly and release. In one study, 57 previous nonresponders or partial responders infected with HCV genotype 1 were treated with celgosivir (400 mg daily) and peg-IFN with or without ribavirin for 12 weeks. Among nonresponders, a greater decrease in HCV RNA (1.2 $\log_{10}$, versus 0.4 $\log_{10}$) and more frequent early viral response (33%, versus 10%) occurred in those receiving celgosivir with peg-IFN and ribavirin than in those receiving dual peg-IFN and ribavirin alone. Celgosivir combination therapy has been reportedly well tolerated and resulted in no significant adverse events, although those receiving celgosivir had an increased frequency of diarrhea and flatulence.

Nitazoxanide. Nitazoxanide, an oral thiazolide, has activity against anaerobic bacteria, protozoa, and viruses and is approved in the United States (Alinia) for treatment of *Cryptosporidium* and *Giardia lamblia* infections. It has activity against HCV, although its mechanism of action is not yet known. In replicon studies, nitazoxanide selectively reduces intracellular HCV replication in AVA5 cells. This activity is synergistic with both IFN-α2b and an NS5B polymerase inhibitor (126). Nitazoxanide is also active against viral strains which had resistance to telaprevir and the NS5B polymerase inhibitor 2′-C-methylcytidine, suggesting an alternative mechanism of action. In a study examining nitazoxanide either with or without peg-IFN and ribavirin in genotype 4-infected, treatment-naïve patients, preliminary results showed that subjects receiving nitazoxanide monotherapy for 12 weeks followed by the triple combination for 36 weeks are more likely to have an undetectable viral load at 12 weeks after completing therapy than are those receiving dual peg-IFN and ribavirin for 48 weeks (79%, versus 43%).

Antiviral Agents for HBV

See chapter 5 on viral hepatitis and chapter 31 on HBV for additional information.

IFNs

In chronic HBV, approximately one-third of patients respond to peg-IFN administered at 52 μg/week for 52 weeks as reflected by loss of HBV e antigen (HBeAg) (115). Fewer than 10% of subjects, however, have an undetectable HBV DNA level or a loss of HBV surface antigen (HBsAg) at the end of follow-up (115, 175). The remissions with HBV are typically sustained, and the response to therapy is most strongly predicted by the pretreatment level of HBV DNA and HBV genotype (115, 175). Nonresponders to IFN therapy may benefit from the combination of IFN with HBsAg vaccination. Trials of combination therapy of HBV with lamivudine and IFN have been disappointing (115), and IFN treatment of HBV infection has been largely supplanted by the availability of a number of specific orally potent agents (see below).

Lamivudine

Clinical Use

In addition to its utility in the treatment of HIV (see chapter 11 on antiretroviral agents), lamivudine is effective in the treatment of chronic HBV infection. Similar to its mechanism against HIV, lamivudine inhibits HBV DNA polymerase-reverse transcriptase (Fig. 4; Tables 1 and 5). Treatment with 100 mg of lamivudine daily for 12 months normalizes the serum ALT level and improves histologic inflammatory scores in 50 to 70% of patients (131). A loss of HBeAg is seen in up to 30% of patients treated with lamivudine, and HBeAg seroconversion, defined as the loss of HBeAg, undetectable levels of serum HBV DNA, and the appearance of antibodies against HBeAg, is seen in up to 20% of patients (199). HBeAg seroconversion is associated with durable antiviral responses. For several years, lamivudine was recommended for the initial treatment of individuals with chronic HBV infection who had active virus replication and active liver disease, defined as a positive serum HBV DNA and elevated serum ALT level with evidence of moderate to severe hepatitis on liver biopsy. With growing concern about resistance, however (see below), and the development of alternative agents with higher barriers to resistance, monotherapy with lamivudine is now discouraged. Lamivudine is effective in the treatment of IFN-α2b nonresponders and in the prophylaxis of HBV recurrence in liver transplant patients (164). The combination of lamivudine with IFN-α for the treatment of chronic HBV infection has been disappointing, with most trials showing that the combination offers no benefit over either agent alone (115). Lamivudine is also being studied in combination with other antiviral agents such as tenofovir and in combination with immunomodulatory agents. In HIV-negative patients, lamivudine should be used at 100 mg daily; however, HIV-infected patients should generally receive the standard 150-mg-b.i.d. or 300-mg-once-daily dosage utilized for the treatment of HIV in combination with other antiretroviral agents. Such regimens should also include two agents active against HBV to try to prevent the emergence of HBV resistance.

Resistance

Resistance of HBV to lamivudine develops with prolonged therapy and is a major impediment to successful treatment. The frequency of genotypic resistance mutations increases from 24% of isolates after the first year to 67% after 4 years of therapy (52). Even higher rates of mutation have been seen in HIV- and HBV-coinfected patients given HIV treatment doses of lamivudine for long periods. The predominant lamivudine resistance mutations in HBV-infected patients are found in the catalytic domain of HBV polymerase in the YMDD motif, principally M204I or M204V (Table 7). These mutations may result in steric hindrance, preventing interaction between lamivudine and HBV polymerase. These mutations appear to decrease viral replication competence, but a frequently associated muta-

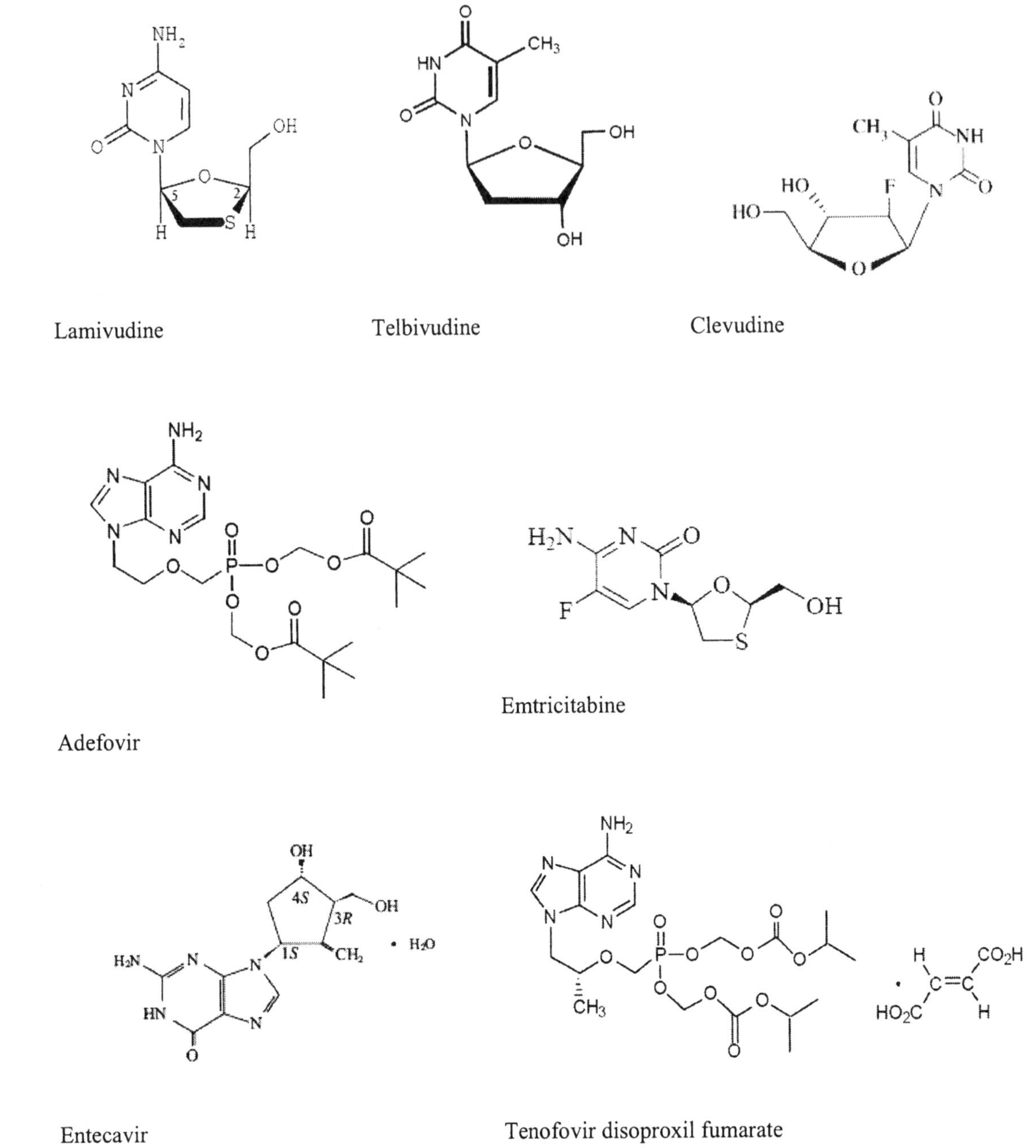

Lamivudine

Telbivudine

Clevudine

Adefovir

Emtricitabine

Entecavir

Tenofovir disoproxil fumarate

FIGURE 4 Chemical structures of anti-HBV agents.

TABLE 7 HBV mutations associated with drug resistance

Drug	Mutations within reverse transcriptase domain
Lamivudine	L80V/I,[a] A181T, V173L,[a] L180M,[a] M204V/I/S
Adefovir	L80I/V, A181V/T, L229W/V, I233V, N236T
Entecavir	I169L, L180M,[b] T184S/A/I/L/F/G, M204V/I,[b] S202C/G/I, M250V/I/L
Telbivudine	L180M,[a] M204I

[a]Secondary or compensatory mutation.
[b]Selected in early steps toward entecavir resistance.

tion, L180M, may restore viral fitness (168). Although withdrawal of therapy results in repopulation with wild-type virus, retreatment with lamivudine results in rapid emergence of resistant strains (140). Failure to achieve a $>1\text{-}\log_{10}$ drop in HBV viral load after 3 months of therapy appears to predict the emergence of lamivudine resistance.

Emtricitabine

Emtricitabine [(−)-β-2′,3′-dideoxy-5-fluoro-3′-thiacytidine; Emtriva] (Fig. 4; Tables 1 and 5) is a 5′-fluorinated derivative of lamivudine with the same mechanism of action and potency (see chapter 11 on antiretroviral agents). Although not FDA approved for the treatment of HBV, several studies have demonstrated the clinical efficacy of emtricitabine in chronic HBV infection. Like with lamivudine, however, resistance develops rapidly when the drug is used in monotherapy and selects the M204I/V mutation in the C domain (YMDD motif) of the HBV DNA polymerase.

Adefovir Dipivoxil

Adefovir dipivoxil [bis-pivaloyloxymethyl-9-(2-phosphonylmethoxyethyl)adenine; Hepsera] (Fig. 4; Tables 1 and 5) is the orally bioavailable prodrug of adefovir, an adenine nucleotide analog.

Spectrum of Activity

Adefovir dipivoxil has activity against several DNA and RNA viruses, including retroviruses, herpesviruses, and hepadnaviruses. It was initially developed for use in HIV-infected individuals, but this use was abandoned because of safety concerns at the dosing levels needed to inhibit HIV. It is active for HBV infection, however, when used at lower doses. The EC_{50} of adefovir for HBV is approximately 0.003 μg/ml, making it 10-fold more potent than tenofovir but half as potent as lamivudine in vitro (246). Because of its low oral bioavailability, however (see below), adefovir is inferior to both lamivudine and tenofovir at doses used clinically.

Mechanism of Action

Once absorbed, adefovir dipivoxil is converted to adefovir, which then undergoes two intracellular phosphorylation steps. The active intracellular metabolite of adefovir, 9-[2-(phosphonomethoxy)ethyl]adenine (PMEA) diphosphate, inhibits viral DNA polymerases by competing with dATP and terminating the DNA chain (39).

Pharmacology

Absorption of adefovir does not appear to be affected by food or stomach pH. About 10% of the absorbed dose is converted intracellularly to the active form, the long elimination $t_{1/2}$ (18 h) of which allows for once-daily dosing. Adefovir is not metabolized by cytochrome P450 enzymes.

Adverse Effects

The toxicities of adefovir at the doses used for treating HBV have been primarily gastrointestinal and hepatic, including nausea and transient increases in transaminase levels. At the higher doses used to treat HIV, gastrointestinal disturbances, elevated liver enzyme levels, and delayed renal effects, including renal tubular dysfunction mimicking the Fanconi syndrome, were seen (166).

Drug Interactions

The activity of adefovir appears to be unaffected or enhanced when the drug is combined with other anti-HBV agents. Adefovir coadministration may decrease delavirdine levels (75).

Resistance

Resistance to adefovir develops more slowly than resistance to lamivudine, with approximately 29% of patients demonstrating genotypic resistance after 5 years of adefovir monotherapy. Of note, however, only 20% of the patients had evidence of viral rebound and 11% had elevations in ALT (i.e., clinical resistance) (90). Several mutations are associated with adefovir resistance, including N236T and A181V (90), and although these mutations decrease susceptibility only 3 to 15% in vitro, hepatic flares and decompensation are seen (80). Primary adefovir resistance has been associated with the I233V mutation, but affected patients appear to remain susceptible to tenofovir and entecavir (37). Adefovir appears to be effective in treating lamivudine-resistant HBV.

Clinical Applications

Adefovir is effective for the treatment of chronic HBV in both HBeAg-positive and HBeAg-negative subjects. After 48 weeks of treatment with adefovir at 10 mg daily, the mean decrease in HBV DNA in HBeAg-positive subjects was 3.52 $\log_{10}$ copies/ml, compared with 0.55 $\log_{10}$ copy/ml in the placebo group (151). Results were similar in the trial of HBeAg-negative subjects (3.91 versus 1.35 $\log_{10}$ copies/ml) (91). Adefovir therapy also resulted in greater improvements in liver histology, decreases in ALT, and, in subjects who were HbeAg positive at the start of the study, higher rates of HBeAg seroconversion. Because of the substantial rates of resistance seen with prolonged adefovir therapy, however, the use of adefovir monotherapy is generally discouraged.

Entecavir

Entecavir {2-amino-1,9-dihydro-9-[(1*S*, 3*R*, 4*S*)-4-hydroxy-3-(hydroxymethyl)-2-methylenecyclopentyl]-6*H*-purin-6-one, monohydrate} (Fig. 4; Tables 1 and 5) is a guanine nucleoside analog.

Spectrum of Activity

Entecavir possesses potent and selective activity against hepadnaviruses. In cell culture, it is between 30- and 1,000-fold more active than lamivudine (104). Preclinical studies originally suggested that entecavir possessed no anti-HIV-1 activity, but in vivo activity resulting in an approximately 1-$\log_{10}$ reduction in plasma HIV-1 RNA level in humans has been described previously (155) (see "Resistance" below).

Mechanism of Action

After it is phosphorylated, entecavir interferes with multiple functions of HBV polymerase, including priming, reverse transcription, and DNA-dependent DNA synthesis (203).

Pharmacology

With once-daily dosing, steady state is achieved after 6 to 10 days. In healthy volunteers receiving 0.5 mg daily for 14 days, the C_{max} averaged 4.2 ng/ml and the elimination $t_{1/2}$ was 130 h (88). The intracellular $t_{1/2}$ for entecavir triphosphate is approximately 15 h. Oral administration of entecavir with a high-fat meal or a light meal results in significant delays in absorption, decreases in C_{max}, and decreases in AUC. Consequently, entecavir should be administered on an empty stomach. Entecavir is primarily eliminated unchanged by the kidneys, and the dosage should be adjusted in subjects with a creatinine clearance of less than 50 ml/min.

Adverse Effects

No significant adverse effects have been described to date.

Drug Interactions

Coadministration of entecavir with adefovir, lamivudine, or tenofovir resulted in no significant interactions (21). No interactions with other medications have been reported.

Resistance

Entecavir resistance rarely emerges in subjects with no prior nucleoside exposure, even after 2 years of monotherapy. Interestingly, although the M204V/I mutation associated with lamivudine resistance does not confer resistance to entecavir, it appears to be a prerequisite for such resistance. When combined with one of the lamivudine resistance mutations (M204V/I and L180M), three known mutations confer entecavir resistance (T184A/I/S, S202C/G, and M250I/L), although alone they are insufficient to cause such resistance (214). To date, prior lamivudine exposure, therefore, appears to be required for the development of entecavir resistance. In a study of lamivudine-refractory subjects treated with entecavir for 2 years, viral rebound occurred in 1% of subjects after 1 year and 9% after 2 years (214).

In preclinical testing, entecavir had no reported anti-HIV activity and was therefore used to treat HIV- and HBV-coinfected patients who did not yet need treatment for their HIV. However, coinfected subjects have developed an M184V mutation in HIV reverse transcriptase despite being on entecavir alone (155). It appears prudent, therefore, to avoid the use of entecavir in coinfected subjects who are not on a completely suppressive anti-HIV regimen.

Clinical Applications

Entecavir monotherapy has been compared to lamivudine in two large trials of HBeAg-positive and HBeAg-negative subjects with elevated ALT, detectable HBV DNA, and evidence of inflammation on liver biopsy. After 52 weeks, entecavir was superior to lamivudine for the frequency of histologic improvement (72% versus 62% in HBeAg-positive subjects [36] and 70% versus 61% in HBeAg-negative subjects [135]). Entecavir was also superior to lamivudine in frequency of undetectable HBV DNA (67% versus 36% in HBeAg-positive subjects and 90% versus 72% in HBeAg-negative subjects). Despite the resistance issues noted above, entecavir has been shown to be effective in HBeAg-positive subjects who are refractory to lamivudine (206), although a dose increase to 1 mg daily is recommended for patients with known resistance to lamivudine.

Telbivudine

Telbivudine (β-L-2′-deoxythymidine) (Fig. 4; Tables 1 and 5), a nucleoside analog, is a recently approved anti-HBV agent.

Spectrum of Activity

Telbivudine is a competitive inhibitor of the HBV DNA polymerase. Telbivudine has no activity against any human viruses other than HBV and does not inhibit human cellular polymerases. Inhibition of human mitochondrial DNA polymerase γ is felt to be the cause of much of the toxicity seen with other nucleoside analogs (e.g., neuropathy, myopathy, and lactic acidosis) (30).

Mechanism of Action

Telbivudine requires biotransformation to the triphosphate form, but unlike lamivudine, it preferentially inhibits anticomplementary (second-strand) DNA (204). Because it lacks a 3′-OH group, it acts as a chain terminator once incorporated into the growing DNA strand.

Pharmacology

In pharmacokinetic studies, the C_{max} following an oral dose of telbivudine was achieved in 0.8 to 2.8 h (134). The C_{max} ranged from 0.20 to 5.46 μg/ml, and the AUC was approximately 26 μg/ml · h. Telbivudine is cleared primarily via the kidneys and elimination is biphasic, with an intracellular $t_{1/2}$ of approximately 14 h and an elimination $t_{1/2}$ of approximately 40 h. Dose adjustments should be made in patients with a creatinine clearance of <50 ml/min.

Adverse Effects

Telbivudine is generally well tolerated. Elevations in serum creatine kinase have been more common in those receiving telbivudine than in those receiving lamivudine, although these were not associated with muscle-related adverse events (132). The package insert for all nucleoside analogs carries a boxed warning for lactic acidosis, though this has not yet been reported with telbivudine specifically.

Drug Interactions

One trial comparing telbivudine, lamivudine, and their combined administration in subjects with HBeAg-positive chronic HBV (133) found that more of the subjects receiving the combination had viral breakthrough and fewer achieved normalization of ALT or loss of HBeAg than those receiving telbivudine alone. Because there was no pharmacokinetic evidence of antagonism, there may be intracellular antagonism or interference between lamivudine and telbivudine.

Resistance

Resistance to telbivudine has developed at less than half the rate of resistance to lamivudine (5.0% versus 11% for HBeAg-positive subjects and 2.3% versus 10.7% for HBeAg-negative subjects) (132). The signature mutation associated with telbivudine resistance has been an M204I substitution in the HBV DNA polymerase (211). Individuals failing lamivudine were found to have either M204I, M204V, or a mixture, 204M/I/V. Telbivudine is active against strains with an isolated M204V mutation but inactive against strains with M204V plus L180M. In vitro, telbivudine remains active against strains resistant to adefovir (211).

Clinical Applications

One large study comparing telbivudine to lamivudine monotherapy showed that telbivudine is not inferior to lamivudine after 52 weeks (132). In the subgroup of HbeAg-positive subjects, telbivudine was superior to lamivudine for the primary endpoint (viral load of <5 $\log_{10}$ copies/ml coupled with normalization of ALT or loss of HBeAg), and both HBeAg-positive and HBeAg-negative subjects achieved greater and faster reductions in HBV DNA if they were receiving telbivudine.

When compared directly with adefovir in HBeAg-positive subjects (35), telbivudine treatment for 52 weeks resulted in a greater mean reduction in HBV DNA than adefovir treatment for 52 weeks or 24 weeks of adefovir followed by 28 weeks of telbivudine. Subjects in the telbivudine-only arm were also significantly less likely to experience primary treatment failure (2%, versus 29% in the adefovir-only arm).

Tenofovir

Tenofovir disoproxil fumarate (Fig. 4; Tables 1 and 5) is an oral prodrug of tenofovir, a nucleotide analog. Approved for the treatment of HIV infection (see chapter 11 on antiretroviral agents), it also has potent activity against HBV. Though not currently FDA approved for this indication, tenofovir shows clinical efficacy in the treatment of chronic HBV (177), particularly in HIV and HBV coinfection, in which it is often given coformulated with emtricitabine (Truvada). Changing to tenofovir often results in excellent viral suppression in subjects resistant to lamivudine who have viral breakthrough on adefovir (225). One pilot study demonstrated viral suppression for 80 weeks with a lower dose of tenofovir (75 mg) (57). When subjects were then changed to adefovir, almost half of them experienced a viral rebound. Combination therapy with lamivudine or emtricitabine may be superior to either drug alone in HIV and HBV coinfection. To date, there have been no reports of HBV variants with resistance to tenofovir.

Clevudine

Clevudine [1-(2-deoxy-2-fluoro-β-L-arabinofuranosyl) thymine] is an investigational nucleoside analog (Fig. 4) with potent activity against HBV. Like telbivudine, it has no effect on human cellular DNA polymerases or mitochondrial function. Clevudine is phosphorylated intracellularly to its active form, clevudine triphosphate. After daily oral dosing (50 mg/day) for 28 days, the C_{max} was 0.4 μg/ml, with a terminal $t_{1/2}$ of 61 h (89). Clevudine produced marked HBV DNA suppression as well as considerable persistent suppression following withdrawal of therapy. This prolonged effect does not occur in cell culture, and the mechanism remains unclear. In woodchucks, however, clevudine suppresses covalently closed circular DNA, resulting in a more sustained viral suppression than with other compounds (250). In a Korean phase III study, clevudine treatment for 24 weeks (30 mg orally daily) produced a profound drop in HBV DNA (5.1 $\log_{10}$, versus 0.27 $\log_{10}$ in the placebo group). Furthermore, those in the clevudine group had sustained viral suppression off therapy (3.73 $\log_{10}$ at week 34 and 2.02 $\log_{10}$ at week 48) (247). Adverse effects were no more common than in the placebo group. Plans for a global phase III registration study are underway.

ANTIVIRAL AGENTS FOR RESPIRATORY VIRUSES

See chapter 42 on influenza virus and chapter 36 on RSV and other paramyxoviruses for additional information.

Amantadine

Amantadine (1-adamantane amine hydrochloride; Symmetrel), a tricyclic amine (Fig. 5; Tables 1 and 8), was approved in the United States in 1966 for the treatment of influenza A. Amantadine belongs to the class of drugs known as adamantanes, which also includes rimantadine.

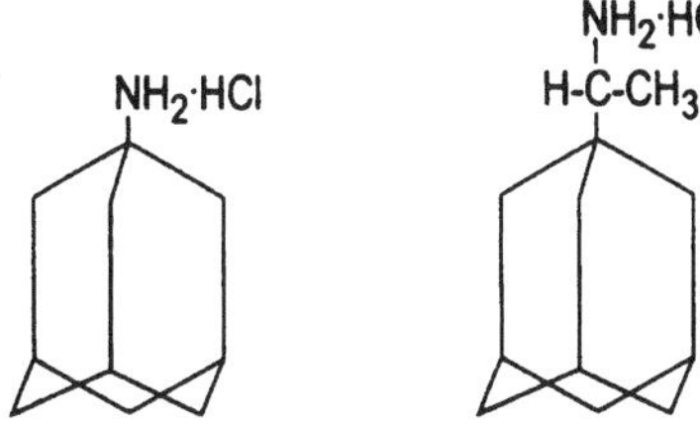

FIGURE 5 Chemical structures of amantadine (left) and rimantadine (right).

Spectrum of Activity

Amantadine is active against influenza A virus strains at clinically achievable concentrations. Inhibitory concentrations of susceptible isolates are generally in the range of 0.1 to 0.4 μg/ml. At approximately 100-fold-higher concentrations, in vitro inhibitory activity against other viral agents, such as influenza B virus and flaviviruses, including dengue virus (125), can be demonstrated, but such concentrations are not achievable in vivo and would be toxic. Amantadine's possible activity against HCV has not been shown to be clinically useful.

Mechanism of Action

Amantadine predominantly inhibits an early step in influenza A virus replication by interfering with the function of the viral M2 protein. Segment 7 of the influenza A virus RNA genome encodes two separate membrane proteins: M1 and M2. In the normal replication cycle, the M2 protein acts as a transmembrane ion channel facilitating the hydrogen ion-mediated dissociation of the matrix protein from the nucleocapsid. M2 also modulates the pH of the *trans*-Golgi network during transport of viral hemagglutinin. Thus, amantadine may act at a later step in the influenza A virus replication cycle by altering hemagglutinin formation.

Pharmacology

Amantadine is well absorbed, reaching the C_{max} in 2 to 4 h following an oral dose. Concentrations in the range of 0.5 to 0.8 μg/ml are typically achieved with the standard dosage of 100 mg b.i.d.; levels in nasal secretions approximate those in plasma (7). The primary route of elimination is renal, and over 90% of the drug is excreted unchanged in the urine. The elimination $t_{1/2}$ is 12 to 18 h in healthy young adults but is substantially prolonged in the setting of renal insufficiency and in the elderly. Dose adjustments are needed for these groups. Patients over the age of 65 years should receive half of the recommended dosage, i.e., 100 mg/day.

Adverse Effects

The major adverse effect of amantadine is neurotoxicity. Generally, CNS effects are minor and include lightheadedness, restlessness, insomnia, and mild cognitive difficulties. Such side effects may occur in up to one-third of patients. More serious neurotoxic reactions, including tremor, seizure, and coma, typically occur in elderly subjects or those with renal failure, situations in which drug can accumulate. The availability of rimantadine in some

TABLE 8 Respiratory virus agents: pharmacokinetics, major toxicities, and drug interaction characteristics

Agent	Oral bioavailability (%)	Effect of food on AUC	$t_{1/2}$ (h) in adults	Major route of elimination	Adjustment for renal insufficiency	Major toxicities	Major drug interactions
Amantadine	90	No	12–18	Over 90% renally excreted unchanged	Yes	Neurotoxicity, nausea, livedo reticularis, orthostatic hypotension, urinary retention	Neurotoxic agents may potentiate amantadine neurotoxic effects; trimethoprim-sulfamethoxazole and triamterene hydrochlorothiazide decrease amantadine excretion.
Rimantadine	>90	?	24–36	Mainly hepatically metabolized; <25% renally excreted unchanged	Yes	Neurotoxicity, nausea, vomiting	Acetaminophen and aspirin decrease rimantadine concentrations; cimetidine decreases rimantadine clearance.
Oseltamivir	>75	No	6–10	Hepatic metabolism to active form; renally eliminated	Yes	Nausea, vomiting; closely monitor for any neuropsychiatric symptoms in children	None
Zanamivir	4–17	NA	2–5	Renal, unchanged	No	Bronchospasm, decreased FEV_1, rash, oropharyngeal edema, headache, cough, nasal symptoms	None
Ribavirin (inhalational)	NA[a]	NA	9	Renal and hepatic	Yes	Bronchospasm, anemia, neurotoxicity; teratogenic, carcinogenic and mutagenic potential	Mitochondrial toxicity with didanosine; ? antagonize zidovudine

[a]NA, not applicable

countries means that it is best to avoid the use of amantadine in patients with a history of seizure disorder or psychosis. Minor gastrointestinal side effects are common, and with prolonged use (such as for Parkinson's disease), livedo reticularis, fluid retention, orthostatic hypotension, and urinary retention may occur, the last of these presumably related to the anticholinergic properties of the drug. Amantadine is teratogenic and therefore should not be used during pregnancy.

Drug Interactions

The major drug-drug interactions are those that potentiate the neurotoxic side effects. Therefore, drugs with antihistaminic or anticholinergic activity should be avoided, particularly in older subjects. Drugs which have been reported to decrease the excretion of amantadine include trimethoprim-sulfamethoxazole, triamterene, and hydrochlorothiazide (169).

Resistance

Diminished susceptibility (>100-fold changes) to amantadine is mediated by specific mutations in the M2 coding region of influenza A virus at codons 27, 30, 31, and 34 (19). Resistant isolates have been recovered readily from persons exposed to the drug. Amantadine-resistant strains can be isolated from 30% of treated subjects within 2 to 5 days, and resistant isolates are transmissible to household or institutional contacts. Although immunocompetent subjects from whom resistant strains are isolated have been reported to resolve their illness in the usual time frame when receiving amantadine, the transmission of resistant isolates to contacts abrogates the usefulness of amantadine prophylaxis. Prolonged shedding of resistant variants occurs in immunocompromised hosts.

In recent years, a dramatic increase in resistance to the adamantanes has developed in circulating H3N2 and, more recently, H1N1 viruses. Beginning in 2003, resistance prevalence rose from 1 to 3% to more than 70% in China and Hong Kong during a surveillance of H3N2 influenza viruses globally. Subsequently, an increase in resistant influenza A virus strains was observed in numerous countries (167). In the United States, the frequency of resistance among the H3N2 isolates rose from 1 to 2% to approximately 14% during the 2004–2005 season, increased to more than 92% during the 2005–2006 season, and was 99% during the 2007–2008 season, with resistance also observed in 8% of H1N1 subtype isolates (34). Adamantane-resistant influenza A virus strains typically possess a mutation in the M2 gene that leads to a Ser31Asn change and confers full cross-resistance to rimantadine but does not affect susceptibility to neuraminidase inhibitors (97, 192). Other mutations observed among H3N2 and H1N1 viruses isolated globally include Ala30Thr encoded by the M2 gene, which confers resistance to the adamantine class, along with Leu26Phe, Val27Ile, Val28Ile, Ala29Thr, and Ala29Val, which are not associated with resistance to the adamantanes. Hemagglutinin phylogenetic analysis of the H3N2 and H1N1 viral isolates showed that resistant viruses were introduced into human populations by at least two independent pathways, giving rise to distinct subclades (59).

In addition, clade 1 influenza A (H5N1) viruses found in Vietnam, Cambodia, and Thailand are consistently resistant to amantadine. In contrast, clade 0 H5N1 strains from Hong Kong in 1997 and, most recently, clade 2 H5N1 viruses, except for clade 2.1 viruses from Indonesia, have usually retained susceptibility to the adamantanes (97).

Clinical Applications

Amantadine is approved for prophylaxis and treatment of influenza A virus infections, but its use is currently discouraged because of widespread resistance (see chapter 42 on influenza virus). When this drug is given at the standard dosage of 200 mg/day, the prophylactic efficacy of this agent has been consistently reported to be in the range of 70 to 90% for susceptible strains (60). Efficacy has also been shown for postcontact prophylaxis in households and in outbreak control in closed populations. Amantadine treatment begun promptly after symptom onset can decrease the duration of fever and other symptoms by 24 to 48 h (60). Its usefulness in reducing complications of influenza virus infection or in the management of established influenza A pneumonia is unproven.

Because of the recent rise in resistance to amantadine and rimantadine, this class of antiviral agents is currently not recommended for influenza treatment or prophylaxis by the CDC. Instead, oseltamivir and zanamivir are recommended for these indications. This highlights the importance of annual surveillance for adamantane resistance in circulating influenza virus strains.

Amantadine has also been reported to be useful in the treatment of bipolar depression in individuals with evidence of Borna disease virus, but it is not clear if improvement is due to antiviral effects of amantadine or its inherent antidepressive effects (23).

Rimantadine

Rimantadine (alpha-methyl-1-adamantane methylamine hydrochloride; Flumadine, Roflual) (Fig. 5; Tables 1 and 8) is a tricyclic amine which is closely related structurally to amantadine.

Spectrum of Activity

The activity of rimantadine is exclusively against influenza A viruses at clinically achievable drug concentrations. It is up to 10-fold more active in vitro, with inhibitory concentrations ranging from 0.01 to 0.1 μg/ml (224). Rimantadine has an inhibitory effect on flaviviruses at higher concentrations in vitro, but this has not been shown to correlate with clinical efficacy (77).

Mechanism of Action

The mechanism of action of rimantadine against influenza A virus is identical to that of amantadine.

Pharmacology

Rimantadine, like amantadine, is well absorbed from the gastrointestinal tract, achieving a C_{max} of 0.4 to 0.5 μg/ml after repeated dosing (240). However, the two drugs differ in a number of important pharmacokinetic characteristics. In contrast to amantadine, rimantadine is concentrated in nasal secretions at a maximal achievable ratio of 1.75:1 (215). The elimination $t_{1/2}$ of rimantadine in plasma is 24 to 36 h, substantially longer than that of amantadine, and only 15 to 20% of an administered dose is excreted unchanged in the urine. The remainder is hepatically metabolized to ortho-, para-, and meta-hydroxy metabolites, which have 100- to 300-fold-less inhibitory activity than the parent compound (242), and then renally excreted. Older individuals have higher plasma drug levels than young adults when given the same dosage of 200 mg/day. Thus, the dosage should be halved in individuals older than 65 years. In patients with advanced liver or renal disease, the dosage should also be reduced by 50%.

Adverse Effects

The frequency of neurotoxic side effects is lower for rimantadine than amantadine, with treatment cessation rates in clinical trials averaging less than 5%. However, insomnia, minor cognitive difficulties, and, rarely, seizures have occurred. Minor gastrointestinal side effects (e.g., nausea) are common. Rimantadine is teratogenic and is classified as a pregnancy category C drug.

Drug Interactions

Only a few drugs have been studied carefully with respect to their effects on rimantadine clearance. Acetaminophen and aspirin decrease rimantadine clearance by 10 and 11%, respectively, and cimetidine increases clearance by 18%; however, adjustment of the rimantadine dosage is not necessary. As with amantadine, any other drug with neurotoxic potential should be used with caution in rimantadine-treated subjects.

Resistance

The mechanism of resistance to rimantadine is identical to that of amantadine (see above), and complete cross-resistance between these two agents exists. Amantadine- and rimantadine-resistant isolates remain susceptible to ribavirin and to the neuraminidase inhibitors.

Animal studies evaluating combination therapy with rimantadine and oseltamivir in avian H5N1 influenza viruses show increased antiviral effects and survival rates compared to treatment with each drug alone for adamantane-susceptible strains. Combination therapy with an adamantane and a neuraminidase inhibitor may decrease the development of drug resistance in such models (103). Combination treatment with amantadine and oseltamivir in a murine study was superior to single-drug therapy in H5N1 infection, with a 60 to 90% survival rate. The combination regimen was effective in preventing viral spread from the respiratory tract to the CNS. No mutations in the hemagglutinin, neuraminidase, and M2 proteins were seen with the combination therapy (103). One clinical trial assessing the efficacy of aerosolized zanamivir in combination with rimantadine found no resistance to rimantadine in those subjects who received combination therapy in contrast to rimantadine monotherapy (107). Further studies of combination therapy including ribavirin with a neuraminidase inhibitor or dual neuraminidase inhibitors are warranted.

Clinical Applications

Rimantadine, in general, has an efficacy comparable to that of amantadine for either prophylaxis or treatment of uncomplicated influenza A virus infections, and the indications for its use are similar to those discussed above. However, the improved side effect profile and tolerance of rimantadine make it the preferred agent for these indications in elderly and high-risk persons. As with amantadine, rimantadine is currently not recommended for influenza treatment and prevention given the significant increase in resistance in recent years. Clinical studies of rimantadine for refractory HCV infection have been disappointing (77).

Zanamivir

Zanamivir (5-acetylamino-4-[aminoiminomethylamino]-2,[iw-1]6-anhydro-3,4,5-trideoxy-D-glycero-D-galacto-non-2-enonic[ol0] acid; Relenza) (Fig. 6; Tables 1 and 8), an influenza virus neuraminidase inhibitor, was approved in the United States for the treatment of influenza A and B virus infections in 1999 and for prophylaxis in 2006.

Spectrum of Activity

Zanamivir is the first of a class of anti-influenza agents that potently and selectively reduce the replication of influenza

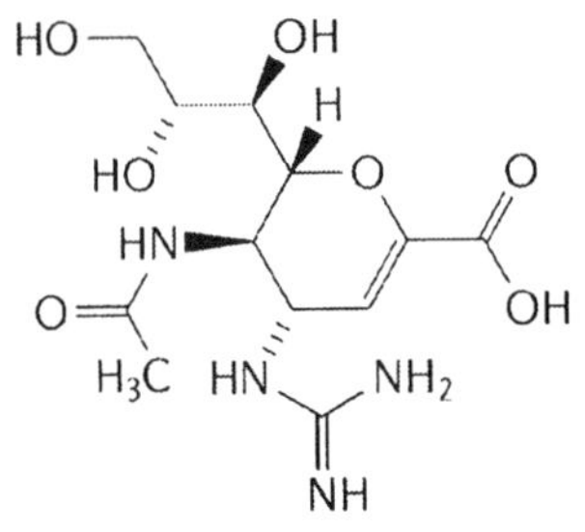

Zanamivir

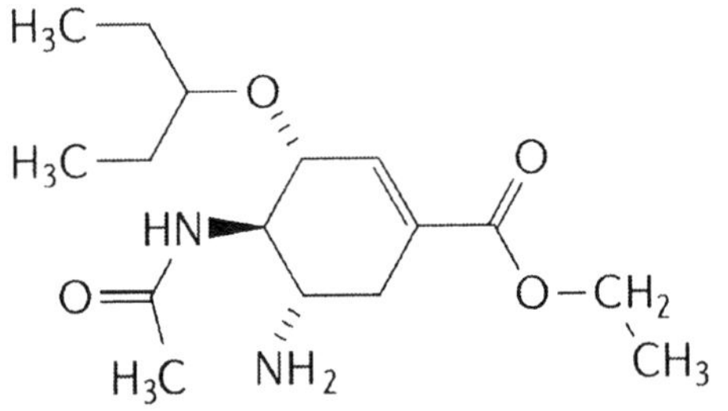

Oseltamivir

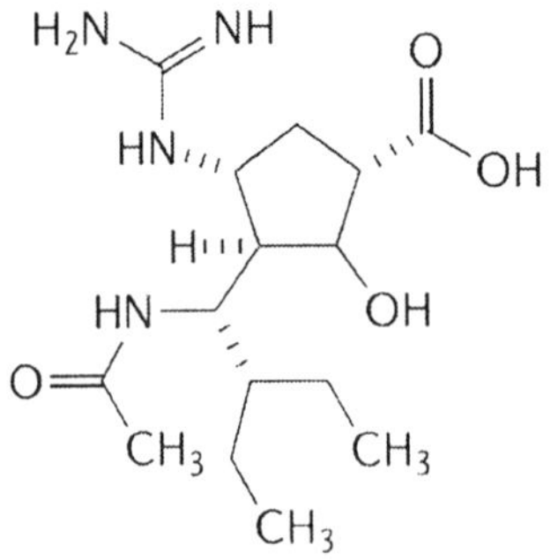

Peramivir

FIGURE 6 Chemical structures of anti-influenza virus agents.

A and B viruses through inhibition of influenza virus neuraminidase activity. Its IC_{50} for influenza A virus neuraminidase averages 0.9 ng/ml but ranges substantially among different neuraminidases. It has no activity against other viral neuraminidases or influenza C virus.

Mechanism of Action

Zanamivir was specifically designed to bind to the highly conserved active enzyme site of influenza virus neuraminidase. It interacts somewhat differently than oseltamivir with viral neuraminidase and consequently has a different spectrum of antiviral activity. Inhibition of influenza virus neuraminidase prevents the cleavage of silica acid residues, interfering with progeny virus dispersion and reducing infectivity.

Pharmacology

Zanamivir is available only as a dry-powder oral inhalation, since the absolute oral bioavailability is low, at 4 to 17%. Following a 10-mg dose of zanamivir, the C_{max} is achieved within 1 to 2 h and ranges from 17 to 142 ng/ml. Binding of zanamivir to human plasma protein is low (<10%). The elimination $t_{1/2}$ varies from 2.5 to 5.1 h. The increased drug exposure in individuals with severe renal impairment is not considered clinically relevant; no dosage adjustment is recommended for renal insufficiency or people older than 65 years. Elderly patients, especially those with cognitive impairment, may experience difficulty in using the inhaler device.

The safety and efficacy of intravenously administered zanamivir are of investigative interest, in part given its spectrum of activity against many oseltamivir-resistant variants and the current lack of a parenteral anti-influenza drug. Intravenously administered zanamivir provides high levels in blood, is distributed to the respiratory mucosa, and protects against infection and disease after challenge with experimental human influenza A virus. Clinical development of intravenously administered zanamivir is warranted.

Adverse Effects

Bronchospasm, decreased forced expiratory volume in 1 s (FEV_1), and decreased peak expiratory flow rates have been seen uncommonly in individuals treated with orally inhaled zanamivir. Severe respiratory distress, particularly in influenza virus-infected patients with preexisting lung disease, may lead to hospitalization and, rarely, death. As a result, zanamivir is not recommended for use in individuals with severe underlying airway disease, although the use of zanamivir in influenza patients with mild or moderate asthma appears to be safe (33). Other adverse events include headache, bronchitis, nausea, vomiting, and diarrhea, all of which occurred in no more than 3% of treated subjects, comparable to the effects of placebo. Allergic reactions, including oropharyngeal edema and skin rashes, occur rarely with zanamivir. Zanamivir is a pregnancy category C drug. Gravid rats given 1,000 times the human dose of zanamivir produced offspring with a variety of skeletal alterations. There are insufficient data concerning the safety of zanamivir in pregnant women.

Drug Interactions

Drug interactions with zanamivir are unlikely. Zanamivir is not an inducer or inhibitor of cytochrome P450 isoenzymes, is not metabolized by the liver, and does not affect drug metabolism in human liver microsomes. Protein binding is low. Inhaled zanamivir does not affect the humoral response to injected influenza vaccine.

Resistance

Clinical isolates resistant to zanamivir are very uncommon and were initially found in immunocompromised individuals (245). Prolonged treatment of one immunocompromised child with influenza B resulted in the emergence of a dual hemagglutinin and neuraminidase mutant (position 152) virus with reduced sensitivity (86). An immunosuppressed child with influenza B virus infection had an Asp198Asn mutation, with decreased sensitivity to both oseltamivir and zanamivir (108). Resistance has also been observed infrequently in community isolates of influenza B virus. In a Japanese study examining 74 children with influenza B virus infection who had received oseltamivir treatment, 1 (1.4%) had a viral isolate with decreased sensitivity to the neuraminidase inhibitors with a Gly402Ser mutation. Among 422 children and adults with untreated influenza virus infection, 7 had isolates with reduced susceptibility to oseltamivir and zanamivir with Asp198Asn, Ile222Thr, or Ser250Glu mutations (93). During the first 3 years of neuraminidase inhibitor use, from 1999 to 2002, two (<0.1%) A (H1N1) viral isolates showed >10-fold-decreased susceptibility to zanamivir (159). Oseltamivir-resistant variants with His274Tyr in N1 and Glu119Val or Arg292Lys in N2 remained sensitive to zanamivir. Zanamivir resistance was not observed in other subtypes during the same period (34).

Clinical Applications

Inhaled zanamivir is effective in the treatment of influenza A and B virus infections if given within 48 h of the onset of symptoms (160). In these studies, zanamivir reduced the duration of symptoms by 1 to 3 days (160). Early treatment with zanamivir also reduces antibiotic usage in adults and adolescents with influenza (116), but there are insufficient data to suggest that zanamivir prevents serious complications of influenza. Zanamivir, given at the usual adult dosage of 10 mg b.i.d., is safe and effective in children aged 5 to 12 years. Because of a low estimated treatment effect and inadequate inhalation technique in children aged 5 to 7 years, zanamivir treatment is approved by the FDA only for children older than 7 years. Zanamivir prophylaxis is approved for children older than 5 years.

The protective efficacy of zanamivir was approximately 79% in a number of large multicenter studies of postexposure prophylaxis (96). Postexposure prophylaxis with zanamivir for amantadine-resistant influenza A virus has also been demonstrated to be safe and efficacious (141). Zanamivir therapy does not affect antibody responses to influenza vaccination and may safely be given in combination with the vaccine (235).

In animal models and in vivo, zanamivir is active against influenza A virus (H5N1), including oseltamivir-resistant strains with the H274Y mutation; however, use of zanamivir for H5N1 in humans has not been directly assessed (201). A WHO panel weakly endorsed use of zanamivir to treat H5N1 infection because of a lack of data (201). Concerns about the effectiveness of zanamivir in treating influenza A virus (H5N1) infection in humans include inhaler dosing and systemic absorption.

Oseltamivir

Oseltamivir [ethyl(3*R*,4*R*,5*S*)-4-acetomido-5-amino-3-(1-ethylpropoxy)-1-cyclohexene-1-carboxylate; Tamiflu] (Fig. 6; Tables 1 and 8), a neuraminidase inhibitor, was approved for treatment of influenza in the United States in 1999 and for prevention of influenza in 2000.

Spectrum of Activity

Oseltamivir carboxylate (GS4071) is a potent inhibitor of influenza virus neuraminidase activity. It is specific for influenza A and B virus neuraminidases, and no clinically relevant activity is seen against other viral neuraminidases. Differences in levels of susceptibility to oseltamivir have been demonstrated among influenza A and B viruses, with a lower inhibitory effect of the drug on influenza B virus. In one study, the mean IC_{50}s for influenza A virus clinical isolates in neuraminidase inhibition assays ranged from 0.67 to 1.53 nM, whereas the mean IC_{50}s for influenza B virus clinical isolates varied from 10.01 to 11.53 nM (24). Similarly, in another study, the median IC_{50}s for influenza A virus H1N1 and H3N2 strains were 0.45 and 0.37 nM, respectively, while the median IC_{50} for influenza B virus was 8.50 nM (87). These differences in susceptibility may explain the reduced efficacy of oseltamivir in treating influenza B virus infection in children. Influenza C virus lacks a true neuraminidase and therefore is not inhibited by oseltamivir. Oseltamivir also has an immunosuppressive effect by blocking endogenous sialidase activity in host lung mononuclear cells, as sialidases are involved in modulating T-cell activation and cytokine production. One study showed that oseltamivir decreased $CD8^+$ T-cell-mediated immunity to RSV infection (161).

Mechanism of Action

Influenza virus neuraminidase catalyzes cleavage of the terminal sialic acid residues attached to glycoproteins and glycolipids, a process necessary for release of influenza virus virions from host cell surfaces and for spread of the virus through respiratory mucus. Oseltamivir is the orally available ethyl ester prodrug of GS4071, oseltamivir carboxylate, a highly potent influenza virus neuraminidase inhibitor. GS4071 is a carbocyclic transition state analog of sialic acid which binds to conserved residues within the active sites of influenza A and B virus neuraminidases and dissociates very slowly, effectively inhibiting enzymatic function (118). In preclinical studies, influenza virus neuraminidase cleaves sialic acid from pulmonary cells to expose receptors for *Streptococcus pneumoniae* adherence; neuraminidase inhibitors can inhibit this effect and reduce the mortality of secondary bacterial pneumonia.

Pharmacology

After oral administration, oseltamivir phosphate is readily absorbed from the gastrointestinal tract and converted to its active carboxylate metabolite with a bioavailability of at least 75%. The carboxylate is detectable in plasma within 30 min of administration, and a C_{max} of 348 to 551 ng/ml is reached within 3 to 4 h of a standard 75-mg dose. Administration of food has no significant effect on peak levels. In rat models, peak levels of drug within bronchoalveolar lining fluid are approximately the same as those in plasma and decline more slowly (66). Oseltamivir phosphate is converted into its active metabolite in the liver. Neither compound interacts with cytochrome P450 mixed-function oxidases or glucuronosyltransferases (99). The active metabolite is cleared unchanged by glomerular filtration and active tubular secretion in the kidneys, with a $t_{1/2}$ in plasma of 6 to 10 h in healthy young adults.

Exposure to both oseltamivir and its active metabolite is increased in elderly patients by approximately 25%, but no dose adjustment is necessary for this group. Young children (aged 1 to 12 years) clear oseltamivir faster than do older children and adults, and it is recommended that children up to the age of 12 years (or weighing up to 40 kg) receive approximately 2 mg/kg in unit doses of 30, 45, and 60 mg b.i.d. depending on their age and weight. Because clearance of the drug depends on renal function, individuals with creatinine clearances lower than 30 ml/min should be given 75 mg/day, half the usual daily dosage (99). In one study examining the safety and pharmacokinetics of oseltamivir and its active carboxyl metabolite in persons with mild and moderate hepatic disease, the C_{max} of oseltamivir was ≤6% lower in persons with hepatic impairment than that in healthy subjects, while the C_{max} of oseltamivir carboxylate was ≤19% lower. The mean AUC of oseltamivir was 33% higher than that in healthy subjects, whereas the mean AUC of the active metabolite was ≤19% lower. Other parameters, including time to C_{max}, $t_{1/2}$, and oral clearance, were comparable between hepatically impaired and healthy subjects. Oseltamivir was well tolerated by both groups. Therefore, no dose adjustment of oseltamivir is likely needed in persons with hepatic impairment.

Adverse Effects

Oseltamivir is generally well tolerated. The most common adverse effects are nausea and vomiting, which occur in 3 to 15% of subjects (99). Diarrhea, abdominal pain, dizziness, and headache were reported to occur in 2 to 20% of subjects, rates comparable to those for patients given placebo (99). Administration of oseltamivir with food decreases the risk of gastrointestinal side effects. Serious reactions such as aggravation of diabetes, arrhythmia, confusion, seizures, orofacial edema, toxic epidermal necrolysis, and unstable angina occur with a frequency of less than 1%, although a direct causal relationship is not proven (162). Oseltamivir is a pregnancy category C drug. In a rabbit model, a maternal dosage of 150 to 500 mg/kg/day resulted in a dose-dependent increase in minor skeletal abnormalities.

Serious neuropsychiatric adverse events related to oseltamivir therapy in adolescents were reported in Japan in 2007, prompting Japanese authorities to recommend against prescribing oseltamivir to persons aged 10 to 19 years in that country. In November 2007, the U.S. FDA recommended that revised precautions about serious neuropsychiatric events associated with pediatric oseltamivir use be included in package labeling for the drug. Physicians are advised to closely monitor patients for symptoms of abnormal behavior during oseltamivir treatment, and to assess the risks and benefits of continuing therapy in patients who develop these symptoms. More recently, the Japanese Ministry for Health, Labour and Welfare issued a preliminary analysis concluding no causal relationship between oseltamivir therapy and occurrence of severe neuropsychiatric events.

Drug Interactions

Neither oseltamivir nor its carboxylate interacts with cytochrome P450 enzymes. Both compounds have low protein binding. Coadministration of oseltamivir with cimetidine, an inhibitor of cytochrome P450 and competitor for renal tubular excretion, resulted in no effect on the levels of oseltamivir or its metabolite in plasma. Probenecid coadministration results in a twofold increase in oseltamivir exposure, but no dose adjustments are required due to the safety margin of oseltamivir. One in vitro study suggested that concurrent clopidogrel may reduce the antiviral activity of oseltamivir by inhibiting its hydrolysis to the carboxylate form; the clinical relevance of this effect is unproven (207).

Resistance

Oseltamivir treatment uncommonly results in the development of neuraminidase active-site mutations that confer drug resistance. Various neuraminidase mutations have been recognized in clinical isolates, most commonly Arg292Lys or Glu119Val in A (H3N2) virus, His274Tyr in A (H1N1) and A (H5N1) viruses, Asn294Ser in A (H5N1) virus, and Asp198Asn or Ile222Thr in B virus (184). Cross-resistance between oseltamivir and zanamivir is variable and depends on the specific mutation observed. Resistance to oseltamivir occurs more frequently in children than in adults. This may be explained by higher viral titers and longer periods of viral shedding in children (97). Influenza viruses resistant to oseltamivir have mostly remained sensitive to zanamivir and A-315675, an investigational neuraminidase inhibitor, and are partially sensitive to peramivir (97).

Global surveillance results from the Neuraminidase Inhibitor Susceptibility Network during the first 3 years of clinical use of the drug class showed a >10-fold decline in oseltamivir sensitivity in 8 (0.33%) of 2,287 influenza virus clinical isolates. None of these isolates were from persons who had previously received treatment with neuraminidase inhibitors (159). No oseltamivir resistance has been observed in recent influenza B virus strains or A (H3N2) isolates in the United States (34). However, during the 2007–2008 season, the His274Tyr mutation was found in variable proportions (0 to >60%) of H1N1 isolates in multiple countries, including an 8 to 10% prevalence in the United States, in the apparent absence of selective drug pressure. This mutation leads to a >400-fold reduction in susceptibility to oseltamivir (97). This mutation has also emerged in two of eight influenza A virus (H5N1)-infected patients given oseltamivir, both of whom died (56).

Clinical Applications

Oseltamivir is effective for treatment of influenza A and B virus infections in ambulatory adults if given within 36 h of the onset of symptoms and in children if given within 48 h. Treatment reduces the risk of complications leading to antibiotic use, including otitis media and perhaps pneumonia in children (237). Oseltamivir is associated with a lower rate of lower respiratory tract complications necessitating antibiotic therapy and a lower rate of hospitalization (162).

Postexposure prophylaxis of household contacts with oseltamivir (75 mg once daily) is protective, with an efficacy of 89% (236). Long-term prophylaxis with oseltamivir (75 mg daily or b.i.d.) for 6 weeks during peak influenza virus activity resulted in a protective efficacy of 74 to 82% depending upon the rate of influenza virus infection in the area (95). Oseltamivir therapy does not appear to interfere with antibody responses to natural infection or influenza vaccination.

Early initiation of oseltamivir to treat H5N1 infection is recommended, as it has been shown in several observational studies to reduce the mortality rate. Survival benefit was observed in persons with oseltamivir treatment compared to those with no treatment (29 to 67% survival rate, versus 0 to 33%). It is also recommended that persons with H5N1 infection who present at a late clinical stage be treated with oseltamivir, given that viral replication is often prolonged. Even with oseltamivir treatment, the mortality rate for H5N1 infection is high. Factors associated with poor prognosis are late initiation of treatment and persistence of viral replication after completion of standard therapy. It is unclear if severe diarrhea and gastric paresis experienced by persons with H5N1 infection affect drug absorption and bioavailability (244). A standard 5-day course of oseltamivir is advised. Modified treatment options, such as higher dosages of oseltamivir (150 mg b.i.d. in adults), prolonged duration (course increased to a total of 10 days), and combination regimen with the adamantanes, should be guided on a case-by-case basis. (244a).

Investigational Influenza Virus Agents

Peramivir

Peramivir (BCX-1812) (Fig. 6; Table 9) is a novel cyclopentane compound designed, using X-ray crystallography and structure-based drug design, to inhibit the active site of influenza virus neuraminidase.

Peramivir has a very low oral bioavailability (≤3%), a finding that led to abandonment of the oral formulation, and currently is under study using intravenous and intramuscular dosing routes. Peramivir is renally excreted, and the $t_{1/2}$ in plasma is estimated at 18 to 20 h in humans. It manifests a prolonged dissociation $t_{1/2}$ from influenza virus neuraminidase and is active in some animal models with single intramuscular dosing (16). In addition to intramuscular administration, testing of an intravenous peramivir formulation is currently in a phase I clinical trial.

A-315675

A-315675, a pyrrolidine-based compound, is a novel neuraminidase inhibitor that shows activity against influenza A virus strains similar to that of oseltamivir but is more potent against influenza B virus strains (1). Its isopropyl ester prodrug, A-322278, is active given orally in immunocompromised murine models of influenza (23a). Its antiviral spectrum is encouraging, but no clinical data regarding its safety and efficacy are currently available.

Other Neuraminidase Inhibitors

Long-acting neuraminidase inhibitors (LANI's) are second-generation neuraminidase inhibitors that display prolonged activity in the respiratory tract after inhaled administration. The long-lasting effects of LANI's permit once-weekly administration in animal models (234). Other investigational influenza agents are listed in Table 9.

Ribavirin

Ribavirin (1-β-D-ribofuranosyl-1,2,4-triazole-3-carboxamide, Virazole) (Fig. 2; Tables 1 and 8) is a synthetic nucleoside analog of guanosine approved in the United States for treatment of RSV infection and in combination with IFN-α for treatment of HCV (see "Antiviral Agents for HCV" above).

TABLE 9 Investigational respiratory viral agents

Agent or class	Mechanism of action	Phase	Remarks
Influenza virus			
Peramivir	Neuraminidase inhibitor	II	Phase II and III trials of oral peramivir did not show statistically significant improvement in time to relief of symptoms; intramuscular and intravenous formulations are currently being investigated.
A-315675 (A-322278 prodrug)	Neuraminidase inhibitor	Preclinical	Has activity against influenza A and B, limited cross-resistance between A-315675 and oseltamivir in vitro
Long-acting neuraminidase inhibitors	Neuraminidase inhibitor	Preclinical and II	Class includes CS-8958 and FLUNET, which are multimeric derivatives of zanamivir with prolonged activity in the respiratory tract after inhaled administration, permitting once-weekly dosing
Small interfering RNAs	Silent expression of virus M2 and nucleocapsid protein NP genes	Preclinical	Provide inhibition of virus-specific genes and do not affect cellular gene expression to a significant degree
Cyanovirin-N	Targets hemagglutinin	Preclinical	Has activity against influenza A and B strains resistant to neuraminidase inhibitors
T-705	Viral polymerase inhibitor	Preclinical	Oral administration; has activity against influenza A, B, and C in murine models; has high selectivity against viral replication without significant effects on cellular DNA and RNA synthesis
RSV			
JNJ-2408068	Fusion inhibitor	Preclinical	IC_{50}s of 2.1 nM in vitro and 0.9 nM in cell fusion assays
TMC353121	Fusion inhibitor	Preclinical	
Antisense oligodeoxynucleotides	Binds to complementary mRNA regions	Preclinical	
ALN-RSV01	Small interfering RNA	II	Phase I trials showed intranasal ALN-RSV01 to be well tolerated. A 38% decrease in RSV infection rate was observed.
RSV604	Inhibits N protein involved in RSV replication	II	Favorable pharmacokinetics with once-a-day oral dosing
Rhinovirus			
Pleconaril	Causes conformational changes in viral capsid	II	Oral pleconaril not approved by the U.S. FDA in 2002 because of hepatic CYP3A enzyme induction and drug interactions; currently being investigated as an intranasal formulation to prevent asthma exacerbations

Controversy exists about the precise role of ribavirin for treatment of lower respiratory tract RSV infections in children (see chapter 36 on RSV), because studies have not consistently shown virologic and/or clinical benefit for ribavirin recipients, and some have been criticized for design flaws (32). Ribavirin is also used to treat serious RSV infections in immunocompromised adults.

Intravenous ribavirin appears to be effective for the treatment of Lassa fever, hantavirus hemorrhagic fever with renal syndrome, and possibly Crimean-Congo hemorrhagic fever. Oral ribavirin may be an effective prophylaxis for Lassa fever, Crimean-Congo hemorrhagic fever, Rift Valley fever, and sandfly virus fever. Ribavirin has been used in treatment of influenza virus, parainfluenza virus, measles virus, adenovirus, human papillomavirus, and West Nile virus infections; however, its role remains unclear in these situations. Ribavirin is active against human metapneumovirus in vitro and in animal studies, and one case report indicated a successful outcome with intravenous ribavirin treatment in a lung transplant recipient with human metapneumovirus pneumonia complicated by respiratory failure and sepsis (182).

Ribavirin along with corticosteroids was used extensively as an empirical regimen during the early stages of the global outbreak of severe acute respiratory syndrome (SARS) caused by SARS-associated coronavirus but was later shown to lack in vitro activity against the virus.

Investigational RSV Agents

There are several different classes of investigational agents with activity against RSV in preclinical and early clinical development (Table 9). The fusion event of RSV is mediated by the viral F glycoprotein, which is made up of F1 and F2 subunits. The F1 subunit has two heptad repeat regions, HR1 and HR2. When the F protein changes shape, a stable HR1/HR2 six-helix structure is formed which leads to the fusion of viral and cellular membranes. JNJ-2408068, a benzimidazole compound, is a small molecule that binds to the F protein and interacts with HR1 and HR2 (1). TMC353121 is an RSV fusion inhibitor derived from the small molecule R170591 that had picomolar antiviral activity but was limited by its long elimination $t_{1/2}$ from several tissues, including the lungs (26).

Antisense oligodeoxynucleotides are short single-stranded molecules consisting of 18 to 25 nucleotides that bind to complementary mRNA regions. Endogenous ribonuclease H cleaves the RNA part of the newly formed RNA-DNA complex, causing degradation and preventing protein translation. A phosphorothioate oligodeoxynucleotide targeting RSV regions has exhibited potent in vitro activity (1). More recently, ALN-RSV01, a small interfering RNA directed against the mRNA encoding the viral nucleocapsid protein or N protein of RSV, was effective in decreasing viral replication in respiratory tissue in animal models. Two phase I clinical studies of intranasal administration of ALN-RSV01 showed the drug to be well tolerated, with mild to moderate side effects that were comparable in frequency and severity to those of the placebo group. Low systemic absorption of the drug was observed (58). Five-day treatment with intranasal ALN-RSV01 has shown antiviral activity in an adult volunteer model of experimentally induced RSV infection.

RSV604, formerly known as A-60444, is a novel compound that inhibits the N protein involved in RSV replication. Phase I data from healthy volunteers showed that the oral drug was well tolerated, without significant adverse effects. Phase II studies are currently in progress to evaluate use of the drug to treat RSV infections in stem cell transplant patients.

REFERENCES

1. **Abed, Y., and G. Boivin.** 2006. Treatment of respiratory virus infections. *Antivir. Res.* **70:**1–16.
2. **Andrei, G., J. Balzarini, P. Fiten, E. De Clercq, G. Opdenakker, and R. Snoeck.** 2005. Characterization of herpes simplex virus type 1 thymidine kinase mutants selected under a single round of high-dose brivudin. *J. Virol.* **79:**5863–5869.
3. **Andrei, G., E. De Clercq, and R. Snoeck.** 2004. In vitro selection of drug-resistant varicella-zoster virus (VZV) mutants (OKA strain): differences between acyclovir and penciclovir? *Antivir. Res.* **61:**181–187.
4. **Anonymous.** 1992. Mortality in patients with the acquired immunodeficiency syndrome treated with either foscarnet or ganciclovir for cytomegalovirus retinitis. Studies of Ocular Complications of AIDS Research Group, in collaboration with the AIDS Clinical Trials Group. *N. Engl. J. Med.* **326:**213–220.
5. **Anonymous.** 2002. A randomized controlled clinical trial of intravitreous fomivirsen for treatment of newly diagnosed peripheral cytomegalovirus retinitis in patients with AIDS. *Am. J. Ophthalmol.* **133:**467–474.
6. **Anonymous.** 2002. Randomized dose-comparison studies of intravitreous fomivirsen for treatment of cytomegalovirus retinitis that has reactivated or is persistently active despite other therapies in patients with AIDS. *Am. J. Ophthalmol.* **133:**475–483.
7. **Aoki, F. Y., and D. S. Sitar.** 1988. Clinical pharmacokinetics of amantadine hydrochloride. *Clin. Pharmacokinet.* **14:**35–51.
8. **Aoki, F. Y., S. Tyring, F. Diaz-Mitoma, G. Gross, J. Gao, and K. Hamed.** 2006. Single-day, patient-initiated famciclovir therapy for recurrent genital herpes: a randomized, double-blind, placebo-controlled trial. *Clin. Infect. Dis.* **42:**8–13.
9. **Ashley, R. L., and L. Corey.** 1984. Effect of acyclovir treatment of primary genital herpes on the antibody response to herpes simplex virus. *J. Clin. Investig.* **73:**681–688.
10. **Aweeka, F., J. Gambertoglio, J. Mills, and M. A. Jacobson.** 1989. Pharmacokinetics of intermittently administered intravenous foscarnet in the treatment of acquired immunodeficiency syndrome patients with serious cytomegalovirus retinitis. *Antimicrob. Agents Chemother.* **33:** 742–745.
11. **Aweeka, F. T., J. G. Gambertoglio, F. Kramer, C. van der Horst, B. Polsky, A. Jayewardene, P. Lizak, L. Emrick, W. Tong, and M. A. Jacobson.** 1995. Foscarnet and ganciclovir pharmacokinetics during concomitant or alternating maintenance therapy for AIDS-related cytomegalovirus retinitis. *Clin. Pharmacol. Ther.* **57:**403–412.
12. **Aweeka, F. T., J. G. Gambertoglio, C. van der Horst, R. Raasch, and M. A. Jacobson.** 1992. Pharmacokinetics of concomitantly administered foscarnet and zidovudine for treatment of human immunodeficiency virus infection (AIDS Clinical Trials Group protocol 053). *Antimicrob. Agents Chemother.* **36:**1773–1778.
13. **Aweeka, F. T., M. Kang, J. Y. Yu, P. Lizak, B. Alston, and R. T. Chung.** 2007. Pharmacokinetic evaluation of the effects of ribavirin on zidovudine triphosphate formation: ACTG 5092s Study Team. *HIV Med.* **8:**288–294.
14. **Bain, V. G., K. D. Kaita, E. M. Yoshida, M. G. Swain, E. J. Heathcote, A. U. Neumann, M. Fiscella, R. Yu,**

B. L. Osborn, P. W. Cronin, W. W. Freimuth, J. G. McHutchison, and G. M. Subramanian. 2006. A phase 2 study to evaluate the antiviral activity, safety, and pharmacokinetics of recombinant human albumin-interferon alfa fusion protein in genotype 1 chronic hepatitis C patients. *J. Hepatol.* **44:**671–678.

15. **Balfour, H. H., Jr., C. Benson, J. Braun, B. Cassens, A. Erice, A. Friedman-Kien, T. Klein, B. Polsky, and S. Safrin.** 1994. Management of acyclovir-resistant herpes simplex and varicella-zoster virus infections. *J. Acquir. Immune Defic. Syndr.* **7:**254–260.
16. **Bantia, S., C. S. Arnold, C. D. Parker, R. Upshaw, and P. Chand.** 2006. Anti-influenza virus activity of peramivir in mice with single intramuscular injection. *Antivir. Res.* **69:**39–45.
17. Reference deleted.
18. **Bell, W. R., J. D. Chulay, and J. E. Feinberg.** 1997. Manifestations resembling thrombotic microangiopathy in patients with advanced human immunodeficiency virus (HIV) disease in a cytomegalovirus prophylaxis trial (ACTG 204). *Medicine* (Baltimore) **76:**369–380.
19. **Belshe, R. B., M. H. Smith, C. B. Hall, R. Betts, and A. J. Hay.** 1988. Genetic basis of resistance to rimantadine emerging during treatment of influenza virus infection. *J. Virol.* **62:**1508–1512.
20. **Bernstein, D. I., S. L. Spruance, S. S. Arora, J. L. Schroeder, and T. C. Meng.** 2005. Evaluation of imiquimod 5% cream to modify the natural history of herpes labialis: a pilot study. *Clin. Infect. Dis.* **41:**808–814.
21. **Bifano, M., J. H. Yan, R. A. Smith, D. Zhang, D. M. Grasela, and F. Lacreta.** 2007. Absence of a pharmacokinetic interaction between entecavir and adefovir. *J. Clin. Pharmacol.* **47:**1327–1334.
22. **Biron, K. K., R. J. Harvey, S. C. Chamberlain, S. S. Good, A. A. Smith III, M. G. Davis, C. L. Talarico, W. H. Miller, R. Ferris, R. E. Dornsife, S. C. Stanat, J. C. Drach, L. B. Townsend, and G. W. Koszalka.** 2002. Potent and selective inhibition of human cytomegalovirus replication by 1263W94, a benzimidazole L-riboside with a unique mode of action. *Antimicrob. Agents Chemother.* **46:**2365–1272.
23. **Bode, L., D. E. Dietrich, R. Stoyloff, H. M. Emrich, and H. Ludwig.** 1997. Amantadine and human Borna disease virus in vitro and in vivo in an infected patient with bipolar depression. *Lancet* **349:**178–179.

23a. **Boivin, G., M. Baz, and Y. Abed.** 2007. Abstr. F1-946. *Abstr. 47th Intersci. Conf. Antimicrob. Agents Chemother.*

24. **Boivin, G., and N. Goyette.** 2002. Susceptibility of recent Canadian influenza A and B virus isolates to different neuraminidase inhibitors. *Antivir. Res.* **54:**143–147.
25. **Boivin, G., N. Goyette, C. Gilbert, and E. Covington.** 2005. Analysis of cytomegalovirus DNA polymerase (UL54) mutations in solid organ transplant patients receiving valganciclovir or ganciclovir prophylaxis. *J. Med. Virol.* **77:**425–429.
26. **Bonfanti, J. F., C. Meyer, F. Doublet, J. Fortin, P. Muller, L. Queguiner, T. Gevers, P. Janssens, H. Szel, R. Willebrords, P. Timmerman, K. Wuyts, P. van Remoortere, F. Janssens, P. Wigerinck, and K. Andries.** 2008. Selection of a respiratory syncytial virus fusion inhibitor clinical candidate. 2. Discovery of a morpholinopropylaminobenzimidazole derivative (TMC353121). *J. Med. Chem.* **51:**875–896. [Epub ahead of print.]
27. **Boon, R., J. J. Goodman, J. Martinez, G. L. Marks, M. Gamble, and C. Welch for the Penciclovir Cream Herpes Labialis Study Group.** 2000. Penciclovir cream for the treatment of sunlight-induced herpes simplex labialis: a randomized, double-blind, placebo-controlled trial. *Clin. Ther.* **22:**76–90.
28. **Boon, R. J., and D. R. Griffin.** 1995. Efficacy of famciclovir in the treatment of herpes zoster: reduction of pain associated with zoster. *Neurology* **45:**S76–S77.
29. **Bray, M., M. Martinez, D. Kefauver, M. West, and C. Roy.** 2002. Treatment of aerosolized cowpox virus infection in mice with aerosolized cidofovir. *Antivir. Res.* **54:**129–142.
30. **Brinkman, K., J. A. Smeitink, J. A. Romijn, and P. Reiss.** 1999. Mitochondrial toxicity induced by nucleoside-analogue reverse-transcriptase inhibitors is a key factor in the pathogenesis of antiretroviral-therapy-related lipodystrophy. *Lancet* **354:**1112–1115.
31. **Butt, A. A.** 2003. Fatal lactic acidosis and pancreatitis associated with ribavirin and didanosine therapy. *AIDS Read.* **13:**344–348.
32. **Carmack, M. A., and C. G. Prober.** 1995. Respiratory syncytial virus: antiviral therapy, p. 357–390. *In* D. J. Jeffries and E. DeClerq (ed.), *Antiviral Chemotherapy*. John Wiley & Sons, Ltd., Chichester, United Kingdom.
33. **Cass, L. M., K. A. Gunawardena, M. M. Macmahon, and A. Bye.** 2000. Pulmonary function and airway responsiveness in mild to moderate asthmatics given repeated inhaled doses of zanamivir. *Respir. Med.* **94:**166–173.
34. **Centers for Disease Control and Prevention.** 2008. Update: influenza activity—United States, September 30, 2007–February 9, 2008. *Morb. Mortal. Wkly. Rep.* **57:**1–5.
35. **Chan, H. L., E. J. Heathcote, P. Marcellin, C. L. Lai, M. Cho, Y. M. Moon, Y. C. Chao, R. P. Myers, G. Y. Minuk, L. Jeffers, W. Sievert, N. Bzowej, G. Harb, R. Kaiser, X. J. Qiao, and N. A. Brown.** 2007. Treatment of hepatitis B e antigen positive chronic hepatitis with telbivudine or adefovir: a randomized trial. *Ann. Intern. Med.* **147:**745–754.
36. **Chang, T. T., R. G. Gish, R. de Man, A. Gadano, J. Sollano, Y. C. Chao, A. S. Lok, K. H. Han, Z. Goodman, J. Zhu, A. Cross, D. DeHertogh, R. Wilber, R. Colonno, and D. Apelian.** 2006. A comparison of entecavir and lamivudine for HBeAg-positive chronic hepatitis B. *N. Engl. J. Med.* **354:**1001–1010.
37. **Chang, T. T., and C. L. Lai.** 2006. Hepatitis B virus with primary resistance to adefovir. *N. Engl. J. Med.* **355:**322–323. (Author's reply, **355:**323.)
38. **Cherrington, J. M., M. D. Fuller, P. D. Lamy, R. Miner, J. P. Lalezari, S. Nuessle, and W. L. Drew.** 1998. In vitro antiviral susceptibilities of isolates from cytomegalovirus retinitis patients receiving first- or second-line cidofovir therapy: relationship to clinical outcome. *J. Infect. Dis.* **178:**1821–1825.
39. **Cherrington, J. M., A. S. Mulato, M. D. Fuller, and M. S. Chen.** 1996. Novel mutation (K70E) in human immunodeficiency virus type 1 reverse transcriptase confers decreased susceptibility to 9-[2-(phosphonomethoxy) ethyl]adenine in vitro. *Antimicrob. Agents Chemother.* **40:**2212–2216.
40. **Chosidow, O., Y. Drouault, F. Leconte-Veyriac, M. Aymard, J. P. Ortonne, F. Pouget, J. Revuz, J. M. Decazes, and J. E. Malkin.** 2001. Famciclovir vs. aciclovir in immunocompetent patients with recurrent genital herpes infections: a parallel-groups, randomized, double-blind clinical trial. *Br. J. Dermatol.* **144:**818–824.
41. **Chou, S., and G. I. Marousek.** 2006. Maribavir antagonizes the antiviral action of ganciclovir on human cytomegalovirus. *Antimicrob. Agents Chemother.* **50:**3470–3472.
42. **Chou, S., L. C. Wechel, and G. I. Marousek.** 2007. Cytomegalovirus UL97 kinase mutations that confer maribavir resistance. *J. Infect. Dis.* **196:**91–94.

43. **Clark, J. L., L. Hollecker, J. C. Mason, L. J. Stuyver, P. M. Tharnish, S. Lostia, T. R. McBrayer, R. F. Schinazi, K. A. Watanabe, M. J. Otto, P. A. Furman, W. J. Stec, S. E. Patterson, and K. W. Pankiewicz.** 2005. Design, synthesis, and antiviral activity of 2′-deoxy-2′-fluoro-2′-C-methylcytidine, a potent inhibitor of hepatitis C virus replication. *J. Med. Chem.* **48:**5504–5508.
44. Reference deleted.
45. **Coen, D. M.** 1991. The implications of resistance to antiviral agents for herpesvirus drug targets and drug therapy. *Antivir. Res.* **15:**287–300.
46. **Coen, D. M., and P. A. Schaffer.** 2003. Antiherpesvirus drugs: a promising spectrum of new drugs and drug targets. *Nat. Rev. Drug Discov.* **2:**278–288.
47. **Corey, L., A. J. Nahmias, M. E. Guinan, J. K. Benedetti, C. W. Critchlow, and K. K. Holmes.** 1982. A trial of topical acyclovir in genital herpes simplex virus infections. *N. Engl. J. Med.* **306:**1313–1319.
48. **Cundy, K. C., B. G. Petty, J. Flaherty, P. E. Fisher, M. A. Polis, M. Wachsman, P. S. Lietman, J. P. Lalezari, M. J. Hitchcock, and H. S. Jaffe.** 1995. Clinical pharmacokinetics of cidofovir in human immunodeficiency virus-infected patients. *Antimicrob. Agents Chemother.* **39:**1247–1252.
49. **Curran, M., and S. Noble.** 2001. Valganciclovir. *Drugs* **61:**1145–1150; discussion, 1151–1152.
50. **Dal Pero, F., K. H. Tang, M. Gerotto, G. Bortoletto, E. Paulon, E. Herrmann, S. Zeuzem, A. Alberti, and N. V. Naoumov.** 2007. Impact of NS5A sequences of hepatitis C virus genotype 1a on early viral kinetics during treatment with peginterferon-alpha 2a plus ribavirin. *J. Infect. Dis.* **196:**998–1005.
51. **Darnell, J. E., Jr., I. M. Kerr, and G. R. Stark.** 1994. Jak-STAT pathways and transcriptional activation in response to IFNs and other extracellular signaling proteins. *Science* **264:**1415–1421.
52. **Das, K., X. Xiong, H. Yang, C. E. Westland, C. S. Gibbs, S. G. Sarafianos, and E. Arnold.** 2001. Molecular modeling and biochemical characterization reveal the mechanism of hepatitis B virus polymerase resistance to lamivudine (3TC) and emtricitabine (FTC). *J. Virol.* **75:**4771–4779.
53. **Davis, J. L., I. Taskintuna, W. R. Freeman, D. V. Weinberg, W. J. Feuer, and R. E. Leonard.** 1997. Iritis and hypotony after treatment with intravenous cidofovir for cytomegalovirus retinitis. *Arch. Ophthalmol.* **115:**733–737.
54. **De Clercq, E.** 2004. Discovery and development of BVDU (brivudin) as a therapeutic for the treatment of herpes zoster. *Biochem. Pharmacol.* **68:**2301–2315.
55. **De Clercq, E.** 1986. Towards a selective chemotherapy of virus infections. Development of bromovinyldeoxyuridine as a highly potent and selective antiherpetic drug. *Verh. K. Acad. Geneeskd. Belg.* **48:**261–290.
56. **de Jong, M. D., T. T. Tran, H. K. Truong, M. H. Vo, G. J. Smith, V. C. Nguyen, V. C. Bach, T. Q. Phan, Q. H. Do, Y. Guan, J. S. Peiris, T. H. Tran, and J. Farrar.** 2005. Oseltamivir resistance during treatment of influenza A (H5N1) infection. *N. Engl. J. Med.* **353:**2667–2672.
57. **Del Poggio, P., M. Zaccanelli, M. Oggionni, S. Colombo, C. Jamoletti, and V. Puhalo.** 2007. Low-dose tenofovir is more potent than adefovir and is effective in controlling HBV viremia in chronic HBeAg-negative hepatitis B. *World J. Gastroenterol.* **13:**4096–4099.
58. **DeVincenzo, J., J. E. Cehelsky, R. Alvarez, S. Elbashir, J. Harborth, I. Toudjarska, L. Nechev, V. Murugaiah, A. Van Vliet, A. K. Vaishnaw, and R. Meyers.** 2008. Evaluation of the safety, tolerability and pharmacokinetics of ALN-RSV01, a novel RNAi antiviral therapeutic directed against respiratory syncytial virus (RSV). *Antivir. Res.* **77:**225–231.
59. **Deyde, V. M., X. Xu, R. A. Bright, M. Shaw, C. B. Smith, Y. Zhang, Y. Shu, L. V. Gubareva, N. J. Cox, and A. I. Klimov.** 2007. Surveillance of resistance to adamantanes among influenza A(H3N2) and A(H1N1) viruses isolated worldwide. *J. Infect. Dis.* **196:**249–257.
60. **Douglas, R. G., Jr.** 1990. Prophylaxis and treatment of influenza. *N. Engl. J. Med.* **322:**443–450.
61. **Drew, W. L.** 1992. Cytomegalovirus infection in patients with AIDS. *Clin. Infect. Dis.* **14:**608–615.
62. **Drew, W. L., R. C. Miner, D. F. Busch, S. E. Follansbee, J. Gullett, S. G. Mehalko, S. M. Gordon, W. F. Owen, Jr., T. R. Matthews, W. C. Buhles, et al.** 1991. Prevalence of resistance in patients receiving ganciclovir for serious cytomegalovirus infection. *J. Infect. Dis.* **163:**716–719.
63. **Drew, W. L., R. C. Miner, G. I. Marousek, and S. Chou.** 2006. Maribavir sensitivity of cytomegalovirus isolates resistant to ganciclovir, cidofovir or foscarnet. *J. Clin. Virol.* **37:**124–127.
64. **Earnshaw, D. L., T. H. Bacon, S. J. Darlison, K. Edmonds, R. M. Perkins, and R. A. Vere Hodge.** 1992. Mode of antiviral action of penciclovir in MRC-5 cells infected with herpes simplex virus type 1 (HSV-1), HSV-2, and varicella-zoster virus. *Antimicrob. Agents Chemother.* **36:**2747–2757.
65. **Eid, A. J., S. K. Arthurs, P. J. Deziel, M. P. Wilhelm, and R. R. Razonable.** 2008. Emergence of drug-resistant cytomegalovirus in the era of valganciclovir prophylaxis: therapeutic implications and outcomes. *Clin. Transplant.* **22:**162–170.
66. **Eisenberg, E. J., A. Bidgood, and K. C. Cundy.** 1997. Penetration of GS4071, a novel influenza neuraminidase inhibitor, into rat bronchoalveolar lining fluid following oral administration of the prodrug GS4104. *Antimicrob. Agents Chemother.* **41:**1949–1952.
67. **Elion, G. B.** 1982. Mechanism of action and selectivity of acyclovir. *Am. J. Med.* **73:**7–13.
68. **Erice, A.** 1999. Resistance of human cytomegalovirus to antiviral drugs. *Clin. Microbiol. Rev.* **12:**286–297.
69. **Fardeau, C., M. Langlois, B. Mathys, P. Rafales, F. Nugier, V. Godard, M. Aymard, and J. Denis.** 1991. Emergence of cross-resistant herpes simplex virus following topical drug therapy in rabbit keratitis. *Curr. Eye Res.* **10(Suppl.):**151–158.
70. **Farrar, M. A., and R. D. Schreiber.** 1993. The molecular cell biology of interferon-gamma and its receptor. *Annu. Rev. Immunol.* **11:**571–611.
71. **Feldstein, T. J., J. L. Swegarden, G. F. Atwood, and C. D. Peterson.** 1995. Ribavirin therapy: implementation of hospital guidelines and effect on usage and cost of therapy. *Pediatrics* **96:**14–17.
72. **Field, A. K., M. E. Davies, C. DeWitt, H. C. Perry, R. Liou, J. Germershausen, J. D. Karkas, W. T. Ashton, D. B. Johnston, and R. L. Tolman.** 1983. 9-([2-Hydroxy-1-(hydroxymethyl)ethoxy]methyl)guanine: a selective inhibitor of herpes group virus replication. *Proc. Natl. Acad. Sci. USA* **80:**4139–4143.
73. **Fife, K. H., R. A. Barbarash, T. Rudolph, B. Degregorio, and R. Roth for The Valaciclovir International Herpes Simplex Virus Study Group.** 1997. Valaciclovir versus acyclovir in the treatment of first-episode genital herpes infection: results of an international, multicenter, double-blind, randomized clinical trial. *Sex. Transm. Dis.* **24:**481–486.
74. **Filer, C. W., G. D. Allen, T. A. Brown, S. E. Fowles, F. J. Hollis, E. E. Mort, W. T. Prince, and J. V. Ramji.**

1994. Metabolic and pharmacokinetic studies following oral administration of 14C-famciclovir to healthy subjects. *Xenobiotica* **24**:357–368.

75. **Fletcher, C. V., E. P. Acosta, H. Cheng, R. Haubrich, M. Fischl, R. Raasch, C. Mills, X. J. Hu, D. Katzenstein, R. P. Remmel, and R. M. Gulick.** 2000. Competing drug-drug interactions among multidrug antiretroviral regimens used in the treatment of HIV-infected subjects: ACTG 884. *AIDS* **14**:2495–2501.
76. **Flisiak, R. H., A. Horbans, P. Gallay, M. Bobardt, S. Selvarajah, A. Wiercinska-Drapalo, E. Siwak, I. Cielniak, J. Kierkus, J. Higersberger, C. Aeschlimann, P. Grosgurin, V. Nicolas-Métral, J.-M. Dumont, H. Porchet, R. Crabbé, and P. Scalfaro.** 2008. The cyclophilin inhibitor Debio-025 shows potent anti-hepatitis C effect in patients coinfected with hepatitis and human immunodeficiency virus. *Hepatology* **47**:817–826.
77. **Fong, T. L., M. W. Fried, and J. Clarke-Platt.** 1999. A pilot study of rimantadine for patients with chronic hepatitis C unresponsive to interferon therapy. *Am. J. Gastroenterol.* **94**:990–993.
78. **Fried, M. W., M. L. Shiffman, K. R. Reddy, C. Smith, G. Marinos, F. L. Goncales, Jr., D. Haussinger, M. Diago, G. Carosi, D. Dhumeaux, A. Craxi, A. Lin, J. Hoffman, and J. Yu.** 2002. Peginterferon alfa-2a plus ribavirin for chronic hepatitis C virus infection. *N. Engl. J. Med.* **347**:975–982.
79. **Funch, D. P., A. M. Walker, G. Schneider, N. J. Ziyadeh, and M. D. Pescovitz.** 2005. Ganciclovir and acyclovir reduce the risk of post-transplant lymphoproliferative disorder in renal transplant recipients. *Am. J. Transplant.* **5**:2894–2900.
80. **Fung, S. K., P. Andreone, S. H. Han, K. Rajender Reddy, A. Regev, E. B. Keeffe, M. Hussain, C. Cursaro, P. Richtmyer, J. A. Marrero, and A. S. Lok.** 2005. Adefovir-resistant hepatitis B can be associated with viral rebound and hepatic decompensation. *J. Hepatol.* **43**: 937–943.
81. **Fyfe, J. A.** 1982. Differential phosphorylation of (E)-5-(2-bromovinyl)-2′-deoxyuridine monophosphate by thymidylate kinases from herpes simplex viruses types 1 and 2 and varicella zoster virus. *Mol. Pharmacol.* **21**:432–437.
82. **Gilbert, C., J. Bestman-Smith, and G. Boivin.** 2002. Resistance of herpesviruses to antiviral drugs: clinical impacts and molecular mechanisms. *Drug Resist. Updates* **5**: 88–114.
83. **Gish, R. G.** 2006. Treating HCV with ribavirin analogues and ribavirin-like molecules. *J. Antimicrob. Chemother.* **57**:8–13.
84. **Gish, R. G., S. Arora, K. Rajender Reddy, D. R. Nelson, C. O'Brien, Y. Xu, and B. Murphy.** 2007. Virological response and safety outcomes in therapy-naive patients treated for chronic hepatitis C with taribavirin or ribavirin in combination with pegylated interferon alfa-2a: a randomized, phase 2 study. *J. Hepatol.* **47**:51–59.
85. **Griffiths, P. D., J. E. Feinberg, J. Fry, C. Sabin, L. Dix, D. Gor, A. Ansari, and V. C. Emery for the AIDS Clinical Trials Group Protocol 204/Glaxo Wellcome 123-014 International CMV Prophylaxis Study Group.** 1998. The effect of valaciclovir on cytomegalovirus viremia and viruria detected by polymerase chain reaction in patients with advanced human immunodeficiency virus disease. *J. Infect. Dis.* **177**:57–64.
86. **Gubareva, L. V., M. N. Matrosovich, M. K. Brenner, R. C. Bethell, and R. G. Webster.** 1998. Evidence for zanamivir resistance in an immunocompromised child infected with influenza B virus. *J. Infect. Dis.* **178**:1257–1262.
87. **Gubareva, L. V., R. G. Webster, and F. G. Hayden.** 2001. Comparison of the activities of zanamivir, oseltamivir, and RWJ-270201 against clinical isolates of influenza virus and neuraminidase inhibitor-resistant variants. *Antimicrob. Agents Chemother.* **45**:3403–3408.
88. **Hadziyannis, S. J.** 2006. New developments in the treatment of chronic hepatitis B. *Expert Opin. Biol. Ther.* **6**:913–921.
89. **Hadziyannis, S. J., H. Sette, Jr., T. R. Morgan, V. Balan, M. Diago, P. Marcellin, G. Ramadori, H. Bodenheimer, Jr., D. Bernstein, M. Rizzetto, S. Zeuzem, P. J. Pockros, A. Lin, and A. M. Ackrill.** 2004. Peginterferon-alpha2a and ribavirin combination therapy in chronic hepatitis C: a randomized study of treatment duration and ribavirin dose. *Ann. Intern. Med.* **140**:346–355.
90. **Hadziyannis, S. J., N. C. Tassopoulos, E. J. Heathcote, T. T. Chang, G. Kitis, M. Rizzetto, P. Marcellin, S. G. Lim, Z. Goodman, J. Ma, S. Arterburn, S. Xiong, G. Currie, and C. L. Brosgart.** 2005. Long-term therapy with adefovir dipivoxil for HBeAg-negative chronic hepatitis B. *N. Engl. J. Med.* **352**:2673–2681.
91. **Hadziyannis, S. J., N. C. Tassopoulos, E. J. Heathcote, T. T. Chang, G. Kitis, M. Rizzetto, P. Marcellin, S. G. Lim, Z. Goodman, M. S. Wulfsohn, S. Xiong, J. Fry, and C. L. Brosgart.** 2003. Adefovir dipivoxil for the treatment of hepatitis B e antigen-negative chronic hepatitis B. *N. Engl. J. Med.* **348**:800–807.
92. **Hardy, D., S. Spector, B. Polsky, C. Crumpacker, C. van der Horst, G. Holland, W. Freeman, M. H. Heinemann, G. Sharuk, J. Klystra, et al.** 1994. Combination of ganciclovir and granulocyte-macrophage colony-stimulating factor in the treatment of cytomegalovirus retinitis in AIDS patients. The ACTG 073 Team. *Eur. J. Clin. Microbiol. Infect. Dis.* **13**(Suppl. 2): S34–S40.
93. **Hatakeyama, S., N. Sugaya, M. Ito, M. Yamazaki, M. Ichikawa, K. Kimura, M. Kiso, H. Shimizu, C. Kawakami, K. Koike, K. Mitamura, and Y. Kawaoka.** 2007. Emergence of influenza B viruses with reduced sensitivity to neuraminidase inhibitors. *JAMA* **297**:1435–1442.
94. **Hatziioannou, T., D. Perez-Caballero, S. Cowan, and P. D. Bieniasz.** 2005. Cyclophilin interactions with incoming human immunodeficiency virus type 1 capsids with opposing effects on infectivity in human cells. *J. Virol.* **79**:176–183.
95. **Hayden, F. G., R. L. Atmar, M. Schilling, C. Johnson, D. Poretz, D. Paar, L. Huson, P. Ward, and R. G. Mills.** 1999. Use of the selective oral neuraminidase inhibitor oseltamivir to prevent influenza. *N. Engl. J. Med.* **341**:1336–1343.
96. **Hayden, F. G., L. V. Gubareva, A. S. Monto, T. C. Klein, M. J. Elliot, J. M. Hammond, S. J. Sharp, and M. J. Ossi for The Zanamivir Family Study Group.** 2000. Inhaled zanamivir for the prevention of influenza in families. *N. Engl. J. Med.* **343**:1282–1289.
97. **Hayden, F. G., and A. T. Pavia.** 2006. Antiviral management of seasonal and pandemic influenza. *J. Infect. Dis.* **194**(Suppl. 2):S119–S126.
98. **Hazari, S., L. Taylor, S. Haque, R. F. Garry, S. Florman, R. Luftig, F. Regenstein, and S. Dash.** 2007. Reduced expression of Jak-1 and Tyk-2 proteins leads to interferon resistance in hepatitis C virus replicon. *Virol. J.* **4**:89.
99. **He, G., J. Massarella, and P. Ward.** 1999. Clinical pharmacokinetics of the prodrug oseltamivir and its active metabolite Ro 64-0802. *Clin. Pharmacokinet.* **37**:471–484.
100. **Hengge, U. R., N. H. Brockmeyer, R. Malessa, U. Ravens, and M. Goos.** 1993. Foscarnet penetrates the

blood-brain barrier: rationale for therapy of cytomegalovirus encephalitis. *Antimicrob. Agents Chemother.* **37:** 1010–1014.

101. **Ho, H. T., K. L. Woods, J. J. Bronson, H. De Boeck, J. C. Martin, and M. J. Hitchcock.** 1992. Intracellular metabolism of the antiherpes agent (S)-1-[3-hydroxy-2-(phosphonylmethoxy)propyl]cytosine. *Mol. Pharmacol.* **41:**197–202.
102. **Holland, G. N., R. D. Levinson, and M. A. Jacobson for the AIDS Clinical Trials Group Protocol 915 Team.** 1995. Dose-related difference in progression rates of cytomegalovirus retinopathy during foscarnet maintenance therapy. *Am. J. Ophthalmol.* **119:**576–586.
103. **Ilyushina, N. A., N. V. Bovin, R. G. Webster, and E. A. Govorkova.** 2006. Combination chemotherapy, a potential strategy for reducing the emergence of drug-resistant influenza A variants. *Antivir. Res.* **70:**121–131.
104. **Innaimo, S. F., M. Seifer, G. S. Bisacchi, D. N. Standring, R. Zahler, and R. J. Colonno.** 1997. Identification of BMS-200475 as a potent and selective inhibitor of hepatitis B virus. *Antimicrob. Agents Chemother.* **41:** 1444–1448.
105. **Inoue, K., K. Sekiyama, M. Yamada, T. Watanabe, H. Yasuda, and M. Yoshiba.** 2003. Combined interferon alpha2b and cyclosporin A in the treatment of chronic hepatitis C: controlled trial. *J. Gastroenterol.* **38:**567–572.
106. **Inoue, K., T. Umehara, U. T. Ruegg, F. Yasui, T. Watanabe, H. Yasuda, J. M. Dumont, P. Scalfaro, M. Yoshiba, and M. Kohara.** 2007. Evaluation of a cyclophilin inhibitor in hepatitis C virus-infected chimeric mice in vivo. *Hepatology* **45:**921–928.
107. **Ison, M. G., J. W. Gnann, Jr., S. Nagy-Agren, J. Treannor, C. Paya, R. Steigbigel, M. Elliott, H. L. Weiss, and F. G. Hayden.** 2003. Safety and efficacy of nebulized zanamivir in hospitalized patients with serious influenza. *Antivir. Ther.* **8:**183–190.
108. **Ison, M. G., L. V. Gubareva, R. L. Atmar, J. Treanor, and F. G. Hayden.** 2006. Recovery of drug-resistant influenza virus from immunocompromised patients: a case series. *J. Infect. Dis.* **193:**760–764.
109. **Jabs, D. A., C. Enger, M. Forman, and J. P. Dunn for The Cytomegalovirus Retinitis and Viral Resistance Study Group.** 1998. Incidence of foscarnet resistance and cidofovir resistance in patients treated for cytomegalovirus retinitis. *Antimicrob. Agents Chemother.* **42:** 2240–2244.
110. **Jabs, D. A., and P. D. Griffiths.** 2002. Fomivirsen for the treatment of cytomegalovirus retinitis. *Am. J. Ophthalmol.* **133:**552–556.
111. **Jacobson, M. A., J. Gallant, L. H. Wang, D. Coakley, S. Weller, D. Gary, L. Squires, M. L. Smiley, M. R. Blum, and J. Feinberg.** 1994. Phase I trial of valaciclovir, the L-valyl ester of acyclovir, in patients with advanced human immunodeficiency virus disease. *Antimicrob. Agents Chemother.* **38:**1534–1540.
112. **Jacobson, M. A., F. Kramer, Y. Bassiakos, T. Hooton, B. Polsky, H. Geheb, J. J. O'Donnell, J. D. Walker, J. A. Korvick, and C. van der Horst.** 1994. Randomized phase I trial of two different combination foscarnet and ganciclovir chronic maintenance therapy regimens for AIDS patients with cytomegalovirus retinitis: AIDS Clinical Trials Group Protocol 151. *J. Infect. Dis.* **170:** 189–193.
113. **Jacobson, M. A., and J. Mills.** 1988. Serious cytomegalovirus disease in the acquired immunodeficiency syndrome (AIDS). Clinical findings, diagnosis, and treatment. *Ann. Intern. Med.* **108:**585–594.
114. **Jacobson, M. A., S. Wilson, H. Stanley, C. Holtzer, J. Cherrington, and S. Safrin.** 1999. Phase I study of combination therapy with intravenous cidofovir and oral ganciclovir for cytomegalovirus retinitis in patients with AIDS. *Clin. Infect. Dis.* **28:**528–533.
115. **Janssen, H. L., M. van Zonneveld, H. Senturk, S. Zeuzem, U. S. Akarca, Y. Cakaloglu, C. Simon, T. M. So, G. Gerken, R. A. de Man, H. G. Niesters, P. Zondervan, B. Hansen, and S. W. Schalm.** 2005. Pegylated interferon alfa-2b alone or in combination with lamivudine for HBeAg-positive chronic hepatitis B: a randomised trial. *Lancet* **365:**123–129.
116. **Kaiser, L., C. E. Crump, and F. G. Hayden.** 2000. In vitro activity of pleconaril and AG7088 against selected serotypes and clinical isolates of human rhinoviruses. *Antivir. Res.* **47:**215–220.
117. **Karupiah, G., Q. W. Xie, R. M. Buller, C. Nathan, C. Duarte, and J. D. MacMicking.** 1993. Inhibition of viral replication by interferon-gamma-induced nitric oxide synthase. *Science* **261:**1445–1448.
118. **Kati, W. M., A. S. Saldivar, F. Mohamadi, H. L. Sham, W. G. Laver, and W. E. Kohlbrenner.** 1998. GS4071 is a slow-binding inhibitor of influenza neuraminidase from both A and B strains. *Biochem. Biophys. Res. Commun.* **244:**408–413.
119. **Keam, S. J., T. M. Chapman, and D. P. Figgitt.** 2004. Brivudin (bromovinyl deoxyuridine). *Drugs* **64:**2091–2097; discussion, 2098–2099.
120. **Kempf, D. J., C. Klein, H. J. Chen, L. L. Klein, C. Yeung, J. T. Randolph, Y. Y. Lau, L. E. Chovan, Z. Guan, L. Hernandez, T. M. Turner, P. J. Dandliker, and K. C. Marsh.** 2007. Pharmacokinetic enhancement of the hepatitis C virus protease inhibitors VX-950 and SCH 503034 by co-dosing with ritonavir. *Antivir. Chem. Chemother.* **18:**163–167.
121. **Kinghorn, G. R., E. B. Turner, I. G. Barton, C. W. Potter, C. A. Burke, and A. P. Fiddian.** 1983. Efficacy of topical acyclovir cream in first and recurrent episodes of genital herpes. *Antivir. Res.* **3:**291–301.
122. **Kirsch, L. S., J. F. Arevalo, E. Chavez de la Paz, D. Munguia, E. de Clercq, and W. R. Freeman.** 1995. Intravitreal cidofovir (HPMPC) treatment of cytomegalovirus retinitis in patients with acquired immune deficiency syndrome. *Ophthalmology* **102:**533–542; discussion, 542–543.
123. **Klumpp, K., V. Leveque, S. Le Pogam, H. Ma, W. R. Jiang, H. Kang, C. Granycome, M. Singer, C. Laxton, J. Q. Hang, K. Sarma, D. B. Smith, D. Heindl, C. J. Hobbs, J. H. Merrett, J. Symons, N. Cammack, J. A. Martin, R. Devos, and I. Najera.** 2006. The novel nucleoside analog R1479 (4′-azidocytidine) is a potent inhibitor of NS5B-dependent RNA synthesis and hepatitis C virus replication in cell culture. *J. Biol. Chem.* **281:** 3793–3799.
124. **Knox, K. K., W. R. Drobyski, and D. R. Carrigan.** 1991. Cytomegalovirus isolate resistant to ganciclovir and foscarnet from a marrow transplant patient. *Lancet* **337:**1292–1293.
125. **Koff, W. C., J. L. Elm, Jr., and S. B. Halstead.** 1980. Inhibition of dengue virus replication by amantadine hydrochloride. *Antimicrob. Agents Chemother.* **18:**125–129.
126. **Korba, B. E., A. B. Montero, K. Farrar, K. Gaye, S. Mukerjee, M. S. Ayers, and J. F. Rossignol.** 2007. Nitazoxanide, tizoxanide and other thiazolides are potent inhibitors of hepatitis B virus and hepatitis C virus replication. *Antivir. Res.* **77:**56–63.
127. **Krawitt, E. L., T. Ashikaga, S. R. Gordon, N. Ferrentino, M. A. Ray, and S. D. Lidofsky.** 2005. Peginter-

feron alfa-2b and ribavirin for treatment-refractory chronic hepatitis C. *J. Hepatol.* **43:**243–249.

128. **Krosky, P. M., M. C. Baek, and D. M. Coen.** 2003. The human cytomegalovirus UL97 protein kinase, an antiviral drug target, is required at the stage of nuclear egress. *J. Virol.* **77:**905–914.
129. **Krown, S. E.** 1987. The role of interferon in the therapy of epidemic Kaposi's sarcoma. *Semin. Oncol.* **14:**27–33.
130. **Kuppermann, B. D., J. I. Quiceno, M. Flores-Aguilar, J. D. Connor, E. V. Capparelli, C. H. Sherwood, and W. R. Freeman.** 1993. Intravitreal ganciclovir concentration after intravenous administration in AIDS patients with cytomegalovirus retinitis: implications for therapy. *J. Infect. Dis.* **168:**1506–1509.
131. **Lai, C.-L., R.-N. Chien, N. W. Y. Leung, T.-T. Chang, R. Guan, D.-I. Tai, K.-Y. Ng, P.-C. Wu, J. C. Dent, J. Barber, S. L. Stephenson, and D. F. Gray for the Asia Hepatitis Lamivudine Study Group.** 1998. A one-year trial of lamivudine for chronic hepatitis B. *N. Engl. J. Med.* **339:**61–68.
132. **Lai, C. L., E. Gane, Y. F. Liaw, C. W. Hsu, S. Thongsawat, Y. Wang, Y. Chen, E. J. Heathcote, J. Rasenack, N. Bzowej, N. V. Naoumov, A. M. Di Bisceglie, S. Zeuzem, Y. M. Moon, Z. Goodman, G. Chao, B. F. Constance, and N. A. Brown.** 2007. Telbivudine versus lamivudine in patients with chronic hepatitis B. *N. Engl. J. Med.* **357:**2576–2588.
133. **Lai, C. L., N. Leung, E. K. Teo, M. Tong, F. Wong, H. W. Hann, S. Han, T. Poynard, M. Myers, G. Chao, D. Lloyd, and N. A. Brown.** 2005. A 1-year trial of telbivudine, lamivudine, and the combination in patients with hepatitis B e antigen-positive chronic hepatitis B. *Gastroenterology* **129:**528–536.
134. **Lai, C. L., S. G. Lim, N. A. Brown, X. J. Zhou, D. M. Lloyd, Y. M. Lee, M. F. Yuen, G. C. Chao, and M. W. Myers.** 2004. A dose-finding study of once-daily oral telbivudine in HBeAg-positive patients with chronic hepatitis B virus infection. *Hepatology* **40:**719–726.
135. **Lai, C. L., D. Shouval, A. S. Lok, T. T. Chang, H. Cheinquer, Z. Goodman, D. DeHertogh, R. Wilber, R. C. Zink, A. Cross, R. Colonno, and L. Fernandes.** 2006. Entecavir versus lamivudine for patients with HBeAg-negative chronic hepatitis B. *N. Engl. J. Med.* **354:**1011–1020.
136. **Lalezari, J., T. Schacker, J. Feinberg, J. Gathe, S. Lee, T. Cheung, F. Kramer, H. Kessler, L. Corey, W. L. Drew, J. Boggs, B. McGuire, H. S. Jaffe, and S. Safrin.** 1997. A randomized, double-blind, placebo-controlled trial of cidofovir gel for the treatment of acyclovir-unresponsive mucocutaneous herpes simplex virus infection in patients with AIDS. *J. Infect. Dis.* **176:**892–898.
137. **Lalezari, J. P., J. A. Aberg, L. H. Wang, M. B. Wire, R. Miner, W. Snowden, C. L. Talarico, S. Shaw, M. A. Jacobson, and W. L. Drew.** 2002. Phase I dose escalation trial evaluating the pharmacokinetics, anti-human cytomegalovirus (HCMV) activity, and safety of 1263W94 in human immunodeficiency virus-infected men with asymptomatic HCMV shedding. *Antimicrob. Agents Chemother.* **46:**2969–2976.
138. **Lalezari, J. P., W. L. Drew, E. Glutzer, C. James, D. Miner, J. Flaherty, P. E. Fisher, K. Cundy, J. Hannigan, J. C. Martin, et al.** 1995. (S)-1-[3-hydroxy-2-(phosphonylmethoxy)propyl]cytosine (cidofovir): results of a phase I/II study of a novel antiviral nucleotide analogue. *J. Infect. Dis.* **171:**788–796.
139. **Lalezari, J. P., G. N. Holland, F. Kramer, G. F. McKinley, C. A. Kemper, D. V. Ives, R. Nelson, W. D. Hardy, B. D. Kuppermann, D. W. Northfelt, M. Youle, M. Johnson, R. A. Lewis, D. V. Weinberg, G. L. Simon, R. A. Wolitz, A. E. Ruby, R. J. Stagg, and H. S. Jaffe.** 1998. Randomized, controlled study of the safety and efficacy of intravenous cidofovir for the treatment of relapsing cytomegalovirus retinitis in patients with AIDS. *J. Acquir. Immune Defic. Syndr. Hum. Retrovirol.* **17:**339–344.
140. **Lau, D. T., M. F. Khokhar, E. Doo, M. G. Ghany, D. Herion, Y. Park, D. E. Kleiner, P. Schmid, L. D. Condreay, J. Gauthier, M. C. Kuhns, T. J. Liang, and J. H. Hoofnagle.** 2000. Long-term therapy of chronic hepatitis B with lamivudine. *Hepatology* **32:**828–834.
141. **Lee, C., M. Loeb, A. Phillips, J. Nesbitt, K. Smith, and M. Fearon.** 2000. Zanamivir use during transmission of amantadine-resistant influenza A in a nursing home. *Infect. Control Hosp. Epidemiol.* **21:**700–704.
142. **Leeds, J. M., S. P. Henry, L. Truong, A. Zutshi, A. A. Levin, and D. Kornbrust.** 1997. Pharmacokinetics of a potential human cytomegalovirus therapeutic, a phosphorothioate oligonucleotide, after intravitreal injection in the rabbit. *Drug Metab. Dispos.* **25:**921–926.
143. **Leone, P. A., S. Trottier, and J. M. Miller.** 2002. Valacyclovir for episodic treatment of genital herpes: a shorter 3-day treatment course compared with 5-day treatment. *Clin. Infect. Dis.* **34:**958–962.
144. **Li, K., E. Foy, J. C. Ferreon, M. Nakamura, A. C. Ferreon, M. Ikeda, S. C. Ray, M. Gale, Jr., and S. M. Lemon.** 2005. Immune evasion by hepatitis C virus NS3/4A protease-mediated cleavage of the Toll-like receptor 3 adaptor protein TRIF. *Proc. Natl. Acad. Sci. USA* **102:**2992–2997.
145. **Limaye, A. P., L. Corey, D. M. Koelle, C. L. Davis, and M. Boeckh.** 2000. Emergence of ganciclovir-resistant cytomegalovirus disease among recipients of solid-organ transplants. *Lancet* **356:**645–649.
146. Reference deleted.
147. **Lin, C.-C., D. Lourenco, G. Xu, and L.-T. Yeh.** 2004. Disposition and metabolic profiles of [^{14}C]viramidine and [^{14}C]ribavirin in rat and monkey red blood cells and liver. *Antimicrob. Agents Chemother.* **48:**1872–1875.
148. **Ljungman, P.** 2001. Prophylaxis against herpesvirus infections in transplant recipients. *Drugs* **61:**187–196.
149. **Manns, M. P., J. G. McHutchison, S. C. Gordon, V. K. Rustgi, M. Shiffman, R. Reindollar, Z. D. Goodman, K. Koury, M. Ling, and J. K. Albrecht.** 2001. Peginterferon alfa-2b plus ribavirin compared with interferon alfa-2b plus ribavirin for initial treatment of chronic hepatitis C: a randomised trial. *Lancet* **358:**958–965.
150. **Marcelletti, J. F.** 2002. Synergistic inhibition of herpesvirus replication by docosanol and antiviral nucleoside analogs. *Antivir. Res.* **56:**153–166.
151. **Marcellin, P., T. T. Chang, S. G. Lim, M. J. Tong, W. Sievert, M. L. Shiffman, L. Jeffers, Z. Goodman, M. S. Wulfsohn, S. Xiong, J. Fry, and C. L. Brosgart.** 2003. Adefovir dipivoxil for the treatment of hepatitis B e antigen-positive chronic hepatitis B. *N. Engl. J. Med.* **348:**808–816.
152. **Marfori, J. E., M. M. Exner, G. I. Marousek, S. Chou, and W. L. Drew.** 2007. Development of new cytomegalovirus UL97 and DNA polymerase mutations conferring drug resistance after valganciclovir therapy in allogeneic stem cell recipients. *J. Clin. Virol.* **38:**120–125.
153. **Markham, A., and D. Faulds.** 1994. Ganciclovir. An update of its therapeutic use in cytomegalovirus infection. *Drugs* **48:**455–484.
154. **Martin, D. F., B. D. Kuppermann, R. A. Wolitz, A. G. Palestine, H. Li, and C. A. Robinson for The Roche Ganciclovir Study Group.** 1999. Oral ganciclovir for

patients with cytomegalovirus retinitis treated with a ganciclovir implant. *N. Engl. J. Med.* **340:**1063–1070.

155. **McMahon, M. A., B. L. Jilek, T. P. Brennan, L. Shen, Y. Zhou, M. Wind-Rotolo, S. Xing, S. Bhat, B. Hale, R. Hegarty, C. R. Chong, J. O. Liu, R. F. Siliciano, and C. L. Thio.** 2007. The HBV drug entecavir—effects on HIV-1 replication and resistance. *N. Engl. J. Med.* **356:**2614–2621.
156. **Mercorelli, B., E. Sinigalia, A. Loregian, and G. Palù.** 2008. Human cytomegalovirus DNA replication: antiviral targets and drugs. *Rev. Med. Virol.* **18:**177–210.
157. **Meurs, E., K. Chong, J. Galabru, N. S. Thomas, I. M. Kerr, B. R. Williams, and A. G. Hovanessian.** 1990. Molecular cloning and characterization of the human double-stranded RNA-activated protein kinase induced by interferon. *Cell* **62:**379–390.
158. **Meylan, E., J. Curran, K. Hofmann, D. Moradpour, M. Binder, R. Bartenschlager, and J. Tschopp.** 2005. Cardif is an adaptor protein in the RIG-I antiviral pathway and is targeted by hepatitis C virus. *Nature* **437:** 1167–1172.
159. **Monto, A. S., J. L. McKimm-Breschkin, C. Macken, A. W. Hampson, A. Hay, A. Klimov, M. Tashiro, R. G. Webster, M. Aymard, F. G. Hayden, and M. Zambon.** 2006. Detection of influenza viruses resistant to neuraminidase inhibitors in global surveillance during the first 3 years of their use. *Antimicrob. Agents Chemother.* **50:**2395–2402.
160. **Monto, A. S., A. Webster, and O. Keene.** 1999. Randomized, placebo-controlled studies of inhaled zanamivir in the treatment of influenza A and B: pooled efficacy analysis. *J. Antimicrob. Chemother.* **44**(Suppl. B):23–29.
161. **Moore, M. L., M. H. Chi, W. Zhou, K. Goleniewska, J. F. O'Neal, J. N. Higginbotham, and R. S. Peebles, Jr.** 2007. Cutting edge: oseltamivir decreases T cell GM1 expression and inhibits clearance of respiratory syncytial virus: potential role of endogenous sialidase in antiviral immunity. *J. Immunol.* **178:**2651–2654.
162. **Moscona, A.** 2005. Neuraminidase inhibitors for influenza. *N. Engl. J. Med.* **353:**1363–1373.
163. **Mulamba, G. B., A. Hu, R. F. Azad, K. P. Anderson, and D. M. Coen.** 1998. Human cytomegalovirus mutant with sequence-dependent resistance to the phosphorothioate oligonucleotide fomivirsen (ISIS 2922). *Antimicrob. Agents Chemother.* **42:**971–973.
164. **Naoumov, N. V., A. R. Lopes, P. Burra, L. Caccamo, R. M. Iemmolo, R. A. de Man, M. Bassendine, J. G. O'Grady, B. C. Portmann, G. Anschuetz, C. A. Barrett, R. Williams, and M. Atkins.** 2001. Randomized trial of lamivudine versus hepatitis B immunoglobulin for long-term prophylaxis of hepatitis B recurrence after liver transplantation. *J. Hepatol.* **34:**888–894.
165. **Neyts, J., R. Snoeck, J. Balzarini, and E. De Clercq.** 1991. Particular characteristics of the anti-human cytomegalovirus activity of (S)-1-(3-hydroxy-2-phosphonylmethoxypropyl)cytosine (HPMPC) in vitro. *Antivir. Res.* **16:**41–52.
166. **Noble, S., and K. L. Goa.** 1999. Adefovir dipivoxil. *Drugs* **58:**479–487; discussion, 488–489.
167. **Ong, A. K., and F. G. Hayden.** 2007. John F. Enders lecture 2006: antivirals for influenza. *J. Infect. Dis.* **196:** 181–190.
168. **Ono, S. K., N. Kato, Y. Shiratori, J. Kato, T. Goto, R. F. Schinazi, F. J. Carrilho, and M. Omata.** 2001. The polymerase L528M mutation cooperates with nucleotide binding-site mutations, increasing hepatitis B virus replication and drug resistance. *J. Clin. Investig.* **107:**449–455.
169. **Oxford, J. S., and A. Galbraith.** 1980. Antiviral activity of amantadine: a review of laboratory and clinical data. *Pharmacol. Ther.* **11:**181–262.
170. **Paeshuyse, J., A. Kaul, E. De Clercq, B. Rosenwirth, J. M. Dumont, P. Scalfaro, R. Bartenschlager, and J. Neyts.** 2006. The non-immunosuppressive cyclosporin DEBIO-025 is a potent inhibitor of hepatitis C virus replication in vitro. *Hepatology* **43:**761–770.
171. **Painter, G. R., and K. Y. Hostetler.** 2004. Design and development of oral drugs for the prophylaxis and treatment of smallpox infection. *Trends Biotechnol.* **22:**423–427.
172. **Patel, R., N. J. Bodsworth, P. Woolley, B. Peters, G. Vejlsgaard, S. Saari, A. Gibb, and J. Robinson.** 1997. Valaciclovir for the suppression of recurrent genital HSV infection: a placebo controlled study of once daily therapy. International Valaciclovir HSV Study Group. *Genitourin. Med.* **73:**105–109.
173. **Pavlovic, J., T. Zurcher, O. Haller, and P. Staeheli.** 1990. Resistance to influenza virus and vesicular stomatitis virus conferred by expression of human MxA protein. *J. Virol.* **64:**3370–3375.
174. **Perni, R. B., S. J. Almquist, R. A. Byrn, G. Chandorkar, P. R. Chaturvedi, L. F. Courtney, C. J. Decker, K. Dinehart, C. A. Gates, S. L. Harbeson, A. Heiser, G. Kalkeri, E. Kolaczkowski, K. Lin, Y. P. Luong, B. G. Rao, W. P. Taylor, J. A. Thomson, R. D. Tung, Y. Wei, A. D. Kwong, and C. Lin.** 2006. Preclinical profile of VX-950, a potent, selective, and orally bioavailable inhibitor of hepatitis C virus NS3-4A serine protease. *Antimicrob. Agents Chemother.* **50:**899–909.
175. **Perrillo, R. P., E. R. Schiff, G. L. Davis, H. C. Bodenheimer, Jr., K. Lindsay, J. Payne, J. L. Dienstag, C. O'Brien, C. Tamburro, I. M. Jacobson, et al.** 1990. A randomized, controlled trial of interferon alfa-2b alone and after prednisone withdrawal for the treatment of chronic hepatitis B. The Hepatitis Interventional Therapy Group. *N. Engl. J. Med.* **323:**295–301.
176. **Pescovitz, M. D., J. Rabkin, R. M. Merion, C. V. Paya, J. Pirsch, R. B. Freeman, J. O'Grady, C. Robinson, Z. To, K. Wren, L. Banken, W. Buhles, and F. Brown.** 2000. Valganciclovir results in improved oral absorption of ganciclovir in liver transplant recipients. *Antimicrob. Agents Chemother.* **44:**2811–2815.
177. **Peters, M. G., J. Andersen, P. Lynch, T. Liu, B. Alston-Smith, C. L. Brosgart, J. M. Jacobson, V. A. Johnson, R. B. Pollard, J. F. Rooney, K. E. Sherman, S. Swindells, and B. Polsky.** 2006. Randomized controlled study of tenofovir and adefovir in chronic hepatitis B virus and HIV infection: ACTG A5127. *Hepatology* **44:**1110–1116.
178. **Pfeiffer, J. K., and K. Kirkegaard.** 2005. Ribavirin resistance in hepatitis C virus replicon-containing cell lines conferred by changes in the cell line or mutations in the replicon RNA. *J. Virol.* **79:**2346–2355.
179. **Polis, M. A., K. M. Spooner, B. F. Baird, J. F. Manischewitz, H. S. Jaffe, P. E. Fisher, J. Falloon, R. T. Davey, Jr., J. A. Kovacs, R. E. Walker, S. M. Whitcup, R. B. Nussenblatt, H. C. Lane, and H. Masur.** 1995. Anticytomegaloviral activity and safety of cidofovir in patients with human immunodeficiency virus infection and cytomegalovirus viruria. *Antimicrob. Agents Chemother.* **39:**882–886.
180. **Prongay, A. J., Z. Guo, N. Yao, J. Pichardo, T. Fischmann, C. Strickland, J. Myers, Jr., P. C. Weber, B. M. Beyer, R. Ingram, Z. Hong, W. W. Prosise, L. Ramanathan, S. S. Taremi, T. Yarosh-Tomaine, R. Zhang, M. Senior, R. S. Yang, B. Malcolm, A. Arasappan, F. Bennett, S. L. Bogen, K. Chen, E. Jao, Y. T. Liu, R. G.

Lovey, A. K. Saksena, S. Venkatraman, V. Girijavallabhan, F. G. Njoroge, and V. Madison. 2007. Discovery of the HCV NS3/4A protease inhibitor (1R,5S)-N-[3-amino-1-(cyclobutylmethyl)-2,3-dioxopropyl]-3-[2(S)-[[[(1,1-dimethylethyl)amino]carbonyl]amino]-3,3-dimethyl-1-oxobutyl]-6,6-dimethyl-3-azabicyclo[3.1.0]hexan-2(S)-carboxamide (Sch 503034). II. Key steps in structure-based optimization. *J. Med. Chem.* **50:**2310–2318.

181. **Ptak, R. G., P. A. Gallay, D. Jochmans, A. P. Halestrap, U. T. Ruegg, L. A. Pallansch, M. D. Bobardt, M.-P. de Béthune, J. Neyts, E. De Clercq, J.-M. Dumont, P. Scalfaro, K. Besseghir, R. M. Wenger, and B. Rosenwirth.** 2008. Inhibition of human immunodeficiency virus type 1 replication in human cells by Debio-025, a novel cyclophilin binding agent. *Antimicrob. Agents Chemother.* **52:**1302–1317.

182. **Raza, K., S. B. Ismailjee, M. Crespo, S. M. Studer, S. Sanghavi, D. L. Paterson, E. J. Kwak, C. R. Rinaldo, Jr., J. M. Pilewski, K. R. McCurry, and S. Husain.** 2007. Successful outcome of human metapneumovirus (hMPV) pneumonia in a lung transplant recipient treated with intravenous ribavirin. *J. Heart Lung Transplant.* **26:**862–864.

183. **Read, R. C., F. J. Vilar, and T. L. Smith.** 1998. AIDS-related herpes simplex virus encephalitis during maintenance foscarnet therapy. *Clin. Infect. Dis.* **26:**513–514.

183a. **Reddy, R., M. Rodriguez-Torres, E. Gane, R. Robson, J. Lalezari, G. T. Everson, E. DeJesus, J. G. McHutchinson, H. E. Vargas, A. Beard, C. A. Rodriguez, G. Z. Hill, W. T. Symonds, and M. M. Berry.** 2007. Abstr. LB9. *Abstr. 58th Annu. Meet. Am. Assoc. Study Liver Dis.*

184. **Reece, P. A.** 2007. Neuraminidase inhibitor resistance in influenza viruses. *J. Med. Virol.* **79:**1577–1586.

185. **Reed, E. C., J. L. Wolford, K. J. Kopecky, K. E. Lilleby, P. S. Dandliker, J. L. Todaro, G. B. McDonald, and J. D. Meyers.** 1990. Ganciclovir for the treatment of cytomegalovirus gastroenteritis in bone marrow transplant patients. A randomized, placebo-controlled trial. *Ann. Intern. Med.* **112:**505–510.

186. **Reesink, H. W., S. Zeuzem, C. J. Weegink, N. Forestier, A. van Vliet, J. van de Wetering de Rooij, L. McNair, S. Purdy, R. Kauffman, J. Alam, and P. L. Jansen.** 2006. Rapid decline of viral RNA in hepatitis C patients treated with VX-950: a phase Ib, placebo-controlled, randomized study. *Gastroenterology* **131:**997–1002.

187. **Reichman, R. C., D. Oakes, W. Bonnez, D. Brown, H. R. Mattison, A. Bailey-Farchione, M. H. Stoler, L. M. Demeter, S. K. Tyring, L. Miller, et al.** 1990. Treatment of condyloma acuminatum with three different interferon-alpha preparations administered parenterally: a double-blind, placebo-controlled trial. *J. Infect. Dis.* **162:**1270–1276.

188. **Reusser, P., H. Einsele, J. Lee, L. Volin, M. Rovira, D. Engelhard, J. Finke, C. Cordonnier, H. Link, and P. Ljungman.** 2002. Randomized multicenter trial of foscarnet versus ganciclovir for preemptive therapy of cytomegalovirus infection after allogeneic stem cell transplantation. *Blood* **99:**1159–1164.

189. **Rooney, J. F., S. E. Straus, M. L. Mannix, C. R. Wohlenberg, D. W. Alling, J. A. Dumois, and A. L. Notkins.** 1993. Oral acyclovir to suppress frequently recurrent herpes labialis. A double-blind, placebo-controlled trial. *Ann. Intern. Med.* **118:**268–272.

190. **Sacks, S. L., R. A. Thisted, T. M. Jones, R. A. Barbarash, D. J. Mikolich, G. E. Ruoff, J. L. Jorizzo, L. B. Gunnill, D. H. Katz, M. H. Khalil, P. R. Morrow, G. J. Yakatan, L. E. Pope, and J. E. Berg.** 2001. Clinical efficacy of topical docosanol 10% cream for herpes simplex labialis: a multicenter, randomized, placebo-controlled trial. *J. Am. Acad. Dermatol.* **45:**222–230.

191. **Safrin, S., T. Assaykeen, S. Follansbee, and J. Mills.** 1990. Foscarnet therapy for acyclovir-resistant mucocutaneous herpes simplex virus infection in 26 AIDS patients: preliminary data. *J. Infect. Dis.* **161:**1078–1084.

192. **Saito, R., D. Li, Y. Suzuki, I. Sato, H. Masaki, H. Nishimura, T. Kawashima, Y. Shirahige, C. Shimomura, N. Asoh, S. Degawa, H. Ishikawa, M. Sato, Y. Shobugawa, and H. Suzuki.** 2007. High prevalence of amantadine-resistance influenza a (H3N2) in six prefectures, Japan, in the 2005–2006 season. *J. Med. Virol.* **79:**1569–1576.

193. **Sarisky, R. T., T. H. Bacon, R. J. Boon, K. E. Duffy, K. M. Esser, J. Leary, L. A. Locke, T. T. Nguyen, M. R. Quail, and R. Saltzman.** 2003. Profiling penciclovir susceptibility and prevalence of resistance of herpes simplex virus isolates across eleven clinical trials. *Arch. Virol.* **148:**1757–1769.

194. **Sarrazin, C., T. L. Kieffer, D. Bartels, B. Hanzelka, U. Muh, M. Welker, D. Wincheringer, Y. Zhou, H. M. Chu, C. Lin, C. Weegink, H. Reesink, S. Zeuzem, and A. D. Kwong.** 2007. Dynamic hepatitis C virus genotypic and phenotypic changes in patients treated with the protease inhibitor telaprevir. *Gastroenterology* **132:**1767–1777.

195. **Sarrazin, C., R. Rouzier, F. Wagner, N. Forestier, D. Larrey, S. K. Gupta, M. Hussain, A. Shah, D. Cutler, J. Zhang, and S. Zeuzem.** 2007. SCH 503034, a novel hepatitis C virus protease inhibitor, plus pegylated interferon alpha-2b for genotype 1 nonresponders. *Gastroenterology* **132:**1270–1278.

196. **Schacker, T. W., M. Conant, C. Thoming, T. Stanczak, Z. Wang, and M. Smith.** 2002. Imiquimod 5-percent cream does not alter the natural history of recurrent herpes genitalis: a phase II, randomized, double-blind, placebo-controlled study. *Antimicrob. Agents Chemother.* **46:**3243–3248.

197. **Schaeffer, H. J., L. Beauchamp, P. de Miranda, G. B. Elion, D. J. Bauer, and P. Collins.** 1978. 9-(2-hydroxyethoxymethyl) guanine activity against viruses of the herpes group. *Nature* **272:**583–585.

198. **Scheidel, L. M., R. K. Durbin, and V. Stollar.** 1987. Sindbis virus mutants resistant to mycophenolic acid and ribavirin. *Virology* **158:**1–7.

199. **Schiff, E., J. Cianciara, and S. Karayalcin.** 2000. Durable HBeAg and HBsAg seroconversion after lamivudine for chronic hepatitis B. *J. Hepatol.* **32**(Suppl. 2)**:**99A.

200. **Schultheiss, M., and R. Thimme.** 2007. Toll like receptor 7 and hepatitis C virus infection. *J. Hepatol.* **47:**165–167.

201. **Schunemann, H. J., S. R. Hill, M. Kakad, R. Bellamy, T. M. Uyeki, F. G. Hayden, Y. Yazdanpanah, J. Beigel, T. Chotpitayasunondh, C. Del Mar, J. Farrar, T. H. Tran, B. Ozbay, N. Sugaya, K. Fukuda, N. Shindo, L. Stockman, G. E. Vist, A. Croisier, A. Nagjdaliyev, C. Roth, G. Thomson, H. Zucker, and A. D. Oxman.** 2007. WHO Rapid Advice Guidelines for pharmacological management of sporadic human infection with avian influenza A (H5N1) virus. *Lancet Infect. Dis.* **7:**21–31.

202. **Seale, L., C. J. Jones, S. Kathpalia, G. G. Jackson, M. Mozes, M. S. Maddux, and D. Packham.** 1985. Prevention of herpesvirus infections in renal allograft recipients by low-dose oral acyclovir. *JAMA* **254:**3435–3438.

203. **Seifer, M., R. K. Hamatake, R. J. Colonno, and D. N. Standring.** 1998. In vitro inhibition of hepadnavirus polymerases by the triphosphates of BMS-200475 and lobucavir. *Antimicrob. Agents Chemother.* **42:**3200–3208.
204. **Seifer, M., A. Patty, D. Duldlan, G. Gosselin, J. L. Imbach, J. P. Sommadossi, M. Bryant, and D. Standring.** 2005. Telbivudine (LdT) preferentially inhibits second (+) strand HBV DNA synthesis. *J. Hepatol.* **42:** 151.
205. **Sen, G. C., and R. M. Ransohoff.** 1993. Interferon-induced antiviral actions and their regulation. *Adv. Virus Res.* **42:**57–102.
205a. **Sherman, K. E.** 2007. Clinical need and therapeutic targets for new HCV agents, p. 1–18. *In The Future of HCV: Small Molecules in Development for Chronic Hepatitis C.* Clinical Care Options Hepatitis, Reston, VA. http://www.clinicaloptions.com/Hepatitis/Treatment%20Updates/Small%20Molecule%20HCV%20Agents.aspx. Accessed 16 July 2008.
206. **Sherman, M., C. Yurdaydin, J. Sollano, M. Silva, Y. F. Liaw, J. Cianciara, A. Boron-Kaczmarska, P. Martin, Z. Goodman, R. Colonno, A. Cross, G. Denisky, B. Kreter, and R. Hindes.** 2006. Entecavir for treatment of lamivudine-refractory, HBeAg-positive chronic hepatitis B. *Gastroenterology* **130:**2039–2049.
207. **Shi, D., J. Yang, D. Yang, E. L. LeCluyse, C. Black, L. You, F. Akhlaghi, and B. Yan.** 2006. Anti-influenza prodrug oseltamivir is activated by carboxylesterase human carboxylesterase 1, and the activation is inhibited by antiplatelet agent clopidogrel. *J. Pharmacol. Exp. Ther.* **319:**1477–1484.
208. **Shigeta, S., T. Yokota, T. Iwabuchi, M. Baba, K. Konno, M. Ogata, and E. De Clercq.** 1983. Comparative efficacy of antiherpes drugs against various strains of varicella-zoster virus. *J. Infect. Dis.* **147:**576–584.
209. **Small, L. N., J. Lau, and D. R. Snydman.** 2006. Preventing post-organ transplantation cytomegalovirus disease with ganciclovir: a meta-analysis comparing prophylactic and preemptive therapies. *Clin. Infect. Dis.* **43:**869–880.
210. **Spruance, S. L., N. Bodsworth, H. Resnick, M. Conant, C. Oeuvray, J. Gao, and K. Hamed.** 2006. Single-dose, patient-initiated famciclovir: a randomized, double-blind, placebo-controlled trial for episodic treatment of herpes labialis. *J. Am. Acad. Dermatol.* **55:**47–53.
211. **Standring, D., M. Seifer, and A. Patty.** 2006. HBV resistance determination from the telbivudine GLOBE registration trial. *J. Hepatol.* **44**(Suppl. 2)**:**191.
212. **Sullivan, F. M., I. R. Swan, P. T. Donnan, J. M. Morrison, B. H. Smith, B. McKinstry, R. J. Davenport, L. D. Vale, J. E. Clarkson, V. Hammersley, S. Hayavi, A. McAteer, K. Stewart, and F. Daly.** 2007. Early treatment with prednisolone or acyclovir in Bell's palsy. *N. Engl. J. Med.* **357:**1598–1607.
213. **Swan, S. K., W. B. Smith, T. C. Marbury, M. Schumacher, C. Dougherty, B. A. Mico, and S. A. Villano.** 2007. Pharmacokinetics of maribavir, a novel oral anti-cytomegalovirus agent, in subjects with varying degrees of renal impairment. *J. Clin. Pharmacol.* **47:**209–217.
214. **Tenney, D. J., R. E. Rose, C. J. Baldick, S. M. Levine, K. A. Pokornowski, A. W. Walsh, J. Fang, C. F. Yu, S. Zhang, C. E. Mazzucco, B. Eggers, M. Hsu, M. J. Plym, P. Poundstone, J. Yang, and R. J. Colonno.** 2007. Two-year assessment of entecavir resistance in lamivudine-refractory hepatitis B virus patients reveals different clinical outcomes depending on the resistance substitutions present. *Antimicrob. Agents Chemother.* **51:** 902–911.
215. **Tominack, R. L., R. J. Wills, L. E. Gustavson, and F. G. Hayden.** 1988. Multiple-dose pharmacokinetics of rimantadine in elderly adults. *Antimicrob. Agents Chemother.* **32:**1813–1819.
216. **Tong, X., R. Chase, A. Skelton, T. Chen, J. Wright-Minogue, and B. A. Malcolm.** 2006. Identification and analysis of fitness of resistance mutations against the HCV protease inhibitor SCH 503034. *Antivir. Res.* **70:** 28–38.
217. **Torriani, F. J., M. Rodriguez-Torres, J. K. Rockstroh, E. Lissen, J. Gonzalez-Garcia, A. Lazzarin, G. Carosi, J. Sasadeusz, C. Katlama, J. Montaner, H. Sette, Jr., S. Passe, J. De Pamphilis, F. Duff, U. M. Schrenk, and D. T. Dieterich.** 2004. Peginterferon alfa-2a plus ribavirin for chronic hepatitis C virus infection in HIV-infected patients. *N. Engl. J. Med.* **351:**438–450.
218. **Tricot, G., E. De Clercq, M. A. Boogaerts, and R. L. Verwilghen.** 1986. Oral bromovinyldeoxyuridine therapy for herpes simplex and varicella-zoster virus infections in severely immunosuppressed patients: a preliminary clinical trial. *J. Med. Virol.* **18:**11–20.
219. **Tyring, S., R. A. Barbarash, J. E. Nahlik, A. Cunningham, J. Marley, M. Heng, T. Jones, T. Rea, R. Boon, and R. Saltzman for The Collaborative Famciclovir Herpes Zoster Study Group.** 1995. Famciclovir for the treatment of acute herpes zoster: effects on acute disease and postherpetic neuralgia. A randomized, double-blind, placebo-controlled trial. *Ann. Intern. Med.* **123:**89–96.
220. **Tyring, S., R. Engst, C. Corriveau, N. Robillard, S. Trottier, S. Van Slycken, R. A. Crann, L. A. Locke, R. Saltzman, and A. G. Palestine.** 2001. Famciclovir for ophthalmic zoster: a randomised aciclovir controlled study. *Br. J. Ophthalmol.* **85:**576–581.
221. **Tyring, S. K., D. Baker, and W. Snowden.** 2002. Valacyclovir for herpes simplex virus infection: long-term safety and sustained efficacy after 20 years' experience with acyclovir. *J. Infect. Dis.* **186**(Suppl. 1)**:**S40–S46.
222. **Tyring, S. K., K. R. Beutner, B. A. Tucker, W. C. Anderson, and R. J. Crooks.** 2000. Antiviral therapy for herpes zoster: randomized, controlled clinical trial of valacyclovir and famciclovir therapy in immunocompetent patients 50 years and older. *Arch. Fam. Med.* **9:** 863–869.
223. **Tyring, S. K., J. M. Douglas, Jr., L. Corey, S. L. Spruance, and J. Esmann for the Valaciclovir International Study Group.** 1998. A randomized, placebo-controlled comparison of oral valacyclovir and acyclovir in immunocompetent patients with recurrent genital herpes infections. *Arch. Dermatol.* **134:**185–191.
224. **Valette, M., J. P. Allard, M. Aymard, and V. Millet.** 1993. Susceptibilities to rimantadine of influenza A/H1N1 and A/H3N2 viruses isolated during the epidemics of 1988 to 1989 and 1989 to 1990. *Antimicrob. Agents Chemother.* **37:**2239–2240.
225. **van Bommel, F., B. Zollner, C. Sarrazin, U. Spengler, D. Huppe, B. Moller, H. H. Feucht, B. Wiedenmann, and T. Berg.** 2006. Tenofovir for patients with lamivudine-resistant hepatitis B virus (HBV) infection and high HBV DNA level during adefovir therapy. *Hepatology* **44:**318–325.
226. **Vilcek, J., and G. C. I. Sen.** 1996. Interferons and other cytokines, p. 375–399. *In* B. N. Fields, D. M. Knipe, and P. M. Howley (ed.), *Fields Virology*, 3rd ed. Lippincott-Raven Publishers, Philadelphia, PA.
227. **Wagstaff, A. J., and H. M. Bryson.** 1994. Foscarnet. A reappraisal of its antiviral activity, pharmacokinetic properties and therapeutic use in immunocompromised patients with viral infections. *Drugs* **48:**199–226.

228. **Wald, A., D. Carrell, M. Remington, E. Kexel, J. Zeh, and L. Corey.** 2002. Two-day regimen of acyclovir for treatment of recurrent genital herpes simplex virus type 2 infection. *Clin. Infect. Dis.* **34:**944–948.
229. **Wald, A., J. Zeh, G. Barnum, L. G. Davis, and L. Corey.** 1996. Suppression of subclinical shedding of herpes simplex virus type 2 with acyclovir. *Ann. Intern. Med.* **124:**8–15.
230. **Wang, L. H., R. W. Peck, Y. Yin, J. Allanson, R. Wiggs, and M. B. Wire.** 2003. Phase I safety and pharmacokinetic trials of 1263W94, a novel oral anti-human cytomegalovirus agent, in healthy and human immunodeficiency virus-infected subjects. *Antimicrob. Agents Chemother.* **47:**1334–1342.
231. **Wassilew, S.** 2005. Brivudin compared with famciclovir in the treatment of herpes zoster: effects in acute disease and chronic pain in immunocompetent patients. A randomized, double-blind, multinational study. *J. Eur. Acad. Dermatol. Venereol.* **19:**47–55.
232. **Wassilew, S. W., and P. Wutzler.** 2003. Oral brivudin in comparison with acyclovir for improved therapy of herpes zoster in immunocompetent patients: results of a randomized, double-blind, multicentered study. *Antivir. Res.* **59:**49–56.
233. **Watashi, K., M. Hijikata, M. Hosaka, M. Yamaji, and K. Shimotohno.** 2003. Cyclosporin A suppresses replication of hepatitis C virus genome in cultured hepatocytes. *Hepatology* **38:**1282–1288.
234. **Watson, K. G., R. Cameron, R. J. Fenton, D. Gower, S. Hamilton, B. Jin, G. Y. Krippner, A. Luttick, D. McConnell, S. J. MacDonald, A. M. Mason, V. Nguyen, S. P. Tucker, and W. Y. Wu.** 2004. Highly potent and long-acting trimeric and tetrameric inhibitors of influenza virus neuraminidase. *Bioorg. Med. Chem. Lett.* **14:**1589–1592.
235. **Webster, A., M. Boyce, S. Edmundson, and I. Miller.** 1999. Coadministration of orally inhaled zanamivir with inactivated trivalent influenza vaccine does not adversely affect the production of antihaemagglutinin antibodies in the serum of healthy volunteers. *Clin. Pharmacokinet.* **36**(Suppl. 1)**:**51–58.
236. **Welliver, R., A. S. Monto, O. Carewicz, E. Schatteman, M. Hassman, J. Hedrick, H. C. Jackson, L. Huson, P. Ward, and J. S. Oxford.** 2001. Effectiveness of oseltamivir in preventing influenza in household contacts: a randomized controlled trial. *JAMA* **285:**748–754.
237. **Whitley, R. J., F. G. Hayden, K. S. Reisinger, N. Young, R. Dutkowski, D. Ipe, R. G. Mills, and P. Ward.** 2001. Oral oseltamivir treatment of influenza in children. *Pediatr. Infect. Dis. J.* **20:**127–133.
238. **Whitley, R. J., and B. Roizman.** 2001. Herpes simplex virus infections. *Lancet* **357:**1513–1518.
239. **Wilhelmus, K. R., L. Gee, W. W. Hauck, N. Kurinij, C. R. Dawson, D. B. Jones, B. A. Barron, H. E. Kaufman, J. Sugar, R. A. Hyndiuk, et al.** 1994. Herpetic Eye Disease Study. A controlled trial of topical corticosteroids for herpes simplex stromal keratitis. *Ophthalmology* **101:**1883–1895; discussion, 1895–1896.
240. **Wills, R. J., R. Belshe, D. Tomlinsin, F. De Grazia, A. Lin, S. Wells, J. Milazzo, and C. Berry.** 1987. Pharmacokinetics of rimantadine hydrochloride in patients with chronic liver disease. *Clin. Pharmacol. Ther.* **42:**449–454.
241. **Winston, D. J., J. A. Young, V. Pullarkat, G. A. Papanicolaou, R. Vij, E. Vance, G. J. Alangaden, R. F. Chemaly, F. Petersen, N. Chao, J. Klein, K. Sprague, S. A. Villano, and M. Boeckh.** 2008. Maribavir prophylaxis for prevention of cytomegalovirus infection in allogeneic stem-cell transplant recipients: a multicenter, randomized, double-blind, placebo-controlled, dose-ranging study. *Blood* **111:**5403–5410.
242. **Wintermeyer, S. M., and M. C. Nahata.** 1995. Rimantadine: a clinical perspective. *Ann. Pharmacother.* **29:**299–310.
243. **Wood, M. J., R. Kay, R. H. Dworkin, S. J. Soong, and R. J. Whitley.** 1996. Oral acyclovir therapy accelerates pain resolution in patients with herpes zoster: a meta-analysis of placebo-controlled trials. *Clin. Infect. Dis.* **22:**341–347.
244. **Writing Committee of the Second World Health Organization Consultation on Clinical Aspects of Human Infection with Avian Influenza (H5N1) Virus.** 2008. Update on avian influenza A (H5N1) virus infection in humans. *N. Engl. J. Med.* **358:**261–273.

244a. **The Writing Committee of the World Health Organization (WHO) on Human Influenza A/H5.** 2005. Avian influenza A (H5N1) infection in humans. *N. Engl. J. Med.* **353:**1374–1385. (Erratum, **354:**884, 2006.)

245. **Yen, H.-L., N. A. Ilyushina, R. Salomon, E. Hoffmann, R. G. Webster, and E. A. Govorkova.** 2007. Neuraminidase inhibitor-resistant recombinant A/Vietnam/1203/04 (H5N1) influenza viruses retain their replication efficiency and pathogenicity in vitro and in vivo. *J. Virol.* **81:**12418–12426.
246. **Ying, C., E. De Clercq, and J. Neyts.** 2000. Lamivudine, adefovir and tenofovir exhibit long-lasting anti-hepatitis B virus activity in cell culture. *J. Viral Hepat.* **7:**79–83.
247. **Yoo, B. C., J. H. Kim, Y. H. Chung, K. S. Lee, S. W. Paik, S. H. Ryu, B. H. Han, J. Y. Han, K. S. Byun, M. Cho, H. J. Lee, T. H. Kim, S. H. Cho, J. W. Park, S. H. Um, S. G. Hwang, Y. S. Kim, Y. J. Lee, C. Y. Chon, B. I. Kim, Y. S. Lee, J. M. Yang, H. C. Kim, J. S. Hwang, S. K. Choi, Y. O. Kweon, S. H. Jeong, M. S. Lee, J. Y. Choi, D. G. Kim, Y. S. Kim, H. Y. Lee, K. Yoo, H. W. Yoo, and H. S. Lee.** 2007. Twenty-four-week clevudine therapy showed potent and sustained antiviral activity in HBeAg-positive chronic hepatitis B. *Hepatology* **45:**1172–1178.
248. **Young, K. C., K. L. Lindsay, K. J. Lee, W. C. Liu, J. W. He, S. L. Milstein, and M. M. Lai.** 2003. Identification of a ribavirin-resistant NS5B mutation of hepatitis C virus during ribavirin monotherapy. *Hepatology* **38:**869–878.
249. **Yuen, G. J., G. L. Drusano, C. Fletcher, E. Capparelli, J. D. Connor, J. P. Lalezari, L. Drew, S. Follansbee, D. Busch, M. Jacobson, S. A. Spector, K. Squires, and W. Buhles.** 1995. Population differences in ganciclovir clearance as determined by nonlinear mixed-effects modelling. *Antimicrob. Agents Chemother.* **39:**2350–2352.
250. **Zhu, Y., T. Yamamoto, J. Cullen, J. Saputelli, C. E. Aldrich, D. S. Miller, S. Litwin, P. A. Furman, A. R. Jilbert, and W. S. Mason.** 2001. Kinetics of hepadnavirus loss from the liver during inhibition of viral DNA synthesis. *J. Virol.* **75:**311–322.

Diagnosis of Viral Infections*

GUY BOIVIN, TONY MAZZULLI, MARTIN PETRIC, AND MICHEL COUILLARD

13

The clinical virology laboratory has emerged as an important and leading component of general microbiology that can now provide significant benefit to patient care. The traditional epidemiological and academic reasons for diagnosis of viral infections have been expanded by rapid, often quantitative assays that can impact on therapeutic management and public health decisions. Such change is the result of many advances in diagnostic virology, including improvement in cell culture (shell vial assays, mixed cell cultures, and genetically engineered cell lines), availability of specific reagents such as monoclonal antibodies, and, most importantly, the introduction of molecular techniques mostly based on PCR which allow the sensitive and rapid detection of slowly growing or uncultivable viruses. The impact of PCR is illustrated by the recent identification of several respiratory viruses, including the human metapneumovirus (136); multiple coronaviruses, including the severe acute respiratory syndrome (SARS) coronavirus (31); and human bocavirus (3).

Apart from technological advances, the expanded role of the diagnostic virology laboratory can also be attributed to the increased pool of immunocompromised patients (e.g., human immunodeficiency virus [HIV]-infected individuals and transplant recipients) at risk of serious opportunistic viral infections and the increasing number of antiviral agents available for herpesviruses, HIV, influenza viruses, and hepatitis viruses. These factors have driven the development of rapid, sometimes point-of-care, diagnostic methods and new diagnostic approaches, including viral load measurement, antiviral drug susceptibility testing, and determination of viral genotypes.

Despite the recent advances in molecular techniques, the clinical virology laboratory still relies on multiple methods for detecting viral infections. Viral culture, electron microscopy (EM), histopathology, and detection of viral antigens and nucleic acids can be used to detect active viral infection, whereas serologic testing is performed to assess the presence of virus-specific immune responses. Such a diversity of methods has made it increasingly more complex for physicians to request the right procedure and to interpret the result. This necessitates excellent and frequent communication between the physician and the virology laboratory for the optimal use of diagnostic tests.

SPECIMENS

The performance of viral diagnosis can never exceed the quality of the specimen that is received in the laboratory. Detection of viral pathogens is highly dependent on three important variables: (i) obtaining the specimen from the appropriate site, (ii) proper timing of specimen collection relative to onset of symptoms, and (iii) effective and timely processing of sufficient specimen. The specimen site should be determined by the clinical syndrome and the suspected virus(es). The specific procedures for collecting clinical specimens are addressed in clinical laboratory manuals (42). The physician should be advised that the selection of some clinical specimens could strongly affect the performance of a diagnostic test. This is particularly true for the diagnosis of respiratory virus infections for which nasopharyngeal aspirates or nasal washes are generally preferred to nasal or throat swabs. Also, the type of materials used for specimen collection could have an impact on the test result. For example, Dacron or rayon swabs are recommended in the case of vesicular lesions, since both herpes simplex virus (HSV) and varicella-zoster virus (VZV) have been shown to be inactivated by cotton and calcium alginate swabs (10, 88).

For many acute virus infections, viral shedding begins shortly before the symptoms, peaks rapidly after the onset of symptoms, and then declines steadily as illness resolves. Thus, in general, specimens should be collected as soon as possible after the onset of symptoms. However, there are some exceptions, such as SARS coronavirus infections in which viral load in respiratory specimens peaked at week 2 after the onset of symptoms (22).

Transport to the laboratory should be accomplished as soon as possible after collection of the specimen to ensure its integrity. This point is critical for cell culture procedures which require viable cells but may be less relevant for detection of viral antigens or nucleic acids. In general, nonenveloped viruses (e.g., adenoviruses and enteroviruses) are more stable than viruses surrounded by a lipid envelope (e.g., VZV and respiratory syncytial virus [RSV]). Specimens other than blood should usually be kept at 4°C (wet ice) during transport, especially if transport will require

*This chapter is based in part on chapter 12 from the second edition by S. Specter, R. L. Hodinka, D. L. Wiedbrauk, and S. A. Young.

more than 1 h. If a delay of >24 h is anticipated, the specimen should generally be frozen at a temperature of −70°C or lower (dry ice). However, freezing in a standard freezer (−20°C) is generally associated with a greater loss of infectivity than holding at 4°C for several days and should be avoided. Swabs and tissue specimens should be placed in a viral transport medium (VTM) to preserve the quality of the sample. Many VTM formulations exist; they generally contain a salt solution to ensure proper ionic concentrations, a buffer to maintain pH, a source of protein for virus stability, and antibiotics or antifungals to prevent microbial contamination. Some nucleic acid tests (NATs) have their own special VTM, which have been optimized for specific specimens.

Laboratories should receive specimens after proper storage and transport and with relevant clinical information on an appropriate requisition form. Such a form should contain key information about the sampling site and when the specimen was collected, the diagnostic concerns of the physician, and key identifying information for the patient.

CELL CULTURE

All methods used for viral isolation require living cells because viruses are obligate intracellular parasites. Historically, the systems used to isolate viruses of medical importance consisted of laboratory animals, embryonated eggs, and cultured cells. However, most diagnostic virology laboratories no longer routinely perform viral isolation in either laboratory animals or embryonated eggs but now rely solely on cell culture. Although it is gradually being replaced by immunologic and molecular methods, cell culture retains the following advantages for viral diagnosis. (i) The method is relatively sensitive based on the natural amplification of virus during the replication process and is specific in that only virus will be amplified. (ii) Viral culture has the potential to detect many different viruses if a sufficient number of sensitive cell lines are available to the laboratory. Therefore, one of the most important principles of designing a virus isolation protocol is the selection of cell lines that propagate important viruses from each sample type received by the laboratory. (iii) Culture provides a viral isolate that can be further characterized if necessary (e.g., serotyping, genotyping, and antiviral drug susceptibility testing).

There are also limitations to viral isolation for the diagnostic laboratory. (i) Certain viruses do not grow or grow very slowly in available cell lines, so the result is not clinically useful. (ii) Techniques for detecting a viral infection in lieu of virus isolation are more cost-effective. (iii) Successful culture depends on the viability of the virus in the specimen. However, several new approaches (enhanced cell culture) have shortened the time of virus isolation to more clinically useful time frames, and they are discussed below.

Standard Cell Cultures

The utility of cell culture in viral isolation was pioneered by two important discoveries. First was the work of Gey, who developed monolayer cell culture techniques (44). This was followed by the work of Enders, Weller, and colleagues who demonstrated that vaccinia virus (41) and polioviruses (35) could be grown and detected in roller tube cell cultures. Previously, the systems used for viral isolation had been either animal or embryonated-egg inoculation. Following this landmark discovery, the number and type of cell lines that are useful for viral isolation have continued to expand and change.

The types of cell culture routinely used for viral isolation can be placed in one of three categories: primary cells, diploid (also called semicontinuous) cell lines, and heteroploid cell lines. Primary cells (e.g., monkey cells and chicken embryo cells) are derived from tissue and have been propagated in vitro for the first time. These cells have the same chromosome number as the parental tissue and generally can be subcultured only once or twice. Diploid cell lines (e.g., human embryonic lung fibroblasts) develop during subculture of primary cells. A diploid cell line will consist of 75 to 100% of the cells having the same karyotype as cells from the species of origin and can be subcultured 20 to 50 times prior to cell death. Heteroploid, or continuous, cell lines (e.g., HEp-2 and HeLa cells) exist as a population of cells with less than 75% of the population having a diploid chromosome constitution. The most important feature of this type of cell line is the ability of indefinite passages due to cell immortalization, which facilitates continuous access to cells for virus isolation. The two issues that have fostered the development of additional cell culture lines for viral isolation are susceptibility (Table 1) and speed of replication (Table 2). Each cell culture type displays a differential susceptibility to each group or member of the virus families. Thus, multiple cell lines are required for a given sample type to detect the families of viruses capable of infecting a given organ system. In addition, isolation of viruses does not always use cell culture in monolayers. Suspension cultures of lymphocytes are used for isolation of retroviruses such as HIV type 1 (HIV-1) and HIV-2, and several herpesviruses such as Epstein-Barr virus (EBV) and human herpesviruses 6 and 7 (HHV-6 and HHV-7).

TABLE 1 Susceptibility of cell culture types to commonly isolated human viruses[a]

Culture type	Virus(es) propagated
Primary	
Monkey kidney	Influenza virus, parainfluenza virus, enteroviruses
Rabbit kidney	HSV
Human embryonic kidney	Enteroviruses, adenoviruses
Diploid	
Fibroblast	CMV, VZV, HSV, adenoviruses, rhinoviruses, enteroviruses (some)
Continuous	
HEp-2	RSV, adenoviruses, HSV, enteroviruses (some)
A549	Adenoviruses, HSV, enteroviruses (some)
LLC-MK2	Parainfluenza virus, human metapneumovirus
MDCK	Influenza virus
RD	Echoviruses
Buffalo green monkey kidney	Coxsackieviruses

[a] Modified from reference 128a with permission of Elsevier.

TABLE 2 Times required to detect viruses in cell culture[a]

Virus	No. of isolates	Earliest day positive	Day when 50% were positive	Day when 90% were positive
HSV	512	1	1	3
VZV	30[b]	3	7	13
CMV	116[c]	3	13	20
Adenovirus	125[d]	1	4	11
Enteroviruses	85	1	4	10
RSV	70[e]	2	4	7
Influenza virus	61[f]	2	4	7
Parainfluenza virus	104[g]	1	6	12
Rhinovirus	130	1	6	12

[a] Reproduced from reference 128a with permission of Elsevier. Data are from St. Louis Children's Hospital Virology Laboratory, 1997.
[b] A total of 12 of these were also detected on day 2 by shell vial assay.
[c] A total of 462 additional isolates were detected on day 1 or 2 by shell vial assay.
[d] A total of 18 of these were detected on day 1 by fluorescent-antibody staining.
[e] A total of 734 additional specimens were positive on day 1 by fluorescent-antibody staining or EIA.
[f] A total of 61 additional specimens were positive on day 1 by fluorescent-antibody staining.
[g] A total of 30 additional specimens were positive on day 1 by fluorescent-antibody staining.

The cell culture systems used for viral isolation will in general depend on the type of specimen submitted to the laboratory. Traditionally, three cell types have been used for viral isolation: a primary cell culture such as rhesus monkey kidney, a diploid line such as human embryonic lung, and a heteroploid line such as HEp-2. While this may still be a reasonable approach for some specimen types, it is no longer feasible or desirable for all virus isolations. Due to cost and cell access considerations, some laboratories have replaced primary cells with a panel of continuous cell lines. It is also reasonable, both scientifically and financially, to use a single cell line when a specimen is submitted only for isolation of selected viruses like HSV, cytomegalovirus (CMV), and VZV. The selection and types of cell cultures used in a laboratory offering virus isolation will depend on many factors, including the clinical or epidemiological need for viral isolation, the common specimen types received, the cost to prepare or purchase the needed cell lines, and the availability of experienced personnel.

The general procedure for viral isolation starts with the processing of the clinical specimen. In most cases, this consists of the addition of antibiotics to the sample prior to inoculation of the appropriate cell lines. Each cell line to be inoculated should be visually inspected prior to inoculation, and only recently prepared cells should be used since older cell cultures are less susceptible to virus replication. The standard tube used for cell culture is a 16- by 125-mm screw-cap tube. These tubes facilitate incubation following sample adsorption either in a roller drum or in stationary racks. In either case, the system must slant the tubes at a 5 to 7° angle. In general, the inoculated tubes are incubated at 35 to 37°C, but lower temperatures (33°C) facilitate the isolation of some viruses (e.g., rhinoviruses). Some laboratories have replaced tubes with microwell plates for cell culture, which facilitate the use of multiple cell lines for optimal recovery of several viruses.

Cytopathic Effect

Each inoculated cell culture tube is examined with a light microscope to detect morphological changes typically daily for the first week and less frequently thereafter for up to 21 days. Morphological changes that are the result of viral replication are termed cytopathic effects (CPE). The inoculated cell culture must be compared to sham-inoculated control monolayers from the same batch of cells. The CPE observed in cell culture may be characterized by the following: cell rounding, refractile cells, cell clumping, vacuolation, granulation, giant cells, syncytium formation, and cell destruction. The type of specimen, the cell line displaying CPE, and the type of CPE may be used as preliminary evidence for identification of the replicating virus. For example, a respiratory sample inoculated into HEp-2 cells displaying large syncytia is consistent with the presence of RSV. A cerebrospinal fluid (CSF) sample inoculated into rhabdomyosarcoma (RD) cells displaying cell rounding and destruction is consistent with an echovirus. A urine sample inoculated into fibroblasts displaying isolated foci of swollen cells is consistent with CMV (Fig. 1).

The replication of certain viruses in cell culture may not produce any CPE. The replication of these agents can be detected by alternative techniques such as hemadsorption or interference assays. Hemadsorption is commonly used to detect the replication of orthomyxoviruses and some paramyxoviruses. Influenza viruses, parainfluenza viruses, and mumps and measles viruses insert viral glycoproteins (hemagglutinin and hemagglutinin-neuraminidase) into the host cell membrane to facilitate the maturation process of replication. The viral glycoproteins promote attachment of certain species of red blood cells (RBC) (e.g., guinea pig RBC) to the infected cell membrane. Hemadsorption can be observed with a light microscope and, like CPE, is preliminary evidence that one of these viruses is replicating in the cell culture. Some other viruses, notably rubella virus, can be detected by taking advantage of the phenomenon of interference. For instance, when rubella virus grows in primary monkey kidney cells, they become resistant to challenge with an echovirus type 2 strain.

Identifying a virus replicating in a cell culture is confirmed using more definitive criteria of reaction with monospecific or monoclonal antibodies. Generally, these reagents are chemically conjugated to fluorochromes so that the reaction with a specific antibody can be determined by fluorescent microscopy. The immunofluorescence technique can be either indirect or direct. The indirect technique uses an unconjugated primary antibody to react with the infected cells, followed by a fluorochrome-

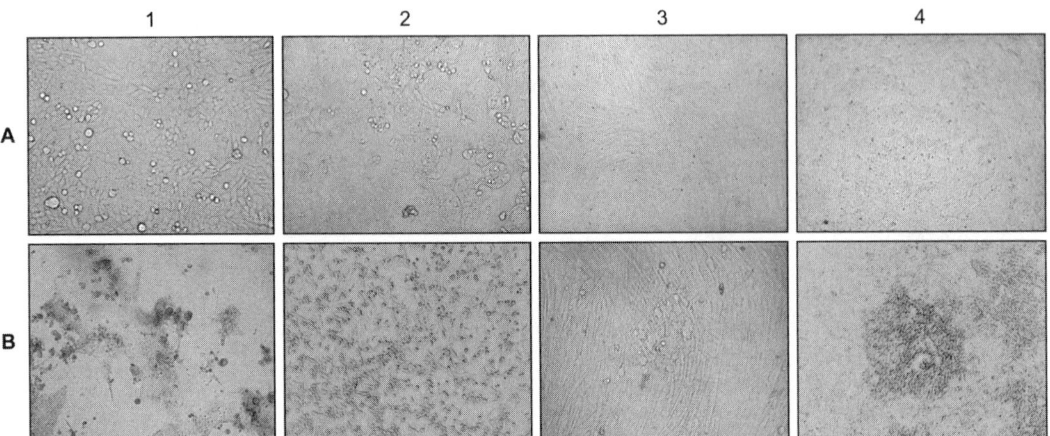

FIGURE 1 CPE induced by some viruses. Row A shows uninfected cell lines, including HEp-2 cells (1), RD cells (2), fibroblasts (3), and Vero cells (4). Row B shows the same cell lines infected with RSV (1), enterovirus (2), CMV (3), and HSV (4).

conjugated secondary antibody usually directed against the species specificity of the primary antibody. The direct technique consists of the primary antibody that is conjugated to a fluorochrome so that only a single step of staining and washing of the infected cells is necessary. Alternatively, some virology laboratories may use monospecific or pooled antisera to prevent the infection of susceptible cells, a process known as neutralization. Most virology laboratories use an immunofluorescence microscopy method for viral identification, whereas the neutralization method is primarily used to determine enterovirus serotypes.

In some clinical situations, the process of observing cells for CPE and then confirming that the CPE can be attributed to viral replication occurs too slowly. Over the last 2 decades, several enhanced cell culture methods have facilitated more rapid detection of viral replication.

Shell Vial Culture

The ability to detect viral infection prior to the development of CPE was first demonstrated with CMV (47). The shell vial culture method uses low-speed centrifugation to enhance the infection of human diploid embryonic fibroblasts (MRC-5) by CMV, followed by overnight incubation to amplify CMV-specific proteins in the nucleus and, finally, an immunofluorescent staining procedure specific for an immediate-early CMV protein. A shell vial is a vial containing a coverslip onto which a monolayer of cells has grown. After centrifugation and incubation for 18 to 48 h, immunofluorescent staining is performed on the cells on the coverslip using monoclonal antibodies recognizing proteins that are expressed very early in the CMV replicative cycle. The speed and relative sensitivity of the shell vial system for CMV stimulated the development of shell vial systems for other viruses, such as HSV, VZV, adenoviruses, and respiratory viruses. The detection of respiratory viruses requires inoculation of a greater number of shell vials with different cell types, increasing the incubation times, and using pools or cocktails of monoclonal antibodies capable of detecting each respiratory virus. Each antibody in the pool for detecting respiratory viruses has a unique staining pattern that can be used as a means to give a preliminary identification of the virus present in the shell vial monolayer. A second shell vial can then be stained with a single monoclonal antibody to confirm the preliminary identification.

Mixed Cell Cultures

A recent development in viral isolation is use of the shell vial cell culture assay with a mixture of cells in the monolayer. A mixture of cell types provides more susceptible cell types for a number of viruses, the low-speed centrifugation enhances infectivity, cell culture amplifies the signal, and immunofluorescent staining facilitates rapid detection of virus replication. The mixed-cell systems have been developed to target viruses from specific types of specimens. The rapid respiratory virus mix, R-Mix (Diagnostic Hybrids Inc.), is a combination of mink lung cells and A549 cells (60) for detection of RSV, parainfluenza viruses, influenza viruses, and adenoviruses. An H and V mix is a combination of CV-1 and MCR-5 cells for detection of HSV, CMV, and VZV. The E-mix is a combination of BGMK (buffalo African green monkey kidney) and A549 cells for detection of enteroviruses and other viral agents. The R-Mix with immunofluorescent staining performs comparably with either conventional tube culture or single-cell shell vial culture with immunofluorescent staining (33). This system is a reasonable approach for laboratories that want to continue using shell vials for viral detection.

Genetically Engineered Cell Lines

Genetically engineered cell lines to be used for virus isolation were first developed for HSV (126). A baby hamster kidney cell line (BHK-21) was stably transformed with an HSV-inducible promoter (UL39 gene) attached to a functional *Escherichia coli* beta-galactosidase gene. Infection of this cell line by either HSV type 1 (HSV-1) or HSV-2 (most specifically, HSV proteins ICP0 and VP16) induces beta-galactosidase enzyme activity. The addition of a substrate, 5-bromo-4-chloro-3-indolyl-β-D-glactopyranoside (X-Gal), for this enzyme results in the formation of a colored product in the HSV-infected cells. This system is now commercially available as the enzyme-linked virus-inducible system (ELVIS HSV ID; Diagnostic Hybrids Inc.). The advantages of this system include rapid detection, with a result available after overnight incubation and treatment with the substrate; visual signal by detection of CPE and/or the blue color; adaptability to large-volume laboratories; and potential automation. A modification of the ELVIS system now allows subsequent staining directly on the monolayer with type-specific, fluorescently labeled HSV monoclonal antibodies. The concept of virus-specific indicator cell lines may be feasible for other viruses (106), and a format has been developed for rapid HSV antiviral susceptibility testing (130).

ANTIVIRAL SUSCEPTIBILITY TESTING

In the past 2 decades, safe and effective antiviral drugs have been developed for the treatment of many acute and chronic viral infections (see chapters 11 and 12). Not surprisingly, the increased and prolonged use of these drugs, most notably in immunocompromised patients, has been accompanied by the emergence of drug-resistant viruses. However, clinical failure may be due to the presence of a drug-resistant virus or to factors such as the patient's immunologic status and compliance and the pharmacokinetics of the drug in that patient. Examples of clinical situations which warrant the use of antiviral susceptibility testing for herpesviruses include failure of HSV or VZV cutaneous lesions to resolve or the appearance of new lesions while the patient is on acyclovir (valacyclovir or famciclovir) therapy (15, 122) and progressive retinal or visceral CMV disease during ganciclovir (valganciclovir) therapy (14, 46). Ganciclovir-resistant CMV infections were first reported among HIV-infected subjects with CD4 T-cell counts of $<50 \times 10^9$/liter (37) and are now an emerging problem in hematopoietic stem cell transplant and solid-organ transplant recipients, particularly in the context of a primary infection after organ transplantation (CMV-seropositive donor and CMV-seronegative recipient) (17, 89). Also, continuous influenza virus shedding during therapy with amantadine or rimantadine or neuraminidase (NA) inhibitors (oseltamivir and zanamivir) in immunocompromised patients should lead to suspicion of antiviral drug resistance and may warrant antiviral testing (7, 63). Resistance testing for clinical management of HIV-1 infection is now recommended by most experts in the case of treatment failure (worsening clinical disease, increase in viral load, and decrease in CD4 T lymphocytes), primary infection, and pregnancy (57, 149).

Phenotypic Assays

Phenotypic assays measure the effect of an antiviral drug on the growth of a virus, which can be measured by infectivity (e.g., plaque or yield reduction) assays, viral antigen or viral nucleic acid production, and enzyme activity. Such assays directly measure and quantify the effect of antiviral drugs on viral growth. However, they generally require isolation and passage of the virus in cell culture, followed by viral titration before antiviral drug testing begins. Thus, these tests tend to be slow, labor-intensive, and difficult to standardize. Phenotypic results are typically expressed as the drug concentration that inhibits 50 or 90% of viral growth relative to a no-drug control (IC_{50} or IC_{90}). Importantly, because these assays have been difficult to standardize, resistant and susceptible control strains should be tested with each batch of clinical isolates. Phenotypic antiviral susceptibility assays are currently in use for herpesviruses (HSV, VZV, and CMV), influenza viruses, and HIV-1. A standard procedure for HSV antiviral susceptibility testing by plaque reduction assay (PRA) was approved by the Clinical and Laboratory Standards Institute (formerly NCCLS) in 2004 (103a). A similar PRA has been described for CMV (81).

The PRA has classically been the standard method of susceptibility testing to which new methods are compared. In this assay, a standardized viral inoculum is added into multiple wells of a plate containing susceptible cells and serial concentrations of an antiviral agent. A solidifying agent such as agarose is usually added to the cell culture medium to allow the formation of discrete viral plaques. Following an incubation period (which varies according to the virus), the plates are fixed and stained with a dye (crystal violet) and the plaques are counted. The IC_{50} and sometimes the IC_{90} are determined and compared to those obtained for susceptible and resistant control strains. Breakpoint resistance values have been proposed for HSV and CMV (Table 3), although it should be emphasized that many variables can affect the results, such as the cell line, the viral inoculum, the incubation period, etc. For a slow-growing virus such as CMV, the time involved for initial growth, viral stock preparation, and antiviral susceptibility testing is >6 to 8 weeks, whereas it can take <2 weeks in the case of HSV. Another drawback of the PRA is the possibility of selecting some genotypes in a mixed viral population ("quasispecies") during the initial passages in cell culture in the absence of a drug (45).

Other phenotypic assays (see more detailed procedures in reference 5) include the dye uptake assay for susceptibility testing of HSV (100). This is a colorimetric method that involves the quantification of a vital dye (neutral red) by viable cells but not by infected (nonviable) cells. The assay is semiautomated and is reproducible with the use of 96-well microtiter plates and a spectrophotometer. A DNA hybridization assay (Hybriwix assay; Diagnostic Hybrids Inc.) was developed to measure HSV, CMV, and VZV drug susceptibilities (28), but this assay is no longer commercially available. After appropriate incubation of the virus in the presence of various concentrations of antivirals, the cells were lysed and the DNA was transferred to wicks of nitrocellulose paper. The DNA immobilized on the wicks was then hybridized to a virus-specific radiolabeled probe.

For testing of influenza virus phenotypic susceptibility to NA inhibitors (zanamivir and oseltamivir), the currently preferred method consists of directly measuring inhibition of NA activity (113). After incubation of the viral NA with different concentrations of NA inhibitors, a fluorescent or chemiluminescent substrate is added and then fluorescence or chemiluminescence is quantitated. Of note, the NA assay cannot detect drug resistance caused by the presence of hemagglutinin mutations, which have been less commonly reported than NA mutations (99).

TABLE 3 IC_{50} cutoffs for HSV and CMV antiviral resistance using PRA

Virus	Drug	IC_{50} (μM)		
		Susceptible	Intermediate	Resistant
HSV	Acyclovir	<8		≥8
	Foscarnet	<330		≥330
CMV	Ganciclovir	≤6	6–12	>12
	Foscarnet	≤400		>400

Phenotypic assays for susceptibility testing of HIV-1 were traditionally performed in cell culture using primary peripheral blood mononuclear cells from HIV-1-negative donors (66). In this assay, virus replication in the presence or absence of an antiretroviral drug is monitored by quantifying HIV-1 p24 antigen using enzyme immunoassay (EIA). More recently developed recombinant virus phenotypic assays (18) involve insertion of the reverse transcriptase and polymerase genes of HIV from a patient into a vector consisting of a rapidly replicating laboratory viral strain that also contains a reporter gene (e.g., the luciferase gene) to measure viral growth in the presence of a drug compared to that of a wild-type virus. Some recombinant virus assays have been developed commercially, such as the PhenoSense assay (Virologic Inc.) and the Antivirogram assay (Tibotec-Virco) (112). Other types of phenotypic assays beyond the scope of this chapter include the yield reduction assay (83), EIA-based tests (9), and flow cytometry testing (101).

Genotypic Assays

Genotypic assays allow the rapid detection of genetic mutations associated with antiviral drug resistance. Most of these tests first involve a round of nucleic acid amplification for the specific viral genes implicated in resistance to a certain drug, followed by direct sequencing of the amplified product, and, finally, comparison of the viral sequence to that of a pretherapy isolate or a reference strain. These assays are particularly useful for detecting evidence of resistance when a discrete number of known resistance mutations are known. Genotypic assays have been most widely used for detecting ganciclovir-resistant CMV or antiretroviral-refractory HIV-1 infections, since phenotypic assays for these viruses are slow and tedious. However, such tests have also been used to distinguish genetic variants of hepatitis B virus (HBV) associated with lamivudine resistance (52), M2 mutants associated with influenza A virus resistance to amantadine (75), NA and/or hemagglutinin influenza virus mutations associated with resistance to NA inhibitors (1, 54), and HSV or VZV mutations conferring resistance to acyclovir (15, 122). In the last case, development of genotypic assays has been hampered by the facts that the thymidine kinase and DNA polymerase genes of herpesviruses are highly polymorphic and that drug resistance mutations are scattered throughout the gene. Also, phenotypic assays for HSV are generally more convenient due to the rapid growth of this virus (typically 24 to 48 h).

Genotypic assays for CMV have been developed mainly to detect UL97 (protein kinase) and also UL54 (DNA polymerase) mutations associated with ganciclovir (or valganciclovir) resistance (Fig. 2). PCR amplification of a short fragment of the UL97 gene followed by either restriction endonuclease digestion or direct sequencing has been used to detect the most frequent ganciclovir resistance mutations, at codons 460, 520, 594, and 595, which are responsible for approximately 80% of resistance cases (16, 23). The major advantage of this method consists of its rapidity, since resistance-associated mutations can be detected directly in clinical samples such as whole blood, leukocytes, plasma, urine, etc., within a few days after sample collection (14). For more comprehensive analysis of ganciclovir resistance but also to detect CMV resistance to cidofovir and foscarnet, PCR amplification and DNA sequencing of the catalytic regions of the UL54 gene must also be undertaken. However, the genetic map of CMV UL54 mutations associated with drug resistance has not been completed yet, and an important problem consists of discriminating between polymorphic mutations (natural variations) and resistance mutations. Marker transfer experiments must be performed to definitively determine that a particular mutation is associated with drug resistance (24, 96), which is beyond the scope of the general virology laboratory.

The development of HIV resistance to all antiretroviral agents is currently a significant clinical problem. Direct sequencing of PCR-amplified reverse transcriptase or protease genes is considered to be the "gold standard" for assessing HIV-1 drug resistance (reviewed in references 144 and 149). The clinical utility of resistance testing has been demonstrated in a number of randomized prospective studies, and HIV resistance testing is now recommended by various international AIDS societies (57, 124). Commercially available sequencing-based methods for HIV genotyping include the Trugene HIV-1 (Visible Genetics/Siemens Diagnostics), ViroSeq HIV-1 (Celera Diagnostics/Abbott Laboratories), Virco Type HIV-1 (Virco BVBA), GenSeq (Monogram), and GenoSure Plus (LabCorp). The first two assays have been approved by the FDA. The two systems are similar with respect to the complexity of the assays and have a detection limit of ≈20% for minor quasispecies according to the manufacturers' instructions. Hybridization techniques, as an alternative to complete sequencing, may be used to detect specific mutations associated with drug resistance. In the INNO-LiPA HIV-1 line probe assay (Murex Innogenetics/Bayer Diagnostics), codon-specific oligonucleotide probes are applied as discrete lines on a nitrocellulose membrane in a strip format. Hybridization of biotin-labeled test isolate amplicons with

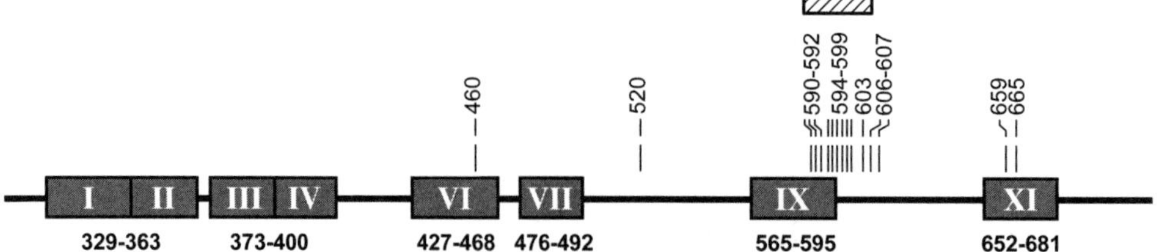

FIGURE 2 CMV UL97 mutations associated with ganciclovir resistance. CMV UL97 conserved regions are represented by shaded boxes. Numbers under the boxes indicate the positions (codon numbers) of these conserved regions. Vertical bars indicate the presence of amino acid substitutions, while the hatched box indicates a region (codons 590 to 607) in which diverse deletions (from 1 to 17 codons) have been reported.

the probes for specific codons (wild type and mutants) leads to the production of color in the presence of an avidin-enzyme complex and a substrate. Some researchers have concluded that the clinical utility of LiPA is limited by the high rate of indeterminate results (134), and this test is currently available for research use only. In another hybridization method, the microarray chip-based technology, over 16,000 unique oligonucleotide probes are used for hybridization with fluorescein-labeled target nucleic acid (HIV PRT GenChip; Affymetrix). This method was shown to be less reliable than dideoxynucleotide sequencing and is no longer commercially available (53). The final step in the process of genotypic resistance testing is the analysis of generated sequences. Interpretation of the genotype can be based either on rule-based algorithms or on "virtual phenotypes." The sequences may be aligned using different software programs included in commercially available genotypic assays or with online databases. In "virtual" phenotyping, the genotypic mutation profile of a viral strain is compared with the available paired genotypes and phenotypes in the database (VircoGEN; VircoLab).

In summary, phenotypic or genotypic assays can be used depending on the virus and the clinical situation. Phenotypic assays offer the advantage of providing a direct measurement of viral susceptibility to any antiviral drugs and of quantifying the level of resistance. On the other hand, genotypic assays offer the distinct advantages of greater speed and efficiency in analyzing large numbers of viral strains but only identify known drug resistance mutations. Discordance between phenotypic and genotypic assays can result from the presence of viral quasispecies (genotypic mixture of wild-type and mutant viruses) and the presence of complex patterns of mutations (resistance and compensatory mutations).

DIRECT DETECTION OF VIRUS OR VIRAL ANTIGEN

Electron Microscopy

In most diagnostic laboratories, EM for the diagnosis of viral infections has been supplanted by other methods, and many reviews of specific diagnostic recommendations fail to even mention the potential role of EM (128). Although EM is no longer the method of choice for the diagnosis of any viral infection, it remains an important and often rapid method for detecting viruses in clinical samples (11, 27). For example, many laboratories use EM for screening stool samples for viruses associated with acute gastroenteritis because of the wide array of potential viral pathogens that may be detected and the lack of a simple, single assay for the multiple viral pathogens (95, 108). EM continues to play an important role in the detection of BK polyomavirus in tissue biopsy samples and urine samples from renal transplant patients with suspected BK virus-associated nephropathy (30, 56).

Virtually any specimen type can be examined by EM for viruses, although sample preparation may vary with different types of specimens. In general, liquid samples such as CSF, saliva, tears, urine, and vesicle fluid may be used directly, while others may need to be rehydrated (e.g., dried tissue samples) or clarified (e.g., fecal material) before examination by EM. Specimens to be examined by EM must be adsorbed onto a thin plastic and/or carbon film applied to the surface of an electron microscope grid before staining (27, 55). In order to improve the sensitivity of EM, either pooled human immunoglobulins (Igs) or specific antibodies during the adsorption step can be used (e.g., solid-phase immunoelectron microscopy). In addition, ultracentrifugation of the original sample followed by resuspension in a smaller volume or direct centrifugation of the sample onto the electron microscope grid may also help increase the probability of detecting virus particles by EM. Once the grid has been prepared with the specimen, it is subjected to either positive or negative staining. Both methods use heavy metal ions (e.g., lead, tungsten, and uranium ions) to generate sufficient image contrast and resolution (55). Because positive staining is technically more demanding and requires considerably more time to perform, it is impractical for routine clinical specimens and has been replaced by negative staining. The most common negative stains are 1% aqueous uranyl acetate and 1% phosphotungstic acid. These electron-dense stains penetrate the virion and provide contrast for visualization of the surface detail of virus particles. Negative staining allows for examination and morphological detection of viruses in a sample within 10 min (55). Based on the unique morphologies of different virus families and measurement of the size of the virus particle, EM allows for a virus to be classified into a particular family relatively easily.

Key advantages of EM in diagnostic virology include the speed with which a sample can be screened for virus particles and the ability to search for unknown viral agents within a sample. These features make EM well suited for investigation of potential outbreaks due to new and emerging viruses and possible bioterrorism events (27, 55, 64, 114). EM is far less prone to cross-contamination, as may occur with molecular diagnostic techniques. Furthermore, no virus-specific reagents (e.g., monoclonal antibodies and primers) are needed for performing negative-staining EM.

Many limitations to EM exist, so it is usually available only in reference centers. The availability of EM is limited by the cost of the instrument and the need for expertise in reading grids. EM is not well suited for screening large numbers of routine samples, as may be required in a clinical diagnostic laboratory. Estimates on the amount of virus needed in order to be detectable by EM have ranged from 10^5 to 10^8 particles/ml, and thus EM is far less sensitive than other techniques (11, 55). However, despite its limited sensitivity, EM will occasionally detect viruses not detected by molecular diagnostic techniques because of the genetic diversity of some viruses (95).

Histopathology and Cytopathology

Standard light microscopy examination of stained clinical material may identify direct cellular changes which may be the first evidence of a viral infection. For some viruses, infected cells and tissues may exhibit cytological alterations that are pathognomonic for a specific virus (Table 4), while for others, the changes may be nonspecific and simply raise the possibility of a viral infection. Some stains allow for the detection of viral inclusions but cannot provide a definitive identification of the specific viral agent.

None of the usual cytological stains (e.g., hematoxylin and eosin, Wright-Giemsa, Giemsa [Tzanck preparation], or Papanicolaou [Pap]) is specific for detecting the presence of a viral infection, and all lack sensitivity. For example, the classic Tzanck preparation cannot be used to distinguish HSV from VZV infections, an important clinical

TABLE 4 Cytological changes associated with selected viral infections

Virus	Clinical presentation	Cytological findings
Adenovirus	Upper respiratory tract infections, pneumonia, acute keratoconjunctivitis	Small multiple eosinophilic intranuclear inclusions (early); large, single dense basophilic intranuclear inclusions ("smudge cells," late)
	Hemorrhagic cystitis	Dense basophilic intranuclear inclusions in transition cells
BK virus	Urethral stenosis (renal transplant patients) and interstitial nephritis (immunosuppressed patients)	Large full mucoid intranuclear inclusions (early); dense full basophilic inclusions bulging from cytoplasm (late)
CMV	Pneumonia	Cytomegaly; large, single amphophilic intranuclear inclusions (Cowdry A); small basophilic intracytoplasmic inclusions
HSV	Herpes genitalis, tracheobronchitis, corneal vesicle or ulcer	Large ground-glass nucleus (early); eosinophilic intranuclear inclusions (late) with peripheral chromatin condensation; multinuclearity with nuclear molding
	Generalized infection or local cystitis	Ground-glass nuclei (early); eosinophilic intranuclear inclusions (late); multinuclearity; may be part of tubular cast
HPV	Condyloma acuminatum, cervical dysplasia	Enlarged hyperchromatic nucleus; rare basophilic intranuclear inclusions; perivascular cytoplasmic clearing and vacuolar degeneration (koilocytic change)
Human polyomavirus	Progressive multifocal leukoencephalopathy	Enlarged oligodendrocytes with enlarged nuclei containing large basophilic inclusions
	Polyomavirus-associated nephropathy	Enlarged basophilic inclusions and displaced chromatin in renal tubular epithelium and urothelium; basophilic ground-glass nuclear inclusions in epithelial cells ("decoy cells") in urine
Measles virus	Prodromal	Mulberry-like clusters of lymphocytic nuclei in nasal secretions
	Measles with exanthema	Multinucleated giant cells with intracytoplasmic and intranuclear inclusions
Molluscum contagiosum	Reddish papular lesions of eyelid or conjunctiva	Large dense basophilic intracytoplasmic inclusions displacing the nucleus
	Vaginal, penile, or perineal papule with central umbilication	Large dense basophilic intracytoplasmic inclusions displacing the nucleus; squamous cells often bean shaped
Nipah virus	Encephalitis	Intracytoplasmic eosinophilic inclusions
Parainfluenza virus	Bronchitis	Cytomegaly; single or multiple nuclei; small eosinophilic intracytoplasmic inclusions
Parvovirus B19	Aplastic crisis, hydrops fetalis	Nuclear inclusions in erythroid precursor cells, bone marrow, or liver (fetus)
RSV	Tracheobronchitis, pneumonia	Large multinucleated cells; intracytoplasmic basophilic inclusions with prominent halos
VZV	Vesicular eruptions in dermatome (shingles) or accompanying varicella	Multinucleated cells with intranuclear eosinophilic inclusions

distinction required for proper management, infection control, and counseling of patients.

One of the key areas where cytological examination plays an important role has been the Pap smear for cervical scrapings as part of screening for early changes of cervical cancer. Virtually all cervical cancers are associated with specific oncogenic subtypes of human papillomavirus (HPV). Thus, examination for the presence of atypical squamous cells of undetermined significance and atypical glandular cells of undetermined significance coupled with newer molecular tests which can detect the presence of most of the oncogenic subtypes of HPV is rapidly becoming the standard for cervical cancer prevention.

Up to 10% of renal transplant patients may develop polyomavirus nephropathy which may result in loss of the renal graft. Histologic diagnosis using light microscopy plays an important role for these patients (30). However, because the pathological changes of polyomavirus nephropathy are heterogeneous and the intranuclear viral inclusions are indistinguishable from those of other viruses such as adenovirus and herpesviruses, immunohistochemical staining, EM, or molecular testing is required for making a definitive diagnosis. Similarly, although cytological examination of cells shed in urine may identify "decoy cells," which are cells containing intranuclear inclusions, it cannot distinguish between the different types of polyomavirus (e.g., BK versus JC) or adenovirus-infected cells (115).

Cytological examination may also play a role in distinguishing viral shedding from active infection in some clinical situations. For example, the presence of cytological changes, including the presence of cytomegalic inclusion bodies in a bronchoalveolar lavage sample, is more suggestive of active CMV infection than is detection of CMV in the same sample without evidence of cytological changes.

Immunoassays

A large number of immunoassays exist for the detection of viruses directly within clinical specimens. These assays utilize antibodies (antisera), which may be monoclonal or polyclonal, directed against a specific viral antigen or antigens (21). The resulting antibody-antigen complexes can be detected using a number of different techniques, ranging from direct visualization methods to those that detect viral antigens using solid-phase immunoassays (SPIA) such as EIAs and enzyme-linked immunosorbent assays (ELISA).

Direct Visualization Immunoassays

Visualization of viral antigens is most commonly achieved by either direct or indirect staining methods. In the direct method, the antibody (antiserum) directed against the virus of interest is conjugated with either an enzyme (e.g., horseradish peroxidase) or a fluorescent label (e.g., fluorescein isothiocyanate [FITC]). Once the antibody-antigen reaction is allowed to occur on a glass slide, a substrate is added for the conjugated enzyme; action of the substrate upon the enzyme results in a color reaction that is visible using a light microscope. If the antibody label used was FITC, the antibody-antigen complexes can be visualized using an immunofluorescence microscope set at the appropriate wavelength. In the indirect method, the initial antibody (e.g., mouse antibody) directed against the virus of interest is not conjugated to an enzyme or a fluorescent label. Therefore, after it is allowed to bind to the virus of interest, a second conjugated or labeled antibody directed against the first (e.g., goat anti-mouse antibody) is allowed to bind to the antibody within the antigen-antibody complex. Visualization is then performed as for the direct method. The advantage of the indirect method is that it can "amplify" the signal because many secondary antibodies may bind to the initial antibody, resulting in a stronger fluorescence signal.

Fluorescent-antibody immunoassays, including direct immunofluorescence (DFA) and indirect immunofluorescence (IFA) microscopy, have become widely used in diagnostic virology because they are relatively easy to perform and inexpensive (Table 5). They are applicable to a wide variety of specimen types and can be used for the detection of numerous different viral pathogens with high specificity, particularly when monoclonal antibodies are used. As well, pooling of monoclonal antibodies, each labeled with different fluorescence molecules, allows for the simultaneous detection of different viruses in the same sample. For example, a pool of monoclonal antibodies directed against influenza viruses A and B, RSV, parainfluenza viruses 1, 2, and 3, and adenovirus is often used to screen respiratory specimens such as nasopharyngeal washings. If the screen is positive, then individual slides can be prepared and stained individually to identify the specific virus present in the specimen. Fluorescent-antibody staining is used in many laboratories as the initial screening for HSV and VZV in skin and mucous membrane samples and for respiratory viruses in respiratory specimens (80, 128). Detection of CMV pp65 antigens using direct immunofluorescent staining of peripheral blood leukocytes is used in many centers as an alternative to molecular techniques for monitoring patients after organ and bone marrow transplantation (125).

TABLE 5 Detection of viral antigens by DFA staining

Clinical presentation	Possible viral agents detectable by DFA	Specimen type or source
Colorado tick fever	Colorado tick fever virus	Blood (RBC)
Congenital infections	Rubella virus, CMV, HSV	Nasopharynx, throat, lesion scrapings, tissue
Conjunctivitis, keratitis	HSV, adenovirus, measles virus	Conjunctival cells, corneal scrapings
Disseminated disease (immunocompromised host)	HSV, CMV, VZV, EBV	Tissues, lesion scrapings
Encephalitis	HSV	Brain biopsy sample
	Rabies virus	Brain tissue
	Mumps virus	Throat, urine sediment
Macular or maculopapular exanthems	Measles virus, rubella virus, mumps virus, adenovirus	Nasopharynx, throat, urine sediment
Mucocutaneous vesicles or ulcers	HSV, VZV, adenovirus	Scrapings from base of the lesion, mucosal cells
Respiratory infection	Influenza A and B viruses, parainfluenza viruses, adenovirus, RSV, human metapneumovirus, measles virus, mumps virus	Nasopharyngeal swabs, washes, or aspirates; throat swab; lung biopsy sample; bronchoalveolar lavage or brushing

SPIA

SPIA for the detection of viral antigens directed against specific viruses include EIA, ELISA, latex agglutination (LA), and radioimmunoassay (RIA) (21). In many laboratories, EIAs and ELISAs have become the predominant SPIA techniques used for viral diagnosis. EIAs and ELISAs have been automated, which improves consistency in the performance of these tests and objectivity in the interpretation of the results, as well as increasing throughput. Although the terms EIA and ELISA have slightly different meanings, they are often used interchangeably to denote any assay that utilizes an enzyme label. For simplicity, "ELISA" is used in the remainder of this section.

ELISAs, like the other methods noted above, can be used to detect either antigens or antibodies in a clinical sample (79). For detection of viral antigens, the surface of a solid phase (e.g., the well of a microtiter plate) is coated with antibodies directed against the antigen of interest. When the sample is added to the solid phase, the antigen, if present, will bind to the antibody, forming an antigen-antibody complex. Once the excess sample is removed by several washing steps, a second antibody is added that will bind to the antigen-antibody complex. Detection can be achieved either by having the secondary antibody conjugated with an enzyme followed by addition of a substrate (appropriate for the enzyme) which results in a color reaction or by use of a third antibody which is conjugated with an enzyme followed by addition of the substrate. Different enzymes have been used, including horseradish peroxidase, alkaline phosphatase, beta-glucosidase, and others. The presence and intensity of the color reaction are usually read using a spectrophotometer, which yields a result as an optical density. It should be noted that most assays are qualitative, and one cannot assume that a high optical density correlates with the presence of more antigen in the patient's sample. Some assays include quantitation standards that can be used to generate a standard curve for quantifying the amount of antigen in a patient's sample.

The solid phase can be a membrane rather than a microtiter plate. This format has been developed for detection of such viral antigens as influenza virus, RSV, and rotavirus (62). Tiny beads (microparticles) have also been used as the solid phase in order to increase the surface area for the coating of antigens or antibodies. These methods can decrease the reaction time and provide a result within approximately 30 min or less. ELISAs may be noncompetitive ("sandwich assays," which is the format described above) or competitive assays. In the latter, the solid phase is coated with the antigen of interest and the patient sample and secondary specific antibody are added simultaneously. The remainder of the assay is completed as for the sandwich assay. If the patient's sample contains the antigen of interest, the specific antibody will bind to it, leaving fewer specific antibodies to bind to the antigen used to coat the solid phase. This results in a decrease in the intensity of the color reaction, which, in turn, is inversely proportional to the amount of antigen present in the patient's sample.

ELISAs are extremely sensitive and are capable of detecting antigens at the picomolar to nanomolar range (10^{-12} to 10^{-9} mol/liter) (79). They have been developed for the detection of numerous different viral antigens. However, most assays have been developed and validated using a limited number of different sample types. Nonspecific reactions or cross-reactions can occur with ELISAs depending on whether the antibodies used in the assay are monoclonal or polyclonal. Despite these limitations, ELISAs have come into widespread use in the clinical diagnostic virology laboratory and are the mainstay for the laboratory diagnosis of numerous different viral infections (80).

NUCLEIC ACID DETECTION

Identification of viral nucleic acids is based on relatively conserved and unique nucleotide sequences which can be copied into complementary oligonucleotides by polymerases, cut at defined sequence-specific sites by restriction endonucleases, and differentially annealed to complementary sequences under defined conditions. The relatively short length of viral genomes makes viruses ideal candidates for nucleic acid-based diagnosis.

NATs were used to a limited extent before the advent of current amplification assays such as PCR. These consisted of simple hybridization assays, such as in the case of the HPVs (74), as well as detection of defined size segments of viral genome either present endogenously, in the case of rotavirus, or resulting from restriction endonuclease digestion, as in the case of herpesviruses and adenoviruses (19, 111). With the advent of the PCR assay, NAT-based diagnosis has been extended to nearly all recognized viruses. The PCR assay has evolved from conventional PCR, in which products are identified by agarose gel electrophoresis, to real-time PCR, in which products are identified using probes or intercalating dyes within the reaction, and has now progressed to the development of microarray-based assays in either chip- or bead-based formats. Finally, PCR assays have been adapted for quantitation of specific viruses in a specimen.

PCR Assay

The development of the PCR assay for DNA virus detection, combined with the preceding reverse transcriptase step for RNA viruses, was a major breakthrough in diagnostic virology. This methodology allows for greatly enhanced levels of viral detection, because for every infectious unit, there are numerous defective or otherwise noninfectious particles, all containing the target genome. As shown in Fig. 3, the PCR assay is based on cycling a mixture of specimen DNA, virus-specific oligonucleotide primers in high excess, a thermostable polymerase, and nucleotide triphosphates at a high temperature at which the target DNA strands separate, a low temperature at which the primers anneal to their complementary sites, and an intermediate temperature optimal for the polymerase to elongate the complementary strand as an extension from the primers (119). Each time the cycle is repeated, the number of copies, or amplicons, doubles such that after 20 cycles there are potentially over one million amplicons from a single target molecule.

Primers are the major determinant of the sensitivity and specificity of each PCR assay. Since the sequences of most viral genomes are known, at least at the genus level, identifying oligonucleotide primers to conserved regions of the virus genome is feasible. While primers for in-house assays are known, those for commercial assays may not be readily available. In PCR assays for RNA viruses, a virus-specific primer or a random hexamer primer has been found to be acceptable for the initial reverse transcriptase reaction to produce the cDNA product for amplification. The sensi-

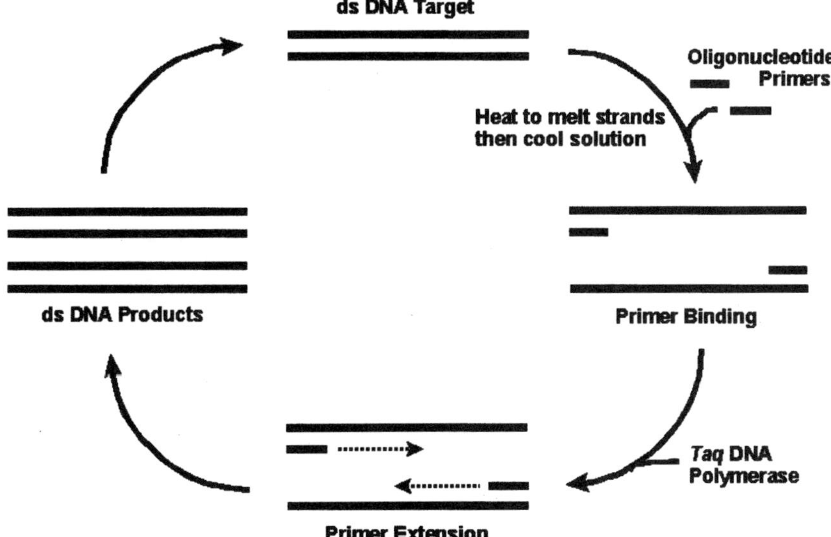

FIGURE 3 PCR. The strands of the target DNA are separated by heating (melting), and on cooling they anneal with the complementary primers present in excess. The thermostable DNA polymerase extends the primers, forming two double-stranded DNA molecules. On subsequent heating, the strands separate and each anneals with the complementary primer. The cycling of temperature among melting, annealing, and primer extension is repeated multiple times, and the number of product strands is doubled with each cycle. (Reprinted from reference 141a with permission.)

tivity and specificity of these assays are also influenced by the enzymes, buffers, and cycling temperatures, and these must be optimized for each specific assay.

Extraction of Nucleic Acid from Specimens

Because of their sensitivity, NATs such as PCR are less fastidious as to the nature of the specimen, such as the need for infectious virus for isolation or intact, infected cells for immunofluorescence microscopy. Nucleic acids are generally extracted using commercial kits which are based on the differential binding of the nucleic acid to silica under conditions of different ionic strengths. Extracted DNA is stable in EDTA solutions which chelate the magnesium required for DNase activity. RNA, which is less stable, can be preserved using an RNase inhibitor. Likewise, extracted RNAs and DNAs are stable when frozen at −80°C. Automated extractors allow for scaled-up extractions of specimens.

Detection of Amplicons

Conventional detection of amplicons has been achieved by agarose gel electrophoresis with staining by ethidium bromide. Other DNA intercalating dyes such as SYBR green are an option, as they are less toxic and easier to dispose of, but they are also more expensive. Digestion of the amplicon preparation with restriction endonucleases before electrophoresis enhances the specificity of the assay and allows for more precise identification of the virus at the level of genus and type (68). For enhanced detection, the amplicons resolved on gel electrophoresis can be transferred to a membrane and probed by Southern blotting (132). This can also be accomplished by performing the hybridization of the PCR products in a microtiter plate format, which allows for final analysis with a plate reader, an approach utilized in commercial kits.

Multiplex PCR

Multiple viruses can be responsible for the same clinical presentation, such as in a respiratory infection. Detection based on a single specimen can be performed by a PCR assay that can detect multiple genome targets. Such multiplex assays, though feasible, require careful design to ensure that the primers chosen have similar annealing temperatures and do not react with other primers to reduce the sensitivity and that the amplicons can readily be detected based on their size or by probes specific for each viral amplicon sequence (131). Multiplexing has been elegantly addressed in recently developed commercial respiratory virus assays. In such an assay, any RNA viral genomes are reverse transcribed to cDNA using random primers (92). The preparation is then subjected to a multiplex PCR with primers to all target virus sequences. The PCR products are then subjected to a multiplex target-specific extension reaction using primers specific for the viral cDNA sequences, which also have respective proprietary target-specific oligonucleotide tags at the 5′ end, in a reaction mixture that contains biotinylated deoxyribonucleoside triphosphates. The products of this extension reaction are reacted with microbeads with covalently attached antitag sequences unique to each virus type to which the complementary tagged sequences hybridize. The preparation is then analyzed by passage through the Luminex flow cell, where the unique signals of each bead type and the common signal from the biotin-streptavidin-phycoerythrin conjugate are measured as illustrated in Fig. 4.

Real-Time PCR

Real-time PCR is an enhancement of the conventional PCR in which amplicons are detected in a closed system after each cycle. This initially involved the detection of

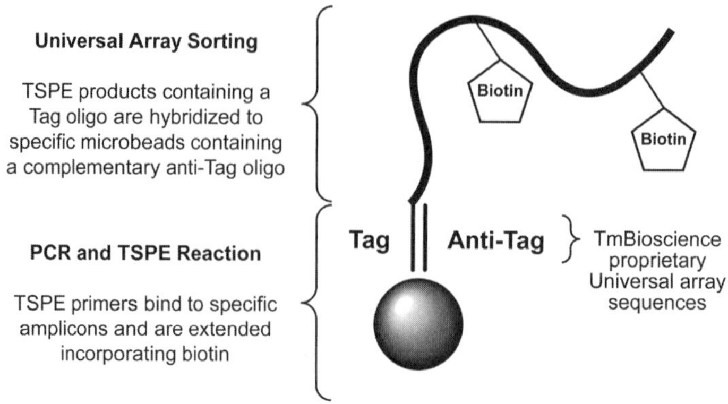

FIGURE 4 RVP assay (Luminex Molecular Diagnostics Inc.). Identification of the target-specific primer extension (TSPE) reaction that has been captured on the microbead is achieved through the oligonucleotide tag. Sorting of the microbeads occurs in the Luminex 100 flow cell instrument, which identifies colored beads with one laser and a phycoerythrin signal on the attached extended amplicon with a second laser.

fluorescence of the SYBR green dye that had intercalated into the amplicons before each melting step of the cycle (145). Subsequent detection systems incorporate the energy transfer reactions between fluorescent dyes in a process called fluorescence resonance energy transfer. This consists of two dyes, one of which is called the donor dye and the other of which is called the acceptor dye. When they are brought close together through the annealing of two adjacent primers to the target, the upstream one labeled at the 3′ end with the donor dye (for example, fluorescein) and the downstream one labeled at the 5′ end with the acceptor dye (for example, Cy5), light is absorbed by the donor dye and emitted by the acceptor dye, thereby creating a signal (20).

An alternative configuration is a single probe labeled at the 5′ end by a reporter dye and at the 3′ end by a quencher dye (90). The probe exhibits minimal fluorescence in the unhybridized state when the oligonucleotide is variably folded on itself, but it exhibits strong fluorescence at defined wavelengths when the quencher becomes separated from the reporter fluorophore, i.e., when the probe is linearized by hybridization to a target sequence. Such structures are called a molecular beacon (69). Alternatively, the reporter fluorophore and quencher, both of which are linked to the probe, may be separated after the probe hybridizes to the amplicon by the 5′ exonuclease action of the thermostable polymerase in the TaqMan platform, as illustrated in Fig. 5 (102). In this case, the fluorophore accumulates in the reaction mixture in increasing quantities with each cycle.

Real-time PCR has a number of advantages: it is more rapid than conventional PCR, does not include postamplification processing (thereby minimizing amplicon contamination), and is applicable to quantitative assays. Disadvantages include the inherent difficulty of readily monitoring for amplicon size (which precludes the utilization of digestion with restriction endonucleases as a control), difficulty of performing nested PCR, and limitations on the sizes of amplicons and probes. Furthermore, a mutation occurring in the sequence targeted by the probe would preclude the detection of the amplicon, in contrast to it still being detected by analysis of the products by gel electrophoresis. Nevertheless, the advantages of speed, sensitivity, and reduction of amplicon contamination have made real-time PCR the platform of choice in diagnostic virology.

Non-PCR-Based Nucleic Acid Amplification Systems

Nucleic acid amplification can be performed using approaches other than PCR.

Strand Displacement Amplification

Strand displacement amplification is based on the use of oligonucleotide primers containing a restriction endonuclease cleavage site, a DNA polymerase deficient in 5′ exo-

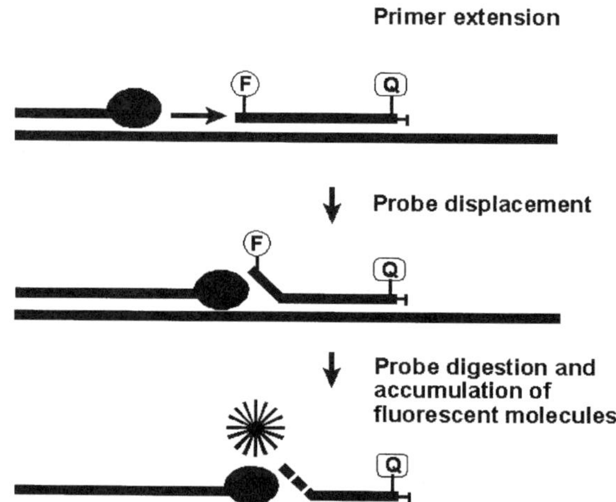

FIGURE 5 Real-time PCR (TaqMan process). In this thermocycling reaction, the internal probe, which is conjugated to the fluorescent dye (F) and the quencher dye (Q), hybridizes with the denatured target DNA. When these two dyes are present in close proximity on the probe, the fluorescence of the F dye is quenched. When the new strand being synthesized as an extension of the terminal primers reaches the probe, it is digested by the 5′ exonuclease activity of the thermostable polymerase, liberating the F dye and resulting in the generation of a fluorescent signal. (Reprinted from reference 141a with permission.)

nuclease activity, the cognate restriction endonuclease, and nucleotide triphosphates, of which dCTP has an alpha-thiol group (138). In the reaction, the primer binds to the target sequence on the viral genome, and the polymerase synthesizes a double-stranded product with the endonuclease cleavage site at the 5′ end of the new strand. The restriction endonuclease introduces a nick in the primer site of the new amplicon but not in the complementary strand that has the thiolated dCTP. The nick is recognized by the DNA polymerase, which extends the oligonucleotide downstream from the nick and displaces the nicked strand. Annealing of the antisense primer, also containing the restriction endonuclease site, allows the process to continue on the newly synthesized strand. As shown in Fig. 6, this process results in an exponential amplification of the area bracketed by the primers under isothermal conditions. The BDProbeTec (Becton Dickinson) is an example of an automated platform utilizing this method. The assay has a sensitivity of 5 to 50 genome copies per ml and requires approximately 1 h for completion.

Ligase Chain Reaction

The principle of the ligase chain reaction assay, illustrated in Fig. 7, involves thermal cycling with the polymerase replaced by a thermostable ligase (143). The assay involves

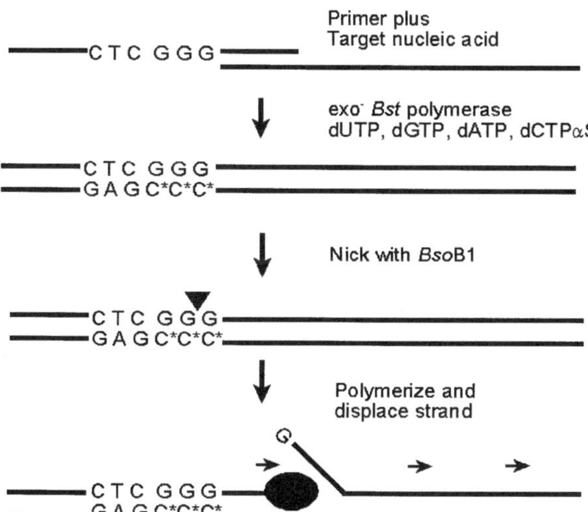

FIGURE 6 Strand displacement amplification. This isothermal amplification assay is based on four requirements, namely, primers which include an upstream restriction endonuclease site (BsoB1), the cognate enzyme (BsoB1), a DNA polymerase lacking 5′ exonuclease activity, and nucleoside triphosphates, of which one has been modified to contain an alpha-thiol group (dCTPαS). In this reaction, the target DNA anneals with the primers and is converted to a double-stranded form by the polymerase. The restriction endonuclease introduces a cleavage in the primer sequence, and the polymerase synthesizes a new strand from this site and displaces the existing strand. The restriction endonuclease is not able to cut the newly synthesized strands because of the modified nucleotides and can only introduce cuts in the sites present in the primers. Restriction site-bearing primers are designed to anneal to sequences of both strands of the target DNA, resulting in an exponential synthesis of displaced strands. (Adapted from reference 141a with permission.)

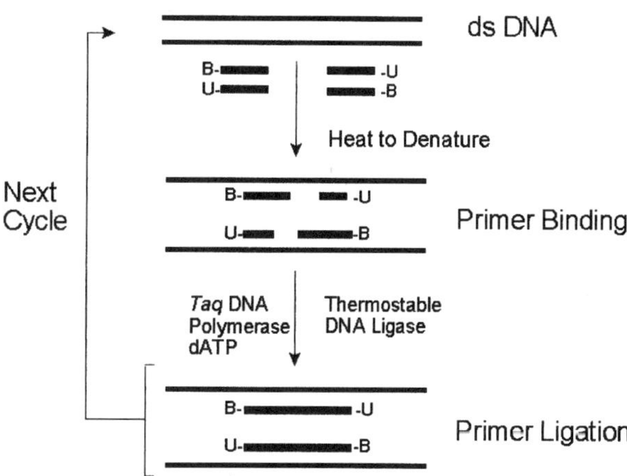

FIGURE 7 Ligase chain reaction. This reaction includes two pairs of primers, each pair annealing to one strand of heat-denatured target DNA with a gap of 2 to 7 nucleotides between. The primers are designed to bind so that the gap between them consists of a single nucleotide type. The reaction also contains the relevant nucleotide triphosphates, a thermostable DNA polymerase, and a thermostable DNA ligase. Once the gap is filled by the polymerase, the ligase joins the last nucleotide to the downstream primer. The temperature is then raised to denature the product and then lowered to allow further primer binding. The cycle is repeated so that additional primer pairs can be ligated. By having the upstream primer labeled at the 5′ end with biotin (B) and the downstream primer labeled at the 3′ end with a fluorescent label, the products can be captured on a solid phase and tested for the presence of the fluorescent label. (Reprinted from reference 141a with permission.)

the ligation of a pair of primers complementary to the full length of the target sequence of each strand that hybridize at adjacent positions and are joined by the ligase. Increasing the temperature results in the dissociation of the primer-derived strands, to which new primers can anneal at reduced temperature and allow the reaction to continue, with the formation of the ligated primers as the end product. The assay has a sensitivity of 5 to 50 genome copies per ml and is reported to be minimally susceptible to inhibitors in the specimen.

Nucleic Acid Sequence-Based Amplification

Nucleic acid sequence-based amplification (NASBA), an isothermal assay, is based on the amplification of predominantly RNA genome targets using two primers, one of which has a T7 promoter sequence at the 5′ end, a reverse transcriptase, a T7 DNA-dependent RNA polymerase, and RNase H, along with the deoxynucleotide triphosphates (50). In the assay, the primer with the T7 promoter hybridizes to the RNA template and is extended by the reverse transcriptase. The RNA portion of the heteroduplex is digested by RNase H, and the reverse primer hybridizes to the new DNA strand and is extended by the reverse transcriptase to produce a double-stranded DNA. The T7 polymerase copies multiple RNA strands off the DNA template in a primer-independent manner. Each of these can bind the primers and repeat the entire process. These reactions are illustrated in Fig. 8. A closely related approach, transcription-mediated amplification, initially called self-sustained sequence replication, is very similar; it differs

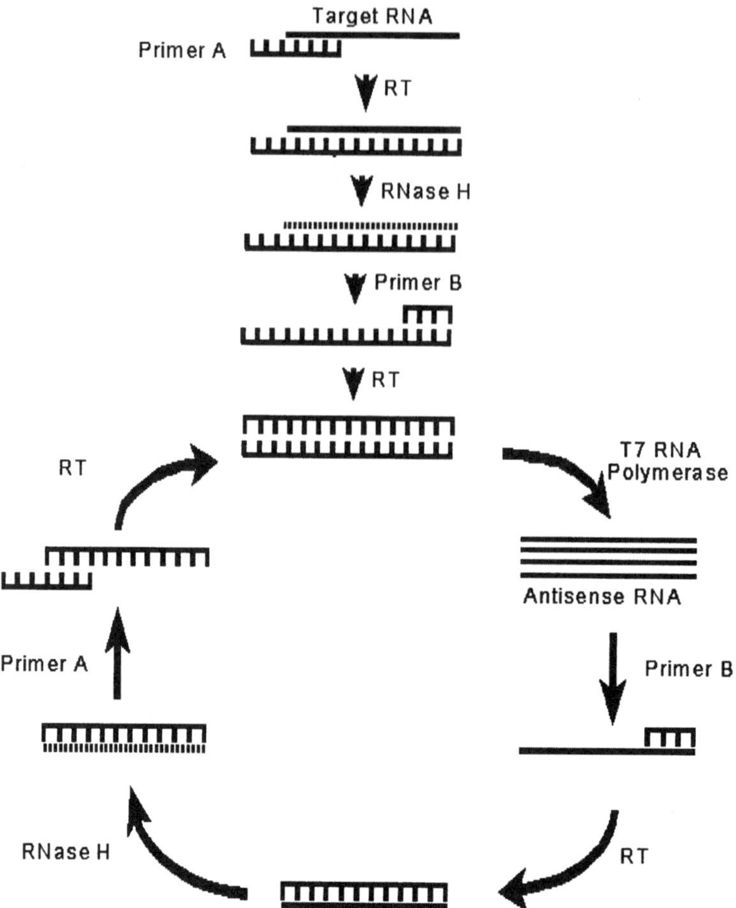

FIGURE 8 NASBA. This procedure is particularly well adapted to the detection of RNA. The reaction mixture consists of one primer which contains the sequence for the T7 RNA polymerase promoter at its 5′ end, a second primer at the downstream end of the sequence to be amplified, T7 RNA polymerase, reverse transcriptase, and RNase H as well as the ribo- and deoxyribonucleotide triphosphates. When the primer containing the T7 promoter anneals to the target RNA, the reverse transcriptase synthesizes the complementary DNA strand and the RNA portion of this duplex is digested by the RNase H. After binding of the downstream primer, the reverse transcriptase synthesizes a double-stranded DNA with a T7 promoter at one end which serves as a template for the T7 RNA polymerase, which synthesizes approximately 1,000 copies of antisense RNA in a promoter-dependent manner. This RNA can be further reverse transcribed to double-stranded DNA which can serve as a template on which the RNA polymerase can synthesize multiple antisense RNA copies. (Reprinted from reference 141a with permission.)

only in that conditions are set so that the endogenous RNase H activity of the reverse transcriptase is able to substitute for the exogenously added RNase H (39). This platform has been adopted in kits such as those from GenProbe Inc. and BioMérieux Inc. The assay is reported to have a sensitivity of 5 to 50 genome copies per ml.

Hybridization-Based Assays

Hybridization with labeled probes has long been used for detection of viral genomes. This has been refined to a high sensitivity in the branched-chain DNA assay, which is based on signal amplification (135). In this process, shown in Fig. 9, the genome is hybridized to a primary probe of complementary sequence which is immobilized on a solid phase. The genome then further hybridizes to secondary probes, which then hybridize with an amplification multimer. The latter hybridizes further with labeled probes that allow for detection of the branched-chain structure. Branched-chain DNA assays have a sensitivity of 50 to 500 genome copies per ml. An alternative approach exemplified by the hybrid capture assay involves hybridization in solution between a denatured DNA target and cRNA probes, resulting in the formation of a DNA-RNA hybrid. This structure is recognized by an antibody which is then detected by an immunoassay detection system. Such an approach has been commercially applied in the Digene Corporation hybrid capture assays. Hybridization assays, while not as sensitive as nucleic acid amplification (i.e., limit of detection of 500 to 1,000 genome copies per ml), have an ability to quantitate the amount of genome pres-

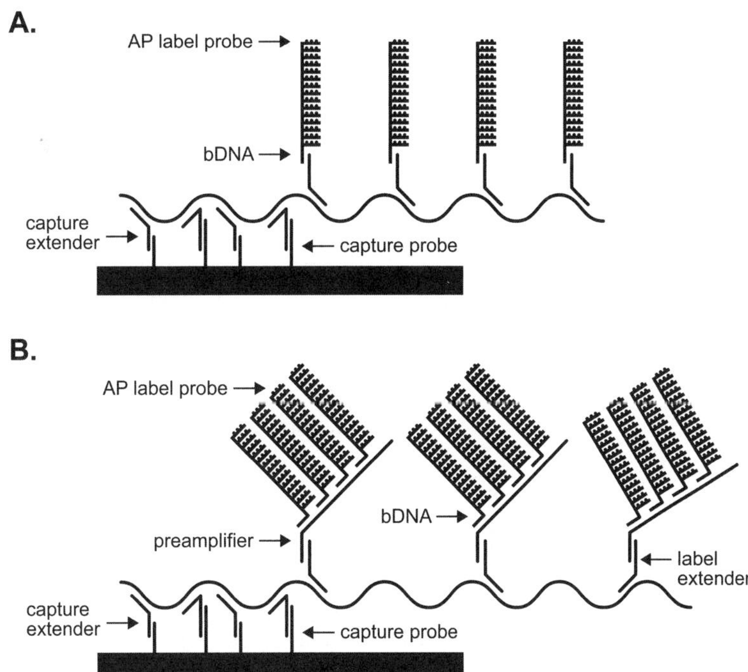

FIGURE 9 Branched-chain DNA (bDNA) assay of first (A) and third (B) generations. Target DNA hybridizes to capture probes linked to a solid phase. A short oligonucleotide called the label extender hybridizes with complementary sequences on the target DNA and with either the amplifier oligonucleotide shown in panel A or a longer oligonucleotide called the preamplifier that contains multiple repeat sequences, shown in panel B. Amplifier oligonucleotides then hybridize to the alkaline phosphatase-linked probes shown in panel A as well as the preamplifier sites shown in panel B. Alkaline phosphatase is detected by standard reagents for the enzyme.

ent in the specimen. These have been successfully adapted to the quantitation of HCV RNA (65).

Quantitative NATs

Initially, quantitation by PCR assays was accomplished by performing the assay on serial dilutions of the specimen. Currently, quantitative PCR assays contain an internal standard target of defined concentration that serves as a reference on which the calculations of concentrations of the analyte nucleic acid are based. Due to inherent variability, most commercial assays claim an accuracy within 0.5 $\log_{10}$, or approximately threefold. These approaches are based on the assumption that the amplification efficiencies of the standard and the target are nearly equivalent. Quantitation can also be achieved by NASBA and branch-chain DNA assay (117). The latter, being a signal amplification assay, is considered less variable but also less sensitive than target amplification assays. NASBA and PCR assays have been optimized to detect the product in the log phase of the amplification rather than at the end, thereby increasing the dynamic range.

Controls

Controls are critical in NATs, because the analytical sensitivity is high and because the amplicons generated in the PCRs are relatively stable and serve as a potential source of contamination. Efforts to overcome this problem include the use of assays that do not create DNA amplicons, such as NASBA, branched-chain DNA, and real-time PCR, which does not involve opening the tube with amplified products. The addition of dUTP together with uracil DNA glycosylase to the PCR, which destroys the amplicon sequence at the end of the assay (91), is commonly used. Fastidious adherence to the design of the laboratories so that amplicon contamination is avoided by restriction of movement among clean and dirty rooms is essential. Amplicon contamination of the environment can be further reduced by wiping the surfaces with household bleach, exposing working surfaces to short UV light, and working in laminar-flow biological safety cabinets with appropriate clothing and use of gloves.

NATs require numerous controls to ensure that the amplification reactions did occur and that they were free of any contamination. These include amplification controls or target-related oligonucleotides, such as genomes of related viruses with sequences complementary to the same probes, genomes of other viruses for which probes are provided, DNA of defined sequences in plasmid vectors, or RNA produced by T7 polymerase from a recombinant DNA target with a T7 promoter. It is particularly important to protect the RNA controls from endogenous RNases by including RNase inhibitors or by encapsidating the controls into proteins such as that of MS1 phage, as in the case of "armored RNA" (110). Controls are also added to the specimen or aliquot thereof before extraction to serve as extraction controls. Water, free of any target, is an essential negative control. Finally, a sample quality control consisting of a common gene, such as the beta-globin or RNase P gene, helps to validate that the specimen contained adequate tissue for testing.

Application of NAT in Virology

The very high sensitivity of NAT has greatly improved the ability to obtain an accurate viral diagnosis but has also created a need for enhanced insight into the interpretation of the test results and the need to more thoroughly understand the pathogenesis of viral infections. Applications of NAT include detection of the virus in the patient specimen in acute and chronic infections and the potential to subtype the virus to the level of its genome sequence; to quantitate the concentration of the virus to determine the extent of the infection, the likelihood for transmission, and the response to antiviral therapy; and to monitor for the development of strains resistant to antiviral agents.

Routine Diagnosis of Viral Infection

Detection of most common viruses can now be performed by NAT within comparable or superior turnaround times and with substantially increased sensitivity relative to those of conventional methods. Using real-time PCR, most of these viruses can be identified in patient specimens on a same-day to next-day basis, making the diagnosis relevant for patient management. In addition, the development of multiplex assays has allowed for an unprecedented breadth of testing for all known respiratory viruses in a patient specimen within a working day using a single test (92). Likewise, nucleic acid microarray technology is believed to have a similar potential (139).

Real-time PCR has been successfully applied to same-day testing for HSV in either in-house or commercially marketed assays (38). The detection of noroviruses by NAT is more efficient and reliable than by ELISA or EM (70). While enteroviruses have conventionally been detected by isolation in cell culture, NAT is substantially more sensitive, an important consideration in the diagnosis of infection with neurotropic viruses (118). Accordingly, laboratories are becoming increasingly reliant on NAT for routine virus detection, a trend that is likely to continue as the costs of these tests decrease with increased volumes of use and the implementation of further automation.

Diagnosis of Novel and Emerging Viral Infections

NAT is particularly suitable for the diagnosis of novel and emerging infections. The two that stand out in recent times are the diagnosis of the Sin Nombre hantavirus infections in 1993 and the diagnosis of SARS coronavirus infections in 2003 (104, 140). A major advantage of NAT in the workup for novel agents of an as-yet-unknown risk or those associated with high morbidity and mortality is that much of the investigation does not need to be performed under biosafety level 3 (BSL-3) conditions. The risk of working with extracted nucleic acids is minimal under BSL-2 conditions. Group-specific PCR assays based on conserved sequences can provide evidence as to the identity of the virus at the family level, and the virus can be further characterized by sequencing of the amplicons. Similarly, amplicons from randomly primed PCRs can be characterized by shotgun sequencing. In designing tests for pandemic influenza virus, NAT reagents are expected to be readily available, the primer sequences will be quickly identified and communicated to laboratories, the extraction and NATs can readily be scaled up 10-fold, and testing can be performed in BSL-2 laboratories, with perhaps specimen extraction being the only risky step.

Diagnosis of Chronic Viral Infections

Primary diagnosis of chronic viral infections such as with HIV, HBV, and HCV is generally accomplished by serology, but NAT has an important role in the follow-up of these infections. With NAT, one can differentiate between a chronic HCV infection, which is present in approximately 75% of seropositive patients, and successful resolution of the infection in the remainder (133). NAT is used to determine whether a child born of an HIV-seropositive mother is infected or whether the antibody in his or her serum comes from passive maternal transfer (32). NAT can help resolve conundrums in HBV serology and establish or rule out infectivity. Likewise, NAT is used for testing blood donors to prevent the use of the very rare infected unit that cannot be identified by serology or other screening methods. Finally, NAT is often the only realistic test to use to investigate infection in immunocompromised patients unable to mount a humoral immune response.

NATs that can assess the concentration of virus in the blood have proven valuable, as the viral load correlates with the risk of transmission. Pregnant mothers with HIV are treated with antiviral drugs to suppress the viral load, which can be monitored (32). Likewise, the viral load correlates directly with the risk of transmission in HIV-discordant couples (49). Finally, for health care workers with chronic HBV infections, a high viral load can be used to exclude them from certain procedures.

Viral Diagnosis in Management of Immunocompromised Patients

Patients immunocompromised through infection or malignancy or iatrogenically, such as those having undergone transplants, are subject to many life-threatening viral infections. Infections of particular concern to such patients are those of the herpesviruses, EBV, and CMV (73). Monitoring the viral load in the blood of transplant patients, especially those in the pediatric group, and either modulating immunosuppression or using antiviral drugs such as ganciclovir are critical for their survival. Likewise, monitoring the presence of adenoviruses and the human polyomavirus BK in the blood and urine is important in transplant patients, and this is most commonly done by NAT (29, 30).

Monitoring Response to Antiviral Therapy and Antiviral Drug Resistance

In HCV-infected individuals, the duration of antiviral therapy with interferon and ribavirin is determined by the genotype of the virus and the efficacy of the treatment on the viremia (40). The viral genotype is obtained by characterizing the amplified 5′ untranslated region of the genome either by sequence analysis or by hybridization to probes immobilized as lines on a solid phase (line blot). The response of specific genotypes to treatment is monitored by quantitative assays such as branched-chain DNA and quantitative PCR. These are vital assays for HCV treatment, the utilization of which is dependent on a brisk fall in viremia and the absence of detectable virus at the end of treatment. Likewise, HBV viral load can be quantitated by branched-chain DNA or PCR assays and used to monitor the response to antiviral drugs.

The capacity to accurately assess the viral load is essential in the management of HIV infections, in which there is a relationship between viral load, the CD4 cell count, and disease progression (61). When patients are undergoing antiviral treatment, the goal is to maintain the viral load at levels below 50 genome copies per ml of plasma, the lower limit of detection of quantitative assays (34). In another application, an increased viral load in a patient receiving antiviral therapy may suggest the development of viral resistance, which can be confirmed by specific phenotypic or genotypic resistance assays.

Nucleic Acid Sequencing

DNA sequencing has evolved from a research tool to become an expected part of diagnostic virology. It has proven its value by greatly simplifying the typing of enteroviruses and adenoviruses (105, 120). It allows for identifying specific genotypes of noroviruses and rotaviruses (70, 77) and for monitoring the drift of influenza A viruses at the nucleotide level over time (2). Newer sequencing technologies such as pyrosequencing and techniques such as shotgun sequencing allow for even more effective application of sequencing to diagnostics and are indicative of the future directions of these technologies in viral diagnosis (78).

SERODIAGNOSIS OF VIRAL DISEASES

Viral serologic assays contribute significantly to the indirect diagnosis of acute, recent, or chronic viral infections and are used widely for determining the immune status of a person or group of individuals with regard to a specific virus or to verify the immune response to vaccination (Table 6). Rapid determination of immune status in a hospital setting may aid in the prevention of nosocomial spread of certain viruses to nonimmune patients or in the application of prophylactic treatment to health care workers following needlestick injuries. Safety of the blood supply requires testing for virus-specific antibodies in all blood units to minimize the risk of acquisition of blood-borne infections. Knowing the serologic status of organ donors and recipients prior to transplantation is important when

TABLE 6 Utility of serologic determinations in clinical virology

Application	Most common virus(es)[a]
Diagnosis of recent or chronic infections	
Hepatitis	HAV–HEV, HGV, CMV, EBV, HSV, VZV, HIV, coxsackievirus B, adenovirus, yellow fever virus
CNS	HSV, CMV, VZV, EBV, HHV-6, enteroviruses, WNV and other arboviruses, measles virus, mumps virus, rubella virus, rabies virus, HIV, LCMV
Congenital/perinatal	CMV, HSV, VZV, rubella virus, HBV, HCV, parvovirus B19, LCMV
Exanthems	Measles virus, rubella virus, parvovirus B19, HHV-6, HHV-7, arboviruses
Myocarditis/pericarditis	Coxsackievirus B types 1–5, influenza virus types A and B, CMV
Infectious mononucleosis	
Heterophile antibody positive	EBV
Heterophile antibody negative	EBV,[b] CMV, HIV, rubella virus, HHV-6
Nonspecific febrile illness	CMV, EBV, HHV-6, HHV-7, parvovirus B19, HIV, dengue virus, Colorado tick fever virus
T-cell leukemia	HTLV-1 and -2
Hemorrhagic fever	Filoviruses, arenaviruses, flaviviruses, bunyaviruses
Hantavirus pulmonary syndrome	Sin Nombre virus, other hantaviruses
Screening for immune status	
Preemployment	VZV, rubella virus, measles virus, HBV
Prenatal	Rubella virus, CMV, HSV, VZV, parvovirus B19, HBV, HCV, HIV
Pretransplant	CMV, HSV, EBV, VZV, HBV, HCV, HIV
Blood donation	HIV, HBV, HCV, HTLV-1 and -2
Postexposure	HIV, HAV, HBV, HCV, VZV
Epidemiology and surveillance	All viruses
Verification response to vaccination	HAV, HBV, HPV, VZV, measles virus, mumps virus, rubella virus

[a] Abbreviations: LCMV, lymphocytic choriomeningitis virus; WNV, West Nile virus.

[b] A comprehensive panel of EBV-specific serologic tests should be performed for patients with heterophile-negative infectious mononucleosis, since only 60% of individuals will have heterophile antibodies by the second week of EBV mononucleosis and the test is usually negative for children ≤4 years of age. Commercial EIA and IFA EBV serologic tests allow for the simultaneous titration of virus-specific antibodies to the viral capsid and the early and nuclear antigens of the virus. Interpretation of the panel permits identification of current or recent primary infection, recurrent or chronic infection, or past infection with EBV.

considering the type of donor and blood products to be given, in preventing transmission of blood-borne viruses to individuals at high risk for severe disease, and in determining the treatment or prophylaxis to be used following transplantation. Prenatal antibody screening can supply useful information on the risk for contracting certain viral infections during pregnancy and be a determinant in establishing prognosis and prevention of perinatal transmission for seropositive parturient women.

Identification and measurement of virus-specific antibodies in a patient's serum also may be the only means of making a viral diagnosis under certain circumstances. A number of viruses are impossible, difficult, or even hazardous to grow in culture or difficult to detect by other methods. Proper specimens for culture or direct detection assays may be difficult to obtain or may not be obtained because viremia or virus shedding has subsided to undetectable levels when symptoms occur. Serodiagnosis is often the last resort when an investigation is undertaken retrospectively or too late in the course of the disease. Sometimes, a virus identified in a direct assay may have an uncertain role in the current disease process, and serology may assist in establishing a causal relationship. Serology is also an invaluable tool in the public health domain, whether to assess the incidence and prevalence of viral diseases for epidemiological studies, surveillance systems, or evaluation of the efficacy of prevention and control programs.

Although traditional methods of viral serodiagnosis are still in use, automated technologies are the mainstream of serologic testing in clinical laboratories. Use of recombinant antigens and synthetic peptides representing immunodominant regions has improved test sensitivity and specificity for detecting and confirming the presence of virus-specific antibodies. At the same time, the introduction of simple-to-use commercial tests or devices aimed at analyzing single specimens answers the growing need for rapid point-of-care testing.

Antibody Response to Viral Infections

Igs as markers of humoral response are more useful and reliable than cell-mediated immunity for diagnostic purposes because of historical and practical reasons. Antibodies can be detected and measured as they develop in response to an invading virus or to immunization (Fig. 10). Because of the transient nature of the IgM antibody response, its presence is generally indicative of current or recent viral infection. A significant rise in IgG antibody concentration over time is also accepted as evidence of a contemporary infection. In some instances, measurement of antibody avidity can help in estimating the time of occurrence of an infection, the rationale being that low-avidity antibodies are present in the early phase of infection, while high-avidity antibodies are a reflection of antibody maturation. Hence, a low avidity is likely to point to a recent primary infection (13). Accurate diagnosis of rubella virus and CMV infection during pregnancy may require an estimation of IgG avidity to rule out a recent infection. The role, onset, level, and duration of IgA, IgD, and IgE antibodies are less predictable than those of either IgM or IgG, and serologic tests for these isotypes

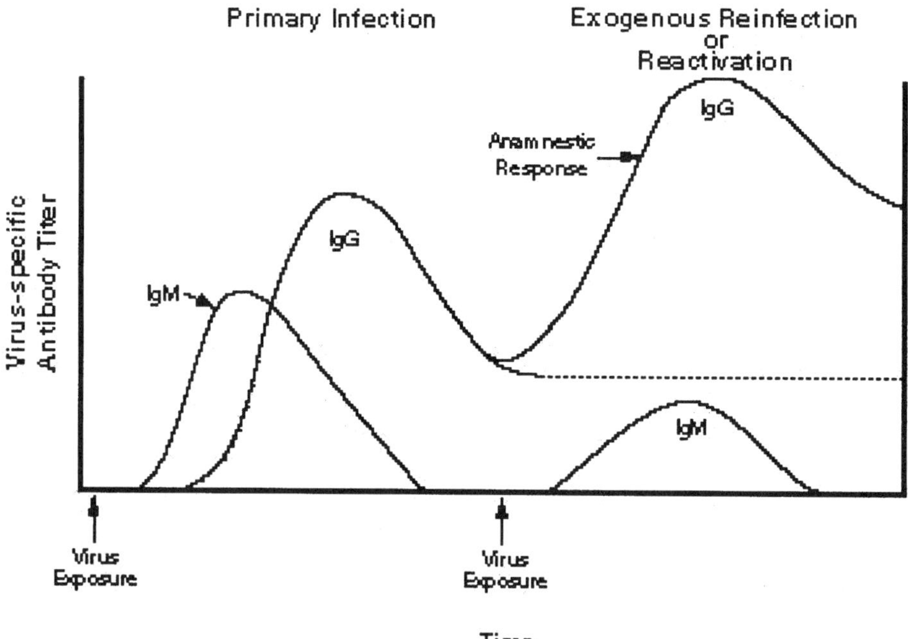

FIGURE 10 Diagram depicting the typical IgM and IgG antibody responses following primary viral infection, reactivation, or reinfection. During primary infection, IgM appears within several days after onset of symptoms, peaks at 7 to 10 days, and normally declines to undetectable levels within 1 to 3 months. Following natural viral infection or successful immunization, IgG antibodies appear several days after the production of IgM, reach higher levels than IgM, and can persist for years, even lifelong, in lower quantities. During reactivation or exogenous reinfection, an anamnestic response in IgG antibodies will occur and an IgM response may or may not be observed.

are generally not performed routinely in diagnostic laboratories.

Specimens for Serodiagnosis

Serum is the specimen of choice for most serologic assays; plasma can be used in some instances but is not suitable for all antibody tests unless specified by the manufacturer of the assay. For adults, 4 to 7 ml of blood obtained by venipuncture in a collection tube containing no additive is usually sufficient for most testing. If necessary, the laboratory will accept smaller volumes of blood, particularly from infants and young children or when few tests are being requested. Whole blood collected and dried on filter paper has been studied as a practical and effective substitution for obtaining serum by venipuncture, especially when screening for antibody to HIV (12). A consumer-controlled home collection kit using whole blood has been licensed for HIV-1 testing. Dried blood specimens have also been used for HBV and HCV and measles, mumps, and rubella virus antibody screening either because phlebotomy was resisted by the patient or because transport and long-term storage of serum and plasma specimens were logistically difficult (25, 109).

Whole blood should be allowed to clot for 30 to 60 min at room temperature. A centrifugation step allows separation of the serum from the remainder of the blood components to prevent hemolysis. Collected blood should not be frozen or transported to a remote laboratory in its collection tube, since this causes hemolysis and may render the specimen unusable for serologic testing. Icteric, lipemic, or heat-inactivated sera may also cause erroneous test results and should be avoided, if possible. Serum should be refrigerated at 4°C shortly after collection and during transport to the laboratory. If an extended delay in transport of a specimen is anticipated (e.g., holding an acute-phase serum until the convalescent-phase serum is collected), freezing the serum to at least −20°C is advised.

A single serum specimen is required to determine the immune status of an individual or to detect IgM-specific antibody. With few exceptions (e.g., EBV mononucleosis), paired serum specimens, collected 10 to 14 days apart, are required for the diagnosis of current or recent viral infections when specimens are tested for IgG antibody. The acute-phase serum should be obtained as soon as possible during the course of the illness, and no later than 5 to 7 days after onset. The most useful results are obtained by testing acute- and convalescent-phase sera simultaneously in a single laboratory. Evaluation of serum for antibodies to so-called TORCH agents associated with congenital and peripartum infections (i.e., *Toxoplasma gondii*, other agents, rubella virus, CMV, and HSV) requires that two serum specimens be submitted for testing: one from the mother and the other from her infant. To identify congenital infection, the newborn should be younger than 3 weeks when the specimen is obtained.

CSF may be tested for viral antibodies in patients with viral central nervous system (CNS) disease and may be superior to NAT detection for some infections (e.g., West Nile virus). For herpesviruses and some respiratory viruses that may cause neurologic disease, both CSF and serum specimens should be collected and paired for accurate measurement of virus-specific intrathecal antibody synthesis (4). Simply the presence of virus-specific IgG antibody to these agents in the CSF is not diagnostic of CNS infection because of the expected passage of Ig from blood to CSF. The normal ratio of Ig in blood to CSF is about 250:1.

Whole saliva, oral mucosal transudates rich in gingival crevicular fluid, and urine, which are collected by noninvasive means, have been advocated as alternatives to blood for the detection of antibodies to a number of different viruses (72). Particular attention has been paid to the value of oral fluids and urine for the diagnosis of infections with HIV (48, 59, 97). Accuracy of saliva for HIV antibody detection was shown to be equivalent to that of serum for clinical usage as well as epidemiological surveillance (72). The sensitivity and specificity of urine tests are inferior to those of blood and oral fluid tests. FDA-approved HIV oral fluid and urine tests are commercially available. Accordingly, several commercial devices have been developed for the collection of oral mucosal transudate specimens. The devices provide a homogeneous specimen rich in plasma-derived IgG and IgM that is passively transferred to the mouth across the mucosa and through the gingival crevices (67). Lastly, vitreous humor has been used for the detection of antibodies to HSV or VZV in individuals having eye infections due to these agents (121, 129).

Procedures for Detecting Viral Antibodies

A variety of methods are available for serodiagnosis of viral infections (reviewed in references 21, 26, 58, 85, and 93). The more traditional assays include complement fixation (CF), hemagglutination inhibition (HI), neutralization, immune adherence hemagglutination (IAHA), anticomplement immunofluorescence (ACIF), and IFA. With the exception of some commercial IFA kits, these are in-house assays and rarely done outside of specialized reference or public health laboratories. Nowadays, most clinical laboratories use commercially manufactured assays, including SPIA, passive latex agglutination (PLA), immunoblotting (IB), and immunochromatographic (IC) tests. The selection of which tests to perform will depend on the patient population and clinical situation, the number of specimens to be tested, turnaround time, ease of testing, and the resources and capabilities of the individual laboratory. Critical clinical information such as the date of onset of disease symptoms, recent travel history, immunization, or medical antecedents may also influence the choice of an adequate analytical strategy. Qualitative measurements of virus-induced antibody can be performed when it is useful to know simply that a specific antibody is present or absent. Quantitation is essential when it is important to know the amount of antibody present, particularly when measuring virus-specific IgG antibodies.

Complement Fixation

For many years, CF was one of the most widely used serologic assays in clinical virology. The assay can be used for measuring antibodies against virtually any cultivable virus, and it has the distinct advantage of assessing significant rises in antibody levels during viral infections (127). The CF method uses the cytolytic property of the complement system as an indirect marker for the antigen-antibody reaction. When virus-specific antibody is present in a patient's serum, it will complex with its corresponding antigen and fix guinea pig complement, thereby preventing lysis of sheep RBC complexed with anti-RBC antibodies. Conversely, an absence of antibody results in activation of the complement cascade, causing lysis of sensitized RBC. Although inexpensive in material and reagents, the method is technically demanding, requires rigid standardization and titration of reagents, and has a long turnaround time. The CF test is also less sensitive than other methods, making the assay unsuitable for use as a screening tool for immune status. Invalid results can occur with sera possessing anticomplementary activity due to nonspecific binding of serum components to the complement used in the assay. For these reasons, the CF test is used mainly for viral agents for which no other commercial reagents are available.

Hemagglutination Inhibition

HI has been applied to the detection of antibodies to viruses possessing surface proteins that can agglutinate RBC (148), particularly to detect antibodies to influenza, parainfluenza, measles, mumps, and rubella viruses and sometimes to the arboviruses, adenoviruses, and polyomaviruses. Antiviral antibodies in a patient serum can inhibit the agglutination of RBC by a viral antigen. The assay is technically demanding and requires appropriate quality control. The specific virus or antigen used as the source of hemagglutinin requires accurate titration for assay performance. Nonspecific inhibitors and natural agglutinins need to be removed from some serum specimens before virus-specific antibodies can be detected. The specificity of HI also varies with the virus, being highly specific for influenza and parainfluenza viruses but less so for arboviruses. Detection of HI antibodies is the current standard for assessing the immunogenicity of seasonal influenza vaccines and is often used for retrospective diagnosis of individual infections. The HI assay is also commonly used for subtyping and antigenic characterization of influenza virus isolates by reference laboratories.

Neutralization

In the neutralization assay, virus-specific antibodies are detected by their ability to neutralize or block the infectivity and replication of a given virus within a cell culture system (6). Neutralization titer is usually expressed as the reciprocal of the highest serum dilution resulting in a 90% reduction in the number of infected foci or plaques produced by a virus on a cell monolayer. The assay results are also biologically relevant, since the production of neutralizing antibodies is important in establishing protective immunity in response to a viral infection or vaccination. However, the assay is cumbersome, expensive, and time-consuming, and in the case of highly pathogenic viruses, it needs to be performed under high biosafety conditions (e.g., BSL-3 for West Nile virus and avian influenza A [H5N1] viruses). Similar to the case with HI, the quantity of virus used in the system must be carefully determined to obtain accurate results. The neutralization assay remains the method of choice for detection of antibodies to enteroviruses and the most specific test for confirmation of infection with West Nile virus and other arthropod-borne flaviviruses.

Immune Adherence Hemagglutination

The IAHA method uses the hemagglutinating property of the C3b fragment of the complement following attachment to C3b receptors on human type O RBC as an indirect marker for the antigen-antibody reaction (87). Virus-specific antibodies in a test serum are detected when complement binds to antibody-antigen complexes that have formed instead of RBC, thereby hampering hemagglutination. The assay is simple and has a sensitivity and specificity that are better than those of CF and comparable to those of IFA; IAHA is only slightly less sensitive than SPIA. IAHA is reliable for immune status testing and quantitative measurements of antibody titers. IgM can be detected after fractionation from IgG antibodies. Special attention has to be given to find an adequate supply of human type O erythrocytes and to qualify commercial antigen preparations. A prozone effect may occur with an excess of virus-specific antibody in the test serum. IAHA has been described for detection of antibodies in many viral infections (e.g., rabies and hepatitis viruses and VZV). Nowadays, it is rarely used in clinical virology laboratories.

Immunofluorescence Assays

IFAs are very useful and inexpensive methods that offer the advantages of speed and simplicity for the qualitative and quantitative detection of either IgM or IgG antiviral antibodies from clinical specimens (123). Commercial kits or antigen-coated slides are readily available for many of the common viruses, and labeled secondary antibodies can be purchased separately. Antibody is usually detected by either IFA or ACIF. In IFA, dilutions of serum are incubated with virus-infected cells that have been fixed to a glass microscope slide; specific antibody-antigen complexes that form are then detected using an anti-human antibody conjugated with a fluorochrome, most often FITC. A variation of this procedure called monoclonal antibody-enhanced IFA has been designed to increase the sensitivity of the fluorescent signal. It is a three-step procedure using an anti-human Ig mouse monoclonal antibody allowed to react with antibody-antigen complexes before an anti-mouse labeled antibody is used in the detection step (86). ACIF differs in that following incubation of test serum with virus-infected cells on glass slides, fresh complement is added and bound by any specific antigen-antibody complexes that have formed. A fluorescein-labeled anticomplement antibody is then added and binds to the C3 component of complement. ACIF amplifies the fluorescence signal, allowing for the detection of small amounts of antibody or antibodies of low avidity. This method is routinely used to detect antibodies to the nuclear antigen of EBV.

The disadvantages of IFA are that it requires a fluorescence microscope and darkroom for examining slides, and extensive training and critical evaluation are needed to read and reliably interpret the test results. The number of positively fluorescing cells, as well as the quality and intensity of the fluorescence, must be carefully examined and compared to those of cells reacted with positive and negative control sera. Most manufacturers of commercial kits provide antigen slides in which only 20 to 40% of the cells express viral antigens. Therefore, nonspecific binding of antibodies to the cells is easily discerned, since the staining produced by these antibodies involves all of the cells.

Solid-Phase Immunoassays

The term SPIA encompasses a large variety of methods and platforms aimed at detecting immobilized antigen-antibody complexes by means of a reporter signal. They have become the methods of choice for the detection of many virus-specific antibodies because of their speed, convenience, relative simplicity, and excellent sensitivity and specificity. The assay format is quite versatile, has evolved from polypropylene test tubes to microscopic spheres, and is applicable to many viruses and large numbers of specimens at a relatively low cost. EIAs are the most popular

SPIA used in clinical virology laboratories; they offer the advantages of using highly standardized and stable immunoreagents, especially those using recombinant antigens and synthetic peptides. EIAs that detect IgG or IgM antibodies to a number of different viruses are available from a variety of commercial sources. A newer generation of assays even provides simultaneous detection of antigen and antibody, thereby improving the early detection of HIV and HCV (51, 82).

Both noncompetitive and competitive assays have been described, and the results can be evaluated either qualitatively or quantitatively (21). The basic principle of the noncompetitive EIA is that viral antigen immobilized on a solid phase is used to capture free virus-specific antibody from a clinical specimen. The antigen-antibody complexes that form are then detected with the addition of an enzyme-labeled anti-human antibody that binds to the complexes and reacts with a chromogenic substrate to produce a color change. The intensity of the color generated is measured in a spectrophotometer and is usually proportional to the amount of virus-specific antibody in the specimen. Antibody content can be calculated from a standard curve equation established from serial dilutions of a reference antibody. Horseradish peroxidase and alkaline phosphatase are common enzyme labels. Fluorochrome labels such as fluorescein, rhodamine, and Texas red and chemiluminescent substrates have also been used.

In a competitive EIA, enzyme-labeled antiviral antibody is mixed with test serum, and virus-specific antibodies in the specimen will compete with the labeled antibody for a limited number of viral antigen binding sites on the solid phase. The activity of labeled antibody activity is then measured as described above. The decrease in detectable labeled antibody is inversely proportional to the quantity of antibody present in the sample. Competitive antibody assays are often used to provide greater specificity than noncompetitive assays; commercial tests are available for the detection of total antibodies to HAV and HBV core antigen.

RIAs using radioactive iodine as a label were developed in the 1970s (103). RIAs are less appealing because of the precautions and regulations needed to work with radioisotopes and dispose of these hazardous materials. Consequently, RIA has been largely replaced by EIA, especially since there is little difference in the sensitivities and specificities between the two methods. Today, RIA commercial reagents are available mainly for the detection of antibodies to HBV.

Microbead-based liquid arrays combine SPIA with flow cytometry to allow simultaneous detection of multiple antibodies (43, 94). The system uses 5.6-μm-diameter polystyrene microspheres, each containing a unique spectral address determined by varying the concentrations of red and infrared fluorochromes. Each bead, coated with carboxyl groups, is covalently linked to peptides or proteins. Antiviral antibodies are then allowed to bind to their respective target antigens labeled with a fluorescent reporter molecule. Detection is performed by means of a flow cytometer composed of a dual-beam laser detection system. A microfluidic device drives the microspheres into the laser beams. A red laser classifies the bead based on its internal color corresponding to a given antigen. A green laser measures fluorescence intensity corresponding to the reaction of antibodies with the antigen-reporter molecule complex. Microsphere immunoassays can detect up to 100 different viral antigens in a single well in less than 30 s per well and require only small sample volumes. They have been applied successfully to the detection of antibodies to HIV, respiratory viruses, arboviruses, EBV, and HPV (8, 76, 98, 107, 146).

A number of semiautomated and fully automated immunoassay analyzers for SPIA are now commercially available. These systems have found particular utility in the area of blood banking and clinical virology, where extensive test menus now exist for the automated performance of serologic assays for antibodies to HIV, hepatitis viruses, viral agents causing congenital infection, and other viruses of clinical importance. The majority of the automated immunoassay analyzers provide walk-away simplicity to perform assays from sample processing through interpretation of results. Most manufacturers of automated instruments also provide software for the analysis and management of patient data and for monitoring the quality of the testing being performed. Many of the instruments also can interface with computer-based hospital laboratory information systems for seamless reporting of results. Automation of viral serologic assays can be advantageous to laboratories that have a shortage of trained medical technologists or that need to reduce costs or improve the turnaround time for test results.

Passive Latex Agglutination Assays

PLA is an uncomplicated, convenient, and inexpensive method that it is best suited for testing small numbers of specimens. A suspension of latex particles coated with viral antigens is mixed with a clinical specimen and allowed to incubate with rotation for a short time (71). The antigen-coated particles will clump and produce agglutination in the presence of virus-specific antibody. The agglutination is visible to the naked eye. The test can be completed within 10 min and requires limited equipment and technical ability. Both IgG and IgM antibodies are detected without differentiation, and the sensitivity and specificity of PLA are reported to be comparable to those observed for EIA and IFA. However, reading an agglutination reaction by PLA can be subjective, and the results may be difficult to interpret. Also, a prozone or reduction in the degree of agglutination can occur with sera that have high levels of specific antibody, resulting in the need to dilute negative specimens and repeat the assay. Commercial PLA kits are currently available for the detection of antibodies to CMV, VZV, and rubella virus. PLA is best suited for qualitative determinations of viral antibody, but quantitation can also be performed. An automated particle counting technology has been developed which allows objective reading of the agglutination reaction (147). When RBC are coated with viral antigen, the procedure described for PLA is termed passive hemagglutination.

IB Assays

IB is a distinct type of SPIA using nitrocellulose or polyvinylidene fluoride membranes as the physical support for the detection of antibodies to specific viral antigens (84). The classic example is the Western blot, an assay widely used for confirmation of positive HIV antibody results obtained in a screening test. In the Western blot assay, whole-virus lysates of inactivated and disrupted viral proteins are separated by electrophoresis according to their molecular weight or relative mobility as they migrate through a polyacrylamide gel in the presence of sodium dodecyl sulfate. The resolved protein bands are then transferred onto a membrane in order to make the antigens accessible to antibody detection. The membrane is then cut into strips that are reacted with serum specimens. If virus-specific antibody is present in the serum, binding of antibody occurs in bands corresponding to the presence of the separated viral proteins. The bands are directly visualized by using an enzyme-labeled anti-human antibody followed by a chromogenic substrate.

Strip IB assays, also known as line immunoassays, are similar to Western blot assays except for the preparation of the membrane strip (26). They use the same general procedure for incubation and readout of a chromogenic enzymatic product at the site of binding of a virus-specific antibody. However, strip IB utilizes recombinantly derived proteins and synthetic peptides of a virus that are directly deposited and immobilized at predetermined positions on the membrane. These artificial antigens reduce the presence of contaminating material derived from whole-virus lysates and cell culture, which may interfere with the assay. Strip IB assays are used mainly as confirmatory or supplemental tests to help verify the specificity of positive results obtained from SPIA used to initially screen for virus-specific antibodies. Commercial kits are available for HSV-1, HSV-2, HIV-1, HIV-2, HCV, human T-cell lymphotropic virus type 1 (HTLV-1), and HTLV-2. These assays are less sensitive than EIA screening assays but more specific, with fewer indeterminate results than with Western blotting. However, they are relatively expensive and can be subject to interpretation.

IC Assays

IC tests, also known as lateral-flow tests, are a combination of SPIA and IB. In most assays, blood or diluted serum is deposited at the bottom of a membrane. Virus-specific antibodies bind to a solid phase composed of recombinant viral antigens or peptides and a detector reagent. As this solid phase migrates across the membrane by capillary flow, it interacts with antibody capture lines deposited across the membrane. A built-in control line confirms proper functioning of the device after addition of the patient's sample and adequate procedural application. The result is read visually. The advantages of these qualitative assays are that they are simple to use, do not usually require special instrumentation, allow quick turnaround time, are easy to interpret, and are applicable to urgent, field, and point-of-care testing (137). Commercial devices have been developed in recent years, notably for HIV, with sensitivities comparable to those of conventional EIA.

IgM Antibody Determination

Virus-specific IgM antibodies are most commonly detected using SPIA and IFA (36). The methods are similar to those used for detecting IgG antibodies, except that IgM bound to viral antigen on the solid phase is detected using secondary anti-human IgM antibodies labeled with suitable markers. Assays to detect virus-specific IgM have been developed for most human viruses, and commercial reagents and complete diagnostic kits are available for a number of the agents (Table 7). However, false-positive and false-negative reactions are major concerns when measuring virus-specific IgM antibodies (36). False-negative reactions are the result of high levels of specific IgG antibodies competitively blocking the binding of IgM to the viral antigen placed on the solid phase. False-positive reactions occur when sera contain unusually high levels of rheumatoid factor (RF) or other interfering substances. RF is an IgM class Ig that reacts with IgG and is produced in some rheumatologic, vasculitic, and viral diseases. In the presence of virus-specific IgG antibodies, RF will form a complex with the IgG molecules. The IgG can then bind to the viral antigen on the solid phase, carrying nonviral IgM antibody with it and resulting in a false-positive result. The incidence of these false-negative and false-positive results can be minimized by separation of IgG and IgM from sera before testing.

TABLE 7 Examples of viruses for which IgM serologic determinations are useful and commercial reagents and/or kits are available

Measles virus	Dengue virus
Mumps virus	Hantavirus
Rubella virus	CMV
Parvovirus B19	EBV
Hepatitis A virus	VZV
Hepatitis B virus	HHV-6 and -7
West Nile virus	HSV-1 and -2

A variety of methods have been developed for the removal of interfering RF and IgG molecules from serum, resulting in more reliable IgM tests (142). IgG and IgM antibodies can be physically separated using gel filtration, ion-exchange chromatography, affinity chromatography, or sucrose density gradient centrifugation. Although such techniques are effective for separation of IgG and IgM, they are not very practical for clinical use. More rapid and simple procedures have been used for the selective absorption and removal of the IgG fraction from serum using hyperimmune anti-human IgG, staphylococcal protein A, or recombinant protein G from group G streptococci. These pretreatment methods are readily available and are incorporated within most commercial IgM detection kits.

Reverse-capture solid-phase IgM or μ capture assays have been developed as an alternative to the physical fractionation of serum. In this method, the solid phase is coated with an anti-human IgM antibody that is used to capture the virus-specific IgM from the serum specimen. This is followed by washing to remove competing IgG antibody and immune complexes that may interfere with the accuracy of the test. A specific viral antigen is then added and allowed to bind to the captured IgM. The antigen-antibody complexes are detected by adding an enzyme-conjugated secondary antibody followed by a chromogenic substrate. IgM capture assays are very sensitive and specific and are considered superior to other IgM assay formats. An additional background subtraction step can further reduce nonspecific reactivity from interfering substances in serum (116).

Interpretation of Serology Test Results

Interpretation of results for virus-specific antibodies in clinical virology is summarized in Table 8. Demonstration of a seroconversion from a negative to a positive IgG antibody response or the presence of virus-specific IgM can be diagnostic of primary viral infection. Differences in antibody titers between acute- and convalescent-phase sera may support a recent viral infection due to reactivation or reinfection, although such testing is retrospective and has a limited impact on patient care. A significant change is defined as a $\geq$4-fold rise in IgG for methods yielding results in serial dilution endpoints. Interpretation of a significant

TABLE 8 Interpretation of results for virus-specific antibodies in clinical virology

Context	Result	Interpretation
Immune status	IgG present	Past exposure or immunization
	IgG absent	Past exposure unlikely
Diagnosis of acute infection	IgM present	Primary or recent viral infection likely
	IgG seroconversion	
	Fourfold rise in IgG titers	
	Absence of IgM or IgG	Excludes viral infection
	IgG present, single or stable titer	Past exposure
CSF infection	IgM present	Strong evidence of CNS infection
	IgG seroconversion	
Congenital infection	IgM in infant	Evidence of congenital infection
	Absence of IgM or IgG in mother and infant	Suspected infection unlikely
	IgG in infant < IgG in mother	Passive antibody transfer
	IgG in infant = IgG in mother	Retesting in 1 to 2 mo required
	IgG in infant > IgG in mother	Suggests congenitally or perinatally acquired infection
Immunocompromised individual	IgM and/or IgG absent	Possible delay in production of serum antibodies

difference must rely on objective criteria specified by the laboratory or manufacturer when results of assays such as SPIA are expressed in optical density, relative luminescence, or index values. Fourfold decreases in titer are seldom observed early enough to be useful for laboratory diagnosis, since antibody levels tend to decline slowly over several months after infection. Detection of virus-specific IgG in a single serum specimen or no change in antibody levels between acute- and convalescent-phase sera indicates exposure to a virus some time in the past. Negative serum antibody titers may exclude viral infection.

The identification of intrathecal virus-specific antibody production in CSF can confirm the diagnosis of viral CNS infection (4). Finding virus-specific IgM antibodies in CSF is strong evidence for CNS disease caused by arboviruses and lymphocytic choriomeningitis, measles, mumps, and rubella viruses. Similar to the case with serum, fourfold rises in virus-specific CSF IgG titers can also be diagnostic for these agents, but they are less practical because of the need for and delay in testing acute- and convalescent-phase CSF specimens. The detection of any virus-specific antibodies to rabies virus in the CSF is diagnostic of active infection.

In assessment of a newborn for congenital viral infections, the presence of IgM in the infant strongly suggests infection, since IgM antibodies do not cross the placenta. Seronegative results for both the mother and infant indicate that the suspected viral agent is very unlikely to have infected the infant. Comparison of virus-specific IgG antibody titers of the infant and the mother is essential; a lower titer in the infant reflects passive antibody transfer, whereas higher antibody titers in the infant than in the mother may reflect active antibody production. If maternal and infant serum antibody titers are the same, additional serum from the infant should be obtained 1 to 2 months later and periodically thereafter for 6 to 9 months, to be tested for comparison with the earlier antibody titer. These sera should show a decrease in virus-specific antibody relative to the first specimen, if the infant has not been congenitally or perinatally infected with the tested agent.

The results of serologic tests for the detection of virus-specific antibodies must be interpreted with caution, because measurements of an antibody response to viral infections can be complicated by a number of factors. There may be a lack of or delay in production of serum IgM or IgG antibodies, particularly in newborns, the elderly, and immunocompromised hosts. IgM antibodies also may persist for extended periods after primary infection and can be present during reactivation of latent viral infections. IgM may be undetectable during acute disease for individuals who were previously immunized but unsuccessfully protected. Significant rises in IgG antibodies do not always occur as a result of recurrent infections or exogenous reinfection. Virus-specific IgG antibodies may be present in recipients of intravenous Ig, newborn infants possessing passively acquired maternal antibody, or patients who have received recent blood transfusions, making it difficult to interpret IgG tests. Rises in the titers of either IgM or IgG antibody to certain viruses also may be nonspecific and in response to recent infections with other viruses. Accordingly, the possibility of a false-positive IgM result should be considered when the incidence of the virus under investigation is low. Indeterminate results inherent to some immunoassays may represent additional patient visits, venipuncture, and repeated serologic testing. Accuracy of antibody detection assays is critical when follow-up care decisions are based on test results. For this reason, serologic assays producing fewer inaccurate or indeterminate results than others are likely to be more cost-effective. Finally, failure to establish an accurate serologic diagnosis frequently results from the inability to submit an adequate pair of serum samples.

For neurologic viral diseases, the appearance of virus-specific antibody in the CSF may be delayed for 2 to 4 weeks. Also, for certain viruses, the presence of virus-specific antibody in the CSF may represent the passive transfer of serum antibodies across a damaged blood-brain barrier. Methods must be performed to determine and compare the CSF/serum ratio of virus-specific antibody to the CSF/serum ratio of albumin, particularly for the herpesviruses (4). Since albumin is not synthesized in the CNS, its presence in high concentrations within the CSF reflects the presence of contaminating serum proteins and an interruption of the blood-brain barrier. Demonstration of an intact blood-brain barrier in the presence of high levels of detectable virus-specific CSF antibody represents intrathecal production of antibody and is considered evidence of viral infection of the CNS.

In the diagnosis of an infant with suspected viral congenital disease, measuring the titers of IgG antibody to the common agents rarely results in a definitive diagnosis and is more useful for excluding infection. Detecting a single elevated titer of IgG antibody to a specific viral agent is not useful, and testing for HSV-specific antibody is of limited value. Negative antibody titers in the mother and child also may be the result of the mother having a primary infection of recent onset without immediate production of virus-specific antibodies. Appropriate follow-up studies are essential. Because of the many caveats associated with serologic diagnoses of viral infections, antibody determinations should be confirmed by isolation of the virus in culture or by using direct methods of detecting viral antigens or nucleic acids. The results should also be interpreted with careful consideration of the patient's symptoms and history.

QUALITY ASSURANCE AND QUALITY CONTROL

Quality management, assurance, and control and continuous improvement are key elements of a complete quality assessment system ensuring that all steps from specimen collection to result reporting are performed correctly. The goal of maintaining a quality system in a diagnostic laboratory is that the right test is performed on the right specimen, and that the right result and interpretation are delivered timely to the right individual.

Quality Assurance

Quality assurance is a broad term used to describe administrative and technical procedures for monitoring quality in the laboratory. Licensed, certified, or accredited clinical virology laboratories must comply with specific requirements of comprehensive quality assurance programs that are issued by regulatory and accreditation agencies. In the United States, some minimal requirements are supported by legislative measures. In other countries, their scope may vary depending on local or regional jurisdictions. Quality assurance requires active participation by all members of the institution. Standard operating procedures specify how preanalytical, analytical, and postanalytical activities are to be performed. These procedures are revised periodically and updated when necessary. Internal audits performed at regular intervals monitor compliance. Record keeping, equipment calibration and preventive maintenance, personnel training and competence assessment, and internal and external proficiency testing are all part of a quality assurance program (141). Ultimately, quality assurance leads to improvement of all aspects of laboratory services so that patient health care will benefit.

Quality Control

Quality control focuses on monitoring the testing process itself in order to ensure test system performance. Variables affecting the quality of results are adequacy of training of laboratory personnel, sample type and condition, assay reagents, equipment performance, testing procedure deviance, and interpretation, transcription, and reporting of test results. Key elements of quality control include a set of written procedures specifying the elements to verify prior to, during, and after the testing process. Major issues to be considered in this regard are documenting instrument conditions (e.g., temperature), calibration, and use; reagent labeling regarding receipt, storage, and use prior to expiration date; storage of materials; hazardous material labeling and use; comparison of new methods to prior standards; and satisfactory performance of kits. Initial qualification of new lots of kits and reagents using known standard panels and insertion of control samples on each test run ensure that the kit, device, or equipment is performing within specifications and that the results generated are correct. For in-house assays, performance characteristics must be established. These include repeatability and reproducibility, cutoffs for qualitative assays, and linearity, including lower and upper limits of quantification for quantitative and semiquantitative assays.

Monitoring test performance may allow detection of factors affecting assay quality and, ultimately, reliability of results. Analyzing data for trends can establish deviation in test results over time (e.g., drift in the performance of a manufactured diagnostic kit). Investigation of a faulty test or run is facilitated when ancillary information is documented and thus traceable throughout the procedure. If a result is not obtained according to procedure, or a specific instrument or reagent has failed to meet prescribed criteria, a nonconformity to a test procedure as well as the corrective action that is put in place to remedy the problem should be documented. This compilation is essential, as it can identify a weakness in assay performance that otherwise may go unnoticed.

Analyzers and robotic platforms interfaced with computers are more common now in the virology laboratory, especially for antigen, antibody, and nucleic acid detection assays. Bar-coded clinical specimens and reagents limit errors and facilitate monitoring and documentation of test parameters. Users have the responsibility to assess the performance of these automated instruments. As test results are required rapidly to ensure prompt medical decisions, the diagnostics industry has been responding with point-of-care devices or tests, such as for influenza virus, RSV, and HIV. These assays are aimed to be used outside of the strictly controlled laboratory realm and constitute a new challenge for quality control in clinical virology. Development of adequate built-in controls may help to ensure the accuracy of the kit result. However, deficiencies regarding basic documentation, training, conformity of testing to the manufacturer's package insert, respect of expiration dates, and knowledge of the limits of the test may affect result quality and interpretation. The consequences of an inaccurate result may include inappropriate medical decisions, unnecessary interventions, and worry for the patient. Therefore, personnel performing point-of-care tests should comply with documented protocols for specimen collection, processing, and testing, including adherence to established guidelines for confirmatory testing. It may also be considered to retest negative samples with an alternative assay when point-of-care testing is used to support prophylactic decisions (e.g., with HIV). Finally, users should initiate corrective action when deviations from established parameters are detected.

Practical aspects of quality assurance programs and quality control in the clinical laboratory can be found in several American Society for Microbiology documents, including the *Clinical Microbiology Procedures Handbook* and *Cumitechs* (http://www.asm.org/). The Clinical and Laboratory Standards Institute has also published guideline documents addressing quality assurance and quality control issues for viral culture, immunoassays, point-of-care testing, and molecular diagnostic methods (http://www.clsi.org/).

REFERENCES

1. **Abed, Y., A. M. Bourgault, R. J. Fenton, P. J. Morley, D. Gower, I. J. Owens, M. Tisdale, and G. Boivin.** 2002. Characterization of 2 influenza A(H3N2) clinical isolates with reduced susceptibility to neuraminidase inhibitors due to mutations in the hemagglutinin gene. *J. Infect. Dis.* **186:**1074–1080.
2. **Abed, Y., I. Hardy, Y. Li, and G. Boivin.** 2002. Divergent evolution of hemagglutinin and neuraminidase genes in recent influenza A:H3N2 viruses isolated in Canada. *J. Med. Virol.* **67:**589–595.
3. **Allander, T., M. T. Tammi, M. Eriksson, A. Bjerkner, A. Tiveljung-Lindell, and B. Andersson.** 2005. Cloning of a human parvovirus by molecular screening of respiratory tract samples. *Proc. Natl. Acad. Sci. USA* **102:** 12891–12896.
4. **Andiman, W. A.** 1991. Organism-specific antibody indices, the cerebrospinal fluid-immunoglobulin index and other tools: a clinician's guide to the etiologic diagnosis of central nervous system infection. *Pediatr. Infect. Dis. J.* **10:**490–495.
5. **Arens, M. Q., and E. M. Swierkosz.** 2007. Susceptibility test methods: viruses, p. 1705–1718. *In* P. R. Murray, E. J. Baron, J. H. Jorgensen, M. L. Landry, and M. A. Pfaller (ed.), *Manual of Clinical Microbiology*, 9th ed. ASM Press, Washington, DC.
6. **Ballew, H. C.** 2000. Neutralization, p. 127–134. *In* S. C. Specter, R. L. Hodinka, and S. A. Young (ed.), *Clinical Virology Manual*, 3rd ed. ASM Press, Washington, DC.
7. **Baz, M., Y. Abed, J. McDonald, and G. Boivin.** 2006. Characterization of multidrug-resistant influenza A/H3N2 viruses shed during 1 year by an immunocompromised child. *Clin. Infect. Dis.* **43:**1555–1561.
8. **Bellisario, R., R. J. Colinas, and K. A. Pass.** 2001. Simultaneous measurement of antibodies to three HIV-1 antigens in newborn dried blood-spot specimens using a multiplexed microsphere-based immunoassay. *Early. Hum. Dev.* **64:**21–25.
9. **Belshe, R. B., B. Burk, F. Newman, R. L. Cerruti, and I. S. Sim.** 1989. Resistance of influenza A virus to amantadine and rimantadine: results of one decade of surveillance. *J. Infect. Dis.* **159:**430–435.
10. **Bettoli, E. J., P. M. Brewer, M. J. Oxtoby, A. A. Zaidi, and M. E. Guinan.** 1982. The role of temperature and swab materials in the recovery of herpes simplex virus from lesions. *J. Infect. Dis.* **145:**399.
11. **Biel, S. S., and H. R. Gelderblom.** 1999. Diagnostic electron microscopy is still a timely and rewarding method. *J. Clin. Virol.* **13:**105–119.
12. **Biggar, R. J., W. Miley, P. Miotti, T. E. Taha, A. Butcher, J. Spadoro, and D. Waters.** 1997. Blood collection on filter paper: a practical approach to sample collection for studies of perinatal HIV transmission. *J. Acquir. Immune Defic. Syndr. Hum. Retrovirol.* **14:**368–373.
13. **Blackburn, N. K., T. G. Besselaar, B. D. Schoub, and K. F. O'Connell.** 1991. Differentiation of primary cytomegalovirus infection from reactivation using the urea denaturation test for measuring antibody avidity. *J. Med. Virol.* **33:**6–9.
14. **Boivin, G., S. Chou, M. R. Quirk, A. Erice, and M. C. Jordan.** 1996. Detection of ganciclovir resistance mutations and quantitation of cytomegalovirus (CMV) DNA in leukocytes of patients with fatal disseminated CMV disease. *J. Infect. Dis.* **173:**523–528.
15. **Boivin, G., C. K. Edelman, L. Pedneault, C. L. Talarico, K. K. Biron, and H. H. Balfour, Jr.** 1994. Phenotypic and genotypic characterization of acyclovir-resistant varicella-zoster viruses isolated from persons with AIDS. *J. Infect. Dis.* **170:**68–75.
16. **Boivin, G., C. Gilbert, A. Gaudreau, I. Greenfield, R. Sudlow, and N. A. Roberts.** 2001. Rate of emergence of cytomegalovirus (CMV) mutations in leukocytes of patients with acquired immunodeficiency syndrome who are receiving valganciclovir as induction and maintenance therapy for CMV retinitis. *J. Infect. Dis.* **184:**1598–1602.
17. **Boivin, G., N. Goyette, C. Gilbert, A. Humar, and E. Covington.** 2005. Clinical impact of ganciclovir-resistant cytomegalovirus infections in solid organ transplant patients. *Transplant Infect. Dis.* **7:**166–170.
18. **Boucher, C. A., W. Keulen, T. van Bommel, M. Nijhuis, D. de Jong, M. D. de Jong, P. Schipper, and N. K. Back.** 1996. Human immunodeficiency virus type 1 drug susceptibility determination by using recombinant viruses generated from patient sera tested in a cell-killing assay. *Antimicrob. Agents Chemother.* **40:**2404–2409.
19. **Brown, M., M. Petric, and P. J. Middleton.** 1984. Silver staining of DNA restriction fragments for the rapid identification of adenovirus isolates: application during nosocomial outbreaks. *J. Virol. Methods* **9:**87–98.
20. **Cane, P. A., P. Cook, D. Ratcliffe, D. Mutimer, and D. Pillay.** 1999. Use of real-time PCR and fluorimetry to detect lamivudine resistance-associated mutations in hepatitis B virus. *Antimicrob. Agents Chemother.* **43:**1600–1608.
21. **Carpenter, A. B.** 2007. Immunoassays for the diagnosis of infectious diseases, p. 257–270. *In* P. R. Murray, E. J. Baron, M. A. Pfaller, F. C. Tenover, and R. H. Yolken (ed.), *Manual of Clinical Microbiology*, 9th ed. ASM Press, Washington, DC.
22. **Chan, P. K., W. K. To, K. C. Ng, R. K. Lam, T. K. Ng, R. C. Chan, A. Wu, W. C. Yu, N. Lee, D. S. Hui, S. T. Lai, E. K. Hon, C. K. Li, J. J. Sung, and J. S. Tam.** 2004. Laboratory diagnosis of SARS. *Emerg. Infect. Dis.* **10:**825–831.
23. **Chou, S., S. Guentzel, K. R. Michels, R. C. Miner, and W. L. Drew.** 1995. Frequency of UL97 phosphotransferase mutations related to ganciclovir resistance in clinical cytomegalovirus isolates. *J. Infect. Dis.* **172:**239–242.
24. **Chou, S., N. S. Lurain, K. D. Thompson, R. C. Miner, and W. L. Drew.** 2003. Viral DNA polymerase mutations associated with drug resistance in human cytomegalovirus. *J. Infect. Dis.* **188:**32–39.
25. **Condorelli, F., G. Scalia, A. Stivala, R. Gallo, A. Marino, C. M. Battaglini, and A. Castro.** 1994. Detection of immunoglobulin G to measles virus, rubella virus, and mumps virus in serum samples and in microquantities of whole blood dried on filter paper. *J. Virol. Methods* **49:** 25–36.
26. **Constantine, N. T., R. Saville, and E. Dax.** 2005. *Retroviral Testing and Quality Assurance: Essentials for Laboratory Diagnosis*. Malloy Printers.
27. **Curry, A., H. Appleton, and B. Dowsett.** 2006. Application of transmission electron microscopy to the clinical study of viral and bacterial infections: present and future. *Micron* **37:**91–106.
28. **Dankner, W. M., D. Scholl, S. C. Stanat, M. Martin, R. L. Sonke, and S. A. Spector.** 1990. Rapid antiviral DNA-DNA hybridization assay for human cytomegalovirus. *J. Virol. Methods* **28:**293–298.
29. **de Mezerville, M. H., R. Tellier, S. Richardson, D. Hebert, J. Doyle, and U. Allen.** 2006. Adenoviral infections

in pediatric transplant recipients: a hospital-based study. *Pediatr. Infect. Dis. J.* **25:**815–818.

30. **Drachenberg, C. B., H. H. Hirsch, E. Ramos, and J. C. Papadimitriou.** 2005. Polyomavirus disease in renal transplantation: review of pathological findings and diagnostic methods. *Hum. Pathol.* **36:**1245–1255.
31. **Drosten, C., S. Gunther, W. Preiser, S. van der Werf, H. R. Brodt, S. Becker, H. Rabenau, M. Panning, L. Kolesnikova, R. A. Fouchier, A. Berger, A. M. Burguiere, J. Cinatl, M. Eickmann, N. Escriou, K. Grywna, S. Kramme, J. C. Manuguerra, S. Muller, V. Rickerts, M. Sturmer, S. Vieth, H. D. Klenk, A. D. Osterhaus, H. Schmitz, and H. W. Doerr.** 2003. Identification of a novel coronavirus in patients with severe acute respiratory syndrome. *N. Engl. J. Med.* **348:**1967–1976.
32. **Dunn, D. T., C. D. Brandt, A. Krivine, S. A. Cassol, P. Roques, W. Borkowsky, A. De Rossi, E. Denamur, A. Ehrnst, and C. Loveday.** 1995. The sensitivity of HIV-1 DNA polymerase chain reaction in the neonatal period and the relative contributions of intra-uterine and intra-partum transmission. *AIDS* **9:**F7–11.
33. **Dunn, J. J., R. D. Woolstenhulme, J. Langer, and K. C. Carroll.** 2004. Sensitivity of respiratory virus culture when screening with R-Mix fresh cells. *J. Clin. Microbiol.* **42:**79–82.
34. **Dybul, M., A. S. Fauci, J. G. Bartlett, J. E. Kaplan, and A. K. Pau.** 2002. Guidelines for using antiretroviral agents among HIV-infected adults and adolescents. Recommendations of the Panel on Clinical Practices for Treatment of HIV. *Morb. Mortal. Wkly. Rep. Recomm. Rep.* **51:**1–55.
35. **Enders, J. F., T. H. Weller, and F. C. Robbins.** 1949. Cultivation of the Lansing strain of poliomyelitis virus in cultures of various human embryonic tissues. *Science* **109:** 85–87.
36. **Erdman, D. D.** 2000. Immunoglobulin M determinations, p. 146–153. *In* S. C. Specter, R. L. Hodinka, and S. A. Young (ed.), *Clinical Virology Manual*, 3rd ed. ASM Press, Washington, DC.
37. **Erice, A., S. Chou, K. K. Biron, S. C. Stanat, H. H. Balfour, Jr., and M. C. Jordan.** 1989. Progressive disease due to ganciclovir-resistant cytomegalovirus in immunocompromised patients. *N. Engl. J. Med.* **320:**289–293.
38. **Espy, M. J., J. R. Uhl, P. S. Mitchell, J. N. Thorvilson, K. A. Svien, A. D. Wold, and T. F. Smith.** 2000. Diagnosis of herpes simplex virus infections in the clinical laboratory by LightCycler PCR. *J. Clin. Microbiol.* **38:** 795–799.
39. **Fahy, E., D. Y. Kwoh, and T. R. Gingeras.** 1991. Self-sustained sequence replication (3SR): an isothermal transcription-based amplification system alternative to PCR. *PCR Methods Appl.* **1:**25–33.
40. **Feld, J. J., and J. H. Hoofnagle.** 2005. Mechanism of action of interferon and ribavirin in treatment of hepatitis C. *Nature* **436:**967–972.
41. **Feller, A. E., J. F. Enders, and T. H. Weller.** 1940. The prolonged coexistence of vaccinia virus in high titre and living cells in roller tube cultures of chick embryonic tissues. *J. Exp. Med.* **72:**367–388.
42. **Forman, M. S., and A. Valsamakis.** 2007. Specimen collection, transport, and processing: virology, p. 1284–1296. *In* P. R. Murray, E. J. Baron, J. H. Jorgensen, M. L. Landry, and M. A. Pfaller (ed.), *Manual of Clinical Microbiology*, 9th ed. ASM Press, Washington, DC.
43. **Fulton, R. J., R. L. McDade, P. L. Smith, L. J. Kienker, and J. R. Kettman, Jr.** 1997. Advanced multiplexed analysis with the FlowMetrix system. *Clin. Chem.* **43:**1749–1756.
44. **Gey, G. O.** 1933. An improved technique for massive tissue culture. *Am. J. Cancer* **17:**752–756.
45. **Gilbert, C., and G. Boivin.** 2003. Discordant phenotypes and genotypes of cytomegalovirus (CMV) in patients with AIDS and relapsing CMV retinitis. *AIDS* **17:**337–341.
46. **Gilbert, C., J. Handfield, E. Toma, R. Lalonde, M. G. Bergeron, and G. Boivin.** 1998. Emergence and prevalence of cytomegalovirus UL97 mutations associated with ganciclovir resistance in AIDS patients. *AIDS* **12:**125–129.
47. **Gleaves, C. A., T. F. Smith, E. A. Shuster, and G. R. Pearson.** 1984. Rapid detection of cytomegalovirus in MRC-5 cells inoculated with urine specimens by using low-speed centrifugation and monoclonal antibody to an early antigen. *J. Clin. Microbiol.* **19:**917–919.
48. **Gottfried, T. D., J. C. Sturge, and H. B. Urnovitz.** 1999. A urine test system for HIV-1 antibodies. *Am. Clin. Lab.* **18:**4.
49. **Gray, R. H., M. J. Wawer, R. Brookmeyer, N. K. Sewankambo, D. Serwadda, F. Wabwire-Mangen, T. Lutalo, X. Li, T. vanCott, and T. C. Quinn.** 2001. Probability of HIV-1 transmission per coital act in monogamous, heterosexual, HIV-1-discordant couples in Rakai, Uganda. *Lancet* **357:**1149–1153.
50. **Guatelli, J. C., K. M. Whitfield, D. Y. Kwoh, K. J. Barringer, D. D. Richman, and T. R. Gingeras.** 1990. Isothermal, in vitro amplification of nucleic acids by a multienzyme reaction modeled after retroviral replication. *Proc. Natl. Acad. Sci. USA* **87:**1874–1878.
51. **Gürtler, L., A. Mühlbacher, U. Michl, H. Hofmann, G. G. Paggi, V. Bossi, R. Thorstensson, R. G. Villaescusa, A. Eiras, J. M. Hernandez, W. Melchior, F. Donie, and B. Weber.** 1998. Reduction of the diagnostic window with a new combined p24 antigen and human immunodeficiency virus antibody screening assay. *J. Virol. Methods* **75:**27–38.
52. **Gutfreund, K. S., M. Williams, R. George, V. G. Bain, M. M. Ma, E. M. Yoshida, J. P. Villeneuve, K. P. Fischer, and D. L. Tyrrel.** 2000. Genotypic succession of mutations of the hepatitis B virus polymerase associated with lamivudine resistance. *J. Hepatol.* **33:**469–475.
53. **Hanna, G. J., V. A. Johnson, D. R. Kuritzkes, D. D. Richman, J. Martinez-Picado, L. Sutton, J. D. Hazelwood, and R. T. D'Aquila.** 2000. Comparison of sequencing by hybridization and cycle sequencing for genotyping of human immunodeficiency virus type 1 reverse transcriptase. *J. Clin. Microbiol.* **38:**2715–2721.
54. **Hayden, F., A. Klimov, M. Tashiro, A. Hay, A. Monto, J. McKimm-Breschkin, C. Macken, A. Hampson, R. G. Webster, M. Amyard, and M. Zambon.** 2005. Neuraminidase Inhibitor Susceptibility Network position statement: antiviral resistance in influenza A/H5N1 viruses. *Antivir. Ther.* **10:**873–877.
55. **Hazelton, P. R., and H. R. Gelderblom.** 2003. Electron microscopy for rapid diagnosis of infectious agents in emergent situations. *Emerg. Infect. Dis.* **9:**294–303.
56. **Herrera, G. A., R. Veeramachaneni, and E. A. Turbat-Herrera.** 2005. Electron microscopy in the diagnosis of BK-polyoma virus infection in the transplanted kidney. *Ultrastruct. Pathol.* **29:**469–474.
57. **Hirsch, M. S., F. Brun-Vezinet, B. Clotet, B. Conway, D. R. Kuritzkes, R. T. D'Aquila, L. M. Demeter, S. M. Hammer, V. A. Johnson, C. Loveday, J. W. Mellors, D. M. Jacobsen, and D. D. Richman.** 2003. Antiretroviral drug resistance testing in adults infected with human immunodeficiency virus type 1: 2003 recommendations of an International AIDS Society-USA Panel. *Clin. Infect. Dis.* **37:**113–128.

58. **Hodinka, R. L.** 1999. Serological tests in clinical virology, p. 195–211. *In* E. H. Lennette and T. F. Smith (ed.), *Laboratory Diagnosis of Viral Infections*, 3rd ed. Marcel Dekker, Inc., New York, NY.
59. **Hodinka, R. L., T. Nagashunmugam, and D. Malamud.** 1998. Detection of human immunodeficiency virus antibodies in oral fluids. *Clin. Diagn. Lab. Immunol.* **5:**419–426.
60. **Huang, Y. T., and B. M. Turchek.** 2000. Mink lung cells and mixed mink lung and A549 cells for rapid detection of influenza virus and other respiratory viruses. *J. Clin. Microbiol.* **38:**422–423.
61. **Hughes, M. D., V. A. Johnson, M. S. Hirsch, J. W. Bremer, T. Elbeik, A. Erice, D. R. Kuritzkes, W. A. Scott, S. A. Spector, N. Basgoz, M. A. Fischl, and R. T. D'Aquila for the ACTG 241 Protocol Virology Substudy Team.** 1997. Monitoring plasma HIV-1 RNA levels in addition to $CD4^+$ lymphocyte count improves assessment of antiretroviral therapeutic response. *Ann. Intern. Med.* **126:**929–938.
62. **Hurt, A. C., R. Alexander, J. Hibbert, N. Deed, and I. G. Barr.** 2007. Performance of six influenza rapid tests in detecting human influenza in clinical specimens. *J. Clin. Virol.* **39:**132–135.
63. **Ison, M. G., L. V. Gubareva, R. L. Atmar, J. Treanor, and F. G. Hayden.** 2006. Recovery of drug-resistant influenza virus from immunocompromised patients: a case series. *J. Infect. Dis.* **193:**760–764.
64. **Itoh, Y., M. Takahashi, M. Fukuda, T. Shibayama, T. Ishikawa, F. Tsuda, T. Tanaka, T. Nishizawa, and H. Okamoto.** 2000. Visualization of TT virus particles recovered from the sera and feces of infected humans. *Biochem. Biophys. Res. Commun.* **279:**718–724.
65. **Jacob, S., D. Baudy, E. Jones, L. Xu, A. Mason, F. Regenstein, and R. P. Perrillo.** 1997. Comparison of quantitative HCV RNA assays in chronic hepatitis C. *Am. J. Clin. Pathol.* **107:**362–367.
66. **Japour, A. J., D. L. Mayers, V. A. Johnson, D. R. Kuritzkes, L. A. Beckett, J. M. Arduino, J. Lane, R. J. Black, P. S. Reichelderfer, R. T. D'Aquila, C. S. Crumpacker, the RV-43 Study Group, and the AIDS Clinical Trials Group Virology Committee Resistance Working Group.** 1993. Standardized peripheral blood mononuclear cell culture assay for determination of drug susceptibilities of clinical human immunodeficiency virus type 1 isolates. *Antimicrob. Agents Chemother.* **37:**1095–1101.
67. **Jayashree, S., M. K. Bhan, R. Kumar, P. Raj, R. Glass, and N. Bhandari.** 1988. Serum and salivary antibodies as indicators of rotavirus infection in neonates. *J. Infect. Dis.* **158:**1117–1120.
68. **Johnson, G., S. Nelson, M. Petric, and R. Tellier.** 2000. Comprehensive PCR-based assay for detection and species identification of human herpesviruses. *J. Clin. Microbiol.* **38:**3274–3279.
69. **Jordens, J. Z., S. Lanham, M. A. Pickett, S. Amarasekara, I. Abeywickrema, and P. J. Watt.** 2000. Amplification with molecular beacon primers and reverse line blotting for the detection and typing of human papillomaviruses. *J. Virol. Methods* **89:**29–37.
70. **Kageyama, T., S. Kojima, M. Shinohara, K. Uchida, S. Fukushi, F. B. Hoshino, N. Takeda, and K. Katayama.** 2003. Broadly reactive and highly sensitive assay for Norwalk-like viruses based on real-time quantitative reverse transcription-PCR. *J. Clin. Microbiol.* **41:**1548–1557.
71. **Kasahara, Y.** 1997. Agglutination immunoassays, p. 7–12. *In* N. R. Rose, E. Conway de Macario, J. D. Folds, E. C. Lane, and M. Nakamura (ed.), *Manual of Clinical Laboratory Immunology*, 5th ed. ASM Press, Washington, DC.
72. **Kaufman, E., and I. B. Lamster.** 2002. The diagnostic applications of saliva—a review. *Crit. Rev. Oral Biol. Med.* **13:**197–212.
73. **King, S. M., M. Petric, R. Superina, N. Graham, and E. A. Roberts.** 1990. Cytomegalovirus infections in pediatric liver transplantation. *Am. J. Dis. Child.* **144:**1307–1310.
74. **Kiviat, N. B., L. A. Koutsky, C. W. Critchlow, D. A. Galloway, D. A. Vernon, M. L. Peterson, P. E. McElhose, S. J. Pendras, C. E. Stevens, and K. K. Holmes.** 1990. Comparison of Southern transfer hybridization and dot filter hybridization for detection of cervical human papillomavirus infection with types 6, 11, 16, 18, 31, 33, and 35. *Am. J. Clin. Pathol.* **94:**561–565.
75. **Klimov, A. I., E. Rocha, F. G. Hayden, P. A. Shult, L. F. Roumillat, and N. J. Cox.** 1995. Prolonged shedding of amantadine-resistant influenza A viruses by immunodeficient patients: detection by polymerase chain reaction-restriction analysis. *J. Infect. Dis.* **172:**1352–1355.
76. **Klutts, J. S., R. S. Liao, W. M. Dunne, Jr., and A. M. Gronowski.** 2004. Evaluation of a multiplexed bead assay for assessment of Epstein-Barr virus immunologic status. *J. Clin. Microbiol.* **42:**4996–5000.
77. **Kostouros, E., K. Siu, E. L. Ford-Jones, M. Petric, and R. Tellier.** 2003. Molecular characterization of rotavirus strains from children in Toronto, Canada. *J. Clin. Virol.* **28:**77–84.
78. **Kramski, M., H. Meisel, B. Klempa, D. H. Kruger, G. Pauli, and A. Nitsche.** 2007. Detection and typing of human pathogenic hantaviruses by real-time reverse transcription-PCR and pyrosequencing. *Clin. Chem.* **53:**1899–1905.
79. **Lai, Y., K. L. Feldman, and R. S. Clark.** 2005. Enzyme-linked immunosorbent assays (ELISAs). *Crit. Care Med.* **33:**S433–S434.
80. **Landry, M. L., A. M. Caliendo, Y. W. Tang, and A. Valsamakis.** 2007. Algorithms for detection and identification of viruses, p. 1304–1307. *In* P. R. Murray, E. J. Baron, J. H. Jorgensen, M. L. Landry, and M. A. Pfaller (ed.), *Manual of Clinical Microbiology*, 9th ed. ASM Press, Washington, DC.
81. **Landry, M. L., S. Stanat, K. Biron, D. Brambilla, W. Britt, J. Jokela, S. Chou, W. L. Drew, A. Erice, B. Gilliam, N. Lurain, J. Manischewitz, R. Miner, M. Nokta, P. Reichelderfer, S. Spector, A. Weinberg, B. Yen-Lieberman, and C. Crumpacker.** 2000. A standardized plaque reduction assay for determination of drug susceptibilities of cytomegalovirus clinical isolates. *Antimicrob. Agents Chemother.* **44:**688–692.
82. **Laperche, S., N. Le Marrec, A. Girault, F. Bouchardeau, A. Servant-Delmas, M. Maniez-Montreuil, P. Gallian, T. Levayer, P. Morel, and N. Simon.** 2005. Simultaneous detection of hepatitis C virus (HCV) core antigen and anti-HCV antibodies improves the early detection of HCV infection. *J. Clin. Microbiol.* **43:**3877–3883.
83. **Leary, J. J., R. Wittrock, R. T. Sarisky, A. Weinberg, and M. J. Levin.** 2002. Susceptibilities of herpes simplex viruses to penciclovir and acyclovir in eight cell lines. *Antimicrob. Agents Chemother.* **46:**762–768.
84. **Ledue, T. B., and D. E. Garfin.** 1997. Immunofixation and immunoblotting, p. 54–64. *In* N. R. Rose, E. Conway de Macario, J. D. Folds, E. C. Lane, and R. M. Nakamura (ed.), *Manual of Clinical Laboratory Immunology*, 5th ed. ASM Press, Washington, DC.
85. **Leland, D. S.** 1996. Concepts of immunoserological and molecular techniques, p. 21–49. *In* D. S. Leland (ed.), *Clinical Virology*. The W. B. Saunders Co., Philadelphia, PA.

86. **Lennette, E. T., D. J. Blackbourn, and J. A. Levy.** 1996. Antibodies to human herpesvirus type 8 in the general population and in Kaposi's sarcoma patients. *Lancet* **348:**858–861.
87. **Lennette, E. T., and D. A. Lennette.** 2000. Immune adherence hemagglutination, p. 140–145. *In* S. C. Specter, R. L. Hodinka, and S. A. Young (ed.), *Clinical Virology Manual*, 3rd ed. ASM Press, Washington, DC.
88. **Levin, M. J., S. Leventhal, and H. A. Masters.** 1984. Factors influencing quantitative isolation of varicella-zoster virus. *J. Clin. Microbiol.* **19:**880–883.
89. **Limaye, A. P.** 2002. Ganciclovir-resistant cytomegalovirus in organ transplant recipients. *Clin. Infect. Dis.* **35:**866–872.
90. **Livak, K. J., S. J. Flood, J. Marmaro, W. Giusti, and K. Deetz.** 1995. Oligonucleotides with fluorescent dyes at opposite ends provide a quenched probe system useful for detecting PCR product and nucleic acid hybridization. *PCR Methods Appl.* **4:**357–362.
91. **Longo, M. C., M. S. Berninger, and J. L. Hartley.** 1990. Use of uracil DNA glycosylase to control carry-over contamination in polymerase chain reactions. *Gene* **93:**125–128.
92. **Mahony, J., S. Chong, F. Merante, S. Yaghoubian, T. Sinha, C. Lisle, and R. Janeczko.** 2007. Development of a respiratory virus panel test for detection of twenty human respiratory viruses by use of multiplex PCR and a fluid microbead-based assay. *J. Clin. Microbiol.* **45:**2965–2970.
93. **Mahony, J. B., and M. A. Chernesky.** 1999. Immunoassays for the diagnosis of infectious diseases, p. 202–214. *In* P. R. Murray, E. J. Baron, M. A. Pfaller, F. C. Tenover, and R. H. Yolken (ed.), *Manual of Clinical Microbiology*, 7th ed. ASM Press, Washington, DC.
94. **Mandy, F. F., T. Nakamura, M. Bergeron, and K. Sekiguchi.** 2001. Overview and application of suspension array technology. *Clin. Lab. Med.* **21:**713–729.
95. **Marshall, J. A., and L. D. Bruggink.** 2006. Laboratory diagnosis of norovirus. *Clin. Lab.* **52:**571–581.
96. **Martin, M., C. Gilbert, E. Covington, and G. Boivin.** 2006. Characterization of human cytomegalovirus (HCMV) UL97 mutations found in a valganciclovir/oral ganciclovir prophylactic trial by use of a bacterial artificial chromosome containing the HCMV genome. *J. Infect. Dis.* **194:**579–583.
97. **Martínez, P. M., A. R. Torres, R. Ortiz de Lejarazu, A. Montoya, J. F. Martin, and J. M. Eiros.** 1999. Human immunodeficiency virus antibody testing by enzyme-linked fluorescent and Western blot assays using serum, gingival-crevicular transudate, and urine samples. *J. Clin. Microbiol.* **37:**1100–1106.
98. **Martins, T. B.** 2002. Development of internal controls for the Luminex instrument as part of a multiplex seven-analyte viral respiratory antibody profile. *Clin. Diagn. Lab. Immunol.* **9:**41–45.
99. **McKimm-Breschkin, J. L.** 2000. Resistance of influenza viruses to neuraminidase inhibitors—a review. *Antivir. Res.* **47:**1–17.
100. **McLaren, C., M. N. Ellis, and G. A. Hunter.** 1983. A colorimetric assay for the measurement of the sensitivity of herpes simplex viruses to antiviral agents. *Antivir. Res.* **3:**223–234.
101. **McSharry, J. M., N. S. Lurain, G. L. Drusano, A. Landay, J. Manischewitz, M. Nokta, M. O'Gorman, H. M. Shapiro, A. Weinberg, P. Reichelderfer, and C. Crumpacker.** 1998. Flow cytometric determination of ganciclovir susceptibilities of human cytomegalovirus clinical isolates. *J. Clin. Microbiol.* **36:**958–964.
102. **Morris, T., B. Robertson, and M. Gallagher.** 1996. Rapid reverse transcription-PCR detection of hepatitis C virus RNA in serum by using the TaqMan fluorogenic detection system. *J. Clin. Microbiol.* **34:**2933–2936.
103. **Mushahwar, I. K., and T. A. Brawner.** 2000. Radioimmunoassay, p. 79–92. *In* S. C. Specter, R. L. Hodinka, and S. A. Young (ed.), *Clinical Virology Manual*, 3rd ed. ASM Press, Washington, DC.
103a. **NCCLS.** 2004. Antiviral susceptibility testing: herpes simplex virus by plaque reduction assay. Standard M33-A. NCCLS, Wayne, PA.
104. **Nichol, S. T., C. F. Spiropoulou, S. Morzunov, P. E. Rollin, T. G. Ksiazek, H. Feldmann, A. Sanchez, J. Childs, S. Zaki, and C. J. Peters.** 1993. Genetic identification of a hantavirus associated with an outbreak of acute respiratory illness. *Science* **262:**914–917.
105. **Oberste, M. S., K. Maher, D. R. Kilpatrick, M. R. Flemister, B. A. Brown, and M. A. Pallansch.** 1999. Typing of human enteroviruses by partial sequencing of VP1. *J. Clin. Microbiol.* **37:**1288–1293.
106. **Olivo, P. D.** 1996. Transgenic cell lines for detection of animal viruses. *Clin. Microbiol. Rev.* **9:**321–334.
107. **Opalka, D., C. E. Lachman, S. A. MacMullen, K. U. Jansen, J. F. Smith, N. Chirmule, and M. T. Esser.** 2003. Simultaneous quantitation of antibodies to neutralizing epitopes on virus-like particles for human papillomavirus types 6, 11, 16, and 18 by a multiplexed Luminex assay. *Clin. Diagn. Lab. Immunol.* **10:**108–115.
108. **Otsu, R., A. Ishikawa, and K. Mukae.** 2000. Detection of small round structured viruses in stool specimens from outbreaks of gastroenteritis by electron microscopy and reverse transcription-polymerase chain reaction. *Acta Virol.* **44:**53–55.
109. **Parker, S. P., W. D. Cubitt, and A. E. Ades.** 1997. A method for the detection and confirmation of antibodies to hepatitis C virus in dried blood spots. *J. Virol. Methods* **68:**199–205.
110. **Pasloske, B. L., C. R. Walkerpeach, R. D. Obermoeller, M. Winkler, and D. B. DuBois.** 1998. Armored RNA technology for production of ribonuclease-resistant viral RNA controls and standards. *J. Clin. Microbiol.* **36:**3590–3594.
111. **Peterson, E., O. W. Schmidt, L. C. Goldstein, R. C. Nowinski, and L. Corey.** 1983. Typing of clinical herpes simplex virus isolates with mouse monoclonal antibodies to herpes simplex virus types 1 and 2: comparison with type-specific rabbit antisera and restriction endonuclease analysis of viral DNA. *J. Clin. Microbiol.* **17:**92–96.
112. **Petropoulos, C. J., N. T. Parkin, K. L. Limoli, Y. S. Lie, T. Wrin, W. Huang, H. Tian, D. Smith, G. A. Winslow, D. J. Capon, and J. M. Whitcomb.** 2000. A novel phenotypic drug susceptibility assay for human immunodeficiency virus type 1. *Antimicrob. Agents Chemother.* **44:**920–928.
113. **Potier, M., L. Mameli, M. Belisle, L. Dallaire, and S. B. Melancon.** 1979. Fluorometric assay of neuraminidase with a sodium (4-methylumbelliferyl-alpha-D-*N*-acetylneuraminate) substrate. *Anal. Biochem.* **94:**287–296.
114. **Pugliese, A., T. Beltramo, and D. Torre.** 2007. Emerging and re-emerging viral infections in Europe. *Cell Biochem. Funct.* **25:**1–13.
115. **Randhawa, P., A. Vats, and R. Shapiro.** 2005. Monitoring for polyomavirus BK and JC in urine: comparison of quantitative polymerase chain reaction with urine cytology. *Transplantation* **79:**984–986.
116. **Rawlins, M. L., E. M. Swenson, H. R. Hill, and C. M. Litwin.** 2007. Evaluation of an enzyme immunoassay for detection of immunoglobulin M antibodies to West Nile

virus and the importance of background subtraction in detecting nonspecific reactivity. *Clin. Vaccine Immunol.* **14:**665–668.

117. **Revets, H., D. Marissens, S. de Wit, P. Lacor, N. Clumeck, S. Lauwers, and G. Zissis.** 1996. Comparative evaluation of NASBA HIV-1 RNA QT, AMPLICOR-HIV Monitor, and QUANTIPLEX HIV RNA assay, three methods for quantification of human immunodeficiency virus type 1 RNA in plasma. *J. Clin. Microbiol.* **34:**1058–1064.
118. **Rotbart, H. A.** 1991. Nucleic acid detection systems for enteroviruses. *Clin. Microbiol. Rev.* **4:**156–168.
119. **Saiki, R. K., S. Scharf, F. Faloona, K. B. Mullis, G. T. Horn, H. A. Erlich, and N. Arnheim.** 1992. Enzymatic amplification of beta-globin genomic sequences and restriction site analysis for diagnosis of sickle cell anemia. 1985. *Biotechnology* **24:**476–480.
120. **Sarantis, H., G. Johnson, M. Brown, M. Petric, and R. Tellier.** 2004. Comprehensive detection and serotyping of human adenoviruses by PCR and sequencing. *J. Clin. Microbiol.* **42:**3963–3969.
121. **Sarkies, N., Z. Gregor, T. Forsey, and S. Darougar.** 1986. Antibodies to herpes simplex virus type I in intraocular fluids of patients with acute retinal necrosis. *Br. J. Ophthalmol.* **70:**81–84.
122. **Schmit, I., and G. Boivin.** 1999. Characterization of the DNA polymerase and thymidine kinase genes of herpes simplex virus isolates from AIDS patients in whom acyclovir and foscarnet therapy sequentially failed. *J. Infect. Dis.* **180:**487–490.
123. **Schutzbank, T. A., and R. McGuire.** 2000. Immunofluorescence, p. 69–78. *In* S. C. Specter, R. L. Hodinka, and S. A. Young (ed.), *Clinical Virology Manual*, 3rd ed. ASM Press, Washington, DC.
124. **Shafer, R. W.** 2002. Genotypic testing for human immunodeficiency virus type 1 drug resistance. *Clin. Microbiol. Rev.* **15:**247–277.
125. **Small, L. N., J. Lau, and D. R. Snydman.** 2006. Preventing post-organ transplantation cytomegalovirus disease with ganciclovir: a meta-analysis comparing prophylactic and preemptive therapies. *Clin. Infect. Dis.* **43:** 869–880.
126. **Stabell, E. C., and P. D. Olivo.** 1992. Isolation of a cell line for rapid and sensitive histochemical assay for the detection of herpes simplex virus. *J. Virol. Methods* **38:** 195–204.
127. **Stark, L. M., and A. L. Lewis.** 2000. Complement fixation test, p. 112–126. *In* S. C. Specter, R. L. Hodinka, and S. A. Young (ed.), *Clinical Virology Manual*, 3rd ed. ASM Press, Washington, DC.
128. **Storch, G. A.** 2000. Diagnostic virology. *Clin. Infect. Dis.* **31:**739–751.

128a. **Storch, G. A. (ed.).** 2000. *Essentials of Diagnostic Virology*. Churchill Livingstone, New York, NY.

129. **Suttorp-Schulten, M. S., M. J. Zaal, L. Luyendijk, P. J. Bos, A. Kijlstra, and A. Rothova.** 1989. Aqueous chamber tap and serology in acute retinal necrosis. *Am. J. Ophthalmol.* **108:**327–328.
130. **Tebas, P., E. C. Stabell, and P. D. Olivo.** 1995. Antiviral susceptibility testing with a cell line which expresses beta-galactosidase after infection with herpes simplex virus. *Antimicrob. Agents Chemother.* **39:**1287–1291.
131. **Templeton, K. E., S. A. Scheltinga, M. F. Beersma, A. C. Kroes, and E. C. Claas.** 2004. Rapid and sensitive method using multiplex real-time PCR for diagnosis of infections by influenza A and influenza B viruses, respiratory syncytial virus, and parainfluenza viruses 1, 2, 3, and 4. *J. Clin. Microbiol.* **42:**1564–1569.
132. **Theilmann, L., M. Fischer, P. R. Galle, and M. Nassal.** 1989. Detection of HBV DNA in HBsAg-positive sera after amplification using the polymerase chain reaction. *Liver* **9:**322–328.
133. **Thomas, D. L., J. Astemborski, R. M. Rai, F. A. Anania, M. Schaeffer, N. Galai, K. Nolt, K. E. Nelson, S. A. Strathdee, L. Johnson, O. Laeyendecker, J. Boitnott, L. E. Wilson, and D. Vlahov.** 2000. The natural history of hepatitis C virus infection: host, viral, and environmental factors. *JAMA* **284:**450–456.
134. **Tsongalis, G. J., T. Gleeson, M. Rodina, D. Anamani, J. Ross, I. Joanisse, L. Tanimoto, and R. Ziermann.** 2005. Comparative performance evaluation of the HIV-1 LiPA protease and reverse transcriptase resistance assay on clinical isolates. *J. Clin. Virol.* **34:**268–271.
135. **Urdea, M. S.** 1993. Synthesis and characterization of branched DNA (bDNA) for the direct and quantitative detection of CMV, HBV, HCV, and HIV. *Clin. Chem.* **39:**725–726.
136. **van den Hoogen, B. G., J. C. de Jong, J. Groen, T. Kuiken, R. de Groot, R. A. Fouchier, and A. D. Osterhaus.** 2001. A newly discovered human pneumovirus isolated from young children with respiratory tract disease. *Nat. Med.* **7:**719–724.
137. **von Lode, P.** 2005. Point-of-care immunotesting: approaching the analytical performance of central laboratory methods. *Clin. Biochem.* **38:**591–606.
138. **Walker, G. T., J. G. Nadeau, P. A. Spears, J. L. Schram, C. M. Nycz, and D. D. Shank.** 1994. Multiplex strand displacement amplification (SDA) and detection of DNA sequences from Mycobacterium tuberculosis and other mycobacteria. *Nucleic Acids Res.* **22:**2670–2677.
139. **Wang, D., L. Coscoy, M. Zylberberg, P. C. Avila, H. A. Boushey, D. Ganem, and J. L. DeRisi.** 2002. Microarray-based detection and genotyping of viral pathogens. *Proc. Natl. Acad. Sci. USA* **99:**15687–15692.
140. **Wang, D., A. Urisman, Y. T. Liu, M. Springer, T. G. Ksiazek, D. D. Erdman, E. R. Mardis, M. Hickenbotham, V. Magrini, J. Eldred, J. P. Latreille, R. K. Wilson, D. Ganem, and J. L. DeRisi.** 2003. Viral discovery and sequence recovery using DNA microarrays. *PLoS Biol.* **1:**E2.
141. **Warford, A.** 2000. Quality assurance in clinical virology, p. 3–10. *In* S. C. Specter, R. L. Hodinka, and S. A. Young (ed.), *Clinical Virology Manual*, 3rd ed. ASM Press, Washington, DC.

141a. **Wiedbrauk, D. L.** 2000. Nucleic acid amplification methods, p. 188–197. *In* S. C. Specter, R. L. Hodinka, and S. A. Young (ed.), *Clinical Virology Manual*, 3rd ed. ASM Press, Washington, DC.

142. **Wiedbrauk, D. L., and H. Y. K. Chuang.** 1988. Managing IgM serologies: getting the IgG out. *Lab. Manag.* **26:**24–27.
143. **Wiedmann, M., W. J. Wilson, J. Czajka, J. Luo, F. Barany, and C. A. Batt.** 1994. Ligase chain reaction (LCR)—overview and applications. *PCR Methods Appl.* **3:**S51–S64.
144. **Wittek, M., M. Sturmer, H. W. Doerr, and A. Berger.** 2007. Molecular assays for monitoring HIV infection and antiretroviral therapy. *Expert Rev. Mol. Diagn.* **7:** 237–246.
145. **Wittwer, C. T., M. G. Herrmann, A. A. Moss, and R. P. Rasmussen.** 1997. Continuous fluorescence monitoring of rapid cycle DNA amplification. *BioTechniques* **22:**130–131, 134–138.

146. **Wong, S. J., R. H. Boyle, V. L. Demarest, A. N. Woodmansee, L. D. Kramer, H. Li, M. Drebot, R. A. Koski, E. Fikrig, D. A. Martin, and P. Y. Shi.** 2003. Immunoassay targeting nonstructural protein 5 to differentiate West Nile virus infection from dengue and St. Louis encephalitis virus infections and from flavivirus vaccination. *J. Clin. Microbiol.* **41:**4217–4223.
147. **Yamaguchi, K., Y. Yonemura, H. Okabe, Y. Takahama, S. Nagai, H. Yamaguchi, and K. Hirai.** 2003. Detection of anti-human T-lymphotropic virus type I antibody in whole blood by a novel counting immunoassay. *Clin. Chem.* **49:**275–280.
148. **Young, S. A., and L. C. McLaren.** 2000. Hemagglutination inhibition and hemadsorption, p. 135–139. *In* S. C. Specter, R. L. Hodinka, and S. A. Young (ed.), *Clinical Virology Manual,* 3rd ed. ASM Press, Washington, DC.
149. **Zolopa, A. R.** 2006. Incorporating drug-resistance measurements into the clinical management of HIV-1 infection. *J. Infect. Dis.* **194**(Suppl. 1)**:**S59–S64.

Immune Responses to Viruses

JONATHAN W. YEWDELL, THEODORE C. PIERSON, AND JACK R. BENNINK

14

OVERVIEW OF THE IMMUNE SYSTEM

Threat and Response

Viruses pose a constant danger to living organisms. A glimpse at the later chapters of this book will reveal the astounding variety of viruses recognized as human pathogens. This list only lengthens as humans come into more intimate contact with animal reservoirs harboring novel viruses capable "off the shelf" of infecting humans and new technologies reveal human viruses that have previously escaped detection. Human viruses, of course, constitute a minute fraction of all virus species. And while the vast majority of virus species are innocuous, due to their inability to infect or damage human cells, this defect can be overcome in some circumstances by mutation and natural selection. Two characteristics of viruses greatly accelerate their evolution relative to that of higher organisms. First, they produce progeny with great rapidity (each infected cell generally produces from 100 to 1,000 virions, generally in less than a day and in some cases as rapidly as a few hours), and second, they have extremely high intrinsic mutation rates.

The vertebrate immune system evolved in response to the threat posed by viruses. The importance of the immune system in protection against lethal viral infections becomes obvious in innate or acquired immunodeficiencies, in which depression of one or more elements of the system results in death from a typically self-limited viral infection, or in the success of vaccines in preventing dangerous viral infections and, in one case, even apparently causing the extinction of a virus species (variola virus, the cause of smallpox). The immune system (like every biological system) is not perfect, and overzealous antiviral responses can contribute to viral diseases and even, in some cases, mortality.

Viruses also continuously evolve in response to the threat posed by the host immune system. Every virus has to counter the mechanisms employed by every cell type in an organism to block virus replication. A number of viruses have evolved gene products for subverting specific elements of the immune system.

The adaptive elements of the immune system (discussed below) can be viewed as the evolutionary response of vertebrates to the formidable mutability of viruses and other pathogens, allowing the host to mutate its specific defense molecules at a rate sufficient to cope with the genesis of novel antigens not previously encountered in evolution. As originally noted by Ehrlich at the turn of the 20th century, the discriminatory power of this system is nothing short of amazing, for in addition to having to recognize and destroy pathogens numbering in the tens of thousands of species, it must do so without harming the host. This task is particularly daunting in the case of viruses, which are composed of material produced by host cells and typically do not betray their existence by display of evolutionarily distinct compounds generated by enzymatic activities not encoded by hosts (e.g., uniquely constituted glycolipids present in the bacterial cell wall).

Specific and Nonspecific Immune Elements

The immune system can be broadly (and somewhat arbitrarily) divided into specific and nonspecific components, with "specific" referring to the degree to which the immune response is restricted to a given agent. "Nonspecific" elements, are not, of course, entirely so, but rather are specific for features that are shared by given classes of pathogens. A similar array of nonspecific elements are called into play against virtually all viruses, while the specific components generally demonstrate a very limited reactivity to a single virus and its close relatives.

An aspect critical to nonspecific immunity (also known as innate or natural immunity) is its lack of memory. While the aggregate activities of nonspecific immune mechanisms wax and wane over time, reexposure to a previously encountered virus does not directly trigger a more vigorous immune response from nonspecific elements than the initial encounter, although this "rule" of immunology (like many others) may have to be reconsidered (33). Nonspecific elements include the following:

1. Phagocytic cells (macrophages and neutrophils) that engulf and destroy viruses
2. Cells (macrophages, neutrophils, mast cells, and basophils) that release cytokines, chemokines, defensins, or other molecules with antiviral or immunoregulatory activities (Table 1)
3. Cells (natural killer [NK]) that recognize virus-infected cells based on alterations common to many virus infections and either destroy the cells or release cytokines

TABLE 1 Cytokines used in anti-inflammatory immune responses

Cytokine[a]	Source	Function
IFN-γ	T cells, NK cells	Antiviral, ↑ class I and class II antigen processing and presentation, macrophage activation, ↓ Th2
IFN-α	Leukocytes, T cells	Antiviral, ↑ class I antigen processing and presentation
IFN-β	Fibroblasts, T cells	Antiviral, ↑ class I antigen processing and presentation
TNF-α	Macrophages	Inflammatory, endothelial activation, pyretic
TNF-β	T and B cells	Cytotoxic, endothelial activation
TGF-β	T cells, monocytes, and chondrocytes	Anti-inflammatory, inhibits cell growth
GM-CSF	T cells, macrophages, fibroblasts, and endothelial cells	Myelomonocytic cell growth and differentiation
G-CSF	Macrophages, fibroblasts, endothelial cells, and bone marrow stroma	Growth, differentiation, and activation of neutrophils
M-CSF	Lymphocytes, monocytes, fibroblasts, epithelial cells, endothelial cells, myoblasts, and osteoblasts	Survival, growth, differentiation, and activation factor for macrophages
MIF	T cells	Macrophage migration inhibition
LIF	T cells, myelomonocytic cells, fibroblasts, liver, heart, and myeloma	Proliferation of hematopoietic stem cells
PBSF	Fibroblasts, bone marrow stromal cells	Growth factor for pre-B cells
OSM	T cells and monocytes	Inhibits cell growth and proliferation and cytokine release
VEGF	Monocytes/macrophages, pituitary, smooth muscle, and keratinocytes	Activates and chemoattracts monocytes, enhances blood vessel permeability, and is a proaggulant
IL-1α	T and B cells, monocytes, macrophages, and epithelial cells	Multiple effects on T and B cells and monocytes, acute-phase reaction
IL-1β	T and B cells, monocytes, macrophages, and epithelial cells	Multiple effects on T and B cells and monocytes, acute-phase reaction
IL-2	T cells	Growth and differentiation of T and B cells, NK cells, monocytes, and macrophages
IL-3	T cells and thymic epithelial cells	Hematopoietic growth factor
IL-4	T cells, mast cells, bone marrow	Multiple effects on B and T cells, monocytes, endothelial cells, and fibroblasts
IL-5	T cells, mast cells, and eosinophils	Stimulates eosinophil colony formation and differentiation
IL-6	T and B cells and macrophages	Regulates B- and T-cell function and hematopoiesis
IL-7	Bone marrow, thymic stroma	Pre-B-cell and pre-T-cell growth, T-cell proliferation, and differentiation
IL-8	Macrophages, epithelial cells, and endothelial cells	Neutrophil chemotaxis

IL-9	T cells	↑ Mast cell activity and T-cell proliferation
IL-10	T and B cells, macrophages, monocytes, and keratinocytes	↓ Cytokine synthesis in macrophages, Th1, and NK cells; ↑ proliferation of B cells, thymocytes, mast cells; ↓ Th1
IL-11	Fibroblasts, bone marrow	IL-3 and IL-4 hematopoiesis synergist
IL-12	B cells, macrophages	Activates NK cells, induces Th1 response
IL-13	T cells	↑ B-cell proliferation, ↑ MHC class II expression, ↓ macrophage function, inflammatory cytokine production
IL-15	T cells, monocytes, and epithelial and many other cells	↑ T-cell proliferation, induces NK cells
IL-16	T-$_{CD8^+}$	Lymphocyte chemoattractant
IL-17	T-$_{CD4^+}$	↑ ICAM-1, induces inflammatory cytokines
IL-18	Monocytes and macrophages	Th1 and IFN-γ induction
IL-19	Monocytes	Potential immunosuppressive for proinflammatory cytokine release; up-regulates thymocytes, B cells, and mast cells
IL-20	Skin, keratinocytes, trachea, other tissues	Epidermal differentiation, potential role in psoriasis
IL-21	T cells	NK cell expansion, B- and T-cell proliferation
IL-22	T cells	Activates STAT1, -3, and -5; modest inhibition of IL-4 production
IL-23	DCs	Stimulates IFN-γ production and T-cell proliferation
IL-24	Monocytes, macrophages, and Th2	Enhances cell survival and controls proliferation; tumor suppressive and active in wound healing and psoriasis
IL-25	Th2	Induces IL-4, IL-5, and IL-13 and stimulates eosinophil production
IL-26	T cells	Induces IL-10 and IL-8 secretion and CD54 expression on epithelial cells
IL-27	Activated APC	Activates naïve CD4 T cells
IL-28	Peripheral blood mononuclear cells (IFN-γ2 and -γ3)	Antiviral, ↑ MHC class I expression
IL-29	Peripheral blood mononuclear cells (IFN-γ1)	Antiviral, ↑ MHC class I expression
IL-31	T cells	Induces dermatitis and epithelial responses
IL-32	NK cells, lymphocytes	Induces monocytes and macrophages to secrete TNF-α, IL-8, and CXCL2
IL-33	Epithelial cells, fibroblasts, smooth muscle	Anti-inflammatory, Th2 regulatory activity

[a] TGF-β, transforming growth factor β; MIF, macrophage inhibitory factor; LIF, leukemia inhibitory factor; PBSF, pre-B-cell growth-stimulating factor; OSM, oncostatin M; VEGF, vesicular endothelial growth factor.

4. Components in body fluids that neutralize viral infectivity independently or in conjunction with antibodies

Despite its importance, natural immunity was only a peripheral topic of interest for the century following Metchnikoff's brilliant discoveries of macrophages, their capacity to phagocytose foreign material (including pathogenic bacteria), and the enhancing effects of coating bacteria with antibodies (having been only recently described by von Behring). It was only in the past decade that innate immune mechanisms became a topic of intense research (2, 20). This has led to an explosion of knowledge, including the discovery of structurally diverse sensors with the capacity to recognize specific foreign substances and initiate immune responses. This work has extended immune recognition to include all cells in multicellular organisms, and it has particular importance for viral infections.

The specific arm of the immune system consists of B and T cells. Both types of cells express receptors on their surface in a clonally restricted manner that interact in a highly specific way with a limited set of related substances. Substances capable of interacting with these receptors in a biologically relevant manner are termed antigens. Most antigens are also immunogenic; i.e., they are capable of eliciting a response from a specific set of B or T cells, or both B and T cells. For both B and T cells, the variable antigen-specific receptors exist in a complex on the cell surface with invariant components that transfer information of antigen interaction to the cytosol and, ultimately, the nucleus.

The antigen-specific receptor present on the surface of B cells (named for their development in the bursa, an avian organ with no precise anatomic correlate in mammals) is immunoglobulin (Ig), originally termed "antikorper" (antibodies). Antibodies were the first specific element of the immune system to be discovered. Antibodies are a particular favorite of the Nobel Prize committee, the initial prize in Medicine and Physiology awarded in 1901 to von Behring for his discovery of antitoxins, with no fewer than four subsequent Nobel Prizes given for discoveries related to antibody formation. B cells secrete large quantities of Ig into body fluids. Ig interacts with extracellular virus and inhibits viral infectivity. The induction of such virus "neutralizing" antibodies is the goal of most vaccination strategies. T cells (named for their development in the thymus, an organ present in all jawed vertebrates) express a surface antigen receptor termed the T-cell receptor (TCR) that is structurally and genetically similar to Ig. The TCR enables T cells to recognize cells expressing fragments of viral proteins on their surfaces (termed antigen-presenting cells [APCs]) and to respond at a local level. Antigenic peptides are tethered to the APC surface through their interaction with integral membrane glycoproteins encoded by the major histocompatibility complex (MHC). Depending on the type of T cell and the type of APC, possible outcomes include the destruction of the virus-infected cell or enhancement of the ability of B cells to produce antiviral antibodies. Note that unlike for B cells, whose trigger and effector functions (mediated by the Ig clonotype they secrete) are both antigen specific, the triggering of T cells is antigen specific, but most of their effector functions are not. Thus, T-cell responses can be viewed as a means of localizing nonspecific immune responses to a specific site.

In many respects, Ig and the TCR represent the jewels in the evolutionary crown of the immune system. Uniquely among the various cell types that constitute an organism, the precise type of Ig and TCR produced by any given B or T cell is determined by random genetic events that occur during the growth and differentiation of the cells. As a result, B- and T-cell populations within an individual consist of an extremely heterogeneous mixture of clones, with each clone consisting of a relatively small number of cells expressing a receptor unique to that clone. Humans possess $\sim 10^{11}$ and 10^{8} different B- and T-cell clonotypes, respectively (note that the B-cell estimate is very rough), while mice exhibit approximately 10-fold-less diversity in each compartment.

While different receptors may react equally strongly with a given antigen, the interaction of individual receptors with the universe of potential antigens is unique. Following the interaction of the clone with an antigen that binds sufficiently strongly to the surface antigen receptor to trigger activation, the clone expands to provide a sufficient number of cells to exert an antiviral effect. In the case of B cells, the initial activation steps induce the clone to further mutate its receptor, resulting in the production of a high percentage of progeny with novel antigen receptors (this process is known as somatic mutation). Clones that bind antigen more tightly than their parent will receive greater stimulation and divide more rapidly. After the virus infection is cleared, portions of the expanded clones persist for long periods as memory cells. B-cell clones can persist for a lifetime and constitutively secrete sufficient amounts of antibodies to provide lifelong protection against reinfection. Memory T-cell clones may be somewhat shorter-lived but still persist for years. Upon reexposure to antigen, the increased number of cells responsive to the antigen, in combination with the improved quality of their antigen receptors (for B cells) and relaxed requirements for antigen-induced triggering, results in a more rapid response of increased effectiveness. Thus, unlike nonspecific immune elements, antigen-specific elements demonstrate memory.

It would be difficult to overemphasize that distinct elements of the adaptive and innate immune systems are often involved in preventing, limiting, and eradicating viral infections. The innate immune system plays an essential role in limiting virus replication in the first days following infection. For most viruses, Ig plays an essential role in preventing infections. While Ig can also play an important role in eradicating existing infections, T-cell responses are often required for a rapid and complete recovery. Thus, the most relevant immune component to target for therapeutic intervention varies depending on whether the goal is preventing or treating infection.

Limitations

Human immunology is a difficult experimental science. Ethical concerns greatly restrict the latitude to perform many important experiments. There is only limited access to peripheral (lymph nodes and spleen) and central (thymus and bone marrow) lymphatic organs of infected individuals, which typically limits experiments to peripheral blood lymphocytes (PBLs). In experimental animals, the activities of PBLs (difficult to obtain in quantity from mice) are often different from those of cells obtained from the spleen or lymph nodes, which themselves can also display large differences in immune functions. The outbred nature of human populations further hinders comparison between individuals (though widespread sequence nucleotide polymorphism phenotyping of patient populations will pave the way to discovering the very large number of genes that are bound to contribute to disease resistance or susceptibility and immune responsiveness) and, as described below, makes characterization of T-cell responses particularly difficult.

Due to these formidable obstacles, most of the present knowledge concerning immune responses to viruses was obtained using experimental animals, and virtually all of our knowledge of cellular immune responses was obtained using inbred mice. While the value of these experimental models is indisputable, it should still be appreciated that there are liable to be major differences between the immune responses of mice and humans to some, and perhaps even many, antigens. This problem is particularly acute with responses to viral infections. Most viruses have a highly limited capacity to infect other species. When human viruses infect animals, the features of infection differ enormously. The practical consequence is that it is difficult to impossible to find accurate animal models for human viral diseases. For immunologists it is crucial to recognize that different elements of the immune system may be used for combating infections with the same virus in different species. Moreover, molecules that evolve to interfere with host responses may be highly species specific and may even interact with different target molecules in heterologous species.

Achieving a thorough understanding of the relative importance and interactions of the various immune effector functions remains a challenging task, even when studying simple experimental animal models. The complexity of the immune system is considerable in comparison to the capacity of our brains to process information. The sheer number of known cytokines (13 distinct genes encode alpha interferon [IFN-α] alone), chemokines, and their receptors is daunting, though now that the human genome is sequenced, we have an accurate idea of the number of gene products binned into each family. These substances have spectra of activities that overlap considerably with each other (Tables 1 and 2), and the net effect of all acting in concert may require unachievable computational abilities. The other vertebrate system of great complexity, the nervous system, probably plays a major role in modulating these activities, a highly fertile topic of research that has barely been explored.

One of the hallmarks of the immune response to complex and dangerous antigens such as viruses is its redundancy. Selective ablation of a given component of an immune response by targeted genetic deletion or by administration of a suitable antibody may have little discernible effect on the resistance of the host to the virus, even though that component plays an important physiological role and may be critical in inducing maximally protective responses following vaccination. Different components of the immune response often have overlapping functions. Thus, just as balance is important in the immune response itself, it is important to study immune responses using a balanced and open-minded approach combining negative and positive manipulation of individual components.

Given this state of ignorance regarding the immune system in general and human immune responses in particular, the reader should appreciate that we are just beginning to understand the human immune response to viruses, and that many of the "facts" that follow (and are inscribed in other textbooks) are frequently not much more than intelligent guesses.

INNATE IMMUNITY

General Considerations

In the initial encounter with a virus, nonspecific immune effector mechanisms play a crucial holding action in preventing massive tissue destruction and virus dissemination. Some viruses are capable of completing an infectious cycle in just a few hours, resulting in the release of 1,000 infectious progeny. With such celerity, 10^{11} virions can potentially be produced in the first day alone, an impressive number considering that humans are composed of $\sim 10^{14}$ of their own cells (and 10^{15} bacteria). Since adaptive immune mechanisms (B- and T-cell responses) require 3 to 4 days to reach even minimally effective levels, the potential for damage is enormous. Depending on the virus, natural immune mechanisms play a crucial role in initial responses to many virus infections. While natural immunity is usually not capable of clearing a virus infection on its own, it often works in concert with specific immune mechanisms in the later phase of viral clearance to achieve this result.

Nonspecific immune mechanisms can be triggered by cellular sensing of viral invasion, viral destruction of cells, recognition of infected cells by NK cells, or direct interaction of complement with virions. These initiate cytokine release, activation of complement and kinin cascades, and recruitment of cytokine-spewing monocytes and neutrophils. This triggers increased blood flow and capillary permeability at the site of infection, resulting in the increased delivery of high-molecular-weight serum proteins and recruitment of additional immune cells that make their own contributions to the cytokine cocktail. Together these changes at the site of infection are recognized as a local inflammation, which if present in the skin can be observed as a rash.

When cytokines (particularly interleukin 1 [IL-1] and IL-6) and other substances produced at the site of the inflammation reach a sufficient concentration in the serum, an acute-phase response is triggered. This is a global response of the host induced by trauma or infection with either viruses or uni- or multicellular pathogens. Neutrophils are mobilized from the bone marrow and enter the circulation in large numbers. Hepatocytes shift their biosynthetic resources from producing albumin to secreting greater amounts of a group of serum proteins known as acute-phase proteins, whose concentrations rise approximately 10-fold. Acute-phase proteins participate in or abet immune responses, sequester factors needed for microbial growth, or function to minimize tissue damage by proteases or oxidants released at the inflammation site. The neuroendocrine system is triggered to increase body temperature and shift overall metabolism to a catabolic state that helps marshal body resources to fend off infection. These changes are reflected in the common clinical syndrome (fever, anorexia, and fatigue) associated with many acute virus infections. This unsettling reminder of the active status of our immune system probably contributes to the antiviral response directly (increasing the body temperature 1 or 2°C enhances many cellular immune functions and also disfavors viral replication in many circumstances) or indirectly (minimizing physical and digestive activity de-

TABLE 2 Chemokines used in anti-inflammatory immune responses

Chemokine	Protein	Source	Function
GROα/MGSAα	CXCL1	Monocytes, macrophages, fibroblasts, endothelial cells, and melanoma cells	Chemoattractant and activator for neutrophils, basophils, and T cells; proliferation of fibroblasts, endothelial cells, and melanoma cells
GROβ/MGSAβ	CXCL2	Monocytes, macrophages, fibroblasts, endothelial cells, and melanoma cells	Chemoattractant and activator for neutrophils, basophils, and T cells; proliferation of fibroblasts, endothelial cells, and melanoma cells
GROγ/MGSAδ	CXCL3	Monocytes, macrophages, fibroblasts, endothelial cells, and melanoma cells	Chemoattractant and activator for neutrophils, basophils, and T cells; proliferation of fibroblasts, endothelial cells, and melanoma cells
PF4	CXCL4	Activated T cells and platelets	Angiostatic procoagulant
ENA-78	CXCL5	Monocytes, macrophages, keratinocytes, fibroblasts, endothelial cells, and smooth muscle cells	Neutrophil attractant, angiogenesis
GCP-2	CXCL6	Osteosarcoma cells	Chemoattractant for neutrophils and endothelial cells
NAP-2	CXCL7	Platelets	Chemoattractant for neutrophils and clot resorption
IL-8	CXCL8	Leukocytes, fibroblasts, endothelial cells, epithelial cells, hepatocytes, keratinocytes, mesangial cells, and chondrocytes	Neutrophil, basophil, and T-cell chemotaxis
Mig	CXCL9	Monocytes and hepatocytes	Chemotactic for activated T cells and NK cells, angiostatic
IP-10	CXCL10	T cells, monocytes, keratinocytes, endothelial cells, and fibroblasts	Chemoattractant for monocytes, NK cells, and activated T cells; angiostatic
I-TAC	CXCL11	Astrocytes, monocytes, and T cells	T-cell attractant, bacterial resistance
SDF-1α/β	CXCL12	Bone marrow stroma, astrocytes, and many other cell types	T-cell attractant, B-cell development; attracts $CD34^+$ cells, B cells, endothelial cells, progenitor cells, and megakaryocytes; cerebellum, cardiac, and gastric development
BCA-1	CXCL13	Spleen, lymph node, liver, and appendix	Attracts B cells and subsets of $CD45RO^+$, IL-2 receptor $A\alpha^+$ T cells; B-cell homing
BRAK/bolekine	CXCL14	Squamous epithelium, B cells, monocytes, and peripheral blood mononuclear cells	Inflammatory cell up-regulated, NK cell migration
	CXCL16	DCs in lymphoid organ T-cell zones and cells in splenic red pulp, thymic medulla cells, and other nonlymphoid tissues	Activated T-cell and NK cell attractant, thymic development and T-cell trafficking
DMC	CXCL17	Lung cells	DC and monocyte attractant
NAP-4		Platelets	Neutrophil attractant
Lymphotactin α	XCL1	T cells and NK cells	Attractant for DCs, T cells, NK cells, and thymocytes
SCM-1β	XCL2	T cells and NK cells	Attractant for DCs, T cells, NK cells, and thymocytes
Fractalkine	CX_3CL1	Macrophages, endothelial cells, and microglial cells	Attractant for T cells, monocytes, NK cells, and neutrophils

I-309	CCL1	T cells and mast cells	Monocyte chemoattractant
MCP-1/MCAF	CCL2	Macrophages, monocytes, T cells, endothelium, smooth muscle, and keratinocytes	Monocyte chemotaxis
MIP-1α/LD78α	CCL3	Macrophages and Langerhans cells	Inhibitor of stem cell proliferation; chemoattractant for eosinophils, monocytes, and B and T cells
LD78β	CCL3L1	Macrophages and Langerhans cells	Inhibitor of stem cell proliferation; chemoattractant for eosinophils, monocytes, and B and T cells
MIP-1β	CCL4	Activated T cells, platelets, and many other cell types	Chemotactic for monocytes and memory Th cells, basophil histamine release, and activation of eosinophils
RANTES	CCL5	T cells, fibroblasts, and macrophages	Stimulatory effects on myelopoietic cell growth and leukocyte chemoattractant, activates T cells and macrophages
MCP-3	CCL7	Monocytes, endothelial cells, peripheral blood mononuclear cells, and astrocytes	Activates macrophages, basophils, and mast cells, releases histamines and induces anti-tumor activity
MCP-2	CCL8	Small intestine, heart, peripheral blood mononuclear cells, astrocytes, lung, skeletal muscle, pancreas, thymus, mesenchymal cells	Activates macrophages, releases histamines, attracts basophils and eosinophils
Eotaxin	CCL11	Monocytes, macrophages, endothelial cells, lymph node, lungs, and epithelial cells	Chemotactic for eosinophils, T cells, and basophils
MCP 4/HCC-2	CCL13	Macrophages, small intestine, colon, and endothelial cells	Releases histamines; attracts eosinophils and mast cells
HCC-1	CCL14	Wide distribution (lymphoid tissues, muscles, and bone marrow)	Bone marrow progenitor proliferation
MIP-1δ/HCC-2	CCL15	Monocytes, liver, small intestine, colon, and fetal liver	Attracts T cells and eosinophils; inhibits bone marrow proliferation
LEC/HCC-4	CCL16	Liver and monocytes	Attracts T cells; inhibits bone marrow progenitor cell proliferation
TARC	CCL17	DCs, thymic DCs, lung, colon, and endothelial cells	Mononuclear chemotaxis; favors Th2 response
PARC/DC-CK1	CCL18	Thymus, lymph nodes, monocytes, and lungs	Mononuclear chemotaxis (T cells)
MIP-3β/ELC	CCL19	Monocytes, thymus, lymph node, and spleen	Attracts T cells, monocytes, and neutrophils
MIP-3α/LARC	CCL20	Monocytes, DCs, liver, lung, and lymphoid tissue	Inflammatory activator; DC chemoattractant
SLC, 6CKine	CCL21	Spleen, lymph node, and intestine	T-cell and DC homing
MDC/STPC-1	CCL22	Monocyte-derived DCs, thymus, lymph node, appendix, and mature macrophages	Attracts myeloid DC and activates NK cells and Th2 responses
MPIF 1/Ckβ8	CCL23	Aortic endothelial cells, lung, liver, bone marrow, placenta, and macrophages	Inhibits bone marrow progenitor cell proliferation; attracts activated monocytes
Eotaxin 2, MPIF-2	CCL24	Activated T cells and macrophages	Eosinophil attractant, induction of histamines, bone marrow progenitor cell proliferation, LTC4 from basophils
TECK	CCL25	Thymus, DCs, and thymic progenitors	T-cell development in fetal liver, attracts monocytes, splenic DCs, and thymocytes
Eotaxin 3	CCL26	Heart, ovary, dermal fibroblasts, and keratinocytes	Eosinophil and basophil chemotaxis
CTACK/ILC	CCL27	Keratinocytes	Attracts cutaneous T cells; has role in skin homeostasis and inflammation
MEC	CCL28	Salivary gland, mucosal sites (colon, trachea, and mammary gland), and epithelial cells	Attractant for transfected lymphoid cells; attracts eosinophils and memory lymphocytes

creases overall metabolic demands, allowing the host to devote maximal effort to the immune response).

Sensing Viral Infections

The most critical facet of natural viral immunity is the innate capacity of vertebrate cells to detect and resist incoming pathogens (11, 37). Infection of cells with unrelated virus types can result in the induction of an "antiviral state" that functions to limit viral replication and spread, often to the detriment of the infected cell. Innate immunity relies on the detection of molecular signatures shared by classes of pathogens. These so-called pathogen-associated molecular patterns (PAMPs) are chemically diverse molecules (polypeptide, lipid, carbohydrate, or nucleic acid) that are present in bacterial, fungal, or viral pathogens or are products of their replication cycle. Recognition of PAMPs is mediated by a group of structurally unrelated pattern recognition receptors (PRRs) that survey different compartments of the cell, including the sites of entry and replication of many viruses. While several distinct detection and signaling systems are employed by cells to sound the alarm at the outset of viral infection, they represent complementary and overlapping pathways that typically converge on the production of type I IFNs.

Type I IFNs are a group of structurally related cytokines capable of inhibiting or "interfering" with virus replication. Type I IFNs include IFN-α (13 subtypes), IFN-β, and at least three other gene products (IFN-ω, -ε, and -κ) that exert their effects by engaging a shared receptor composed of two chains (IFNAR1 and -2). Signal transduction through the IFN-α/β receptor is initiated by IFN-mediated dimerization, resulting in the recruitment of Janus-activated kinases (JAK) or tyrosine kinase 2 (TYK2) via interactions with the cytoplasmic tail of the IFN receptor. These proteins then phosphorylate signal transducers and activators of transcription 1 and 2 (STAT1 and STAT2). Phosphorylated STAT proteins assemble as dimers and translocate into the nucleus to enhance transcription of genes that contain IFN-stimulated response elements or IFN-γ-activated sites within their promoters. This pathway results in the induction of hundreds of IFN-stimulated genes. Well-characterized IFN-stimulated genes involved in innate defense against viruses include (i) myxovirus resistance protein (Mx), (ii) double-stranded-RNA (dsRNA)-dependent protein kinase (PKR), (iii) adenosine deaminase (ADAR1), and (iv) proteins involved in the 2′-5′ oligoadenylate system (22).

Type I IFN expression is controlled at the transcriptional level through the regulated activity of NF-κB and members of the IFN regulatory factor (IRF) transcription factor family. IRF-3 is a constitutively expressed transcription factor that regulates IFN-β and IFN-α4 expression. IRF-3 activity is regulated by phosphorylation events at the carboxy terminus that induce conformational changes inducing oligomerization, relocation to the nucleus, and association with the transcriptional coactivator CBP/300. IRF-7 is a structurally related protein that controls the expression of most of the IFN-α gene products. Unlike IRF-3 (with the exception of a subset of dendritic cells [DCs]), IRF-7 expression is not constitutive and instead is induced by virus infection and IFN. A key element of IRF-7 function is its relatively short half-life, which enables cells to return to a nonviral state once the danger has passed. Together, IRF-3 and IRF-7 play a central role in regulating IFN expression and mediate in part the feedback loops responsible for induction of type I IFNs in response to viral infection (17).

TLRs: Surveying the Borders

Toll-like receptors (TLRs) are vertebrate homologs of the *Drosophila* embryonic patterning protein Toll. TLRs function as PRRs capable of sensing infections at cellular portals commonly exploited by pathogens to gain access to intracellular compartments. TLRs are type I transmembrane proteins that contain an amino-terminal leucine-rich repeat somehow involved in ligand recognition (the structural basis of ligand recognition is poorly understood at present). TLRs possess a common cytoplasmic signaling structure called the Toll–IL-1 receptor (TIR) domain that mediates homotypic interactions with a family of five distinct TIR domain-containing adaptors that orchestrate distinct signaling cascades from different TLRs. More than a dozen vertebrate TLRs have been identified to date. Innate antiviral immunity is thought to be initiated primarily through the activities of TLRs capable of binding dsRNA (TLR-3), single-stranded RNA (TLR-7/8), nonmethylated DNA (TLR-9), and even the envelope proteins of several different viruses (TLR-2 and -4). TLRs are expressed broadly and in various combinations on the plasma membrane and subcellular compartments of endothelial, epithelial, and hematopoietic cell types. Localization of TLRs specific for nucleic acids is largely restricted to the endosome, presumably to intercept viral and bacterial pathogens during the entry process. Endosomal localization may also reflect a requirement to compartmentalize these PRRs to avoid recognition of "self" molecules.

Considerable progress has been made in elucidating TLR signaling pathways and the programming of pathogen-specific gene expression programs (25). As illustrated below, many of these pathways converge on common transcription factors that regulate type I IFN expression. Signaling from TLRs is initiated by ligand-mediated dimerization, resulting in conformational changes required for the recruitment of TIR domain-containing adaptor proteins. A key component of TLR signaling is the adaptor protein called myeloid differentiation primary response protein 88 (MyD88). MyD88 interacts with oligomeric TLR-7 (or TLR-9) and recruits members of the IL-1 receptor-associated kinase (IRAK) family. IRAKs, in concert with tumor necrosis factor (TNF) receptor-associated factor (TRAF) proteins, activate NF-κB. NF-κB, in turn, stimulates transcription of a variety of proinflammatory cytokines (e.g., IL-6 and IL-12). This pathway is also capable of activating IRF-7, when present, resulting in induction of type I IFN transcription. As discussed below, IRF-7 is expressed only in a subset of cell types, illustrating that the outcome of TLR-7 and TLR-9 signaling can vary markedly between different cell types of the host. Importantly, not all TLRs signal in a MyD88-dependent fashion. Engagement of TLR-3 by dsRNA results in the recruitment of TIR domain-containing adaptor inducing IFN-β (TRIF), which leads to the activation of IRF-3, AP-1, and NF-κB via the activities of the TRAF family-member-associated NF-κB activator binding kinase (TBK-1). Phosphorylated IRF-3 then promotes expression of IFN-α4 and IFN-β. This signaling cascade may be amplified by a feedback loop established by IFN signaling. IFN promotes expression of IRF-7, which, in turn, is capable of activating transcription of a large number of IFN-α genes.

Internal Sensors for Viral RNA

In recent years, two cytoplasmic RNA sensors have been identified that play a significant role in antiviral immunity (31). Retinoic acid-inducible gene I (RIG-I) and melanoma differentiation-associated gene 5 (MDA5) are RNA helicases that detect viral RNAs and orchestrate a signal transduction cascade resulting in NF-κB and IRF-3 activation. RIG-I signaling and MDA5 signaling converge upon a single adaptor protein named IPS-1 (also called CARDIF, MAVS, or VISA) that binds RIG-I and MDA5. Interestingly, IPS-1 function depends on its localization to the mitochondrial outer membrane, suggesting the potential involvement of mitochondrial factors and the potential for cross talk between IFN induction and mitochondrial functions (e.g., apoptosis, energy generation, etc.). A third RIG-I-like helicase called Lgp2 has been identified and may function as a negative regulator of RIG-I and/or MDA5 signaling. Lgp2 binds dsRNA but lacks the CARD domain required for interactions with IPS-1 and thus may sequester RNA from RIG-I and MDA5.

Studies with RIG-I- and MDA5-deficient animals suggest that RIG-I and MDA5 play complementary roles in innate antiviral responses. RIG-I participates in the initiation of innate defense against a diverse and unrelated group of viruses, including paramyxoviruses, orthomyxoviruses, rhabdoviruses, and flaviviruses, whereas MDA5 appears to primarily mediate responses to picornaviruses. However, some viruses, such as dengue and West Nile viruses, appear to contain structures that are recognized by both helicases. These molecules distinguish cellular from viral RNAs in the cytosol. RIG-I binds single-stranded RNAs or dsRNAs containing 5′ triphosphate termini or complex secondary structures. Cellular RNAs typically do not display 5′ phosphates as a result of the 7-methyl guanosine capping reaction, cleavage, or other modifications, although there are exceptions. The precise ligand for MDA5 is unidentified but is thought to involve complex secondary structures of RNA such as those present in picornaviruses. MDA5 also recognizes synthetic RNAs composed of stretches of annealed inosine and cytosines [poly(I)·poly(C)].

pDCs: Professional Sensors of Virus Infection

Plasmacytoid DCs (pDCs) are bone marrow-derived cells that are the source for most of the initial wave of type I IFNs induced by many viruses (7, 15). These cells reside in the T-cell regions of the spleen and lymph nodes and can be activated by noninfectious forms of viruses. Within 4 h of activation they begin to synthesize predominantly IFN-α and rapidly reach maximum levels of production. Their rate of secretion of IFNs is on the same order as plasma secretion of antibodies (~3,000 molecules per minute), accounting for their plasma cell-like morphology, which features extensive rough endoplasmic reticulum (ER) used for synthesizing IFN. The rate of secretion is 100- to 1,000-fold higher than that of other cells, which seems to enable this small subset of cells to produce the lion's share of systemic IFN.

pDCs employ TLR- and MyD88-dependent pathways to control activation of type I IFNs. A distinguishing feature of pDCs is their constitutive high-level expression of IRF-7 and TLR-9, which confers rapid and robust responses to TLR signals. IRF-7 is thought to complex with TLR-9, MyD88, and TRAF6 in pDCs. The formation of this signaling complex at endosomes appears to result in retaining the bound PAMP and may play an important role in sustained IFN production. IRF-8 may also play a critical role in feedback circuits required for high levels of IFN-α production. pDCs do not express TLR-3 or the RIG-I helicase, and IRF-3 is dispensable for IFN induction in this cell type. In contrast to that from pDCs, IFN-α production from conventional DCs is mediated primarily via TLR-3- and RNA helicase-dependent pathways such as the RIG-I pathway. TLR-9-dependent processes do occur in conventional DCs but signal through IRF-1 or IRF-5 and result in the production of IFN-β and a variety of inflammatory cytokines rather than IFN-α.

A curious feature of TLR-dependent antiviral responses is the detection of viral nucleic acids that are thought to be inaccessible in intact incoming virus particles. The genomes of viruses are often introduced directly into the cytoplasm during the virus entry pathway. While it is certainly possible that the ligands of these PRRs represent materials taken up from adjacent cells succumbing to the cytopathic effects of viral infection (cross-priming for the innate immune response), some cell types may possess a more deliberate solution. pDCs may degrade a fraction of incoming viruses to facilitate access to viral nucleic acid PAMPs. Autophagy describes three homeostatic regulated cellular pathways that deliver intracellular cargo to the lysosome for degradation (27, 44). In pDCs, autophagy may be an important mechanism to expose TLRs to viral ligands. TLR-7-dependent activation of IFN-α by pDCs does not occur following vesicular stomatitis virus or Sendai virus infection when autophagy is compromised (24). Autophagy, however, does not appear to be a universal requirement for antiviral TLR pDC activation, since HSV-triggered activation is unaffected by inhibiting autophagy.

Interactions between Innate and Adaptive Immune Systems

Signals transduced through recognition of PRRs at the onset of innate responses critically impact the development of adaptive immune responses. Engagement of TLR proteins on DCs results in "maturation" and the up-regulation of costimulatory molecules required for efficient T-cell activation, including CD40, CD80, and CD86. These processes reflect not only TLR-mediated NF-κB activation but also IFN-induced effects (41). The release of cytokines and IFN by DCs stimulated through one or more TLRs is required for T-cell activation and differentiation, as well as NK cell activation. A role for TLR signals in several facets of B-cell activation, including germinal-center formation, has also been suggested. TLR signals also have the ability to impact antigen processing by DCs by regulating the ability of these cells to capture antigen via endo- and phagocytosis, modulating protein translation and turnover, and influencing MHC class II expression.

Humoral Effector Mechanisms

Directly Acting Antiviral Substances

Viruses are "nonspecifically" inhibited by high concentrations of serum or plasma. In only a few instances are the responsible substances characterized (e.g., sialic acid-containing glycoproteins that competitively block influenza virus binding to cellular sialic acids). While the relevance of such nonspecific inhibition is uncertain, large doses of infectious virus are often needed to initiate experimental infections in animals or to successfully immunize humans with attenuated virus vaccines. Perhaps this is in part due to the action of humoral antiviral factors. Possible contributors include the following.

1. Abundant antibodies that bind to viruses with low avidity (32). Such antibodies may have been induced by prior exposure to cross-reactive antigens, or they might be naturally produced by the immune system in the absence of specific antigenic stimulation due to their general protective properties. "Natural antibodies" are IgM (see below) antibodies produced from antibody genes that have been rearranged but not further altered by somatic mutation. A special category of antiviral antibodies produced by humans and other primates are specific for terminal galactose residues linked to a penultimate galactose by a 1-3α bond. This oligosaccharide is absent in humans and other primates but is present in gut bacteria, which induce the antibody response. Importantly, nonprimate mammals and insects generate this oligosaccharide linkage, with the consequence that membrane viruses produced by these species may express surface glycoproteins with the oligosaccharide. Such antibodies appear to protect humans from infection by a number of viruses transmitted by these organisms.

2. Complement components. The complement system is comprised of a group of more than 30 proteins, up to 10% of serum proteins, that play myriad roles in the immune response, including immunoregulation, phagocytosis, membrane lysis, and inflammation. Complement components are induced in the acute-phase response. Some viruses may be directly neutralized by complement, particularly membrane viruses that can potentially be inactivated by insertion of pores formed by the complement membrane attack complex. This would appear, however, to be a minor contribution relative to the enhancing function that complement has on antibody-mediated neutralization and phagocytosis.

3. Collectins. Collectins (including complement protein C1q) are carbohydrate-binding molecules present in serum (where they are also acute-phase proteins) and the alveolar surface. Type II alveolar cells produce at least two collectins (surfactant proteins A and D) that can bind to oligosaccharides present on the proteins or lipids of respiratory viruses and enhance their phagocytosis by alveolar macrophages.

There are other substances with direct antiviral activity that could diminish viral infectivity in vivo. Human saliva contains factors (including lactoferrin, mucins, and serum leukocyte protein inhibitor) that inhibit in vitro infection with human immunodeficiency virus (HIV) through mostly undefined mechanisms; this may contribute to the infrequent oral transmission of HIV. Neutrophils, Paneth cells of the small intestine, and macrophages secrete a variety of small (<40 residues) positively charged peptides (collectively known as defensins) that intercalate into membranes. Defensins appear to primarily function to inhibit bacterial replication, but they have also been shown to neutralize viruses (23).

Cellular Immune Effector Functions

NK Cells

NK cells are cells derived from the lymphoid lineage from hematopoietic stem cells. They develop in a thymus-independent manner. Their numbers were not thought to be influenced by prior exposure to antigens, but recent evidence calls into question this conclusion (33). They do not express either Ig or TCR-like molecules, and they demonstrate limited clonal diversity relative to T or B cells.

The induction of NK activity is an early and prominent feature of the immune response to many viruses. NK cells appear to play a particularly important role in controlling primary infections with members of the *Herpesviridae* family, since patients with a deficiency in NK cell activity suffer from severe primary infections with a variety of herpesviruses (34). More recently, two syndromes were identified at the genetic and molecular levels in which severe herpesvirus infections were associated with defects in NK cell lytic activity (28, 65).

The activity of NK cells is increased up to 100-fold by exposure to IL-2, IL-12, or IFN-α, -β, or -γ. As many virus-infected nonlymphoid cells secrete IFN-β, this is likely to be a major stimulus of initial NK responses to virus infections. NK cells are deactivated by transforming growth factor β, a cytokine produced by activated macrophages. Since $CD4^+$ T cells (T_{CD4^+}) play an important role in activating macrophages, this may contribute to the characteristic decay in NK cell activity as T_{CD4^+} responses rise. Triggering of NK cells by antigen recognition results in the rapid release of presynthesized cytokines residing in secretory vesicles, particularly IFN-γ granulocyte-macrophage colony-stimulating factor (GM-CSF), and TNF. IFN-γ appears to be particularly important in the antiviral activity of NK cells. These cytokines activate macrophages and favor the development of T helper 1 (Th1) cells (described below). Thus, NK activation may be an important factor in the tilting of antiviral responses to the Th1 type.

NK cells can directly interfere with viral reproduction by releasing cytokines with antiviral activity or by lysing virus-infected cells. Lysis is usually mediated by the perforin/granzyme mechanism used by T_{CD8^+} (described below). Virus-infected cells can also be lysed by NK cells targeted to viral antigens by antibodies bound to an Fc receptor on the NK cell surface (this is termed antibody-dependent cellular cytotoxicity [ADCC]). The importance of NK-mediated ADCC in virus infections is uncertain, and this ADCC would have no role in the early response to a newly encountered virus, when virus-specific antibodies have yet to be produced.

In the last 10 years there has been tremendous progress in delineating the NK cell receptors used to detect alterations in virus-infected cells (21, 26, 63). In brief, NK cells usually express both positive and negative receptors, i.e., those that trigger and inhibit activation, respectively. Many of these receptors are expressed by $\gamma\delta$ T cells and by activated $\alpha\beta$ T cells, especially T_{CD8^+}, although the functional significance of this is unknown.

Two distinct classes of negative signaling receptors recognize MHC class I molecules (described in the next section). Killing inhibitory receptors (KIR) are a family of receptors whose individual members recognize HLA-A, HLA-B, HLA-C, or HLA-G molecules. Occupation of the peptide binding groove of class I molecules seems to be essential for proper signaling of the inhibitory NK receptor. KIR class I receptors can discriminate between peptides but do not appear to distinguish between self-peptides and foreign peptides, and the significance of their peptide specificity is unclear. NK cells typically express zero to three different KIR genes. Mice do not possess KIR-like genes and instead use Ly49 gene family members (missing from humans) to perform a similar function. Both KIR and Ly49 genes are highly polymorphic, and individuals can vary widely in the numbers of family member genes present in their genomes.

A number of KIR and Ly49 gene products have homologs with differences in their cytoplasmic tails that convert them to activating NK receptors. These activating homologs also seem to recognize classical MHC class I molecules. The activating CD94/NKG2A heterodimeric receptor recognizes the nonclassical class I molecule HLA-E in humans and Qa-1 in mice. Both of these molecules preferentially present leader sequences from classical class I molecules, providing NK cells with a method for monitoring the synthesis of class I molecules by target cells.

Class I surveillance is a major function of NK cells. Some viruses deliberately interfere with class I expression to evade T_{CD8^+} immunosurveillance; others decrease class I expression as a consequence (probably unintended) of inhibiting host protein synthesis. Viruses can also interfere with the production or presentation of a specific set of host peptides recognized in association with MHC class I molecules by NK cell receptors. This might be a global effect due to increased competition from viral peptides. More likely, however, is that the essential host peptides are produced from proteins whose synthesis or processing is sensitive to viral infections.

NK cells utilize class I-independent strategies for detecting virus-infected cells. NKG2D is an NK receptor that is activated by interaction with a number of target cell surface molecules induced by stress, including that of viral infection. One group of ligands are the human MICA and MICB MHC class Ib molecules. Two activating receptors, NKp46 and NKp44 (NCR1 and NCR2, respectively, in mice), recognize viral proteins with sialic acid binding activity. Numerous viruses, including influenza virus, use terminal sialic acids as a cell surface receptor, and mice lacking NCR1 demonstrated increased mortality following influenza (12).

NKR-P1 is a family of activating and inhibiting C-type lectin-like receptors that recognize a group of C-type lectin-like ligands in the Clec2 family. The genes encoding the receptor and its ligands are intertwined in the genome, guaranteeing coinheritance of these protagonists. Rat cytomegalovirus (CMV) activates NKR-P1 by inhibiting expression of its inhibitory Clec2 ligand, but only when the virus lacks a decoy protein that replaces the Clec2 ligand (54). Poxviruses express similar proteins that may also subvert NKR-P1 recognition.

NK cells function not only to kill but also as early responders that help generate the proper cytokine response to generate a beneficial inflammatory response at a site of infection. While exhibiting nowhere near the magnitude of diversity of lymphocytes, NK cells demonstrate considerable diversity in their receptor expression, and different NK cell clones clearly demonstrate specificity at the level of recognizing cells infected with different viruses. The dogma that NK cells demonstrate no memory is probably incorrect, although the relevance of this finding to viral immunity remains to be established, as does the duration of the NK cell memory. Still, NK cells may contribute to memory responses and thus need to be considered in devising rational cellular-immunity-based vaccines.

Macrophages and Neutrophils

There is only limited information on the role of macrophages in viral infections, in contrast to bacterial immunity, where macrophages clearly play a central role. In mice, depletion of macrophages increases the severity of infection with a number of viruses, but the mechanism is largely undetermined. Macrophages potentially play an important role in lymphocyte activation. Macrophages that express MHC class II molecules are efficient activators of T_{CD4^+}. Although they are not believed to play much of a role in activating T_{CD8^+}, macrophages are as efficient in priming T_{CD8^+} responses as DCs under some in vivo conditions (39). In fact, the relative roles of macrophages and DCs in priming of antiviral T cells are uncertain.

Macrophages recruited to the site of infection likely function to establish and maintain the local inflammation by cytokine secretion and, later, to dispose of debris from cells destroyed by virus or host effector mechanisms. Macrophages also play a role in the destruction of antibody-coated virions, via Fc receptor-mediated internalization of immune complexes into lysosomes.

The role of neutrophils in viral immunity is very poorly defined, even though neutrophils, like macrophages, are highly abundant phagocytic cells with Fc receptors and are recruited in large numbers to sites of viral infection. Neutropenia is a feature of many viral infections, and like macrophages, neutrophils can be infected by viruses. Recent work on the interaction of the herpesvirus Epstein-Barr virus with macrophages and neutrophils (43) clearly demonstrates the great opportunities for discoveries in this neglected area of antiviral innate immunity.

pDCs and Mast Cells

pDCs are bone marrow-derived cells that are the source for most of the initial wave of type I IFNs induced by many viruses as discussed above (7, 15). Mast cells are abundant cells that reside in most (if not all) tissues in close proximity to blood vessels and nerves. Their major defined function is to release histamine upon binding IgE complexed to antigens via the IgE Fc receptor, but they also express IgG Fc receptors and are able to secrete a wide variety of cytokines. Mast cells can be chronically infected by HIV and dengue virus and secrete cytokines upon infection (29). More studies of mast cell functions in virus model systems using knockout mice lacking mast cells and drugs that selectively inhibit mast cells are awaited.

$\gamma\delta$ T Cells

A subset of T cells expressing $\gamma\delta$ TCR chains (described below) are prominent in mucosal epithelium and skin. Although they are difficult to enumerate accurately due to difficulties in recovering them from these tissues, they might be the most abundant T cells in mice and humans. $\gamma\delta$ T cells express highly limited TCR variability, and these relatively invariant receptors delineate functional and anatomic subsets of the cell. Distinct receptor subsets are used for different viruses. Many $\gamma\delta$ T cells mature in a thymus-independent manner, further distinguishing them from classic $\alpha\beta$ T cells.

$\gamma\delta$ T cells participate in immune responses to many viruses (38). Although the antiviral effector mechanisms in vivo are poorly defined, freshly isolated $\gamma\delta$ T cells are typically not cytotoxic and are frequently found to release IFN-γ. Under some circumstances, however, $\gamma\delta$ cells exhibit NK-like cytotoxicity and express NK cell receptors. Antiviral $\gamma\delta$ T cells straddle the border between innate and adaptive immune responses. $\gamma\delta$ T cells typically recognize general virus-induced alterations in infected cells (e.g., increased expression of stress proteins or class Ib molecules) but can also be activated by interacting with specific viral gene products.

Much remains to be learned about this important group of cells, which has been like an ignored stepchild in the T-cell family.

SPECIFIC EFFECTOR MECHANISMS

Humoral Immunity

Antibodies

Polyclonal Sera and MAbs

The early discovery and characterization of antibodies were facilitated by their direct mode of action (often binding to antigen is sufficient to inactivate the antigen's biological activity), their high concentrations in serum (total Ig is present at 10 mg/ml; peak antigen-specific responses generally range from 0.1 to 1 mg/ml), their high avidity for antigen (usually between 10^8 and 10^{11} liters/mol for viral antigens), and their stability after removal from the body (many decades at 4°C). Serum antibodies consist of an extremely heterogeneous mixture of closely related proteins, with each distinct clone of B cells synthesizing a unique protein (hence the term polyclonal antiserum). Through the technique of cell fusion with myeloma cells, it is possible to produce permanent cell lines ("hybridomas," since the cells are somatic cell hybrids) secreting a single type of antibody (monoclonal antibody [MAb]). Antiviral MAbs have proven indispensable for characterizing the antigenic structure of viral proteins, understanding virus neutralization, and studying the folding, structure, function, and intracellular trafficking of viral proteins. MAbs are also important clinically, where they are presently employed for diagnosis and epidemiological surveillance and are replacing polyclonal antibodies for passive antiviral immunization.

Ig Generation and Structure

The five types of human Igs are termed IgA, IgD, IgE, IgG, and IgM. The basic structure of each is a disulfide-linked homodimer, with each subunit consisting of a longer glycoprotein (heavy chain) linked by a disulfide bond to a protein (light chain) of approximately half the size. The NH_2 terminus of each chain is variable, while the COOH terminus is constant among the different classes (the constant region is termed "Fc" since it crystallizes relatively easily when proteolytically released from the variable region). All the residues within the heavy- and light-chain variable regions can vary among Igs, with three clusters of residues on each chain displaying hypervariability. As might be expected, these hypervariable regions (termed complementary determining regions [CDRs]) play a critical role in antibody specificity, and examination of the structure of antigen-antibody complexes by X-ray crystallography reveals that they occupy positions in the contact regions between antibody and antigen.

The immune system is capable of generating over 10^{11} distinct antibody variable regions. Underlying this phenomenal achievement are several distinct mechanisms (18):

1. In the germ line of mammals are between 200 and 1,000 genes encoding variable regions for light and heavy chains (each type of chain with its own set of variable genes).

2. During the genetic recombination of variable segments with light- and heavy-chain constant segments, further shuffling occurs. One of five or six small regions (termed J for joining) is inserted at the junction of the third CDR with the constant region. In the case of heavy chains, 1 of 20 or more additional even smaller regions (termed D for diversity) is inserted between the J segment and variable region.

3. During the course of an immune response, "somatic mutation" occurs, resulting in the random mutagenesis of the variable region gene expressed by a responding B cell (0.5 substitution/cell division, on average).

If the recombination process were truly random, and all heavy and light chains produced genetically could properly assemble and fold in the B cell, the potential diversity calculated combinatorially by the first two mechanisms alone would be enormous (on the order of 10^{11}). Since *only* 10^7 specificities are believed to be generated by all three processes acting together, there obviously are constraints on the generating process, most of which probably occur at the protein folding level.

At the other (COOH-terminal) end of Ig is the constant region. Initially, all B cells express surface-anchored IgM, and the initial Ig secreted upon antigen stimulation is IgM (naïve B cells also express the same variable region on another membrane-anchored heavy chain, termed IgD, that is rarely secreted; why two heavy chains are required is unclear). Unique among Igs, individual IgM molecules can be disulfide linked into pentameric structures that contain 10 antigen-binding sites (compared to 2 sites per normal Ig). The pentameric structure of IgM greatly increases its ability to bind a multimeric antigen such as a virus, since the chance of the entire molecule dissociating from antigen is lowered considerably when it can be bound via 10 independent sites (the binding of multivalent receptors to multivalent ligands is termed avidity, as opposed to affinity [or intrinsic affinity], which refers to monovalent binding). High avidity is critical in primary responses, since the affinities of most primary antibodies for antigen will be relatively low due to limited clonal selection and the absence of somatic mutation.

As T cells respond to infection, those of the helper class (Th) intimately associate with B cells producing antiviral antibodies, and they signal B cells to alter their response in three ways. First, Ig heavy-chain genes are rearranged such that the same variable region is now attached to a different heavy chain. Second, B cells are induced to divide and undergo somatic mutation. Third, a subset of each B-cell clone producing the best-binding antibodies at the peak of the primary response differentiates into very long-lived plasma cells or memory cells. The former continuously secrete large amounts of antibodies, while the latter are rapidly reactivated when reexposed to antigen following reinfection, proliferate, and undergo further affinity maturation; they also generate a second batch of memory B cells and plasma cells.

Affinity maturation of B cells predominantly occurs in lymphoid tissues (lymph nodes, tonsils, and spleen) in discrete areas known as germinal centers, which form approximately a week after significant levels of antigen are present. B cells that have received help from T cells in other regions of lymphoid tissues can differentiate terminally outside of germinal centers into plasma cells, which produce the bulk of the early IgG response. Alternatively, activated B cells can migrate to primary follicles in lymphoid tissue and form a germinal center. B cells can also capture immune complexes, viruses, or particulate antigens from subcapsular sinus macrophages that project large processes across the subcapsular sinus into the germinal center (19, 36). A critical feature of germinal centers is the presence of follicular DCs, which have a unique capacity to collect and retain intact antigens on their surfaces for extremely long periods (perhaps years) and also possess surface molecules (CD23 and probably others) that induce B-cell division and somatic mutation. (CD is acronymic for "cluster of differentiation," the terminology used for designating proteins detected at the surface of human leukocytes using MAbs. Most of the surface molecules used by immune cells have been given CD numbers, but there are a few exceptions described below.) B cells deliver immune complexes to the follicular DCs through a complement receptor expression-dependent mechanism. The cells then produce immune complexes that are shed as small membrane fragments (iccosomes) that are efficiently processed by B cells for presentation to T cells in the germinal center, which respond by producing cytokines necessary for B-cell differentiation. Competition by B cells for the small amounts of antigen present on follicular DCs drives the somatic mutation process by selecting for those cells with the highest-affinity Ig. Competition for antigen is enhanced further by the presence of increasing amounts of soluble antibodies of increasing affinity. Those B cells that survive the selection process differentiate to either plasma cells or memory cells.

This basic biology of the B-cell response accounts for the humoral response following infection with virtually all viruses. An initial IgM response of low affinity gradually becomes an IgG response of increasing affinity over a period of several weeks. Following reinfection, a rapid IgG response of high affinity is produced to add to low but significant levels of circulating IgG produced by plasma cells from the initial infection.

Heavy-Chain Classes

The different constant regions present in human Igs possess distinct biological activities. The composition of Ig classes that respond to each antigen is tailored by the immune system, probably by the nature of the T-cell response. The major properties of each heavy-chain class are summarized in Table 3. No doubt there are additional unique features of class that play an important role in the response to some viruses.

Some features of heavy-chain constant regions are worthy of special note. First, both IgM (occasionally) and IgA (usually) possess an additional disulfide-linked polypeptide ("J" chain) that targets the Igs to specific receptors expressed on the basolateral surface of hepatocytes and many epithelial cells. Igs are then internalized and transported across the cell and delivered to the apical surface, which forms the inner lining of various body cavities (lungs, gut, bile ducts, gall bladder, bladder, uterus, etc.). This mechanism is also used by salivary, tear, and lactating mammary glands. Part of the receptor (the "secretory component") remains attached to the antibody, possibly to provide additional protection against proteolysis (antibodies are already quite resistant to many proteases). Since in many circumstances the initial encounter between a virus and the host occurs on a mucosal surface, secretory antibodies often play a critical role in preventing viral infections. The importance of the secretory immune system snaps into focus when it is considered that the gut mucosa (which has a surface area on the order of 250 m^2) contains 80% of all Ig-producing B cells, with daily secretion of IgA into the gut alone being greater than secretion of IgG into internal body fluids.

Second, IgM and, to a lesser extent, some of the IgG subclasses are able to activate the complement system. Components of the complement system can enhance antibody neutralization of viral infectivity by direct attack of the lipid bilayer of enveloped viruses; by increasing steric inference of virus-surface protein function; by aggregating virions, thereby reducing the number of infectious units; by increasing antibody avidity by cross-linking antibodies; and by targeting antibody-antigen complexes to macrophages via complement receptors. Complement components can also bind to the surface of some enveloped viruses, directly exerting an antiviral effect. Additionally, complement can lyse virus-infected cells in the event of antibody binding to viral proteins expressed on the infected cell surface. Complement plays an important role in inducing inflammation at sites of infection and is required for optimal activation of B cells. At least three virus families (*Poxviridae*, *Herpesviridae*, and *Flaviviridae*) express gene products that interfere with the effector functions of the complement cascade. Thus, for these viruses, complement has the potential to diminish viral replication sufficiently to drive selection for complement-resistant variants.

TABLE 3 Properties of human Ig subclasses

Property	Value for[a]:								
	IgD	IgM	IgE	IgA1	IgA2	IgG1	IgG2	IgG3	IgG4
Level in serum (mg/ml)	0.003–0.3	0.5–2.0	0.0001–0.0007	0.8–3.4	0.2–0.6	5–10	1.8–3.5	0.6–1.2	0.3–0.6
Half-life in serum (days)	3	5	2.5	6	6	12–21	12–21	7–8	11–21
Catabolic rate (%/day)	37	8.8–18.8	62–71	25	25	7	7	17	7
Complement activation	–	++++	–	+	+	++	+	++	–
Opsonization	–	–	–	+	+	+++	–	++	+
ADCC	–	–	–	–	–	++	–	++	–
Mast cell activation	–	–	++++	–	–	–	–	–	–
Traverses placenta	–	–	–	–	–	+	+	+	+
Diffusion into extravascular sites	–	–	++	+	+	++	++	++	++
Traverses epithelia	–	+	–	+++	+++	–	–	–	–

[a] –, no biological activity; + to ++++, increasing biological activities.

Third, two of the IgG subclasses are recognized by Fc receptors on the surface of NK cells. Thus, if the antibodies bind viral proteins expressed on infected cells, the NK cells can lyse the cells (termed ADCC).

Fourth, the different tendencies of the various heavy-chain subclasses to aggregate can influence the ability of the antibodies to form multivalent interactions with multivalent antigens such as viruses. As discussed above with regard to the multivalency of IgM, this can greatly enhance the strength of the antibody-virus interaction.

The Nature of Antigenic Determinants Recognized by Antibodies

Following viral infection, any viral protein, structural or nonstructural, may induce an antibody response. For reasons that are usually unclear, some viral proteins induce weak or undetectable responses. Even on highly antigenic proteins, only a few regions will usually elicit antibody responses. Numerous factors can potentially contribute to this:

1. Quantities of a given protein sufficient to elicit a response may not encounter B cells. This could be due to low expression of the protein, digestion of the protein by serum proteases, or the physical disposition of the protein (e.g., an internal viral structural protein that is rarely exposed). Within individual proteins, many potentially antigenic regions are probably never sufficiently exposed to solvent to allow for binding to the B-cell surface.
2. The protein may not be presented to B cells in a manner that allows for T cells to augment responses (discussed below).
3. The protein may simply not have any regions that can be recognized by antibodies expressed by primary B cells. This could be due to a natural hole in the antibody repertoire or one created by the deletion of self-reactive B cells.

Solution of the three-dimensional structure of antibodies complexed to protein antigens (including several viral antigens (Color Plate 25) reveals an extensive area of interaction between the surface of the antibody and antigen (6, 64). Approximately 20 residues on each partner are in close proximity, covering an area of 700 Å^2. Given this large surface area and the potential for numerous interactions between residues, what is most surprising in thermodynamic terms is not how tightly most antibodies bind antigen but how weakly. A typical high-affinity antiviral antibody binds with a K_a of 10^{10} liters/mol. This is equivalent to 10 kcal/mol, or just 10 hydrogen bonds. Paradoxically, crystallographers can identify upwards of 100 hydrogen bonds between the two ligands, as well as numerous hydrophobic interactions and salt bridges. Thus, in addition to these interactions thermodynamically favoring association, there must be a very nearly equal number of interactions disfavoring association (entropy decreases that accompany binding also disfavor binding). Thus, a slight thermodynamic plurality with even small amounts of an antibody of sufficiently high affinity for a virus surface protein can provide complete protection from infection.

The subtlety of the antigen-antibody interaction provides an answer to antigenic variation, which is one of the most important aspects of the humoral response to viruses (3). Numerous viruses undergo gradual antigenic evolution in their surface proteins such that they no longer interact with antibodies against the original strain introduced into a population, creating serotypes. This phenomenon, which is termed antigenic drift when it occurs rapidly, was first noted in influenza virus more than 60 years ago, and it remains a barrier to producing a durably effective influenza vaccine. Rapid antigenic variation is also a feature of HIV and hepatitis C virus (HCV). Studies using MAbs with virus neutralizing activity to select in vitro for neutralization-resistant mutants of numerous types of virus (also termed escape mutants or antigenic variants) revealed that a single amino acid substitution is sufficient to reduce antibody affinity to a point where it is no longer biologically effective. X-ray crystallographic studies show that the effect of the substitution is strictly local; one side chain is simply substituted for the other without any alterations in surrounding residues. However, crystallography provides a static snapshot of highly dynamic structures, and it seems very likely that amino acid substitutions have significant effects on protein dynamics.

The large area of the antibody-antigen interaction combined with the globular nature of most viral proteins explains why the vast majority of antiviral antibodies with biological activity bind only to native viral proteins. The antigenic determinants recognized by these antibodies (termed epitopes, with "epi-" referring to their presence on the surface of native proteins) are formed by residues derived from different regions of the unfolded polypeptide chain that form a continuous surface when the protein folds. These determinants, designated conformational (or discontinuous) determinants, should be distinguished from linear (or sequential) determinants, such as those formed by short synthetic peptides. If such peptides, which have low intrinsic immunogenicity due to their inability to elicit T-cell responses, are administered in a manner that enables delivery of T-cell help, they can elicit reasonably robust antibody responses. Antibodies raised in this manner bind well to the immunogen and unfolded full-length protein and are of great value for techniques such as immunoblotting. Usually, however, antipeptide antibodies bind to native viral surface antigens with such low affinity that they do not exhibit biological activity. To date, the use of synthetic peptides to elicit protective antibody responses to viruses has proven to be a great disappointment.

Defining the Antigenic Structure of Viral Proteins

Antigens are defined by the immune system. The antigenic structure of a protein is strictly a relative term that is defined by the conditions used to elicit an immune response. Consequently, there is no one antigenic structure to a protein, although antibody responses by many mammalian species elicited by administration of a protein in various guises will often focus on selected regions of the protein. An important variable in defining the antigenic structure is the method used to detect antibody interaction. If, for example, virus neutralization is used to measure antibody binding, then only those regions of the protein on virions that are accessible to antibody and whose binding blocks viral infectivity will be scored as antigenic. If immunoblotting is used, then almost all of the antigenic sites scored will be of the sequential type. Thus, the antigenicity of a protein is by definition operational, depending on the nature of the antibodies and the aspect of virus function or structure in question.

Antiviral Antibody Effector Mechanisms

For most viruses, the most important role for antibody in immunity is preventing viral infection of host cells.

When viruses initiate infection of the host, most are vulnerable to antibodies present in serum or on mucosae (the exceptions being viruses transferred between individuals via infected cells that can transmit the virus to the new host cells by direct contact, as has been proposed for HIV). Viruses released from the host cell remain susceptible to antibodies until a new cell internalizes them. Viruses that spread between adjacent cells are less susceptible to antibodies, particularly those viruses that induce fusion between infected and uninfected cells (such fused cells are termed syncytia). The goal of most immunization schemes is, in fact, to induce permanent secretion of neutralizing antibody (5). Antibodies can neutralize virions via a number of mechanisms:

1. Prevent virus attachment by steric or, less commonly, allosteric effects.
2. Prevent viral penetration by blocking the function of proteins responsible for fusion of host and viral membranes (enveloped viruses) or for breaching cellular membranes (nonenveloped viruses).
3. Target complement to lyse the membrane of enveloped viruses, or to deliver virus to phagocytic cells via complement receptors.
4. Direct virus to cells with Fc receptors capable of disposing of the virus in lysosomes (for viruses like dengue virus that can infect such cells, however, this may actually enhance infectivity in vivo).

In addition to neutralization, antibodies exert other antiviral activities, although these are usually of much less significance:

1. Antibodies specific for viral proteins expressed on the surface of infected cells can direct complement or NK cells to lyse infected cells (depending, of course, on their heavy-chain class). This generally requires fairly large quantities of antibody. Since recognition by T cells is earlier and far more sensitive, these mechanisms will play a role only in cases where T-cell recognition is limited.
2. Antibodies can prevent release of virus from the infected cell. Newly budded influenza virus, for example, remains attached to the cell in the presence of antibodies that block the ability of the viral neuraminidase to cleave sialic acids present on the host cell surface that serve as a receptor for the viral attachment protein (such antibodies will also prevent the virus from detaching itself from noncellular, sialic acid-containing substrates).
3. Antibodies specific for alphavirus have been found to abort an ongoing infection in neuronal cells. The mechanism for this fascinating phenomenon is uncertain, and the extent to which this applies to nonneuronal cells or other viruses remains to be established.
4. In the case of viruses that spread by syncytium formation, antibodies can bind viral proteins expressed at the cell surface and prevent the intracellular adherence or fusion of membranes.

Antigenic Variation in Viral Proteins

Since single amino acid substitutions can often reduce antibody binding to biologically insignificant levels, the degree of variation observed among the various viral proteins provides an important clue to the effectiveness of antibody-mediated antiviral activities (assuming, of course, that various viral proteins exhibit equal abilities to accept substitutions that alter antigenicity). This reveals that the surface proteins of viruses vary considerably more than the internal proteins. Indeed, for diagnostic purposes, antibodies to surface proteins are generally used for determining the virus strain, while antibodies to internal proteins are used to determine the virus type. Among surface proteins, variation clusters in the antigenic determinants bound by neutralizing antibodies, providing a genetic exclamation point to the relative importance of antibody-mediated virus neutralization in the immune response to many viruses.

It remains uncertain why some viruses exhibit enormous antigenic variability and others exhibit almost none. The surface proteins of the influenza virus demonstrate two types of variation, termed antigenic shift and antigenic drift (see chapter 42). The former represents the occasional reshuffling of a distantly related gene into the segmented virus genome (due in some cases to recombination between animal and human influenza viruses) and results in a novel virus which can be completely non-cross-reactive antigenically to circulating strains. Antigenic drift results from point mutations. The rapid drift of influenza virus cannot be attributed simply to a high frequency of producing antigenic variants, since other antigenically invariant viruses generate variants at a similar frequency when virus is grown in cultured cells. Nor can it be that single substitutions in influenza virus have a greater effect on overall variation, since the hemagglutinin (HA), like other viral proteins, possesses multiple antigenic sites bound by neutralizing antibodies and produces variants that differ one antigenic site at a time. Thus, there may be something unique about the biology of influenza virus infection, such that selection is allowed to occur sequentially, due perhaps to virus sequestration in a compartment producing antibody specific for a single antigenic site.

Cellular Immunity

Overview of T-Cell Recognition and Function

Enumerating T Cells

Formerly, enumerating T-cell responses was based on relatively clumsy assays that provided a very imprecise measure of numbers of responding cells, e.g., cytolysis of target cells and amounts of cytokines released. The introduction of three new technologies has changed this circumstance. The first is class I peptide tetramers, which enable direct identification of T_{CD8^+} specific for a given class I peptide complex and provide a measure of TCR affinity for its cognate MHC-peptide complex. The second is intracellular cytokine staining, which uses flow cytometry to identify activated T_{CD8^+} or T_{CD4^+} based on the induction and intracellular accumulation of cytokines (usually IFN-γ or TNF-α). The last is enzyme-linked immunospot assay, based on the local trapping of secreted cytokines by antibody bound to plastic. These methods demonstrated that previous estimates of responding T_{CD8^+} were 10- to 100-fold too low and have enabled quantitative studies of antigen-specific T-cell responses.

T-Cell Function

T cells play two roles in viral immunity. First, through the release of the appropriate lymphokines, they orchestrate the immune response by controlling the types of antibodies secreted by B cells, regulating the inflammation at the site of infection, and aiding the development of T cells with antiviral activity. Second, they are able to specifically recognize virus-infected cells, and they either destroy the cell before progeny virus are released or deliver lymphokines that modulate virus replication.

These functions hinge on the recognition of viral antigens on the surface of APCs. Since the APCs either are not actually infected by the virus or are infected by viruses that need not betray their existence by the expression of proteins at the cell surface, a novel system had to evolve that allowed for recognition of cells either exposed to viral antigens or experiencing the initial events in viral replication. This resulted in the evolution of two types of proteins. One is a peptide-binding membrane protein encoded by the MHC that samples proteins in the cytosol and endosomal compartments and displays short peptides derived from these proteins on the surface of APCs. The other is the TCR, a close relative of Igs, which recognizes the MHC-peptide complex and activates T-cell function.

TCR Structure and Function

Like B cells, each T-cell clone expresses a unique antigen receptor on its surface. The TCR consists of a heterodimer of two integral membrane proteins, termed the α and β chains. Each chain consists of a constant, membrane-proximal COOH-terminal region and a variable NH_2-terminal domain. As with Ig, the variable region is attached to the constant region by genetic rearrangement, with additional combinatorial diversity generated in CDR3 (as with Ig, located at the junction of variable constant regions) by the insertion of one (for α chains) or two (for β chains) additional small segments. Thus, as with Ig, most of the diversity in the TCR occurs in CDR3, which typically is in direct contact with the peptide bound by the MHC molecule. The other CDRs contact the α-helices that form the ridges of the MHC-peptide binding pocket. This provides the structural basis for the phenomenon of MHC restriction (10). Note that the area of TCR contact with the MHC-peptide complex is similar in size to the antibody-antigen interface and that the antigen specificity of the interaction is largely based on the interaction with just a few residues from the bound peptide that point toward the TCR, since peptide binding has only subtle conformation effects on MHC structure. Consequently, the degree of specificity of TCR antigen recognition is expected to be significantly less than that of Ig antigen recognition.

Unlike B cells, T cells do not alter the constant region of the antigen receptor, which is understandable since the receptor serves a single purpose, signaling for T-cell activation. The TCR is believed not to undergo somatic mutation during the course of an immune response. Thus, while the number of responding T cells increases during a response, the quality of the response can apparently be altered only by recruiting new clonotypes or modulating the numbers of or sensitivity of responding clones (56).

A substantial population of human T cells, often prevalent in epithelia, expresses a TCR heterodimer consisting of $\gamma\delta$ chains. These are closely related to $\alpha\beta$ chains and are generated in a highly similar manner, utilizing their own V region genes. The extent of diversity exhibited by $\gamma\delta$ TCRs is often much less than that of $\alpha\beta$ TCRs, and $\gamma\delta$ T cells present in a given epithelial site often possess similar or identical TCRs. The function of $\gamma\delta$-bearing T cells has remained elusive. They appear to recognize viral proteins expressed on the target cell surface or stress proteins induced by viral infection. The role of these cells and the nature of their interaction with APCs remain major challenges for immunologists.

The MHC and Its Gene Products

The mode of discovery of the MHC is betrayed by its name, which was bestowed by pioneering mouse geneticists studying the rejection of transplanted tissues and tumors. The critical role of the MHC in transplantation is probably incidental to its true function, which is the presentation of peptides from pathogenic organisms to T cells. The human MHC (termed HLA) encompasses more than 50 genes (Fig. 1), which include ones encoding the molecules that present antigen to T cells, termed class I and class II molecules. Class I molecules consist of a highly polymorphic integral membrane protein (α chain) noncovalently bound to a small soluble subunit (β_2-microglobulin [β_2m]) encoded by a gene located on a different chromosome. Class II molecules consist of two highly polymorphic, noncovalently bound integral membrane proteins, termed α and β chains. While the sequences of class I and II molecules are only distantly related, their three-dimensional structures are extraordinarily similar, particularly in the site at the distal portion of the molecule (relative to the cell surface) that binds short peptides (Color Plates 26 and 27). The HLA complex encodes three distinct class I α chains (HLA-A, -B, and -C) and three pairs of class II $\alpha\beta$ heterodimers (HLA-DP, HLA-DQ, and HLA-DR) that preferentially bind to one another (one of the pairs encodes an extra β chain, so each chromosome can produce four distinct class II molecules).

Class I and II genes are the most polymorphic genes known in humans; for any given gene at least hundreds of alleles exist in human populations at significant frequencies. The offspring of parents with completely different alleles produce 6 distinct class I molecules and potentially 14 or more distinct class II molecules (since various α and β alleles contained by loci on different chromosomes can often associate to some extent, and some cross-locus pair-

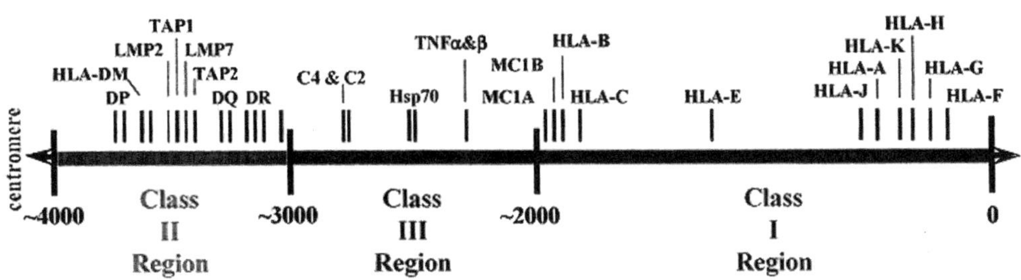

FIGURE 1 Genetic map of the HLA complex.

ing can also occur). The various class I and II alleles contained by any given locus are frequently as different from each other as alleles contained by different loci. Thus, it is useful to refer to all of the various alleles contained by class I or class II loci as class I or class II allomorphs.

Most of the polymorphic residues in class I and class II allomorphs are located in and about the peptide-binding region, which results in each of the distinct alleles binding a different spectrum of peptides. By encoding multiple copies of class I and II molecules, an individual broadens the spectrum of foreign peptides presented to the immune system. On the population level, the presence of numerous alleles minimizes the risk of a pathogen mutating its antigenic peptides to avoid T-cell recognition.

In addition to classical class I genes, the MHC contains class I genes with limited polymorphism. The corresponding molecules, known as class Ib or nonclassical class I molecules, are highly similar in structure to class I molecules. Unlike that of class I molecules, their expression is typically limited to a few tissues. Humans possess at least three such molecules, termed HLA-E, -F, and -G, with close homology to class Ia molecules, and two additional molecules (termed MIC for MHC class I chain related) encoded in the MHC with clear, but more distant, homology to class Ia molecules (MIC molecules are more polymorphic than other class Ib molecules). All of these molecules likely present ligands to the immune system, but their function is poorly understood. Their lack of polymorphism is consistent with the idea that they present self-peptides whose production is triggered by alterations in cellular physiology related to the presence of pathogens. In some cases, these complexes may be recognized by $\gamma\delta$-bearing T cells that display little TCR diversity. MIC molecules activate NK cells via interaction with NKG2 and are induced by virus infections (13). CMV has evolved several mechanisms to avoid detection in this manner, including expression of micro-RNA that targets MIC RNA for degradation (49). Other class Ib molecules are encoded outside the MHC. Four of these molecules (CD1a to CD1d) are highly related and are encoded by a cluster of genes on chromosome 1. CD1 molecules typically present lipids and appear to principally be involved in antibacterial immunity, but they could detect virus-induced alterations in host lipid metabolism, which are known to occur.

In addition to genes encoding class I and II molecules, numerous other genes are located in the MHC, and some are intimately involved with antigen processing. These genes encode the subunits of TAP (acronym for transporter associated with antigen processing), a membrane protein that transports cytosolic peptides across the membrane of the ER to newly synthesized class I molecules. Interdigitated between the TAP genes are two genes termed the LMP2 (β1i) and LMP7 (β5i) genes that encode subunits of a subset of proteasomes. Proteasomes are abundant cytosolic macromolecular proteases essential to cell viability that function to degrade defective or unwanted cellular proteins. LMP2 and LMP7, along with another subunit termed MECL1 (β2i) encoded by another chromosome, replace constitutively synthesized counterparts to form "immunoproteasomes." Of the 14 unique subunits that constitute proteasomes, only the β1, β2, and β5 subunits (and their immunoreplacements) are known to exhibit catalytic activity. Inclusion of the immunosubunits alters proteasome specificity to modify the repertoire of antigen peptides displayed by class I molecules.

Also encoded in the MHC are a number of molecules dedicated to assisting the intracellular trafficking or peptide loading of class I and class II molecules. These include tapasin, which is used to tether class I molecules to TAP; HLA-DM α and β chains, which facilitate class II trafficking and peptide loading; and HLA-DO α and β chains, which play a similar role but predominantly in a subset of professional APCs (pAPCs).

T-Cell Development

The final differentiation of most T cells occurs in the thymus, which is responsible for ensuring that mature T cells can recognize self-MHC molecules with foreign peptide antigens but not self-peptide antigens. This involves both positive and negative selection steps and results in the death of the vast majority of immature thymocytes (on the order of 98%). Late in the course of thymic maturation, most T cells express either the CD4 or CD8 cell surface glycoprotein. These molecules bind class II or class I molecules of the MHC, respectively, and while the bimolecular interaction is relatively weak, it is required for the positive selection of T cells. Consequently, T_{CD8^+} recognize peptides in association with class I molecules, while T_{CD4^+} recognize peptides in association with class II molecules.

T cells can also develop in extrathymic sites, particularly in the gut, where they may provide a substantial fraction of intraepithelial T cells. The specificity and function of extrathymic T cells, which are of great interest, are uncertain.

Division of Labor

T_{CD8^+} and T_{CD4^+} have different roles in the immune response to viruses. T_{CD4^+} function largely as immune regulators by recruiting nonspecific immune cells to the site of infection, stimulating the quantity and quality of antiviral Igs secreted by B cells, and augmenting T_{CD8^+} responses. By contrast, T_{CD8^+} play a more direct role in mediating antiviral effects, either by directly lysing virus-infected cells or by releasing substances with antiviral activities. These distinct duties result in major differences in the types of cells that present antigens to T_{CD4^+} and T_{CD8^+} and in the types of peptides presented.

T_{CD8^+} must be able to recognize virtually any cell type, since every cell is susceptible to virus infection. By contrast, T_{CD4^+} focus on detecting viral antigen in extracellular fluids and interact with cells specially adapted to internalizing foreign substances. These include monocytes/macrophages, follicular DCs, DCs, and B cells (particularly those producing Ig specific for the viral antigen), which together are termed pAPCs. In keeping with the recognition of extracellular antigens by T_{CD4^+}, class II molecules bind peptides generated in endosomal compartments from pinocytosed or endocytosed material. Conversely, taking advantage of the necessity for every virus to replicate its proteins on host cell ribosomes, which are located in the cytosol, class I molecules acquire most of their peptides from a cytosolic antigen pool. Consistent with these roles, class I molecules are constitutively expressed by numerous cell types, while constitutive expression of class II molecules is restricted largely to pAPCs.

An important practical ramification of this split system is that T_{CD4^+} responses can be elicited by simply introducing viral antigens into extracellular body fluids where they will be internalized, processed, and presented by pAPCs, while induction of T_{CD8^+} responses requires delivery of the antigens to the cytosol of an appropriate APC. While most APCs can trigger activated T cells, specialized APCs are required to activate naïve T_{CD8^+} (discussed below). Thus, while T_{CD4^+} responses are elicited by immunization with either infectious virus or many types of noninfectious preparations of viral antigens (including native and denatured proteins), induction of T_{CD8^+} occurs most efficiently with infectious virus. Noninfectious viral antigens can be used to elicit T_{CD8^+} responses, but the antigens must be able to reach the cytosol of a pAPC.

Antigen Processing

Class I Pathway

Class I structure and peptide specificity. Class I molecules consist of a COOH-terminal short cytosolic domain, a typical transmembrane hydrophobic region, and a large extracellular domain comprised of three regions. The three-dimensional structures of the extracellular domains of numerous class I allomorphs have been determined by X-ray crystallography (Color Plates 26 and 27).

The binding of peptides to class I molecules displays two important features. First, main-chain atoms at the COOH and NH_2 termini of the peptide make important bonds with invariant residues in the groove. Elongation of peptides past this point prevents these interactions, and as a result, class I peptides exhibit little size heterogeneity, with perhaps 90% of the peptides recovered from class I molecules falling within the range of 8 to 10 residues in length, depending on the class I allomorph and the ability of peptides to bend in the groove. Second, the residues that demonstrate the most polymorphism among allomorphs form two or three deep pockets in the bottom of the groove that accommodate a highly restricted set of amino acids from bound peptides. As a consequence, each class I molecule demonstrates a distinct preference for peptides that possess the complementary "anchor" residues, one of which is usually located at the COOH terminus (Table 4).

Many of the dominant anchor residues of peptides bound by numerous HLA class I allomorphs have been determined by Edman sequencing of peptide pools recovered from purified molecules (the exact sequence of peptides of sufficient abundance can be determined directly by mass spectroscopy). If antiviral T_{CD8^+} are known to be specific for a given viral protein presented by an allomorph with defined anchor residues, it is possible to identify a reasonably small number of candidate peptides from the protein (depending on the size of the viral protein, there are usually two to five such peptides). These peptides can then be synthesized and used to determine the precise peptide recognized by virus-specific T_{CD8^+}. This method is used routinely and is able to identify ~50 to 75% of the determinants recognized by antiviral T_{CD8^+}. Peptides that fail to be identified may either not fit the predictive motif or possess posttranslational modifications (e.g., phosphorylation) needed for recognition.

Many peptides bind to class I molecules quite snugly, and once assembled they may not dissociate until the entire molecule is disposed of, which often occurs only after 10 or more hours. It is likely that a substantial portion of peptides bind class I molecules less stably, however. Once these peptides dissociate from cell surface class I molecules, class I molecules are unstable and unfold with a half-life of ~15 min. In this interval, however, the class I molecules are able to bind peptides present in extracellular fluids, particularly if β_2m is also present in sufficient quantities, as it is in human plasma. While free peptides are probably rarely present in sufficient concentrations in vivo during a virus infection, this mechanism accounts for the ability of cells to present synthetic peptides in vitro. This is the basis for using synthetic peptides to either sensitize cells for lysis by T_{CD8^+} or stimulate secondary in vitro responses (an oft-used method to generate T_{CD8^+} specific for a known peptide and an alternative method for determining which peptides are recognized by T_{CD8^+}). It might also be exploited for vaccine purposes.

The class I antigen processing pathway. The process by which peptides are derived from proteins and delivered to MHC class I or class II molecules is termed antigen processing. The class I antigen processing pathway begins in the cytosol. For most viruses it is likely that proteins biosynthesized by infected APCs are the primary source of peptides. If, however, sufficient quantities of viral proteins are introduced into the cytosol by incoming virions, they too can serve as a source of peptides. This may particularly apply to abundant structural proteins (42). In large viruses, even single virion core delivered to the cytosol can be sufficient for T-cell recognition. Note that pAPCs have the ability to transfer phagocytosed virions or infected cell material to the cytosol and "cross-present" the material to T_{CD8^+}.

Antigenic peptides can be derived from any type of viral protein, including cytosolic, membrane, secreted, nuclear, structural, or nonstructural proteins. Most viral peptides are derived from defective ribosomal products (DRiPs), rapidly degraded forms of newly synthesized proteins, presumably so degraded because they are defective in some way (62). This enables the rapid presentation of viral antigens even from highly stable viral proteins. In experimental systems, presentation to T_{CD8^+} can frequently be detected less than 1 h after the initiation of viral infection. Viral proteins are typically highly stable (half-life in days). If antigenic peptides were derived from standard turnover of these proteins, even for the most abundant viral proteins, it would take many hours to generate enough peptides to compete with peptides from the billions of cellular proteins present at the time of infection that are degraded with similar (or faster) kinetics. Additionally, using DRiPs as a source of peptides provides a mechanism for monitoring expression of the ~25% of cellular gene products (and many viral proteins) that are targeted to the ER for secretion or cell surface display and are ultimately degraded by extracytosolic proteases.

The proteasome is the principal cytosolic protease involved in generating antigenic peptides or their precursors. Proteasomes come in multiple forms. Indeed, the initial evidence implicating proteasomes in antigen processing was the discovery of the MHC-encoded proteasome subunits and that their expression (and that of a third subunit) is controlled by cytokines (IFN-γ and TNF-α) principally released by activated T cells and NK cells. When induced, these subunits replace constitutively expressed subunits in newly assembled proteasomes to create 20S immunoproteasomes, which appear to be somewhat more adept at producing peptides favored by MHC class I molecules. At the same time, some class I-binding peptides are less efficiently generated by immunoproteasomes. Immunoproteasomes

TABLE 4 Human MHC class I-binding peptide motifs

HLA molecule[a]	Residue(s)[b] at position:								
	1	2	3	4	5	6	7	8	9
HLA-A1		T,S	D,E				L		Y
HLA-A*0201		L,M				V			V,L
HLA-A*0202		L							L,V
HLA-A*0204		L							L
HLA-A*0205		V,L,I,M				I,V,L,A			L
HLA-A*0206		V							V
HLA-A*0207		L	D						L
HLA-A*0214		V,Q,L				I,L,V,F			L
HLA-A*0217		L	P						L
HLA-A*03		L,V,M	F,Y			I,M,F,V,L	I,L,M,F		K,Y,F
HLA-A*1101		V,I,F,Y	M,L,F,V,I,A				L,I,Y,V,F		K,R
HLA-A*24		Y			I,V	F			I,L,F
HLA-A*2402		Y,F							L,F,I
HLA-A*2601,2		V,T,I,L,F				I,L,V			Y,F
HLA-A*2603	E	V,T,I,L,F				F,I,L,V,Y			Y,F,M,L
HLA-A*2902		E	F						Y
HLA-A*3001		Y,F							L
HLA-A*3002		Y,F,L,V							Y
HLA-A*3003		F,Y,I,V,L							Y
HLA-A*3004		V,Y,T,Q,M,I,F							Y,M,L
HLA-A*3101		L,V,Y,F	F,L,Y,W			L,F,V,I			R
HLA-A*3303		A,I,L,F,Y,V							R
HLA-A*6601	E,D	T,V							R,K
HLA-A*6801	D,E	V,T							R,K
HLA-A*6901		V,T,A	I,F,L,M			I,F,L			V,L
HLA-B*07		P	R						L,F
HLA-B*0702		P							L
HLA-B*0703		P	R					E	L
HLA-B*0705		P							L
HLA-B*08			K		K,R				K
HLA-B*0801			K						
HLA-B*0802			K		K				
HLA-B*14		R,K	L,Y,F		R,H	I,L			L
HLA-B*1501(B62)		Q,L			I,V				F,Y
HLA-B*1502		Q,L,V,P							F,Y,M
HLA-B*1503		Q,K							Y,F
HLA-B*1508		P,A							Y,F
HLA-B*1509		H							L,F,M
HLA-B*1510		H							L
HLA-B*1512		Q							Y,F
HLA-B*1513		L,I,Q,V,P,M							W
HLA-B*1516		S,T	P						I,V,Y,F
HLA-B*1517		T,S						L	Y,F,L,I
HLA-B*1518		H							Y
HLA-B*1801	D	E			L				F,Y
HLA-B*27		R							
HLA-B*2701		R,Q							Y
HLA-B*2702		R							F,Y,I,L,W
HLA-B*2703		R							Y,F
HLA-B*2704		R							Y,L,F
HLA-B*2705		R							L,F
HLA-B*2706		R							L
HLA-B*2707		R	F						L,F
HLA-B*2902		E							Y
HLA-B*35		P							Y,F,M,L,I
HLA-B*3501		P							Y,F,M,L,I
HLA-B*3503		P							M,L
HLA-B*3701		D,E		V,I				F,M,L	I,L
HLA-B*3801		H	D,E						F,L

(Continued on next page)

TABLE 4 Human MHC class I-binding peptide motifs *(Continued)*

HLA molecule[a]	Residue(s)[b] at position:								
	1	2	3	4	5	6	7	8	9
HLA-B*3901		R,H			I,V,L				L
HLA-B*3902		K,Q			I,L,F,V				L
HLA-A*3909		R,H							L,F
HLA-B*40		E	F,I,V						L,W,M,A,T,R
HLA-B*4001(B60)		E					I,V		L
HLA-B*4006(B61)		E	F,I,L,V,Y,W				I		V
HLA-B*44		E							Y
HLA-B*4402		E							F,Y
HLA-B*4403		E							Y,F
HLA-B*4601		M							Y
HLA-B*4801		Q,K							L
HLA-B*5101		A,P,G							V,I
HLA-B*5102		P,A,G	Y						I,V
HLA-B*5103		A,P,G	Y						V,I,F
HLA-B*5201		Q	F,Y,W		L,I,V			I,V	I,V
HLA-B*5301		P							W,F,L
HLA-B*5401		P							
HLA-B*5501		P							
HLA-B*5502		P							
HLA-B*5601	A	P	Y						A
HLA-B*5701		A,T,S							F,W,Y
HLA-B*5702		A,T,S							F,W
HLA-B*5801		A,S,T	P,E,K	V,I,L,M,F					F,W
HLA-B*5802		S,T				R			F
HLA-B*6701		P							
HLA-B*7301		R							P
HLA-B*7801		P,A,G				I,L,F,V			A
HLA-Cw*0102		A,L							L
HLA-Cw*0301			V,I,Y,L,M	P		F,Y			L,F,M,I
HLA-Cw*0304		A	V,I,P,Y,M,A	P,E,D			M,E		L,M
HLA-Cw*0401		Y,P,F				V,I,L			L,F,M
HLA-Cw*06					I,L,F,M	V,I,L			L,I,V,Y
HLA-Cw*0601					I,L,F,M	V,I,L			L,I,V,Y
HLA-Cw*0602					I,L,F,M	V,I,L			L,I,V,Y
HLA-Cw*0702		Y,P			V,Y,I,L,F,M	V,I,L,M			Y,F,L
HLA-G	I,L	P							L

[a] Human MHC molecules are termed HLAs. There are three loci encoding class I molecules HLA-A, -B, and -C. Originally HLA molecules were typed serologically; such antigenically defined gene products are identified by one or two digits. At present, HLA gene products are identified indirectly by genotyping. This provides much greater precision and has revealed that previously identified alleles comprised a number of closely related genes. HLA genes (as opposed to gene products) are designated by an asterisk and are numbered with up to seven digits. Closely related alleles share the first two digits and are discriminated by the last two digits (the remaining three digits are used to designate synonymous alterations in coding regions, or changes in noncoding regions). For example, there are 30 known genes closely related to the canonical HLA-A2; these are numbered A0201 through A0230. HLA-C genes are given a gratuitous "w" to avoid confusion with complement components.

[b] Due to the nature of the peptide binding groove, only the few peptide side chains that point into the groove intimately interact with MHC class I molecules, which feature pockets that interact with two or three "anchor" residues indicated. The chemical nature of these pockets dictates the type of residues that will interact with high affinity. The anchor residues are defined empirically from pooled sequencing of peptides eluted from purified class I molecules (40). The presence of anchor residues at consecutive positions at the COOH terminus reflects heterogeneity in peptide length, and not consecutive anchor positions. The underlined amino acids are auxiliary anchor residues. Using these rules and refined computer algorithms, it is possible to predict a high percentage of viral peptides that induce class I-restricted responses.

are constitutively expressed by many bone marrow-derived cells, and antigen processing may not be their most important function. Mice lacking individual immunoproteasome subunits demonstrate intrinsic alterations in T cells that are probably unrelated to alterations in class I peptide ligand production. Cytokine-exposed cells also produce 11S regulators, which take the place of 19S regulators at one or both ends of the 20S proteasome and favor antigen presentation through an undefined mechanism.

Proteasomes can generate the precise peptides presented by MHC class I molecules, but they also produce precursors of MHC class I ligands that are trimmed by other proteases. Peptides can be trimmed by aminopeptidases in the cytosol and particularly in the ER (the home of an aminopeptidase dedicated to antigen processing), whereas carboxypeptidase trimming seems to be highly unusual. ER trimming is possible because TAP, the MHC-encoded heterodimer that transports peptides across the ER membrane to nascent MHC class I molecules, transports peptides of 8 to ~17 residues with similar efficiency.

Cytosolic proteases do not have an unlimited ability to liberate peptide from all contexts, since the sequences flanking a given determinant can block antigen presentation. It appears that the immediate flanking residues (five or fewer on each terminus) have the greatest effect on blocking peptide liberation. Algorithms have been developed for predicting peptides liberated by proteasomes, but to date they have been of limited use in predicting viral determinants.

Peptides are transported from the cytosol into the ER via TAP, a member of a large family of prokaryotic and eukaryotic proteins that function in the transmembrane transport of a wide variety of substrates. As with other family members, TAP-mediated peptide transport is driven by hydrolysis of ATP or other trinucleotides. TAP preferentially transports the types of peptides preferred by class I molecules, particularly in its requirements that peptides be at least eight residues in length. The upper limit of peptide length is messier, but the efficiency drops off when peptides are longer than 17 residues or so. TAP also demonstrates a marked preference for the types of COOH termini preferred by class I molecules (in humans, hydrophobic or positively charged residues, depending on the allomorph; in mice, hydrophobic residues). Thus, most of the longer peptides transported into the ER probably possess extensions at the NH_2 terminus that are trimmed by aminopeptidases. It is unclear whether such trimming occurs prior to peptide association with class I molecules or when loosely tethered by their COOH termini.

While human TAP genes do display limited polymorphism, the known alleles do not appear to differ greatly in their peptide specificities, and no information is available on potential differences between alleles in terms of the function of the class I assembly complex or the ability of viral proteins to modify TAP function. As mentioned above, class I molecules are bound to TAP (via tapasin) until released by peptide binding. It is thought that this facilitates their association with peptides transported by the same complex, thereby greatly increasing the effective peptide concentration. TAP is not, however, essential for peptide loading onto class I molecules. Peptides targeted to the ER are able to efficiently associate with class I molecules in cells lacking TAP. Indeed, in studies using recombinant vaccinia virus expressing various forms of a peptide antigen, peptides targeted to the ER have been found to be more immunogenic in mice than cytosolic peptides biosynthesized in similar amounts or the full-length gene viral protein products that are the natural source of the peptides. Cytosolic antigens can be presented to a limited extent in a TAP-independent manner by an unknown mechanism. While these exceptions are interesting and possibly of practical importance (using ER-targeted peptides for vaccination), it should be emphasized that TAP plays a critical role in the presentation of most viral determinants, at least in model systems. TAP is also crucial for T-cell development, since TAP-deficient individuals demonstrate greatly decreased levels of T cells. Curiously, TAP-deficient patients suffer not from viral infections but from bacterial infections of the lungs and upper airway, probably related to alterations in innate immune responses (TAP is heavily involved in NK cell function, since these cells also recognize class I molecules) rather than to the involvement of the class I pathway in antibacterial immunity.

Regulation of antigen presentation. Since peptides associate with newly synthesized class I molecules, the efficiency of antigen presentation is related to the rate of class I biosynthesis and transport to the cell surface and not the steady-state levels of class I molecules present at the cell surface. Thus, the observation that a certain cell type expresses detectable levels of surface class I molecules does not guarantee that upon viral infection it can efficiently present viral peptides to T_{CD8^+}. The situation is further complicated by the essential role that TAP plays in the presentation of most viral antigens. Tissue-specific expression of TAP appears to be quite low in some tissues. Indeed, one of the earliest responses to viral infection is the release of IFNs by infected cells and by activated NK cells, which also release TNF-α. A major effect of type I and type II IFNs and TNF-α on numerous cell types is the enhanced expression of class I molecules, TAP, and MHC-encoded proteasome components.

Class II Pathway

Class II structure and specificity. The structure of the extracellular domain of class II molecules as revealed by X-ray crystallography shows an astonishing similarity to class I molecules (which differ considerably in amino acid sequence), with one of the domains of the α chain taking the place of β_2m. The most important difference between class I and class II molecules occurs in the peptide binding groove: the class II groove does not make critical bonds with the main-chain atoms of the peptide termini, and as a result, the peptides in class II molecules can be extended at little or no thermodynamic cost. As a consequence, peptides bound to class II molecules demonstrate much greater heterogeneity in length than class I-bound peptides. This has confounded attempts to determine class II binding motifs by sequencing of pooled peptides recovered from purified molecules, although this has been accomplished for some allomorphs (Table 5). As with class I molecules, the motifs reflect the presence of pockets in the class II groove formed by highly polymorphic residues, although the pockets accommodate a broader spectrum of residues than class I pockets. The net result of these differences is that class II molecules bind a wider array of peptide than class I molecules, with regard to both length and composition.

Class II assembly and surface expression. The assembly and transport of class II molecules appear to be more complicated than those of class I molecules. After initial association with calnexin and possibly other molecular chaperones, α and β chains form heterotrimers that bind to trimers of invariant chain (Ii), a non-MHC-encoded molecule (which itself transiently associates with calnexin). Ii serves to reduce class II binding to peptides in the ER and diverts class II molecules from the trans-Golgi network to an endolysosomal compartment where Ii is cleaved by cathepsins to leave a fragment of Ii (CLIP) in the class II groove. Class II molecules bearing CLIP are then delivered to a specialized antigen processing compartment, the class II-containing compartment (MIIC). MIIC is mildly acidic (pH 5.5) and contains numerous acid proteases. CLIP is removed through the action of HLA-DM, a heterodimer consisting of two MHC-encoded subunits (DM A and DM B) homologous to class II molecules. HLA-DM also seems to play a direct role in loading peptides onto class II molecules and provides peptide editing functions to favor the association of peptides that bind with higher affinity. Following peptide association, class II molecules are transported to the cell surface for recognition by T_{CD4^+}. B cells and thymic epithelial cells express another class II-like molecule (HLA-DO or H-2O) that as-

TABLE 5 Human MHC class II-binding peptide motifs[a]

HLA molecule	Residue(s) at position: 1	2	3	4	5	6	7	8	9	10
HLA-DPA1*0102/DPB1*0201	F,L,M,V, W,Y				F,L,M,Y			I,A,M,V		
HLA-DPA1*0201/DPB1*0401	F,L,Y,M,I, V,A						F,L,Y,M,V, I,A			V,Y,I,A,L
HLA-DQA1*0301/DQB1*0301(DQ3.1)	D,E,W			A,G,S,T		A,C,L,M				
HLA-DQA1*0301/DQB1*0302(DQ8)	T,S,W								R,E	
HLA-DQA1*0501/DQB1*0201(DQ2)	F,W,Y,I, L,V			D,E,L,V, I,H		P,D,E,H, P,A	D,E		F,W,Y,I,L, V,M	
HLA-DQA1*0501/DQB1*0301(DQ7)	W,Y,A,V,M			A		A,I,V,T,S			Q,N	
HLA-DQB1*0602	L,N,A,F,C, I,M,Q,S,T, V,W,Y,D,E		A,G,F,I,L, M,N,Q,S,T, V,W,Y,C, D,E	T,S,A,F,G, I,L,M,N,Q, S,V,W,Y		R,I,L,V,A, P,S,T			Q,L,A,S,T, G,I,V,P	
HLA-DRB1*0101	Y,V,L,F,I, A,M,W			L,A,I,V,M, N,Q		A,G,S,T, C,P			L,A,I,V,N, F,Y	
HLA-DRB1*0102	I,Y,V,M			A,L,M		A,G,S,T,P			I,L,A,M, Y,W	
HLA-DRB1*03	V,I,L,M, V,F		D,N,E			K,R,N,Q,E			L,Y,F,M,I	
HLA-DRB1*0301(DR17)	L,I,F,M,V			D		K,R,E,Q,N			Y,L,F	
HLA-DRB1*0401(DR4Dw4)	F,Y,W,I, L,V,M			P,W,I,L,V, A,D,E		N,S,T,Q, H,R	D,E,H,K,N, Q,R,S,T,Y		D,E,H,K,N, Q,R,S,T,Y	

HLA-DRB1*0402(DR4Dw10)	V,I,L,M		Y,F,W,I,L, M,R,N	N,Q,S,T,K	R,K,H,N, Q,P	D,E,H,L,N, Q,R,S,T,Y, C,I,M,V,A
HLA-DRB1*0404(DR4Dw14)	V,I,L,M		F,Y,W,I,L, V,M,A,D,E	N,T,S,Q,R		K
HLA-DRB1*0405(DR4Dw15)	F,Y,W,V,I, L,M		V,I,L,M, D,E	N,S,T,Q, K,D		D,E,Q
HLA-DRB1*0407(DR4Dw13)	F,Y,W		A,V,K	N,T,D,S		Q,N
HLA-DRB1*0701	F,Y,W,I, L,V		D,E,H,K,N, Q,R,S,T	N,S,T		V,I,L,Y,F
HLA-DRB1*0901	W,Y,F,L		A,V,S			
HLA-DRB1*1101	W,Y,F		L,V,M,A, F,Y	R,K,H		A,G,S,P
HLA-DRB1*1104	I,L,V		L,V,M,A, F,Y	R,K,H		A,G,S,P
HLA-DRB1*1201	I,L,F,Y,V	L,M,N,V,A		V,Y,F,I, N,A		Y,F,M,I,V
HLA-DRB1*1301	I,L,V		L,V,M,A, W,Y	R,K		Y,F,A,S,T
HLA-DRB1*1302	Y,F,V,A,I		L,V,M,A, W,Y	R,K		Y,F,A,S,T
HLA-DRB1*1501 (DR2b)	L,V,I		F,Y,I		I,L,V,M,F	
HLA-DRB3*0202(DR52Dw25)	Y,F,I,L		N	A,S,P,D,E		L,V,I,S,G
HLA-DRB3*0301(DR52Dw26)	I,L,V		N	A,S,P,D,E		I,L,V
HLA-DRB5*0101(DR2a)	F,Y,L,M		Q,V,I,M			R,K

[a] The anchor residues that favor binding to various human class II allomorphs as determined by pooled sequencing of peptides eluted from purified class II molecules using the location of expected anchor residues to align the heterogeneously sized peptides recovered.

sociates with HLA-DM and influences peptide binding in ways that remain to be clearly elucidated.

Class II antigen processing. Most class II-associated antigens are derived from exogenous proteins delivered to the MIIC by endosomal trafficking. The presence of a ligand on the cell surface capable of delivering the antigen to the MIIC by adsorptive endocytosis greatly increases the efficiency of antigen presentation. Indeed, this is a key mechanism utilized by B cells, which by binding antigen through surface Ig can present antigens at extremely high efficiency to T_{CD4^+}. Adsorptive endocytosis is also utilized in a number of other circumstances to present antigen to T_{CD4^+} in the course of a viral infection. First, the virus may bind to the APCs. This may result from a highly specific interaction (e.g., binding of Epstein-Barr virus to the complement receptor on B cells) or a more general interaction (binding of influenza virus to sialic acids). Second, virus-antibody complexes may bind to Fc receptors on macrophages. Third, complement-coated virus may bind to complement receptors.

Although it has been known for some time that class II-associated peptides are produced in an endosomal compartment, and numerous endosomal proteases have been characterized, there is little information regarding the specific proteases that contribute to antigen processing. Cathepsins L and S are required for proper proteolytic processing of Ii. It is likely that there is considerable redundancy in the ability of lysosomal proteases to participate in antigen processing, making it difficult to experimentally discern the role of individual proteases. Since many extracellular proteins are resistant to proteolysis until they are unfolded, it is likely that protein unfolding is a key step in the processing of some antigens. Unfolding of proteins with disulfide bonds is catalyzed by GILT (IFN-γ-inducible lysosomal thiol reductase), which reduces disulfide bonds and exposes residues that can be cleaved by endoproteases. GILT is expressed constitutively by APCs and in an IFN-γ-inducible manner by other cells.

While class II antigen processing is clearly designed to present extracellular antigens, the system is capable of presenting antigens biosynthesized by the APCs. In some circumstances, biosynthesized antigens can be the major source of antigenic peptides. With influenza virus, for example, some determinants derived from the viral glycoproteins are not efficiently created by endosomal processing and are much more efficiently derived from newly synthesized viral antigens. Presumably, these peptides are derived from the viral glycoproteins present in the secretory pathway in a compartment not accessible to extracellular virus, or the peptides are derived from an alternative form of the glycoproteins not present in virions. Class II-associated peptides can also be derived from cytosolic viral antigens. TAP does not seem to be involved in this process; the delivery of cytosolic antigens to the MIIC may occur by autophagy, the process by which regions of the cytoplasm are enclosed by a membrane and delivered to the endosomal-lysosomal system. In addition, antigens delivered to the cytosol of DCs via the cross-presentation pathway can be processed by proteasomes and delivered to the secretory pathway by TAP, possibly directly to early endosomes themselves, since the peptides appear to associate not with nascent class II but with class II molecules that recycle from the cell surface into an early endosomal compartment (50).

One curious feature of class II molecules is that they are expressed on activated human T cells but not activated mouse cells. Activated human T cells also express B7 (now termed CD80) and adhesion molecules and can activate naïve T_{CD4^+} (the requirements for T-cell activation, as discussed below). The biological significance of class II-restricted presentation by activated T cells is unknown. Possibly it is related to immunoregulation, since activated T cells seem to preferentially induce T_{CD4^+} with cytolytic activity, which may destroy the activated APCs. Alternatively, the induction of cytolytic T_{CD4^+} responses might result from evolutionary selection by human viruses tropic for activated T cells, enhancing the destruction of infected, activated T cells. In this case, the species-related difference need not reflect large differences between human and mouse immune responses. On the other hand, it is possible that such differences do exist, which should engender caution in facile transposition of results obtained in mouse model systems to human responses.

Predicting T-Cell Responses to Individual Determinants

Antigenic peptides can be derived from virtually any type of viral protein. For class I-restricted responses it is possible to rapidly narrow down potential peptides, since the size and sequence requirements for binding to class I molecules are relatively rigorous. Merely identifying a class I-binding peptide in a viral peptide does not, however, guarantee that the peptide is recognized by antiviral T_{CD8^+}. Indeed, most T_{CD8^+} responses focus on only a few viral peptides. For even quite large viral proteins, no peptides may be immunogenic for any given class I allomorph. This phenomenon is known as immunodominance.

Several factors limit the immunogenicity of class I-binding peptides present in viral proteins. First, flanking sequences can prevent peptide liberation. Second, cytosolic proteases may destroy the peptide. Third, TAP may not be able to efficiently transport the peptide. Fourth, the peptide may preferentially bind another protein. Fifth, there may not be T_{CD8^+} capable of recognizing the peptide due to a hole in the TCR repertoire or deletion of the clones by a cross-reactive self-peptide. Finally, the presence of a highly immunogenic peptide within a protein suppresses the immunogenicity of other peptides in the protein, possibly due to competition of T cells for APCs. All of these factors contribute to immunodominance (59).

T-Cell Function

Triggering

Naïve versus Activated Cells

A central feature of the immune system is that it is more difficult to trigger naïve lymphocytes than activated lymphocytes. In addition to the appropriate antigen, stimulation of naïve cells requires additional signaling events through lymphocyte cell surface molecules whose ligands are expressed only on pAPCs. In fact, antigenic stimulation of T cells in the absence of these costimulatory signals often results in prolonged T-cell anergy, i.e., a state in which the cell is refractory to subsequent stimulation even by pAPCs. Since the thymus cannot express every self-peptide, the stringent requirements for T-cell activation play an important role in preventing T-cell recognition of self-antigens in nonthymic tissue. Once a cell has been activated, however, its effector function can be triggered by exposure to the appropriate antigen. In practical terms, in the case of virus-infected cells, expression of costimulatory molecules is not required for activated T cells to exert antiviral activity.

Site and Nature of Naïve T-Cell Stimulation

The requirement for pAPCs in stimulating responses means that under most circumstances stimulation of naïve T cells will occur not at the site of infection but in a peripheral lymphoid organ (spleen for blood-borne viruses, Peyer's patches or tonsils for enteric viruses, and draining nodes for peripheral infections). To increase the likelihood that naïve T cells will encounter viral antigens, the cells continuously circulate through the lymph nodes via the blood and lymphatic systems.

There are three major APCs in lymphoid organs: B cells, macrophages, and DCs (related to the follicular DCs involved in B-cell stimulation only in sharing a branched morphology). During the initial encounter with a virus, the number of virus-specific B cells will be minimal, leaving the antigen-presenting chores to macrophages and DCs. Moreover, B cells must be activated to express the proper costimulatory molecules. The same holds for macrophages, which are usually activated either by activated T_{CD4^+} or by the surface properties of bacteria, neither of which is applicable in primary viral infections. Thus, although direct experimental evidence is limited, it is expected that DCs are the most important APCs in many viral infections.

DCs originate from either myeloid or lymphoid progenitor cells and are present in substantial numbers in lymphoid organs. They constitutively express high levels of both MHC molecules and the surface molecules used to adhere to and costimulate T cells. In many experimental systems, they are the most potent stimulators of naïve T cells. Large numbers of a special type of DC known as a Langerhans cell are present in the epidermis (3% of all cells in the epidermis). Classical DCs are also present in the dermis. DC precursors are thought to be present in significant numbers in most other organs. Such precursor cells lack costimulatory activity until they are activated. Class II molecules are sequestered in endosomal or lysosomal compartments awaiting activation. Immature DCs express cystatin C, which blocks the action of cathepsins on Ii.

Viruses can access immune tissues either by directly infecting cells in the immune tissue or by infecting DCs that traffic to the immune tissue. Recent findings indicate that viruses can be rapidly delivered to lymph nodes, where they infect macrophages and DCs residing just beneath the subcapsular sinus (16). T_{CD8^+} are recruited to infected DCs located between B-cell follicles and become activated in situ. These findings were made after injecting mice subcutaneously with relatively large amounts of virus. It is likely that when virus is present in limiting amounts in tissues, DCs infected in the tissue that migrate into the nodes play an important role in T_{CD8^+} activation.

An alternative mechanism termed cross-priming probably also plays an important role in T_{CD8^+} priming. Cross-priming, discovered shortly after the revelation of MHC restriction, is based on the acquisition of antigens by DCs from other cells. This mechanism would enable the immune system to mount a T_{CD8^+} response to viruses unable to infect APCs. It limits the ability of viruses to evade T_{CD8^+} immunosurveillance by evolving to not penetrate or otherwise express their proteins in pAPCs. Cross-priming has been shown to occur in virus infection. The relative role of cross-priming versus direct priming probably varies considerably depending on the virus, the protein, and even the peptide itself.

The nature of the cross-priming factor is uncertain. A considerable effort has been made to test the "chaperoned peptide" hypothesis that cross-priming of T_{CD8^+} responses is based on the transfer of molecular chaperones (particularly heat shock protein 90 [HSP90] and HSP70 family members) bearing oligopeptides. Recent results suggest that the role of molecular chaperones is limited to providing activation signals to APCs and not to convey preprocessed peptides. Rather, cross-priming appears to be based on the transfer of intact proteins to DCs, probably as components of dead cells that are phagocytosed by DCs (45). DCs (and macrophages) have the capacity to transfer phagocytosed material to the cytosol, probably following the fusion of phagosomes with a subdomain of the ER (the fusion of phagosomes with the ER is contentious). Transfer appears to follow the same route as used to target misfolded ER proteins for degradation by proteasomes (14).

Cell Surface Molecules Involved in Triggering

To be optimally triggered, a naïve T cell must make five crucial interactions with the same pAPC:

1. The TCR must bind a peptide-MHC complex with sufficient avidity.
2. CD4 or CD8 molecules in a complex with the TCR must contact the same MHC-peptide complex as bound by the TCR.
3. The T-cell surface glycoprotein CD28 must contact CD80 (B7-1) or CD86 (B7-2) glycoprotein on the pAPC surface. Virus infections typically induce expression of pAPC costimulatory molecules, while for other antigens, pAPCs must be activated by T_{CD4^+}. This is believed to account for T_{CD4^+} independence of antiviral T_{CD8^+} responses.
4. The CD137 (4-1BBL) glycoprotein on T_{CD8^+} must contact its ligand.
5. CD40L and CD134 (Ox40) glycoproteins on T_{CD4^+} should contact their ligands.

In addition, other interactions between T-cell surface molecules and complementary ligands on the APC surface enhance the interaction. T cells may initially contact an APC through the weak interaction of T-cell LFA-1 with APC ICAM-3. If the TCR then binds sufficiently tightly to MHC molecules on the APC, this triggers an intracellular signal that induces conformational alterations in LFA-1 that increase its affinity for ICAM-3. TCR binding also triggers conformational alterations in CD8 that increase its affinity for class I molecules.

Appropriate liganding of the TCR results ultimately in the activation of protein kinase C, which acts on DNA binding proteins that, in turn, modify T-cell gene expression and allow T cells to enter the G_1 phase of the cell cycle. Activation of protein kinase C is achieved through the action of numerous accessory proteins. One (ζ chain) is disulfide linked as a dimer to the TCR. Three additional proteins comprise the CD3 complex, which is noncovalently associated with the TCR. Associated with the cytosolic domains of ζ and CD4, respectively, are two protein kinases (Lck and Fyn) that require CD45, another surface glycoprotein, for activation. Activated Fyn, working in conjunction with another kinase (ZAP-70) recruited to ζ

by the concerted actions of Lck and Fyn, then activates protein kinase C to kick off the cascade. This brief description is painted in the broadest possible strokes and is meant only to convey some of the complexity of the process. Adding to the complexity, the spatial organization at the region of contact between the APC and T cell (termed the immunologic synapse) is a key part of the activating process. Through carefully choreographed alterations in cytoskeleton organization, the TCR and cognate MHC-peptide complexes occupy an elevated bull's-eye surrounded by a trench containing interacting adhesion molecules.

The most important result of TCR stimulation of naïve T cells is the increase in the transcription of IL-2 and the IL-2 receptor. IL-2 transcription is further stimulated by the interaction of CD28 with B7. The more significant effect of CD28 stimulation, however, is on the stabilization of IL-2 mRNA, which, like most lymphokine mRNAs, is rapidly degraded. The net result of CD28 cosignaling is a 100-fold increase in IL-2 secretion. IL-2 can act in either an autocrine or paracrine manner. IL-2, while an extremely important cytokine for T-cell activation, is not absolutely essential, as it can be replaced by IL-15, which is produced by monocytes and other inflammatory cells. The signals imparted by the two cytokines are not identical, however, and the immune system uses them in a discriminating manner to optimize T-cell activation, apoptosis, and memory.

Stimulation of naïve cells to an activated state (termed armed effector cells) is accompanied by a number of additional alterations that facilitate triggering of their effector functions. The most critical functional aspect is that activated cells no longer need costimulation for triggering. Additionally, they demonstrate the following characteristics:

1. Reorganization of the TCR complex, resulting in greater sensitivity (i.e., fewer peptide-MHC complexes needed for triggering)
2. Expression of a higher-affinity B7 ligand (CTLA4), which may have an opposing effect on CD28 stimulation of IL-2 production and have a role in creating memory T cells
3. Increased expression of cell adhesion molecules LFA-1 and CD2, resulting in tighter binding to APCs
4. Substitution of L-selectin surface protein with the VLA-4 surface protein, which retargets cells from recirculating between lymphoid organs to the vascular endothelium located at the sites of infection

Effector Functions of T Lymphocytes

Localized Secretion

The major function of the cellular immune system is the local delivery of immune effector molecules and signals. Concordant with this role, triggering of T-cell functions requires interaction with APCs and not free antigen. T cells demonstrate a further specialization that allows for secreted molecules to be targeted precisely to the APCs, thereby maximizing effects on the appropriate APCs while minimizing effects on surrounding cells. Triggering through the TCR results in a cytoskeletal reorganization that repositions the secretory apparatus toward the site of the interaction with the APC. Molecules are then secreted in a polarized manner into the interface between the T cell and APC, much as neurons release neurotransmitters only at axon terminals.

T_{CD8^+}

T_{CD8^+} play a critical role in the immune response to many viruses. They exert their antiviral activities by two general mechanisms, directly lysing virus-infected cells, thereby preventing additional virus replication, and releasing lymphokines that either modify cellular physiology to discourage virus replication or enhance the local inflammatory response. In both cases, the relevant T-cell effector molecules are stored in secretory granules, so release upon triggering is rapid.

Lysis of target cells is believed to be a two-step process, involving two types of proteins secreted by triggered T_{CD8^+}: perforin and granzymes (for granule-associated enzymes, a group of seven or more distinct serine proteases). Perforin inserts into the APC membrane, where it assembles into a pore that allows granzymes access to the cytosol, where they trigger apoptosis of the APCs. One of the earliest events in apoptosis is the induction of DNase activity that fragments host DNA, and it is thought that this may play a crucial role in destroying viral DNA as well. Undoubtedly, other, yet-to-be-discovered features of apoptosis have evolved with the precise goal of minimizing viral replication.

Apoptosis of APCs can also be induced in a different manner, involving the interaction of a T-cell surface protein (Fas ligand) with an APC surface protein (Fas). While Fas is widely expressed among cells in various tissues, its relative importance in viral immunity has not been clearly established. T-cell Fas ligand may be used predominantly for interactions with other cells of immune lineage and not for triggering apoptosis in virus-infected nonimmune cells.

The second manner via which T_{CD8^+} exert antiviral activity is through the release of cytokines. Probably the most important in many viral infections is IFN-γ, which induces an antiviral state in cells and increases the expression of MHC molecules, TAP, the LMP proteasome subunits and numerous other gene products in cells. T_{CD8^+} also release TNF-α, which can have direct cytotoxic and antiviral activities, particularly when acting in concert with IFN-γ. For example, cytokine release appears to play a particularly important role in responding to hepatic viral infections; cytotoxic-T-lymphocyte-mediated lysis of hepatocytes is associated with hepatitis. Other cytokines released by T_{CD8^+} may have effects on the replication of given viruses, but at present little specific information is available.

T_{CD4^+}

Th1 and Th2. Activation of T_{CD4^+} results in the generation of cells that can secrete a variety of cytokines. Unlike T_{CD8^+}, which have stores of effector molecules in secretory vesicles that are released within seconds upon signaling, many T_{CD4^+} have only small amounts of cytokines in storage, and cytokines must be synthesized before they can be released in significant amounts. Although the profiles of cytokines released by various T_{CD4^+} clones exist in a continuum, many cells fall into one of two patterns of secretion, termed Th1 and Th2. Th1 produce and secrete IFN-γ, TNF-β, and IL-2, while Th2 secrete IL-4, IL-5, IL-6, and IL-10; additionally, both types secrete other cytokines in common. As result of the biological activities of the individual cytokines and the complex effects resulting from their synergistic effects, Th1 favor activation of macrophages and NK cells, while Th2 favor antibody production by B cells and activation of mast cells and eosinophils. Additionally, some of the cytokines produced by each subset reciprocally inhibit the activity of the opposing set. The factors that favor the induction of Th1 versus Th2 during the course of the immune response are just being delineated: the density of antigen on the APC plays a role, as do the mixture of cytokines released by accessory cells and the nature of costimulation provided by APCs. At the risk of gross oversimplification, it appears that in most virus infections, Th1 responses are the most beneficial and generally predominate.

Other classes of Th cells are likely to be defined in the coming years, as shown by the definition of a novel class of class II-restricted T cells (Th17) that secrete IL-17. The contributions of Th17 to antiviral immunity is undergoing active study.

Antiviral activity of T_{CD4^+}. Most of the antiviral activities of T_{CD4^+} are mediated through effects on B cells, macrophages, and T_{CD8^+}. T_{CD4^+} are also capable of direct antiviral activity. First, they can release cytokines (such as IFN-γ) with antiviral activity. Second, both Th1 and Th2 can lyse virus-infected cells expressing class II molecules. Although constitutive expression of class II molecules is largely limited to cells of immune lineage, many cell types synthesize and express class II molecules in response to IFN-γ (but not IFN-α or IFN-β), and it is believed that for some viruses, such cytotoxic T_{CD4^+} play a role in clearance. Cytotoxicity is perforin independent and appears to be mediated by two major mechanisms, one the coordinate action of IFN-γ and TNF-β and the other unknown (possibly Fas mediated).

Interactions between Cellular Subsets

Collaboration between B and T Cells

As mentioned above, the interaction of viruses with antigen-specific Ig on the B-cell surface greatly enhances the ability of B cells to present antigens to T_{CD4^+}. The antigens recognized by the B and T cells need not be identical; indeed, antibody binding probably hinders the processing of the bound region of antigen, preventing its recognition by T_{CD4^+}. The essential feature is that presentation of all proteins physically linked to the antigen recognized by surface Ig will be enhanced. B cells specific for a surface viral glycoprotein can internalize an intact virion and present peptides from an internal virion protein that are liberated during antigen processing. Similarly, B cells specific for internal viral proteins can internalize fragmented virions and present determinants from viral surface proteins to T cells. Thus, T_{CD4^+} induced by immunizing individuals with internal viral components can enhance production of neutralizing antibodies specific for viral surface proteins upon exposure to the virus.

The interplay of T_{CD4^+} and B cells is intricate, involving numerous interactions between cell surface molecules and secreted lymphokines. T cells provide two crucial events for B-cell stimulation. First, gp39 on T_{CD4^+} binds CD40 present on the B-cell surface. Second, T cells secrete cytokines that induce B cells to divide and to switch Ig production from the IgM heavy chain to other heavy-chain classes. The precise mixture and timing of cytokines secreted by T_{CD4^+} (which are greatly influenced by the balance of Th1 versus Th2 induced) regulate the class of Ig secreted and the final differentiation state of the B cell. B-cell activation is at least as complicated as T-cell activation, involving interactions between numerous kinases and cofactors.

If B cells presenting antigens to T_{CD4^+} express the B7 cell surface molecule, stimulatory signals are provided to T cells via CD28 (the B7 receptor), resulting in T-cell activation. Since B7 expression occurs only upon B-cell activation, this is more likely to occur in the later phases of the immune response to viruses, or upon secondary exposure to virus.

Interaction between T-Cell Subsets

The requirement for T_{CD4^+} involvement in the generation of mouse T_{CD8^+} varies considerably among viruses, possibly related to the ability of the virus to fully activate DCs that present to naïve T_{CD8^+}. Help is delivered by T_{CD4^+} recognizing the same APCs as the T_{CD8^+}. Two mechanisms have been proposed: IL-2 secretion by T_{CD4^+} or T_{CD4^+}-mediated alterations of the APC surface which then provide a costimulatory signal to T_{CD8^+}. Additionally, activated T_{CD8^+} can provide help for naïve T_{CD8^+}, probably by secretion of IL-2.

Memory

Importance

Memory is one of the most important aspects of specific immune responses to viral antigens. Whether induced by a natural viral infection or by vaccination, immunologic memory can provide lifelong protection against infection, either by completely preventing infection through antibody neutralization of virus or by mounting responses of sufficient magnitude and rapidity that infection is limited to a few rounds of replication.

B-Cell Memory

The initial exposure to a virus generally results in the production of memory B cells that remain for the life of the individual. Memory B cells have already undergone heavy-chain class switching and affinity maturation, which account for the increased affinity and heavy skewing of the response from IgM to IgA and IgG. These cells, which may be located predominantly in the bone marrow, continuously produce virus-specific antibodies that, if of high neutralizing capacity, can provide complete protection against reinfection. Reinfection with the virus results in the rapid production of additional amounts of high-affinity antibodies. The relationship between memory cells constitutively producing antibodies and those recruited by reinfection is uncertain. It is also unclear to what extent memory B cells owe their continued existence to episodic reexposure to or the prolonged presence of viral antigens, though there is clear evidence in mice that persistence is not absolutely required to maintain memory B cells (30). Viral antigens may persist due to prolonged, indolent replication of virus in a small number of cells or to the retention of antigen by follicular DCs or other antigen reservoirs. Even classically "acute" viruses may persist in infected organisms at a low level, at least with regard to gene expression (47, 52).

Not uncommonly, upon exposure to a virus serologically related to a previously encountered virus, individuals produce antibodies with higher affinity to the priming virus. This phenomenon, termed original antigenic sin, was first noted in studies of responses to influenza virus vaccines. It is thought that stimulation of naïve B cells with new specificities may be inhibited by three mechanisms:

1. Trapping of limiting amounts of antigen by preexisting B cells

2. Binding of immune complexes to Fc receptors that negatively signal naïve, but not memory, B cells

3. Suppressive effects mediated by T_{CD8^+} acting in an undefined manner

T-Cell Memory

Viral infections result in the generation of memory T_{CD8^+} and T_{CD4^+}, whose maintenance does not appear to require persistent antigen (though it is difficult to eliminate the persistence of low levels of viruses). Memory T_{CD8^+} appear to persist longer than memory T_{CD4^+}. IL-7 and IL-15 appear to play a critical role in maintaining memory T cells. With the elimination of smallpox from human populations, it is possible to study the persistence of memory cells in the absence of reinfection by studying individuals infected once with vaccinia virus. This revealed that anti-vaccinia virus T_{CD8^+} decay with a half-life of ~10 years (1).

Until recently it was believed that T cells do not demonstrate affinity maturation. It now appears that there is selection for clones bearing TCRs with higher affinity for peptide-MHC complexes (53). This results in a modest increase in average TCR affinity for cognate peptide-MHC complexes, as contrasted with the >1,000-fold increases in affinity that can be generated by B-cell somatic mutation. TCR affinity is probably limited by the structural constraints of self- versus non-self-discrimination between MHC molecules bearing foreign peptides versus self-peptides, with the very small contribution to binding affinity provided by the peptide, which offers only a few side chains to the TCR footprint.

Secondary T-cell responses measured in immune organs (spleen and nodes) are generally of greater magnitude due to expansion of the number of responding cells. Such central memory T cells also respond more rapidly following infection than naïve cells. On average, a secondary response occurs a few days earlier than a primary response. Another population of memory T cells (effector memory T cells) is present in peripheral organs in an effector-ready state. These T cells may play an important role in providing immediate effector function against repeat infection.

An important aspect of secondary responses to viruses is that antibodies often sufficiently neutralize viral infectivity to prevent induction of a detectable T_{CD8^+} response. Neutralizing antibodies may be preexisting or result from secondary B-cell stimulation. Since activated B cells are excellent T_{CD4^+} stimulators, induction of T_{CD4^+} responses is not compromised by antibodies. Note that this applies only when neutralizing antibodies are serologically cross-reactive between the priming and restimulating virus. A stimulating virus possessing all of the T_{CD8^+} peptides of the priming virus but none of the neutralizing epitopes can be used as a booster immunogen if the goal is to maximize T_{CD8^+} responses.

Preexisting T cells themselves also can inhibit the induction of naïve T cells upon antigen reexposure. This effect is poorly characterized but may simply result from the rapid clearance of virus preventing a sufficient accumulation of viral antigens to activate naïve T cells.

Immunoregulation

One of the most obvious features of the immune response to infection with all but a few viruses is its transience. One factor that contributes to the decline in immune effector functions is the decrease in viral antigen resulting from an effective immune response. This may be the major, or even sole, factor for the decline in responses to some viruses. However, in some circumstances, T-cell-mediated suppression is a contributing factor. While it proved difficult to produce stable T-cell lines or clones that maintained suppressive capacity, numerous labs repeatedly demonstrated the phenomenon of suppression in different systems.

In the past decade, suppression has been resurrected with the discovery of regulatory T cells (T_{reg}). These are $CD4^+$ T cells that constitutively express the IL-2 receptor α chain (CD25) and the transcription factor Foxp3, which plays an important role in their differentiation. T_{reg} inhibit both T_{CD4^+} and T_{CD8^+} through a mechanism that remains to be established, but it appears to require direct contact or close proximity of the T_{reg} to the regulated T cell. T_{reg} influence antiviral immunity and inhibition of T_{CD8^+} responses in mice and represent an intriguing area of future research with potentially important practical applications.

The central nervous system plays a poorly understood role in antiviral immunity, and the nervous system and immune system are intimately intertwined anatomically and functionally. For IL-1 and IL-6 (and probably others), designation as cytokines versus neural hormones is arbitrary, since they act through the central nervous system to control body temperature and the acute-phase response. Probably all immune cells have receptors for neurotransmitters and other neuronal messengers. Lymphoid organs are richly innervated by sympathetic nerves. Viruses are known to activate the sympathetic nervous system and can also activate the hypothalamus-pituitary axis, resulting in glucocorticoid secretion.

MUCOSAL IMMUNITY

Most viruses enter the body through mucosal surfaces. Due to their roles as potential portals for microbial invasion, mucosae are endowed with their own semiautonomous immune systems. As most antigens encounter the immune system at the mucosal surface, this system is more important than the more widely studied systemic immune system. The efficacy of oral and nasal vaccines is based on protection provided through the mucosal immune system. Moreover, while optimal protection against a particular virus follows infections with the identical or closely related virus, the role of specifically activating the mucosal immune system is underappreciated. The immune system tailors its armamentarium of effector mechanisms to take advantage of special features of infecting organisms. Indeed, increased understanding of mucosal immunity will pay enormous dividends in generating better vaccines.

Anatomically, the most striking feature of the mucosal immune system is the mucosa-associated lymphoid tissue (MALT), which is present in the intestines, bronchial tree, nasopharynx, mammary gland, salivary and lacrimal glands, genitourinary tract, and inner ear. MALT is comprised of lymphocytes scattered among epithelial cells (intraepithelial lymphocytes [IELs]) and lamina propria (lamina propria lymphocytes [LPLs]), as well as local aggregations of nonencapsulated lymphoid tissue. In humans the local aggregations are particularly prominent in the nasopharynx-associated lymphoid tissue and gut-associated lymphoid tissue. In the small intestine, these structures are known as Peyer's patches. They function much like lymph nodes in providing a site for antigen concentration and intercellular interactions. A prominent feature is the presence of microfold cells, specialized epithelial cells that transport antigens via transcytosis (transport of antigens in endocytic vesicles from the apical surface to the basal surface) from the lumen of the relevant organ to APCs (macrophages and DCs) present in the dome region of the aggregation. The dome region also contains T cells (largely T_{CD4^+}) that can be activated by the APCs. Beneath the dome region are germinal centers, in which the growth and selection of B cells occur. Most of the B cells present in the germinal centers produce IgA, with a significant minority secreting IgM. Plasma cells are rarely observed in the aggregations, with the vast majority being present in the lamina propria, where they constitute up to 50% of the LPLs. Much of the IgM and IgA produced possess J chain, which allows for their active secretion into the organ lumen by epithelial cells. Additionally, IgA can also be delivered to the gut via uptake from the blood by biliary epithelial cells and hepatocytes and subsequent secretion into bile.

The IELs consist largely of T lymphocytes, while the LPLs are comprised of roughly equal amounts of B and T cells. The majority of T cells in both compartments appear to be activated. In comparison to other sites, the ratio of $\gamma\delta$- and $\alpha\beta$-expressing IELs is unusually high, varying considerably depending on the organ (the colon is the richest source of $\gamma\delta$ T cells, which represent more than 50% of IELs). T_{CD8^+} predominate among IELs, while T_{CD4^+} comprise the majority of LPLs. At least some of the $\alpha\beta$ T_{CD8^+} IELs recovered from mice responding to primary intestinal virus infections are typical T_{CD8^+} capable of responding to viral antigens in a class I-restricted manner. The function of the $\gamma\delta$ cells in mice as well as humans is largely mysterious.

An important feature of mucosal immunity is that MALT-derived antigen-specific B and T cells leave their sites of induction and preferentially seed MALT in other locales via the interaction of cell surface molecules with specific ligands on endothelial cells that direct them to MALT. Thus, a localized respiratory infection often leads to induction of IgA responses in other mucosal organs, although responses are usually less intense than at the site of infection. This suggests that some evolutionarily significant pathogens can initiate infections through different organs.

MALT does not operate completely independently of other lymphoid tissues. Mucosal immunization results in dissemination of MALT lymphocytes to the following route: MALT → regional lymph nodes → thoracic duct → blood → spleen, bone marrow, or other lymph nodes. Immunization via nonmucosal routes leads to deposition of T cells and, particularly, B cells in MALT. Moreover, serum antibodies are capable of reaching mucosal surfaces (through an uncertain mechanism), which probably accounts for the ability of parenterally administered antibodies in some circumstances to provide complete protection against infection with viruses that enter through mucosae. IgA represents the bulk of antibodies in the gastrointestinal tract, nose, and eyes and about half of antibodies in the airway and urinary tract. The bulk of secreted antibodies are produced locally. When the epithelial barrier is breached during the course of infection and inflammation, however, serum antibodies have free access to the site of infection and therefore can play an important role in limiting virus dissemination and in recovery.

Despite the extensive interconnections of MALT with the rest of the immune system, increased protection against a virus that enters through a mucosal surface is often provided by mucosal immunization. This could play an important role in the enhanced protection against enteric and respiratory viruses observed following natural infection or enteric vaccination relative to intramuscular vaccination (with the drawback that the antigen preparation must be formulated to survive the acidic journey through the stomach and resist proteolysis in the gut). Indeed, local immunity may be an important factor in vaccination, as recent evidence suggests that optimal immunization should be targeted to the relevant organ (4). Although direct evidence obtained in humans is lacking, indirect studies and animal models suggest that secreted IgA plays a crucial role in protection against reinfection with some viruses. Since IgA responses often fall to less-than-detectable levels within 3 months following primary infections (in contrast to lifelong maintenance of serum IgG levels), it has been suggested that this accounts for the relatively high frequency of reinfection of individuals with some viruses (respiratory syncytial virus, for example). Such reinfections are usually mild (often subclinical), due to either MALT memory or the involvement of serum IgG.

Interestingly, humans lack the enzyme required to transfer galactose to the terminus of oligosaccharides via α-bonds. This linkage is ubiquitous elsewhere in nature, including the bacteria that colonize the gut. Lacking tolerance, humans produce prodigious amounts of antibodies specific for α-galactose-containing oligosaccharides. A special consequence for viral immunology is that these antibodies can neutralize enveloped viruses with glycoproteins synthesized by other species that possess this enzyme.

In addition to specific B- and T-cell responses, MALT possesses nonspecific immune mechanisms. Macrophages and mast cell precursors are abundant throughout the mucosa. Of particular note are the Paneth cells of the small intestine, which secrete numerous bioactive peptides, including TNF and numerous peptides with direct antibacterial activity. It is almost to be expected that peptides with antiviral activity are also secreted.

PEDIATRIC IMMUNITY TO VIRUSES

Children are more susceptible to most virus infections than adults. Even in the developed world, children still average 10 clinically significant virus infections/year until their third to fifth year, when they reach adult rates of 1 or 2 infections per year. In large part, the greater toll of infectious diseases exacted on children simply stems from their naïve immune status with regard to the pathogen. It is also possible that the ongoing maturation of the immune system increases susceptibility to some viruses. Given the increased risk of infectious diseases faced by children, and that the vast majority of vaccines are administered to children, there is surprising ignorance regarding the postnatal development of the human immune system.

The immune systems of children, particularly those less than 2 years old, are less capable of effectively responding to virus infections than those of adults. Newborns can produce only limited amounts of antibody, and until 3 to 6 months of age, responses are limited almost entirely to IgM, possibly due to low levels of T_{CD4^+} activity. This may be due either to intrinsic properties of neonatal T_{CD4^+} or to decreased APC function. B cells (but not T cells) appear intrinsically less capable of generating a diverse antibody response; NK cell activity also appears to be diminished in neonates.

Maternal IgG antibodies of all subclasses are actively transferred to the fetus. At birth, fetal levels of serum IgG are often 10 to 15% higher than maternal values. The lack of IgG becomes important from 3 to 6 months after birth, as maternal antibodies present in the serum are catabolized. Maternal antibodies confer resistance to some viral diseases and can interfere with immunization, presumably by competing with B cells for antigen. This is one reason why immunization is delayed until 6 months following birth (posing a major problem for vaccination against viruses that infect infants once maternal IgG levels decay). Immunization during pregnancy can induce resistance via transfer of antibody or, less frequently, transfer of antigen, which can lead to a fetal IgM response.

IgA is present in human milk in high concentrations and includes antibodies specific for viruses that infect both the gastrointestinal and respiratory systems. Active maternal humoral responses to mucosal pathogens result in transfer of IgA antibodies specific for the pathogen, which is also likely to infect the infant. Breast milk (particularly colostrum) also contains macrophages, T_{CD4^+}, and T_{CD8^+}. Whether these cells contribute to neonatal immunity is uncertain. Equally uncertain are the roles of cytokines (including IL-1, TNF-α, and IL-6) present in milk.

VIRAL INTERFERENCE WITH HOST IMMUNITY

The Delicate Balance

For a virus and host to coexist, a balance must be reached. An advantage gained by one side must be parried by the other, lest one party (or both parties) become extinct. Clearly, the existence of some vertebrate species over the course of millions of years indicates that some hosts can withstand the onslaught of viruses and other pathogens for extended periods. However, it is uncertain to what extent infectious organisms contribute to the relatively rapid extinction experienced by most species over the course of evolution.

From the limited temporal perspective of human experience, most viruses and hosts exist in the delicate balance of mutual existence. For some viruses this balance can be achieved by expression of relatively few genes, none of which specifically impairs the immune system. For others, hundreds of genes may evolve, many of which may be devoted to modifying host responses. Increasing complexity is not necessarily accompanied by increased pathogenicity. Ebola virus, expressing only seven genes, causes fulminant hemorrhagic fever leading to rapid death. Members of the *Herpesviridae* family, which often express over 200 gene products, many devoted to interfering with host immunity, generally cause benign self-limited or inapparent infections.

Recent years have witnessed an exponentially growing awareness of the mechanisms by which viruses deliberately perturb immune defenses. A list of many known factors and their proposed modes of action is given in Table 6, but the list is constantly growing. This topic is of great practical importance in producing attenuated vaccine strains and also of great theoretical interest to immunologists, since it provides a new means of studying the complex interplay between viruses and the multifaceted immune system. There are four major strategies that viruses use to disable the immune system: interfering with cellular regulation, interfering with antigen presentation or recognition, infecting and disabling cells of the immune cells, and modifying antigenic proteins.

Mechanisms of Interference

Interfering with Cellular Regulation

Most viral genes dedicated to interfering with host immunity have been discovered in large DNA viruses. Most that interfere with cellular regulation have been clearly hijacked from the host genome. They can be sorted into several categories based on their mode of action.

1. Secreted substances that act as cytokine agonists or antagonists (virokines)
2. Membrane-bound cytokine receptors that amplify or counteract activity of natural receptors (viroceptors)
3. Intracellular proteins that interfere with cytokine-mediated signals

Many of these viral genes are potentially of great practical importance, since they point the way toward development of drugs for interfering with or augmenting immune effector mechanisms. They also provide clues to the facets of the immune response that are most relevant to a given virus. For example, adenovirus has no fewer than three known proteins that apparently function to interfere with the effects of TNF.

Host interference genes do not necessarily enhance viral pathogenicity; indeed, they often have the opposite effect. It is crucial to always remember that viruses evolve to maximize transmission between hosts and not to incapacitate or eliminate their hosts. Since many viruses are host specific, efficient elimination of the host will eliminate the virus too. Fortunately, viral evolution makes it rather difficult for a virus to be both highly transmissible and highly lethal (among human viruses, only variola virus managed this balancing act).

Interfering with Antigen Presentation or Recognition

Modifying Assembly of MHC Molecules

A number of DNA viruses possess proteins that actively interfere with MHC class I assembly or transport. Some adenovirus serotypes express a glycoprotein that binds class I molecules and retains them in the ER, thus preventing presentation of virus-derived peptides. Other adenovirus serotypes lacking this protein express proteins that reduce expression class I molecules and antigen processing proteins at the transcriptional level. Many members of the *Herpesviridae* family are known to interfere with class I presentation. Herpes simplex virus, CMV, and varicella-zoster virus express proteins that block the function of TAP by acting on either the cytosolic or luminal side. CMV expresses two proteins that degrade newly synthesized class I molecules, one of which also acts on class II molecules. CMV also expresses a protein that enhances expression of HLA-E, apparently to thwart recognition by NK cells. Epstein-Barr virus expresses a protein crucial for latency (EBNA-1) that expresses a repeat sequence that confers resistance to proteasomal degradation. Originally believed to interfere with antigen presentation through this mechanism, it now appears that the repeat acts to reduce antigen presentation as a *cis*-acting translation inhibitor and does not prevent the processing of EBNA-1 DRiPs (8). Flaviviruses actually increase class I expression, apparently by increasing the supply of peptides in the ER, an effect

TABLE 6 Viral proteins that interfere with host immunity[a]

Modulator protein	Source virus
Antigen processing modulators	
E1A, inhibits MHC class II up-regulation (prevents activation of IFN transcription factors)	Adenovirus
E3-19K, binds and retains MHC class I in ER	Adenovirus
BZLF2, may inhibit MHC class II antigen presentation	Epstein-Barr virus
EBNA-1, refractory to proteolysis	Epstein-Barr virus
ICP47, inhibits TAP-mediated peptide transport	Herpes simplex virus
ORF14, inhibits class II binding	Herpes simplex virus
Unknown, inhibits class II function	Herpes simplex virus
K3, down-regulates MHC class I expression	Human herpesvirus 8
IE/E, inhibits MHC class II up-regulation (prevents activation of IFN transcription factors)	Human CMV
pp65, inhibits generation of antigenic peptides from a 72-kDa transcription factor	Human CMV
US2, targets MHC class I heavy chains and class II molecules for degradation	Human CMV
US3, retains class I molecules in ER	Human CMV
US6, inhibits TAP	Human CMV
US11, targets MHC class I heavy chains for degradation	Human CMV
UL18, inhibits NK cell lysis as a class I homolog	Human CMV
UL40, may inhibit NK killing through up-regulation of HLA-E	Human CMV
Unknown, inhibits class II up-regulation through IFN transduction cascade	Human and mouse CMV
M4, binds MHC class I molecules	Mouse CMV
M6, targets class I molecules for lysosomal degradation	Mouse CMV
M144, inhibits NK cell lysis as a class I homolog	Mouse CMV
M152, retains MHC class I molecules in ERGIC	Mouse CMV
r144, may inhibit NK cell lysis as a class I homolog	Rat CMV
Nef, causes endocytosis of cell surface MHC class I and CD4 and interferes with class II processing	HIV
Vpu, destabilizes newly synthesized class I molecules and targets CD4 for degradation	HIV
MC80R, may inhibit MHC class II presentation	Molluscum contagiosum virus
K5, down-regulates MHC class I expression	Mouse herpesvirus strain 68
E5, may inhibit MHC class II processing (acidification of endosomal vesicles)	Papillomavirus
E6, may inhibit MHC class II processing (interaction with adaptor protein complex)	Papillomavirus
Complement and antibody response modulators	
S peplomer, IgG Fc receptor homolog	Coronaviruses
Unknown, C3 inactivation	Epstein-Barr virus
gC, CR1 homolog and complement C3 binding receptor	Herpes simplex virus types 1 and 2
gE-gI/gE, IgG Fc receptor homolog	Herpes simplex virus types 1 and 2
HVS-CCPH, complement C3 convertase homolog	Herpesvirus saimiri
ORF4, CD46 and CD55 homologs	Herpesvirus saimiri
ORF15, terminal complement inhibitor CD59 homolog	Herpesvirus saimiri
CCPH, C4bp, CD46, and CD55 homologs	Human herpesvirus 8
gp120-gp41, recruitment of factor H	HIV
NP, ligation of Fcγ receptor II	Measles virus
Fcr1, IgG Fc receptor homolog	Mouse CMV
MγHV68-ORF4, C4bp homolog	Mouse herpesvirus strain 68
VCP/C2IL, IMP, complement C4bp homolog	Poxviruses
gE-gI, IgG Fc receptor homolog	Pseudorabies virus
SPICE, complement C4bp homolog	Variola (smallpox) virus
gE-gI, IgG Fc receptor homolog	Varicella-zoster virus
B5R, contains homology with family of complement control proteins	Vaccinia virus
Incorporation of CD59, CD55, and CD46 proteins into virus envelope	Vaccinia virus, HIV, lymphotrophic virus, and CMV
Cytokine, transcription, and apoptosis modulators	
E1A, inhibits IFN-induced JAK/STAT pathway and decreases STAT 1 and p48	Adenovirus
E1B-19K, inhibits apoptosis as a Bcl-2 homolog	Adenovirus
E1B-55K, inhibits apoptosis by binding and inactivating p53	Adenovirus
E3-10.4K/14.5, inhibits TNF cytolysis and activation of $cPLA_2$	Adenovirus
E3-10.4/14.5K-RID complex, internalization and lysosomal destruction of Fas	Adenovirus
E3-14.7K, inhibits apoptosis through caspase 8 and inhibits TNF cytolysis and activation of $cPLA_2$	Adenovirus
E4 orf6, inhibits apoptosis by binding and inactivating p53	Adenovirus

(Continued on next page)

TABLE 6 Viral proteins that interfere with host immunity[a] *(Continued)*

Modulator protein	Source virus
VAI-RNA, inhibits IFN activation of PKR (dsRNA-dependent protein kinase)	Adenovirus
A224L/4CL, IAP homolog that inhibits apoptosis through caspases	African swine fever virus
A238L, inhibits NF-κB/NFAT signaling	African swine fever virus
EP402R, 8DR, vCD2, immunosuppressive, erythrocyte hemadsorption adhesion molecules	African swine fever virus
AHV-SEMA, semaphorin homolog	Alcelaphine herpesvirus
IAP, inhibits apoptosis through caspases	Baculovirus
P35, inhibits apoptosis through caspases	Baculovirus
PK2, binds to and inhibits PKR	Baculovirus
Q2/3L, G-protein coupled CC chemokine receptor homolog	Capripox virus
Unknown, induces RNase L inhibitor and antagonizes 2′, 5′-OA binding to RNase L	Encephalomyocarditis virus
BARF1, CSF-1R homolog, secreted protein that sequesters CSF-1	Epstein-Barr virus
BCRF1, IL-10 homolog, antagonizes Th1 responses	Epstein-Barr virus
EBER I RNA, blocks PKR activity	Epstein-Barr virus
EBNA-2, inhibits IFN-stimulated transcription	Epstein-Barr virus
LMP-1, inhibits apoptosis by up-regulating Bcl-2 and induces signals of TNF receptor/CD40 pathway	Epstein-Barr virus
E1, binds eotaxin	Equine herpesvirus 2
E6, unknown function, chemokine receptor homolog?	Equine herpesvirus 2
EHVIL-10, IL-10 homolog; may antagonize Th1 responses	Equine herpesvirus 2
Capsid protein, inhibits MxA gene expression	HBV
Terminal protein, blocks IFN signaling	HBV
pX, possible interaction with proteasome, NF-κB activation	HBV
E2, inhibits type I IFN-induced PKR activation	HCV
NS5A, binds to and inhibits PKR	HCV
GI/23NL, homolog to GADD34 that has cellular growth arrest and damage functions	Herpesviruses
K13/ORF71/E8/BORFE2/MC159/MC160, FLIP homolog; inhibits apoptosis through caspases	Herpesviruses
ORF16/M11/BHRF1/BALF1/A9/BORF-B2/5HL/A179L, inhibits apoptosis as a Bcl-2 homolog	Herpesviruses
ORF74, constitutively secreted and active, binds CC and CXC chemokines	Herpesviruses
ECRF3, CXC chemokine receptor homolog	Herpesvirus saimiri
ORF13, IL-17 homolog; possible T-cell mitogen	Herpesvirus saimiri
2′, 5′-OA, RNA analog that inhibits RNase L	Herpes simplex virus
$\gamma_1$34.5, inhibits apoptosis of neuronal cells	Herpes simplex virus
ICP34.5, redirects protein phosphatase I to dephosphorylate and reactivate eIF-2α	Herpes simplex virus
US3, unknown inhibitor of apoptosis, serine/threonine kinase	Herpes simplex virus
US11, binds to and inhibits PKR	Herpes simplex virus
Unknown, synthesis of 2′, 5′-OA antagonists	Herpes simplex virus
1E1/1E2, inhibits apoptosis by blocking TNF-α	Human CMV
UL37, localizes in mitochondria and blocks apoptosis	Human CMV
UL111a, IL-10 homolog	Human CMV
UL144, TNF receptor homolog	Human CMV
UL146/vCXC-1, CXC chemokine agonist and monocyte chemoattractant	Human CMV
UL147vCXC-2, undefined chemokine effects	Human CMV
US27, G-coupled protein, unknown function, chemokine receptor homolog?	Human CMV
US28, MIP-1α receptor homolog (CC chemokine receptor)	Human CMV
Unknown, reduces JAK1 and p48, proteasome involvement	Human CMV
UL33/M33/R33, CC chemokine receptor homolog	Human, mouse, and rat CMV
UL78/M78, binds CC and CXC chemokines	Human and mouse CMV
MCK-1/MCK-2(m131/129), chemokine homolog that promotes virus dissemination	Mouse CMV
U83, CC or CX3C chemokine homolog	Human herpesvirus 6
U12, CC chemokine receptor homolog	Human herpesviruses 6 and 7
U51, CC and CXC chemokine receptor homolog	Human herpesviruses 6 and 7
K2, IL-6 homolog; increases angiogenesis and hematopoiesis, B-cell growth factor	Human herpesvirus 8
vIRF-2, may affect expression of early inflammatory gene products	Human herpesvirus 8
vIRF-K9, IRF homolog; blocks IFN-induced transcription activation	Human herpesvirus 8

(Continued on next page)

TABLE 6 *(Continued)*

Modulator protein	Source virus
vMIP-1, MIP-1 homolog, CCR8 agonist, and TH2 chemoattractant; angiogenic activity	Human herpesvirus 8
vMIP-II, MIP-II homolog; C, CC, CXC, and CX3C chemokine antagonist	Human herpesvirus 8
vMIP-III, MIP III homolog	Human herpesvirus 8
TAR RNA, recruits cellular PKR inhibitor TRBP	HIV
Tat, binds to and inhibits PKR	HIV
Unknown, induces RNase L inhibitor and antagonizes 2′, 5′-OA binding to RNase L	HIV
Unknown, targets STAT2 for degradation	Human parainfluenza 2 virus
Unknown, blocks STAT1 phosphorylation	Human parainfluenza 3 virus and Sendai virus
E6, inhibits apoptosis by targeting p53 for degradation	Human papillomavirus
E7, binds to p48	Human papillomavirus 16
Tax, possible interaction with proteasome, NF-κB activation	Human T-cell lymphotrophic virus
NS1, binds dsRNA and blocks PKR activation, blocks 2′, 5′-OS/RNase L	Influenza virus
Unknown, inhibits PKR by inducing p58IPK	Influenza virus
MEQ, transcription factor inhibiting apoptosis by TNF-α ceramide	Marek's disease virus
HA, binds CD46 and inhibits IL-12 production	Measles virus
MC53, protein that binds and inhibits IL-18	Molluscum contagiosum virus
MC54, protein that binds and inhibits IL-18	Molluscum contagiosum virus
MC66, inhibits apoptosis as glutathione peroxidase homolog	Molluscum contagiosum virus
MC148/MCC-I, MIP-1β homolog and chemokine receptor 8 antagonist	Molluscum contagiosum virus
M3/vCKBP-III, secreted protein that binds CC, CXC, C, and CX3C chemokines	Mouse gamma herpesvirus 68
T antigen, binds to and inactivates JAK1	Murine polyomavirus
M11L, targeted to the mitochondria and inhibits apoptosis of monocytes	Myxoma virus
M-T4, inhibits apoptosis and is retained in ER	Myxoma virus
SERP-1, secreted serpin that has potent anti-inflammatory activity	Myxoma virus
Unknown, induces degradation of PKR	Poliovirus
A2R, a VEGF homolog with angiogenic factor activity	Orf virus
GIF, secreted protein that binds GM-CSF and IL-2	Orf virus
OV IL10, IL-10 homolog; may antagonize Th1 responses	Orf virus
A39R, binds semaphorin receptor VESPR and up-regulates ICAM-1 and cytokine production	Poxviruses
B15R, IL-1β receptor homolog	Poxviruses
C11R/MGF, TGF-α homolog that stimulates cell growth and EGF analog	Poxviruses
CrmA/SPI-2/B22R/B13R2/SERP-2, inhibits apoptosis by caspases 8 and 1 and granzyme B	Poxviruses
CrmB, TNFR homolog; inhibits apoptosis by neutralizing TNF-α and LTα	Poxviruses
CrmC, TNFR homolog; inhibits apoptosis by neutralizing TNF-α	Poxviruses
CrmD, TNFR homolog; inhibits apoptosis by neutralizing TNF-α and LTα	Poxviruses
CrmE, TNFR homolog; inhibits apoptosis by neutralizing TNF-α	Poxviruses
D7L/vCKBP-II, secreted protein that binds and inhibits IL-18	Poxviruses
E3L/OV20.0L, binds dsRNA and inhibits IFN-dependent PKR activation and blocks 2′, 5′-OS/RNase L	Poxviruses
M-T1/H5R/CCI/G3R/B29R/S-T1, secreted protein that sequesters CC chemokines	Poxviruses
M-T7/B8R/vCKBP-I, secreted IFN-γ receptor homolog; binds C, CC, and CXC by heparin-binding site	Poxviruses
p28/N1R, prevents UV-induced apoptosis	Poxviruses
p35, secreted protein that binds CC chemokines	Poxviruses
T2, TNFR homolog; prevents apoptosis by binding and inhibiting TNF	Poxviruses
S3, dsRNA binding and inhibitor of eIF2α phosphorylation, blocks 2′, 5′-OS/RNase L	Reovirus
NSP3, binds dsRNA and blocks PKR activation, blocks 2′, 5′-OS/RNase L	Rotavirus
Large T antigen, inhibits apoptosis by binding and inactivating p53 and pRb	Simian virus 40
V protein, targets STAT1 for proteasome-mediated degradation	Simian virus 5
K2R, IL-8 chemokine receptor homolog	Swinepox virus
Unknown 35-kDa protein, sequesters IFN-γ, IL-2, and IL-5	Tanapox
B13R, inhibits IL-1β converting enzyme and other caspases	Vaccinia virus
B18R, inhibits IFN as a secreted type I IFN-α/β receptor homolog	Vaccinia virus
K3L, inhibits dsRNA-activated protein kinase; eIF2α homolog that prevents phosphorylation	Vaccinia virus
SalF7L/3β-HSD, 3-β-hydroxysteroid dehydrogenase, immunosuppressive activity	Vaccinia virus
Unknown, TNF receptor homolog on surface of infected cells	Vaccinia virus

[a] Gene products in this table are reviewed in references 35, 51, 55, 60, and 61. 2′, 5′-OA, 2′, 5′-oligoadenylate; 2′, 5′-OS, 2′, 5′-oligoadenylatesynthetase.

that may function to delay NK cell recognition of infected cells. Herpesviruses express a number of proteins that bind to class I molecules and interfere with their intracellular trafficking.

Modifying the Action of Complement Components

Members of both the *Herpes-* and *Poxviridae* families express proteins that inhibit the complement pathway. The poxvirus proteins are secreted from infected cells and are believed to inhibit the enhancing effect of complement on antibody-mediated neutralization of viral infectivity. Some of the complement-interacting proteins expressed by *Herpesviridae* are expressed on the surface of cells and virions. Possible functions of these proteins include deactivation of complement components that target virions to virus-destroying cells bearing complement receptors, inhibition of complement-mediated destruction of virions, and inhibition of complement-targeted opsonization.

Modifying the Action of Antibodies

Herpes simplex virus encodes a protein with Fc binding activity (gpD) that is expressed on the surface of virions and infected cells. The protein may bind to the Fc region of antibody bound to other viral surface proteins, thereby blocking the action of complement- or Fc receptor-mediated opsonization. The Fc binding activity is relatively weak, however, and it is possible that the true ligand is not antibody but another member of the Ig superfamily.

Another strategy is employed by flaviviruses, which utilize antibodies or antibodies associated with complement component C3, to target the virus via association either with Fc or with C3 receptors, respectively. This mechanism is thought to contribute to enhanced pathogenicity of dengue virus in some individuals previously infected with a different viral serotype (such cross-reactive antibodies often bind virus without blocking its infectivity) or in the infants of dengue virus-immune mothers.

Disabling Immune Cells

A large number of viruses infect cells of the immune system. The most important of these is HIV, which infects large numbers of T_{CD4^+} cells and macrophages, leading directly (through cytopathogenicity) or indirectly (via immune recognition) to their destruction. Immediately following infection, T_{CD4^+} number and activity in PBLs declines, but it rapidly recovers. From the onset of AIDS, the virus multiplies furiously within lymphatic tissue, but T_{CD4^+} function is not greatly compromised, and the antibody and T_{CD8^+} immune responses to HIV are actually robust. Eventually, T_{CD4^+} cannot be repleted and the host dies, usually not from the unchecked reproduction of HIV but from an opportunistic pathogenic virus or fungus. Thus, even in the case of HIV, the importance to virus dissemination of partially disabling the immune response by killing large numbers of T_{CD4^+} (and possibly macrophages as well) is uncertain.

Many members of the *Herpesviridae* family infect lymphoid cells, where they persist in a latent state for the life of the host. There is little evidence that modification of the immune status by infection contributes to the maintenance of latency. Similarly, for other viruses, the importance of infection of lymphoid cells to enhancing virus transmission or persistence is not known.

Modifying Antigenic Proteins

Neutralizing antibodies can exert considerable selection pressure on viruses, resulting in the appearance of mutations with alterations that decrease the affinity of virus with the neutralizing antibody. Most commonly, mutations result in single amino acid substitutions in an epitope that reduce antibody binding. Less frequently, glycoproteins may acquire a site for N-linked glycosylation that sterically blocks antibody binding. While Ig can recognize oligosaccharides (most antibacterial responses are directed to saccharides), the N-linked oligosaccharides on viruses are identical to those present on host proteins and are not immunogenic. Indeed, a number of viral glycoproteins (most notably HIV gp160) are heavily glycosylated, possibly to minimize the area exposed to antibody recognition. Even less frequently, mutations distant from a given epitope may result in allosteric alterations that reduce antibody binding. Additionally, mutations can increase the avidity of viral receptor proteins for the host cell to tip the scales in favor of virus attachment when levels of neutralizing antibodies are present in limiting amounts.

There is little evidence supporting T_{CD4^+} selection of antigenic variants. Since MHC class II-associated presentation is usually unrelated to the virus life cycle, variation in T_{CD4^+} determinants is likely not of much biological significance. In contrast, antigenic variants could be selected by T_{CD8^+}, which exert direct antiviral activity. Variants with alterations in class I-associated antigenic peptides have been experimentally selected in vivo and in vitro by T_{CD8^+} clones. Variants of HIV, Epstein-Barr virus, and HBV have been isolated from chronically infected patients with alterations in antigenic peptides that prevent recognition by the patient's own T_{CD8^+}. T_{CD8^+} selection of escape variants may even occur in acute infections like influenza virus infection.

Most fascinating are HIV and HBV variants with mutations in antigenic peptides that convert the peptide from a T-cell agonist to a T-cell antagonist. Cells expressing both wild-type and mutant peptides are thus protected from T_{CD8^+}-mediated destruction. This allows for persistence of virus in cells expressing both parent and mutant viruses and for spread of the antigenic variant until the ensuing induction of T_{CD8^+} specific for the variant peptide.

While antigenic variants may contribute to viral persistence in an individual, their epidemiological significance is uncertain, since HLA polymorphism will limit their selective advantage in populations, unless a population consists of a high percentage of individuals with the same HLA allele (indeed this may be one of the driving forces for class I polymorphism).

IMMUNOPATHOLOGY

The effector mechanisms of the immune system to clear virus infections have the capacity to do grave, even lethal, damage to the host. At the end of the last century, it was widely thought that inflammation associated with infections reflected attempts by microorganisms to inflict maximal damage to the host. For viruses that cause limited or no cell destruction, the effects of the immune response can be far worse than having no response at all. Even in the case of normal immune responses, it is difficult to know which elements of the response are essential to viral clearance and recovery and which are excessive. It is difficult to believe that precise immune responses to infections occur routinely; the immune system would likely want to err on the vigorous side.

Immunopathological responses to viruses can be divided into three major categories: humoral, cellular, and autoimmune. Humoral antiviral immunopathology corresponds to type III hypersensitivity reactions (using the classical immunology terminology), in which damage is attributable to immune complexes between antibodies and viral antigens. Such complexes can form when neither component is present in excess amounts. Immune complexes can be deposited in blood vessels, kidneys, or other end organs, where ADCC or complement fixation activates a cascade leading to local inflammation and tissue destruction. This is not a common occurrence in viral infections but can occur with chronic HBV infection, where large amounts of a viral antigen are continuously synthesized in the presence of an antibody response.

Cellular antiviral immunopathology corresponds to type IV hypersensitivity (also known as delayed-type hypersensitivity). Here, damage is due to inappropriate T-cell function. This is thought to account for much of the liver destruction observed in acute fulminant hepatitis and also in chronic active hepatitis, in which individuals with active HBV-specific T_{CD8^+} responses seem to fare worse than those whose immune systems choose to ignore persistently infected hepatocytes. It has also been proposed that much of the loss of T_{CD4^+} in HIV infections results from destruction of infected cells by T_{CD8^+} and T_{CD4^+} (recall that activated human T_{CD4^+} express class II MHC molecules). Another possible example of T-cell-induced immunopathology was the unfortunate potentiation of diseases observed following immunization of children with inactivated respiratory syncytial virus. Experiments in mouse models suggest that priming with inactivated virus shifts the T_{CD4^+} response to infectious virus to a Th1-type response, leading to severe pulmonary inflammation.

The induction of autoimmunity by viruses has long been proposed but has never been convincingly substantiated. In theory, autoimmunity could result from the following:

1. Initiation of an immune response to self-antigens cross-reactive with viral antigens that persists after the virus is cleared
2. Destruction or modification of virus-infected cells such that self-antigens now stimulate an immune response due to enhanced presentation, or additional help provided by T_{CD4^+} specific for viral antigens. Again, the response persists after the virus is gone, reflecting the basic property of the immune response that it is more difficult to initiate a response than to maintain it.
3. A viral protein acting as a "superantigen" that activates T cells by binding the TCR directly in a non-MHC-associated manner. Activated T cells may be self-reactive or could provide nonspecific help to self-reactive B or T cells.
4. Activation of self-reactive B or T cells following infection with lymphotropic, noncytolytic viruses
5. Induction of "anti-idiotypic" B or T cells (i.e., those specific for variable regions of the antiviral B or T cells) that react with self-antigens

SUMMARY: A TYPICAL ANTIVIRAL IMMUNE RESPONSE

In summary, immune responses to viruses are complex and incompletely understood. This chapter concludes by describing in rough sequential order the events comprising a typical immune response to a generic virus (Color Plate 28).

1. The evening following the third day of the new school year, your child sneezes in close proximity to you, delivering numerous infectious particles of a respiratory virus. Upon reaching epithelial cells in the upper airway, the virus replicates unchecked for one to several infectious cycles, each cycle increasing the amount of infectious virions 100- to 1,000-fold.
2. The initial signal to the immune system of the infection may be the release of IFN-β by infected epithelial cells or release of IFN-α or IL-1 by tissue macrophages (if infectible by the virus). IFN is first detected 2 days postinfection, coinciding with the peak of infectious virus, but is probably first released within hours of infection. IFN levels peak 1 day later and diminish to undetectable levels over the next 5 days. IFN activates NK cells, first detected 3 days postinfection and reaching peak levels 1 day later. NK cells release IFN-γ and other cytokines that recruit additional inflammatory cells to the site of infection. Two to three days after infection, cytokines reach sufficient levels to trigger an acute-phase response, which coincides with the onset of clinical symptoms.
3. While the nonspecific immune mechanisms are coping with the virus in the first few days of infection, DCs in MALT and in regional lymph nodes (in the latter case, migrating from the site of infection) present antigens to T cells, resulting in detectable T_{CD4^+} and T_{CD8^+} responses 4 and 6 days, respectively, following infection. T cells are recruited to the site of infection by alterations in local endothelium induced by the inflammatory process.
4. Mucosal IgA responses may be detected 3 days following infection, while IgM responses in the serum are first detected 5 to 6 days after exposure, with IgG responses lagging 2 to 3 days behind. Both the amount and avidity of the Ig responses increase over the next few weeks.
5. Ig and T_{CD8^+} work together to eradicate remaining infectious virus. Virus is generally no longer detected 7 or 8 days after infection. T_{CD8^+} responses peak at this time and decline over the next 7 days to undetectable levels.
6. IgA responses decline to undetectable levels over the next 3 to 6 months, while serum IgG levels persist for the life of the individual. Memory T_{CD8^+} and T_{CD4^+} may also persist for the life of the individual. Serum IgG usually provides complete or partial protection against infection. If reinfection does occur, all aspects of B- and T-cell responses are swift and merciless, often confining the infection to subclinical levels.

We are indebted to Dean Madden (Max Planck-Institut für Medizinische Forschung, Heidelberg, Germany), and Ian Wilson and Robyn Stanfield (Scripps Institute, La Jolla, CA) for providing the color images of the three-dimensional structures of MHC class I and class II molecules and HA-antibody complexes.

REFERENCES

1. **Amanna, I. J., M. K. Slifka, and S. Crotty.** 2006. Immunity and immunological memory following smallpox vaccination. *Immunol. Rev.* **211:**320–337.
2. **Beutler, B., Z. Jiang, P. Georgel, K. Crozat, B. Croker, S. Rutschmann, X. Du, and K. Hoebe.** 2006. Genetic analysis of host resistance: Toll-like receptor signaling and immunity at large. *Annu. Rev. Immunol.* **24:**353–389.

3. **Bizebard, T., C. Barbey-Martin, D. Fleury, B. Gigant, B. Barrere, J. J. Skehel, and M. Knossow.** 2001. Structural studies on viral escape from antibody neutralization. *Curr. Top. Microbiol. Immunol.* **260:**55–64.
4. **Brandtzaeg, P.** 2007. Induction of secretory immunity and memory at mucosal surfaces. *Vaccine* **25:**5467–5484.
5. **Burton, D. R.** 2002. Antibodies, viruses and vaccines. *Nat. Rev. Immunol.* **2:**706–713.
6. **Burton, D. R., R. C. Desrosiers, R. W. Doms, W. C. Koff, P. D. Kwong, J. P. Moore, G. J. Nabel, J. Sodroski, I. A. Wilson, and R. T. Wyatt.** 2004. HIV vaccine design and the neutralizing antibody problem. *Nat. Immunol.* **5:** 233–236.
7. **Cao, W., and Y. J. Liu.** 2007. Innate immune functions of plasmacytoid dendritic cells. *Curr. Opin. Immunol.* **19:** 24–30.
8. **Fahraeus, R.** 2005. Do peptides control their own birth and death? *Nat. Rev. Mol. Cell Biol.* **6:**263–267.
9. **Fremont, D. H., M. Matsumara, E. A. Stura, P. A. Peterson, and I. A. Wilson.** 1992. Crystal structures of two viral peptides in complex with murine MHC class I H-2Kb. *Science* **257:**919–926.
10. **Garcia, K. C., and E. J. Adams.** 2005. How the T cell receptor sees antigen—a structural view. *Cell* **122:**333–336.
11. **Garcia-Sastre, A., and C. A. Biron.** 2006. Type 1 interferons and the virus-host relationship: a lesson in detente. *Science* **312:**879–882.
12. **Gazit, R., R. Gruda, M. Elboim, T. I. Arnon, G. Katz, H. Achdout, J. Hanna, U. Qimron, G. Landau, E. Greenbaum, Z. Zakay-Rones, A. Porgador, and O. Mandelboim.** 2006. Lethal influenza infection in the absence of the natural killer cell receptor gene Ncr1. *Nat. Immunol.* **7:**517–523.
13. **Gonzalez, S., V. Groh, and T. Spies.** 2006. Immunobiology of human NKG2D and its ligands. *Curr. Top. Microbiol. Immunol.* **298:**121–138.
14. **Guermonprez, P., and S. Amigorena.** 2005. Pathways for antigen cross presentation. *Springer Semin. Immunopathol.* **26:**257–271.
15. **Haeryfar, S. M. M.** 2005. The importance of being a pDC in antiviral immunity: the IFN mission versus Ag presentation? *Trends Immunol.* **26:**311–317.
16. **Hickman, H. D., K. Takeda, C. N. Skon, F. R. Murray, S. E. Hensley, J. Loomis, G. N. Barber, J. R. Bennink, and J. W. Yewdell.** 2008. Direct priming of anti-viral $CD8^+$ T cells in the peripheral interfollicular region of lymph nodes. *Nat. Immunol.* **9:**155–163.
17. **Hiscott, J.** 2007. Triggering the innate antiviral response through IRF-3 activation. *J. Biol. Chem.* **282:**15325–15329.
18. **Jung, D., C. Giallourakis, R. Mostoslavsky, and F. W. Alt.** 2006. Mechanism and control of V(D)J recombination at the immunoglobulin heavy chain locus. *Annu. Rev. Immunol.* **24:**541–570.
19. **Junt, T., E. A. Moseman, M. Iannacone, S. Massberg, P. A. Lang, M. Boes, K. Fink, S. E. Henrickson, D. M. Shayakhmetov, N. C. Di Paolo, N. van Rooijen, T. R. Mempel, S. P. Whelan, and U. H. von Andrian.** 2007. Subcapsular sinus macrophages in lymph nodes clear lymph-borne viruses and present them to antiviral B cells. *Nature* **450:**110–114.
20. **Kabelitz, D., and R. Medzhitov.** 2007. Innate immunity—cross-talk with adaptive immunity through pattern recognition receptors and cytokines. *Curr. Opin. Immunol.* **19:**1–3.
21. **Karre, K.** 2002. NK cells, MHC class I molecules and the missing self. *Scand. J. Immunol.* **55:**221–228.
22. **Katze, M. G., Y. He, and M. Gale, Jr.** 2002. Viruses and interferon: a fight for supremacy. *Nat. Rev. Immunol.* **2:** 675–687.
23. **Klotman, M. E., and T. L. Chang.** 2006. Defensins in innate antiviral immunity. *Nat. Rev. Immunol.* **6:**447–456.
24. **Lee, H. K., J. M. Lund, B. Ramanathan, N. Mizushima, and A. Iwasaki.** 2007. Autophagy-dependent viral recognition by plasmacytoid dendritic cells. *Science* **315:** 1398–1401.
25. **Lee, M. S., and Y. J. Kim.** 2007. Signaling pathways downstream of pattern-recognition receptors and their cross talk. *Annu. Rev. Biochem.* **76:**447–480.
26. **Lee, S. H., T. Miyagi, and C. A. Biron.** 2007. Keeping NK cells in highly regulated antiviral warfare. *Trends Immunol.* **28:**252–259.
27. **Levine, B., and V. Deretic.** 2007. Unveiling the roles of autophagy in innate and adaptive immunity. *Nat. Rev. Immunol.* **7:**767–777.
28. **Marcenaro, S., F. Gallo, S. Martini, A. Santoro, G. M. Griffiths, M. Aricó, L. Moretta, and D. Pende.** 2006. Analysis of natural killer-cell function in familial hemophagocytic lymphohistiocytosis (FHL): defective CD107a surface expression heralds Munc13-4 defect and discriminates between genetic subtypes of the disease. *Blood* **108:** 2316–2323.
29. **Marshall, J. S., C. A. King, and J. D. McCurdy.** 2003. Mast cell cytokine and chemokine responses to bacterial and viral infection. *Curr. Pharm. Des.* **9:**11–24.
30. **Maruyama, M., K. P. Lam, and K. Rajewsky.** 2000. Memory B-cell persistence is independent of persisting immunizing antigen. *Nature* **407:**636–642.
31. **Meylan, E., and J. Tschopp.** 2006. Toll-like receptors and RNA helicases: two parallel ways to trigger antiviral responses. *Mol. Cell* **22:**561–569.
32. **Ochsenbein, A. F., and R. M. Zinkernagel.** 2000. Natural antibodies and complement link innate and acquired immunity. *Immunol. Today* **21:**624–630.
33. **O'Leary, J. G., M. Goodarzi, D. L. Drayton, and U. H. Von Andrian.** 2006. T cell- and B cell-independent adaptive immunity mediated by natural killer cells. *Nat. Immunol.* **7:**507–516.
34. **Orange, J. S., and Z. K. Ballas.** 2006. Natural killer cells in human health and disease. *Clin. Immunol.* **118:**1–10.
35. **Orange, J. S., M. S. Fassett, L. A. Koopman, J. E. Boyson, and J. L. Strominger.** 2002. Viral evasion of natural killer cells. *Nat. Immunol.* **3:**1006–1012.
36. **Phan, T. G., I. Grigorova, T. Okada, and J. G. Cyster.** 2007. Subcapsular encounter and complement-dependent transport of immune complexes by lymph node B cells. *Nat. Immunol.* **8:**992–1000.
37. **Pichlmair, A., and C. Reis e Sousa.** 2007. Innate recognition of viruses. *Immunity* **27:**370–383.
38. **Poccia, F., C. Agrati, F. Martini, M. R. Capobianchi, M. Wallace, and M. Malkovsky.** 2005. Antiviral reactivities of $\gamma\delta$ T cells. *Microbes Infect.* **7:**518–528.
39. **Pozzi, L. A., J. W. Maciaszek, and K. L. Rock.** 2005. Both dendritic cells and macrophages can stimulate naive CD8 T cells in vivo to proliferate, develop effector function, and differentiate into memory cells. *J. Immunol.* **175:**2071–2079.
40. **Rammensee, H., J. Bachmann, N. P. Emmerich, O. A. Bachor, and S. Stevanovic.** 1999. SYFPEITHI: database for MHC ligands and peptide motifs. *Immunogenetics* **50:** 213–219.
41. **Reis e Sousa, C.** 2004. Toll-like receptors and dendritic cells: for whom the bug tolls. *Semin. Immunol.* **16:**27–34.
42. **Sacha, J. B., C. Chung, E. G. Rakasz, S. P. Spencer, A. K. Jonas, A. T. Bean, W. Lee, B. J. Burwitz, J. J.**

Stephany, J. T. Loffredo, D. B. Allison, S. Adnan, A. Hoji, N. A. Wilson, T. C. Friedrich, J. D. Lifson, O. O. Yang, and D. I. Watkins. 2007. Gag-specific CD8+ T lymphocytes recognize infected cells before AIDS-virus integration and viral protein expression. *J. Immunol.* **178:**2746–2754.

43. **Savard, M., and J. Gosselin.** 2006. Epstein-Barr virus immunosuppression of innate immunity mediated by phagocytes. *Virus Res.* **119:**134–145.
44. **Schmid, D., and C. Munz.** 2007. Innate and adaptive immunity through autophagy. *Immunity* **27:**11–21.
45. **Shen, L., and K. L. Rock.** 2006. Priming of T cells by exogenous antigen cross-presented on MHC class I molecules. *Curr. Opin. Immunol.* **18:**85–91.
46. **Shibata, K. I., M. Imarai, G. M. Van Bleek, S. Joyce, and S. G. Nathenson.** 1992. Vesicular stomatitis virus antigenic octapeptide N52-59 is anchored into the groove of the H-2Kb molecule by the side chains of three amino acids and the main-chain atoms of the amino terminus. *Proc. Natl. Acad. Sci. USA* **89:**3135–3139.
47. **Simon, I. D., J. Publicover, and J. K. Rose.** 2007. Replication and propagation of attenuated vesicular stomatitis virus vectors in vivo: vector spread correlates with induction of immune responses and persistence of genomic RNA. *J. Virol.* **81:**2078–2082.
48. **Stern, L. J., J. H. Brown, T. S. Jardetzky, J. C. Gorga, R. G. Urban, J. L. Strominger, and D. C. Wiley.** 1994. Crystal structure of the human class II MHC protein HLA-DR1 complexed with an influenza virus peptide. *Nature* **368:**215–221.
49. **Stern-Ginossar, N., N. Elefant, A. Zimmermann, D. G. Wolf, N. Saleh, M. Biton, E. Horwitz, Z. Prokocimer, M. Prichard, G. Hahn, D. Goldman-Wohl, C. Greenfield, S. Yagel, H. Hengel, Y. Altuvia, H. Margalit, and O. Mandelboim.** 2007. Host immune system gene targeting by a viral miRNA. *Science* **317:**376–381.
50. **Tewari, M. K., G. Sinnathamby, D. Rajagopal, and L. C. Eisenlohr.** 2005. A cytosolic pathway for MHC class II-restricted antigen processing that is proteasome and TAP dependent. *Nat. Immunol.* **6:**287–294.
51. **Tortorella, D., B. E. Gewurz, M. H. Furman, D. J. Schust, and H. L. Ploegh.** 2000. Viral subversion of the immune system. *Annu. Rev. Immunol.* **18:**861–926.
52. **Turner, D. L., L. S. Cauley, K. M. Khanna, and L. Lefrancois.** 2007. Persistent antigen presentation after acute vesicular stomatitis virus infection. *J. Virol.* **81:**2039–2046.
53. **van den Boorn, J. G., I. C. Le Poole, and R. M. Luiten.** 2006. T-cell avidity and tuning: the flexible connection between tolerance and autoimmunity. *Int. Rev. Immunol.* **25:**235–258.
54. **Voigt, S., A. Mesci, J. Ettinger, J. H. Fine, P. Chen, W. Chou, and J. R. Carlyle.** 2007. Cytomegalovirus evasion of innate immunity by subversion of the NKR-P1B:Clr-b missing-self axis. *Immunity* **26:**617–627.
55. **Weber, F., and O. Haller.** 2007. Viral suppression of the interferon system. *Biochimie* **89:**836–842.
56. **Whitton, J. L., M. K. Slifka, F. Liu, A. K. Nussbaum, and J. K. Whitmire.** 2004. The regulation and maturation of antiviral immune responses. *Adv. Virus Res.* **63:**181–238.
57. **Wiley, D. C., and J. J. Skehel.** 1987. The structure and function of the hemagglutinin membrane glycoprotein of influenza virus. *Annu. Rev. Biochem.* **56:**365–394.
58. **Wilson, I. A., and N. J. Cox.** 1990. Structural basis of immune recognition of influenza virus hemagglutinin. *Annu. Rev. Immunol.* **214:**737–771.
59. **Yewdell, J. W.** 2006. Confronting complexity: real-world immunodominance in antiviral CD8+ T cell responses. *Immunity* **25:**533–543.
60. **Yewdell, J. W., and J. R. Bennink.** 1999. Mechanisms of viral interference with MHC class I antigen processing and presentation. *Annu. Rev. Cell Dev. Biol.* **15:**579–606.
61. **Yewdell, J. W., and A. B. Hill.** 2002. Viral interference with antigen presentation. *Nat. Immunol.* **3:**1019–1025.
62. **Yewdell, J. W., and C. V. Nicchitta.** 2006. The DRiP hypothesis decennial: support, controversy, refinement and extension. *Trends Immunol.* **27:**368–373.
63. **Yokoyama, W. M.** 2005. Specific and non-specific natural killer cell responses to viral infection. *Adv. Exp. Med. Biol.* **560:**57–61.
64. **Zhou, T., L. Xu, B. Dey, A. J. Hessell, D. Van Ryk, S. H. Xiang, X. Yang, M. Y. Zhang, M. B. Zwick, J. Arthos, D. R. Burton, D. S. Dimitrov, J. Sodroski, R. Wyatt, G. J. Nabel, and P. D. Kwong.** 2007. Structural definition of a conserved neutralization epitope on HIV-1 gp120. *Nature* **445:**732–737.
65. **zur Stadt, U., S. Schmidt, B. Kasper, K. Beutel, A. S. Diler, J.-I. Henter, H. Kabisch, R. Schneppenheim, P. Nürnberg, G. Janka, and H. C. Hennies.** 2005. Linkage of familial hemophagocytic lymphohistiocytosis (FHL) type-4 to chromosome 6q24 and identification of mutations in syntaxin 11. *Hum. Mol. Genet.* **14:**827–834.

Immunization against Viral Diseases

JULIE E. MARTIN AND BARNEY S. GRAHAM

15

Vaccines to prevent viral infections are perhaps the greatest of all biomedical achievements for preventing disease and improving the public health. The most notable example is the success of smallpox vaccination. The practice of variolization (mechanical attenuation and intentional low-dose infection) to reduce the virulence of subsequent smallpox infection was started more than 1,000 years ago in India and China. However, smallpox vaccination was first performed by Jenner in 1796. This event marked the beginning of modern vaccine development and was the first clinical test of vaccine efficacy. An expansive world health effort with global cooperation and leadership in combination with persistence and creative approaches, like the ring vaccination campaign, resulted in the 1980 WHO declaration that naturally occurring smallpox had been eradicated. Numerous other vaccines have made a significant impact on the severity and frequency of viral diseases, and many previously common viral illnesses are rarely encountered in modern clinical care (Table 1). In particular, vaccines against hepatitis A and B, poliovirus, measles, mumps, and rubella have markedly reduced the frequency of these infections in developed countries. Unfortunately, many of these infections remain major health problems in other parts of the world. A description of viral vaccines available for use in the United States is given in Table 2.

Effective immunization safely induces a vaccine-specific host immune response capable of either preventing infection or attenuating illness. Historically, viral vaccine immunogens were created by either inactivating or attenuating whole virus and were tested empirically with a rudimentary understanding of the basic viral pathogenesis or protective immune responses. Newer generations of viral vaccines often involve a detailed understanding of the virology and immunology specific to the pathogen and utilize molecular biology approaches to produce vaccine antigens. This chapter reviews current viral vaccine practices and concepts and indicates future directions for vaccine research and development.

GOALS OF VACCINATION

The goal of immunization against viruses is to improve both individual and public health by preventing or modifying virus-induced disease in the person and preventing or reducing the spread of infection in a population. When individuals do not participate in vaccination efforts against epidemic diseases, there are potential consequences for the person but greater consequences for public health. Vaccination is one of the few opportunities for a personal health benefit to be amplified as a benefit to the greater population.

Prevention of Infection or Disease

Active and Passive Immunization

Immunization is defined as induction of an antigen-specific host immune response by exposing the host to antigens representing, or comprised of those in, the wild-type pathogen. "Active immunization" to a virus can be induced through natural infection or by vaccination. The term implies an induction of immunologic memory. "Passive immunization" refers to a transfer of temporary immunity to the host, which will not provide immunologic memory but provides transient immune-mediated protection from infection or disease. The most common example of passive immunization is the transfer of disease-specific immunoglobulins into a host. In the cases of rabies and hepatitis B exposure, passive (immunoglobulin) and active (vaccine) immunizations are commonly used together to induce both rapid and long-lasting protection.

Prophylactic Vaccination

Most vaccines are designed to prevent virus infection in the individual. In most circumstances, vaccine-induced immunity does not completely block infection but prevents disease by rapidly clearing or aborting infection through blocking transmission of virus to the target organ or preventing the indirect consequences of virus infections. Incomplete protection from infection has no clinical consequences for viruses that are typically self-limited and do not persist. For example, the inactivated polio (Salk) vaccine prevents dissemination of the virus to the anterior horn cells but does not prevent replication and shedding of poliovirus in the gut. The licensed hepatitis B virus (HBV) and human papillomavirus (HPV) vaccines have as a major goal the prevention of a remote clinical consequence of viral infection, cancers of the liver and cervix, respectively (1, 4). For viruses like herpes simplex virus (HSV), HCV, or human immunodeficiency virus (HIV)

TABLE 1 Impact of licensed vaccines on annual prevalence of selected viral diseases reported in the United States

Viral disease	Peak year(s)	Peak prevalence	Recent prevalence	% Reduction
Hepatitis A	1971	59,606	4,488[a,b]	92.5
Hepatitis B	1985	26,654	5,494[a,b]	79.4
Measles	1958–1962	503,282	45[c,d]	>99.9
Mumps	1967	185,691	197[d,e]	99.9
Polio	1951–1954	16,316	0	100
Rubella	1966–1968	47,745	8[d,f]	>99.9
Congenital rubella	1966–1968	823	1[d,f]	99.9
Smallpox	1900–1904	48,164	0	100

[a] Source: http://www.cdc.gov/ncidod/diseases/hepatitis/resource/PDFs/disease_burden.pdf.
[b] 2005 data.
[c] 2006 data.
[d] Source: http://www.who.int/immunization_monitoring/en/globalsummary/timeseries/tsincidencemum.htm.
[e] 2004 data. See text for description of the 2006 mumps outbreak.
[f] All cases were imported.

that can become persistent or latent, the control or prevention of virus infection needs to be more stringent and occur as early as possible. This is one of the great challenges in developing vaccines against these types of viruses.

Postexposure Vaccination

In some cases, vaccine can be effective even when administered after exposure, as for rabies and hepatitis B. Notably, individuals can be protected against a fatal outcome if vaccinia virus vaccine is administered up to 4 days after exposure to variola virus, which has a more rapidly progressive disease course. For postexposure immunization to work, the vaccine must be highly immunogenic, and success is more likely when the pathogenesis involves a relatively long incubation period between infection and disease onset.

Therapeutic Vaccination

Some vaccines can also be used therapeutically after virus-induced disease has occurred. The best example and only licensed vaccine for this indication is against varicella-zoster virus (VZV). Immunization of elderly adults with live attenuated VZV vaccine during latency reduces the incidence of herpes zoster and postherpetic neuralgia (56). Diseases like those caused by HSV type 1 (HSV-1), HSV-2, HCV, or HPV, which produce latent or persistent infection with periodic clinical flares or long-term clinical consequences, are candidates for therapeutic vaccine development. HIV type 1 (HIV-1) is also a target for therapeutic vaccine development, but the task will be more difficult for viruses, like HIV, that cause immunologic impairment as a direct result of infection. Even for viruses like HPV, which has an effective prophylactic vaccine, the efficacy of therapeutic vaccination may be difficult to achieve.

Herd Immunity

As an increasingly large fraction of a population is immunized against a particular pathogen, a beneficial effect occurs that is greater than anticipated relative to vaccination rates. "Herd immunity" occurs as both transmitters and susceptible persons are reduced in the population, resulting in a greater-than-expected decrease in the prevalence of infection. Fewer incident cases of infection will occur in the unprotected portion of the population. This also means that if only a few individuals are not immunized, they will benefit from the immunity of those around them. This is an important consideration in the protection of individuals who have impaired immune systems and may not have the capacity to respond to vaccination. Rubella immunization is a practical example of herd immunity. The major goal is to prevent fetal abnormalities caused by intrauterine infection. Therefore, both males and females are immunized in the United States, even though immunization has little direct benefit to males other than prevention of a relatively mild illness. Another type of herd immunity occurs when persons receiving live virus vaccines transmit the attenuated vaccine strain to other susceptible contacts.

Disease Eradication by Vaccination

The ultimate goal of vaccination is to achieve disease eradication. This is theoretically possible for viruses (like variola) that have no animal reservoir, do not cause persistent or latent infection, do not undergo major antigenic change, and exhibit distinctive clinical signs of disease. Polio and measles meet these criteria, and significant progress has been made in ongoing efforts to eradicate these diseases through vaccination. Beyond those two diseases, there are no viral diseases that are immediate candidates for eradication. With the ever-increasing capability in genome sequencing and molecular biology, even if a virus can be eradicated from nature, there will be full-length genome sequences and laboratory reservoirs that will never be eradicated.

IMMUNOLOGIC BASIS OF VACCINATION AGAINST VIRAL DISEASES

Innate immune responses are an important component of the immune system and provide an early, rapid-onset defense against pathogens. These responses do not require previous exposure, are not antigen specific, and do not confer immunologic memory. The innate immune system is universal, and all cells possess some inherent capacity for protection. In contrast, adaptive immunity is antigen specific and requires an activation and amplification phase as it responds to a primary antigen exposure. This is accomplished primarily through specialized B and T lymphocytes and is characterized by immunologic memory with the capacity for rapid, specific effector responses upon reexposure to a previously recognized antigen. Many aspects of innate immunity intersect with elements of the adaptive immune response by providing mechanisms for recognizing

TABLE 2 Vaccines licensed for use in the United States against viral diseases

Virus target	Vaccine type	Route of administration[a]	Cell substrate	Trade name/sponsor[b]	Comments[c]
Adenovirus	Live	p.o.	Human diploid fibroblasts	N/A	Types 4 and 7 (not currently available). Newer formulation being evaluated by U.S. Army
Hepatitis A	Inactivated	i.m.	Human diploid fibroblasts	Havrix/GSK VAQTA/Merck Twinrix (hepatitis A and B combination)/GSK	
Hepatitis B	Recombinant subunit	i.m.	Yeast	Recombivax HB/Merck Energix-B/GSK Twinrix (hepatitis A and B combination)/GSK	
HPV	Recombinant, virus-like particles	i.m.	Yeast	Gardasil/Merck	Types 6, 11, 16, and 18
Japanese encephalitis	Inactivated	s.c.	Mouse brain	JE-Vax/Research Foundation for Microbial Diseases of Osaka University	
Influenza A and B	Inactivated[d] or live	i.m. or i.n.	Embryonated hen eggs	FluLaval/ID Biomedical Corp. of Quebec Fluarix/GSK Fluvirin/Novartis Fluzone/Sanofi Flumist (live)/MedImmune Vaccines	Specific H3N2, H1N1, and B strains selected annually
Influenza H5N1	Inactivated	i.m.	Embryonated hen eggs	No trade name/Sanofi	Based on the Vietnam strain of H5N1; for national stockpile only
Measles	Live	s.c.	Chicken embryo fibroblasts	Attenuvax/Merck M-M-R II (measles, mumps, and rubella combination)/Merck Proquad (measles, mumps, rubella, and varicella combination)/Merck	
Mumps	Live	s.c.	Embryonated hen eggs and chicken embryo fibroblasts	Mumpsvax/Merck M-M-R II (measles, mumps, and rubella combination)/Merck Proquad (measles, mumps, rubella, and varicella combination)/Merck	
Poliovirus (IPV)	Inactivated	s.c.	Vero monkey kidney cells	IPOL/Sanofi	Serotypes 1, 2, and 3
Poliovirus (OPV)	Live	p.o.	Monkey kidney cells	NA	No longer distributed in the United States
Rabies	Inactivated	i.m. or i.d.	Human diploid fibroblasts or chicken fibroblasts	Imovax/Sanofi RabAvert/Novartis	Two formulations in the United States. Purified chicken embryo cell culture formulations are contraindicated in egg-allergic patients.

(Continued on next page)

TABLE 2 Vaccines licensed for use in the United States against viral diseases *(Continued)*

Virus target	Vaccine type	Route of administration[a]	Cell substrate	Trade name/sponsor[b]	Comments[c]
Rotavirus	Live	p.o.	Vero monkey kidney cells	RotaTeq/Merck	Bovine, pentavalent vaccine available for use in the United States
Rubella	Live	s.c.	Human diploid fibroblasts	Meruvax II/Merck M-M-R II (measles, mumps, and rubella combination)/ Merck Proquad (measles, mumps, rubella, and varicella combination)/Merck	
Smallpox, live	Live	i.d. scarification	Vero monkey kidney cells	ACAM2000/Acambis Inc.	FDA approved in 2007
Smallpox, live, dried	Live	i.d. scarification	Dried calf lymph	Dryvax/Wyeth Pharmaceuticals	Limited availability through DoD or DHHS
Varicella	Live	s.c.	Human diploid fibroblasts	Varivax/Merck	
Yellow fever	Live	s.c.	Embryonated hen eggs	YF-Vax/Sanofi	
Herpes zoster	Live	s.c.	Human diploid fibroblasts	Zostavax/Merck	

[a] p.o., per os; s.c., subcutaneous; i.n., intranasal.
[b] NA, not applicable; GSK, GlaxoSmithKline Biologicals; Merck, Merck & Co.; Novartis, Novartis Vaccines and Diagnostics Ltd.; Sanofi, Sanofi Pasteur, SA.
[c] DoD, Department of Defense; DHHS, Department of Health and Human Services.
[d] Inactivated influenza vaccine is administered i.m.

threats, amplifying the engagement and activation of adaptive responses, and even sharing effector mechanisms.

Antiviral immunity is mediated by both innate and adaptive immune responses. Innate immune responses influence the initial stages of virus infection and thereby alter the severity and characteristics of disease. Most viruses have mechanisms to evade innate immune responses, particularly pathways involving interferons (IFNs), indicating their importance in host defense. However, vaccine-induced immunity depends on immunologic memory, which is an inherent property of adaptive immune responses. Vaccination establishes preexisting antibody and memory populations of T cells that change the next encounter of the host with a particular virus. Preexisting antibody can reduce the initial number of infected cells and pace of viral replication, resulting in an attenuated disease course. A higher precursor frequency of virus-specific T cells can also attenuate disease through subtle changes in the timing and magnitude of responses. Vaccine design, formulation, and delivery will influence the specificity, quality, and location of T-cell responses and change the clinical expression of a subsequent virus infection. While it is the effector mechanisms of the adaptive immune response that are responsible for directly mediating vaccine-induced antiviral immunity, innate immune mechanisms are relevant to the pattern and quality of virus-specific responses that are predestined during the time immediately after vaccination.

Innate Immunity

The innate immune system is designed to rapidly recognize and respond to pathogens. Major cellular components of the innate immune system involved in initiating and molding the response to vaccination include dendritic cells (DCs), macrophages, monocytes, natural killer cells, and neutrophils. The most important, from the standpoint of vaccine-induced immune responses, are the so-called professional antigen-presenting cells (APCs): DCs, macrophages, and monocytes.

Pathogen Recognition

Medzhitov and Janeway predicted that the immune system had mechanisms to recognize molecular patterns associated with pathogens and coined the term pathogen-associated molecular patterns (46). That hypothesis has been realized through the discovery and description of Toll-like receptors (TLRs) that recognize a variety of molecules typically associated with microbial pathogens (5) (Fig. 1). Some of these TLRs appear to have specifically evolved to recognize molecules within endosomes associated with viruses, including double-stranded RNA (TLR-3) and single-stranded RNA (TLR-7 and TLR-8). Other pathogen recognition receptors have evolved to recognize double-stranded RNA in the cytosol like the RNA helicases, retinoic acid-inducible gene I and melanoma differentiation-associated gene 5, or protein kinase receptor (8). Occasional TLRs have been noted to detect viral proteins, like the TLR-4 recognition of the respiratory syncytial virus (RSV) F glycoprotein (39). Triggering TLRs and other pathogen recognition receptors leads to an integrated set of responses by APCs through IFN regulatory factors and NF-κB transcription factors that control the induction of genes involved in the antiviral response. The process of pathogen recognition is an important consider-

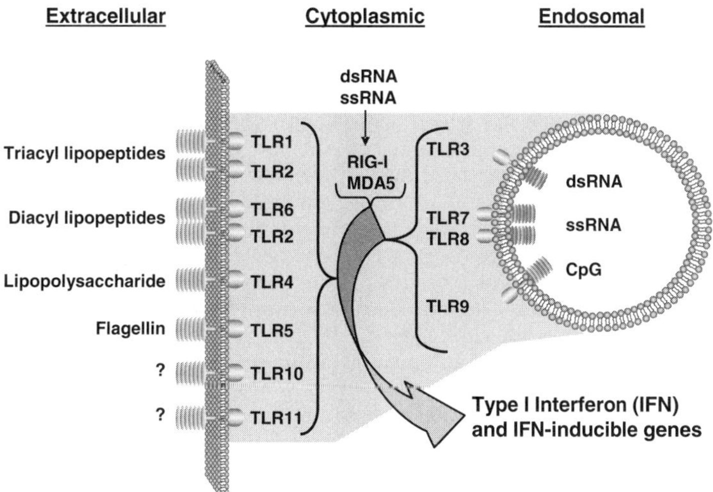

FIGURE 1 Recognition of viral pathogens. Eukaryotes have evolved mechanisms to detect potential microbial pathogens as they encounter the plasma membrane or penetrate the endosomal or cytoplasmic compartment of the cell. The molecules that interact with microbe-derived ligands trigger signaling pathways that lead to inflammatory responses. Harnessing the coordinated regulation of immune responses elicited by TLRs and helicases is a major focus of new adjuvant development for vaccines.

ation when designing the adjuvant and delivery vehicles used in vaccine formulations. These activating stimuli prepare the immune system for recognizing specific antigenic sites on the virus that can be targeted by adaptive immune responses.

Antigen Presentation

The principal APCs for initiating adaptive immune responses are DCs. The function of DCs varies as they progress through successive stages of maturation, the immature state generally being better for phagocytosis and the mature state better for antigen presentation. In addition, there are subpopulations of DCs that have distinct properties. In the future it may be possible to engage selected DC subpopulations and direct the patterns of immune activation. For example, plasmacytoid DCs (pDCs) are characterized by expressing TLR-9 and are a major source of type I IFN production. Activating pDCs during vaccination might be expected to induce strong $CD8^+$ T-cell responses because of the known association of IFN-α and memory $CD8^+$ T cells (40). It may be possible to augment pDC activation with CpGs, which are short palindromic sequences in bacterial DNA that serve as a ligand for TLR-9. DCs usually first encounter antigen in tissue during an inflammatory event. After phagocytosis of the antigen or an apoptotic cell containing antigen, they become mobile and traffic to regional lymph nodes. The mature DC in the lymph node presents processed antigen as peptides in the context of major histocompatibility complex (MHC) class I or II molecules in combination with costimulatory molecules to activate epitope-specific $CD8^+$ and $CD4^+$ T cells, respectively. Therefore, DCs are important for the initial immunization event and are important again after exposure to a viral pathogen occurs to rapidly carry the viral antigen to lymph nodes so that the vaccine-induced memory T cells can be activated and expanded in response to infection.

Immune Modulation

Immune modulation refers to altering the pattern of the immune response. This could involve the balance of response at various levels of specificity. For example, immune responses can be focused more on antibody or T-cell responses, $CD4^+$ or $CD8^+$ T-cell responses, or Th1 or Th2 $CD4^+$ T-cell responses. The patterns and characteristics of the immune response are often determined by the milieu of cytokines and chemokines and innate immune responses present at the time of the initial antigen encounter (72). Therefore, vaccines are a powerful way to direct the pattern of subsequent immune responses to viral pathogens. For example, alum adjuvant protein vaccines are more likely to induce Th2 $CD4^+$ T cells that produce interleukin 4 (IL-4), and gene-based vector vaccines are more likely to induce Th1 $CD4^+$ T cells and $CD8^+$ T cells that produce IFN-γ.

Adaptive Immunity

Adaptive immunity involves the capacity for immunologic memory and for evolving improved antigen recognition and effector functions after subsequent exposures to antigen. The major cellular components of the adaptive immune response include B and T lymphocytes. The relative importance of these two arms of the immune response varies with the particular viral infection. In general, antibodies are the major mediator of resistance to reinfection with virus, and $CD8^+$ T cells are the major mediator of clearing virus-infected cells. $CD4^+$ T cells are critical for the induction of robust antibody responses and important for "helping" $CD8^+$ T-cell responses; they also have potential for direct antiviral effector functions.

Antibody

Antibody is established as the key vaccine-induced effector mechanism for protection against virus diseases. The importance of antibody in protection against virus diseases has been demonstrated by the efficacy of passively administered antibody. Successful antibody prophylaxis has heralded subsequent vaccine development for polio, measles, varicella, hepatitis A, and hepatitis B. Passive antibody prophylaxis can also modulate some diseases for which no vaccine is available, like RSV disease and cytomegalovirus disease, suggesting that active vaccination for these diseases may also be possible.

Antibodies are thought to protect by "neutralizing" viral infectivity. Neutralization specifically refers to the property of reducing the number of infectious virus particles. Viruses are neutralized in vitro by antibodies using a wide variety of mechanisms. Antibodies can cause viral aggregation to effectively reduce the number of infectious units, inhibit virus attachment to cells, inhibit virus entry after attachment by inhibition of virus-cell fusion, or inhibit the release of newly formed virions from infected cells. There are both quantitative and qualitative features of antibody that affect neutralization potency. These include concentration, antibody-to-virus ratio, valency, state of polymerization, affinity, avidity, isotype, ability to bind the polyimmunoglobulin receptor, ability to fix complement, and specificity for a particular antigenic site (22). Recently, in vivo studies of neutralizing antibody protection against a chimeric SIV-HIV (SHIV) challenge suggested that the presence of the Fc receptor is needed for optimal virus neutralization and may be more important than complement binding (27).

Ideally, vaccine-induced protection will be mediated by antibody that has the right functional properties, magnitude, and specificity to completely neutralize virus and provide "sterilizing" immunity. Antibodies are a unique effector element of the adaptive immune response that can be maintained at protective levels prior to infection without causing harmful inflammation. Antibody is especially effective when the target organ for disease is distinct from the initial site of infection. For example, in measles, polio, hepatitis, or the viral encephalitides, in which viremia is required to cause significant clinical disease, vanishingly small amounts of preexisting antibody can protect. However, it is rarely possible to elicit sufficient antibody through vaccination to fully prevent virus infection. Therefore, vaccines that can induce both antibodies and virus-specific CD8$^+$ T cells (cytotoxic T cells) to rapidly eliminate residual virus-infected cells provide an extra measure of certainty that virus-mediated disease will be attenuated.

Specific antigen bound to the B-cell receptor triggers the B cell to proliferate and differentiate into antibody-producing plasma cells. Most plasma cells live for days to weeks, but some survive longer and are able to maintain levels of virus-specific antibody in serum for years. B cells can also undergo differentiation to become long-lived memory B cells. While these memory cells do not secrete significant amounts of antibody, they reside in the germinal centers of lymph nodes and express surface immunoglobulin that allows them to quickly respond to a subsequent encounter with a specific antigen.

Immunization can influence antibody-mediated immunity in many ways. First, by increasing the repertoire and the frequency of immunoglobulin receptors on memory B cells capable of recognizing a particular antigen, the kinetics of antibody production on subsequent exposure will be more rapid. Second, somatic hypermutation and B-cell selection result in antibodies of successively higher affinities, so repeated virus infection or immunization will cause affinity maturation. Therefore, multidose vaccine regimens or vaccination prior to primary infection will improve the affinity, magnitude, and duration of antibody persistence. Third, immunization with a vaccine formulation that promotes IFN-γ production will increase the production of the immunoglobulin G1 (IgG1) and IgG3 subclasses. Complement fixation is mediated by the CH2 region of the antibody Fc domain of IgM, IgG1, and IgG3, and complement binding can sometimes improve the neutralization potency of antibody. In contrast, IL-4 promotes IgE production and IgG4 production, which are less desirable responses to vaccination and can lead to allergic reactions. Finally, repeated immunization can improve the breadth of antibody responses to a particular virus by recruiting new responses to different antigenic regions. For example, there are five major antibody binding domains in influenza H3 hemagglutinin (HA) involved in virus neutralization. Repeated exposures to HA are needed to induce antibody to all domains (9).

CD8$^+$ T Cells

T-cell responses (cell-mediated immunity) are essential components of a successful immune response for many pathogens, especially for viruses. T cells express T-cell receptors (TCRs), which recognize specific peptide epitopes bound to MHC proteins on the surface of APCs. The cytotoxic-T-lymphocyte (CTL) TCR recognizes a short (8- to 10-amino-acid) peptide derived from an endogenously produced viral protein in the context of the MHC class I β_2-microglobulin heterodimer. Virtually all cells express MHC class I molecules and can be recognized by CTLs if they become infected by a virus. However, not all cells are equipped to effectively initiate a CTL response. For vaccine induction of virus-specific CD8$^+$ T cells, the antigen containing the relevant epitopes must be present in the cytosolic compartment of a DC that can process the antigen, liberate the epitope by proteolysis, and transport the peptide into the endoplasmic reticulum, where it can associate with the appropriate MHC class I molecule. Antigen presentation must then be accompanied by costimulatory signals that can activate T cells with relevant TCRs to proliferate and differentiate into effector and memory cells.

The importance of CTLs in recovery from viral infection is demonstrated by the frequency of severe viral infections associated with cellular immunodeficiencies and by the diverse strategies viruses use to escape CTL killing (63). Herpesviruses, poxviruses, and lentiviruses in particular have evolved mechanisms for interfering with antigen presentation or effector molecules required for CTL activity. The influence of CD8$^+$ CTL memory on the outcome of a subsequent virus exposure can be subtle and may depend on the absence or presence of other components of the immune response. The impact of the CTL response is critically dependent on the timing of response and the efficiency and specificity of cytolytic activity. The immune response gains advantage in cases in which virus replication and spread are slower or when the immune response is accelerated. More targeted, rapid killing of virus-infected cells and less bystander killing will reduce immunopathology and generally improve the clinical outcome.

No vaccine based on induction of CTL has ever been licensed, and this is generally a secondary goal to antibody induction in vaccine development. However, for viruses that effectively elude neutralizing antibody (e.g., HIV-1),

CD8$^+$ CTLs became the primary immunogenicity goal in current development programs. New technologies such as polychromatic flow cytometry (57) have made it possible to define functional subsets of T cells with more precision (17) and may provide the necessary tools for effectively targeting CTL induction in the future. Nevertheless, the hypothesis that a CTL-based viral vaccine will be effective in humans remains to be proven.

CD4$^+$ T Cells

CD4$^+$ T cells recognize peptide epitopes associated with the $\alpha\beta$ heterodimeric MHC class II molecules present on professional APCs. They have been categorized into an increasingly complex array of subpopulations (19, 52, 65). These include not only traditional T helper (Th) cells but also cells involved in regulating inflammatory cytokine responses (Th17 cells) and other T-cell responses (T regulatory cells). These subpopulations are important in molding the overall pattern of the subsequent immune response to viral infection and can be influenced by vaccine design and formulation. Th cells are CD4$^+$ T cells that provide help to B cells and CD8$^+$ T cells, thereby augmenting the two major effector mechanisms of the adaptive immune response. For example, Th1 cells are important for creating an IFN-γ-rich environment that promotes better cytolytic activity in CTLs and switching to more potent subclasses of antibody. Th2 cells produce IL-4, IL-5, IL-9, IL-10, and IL-13, which promote B-cell growth and differentiation but can also be associated with allergic inflammation. Antigen-specific Th1 and Th2 cells can be detected following vaccination (18, 45). Th cells can also provide direct antiviral activity in vivo (26, 44, 49, 67), although the contribution is less than that of CTLs, which is consistent with the limited distribution of MHC class II.

CD4$^+$ T-cell epitopes are more numerous on viral proteins than CTL epitopes (38), and some responses can induce a protective immune response in the absence of B cells or CTLs (44). CD4$^+$ T cells secrete IFN-γ, tumor necrosis factor alpha, and other soluble factors with direct antiviral activity. Interestingly, the processes involved in establishing CD4$^+$ T-cell memory are distinct from those involved in CD8$^+$ T-cell memory responses (76). Antigen processing and presentation, unlike for CD8$^+$ T cells, occur through the endocytic pathway, so induction can be achieved by killed virus vaccines or even purified proteins and does not require live virus or gene delivery approaches for cytosolic processing. CD4$^+$ T cells do not proliferate to the same extent as CD8$^+$ T cells during primary infection, and those producing IFN-γ only do not survive as long-lived memory cells (77). In addition, inducing antigen-specific CD4$^+$ CD25$^+$ T regulatory cells may dampen other components of the adaptive immune response and diminish the effector T-cell mechanism upon subsequent exposure to virus (7). Therefore, the pattern of CD4$^+$ T-cell induction is an important consideration in vaccine design.

Mucosal Immunity

Mucosal immunity refers to the local adaptive immune response at mucosal surfaces, including oral, upper and lower respiratory tract, gastrointestinal tract, and vaginal mucosae. The mucosal surface is the primary portal of entry for most viruses, and antigen-specific humoral and cellular immune responses can be found at those surfaces. Theoretically, when antigen-specific immunity can be induced at the mucosal site at risk for future virus exposure, in addition to induction of systemic responses, overall protection should be improved. The live attenuated nasally administered seasonal influenza vaccine is based on this principle. Poliovirus vaccines provide an example of how mucosal immunity influences wild-type virus replication patterns. The inactivated (Salk) poliovirus vaccine given parenterally produces antibody responses that block transmission of poliovirus from the gut via the circulation to anterior horn cells. This vaccine is highly efficacious for preventing paralysis but does not prevent infection and replication in the intestinal mucosa. In contrast, the live attenuated (Sabin) poliovirus vaccine protects against infection and prevents virus shedding. The importance of measurable evidence of mucosal immunity for vaccine-induced protection against other viruses is controversial.

The hallmark of mucosal immunity is the presence of IgA. Dimeric IgA present in plasma or produced locally is trancytosed through mucosal epithelium and when associated with J chain binds the polymeric immunoglobulin receptor prior to secretion. IgA is thought to be particularly important for defense against pathogens limited to mucosal surfaces. IgG antibody present in the systemic circulation often cannot fully protect against mucosal pathogens unless present at very high titers allowing for transudation. In general, the lung is more permissive to transudation of IgG than the nasopharynx, and the intestinal tract is even more resistant. IgA can be present at high concentrations in mucosal fluid and is more resistant to proteolysis in that environment. The concept of a common mucosal immune system in which mucosal immunity at one site confers protection at other mucosal sites has been demonstrated experimentally. However, in general, directly immunizing the mucosal surface at greatest risk of exposure will improve protection at that site. Although not well understood, this phenomenon may be related to observations that suggest that some effector cells can remain in tissue for long periods at the site of a prior infection or antigen exposure (80).

FORMULATION, ANTIGEN CONTENT, AND DELIVERY OF VIRAL VACCINES

Most licensed and investigational viral vaccines fall into one of seven categories: live attenuated vaccines, inactivated vaccines, subunit vaccines, virus-like particles, live or replication-defective vectors, or DNA plasmid vaccines (Table 3). The type of vaccine used for a particular viral pathogen and its formulation or adjuvant properties, antigen selection, schedule, and route of administration will all have profound effects on the types of immunologic effectors induced. Therefore, vaccine design should be informed by an understanding of the pathogenesis and the optimal form of immunity to a particular viral pathogen.

Adjuvants

Adjuvants are used to improve the magnitude, composition, quality, and duration of vaccine-induced humoral and cellular immune responses to viral antigens, Adjuvants have typically been empirically derived from natural products with immunostimulating properties. For example, the classical Freund's adjuvant is a derivative of mycobacterial cell walls. Analysis of Freund's adjuvant led to more distilled products like monophosphoryl lipid A and MF59, an

TABLE 3 Characteristics of vaccine approaches used to prevent viral diseases

Vaccine type	Prototype(s)	Induction of protective antibody	Induction of CD8$^+$ T-cell responses	Potential for mucosal delivery
Live attenuated virus	Sabin polio vaccine (OPV) or Flumist influenza vaccine	+++	+++	+++
Whole killed or inactivated virus	Salk polio vaccine (IPV) or traditional influenza vaccine	+++	+/−	+
Subunit or purified viral protein(s)	HBsAg—Recombivax HB, Energix-B, Twinrix	+++	+/−	+
Virus-like particles	HPV—Gardasil	+++	+	++
Live or replication-defective vectors[a]	Recombinant poxvirus or adenovirus vectors	++	+++	+++
DNA plasmids[a]	Naked DNA	+	+++	+

[a] Investigational approach in humans, although licensed veterinary vaccines utilize this technology.

oil-in-water emulsion. The active component in immune stimulating complexes derived from extracts of the soap bark tree (*Quillaja saponaria* Molina) was found in the 21st high-performance liquid chromatography peak of the bark extract, hence the name QS21.

The underlying mechanism of adjuvants has not been well understood. Traditional adjuvant concepts suggesting the importance of particulate antigen complexes, creation of antigen depots to prolong antigen persistence, or induction of nonspecific inflammation have given way to a more precise understanding of how the innate and adaptive immune responses are linked. The discovery of TLRs and their importance in pathogen recognition and immune activation has invigorated adjuvant development and will lead to new options for vaccine formulations. TLR ligands trigger signaling pathways that change the functional state of APCs and thereby control the pattern and timing of cytokine production, mobility, and expression of costimulatory molecules. Selecting individual cytokines or costimulatory molecules as vaccine adjuvants underestimates the complexity of the milieu and the importance of the timing involved in nascent immune responses. Using TLR ligands as vaccine adjuvants avoids the unanticipated problems that arise when using individual molecular adjuvants in isolation (47) and provides a more authentic stimulus for generating primary immune responses. Many empirically discovered adjuvants are now understood to be TLR ligands. For example, muramyl dipeptide derivatives and monophosphoryl lipid A stimulate TLR-2 and TLR-4, respectively. Imidazoquinoline compounds like imiquimod and resiquimod have been found to be agonists for TLR-7 and TLR-8 that are designed to recognize single-stranded RNA. Palindromic CpG sequences found in bacterial DNA are recognized by TLR-9. Using TLR ligands as adjuvants (43) or conjugates (74) will be an important thrust of future vaccine development.

Antigen Targets

The antigenic content in the vaccine confers specificity to the immune responses. For antibody-mediated protection, the surface glycoproteins and capsid proteins of viruses are the primary antigens to target in a vaccine-induced immune response. These are the proteins associated with tissue tropism, attachment, and entry. Most neutralizing antibodies recognize conformational epitopes, so in most cases it is important to mimic the native structure as much as possible. In some cases (e.g., HIV-1) this is extremely challenging because of the need for oligomeric structures, conformational flexibility and masking, variable glycosylation patterns, highly antigenic regions that are functionally unimportant that divert the recognition of functionally important epitopes, and genetic variation (16, 78). There is usually more than one antigenic site in a virus, and to reduce the risk of immune escape, antibody to multiple sites should be elicited.

Antigen selection for inducing CD8$^+$ T-cell responses involves a different set of considerations. CTLs recognize processed peptide epitopes in MHC class I molecules. Therefore, all viral proteins (surface proteins, internal structural proteins, and regulatory proteins) can serve as antigens because they are all produced in the cytoplasm and are susceptible to proteasomal degradation. Including a large portion of the viral antigenic content allows the APC to select the appropriate epitopes for association with the host MHC class I. Theoretically, another approach would be to build designer proteins with a high density of CTL epitopes separated by flanking sequences susceptible to processing. There are also theoretical advantages to using antigens that are produced in high abundance and early in the virus life cycle. This might allow earlier recognition of the virus-infected cell and more rapid clearance. In addition, there may also be advantages to using internal viral proteins because they are typically more conserved in viruses capable of genetic variation. The principles for developing vaccines based on CTL-mediated protection are not well established at this time, and no vaccine has ever been licensed based purely on its ability to induce a T-cell response.

Vaccine Delivery

The location and durability of vaccine-induced immune responses are affected by route and schedule of vaccine delivery. Currently licensed live virus vaccines are given on mucosal surfaces orally (rotavirus and polio) or by intranasal spray (influenza). They are also given by needle and syringe (measles-mumps-rubella [MMR] and varicella) or bifurcated needle in the case of vaccinia. Delivery of vaccines by needle and syringe intradermally (i.d.) may provide dose sparing. Seasonal influenza vaccine induces similar or improved immunogenicity when delivered i.d. at one-fifth the standard dose delivered intramuscularly (i.m.) (3, 15, 35). A similar finding has also been demonstrated with the licensed hepatitis B vaccine. Large-scale safety and immunogenicity studies were conducted by the U.S. Army to evaluate the dose-sparing potential of i.d. delivery for the licensed HBV vaccine. Delivery of the HBV vaccine by the i.d. route was safe and induced humoral immunogenicity at a lower magnitude (approximately 50% reduction) and a slightly lower frequency of immune response than traditional i.m. delivery (59). As new vaccine technologies emerge, new delivery approaches may include microneedles (6) or, for DNA vaccines, needle-free injection systems like Biojector or Powderject, or electroporation devices that have been reported to improve antigen expression and immunogenicity (42, 55).

Delivery vehicles can provide mechanisms to codeliver mixtures of antigens and adjuvant, protect antigens from a harsh environment, control the timing of antigen release, or carry antigens into subcellular compartments. A number of carriers for delivery of vaccine antigens are in development. For example, virus-derived proteins inserted into liposomal membranes are referred to as virosomes. Virosomes containing the HA of influenza virus are used in licensed products (non-U.S. products) to deliver vaccine antigens for influenza and hepatitis A (17). Immune stimulating complexes (ISCOMs) are 40-nm cage-like structures composed of lipids and saponins that can deliver viral antigens to the cytoplasmic compartment for processing and CTL activation (36). Microparticles or nanoparticles produced from synthetic polymers can be formulated with viral antigens or gene-based vectors for controlled release or delivery to selected cells (24, 79). Conjugates with carrier proteins also allow access to the cytoplasmic compartment of the APC.

Schedule of Immunization

The schedule of vaccine delivery and the concept of boosting are critical for establishing durable immunologic memory for many vaccines. In general, inactivated vaccines require at least two doses in a naïve host to establish a significant immune response. Even live viral vaccines benefit from booster doses (e.g., measles booster in adolescents). Boosting prolongs the duration of the memory immune response, and it may alter the character or breadth of the response by expanding the repertoire of antigens that stimulate an immune response (10, 30, 45, 60, 73). The classic indication of memory induction of the humoral immune response is isotype switching from antigen-specific IgM to IgG production, detected in the serum. Antigen-specific memory T cells may be present even in the absence of a detectable antibody response, as in the case of hepatitis B vaccine nonresponders (those with a negative HBV titer following the last vaccination in the series) (31). Homologous boosting with the same vaccine is used for most licensed vaccines (e.g., hepatitis A or B). Heterologous boosting or the concept of using one vaccine approach for priming and an alternative vaccine approach for boosting (prime-boost) may be important in the development of vector-based vaccines (61, 75) or for focusing the immune response on a particular antigenic site (28). Empirically it has been observed that as the interval between priming and boosting increases, the magnitude of the immune response improves (25). Considerations must be balanced between lengthening the vaccination schedule for potentially improved efficacy and shortening the schedule for efficiency, compliance, and earlier protection. Some insight into the value of lengthening the prime-boost interval has been gained by understanding the basic biology of T-cell memory. After immune stimulation, lymphocytes evolve through an activation phase in which cells are highly functional but susceptible to apoptosis from excessive stimulation. As the acute phase of the response resolves, a population of memory lymphocytes is established with the capacity for rapid expansion rather than apoptosis after antigen stimulation (23). As the tools for immune assessment improve, the rules for the prime-boost interval may be better tailored for each vaccine modality and be supported with a stronger scientific basis.

LICENSED VACCINES FOR VIRAL DISEASES

There are now licensed vaccines for preventing disease caused by 14 viral pathogens and 27 viral subtypes in the United States (Table 2). They can be divided into live viral vaccines and nonreplicating viral vaccines.

Live Virus Vaccines

Viral vaccines that contain live or replication-competent forms of the targeted viral agent are referred to as "live virus vaccines." In live virus vaccines, the infectious virus is attenuated to reduce virulence. Attenuated viruses are sometimes derived from naturally occurring isolates found to have low virulence or altered tropism (e.g., poliovirus 2). In most cases they are generated by performing serial passages of the virus in cell lines from an unnatural host. The underlying mechanism responsible for attenuating a pathogen during serial passage consists of spontaneous mutations that are selected by adaptation to the conditions of repeated passage in embryonated eggs or cell culture. Some of these mutations are associated with diminished pathogenicity in humans. Another source of live attenuated vaccine viruses comes from the "Jennerian" approach. Related viruses that have another species as a natural host are often highly attenuated in human hosts (e.g., rhesus or bovine rotavirus vaccines). Live virus vaccines induce immune responses that closely mimic responses to wild-type virus, including more authentic structures. Live virus vaccines typically activate all components of the immune response. Both antibody responses and virus-specific T-cell responses (including $CD8^+$ T-cell responses) to the potentially protective antigens contained in the virus are induced. The entire antigenic content of the pathogen is delivered by the live virus vaccine approach, and the antigen load is amplified by replication. Another advantage of live virus vaccines is that they can often be delivered to susceptible mucosal surfaces and elicit mucosal immune responses. Live virus vaccines are also associated with more durable immune responses and generally require fewer and less frequent booster vaccinations (54, 71). While there may be immunologic and protective advantages to the live virus vaccine approach, live vaccines may also have increased potential for adverse events. In rare cases, live vaccines may induce a mild or attenuated form of disease. Live virus vaccines are generally contraindicated in immunocompromised patients or in patients in close contact with immunocompromised individuals due to the risk of viral shedding and transmission in the postvaccination period (69). While live virus vaccines are generally easy to manufacture, production in mammalian cell substrates could introduce unexpected contaminants, virulence properties can change, and these vaccines are more susceptible to adverse storage conditions.

Nonreplicating Viral Vaccines

Many killed or inactivated and subunit viral vaccines have also been licensed for the prevention of viral diseases. These vaccines generally require at least two doses to invoke the optimal immune response, and they are generally safe and well tolerated. The major advantage of inactivated vaccines is that there is no risk of infection in the vaccinated patient or of transmission of live virus to potentially immunocompromised close contacts of vaccinees. A disadvantage of inactivated or killed vaccines is that they typically require multiple booster injections in the primary series or later in life to maintain a protective immune response in the majority of individuals. Inactivated influenza vaccines grown in eggs have been used since the 1940s. Hepatitis A vaccine is an example of an inactivated virus vaccine for which formulations are produced by infecting human diploid fibroblast lines (MRC-5) with HAV strains that have been found to be attenuated in humans. Virus from the infected cell line is formalin inactivated to produce a nonlive vaccine product (2). Hepatitis B vaccine represents a nonlive subunit vaccine formulation. Subunit HBV surface antigen (HbsAg) vaccine is produced in yeast cells by recombinant DNA technology (64). The vaccine is noninfectious but can induce transient serum HBsAg positivity (41). The vaccine is given in a three-dose schedule to infants, adolescents, or adults and results in seroconversion in >90% of patients who receive the three-dose regimen (1).

Recently Licensed Vaccines

Rotavirus Vaccine

Rotavirus is the most common cause of infant viral gastroenteritis worldwide and causes about 600,000 deaths in children <5 years of age per year. In 2006, an oral, live, pentavalent human-bovine reassortant rotavirus vaccine was licensed for use in the United States as a three-dose infant vaccine. The vaccine was found to be 63 to 98% efficacious in a phase III vaccine clinical trial of almost 70,000 infants worldwide (70) and is now routinely administered to infants in the United States as part of the recommended childhood vaccination schedule. Importantly, the first immunization with the vaccine should occur before 3 months of age to diminish the risk of intussusception.

HPV Vaccine

A vaccine for the prevention of disease caused by HPV types 6, 11, 16, and 18 was licensed for use in women in the United States in 2006. HPV types 6, 11, 16, and 18 are the etiologic agents responsible for 70% of HPV cases leading to cervical dysplasia and cervical cancer and 90% of cases of genital warts (4, 21). Vaccine efficacy was specifically demonstrated in women, and the product is licensed for women and girls 9 to 26 years of age. Further HPV vaccines representing these and other types of the virus are in development and undergoing clinical trials. The currently approved vaccine represents an important step toward the prevention of a sexually transmitted virus responsible for the majority of cases of cervical cancer. Another HPV vaccine in the final stages of clinical testing includes HPV types 16 and 18. Thus far, HPV vaccination has not been shown to be an effective therapeutic option for preexisting HPV infection (29).

Varicella-Zoster Therapeutic Vaccine

Live attenuated varicella-zoster vaccine has been effectively used to prevent chickenpox in children since 1995. In subsequent studies the vaccine was found to diminish cases of shingles caused by reactivation of latent varicella-zoster (56). The zoster vaccine is prepared as a lyophilized product and licensed for subcutaneous delivery in a single dose of 0.65 ml (19,400 PFU). It is indicated for the prevention but not for the treatment of herpes zoster in immunocompetent adults age 60 years and older (48).

Substrates and Additives in Vaccine Manufacturing

Viral vaccines are regulated by the U.S. Food and Drug Administration (FDA), Center for Biologics Evaluation and Research (CBER). Most viral vaccines are produced in cell substrates that involve mammalian, avian, insect, or bacterial cell culture. Good manufacturing practice requires rigorous record keeping and validated standard operating procedures that minimize the risk of contaminants or adventitious agents (http://www.fda.gov/cber/gdlns/vaccsubstrates.htm). Vaccine preparations are produced in bulk and stored or are formulated with diluents, adjuvants, and preservatives before packaging. Each step in the process in highly regulated, but biological products are complex and raise many theoretical issues that may require clinical consideration and must be balanced for each individual against the personal and public health benefits of vaccination. For example, the preservative thimerosal is an organomercurial compound used in trace or small amounts in some vaccine preparations (http://www.fda.gov/cber/vaccine/thimerosal.htm). Thimerosal is metabolized to ethylmercury but has been controversial because of the neurotoxicity associated with methylmercury. Ethylmercury is more rapidly excreted than methylmercury, and thimerosal has been given to animals and humans at doses well above 1 mg/kg of body weight without evidence of toxicity. The highest ethylmercury content in a 0.5-ml dose of any currently licensed vaccine is ~25 μg, and extensive clinical studies have not shown a causal relationship between thimerosal and neurologic events (66). However, because of ongoing public perception that it may be associated with neurocognitive or neurotoxic events and conditions such as autism, and ongoing efforts to improve vaccine safety and confidence, thimerosal has been removed from most licensed viral vaccines, especially childhood vaccines.

CLINICAL MANAGEMENT OF VACCINATION

Vaccination Schedules

The childhood and adult viral vaccine dosing schedules are routinely updated and listed in complete form by the Centers for Disease Control and Prevention (CDC) at http://www.cdc.gov/vaccines/recs/schedules/default.htm and by the WHO at http://www.who.int/topics/immunization/en/index.html.

When a vaccine regimen is given as a series of doses, the question may arise of what to do in the case of missed or delayed doses. In general, it is not recommended or immunologically necessary to repeat or restart a vaccination regimen or schedule. The vaccine schedule should be continued where it was left off, regardless of the length of time since prior vaccination. If there is concern regarding compliance and immune response, following the last dose of vaccine in a series, an antigen-specific antibody titer can be measured in patient serum to determine if the patient has developed an appropriate immune response. For example, in the case of the licensed hepatitis B vaccine, an anti-HBs antibody titer of ≥10 mIU/ml, determined by a commercially available immunoassay, correlates with protection from infection.

Live and killed viral vaccines can be administered simultaneously as recommended in published vaccination schedules (http://www.cdc.gov/vaccines/recs/schedules/default.htm). The general recommendation for administering multiple live vaccines is to administer them on the same day or, if that is not possible, to separate live vaccines by at least 4 weeks to allow for an optimal immune response to each vaccine. The recommendation is based on the premise that in the acute period of immune response to a live vaccine, additional immune responses to other live vaccines could be diminished because of innate immunity. Combination vaccines, with multiple vaccines coformulated and therefore coadministered, have become increasingly common, both for ease of administration and for improved compliance. Only licensed combination vaccine products that have been rigorously tested for safety, stability, and immunogenicity in combination with other vaccine(s) should be coadministered in a single syringe. Health care providers should follow manufacturers' guidance and label information and should not prepare off-label formulations or combinations of vaccines by combining separate vaccines into a single syringe at the time of vaccination. The formulations of different vaccine products may be incompatible or antagonistic and significantly alter the chemical and antigenic properties of the vaccine products. This type of off-label practice could potentially lead to adverse events or reduction of the vaccine-induced immune response.

It is important to review the recommended vaccine schedule on a routine basis. The recommendations change periodically in response to outbreaks of disease or newly available vaccine products. For example, after several years of fewer than 300 reported cases of mumps per year, there was a multistate outbreak in 2006 with 6,339 cases reported. These were primarily in college age students with a median age of 21 (13). The surge in U.S. mumps cases was preceded by a large increase in mumps cases in the United Kingdom in 2005. Many of the infected persons had been vaccinated, but it is likely that waning immunity, particularly in persons who had not received at least two doses of MMR vaccine, was in part responsible. Adolescents should receive a booster dose of MMR vaccine, especially if they plan to attend college or live in settings, like dormitories, where crowding may exist. Vaccine-induced immunity is not as long lasting as immunity induced by natural infection, and as infection dynamics evolve, vaccination schedules and clinicians will need to adapt.

Adverse Effects of Vaccination

Expected Adverse Events

Vaccines are an important public health measure and provide a safe and effective method to prevent infectious disease. Occasionally, vaccines have been linked to adverse events. Vaccine-related adverse events may be expected with systemic or local reactogenicity, as manifested by mild fever, myalgia, malaise, or vaccination site pain, tenderness, and erythema. In rare cases, unexpected adverse events may occur, including anaphylaxis resulting from an allergy to a vaccine component. Potential causes of vaccine-related anaphylaxis include reactions to residual egg or chicken protein in vaccines grown in chicken embryo fibroblasts or reactions to gelatin, which is a preservative in many vaccine formulations. Viral vaccines which may contain trace amounts of egg or chicken protein and therefore are contraindicated in egg-allergic patients include yellow fever vaccine, inactivated influenza vaccine, live attenuated intranasal influenza vaccine, and one formulation of the rabies vaccine. Although produced in a chicken embryo fibroblast substrate, MMR vaccine is not contraindicated in egg-allergic patients due to a lack of egg or chicken residual proteins in the final vaccine product.

Measles, mumps, rubella, varicella, Japanese encephalitis, yellow fever, and smallpox vaccines contain gelatin as a preservative and are contraindicated in individuals with a history of gelatin allergy. Once a patient has had an allergic reaction to a vaccine, or combination of vaccines, further vaccination with those vaccines or with vaccines containing the same components should be avoided and reconsidered only after a careful allergy evaluation is performed. Consultation with an allergist is indicated if allergy to a vaccine or to vaccine components is suspected.

The National Childhood Vaccine Injury Act of 1986 and The Vaccine Injury Compensation Program (VICP) (established in 1988) were established by the U.S. Congress as a "no fault" alternative to financially compensate patients or the families of patients who suffer from vaccine-related injuries. Viral vaccines covered by the VICP include hepatitis A, hepatitis B, HPV, seasonal influenza, measles, mumps, rubella, polio, rotavirus, and varicella. The VICP Vaccine Injury Table details the covered adverse events and time intervals from vaccination for each of the vaccines (http://www.hrsa.gov/vaccinecompensation/). Included in the table are anaphylaxis for most vaccines, encephalitis for MMR vaccine, chronic arthritis for rubella vaccine, and thrombocytopenic purpura for measles vaccine. While rare, if these adverse events occur within a specified time period after vaccination, and no other cause for the event can be identified, the patient may have a claim.

Prior to vaccination, health care providers should provide the patient or their guardian with a CDC Vaccine Information Statement (VIS) (http://www.cdc.gov/vaccines/pubs/vis/default.htm). This is required under U.S. federal law for all vaccines covered by the VICP. It is strongly recommended for all other vaccines. The CDC routinely updates current VIS forms on the CDC website to be printed by providers and their staff. The provider should document the date and version of the VIS form and note that the VIS was provided in the medical record for each vaccination.

Rare or Idiosyncratic Adverse Events Related to Vaccination

Routine smallpox vaccinations in the U.S. civilian population were discontinued in 1972 but were continued in the U.S. military until 1990. Due to concerns about the possible risks of bioterrorism attacks, the U.S. military and a portion of the U.S. civilian population began to receive smallpox vaccination again in the winter of 2002–2003. Although individuals at increased risk of predictable vaccine-related adverse events were excluded, an unexpected adverse event, myopericarditis, was seen in approximately 1 in 12,000 primary vaccinees (usually within 30 days) following Dryvax vaccination (12). This finding, along with previously documented risks of adverse events, has led to multiple contraindications for prophylactic smallpox vaccination, including past or present atopic dermatitis, compromised immune system (HIV/AIDS, autoimmune disease, most malignancies, and immunosuppressive medications), known or possible coronary artery disease, cerebral vascular disease, pregnancy, and breastfeeding. In the event of a smallpox outbreak or exposure, these contraindications would likely be disregarded and public health officials would make revised recommendations at that time.

A formalin-inactivated whole-virus RSV vaccine (FI-RSV) was studied in infants and children in the 1960s, when Tween-ether and formalin-inactivated measles virus was still being used. The RSV vaccine did not prevent infection and was associated with enhanced disease that was particularly severe in the youngest age group, those <6 months (14, 20). Both FI-RSV-enhanced illness and atypical measles, an aberrant illness caused by infection several years after vaccination with inactivated measles vaccine when neutralizing antibody activity had waned, are thought to be consequences of similar combinations of immunologic events. First, enhanced illness occurred when vaccine-induced antibody did not have significant neutralizing or fusion-inhibiting activity and did not prevent infection (51). Second, vaccine-induced antibody had complement-fixing properties, and immune complex deposition could be demonstrated in affected tissue (58). Third, there was an exaggerated $CD4^+$ T-cell response associated with eosinophilia (14, 37). Animal models of FI-RSV and measles suggest that this was caused by a Th2 (58)-biased response, with production of IL-4, IL-5, and IL-13 and eosinophilia (32).

An oral tetravalent rotavirus vaccine (Rotashield) was licensed for use in the United States in 1998 but was withdrawn from use due to a possible link to intussusception (53). The vaccine was associated with an increased rate of intussusception in up to 1 per 2,500 vaccinees, primarily following the first dose of vaccine (50). Subsequent epidemiological studies led to a significant decrease in the estimates and suggested that the early period of increase in intussusception seen after the first dose was compensated by lower rates after subsequent doses, resulting in no net overall increase in the number of cases in vaccinees less than 1 year of age (50). The cases occurred predominantly when the vaccine was started in children 3 months of age or older, rather than in children who received the recommended schedule (2, 4, and 6 months of age) (22, 33, 62).

Adverse events (local and systemic reactogenicity) related to seasonal influenza vaccines are generally mild, including localized redness or swelling or mild fever and muscle aches. Intranasal live attenuated influenza vaccine can also be associated with mild rhinitis-like symptoms, headache, muscle aches, and fever. There have been rare moderate to severe, unexpected adverse events associated with influenza vaccines. In 1976 the influenza vaccine (swine flu vaccine) was associated with Guillain-Barré syndrome (GBS) at a very low rate (~1 to 10 per 1 million persons vaccinated). A causal relationship between influenza vaccine and GBS was not clearly identified, but due to the historical association, influenza vaccine is contraindicated in individuals with a history of GBS.

Reporting Vaccine-Related Adverse Events

Following licensure of a vaccine, adverse events which are clinically significant or unexpected, as well as events listed in the Reportable Events Table (http://vaers.hhs.gov/pdf/ReportableEventsTable.pdf) and in the manufacturers' package insert, should be reported to the Vaccine Adverse Event Reporting System (VAERS) (http://vaers.hhs.gov/). VAERS is a passive surveillance cooperative program between the CDC and the FDA. Any possibly related or temporally related vaccine side effects may be reported by any health care provider, patient, or patient guardian or representative. VAERS is public and represents unverified reports of possible vaccine-related adverse events. VAERS allows public health experts to identify rare adverse events that may not be discovered during vaccine clinical trials due to their low rates of occurrence (68). Potential vaccine-related concerns in the VAERS database are further investigated and/or verified by the CDC Vaccine Safety Datalink Project (http://www.cdc.gov/od/science/iso/research_activities/vsdp.htm).

Contraindications to Vaccination

Prior to each vaccination the health care provider should assess the patient for possible contraindications to vaccination, including a history of adverse or allergic reactions to a previous vaccination, underlying illness, or allergy. For live-vaccine administration the provider should assess the possibility of immunodeficiency or the potential for patient contact with an immunocompromised individual. Vaccination is contraindicated if there is a known hypersensitivity to the vaccine or to any of the vaccine components. Egg and gelatin allergies are important considerations due to the potential for reactions to vaccines containing them and the prevalence of sensitivity to those components. Allergy consultation is recommended if vaccination is necessary and there is concern about a potential vaccine or vaccine component allergy.

Vaccination of Immunocompromised Individuals

The issue of which viral vaccines should be administered to immunocompromised individuals is complex. Factors that affect the decision include the degree and type of immunosuppression, the overall state of health of the patient, and the type of vaccine to be administered. In general, the most effective way of protecting people with immunodeficiencies from vaccine-preventable diseases is to make sure the people around them are well vaccinated and are not transmitters of infection. If immunization is necessary, the focus should be on nonreplicating vaccines. Schedules for vaccinating selected subgroups of immunocompromised individuals can be found on the second page of the Recommended Adult Immunization Schedule Table at the CDC website (http://www.cdc.gov/vaccines/) by following the link to "immunization schedules."

Live viral vaccines are generally contraindicated in immunocompromised patients and in some cases if the patient has close contact with an immunocompromised person (e.g., smallpox vaccine). Patients undergoing chemotherapy or radiation treatment should avoid live viral vaccines, but in some cases (e.g., varicella) their close contacts should be vaccinated to protect the immunocompromised patient. Measles and varicella vaccines can be administered following cessation of chemotherapy (>3 months or later for measles), if no other contraindication exists. Live viral vaccines, such as varicella or smallpox vaccine, are contraindicated in severely immunosuppressed individuals because there is a risk of disseminated infection with the vaccine virus that can be severe in these patients. Disorders associated with T-cell immunodeficiency are associated with severe disease more often than immunoglobulin disorders. An exception to this is severe enterovirus infection (including poliovirus) in persons with immunoglobulin deficiency.

Nonreplicating viral vaccines do not pose an increased risk to immunocompromised individuals, although the response to a vaccine may be diminished or absent depending on the ability of the adaptive immune system to recognize and respond to the vaccine antigens. For example, the immune response to influenza vaccine has been shown to be reduced in some children with malignancy (11). Persons with renal failure on dialysis often do not make a sufficient antibody to hepatitis B vaccines that are otherwise extremely immunogenic (34). As noted, it is best to vaccinate when host responses are intact and to otherwise follow the national guidance for immunization of persons with selected immunodeficiencies.

LICENSED PRODUCTS FOR PASSIVE IMMUNIZATION

When active immunization is not possible, transient protection from disease or infection can be passively acquired by administration of human polyclonal immune globulin known to have a high titer of antibody against a specific viral pathogen, or virus-specific humanized monoclonal antibodies. Like vaccines, licensed immune globulin products for use in humans are regulated by the FDA, CBER. Human immune globulins are licensed for use in the United States against cytomegalovirus, RSV, vaccinia, varicella-zoster, rabies, and hepatitis B.

Preexposure Prophylaxis

In the past, prophylactic immune globulin was used for protecting travelers against hepatitis A, but it has since been replaced by an effective vaccine. Currently, the only passive antibody prophylaxis in widespread use is for RSV. RSV immune globulin (RespiGam) was indicated for the prevention of serious respiratory disease from RSV infection in high-risk children <2 years of age, but it is no longer in use. A humanized monoclonal antibody against the F glycoprotein of RSV (palivizumab; trade name, Synagis) is indicated for the prevention of serious respiratory disease from RSV infection in high-risk children <2 years of age. Risk factors for severe respiratory disease from RSV include bronchopulmonary dysplasia, premature birth (≤35 weeks), and hemodynamically significant congenital heart disease.

Postexposure Prophylaxis

Rabies immune globulin is given to nonimmune individuals in conjunction with active rabies vaccination following potential or confirmed rabies exposure, such as in the case of animal bites. The wound should be infiltrated with immune globulin at the time of or within 8 days of the first dose of rabies vaccine. Hepatitis B immune globulin is administered to nonimmune individuals exposed to hepatitis B as postexposure prophylaxis, and in that setting it is usually given in association with hepatitis B vaccination. It should be administered within 24 h of exposure to hepatitis B by needlestick, ocular, or mucosal exposure or within 14 days of a potential sexual exposure. Hepatitis B immune globulin is given to newborns of infected mothers (HBsAg positive) within 12 h of birth and again at 3 months of age. Hepatitis B immune globulin is indicated only for prophylaxis and not for the treatment of hepatitis B (active or chronic). Vaccinia immune globulin is indicated for the treatment of smallpox vaccine-related complications, including eczema vaccinatum, progressive vaccinia, and severe generalized vaccinia. Varicella-zoster immune globulin (VariZIG) is an investigational agent which may be useful for the prevention of VZV infection in immunocompromised individuals exposed to VZV. It can be obtained from the manufacturer, under an Investigational New Drug application with the FDA, in affiliation with the CDC and in conjunction with informed consent and local institutional review board approvals.

Adverse Effects and Contraindications to Passive Antibody

Human immune globulin products may contain trace amounts of human IgA. IgA deficiency is the most common cause of primary immunodeficiency, affecting approximately 1 in 500 people, and is often undiagnosed. In rare cases, individuals with IgA deficiency can develop IgE against IgA and experience anaphylaxis upon exposure to human blood products containing IgA, including immune globulins. IgA deficiency is a relative contraindication to receipt of human immune globulin products, and this should be considered prior to administration.

Immune globulin can inhibit the immune response induced by some live viral vaccines. This may occur because virus-specific serum antibody binds to and inhibits live virus vaccine replication and therefore prevents the intended immune response. Varicella vaccination can be inhibited up to 5 months following administration of human immune globulin containing antivaricella antibodies, and rubella vaccination can be affected up to 3 months following immune globulin administration. Ideally, vaccination with varicella and rubella vaccines should be delayed by 5 and 3 months, respectively, following the administration of immune globulin. In cases in which immune globulin is administered to a patient within 3 weeks after MMR or varicella vaccination, the immune response to those live vaccines may be blunted. In that situation, revaccination after 3 to 5 months is recommended if there are no other contraindications. Hepatitis B vaccine can be administered at the same time as hepatitis B immune globulin, or ≥1 month following the administration of immune globulin. The immune response to yellow fever vaccine does not appear to be inhibited by the presence of immune globulin at the time of or following vaccination.

VACCINE DEVELOPMENT AND FUTURE DIRECTIONS

Vaccine development in the 21st century promises new paradigms for design, manufacturing, immune response evaluation, and time lines. While empiricism will always contribute to scientific advances, vaccine development in the future will be guided more by rational design and a deeper understanding of the underlying molecular pathogenesis of disease. The best example of this will be adjuvant developments based on new discoveries and understanding of TLRs. Sequencing technology and advances in molecular virology have allowed rapid identification of new pathogens and flexibility in vaccine design. In addition to the traditional platforms of live attenuated, whole inactivated, and protein subunit vaccines, there are a variety of gene-based delivery approaches using DNA, RNA, or microbial vectors and virus-like particles that will become part of the repertoire of licensed vaccines. Vector-based vaccines and DNA vaccines using gene delivery of vaccine antigens have already been approved for veterinary use for several viral diseases. The capacity to perform more high-throughput structural analyses of proteins and improved methods for carbohydrate analysis have opened the possibility for a structure-based approach to vaccine design and a more precise understanding of immune mechanisms of protection. New technologies have allowed the evaluation of functional immune responses at the level of individual cells and prompted the development and evaluation of T-cell-based vaccine concepts in addition to the traditional concepts of immunity based on antibody responses. Rapid advances in human genetics have created the possibility of designer vaccines that can take advantage of certain host polymorphisms to improve immunity and avoid others to reduce side effects.

Significant biological hurdles still exist for developing effective vaccines to prevent viral infections with large disease burdens like HIV-1, RSV, dengue virus, and HSV, and there is great effort to find effective vaccines for these viruses using modern, highly technical approaches. For viral infections with the potential for sporadic epidemics or intentional release and high disease severity like orthopoxviruses, influenza viruses, filoviruses, and flaviviruses, the challenges are both biological and strategic. The same is true for emerging pathogens with the potential for pandemic spread, like influenza A (H5N1) virus or severe acute respiratory syndrome coronavirus, for which the probability of an outbreak is uncertain. One approach for addressing the strategic issues involving emerging infections and biodefense has been to establish a stockpile of available vaccines and other prophylactic and therapeutic agents under Project Bioshield (http://www.hhs.gov/aspr/barda/bioshield/). Additional research and development are also needed to establish platform vaccine technologies that can be rapidly adapted and deployed against new viral pathogens that will inevitably emerge. Finally, overcoming the political and social obstacles that restrict the distribution and delivery of existing vaccines to regions of the world where they are not widely utilized would dramatically improve global health.

REFERENCES

1. **Andre, F. E.** 1990. Overview of a 5-year clinical experience with a yeast-derived hepatitis B vaccine. *Vaccine* **8**(Suppl.)**:**S74–S78; discussion, S79–S80.
2. **Armstrong, M. E., P. A. Giesa, J. P. Davide, F. Redner, J. A. Waterbury, A. E. Rhoad, R. D. Keys, P. J. Provost, and J. A. Lewis.** 1993. Development of the formalin-inactivated hepatitis A vaccine, VAQTA from the live attenuated virus strain CR326F. *J. Hepatol.* **18**(Suppl. 2)**:** S20–S26.
3. **Auewarakul, P., U. Kositanont, P. Sornsathapornkul, P. Tothong, R. Kanyok, and P. Thongcharoen.** 2007. Antibody responses after dose-sparing intradermal influenza vaccination. *Vaccine* **25:**659–663.
4. **Ault, K. A.** 2007. Effect of prophylactic human papillomavirus L1 virus-like-particle vaccine on risk of cervical intraepithelial neoplasia grade 2, grade 3, and adenocarcinoma in situ: a combined analysis of four randomised clinical trials. *Lancet* **369:**1861–1868.
5. **Barton, G. M.** 2007. Viral recognition by Toll-like receptors. *Semin. Immunol.* **19:**33–40.
6. **Beasley, D. W., C. T. Davis, M. Whiteman, B. Granwehr, R. M. Kinney, and A. D. Barrett.** 2004. Molecular determinants of virulence of West Nile virus in North America. *Arch. Virol. Suppl.* **2004:**35–41.
7. **Belkaid, Y., and B. T. Rouse.** 2005. Natural regulatory T cells in infectious disease. *Nat. Immunol.* **6:**353–360.
8. **Bowie, A. G., and K. A. Fitzgerald.** 2007. RIG-I: tri-ing to discriminate between self and non-self RNA. *Trends Immunol.* **28:**147–150.
9. **Brecht, H., U. Hammerling, and R. Rott.** 1971. Undisturbed release of influenza virus in the presence of univalent antineuraminidase antibodies. *Virology* **46:**337–343.
10. **Brinkman, D. M., C. M. Jol-van der Zijde, M. M. ten Dam, J. M. Vossen, A. D. Osterhaus, F. P. Kroon, and M. J. van Tol.** 2003. Vaccination with rabies to study the humoral and cellular immune response to a T-cell dependent neoantigen in man. *J. Clin. Immunol.* **23:**528–538.
11. **Brydak, L. B., R. Rokicka-Milewska, M. Machala, T. Jackowska, and B. Sikorska-Fic.** 1998. Immunogenicity of subunit trivalent influenza vaccine in children with acute lymphoblastic leukemia. *Pediatr. Infect. Dis. J.* **17:** 125–129.
12. **Cassimatis, D. C., J. E. Atwood, R. M. Engler, P. E. Linz, J. D. Grabenstein, and M. N. Vernalis.** 2004. Smallpox vaccination and myopericarditis: a clinical review. *J. Am. Coll. Cardiol.* **43:**1503–1510.
13. **Centers for Disease Control and Prevention.** 18 May 2006, posting date. Update: multistate outbreak of mumps—United States, January 1–May 2, 2006. http://www.cdc.gov/vaccines/vpd-vac/mumps/outbreak/default.htm.
14. **Chin, J., R. Magoffin, L. Shearer, J. Schieble, and E. Lennett.** 1969. Field evaluation of a respiratory syncytial virus vaccine and a trivalent parainfluenza virus vaccine in a pediatric population. *Am. J. Epidemiol.* **89:**449–463.
15. **Chiu, S. S., J. S. Peiris, K. H. Chan, W. H. Wong, and Y. L. Lau.** 2007. Immunogenicity and safety of intradermal influenza immunization at a reduced dose in healthy children. *Pediatrics* **119:**1076–1082.
16. **Decker, J. M., F. Bibollet-Ruche, X. Wei, S. Wang, D. N. Levy, W. Wang, E. Delaporte, M. Peeters, C. A. Derdeyn, S. Allen, E. Hunter, M. S. Saag, J. A. Hoxie, B. H. Hahn, P. D. Kwong, J. E. Robinson, and G. M. Shaw.** 2005. Antigenic conservation and immunogenicity of the HIV coreceptor binding site. *J. Exp. Med.* **201:** 1407–1419.
17. **De Rosa, S. C., F. X. Lu, J. Yu, S. P. Perfetto, J. Falloon, S. Moser, T. G. Evans, R. Koup, C. J. Miller, and M. Roederer.** 2004. Vaccination in humans generates broad T cell cytokine responses. *J. Immunol.* **173:**5372–5380.
18. **Dhiman, N., I. G. Ovsyannikova, J. E. Ryan, R. M. Jacobson, R. A. Vierkant, V. S. Pankratz, S. J. Jacobsen, and G. A. Poland.** 2005. Correlations among measles virus-specific antibody, lymphoproliferation and Th1/Th2 cytokine responses following measles-mumps-rubella-II (MMR-II) vaccination. *Clin. Exp. Immunol.* **142:**498–504.
19. **Douek, D. C., L. J. Picker, and R. A. Koup.** 2003. T cell dynamics in HIV-1 infection. *Annu. Rev. Immunol.* **21:**265–304.

20. **Dudas, R. A., and R. A. Karron.** 1998. Respiratory syncytial virus vaccines. *Clin. Microbiol. Rev.* **11:**430–439.
21. **FUTURE II Study Group.** 2007. Quadrivalent vaccine against human papillomavirus to prevent high-grade cervical lesions. *N. Engl. J. Med.* **356:**1915–1927.
22. **Graham, B. S., and J. E. Crow.** 2007. Immunization against viral diseases, p. 487–538. *In* D. M. Knipe, P. M. Howley, D. E. Griffin, R. A. Lamb, M. A. Martin, B. Roizman, and S. E. Straus (ed.), *Fields Virology*, 5th ed., vol. 1. Lippincott Williams & Wilkins, Philadelphia, PA.
23. **Grayson, J. M., L. E. Harrington, J. G. Lanier, E. J. Wherry, and R. Ahmed.** 2002. Differential sensitivity of naive and memory CD8+ T cells to apoptosis in vivo. *J. Immunol.* **169:**3760–3770.
24. **Greenland, J. R., and N. L. Letvin.** 2007. Chemical adjuvants for plasmid DNA vaccines. *Vaccine* **25:**3731–3741.
25. **Hadler, S. C., M. A. de Monzon, D. R. Lugo, and M. Perez.** 1989. Effect of timing of hepatitis B vaccine doses on response to vaccine in Yucpa Indians. *Vaccine* **7:**106–110.
26. **Hasenkrug, K. J., D. M. Brooks, and U. Dittmer.** 1998. Critical role for CD4+ T cells in controlling retrovirus replication and spread in persistently infected mice. *J. Virol.* **72:**6559–6564.
27. **Hessell, A. J., L. Hangartner, M. Hunter, C. E. Havenith, F. J. Beurskens, J. M. Bakker, C. M. Lanigan, G. Landucci, D. N. Forthal, P. W. Parren, P. A. Marx, and D. R. Burton.** 2007. Fc receptor but not complement binding is important in antibody protection against HIV. *Nature* **449:**101–104.
28. **Hijnen, M., D. J. van Zoelen, C. Chamorro, P. van Gageldonk, F. R. Mooi, G. Berbers, and R. M. Liskamp.** 2007. A novel strategy to mimic discontinuous protective epitopes using a synthetic scaffold. *Vaccine* **25:**6807–6817.
29. **Hildesheim, A., R. Herrero, S. Wacholder, A. C. Rodriguez, D. Solomon, M. C. Bratti, J. T. Schiller, P. Gonzalez, G. Dubin, C. Porras, S. E. Jimenez, and D. R. Lowy.** 2007. Effect of human papillomavirus 16/18 L1 viruslike particle vaccine among young women with preexisting infection: a randomized trial. *JAMA* **298:**743–753.
30. **Holodniy, M.** 2006. Prevention of shingles by varicella zoster virus vaccination. *Expert Rev. Vaccines* **5:**431–443.
31. **Jarrosson, L., M. N. Kolopp-Sarda, P. Aguilar, M. C. Bene, M. L. Lepori, M. C. Vignaud, G. C. Faure, and C. Kohler.** 2004. Most humoral non-responders to hepatitis B vaccines develop HBV-specific cellular immune responses. *Vaccine* **22:**3789–3796.
32. **Johnson, T. R., R. A. Parker, J. E. Johnson, and B. S. Graham.** 2003. IL-13 is sufficient for respiratory syncytial virus G glycoprotein-induced eosinophilia after respiratory syncytial virus challenge. *J. Immunol.* **170:**2037–2045.
33. **Kapikian, A. Z., L. Simonsen, T. Vesikari, Y. Hoshino, D. M. Morens, R. M. Chanock, J. R. La Montagne, and B. R. Murphy.** 2005. A hexavalent human rotavirus-bovine rotavirus (UK) reassortant vaccine designed for use in developing countries and delivered in a schedule with the potential to eliminate the risk of intussusception. *J. Infect. Dis.* **192**(Suppl. 1)**:**S22–S29.
34. **Karahocagil, M. K., T. Buzgan, H. Irmak, H. Karsen, H. Akdeniz, and N. Akman.** 2006. Comparison of intramuscular and intradermal applications of hepatitis B vaccine in hemodialysis patients. *Renal Fail.* **28:**561–565.
35. **Kenney, R. T., S. A. Frech, L. R. Muenz, C. P. Villar, and G. M. Glenn.** 2004. Dose sparing with intradermal injection of influenza vaccine. *N. Engl. J. Med.* **351:**2295–2301.
36. **Khurana, S., J. Needham, S. Park, B. Mathieson, M. P. Busch, G. Nemo, P. Nyambi, S. Zolla-Pazner, S. Laal, J. Mulenga, E. Chomba, E. Hunter, S. Allen, J. McIntyre, I. Hewlett, S. Lee, S. Tang, E. Cowan, C. Beyrer, M. Altfeld, X. G. Yu, A. Tounkara, O. Koita, A. Kamali, N. Nguyen, B. S. Graham, D. Todd, P. Mugenyi, O. Anzala, E. Sanders, N. Ketter, P. Fast, and H. Golding.** 2006. Novel approach for differential diagnosis of HIV infections in the face of vaccine-generated antibodies: utility for detection of diverse HIV-1 subtypes. *J. Acquir. Immune Defic. Syndr.* **43:**304–312.
37. **Kim, H. W., S. L. Leikin, J. Arrobio, C. D. Brandt, R. M. Chanock, and R. H. Parrott.** 1976. Cell-mediated immunity to respiratory syncytial virus induced by inactivated vaccine or by infection. *Pediatr. Res.* **10:**75–78.
38. **Kundig, T. M., I. Castelmur, M. F. Bachmann, D. Abraham, D. Binder, H. Hengartner, and R. M. Zinkernagel.** 1993. Fewer protective cytotoxic T-cell epitopes than T-helper-cell epitopes on vesicular stomatitis virus. *J. Virol.* **67:**3680–3683.
39. **Kurt-Jones, E. A., L. Popova, L. Kwinn, L. M. Haynes, L. P. Jones, R. A. Tripp, E. E. Walsh, M. W. Freeman, D. T. Golenbock, L. J. Anderson, and R. W. Finberg.** 2000. Pattern recognition receptors TLR4 and CD14 mediate response to respiratory syncytial virus. *Nat. Immunol.* **1:**398–401.
40. **Lore, K., W. C. Adams, M. J. Havenga, M. L. Precopio, L. Holterman, J. Goudsmit, and R. A. Koup.** 2007. Myeloid and plasmacytoid dendritic cells are susceptible to recombinant adenovirus vectors and stimulate polyfunctional memory T cell responses. *J. Immunol.* **179:**1721–1729.
41. **Lunn, E. R., B. J. Hoggarth, and W. J. Cook.** 2000. Prolonged hepatitis B surface antigenemia after vaccination. *Pediatrics* **105:**E81.
42. **Luxembourg, A., D. Hannaman, B. Ellefsen, G. Nakamura, and R. Bernard.** 2006. Enhancement of immune responses to an HBV DNA vaccine by electroporation. *Vaccine* **24:**4490–4493.
43. **Ma, R., J. L. Du, J. Huang, and C. Y. Wu.** 2007. Additive effects of CpG ODN and R-848 as adjuvants on augmenting immune responses to HBsAg vaccination. *Biochem. Biophys. Res. Commun.* **361:**537–542.
44. **Manickan, E., M. Francotte, N. Kuklin, M. Dewerchin, C. Molitor, D. Gheysen, M. Slaoui, and B. T. Rouse.** 1995. Vaccination with recombinant vaccinia viruses expressing ICP27 induces protective immunity against herpes simplex virus through CD4+ Th1+ T cells. *J. Virol.* **69:**4711–4716.
45. **McElhaney, J. E., J. W. Hooton, N. Hooton, and R. C. Bleackley.** 2005. Comparison of single versus booster dose of influenza vaccination on humoral and cellular immune responses in older adults. *Vaccine* **23:**3294–3300.
46. **Medzhitov, R., and C. A. Janeway, Jr.** 2002. Decoding the patterns of self and nonself by the innate immune system. *Science* **296:**298–300.
47. **Mehrishi, J. N., M. Szabo, and T. Bakacs.** 2007. Some aspects of the recombinantly expressed humanised superagonist anti-CD28 mAb, TGN1412 trial catastrophe lessons to safeguard mAbs and vaccine trials. *Vaccine* **25:**3517–3523.
48. **Merck & Co., Inc.** 2006, posting date. http://www.zostavax.com. Product information.
49. **Mozdzanowska, K., M. Furchner, K. Maiese, and W. Gerhard.** 1997. CD4+ T cells are ineffective in clearing a pulmonary infection with influenza type A virus in the absence of B cells. *Virology* **239:**217–225.

50. **Murphy, B. R., D. M. Morens, L. Simonsen, R. M. Chanock, J. R. La Montagne, and A. Z. Kapikian.** 2003. Reappraisal of the association of intussusception with the licensed live rotavirus vaccine challenges initial conclusions. *J. Infect. Dis.* **187:**1301–1308.
51. **Murphy, B. R., G. A. Prince, E. E. Walsh, H. W. Kim, R. H. Parrott, V. G. Hemming, W. J. Rodriguez, and R. M. Chanock.** 1986. Dissociation between serum neutralizing and glycoprotein antibody responses of infants and children who received inactivated respiratory syncytial virus vaccine. *J. Clin. Microbiol.* **24:**197–202.
52. **Murphy, K. M., and S. L. Reiner.** 2002. The lineage decisions of helper T cells. *Nat. Rev. Immunol.* **2:**933–944.
53. **Murphy, T. V., P. M. Gargiullo, M. S. Massoudi, D. B. Nelson, A. O. Jumaan, C. A. Okoro, L. R. Zanardi, S. Setia, E. Fair, C. W. LeBaron, M. Wharton, and J. R. Livengood.** 2001. Intussusception among infants given an oral rotavirus vaccine. *N. Engl. J. Med.* **344:**564–572.
54. **Ogra, P. L.** 1995. Comparative evaluation of immunization with live attenuated and inactivated poliovirus vaccines. *Ann. N. Y. Acad. Sci.* **754:**97–107.
55. **Otten, G. R., M. Schaefer, B. Doe, H. Liu, J. Z. Megede, J. Donnelly, D. Rabussay, S. Barnett, and J. B. Ulmer.** 2006. Potent immunogenicity of an HIV-1 gag-pol fusion DNA vaccine delivered by in vivo electroporation. *Vaccine* **24:**4503–4509.
56. **Oxman, M. N., M. J. Levin, G. R. Johnson, K. E. Schmader, S. E. Straus, L. D. Gelb, R. D. Arbeit, M. S. Simberkoff, A. A. Gershon, L. E. Davis, A. Weinberg, K. D. Boardman, H. M. Williams, J. H. Zhang, P. N. Peduzzi, C. E. Beisel, V. A. Morrison, J. C. Guatelli, P. A. Brooks, C. A. Kauffman, C. T. Pachucki, K. M. Neuzil, R. F. Betts, P. F. Wright, M. R. Griffin, P. Brunell, N. E. Soto, A. R. Marques, S. K. Keay, R. P. Goodman, D. J. Cotton, J. W. Gnann, Jr., J. Loutit, M. Holodniy, W. A. Keitel, G. E. Crawford, S. S. Yeh, Z. Lobo, J. F. Toney, R. N. Greenberg, P. M. Keller, R. Harbecke, A. R. Hayward, M. R. Irwin, T. C. Kyriakides, C. Y. Chan, I. S. Chan, W. W. Wang, P. W. Annunziato, and J. L. Silber.** 2005. A vaccine to prevent herpes zoster and postherpetic neuralgia in older adults. *N. Engl. J. Med.* **352:**2271–2284.
57. **Perfetto, S. P., P. K. Chattopadhyay, and M. Roederer.** 2004. Seventeen-colour flow cytometry: unravelling the immune system. *Nat. Rev. Immunol.* **4:**648–655.
58. **Polack, F. P., M. N. Teng, P. L. Collins, G. A. Prince, M. Exner, H. Regele, D. D. Lirman, R. Rabold, S. J. Hoffman, C. L. Karp, S. R. Kleeberger, M. Wills-Karp, and R. A. Karron.** 2002. A role for immune complexes in enhanced respiratory syncytial virus disease. *J. Exp. Med.* **196:**859–865.
59. **Ronish, R. H., B. M. Diniega, P. W. Kelley, M. H. Sjogren, D. R. Arday, N. E. Aronson, C. H. Hoke, and B. P. Petruccelli.** 1991. Immunogenicity achieved by the intradermal hepatitis B vaccination programme for US Army soldiers in Korea. *Vaccine* **9:**364–368.
60. **Schmidtke, P., P. Habermehl, M. Knuf, C. U. Meyer, R. Sanger, and F. Zepp.** 2005. Cell mediated and antibody immune response to inactivated hepatitis A vaccine. *Vaccine* **23:**5127–5132.
61. **Seaman, M. S., L. Xu, K. Beaudry, K. L. Martin, M. H. Beddall, A. Miura, A. Sambor, B. K. Chakrabarti, Y. Huang, R. Bailer, R. A. Koup, J. R. Mascola, G. J. Nabel, and N. L. Letvin.** 2005. Multiclade human immunodeficiency virus type 1 envelope immunogens elicit broad cellular and humoral immunity in rhesus monkeys. *J. Virol.* **79:**2956–2963.
62. **Simonsen, L., C. Viboud, A. Elixhauser, R. J. Taylor, and A. Z. Kapikian.** 2005. More on RotaShield and intussusception: the role of age at the time of vaccination. *J. Infect. Dis.* **192**(Suppl. 1)**:**S36–S43.
63. **Spriggs, M. K.** 1996. One step ahead of the game: viral immunomodulatory molecules. *Annu. Rev. Immunol.* **14:**101–130.
64. **Stephenne, J.** 1990. Development and production aspects of a recombinant yeast-derived hepatitis B vaccine. *Vaccine* **8**(Suppl.)**:**S69–S73; discussion, S79–S80.
65. **Stockinger, B., G. Kassiotis, and C. Bourgeois.** 2004. CD4 T-cell memory. *Semin. Immunol.* **16:**295–303.
66. **Thompson, W. W., C. Price, B. Goodson, D. K. Shay, P. Benson, V. L. Hinrichsen, E. Lewis, E. Eriksen, P. Ray, S. M. Marcy, J. Dunn, L. A. Jackson, T. A. Lieu, S. Black, G. Stewart, E. S. Weintraub, R. L. Davis, and F. DeStefano.** 2007. Early thimerosal exposure and neuropsychological outcomes at 7 to 10 years. *N. Engl. J. Med.* **357:**1281–1292.
67. **Topham, D. J., and P. C. Doherty.** 1998. Clearance of an influenza A virus by $CD4^+$ T cells is inefficient in the absence of B cells. *J. Virol.* **72:**882–885.
68. **Varricchio, F., J. Iskander, F. Destefano, R. Ball, R. Pless, M. M. Braun, and R. T. Chen.** 2004. Understanding vaccine safety information from the Vaccine Adverse Event Reporting System. *Pediatr. Infect. Dis. J.* **23:**287–294.
69. **Vesikari, T., A. Karvonen, T. Korhonen, K. Edelman, R. Vainionpaa, A. Salmi, M. K. Saville, I. Cho, A. Razmpour, R. Rappaport, R. O'Neill, A. Georgiu, W. Gruber, P. M. Mendelman, and B. Forrest.** 2006. A randomized, double-blind study of the safety, transmissibility and phenotypic and genotypic stability of cold-adapted influenza virus vaccine. *Pediatr. Infect. Dis. J.* **25:**590–595.
70. **Vesikari, T., D. O. Matson, P. Dennehy, P. Van Damme, M. Santosham, Z. Rodriguez, M. J. Dallas, J. F. Heyse, M. G. Goveia, S. B. Black, H. R. Shinefield, C. D. Christie, S. Ylitalo, R. F. Itzler, M. L. Coia, M. T. Onorato, B. A. Adeyi, G. S. Marshall, L. Gothefors, D. Campens, A. Karvonen, J. P. Watt, K. L. O'Brien, M. J. DiNubile, H. F. Clark, J. W. Boslego, P. A. Offit, and P. M. Heaton.** 2006. Safety and efficacy of a pentavalent human-bovine (WC3) reassortant rotavirus vaccine. *N. Engl. J. Med.* **354:**23–33.
71. **Vessey, S. J., C. Y. Chan, B. J. Kuter, K. M. Kaplan, M. Waters, D. P. Kutzler, P. A. Carfagno, J. C. Sadoff, J. F. Heyse, H. Matthews, S. Li, and I. S. Chan.** 2001. Childhood vaccination against varicella: persistence of antibody, duration of protection, and vaccine efficacy. *J. Pediatr.* **139:**297–304.
72. **Wang, R., K. M. Murphy, D. Y. Loh, C. Weaver, and J. H. Russell.** 1993. Differential activation of antigen-stimulated suicide and cytokine production pathways in $CD4^+$ T cells is regulated by the antigen-presenting cell. *J. Immunol.* **150:**3832–3842.
73. **Watson, B., E. Rothstein, H. Bernstein, A. Arbeter, A. Arvin, S. Chartrand, D. Clements, M. L. Kumar, K. Reisinger, M. Blatter, et al.** 1995. Safety and cellular and humoral immune responses of a booster dose of varicella vaccine 6 years after primary immunization. *J. Infect. Dis.* **172:**217–219.
74. **Wille-Reece, U., B. J. Flynn, K. Lore, R. A. Koup, A. P. Miles, A. Saul, R. M. Kedl, J. J. Mattapallil, W. R. Weiss, M. Roederer, and R. A. Seder.** 2006. Toll-like receptor agonists influence the magnitude and quality of memory T cell responses after prime-boost immunization in nonhuman primates. *J. Exp. Med.* **203:**1249–1258.

75. **Woodland, D. L.** 2004. Jump-starting the immune system: prime-boosting comes of age. *Trends Immunol.* **25:**98–104.
76. **Wu, C. Y., J. R. Kirman, M. J. Rotte, D. F. Davey, S. P. Perfetto, E. G. Rhee, B. L. Freidag, B. J. Hill, D. C. Douek, and R. A. Seder.** 2002. Distinct lineages of T(H)1 cells have differential capacities for memory cell generation in vivo. *Nat. Immunol.* **3:**852–858.
77. **Zhang, X., T. Brunner, L. Carter, R. W. Dutton, P. Rogers, L. Bradley, T. Sato, J. C. Reed, D. Green, and S. L. Swain.** 1997. Unequal death in T helper cell (Th)1 and Th2 effectors: Th1, but not Th2, effectors undergo rapid Fas/FasL-mediated apoptosis. *J. Exp. Med.* **185:**1837–1849.
78. **Zhou, T., L. Xu, B. Dey, A. J. Hessell, D. Van Ryk, S. H. Xiang, X. Yang, M. Y. Zhang, M. B. Zwick, J. Arthos, D. R. Burton, D. S. Dimitrov, J. Sodroski, R. Wyatt, G. J. Nabel, and P. D. Kwong.** 2007. Structural definition of a conserved neutralization epitope on HIV-1 gp120. *Nature* **445:**732–737.
79. **Zhou, X., X. Zhang, X. Yu, X. Zha, Q. Fu, B. Liu, X. Wang, Y. Chen, Y. Chen, Y. Shan, Y. Jin, Y. Wu, J. Liu, W. Kong, and J. Shen.** 2008. The effect of conjugation to gold nanoparticles on the ability of low molecular weight chitosan to transfer DNA vaccine. *Biomaterials* **29:**111–117.
80. **Zhu, J., D. M. Koelle, J. Cao, J. Vazquez, M. L. Huang, F. Hladik, A. Wald, and L. Corey.** 2007. Virus-specific $CD8^+$ T cells accumulate near sensory nerve endings in genital skin during subclinical HSV-2 reactivation. *J. Exp. Med.* **204:**595–603.

Gene Therapy and Viruses

DONALD B. KOHN, BARRIE J. CARTER, PAOLO GRANDI, AND JOSEPH C. GLORIOSO

16

Gene therapy is an emerging medical approach which seeks to apply molecular techniques to attack diseases at the fundamental level of the genes. Discussion of gene therapy within a textbook on viruses is especially appropriate because the adaptation of viruses to serve as gene delivery vehicles has been central to the majority of gene therapy investigations. Originally, gene therapy was conceived for the treatment of inherited disorders, where a normal version of the defective gene would be introduced into a patient's cells. Subsequently, a wide array of acquired conditions have been considered for gene therapy, including oncological, cardiovascular, neurologic, and infectious disorders (Table 1). At present, gene therapy is a nascent field, in which basic laboratory research continues on the development of methods for effective gene delivery and expression, while initial clinical trials have begun to test the potential efficacy of gene therapy approaches.

The first techniques which were developed for genetic manipulation of mammalian cells involved direct introduction of genes in the forms of expression plasmids by physical methods (Table 2) (28). Highly polar, negatively charged DNA molecules can be moved across cell membranes by coating the DNA with calcium ions or with positively charged cationic lipids for transfection, or by microinjection, electroporation, or particle-mediated bombardment. Synthetic nucleic acid analogs, such as phosphorothioates, morpholino-derivatives, and peptide nucleic acids, can be used to make molecules containing the same information content as standard oligonucleotides, but possessing more favorable pharmacological properties, such as stability, permeance, and bioavailability.

In general, nonviral gene delivery methods lead to only a transient presence of the nucleic acid moiety. For some clinical purposes, transient expression of an introduced gene may be sufficient to achieve an intended therapeutic purpose, for example, to produce an immunogenic protein for vaccination. Nonviral gene delivery methods typically lead to relatively lower levels of gene expression than do viral methods, although these levels of expression may be biologically relevant for highly potent molecules, such as cytokines or immunogens. In addition to expression plasmids to produce a specific protein, oligonucleotides may be used directly as antisense DNA or RNA, ribozymes, small interfering RNA, or molecular decoys for transcriptional factors to suppress expression of a specific gene, and as mediators of homologous recombination for gene repair.

However, other gene therapy applications require stable persistence of the transferred gene in the target cells, so that the gene will be retained with each cell division and inherited by all progeny cells. While the rare cells into which stable gene integration has been achieved by DNA transfection methods may be selected and expanded in vitro, this low efficiency would be unacceptable with primary cells of limited number. Thus, the use of viruses capable of gene delivery in a stable, persistent manner has been a major focus of research. The viruses which have been adapted and most widely studied for gene transfer include retroviruses, adenovirus (Ad), adeno-associated virus (AAV), herpesviruses, and, most recently, lentiviruses.

While the use of viruses as gene delivery vectors takes advantage of their innate ability to insert genetic material into cells, their major disadvantage is their potential for causing significant side effects. Vectors which integrate into the cellular chromosomal DNA, such as retroviruses, lentiviruses, and AAV, can cause insertional oncogenesis if they insert in or near cellular genes, such as oncogenes or tumor suppressor genes, and alter their expression. Because these vectors have been developed to be replication incompetent, the numbers of integration events should be finite, limiting but not eliminating the risk of insertional oncogenesis. However, if replication-competent viruses emerge by recombination of the viral elements used to package the vectors, the potential would exist for recurrent infections to occur, leading to significantly higher numbers of viral integration events, increasing proportionately the risk of insertional oncogenesis. Replication-competent vector recombinants may also be capable of causing other pathologies, such as immune deficiency, or other organ toxicities. Vectors administered in vivo may be inflammatory and induce immunologic responses, with the potential for damage to transduced tissues by immunologically mediated cytopathicity. The safety profile of each type of vector will vary based upon the specific viral elements which are retained in the vector. Thus, each new vector must be evaluated with careful preclinical toxicity studies followed by well-designed clinical trials, with the first end point being evaluation of toxicities.

TABLE 1 Clinical applications of gene therapy

Genetic diseases
Add functioning copy of relevant gene
Mediate correction of endogenous genetic mutation
Malignant diseases
Replace tumor suppressor gene
Suppress oncogene (e.g., siRNA[a])
Insert "suicide" gene
Add immunostimulatory gene(s)
Add chimeric or T-cell antigen receptor
Decrease therapeutic toxicity from chemotherapy
Infectious diseases
Stimulate immunity to infectious organism
Confer intracellular resistance to infectious organism
Cardiovascular diseases
Suppress inflammation
Induce neoangiogenesis, tissue repair
Neurologic diseases
Express neurotrophins
Provide neurotransmitters
Produce analgesia

[a] siRNA, small interfering RNA.

RNA VIRUSES

Retroviral Vectors

Retroviral Replication

Vector systems have been derived from the three major subgroups of the *Retroviridae* family, including simple retroviruses, lentiviruses, and spumaviruses. The first of these vector systems to be developed used gammaretroviruses (e.g., Moloney murine leukemia virus [MLV]) and are generally granted the name "retroviral vectors," while the vectors produced subsequently are referred to as lentiviral and spumaviral vectors.

The replication cycle of all retroviruses includes an obligatory step in which the viral genome integrates into the chromosomal DNA of the infected target cell. Once the provirus has integrated, it remains as a permanent genetic element and is replicated along with the cellular genes, allowing inheritance by both progeny upon cell division. Retroviral vectors make use of this step in the retroviral replication cycle to achieve permanent genetic modification of target cells. Cloning a gene of interest into a retroviral genome allows the exogenous gene to be carried by the virus into the target cell. The efficiency of stable retrovirus-mediated gene transduction greatly exceeds that of most other physical methods and may reach as high as 50 to 80% with primary cells such as fibroblasts, T lymphocytes, and bone marrow progenitor cells.

The essential regulatory portions of the retrovirus genome that must be retained for a vector are the 5′ and 3′ long terminal repeats (LTR) and the 5′ leader region that contains the packaging or encapsidation sequence (ψ^+) (Fig. 1). The proteins of the retrovirus are encoded as three polyproteins by the *gag, pol,* and *env* genes. The Gag proteins form the internal viral core of the virion. The *pol* region encodes three enzymatic functions: reverse transcriptase, which is an RNA-directed DNA polymerase; the protease, which cleaves the viral polyproteins into individual subunits; and the integrase, which mediates the crossover and covalent linkage between the ends of the LTR and the target cell DNA. The Env proteins, which are embedded in the viral envelope derived from the host cell membrane, mediate binding to receptors on the target cell and ingress across the target cell membrane.

The integration of retroviruses into the genomes of target cells is relatively random, although some distinctive patterns for each subclass of virus have been elucidated (6). Integration of the transcriptionally active retroviral sequences can lead to transcriptional activation (or inactivation) of adjacent cellular genes, and this "insertional oncogenesis" is an underlying mechanism by which they may be transforming, in both nature and clinical applications.

Brief Description of Vectors

The first retroviral vectors contained all or most of the wild-type viral genome, with a portion replaced by the passenger gene (3, 129). This structure is reminiscent of the acutely transforming retroviruses found in nature that carry cell-derived oncogenes. Because these vectors retain the genes encoding the retroviral proteins, they may be replication-competent retroviruses (RCR), which can cause a spreading infection in target cells. The presence of RCR (also known as "helper virus") in vector preparations would allow mobilization of vector sequences from coinfected cells, confounding lineage-marking studies, and could lead to an increased risk of insertional mutagenesis if applied to human subjects.

With the development of packaging cell lines to provide the viral protein in *trans* (see below), it became possible to include in a retroviral vector only genes of

TABLE 2 Comparison of genetic vectors

Genetic vector	Insert size (kb)	Persistence	Advantage(s)	Disadvantage(s)
Nonviral	Unlimited	Transient	No viral sequences, large capacity	Low-efficiency entry, transient persistence
Retrovirus	1–6	Stable	Efficient cell entry, stable integration	Target cell division required, insertional oncogenesis
Lentivirus	1–8	Stable	Transduces, nondividing	Biosafety profile unproven
AAV	4 (±5%)	Stable	Efficient cell entry, long-term persistence	Limited capacity, vector immunogenicity
Ad	2–35	Transient	Efficient in vivo gene delivery	Transient, inflammatory
HSV	Unknown (genome, 150 kb)	Stable in neurons	Neurotropic, large capacity	Production complex

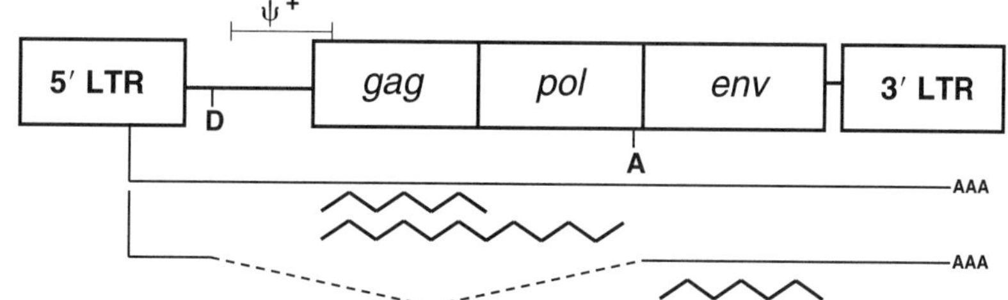

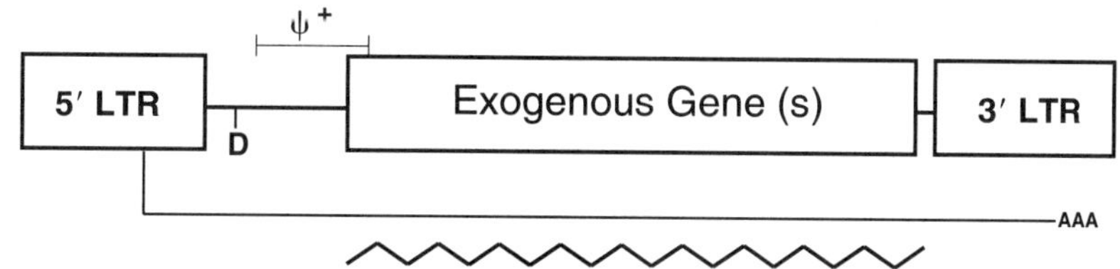

FIGURE 1 Diagrams of typical simple retrovirus and retroviral vector. (Top) Retroviruses have LTR at each end, the psi encapsidation sequences (ψ^+), and regions encoding the Gag, Pol, and Env polyproteins. Splice donor (D) and acceptor (A) sites allow some of the vector transcripts to be spliced to generate subgenomic RNA for translation of the *env* gene. (Bottom) Retrovirus vectors contain the LTR and ψ^+ regions of the retrovirus with the exogenous gene(s) sequences cloned between.

experimental or therapeutic interest. Essentially, all that is required from the retrovirus in a vector are the 5′ and 3′ LTR and the ψ packaging sequence. Between these termini, exogenous gene sequences (approximately 1 to 6 kb) may be placed that will then be carried by the vector (Fig. 1). Vectors lacking the genes encoding the retroviral proteins are replication defective and should not be capable of any replication after transduction of target cells. Although retroviral vectors have been made from a number of different simple retroviruses that infect murine, avian, and other species, the vast majority of the retroviral vectors that have been used for gene therapy studies are derived from MLV.

Helper-Free Vector Packaging Cell Lines

Removal of the genes for the retroviral structural and enzymatic proteins (Gag, Pol, and Env) from the recombinant vector genomes necessitates that these proteins be supplied in *trans*. The initial approach to supplying these viral proteins to package replication-defective vectors involved coinfection of cells containing the vector provirus with wild-type, infectious MLV. The MLV genome produces the Gag, Pol, and Env proteins, which can then package the wild-type MLV genomes as well as pseudotype the recombinant vector genomes. Unfortunately, this pseudotyping approach results in the presence of RCR in vector preparations.

The potential complications that may ensue from exposing patients to RCR were highlighted in a preclinical study in which monkeys were given transplantations with bone marrow transduced by a preparation of retroviral vectors that contained high levels of RCR (23). In the face of the immune deficiency engendered by the total-body irradiation given to the animals prior to transplantation, the RCR was able to freely replicate and led to the development of lymphoma in three of eight recipients, likely due to insertional oncogenesis.

The single most important advance that has allowed the use of retroviral vectors for experimental and clinical applications was the development of packaging cell lines that could produce retroviral vectors free of contaminating RCR (81). The identification of the ψ packaging signal, which is necessary and sufficient for efficient inclusion of RNA into retroviral virions, allowed development of a binary system in which the genetic information encoding the virion structural and regulatory proteins is separate from the vector carrying the intended therapeutic gene(s). "Packaging plasmids" can be constructed from the MLV genome, in which the ψ region is deleted (Fig. 2). The RNA produced by this plasmid is capable of expressing the Gag, Pol, and Env proteins of the virus, but the RNA is not packaged into the virion because it lacks the ψ packaging sequence (Fig. 3A) (74). Stable packaging cell clones (based on 3T3 fibroblasts or other cell types) containing the packaging genome produce, in effect, empty virus particles, lacking any RNA genomes. If a retroviral vector plasmid is transfected into the packaging cells, the RNA produced by transcription of the vector plasmid (which does contain the ψ region) will be packaged into the virion. These retroviral vector particles are capable of a single round of transduction of target cells, resulting in integration of the vector genome into the target cell chromosome. However, no further virus is made in the target cell because the genetic information needed to make new virion structural and regulatory proteins does not leave the packaging cell.

Subsequent improvements were achieved in the design of packaging plasmids to decrease the potential for them to recombine with vector sequences to produce RCR that can undergo repeated cell-to-cell infection. A major

1st Generation: ψ-deleted

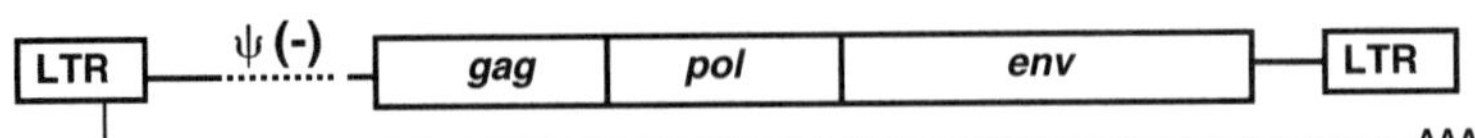

2nd Generation: Multi-deleted

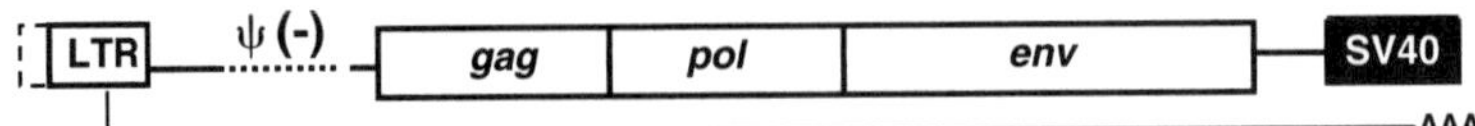

3rd Generation: Split expression plasmids

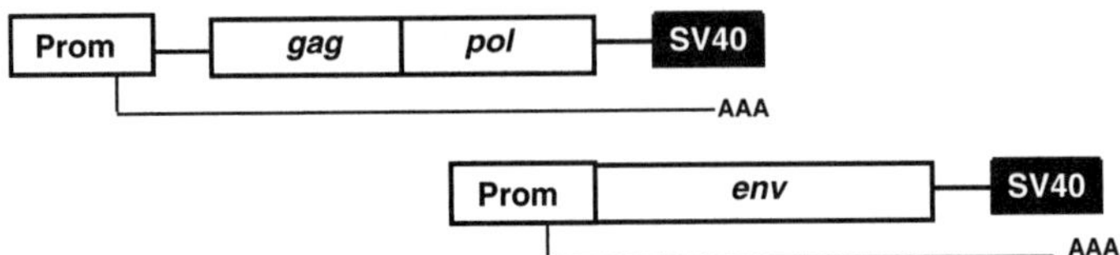

FIGURE 2 Retroviral vector packaging constructs. First-generation packaging constructs had the packaging region deleted to prevent packaging of the transcripts encoding the viral proteins. Second-generation packaging constructs were further altered to minimize the potential for generation of RCR through recombination with sequences in the vector. The 5′ end of the 5′ LTR was deleted and the entire 3′ LTR was replaced with an exogenous polyadenylation signal. Third-generation packaging systems had the open reading frames for Gag-Pol and Env placed on separate plasmids to further minimize the potential for recombination to generate RCR. SV40, simian virus 40.

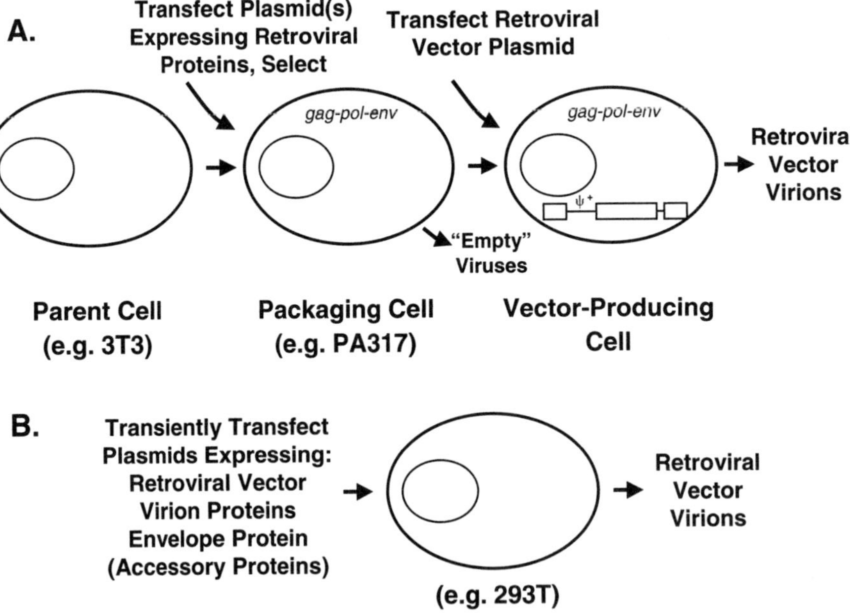

FIGURE 3 Production of lentiviral vectors from stable packaging cell lines and by transient transfection. (A) Stable packaging cell lines can be developed by stable transfection of a cell line to express the Gag, Pol, and Env proteins. Subsequent transfection of the plasmid encoding a retrovirus vector allows the vector genomic RNA to be packaged by the retroviral proteins. (B) Retroviral vectors can be produced by transient transfection of a susceptible cell line, such as 293T, with all of the plasmids encoding the vector, the virion proteins, and an envelope protein.

requirement of the U.S. Food and Drug Administration (FDA) for the use of retroviral vectors in clinical applications is extensive testing to ensure the absence of RCR (2). Under these guidelines, more than 1,000 human subjects have received retroviral vectors, with no evidence of RCR in any subject.

An alternate method to the use of stable packaging cell lines to produce retroviral vectors is the use of transient transfection of plasmids encoding the vector and the packaging proteins (Gag, Pol, and Env) into a cell, which then produces vector particles for a few days (Fig. 3B). A cell line that is efficiently transfected, such as the 293 human embryonic kidney cell line, can yield vectors at titers in the same range as are produced from typical stable packaging cell lines (92, 97, 120). Production of vector by transient transfection is much quicker than the relatively laborious process involved in establishing and screening stable producer cell clones, although it requires production of large quantities of high-quality (i.e., low-endotoxin) plasmids. Vectors encoding cytotoxic or cytostatic gene products, and thereby preventing derivation of stable producer cells, can often be produced transiently.

Alternative Envelopes for Retroviral Vectors

The envelope glycoprotein molecule of a retroviral vector binds to a specific cellular surface protein that acts as the viral receptor. The distribution of the cellular receptor determines the cell types that a vector with a specific envelope protein may transduce. Wild-type MLV has an envelope that binds to a cell surface protein present only on murine cells. Thus, vectors with this envelope protein are "ecotropic," transducing only cells of the home, in this case murine, species. A variant of MLV was isolated from feral mice in California that contained a variant envelope protein binding to a protein present on most mammalian cells (106). Vectors containing this "amphotropic" envelope can transduce cells from most mammals, including mice, rats, cats, dogs, sheep, pigs, monkeys, and humans, and have been widely used for preclinical and clinical studies. The envelope proteins derived from other retroviruses, such as gibbon ape leukemia virus or RD114 feline leukemia virus, or from other viruses, such as Ross River virus or baculovirus (gp64), have also been used to attempt to increase gene transfer via highly abundant cellular receptors (58, 101, 111).

An important innovation is the use of the G surface glycoprotein of vesicular stomatitis virus (VSV) in retroviral vectors (26). The receptor for the VSV G protein (which may be a glycolipid) is widely distributed across species and has allowed the introduction of MLV-based vectors into the genomes of nonmammalian vertebrate species, such as zebrafish (68). The VSV-G receptor does not saturate like receptors for other envelope proteins often do, and it thus allows more efficient gene transfer. Additionally, virions containing the VSV G protein are physically stable, and VSV packaged virions may be readily concentrated by gradient centrifugation, resulting in titers 2 or 3 orders of magnitude higher than those typically seen with "raw" retroviral vectors. A very high vector titer is especially useful for applications involving in vivo delivery into tissues where the volume that may be administered is limited. One drawback to VSV-coated viruses is that sustained expression of the VSV G protein is toxic to packaging cells, and therefore, it has not been possible to establish permanent VSV-packaging cell lines. Instead, a transient transfection of a plasmid encoding the VSV G protein must be performed to produce each batch of vector.

Extensive attempts have been made to target retroviral vectors to transduce specific cell types. Potentially, targeted vectors could be used for in vivo gene therapy; systemically administered vectors would seek out and preferentially transduce only the tissues containing targeted receptors. A fusion protein was made between the ecotropic Env of MLV and human erythropoietin, and the resulting virions containing the erythropoietin ligand were able to specifically transduce cells expressing the erythropoietin receptor, although with quite low efficiency (59). Other efforts at producing retroviral envelopes containing targeting moieties have been unsuccessful, as the modifications interfere with envelope protein activities involved in fusion into the target cell membrane. Recently, incorporation of both a targeting moiety (e.g., monoclonal antibody) and a fusogenic moiety (e.g., modified Sendai virus surface protein) into virions succeeded in achieving vectors that show efficient, targeted transduction (134).

In summary, the "life cycle" of retroviral vectors begins from a plasmid constructed to contain essential viral elements and the transgene(s), proceeds through the packaging stage in a cell line by coexpression of the essential viral structural and enzymatic proteins to produce transduction-competent, but not replication-competent, virions, and ends with the stable integration of the vector provirus into the chromosomal DNA of target cells, with expression of the transgene product (Fig. 4).

Clinical Applications with Retroviral Vectors

Since 2000, there have been several reports of clinical benefit with gene therapy using retroviral vectors. Patients with severe combined immune deficiency (SCID), both the X-linked and adenosine deaminase-deficient forms, and with the neutrophil defect chronic granulomatous disease have realized clinically relevant immune restoration (1, 13, 33, 34, 39, 95). Retroviral vectors carrying the relevant cDNA were used to transduce $CD34^+$ hematopoietic progenitor cells from bone marrow or peripheral blood and reinfused into the patients. The majority of the subjects have shown clinical benefit for more than 5 to 7 years at this point.

The successful treatment of these forms of congenital immune deficiencies by gene therapy using retroviral vectors represents a major milestone in the treatment of primary immune deficiency diseases. However, a dire complication has ensued in one study, in that 4 of 10 treated infants with X-linked SCID developed a T-cell lymphoproliferative disease 2 to 5 years after gene therapy, which was fatal in one case (40). This complication has been attributed to insertional oncogenesis from transactivation of a cellular transgene (LMO-2) by the integrated retroviral vector likely combining, with subtle proliferative effects from constitutive expression of the γC cytokine receptor gene (the therapeutic transgene for X-linked SCID) by the vector (24). This complication has not been observed to date in another cohort of X-linked SCID patients treated or in any of the adenosine deaminase-deficient SCID patients. In the patients with chronic granulomatous disease, there has been an oligoclonal expansion of cells containing the retroviral vector integrated near three cellular genes that are involved in myeloid cell proliferation, but no frank myeloproliferation to date (95).

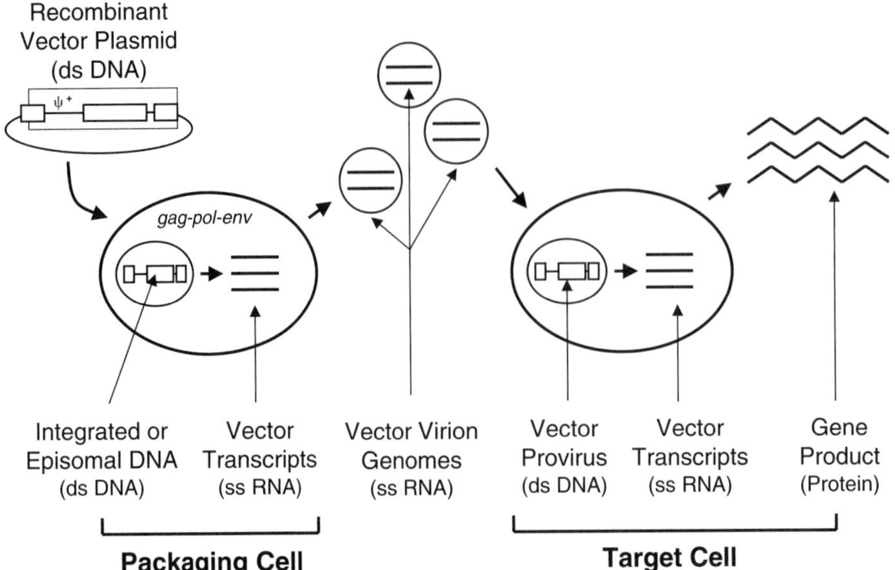

FIGURE 4 Life cycle of a retroviral vector. Retroviral vectors are constructed as plasmids to contain the essential retroviral elements (LTR and psi region) and the transgene and other expression regulatory elements. The plasmid is transfected into a cell for packaging, with either stable or transient coexpression of the necessary retroviral proteins in *trans*. The vector transcripts serve as the virion genome and are packaged into virions and released from the cell. The vector virions can then be used to transduce a target cell, where the vector RNA genome is reverse transcribed into double-stranded (ds) DNA and integrated into the target cell chromosomes as a provirus. The proviral sequences can be transcribed into mRNA that is translated to make the transgene product. ss, single stranded.

Insertional oncogenesis is known to be a primary mechanism by which wild-type murine retroviruses cause leukemia when they repeatedly infect cells in neonatal mice, leading to millions of integration events, some of which transactivate cellular oncogenes (Fig. 5). A common observation in studies characterizing insertional oncogenesis in experimental murine models is that tumors usually contain multiple proviral integrants that lead to transactivation of genes from several different signaling pathways, indicating the need for cooperative transactivation for transformation (24).

These observations spurred investigations into vector integration sites, facilitated by the twin developments of robust techniques for recovering integrated vectors along with flanking genomic DNA sequences (e.g., linear amplification-mediated PCR) and the sequencing of the human genome, which allows the flanking fragments to be mapped to chromosomal sites of integration. These vector integration studies have demonstrated that each specific method for gene delivery has a characteristic pattern of integration site preferences. For example, MLV-based vectors have a strong preference for integrating near the 5′ region of genes (131), and human immunodeficiency virus type 1 (HIV-1)-based vectors target gene-rich regions (114). Human foamy virus-based vectors do not integrate preferentially within genes, despite a modest preference for integration near transcription start sites and a significant preference for CpG islands (126). Avian sarcoma-lymphoma virus-based vectors show only a weak preference for active genes and no preference for transcription start regions (83). Although reduced integration into genes is beneficial for avoidance of tumor suppressor genes, it is not clear if a reduced bias for integration into active genes actually lowers the risk of insertional oncogenesis, as transactivation may occur over relatively long distances, of 1 to 100 kb. However, vector design can influence and counteract transactivation, e.g., by use of promoters with relatively weak enhancers to minimize transactivation, or, possibly, by the use of insulators to block transactivation by the vector enhancers on cellular genes.

Lentiviral Vectors

Lentivirus is a genus of the *Retroviridae* family, and its members share the general genomic organization pattern of other retroviruses (5′ LTR-*ψ-gag-pol-env*-3′ LTR). Lentiviruses also have one or more additional genes that act in a regulatory capacity to modulate viral replication. Additionally, lentiviruses can infect nondividing cells because they have multiple mechanisms for facilitating entry of their genomic preintegration complex through the intact nuclear membrane to achieve genomic integration in nondividing cells (8, 31). In contrast, simple retroviruses require their target cells to undergo mitosis with nuclear membrane breakdown for their genomes to reach the cellular chromosomes for integration (66).

Transfer of foreign genes using lentiviruses was first demonstrated with HIV-1 genomes that carried replacements of nonessential regulatory genes, such as *nef*, with reporter genes (e.g., the luciferase gene) (9, 102, 117). These vectors retained the HIV-1 structural genes and therefore represented replication-competent lentiviruses (RCL), capable of causing an active infection. These early vectors also carried the HIV-1 *env* gene and thus were only able to transduce cells carrying the $CD4^+$ surface protein (e.g., $CD4^+$ T lymphocytes and monocytic cells).

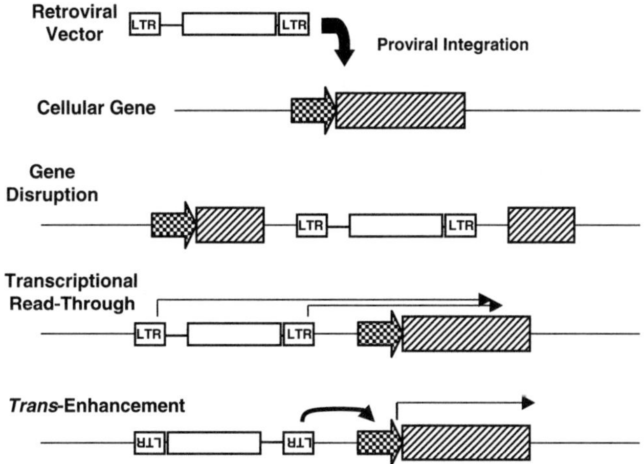

FIGURE 5 Potential mechanisms of insertional oncogenesis by retroviral vectors. Retroviral vectors integrate into the target cell chromosomes and may affect the expression of nearby cellular genes. Gene disruption may occur if the retroviral vector integrates within the cellular gene; tumor suppressor genes may be inactivated by this process. Transcriptional read-through may occur from integrated vector proviruses into downstream cellular genes in the same orientation; inappropriate expression of cellular oncogenes may occur by this process. *trans* Enhancement of expression of cellular genes may occur if strong enhancer elements of the vectors activate expression from the promoters of nearby cellular genes, independently of the relative orientation of the vector (depicted as an upside-down vector in reverse transcriptional orientation relative to the cellular gene). (Figure kindly provided by Erin Weber, U.S.C. Keck School of Medicine.)

Subsequently, lentivirus-based vectors have been developed in which large portions of the HIV-1 genome are deleted and the essential viral proteins (Gag and Pol) are supplied in *trans* by a packaging genome (91). In these vectors the HIV-1 *env* gene is deleted and replaced functionally by the VSV G protein, which is expressed from a separate plasmid. As described in the previous section on retroviral vectors, VSV G protein confers a broad tropism on vectors, significantly expanding the range of target cells beyond $CD4^+$ cells transduced by vectors using only the natural HIV-1 gp120 Env. Additionally, the physical stability of the VSV G protein allows the vectors to be concentrated to relatively high titers, i.e., 10^9 to 10^{10} transducing units/ml.

These HIV-1-based lentiviral vectors have been shown to be significantly superior to oncoretroviral vectors for gene transfer to growth-arrested fibroblasts, nondividing neurons of the brain and retina, liver cells, muscle cells, primitive human hematopoietic progenitor cells, and respiratory epithelial cells (53, 57, 84, 90, 91, 124). The improved ability to transduce these clinically relevant cell types that have been difficult to stably modify using other gene transfer methods should have numerous applications for gene transfer for experimental or therapeutic purposes. Further studies are needed to define the limits of transduction by lentiviral vectors to reveal their ultimate usefulness for clinical applications.

Human foamy virus, from the *Spumavirus* genus of the *Retroviridae* family, has also been developed into a gene vector system (127). Potentially important advantages of foamy viruses are that they perform reverse transcription of their genome in an early stage of infection and that target host cell factors in quiescent cells may not be limiting, as they appear to be for lentiviral vectors (21). Recent data obtained using foamy virus vectors in experimental models of gene therapy via bone marrow transplantation in a canine model suggest that they may have sufficient gene transfer efficacy for clinical utility (61).

Improved Lentiviral Systems

Following the initial description of the lentiviral vectors lacking HIV-1 coding sequences, a series of additional modifications was made to both the vector and the packaging plasmids to improve their effectiveness or biosafety (25, 132, 142). Further deletions from the vector backbone of nonessential HIV-1 sequences have been made to minimize risks of RCL generation due to recombination between vector and packaging sequences. The vectors carry no HIV-1 open reading frames, which should also obviate immunologic responses to viral proteins in transduced cells.

Vectors can be made that lack the enhancers of the LTR using the same aspects of genome production that produce double copies of LTR inserts (Fig. 6). When these "self-inactivating" (SIN) vectors are constructed, the enhancer region is removed from the 3′ LTR of the vector plasmid. Transfection of this plasmid into a packaging cell yields a transcript from the complete 5′ LTR. When the 5′ LTR re-forms its 5′ terminus during reverse transcription in the target cell by copying the 3′ LTR, it acquires the enhancer deletion. Both LTR are now transcriptionally inactive, and only internal promoters will be active. SIN lentiviral vectors have been produced to increase their biosafety, by eliminating the potential for transcription from the LTR of a potential RCL recombinant and by reducing the risk of transcription of cellular genes downstream from the site of vector integration (141).

Importantly, lentiviral vectors tolerate complex genetic elements better than do retroviral vectors, possibly aided by the Rev/Rev response element-mediated mechanism for nuclear-to-cytoplasmic export of HIV-1 transcripts. A min-

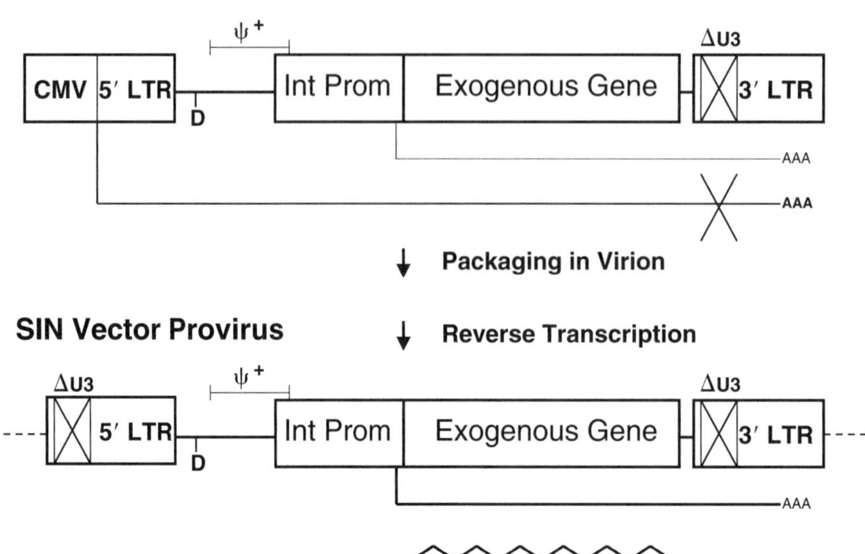

FIGURE 6 SIN lentiviral vectors. The SIN vector plasmid contains deletion of the enhancer and promoter of the 3′ LTR, which are not needed for expression from the plasmid in a packaging cell line. Following packaging of the vector and reverse transcription of the vector genome in a target cell, the 3′ LTR with the deletions of the enhancer and promoter is used as the template for the analogous region of the 5′ LTR, leading to a provirus with both LTR being transcriptionally inactive. Expression of the exogenous gene will then be driven from the internal promoter (Int Prom), which may be lineage specific or have other useful expression patterns. CMV, cytomegalovirus.

ilocus for regulated expression of human β-globin that was not carried intact in retroviral vectors can be transferred with high efficiency and stability into murine bone marrow stem cells by a SIN lentiviral vector; for the first time, a physiological impact on the anemia of β-thalassemia in a murine model has been attained by gene transfer into hematopoietic stem cells (78).

As with the lentiviral vectors, lentiviral packaging plasmids have been progressively improved to optimize activity and safety. Packaging systems in which there is no overlap in sequences of any of the multiple HIV-1-derived components have been produced; the amount of HIV-1 genome remaining in these vectors is significantly less than in vaccine candidates. To date, no publications have reported the inadvertent generation of replication-competent lentiviral vectors during production, in either many research-scale batches or clinical-grade production runs.

Safety

While lentiviral vectors have been superior to retroviral vectors for many cell targets and at least equivalent in other applications, an obvious concern raised is their biosafety. HIV-1 is a known human pathogen that is nearly uniformly fatal, and the magnitude of the worldwide AIDS epidemic attests to its potential for spread. Thus, there may be negative reactions to consideration of its use as a vector, despite the multiple steps taken to prevent generation of replication-competent viruses and the complete absence of the HIV-1 envelope and accessory proteins thought to underlie most aspects of pathogenicity.

As an alternative to HIV-1-based vectors, lentiviruses that infect other mammalian species and that do not normally infect humans have been developed. Vectors have been produced from feline immunodeficiency virus, equine infectious anemia virus, and simian immunodeficiency virus (73, 94, 100). As with vectors derived from HIV-1, these nonhuman lentiviral vectors have also been shown to have the ability to transduce nondividing cells. There have not been any reports of direct comparisons between HIV-1-based vectors and those based on nonhuman lentiviruses to determine whether they possess equivalent efficacies for transduction of clinically relevant primary human cells. Possibly, there are interactions with cellular proteins that occur for viruses adapted to a specific species. While HIV-1 is a human pathogen, there also exists an array of clinically effective antiretroviral drugs that inhibit HIV-1 replication, at least in the short term. The efficacy of these drugs against possible recombinants of nonhuman lentiviruses is unknown.

Lentiviral vectors have entered the clinic in a trial with HIV-1-infected subjects (65). This study targeted mature T cells collected by apheresis for ex vivo transduction with a lentiviral vector encoding antisense RNA to HIV-1 *env* sequences. Gene delivery to the T cells was relatively effective, with ongoing detection of gene-modified T cells for more than 1 year in two of the subjects. Follow-up over 2 years has not detected any adverse clinical effects. Clinical trials are currently in development for treatment of β-thalassemia and sickle cell disease, HIV-1 infection, leukodystrophies, Wiskott-Aldrich syndrome, and Fanconi anemia.

DNA VIRUSES

Retrovirus vectors are suitable for ex vivo gene transfer but are not efficient or feasible for the transfer of genetic material to nondividing or terminally differentiated cells, such as those of the brain, liver, muscle, or respiratory tract. However, DNA virus vectors such as AAV, Ad, and herpes simplex virus (HSV) do not require host cell proliferation for effective gene expression.

AAV vectors exhibit a unique mechanism of persistence of the vector genome as an unintegrated, circular episome and are particularly well suited for long-term gene expression requiring infrequent vector administration. Ad vectors, which also do not integrate, persist much less well but can provide rapid, high-level gene expression and may be useful for cancer or in cardiovascular applications to induce neoangiogenesis. HSV vectors also may be useful for persistent gene expression in some tissues based upon their neurotropism and latency.

Adeno-Associated Virus

AAV is a small (20- to 30-nm) particle comprising a protein capsid enclosing a 4.7-kb single-stranded, linear DNA genome (12). Most of the molecular biology of AAV was established using AAV serotype 2. Generally, the AAV genome consists of two genes: the *rep* gene, which is required for replication and encapsidation of AAV genomes, and the *cap* gene, which encodes the capsid proteins (Fig. 7A). The viral genes are flanked on either side by the inverted terminal repeats (ITR), which act in *cis* as origins of replication and for encapsidation of viral DNA.

Even though it has its own replication gene, AAV is replication defective. In the productive life cycle, AAV requires coinfection with a second helper virus (usually an Ad or a herpesvirus) for AAV replication to occur (Fig. 8). In cultured cells in vitro, in the absence of any helper virus, wild-type AAV can persist by undergoing integration into the host cell genome at a specific site, AAVS1, on human chromosome 19 (62). Infection by Ad of cells containing an integrated AAV genome leads to rescue and replication of the AAV genome in a process that is mediated by interaction of the Rep protein with the AAV ITR regions. This forms the basis of all procedures for production of AAV vectors as described below (12). Nevertheless, recent evidence suggests that naturally occurring AAV genomes present in human tissues such as tonsils persist mainly as unintegrated circular episomes (113).

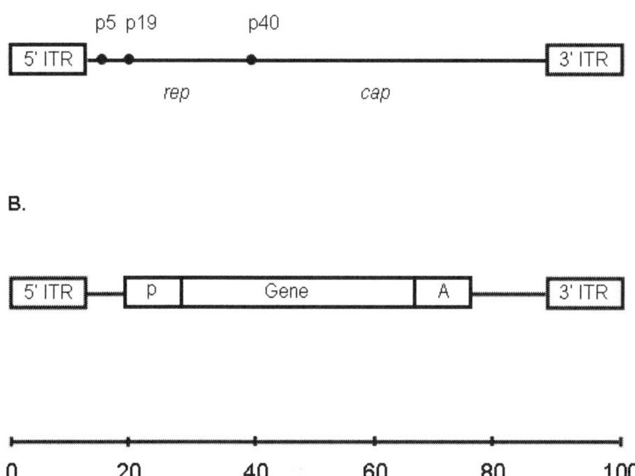

FIGURE 7 Maps of the genomes of wild-type AAV serotype 2 and AAV vector. (A) The AAV serotype 2 genome is 4,681 nucleotides long and is shown on a linear scale of 100 map units. The open boxes show the ITR. The closed circles show the transcription promoters at 5, 19, and 40 map units. The *rep* gene is transcribed from both the p5 and p19 promoters. The *cap* gene is transcribed from the p40 promoter. (B) Schematic diagram of an AAV vector. The entire AAV coding sequence, including the *rep* and *cap* genes, is removed, leaving only the ITR that are required for the origin of replication and for encapsidation. The gene of interest, with appropriate regulatory sequences such as transcription promoter (p) and polyadenylation site (A), is inserted between the ITR.

AAV Vectors

AAV has many advantages as a gene therapy vector because it is not a recognized pathogen and is replication defective. Wild-type AAV replicates in vitro to yield a very large burst size, of more than 100,000 particles per cell, and production systems that are scalable for eventual commercial production and give high yields of AAV vectors are now available (12).

Generation of vectors was enabled by the observation that molecular cloning of double-stranded AAV DNA into bacterial plasmids followed by transfection into helper virus-infected mammalian cells results in rescue and replication of the AAV genome free of any plasmid DNA sequence to yield a burst of infectious AAV particles (12). Vector plasmids are generated by deleting all of the *rep* and *cap* gene sequences and inserting a gene and expression cassette between the *cis*-acting 145-bp ITR at either end of the genome (Fig. 7B). To encapsidate the AAV vector genome into AAV particles, the vector plasmid is introduced into producer cells that are rendered permissive by expression of helper virus (e.g., Ad) functions and that also are complemented with the AAV *rep* and *cap* genes on a separate plasmid.

DNA transfection-based AAV vector production has been improved, and new cell-based AAV production systems have been developed (12, 98). For DNA transfection-based production, Ad can be replaced by a plasmid containing only the Ad E2A, E4, and VA genes, which, together with the E1A genes supplied by 293 cells, provide a complete helper function in the absence of Ad production. For mammalian-cell-based production, AAV vector-packaging cell lines containing the *rep* and *cap* gene cassettes but having deletions of AAV ITR have been developed. Infection of these cells with Ad activates *rep* and *cap* gene expression. The vector plasmid can be stably incorporated into the packaging cells to yield AAV vector producer cell lines which need only be infected with Ad to generate vectors. Improvements in purification procedures have led to much higher-quality AAV vectors which are critical for preclinical studies and clinical trials. The original CsCl centrifugation technique has now been largely abandoned, and purification procedures are generally based on chromatographic procedures (98). Also, the analytical procedures used to characterize AAV vectors are becoming much more highly developed (12).

AAV vector genomes usually contain the ITR of serotype 2, whereas the capsid may be derived from one of the many known AAV serotypes or clades by replacement of the relevant *cap* gene sequence in the production system. The AAV capsid determines many biological properties of AAV vectors. The packaging limit of about 5 kb of DNA

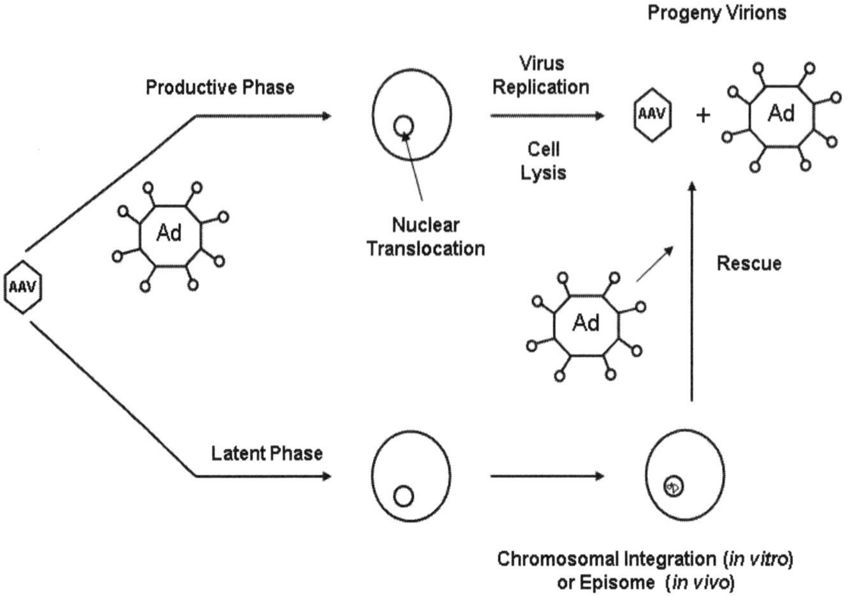

FIGURE 8 AAV life cycle. In the absence of helper virus, AAV enters a latent phase. In cultured cells in vitro, this latent phase leads to chromosomal integration of the AAV genome (see text). In vivo, such as in humans, latency may involve persistence of the AAV genome as an episome. The productive phase occurs if helper virus is present and coinfects the host cells. If latently infected cells in vitro are later infected with helper virus, the AAV DNA can be rescued from the host cell genome by replication. This rescue and amplification of AAV from latently infected cells in vitro together form the basis for production of AAV vectors as discussed in the text.

places some constraints on expression of very large cDNAs. Except for the packaging size, there are no obvious limitations on the design of gene cassettes in AAV vectors; tissue-specific promoters retain specificity, more than one promoter and gene cassette can be inserted into the same vector, and transcription generally is not susceptible to in vivo silencing.

AAV has a broad host range, and different AAV serotypes infect and grow in vitro in many human cell lines. However, the in vivo transduction efficiencies of vectors having capsids from different serotypes (pseudotyped AAV vectors) vary widely depending on the tissue or cell type. This reflects differences in receptors that mediate AAV entry and other trafficking properties of different AAV serotypes (12, 88). Further studies may allow a more optimal matching or mutational modification of the vector capsid for particular target tissues (88).

AAV vectors have several other advantages. In vivo, nondividing cells are the preferred target and host cell proliferation is not required for gene expression. Vectors administered in vivo can provide persistent gene expression for very prolonged periods, of months or years (52). This persistence involves formation of multimeric duplex AAV genomes that are predominantly episomal concatemers with only a small fraction, if any, becoming integrated (112). This process occurs by intermolecular recombination and may be initiated over several days or weeks.

AAV vectors may be used mainly for clinical applications requiring only infrequent delivery, but potential humoral immune responses against the viral capsid, either preexisting or induced by vector administration, must be considered (12). Induction of anti-AAV capsid antibody responses after vector administration may reduce the efficiency of transduction upon readministration (15, 43), but this also depends upon the route of administration (133). In some animal models, readministration of AAV vectors to the lungs can be inhibited by an antibody response to the capsid (42), but other studies indicate that immune responses are greatly reduced following airway administration of AAV (5). It remains to be determined whether preexisting or induced neutralizing antibody responses to AAV vector capsids will impact clinical applications of AAV vectors.

All the viral gene sequences are deleted from the AAV vectors, which may decrease the risk of cellular immune responses to viral proteins. Administration of AAV vectors in animals does not appear to induce innate immune responses or proinflammatory cytokines, and cellular immune responses against the viral capsid have not been readily observed in rodents, rabbits, dogs, or nonhuman primates (47). Nevertheless, in view of the potential elimination of AAV-transduced hepatocytes in a hemophiliac subject (75), this is being examined further.

Applications of AAV Vectors

About a decade ago, AAV vectors were introduced into clinical trials for treatment of cystic fibrosis (CF). Since then, at least 19 different AAV vectors have been tested in at least 27 clinical trials employing various routes of delivery, including inhaled aerosol, intramuscular injection, intra-articular injection, intrahepatic infusion, and intracranial stereotactic injection (10). Most of these trials are phase I studies, but more than 500 subjects have been administered AAV vectors with good safety profiles. There are some observations of biological activity, although there are no firmly established demonstrations of clinical benefit. The clinical trials that have been most extensively described were for two genetic diseases, CF and hemophilia B (factor IX deficiency).

CF appeared to be an attractive target for gene therapy, and extensive preclinical studies of the safety and toxicity of an AAV-CFTR vector (AAV vector containing the cDNA of the CF transmembrane regulator [CFTR] gene) were performed by delivery of vector particles directly to the lungs in rabbits and nonhuman primates (16). The vector persisted and was expressed for up to 6 months, no toxicity was observed, and there was no indication of T-cell infiltration or inflammatory responses. There was minimal biodistribution of the vector to organs outside of the lungs, and the vector could not be mobilized, suggesting a low probability of shedding or transmission to others.

This AAV-CFTR vector was tested in a series of clinical trials in CF patients involving administration by various routes, including direct instillation of the vector in the lungs, and maxillary sinus and by aerosol inhalation to the whole lung (10). The administration of the vector was safe and well tolerated in all of these studies. A phase II randomized, placebo-controlled, double-blinded study in 37 subjects who were administered by whole-lung aerosol with three doses (10^{13} vector genomes per dose) at monthly intervals suggested that there was improved pulmonary function as measured by spirometry, and a decrease in the level of the proinflammatory cytokine interleukin 8 (IL-8) in the sputum (85). However, a second phase IIb trial conducted in 100 CF subjects failed to confirm effects on lung function or IL-8 (86) and highlighted an emerging general problem in many trials in CF patients. The behavior of placebo arms is unpredictable, and coupled with the difficulty of evaluating gene expression in small airways, this makes development of any gene therapy for CF a daunting task.

AAV vectors containing factor IX cDNA were tested in clinical trials for treatment of hemophilia B. AAV vectors administered by injection to muscle or by direct intrahepatic injection showed prolonged expression, for months or years, of factor IX protein at therapeutic levels in several animal species, including mice and dogs with hemophilia B (48, 89). A phase I dose escalation trial of an AAV-factor IX vector in eight subjects with hemophilia B was conducted by injection of the vector at multiple sites in the muscles of one or both legs. The vector was well tolerated and expression of factor IX protein was detected at the muscle injection sites, remarkably, up to 40 months later, but there was little or no secretion into the serum (52). In a second phase I trial, the AAV2-factor IX vector was administered to hemophilia B patients at three dose levels, 10^{11}, 10^{12}, and 2×10^{13} vector genomes, by direct injection into the hepatic artery (75). Several unexpected observations were made. First, for some subjects, vector sequences were detected in the semen for several weeks after administration. Subsequent extensive testing in multiple animal species showed a dose-dependent biodistribution of the vector to gonad tissue that waned over time. Importantly, sperm is generally negative for vector sequences, which diminishes the likelihood of modifying germ line cells (115). At the highest dose administered, in one subject there was expression of factor IX protein in serum at 11% of the normal level, which, if maintained, would be a therapeutic level. However, after 5 to 6 weeks, expression was abruptly lost and there was a contemporaneous transient rise in serum transaminase levels. Although suggestive of a cytotoxic T-lymphocyte response, the mechanism underlying this observation is not understood (82).

Clinical trials of AAV vectors which are now under way include administration to muscle for expression of alpha-1-antitrypsin for emphysema (7), expression of HIV antigens for an AIDS vaccine (55), intra-articular injection for expression of a soluble anti-tumor necrosis factor alpha inhibitor for inflammatory joint disease (110), and intracranial injection for a number of neurodegenerative diseases, including Parkinson, Alzheimer, Batten, and Canavan diseases (10, 11).

Adenovirus

The replication cycle of Ad is described in chapter 26. Initially, most Ad vectors were based on Ad serotype 2 (Ad2) and Ad5, which have very similar DNA genomes. Many of the more than 40 human serotypes and Ad strains isolated from chimpanzees are now being developed as vectors (4, 56, 79). Ad strains infect and grow in dividing or nondividing cells and naturally may persist for prolonged periods in adenoids and tonsils, but the mechanism of this persistence is poorly understood.

Ad particles are nonenveloped icosahedral particles about 80 nm in diameter. They have a complex structure with a 35-kb, linear duplex DNA genome that codes for 40 to 50 proteins, at least 12 of which are structural proteins (79). The number and complexity of the protein components of Ad have important implications both for generation of vectors in complementation systems and for eliciting host responses. Nearly all of the Ad genes are required either for genome replication or for generation of Ad particles, and this presents a complex complementation problem. Ad particles have strong adjuvant effects and may elicit significant innate immune responses as well as humoral responses to the protein components of the particles (79, 87). Also, most Ad vectors contain a large number of viral genes which may be expressed and elicit undesirable cellular immune responses in vivo. Ad vectors introduced into many organs can mediate rapid, high-level, but transient gene expression (41). This shutdown of gene expression may reflect the absence of a specific mechanism for Ad DNA persistence as well as the induction of innate and adaptive host immune responses (79). Although Ad vectors were first considered to treat genetic diseases, they may be better suited for some applications in cancer therapy (56) or as vectors for viral vaccines (4) where the immunologic adjuvant effects may be advantageous, or at least not deleterious. Ad vectors may also have utility for certain cardiovascular applications where one-time administration and short-term expression are aimed at inducing therapeutic angiogenesis (107).

Ad Vectors

The first production systems for Ad vectors were all based on use of the human 293 cell line, which expresses the Ad5 E1A and E1B proteins and can complement $E1^-$ Ad (41). First-generation Ad vectors ($E1^-$) contain the transgene cassette in place of the E1 gene, but three problems limit the use of this system. First, replication-competent Ad (RCA) is generated by recombination between the vector and Ad sequences in the 293 cell line. Second, the vectors are relatively crippled for replication but still express significant amounts of Ad early (E) and late (L) genes that induce strong cellular immune responses. Third, the packaging capacity is limited to about 4 to 5 kb. Several different approaches have been employed to alter the vector design or to generate alternate packaging cell lines (41, 56).

RCA is undesirable because Ad strains are human pathogens. Currently, the U.S. FDA requires clinical lots of Ad vectors to contain very low levels of RCA per patient dose, and this has placed limitations on dosing in clinical trials. One way to decrease RCA is to avoid direct overlapping homology with the E1A and surrounding sequences in 293 cells (46) or to design new complementing lines containing only the E1 gene, with no Ad flanking sequences (27).

The packaging capacity is increased by 2.5 kb by deleting the E3 region, but this has engendered some debate because the E3 proteins may help suppress the likelihood of immune responses to the vector (79, 87). Other efforts have been spent in designing complementation systems to increase packaging size and decrease immune responses by supplying additional complementing Ad genes such as E2A and E4 from cell lines. Several groups have attempted to generate helper-dependent (HD) mini-Ad or gutted Ad vectors that have deletions of most viral genes (56) but include a helper Ad which may have deletions of E1 and packaging signals, but these HD systems still generate significant levels of RCA or helper virus. The classical method for purification of Ad particles, like AAV, generally involves ultracentrifugation to equilibrium in CsCl gradients, but more current approaches to purifying vectors, especially for Good Manufacturing Practice production, employ column chromatography and filtration (71).

The efficacy and safety of Ad vectors have been significantly impaired by the innate and adaptive host responses. The viral capsid proteins of Ad are highly immunogenic and elicit active immune responses from the host which are exacerbated because recombinant Ad strains may continue to express these proteins and evoke host cytotoxic T-lymphocyte responses in addition to neutralizing antibody responses (136, 139). The current efforts under way to design HD or gutted Ad vectors may minimize the cellular immune response and lead to vectors that are expressed for much longer periods in vivo (56).

Many genes have been expressed from Ad vectors (79), including the Ad-CFTR vectors for CF, p53, factor IX, ornithine transcarbamylase (OTC), vascular endothelial growth factor, and minidystrophin and the HSV thymidine kinase genes. In these studies, a variety of cell types have been transduced both in vitro and in vivo with the Ad vectors, including respiratory epithelium, submucosal gland, liver, skeletal, cardiac, smooth muscle, and blood vessel endothelium cells and neurons. However, in the in vivo animal models, gene expression is often rapidly attenuated, within a month. This absence of persistent expression was seen also in the series of clinical trials conducted with Ad-CFTR vectors. In addition, most of these Ad vectors induced significant inflammatory responses and cellular immune responses and were limited for readministration by humoral immune responses (41).

Applications of Ad Vectors

The first clinical indication for which Ad vectors were tested was to introduce the CFTR gene to airway epithelium of patients with CF, but this disease now appears to be a less ideal target for Ad vectors with respect to both the short duration of expression and the indication of potentially significant inflammatory responses (19). Even single administration of Ad vectors may result in severe consequences, as occurred in the only clinical trial conducted to treat a metabolic disease. This was a single-administration, dose escalation trial in adult patients with a deficiency in the urea cycle enzyme OTC, either female carriers or males with mild disease. The patients were infused via the hepatic artery with increasing doses of an Ad vector that expressed the gene for OTC. An 18-year-old male in the sixth and highest-dose cohort died 4 days after receiving the vector infusion (105). Subsequent analysis, and additional studies in animals, indicated that this appeared to involve an initial high level of entry of the vector into nonparenchymal Kuppfer cells in the liver and vector interactions with the reticuloendothelial system (118) which led to a disseminated intravascular coagulopathy and proinflammatory cytokines in the blood and then acute respiratory distress syndrome and multiorgan failure (105). The toxicities involving disseminated intravascular coagulopathy and the proinflammatory cytokines appeared to be dose dependent and linked and to occur at similar doses of vector.

The current Ad vectors may not be suitable for treating genetic diseases but may be suitable for some cancer applications where inducing a destructive immune response against the cell may be an advantage and where the toxicity profile may be more acceptable relative to the disease. A large number of clinical trials are now testing Ad vectors in cancer patients, and delivery of the tumor suppressor p53 gene has now moved to phase III trials with head and neck cancer patients in the United States (60). In addition, an Ad expressing a p53 gene has been approved for use in China, but the circumstances and clinical trial data on which this product was approved have not been fully described (99). Ad vectors are also being tested in clinical trials to treat cardiovascular disease, and these trials have advanced to phase II and phase III. These applications seek to induce therapeutic angiogenesis by delivery of vectors expressing growth factors such as vascular endothelial growth factor or platelet-derived growth factor vessels in the ischemic heart or in peripheral artery disease (72, 107). Ad vectors may also be useful as vectors for antiviral vaccines, and this approach is now in proof-of-concept trials of candidate HIV-1 vaccines with doses in the range of 10^{11} vector genomes in several thousand study subjects.

Herpes Simplex Virus

HSV type 1 (HSV-1) has been extensively engineered as a gene transfer vector, and much is known about its gene functions and molecular biology (see chapter 19). For use in gene transfer, its most important features are its abilities to infect cells with high efficiency and to deliver a large transgene "payload." Indeed, almost the entire genome can be replaced by non-HSV DNA and packaged into infectious particles. Of particular interest for vector engineering is the ability of HSV to persist in neurons as an episomal element; in human infections and animal models, this state of latency appears to remain for the life of the host. During latent infection, there is little detectable expression of immediate-early (IE), E, or L viral proteins. Expression is limited to a set of nontranslated RNA species known as latency-associated transcripts (18, 108, 122, 123). A portion of the promoter regulating expression of latency-associated transcripts, LAP2, has been used for constructing HSV-1 vectors that allow long-term transgene expression in neurons. The LAP2 element is capable of driving expression of therapeutic transgenes in both the central and peripheral nervous systems (14, 103). For many gene therapy applications that involve nervous system disease, the vector can serve as a platform for therapeutic gene expression at the site where therapy is needed and transgene expression can be short or long term depending on the vector promoter employed. For cancer applications, this biology is less important since the goal is to destroy tumor cells, and thus targeting virus infection to the tumor becomes the paramount task. Although the majority of experience and greatest expectations for success utilize replication-competent lytic vectors, especially for treatment of brain tumors, other vector types may prove important, and their testing in patients is anticipated.

HSV Vector Designs

Two HSV vector systems have been developed: genomic vectors and amplicons. Genomic HSV vectors (replication-competent or replication-defective vectors) are mutated in nonessential and essential genes that compromise virus growth in some or all cell types. Replication-competent vectors are mutant viruses with deletions of nonessential genes that replicate in specific cell types (Fig. 9A). Their selectivity can be substantial and is often related to whether the targeted cells are actively dividing and on the particular genetic and cellular backgrounds. Most often the targeted cell types are malignant. Replication-defective vectors can be created by deletion of any essential gene requiring specialized cells that complement the defective gene(s) in *trans* for vector production (Fig. 9B). Typically IE essential genes are deleted, thereby blocking the subsequent expression of E and L gene functions. Because several of these IE genes are cytotoxic, their complete deletion renders the virus harmless to cells while retaining transgene expression capability (54, 63, 109) and vector persistence in neuronal and nonmitotic somatic cells (130).

HSV amplicon vectors consist of plasmids bearing an HSV origin of DNA replication *(ori)* and packaging signal *(pac)* which allows the amplicon DNA to be replicated and packaged as a concatenate into HSV virions in the presence of HSV helper functions (35, 36, 67, 121) (Fig. 9C). These vectors can be packaged concomitantly with replication-competent HSV helper virus or produced free of helper virus. The latter can be accomplished by vector cotransfection with an HSV genome with deletions of *pac* signals and also either mutated in or having a deletion(s) of an essential HSV gene(s) or engineered to be too large for incorporation into the virus capsid (64, 93). The advantages of amplicon vectors are essentially no toxicity or antigenicity, as they express no virus proteins; a very large transgene capacity (up to 150 kb) (128); relatively high titers (~10^8 transducing units/ml); and long-term retention in nondividing cells. Disadvantages include difficulty in producing large quantities of clinical-grade vector and lack of retention in dividing cells. A variation of the HSV-1 vector platform is similar to the amplicon approach except that instead of using seven overlapping cosmids to

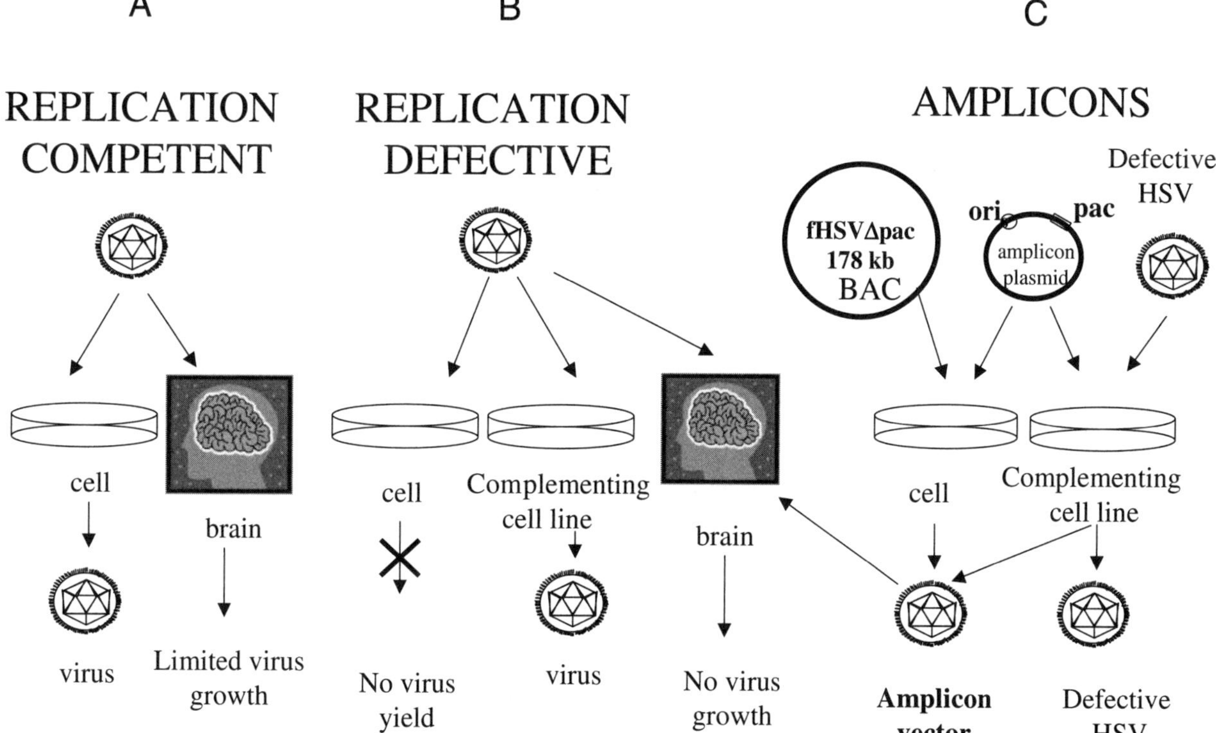

FIGURE 9 Generation of three major types of HSV vectors on the basis of the genes targeted for deletion. (A) Replication-competent vectors are generated by deletion of accessory genes to replicate in tumor cells preferentially over normal cells; (B) replication-defective vectors are generated by deletion of an essential gene(s) to block virus growth; (C) amplicon vectors are generated using plasmids bearing the HSV origin of DNA replication.

comprise the HSV-1 genome, the entire genome is cloned into a bacterial artificial chromosome.

Clinical Applications of HSV Vectors

Cancer Therapies

Knowledge of the biology of HSV-1, the molecular biology of tumor cells, and the novel interactions of these genetically altered cells with HSV provides a unique opportunity to engineer HSV-1 as a highly selective and potent anticancer vector potentially tailored to individual patient tumors. The use of viruses with improved initial intratumoral distribution and carrying genes that both overcome innate immune responses and promote an intracellular proapoptotic state should improve the potency of HSV cancer gene therapy vectors without compromising safety. Oncolytic viruses have been used in early-phase clinical trials for a variety of tumors, including colorectal cancer metastatic to the liver (76, 116) and glioblastoma multiforme (22, 32, 69, 77, 96, 104). Recent trials have been encouraging, showing these viruses to be relatively nontoxic for normal cells but remaining lytic in tumor cells. The targeting of tumor cells has not been absolute, but it may be possible to improve tumor specificity by retargeting infection to tumor cell surface receptors that are more abundant in or specific to the tumor cell membrane. Brain tumors are particularly good targets for HSV oncolytic vectors because of the vector neurotropism and their remarkable ability to be engineered for replication within these tumors without toxicity for normal brain. In addition, the nonreplicative HSV vectors and amplicon-based systems should also add to the arsenal of potential treatment vehicles. These vectors might be used in combination with the replicative vectors to modify the local environment to discourage tumor metastasis, for example, or under circumstances where vector gene expression is intended for the induction of anticancer immunity. Finally, multimodal therapies will probably be essential for successful treatment of solid tumors even where there is infiltration into normal tissue.

Chronic Pain Therapies

HSV vectors have been used extensively for gene therapy in animal models of pain. Nonreplicating HSV vectors that can be introduced into the skin, where vector particles enter nerve terminals, are transported along axons to the neuronal perikaryon in the dorsal root ganglia, and vector genomes serve as a platform for expression of therapeutic gene products. Thus, by selection of the dermatome where pain is present, the vector can be targeted to the appropriate ganglion and the analgesic gene products can be expressed precisely at the site where therapy is needed. Such targeting and limited exposure of therapeutic molecules provide a considerable advantage to gene therapy using HSV, particularly since it is the only vector with this novel transport mechanism in humans.

An HSV vector with a *tk* deletion and containing the proenkephalin gene reduced hyperalgesia (38). Gene therapy for pain can be used without the induction of tolerance, and the vector has been capable of repeat administration with the reestablishment of the analgesic state (38). The use of enkephalin gene therapy has been extended in a mouse model of bone cancer pain (37), bladder irritation (138), craniofacial pain (80), and pancreatitis (70). Together, these data provide proof of principle that the HSV vector-mediated delivery of enkephalin can provide an analgesic effect in several different models of pain, and they set the stage for a human trial to treat chronic pain using HSV vector-expressed enkephalin. Other genes eliciting specific analgesic responses that have been transferred using herpesvirus vectors include the genes for endomorphin 2, a potent analgesic peptide (119, 140); human glutamic acid decarboxylase (GAD67) (45); glial derived neurotrophic factor; IL-4 (44); the voltage-gated sodium channel NaV1.7; and the peptide neurotransmitter calcitonin gene-related peptide (137).

HSV Gene Therapy for Treatment of Neuropathy

HSV-based vectors have been administered by subcutaneous inoculation to deliver and express neurotrophic factors in dorsal root ganglion neurons to protect against peripheral nerve degeneration in models of neuropathy. Expression of neurotrophin 3 or nerve growth factor was effective in the treatment of nerve loss in a pyridoxine intoxication model of large-fiber sensory neuropathy and in a streptozotocin model of diabetic neuropathy (38). A similar protective effect was shown following administration of the chemotherapeutic drug cisplatin (45). Treatment of induced sensory nerve degeneration by chemotherapy may well provide a suitable first human trial for gene therapy of neuropathy.

NOVEL VECTORS

A long list of other viruses is under study for their potential utility for gene delivery. Among these are vectors which may persist by chromosomal integration (foamy virus and parvovirus) or as episomes (simian virus 40 and Epstein-Barr virus) and vectors which may be present only transiently for expression of immunogenic proteins (vaccinia virus, alphaviruses, and canarypox virus) or for cytopathicity (conditionally replicating Ad and VSV). In evaluating the utility of a new vector system, considerations include the target range (species, cell types, and cell activation status requirements), the vector carrying capacity, the intrinsic gene transfer efficiency, the duration of persistence of the vector, the achievable gene expression level, the immunogenicity of the vector, the toxicity and safety profile, and the logistics of production and testing.

In the past few years, gene integration systems have been developed that may be described as semiviral. They use recombinase proteins from transposons or bacteriophage to mediate chromosomal integration of gene expression units, such as expression plasmids. These recombinase-based systems may lead to patterns of chromosomal integration sites that have reduced potential for transactivation of cellular genes compared to the retro- and lentiviral vectors that have strong predilections to integrate near genes that are actively expressed. The Sleeping Beauty system was developed by reanimating the devolved transposase gene from a long-dormant transposon in fish genomes (51). The transposase acts on the ITR of the transposon to mediate recombination into target DNA, with minimal target sequence specificity or chromosomal status. The Sleeping Beauty transposase system has been shown to mediate high-efficiency integration of plasmids transfected or electroporated into cells in culture or by direct in vivo injection of the plasmids carrying the transposase and bearing the Sleeping Beauty ITR (49, 50, 135).

Another system was developed based on the recombinase from the bacteriophage PhiC31, which mediates site-specific integration of the bacteriophage DNA genome into the host bacterial chromosome (125). In mammalian cells, the PhiC31 recombinase mediates integration of expression plasmids carrying the bacterial integration *(attB)* sequence into several preferred sites of the host cell chromosome that have some degree of homology to the bacteriophage integration sequence *(attP)*. Vector integration restricted to a lower number of sites may be safer than more wide-ranging and random integration, although it depends on the specific nature of the recurrent integration sites.

Hybrid vectors have been developed that contain elements from different viruses and/or nonviral gene delivery systems to take advantage of their respective attributes. For example, the high initial gene transfer efficiency of Ad strains or herpesviruses can be used to deliver the genes needed to produce a persisting vector, such as a retrovirus, AAV, or transposons (17, 29, 30). Targeting moieties, such as ligands for surface receptors or single-chain antibodies, can be included in viruses to modify their tropism (20, 134). Ad proteins can be mixed with nonviral components, such as cationic lipids, to improve binding to cell surface molecules or to assist with intracellular gene delivery.

REFERENCES

1. **Aiuti, A., S. Slavin, M. Aker, F. Ficara, S. Deola, A. Mortellaro, S. Morecki, G. Andolfi, A. Tabucchi, F. Carlucci, E. Marinello, F. Cattaneo, S. Vai, P. Servida, R. Miniero, M. G. Roncarolo, and C. Bordignon.** 2002. Correction of ADA-SCID by stem cell gene therapy combined with nonmyeloablative conditioning. *Science* **296:** 2410–2413.
2. **Anderson, W. F., G. J. McGarrity, and R. C. Moen.** 1993. Report to the NIH Recombinant DNA Advisory Committee on murine replication-competent retrovirus (RCR) assays. *Hum. Gene Ther.* **4:**311–321.
3. **Bandyopadhyay, P. K., and H. M. Temin.** 1984. Expression of complete chicken thymidine kinase gene inserted in a retrovirus vector. *Mol. Cell Biol.* **4:**749–754.
4. **Barouch, D. H., and G. J. Nabel.** 2005. Adenovirus vector based vaccines for human immunodeficiency virus type 1. *Hum. Gene Ther.* **16:**149–156.
5. **Beck, S. E., L. A. Jones, K. Chesnut, S. Walsh, T. Reynolds, B. J. Carter, F. B. Askin, T. R. Flotte, and W. B. Guggino.** 1999. Repeated delivery of adeno-associated virus vectors to rabbit airway. *J. Virol.* **73:** 9446–9455.
6. **Berry, C., S. Hannenhalli, J. Leipzig, and F. D. Bushman.** 2006. Selection of target sites for mobile DNA integration in the human genome. *PLoS Comput. Biol.* **2:** e157.
7. **Brantly, M. L., L. T. Spencer, M. Humphries, T. J. Conlon, C. T. Spencer, A. Poirier, W. Garlington, D. Baker, S. Song, K. I. Berns, N. Muzyczka, R. O. Snyder, B. J. Byrne, and T. R. Flotte.** 2006. Phase I trial of intramuscular injection of a recombinant adeno-associated virus serotype 2 α1-antitrypsin (AAT) vector in AAT-deficient adults. *Hum. Gene Ther.* **17:**1177–1186.
8. **Bukrinsky, M. I., N. Sharova, M. P. Dempsey, T. L. Stanwick, A. G. Bukrinskaya, S. Haggerty, and M. Stevenson.** 1992. Active nuclear import of human immunodeficiency virus type 1 preintegration complexes. *Proc. Natl. Acad. Sci. USA* **89:**6580–6584.
9. **Carroll, R., J. T. Lin, E. J. Dacquel, J. D. Mosca, D. S. Burke, and D. C. St. Louis.** 1994. A human immunodeficiency virus type 1 (HIV-1)-based retroviral vector system utilizing stable HIV-1 packaging cell lines. *J. Virol.* **68:**6047–6051.
10. **Carter, B. J.** 2005. Adeno-associated virus vectors in clinical trials. *Hum. Gene Ther.* **16:**541–550.
11. **Carter, B. J.** 2006. Clinical development with adeno-associated virus vectors, p. 499–510. *In* J. R. Kerr, S. F. Cotmore, M. E. Bloom, R. M. Linden, and C. R. Parrish (ed.), *Parvoviruses*. Hodder Arnold, London, United Kingdom.
12. **Carter, B. J., H. Burstein, and R. W. Peluso.** 2004. Adeno-associated virus and AAV vectors for gene delivery, p. 71–101. *In* N. S. Templeton (ed.), *Gene Therapy: Therapeutic Mechanisms and Strategies*, 2nd ed. Marcel Dekker, New York, NY.
13. **Cavazzana-Calvo, M., S. Hacein-Bey, G. de Saint Basile, F. Gross, E. Yvon, P. Nusbaum, F. Selz, C. Hue, S. Certain, J. L. Casanova, P. Bousso, F. Le Deist, and A. Fischer.** 2000. Gene therapy of human severe combined immunodeficiency (SCID)-X1 disease. *Science* **288:**669–672.
14. **Chattopadhyay, M., D. Wolfe, M. Mata, S. Huang, J. C. Glorioso, and D. J. Fink.** 2005. Long-term neuroprotection achieved with latency-associated promoter-driven herpes simplex virus gene transfer to the peripheral nervous system. *Mol. Ther.* **12:**307–313.
15. **Chirmule, N., W. Xiao, A. Truneh, M. Schnell, J. V. Hughes, P. Zoltich, and J. M. Wilson.** 2000. Humoral immunity to adeno-associated virus type 2 vectors following administration to murine and non-human primate muscle. *J. Virol.* **74:**2420–2425.
16. **Conrad, C. K., S. S. Allen, S. A. Afione, T. C. Reynolds, S. E. Beck, M. Fee-Maki, X. Barrazza-Ortiz, R. Adams, F. B. Askin, B. J. Carter, W. B. Guggino, and T. R. Flotte.** 1996. Safety of single-dose administration of an adeno-associated virus (AAV-CFTR) vector in the primate lung. *Gene Ther.* **3:**658–668.
17. **Costantini, L. C., D. R. Jacoby, S. Wang, C. Fraefel, X. O. Breakefield, and O. Isacson.** 1999. Gene transfer to the nigrostriatal system by hybrid herpes simplex virus/adeno-associated virus amplicon vectors. *Hum. Gene Ther.* **10:**2481–2494.
18. **Croen, K. D., J. M. Ostrove, L. J. Dragovic, J. E. Smialek, and S. E. Straus.** 1987. Latent herpes simplex virus in human trigeminal ganglia. Detection of an immediate early gene "anti-sense" transcript by in situ hybridization. *N. Engl. J. Med.* **317:**1427–1432.
19. **Crystal, R. G., N. G. McElvaney, M. A. Rosenfeld, C. S. Chu, A. Mastrangeli, J. G. Hay, S. L. Brody, H. A. Jaffe, N. T. T. Eissa, and C. Danel.** 1994. Administration of an adenovirus containing the human CFTR CDNA to the respiratory tract of individuals with cystic fibrosis. *Nat. Genet.* **8:**42–51.
20. **Curiel, D. T.** 1999. Strategies to adapt adenoviral vectors for target delivery. *Ann. N.Y. Acad. Sci.* **886:**158–171.
21. **Delelis, O., A. Saib, and P. Sonigo.** 2003. Biphasic DNA synthesis in spumaviruses. *J. Virol.* **77:**8141–8161.
22. **Detta, A., J. Harland, I. Hanif, S. M. Brown, and G. Cruickshank.** 2003. Proliferative activity and in vitro replication of HSV1716 in human metastatic brain tumours. *J. Gene Med.* **5:**681–689.
23. **Donahue, R. E., S. W. Kessler, D. Bodine, K. McDonagh, C. Dunbar, S. Goodman, B. Agricola, E. Byrne, M. Raffeld, R. Moen, J. Bacher, K. M. Zsebo, and A. W. Nienhuis.** 1992. Helper virus induced T cell lymphoma in nonhuman primates after retroviral mediated gene transfer. *J. Exp. Med.* **176:**1125–1135.
24. **Du, Y., S. E. Spence, N. A. Jenkins, and N. G. Copeland.** 2005. Cooperating cancer-gene identification

through oncogenic-retrovirus-induced insertional mutagenesis. *Blood* **106:**2498–2505.

25. **Dull, T., R. Zufferey, M. Kelly, R. J. Mandel, M. Nguyen, D. Trono, and L. Naldini.** 1998. A third-generation lentivirus vector with a conditional packaging system. *J. Virol.* **72:**8463–8471.
26. **Emi, N., T. Friedmann, and J. K. Yee.** 1991. Pseudotype formation of murine leukemia virus with the G protein of vesicular stomatitis virus. *J. Virol.* **65:**1202–1207.
27. **Fallaux, F. J., A. Bout, I. van der Velde, D. J. van den Wollenberg, K. M. Hehir, J. Keegan, C. Auger, S. J. Cramer, H. van Ormondt, A. J. vander Eb, D. Valerio, and R. C. Hoeben.** 1998. New helper cells and matched early region 1-deleted adenovirus vectors to prevent generation of replication-competent adenoviruses. *Hum. Gene Ther.* **9:**1909–1917.
28. **Felgner, P. L.** 1997. Nonviral strategies for gene therapy. *Sci. Am.* **276:**102–106.
29. **Feng, M., W. H. Jackson, C. K. Goldman, C. Rancourt, M. Wang, S. K. Dusing, G. Siegal, and D. T. Curiel.** 1997. Stable in vivo gene transduction via a novel adenoviral/retroviral chimeric vector. *Nat. Biotechnol.* **15:**866–870.
30. **Fisher, K. J., W. M. Kelley, J. F. Burda, and J. M. Wilson.** 1996. A novel adenovirus-adeno-associated virus hybrid vector displays efficient rescue and delivery of the AAV genome. *Hum. Gene Ther.* **7:**2079–2087.
31. **Gallay, P., S. Swingler, C. Aiken, and D. Trono.** 1995. HIV-1 infection of nondividing cells: C-terminal tyrosine phosphorylation of the viral matrix protein is a key regulator. *Cell* **80:**379–388.
32. **Ganly, I., D. S. Soutar, and S. B. Kaye.** 2000. Current role of gene therapy in head and neck cancer. *Eur. J. Surg. Oncol.* **26:**338–343.
33. **Gaspar, H. B., K. L. Parsley, S. Howe, D. King, K. C. Gilmour, J. Sinclair, G. Brouns, M. Schmidt, C. Von Kalle, T. Barington, M. A. Jakobsen, H. O. Christensen, A. Al Ghonaium, H. N. White, J. L. Smith, R. J. Levinsky, R. R. Ali, C. Kinnon, and A. J. Thrasher.** 2004. Gene therapy of X-linked severe combined immunodeficiency by use of a pseudotyped gammaretroviral vector. *Lancet* **364:**2181–2187.
34. **Gaspar, H. B., E. Bjorkegren, K. Parsley, K. C. Gilmour, D. King, J. Sinclair, F. Zhang, A. Giannakopoulos, S. Adams, L. D. Fairbanks, J. Gaspar, L. Henderson, J. H. Xu-Bayford, E. G. Davies, P. A. Veys, C. Kinnon, and A. J. Thrasher.** 2006. Successful reconstitution of immunity in ADA-SCID by stem cell gene therapy following cessation of PEG-ADA and use of mild preconditioning. *Mol. Ther.* **14:**505–513.
35. **Geller, A., and X. Breakefield.** 1988. A defective HSV-1 vector expresses Escherichia coli β-galactosidase in cultured peripheral neurons. *Science* **241:**1667–1669.
36. **Geller, A., K. Keyomarsi, J. Bryan, and A. Pardee.** 1990. An efficient deletion mutant packaging system for defective herpes simplex virus vectors: potential applications to human gene therapy and neuronal physiology. *Proc. Natl. Acad. Sci. USA* **87:**8950–8954.
37. **Goss, J. R., C. F. Harley, M. Mata, M. E. O'Malley, W. F. Goins, X. Hu, J. C. Glorioso, and D. J. Fink.** 2002. Herpes vector-mediated expression of proenkephalin reduces bone cancer pain. *Ann. Neurol.* **52:**662–665.
38. **Goss, J. R., M. Mata, W. F. Goins, H. H. Wu, J. C. Glorioso, and D. J. Fink.** 2001. Antinociceptive effect of a genomic herpes simplex virus-based vector expressing human proenkephalin in rat dorsal root ganglion. *Gene Ther.* **8:**551–556.
39. **Hacein-Bey-Abina, S., F. Le Deist, F. Carlier, C. Bouneaud, C. Hue, J. P. De Villartay, A. J. Thrasher, N. Wulffraat, R. Sorensen, S. Dupuis-Girod, A. Fischer, E. G. Davies, W. Kuis, L. Leiva, and M. Cavazzana-Calvo.** 2002. Sustained correction of X-linked severe combined immunodeficiency by ex vivo gene therapy. *N. Engl. J. Med.* **346:**1185–1193.
40. **Hacein-Bey-Abina, S., C. Von Kalle, M. Schmidt, M. P. McCormack, N. Wulffraat, P. Leboulch, A. Lim, C. S. Osborne, R. Pawliuk, E. Morillon, R. Sorensen, A. Forster, P. Fraser, J. L. Cohen, G. de Saint Basile, I. Alexander, U. Wintergerst, T. Frebourg, A. Aurias, D. Stoppa-Lyonnet, S. Romana, I. Radford-Weiss, F. Gross, F. Valensi, E. Delabesse, E. Macintyre, F. Sigaux, J. Soulier, L. E. Leiva, M. Wissler, C. Prinz, T. H. Rabbitts, F. Le Deist, A. Fischer, and M. Cavazzana-Calvo.** 2003. LMO2-associated clonal T cell proliferation in two patients after gene therapy for SCID-X1. *Science* **302:**415–419.
41. **Hackett, N. R., and R. G. Crystal.** 2004. Adenovirus vectors for gene therapy, p. 17–41. *In* N. S. Templeton (ed.), *Gene Therapy,Therapeutic Mechanisms and Strategies*, 2nd ed. Marcel Dekker, New York, NY.
42. **Halbert, C., T. A. Standaert, C. B. Wilson, and A. D. Miller.** 1998. Successful readministration of adeno-associated virus vectors to the mouse lung requires transient immunosuppression during the initial exposure. *J. Virol.* **72:**9795–9805.
43. **Halbert, C. L., A. D. Miller, A. McNamara, J. Emerson, R. L. Gibson, B. Ramsey, and M. L. Aitken.** 2006. Prevalence of neutralizing antibodies against adeno-associated virus (AAV) types 2, 5, and 6 in cystic fibrosis and normal populations: implications for gene therapy using AAV vectors. *Hum. Gene Ther.* **17:**440–447.
44. **Hao, S., M. Mata, J. C. Glorioso, and D. J. Fink.** 2007. Gene transfer to interfere with TNFalpha signaling in neuropathic pain. *Gene Ther.* **14:**1010–1016.
45. **Hao, S., M. Mata, D. Wolfe, S. Huang, J. C. Glorioso, and D. J. Fink.** 2003. HSV-mediated gene transfer of the glial cell-derived neurotrophic factor provides an antiallodynic effect on neuropathic pain. *Mol. Ther.* **8:**367–375.
46. **Hehir, K., D. M. Armentano, L. M. Cardoza, T. L. Choquette, P. B. Berthelette, G. A. White, L. A. Couture, M. B. Everton, J. Keegan, J. M. Martin, D. A. Pratt, M. P. Smith, A. E. Smith, and S. C. Wadsworth.** 1996. Molecular characterization of replication-competent variants of adenovirus vector and genome modifications to prevent their occurrence. *J. Virol.* **70:**8459–8467.
47. **Hernandez, Y. J., J. Wang, W. G. Kearns, S. Loiler, A. Poirier, and T. R. Flotte.** 1999. Latent adeno-associated virus infection elicits humoral but not cell-mediated immune responses in a nonhuman primate model. *J. Virol.* **73:**8549–8558.
48. **Herzog, R. W., J. N. Hagstrom, S. H. Jung, S. J. Tai, J. M. Wilson, K. J. Fisher, and K. A. High.** 1997. Stable gene transfer and expression of human blood coagulation factor IX after intramuscular injection of recombinant adeno-associated virus. *Proc. Natl. Acad. Sci. USA* **94:**5804–5809.
49. **Hollis, R. P., S. J. Nightingale, X. Wang, K. A. Pepper, X. J. Yu, L. Barsky, G. M. Crooks, and D. B. Kohn.** 2006. Stable gene transfer to human CD34(+) hematopoietic cells using the Sleeping Beauty transposon. *Exp. Hematol.* **34:**1333–1343.
50. **Huang, X., A. C. Wilber, L. Bao, D. Tuong, J. Tolar, P. J. Orchard, B. L. Levine, C. H. June, R. S. McIvor, B. R. Blazar, and X. Zhou.** 2006. Stable gene transfer

and expression in human primary T cells by the Sleeping Beauty transposon system. *Blood* **107:**483–491.

51. **Ivics, Z., P. B. Hackett, R. H. Plasterk, and Z. Izsvák.** 1997. Molecular reconstruction of Sleeping Beauty, a Tc1-like transposon from fish, and its transposition in human cells. *Cell* **91:**501–510.
52. **Jiang, H., G. F. Pierce, M. C. Ozelo, E. V. de Paula, J. A. Vargas, P. Smith, J. Sommer, A. Luk, C. S. Manno, K. A. High, and V. R. Arruda.** 2006. Evidence of multiyear factor IX expression by AAV-mediated gene transfer to skeletal muscle in an individual with severe hemophilia B. *Mol. Ther.* **14:**452–455.
53. **Johnson, L. G., J. C. Olsen, L. Naldini, and R. C. Boucher.** 2000. Pseudotyped human lentiviral vector-mediated gene transfer to airway epithelia in vivo. *Gene Ther.* **7:**568–574.
54. **Johnson, P., M. Wang, and T. Friedmann.** 1994. Improved cell survival by the reduction of immediate-early gene expression in replication-defective mutants of herpes simplex virus type 1 but not by mutation of the virion host shutoff function. *J. Virol.* **68:**6347–6362.
55. **Johnson, P. R., B. C. Schnepp, M. J. Connell, D. Rohne, S. Robinson, G. R. Krivulka, C. I. Lord, R. Zinn, D. C. Montefiori, N. L. Letvin, and K. R. Clark.** 2005. Novel adeno-associated virus vector vaccine restricts replication of simian immunodeficiency virus in macaques. *J. Virol.* **79:**955–965.
56. **Jolly, D., E. Aguilar-Cordova, and L. K. Aguilar.** 2008. Adenovirus vectors: history and perspective, p. 39–59. *In* B. Dropulic and B. J. Carter (ed.), *Current Concepts in Genetic Medicine*. John Wiley & Sons, New York, NY.
57. **Kafri, T., U. Blömer, D. A. Peterson, F. H. Gage, and I. M. Verma.** 1997. Sustained expression of genes delivered directly into liver and muscle by lentiviral vectors. *Nat. Genet.* **17:**314–317.
58. **Kang, Y., C. S. Stein, J. A. Heth, P. L. Sinn, A. K. Penisten, P. D. Staber, K. L. Ratliff, H. Shen, C. K. Barker, I. Martins, C. M. Sharkey, D. A. Sanders, P. B. McCray, Jr., and B. L. Davidson.** 2002. In vivo gene transfer using a nonprimate lentiviral vector pseudotyped with Ross River virus glycoproteins. *J. Virol.* **76:**9378–9388.
59. **Kasahara, N., A. M. Dozy, and Y. W. Kan.** 1994. Tissue-specific targeting of retroviral vectors through ligand-receptor interactions. *Science* **266:**1373–1376.
60. **Khuri, F. R., J. Nemunaitis, I. Ganly, J. Arseneau, I. F. Tannock, L. Romel, M. Gore, J. Ironside, R. H. MacDougall, C. Heise, B. Randlev, A. M. Gillenwater, P. Bruso, S. B. Kaye, W. K. Hong, and D. H. Kirn.** 2000. A controlled trial of intratumoral ONYX-015, a selectively replicating adenovirus, in combination with cisplatin and 5-fluorouracil in patients with recurrent head and neck cancer. *Nat. Med.* **6:**879–885.
61. **Kiem, H. P., J. Allen, G. Trobridge, E. Olson, K. Keyser, L. Peterson, and D. W. Russell.** 2007. Foamy-virus-mediated gene transfer to canine repopulating cells. *Blood* **109:**65–70.
62. **Kotin, R. M., M. Siniscalo, R. J. Samulski, X. D. Zhy, L. Hunter, C. A. Laughlin, S. Mclaughlin, N. Muzyczka, M. Rocchi, and K. I. Berns.** 1990. Site-specific integration by AAV. *Proc. Natl. Acad. Sci. USA* **87:**2211–2215.
63. **Krisky, D. M., D. Wolfe, W. F. Goins, P. C. Marconi, R. Ramakrishnan, M. Mata, R. J. D. Rouse, D. J. Fink, and J. C. Glorioso.** 1998. Deletion of multiple immediate early genes from herpes simplex virus reduces cytotoxicity and permits long-term gene expression in neurons. *Gene Ther.* **5:**1593–1603.
64. **Kubo, S., Y. Saeki, E. A. Chiocca, and K. Mitani.** 2003. An HSV amplicon-based helper system for helper-dependent adenoviral vectors. *Biochem. Biophys. Res. Commun.* **307:**826–830.
65. **Levine, B. L., L. M. Humeau, J. Boyer, R. R. MacGregor, T. Rebello, X. Lu, G. K. Binder, V. Slepushkin, F. Lemiale, J. R. Mascola, F. D. Bushman, B. Dropulic, and C. H. June.** 2006. Gene transfer in humans using a conditionally replicating lentiviral vector. *Proc. Natl. Acad. Sci. USA* **103:**17372–17377.
66. **Lewis, P. F., and M. Emerman.** 1994. Passage through mitosis is required for oncoretroviruses but not for the human immunodeficiency virus. *J. Virol.* **68:**510–516.
67. **Lim, F., D. Hartley, P. Starr, P. Lang, S. Song, L. Yu, Y. Wang, and A. I. Geller.** 1996. Generation of high-titer defective HSV-1 vectors using an IE 2 deletion mutant and quantitative study of expression in cultured cortical cells. *BioTechniques* **20:**460–469.
68. **Lin, S., N. Gaiano, P. Culp, J. C. Burns, T. Friedmann, J. K. Yee, and N. Hopkins.** 1994. Integration and germ-line transmission of a pseudotyped retroviral vector in zebrafish. *Science* **265:**666–669.
69. **Liu, B. L., M. Robinson, Z. Q. Han, R. H. Branston, C. English, P. Reay, Y. McGrath, S. K. Thomas, M. Thornton, P. Bullock, C. A. Love, and R. S. Coffin.** 2003. ICP34.5 deleted herpes simplex virus with enhanced oncolytic, immune stimulating, and anti-tumour properties. *Gene Ther.* **10:**292–303.
70. **Lu, Y., T. A. McNearney, W. Lin, S. P. Wilson, D. C. Yeomans, and K. N. Westlund.** 2007. Treatment of inflamed pancreas with enkephalin encoding HSV-1 recombinant vector reduces inflammatory damage and behavioral sequelae. *Mol. Ther.* **15:**1812–1819. [Epub ahead of print.]
71. **Lusky, M.** 2005. Good manufacturing practice production of adenoviral vectors for clinical trials. *Hum. Gene Ther.* **16:**281–291.
72. **Mack, C. A., S. R. Patel, E. A. Schwarz, P. Zanzonico, R. T. Hahn, A. Ilercil, R. B. Devereux, S. J. Goldsmith, T. F. Christian, T. A. Sandborn, I. Kovesdi, N. Hackett, R. W. Isom, R. G. Crystal, and T. K. Rosengart.** 1998. Biologic bypass with the use of adenovirus-mediated gene transfer of the complementary DNA for vascular endothelial growth factor 121 improves myocardial perfusion and function in the ischemic porcine heart. *J. Thorac. Cardiovasc. Surg.* **115:**168–176.
73. **Mangeot, P.-E., D. Nègre, B. Dubois, A. J. Winter, P. Leissner, M. Mehtali, D. Kaiserlian, F.-L. Cosset, and J.-L. Darlix.** 2000. Development of minimal lentivirus vectors derived from simian immunodeficiency virus (SIVmac251) and their use for gene transfer into human dendritic cells. *J. Virol.* **74:**8307–8315.
74. **Mann, R., R. C. Mulligan, and D. Baltimore.** 1983. Construction of a retrovirus packaging mutant and its use to produce helper-free defective retrovirus. *Cell* **33:**153–159.
75. **Manno, C. S., V. R. Arruda, G. F. Pierce, B. Glader, M. Ragni, J. Rasko, M. C. Ozelo, K. Hoots, P. Blatt, B. Konkle, M. Dake, R. Kaye, M Razavi, A. Zajko, J. Zehneder, H. Nakai, A. Chew, D. Leonard, J. F. Wright, R. S. Lessard, J. M. Sommer, M.Tigges, D. Sabatino, A. Luk, H. Jiang, F. Mingozzi, L. Couto, H. C. Ertl, K. A. High, and M. A. Kay.** 2006. Successful transduction of liver in hemophilia by AAV-factor IX and limitations imposed by the host immune response. *Nat. Med.* **12:**342–347.
76. **Markert, J. M., G. Y. Gillespie, R. R. Weichselbaum, B. Roizman, and R. J. Whitley.** Genetically engineered

HSV in the treatment of glioma: a review. *Rev. Med. Virol.* **10:**17–30.

77. **Markert, J. M., M. D. Medlock, S. D. Rabkin, G. Y. Gillespie, T. Todo, W. D. Hunter, C. A. Palmer, F. Feigenbaum, C. Tornatore, F. Tufaro, and R. L. Martuza.** 2000. Conditionally replicating herpes simplex virus mutant, G207 for the treatment of malignant glioma: results of a phase I trial. *Gene Ther.* **7:**867–874.
78. **May, C., S. Rivella, J. Callegari, G. Heller, K. M. Gaensler, L. Luzzatto, and M. Sadelain.** 2000. Therapeutic haemoglobin synthesis in beta-thalassaemic mice expressing lentivirus-encoded human beta-globin. *Nature* **406:** 82–86.
79. **McConnell, M. J., and M. J. Imperiale.** 2004. Biology of adenovirus and its use as a vector for gene therapy. *Hum. Gene Ther.* **15:**1022–1033.
80. **Meunier, A., A. Latremoliere, A. Mauborgne, S. Bourgoin, V. Kayser, F. Cesselin, M. Hamon, and M. Pohl.** 2005. Attenuation of pain-related behavior in a rat model of trigeminal neuropathic pain by viral-driven enkephalin overproduction in trigeminal ganglion neurons. *Mol. Ther.* **11:**608–616.
81. **Miller, A. D.** 1990. Retrovirus packaging cells. *Hum. Gene Ther.* **1:**5–14.
82. **Mingozzi, F., M. V. Maus, D. J. Hiu, D. E. Sabatino, S. L. Murphy, J. E. Rasko, M. V. Ragni, C. S. Manno, J. Sommer, H. Jiang, G. F. Pierce, H. C. J. Ertl, and K. A. High.** 2007. CD8+ T-cell responses to adeno-associated virus capsid in humans. *Nat. Med.* **13:**419–422.
83. **Mitchell, R. S., B. F. Beitzel, A. R. Schroder, P. Shinn, H. Chen, C. C. Berry, J. R. Ecker, and F. D. Bushman.** 2004. Retroviral DNA integration: ASLV, HIV, and MLV show distinct target site preferences. *PLoS Biol.* **2:**E234.
84. **Miyoshi, H., K. A. Smith, D. E. Mosier, I. M. Verma, and B. E. Torbett.** 1999. Transduction of human CE34+ cells that mediate long-term engraftment of NOD/SCID mice by HIV vectors. *Science* **283:**682–686.
85. **Moss, R. B., D. Rodman, L. T. Spencer, M. L. Aitken, P. L. Zeitlen, D. Waltz, C. Milla, A. S. Brody, J. P. Clancy, B. Ramsey, N. Hamblett, and A. E. Heald.** 2004. Repeated adeno-associated virus serotype 2 aerosol-mediated cystic fibrosis transmembrane regulator gene transfer to the lungs of patients with cystic fibrosis. *Chest* **125:**509–521.
86. **Moss, R. B., C. Milla, J. Colombo, F. Accurso, P. L. Zeitlin, J. P. Clancy, L. T. Spencer, J. Pilewski, D. A. Waltz, H. Dorkin, T. Ferkol, M. Pian, B. Ramsey, B. J. Carter, D. Martin, and A. E. Heald.** 2007. Repeated aerosolized AAV-CFTR for treatment of cystic fibrosis. A randomized placebo-controlled phase 2B trial. *Hum. Gene Ther.* **18:**726–732.
87. **Muruve, D.** 2004. The innate immune response to adenovirus vectors. *Hum. Gene Ther.* **15:**1157–1166.
88. **Muzyczka, N., and K. H. Warrington.** 2005. Custom adeno-associated virus capsids: the next generation of recombinant vectors with novel tropism. *Hum. Gene Ther.* **16:**408–416.
89. **Nakai, H., R. W. Herzog, J. Hagstrom, J. Walter, S. H. Kung, E. Y. Yang, S. J. Tsai, Y. Iwaki, G. Kurtzman, K. J. Fisher, P. Colosi, L. B. Couto, and K. A. High.** 1998. Adeno-associated viral vector-mediated gene transfer of human blood coagulation factor IX into mouse liver. *Blood* **91:**4600–4607.
90. **Naldini, L., U. Blömer, F. H. Gage, D. Trono, and I. M. Verma.** 1996. Efficient transfer, integration, and sustained long-term expression of the transgene in adult rat brains injected with a lentiviral vector. *Proc. Natl. Acad. Sci. USA* **93:**11382–11388.
91. **Naldini, L., U. Blömer, P. Gallay, D. Ory, R. Mulligan, F. H. Gage, I. M. Verma, and D. Trono.** 1996. In vivo gene delivery and stable transduction of nondividing cells by a lentiviral vector. *Science* **272:**263–267.
92. **Naviaux, R. K., E. Costanzi, M. Haas, and I. M. Verma.** 1996. The pCL vector system: rapid production of helper-free, high-titer, recombinant retroviruses. *J. Virol.* **70:**5701–5705.
93. **Oehmig, A., C. Fraefel, X. O. Breakefield, and M. Ackermann.** 2004. Herpes simplex virus type 1 amplicons and their hybrid virus partners, EBV, AAV, and retrovirus. *Curr. Gene Ther.* **4:**385–408.
94. **Olsen, J. C.** 1998. Gene transfer vectors derived from equine infectious anemia virus. *Gene Ther.* **5:**1481–1487.
95. **Ott, M. G., M. Schmidt, K. Schwarzwaelder, S. Stein, U. Siler, U. Koehl, H. Glimm, K. Kuhlcke, A. Schilz, H. Kunkel, S. Naundorf, A. Brinkmann, A. Deichmann, M. Fischer, C. Ball, I. Pilz, C. Dunbar, Y. Du, N. A. Jenkins, N. G. Copeland, U. Luthi, M. Hassan, A. J. Thrasher, D. Hoelzer, C. von Kalle, R. Seger, and M. Grez.** 2006. Correction of X-linked chronic granulomatous disease by gene therapy, augmented by insertional activation of MDS1-EVI1, PRDM16 or SETBP1. *Nat. Med.* **12:**401–409.
96. **Papanastassiou, V., R. Rampling, M. Fraser, R. Petty, D. Hadley, J. Nicoll, J. Harland, R. Mabbs, and M. Brown.** 2002. The potential for efficacy of the modified (ICP 34.5(−)) herpes simplex virus HSV1716 following intratumoural injection into human malignant glioma: a proof of principle study. *Gene Ther.* **9:**398–406.
97. **Pear, W. S., G. P. Nolan, M. L. Scott, and D. Baltimore.** 1993. Production of high-titer helper-free retroviruses by transient transfection. *Proc. Natl. Acad. Sci. USA* **90:**8392–8396.
98. **Peluso, R. W.** 2008. The manufacture of adeno-associated viral vectors, p. 245–252. *In* B. Dropulic and B. J. Carter (ed.), *Current Concepts in Genetic Medicine.* John Wiley & Sons, New York, NY.
99. **Peng, Z.** 2005. Current status of gendicine in China: recombinant human Ad-p53 for treatment of cancers. *Hum. Gene Ther.* **16:**1016–1027.
100. **Poeschla, E. M., F. Wong-Staal, and D. J. Looney.** 1998. Efficient transduction of nondividing human cells by feline immunodeficiency virus lentiviral vectors. *Nat. Med.* **4:**354–357.
101. **Porter, C. D., M. K. Collins, C. S. Tailor, M. H. Parkar, F. L. Cosset, R. A. Weiss, and Y. Takeuchi.** 1996. Comparison of efficiency of infection of human gene therapy target cells via four different retroviral receptors. *Hum. Gene Ther.* **7:**913–919.
102. **Poznansky, M., A. Lever, L. Bergeron, W. Haseltine, and J. Sodroski.** 1991. Gene transfer into human lymphocytes by a defective human immunodeficiency virus type 1 vector. *J. Virol.* **65:**532–536.
103. **Puskovic, V., D. Wolfe, J. Goss, S. Huang, M. Mata, J. C. Glorioso, and D. J. Fink.** 2004. Prolonged biologically active transgene expression driven by HSV LAP2 in brain in vivo. *Mol. Ther.* **10:**67–75.
104. **Rampling, R., G. Cruickshank, V. Papanastassiou, J. Nicoll, D. Hadley, D. Brennan, R. Petty, A. MacLean, J. Harland, E. McKie, R. Mabbs, and M. Brown.** 2000. Toxicity evaluation of replication-competent herpes simplex virus (ICP 34.5 null mutant 1716) in patients with recurrent malignant glioma. *Gene Ther.* **7:**859–866.
105. **Raper, S. E., N. Chirmule, F. S. Lee, N. A. Wivel, A. Bagg, G. P. Gao, J. M. Wilson, and M. L. Batshaw.**

2003. Fatal systemic inflammatory response syndrome in a *[sic]* ornithine transcarbamylase deficient patient following adenoviral gene transfer. *Mol. Genet. Metab.* **80:** 148–158.

106. **Rasheed, S., M. B. Gardner, and E. Chan.** 1976. Amphotropic host range of naturally occurring wild mouse leukemia viruses. *J. Virol.* **19:**13–18.

107. **Rissanen, T. T., and S. Yla-Herttuala.** 2007. Current status of cardiovascular gene therapy. *Mol. Ther.* **15:** 1233–1247.

108. **Rock, D. L., A. B. Nesburn, H. Ghiasi, J. Ong, T. L. Lewis, J. R. Lokensgard, and S. L. Wechsler.** 1987. Detection of latency-related viral RNAs in trigeminal ganglia of rabbits latently infected with herpes simplex virus type 1. *J. Virol.* **61:**3820–3826.

109. **Samaniego, L. A., L. Neiderhiser, and N. A. DeLuca.** 1998. Persistence and expression of the herpes simplex virus genome in the absence of immediate-early proteins. *J. Virol.* **72:**3307–3320.

110. **Sandalon, Z., E. M. Bruckheimer, K. H. Lustig, and H. Burstein.** 2007. Long-term suppression of experimental arthritis following intramuscular administration of a pseudotyped AAV2/TNFR:Fc vector. *Mol. Ther.* **15:**264–269.

111. **Schauber-Plewa, C., A. Simmons, M. J. Tuerk, C. D. Pacheco, and G. Veres.** 2005. Complement regulatory proteins are incorporated into lentiviral vectors and protect particles against complement inactivation. *Gene Ther.* **12:**238–245.

112. **Schnepp, B. C., K. R. Clark, D. L. Klemanski, C. A. Pacak, and P. R. Johnson.** 2003. Genetic fate of recombinant adeno-associated virus vector genomes in muscle. *J. Virol.* **77:**3495–3504.

113. **Schnepp, B. C., R. L. Jensen, C. L. Chen, P. R. Johnson, and K. R. Clark.** 2005. Characterization of adeno-associated genomes isolated from human tissues. *J. Virol.* **79:**14793–14803.

114. **Schroder, A. R., P. Shinn, H. Chen, C. Berry, J. R. Ecker, and F. Bushman.** 2002. HIV-1 integration in the human genome favors active genes and local hotspots. *Cell* **110:**521–529.

115. **Schuettrumpf, J., J. H. Liu, L. B. Couto, K. Addya, D. G. B. Leonard, Z. Zhen, J. Sommer, and V. R. Arruda.** 2006. Inadvertent germline transmission of AAV2 vector: findings in a rabbit model correlate with those in a human clinical trial. *Mol. Ther.* **13:**1064–1073.

116. **Shen, Y., and J. Nemunaitis.** 2006. Herpes simplex virus 1 (HSV-1) for cancer treatment. *Cancer Gene Ther.* **13:** 975–992.

117. **Shimada, T., H. Fujii, H. Mitsuya, and A. W. Nienhuis.** 1991. Targeted and highly efficient gene transfer into CD34+ cells by a recombinant human immunodeficiency virus retroviral vector. *J. Clin. Invest.* **88:** 1043–1047.

118. **Smith, J. S., J. Tian, J. N. Lozier, and A. P. Byrnes.** 2004. Severe pulmonary pathology after intravenous administration of adenovirus vectors in cirrhotic rats. *Mol. Ther.* **9:**932–941.

119. **Soignier, R. D., A. L. Vaccarino, A. M. Brennan, A. J. Kastin, and J. E. Zadina.** 2000. Analgesic effects of endomorphin-1 and endomorphin-2 in the formalin test in mice. *Life Sci.* **67:**907–912.

120. **Soneoka, Y., P. M. Cannon, E. E. Ramsdale, J. C. Griffiths, G. Romano, S. M. Kingsman, and A. J. Kingsman.** 1995. A transient three-plasmid expression system for the production of high titer retroviral vectors. *Nucleic Acids Res.* **23:**628–633.

121. **Spaete, R., and N. Frenkel.** 1982. The herpes simplex virus amplicon: a new eucaryotic defective-virus cloning amplifying vector. *Cell* **30:**295–304.

122. **Spivack, J. G., and N. W. Fraser.** 1987. Detection of herpes simplex virus type 1 transcripts during latent infection in mice. *J. Virol.* **61:**3841–3847.

123. **Stevens, J. G., E. K. Wagner, G. B. Devi-Rao, M. L. Cook, and L. T. Feldman.** 1987. RNA complementary to a herpesvirus alpha gene mRNA is prominent in latently infected neurons. *Science* **235:**1056–1059.

124. **Sutton, R. E., H. T. Wu, R. Rigg, E. Bohnlein, and P. O. Brown.** 1998. Human immunodeficiency virus type 1 vectors efficiently transduce human hematopoietic stem cells. *J. Virol.* **72:**5781–5788.

125. **Thyagarajan, B., E. C. Olivares, R. P. Hollis, D. S. Ginsburg, and M. P. Calos.** 2001. Site-specific genomic integration in mammalian cells mediated by phage phiC31 integrase. *Mol. Cell. Biol.* **21:**3926–3934.

126. **Trobridge, G. D., D. G. Miller, M. A. Jacobs, J. M. Allen, H. P. Kiem, R. Kaul, and D. W. Russell.** 2006. Foamy virus vector integration sites in normal human cells. *Proc. Natl. Acad. Sci. USA* **103:**1498–1503.

127. **Trobridge, G. D., and D. W. Russell.** 1998. Helper-free foamy virus vectors. *Hum. Gene Ther.* **9:**2517–2525.

128. **Wade-Martins, R., Y. Saeki, and E. A. Chiocca.** 2003. Infectious delivery of a 135-kb LDLR genomic locus leads to regulated complementation of low-density lipoprotein receptor deficiency in human cells. *Mol. Ther.* **7:**604–612.

129. **Willis, R. C., D. J. Jolly, A. D. Miller, M. M. Plent, A. C. Esty, P. J. Anderson, H. C. Chang, O. W. Jones, J. E. Seegmiller, and T. Friedmann.** 1984. Partial phenotypic correction of human Lesch-Nyhan (hypoxanthine-guanine phosphoribosyltransferase-deficient) lymphoblasts with a transmissible retroviral vector. *J. Biol. Chem.* **259:**7842–7849.

130. **Wolfe, D., W. F. Goins, T. J. Kaplan, S. V. Capuano, J. Fradette, M. Murphey-Corb, J. B. Cohen, P. D. Robbins, and J. C. Glorioso.** 2001. Systemic delivery of nerve growth factor following herpesvirus gene transfer. *Mol. Ther.* **3:**61–69.

131. **Wu, X., Y. Li, B. Crise, and S. M. Burgess.** 2003. Transcription start regions in the human genome are favored targets for MLV integration. *Science* **300:**1749–1751.

132. **Wu, X., J. K. Wakefield, H. Liu, H. Xiao, R. Kralovics, J. T. Prchal, and J. C. Kappes.** 2000. Development of a novel trans-lentiviral vector that affords predictable safety. *Mol. Ther.* **2:**47–55.

133. **Xiao, W., N. Chirmule, M. A. Schnell, J. Tazelaar, J. V. Hughes, and J. M. Wilson.** 2000. Route of administration determines induction of T-cell independent humoral responses to adeno-associated virus vectors. *Mol. Ther.* **1:**323–329.

134. **Yang, L., L. Bailey, D. Baltimore, and P. Wang.** 2006. Targeting lentiviral vectors to specific cell types in vivo. *Proc. Natl. Acad. Sci. USA* **103:**11479–11484.

135. **Yant, S. R., L. Meuse, W. Chiu, Z. Ivics, Z. Izsvak, and M. A. Kay.** 2000. Somatic integration and long-term transgene expression in normal and haemophilic mice using a DNA transposon system. *Nat. Genet.* **25:** 35–41.

136. **Yei, S., N. Mittereder, K. Tang, C. O. Sullivan, and B. C. Trapnell.** 1994. Adenovirus-mediated gene transfer for cystic fibrosis: quantitative evaluation of repeated in vivo vector administration to the lung. *Gene Ther.* **1:** 192–200.

137. **Yeomans, D. C., S. R. Levinson, M. C. Peters, A. G. Koszowski, A. Z. Tzabazis, W. F. Gilly, and S. P. Wilson.** 2005. Decrease in inflammatory hyperalgesia by herpes vector-mediated knockdown of Nav1.7 sodium channels in primary afferents. *Hum. Gene Ther.* **16:**271–277.

138. **Yoshimura, N., M. E. Franks, K. Sasaki, W. F. Goins, J. Goss, T. Yokoyama, M. O. Fraser, S. Seki, J. Fink, J. Glorioso, W. C. de Groat, and M. B. Chancellor.** 2001. Gene therapy of bladder pain with herpes simplex virus (HSV) vectors expressing preproenkephalin (PPE). *Urology* **57:**116.

139. **Zabner, J., D. M. Petersen, A. P. Puga, S. M. Graham, L. A. Couture, L. D. Keyes, M. J. Lukason, J. A. St. George, R. J. Gregory, and A. E. Smith.** 1994. Safety and efficacy of repetitive adenovirus-mediated gene transfer of CFTR cDNA to airway epithelia of primates and cotton rats. *Nat. Genet.* **6:**75–83.

140. **Zadina, J. E.** 2002. Isolation and distribution of endomorphins in the central nervous system. *Jpn. J. Pharmacol.* **89:**203–208.

141. **Zufferey, R., T. Dull, R. J. Mandel, A. Bukovsky, D. Quiroz, L. Naldini, and D. Trono.** 1998. Self-inactivating lentivirus vector for safe and efficient in vivo gene delivery. *J. Virol.* **72:**9873–9880.

142. **Zufferey, R., D. Nagy, R. J. Mandel, L. Naldini, and D. Trono.** 1997. Multiple attenuated lentiviral vectors achieve efficient gene delivery in vivo. *Nat. Biotechnol.* **15:**871–875.

Chronic Fatigue and Postinfective Fatigue Syndromes

ANDREW R. LLOYD, IAN HICKIE, AND DENIS WAKEFIELD

17

Chronic fatigue syndrome is the label that has been applied to a symptom complex characterized by unexplained, persistent fatigue when no clear implication of an infective or other cause for the prolonged illness can be inferred (37). Constitutional symptoms, including myalgia, arthralgia, sore throat, headache, and tender lymph nodes, are also common. In addition, complaints of unrefreshing sleep, irritability, and neurocognitive abnormalities, like short-term memory impairment and concentration difficulty, are typical (37).

However, fatigue is a subjective and nonspecific symptom, present in at least 15 to 30% of patients in primary-care settings (26, 72), where it is predominantly associated with minor psychiatric morbidity and transient infective illnesses (63). The relationships and boundaries between the ubiquitous symptom of fatigue in the community, the broadly inclusive symptom complex designated as chronic fatigue syndrome, and the more discrete entity of postinfective fatigue syndrome are often blurred. Patients with postinfective fatigue represent a subset of those with chronic fatigue syndrome, although the size of this subgroup is uncertain, as many acute infections are subclinical and are not investigated and the causative agent for an apparent infective trigger for a fatigue syndrome is often not identified. In addition, the case definition for chronic fatigue syndrome stipulates 6 months or more of disabling illness; although postinfective fatigue states are comparable in both symptom profile and functional impairment to chronic fatigue syndrome, the majority of episodes are of shorter duration (50).

Individuals suffering from acute infective illnesses typically develop a constellation of systemic symptoms, including feverishness, myalgia, arthralgia, and headache, as well as fatigue (46). In both humans and animals, infections are also accompanied by increased slow-wave sleep and stereotyped behavioral responses, including reduced motor activity, social withdrawal, and anorexia (46). These characteristic physical and behavioral correlates of infection result primarily from the host response to the pathogen, as they are reproduced in infections resulting from a wide range of microbiological agents (126). In a minority of cases, selected symptom domains from the acute phase of the illness persist and cause protracted ill health, marked by fatigue and disability. Prospective evaluation of such symptoms following serologically documented Epstein-Barr virus (EBV) infection indicates that illness extending over several months, marked by fatigue, is common (Fig. 1).

Chronic fatigue syndrome and, more recently, postinfective fatigue syndrome have been the focus of considerable research interest, including epidemiological studies; investigations of microbiological, immunologic, neuroendocrine, metabolic, and psychological hypotheses of etiology; and treatment interventions (reviewed in references 1 and 100).

A HISTORICAL PERSPECTIVE

A review of the history of the modern-day phenomenon of chronic fatigue syndrome indicates that the disorder is unlikely to be new (113). Perhaps the earliest description comes from Sir Richard Manningham in 1750, who described "febricula," or little fever, as "listlessness with great lassitude and weariness all over the body. . ." (81). Other features included fleeting muscle and joint pains, as well as neurocognitive disturbance: "sometimes the patient is a little delirious and forgetful" (81).

The most widely known predecessor to the current label of chronic fatigue syndrome is the disorder termed "neurasthenia," which was first delineated by George Beard, an American neurologist, in 1869 (5). This disorder was best described by Cobb in 1920: "Neurasthenia is a condition of nervous exhaustion, characterized by undue fatigue on slightest exertion, both physical and mental, with which are associated symptoms of abnormal functioning, mainly referable to disorders of the vegetative nervous system. The chief complaints are headache, gastrointestinal disturbances and subjective sensations of all kinds" (24).

Despite these vivid historical references, precise parallels cannot be drawn with any confidence between the current label of chronic fatigue syndrome (which requires systematic clinical and laboratory evaluations to exclude alternative diagnoses) and disorders such as the febricula or neurasthenia of earlier centuries. The term neurasthenia, for instance, was used in a variety of different contexts, including as a synonym for general nervousness and evolving psychosis, as the male equivalent of hysteria in women, as an alternative label for minor depression, and as a diagnosis of fatigue states in patients who were not apparently depressed (113).

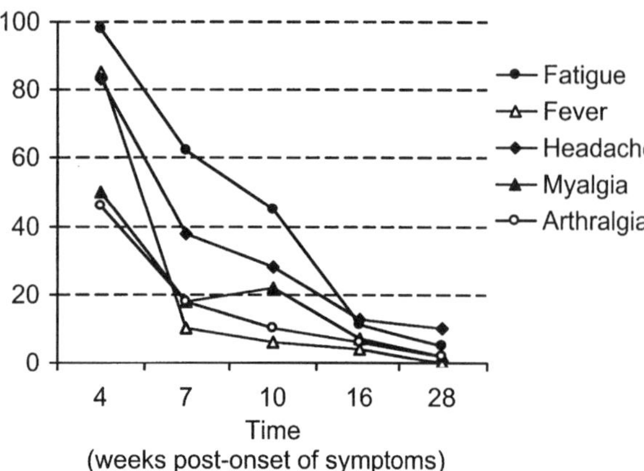

FIGURE 1 Time to resolution of symptoms in 50 patients monitored prospectively from the time of diagnosis of serologically documented acute EBV infection. The vertical axis indicates the percentage of the group reporting the symptom (50; A. R. Lloyd, unpublished data).

Although even the first descriptions of neurasthenia included a link with febrile illness, the observation that specific infectious diseases precipitated a subsequent fatigue state came with the microbiological revolution of the late 19th and early 20th centuries. Notable among the infections linked to postinfective fatigue were influenza (56), brucellosis (34), and EBV infection (57) (Table 1). This association of a largely subjective syndrome of chronic fatigue with discrete infections, like influenza and brucellosis, sparked considerable controversy. Studies conducted in the 1950s provided evidence that much of the continued morbidity was attributable to psychological disorders. Retrospective studies following up patients after acute brucellosis failed to find bacteriological evidence of continued infection but did document substantial psychological abnormalities (114). However, sensitive detection techniques such as PCR to identify low levels of persistent nucleic acids of the microorganisms, or immunoassays to identify microbial antigens, were not available. The critical issue of whether the fatiguing illness led to psychological disorder or, conversely, whether such disorder resulted from chronic ill health was studied in a prospective evaluation of military personnel before the Asian influenza epidemic of 1957 (56). This study pointed to premorbid psychological vulnerability as an important determinant of protracted recovery after infection, although it should be noted that the number of cases available for this analysis was very small.

TABLE 1 Infectious diseases putatively linked to fatigue syndromes[a]

Infection, categorized by type of agent implicated (1869–2007)		
Viruses	Bacteria	Parasites
Influenza	Typhoid fever	Malaria
St. Louis encephalitis	Streptococcal infection	Schistosomiasis
Epstein-Barr virus infection	Brucellosis	Toxoplasmosis
Hepatitis A	Lyme disease	
Yellow fever	Q fever	
Varicella	Leptospirosis	
Coxsackie B		
Cytomegalovirus infection		
HHV-6 infection		
RRV infection		
Mumps		
Retrovirus infection		
HHV-7 infection		
Borna disease virus infection		
Parvovirus infection		
Dengue fever		

[a] Modified from reference 51.

These controversies of microbiological versus psychological determinants of postinfective fatigue have continued to the present. The first prospective evaluation of patients monitored from mononucleosis illnesses suggested that both concepts are valid (135–137). In this study, 245 patients were enrolled with either infectious mononucleosis (77%) or upper respiratory tract infection (23%). Of these, 101 (41%) had a fatigue syndrome associated with significant functional impairment at the time of enrollment. The fatigue state persisted for 1 month or more in 71 individuals from this group (73%), for 2 months or more in 43 (43%), and for 6 months or more in 9 (9%). The fatigue syndrome was most prevalent in those with mononucleosis documented to be due to EBV infection and was shown to be essentially independent of psychiatric diagnoses (137). By contrast, a well-controlled longitudinal study in general practice found that patients presenting with minor symptomatic infections, such as gastroenteritis, were not more likely to subsequently report chronic fatigue than patients presenting for other noninfective reasons (134). More recently, a prospective cohort study monitoring individuals from the time of onset of serologically documented infection identified a stereotyped postinfective fatigue syndrome following varied infective triggers (50). This study enrolled individuals after onset of infection with one of three microbiologically distinct pathogens: EBV, a large DNA virus with recognized latency; Ross River virus (RRV), a small, mosquito-borne RNA virus prevalent in Australia; and *Coxiella burnetii*, the intracellular bacterium which is the causative agent of Q fever (50). The study documented that of 253 subjects enrolled, 29 (12%) experienced a prolonged illness characterized by fatigue, musculoskeletal pain, neurocognitive difficulties, and mood disturbance lasting 6 months or more and 28 (11%) met the diagnostic criteria for chronic fatigue syndrome after systematic assessment to exclude alternative medical and psychiatric explanations for the ongoing illness. The advent of a postinfective fatigue syndrome was predicted largely by the severity of the acute illness and not by demographic, psychological, or individual microbiological factors. The fatigue state was present from the time of onset of symptoms of the acute infection and was stable in character over time, suggesting that the genesis of the postinfective fatigue syndrome is intrinsically linked to the host-pathogen interactions in the acute infection phase (50).

EPIDEMIOLOGY AND NATURAL HISTORY

Chronic fatigue syndrome is a relatively common condition in the community. The disorder predominantly affects young adults, with a peak age of onset of 20 to 40 years, often following a documented, or an apparent, infectious illness (58, 71, 78, 115). Chronic fatigue syndrome does not preferentially affect individuals from upper socioeconomic groups (contrary to the notion of "yuppie flu"); rather, some studies suggest that fatigue syndromes are more common in people from more socially disadvantaged groups (52, 58). Estimates of the prevalence of chronic fatigue syndrome in the general community range from 0.1 to 0.7% (i.e., 100 to 700 cases per 100,000 population) (58, 71, 103, 115). Studies in primary-care settings (which record the cases only among those attending medical practice and are therefore subject to selection bias) suggest prevalence rates ranging from 0.04 to 2.6% (14, 52, 58, 103). These differences in prevalence rates result from differences in the method of ascertainment (e.g., self-report or physician report) and in the case definitions used for the syndrome, notably, in the extent of the assessments undertaken to exclude alternative medical and psychiatric diagnoses (79). Preliminary estimates of the incidence of chronic fatigue syndrome in primary care suggest annual rates of approximately 0.2 to 0.4% (39, 71, 103).

The long-term outcome for patients with chronic fatigue syndrome has been evaluated predominantly in tertiary referral settings, where the patient populations are intrinsically biased towards chronicity and disability. In one such study, 65 of 103 patients (63%) who had longstanding symptoms and who had been enrolled in treatment trials reported improvement in symptoms and functional capacity at follow-up approximately 3 years later (139). Complete recovery was uncommon (6%). By contrast, spontaneous recovery in cases of fatigue of shorter duration in primary care appears to be high (10, 33, 104). Prospective, community-based studies suggest that the prognosis for recovery is good when the illness is abrupt in onset (potentially indicating an infective trigger) and of short duration (6 to 12 months) but declines substantively when the illness has been present for several years (15, 109, 122). Similarly, the prognosis for recovery in postinfective fatigue syndrome is good, even after 6 months of illness has passed (50).

DIAGNOSTIC CRITERIA

The modern era of research in relation to chronic fatigue syndrome has been marked by the formulation of diagnostic criteria. Initially, Australian (77), American (54), and British (112), researchers separately developed consensus criteria for the case definition of the disorder. The Centers for Disease Control and Prevention (108) then proposed the term chronic fatigue syndrome to replace numerous previous eponyms, in particular, because this name removed the presumption of a postinfective or any other inflammatory etiology (as was implied in the earlier British nomenclature "myalgic encephalomyelitis"). In 1994, the Centers for Disease Control and Prevention convened an international study group to reformulate the now widely accepted diagnostic criteria (37) (Table 2). The criteria define persons with chronic fatigue syndrome as presenting with unexplained persistent or relapsing fatigue of at least 6 months' duration that is not relieved by rest, results in disability, and is accompanied by at least four of eight core symptoms (postexertional fatigue, impaired memory or concentration, unrefreshing sleep, headaches, muscle pain, multijoint pain, sore throat, and tender cervical/axillary lymph nodes). With these criteria an epidemiological perspective was provided for research into fatigue states. This perspective recognized that although prolonged fatigue syndromes are common and are associated with increased health care utilization, such syndromes are likely to be heterogeneous with regard to etiology and possibly also pathophysiology (49, 141). Although not derived empirically, these criteria are consistent with symptom constructs described in both population-based samples and clinic studies (49, 59, 90, 91).

TABLE 2 Diagnostic criteria for chronic fatigue syndrome[a]

A. Clinically evaluated, unexplained, persistent or relapsing fatigue that is of new or definite onset; is not the result of ongoing exertion; is not substantially alleviated by rest; and results in substantial reduction in previous levels of occupational, educational, social, or personal activities

and

B. Four or more of the following concurrent and persistent symptoms:

Impaired short-term memory or concentration
Sore throat
Tender cervical or axillary lymph nodes
Muscle pain
Multijoint pain without arthritis
Headaches of a new type, pattern, or severity
Unrefreshing sleep
Postexertional malaise lasting more than 24 h

[a] Data from reference 37.

PROPOSED ETIOLOGIES

The leading hypotheses for the pathophysiological basis of chronic fatigue syndrome include a unique pattern of infection with a recognized or novel pathogen, an abnormal immune response to a recognized pathogen, a psychologically determined response to infection or other stimulus occurring in "vulnerable" individuals, a metabolic or neuroendocrine disturbance initiated by an unknown trigger, and a neuroimmune disturbance triggered by acute infection (reviewed in references 1 and 100). Interactions and overlaps among these alternatives are also possible. In addition, a myriad of less extensively evaluated hypotheses exist.

Infection

The potential role of infectious agents in producing chronic fatigue is the possibility that has been most closely examined. This notion arose naturally from the historical observations linking specific infections such as brucellosis to a subsequent fatigue state. Further support for this possibility comes from the anecdotal histories that patients with chronic fatigue syndrome give. These recollections typically describe a "flu-like" illness demarcating the patient's prior good health from the subsequent chronic fatigue state. Unfortunately, these associations are frequently retrospective attributions with uncertain validity, as the expected incidence of symptomatic viral infections in the general population is approximately four annually (25), making chance associations likely. In addition, many reported case series are confounded by the selection bias of referral to specialty clinics because of the history of an infective illness (55). Nevertheless, the recent prospective studies monitoring patients from the onset of acute EBV and other infections provide clear support for the hypothesis that a discrete postinfective fatigue syndrome can be precipitated by specific pathogens (50, 135–137). Several other viral, and some nonviral, agents have been implicated as apparent triggers for a postinfective fatigue syndrome (Table 1). A noteworthy inclusion in this list is the so-called "post-Lyme borreliosis syndrome" or "chronic Lyme disease," which features fatigue, musculoskeletal pain, and neurocognitive difficulties lasting months or years after primary infection (16) and is unresponsive to prolonged antibiotic therapy (61, 66, 68).

Hypothetically, abnormal persistence of the triggering pathogen may underpin postinfective fatigue syndromes. Several early studies examined this possibility in patients with chronic fatigue syndrome without consideration of the (likely) heterogeneous nature of the triggering agents in such patient groups. Although initial reports suggested "elevated" titers of antibodies directed against organisms such as EBV and human herpesvirus 6 (HHV-6) (perhaps implying persistent antigenic stimulation), these findings were refuted in suitably designed case control studies and discordant-twin studies (reviewed in references 1 and 100).

However, the notion of persistence of the microorganism as a key component of the pathogenesis of postinfective fatigue has been supported by the report of persistent microbial nucleic acids in patients with postinfective fatigue following serologically documented and appropriately treated Q fever (45). Coxiella DNA sequences were amplified from blood samples by PCR in 4 of 30 cases and none of the 18 control samples. PCR amplification of coxiella sequences was also positive for 11 of 20 bone marrow aspirate samples and 2 of 14 liver biopsy samples from the patients. The amplicons were sequenced in four of the positive results, confirming complete identity with the *C. burnetii* genome sequence in all cases. By contrast, attempted PCR amplification of spirochetal DNA from the blood of 1,800 patients with post-Lyme borreliosis syndrome was uniformly negative (132). Although EBV persists naturally in all subjects following primary infection by establishment of latency in B lymphocytes, the possibility of alterations in viral titer during or following the acute illness was examined in a case control series of subjects with infectious mononucleosis who developed a postinfective fatigue syndrome in comparison to those who recovered promptly; no difference in cell-associated viral load in the peripheral blood was detected at any time point (17). Thus, there is a growing body of evidence against the role of ongoing, active infection with the triggering pathogen in postinfective fatigue syndrome.

In relation to chronic fatigue syndrome, the possibility of reactivation of latent HHV-6 infection as a driver for an ongoing immune response and hence ongoing symptoms has been examined in several studies, with inconclusive results. The initial positive report, based on viral cultures augmented by immunofluorescence and PCR detection, demonstrated the presence of HHV-6 in peripheral blood mononuclear cells in a substantially greater proportion of patients than control subjects (12). However, other case control studies using both serologic and PCR techniques have yielded conflicting evidence for HHV-6 reactivation (including specific examination of HHV-6A and -6B) in patients with chronic fatigue syndrome (20, 31, 142).

An association between enteroviral infection and chronic fatigue syndrome was first considered in relation to several of the apparent epidemics of the disorder. Virologic and serologic studies suggested persistence of the enteroviral antigen VP1 and of enteroviral RNA in muscle biopsy samples of a subset of patients with chronic fatigue syndrome (2, 7). Subsequent reports, including one from the same research group, failed to confirm the initial positive findings (44, 84, 121). Similarly, searches for a novel pathogen in patients with chronic fatigue syndrome have been fruitless, with initial positive findings failing to pass the subsequent hurdle of independent confirmation, including in relation to retroviruses (29, 40, 43, 64) and Borna virus (35, 65). Given the diversity of specific infections now clearly linked temporally with the onset of a chronic fatigue syndrome, and the essentially negative findings for occult pathogens to date, it is unlikely that any single infectious agent will be identified as the cause of chronic fatigue syndrome.

Immunologic Disturbance

The clinical course of most acute infections ranges from asymptomatic to severe, incapacitating illness. This spectrum of disease is at least partially due to the magnitude of the immune response induced to control the invading organism, rather than a direct effect of microbial replication. Cytokines, such as interleukin 1 (IL-1), IL-6, tumor necrosis factor alpha, and the interferons, are released in a cascade of cellular activation induced by microbial antigens. In the context of acute infection, the classical sign of this host response, which is fever, has been shown to be induced by the action of proinflammatory cytokines on receptors within the brain (46). More recently, the severity of the neurobehavioral manifestations of the acute sickness response, including fatigue, musculoskeletal pain, anorexia, somnolence, and mood disturbance, was shown to correlate with production of proinflammatory cytokines (127).

Accordingly, the immunologic hypothesis for postinfective fatigue syndrome is that an aberrant and persistent cellular immune response to precipitating infectious agents results in chronic cytokine production, which may directly mediate protracted symptoms (125). Studies of cellular immunity in patients with chronic fatigue syndrome have produced widely varied results (reviewed in reference 80). The most consistent findings are of alterations in T-cell responses and reduced natural killer cell activity, but these changes have rarely correlated with the clinical condition. Given the diversity of infective and other triggers for the onset and persistence of chronic fatigue syndrome, these inconclusive findings may reflect underlying heterogeneity in the condition (49, 141). The first comprehensive examination of antigen-specific immune responses against the pathogen documented to trigger the onset of postinfective fatigue syndrome has recently been reported for a longitudinal case control series of subjects monitored from acute EBV infection either into a postinfective fatigue syndrome or to prompt resolution of clinical illness. Although minor differences in the kinetics of both humoral and T-cell responses against latent EBV antigens were documented, these changes did not correlate with the course of illness (17).

Numerous studies of cytokine production have been conducted for patients with chronic fatigue syndrome, with no consistent alteration in serum or cerebrospinal fluid cytokine levels detected (73, 75, 93, 118). The possibility of aberrant, exercise-induced cytokine production has also been evaluated, with negative findings (18, 76). The opportunity to examine cytokine production in response to antigens derived from the microbe believed to have precipitated the postinfective fatigue syndrome has been provided by the recognition of a post-Q fever fatigue syndrome. The initial report suggested that increased production of IL-6 was evident in samples from subjects with post-Q fever fatigue compared to that in samples from subjects who recovered uneventfully from acute Q fever (94). However, a larger and more comprehensive examination of serum cytokine levels and ex vivo production of cytokines in patients with postinfective fatigue syndrome and matched control subjects who recovered promptly after EBV, RRV, or Q fever did not reveal any significant alterations in cytokine production in those with postinfective fatigue. The possibility of an immunologic disturbance restricted to the central nervous system triggered by the insult of acute infection has not been formally examined.

In summary, although there is evidence of minor disturbances in cellular immunity in patients with chronic fatigue syndrome, the changes do not correlate with disease severity or course and are not associated with clinically significant consequences such as infection or malignancy. Cytokine levels do correlate with illness manifestations, including fatigue in the context of acute infection, but there is no evidence for ongoing cytokine production in the circulation in patients with postinfective fatigue. Given these findings, there is no role for immunologic testing as a diagnostic tool in the assessment of patients with chronic fatigue syndrome (37), other than for the detection of alternative medical conditions (Fig. 2 and Table 3).

Psychological Disturbance

Approximately 30 to 70% of patients with chronic fatigue syndrome also meet criteria for the diagnosis of major depression (28, 48, 67; reviewed in references 1 and 100). This high degree of comorbidity with depression is, in part, an artifact of overlapping symptoms (both disorders list fatigue, sleep disturbance, psychomotor change, cognitive impairment, and mood change as characteristic features). Furthermore, major depression is a common accompaniment of most chronic, disabling medical disorders. Some characteristic clinical features of depression may help differentiate it from chronic fatigue syndrome (if present), including weight loss, feelings of guilt, suicidal ideation, and observable psychomotor slowing. The mood disturbance described by patients with chronic fatigue syndrome tends to be of irritability and transient depression rather than the profound loss of interest in and pleasure from daily activities (i.e., persistent anhedonia), which is the hallmark of a primary major depression.

The presence of concurrent mood disturbance does not demonstrate that depression is the cause of chronic fatigue syndrome. Studies have therefore sought to determine the premorbid rate of psychiatric disorder and also compared patients with chronic fatigue syndrome with subjects suffering from other relevant psychiatric, neurologic, and chronic medical illnesses (133). Patients with chronic fatigue syndrome appear to occupy an intermediate status, having more premorbid and current psychopathology than patients with medical illnesses, but less than patients with overt psychiatric disorders.

The most contentious area of psychiatric comorbidity concerns "somatoform disorders" (i.e., psychological disturbances presenting with physical complaints). Patients with typical somatization disorder complain of a wide range of nonspecific medical symptoms, demonstrate a lifelong pattern of excessive medical treatment, and reject psychological interpretations of their illness. Analyses of the symptoms presented by patients with chronic fatigue syndrome in tertiary referral settings suggest that 30% of patients have a form of somatization (21, 70).

In relation to postinfective fatigue syndrome, the prospective cohort studies have not found a premorbid (i.e., preinfection) history of depression to be a risk factor for a subsequent fatigue syndrome (50, 137). In addition, formal psychiatric assessment of patients with postinfective fatigue at 6 months after onset of infection revealed comorbid depression to be rare (50). In combination with the studies of chronic fatigue syndrome, these data suggest that there may be more than one pathway into chronic fatigue syndrome—one via infection and another potentially via mood disorder. Whether the biological processes underlying these proposed pathways are shared or divergent is unknown.

Metabolic or Neuroendocrine Disturbances

Evidence has been presented for several other pathophysiological disturbances in chronic fatigue syndrome, including impaired hypothalamic-pituitary-adrenal (HPA) axis activation (6, 22, 30, 60), primary sleep disorder (4, 13, 36, 129), and neurally mediated hypotension (11, 97, 101, 106). In the most exhaustive neuroendocrine study, lower mean urinary free cortisol and basal evening glucocorticoid levels were found in patients with chronic fatigue syndrome than in healthy control subjects. In addition, the patients were shown to have an increased adrenocortical sensitivity to administered adrenocorticotropin, but a blunted response to corticotropin releasing hormone, consistent with a mild hypothalmic defect in the regulation of adrenal function (30). Other studies show generally concordant findings (reviewed in reference 23). The alterations in HPA axis performance were shown to differ in patients with major depression (in whom relative hypercortisolism and resistance to dexamethasone suppression are evident) and those with chronic fatigue syndrome (22). The available evidence suggests that these changes are a consequence of the chronic illness rather than the cause, as they are absent early in the course of illness and improve following unrelated treatment interventions such as cognitive-behavioral therapy (see below) (23).

The complaint of unrefreshing sleep is a universal one in patients with chronic fatigue syndrome, often associated with either hypersomnia or insomnia. Disturbances of sleep maintenance (i.e., frequent awakenings) are prevalent, and circadian rhythm may also be disturbed (3). The report of a characteristic sleep abnormality with the intrusion of high-amplitude alpha waves into the delta pattern of stage III to IV non-REM sleep has not been reliably demonstrated, nor is it specific to chronic fatigue syndrome (82, 123). Other reports have highlighted the importance of excluding alternative sleep pathologies such as obstructive sleep apnea before applying the label of chronic fatigue syndrome (13, 86).

The potential role of altered autonomic reflexes manifesting as neurally mediated hypotension in the development of chronic fatigue syndrome has also been examined (11, 97, 101, 106). In the initial study, patients were evaluated using a three-stage tilt-table test with the admin-

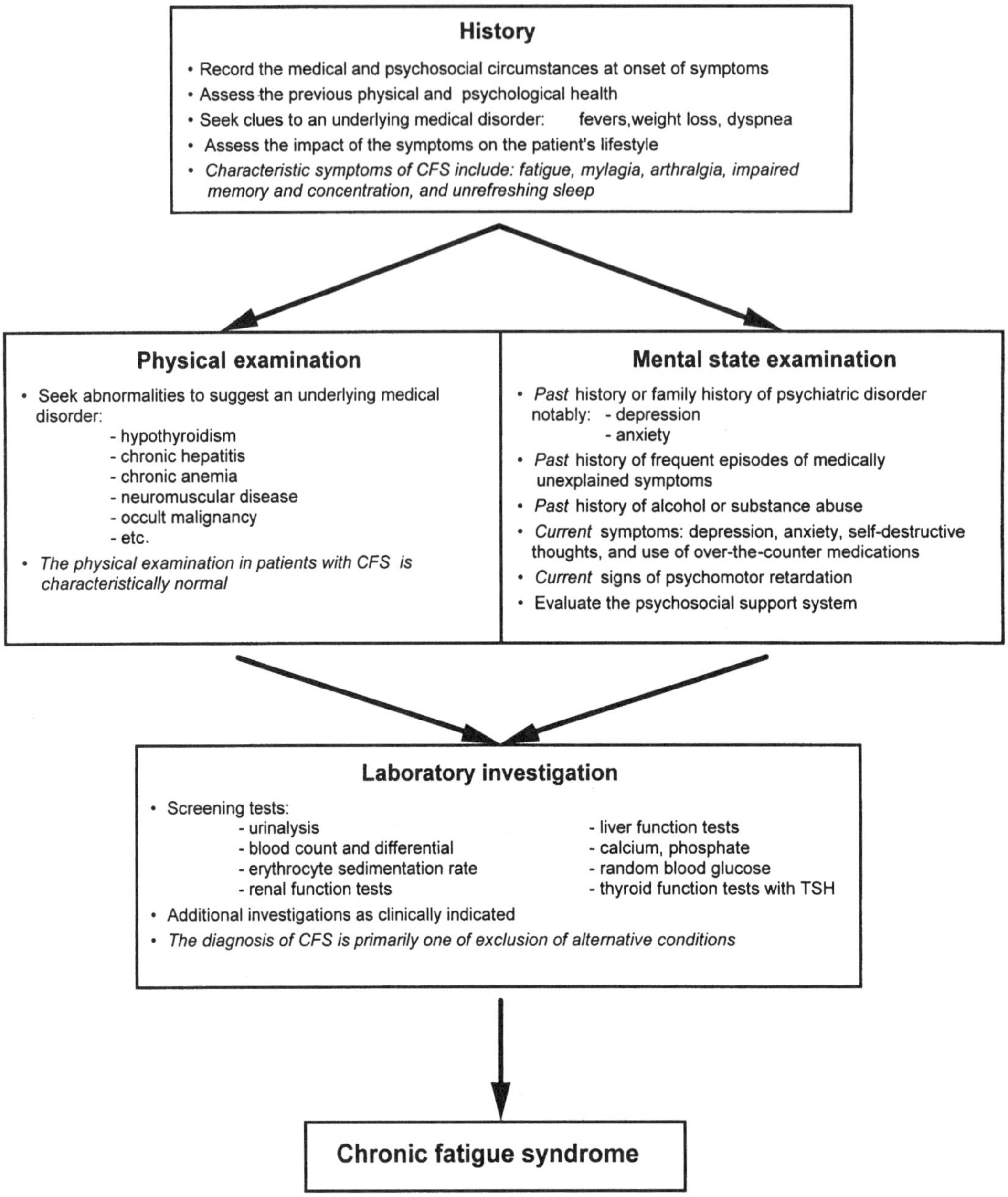

FIGURE 2 Approach to the assessment of chronic fatigue. CFS, chronic fatigue syndrome; TSH, thyroid-stimulating hormone. (Adapted from reference 51 with permission.)

istration of isoprotenerol. An abnormal response was documented for 22 of 23 patients (96%), in comparison to 4 of 14 healthy control subjects (29%). Subsequent studies have generally confirmed that a subset of patients with chronic fatigue syndrome also display features of neurally mediated hypotension (69, 110). It is unlikely that this phenomenon is causative in chronic fatigue syndrome, as studies in identical twin pairs discordant for the illness have revealed comparable evidence for altered regulation of vasomotor control in the unaffected siblings (97). In addition, appropriate treatment for this condition in the form of mineralocorticoid supplementation with fludrocortisone to promote salt and water retention has been shown to be ineffective in resolving the major symptoms of the disorder (see below) (107).

CLINICAL AND LABORATORY ASSESSMENTS

Until a reliable biological marker for the syndrome is available, the key to evaluation of patients presenting with chronic fatigue will continue to include a thorough medical history, physical examination, and detailed assessment of psychological factors (Fig. 2) (51, 102). The medical interview should specifically determine (i) whether the fatigue is of recent and discrete onset, (ii) the medical and psychosocial circumstances at onset, and (iii) the presence

TABLE 3 Causes of chronic fatigue

Physiological	Infectious diseases
Increased physical exertion	Infectious mononucleosis
Inadequate rest	HIV[a]/AIDS
Sedentary lifestyle	Chronic hepatitis B or C
Environmental stress (e.g., heat)	Lyme disease
Drugs	Syphilis
Medications (e.g., beta blockers)	Tuberculosis
Alcohol dependence	Subacute bacterial endocarditis
Other substance abuse	Chronic parasitic infection
Drug withdrawal	Invasive fungal disease
Psychosocial	Cardiorespiratory disorders
Depression	Chronic airflow limitation
Anxiety disorder	Cardiac failure
Somatization disorder	Silent myocardial infarction
Dysthymia and grief	Cardiac arrthymias
Pregnancy	Mitral valve disease
Autoimmune disorders	Hematologic disorders
Systemic lupus erythematosis	Anemia
Multiple sclerosis	Myeloproliferative disorders
Rheumatoid arthritis	Occult malignancy
Vasculitides (e.g., Wegener's granulomatosis)	Sleep disorders
Sarcoidosis	Obstructive sleep apnea
Endocrine disorders	Narcolepsy
Hypothyroidism	Neuromuscular disorders
Hyperthyroidism	Myopathic diseases
Hyperparathyroidism	Muscular dystrophies
Adrenal insufficiency	Myasthenia gravis
Cushing's syndrome	Guillain-Barré syndrome
Hyopituitarism	Syndromes of uncertain etiology
Diabetes mellitus	Chronic fatigue syndrome
Metabolic disorders	Fibromyalgia (fibrositis)
Hypocalcemia	
Hypokalemia	
Hyponatremia	
Chronic renal failure	
Chronic liver disease, e.g., alcohol related	

[a] HIV, human immunodeficiency virus.

of symptoms suggestive of an underlying medical condition (e.g., documented fever, weight loss, or arthritis) (37). It is important to distinguish the characteristics of the phenomenon of fatigue—to verify that the primary complaint is not muscle weakness, somnolence, or motivational loss. Patients with chronic fatigue syndrome characteristically describe profound fatigue which is precipitated by physical tasks previously achieved with ease and is associated with a protracted recovery period extending over hours or even days.

The physical examination should similarly be directed at detection of signs of unrecognized medical disorders (e.g., goiter, stigmata of chronic liver disease, and neurologic signs of myopathy or multiple sclerosis). The physical examination in patients with chronic fatigue syndrome should be normal. The psychological evaluation should directly assess current mood, cognitive function, and illness attitudes. Particular attention should be directed towards the identification of serious and treatable anxiety or depressive disorders. Other important historical features include a personal or family history of psychiatric disorder, previous episodes of medically unexplained syndromes and excessive health care utilization (suggesting a diagnosis of somatization disorder), and excessive use of alcohol or other substances.

Medical causes of chronic fatigue that should be ruled out include hypothyroidism, chronic hepatitis, anemia, sleep apnea, and side effects of prescribed medications, although many other causes are possible (Table 3). Patients diagnosed as having "fibromyalgia" have essentially a disorder synonymous with chronic fatigue syndrome, differing principally in the prevalence and severity of musculoskeletal pain (42). Psychiatric disorders that commonly present with chronic fatigue include major depression, somatoform disorders, panic and other anxiety disorders, alcohol and substance abuse, and eating disorders.

Despite the wide range of hematologic, immunologic, virologic, psychometric, and neuroimaging investigations that have been conducted, no specific diagnostic test for chronic fatigue syndrome has emerged. In fact, the clinical heterogeneity of patients diagnosed as having chronic fatigue syndrome makes it highly unlikely that any specific test could emerge (49, 141). Examples of specific tests that do not confirm, or exclude, the diagnosis of chronic fatigue syndrome include serologic tests for EBV, HHV-6, enteroviruses, and *Candida albicans*; detection of nucleic acids of

Mycoplasma or other microorganisms by PCR; tests of immunity, including T-lymphocyte phenotype and functional assays; and neuroimaging studies, including cerebral magnetic resonance imaging scans and radionuclide studies. The limited number of screening laboratory tests which are recommended are intended for the detection of underlying medical conditions (Fig. 3) (37). If alternative diagnoses are suggested by the clinical history or examination (e.g., sleep apnea or multiple sclerosis), then further directed investigations (e.g., overnight sleep study or magnetic resonance imaging, respectively) may be warranted. Similarly, if the mental status examination raises the issue of psychiatric disorder, then referral for specialist psychiatric opinion should be sought.

TREATMENT

A wide range of antiviral immunoregulatory, neuroendocrine, metabolic, and antidepressant therapies have been evaluated in randomized, placebo-controlled trials (8, 9, 47, 53, 62, 74, 85, 88, 89, 92, 95, 96, 105, 107, 116, 117, 119, 124, 130, 131) and reviewed elsewhere (1, 32, 51, 100, 138). While some positive outcomes have been reported, to date no pharmacological agent has consistently demonstrated efficacy in repeated, well-designed studies. Nine of the trials have compared an immunologic therapy to placebo and have failed to show reproducible evidence of benefit. The single antiviral drug trial evaluated acyclovir and failed to show benefit, although subjects with postinfective fatigue which had been triggered by well-documented EBV infection were not specifically included. Antimicrobial therapy for post-Lyme borreliosis also did not show benefit (61, 66, 68).

Four of the placebo-controlled trials evaluated a pharmacological therapy directed at the HPA axis disturbance by administration of corticosteroids—fludrocortisone and hydrocortisone. Two placebo-controlled trials involving a total of 105 patients suggested that low-dose glucocorticoids (hydrocortisone) may improve subjective fatigue or sense of wellness, but at the expense of potentially harmful suppression of adrenal function and risk of long-term adverse effects. The two placebo-controlled trials of mineralocorticoids (fludrocortisone) showed no benefit in improving symptoms or functional outcomes. One of these two trials was specifically limited to patients with chronic fatigue syndrome associated with documented neurally mediated hypotension.

Although antidepressant therapies are commonly suggested for the treatment of chronic fatigue syndrome, the empirical evidence for their utility is very limited. Five placebo-controlled trials of antidepressant therapy in patients with chronic fatigue syndrome have been reported. None of these studies demonstrated a substantive or sustained benefit from the agents studied, which included the monoamine oxidase inhibitors phenelzine, selegiline, and moclobemide, as well as the serotonin reuptake inhibitor fluoxetine. Studies with patients with the overlapping clinical syndrome of fibromyalgia have demonstrated the benefit of a combination of a low-dose tricyclic antidepressant and a nonsteroidal anti-inflammatory agent, where effects on muscle pain and sleep disturbance are notable (41), arguing for a similar therapeutic trial in patients with chronic fatigue syndrome in whom pain and sleep disturbance are prominent. A recent review of the evidence base for management of fibromyalgia (19) endorsed the use of pharmacological agents for pain (antidepressants and tramadol) and nonpharmacological interventions (graded exercise and heated pool), consistent with the principles of management of chronic fatigue syndrome.

Patient cohorts in such drug treatment trials are likely to be heterogeneous, as a simple consequence of the subjective, prevalent, and nonspecific symptom criteria used to make the diagnosis of chronic fatigue syndrome. Consequently, any treatment that claims to cure the majority of patients with chronic fatigue syndrome is likely to be acting via a nonspecific mechanism. As is true in other chronic medical conditions, at least 30% of patients with chronic fatigue syndrome generally demonstrate improvement in the nonspecific treatment arm of controlled trials (140).

Specific cognitive-behavioral (27, 83, 99, 111, 120) and graded physical exercise (38, 87, 98, 128) strategies have been evaluated in patients with chronic fatigue syndrome. These management approaches link the principles of good clinical management with various degrees of psychological intervention and graded physical and cognitive activities. The initial uncontrolled study suggested a benefit from a cognitive-behavioral approach in conjunction with antidepressant therapy. Several subsequent controlled studies evaluated cognitive-behavioral therapy in comparison with standard, supportive clinical management (either standard medical care, relaxation, or counseling) or no treatment. Although not all of these studies showed a beneficial effect of cognitive-behavioral therapy, it is likely that the discrepant results relate to the intensity and duration of the cognitive-behavioral intervention. In addition, the nature of the standard clinical management of patients in the control arm may have been confounding, as this may approximate the beneficial effect of the treatment.

Given the likelihood of spontaneous improvement in patients with chronic fatigue, controlled treatment trials are essential for all proposed therapeutic modalities. Prevention of secondary medical and psychological morbidity due to prolonged rest and social isolation should be emphasized. Nonspecific aspects of good clinical management are highly effective and include careful medical and psychological evaluation, judicious use of investigations and specialist referral, consistent and empathic interactions with the patient over the course of the illness, and the encouragement of a graded rehabilitation approach. Irrespective of attitudes to etiology, the patient should be encouraged to incorporate the widest possible view of the roles of psychosocial, medical, and rehabilitative strategies to promote recovery.

REFERENCES

1. **Afari, N., and D. Buchwald.** 2003. Chronic fatigue syndrome: a review. *Am. J. Psychiatry* **160:**221–236.
2. **Archard, L. C., N. E. Bowles, P. O. Behan, E. J. Bell, and D. Doyle.** 1988. Postviral fatigue syndrome: persistence of enterovirus RNA in muscle and elevated creatine kinase. *J. R. Soc. Med.* **81:**326–329.
3. **Armitage, R., C. Landis, R. Hoffmann, M. Lentz, N. F. Watson, J. Goldberg, and D. Buchwald.** 2007. The impact of a 4-hour sleep delay on slow wave activity in twins discordant for chronic fatigue syndrome. *Sleep* **30:**657–662.
4. **Ball, N., D. S. Buchwald, D. Schmidt, J. Goldberg, S. Ashton, and R. Armitage.** 2004. Monozygotic twins discordant for chronic fatigue syndrome: objective measures of sleep. *J. Psychosom. Res.* **56:**207–212.

5. **Beard, G.** 1869. Neurasthenia, or nervous exhaustion. *Boston Med. Surg. J.* **3:**217–221.
6. **Bearn, J., T. Allain, P. Coskeran, N. Munro, J. Butler, A. McGregor, and S. Wessely.** 1995. Neuroendocrine responses to d-fenfluramine and insulin-induced hypoglycemia in chronic fatigue syndrome. *Biol. Psychiatry* **37:** 245–252.
7. **Behan, P. O., W. M. Behan, and E. J. Bell.** 1985. The postviral fatigue syndrome—an analysis of the findings in 50 cases. *J. Infect.* **10:**211–222.
8. **Behan, P. O., W. M. Behan, and D. Horrobin.** 1990. Effect of high doses of essential fatty acids on the postviral fatigue syndrome. *Acta Neurol. Scand.* **82:**209–216.
9. **Blacker, C. V. R., D. T. Greenwood, K. A. Wesnes, R. Wilson, C. Woodward, I. Howe, and T. Ali.** 2004. Effect of galantamine hydrobromide in chronic fatigue syndrome: a randomized controlled trial. *JAMA* **292:**1195–1204.
10. **Bonner, D., M. Ron, T. Chalder, S. Butler, and S. Wessely.** 1994. Chronic fatigue syndrome: a follow up study. *J. Neurol. Neurosurg. Psychiatry* **57:**617–621.
11. **Bou-Holaigah, I., P. C. Rowe, J. Kan, and H. Calkins.** 1995. The relationship between neurally mediated hypotension and the chronic fatigue syndrome. *JAMA* **274:** 961–967.
12. **Buchwald, D., P. R. Cheney, D. L. Peterson, B. Henry, S. B. Wormsley, A. Geiger, D. V. Ablashi, S. Z. Salahuddin, C. Saxinger, R. Biddle, et al.** 1992. A chronic illness characterized by fatigue, neurologic and immunologic disorders, and active human herpesvirus type 6 infection. *Ann. Intern. Med.* **116:**103–113.
13. **Buchwald, D., R. Pascualy, C. Bombardier, and P. Kith.** 1994. Sleep disorders in patients with chronic fatigue. *Clin. Infect. Dis.* **18**(Suppl. 1):S68–S72.
14. **Buchwald, D., P. Umali, J. Umali, P. Kith, T. Pearlman, and A. L. Komaroff.** 1995. Chronic fatigue and the chronic fatigue syndrome: prevalence in a Pacific Northwest health care system. *Ann. Intern. Med.* **123:**81–88.
15. **Cairns, R., and M. Hotopf.** 2005. A systematic review describing the prognosis of chronic fatigue syndrome. *Occup. Med.* (Oxford) **55:**20–31.
16. **Cairns, V., and J. Godwin.** 2005. Post-Lyme borreliosis syndrome: a meta-analysis of reported symptoms. *Int. J. Epidemiol.* **34:**1340–1345.
17. **Cameron, B., M. Bharadwaj, J. Burrows, C. Fazou, D. Wakefield, I. Hickie, R. Ffrench, R. Khanna, and A. Lloyd, for the Dubbo Infection Outcomes Study.** 2006. Prolonged illness after infectious mononucleosis is associated with altered immunity but not with increased viral load. *J. Infect. Dis.* **193:**664–671.
18. **Cannon, J. G., J. B. Angel, L. W. Abad, E. Vannier, M. D. Mileno, L. Fagioli, S. M. Wolff, and A. L. Komaroff.** 1997. Interleukin-1 beta, interleukin-1 receptor antagonist, and soluble interleukin-1 receptor type II secretion in chronic fatigue syndrome. *J. Clin. Immunol.* **17:** 253–261.
19. **Carville, S. F., S. Arendt-Nielsen, H. Bliddal, F. Blotman, J. C. Branco, D. Buskila, J. A. Da Silva, B. Danneskiold-Samsøe, F. Dincer, C. Henriksson, K. Henriksson, E. Kosek, K. Longley, G. M. McCarthy, S. Perrot, M. J. Puszczewicz, P. Sarzi-Puttini, A. Silman, M. Späth, and E. H. Choy.** 2008. EULAR evidence based recommendations for the management of fibromyalgia syndrome. *Ann. Rheum. Dis.* **67:**536–541.
20. **Chapenko, S., A. Krumina, S. Kozireva, Z. Nora, A. Sultanova, L. Viksna, and M. Murovska.** 2006. Activation of human herpesviruses 6 and 7 in patients with chronic fatigue syndrome. *J. Clin. Virol.* **37**(Suppl. 1): S47–S51.
21. **Clark, M., and W. Katon.** 1994. The relevance of psychiatric research on somatization to the concept of chronic fatigue syndrome, p. 329–349. In S. Straus (ed.), *Chronic Fatigue Syndrome*. Marcel Dekker, New York, NY.
22. **Cleare, A. J., J. Bearn, T. Allain, A. McGregor, S. Wessely, R. M. Murray, and V. O'Keane.** 1995. Contrasting neuroendocrine responses in depression and chronic fatigue syndrome. *J. Affect. Disord.* **34:**283–289.
23. **Cleare, A. J.** 2004. The HPA axis and the genesis of chronic fatigue syndrome. *Trends Endocrinol. Metab.* **15:** 55–59.
24. **Cobb, I.** 1920. *A Manual of Neurasthenia (Nervous Exhaustion)*. Balliere, Tindall and Cox, London, United Kingdom.
25. **Cox, B., and M. Baxter.** 1987. *The Health and Lifestyle Survey*. Health Promotion Research Trust, London, United Kingdom.
26. **David, A., A. Pelosi, E. McDonald, D. Stephens, D. Ledger, R. Rathbone, and A. Mann.** 1990. Tired, weak, or in need of rest: fatigue among general practice attenders. *BMJ* **301:**1199–1202.
27. **Deale, A., T. Chalder, I. Marks, and S. Wessely.** 1997. Cognitive behavior therapy for chronic fatigue syndrome: a randomized controlled trial. *Am. J. Psychiatry* **154:**408–414.
28. **Deale, A., and S. Wessely.** 2000. Diagnosis of psychiatric disorder in clinical evaluation of chronic fatigue syndrome. *J. R. Soc. Med.* **93:**310–312.
29. **DeFreitas, E., B. Hilliard, P. R. Cheney, D. S. Bell, E. Kiggundu, D. Sankey, Z. Wroblewska, M. Palladino, J. P. Woodward, and H. Koprowski.** 1991. Retroviral sequences related to human T-lymphotropic virus type II in patients with chronic fatigue immune dysfunction syndrome. *Proc. Nat. Acad. Sci. USA* **88:**2922–2926.
30. **Demitrack, M. A., J. K. Dale, S. E. Straus, L. Laue, S. J. Listwak, M. J. Kruesi, G. P. Chrousos, and P. W. Gold.** 1991. Evidence for impaired activation of the hypothalamic-pituitary-adrenal axis in patients with chronic fatigue syndrome. *J. Clin. Endocrinol. Metab.* **73:** 1224–1234.
31. **Di Luca, D., M. Zorzenon, P. Mirandola, R. Colle, G. A. Botta, and E. Cassai.** 1995. Human herpesvirus 6 and human herpesvirus 7 in chronic fatigue syndrome. *J. Clin. Microbiol.* **33:**1660–1661.
32. **Edmonds, M., H. McGuire, and J. Price.** 2004. Exercise therapy for chronic fatigue syndrome. *Cochrane Database of Systematic Reviews* CD003200.
33. **Elnicki, D., W. Shockcor, J. Brick, and D. Beynon.** 1992. Evaluating the complaint of fatigue in primary care: diagnoses and outcomes. *Am. J. Med.* **93:**303–306.
34. **Evans, A.** 1934. Chronic brucellosis. *JAMA* **103:**665.
35. **Evengard, B., T. Briese, G. Lindh, S. Lee, and W. I. Lipkin.** 1999. Absence of evidence of Borna disease virus infection in Swedish patients with chronic fatigue syndrome. *J. Neurovirol.* **5:**495–499.
36. **Fischler, B., O. Le Bon, G. Hoffmann, R. Cluydts, L. Kaufman, and K. De Meirleir.** 1997. Sleep anomalies in the chronic fatigue syndrome. A comorbidity study. *Neuropsychobiology* **35:**115–122.
37. **Fukuda, K., S. E. Straus, I. Hickie, M. C. Sharpe, J. G. Dobbins, A. Komaroff, and International Chronic Fatigue Syndrome Study Group.** 1994. The chronic fatigue syndrome: a comprehensive approach to its definition and study. *Ann. Intern. Med.* **121:**953–959.
38. **Fulcher, K. Y., and P. D. White.** 1997. Randomised controlled trial of graded exercise in patients with the chronic fatigue syndrome. *BMJ* **314:**1647–1652.
39. **Gallagher, A. M., J. M. Thomas, W. T. Hamilton, and P. D. White.** 2004. Incidence of fatigue symptoms and

diagnoses presenting in UK primary care from 1990 to 2001. *J. R. Soc. Med.* **97:**571–575.

40. **Gelman, I. H., E. R. Unger, A. C. Mawle, R. Nisenbaum, and W. C. Reeves.** 2000. Chronic fatigue syndrome is not associated with expression of endogenous retroviral p15E. *Mol. Diagn.* **5:**155–156.
41. **Goldenberg, D., D. Felson, and H. Dinerman.** 1986. A randomized controlled trial of amitriptyline and naproxen in the treatment of patients with fibromyalgia. *Arthritis Rheum.* **29:**1371–1377.
42. **Goldenberg, D. L., R. W. Simms, A. Geiger, and A. L. Komaroff.** 1990. High frequency of fibromyalgia in patients with chronic fatigue seen in a primary care practice. *Arthritis Rheum.* **33:**381–387.
43. **Gow, J. W., K. Simpson, A. Schliephake, W. M. Behan, L. J. Morrison, H. Cavanagh, A. Rethwilm, and P. O. Behan.** 1992. Search for retrovirus in the chronic fatigue syndrome. *J. Clin. Pathol.* **45:**1058–1061.
44. **Gow, J. W., W. M. Behan, K. Simpson, F. McGarry, S. Keir, and P. O. Behan.** 1994. Studies on enterovirus in patients with chronic fatigue syndrome. *Clin. Infect. Dis.* **18**(Suppl. 1)**:**S126–S129.
45. **Harris, R. J., P. A. Storm, A. Lloyd, M. Arens, and B. P. Marmion.** 2000. Long-term persistence of Coxiella burnetii in the host after primary Q fever. *Epidemiol. Infect.* **124:**543–549.
46. **Hart, B. L.** 1988. Biological basis of the behavior of sick animals. *Neurosci. Biobehav. Rev.* **12:**123–137.
47. **Hartz, A. J., S. Bentler, R. Noyes, J. Hoehns, C. Logemann, S. Sinift, Y. Butani, W. Wang, K. Brake, M. Ernst, and H. Kautzman.** 2004. Randomized controlled trial of Siberian ginseng for chronic fatigue. *Psychol. Med.* **34:**51–61.
48. **Hickie, I., A. Lloyd, D. Wakefield, and G. Parker.** 1990. The psychiatric status of patients with the chronic fatigue syndrome. *Br. J. Psychiatry* **156:**534–540.
49. **Hickie, I., A. Lloyd, D. Hadzi-Pavlovic, G. Parker, K. Bird, and D. Wakefield.** 1995. Can the chronic fatigue syndrome be defined by distinct clinical features? *Psychol. Med.* **25:**925–935.
50. **Hickie, I., T. Davenport, D. Wakefield, U. Vollmer-Conna, B. Cameron, S. D. Vernon, W. C. Reeves, and A. Lloyd for the Dubbo Infection Outcomes Study Group.** 2006. Post-infective and chronic fatigue syndromes precipitated by viral and non-viral pathogens: prospective cohort study. *BMJ* **333:**575.
51. **Hickie, I. B., A. R. Lloyd, and D. Wakefield.** 1995. Chronic fatigue syndrome: current perspectives on evaluation and management. *Med. J. Aust.* **163:**314–318.
52. **Hickie, I. B., A. W. Hooker, D. Hadzi-Pavlovic, B. K. Bennett, A. J. Wilson, and A. R. Lloyd.** 1996. Fatigue in selected primary care settings: sociodemographic and psychiatric correlates. *Med. J. Aust.* **164:**585–588.
53. **Hickie, I. B., A. J. Wilson, J. M. Wright, B. K. Bennett, D. Wakefield, and A. R. Lloyd.** 2000. A randomized, double-blind placebo-controlled trial of moclobemide in patients with chronic fatigue syndrome. *J. Clin. Psychiatry* **61:**643–648.
54. **Holmes, G., J. Kaplan, N. Gantz, A. Komaroff, L. Schonberger, S. Straus, J. Jones, R. Dubois, C. Cunningham-Rundles, and S. Pahwa.** 1989. Chronic fatigue syndrome: a working case definition. *Ann. Intern. Med.* **108:**387–389.
55. **Hotopf, M. H., and S. Wessely.** 1994. Viruses, neurosis and fatigue. *J. Psychosom. Res.* **38:**499–514.
56. **Imboden, J., A. Cantor, and L. Cluff.** 1961. Convalescence from influenza. A study of the psychological and clinical determinants. *Arch. Intern. Med.* **108:**393–398.
57. **Isaacs, R.** 1948. Chronic infectious mononucleosis. *Blood* **3:**858–861.
58. **Jason, L. A., J. A. Richman, A. W. Rademaker, K. M. Jordan, A. V. Plioplys, R. R. Taylor, W. McCready, C. F. Huang, and S. Plioplys.** 1999. A community-based study of chronic fatigue syndrome. *Arch. Intern. Med.* **159:**2129–2137.
59. **Jason, L. A., R. R. Taylor, C. L. Kennedy, K. Jordan, C.-F. Huang, S. Torres-Harding, S. Song, and D. Johnson.** 2002. A factor analysis of chronic fatigue symptoms in a community-based sample. *Soc. Psychiatry Psychiatr. Epidemiol.* **37:**183–189.
60. **Jerjes, W. K., A. J. Cleare, S. Wessely, P. J. Wood, and N. F. Taylor.** 2005. Diurnal patterns of salivary cortisol and cortisone output in chronic fatigue syndrome. *J. Affect. Disord.* **87:**299–304.
61. **Kaplan, R. F., R. P. Trevino, G. M. Johnson, L. Levy, R. Dornbush, L. T. Hu, J. Evans, A. Weinstein, C. H. Schmid, and M. S. Klempner.** 2003. Cognitive function in post-treatment Lyme disease: do additional antibiotics help? *Neurology* **60:**1916–1922.
62. **Kaslow, J. E., L. Rucker, and R. Onishi.** 1989. Liver extract-folic acid-cyanocobalamin vs placebo for chronic fatigue syndrome. *Arch. Intern. Med.* **149:**2501–2503.
63. **Katon, W., and E. Walker.** 1993. The relationship of chronic fatigue to psychiatric illness in community, primary care and tertiary care samples. *Ciba Found. Symp.* **173:**193–204.
64. **Khan, A. S., W. M. Heneine, L. E. Chapman, H. E. Gary, Jr., T. C. Woods, T. M. Folks, and L. B. Schonberger.** 1993. Assessment of a retrovirus sequence and other possible risk factors for the chronic fatigue syndrome in adults. *Ann. Intern. Med.* **118:**241–245.
65. **Kitani, T., H. Kuratsune, I. Fuke, Y. Nakamura, T. Nakaya, S. Asahi, M. Tobiume, K. Yamaguti, T. Machii, R. Inagi, K. Yamanishi, and K. Ikuta.** 1996. Possible correlation between Borna disease virus infection and Japanese patients with chronic fatigue syndrome. *Microbiol. Immunol.* **40:**459–462.
66. **Klempner, M. S., L. T. Hu, J. Evans, C. H. Schmid, G. M. Johnson, R. P. Trevino, D. Norton, L. Levy, D. Wall, J. McCall, M. Kosinski, and A. Weinstein.** 2001. Two controlled trials of antibiotic treatment in patients with persistent symptoms and a history of Lyme disease. *N. Engl. J. Med.* **345:**85–92.
67. **Kruesi, M. J., J. Dale, and S. E. Straus.** 1989. Psychiatric diagnoses in patients who have chronic fatigue syndrome. *J. Clin. Psychiatry* **50:**53–56.
68. **Krupp, L. B., L. G. Hyman, R. Grimson, P. K. Coyle, P. Melville, S. Ahnn, R. Dattwyler, and B. Chandler.** 2003. Study and treatment of post Lyme disease (STOP-LD): a randomized double masked clinical trial. *Neurology* **60:**1923–1930.
69. **LaManca, J. J., A. Peckerman, J. Walker, W. Kesil, S. Cook, A. Taylor, and B. H. Natelson.** 1999. Cardiovascular response during head-up tilt in chronic fatigue syndrome. *Clin. Physiol.* **19:**111–120.
70. **Lane, T. J., P. Manu, and D. A. Matthews.** 1991. Depression and somatization in the chronic fatigue syndrome. *Am. J. Med.* **91:**335–344.
71. **Lawrie, S. M., D. N. Manders, J. R. Geddes, and A. J. Pelosi.** 1997. A population-based incidence study of chronic fatigue. *Psychol. Med.* **27:**343–353.
72. **Lewis, S., and S. Wessely.** 1991. The epidemiology of fatigue: more questions than answers. *J. Epidemiol. Community Health* **46:**92–97.
73. **Linde, A., B. Andersson, S. B. Svenson, H. Ahrne, M. Carlsson, P. Forsberg, H. Hugo, A. Karstorp, R. Lenkei, A. Lindwall, et al.** 1992. Serum levels of lymphokines

and soluble cellular receptors in primary Epstein-Barr virus infection and in patients with chronic fatigue syndrome. *J. Infect. Dis.* **165**:994–1000.

74. **Lloyd, A., I. Hickie, D. Wakefield, C. Boughton, and J. Dwyer.** 1990. A double-blind, placebo-controlled trial of intravenous immunoglobulin therapy in patients with chronic fatigue syndrome. *Am. J. Med.* **89**:561–568.
75. **Lloyd, A., I. Hickie, A. Brockman, J. Dwyer, and D. Wakefield.** 1991. Cytokine levels in serum and cerebrospinal fluid in patients with chronic fatigue syndrome and control subjects. *J. Infect. Dis.* **164**:1023–1024.
76. **Lloyd, A., S. Gandevia, A. Brockman, J. Hales, and D. Wakefield.** 1994. Cytokine production and fatigue in patients with chronic fatigue syndrome and healthy control subjects in response to exercise. *Clin. Infect. Dis.* **18**(Suppl. 1):S142–S146.
77. **Lloyd, A. R., D. Wakefield, C. Boughton, and J. Dwyer.** 1988. What is myalgic encephalomyelitis? *Lancet* **i**:1286–1287.
78. **Lloyd, A. R., I. Hickie, C. R. Boughton, O. Spencer, and D. Wakefield.** 1990. Prevalence of chronic fatigue syndrome in an Australian population. *Med. J. Aust.* **153**: 522–528.
79. **Lloyd, A. R.** 1998. Chronic fatigue and chronic fatigue syndrome: shifting boundaries and attributions. *Am. J. Med.* **105**:7S–10S.
80. **Lyall, M., M. Peakman, and S. Wessely.** 2003. A systematic review and critical evaluation of the immunology of chronic fatigue syndrome. *J. Psychosom. Res.* **55**:79–90.
81. **Manningham, R.** 1750. *The Symptoms, Nature and Causes of the Febricula or Little Fever: Commonly Called Nervous or Hysteric Fever; the Fever on the Spirits; Vapours, Hypo or Spleen*, 2nd ed. J. Robinson, London, United Kingdom.
82. **Manu, P., T. J. Lane, D. A. Matthews, R. J. Castriotta, R. K. Watson, and M. Abeles.** 1994. Alpha-delta sleep in patients with a chief complaint of chronic fatigue. *South. Med. J.* **87**:465–470.
83. **Marlin, R. G., H. Anchel, J. C. Gibson, W. M. Goldberg, and M. Swinton.** 1998. An evaluation of multidisciplinary intervention for chronic fatigue syndrome with long-term follow-up, and a comparison with untreated controls. *Am. J. Med.* **105**:110S–114S.
84. **McArdle, A., F. McArdle, M. J. Jackson, S. F. Page, I. Fahal, and R. H. Edwards.** 1996. Investigation by polymerase chain reaction of enteroviral infection in patients with chronic fatigue syndrome. *Clin. Sci.* **90**: 295–300.
85. **McKenzie, R., A. O'Fallon, J. Dale, M. Demitrack, G. Sharma, M. Deloria, D. Garcia-Borreguero, W. Blackwelder, and S. E. Straus.** 1998. Low-dose hydrocortisone for treatment of chronic fatigue syndrome: a randomized controlled trial. *JAMA* **280**:1061–1066.
86. **Morriss, R., M. Sharpe, A. L. Sharpley, P. J. Cowen, K. Hawton, and J. Morris.** 1993. Abnormalities of sleep in patients with the chronic fatigue syndrome. *BMJ* **306**: 1161–1164.
87. **Moss-Morris, R., C. Sharon, R. Tobin, and J. C. Baldi.** 2005. A randomized controlled graded exercise trial for chronic fatigue syndrome: outcomes and mechanisms of change. *J. Health Psychol.* **10**:245–259.
88. **Natelson, B. H., J. Cheu, J. Pareja, S. P. Ellis, T. Policastro, and T. W. Findley.** 1996. Randomized, double blind, controlled placebo-phase in trial of low dose phenelzine in the chronic fatigue syndrome. *Psychopharmacology* **124**:226–230.
89. **Natelson, B. H., J. Cheu, N. Hill, M. Bergen, L. Korn, T. Denny, and K. Dahl.** 1998. Single-blind, placebo phase-in trial of two escalating doses of selegiline in the chronic fatigue syndrome. *Neuropsychobiology* **37**:150–154.
90. **Nisenbaum, R., M. Reyes, A. C. Mawle, and W. C. Reeves.** 1998. Factor analysis of unexplained severe fatigue and interrelated symptoms: overlap with criteria for chronic fatigue syndrome. *Am. J. Epidemiol.* **148**:72–77.
91. **Nisenbaum, R., M. Reyes, E. R. Unger, and W. C. Reeves.** 2004. Factor analysis of symptoms among subjects with unexplained chronic fatigue: what can we learn about chronic fatigue syndrome? *J. Psychosom. Res.* **56**:171–178.
92. **Olson, L. G., A. Ambrogetti, and D. C. Sutherland.** 2003. A pilot randomized controlled trial of dexamphetamine in patients with chronic fatigue syndrome. *Psychosomatics* **44**: 38–43.
93. **Patarca, R.** 2001. Cytokines and chronic fatigue syndrome. *Ann. N.Y. Acad. Sci.* **933**:185–200.
94. **Penttila, I. A., R. J. Harris, P. Storm, D. Haynes, D. A. Worswick, and B. P. Marmion.** 1998. Cytokine dysregulation in the post-Q-fever fatigue syndrome. *QJM* **91**:549–560.
95. **Peterson, P. K., J. Shepard, M. Macres, C. Schenck, J. Crosson, D. Rechtman, and N. Lurie.** 1990. A controlled trial of intravenous immunoglobulin G in chronic fatigue syndrome. *Am. J. Med.* **89**:554–560.
96. **Peterson, P. K., A. Pheley, J. Schroeppel, C. Schenck, P. Marshall, A. Kind, J. M. Haugland, L. J. Lambrecht, S. Swan, and S. Goldsmith.** 1998. A preliminary placebo-controlled crossover trial of fludrocortisone for chronic fatigue syndrome. *Arch. Intern. Med.* **158**:908–914.
97. **Poole, J., R. Herrell, S. Ashton, J. Goldberg, and D. Buchwald.** 2000. Results of isoproterenol tilt table testing in monozygotic twins discordant for chronic fatigue syndrome. *Arch. Intern. Med.* **160**:3461–3468.
98. **Powell, P., R. P. Bentall, F. J. Nye, and R. H. Edwards.** 2001. Randomised controlled trial of patient education to encourage graded exercise in chronic fatigue syndrome. *BMJ* **322**:387–390.
99. **Prins, J. B., G. Bleijenberg, E. Bazelmans, L. D. Elving, T. M. de Boo, J. L. Severens, G. J. van der Wilt, P. Spinhoven, and J. W. van der Meer.** 2001. Cognitive behaviour therapy for chronic fatigue syndrome: a multicentre randomised controlled trial. *Lancet* **357**:841–847.
100. **Prins, J. B., J. W. M. van der Meer, and G. Bleijenberg.** 2006. Chronic fatigue syndrome. *Lancet* **367**:346–355.
101. **Razumovsky, A. Y., K. DeBusk, H. Calkins, S. Snader, K. E. Lucas, P. Vyas, D. F. Hanley, and P. C. Rowe.** 2003. Cerebral and systemic hemodynamics changes during upright tilt in chronic fatigue syndrome. *J. Neuroimaging* **13**:57–67.
102. **Reeves, W. C., A. Lloyd, S. D. Vernon, N. Klimas, L. A. Jason, G. Bleijenberg, B. Evengard, P. D. White, R. Nisenbaum, E. R. Unger, and the International Chronic Fatigue Syndrome Study Group.** 2003. Identification of ambiguities in the 1994 chronic fatigue syndrome research case definition and recommendations for resolution. *BMC Health Services Res.* **3**:25.
103. **Reyes, M., R. Nisenbaum, D. C. Hoaglin, E. R. Unger, C. Emmons, B. Randall, J. A. Stewart, S. Abbey, J. F. Jones, N. Gantz, S. Minden, and W. C. Reeves.** 2003. Prevalence and incidence of chronic fatigue syndrome in Wichita, Kansas. *Arch. Intern. Med.* **163**:1530–1536.
104. **Ridsdale, L., A. Evans, W. Jerrett, S. Mandalia, K. Osler, and H. Vora.** 1993. Patients with fatigue in general practice: a prospective study. *BMJ* **307**:103–106.
105. **Rowe, K. S.** 1997. Double-blind randomized controlled trial to assess the efficacy of intravenous gammaglobulin for the management of chronic fatigue syndrome in adolescents. *J. Psychiatr. Res.* **31**:133–147.

106. **Rowe, P. C., and H. Calkins.** 1998. Neurally mediated hypotension and chronic fatigue syndrome. *Am. J. Med.* **105:**15S–21S.
107. **Rowe, P. C., H. Calkins, K. DeBusk, R. McKenzie, R. Anand, G. Sharma, B. A. Cuccherini, N. Soto, P. Hohman, S. Snader, K. E. Lucas, M. Wolff, and S. E. Straus.** 2001. Fludrocortisone acetate to treat neurally mediated hypotension in chronic fatigue syndrome: a randomized controlled trial. *JAMA* **285:**52–59.
108. **Schluederberg, A., S. E. Straus, P. Peterson, S. Blumenthal, A. L. Komaroff, S. B. Spring, A. Landay, and D. Buchwald.** 1992. NIH conference. Chronic fatigue syndrome research. Definition and medical outcome assessment. *Ann. Intern. Med.* **117:**325–331.
109. **Schmaling, K. B., J. I. Fiedelak, W. J. Katon, J. O. Bader, and D. S. Buchwald.** 2003. Prospective study of the prognosis of unexplained chronic fatigue in a clinic-based cohort. *Psychosom. Med.* **65:**1047–1054.
110. **Schondorf, R., J. Benoit, T. Wein, and D. Phaneuf.** 1999. Orthostatic intolerance in the chronic fatigue syndrome. *J. Auton. Nerv. Sys.* **75:**192–201.
111. **Sharpe, M., K. Hawton, S. Simkin, C. Surawy, A. Hackmann, I. Klimes, T. Peto, D. Warrell, and V. Seagroatt.** 1996. Cognitive behaviour therapy for the chronic fatigue syndrome: a randomized controlled trial. *BMJ* **312:**22–26.
112. **Sharpe, M. C., L. C. Archard, J. E. Banatvala, L. K. Borysiewicz, A. W. Clare, A. David, R. H. Edwards, K. E. Hawton, H. P. Lambert, R. J. Lane, et al.** 1991. A report—chronic fatigue syndrome: guidelines for research. *J. R. Soc. Med.* **84:**118–121.
113. **Shorter, E.** 1993. Chronic fatigue in historical perspective. *Ciba Found. Symp.* **173:**6–16.
114. **Spink, W.** 1951. What is chronic brucellosis? *Ann. Intern. Med.* **35:**358–374.
115. **Steele, L., J. G. Dobbins, K. Fukuda, M. Reyes, B. Randall, M. Koppelman, and W. C. Reeves.** 1998. The epidemiology of chronic fatigue in San Francisco. *Am. J. Med.* **105:**83S–90S.
116. **Steinberg, P., B. E. McNutt, P. Marshall, C. Schenck, N. Lurie, A. Pheley, and P. K. Peterson.** 1996. Double-blind placebo-controlled study of the efficacy of oral terfenadine in the treatment of chronic fatigue syndrome. *J. Allergy Clin. Immunol.* **97:**119–126.
117. **Straus, S. E., J. K. Dale, M. Tobi, T. Lawley, O. Preble, R. M. Blaese, C. Hallahan, and W. Henle.** 1988. Acyclovir treatment of the chronic fatigue syndrome. Lack of efficacy in a placebo-controlled trial. *N. Engl. J. Med.* **319:**1692–1698.
118. **Straus, S. E., J. K. Dale, J. B. Peter, and C. A. Dinarello.** 1989. Circulating lymphokine levels in the chronic fatigue syndrome. *J. Infect. Dis.* **160:**1085–1086.
119. **Strayer, D. R., W. A. Carter, I. Brodsky, P. Cheney, D. Peterson, P. Salvato, C. Thompson, M. Loveless, D. E. Shapiro, W. Elsasser, et al.** 1994. A controlled clinical trial with a specifically configured RNA drug, poly(I)·poly(C12U), in chronic fatigue syndrome. *Clin. Infect. Dis.* **18**(Suppl. 1)**:**S88–S95.
120. **Stulemeijer, M., L. W. A. M. de Jong, T. J. W. Fiselier, S. W. B. Hoogveld, and G. Bleijenberg.** 2005. Cognitive behaviour therapy for adolescents with chronic fatigue syndrome: randomised controlled trial. *BMJ* **330:**14.
121. **Swanink, C. M., W. J. Melchers, J. W. van der Meer, J. H. Vercoulen, G. Bleijenberg, J. F. Fennis, and J. M. Galama.** 1994. Enteroviruses and the chronic fatigue syndrome. *Clin. Infect. Dis.* **19:**860–864.
122. **Taylor, R. R., L. A. Jason, and C. J. Curie.** 2002. Prognosis of chronic fatigue in a community-based sample. *Psychosom. Med.* **64:**319–327.
123. **Van Hoof, E., P. De Becker, C. Lapp, R. Cluydts, and K. De Meirleir.** 2007. Defining the occurrence and influence of alpha-delta sleep in chronic fatigue syndrome. *Am. J. Med. Sci.* **333:**78–84.
124. **Vollmer-Conna, U., I. Hickie, D. Hadzi-Pavlovic, K. Tymms, D. Wakefield, J. Dwyer, and A. Lloyd.** 1997. Intravenous immunoglobulin is ineffective in the treatment of patients with chronic fatigue syndrome. *Am. J. Med.* **103:**38–43.
125. **Vollmer-Conna, U., A. Lloyd, I. Hickie, and D. Wakefield.** 1998. Chronic fatigue syndrome: an immunological perspective. *Aust. N.Z. J. Psychiatry* **32:**523–527.
126. **Vollmer-Conna, U.** 2001. Acute sickness behaviour: an immune system-to-brain communication? *Psychol. Med.* **31:**761–767.
127. **Vollmer-Conna, U., C. Fazou, B. Cameron, H. Li, C. Brennan, L. Luck, T. Davenport, D. Wakefield, I. Hickie, and A. Lloyd.** 2004. Production of pro-inflammatory cytokines correlates with the symptoms of acute sickness behaviour in humans. *Psychol. Med.* **34:**1289–1297.
128. **Wallman, K. E., A. R. Morton, C. Goodman, R. Grove, and A. M. Guilfoyle.** 2004. Randomised controlled trial of graded exercise in chronic fatigue syndrome. *Med. J. Aust.* **180:**444–448.
129. **Watson, N. F., V. Kapur, L. M. Arguelles, J. Goldberg, D. F. Schmidt, R. Armitage, and D. Buchwald.** 2003. Comparison of subjective and objective measures of insomnia in monozygotic twins discordant for chronic fatigue syndrome. *Sleep* **26:**324–328.
130. **Wearden, A. J., R. K. Morriss, R. Mullis, P. L. Strickland, D. J. Pearson, L. Appleby, I. T. Campbell, and J. A. Morris.** 1998. Randomised, double-blind, placebo-controlled treatment trial of fluoxetine and graded exercise for chronic fatigue syndrome. *Br. J. Psychiatry* **172:**485–490.
131. **Weatherley-Jones, E., J. P. Nicholl, K. J. Thomas, G. J. Parry, M. W. McKendrick, S. T. Green, P. J. Stanley, and S. P. J. Lynch.** 2004. A randomised, controlled, triple-blind trial of the efficacy of homeopathic treatment for chronic fatigue syndrome. *J. Psychosom. Res.* **56:**189–197.
132. **Weinstein, A. W., and M. Klempner.** 2001. Treatment of patients with persistent symptoms and a history of Lyme disease. *N. Engl. J. Med.* **345:**1424–1425.
133. **Wessely, S., and R. Powell.** 1989. Fatigue syndromes: a comparison of chronic 'postviral' fatigue with neuromuscular and affective disorders. *J. Neurol. Neurosurg. Psychiatry* **52:**940–948.
134. **Wessely, S., T. Chalder, S. Hirsch, T. Pawlikowska, P. Wallace, and D. J. Wright.** 1995. Postinfectious fatigue: prospective cohort study in primary care. *Lancet* **345:**1333–1338.
135. **White, P. D., S. A. Grover, H. O. Kangro, J. M. Thomas, J. Amess, and A. W. Clare.** 1995. The validity and reliability of the fatigue syndrome that follows glandular fever. *Psychol. Med.* **25:**917–924.
136. **White, P. D., J. M. Thomas, J. Amess, S. A. Grover, H. O. Kangro, and A. W. Clare.** 1995. The existence of a fatigue syndrome after glandular fever. *Psychol. Med.* **25:**907–916.
137. **White, P. D., J. M. Thomas, J. Amess, D. H. Crawford, S. A. Grover, H. O. Kangro, and A. W. Clare.** 1998. Incidence, risk and prognosis of acute and chronic fatigue syndromes and psychiatric disorders after glandular fever. *Br. J. Psychiatry* **173:**475–481.
138. **Whiting, P., A. M. Bagnall, A. J. Sowden, J. E. Cornell, C. D. Mulrow, and G. Ramirez.** 2001. Interventions for the treatment and management of chronic

fatigue syndrome: a systematic review. *JAMA* **286:**1360–1368.

139. **Wilson, A., I. Hickie, A. Lloyd, D. Hadzi-Pavlovic, C. Boughton, J. Dwyer, and D. Wakefield.** 1994. Longitudinal study of outcome of chronic fatigue syndrome. *BMJ* **308:**756–769.
140. **Wilson, A., I. Hickie, A. Lloyd, and D. Wakefield.** 1994. The treatment of chronic fatigue syndrome: science and speculation. *Am. J. Med.* **96:**544–550.
141. **Wilson, A., I. Hickie, D. Hadzi-Pavlovic, D. Wakefield, G. Parker, S. E. Straus, J. Dale, D. McCluskey, G. Hinds, A. Brickman, D. Goldenberg, M. Demitrack, T. Blakely, S. Wessely, M. Sharpe, and A. Lloyd.** 2001. What is chronic fatigue syndrome? Heterogeneity within an international multicentre study. *Aust. N. Z. J. Psychiatry* **35:**520–527.
142. **Yalcin, S., H. Kuratsune, K. Yamaguchi, T. Kitani, and K. Yamanishi.** 1994. Prevalence of human herpesvirus 6 variants A and B in patients with chronic fatigue syndrome. *Microbiol. Immunol.* **38:**587–590.

The Agents

SECTION II

Poxviruses

R. MARK BULLER AND FRANK FENNER

18

VIROLOGY

Classification and History

The poxviruses (family *Poxviridae*) are the largest and most complex of all viruses (25, 98). The subfamily *Chordopoxvirinae* (poxviruses of vertebrates) contains eight genera (15). Human infections are caused by 11 poxvirus species belonging to four genera, the majority of which cause zoonotic infections (Table 1). The orthopoxvirus pathogens are the best studied, and variola virus (VARV) is the most important species, as it caused a severe generalized human disease known as smallpox. Smallpox was eliminated from the human population in 1977, which resulted in drawdown of vaccine stockpiles and cessation of childhood vaccination programs. These steps increased the vulnerability of the human population to a devastating smallpox epidemic and increased the value of VARV as bioweapon. This unintended consequence of the most successful vaccination program in history was exploited by the former Soviet Union, which weaponized VARV in contradiction of the 1972 Biological and Toxin Weapons Convention (1, 58). This occurrence raised concerns that other rogue nations or terrorist groups could also develop VARV or monkeypox virus (MPXV) as a bioweapon.

Monkeypox is a disease that is clinically almost identical to smallpox. MPXV was discovered as a disease-causing agent of laboratory primates in Copenhagen, Denmark, in 1958 (137), and it caused several other outbreaks in captive primates before it was recognized as the cause of a smallpox-like zoonotic disease in West and central Africa in 1970. The incidence of monkeypox is on the rise in central Africa (109).

Vaccinia virus (VACV) and cowpox virus (CPXV) are distinct orthopoxviruses that cause human infections, and one is not a synonym for the other. CPXV is the agent that Jenner used to prove the efficacy of vaccination against smallpox; however, VACV was subsequently used for at least the last 100 years to vaccinate against smallpox. Human CPXV infections are rare and are usually acquired from the domestic cat. The source of human infections with VACV is contact with vaccinees or domestic animals persistently infected with VACV as a result of the smallpox eradication (cantagalo and buffalopox viruses) (86, 99, 100). VACV and two members of the genus *Avipoxvirus* (fowlpox virus and canarypox virus) have been used as vectors for the production of novel vaccines and for gene therapy (see chapter 16).

The remaining human poxvirus pathogens belong to three genera: four in *Parapoxvirus*, two in *Yatapoxvirus*, and one in *Molluscipoxvirus* (Table 1). Orf virus (ORFV) causes orf (synonyms: contagious pustular dermatitis, contagious ecthyma, and scabby mouth), a disease of sheep. Pseudocowpox (PCPV; synonyms: milker's nodule and paravaccinia) and bovine pustular stomatitis (BPSV) viruses cause diseases of cattle (117). Very rarely, humans may be infected with seal parapoxvirus (60). Tanapox virus (TANV) and Yaba monkey tumor poxvirus (YMTV) are rare causes of zoonotic diseases mainly in Africa. Molluscum contagiosum virus (MCV) causes a common cosmopolitan human disease and is the only poxvirus currently maintained in the human population without a zoonotic host (13).

Structure of Virus

Poxvirus virions appear to be oval or brick-shaped structures of about 200 to 400 nm in length with axial ratios of 1.2 to 1.7. The structure of VACV (Fig. 1A and D) is characteristic of that of all the poxviruses that infect humans except those belonging to the genus *Parapoxvirus* (Fig. 1B and E). The outer membrane of orthopoxviruses consists of tubular lipoprotein subunits arranged rather irregularly, whereas parapoxviruses have a regular spiral structure. The membrane encloses a dumbbell-shaped core and two "lateral bodies." The core contains the viral DNA and associated proteins.

The double-stranded DNA poxvirus genome is 130 to 375 kbp in length and codes for 150 to 300 proteins, depending on the species. The genomes of a large number of poxvirus species, including 55 isolates of VARV, have been completely sequenced (http://www.vbrc.org). The genomic organization of the prototypic orthopoxvirus, VACV, is displayed in Color Plate 29. Orthopoxvirus virions contain a hemagglutinin, and estimates of virus phylogeny based on hemagglutinin and A-type inclusion body protein gene sequences agree well with those based on restriction endonuclease maps, permitting the use of PCR analyses of these genes as the assay of choice for identifying orthopoxvirus species (94, 104, 118). Assignment of a pox-

TABLE 1 Poxviruses that can cause disease in humans

Genus	Species	Distribution	Reservoir	Disease in humans
Orthopoxvirus	Variola virus	Was worldwide	Humans (before 1977)	Smallpox, specifically human, generalized disease
	Monkeypox virus	Central and West Africa	Squirrels, monkeys	Smallpox-like disease; a zoonosis
	Vaccinia virus	Worldwide	Laboratory virus	Used for smallpox vaccination, localized lesions
	Buffalopox virus, variant of vaccinia virus	India (Egypt, Indonesia)	Buffaloes, rodents	Localized pustular skin lesions
	Cantagalo virus, variant of vaccinia virus	Brazil	Cattle	Localized pustular skin lesions
	Cowpox virus	Europe, western Asia	Wild rodents	Localized pustular skin lesions; a rare zoonosis
Parapoxvirus	Orf virus	Worldwide	Sheep	Localized nodular skin lesions; a rare zoonosis
	Bovine papular stomatitis virus	Worldwide	Cattle	Localized nodular skin lesions; a rare zoonosis
	Pseudocowpox virus	Worldwide	Cows	Localized nodular skin lesions; a rare zoonosis
	Sealpox virus	Worldwide	Seals	Localized nodular skin lesions; a rare zoonosis
Yatapoxvirus	Tanapoxvirus	Tropical Africa	Unknown	Localized nodular skin lesions; a rare zoonosis
	Yaba monkey tumor virus	West Africa	Unknown, possibly monkeys	Localized nodular skin lesions; rare accidental infections
Molluscipoxvirus	Molluscum contagiosum virus	Worldwide	Humans	Few or many nodular lesions; worse in AIDS cases

virus to a particular taxonomic group is based on extensive analyses of virus genomic sequences.

There is extensive cross-neutralization and cross-protection between viruses belonging to the same genus, but little to none between viruses of different genera; in laboratory experiments genetic recombination occurs readily between viruses of the same genus but rarely between those of different genera (40).

Biology

Replication Strategy

Replication of poxviruses occurs in the cytoplasm, and poxviruses encode dozens of enzymes required for transcription and replication of the viral genome, several of which [including DNA-dependent RNA polymerase, poly(A) polymerase, capping enzyme, methylating enzymes, and transcription factor] are carried in the virion itself (98). The viral core is released into the cytoplasm after fusion of the virion with the plasma membrane through a mechanism that is not fully understood (Fig. 2). Transcription is initiated by the viral transcriptase, and functional capped and polyadenylated mRNAs are produced minutes after infection. The polypeptides produced by translation of these mRNAs complete the uncoating of the core, and transcription of about 100 early genes, distributed throughout the genome, occurs before viral DNA synthesis begins. Early proteins include DNA polymerase, thymidine kinase, and several other enzymes required for replication of the genome.

With the onset of viral DNA replication there is a dramatic shift in gene expression. Transcription of intermediate and late genes is controlled by binding of specific viral proteins to characteristic promoter sequences. Virion assembly occurs in circumscribed areas of the cytoplasm, where spherical immature particles assembling on cellular membranes can be visualized by electron microscopy. The immature particle incorporates DNA and additional proteins during morphogenesis to the mature virus. Most mature virus remains in the cytoplasm and is released on cell death; however, some moves to the Golgi complex, where it is wrapped in a double membrane, transported to the plasma membrane, and released by exocytosis with the loss of one of the Golgi acquired membranes to produce extracellular enveloped virus. Both mature virus and extracellular enveloped virus particles are infectious, but extracellular enveloped virus particles appear to be important in virus spread through the body.

Poxviruses encode a large number of proteins that enhance the ability of the virus to replicate efficiently and spread within the animal host (98). A number of these gene products are important for optimal replication in differentiated and nondividing cell types, and some are involved in the blockade of cellular apoptosis pathways (131). Others are immunosubversive proteins that are se-

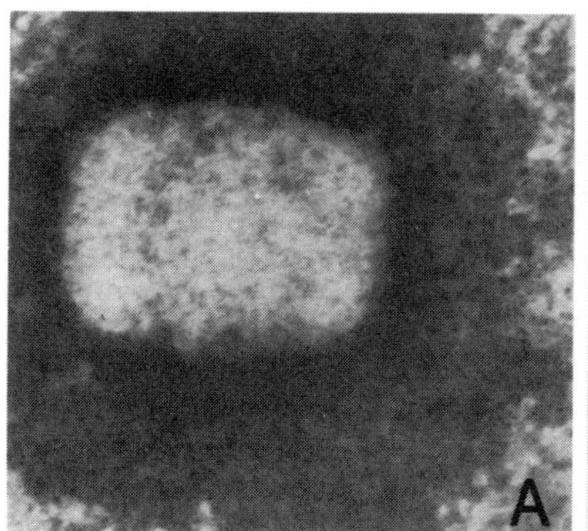

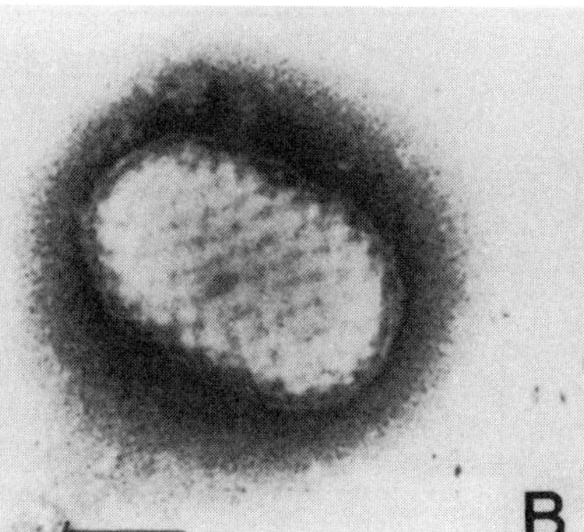

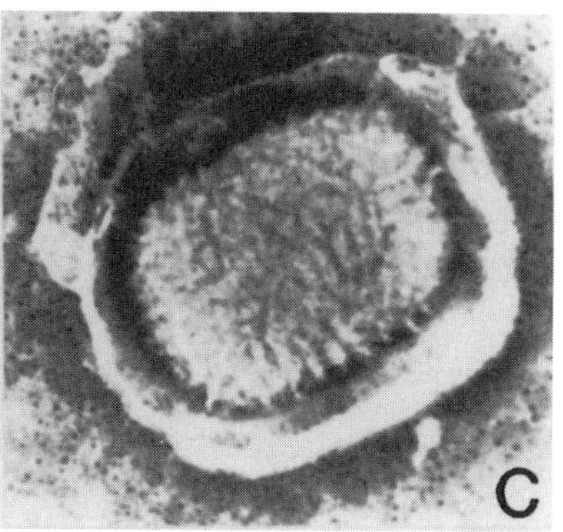

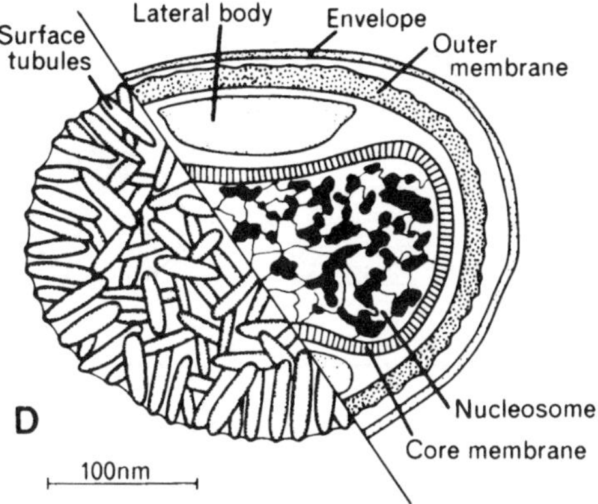

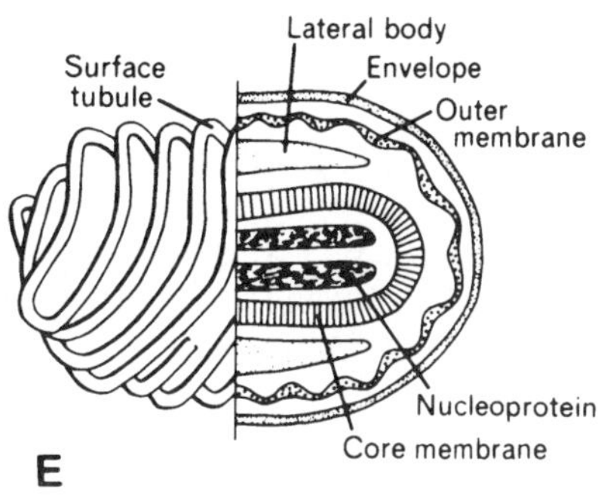

FIGURE 1 Structure of virions of poxviruses that cause human infections. Shown are negatively stained preparations of orthopoxvirus virions (cowpox, monkeypox, vaccinia, and variola viruses) (A), parapoxvirus virions (ORFV, BPSV, PCPV, and sealpox viruses) (B), and yatapoxvirus virions (TANV and YMTV) (C). The virions of orthopoxviruses and yatapoxviruses have similar morphologies, but those of yatapoxviruses always have two membranes. Virions of the parapoxviruses are smaller and have a distinctive regular surface structure. (D) Diagram of the structure of the virion of VACV. The viral DNA and several proteins within the core are organized as a nucleosome. The core has a 9-nm-thick shell with a regular subunit structure. Within the virion, the core assumes the shape of a dumbbell because of the large lateral bodies, which are, in turn, enclosed within a protein shell about 12 nm thick—the first membrane, the surface of which appears to consist of irregularly arranged surface tubules, which, in turn, consist of small globular subunits. Mature virus released by exocytosis (extracellular enveloped virus) is enclosed within a second membrane (envelope) acquired from the Golgi. This membrane contains host cell lipids and several unique virus-specific polypeptides not found in the intracellular mature virus outer membrane. Most virions remain cell associated and are released by cellular disruption, without the second membrane. (E) Diagram of the structure of the virion of ORFV. The first membrane consists of a single long tubule that appears to be wound around the particle. In negatively stained preparations (B) both sides are visible, giving a characteristic criss-cross appearance. The second membrane is usually closely applied to the surface of the first membrane. Bar = 100 nm. (Reprinted from reference 39a with permission.)

creted mimics of host ligands, regulators, or receptors. These include homologs of epidermal growth factor and binding proteins for complement regulatory proteins C3 and C4, interleukin 1, interleukin 18, tumor necrosis factors alpha and beta, and type I and type II interferons (89).

Host Range

The animal host range of poxviruses that infect humans is narrow for VARV and MCV and relatively broad for VACV, CPXV, and MPXV. VARV has not been shown to cause significant disease in tested immunocompetent animal models except in nonhuman primates, in which lethal infections can be obtained under nonphysiological conditions. The challenge of cynomolgus macaques with up to $10^{8.5}$ PFU of VARV in aerosols resulted in an inapparent infection (65); however, lethal disease could be achieved 3 to 6 days following intravenous administration of 10^9 PFU. This model does not recapitulate the natural pathogenesis of VARV, which is initiated by deposition of a small number of virions on the respiratory mucosa, the appearance of rash (10 to 12 days later), and death (20 to 22 days later) or recovery.

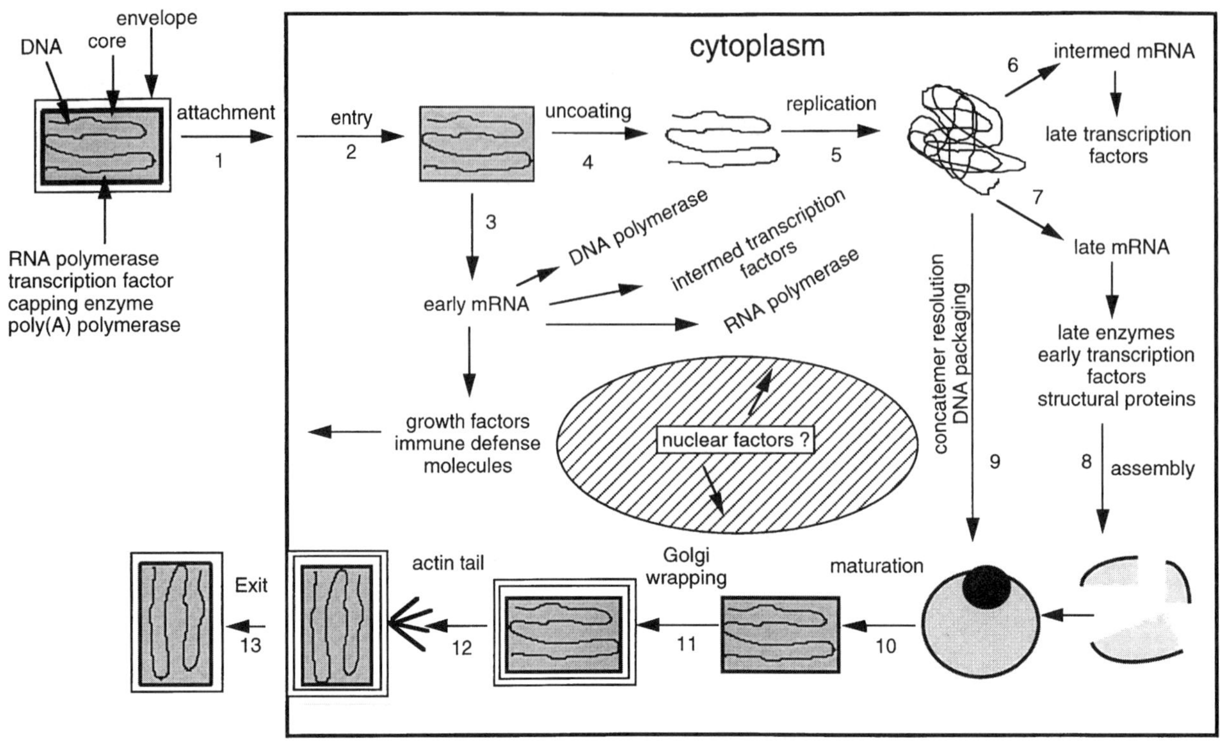

FIGURE 2 Diagram illustrating the replication cycle of vaccinia virus, the prototype orthopoxvirus. (Reprinted from reference 98 with permission.)

The ecology of MPXV is still not completely understood with respect to reservoir and incidental hosts (109). Seroprevalence studies suggest that there may be no one reservoir of MPXV; rather, several animal species may support MPXV in nature. For example, two genera and six species of squirrels and five genera and nine species of nonhuman primates were observed to have MPXV-specific antibodies (109). Virus has been isolated from an animal in nature only once, and the source was a diseased squirrel of the species *Funisciurus anerythrus* (75); however, in a 2003 shipment of African rodents to the United States cell culture and/or PCR assays demonstrated MPXV in two *Funisciurus* spp. (rope squirrel), one *Cricetomys* sp. (giant pouched rat), and three *Graphiurus* spp. (African dormouse) (54). These observations suggest the natural life cycle to be a complex interaction of reservoir hosts and incidental species. This broad host range is a cause for concern, as it may facilitate the adaptation of MPXV to new hosts in new regions. Laboratory studies have demonstrated that cynomolgus macaques (147), prairie dogs (144), and ground squirrels (132) can be employed as experimental hosts.

CPXV has a very broad host range in nature. The virus is maintained in wild rodents in western Eurasia, in particular, voles and wood mice. Short-tailed field voles have been demonstrated conclusively to be the reservoir host in Great Britain (19). Cows are merely incidental hosts, as are rats, dogs, zoo animals (lions, cheetahs, pumas, panthers, and jaguars), and domestic cats (4, 88). The domestic cat is the frequent liaison host of human infections (5). In the laboratory, the mouse model is most often used to study CPXV.

VACV may originally have been maintained in nature in horses, as a recent comparative genome sequencing study placed a poxvirus isolated in 1976 from a diseased Mongolian horse as a member of the VACV clade of orthopoxviruses (135). VACV infects domesticated livestock species, possibly as a result of the smallpox vaccination campaign in which various animals were purposely used for vaccine production or inadvertently infected by contact with vaccinees (134). In Holland in 1963, 8 out of 36 outbreaks of "cowpox" in milking cows were found to be caused by VACV, and the rest were caused by authentic CPXV (27). In 1985, VACV was isolated from scabs taken from pox lesions on buffaloes in five different districts of Maharashtra State, India (34), and was also observed in Egypt and Indonesia, where water buffaloes (*Bubalus bubalis*) are used as domestic animals (78). Buffalopox outbreaks continued through 1996, with human infections and possible subclinical disease in areas of endemicity (78). In addition, since 1999, VACV has been causing increasing numbers of infectious outbreaks in cattle and dairy workers based in Minas Gerais State, Brazil (83). Similarly, in 1932, VACV appeared to adapt to a rabbit host, causing a new disease that was highly lethal and transmissible to contact rabbits by airborne infection (53). The isolated agent was named rabbitpox virus, and recent sequencing of its genome confirmed it as a strain of VACV (84). VACV replicates to various degrees in most tested animal models.

MCV has the narrowest host range of any poxvirus and has similarities in this regard to human papillomavirus (see chapter 28). MCV appears to replicate only in the human keratinocyte and has yet to be cultivated in cultured cells.

Although MCV from skin lesions has been propagated in human foreskin xenografts (14), no experimental animals have been shown to support its growth.

Growth in Cell Culture

Although the host range of human poxvirus pathogens can be quite narrow, all the orthopoxviruses replicate in a broad range of fibroblast or epithelial cell lines, including HeLa, BS-C-1, and Vero cells. Infection causes the cell to round and detach from the substrate, which is the basis for the plaque assay used to measure virus infectivity. Cytoplasmic inclusion bodies can be detected with appropriate histologic stains.

Inactivation by Physical and Chemical Agents

Poxvirus infectivity is relatively stable in the environment compared to the infectivities of other enveloped viruses, although stability is measured in days or weeks, not years (41). Since all poxvirus species likely share similar sensitivities to physical and chemical agents, data acquired with one poxvirus species can be applied to another. VACV viability is adversely affected by both high temperatures and high humidity. VACV sprayed in aerosols at room temperature (21 to 23°C) maintained 46 and 24% of the initial infectivity in 18 to 19% and 82 to 84% relative humidity, respectively, over a 4-h period (57). For the same period at 31.5 to 33.5°C, infectivity at low humidity was unaffected, whereas infectivity dropped from 24 to 5.9% at 82 to 84% relative humidity. Since orthopoxviruses are highly infectious, and it takes only a small number of virions to initiate infection (109), the physical environment occupied by a person with poxvirus disease must be appropriately decontaminated. There are a number of disinfectants that show good activity against poxviruses. Using the orthopoxvirus ectromelia virus, White and Fenner examined a range of chemical treatments for surface decontamination (140). For example, a 10-min treatment with 2% phenol or 40% alcohol was sufficient to destroy virus infectivity completely. Sterilization of surfaces can be achieved with formaldehyde gas or a range of commercially available contact sterilants, including fresh solutions of 10% bleach, Spor-Klenz, or Envirocide.

EPIDEMIOLOGY

Distribution

Smallpox has long been known as a severe generalized human disease (41, 61). Already endemic in India 2,000 years ago, smallpox had spread to China and Japan in the east and Europe and North Africa in the west by about 700 A.D. It was introduced to the Caribbean with the African slave trade in 1518 and thence to Mexico in 1520, taking a terrible toll on the totally nonimmune Amerindians. Repeated introductions from Europe and, to a lesser extent, from Africa into North America occurred from 1617 onward. With the discovery of vaccination by Jenner in the latter part of the 18th century, the disease was brought under control first by local initiatives, which became national and finally global. The world was certified free of smallpox by the World Health Assembly in May 1980 (41).

Monkeypox is now the most frequent human orthopoxvirus infection (109). Because monkeypox is clinically difficult to distinguish from smallpox, it was not identified as a distinct disease until smallpox was no longer endemic. Monkeypox is found mainly among the inhabitants of small villages in the tropical rain forests of West and central Africa, with occasional outbreaks elsewhere (40, 59, 67). In 2003 and 2005 there were outbreaks in the United States and Sudan, respectively (26, 116). The U.S. importation was traced to a shipment of pocket pets from Ghana destined for the pet trade (116). Human cowpox is restricted to a region bounded by Norway, northern Russia, Turkmenistan, France, and Great Britain because of the limited ability to remain enzootic except in particular species of rodents. Zoonotic VACV infections are currently confined to Brazil and India, and contact infections from subjects receiving the smallpox vaccine are limited to countries which vaccinate their military or first responders to infectious disease outbreaks.

Of the remaining human poxvirus infections, ORFV has worldwide distribution. PCPV and BPSV are maintained in dairy herds derived from European herds in all parts of the world. In Great Britain, PCPV infection is enzootic in cattle and, in contrast to CPXV, persists in relatively small herds (51). Tanapox was first observed as an acute febrile illness associated with localized skin lesions, occurring in epidemics in 1957 and 1962 among people living in the flood plain of the Tana River in Kenya (33). It is endemic in this area, in the Democratic Republic of Congo (DRC, former Zaire), and probably elsewhere in tropical Africa (68). Molluscum contagiosum has a worldwide distribution and is very common in certain areas.

Subclinical Infection Rate

VARV subclinical infections of vaccinated subjects were documented in the smallpox eradication program, which is perhaps not surprising (41); however, it was more difficult to study this issue in naïve subjects. This was not the case with studies of human monkeypox carried out in Zaire between 1981 and 1986, as smallpox vaccination had ceased in 1970s. Of 774 unvaccinated contacts of monkeypox patients, 136 showed serologic evidence of infection. Twenty-seven of 136 (20%) persons gave no history of illness, residual skin lesions, or other changes suggestive of monkeypox, and therefore were classified as having subclinical infections (67). Subclinical infections are probably universal for poxviruses, as multiple strains of mice can be infected subclinically with ectromelia virus and act as "silent" reservoirs of infectious virus for contact mice (16).

Epidemic Patterns

Except for VARV and MPXV infections, in which case fatality rates range from 1 to 30%, poxvirus infections of healthy individuals do not result in death. In 1981, a study was carried out to determine prevalence of monkeypox in central and West Africa. Thirteen percent of West African children (Ivory Coast and Sierra Leone) and 19% of central African children (DRC) were positive for hemagglutinin-inhibiting (orthopoxvirus) antibodies among 10,300 unvaccinated children. As a follow-up test, a less sensitive but more specific radioimmunoassay adsorption test for MPXV antibodies was utilized. This test indicated that 17% of the sera positive for hemagglutinin inhibition contained MPXV-specific antibodies (59, 67). A more recent study with a less specific assay reported similar results, with 1.7% of 994 specimens positive for orthopoxvirus immunoglobulin M in the Likouala region of the DRC (82).

In Africa, just over 400 cases of monkeypox were diagnosed between 1970 and 1986, the great majority in parts of Zaire where intensive surveillance supported by the WHO was in operation from 1980 to 1986. The case fatality rate was about 10%. Person-to-person transmission was uncommon and accounted for about 30% of the observed cases in the Zaire survey. Additional outbreaks were reported in the DRC between 1996 and 1998, but there were concurrent outbreaks of chickenpox and investigations were hampered by an ongoing civil war (64). In a review by the WHO in 1999, however, it was estimated that about half of the 800 suspected cases in the Kasai Oriental for which onset was reported between February 1996 and July 1998 were monkeypox (143). Cases appeared to be no more severe than in the 1980s, but the numbers of index cases and the proportion of secondary cases have increased in recent years (109).

In 2003 in the Midwest of the United States, an MPXV outbreak occurred in prairie dogs housed in proximity to MPXV-infected African rodents; the prairie dogs acted as an amplifying host for the documented human infections. A majority of the infections (19 of 34, 56%) occurred after close contact with MPXV-infected prairie dogs (63), but a significant number of cases appeared to result from indirect exposure to the virus through fomites or aerosols.

The incidence of other orthopoxvirus infections is far less than that of human monkeypox, with ~54 cases of cowpox reported in Europe from 1969 to 1993 (5). Cowpox has been known in Europe for hundreds of years as a disease of cows, manifesting as ulcers on the teats (40). Occasionally, contact with such lesions produced pustular lesions on the hands of milkers. The cow is an accidental and occasional host of CPXV, but cows, cats, and zoo animals can be infected from a rodent reservoir host. Humans may be infected by contact with a wildlife source or with accidentally infected animals of several species, especially domestic cats (Fig. 3).

Natural infections with VACV result from epizootics based on virus reservoirs in buffalo and cattle. Buffalopox virus has persisted in India since the cessation of human vaccination (99) and is characterized by pustular lesions on the teats and udders of milking buffaloes; occasionally a generalized disease is seen, especially in calves. Sometimes humans in contact with diseased buffaloes are infected (Fig. 3); thus, lesions may occur on the hands and face of milkers. Most strains have restriction maps somewhat different from those of the VACV strains used in India in the days of smallpox vaccination (34). In Brazil, a strain of VACV maintained in cattle is similarly causing zoonotic infections (28).

Human infections with parapoxviruses are an occupational hazard. ORFV, PCPV, and BPSV cause the so-called "barnyard" poxvirus infections, with ORFV infections being the most common. The papules and vesicles on the skin of the lips (scabby mouth) and sometimes around the nostrils and eyes of infected animals serve as a source for human infection. Persistence of the virus in flocks is due in large part to the persistent infectivity of virions in scabs that fall on pasture plants or the soil.

TANV infects both sexes and all age groups and occurs most frequently among persons who work or play close to the Tana River (68). There has been one case of human-to-human transmission reported in the United States (52). The same virus, described variously as Yaba-like disease virus, Yaba-related disease virus, and Oregon "1211" poxvirus, gave rise to epizootics in macaque monkeys in three primate centers in the United States in 1966, in which some of the animal handlers were infected (90). YMTV was first recovered from subcutaneous tumors that occurred in a colony of rhesus (Asian) monkeys in Nigeria (103). Infections of humans with YMTV have not been found in the field in Africa.

Molluscum contagiosum is endemic throughout the world to various degrees. There are four subtypes (101), but although the subtype restriction patterns differ considerably, cross-hybridization revealed that all had similar nucleotide sequences. All subtypes produce similar clinical disease. In the United States, 98% of cases are caused by MCV genotype 1 (13). Molluscum contagiosum is very common in Fiji, where 4.5% of a village population bore lesions (113), and in Papua New Guinea (130). A study

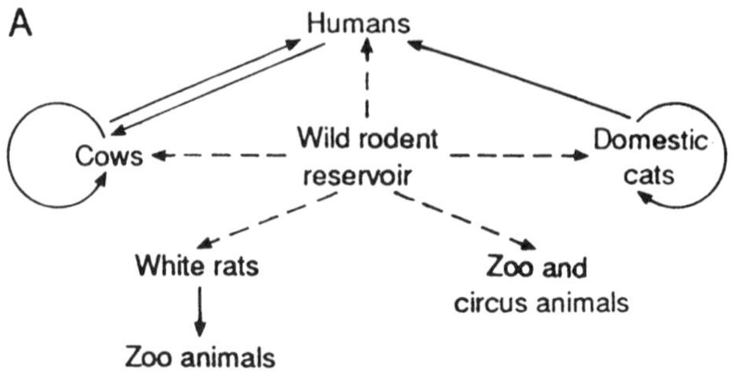

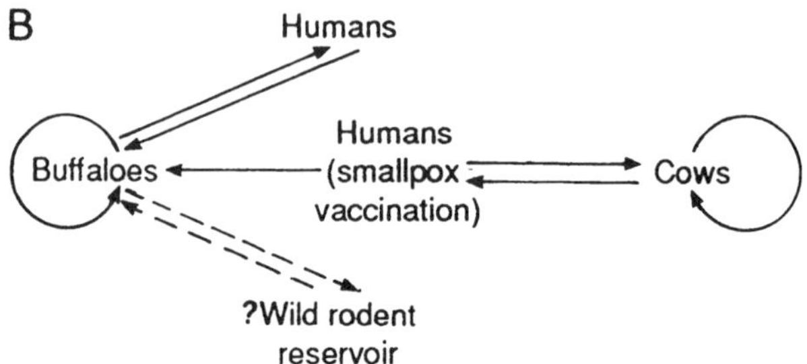

FIGURE 3 Diagram illustrating the epidemiology of cowpox and buffalopox. Solid lines represent known paths of transmission; broken lines represent presumed or possible paths of transmission. (A) Identified wild-rodent reservoir hosts of cowpox include bank voles, wood mice, and short-tailed voles in Great Britain and probably elsewhere in Europe, lemmings in Norway, and susliks and gerbils in Turkmenistan. The traditional liaison hosts from which humans were infected were cows, but currently the most common liaison hosts are domestic cats. White rats, the source of disastrous outbreaks in animals in the Moscow Zoo in 1973 and 1974 (88), probably acquired infection from wild-rodent-contaminated straw or other bedding material. (B) In India, Egypt, and Indonesia, in the days of smallpox vaccination, buffaloes were sometimes infected with vaccinia virus from recently vaccinated humans, causing what was called buffalopox. Buffalopox seems to have disappeared in Indonesia and Egypt but is still a problem in several states of India. Since the cessation of vaccination, infected buffaloes constitute a source of infection of humans. It is possible that the virus can be maintained by serial transmission in buffaloes, but on the analogy of cowpox in Europe, it is possible that there is an unknown rodent reservoir. (Reprinted from reference 140 with permission.)

in The Netherlands found the cumulative incidence of childhood molluscum contagiosum to be about 17% in persons 15 years of age (30). In Australia, 357 sera from a representative cross-section of the population showed a seroprevalence of 23% (30).

Age-Specific Attack Rates

Information on age-specific attack rates of unvaccinated contacts is available for smallpox, monkeypox, and molluscum contagiosum. For smallpox and monkeypox, the contacts <15 years of age showed the greatest risk of infection; this probably reflects the intimacy of physical contact, which is highest among the youngest siblings in a family, which proved to be the most important focus for person-to-person transmission. For monkeypox in Africa, the primary attack rate reflects the probability of developing the disease after exposure to an animal source. For molluscum contagiosum, studies in New Guinea, Japan, The Netherlands, and the United States found the peak incidence to be in individuals <10 years of age (30).

Risk Factors and High-Risk Groups

Persons of all ages were susceptible to VARV, but the mortality rates were highest in the very young, the elderly, pregnant women, and immunosuppressed individuals. A similar pattern is likely to exist for monkeypox.

Severely immunosuppressed patients have more severe disease with all poxvirus infections, and this has been documented for MCV (123) and ORFV (50). Individuals with atopic dermatitis are probably predisposed to poxvirus diseases of greater severity, especially at the sites of dermatitis. This has been documented for infections with VACV, ORFV, and MCV (7, 30, 35). In the case of molluscum contagiosum, 24% of patients were diagnosed with atopic dermatitis (30). At least two fatal case of cowpox have been documented for persons suffering from atopic dermatitis (122).

Other factors were also involved depending on the poxvirus. Observed sex differences in smallpox and monkeypox are more likely attributed to factors that differ in importance in different studies but do not represent an intrinsic infection susceptibility or disease severity difference based on sex. For example, although female and male household contacts of monkeypox patients had a 4.2 and 3.3% risk of acquiring the disease, this difference was likely due to the close contact between the patient and the female relatives, who most often provided the care. The lack of vaccination immunity is by far the most important risk factor for severe disease in smallpox and monkeypox. The risk of human cowpox increases with ownership of a cat that has access to infected rodent populations. The risk of parapoxvirus infection is occupational.

Reinfections

Recovery from VARV, MPXV, and VACV yields long-lived to lifelong protection from severe disease following reinfection, whereas the generated immunity to CPXV is shorter-lived or is unable to block reinfection with CPXV (66). Reinfection with MCV or further spread of the virus to other areas of an infected individual can be common.

Seasonality

In the tropics, smallpox was most prevalent in the cool, dry season. Monkeypox in Africa shows no clear evidence of a seasonal pattern (67).

Transmission

Routes

Human poxvirus infections can be acquired through multiple routes. VARV was spread by the respiratory route, usually requiring close (household) contact. MPXV infection from the zoonotic host probably occurs through puncture wounds or microbreaks in the skin. MPXV human-to-human transmission is likely to occur via the respiratory route. CPXV and parapoxvirus infections are a consequence of the introduction of virus either directly or indirectly into breaks in the skin. MCV is spread by fomites or close contact among children and is sexually transmitted among adults.

Risk of Infection after Specific Exposures

The risk of MPXV infection may be considered multifactorial. Primary MPXV infection is associated with adult male activities such as hunting and carcass preparation, whereas female caregivers are more at risk for human-to-human infections. In general, Africans may be more susceptible to severe disease due to poor nutrition or coinfections with other pathogens. Two reports have documented coinfections of MPXV and varicella-zoster virus, with one fatal outcome (64, 93). It is known that AIDS increases the morbidity and mortality of humans when they are concurrently infected with *Mycobacterium tuberculosis* (92, 126), and a similar effect would be expected following coinfection with MPXV.

Parapoxvirus infections occur through occupational exposure. For example, marine mammal technicians are at risk for sealpox through bites from seals or sea lions (24).

Sexual activity is a risk factor for molluscum contagiosum in adults. Genital molluscum has become a much more common infection in the last two decades and can be an epidemiological marker for sexually transmitted diseases. The disease can be a troublesome complication of AIDS in western countries, especially in homosexual men (6).

Nosocomial Infection

VARV and MPXV, which can be transmitted by respiratory droplets, can cause nosocomial infections. In 1970, a smallpox patient maintained in an isolation ward in a general hospital in Meschede, Germany, infected 17 contacts at a distance in the hospital (139). In 2003, extended interhuman transmission of MPXV was documented in a community hospital in the DRC (81).

Duration of Infectiousness

The ability of human poxvirus infections to transmit infectious virus is dependent on the generation of a lesion in the cornified or mucosal epithelium that ulcerates, releasing virus into the environment. For VACV, CPXV, parapoxviruses, and MCV, the lesions are usually in the cornified epithelium and are likely infectious until scab formation or reabsorption. For smallpox and probably monkeypox acquired from human index cases, the mucosal lesions of the respiratory tract are a greater source of infectious virus than lesions of the cornified skin and are more important in the natural life cycle of the virus. A number of studies have measured VARV in oropharyngeal secretions of smallpox patients, and virus is detected 2 to 4 days following the onset of fever and reaches the highest level on the third and fourth days of disease (i.e., just after rash appearance). As one might expect, the level of virus was greatest and persisted the longest in cases that had confluent ordinary-type (lesions on face or extremities are confluent) or flat-type smallpox. High levels of virus in secretions correlated with infectiousness of the patient, a period that usually lasted for the first week of the rash.

PATHOGENESIS IN HUMANS

Incubation Period

The incubation period for human poxvirus infections has been thoroughly documented only for smallpox, for which it was 10 to 14 days (41). A limited number of case studies of human-to-human transmission of MPXV suggest a similar incubation period (67).

Patterns of Virus Replication and Spread

Our understanding of the pathogenesis of smallpox is based on studies on animal systems: ectromelia virus in mice (37, 38; Fig. 4) and MPXV in monkeys (23). Based on these models and observations on the epidemiology of smallpox, infection with VARV usually occurred by the inhalation of virus released from lesions in the oropharynx into the oropharyngeal secretions during the first week of the rash in the index case. After infection of cells in the upper or lower respiratory tract of contacts, macrophages became infected and entered the lymphatics. Infected white blood cells sometimes entered the bloodstream at this stage, or in any case by about the fourth day. Lymphoid tissue and internal organs were infected following this primary viremia. The initial stages of infection produced neither symptoms nor a local lesion, and patients were not infectious during the incubation period. By analogy to animal models, ~8 to 10 days following infection, cell-associated virus produced from infected internal organs (secondary viremia) localized in small vessels of the dermis and led to infection of the underlying dermis of the mucosal and cornified epithelium. The rash was detected ~10 days after infection, evolved through a number of distinct stages, and resolved with scab separation ~32 days following infection. Virus was difficult to detect in blood from cases of ordinary-type smallpox at all times during disease; however, this was not the case with hemorrhagic-type smallpox, in which high titers were readily detectable in blood of all cases. The outcome of the infection was either death, which was said to be usually due to "toxemia," or recovery, with complete elimination of the virus but sometimes with sequelae. The most common sequelae were pockmarks, which could occur all over the body but were usually most profuse on the face (9). Blindness was an important but rare complication. Recovery was accompanied by prolonged immunity to reinfection.

The pathogenesis of monkeypox probably follows at least two distinct courses dependent on the route of inoculation. Inhalation of MPXV, which is likely the mechanism of infection between an index case and contacts, is likely very similar or identical to that of the smallpox virus. Infections from an animal source may occur through additional routes of exposure via puncture wounds or small lesions on the skin or the oropharynx. Infections through the skin likely have a distinct pattern of pathogenesis compared to that following a respiratory infection. This supposition is based on the fact that the smallpox case fatality rate was 20 to 30% following inhalation but was dramatically lower, at 0.5 to 2%, if virus was introduced into the cornified epithelium (variolation; see below).

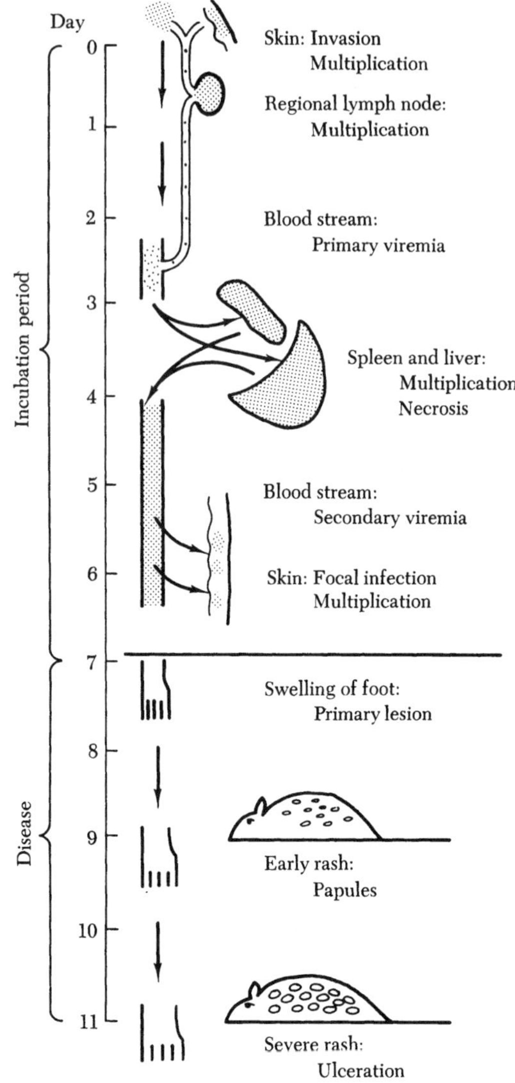

FIGURE 4 Diagrammatic representation of the mode of spread of ectromelia virus through the body in mousepox. (Reprinted from reference 38 with permission.)

Except for VARV and MPXV, poxvirus infections of humans are most often through the cornified epithelium. The introduction of CPXV, VACV, or parapoxviruses into the skin causes localized distinct pustular lesions at the site of introduction that have species-specific distinctions. In immunocompetent individuals, systemic infections occur at a low frequency following VACV infection (Table 2, generalized vaccinia) and are extremely rare for CPXV or other human zoonotic poxvirus infections. The primary lesions heal over in 3 to 6 weeks following infection.

Factors in Disease Production

Characteristic Histopathological Changes

The secondary skin lesion of smallpox develops through a series of characteristic stages that presumably begin with a virus-infected cell entering into the dermis through dia-

TABLE 2 Complications of smallpox vaccination in the United States in 1968

Status and age	No. of vaccinations	Complication rate (cases per million)				
		Postvaccinial encephalitis	Progressive vaccinia	Eczema vaccinatum	Generalized vaccinia	Other[a]
National survey[b]						
Primary vaccination						
<1 yr	614,000	6.5	0	8.1	70.0	27.7
1–4 yr	2,733,000	2.2	0.4	11.3	17.2	47.9
>5 yr	2,247,000	2.7	1.8	9.3	16.9	23.6
Revaccination						
<1 yr	0					
1–4 yr	478,000	0	0	2.1	0	4.2
>4 yr	8,096,000	0	0.7	0.9	1.2	1.7
Ten-state survey[c]						
Primary vaccination						
<1 yr	71,000	42	0	14	394	1,099
1–4 yr	317,000	9.5	3.2	44	233	972
>4 yr	262,000	7.6	0	34	149	748
Revaccination						
<1 yr	0					
1–4 yr	55,000	0	0	0	0	200
>4 yr	943,000	2.1	3.2	3.2	9.5	81

[a] Includes accidental infection, erythema multiforme, bacterial infections, and severe "normal" reactions requiring medical care.
[b] Data from reference 79.
[c] Data from reference 80.

pedesis, which is followed by local replication. The focus of infection becomes mildly inflamed due to the local release of cytokines and chemokines, which attract circulating inflammatory cells. Virus replication spreads from the dermis into the epidermis. Cells in the epidermis become swollen and vacuolated and stain for the characteristic B-type (Guarnieri) inclusion bodies. The rupturing cells contribute to early vesicle formation. Lesions evolve from macules to papules and into pustules through the migration of polymorphonuclear leukocytes from the subpapillary vessels into the epidermal lesion. The pustule umbilicates, and with the development of an effective immune response, the healing process commences and results in regeneration of the epidermis and the start of scab formation at ~16 days postinfection.

The evolution of the rash in monkeypox in central Africa is similar to that of smallpox. The rash is most severe on the extremities, and the lesions evolve as a group. This is in contrast to the disease observed in the 2003 U.S. outbreak, in which distinct differences were noted in the morphology, evolution, and absolute numbers of skin lesions. In the U.S. outbreak the lesion morphology varied from case to case and even within a family, and the lesions healed with a distinctive and prominent hemorrhagic crust (85).

The earliest histologic changes observed in VACV lesions following vaccination were cytoplasmic and perinuclear vacuolation in the epithelium, which were accompanied by coagulation necrosis, intercellular edema, and vesicle formation (41). By 48 h postvaccination, a cup-shaped vesicle traversed by an eosinophilic reticular network had appeared with the roof and floor formed by the stratum corneum and dermis, respectively. The region was characterized by edema, free erythrocytes, and a progressive infiltration of mononuclear and polymorphonuclear cells, which with time formed a dense, homogeneous, deeply staining reticulum that formed the crust beneath which epithelial outgrowth occurred.

In contrast to lesions of smallpox and monkeypox, parapoxvirus lesions are markedly proliferative (76). Changes that occur early in the proliferating keratinocytes include nucleolar enlargement and focal lysis of keratin fibrils. Extreme swelling of the cells results in ballooning degeneration which, when accompanied by B-type cytoplasmic inclusion bodies and nuclear shrinkage, is pathognomonic of ORFV lesions. Dermal infiltration with monocytes and lymphoid cells is prominent around hyperemic capillaries and venules, and infection of the endothelial cells may produce endothelial proliferation.

Tanapox lesions histologically show some typical features of an orthopoxvirus skin lesion, i.e., marked thickening of the epidermis with extensive ballooning degeneration of the prickle cell layer. The cytoplasm of swollen epidermal cells is filled with large, pleomorphic, granular, eosinophilic, B-type inclusion bodies. YMTV produces tumors in monkeys and humans after subcutaneous or intradermal inoculation. These are composed of masses of histiocytes which are later infiltrated with lymphocytes and polymorphonuclear cells. No true neoplastic proliferation occurs, and the lesions regress as the immune response develops (128).

The typical molluscum contagiosum lesion consists of a localized mass of hypertrophied and hyperplastic epidermis extending down into the underlying dermis and projecting above the adjacent skin as a visible tumor. Each infected keratinocyte is many times larger than normal, and the cytoplasm is filled with a large hyaline acidophilic granular mass known as the molluscum body (Fig. 5), which pushes the nucleus to the edge of the cell. The core of the lesion consists of degenerating epidermal cells with inclusion bodies and keratin, which uninfected cells continue to produce. Unlike with orthopoxvirus lesions, there is no vesicle

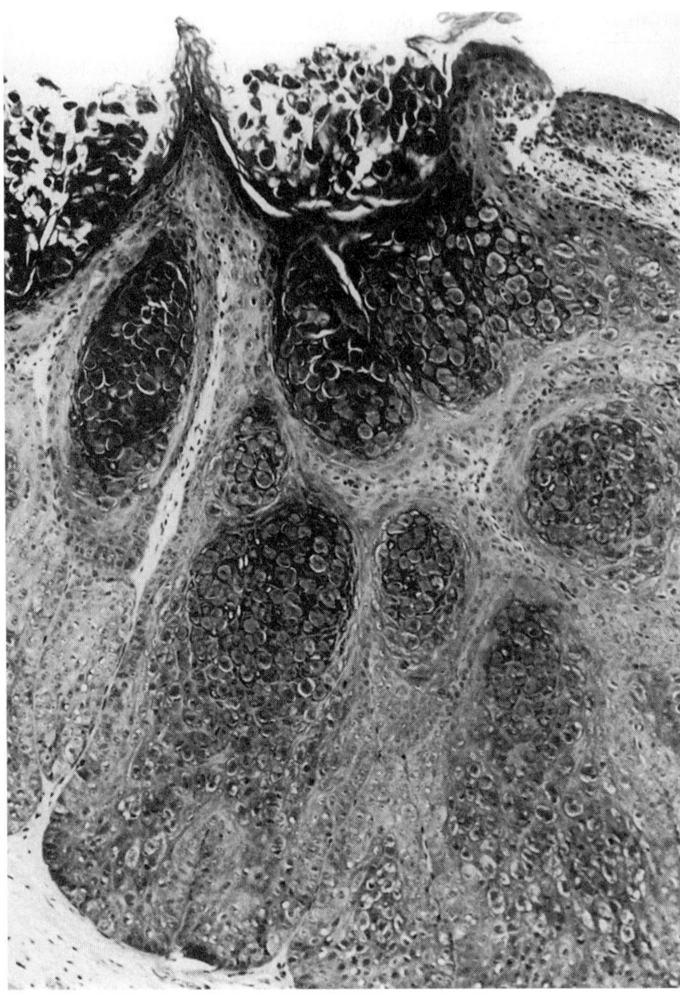

FIGURE 5 Section of a skin lesion of molluscum contagiosum. (Courtesy of D. Lowy.)

formation or inflammatory reaction unless secondary bacterial infection has occurred. The lack of inflammation is due to the restricted replication of the virus to the keratinocyte of the epidermis, the release of little antigenic material or virus from infected cells, and the expression of immunosuppressive proteins (97).

Immune Responses

Innate Responses

Innate responses have not been studied in human poxvirus infections but can be inferred from our knowledge of experimental mousepox (37). Infection with necrosis initiates a cascade of cytokines and chemokines and cellular activation. The cascade is further amplified by the autocrine and paracrine proinflammatory activities of the resident and infiltrating cells (monocytes, granulocytes, and natural killer cells) as well as the vascular endothelial cells. In MCV this process is absent or transient in nature.

Adaptive Immunity

The adaptive response is characterized by the production of cytotoxic and cytokine-secreting T cells and antibody-secreting B cells. The cytotoxic T cells kill cells prior to the completion of the virus replication cycle by recognizing viral peptides in the context of antigens from the HLA complex. In animal models the humoral response plays a major role along with T cells in recovery from primary infection and is critical for protection from reinfection (20, 107). The most important targets of neutralizing antibodies are unique proteins found on the surface of mature virus and extracellular enveloped virus (43).

Infections with VARV, CPXV, and VACV produce strong long-term immunity. MCV, however, provokes little immunity, and in individual patients the lesions may persist for as little as 2 weeks or as long as 2 years, without any sign of inflammation. Reinfections are relatively common (105). The lesions are noteworthy for the absence of reactive cells, and virus-specific antibodies are demonstrable in only about 70% of patients (124).

Correlates of Immune Protection

The presence of scars from VARV, MPXV, or VACV lesions is considered a correlate of immune protection.

Correlates of Disease Resolution

In human poxvirus infections, scab separation of the last active lesion indicates disease resolution. In smallpox, this separation occurred at ~32 days following infection.

CLINICAL MANIFESTATIONS

Major Clinical Syndromes

There were two clinical types of smallpox caused by two viral variants, variola major and variola minor (alastrim) (41). Variola major had a case fatality rate of 20 to 30% in unvaccinated persons, and variola minor had a case fatality rate of about 1%. The onset was acute, with fever, malaise, headache, and backache. Three or four days after the onset of symptoms the characteristic rash appeared, first on the buccal and pharyngeal mucosa and then on the face, forearms, and hands. The lesions began as macules which soon became firm papules and then vesicles which quickly became opaque and pustular. About 8 or 9 days after the onset, the pustules became umbilicated and dried up. The distribution of the rash, as well as its evolution, was highly characteristic, being usually most profuse on the face and more abundant on the forearms than the upper arms and the lower legs than the thighs, and relatively sparse on the trunk, especially the abdomen (Fig. 6, left panel).

The clinical features of monkeypox are indistinguishable from those of ordinary-type smallpox, except that enlargement of cervical and often the inguinal lymph nodes is much more pronounced than in smallpox (Fig. 6, middle and right panels). Although like smallpox, monkeypox is clinically distinct from chickenpox, misdiagnosis of monkeypox for chickenpox and chickenpox for monkeypox is quite common (69).

Recent studies have determined that there are at least two distinctive clades of MPXV, one found in West Africa and the other in central Africa (21, 85). Epidemiological studies and studies of representative viruses in nonhuman primates suggest that the West African isolates are less virulent than those from central Africa. The lesion character in the 2003 U.S. outbreak was distinct from that of classic African monkeypox, and infected patients had, on average, fewer lesions (85). Patients also presented with a broad range of nonspecific signs and symptoms, with and without rash (56, 63). Interestingly, no deaths were reported, perhaps due to the fact that the virus was the less virulent West African strain (116).

CPXV lesions are often found on the thumbs, the first interdigital cleft, and the forefinger. The lesions are quite distinctive (Fig. 7A and B); CPXV causes pustular lesions like those of VACV, and the parapoxviruses produce nonulcerating nodules. The CPXV lesions pass through stages of vesicle and pustule before a deep-seated, hard black eschar forms 2 weeks later. Cowpox was traditionally associated with the milking of cows, but many cases involve no such history, and domestic cats now constitute a more important source of human infection.

Figure 8 shows a primary response to VACV vaccination. VACV infection via vaccination caused a papule to appear at the vaccination site 4 to 5 days after vaccination; 2 to 3 days later, this became vesicular and constituted the umbilicated and multilocular "Jennerian vesicle." The contents rapidly became turbid because of the infiltration of inflammatory cells, and the central lesion was surrounded by erythema and induration, which reached their maximum diameter on the 9th or 10th day. At this time the draining lymph nodes in the axilla were enlarged and tender, and many patients had a mild fever. The pustule dried from the center outward, and the brown scab fell off

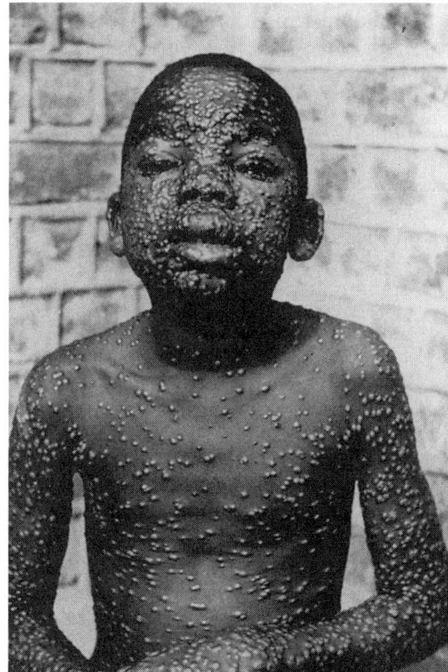
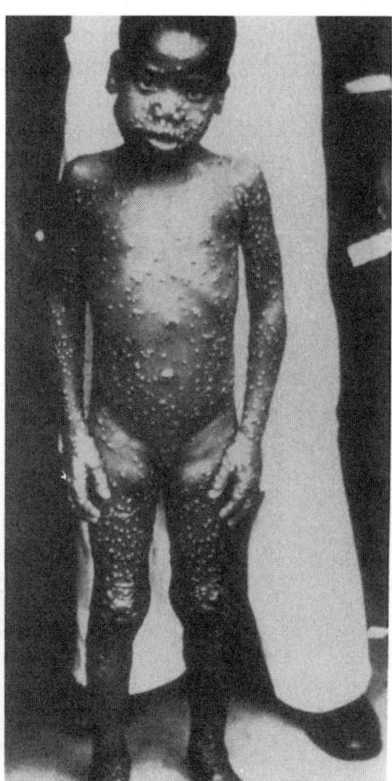
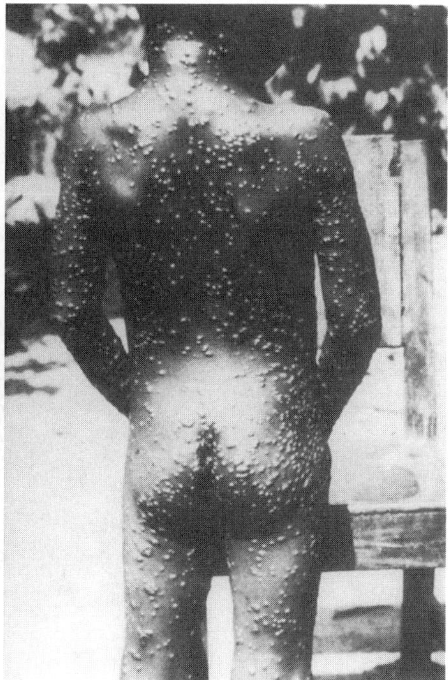

FIGURE 6 Clinical features of smallpox and monkeypox. (Left) The rash of smallpox in a boy in Zaire. (Middle and right) Front and rear views of a 7-year-old girl from Zaire with monkeypox, on the eighth day after the appearance of the rash. Note the enlargement of the cervical and inguinal lymph nodes, a feature not seen in smallpox. (Middle and right panels reprinted from reference 11 with permission.)

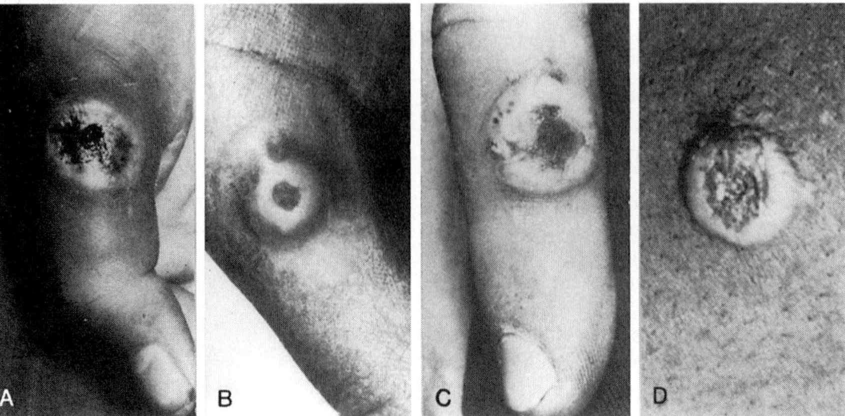

FIGURE 7 Localized zoonotic infections with poxviruses. (A and B) Lesions on hands acquired by milking infected cows: cowpox, caused by an orthopoxvirus (A), and milker's nodes, caused by a parapoxvirus, PCPV (B). (C) Parapoxvirus lesion of ORFV, acquired by handling sheep or goats suffering from contagious pustular dermatitis. (D) Lesion of tanapox on an arm of a child in the DRC. The virus was transmitted mechanically by mosquitoes from an animal reservoir host. (Panels A and B courtesy of D. Baxby; panel C courtesy of J. Nagington; panel D courtesy of Z. Jezek.)

after about 3 weeks, leaving a scar by which previous vaccination could be recognized for many years.

Parapoxvirus infections are occupational diseases. Orf and milker's nodules are acquired by contact with infected sheep and cows, respectively. The infection occurs through abrasions of the skin, and localized lesions are usually found on the hands. The lesions of orf are rather large nodules that may be multiple, and the surrounding skin is inflamed (Fig. 7C). There may be a low fever and swelling of the draining lymph nodes; the local lesion is rather painful. The lesions of milker's nodule (Fig. 7B) are hemispherical, highly vascular papules which appear 5 to 7 days after exposure and gradually enlarge into purple, hemispherical nodules up to 2 cm in diameter. They are relatively painless but may itch, but they do not ulcerate. The granulation tissue that makes up the mass of the nodule gradually becomes absorbed, and the lesions disappear after 4 to 6 weeks. The only evidence of systemic infection is occasional slight swelling of the draining lymph nodes. Human infections with BPSV are less common than with the other two parapoxviruses that infect humans, probably because contact between animal handlers and lesions of BPSV are less common than those of shearers with orf and milkers with milker's nodules (17, 18). The BPSV lesions appear as circumscribed wart-like nodules that gradually enlarge until they are 3 to 8 mm in diameter.

The first symptoms following a TANV infection are a mild preeruptive fever, sometimes accompanied by severe headache, backache, and myalgia, often with itching at the site where the skin lesion develops (29, 32, 68). Two to four days following onset of fever, a usually solitary erythematous macule appears on the skin. Initially there is a small nodule, which soon becomes papular and reaches a maximum diameter of about 15 mm by the end of the second week. The appearance of the skin lesion of tanapox is illustrated in Fig. 7D. The nodule is surrounded by an

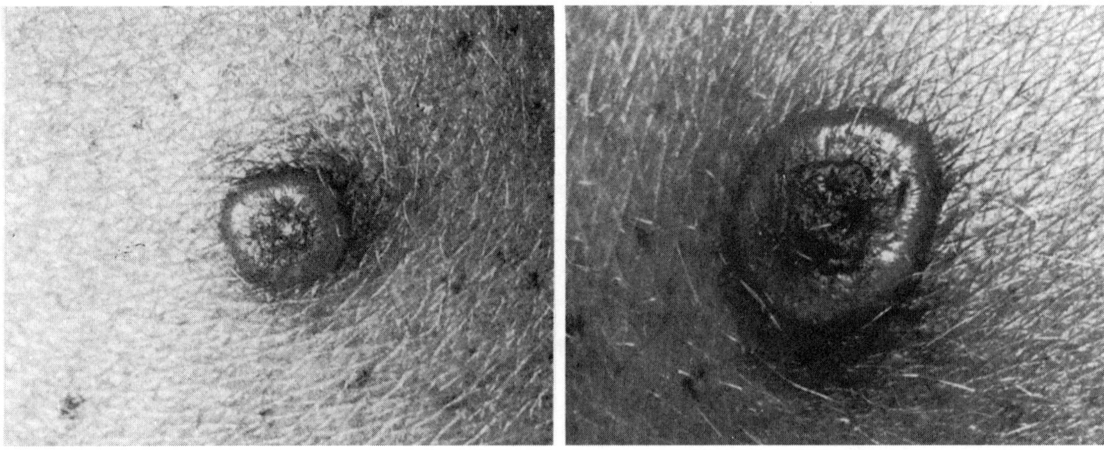

FIGURE 8 Primary response to vaccination; typical vesiculo-pustular response, maximal at 8 to 11 days. (Left) Response at 7 days; (right) response at 11 days. (Courtesy of J. R. L. Forsyth.)

edematous zone and a large erythematous areola. The draining lymph nodes are enlarged and tender from about the fifth day. The skin lesion usually ulcerates during the third week and then gradually heals within 5 to 6 weeks, leaving a scar. In Kenya, the lesions were almost always solitary and on the upper arm, face, neck, and trunk (33), but in the DRC, 22% of patients had multiple lesions (68). YMTV produces large protuberant tumors in monkeys, which are histiocytomas in which poxvirus particles can be seen by electron microscopy (120, 128). Rarely, similar lesions may be produced in humans by accidental contact with infected monkeys or after inoculation.

Molluscum contagiosum is characterized by multiple, small, noninflamed lumps in the skin scattered over the body or, in adults, usually in the genital or anal region (Fig. 9A) (13). The lesions of molluscum contagiosum are pearly, flesh-colored, raised, umbilicated nodules in the epidermal layer of the skin, usually 2 to 5 mm in diameter. Rarely, lesions will present as a large lesion called giant molluscum (>5 mm in diameter). The incubation period varies from 14 to 50 days. The nodules are painless, and at the top of each there is often an opening through which a small white core can be seen (Fig. 9B). The lesions often persist for months but ultimately resolve spontaneously or following trauma or bacterial infection.

Prodrome

In the case of smallpox or classic monkeypox, a spiking fever, malaise, and possibly headache were followed by the development of a rash (41, 67). In the case of cowpox, fever and myalgia can also be associated with the prodrome, but with less severity compared to that of smallpox and monkeypox. In the first 6 days following vaccination with VACV (Dryvax), fever, headache, muscle aches, chills, nausea, and fatigue were reported in 3, 44, 39, 13.5, 19, and 53% of 665 subjects, respectively (46). In tanapox the first signs of infection were mild fever, headache, and myalgia. There were few, if any, signs or symptoms of MCV and the parapoxvirus (except occasional fever) infections prior to development of the primary lesion.

Age-Related Differences

In smallpox and monkeypox the young were more likely to be infected than the old, and the disease was most severe in the young and old. The exception was the 2003 U.S. monkeypox outbreak, in which the majority of the cases were in adults (63); however, the pediatric patients were more likely to be hospitalized in an intensive care unit. Cowpox in children was usually more severe than the usual response to vaccination (5, 19).

Complications

Three other clinical types of smallpox were recognized. The rare hemorrhagic-type smallpox, most common in pregnant women, was associated with petechiae in the skin and bleeding from the conjunctiva and mucous membranes, very severe toxemia, and early death. Flat-type smallpox was characterized by intense toxemia and slow evolution of the skin lesions, which were usually flat and soft; most such cases were fatal. Modified-type smallpox was seen in persons who had been vaccinated, usually many years earlier; the disease was mild and the skin lesions evolved quickly and were often sparse.

Smallpox immunizations with VACV result in occasional serious complications (Fig. 10; Table 2) (49, 79, 80). Vaccination against smallpox is undoubtedly associated with a worse reaction and more and worse complications than any other of the commonly used vaccines (141). Progressive vaccinia (Fig. 10B) occurs only in persons with deficiencies of the cell-mediated immune system. Vaccinated subjects with agammaglobulinemia but a normal cell-mediated response recovered normally (45, 47). Eczema vaccinatum (Fig. 10A) occurs only in persons who suffered from eczema. Generalized vaccinia comprises a generalized vaccinial rash, sometimes covering the whole body (Fig. 10C), occurring 6 to 9 days after vaccination.

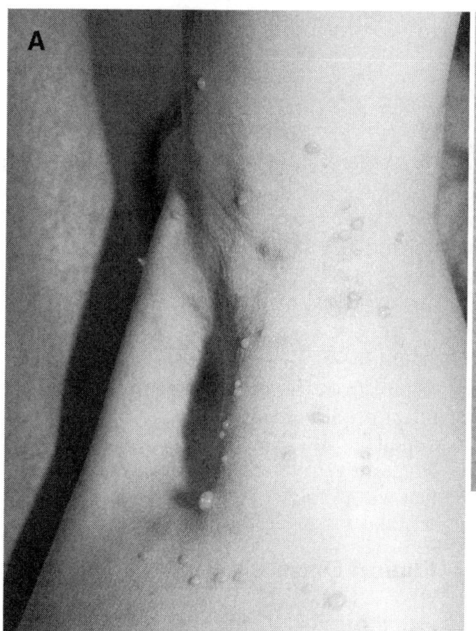

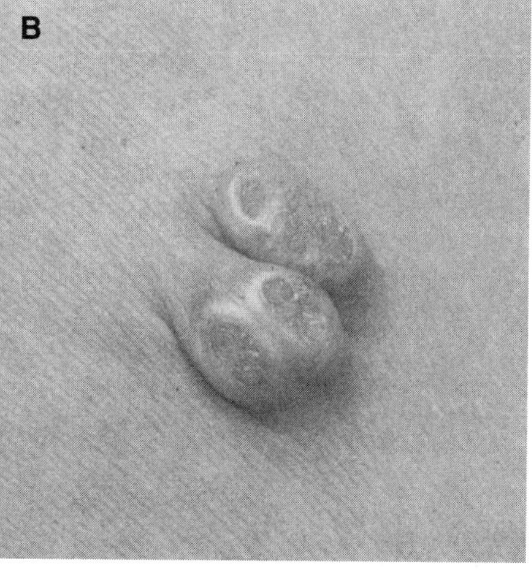

FIGURE 9 Molluscum contagiosum lesions. (Courtesy of E. C. Siegfried.)

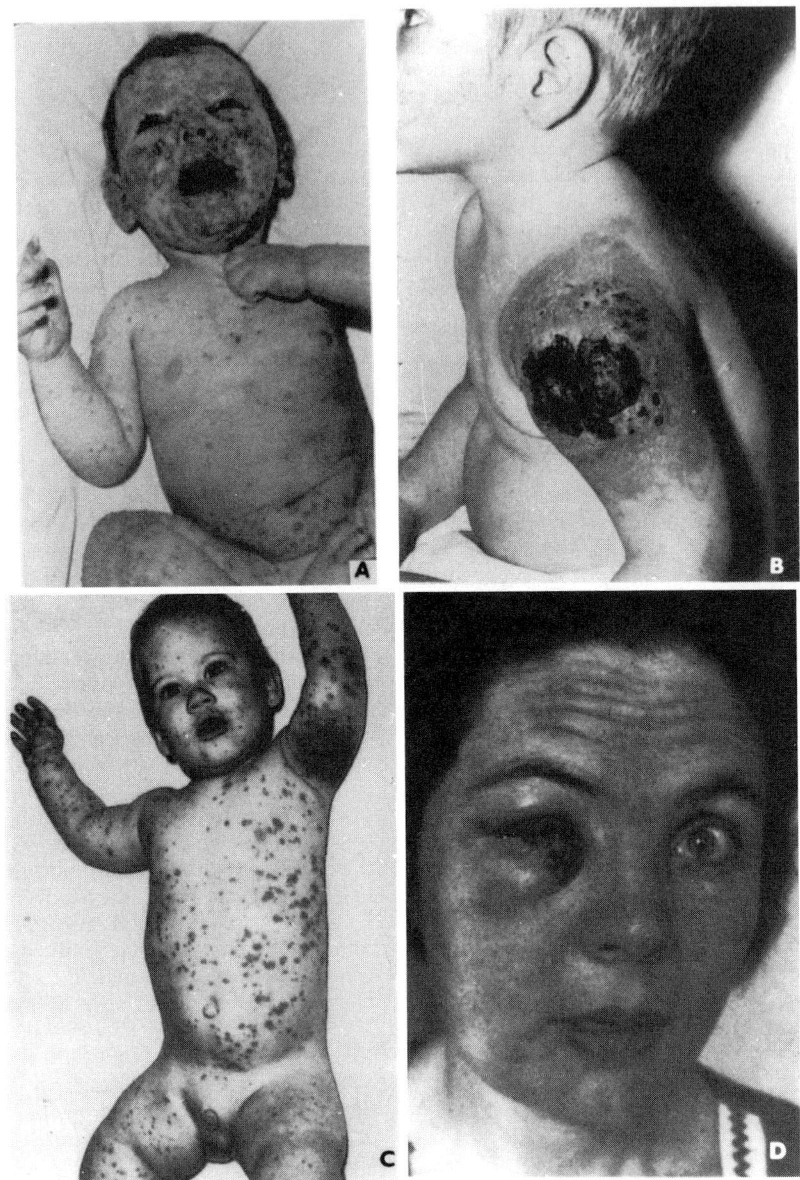

FIGURE 10 Severe complications of vaccination. (A) Eczema vaccinatum in an unvaccinated sibling of a vaccinated individual. (B) Progressive vaccinia (vaccinia gangrenosum), which was fatal in a child with a congenital defect in cell-mediated immunity. (C) Generalized vaccinia, 10 days after primary vaccination; benign course, no scarring. (D) Ocular vaccinia after autoinoculation. (Reprinted from reference 41 with permission.)

It is not associated with immunodeficiency, and the prognosis is good. Postvaccinial encephalitis is an unpredictable complication (70). In children less than 2 years old there is very occasionally a general encephalopathy associated with demonstrable viremia that occurs 6 to 10 days after immunization and is characterized often by convulsion, hemiplegia, and aphasia (127). In subjects over 2 years of age the complication occurs ~11 to 15 days after immunization. The onset of disease is marked by fever, vomiting, and other symptoms of cerebral involvement. The pathological findings resemble those of other postinfectious encephalitides, and the case fatality rate is ~45% (70). Perivenular inflammation and demyelination are the principal lesions. Accidental infection of some part of the body distant from the inoculation site is the most common complication. Over the period from 1963 to 1968, ocular vaccinia (Fig. 10D) was found to have occurred in 348 persons (including 259 vaccinees and 66 contacts) (121). The cornea was involved in 22 of these cases, and 11 persons had residual visual defects.

Clinical Diagnosis

When smallpox was endemic, the diagnosis of most cases could be made easily from the distribution and evolution of the rash. Where their occurrence was not expected, modified-type variola major and variola minor were often confused with chickenpox, but the evolution and distribution of the rash in the two diseases were usually distinctive. In smallpox, lesions developed simultaneously all over the body, most obviously on the face and limbs rather than the trunk, whereas in chickenpox, the skin lesions were more superficial and appeared in "crops," more apparent on the trunk than on the face and extremities.

The diagnosis of zoonotic poxvirus infections facilitated by the geographic location and epidemiological features of cases can be of help in the differential diagnosis, unless the disease appears in a nonenzootic region, as in the case of importation of MPXV into the United States in 2003. Like smallpox, monkeypox can be misdiagnosed as chickenpox. Poxvirus infections acquired from contact with cows must be differentiated from among CPXV, PCPV, and BPSV. If the infection is acquired from sheep, it is likely ORFV. Tanapox is known to occur in animal attendants in contact with monkeys infected with TANV or YMTV or wild animals in regions of Africa where these viruses are endemic.

A problem of diagnosis of a VACV infection arises only in subjects infected by contact with a vaccinee. The history of contact with a recently vaccinated person or with a laboratory source of VACV, or with a buffalo with buffalopox or cattle infected with cantagalo virus, should arouse suspicion; the diagnosis can be confirmed by recovery and characterization of the virus.

Molluscum contagiosum is endemic in most human populations. The diagnosis can be made clinically from the appearance of the lesions and their chronic nature. Occasionally, solitary lesions on the face or neck may be misdiagnosed as basal cell carcinoma. Cutaneous cryptococcosis can mimic molluscum lesions in patients with AIDS.

LABORATORY DIAGNOSIS

The major diagnostic criteria for poxvirus infections are the size and morphology of the poxvirus virion in negatively stained preparations viewed with an electron microscope (Fig. 1). This approach is giving way to PCR.

Virus Isolation

Optimal Specimen Types

Specimens are usually fluid from primary or secondary vesicles or scabs, all of which contain sufficient viral material to be used for PCR identification.

Cell Culture

Historically, species diagnosis was made by observation of the characteristic pocks on the chorioallantoic membrane of the developing chicken embryo. In combination with growth ceiling temperature, the careful diagnostic technician could use the observation of pocks to differentiate CPXV, VACV, MPXV, and VARV. More recently, tissue culture in combination with antigen staining has been used as a confirmatory assay for electron microscopy. Orthopoxviruses produce cytopathic effect in Vero cells. Parapoxviruses from human lesions grow in primary bovine or ovine embryo kidney or testis cells or primary human amnion cells. Once isolated, they grow well in human embryonic fibroblasts and LLC-MK2 cells. Yatapoxviruses grow in human thyroid cells; vervet monkey and patas monkey kidney cells; and WI-38, HEp-2, and Vero cells, producing focal lesions characterized by intense granularity followed by rounding up of the cells (33).

Antigen Detection

Historically, antigen detection protocols rarely could differentiate poxviruses at the species level. Thus, VACV could not be discriminated from MPXV or VARV. This approach is rarely used since the development of PCR.

Histology

Molluscum contagiosum can be diagnosed solely on clinical grounds based on the gross appearance of lesions and their chronic nature; however, giant molluscum can be confused with other disorders. The differential diagnosis is readily confirmed by hematoxylin and eosin staining of biopsy material, and the presence of "molluscum" or Henderson-Patterson bodies is pathognomonic for disease. Electron microscopy and PCR can also be used for diagnosis, but these are usually not warranted (133).

Nucleic Acid Detection

The requirement of specific banks of tissue culture cells for poxvirus isolation and the long time to generate assay endpoints spurred the development of the PCR assay as the mainstay diagnostic method. PCR has become the method of choice to distinguish 11 species of *Orthopoxvirus* from each other and variola major virus from variola minor virus (104), four species of *Parapoxvirus* (102), MCV (133), and three species of *Yatapoxvirus* (29, 148).

Serologic Assays

Presently, there are no sensitive, specific, and reliable serologic assays that retrospectively differentiate among orthopoxvirus infections. Also, following ORFV, PCPV, and MCV infections, antibodies have not always been detected or persist only transiently. Recently, an immunoglobulin M capture enzyme-linked immunosorbent assay (ELISA) using VACV antigen has been developed as an epidemiological tool; however, this assay cannot directly differentiate among antibodies induced by orthopoxvirus species (71). The lack of a single species-specific ELISA for orthopoxvirus infections can be overcome by the use of an ELISA based on antigens of the orthopoxvirus species that need to be differentiated, and comparison of titers in serum using these antigens along with known serologic standards (55). For example, in the 2003 monkeypox outbreak the serologic assay needed to discriminate between an acute MPXV infection, residual immunity from smallpox vaccination in an uninfected subject, and MPXV infection of an individual with residual vaccine immunity.

PREVENTION

General

Environmental

Environmental surroundings can be contaminated from lesional sources of poxvirus. For VARV and possibly other orthopoxviruses, this contamination is not usually of epidemiological significance, as the virions are locked in inspissated, pustular fluid that is difficult to resuspend into the air in a respirable form. In contrast, transmissions of MCV and parapoxvirus infections have been documented with a large number of fomites (114, 117). Thus, environmental surfaces potentially exposed to poxviruses must be thoroughly disinfected.

Behavioral

Of the human poxvirus infections, only MCV has a behavioral component. The majority of adult MCV infections are the result of sexual contact (12).

Isolation of Infected Persons

Historically, the quarantine of communities and the isolation of infected individuals or their contacts have been practiced for smallpox and, to a certain extent, human monkeypox because the virions can be transmitted by respiratory droplets. Vaccinees are counseled to avoid contact with the extremely young, with pregnant women, and with persons with atopic dermatitis or an immunosuppressed immune system.

Passive Immunoprophylaxis

Intramuscular administration of vaccinia immunoglobulin (VIG), a product derived from the pooled plasma of vaccinated individuals, is indicated for treatment of generalized vaccinia, progressive vaccinia (vaccinia necrosum), eczema vaccinatum, and certain autoinoculations, although efficacy has not been demonstrated through controlled clinical trials (142). VIG was reported to halt formation of new lesions and to cause rapid clinical improvement in cases of generalized vaccinia and eczema vaccinatum (10). One large study suggested that postexposure treatment of contacts of patients with smallpox with vaccination and VIG appeared to be more efficacious than vaccination alone. Smallpox developed in 5 of 326 contacts who received VIG, compared to 21 of 379 controls, for a relative efficacy of 70% in preventing smallpox (74, 119). In 2005, the Food and Drug Administration (FDA) approved the manufacture of new stocks of VIG by DynPort Vaccine Company LLC. The lack of a reproducible and clear-cut benefit of VIG may be due to the low potency of the antivaccinia antibodies present in the product. A highly potent cocktail of monoclonal antibodies generated against key neutralizing epitopes on surface proteins of intracellular mature virus and extracellular enveloped virus has shown promise in nonhuman primate and mouse studies (22, 87).

Active Immunization

Vaccination has a long history with poxvirus infections. As early as the 10th century in Asia, the inoculation of pustule fluid or scab material into the skin ("inoculation" or "variolation") was shown to protect against "natural" smallpox, with case fatality rates of 0.5 to 2% instead of 20 to 30%. Variolation was introduced into Europe early in the 18th century, and in some countries, notably England, it was practiced on a large scale.

In 1796 Edward Jenner showed that persons who had been inoculated with a related orthopoxvirus, CPXV, were completely resistant to smallpox (66). Vaccination (named from *vacca*, cow) led to a great decline in the incidence of smallpox in many countries. By the early 1950s many of the industrialized countries had eliminated endemic smallpox, and in 1958 the World Health Assembly accepted the concept of global eradication of smallpox. Realization of this goal faltered for several years, but in 1967 a Smallpox Eradication Unit was established at WHO headquarters, and the goal of global eradication within a decade was pursued with vigor and enthusiasm. Helped by the availability of adequate amounts of potent and stable freeze-dried vaccine, a change in strategy from reliance on mass vaccination alone to mass vaccination supported by surveillance and containment, and a new and simple inoculation device (the bifurcated needle), the WHO program achieved its target in October 1977, and the world was certified free of smallpox by the World Health Assembly in May 1980 (41).

The traditional smallpox vaccine could be given as late as 4 days postinfection (96) and still modify the disease course. When the vaccine was administered optimally, complete protection against smallpox was maintained for about 5 years, and various degrees of protection were maintained after that. This vaccine was estimated to be ≥85% effective against severe monkeypox disease (67). As with smallpox, individuals who had been vaccinated as children were still infected with MPXV during the 2003 U.S. outbreak, but they presented with mild or no disease (55, 72). The smallpox vaccine is likely efficacious to various degrees against other orthopoxviruses but not poxviruses from other genera.

Due to the threat of bioterrorism, the United States developed a new smallpox vaccine, ACAM2000, as a replacement for the limited and aging stocks of Dryvax. This vaccine was developed from Dryvax and is administered by bifurcated needle, as is Dryvax. In three phase I clinical trials, ACAM2000 produced major cutaneous reactions, evoked neutralizing antibody and cell-mediated responses, and had a reactogenicity profile similar to that of Dryvax (95). Similarly, phase II randomized, double-blinded, controlled trials found ACAM2000 to be equivalent to Dryvax in terms of cutaneous response rate, antibody responses, and safety (3). In phase III clinical trials, three cases of myo/pericarditis were observed with ACAM2000, although this was not unexpected, as several cases of myo/pericarditis were identified after smallpox vaccination in three Dryvax and one ACAM2000 phase II clinical trial held in 2003 (112).

A significant proportion of the American population is contraindicated for vaccination with Dryvax or ACAM2000, as they are immunosuppressed through infection with human immunodeficiency virus or as a result of immunosuppressive drugs for cancer chemotherapy and anti-organ rejection therapy. For this reason, modified Ankara virus (MVA) vaccine is under evaluation. From 1968, MVA has been safely used in more than 100,000 humans without documentation of any of the adverse reactions associated with other VACV vaccines. Following prophylactic intramuscular or subcutaneous immunization, mice and cynomolgus monkeys are protected from intranasal VACV (36, 91) and intravenous MPXV (36, 129) challenges, respectively. IMVAMUNE, an MVA vaccine (strain BN; Bavarian Nordic GmbH), has been tested for safety and immunogenicity in human volunteers (110, 136), and has been approved for licensure. Because the MVA virus does not replicate efficiently in human cells, one or two vaccine doses containing ~100 times more MVA virus than Dryvax may be required to induce equivalent immune responses and protection, making this a potentially expensive vaccine in the absence of adjuvants.

Dryvax, ACAM2000, and MVA induced cell-mediated and antibody responses against many viral antigens (108). Animal models suggest that antibodies targeting a limited number of antigens on the surface of intracellular mature virus and extracellular enveloped virus may be sufficient for protection from disease on challenge, as they protect against dissemination of virions through the body (8, 44, 111).

Currently, vaccination is recommended for laboratory workers who directly handle cultures or animals infected with VACV or recombinant VACV or other orthopoxviruses that infect humans (48; http://www.bt.cdc.gov/). Stocks of VACV vaccine for immunization of laboratory personnel are available from the Centers for Disease Control and Prevention in Atlanta, GA. To prevent accidental infection of unvaccinated subjects, especially those immunosuppressed or suffering from atopic dermatitis, the scarified area is "sealed" with an occlusive bandage.

Antiviral Chemoprophylaxis

Cidofovir (CDV), a DNA polymerase inhibitor currently used to treat cytomegalovirus retinitis in AIDS patients, has been approved to treat complications from vaccination under an investigational new-drug protocol; however, it must be given intravenously and has nephrotoxicity (http://www.bt.cdc.gov). This drug has been used off-license (146) to treat ORFV (50) and MCV (42) infections.

Management of Outbreaks

The approach to control a human orthopoxvirus that infects via respiratory droplets would depend to a large extent on the size of the initial focus and the reproduction rate of the agent (i.e., the average number of secondary cases generated by a typical primary case in a susceptible population). Although the transmission chains are becoming longer, MPXV still cannot maintain itself in the human population without constant reintroduction from zoonotic hosts. A natural outbreak, or bioterrorist release, of MPXV could be adequately contained with the traditional tracing and vaccination of contacts ("ring vaccination") and the isolation of symptomatic cases. The response to a bioterrorist release of VARV could also be a ring vaccination or the vaccination of large segments of the population and the restriction of civil liberties, depending on the initial burden of cases and the reproduction rate.

TREATMENT

Symptomatic

For nonsystemic zoonotic poxvirus infections, excluding MPXV, supportive care is provided on an outpatient basis.

Role of End-Organ Support in Severe Disease

Systemic disease such as monkeypox requires hospitalization in severe cases. In the 2003 U.S. outbreak, 9 of 34 patients with laboratory-confirmed monkeypox and no pre-existing medical conditions were hospitalized as inpatients. Two were held in the intensive care unit with respiratory complications (63).

Antiviral Treatment

During the smallpox eradication program, a number of compounds were shown to have efficacy against orthopoxvirus infections in tissue culture, and some were actually tested in field conditions. Thiosemicarbazone and metisazone were administered prophylactically in a series of trials in India and showed some protective effect; however, their administration was often associated with severe nausea and vomiting (41). Cytosine arabinoside and adenine arabinoside were also used to treat variola major and variola minor, but they failed to affect the case mortality rate or the clinical progression of disease. Rifampin showed antiviral activity against VACV in a mouse model but was never tested clinically against VARV.

Two orally available antivirals have been developed and have entered phase I or II clinical testing. As of 2007, Chimerix and SIGA Inc. have received investigational new-drug status for compounds CMX001 and ST-246, respectively. CMX001 is a hexadecyloxypropyl (HDP)-CDV salt synthesized by covalently coupling CDV to an alkoxyalkanol to form a prodrug of CDV (106). Eighty-eight percent of HDP-CDV is bioavailable and is distributed hematogenously to tissues without significant concentration in the kidneys and would be predicted to lack nephrotoxicity. Most importantly, CDV and HDP-CDV have broad-spectrum activity against viruses that encode DNA polymerases, including all poxviruses known to infect humans, adenoviruses, and many herpesviruses (62).

ST-246 is active against multiple species of orthopoxviruses, including two strains of VARV (145). Resistance mapping studies indicate that ST-246 targets the VACV F13L gene, which is conserved in orthopoxviruses. The F13L gene encodes a major envelope protein, p37, which is required for production of extracellular, but not intracellular, virus. Thus, ST-246 does not affect the actual production of infectious virus, only its efficient egress from cells. Because CMX001 and ST-246 target different stages in the virus replication cycle, they show potent synergy in standard mouse orthopoxvirus infection models (115).

Both of these antivirals will likely treat all human orthopoxvirus infections, and CMX001 should be effective against the remaining human poxviruses, because the DNA polymerase is highly conserved. Consistent with this, CDV diphosphate, which is the active metabolite for both CDV and HDP-CDV, was shown to have activity against MCV DNA polymerase (138). The effectiveness of the egress inhibitor ST-246 against poxviruses of other genera will depend on the importance of the cell-to-cell spread of virus in the disease process.

Resistance Emergence and Its Implications

The only data available on the emergence of resistance to antiviral treatment come from animal models. Resistance to CDV can be generated after successive tissue culture passage in the presence of drug or through the introduction of mutations through recombinant DNA technology (2, 77, 125). The mutations necessary to make the poxvirus polymerase resistant to CDV in tissue culture appear to reduce the virulence of the virus in tested animal models. Because human orthopoxvirus infections are acute in nature, and drug treatment course will be short, resistance to antivirals will likely not be a problem in the clinic.

Invasive Procedures

Invasive treatment procedures are applicable only to MCV and will become less important with the availability of efficacious topical or systemic antiviral treatment options. For MCV the umbilicated core can be removed surgically or the lesions may be treated by cryotherapy. These approaches are not appropriate for large numbers of lesions. Cantharidin and topical imiquimod are also commonly utilized agents, although efficacy has not been demonstrated in randomized double-blinded clinical trials (30). Lesions in children tend to disappear as they grow older. In immunosuppressed AIDS patients, lesions persist in the anogenital area and on the head and neck.

REFERENCES

1. **Alibek, K., and S. Handelman**. 1999. *Biohazard*. Random House, London, United Kingdom.
2. **Andrei, G, D. B. Gammon, P. Fiten, E. De Clercq, G. Opdenakker, R. Snoeck, and D. H. Evans.** 2006. Cidofovir resistance in vaccinia virus is linked to diminished virulence in mice. *J. Virol.* **80:**9391–9401.
3. **Artenstein, A. W., C. Johnson, T. C. Marbury, D. Morrison, P. S. Blum, T. Kemp, R. Nichols, J. P. Balser, M. Currie, and T. P. Monath**. 2005. A novel, cell culture-derived smallpox vaccine in vaccinia-naive adults. *Vaccine* **23:**3301–3309.
4. **Baxby, D**. 1982. An outbreak of cowpox in captive cheetahs: virological and epidemiological studies. *J. Hyg. Camb.* **89:**365–372.
5. **Baxby, D., M. Bennett, and B. Getty.** 1994. Human cowpox 1969–93: a review based on 54 cases. *Br. J. Dermatol.* **131:**598–607.
6. **Birthistle, K., and D. Carrington.** 1997. Molluscum contagiosum virus. *J. Infect.* **34:**21–28.
7. **Blackford, S., D. L. Roberts, and P. D. Thomas.** 1993. Cowpox infection causing a generalized eruption in a patient with atopic dermatitis. *Br. J. Dermatol.* **129:**628–629.
8. **Boulter, E. A., and G. Appleyard.** 1973. Differences between extracellular and intracellular forms of poxvirus and their implications. *Prog. Med. Virol.* **16:**86–108.
9. **Bras, G.** 1952. Observations on the formation of smallpox scars. *Arch. Pathol.* **54:**149–156.
10. **Bray, M.** 2003. Pathogenesis and potential antiviral therapy of complications of smallpox vaccination. *Antivir. Res.* **58:**101–114.
11. **Breman, J. G., Kalisa-Ruti, M. V. Steniowski, E. Zanotto, A. I. Gromyko, and I. Arita.** 1980. Human monkeypox, 1970–79. *Bull. W. H. O.* **58:**165–182.
12. **Brown, S. T., J. F. Nalley, and S. J. Kraus.** 1981. Molluscum contagiosum. *Sex. Trans. Dis.* **8:**227–234.
13. **Bugert, J. J., and G. Darai.** 1997. Recent advances in molluscum contagiosum research. *Arch. Virol. Suppl.* **13:** 35–47.
14. **Buller, R. M., J. Burnett, W. Chen, and J. Kreider.** 1995. Replication of molluscum contagiosum virus. *Virology* **213:**655–659.
15. **Buller, R. M., B. M. Arif, D. N. Black, K. R. Dumbell, J. J. Esposito, E. J. Lefkowitz, G. McFadden, B. Moss, A. A. Mercer, R. W. Moyer, M. A. Skinner, and D. N. Tripathy.** 2005. *Poxviridae*, p. 117–133. *In* C. M. Fauquet, M. A. Mayo, J. Maniloff, U. Desselberger, and L. A. Ball (ed.), *Virus Taxonomy: Classification and Nomenclature of Viruses. Eighth Report of the International Committee on Taxonomy of Viruses*. Elsevier Academic Press, San Diego, CA.
16. **Buller, R. M. L., and F. Fenner.** 2007. *Mousepox*, p. 67–92. *In* J. G. Fox, S. W. Barthold, M. T. Davisson, C. E. Newcomer, F. W. Quimby, and A. L. Smith (ed.), *The Mouse in Biomedical Research*, 2nd ed., vol. 2. Elsevier, New York, NY.
17. **Carson, C. A., and K. M. Kerr.** 1967. Bovine papular stomatitis with apparent transmission to man. *J. Am. Vet. Med. Assoc.* **151:**183–187.
18. **Carson, C. A., K. M. Kerr, and I. C. Grumbles.** 1968. Bovine papular stomatitis: experimental transmission from man. *Am. J. Vet. Res.* **29:**1783–1790.
19. **Chantrey, J., H. Meyer, D. Baxby, M. Begon, K. J. Bown, S. M. Hazel, T. Jones, W. I. Montgomery, and M. Bennett.** 1999. Cowpox: reservoir hosts and geographic range. *Epidemiol. Infect.* **122:**455–460.
20. **Chaudhri, G., V. Panchanathan, H. Bluethmann, and G. Karupiah.** 2006. Obligatory requirement for antibody in recovery from a primary poxvirus infection. *J. Virol.* **80:**6339–6344.
21. **Chen, N., G. Li, M. K. Liszewski, J. P. Atkinson, P. B. Jahrling, Z, Feng, J. Schriewer, C. Buck, C. Wang, E. J. Lefkowitz, J. J. Esposito, T. Harms, I. K. Damon, R. L. Roper, C. Upton, and R. M. L. Buller.** 2005. Virulence differences between monkeypox virus isolates from West Africa and the Congo basin. *Virology* **340:**46–63.
22. **Chen, Z., P. Earl, J. Americo, I. Damon, S. K. Smith, F. Yu, A. Sebrell, S. Emerson, G. Cohen, R. J. Eisenberg, I. Gorshkova, P. Schuck, W. Satterfield, B. Moss, and R. Purcell.** 2007. Characterization of chimpanzee/human monoclonal antibodies to vaccinia virus A33 glycoprotein and its variola virus homolog in vitro and in a vaccinia virus mouse protection model. *J. Virol.* **81:**8989–8995.
23. **Cho, C. T., and H. A. Wenner.** 1973. Monkeypox virus. *Bacteriol. Rev.* **37:**1–18.
24. **Clark, C., P. G. McIntyre, A. Evans, C. J. McInnes, and S. Lewis-Jones.** 2005. Human sealpox resulting from a seal bite: confirmation that sealpox virus is zoonotic. *Br. J. Dermatol.* **152:**791–793.
25. **Damon, I.** 2007. Poxviruses, p. 2947–2975. *In* D. M. Knipe, P. M. Howley, D. E. Griffin, R. A. Lamb, M. A. Martin, B. Roizman, and S. E. Straus (ed.), *Fields Virology*, 5th ed. Lippincott Williams & Wilkins, Philadelphia, PA.
26. **Damon, I. K., C. E. Roth, and V. Chowdhary.** 2006. Discovery of monkeypox in the Sudan. *N. Engl. J. Med.* **355:**969–973.
27. **Dekking, F.** 1964. Cowpox and vaccinia, p. 411–418. *In* J. van der Hoeden (ed.), *Zoonoses*. Elsevier, Amsterdam, The Netherlands.
28. **de Souza Trindade, G., B. P. Drumond, M. I. M. C. Guedes, J. A. Leite, B. E. F. Mota, M. A. Campos, F. G. da Fonseca, M. L. Nogueira, Z. I. P. Lobato, C. A. Bonjardim, P. C. P. Ferreira, and E. G. Kroon.** 2007. Zoonotic vaccinia virus infection in Brazil: clinical description and implications for health professionals. *J. Clin. Microbiol.* **45:**1370–1372.
29. **Dhar, A. D., A. E. Werchniak, Y. Li, J. B. Brennick, C. S. Goldsmith, R. Kline, I. Damon, and S. N. Klaus.** 2004. Tanapox infection in a college student. *N. Engl. J. Med.* **350:**361–366.
30. **Dohil, M. A., P. Lin, J. Lee, A. W. Lucky, A. S. Paller, and L. F. Eichenfield.** 2006. The epidemiology of molluscum contagiosum in children. *J. Am. Acad. Dermatol.* **54:**47–54.
31. **Downie, A. W.** 1939. A study of the lesions produced experimentally by cowpox virus. *J. Pathol. Bacteriol.* **48:** 361–379.
32. **Downie, A. W., and C. Espana.** 1973. A comparative study of Tanapox and Yaba viruses. *J. Gen. Virol.* **19:**37–49.
33. **Downie, A. W., C. H. Taylor-Robinson, A. E. Caunt, G. S, Nelson, P. E. Manson-Bahr, and T. C. Matthews.** 1971. Tanapox: a new disease caused by a poxvirus. *Br. Med. J.* **1:**363–368.
34. **Dumbell, K., and M. Richardson.** 1993. Virological investigations of specimens from buffaloes affected by buffalopox in Maharashtra State, India between 1985 and 1987. *Arch. Virol.* **128:**257–267.
35. **Dupre, A., B. Christol, J. L. Bonafe, and J. Lassere.** 1981. Orf and atopic dermatitis. *Br. J. Dermatol.* **105:** 103–104.
36. **Earl, P. L., J. L. Americo, L. S. Wyatt, L. A. Eller, J. C. Whitbeck, G. H. Cohen, R. J. Eisenberg, C. J. Hartmann, D. L. Jackson, D. A. Kulesh, M. J. Martinez,**

D. M. Miller, E. M. Mucker, J. D. Shamblin, S. H. Zwiers, J. W. Huggins, P. B. Jahrling, and B. Moss. 2004. Immunogenicity of a highly attenuated MVA smallpox vaccine and protection against monkeypox. *Nature* **428:**182–185.

37. **Esteban, D. J., and R. M. Buller.** 2005. Ectromelia virus: the causative agent of mousepox. *J. Gen. Virol.* **86:**2645–2659.

38. **Fenner, F.** 1948. The pathogenesis of the acute exanthems. *Lancet* **ii:**915–920.

39. **Fenner, F.** 1949. Mouse pox (infectious ectromelia of mice): a review. *J. Immunol.* **63:**341–373.

39a. **Fenner, F., and J. H. Nakano.** 1988. *Poxviridae:* the poxviruses, p. 177–210. *In* E. H. Lennette, P. Halonen, and F. A. Murphy (ed.), *The Laboratory Diagnosis of Infectious Diseases: Principles and Practice*, vol. II. *Viral, Rickettsial and Chlamydial Diseases*. Springer-Verlag, New York, NY.

40. **Fenner, F., R. Wittek, and K. R. Dumbell.** 1989. *The Orthopoxviruses*. Academic Press, San Diego, CA.

41. **Fenner, F., D. A. Henderson, I. Arita, Z. Jezek, and I. D. Ladnyi.** 1988. *Smallpox and Its Eradication*. World Health Organization, Geneva, Switzerland.

42. **Fery-Blanco, C., F. Pelletier, P. Humbert, and F. Aubin.** 2007. Disseminated molluscum contagiosum during topical treatment of atopic dermatitis with tacrolimus: efficacy of cidofovir. *Ann. Dermatol. Venereol.* **134:**457–459.

43. **Fogg, C., S. Lustig, J. C. Whitbeck, R. J. Eisenberg, G. H. Cohen, and B. Moss.** 2004. Protective immunity to vaccinia virus induced by vaccination with multiple recombinant outer membrane proteins of intracellular and extracellular virions. *J. Virol.* **78:**10230–10237.

44. **Fogg, C. N., J. L. Americo, S. Lustig, J. W. Huggins, S. K. Smith, I. Damon, W. Resch, P. L. Earl, D. M. Klinman, and B. Moss.** 2007. Adjuvant-enhanced antibody responses to recombinant proteins correlates with protection of mice and monkeys to orthopoxvirus challenges. *Vaccine* **25:**2787–2799.

45. **Freed, E. R., J. D. Richard, and M. R. Escobar.** 1972. Vaccinia necrosum and its relationship to impaired immunologic responsiveness. *Am. J. Med.* **52:**411–420.

46. **Frey, S. E., R. B. Couch, C. O. Tacket, J. J. Treanor, M. Wolff, F. K. Newman, R. L. Atmar, R. Edelman, C. M. Nolan, and R. B. Belshe.** 2002. Clinical responses to undiluted and diluted smallpox vaccine. *N. Engl. J. Med.* **346:**1265–1274.

47. **Fulginiti, V. A., C. H. Kempe, W. E. Hathaway, D. S. Perlman, O. F. Serber, J. J. Eller, J. J. Joyner, Sr., and A. Robinson.** 1968. Progressive vaccinia in immunologically deficient individuals. *Birth Defects* **4:**129–145.

48. **Fulginiti, V. A., A. Papier, J. M. Lane, J. M. Neff, and D. A. Henderson.** 2003. Smallpox vaccination: a review, part I. Background, vaccination technique, normal vaccination and revaccination, and expected normal reactions. *Clin. Infect. Dis.* **37:**241–250.

49. **Fulginiti, V. A., A. Papier, J. M. Lane, J. M. Neff, and D. A. Henderson.** 2003. Smallpox vaccination: a review, part II. Adverse events. *Clin. Infect. Dis.* **37:**251–271.

50. **Geerinck, K., G. Lukito, R. Snoeck, R. De Vos, E. De Clercq, Y. Vanrenterghem, H. Degreef, and B. Maes.** 2001. A case of human orf in an immunocompromised patient treated successfully with cidofovir cream. *J. Med. Virol.* **64:**543–549.

51. **Gibbs, E. P. J., and A. D. Osborne.** 1974. Observations on the epidemiology of pseudocowpox in south-west England and south Wales. *Br. Vet. J.* **130:**150–159.

52. **Grace, J. T., Jr., and E. A. Mirand.** 1963. Human susceptibility to a simian tumor virus. *Ann. N. Y. Acad. Sci.* **108:**1123–1128.

53. **Greene, H. S. N.** 1933. A pandemic of rabbit-pox. *Proc. Soc. Exp. Biol. Med.* **30:**892–894.

54. **Guarner, J., B. J. Johnson, C. D. Paddock, W. J. Shieh, C. S. Goldsmith, M. G. Reynolds, I. K. Damon, R. L. Regnery, and S. R. Zaki.** 2004. Monkeypox transmission and pathogenesis in prairie dogs. *Emerg. Infect. Dis.* **10:** 426–431.

55. **Hammarlund, E., M. W. Lewis, S. V. Carter, I. Amanna, S. G. Hansen, L. I. Strelow, S. W. Wong, P. Yoshihara, J. M. Hanifin, and M. K. Slifka.** 2005. Multiple diagnostic techniques identify previously vaccinated individuals with protective immunity against monkeypox. *Nat. Med.* **11:**1005–1011.

56. **Hammarlund, E., J. M. Hanifin, and M. K. Slifka.** 2007. Monkeypox without exanthema. *N. Engl. J. Med.* **356:** 2112–2114.

57. **Harper, G. J.** 1961. Airborne micro-organisms: survival tests with four viruses. *J. Hyg.* **59:**479–486.

58. **Henderson, D. A.** 1998. Bioterrorism as a public health threat. *Emerg. Infect. Dis.* **4:**488–492.

59. **Heymann, D. L., M. Szczeniowski, and K. Esteves.** 1998. Re-emergence of monkeypox in Africa: a review of the past six years. *Br. Med. Bull.* **54:**693–670.

60. **Hicks, B. D., and G. A. J. Worthy.** 1987. Sealpox in captive grey seals *(Halichoerus grypus)* and their handlers. *J. Wildl. Dis.* **23:**1–6.

61. **Hopkins, D. R.** 1983. *Princes and Peasants. Smallpox in History*. Chicago University Press, Chicago, IL.

62. **Hostetler, K. Y.** 2007. Synthesis and antiviral evaluation of broad spectrum, orally active analogs of cidofovir and other acyclic nucleoside phosphonates, p. 167–184. *In* E. De Clercq (ed.), *Advances in Antiviral Drug Design*, vol. 5. Elsevier, Amsterdam, The Netherlands.

63. **Huhn, G. D., A. M. Bauer, K. Yorita, M. B. Graham, J. Sejvar, A. Likos, I. K. Damon, M. G. Reynolds, and M. J. Kuehnert.** 2005. Clinical characteristics of human monkeypox and risk factors for severe disease. *Clin. Infect. Dis.* **41:**1742–1751.

64. **Hutin, Y. J., R. J. Williams, P. Malfait, R. Pebody, V. N. Loparev, S. L. Ropp, M. Rodriguez, J. C. Knight, F. K. Tshioko, A. S. Khan, M. V. Szczeniowski, and J. J. Esposito.** 2001. Outbreak of human monkeypox, Democratic Republic of Congo, 1996 to 1997. *Emerg. Infect. Dis.* **7:**434–438.

65. **Jahrling, P. B., L. E. Hensley, M. J. Martinez, J. W. Leduc, K. H. Rubins, D. A. Relman, and J. W. Huggins.** 2004. Exploring the potential of variola virus infection of cynomologus macaques as a model for human smallpox. *Proc. Natl. Acad. Sci. USA* **101:**15196–15200.

66. **Jenner, E.** 1798. An inquiry into the causes and effects of the variolae vaccinae, a disease discovered in some of the western counties of England, particularly Gloucestershire, and known by the name of the cow pox. *Reprinted in* C. N. B. Camac (ed.), *Classics of Medicine and Surgery*, p. 213–240, 1959. Dover, New York, NY.

67. **Jezek, Z., and F. Fenner.** 1988. *Human monkeypox. Virol. Monogr.* **17:**1–140.

68. **Jezek, Z., I. Arita, M. Szczeniowski, K. M. Paluku, K. Ruti, and J. H. Nakano.** 1985. Human tanapox in Zaire: clinical and epidemiological observations on cases confirmed by laboratory studies. *Bull. W. H. O.* **63:**1027–1035.

69. **Jezek, Z., M. Szczeniowski, K. M. Paluku, M. Mutombo, and B. Grab.** 1988. Human monkeypox: confusion with chickenpox. *Acta Trop.* **45:**297–307.

70. **Johnson, R. T.** 1982. *Viral Infections of the Nervous System*. Raven Press, New York, NY.

71. **Karem, K. L., M. Reynolds, Z. Braden, G. Lou, N. Bernard, J. Patton, and I. K. Damon.** 2005. Characterization

of acute-phase humoral immunity to monkeypox: use of immunoglobulin M enzyme-linked immunosorbent assay for detection of monkeypox infection during the 2003 North American outbreak. *Clin. Diagn. Lab. Immunol.* **12:**867–872.

72. **Karem, K. L., M. Reynolds, C. Hughes, Z. Braden, P. Nigam, S. Crotty, J. Glidewell, R. Ahmed, R. Amara, and I. K. Damon.** 2007. Monkeypox-induced immunity and failure of childhood smallpox vaccination to provide complete protection. *Clin. Vaccine Immunol.* **14:**1318–1327.
73. **Kempe, C. H.** 1960. Studies on smallpox and complications of smallpox vaccination. *Pediatrics* **26:**176–189.
74. **Kempe, C. H., C. Bowles, G. Meiklejohn, T. O. Berge, L. St. Vincent, B. V. Babu, S. Govindarajan, N. R. Ratnakannan, A. W. Downie, and V. R. Murthy.** 1961. The use of vaccinia hyperimmune gamma-globulin in the prophylaxis of smallpox. *Bull. W. H. O.* **25:**41–48.
75. **Khodakevich, L., Z. Jezek, and K. Kinzanzka.** 1986. Isolation of monkeypox virus from wild squirrel infected in nature. *Lancet* **i:**98–99.
76. **Kluge, J. P., N. F. Cheville, and T. M. Peery.** 1972. The pathogenesis of contagious ecthyma. *Am. J. Vet. Res.* **33:** 1191–2000.
77. **Kornbluth, R. S., D. F. Smee, R. W. Sidwell, V. Snarsky, D. H. Evans, and K. Y. Hostetler.** 2006. Mutations in the E9L polymerase gene of cidofovir-resistant vaccinia virus strain WR are associated with the drug resistance phenotype. *Antimicrob. Agents Chemother.* **50:**4038–4043.
78. **Lal, S. M., and I. P. Singh.** 1977. Buffalopox—a review. *Trop. Anim. Health Prod.* **9:**107–112.
79. **Lane, J. M., F. L. Ruben, J. M. Neff, and J. D. Millar.** 1969. Complications of smallpox vaccination 1968; national survey in the United States. *N. Engl. J. Med.* **281:** 1201–1208.
80. **Lane, J. M., F. L. Ruben, J. M. Neff, and J. D. Millar.** 1970. Complications of smallpox vaccination 1968; results of ten statewide surveys. *J. Infect. Dis.* **122:**303–309.
81. **Learned, L. A., M. G. Reynolds, D. W. Wassa, Y. Li, V. A. Olson, K. Karem, L. L. Stempora, Z. H. Braden, R. Kline, A. Likos, F. Libama, H. Moudzeo, J. D. Bolanda, P. Tarangonia, P. Boumandoki, P. Formenty, J. M. Harvey. and I. K. Damon.** 2005. Extended interhuman transmission of monkeypox in a hospital community in the Republic of the Congo, 2003. *Am. J. Trop. Med. Hyg.* **73:**428–434.
82. **Lederman, E. R., M. G. Reynolds, K. Karem, Z. Braden, L. A. Learned-Orozco, D. Wassa-Wassa, O. Moundeli, C. Hughes, J. Harvey, R. Regnery, J. V. Mombouli, and I. K. Damon.** 2007. Prevalence of antibodies against orthopoxviruses among residents of Likouala region, Republic of Congo: evidence for monkeypox virus exposure. *Am. J. Trop. Med. Hyg.* **77:**1150–1156.
83. **Leite, J. A., B. P. Drumond, G. S. Trindade, Z. I. Lobato, F. G. da Fonseca, S. J. Dos, M. C. Madureira, M. I. Guedes, J. M. Ferreira, C. A. Bonjardim, P. C. Ferreira, and E. G. Kroon.** 2005. Passatempo virus, a vaccinia virus strain, Brazil. *Emerg. Infect. Dis.* **11:**1935–1938.
84. **Li, G., N. Chen, R. L. Roper, Z. Feng, A. Hunter, M. Danila, E. J. Lefkowitz, R. M. Buller, and C. Upton.** 2005. Complete coding sequences of the rabbitpox virus genome. *J. Gen. Virol.* **86:**2969–2977.
85. **Likos, A. M., S. A. Sammons, V. A. Olson, A. M. Frace, Y. Li, M. Olsen-Rasmussen, W. Davidson, R. Galloway, M. L. Khristova, M. G. Reynolds, H. Zhao, D. S. Carroll, A. Curns, P. Formenty, J. J. Esposito, R. L. Regnery, and I. K. Damon.** 2005. A tale of two clades: monkeypox viruses. *J. Gen. Virol.* **86:**2661–2672.
86. **Lum, G. S., F. Soriano, A. Trejos, and J. Llerena.** 1967. Vaccinia epidemic and epizootic in El Salvador. *Am. J. Trop. Med. Hyg.* **16:**332–338.
87. **Lustig, S., C. Fogg, J. C. Whitbeck, R. J. Eisenberg, G. H. Cohen, and B. Moss.** 2005. Combinations of polyclonal or monoclonal antibodies to proteins of the outer membranes of the two infectious forms of vaccinia virus protect mice against a lethal respiratory challenge. *J. Virol.* **79:**13454–13462.
88. **Marennikova, S. S., N. N. Maltseva, V. I. Koreeva, and N. M. Garanina.** 1977. Outbreak of pox disease among carnivora (Felidae) and Edentata. *J. Infect. Dis.* **135:**358–366.
89. **McFadden, G., A. Lalani, H. Everett, P. Nash, and X. Xu.** 1998. Virus-coded receptors for cytokines and chemokines. *Semin. Cell Dev. Biol.* **9:**359–368.
90. **McNulty, W. P., Jr., W. C. Lobitz, F. Hu, C. A. Maruffo, and A. S. Hall.** 1968. A pox disease in monkeys transmitted to man. Clinical and histological features. *Arch. Dermatol.* **97:**286–293.
91. **Meseda, C. A., A. D. Garcia, A. Kumar, A. E. Mayer, J. Manischewitz, L. R. King, H. Golding, M. Merchlinsky, and J. P. Weir.** 2005. Enhanced immunogenicity and protective effect conferred by vaccination with combinations of modified vaccinia virus Ankara and licensed smallpox vaccine Dryvax in a mouse model. *Virology* **339:**164–175.
92. **Mets, T., P. Ngendahayo, P. Van de Perre, and A. Mutwewingabo.** 1989. HIV infection and tuberculosis in Central Africa. *N. Engl. J. Med.* **321:**542–543.
93. **Meyer, H., M. Perrichot, M. Stemmler, P. Emmerich, H. Schmitz, F. Varaine, R. Shunqu, F. Tshioko, and P. Formenty.** 2002. Outbreaks of disease suspected of being due to human monkeypox virus infection in the Democratic Republic of Congo in 2001. *J. Clin. Microbiol.* **40:**2919–2921.
94. **Meyer, H. P., M. Pfeffer, and H. J. Rziha.** 1994. Sequence alterations within and downstream of the A-type inclusion protein genes allow differentiation of Orthopoxvirus species by polymerase chain reaction. *J. Gen. Virol.* **75:**1975–1981.
95. **Monath, T. P., J. R. Caldwell, W. Mundt, J. Fusco, C. S. Johnson, R. M. Buller, J. Liu, B. Gardner, G. Downing, P. S. Blum, T. Kemp, R. Nichols, and R. Weltzin.** 2004. ACAM2000 clonal Vero cell culture vaccinia virus (New York City Board of Health strain)—a second-generation smallpox vaccine for biological defense. *Int. J. Infect. Dis.* **8**(Suppl. 2)**:**S31–S44.
96. **Mortimer, P. P.** 2003. Can postexposure vaccination against smallpox succeed? *Clin. Infect. Dis.* **36:**622–629.
97. **Moss, B., J. L. Shisler, Y. Xian, and T. G. Senkevich.** 2000. Immune-defense molecules of molluscum contagiosum virus, a human poxvirus. *Trends Microbiol.* **8:** 473–477.
98. **Moss, B.** 2007. *Poxviridae:* the viruses and their replication, p. 2906–2945. *In* D. M. Knipe, P. M. Howley, D. E. Griffin, R. A. Lamb, M. A. Martin, B. Roizman, and S. E. Straus (ed.), *Fields Virology*, 5th ed. Lippincott Williams & Wilkins, Philadelphia, PA.
99. **Muraleedharan, K., R. Raghavan, G. V. K. Murthy, V. S. S. Murthy, K. G. Swamy, and T. Prasanna.** 1989. An investigation on the outbreaks of pox in buffaloes in Karnataka. *Curr. Res. Univ. Agric. Sci.* **18:**26–27.
100. **Murphy, F. A., E. P. J. Gibbs, M. C. Horzinek, and M. J. Studdert.** 1999. *Poxviridae*, p. 277–291. *In Veterinary Virology*, 3rd ed. Academic Press, San Diego, CA.
101. **Nakamura, J., J. Muraki, M. Yamada, Y. Hatano, and S. Nii.** 1995. Analysis of molluscum contagiosum virus genomes isolated in Japan. *J. Med. Virol.* **46:**339–348.
102. **Nitsche, A., M. Buttner, S. Wilhelm, G. Pauli, and H. Meyer.** 2006. Real-time PCR detection of parapoxvirus DNA. *Clin. Chem.* **52:**316–319.

103. **Niven, J. S. F., J. A. Armstrong, C. H. Andrewes, H. G. Pereira, and R. C. Valentine.** 1961. Subcutaneous "growths" in monkeys produced by a poxvirus. *J. Pathol. Bacteriol.* **81:**1–14.
104. **Olson, V. A., T. Laue, M. T. Laker, I. V. Babkin, C. Drosten, S. N. Shchelkunov, M. Niedrig, I. K. Damon, and H. Meyer.** 2004. Real-time PCR system for detection of orthopoxviruses and simultaneous identification of smallpox virus. *J. Clin. Microbiol.* **42:**1940–1946.
105. **Overfield, T. M., and J. A. Brody.** 1966. An epidemiologic study of molluscum contagiosum in Anchorage, Alaska. *J. Pediatr.* **69:**640–642.
106. **Painter, G. R., and K. Y. Hostetler.** 2004. Design and development of oral drugs for the prophylaxis and treatment of smallpox infection. *Trends Biotechnol.* **22:**423–427.
107. **Panchanathan, V., G. Chaudhri, and G. Karupiah.** 2006. Protective immunity against secondary poxvirus infection is dependent on antibody but not on CD4 or CD8 T-cell function. *J. Virol.* **80:**6333–6338.
108. **Panchanathan, V., G. Chaudhri, and G. Karupiah.** 2008. Correlates of protective immunity in poxvirus infection: where does antibody stand? *Immunol. Cell Biol.* **86:**80–86.
109. **Parker, S., A. Nuara, R. M. Buller, and D. A. Schultz.** 2007. Human monkeypox: an emerging zoonotic disease. *Future Med.* **2:**17–34.
110. **Parrino, J., L. H. McCurdy, B. D. Larkin, I. J. Gordon, S. E. Rucker, M. E. Enama, R. A. Koup, M. Roederer, R. T. Bailer, Z. Moodie, L. Gu, L. Yan, and B. S. Graham.** 2007. Safety, immunogenicity and efficacy of modified vaccinia Ankara (MVA) against Dryvax™ challenge in vaccinia-naïve and vaccine-immune individuals. *Vaccine* **25:**1513–1525.
111. **Payne, L.** 1980. Significance of extracellular enveloped virus in the *in vitro* and *in vivo* dissemination of vaccinia. *J. Gen. Virol.* **50:**89–100.
112. **Poland, G. A., J. D. Grabenstein, and J. M. Neff.** 2005. The US smallpox vaccination program: a review of a large modern era smallpox vaccination implementation program. *Vaccine* **23:**2078–2081.
113. **Postlethwaite, R., J. A. Watt, T. G. Hawley, I. Simpson, and H. Adam.** 1967. Features of molluscum contagiosum in the northeast of Scotland and in Fijian village settlements. *J. Hyg.* **65:**281–291.
114. **Postlethwaite, R.** 1970. Molluscum contagiosum virus. *Arch. Environ. Health* **21:**432–452.
115. **Quenelle, D. C., M. N. Prichard, K. A. Keith, D. E. Hruby, R. Jordan, G. R. Painter, A. Robertson, and E. R. Kern.** 2007. Synergistic efficacy of the combination of ST-246 with CMX001 against orthopoxviruses. *Antimicrob. Agents Chemother.* **51:**4118–4124.
116. **Reed, K. D., J. W. Melski, M. B. Graham, R. L. Regnery, M. J. Sotir, M. V. Wegner, J. J. Kazmierczak, E. J. Stratman, Y. Li, J. A. Fairley, G. R. Swain, V. A. Olson, E. K. Sargent, S. C. Kehl, M. A. Frace, R. Kline, S. L. Foldy, J. P. Davis, and I. K. Damon.** 2004. The detection of monkeypox in humans in the Western Hemisphere. *N. Engl. J. Med.* **350:**342–350.
117. **Robinson, A. J., and D. J. Lyttle.** 1992. Parapoxviruses: their biology and potential as recombinant vaccines, p. 285–327. *In* M. M. Binns and G. L. Smith (ed.), *Recombinant Poxviruses*. CRC Press, Boca Raton, FL.
118. **Ropp, S. L., Q. Jin, J. C. Knight, R. F. Massung, and J. J. Esposito.** 1995. PCR strategy for identification and differentiation of smallpox and other orthopoxviruses. *J. Clin. Virol.* **33:**2069–2076.
119. **Rosenthal, S. R., M. Merchlinsky, C. Kleppinger, and K. L. Goldenthal.** 2001. Developing new smallpox vaccines. *Emerg. Infect. Dis.* **7:**920–926.
120. **Rouhandeh, H.** 1988. Yaba virus, p. 1–15. *In* G. Darai (ed.), *Virus Diseases in Laboratory and Captive Animals*. Martinus Nijhoff, Boston, MA.
121. **Ruben, F. M., and J. M. Lane.** 1970. Ocular vaccinia. An epidemiologic analysis of 348 cases. *Arch. Ophthalmol.* **84:**45–48.
122. **Schupp, P., M. Pfeffer, H. Meyer, G. Burck, K. Kolmel, and C. Neumann.** 2001. Cowpox in a 12-year-old boy: rapid identification by an orthopoxvirus-specific polymerase chain reaction. *Br. J. Dermatol.* **145:**146–150.
123. **Schwartz, J. J., and P. L. Myskowski.** 1992. Molluscum contagiosum in patients with human immunodeficiency virus infection. *J. Am. Acad. Dermatol.* **27:**583–588.
124. **Shirodaria, P. V., R. S. Matthews, and M. Samuel.** 1979. Virus-specific and anticellular antibodies in molluscum contagiosum. *Br. J. Dermatol.* **101:**133–140.
125. **Smee, D. F., M. K. Wandersee, K. W. Bailey, K. Y. Hostetler, A. Holy, and R. W. Sidwell.** 2005. Characterization and treatment of cidofovir-resistant vaccinia (WR strain) virus infections in cell culture and in mice. *Antivir. Chem. Chemother.* **16:**203–211.
126. **Sonnet, J., J. Prignot, F. Zech, and J. C. Willame.** 1987. High prevalence of tuberculosis in HIV infected black patients from Central Africa. *Ann. Soc. Belg. Med. Trop.* **67:**299–300.
127. **Spillane, J. D., and C. E. Wells.** 1964. The neurology of Jennerian vaccination. A clinical account of the neurological complications which occurred during the smallpox epidemic in South Wales in 1962. *Brain* **87:**1–44.
128. **Sproul, E. E., R. S. Metzgar, and J. T. Grace, Jr.** 1963. The pathogenesis of Yaba virus-induced histiocytomas in primates. *Cancer Res.* **23:**671–675.
129. **Stittelaar, K. J., G. van Amerongen, I. Kondova, T. Kuiken, R. F. van Lavieren, F. H. Pistoor, H. G. Niesters, G. van Doornum, B. A. van der Zeijst, L. Mateo, P. Chaplin, and A. D. Osterhaus.** 2005. Modified vaccinia virus Ankara protects macaques against respiratory challenge with monkeypox virus. *J. Virol.* **79:**7845–7851.
130. **Sturt, R. J., H. K. Muller, and G. D. Francis.** 1971. Molluscum contagiosum in villages of the West Sepik district of New Guinea. *Med. J. Aust.* **2:**751–754.
131. **Taylor, J. M., and M. Barry.** 2006. Near death experiences: poxvirus regulation of apoptotic death. *Virology* **344:**139–150.
132. **Tesh, R. B., D. M. Watts, E. Sbrana, M. Siirin, V. L. Popov, and S. Xiao.** 2004. Experimental infection of ground squirrels (*Spermophilus tridecemlineatus*) with monkeypox virus. *Emerg. Infect. Dis.* **10:**1563–1567.
133. **Thompson, C. H.** 1997. Identification and typing of molluscum contagiosum virus in clinical specimens by polymerase chain reaction. *Virology* **197:**328–338.
134. **Topciu, V., I. Luca, E. Moldovan, V. Stoianovici, L. Plavosin, D. D. Milin, and E. Welter.** 1976. Transmission of vaccinia virus from vaccinated milkers to cattle. *Virologie* **27:**279–282.
135. **Tulman, E. R., G. Delhon, C. L. Afonso, Z. Lu, L. Zsak, N. T. Sandybaev, U. Z. Kerembekova, V. L. Zaitsev, G. F. Kutish, and D. L. Rock.** 2006. Genome of horsepox virus. *J. Virol.* **80:**9244–9258.
136. **Vollmar, J., N. Arndtz, K. M. Eckl, T. Thomsen, B. Petzold, L. Mateo, B. Schlereth, A. Handley, L. King, V. Hulsemann, M. Tzatzaris, K. Merkl, N. Wulff, and P. Chaplin.** 2006. Safety and immunogenicity of IMVAMUNE, a promising candidate as a third generation smallpox vaccine. *Vaccine* **24:**2065–2070.
137. **von Magnus, P., E. K. Andersen, K. B. Petersen, and A. Birch-Andersen.** 1959. A pox-like disease in cyno-

molgus monkeys. *Acta Pathol. Microbiol. Scand.* **46:**156–176.

138. **Watanabe, T., and K. Tamaki.** 15 November 2007. Cidofovir diphosphate inhibits molluscum contagiosum virus DNA polymerase activity. *J. Investig. Dermatol.* [Epub ahead of print.]
139. **Wehrle, P. F., J. Posch, K. H. Richter, and D. A. Henderson.** 1970. An airborne outbreak of smallpox in a German hospital and its significance with respect to other recent outbreaks in Europe. *Bull. W. H. O.* **43:** 669–679.
140. **White, D. O., and F. Fenner.** 1994. *Medical Virology*, 4th ed., p. 355. Academic Press, San Diego, CA.
141. **Wilson, G. S.** 1967. *The Hazards of Immunization*. Athlone Press, London, United Kingdom.
142. **Wittek, R.** 2006. Vaccinia immune globulin: current policies, preparedness, and product safety and efficacy. *Int. J. Infect. Dis.* **10:**193–201.
143. **World Health Organization Technical Advisory Group on Human Monkeypox.** 1999. Report of a WHO Meeting 11–12 January 1999 (WFH/CDS/CSR/APH/99.5). World Health Organization, Geneva, Switzerland.
144. **Xiao, S., E. Sbrana, D. M. Watts, M. Siirin, A. Travassos da Rosa, and R. B. Tesh.** 2005. Experimental infection of prairie dogs with monkeypox virus. *Emerg. Infect. Dis.* **11:**539–545.
145. **Yang, G., D. C. Pevear, M. H. Davies, M. S. Collett, T. Bailey, S. Rippen, L. Barone, C. Burns, G. Rhodes, S. Tohan, J. W. Huggins, R. O. Baker, R. M. Buller, E. Touchette, K. Waller, J. Schriewer, J. Neyts, E. DeClercq, K. Jones, D. Hruby, and R. Jordan.** 2005. An orally bioavailable antipoxvirus compound (ST-246) inhibits extracellular virus formation and protects mice from lethal orthopoxvirus challenge. *J. Virol.* **79:**13139–13149.
146. **Zabawski, E. J., Jr., and C. J. Cockerell.** 1998. Topical and intralesional cidofovir: a review of pharmacology and therapeutic effects. *J. Am. Acad. Dermatol.* **39:**741–745.
147. **Zaucha, G. M., P. B. Jahrling, T. W. Geisbert, J. R. Swearengen, and L. Hensley.** 2001. The pathology of experimental aerosolized monkeypox virus infection in cynomolgus monkeys (Macaca fascicularis). *Lab. Investig.* **81:**1581–1600.
148. **Zimmermann, P., I. Thordsen, D. Frangoulidis, and H. Meyer.** 2005. Real-time PCR assay for the detection of tanapox virus and yaba-like disease virus. *J. Virol. Methods* **130:**149–153.

Herpes Simplex Viruses

RICHARD J. WHITLEY AND BERNARD ROIZMAN

19

Herpes simplex virus (HSV) infections of humans have been documented since the advent of writing. Genital herpes has been described in Sumerian literature (127). Greek scholars, particularly Hippocrates, used the word "herpes," meaning to creep or crawl, to describe the spreading nature of skin lesions (158). Herodotus associated mouth ulcers and lip vesicles with fever and called it "herpes febrilis." Many of these original observations likely emanated from Galen's deduction that the appearance of lesions was an attempt by the body to rid itself of evil humors, leading to the description "herpes excretins" (158). These original descriptions of skin lesions probably bear little resemblance to reports of the 19th and 20th centuries.

As noted by Wildy (158), Shakespeare wrote of recurrent HSV labial lesions. In *Romeo and Juliet,* Queen Mab, the midwife of the fairies, stated: "O'er ladies lips, who straight on kisses dream, which oft the angry Mab with blisters plagues, because their breaths with sweetmeats tainted are." In the 18th century, Astruc, physician to King Louis XIV, associated herpetic lesions with genital infection. By the early 19th century, the vesicular nature of lesions associated with herpetic infections was well characterized. However, it was not until 1893 that Vidal specifically recognized person-to-person transmission of HSV infections (158).

By the beginning of the 20th century, histopathological studies described multinucleated giant cells associated with infection, and the infectivity of HSV was established by transmission of virus from humans to the cornea of the rabbit, resulting in keratitis. Reports through the 1960s focused on the biological manifestations of HSV infection and the natural history of human disease. The host range of HSV was expanded to include a variety of laboratory animals, chicken embryos, and cell culture systems. Expanded animal studies demonstrated that not only could human virus be transmitted to the rabbit, as noted above, but also transmission of human virus could lead to infections of the skin or the central nervous system (CNS) (151, 154).

Host immune responses to HSV defined the presence of neutralizing antibodies to HSV in the serum of newly and previously infected children and adults (40). Subsequently, some seropositive individuals developed recurrent labial lesions, albeit less severe than those associated with the initial episode. This observation led to the recognition of a unique biological property of HSV, namely, the ability of these viruses to recur in the presence of humoral immunity—a characteristic known as reactivation of latent infection. The spectrum of disease was expanded to include primary and recurrent infections of mucous membranes (e.g., gingivostomatitis, herpes labialis, and genital HSV infections), keratoconjunctivitis, neonatal HSV infection, visceral HSV infections of the immunocompromised host, HSV encephalitis, Kaposi's varicella-like eruption, and an association with erythema multiforme.

Among many important laboratory advances was the detection of antigenic differences between HSV types (95). HSV type 1 (HSV-1) was more frequently associated with nongenital infection (infection above the belt), while HSV-2 was associated with genital disease (infection below the belt). This knowledge provided a foundation for many of the studies performed during the latter part of the 20th century. Interestingly, over the past decade, HSV-1 and -2 have been found in both the mouth and the genital tract.

INFECTIOUS AGENT

Virion Structure

HSVs belong to the family *Herpesviridae*. The >100 known members of this family share the structure of their virions, general features of their reproductive cycle, and the capacity to remain latent. They differ, however, in many respects, and they have been classified into three subfamilies with respect to the details of their replication, the cells in which they remain latent, gene content, and gene organization. HSVs belong to the subfamily *Alphaherpesvirindae* (119).

The HSV virion consists of four concentric components; from the center out, these are (i) an electron-dense core containing viral DNA, (ii) an icosadeltahedral capsid consisting of capsomeres (114), (iii) an amorphous layer of proteins designated tegument and which surrounds the capsid, and (iv) an envelope containing lipid and polyamines and studded with at least 10 viral glycoproteins and several nonglycosylated membrane proteins. HSVs are members of a family of viruses whose genomes consist of a single large double-strand molecule (114, 116). The HSV genome has a molecular mass of approximately 10^8 Da and consists of an excess of 152 kb (depending on the number of terminal repeats). The base composition of G+C is 68% for HSV-1 and 69% for HSV-2. The HSV-1 and HSV-2 genomes encode at least 84 different polypeptides (87, 114). The DNAs consist of two covalently linked components, long and short (L and S), each consisting of stretches of unique sequences designated U_L and U_S flanked by the inverted repeats ab and ca, respectively. The two components invert relative to each other to yield four populations of molecules differing solely in the relative orientation of these DNA sequences (57).

HSV encodes at least 90 transcripts, of which 84 are translated into unique proteins. Of this number, 46 are dispensable for viral replication in at least some cultivated cells in vitro. The function of many of these dispensable genes is to render viral replication and spread more efficient or to block host responses to infection (114, 115). Importantly, these genes are not truly dispensable, since viruses lacking these genes have not been isolated from humans. Viruses from which these genes have been deleted by genetic engineering frequently exhibit a reduced capacity to multiply and spread in experimental animals (114, 115). Indeed, the observation that so many HSV genes are dispensable and can be replaced by non-HSV genes sustains the expectation that a live attenuated vaccine capable of acting as a vector for foreign gene expression is feasible.

Since viral proteins studied to date have been found to perform several functions, it is likely that HSV encodes several hundred functions expressed by adjacent or overlapping amino acid blocks. Each function is performed at a particular time during replication and at an intracellular location that may be determined by posttranslational modifications and protein partners with differential affinity of the modified proteins. Modifications include phosphorylation by cellular (e.g., cdc2) or viral (U_L13 and U_S3) protein kinases, nucleotidylation by casein kinase 2, poly(ADD-ribosyl)ation, and others. U_L13, a key viral protein kinase, is homologous to the U_L97 protein kinase of human cytomegalovirus and a potential target of antiviral chemotherapy.

Although they differ with respect to nucleotide sequence, restriction endonuclease cleavage sites, and apparent sizes of many viral proteins they encode, the HSV-1 and HSV-2 genomes are collinear and readily form intertypic recombinants in the laboratory (57).

Viral Replication

To initiate infection, HSV must attach to cell surface receptors, fuse its envelope to the plasma membrane, and allow the de-enveloped core to be transported to the nuclear pores. Viral surface glycoproteins mediate attachment and penetration of the virus into cells. They also elicit a protective host immune response to the virus. Currently, there are 12 viral glycoproteins, designated gB, gC, gD, gE, gG, gH, gI, gJ, gK, gL, gM, and gN. Of these, gB and gC are required for the initial interaction of the virion with heparin-sulfated proteoglycans, gD is required for the subsequent interaction with its receptor, and gB, gD, gH, and gL mediate the fusion of the envelope with the plasma membrane. gE and gI form a portion of the Fc receptor. The function of other glycoproteins is not fully understood. To date, three cellular receptors have been described. These are HveA, a member of the tumor necrosis factor alpha receptor family; Nectin1, a member of the extended immunoglobulin family; and a modified heparin-sulfated proteoglycan. Of the three, HveA is the major receptor enabling infection of human cells with HSV (49, 114).

At the nuclear pore, the DNA is released into the nucleus. The key events in viral replication (transcription, DNA synthesis, capsid assembly, DNA packaging, and envelopment) take place in the nucleus (Fig. 1) (114). The stage for effective viral replication is set by the tegument protein. Of these, one (α-TIF or VP16) enhances the transcription of α or immediate-early genes, the first set of viral genes expressed after infection. A second protein induces the degradation of mRNA during the early stages of viral replication, thereby blocking the induction of cellular genes during infection. Of the six α proteins, five regulate viral gene expression and, at the same time, modify many key functions of the host cell, whereas one blocks the presentation of antigenic peptides on infected cell surfaces. Functional α proteins are required for the second and third rounds of transcription of the viral genome, yielding β (early) and γ (late) proteins, respectively.

Most of the β proteins function to assist viral nucleic acid metabolism. Thus, at least seven viral proteins and most likely additional host factors are required for the synthesis of viral DNA by a rolling-circle mechanism which yields endless, head-to-tail concatemers. Other viral proteins increase the pool of deoxyribonucleotides, repair viral DNA, and perform other functions. Still other members of this class of proteins, particularly viral protein kinases, posttranslationally alter viral proteins primarily to modify their function (114). β proteins are the main target of antiviral chemotherapy. Thus, viral thymidine kinase selectively phosphorylates most antiviral nucleoside analogs, and these and other nucleoside triphosphates block or reduce the capacity of the viral DNA polymerase to synthesize viral DNA.

The genes expressed next encode proteins involved primarily in the assembly of virions, packaging of DNA, and egress from the infected cell (114). Capsid assembly takes place in steps. First, a procapsid is formed from scaffolding proteins (a protease and its substrate) and capsid proteins. Next, the newly synthesized DNA is packaged and cleaved into unit length molecules. In the process, the scaffolding protein is cleaved and extruded from the capsid. Envelopment favors capsids containing DNA. Capsids containing DNA attach to the nuclear surface of the inner nuclear membrane and are rapidly enveloped and released into the space between the inner and outer nuclear membranes. The mechanism by which the virus is transported through the cytoplasm is a subject of intense debate. The single-envelopment theory is that virions become enveloped at two sites. Early in infection, capsids are enveloped at the inner nuclear membrane and are transported through the Golgi network in vesicles derived from the outer nuclear membrane. Later in infection, the nuclear pore becomes enlarged and capsids in large numbers are transported through the nuclear pore and are enveloped at cytoplasmic vesicles. The double-envelopment theory holds that the virions enveloped at the inner nuclear membrane become de-enveloped at the outer membrane and are then re-enveloped in the cytoplasm. Exocytosis is aided by the development of multivesicular bodies. Viral replication takes approximately 18 h.

Viral replication is highly deleterious to the integrity of the infected cell. Thus, cellular chromosomes are marginated to the nuclear membrane and degraded, the nucleolus falls apart, the Golgi complex is fragmented and dispersed,

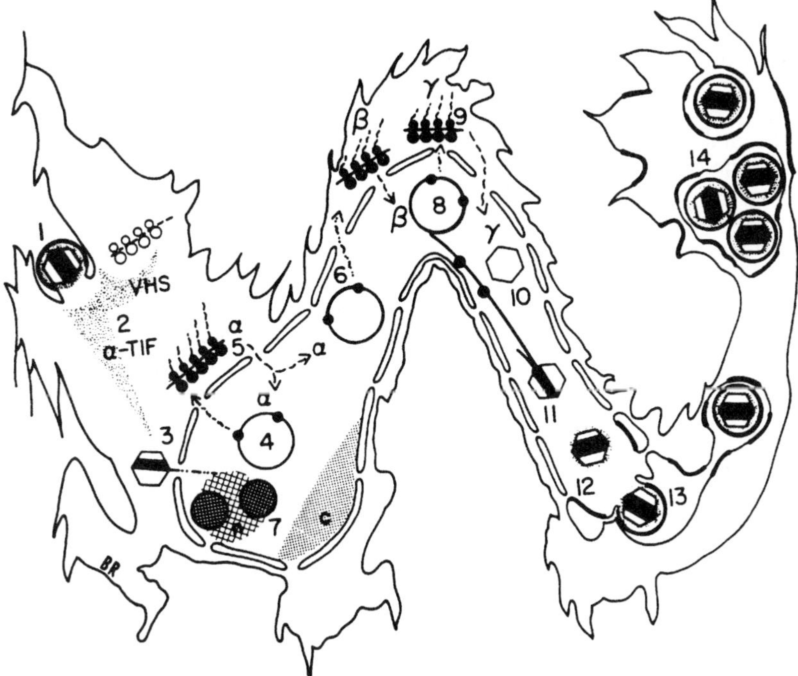

FIGURE 1 Schematic representation of the replication of HSVs in susceptible cells. 1, The virus initiates infection by fusion of the viral envelope with the plasma membrane following attachment to the cell surface. 2, Fusion of the membranes releases two proteins from the virion. VHS shuts off protein synthesis (broken RNA in open polyribosomes). α-TIF (the α gene *trans*-inducing factor) is transported to the nucleus. 3, The capsid is transported to the nuclear pore, where viral DNA is released into the nucleus and immediately circularizes. 4, The transcription of α genes by cellular enzymes is induced by α-TIF. 5, The five α mRNAs are transported into the cytoplasm and translated (filled polyribosome); the proteins are transported into the nucleus. 6, A new round of transcription results in the synthesis of β proteins. 7, At this stage in the infection, the chromatin (c) is degraded and displaced toward the nuclear membrane, whereas the nucleoli (round hatched structures) become disaggregated. 8, Viral DNA is replicated by a rolling-circle mechanism which yields head-to-tail concatemers of unit length viral DNA. 9, A new round of transcription/translation yields the γ proteins, consisting primarily of structural proteins of the virus. 10, The capsid proteins form empty capsids. 11, Unit length viral DNA is cleaved from concatemers and packaged into the preformed capsids. 12, Capsids containing viral DNA acquire a new protein. 13, Viral glycoproteins and tegument proteins accumulate and form patches in cellular membranes. The capsids containing DNA and the additional protein attach to the underside of the membrane patches containing viral proteins and are enveloped. 14, The enveloped proteins accumulate in the endoplasmic reticulum and are transported into the extracellular space. BR, Bernard Roizman. (Reprinted from reference 118 with permission.)

and the microtubules are rearranged. All of these events are designed to provide the precursors necessary for viral DNA synthesis to prevent a host response to infection and to enhance the capacity of the infected cell to export virions (114).

Several aspects of the viral replication cycle are relevant to the pathogenesis of human disease and to the present and future developments for antiviral chemotherapy (114). Specifically, HSV-1 and HSV-2 bring into cells at least 12 viral proteins (the tegument) whose function is to enable viral replication and shutoff of host responses to infection. The transcription of α genes, as noted above, is enhanced by the interaction of the tegument protein VP16 (α-TIF) with cellular transcriptional factors Oct1 and HCF1. Another tegument protein, virion host shutoff (VHS) encoded by the UL41 gene, acts as an RNase to selectively degrade mRNAs. The basis of the selectivity is not known, but the targets of the RNase appear to be mRNAs of housekeeping genes and of genes activated by host responses to infection. The six α proteins regulate viral replication and block host responses to infection. ICP4 acts as a repressor by binding to the transcription initiation sites of selected genes and as a transcriptional activator by a mechanism that remains to be fully understood. ICP0 has at least two sets of major functions. Early in infection, it blocks CoREST/REST/HDAC1 or -2, a major cellular repressor system, from silencing viral DNA. At the same time, it acts as a ubiquitin ligase to degrade several SP100, DNA-dependent protein kinases, and the summoylated forms of promyelocytic leukemia protein and disperse the ND10 nuclear bodies. At least one objective of this function is to block exogenous interferon from blocking viral replication—a function mediated by the ND10 bodies. ICP22 and $U_S1.5$ also perform several functions. The key apparent function is to enable efficient synthesis of late proteins. ICP27 performs at least two functions. Early in infection, ICP27 interferes with RNA splicing, and consequently, unspliced mRNAs are transported to the cytoplasm but are not translated. Late in infection, ICP27 shuttles viral mRNA from the nucleus to the cytoplasm. Lastly, cells frequently target a large fraction of newly made protein to proteasomal degradation. The peptide products of proteasomal proteolysis are transported to the endoplasmic reticulum, where they are loaded onto major histocompatibility complex class I molecules and presented to the immune system. Another α protein, encoded by the α47 gene, blocks the transport of peptide into the endoplasmic reticulum by binding to the TAP1 and TAP2 transport proteins.

Several proteins made later in infection are of particular interest. Of the HSV proteins involved in nucleic metabolism, thymidine kinase (TK), ribonucleotide reductase, dUTPase, and uracyl DNA glucosylase are dispensable for viral replication in dividing cells but are required for viral DNA synthesis in nondividing cells. Of this group, polymerase and TK are the targets of current antiviral chemotherapeutic agents. Other genes, notably, the ribonucleotide reductase gene, have been deleted in vectors designed for oncolysis of CNS tumors. The group of proteins involved in packaging DNA, most notably, the protease, its substrate, and the proteins encoded by U_L15 and U_L28, are candidates for targeting of the next generation of nonnucleoside antiviral drugs.

Enhanced expression of late genes after the onset of viral DNA synthesis results in activation of protein kinase R (PKR), possibly as a result of accumulation of double-stranded RNA. A consequence of activation of PKR is the phosphorylation of the translation initiation factor eIF2α and total shutoff of protein synthesis. A viral protein, $\gamma_1$34.5, recruits phosphatase 1α to dephosphorylate eIF2α, enabling uninterrupted protein synthesis. One function of activated PKR is to activate NF-κB. Current evidence suggests that while activation of NF-κB results in the synthesis of proteins that enhance viral replication, a vast majority of the transcripts induced by the activated NF-κB are degraded by the VHS RNase.

gD and gJ and the protein kinase encoded by the U_S3 gene each in its own way block activation of programmed cell death. Thus, viral entry by endocytosis can trigger discharge of lysosomal enzymes. At a high multiplicity of infection, the lysosomal discharge causes apoptosis. gD blocks the discharge, as does chloroquine or overexpression of cation-independent 6 mannose receptor. Independently, apoptosis is also induced by an absence of late gene expression, as in cells infected with mutants lacking ICP4 or ICP27. Overexpression of U_S3 protein kinase blocks apoptosis induced by defective viruses as well as overexpression of proapoptotic genes, hyperthermia, osmotic shock, etc.

The remarkable features of HSV replication are the number and diversity of viral functions designed to block host innate and adaptive immunity; for example, the interferon pathways are blocked by ICP0, ICP27, VHS RNase, the U_S3 kinase, and the $\gamma_1$34.5 gene product. Each of the corresponding genes targets a different component of the interferon pathways. As noted in this brief introduction to the biology of HSV, the virus also blocks silencing of viral DNA by host chromatin modifiers (VP16, ICP0, and U_S3 kinase), blocks the synthesis of proteins potentially inimical to viral replication (VHS RNase and ICP27), blocks attempts by the cell to commit suicide (apoptosis) to preclude viral replication (U_S3, gD, and gJ), degrades potentially inimical host proteins (ICP0), and blocks presentation of antigenic peptides to the cell surface (ICP47). The most remarkable aspect of this list is that it is based on intense studies of just a handful of viral proteins. We still do not know the function of many proteins and noncoding RNAs encoded by the virus.

Neurovirulence and Latency

HSV-1 and HSV-2 exhibit two unique biological properties that influence human disease. These viruses have the capacity to invade and replicate in the CNS and the capacity to establish a latent infection. Alphaherpesviruses, including HSV and varicella-zoster virus, establish latent infection in dorsal root ganglia (116).

The term neurovirulence encompasses both neuroinvasiveness from peripheral sites and replication in neuronal cells. When paired isolates (brain and lip) from patients with HSV encephalitis are evaluated by PFU/50% lethal dose ratios following direct intracerebral inoculation in mice, the encephalitis isolates are found to have lower PFU/50% lethal dose ratios than isolates from lip lesions. Neurovirulence appears to be the function of numerous genes (114). In fact, deletion of virtually any of the genes dispensable for viral replication in cell culture reduces the capacity of the virus to invade and replicate in the CNS. Mutations affecting neuroinvasiveness have also been mapped in genes encoding glycoproteins. Access to neuronal cells from usual portals of entry into the body requires postsynaptic transmission of virus and, therefore, a particularly vigorous capacity to multiply and to direct the virions to appropriate membranes. In addition, since neuronal cells are terminally differentiated and do not make cellular DNA, they lack the precursors for viral DNA synthesis that are also encoded by the viral genes dispensable for growth in cell culture. Of particular interest, however, is the role of the $\gamma_1$34.5 gene in neurovirulence (28, 29, 59, 152). Although $\gamma_1$34.5 deletion mutants multiply well in a variety of cells in culture, they are among the most avirulent mutants identified to date in vivo.

Latency has been recognized biologically since the beginning of the 20th century (8, 9, 138) and has been extensively reviewed (98, 114, 117). Following entry, both HSV-1 and HSV-2 infect nerve endings and translocate by retrograde transport to the nuclei of sensory ganglia. The virus multiplies in a small number of sensory neurons, which are ultimately destroyed. In the vast majority of the infected neurons, the viral genome remains for the entire life of the individual in an episomal state. In a fraction of individuals, the virus reactivates and is moved by anterograde transport to a site at or near the portal of entry. Reactivations occur following a variety of local or systemic stimuli.

Patients treated for trigeminal neuralgia by sectioning a branch of that nerve develop herpetic lesions along the innervated areas of the sectioned branch (25, 38, 52, 105). Reactivation of latent virus appears to be dependent upon an intact anterior nerve route and peripheral nerve pathways. Latent virus can be retrieved from the trigeminal, sacral, and vagal ganglia of humans either unilaterally or bilaterally (9). The recovery of virus by in vitro cultivation of trigeminal ganglia helps explain the observation of vesicles that recur at the same site in humans, usually the vermilion border of the lip. Recurrences occur in the presence of both cell-mediated and humoral immunity. Recurrences are spontaneous, but there is an association with physical or emotional stress, fever, and exposure to UV light, tissue damage, and immunosuppression. Recurrent herpes labialis is three times more frequent in febrile patients than in nonfebrile controls (8, 117, 128).

Little is known regarding the mechanisms by which the virus establishes and maintains a latent state or is reactivated. There are in fact disagreements on the fate of neurons in which latent virus became reactivated. The relevant issues can be summarized as follows.

1. Sensory neurons harboring virus contain nuclear transcripts arising from approximately 8.5 kbp of the sequences flanking the U_L sequence. These transcripts are known as the latency-associated transcripts (LATs). A shorter region is more abundantly represented in the nuclei. The RNA transcribed from this region forms two populations, 2 and 1.5 kbp, and represents stable introns of an unknown and relatively unstable transcript. The abundant 2.5- and 1.5-kbp RNAs play no role in the establishment or maintenance of the latent state, although they may play a role in reactivation. These LATs appear to block the death of neurons harboring latent virus. The mechanism by which LATs maintain the viability of latently infected neurons is unclear. The hypothesis that the RNAs silence viral gene expression is consistent with some, but not all, published data.

Since latency is established and the virus reactivates only in sensory neurons, at least a portion of the genetic information resides in these cells. A prevailing hypothesis is that at the time of entry of the virus into neurons, a fraction of the neurons express LATs and silence all viral gene expression except the synthesis of LATs. Consistent with this model, all of the deletion mutants tested to date establish latency, but not all reactivate. In contrast to the viral requirements for the establishment of latency, the activation of viral gene expression that leads to viral replication does require a full complement of viral genes.

2. There are three fundamental issues that are central to a better understanding of the establishment and reactivation of virus from the latent state. The first concerns the observation that not all neurons reactivate at once as in the case of zoster. Asynchronous reactivation would be expected following activation of sensory neurons by exposure of skin to UV light but not after systemic activation (e.g., hormones and menstruation). The second issue stems from the observation that, at least in cell culture, the virus destroys the cells in which it replicates. The hallmark of cutaneous HSV infection is tissue destruction. Nevertheless, HSV reactivates frequently at the same site. Furthermore, studies on genital tissues in women confirmed a long-standing view that the number of clinically inapparent reactivations far exceeds the number of clinically proven recrudescences. Frequent destruction of sensory neurons would result in anesthesia of the sites of frequent recurrences, but this is not the case. These observations raised the question of whether, in contrast to cutaneous or CNS lesions, infected neurons survive reactivation. Lastly, a legitimate question raised in at least one study is whether the frequency of reactivations is genetically determined by the host. The affirmative conclusion will no doubt be revisited in the future.

EPIDEMIOLOGY

Orolabial HSV Infections

Although HSV-1 and HSV-2 are usually transmitted by different routes and may involve different body sites, there is a great deal of overlap between their epidemiology and clinical manifestations. These viruses are distributed worldwide and occur in both developed and underdeveloped countries, including among remote Brazilian tribes (13). Animal vectors for human HSV infections have not been described; therefore, humans remain the sole reservoir for transmission to other humans. Virus is transmitted from infected to susceptible individuals during close personal contact. There is no seasonal variation in the incidence of infection. Because infection is rarely fatal and HSV becomes latent, over one-third of the world's population have recurrent HSV infections and, therefore, the capability of transmitting HSV during episodes of productive infection.

Geographic location, socioeconomic status, and age influence the prevalence of HSV-1 infection (40, 126). In developing countries, infection indicated by seroconversion occurs early in life. Among Brazilian Indians and children of New Orleans, LA, HSV antibodies develop in over 95% of children by the age of 15 (6). In populations with a lower socioeconomic status, approximately one-third of children seroconvert by 5 years of age; this frequency increases to 70 to 80% by early adolescence. Middle-class individuals of industrialized societies acquire antibodies later in life such that seroconversion over the first 5 years occurs in 20% of children, followed by no significant increase until the second and third decades of life, at which time the prevalence of antibodies increases to 40 and 60%, respectively (51). Seroconversion of susceptible university students occurs at an annual frequency of approximately 5 to 10% (51).

Data on the seroprevalence of HSV-1 and HSV-2 infections in the United States are illuminating (Fig. 2) (65, 97). By the age of 5, over 35% of African-American children, versus 18% of Caucasian children, were found to be infected by HSV-1. Through adolescence, African-Americans had approximately a twofold-higher prevalence of antibodies to HSV-1 than Caucasians, and females had a slightly higher prevalence of HSV-1 antibodies than males. By the age of 40, African-Americans and Caucasians had similar prevalences of antibodies. The high prevalence of antibodies appearing later in life may be the consequence of a cohort effect; namely, these individuals had a higher rate of acquisition of HSV-1 earlier in life.

Seroprevalence worldwide shows a high rate of geographic variation. An HSV-1 antibody prevalence of less than 70% is found in populations residing in Pittsburgh, PA; Birmingham, AL; Atlanta, GA; Japan; Lyon, France; and Sweden and among Caucasian Americans (U.S. National Health and Nutrition Examination Survey [NHANES] participants). Antibody prevalence in excess of 95% has been detected in Spain, Italy, Rwanda, Zaire, Senegal, China, Taiwan, Haiti, Jamaica, and Costa Rica for adults between the ages of 20 and 40. The largest reservoir of HSV infections in the community is recurrent herpes labialis. A positive history of recurrent herpes labialis was noted in 38% of 1,800 graduate students in Philadelphia, PA (130). New lesions occurred at a frequency of one per month in 5% of the students and at intervals of 2 to 11 months in 34% of the students. Recurrences of one per year or less often were found in 61%. Over the past several

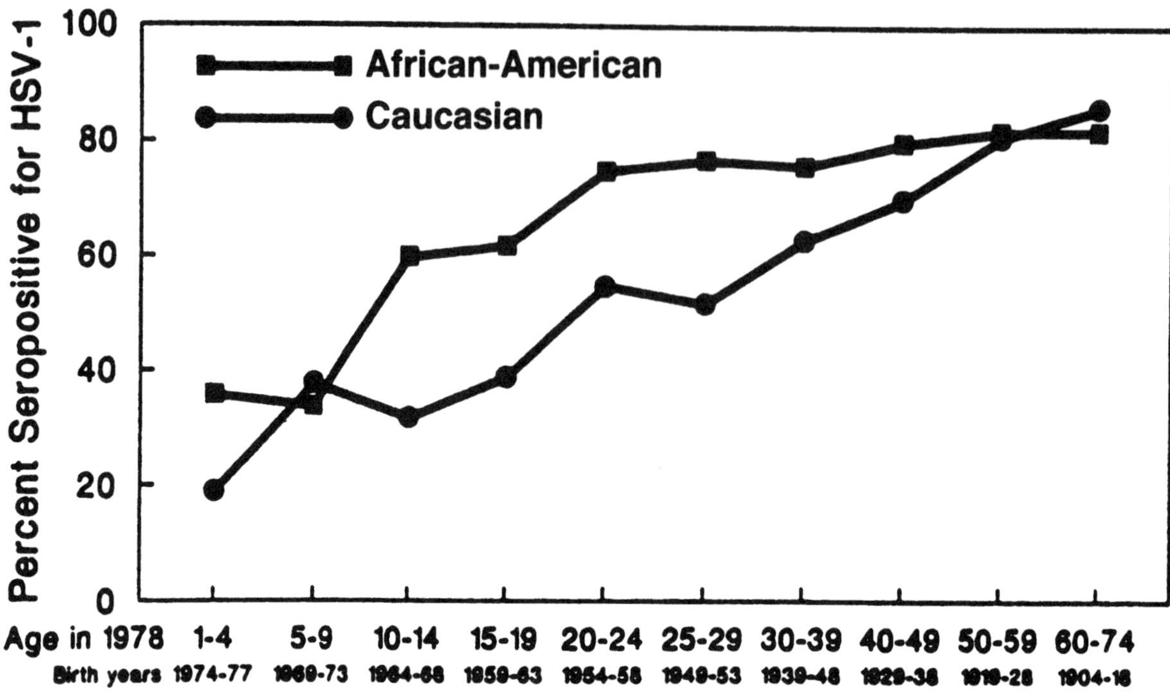

FIGURE 2 Seroprevalence of HSV-1 and HSV-2 by age.

years, HSV-2 infections of the oropharynx have been recognized in both immunocompetent and immunocompromised hosts (162).

Outbreaks of HSV-1

Clustered human outbreaks of HSV infections have been reported (126), but there is no indication from either clinical or molecular epidemiological studies that HSV causes epidemics. Most of the studies involve families in which several individuals suffer from HSV infection at approximately the same time, perhaps through exposure to recurrent labial lesions of one family member. While hospital outbreaks have occurred, no commonality can be determined. An outbreak of eczema herpeticum was reported to occur in a large group of hospitalized patients within an 8-day period; in this case, the lack of attention to infection control procedures (e.g., handwashing) was incriminated as being responsible for virus transmission. Outbreaks of herpetic stomatitis have been reported to occur in a dentist's office and within orphanages (54), where attack rates for apparent infection were approximately 75% among susceptible children. Increased transmission of HSV in day care centers has not yet been reported (125).

Genital HSV Infections

Because genital HSV infections are usually acquired through sexual contact, antibodies to HSV-2, at least, are rarely found before the age of onset of sexual activity (66). Although most recurrent genital HSV infections are caused by HSV-2, an ever-increasing proportion of primary acquisition is attributable to HSV-1 (32). The differentiation in virus type is significant, since genital HSV-1 infections are usually both less severe clinically and significantly less prone to recur (32, 112). The number of new cases of genital HSV infections has been conservatively estimated to be approximately 500,000 annually. Predicated upon newer serologic methods for detection of prior HSV-2 infection, a range of 40 million to 60 million Americans are infected with HSV-2 (80).

Seroprevalence of HSV-2 increases from 5.6% between 12 and 19 years of age to 24.3% by the age of 60. Analysis by race shows that 4.5 and 8.7% of Caucasians and 18.2 and 76.8% of African-Americans in the 12 to 19 and >20 age groups, respectively, had HSV-2 antibodies. Factors found to influence acquisition of HSV-2 include gender (women greater than men), race (blacks more than whites), marital status (divorced more than single or married), and place of residence (city more than suburb) (46). These data represent a 20% increase in genital herpes between NHANES II (1976 to 1980) and NHANES III (1988) (Fig. 3). A more recent study (NHANES IV) indicates slightly lower HSV-2 seroprevalence rates, but the difference is not of great significance (159). Seroprevalence studies indicated that the highest prevalence of antibodies to HSV-2 in the United States is in female prostitutes (75%) and that the seroprevalence is virtually identical to that of prostitutes in Tokyo, Japan (16, 72, 97, 122). Seropositivity among female prostitutes in Dakar, Senegal, was even higher, 95.7%, in 1985. Homosexual men have HSV-2 seroprevalence rates varying from a high of 83.1% in San Francisco, CA (1985–1986), to lows of 21.6% in Seville, Spain (1985–1986); 24.2% in Tokyo (1988); and 50.0% in Amsterdam, The Netherlands (1986).

The number of different sexual partners correlates directly with acquisition of HSV-2 (Fig. 4). For heterosexual women living in the United States with one partner, the probability of acquisition of HSV-2 is less than 10%, but it increases to 40, 62, and greater than 80% as the number of lifetime sexual partners increases to 2 to 10, 11 to 50, and greater than 50, respectively. For heterosexual men, similar data are 0% for one lifetime sexual partner and 20,

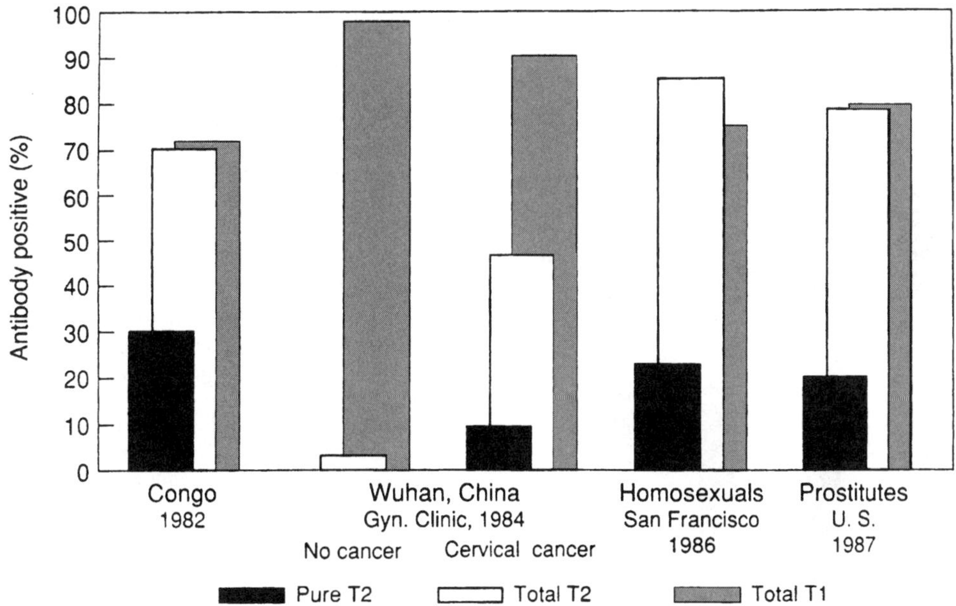

FIGURE 3 Seroprevalence of HSV-1 and HSV-2 by selected country. T2, HSV-2 antibodies; T1, HSV-1 antibodies. (Reprinted from reference 97 with permission.)

35, and 70% for each of the three risk groups, respectively. In contrast, for homosexual men, seroprevalence increases from greater than 60 to 90% for those with 11 to 50 and greater than 50 partners. Thus, having multiple sexual partners, irrespective of sexual preference, correlates directly with acquisition of HSV-2 infection (97). As with HSV-1 infections of the mouth, HSV-2 is excreted more frequently in the absence of symptoms at the time of primary, initial, or recurrent infection (44, 111, 146), providing a silent reservoir for transmission. The frequency of clinical recurrences varies somewhat between males and females, with rates of 2.7 and 1.9 per 100 days, respectively (32). Recurrences are most frequent in the year immediately following acquisition and tend to decrease somewhat over subsequent years. Several studies have implicated a frequency of clinical recurrences as high as 60%. Genital infections by HSV-1 recur less frequently than those caused by HSV-2 (75, 112). Following the first episode of genital herpes, asymptomatic shedding was detected in approximately 12, 18, and 23% of women with primary HSV-1, primary HSV-2, and nonprimary HSV-2 infection, respectively (70). For women with established genital HSV-2 infection, asymptomatic shedding was detected on 1% of all days cultures were obtained (17, 146). However, more contemporary studies indicate that only 20 to 25% of women who are HSV-2 seropositive have symptoms of genital herpes (73, 74). With the application of PCR to the serial evaluation of genital swabs from women with genital infection, the frequency of shedding of HSV DNA is even higher, suggesting that HSV is a chronic infection rather than an intermittent one (145). Indeed, HSV DNA can be detected on up to 20% of all days for women with HSV-2 infection. Similar shedding data will be found for HSV-1 oropharyngeal infection (162).

Prospective studies of the incidence of HSV-2 infection indicate that among low-risk individuals, namely, college students, the rate of acquisition was approximately 2% per year over 4 years, compared to 4% per year for homosexual men in San Francisco (97). The incidence of HSV-2 infection during pregnancy is about 2.5% per gestation but may be as low as 0.58%. The rate of acquisition of HSV-2 infection between monogamous sexual partners with discordant infection status is 10 to 15% yearly (90).

HSV-2 infection, by the nature of being an ulcerative disease, is associated with acquisition of HIV-1. Most case control studies performed in the United States and Central Africa indicate increased relative risks by a factor of 1.5 to >2 (60, 61, 97, 134). Further, concomitant infection is associated with higher plasma human immunodeficiency virus (HIV) RNA levels that can be decreased with HSV therapy (86, 124). The association between acquisition of HIV and HSV-2 was also documented for heterosexual populations (61).

Genital HSV infection in pregnant women is not uncommon but must be considered separately from that in nonpregnant populations because of the risk to the fetus and newborn. Recurrent infection is the most common form of infection during pregnancy. Transmission of infection to the fetus is related to shedding of virus at the time of delivery. The prevalence of viral excretion, as determined by culture, at delivery is 0.01 to 0.39% for all women, irrespective of history (111), with rates as high as 0.6% (18). In a predominantly white, middle-class population, documented recurrent infection occurred in 84% of pregnant women with a history of recurrent disease. Asymptomatic viral shedding occurred in at least 12% of the recurrent episodes. Viral shedding from the cervix occurred in 0.56% of symptomatic infections, versus 0.66% of asymptomatic infections (111). The prevalence of cervical shedding in pregnant women with asymptomatic HSV infection averages approximately 3%. However, the observed rate for these women varies more than that among nonpregnant women (from 0.2 to 7.4%), depending upon the study population and trial design (53, 111).

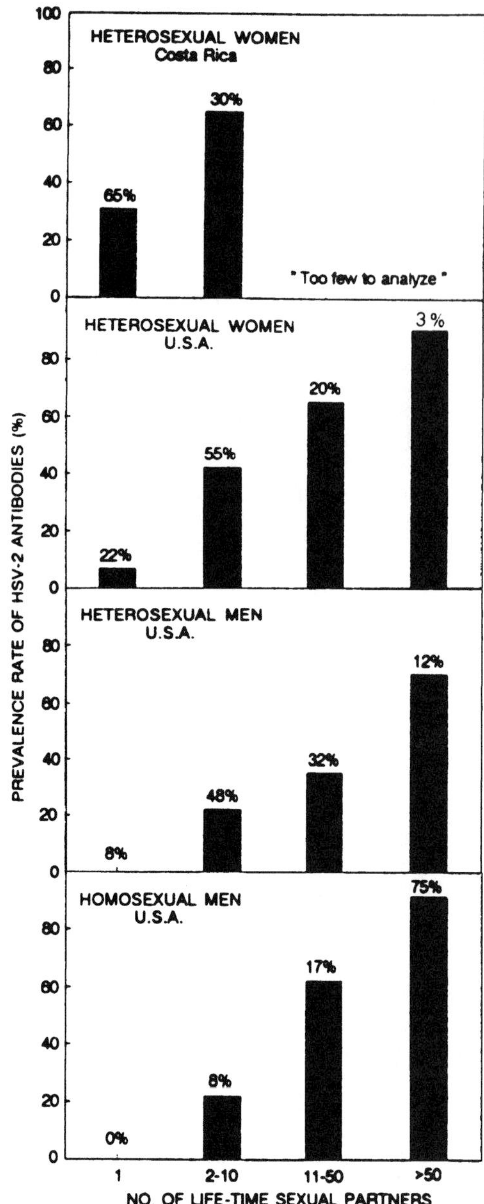

FIGURE 4 Seroprevalence of HSV-2 as a function of the number of sexual partners. Numbers above bars indicate percentages of population. (Reprinted from reference 97 with permission.)

PATHOLOGY AND PATHOGENESIS

Pathology

The histopathological characteristics of a primary or recurrent HSV infection (Fig. 5) reflect virus-mediated cellular death and associated inflammatory response. Viral infection induces ballooning of cells with condensed chromatin within the nuclei of cells, followed by nuclear degeneration, generally within parabasal and intermediate cells of the epithelium. Cells lose intact plasma membranes and form multinucleated giant cells. With cell lysis, a clear (referred to as vesicular) fluid containing large quantities of virus appears between the epidermis and dermal layer. The vesicular fluid contains cell debris, inflammatory cells, and, often, multinucleated giant cells. In dermal substructures there is an intense inflammatory response, usually in the corium of the skin, more so with primary infection than with recurrent infection. With healing, the vesicular fluid becomes pustular with the recruitment of inflammatory cells and scabs. Scarring is uncommon. When mucous membranes are involved, vesicles are replaced by shallow ulcers.

Pathogenesis

The transmission of human infection is dependent upon intimate, personal contact between a susceptible seronegative individual with someone excreting HSV. Virus must come in contact with mucosal surfaces or abraded skin for infection to be initiated. With viral replication at the site of infection, either an intact virion or, more simply, the capsid is transported retrograde by neurons to the dorsal root ganglia, where, after another round of viral replication, latency is established (Fig. 6). The more severe the primary infection, as reflected by the size, number, and extent of lesions, the more likely it is that recurrences will ensue. Although replication sometimes leads to disease and infrequently results in life-threatening infection (e.g., encephalitis), the host-virus interaction leading to latency predominates. After latency is established, a proper stimulus causes reactivation; virus becomes evident at mucocutaneous sites, appearing as skin vesicles or mucosal ulcers (Fig. 7).

Infection with HSV-1 generally occurs in the oropharyngeal mucosa. The trigeminal ganglion becomes colonized and harbors latent virus. Acquisition of HSV-2 infection is usually the consequence of transmission by genital contact; however, genital oral spread is increasingly common and results in alternative modes of transmission from mucous membrane to mucous membrane. Virus replicates in the genital, perigenital, or anal skin sites with seeding of the sacral ganglia (Fig. 8).

Operative definitions of the nature of the infection are of pathogenic relevance. Susceptible individuals (namely, those without preexisting HSV antibodies) develop primary infection after the first exposure to either HSV-1 or HSV-2. A recurrence of HSV is known as recurrent infection. Initial infection occurs when an individual with preexisting antibodies to one type of HSV (namely, HSV-1 or HSV-2) can experience a first infection with the opposite virus type (namely, HSV-2 or HSV-1, respectively). Reinfection with a different strain of HSV can occur, albeit extremely uncommonly in the healthy host, and is called exogenous reinfection.

Exogenous Reinfection

Cleavage of HSV DNA by restriction endonuclease enzymes yields a characteristic pattern of subgenomic products. Analyses of numerous HSV-1 and HSV-2 isolates from a variety of clinical situations and widely divergent geographic areas demonstrate that epidemiologically unrelated strains yield distinct HSV DNA fragment patterns. In contrast, fragments of HSV DNA derived from the same individual obtained years apart, from monogamous sexual partners, or following short and long passages in vitro have identical fragments after restriction endonuclease cleavage (21). As determined by utilizing endonuclease technology, the rate of exogenous reinfection is exceedingly low in immunocompetent hosts.

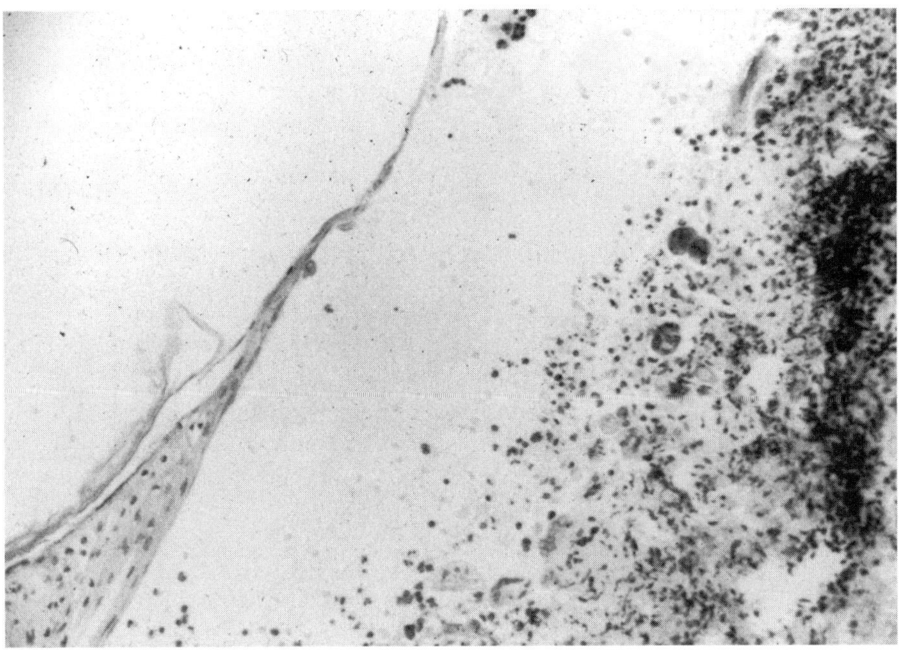

FIGURE 5 Histopathology of HSV infection.

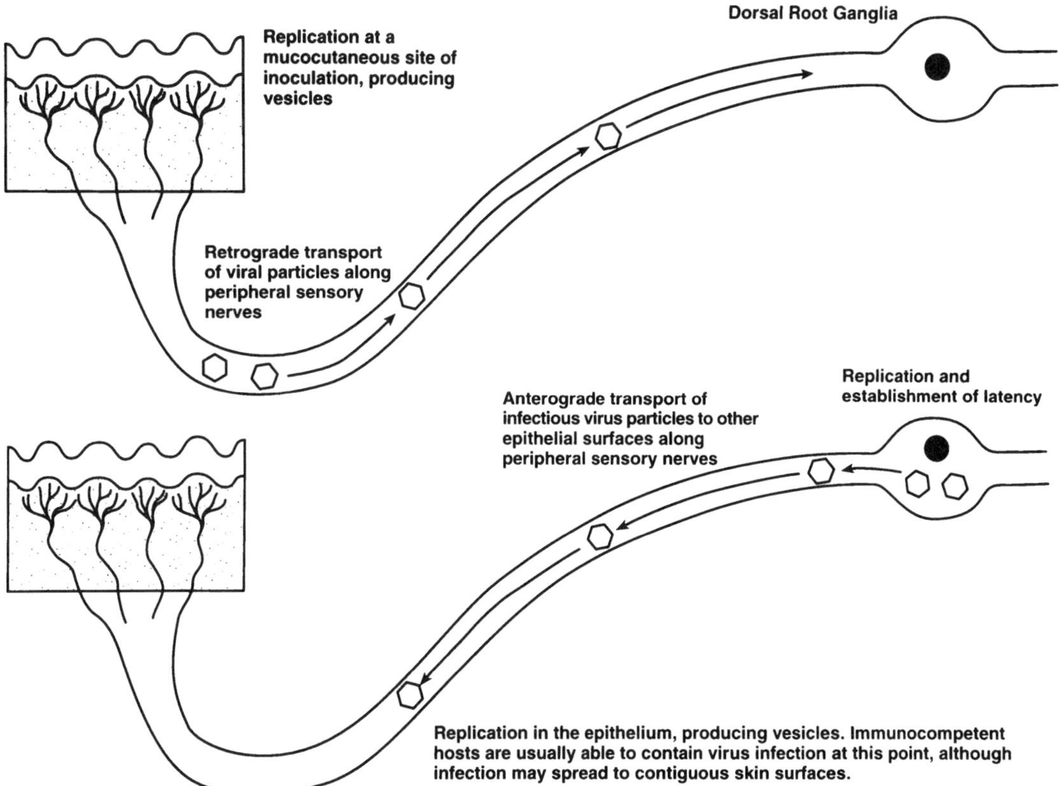

FIGURE 6 Schematic diagram of primary HSV infection. (Reprinted from reference 93a with permission of Elsevier.)

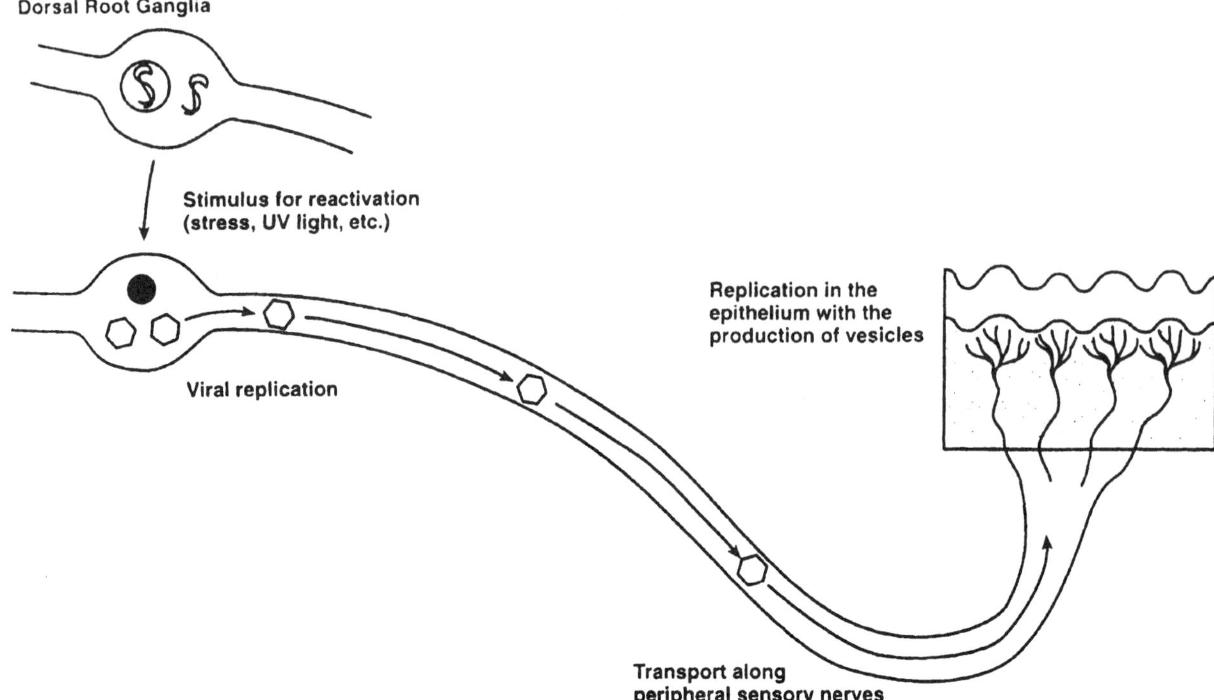

FIGURE 7 Schematic diagram of latency and reactivation. (Reprinted from reference 93a with permission of Elsevier.)

IMMUNOLOGIC RESPONSES TO HSV INFECTION

The natural history of HSV infections is influenced by both specific and nonspecific host defense mechanisms (79). With the appearance of nonspecific inflammatory changes, paralleling a peak in viral replication, specific host responses can be quantitated but vary from one animal system to the next. In the mouse, delayed-type hypersensitivity responses are identified within 4 to 6 days after disease onset, followed by a cytotoxic T-cell response and by the appearance of both immunoglobulin M (IgM)- and IgG-specific antibodies. Host responses in humans are de-

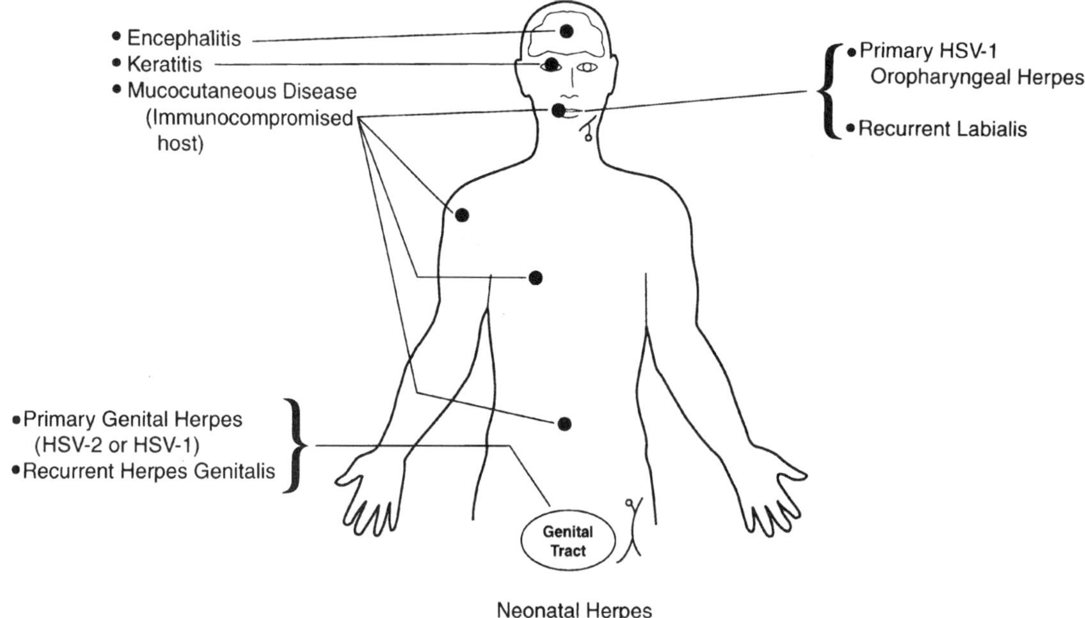

FIGURE 8 Sites of HSV infection and disease.

layed, developing approximately 7 to 10 days later. Immunodepletion studies have identified the importance of cytotoxic T-cells in resolving cutaneous disease. Adoptive transfer of $CD8^+$ or HSV-immune $CD4^+$ T cells also reduces viral replication and confers protection with challenge.

T-cell lymphocyte subsets have been examined for host susceptibility to infection, including those cells responsible either for H2-restricted cytotoxicity or for in vitro or adoptive transfer of delayed-type hypersensitivity (71). The latter cells have a requirement for both the IA and H2 K/D regions (99). Studies utilizing a specific infected cell polypeptide product (ICP4) have identified its requirement for mediation of T cells (85). Prior immune responses to HSV-1 infection have a protective effect on the acquisition of HSV-2 infection (90). Polyclonal antibody therapy will decrease mortality rates in the newborn mouse (18). In addition, administration of these antibodies can limit progression of both neurologic and ocular disease. Protection can be achieved with monoclonal antibodies to specific viral polypeptides, especially the envelope glycoproteins. Such results have been accomplished with both neutralizing and nonneutralizing antibodies. Antibody-dependent cell-mediated cellular cytotoxic host responses also correlate with improved clinical outcome, as is noted below for neonatal HSV infections.

Numerous reports have incriminated or refuted HLA associations with human HSV infections. For recurrent fever blisters, these studies have included HLA-A1, HLA-A2, HLA-A9, HLA-BW16, and HLA-CW2. Recurrent ocular HSV infections have been associated with HLA-A1, HLA-A2, HLA-A9, and HLA-DR3. These conflicting associations can be faulted by population selection bias.

Humoral antibody responses of humans parallel those following systemic infection of mice and rabbits. IgM antibodies appear transiently and are followed by IgG and IgA antibodies, which persist over time. Neutralizing and antibody-dependent cellular cytotoxic antibodies generally appear 2 to 6 weeks after infection and persist for the lifetime of the host. Immunoblot and immunoprecipitation antibody responses have defined the host response to infected cell polypeptides and correlated these responses with the development of neutralizing antibodies (11, 43). After the onset of infection, antibodies appear which are directed against gD, gB, ICP4, gE, gG-1 or gG-2, and gC. Both IgM and IgG antibodies can be demonstrated, depending upon the time of assessment.

Lymphocyte blastogenesis responses develop within 4 to 6 weeks after the onset of infection and sometimes as early as 2 weeks (35, 121, 141). With recurrences, boosts in blastogenic responses can be defined promptly; however, these responses, as after primary infection, decrease with time. Nonspecific blastogenic responses do not correlate with a history of recurrences.

The host response of the newborn to HSV differs from that of older individuals. Impairment of host defense mechanisms contributes to the increased severity of some infectious agents in the fetus and the newborn. Factors which must be considered in defining the host response of the newborn include the mode of transmission of the agent (viremia versus mucocutaneous infection without blood-borne spread) and time of acquisition of infection.

Humoral immunity does not prevent either recurrences or exogenous reinfection. Thus, it is not surprising that transplacentally acquired antibodies from the mother are not totally protective against newborn infection (71, 141). The quantity of neutralizing antibodies is higher in those newborns who do not develop infection when exposed to HSV at delivery (108). Transplacentally acquired neutralizing antibodies either prevent or ameliorate infection in exposed newborns, as do antibody-dependent cell-mediated cytotoxicity antibodies (108). Nevertheless, the presence of antibodies at the time of disease presentation does not necessarily influence the subsequent outcome (151, 155).

Infected newborns produce IgM antibodies (as detected by immunofluorescence) specific for HSV within the first 3 weeks of infection; these antibodies increase rapidly during the first 2 to 3 months and are detectable for as long as 1 year after infection. The most reactive immunodeterminants are the surface viral glycoproteins, particularly gB and gD (141).

Newborns infected by HSV have a delayed T-lymphocyte proliferative response compared to that of older individuals (141). Most infants have no detectable T-lymphocyte responses to HSV 2 to 4 weeks after the onset of clinical symptoms (110, 141). These delayed responses may be associated with disease progression (141).

Infected newborns have decreased alpha interferon (IFN-α) production in response to HSV antigen compared to that of adults with primary HSV infection (141). Lymphocytes from infected babies also have decreased responses to IFN-α generation (141).

Genetic susceptibility to HSV infections is attracting increasing attention. Recently, a polymorphism resulting in an IFN-γ defect has been reported for two children with herpes encephalitis. Its implications warrant further scrutiny (26).

CLINICAL MANIFESTATIONS OF DISEASE

Oropharyngeal Disease

Great variability exists in the clinical symptomatology of primary HSV-1 infections. Asymptomatic infection is the rule rather than the exception. Manifestations of disease range from a total absence of symptoms to combinations of fever, sore throat, ulcerative and vesicular lesions, gingivostomatitis, edema, localized lymphadenopathy, anorexia, and malaise. The incubation period ranges from 2 to 12 days, with a mean of approximately 4 days. Importantly, asymptomatic infection occurs twice as often as symptomatic disease.

Primary HSV-1 infection results in oral shedding of virus in mouth for as long as 23 days (average of 7 to 10 days). Notably, the natural history of HSV-2 infection of the oropharynx is not well characterized. Neutralizing antibodies appear between days 4 and 7 after onset of disease and peak in approximately 3 weeks (40). Virus can also be isolated from the saliva of approximately 20% of asymptomatic children between 7 months and 2 years of age (22). Virus shedding in children less than 6 months of age is uncommon. In older children, 3 to 14 years of age, presumed asymptomatic shedding has been documented for 18% of volunteers. Virus retrieval decreases with advancing age; over 15 years of age, the frequency of excretion is 2.7%, similar to the values in contemporary cross-sectional surveys, which range from 2 to 5% (27, 78, 137, 161). Among the 18,730 Yugoslavian children attending outpatient clinics, evidence of oral herpetic infection was found in approximately 13% over a 10-year period. Children between 1 and 2 years of age were most commonly afflicted, accounting for over half of all cases. No differences in gender or seasonal variation were detected. In a study of 70 seronegative children who had primary infection, only 6 (less than 10%) had clinical symptoms associated with illness. (27). In an Australian study, 67.4% of seronegative children (29 of 43) developed HSV antibodies over a period of 1 year; 69% had asymptomatic infection. Recurrent infection may be asymptomatic, occurring at about 1% in children and 1 to 5% in immunocompetent adults (27, 51, 55, 56, 78). Nearly 1% of pregnant women and nursery personnel excrete HSV at any time (56) and are sources of virus for transmission to the newborn. Asymptomatic excretion of virus is not limited to the healthy adult, as excretion of HSV in renal transplant recipients without signs or symptoms of disease occurs in nearly one-third of seropositive patients (103).

Symptomatic disease in children is characterized by involvement of the buccal and gingival mucosa (Fig. 9). The duration of illness is 2 to 3 weeks, with fever ranging between 101 and 104°F. Often, children with symptomatic primary infection are unable to swallow liquids because of the associated pain. Lesions within the mouth evolve from vesicles to shallow ulcerations on an erythematous base before healing. Submandibular lymphadenopathy is common with primary gingivostomatitis but rare with recurrent infections. Other findings include sore throat and mouth, malaise, tender cervical lymphadenopathy, and an inability to eat. A clinical distinction should be drawn between intraoral gingival lesions and lip lesions indicative of presumed primary and recurrent infections, respectively.

Primary HSV infections of adolescents and adults cause both pharyngitis and a mononucleosis syndrome (51). The differential diagnosis of both primary HSV gingivostomatitis and pharyngitis includes herpangina (usually caused by the coxsackieviruses), candidal infections of the mouth, Epstein-Barr virus-induced mononucleosis, lesions induced by chemotherapy or radiation therapy, and Stevens-Johnson syndrome.

The onset of recurrent orolabial lesions is heralded by a prodrome of pain, burning, tingling, or itching, which generally lasts for 6 h, followed by vesicles (132, 161). Vesicles appear most commonly at the vermilion border of the lip and persist for only 48 h on average (Fig. 10). Vesicles generally number three to five. The total area of involvement usually is localized, and lesions progress to the pustular or ulcerative and crusting stage within 72 to 96 h. Pain is most severe at the outset and resolves quickly over 96 to 120 h. Similarly, the loss of virus from lesions decreases with progressive healing over 2 to 3 days (6, 132). Healing is rapid, generally being complete in 8 to 10 days. The frequency of recurrences varies among individuals (132).

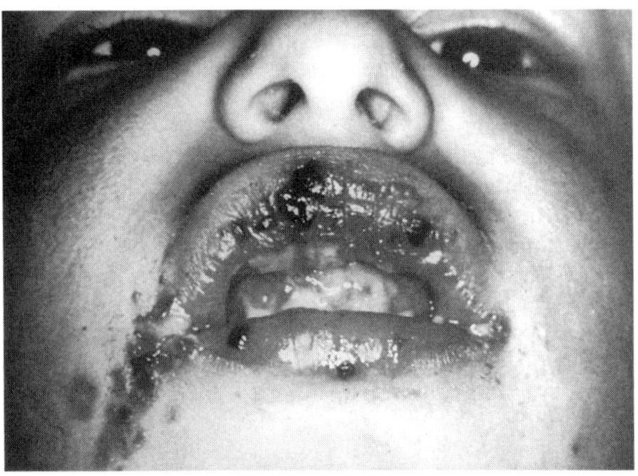

FIGURE 9 Herpes simplex gingivostomatitis.

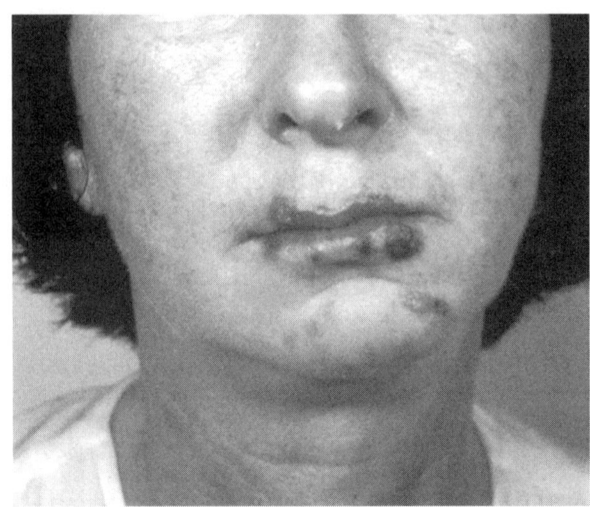

FIGURE 10 Recurrent herpes simplex labialis.

Genital Disease

Primary genital herpes is manifested by macules and papules, followed by vesicles, pustules, and ulcers. Lesions persist for about 3 weeks (31, 32). Primary infection is associated with larger quantities of virus replicating in the genital tract (>10^6 viral particles per 0.2 ml of inoculum) and a period of viral excretion which may persist for 3 weeks. Systemic complications in the male are relatively uncommon; however, aseptic meningitis can develop. Paresthesias and dysesthesias which involve the lower extremities and perineum can result from genital herpetic infection.

Primary infections are usually associated with fever, dysuria, localized inguinal adenopathy, and malaise in both men and women. The severity of primary infection and its association with complications are statistically higher in women than in men (20, 32). Systemic complaints are common in both sexes, approaching 70% of all cases. The most common complications include aseptic meningitis and extragenital lesions.

In women with primary infection, lesions appear on the vulva and are usually bilateral, as shown in Fig. 11, with the cervix invariably involved. The actual frequency of primary cervical infection in the absence of vulvar infection is unknown. Lesions usually are excruciatingly painful, associated with inguinal adenopathy and dysuria, and may involve the vulva, perineum, buttocks, cervix, and vagina. A urinary retention syndrome occurs in 10 to 15% of female patients, and as many as 25% of women will develop aseptic meningitis.

In males, primary genital HSV infections are most often associated with vesicular lesions superimposed upon an erythematous base, usually appearing on the glans penis or the penile shaft, as shown in Fig. 12. The total number of lesions can vary significantly, from 6 to 10 to many more.

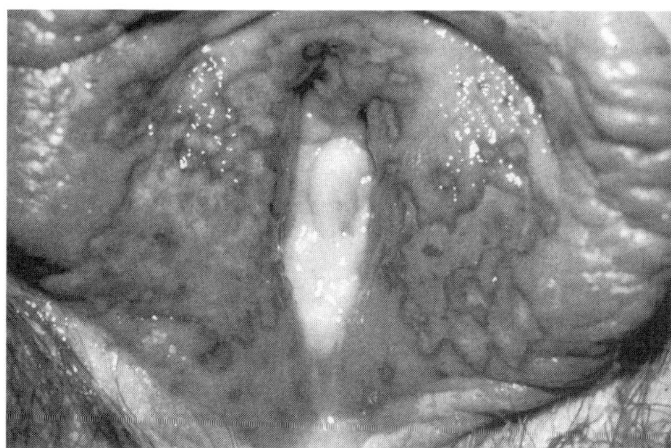

FIGURE 11 Genital HSV infection (female). (Reprinted from reference 93b with permission of Elsevier.)

Extragenital lesions of the thigh, buttocks, and perineum can occur.

Complications following primary genital herpetic infection have included sacral radioculomyelitis, which can lead to urinary retention, neuralgias, and meningoencephalitis. Primary perianal and anal HSV-2 infections, as well as associated proctitis, are more common in male homosexuals. As with HSV-1 infections, as many as two-thirds of HSV-2 infections are subclinical, involving the mouth (54) or the uterine cervix (66, 73, 74). Nonprimary, initial genital infection is less severe symptomatically and heals more quickly. The duration of infection is usually 2 weeks. The number of lesions, severity of pain, and likelihood of complications are significantly decreased. Preexisting antibodies to HSV-1 have an ameliorative effect on the severity of HSV-2 disease (75).

With recurrent genital herpetic infection, a limited number of vesicles, usually three to five, appear on the shaft of the penis of the male or as simply a vulvar irritation in the female. The duration of disease parallels that encountered with recurrent HSV labialis, approximately 7 to 10 days. Neurologic or systemic complications are uncommon with recurrent disease; however, paresthesias and dysesthesias occur. Virus is shed for an average of 2 to 5 days and at lower concentrations (approximately 10^2 to 10^3 per 0.2 ml of inoculum in tissue culture systems) in women with recurrent genital infection. Recurrent genital herpetic infection in both men and women is characterized by prodrome, which is a useful marker for therapeutic trials, and by localized irritation.

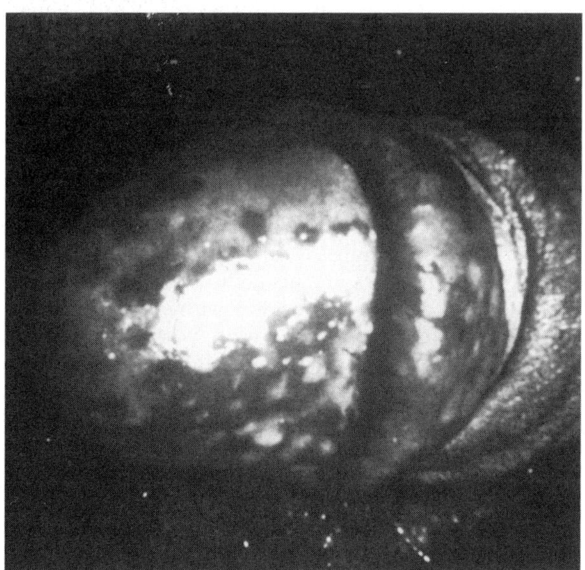

FIGURE 12 Genital HSV infection (male).

The frequency of recurrences varies from one individual to the next. As noted above, recurrences are more frequent in the first year after primary infection. The severity of primary infection appears to correlate with the frequency of recurrences; that is, the more severe the primary infection is, the more likely and frequent recurrences are. One-third of infected individuals are estimated to have recurrences in excess of eight or nine per year, one-third will have two to three per year, and the remaining one-third will have between four and seven (32). Individuals can transmit infection to sexual partners with symptomatic or, more commonly, asymptomatic recurrences. Recent studies suggest a high frequency of HSV DNA as detected by PCR in genital secretions between clinical recurrences (30). Many recurrences may only be hours in duration (67). The implications of these data require the education of patients, including behavioral interventions and use of condoms to prevent transmission of infection.

Pregnancy and Neonatal Infection

An uncommon problem encountered with HSV infections during pregnancy is that of widely disseminated disease (160), involving multiple visceral sites, in addition to cutaneous dissemination. Dissemination after primary oropharyngeal or genital infection has led to necrotizing hepatitis with or without thrombocytopenia, disseminated intravascular coagulopathy, and encephalitis. The mortality among pregnant women is reported to be greater than 50%. Fetal deaths have also occurred in more than 50% of cases, although mortality did not necessarily correlate with the death of the mother. Cumulative experience suggests that factors associated with pregnancy may place both the mother and fetus at increased risk for severe infection, possibly because of altered cell-mediated immunity.

The major risk to the fetus is with primary or initial genital HSV infection of the mother (18, 74). Thus, identification of the woman at risk for primary infection is of paramount importance. Serologic discordance such that the mother is HSV-2 seronegative and her partner is HSV-2 seropositive averages 15 to 20%. The risk for transmission from the father is 10 to 15%.

Maternal primary infection prior to 20 weeks' gestation in some women has been associated with spontaneous abortion (96) that was thought to occur in as many as 20% of cases. The contribution of primary maternal genital infection to spontaneous abortion must be weighed above that of a routine rate of fetal loss of approximately 20%. Infection which develops later in gestation has not been associated with the termination of pregnancy, but morbidity of the fetus born to a woman with primary infection was documented with manifestations of neonatal HSV disease, severe intrauterine growth retardation, or premature termination of gestation compared to that in controls (19).

Neonatal Disease

Background

The estimated incidence of neonatal HSV is approximately 1 in 2,000 to 1 in 5,000 deliveries per year. An increase in the number of cases of neonatal HSV infection was noted in some areas, with rates approaching 1 in 1,500 deliveries. Four factors appear to influence transmission of infection from mother to fetus. First, the risk of transmission is 30 to 50% with maternal primary or initial infection, compared to 3% or less with recurrent infection (18, 31, 32). Second, paralleling the type of maternal infection, the mother's antibody status prior to delivery influences both the severity of infection and the likelihood of transmission. Transplacental maternal neutralizing and antibody-dependent cell-mediated cytotoxic antibodies have at least an ameliorative effect on acquisition of infection for babies inadvertently exposed to virus at delivery (108). Third, prolonged rupture of membranes (greater than 6 h) increases the risk of acquisition of infection as a consequence of ascending infection from the cervix. Fourth, fetal scalp monitors can be a site of inoculation of virus. Such devices should be relatively contraindicated in women with a history of recurrent genital HSV infection.

Infection of the newborn can be acquired at one of three times, and in all cases, the mother is the most common source of infection. First, in utero infection is rare and requires (64) stringent diagnostic criteria (namely, identification of infected babies within the first 48 h of life who have virologic confirmation of infection). The second route of infection is that of intrapartum contact of the fetus with infected maternal genital secretions. Approximately 75 to 80% of babies possibly acquire HSV infection by this route. The third route of transmission is postnatal acquisition. While HSV-1 is associated with genital lesions, postnatal transmission of HSV is increasingly suggested in that 15 to 20% of neonatal HSV infections are caused by this type (151). Relatives and hospital personnel with orolabial herpes can be a reservoir for HSV infection of the newborn. The documentation of postnatal transmission of HSV has focused attention on such sources of virus for neonatal infection (48). The presence of identical isolates, as demonstrated by restriction endonuclease technology, from babies born to different mothers in a nursery is rare. Postnatal transmission from mother to child as a consequence of nursing on an infected breast has been documented. Father-to-baby transmission from lesions of herpes labialis has also been documented.

Clinical Presentation

Neonatal HSV infection is almost invariably symptomatic and frequently lethal. Babies with congenital infection should be identified within 48 h following birth. Those babies who are infected intrapartum or postnatally with HSV infection can be divided into three categories: those with (i) disease localized to the skin, eye, and mouth; (ii) encephalitis with or without skin involvement; and (iii) disseminated infection which involves multiple organs, including the CNS, lungs, liver, adrenals, skin, eyes, and/or mouth (157).

Intrauterine Infection

Intrauterine infection is apparent at birth and is characterized by the triad of skin vesicles or skin scarring, eye disease, and the far more severe manifestations of microcephaly or hydranencephaly. Often, retinitis alone or in combination with other eye findings, such as keratoconjunctivitis, is a component of the clinical presentation. The frequency of occurrence of these manifestations is estimated to be 1 in 200,000 deliveries.

Disseminated Infection

Babies with the highest mortality present for therapy between 9 and 11 days of age. However, signs of infection usually begin on an average of 4 to 5 days earlier. With the early introduction of antiviral therapy, about 23% of babies with neonatal HSV infection have disseminated disease. The principal organs involved are the liver, lungs, and adrenals, but other involved organs include the larynx, trachea, esophagus, stomach, gastrointestinal tract, spleen, kidneys, pancreas, and heart. Constitutional signs and symptoms include irritability, seizures, respiratory distress, jaundice, bleeding diatheses, shock, and, frequently, the characteristic vesicular exanthem which is often considered pathognomonic for infection. Encephalitis appears to be a common component of disseminated infection, occurring in about 60 to 75% of children. The vesicular rash, as described below, is particularly important in the diagnosis of HSV infection. However, over 20% of these children do not develop skin vesicles during the course of illness (3, 151). Mortality in the absence of therapy exceeds 80%; all but a few survivors are impaired. The most common cause of death in babies with disseminated disease is either HSV pneumonitis or disseminated intravascular coagulopathy.

Encephalitis

Babies with infection of the CNS alone or in combination with disseminated disease present with the findings indicative of encephalitis in the newborn. Brain infection occurs in one of two fashions—namely, either as a component of multiorgan disseminated infection or only as encephalitis with or without skin, eye, and mouth involvement. Nearly one-third of all babies with neonatal HSV infection have encephalitis. The modes of pathogenesis of these two forms of brain infection are likely different. Babies with disseminated infection probably seed the brain by a blood-borne route, resulting in multiple areas of cortical hemorrhagic necrosis. In contrast, babies who present with only encephalitis likely develop brain disease as a consequence of retrograde axonal transport of virus to the CNS. Two pieces of data support this contention. Babies with disseminated disease have documented viremia and are hospitalized earlier in life than those with only encephalitis, at 9 to 10 days versus 16 to 17 days. Babies with encephalitis are more likely to receive transplacental neutralizing antibodies from their mothers which may prevent viremia, allowing for only intraneuronal transmission of virus to the brain.

Clinical manifestations of either encephalitis (alone or in association with disseminated disease) include seizures (both focal and generalized), lethargy, irritability, tremors, poor feeding, temperature instability, bulging fontanelle, and pyramidal tract signs. Children with encephalitis without disseminated disease have skin vesicles in approximately 60% of cases at any time during the disease course (3, 151). Virus can be cultured from cerebrospinal fluid in 25 to 40% of all cases. Anticipated findings on cerebrospinal fluid examination include pleocytosis and proteinosis (as high as 500 to 1,000 mg/dl), although a few babies with CNS infection have no abnormalities of cerebrospinal fluid. Death occurs in 50% of babies with CNS disease who are not treated and is usually related to brain stem involvement. With rare exceptions, survivors are left with severe neurologic impairment.

The long-term prognosis, following either disseminated infection or encephalitis, is particularly poor. As many as 50% of surviving children have some degree of psychomotor retardation, often in association with microcephaly, hydrancephaly, porencephalic cysts, spasticity, blindness, retinitis, or learning disabilities.

A comment regarding the diagnosis of encephalitis is indicated. For children with disease localized to the CNS, skin vesicles, the classic sign of disease, may not be present in as many as 40% of babies. Thus, for the baby with cells and protein in the cerebrospinal fluid at 2 to 3 weeks of life, other diagnostic clues, such as skin vesicles, may not be present. For the neonate with cerebrospinal fluid findings indicative of infection, HSV must be considered along with bacterial pathogens (e.g., group B streptococci or *Escherichia coli*). A reasonable diagnostic approach, if all antigen and Gram stain studies are negative, would be serial cerebrospinal fluid examinations to document progression in protein and mononuclear cell counts.

Skin, Eye, and/or Mouth Infection

Infection localized to the skin, eyes, and/or mouth is associated with morbidity and not mortality. When infection is localized to the skin, the presence of discrete vesicles remains the hallmark of disease. Clusters of vesicles often appear initially on the part of the body which was in direct contact with the virus during birth. With time, the rash progresses to involve other areas of the body as well, particularly if viremia occurs. Vesicles occur in 90% of children with skin, eye, or mouth infection. Children with disease localized to the skin, eyes, or mouth generally present at about 10 to 11 days of life. Babies with skin lesions invariably will suffer from recurrences over the first 6 months (and longer) of life, regardless of whether therapy was administered. Approximately 30% of these children eventually develop evidence of neurologic impairment in the absence of therapy (154). The skin vesicles (Fig. 13) usually erupt from an erythematous base and are usually 1 to 2 mm in diameter. Other manifestations of skin lesions include a zosteriform eruption. Infections involving the eyes manifest as keratoconjunctivitis or, later, as retinitis. The eyes can be the only site of HSV involvement in the newborn.

Long-term neurologic impairment has been documented to occur in children whose disease appeared localized to the skin, eyes, and/or mouth. The significant findings include spastic quadriplegia, microcephaly, and blindness. Despite normal clinical examinations in these children, neurologic impairment has become apparent between 6 months and 1 year of life.

Prognostic Factors

Babies with the most severe disease have the worst outcome, as identified by disease classification (150). Level of consciousness also predicted a poor prognosis. By disease classification, the poorest prognostic factors for babies with disseminated disease were, in addition to the above, the development of HSV pneumonia or disseminated intravascular coagulopathy. With encephalitis, prematurity and seizures predicted a poor outcome. Finally, for babies with skin, eye, or mouth disease, frequently recurrent HSV-2 cutaneous lesions defined a group at risk for a poor neurologic outcome.

Herpes Simplex Keratoconjunctivitis

Viral infections of the eyes beyond the newborn age are usually caused by HSV-1 (12). Approximately 300,000 cases of HSV infections of the eyes are diagnosed annually in the United States, where these infections are second only to trauma as the cause of corneal blindness. Herpetic keratoconjunctivitis is associated with either unilateral or bilateral conjunctivitis which can be follicular in nature, followed soon thereafter by preauricular adenopathy. Eye infection is also associated with photophobia, tearing, eyelid edema, and chemosis, accompanied by the pathognomonic findings of branching dendritic lesions. Less commonly, with advanced disease the infection is associated with a geographic ulcer of the cornea. Healing of the cornea can take as long as 1 month, even with appropriate antiviral therapy.

Recurrences parallel that which was described for herpes labialis. Most frequently, they are unilateral in involve-

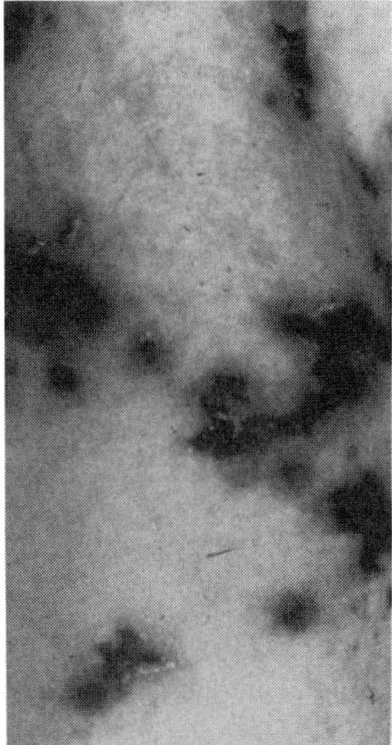
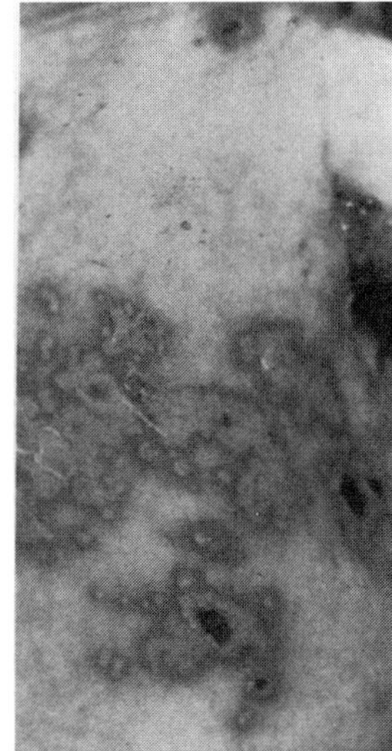
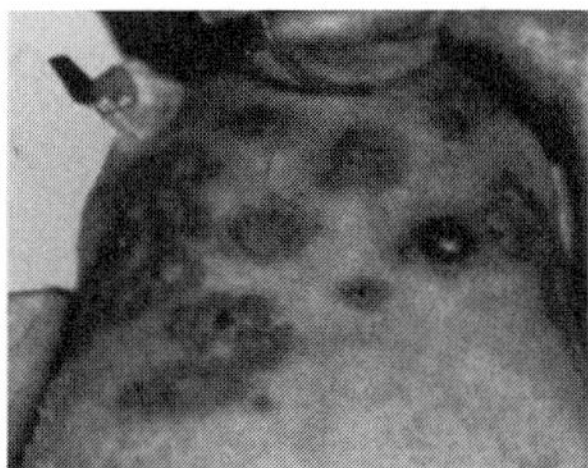

FIGURE 13 Vesicular rash of neonatal HSV infection.

ment, but a small percentage of cases involve both eyes. Characteristically, either dendritic ulceration or stromal involvement occurs. Visual acuity is decreased in the presence of the ulcers; and with progressive stromal involvement, opacification of the cornea may occur. Progressive disease can result in visual loss and even rupture of the globe.

Skin Infections

Skin infections caused by HSV generally manifest as eczema herpeticum in patients with underlying atopic dermatitis. Lesions can either be localized, resembling herpes zoster, or disseminated, as occurs with Kaposi's varicella-like eruption. Infections of the digits, known as herpetic whitlow, are particularly common among medical and dental personnel. The estimated incidence is 2.4 cases per 100,000 population per year, caused by HSV-1 or HSV-2. An increasing incidence of HSV-2 herpetic whitlow has been reported (50).

The prevalence of HSV skin infections in Skaraborg, Sweden, was assessed among approximately 7,500 individuals over 7 years of age and was found to be about 1%. In another Swedish study performed in dermatology clinics, 2% of men and 1.5% of women attending clinics in Gothenburg over a 6-year period had evidence of herpetic skin infections. In addition to individuals with atopic disease, patients with skin abrasions or burns appear to be particularly susceptible to HSV-1 and HSV-2 infections, and some develop disseminated infection (47). Disseminated HSV infections have been reported among wrestlers (herpes gladitorium) (148). Other skin disorders associated with extensive cutaneous lesions include Darier's disease and Sézary's syndrome. As would be predicted, localized recurrences followed by a second episode of dissemination were observed. HSV infections of either type can trigger erythema multiforme (147). The rate of detection of HSV DNA in skin lesions of erythema multiforme is as high as 80%.

Infections of the Immunocompromised Host

Patients compromised by immune therapy, underlying disease, or malnutrition are at increased risk for severe HSV infection. Renal, hepatic, bone marrow, and cardiac transplant recipients are all at high risk for increased severity of HSV infection (94). An example of cutaneous dissemination following shaving in a renal transplant recipient is shown in Fig. 14. Virus was likely autoinoculated to multiple skin sites. In organ transplant recipients, the presence of antibodies to HSV prior to treatment predicts the individual at greatest risk for recurrence (103). These patients may develop progressive disease involving the respiratory tract, esophagus, or even the gastrointestinal tract. The severe nature of progressive disease in these patients appears to be directly related to the degree of immunosuppressive therapy employed. Esophagitis is a common occurrence in the immunocompromised host and can be caused by HSV, cytomegalovirus, or *Candida albicans*. Notably, acyclovir-resistant HSV disease can occur in the immunocompromised host and be progressive. Reactivation of latent HSV infections in these patients can occur at multiple sites, and healing occurs over an average of 6 weeks (153).

Since the first reports of AIDS, the severity of HSV clinical disease in hosts rendered severely immunocompromised by this disease was noted (81). Disease is more frequent and severe. Because of persistent and high-level viral replication, resistance to antiviral therapy can develop. Asymptomatic excretion of HSV can occur even in the immunocompromised host. Parenthetically, acquisition of HSV infection from a transplanted organ (kidney) has been reported (42).

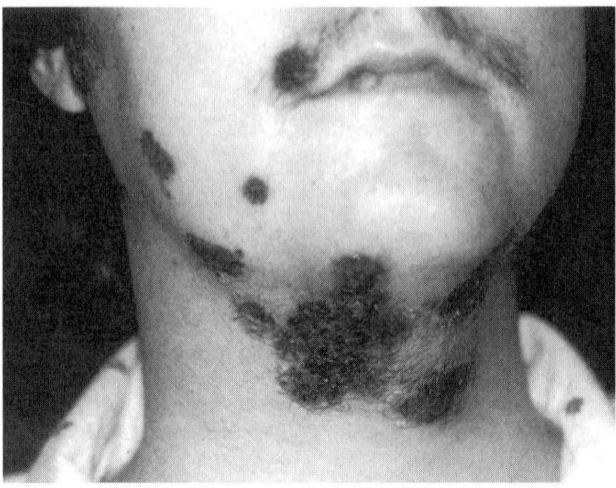

FIGURE 14 Cutaneous dissemination of HSV infection in an immunosuppressed host.

Infections of the CNS

Herpes simplex encephalitis is the most devastating of all HSV infections (Fig. 15) and is considered the most common cause of sporadic, fatal encephalitis (102). From data collected prospectively, the incidence of severe hemorrhagic focal encephalitis is approximately 1 in 200,000 individuals per year, for a national annual rate of approximately 1,250 cases in the United States.

The manifestations of HSV encephalitis in the older child and adult are indicative of the areas of the brain affected. These include primarily a focal encephalitis associated with fever, altered consciousness, bizarre behavior, disordered mentation, and localized neurologic findings. Clinical signs and symptoms reflect localized temporal lobe disease (156, 157). No signs are pathognomonic for HSV; however, a progressively deteriorating level of consciousness, expressive aphasia, bizarre behavior, fever, an abnormal cerebrospinal fluid formula, and focal neurologic findings in the absence of other causes should lead to a high degree of suspicion of this disease. Diagnostic evaluations should be initiated immediately, since other treatable diseases mimic HSV encephalitis. Mortality in untreated patients is in excess of 70%, and only 2.5% of untreated patients return to normal neurologic functions.

Standard neurodiagnostic procedures include cerebrospinal fluid examination, electroencephalogram, and one or more scanning procedures such as computed tomography or magnetic resonance imaging. Characteristic abnormalities of the cerebrospinal fluid include elevated levels of cells (usually mononuclear) and protein. Red blood cells are found in most (but not all) cerebrospinal fluid samples obtained from patients with HSV encephalitis. Upon serial cerebrospinal fluid examination, protein and cell counts rise dramatically. The electroencephalogram generally localizes spike and slow-wave activity to the temporal lobe. A burst suppression pattern is characteristic of HSV encephalitis. Imaging will allow for localization of disease to the temporal lobe. Early after onset, only evidence of

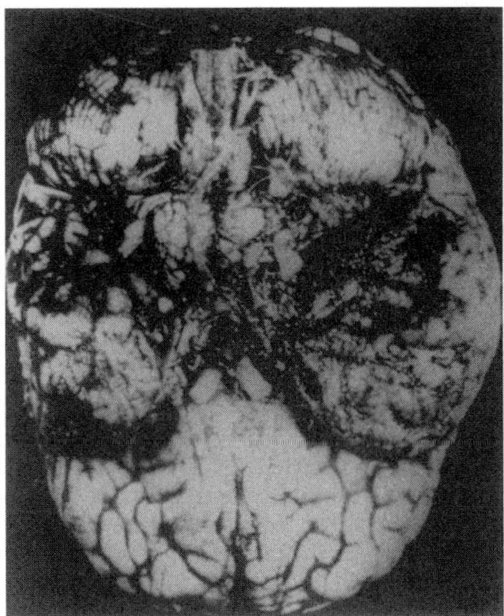
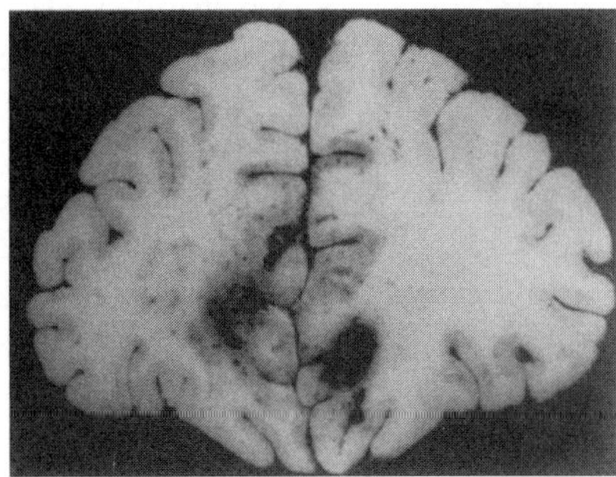

FIGURE 15 Coronal sections of brain from a patient with herpes simplex encephalitis.

edema is detectable, if anything. This finding is followed by evidence of hemorrhage and midline shift in the cortical structures. Specific diagnostic assays are delineated below.

Other Neurologic Syndromes

In addition to encephalitis, HSV can involve virtually all anatomic areas of the nervous system, including meningitis, myelitis, and radiculitis, among others. Aseptic meningitis is a common occurrence in individuals with primary genital HSV infections.

Other Forms of Infection

Other forms of infection should be noted briefly. HSV was isolated from the respiratory tract of adults with adult respiratory distress syndrome and acute-onset bronchospasm (142). Both were associated with increased mortality and morbidity.

DIAGNOSIS

Tissue Culture

The appropriate utilization of laboratory tools is essential if a diagnosis of HSV infection is to be achieved. Virus isolation remains a definitive diagnostic method. If skin lesions are present, a scraping of skin vesicles should be made and transferred in an appropriate virus transport medium to a diagnostic virology laboratory. Clinical specimens should be shipped on ice for inoculation onto cell cultures (e.g., human foreskin fibroblasts or Vero cells) which are susceptible to cytopathic effects characteristic of HSV replication. Cytopathic effect usually develops within 24 to 48 h after inoculation of specimens containing infectious virus. The shipping and processing of specimens should be expedited. In addition to skin vesicles, other sites from which virus may be isolated include the cerebrospinal fluid, stool, urine, throat, nasopharynx, and conjunctivae. Duodenal aspirates from infants with hepatitis or other gastrointestinal abnormalities are useful for HSV isolation. Since outcome with treatment does not appear to be related to the virus type, identification is only of epidemiological and pathogenetic importance and, therefore, not usually necessary.

Every effort should be made to confirm infection by viral isolation. Cytological examination of cells from the maternal cervix or from the infant's skin, mouth, conjunctivae, or corneal lesions is of low sensitivity, approximately 60 to 70% (98). Cellular material obtained by scraping the periphery of the base of lesions should be smeared on a glass slide and promptly fixed in cold ethanol. The slide can be stained according to the methods of Papanicolaou, Giemsa, or Wright before examination by a trained cytologist. Giemsa or Tzanck smears likely will not demonstrate the presence of intranuclear inclusions. The presence of intranuclear inclusions and multinucleated giant cells is indicative, but not diagnostic, of HSV infection. Electron microscopic assays are available but impractical.

Serologic Assessment

Serologic diagnosis of HSV infection is of little clinical value. Therapeutic decisions cannot await the results of serologic studies. Serologic assays that distinguish HSV-1 from HSV-2 are commercially available. The use of enzyme-linked immunosorbent assays only allows definition of past infection or seroconversion and cannot distinguish HSV-1 from HSV-2. Other commonly used tests for measurement of HSV antibodies are complement fixation, passive hemagglutination, neutralization, and immunofluorescence. The more recently developed type-specific antibody assays will likely replace many of the older systems.

PCR

PCR is the diagnostic method of choice for HSV infections of the CNS (5, 120) and may well replace culture for routine skin infections because of its sensitivity. Primers from an HSV DNA sequence which was common to both HSV-1 and HSV-2 (either the gB domain or HSV DNA polymerase) identify HSV DNA in cerebrospinal fluid. The evaluation of cerebrospinal fluid specimens obtained from patients with biopsy-proven herpes simplex encephalitis and those with proven other diseases indicates a sensitivity of >95% at the time of clinical presentation and a specificity which approaches 100% (5, 76). False-negative assessments can be found when there is hemoglobin contamination in the cerebrospinal fluid or the presence of inhibitors, such as heparin. Likely, PCR analyses of cerebrospinal fluid specimens continue to reinforce the focal presentation of HSV infections of the CNS. Importantly, PCR evaluation of cerebrospinal fluid can be utilized to monitor therapeutic outcome in patients with herpes simplex encephalitis. Persistence of HSV DNA in the cerebrospinal fluid of newborns with suspected herpes simplex encephalitis predicts a poor outcome.

PROPHYLAXIS

Education

Because of awareness of the increasing incidence of genital herpes and neonatal herpes and their association with acquisition of HIV infection, every effort should be made to prevent HSV-2 infection. Until a vaccine is proven effective, educational efforts must be developed for adolescents and adults at greatest risk. The utilization of condoms should be promoted.

Prevention

Neonatal HSV Infection

Surgical abdominal delivery will decrease transmission of infection when membranes are ruptured less than 4 h, but cesarean section has not been proven efficacious when membranes are ruptured for longer periods. Nevertheless, cesarean section is recommended when membranes are ruptured up to 24 h in the presence of active lesions. Although the recommendation seems logical, no data exist to support it.

For women with a history of genital HSV infection, a careful vaginal examination at presentation to the delivery suite is of paramount importance. While visualization of the cervix is often difficult, speculum examination for documentation of recurrent lesions is extremely important and should be attempted in all mothers at delivery. A culture for HSV obtained at the time of delivery can be of great importance in establishing whether excretion can lead to transmission of infection to the fetus.

Clearly, identifying women who excrete HSV at delivery and then optimizing either prophylaxis with safe and acceptable antivirals or delivery by cesarean section remains the optimal management of genital infection at delivery. The detection of type-specific antibodies to gG-2 will be of value in identifying those women at greatest risk. Documentation of discordant serologic status between sexual partners may assist in prevention of maternal primary infection. Clearly, male partners who are seropositive should be educated regarding HSV transmission.

Nosocomial Transmission

At many institutions, a policy which requires transfer or provision of medical leave for nursery personnel who have a labial HSV infection is impractical and causes an excessive burden on those attempting to provide adequate care. Temporary removal of personnel who have cold sores has been suggested. As noted previously, individuals with herpetic whitlow shed virus. These individuals should be removed from the care of newborns at risk for acquiring neonatal HSV infection, since even gloves may not prevent transmission of infection. Education regarding the risks of transmission of virus and the importance of hand washing when lesions are present should be repeatedly emphasized to health care workers. In addition, hospital personnel should wear masks when active lesions are present.

Vaccine Development

Vaccination remains the ideal method for prevention of viral infection; however, prevention of HSV infections introduces unique problems because of recurrences in the presence of humoral immunity. Nevertheless, protection from life-threatening disease can be achieved in animal models with avirulent, inactivated, or even subunit glycoprotein vaccines. Excellent reviews summarize HSV vaccine development (23, 135).

Wild-Type Virus Vaccines

Numerous clinical investigators have attempted to alter the pattern of recurrences by inoculation of (i) autologous virus, (ii) virus from another infected individual, or (iii) virus recovered from an experimentally infected rabbit. In each circumstance, the inoculation of virus led to infection at the site of injection in as many as 40 to 80% of patients. Efficacy was reported but without the utilization of matched controls. In some of these cases, inoculation led to recurrences of latent infection (14). This approach is considered unacceptable.

Inactivated (Killed) Virus Vaccines

Killed viruses have been used as vaccines in a variety of animal model systems, often with good results. When these vaccines were administered to patients with preexisting HSV infection in order to alleviate recurrences, most studies failed to include an appropriate control group. Significant bias was introduced, since patients may experience a 30 to 70% decrease in the frequency of recurrent lesions as well as improvement in severity, simply from having received placebo.

The initial inactivated vaccines were made from phenol-treated tissues obtained from infected animals (15). Because of the potential for demyelination following the administration of animal proteins, these vaccines attracted little biomedical attention. Viral antigens obtained from amniotic or allantoic fluid, chorioallantoic membranes, chick cell cultures, sheep kidney cells, and rabbit kidney cells, which were inactivated by either formalin, UV light, or heat, have been used as vaccines in thousands of patients. With one exception, each of these studies reported significant improvement in as many as 60 to 80% of patients. Notably, however, no controls were employed.

Few studies utilizing inactivated vaccines have been placebo controlled. The results from these studies differ widely, even when the same vaccine was utilized. A conclusion from these investigations was that there may be some initial benefit for patients with recurrent infection; however, long-term benefit could not be established.

The only prospective study of prevention of HSV infections by vaccination was performed by Anderson and coworkers with children living in an orphanage (1). In this study, 10 children received vaccine and 10 received the placebo; nevertheless, HSV gingivostomatitis was found to have developed in equal numbers of patients in these groups on long-term follow-up.

Subunit Vaccines

Subunit vaccines evolved from attempts to remove viral DNA to eliminate the potential for cellular transformation, enhance antigenic concentration, induce stronger immune responses, and exclude any possibility of contamination with residual live virus. Subunit vaccines were prepared using a variety of methods for antigen expression or extraction from infected cell lysates by detergent and subsequent purification.

The immunogenicity of envelope glycoproteins, free of viral DNA, was demonstrated in animals. Envelope glycoproteins do not appear to confer protection on uninfected sexual partners of individuals with genital infection, but results are preliminary (4).

Subunit vaccines have been produced by cloning specific glycoproteins in yeasts or Chinese hamster ovary cells (10) or by other methods. For a cloned vaccine, performed by Biocine/Chiron investigators, a gD-2 gene was truncated to yield a mature protein containing 348 gD-2 residues. A similar gB-2 vaccine was prepared. These subunit vaccines, as well as others, have been studied in a variety of animal model systems, including mice, guinea pigs, and rabbits. Neutralizing and enzyme-linked immunosorbent assay antibodies can be detected in these systems in various amounts. The quantity of neutralizing antibody appears to correlate with the degree of protection upon challenge in experimental models such as mice (22), rabbits (24), and guinea pigs. Each of these systems utilized a variety of different routes of challenge as well as dosages (77).

In a study of the Merck glycoprotein envelope subunit vaccine carried out with sexual partners of patients known to have genital herpes, the number of individuals developing herpetic infection was nearly the same for both placebo and vaccine recipients, indicating that the vaccine was not effective (4).

Two clinical trials of subunit vaccines have been reported. A vaccine combining gB and gD with the adjuvant MF-59 failed to either provide protection to seronegative volunteers or reduce recurrences in infected individuals (34). However, a parallel vaccine trial with gD alone and a proprietary adjuvant protected seronegative women but had no effect on either men or HSV-1-seropositive women. These findings are being assessed in a large National Institute of Allergy and Infectious Diseases clinical trial (136).

Genetically Engineered HSV

The technology developed by Post and Roizman (107) has been used to construct recombinant HSV as a prototype of herpes vaccines (88). The genome of the HSV-1(F) strain was deleted in the domain of the viral TK gene and in the junction region of the U_L and U_S segments in order to excise some of the genetic loci responsible for neurovirulence, as well as to create convenient sites and space within the genome for insertion of other genes. An HSV-2 DNA fragment encoding gD, gG, and gI was inserted in place of the internal inverted repeat. This virus expresses TK; thus, it is susceptible to antiviral chemotherapy with acyclovir. When evaluated in rodent models, the constructs were attenuated in pathogenicity and ability to establish latency and were capable of inducing protective immunity. The recombinants neither regained virulence nor had altered DNA restriction enzyme cleavage patterns when subjected to serial passages in mouse brain (88). These results were corroborated by studies with owl monkeys (*Aotus trivirgatus*) (107). While 100 PFU of wild-type virus administered by peripheral routes was fatal to the monkeys, recombinants given by various routes in amounts at least 10^5-fold greater were innocuous or produced mild infections, even in the presence of immunosuppression by total lymphoid irradiation (89). When this candidate vaccine was evaluated in humans, low-level immune responses were elicited. Unfortunately, production difficulties precluded the administration of higher dosages of vaccine.

The ideal genetically engineered virus is an attenuated virus that exhibits limited replication at peripheral sites but cannot be transported anterograde to either the CNS or dorsal root ganglia. Lack of knowledge of the mechanisms by which HSV is transported retrograde to the CNS has led to the design of attenuated virus that suffers from a limited ability to replicate not only in humans but also in cultured cells. The accrual of information on viral functions responsible for neuroinvasiveness will ultimately lead to a level of attenuation appropriate to induce a strong immune response without the risk of colonization of dorsal root ganglia or invasion of the CNS.

GENE THERAPY

Genetically engineered HSVs have undergone extensive preclinical studies and are now in clinical tests to assess their oncolytic effects in gene therapy studies. Viruses lacking the $\gamma_1 34.5$ gene are incapable of replicating in postmitotic cells of the brain. Such viruses do not induce encephalitis upon intratumoral inoculation in patients with glioblastoma multiforme (82, 83). Viruses lacking this and other genes are in preclinical studies for use as vectors for foreign-gene expression. Other useful mutants for cancer therapy lack the internal inverted repeats flanking U_L and U_S. Mutants with more extensive deletions of essential genes are in various stages of development to serve as vectors for delivery to the CNS of cellular genes that are missing or damaged. Such mutants could be expected to establish latency and express the cellular gene for long periods. The use of HSV for gene therapy heralds a new era of herpes biology, the conversion of a hazardous foe into a user-friendly surgical tool. A recent review summarizes these data (84).

TREATMENT

Acyclovir (9-[2-hydroxyethoxymethyl] guanine) has become the standard of systemic therapy of HSV infections. This drug, a synthetic acyclic purine nucleoside analog, is described in detail in chapter 11. Valacyclovir is a prodrug of acyclovir. When administered at 1 g every 8 h, resulting levels in plasma are similar to those with 5 mg of acyclovir per kg of body weight given intravenously. Famciclovir is the prodrug of penciclovir. Valacyclovir and famciclovir are licensed and provide enhanced oral bioavailability compared to that of acyclovir (2, 7, 159).

Genital Herpes

Initial genital HSV infection can be treated with oral or intravenous acyclovir. While topical application of acyclovir reduces the duration of viral shedding and the length of time before all lesions become crusted, it is less effective than oral or intravenous therapy (33). Intravenous acyclovir is the most effective treatment for first-episode genital herpes and results in a significant reduction in the median duration of viral shedding (Fig. 16), pain, and length of time to complete healing (8 versus 14 days) (106). Since intravenous acyclovir therapy usually requires hospitaliza-

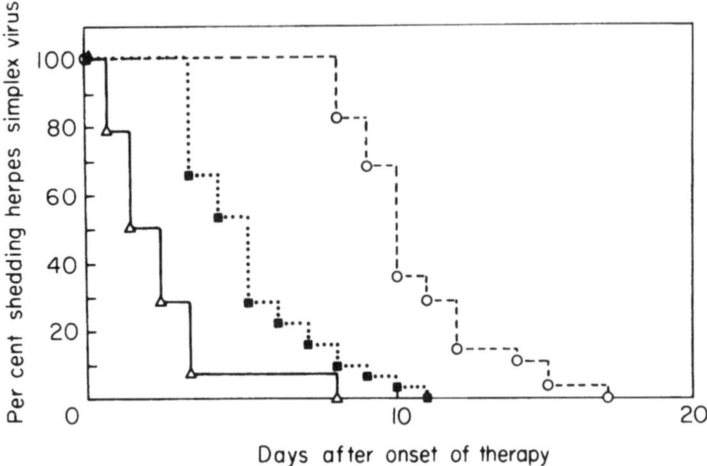

FIGURE 16 Clearance of virus from patients with primary genital HSV infection, according to the route of drug delivery. Δ, intravenous acyclovir; ■, oral acyclovir; ○, topical acyclovir. (Reprinted from reference 33 with permission.)

tion, it should be reserved for patients with severe local disease or systemic complications. Oral therapy (200 mg five times daily) is nearly as effective as intravenous acyclovir for initial genital herpes (20, 91) and has become the standard treatment (Table 1). Neither intravenous nor oral acyclovir treatment of acute HSV infection reduces the frequency of recurrences (2, 91, 106).

Recurrent genital herpes is less severe and resolves more rapidly than primary infection; thus, there is less time to introduce antiviral chemotherapy successfully. Oral acyclovir therapy shortens both the duration of viral shedding and the length of time to healing (6 versus 7 days) when initiated early (within 24 h of onset), but the duration of symptoms and length of time to recurrence are not affected (100, 113). Valacyclovir and famciclovir provide added benefit, particularly with short-course therapy as described in chapter 12 (2, 39, 104, 159).

Long-term oral administration of acyclovir effectively suppresses genital herpes in patients who have frequent recurrences (41, 92, 140). Daily administration of acyclovir reduces the frequency of recurrences by up to 80%, and 25 to 30% of patients have no further recurrences while taking acyclovir (92). Successful suppression for as long as 3 years has been reported, with no evidence of significant adverse effects. Titration of the dose of acyclovir (400 mg twice daily or 200 mg two to five times daily) may be required to establish the minimal dose that is most effective and economical. Treatment should be interrupted every 12 months to reassess the need for continued suppression. The emergence of acyclovir-resistant strains of HSV appears to be infrequent in immunologically normal individuals (101). Importantly, asymptomatic shedding of virus can continue despite clinically effective suppression with acyclovir, so the possibility of person-to-person transmission persists (139).

Valacyclovir and famciclovir are also efficacious in the treatment of recurrent genital herpes or for suppression. Valacyclovir for treatment is administered at a dosage of 500 mg twice daily for 5 to 7 days and for suppression at 500 mg or 1 g daily. Famciclovir is administered at 250 mg thrice daily for treatment and suppression.

Recently, valacyclovir was proven to decrease person-to-person transmission when administered to the seropositive partner (36).

Herpes Labialis

Topical therapy is of no value. Orally administered acyclovir (at a dosage of 200 mg five times daily for 5 days) reduces the length of time to the loss of crusts by approximately 1 day (7 versus 8 days) but does not alter the duration of pain or the length of time to complete healing (109). If the dosage is increased to 400 mg five times daily for 5 days, treatment started during the prodromal or erythematous stage of infection reduces the duration of pain by 36% and the length of time to the loss of crusts by 27% (133). Thus, oral acyclovir has modest clinical benefit only if initiated very early after recurrence.

Oral administration of acyclovir can alter the severity of sun-induced reactivation of labial HSV infections. The administration of 200 mg five times daily to skiers did not decrease the frequency of recurrent labial infections compared with placebo, but significantly fewer lesions formed on days 5 to 7 among acyclovir recipients. Short-term prophylactic therapy with acyclovir may benefit some patients with recurrent herpes labialis who anticipate engaging in a high-risk activity (e.g., intense exposure to sunlight). The intermittent administration of acyclovir does not alter the frequency of subsequent recurrences. No data support the use of long-term treatment with acyclovir for the prevention of herpes labialis.

Mucocutaneous HSV Infections in Immunocompromised Patients

HSV infections of the lip, mouth, skin, perianal area, or genitals may be much more severe in immunocompromised patients than in healthy hosts. In the former, the lesions tend to be more invasive, slower to heal, and associated with prolonged viral shedding. Intravenous acyclovir therapy is very beneficial in such patients (144). Immunocompromised patients receiving acyclovir had a shorter duration of viral shedding and more rapid healing of lesions than patients receiving placebo (Fig. 17) (93). Oral acy-

TABLE 1 Indications for acyclovir therapy

Type of infection	Route and dosage[a]	Comment
Genital HSV		
Initial episode		
Acyclovir	200 mg p.o. five times/day for 7–10 days	Preferred route in healthy host
	5 mg/kg i.v. every 8 h for 5–7 days	Reserved for severe cases
	400 mg p.o. t.i.d.	
Valacyclovir	1 g p.o. b.i.d. for 7–10 days	
Famciclovir	250 mg p.o. t.i.d. for 5–10 days	
Recurrent episode		
Acyclovir	400 mg p.o. b.i.d. for 5 days	Limited clinical benefit
Valacyclovir	500 mg p.o. b.i.d. for 5 days	
Famciclovir	125–250 mg p.o. b.i.d. for 5 days	
Suppression		
Acyclovir	400 mg p.o. b.i.d.	Titrate dose as required
Valacyclovir	500 or 1,000 mg p.o. once/day	
Famciclovir	250 mg p.o. b.i.d.	
Mucocutaneous HSV in an immunocompromised patient		
Acyclovir	200–400 mg p.o. five times/day for 10 days	For minor lesions only
	5 mg/kg i.v. every 8 h for 7–14 days	
	400 mg p.o. five times/day for 7–14 days	
Valacyclovir	500 mg p.o. b.i.d.	
Famciclovir	250 mg p.o. t.i.d.	
HSV encephalitis		
Acyclovir	10–15 mg/kg i.v. every 8 h for 14–21 days	
Neonatal HSV[b]		
Acyclovir	20 mg/kg i.v. every 8 h for 14–21 days	

[a] The doses are for adults with normal renal function unless otherwise noted. p.o., orally; i.v., intravenously; t.i.d., thrice daily, b.i.d., twice daily.
[b] Not currently approved by the FDA.

clovir therapy is also very effective in immunocompromised patients (129).

Acyclovir prophylaxis of HSV infections is of clinical value in severely immunocompromised patients, especially those undergoing induction chemotherapy or transplantation. Intravenous or oral administration of acyclovir reduces the incidence of symptomatic HSV infection from about 70% to 5 to 20% (123). A sequential regimen of intravenous acyclovir followed by oral acyclovir, valacycovir, or famciclovir for 3 to 6 months can virtually eliminate symptomatic HSV infections in organ transplant recipients. A variety of oral dosing regimens, ranging from 200 mg three times daily to 800 mg twice daily, have been used successfully. Among bone marrow transplant recipients and patients with AIDS, acyclovir-resistant HSV isolates have been identified more frequently after therapeutic acyclovir administration than during prophylaxis. Acyclovir has become a therapeutic mainstay for treatment and suppression of herpesvirus infections in immunocompromised patients.

Herpes Simplex Encephalitis

Herpes simplex encephalitis is associated with substantial morbidity and mortality despite the use of antiviral therapy (131, 149). The administration of acyclovir at a dosage of 10 mg/kg every 8 h for 10 to 14 days reduced mortality at 3 months to 19%, compared with approximately 50% among patients treated with vidarabine (Fig. 18) (149). Furthermore, 38% of the patients treated with acyclovir regained normal function. Patients with a Glasgow coma score of less than 6, those over 30 years of age, and those with encephalitis longer than 4 days had a poor outcome. For the most favorable outcome, therapy must be instituted before semicoma or coma develops.

Neonatal HSV Infections

Newborns with HSV infections can be classified as having disease that is localized to the skin, eyes, and mouth; affects the CNS; or is disseminated. Babies with CNS or disseminated disease when treated with 20 mg/kg every 8 h for 21 days have mortality rates of 5 and 25%, compared to historical rates of 10 and 55%, respectively. Among those survivors, 35 and 80% of babies develop normally, respectively (68, 69). No baby with disease localized to the skin, eyes, or mouth died. Of note, PCR assessment of the cerebrospinal fluid should be utilized to classify the extent of disease (i.e., CNS involvement), as well as identify babies with skin, eye, and/or mouth disease who have asympto-

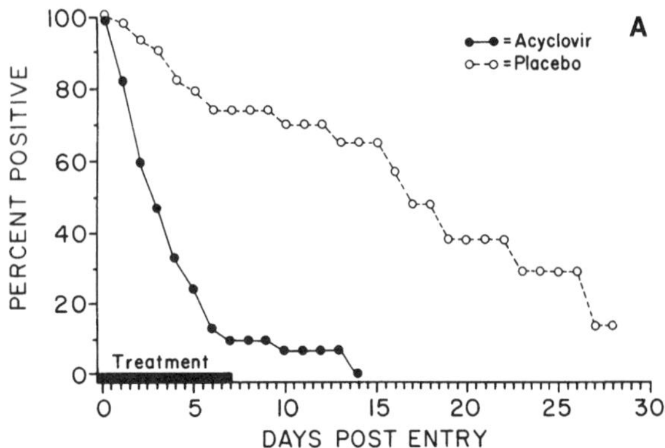

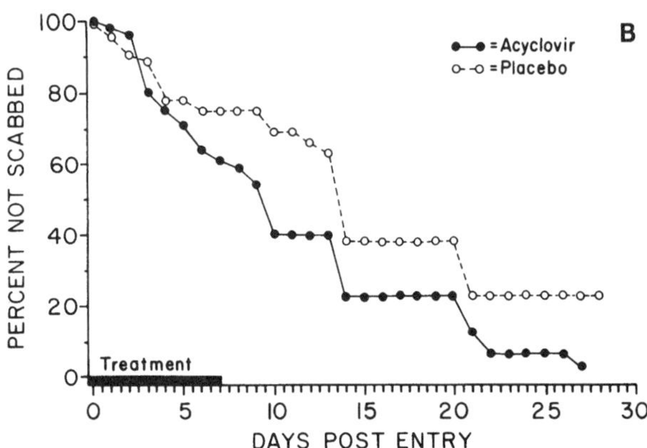

FIGURE 17 Acyclovir therapy of mucocutaneous HSV infections in immunocompromised patients, according to the clearance of virus (A) and the extent of healing (B). (Reprinted from reference 93a with permission of Elsevier.)

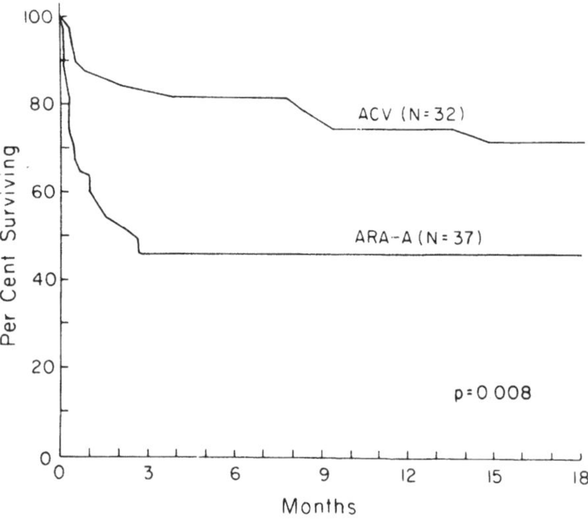

FIGURE 18 Comparison of survival in patients with biopsy-proven herpes simplex encephalitis treated with vidarabine (ARA-A) or acyclovir (ACV). (Reprinted from reference 93a with permission of Elsevier.)

TABLE 2 Investigational uses of acyclovir

Herpes labialis (prophylaxis)
HSV keratitis
Suppression of HSV infections in immunocompromised patients
Disseminated or visceral HSV infections (e.g., hepatitis)

matic CNS involvement. Furthermore, an end-of-therapy assessment should be considered.

Other HSV Infections

Case reports have described the successful use of acyclovir in the treatment of other HSV infections such as hepatitis, pulmonary infections, herpetic esophagitis, proctitis, eczema herpeticum, erythema multiform, and herpetic whitlow (Table 2). Topical therapy with acyclovir for HSV ocular infections is effective but probably not superior to trifluridine (58, 62).

Viral Resistance

HSV can develop resistance to acyclovir through mutations in the viral gene encoding TK: through the generation of TK-deficient mutants or through the selection of mutants possessing a TK that is unable to phosphorylate acyclovir (37). Clinical isolates resistant to acyclovir are almost uniformly deficient in TK, although isolates with altered DNA polymerase have been recovered from HSV-infected patients. Drug resistance was considered rare and resistant isolates were thought to be less pathogenic until a series of acyclovir-resistant HSV isolates from patients with AIDS were characterized (45). These resistant mutants were deficient in TK. Although acyclovir-resistant HSV is sensitive to vidarabine and foscarnet in vitro, only foscarnet has been shown to be effective in the treatment of acyclovir-resistant HSV. Acyclovir-resistant HSV isolates have been identified as the cause of pneumonia, encephalitis, esophagitis, and mucocutaneous infections in immunocompromised patients.

Toxicity

Acyclovir, valacyclovir, and famciclovir therapy is associated with very few adverse effects. Renal dysfunction has been reported, especially for patients given large doses of acyclovir by rapid intravenous infusion, but it appears to be uncommon and is usually reversible. The risk of nephrotoxicity can be minimized by administering acyclovir by slow infusion and ensuring adequate hydration. Oral acyclovir therapy, even at dosages of 800 mg five times daily, has not been associated with renal dysfunction (63). A few reports have linked intravenous administration of acyclovir with disturbances of the CNS, including agitation, hallucinations, disorientation, tremors, and myoclonus (143).

The Acyclovir in Pregnancy Registry has gathered data on prenatal exposure to acyclovir. No increase in the risk to the mother or fetus has been documented, but the total number of monitored pregnancies is too small to detect any low-frequency events (1a). Since acyclovir crosses the placenta and is concentrated in amniotic fluid, there is concern about the potential for fetal nephrotoxicity, although none has been observed.

Studies performed by us were initiated and supported under a contract (NO1-AI-62554) from the Antiviral Research Branch of the National Institute of Allergy and Infectious Diseases (NIAID)

(R.J.W.), a Program Project Grant (PO1 AI 24009)(B.R. and R.J.W.), an Outstanding Investigator Award (2R35 CA 47451-08)(B.R.), Unrestricted Grants in Infectious Diseases from Bristol-Myers Squibb (B.R. and R.J.W.), and grants from the General Clinical Research Center Program (RR-032) and the State of Alabama.

REFERENCES

1. **Anderson, S. G., J. Hamilton, and S. Williams.** 1950. An attempt to vaccinate against herpes simplex. *Aust. J. Exp. Biol. Med. Sci.* **28:**579–584.

1a. **Andrews, E. B., H. H. Tilson, B. A. Hurin, F. R. C. Path, and J. F. Cordero.** 1988. Acyclovir in pregnancy registry. An observational epidemiological approach. *Am. J. Med.* **85**(Suppl. 2A)**:**123–128.

2. **Aoki, F. Y., S. Tyring, F. Diaz-Mitoma, G. Gross, J. Gao, and K. Hamed.** 2006. Single-day, patient-initiated famciclovir therapy for recurrent genital herpes: a randomized, double-blind, placebo-controlled trial. *Clin. Infect. Dis.* **42:**8–13.

3. **Arvin, A. M., A. S. Yeager, F. W. Bruhn, and M. Grossman.** 1982. Neonatal herpes simplex infection in the absence of mucocutaneous lesions. *J. Pediatr.* **100:**715–721.

4. **Ashley, R., G. J. Mertz, and L. Corey.** 1987. Detection of asymptomatic herpes simplex virus infections after vaccination. *J. Virol.* **61:**264–268.

5. **Aurelius, E., B. Johansson, B. Skoldenberg, A. Staland, and M. Forsgren.** 1991. Rapid diagnosis of herpes simplex encephalitis by nested polymerase chain reaction assay of cerebrospinal fluid. *Lancet* **337:**189–192.

6. **Bader, C., C. S. Crumpacker, L. E. Schnipper, B. Ransel, J. E. Clark, K. Arndt, and I. M. Freedberg.** 1978. The natural history of recurrent facial-oral infection with herpes simplex virus. *J. Infect. Dis.* **138:**897–905.

7. **Balfour, H. H., Jr.** 1999. Antiviral drugs. *N. Engl. J. Med.* **340:**1255–1268.

8. **Baringer, J. R., and P. Swoveland.** 1973. Recovery of herpes simplex virus from human trigeminal ganglions. *N. Engl. J. Med.* **288:**648–650.

9. **Bastian, F. O., A. S. Rabson, and C. L. Yee.** 1972. Herpesvirus hominis: isolation from human trigeminal ganglion. *Science* **178:**306.

10. **Berman, P. W., T. Gregory, D. Crase, and L. A. Lasky.** 1985. Protection from genital herpes simplex virus type 2 infection by vaccination with cloned type 1 glycoprotein D. *Science* **227:**1490–1492.

11. **Bernstein, D. I., E. Garratty, M. A. Lovett, and Y. J. Bryson.** 1985. Comparison of Western blot analysis to microneutralization for the protection of type-specific herpes simplex virus antibodies. *J. Med. Virol.* **15:**223–230.

12. **Binder, P. S.** 1977. Herpes simplex keratitis. *Surv. Ophthalmol.* **21:**313–331.

13. **Black, F. L.** 1975. Infectious diseases in primitive societies. *Science* **187:**515–518.

14. **Blank, H., and H. G. Haines.** 1973. Experimental human reinfection with herpes simplex virus. *J. Investig. Dermatol.* **61:**223–225.

15. **Brain, R. T.** 1936. Biological therapy in virus diseases. *Br. J. Dermatol. Syph.* **48:**21–26.

16. **Breinig, M. K., L. A. Kingsley, J. A. Armstrong, D. J. Freeman, and M. Ho.** 1990. Epidemiology of genital herpes in Pittsburgh: serologic, sexual, and racial correlates of apparent and inapparent herpes simplex infections. *J. Infect. Dis.* **162:**299–305.

17. **Brock, B. V., S. Selke, J. Benedetti, J. M. Douglas, Jr., and L. Corey.** 1990. Frequency of asymptomatic shedding of herpes simplex virus in women with genital herpes. *JAMA* **263:**418–420.

18. **Brown, Z. A., J. Benedetti, R. Ashley, S. Burchett, S. Selke, S. Berry, L. A. Vontver, and L. Corey.** 1991. Neonatal herpes simplex virus infection in relation to asymptomatic maternal infection at the time of labor. *N. Engl. J. Med.* **324:**1247–1252.

19. **Brown, Z. A., L. A. Vontver, J. Benedetti, C. W. Critchlow, C. J. Sells, S. Berry, and L. Corey.** 1987. Effects on infants of a first episode of genital herpes during pregnancy. *N. Engl. J. Med.* **317:**1246–1251.

20. **Bryson, Y. J., M. Dillon, M. Lovett, G. Acuna, S. Taylor, J. Cherry, L. Johnson, E. Wiesmeier, W. Growdon, T. Creagh-Kirk, and R. Keeney.** 1983. Treatment of first episodes of genital herpes simplex virus infection with oral acyclovir: a randomized double-blind controlled trial in normal subjects. *N. Engl. J. Med.* **308:**916–921.

21. **Buchman, T. G., B. Roizman, G. Adams, and B. H. Stover.** 1978. Restriction endonuclease fingerprinting of herpes simplex DNA: a novel epidemiological tool applied to a nosocomial outbreak. *J. Infect. Dis.* **138:**488–498.

22. **Buddingh, G. H., D. I. Schrum, J. C. Lanier, and D. J. Guidy.** 1953. Studies of the natural history of herpes simplex infections. *Pediatrics* **11:**595.

23. **Burke, R. L.** 1991. Development of a herpes simplex virus subunit glycoprotein vaccine for prophylactic and therapeutic use. *Rev. Infect. Dis.* **13:**S906–S911.

24. **Carter, C. A., C. E. Hartley, G. R. B. Skinner, S. P. Turner, and D. L. Easty.** 1981. Experimental ulcerative herpetic keratitis. IV. Preliminary observations on the efficacy of a herpes simplex subunit vaccine. *Br. J. Ophthalmol.* **65:**679–682.

25. **Carton, C. A., and E. D. Kilbourne.** 1952. Activation of latent herpes simplex by trigeminal sensory-root section. *N. Engl. J. Med.* **246:**172–176.

26. **Casrouge, A., S. Y. Zhang, C. Eidenschenk, E. Jouanguy, A. Puel, K. Yang, A. Alcais, C. Picard, N. Mahfoufi, N. Nicolas, L. Lorenzo, S. Plancoulaine, B. Senechal, F. Geissmann, K. Tabeta, K. Hoebe, X. Du, R. L. Miller, B. Heron, C. Mignot, T. B. de Villemeur, P. Lebon, O. Dulac, F. Rozenberg, B. Beutler, M. Tardieu, L. Abel, and J. L. Casanova.** 2006. Herpes simplex virus encephalitis in human unc-93b deficiency. *Science* **314:**308–312.

27. **Cesario, T. C., J. D. Poland, H. Wulff, T. D. Chin, and H. A. Wenner.** 1969. Six years experiences with herpes simplex virus in a children's home. *Am. J. Epidemiol.* **90:**416–422.

28. **Chou, J., E. R. Kern, R. J. Whitley, and B. Roizman.** 1990. Mapping of herpes simplex virus-1 neurovirulence to gamma $_1$34.5, a gene nonessential for growth in culture. *Science* **250:**1262–1266.

29. **Chou, J., and B. Roizman.** 1986. The terminal a sequence of the herpes simplex virus genome contains the promoter of a gene located in the repeat sequences of the L component. *J. Virol.* **57:**629–637.

30. **Cone, R. W., A. C. Hobson, Z. Brown, R. Ashley, S. Berry, C. Winter, and L. Corey.** 1994. Frequent detection of genital herpes simplex virus DNA by polymerase chain reaction among pregnant women. *JAMA* **272:**792–796.

31. **Corey, L.** 1982. The diagnosis and treatment of genital herpes. *JAMA* **248:**1041–1049.

32. **Corey, L., H. G. Adams, Z. A. Brown, and K. K. Holmes.** 1983. Genital herpes simplex virus infections: clinical manifestations, course and complications. *Ann. Intern. Med.* **98:**958–972.

33. **Corey, L., J. Benedetti, C. Critchlow, G. Mertz, J. Douglas, K. Fife, A. Fahnlander, M. L. Remington, C. Winter, and J. Dragavon.** 1983. Treatment of primary first

episode genital herpes simplex virus infections with acyclovir: results of topical, intravenous, and oral therapy. *J. Antimicrob. Chemother.* **12:**79–88.

34. **Corey, L., A. G. Langenberg, R. Ashley, R. E. Sekulovich, A. E. Izu, J. M. Douglas, Jr., H. H. Handsfield, T. Warren, L. Marr, S. Tyring, R. DiCarlo, A. A. Adimora, P. Leone, C. L. Dekker, R. L. Burke, W. P. Leong, and S. E. Straus for the Chiron HSV Vaccine Study Group.** 1999. Recombinant glycoprotein vaccine for the prevention of genital HSV-2 infection: two randomized controlled trials. *JAMA* **282:**331–340.
35. **Corey, L., W. C. Reeves, and K. K. Holmes.** 1978. Cellular immune response in genital herpes simplex virus infection. *N. Engl. J. Med.* **299:**986–991.
36. **Corey, L., A. Wald, R. Patel, S. L. Sacks, S. K. Tyring, T. Warren, J. M. Douglas, Jr., J. Paavonen, R. A. Morrow, K. R. Beutner, L. S. Stratchounsky, G. Mertz, O. N. Keene, H. A. Watson, D. Tait, and M. Vargas-Cortes.** 2004. Once-daily valacyclovir to reduce the risk of transmission of genital herpes. *N. Engl. J. Med.* **350:** 11–20.
37. **Crumpacker, C. S., L. E. Schnipper, S. I. Marlowe, P. N. Kowalsky, B. J. Hershey, and M. J. Levin.** 1982. Resistance to antiviral drugs of herpes simplex virus isolated from a patient treated with acyclovir. *N. Engl. J. Med.* **305:**343–346.
38. **Cushing, H.** 1905. Surgical aspects of major neuralgia of trigeminal nerve: report of 20 cases of operation upon the Gasserian ganglion with anatomic and physiologic notes on the consequences of its removal. *JAMA* **44:**773–779, 860–865, 920–929, 1002–1008.
39. **Diaz-Mitoma, F., R. G. Sibbald, S. D. Shafran, R. Boon, and R. L. Saltzman for the Collaborative Famciclovir Genital Herpes Research Group.** 1998. Oral famciclovir for the suppression of recurrent genital herpes; a randomized controlled trial. *JAMA* **280:**887–892.
40. **Dodd, K., L. M. Johnston, and G. J. Buddingh.** 1938. Herpetic stomatitis. *J. Pediatr.* **12:**95.
41. **Douglas, J. M., C. Critchlow, J. Benedetti, G. J. Mertz, J. D. Connor, M. A. Hintz, A. Fahnlander, M. Remington, C. Winter, and L. Corey.** 1984. A double-blind study of oral acyclovir for suppression of recurrences of genital herpes simplex virus infection. *N. Engl. J. Med.* **310:**1551–1556.
42. **Dummer, J. S., J. Arnstrong, J. Somers, S. Kusne, B. J. Carpenter, J. T. Rosenthal, and M. Ho.** 1987. Transmission of infection with herpes simplex virus by renal transplantation. *J. Infect. Dis.* **155:**202–206.
43. **Eberle, R., R. G. Russell, and B. T. Rouse.** 1981. Cell-mediated immunity to herpes simplex virus: recognition of type-specific and type-common surface antigens by cytotoxic T cell populations. *Infect. Immun.* **34:**795–803.
44. **Ekwo, E., Y. W. Wong, and M. Myers.** 1979. Asymptomatic cervicovaginal shedding of herpes simplex virus. *Am. J. Obstet. Gynecol.* **134:**102–103.
45. **Erlich, K. S., J. Mills, P. Chatis, G. J. Mertz, D. F. Busch, S. E. Follansbee, R. M. Grant, and C. S. Crumpacker.** 1989. Acyclovir-resistant herpes simplex virus infections in patients with the acquired immunodeficiency syndrome. *N. Engl. J. Med.* **320:**293–296.
46. **Fleming, D. T., G. M. McQuillan, R. E. Johnson, A. J. Nahmias, S. O. Aral, F. K. Lee, and M. E. St. Louis.** 1997. Herpes simplex virus type 2 in the United States, 1976–1994. *N. Engl. J. Med.* **337:**1105–1111.
47. **Foley, F. D., K. A. Greenwald, G. Nash, and B. A. Pruitt.** 1970. Herpesvirus infection in burned patients. *N. Engl. J. Med.* **282:**652–656.
48. **Francis, D. P., K. L. Hermann, and J. R. MacMahon.** 1975. Nosocomial and maternally acquired herpesvirus hominis infections. *Am. J. Dis. Child.* **129:**889–893.
49. **Fricker, J.** 1996. Herpes vaccines: spinning a new disc. *Lancet* **348:**1576.
50. **Gill, M. J., J. Arlette, and K. Buchan.** 1988. Herpes simplex virus infection of the hand. A profile of 79 cases. *Am. J. Med.* **84:**89–93.
51. **Glezen, W. P., G. W. Fernald, and J. A. Lohr.** 1975. Acute respiratory disease of university students with special references to the etiologic role of herpesvirus hominis. *Am. J. Epidemiol.* **101:**111–121.
52. **Goodpasture, E. W.** 1929. Herpetic infections with special reference to involvement of the nervous system. *Medicine* **8:**223–243.
53. **Guinan, M. E., J. MacCalman, E. R. Kern, J. C. Overall, and S. L. Spruance.** 1981. The course of untreated recurrent genital herpes simplex infection in 27 women. *N. Engl. J. Med.* **304:**759–763.
54. **Hale, B. D., R. C. Reindtorff, L. C. Walker, and A. N. Roberts.** 1953. Epidemic herpetic stomatitis in an orphanage nursery. *JAMA* **183:**1068.
55. **Hatherley, L. I., K. Hayes, E. M. Hennessy, and I. Jack.** 1980. Herpesvirus in an obstetric hospital. I. Herpetic eruptions. *Med. J. Aust.* **2:**205–208.
56. **Hatherley, L. I., K. Hayes, and I. Jack.** 1980. Herpesvirus in an obstetric hospital. II. Asymptomatic virus excretion in staff members. *Med. J. Aust.* **2:**273–275.
57. **Hayward, G. S., R. J. Jacob, S. C. Wadsworth, and B. Roizman.** 1975. Anatomy of herpes simplex virus DNA. Evidence for four populations of molecules that differ in the relative orientations of their long and short components. *Proc. Natl. Acad. Sci. USA* **72:**4243–4247.
58. **Herpetic Eye Disease Study Group.** 2000. Oral acyclovir herpes simplex virus eye disease: effect on prevention of epithelial keratitis and stromal keratitis. *Arch. Ophthalmol.* **118:**1030–1036.
59. **Hesselgesser, J., and R. Horuk.** 1999. Chemokine and chemokine receptor expression in the central nervous system. *J. Neurovirol.* **5:**13–26.
60. **Holmberg, S. D., J. A. Stewart, A. R. Gerber, R. H. Byers, F. K. Lee, P. M. O'Malley, and A. J. Nahmias.** 1988. Prior herpes simplex virus type 2 infection as a risk factor for HIV infection. *Am. J. Med.* **259:**1048–1050.
61. **Hook, E., R. Cannon, A. J. Nahmias, F. Lee, C. Campbell, D. Glasser, and T. Quinn.** 1992. Herpes simplex virus infection as a risk factor for human immunodeficiency virus infection in heterosexuals. *J. Infect. Dis.* **165:** 251–255.
62. **Hovding, G.** 1989. A comparison between acyclovir and triflurothymidine ophthalmic ointment in the treatment of epithelial dendritic keratitis: a double-blind, randomized parallel group trial. *Acta Ophthalmol.* **67:**51–54.
63. **Huff, J. C., B. Bean, H. H. Balfour, Jr., O. L. Laskin, J. D. Connor, L. Corey, Y. J. Bryson, and P. W. McGuirt.** 1988. Therapy of herpes zoster with oral acyclovir. *Am. J. Med.* **85:**84–89.
64. **Hutto, C., A. Arvin, R. Jacobs, R. Steele, S. Stagno, R. Lyrene, L. Willett, D. Powell, R. Anderson, J. Wetherman, G. Ratliff, A. J. Nahmias, and R. J. Whitley.** 1987. Intrauterine herpes simplex virus infections. *J. Pediatr.* **110:**97–101.
65. **Johnson, R. E., A. J. Nahmias, L. S. Magder, F. K. Lee, C. Brooks, and C. Snowden.** 1989. A seroepidemiologic survey of the prevalence of herpes simplex virus type 2 infection in the United States. *N. Engl. J. Med.* **321:**7–12.
66. **Josey, W. E.** 1968. Genital infection with type-2 herpesvirus hominis. *Am. J. Obstet. Gynecol.* **101:**718.
67. **Kimberlin, D. W., E. P. Acosta, P. J. Sánchez, S. Sood, V. Agrawal, J. Homans, R. F. Jacobs, D. Lang, J. R. Romero, J. Griffin, G. A. Cloud, F. D. Lakeman, and**

R. J. Whitley for the National Institute of Allergy and Infectious Diseases Collaborative Antiviral Study Group. 2008. Pharmacokinetic and pharmacodynamic assessment of oral valganciclovir in the treatment of symptomatic congenital cytomegalovirus disease. *J. Infect. Dis.* **197:**836–845.

68. **Kimberlin, D. W., C.-Y. Lin, R. F. Jacobs, D. A. Powell, L. Corey, W. C. Gruber, M. Rathore, J. Bradley, P. S. Diaz, M. Kumar, A. M. Arvin, K. Gutierrez, M. Shelton, L. B. Weiner, J. W. Sleasman, T. M. de Sierra, S. Weller, and S.-J. Soong.** 2001. The safety and efficacy of high-dose intravenous acyclovir in the management of neonatal herpes simplex virus infections. *Pediatrics* **108:** 230–238.

69. **Kimberlin, D. W., C.-Y. Lin, R. F. Jacobs, D. A. Powell, F. L, W. Gruber, M. Rathore, J. Bradley, P. S. Diaz, M. Kumar, A. M. Arvin, K. Gutierrez, M. Shelton, L. B. Weiner, J. W. Sleasman, T. M. de Sierra, S.-J. Soong, F. D. Lakeman, R. J. Whitley, and the National Institute of Allergy and Infectious Diseases Collaborative Antiviral Study Group.** 2001. Natural history of neonatal herpes simplex virus infections in the acyclovir era. *Pediatrics* **108:**223–229.

70. **Koelle, D. M., J. Genedetti, A. Langenberg, and L. Corey.** 1992. Asymptomatic reactivation of herpes simplex virus in women after the first episode of genital herpes. *Ann. Intern. Med.* **116:**433–437.

71. **Kohl, S., M. S. West, C. G. Prober, W. M. Sullender, L. S. Loo, and A. M. Arvin.** 1989. Neonatal antibody-dependent cellular cytoxic antibody levels are associated with the clinical presentation of neonatal herpes simplex virus infection. *J. Infect. Dis.* **160:**770–776.

72. **Koutsky, L. A., R. L. Ashley, K. K. Holmes, C. E. Stevens, C. W. Critchlow, N. Kiviat, C. M. Lipinski, P. Wolner-Hanssen, and L. Corey.** 1990. The frequency of unrecognized type 2 herpes simplex virus infection among women. Implications for the control of genital herpes. *Sex. Transm. Dis.* **17:**90–94.

73. **Koutsky, L. A., C. E. Stevens, K. K. Holmes, R. L. Ashley, N. B. Kiviat, C. W. Critchlow, and L. Corey.** 1992. Underdiagnosis of genital herpes by current clinical and viral-isolation procedures. *N. Engl. J. Med.* **326:** 1533–1539.

74. **Kulhanjian, J. A., V. Soroush, D. S. Au, R. N. Bronzan, L. L. Yasukawa, L. E. Weylman, A. M. Arvin, and C. G. Prober.** 1992. Identification of women at unsuspected risk of primary infection with herpes simplex virus type 2 during pregnancy. *N. Engl. J. Med.* **326:**916–920.

75. **Lafferty, W. E., R. W. Coombs, J. Benedetti, C. Critchlow, and L. Corey.** 1987. Recurrences after oral and genital herpes simplex virus infection. Influence of site of infection and viral type. *N. Engl. J. Med.* **316:**1444–1449.

76. **Lakeman, F. D., R. J. Whitley, and the National Institute of Allergy and Infectious Diseases Collaborative Antiviral Study Group.** 1995. Diagnosis of herpes simplex encephalitis: application of polymerase chain reaction to cerebrospinal fluid from brain biopsied patients and correlation with disease. *J. Infect. Dis.* **172:**857–863.

77. **Langenberg, A. G. M., L. Corey, R. L. Ashley, W. P. Leong, and S. E. Straus for the Chiron HSV Vaccine Study Group.** 1999. A prospective study of new infections with herpes simplex virus type 1 and type 2. *N. Engl. J. Med.* **341:**1432–1438.

78. **Lindgren, K. M., R. G. Douglas, Jr., and R. B. Couch.** 1968. Significance of herpesvirus hominis in respiratory secretions of man. *N. Engl. J. Med.* **276:**517–523.

79. **Lopez, C., A. M. Arvin, and R. Ashley.** 1993. Immunity to herpesvirus infections in humans, p. 397–425. *In* B. Roizman, R. J. Whitley, and C. Lopez (ed.), *The Human Herpesviruses*. Raven Press, New York, NY.

80. **Magder, L. S., A. J. Nahmias, R. E. Johnson, F. K. Lee, C. Brooks, and C. Snowden.** 1989. The prevalence and distribution of herpes simplex virus type 1 and 2 antibodies in the United States population. *N. Engl. J. Med.* **321:** 7–12.

81. **Mann, S. L., J. D. Meyers, K. L. Holmes, and L. Corey.** 1984. Prevalence and incidence of herpesvirus infections among homosexually active men. *J. Infect. Dis.* **149:** 1026–1027.

82. **Markert, J. M., Y. G. Gillespie, R. R. Weichselbaum, B. Roizman, and R. J. Whitley.** 2000. Genetically engineered HSV in the treatment of glioma: a review. *Rev. Med. Virol.* **10:**17–30.

83. **Markert, J. M., M. D. Medlock, S. D. Rabkin, G. Y. Gillespie, T. Todo, W. D. Hunter, C. A. Palmer, F. Feigenbaum, C. Tornatore, F. Tufaro, and R. L. Martuza.** 2000. Conditionally replicating herpes simplex virus mutant, G207 for the treatment of malignant glioma: results of a phase I trial. *Gene Ther.* **7:**867–874.

84. **Markert, J. M., J. N. Parker, D. J. Buchsbaum, W. E. Grizzle, G. Y. Gillespie, and R. J. Whitley.** 2006. Oncolytic HSV-1 for the treatment of brain tumours. *Herpes* **13:**66–71.

85. **Martin, S., R. J. Courtney, G. Fowler, and B. T. Rouse.** 1988. Herpes simplex virus type 1-specific cytotoxic T lymphocytes recognize virus nonstructural proteins. *J. Virol.* **62:**2265–2273.

86. **Martinez, V., and E. Caumes.** 2007. HSV therapy and HIV-1 reduction. *N. Engl. J. Med.* **356:**2323. (Author's reply, **356:**2324.)

87. **McGeoch, D. J., M. A. Dalrymple, A. J. Davison, A. Dolan, M. C. Frame, D. McNab, L. J. Perry, J. E. Scott, and P. Taylor.** 1988. The complete DNA sequence of the long unique region in the genome of herpes simplex virus type 1. *J. Gen. Virol.* **69:**1531–1574.

88. **Meignier, B., R. Longnecker, and B. Roizman.** 1988. In vivo behavior of genetically engineered herpes simplex virus R7017 and R7020. Construction and evaluation in rodents. *J. Infect. Dis.* **158:**602–614.

89. **Meignier, B., B. Martin, R. Whitley, and B. Roizman.** 1990. In vivo behavior of genetically engineered herpes simplex viruses R7017 and R7020. II. Studies in immunocompetent and immunosuppressed owl monkeys *(Aotus trivirgatus)*. *J. Infect. Dis.* **162:**313–321.

90. **Mertz, G. J., J. Benedetti, R. Ashley, S. Selke, and L. Corey.** 1992. Risk factors for the sexual transmission of genital herpes. *Ann. Intern. Med.* **116:**197–202.

91. **Mertz, G. J., C. W. Critchlow, J. Benedetti, R. C. Reichman, R. Dolin, J. Connor, D. C. Redfield, M. C. Savoia, D. D. Richman, D. L. Tyrrell, L. Miedzinski, J. Portnoy, R. E. Keeney, and L. Corey.** 1984. Double-blind placebo-controlled trial of oral acyclovir in first-episode genital herpes simplex virus infection. *JAMA* **252:**1147–1151.

92. **Mertz, G. J., C. C. Jones, J. Mills, and S. M. Lemon.** 1988. Long-term acyclovir suppression of frequently recurring genital herpes simplex virus infection. *JAMA* **260:**201–206.

93. **Meyers, J. D., J. C. Wade, C. D. Mitchell, R. Saral, P. S. Lietman, D. T. Durack, M. J. Levin, A. C. Segreti, and H. H. Balfour, Jr.** 1982. Multicenter collaborative trial of intravenous acyclovir for treatment of mucocutaneous herpes simplex virus infection in the immunocompromised host. *Am. J. Med.* **73:**229–235.

93a. **Middlebrooks, M., and R. J.Whitley.** 1991. Herpes simplex virus infections, p. 1831–1835. *In* J. P. Wyngaarden, L. H. Smith, and J. C. Bennett (ed.), *Cecil Textbook of Medicine*, 19th ed. The W. B. Saunders Co., Philadelphia, PA.

93b. **Middlebrooks, M., and R. J. Whitley.** 1991. Herpesviruses, p. 865–879. *In* S. Baron (ed.), *Medical Microbiology*, 3rd ed. Churchill Livingstone, Inc., New York, NY.
94. **Muller, S. A., F. C. Hermann, and R. K. Winkelman.** 1972. Herpes simplex infections in hematologic malignancies. *Am. J. Med.* **52:**102–114.
95. **Nahmias, A. J., and W. R. Dowdle.** 1968. Antigenic and biologic differences in herpesvirus hominis. *Prog. Med. Virol.* **10:**110–159.
96. **Nahmias, A. J., W. E. Josey, Z. M. Naib, M. G. Freeman, R. J. Fernandez, and J. H. Wheeler.** 1971. Perinatal risk associated with maternal genital herpes simplex virus infection. *Am. J. Obstet. Gynecol.* **110:**825–836.
97. **Nahmias, A. J., F. K. Lee, and S. Bechman-Nahmias.** 1990. Sero-epidemiological and sociological patterns of herpes simplex virus infection in the world. *Scand. J. Infect. Dis.* **69:**19–36.
98. **Nahmias, A. J., and B. Roizman.** 1973. Infection with herpes simplex viruses 1 and 2. *N. Engl. J. Med.* **289:**667–674, 719–725, 781–789.
99. **Nash, A. A., J. Phelan, and P. Wildy.** 1981. Cell-mediated immunity to herpes simplex virus-infected mice: H-2 mapping of the delayed-type hypersensitivity response and the antiviral T-cell response. *J. Immunol.* **126:**1260–1262.
100. **Nilsen, A. E., T. Aasen, A. M. Halsos, B. R. Kinge, E. A. L. Tjotta, K. Wikstrom, and A. P. Fiddian.** 1982. Efficacy of oral acyclovir in the treatment of initial and recurrent genital herpes. *Lancet* **ii:**571–573.
101. **Nusinoff-Lehrman, S., J. M. Douglas, L. Corey, and D. W. Barry.** 1986. Recurrent genital herpes and suppressive oral acyclovir therapy. *Ann. Intern. Med.* **104:**786–790.
102. **Olson, L. C., E. L. Buescher, M. S. Artenstein, and P. D. Parkman.** 1967. Herpesvirus infections of the human central nervous system. *N. Engl. J. Med.* **277:**1271–1277.
103. **Pass, R. F., R. J. Whitley, J. D. Whelchel, A. G. Diethelm, D. W. Reynolds, and C. A. Alford.** 1979. Identification of patients with increased risk of infection with herpes simplex virus after renal transplantation. *J. Infect. Dis.* **140:**487–492.
104. **Patel, R., N. J. Bodsworth, P. Woolley, B. Peters, G. Vejlsgaard, S. Saari, A. Gibb, J. Robinson, and the International Valaciclovir HSV Study Group.** 1997. Valaciclovir for the suppression of recurrent genital HSV infection: a placebo controlled study of once daily therapy. *Genitourin. Med.* **73:**105–109.
105. **Pazin, G. J., M. Ho, and P. J. Jannetta.** 1978. Reactivation of herpes simplex virus after decompression of the trigeminal nerve root. *J. Infect. Dis.* **138:**405–409.
106. **Peacock, J. E., L. G. Kaplowitz, P. F. Sparling, D. T. Durack, J. W. Gnann, and R. J. Whitley.** 1988. Intravenous acyclovir therapy of first episodes of genital herpes: a multicenter double-blind, placebo-controlled trial. *Am. J. Med.* **85:**301–306.
107. **Post, L. E., and B. Roizman.** 1981. A generalized technique for deletion of specific genes in large genomes: alpha gene 22 of herpes simplex virus 1 is not essential for growth. *Cell* **25:**227–232.
108. **Prober, C. G., W. M. Sullender, L. L. Yasukawa, D. S. Au, A. S. Yeager, and A. M. Arvin.** 1987. Low risk of herpes simplex virus infections in neonates exposed to the virus at the time of vaginal delivery to mothers with recurrent genital herpes simplex virus infections. *N. Engl. J. Med.* **316:**240–244.
109. **Raborn, G. W., W. T. McGaw, M. Grace, L. D. Tyrrell, and S. M. Samuels.** 1987. Oral acyclovir and herpes labialis: a randomized, double-blind, placebo-controlled study. *J. Am. Dent. Assoc.* **115:**38–42.
110. **Rasmussen, L., and T. C. Merigan.** 1978. Role of T-lymphocytes in cellular immune responses during herpes simplex virus infection in humans. *Proc. Natl. Acad. Sci. USA* **75:**3957–3961.
111. **Rattray, M. C., L. Corey, W. C. Reeves, L. A. Vontver, and K. K. Holmes.** 1978. Recurrent genital herpes among women: symptomatic versus asymptomatic viral shedding. *Br. J. Vener. Dis.* **54:**262–265.
112. **Reeves, W. C., L. Corey, H. G. Adams, L. A. Vontver, and K. K. Holmes.** 1981. Risk of recurrence after first episodes of genital herpes: relation to HSV type and antibody response. *N. Engl. J. Med.* **305:**315–319.
113. **Reichman, R. C., G. J. Badger, G. J. Mertz, and L. Corey.** 1984. Treatment of recurrent genital herpes simplex infection with oral acyclovir. Controlled trial. *JAMA* **251:**2103–2107.
114. **Roizman, B., and D. M. Knipe.** 2001. Herpes simplex viruses and their replication, p. 2399–2459. *In* B. N. Fields and D. M. Knipe (ed.), *Fields Virology*, 4th ed. Lippincott Williams & Wilkins, Philadelphia, PA.
115. **Roizman, B., D. M. Knipe, and R. Whitley.** 2007. The replication of herpes simplex viruses, p. 2501–2601. *In* D. M. Knipe, P. M. Howley, D. E. Griffin, R. A. Lamb, M. A. Martin, B. Roizman, and S. E. Straus (ed.), *Fields Virology*, 5th ed. Lippincott Williams & Wilkins, Philadelphia, PA.
116. **Roizman, B., and P. E. Pellett.** 2001. Herpesviridae, p. 2381–2397. *In* B. N. Fields and D. M. Knipe (ed.), *Fields Virology*, 4th ed. Lippincott Williams & Wilkins, Philadelphia, PA.
117. **Roizman, B., and A. Sears.** 1987. An inquiry into the mechanisms of herpes simplex virus latency. *Annu. Rev. Microbiol.* **41:**543–571.
118. **Roizman, B., and A. E. Sears.** 1996. Herpes simplex viruses and their replication, p. 2231–2295. *In* B. N. Fields, D. M. Knipe, P. M. Howley, R. M. Chanock, J. L. Melnick, T. P. Monath, B. Roizman, and S. E. Straus (ed.), *Fields Virology*, 3rd ed. Lippincott-Raven Publishers, Philadelphia, PA.
119. **Roizman, B., and B. Taddeo.** 2007. The strategy of viral replication and takeover of the host cell, p. 163–173. *In* A. Arvin, G. Campadelli-Fiume, E. Mocarski, P. S. Moore, B. Roizman, R. Whitley, and K. Yamanishi (ed.), *Human Herpesviruses: Biology, Therapy, and Immunoprophylaxis*. Cambridge University Press, Cambridge, England.
120. **Rowley, A., F. Lakeman, R. Whitley, and S. Wolinsky.** 1990. Rapid detection of herpes simplex virus DNA in cerebrospinal fluid of patients with herpes simplex encephalitis. *Lancet* **335:**440–441.
121. **Russell, A. S.** 1974. Cell-mediated immunity to herpes simplex virus in man. *J. Infect. Dis.* **129:**142–146.
122. **Sanchez-Martinez, D., D. S. Schmid, W. Whittington, D. Brown, W. C. Reeves, S. Chatterjee, R. J. Whitley, and P. Pellett.** 1991. Evaluation of a test based on baculovirus-expressed glycoprotein G for detection of herpes simplex virus type specific antibodies. *J. Infect. Dis.* **164:**1196–1199.
123. **Saral, R., W. H. Burns, O. L. Laskin, G. W. Santos, and P. S. Leitman.** 1981. Acyclovir prophylaxis of herpes simplex virus infections: a randomized, double-blind, controlled trial in bone-marrow-transplant recipients. *N. Engl. J. Med.* **305:**63–67.
124. **Schacker, T., J. Zeh, H. Hu, M. Shaughnessy, and L. Corey.** 2002. Changes in plasma human immunodeficiency virus type 1 RNA associated with herpes simplex

virus reactivation and suppression. *J. Infect. Dis.* **186:** 1718–1725.

125. **Schmitt, D. L., D. W. Johnson, and F. W. Henderson.** 1991. Herpes simplex type 1 infections in group day care. *Pediatr. Infect. Dis. J.* **10:**729–734.
126. **Scott, T. F., A. J. Steigman, and J. H. Convey.** 1941. Acute infectious gingivostomatitis: etiology, epidemiology, and clinical pictures of a common disorder caused by the virus of herpes simplex. *JAMA* **117:**999.
127. **Scurlock, J., and B. R. Andersen.** 2005. *Diagnosis in Assyrian and Babylonian Medicine*. University of Illinois Press, Champaign.
128. **Selling, B., and S. Kibrick.** 1964. An outbreak of herpes simplex among wrestlers (herpes gladiatorum). *N. Engl. J. Med.* **270:**979–982.
129. **Shepp, D. H., B. A. Newton, P. S. Dandliker, N. Flornoy, and J. D. Meyers.** 1985. Oral acyclovir therapy for mucocutaneous herpes simplex virus infections in immunocompromised marrow transplant recipients. *Ann. Intern. Med.* **102:**783–785.
130. **Ship, I. I., A. L. Morris, R. T. Durocher, and L. W. Burket.** 1960. Recurrent aphthous ulcerations and recurrent herpes labialis in a professional school student population. I. Experience. *Oral Surg. Oral Med. Oral Pathol.* **13:**1191–1202.
131. **Skoldenberg, B., M. Forsgren, K. Alestig, T. Bergstrom, L. Burman, E. Dahlqvist, A. Forkman, A. Fryden, K. Lovgren, K. Norlin, R. Norrby, E. Olding-Stenkvist, G. Stiernstedt, I. Uhnoo, and K. deVahl.** 1984. Acyclovir versus vidarabine in herpes simplex encephalitis: a randomized multicentre study in consecutive Swedish patients. *Lancet* **ii:**707–711.
132. **Spruance, S. L., J. C. Overall, Jr., E. R. Kern, G. G. Krueger, V. Pliam, and W. Miller.** 1977. The natural history of recurrent herpes simplex labialis—implications for antiviral therapy. *N. Engl. J. Med.* **297:** 69–75.
133. **Spruance, S. L., J. C. B. Stewart, N. H. Rowe, M. B. McKeough, G. Wenerstrom, and D. J. Freeman.** 1990. Treatment of recurrent herpes simplex labialis with oral acyclovir. *J. Infect. Dis.* **161:**185–190.
134. **Stamm, W. E., H. H. Handsfield, A. M. Rompalo, R. L. Ashley, P. L. Roberts, and L. Corey.** 1988. The association between genital ulcer disease and acquisition of HIV infection in homosexual men. *JAMA* **260:**1429–1433.
135. **Stanberry, L., D. Koelle, and R. Whitley.** Herpes simplex vaccines. *In* G. D. M. Levine, M. Good, M. Liu, G. Nabel, J. Nataro, and R. Rappuoli (ed.), *New Generation Vaccines*, in press. Informa Healthcare, New York, NY.
136. **Stanberry, L. R., S. L. Spruance, A. L. Cunningham, D. I. Bernstein, A. Mindel, S. Sacks, S. Tyring, F. Y. Aoki, M. Slaoui, M. Denis, P. Vandepapeliere, and G. Dubin for the GlaxoSmithKline Herpes Vaccine Efficacy Study Group.** 2002. Glycoprotein-D–adjuvant vaccine to prevent genital herpes. *N. Engl. J. Med.* **347:** 1652–1661.
137. **Stern, H., S. D. Elek, D. M. Miller, and H. F. Anderson.** 1959. Herpetic whitlow, a form of cross-infection in hospitals. *Lancet* **ii:**871.
138. **Stevens, J. G., and M. L. Cook.** 1971. Latent herpes simplex virus in spinal ganglia. *Science* **173:**843–845.
139. **Straus, S. E., M. Seidin, H. E. Takiff, J. F. Rooney, J. M. Felser, H. A. Smith, P. Roane, F. Johnson, C. Hallahan, and J. M. Ostrove.** 1989. Effect of oral acyclovir treatment on symptomatic and asymptomatic shedding in recurrent genital herpes. *Sex. Transm. Dis.* **16:**107–113.
140. **Straus, S. E., H. E. Takiff, M. Seidlin, S. Bachrach, L. Lininger, J. J. DiGiovanna, K. A. Western, H. A. Smith, S. N. Lehrman, T. Creagh-Kirk, and D. W. Alling.** 1984. Suppression of frequently recurring genital herpes: placebo-controlled double-blind trial of oral acyclovir. *N. Engl. J. Med.* **310:**1545–1550.
141. **Sullender, W. M., J. L. Miller, L. L. Yasukawa, J. S. Bradley, S. Black, A. S. Yeager, and A. M. Arvin.** 1987. Humoral and cell-mediated immunity in neonates with herpes simplex virus infection. *J. Infect. Dis.* **155:** 28–37.
142. **Tuxen, D. V., J. F. Cade, M. I. McDonald, M. R. Buchanan, R. J. Clark, and M. C. Pain.** 1982. Herpes simplex virus from the lower respiratory tract in adult respiratory distress syndrome. *Am. Rev. Respir. Dis.* **126:** 416–419.
143. **Wade, J. C., and J. D. Meyers.** 1982. Neurologic symptoms associated with parenteral acyclovir treatment after marrow transplantation. *Ann. Intern. Med.* **98:**921–925.
144. **Wade, J. C., B. Newton, C. McLaren, N. Flournoy, R. E. Keeney, and J. D. Meyers.** 1982. Intravenous acyclovir to treat mucocutaneous herpes simplex virus infection after marrow transplantation: double-blind trial. *Ann. Intern. Med.* **96:**265–269.
145. **Wald, A., G. Barnum, S. Selke, G. Davis, J. Zeh, and L. Corey.** 1995. Acyclovir suppresses asymptomatic shedding of HSV-2 in the genital tract. *N. Engl. J. Med.* **326:**770–775.
146. **Wald, A., J. Zeh, S. Selke, A. Ryncarz, R. Ashley, J. N. Krieger, and L. Corey.** 2000. Reactivation of genital herpes simplex virus type 2 infection in asymptomatic seropositive persons. *N. Engl. J. Med.* **342:**844–850.
147. **Weston, W. L., S. L. Brice, J. D. Jester, A. T. Lane, S. Stockert, and J. C. Huff.** 1992. Herpes simplex virus in childhood erythema multiforme. *Pediatrics* **89:**32–34.
148. **Wheeler, C. E., Jr., and W. H. Cabaniss, Jr.** 1965. Epidemic cutaneous herpes simplex in wrestlers (herpes gladiatorum). *JAMA* **194:**993–997.
149. **Whitley, R. J., C. A. Alford, Jr., M. S. Hirsch, R. T. Schooley, J. P. Luby, F. Y. Aoki, D. Hanley, A. J. Nahmias, S.-J. Soong, and the National Institute of Allergy and Infectious Diseases Collaborative Antiviral Study Group.** 1986. Vidarabine versus acyclovir therapy in herpes simplex encephalitis. *N. Engl. J. Med.* **314:**144–149.
150. **Whitley, R. J., A. Arvin, C. Prober, L. Corey, S. Burchett, S. Plotkin, S. E. Starr, R. F. Jacobs, D. A. Powell, A. J. Nahmias, C. Sumaya, C. Edwards, C. Alford, G. Caddell, S. J. Soong, and the National Institute of Allergy and Infectious Diseases Collaborative Antiviral Study Group.** 1991. Predictors of morbidity and mortality in neonates with herpes simplex virus infections. *N. Engl. J. Med.* **324:**450–454.
151. **Whitley, R. J., L. Corey, A. Arvin, F. D. Lakeman, C. V. Sumaya, P. F. Wright, L. M. Dunkle, R. W. Steele, S. J. Soong, A. J. Nahmias, and the National Institute of Allergy and Infectious Diseases Collaborative Antiviral Study Group.** 1988. Changing presentation of herpes simplex virus infection in neonates. *J. Infect. Dis.* **158:**109–116.
152. **Whitley, R. J., E. R. Kern, S. Chatterjee, J. Chou, and B. Roizman.** 1993. Replication, establishment of latency, and induced reactivation of herpes simplex virus γ_1 34.5 deletion mutants in rodent models. *J. Clin. Investig.* **91:**2837–2843.
153. **Whitley, R. J., M. Levin, N. Barton, B. J. Hershey, G. Davis, R. E. Keeney, J. Welchel, A. G. Diethelm, P. Kartus, and S. J. Soong.** 1984. Infections caused by her-

pes simplex virus in the immunocompromised host: natural history and topical acyclovir therapy. *J. Infect. Dis.* **150:**323–329.

154. **Whitley, R. J., A. J. Nahmias, S.-J. Soong, G. G. Galasso, C. L. Fleming, C. A. Alford, Jr., and the National Institute of Allergy and Infectious Diseases Collaborative Antiviral Study Group.** 1980. Vidarabine therapy of neonatal herpes simplex virus infection. *Pediatrics* **66:** 495–501.
155. **Whitley, R. J., A. J. Nahmias, A. M. Visitine, C. L. Fleming, C. A. Alford, Jr., and the National Institute of Allergy and Infectious Diseases Collaborative Antiviral Study Group.** 1980. The natural history of herpes simplex virus infection of mother and newborn. *Pediatrics* **66:**489–494.
156. **Whitley, R. J., S.-J. Soong, R. Dolin, G. J. Galasso, L. T. Chien, C. A. Alford, Jr., and the National Institute of Allergy and Infectious Diseases Collaborative Antiviral Study Group.** 1977. Adenine arabinoside therapy of biopsy-proved herpes simplex encephalitis: National Institute of Allergy and Infectious Diseases Collaborative Antiviral study. *N. Engl. J. Med.* **297:** 289–294.
157. **Whitley, R. J., S.-J. Soong, M. S. Hirsch, A. W. Karchmer, R. Dolin, G. Galasso, J. K. Dunnick, C. A. Alford, Jr., and the National Institute of Allergy and Infectious Diseases Collaborative Antiviral Study Group.** 1981. Herpes simplex encephalitis: vidarabine therapy and diagnostic problems. *N. Engl. J. Med.* **304:** 313–318.
158. **Wildy, P.** 1973. Herpes: history and classification, p. 1–25. *In* A. S. Kaplan (ed.), *The Herpesviruses*. Academic Press, New York, NY.
159. **Xu, F., M. R. Sternberg, B. J. Kottiri, G. M. McQuillan, F. K. Lee, A. J. Nahmias, S. M. Berman, and L. E. Markowitz.** 2006. Trends in herpes simplex virus type 1 and type 2 seroprevalence in the United States. *JAMA* **296:**964–973.
160. **Young, E. J., A. P. Killam, and J. F. Greene.** 1976. Disseminated herpesvirus infection associated with primary genital herpes in pregnancy. *JAMA* **235:**2731–2733.
161. **Young, S. K., N. H. Rowe, and R. A. Buchanan.** 1976. A clinical study for the control of facial mucocutaneous herpes virus infections. I. Characterization of natural history in a professional school population. *Oral Surg. Oral Med. Oral Pathol.* **41:**498–507.
162. **Zuckerman, R. A., A. Lucchetti, W. L. Whittington, J. Sanchez, R. W. Coombs, R. Zuniga, A. S. Magaret, A. Wald, L. Corey, and C. Celum.** 2007. Herpes simplex virus (HSV) suppression with valacyclovir reduces rectal and blood plasma HIV-1 levels in HIV-1/HSV-2-seropositive men: a randomized, double-blind, placebo-controlled crossover trial. *J. Infect. Dis.* **196:**1500–1508.

Cercopithecine Herpesvirus 1 (B Virus)

RICHARD J. WHITLEY

20

B virus, endemic in macaques, has the unique distinction of being the only one of nearly 35 identified nonhuman primate herpesviruses that is highly pathogenic for humans. Infection has resulted in over 50 cases, with a mortality rate in excess of 80%, since its discovery. The unique biology of B virus includes its neurotrophism and neurovirulence. Because untreated B virus infections are associated with a high mortality rate in humans, individuals handling macaques or macaque cells and tissues are at risk for infection. Human infection is associated with a breach of skin or mucosa and subsequent infection with virus. Fomites and contaminated particulates or surfaces can serve as a source of virus infection as well. In one case, human-to-human transmission was attributed to a shared tube of antiviral medication that was applied to treat a patient's bite wound. Later, the same patient autoinoculated an eye. Prior to the advent of antiviral therapy, the mortality rate was 80%. However, since the early 1980s, 80% of infected individuals have survived. Timely antiviral intervention is the only effective means of reducing B virus-associated morbidity and preventing a fatal outcome.

HISTORY

In 1932, a young physician (W.B.) was bitten by a monkey and later developed localized erythema at the site of the bite. This apparent localized infection was followed by lymphangitis, lymphadenitis, and, ultimately, a transverse myelitis with demise ascribed to respiratory failure. Autopsy tissue specimens from W.B. were obtained for laboratory investigation by Gay and Holden, who reported that an ultrafilterable agent recovered from neurologic tissues caused a cytopathic effect in tissue culture similar to herpes simplex virus (HSV) (48). The isolate was initially designated W virus. Gay and Holden noted that it caused similar disease in rabbits infected by either the intradermal or intracranial route. Importantly, a rhesus macaque exposed to this virus showed no evidence of illness but developed antibodies, indicating asymptomatic infection.

Within a year of this first report, Sabin and Wright independently also found an ultrafilterable agent in the tissue of this index patient. They identified this as B virus (101), naming the virus by the initial of the patient's last name. Thus, the virus subsequently has been called herpes B virus, herpesvirus simiae, cercopithecine herpesvirus 1, or, more simply, B virus. The lethality of B virus infection in rabbits was also described by Sabin and Wright, who showed that infectivity was independent of the route of inoculation. Experimentally infected dogs, mice, and guinea pigs showed no susceptibility to infection, regardless of the route of inoculation (101). In another study, Sabin observed that B virus induced immunologic responses in an infected host similar to HSV (97). The virus was also noted to share similarity with pseudorabies, among other viruses, including SA8 and two additional nonhuman primate alphaherpesviruses recently described, HPV-2 and Langur herpesvirus (20, 21, 39, 97–99).

By 1959, B virus had resulted in 12 cumulative fatalities, with 5 recognized survivors (18, 68, 91), suggesting that this infection may not always be fatal. While B virus antibodies were detected in a number of individuals who had no clinical symptoms but a history of working with macaques (113), the early serologic assays could not distinguish between HSV and B virus infection. Once differentiation of humoral immune responses to these viruses was possible, a high-risk group of 325 subjects rarely, if ever, had antibodies in the absence of clinical symptoms.

During the decades since the initial reports of B virus infection, investigators have defined the molecular biology of this virus and the resultant illness in humans and nonhuman primates, including its natural host, the macaque. Because of its neurovirulence in a foreign host, B virus is considered by some to be one of the most dangerous occupational hazards for those who work directly with macaques or their tissues or with monkeys who have been in contact with macaques.

DISTRIBUTION IN NATURE

As stated above, B virus is endemic in macaques, one of the Old World monkeys widely distributed throughout Asia. All species of macaques tested thus far serve as natural hosts. The virus can infect other nonhuman primates, but in such cases, the infected animal is considered a foreign host, and infection generally results in death within a relatively short time. Transmission of virus can occur by direct contact between members of the *Macaca* genus, from infected animal to human, from virus-contaminated surfaces, or, in one case, from human to human, as reviewed previously (27, 35, 41–44, 64, 69, 70, 73, 74, 90, 117, 122).

Prevalence estimations of B virus infection, using different serologic methods and sampling approaches in both wild and captive macaque colonies, indicate wide variability (118). Spread of infection correlates with onset of sexual activity, which facilitates transmission of the virus among animals (106, 120). Crowding of animals during transportation accelerates the spread of infection as well (106).

B virus infection in macaques rarely causes disease, and if so, it is in the form of mild ulcerative lesions. Infection in macaques is seldom associated with death, unless conditions prevail that facilitate generalized systemic infections (29). Asymptomatic excretion of virus occurs in slightly more than 2% of antibody-positive animals from mucosal sites and the eye. These observations suggest that reactivation is only transient (15, 45, 65, 77, 82, 106, 114–116, 118, 120).

THE VIRUS

Isolation and Growth Properties of B Virus

Because B virus causes fatal human disease in 80% of untreated cases, the Centers for Disease Control and Prevention (CDC) has published agent summary statements for laboratory studies. Growth of the virus is recommended in a biosafety level 3 (BSL-3) laboratory, whereas propagation should be strictly confined to a BSL-4 facility (112). While the initial isolation of B virus was achieved using rabbits for passage of the virus (47, 48, 101), shortly thereafter, virus was grown on chorioallantoic membranes of embryonated eggs as well (20).

In 1954, B virus was isolated from rhesus kidney tissue that was used for preparation of poliomyelitis vaccines (124) and from rhesus central nervous system tissue (84). Subsequently, cultured cells, derived from monkey kidney and chicken embryo, were found to support the replication of B virus (78, 94). The virus is stable in cell culture medium stored at 4°C and can be maintained for years at −80°C but not at −20°C.

The replication kinetics of B virus follows a time course similar to that of HSV in vitro, with Vero cells being the best system for propagation (20, 97–100, 102). Virus adsorbs to the surface of a susceptible cell within 30 to 60 min after infection. Host cell machinery ceases once virus enters the cell. An eclipse of cell and viral activities is noted during the first 2 to 3 h after infection, followed by synthesis of polypeptides early during infection. By 4 h after infection, DNA synthesis increases dramatically and in parallel with the synthesis of viral polypeptides. Morphogenesis is also similar to that of HSV, as shown by electron microscopic studies (96). Infectious virus is detectable within 6 to 10 h after infection, and both extracellular and intracellular virus levels plateau about 24 to 28 h after infection, declining thereafter (56, 94). B virus, like HSV, has been observed to express sequential classes of proteins, that is, immediate-early, early, and late proteins (56), and to possess glycoproteins and other structural proteins that were studied in detail with respect to their antigenic relatedness to HSV and later to other nonhuman primate alphaherpesviruses (36, 55, 81, 88). B virus replicates to high titers in cell lines of Old World monkeys, particularly in Vero, African green monkey, and vervet kidney cell lines, as well as rabbit kidney, BSC-1, and LLC-RK cells (62, 65). Although B virus replication in cultured cells usually results in syncytium formation, as shown in Fig. 1, some primary isolates produce cell rounding. Generally, cells balloon, fusing into polykaryocytes that expand outwardly as more cells become infected. In this manner, virus infection spreads through the entire cell monolayer, destroying cells. Eosinophilic intranuclear inclusions (Cowdry type A) can be visualized after fixation and staining of infected cell monolayers; however, these inclusions are not observed either in infected animals or in some humans with zoonotic infection (34, 61). Thus, the presence of characteristic intranuclear inclusion bodies is not a reliable diagnostic marker of infection.

The B Virus Genome

B virus contains a double-stranded DNA genome of about 162 kb. One strain of virus originating from a cynomolgus monkey has been mapped and subcloned (52). The genome contains two unique regions (UL and US) flanked by a pair of inverted repeats, two of which are at the termini and two internally located, an arrangement that results in four sequence-orientated isomeric forms, as occurs with HSV. Figure 2 shows the comparative genome organizations of B virus and HSV type 1 (HSV-1), as established by using HSV-1 genes to identify and locate specific B virus homologs (52). The overall size of the genome is slightly larger than those of HSV-1 (152 kb) and HSV-2 (155 kb). The guanosine-plus-cytosine (G+C) content of the DNA has been calculated to be 75% based on the buoyant density of viral DNA. There is genome homology between B virus and HSV-1 and HSV-2 for the gB, gC, gD, gE, and gG genes (38). Further examination of the sequences of the nine major glycoproteins showed that the 75% G+C content is conserved within most glycoproteins. Additionally, the locations of genes within the UL regions of HSV and B virus are collinear (52). One gene rearrangement was described for an isolate from a cynomolgus macaque. Homologs of the HSV *US9* and *US10* genes are located upstream of the US glycoprotein gene cluster. This is in contrast to the downstream location of these genes in the HSV US region (52). Sequence analysis of the prototype strain (E2490), which originated from a rhesus macaque, however, showed that B virus DNA is collinear in these regions with the HSV-1 genomic arrangement.

To date, sequences for only a few B virus genes have been submitted to GenBank—homologs of the gB, gD, gC, gG, gI, and gL genes—largely covering the sequence of the US region (9, 76, 108). Each of the glycoproteins for which sequence information is available, except gG, has about 50% identity with HSV, slightly higher for HSV-2 than HSV-1. B virus gG is a homolog of HSV-2 gG and is closer in size to gG-2 (699 kb) than gG-1 (238 kb) (108). Glycoprotein sequences demonstrate that all cysteines are conserved, as are most glycosylation sites. This conservation suggests that B virus glycoproteins have a secondary structure similar to that of HSV. Sequence analyses also suggest that B virus and HSV-1 and -2 probably diverged from a common ancestor during the evolution of these pathogens.

Using restriction length polymorphisms as a guide, several investigators have shown intrastrain variation among both human- and nonhuman-primate-derived isolates, the significance of which remains to be defined (57, 59, 109), but is common with HSV-1 and -2. Eberle and colleagues (40) postulated the possible existence of B virus isolates which vary with respect to pathogenicity for nonmacaque species, based on the existence of three distinct B virus genotypes. These genotypes were identified when collected

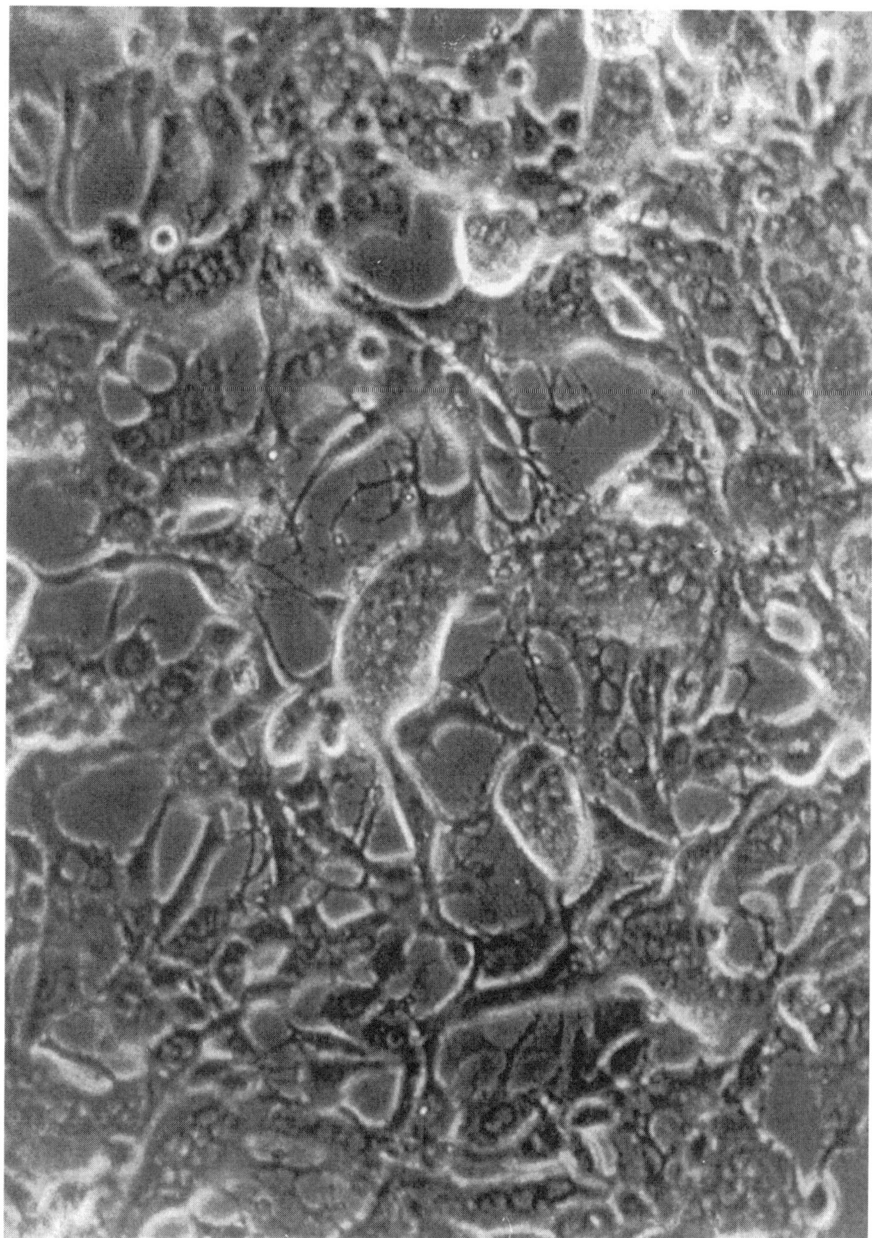

FIGURE 1 Vero cell monolayer infected with B virus.

data were analyzed phylogenetically; however, this postulate must be studied in a suitable animal model. Published case summaries that implicate other macaque species, and in one case a baboon, are difficult, if not impossible, to confirm (90).

Synthesis of Viral Proteins

More than 50 different polypeptides have been identified by immunoblot analysis. Each has been assigned an infected-cell polypeptide number as an initial reference point (56). This number may be an underestimate of the total synthesized, but it serves as a basis for comparison in ongoing studies. The sizes of these infected-cell polypeptides range from about 10,000 to 250,000 Da. More than 75% of the expected coding capacity of the viral DNA is accounted for by these infected-cell polypeptides. Many of these glycoproteins have been cloned and sequenced recently by two laboratory groups (9, 10, 40). The proteins encoded were mapped to genes by the US region, which was largely collinear to the HSV glycoproteins gD, gI, gJ, and gG, as previously described. Sequence analysis of selected genes showed that B virus is most closely related to herpesvirus papio 2 (37). Although there are protein homologs in herpesviruses of New World monkeys, very little, if any, cross-reactivity exists between B virus and the New World monkey herpesviruses.

The kinetics of protein and glycoprotein synthesis in infected cell culture are similar to that observed for HSV, although infectious virus is detected earlier, appearing 6 h after infection. Both host cell DNA and protein synthetic

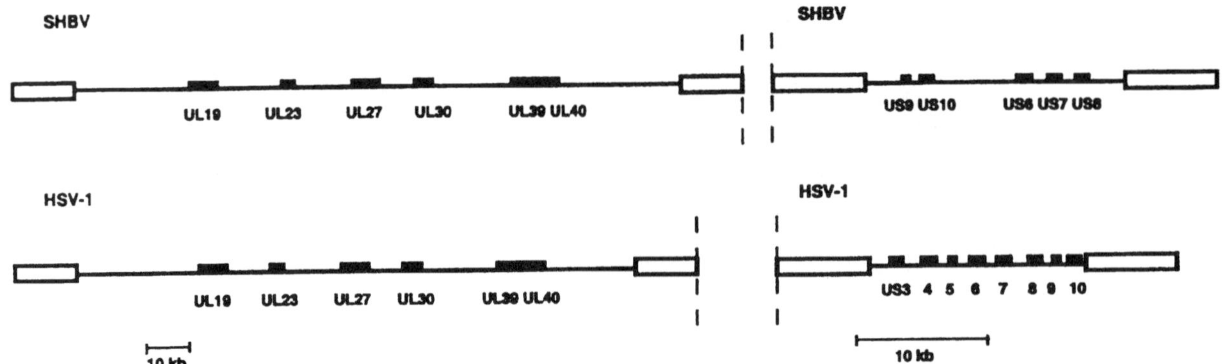

FIGURE 2 Physical map of B virus as proposed by Harrington and colleagues (52). (Reprinted from reference 52 with permission.)

activities appeared to be curtailed during the first 4 h after infection. The polypeptides of B virus-infected cells, summarized in Table 1, may represent an overestimate of the primary gene products of the virus; however, this summary should serve as a fairly complete listing of B virus-induced polypeptides for future reference. As for glycoproteins, only glucosamine and some mannose are incorporated during the infection in vitro. B virus polypeptides and glycoproteins can be grouped into classes that differ in their relative rates of synthesis at different times throughout the virus replication cycle, as is characteristic of alphaherpesviruses (56).

PATHOLOGY AND PATHOGENESIS

During the course of B virus infection, several observations are common to the natural host, the experimentally infected host, and infected humans. First, pathogenetic outcome varies according to infected host. The route of inoculation predicts differences in the time course of infection, development, and spread through the central nervous system and visceral organs (e.g., the spleen, adrenals, kidneys, and, in some cases, even the heart). These routes of infection are unique to the mode of infection: natural, experimentally infected, and human zoonotic infections. For example, venereal transmission of the virus is common in macaque hosts, whereas an intranasal route of virus delivery defines the experimental rabbit model or, in the case of human zoonotic exposure, accidental aerosolization of virus. However, these routes share one common feature: all require exposure of mucosal membranes to infectious virus.

The cells that come into contact with the virus initially are also important to the permissiveness of infection. For example, the nasal mucosa is a less ideal site for virus replication than the lungs (6–8, 28, 69). Another important consideration in B virus infection is the quantity of the virus introduced initially into a host. For example, a far greater quantity of virus is required to infect rabbits by aerosolization than by an intradermal route of inoculation, although practically, whether these routes and doses influence human or nonhuman primate infection is unconfirmed. Also, the dose is likely an important factor in determining associated morbidity and mortality. Another common feature of natural, experimental, or zoonotic infection is that B virus can be found in the central nervous system shortly after the onset of acute infection. But the distribution of virus and its consequences differ widely in natural infection compared with infection failure in susceptible foreign hosts.

TABLE 1 Hybridization of plasmids containing HSV-1 DNA fragments to simian herpes B virus DNA blot membranes

Probe DNA			SHBV[a] fragment(s) to which probe hybridized	
HSV-1 KpnI clone	Fragment	Gene function	BamHI	SalI
h	SstI	Glycoprotein D (HSV US6)	g	i
h	SstI	Glycoprotein E (HSV US8)	g	p′n′
h	SstI	Glycoprotein I (HSV US7)	g	ip′
h	BamHI	Tegument phosphoprotein (HSV US9)	r	c′
h	BamHI	Virion protein (HSV US10)	r	c′
n	XhoI/AspI	Glycoprotein B (HSV US27)	d	pz
a′	NotI	DNA polymerase (HSV US30)	z	e′f
i	BstX	Major capsid protein (HSV US19)	j	s, y
s	KpnI/BglI	Ribonucleotide reductase 1 (HSV US39)	m	t
s	KspI/KpnI	Ribonucleotide reductase 2 (HSV US40)	p	t

[a] SHBV, simian herpes B virus.

The Natural Host

The macaque suffers little or no morbidity as a consequence of infection. Exceptions occur rarely and appear to involve specific accompanying factors, such as immunosuppression or stress (29, 107, 125). Infection is self-limiting (1, 11, 73, 74, 120, 121). Virus replicates at the site of inoculation and induces a localized erythema. There is also evidence of limited focal infection of the liver and kidneys in some macaques (73, 74). Virus travels through the peripheral nerves from the site of inoculation to the representative sensory ganglia. Latent infection is established in the ganglia, with intermittent reactivation of the virus throughout the life of the macaque (14, 15, 43, 79, 102, 115, 118). In rare cases, viremia has been observed (22, 83, 107). Virus has also been recovered from urine as well as multiple organs of animals. Reactivation from latency occurs in the natural host as judged by increasing antibody titers, recovery of virus by cocultivation of sensory ganglia, and isolation of virus in the absence of detectable lesions (29, 51, 82).

During active B virus replication, isolation of virus is readily accomplished from buccal, conjunctival, or genital mucosa sites (1, 33). The frequency of active infection among seropositive macaques is low, with relatively short periods for successful virus recovery from mucosal sites (118, 120).

Mucosal ulcers, if present, extend down to the papillary layer of the dermis. Two distinct zones have been described, namely, a central area of necrosis and a surrounding zone of ballooning degeneration. Around the lesion, "normal" epithelium exists. An eosinophilic polymorphonuclear infiltration characterizes the histopathology of the lesion. Postmortem histopathological examination of monkey tissues from animals euthanized at the time of active virus shedding reveals perivascular lymphocytic cuffing in sections of spinal cord. Examinations of latently infected but healthy animals failed to detect virus excretion from peripheral sites routinely, but virus can still be recovered from sensory ganglia (14).

Experimental Infections

Rabbits, mice, rats, guinea pigs, and chickens have been studied as B virus models, as previously mentioned (47, 97, 102). Disease is not a uniform consequence following B virus inoculation into mice and guinea pigs; however, several strains of B virus that have increased virulence for the mouse have been identified. One strain, identified as E2490, was avirulent for white rats and chickens; nonetheless, antibody developed after infection (64). Cotton rats infected by the intraperitoneal, subcutaneous, or intracerebral route succumbed to infection with selected strains. Rats had typical hind-leg paralysis secondary to transverse myelitis, similar to symptoms in the rabbit. Serial passages of human B virus strains are capable of infecting mice, hamsters, and white chicks (92, 93). With respect to experimental infections, the rabbit is the most useful small-animal model because virus replicates to high titers, making it a particularly good model for testing antiviral agents.

Using the rabbit or the mouse model, investigators have demonstrated that the viral dose is important, depending on the route of inoculation, as would be predicted. Experimentally infected animals inoculated with low doses of virus intradermally developed only erythema that disappeared within a few days and was not associated with further apparent symptoms. In contrast, animals receiving a larger dose developed a necrotic lesion that was generally followed by central nervous system invasion (49, 50). B virus subsequently appeared in the regional lymph nodes late after infection. These nodes drained the area of initial infection, and with time, necrosis of the infected nodes occurred, as seen upon postmortem examination. In the central nervous system, focal lesions are evident in pons, medulla, and spinal cord virus. While virus spread through peripheral nerves is most common, in rare cases, hematogenous spread in experimentally or inadvertently infected hosts occurs (29, 49, 50, 99, 111).

The cervical spinal cord and medulla oblongata are the primary sites of postmortem virus recovery. With time after infection, virus is also found in olfactory regions of the brain, possibly as a consequence of movement of the virus centripetally through the nerves innervating the nasal mucosa. Perivascular cuffing and glial infiltration are characteristic histopathological findings upon examination of brain tissue. Hepatic congestion is accompanied by infiltration of polymorphonuclear and mononuclear cells seen in the periportal areas of the liver. Scattered foci of necrosis can be found throughout the lobes of the liver. The presence of inclusions is visualized mainly in the regions of inflammation, around pyknotic or karyorrhetic hepatocytes. When lesions are present on skin, the depth of the involved tissue is significantly greater than that of mucous membranes, explaining perhaps why B virus can be recovered weeks or months later from these sites (34, 60, 61).

Human Infection

Human B virus infection generally occurs through an occupational exposure to a macaque shedding virus at a site that comes into contact with broken skin or mucosal membranes of the susceptible human. Several cases in which monkey contact had not occurred in years suggest that virus can be reactivated.

Review of all confirmed cases of B virus in humans can be summarized as follows. The most striking characteristic of human B virus infection is the involvement of the central nervous system, specifically the upper spinal cord and brain stem. These areas are the principal sites for virus replication. Initially, the infected individual experiences an influenza-like syndrome followed by numbness or paresthesia around the site of inoculation. An ascending transverse myelitis occurs during the final stages of the infection in humans, resulting ultimately in respiratory failure. Virus can be recovered at skin sites of inoculation for extended periods, and viral DNA can be detected generally in cerebrospinal fluid (CSF) by the time neurologic symptoms are experienced. CSF antibodies can also be detected. Cutaneous vesicular lesions are a source of virus isolation, even late in infection (85). Edema and degeneration of motor neurons are prominent. Even with advanced disease, Cowdry type A eosinophilic intranuclear inclusions can be found in only a few cases, and certainly not uniformly. Gliosis and astrocytosis are late histopathological findings; thus, there can be evidence of myelitis, encephalomyelitis, or encephalitis, or combinations of each of these conditions (90).

Surviving patients have various degrees of morbidity, ranging from little or no neurologic impairment to more extensive central nervous system involvement (2, 18, 19, 46). Some survivors experience slow neurologic decline, whereas others report few, if any, long-term effects. Several infected individuals have subsequently given birth to healthy children, with no ill effects in either the mother or infant. Monitoring of the vaginal canal for virus shedding in these individuals before delivery has produced negative results. Ocular disease has been reported (86, 95). Histopathological examination of the eye revealed a multifocal necrotizing retinitis associated with vitritis, optic neuritis, and prominent panuveitis. Herpes-like viral particles were identified in the involved retina by electron microscopy in one case. Postmortem vitreous cultures taken from both eyes and retinal cultures taken from the right eye in the latter case were positive for B virus. Thus, B virus can infect and destroy retinal tissue in a manner similar to that of other herpesviruses. Ophthalmic zoster-like symptoms have been reported as well (45), and in one particular case, reactivation of latent infection was postulated.

To summarize human pathogenesis, the tissues and organs that become infected by B virus vary, likely according to the route of inoculation. If skin is the primary site of infection, the virus usually, but not always, replicates in the skin, resulting in localized erythema. Knowledge of the site of initial replication is useful for the development of guidelines for disease prevention and also for retrieval of a virus isolate that then allows unequivocal diagnosis. Subsequently, lymphangitis and lymph node involvement are observed. Although viremia has been documented to occur in rabbits and monkeys, it has not been proved to occur in humans, although with the application of more sensitive assays (e.g., PCR), more details of infection can be uncovered. Certainly, with lymphatic involvement, virus can spread, particularly to abdominal viscera, where it has been isolated. Nevertheless, spread through neuronal routes is the fundamental route of transmission of the virus, as it is with HSV, given the involvement of the spinal cord and central nervous system. Visceral organs, including the heart, liver, spleen, lungs, kidneys, and adrenals, demonstrate congestion and focal necrosis, with variations in the extent of involvement from patient to patient. Recent human cases failed to demonstrate necrosis, but virus was isolated from adrenal, kidney, lung, and liver tissue collected at autopsy (34, 61). In cases in which B virus infection is suspected, medical personnel should follow published guidelines at the time of injury or observation of symptoms of possible infection (23–26).

LATENCY

A characteristic of all herpesviruses is the ability to establish latency and to reactivate when provoked by the proper stimulus. B virus is no exception. Reactivation has been described for both wild macaques and established captive colonies (82, 117–120). Unequivocal evidence of latent B virus infection in macaques came with studies on frequency of recovery of virus in monkey kidney cell culture systems. Wood and Shimada obtained six isolates from 650 pools of monkey kidneys, suggesting that at least 1% of macaque kidneys contain latent virus that can be reactivated in cell culture (124). Virus was also isolated from rhesus tissues (14, 15) as well as by cocultivation from a variety of neuronal tissues, including gasserian ganglia, trigeminal ganglia, dorsal route ganglia, and spinal cord (116). Latent virus has been isolated by cocultivation of tissues from experimentally infected rabbits (116), further supporting the rabbit as a potentially acceptable animal model for B virus infections. Latency likely occurs after human infection.

As with human HSV infections, a prominent factor associated with reactivation of B virus in macaques appears to be stress, particularly that associated with the capture and shipment of animals from the wild to captivity. Shedding of virus after reactivation also occurs with illness and during the breeding season of the natural host. No information is yet available on the state of the viral DNA during latency or on the molecular or biochemical events associated with the establishment and reactivation of latent virus.

EPIDEMIOLOGY

Natural Hosts

Macaques

Most adult wild macaques are seropositive for B virus (106). However, colonies of animals exist in the wild that have been found to be predominantly seronegative. More recently, colonies have been established apart from original natural habitats to meet escalating needs for seronegative animals by the scientific community. The seroprevalence in wild macaques, in addition to the noted high infectivity (118) and low morbidity within captive colonies (20), confirmed the macaque as the natural host. Recent studies among macaques belonging to captive breeding colonies reveal a high seroprevalence, in fact one that increases after the onset of puberty (118, 119). Increasing seroprevalence appears to be associated with sexual transmission within the colony (111, 119). Infants and juveniles have a very low incidence of infection, judged by low prevalence of specific B virus antibodies (118). There is evidence of transplacental antibody transmission. Importantly, all age groups have been found to be virus positive, indicating that routes of transmission other than sexual activity exist (1).

No particular species of macaque appears to be excluded as a natural host for B virus infection, although there are minimal or no data available for certain species. While detection of antibodies has been confirmed in most macaque species, there has been speculation that virus isolated from certain species is less neurovirulent or less neurotropic than virus shed by rhesus macaques (12).

Virus shedding during either primary or recurrent infections has been noted to occur. In general, macaques shed virus for a longer duration during primary infection and for short periods, even hours, with recurrent infections. Levels of virus, as measured from mucosal swabs, range from 10^2 to 10^3 PFU.

Humans

B virus is an infection that humans rarely contract, but when they do, 80% of untreated cases result in death, as noted previously. Epidemiological analysis indicates B virus is usually acquired through zoonotic transmission from either a macaque or infected cells or tissues from the animal. There is, however, one documented case of transmission from human to human, as noted above, supporting the assumption that B virus can be transmitted in a fashion similar to that of HSV. A recent fatal case resulted from exposure of ocular membranes to virus from a monkey in the process of being transported. This tragedy has refocused attention on an earlier report implicating this type of transmission in the epidemiological analysis of zoonotic transmission of the virus (78). Interestingly, current case analyses suggest that categorization of risk levels with regard to the severity of injury is not useful. The low incidence of B virus infection in humans makes it difficult to reach statistical conclusions, but analyses of cases occurring during the 1990s supported the observation that immediate medical attention ameliorates, if not prevents, disease. Only minimal disruption of the protective skin layer or instillation directly to a mucosal membrane can result in initiation of infection. The level of virus required to initiate infection in humans remains unknown. Where data are available, rhesus macaques were most frequently implicated as the source of infectious virus in the known human cases, but alone, this is insufficient to conclude that rhesus-derived virus is uniquely important in the establishment of zoonotic infections. Other species of macaques, including baboons, have been linked to fatal zoonotic infections (90).

The incidence of zoonotic infections has been correlated retrospectively with periods of increased usage of macaques for biomedical research. Evaluation of past cases underscores that transmission of the virus is often associated with no more than a superficial scratch or puncture, suggesting that once virus gains entry into a host, the ability to initiate disease is perhaps dose independent, at least in some cases.

HOST IMMUNE RESPONSE

B virus antibodies have been studied in both natural and foreign hosts by a variety of methods, including serum neutralization with or without complement, competitive radioimmunoassay (RIA), multiple types of enzyme-linked immunosorbent assay (ELISA), including competition ELISA, and Western blotting. Limited serial observations have been available from both the natural and foreign host, but comparison of available data has been useful in that a relatively consistent response is induced in both types of hosts (3–5, 63, 66, 67). The natural history of antibody development has been measured in wild macaques, captive colony populations, individually imported animals, experimentally infected macaques, zoonotically infected humans, and even vaccine trial recipients. The ELISA methodologies provide a rapid diagnostic tool with increased sensitivities of detection and with enhanced specificity when competition protocols are used. Host humoral responses to B virus infections in both humans and nonhuman primates neutralize HSV-1 and HSV-2 as well as nonhuman primate alphaherpesviruses. Interestingly, HSV antibodies do not neutralize B virus, indicating the presence of virus-specific antigens unique to B virus (16, 103). Sequence data have been useful in confirming the existence of B virus-specific epitopes (9, 76, 108).

The humoral immune response to B virus infection has a characteristic pattern (34, 61, 79). The glycoproteins induce antibodies early in the course of infection. Antibodies begin to appear within 7 to 10 days after the infection and consist of immunoglobulin M. Within 14 to 21 days after the onset of acute infection, immunoglobulin G antibodies are present. In rare cases, the infected host remains persistently antibody negative despite virus isolation. The pattern of the immune response is somewhat altered in the cases of humans who have had a previous infection with HSV-1 or HSV-2, because viral antigens that are shared among the three viruses induce an anamnestic response toward shared protein or glycoprotein sequences. Neutralizing antibodies develop in both the natural and foreign host, but at significantly lower levels in the foreign host. The nature and specificity of the humoral responses make it possible to design enhanced serologic testing strategies to identify detectable antibodies rapidly and to provide the basis for future diagnostic strategies.

CLINICAL MANIFESTATIONS

Observations of the clinical pattern of disease are important for rapid diagnosis of B virus infection in both macaques and humans. In the natural host, recognition of early infection allows removal of infected monkeys from captive colonies that are being established as B virus free. In B virus-free colonies, it is important to remove seropositive animals and isolate animals with equivocal results to prevent infection of other colony members, or in seropositive colonies to minimize risk to humans who handle them. Macaques are not treated with antivirals because the high prevalence of infection makes it cost prohibitive. In the case of human illness, early recognition of disease facilitates treatment with antivirals, principally such nucleoside analogs as acyclovir, valacyclovir, and famciclovir, a course that appears to lower the morbidity and mortality (34, 61). Immunosuppression (e.g., administration of corticosteroids) is often associated with reactivation, often mild, in the natural host (125), whereas other agents appear to be capable of facilitating systemic B virus disease culminating in death (27).

Humans exposed to B virus demonstrate clinically variable signs of disease. Most often, illness is apparent within days to weeks, but in some cases, there appears to be a delay in development of acute disease. The reasons for this delay are unknown, and although rare, delays may even range from months to years, making diagnosis difficult. Once symptoms appear, the clinical progression is associated with relatively consistent symptoms, including influenza-like illness, lymphadenitis, fever, headache, vomiting, myalgia, cramping, meningeal irritation, stiff neck, limb paresthesias, and urinary retention with an ascending paralysis culminating in respiratory failure, requiring ventilatory support. Cranial nerve signs, such as nystagmus and diplopia, are common in most published cases. Sinusitis and conjunctivitis have been observed in some (34, 61). The array of symptoms may be related to the dose of virus with which the individual was infected or the route of inoculation. A summary of descriptions of human cases can be found in two comprehensive reviews (90, 117).

The highest percentage of deaths occurs within a few weeks after onset of disease. In some cases, however, life was prolonged artificially for months or years. Incubation times from identifiable exposures to onset of clinical symptoms range from days to years, but most cases occur within days to months. Virus has been recovered from throat, buccal, and conjunctival sites as well as from lesions, vesicles, or injury sites as late as weeks to months after infection. Most clinical cases are associated with bites (50%), fomites, (8%) saliva (<5%), and aerosols (10%).

DIAGNOSIS

Nonhuman Primates

Macaques

B virus infection in macaques is identified by virus isolation, the presence of specific antibodies, or both (30, 59,

75). The neutralization antibody test was the predominant diagnostic tool in macaques and humans for many decades. The time required for the results of this test was often a drawback, necessitating a more rapid test. Thus, the dot blot, RIA, ELISA, and Western blot were developed (13, 32, 53, 54, 71, 72, 87). Three of these techniques (dot blot, ELISA, and Western blot) rely on the use of monoclonal antibody. The results of these tests can be acquired in less than 1 day. These tests are available through commercial laboratories as well as through a national resource laboratory subsidized through the National Institutes of Health (NIH) National Center for Research Resources. All of these assays use B virus-infected cells for antibody detection, making such tests more effective than other types of assays that rely on HSV-1 (89). This is a particularly important point with respect to diagnostic tools used to identify signs of infection for the establishment of B virus-free colonies. Tests dependent on monoclonal antibodies or recombinant reagents have defined sensitivity and specificity for each macaque species to be tested. Finally, evaluation of a macaque is optimal only when analysis is performed on multiple samples on different dates, especially in cases in which the antibody titer is low (less than 1:50). A constellation of different tests for deployment at various points after infection may be necessary in some cases to determine correctly the status of an animal with a very low antibody titer, particularly when such an animal is housed in a B virus-free colony (58).

Virus isolation is the "gold standard" for diagnosis of infected macaques. Unfortunately, virus isolation is not a particularly sensitive diagnostic tool, with the possibility of many false-negative results. Nonetheless, standard cell culture for virus isolation remains a valuable tool for the colony manager and for the veterinarian. Virus-positive cultures can be easily recognized by the unique cytopathic effect, but unequivocal confirmation requires either electrophoretic analysis of infected-cell polypeptides or restriction endonuclease-digested DNA. Several PCR tests have been described that can be used to verify the identity of the virus; however, this diagnostic tool for colony management is costly. Nonetheless, when a possible zoonotic infection must be confirmed, PCR may be beneficial for identification of B virus in macaques.

Nonmacaques

Other species of monkeys infrequently become infected with B virus, as discussed above. These are usually animals that have been cohoused or housed in close proximity to B virus-infected macaques at some time. Because many, if not all, nonhuman primates harbor indigenous alphaherpesviruses, the important diagnostic point is to differentiate specific antibodies from cross-reactive ones. Euthanasia is generally advised in the case of a B virus infection in a nonmacaque because it is likely that the animal will succumb and, in the meantime, would pose a great risk to anyone attempting to treat the infection. B virus has been identified in the patas monkey and colobus monkey (80, 110, 123). In each case, there is a major concern for the people responsible for care of the animal, particularly because these animals often have severe morbidity and shed virus. Currently, the most effective assay for diagnosis of B virus in a nonmacaque is a competition ELISA to facilitate discrimination between specific and cross-reactive antibodies, similar to the challenge faced when diagnosing infection in humans.

Humans

The evaluation of clinical symptoms associated with an antibody- or virus-positive case is the gold standard for diagnosis of B virus infection in an exposed individual. Both serologic and virologic techniques are available for diagnosis of B virus-infected humans. The CDC has published specific guidelines for recognition and treatment of such infections (61). In the case of a suspected infection, several emergency resources are available. Contact with the CDC or laboratories recommended by the CDC (see guidelines) can expedite laboratory assistance for the clinician suspecting B virus infection. Generally, a rise in B virus-specific antibodies over several days during acute infection substantiates B virus as the etiologic agent. However, in other cases, data are equivocal, and decisions with regard to patient management must be based on a complex decision table collectively using all diagnostic tools, including clinical symptoms. Virus isolation remains the gold standard for diagnosis; however, virus isolation is frequently not possible even under the best of circumstances. Serologic diagnosis of B virus in humans is a complex task when an individual with a suspected infection has detectable antibodies as a result of a previous HSV infection. As discussed above, significant cross-reactivity of host response exists among these viruses. In the absence of these cross-reactive antibodies, diagnosis is rapid and straightforward, with confirmation using the neutralization assay, Western blot, or both. This was not the case before the development of rapid diagnostic competitive ELISAs and RIAs (71, 72). The diagnostic tests for humans are performed currently by only a few facilities that have been licensed and have access to BSL-4 containment laboratories for the preparation of B virus antigen.

Virus identification can be accomplished by isolation using conventional cell culture and, in clinical emergencies, by PCR (104). The identity of isolates should be confirmed by electrophoretic analysis of infected-cell polypeptides or restriction endonuclease-digested DNA (56). The application of PCR is most helpful for the symptomatic patient if virus cannot be recovered. PCR is also a useful tool for monitoring the efficacy of antiviral interventions.

CONTROL OF B VIRUS INFECTION

Multiple levels of prevention are used to prevent B virus infection in both humans and nonhuman primates, ranging from attempts to eliminate virus from colonies to designing methods to work safely in environments where there is an increased risk for contracting this agent. The CDC has published detailed guidelines for maximizing protection of individuals working with macaques (23, 25). Further, the NIH National Center for Research Resources has funded the development of B virus-free colonies for NIH-funded research involving these animals in an attempt to eliminate this virus from colonies used for biomedical research. Nonetheless, B virus-infected monkeys are plentiful and require handling that can be done safely if strict guidelines are followed, including barrier precautions.

When B virus is detected, inactivation is accomplished with either heat or formaldehyde (91). Other virus inactivators include detergents and bleach, but individuals working in a decontaminated area should still be alert for injury prevention. Minimizing fomites decreases worker risk and reduces virus spread among animals. One B virus infection in a human was acquired from a cage after the person sustained a scratch (61), underscoring that surface decontamination can play an important role in infection control.

As early as the 1930s, attempts were made to identify an effective vaccine for protection of individuals who could be exposed to this virus while working with macaques or their cells or tissues. Limited vaccine trials have been performed in human volunteers (66, 67), and although short-term antibodies were induced, they waned quickly. Thus, the vaccine was not pursued further. Recently, a recombinant vaccine was tested and found to induce antibodies in macaques, but the duration of antibody persistence and efficacy remain to be assessed (10).

Antiviral therapy is recognized as an effective prophylactic for prevention of infection in human and animal trials, when administered early after exposure (17, 31, 34, 61, 126). Acyclovir and the related family of nucleoside analogs were noted to be effective when given in high dosages (60), for example, acyclovir at 10 mg/kg of body weight intravenously three times daily for 14 to 21 days. Efficacy of therapy in cases of infection in humans has been monitored by inhibition of peripheral virus shedding in some cases and by reduction in CSF antibodies or viral DNA load in others (34, 61, 105). Some physicians follow intravenous therapy with long-term oral suppression (acyclovir, valacyclovir, or famciclovir). Ganciclovir has a greater efficacy in vitro and thus was used in a few cases since 1989 with success. Interestingly, before 1987, in at least five retrospectively analyzed cases, individuals fared well in the absence of antiviral therapy, but the use of one of these nucleoside analogs is recommended by CDC. Antiviral therapy is uniformly used in humans with clinical disease. Moreover, it is also used by an increasing number of facilities for postinjury prophylaxis or after laboratory results indicate that an animal may have been actively infected around the time of the exposure. Postinjury prophylaxis has been performed with famciclovir or valacyclovir, and both have demonstrated efficacy in vitro. Recommendations and guidelines have been published by the CDC, as discussed above, and can be readily accessed (60). Only a handful of physicians have had experience in the treatment of B virus zoonosis, and their participation and expertise have been important in the development of the CDC guidelines. There are other compounds that show a high degree of efficacy against B virus in vitro, but their clinical usefulness in the treatment of infections in humans must be further investigated owing to the toxicity of the compounds. Toxicity may be averted by lower doses of these compounds, but safety trials in animals are not complete.

Finally, with respect to prevention, first aid after a potential exposure due to a bite, scratch, splash, or other suspicious injury is very important. Guidelines for wound cleaning are described in detail by the CDC. Every institution working with macaques should have an injury protocol with immediate availability of first aid, a secondary care plan, and, last but not least, an infectious-disease specialist who is a member of the institution's prevention and care response team.

CONCLUSIONS

B virus is usually a rapidly progressive, devastating disease that can be interrupted by effective use of antiviral therapies if deployed sufficiently soon after infection. The guidelines for treatment and prevention are widely published and can be rapidly accessed through either the CDC or the diagnostic resource using the World Wide Web address http://www.gsu.edu/bvirus. Other websites are beginning to spring up as well and can be useful in learning more about B virus infections in both humans and nonhuman primates. Diagnostic techniques are rapidly improving to support clinical diagnosis and information regarding sample collection. Evaluation is available at any time to clinical care centers in case of emergencies.

With the newer diagnostic techniques, the sensitivity of detection is improving, and the barriers posed by the high degree of cross-reactivity among this family of viruses are rapidly being diminished.

Because of the risk of human disease, precautionary methods must be followed in the workplace. Proper attention to the details of housing, management, and handling of macaques and organized exposure response measures using the CDC guidelines can minimize B virus zoonotic infections. Rapid identification of infection is essential for early initiation of antiviral drug therapy, which can prevent further mortality associated with this very interesting alphaherpesvirus.

Studies performed by me were initiated and supported under a contract (NO1-AI-62554) from the Antiviral Research Branch of the National Institute of Allergy and Infectious Diseases (NIAID), a Program Project Grant (PO1 AI 24009), an Outstanding Investigator Award (2R35 CA 47451-08), Unrestricted Grants in Infectious Diseases from Bristol-Myers Squibb, and grants from the General Clinical Research Center Program (RR-032) and the State of Alabama.

REFERENCES

1. **Anderson, D. C., R. B. Swenson, J. L. Orkin, S. S. Kalter, and H. M. McClure.** 1994. Primary herpesvirus simiae (B-virus) infection in infant macaques. *Lab. Anim. Sci.* **44:**526–530.
2. **Artenstein, A. W., C. B. Hicks, B. S. Goodwin, and J. K. Hilliard.** 1991. Human infection with B virus following a needlestick injury. *Rev. Infect. Dis.* **13:**288–291.
3. **Benda, R.** 1965. Active immunization against an infection caused by the B virus (herpesvirus simiae). I. Experience with the preparation and evaluation of Hull's formaldehyde vaccine. *Cesk. Epidemiol. Mikrobiol. Imunol.* **14:**330–338.
4. **Benda, R.** 1965. Active immunization against infection caused by B virus (herpesvirus simiae). II. Dynamics of neutralizing antibodies in rabbits immunized with inactivated vaccine and challenged with live virus. Attempts to obtain highly active antiserum against B virus. *J. Hyg. Epidemiol. Microbiol. Immunol.* **9:**487–499.
5. **Benda, R.** 1966. Active immunization against infection caused by B virus (herpesvirus simiae). III. Immunoprophylaxis of inhalation infection in rabbits. *J. Hyg. Epidemiol. Microbiol. Immunol.* **10:**105–108.
6. **Benda, R., M. Fuchsova, and V. Hronovský.** 1969. Course of air-borne infection caused by B virus (herpesvirus simiae). II. Distribution of B virus in the organism of rabbits and histopathological changes in the organs. *J. Hyg. Epidemiol. Microbiol. Immunol.* **13:**214–226.
7. **Benda, R., and V. Hronovský.** 1969. Course of air-borne infection caused by B virus (herpesvirus simiae). IV. Role of alveolar macrophages of the lungs in inhalation B-virus infection of rabbits. *J. Hyg. Epidemiol. Microbiol. Immunol.* **13:**493–502.

8. **Benda, R., and F. Polomik.** 1969. Course of air-borne infection caused by B virus (herpesvirus simiae). I. Lethal inhalation dose of B virus for rabbits. *J. Hyg. Epidemiol. Microbiol. Immunol.* **13:**24–30.
9. **Bennett, A. M., L. Harrington, and D. C. Kelly.** 1992. Nucleotide sequence analysis of genes encoding glycoproteins D and J in simian herpes B virus. *J. Gen. Virol.* **73:** 2963–2967.
10. **Bennett, A. M., M. J. Slomka, D. W. Brown, G. Lloyd, and M. Mackett.** 1999. Protection against herpes B virus infection in rabbits with a recombinant vaccinia virus expressing glycoprotein D. *J. Med. Virol.* **57:**47–56.
11. **Benson, P. M., S. L. Malane, R. Banks, C. B. Hicks, and J. K. Hilliard.** 1989. B virus (herpesvirus simiae) and human infection. *Arch. Dermatol.* **125:**1247–1248.
12. **Blewett, E. L., D. Black, and R. Eberle.** 1996. Characterization of virus-specific and cross-reactive monoclonal antibodies to herpesvirus simiae (B virus). *J. Gen. Virol.* **77**(11)**:**2787–2793.
13. **Blewett, E. L., J. T. Salifi, and R. Eberle.** 1999. Development of a competitive ELISA for detection of primates infected with monkey B virus (herpesvirus simiae). *J. Virol. Methods* **77:**59–67.
14. **Boulter, E. A.** 1975. The isolation of monkey B virus (herpesvirus simiae) from the trigeminal ganglia of a healthy seropositive rhesus monkey. *J. Biol. Stand.* **3:**279–280.
15. **Boulter, E. A., and D. P. Grant.** 1977. Latent infection of monkeys with B virus and prophylactic studies in a rabbit model of this disease. *J. Antimicrob. Chemother.* **3**(Suppl. A)**:**107–113.
16. **Boulter, E. A., S. S. Kalter, R. L. Heberling, J. E. Guajardo, and T. L. Lester.** 1982. A comparison of neutralization tests for the detection of antibodies to herpesvirus simiae (monkey B virus). *Lab. Anim. Sci.* **32:**150–152.
17. **Boulter, E. A., B. Thornton, E. J. Bauer, and A. Bye.** 1980. Successful treatment of experimental B virus (herpesvirus simiae) infection with acyclovir. *Br. Med. J.* **280:** 681–683.
18. **Breen, G. E., S. G. Lamb, and A. T. Otaki.** 1958. Monkey bite encephalomyelitis: report of a case with recovery. *Br. Med. J.* **2:**22–23.
19. **Bryan, B. L., C. D. Espana, R. W. Emmons, N. Vijayan, and P. D. Hoeprich.** 1975. Recovery from encephalomyelitis caused by herpesvirus simiae: report of a case. *Arch. Intern. Med.* **135:**868–870.
20. **Burnet, F. M., D. Lush, and A. V. Jackson.** 1939. The propagation of herpes B and pseudorabies viruses on the chorioallantois. *Aust. J. Exp. Biol. Med. Sci.* **17:**35–52.
21. **Burnet, F. M., D. Lush, and A. V. Jackson.** 1939. The relationship of herpes and B viruses: immunological and epidemiological considerations. *Aust. J. Exp. Biol. Med. Sci.* **17:**41–51.
22. **Carlson, C. S., M. G. O'Sullivan, M. J. Jayo, D. K. Anderson, E. S. Harver, W. G. Jerome, B. C. Bullock, and R. L. Heberling.** 1997. Fatal disseminated Cercopithecine herpes virus 1 (herpes B) infection in cynomolgus monkeys *(Macaca fascicularis)*. *Vet. Pathol.* **34:**405–414.
23. **Centers for Disease Control.** 1987. Guidelines for prevention of herpesvirus simiae (B virus) infection in monkey handlers. *Morb. Mortal. Wkly. Rep.* **36:**680–687.
24. **Centers for Disease Control.** 1987. Leads from the MMWR. Guidelines for prevention of herpesvirus simiae (B virus) infection in monkey handlers. *JAMA* **258:** 3493–3495.
25. **Centers for Disease Control.** 1995. Publication of guidelines for the prevention and treatment of B virus infections in exposed persons. *Morb. Mortal. Wkly. Rep.* **44:** 96–97.
26. **Centers for Disease Control and Prevention.** 1998. Fatal Cercopithecine herpesvirus 1 (B virus) infection following a mucocutaneous exposure and interim recommendations for worker protection. *Morb. Mortal. Wkly. Rep.* **47:**1073–1076.
27. **Chapman, L. E., and C. J. Peter.** 1987. Human infections caused by simian herpesviruses, p. 1508–1509. *In* D. J. Weatherall, J. G. G. Ledingham, and D. A. Warrell (ed.), *Oxford Textbook of Medicine*, 2nd ed. Oxford University Press, Headington, United Kingdom.
28. **Chappell, W. A.** 1960. Animal infectivity of aerosols of monkey B virus. *Ann. N. Y. Acad. Sci.* **851:**931–934.
29. **Chellman, G. J., V. S. Lukas, E. M. Eugui, K. P. Altera, S. J. Almquist, and J. K. Hilliard.** 1992. Activation of B virus (herpesvirus simiae) in chronically immunosuppressed cynomolgus monkeys. *Lab. Anim. Sci.* **42:**146–151.
30. **Cole, W. C., R. E. Bostrom, and R. A. J. Whitney.** 1968. Diagnosis and handling of B virus in a rhesus monkey. *J. Am. Vet. Med. Assoc.* **153:**894–898.
31. **Collins, P.** 1983. The spectrum of antiviral activities of acyclovir *in vitro* and *in vivo*. *J. Antimicrob. Chemother.* **12**(Suppl. B)**:**19–27.
32. **Cropper, L. M., D. N. Lees, R. Patt, I. R. Sharp, and D. Brown.** 1992. Monoclonal antibodies for the identification of herpesvirus simiae (B virus). *Arch. Virol.* **123:** 266–277.
33. **Daniel, M. D., F. G. Garcia, L. V. Melendez, R. D. Hunt, J. O'Connor, and D. Silva.** 1975. Multiple herpesvirus simiae isolation from a rhesus monkey which died of cerebral infarction. *Lab. Anim. Sci.* **25:**303–308.
34. **Davenport, D. S., D. R. Johnson, G. P. Holmes, D. Jewitt, S. C. Ross, and J. K. Hilliard.** 1994. Diagnosis and management of human B virus (herpesvirus simiae) infections in Michigan. *Clin. Infect. Dis.* **19:**33–41.
35. **Davidson, W. L., and K. Hummeler.** 1960. B virus infection in man. *Ann. N. Y. Acad. Sci.* **85:**970–979.
36. **Eberle, R., D. Black, and J. K. Hilliard.** 1989. Relatedness of glycoproteins expressed on the surface of simian herpes-virus virions and infected cells to specific HSV glycoproteins. *Arch. Virol.* **109:**233–252.
37. **Eberle, R., D. H. Black, S. Lipper, and J. K. Hilliard.** 1995. Herpesvirus papio 2, an SA8-like alphaherpesvirus of baboons. *Arch. Virol.* **140:**529–545.
38. **Eberle, R., and J. Hilliard.** 1989. Serological evidence for variation in the incidence of herpesvirus infections in different species of apes. *J. Clin. Microbiol.* **27:**1357–1366.
39. **Eberle, R., and J. Hilliard.** 1995. The simian herpesviruses. *Infect. Agents Dis.* **45:**55–70.
40. **Eberle, R., B. Tanamachi, D. Black, E. L. Blewett, M. Ali, H. Openshaw, and E. M. Cantin.** 1997. Genetic and functional complementation of the HSV1 UL27 gene and gB glycoprotein by simian alpha-herpesvirus homologs. *Arch. Virol.* **142:**721–736.
41. **Endo, M., T. Kamimura, Y. Aoyama, T. Hayashida, T. Kinyo, Y. Ono, S. Kotera, K. Suzuki, Y. Tajima, and K. Ando.** 1960. Etude du virus B au Japon. 1. Recherche des anticorps neutralisant le irus B chez les singes d'origine Japonaise et les singes etrangers au Japon. *Jpn. J. Exp. Med.* **30:**227–233.
42. **Endo, M., T. Kamimura, N. Kusano, K. Kawai, Y. Aoyama, K. Suzuki, and S. Kotera.** 1960. Etude du virus B au Japon. II. Le premier insolement du virus B au Japon. *Jpn. Exp. Med.* **30:**385–392.
43. **Espana, C.** 1973. Herpesvirus simiae infection in Macaca radiata. *Am. J. Phys. Anthropol.* **38:**447–454.
44. **Espana, C.** 1974. Viral epizootics in captive nonhuman primates. *Lab. Anim. Sci.* **24:**167–176.

45. **Fierer, J., P. Bazeley, and A. E. Braude.** 1973. Herpes B virus encephalomyelitis presenting as ophthalmic zoster. *Ann. Intern. Med.* **79:**225–228.
46. **Freifeld, A. G., J. Hilliard, J. Southers, M. Murray, B. Savarese, J. M. Schmitt, and S. E. Straus.** 1995. A controlled seroprevalence survey of primate handlers for evidence of asymptomatic herpes B virus infection. *J. Infect. Dis.* **171:**1031–1034.
47. **Gay, F. P., and M. Holden.** 1933. The herpes encephalitis problem. *J. Infect. Dis.* **53:**287–303.
48. **Gay, F. P., and M. Holden.** 1933. Isolation of herpes virus from several cases of epidemic encephalitis. *Proc. Soc. Exp. Biol. Med.* **30:**1051–1053.
49. **Gosztonyi, G., D. Falke, and H. Ludwig.** 1992. Axonal and transsynaptic (transneuronal) spread of herpesvirus simiae (B virus) in experimentally infected mice. *Histol. Histopathol.* **7:**63–74.
50. **Gosztonyi, G., D. Falke, and H. Ludwig.** 1992. Axonal-transsynaptic spread as the basic pathogenetic mechanism in B virus infection of the nervous system. *J. Med. Primatol.* **21:**42–43.
51. **Gralla, E. J., S. J. Ciecura, and C. S. Delahunt.** 1966. Extended B-virus antibody determinations in a closed monkey colony. *Lab. Anim. Sci.* **16:**510–516.
52. **Harrington, L., L. V. Wall, and D. C. Kelly.** 1992. Molecular cloning and physical mapping of the genome of simian herpes B virus and comparison of genome organization with that of herpes simplex virus type 1. *J. Gen. Virol.* **73:**1217–1226.
53. **Heberling, R. L.** 1986. Dot immunobinding assay of viral antigens and antibodies. *Dev. Biol. Stand.* **64:**199–203.
54. **Heberling, R. L., and S. S. Kalter.** 1987. A dot-immunoblotting assay on nitrocellulose with psoralen inactivated herpesvirus simiae (B virus). *Lab. Anim. Sci.* **37:** 304–308.
55. **Hilliard, J. K., D. Black, and R. Eberle.** 1989. Simian alphaherpesviruses and their relation to the human herpes simplex viruses. *Arch. Virol.* **109:**83–102.
56. **Hilliard, J. K., R. Eberle, S. L. Lipper, R. M. Monoz, and S. A. Weiss.** 1987. Herpesvirus simiae (B virus): replication of the virus and identification of viral polypeptides in infected cells. *Arch. Virol.* **93:**185–198.
57. **Hilliard, J. K., R. M. Munoz, S. L. Lipper, and R. Eberle.** 1986. Rapid identification of herpesvirus simiae (B virus) DNA from clinical isolates in nonhuman primate colonies. *J. Virol. Methods* **13:**55–62.
58. **Hilliard, J. K., and J. A. Ward.** 1999. B virus specific-pathogen-free breeding colonies of macaques *(Macaca mulatta)*: retrospective study of seven years of testing. *Lab. Anim. Sci.* **49:**144–148.
59. **Hilliard, J. K., and B. J. Weigler.** 1999. The existence of differing monkey B virus genotypes with possible implications for degree of virulence in humans. *Lab. Anim. Sci.* **49:**10–11.
60. **Holmes, G. P., L. E. Chapman, J. E. Stewart, S. E. Straus, J. K. Hilliard, D. S. Davenport, and the B Virus Working Group.** 1995. Guidelines for preventing and treating B virus infections in exposed persons. *Clin. Infect. Dis.* **20:**421–439.
61. **Holmes, G. P., J. K. Hilliard, and K. C. Klontz.** 1990. B virus (herpes virus simiae) infection in humans: epidemiologic investigation of a cluster. *Ann. Intern. Med.* **112:**833–839.
62. **Hopps, H. E., B. C. Bernheim, A. Nisalak, J. H. Tijo, and J. E. Smadel.** 1963. Biologic characteristics of a continuous kidney cell line derived from the African green monkey. *J. Immunol.* **91:**416–424.
63. **Hull, R. N.** 1971. B virus vaccines. *Lab. Anim. Sci.* **21:** 1068–1071.
64. **Hull, R. N.** 1973. The simian herpesviruses, p. 389–425. *In* A. S. Kaplan (ed.), *The Herpesviruses*. Academic Press, New York, NY.
65. **Hull, R. N., J. R. Minner, and C. C. Mascoli.** 1958. New viral agents recovered from tissue cultures of monkey kidney cells. III. Recovery of additional agents both from cultures of monkey tissues and directly from tissues and excreta. *Am. J. Hyg.* **68:**31–44.
66. **Hull, R. N., and J. C. Nash.** 1960. Immunization against B virus infection. I. Preparation of an experimental vaccine. *Am. J. Hyg.* **71:**15–28.
67. **Hull, R. N., F. B. Peck, Jr., T. G. Ward, and J. C. Nash.** 1962. Immunization against B virus infection. II. Further laboratory and clinical studies with an experimental vaccine. *Am. J. Hyg.* **76:**239–251.
68. **Hummeler, K., W. L. Davidson, W. Henle, A. C. LaBoccetta, and H. G. Rush.** 1959. Encephalomyelitis due to infection with herpesvirus simiae (herpes B virus): a report of two fatal, laboratory acquired cases. *N. Engl. J. Med.* **261:**64–68.
69. **Jainkittivong, A., and R. P. Langlais.** 1998. Herpes B virus infection. *Oral Surg. Oral Med. Oral Pathol. Oral Radiol. Endod.* **85:**399–403.
70. **Kalter, S. S., and R. L. Heberling.** 1971. Comparative virology of primates. *Bacteriol. Rev.* **35:**310–364.
71. **Katz, D., J. K. Hilliard, R. Eberle, and S. L. Lipper.** 1986. ELISA for detection of group-common and virus-specific antibodies in human and simian sera induced by herpes simplex and related simian viruses. *J. Virol. Methods* **14:**99–109.
72. **Katz, D., J. K. Hilliard, R. R. Mirkovic, and R. A. Word.** 1986. ELISA for detection of IgG and IgM antibodies to HSV-1 and HSV-2 in human sera. *J. Virol. Methods* **14:**43–55.
73. **Keeble, S. A.** 1960. B virus infection in monkeys. *Ann. N. Y. Acad. Sci.* **85:**960–969.
74. **Keeble, S. A., G. J. Christofinis, and W. Wood.** 1958. Natural virus B infection in rhesus monkeys. *J. Pathol. Bacteriol.* **76:**189–199.
75. **Kessler, M. J., and J. K. Hilliard.** 1990. Seroprevalence of B virus (herpesvirus simiae) antibodies in a naturally formed group of rhesus macaques. *J. Med. Primatol.* **19:** 155–160.
76. **Killeen, A. M., L. Harrington, L. V. Wall, and D. C. Kelly.** 1992. Nucleotide sequence analysis of a homologue of herpes simplex virus type 1 gene US9 found in the genome of simian herpes B virus. *J. Gen. Virol.* **73:**195–199.
77. **Kohn, A.** 1975. Latency of simian herpes in rabbits. *Harefuah* **89:**430.
78. **Krech, U., and L. J. Lewis.** 1954. Propagation of B virus in tissue culture. *Proc. Soc. Exp. Biol. Med.* **87:**174–178.
79. **Lees, D. N.** 1991. Herpesvirus simiae (B virus) antibody response and virus shedding in experimental primary infection of cynomolgus monkeys. *Lab. Anim. Sci.* **41:**360–364.
80. **Loomis, M. R., T. O'Neill, M. Bush, and R. J. Montali.** 1981. Fatal herpesvirus infection in patas monkeys and a black and white colobus monkey. *J. Am. Vet. Med. Assoc.* **179:**1236–1239.
81. **Ludwig, H., G. Pauli, B. Norrild, B. F. Vestergaard, and M. D. Daniel.** 1978. Immunological characterization of a common antigen present in herpes simplex virus, bovine mammillitis virus and herpesvirus simiae (B virus). *IARC Sci. Publ.* **24:**235–241.
82. **McCarthy, K., and F. A. Tosolini.** 1975. A review of primate herpes viruses. *Proc. R. Soc. Med.* **68:**145–150.
83. **McClure, H. M., B. Olberding, and L. M. Strozier.** 1973. Disseminated herpesvirus infection in a rhesus monkey *(Macaca mulatta)*. *J. Med. Primatol.* **2:**190–194.

84. **Melnick, J. L., and D. D. Banker.** 1954. Isolation of B virus (herpes group) from the central nervous system of a rhesus monkey. *J. Exp. Med.* **100:**181–194.
85. **Nagler, F. P., and M. Klotz.** 1958. A fatal B virus infection in a person subject to recurrent herpes labialis. *Can. Med. Assoc. J.* **79:**743–745.
86. **Nanda, M., V. T. Curtin, J. K. Hilliard, N. D. Bernstein, and R. D. Dix.** 1990. Ocular histopathologic findings in a case of human herpes B virus. *Arch. Ophthalmol.* **108:**713–716.
87. **Norcott, J. P., and D. W. Brown.** 1993. Competitive radioimmunoassay to detect antibodies to herpes B virus and SA8 virus. *J. Clin. Microbiol.* **31:**931–935.
88. **Norrild, B., H. Ludwig, and R. Rott.** 1978. Identification of a common antigen of herpes simplex virus, bovine herpes mammillitis virus, and B virus. *J. Virol.* **26:** 712–717.
89. **Ohsawa, K., T. W. Lehenbauer, and R. Eberle.** 1999. Herpesvirus papio 2: alternative antigen for use in monkey B virus diagnostic assays. *Lab. Anim. Sci.* **49:**605–616.
90. **Palmer, A. E.** 1987. B virus, herpesvirus simiae: historical perspective. *J. Med. Primatol.* **16:**99–130.
91. **Pierce, E. C., J. D. Pierce, and R. N. Hull.** 1958. B virus: its current significance, description and diagnosis of a fatal human infection. *Am. J. Hyg.* **68:**242–250.
92. **Reagan, R. L., W. C. Day, M. P. Harmon, and A. L. Bruecker.** 1952. Adaptation of 'B' virus to the Swiss albino mouse. *J. Gen. Microbiol.* **7:**827–828.
93. **Reagan, R. L., W. C. Day, M. P. Harmon, and A. L. Bruecker.** 1952. Effect of "gb" virus (strain no. 1) in the Syrian hamster. *Am. J. Trop. Med. Hyg.* **1:**987–989.
94. **Reissig, M., and J. L. Melnick.** 1955. The cellular changes produced in tissue cultures by herpes B virus correlated with concurrent multiplication of the virus. *J. Exp. Med.* **101:**341–351.
95. **Roth, A. M., and T. W. Purcell.** 1977. Ocular findings associated with encephalomyelitis caused by herpesvirus simiae. *Am. J. Ophthalmol.* **84:**345–348.
96. **Ruebner, B. H., D. Kevereux, M. Rorvik, C. Espana, and J. F. Brown.** 1975. Ultrastructure of herpesvirus simiae (herpes B virus). *Exp. Mol. Pathol.* **22:**317–325.
97. **Sabin, A. B.** 1934. Studies on the B virus. I. The immunological identity of a virus isolated from a human case of ascending myelitis associated with visceral necrosis. *Br. J. Exp. Pathol.* **15:**248–268.
98. **Sabin, A. B.** 1934. Studies on the B virus. II. Properties of the virus and pathogenesis of the experimental disease in rabbits. *Br. J. Exp. Pathol.* **15:**269–279.
99. **Sabin, A. B.** 1934. Studies on the B virus. III. The experimental disease in macacus rhesus monkeys. *Br. J. Exp. Pathol.* **15:**321–334.
100. **Sabin, A. B.** 1949. Fatal B virus encephalomyelitis in a physician working with monkeys. *J. Clin. Investig.* **28:** 808.
101. **Sabin, A. B., and M. W. Wright.** 1934. Acute ascending myelitis following a monkey bite, with the isolation of a virus capable of reproducing the disease. *J. Exp. Med.* **59:**115–136.
102. **Sabin, A. B., and W. E. Hurst.** 1935. Studies on the B virus. IV. Histopathology of the experimental disease in rhesus monkeys and rabbits. *Br. J. Exp. Pathol.* **16:**133–148.
103. **Sasagawa, A.** 1986. Herpes simplex virus complement fixing antibody and herpes B virus serum neutralizing antibody in sera of wild and laboratory-bred cynomolgus monkeys. *Jikken Dobutsu* **35:**59–63.
104. **Scinicariello, F., R. Eberle, and J. K. Hilliard.** 1993. Rapid detection of B virus (herpesvirus simiae) DNA by polymerase chain reaction. *J. Infect. Dis.* **168:**747–750.
105. **Scinicariello, F., W. J. English, and J. Hilliard.** 1993. Identification by PCR of meningitis caused by herpes B virus. *Lancet* **341:**1660–1661. (Letter.)
106. **Shah, K. V., and C. H. Southwick.** 1965. Prevalence of antibodies to certain viruses in sera of free-living rhesus and of captive monkeys. *Indian J. Med. Res.* **35:**488–500.
107. **Simon, M. A., M. D. Daniel, D. Lee-Parritz, N. W. King, and D. J. Ringler.** 1993. Disseminated B virus infection in a cynomolgus monkey. *Lab. Anim. Sci.* **43:** 545–550.
108. **Slomka, M. J., L. Harrington, C. Arnold, J. P. Norcott, and D. W. Brown.** 1995. Complete nucleotide sequence of the herpesvirus simiae glycoprotein G gene and its expression as an immunogenic fusion protein in bacteria. *J. Gen. Virol.* **76:**2161–2168.
109. **Smith, A. L., D. H. Black, and R. Eberle.** 1998. Molecular evidence for distinct genotypes of monkey B virus (herpesvirus simiae) which are related to the macaque host species. *J. Virol.* **72:**9224–9232.
110. **Thompson, S. A., J. K. Hilliard, D. Kittel, J. Foster, S. Lipper, W. E. Giddens, Jr., D. H. Black, and R. Eberle.** 2000. Retrospective analysis of an outbreak of B virus in a colony of DeBrazza's monkeys. *Comp. Med.* **50:**649–657.
111. **Tribe, G. W.** 1982. The pathogenesis and epidemiology of B-virus. *J. Inst. Anim. Tech.* **33:**1–4.
112. **U.S. Department of Health and Human Services, Centers for Disease Control and Prevention.** 1999. *Biosafety in Microbiological and Biomedical Laboratories*, 4th ed. U.S. Government Printing Office, Washington, D.C.
113. **van Hoosier, G. L., and J. L. Melnick.** 1961. Neutralizing antibodies in human sera to herpesvirus simiae. *Tex. Rep. Biol. Med.* **19:**376–380.
114. **Vizoso, A. D.** 1974. Heterogeneity in herpes simiae (B virus) and some antigenic relationship in the herpes group. *Br. J. Exp. Pathol.* **55:**471–477.
115. **Vizoso, A. D.** 1975. Latency of herpes simiae (B virus) in rabbits. *Br. J. Exp. Pathol.* **56:**489–494.
116. **Vizoso, A. D.** 1975. Recovery of herpesvirus simiae (B virus) from both primary and latent infections in rhesus monkeys. *Br. J. Exp. Pathol.* **56:**485–488.
117. **Weigler, B. J.** 1992. Biology of B virus in macaques and human hosts: a review. *Clin. Infect. Dis.* **14:**555–567.
118. **Weigler, B. J., D. W. Hird, J. K. Hilliard, N. W. Lerche, J. A. Roberts, and L. M. Scott.** 1993. Epidemiology of Cercopithecine herpesvirus 1 (B virus) infection and shedding in a large breeding cohort of rhesus macaques. *J. Infect. Dis.* **167:**257–263.
119. **Weigler, B. J., J. A. Roberts, D. W. Hird, N. W. Lerche, and J. K. Hilliard.** 1990. A cross sectional survey for B virus antibody in a colony of group housed rhesus macaques. *Lab. Anim. Sci.* **40:**257–261.
120. **Weigler, B. J., F. Scinicariello, and J. K. Hilliard.** 1995. Risk of venereal B virus (cercopithecine herpesvirus 1) transmission in rhesus monkeys using molecular epidemiology. *J. Infect. Dis.* **171:**1139–1143.
121. **Weir, E. C., P. N. Bhatt, R. O. Jacoby, J. K. Hilliard, and S. Morgenstern.** 1993. Infrequent shedding and transmission of herpesvirus simiae from seropositive macaques. *Lab. Anim. Sci.* **43:**541–544.
122. **Weller, T. H., and R. Pearson.** 1972. Herpes-like simian viruses: retrospective and prospective considerations. *J. Natl. Cancer Inst.* **49:**209–211.
123. **Wilson, R. B., M. A. Holscher, T. Chang, and J. R. Hodges.** 1990. Fatal herpesvirae simiae (B virus) infection in a patas monkey *(Erythrocebus patas)*. *J. Vet.*

Diagn. Investig. **2:**242–244.
124. **Wood, W., and F. T. Shimada.** 1954. Isolation of strains of virus B from tissue cultures of cynomolgus and rhesus kidney. *Can. J. Public Health* **45:**509–518.
125. **Zwartouw, H. T., and E. A. Boulter.** 1984. Excretion of B virus in monkeys and evidence of genital infection. *Lab. Anim.* **18:**65–70.
126. **Zwartouw, H. T., C. R. Humphreys, and P. Collins.** 1989. Oral chemotherapy of fatal B virus (herpesvirus simiae) infection. *Antivir. Res.* **11:**275–283.

Varicella-Zoster Virus

ANNE A. GERSHON AND SAUL J. SILVERSTEIN

21

Varicella-zoster virus (VZV) is the etiologic agent of two diseases, varicella (chickenpox) and zoster (shingles). Varicella, which occurs after the initial encounter with VZV, is a disease manifested by a pruritic rash accompanied by fever and other systemic signs and symptoms that are usually mild to moderate in nature. Most often, but not always, varicella is a self-limited infection of childhood. Live attenuated varicella vaccine was licensed for routine use in the United States in 1995, which after more than 13 years of use has changed the epidemiology of the disease, as the incidences of varicella and its complications have now significantly declined (44, 111).

Zoster is mainly a disease of adults. A prerequisite for developing zoster is a prior episode of varicella, which on occasion may have been subclinical or following varicella vaccination. During primary infection, VZV establishes a latent infection in sensory and cranial neurons; zoster results when the latent virus reactivates and returns from the neuron to infect the skin. Most often VZV reactivates in the setting of relative immunologic compromise, particularly of cell-mediated immunity (CMI), as occurs with aging, or following disease or various treatments such as steroids, cancer chemotherapy, transplantation, and irradiation (99).

Varicella was distinguished clinically from smallpox in the mid-18th century. The origin of the name chickenpox is uncertain, but it may have been derived from the French pois chiche (chick pea), or from the domestic fowl (in Old English cicen and Middle High German kuchen). Herpes is derived from the Greek word meaning to creep; zoster comes from the Greek word for belt, and the word shingles is derived from the Latin word (cingulus) for girdle (44).

The delineation of the link between varicella and zoster is of virologic, medical, and historical interest. In 1888 Bokay recognized that cases of varicella often occurred following an exposure to patients with zoster and postulated that there was a relationship between the two diseases (44). In early attempts to develop a vaccine against varicella, medical investigators inoculated vesicular fluid from zoster patients into varicella-susceptible children, who subsequently manifested chickenpox (44). Weller and Stoddard performed the first successful in vitro studies and showed that viruses isolated from patients with varicella and zoster are immunologically similar (132). In the mid-1940s a possible analogy with herpes simplex virus (HSV) infection was recognized, and it was proposed that zoster was due to reactivation of latent VZV (44). Hope-Simpson was the first to recognize the importance of the immune system in controlling manifestations of zoster; he postulated that zoster resulted from waning immunity to VZV in the years following varicella, permitting the latent virus to emerge (63). More recently the importance of declining cellular immunity to VZV was recognized in the pathogenesis of zoster (44). Using molecular techniques for DNA analysis, it was demonstrated that latent VZV is present in sensory neurons of individuals with a history of varicella (19, 24, 26, 59, 71, 89, 90). VZV DNA from zoster isolates was shown to be similar to the DNA of the virus which caused the primary VZV infection or the DNA of the virus used for vaccination, proving that zoster results from reactivation of latent VZV (44). It is now therefore widely accepted that zoster is not acquired from contact with patients with chickenpox; in a placebo-controlled study of vaccination against zoster in the elderly, the vaccine recipients were not predisposed to develop early zoster compared to controls (99).

VIROLOGY

Classification

There is only one serotype of VZV; no differences in antigenicity among virus isolates have been identified. There are minor differences in DNA sequence among VZV isolates, and at least seven genotypes have now been identified, which on the basis of single nucleotide polymorphisms are classified as European, Japanese, or Mosaics (44). Analysis of 130 circulating VZV strains from the United States in 2001 and 2002 indicated that 81.5, 3, and 15.5% were of the European, Japanese, and Mosaics genotypes, respectively (110). The Oka strain has not been demonstrated to circulate.

The genomes of the parental (wild-type) and vaccine Oka strains have been fully sequenced; there are numerous differences between the parent and vaccine strains, especially within open reading frame (ORF) 62 (44). Fifteen of 42 (36%) base differences between vaccine and wild-type VZV were present in ORF 62 (140).

The wild-type VZV DNA sequence is readily distinguished from that of vaccine virus by restriction enzyme analysis of DNA from cultured virus and/or by PCR. In countries other than Japan, a useful marker for the vaccine strain is the absence of a PstI restriction site in ORF 38 (44); however, this assay may become less useful should there be significant circulation of Japanese wild-type VZV in the United States. The presence of SmaI and NaeI restriction sites in ORF 62 clearly discriminates between the Oka vaccine strain and all wild-type strains, including Japanese wild-type virus (44). Using DNA sequence analysis of a single nucleotide polymorphism at 106262 in ORF 62, it is possible to distinguish rapidly between vaccine and wild-type VZVs (101). Molecular assays are useful for identification of adverse events temporally associated with varicella vaccine (44, 87).

Composition of the Virus

Enveloped virions are 150 to 200 nm in diameter, with a central DNA core. The inner viral nucleocapsid has an approximate diameter of 100 nm, consisting of 162 hexagonal capsomeres with central axial hollows organized as an icosahedron with 5:3:2 axial symmetry (44). Consistent with the morphological structure of other herpesvirus virions, a biologically important coat, the tegument, surrounds the nucleocapsid, which is, in turn, surrounded by an envelope derived in part from cellular membranes.

The genome of VZV is composed of approximately 125,000 bp. It contains 74 ORFs, which account for 71 different gene products (44). The linear double-stranded DNA consists of a long unique segment of approximately 100 kbp and a short unique sequence of approximately 5.4 kbp, flanked by internal and terminal repeats of 6.8 kbp (Color Plate 30) (29). It exists in four isomers; the predominant ones account for 95% of the population (44).

By analogy with HSV, VZV is thought to replicate via a temporally regulated cascade of gene expression, consisting in general of synthesis of immediate-early (IE), early (E), and, lastly, late (L) genes. Expression of L genes culminates in lytic, productive viral infection. Interruption of the cascade, particularly at the IE/E stage, can result in failure to synthesize infectious virus and may result in latent infection (59). IE genes are for the most part regulatory, E genes may be regulatory or structural, and L genes encode structural elements of the virion. Some of the IE regulatory gene products that also encode structural elements of the virion, such as the regulatory ORFs 62, 4, and 63, are also found in purified virions (73) (Table 1). Gene products of ORFs 21 and 29 are lytic-cycle genes expressed early in infection. The ORF 62 protein acts as a transcriptional activator or as a repressor and is required for further latent or lytic viral synthesis because IE gene 62 is thought to initiate the cascade of gene expression of VZV (59). Gene 61 is a transcriptional repressor (59) that encodes regulatory proteins; however, unlike the ORF 62 protein, the ORF 61 protein is not present in the virion (73).

The functions and biochemical characteristics of most VZV proteins are still unknown. Many are nonstructural proteins involved in different aspects of viral replication. About 30 polypeptides have been detected in VZV, at least 8 of which are glycosylated (59). The virus-encoded glycoproteins are named alphabetically, corresponding to those of HSV, as follows: gB, gC, gE, gH, gI, gK, gL, and gM. There is no VZV equivalent of gD, importantly, which is the major glycoprotein of HSV. Some are essential to viral synthesis (such as gE), and others are less essential (such as gC). Some glycoproteins contain amino acid signal sequences or acid-rich patches in their cytoplasmic tails that are trafficking motifs, which direct their movement, required for envelopment, to structures such as the *trans*-Golgi network and the plasma membrane (128, 129, 145, 146).

TABLE 1 Summary of genetic information on VZV

Protein	ORF(s)	Comments on likely importance
gB	31	Fusion, entry, egress
gC	14	Adhesion, cell entry
gE	68	Most abundant; essential for replication, envelopment, spread
gH	37	Fusion, entry, egress
gI	67	Travels with gE; needed for proper envelopment
gK	5	Essential
gL	60	Travels with gH
gM	50	
Nucleocapsid	20, 40	
	10	Tegument, transactivator
	61	Transcriptional repressor
	28	DNA polymerase
Latency associated		
IE		
	63	Major protein; down-regulates transcription of IE gene 62; tegument
	4	Tegument, transcriptional activator
	62	Tegument, transcriptional activator or repressor
E		
	21	Nucleocapsid protein
	29	DNA binding protein
	66	Protein kinase

gE is the most abundant glycoprotein of VZV; encoded by ORF 68, it is essential for production of infectious virus (91). This glycoprotein exists as several glycopeptides in different maturational stages with molecular masses ranging from 60 to 98 kDa (97). gE is highly immunogenic; it is a phosphorylated high-mannose O-linked and N-linked complex-type glycan which, in concert with gI, binds to the Fc fragment of human immunoglobulin G (IgG) (97, 98). gE and gI are covalently linked and act as an Fc receptor on infected cells. They play an important role in cell-to-cell spread of virus and are also essential for envelopment (129, 141). They are interdependent for viral maturation and for transportation of other glycoproteins to the cell surface (92, 129). gE contains trafficking sequences that mediate assembly of viral proteins and envelopment in the *trans*-Golgi network (145, 146). gE (along with gI) acts as a navigator, directing additional glycoproteins to the cell surface and back to the *trans*-Golgi network, where final envelopment of virions occurs (129). A variant VZV with a mutated gE has been isolated from five individuals (44, 53). These viruses are thought to be escape mutants, and their biological significance needs further study.

The second most abundant glycoprotein is gB, a heterodimeric glycopeptide linked by disulfide bonds. It too plays important roles in viral entry, envelopment, and egress from cells (61). gH is thought to have an important role in virus entry, egress, and cell-to-cell spread in VZV infection (117). gH exists as a single-species glycopeptide with a molecular mass of 118 kDa (116); it is a high-mannose N-linked glycopeptide which does not contain O-linked oligosaccharides. gI is a 60-kDa glycopeptide with both N-linked and O-linked oligosaccharides; it is nonessential for growth of VZV in fibroblasts, but mutants lacking it replicate poorly in cell culture (92, 129). gC is a heterogeneous 95- to 105-kDa glycopeptide that contains N-linked oligosaccharides and possibly O-linked oligosaccharides (52). Antibodies to gE, gI, gB, and gH have neutralizing activity and are therefore hypothesized to be critical for viral spread, particularly attachment and penetration (36, 116, 117, 139).

Biology

Entry of cell-free VZV particles appears to be dependent upon several factors. These include cell surface heparan sulfate proteoglycan (144), calcium-independent mannose 6-phosphate receptors (MPR^{ci}) (21, 144), and the cellular insulin-degrading enzyme, which is a receptor for gE (84, 85). Insulin-degrading enzyme is also critical for cell-to-cell spread of VZV (84, 85). Entry of cell-free enveloped virions into cells is highly cholesterol dependent and occurs mainly by clathrin-mediated endocytosis (Fig. 1) (56).

After uncoated viral particles reach the nucleus, VZV commences replication, synthesizing its DNA core and capsid. The capsid receives a temporary envelope from the inner lamella of the nuclear membrane; in order for it to receive a tegument it is de-enveloped by passing through the rough endoplasmic reticulum into the cytoplasm as a naked nucleocapsid (46). Nucleocapsids and glycoproteins are transferred independently to the *trans*-Golgi network, where the tegument is added and final envelopment occurs (Fig. 2). Additionally, it has been postulated that due to the presence of mannose 6-phosphate in VZV glycoproteins, there is an interaction between MPR^{ci} and VZV that results in the inclusion of virions into endosomes, where they are exposed to lysosomal enzymes and an acid environment and the infectivity of the virions thus becomes compromised (21). Most VZV synthesis occurs by this manner, in vitro and in vivo. In cell cultures, infectious VZV is not released into media. In contrast, in human skin, during the natural maturation of superficial epidermal cells, MPR^{ci}s are lost, along with the lysosomal pathway. In patients infected with VZV, free virions are produced in these cells and are released into skin vesicles during acute varicella and zoster. These 200-nm particles probably play roles in airborne transmission of VZV and establishment of latent infection in neurons (45). If this hypothesis regarding MPR^{ci}s is correct, it may explain why infectious virions are not released into supernatant media in cell cultures and in vivo in cells where MPRs are abundant. In contrast, in vivo in the superficial epidermis, the lysosomal pathway is circumvented and infectious cell-free VZV is released into human skin lesions, accounting for the high degree of infectivity of varicella and establishment of latent infection by infection of neurons, with axons present in the area of the epidermis where the cell-free virions are present (21).

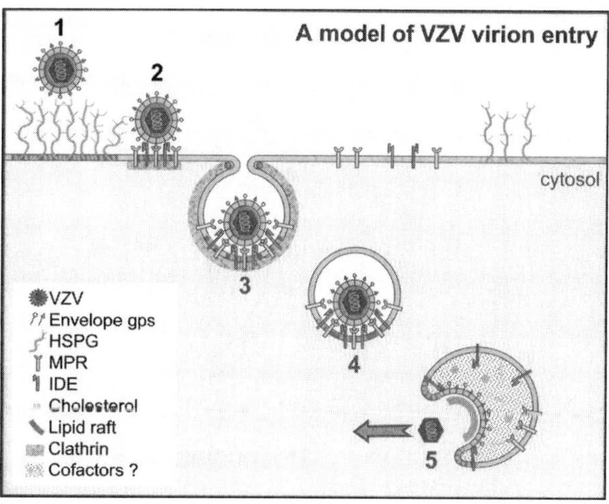

FIGURE 1 A suggested mechanism of VZV virion entry. (1) The incoming virion initially attaches to cellular heparan sulfate proteoglycan (HSPG), facilitating specific interaction with cellular receptor, e.g., MPR^{ci} (2). This leads to receptor-mediated (clathrin-dependent) endocytosis (3) and delivery to an endosomal compartment (4). Within this structure, the virion is exposed to cofactors for membrane fusion, possibly including the insulin-degrading enzyme (IDE) and/or altered pH. (5) Following triggered membrane fusion, the VZV nucleocapsid is delivered to the cytoplasm. Cholesterol may play a role at each stage. (Reprinted from reference 56 with permission.)

VZV appears to spread, therefore, in two ways (45). It can spread from one infected cell to another cell by fusion of the two cells; fusion is mediated in all probability by gE, gI, gH, and gB on the membrane of the infected cell. This form of spread does not require envelopment of virions. In mutant VZVs lacking gI, cell-to-cell spread takes place, although proper viral envelopment does not occur (129). Cell-to-cell spread is thought to be the major means of spread of VZV in the body and would explain the importance of cellular immunity rather than antibodies in host defense against this virus. The other form of spread, described above in the discussion of viral entry, is by cell-

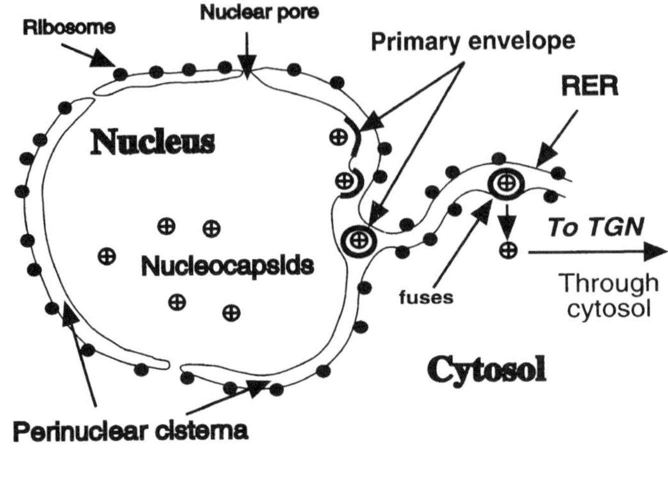

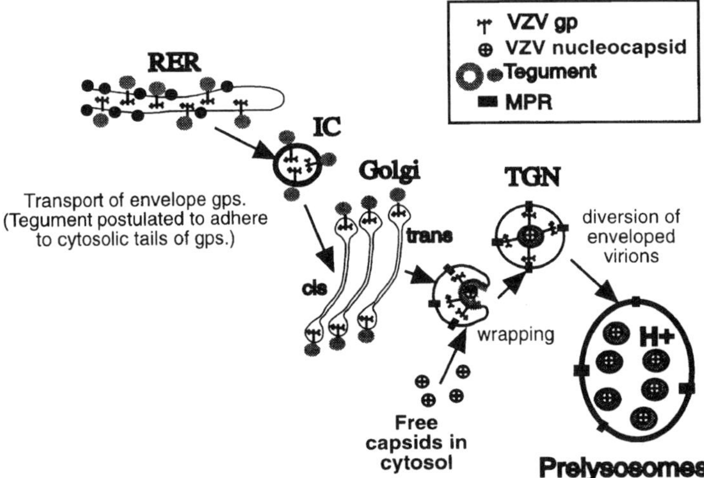

FIGURE 2 Putative route of intracellular transport and maturation of VZV in human embryonic lung fibroblasts. Structures are not drawn to scale. (Top) Nucleocapsids assemble in the nuclei of infected cells and bud through the nuclear envelope to reach the perinuclear cisterna-rough endoplasmic reticulum (RER). A temporary, primary viral envelope is acquired from the inner nuclear membrane. This envelope fuses with the RER, delivering unenveloped nucleocapsids to the cytosol. The nucleocapsids move through the cytosol to reach the *trans*-Golgi network (TGN). (Bottom) The glycoproteins (gps) of the viral envelope are synthesized in the RER independently of the nucleocapsids and are integral membrane proteins. Tegument proteins are probably synthesized by free ribosomes and are transported to the Golgi stack, as are the gps. Virions receive their final envelope by wrapping the TGN-derived sac and are delivered to acidic structures, identified as prelysosomes. (Reprinted from reference 46 with permission.)

free virus. It is hypothesized that synthesis of cell-free VZV occurs only in skin vesicles, because MPRs are not formed in the superficial epidermis and therefore infectious enveloped virions are not exposed to the acid environment of endosomes, so they are released from infected epidermal cells in an infectious form (21). Cell-free VZV in skin vesicles can be aerosolized and thus spread to persons susceptible to varicella. Cell-free virions are also able to establish latent VZV infection in an in vitro neuronal animal model (45).

Latency of VZV differs markedly from latency of HSV. While early information suggested that latency might occur in various cells, it is now widely accepted that latent VZV infection occurs primarily, and probably exclusively, in neurons (70, 72, 88). At least six VZV genes are expressed during latent VZV infection; these are mostly IE genes (ORFs 4, 62, and 63); the IE ORF 61, however, is not expressed in latent infection. ORF 63 protein, the predominant latency protein, interestingly inhibits apoptosis of neurons infected with VZV in vitro (62). Some E genes are also expressed in latent infection (ORFs 21, 29, and 66), but L genes are not; their expression indicates lytic rather than latent infection (19, 23, 25, 26, 45, 59, 71, 89, 90). All of the VZV latency genes have HSV type 1 counterparts; however, none of these genes are expressed in HSV latency. In contrast to VZV, during HSV latency only one region of the genome, termed latency-associated transcripts, is expressed (44). During VZV latency, it is hypothesized that the cascade of viral synthesis is interrupted and that there is a block in the synthetic cascade, perhaps at the level of expression of ORF 61 (59). VZV latency-associated proteins are only cytoplasmic. The mechanism responsible for this aberrant cell localization is poorly understood. At least one latency-associated protein, ORF 29 protein, however, can be made to enter the nuclei of latently infected neurons in response to inhibition of the proteasome or ectopic expression of ORF 61p (114). Dephosphorylation of ORF 62 protein causes this cytoplasmic protein to translocate to the nucleus (74). Reactivation of VZV in human dorsal root neurons was visualized using in situ hybridization to identify VZV DNA in autopsy specimens (88).

There are currently two general hypotheses concerning how latent infection is established. One is that a nerve is infected by cutaneous VZV and that a certain level of viral multiplication takes place prior to VZV becoming latent in a neuron (143). The other posits that cell-free virions from the skin are transported to a neuron, and latency is established but multiplication does not occur. HSV is thought to establish latency without viral replication (109), although this model fails to account for the rather high number of genomes that are present in each latently infected cell. In an experimental in vitro model of VZV latency in guinea pig enteric neurons, following infection with cell-free VZV there is no viral replication, latency results, and the neuron survives in vitro for weeks. Infection of neurons with cell-associated VZV, in contrast, results in replication with rapid neuronal death, despite the presence of ORF 63 protein, which becomes nuclear (19, 45).

Reactivation with production of infectious VZV and rapid neuronal death has been demonstrated in the in vitro guinea pig neuron model of latency (45; J. J. Chen, S. Wan, S. Bischoff, S. J. Silverstein, A. A. Gershon, and M. D. Gershon, presented at the Conference on the Enteric Nervous System, Banff, British Columbia, Canada, 2003). Reactivation of latent VZV is induced by infection with an adenovirus vector carrying VZV ORF 61.

Other important observations with regard to VZV latency include the following. Patients with impaired CMI to VZV have an increased incidence of herpes zoster, which is consistent with the hypothesis that at least some aspects of suppression of VZV infectivity are under immunologic control (99). Various rodent animal models of VZV latency have been developed, although reactivation has not been induced (44, 142).

VZV has an extremely limited host range, infecting mostly primates. Hairless guinea pigs may be infected with VZV that has been adapted in tissue culture to cells from this species. The illness produced is extremely mild, and latent infection occurs only infrequently, but specific immune responses can be demonstrated (44).

In vitro, VZV spreads rather slowly, from one cell to another, as described above. After inoculation of diploid human cell cultures such as human embryonic lung fibroblasts, focal cytopathic effect (CPE) is not observed until at least 48 h after infection (Fig. 3). VZV is best propagated at 32°C (44). The CPE of VZV in cell culture is characteristically focal, the result of cell-to-cell spread. Characteristic CPE consists of foci of swollen refractile cells in a spindle-shaped configuration. Foci of infected cells enlarge and may slowly involve much of the monolayer, but infectious virions are not released from cells. Diploid human cell cultures are the most convenient host system for virus isolation; primary and heteroploid cell lines such as MeWo cells can also be used (52).

There is little available information on the stability of VZV, but it is usually classified as a rather labile agent. Virus obtained from vesicular fluid is stable for years when frozen in sterile fat-free milk at −70°C. Cell-free VZV obtained by sonication of infected cells can be stored at −70°C in tissue culture medium containing fetal bovine serum with sorbitol at a final concentration of 10%. Infected cells can be preserved at −70°C or in liquid nitro-

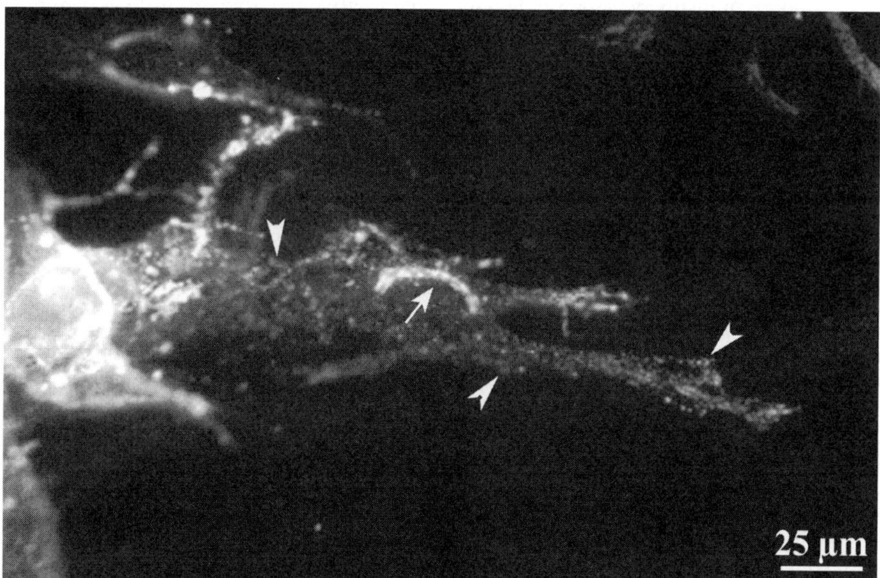

FIGURE 3 VZV propagated in human embryonic lung fibroblasts after several days in culture. The specimen was stained with fluorescein-tagged monoclonal antibodies to gE of VZV. The arrow indicates gE in the *trans*-Golgi network, and the arrowheads indicate gE at the cell surface.

gen in medium containing 10% fetal bovine serum and 10% dimethyl sulfoxide.

EPIDEMIOLOGY

Distribution, Geography, and Seasonality

VZV infections occur worldwide. The virus spreads less readily in countries with tropical climates than in those with temperate climates (44), resulting in a higher rate of susceptibility to varicella in adults in tropical countries than in countries with cooler climates. It is possible that spread of VZV is inhibited at high temperatures because the virus is labile. In the prevaccine era, about 4 million cases of chickenpox, an entire annual birth cohort, were estimated to occur yearly in the United States. The disease affects males and females equally. Varicella is most common in the winter and early spring. In contrast, zoster occurs at equal rates during all seasons of the year.

Incidence and Prevalence of Varicella

Varicella is one of the most contagious of infectious diseases (106). Reported secondary attack rates of varicella following household exposure of susceptible contacts range from 61 to 100% (44, 106). Secondary varicella cases in a family are usually more severe than primary cases (106), presumably due to the intensity of exposure in that setting resulting in a higher viral inoculum. The first child developing varicella in a family thus usually has a milder infection than subsequent family members who become ill.

About three-fourths of U.S. adults with no history of varicella have detectable antibodies to VZV (78), indicating that subclinical varicella can occur. In an epidemiological study in which parents with no history of varicella were exposed to their children with chickenpox and did not contract it themselves, it was estimated that the incidence of subclinical varicella is approximately 5% (106).

In countries with temperate climates where vaccine is not being used universally, varicella is a disease of childhood; most cases occur in children before they are 10 years old, with 8 to 9% of children annually developing disease between the ages of 1 and 9 years (44). These data were representative of children in the United States before many began to attend day care facilities; it is possible that exposures to VZV in the day care setting lead to an earlier acquisition of disease. The effect of day care, however, on the epidemiology of varicella may never be fully known because live attenuated varicella vaccine was licensed for use in all varicella-susceptible children in 1995 in the United States.

Second attacks of varicella are uncommon but have been reported (44). Second attacks may be more frequent in immunocompromised hosts than in healthy individuals. One hypothesis that has been proposed for incomplete protection against varicella in some individuals is that VZV antibodies are of lower avidity in patients with recurrent cases. An absence of antibodies directed at gE, gB, and gH does not account for reinfections (79). There is considerable humoral immunologic boosting to VZV upon exposure of varicella-immune subjects to patients with VZV infections (44). In one study, 32% of parents exposed to their children with varicella manifested either transient IgM antibodies or an increase in antibody titer or both (48). Whether boosting of CMI also occurs after an exposure is not known, but boosting of CMI by immunization years following natural infection has been demonstrated (99). Whether immunologic boosting is required for long-term maintenance of immunity to VZV is not known.

Nosocomial Varicella

Nosocomial varicella can be a serious and expensive problem in hospitals, where both patients and employees may be susceptible to chickenpox (44). With the availability of varicella vaccine for adults and children since 1995, nosocomial varicella apprears to be less of a problem than it was formerly in the United States. Because varicella-susceptible hospital employees may serve as vectors for spread of VZV to susceptible patients, it is now common to test employees for immunity to chickenpox serologically and to offer vaccine to those who are susceptible. Passive immunization (with preformed antibodies) is not useful to terminate potential nosocomial varicella outbreaks, but it is useful to protect varicella-susceptible immunocompromised patients who have been exposed to VZV (see below).

The risk of horizontal transmission of VZV in maternity wards or the newborn nursery after a hospital exposure to an adult or child is extremely low, which has been attributed to several factors (44). Many hospitalized newborn infants are in isolettes, and most hospital employees and mothers and their newborn infants have antibodies to VZV and are at reduced risk of developing clinical illness. Because IgG antibodies to VZV cross the placenta, newborns of immune mothers are at least partially protected. Even in low-birth-weight infants, serum antibodies to VZV are usually detectable (44). Nevertheless, a few episodes of transmission of varicella in the newborn nursery have been reported. Many more instances of an absence of transmission following exposures in this setting, however, have been recorded (38).

Incidence and Prevalence of Zoster

Zoster is traditionally a disease of adults. Patients who have zoster usually have a history of a previous attack of varicella or vaccination (44, 63). Zoster is rare in childhood, but there is an increased incidence in young children who had varicella either in utero or before reaching their second birthday (38). Chickenpox in the first year of life increases the risk of childhood zoster, by a relative factor between roughly 3 and 21 (44), possibly due to immaturity of the immune response to VZV in young infants. Latent infection is also extremely common in infants with congenital varicella syndrome; zoster may occur in over 20% of affected infants (38).

Over a lifetime, zoster occurs in approximately 15 to 20% of individuals. The incidence of zoster in a population begins to increase sharply at about the age of 50 years; the incidence during the fifth decade, approximately 5 per 1,000 person-years annually, is almost double that of the previous decade (28, 63). During the eighth decade the incidence more than doubles again, to 14 per 1,000 person-years annually (28). The increased incidence of zoster with advancing age is attributed to a relative loss of CMI to VZV that occurs naturally with aging (44).

Zoster occurs with increased frequency in immunocompromised patients; those who are severely immunocompromised may also develop disseminated VZV infection with viremia (33). Zoster may be particularly frequent and severe following bone marrow transplantation, after which as many as 35% of patients develop it within a year (44). Spinal trauma, irradiation, and corticosteroid therapy may also be precipitating factors. The distribution of lesions in chickenpox, which primarily involves the trunk and head, is reflected in a proportionately greater representation of these regions in the dermatomal lesions of zoster (44). Zoster may recur, either in the same dermatome or in a different dermatome; however, the chance of developing recurrent zoster seems to be low in healthy individuals (63). The reported incidence of zoster in various groups is shown in Table 2 (44).

Mortality

The mortality rates for varicella and zoster are low, but the rates increase with advancing age, pregnancy, and decreasing immunocompetence. For varicella, the reported case fatality rate is lowest in children aged 1 to 14 years (0.75 per 100,000). The reported case fatality rate in infants less than 1 year old is 6.23 per 100,000, in those aged 15 to 19 it is 2.7 per 100,000, and in those 30 to 49 years old it is 25.2 per 100,000 (104). In the prevaccine era 100 to 150 annual deaths were reported in the United States (44). Pregnancy, particularly when varicella occurs in the third trimester, may increase morbidity and mortality (38, 44, 58, 102). In a report of 44 consecutive cases of varicella during pregnancy, varicella pneumonia occurred in 9% of women, with one fatality (2.4%) (102). In a more recent collaborative study, however, involving 347 pregnant women who were consecutively monitored, there were no fatalities, although 5% developed varicella pneumonia (58). The mortality rate for varicella in leukemic children receiving chemotherapy is reported as 1,000 times higher than that in healthy children (44). A fatality rate of 7% was reported for leukemic children with chickenpox in the preantiviral drug era (34). Epidemiological data from the 1990s suggest that the incidence of severe varicella in healthy hosts was underestimated by a factor of 5 (22). Mortality related to zoster is due primarily to pneumonia; the overall risk of fatal infection is lower than that for varicella in immunocompromised patients, less than 1% (9). Zoster also has a lower mortality rate than varicella in otherwise healthy middle-aged or elderly adults (44).

Transmission

Varicella a highly contagious disease, particularly in the early stages of the illness; VZV is spread by the airborne route (44). It was long thought that the source of transmitted virus was the respiratory tract of infected individuals. Spread of VZV in closed communities that were attributed to exposure to an index case prior to development of rash has been occasionally reported, suggesting that respiratory transmission occurs (13). It is possible, however, that an early insignificant rash went unnoticed in these patients. Studies utilizing PCR identified VZV DNA in the nasopharynx of children during preeruptive and early varicella, although the rates have been inconsistent (44). The presence of VZV DNA, however, does not necessarily indicate the presence of infectious virus. For example, VZV DNA was recovered from room dust 2 weeks after a patient was discharged, long after the virus could remain infectious (44).

Evidence suggests that cell-free virions in vesicular skin lesions of patients with VZV are the major source of infectious virus (21). Secondary to the loss of MPRs in the superficial epidermis, high concentrations of cell-free, 200-nm particles of VZV develop in skin vesicles; these may be aerosolized and thus transmit the virus to others by the airborne route (21). Presumably airborne virus infects the respiratory tract of varicella-susceptible individuals. Clinical studies of transmission of VZV in leukemic vaccinees (122) and immunocompetent children (17, 112) have implicated skin lesions as the source of infectious virus. There was a direct relationship between the number of skin lesions and viral transmission (112, 122). In a recent study from China, an outbreak among schoolchildren became controlled only after children with rash were excluded from attendance (17). There is one report of transmission of VZV to others during an autopsy of a patient with varicella; obviously the virus was not spread from the respiratory tract (103).

Studies of isolation of VZV from patients with varicella also implicate the skin as the source of infectious virus rather than the respiratory tract. VZV is readily isolated in cell culture from skin lesions, but it is extremely difficult to isolate the virus from the respiratory tract. Searches for infectious VZV in throat secretions of immunocompetent patients during the incubation period of varicella have proved largely negative (51, 100, 121). There is, however, one report of isolation of VZV from nasal swabs from 3 of 23 (13%) children and from pharyngeal swabs from 2 of 22 (9%) children on days 2 and 3 after the onset of rash (121). It is possible that there may have been vesicles on the mucous membranes in these children, and also it is not clear whether any of them were immunocompromised. In contrast, VZV can readily be cultured from vesicular lesions in patients with varicella and zoster. Isolation of VZV was successful in 23 of 25 (92%) cases when vesicle fluid was cultured within 3 days after the onset of rash in one study (51) and in 12 of 17 (71%) cases in another study (121). Vesicular fluid specimens collected from 4 to 8 days after onset, however, yielded VZV in only one of seven instances (51). VZV may persist longer in vesicles of zoster patients (44). In general it may be conservatively presumed that varicella is transmissible to others from 1 to 2 days prior to the onset of rash and during the first few days of rash. Skin lesions due to either varicella or zoster are unlikely to harbor infectious virus once they are dry. Taken together, these observations suggest that VZV spreads predominately from skin lesions and that within several days after the onset of rash patients with varicella are no longer contagious to others. In contrast, zoster may be infectious for a somewhat longer period.

Zoster is not transmissible to others as such, but the vesicular lesions contain infectious VZV and are therefore potentially contagious to others as varicella (44). Even patients with localized zoster may transmit VZV to varicella-susceptible individuals, and therefore these patients should

TABLE 2 Reported approximate incidence of zoster in various populations per 1,000 person-years of observation[a]

Adults (all ages): 2–4 (63)*
Adults, age 70–79: 11 (99)
Adults, middle aged, vaccinated against varicella: 0.9 (55)*
Children with leukemia in remission (prior varicella) 25 (57)**
Children with leukemia, vaccinated: 8 (57)**
Adults with HIV (prior varicella): 51 (44)
Children with HIV (prior varicella): 163 (41)***
Children with HIV, vaccinated: 0–3 (Son et al., unpublished)***

[a] Numbers in parentheses are reference numbers. *, trend due only to wide confidence limits; **, significantly different values; ***, significantly different values.

be isolated when hospitalized. Whether VZV is spread from the respiratory tract in zoster is unknown, but it seems unlikely. Based on scant information regarding household transmission of VZV from zoster patients to varicella-susceptible contacts, zoster was estimated to be only about half as contagious as varicella (44).

PATHOGENESIS IN HUMANS

Incubation Period, Patterns of Virus Replication, and Factors in Disease Production

The incubation period of varicella ranges from 10 to 23 days, with an average of 14 days (44). During the incubation period, VZV is thought to spread to regional lymph nodes, undergo multiplication, and cause a primary low-grade viremia about 5 days later (54) (Fig. 4).

In varicella, two viremic phases have been hypothesized to occur, based on studies with the virus that causes mousepox (54). Following a putative early viremia that spreads the virus to the reticuloendothelial system, there is local replication of VZV. This results in the second and greater viremia, which delivers the virus to the skin; there it causes the characteristic skin rash, in which "crops" of lesions develop, possibly reflecting several viremic episodes (54) (Fig. 4).

An alternative proposal for pathogenesis is based in part on studies of mice with severe combined immunodeficiency disease engrafted with various human tissues (SCID hu mouse model) infected with VZV (75). Following exposure of susceptible contacts, VZV infects tonsillar T cells as cell-free virus and multiplies in the respiratory mucosa, and then T lymphocytes are infected. In VZV-infected SCID hu mice, these T cells deliver VZV promptly to implanted skin. In infected individuals, only limited viral multiplication in the skin takes place at first, due to the innate immune response. Innate immunity is eventually overcome as the incubation period of the disease comes to an end. Due to circulation of infected T cells, there is a low-grade viremia for a week or so after infection, but as more and more T cells and keratinocytes are infected, the viremia increases, innate immunity is overcome, and the rash develops. At that time adaptive immunity develops, and within a week or so the pathogen is controlled and the patient recovers. VZV has been isolated from blood cultures either a few days before onset of rash or within 1 to 2 days after rash onset in immunocompetent children (7). VZV has also been isolated from blood obtained from immunocompromised patients with varicella or zoster (44). Experiments in SCID hu mice and human skin cellular implants indicate that human CD4 and CD8 lymphocytes are infected with VZV (96).

A number of strategies for immune evasion of VZV by host cells that facilitate VZV multiplication have been described, some unique to this herpesvirus (1–3, 108). For example, in infected fibroblasts, VZV down-regulates major histocompatibility complex (MHC) class I antigens and thereby interferes with antigen presentation to cytotoxic T cells. Additionally, MHC class II expression can be blocked by VZV gene products, resulting in a decreased gamma interferon response. Immune evasion is thought to play an important role, particularly in viral multiplication that occurs during the incubation period of varicella.

The skin lesions of varicella begin as macules and progress rapidly to papules, vesicles, pustules, and scabs. Vesicles are located in the superficial epidermis. With time, the fluid changes from clear to cloudy, as polymorphonuclear leukocytes (PMNs) reach the site. Interferon is pres-

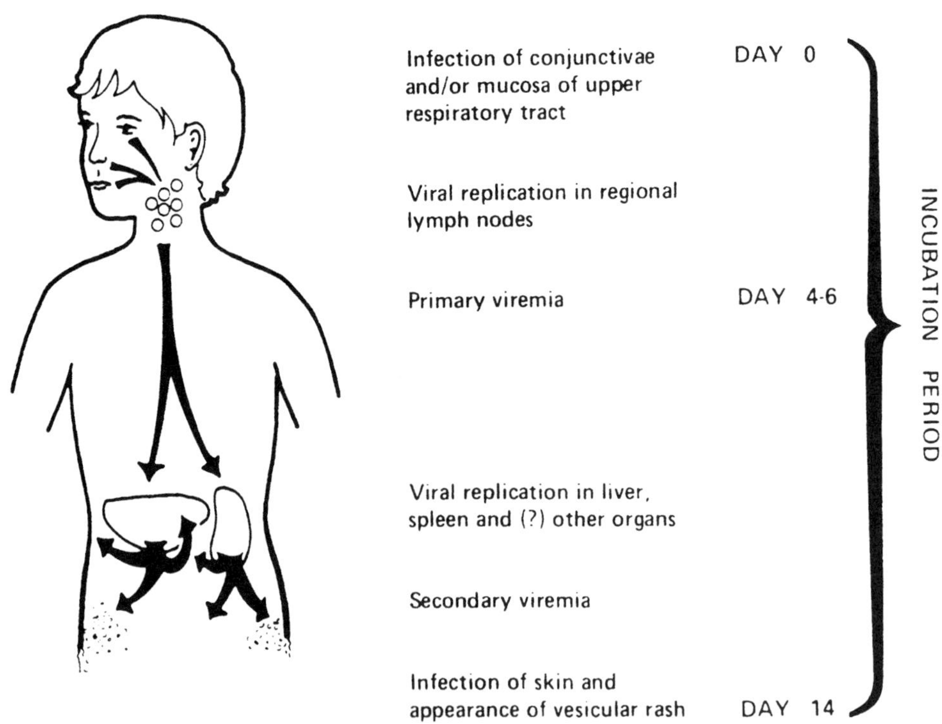

FIGURE 4 Diagram showing proposed pathogenesis of varicella regarding events during the incubation period. (Reprinted from reference 54 with permission.)

ent in vesicular fluid, reflecting the adaptive cell-mediated immune response of the host (93). The predominant cell in vesicular lesions is the PMN, which may play a role in generating interferon in vesicular lesions and play a role in recovery (44). In vitro data also suggest that the PMN plays a role in host defense against VZV, possibly by mediating antibody-dependent cellular cytotoxicity (ADCC) (44). Cytotoxic CD4 and CD8 lymphocytes, however, represent the major host response that controls VZV infection (44).

Histologic changes in the skin vesicles are similar for chickenpox and zoster. The hallmarks of each are multinucleated giant cells and intranuclear inclusions. In varicella these are primarily localized in the epidermis, where ballooning degeneration of cells in the deeper layers is accompanied by intercellular edema. As edema progresses, the cornified layers and basal layers separate to form a thin-roofed vesicle. An exudate of mononuclear cells is seen in the dermis without characteristic nuclear changes of epithelial cells in this region (Fig. 5) (133).

In zoster, in addition to skin lesions that resemble those of varicella, the dorsal root ganglion of the affected dermatome exhibits a mononuclear inflammatory infiltrate. There may also be necrosis of ganglion cells and demyelination of the corresponding axon (32, 88).

Latent VZV is present in human sensory dorsal root and cranial nerve ganglia in human autopsy specimens in persons who have had varicella. Prior to development of zoster, VZV reactivates in the neuron, resulting in lytic infection, and then it travels down the affected sensory nerves to the skin, causing a characteristic unilateral vesicular rash (Fig. 6). Zoster may last for several weeks, particularly in immunocompromised patients, who not only are at increased risk of developing this disease due to low levels of CMI to VZV but also may require long times to recover for the same reason.

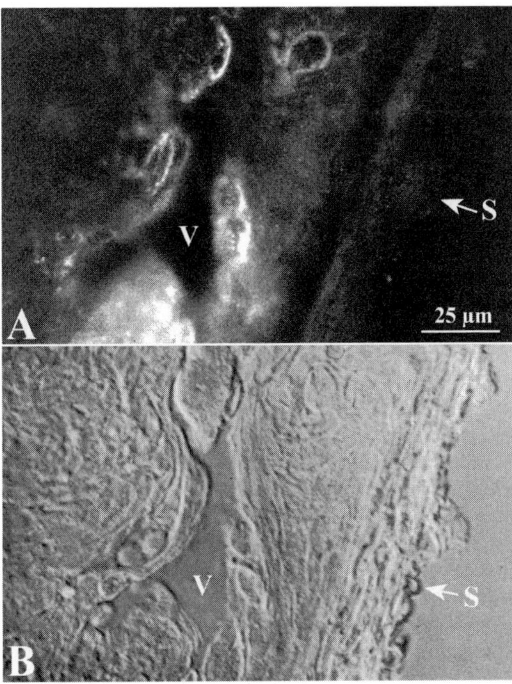

FIGURE 5 Skin vesicle from a patient in the early stages of varicella. The vesicle has not been unroofed. (A) The specimen was stained with fluorescein-tagged monoclonal antibodies to gE of VZV. (B) Same specimen as in panel A, viewed by Nomarski interference contrast microscopy. V, vesicular space; S, outer surface of epidermis.

Immune Responses

Both humoral and cell-mediated adaptive immune responses to VZV develop within a few days after onset of varicella. Peak antibody levels are attained after 4 to 8 weeks, remain high for about 6 months, and then decline. IgG antibody to VZV is detected in healthy adults for decades after varicella (44). After active immunization against varicella, antibody titers are lower than after natural infection but may persist for as long as 20 years (8). Because doses of varicella vaccine used in different countries and made by different companies vary in composition and dosage, persistence of antibodies after vaccination may vary in different locations. Serum IgG, IgA, and IgM develop after both varicella and zoster. Zoster occurs in the face of high levels of specific antibodies, but significantly higher titers develop during convalescence, reflecting the anamnestic response to this reactivation infection (44).

CMI plays the major role in host defense against VZV, probably because the virus spreads almost entirely in the body as an intracellular pathogen. CMI can be demonstrated by stimulation of lymphocytes in vitro with VZV antigens (60, 83), by an intradermal skin test (78), and by specific lysis of histocompatible target cells by cytotoxic T cells (6). Natural killer (NK) cells and ADCC against VZV have also been described (66). CMI reactions can be detected for years after varicella, although this response may wane in many individuals after age 50 (44).

Exactly how immunity to varicella and zoster is mediated, however, is still unclear. It is generally agreed that CMI, in the form of T-cell cytotoxicity, is more important than humoral immunity in recovery from infection. For example, children with isolated agammaglobulinemia are not at increased risk of developing severe varicella. CMI is probably crucial during chickenpox because spread of VZV within the body is almost exclusively by the intracellular route, rather than by release of cell-free virus, as occurs in vesicular fluid.

The response that prevents clinical illness after reinfection with VZV is not known for certain, although it is presumed to be some form of CMI, perhaps at times in concert with antibodies. Patients with agammaglobulinemia are not subject to recurrent varicella. On the other hand, elderly adults, who often have low CMI or an absence of CMI to VZV, are not particularly subject to second attacks of varicella; presumably, their antibodies protect them from recurrent chickenpox. Specific antibodies may play a role in immunity because passive immunization can be used to prevent or modify varicella in exposed susceptible individuals. It may be that antibodies are particularly effective right after infection occurs due to a brief period of multiplication in tonsils in which cell-free VZV, which can be neutralized, is produced. It is thus possible that passive immunization lowers the initial viral load, resulting in modified or asymptomatic infection. Certain antibodies, particularly those to gH, moreover, may impede cell-to-cell spread of the virus (117). Young infants, however, can develop varicella after exposure despite detectable transplacental antibody titers, but usually the illness is attenuated (38). Vaccinated leukemic children

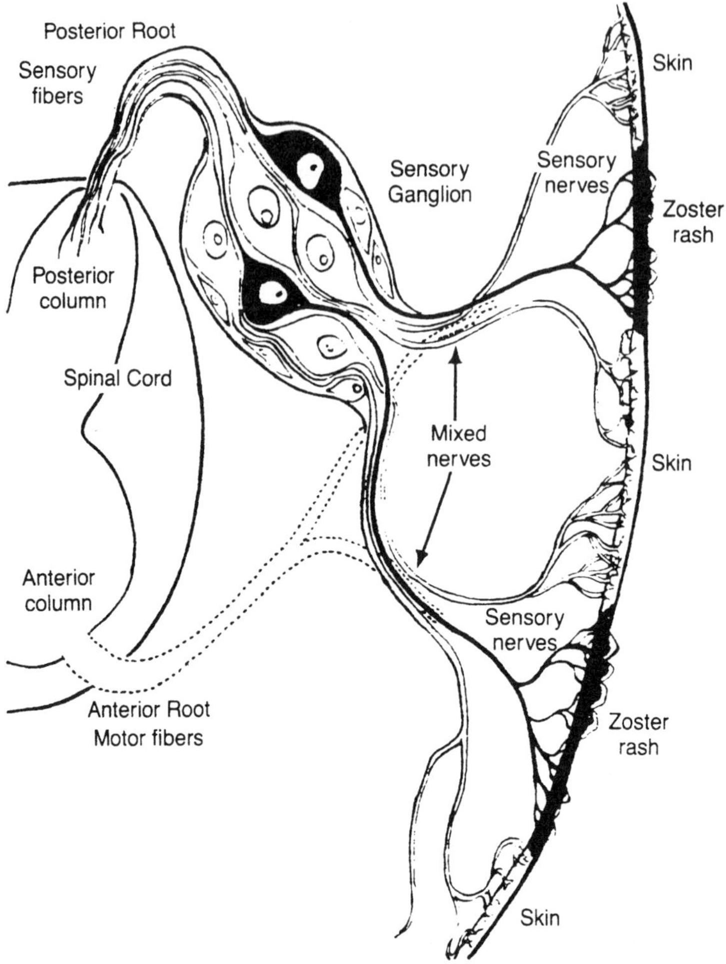

FIGURE 6 Proposed pathogenesis of zoster. (Reprinted from reference 63 with permission.)

have developed modified cases of breakthrough varicella despite detectable VZV antibodies or positive CMI responses as measured by lymphocyte stimulation at exposure to VZV, but they do not have normal immune systems (44). They are, however, highly likely to be protected if they have both humoral and cellular immunity to VZV at exposure (40). Healthy individuals with detectable humoral immunity at exposure to VZV are far less likely to develop clinical illness than those lacking these responses (94). Both antibodies and CMI seem to participate in various aspects of protection against VZV, suggesting that redundancy in the adaptive immune response may provide the best strategy against the virus for the host.

VARICELLA

Clinical Manifestations

Varicella is a highly contagious, usually self-limited systemic infection, characterized by fever and a generalized pruritic rash, lasting about 5 days (Fig. 7). A prodromal phase in children is unusual, but it is not uncommon for adults to experience a prodrome of malaise and fever for 1 to 2 days prior to onset of the rash (44). The rash is characteristically more concentrated on the trunk and head than on the extremities, and it typically evolves as a series of "crops" over 1 to 2 days in healthy hosts. Most children with varicella develop from 250 to 500 skin lesions, many of which are vesicular (106). In many cases a few lesions may develop in the mouth or conjunctiva or on other mucosal sites. Rarely, the skin lesions may be bullous or hemorrhagic. Residual scarring is exceptional, but depigmented areas of skin may result and be persistent. Constitutional symptoms may be mild despite an extensive exanthem, but usually the extent of rash reflects the severity of the illness. It is not uncommon to observe a transient increase in hepatic aminotransferase levels without jaundice during varicella, but this is not considered a complication of the disease (44). Adults are more likely to develop severe varicella than children. Presumably this is due to lower CMI responses to VZV in adults than in children (44). Newborn infants who acquire varicella from their mothers in the few days prior to delivery are also at risk of developing severe varicella, presumably due to immaturity of the CMI response in very young babies in the absence of specific maternal antibodies (44).

Clinical Diagnosis

It is usually not difficult to make a clinical diagnosis of varicella because the vesicular pruritic rash is so characteristic. In questionable cases, epidemiological information

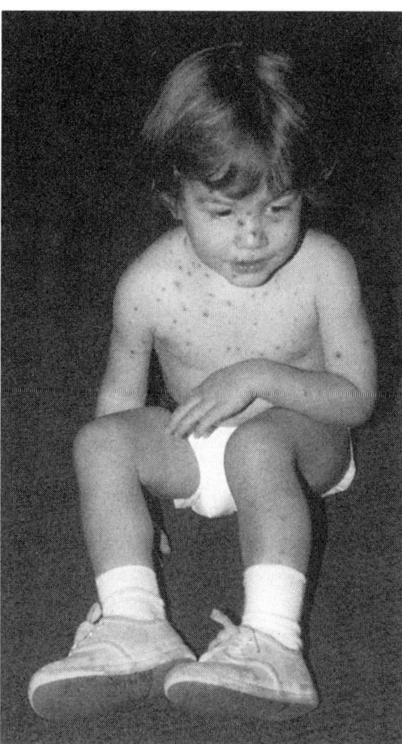

FIGURE 7 Varicella on day 5 in an otherwise healthy 2-year-old boy, showing the typical distribution of skin lesions.

may be useful, such as a history of recent exposure to varicella or zoster and subsequent transmission of varicella to another person. The differential diagnosis of varicella includes generalized HSV infection, rickettsial pox, impetigo, allergic reactions (including Stevens-Johnson syndrome), poison ivy, and insect bites. In locations where vaccine is being used, laboratory confirmation of mild breakthrough varicella in an immunized child (see below) may be required.

Complications

The most frequent complication of varicella in healthy hosts is bacterial superinfection of the skin, lungs, or bones. Severe morbidity and even mortality involving group A beta-hemolytic streptococcal superinfections have been reported (137). Central nervous system complications which may precede or follow varicella in healthy hosts include transient cerebellar ataxia, a severe form of cerebral encephalitis, aseptic meningitis, transverse myelitis, and stroke. Because aspirin is no longer recommended for children with varicella, encephalopathy due to Reye syndrome has become rare. Meningoencephalitis and cerebellar ataxia, which usually occur between 2 and 6 days after onset of the rash, may also occur during the incubation period (44, 115). With these complications, the cerebrospinal fluid (CSF) may be normal or may exhibit a mild lymphocytic pleocytosis (<100 cells/ml), a moderate elevation of protein (<200 mg), and normal glucose. VZV encephalitis can be life threatening; symptoms may reverse rapidly or gradually improve. Chronic neurologic or developmental sequelae may occur (67). Cerebellar ataxia may persist for days to weeks but is almost invariably self-limited. Strokes after varicella are unusual, have only recently been recognized as a complication of the infection, and are hypothesized to be secondary to vasculitis provoked by VZV (95).

Varicella may rarely cause neutropenia and thrombocytopenia with hemorrhagic complications 1 to 2 weeks after the initial infection (35). Arthritis is an infrequent, transient complication; VZV has on occasion been isolated from joint fluid. Vesicular lesions that involve the eyelids and conjunctivae rarely cause serious ocular complications (31). Other rare complications of varicella include renal failure, myocarditis, pericarditis, pancreatitis, orchitis, and purpura fulminans (44, 113, 133).

Varicella may be severe and even fatal in immunocompromised patients. These include persons with an underlying malignancy; congenital or acquired deficits in CMI, such as those who have undergone organ transplantation or have underlying human immunodeficiency virus (HIV) infection; and individuals receiving high doses of corticosteroids for any reason (44). Patients with deficiencies in CMI may manifest progressive varicella, with continuing fever and development of new vesicular lesions for as long as 2 weeks (Fig. 8). Their characteristic skin lesions are often large, umbilicated, and hemorrhagic; primary varicella pneumonia is a frequent complication. Alternatively, some immunocompromised patients develop an acute form of varicella with disseminated intravascular coagulation that is rapidly fatal (44). A rate of visceral disease of 30% and a fatality rate of 7% were reported for leukemic children who developed chickenpox prior to the availability of antiviral drugs (34). Severe varicella has been observed in children with underlying infection with HIV, especially those who have clinical evidence of AIDS, but most HIV-infected children develop mild to moderate forms of varicella. The illness in this population is not potentially as severe as in children with leukemia (41). However, because it is difficult to predict in advance whether a child with HIV infection will develop severe varicella, most physicians routinely elect to treat them at onset with antiviral drugs. Varicella does not seem to be a cofactor for clinical progression of HIV infection to AIDS, but chronic infections with wart-like hyperkeratotic lesions with occasional virus dissemination may develop in these patients (5) (Fig. 9). These lesions appear to be a persistent form of VZV infection rather than classic zoster.

Primary varicella pneumonia accounts for many of the fatalities ascribed to varicella (Fig. 10). It most commonly occurs in immunocompromised patients, adults, and neonates with chickenpox (44). In a chest X-ray study of military recruits with varicella, radiographic evidence of pneumonia was found in 16%, although only one quarter of these patients had pulmonary symptoms (130). Pneumonia usually occurs within several days after the onset of rash, but sometimes this interval may be longer. Symptoms include fever and cough in almost all cases and dyspnea in more than 70%. Other common symptoms and signs include cyanosis, rales, hemoptysis, and chest pain. The chest X-ray typically reveals a diffuse nodular or miliary pattern, most pronounced in the perihilar regions (120). The availability of antiviral chemotherapy has greatly improved the outcome of varicella pneumonia.

ZOSTER

Clinical Manifestations

Zoster usually begins as a localized skin eruption involving one to three dermatomal segments. The characteristic dis-

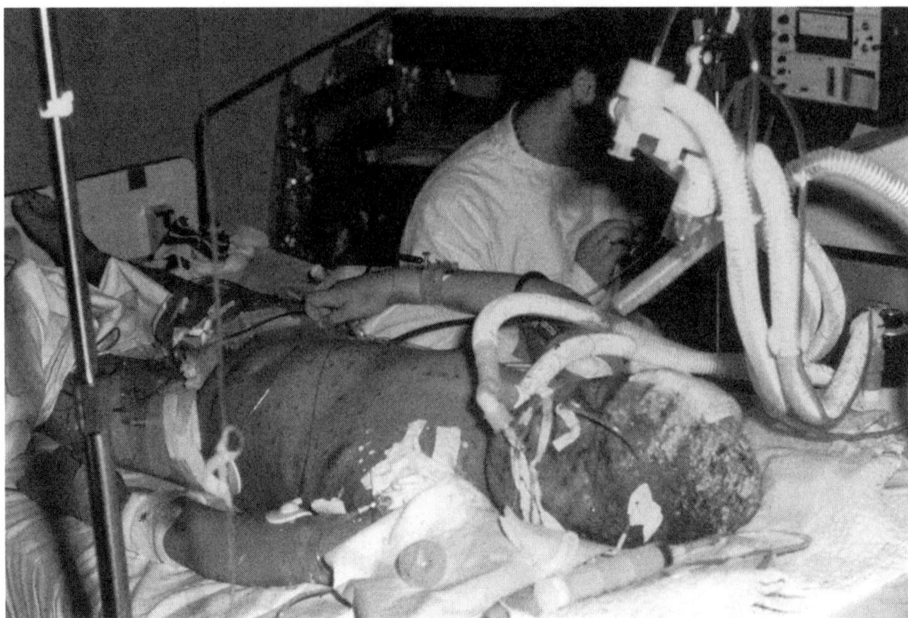

FIGURE 8 Hemorrhagic fatal varicella in a child with underlying lymphoma.

tribution of the unilateral rash reflects its pathogenesis, reactivation of latent VZV from dorsal root or cranial nerve ganglia (Fig. 11). The skin lesions resemble those of varicella but tend more toward confluence. Zoster usually develops in patients who are at least somewhat immunodeficient, due to disease, chemotherapy, or radiotherapy or as a result of aging. On occasion, however, healthy young adults who are not immunocompromised may develop zoster, presumably resulting from a transient decrease in CMI to VZV due to a stimulus such as another viral infection or stress. Because most immunocompromised persons do not develop zoster, deficiency of CMI to VZV is necessary but not sufficient to develop this illness. It is likely that reactivation of VZV first occurs and that then clinical zoster results when the CMI response is deficient.

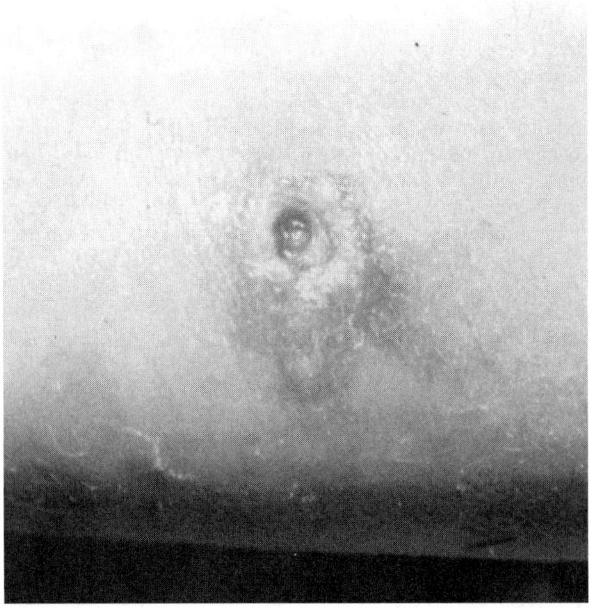

FIGURE 9 Chronic VZV skin lesion in a child with underlying HIV infection.

There is a spectrum of clinical manifestations of zoster. Zoster with no rash but with dermatomal pain has been described (zoster sine herpete) (49), as has visceral zoster without skin rash (27). Increases in VZV antibody titer in the absence of an exposure to the virus have been ascribed to silent reactivation of VZV (44). Subclinical viremia in patients after bone marrow transplantation has been demonstrated by PCR (136). Shedding of infectious VZV from asymptomatic individuals has not been documented as it has for HSV.

Clinical Diagnosis

It is usually not difficult to make a clinical diagnosis of zoster because the unilateral dermatomal rash is so characteristic. In one study, however, 13% of cases clinically diagnosed as zoster were proven by culture to be due to HSV infection (69). HSV should particularly be considered in the differential diagnosis when the rash is in the trigeminal/maxillary, breast (T4), or sacral distribution, and especially if the rash is recurrent. The unilateral rash of zoster most often involves the thoracic and cervical areas, followed by the face. Laboratory verification is becoming of greater importance in the vaccine era, when it may be of clinical interest to determine if a zosteriform rash is due to VZV and if it is wild or vaccine type.

Self-limited meningitis indicated by abnormalities of the CSF, including pleocytosis (predominantly of mononuclear cells) and elevated protein, may develop in many patients with zoster (44). Complete healing of the rash usually occurs within 2 weeks but may require 4 to 6 weeks, especially in immunocompromised patients. Segmental pain and/or itching are common symptoms in zoster. These sensations may precede the onset of rash. Other causes of acute segmental pain such as myocardial infarction, acute

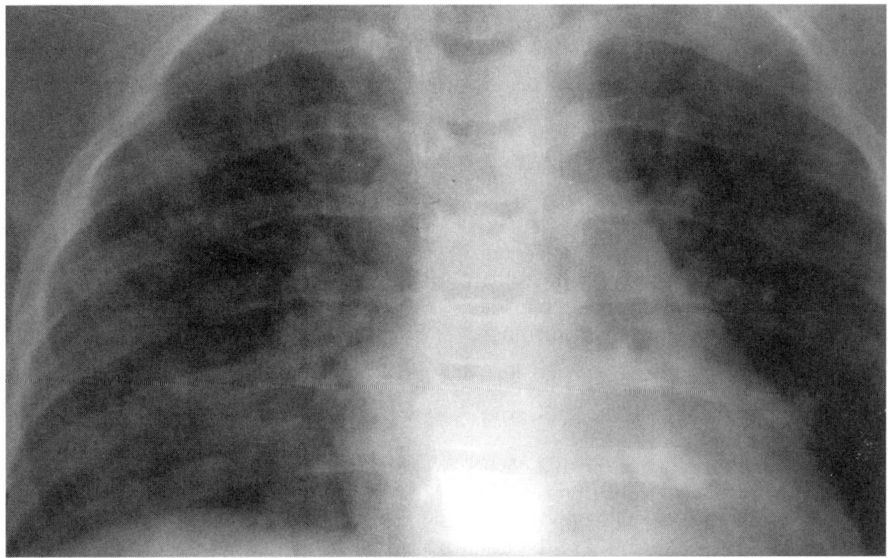

FIGURE 10 Chest radiograph of a patient with primary varicella pneumonia. (Courtesy of Walter Berdon.)

abdomen, and pleurisy may need to be excluded in patients with preeruptive zoster pain or zoster sine herpete.

Complications

From 25 to 50% of persons over the age of 50 who develop zoster may develop protracted pain, or postherpetic neuralgia (PHN), following healing of the rash. Treatment with antiviral drugs has not led to a decrease in the incidence of PHN, although therapy may decrease the duration of pain (44). Pain may persist for months to years and is described as aching, jabbing, burning, or boring. Abnormal sensations may also occur, such as pain after a minimal nonpainful stimulus (allodynia) and severe pain after a mild pain stimulus (hyperalgesia). The precise cause of PHN is unknown. Hypotheses include an aberrant immune response to the virus in the neuron, pain resulting from repair of neuronal damage, and continuing low-level multiplication of virus in the ganglion, with nerve damage from inflammation and hemorrhage. Against the last hypothesis is the observed usual failure of antiviral therapy to relieve PHN. Both the incidence and duration of PHN are directly related to increasing age (50, 99).

Zoster can also involve various cranial nerves. Zoster in the ophthalmic branch of the trigeminal (fifth) nerve may cause dendritic keratitis, anterior uveitis, iridocyclitis with secondary glaucoma, and panophthalmitis (86). Retinitis from VZV is a particular problem for HIV-infected persons (37). Reactivation of VZV involving the maxillary branch results in oral lesions. Motor nerve deficits may also be associated with zoster of the trigeminal nerve. Reactivation in the geniculate ganglion of the seventh (facial) cranial nerve and the eighth (auditory) cranial nerve, termed the Ramsay Hunt syndrome, is associated with facial palsy.

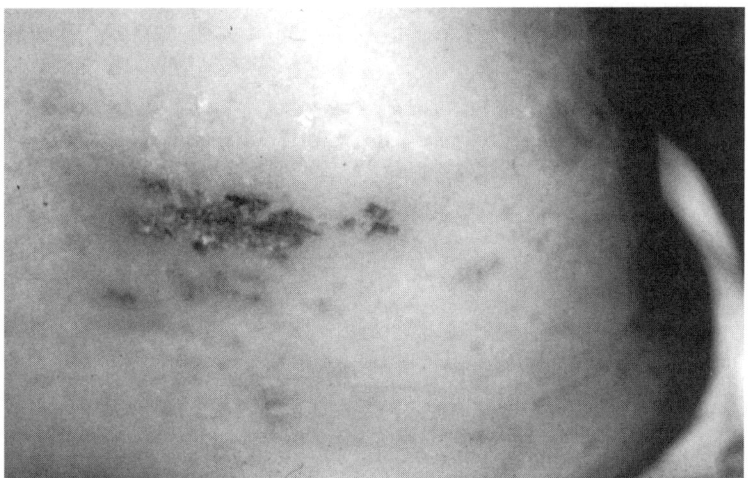

FIGURE 11 Zoster in a 10-year-old boy with underlying leukemia, showing the unilateral lumbar distribution of the skin lesions.

Motor deficits occur in approximately 1% of zoster cases (105). Bladder dysfunction or ileus with intestinal obstruction is an unusual complication of lumbosacral zoster. Partial paralysis of an extremity can also occur after zoster. The prognosis for recovery from these motor deficits is good, although residua may follow in as many as 15% of patients (105). Transverse myelitis is an extremely rare complication with a high mortality rate (50).

Zoster is complicated by clinical encephalitis in an estimated 0.2 to 0.5% of cases. Risk factors include advancing age and cranial nerve involvement. Symptoms, which often occur about a week after onset, include altered state of consciousness, headache, photophobia, and meningismus. The average duration of encephalitic symptoms is about 2 weeks (50, 105).

Granulomatous angiitis resulting in signs and symptoms resembling those of a cerebrovascular hemorrhage or thrombosis is an unusual complication of zoster that occurs particularly in the elderly (50). The central nervous system symptoms characteristically occur on the side opposite the rash, and they may develop months after onset of the rash. There is a high mortality rate, and at autopsy, vascular inflammation with thrombosis and microinfarcts are seen (50).

A syndrome of zoster accompanied by inappropriate secretion of antidiuretic hormone has been described to occur in immunocompromised patients. It may be associated with severe abdominal pain and is associated with a poor prognosis (118, 126).

Visceral zoster with predominant abdominal symptoms, such as pain and even gastrointestinal obstruction, has been described, particularly for immunocompromised patients. Pain may precede the rash by several days, and in some cases, no rash develops (27). Latent VZV in the enteric nervous system of humans has been described, but its consequences as yet are not fully understood (45).

CONGENITAL VARICELLA SYNDROME

Congenital varicella syndrome has a characteristic constellation of developmental abnormalities and was first described in case reports of infants born to mothers who had varicella in early pregnancy. In 1947, LaForet and Lynch described an infant with multiple congenital anomalies after maternal chickenpox during the 8th week of pregnancy (77). The infant had hypoplasia of the right lower extremity with clubfoot and an absence of deep tendon reflexes, cerebral cortical atrophy, cerebellar aplasia, chorioretinitis, torticollis, insufficiency of the anal and vesical sphincters, and scarred cutaneous lesions of the left lower extremity. While initially it was thought that the syndrome occurred after maternal VZV infection in the first trimester of pregnancy, an equal number of reported cases occurred following maternal varicella in the second trimester. Over 100 affected infants have now been reported (38). Almost all of these cases have followed maternal varicella; a few cases following maternal zoster have been described but rarely substantiated (44). If a woman develops varicella in the first or second trimester of pregnancy, it is estimated that there is a 2% chance that her baby will be affected by this syndrome. In the prevaccine era it was estimated that about 40 infants were born annually in the United States with this syndrome (38). Scars of the skin, usually described as cicatricial, are the most prominent stigmata, reported in 70% of cases (Table 3) (38). Other frequent abnormalities include those involving the eyes, such as chorioretinitis, microphthalmia, Horner syndrome, cataract, and nystagmus. Hypoplastic limbs, cortical atrophy and/or mental retardation, and early death are also commonly observed.

LABORATORY DIAGNOSIS

The diagnosis of VZV infection can usually be made clinically, but laboratory diagnosis may be necessary in unusual cases, particularly for vaccinated individuals who develop either possible varicella or zoster. Laboratory diagnosis of active VZV infection is facilitated by the presence of VZV in superficial skin lesions, where it is accessible for testing. Diagnosis is best made by demonstration of VZV DNA or specific viral antigens in vesicular skin lesions. PCR has supplanted viral culture as a diagnostic tool; it has been successfully employed for diagnosis of VZV utilizing skin scrapings, vesicular fluid, respiratory secretions, and CSF (39). PCR can also be used to differentiate between vaccine and wild-type VZV (39) and to demonstrate susceptibility to antiviral drugs (80). VZV antigen may be demonstrated by immunofluorescence (IF), using a commercially available monoclonal antibody to gE of VZV that is conjugated to fluorescein (39). This is a highly sensitive and rapid diagnostic method that can be completed within about an hour and is therefore clinically useful.

The presence of VZV by IF or culture in clinical material obtained from skin or other lesions, or autopsy tissue,

TABLE 3 Clinical data on over 100 reported infants with developmental defects whose mothers had VZV infections (over 95% with varicella) during the first or second trimester of pregnancy between 1947 and 2002[a]

Defect	% of infants with defect
Skin scars	70[b]
Eye abnormalities (chorioretinitis, Horner syndrome/anisocoria, microphthalmia, cataract, nystagmus)	60
Neurologic abnormalities (retardation, seizures, paralysis)	60
Abnormal limb[c] (hypoplasia, equinovarus, abnormal/absent digits)	50
Prematurity, low birth weight	35
Early death	25
Zoster in infancy	20

[a] Modified from reference 38 with permission of Elsevier.
[b] Cicatricial in over 60%.
[c] Fifty percent with hypoplastic limb had mental retardation.

is diagnostic of an active infection because unlike for HSV, there is no known infectious carrier state in asymptomatic individuals. The presence of VZV DNA in specimens such as nervous tissue, however, suggests but does not prove latent VZV infection.

If a culture is to be successfully performed, vesicular fluid should be obtained as early in the course of illness as possible to favor isolation of VZV. Within several days after onset of varicella, vesicular fluid is no longer likely to be infectious, although viable VZV may be present in zoster lesions for a longer period, especially in immunocompromised patients. Isolation of VZV is a relatively slow method, since it takes at least 48 h before the first signs of viral CPE are seen. It is also less sensitive than IF staining, since infectious virus persists for a shorter length of time in vesicles and is more labile than viral antigens. PCR is the most sensitive technique (124). VZV is rarely isolated from CSF, throat, pharyngeal, and conjunctival specimens. Human lung fibroblasts such as WI-38 cells are most frequently utilized to isolate VZV in tissue culture. The Tzanck test provides information only of a nonspecific nature; it has been replaced by more sensitive and specific methods mentioned above.

A number of sensitive serologic tests are available to measure antibodies to VZV. These include the fluorescent antibody to membrane antigen (FAMA) method, latex agglutination, and enzyme-linked immunosorbent assay (39). Antibody to VZV develops within a few days after onset of varicella, persists for many years, and is present before the onset of zoster. VZV infections may be documented by a ≥4-fold rise in VZV antibody titer in acute- and convalescent-phase serum specimens. The presence of specific IgM in one serum specimen suggests recent VZV infection, either varicella or zoster (39). Persistence of VZV antibody in infants beyond 8 months of age is highly suggestive of intrauterine varicella (42). Immunity to varicella is highly likely to be present if a positive titer of antibody (measured by a reliable assay) to VZV is demonstrated with a single serum sample from a child or an adult with no history of disease. Serologic methods, however, particularly commercial enzyme-linked immunosorbent assays, may fail to identify many individuals who have been immunized with live attenuated varicella vaccine (39). While the FAMA assay is the most sensitive test for this purpose, it is not generally available. Latex agglutination is an alternative highly sensitive method and can be recommended for testing of serum obtained after immunization, when performed in an experienced laboratory (43).

The value of serologic procedures for diagnosis of zoster is limited, since heterologous increases in titer of antibody to VZV may occur in patients with HSV infections who have previously had varicella. This phenomenon has been ascribed to antigens common to the two viruses (39).

PREVENTION

VZV is such an infectious agent that general measures are not very useful for prevention of varicella in susceptible individuals. Some protection for hospitalized patients, however, can be accomplished by isolation of patients with moist VZV skin lesions, particularly if they are placed in rooms with negative-pressure ventilation. Hospitalized patients with active VZV infections should be admitted to a private room, and hospital personnel and visitors should wash their hands before and after entering the room and wear masks, gowns, and gloves while in it. Spread of VZV by fomites does not occur. Children with obvious varicella should be excluded from school until the skin lesions are dry. Vaccinated children who develop a few skin vesicles between 2 and 6 weeks after vaccination are unlikely to spread VZV and can attend school if they are otherwise well. Vaccinees with rash 1 to 14 days after immunization are likely to be infected with wild-type VZV. In recently vaccinated patients the development of more than 50 vesicles is highly suggestive of wild-type infection, which unlike the Oka strain is highly transmissible. These patients, therefore, should be excluded from school and if hospitalized should be isolated from other patients.

Prevention of varicella may be accomplished with either active or passive immunization. Varicella-susceptible children at high risk of developing severe chickenpox should be passively immunized if they are closely exposed to someone with either varicella or zoster. Passive immunization usually modifies varicella but may prevent it. Passive immunization may be a life-saving measure for a high-risk susceptible child.

Passive Immunization against Varicella

Varicella-zoster immunoglobulin (VZIG) was approved by the Food and Drug Administration (FDA) for use in 1981. Because the demand for this product decreased sharply after licensure of varicella vaccine in 1995, it is no longer being produced in the United States. It was shown to be most effective when administered up to 3 days after exposure and perhaps helpful for as long as up to 5 days. VZIG has been replaced by a new varicella immunoglobulin product (VariZIG), manufactured in Canada, which is currently available under an investigational new drug application expanded-access protocol (44) (telephone number for requests: 800-843-7477). The dose is 1.25 ml (one vial or 125 U) for each 10 kg of body weight, with a maximum dose of 6 ml (five vials or 625 U) intramuscularly.

The major use of passive immunization is for prevention of severe varicella in persons (usually children) who have been closely exposed to varicella or zoster and are at high risk of developing severe or fatal chickenpox. This includes immunocompromised patients and also newborn infants whose mothers have active varicella at the time of delivery. Passive immunization is customarily readministered to high-risk susceptible persons who are closely reexposed to varicella or zoster 3 weeks following a first exposure for which passive immunization was given.

Infants and children who are listed in the high-risk groups should be considered to be susceptible to varicella if they have no history of having had chickenpox. It is potentially hazardous to withhold passive immunization in an immunocompromised child who has no history of previous clinical varicella based on a positive antibody titer because of the possibility of a false-positive antibody test. Only about 25% of adults with no history of varicella are truly susceptible; therefore, passive immunization should generally be administered to VZV-exposed adults only if they are serologically proven to be susceptible to chickenpox. Presumably, passive immunization is useful for adults, but in contrast to use in children, for whom efficacy has been established, no efficacy studies have been performed in adults. An alternative for healthy varicella-susceptible adults with a known exposure to VZV would be to institute oral antiviral therapy at the very first sign of clinical varicella. The latter approach is considerably less expensive than passive immunization. Susceptible adults who do not develop varicella after a close exposure should be strongly considered for active immunization against varicella (see below).

Patients with HIV infection, especially those with AIDS, are at increased risk of developing severe varicella (44). Their management should be similar to that of other varicella-susceptible immunocompromised children and adults.

Infants whose mothers have active varicella at delivery should receive passive immunization; specifically, this includes infants whose mothers have the onset of chickenpox 5 days or less prior to delivery or within 48 h after delivery. The transplacental route of infection and the immaturity of the immune system probably account for the severity of varicella in these infants (38). The dose of VZIG or VariZIG for newborn infants is 125 U intramuscularly. Attack rates for varicella of up to 50% in infants exposed to mothers who have varicella have been reported, despite administration of VZIG (38). Usually varicella is mild in passively immunized infants; severe varicella after timely administration of VZIG is rare (44). Passively immunized infants should be monitored carefully, but usually these infants can be managed on an outpatient basis even if they develop varicella. They may be given therapeutic oral acyclovir (ACV). The rare passively immunized exposed infant with varicella who develops an extensive skin rash (more than 100 vesicles) or possible pneumonia should be hospitalized and treated with intravenous ACV.

It is unnecessary to passively immunize full-term infants who are exposed to VZV after they are 48 h old. Passive immunization is optional for newborn infants (under 1 week old) if their siblings at home have active varicella, particularly if the mother has no history of chickenpox or if the mother develops varicella. Infants whose mothers have previously had varicella and who are exposed to siblings or others with chickenpox are unlikely to develop severe varicella because they are at least partially protected by transplacental maternal antibody. Infants exposed to mothers with zoster do not require passive immunization because they and their mothers have high titers of antibodies to VZV. Some low-birth-weight infants may have undetectable VZV antibody titers at birth; therefore, it is recommended that newborn infants weighing less than 1,000 g or who are of less than 28 weeks' gestation who are exposed to VZV be passively immunized, even if their mothers had varicella.

Zoster occurs despite humoral immunity to VZV, and patients with zoster have very rapid rises in VZV antibodies; passive immunization is thus not useful to treat or prevent zoster. It is not known whether passive immunization of pregnant varicella-susceptible women who have been closely exposed to VZV will protect the fetus against the congenital varicella syndrome. Passive immunization is potentially useful to prevent severe varicella in varicella-susceptible pregnant women who are exposed to VZV.

Alternatives to VariZIG include intravenous immunoglobulin, 400 mg/kg, and zoster immune plasma (44).

Active Immunization against Varicella

Active immunization against varicella can be successfully accomplished with live attenuated varicella vaccine. This vaccine was developed in Japan in 1974 and was approved by the FDA in the United States in March 1995 for universal administration to healthy children and adults who are susceptible to varicella (119). The vaccine is well tolerated and safe (44). The major complication following vaccination of healthy persons is a vaccine-associated rash occurring in 5% of vaccinees about 1 month later (44). These rashes are usually extremely mild in healthy vaccinees, with an average of five skin lesions that are generalized and/or at the injection site. The risk of transmission of Oka vaccine virus to others is present only while the vaccinee has rash, is exceedingly rare (one transmission per 10 million vaccinees), and is much lower than the rate of transmission after exposure to wild-type VZV (44). The risk to anyone from wild-type VZV is greater than the risk from vaccine-type VZV. Therefore, it is recommended to immunize hospital workers and individuals whose family members are immunocompromised or pregnant, especially if they are susceptible to varicella (15). Highly immunocompromised individuals inadvertently closely exposed to a vaccinee with rash can be passively immunized if they are susceptible to varicella, although this is not considered mandatory.

Vaccinated individuals who develop a rash within 2 to 3 weeks after immunization may have been exposed to wild-type VZV prior to being vaccinated and are likely to have a rash caused by the wild-type virus (44). This should especially be suspected if many lesions occur and are accompanied by systemic symptoms, which are unlikely to be caused by the vaccine-type virus. It is extremely helpful in trying to evaluate such a situation to utilize PCR to differentiate between wild-type and vaccine-type VZV (44).

Live attenuated varicella vaccine is highly protective against chickenpox in healthy and immunocompromised children and in healthy adults. Not all vaccinees, however, are completely protected, particularly after one dose of vaccine (44). Roughly 15% of children may manifest a modified illness, referred to as breakthrough varicella, months to years after receipt of one dose. Varicella vaccine has, however, been over 95% effective in preventing severe varicella (44). Varicella vaccine is less effective in adults than in children; even after two doses of vaccine, only 70% of adults achieve complete protection from varicella following a close exposure to VZV, although the remainder usually have partial protection (4). In contrast, 85% of immunized healthy children are protected after only one dose of vaccine (44, 125). Breakthrough varicella is almost always a modified illness, with fewer than 50 skin lesions and minimal systemic signs. In one study, about two-thirds of cases of breakthrough varicella were classified as mild (<50 skin lesions) (112). Very rarely do vaccinated children who presumably have not responded to vaccine develop severe varicella and succumb (44).

In order to improve protection against breakthrough varicella in healthy child vaccinees, a second routine dose of vaccine was recommended by the Centers for Disease Control and Prevention (CDC) and the American Academy of Pediatrics in June 2006 (44). The second dose may be administered at any time after 1 month following the first dose, but an interval of at least 3 months is preferred. The second dose may be given either as monovalent vaccine or as measles-mumps-rubella-varicella (MMRV) vaccine. When the latter vaccine becomes widely available (16), it may become the preferred vaccine for two doses of all four viral vaccines. In a small efficacy study of monovalent vaccine, two doses of varicella vaccine were somewhat more protective against breakthrough chickenpox than one dose (76). Anamnestic humoral and cellular immune responses to VZV after two doses of vaccine given months or years apart have been reported in several studies (44).

The observation of breakthrough varicella in about 15% of children following one dose of vaccine prompted analyses of whether this phenomenon could be due to primary or secondary immune failure. A result of either or both could be an accumulation of young adults who are susceptible to varicella a decade or so after vaccination. A study of 148 children indicated that the rate of primary vaccine failure was 24%, based on FAMA testing for VZV antibodies in the first 4 months after vaccination (94). An epidemiological study of children in Antelope Valley, CA, indicated that there was an increase in breakthrough varicella with time (over a 9-year period), with increasing severity of breakthrough cases (18). These data were interpreted to represent immunity waning with time (secondary vaccine failure). In contrast, however, a case control study did not reveal any decrease in immunity in years 2 to 8 after immunization (125). The issue of whether waning immunity occurs after receipt of one dose of vaccine is therefore controversial and needs verification. In any case, a recommended second dose of vaccine for all children addresses the possibility of both primary and secondary vaccine failure following one dose.

Varicella vaccine has been used effectively to protect immunocompromised children. It is no longer recommended that leukemic children be vaccinated, due to development of vaccine-associated rash in roughly 50%, often requiring treatment with ACV (47). In contrast, children with HIV infection whose immune function remains relatively intact (more than 15% CD4 lymphocytes) have tolerated varicella vaccine as well as healthy children (81, 82). Two doses at least 1 month apart are recommended for HIV-infected children. Preliminary data indicate that vaccination protects them from varicella and zoster (M. Son, E. Shapiro, P. LaRussa, N. Neu, D. Michalik, M. Meglin, W. Bitar, A. Jurgrou, P. Flynn, and A. Gershon, unpublished data). Vaccination of children prior to renal transplantation has also been highly successful in preventing severe varicella and also zoster (12). Small studies suggest that vaccination after liver transplantation may be safely accomplished (131).

Vaccinated individuals are at risk of developing zoster, but the incidence appears to be lower after vaccination than after natural infection (Fig. 12). Possibly this is because after vaccination there is usually no viremia, the skin is not usually infected, and there is less chance of developing latent infection (57). Children who do develop zoster have usually experienced a rash due to wild-type or vaccine-type VZV and presumably have developed latent infection from skin infection with the virus. This phenomenon has been observed in several studies involving immunocompromised patients (44). A small study of healthy adult vaccinees also suggests similar protection against zoster (55).

Significant progress has been made in development of a vaccine to prevent zoster in the elderly. Interest in this approach was generated by the recognition of immunologic boosting that accompanies reexposure to VZV and the loss of VZV CMI prior to developing zoster (44). In this case, the rationale behind prevention of zoster with vaccination is to minimize reactivation by increasing CMI to VZV in persons who have latent infection.

Zoster can be prevented by immunizing elderly individuals with VZV latent infection due to a prior attack of

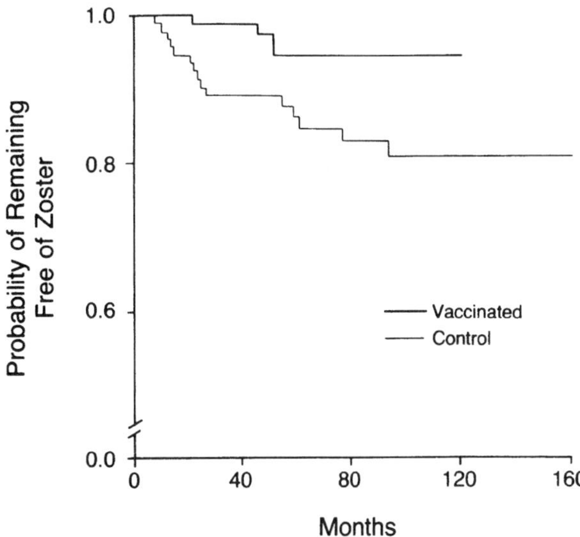

FIGURE 12 Kaplan-Meier product limit analysis of the probability of remaining free of zoster in 96 children with leukemia who had naturally acquired varicella before or after the diagnosis of leukemia. (Reprinted from reference 57 with permission of the Massachusetts Medical Society. All rights reserved.)

varicella. This was shown in a double-blind placebo-controlled study involving 38,546 healthy adults over the age of 60 years, which was conducted from 1999 to 2004 (99). The dose of vaccine used, marketed as Zostavax (Merck and Co.), contains about 14 times the dose of live virus that is present in monovalent varicella vaccine (Varivax) in the United States (not less than 19,400 PFU per 0.65-ml dose). The vaccine proved to be extremely safe; adverse events were similar in vaccinees and placebo recipients, with the exception of transient reactions such as rash or redness at the injection site in 43% of vaccinees, compared to 17% in controls. Although the development of zoster was not the original primary endpoint of this study, a decrease in incidence of zoster of 51% was found in vaccinees compared to placebo recipients. There was better protective efficacy against zoster in vaccinees aged 60 to 69 years (64%) than in vaccinees aged 70 to 79 years (41%). In the original analysis, when development of significant pain, not zoster itself, was the primary endpoint, there was a 61% reduction of significant pain in vaccinees (some vaccinees had mild zoster with only minor or no pain). Vaccination was also highly effective in prevention of PHN, especially in patients aged 70 to 79 years (55% effectiveness). The vaccine against zoster is an important clinical advance, although many questions remain, such as the best age at which to immunize, the duration of the effectiveness of the vaccine, and whether booster doses will be necessary.

Drug Prophylaxis

The antiviral drug ACV has been examined for prevention of varicella in exposed persons (64). Despite apparent prevention of clinical varicella in almost all cases in such studies, the approach is not recommended in countries where passive and active immunization is available. Whether there is long-term maintenance of immunity after prophylactic ACV is not known. The CDC recommends postexposure vaccination for healthy nonpregnant varicella-susceptible individuals who have been exposed to VZV (44).

Long-term ACV therapy as a preventive against development of zoster in patients who have undergone bone marrow transplantation is not routinely recommended, mainly because rebound infections often occur when ACV is stopped and because of concern about development of resistant VZV (14).

TREATMENT

Specific antiviral therapy became available in the mid-1970s. The first drugs used were relatively ineffectual and also toxic. The modern age arrived with the introduction of ACV, which as its triphosphate is an inhibitor of DNA polymerase and a DNA chain terminator that is highly effective against VZV (135). Current recommendations for antiviral therapy for VZV are summarized below, and for additional details, the reader is referred to chapter 12.

ACV is extremely useful for therapy of VZV infections. Patients with severe or potentially severe infections should be treated with the intravenous formulation at dosages of 30 mg/kg/day for adults and adolescents and 1,500 mg/m^2/day for children (both given in three divided doses). Orally administered ACV is less reliable for immunocompromised patients because only about 20% of this formulation is absorbed from the gastrointestinal tract. ACV is excreted by the kidneys; patients with creatinine clearances of less than 50 ml/min/1.73 m^2 should receive one-half to one-third of this dosage. Intravenous ACV is infused over at least 1 h, with maintenance fluids given both before and during the infusion. Adequate hydration is important to prevent precipitation of the drug in the renal tubules, which can result in increases in serum creatinine levels. This complication of ACV has also been associated with bolus administration. Other adverse effects of ACV include phlebitis, rash, nausea, and neurologic manifestations such as headache and tremor. In general, however, ACV is extremely well tolerated.

Because ACV has little associated toxicity, and therapy within 2 to 3 days of onset has been associated with the best outcomes, it is recommended that early therapy be instituted for patients at high risk of developing severe VZV infections, such as leukemic children, in order to prevent dissemination of the virus, as well as patients with ophthalmic zoster (134). Therapy with ACV not only is potentially lifesaving in immunocompromised patients with VZV infections but also it prevents considerable morbidity. In zoster patients, use of intravenous ACV is associated with more rapid healing of skin lesions and resolution of acute pain than if no specific treatment is given (Table 4) (134).

Orally administered ACV may be used for treatment of varicella and zoster in otherwise healthy adults and children, although most of these infections are self-limited. Dosages used are 4 g/day (in five divided doses) for adults and 80 mg/kg/day (in four divided doses) for children. Double-blind placebo-controlled studies with healthy children and adolescents given 80 mg of ACV or placebo per kg a day for 5 days, beginning within 24 h of onset of the varicella rash, revealed that the number of chickenpox skin lesions was reduced by ACV therapy. There was, however, only about 1 day less of fever, and children who were treated with ACV did not return to school any more rapidly than those who received placebo, reflecting a modest benefit conferred by ACV therapy. Therapy with oral ACV did not prevent complications or prevent spread of VZV (30). The therapeutic effect of oral ACV is no more pronounced in adults with varicella than in children (127). Due to the possibility of a therapeutic effect with the use of a very safe drug, however, it has become customary to treat most immunocompetent adolescents and adults who develop varicella with ACV or a related compound.

For zoster, drug efficacy has been shown even if 3 days have elapsed since onset, but the earlier ACV is begun, the greater the therapeutic effect. There is some indication that early ACV therapy may decrease acute pain associated with zoster (65). Therefore, it is recommended that elderly patients with early zoster be given prompt antiviral therapy

TABLE 4 Drugs for treatment of VZV infections[a]

Drug	Dose in treatment of:		Comments
	Varicella	Zoster	
Acyclovir	20 mg/kg QID p.o.[b] for 5 days, 500 mg/m^2 every 8 h i.v.	800 mg 5 times/day p.o. (adult dose) for 7–10 days, 10 mg/kg every 8 h i.v.	i.v. drug of choice for immunocompromised patients; p.o. administration shortens course of varicella by ca. 1 day in children and decreases acute pain of zoster
Valacyclovir (p.o.)	NI	1 g TID for 7 days (adult dose)	High oral bioavailability; decreases ZAP duration; 0.5% of immunocompromised patients develop hemolytic-uremic-like syndrome
Famciclovir (p.o.)	NI	500 mg TID for 7 days (adult dose)	High oral availability; decreases ZAP duration
Foscarnet	180 mg/kg/day in two divided doses (adjust for renal function) i.v.[c]	180 mg/kg/day in two divided doses (adjust for renal function) i.v.[c]	For ACV-resistant VZV infection i.v.[c]

[a] QID, four times a day; TID, three times a day; p.o., orally; i.v., intravenously; NI, not indicated because of lack of supporting data; ZAP, zoster-associated pain (includes PHN).

[b] Maximum per day, 800 mg.

[c] No FDA approval for this indication but may be useful for different patients with drug-resistant VZV.

because the older the patient with this disease, the more likely it is that pain will be a future problem. A recent study showed no difference in outcome in older patients with zoster whether they were treated with ACV for 7 or 21 days (138). In this study, recovery was no more rapid, nor was PHN less likely to occur, if a 3-week course of tapering prednisolone (beginning at 40 mg/day) was given along with ACV.

A newer drug, famciclovir (FCV), is a prodrug of the antiviral penciclovir, to which it is rapidly converted in the body after oral administration. Penciclovir has an antiviral action similar to that of ACV. FCV was approved by the FDA in 1994 for oral therapy of zoster in adults. An advantage of FCV over ACV is that FCV is given three times a day (500 mg per dose) rather than five times a day, which may lead to better patient compliance. One study suggests that FCV given to elderly patients with zoster early in the course of infection decreases the duration of PHN but not its incidence (123). There are no data as to whether varicella may be successfully treated with FCV, nor are there any published data on use of FCV in immunocompromised patients or in children.

The prodrug of ACV, valacyclovir, which is also given orally, reaches levels in blood that are about four times higher than ACV levels after oral administration. Valacyclovir is approved for use in the United States, and one study suggested that it may be superior to ACV in immunocompetent patients with zoster (10). Valacyclovir may not be as effective as intravenous ACV, however, in highly immunocompromised adults, particularly those with AIDS with severe VZV infections (11). The dosage of valacyclovir for immunocompetent adolescents and adults with zoster is 1 g three times a day, orally. As for all antivirals, early therapy (within 3 days of onset of rash) is required for effective results.

Foscarnet is useful for treating VZV infections due to viruses that are resistant to ACV and FCV and was approved by the FDA for this purpose. Foscarnet acts by directly inhibiting the DNA polymerase of VZV (107). Intravenous foscarnet has been used at a dosage of 40 mg/kg every 8 h for HSV infections and 90 to 120 mg/kg every 8 h for retinitis caused by cytomegalovirus in AIDS patients. Its main toxicity is renal. VZV retinitis is a potentially very serious, fortunately rare form of infection. Some forms require treatment with combination antiviral therapy including foscarnet and ganciclovir; consultation with an experienced ophthalmologist is strongly recommended for these patients.

Of concern about the potential widespread use of ACV is that drug resistance may develop and that resistant VZV may spread to others. At present, resistance is less of a problem with VZV than with HSV. As for HSV, however, VZV resistant to ACV has been reported, most commonly for patients with underlying AIDS (68). Rarely, the Oka vaccine strain of VZV has developed resistance to ACV (80).

REFERENCES

1. **Abendroth, A., and A. Arvin.** 2001. Immune evasion mechanisms of varicella-zoster virus. *Arch. Virol. Suppl.* **17:**99–107.
2. **Abendroth, A., I. Lin, B. Slobedman, H. Ploegh, and A. M. Arvin.** 2001. Varicella-zoster virus retains major histocompatibility complex class I proteins in the Golgi compartment of infected cells. *J. Virol.* **75:**4878–4888.
3. **Abendroth, A., B. Slobedman, E. Lee, E. Mellins, M. Wallace, and A. M. Arvin.** 2000. Modulation of major histocompatibility class II protein expression by varicella-zoster virus. *J. Virol.* **74:**1900–1907.
4. **Ampofo, K., L. Saiman, P. LaRussa, S. Steinberg, P. Annunziato, and A. Gershon.** 2002. Persistence of immunity to live attenuated varicella vaccine in healthy adults. *Clin. Infect. Dis.* **34:**774–779.
5. **Aronson, J., G. McSherry, L. Hoyt, M. Boland, J. Oleske, E. Connor, D. Persaud, W. Borkowsky, K. Krasinski, S. Bakshi, J. Pitt, and A. Gershon.** 1992. Varicella in children with HIV infection. *Pediatr. Infect. Dis. J.* **11:**1004–1008.
6. **Arvin, A. M.** 1992. Cell-mediated immunity to varicella-zoster virus. *J. Infect. Dis.* **166:**S35–S41.
7. **Asano, Y., N. Itakura, Y. Hiroishi, S. Hirose, T. Nagai, T. Ozaki, T. Yazaki, Y. Yamanishi, and M. Takahashi.** 1985. Viremia is present in incubation period in nonimmunocompromised children with varicella. *J. Pediatr.* **106:**69–71.
8. **Asano, Y., S. Suga, T. Yoshikawa, H. Kobayashi, T. Yazaki, M. Shibata, K. Tsuzuki, and S. Ito.** 1994. Experience and reason: twenty year follow up of protective immunity of the Oka live varicella vaccine. *Pediatrics* **94:**524–526.
9. **Balfour, H. H.** 1988. Varicella zoster virus infections in immunocompromised hosts. A review of the natural history and management. *Am. J. Med.* **85**(2A)**:**68–73.
10. **Beutner, K. R., D. J. Friedman, C. Forszpaniak, P. L. Andersen, and M. J. Wood.** 1995. Valaciclovir compared with acyclovir for improved therapy for herpes zoster in immunocompetent adults. *Antimicrob. Agents Chemother.* **39:**1546–1553.
11. **Breton, G., M. A. Bouldouyre, A. Gervais, X. Duval, P. Longuet, C. Leport, and J. L. Vildé.** 2004. Failure of valacyclovir for herpes zoster in a moderately immunocompromised HIV-infected patient. *AIDS Patient Care STDS* **18:**255–257.
12. **Broyer, M., M. T. Tete, G. Guest, M. F. Gagnadoux, and C. Rouzioux.** 1997. Varicella and zoster in children after kidney transplantation: long term results of vaccination. *Pediatrics* **99:**35–39.
13. **Brunell, P. A.** 1989. Transmission of chickenpox in a school setting prior to the observed exanthem. *Am. J. Dis. Child.* **143:**1451–1452.
14. **Centers for Disease Control and Prevention.** 2000. Guidelines for preventing opportunistic infections among hematopoietic stem cell transplant recipients. *Morb. Mort. Wkly. Rep.* **49:**1–125.
15. **Centers for Disease Control and Prevention.** 2007. Prevention of varicella. *Morb. Mort. Wkly. Rep.* **56:**1–55.
16. **Centers for Disease Control and Prevention.** 2007. Supply of vaccines containing varicella-zoster virus. *Morb. Mortal. Wkly. Rep.* **56:**146–147.
17. **Centers for Disease Control and Prevention.** 2006. Varicella outbreak among primary school students—Beijing, China, 2004. *Morb. Mortal. Wkly. Rep.* **55:**39–43.
18. **Chaves, S. S., P. Haber, K. Walton, R. P. Wise, H. S. Izureta, O. S. Schmid, and J. F. Seward.** 2008. Safety of varicella vaccine after licensure in the United States: experience from reports to the Vaccine Adverse Event Reporting System, 1995–2005. *J. Infect. Dis.* **197**(Suppl. 2)**:**S170–S177.
19. **Chen, J., A. Gershon, S. J. Silverstein, Z. S. Li, O. Lungu, and M. D. Gershon.** 2003. Latent and lytic infection of isolated guinea pig enteric and dorsal root ganglia by varicella zoster virus. *J. Med. Virol.* **70:**S71–S78.
20. Reference deleted.

21. **Chen, J. J., Z. Zhu, A. A. Gershon, and M. D. Gershon.** 2004. Mannose 6-phosphate receptor dependence of varicella zoster virus infection in vitro and in the epidermis during varicella and zoster. *Cell* **119:**915–926.
22. **Choo, P. W., J. G. Donahue, J. E. Manson, and R. Platt.** 1995. The epidemiology of varicella and its complications. *J. Infect. Dis.* **172:**706–712.
23. **Cohen, J. I., T. Krogmann, J. P. Ross, L. Pesnicak, and E. A. Prikhod'ko.** 2005. Varicella-zoster virus ORF4 latency-associated protein is important for establishment of latency. *J. Virol.* **79:**6969–6975.
24. **Cohrs, R. J., M. Barbour, and D. H. Gilden.** 1996. Varicella-zoster virus (VZV) transcription during latency in human ganglia: detection of transcripts to genes 21, 29, 62, and 63 in a cDNA library enriched for VZV RNA. *J. Virol.* **70:**2789–2796.
25. **Cohrs, R. J., and D. H. Gilden.** 2003. Varicella zoster virus transcription in latently-infected human ganglia. *Anticancer Res.* **23:**2063–2069.
26. **Cohrs, R. J., D. H. Gilden, P. R. Kinchington, E. Grinfeld, and P. G. Kennedy.** 2003. Varicella-zoster virus gene 66 transcription and translation in latently infected human ganglia. *J. Virol.* **77:**6660–6665.
27. **David, D. S., B. R. Tegtmeier, M. R. O'Donnell, I. B. Paz, and T. M. McCarrty.** 1998. Visceral varicella-zoster after bone marrow transplantation: report of a case series and review of the literature. *Am. J. Gasteroenterol.* **93:** 810–813.
28. **Donahue, J. G., P. W. Choo, J. E. Manson, and R. Platt.** 1995. The incidence of herpes zoster. *Arch. Intern. Med.* **155:**1605–1609.
29. **Dumas, A. H., J. L. M. C. Geelen, M. W. Weststrate, P. Werthein, and J. van der Noordaa.** 1981. XbaI, PstI, and BglII restriction enzyme maps of the two orientations of the varicella-zoster virus genome. *J. Virol.* **39:**390–400.
30. **Dunkel, L., A. Arvin, R. Whitley, H. Rotbart, H. Feder, S. Feldman, A. Gershon, M. Levy, G. Hayden, P. McGuirt, J. Harris, and H. Balfour.** 1991. A controlled trial of oral acyclovir for chickenpox in normal children. *N. Engl. J. Med.* **325:**1539–1544.
31. **Edwards, T. S.** 1989. Ophthalmic complications from varicella. *J. Pediatr. Ophthalmol.* **965:**37–44.
32. **Esiri, M., and A. Tomlinson.** 1972. Herpes zoster: demonstration of virus in trigeminal nerve and ganglion by immunofluorescence and electron microscopy. *J. Neurol. Sci.* **15:**35–48.
33. **Feldman, S., S. Chaudhary, M. Ossi, and E. Epp.** 1977. A viremic phase for herpes zoster in children with cancer. *J. Pediatr.* **91:**597–600.
34. **Feldman, S., W. Hughes, and C. Daniel.** 1975. Varicella in children with cancer: 77 cases. *Pediatrics* **80:**388–397.
35. **Fleisher, G., W. Henry, M. McSorley, A. Arbeter, and S. Plotkin.** 1981. Life-threatening complications of varicella. *Am. J. Dis. Child.* **135:**896–899.
36. **Forghani, B., K. W. Dupuis, and N. Schmidt.** 1990. Epitopes functional in neutralization of varicella-zoster virus. *J. Clin. Microbiol.* **28:**2500–2506.
37. **Franco-Paredes, C., T. Bellehemeur, A. Merchant, P. Sanghi, C. DiazGranados, and D. Rimland.** 2002. Aseptic meningitis and optic neuritis preceding varicella-zoster progressive outer retinal necrosis in a patient with AIDS. *AIDS* **16:**1045–1049.
38. **Gershon, A.** 2006. Chickenpox, measles, and mumps, p. 693–737. *In* J. Remington and J. O. Klein (ed.), *Infections of the Fetus and Newborn Infant*, 6th ed. Saunders, Philadelphia, PA.
39. **Gershon, A., J. Chen, P. LaRussa, and S. Steinberg.** 2007. Varicella-zoster virus, p. 1537–1548. *In* P. R. Murray, E. J. Baron, J. H. Jorgensen, M. L. Landry, and M. A. Pfaller (ed.), *Manual of Clinical Microbiology*, 9th ed. ASM Press, Washington, DC.
40. **Gershon, A., P. LaRussa, and S. Steinberg.** 1996. Varicella vaccine: use in immunocompromised patients. *Infect. Dis. Clin. N. Am.* **10:**583–594.
41. **Gershon, A., N. Mervish, P. LaRussa, S. Steinberg, S.-H. Lo, D. Hodes, S. Fikrig, V. Bonagura, and S. Bakshi.** 1997. Varicella-zoster virus infection in children with underlying HIV infection. *J. Infect. Dis.* **176:**1496–1500.
42. **Gershon, A., R. Raker, S. Steinberg, B. Topf-Oldstein, and L. Drusin.** 1976. Antibody to varicella-zoster virus in parturient women and their offspring during the first year of life. *Pediatrics* **58:**692–696.
43. **Gershon, A., S. Steinberg, and P. LaRussa.** 1994. Detection of antibodies to varicella-zoster virus by latex agglutination. *Clin. Diagn. Virol.* **2:**271–277.
44. **Gershon, A., M. Takahashi, and J. Seward.** Varicella vaccine. *In* S. Plotkin and W. Orenstein (ed.), *Vaccines*, 5th ed., in press. Saunders, Philadelphia, PA.
45. **Gershon, A. A., J. Chen, and M. D. Gershon.** 2008. A model of lytic, latent, and reactivating VZV in isolated enteric neurons. *J. Infect. Dis.* **197**(Suppl. 2)**:**S61–S65.
46. **Gershon, A. A., D. L. Sherman, Z. Zhu, C. A. Gabel, R. T. Ambron, and M. D. Gershon.** 1994. Intracellular transport of newly synthesized varicella-zoster virus: final envelopment in the *trans*-Golgi network. *J. Virol.* **68:** 6372–6390.
47. **Gershon, A. A., S. Steinberg, L. Gelb, and NIAID Collaborative Varicella Vaccine Study Group.** 1984. Live attenuated varicella vaccine: efficacy for children with leukemia in remission. *JAMA* **252:**355–362.
48. **Gershon, A. A., S. Steinberg, and NIAID Collaborative Varicella Vaccine Study Group.** 1990. Live attenuated varicella vaccine: protection in healthy adults in comparison to leukemic children. *J. Infect. Dis.* **161:**661–666.
49. **Gilden, D., A. Dueland, M. Devlin, R. Mahlingham, and R. Cohrs.** 1992. Varicella-zoster virus reactivation without rash. *J. Infect. Dis.* **166:**S30–S34.
50. **Gilden, D. H., B. K. Kleinschmidt-DeMasters, J. J. LaGuardia, R. Mahalingam, and R. J. Cohrs.** 2000. Neurologic complications of the reactivation of varicella-zoster virus. *N. Engl. J. Med.* **342:**635–645.
51. **Gold, E.** 1966. Serologic and virus-isolation studies of patients with varicella or herpes zoster infection. *N. Engl. J. Med.* **274:**181–185.
52. **Grose, C.** 1990. Glycoproteins encoded by varicella-zoster virus: biosynthesis, phosphorylation, and intracellular trafficking. *Annu. Rev. Microbiol.* **44:**59–80.
53. **Grose, C., S. Tyler, G. Peters, J. Hiebert, G. M. Stephens, W. T. Ruyechan, W. Jackson, J. Storlie, and G. A. Tipples.** 2004. Complete DNA sequence analyses of the first two varicella-zoster virus glycoprotein E (D150N) mutant viruses found in North America: evolution of genotypes with an accelerated cell spread phenotype. *J. Virol.* **78:**6799–6807.
54. **Grose, C. H.** 1981. Variation on a theme by Fenner. *Pediatrics* **68:**735–737.
55. **Hambleton, S., G. Shapiro, P. LaRussa, S. P. Steinberg, and A. A. Gershon.** 2008. Zoster in adults who received varicella vaccine. *J. Infect. Dis.* **197**(Suppl. 2)**:**S196–S199.
56. **Hambleton, S., S. P. Steinberg, M. D. Gershon, and A. A. Gershon.** 2007. Cholesterol dependence of varicella-zoster virion entry into target cells. *J. Virol.* **81:** 7548–7558.
57. **Hardy, I. B., A. Gershon, S. Steinberg, P. LaRussa, et al.** 1991. The incidence of zoster after immunization with

live attenuated varicella vaccine. A study in children with leukemia. *N. Engl. J. Med.* **325:**1545–1550.

58. **Harger, J. H., J. M. Ernest, G. R. Thurnau, A. Moawad, V. Momirova, M. B. Landon, R. Paul, M. Miodovnik, M. Dombrowski, B. Sibai, and P. Van Dorsten.** 2002. Risk factors and outcome of varicella-zoster virus pneumonia in pregnant women. *J. Infect. Dis.* **185:**422–427.
59. **Hay, J., and W. T. Ruyechan.** 1994. Varicella-zoster virus: a different kind of herpesvirus latency? *Semin. Virol.* **5:**241–248.
60. **Hayward, A. R.** 2001. In vitro measurement of human T cell responses to varicella zoster virus antigen. *Arch. Virol. Suppl.* **17:**143–149.
61. **Heineman, T. C., and S. L. Hall.** 2002. Role of the varicella-zoster virus gB cytoplasmic domain in gB transport and viral egress. *J. Virol.* **76:**591–599.
62. **Hood, C., A. L. Cunningham, B. Slobedman, A. M. Arvin, M. H. Sommer, P. R. Kinchington, and A. Abendroth.** 2006. Varicella-zoster virus ORF63 inhibits apoptosis of primary human neurons. *J. Virol.* **80:**1025–1031.
63. **Hope-Simpson, R. E.** 1965. The nature of herpes zoster: a long term study and a new hypothesis. *Proc. R. Soc. Med.* **58:**9–20.
64. **Huang, Y.-C., T.-Y. Lin, and C.-H. Chiu.** 1995. Acyclovir prophylaxis of varicella after household exposure. *Pediatr. Infect. Dis. J.* **14:**152–154.
65. **Huff, C., B. Bean, H. Balfour, O. Laskin, J. Connor, L. Corey, Y. Bryson, and P. McGuirt.** 1988. Therapy of herpes zoster with oral acyclovir. *Am. J. Med.* **85:**84–89.
66. **Ihara, T., M. Ito, and S. E. Starr.** 1986. Human lymphocyte, monocyte and polymorphonuclear leucocyte mediated antibody-dependent cellular cytotoxicity against varicella-zoster virus-infected targets. *Clin. Exp. Immunol.* **63:**179–187.
67. **Ilias, A., E. Galanakis, M. Raissaki, and M. Kalmanti.** 2006. Childhood encephalitis in Crete, Greece. *J. Child Neurol.* **21:**910–912.
68. **Jacobson, M. A., T. G. Berger, and S. Fikrig.** 1990. Acyclovir-resistant varicella-zoster virus infection after chronic oral acyclovir therapy in patients with the acquired immunodeficiency syndrome. *Ann. Intern. Med.* **112:**187–191.
69. **Kalman, C. M., and O. L. Laskin.** 1986. Herpes zoster and zosteriform herpes simplex virus infections in immunocompetent adults. *Am. J. Med.* **81:**775–778.
70. **Kennedy, P. G.** 2002. Key issues in varicella-zoster virus latency. *J. Neurovirol.* **8**(Suppl. 2)**:**80–84.
71. **Kennedy, P. G.** 2002. Varicella-zoster virus latency in human ganglia. *Rev. Med. Virol.* **12:**327–334.
72. **Kennedy, P. G. E., E. Grinfeld, and J. E. Bell.** 2000. Varicella-zoster virus gene expression in latently infected and explanted human ganglia. *J. Virol.* **74:**11893–11898.
73. **Kinchington, P. R., D. Bookey, and S. E. Turse.** 1995. The transcriptional regulatory proteins encoded by varicella-zoster virus open reading frames (ORFs) 4 and 63, but not ORF 61, are associated with purified virus particles. *J. Virol.* **69:**4274–4282.
74. **Kinchington, P. R., K. Fite, and S. E. Turse.** 2000. Nuclear accumulation of IE62, the varicella-zoster virus (VZV) major transcriptional regulatory protein, is inhibited by phosphorylation mediated by the VZV open reading frame 66 protein kinase. *J. Virol.* **74:**2265–2277.
75. **Ku, C. C., J. Besser, A. Abendroth, C. Grose, and A. M. Arvin.** 2005. Varicella-zoster virus pathogenesis and immunobiology: new concepts emerging from investigations with the SCIDhu mouse model. *J. Virol.* **79:** 2651–2658.
76. **Kuter, B., H. Matthews, H. Shinefield, S. Black, P. Dennehy, B. Watson, K. Reisinger, L. L. Kim, L. Lupinacci, J. Hartzel, and I. Chan.** 2004. Ten year follow-up of healthy children who received one or two injections of varicella vaccine. *Pediatr. Infect. Dis. J.* **23:**132–137.
77. **LaForet, E. G., and L. L. Lynch.** 1947. Multiple congenital defects following maternal varicella. *N. Engl. J. Med.* **236:**534–537.
78. **LaRussa, P., S. Steinberg, M. D. Seeman, and A. A. Gershon.** 1985. Determination of immunity to varicella by means of an intradermal skin test. *J. Infect. Dis.* **152:** 869–875.
79. **LaRussa, P. L., A. A. Gershon, S. Steinberg, and S. Chartrand.** 1990. Antibodies to varicella-zoster virus glycoproteins I, II, and III in leukemic and healthy children. *J. Infect. Dis.* **162:**627–633.
80. **Levin, M. J., K. M. Dahl, A. Weinberg, R. Giller, and A. Patel.** 2003. Development of resistance to acyclovir during chronic Oka strain varicella-zoster virus infection in an immunocompromised child. *J. Infect. Dis.* **188:**954–959.
81. **Levin, M. J., A. A. Gershon, A. Weinberg, S. Blanchard, B. Nowak, P. Palumbo, and C. Y. Chan.** 2001. Immunization of HIV-infected children with varicella vaccine. *J. Pediatr.* **139:**305–310.
82. **Levin, M. J., A. A. Gershon, A. Weinberg, L. Y. Song, T. Fentin, and B. Nowak.** 2006. Administration of live varicella vaccine to HIV-infected children with current or past significant depression of CD4(+) T cells. *J. Infect. Dis.* **194:**247–255.
83. **Levin, M. J., J. G. Smith, R. M. Kaufhold, D. Barber, A. R. Hayward, C. Y. Chan, I. S. Chan, D. J. Li, W. Wang, P. M. Keller, A. Shaw, J. L. Silber, K. Schlienger, I. Chalikonda, S. J. Vessey, and M. J. Caulfield.** 2003. Decline in varicella-zoster virus (VZV)-specific cell-mediated immunity with increasing age and boosting with a high-hose VZV vaccine. *J. Infect. Dis.* **188:**1336–1344.
84. **Li, Q., M. A. Ali, and J. I. Cohen.** 2006. Insulin degrading enzyme is a cellular receptor mediating varicella-zoster virus infection and cell-to-cell spread. *Cell* **127:** 305–316.
85. **Li, Q., T. Krogmann, M. A. Ali, W.-J. Tang, and J. I. Cohen.** 2007. The amino terminus of varicella-zoster virus (VZV) glycoprotein E is required for binding to insulin-degrading enzyme, a VZV receptor. *J. Virol.* **81:** 8525–8532.
86. **Liesegang, T.** 1991. Diagnosis and therapy of herpes zoster ophthalmicus. *Ophthalmology* **98:**1216–1229.
87. **Loparev, V. N., K. McCaustland, B. Holloway, P. R. Krause, M. Takayama, and S. Schmid.** 2000. Rapid genotyping of varicella-zoster virus vaccine and wild type strains with fluorophore-labeled hybridization probes. *J. Clin. Microbiol.* **38:**4315–4319.
88. **Lungu, O., P. Annunziato, A. Gershon, S. Stegatis, D. Josefson, P. LaRussa, and S. Silverstein.** 1995. Reactivated and latent varicella-zoster virus in human dorsal root ganglia. *Proc. Natl. Acad. Sci. USA* **92:**10980–10984.
89. **Lungu, O., C. Panagiotidis, P. Annunziato, A. Gershon, and S. Silverstein.** 1998. Aberrant intracellular localization of varicella-zoster virus regulatory proteins during latency. *Proc. Natl. Acad. Sci. USA* **95:**7080–7085.
90. **Mahalingham, R., M. Wellish, R. Cohrs, S. Debrus, J. Piette, B. Rentier, and D. H. Gilden.** 1996. Expression of protein encoded by varicella-zoster virus open reading frame 63 in latently infected human ganglionic neurons. *Proc. Natl. Acad. Sci. USA* **93:**2122–2124.
91. **Mallory, S., M. Sommer, and A. M. Arvin.** 1998. Analysis of the glycoproteins I and E of varicella-zoster virus (VZV) using deletional mutations of VZV cosmids. *J. Infect. Dis.* **178**(Suppl. 1)**:**S22–S26.

92. **Mallory, S., M. Sommer, and A. M. Arvin.** 1997. Mutational analysis of the role of glycoprotein I in varicella-zoster virus replication and its effects on glycoprotein E conformation and trafficking. *J. Virol.* **71:**8279–8288.
93. **Merigan, T. C., K. Rand, R. Pollard, P. Abdallah, G. W. Jordan, and R. P. Fried.** 1978. Human leukocyte interferon for the treatment of herpes zoster in patients with cancer. *N. Engl. J. Med.* **298:**981–987.
94. **Michalik, D., P. La Russa, S. Steinberg, P. Wright, K. M. Edwards, and A. Gershon.** 2008. Primary vaccine failure after 1 dose of varicella vaccine in healthy children. *J. Infect. Dis.* **197:**944–949.
95. **Miravet, E., N. Danchaivijitr, H. Basu, D. E. Saunders, and V. Ganesan.** 2007. Clinical and radiological features of childhood cerebral infarction following varicella zoster virus infection. *Dev. Med. Child Neurol.* **49:** 417–422.
96. **Moffat, J. F., M. D. Stein, H. Kaneshima, and A. M. Arvin.** 1995. Tropism of varicella-zoster virus for human $CD4^+$ and $CD8^+$ T lymphocytes and epidermal cells in SCID-hu mice. *J. Virol.* **69:**5236–5242.
97. **Montalvo, E. A., R. T. Parmley, and C. Grose.** 1985. Structural analysis of the varicella-zoster virus gp98-gp62 complex: posttranslational addition of N-linked and O-linked oligosaccharide moieties. *J. Virol.* **53:**761–770.
98. **Olson, J. K., and C. Grose.** 1998. Complex formation facilitates endocytosis of the varicella-zoster virus gE:gI Fc receptor. *J. Virol.* **72:**1542–1551.
99. **Oxman, M. N., M. J. Levin, G. R. Johnson, K. E. Schmader, S. E. Straus, L. D. Gelb, R. D. Arbeit, M. S. Simberkoff, A. A. Gershon, L. E. Davis, A. Weinberg, K. D. Boardman, H. M. Williams, J. H. Zhang, P. N. Peduzzi, C. E. Beisel, V. A. Morrison, J. C. Guatelli, P. A. Brooks, C. A. Kauffman, C. T. Pachucki, K. M. Neuzil, R. F. Betts, P. F. Wright, M. R. Griffin, P. Brunell, N. E. Soto, A. R. Marques, S. K. Keay, R. P. Goodman, D. J. Cotton, J. W. Gnann, Jr., J. Loutit, M. Holodniy, W. A. Keitel, G. E. Crawford, S. S. Yeh, Z. Lobo, J. F. Toney, R. N. Greenberg, P. M. Keller, R. Harbecke, A. R. Hayward, M. R. Irwin, T. C. Kyriakides, C. Y. Chan, I. S. Chan, W. W. Wang, P. W. Annunziato, and J. L. Silber.** 2005. A vaccine to prevent herpes zoster and postherpetic neuralgia in older adults. *N. Engl. J. Med.* **352:**2271–2284.
100. **Ozaki, T., Y. Matsui, Y. Asano, T. Okuno, K. Yamanishi, and M. Takahashi.** 1989. Study of virus isolation from pharyngeal swabs in children with varicella. *Am. J. Dis. Child.* **143:**1448–1450.
101. **Parker, S. P., M. Quinlivan, Y. Taha, and J. Breuer.** 2006. Genotyping of varicella-zoster virus and the discrimination of Oka vaccine strains by TaqMan real-time PCR. *J. Clin. Microbiol.* **44:**3911–3914.
102. **Paryani, S. G., and A. M. Arvin.** 1986. Intrauterine infection with varicella-zoster virus after maternal varicella. *N. Engl. J. Med.* **314:**1542–1546.
103. **Paul, N., and M. E. Jacob.** 2006. An outbreak of cadaver-acquired chickenpox in a health care setting. *Clin. Infect. Dis.* **43:**599–601.
104. **Preblud, S. R.** 1981. Age-specific risks of varicella complications. *Pediatrics* **68:**14–17.
105. **Reichman, R. C.** 1978. Neurologic complications of varicella-zoster infections. *Ann. Intern. Med.* **375:**89–96.
106. **Ross, A. H., E. Lencher, and G. Reitman.** 1962. Modification of chickenpox in family contacts by administration of gamma globulin. *N. Engl. J. Med.* **267:**369–376.
107. **Safrin, S., C. Crumpacker, P. Chatis, R. Davis, R. Hafner, J. Rush, H. A. Kessler, B. Landry, and J. Mills.** 1991. A controlled trial comparing foscarnet with vidarabine for acyclovir-resistant mucocutaneous herpes simplex in the acquired immunodeficiency syndrome. *N. Engl. J. Med.* **325:**551–555.
108. **Schaap, A., J.-F. Fortin, M. Sommer, L. Zerboni, S. Stamatis, C.-C. Ku, G. P. Nolan, and A. M. Arvin.** 2005. T-cell tropism and the role of ORF66 protein in pathogenesis of varicella-zoster virus infection. *J. Virol.* **79:**12921–12933.
109. **Sedarati, F., T. Margolis, and J. Stevens.** 1993. Latent infection can be established with drastically reduced transcription and replication of the HSV-1 genome. *Virology* **192:**687–691.
110. **Sergeev, N., E. Rubtcova, V. Chizikov, D. S. Schmid, and V. N. Loparev.** 2006. New mosaic subgenotype of varicella-zoster virus in the USA: VZV detection and genotyping by oligonucleotide-microarray. *J. Virol. Methods* **136:**8–16.
111. **Seward, J. F., B. M. Watson, C. L. Peterson, L. Mascola, J. W. Pelosi, J. X. Zhang, T. J. Maupin, G. S. Goldman, L. J. Tabony, K. G. Brodovicz, A. O. Jumaan, and M. Wharton.** 2002. Varicella disease after introduction of varicella vaccine in the United States, 1995–2000. *JAMA* **287:**606–611.
112. **Seward, J. F., J. X. Zhang, T. J. Maupin, L. Mascola, and A. O. Jumaan.** 2004. Contagiousness of varicella in vaccinated cases: a household contact study. *JAMA* **292:** 704–708.
113. **Sharman, V. L., and F. J. Goodwin.** 1980. Hemolytic uremic syndrome following chicken pox. *Clin. Nephrol.* **14:**49–51.
114. **Stallings, C. L., G. J. Duigou, A. A. Gershon, M. D. Gershon, and S. J. Silverstein.** 2006. The cellular localization pattern of varicella-zoster virus ORF29p is influenced by proteasome-mediated degradation. *J. Virol.* **80:**1497–1512.
115. **Stone, M. J., and C. P. Hawkins.** 2007. A medical overview of encephalitis. *Neuropsychol. Rehabil.* **17:**429–449.
116. **Sugano, T., T. Tomiyama, Y. Matsumoto, S. Sasaki, T. Kimura, B. Forghani, and Y. Mashuho.** 1991. A human monoclonal antibody against varicella-zoster virus glycoprotein III. *J. Gen. Virol.* **72:**2065–2073.
117. **Suzuki, K., Y. Akahori, Y. Asano, Y. Kurosawa, and K. Shiraki.** 2007. Isolation of therapeutic human monoclonal antibodies for varicella-zoster virus and the effect of light chains on the neutralizing activity. *J. Med. Virol.* **79:**852–862.
118. **Szabo, F., N. Horvath, S. Seimon, and T. Hughes.** 2000. Inappropriate antidiuretic hormone secretion, abdominal pain and disseminated varicella-zoster virus infection: an unusual triad in a patient 6 months post mini-allogeneic peripheral stem cell transplant for chronic myeloid leukemia. *Bone Marrow Transplant.* **26:** 231–233.
119. **Takahashi, M., T. Otsuka, Y. Okuno, Y. Asano, T. Yazaki, and S. Isomura.** 1974. Live vaccine used to prevent the spread of varicella in children in hospital. *Lancet* **ii:**1288–1290.
120. **Triebwasser, J. H., R. E. Harris, R. E. Bryant, and E. R. Rhodes.** 1967. Varicella pneumonia in adults. Report of seven cases and a review of the literature. *Medicine* **46:**409–423.
121. **Trlifajova, J., D. Bryndova, and M. Ryc.** 1984. Isolation of varicella-zoster virus from pharyngeal and nasal swabs in varicella patients. *J. Hyg. Epidemiol. Microbiol. Immunol.* **28:**201–206.
122. **Tsolia, M., A. Gershon, S. Steinberg, and L. Gelb.** 1990. Live attenuated varicella vaccine: evidence that the virus is attenuated and the importance of skin lesions

in transmission of varicella-zoster virus. *J. Pediatr.* **116:** 184–189.

123. **Tyring, S., R. A. Barbarash, J. E. Nahlik, A. Cunningham, J. Marley, M. Heng, T. Jones, T. Rea, R. Boon, R. Saltzman, and the Collaborative Famciclovir Herpes Zoster Study Group.** 1995. Famciclovir for the treatment of acute herpes zoster: effects on acute disease and post herpetic neuralgia. *Ann. Intern. Med.* **123:**89–96.
124. **Vazquez, M., P. LaRussa, A. Gershon, S. Steinberg, K. Freudigman, and E. Shapiro.** 2001. The effectiveness of the varicella vaccine in clinical practice. *N. Engl. J. Med.* **344:**955–960.
125. **Vazquez, M., P. S. LaRussa, A. A. Gershon, L. M. Niccolai, C. E. Muehlenbein, S. P. Steinberg, and E. D. Shapiro.** 2004. Effectiveness over time of varicella vaccine. *JAMA* **291:**851–855.
126. **Vinzio, S., B. Lioure, I. Enescu, J. L. Schlienger, and B. Goichot.** 2005. Severe abdominal pain and inappropriate antidiuretic hormone secretion preceding varicella-zoster virus reactivation 10 months after autologous stem cell transplantation for acute myeloid leukaemia. *Bone Marrow Transplant.* **35:**525–527.
127. **Wallace, M. R., W. A. Bowler, N. B. Murray, S. K. Brodine, and E. C. Oldfield.** 1992. Treatment of adult varicella with oral acyclovir. A randomized, placebo-controlled trial. *Ann. Intern. Med.* **117:**358–363.
128. **Wang, Z.-H., M. D. Gershon, O. Lungu, Z. Zhu, and A. A. Gershon.** 2000. Trafficking of varicella-zoster virus glycoprotein gI: T^{338}-dependent retention in the *trans*-Golgi network, secretion, and mannose 6-phosphate-inhibitable uptake of the ectodomain. *J. Virol.* **174:**6600–6613.
129. **Wang, Z.-H., M. D. Gershon, O. Lungu, Z. Zhu, S. Mallory, A. M. Arvin, and A. A. Gershon.** 2001. Essential role played by the C-terminal domain of glycoprotein I in envelopment of varicella-zoster virus in the *trans*-Golgi network: interactions of glycoproteins with tegument. *J. Virol.* **75:**323–340.
130. **Weber, D. M., and J. A. Pellecchia.** 1965. Varicella pneumonia: study of prevalence in adult men. *JAMA* **192:**572.
131. **Weinberg, A., S. P. Horslen, S. S. Kaufman, R. Jesser, A. Devoll-Zabrocki, B. L. Fleckten, S. Kochanowicz, K. R. Seipel, and M. J. Levin.** 2006. Safety and immunogenicity of varicella-zoster virus vaccine in pediatric liver and intestine transplant recipients. *Am. J. Transplant.* **6:**565–568.
132. **Weller, T., and M. B. Stoddard.** 1952. Intranuclear inclusion bodies in cultures of human tissue inoculated with varicella vesicle fluid. *J. Immunol.* **68:**311–319.
133. **Weller, T. H.** 1983. Varicella and herpes zoster: changing concepts of the natural history, control, and importance of a not-so-benign virus. *N. Engl. J. Med.* **309:** 1362–1368, 1434–1440.
134. **Whitley, R.** 1992. Therapeutic approaches to varicella-zoster virus infections. *J. Infect. Dis.* **166:**S51–S57.
135. **Whitley, R. J., and S. Straus.** 1993. Therapy for varicella-zoster virus infections: where do we stand? *Infect. Dis. Clin. Pract.* **2:**100–108.
136. **Wilson, A., M. Sharp, C. M. Koropchak, S. F. Ting, and A. M. Arvin.** 1992. Subclinical varicella-zoster virus viremia, herpes zoster, and T lymphocyte immunity to varicella-zoster viral antigens after bone marrow transplantation. *J. Infect. Dis.* **165:**119–126.
137. **Wilson, G., D. Talkington, W. Gruber, K. Edwards, and T. Dermody.** 1995. Group A streptococcal necrotizing fasciitis following varicella in children: case reports and review. *Clin. Infect. Dis.* **20:**1333–1338.
138. **Wood, M. J., R. W. Johnson, M. W. McKendrick, J. Taylor, B. K. Mandal, and J. Crooks.** 1994. A randomized trial of acyclovir for 7 days or 21 days with and without prednisolone for treatment of acute herpes zoster. *N. Engl. J. Med.* **330:**896–900.
139. **Wu, L., and B. Forghani.** 1997. Characterization of neutralizing domains on varicella-zoster virus glycoprotein E defined by monoclonal antibodies. *Arch. Virol.* **142:** 349–362.
140. **Yamanishi, K.** 2008. Molecular analysis of varicella-zoster virus (VZV) vaccine. *J. Infect. Dis.* **197**(Suppl. 2)**:** S45–S48.
141. **Yao, Z., and C. Grose.** 1994. Unusual phosphorylation sequence in the gpIV (gI) component of the varicella-zoster virus gpI-gpIV glycoprotein complex (VZV gE-gI complex). *J. Virol.* **68:**4204–4211.
142. **Zerboni, L., C. C. Ku, C. D. Jones, J. L. Zehnder, and A. M. Arvin.** 2005. Varicella-zoster virus infection of human dorsal root ganglia in vivo. *Proc. Natl. Acad. Sci. USA* **102:**6490–6495.
143. **Zerboni, L., M. Reichelt, C. D. Jones, J. L. Zehnder, H. Ito, and A. M. Arvin.** 2007. From the cover: aberrant infection and persistence of varicella-zoster virus in human dorsal root ganglia in vivo in the absence of glycoprotein I. *Proc. Natl. Acad. Sci. USA* **104:**14086–14091.
144. **Zhu, Z., M. D. Gershon, C. Gabel, D. Sherman, R. Ambron, and A. A. Gershon.** 1995. Entry and egress of VZV: role of mannose 6-phosphate, heparan sulfate proteoglycan, and signal sequences in targeting virions and viral glycoproteins. *Neurology* **45:**S15–S17.
145. **Zhu, Z., M. D. Gershon, Y. Hao, R. T. Ambron, C. A. Gabel, and A. A. Gershon.** 1995. Envelopment of varicella-zoster virus: targeting of viral glycoproteins to the trans-Golgi network. *J. Virol.* **69:**7951–7959.
146. **Zhu, Z., Y. Hao, M. D. Gershon, R. T. Ambron, and A. A. Gershon.** 1996. Targeting of glycoprotein I (gE) of varicella-zoster virus to the *trans*-Golgi network by an AYRV sequence and an acidic amino acid-rich patch in the cytosolic domain of the molecule. *J. Virol.* **70:**6563–6575.

Cytomegalovirus

PAUL DAVID GRIFFITHS, VINCENT CLIVE EMERY, AND RICHARD MILNE

22

Human cytomegalovirus (HCMV) was first isolated 50 years ago, when the new technology of cell culture became available. It was isolated independently by three different investigators and named after its cytopathic effect (CPE), which produced large, swollen, refractile cells causing "cytomegaly." The virus is ubiquitous, having infected most individuals by early adulthood in developing countries and by late adulthood in developed countries. Most individuals show no symptoms as a result of primary infection, reactivation, or reinfection, showing that the virus is well adapted to its normal host, which commits substantial immune resources to controlling HCMV. However, in individuals whose immune system is either immature (as in the fetus) or compromised by immunosuppressive therapy or human immunodeficiency virus (HIV) infection, HCMV can cause serious end-organ disease (EOD). Furthermore, accumulation of HCMV-specific T cells over decades contributes to immunosenescence. Thus, HCMV acts as an opportunist, damaging the very young and the very old as well as adults and children whose immune systems are impaired.

The pathogenesis of HCMV disease is complex, involving contributions from the host as well as from the virus. Increasing knowledge about the genetic composition of the virus can help to illuminate this complex series of relationships and provide a rational basis for therapeutic intervention and prevention of disease.

VIROLOGY

Classification

HCMV is a member of the *Betaherpesvirinae* subfamily of the *Herpesviridae*. This classification was originally based on its slow growth in vitro and strict species specificity but is now based on genetic sequence homologies among the *Alpha-*, *Beta-*, and *Gammaherpesvirinae* subfamilies. Based on restriction enzyme analysis of virion DNA, there are multiple genetic variants, termed strains. These genetic differences do not allow classification into distinct genotypes. Likewise, the corresponding differences in antigenic constitution do not allow distinct serotypes to be defined. Strains are still best characterized as having an antigenic mosaic, which is recognized broadly by the host cellular and humoral immune responses. Individuals infected with one strain of HCMV thus have cross-reactive immunity against all strains, although the extent to which this provides cross-protection from disease remains to be defined.

The International HCMV Workshop in 1993 agreed upon a nomenclature for the description of HCMV proteins, which is used for this chapter (99). The system designates p for protein, gp for glycoprotein, or pp for phosphoprotein, followed by the genetic locus and any preferred trivial name in parentheses. For example, gpUL55 (gB) is the glycoprotein encoded by the 55th open reading frame (ORF) in the unique long (UL) region, known as glycoprotein B (gB).

Composition

Purified HCMV virions contain about 60 virus-encoded proteins and more than 70 host proteins (113). In common with all herpesviruses, the HCMV virion has three basic structural units.

Capsid

The HCMV capsid has a diameter of 125 nm and, by cryo-electron microscopic (cryo-EM) reconstruction, is made up of 162 capsomeres arranged as an icosahedral lattice with a triangulation number of 16. There are 150 hexons, which comprise 6 copies of the major capsid protein (MCP, encoded by the UL86 gene), 11 pentons (5 copies of the MCP), and, by analogy with herpes simplex virus (HSV), 1 penton that is structurally distinct and acts as the portal for DNA packaging. In HSV, the portal is a dodecamer of the UL6 protein: the HCMV homolog of this is UL104. The capsid provides the architecture to contain the viral genome, a double-stranded DNA molecule.

Tegument

Historically, the tegument has been described as an amorphous layer. Cryo-EM reconstructions of HSV have revealed a more structured protein layer (80), and it seems likely that the HCMV tegument has a broadly similar appearance. Structurally, the tegument is a link between capsid and envelope and may play a pivotal role in particle assembly. Functionally, the tegument contains key regulatory proteins, pp65 and pp71, that are delivered in significant amounts to the host cell.

pp65

pp65 (ppUL83) is the most abundant virion protein, accounting for about 15% of the total virion protein (and in excess of 90% of the dense body protein). It is the antigen that is detected in the diagnostic antigenemia assay and is also the major component of dense bodies. The latter are noninfectious particles comprising a core of tegument proteins enclosed in a lipid envelope, which are formed during HCMV infection. pp65 is trafficked to the nucleus very early in the infection via an unusual bipartite nuclear localization signal. pp65 is a multifunctional protein that is required for various immunomodulatory roles: affecting presentation of immediate-early (IE) peptides (64), down-regulation of HLA-DR (116), and inhibiting NK cell responses (8). The protein also binds another tegument component, the viral protein kinase UL97 (90). Immunologically, pp65 is a significant target for CD4 and CD8 T-cell responses (158). Remarkably, a virus mutant lacking pp65 has no growth defect in vitro, although no dense bodies are formed (140).

pp71

pp71 (ppUL82) is rapidly translocated to the nucleus after virus entry. It is a transcriptional transactivator, recognizing promoters with AP1 or ATF sites in their regulatory regions, particularly the major IE promoter (MIEP) (27). This transactivation is enhanced by an interaction with another tegument protein, ppUL35. As a potent transactivator, pp71 is analogous to the VP16 virion transactivator protein of HSV. In addition to its role as a transcriptional transactivator, pp71 overcomes hDaax-mediated suppression of HCMV replication and is thus essential for the onset of productive replication (29). Like pp65, pp71 appears to have an immunomodulatory role, disrupting major histocompatibility complex class I expression (162).

pp150

The basic phosphoprotein ppUL32 (pp150) accumulates late in infection at the putative sites of virus assembly, and a UL32-negative virus fails to complete the cytoplasmic stages of egress, consistent with a role in envelopment (9). The tight physical association of pp150 with capsids (13) emphasizes the presumed structural role of tegument in linking capsid with envelope and, perhaps, in driving virus assembly. pp150 is an immunodominant B-cell target.

Envelope

The viral envelope is a host-derived lipid bilayer, termed the envelope, which contains viral glycoproteins. Envelopment is thought to occur in the endoplasmic reticulum (ER)-Golgi intermediate compartment (137), and the envelope is thus most likely derived from membranes in this region of the cell (see below). The HCMV genome codes for in excess of 50 predicted glycoproteins; 19 of these were detected in mass spectrometric analysis of purified virions (166). The envelope glycoproteins represent the main point of contact between intact virus and host, and as such they are important inducers of neutralizing antibodies.

An important subset of envelope glycoproteins mediate virus entry (Table 1). The entry glycoproteins fall into two groups: those that are conserved throughout herpesviruses, i.e., gpUL55 (gB), gH, gL, gM, and gN, and those limited to betaherpesviruses, i.e., gO, gUL128, gpUL130, and gpUL131. The latter are thought to modulate entry and to determine cell tropism by differential receptor binding.

TABLE 1 HCMV envelope glycoproteins

Complex in envelope	Constituent protein(s)	Mapped ORF
gCI	gB homodimer	gpUL55
gCII	gM	gpUL100
	gN	gpUL73
gCIII	gH	gpUL75
	and	
	gL	gpUL115
	plus	
	gO	gpUL74
		gpUL128
		gpUL130
		gpUL131A

The HCMV envelope glycoproteins appear to exist in three distinct complexes: gCI, gCII, and gCIII (69). gCI is made up of oligomers of gB which are thought to have a role in attachment, fusion, and receptor binding (see below). The gB monomer (Fig. 1) comprises two subunits, gp116 and gp55, derived by furin cleavage of a precursor. This cleavage is not essential for virus infectivity in vitro (157). The protein dimerizes rapidly after synthesis but subsequently undergoes further processing and oligomerization (16). Studies of the crystal structure of HSV gB have shown a homotrimer, and HCMV gB probably shares this overall structure, although biochemical data have shown a homodimer.

gCII comprises heterodimers of gM (UL100) and gN (UL73). This complex plays a role in virus attachment via the host cell proteoglycan-binding activity of gN. Both components also have roles in assembly (28).

gCIII is based on the disulfide-linked heterodimer of gH (UL75) and gL (UL115). This, in turn, interacts with gO (UL74) or with gpUL128, gpUL130, and gpUL131A, forming two or more distinct complexes (2). Virus-free fusion assays have implicated gH/gL alone as a fusogenic complex (96).

A number of other envelope glycoproteins have been recognized. gpUL4 is a glycoprotein of unknown function that is expressed with early kinetics. HCMV encodes four chemokine receptor homologs, US27, US28, UL33, and UL78. Two (UL33 and US27) are known to be in the virion (105). In contrast to most host receptors, the viral CCR homologs are constitutively activated. Those in the virion are theoretically able to signal as soon as they become incorporated into host membranes following virus entry. US28 induces migration of smooth muscle cells (155), and this is perhaps significant in terms of an association of HCMV with vascular disease.

Viral Genome

The most accurate representation of the HCMV genome has come from comparisons of the complete genomic sequence of a minimally passaged strain, Merlin, with partial sequences from other strains, including some obtained directly from clinical material (46). Gene assignments have been strengthened by comparison with the colinear sequence of chimpanzee CMV. HCMV genomic analyses have been complicated by the tendency of the virus to lose a 22-kb segment of the genome, termed ULb′, rapidly upon isolation and passage in fibroblasts (31). The ULb′ seg-

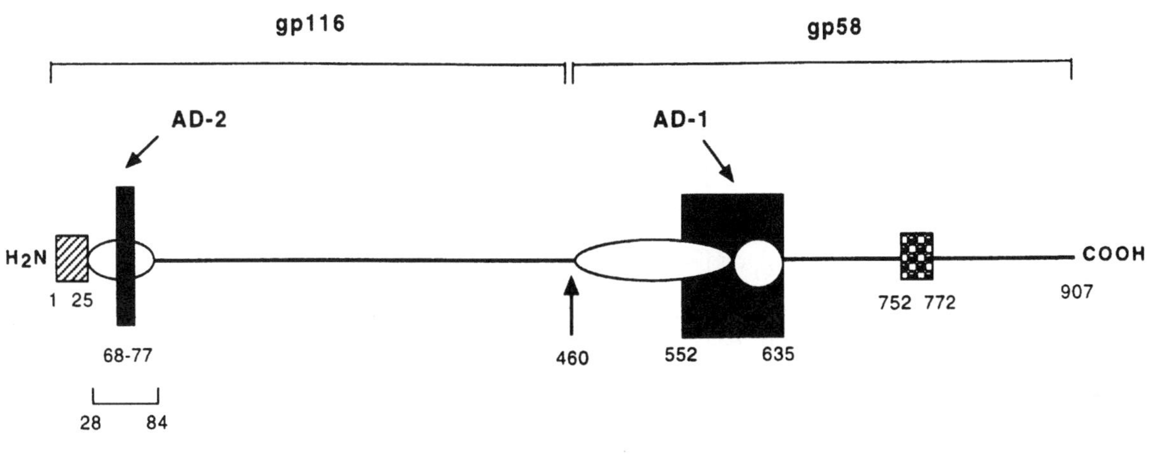

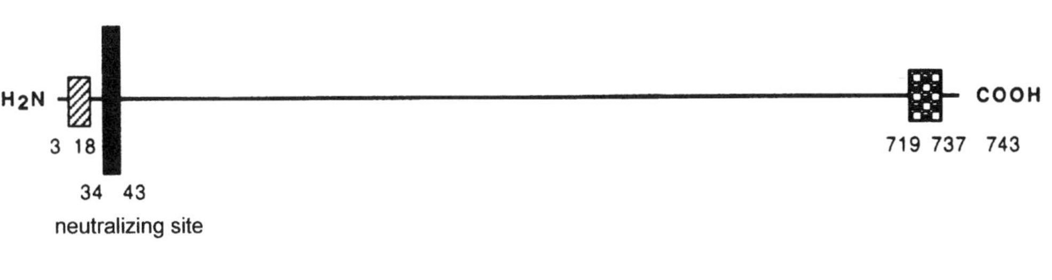

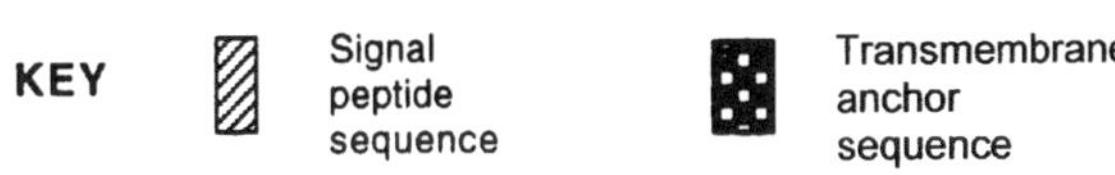

FIGURE 1 Schematic representation of epitopes identified on gpUL55 (gB) and gpUL75 (gH). Numbers represent codons.

ment contains genes that are not essential for replication in vitro but ones that play key roles in immune evasion and in determining cell tropism.

The HCMV Merlin genome is a 235,645-bp linear double-stranded DNA molecule with a coding capacity of 165 genes (46). It is the largest genome among the human herpesviruses. The genome comprises two unique regions, termed UL and unique short (US), flanked by repeated sequences. Inversions of the unique regions give rise to four isomeric forms of virion DNA present in equimolar amounts. No pathological significance has been attributed to these isomers.

The structure of the Merlin genome is shown in Color Plate 31. The central section of the genome contains the core genes: some 40 genes that are conserved throughout the *Alpha-*, *Beta-*, and *Gammaherpesvirinae*. Many of the other genes are grouped into families of related genes (Color Plate 31) thought to have evolved by duplication events. There are numerous spliced genes. MicroRNAs have been detected across the genome encoded by both strands (51, 70, 122). A functional RNA is encoded that regulates mitochondrion-induced cell death (131). Two proteins are also known to block apoptosis by inhibiting activation of caspase 8 (UL36) and inhibiting mitochondrial activation (UL37 exon 1).

Sequence variation occurs across the genome but appears to be highest at either end of the UL segment. A number of genes, notably UL146, which encodes a functional alpha chemokine, as well as UL73, UL74, and UL144, show a remarkable level of sequence variation (82). The functional significance of this variation is not known.

Virus Replication Cycle

Virus Entry

In common with other herpesviruses, primary attachment of HCMV is mediated by interactions between virion glycoproteins and sulfated proteoglycans on the host cell surface (38). This primary attachment serves to bring the virus into close association with the target cell to allow receptor binding. HCMV entry can occur by direct fusion between the virion envelope and the plasma membrane or via endocytosis followed by fusion from within the endosome (17, 37). The latter fusion step is facilitated by endosome acidification. The cellular and viral factors contributing to the choice of pathway are not known. Three glycoproteins—gB, gH, and gL—constitute the core herpesvirus entry machinery. The roles played by each protein in the entry process remain unknown.

The crystal structure of HSV gB shows convincing similarities to the G protein of vesicular stomatitis virus, a known fusion protein (84). HCMV gB appears to be fusogenic when stably expressed in U373 cells, although fusion assays have shown that HCMV gH/gL alone can mediate fusion (96), and HSV gH/gL has certain characteristics that resemble fusion proteins. Regardless of the detailed roles played by each protein, it is clear that they cooperate closely to mediate fusion. Indeed, coimmunoprecipitation studies show that HCMV gB and gH interact transiently during virus entry (121).

The gH/gL heterodimer is found in at least two distinct complexes (Table 1), one with gO and one with glycoproteins encoded by members of the genes from UL128 to UL131. The latter have been shown to have a role in mediating entry to endothelial cell types, but not fibroblasts (169), and blocking studies with soluble UL128 protein suggest that this may bind a receptor on endothelial cells (121). The use of different forms of gH/gL complex as a means of regulating host cell tropism is an emerging theme in the beta- and gammaherpesviruses (22).

The virus cell contacts that are a precursor to entry induce a range of signaling events, but their role in the context of virus entry is not clear. Various candidate receptors for gB and gH/gL have been proposed, but there is, as yet, no consensus as to their role in entry.

Transport to the Nucleus

After entry, the tegument and capsid are released into the cytoplasm. Transport of the capsid to the nucleus occurs in a microtubule-dependent manner, and capsids appear to retain some tegument throughout this process (117). The viral genome is released from capsids when they reach the nuclear pores. The mechanism underlying localization and release of the genome is unknown, although recent data implicate the UL47 tegument protein in this process (14).

Transcription and Gene Expression

HCMV gene expression, in common with gene expression in other herpesviruses, occurs in three phases termed IE, early (E), and late (L). In general, IE genes encode regulatory proteins, E genes encode replication proteins, and L genes encode structural proteins. The IE genes are the first to be transcribed in the replication cycle. A defining characteristic is that they are transcribed in the absence of viral protein synthesis. There are five IE transcription loci in the genome: UL36-37, UL122/123 (IE1 and IE2), UL119-115, US3, and TRS1. The most abundant, and by far the best studied, transcripts are those arising from the major IE locus: UL122/123. Expression of these genes is controlled by the MIEP, well known from its widespread use in expression plasmids. The MIEP is complex, with multiple transcription factor binding sites in the upstream enhancer element. This combination of sites may well play a role in allowing IE gene expression to occur in a diverse array of cell types, perhaps containing a varied repertoire of transcription factors. Broadly speaking, the MIEP is active in differentiated cell types and is repressed in undifferentiated cell types. This differential activity appears to be a significant regulator of latency and reactivation.

Though numerous gene products are produced through intricate patterns of splicing, the two major products are the IE1 (IE72) and IE2 (IE86) proteins (Fig. 2). These two proteins have a common N-terminal region, corresponding to exons 2 and 3 of the gene locus; they differ in the C-terminal region, IE1 corresponding to exon 4 and IE2 corresponding to exon 7.

MIEP-driven transcription is favored by events that occur concurrently with virus entry. Cell surface binding by gB and gH induces NF-κB and Sp1 expression (177). This signaling is mediated in part by binding of gB to the epidermal growth factor receptor. The MIEP enhancer contains multiple recognition sites for both these transcription factors. Additionally, the MIEP is specifically transactivated by the tegument protein pp71, which is released as soon as incoming virions are uncoated (27). Thus, HCMV employs multiple methods independent of de novo viral gene expression to induce an intracellular milieu favorable to the initiation of IE gene transcription.

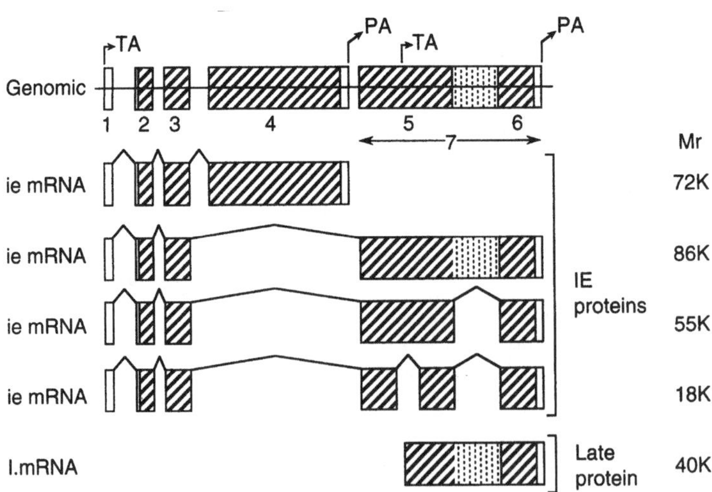

FIGURE 2 The major IE region of HCMV showing the splicing events that produce distinct proteins. TA, transcriptional activation; PA, polyadenylation; l.mRNA, late mRNA.

The detailed functions of the IE1 and IE2 proteins have been recently reviewed (114). IE1 binds PML and disrupts ND10 (171). An IE1-negative virus is viable at a high multiplicity of infection but fails to replicate at a low multiplicity of infection. This deficit can be overcome by histone deacetylase (HDAC) inhibitors (115), highlighting the importance of these molecules in the regulation of MIEP activity (see below). Binding of IE1 to HDAC3 promotes transcription by antagonizing histone deacetylation, altering the acetylation state of the MIEP and thus favoring transcription (115). IE1 is also capable of direct transactivation (83).

IE2 is essential for virus replication. It has dual roles in regulating expression of viral and cellular genes and negatively autoregulating the MIEP via an upstream *cis*-acting repressive sequence (Fig. 3). IE2 also binds HDAC3, potentially resulting in an effect similar to that of IE1 (115). IE2 localizes to ND10-like structures in association with the viral genome. These foci develop into replication compartments, consistent with a role for IE2 in the early stages of genome replication (147). Indeed, IE2 binds a promoter in the lytic origin of replication in complex with the E protein UL84 (see below).

Switch to E and L Viral Gene Expression

Both IE1 and IE2 activate E and L gene expression. E genes are defined as those genes that (i) require prior expression of the IE genes for transcription and (ii) can be expressed in the presence of inhibitors of DNA replication, such as ganciclovir and foscarnet.

DNA Replication, Capsid Assembly, and DNA Packaging

In contrast to transcription, for which the virus relies on cellular machinery, the virus encodes its own DNA replication apparatus. Thus, viral DNA replication is a key target for the development of antiviral drugs. HCMV also stimulates progression of the host cell cycle toward S phase yet suppresses host DNA synthesis, thus ensuring a cellular environment suitable for viral DNA replication (10). Upon delivery to the nucleus, genomes are deposited at ND10 sites, where transcription and DNA replication both occur (88).

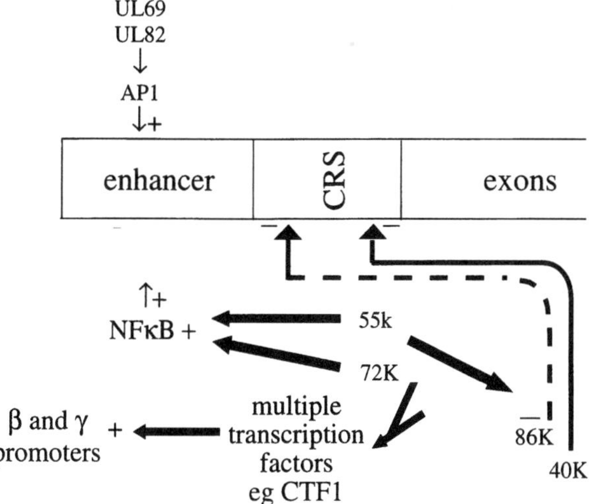

FIGURE 3 Regulation of the major IE region of HCMV. CRS, *cis* repression sequence.

The input genome is thought to be circularized independently of viral gene expression. Circularization is consistent with a rolling-circle mode of replication, but this has not been proven for HCMV. Indeed, HCMV genome replication intermediates are more complex than would be produced by this method (4).

Transient replication assays have shown that 11 loci (Table 2) are required for HCMV genome replication (118). The core replication proteins corresponding to UL54 (DNA polymerase), UL44 (DNA polymerase accessory protein), UL57 (single-stranded DNA binding protein), UL105 (helicase), UL70 (primase), and UL102 (primase-associated factor), which are present in all herpesviruses, provide the basic DNA replication machinery. However, the details of their function and interactions are unknown (36).

The origin of replication, *ori*Lyt, is adjacent to the UL57 gene, essential for virus replication, and distinct from other viral origins (21). It is structurally complex and contains numerous short repeated sequences, including transcription factor binding sites, and has an overall asymmetry of nucleotide distribution, being AT rich on the left side but GC rich on the other (5). Transcripts are produced within *ori*Lyt (87), and two viral RNAs are present as RNA/DNA hybrids within the region in packaged genomes (127). Given the absence of an obvious origin binding protein in HCMV, it seems likely that these are in some way involved in initiation of replication (127); indeed, the UL84 protein, which is required for genome replication, binds stably to this region of *ori*Lyt (36). The initiation of L gene expression, which is, presumably, in some way regulated by the onset of DNA replication, is not understood.

Capsid Assembly

Based on their structural similarities, assembly of HCMV capsids is likely to resemble that of HSV capsids. The MCPs are conserved throughout the herpesviruses.

A transient internal scaffold coordinates assembly of the nascent capsid (100). This scaffold contains two major components encoded by the UL80 gene region: the protease precursor (UL80) and the assembly protein, pAP (UL80.5), which comprises the C-terminal half of the protease. The first steps in capsid assembly occur in the cy-

TABLE 2 Eleven loci required for HCMV replication[a]

Protein(s)	Locus
DNA polymerase	UL54
Polymerase-associated protein	UL44
ssDNA[b] binding protein	UL57
Helicase-primase	UL70 UL105 UL101–102
Transactivators	UL36–38 IRS1 (or TRS1) IE1/2
Unknown functions	UL84 UL112–113

[a] Reprinted from reference 117a with permission.
[b] ssDNA, single-stranded DNA.

toplasm, where pAP interacts with itself and with the MCP and causes the translocation of these capsid protomers to the nucleus (124). Once in the nucleus, pAP associates with the protease precursor and other capsid components are recruited to the protomers, giving rise to procapsids. Autoproteolysis of the protease then liberates the scaffold components from the nascent capsid (30).

Capsid maturation is coupled to DNA packaging. Based on data from HSV, DNA is packaged through a unique vertex containing the portal protein (UL6 in HSV). The HCMV portal homolog, UL104, forms high-molecular-weight complexes and binds DNA in a sequence-independent manner (45). HSV UL6 is thought to act as a nucleation factor for capsid assembly, explaining its asymmetric localization in the capsid.

DNA packaging requires *pac* signals located at the genome termini. These are recognized by the viral terminase complex, made up of UL56 and UL89 (160), which likely interacts with the portal protein.

Egress

The broadly accepted model for HCMV egress is the envelopment–de-envelopment–re-envelopment model. Mature capsids bud through the inner nuclear membrane (INM), acquiring a primary envelope. The resulting perinuclear enveloped virions then fuse with the outer nuclear membrane, liberating capsids to the cytoplasm. These traffic to the site of envelopment, where they acquire tegument and the final envelope. Mature virions are released from the cell by exocytosis or lysis. However, much of this pathway is inferred from studies of other herpesviruses, and some aspects of the pathway remain controversial.

The earliest step is recruitment of capsids to the INM. For HSV, the UL31 and UL34 proteins play a role in this recruitment. The HCMV homologs of these proteins, UL53 and UL50, are thought to have a similar function, and UL53 colocalizes with lamin B at the INM, consistent with a role in nuclear egress (42). Primary envelopment likely occurs by budding into large infoldings of the INM. It is not clear whether all of the tegument proteins are present in these particles. Cryo-EM tomogram images of perinuclear enveloped HSV show that the tegument is distinct from that in mature virions, suggesting that a subset of tegument proteins may be included in these particles, although not all HCMV tegument proteins have been detected in the nucleus. The primary envelope is then lost by fusion between the primary enveloped virion and the outer nuclear membrane, giving rise to naked cytoplasmic capsids.

Using confocal microscopic analysis, the site of final assembly has been defined as a secretory vacuolar structure that expresses Rab 3, TGN 46, and mannosidase II (86). Data also support a role for endocytic compartments in assembly and final envelopment. A fluid phase marker colocalizes with sites of virus budding, and cell surface biotinylation of infected cells leads to incorporation of biotinylated gB into virions (128).

Some tegument proteins may play a key role in driving the last stages of virus assembly, including the secondary envelopment step. A pp28-negative virus has cytoplasmic accumulations of nonenveloped tegumented capsids (141); accumulation of other viral proteins in the Golgi-associated assembly region is not affected. Additionally, both gM and gN (which form a heterodimer in the virion) have roles in assembly.

The involvement of cellular machinery in the later stages of virus assembly has been less well defined. An interaction between phosphorylated gB and the host trafficking protein PACS-1 is involved in recruitment of this protein to the site of assembly, and blocking of PACS-1 function has a modest effect on progeny titers (40). The endosomal sorting protein VPS4 has been shown to have a role in HSV secondary envelopment and budding (41). EM studies have shown an association of HCMV glycoproteins and budding particles with cytoplasmic multivesicular bodies, and depletion of VPS4 using small interfering RNA technology leads to enhanced release of HCMV particles and implicates the multivesicular bodies as components in viral degradation (62).

Latency and Reactivation

A defining characteristic of herpesviruses is the establishment and maintenance of a latent state from which the virus can periodically reactivate to undergo productive replication.

Sensitive PCR analyses show that peripheral blood monocytes are a major site of carriage of HCMV DNA in healthy individuals (159). Monocytes arise from bone marrow resident pluripotent $CD34^+$ stem cells, and this cell population appears to be a site of HCMV latency, although it is not clear if this is the only one.

$CD34^+$ precursor cells are a self-renewing population, but it is not clear whether successive generations of cells are reinfected by virus produced from infected bone marrow stromal cells or circulating infected endothelial cells or whether the HCMV genome is maintained in this population by some form of replication, perhaps analogous to the maintenance of the latent Epstein-Barr virus (EBV) genome in replicating B cells (142). The HCMV genome in $CD14^+$ peripheral blood mononuclear cells is in a circular plasmid form (18), but there is no evidence of a latent origin of replication or of genes homologous to those required for EBV genome maintenance (142).

$CD34^+$ monocytic precursors spend a relatively short time in the bone marrow before differentiating and moving to the peripheral blood. The regulation and initiation of reactivation appear to be governed largely by differentiation-dependent chromatin remodelling around the MIEP. Studies of the MIEP in latently infected $CD34^+$ cells and monocytes from healthy donors show that it is associated with heterochromatin protein 1 (HP-1) and nonacetylated histones, both markers of transcriptional repression. Differentiation of these cells led to loss of HP-1 and histone acetylation, providing an environment consistent with transcriptional activation. This was correlated with recovery of infectious virus, showing that HCMV reactivation is associated directly with the chromatin remodelling that occurs with differentiation (132).

Various viral transcripts have been associated with latent infection, including those from IE1/2, the viral interleukin 10 (IL-10) gene (UL111A), UL138, and an antisense transcript from the UL81-UL82 locus containing a 133-amino-acid ORF product (15). The role of these transcripts in latency, and of any proteins encoded by the transcripts, is currently unknown.

HLA Modulation

HCMV has evolved to contain a series of genes which are capable of interfering with the immune response (see chapter 14). Most of these are proteins, but one is a microRNA, and HCMV also recruits some cellular proteins, in the form of complement control proteins, to help avoid innate immune responses (Table 3). The presence of these multiple genes presumably allows HCMV to persist in multiple sanctuary sites throughout the body.

Several proteins have been shown to be responsible for down-regulating the cell surface display of mature class I complexes (Fig. 4). At IE times, pUS3 binds to HLA heavy chains in the lumen of the ER and sequesters them. At E times, pUS6 blocks TAP, the transporter associated with antigen presentation. At E times also, pUS2 and pUS11 reexport mature complexes back from the ER to the cytosol, where they are degraded in the proteasome. The coordinated action of these proteins produces a dramatic down-regulation of mature class I HLA complexes, blocking the ability of cytotoxic T lymphocytes (CTLs) to recognize the virus-infected cell. However, the cell would then be susceptible to lysis by NK cells, which recognize the absence of negative signals provided by non-antigen-specific HLA molecules. Accordingly, HCMV encodes two other proteins able to mimic these negative signals: gpUL18 and gpUL40 (Fig. 4). The latter protein encodes a canonical ligand within its leader sequence for HLA-E that is identical to the HLA-Cw03 signal sequence peptide. Expression of gpUL40 in HLA-E-positive cells confers resistance to NK cell lysis via the CD94/NKG2A receptor. The generation of the gpUL40 peptide ligand does not require the TAP system, and the mature gpUL40 can up-regulate expression of HLA-E.

HCMV also contains other genes that interfere with the stress response of the cell, which would normally activate NK cells to destroy the cell (Fig. 4). These include the proteins encoded by UL16, UL141, and UL142, which inhibit the action of the "UL binding proteins," CD155, and an unknown stimulatory molecule. In addition, a microRNA also blocks one of the UL binding proteins (154).

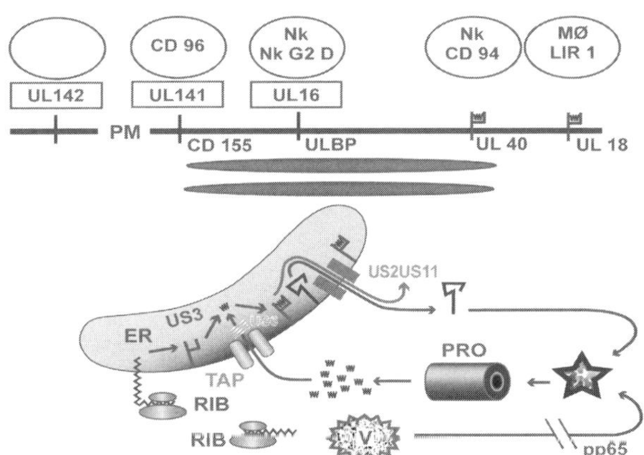

FIGURE 4 Effect of HCMV proteins on display of mature HLA complexes at the plasma membrane (PM). TAP, transporter associated with antigen presentation; RIB, ribosome; PRO, proteasome. The empty oval represents unknown binding factor.

EPIDEMIOLOGY

Prevalence and Incidence

HCMV infects both vertically and horizontally and can be transmitted by either route during primary infection, reinfection, or reactivation. It is frequently shed in saliva, semen, and cervico-vaginal secretions in the absence of symptoms, enabling transmission to others. Between 2 and 10% of infants are infected by the age of 12 months in all parts of the world. In later childhood, close contact facilitates transmission, so family groups, particularly those crowded together in unhygienic circumstances, have a high prevalence of infection.

In populations with good social circumstances, approximately 40% of adolescents are seropositive, and this figure thereafter increases by approximately 1% annually (72) (Fig. 5). Approximately 70% of adults under good socioeconomic conditions and 90% under poor conditions eventually become infected with HCMV. HCMV infection is distributed worldwide, with geographic differences explained by socioeconomic differences of exposure.

Following primary infection, HCMV persists either in a true latent form or in a state of low-level replication made possible by the immune evasion genes described above. Thus, individual cells could exhibit HCMV latency, while particular organs could always have some cells producing virus particles. Occasional reactivations of HCMV are almost always asymptomatic but presumably allow HCMV to spread horizontally. Reactivations also transmit vertically, so congenital HCMV infection is found most frequently in the poorest communities in the world (47).

Reinfection with another, or possibly the same, strain of HCMV can also occur; comparison of virion DNA samples by restriction enzyme analysis or by sequencing can differentiate between strains. The term recurrent infection is often used when infection is nonprimary but it has not been possible to differentiate reactivation from reinfection. Given all of these possible routes of infection, it should be clear why there is no seasonal pattern.

TABLE 3 HCMV immune evasion genes

Immune defense	Viral genes or host proteins
Complement	CD46, CD55, CD59
Chemokines	UL146, UL147, UL128
Chemokine receptors	UL33, UL78, US27, US28
Interferon	UL83, UL122, UL123, TRS1/IRS1
Fc receptors	UL118/119, IRL 11
IL-10	UL111.5 (vil-10)
CTLs	UL83, US6, US3, US2, US11
NK cells	UL18, UL40, UL16, UL141, UL142 MicroRNA miR-UL112

Transmission

Routes of Primary Infection

Intrauterine

Intrauterine infection presumably follows maternal viremia and associated placental infection. Intrauterine transmission of HCMV occurs in approximately 37% of pregnant women with primary infection. CMV-specific cell-mediated and neutralizing antibody levels would be expected to develop more rapidly in nontransmitters than transmitters, but the significance of detecting early responses in pregnancy is confounded by gestational stage (19). Approximately 1% of seropositive women transmit

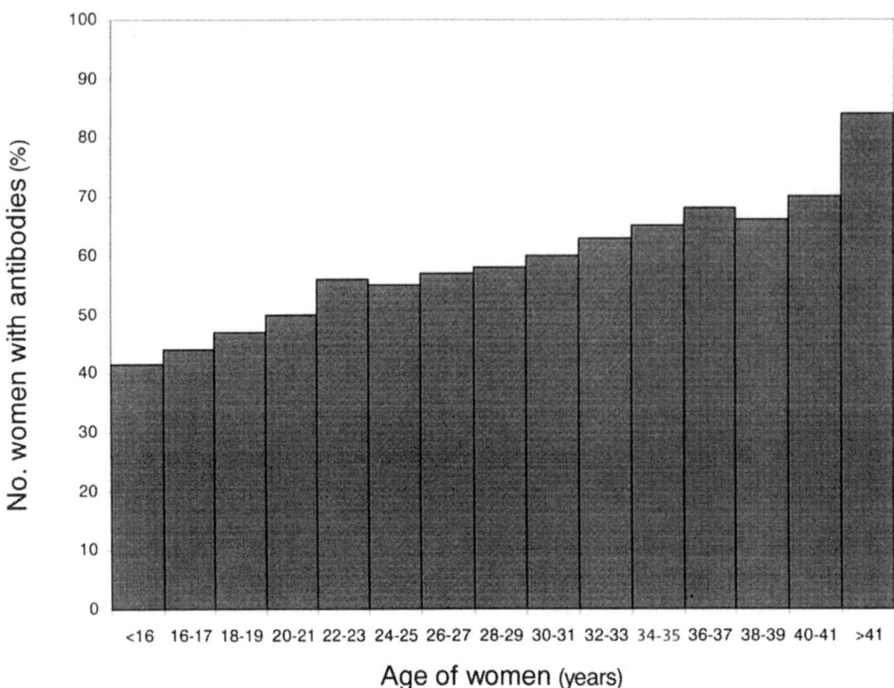

FIGURE 5 Age-specific prevalence of IgG antibodies against HCMV.

HCMV in utero, but at present there are no laboratory markers to identify those most at risk.

Perinatal

Perinatal infection can be acquired from infected maternal genital secretions or breast milk. Milk is a plausible source of HCMV, because perinatal infection has occurred only when breast-feeding has taken place, not when infected women gave bottle feeds to the infants.

Postnatal

The asymptomatic nature of most postnatal HCMV infections precludes identification of the routes of transmission, but exposure to saliva or genital secretions during sexual contact is suspected, because these contain infectious virus. HCMV transmission occurs from child to child in day care centers. This is most common among young children, especially if one is known to be excreting HCMV. Transmission via fomites, such as toys contaminated by saliva, has been implicated. Infection in children is usually asymptomatic, but infectious toddlers may transmit virus to adult staff or to mothers (120). There is a risk of fetal damage in pregnant women, especially when seronegative. Because the major risk to the fetus follows primary maternal infection during pregnancy, changes in child-rearing practices could affect the incidence of disease attributable to congenital HCMV. Typically, middle-class seronegative women are at potential risk when they send their children to child care centers with young children excreting HCMV (152). Considerable anxiety may be induced in both mothers and day care workers because HCMV infection is usually asymptomatic and excretion is prolonged. Because professionally trained nursing staff are not at increased risk of acquiring HCMV infection from patients (11), routine precautions such as hand washing must be sufficient to protect against transmission. Consequently, day care centers should be advised to review and improve their general hygiene standards. The same advice should be given to female staff, irrespective of their serologic status; humoral immunity in these women cannot guarantee that the fetus will be protected from infection, although it should reduce the chance of disease.

HCMV seroprevalence is 90 to 100% among patients attending clinics for sexually transmitted disease and among male homosexuals. Individuals linked epidemiologically by sexual contact have been shown to excrete strains of HCMV on the cervix and in semen that are indistinguishable by restriction enzyme typing. While these findings are consistent with the sexual transmission of HCMV, formal studies have not quantified the risk of acquiring HCMV by seronegative or seropositive contacts from particular sexual practices. Individuals can be infected with more than one strain of HCMV (35).

Blood Transfusion

The introduction of extracorporeal blood perfusion in the 1960s led to a syndrome of leukopenia, pyrexia, and atypical leukocytosis, termed postperfusion syndrome, caused by primary HCMV infection. The failure to isolate HCMV from blood suggests that the virus exists in a latent state, presumably within leukocytes, and is reactivated when cells encounter an allogeneic stimulus. Allogeneic stimulation of macrophages containing latent HCMV reactivates virus, which can subsequently infect and replicate in fibroblasts (146).

Although HCMV can be transmitted by blood transfusion, this is an uncommon event, occurring in only 1 to 5% of seronegative recipients exposed to seropositive blood. The risk is reduced to zero where filters are used routinely to remove leukocytes. No laboratory tests have been shown to identify donors at high risk of transmitting HCMV.

Organ Transplantation

Seronegative patients undergoing solid-organ transplantation are at no risk of primary infection from seronegative donors, whereas a seropositive organ transmits the virus in 60 to 80% of donations. Both kidneys from a single donor are usually concordant for transmission; however, it is not clear whether parenchymal cells of the organ or infiltrating leukocytes are the source of the infectious virus. Reinfection also occurs with transmission from a seropositive donor to a seropositive recipient. In contrast, typing of strains by restriction enzyme analysis of DNA demonstrates that the virus causing disease after bone marrow transplantation is derived from the recipient (174). Indeed, seropositive donors may be chosen preferentially for seropositive recipients because they can adoptively transfer some immunity into the recipient (77).

PATHOGENESIS

HCMV replication occurs widely in multiple tissues, as illustrated by isolation from autopsy material from AIDS patients (Table 4). During life, biopsy samples of lung, liver, esophagus, colon, and kidney are frequently found to contain HCMV. Replication has been demonstrated in polymorphonuclear leukocytes, monocytes, T lymphocytes ($CD4^+$ and $CD8^+$), and B lymphocytes (111). Thus, HCMV is a systemic infection. As described above, this ability to replicate in multiple tissues is consistent with the presence of many isoforms of transactivating proteins potentially able to function in many cell types. However, it is not consistent with the restricted range of cell types that can be infected in vitro. The latter finding is probably an artifact resulting from the inability to propagate and maintain in the laboratory the fully differentiated cells preferred by HCMV. An incubation period of 4 to 8 weeks can be estimated from four distinct informative clinical settings. They are perinatal infection, transmission by organ allograft, transmission by blood transfusion, and intrauterine transmission following primary infection in the mother.

TABLE 4 Site of HCMV detection by cell culture in 47 AIDS patient autopsies[a]

Site	No. (%) of cases
Esophagus	3 (6)
Stomach	3 (6)
Small bowel	5 (11)
Large bowel	7 (15)
Liver	6 (13)
Pancreas	3 (6)
Spleen	2 (4)
Trachea	4 (9)
Lung	19 (40)
Heart	5 (11)
Adrenal	17 (36)
Thyroid	4 (9)
Salivary gland	6 (13)
Brain	8 (17)
Spinal cord	1 (2)
Ganglion	2 (4)

[a] Reprinted from reference 123 with permission.

Factors in Disease Production

Primary Infection

Infection in an immunologically unprimed individual represents the greatest risk of disease in pregnant women (60) and recipients of solid-organ transplants (78), but this effect is not absolute. Some patients with primary infection do not have disease, whereas some with reinfection get disease. HCMV reinfection of seropositive renal transplant patients represents more of a risk for disease than reactivation of latent virus (78). In contrast to the case with solid-organ recipients, reactivation represents the major source of HCMV disease in bone marrow transplant patients (174). Likewise, HIV-positive patients rarely experience primary HCMV infection; their disease results from either reactivation of latent infection or reinfection.

Viremia

In recipients of solid-organ transplants or bone marrow, the detection of active infection in saliva or urine using conventional cell culture or PCR has a relative risk of approximately 2 for future HCMV disease (170). In contrast, the detection of HCMV in the blood has a relative risk of 5 to 7, irrespective of methods of detection employed (170). This provides the scientific basis for administering antiviral drugs to patients with active HCMV infection before they develop symptoms. For patients with viremia, the term preemptive therapy is used, whereas the term suppression has been used for those with viruria. Viremia is not an absolute marker of disease but has a strong positive predictive value (Table 5). Presumably, viremia indicates that innate immune responses at local sites of infection have been inadequate. Viremia allows HCMV to seed multiple organs, but some transplant patients can presumably mount adequate regional innate or adaptive responses to prevent HCMV disease. This high risk for HCMV disease indicates that preemptive therapy should be considered in patients with viremia (135). Note that in the special case of HCMV pneumonitis in transplant patients, especially bone marrow transplant patients, the HCMV immune response contributes to disease (i.e., HCMV pneumonitis may be an immunopathological condition that, once initiated, does not respond well to effective anti-HCMV therapy) (79). Nevertheless, the incidence of such disease can be reduced significantly if antiviral therapy is given as suppression (67), preemptively (139), or as prophylaxis (126). This emphasizes the importance of targeting of antiviral drugs at the earliest possible stage of infection, rather than when the patient has disease.

Virus Load

In 1975, Stagno and colleagues (152) showed that among neonates with congenital HCMV, the titer of viruria was

TABLE 5 Comparison of PCR and culture for 150 immunocompromised patients[a]

Assay	Value in blood[b]				
	Sensitivity	Specificity	PPV	NPV	RR
Culture	0.26	0.93	0.5	0.82	3.4
PCR	0.8	0.86	0.62	0.94	5.84

[a] Reprinted from reference 94 with permission of Lippincott Williams & Wilkins.

[b] PPV, positive predictive value; NPV, negative predictive value; RR, relative risk.

significantly increased among those with disease or those destined to develop disease (Fig. 6). The kidney is not a target organ for HCMV disease in neonates, so the quantity of viruria presumably reflects systemic infection in which viral production in the kidney acts as a marker for replication in the target organs, which are less clinically accessible (brain and inner ear) (76). In the case of the neonate, this observation is even more remarkable, given that the urine is sampled after birth, yet infection may have occurred months earlier in utero (60). Nevertheless, by 3 months of age, the significant difference between viral loads in the two groups of neonates is no longer present (152), presumably reflecting the ability of the neonate's immune response to control active replication.

The advent of PCR has enabled greater sensitivity of detection of HCMV to be achieved, and quantitative-competitive PCR or quantification by real-time PCR can be used to determine HCMV load and thereby gain insight into HCMV pathogenesis in transplant patients (61). For example, in renal transplant patients, the peak level of viruria and risk of HCMV disease are clearly related ($P < 0.01$) (Fig. 7). The difference between the median values in those with and without disease is approximately 2 logs, very similar to the difference found in the neonates using cell culture methods (152). Among three factors associated with HCMV disease (i.e., high viral load, viremia, and recipient serostatus), only viral load remains a significant independent risk factor in a multivariate model (Table 6). Furthermore, a plot of peak viral load against the probability of HCMV disease has a sigmoidal shape (Fig. 8), showing that HCMV infection is well tolerated clinically until very high levels are reached. Viral load measurements in stored neonatal dried blood spots from children who subsequently developed hearing loss have also confirmed the threshold relationship (168). This sigmoidal relationship suggests that antiviral interventions and vaccination strategies should be designed to prevent viral loads rising into the critical high range of $>10^3$ to 10^4 genomes/ml of whole blood (or 10^2 genomes/semicircle of dried blood spot). Furthermore, the shape of the curve implies that a marked effect on HCMV disease could be achieved with a modest reduction in peak viral load. In AIDS Clinical Trials Group protocol 204, in which 1,227 AIDS patients were randomized to receive valacyclovir at 2 g daily or one

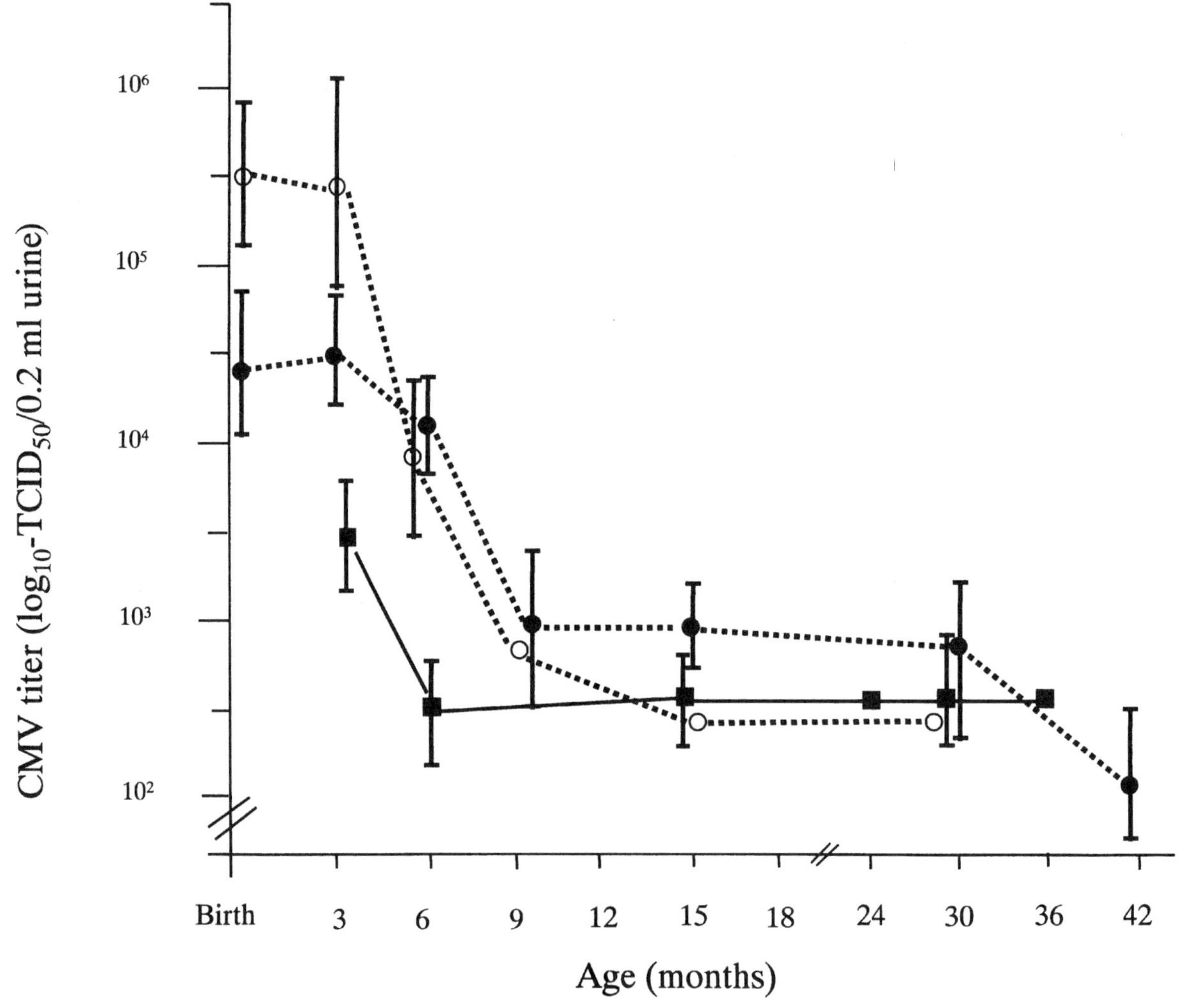

FIGURE 6 CMV load in the urine of neonates. $TCID_{50}$, 50% tissue culture infective dose. Symbols: ○, symptomatic congenital infection; ●, asymptomatic; ■, natal infection. Error bars indicate standard errors of the means.

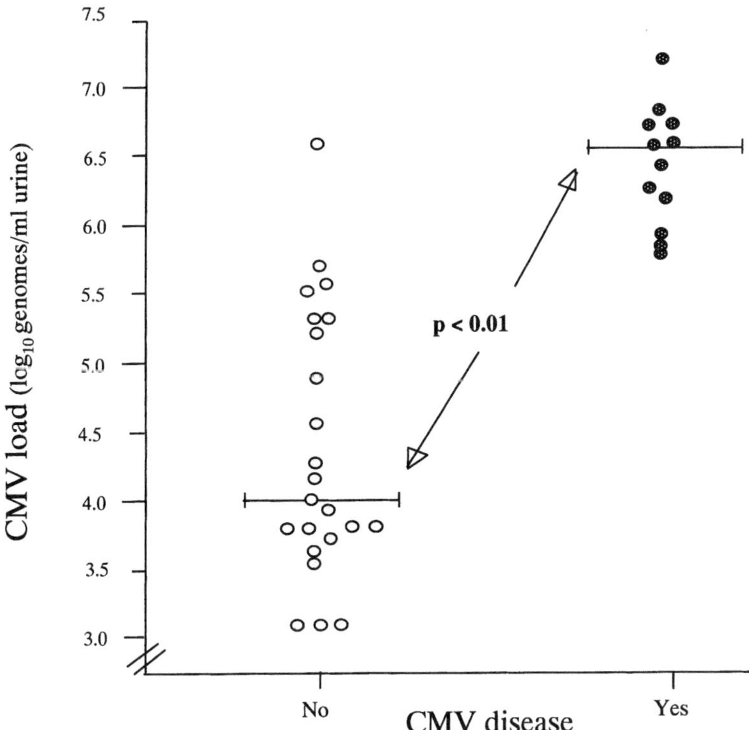

FIGURE 7 CMV load in the urine of renal transplant recipients.

of two doses of acyclovir, the higher of which had been shown to be ineffective in controlling HCMV disease, it was found that valacyclovir significantly reduced HCMV disease despite a relatively modest reduction in HCMV load from baseline (median, 1.3 logs) (55). The serial measures of virus load in blood have also revealed the dynamic process of HCMV replication in its host, with an average doubling time (viral load increasing) or half-life (viral load decreasing) of approximately 1 day (53). Furthermore, serial measures of viral load can provide estimates of the efficacy of antiviral drugs, such as ganciclovir, required to bring HCMV replication under control (54).

Imbalance between the rate of production of HCMV at sites of infection and its effective rate of immune clearance may produce viremia. Subsequently, viremia seeds target organs, which may or may not have sufficient local defenses to prevent viral disease. The amount of HCMV required to cause disease is predicted to vary considerably, depending on the precise details of the pathogenic mechanisms. Thus, immunopathology may be triggered at low viral loads but remain present at high loads. Moderate loads may cause disease through cell lysis secondary to viral replication. Finally, very high viral loads might damage target cells when HCMV binds to them, a process we term direct toxicity. This hypothetical scenario will become increasingly susceptible to investigation using measures of viral dynamics. Because HCMV DNA can also be detected in the plasma of patients (149), it will be important to determine if plasma viremia marks a distinct phase of pathogenesis.

Differences among Groups of Immunocompromised Patients

Table 7 provides an overview of the relative importance of HCMV disease in different patient groups. The phrase "HCMV infection in the immunocompromised host" obscures the great diversity among the various patient groups. The pathogenesis of bone marrow failure after bone marrow transplantation is thought to follow HCMV infection of stromal cells releasing cytokines and so producing a milieu unfavorable for hematopoiesis (7).

TABLE 6 Univariate and multivariate assessment of prognostic factors for HCMV disease in renal allograft recipients[a]

Parameter	Univariate[b] factor			Multivariate[b] factor		
	OR	95% CI	*P*	OR	95% CI	*P*
Viral load (per 0.25 log)	2.79	1.22–6.39	0.02	2.77	1.07–7.18	0.04
Viremia	23.75	3.69–153	0.0009	34.54	0.75–1599	0.07
R^+ serostatus	0.22	0.05–0.95	0.05	0.92	0.002–446	0.98

[a] Reprinted from reference 39 with permission of Wiley-Liss, Inc., a subsidiary of John Wiley & Sons, Inc. The results demonstrate that virus load is a major determinant of disease and that viremia and recipient serostatus are markers of disease because of their statistical association with high viral load.

[b] OR, odds ratio; CI, confidence interval.

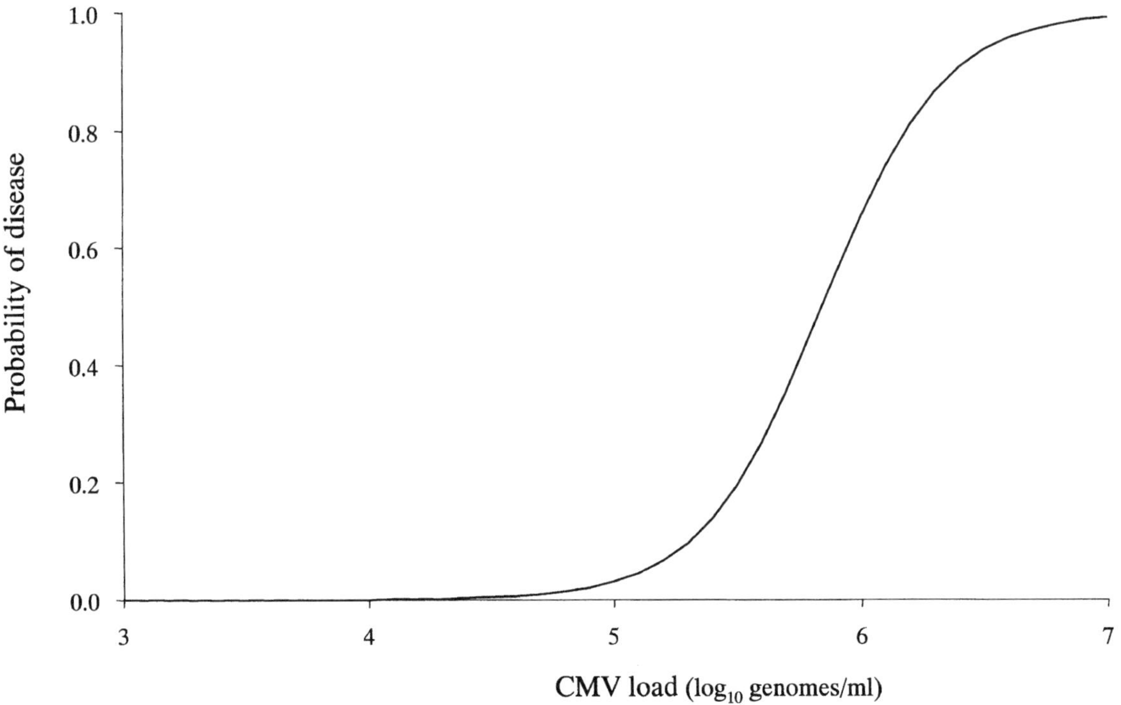

FIGURE 8 Threshold concept of CMV pathogenesis.

CMV Pneumonitis

HCMV pneumonitis after bone marrow transplantation may be immunopathologically mediated (79). This hypothesis explains the timing of pneumonitis, because it only occurs once patients have engrafted their bone marrow, arguing that a host immune response is required for disease. It also explains why AIDS patients do not appear to suffer from HCMV pneumonitis, although HCMV is frequently found in their lungs. Presumably, they cannot mount the immunopathological response required to cause disease. Patients with HIV seroconversion illness may, however, get HCMV pneumonitis, presumably because their cell-mediated immune response has not been sufficiently abrogated at this stage (151). The precise nature of the immunopathological response has not been identified, although the histologic appearance (Fig. 9) suggests that it is probably mediated by cytokines attracting leukocytes to the lung interstitium and so increasing the distance required for gas diffusion from alveoli to blood. If so, it is perhaps surprising that cases of HCMV pneumonitis have not been seen in patients given highly active antiretroviral therapy (HAART), in whom the regenerating immune system could recognize HCMV-infected target cells and trigger immunopathology. Perhaps HAART provides protective cell-mediated immune responses able to control HCMV in the lungs.

TABLE 7 HCMV diseases in immunocompromised persons

Symptom	Symptom in patients with[a]:		
	Solid-organ transplant	Bone marrow transplant	AIDS
Direct effects			
Fever/hepatitis	++	+	+
Gastrointestinal	+	+	+
Retinitis	+	+	++
Pneumonitis	+	++	
Myelosuppression		+	
Encephalopathy			+
Polyradiculopathy			+
Addisonian			+
Indirect effects			
Immunosuppression	+		
Rejection/GVHD	+	?	
Atherosclerosis	+		
Death		+	+

[a] +, symptom occurs; ++, symptom most common.

CMV Retinitis

The dramatically increased proportion of HCMV retinitis found in AIDS patients compared to transplant patients remains unexplained but may result from prolonged exposure to high levels of viremia. Another new disease has occurred in AIDS patients given HAART which has all the hallmarks of immunopathology. Patients with a history of HCMV retinitis, which is typically now clinically silent, can nevertheless develop an inflammatory vitritis due to the infiltration of $CD8^+$ T cells specific for HCMV. Usually, vitreous fluid does not contain viral DNA detectable by PCR, implying that these CD8 cells do not recognize HCMV virions.

CMV Encephalitis

In AIDS patients, viremia can disseminate HCMV to the brain in two distinct ways. The first seeds virus to the brain endothelial cells, allowing HCMV to spread to contiguous astrocytes and then to neurons. The histopathologic cor-

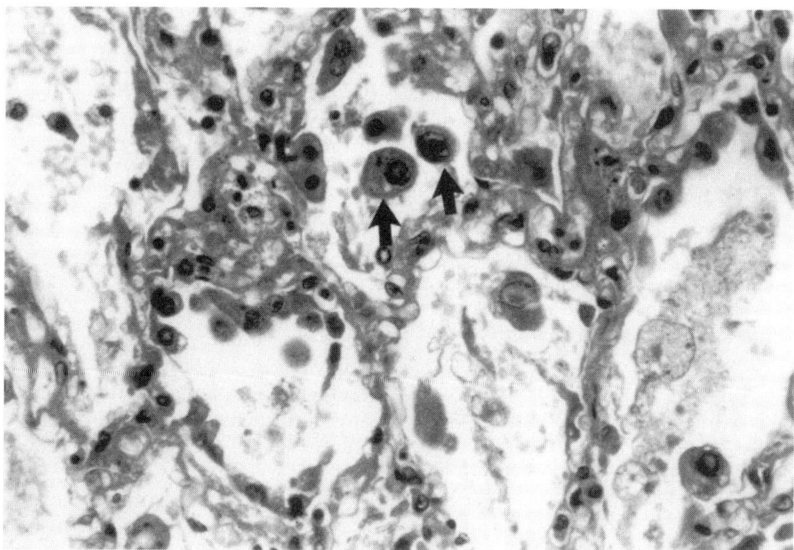

FIGURE 9 Histologic section of a lung sample from a patient with HCMV pneumonitis following bone marrow transplantation. Arrows show alveolar macrophages bearing the typical intranuclear inclusions of HCMV. An interstitial mononuclear cell infiltrate is seen. (Courtesy of J. E. McLoughlin [from a patient under the care of H. G. Prentice, Royal Free and University College Medical School].)

relates of this route of infection include endothelial cell infection, with or without thrombosis, and multiple areas of glial nodular encephalitis (167). The second seeds virus to the choroid plexus epithelial cells and thence to the cerebrospinal fluid (CSF). Transmission to ependymal surfaces produces necrotizing ventricular encephalitis.

CMV Polyradiculopathy

Viremic dissemination seeds CMV to peripheral nerves and the cauda equina.

Other Syndromes

In addition to these EODs, HCMV is associated with a variety of conditions, collectively called indirect effects (136). Although HCMV has been shown for many years to be associated with these conditions, it is only recently that the results of controlled clinical trials have demonstrated that the associations are causal. The precise mechanisms whereby HCMV causes these effects have not been demonstrated, although there are several candidates, not least of which is the possibility that HCMV perturbs normal immune functions. In addition, in the case of graft rejection, HCMV may act like a minor transplantation antigen, may up-regulate cellular class I molecules bearing donor epitopes in adjacent noninfected cells, or may express the UL18 class I homolog. Fungal superinfections may reflect HCMV-induced immunosuppression, although there is no immunologic marker of this. Finally, HCMV may trigger post-cardiac allograft coronary atherosclerosis because (i) pUS28 confers chemotactic mobility on smooth muscle cells; (ii) IE72 binds p53 in the same cells, preventing their apoptosis; or (iii) HCMV activates cyclooxygenase, so producing reactive lipoprotein peroxides.

In AIDS patients, clinically silent HCMV infection may similarly interact in multiple ways with HIV to increase its pathogenicity (i.e., act as a cofactor for progression of HIV disease) (71). This subject is controversial but is supported by data showing that HCMV can transactivate the HIV long terminal repeat in vitro and can provide an alternative receptor for HIV by inducing an Fc receptor (108). HCMV is widely disseminated at autopsy, being found in most tissues (Table 4). HCMV-HIV coinfection of individual cells or organs has also been described. The risk of AIDS is increased among male homosexuals with persistent HCMV excretion in semen, even after allowing for differences in baseline CD4 counts (44). Cohorts of patients develop AIDS more rapidly if they are coinfected with HCMV. Furthermore, high levels of HCMV viremia are significantly associated with the death of AIDS patients (26). This effect is stronger than the association of HIV viral load with death (148) and persists in the era of HAART (43). Patients given intraocular treatment for HCMV retinitis had a survival benefit if they were also given systemic treatment (91). Overall, it is difficult to avoid the conclusion that HCMV adversely affects the outcome in AIDS patients but that this effect is clinically inapparent and can only be documented by appropriate laboratory studies. Overall, while these results are consistent with the possibility that HCMV may play a cofactor role, extensive controlled investigations would be required to establish this conclusively.

Immune Responses

The major targets for CD8 T cells against HCMV are ppUL83 (pp65) and the IE2 protein. However, many epitopes of HCMV are recognized by the host, so the human immune system commits more resources to controlling HCMV than to controlling any other virus (158). Using conventional limiting dilutional analysis, frequencies of CD8 T cells against pp65 were approximately 1:5,000, but more recent measurements of responding CD8 T cells show that the frequency of CD8 T cells against HCMV is much higher than previously thought. For example, using class I HLA tetramers in immunocompetent and immunocompromised patients with or without active replication, frequencies of CD8 T cells against epitopes within pp65 comprise approximately 1% in healthy seropositive individuals and up to 10% in patients experiencing active HCMV replication (57).

Prior exposure to HCMV can ameliorate the pathological potential of HCMV in some, but not all, patients. In pregnant women, the risk of damage to the fetus and the severity of that damage are clearly decreased in women who were "immune" before they became pregnant (59), suggesting that prior immunity in the mother can reduce the inoculum of HCMV received by the fetus. In women experiencing primary infection during pregnancy, an increased titer of neutralizing antibody and its avidity correlate with reduced risk of disease in the neonate (19).

The results for bone marrow transplant patients are distinct because reactivation of the recipient virus represents the source of HCMV-causing disease. Nevertheless, among seropositive recipients, those receiving marrow from immune donors have a reduced risk of disease (77). Direct evidence for adoptive transfer of immunity from the donor into the recipient was found by immunizing donors or recipients (or both, or neither) with tetanus toxoid (172). Note that this beneficial effect of donor seropositivity is not seen unless the donor is depleted of mature T cells as prophylaxis against graft-versus-host disease (GVHD). Without this manipulation, the donor marrow may be a source of HCMV infection, as is donor blood. This observation suggests two conclusions: first, the marrow cells that contain HCMV are removed by the process of T-cell depletion, and second, the adoptive transfer is of non-T origin. Although cell-mediated immunity is clearly the major response capable of containing HCMV infection, the possibility that HCMV disease may be controlled by other responses such as humoral immunity has been incompletely investigated. A threshold effect for the quantity of HCMV required to cause disease in renal transplant patients (Fig. 8) could explain these findings in bone marrow transplant patients. Humoral immunity could reduce the level of HCMV replication and reduce disease without being able to eliminate infection entirely. Humoral immune responses are directed against multiple CMV proteins, including surface glycoproteins, phosphoproteins of the tegument, and structural proteins of the capsid. Much of the antibody which neutralizes infectivity in vitro can be absorbed from sera with recombinant soluble gB, showing that this is the major target of the neutralizing response, but additional neutralizing epitopes are also found on gH, gL, and gN.

CLINICAL MANIFESTATIONS

Congenital Infection

Results from a recent systematic review of published prospective case series are discussed in this section (47). A total of 12.7% of congenitally infected babies are born with "cytomegalic inclusion disease" (Table 8). The remaining 87.3% appear to be normal at birth, but a proportion are found to have developed sequelae on follow-up as described below.

In those symptomatic at birth, most of the non-central nervous system (non-CNS) disease is self-limiting, although severe thrombocytopenic purpura, hepatitis, pneumonitis, and myocarditis may occasionally be life threatening (Table 8). A total of 0.5% of these patients die during infancy, and 50% of the survivors have permanent serious abnormalities. Brain damage may present as microcephaly, mental retardation, spastic diplegia or seizures, and perceptual organ damage such as optic atrophy, blindness, or deafness. These abnormalities may occur alone or in combination.

TABLE 8 Clinical features of cytomegalic inclusion disease

Intrauterine growth retardation
Jaundice
Hepatosplenomegaly
Thrombocytopenia
Microcephaly
Intracranial calcifications
Retinitis

Among those asymptomatic at birth, approximately 13.5% will develop hearing defects or impaired intellectual performance (Table 9). Twice as many children who come from the group who appear to be normal at birth are ultimately damaged by congenital HCMV, compared to those born with classical symptoms. This helps to explain why the burden of disease is underestimated for this infection.

A plausible pathogenesis for progressive hearing loss is apparent from the histologic preparation of inner ear structures from a patient with a fatal case of congenital HCMV infection (Fig. 10). The virus spread by the cell-to-cell route to produce a focus of infection surrounded by inflammation. This may represent stages of the infectious process in the inner ear, explaining how progressive damage to the organ of Corti could occur.

Perinatal Infection

Neonates acquiring perinatal infection can start to excrete CMV in the urine from 3 weeks of age onwards. Most perinatally infected infants do not develop acute symptoms, although occasional cases of infantile pneumonitis develop, making HCMV a frequent pathogen in those few children presenting with an appearance of sepsis in the first 3 months of life (138). Perinatal infection may be severe in such premature neonates because they do not benefit from transplacental passage of maternal immunoglobulin G (IgG) antibodies.

Postnatal Infection

Primary infection in the immunocompetent child or adult is almost always asymptomatic, except for occasional cases

TABLE 9 Disease outcome in 1,000 babies born with congenital HCMV infection[a]

Outcome	No. (%)
Born with symptoms of CID[b]	127 (12.7%)
Die during infancy	5 (0.5%)
	122
50% Develop long-term handicap	61
Born without symptoms of CID	873
Develop handicap	118 (13.5%)
Total damaged	179 (18%)

[a] Adapted from reference 47 with permission.
[b] CID, cytomegalic inclusion disease.

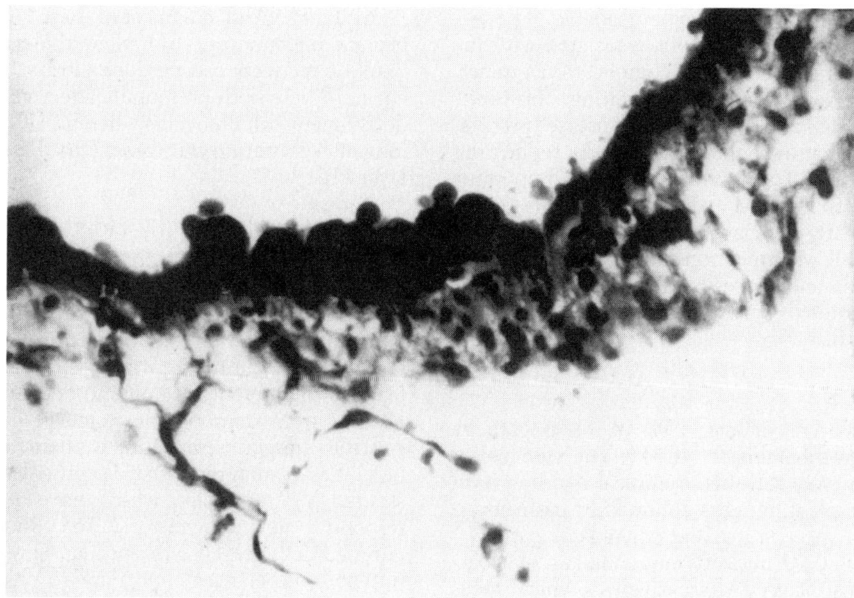

FIGURE 10 Histologic appearance of the inner ear in a patient with a fatal case of cytomegalic inclusion disease. Note the focus of large inclusion-bearing cells and accompanying inflammation. (Courtesy of S. Stagno. Reprinted from reference 71a with permission.)

of infectious mononucleosis. The patient presents with a fever with few localizing symptoms; pharyngitis, lymphadenopathy, and splenomegaly are less common than in EBV mononucleosis. Laboratory tests reveal biochemical hepatitis, with moderately raised transaminases, lymphocytosis with atypical mononuclear cells, and a negative result for heterophile agglutinins. The condition resolves spontaneously, with a mean of 19 days' fever in one large study (97). Guillain-Barré syndrome has been described as a complication of postnatal primary HCMV infection. Rare cases of CMV EOD have been described among patients who are immunocompetent, including hepatitis, gastrointestinal ulceration with or without hemorrhage, and pneumonitis. It is assumed that these individuals have received a larger-than-average inoculum of CMV to explain their severe outcome.

Immunocompromised Patients

Active HCMV infection causes a wide spectrum of disease, ranging from life threatening to asymptomatic and involving specific organs or causing constitutional disturbances. The systemic nature of HCMV infection and the factors associated with disease are described in "Pathogenesis" above.

Fever is a common component of all HCMV diseases in all immunocompromised hosts. Typically, this follows a spiking pattern, with temperatures in the range of 38 to 40°C, followed by precipitous declines below 37°C. During the fever, the patient complains of malaise and lethargy and may develop myalgia or arthralgia. This systemic phase of HCMV may resolve spontaneously or may herald particular clinical syndromes (EOD due to viremic dissemination of virus) that vary in incidence according to the underlying cause of the immunocompromised state (Table 7). The most common clinical presentations for each patient group are illustrated in Table 7, but any can occur in any patient group. HCMV disease typically manifests when the patient is most profoundly immunocompromised, that is, in the first and second months posttransplantation or, in AIDS patients, once the CD4 count has declined below 50 cells/μl. Indeed, successful institution of HAART reverses these changes and leads to immune-mediated control of HCMV viremia and prevention of EOD.

Recipients of Solid-Organ Allografts

Leukopenia is common and may be profound. If leukopenia persists, it is associated with the development of secondary fungal and bacterial infections (32). Biochemical evidence of hepatitis is often found, with transaminase levels raised two to three times the upper limit of normal. Thrombocytopenia may occur, with serial daily platelet counts below 100,000. All of these features usually respond to therapy with intravenous ganciclovir or its prodrug, valganciclovir.

Pneumonitis with interstitial infiltrates may occur, especially in recipients of lung (or heart-lung) transplants. Despite prolonged treatment, obliterative bronchiolitis may supervene (50), showing that HCMV plays an important role in the etiology of this chronic rejection process. Likewise, HCMV has been implicated in the development of accelerated atherosclerosis after cardiac transplantation (98) or graft rejection and graft atherosclerosis (49, 68). These conditions present as dysfunction of the transplanted organ with no clinical symptoms or signs to reveal the underlying contribution from HCMV. Yet, approximately 50% of acute biopsy-proven renal allograft rejections can be prevented by anti-HCMV prophylaxis with valacyclovir (101). Thus, the conventional diagnostic conundrum in the febrile allograft recipient of "rejection or HCMV" should be replaced with "rejection and HCMV."

Recipients of Bone Marrow Grafts

Pneumonitis is the major life-threatening presentation of HCMV, occurring in 10 to 20% of bone marrow allograft patients before antiviral drugs became available. The patient presents with fever and hypoxia, associated with interstitial infiltrates of the lung. This complication is much less common (less than 5%) after autografting, consistent with a postulated immunopathological disease process. HCMV may delay marrow engraftment (7) by replicating in bone marrow stromal supporting cells. An important clinical feature is that HCMV disease, especially pneumonitis, is statistically associated with GVHD (23). It is not clear whether HCMV infection can precipitate GVHD or whether the immunosuppressive nature of GVHD, or the treatment required for its suppression, facilitates HCMV reactivation.

Patients with AIDS

In the pre-HAART era, at least 25% of AIDS patients developed disease attributable to HCMV. The vast majority (85%) of cases were retinitis, a clinical manifestation that is rare in transplant patients, followed by gastrointestinal involvement, encephalitis, and polyradiculopathy.

The patient with CMV retinitis may complain of "floaters" or loss of visual acuity. Alternatively, a typical focus of retinitis may be recognized at routine follow-up visits. Early lesions may be white due to edema, necrosis, or both (see figures in chapter 10). Without treatment, the focus of infection spreads to involve neighboring cells (25), leaving white necrosis at the advancing border. There is hemorrhage, often flame shaped, surrounding blood vessels, with or without perivascular sheathing. It may be accompanied by anterior uveitis, retinal edema, or retinal detachment (161).

HCMV may also involve the gastrointestinal tract to cause ulcers deep in the submucosal layers. Clinical features vary with the anatomic site involved. Odynophagia is a common presentation of HCMV esophagitis, whereas abdominal pain and hematochezia frequently occur with HCMV colitis. Ulceration at these sites may cause perforation or hemorrhage.

HCMV causes encephalitis of two types in AIDS patients that mirror the pathology described above. The first is difficult to differentiate clinically from HIV dementia and manifests as subacute or chronic symptoms of confusion and disorientation attributable to cortical involvement. Focal signs can be attributed to lesions in the brain stem. The second manifests as defects in cranial nerves, nystagmus, and increasing ventricular size (89), which progress rapidly to a fatal outcome.

HCMV also causes polyradiculopathy. Patients subacutely present with weakness of legs and numbness, progressing to flacid paraparesis, often with pain in the legs and perineum, bladder dysfunction, or both. The CSF shows a remarkable preponderance of polymorphonuclear leukocytes.

In the HAART era, most of these HCMV diseases have become uncommon (161). Nevertheless, HAART-induced immune recovery can produce vitritis and cystoid macular edema. These both profoundly affect vision, as does retinal detachment, which occurs when an HCMV-infected retina loses its substratum attachment to the underlying choroid layer (161).

The Apparently Healthy Elderly

Immunosenescence is a major underlying contributor to morbidity and mortality (reviewed in reference 156). Immunosenescence is significantly increased in elderly patients with HCMV antibodies compared to HCMV-seronegative controls, although there are no clinical features to differentiate immunosenescence associated with HCMV from immunosenescence in HCMV-seronegative controls. Immunosenescence is characterized by an excess of clones of differentiated T cells, detected by their restricted Vβ repertoire, which have a reduced ability to respond to new antigens. (92, 163). Many clones of differentiated cells are HCMV specific, have an activated phenotype, and so may contribute to chronic inflammatory conditions, including atherosclerosis, potentially explaining why HCMV antibodies represent a significant risk factor for imminent death in the elderly (156). Direct evidence for the adverse functional consequences of HCMV-associated immunosenescence includes the fact that HCMV-seropositive persons aged 65 to 99 were less likely to produce a fourfold rise in hemagglutination-inhibiting antibodies to influenza virus when given influenza vaccine than were HCMV-seronegative individuals (163).

LABORATORY DIAGNOSIS

Detection of Virus

The characteristics of the assays used frequently in the identification of active HCMV infection vary widely among laboratories (Table 10). While the precise methodological details vary, all diagnostic virology laboratories should offer a service for rapid HCMV detection. The clinician should inquire about the positive and negative predictive values of particular tests and whether day-to-day results have been audited to ensure that appropriate targets are achieved.

Selection of Sites for Examination

Urine or saliva samples are usually collected to diagnose congenital or perinatal infection. If lumbar puncture or liver biopsy is indicated clinically, then samples can be processed, but the detection of HCMV at these sites does not have prognostic value for these children.

TABLE 10 HCMV detection in body fluids

Method	Sensitivity	Specificity	Reliability	Rapidity	Proven prognostic value
Conventional cell culture	++	+++	++		+
Detection of early-antigen fluorescent foci (shell vial)	+	+++	++	+	+
Antigenemia	++	+++	++	++	++
PCR	+++	+++	++	+	+++

For adults with mononucleosis or hepatitis, urine and blood are the best samples. HCMV viruria might be coincidental, but the detection of viremia strongly supports the diagnosis. Pregnant women with symptoms should be investigated as for other adults. The investigation of asymptomatic women has not been shown to identify those who will have babies with congenital infection and so is not recommended.

Transplant patients should have surveillance samples of blood taken at least weekly from the time of transplantation. In the past, urine and saliva samples were also collected, but this has been superseded by assays using blood. Whole blood is the most sensitive for PCR (129). HCMV excretion from urine and saliva is very common but only doubles the relative risk for future disease. In contrast, viremia is detected less frequently in allograft patients but increases the relative risk to about 6 (Table 5). These different risks are used to define distinct treatment strategies discussed below.

Patients who are HIV positive follow the same basic principles of HCMV natural history in the pre-HAART era, and these principles may become relevant again as individuals start to exhaust the salvage antiretroviral options in the post-HAART era. Individual AIDS patients with suspected CMV infection can be investigated for CMV viremia and by examining CSF by PCR when encephalitis or polyradiculopathy is suspected.

Laboratory Assays

Real-time PCR has become the new "gold standard" for detection of HCMV, in part because cell culture results can be misleading (Table 11).

PCR

Because HCMV persists for the lifetime of infected individuals, a very sensitive technique such as nested PCR could potentially detect latent HCMV or virus that was replicating at such a low level that it had no clinical consequences. Four approaches have been taken to avoid this disadvantage.

Minimization of Latent Viral DNA Detection

A non-nested PCR method with high sensitivity but only using a small quantity of sample nucleic acid for analysis (i.e., 5 μl of urine or 30 ng of DNA from peripheral whole blood) has correlated well with conventional cell culture and provided useful prognostic information (Table 5) (94). In practice, the presence of two consecutive positive PCR results has been used to identify high-risk patients.

Plasma PCR

Because the latent DNA of HCMV persists in the cellular fraction of blood, the detection of HCMV DNA in plasma should reflect active infection (149). An FDA-approved commercial assay is now available (Roche Amplicor).

RT-PCR and NASBA

Reverse transcription-PCR (RT-PCR) should detect only cells in which HCMV is replicating, since the target is mRNA. A nucleic acid sequence-based amplification NASBA assay for the detection of a late gene transcript (pp67) appears to be sensitive and specific and is available commercially (Biomerieux Nuclisens). However, there is no evidence that this assay offers any advantages over standard PCR.

Real-Time PCR

With the advent of Taqman and related technologies, it is now possible to offer assessments of HCMV load in real time. While such assays usually do not incorporate quantitative-competitive formats to identify possible inhibitors of PCR in the clinical sample, the results represent an important contribution toward controlling HCMV disease. The viral load found in the first available sample correlates with the peak viral load (56). The rate of increase in viral load can be estimated by back-projecting from the initial load to the last available PCR-negative sample from that patient. In multivariate models, the parameters of initial viral load and rate of increase are independent of each other, so both parameters can be used in combination to estimate an individual's risk of future HCMV disease (56). Serial results from real-time PCR are frequently used to decide when to initiate preemptive therapy and to monitor the response to this treatment.

In addition to testing blood, PCR has become invaluable for the investigation of CNS involvement in AIDS patients. A very sensitive nested PCR is required because the amount of HCMV DNA in the CSF is small.

Antigenemia

Monoclonal antibodies can be used to detect HCMV antigens directly in leukocytes from the blood of immunocompromised patients. The monoclonal antibodies react with pp65, the product of UL83. These monoclonal anti-

TABLE 11 Misleading concepts about HCMV derived from propagation of the virus in fibroblast cultures

Concept	Fact	Reference(s)
In vitro strains are genetically representative of those found in vivo	Strain Ad169 has 22 missing ORFs; Towne has 19 missing ORFs	31
A live attenuated vaccine can be prepared in fibroblasts	No protection against HCMV infection from Towne strain, although severity of disease is reduced	125
In vitro assays correctly identify the susceptibility of HCMV to antivirals	Failed to detect clinically important susceptibility to acyclovir	12, 101, 104
HCMV is a slowly replicating virus	HCMV replicates rapidly	53
Strains of HCMV resistant to ganciclovir occur infrequently in immunocompromised patients	Resistance is more common; cell cultures select against detection of resistant strains	54

bodies stain polymorphonuclear cells, monocytes, and endothelial cells from the peripheral circulation. The advantages of this technique are that it takes only a few hours and does not require facilities for cell culture or for PCR. The disadvantages are that it is subjective and samples can deteriorate rapidly. The antigenemia assay is therefore used by laboratories situated close to clinical facilities. It is possible to count the stained cells to provide a semiquantitative assessment of viral load. In general, antigenemia is being replaced by real-time PCR in many laboratories.

Histopathology

Biopsies are often taken to confirm organ involvement. HCMV is recognized by its characteristic intranuclear "owl's eye" inclusions, which have a surrounding halo and marginated chromatin. They occur in kidney tubules, bile ducts, lung and liver parenchyma, and the gut, inner ear, and salivary gland but are less prominent in brain tissue (Fig. 9 and 10). Cytoplasmic inclusions can also be seen in infected cells, particularly when stained with CMV-specific monoclonal antibodies. Histopathology provides a specific diagnosis which is insensitive (Fig. 11) compared to viral load measurements made by PCR in the same organs (107).

Virus Isolation

Human fibroblasts (typically from foreskins or embryo lungs) are used to support HCMV replication in vitro. For the detection of viremia, buffy coat or unseparated heparinized blood can be inoculated into cell cultures. If toxicity is observed, denuded areas of the monolayer can be repaired by the addition of fresh fibroblasts.

All cultures should be observed at least twice weekly for the typical focal CPE of HCMV (Fig. 12). Occasionally, urine samples from patients with congenital infection produce widespread CPE within 24 to 48 h that resembles that of HSV. More usually, the CPE evolves only slowly, typically becoming apparent at 14 to 16 days, so the cultures must be maintained for a minimum of 21 days before being reported as negative.

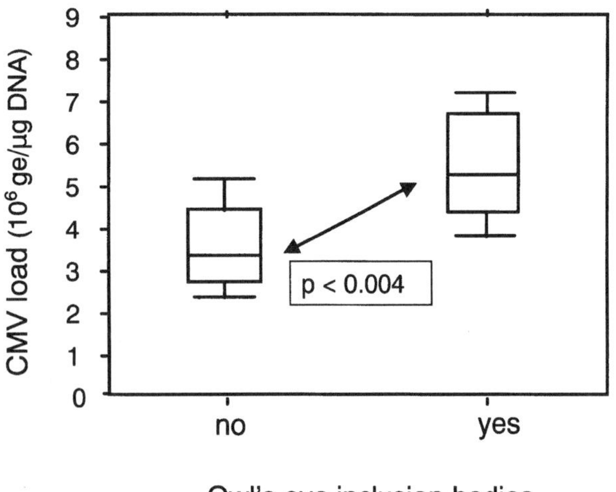

FIGURE 11 Correlation between high HCMV load and detection of intranuclear inclusions. ge, genomes.

The advent of monoclonal antibodies against the major IE and other E proteins of HCMV provided reagents that could be used to detect the virus in cell cultures within 48 h before CPE had become apparent. Two techniques were developed independently in the United States and in the United Kingdom; the former (65) was termed the shell vial assay (after the name of the container), and the latter (75) was termed the DEAFF test (for detection of early antigen fluorescent foci). Although not as sensitive as conventional cell culture, these assays were a great improvement in their day due to the rapid availability of results but have now been replaced by real-time PCR (see above) for testing surveillance samples.

Serologic Assays

IgG Antibody as a Marker of Past Infection

Many assays can detect HCMV IgG antibodies. The presence of IgG antibodies against HCMV is indicative of infection sometime in the past. Because the seropositive individual is liable to experience reactivations of his or her latent infection, the presence of IgG antibodies against HCMV is a marker of potential infectivity; however, immunologic responses do not imply complete protection from endogenous or exogenous infection.

IgG Antibody as a Marker of Recent Infection

IgG antibody detection may be used to identify infections in populations, such as pregnant women, in whom the availability of avidity assays offers a practical way of detecting asymptomatic primary HCMV infections. Typically, it takes 16 to 20 weeks for IgG avidity to mature to high levels, and the reproducibility and specificity of the commercial assays appear to be superior to those of IgM assays. For pregnant women found on routine screening to be IgM positive, avidity assays can be used to triage them into groups with primary infection or recurrent infection and so reduce the number of terminations of pregnancy that might be undertaken based on the results of IgM testing alone (81).

To detect serologic responses due to native virus infection after immunization with candidate vaccines, sera can be preabsorbed with the immunogen to ensure that responses to this component of the vaccine are not mistaken for seroconversion (178).

Immunocompromised patients most at risk of HCMV disease may be those least able to mount prompt immune responses. In addition, false-positive *interpretations* are frequently seen when patients receive blood or blood products. Note that these are not false-positive *reactions*, as the patients do truly have HCMV IgG antibodies in their blood but these have come from an exogenous source. Thus, serial serologic testing is not recommended for monitoring individual immunocompromised patients; instead, rapid tests for virus should be used to allow the option of antiviral chemotherapy to be considered.

IgM Antibody as a Marker of Current Infection

IgM antibodies can also be used to detect infection in immunocompetent patients such as those with HCMV mononucleosis, but this approach is not recommended for the immunocompromised individual, in whom rapid detection of CMV is preferred.

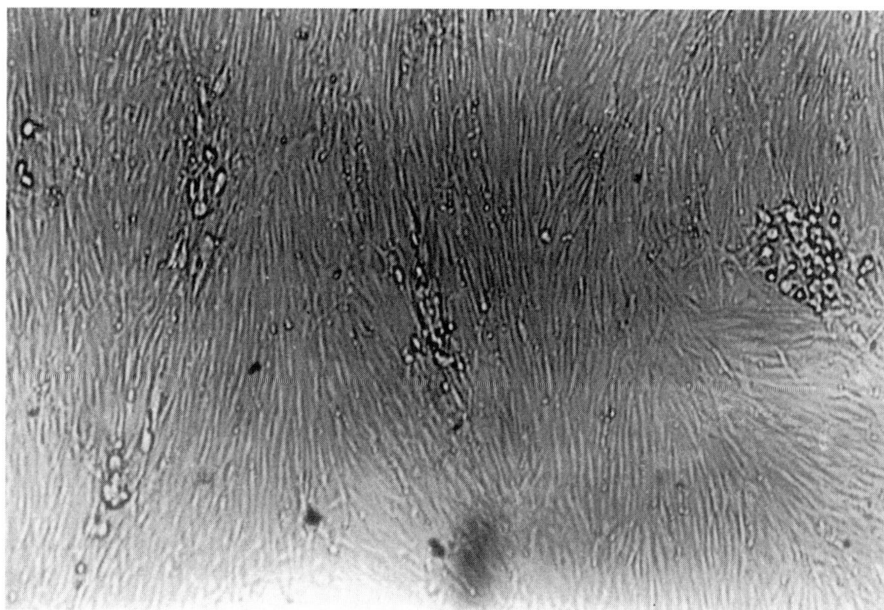

FIGURE 12 Photograph of human embryonic lung fibroblasts showing the focal CPE of HCMV. (Figure prepared by J. A. Bishop.)

PREVENTION

HCMV infection can be prevented in some patients by screening of blood products. Blood from donors who are seronegative should ideally be used for intrauterine transfusion, for pregnant women, and for immunocompromised patients, irrespective of whether the recipients are CMV seronegative or seropositive. Because such blood is in short supply, an alternative is to pass the blood through in-line filters capable of retaining leukocytes (63).

In the solid-organ transplantation setting, HCMV disease could be potentially reduced by matching donors and recipients, so that organs from seropositive donors are not given to seronegative recipients. However, in practice, this would reduce the likelihood of achieving the best available HLA match and would delay transplants for many recipients whose medical condition may deteriorate while they wait for a seronegative donor. Furthermore, because donor organs are in such short supply, there is pressure not to reject donations unless absolutely necessary. As a result, donor-recipient matching is generally required only by some centers where the risk for HCMV disease is considered especially high, such as for seropositive donors of lungs destined for seronegative recipients. In the remaining patients, various strategies with antiviral drugs can be employed to reduce HCMV disease.

Active Immunization

Pioneering work with live attenuated vaccine strains by Plotkin and colleagues showed in volunteers that the Towne strain was truly attenuated compared to the virulent Toledo strain. A controlled trial in dialysis patients who were candidates for renal transplantation showed no reduction in the proportions of patients who became infected or ill due to CMV after transplantation, but the trial demonstrated a significant reduction in the severity of disease (125). The Towne vaccine did not provide protection against primary infection in parents of children attending day care centers (3). Overall, the effects seen were not sufficiently encouraging to allow further development of this vaccine but provided a useful framework for the evaluation of future preparations. Phase I studies are underway to administer Towne vaccine together with IL-12 as a way of improving immunogenicity. The Towne strain of HCMV lacks 19 genes found in strain Toledo (31), and it is possible that some of these genes could provide protection against wild-type HCMV if they were incorporated into a vaccine. Accordingly, recombinants between Towne and Toledo have been prepared which include all 19 genes incorporated into the Towne attenuated background. Vaccine candidates have shown safety and immunogenicity in a phase I study but are no longer in development.

Recombinant vaccines based upon gB have been developed. This protein was chosen because it can adsorb most of the neutralizing antibody from sera and also contains T-helper epitopes. Cells infected with a vaccinia virus gB recombinant adsorb between 40 and 88% of the total serum neutralizing activity in individuals who are either naturally immune or vaccinated with the Towne vaccine strain of HCMV. Purified and recombinant preparations of gB induce humoral immunity in experimental animals and can reduce the fetal loss and congenital infection which results from inoculation of guinea pig HCMV. Antibodies generated by Towne gB cloned into an adenovirus 5 vector under the control of the adenovirus E3 promoter correlate significantly with serum neutralizing activity in hamsters. Intranasal inoculation of hamsters induced antibodies that neutralized HCMV in vitro.

gB also possesses T-helper epitopes, although humans of particular HLA types have been shown to be low responders. A canarypox virus vector that incorporates the ppUL83 (pp65) gene, which is the major target for cell-mediated T-cytotoxic responses, was immunogenic in phase I studies, although no humoral immunity was induced. A DNA vaccine containing gB and ppUL83 (pp65) has been used in mice and shown to elicit good antibody levels and CTLs against ppUL83. Phase I trials of a DNA

TABLE 12 Vaccine candidates studied clinically

Preparation	Type	Status
Towne	Live attenuated	Development continuing with prime-boost using DNA plasmids
gB	Soluble recombinant	Phase II
Towne/Toledo recombinant	Live attenuated	Phase I; discontinued
Canarypox virus pp65	Live, single cycle, heterologous	Phase I
pp65, gB	DNA plasmids	Phase I
Alphavax	Live, single cycle, heterologous	Phase I

vaccine for HCMV in humans provide evidence of priming of the immune system. An alphavirus recombinant expressing gB has been shown to be well tolerated and immunogenic in a phase I study (Table 12).

Most clinical experience to date has been with a truncated form of gB expressed in mammalian cells and used to immunize volunteers in phase I and phase II studies. This prototype vaccine was immunogenic in seronegative healthy volunteers and induced neutralizing antibody titers greater than those found in seropositive persons (119). The novel adjuvant MF59 gave antibody titers superior to those obtained with the conventional adjuvant, alum, and the optimum immunization schedule was to give vaccine at 0, 1, and 6 months (119). Although antibody levels declined with time after this primary course of three vaccine doses, a prompt anamnestic response to a booster dose given at 12 months was seen (119). This vaccine produced very high neutralizing titers when given to seronegative toddlers and also boosted the titer of neutralizing antibodies when given to seropositive individuals. This gB/MF59 vaccine is currently undergoing phase II studies. Controlled studies are in progress in postpartum seronegative women to determine if the rate of maternal infection, or the quantity or duration of viremia, can be decreased. Seronegative adolescents and seronegative or seropositive recipients of a kidney or a liver transplant will be studied in the same way.

A summary of HCMV vaccine candidates is shown in Table 12, and a list of possible volunteers for immunogenicity and phase III protection studies is shown in Table 13. One theoretical concern that has been raised about widespread introduction of an HCMV vaccine is that alterations in herd immunity could lead to more women acquiring primary infection during pregnancy. This was also a concern during the development of rubella vaccine and is relevant because all vaccines increase the average age at which unvaccinated individuals acquire natural infection. Mathematical modelling shows that such a phenomenon will not produce a problem for HCMV vaccinees in a typical developed country because the average age of infection is already greater than the average age at which pregnancies occur (Fig. 13) (74). The results of this modelling also demonstrate that the basic reproductive number of HCMV in such a population is similar to that of smallpox, so, by reducing the number of infectious individuals in a society, herd immunity could reduce the incidence of reinfections as well as primary infections (Fig. 14). Because reinfections are a more important cause of disease than reactivations in transplant patients (78) and, probably, in pregnant women as well (20), this prediction provides encouragement for the ultimate eradication of HCMV infection, although several generations of people would need to be immunized and eradication would take longer in communities where HCMV is acquired earlier in life. Nevertheless, we continue to hypothesize that control of initial HCMV infection could impair its ability to establish sanctuary sites protected by its immune evasion genes, so that individuals become less contagious to others. This optimistic scenario has already been proven true for other infections which persist in humans (hepatitis B virus, varicella-zoster virus, and human papillomavirus), so hopefully, one or more of the current HCMV vaccine candidates will demonstrate the modest degree of protection required to allow this hypothesis to be tested.

TREATMENT

Transplant Patients

Before antiviral drugs became available, an important therapeutic decision in transplant patients with active HCMV

TABLE 13 Populations in whom efficacy of HCMV vaccines could be evaluated by using virologic endpoints

Population given vaccine/placebo	Outcome
Seronegative postpartum women[a] Seronegative workers at day care centers[a] Seronegative women with children at day care centers[a] Adolescents[a] Toddlers	Reduced primary HCMV infection
Seronegative patients on waiting list for receipt of solid organs Seropositive patients on waiting list for receipt of solid organs Seropositive or seronegative recipients of stem cells Seronegative or seropositive donors of stem cells to seropositive recipients (adoptive transfer)	Reduced HCMV viremia/need for preemptive therapy

[a] Females in this population who became pregnant may show a reduced rate of congenital transmission to their offspring.

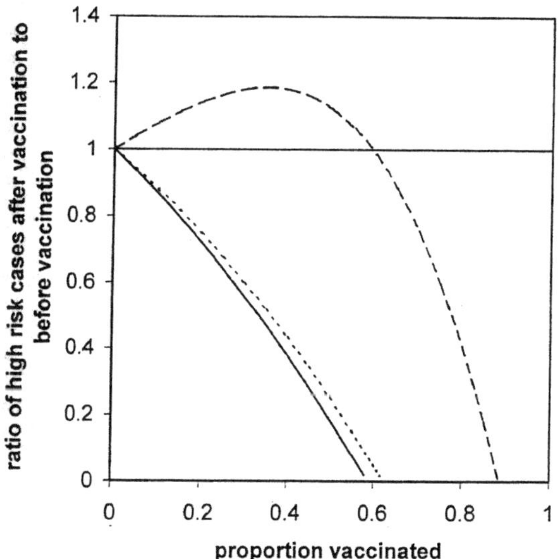

FIGURE 13 Herd immunity for HCMV or rubella. ____, CMV study 1; ...., CMV study 2; ----, rubella.

infection was to reduce the dose of immunosuppressive drugs. This should remain a component of the management of HCMV infection, supported by the administration of specific antiviral drugs. In transplant patients, the availability of surveillance samples allows treatment options in addition to those of prophylaxis and treatment of established disease. Drugs with activity against HCMV could potentially be used in four main ways, depending in part on their toxicity profiles (Table 14). Sixteen double-blind, placebo-controlled, randomized trials conducted for HCMV are summarized in Table 15 according to four main criteria of success: prevention of HCMV infection, prevention of HCMV disease, reduction in mortality rate, and decreased indirect effects. In addition to ganciclovir, several agents, including acyclovir, alpha interferon, and valacyclovir, have activity against HCMV in vivo (Table 15). In contrast to their relatively low potency when tested against HCMV in vitro, all treatments significantly reduced HCMV excretion, except immunoglobulin (Table 15). Quantitative virologic assessments were not done, but this suggests that any beneficial effect observed from the use of immunoglobulin is not necessarily mediated through a reduction in HCMV infection.

Only some of the studies have shown that control of HCMV infection leads to a reduction in HCMV disease (Table 15). The most consistent results come from the trials of ganciclovir, which clearly can markedly reduce HCMV disease in some groups (like stem cell transplant patients) but not in others (an effect was seen in heart transplant patients for reactivation but not for primary HCMV infection in one study, whereas the converse was true in a second study). The apparent discrepancies among clinical trials (no significant effect for ganciclovir in one of two bone marrow transplant studies, an effect of acyclovir in renal transplant but not bone marrow transplant patients, and benefit in only two of the three alpha interferon trials), can be explained by relatively small sample

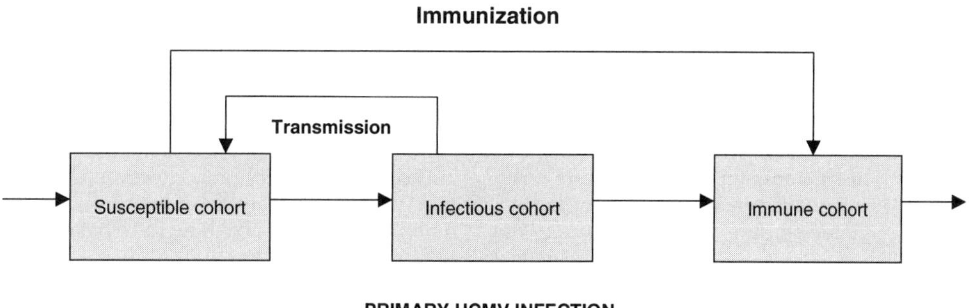

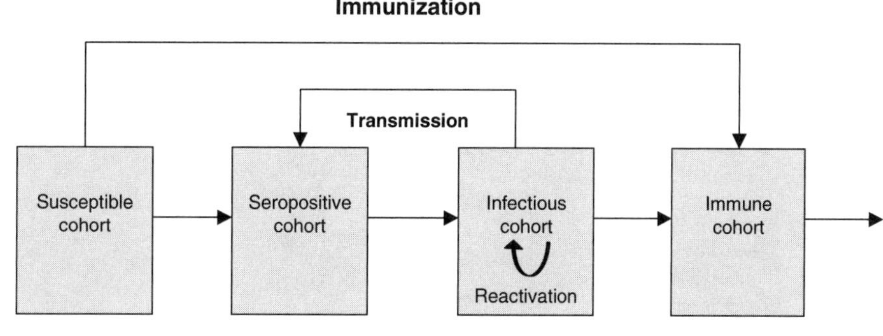

FIGURE 14 Standard population models of susceptible, infectious, and immune individuals, modified to include seropositive individuals who act as a source of HCMV for reinfections.

TABLE 14 Strategies for chemotherapy of HCMV

Term used	Time when drug is given	Risk of disease	Acceptable toxicity	Agent responsible for treatment decision
True prophylaxis	Before active infection	Low	None	Clinician
Delayed prophylaxis	When there is increased risk, but before active infection and after rejection	Medium	Low	Clinician
Suppression	After peripheral detection of virus	Medium	Low	Laboratory
Preemptive therapy	After systemic detection of virus	High	Medium	Laboratory
Treatment	Once disease is apparent	Established	High	Clinician and laboratory

sizes. Each trial showed trends in favor of a reduction in HCMV disease.

When the parameter of clinical benefit was survival, only three studies showed a positive result (Table 15). Ganciclovir given to patients already excreting HCMV was lifesaving, but the same was not true in either of two studies that evaluated prophylactic ganciclovir in bone marrow transplant recipients. These studies showed that the bone marrow toxicity of ganciclovir, manifested as neutropenia, was associated with bacterial superinfection (66, 174). Because all patients in this prophylaxis study were exposed to potentially fatal side effects but only some benefited from a reduced mortality rate associated with HCMV, these two effects cancelled each other out. In contrast, when ganciclovir was used in the suppressive mode, a major benefit was achieved while exposure to drug toxicity was minimized. Acyclovir use in the same patient population provides an interesting contrast. Although this drug is less potent than ganciclovir, patients showed a survival benefit overall because there was no serious toxicity to offset its moderate efficacy (126).

When the parameter assessed is the ability to control the indirect effects of HCMV, both ganciclovir and valacyclovir show significant benefits. In the original study by Merigan et al. (109), heart transplant recipients were randomized to receive intravenous ganciclovir at 5 mg/kg of body weight twice daily for 14 days, followed by 6 mg/kg once daily only on weekdays for the next 2 weeks. Given our improved understanding of the dynamics of HCMV, this regimen would nowadays be seen as suboptimal, in terms of both dose and duration. Indeed, the trial reported that HCMV disease was reduced among seropositive but not seronegative recipients, who we now know have high viral loads. Nevertheless, this suboptimal regimen produced significantly reduced risks of fungal superinfections and accelerated atherosclerosis during long-term follow-up (165). In renal allograft patients randomly allocated valacyclovir, 2 g four times daily for 90 days, or matching placebo, seronegative recipients showed a 50% reduced risk of biopsy-proven acute graft rejections (101). Taken together, these results strongly implicate HCMV as a cause of the indirect effects listed in Table 7.

In addition to the double-blind, placebo-controlled, randomized trials discussed above, other trials of antiviral chemotherapy have been conducted to provide important supporting information. Meyers et al. (112) were the first to study acyclovir prophylaxis in bone marrow transplant patients. Among HCMV-seropositive patients, those who were also HSV seropositive received high-dose intravenous acyclovir, while HSV-seronegative individuals received placebo. The results showed a marked reduction in HCMV disease and mortality rate. However, these encouraging results were not widely accepted, probably because at that time, acyclovir was not thought to have useful anti-HCMV

TABLE 15 Double-blind, placebo-controlled, randomized trials for HCMV

Strategy	Drug	Reference to trial of drug use in:			
		Bone marrow transplant	Renal transplant	Heart transplant	Liver transplant
Treatment	Ganciclovir	130[a]			
Preemptive therapy					121a[a,b]
Suppressive	Ganciclovir	67[a,b,c]			
Prophylaxis	Interferon		33[a] 85[a,b] 102[a]		
	Acyclovir	126[a,c]	12[a,b]		
	Valacyclovir		101[a,b,d]		
	Immunoglobulin		110[c]		145[b]
	Ganciclovir	174[a] 66[a,b]		109[a,b,d] 103[a,b]	62a[a,b]

[a] Reported significant benefit for HCMV infection.
[b] Reported significant benefit for HCMV disease.
[c] Reported significant benefit for survival.
[d] Reported significant benefit for indirect effects (including follow-up studies).

activity. The 50% effective dose in vitro was typically 60 to 100 μM, and HCMV was known not to contain a gene homologous to the thymidine kinase gene of HSV. However, HCMV is now known to contain a gene, UL97, whose product can phosphorylate acyclovir, in addition to ganciclovir. A subsequent trial (126) based upon the protocol used by Meyers et al. (112) confirmed that acyclovir reduces the mortality rate in this patient group.

Among bone marrow transplant patients, Schmidt et al. (139) performed routine bronchoalveolar lavage on day 35 in asymptomatic patients and used the shell vial technique to detect HCMV infection. HCMV-infected patients were then randomized to receive ganciclovir or to be observed. A marked reduction in HCMV pneumonitis following ganciclovir therapy was seen, which contrasts with the failure of ganciclovir to improve survival once HCMV pneumonitis was established in these patients. This apparent contradiction is consistent with the hypothesis that HCMV pneumonitis is an immunopathological condition (79), presumably prevented by preemptive therapy (139). Routine bronchoalveolar lavage at day 35 did not identify all patients who were destined to develop HCMV pneumonitis. It is not clear whether HCMV is present in the lungs of all those at risk by day 35. Either methods more sensitive than shell vial are required to detect this or some patients reactivate HCMV in the lung later than day 35, in which case a second bronchoalveolar lavage would be routinely required. Bronchoalveolar lavage has now been replaced by routine detecton of viremia as a less invasive way of identifying patients in need of preemptive therapy. Meanwhile, open studies of a combination of ganciclovir plus immunoglobulin suggest that better, but not excellent, control of established HCMV pneumonitis can be achieved in this patient group (52, 130). Presumably, the immunoglobulin component has an immunomodulatory effect on HCMV immunopathological pneumonitis, whereas ganciclovir reduces the chance that neighboring lung cells will be recruited by HCMV to stimulate further immunopathology. It seems likely that an immunomodulatory effect of immunoglobulin would be nonspecific, and there is support for this from a rat experimental model (153). Thus, there is little evidence that immunoglobulin prepared from HCMV-positive donors has any advantage over immunoglobulin from unrelated donors, but a comparative trial to test this formally would seem worthwhile. Foscarnet was equipotent to ganciclovir when used for preemptive therapy in bone marrow transplant patients (134). The combination of foscarnet plus ganciclovir (each at half dose) can be used to reduce toxicity without evidence of synergy (106).

In a controlled trial, low-dose intravenous ganciclovir prophylaxis was superior to high-dose oral acyclovir in liver transplant patients (175). In contrast to the case with bone marrow transplant patients, ganciclovir prophylaxis can be used safely in liver transplant patients, partly because of the lower dose chosen and partly because bone marrow toxicity may be a particular problem in bone marrow transplant patients. This trial illustrates that lessons learned from one patient group cannot be applied directly to others.

Following the widespread introduction of antiviral prophylaxis in transplant patients, late-onset disease has emerged as a clinical problem that develops once patients stop their antiviral prophylaxis. Some patients develop disease due to ganciclovir-resistant mutants, and there have been serious cases of EOD, including death. Such late-onset disease is not seen in centers that use preemptive therapy (143). One plausible explanation is that low-level antigen presentation as part of preemptive therapy may stimulate the immune system to control long-term HCMV infection, analogous to "endogenous immunization." Alternatively, ganciclovir may interfere with the division of T cells, thus impairing their ability to form the most potent clonal derivatives. An important question for the field is whether prophylaxis per se selects for this immunologic problem or whether it is an adverse outcome of using ganciclovir prophylaxis. The results with maribavir for prophylaxis are therefore awaited with interest.

Both prophylaxis and preemptive therapy are effective strategies for preventing HCMV disease in transplant recipients, as supported by meta-analyses of the published trials. In addition, two randomized clinical trials have directly compared prophylaxis and preemptive therapy in renal transplant patients. One compared prophylactic valganciclovir with preemptive valganciclovir (93), while the other compared prophylactic valacyclovir with preemptive valganciclovir (133). Both studies reported no significant differences in the incidence of HCMV disease. Thus, while the relative merits of both strategies are hotly debated (143, 144), clinicians can use whichever strategy they find convenient for their transplant center.

AIDS Patients

In contrast to the logical approach to treatment described above for transplant patients, drug evaluation in HIV-positive patients has been largely empirical. Studies have focused on the clinical problem of established HCMV retinitis, rather than targeting HCMV itself based upon knowledge of the natural history of infection.

The trial of the Studies of Ocular Complications of AIDS Research Group recruited patients with first-episode HCMV retinitis and randomly allocated them to receive either ganciclovir for induction and maintenance or foscarnet for induction and maintenance (6). The drugs were equally effective at delaying the time to recurrence of HCMV retinitis, but survival was significantly improved with foscarnet, despite the fact that treatment toxicity necessitating a switch to the alternate treatment was more common in those receiving foscarnet. The possible reason for the survival difference may relate to foscarnet's activity against HIV. Another study compared two doses of foscarnet for maintenance and showed that 120 mg/kg/day was preferable.

Two double-blind, controlled, randomized trials were conducted with AIDS patients without HCMV EOD, with the intention of preventing such disease. One trial used oral ganciclovir (150), while the other used oral valacyclovir (58). These trials have been termed prophylaxis, but this refers to prophylaxis for disease and is not synonymous with prophylaxis of infection described above for transplant patients. Indeed, virologic assessment at entry shows that 50% of patients had HCMV infection detectable by PCR in urine, blood, or both. HCMV infection in HIV-positive patients occurs far earlier than has been appreciated by observing HCMV retinitis in AIDS patients. After 12 months, oral ganciclovir reduced HCMV retinitis from 30% in the placebo arm to 16%, whereas the valacyclovir trial reduced HCMV retinitis from 18% in the combined two-dose acyclovir arms to 12%. Ganciclovir showed significant benefit only in the subset who were PCR negative at baseline (i.e., true prophylaxis), whereas valacyclovir showed significant benefit for both preemptive therapy and prophylaxis (55, 73). This difference probably relates to the doses of the drugs administered rather than to their inherent potencies. Despite its known toxicity, ganciclovir was fairly well tolerated in these patients, partly because poor oral bioavailability may have limited the potential for toxicity. Valacyclovir at the high dosage chosen, 8 g/day, was poorly tolerated by AIDS patients, many of whom stopped therapy prematurely. Thus, the efficacy figures given above for the intention-to-treat analyses should be reviewed with the knowledge that many patients stopped treatment during the trial.

The results from these two trials are encouraging, but there remains much room for improvement. Drugs can now be targeted to reduce HCMV infection and decrease the chance of seeding the retina. One possible approach would be to monitor HIV-positive patients for evidence of HCMV infection by PCR and randomize them to receive preemptive therapy or matching placebo when patients became PCR positive. This protocol was used in ACTG protocol A5030, in which patients whose plasma PCR was positive on a single occasion were given valganciclovir or placebo. No significant benefit was reported, although the study was seriously underpowered because of the difficulties of identifying individuals positive for HCMV as determined by PCR in the era of HAART (D. A. Wohl, M. A. Kendall, J. Andersen, C. Crumpacker, S. Spector, B. Alston-Smith, S. Owens, S. Chafey, M. Marco, S. Maxwell, N. Lurain, D. Jabs, and M. A. Jacobson, unpublished data).

The main strategy to prevent HCMV retinitis in AIDS patients is treatment with HAART regimens that maintain the CD4 count above 100. Indeed, patients who present with HCMV retinitis can have valganciclovir maintenance therapy stopped if their CD4 count rises above 100 and persists at that level for at least 3 months, showing that recovery of preexisting HCMV-specific immunity is sufficient to control progression of this EOD.

Neonates

Important results have been reported from a randomized trial in neonates with congenital HCMV and CNS symptoms or signs conducted by the Collaborative Antiviral Study Group (CASG), demonstrating significant control over progressive hearing loss from ganciclovir at 6 mg/kg twice daily given intravenously for 6 weeks (95). This benefit is consistent both with the increased viral load found in such neonates by Stagno and colleagues (152) and with the clinical observation that much of the hearing loss is acquired progressively after birth. The developmental damage caused by HCMV can also be slowed by this 6-week course of treatment. Six weeks of treatment with intravenous ganciclovir is now established as the standard of care for neonates born with CNS symptoms of congenital HCMV infection which would have made them eligible for the CASG trial described by Kimberlin et al. (95). Of note, ganciclovir has important toxicity (acute neutropenia and thrombocytopenia plus carcinogenicity in rodents at less than the human anticipated exposure), so evaluation of this drug should proceed with caution. Valganciclovir has been shown to be bioavailable orally in neonates (1), and a new CASG trial will randomize congenitally infected neonates to receive 6 weeks versus 6 months of valganciclovir therapy.

Resistance

Strains of HCMV resistant to ganciclovir have been found in AIDS patients receiving maintenance therapy for retinitis. Approximately 8% of urine samples contained resistant virus once patients had been treated for at least 3 months (48), which is probably an underestimate of the true situation in vivo because the long time taken to propagate HCMV in cell cultures allows the wild type to outcompete the resistant strain in vitro.

Most HCMV strains acquire resistance through mutations in the UL97 gene, although occasional mutations in DNA polymerase have been described. A range of mutations have been identified in UL54 which give rise to resistance to the antiviral drugs ganciclovir, foscarnet, and cidofovir. Some of these mutations, such as D301N, give rise to cross-resistance to all of the aforementioned nucleoside analogs. Unlike the situation with UL97, a number of mutations have been detected throughout the UL54 ORF following in vitro passage in the presence of antiviral drugs and in strains derived from patients undergoing drug therapy. It is unlikely that targeted approaches to identify resistance within this gene will be successful, and sequence analysis of the entire ORF will be required to allow the detection of drug resistance at this locus in a clinical setting.

Genetic changes in UL97 have been described, including those proven by site-directed mutagenesis to confer resistance when introduced back into a laboratory-adapted strain (Fig. 15). Most of these strains can be detected by molecular biological techniques in vitro, and others have developed point mutation assays to detect key mutations (34). In a cohort of AIDS patients receiving oral ganciclovir maintenance therapy, 22% had resistance detected in vivo by genotyping (24). None of the patients with resistance responded to reintroduction of ganciclovir, arguing that the laboratory results are clinically relevant. Knowledge of the rapid dynamics of HCMV replication in vivo has been used to explain and predict the development of resistance in AIDS patients (54). At present, resistance is not a major clinical problem because HCMV is controlled indirectly by HAART, but we anticipate further cases in the post-HAART era, and the principles discussed above should be reapplied. Specifically, patients who had genotypically resistant HCMV in the past may present again with HCMV disease poorly responsive to ganciclovir.

Increasing cases of resistance have been reported as antiviral prophylaxis has been used frequently in transplant patients. Mutations identical to those seen in AIDS patients develop. Late-onset HCMV disease, occurring after antiviral prophylaxis has been stopped, has emerged as a major clinical problem and is frequently caused by resistant strains.

Novel Antiviral Targets

Fomivirsen is a licensed treatment for HCMV retinitis, although it is no longer marketed because of the diminishing number of cases of HCMV retinitis. It is an antisense oligonucleotide containing modified bases to reduce nuclease susceptibility. The drug interferes with the IE86 transactivator (Fig. 2) and has to be given by intravitreal injection.

Maribavir is an inhibitor of UL97; the compound is based upon the benzimidazole riboside nucleus. Although strongly protein bound, sufficient drug can be administered to allow the free compound to inhibit HCMV replication. In a phase II study, maribavir prophylaxis was more likely

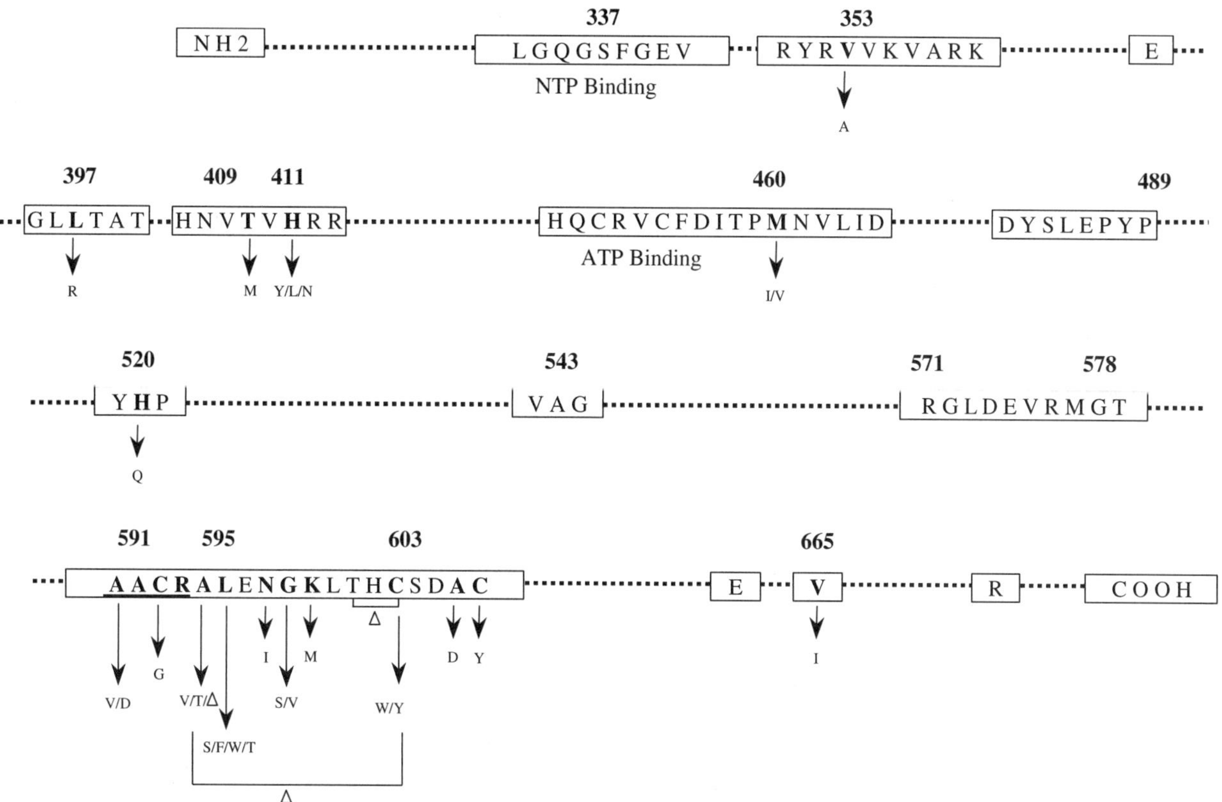

FIGURE 15 Schematic representation of the UL97 gene showing mutations at particular codons that have been proven to cause resistance to ganciclovir in vivo or which are associated with maribavir resistance in vitro. Bold letters indicate mutations confirmed by site-directed mutagenesis. Mutations 460 to 607 concern ganciclovir; mutations 353 to 411 concern maribavir. (Data from reference 33a.)

to prevent the need for preemptive therapy in stem cell transplant patients than was placebo (173). In 2007, maribavir entered phase III clinical trials for prophylaxis in stem cell transplant recipients and in liver transplant patients. Maribavir is active against UL97 mutants and also against UL54 mutants resistant to ganciclovir, foscarnet, or cidofovir. However, because of its inhibition of UL97, maribavir results in a 13-fold increase in the 50% inhibitory concentration for ganciclovir, and consequently, combination therapy with maribavir and ganciclovir will not be possible. No strains of CMV resistant to maribavir have yet been detected in humans, but the genetic changes in UL97 which confer resistance in vitro are summarized in Fig. 15.

The terminase complex cleaves concatemeric DNA into unit length molecules as packaging proceeds by a "head-full" mechanism. Compounds such as BAY-4766 are at the phase I stage of clinical development. Nonnucleoside inhibitors of HCMV DNA polymerase have been identified by screening but are at the preclinical stage.

The HCMV protease is an attractive target, especially since this class of inhibitor has been successfully developed for HIV. However, despite the availability of a three-dimensional structure since 1997, the search for inhibitors has been slow. This is partly compounded by the complexity of the enzyme and partly because the substrate binding groove is shallow, reducing the opportunities for small molecules to bind with high affinity.

REFERENCES

1. **Acosta, E. P., R. C. Brundage, J. R. King, P. J. Sanchez, S. Sood, V. Agrawal, J. Homans, R. F. Jacobs, D. Lang, J. R. Romero, J. Griffin, G. Cloud, R. Whitley, and D. W. Kimberlin.** 2007. Ganciclovir population pharmacokinetics in neonates following intravenous administration of ganciclovir and oral administration of a liquid valganciclovir formulation. *Clin. Pharmacol. Ther.* **81:** 867–872.
2. **Adler, B., L. Scrivano, Z. Ruzcics, B. Rupp, C. Sinzger, and U. Koszinowski.** 2006. Role of human cytomegalovirus UL131A in cell type-specific virus entry and release. *J. Gen. Virol.* **87:**2451–2460.
3. **Adler, S. P., S. E. Starr, S. A. Plotkin, S. H. Hempfling, J. Buis, M. L. Manning, and A. M. Best.** 1995. Immunity induced by primary human cytomegalovirus infection protects against secondary infection among women of childbearing age. *J. Infect. Dis.* **171:**26–32.
4. **Anders, D. G., J. A. Kerry, and G. S. Pari.** 2007. DNA synthesis and late viral gene expression, p. 295–310. *In* A. Arvin (ed.), *Human Herpesviruses: Biology, Therapy and Immunoprophylaxis*. Cambridge University Press, Cambridge, United Kingdom.
5. **Anders, D. G., M. A. Kacica, G. Pari, and S. M. Punturieri.** 1992. Boundaries and structure of human cytomegalovirus *ori*Lyt, a complex origin for lytic-phase DNA replication. *J. Virol.* **66:**3373–3384.
6. **Anonymous.** 1992. Mortality in patients with the acquired immunodeficiency syndrome treated with either

foscarnet or ganciclovir for cytomegalovirus retinitis. Studies of Ocular Complications of AIDS Research Group, in collaboration with the AIDS Clinical Trials Group. *N. Engl. J. Med.* **326:**213–220. (Erratum, **326:** 1172.)

7. **Apperley, J. F., C. Dowding, J. Hibbin, J. Buiter, E. Matutes, P. J. Sissons, M. Gordon, and J. M. Goldman.** 1989. The effect of cytomegalovirus on hemopoiesis: in vitro evidence for selective infection of marrow stromal cells. *Exp. Hematol.* **17:**38–45.
8. **Arnon, T. I., H. Achdout, O. Levi, G. Markel, N. Saleh, G. Katz, R. Gazit, T. Gonen-Gross, J. Hanna, E. Nahari, A. Porgador, A. Honigman, B. Plachter, D. Mevorach, D. G. Wolf, and O. Mandelboim.** 2005. Inhibition of the NKp30 activating receptor by pp65 of human cytomegalovirus. *Nat. Immunol.* **6:**515–523.
9. **AuCoin, D. P., G. B. Smith, C. D. Meiering, and E. S. Mocarski.** 2006. Betaherpesvirus-conserved cytomegalovirus tegument protein ppUL32 (pp150) controls cytoplasmic events during virion maturation. *J. Virol.* **80:** 8199–8210.
10. **Bain, M., and J. Sinclair.** 2007. The S phase of the cell cycle and its perturbation by human cytomegalovirus. *Rev. Med. Virol.* **17:**423–434.
11. **Balcarek, K. B., R. Bagley, G. A. Cloud, and R. F. Pass.** 1990. Cytomegalovirus infection among employees of a children's hospital. No evidence for increased risk associated with patient care. *JAMA* **263:**840–844.
12. **Balfour, H. H., Jr., B. A. Chace, J. T. Stapleton, R. L. Simmons, and D. S. Fryd.** 1989. A randomized, placebo-controlled trial of oral acyclovir for the prevention of cytomegalovirus disease in recipients of renal allografts. *N. Engl. J. Med.* **320:**1381–1387.
13. **Baxter, M. K., and W. Gibson.** 2001. Cytomegalovirus basic phosphoprotein (pUL32) binds to capsids in vitro through its amino one-third. *J. Virol.* **75:**6865–6873.
14. **Bechtel, J. T., and T. Shenk.** 2002. Human cytomegalovirus UL47 tegument protein functions after entry and before immediate-early gene expression. *J. Virol.* **76:** 1043–1050.
15. Reference deleted.
16. **Billstrom, M. A., and W. J. Britt.** 1995. Postoligomerization folding of human cytomegalovirus glycoprotein B: identification of folding intermediates and importance of disulfide bonding. *J. Virol.* **69:**7015–7022.
17. **Bodaghi, B., M. E. Slobbe-van Drunen, A. Topilko, E. Perret, R. C. Vossen, M. C. van Dam-Mieras, D. Zipeto, J. L. Virelizier, P. Lehoang, C. A. Bruggeman, and S. Michelson.** 1999. Entry of human cytomegalovirus into retinal pigment epithelial and endothelial cells by endocytosis. *Investig. Ophthalmol. Vis. Sci.* **40:**2598–2607.
18. **Bolovan-Fritts, C. A., E. S. Mocarski, and J. A. Wiedeman.** 1999. Peripheral blood $CD14^+$ cells from healthy subjects carry a circular conformation of latent cytomegalovirus genome. *Blood* **93:**394–398.
19. **Boppana, S. B., R. F. Pass, and W. J. Britt.** 1993. Virus-specific antibody responses in mothers and their newborn infants with asymptomatic congenital cytomegalovirus infections. *J. Infect. Dis.* **167:**72–77.
20. **Boppana, S. B., L. B. Rivera, K. B. Fowler, M. Mach, and W. J. Britt.** 2001. Intrauterine transmission of cytomegalovirus to infants of women with preconceptional immunity. *N. Engl. J. Med.* **344:**1366–1371.
21. **Borst, E.-M., and M. Messerle.** 2005. Analysis of human cytomegalovirus *ori*Lyt sequence requirements in the context of the viral genome. *J. Virol.* **79:**3615–3626.
22. **Borza, C. M., and L. M. Hutt-Fletcher.** 2002. Alternate replication in B cells and epithelial cells switches tropism of Epstein-Barr virus. *Nat. Med.* **8:**594–599.
23. **Bostrom, L., O. Ringden, B. Sundberg, P. Ljungman, A. Linde, and B. Nilsson.** 1989. Pretransplant herpes virus serology and chronic graft-versus-host disease. *Bone Marrow Transplant.* **4:**547–552.
24. **Bowen, E. F., V. C. Emery, P. Wilson, M. A. Johnson, C. C. Davey, C. A. Sabin, D. Farmer, and P. D. Griffiths.** 1998. Cytomegalovirus polymerase chain reaction viremia in patients receiving ganciclovir maintenance therapy for retinitis. *AIDS* **12:**605–611.
25. **Bowen, E. F., P. Wilson, M. Atkins, S. Madge, P. D. Griffiths, M. A. Johnson, and V. C. Emery.** 1995. Natural history of untreated cytomegalovirus retinitis. *Lancet* **346:**1671–1673.
26. **Bowen, E. F., P. Wilson, A. Cope, C. Sabin, P. Griffiths, C. Davey, M. Johnson, and V. Emery.** 1996. Cytomegalovirus retinitis in AIDS patients: influence of cytomegaloviral load on response to ganciclovir, time to recurrence and survival. *AIDS* **10:**1515–1520.
27. **Bresnahan, W. A., and T. E. Shenk.** 2000. UL82 virion protein activates expression of immediate early viral genes in human cytomegalovirus-infected cells. *Proc. Natl. Acad. Sci. USA* **97:**14506–14511.
28. **Britt, W. J., and L. G. Vugler.** 1992. Oligomerization of the human cytomegalovirus major envelope glycoprotein complex gB (gp55-116). *J. Virol.* **66:**6747–6754.
29. **Cantrell, S. R., and W. A. Bresnahan.** 2006. Human cytomegalovirus (HCMV) UL82 gene product (pp71) relieves hDaxx-mediated repression of HCMV replication. *J. Virol.* **80:**6188–6191.
30. **Casaday, R. J., J. R. Bailey, S. R. Kalb, E. J. Brignole, A. N. Loveland, R. J. Cotter, and W. Gibson.** 2004. Assembly protein precursor (pUL80.5 homolog) of simian cytomegalovirus is phosphorylated at a glycogen synthase kinase 3 site and its downstream "priming" site: phosphorylation affects interactions of protein with itself and with major capsid protein. *J. Virol.* **78:**13501–13511.
31. **Cha, T. A., E. Tom, G. W. Kemble, G. M. Duke, E. S. Mocarski, and R. R. Spaete.** 1996. Human cytomegalovirus clinical isolates carry at least 19 genes not found in laboratory strains. *J. Virol.* **70:**78–83.
32. **Chatterjee, S. N., M. Fiala, J. Weiner, J. A. Stewart, B. Stacey, and N. Warmer.** 1978. Primary cytomegalovirus and opportunistic infections. Incidence in renal transplant recipients. *JAMA* **240:**2446–2449.
33. **Cheeseman, S. H., R. H. Rubin, J. A. Stewart, N. E. Tolkoff-Rubin, A. B. Cosimi, K. Cantell, J. Gilbert, S. Winkle, J. T. Herrin, P. H. Black, P. S. Russell, and M. S. Hirsch.** 1979. Controlled clinical trial of prophylactic human-leukocyte interferon in renal transplantation. Effects on cytomegalovirus and herpes simplex virus infections. *N. Engl. J. Med.* **300:**1345–1349.

33a. **Chou, S.** 2008. Cytomegalovirus UL97 mutations in the era of ganciclovir and maribavir. *Rev. Med. Virol.* **18:**233–246.

34. **Chou, S., A. Erice, M. C. Jordan, G. M. Vercellotti, K. R. Michels, C. L. Talarico, S. C. Stanat, and K. K. Biron.** 1995. Analysis of the UL97 phosphotransferase coding sequence in clinical cytomegalovirus isolates and identification of mutations conferring ganciclovir resistance. *J. Infect. Dis.* **171:**576–583.
35. **Chou, S. W.** 1989. Reactivation and recombination of multiple cytomegalovirus strains from individual organ donors. *J. Infect. Dis.* **160:**11–15.
36. **Colletti, K. S., K. E. Smallenburg, Y. Xu, and G. S. Pari.** 2007. Human cytomegalovirus UL84 interacts with an RNA stem-loop sequence found within the RNA/DNA hybrid region of *ori*Lyt. *J. Virol.* **81:**7077–7085.
37. **Compton, T., R. R. Nepomuceno, and D. M. Nowlin.** 1992. Human cytomegalovirus penetrates host cells by

pH-independent fusion at the cell surface. *Virology* **191:** 387–395.

38. **Compton, T., D. M. Nowlin, and N. R. Cooper.** 1993. Initiation of human cytomegalovirus infection requires initial interaction with cell surface heparan sulfate. *Virology* **193:**834–841.
39. **Cope, A. V., P. Sweny, C. Sabin, L. Rees, P. D. Griffiths, and V. C. Emery.** 1997. Quantity of cytomegalovirus viruria is a major risk factor for cytomegalovirus disease after renal transplantation. *J. Med. Virol.* **52:**200–205.
40. **Crump, C. M., C. H. Hung, L. Thomas, L. Wan, and G. Thomas.** 2003. Role of PACS-1 in trafficking of human cytomegalovirus glycoprotein B and virus production. *J. Virol.* **77:**11105–11113.
41. **Crump, C. M., C. Yates, and T. Minson.** 2007. Herpes simplex virus type 1 cytoplasmic envelopment requires functional Vps4. *J. Virol.* **81:**7380–7387.
42. **Dal, M. P., S. Pignatelli, N. Zini, N. M. Maraldi, E. Perret, M. C. Prevost, and M. P. Landini.** 2002. Analysis of intracellular and intraviral localization of the human cytomegalovirus UL53 protein. *J. Gen. Virol.* **83:**1005–1012.
43. **Deayton, J. R., C. A. Sabin, M. A. Johnson, V. C. Emery, P. Wilson, and P. D. Griffiths.** 2004. Importance of cytomegalovirus viremia in risk of disease progression and death in HIV-infected patients receiving highly active antiretroviral therapy. *Lancet* **363:**2116–2121.
44. **Detels, R., C. T. Leach, K. Hennessey, Z. Liu, B. R. Visscher, J. D. Cherry, and J. V. Giorgi.** 1994. Persistent cytomegalovirus infection of semen increases risk of AIDS. *J. Infect. Dis.* **169:**766–768.
45. **Dittmer, A., and E. Bogner.** 2005. Analysis of the quaternary structure of the putative HCMV portal protein PUL104. *Biochemistry* **44:**759–765.
46. **Dolan, A., C. Cunningham, R. D. Hector, A. F. Hassan-Walker, L. Lee, C. Addison, D. J. Dargan, D. J. McGeoch, D. Gatherer, V. C. Emery, P. D. Griffiths, C. Sinzger, B. P. McSharry, G. W. Wilkinson, and A. J. Davison.** 2004. Genetic content of wild-type human cytomegalovirus. *J. Gen. Virol.* **85:**1301–1312.
47. **Dollard, S. C., S. D. Grosse, and D. S. Ross.** 2007. New estimates of the prevalence of neurological and sensory sequelae and mortality associated with congenital cytomegalovirus infection. *Rev. Med. Virol.* **17:**355–363.
48. **Drew, W. L., R. C. Miner, D. F. Busch, S. E. Follansbee, J. Gullett, S. G. Mehalko, S. M. Gordon, W. F. Owen, Jr., T. R. Matthews, W. C. Buhles, et al.** 1991. Prevalence of resistance in patients receiving ganciclovir for serious cytomegalovirus infection. *J. Infect. Dis.* **163:**716–719.
49. **Dummer, S., A. Lee, M. K. Breinig, R. Kormos, M. Ho, and B. Griffith.** 1994. Investigation of cytomegalovirus infection as a risk factor for coronary atherosclerosis in the explanted hearts of patients undergoing heart transplantation. *J. Med. Virol.* **44:**305–309.
50. **Duncan, S. R., W. F. Grgurich, A. T. Iacono, G. J. Burckart, S. A. Yousem, I. L. Paradis, P. A. Williams, B. A. Johnson, and B. P. Griffith.** 1994. A comparison of ganciclovir and acyclovir to prevent cytomegalovirus after lung transplantation. *Am. J. Respir. Crit. Care Med.* **150:**146–152.
51. **Dunn, W., P. Trang, Q. Zhong, E. Yang, C. van Belle, and F. Liu.** 2005. Human cytomegalovirus expresses novel microRNAs during productive viral infection. *Cell. Microbiol.* **7:**1684–1695.
52. **Emanuel, D., I. Cunningham, K. Jules-Elysee, J. A. Brochstein, N. A. Kernan, J. Laver, D. Stover, D. A. White, A. Fels, B. Polsky, et al.** 1988. Cytomegalovirus pneumonia after bone marrow transplantation successfully treated with the combination of ganciclovir and high-dose intravenous immune globulin. *Ann. Intern. Med.* **109:**777–782.
53. **Emery, V. C., A. V. Cope, E. F. Bowen, D. Gor, and P. D. Griffiths.** 1999. The dynamics of human cytomegalovirus replication in vivo. *J. Exp. Med.* **190:**177–182.
54. **Emery, V. C., and P. D. Griffiths.** 2000. Prediction of cytomegalovirus load and resistance patterns after antiviral chemotherapy. *Proc. Natl. Acad. Sci. USA* **97:**8039–8044.
55. **Emery, V. C., C. Sabin, J. E. Feinberg, M. Grywacz, S. Knight, and P. D. Griffiths for the AIDS Clinical Trials Group 204/Glaxo Wellcome 123-014 International CMV Prophylaxis Study Group.** 1999. Quantitative effects of valacyclovir on the replication of cytomegalovirus (CMV) in persons with advanced human immunodeficiency virus disease: baseline CMV load dictates time to disease and survival. *J. Infect. Dis.* **180:**695–701.
56. **Emery, V. C., C. A. Sabin, A. V. Cope, D. Gor, A. F. Hassan-Walker, and P. D. Griffiths.** 2000. Application of viral-load kinetics to identify patients who develop cytomegalovirus disease after transplantation. *Lancet* **355:** 2032–2036.
57. **Engstrand, M., C. Tournay, M. A. Peyrat, B. M. Eriksson, J. Wadstrom, B. Z. Wirgart, F. Romagne, M. Bonneville, T. H. Totterman, and O. Korsgren.** 2000. Characterization of CMVpp65-specific CD8+ T lymphocytes using MHC tetramers in kidney transplant patients and healthy participants. *Transplantation* **69:**2243–2250.
58. **Feinberg, J. E., S. Hurwitz, D. Cooper, F. R. Sattler, R. R. MacGregor, W. Powderly, G. N. Holland, P. D. Griffiths, R. B. Pollard, M. Youle, M. J. Gill, F. J. Holland, M. E. Power, S. Owens, D. Coakley, J. Fry, and M. A. Jacobson for the AIDS Clinical Trials Group Protocol 204/Glaxo Wellcome 123-014 International CMV Prophylaxis Study Group.** 1998. A randomized, double-blind trial of valaciclovir prophylaxis for cytomegalovirus disease in patients with advanced human immunodeficiency virus infection. *J. Infect. Dis.* **177:**48–56.
59. **Fowler, K. B., S. Stagno, and R. F. Pass.** 2003. Maternal immunity and prevention of congenital cytomegalovirus infection. *JAMA* **289:**1008–1011.
60. **Fowler, K. B., S. Stagno, R. F. Pass, W. J. Britt, T. J. Boll, and C. A. Alford.** 1992. The outcome of congenital cytomegalovirus infection in relation to maternal antibody status. *N. Engl. J. Med.* **326:**663–667.
61. **Fox, J. C., I. M. Kidd, P. D. Griffiths, P. Sweny, and V. C. Emery.** 1995. Longitudinal analysis of cytomegalovirus load in renal transplant recipients using a quantitative polymerase chain reaction: correlation with disease. *J. Gen. Virol.* **76**(Pt. 2)**:**309–319.
62. **Fraile-Ramos, A., A. Pelchen-Matthews, C. Risco, M. T. Rejas, V. C. Emery, A. F. Hassan-Walker, M. Esteban, and M. Marsh.** 2007. The ESCRT machinery is not required for human cytomegalovirus envelopment. *Cell. Microbiol.* **9:**2955–2967.

62a. **Gane, E., F. Saliba, G. J. C. Valdecasas, J. O'Grady, M. D. Pescovitz, S. Lyman, and C. A. Robinson.** 1997. Randomised trial of efficacy and safety of oral ganciclovir in the prevention of cytomegalovirus disease in liver-transplant recipients. The Oral Ganciclovir International Transplantation Study Group. *Lancet* **350:**1729–1733. (Erratum, **351:**454, 1998.)

63. **Gilbert, G. L., K. Hayes, I. L. Hudson, and J. James for the Neonatal Cytomegalovirus Infection Study Group.** 1989. Prevention of transfusion-acquired cytomegalovirus infection in infants by blood filtration to remove leucocytes. *Lancet* **1:**1228–1231.

64. **Gilbert, M. J., S. R. Riddell, B. Plachter, and P. D. Greenberg.** 1996. Cytomegalovirus selectively blocks antigen processing and presentation of its immediate-early gene product. *Nature* **383:**720–722.
65. **Gleaves, C. A., T. F. Smith, E. A. Shuster, and G. R. Pearson.** 1984. Rapid detection of cytomegalovirus in MRC-5 cells inoculated with urine specimens by using low-speed centrifugation and monoclonal antibody to an early antigen. *J. Clin. Microbiol.* **19:**917–919.
66. **Goodrich, J. M., R. A. Bowden, L. Fisher, C. Keller, G. Schoch, and J. D. Meyers.** 1993. Ganciclovir prophylaxis to prevent cytomegalovirus disease after allogeneic marrow transplant. *Ann. Intern. Med.* **118:**173–178.
67. **Goodrich, J. M., M. Mori, C. A. Gleaves, M. C. Du, M. Cays, D. F. Ebeling, W. C. Buhles, B. DeArmond, and J. D. Meyers.** 1991. Early treatment with ganciclovir to prevent cytomegalovirus disease after allogeneic bone marrow transplantation. *N. Engl. J. Med.* **325:**1601–1607.
68. **Grattan, M. T., C. E. Moreno-Cabral, V. A. Starnes, P. E. Oyer, E. B. Stinson, and N. E. Shumway.** 1989. Cytomegalovirus infection is associated with cardiac allograft rejection and atherosclerosis. *JAMA* **261:**3561–3566.
69. **Gretch, D. R., B. Kari, L. Rasmussen, R. C. Gehrz, and M. F. Stinski.** 1988. Identification and characterization of three distinct families of glycoprotein complexes in the envelopes of human cytomegalovirus. *J. Virol.* **62:**875–881.
70. **Grey, F., A. Antoniewicz, E. Allen, J. Saugstad, A. McShea, J. C. Carrington, and J. Nelson.** 2005. Identification and characterization of human cytomegalovirus-encoded microRNAs. *J. Virol.* **79:**12095–12099.
71. **Griffiths, P. D.** 1992. Studies to define viral cofactors for human immunodeficiency virus. *Infect. Agents Dis.* **1:** 237–244.
71a. **Griffiths, P. D.** 2000. Cytomegalovirus, p. 79–115. *In* A. J. Zuckerman, J. E. Banatvala, and J. R. Pattison (ed.), *Clinical Virology*. John Wiley & Sons Ltd., Chichester, United Kingdom.
72. **Griffiths, P. D., and C. Baboonian.** 1984. A prospective study of primary cytomegalovirus infection during pregnancy: final report. *Br. J. Obstet. Gynaecol.* **91:**307–315.
73. **Griffiths, P. D., J. E. Feinberg, J. Fry, C. Sabin, L. Dix, D. Gor, A. Ansari, and V. C. Emery for the AIDS Clinical Trials Group Protocol 204/Glaxo Wellcome 123-014 International CMV Prophylaxis Study Group.** 1998. The effect of valaciclovir on cytomegalovirus viremia and viruria detected by polymerase chain reaction in patients with advanced human immunodeficiency virus disease. *J. Infect. Dis.* **177:**57–64.
74. **Griffiths, P. D., A. McLean, and V. C. Emery.** 2001. Encouraging prospects for immunization against primary cytomegalovirus infection. *Vaccine* **19:**1356–1362.
75. **Griffiths, P. D., D. D. Panjwani, P. R. Stirk, M. G. Ball, M. Ganczakowski, H. A. Blacklock, and H. G. Prentice.** 1984. Rapid diagnosis of cytomegalovirus infection in immunocompromised patients by detection of early antigen fluorescent foci. *Lancet* **2:**1242–1245.
76. **Griffiths, P. D., S. Stagno, R. F. Pass, R. J. Smith, and C. A. Alford, Jr.** 1982. Congenital cytomegalovirus infection: diagnostic and prognostic significance of the detection of specific immunoglobulin M antibodies in cord serum. *Pediatrics* **69:**544–549.
77. **Grob, J. P., J. E. Grundy, H. G. Prentice, P. D. Griffiths, A. V. Hoffbrand, M. D. Hughes, T. Tate, J. Z. Wimperis, and M. K. Brenner.** 1987. Immune donors can protect marrow-transplant recipients from severe cytomegalovirus infections. *Lancet* **i:**774–776.
78. **Grundy, J. E., S. F. Lui, M. Super, N. J. Berry, P. Sweny, O. N. Fernando, J. Moorhead, and P. D. Griffiths.** 1988. Symptomatic cytomegalovirus infection in seropositive kidney recipients: reinfection with donor virus rather than reactivation of recipient virus. *Lancet* **ii:** 132–135.
79. **Grundy, J. E., J. D. Shanley, and P. D. Griffiths.** 1987. Is cytomegalovirus interstitial pneumonitis in transplant recipients an immunopathological condition? *Lancet* **ii:** 996–999.
80. **Grunewald, K., P. Desai, D. C. Winkler, J. B. Heymann, D. M. Belnap, W. Baumeister, and A. C. Steven.** 2003. Three-dimensional structure of herpes simplex virus from cryo-electron tomography. *Science* **302:**1396–1398.
81. **Guerra, B., G. Simonazzi, A. Banfi, T. Lazzarotto, A. Farina, M. Lanari, and N. Rizzo.** 2007. Impact of diagnostic and confirmatory tests and prenatal counseling on the rate of pregnancy termination among women with positive cytomegalovirus immunoglobulin M antibody titers. *Am. J. Obstet. Gynecol.* **196:**221–226.
82. **Hassan-Walker, A. F., S. Okwuadi, L. Lee, P. D. Griffiths, and V. C. Emery.** 2004. Sequence variability of the alpha-chemokine UL146 from clinical strains of human cytomegalovirus. *J. Med. Virol.* **74:**573–579.
83. **Hayhurst, G. P., L. A. Bryant, R. C. Caswell, S. M. Walker, and J. H. Sinclair.** 1995. CCAAT box-dependent activation of the TATA-less human DNA polymerase alpha promoter by the human cytomegalovirus 72-kilodalton major immediate-early protein. *J. Virol.* **69:**182–188.
84. **Heldwein, E. E., H. Lou, F. C. Bender, G. H. Cohen, R. J. Eisenberg, and S. C. Harrison.** 2006. Crystal structure of glycoprotein B from herpes simplex virus 1. *Science* **313:**217–220.
85. **Hirsch, M. S., R. T. Schooley, A. B. Cosimi, P. S. Russell, F. L. Delmonico, N. E. Tolkoff-Rubin, J. T. Herrin, K. Cantell, M. L. Farrell, T. R. Rota, and R. H. Rubin.** 1983. Effects of interferon-alpha on cytomegalovirus reactivation syndromes in renal-transplant recipients. *N. Engl. J. Med.* **308:**1489–1493.
86. **Homman-Loudiyi, M., K. Hultenby, W. Britt, and C. Söderberg-Nauclér.** 2003. Envelopment of human cytomegalovirus occurs by budding into Golgi-derived vacuole compartments positive for gB, Rab 3, trans-Golgi network 46, and mannosidase II. *J. Virol.* **77:**3191–3203.
87. **Huang, L., Y. Zhu, and D. G. Anders.** 1996. The variable 3′ ends of a human cytomegalovirus *ori*Lyt transcript (SRT) overlap an essential, conserved replicator element. *J. Virol.* **70:**5272–5281.
88. **Ishov, A. M., R. M. Stenberg, and G. G. Maul.** 1997. Human cytomegalovirus immediate early interaction with host nuclear structures: definition of an immediate transcript environment. *J. Cell Biol.* **138:**5–16.
89. **Kalayjian, R. C., M. L. Cohen, R. A. Bonomo, and T. P. Flanigan.** 1993. Cytomegalovirus ventriculoencephalitis in AIDS. A syndrome with distinct clinical and pathologic features. *Medicine* (Baltimore) **72:**67–77.
90. **Kamil, J. P., and D. M. Coen.** 2007. Human cytomegalovirus protein kinase UL97 forms a complex with the tegument phosphoprotein pp65. *J. Virol.* **81:**10659–10668.
91. **Kempen, J. H., D. A. Jabs, L. A. Wilson, J. P. Dunn, S. K. West, and J. Tonascia.** 2003. Mortality risk for patients with cytomegalovirus retinitis and acquired immune deficiency syndrome. *Clin. Infect. Dis.* **37:**1365–1373.
92. **Khan, N., N. Shariff, M. Cobbold, R. Bruton, J. A. Ainsworth, A. J. Sinclair, L. Nayak, and P. A. Moss.** 2002. Cytomegalovirus seropositivity drives the CD8 T

cell repertoire toward greater clonality in healthy elderly individuals. *J. Immunol.* **169:**1984–1992.
93. **Khoury, J. A., G. A. Storch, D. L. Bohl, R. M. Schuessler, S. M. Torrence, M. Lockwood, M. Gaudreault-Keener, M. J. Koch, B. W. Miller, K. L. Hardinger, M. A. Schnitzler, and D. C. Brennan.** 2006. Prophylactic versus preemptive oral valganciclovir for the management of cytomegalovirus infection in adult renal transplant recipients. *Am. J. Transplant.* **6:**2134–2143.
94. **Kidd, I. M., J. C. Fox, D. Pillay, H. Charman, P. D. Griffiths, and V. C. Emery.** 1993. Provision of prognostic information in immunocompromised patients by routine application of the polymerase chain reaction for cytomegalovirus. *Transplantation* **56:**867–871.
95. **Kimberlin, D. W., C. Y. Lin, P. J. Sanchez, G. J. Demmler, W. Dankner, M. Shelton, R. F. Jacobs, W. Vaudry, R. F. Pass, J. M. Kiell, S. J. Soong, and R. J. Whitley.** 2003. Effect of ganciclovir therapy on hearing in symptomatic congenital cytomegalovirus disease involving the central nervous system: a randomized, controlled trial. *J. Pediatr.* **143:**16–25.
96. **Kinzler, E. R., and T. Compton.** 2005. Characterization of human cytomegalovirus glycoprotein-induced cell-cell fusion. *J. Virol.* **79:**7827–7837.
97. **Klemola, E., R. Von Essen, G. Henle, and W. Henle.** 1970. Infectious-mononucleosis-like disease with negative heterophil agglutination test. Clinical features in relation to Epstein-Barr virus and cytomegalovirus antibodies. *J. Infect. Dis.* **121:**608–614.
98. **Koskinen, P. K., M. S. Nieminen, L. A. Krogerus, K. B. Lemström, S. P. Mattila, P. J. Häyry, and I. T. Lautenschlager.** 1993. Cytomegalovirus infection and accelerated cardiac allograft vasculopathy in human cardiac allografts. *J. Heart Lung Transplant.* **12:**724–729.
99. **Landini, M. P., and R. R. Spaete.** 1993. Human cytomegalovirus structural proteins: a report of the first nomenclature workshop, p. 65–74. *In* S. Michelson and S. A. Plotkin (ed.), *Multidisciplinary Approach to Understanding Cytomegalovirus Disease*. Elsevier, Amsterdam, The Netherlands.
100. **Loveland, A. N., N. L. Nguyen, E. J. Brignole, and W. Gibson.** 2007. The amino-conserved domain of human cytomegalovirus UL80a proteins is required for key interactions during early stages of capsid formation and virus production. *J. Virol.* **81:**620–628.
101. **Lowance, D., H.-H. Neumayer, C. M. Legendre, J.-P. Squifflet, J. Kovarik, P. J. Brennan, D. Norman, R. Mendez, M. R. Keating, G. L. Coggon, A. Crisp, and I. C. Lee for the International Valacyclovir Cytomegalovirus Prophylaxis Transplantation Study Group.** 1999. Valacyclovir for the prevention of cytomegalovirus disease after renal transplantation. *N. Engl. J. Med.* **340:**1462–1470.
102. **Lui, S. F., A. A. Ali, J. E. Grundy, O. N. Fernando, P. D. Griffiths, and P. Sweny.** 1992. Double-blind, placebo-controlled trial of human lymphoblastoid interferon prophylaxis of cytomegalovirus infection in renal transplant recipients. *Nephrol. Dial. Transplant.* **7:**1230–1237.
103. **Macdonald, P. S., A. M. Keogh, D. Marshman, D. Richens, A. Harvison, A. M. Kaan, and P. M. Spratt.** 1995. A double-blind placebo-controlled trial of low-dose ganciclovir to prevent cytomegalovirus disease after heart transplantation. *J. Heart Lung Transplant.* **14:**32–38.
104. **Mar, E. C., E. S, Huang, Y. C. Cheng, and J. F. Chiou.** 1985. Inhibition of cellular DNA polymerase alpha and human cytomegalovirus-induced DNA polymerase by the triphosphates of 9-(2-hydroxyethoxymethyl)guanine and 9-(1,3-dihydroxy-2-propoxymethyl)guanine. *J. Virol.* **53:**776–780.
105. **Margulies, B. J., and W. Gibson.** 2007. The chemokine receptor homologue encoded by US27 of human cytomegalovirus is heavily glycosylated and is present in infected human foreskin fibroblasts and enveloped virus particles. *Virus Res.* **123:**57–71.
106. **Mattes, F. M., E. G. Hainsworth, A. M. Geretti, G. Nebbia, G. Prentice, M. Potter, A. K. Burroughs, P. Sweny, A. F. Hassan-Walker, S. Okwuadi, C. Sabin, G. Amooty, V. S. Brown, S. C. Grace, V. C. Emery, and P. D. Griffiths.** 2004. A randomized, controlled trial comparing ganciclovir to ganciclovir plus foscarnet (each at half dose) for preemptive therapy of cytomegalovirus infection in transplant recipients. *J. Infect. Dis.* **189:**1355–1361.
107. **Mattes, F. M., J. E. McLaughlin, V. C. Emery, D. A. Clark, and P. D. Griffiths.** 2000. Histopathological detection of owl's eye inclusions is still specific for cytomegalovirus in the era of human herpesviruses 6 and 7. *J. Clin. Pathol.* **53:**612–614.
108. **McKeating, J. A., P. D. Griffiths, and R. A. Weiss.** 1990. HIV susceptibility conferred to human fibroblasts by cytomegalovirus-induced Fc receptor. *Nature* **343:**659–661.
109. **Merigan, T. C., D. G. Renlund, S. Keay, M. R. Bristow, V. Starnes, J. B. O'Connell, S. Resta, D. Dunn, P. Gamberg, R. M. Ratkovec, et al.** 1992. A controlled trial of ganciclovir to prevent cytomegalovirus disease after heart transplantation. *N. Engl. J. Med.* **326:**1182–1186.
110. **Metselaar, H. J., P. H. Rothbarth, R. M. Brouwer, G. J. Wenting, J. Jeekel, and W. Weimar.** 1989. Prevention of cytomegalovirus-related death by passive immunization. A double-blind placebo-controlled study in kidney transplant recipients treated for rejection. *Transplantation* **48:**264–266.
111. **Meyer-Konig, U., A. Serr, L. D. von Laer, G. Kirste, C. Wolff, O. Haller, D. Neumann-Haefelin, and F. T. Hufert.** 1995. Human cytomegalovirus immediate early and late transcripts in peripheral blood leukocytes: diagnostic value in renal transplant recipients. *J. Infect. Dis.* **171:**705–709.
112. **Meyers, J. D., E. C. Reed, D. H. Shepp, M. Thornquist, P. S. Dandliker, C. A. Vicary, N. Flournoy, L. E. Kirk, J. H. Kersey, E. D. Thomas, et al.** 1988. Acyclovir for prevention of cytomegalovirus infection and disease after allogeneic marrow transplantation. *N. Engl. J. Med.* **318:**70–75.
113. **Mocarski, E. S.** 1993. Cytomegalovirus biology and replication, p. 173–226. *In* B. Roizman, R. J. Whitley, and C. Lopez (ed.), *The Human Herpesviruses*. Raven Press, New York, NY.
114. **Mocarski, E. S., T. Shenk, and R. Pass.** 2007. Cytomegalovirus, p. 2701–2772. *In* D. M. Knipe, P. M. Howley, D. E. Griffin, R. A. Lamb, M. A. Martin, B. Roizman, and S. E. Straus (ed.), *Fields Virology*, 5th ed. Lippincott Williams & Wilkins, Philadelphia, PA.
115. **Nevels, M., C. Paulus, and T. Shenk.** 2004. Human cytomegalovirus immediate-early 1 protein facilitates viral replication by antagonizing histone deacetylation. *Proc. Natl. Acad. Sci. USA* **101:**17234–17239.
116. **Odeberg, J., B. Plachter, L. Branden, and C. Soderberg-Naucler.** 2003. Human cytomegalovirus protein pp65 mediates accumulation of HLA-DR in lysosomes and destruction of the HLA-DR alpha-chain. *Blood* **101:**4870–4877.
117. **Ogawa-Goto, K., K. Tanaka, W. Gibson, E. Moriishi, Y. Miura, T. Kurata, S. Irie, and T. Sata.** 2003. Micro-

tubule network facilitates nuclear targeting of human cytomegalovirus capsid. *J. Virol.* **77:**8541–8547.

117a. **Pari, G. S., and D. G. Anders.** 1993. Eleven loci encoding *trans*-acting factors are required for transient complementation of human cytomegalovirus *ori*Lyt-dependent DNA replication. *J. Virol.* **67:**6979–6988.

118. **Pari, G. S., M. A. Kacica, and D. G. Anders.** 1993. Open reading frames UL44, IRS1/TRS1, and UL36-38 are required for transient complementation of human cytomegalovirus *ori*Lyt-dependent DNA synthesis. *J. Virol.* **67:**2575–2582.

119. **Pass, R. F., A. M. Duliege, S. Boppana, R. Sekulovich, S. Percell, W. Britt, and R. L. Burke.** 1999. A subunit cytomegalovirus vaccine based on recombinant envelope glycoprotein B and a new adjuvant. *J. Infect. Dis.* **180:** 970–975.

120. **Pass, R. F., C. Hutto, M. D. Lyon, and G. Cloud.** 1990. Increased rate of cytomegalovirus infection among day care center workers. *Pediatr. Infect. Dis. J.* **9:**465–470.

121. **Patrone, M., M. Secchi, E. Bonaparte, G. Milanesi, and A. Gallina.** 2007. Cytomegalovirus UL131-128 products promote gB conformational transition and gB-gH interaction during entry into endothelial cells. *J. Virol.* **81:** 11479–11488.

121a. **Paya, C. V., J. A. Richardson, M. J. Espy, I. G. Sia, M. J. DeBernardi, T. F. Smith, R. Patel, G. Jenkins, W. S. Harmsen, D. J. Vanness, and R. H. Wiesner.** 2002. Preemptive use of oral ganciclovir to prevent cytomegalovirus infection in liver transplant patients: a randomized, placebo-controlled trial. *J. Infect. Dis.* **185:** 854–860.

122. **Pfeffer, S., A. Sewer, M. Lagos-Quintana, R. Sheridan, C. Sander, F. A. Grasser, L. F. van Dyk, C. K. Ho, S. Shuman, M. Chien, J. J. Russo, J. Ju, G. Randall, B. D. Lindenbach, C. M. Rice, V. Simon, D. D. Ho, M. Zavolan, and T. Tuschl.** 2005. Identification of microRNAs of the herpesvirus family. *Nat. Meth.* **2:**269–276.

123. **Pillay, D., M. C. Lipman, C. A. Lee, M. A. Johnson, P. D. Griffiths, and J. E. McLaughlin.** 1993. A clinicopathological audit of opportunistic viral infections in HIV-infected patients. *AIDS* **7:**969–974.

124. **Plafker, S. M., and W. Gibson.** 1998. Cytomegalovirus assembly protein precursor and proteinase precursor contain two nuclear localization signals that mediate their own nuclear translocation and that of the major capsid protein. *J. Virol.* **72:**7722–7732.

125. **Plotkin, S. A., M. L. Smiley, H. M. Friedman, S. E. Starr, G. R. Fleisher, C. Wlodaver, D. C. Dafoe, A. D. Friedman, R. A. Grossman, and C. F. Barker.** 1984. Towne-vaccine-induced prevention of cytomegalovirus disease after renal transplants. *Lancet* **i:**528–530.

126. **Prentice, H. G., E. Gluckman, R. L. Powles, P. Ljungman, N. Milpied, J. M. Fernandez Rañada, F. Mandelli, P. Kho, L. Kennedy, and A. R. Bell for the European Acyclovir for CMV Prophylaxis Study Group.** 1994. Impact of long-term acyclovir on cytomegalovirus infection and survival after allogeneic bone marrow transplantation. *Lancet* **343:**749–753.

127. **Prichard, M. N., S. Jairath, M. E. Penfold, S. St. Jeor, M. C. Bohlman, and G. S. Pari.** 1998. Identification of persistent RNA-DNA hybrid structures within the origin of replication of human cytomegalovirus. *J. Virol.* **72:**6997–7004.

128. **Radsak, K., M. Eickmann, T. Mockenhaupt, E. Bogner, H. Kern, A. Eis-Hubinger, and M. Reschke.** 1996. Retrieval of human cytomegalovirus glycoprotein B from the infected cell surface for virus envelopment. *Arch. Virol.* **141:**557–572.

129. **Razonable, R. R., R. A. Brown, J. Wilson, C. Groettum, W. Kremers, M. Espy, T. F. Smith, and C. V. Paya.** 2002. The clinical use of various blood compartments for cytomegalovirus (CMV) DNA quantitation in transplant recipients with CMV disease. *Transplantation* **73:**968–973.

130. **Reed, E. C., J. L. Wolford, K. J. Kopecky, K. E. Lilleby, P. S. Dandliker, J. L. Todaro, G. B. McDonald, and J. D. Meyers.** 1990. Ganciclovir for the treatment of cytomegalovirus gastroenteritis in bone marrow transplant patients. A randomized, placebo-controlled trial. *Ann. Intern. Med.* **112:**505–510.

131. **Reeves, M. B., A. A. Davies, B. P. McSharry, G. W. Wilkinson, and J. H. Sinclair.** 2007. Complex I binding by a virally encoded RNA regulates mitochondria-induced cell death. *Science* **316:**1345–1348.

132. **Reeves, M. B., P. A. MacAry, P. J. Lehner, J. G. Sissons, and J. H. Sinclair.** 2005. Latency, chromatin remodeling, and reactivation of human cytomegalovirus in the dendritic cells of healthy carriers. *Proc. Natl. Acad. Sci. USA* **102:**4140–4145.

133. **Reischig, T., P. Jindra, O. Hes, M. Svecová, J. Klaboch, and V. Treska.** 2008. Valacyclovir prophylaxis versus preemptive valganciclovir therapy to prevent cytomegalovirus disease after renal transplantation. *Am. J. Transplant.* **8:**69–77.

134. **Reusser, P., H. Einsele, J. Lee, L. Volin, M. Rovira, D. Engelhard, J. Finke, C. Cordonnier, H. Link, and P. Ljungman.** 2002. Randomized multicenter trial of foscarnet versus ganciclovir for preemptive therapy of cytomegalovirus infection after allogeneic stem cell transplantation. *Blood* **99:**1159–1164.

135. **Rubin, R. H.** 1991. Preemptive therapy in immunocompromised hosts. *N. Engl. J. Med.* **324:**1057–1059.

136. **Rubin, R. H.** 1989. The indirect effects of cytomegalovirus infection on the outcome of organ transplantation. *JAMA* **261:**3607–3609.

137. **Sanchez, V., E. Sztul, and W. J. Britt.** 2000. Human cytomegalovirus pp28 (UL99) localizes to a cytoplasmic compartment which overlaps the endoplasmic reticulum-Golgi-intermediate compartment. *J. Virol.* **74:** 3842–3851.

138. **Schleiss, M. R.** 2006. Acquisition of human cytomegalovirus infection in infants via breast milk: natural immunization or cause for concern? *Rev. Med. Virol.* **16:** 73–82.

139. **Schmidt, G. M., D. A. Horak, J. C. Niland, S. R. Duncan, S. J. Forman, and J. A. Zaia for The City of Hope-Stanford-Syntex CMV Study Group.** 1991. A randomized, controlled trial of prophylactic ganciclovir for cytomegalovirus pulmonary infection in recipients of allogeneic bone marrow transplants. *N. Engl. J. Med.* **324:**1005–1011.

140. **Schmolke, S., H. F. Kern, P. Drescher, G. Jahn, and B. Plachter.** 1995. The dominant phosphoprotein pp65 (UL83) of human cytomegalovirus is dispensable for growth in cell culture. *J. Virol.* **69:**5959–5968.

141. **Silva, M. C., Q. C. Yu, L. Enquist, and T. Shenk.** 2003. Human cytomegalovirus UL99-encoded pp28 is required for the cytoplasmic envelopment of tegument-associated capsids. *J. Virol.* **77:**10594–10605.

142. **Sinclair, J., and P. Sissons.** 2006. Latency and reactivation of human cytomegalovirus. *J. Gen. Virol.* **87:** 1763–1779.

143. **Singh, N.** 2006. Antiviral drugs for cytomegalovirus in transplant recipients: advantages of preemptive therapy. *Rev. Med. Virol.* **16:**281–287.

144. **Snydman, D. R.** 2006. The case for cytomegalovirus prophylaxis in solid organ transplantation. *Rev. Med. Virol.* **16:**289–295.

145. **Snydman, D. R., B. G. Werner, N. N. Dougherty, J. Griffith, R. H. Rubin, J. L. Dienstag, R. H. Rohrer, R. Freeman, R. Jenkins, W. D. Lewis, S. Hammer, E. O'Rourke, G. F. Grady, K. Fawaz, M. M. Kaplan, M. A. Hoffman, A. T. Katz, and M. Doran for The Boston Center for Liver Transplantation CMVIG Study Group.** 1993. Cytomegalovirus immune globulin prophylaxis in liver transplantation. A randomized, double-blind, placebo-controlled trial. *Ann. Intern. Med.* **119:**984–991.

146. **Soderberg-Naucler, C., K. N. Fish, and J. A. Nelson.** 1997. Reactivation of latent human cytomegalovirus by allogeneic stimulation of blood cells from healthy donors. *Cell* **91:**119–126.

147. **Sourvinos, G., N. Tavalai, A. Berndt, D. A. Spandidos, and T. Stamminger.** 2007. Recruitment of human cytomegalovirus immediate-early 2 protein onto parental viral genomes in association with ND10 in live-infected cells. *J. Virol.* **81:**10123–10136.

148. **Spector, S. A., K. Hsia, M. Crager, M. Pilcher, S. Cabral, and M. J. Stempien.** 1999. Cytomegalovirus (CMV) DNA load is an independent predictor of CMV disease and survival in advanced AIDS. *J. Virol.* **73:** 7027–7030.

149. **Spector, S. A., R. Merrill, D. Wolf, and W. M. Dankner.** 1992. Detection of human cytomegalovirus in plasma of AIDS patients during acute visceral disease by DNA amplification. *J. Clin. Microbiol.* **30:**2359–2365.

150. **Spector, S. A., R. Wong, K. Hsia, M. Pilcher, and M. J. Stempien.** 1998. Plasma cytomegalovirus (CMV) DNA load predicts CMV disease and survival in AIDS patients. *J. Clin. Investig.* **101:**497–502.

151. **Squire, S. B., M. C. Lipman, E. K. Bagdades, P. M. Mulvenna, J. E. Grundy, P. D. Griffiths, and M. A. Johnson.** 1992. Severe cytomegalovirus pneumonitis in HIV infected patients with higher than average CD4 counts. *Thorax* **47:**301–304.

152. **Stagno, S., D. W. Reynolds, A. Tsiantos, D. A. Fuccillo, W. Long, and C. A. Alford.** 1975. Comparative serial virologic and serologic studies of symptomatic and subclinical congenitally and natally acquired cytomegalovirus infections. *J. Infect. Dis.* **132:**568–577.

153. **Stals, F. S., S. S. Wagenaar, and C. A. Bruggeman.** 1994. Generalized cytomegalovirus (CMV) infection and CMV-induced pneumonitis in the rat: combined effect of 9-(1,3-dihydroxy-2-propoxymethyl)guanine and specific antibody treatment. *Antivir. Res.* **25:**147–160.

154. **Stern-Ginossar, N., N. Elefant, A. Zimmermann, D. G. Wolf, N. Saleh, M. Biton, E. Horwitz, Z. Prokocimer, M. Prichard, G. Hahn, D. Goldman-Wohl, C. Greenfield, S. Yagel, H. Hengel, Y. Altuvia, H. Margalit, and O. Mandelboim.** 2007. Host immune system gene targeting by a viral miRNA. *Science* **317:**376–381.

155. **Streblow, D. N., C. Soderberg-Naucler, J. Vieira, P. Smith, E. Wakabayashi, F. Ruchti, K. Mattison, Y. Altschuler, and J. A. Nelson.** 1999. The human cytomegalovirus chemokine receptor US28 mediates vascular smooth muscle cell migration. *Cell* **99:**511–520.

156. **Strindhall, J., B. O. Nilsson, S. Löfgren, J. Ernerudh, G. Pawelec, B. Johansson, and A. Wikby.** 2007. No Immune Risk Profile among individuals who reach 100 years of age: findings from the Swedish NONA immune longitudinal study. *Exp. Gerontol.* **42:**753–761.

157. **Strive, T., E. Borst, M. Messerle, and K. Radsak.** 2002. Proteolytic processing of human cytomegalovirus glycoprotein B is dispensable for viral growth in culture. *J. Virol.* **76:**1252–1264.

158. **Sylwester, A. W., B. L. Mitchell, J. B. Edgar, C. Taormina, C. Pelte, F. Ruchti, P. R. Sleath, K. H. Grabstein, N. A. Hosken, F. Kern, J. A. Nelson, and L. J. Picker.** 2005. Broadly targeted human cytomegalovirus-specific CD4+ and CD8+ T cells dominate the memory compartments of exposed subjects. *J. Exp. Med.* **202:** 673–685.

159. **Taylor-Wiedeman, J., J. G. Sissons, L. K. Borysiewicz, and J. H. Sinclair.** 1991. Monocytes are a major site of persistence of human cytomegalovirus in peripheral blood mononuclear cells. *J. Gen. Virol.* **72**(Pt. 9)**:**2059–2064.

160. **Thoma, C., E. Borst, M. Messerle, M. Rieger, J. S. Hwang, and E. Bogner.** 2006. Identification of the interaction domain of the small terminase subunit pUL89 with the large subunit pUL56 of human cytomegalovirus. *Biochemistry* **45:**8855–8863.

161. **Thorne, J. E., D. A. Jabs, J. H. Kempen, J. T. Holbrook, C. Nichols, and C. L. Meinert.** 2006. Causes of visual acuity loss among patients with AIDS and cytomegalovirus retinitis in the era of highly active antiretroviral therapy. *Ophthalmology* **113:**1441–1445.

162. **Trgovcich, J., C. Cebulla, P. Zimmerman, and D. D. Sedmak.** 2006. Human cytomegalovirus protein pp71 disrupts major histocompatibility complex class I cell surface expression. *J. Virol.* **80:**951–963.

163. **Trzonkowski, P., J. Mysliwska, E. Szmit, J. Wieckiewicz, K. Lukaszuk, L. B. Brydak, M. Machala, and A. Mysliwski.** 2003. Association between cytomegalovirus infection, enhanced proinflammatory response and low level of anti-hemagglutinins during the anti-influenza vaccination—an impact of immunosenescence. *Vaccine* **21:**3826–3836.

164. Reference deleted.

165. **Valantine, H. A., S. Z. Gao, S. G. Menon, D. G. Renlund, S. A. Hunt, P. Oyer, E. B. Stinson, B. W. Brown, Jr., T. C. Merigan, and J. S. Schroeder.** 1999. Impact of prophylactic immediate posttransplant ganciclovir on development of transplant atherosclerosis: a post hoc analysis of a randomized, placebo-controlled study. *Circulation* **100:**61–66.

166. **Varnum, S. M., D. N. Streblow, M. E. Monroe, P. Smith, K. J. Auberry, L. Pasa-Tolic, D. Wang, D. G. Camp, K. Rodland, S. Wiley, W. Britt, T. Shenk, R. D. Smith, and J. A. Nelson.** 2004. Identification of proteins in human cytomegalovirus (HCMV) particles: the HCMV proteome. *J. Virol.* **78:**10960–10966.

167. **Vinters, H. V., M. K. Kwok, H. W. Ho, K. H. Anders, U. Tomiyasu, and W. L. Wolfson.** 1989. Cytomegalovirus in the nervous system of patients with the acquired immune deficiency syndrome. *Brain* **112:**245–268.

168. **Walter, S., C. E. Atkinson, M. Sharland, P. Rice, E. Raglan, V. C. Emery, and P. D. Griffiths.** 2008. Congenital cytomegalovirus: association between dried blood spot viral load and hearing loss. *Arch. Dis. Child. Fet. Neonat. Ed.* **93:**F280–F285.

169. **Wang, D., and T. Shenk.** 2005. Human cytomegalovirus virion protein complex required for epithelial and endothelial cell tropism. *Proc. Natl. Acad. Sci. USA* **102:** 18153–18158.

170. **Webster, A., B. Blizzard, D. Pillay, H. G. Prentice, K. Pothecary, and P. D. Griffiths.** 1993. Value of routine surveillance cultures for detection of CMV pneumonitis following bone marrow transplantation. *Bone Marrow Transplant.* **12:**477–481.

171. **Wilkinson, G. W., C. Kelly, J. H. Sinclair, and C. Rickards.** 1998. Disruption of PML-associated nuclear bodies mediated by the human cytomegalovirus major

immediate early gene product. *J. Gen. Virol.* **79**(Pt. 5): 1233–1245.

172. **Wimperis, J. Z., M. K. Brenner, H. G. Prentice, J. E. Reittie, P. Karayiannis, and A. V. Hoffbrand.** 1986. Transfer of a functioning humoral immune system in transplantation of T-lymphocyte-depleted bone marrow. *Lancet* **i**:339–343.
173. **Winston, D. J., J.-A. H. Young, V. Pullarkat, G. A. Papanicolaou, R. Vij, E. Vance, G. J. Alangaden, R. F. Chemaly, F. Petersen, N. Chao, J. Klein, K. Sprague, S. A. Villano, and M. Boeckh.** 2008. Maribavir prophylaxis for prevention of cytomegalovirus infection in allogeneic stem cell transplant recipients: a multicenter, randomized, double-blind, placebo-controlled, dose-ranging study. *Blood* **111**:5403–5410.
174. **Winston, D. J., E. S. Huang, M. J. Miller, C. H. Lin, W. G. Ho, R. P. Gale, and R. E. Champlin.** 1985. Molecular epidemiology of cytomegalovirus infections associated with bone marrow transplantation. *Ann. Intern. Med.* **102**:16–20.
175. **Winston, D. J., D. Wirin, A. Shaked, and R. W. Busuttil.** 1995. Randomized comparison of ganciclovir and high-dose acyclovir for long-term cytomegalovirus prophylaxis in liver-transplant recipients. *Lancet* **346**:69–74.
176. Reference deleted.
177. **Yurochko, A. D., E. S. Hwang, L. Rasmussen, S. Keay, L. Pereira, and E. S. Huang.** 1997. The human cytomegalovirus UL55 (gB) and UL75 (gH) glycoprotein ligands initiate the rapid activation of Sp1 and NF-κB during infection. *J. Virol.* **71**:5051–5059.
178. **Zhang, C., H. Buchanan, W. Andrews, A. Evans, and R. F. Pass.** 2006. Detection of cytomegalovirus infection during a vaccine clinical trial in healthy young women: seroconversion and viral shedding. *J. Clin. Virol.* **35**: 338–342.

Human Herpesvirus 6 and Human Herpesvirus 7

KOICHI YAMANISHI AND YASUKO MORI

23

Human herpesvirus 6 (HHV-6) was first isolated from patients with lymphoproliferative disorders in 1986 and was initially named human B-lymphotropic virus (113). Later it was found to mainly infect and replicate in lymphocytes of T-cell lineage (1). Subsequently, several reports described the isolation of similar viruses mainly from patients with human immunodeficiency virus (HIV) infection/AIDS. Characterization of HHV-6 indicated that the virus is antigenically and genetically distinct from other known human herpesviruses (81, 113). Primary HHV-6 infection occurs during infancy; this virus was recognized as the causative agent of exanthem subitum (ES) in infants in 1988 (148).

Another novel human herpesvirus, human herpesvirus 7 (HHV-7), was isolated in 1990 by Frenkel et al. from $CD4^+$ lymphocytes of a healthy adult (44). Seroepidemiological studies have indicated that primary HHV-7 infection also occurs during childhood, as occurs with HHV-6.

VIROLOGY

Classification

HHV-6 and HHV-7 are members of the *Herpesviridae* family. Genomic analysis supports their classification as in the *Roseolovirus* genus of betaherpesviruses. On the basis of similarity between the amino acid sequences, gene organization, and putative protein functions, human cytomegalovirus (HCMV) is the closest phylogenetic relative of HHV-6 and HHV-7 (11, 76).

HHV-6 strains which were isolated in different regions of the world are closely related to one another. Two distinct variants of HHV-6 exist, as demonstrated by the molecular epidemiological techniques of restriction enzyme analysis, DNA sequencing, and reactivity with monoclonal antibodies (MAbs). These are named HHV-6 variant A (HHV-6A) and variant B (HHV-6B). Virus strains belonging to HHV-6A, including the original isolate (GS strain), are isolated mainly from patients with lymphoproliferative disorders or AIDS. HHV-6B strains are isolated mostly from patients with ES.

HHV-7 cross-hybridizes with some HHV-6 DNA probes. There are no recognized HHV-7 variants to date, but there is significant genetic variation among isolates. Predictably, there is also antigenic cross-reactivity between HHV-6 and HHV-7 (11, 143).

Composition

Virion Structure

Electron microscopic examination of infected cells showed that HHV-6 is an enveloped virion with an icosahedral capsid with 162 capsomeres (Fig. 1) (13). Most of the capsids are in the nucleus and have cores of low density with a diameter of 90 to 110 nm. Enveloped viral particles are observed in cytoplasmic vacuoles as well as extracellularly and have a diameter of 170 to 200 nm. In the nucleus, tubular structures have been occasionally observed (149). Naked particles gradually acquire a full tegument in a nuclear vacuole. The tegument is clearly demonstrable in extracellular particles. Fusion events with the nuclear membranes result in the release of the tegumented capsids into the cytoplasm. The tegumented capsids then undergo envelopment in cytoplasmic vacuoles, yielding mature virions. Fusion of the vacuole membrane with the cell membrane releases the intact virion into the extracellular space.

Ultrastructural analysis of cells infected with HHV-6 revealed the presence of annulate lamellae (AL) in the cell cytoplasm. Their formation correlated with the expression of the late viral glycoprotein gp116. AL serve as a viral glycoprotein storage compartment and are a putative site of O glycosylation (18). HHV-6 does not express viral glycoproteins on the plasma membrane, a finding distinctly different from that of the other members of the herpesvirus family. Immunolabeling with MAbs shows that the viral glycoproteins are undetectable on nuclear membranes. At the inner nuclear membrane, nucleocapsids acquire a primary envelope lacking viral glycoproteins. After de-envelopment, cytoplasmic nucleocapsids acquire a thick tegument and a secondary envelope with viral glycoproteins at the level of newly formed AL or at the *cis* side of the Golgi complex. The newly acquired secondary viral envelopes contain intermediate forms of glycocomponents, suggesting a sequential glycosylation of the virions during their transit through the Golgi area before their final release into the extracellular space. Immunogold labeling also demonstrates that the viral glycoproteins, which are

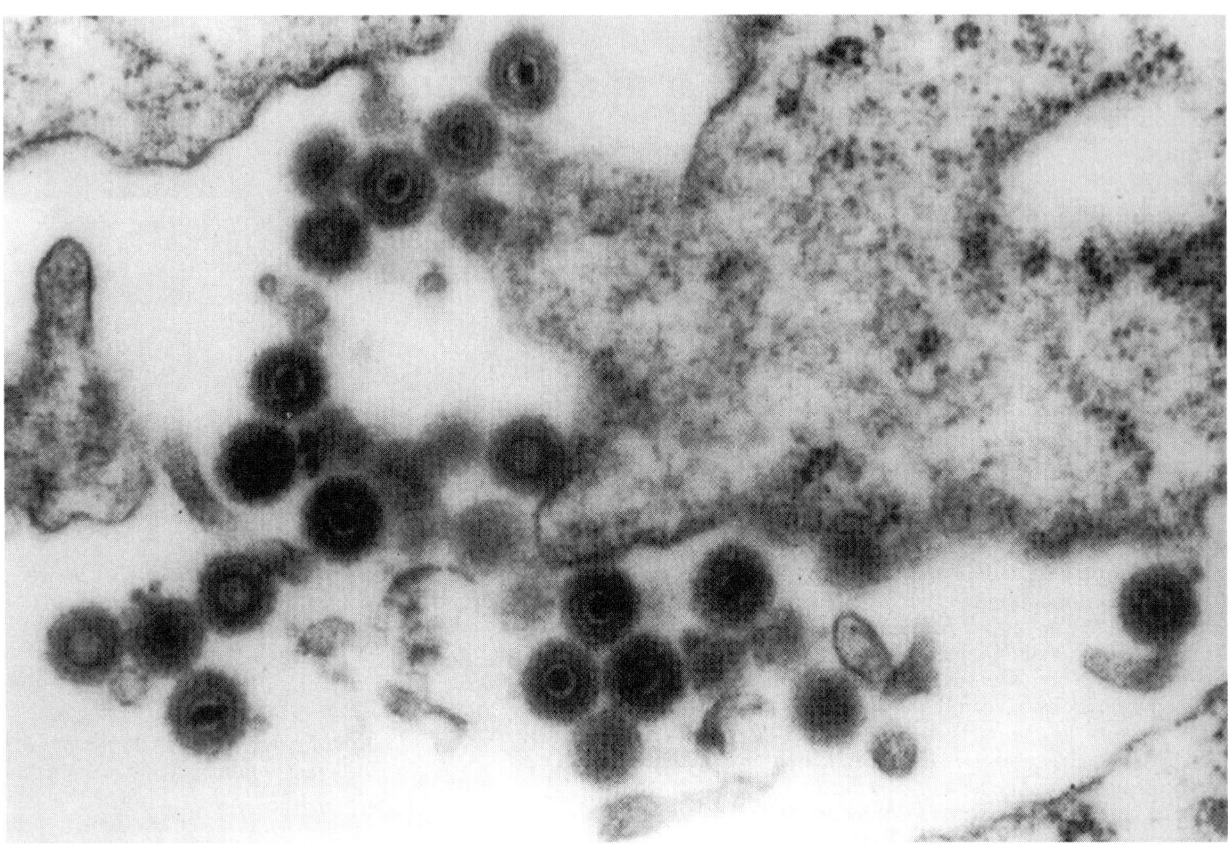

FIGURE 1 Herpesvirus particles seen outside of HHV-6-infected cells.

not involved in the budding process, accumulate in the endosomal/lysosomal compartment (135).

Genomic and Genetic Properties

The HHV-6 genome is a linear, double-stranded DNA molecule with a size of 160 to 170 kbp and is composed of a central segment of a largely unique sequence (U) of approximately 141 kbp, with a sequence of approximately 10 to 13 kbp duplicated in the same orientation at both the left and right genomic termini (DR) (46) (Fig. 2). The DNA length variation maps to the left end of both DR elements, termed the heterogeneous, or *het,* region (79, 107). The left and right termini of the DR contain homologs of the herpesvirus cleavage and packing signals, *pac-1* and *pac-2*, respectively. The mean G+C content of genomic DNA is 43% (79). The entire HHV-6A (U1102 strain) (46), HHV-6B HST (56), and Z29 (33) genomes have been sequenced. HHV-6A and HHV-6B have an overall nucleotide sequence identity of 90% (Fig. 2); the portions of the genomes that span U32 to U77 are highly conserved (95% identity), while the segment spanning U86 to U100 is only 72% identical (33).

HHV-7 also has a linear, double-stranded DNA of 140 to 160 kbp. The complete genomic DNAs of two strains (JI and RK strains) have been sequenced (91, 100). HHV-7 also possesses a similar genome organization, with a single long U flanked by identical direct repeats (DR_L and DR_R), yielding the arrangement DR_L-U-DR_R (116). Furthermore, there are *pac-1* and *pac-2* sequences and repeated sequences of GGGTTA at the end of each DR motif.

Over the conserved domains, roseoloviruses are genetically collinear with cytomegaloviruses, although the cytomegaloviruses contain many genes without roseolovirus counterparts. Within each variant (HHV-6A and HHV-6B) or species (HHV-7), these viruses exhibit relatively little genetic variability. Between HHV-6 and HHV-7, amino acid sequence identities range from 22 to 75%, most being in the vicinity of 50%. There is evidence for subgrouping within the HHV-6B variant at some genomic loci (25) and among HHV-7 isolates (43), but there is no indication that this is anything other than intraspecies allelic variation.

Protein Properties

More than 30 polypeptides with molecular masses ranging from 30 to 200 kDa, including six or seven glycoproteins, are found in HHV-6 virions and in cells infected with HHV-6 (10, 118, 146). Glycoprotein B (gB) and gH are essential for viral replication; gH induces neutralizing antibody and inhibits the penetration of HHV-6 into susceptible human T lymphocytes (40). The HHV-6 gH/gL complex associates with the gQ complex. The gQ complex, made up of the products of the U100 gene, are unique to HHV-6 and HHV-7. The gQ gene products are formed by a complex of gQ1 and gQ2. The gQ2 complex interacts with the gH/gL/gQ1 complex in infected cells and virions to form the gH/gL/gQ1/gQ2 complex (3, 94). The complex is a viral ligand for its cellular receptor, CD46 (97). HHV-6 U47 is a positional homolog of the HCMV gO gene (46) and also associates with the gH/gL complex

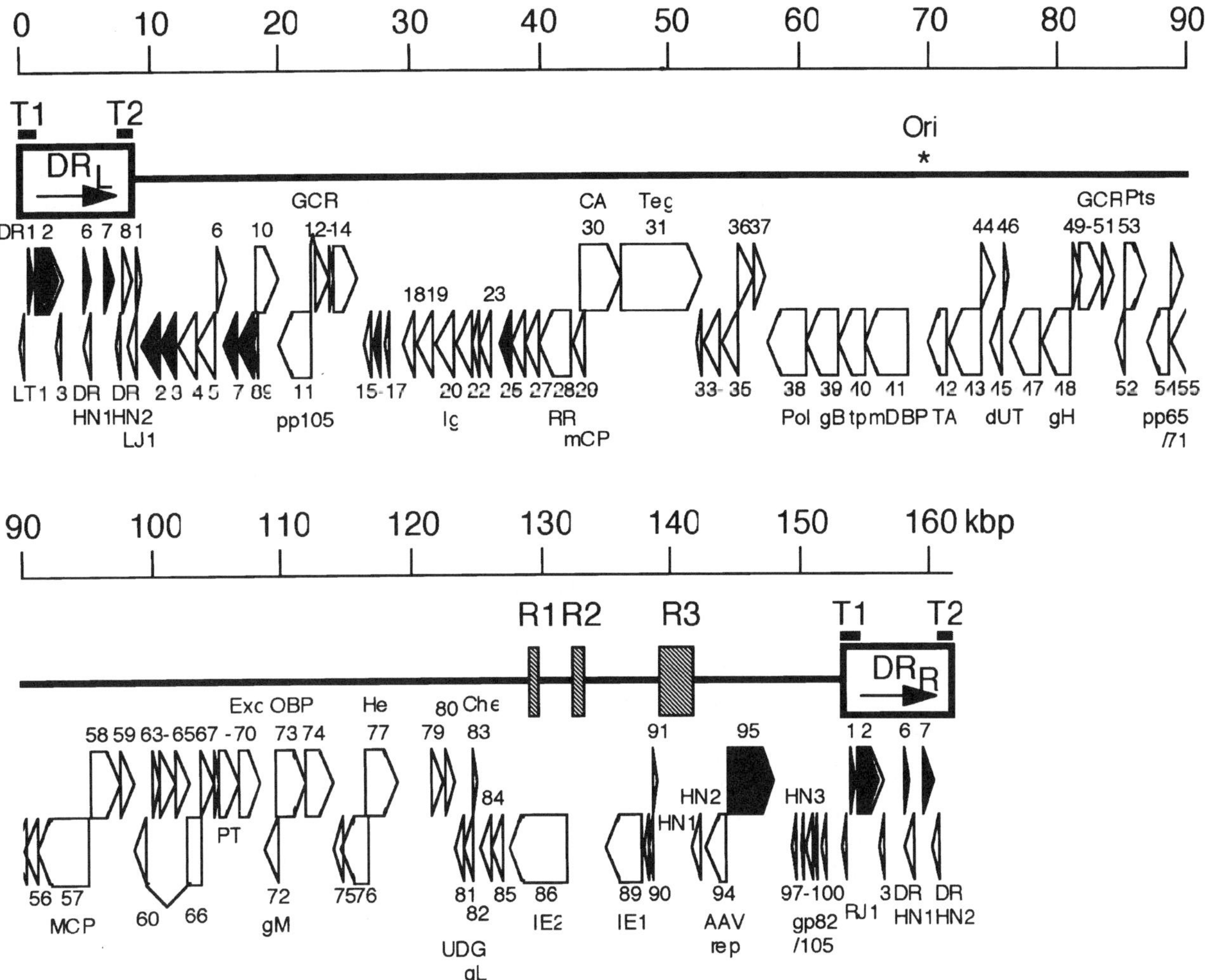

FIGURE 2 Predicted ORF organization of HHV-6 strain HST. Repeat regions (DR_L, DR_R, R1, R2, and R3) are boxed, telomeric repeat regions (T1 and T2) are indicated above the DRs, and UR is indicated by a solid line. Protein coding regions are indicated as open arrows and are numbered DR1, DR2, DR3, DR6, DR7, DR8, DRHN1, and DRHN2 within the direct repeats and HN1, HN2, HN3, and U1 to U100 (excluding U78, U88, U92, U93, and U96) within the UR. The origin of replication (Ori) is indicated by an asterisk. The US22 gene family is shaded. Abbreviations not used in the text: GCR, G-protein-coupled receptor; Ig, Ig immunoglobulin superfamily; RR, large subunit of ribonucleotide reductase; mCP, minor capsid protein; CA, capsid assembly protein; Teg, tegument protein; Pol, DNA polymerase; tp, transport protein; mDBP, major single-stranded DNA binding protein; TA, conserved herpesvirus transactivator; dUT, dUTPase; Pts, protease/assembly protein; pp65/71, phosphoprotein 65/71K; MCP, major capsid protein; PT, phosphotransferase; Exo, exonuclease; OBP, origin binding protein; Hel, helicase; UDG, uracil-DNA glycosylase; Che, chemokine; AAV rep1, adeno-associated virus replication protein homolog. (Reprinted from reference 56 with permission.)

(94). gQ and gO have much greater sequence divergence than do other glycoproteins (76.8 and 72.1% identity, respectively), suggesting that they contribute to the biological differences. HHV-7 gO also associates with the gH/gL complex in infected cells (112). HHV-6 and HHV-7-U21-encoded glycoproteins associate with the major histocompatibility complex class I molecule (45, 54), and the association functions in lysosome sorting, which may reduce recognition of infected cells by cytotoxic T lymphocytes (CTL).

The predominant species immunoreactive with human serum are p100 (HHV-6A) and p101 (HHV-6B) (99). These proteins function as a tegument protein, like HCMV phosphoprotein 150 (pp150). A polypeptide with an approximate molecular mass of 41 kDa is produced early in the replicative cycle (24). The immediate-early proteins (Fig. 2) may transactivate the HIV long terminal repeat (LTR). HHV-6 also encodes virus-specific DNA polymerase, uracil-DNA glycosidase, and alkaline DNase and induces thymidine kinase and dUTP nucleotidohydrolase. The HHV-6B *rep* gene, which is a homolog of adeno-associated virus type 2 *rep* and is unique in the herpesvirus family, was identified previously (95). HHV-6 and HHV-7 encode viral chemokine and chemokine receptor homologs

(57, 153). U83A encoded by HHV-6A binds a human chemokine, CCR-5, and inhibits HIV replication in vitro, suggesting that HHV-6 U83A acts as a novel inhibitor of HHV-6 infection (22).

At least 20 proteins, including 7 glycoproteins, are specific to HHV-7 and range in apparent molecular mass from 136 to 30 kDa (39). Human antibodies raised to HHV-7 are directed predominantly to one or more HHV-7-infected cell proteins with apparent molecular masses of about 85 to 89 kDa. pp85 is considered a major determinant of the human immune response to HHV-7, discriminating HHV-6 from HHV-7 infection. Further, human sera recognize additional epitopes of pp85 that are required for their full reactivity (41, 121). Some MAbs reacted in immunofluorescence assays with HHV-6 antigens to the same degree as with HHV-7 protein (39, 98).

Biology

HHV-6 is isolated only from human mononuclear cells (mainly $CD4^+$ lymphocytes) and propagates predominantly in $CD4^+$ lymphocytes (89, 129). HHV-6 infects a variety of human cells such as T and B lymphocytes of peripheral blood and cell lines of lymphocytes and macrophages in vitro, and it also infects lymphocytes of chimpanzees.

The cytopathic effect (CPE) induced by HHV-6 begins 1 to 2 days postinfection, as evidenced by enlargement of infected lymphocytes. These refractive giant cells usually contain one or two nuclei, and following the development of CPE, lytic degeneration of the cells occurs (Fig. 3). CD46 is a cellular receptor for HHV-6 (114). HHV-6A can induce fusion from without (fusion that does not require viral protein synthesis) in a variety of human cells, dependent on CD46 expression (96), while the HHV-6B variant is less likely to induce fusion from without based on CD46 expression (106). In contrast, HHV-7 uses CD4 as a receptor for infection in T cells (90).

Although all HHV-6 isolates can infect and replicate in human umbilical cord blood mononuclear cells, HHV-6A strains replicate in immature lymphocytes and more rapidly in a variety of established cell lines, including Epstein-Barr virus-positive B cells, continuous T-cell lines, fibroblasts, megakaryocytes, and glioblastoma cells (1). HHV-6B strains fail to replicate in most continuous cell lines (15), with the exception of Molt-3 and MT-4 cells. The different cellular affinities between the two variants may be due to the lack of viral receptors for entry into the cells or a deficiency in gene expression and viral replication. HHV-6B strains replicate in mature lymphocytes. Prior mitogen activation and full progression of the cell cycle are required for efficient replication, particularly for HHV-6B strains. High levels of interleukin 2 (IL-2) can delay or inhibit viral replication (111).

EPIDEMIOLOGY

Seroprevalence of HHV-6 and -7

The prevalence of antibody to HHV-6 is high in most, but not all, areas of the world. An HHV-6 serologic study in Japan found that the incidences of antibody in different age groups were similar, even in those younger than 10 years. From 6 months of age, the number of children having antibodies gradually increased, and almost all children older than 13 months were seropositive, indicating that almost all children are exposed to HHV-6 in the latter half of the first year of life (104). Since most pregnant women have antibody to HHV-6, immunoglobulin G (IgG) antibody is transferred from mother to child across the placenta, and IgG is detectable in infants during the early

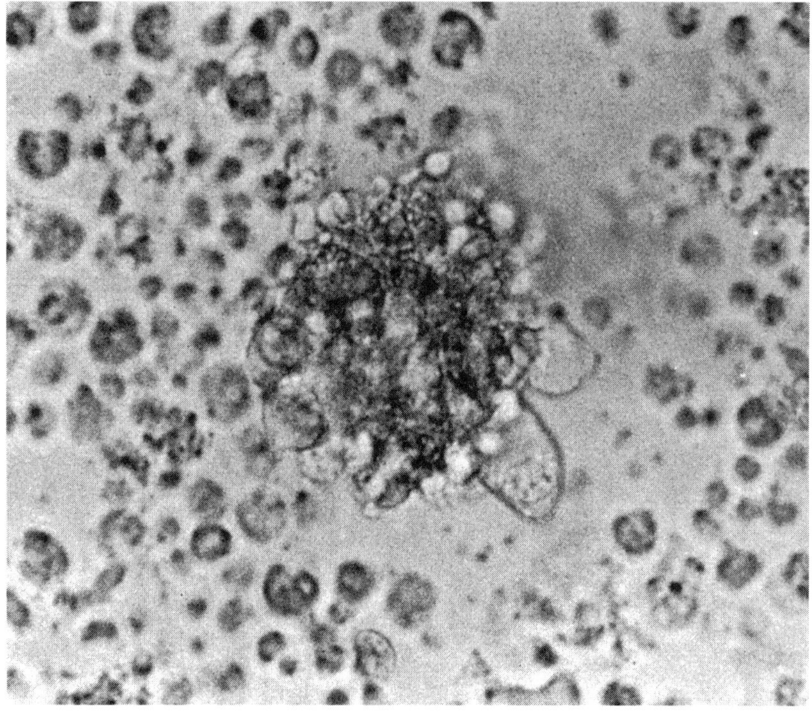

FIGURE 3 CPE by HHV-6. Note the balloon-like cells around clumps of lymphocytes.

months after birth. Very young infants (younger than 6 months) are probably protected against HHV-6 infection by antibody from their mothers.

Infection by HHV-7 occurs slightly later than with HHV-6 (27, 143), although a study in the United Kingdom indicated no difference in the prevalence of antibody to both viruses with respect to age-matched controls (151). No antibody was detectable in children younger than 2 years in the United States (143), but the rate of seropositivity to HHV-7 was 75% in children aged 12 to 23 months in Japan (132).

Mode of Transmission of HHV-6 and -7

The mode of transmission of HHV-6 and -7 to children is not fully understood. No difference has been found in the prevalence rates of HHV-6 infection between breast- and bottle-fed infants (130) or between babies born by cesarean section and those born vaginally. HHV-6 DNA has been detected in saliva and throat swabs from ES patients, as well as in healthy adults, including mothers, by PCR (48, 59, 67). HHV-6 is also present in vaginal secretions of pregnant women (77, 103).

Local spread and seasonal outbreaks of ES are rare, although outbreaks of HHV-6 infection are occasionally observed among institutionalized children (102). Thus, persistent excretion and/or recurrent episodes of shedding of HHV-6 from saliva and cervical secretions of adults suggest that direct close contact is a mode of transmission early in life, mainly from mother to child.

Viral DNA has been detected in fetuses and in the blood of newborns (8, 49, 75). HHV-6 DNA has been detected in 41 to 44% of samples from cervical swabs over a period of 3 to 8 months of pregnancy, which is significantly higher than in the control population (24% of age-matched controls) (31). Specific DNA could be detected in 1 to 1.6% of cord blood specimens from babies born to ostensibly healthy mothers (2, 31). Thus, HHV-6 reactivation seems common during pregnancy, and HHV-6 infection of the fetus may occur. HHV-6 has been found in chromosomes of peripheral blood cells (32, 83), suggesting possible intrauterine infection.

HHV-7 can be frequently isolated from saliva of healthy adults (14, 51, 142), and horizontal transmission of HHV-7 may occur even from grandparents or parents to children through close household contact. Thus, the modes of transmission of HHV-6 and -7 are very similar; however, it is not clear why HHV-7 infection occurs generally later than HHV-6 infection.

PATHOGENESIS

The mechanisms by which HHV-6 induces pathology have not been precisely defined. Immunologic and molecular analyses revealed that $CD4^+$ T lymphocytes are the predominant target cells for HHV-6. Direct viral cytolysis from acute diseases such as ES and heterophil-negative infectious mononucleosis may be responsible. Besides the direct infection of immune cells, indirect pathogenic mechanisms following HHV-6 infection may result from modulation of the immune system. In fact, HHV-6 has been shown to up-regulate CD4 (85) and NK (87) cells and down-regulate CD3 molecules in T cells (86) as well as to induce the release of alpha interferon (IFN-α) (68, 70, 128), IL-1β, and tumor necrosis factor alpha by infected cells (38). Such altered polyclonal cell stimulation and cytokine burst might contribute to the development of lymphoproliferative disorders, including lymphoma and leukemia.

Furthermore, these proinflammatory cytokines can up-regulate HIV replication in vitro and contribute to the pathogenesis of AIDS. Both viruses infect $CD4^+$ T lymphocytes. HHV-6 expression transactivates the HIV type 1 (HIV-1) LTR. HHV-6 infection also induces CD4 molecules on the surfaces of $CD4^-$ $CD8^+$ cells at the transcriptional level, resulting in enhanced susceptibility to HIV-1 infection (36, 53, 85). However, this concept is still controversial, since other reports suggest inhibition of HIV replication in the case of coinfection (19, 78, 81, 108).

As described above, HHV-6 and -7 establish latency after primary infection, but the mechanism is not understood completely. Recently, Jaworska et al. (60) described an immediate-early 1 protein of HHV-6 that inhibits transcription of the IFN-β gene, suggesting a contribution of HHV-6 to latency.

Two HHV-6 (GS) DNA clones induce in vitro tumorigenic transformation of human epidermal keratinocytes (110), but there are no correlates with human tumors to date.

Animal models of HHV-6 or -7 infections are lacking. The transmission of a fever-producing agent to the monkeys inoculated with the serum of a patient during the febrile period of ES has been done (63). Western blotting and immunofluorescent-antibody assay (IFA) demonstrated the presence of HHV-6 antibody in monkeys (52). Chimpanzees are susceptible to productive infection by HHV-6 (88).

CLINICAL MANIFESTATIONS

Acute Infection

Primary HHV-6 infection in early infancy causes ES (roseola infantum), a common illness characterized by high fever for a few days and the appearance of a rash coinciding with subsidence of the fever. The rash appears on the trunk and face and spreads to lower extremities during the subsiding fever (Fig. 4). Human-to-human transmission has been confirmed by experimental inoculation of blood from ES patients into other infants (50, 63). Novel cell culture techniques allowed isolation of the virus (148). HHV-6 infection can occur without clinical symptoms of rash or fever (6, 72, 109, 124, 130). When people escape childhood HHV-6 infection and are infected as adults, they develop a self-limited febrile disease that resembles infectious mononucleosis (12, 121).

The clinical features of primary HHV-7 infection have not been established. In 1994, HHV-7 was isolated from peripheral blood mononuclear cells of two infants with typical ES, and the DNA patterns of the isolated viruses which were digested with various restriction enzymes were very similar to that of the prototype HHV-7 (RK strain) (131). During the convalescent period of one patient, the titer of antibody to HHV-7 increased significantly, whereas the titer of antibody to HHV-6 remained undetectable. In the second patient, who had two independent episodes of ES over 2 months, HHV-6 and -7 were sequentially isolated; HHV-6 seroconversion occurred during the first episode, and HHV-7 seroconversion occurred during the second episode. These results suggest that HHV-7 is also a causative agent of ES. Temporally, isolation of HHV-7 be-

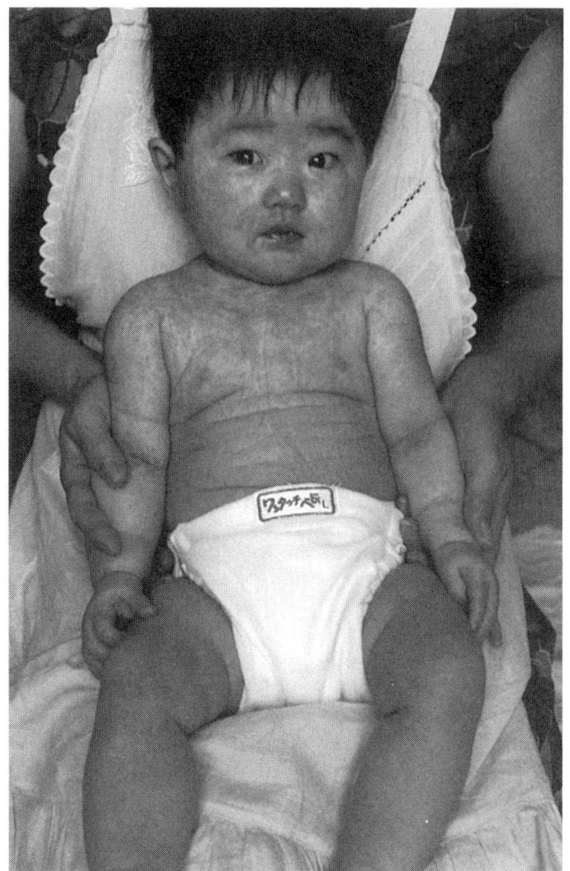

FIGURE 4 Clinical feature (typical rash) of a patient with ES.

fore HHV-6 is uncommon; thus, it is still not completely clear whether HHV-7 causes ES-like symptoms.

ES is a common disease of infancy, and the symptoms are usually mild. Normally, children can recover from this disease after a few days without any complications. However, a few infants show hepatic dysfunction associated with ES (7, 127). Another common complication associated with ES is seizures (93), reported to occur in 0.6 to 50% of patients, but the exact incidence of seizures occurring with ES is difficult to estimate. Thus, ES has been suggested to be a risk factor for recurrent febrile seizures. Encephalitis and other complications of the central nervous system (CNS) have also been reported (21, 58, 152). HHV-6 DNA can be detected in the cerebrospinal fluid of some patients (74). These data suggest that HHV-6 may invade the brain during the acute phase of ES. HHV-6 has also been detected by PCR in brains of normal cadavers and brains of AIDS patients (82). HHV-6 may also cause lymphadenitis (125). Idiopathic thrombocytopenic purpura has been asssociated with primary infection by HHV-6 (69).

Primary HHV-7 infection results in a febrile illness in childhood, complicated by seizures (20), and children with ES can develop CNS disease, including acute hemiplegia (134), suggesting that HHV-7 may also infect the brain. One study with hospitalized children during the first 2 years of life (138) found that 17% of the encephalitis cases were associated with primary infections by HHV-6 and -7 and that the two viruses contributed equally.

Latent Infection and Associated Diseases during HHV-6 and -7 Reactivation

As noted above, after primary infection, both viruses establish latency. They can be reactivated under some conditions, such as the immunosuppressed state. The site of latent infection with HHV-6 is unknown, but HHV-6 antigen has been detected in salivary glands. HHV-6 DNA can be detected in peripheral blood of healthy adults at low frequency, as well as in both monocytes/macrophages and lymphocytes during the acute phase of ES and mainly in monocytes/macrophages of patients in the convalescent phase and of healthy adults (73).

Reactivation of HHV-6 occurs after bone marrow transplantation, solid-organ transplantation, and AIDS as described above. Asymptomatic HHV-6 reactivations appear to be common in allogeneic bone marrow transplant patients (30), but symptomatic HHV-6 reactivation may result in bone marrow suppression (70), encephalitis (35), pneumonitis (29), and acute graft-versus-host disease (4). In fact, HHV-6 DNA is detectable in cerebrospinal fluid of patients after bone marrow and stem cell transplantation (42).

An association between rejection of transplanted kidneys and HHV-6 reactivation has been reported (101). HHV-6 reactivation in liver transplant recipients is associated with severe cytopenia (119, 120). Other associations include interstitial pneumonitis due to HHV-6, life-threatening thrombocytopenia, progressive encephalopathy, and skin rash in adults. HHV-6, HHV-7, and HCMV may contribute to the disease burden by reactivating at the same time during the course of transplantation (66).

The possible role of HHV-6 as a cofactor in HIV infection has been noted, since both viruses can infect $CD4^+$ cells and since HHV-6 can transactivate the LTR of HIV-1. HHV-6 can induce CD4 gene transcription and expression in $CD4^-$ cells. HHV-6A was recently shown to dramatically accelerate progression from HIV infection to full-blown AIDS in monkeys (84). Since HHV-6 is neuroinvasive, as described above, it may contribute to the neuropathogenesis of HIV/AIDS. HHV-6 is extensively disseminated in neural cells in the brains of HIV patients, suggesting a contribution to the pathogenesis of AIDS encephalopathy (71). In contrast, HHV-7 down-regulates CD4, the cellular receptor shared by HIV and HHV-7. HHV-7 suppresses the replication of CCR-5-tropic HIV isolates through CD4 modulation, suggesting that HHV-7 and HIV-1 may interfere in lymphoid tissue in vivo (80).

HHV-6 has been demonstrated in some neoplasms, including non-Hodgkin's lymphoma and Hodgkin's disease. A high prevalence of HHV-6 has been found in oral, particularly salivary gland, carcinoma tissues (144). A possible specific association of HHV-6 with the unusual disorder S100-positive, T-cell chronic lymphoproliferative disease has been reported (17). The frequency of HHV-6 variants in certain tumors suggests that they might serve as cofactors in multistep carcinogenesis, but there has been no conclusive demonstration that HHV-6 plays a causative role in any malignancy.

A reported association between chronic fatigue syndrome (CFS) and HHV-6 infection (61, 137) requires confirmation. More CFS patients than controls had elevated levels of HHV-6 early-antigen-specific IgM, perhaps indicating active replication of HHV-6 in CFS (105). Further work is required to determine whether HHV-6 contributes to the clinical manifestations.

Several studies have suggested an association between HHV-6 and multiple sclerosis (MS). A DNA fragment containing the major DNA binding protein gene of HHV-6 was detected in the brains of patients with MS by representational difference analysis. Examination of 86 brain specimens by PCR demonstrated that HHV-6B was present in the brains of >70% of MS patients and controls. Nuclear staining of oligodendrocytes using MAb against HHV-6 virion protein 101K and DNA binding protein p41 has been observed in samples from MS patients but not from controls. Samples from MS patients showed prominent cytoplasmic staining of neurons in gray matter adjacent to plaques, although neurons expressing HHV-6 were also found in certain controls (23, 47) . One study reported increased IgM serum antibody responses to HHV-6 early antigen (p41/38) in patients with relapsing-remitting MS compared with those with chronic progressive MS or other patients with neurologic disease, autoimmune disease, and healthy controls. However, other groups have not confirmed these findings (37), and further studies are required (28).

Reactivation of HHV-6B, possibly in concert with HHV-7, can contribute to the development of a severe drug-induced hypersensitivity syndrome (126, 133).

Association of pityriasis with HHV-7 infection is a clinical presentation of HHV-7 reactivation (34). No significant differences in DNA and antibody tests are noted between patients and control groups (141). Further experiments are necessary.

LABORATORY DIAGNOSIS

Virus Isolation and Assay of HHV-6 and -7

HHV-6 is easily recovered from the peripheral blood lymphocytes of ES patients on the first and second days of the disease (during the febrile phase of ES), and the isolation rate gradually decreases thereafter. Virus has been isolated on some occasions from saliva, but the isolation rate is extremely low.

An effective method for virus isolation (148) involves use of uninfected cord blood lymphocytes. Cord blood cells are recommended because HHV-6 and -7 may latently infect and reactivate during cultivation in peripheral blood mononuclear cells. CPE, with characteristic balloon-like syncytia, usually appears 2 to 4 days postinfection. Mitogen-stimulated human cord blood mononuclear cells and adult peripheral mononuclear cells are readily infected by HHV-6. HHV-6A also infects cells of HSB-2, an immature T-cell line, and HHV-6B infects several T-cell lines, including MT-4 and Molt-3. Since high concentrations of IL-2 inhibit viral replication (111), culture medium after infection should contain only very low concentrations of IL-2.

IgM antibodies are detected by day 7 and persist for 3 weeks, but they are not detectable in most sera 1 month after the onset of disease. IgG antibody is first detected 7 days after the onset of illness, increases in titer until 3 weeks after onset, and persists for at least 2 months. Interestingly, titers of antibody to HHV-6 are boosted during other virus infections, such as with HHV-7 (62, 145) or measles virus (123).

HHV-7 is isolated sometimes from the peripheral blood of patients of ES and frequently from the saliva of individuals who have antibody to HHV-7. Inoculation of salivary samples onto mitogen-stimulated human cord blood lymphocytes results in CPE by 2 to 4 weeks.

DNA Detection

HHV-6 DNA can be detected by DNA hybridization and by PCR. Southern blot hybridization is useful for rapid screening of large numbers of specimens, but it is generally a less sensitive technique than PCR. Numerous PCR primer sets which are sensitive and specific have been described for HHV-6 DNA, and some of these sets allow easy discrimination of the variants (9, 25, 115, 147). Variant-specific oligonucleotide hybridization is based on the amplification of two distinct regions of the HHV-6 genome, followed by hybridization of amplimers with variant-specific oligonucleotide probes (9). The putative coding region of immediate-early genes of HHV-6A was 2,517 nucleotides long, and two large additional regions, of 108 and 228 bp, were found in HHV-6B. PCR ampflication using primers covering one of these regions results in PCR products with different molecular masses. HHV-6 DNA is easily detectable by PCR in peripheral blood of ES patients during the acute phase, but detection of cell-free virus in serum or plasma by PCR offers the possibility of diagnosing active HHV-6 infections.

A reverse transcription-PCR assay can determine the presence of HHV-6 RNA in clinical specimens. The primers for amplification of mRNA of a major structural gene (gQ), which is expressed as a late gene and whose mRNA has a spliced structure, are employed. Therefore, the amplification of this gene has the advantage of detecting replicating virus and readily distinguishes mRNA from residual DNA contamination. This method showed a low false-positivity rate (1.2%) and a high specificity (98.8%).

A quantitative competitive PCR assay for HHV-6 has demonstrated the persistence of a high HHV-6 load in the absence of apparent disease (26). The primer sequences, based on consensus sequences in the DNA polymerase gene of herpesviruses, can be used for testing for six different herpesviruses simultaneously (92). For detection of HHV-7 DNA in a throat swab or peripheral blood, PCR can also be used directly. The method is essentially the same as for the detection of HHV-6 DNA. Qualitative and quantitative competitive nested PCR assays have also been developed for the detection of HHV-7 DNA. These assays amplify a DNA sequence containing part of the HHV-7 U42 gene (64).

Loop-mediated isothermal amplification is a novel technique that allows rapid detection of HHV-6 DNA using simple and relatively inexpensive equipment already available at most hospitals, making it suitable for rapid diagnosis of roseola (55).

A multiplex PCR method was also developed for the simultaneous detection of HHV-6 and -7 in clinical samples, using primers that amplify a segment of the HHV-6 U67 gene and the HHV-7 U42 gene. Comparison of the multiplex assay with the respective single PCR assays using cloned HHV-6 and HHV-7 sequences as targets for amplification demonstrated equivalent sensitivities and specificities of the assays. This multiplex assay is an efficient and cost-effective approach to the analysis of large numbers of samples to determine the epidemiological importance of HHV-6 and -7 (65).

Since both HHV-6A and -6B have been found integrated into the chromosomes of immunocompetent patients at persistently high levels of viral DNA in blood, sera, and hair follicles (139, 140), PCR should be carefully performed for diagnosis even with cerebrospinal fluid.

Serologic Assays

Several serologic assays are available for HHV-6 studies, including IFA, enzyme-linked immunosorbent assay, neutralization, radioimmunoprecipitation, and immunoblotting. Indirect IFA is presently the most commonly applied method for HHV-6 viral antigen and antibody detection. Separation of serum IgM from IgG and IgA significantly increases the specificity of HHV-6-specific IgM detection. Density gradient columns and protein A absorption and anti-IgG treatment techniques can be applied for removal of interfering substances such as heterotropic cross-reactions, rheumatoid factors, and antinuclear antibodies.

Neutralizing antibody tests using a CPE reading, chemically attached MT-4 cells (T-cell line), or dot blot assays have been reported (5). Neutralizing antibody titers appear to correlate with the antibody titers determined by the indirect IFA test (136).

An enzyme immunoassay, an immunoblot assay, and an indirect IFA have been developed for the detection of HHV-7 antibodies in human serum. Cross-absorption studies with ELISA or IFA using HHV-6 and -7 antigens indicated that most human sera contain cross-reactive HHV-6 and -7 antibodies. The degree of cross-reactivity varies between individual serum specimens. An 85- or 89-kDa protein was identified as an HHV-7-specific serologic marker by immunoblot analysis (122). To detect antibody to HHV-7 specifically and sensitively, the p89/85 proteins, which are encoded by open reading frames U14 (85 kDa) and U11 (86 kDa) of HHV-7, were expressed as recombinant proteins in bacteria and developed for the immunoblotting kit. Of the three assays, the enzyme-linked immunosorbent assay is the most sensitive, while the immunoblot assay is the most specific (16).

TREATMENT AND PREVENTION

Several antiviral drugs are inhibitory for HHV-6, including phosphonoformic acid (PFA), 9-(2-hydroxyethoxymethyl) guanine (ACV; acyclovir), 9-[(1,3-dihydroxy-2-propoxy) methyl]guanine (DHPG; ganciclovir), and (S)-1-[(3-hydroxy-2-phosphonylmethoxy)propyl]cytosine [(S)-HPMPC]. DHPG and (S)-HPMPC were more effective than the others (117). The sensitivity of HHV-7 to the guanine analogs was different from that of HHV-6, suggesting a difference in selectivity of specific viral enzymes (150). Prophylaxis with ACV did not prevent the occurrence of HHV-6-associated CNS disease after allogeneic bone marrow transplantation. IFN-α and IFN-β inhibit HHV-6 replication in vitro (128).

REFERENCES

1. **Ablashi, D. V., S. Z. Salahuddin, S. F. Josephs, F. Imam, P. Lusso, R. C. Gallo, C. Hung, J. Lemp, and P. D. Markham.** 1987. HBLV (or HHV-6) in human cell lines. *Nature* **329:**207.
2. **Adams, O., C. Krempe, G. Kogler, P. Wernet, and A. Scheid.** 1998. Congenital infections with human herpesvirus 6. *J. Infect. Dis.* **178:**544–546.
3. **Akkapaiboon, P., Y. Mori, T. Sadaoka, S. Yonemoto, and K. Yamanishi.** 2004. Intracellular processing of human herpesvirus 6 glycoproteins Q1 and Q2 into tetrameric complexes expressed on the viral envelope. *J. Virol.* **78:**7969–7983.
4. **Appleton, A. L., L. Sviland, J. S. Peiris, C. E. Taylor, J. Wilkes, M. A. Green, A. D. Pearson, P. J. Kelly, A. J. Malcolm, S. J. Proctor, P. J. Hamilton, and A. J. Cant for the Newcastle upon Tyne Bone Marrow Transport Group.** 1995. Human herpes virus-6 infection in marrow graft recipients: role in pathogenesis of graft-versus-host disease. *Bone Marrow Transplant.* **16:**777–782.
5. **Asada, H., S. Yalcin, K. Balachandra, K. Higashi, and K. Yamanishi.** 1989. Establishment of titration system for human herpesvirus 6 and evaluation of neutralizing antibody response to the virus. *J. Clin. Microbiol.* **27:**2204–2207.
6. **Asano, Y., S. Suga, T. Yoshikawa, A. Urisu, and T. Yazaki.** 1989. Human herpesvirus type 6 infection (exanthem subitum) without fever. *J. Pediatr.* **115:**264–265.
7. **Asano, Y., T. Yoshikawa, S. Suga, T. Yazaki, K. Kondo, and K. Yamanishi.** 1990. Fatal fulminant hepatitis in an infant with human herpesvirus-6 infection. *Lancet* **335:**862–863.
8. **Aubin, J. T., L. Poirel, H. Agut, J. M. Huraux, C. Bignozzi, Y. Brossard, N. Mulliez, J. Roume, F. Lecuru, and R. Taurelle.** 1992. Intrauterine transmission of human herpesvirus 6. *Lancet* **340:**482–483.
9. **Aubin, J. T., L. Poirel, C. Robert, J. M. Huraux, and H. Agut.** 1994. Identification of human herpesvirus 6 variants A and B by amplimer hybridization with variant-specific oligonucleotides and amplification with variant-specific primers. *J. Clin. Microbiol.* **32:**2434–2440.
10. **Balachandran, N., R. E. Amelse, W. W. Zhou, and C. K. Chang.** 1989. Identification of proteins specific for human herpesvirus 6-infected human T cells. *J. Virol.* **63:**2835–2840.
11. **Berneman, Z. N., D. V. Ablashi, G. Li, M. Eger-Fletcher, M. S. Reitz, Jr., C. L. Hung, I. Brus, A. L. Komaroff, and R. C. Gallo.** 1992. Human herpesvirus 7 is a T-lymphotropic virus and is related to, but significantly different from, human herpesvirus 6 and human cytomegalovirus. *Proc. Natl. Acad. Sci. USA* **89:**10552–10556.
12. **Bertram, G., N. Dreiner, G. R. Krueger, A. Ramon, D. V. Ablashi, S. Z. Salahuddin, and N. Balachandram.** 1991. Frequent double infection with Epstein-Barr virus and human herpesvirus-6 in patients with acute infectious mononucleosis. *In Vivo* **5:**271–279.
13. **Biberfeld, P., B. Kramarsky, S. Z. Salahuddin, and R. C. Gallo.** 1987. Ultrastructural characterization of a new human B lymphotropic DNA virus (human herpesvirus 6) isolated from patients with lymphoproliferative disease. *J. Natl. Cancer Inst.* **79:**933–941.
14. **Black, J. B., N. Inoue, K. Kite-Powell, S. Zaki, and P. E. Pellett.** 1993. Frequent isolation of human herpesvirus 7 from saliva. *Virus Res.* **29:**91–98.
15. **Black, J. B., K. C. Sanderlin, C. S. Goldsmith, H. E. Gary, C. Lopez, and P. E. Pellett.** 1989. Growth properties of human herpesvirus-6 strain Z29. *J. Virol. Methods* **26:**133–145.
16. **Black, J. B., T. F. Schwarz, J. L. Patton, K. Kite-Powell, P. E. Pellett, S. Wiersbitzky, R. Bruns, C. Muller, G. Jager, and J. A. Stewart.** 1996. Evaluation of immunoassays for detection of antibodies to human herpesvirus 7. *Clin. Diagn. Lab. Immunol.* **3:**79–83.
17. **Braun, D. K., P. E. Pellett, and C. A. Hanson.** 1995. Presence and expression of human herpesvirus 6 in peripheral blood mononuclear cells of S100-positive, T cell

chronic lymphoproliferative disease. *J. Infect. Dis.* **171:** 1351–1355.

18. **Cardinali, G., M. Gentile, M. Cirone, C. Zompetta, L. Frati, A. Faggioni, and M. R. Torrisi.** 1998. Viral glycoproteins accumulate in newly formed annulate lamellae following infection of lymphoid cells by human herpesvirus 6. *J. Virol.* **72:**9738–9746.
19. **Carrigan, D. R., K. K. Knox, and M. A. Tapper.** 1990. Suppression of human immunodeficiency virus type 1 replication by human herpesvirus-6. *J. Infect. Dis.* **162:**844–851.
20. **Caserta, M. T., C. B. Hall, K. Schnabel, C. E. Long, and N. D'Heron.** 1998. Primary human herpesvirus 7 infection: a comparison of human herpesvirus 7 and human herpesvirus 6 infections in children. *J. Pediatr.* **133:**386–389.
21. **Caserta, M. T., C. B. Hall, K. Schnabel, K. McIntyre, C. Long, M. Costanzo, S. Dewhurst, R. Insel, and L. G. Epstein.** 1994. Neuroinvasion and persistence of human herpesvirus 6 in children. *J. Infect. Dis.* **170:**1586–1589.
22. **Catusse, J., C. M. Parry, D. R. Dewin, and U. A. Gompels.** 2007. Inhibition of HIV-1 infection by viral chemokine U83A via high-affinity CCR5 interactions that block human chemokine-induced leukocyte chemotaxis and receptor internalization. *Blood* **109:**3633–3639.
23. **Challoner, P. B., K. T. Smith, J. D. Parker, D. L. MacLeod, S. N. Coulter, T. M. Rose, E. R. Schultz, J. L. Bennett, R. L. Garber, M. Chang, P. A. Schad, P. M. Stewart, R. C. Nowinski, J. P. Brown, and G. C. Burmer.** 1995. Plaque-associated expression of human herpesvirus 6 in multiple sclerosis. *Proc. Natl. Acad. Sci. USA* **92:**7440–7444.
24. **Chang, C. K., and N. Balachandran.** 1991. Identification, characterization, and sequence analysis of a cDNA encoding a phosphoprotein of human herpesvirus 6. *J. Virol.* **65:**2884–2894. (Erratum, **65:**7085.)
25. **Chou, S., and G. I. Marousek.** 1994. Analysis of interstrain variation in a putative immediate-early region of human herpesvirus 6 DNA and definition of variant-specific sequences. *Virology* **198:**370–376.
26. **Clark, D. A., M. Ait-Khaled, A. C. Wheeler, I. M. Kidd, J. E. McLaughlin, M. A. Johnson, P. D. Griffiths, and V. C. Emery.** 1996. Quantification of human herpesvirus 6 in immunocompetent persons and post-mortem tissues from AIDS patients by PCR. *J. Gen. Virol.* **77**(Pt. 9)**:**2271–2275.
27. **Clark, D. A., M. L. Freeland, L. K. Mackie, R. F. Jarrett, and D. E. Onions.** 1993. Prevalence of antibody to human herpesvirus 7 by age. *J. Infect. Dis.* **168:**251–252.
28. **Coates, A. R., and J. Bell.** 1998. HHV-6 and multiple sclerosis. *Nat. Med.* **4:**537–538.
29. **Cone, R. W., R. C. Hackman, M. L. Huang, R. A. Bowden, J. D. Meyers, M. Metcalf, J. Zeh, R. Ashley, and L. Corey.** 1993. Human herpesvirus 6 in lung tissue from patients with pneumonitis after bone marrow transplantation. *N. Engl. J. Med.* **329:**156–161.
30. **Cone, R. W., M. L. Huang, L. Corey, J. Zeh, R. Ashley, and R. Bowden.** 1999. Human herpesvirus 6 infections after bone marrow transplantation: clinical and virologic manifestations. *J. Infect. Dis.* **179:**311–318.
31. **Dahl, H., G. Fjaertoft, T. Norsted, F. Z. Wang, M. Mousavi-Jazi, and A. Linde.** 1999. Reactivation of human herpesvirus 6 during pregnancy. *J. Infect. Dis.* **180:** 2035–2038.
32. **Daibata, M., T. Taguchi, T. Sawada, H. Taguchi, and I. Miyoshi.** 1998. Chromosomal transmission of human herpesvirus 6 DNA in acute lymphoblastic leukaemia. *Lancet* **352:**543–544.
33. **Dominguez, G., T. R. Dambaugh, F. R. Stamey, S. Dewhurst, N. Inoue, and P. E. Pellett.** 1999. Human herpesvirus 6B genome sequence: coding content and comparison with human herpesvirus 6A. *J. Virol.* **73:** 8040–8052.
34. **Drago, F., E. Ranieri, F. Malaguti, E. Losi, and A. Rebora.** 1997. Human herpesvirus 7 in pityriasis rosea. *Lancet* **349:**1367–1368.
35. **Drobyski, W. R., K. K. Knox, D. Majewski, and D. R. Carrigan.** 1994. Brief report: fatal encephalitis due to variant B human herpesvirus-6 infection in a bone marrow-transplant recipient. *N. Engl. J. Med.* **330:**1356–1360.
36. **Ensoli, B., P. Lusso, F. Schachter, S. F. Josephs, J. Rappaport, F. Negro, R. C. Gallo, and F. Wong-Staal.** 1989. Human herpes virus-6 increases HIV-1 expression in co-infected T cells via nuclear factors binding to the HIV-1 enhancer. *EMBO J.* **8:**3019–3027.
37. **Fillet, A. M., P. Lozeron, H. Agut, O. Lyon-Caen, and R. Liblau.** 1998. HHV-6 and multiple sclerosis. *Nat. Med.* **4:**537. (Author reply, **4:**538.)
38. **Flamand, L., J. Gosselin, M. D'Addario, J. Hiscott, D. V. Ablashi, R. C. Gallo, and J. Menezes.** 1991. Human herpesvirus 6 induces interleukin-1 beta and tumor necrosis factor alpha, but not interleukin-6, in peripheral blood mononuclear cell cultures. *J. Virol.* **65:**5105–5110.
39. **Foa-Tomasi, L., E. Avitabile, L. Ke, and G. Campadelli-Fiume.** 1994. Polyvalent and monoclonal antibodies identify major immunogenic proteins specific for human herpesvirus 7-infected cells and have weak cross-reactivity with human herpesvirus 6. *J. Gen. Virol.* **75**(Pt. 10)**:** 2719–2727.
40. **Foa-Tomasi, L., A. Boscaro, S. di Gaeta, and G. Campadelli-Fiume.** 1991. Monoclonal antibodies to gp100 inhibit penetration of human herpesvirus 6 and polykaryocyte formation in susceptible cells. *J. Virol.* **65:** 4124–4129.
41. **Foa-Tomasi, L., M. P. Fiorilli, E. Avitabile, and G. Campadelli-Fiume.** 1996. Identification of an 85 kDa phosphoprotein as an immunodominant protein specific for human herpesvirus 7-infected cells. *J. Gen. Virol.* **77**(Pt. 3)**:**511–518.
42. **Fotheringham, J., N. Akhyani, A. Vortmeyer, D. Donati, E. Williams, U. Oh, M. Bishop, J. Barrett, J. Gea-Banacloche, and S. Jacobson.** 2007. Detection of active human herpesvirus-6 infection in the brain: correlation with polymerase chain reaction detection in cerebrospinal fluid. *J. Infect. Dis.* **195:**450–454.
43. **Franti, M., J. T. Aubin, A. Gautheret-Dejean, I. Malet, A. Cahour, J. M. Huraux, and H. Agut.** 1999. Preferential associations of alleles of three distinct genes argue for the existence of two prototype variants of human herpesvirus 7. *J. Virol.* **73:**9655–9658.
44. **Frenkel, N., E. C. Schirmer, L. S. Wyatt, G. Katsafanas, E. Roffman, R. M. Danovich, and C. H. June.** 1990. Isolation of a new herpesvirus from human $CD4^+$ T cells. *Proc. Natl. Acad. Sci. USA* **87:**748–752.
45. **Glosson, N. L., and A. W. Hudson.** 2007. Human herpesvirus-6A and -6B encode viral immunoevasins that downregulate class I MHC molecules. *Virology* **365:**125–135.
46. **Gompels, U. A., J. Nicholas, G. Lawrence, M. Jones, B. J. Thomson, M. E. Martin, S. Efstathiou, M. Craxton, and H. A. Macaulay.** 1995. The DNA sequence of human herpesvirus-6: structure, coding content, and genome evolution. *Virology* **209:**29–51.
47. **Goodman, A. D., D. J. Mock, J. M. Powers, J. V. Baker, and B. M. Blumberg.** 2003. Human herpesvirus 6 genome and antigen in acute multiple sclerosis lesions. *J. Infect. Dis.* **187:**1365–1376.

48. **Gopal, M. R., B. J. Thomson, J. Fox, R. S. Tedder, and R. W. Honess.** 1990. Detection by PCR of HHV-6 and EBV DNA in blood and oropharynx of healthy adults and HIV-seropositives. *Lancet* **335:**1598–1599.
49. **Hall, C. B., C. E. Long, K. C. Schnabel, M. T. Caserta, K. M. McIntyre, M. A. Costanzo, A. Knott, S. Dewhurst, R. A. Insel, and L. G. Epstein.** 1994. Human herpesvirus-6 infection in children. A prospective study of complications and reactivation. *N. Engl. J. Med.* **331:** 432–438.
50. **Hellstrom, B., and B. Vahlquist.** 1951. Experimental inoculation of roseola infantum. *Acta Paediatr.* **40:**189–197.
51. **Hidaka, Y., Y. Liu, M. Yamamoto, R. Mori, C. Miyazaki, K. Kusuhara, K. Okada, and K. Ueda.** 1993. Frequent isolation of human herpesvirus 7 from saliva samples. *J. Med. Virol.* **40:**343–346.
52. **Higashi, K., H. Asada, T. Kurata, K. Ishikawa, M. Hayami, Y. Spriatna, Y. Sutarman, and K. Yamanishi.** 1989. Presence of antibody to human herpesvirus 6 in monkeys. *J. Gen. Virol.* **70**(Pt. 12)**:**3171–3176.
53. **Horvat, R. T., C. Wood, and N. Balachandran.** 1989. Transactivation of human immunodeficiency virus promoter by human herpesvirus 6. *J. Virol.* **63:**970–973.
54. **Hudson, A. W., D. Blom, P. M. Howley, and H. L. Ploegh.** 2003. The ER-lumenal domain of the HHV-7 immunoevasin U21 directs class I MHC molecules to lysosomes. *Traffic* **4:**824–837.
55. **Ihira, M., S. Akimoto, F. Miyake, A. Fujita, K. Sugata, S. Suga, M. Ohashi, N. Nishimura, T. Ozaki, Y. Asano, and T. Yoshikawa.** 2007. Direct detection of human herpesvirus 6 DNA in serum by the loop-mediated isothermal amplification method. *J. Clin. Virol.* **39:**22–26.
56. **Isegawa, Y., T. Mukai, K. Nakano, M. Kagawa, J. Chen, Y. Mori, T. Sunagawa, K. Kawanishi, J. Sashihara, A. Hata, P. Zou, H. Kosuge, and K. Yamanishi.** 1999. Comparison of the complete DNA sequences of human herpesvirus 6 variants A and B. *J. Virol.* **73:**8053–8063.
57. **Isegawa, Y., Z. Ping, K. Nakano, N. Sugimoto, and K. Yamanishi.** 1998. Human herpesvirus 6 open reading frame U12 encodes a functional beta-chemokine receptor. *J. Virol.* **72:**6104–6112.
58. **Ishiguro, N., S. Yamada, T. Takahashi, Y. Takahashi, T. Togashi, T. Okuno, and K. Yamanishi.** 1990. Meningoencephalitis associated with HHV-6 related exanthem subitum. *Acta Paediatr. Scand.* **79:**987–989.
59. **Jarrett, R. F., D. A. Clark, S. F. Josephs, and D. E. Onions.** 1990. Detection of human herpesvirus-6 DNA in peripheral blood and saliva. *J. Med. Virol.* **32:**73–76.
60. **Jaworska, J., A. Gravel, K. Fink, N. Grandvaux, and L. Flamand.** 2007. Inhibition of transcription of the beta interferon gene by the human herpesvirus 6 immediate-early 1 protein. *J. Virol.* **81:**5737–5748.
61. **Josephs, S. F., B. Henry, N. Balachandran, D. Strayer, D. Peterson, A. L. Komaroff, and D. V. Ablashi.** 1991. HHV-6 reactivation in chronic fatigue syndrome. *Lancet* **337:**1346–1347.
62. **Katsafanas, G. C., E. C. Schirmer, L. S. Wyatt, and N. Frenkel.** 1996. In vitro activation of human herpesviruses 6 and 7 from latency. *Proc. Natl. Acad. Sci. USA* **93:** 9788–9792.
63. **Kempe, C. H., E. B. Shaw, J. R. Jackson, and H. K. Silver.** 1950. Studies on the etiology of exanthema subitum (roseola infantum). *J. Pediatr.* **37:**561–568.
64. **Kidd, I. M., D. A. Clark, M. Ait-Khaled, P. D. Griffiths, and V. C. Emery.** 1996. Measurement of human herpesvirus 7 load in peripheral blood and saliva of healthy subjects by quantitative polymerase chain reaction. *J. Infect. Dis.* **174:**396–401.
65. **Kidd, I. M., D. A. Clark, J. A. Bremner, D. Pillay, P. D. Griffiths, and V. C. Emery.** 1998. A multiplex PCR assay for the simultaneous detection of human herpesvirus 6 and human herpesvirus 7, with typing of HHV-6 by enzyme cleavage of PCR products. *J. Virol. Methods* **70:**29–36.
66. **Kidd, I. M., D. A. Clark, C. A. Sabin, D. Andrew, A. F. Hassan-Walker, P. Sweny, P. D. Griffiths, and V. C. Emery.** 2000. Prospective study of human betaherpesviruses after renal transplantation: association of human herpesvirus 7 and cytomegalovirus co-infection with cytomegalovirus disease and increased rejection. *Transplantation* **69:**2400–2404.
67. **Kido, S., K. Kondo, T. Kondo, T. Morishima, M. Takahashi, and K. Yamanishi.** 1990. Detection of human herpesvirus 6 DNA in throat swabs by polymerase chain reaction. *J. Med. Virol.* **32:**139–142.
68. **Kikuta, H., A. Nakane, H. Lu, Y. Taguchi, T. Minagawa, and S. Matsumoto.** 1990. Interferon induction by human herpesvirus 6 in human mononuclear cells. *J. Infect. Dis.* **162:**35–38.
69. **Kitamura, K., H. Ohta, T. Ihara, H. Kamiya, H. Ochiai, K. Yamanishi, and K. Tanaka.** 1994. Idiopathic thrombocytopenic purpura after human herpesvirus 6 infection. *Lancet* **344:**830.
70. **Knox, K. K., and D. R. Carrigan.** 1992. In vitro suppression of bone marrow progenitor cell differentiation by human herpesvirus 6 infection. *J. Infect. Dis.* **165:**925–929.
71. **Knox, K. K., D. P. Harrington, and D. R. Carrigan.** 1995. Fulminant human herpesvirus six encephalitis in a human immunodeficiency virus-infected infant. *J. Med. Virol.* **45:**288–292.
72. **Kondo, K., Y. Hayakawa, H. Mori, S. Sato, T. Kondo, K. Takahashi, Y. Minamishima, M. Takahashi, and K. Yamanishi.** 1990. Detection by polymerase chain reaction amplification of human herpesvirus 6 DNA in peripheral blood of patients with exanthem subitum. *J. Clin. Microbiol.* **28:**970–974.
73. **Kondo, K., T. Kondo, T. Okuno, M. Takahashi, and K. Yamanishi.** 1991. Latent human herpesvirus 6 infection of human monocytes/macrophages. *J. Gen. Virol.* **72**(Pt. 6)**:**1401–1408.
74. **Kondo, K., H. Nagafuji, A. Hata, C. Tomomori, and K. Yamanishi.** 1993. Association of human herpesvirus 6 infection of the central nervous system with recurrence of febrile convulsions. *J. Infect. Dis.* **167:**1197–1200.
75. **Kositanont, U., C. Wasi, N. Wanprapar, P. Bowonkiratikachorn, K. Chokephaibulkit, S. Chearskul, K. Chimabutra, R. Sutthent, S. Foongladda, R. Inagi, T. Kurata, and K. Yamanishi.** 1999. Primary infection of human herpesvirus 6 in children with vertical infection of human immunodeficiency virus type 1. *J. Infect. Dis.* **180:**50–55.
76. **Lawrence, G. L., M. Chee, M. A. Craxton, U. A. Gompels, R. W. Honess, and B. G. Barrell.** 1990. Human herpesvirus 6 is closely related to human cytomegalovirus. *J. Virol.* **64:**287–299.
77. **Leach, C. T., E. R. Newton, S. McParlin, and H. B. Jenson.** 1994. Human herpesvirus 6 infection of the female genital tract. *J. Infect. Dis.* **169:**1281–1283.
78. **Levy, J. A., A. Landay, and E. T. Lennette.** 1990. Human herpesvirus 6 inhibits human immunodeficiency virus type 1 replication in cell culture. *J. Clin. Microbiol.* **28:**2362–2364.
79. **Lindquester, G. J., and P. E. Pellett.** 1991. Properties of the human herpesvirus 6 strain Z29 genome: G + C content, length, and presence of variable-length directly re-

peated terminal sequence elements. *Virology* **182:**102–110.

80. **Lisco, A., J. C. Grivel, A. Biancotto, C. Vanpouille, F. Origgi, M. S. Malnati, D. Schols, P. Lusso, and L. B. Margolis.** 2007. Viral interactions in human lymphoid tissue: human herpesvirus 7 suppresses the replication of CCR5-tropic human immunodeficiency virus type 1 via CD4 modulation. *J. Virol.* **81:**708–717.
81. **Lopez, C., P. Pellett, J. Stewart, C. Goldsmith, K. Sanderlin, J. Black, D. Warfield, and P. Feorino.** 1988. Characteristics of human herpesvirus-6. *J. Infect. Dis.* **157:**1271–1273.
82. **Luppi, M., P. Barozzi, A. Maiorana, R. Marasca, and G. Torelli.** 1994. Human herpesvirus 6 infection in normal human brain tissue. *J. Infect. Dis.* **169:**943–944.
83. **Luppi, M., P. Barozzi, C. M. Morris, E. Merelli, and G. Torelli.** 1998. Integration of human herpesvirus 6 genome in human chromosomes. *Lancet* **352:**1707–1708.
84. **Lusso, P., R. W. Crowley, M. S. Malnati, C. Di Serio, M. Ponzoni, A. Biancotto, P. D. Markham, and R. C. Gallo.** 2007. Human herpesvirus 6A accelerates AIDS progression in macaques. *Proc. Natl. Acad. Sci. USA* **104:**5067–5072.
85. **Lusso, P., A. De Maria, M. Malnati, F. Lori, S. E. DeRocco, M. Baseler, and R. C. Gallo.** 1991. Induction of CD4 and susceptibility to HIV-1 infection in human $CD8^+$ T lymphocytes by human herpesvirus 6. *Nature* **349:**533–535.
86. **Lusso, P., M. Malnati, A. De Maria, C. Balotta, S. E. DeRocco, P. D. Markham, and R. C. Gallo.** 1991. Productive infection of $CD4^+$ and $CD8^+$ mature human T cell populations and clones by human herpesvirus 6. Transcriptional down-regulation of CD3. *J. Immunol.* **147:**685–691.
87. **Lusso, P., M. S. Malnati, A. Garzino-Demo, R. W. Crowley, E. O. Long, and R. C. Gallo.** 1993. Infection of natural killer cells by human herpesvirus 6. *Nature* **362:**458–462.
88. **Lusso, P., P. D. Markham, S. E. DeRocco, and R. C. Gallo.** 1990. In vitro susceptibility of T lymphocytes from chimpanzees *(Pan troglodytes)* to human herpesvirus 6 (HHV-6): a potential animal model to study the interaction between HHV-6 and human immunodeficiency virus type 1 in vivo. *J. Virol.* **64:**2751–2758.
89. **Lusso, P., P. D. Markham, E. Tschachler, F. di Marzo Veronese, S. Z. Salahuddin, D. V. Ablashi, S. Pahwa, K. Krohn, and R. C. Gallo.** 1988. In vitro cellular tropism of human B-lymphotropic virus (human herpesvirus-6). *J. Exp. Med.* **167:**1659–1670.
90. **Lusso, P., P. Secchiero, R. W. Crowley, A. Garzino-Demo, Z. N. Berneman, and R. C. Gallo.** 1994. CD4 is a critical component of the receptor for human herpesvirus 7: interference with human immunodeficiency virus. *Proc. Natl. Acad. Sci. USA* **91:**3872–3876.
91. **Megaw, A. G., D. Rapaport, B. Avidor, N. Frenkel, and A. J. Davison.** 1998. The DNA sequence of the RK strain of human herpesvirus 7. *Virology* **244:**119–132.
92. **Minjolle, S., C. Michelet, I. Jusselin, M. Joannes, F. Cartier, and R. Colimon.** 1999. Amplification of the six major human herpesviruses from cerebrospinal fluid by a single PCR. *J. Clin. Microbiol.* **37:**950–953.
93. **Moller, K. L.** 1956. Exanthema subitum and febrile convulsions. *Acta Paediatr.* **45:**534–540.
94. **Mori, Y., P. Akkapaiboon, S. Yonemoto, M. Koike, M. Takemoto, T. Sadaoka, Y. Sasamoto, S. Konishi, Y. Uchiyama, and K. Yamanishi.** 2004. Discovery of a second form of tripartite complex containing gH-gL of human herpesvirus 6 and observations on CD46. *J. Virol.* **78:**4609–4616.
95. **Mori, Y., P. Dhepakson, T. Shimamoto, K. Ueda, Y. Gomi, H. Tani, Y. Matsuura, and K. Yamanishi.** 2000. Expression of human herpesvirus 6B *rep* within infected cells and binding of its gene product to the TATA-binding protein in vitro and in vivo. *J. Virol.* **74:**6096–6104.
96. **Mori, Y., T. Seya, H. L. Huang, P. Akkapaiboon, P. Dhepakson, and K. Yamanishi.** 2002. Human herpesvirus 6 variant A but not variant B induces fusion from without in a variety of human cells through a human herpesvirus 6 entry receptor, CD46. *J. Virol.* **76:**6750–6761.
97. **Mori, Y., X. Yang, P. Akkapaiboon, T. Okuno, and K. Yamanishi.** 2003. Human herpesvirus 6 variant A glycoprotein H-glycoprotein L-glycoprotein Q complex associates with human CD46. *J. Virol.* **77:**4992–4999.
98. **Nakagawa, N., T. Mukai, J. Sakamoto, A. Hata, T. Okuno, K. Takeda, and K. Yamanishi.** 1997. Antigenic analysis of human herpesvirus 7 (HHV-7) and HHV-6 using immune sera and monoclonal antibodies against HHV-7. *J. Gen. Virol.* **78**(Pt. 5)**:**1131–1137.
99. **Neipel, F., K. Ellinger, and B. Fleckenstein.** 1992. Gene for the major antigenic structural protein (p100) of human herpesvirus 6. *J. Virol.* **66:**3918–3924.
100. **Nicholas, J.** 1996. Determination and analysis of the complete nucleotide sequence of human herpesvirus. *J. Virol.* **70:**5975–5989.
101. **Okuno, T., K. Higashi, K. Shiraki, K. Yamanishi, M. Takahashi, Y. Kokado, M. Ishibashi, S. Takahara, T. Sonoda, K. Tanaka, K. Baba, H. Yabuuchi, and T. Kurata.** 1990. Human herpesvirus 6 infection in renal transplantation. *Transplantation* **49:**519–522.
102. **Okuno, T., T. Mukai, K. Baba, Y. Ohsumi, M. Takahashi, and K. Yamanishi.** 1991. Outbreak of exanthem subitum in an orphanage. *J. Pediatr.* **119:**759–761.
103. **Okuno, T., H. Oishi, K. Hayashi, M. Nonogaki, K. Tanaka, and K. Yamanishi.** 1995. Human herpesviruses 6 and 7 in cervixes of pregnant women. *J. Clin. Microbiol.* **33:**1968–1970.
104. **Okuno, T., K. Takahashi, K. Balachandra, K. Shiraki, K. Yamanishi, M. Takahashi, and K. Baba.** 1989. Seroepidemiology of human herpesvirus 6 infection in normal children and adults. *J. Clin. Microbiol.* **27:**651–653.
105. **Patnaik, M., A. L. Komaroff, E. Conley, E. A. Ojo-Amaize, and J. B. Peter.** 1995. Prevalence of IgM antibodies to human herpesvirus 6 early antigen (p41/38) in patients with chronic fatigue syndrome. *J. Infect. Dis.* **172:**1364–1367.
106. **Pedersen, S. M., B. Oster, B. Bundgaard, and P. Hollsberg.** 2006. Induction of cell-cell fusion from without by human herpesvirus 6B. *J. Virol.* **80:**9916–9920.
107. **Pellett, P. E., G. J. Lindquester, P. Feorino, and C. Lopez.** 1990. Genomic heterogeneity of human herpesvirus 6 isolates. *Adv. Exp. Med. Biol.* **278:**9–18.
108. **Pietroboni, G. R., G. B. Harnett, T. J. Farr, and M. R. Bucens.** 1988. Human herpes virus type 6 (HHV-6) and its in vitro effect on human immunodeficiency virus (HIV). *J. Clin. Pathol.* **41:**1310–1312.
109. **Pruksananonda, P., C. B. Hall, R. A. Insel, K. McIntyre, P. E. Pellett, C. E. Long, K. C. Schnabel, P. H. Pincus, F. R. Stamey, T. R. Dambaugh, and J. A. Stewart.** 1992. Primary human herpesvirus 6 infection in young children. *N. Engl. J. Med.* **326:**1445–1450.
110. **Razzaque, A.** 1990. Oncogenic potential of human herpesvirus-6 DNA. *Oncogene* **5:**1365–1370.
111. **Roffman, E., and N. Frenkel.** 1990. Interleukin-2 inhibits the replication of human herpesvirus-6 in mature thymocytes. *Virology* **175:**591–594.

112. **Sadaoka, T., K. Yamanishi, and Y. Mori.** 2006. Human herpesvirus 7 U47 gene products are glycoproteins expressed in virions and associate with glycoprotein H. *J. Gen. Virol.* **87:**501–508.

113. **Salahuddin, S. Z., D. V. Ablashi, P. D. Markham, S. F. Josephs, S. Sturzenegger, M. Kaplan, G. Halligan, P. Biberfeld, F. Wong-Staal, B. Kramarsky, and R. C. Gallo.** 1986. Isolation of a new virus, HBLV, in patients with lymphoproliferative disorders. *Science* **234:**596–601.

114. **Santoro, F., P. E. Kennedy, G. Locatelli, M. S. Malnati, E. A. Berger, and P. Lusso.** 1999. CD46 is a cellular receptor for human herpesvirus 6. *Cell* **99:**817–827.

115. **Schirmer, E. C., L. S. Wyatt, K. Yamanishi, W. J. Rodriguez, and N. Frenkel.** 1991. Differentiation between two distinct classes of viruses now classified as human herpesvirus 6. *Proc. Natl. Acad. Sci. USA* **88:**5922–5926.

116. **Secchiero, P., J. Nicholas, H. Deng, T. Xiaopeng, N. van Loon, V. R. Ruvolo, Z. N. Berneman, M. S. Reitz, Jr., and S. Dewhurst.** 1995. Identification of human telomeric repeat motifs at the genome termini of human herpesvirus 7: structural analysis and heterogeneity. *J. Virol.* **69:**8041–8045.

117. **Shiraki, K., T. Okuno, K. Yamanishi, and M. Takahashi.** 1989. Phosphonoacetic acid inhibits replication of human herpesvirus-6. *Antivir. Res.* **12:**311–318.

118. **Shiraki, K., T. Okuno, K. Yamanishi, and M. Takahashi.** 1989. Virion and nonstructural polypeptides of human herpesvirus-6. *Virus Res.* **13:**173–178.

119. **Singh, N., D. R. Carrigan, T. Gayowski, and I. R. Marino.** 1997. Human herpesvirus-6 infection in liver transplant recipients: documentation of pathogenicity. *Transplantation* **64:**674–678.

120. **Singh, N., D. R. Carrigan, T. Gayowski, J. Singh, and I. R. Marino.** 1995. Variant B human herpesvirus-6 associated febrile dermatosis with thrombocytopenia and encephalopathy in a liver transplant recipient. *Transplantation* **60:**1355–1357.

121. **Steeper, T. A., C. A. Horwitz, D. V. Ablashi, S. Z. Salahuddin, C. Saxinger, R. Saltzman, and B. Schwartz.** 1990. The spectrum of clinical and laboratory findings resulting from human herpesvirus-6 (HHV-6) in patients with mononucleosis-like illnesses not resulting from Epstein-Barr virus or cytomegalovirus. *Am. J. Clin. Pathol.* **93:**776–783.

122. **Stefan, A., M. De Lillo, G. Frascaroli, P. Secchiero, F. Neipel, and G. Campadelli-Fiume.** 1999. Development of recombinant diagnostic reagents based on pp85(U14) and p86(U11) proteins to detect the human immune response to human herpesvirus 7 infection. *J. Clin. Microbiol.* **37:**3980–3985.

123. **Suga, S., T. Yoshikawa, Y. Asano, T. Nakashima, I. Kobayashi, and T. Yazaki.** 1992. Activation of human herpesvirus-6 in children with acute measles. *J. Med. Virol.* **38:**278–282.

124. **Suga, S., T. Yoshikawa, Y. Asano, T. Yazaki, and S. Hirata.** 1989. Human herpesvirus-6 infection (exanthem subitum) without rash. *Pediatrics* **83:**1003–1006.

125. **Sumiyoshi, Y., M. Kikuchi, K. Ohshima, M. Takeshita, Y. Eizuru, and Y. Minamishima.** 1993. Analysis of human herpes virus-6 genomes in lymphoid malignancy in Japan. *J. Clin. Pathol.* **46:**1137–1138.

126. **Suzuki, Y., R. Inagi, T. Aono, K. Yamanishi, and T. Shiohara.** 1998. Human herpesvirus 6 infection as a risk factor for the development of severe drug-induced hypersensitivity syndrome. *Arch. Dermatol.* **134:**1108–1112.

127. **Tajiri, H., O. Nose, K. Baba, and S. Okada.** 1990. Human herpesvirus-6 infection with liver injury in neonatal hepatitis. *Lancet* **335:**863.

128. **Takahashi, K., E. Segal, T. Kondo, T. Mukai, M. Moriyama, M. Takahashi, and K. Yamanishi.** 1992. Interferon and natural killer cell activity in patients with exanthem subitum. *Pediatr. Infect. Dis. J.* **11:**369–373.

129. **Takahashi, K., S. Sonoda, K. Higashi, T. Kondo, H. Takahashi, M. Takahashi, and K. Yamanishi.** 1989. Predominant CD4 T-lymphocyte tropism of human herpesvirus 6-related virus. *J. Virol.* **63:**3161–3163.

130. **Takahashi, K., S. Sonoda, K. Kawakami, K. Miyata, T. Oki, T. Nagata, T. Okuno, and K. Yamanishi.** 1988. Human herpesvirus 6 and exanthem subitum. *Lancet* **i:** 1463.

131. **Tanaka, K., T. Kondo, S. Torigoe, S. Okada, T. Mukai, and K. Yamanishi.** 1994. Human herpesvirus 7: another causal agent for roseola (exanthem subitum). *J. Pediatr.* **125:**1–5.

132. **Tanaka-Taya, K., T. Kondo, T. Mukai, H. Miyoshi, Y. Yamamoto, S. Okada, and K. Yamanishi.** 1996. Seroepidemiological study of human herpesvirus-6 and -7 in children of different ages and detection of these two viruses in throat swabs by polymerase chain reaction. *J. Med. Virol.* **48:**88–94.

133. **Tohyama, M., Y. Yahata, M. Yasukawa, R. Inagi, Y. Urano, K. Yamanishi, and K. Hashimoto.** 1998. Severe hypersensitivity syndrome due to sulfasalazine associated with reactivation of human herpesvirus 6. *Arch. Dermatol.* **134:**1113–1117.

134. **Torigoe, S., W. Koide, M. Yamada, E. Miyashiro, K. Tanaka-Taya, and K. Yamanishi.** 1996. Human herpesvirus 7 infection associated with central nervous system manifestations. *J. Pediatr.* **129:**301–305.

135. **Torrisi, M. R., M. Gentile, G. Cardinali, M. Cirone, C. Zompetta, L. V. Lotti, L. Frati, and A. Faggioni.** 1999. Intracellular transport and maturation pathway of human herpesvirus 6. *Virology* **257:**460–471.

136. **Tsukazaki, T., M. Yoshida, H. Namba, M. Yamada, N. Shimizu, and S. Nii.** 1998. Development of a dot blot neutralizing assay for HHV-6 and HHV-7 using specific monoclonal antibodies. *J. Virol. Methods* **73:**141–149.

137. **Wakefield, D., A. Lloyd, J. Dwyer, S. Z. Salahuddin, and D. V. Ablashi.** 1988. Human herpesvirus 6 and myalgic encephalomyelitis. *Lancet* **i:**1059.

138. **Ward, K. N., N. J. Andrews, C. M. Verity, E. Miller, and E. M. Ross.** 2005. Human herpesviruses-6 and -7 each cause significant neurological morbidity in Britain and Ireland. *Arch. Dis. Child.* **90:**619–623.

139. **Ward, K. N., H. N. Leong, E. P. Nacheva, J. Howard, C. E. Atkinson, N. W. Davies, P. D. Griffiths, and D. A. Clark.** 2006. Human herpesvirus 6 chromosomal integration in immunocompetent patients results in high levels of viral DNA in blood, sera, and hair follicles. *J. Clin. Microbiol.* **44:**1571–1574.

140. **Ward, K. N., A. D. Thiruchelvam, and X. Couto-Parada.** 2005. Unexpected occasional persistence of high levels of HHV-6 DNA in sera: detection of variants A and B. *J. Med. Virol.* **76:**563–570.

141. **Watanabe, T., M. Sugaya, K. Nakamura, and K. Tamaki.** 1999. Human herpesvirus 7 and pityriasis rosea. *J. Investig. Dermatol.* **113:**288–289.

142. **Wyatt, L. S., and N. Frenkel.** 1992. Human herpesvirus 7 is a constitutive inhabitant of adult human saliva. *J. Virol.* **66:**3206–3209.

143. **Wyatt, L. S., W. J. Rodriguez, N. Balachandran, and N. Frenkel.** 1991. Human herpesvirus 7: antigenic properties and prevalence in children and adults. *J. Virol.* **65:** 6260–6265.

144. **Yadav, M., M. Arivananthan, A. Chandrashekran, B. S. Tan, and B. Y. Hashim.** 1997. Human herpesvirus-6 (HHV-6) DNA and virus-encoded antigen in oral lesions. *J. Oral Pathol. Med.* **26:**393–401.

145. **Yalcin, S., T. Mukai, K. Kondo, Y. Ami, T. Okawa, A. Kojima, T. Kurata, and K. Yamanishi.** 1992. Experimental infection of cynomolgus and African green monkeys with human herpesvirus 6. *J. Gen. Virol.* **73**(Pt. 7)**:** 1673–1677.

146. **Yamamoto, M., J. B. Black, J. A. Stewart, C. Lopez, and P. E. Pellett.** 1990. Identification of a nucleocapsid protein as a specific serological marker of human herpesvirus 6 infection. *J. Clin. Microbiol.* **28:**1957–1962.

147. **Yamamoto, T., T. Mukai, K. Kondo, and K. Yamanishi.** 1994. Variation of DNA sequence in immediate-early gene of human herpesvirus 6 and variant identification by PCR. *J. Clin. Microbiol.* **32:**473–476.

148. **Yamanishi, K., T. Okuno, K. Shiraki, M. Takahashi, T. Kondo, Y. Asano, and T. Kurata.** 1988. Identification of human herpesvirus-6 as a causal agent for exanthem subitum. *Lancet* **i:**1065–1067.

149. **Yoshida, M., F. Uno, Z. L. Bai, M. Yamada, S. Nii, T. Sata, T. Kurata, K. Yamanishi, and M. Takahashi.** 1989. Electron microscopic study of a herpes-type virus isolated from an infant with exanthem subitum. *Microbiol. Immunol.* **33:**147–154.

150. **Yoshida, M., M. Yamada, S. Chatterjee, F. Lakeman, S. Nii, and R. J. Whitley.** 1996. A method for detection of HHV-6 antigens and its use for evaluating antiviral drugs. *J. Virol. Methods* **58:**137–143.

151. **Yoshikawa, T., Y. Asano, I. Kobayashi, T. Nakashima, T. Yazaki, S. Suga, T. Ozaki, L. S. Wyatt, and N. Frenkel.** 1993. Seroepidemiology of human herpesvirus 7 in healthy children and adults in Japan. *J. Med. Virol.* **41:**319–323.

152. **Yoshikawa, T., T. Nakashima, S. Suga, Y. Asano, T. Yazaki, H. Kimura, T. Morishima, K. Kondo, and K. Yamanishi.** 1992. Human herpesvirus-6 DNA in cerebrospinal fluid of a child with exanthem subitum and meningoencephalitis. *Pediatrics* **89:**888–890.

153. **Zou, P., Y. Isegawa, K. Nakano, M. Haque, Y. Horiguchi, and K. Yamanishi.** 1999. Human herpesvirus 6 open reading frame U83 encodes a functional chemokine. *J. Virol.* **73:**5926–5933.

Epstein-Barr Virus

KATHERINE LUZURIAGA AND JOHN L. SULLIVAN

24

In the century preceding the discovery of Epstein-Barr virus (EBV), physicians speculated on an infectious etiology to explain a common clinical syndrome initially termed glandular fever, characterized by fever, tonsillar adenopathy, splenomegaly, and mononuclear leukocytosis. Downey and McKinlay described the now-classic atypical lymphocytes as a marker for recognizing glandular fever, later renamed infectious mononucleosis (IM) (30). Almost a decade later, Paul and Bunnell described high titers of spontaneously occurring heterophilic antibodies in the sera of patients with IM (88). In March 1961, the British surgeon Denis P. Burkitt gave the first account, outside of Africa, of "The Commonest Children's Cancer in Tropical Africa." This seminar, at Middlesex Hospital in London, England, detailed the geographic relationship between Burkitt's lymphoma (BL) and conditions of temperature, altitude, and rainfall. M. Anthony Epstein attended this seminar and was intrigued with the idea that some biological agent might be involved in the etiology of BL (31). In 1964, the Epstein laboratory analyzed tumor biopsy samples by thin-section electron microscopy and discovered a new, large, icosahedral herpesvirus which could be directly reactivated from in vitro-grown BL cells. The initial findings were reported in *Lancet*, and the virus was later named after Epstein and his graduate student Yvonne Barr (32). Shortly thereafter, two independent groups (48, 89) reported on the ability of EBV to transform primary human B lymphocytes into permanently growing lymphoblastoid cell lines, providing the first concrete evidence to support a causal role for EBV in the establishment of a human cancer. In 1968, Henle et al. made a critical observation when they noted that seroconversion to EBV occurred during the course of acute IM (AIM) in a female laboratory technician (47). Furthermore, an immortalized EBV-carrying lymphoblastoid cell line was established from a peripheral blood leukocyte culture taken during the acute phase of the research technician's illness. Henle et al. followed up this observation with a serologic study on sera provided by Niederman and McCollum of Yale University that were collected from incoming freshmen and later from individuals who had developed AIM. This study, as well as others, revealed EBV-specific antibodies in the sera of all students who developed AIM, thus confirming the etiologic association between EBV and AIM (84).

VIROLOGY

Classification

Taxonomy

EBV is a member of the *Gammaherpesvirinae* subfamily of the family *Herpesviridae* and is the prototype for the *Lymphocryptovirus* genus. In vitro, all gammaherpesviruses replicate in lymphoid cells, and some are capable of lytic replication in epithelial cells and fibroblasts. The host range of the *Lymphocryptovirus* genus is generally restricted to primate B lymphocytes, which are also the site of latent virus infection in vivo. Infection of primate B lymphocytes with lymphocryptoviruses typically results in a latent infection characterized by persistence of the viral genome along with expression of a restricted set of latent gene products which contribute to the transformation process and help drive cell proliferation (62).

Type and Strain Variations

Two types of EBV, EBV-1 and EBV-2, have been identified in most human populations (127). There is extensive homology and restriction endonuclease site conservation throughout most of the EBV-1 and EBV-2 genomes (28). The major identified differences between the EBV-1 and EBV-2 genomes exist in the latent infection cycle nuclear antigen genes for EBV nuclear antigen 2 (EBNA-2); EBNA-LP (28); and EBNA-3A, -3B, and -3C (96) and in the small, nonpolyadenylated RNA EBER-1 and -2 (6). As expected, the differences between EBV-1 and EBV-2 EBNA genes are reflected in type-specific and type-common EBNA epitopes. Immunorecognition of EBV-transformed B lymphoblastoid cells by EBV-specific cytotoxic T lymphocytes is dependent upon the infecting EBV strain (94). The prevalence and geographic distribution of the two EBV strains have been determined by serologic reactivities to EBNA-2. Results indicate that African EBV genomes are almost as frequently type 2 as type 1, which contrasts with American and European EBV genomes, which are 10 times more likely to be type 1 than type 2. Similar serologic findings extend to the EBNA-3A, -3B, and -3C genes (96). Sera from EBV-1-infected patients preferentially react with type 1 EBNA-3A, -3B, and -3C, whereas sera from individuals infected with EBV-2 react preferentially with type 2 EBNA-3 gene products.

With respect to homology, the EBNA gene products share 50 to 85% primary amino acid sequence identity; EBV-1 EBNA-2, -3A, -3B, and -3C differ in predicted primary amino acid sequence from their EBV-2 counterparts by 47, 16, 20, and 28%, respectively (94). Limited genomic divergence between various EBV-1 isolates has also been documented. In one study, 2% nucleotide sequence divergence and 5% amino acid sequence divergence were observed between two EBV-1 latent membrane protein 1 (LMP-1) genes (44).

Composition of Virus and Genome Structure

EBV consists of a toroid-shaped protein core wrapped with linear double-stranded DNA, an icosahedral nucleocapsid containing 162 capsomeres, an amorphous protein tegument surrounding the capsid, and the outer viral envelope, which consists of predominantly a single glycoprotein known as gp350/220 (hereafter referred to as gp350) (62).

The EBV genome was first characterized in 1970 and consists of a linear, 172-kbp, double-stranded DNA molecule. EBV was completely sequenced in the early 1980s (8). The characteristic features of the EBV genome, as depicted in Fig. 1, include a single overall format and gene arrangement, tandemly reiterated 0.5-kbp terminal repeats and tandemly reiterated 3-kbp internal repeats which divide the genome into predominantly unique long and short regions. EBV DNA is linear in the virus particles, but the terminal repeats mediate circularization in infected cells; each infected cell contains 1 to 20 copies of the EBV episome in the nucleus. The characteristic DNA repeat elements serve as important landmarks on the EBV genome, which allow one to distinguish between EBV strains. While various EBV isolates differ in their tandem-repeat frequency, individual EBV isolates tend to contain a constant number of repeats even through serial passage. This is exemplified each time EBV establishes latent infection, in which the virus persists as an episome containing a set number of tandem terminal repeats. This principle is extremely useful in determining whether latently infected cells, such as BL, arise from a single progenitor (92).

There is general conservation of the genetic organization between herpesvirus saimiri, a primate gammaherpesvirus, and EBV; however, there are unique EBV DNA segments that function during latent B-cell infection (82). Antigenic cross-reactivity between EBV and other herpesviruses is rare, even among the proteins encoded by the more conserved genes. In fact, the EBV genes expressed in latent infection as well as several lytic-cycle genes have no detectable homology to other herpesvirus genes, and many believe that they may have arisen in part from cellular DNA (62). In particular, an irregular repeat motif, GGGGCAGGA, present in the latent-cycle EBNA-1, is also interspersed in human cell DNA. Other examples of EBV lytic-cycle genes with significant homology to the human genome, but little homology to other herpesviruses, include BZLF1, BHRF1, and BCRF1. BZLF1 is an immediate-early gene closely related to the *fos* and *jun* transcriptional activators (86). BHRF1 is an EBV early gene with significant homology to the human *bcl-2* gene (23), thought to be involved in preventing B cells and other cells from undergoing apoptosis. Lastly, BCRF1 is an EBV late gene whose product has a primary amino acid sequence and biological activity nearly identical to those of human interleukin 10 (55).

Biology

Host Range and Virus Receptor

The host range of EBV is restricted to humans and certain nonhuman primates, including squirrel monkeys and cotton-top marmosets (76). Related oncogenic herpesviruses have been detected in Old World primate species and, more recently, in New World primates (22).

B lymphocytes are the primary cellular reservoir of EBV infection. The initial stage of infection involves a high-affinity interaction between the major EBV outer envelope glycoprotein, gp350, with CD21 on the surface of B cells (26, 111). Multiple lines of evidence have confirmed CD21, the receptor for the C3d component of complement, as the primary human cellular receptor on B cells: (i) purified CD21 binds to EBV, (ii) virus infection is blocked by antibody directed against the CD21 glycoprotein, and (iii) the expression of CD21 on heterologous cells confers binding to EBV. Currently, gp350 is believed to bind exclusively to the CD21 molecule. Comparison of the primary amino acid sequences of gp350 and C3d has revealed a shared nonapeptide (EDPGFFNVE) which likely explains their common binding properties with CD21 (67).

In addition to infecting B cells, EBV can infect T cells, monocytes, and epithelial cells. CD21 or related molecules are also present on thymocytes and peripheral blood T cells (118). As is discussed below, the primary receptor used for attachment of EBV to epithelial cells is unknown but is not thought to be CD21.

EBV Adsorption, Penetration, and Uncoating

The gp350-CD21 interaction initiates intracellular signaling and endocytosis. Fusion of the EBV envelope with the host cell membrane is initiated by interactions between human leukocyte antigen (HLA) class II on the B-cell sur-

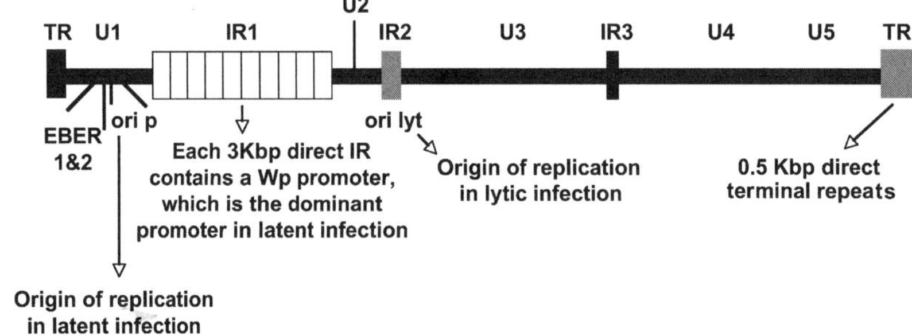

FIGURE 1 Schematic depiction of the linear EBV genome. TR, terminal repeat; IR, internal repeat. (Adapted from reference 62 with permission.)

face and the viral membrane glycoprotein gp42 in complex with the viral glycoproteins gH and gL (123); another EBV glycoprotein, gB (gp110), also appears to be necessary for virus-cell fusion.

While EBV can also infect epithelial cells in vitro and in vivo, the precise role of the epithelium in EBV replication and persistence has been somewhat controversial (56). Interactions between B cells and B cell-epithelial cells may facilitate the infection of epithelial cells (100), but the receptor used by EBV to initiate attachment to epithelial cells remains unknown. Currently available data suggest that EBV may use different CD21-independent mechanisms to enter epithelial cells, depending on the membrane domain (119). Fusion of the EBV envelope with the cell membrane appears to be mediated by an interaction between gH-gL and an unidentified receptor on the surface of epithelial cells.

Dissolution of the viral nucleocapsid and transport of the genome to the cell nucleus are less well understood. Once inside the nucleus, the linear EBV genome circularizes, which precedes, or at least coincides with, the earliest gene expression, directed from the first latent infection promoter Wp (62). The EBV genome is replicated by cellular DNA polymerases during the cell cycle S phase and persists as multiple, extrachromosomal double-stranded EBV episomes, which are organized into nucleosomes similar to chromosomal DNA (62).

Virus Expression in Latent Infection

The hallmark of B-lymphocyte infection with EBV is the establishment of latency, which is characterized by three distinct processes: (i) viral persistence; (ii) restricted virus expression, which alters cell growth and proliferation; and (iii) retained potential for reactivation to lytic replication. Intracellular persistence of the entire viral genome is achieved through circularization of the linear EBV genome present in viral particles and maintenance of multiple copies of this covalently closed episomal DNA (62). The episomes are replicated semiconservatively during cell cycle S phase by cellular DNA polymerases, and equal partitioning of episomes to daughter cells is mediated by interactions between the latent origin of plasmid replication (OriP) and EBNA-1 (62, 64). The 172-kbp EBV genome contains approximately 100 genes, 10 of which are expressed during latency and are thought to be involved in establishing and maintaining the "immortalized" state, including those for six EBV nuclear proteins (EBNA-1, -2, -3A, -3B, -3C, and -LP), two latent membrane proteins (LMP-1 and -2), and two small untranslated, nonpolyadenylated RNAs (EBER-1 and -2) (62). Latency can be disrupted through a variety of cellular activators, resulting in expression of BZLF1 with associated destruction of the host cell (34, 86). A mutation in BZLF1 results in inhibition of the ability to induce lytic replication, but addition of a second factor, BRLF1, partially restores this activity (1).

While only about 10% of the genes of EBV are expressed in latently infected B cells, the transcribed regions encompass a major portion of the viral genome. Transcription of the EBNA and LMP genes is mediated by cell-derived RNA polymerase II, while the EBERs are primarily transcribed by RNA polymerase III (54). EBER genes are the most abundantly transcribed EBV genes in latently infected cells (10^4 to 10^5 copies/cell), distantly followed by the LMP-1 gene, which, in turn, is significantly more abundant than the EBNA and LMP-2 genes. The majority of the genome 3′ of the Wp promoter is transcribed; however, the selection of specific promoters and alternate splicing ultimately determine the levels of latent gene expression (97). Figure 2 depicts the extensive transcription and long-range splicing of the EBV genome, which occur in latently infected B lymphocytes.

Following circularization of the linear EBV genome within the cell nucleus, rightward transcription of the EBNA genes is initiated from the Wp promoter within internal repeat 1, a copy of which is encoded in each 3-kb-long internal repeat. The EBNA mRNAs are assembled by alternative splicing and 3′ processing of a common precursor encoded by more than 100 kb of the genome. EBNA-LP and EBNA-2 are the first EBV proteins expressed during latent infection of B cells and reach their steady-state levels within 24 to 32 h. EBNA-2 is essential to the immortalization process; viruses with EBNA-2 deletions are immortalization incompetent. Restoration of the deleted DNA in defective EBV produces progeny virus with the ability to transform primary human B lymphocytes. EBNA-2 is also required for expression of other EBV latent genes and for the transactivation of EBV genes and cellular genes. EBNA-2 also probably plays a role in promoter switching during the initial stages of latent B-cell infection. By 32 h postinfection, all of the EBNA proteins and LMP-1 can be detected using appropriate antisera. Due to a lack of good-quality antisera, less is known about the onset of expression of LMP-2A and LMP-2B. Concomitant with LMP-1 expression is a further increase in the level of CD23 and the onset of cell DNA synthesis. Expression of the EBNA proteins reaches a steady-state level within 48 h of primary B-cell infection.

Transformation and Latent Proteins

Many of the proteins discussed above are involved in cellular transformation, including the EBNAs and the LMPs.

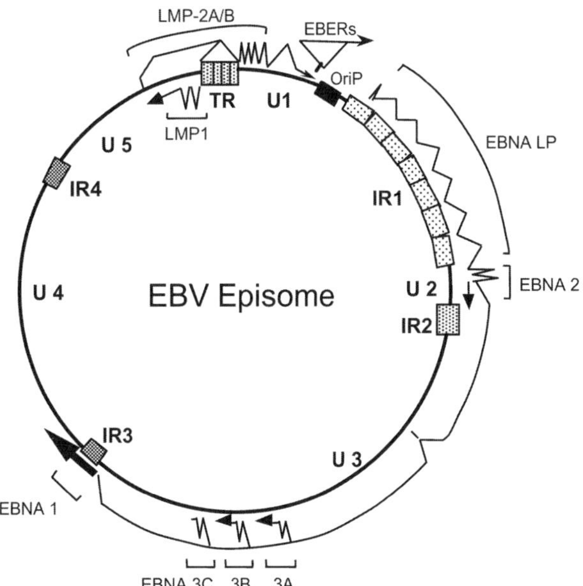

FIGURE 2 Transcription of the EBV episome in latently infected B lymphocytes. TR, terminal repeat; IR, internal repeat. (Adapted from reference 62 with permission.)

EBNA-1

EBNA-1 is required for episome replication and maintenance of the viral genome (35). It is diffusely associated with all chromosomes in the nuclei of latently infected cells and the combined interaction of EBNA-1 with both OriP and chromosomal proteins, which ensures equal partitioning of EBV episomes to progeny cells (77).

EBNA-2

As mentioned above, EBNA-2 mutants have demonstrated that EBNA-2 is essential to the process of B-lymphocyte immortalization and for the expression of EBNA-1 and EBNA-3 (62). Two major strains of EBV exist, EBV-1 and -2, and variations in the EBNA-2 protein impart the most significant biological differences between these two types. In general, EBV-1 transforms normal human B lymphocytes much more efficiently than EBV-2.

The first biochemical evidence for a role for EBNA-2 in B-cell growth transformation came from the demonstration that EBNA-2 specifically transactivates expression of the B-lymphocyte activation marker CD23, which is abundantly expressed on EBV-transformed and antigen-primed B lymphocytes (62). EBNA-2 also up-regulates expression of the EBV receptor CD21 and c-*fgr* and the EBV latent LMP-1 and LMP-2 genes. Thus, most of EBNA-2's role in B-lymphocyte transformation comes from its ability to transactivate cellular and EBV genes.

EBNA-3

EBNA-3 consists of a family of three high-molecular-weight gene products (EBNA-3A, -3B, and -3C) whose genes are located in tandem on the EBV genome (62). Much like the EBNA-2 gene, the EBNA-3 genes are polymorphic and differ according to EBV type. Unlike the difference in transformation phenotype imparted by the EBNA-2 type (1 or 2), the type specificity of the EBNA-3 genes does not affect the ability of the virus to initiate growth transformation, episome maintenance, or lytic replication. Systematic analysis of the transformation capability of EBV recombinants having specific mutations in each of the EBNA-3 genes demonstrated that while EBNA-3B is dispensable for B-lymphocyte growth transformation, mutations in either EBNA-3A or -3C render the virus transformation incompetent (62).

EBNA-LP

EBNA-LP, or leader protein, is actually a set of highly polymorphic proteins. While the function of EBNA-LP remains unclear, some have speculated that it may play a role in RNA processing or associate with some nuclear regulatory protein; alternatively, it may function by up-regulating expression of autocrine factors critical to B-lymphoblastoid cell line (BLCL) growth (62).

LMP-1

The second most abundant EBV mRNA species present in latently infected B lymphocytes (60 copies/cell) is highly stable and encodes a 63-kDa integral membrane protein, LMP-1 (62). The LMP-1 promoter contains an EBNA-2 response element which functions to up-regulate LMP-1 expression. However, LMP-1 is expressed in the absence of EBNA-2 during lytic-cycle activation in BL cells and in nasopharyngeal carcinoma (NPC) tumors.

In vitro, LMP-1 is essential for EBV-induced transformation of B cells into BLCLs and induces many of the activation markers associated with EBV infection of B lymphocytes. The association of LMP-1 with the plasma membrane in patches prompted an exploration of its role in B-lymphocyte growth transformation. Transfer of the LMP-1 gene into continuous rodent fibroblast lines demonstrated multiple transforming effects. Importantly, some of these lines, which are not normally tumorigenic in nude mice, become uniformly tumorigenic when expressing LMP-1; mice expressing the transgene develop B-cell lymphomas (65).

Expression of LMP-1 in EBV-negative BL lines induces many of the changes typically associated with EBV infection or antigen activation of primary B lymphocytes. LMP-expressing cells grow in tight clumps due to increased expression of the homotypic cellular adhesion molecules LFA-1 and ICAM-1. This LMP-1 induction of the adhesion molecules LFA-1, LFA-3, and ICAM-1 promotes interaction between B and T lymphocytes via the LFA-3/CD-2 and LFA-1/ICAM-1 adhesion pathways. These heterotypic adhesions are important, as the in vivo elimination of EBV-transformed B lymphocytes is dependent on conjugate formation with cytotoxic T cells. Indeed, the levels of LFA-3 and ICAM-1 on infected cells influence their susceptibility to cytotoxic-T-lymphocyte lysis by modifying the affinity of effector-target conjugate formation. LMP-1 also induces cell surface expression of a number of B-cell activation molecules, including CD23, CD39, CD40, and CD44. The signaling response induced by LMP-1 mimics that induced by CD40 in B cells (120). LMP-1 protects EBV-infected B cells from programmed cell death (apoptosis), in part via induction of the cellular oncogene *bcl-2* (39, 46). The transforming action of LMP-1 appears to involve the engagement of signaling proteins from the tumor necrosis factor receptor-associated factors (57, 71, 78). LMP-1 mutations that eliminate the association with these factors prevent B-cell growth transformation (57). A second LMP-1 site required for lymphoblastoid cell outgrowth also has been identified which interacts with the tumor necrosis factor receptor-associated death domain protein (58).

LMP-2

LMP-2 is an integral membrane protein containing 12 hydrophobic transmembrane domains which colocalizes with LMP-1 in the plasma membrane of EBV-infected lymphocytes (62). Among the transformation-associated EBV proteins, EBNA-1, LMP-1, and LMP-2 are present most consistently in NPC tumor biopsy samples and EBV-related malignancies. Since both LMP-1 and LMP-2 contain T-cell epitopes, their persistent expression in vivo argues for an important role in the persistence of EBV in the human host.

Functionally, LMP-2 is a substrate for B-lymphocyte *src* family tyrosine kinases and associates with a 70-kDa tyrosine-phosphorylated cellular protein. In view of the prominent roles of tyrosine kinases in growth factor receptor-mediated transmembrane signaling, the association of LMP-2 with a tyrosine kinase is believed to be important in EBV's effects on cell growth. Observations which conflict with this viewpoint include the following: (i) EBV recombinants carrying LMP-2A mutations which do not express LMP-2A protein are capable of initiating and maintaining B-lymphocyte growth transformation in vitro, and surprisingly, (ii) BLCLs derived from the LMP-2A mutants are identical to wild-type EBV-transformed

BLCLs with regard to growth characteristics and permissiveness to lytic infection and virus replication. Transgenic mice expressing the LMP-2 transgene demonstrate the survival of nontransformed B cells in the absence of normal B-cell receptor signaling (15).

EBER-1 and EBER-2

The most abundant EBV transcripts in latently infected B cells are the small (167- to 172-nucleotide), nonpolyadenylated RNAs named EBER-1 and -2 (62). Unlike the other EBV genes expressed during latent infection, the EBERs are also transcribed during lytic infection. EBV-infected cells may express 10^5 EBER copies/cell, and detection of EBERs by in vitro hybridization is a widely used technique to detect EBV-infected cells. The majority of EBERs are localized within the cell nucleus, where they are complexed with the cellular protein La. EBERs' role in infection is unknown; however, EBER sequences are highly conserved across EBV strains, suggesting their importance in the viral life cycle.

EBV DNA Persistence in Latency

During primary infection, EBV uses its different transcription programs (Fig. 3) to activate and trigger the differentiation of B-cell blasts through the germinal-center reaction into resting latently infected memory B cells, the primary reservoir for lifelong persistence of the virus (112, 114). Twenty-five to 50% of peripheral blood memory B cells are latently infected during primary infection; the frequency of latently infected primary B cells falls to 1 in 10^5 to 1 in 10^6 during chronic infection (52). Latently infected memory B cells typically contain 1 to 20 EBV episomes per cell. These latently infected memory B cells are transcriptionally quiescent and express only small amounts of EBNA-1, important for episomal amplification and maintenance upon division (51), and are thus inapparent to immune surveillance. Periodic activation and differentiation of memory B cells into plasma cells initiate the EBV lytic replication cycle (66); EBV-specific CD8$^+$ T cells are likely important in eradicating these cells and controlling new cycles of infection (42).

Lytic Infection and Virus Replication

In vitro, latently infected B cells can be induced to undergo lytic-cycle replication by activation with either phorbol esters or calcium ionophores or by cross-linking cell surface immunoglobulin (Ig) (62). Following induction, cells undergo cytopathic changes characteristic of lytic herpesvirus infection, including chromatin margination, viral DNA synthesis, nucleocapsid assembly at the nucleus periphery, virus budding through the nuclear membrane, and inhibition of host cell protein synthesis. The activation and differentiation of memory B cells into plasma cells initiate the EBV lytic replication cycle in vivo (66).

In lytic EBV infection, immediate-early genes are defined as genes that are transcribed in newly infected cells in the absence of new viral protein synthesis. The key immediate-early transactivators of EBV lytic-cycle genes are the 1-kb BZLR1 mRNA and the 2.8-kb BRLF1 RNA (62). The induction of EBV lytic-cycle replication results in increased episome copy number and suggests that circular episomal DNA replication is a precursor to subsequent DNA replication. Unexpectedly, the EBV DNA polymerase is not required for viral DNA replication associated with episome establishment.

The EBV genes expressed during the late stages of lytic infection mostly encode structural viral proteins, which permit virion maintenance and egress. The viral glycoproteins are all encoded by late genes, which are of potential importance in antibody-mediated immunity to EBV. Two EBV glycoproteins forming important parts of the virus coat are gp350 and gp85 (62). gp350 is the major virus

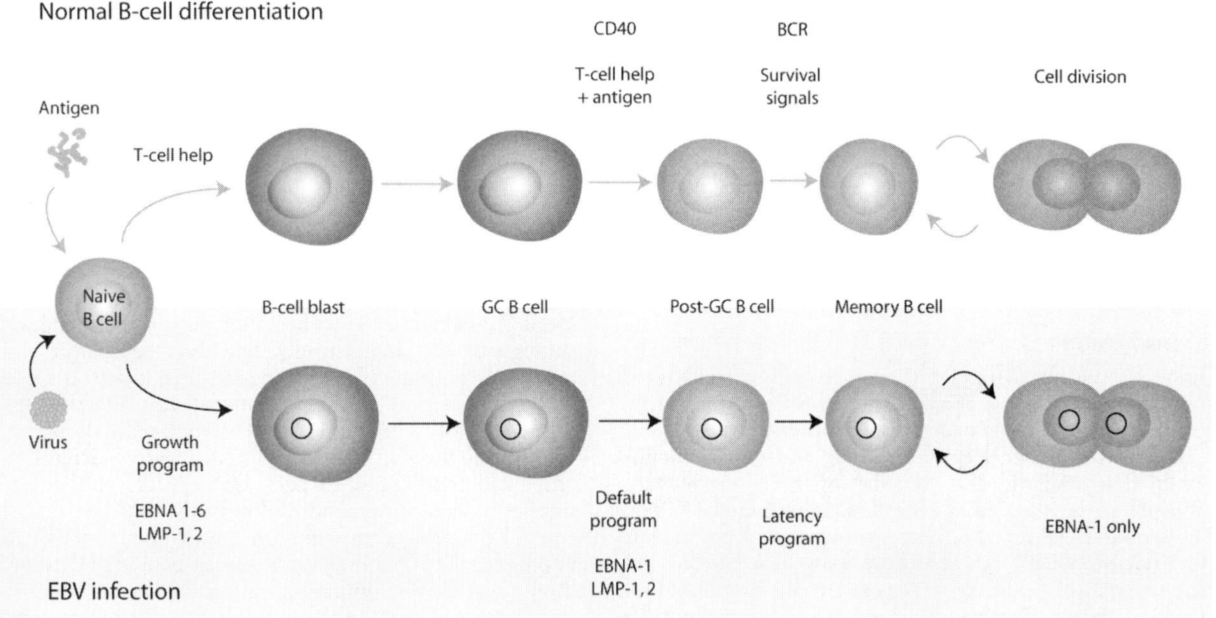

FIGURE 3 EBV manipulates normal B-cell biology to establish a memory B-cell reservoir of infection. GC, germinal center. (Adapted from reference 114; copyright 2004 Massachusetts Medical Society [all rights reserved].)

coat glycoprotein and mediates virus binding to the B-lymphocyte receptor CD21. gp85 is a relatively minor virus component which is functionally involved in the fusion between virus and cell membranes.

EPIDEMIOLOGY

Distribution and Geography

Information on the incidence and prevalence of EBV infection under different environmental and sociological conditions has been obtained primarily through seroepidemiological studies. Antibodies to EBV have been demonstrated in all population groups, and about 90 to 95% of adults worldwide are EBV seropositive. In lower-resource settings, most children acquire EBV infection over the first 2 years of life; for example, 82% of children in Ghana were EBV seropositive by 18 months of age (11). In higher-resource settings, EBV infection typically occurs in late childhood or adolescence. The two strains of EBV, EBV-1 and EBV-2, are widely distributed geographically. While EBV-1 is more commonly found in the United States and Europe, EBV-2 is more common in Africa (127). Immunocompetent as well as immunocompromised individuals can be coinfected with the two strains (27, 99).

Incidence and Prevalence of Infection

The incidence of clinically symptomatic infection (AIM) is greatest when primary EBV infection is delayed until the second decade of life. In the United States and Great Britain, EBV seroconversion occurs before age 5 in about 50% of the population, with a second wave occurring in the middle of the second decade. The overall incidence of AIM in the United States is about 50 cases/100,000 per year, with the highest incidence in the 15- to 24-year age group. In college-aged populations, 30 to 75% of entering freshmen are EBV seronegative (27). Each year, approximately 10 to 15% of susceptible individuals will become infected and 50 to 70% of the infections will be associated with AIM. By contrast, AIM is observed in fewer than 10% of infections in infants and children. No obvious yearly cycles or seasonal changes in incidence are known.

High titers of virus are present in throat washings of patients with AIM (10, 42), and intermittent, asymptomatic oropharyngeal shedding persists at lower levels for the lifetime of infected individuals. Consequently, only a small percentage of patients with AIM recall prior contact with other individuals with AIM, and most infections are acquired from asymptomatic shedders.

Transmission

EBV is transmitted primarily through contact with oropharyngeal secretions. The detection of EBV in the uterine cervix suggests that sexual transmission can occur as well (103). Oropharyngeal epithelial cells and/or B lymphocytes that underlie the tonsillar epithelial crypts are thought to be the initial cells that are infected (4, 59). This productive infection leads to continued production and release of EBV into the oropharyngeal secretions and the infection of additional B cells in the lymphoid-rich areas of the oropharynx. As discussed above, memory B cells are responsible for the dissemination of the infection throughout the lymphoreticular system and are necessary for viral persistence. Total-body lymphoid irradiation may eliminate the EBV carrier state. Individuals lacking B cells due to X-linked agammaglobulinemia do not develop persistent EBV infection.

PATHOGENESIS IN HUMANS

Incubation Period and Early Infection

The propagation of EBV in humans is dependent upon viral replication in the oropharynx and spread of virus to uninfected persons via contact with virus-contaminated saliva. The incubation period from initial exposure to symptoms, coincident with the detection of large numbers of EBV-infected B cells (up to 25 to 50% of circulating memory B cells) in the circulation, is approximately 30 to 50 days.

Figure 4 summarizes the pathogenesis of EBV infection. Infection is initiated in the oropharynx following contact with infected secretions. Viral replication occurs first in epithelial cells or in tonsillar crypt B lymphocytes. EBV infection of B cell blasts and selective viral gene expression result in the differentiation into memory B cells. The cellular immune response, which occurs following EBV infection, is massive, and it is likely that this response not only limits further rounds of viral replication but may also contribute directly or indirectly to the symptoms of AIM. Perturbation of these cellular immune responses may result in uncontrolled EBV infection (as seen in X-linked lymphoproliferative syndrome) or the genesis of an EBV-induced malignancy.

Humoral Immune Response to EBV Infection

Primary EBV infection induces circulating antibodies directed against viral antigens as well as unrelated antigens found on sheep and horse red cells. The latter antibodies, named heterophilic antibodies, are a heterogeneous group of mostly IgM antibodies with either Forssman or Paul and Bunnell specificity, which do not cross-react with EBV antigens. The detection of these heterophilic antibodies is often used to screen patients for AIM. EBV-specific antibody must be used to differentiate primary EBV infection from other diseases presenting with lymphocytosis, fever, lymphadenopathy, and malaise. The diagnosis of EBV infection is based upon the detection of transient levels in serum of IgM against viral capsid antigens (VCA), as well as IgG against VCA, early antigens (EA), and EBNA proteins (25). The transient IgM response to VCA reaches high titers early and disappears within weeks. IgM VCA antibodies are not demonstrable in the general population, and thus, their presence is virtually diagnostic of primary EBV infection. IgG antibody titers to VCA reach peak levels 2 weeks later and thereafter persist at lower levels throughout life. Interestingly, IgG directed against early lytic-cycle proteins (EA-D) tends to appear with the peak IgM response and reaches maximal levels after the IgM response. Lastly, IgG anti-EBNA titers usually do not develop until the convalescent period. Figure 5 depicts the onset and time course of peak EBV-specific antibody responses observed in young adults with AIM.

gp350 is the most abundant viral protein in lytically infected cell plasma membranes, and accordingly, most of the human EBV-neutralizing IgG antibody response is directed against gp350 (85, 115). These neutralizing antibodies reach maximal levels 6 to 7 weeks after the onset of illness, and stable titers persist for life. gp350-specific antibodies can also mediate complement fixation and antibody-dependent cellular cytotoxicity (61). Fortui-

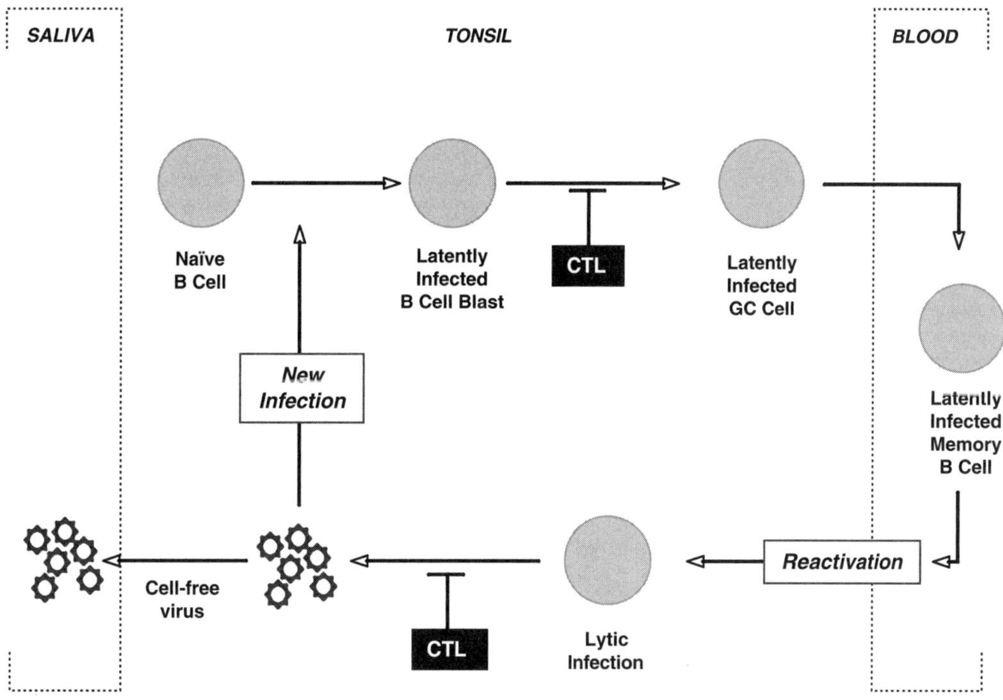

FIGURE 4 Pathogenesis of EBV infection. (Adapted from reference 42 with permission of the American Society of Hematology.)

tously, the gp350 molecule is highly conserved between EBV-1 and -2, and thus, gp350 is considered to be an essential component of any prospective EBV vaccine.

Cellular Immune Response to EBV

A hallmark of primary EBV infection is the appearance of "atypical lymphocytes" in the peripheral blood, which account for 60 to 70% of the total white cell count, averaging 12,000 to 18,000/mm^3. NK cells play a primary role in immune surveillance against virus-infected or -transformed cells, since they do not require priming or prior antigen exposure. NK cells alone are not sufficient to

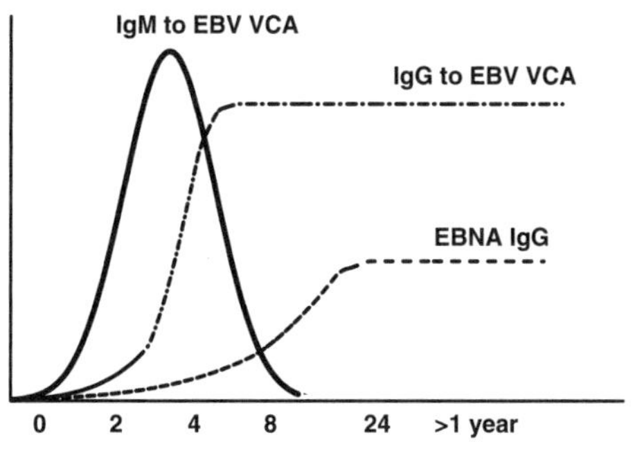

	IgM VCA	IgG VCA	EBNA IgG
Acute infection	+	–	–
Late acute infection	+	+	–
Past infection	–	+	+

FIGURE 5 Characteristic EBV-specific antibody responses observed in young adults with AIM.

prevent the establishment of EBV-transformed B-cell lines in vitro; however, they do contribute to improved BLCL regression in the presence of EBV-specific CD8$^+$ T cells (73). This effect may be due to either direct cytotoxicity or interferon (IFN) production, since EBV and EBV-infected cells induce IFN-γ production by NK cells (5), and IFN-α is known to inhibit EBV-induced B-cell proliferation in vitro (113). However, a patient described by Biron et al. (12) with a complete absence of NK cells experienced an unremarkable EBV infection in the face of life-threatening infections with varicella-zoster virus, cytomegalovirus, and herpes simplex virus, suggesting that NK cells are not necessary for control of primary EBV infection.

Several lines of evidence suggest that EBV-specific CD4$^+$ and CD8$^+$ T-cell responses are important for limiting primary EBV infection and controlling chronic infection. EBV-specific CD4$^+$ and CD8$^+$ T cells can prevent the transformation of B lymphocytes in vitro. The increased incidence of EBV-associated lymphoproliferative disorders or lymphomas in individuals with compromised cell-mediated immunity also suggests that T cells are important for the long-term control of EBV replication. EBV reactivation and a transient AIM syndrome were observed in patients who underwent T-cell depletion after treatment with anti-CD3 antibody (60).

Over the past decade, powerful and precise methods for the enumeration and characterization of virus-specific CD4$^+$ and CD8$^+$ T cells in the peripheral blood have been developed (29, 75). These include the use of labeled major histocompatibility complex-peptide complexes (tetramers) to directly detect, measure, and isolate antigen-specific lymphocytes and assays to detect antigen-specific cytokine-secreting cells following in vitro stimulation (IFN-γ enzyme-linked immunospot assays and flow cytometry-based assays to measure intracellular cytokine secretion). These novel methods have markedly improved our understanding of the strength and breadth of EBV-specific $CD4^+$ and $CD8^+$ T-cell responses over the course of infection.

During primary EBV infection, high frequencies of EBV-specific $CD4^+$ and $CD8^+$ T-cell responses have been detected directly ex vivo (16, 17, 90, 110). EBV-specific $CD8^+$ T-cell responses in primary infection are primarily directed against lytic-cycle antigens; latent antigen-specific responses are detected later and at lower frequencies (17). Up to 44% of peripheral blood $CD8^+$ T cells are EBV specific and express CD45RO, HLA-DR, and CD38, suggesting high-level activation and turnover of these cells in vivo (16). By contrast, early EBV-specific $CD4^+$ T-cell responses target both lytic and latent antigens (90). In chronically infected individuals, EBV-specific $CD8^+$ T cells represent up to 5% of peripheral blood $CD8^+$ T cells, while EBV-specific $CD4^+$ T cells are detected at much lower frequencies.

CLINICAL MANIFESTATIONS

Congenital and Perinatal Infections

Intrauterine infection with EBV appears to be a very rare event. Primary infection during pregnancy is unusual because in most populations, fewer than 5% of pregnant women are susceptible. Isolated cases of infants born with congenital anomalies (biliary atresia, congenital heart disease, hypotonia, micrognathia, cataracts, and thrombocytopenia) have been reported in which some evidence for EBV infection has been presented (38). However, a number of lines of evidence argue against EBV as a significant cause of congenital infection. Studies of large numbers of children with congenital anomalies have failed to disclose evidence of EBV infection. Furthermore, cord blood samples from thousands of infants have failed to yield evidence of EBV-infected or -transformed cells. Finally, prospective studies on seronegative susceptible pregnant women have generally failed to find evidence either of maternal primary EBV infection or of congenital abnormalities in infants of women who develop primary EBV infection during pregnancy (33).

Primary EBV Infection in Infants and Children

Primary EBV infections in young infants and children are frequently asymptomatic. When symptoms do occur, they are usually mild and nonspecific (otitis media, diarrhea, abdominal complaints, and upper respiratory infection); classical symptoms of AIM are rare (40). In one series, blood smears from only 32 of 200 children who presented under 4 years of age with clinical findings compatible with AIM (pharyngitis and significant cervical adenopathy) had more than 50% mononuclear cells and more than 10% atypical lymphocytes (53); respiratory symptoms were frequently prominent, especially in young infants. Heterophilic antibodies were detected in only 25% of infants aged 10 to 24 months but were detected in 75% of children aged 24 to 28 months. IgM antibodies to VCA were also less frequently detected in infants (60%, compared to 100% in older children and young adults); in addition, peak titers of IgG VCA antibodies were lower, and the development of antibodies to EA was less common in infants. Despite the reduction in antibody production, young infants can mount EBV-specific $CD8^+$ T-cell responses during acute EBV infection, and the latent proteins recognized are identical to those recognized by young adults (109).

Acute Infectious Mononucleosis

EBV is a common, but not exclusive, cause of AIM, a syndrome marked by malaise, headache, fever, tonsillitis and/or pharyngitis, and cervical lymph node enlargement and tenderness (25). Affected patients usually have peripheral blood lymphocytosis, composed in large measure of atypical lymphocytes. The lymphadenopathy characteristically is symmetric and involves the posterior cervical chain more than the anterior chain. Tonsillar exudates are a frequent component of the pharyngitis; the exudates can have a white, gray-green, or necrotic appearance. Severe fatigue is often prominent, while other, less common findings include palatal petechiae, periorbital or palpebral edema, and maculopapular and morbilliform rash. Nausea, vomiting, and anorexia are common in patients with IM, probably reflecting the mild hepatitis found in about 90% of infected individuals; however, hepatomegaly and jaundice are uncommon. Splenomegaly is almost universally detected by sonography but is detected in fewer (20 to 50%) AIM patients by palpation.

Most patients with AIM caused by EBV have prominent pharyngeal symptoms. There are, however, several other forms of the illness. Some individuals with AIM present with the so-called glandular form of the disease, in which lymph node enlargement is out of proportion to the pharyngeal symptoms; others develop a systemic form of the infection in which fever and fatigue predominate, while lymphadenopathy and pharyngitis are mild or absent. Some patients have hepatitis in the absence of other typical features of AIM. The vast majority of individuals with AIM recover uneventfully and develop a high degree of durable immunity. Acute symptoms typically resolve in 1 to 2 weeks, but fatigue may persist for months.

Other Manifestations

Numerous other manifestations have been associated with primary EBV infection. Neurologic syndromes can include Guillain-Barré syndrome, facial nerve palsy, meningoencephalitis, aseptic meningitis, transverse myelitis, peripheral neuritis, cerebellitis, and optic neuritis (117). Hematologic abnormalities can include hemolytic anemia, thrombocytopenia, aplastic anemia, thrombotic thrombocytopenic purpura/hemolytic-uremic syndrome, and disseminated intravascular coagulation. EBV can affect virtually any organ system and has been associated with such diverse disease manifestations as pneumonia, myocarditis, pancreatitis, mesenteric adenitis, myositis, glomerulonephritis, and genital ulceration.

Complications and Associated Malignancies

EBV infection is associated with a number of acute complications and, in certain hosts, more delayed effects.

Rash

One of the more common complications of IM is a morbilliform rash following the administration of ampicillin or amoxicillin and, to a lesser extent, penicillin. The incidence initially was reported to be as high as 70 to 90% but is probably lower (45). The mechanism responsible for this rash is not understood but has been thought to involve circulating antibodies to ampicillin. Development of this rash during AIM does not appear to presage a true ampicillin allergy; patients have subsequently tolerated ampicillin without adverse reactions.

Splenic Rupture

Splenic rupture is a rare but potentially life-threatening complication of AIM, estimated to occur in one or two cases per thousand (2). Almost all cases have been in males. Splenic rupture is often the first symptom of AIM that brings the patient to medical attention; it is spontaneous in more than half of the reported cases, with no history of specific injury. Again, splenic enlargement can be detected in most AIM patients sonographically, but splenomegaly is detected in only 20 to 50% of patients. Rupture has occurred between the 4th and 21st days of symptomatic illness and has not correlated with the clinical severity of AIM or with laboratory findings. Despite its life-threatening potential, fatality from this complication is rare. The management of splenic rupture is similar to that of other forms of splenic injury. Nonoperative treatment with intensive supportive care and splenic preservation has been successfully carried out in some cases, while others require splenectomy (7).

Airway Obstruction

Obstruction of the upper airway due to massive lymphoid hyperplasia and mucosal edema has long been recognized as an uncommon and potentially fatal complication of IM. Severe obstruction can be successfully treated by tracheotomy or endotracheal intubation. Alternatively, the use of corticosteroids to reduce pharyngeal edema and lymphoid hypertrophy is advocated for individuals with incipient obstruction.

Lymphoproliferative Disorders

EBV infection is associated with a variety of lymphoproliferative disorders.

Hemophagocytic Lymphohistiocytosis

EBV is one of the recognized causes of sporadic hemophagocytic lymphohistiocytosis, a benign disorder characterized pathologically by generalized histiocytic proliferation and hemophagocytosis (108). Patients with this unusual syndrome present with fever, generalized lymphadenopathy, hepatosplenomegaly, hepatitis, pancytopenia, and coagulopathy.

T-cell proliferation is a primary feature of hemophagocytic lymphohistiocytosis (68, 105). The proposed pathogenesis of this disorder suggests that infection of T cells by EBV selectively up-regulates the expression of tumor necrosis factor alpha, which, in combination with IFN-γ and other cytokines, can activate macrophages. There is anecdotal evidence that acyclovir may be beneficial (108).

Lymphomatoid Granulomatosis

Lymphomatoid granulomatosis is an angiodestructive disorder of the lymphoid system; over 90% of cases have been associated with EBV infection (43, 93, 124). In the majority of cases, EBV-infected B cells are present, and the B-cell proliferation is clonal. Patients often have evidence of immunodeficiency, including congenital and acquired conditions such as human immunodeficiency virus (HIV) infection. The pathogenesis of this disorder is thus likely directly related to transformation of EBV-infected B cells in an environment with impaired T-cell function. Patients with lymphomatoid granulomatosis may respond to IFN-α (124). Clinical features include fever, cough, malaise, and weight loss, with involvement of lung, kidney, liver, skin, and subcutaneous tissue and the central nervous system, with the typical histologic changes.

CAEBV Infection

Chronic active EBV (CAEBV) infection is a rare disorder that is characterized by recurrent fever, lymphadenopathy, and hepatosplenomegaly persisting over several years (25). CAEBV is frequently accompanied by grossly abnormal EBV antibody titers, with titers of IgG antibody to the EBV VCA in excess of 1:5,000. Recent studies by Kimura et al. have demonstrated high EBV viral loads and EBV monoclonality in the majority of individuals with CAEBV (63). Individuals with CAEBV were found to have either EBV-infected T cells or NK cells in the peripheral blood. Those individuals with EBV-infected T cells had a 5-year survival rate of less than 50%, while those with the NK phenotype had a 5-year survival rate of 80%.

XLP Syndrome

X-linked lymphoproliferative (XLP) syndrome is characterized by a selective immunodeficiency to EBV manifested by severe or fatal IM and acquired immunodeficiency (107). Prospective studies with males prior to EBV infection have demonstrated normal cellular and humoral immunity. During acute EBV infection, males with XLP syndrome demonstrate vigorous cytotoxic cellular responses, which predominately involve activated virus-specific $CD8^{+}$ T cells. The gene (SH2D1A) responsible for XLP syndrome has been identified and encodes a 128-amino-acid protein which plays an important role in signal transduction pathways in T lymphocytes (24, 83, 98). Recent studies in an SH2D1A knockout mouse model suggest that the SH2D1A protein plays an important role in signaling CD8 T-cell apoptosis and that the SH2D1A mutation prevents normal activation-induced cell death, resulting in uncontrolled CD8 T-cell proliferation observed in patients with XLP syndrome (21, 106). At this time, with the discovery of the XLP syndrome gene, SH2D1A, the diagnosis of XLP syndrome can be made in the majority of individuals by genetic analysis. In the situation of an affected male with XLP syndrome presenting with acute EBV infection, therapy should be directed at elimination of both activated CD8 T cells and EBV-transformed B lymphocytes. While the use of recently developed monoclonal antibodies directed against T lymphocytes (CAMPATH) and B lymphocytes (CAMPATH and RITUXAN) has not been reported for patients with XLP syndrome, their use in this setting may be warranted. The definitive treatment of XLP syndrome is currently bone marrow or cord blood stem cell transplantation. Ziegner et al. reported on the successful correction of XLP syndrome using transplantation of cord blood stem cells from an unrelated donor (126).

BL

BL is the most common childhood malignancy in equatorial Africa. This unmistakable tumor is typically localized in the jaw of young patients; the majority of endemic cases occur in discrete geographic climates located along the malaria belt across Africa. It is hypothesized that malaria provides a chronic stimulus for proliferation of B lymphocytes, some of which carry latent EBV.

Tumor cells from areas where BL is endemic contain copies of the EBV genome more frequently than tumor cells from patients with sporadic cases of BL from areas of low incidence (>95% versus 15 to 20%). Analysis of the EBV genome terminal-repeat copy number in endemic BLs has demonstrated that the tumors originate in the lineage of a single EBV-infected B cell.

Malignant cells obtained from fresh tumor biopsy samples consistently display a homogeneous surface phenotype including the pan-B-cell marker CD20, the common acute lymphoblastic leukemia antigen (CALLA, CD10), and the BL-associated antigen (CD77). These cells do not express any of the B-cell activation antigens CD23, CD30, CD39, and CD70 or any of the cell adhesion molecules LFA-1 (CD11a/18), ICAM-1 (CD54), and LFA-3 (CD58). Fresh BL tumor cells retain a resting B-cell phenotype and typically express only EBNA-1 and EBERs.

Posttransplant LPD

EBV is associated with lymphoproliferative disorders (LPD) in individuals receiving organ allografts along with immunosuppressive therapy (81). These LPD range from the benign polyclonal B-cell proliferations to malignant B-cell lymphomas. The frequency of posttransplant LPD following receipt of allografts is related to the degree and type of immunosuppression. Reported frequencies of LPD following allografts are given in Table 1.

The most common form of LPD is the benign polyclonal B-cell proliferation frequently observed in individuals experiencing a primary EBV infection following transplant of the allograft. Systemic symptoms of fever and sore throat may be present. Prolonged symptoms and lymphadenopathy usually respond to reduction in immunosuppressive therapy. The development of a monoclonal B-cell lymphoma may be preceded by benign polyclonal B-cell proliferation or by the sudden development of a solid tumor mass in the organ allograft or any other tissue. These lymphomas are polymorphic, with monoclonal B-cell proliferations, and are in general resistant to treatment. The clinical course is usually one of an aggressive lymphoma, with survival less than a year. In severe cases of polyclonal LPD and in some cases of monoclonal B-cell lymphoma, the infusion of donor leukocytes or polyclonal EBV-specific T-cell lines has been successful in treating the LPD (50, 95).

Malignancies and HIV Infection

In the setting of immunodeficiency associated with HIV type 1 infections, non-Hodgkin's lymphomas (NHL) have been shown to occur approximately 60- to 100-fold more frequently than expected (36, 70). A study conducted in Los Angeles County, CA, from 1984 to 1992 showed that EBV was associated with 39 of 59 (66%) HIV-related systemic lymphomas (101). Analysis of EBV terminal repeats in these lymphomas again confirmed their monoclonal origin, and c-*myc* rearrangements were noted in 40%.

TABLE 1 Frequency of EBV-associated posttransplant LPD

Allograft	Frequency of LPD (%)
Bone marrow	1–2
Heart	5–13
Heart-lung	9
Liver	2
Kidney	1–3

Given the profound immune defects in HIV-infected patients, along with the known role of CD8$^+$ T cells in controlling EBV-induced proliferation, it is not surprising that the number of EBV-infected B cells in the peripheral blood of those with HIV infection is higher than in the general population (13).

HIV-associated NHL, usually of B-cell origin, is a relatively late manifestation of HIV infection (70). For unknown reasons, the majority of EBV-associated NHL in HIV-infected patients has presented as primary central nervous system lymphomas (72).

Another EBV-induced disease in HIV-infected individuals is oral hairy leukoplasia, an unusual wart-like disease of the lingual squamous epithelium. Virus replication is evident only in the upper layers of the epithelium and is effectively inhibited by acycloguanosine. Interestingly, the oral hairy leukoplasia lesions, initially thought to be specific for HIV-related immunodeficiency, have now been observed in other immunosuppressed patients and in healthy individuals (102, 122).

EBV and Smooth-Muscle Tumors

Children infected with HIV experience an unusually high incidence of smooth-muscle tumors (leiomyomas and leiomyosarcomas) (18). Ordinarily, the incidence of leiomyomas in children is extremely low. The recent demonstration that EBV can infect smooth-muscle cells in HIV-infected individuals may help explain the role of EBV in the pathogenesis of leiomyomas (74). Additional convincing evidence for an etiologic role of EBV in the development of these neoplastic lesions is provided by the description of smooth-muscle tumors containing clonal EBV, developing in three children after liver transplantation (69).

Hodgkin's Disease

EBV genomic DNA was first reported in Hodgkin's disease (HD) in 1987. Recent evidence supports a role for EBV in the pathogenesis of classical HD (nodular sclerosing and mixed cellularity), where the malignant cells, including Reed-Sternberg cells, contain the EBV genome in up to 50% of "Western" cases (37). As with BL, the association of EBV with HD appears to vary geographically, as 94% of classical HD cases occurring in Peru contain EBV transcripts within Reed-Sternberg cells (19). The type of EBV latency in HD has been evaluated by PCR and in situ hybridization of EBV-specific latent gene transcripts and most resembles the type II latency described in NPC. In Hodgkin's lymphomas, EBNA-1 is expressed from the Qp promoter, while expression of other EBNAs is prevented by the silent Cp and Wp promoters. LMP-1, LMP-2, and EBER transcripts are consistently detected in these EBV-positive Hodgkin's lymphomas, irrespective of the histologic subtype. The EBV genome is invariably detected in cases of HD that appear in individuals with primary immunodeficiency or HIV infection (93, 116).

Nasopharyngeal Carcinoma

Worldwide, NPC is relatively rare; however, it is one of the most common cancers in southern China, with age-adjusted incidence rates of up to 25 to 100 per 100,000 (91). In contrast to BL, the association of EBV with NPC is highly consistent in both low- and high-incidence areas; in fact, EBV is present in every anaplastic NPC cell.

A wealth of evidence continues to strengthen the role of EBV as the primary etiologic agent in the pathogenesis of NPC. The presence of a single clonal form of EBV in pervasive lesions such as nasopharyngeal dysplasia or carcinoma in situ indicates that EBV-induced cellular proliferation precedes the acquisition of invasiveness of these tumors. EBNA-1 is universally detected, while LMP-1 and LMP-2 are detected in about 50% of tumors. While EBNA-2 is essential for the transformation of lymphocytes, its absence in preinvasive neoplasia and NPC indicates that EBNA-2 is not required for altered epithelial cell growth. In light of the described molecular link between LMP-1 and cell growth, the presence of LMP-1 (and possibly LMP-2) in NPC makes it a likely prerequisite to this multistep neoplastic transformation.

T-Cell Lymphoma

Until recently there was little evidence that normal T lymphocytes were susceptible to EBV infection. Studies by Anagnostopoulos et al. have demonstrated EBV infected tonsillar T lymphocytes in individuals with AIM (4). This observation is consistent with the description of T-cell lymphomas in individuals with chronic EBV infection (3). The characterization of an EBV-associated peripheral T-cell lymphoma has demonstrated the expression of EBV latent genes for EBNA-1, LMP-1, and LMP-2 as seen in NPC (20).

TREATMENT

Symptomatic and Anti-Inflammatory

The mainstay of treatment for individuals with AIM is supportive care. Acetaminophen or nonsteroidal anti-inflammatory agents are recommended for the treatment of fever, throat discomfort, and malaise. Provision of adequate fluids and nutrition is also appropriate. Although getting adequate rest is prudent, bed rest per se is unnecessary. Contact sports should be avoided due to the risk of splenic rupture.

The use of corticosteroids in the treatment of EBV-induced AIM has been controversial. Studies looking at the use of steroids have been imperfect, but they do suggest that these agents induce a modest improvement with reduction of lymphoid and mucosal swelling. Thus, a trial of corticosteroids in individuals with impending airway obstruction (manifested clinically by difficulty breathing in the recumbent position) is warranted. In addition, individuals suffering from severe, overwhelming, life-threatening infection (e.g., liver failure) along with individuals who sustain other severe complications such as aplastic anemia should also be considered for corticosteroid therapy, although data supporting benefit in these situations are lacking.

Despite the recommendations of some experienced clinicians that steroids be administered in routine cases of AIM, we do not share this opinion and the literature does not support this approach. The clinical illness of AIM represents the immune response to EBV, an agent, which establishes lifelong latency and which has oncogenic potential. For this reason, the administration of immunomodulating agents such as corticosteroids during primary infection is theoretically contraindicated because of the possibility of altering the immune response and predisposing the patient to a long-term lymphoproliferative complication. Indeed, studies of individuals with AIM who received corticosteroids many weeks earlier have demonstrated diminished number of B cells and T cells, including diminished numbers of CD4 T-helper and CD8 T cytotoxic cells (14); several studies have also documented increased risk of HD in individuals who have experienced AIM. Since no long-term data obtained for individuals who receive steroids during primary EBV infection are available, it would seem prudent, despite the potential of short-term improvement, to withhold such treatment from most individuals given the self-limited nature of this infection in the vast majority of cases.

Antiviral Treatment

Acyclovir is a nucleoside analog which inhibits permissive EBV infection through inhibition of EBV DNA polymerase, but it has no effect on latent infection. Specific therapy of acute EBV infections with intravenous and oral formulations of acyclovir has been studied (121, 125). While short-term suppression of viral shedding can be demonstrated, significant clinical benefit has not been demonstrated. These results are not surprising in view of data documenting that viral load has likely peaked at the time of presentation with AIM and that the manifestations of AIM are more likely due to robust immune responses (42).

In the majority of the EBV-associated malignancies, where the stage of the virus life cycle has been characterized, there is little evidence for permissive (lytic) infection. Since acyclovir is only effective in inhibiting replication of linear EBV DNA, there is little to be gained by its use in diseases associated with latent infection.

There is anecdotal support for the use of acyclovir in EBV-induced histiocytic hemophagocytosis, where evidence of replicating EBV has been demonstrated (108). Anecdotal use of other agents such as interleukin 2, IFN-α, and intravenous Igs in EBV-associated diseases has been reported. No clear-cut benefits of such modalities have been demonstrated thus far.

PREVENTION

Active Immunization

The wealth of evidence implicating EBV in the etiology of a variety of human neoplasms has made the prospect of developing a virus-based vaccine effective against human cancers very appealing. In regions of the world where EBV is endemic, vaccination of infants against EBV would potentially reduce the incidence of BL, while vaccine administration in developed countries would prevent the development of acute AIM in young adults. With the annual incidence of acute AIM estimated at 100,000 cases, EBV causes significantly more illness than mumps, for which a successful vaccination strategy exists.

As discussed above, gp350 is important for B-cell entry; it is one of the most abundant late viral proteins present in lytically infected cell plasma membranes and is the most abundant protein on the outer surface of the virus coat. Passively transferred antibodies are likely important in protecting infants from EBV infection. Since most of the human EBV-neutralizing antibody response is directed against gp350 (115), the gp350 gene is the major EBV lytic-cycle gene being pursued in the development of a subunit vaccine. A phase I trial demonstrated the safety and immunogenicity of a recombinant vaccinia virus-gp350 vaccine in healthy adults and children (41). In this small trial, a trend towards protection of vaccinated infants against the acquisition of infection was reported; however, this vaccine has not undergone further development. Phase I and II trials of an adjuvant recombinant gp350 vaccine demonstrated safety and immunogenicity (80). A phase II randomized, double-blind, placebo-controlled trial of this vaccine was recently completed in healthy, EBV-seronegative young adults (9, 104). More than 90% of vaccinated individuals developed anti-gp350 antibodies. Importantly, the vaccine demonstrated efficacy (78%) in preventing symptomatic primary EBV infection (AIM) but was not effective in preventing asymptomatic infection. Overall, these data justify further development and testing of anti-gp350 vaccines. However, with the recognition that $CD8^+$ T-cell responses are essential for controlling EBV replication and LPD, future vaccine research defining T-cell epitopes for inclusion in EBV vaccines will also be important (79).

REFERENCES

1. **Adamson, A. L., and S. C. Kenney.** 1998. Rescue of the Epstein-Barr virus BZLF1 mutant, Z(S186A), early gene activation defect by the BRLF1 gene product. *Virology* **251:**187–197.
2. **Aldrete, J. S.** 1992. Spontaneous rupture of the spleen in patients with infectious mononucleosis. *Mayo Clin. Proc.* **67:**910–912.
3. **Anagnostopoulos, I., M. Hummel, T. Finn, M. Tiemann, P. Korbjuhn, C. Dimmler, K. Gatter, F. Dallenbach, M. R. Parwaresch, and H. Stein.** 1992. Heterogeneous Epstein-Barr virus infection patterns in peripheral T-cell lymphoma of angioimmunoblastic lymphadenopathy type. *Blood* **80:**1804–1812.
4. **Anagnostopoulos, I., M. Hummel, C. Kreschel, and H. Stein.** 1995. Morphology, immunophenotype, and distribution of latently and/or productively Epstein-Barr virus-infected cells in acute infectious mononucleosis: implications for the interindividual infection route of Epstein-Barr virus. *Blood* **85:**744–750.
5. **Andersson, U., O. Martinez-Maza, J. Andersson, S. Britton, H. Gadler, M. De Ley, and S. Modrow.** 1984. Secretion of gamma-interferon at the cellular level. Induction by Epstein-Barr virus. *Scand. J. Immunol.* **20:**425–432.
6. **Arrand, J. R., L. S. Young, and J. D. Tugwood.** 1989. Two families of sequences in the small RNA-encoding region of Epstein-Barr virus (EBV) correlate with EBV types A and B. *J. Virol.* **63:**983–986.
7. **Asgari, M. M., and D. G. Begos.** 1997. Spontaneous splenic rupture in infectious mononucleosis: a review. *Yale J. Biol. Med.* **70:**175–182.
8. **Baer, R., A. T. Bankier, M. D. Biggin, P. L. Deininger, P. J. Farrell, T. J. Gibson, G. Hatfull, G. S. Hudson, S. C. Satchwell, C. Séguin, et al.** 1984. DNA sequence and expression of the B95-8 Epstein-Barr virus genome. *Nature* **310:**207–211.
9. **Balfour, H. H., Jr.** 2007. Epstein-Barr virus vaccine for the prevention of infectious mononucleosis—and what else? *J. Infect. Dis.* **196:**1724–1726.
10. **Balfour, H. H., Jr., C. J. Holman, K. M. Hokanson, M. M. Lelonek, J. E. Giesbrecht, D. R. White, D. O. Schmeling, C. H. Webb, W. Cavert, D. H. Wang, and R. C. Brundage.** 2005. A prospective clinical study of Epstein-Barr virus and host interactions during acute infectious mononucleosis. *J. Infect. Dis.* **192:**1505–1512.
11. **Biggar, R. J., W. Henle, G. Fleisher, J. Bocker, E. T. Lennette, and G. Henle.** 1978. Primary Epstein-Barr virus infections in African infants. I. Decline of maternal antibodies and time of infection. *Int. J. Cancer* **22:**239–243.
12. **Biron, C. A., K. S. Byron, and J. L. Sullivan.** 1989. Severe herpesvirus infections in an adolescent without natural killer cells. *N. Engl. J. Med.* **320:**1731–1735.
13. **Birx, D. L., R. R. Redfield, and G. Tosato.** 1986. Defective regulation of Epstein-Barr virus infection in patients with acquired immunodeficiency syndrome (AIDS) or AIDS-related disorders. *N. Engl. J. Med.* **314:**874–879.
14. **Brandfonbrener, A., A. Epstein, S. Wu, and J. Phair.** 1986. Corticosteroid therapy in Epstein-Barr virus infection. Effect on lymphocyte class, subset, and response to early antigen. *Arch. Intern. Med.* **146:**337–339.
15. **Caldwell, R. G., J. B. Wilson, S. J. Anderson, and R. Longnecker.** 1998. Epstein-Barr virus LMP2A drives B cell development and survival in the absence of normal B cell receptor signals. *Immunity* **9:**405–411.
16. **Callan, M. F., L. Tan, N. Annels, G. S. Ogg, J. D. Wilson, C. A. O'Callaghan, N. Steven, A. J. McMichael, and A. B. Rickinson.** 1998. Direct visualization of antigen-specific $CD8^+$ T cells during the primary immune response to Epstein-Barr virus in vivo. *J. Exp. Med.* **187:** 1395–1402.
17. **Catalina, M. D., J. L. Sullivan, K. R. Bak, and K. Luzuriaga.** 2001. Differential evolution and stability of epitope-specific $CD8^+$ T cell responses in EBV infection. *J. Immunol.* **167:**4450–4457.
18. **Chadwick, E. G., E. J. Connor, I. C. Hanson, V. V. Joshi, H. Abu-Farsakh, R. Yogev, G. McSherry, K. McClain, and S. B. Murphy.** 1990. Tumors of smooth-muscle origin in HIV-infected children. *JAMA* **263:** 3182–3184.
19. **Chang, K. L., P. F. Albujar, Y. Y. Chen, R. M. Johnson, and L. M. Weiss.** 1993. High prevalence of Epstein-Barr virus in the Reed-Sternberg cells of Hodgkin's disease occurring in Peru. *Blood* **81:**496–501.
20. **Chen, C. L., R. H. Sadler, D. M. Walling, I. J. Su, H. C. Hsieh, and N. Raab-Traub.** 1993. Epstein-Barr virus (EBV) gene expression in EBV-positive peripheral T-cell lymphomas. *J. Virol.* **67:**6303–6308.
21. **Chen, G., A. K. Tai, M. Lin, F. Chang, C. Terhorst, and B. T. Huber.** 2007. Increased proliferation of $CD8^+$ T cells in SAP-deficient mice is associated with impaired activation-induced cell death. *Eur. J. Immunol.* **37:**663–674.
22. **Cho, Y., J. Ramer, P. Rivailler, C. Quink, R. L. Garber, D. R. Beier, and F. Wang.** 2001. An Epstein-Barr-related herpesvirus from marmoset lymphomas. *Proc. Natl. Acad. Sci. USA* **98:**1224–1229.
23. **Cleary, M. L., S. D. Smith, and J. Sklar.** 1986. Cloning and structural analysis of cDNAs for bcl-2 and a hybrid bcl-2/immunoglobulin transcript resulting from the t(14; 18) translocation. *Cell* **47:**19–28.
24. **Coffey, A. J., R. A. Brooksbank, O. Brandau, T. Oohashi, G. R. Howell, J. M. Bye, A. P. Cahn, J. Durham, P. Heath, P. Wray, R. Pavitt, J. Wilkinson, M. Leversha, E. Huckle, C. J. Shaw-Smith, A. Dunham, S. Rhodes, V. Schuster, G. Porta, L. Yin, P. Serafini, B. Sylla, M. Zollo, B. Franco, A. Bolino, M. Seri, A. Lanyi, J. R. Davis, D. Webster, A. Harris, G. Lenoir, G. de St Basile, A. Jones, B. H. Behloradsky, H. Achatz, J. Murken, R. Fassler, J. Sumegi, G. Romeo, M. Vaudin, M. T. Ross, A. Meindl, and D. R. Bentley.** 1998. Host response to EBV infection in X-linked lymphoproliferative disease results from mutations in an SH2-domain encoding gene. *Nat. Genet.* **20:**129–135.
25. **Cohen, J. I.** 2005. Clinical aspects of Epstein-Barr virus infection, p. 35–54. In E. S. Robertson (ed.), *Epstein-Barr Virus*. Caister Academic Press, Norfolk, England.
26. **Cooper, N. R., M. D. Moore, and G. R. Nemerow.** 1988. Immunobiology of CR2, the B lymphocyte receptor for

Epstein-Barr virus and the C3d complement fragment. *Annu. Rev. Immunol.* **6:**85–113.

27. **Crawford, D. H., K. F. Macsween, C. D. Higgins, R. Thomas, K. McAulay, H. Williams, N. Harrison, S. Reid, M. Conacher, J. Douglas, and A. J. Swerdlow.** 2006. A cohort study among university students: identification of risk factors for Epstein-Barr virus seroconversion and infectious mononucleosis. *Clin. Infect. Dis.* **43:**276–282.
28. **Dambaugh, T., K. Hennessy, L. Chamnankit, and E. Kieff.** 1984. U2 region of Epstein-Barr virus DNA may encode Epstein-Barr nuclear antigen 2. *Proc. Natl. Acad. Sci. USA* **81:**7632–7636.
29. **Doherty, P. C.** 1998. The numbers game for virus-specific CD8+ T cells. *Science* **280:**227.
30. **Downey, H., and C. McKinlay.** 1923. Acute lymphadenosis compared with acute lymphatic leukemia. *Arch. Intern. Med.* **32:**82–112.
31. **Epstein, M. A.** 2005. The origins of EBV research: discovery and characterization of the virus, p. 1–14. *In* E. S. Robertson (ed.), *Epstein-Barr Virus*. Caister Academic Press, Norfolk, England.
32. **Epstein, M. A., B. G. Achong, and Y. M. Barr.** 1964. Virus particles in cultured lymphoblasts from Burkitt's lymphoma. *Lancet* **i:**702–703.
33. **Fleisher, G., and R. Bologonese.** 1984. Epstein-Barr virus infections in pregnancy: a prospective study. *J. Pediatr.* **104:**374–379.
34. **Flemington, E., and S. H. Speck.** 1990. Epstein-Barr virus BZLF1 *trans* activator induces the promoter of a cellular cognate gene, c-*fos*. *J. Virol.* **64:**4549–4552.
35. **Gahn, T. A., and C. L. Schildkraut.** 1989. The Epstein-Barr virus origin of plasmid replication, oriP, contains both the initiation and termination sites of DNA replication. *Cell* **58:**527–535.
36. **Gaidano, G., A. Carbone, and R. Dalla-Favera.** 1998. Pathogenesis of AIDS-related lymphomas: molecular and histogenetic heterogeneity. *Am. J. Pathol.* **152:**623–630.
37. **Glaser, S. L., R. J. Lin, S. L. Stewart, R. F. Ambinder, R. F. Jarrett, P. Brousset, G. Pallesen, M. L. Gulley, G. Khan, J. O'Grady, M. Hummel, M. V. Preciado, H. Knecht, J. K. Chan, and A. Claviez.** 1997. Epstein-Barr virus-associated Hodgkin's disease: epidemiologic characteristics in international data. *Int. J. Cancer* **70:**375–382.
38. **Goldberg, G. N., V. A. Fulginiti, C. G. Ray, P. Ferry, J. F. Jones, H. Cross, and L. Minnich.** 1981. In utero Epstein-Barr virus (infectious mononucleosis) infection. *JAMA* **246:**1579–1581.
39. **Gregory, C. D., C. Dive, S. Henderson, C. A. Smith, G. T. Williams, J. Gordon, and A. B. Rickinson.** 1991. Activation of Epstein-Barr virus latent genes protects human B cells from death by apoptosis. *Nature* **349:**612–614.
40. **Grose, C.** 1985. The many faces of infectious mononucelosis: the spectrum of Epstein-Barr virus infection in children. *Pediatr. Rev.* **7:**35–44.
41. **Gu, S. Y., T. M. Huang, L. Ruan, Y. H. Miao, H. Lu, C. M. Chu, M. Motz, and H. Wolf.** 1995. First EBV vaccine trial in humans using recombinant vaccinia virus expressing the major membrane antigen. *Dev. Biol. Stand.* **84:**171–177.
42. **Hadinoto, V., M. Shapiro, T. C. Greenough, J. L. Sullivan, K. Luzuriaga, and D. A. Thorley-Lawson.** 2008. On the dynamics of acute EBV infection and the pathogenesis of infectious mononucleosis. *Blood* **111:**1420–1427.
43. **Haque, A. K., J. L. Myers, S. D. Hudnall, B. B. Gelman, R. V. Lloyd, D. Payne, and M. Borucki.** 1998. Pulmonary lymphomatoid granulomatosis in acquired immunodeficiency syndrome: lesions with Epstein-Barr virus infection. *Mod. Pathol.* **11:**347–356.
44. **Hatfull, G., A. T. Bankier, B. G. Barrell, and P. J. Farrell.** 1988. Sequence analysis of Raji Epstein-Barr virus DNA. *Virology* **164:**334–340.
45. **Haverkos, H. W., Z. Amsel, and D. P. Drotman.** 1991. Adverse virus-drug interactions. *Rev. Infect. Dis.* **13:**697–704.
46. **Henderson, S., M. Rowe, C. Gregory, D. Croom-Carter, F. Wang, R. Longnecker, E. Kieff, and A. Rickinson.** 1991. Induction of bcl-2 expression by Epstein-Barr virus latent membrane protein 1 protects infected B cells from programmed cell death. *Cell* **65:**1107–1115.
47. **Henle, G., W. Henle, and V. Diehl.** 1968. Relation of Burkitt's tumor-associated herpes-type virus to infectious mononucleosis. *Proc. Natl. Acad. Sci. USA* **59:**94–101.
48. **Henle, W., V. Diehl, G. Kohn, H. Zur Hausen, and G. Henle.** 1967. Herpes-type virus and chromosome marker in normal leukocytes after growth with irradiated Burkitt cells. *Science* **157:**1064–1065.
49. **Henle, W., G. E. Henle, and C. A. Horwitz.** 1974. Epstein-Barr virus specific diagnostic tests in infectious mononucleosis. *Hum. Pathol.* **5:**551–565.
50. **Heslop, H. E., and C. M. Rooney.** 1997. Adoptive cellular immunotherapy for EBV lymphoproliferative disease. *Immunol. Rev.* **157:**217–222.
51. **Hochberg, D., J. M. Middeldorp, M. Catalina, J. L. Sullivan, K. Luzuriaga, and D. A. Thorley-Lawson.** 2004. Demonstration of the Burkitt's lymphoma Epstein-Barr virus phenotype in dividing latently infected memory cells in vivo. *Proc. Natl. Acad. Sci. USA* **101:**239–244.
52. **Hochberg, D., T. Souza, M. Catalina, J. L. Sullivan, K. Luzuriaga, and D. A. Thorley-Lawson.** 2004. Acute infection with Epstein-Barr virus targets and overwhelms the peripheral memory B-cell compartment with resting, latently infected cells. *J. Virol.* **78:**5194–5204.
53. **Horwitz, C. A., W. Henle, G. Henle, M. Goldfarb, P. Kubic, R. C. Gehrz, H. H. Balfour, Jr., G. R. Fleisher, and W. Krivit.** 1981. Clinical and laboratory evaluation of infants and children with Epstein-Barr virus-induced infectious mononucleosis: report of 32 patients (aged 10–48 months). *Blood* **57:**933–938.
54. **Howe, J. G., and M. D. Shu.** 1989. Epstein-Barr virus small RNA (EBER) genes: unique transcription units that combine RNA polymerase II and III promoter elements. *Cell* **57:**825–834.
55. **Hsu, D. H., R. de Waal Malefyt, D. F. Fiorentino, M. N. Dang, P. Vieira, J. de Vries, H. Spits, T. R. Mosmann, and K. W. Moore.** 1990. Expression of interleukin-10 activity by Epstein-Barr virus protein BCRF1. *Science* **250:**830–832.
56. **Hutt-Fletcher, L.** 2005. EBV entry and epithelial infection, p. 359–378. *In* E. S. Robertson (ed.), *Epstein-Barr Virus*. Caister Academic Press, Norfolk, England.
57. **Izumi, K. M., K. M. Kaye, and E. D. Kieff.** 1997. The Epstein-Barr virus LMP1 amino acid sequence that engages tumor necrosis factor receptor associated factors is critical for primary B lymphocyte growth transformation. *Proc. Natl. Acad. Sci. USA* **94:**1447–1452.
58. **Izumi, K. M., and E. D. Kieff.** 1997. The Epstein-Barr virus oncogene product latent membrane protein 1 engages the tumor necrosis factor receptor-associated death domain protein to mediate B lymphocyte growth transformation and activate NF-κB. *Proc. Natl. Acad. Sci. USA* **94:**12592–12597.
59. **Karajannis, M. A., M. Hummel, I. Anagnostopoulos, and H. Stein.** 1997. Strict lymphotropism of Epstein-Barr virus during acute infectious mononucleosis in nonimmunocompromised individuals. *Blood* **89:**2856–2862.

60. **Keymeulen, B., E. Vandemeulebroucke, A. G. Ziegler, C. Mathieu, L. Kaufman, G. Hale, F. Gorus, M. Goldman, M. Walter, S. Candon, L. Schandene, L. Crenier, C. De Block, J. M. Seigneurin, P. De Pauw, D. Pierard, I. Weets, P. Rebello, P. Bird, E. Berrie, M. Frewin, H. Waldmann, J. F. Bach, D. Pipeleers, and L. Chatenoud.** 2005. Insulin needs after CD3-antibody therapy in new-onset type 1 diabetes. *N. Engl. J. Med.* **352:**2598–2608.
61. **Khyatti, M., P. C. Patel, I. Stefanescu, and J. Menezes.** 1991. Epstein-Barr virus (EBV) glycoprotein gp350 expressed on transfected cells resistant to natural killer cell activity serves as a target antigen for EBV-specific antibody-dependent cellular cytotoxicity. *J. Virol.* **65:** 996–1001.
62. **Kieff, E., and A. B. Rickinson.** 2007. Epstein-Barr virus and its replication, p. 2603–2654. *In* D. M. Knipe, P. M. Howley, D. E. Griffin, R. A. Lamb, M. A. Martin, B. Roizman, and S. E. Straus (ed.), *Fields Virology*, 5th ed. Lippincott Williams & Wilkins, Philadelphia, PA.
63. **Kimura, H., Y. Hoshino, H. Kanegane, I. Tsuge, T. Okamura, K. Kawa, and T. Morishima.** 2001. Clinical and virologic characteristics of chronic active Epstein-Barr virus infection. *Blood* **98:**280–286.
64. **Kirchmaier, A. L., and B. Sugden.** 1998. Rep*: a viral element that can partially replace the origin of plasmid DNA synthesis of Epstein-Barr virus. *J. Virol.* **72:**4657–4666.
65. **Kulwichit, W., R. H. Edwards, E. M. Davenport, J. F. Baskar, V. Godfrey, and N. Raab-Traub.** 1998. Expression of the Epstein-Barr virus latent membrane protein 1 induces B cell lymphoma in transgenic mice. *Proc. Natl. Acad. Sci. USA* **95:**11963–11968.
66. **Laichalk, L. L., and D. A. Thorley-Lawson.** 2005. Terminal differentiation into plasma cells initiates the replicative cycle of Epstein-Barr virus in vivo. *J. Virol.* **79:** 1296–1307.
67. **Lambris, J. D., V. S. Ganu, S. Hirani, and H. J. Muller-Eberhard.** 1985. Mapping of the C3d receptor (CR2)-binding site and a neoantigenic site in the C3d domain of the third component of complement. *Proc. Natl. Acad. Sci. USA* **82:**4235–4239.
68. **Lay, J. D., C. J. Tsao, J. Y. Chen, M. E. Kadin, and I. J. Su.** 1997. Upregulation of tumor necrosis factor-alpha gene by Epstein-Barr virus and activation of macrophages in Epstein-Barr virus-infected T cells in the pathogenesis of hemophagocytic syndrome. *J. Clin. Investig.* **100:**1969–1979.
69. **Lee, E. S., J. Locker, M. Nalesnik, J. Reyes, R. Jaffe, M. Alashari, B. Nour, A. Tzakis, and P. S. Dickman.** 1995. The association of Epstein-Barr virus with smooth-muscle tumors occurring after organ transplantation. *N. Engl. J. Med.* **332:**19–25.
70. **Levine, A. M.** 1993. AIDS-related malignancies: the emerging epidemic. *J. Natl. Cancer Inst.* **85:**1382–1397.
71. **Liebowitz, D.** 1998. Epstein-Barr virus and a cellular signaling pathway in lymphomas from immunosuppressed patients. *N. Engl. J. Med.* **338:**1413–1421.
72. **MacMahon, E. M., J. D. Glass, S. D. Hayward, R. B. Mann, P. S. Becker, P. Charache, J. C. McArthur, and R. F. Ambinder.** 1991. Epstein-Barr virus in AIDS-related primary central nervous system lymphoma. *Lancet* **338:** 969–973.
73. **Masucci, M. G., M. T. Bejarano, G. Masucci, and E. Klein.** 1983. Large granular lymphocytes inhibit the in vitro growth of autologous Epstein-Barr virus-infected B cells. *Cell. Immunol.* **76:**311–321.
74. **McClain, K. L., C. T. Leach, H. B. Jenson, V. V. Joshi, B. H. Pollock, R. T. Parmley, F. J. DiCarlo, E. G. Chadwick, and S. B. Murphy.** 1995. Association of Epstein-Barr virus with leiomyosarcomas in children with AIDS. *N. Engl. J. Med.* **332:**12–18.
75. **McMichael, A. J., and C. A. O'Callaghan.** 1998. A new look at T cells. *J. Exp. Med.* **187:**1367–1371.
76. **Miller, G., T. Shope, H. Lisco, D. Stitt, and M. Lipman.** 1972. Epstein-Barr virus: transformation, cytopathic changes, and viral antigens in squirrel monkey and marmoset leukocytes. *Proc. Natl. Acad. Sci. USA* **69:**383–387.
77. **Miyashita, E. M., B. Yang, K. M. Lam, D. H. Crawford, and D. A. Thorley-Lawson.** 1995. A novel form of Epstein-Barr virus latency in normal B cells in vivo. *Cell* **80:**593–601.
78. **Mosialos, G., M. Birkenbach, R. Yalamanchili, T. VanArsdale, C. Ware, and E. Kieff.** 1995. The Epstein-Barr virus transforming protein LMP1 engages signaling proteins for the tumor necrosis factor receptor family. *Cell* **80:**389–399.
79. **Moss, D. J., S. R. Burrows, and R. Khanna.** 2005. Developing vaccines against EBV-associated diseases, p. 651–667. *In* E. S. Robertson (ed.), *Epstein-Barr Virus*. Caister Academic Press, Norfolk, England.
80. **Moutschen, M., P. Leonard, E. M. Sokal, F. Smets, M. Haumont, P. Mazzu, A. Bollen, F. Denamur, P. Peeters, G. Dubin, and M. Denis.** 2007. Phase I/II studies to evaluate safety and immunogenicity of a recombinant gp350 Epstein-Barr virus vaccine in healthy adults. *Vaccine* **25:** 4697–4705.
81. **Nalesnik, M. A., L. Makowka, and T. E. Starzl.** 1988. The diagnosis and treatment of posttransplant lymphoproliferative disorders. *Curr. Probl. Surg.* **25:**367–472.
82. **Nicholas, J., K. R. Cameron, H. Coleman, C. Newman, and R. W. Honess.** 1992. Analysis of nucleotide sequence of the rightmost 43 kbp of herpesvirus saimiri (HVS) L-DNA: general conservation of genetic organization between HVS and Epstein-Barr virus. *Virology* **188:**296–310.
83. **Nichols, K. E., D. P. Harkin, S. Levitz, M. Krainer, K. A. Kolquist, C. Genovese, A. Bernard, M. Ferguson, L. Zuo, E. Snyder, A. J. Buckler, C. Wise, J. Ashley, M. Lovett, M. B. Valentine, A. T. Look, W. Gerald, D. E. Housman, and D. A. Haber.** 1998. Inactivating mutations in an SH2 domain-encoding gene in X-linked lymphoproliferative syndrome. *Proc. Natl. Acad. Sci. USA* **95:**13765–13770.
84. **Niederman, J. C., R. W. McCollum, G. Henle, and W. Henle.** 1968. Infectious mononucleosis. Clinical manifestations in relation to EB virus antibodies. *JAMA* **203:** 205–209.
85. **North, J. R., A. J. Morgan, J. L. Thompson, and M. A. Epstein.** 1982. Purified Epstein-Barr virus Mr 340,000 glycoprotein induces potent virus-neutralizing antibodies when incorporated in liposomes. *Proc. Natl. Acad. Sci. USA* **79:**7504–7508.
86. **Packham, G., A. Economou, C. M. Rooney, D. T. Rowe, and P. J. Farrell.** 1990. Structure and function of the Epstein-Barr virus BZLF1 protein. *J. Virol.* **64:**2110–2116.
87. Reference deleted.
88. **Paul, J. R., and W. W. Bunnell.** 1932. The presence of heterophile antibodies in infectious mononucleosis. *Am. J. Med. Sci.* **183:**90–104.
89. **Pope, J. H.** 1968. Establishment of cell lines from Australian leukaemic patients: presence of a herpes-like virus. *Aust. J. Exp. Biol. Med. Sci.* **46:**643–645.
90. **Precopio, M. L., J. L. Sullivan, C. Willard, M. Somasundaran, and K. Luzuriaga.** 2003. Differential kinetics and specificity of EBV-specific $CD4^+$ and $CD8^+$ T cells during primary infection. *J. Immunol.* **170:**2590–2598.

91. **Raab-Traub, N.** 2005. Epstein-Barr virus in the pathogenesis of NPC, p. 71–92. *In* E. S. Robertson (ed.), *Epstein-Barr Virus*. Caister Academic Press, Norfolk, England.
92. **Raab-Traub, N., and K. Flynn.** 1986. The structure of the termini of the Epstein-Barr virus as a marker of clonal cellular proliferation. *Cell* **47:**883–889.
93. **Rezk, S. A., and L. M. Weiss.** 2007. Epstein-Barr virus-associated lymphoproliferative disorders. *Hum. Pathol.* **38:**1293–1304.
94. **Rickinson, A. B., and D. J. Moss.** 1997. Human cytotoxic T lymphocyte responses to Epstein-Barr virus infection. *Annu. Rev. Immunol.* **15:**405–431.
95. **Rooney, C. M., C. A. Smith, C. Y. Ng, S. K. Loftin, J. W. Sixbey, Y. Gan, D. K. Srivastava, L. C. Bowman, R. A. Krance, M. K. Brenner, and H. E. Heslop.** 1998. Infusion of cytotoxic T cells for the prevention and treatment of Epstein-Barr virus-induced lymphoma in allogeneic transplant recipients. *Blood* **92:**1549–1555.
96. **Rowe, M., L. S. Young, K. Cadwallader, L. Petti, E. Kieff, and A. B. Rickinson.** 1989. Distinction between Epstein-Barr virus type A (EBNA 2A) and type B (EBNA 2B) isolates extends to the EBNA 3 family of nuclear proteins. *J. Virol.* **63:**1031–1039.
97. **Sample, J., and E. Kieff.** 1990. Transcription of the Epstein-Barr virus genome during latency in growth-transformed lymphocytes. *J. Virol.* **64:**1667–1674.
98. **Sayos, J., C. Wu, M. Morra, N. Wang, X. Zhang, D. Allen, S. van Schaik, L. Notarangelo, R. Geha, M. G. Roncarolo, H. Oettgen, J. E. De Vries, G. Aversa, and C. Terhorst.** 1998. The X-linked lymphoproliferative-disease gene product SAP regulates signals induced through the co-receptor SLAM. *Nature* **395:**462–469.
99. **Sculley, T. B., A. Apolloni, L. Hurren, D. J. Moss, and D. A. Cooper.** 1990. Coinfection with A- and B-type Epstein-Barr virus in human immunodeficiency virus-positive subjects. *J. Infect. Dis.* **162:**643–648.
100. **Shannon-Lowe, C. D., B. Neuhierl, G. Baldwin, A. B. Rickinson, and H. J. Delecluse.** 2006. Resting B cells as a transfer vehicle for Epstein-Barr virus infection of epithelial cells. *Proc. Natl. Acad. Sci. USA* **103:**7065–7070.
101. **Shibata, D., L. M. Weiss, A. M. Hernandez, B. N. Nathwani, L. Bernstein, and A. M. Levine.** 1993. Epstein-Barr virus-associated non-Hodgkin's lymphoma in patients infected with the human immunodeficiency virus. *Blood* **81:**2102–2109.
102. **Shiramizu, B., B. Herndier, T. Meeker, L. Kaplan, and M. McGrath.** 1992. Molecular and immunophenotypic characterization of AIDS-associated, Epstein-Barr virus-negative, polyclonal lymphoma. *J. Clin. Oncol.* **10:**383–389.
103. **Sixbey, J. W., S. M. Lemon, and J. S. Pagano.** 1986. A second site for Epstein-Barr virus shedding: the uterine cervix. *Lancet* **ii:**1122–1124.
104. **Sokal, E. M., K. Hoppenbrouwers, C. Vandermeulen, M. Moutschen, P. Léonard, A. Moreels, M. Haumont, A. Bollen, F. Smets, and M. Denis.** 2007. Recombinant gp350 vaccine for infectious mononucleosis: a phase 2, randomized, double-blind, placebo-controlled trial to evaluate the safety, immunogenicity, and efficacy of an Epstein-Barr virus vaccine in healthy young adults. *J. Infect. Dis.* **196:**1749–1753.
105. **Su, I. J., and J. Y. Chen.** 1997. The role of Epstein-Barr virus in lymphoid malignancies. *Crit. Rev. Oncol. Hematol.* **26:**25–41.
106. **Sullivan, J. L.** 1999. The abnormal gene in X-linked lymphoproliferative syndrome. *Curr. Opin. Immunol.* **11:**431–434.
107. **Sullivan, J. L., and B. A. Woda.** 1989. X-linked lymphoproliferative syndrome. *Immunodefic. Rev.* **1:**325–347.
108. **Sullivan, J. L., B. A. Woda, H. G. Herrod, G. Koh, F. P. Rivara, and C. Mulder.** 1985. Epstein-Barr virus-associated hemophagocytic syndrome: virological and immunopathological studies. *Blood* **65:**1097–1104.
109. **Tamaki, H., B. L. Beaulieu, M. Somasundaran, and J. L. Sullivan.** 1995. Major histocompatibility complex class I-restricted cytotoxic T lymphocyte responses to Epstein-Barr virus in children. *J. Infect. Dis.* **172:**739–746.
110. **Tan, L. C., N. Gudgeon, N. E. Annels, P. Hansasuta, C. A. O'Callaghan, S. Rowland-Jones, A. J. McMichael, A. B. Rickinson, and M. F. Callan.** 1999. A re-evaluation of the frequency of $CD8^+$ T cells specific for EBV in healthy virus carriers. *J. Immunol.* **162:**1827–1835.
111. **Tanner, J., J. Weis, D. Fearon, Y. Whang, and E. Kieff.** 1987. Epstein-Barr virus gp350/220 binding to the B lymphocyte C3d receptor mediates adsorption, capping, and endocytosis. *Cell* **50:**203–213.
112. **Thorley-Lawson, D. A.** 2001. Epstein-Barr virus: exploiting the immune system. *Nat. Rev. Immunol.* **1:**75–82.
113. **Thorley-Lawson, D. A.** 1981. The transformation of adult but not newborn human lymphocytes by Epstein Barr virus and phytohemagglutinin is inhibited by interferon: the early suppression by T cells of Epstein Barr infection is mediated by interferon. *J. Immunol.* **126:**829–833.
114. **Thorley-Lawson, D. A., and A. Gross.** 2004. Persistence of the Epstein-Barr virus and the origins of associated lymphomas. *N. Engl. J. Med.* **350:**1328–1337.
115. **Thorley-Lawson, D. A., and C. A. Poodry.** 1982. Identification and isolation of the main component (gp350-gp220) of Epstein-Barr virus responsible for generating neutralizing antibodies in vivo. *J. Virol.* **43:**730–736.
116. **Tinguely, M., R. Vonlanthen, E. Muller, C. C. Dommann-Scherrer, J. Schneider, J. A. Laissue, and B. Borisch.** 1998. Hodgkin's disease-like lymphoproliferative disorders in patients with different underlying immunodeficiency states. *Mod. Pathol.* **11:**307–312.
117. **Tselis, A., R. Duman, G. A. Storch, and R. P. Lisak.** 1997. Epstein-Barr virus encephalomyelitis diagnosed by polymerase chain reaction: detection of the genome in the CSF. *Neurology* **48:**1351–1355.
118. **Tsoukas, C. D., and J. D. Lambris.** 1993. Expression of EBV/C3d receptors on T cells: biological significance. *Immunol. Today* **14:**56–59.
119. **Tugizov, S. M., J. W. Berline, and J. M. Palefsky.** 2003. Epstein-Barr virus infection of polarized tongue and nasopharyngeal epithelial cells. *Nat. Med.* **9:**307–314.
120. **Uchida, J., T. Yasui, Y. Takaoka-Shichijo, M. Muraoka, W. Kulwichit, N. Raab-Traub, and H. Kikutani.** 1999. Mimicry of CD40 signals by Epstein-Barr virus LMP1 in B lymphocyte responses. *Science* **286:**300–303.
121. **van der Horst, C., J. Joncas, G. Ahronheim, N. Gustafson, G. Stein, M. Gurwith, G. Fleisher, J. Sullivan, J. Sixbey, S. Roland, et al.** 1991. Lack of effect of peroral acyclovir for the treatment of acute infectious mononucleosis. *J. Infect. Dis.* **164:**788–792.
122. **Walling, D. M., N. M. Clark, D. M. Markovitz, T. S. Frank, D. K. Braun, E. Eisenberg, D. J. Krutchkoff, D. H. Felix, and N. Raab-Traub.** 1995. Epstein-Barr virus coinfection and recombination in non-human immunodeficiency virus-associated oral hairy leukoplakia. *J. Infect. Dis.* **171:**1122–1130.

123. **Wang, X., and L. M. Hutt-Fletcher.** 1998. Epstein-Barr virus lacking glycoprotein gp42 can bind to B cells but is not able to infect. *J. Virol.* **72:**158–163.
124. **Wilson, W. H., D. W. Kingma, M. Raffeld, R. E. Wittes, and E. S. Jaffe.** 1996. Association of lymphomatoid granulomatosis with Epstein-Barr viral infection of B lymphocytes and response to interferon-alpha 2b. *Blood* **87:**4531–4537.
125. **Yao, Q. Y., P. Ogan, M. Rowe, M. Wood, and A. B. Rickinson.** 1989. The Epstein-Barr virus: host balance in acute infectious mononucleosis patients receiving acyclovir anti-viral therapy. *Int. J. Cancer* **43:**61–66.
126. **Ziegner, U. H., H. D. Ochs, C. Schanen, S. A. Feig, K. Seyama, T. Futatani, T. Gross, M. Wakim, R. L. Roberts, D. J. Rawlings, S. Dovat, J. K. Fraser, and E. R. Stiehm.** 2001. Unrelated umbilical cord stem cell transplantation for X-linked immunodeficiencies. *J. Pediatr.* **138:**570–573.
127. **Zimber, U., H. K. Adldinger, G. M. Lenoir, M. Vuillaume, M. V. Knebel-Doeberitz, G. Laux, C. Desgranges, P. Wittmann, U. K. Freese, U. Schneider, et al.** 1986. Geographical prevalence of two types of Epstein-Barr virus. *Virology* **154:**56–66.

Kaposi's Sarcoma-Associated Herpesvirus

PATRICK S. MOORE AND YUAN CHANG

25

Kaposi's sarcoma-associated herpesvirus (KSHV; also called human herpesvirus 8 [HHV-8]) is a large double-stranded DNA herpesvirus that causes Kaposi's sarcoma (KS) as well as some malignant and hyperplastic lymphoid disorders. KSHV belongs to the *Rhadinovirus* genus of the *Gammaherpesvirinae* subfamily of the family *Herpesviridae*. Like all other herpesviruses, KSHV has both latent and lytic replication cycles, and infection is presumed to be lifelong. It is remarkable for its extensive piracy of cellular regulatory genes and its immune evasion strategies that block adaptive and innate immunity at multiple levels. The cancers caused by KSHV are frequently underappreciated as public health problems. KS is now the most common cancer in sub-Saharan Africa (34, 112), driven in large part by the AIDS pandemic. KSHV transmission and reactivation among transplant patients are also major preventable causes of mortality and graft loss.

KS, a spindle cell tumor arising from lymphatic endothelium, was first described by the Austrian dermatologist and dermatopathologist Moriz Kaposi in 1872 (79). The tumor had been suspected to be caused by an infectious agent since the 1950s (130). This was reinforced by the emergence of KS as an AIDS-related tumor and its differential occurrence among different human immunodeficiency virus (HIV) risk groups (6).

KSHV was discovered in 1993 through a PCR-based DNA subtractive hybridization method from AIDS-KS tissues (24). These findings were rapidly extended to show that a post-germinal center B-cell lymphoma, now known as primary effusion lymphoma (PEL), is infected with the virus (20), and cell lines from this tumor provided a source for growing the virus in culture (21, 148). Shortly after the initial description of KSHV, all forms of KS, in both HIV-positive and HIV-negative patients, were found to be infected with the virus, and a second B-cell lymphoproliferative disorder, multicentric Castleman's disease (MCD), was found to be associated with KSHV infection (163). Early serologic studies demonstrated that KSHV was an uncommon infection in developed countries, where it was most commonly associated with homosexual transmission (107). Surveys from other populations revealed areas of hyperendemicity in sub-Saharan Africa (54) and remote regions of South America (7) where viral transmission occurs through nonsexual routes.

More recently, nonneoplastic diseases, including bone marrow failure and some forms of autoimmune hemolytic anemia in the setting of Castleman's disease, have been attributed to KSHV infection (102, 136). The virus was sequenced in 1996 (153) and shown to possess a remarkable array of viral genes homologous to cellular regulatory genes and oncogenes that continue to be a source of investigations into viral causes of cancer.

VIROLOGY

KSHV Structure

Typical herpesvirus virion structures with diameters of approximately 100 nm have been detected in the nuclei of KSHV-infected B-cell lines 24 to 48 h after chemical induction (133, 148) (Fig. 1). Electron cryomicroscopic reconstruction shows that KSHV has a three-dimensional structure similar to those of other herpesviruses. The KSHV capsid shell is composed of 12 pentons, 150 hexons, and 320 triplexes arranged on an icosahedral lattice (174, 184). The primary capsid component is the major capsid protein, which forms both the pentons and the hexons (126). Triplex proteins (open reading frame 62 [ORF62] and ORF26 proteins), a small capsomere-interacting protein (SCIP; ORF65), and the scaffolding protein (ORF17.5) are the other major components of the capsid, giving a total estimated molecular mass for the packed capsid of 300 MDa.

The space between the virus capsid and the viral envelope is filled with an amorphous protein structure called the tegument. The tegument is composed of specific proteins, such as ORF45 and ORF75 proteins (190), that are microinjected into cells after viral membrane fusion with the host cell and prepare it for infection and viral takeover. Remarkably, the tegument also incorporates a number of viral mRNAs (4, 186) that similarly can be immediately translated once injected into a new cell.

While virus is most easily produced from naturally infected tissue culture cell lines, it can been seen directly by electron microscopy in rare spindle cells of KS lesions (133) and may have been seen by electron microscopy as early as 1984 in AIDS-KS lesions (177). The virus rests in a latent state in the majority of KS tumor cells (~95%),

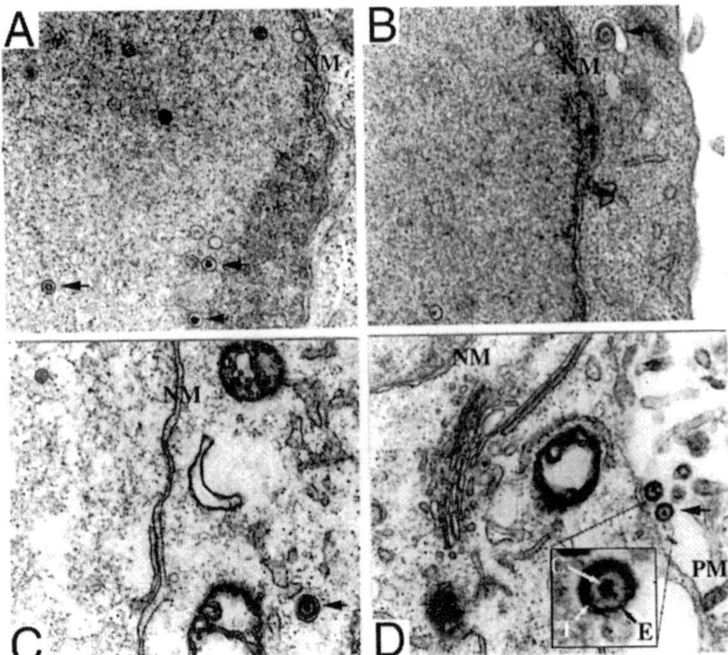

FIGURE 1 Electron photomicrographs of KSHV virion formation and egress in a PEL cell line induced into lytic replication with tetradecanoyl phorbol acetate. (A) Naked virus capsids formed in the nucleus of the cell (nuclear membrane [NM]); (B) virions budding through the nuclear membrane and becoming enveloped viruses; (C) transit of the virus through the cytoplasm (arrow); (D) egress of the fully enveloped virus from the cell plasma membrane (PM). The inset (E) shows a high-magnification image of the virus with the capsid, tegument, and envelope. (Photos courtesy of Antonella Tosoni, University of Milan.)

and only a small percentage of cells undergo lytic virus production.

Classification and Genotyping

In the family *Herpesviridae*, the *Gammaherpesvirinae* contain KSHV and Epstein-Barr virus (EBV, or HHV-4) (Fig. 2). The gammaherpesviruses are, in turn, divided into two genera, *Lymphocryptovirus*, which includes EBV and EBV-related primate viruses, and *Rhadinovirus* (120), which includes KSHV and has members broadly represented among mammals. Genomic analysis suggests that lymphocryptoviruses may have been the ancestral precursor to the gammaherpesviruses (113); in contrast, the distribution of these viruses suggests that EBV-like viruses secondarily emerged from a rhadinoviral ancestor during primate evolution. While EBV and KSHV are highly divergent from each other in terms of gene structure, these two viruses share many similarities, including a trophism for B lymphocytes and the ability to cause human cancers.

Evolutionary studies of KSHV have been particularly useful in understanding the epidemiology of this virus. Early searches for KSHV-like viruses among primates revealed several surprises: KSHV-like rhadinoviruses were also discovered to infect rhesus macaques (152), and similar viruses were later discovered among higher primates (Fig. 3). All Old World and New World primates appear to be infected with KSHV-like rhadinoviruses that have coevolved with their hosts. During this search, however, a second distinct but closely related rhadinovirus lineage was found among rhesus monkeys (37), called rhesus rhadinovirus (RRV). Viruses of this lineage were also found among higher primates (90), leading to the intriguing conclusion that there may be an undiscovered RRV ("HHV-9") infecting and possibly causing disease among humans.

KSHV genotyping has also proved useful in characterizing KSHV transmission (102), and a thorough overview of KSHV molecular typing can be found elsewhere (67). Genotypic diversity among KSHV isolates is highest at the left and right ends of the long unique region (LUR) in ORFs K1 and K15, respectively. The K1 ORF protein displays up to 30% amino acid variability, which has been used to define at least four major viral clades designated A, B, C, and D (alternative nomenclature: clades I, IV, II, and III, respectively). Subtype B is found almost exclusively in KSHV-infected patients from Africa or of African heritage, subtype D is found in Pacific Island populations, subtype C is common in patients from the Middle East and Asia, and both subtypes A and C are seen in North America. To date, no consistent correlation between variability at the K1 locus and biological behavior has been found; however, inferences regarding virus evolution and human migratory patterns have emerged (142, 195).

At the opposite end of the viral genome, the K15 ORF can occur in multiple forms that encode distinct groups of alternatively spliced K15 proteins. These forms, designated as predominant and minor forms (142), apparently arose from rare intertypic recombinations and can be found among all of the KSHV clades. Similar to the case with K1, no correlation between the two forms of K15 and clinical disease exists. The assignment of virus to specific subtypes or forms is not categorical, since additional minor subtypes have been proposed, and mosaic or chimeric vi-

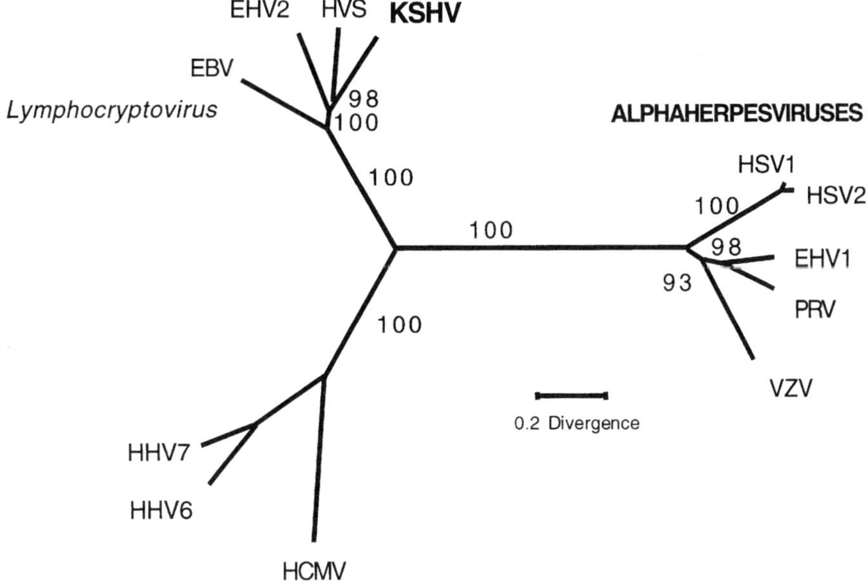

FIGURE 2 Phylogenetic tree showing the alpha-, beta-, and gammaherpevirus subfamilies. KSHV belongs to the genus *Rhadinovirus*, also known as γ-2 herpesviruses, in the lymphotrophic gammaherpesvirus subfamily. Other related gammaherpesviruses are also associated with lymphoproliferative disorders, including EBV in humans and herpesvirus saimiri in New World monkeys. Herpesviruses from the alphaherpesvirus (e.g., herpes simplex virus [HSV] and varicella-zoster virus [VZV]) and betaherpesvirus (e.g., CMV and HHV-6 and -7) subfamilies have not been found to cause tumors in humans. (Reprinted from reference 120 with permission.)

ruses exist (7). Analysis of K1 and K15 genotype patterns has been useful for molecular epidemiological studies, such as confirming virus transmission from one individual to another as a result of organ transplantation.

Finally, internal repeat regions in the latency-associated nuclear antigen 1 (LANA1) gene, ORF73, show strain-to-strain variation in repeat numbers that has been used for genotyping (55). The numbers of terminal repeat sequences also vary, and these sequences are thought to be gained or deleted with each replication cycle. This variability has been used to measure viral monoclonality in KSHV-infected tumors (9).

Replication of KSHV

Like other herpesviruses, KSHV has a double-stranded DNA genome (~165 kb) that is packaged into an icosahedral capsid and enveloped by a lipid bilayer (Fig. 4). KSHV has both lytic and latent life cycles. During lytic replication, the virus expresses its own DNA polymerase, replicates its own DNA, and generates hundreds to thousands of viral particles over a 24- to 72-h period, a process thought to invariably lead to cell death. During latent replication, viral DNA exists as a circular, nuclear episome that relies on host enzymes for genome replication.

Much of what is known about the mechanics of KSHV genome replication, capsid assembly, and egress during lytic replication is based on studies from other herpesviruses. Lytic replicating viruses can be seen as massed nuclear inclusions containing electron-dense cores in KSHV-infected cells. The virus replicates in the cell nucleus and packages its genome into the viral capsid as a linear molecule that acquires an initial membrane envelope by budding through the inner nuclear membrane. Components of this membrane mature as the virus passes through the outer nuclear membrane and transits through the Golgi apparatus, where the virus incorporates specific viral glycoproteins prior to reaching the plasma membrane. The virus can be released from the cell by direct plasma membrane budding, although release through exocytic vesicles is thought to be more common (182).

The lytic viral genome is believed to replicate through a rolling-circle mechanism from the circular latent genome, like the unrolling of a tape, producing a linear strand of concatenated genomes. The KSHV genome concatemer is packaged into the nascent capsid through a portal protein complex (35) and cleaved within the middle of the terminal repeat region so that each linear viral genome has variable numbers of terminal repeat sequences at both ends. Similarities in capsid structure and replication mechanisms between herpesviruses and bacteriophage suggest that herpesviruses may have distantly evolved from these prokaryote phage viruses (42). Lytic viral genome replication is most efficient when cells enter S phase (88,

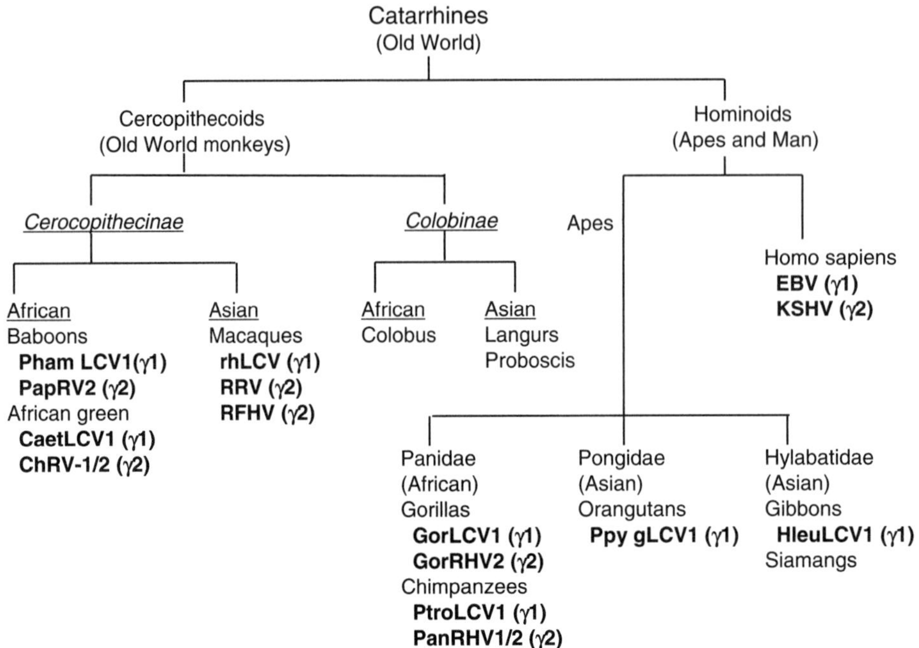

FIGURE 3 Old World primate hosts and their gammaherpesviruses. It is evident from this phylogenetic tree that these are ancient viruses that have coevolved with their hosts. A second rhadinovirus, RRV, has been found to be widely distributed among primates, including chimpanzees. It is likely that a human version of this virus exists but has not yet been found. (Reprinted from reference 33 with permission of Cambridge University Press.)

182), and KSHV genes expressed during lytic replication act to overcome the G_1/S cell cycle checkpoint as well as to disarm host cell innate immune signaling pathways. During late stages of infection, structural component proteins of the capsid are synthesized; the capsid forms on a putative scaffolding that is turned over or incorporated into the capsid as the virus matures.

Rapid viral synthesis after initiation of lytic replication results in partially filled capsids (126), and only a portion of virus produced during lytic replication is fully mature

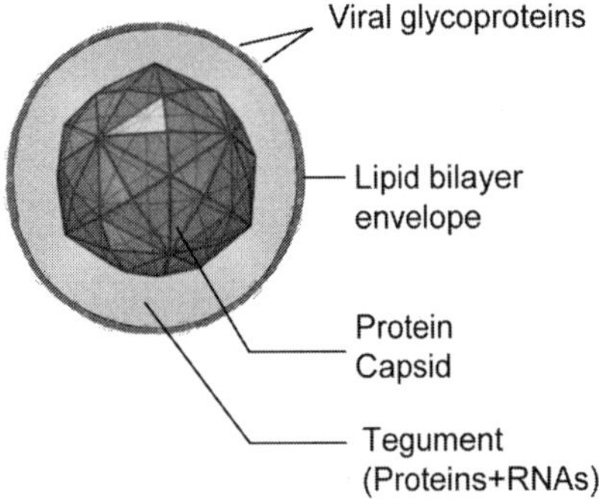

FIGURE 4 Schematic diagram of KSHV enveloped virus structure. The capsid is composed of hexons, pentons, and triplexes arranged in an icosahedral lattice that contains the virus genome. This is surrounded by an amorphous tegument layer composed of viral and cellular proteins and viral RNAs that are microinjected into the cell on infection. The bilayer envelope surrounding the tegument contains viral glycoproteins, such as gB, that act as receptor and entry proteins.

and transmissible. When KSHV lytic replication is initiated, early genes alter cell cycle transit (117, 183) and inhibit cellular mRNA processing and stability to maximize production of viral DNA (65, 128). Simultaneously, nonstructural KSHV gene expression alters the cell to prevent adaptive and innate immune activation. Although antiapoptotic proteins are expressed during lytic virus replication to prolong survival of the infected cell (157), damage caused by host protein synthesis shutoff (58), fragmentation of viral DNA (160), and activation of innate immune signaling (143) pathways probably contributes to cell death during lytic replication.

KSHV also resides as a latent virus in infected cells. In contrast to lytic replication, latent viral gene expression provides proliferation and survival factors that inhibit premature cell death. KSHV and its sister virus, EBV, are the only herpesviruses that have latent tissue culture models which can be readily manipulated, and many general aspects regarding viral latency for other mammalian viruses are inferred from these two agents. During KSHV latency, gene expression is constrained to a few proteins to prevent provoking an immune response, and the virus uses host replication machinery to replicate in tandem with host chromosomes. KSHV genes expressed during latency tend to promote survival by targeting cell cycle arrest and apoptosis signaling pathways. The bulk of KS tumor cells infected with KSHV are in a latent state, and less than 5% of cells are actively undergoing lytic replication at any one time.

A latently infected cell can be induced into lytic replication through activation of protein kinase C and H-Ras (38, 187) signaling pathways using chemical agents. These agents include phorbol esters and histone deacetylase inhibitors, which first induce expression of the key viral regulatory protein RTA, encoded by ORF50, which, in turn, acts as the master regulator for subsequent lytic replication and gene expression (171). RTA in combination with the transcription factor RBP-Jκ activates its own promoter (98), resulting in a positive feedback loop to generate sufficient RTA to initiate the remaining steps in lytic or productive virus replication.

Latent and Lytic Gene Expression

Initiation of lytic replication begins with a highly choreographed cascade of gene expression that determines the sequence of events leading to linear genome replication, virion synthesis, genome packaging, and egress of the virus from the infected cell (172, 191). Initiation of lytic replication begins with immediate-early expression of the replication and transcription activator protein, RTA (100, 171). While the cellular circuits controlling when and how KSHV expresses RTA and initiates lytic replication during natural infection are still being uncovered, evidence suggests that cellular signaling involving extracellular signal-regulated kinase and other pathways activates RTA expression (29, 187).

Latent KSHV gene expression, in contrast, is constitutive and not dependent on the replication status of the virus, although it may be regulated by cell cycle stage or tissue type (39, 150, 158). Individual KSHV genes are often mistakenly referred to as "latent" or "lytic" genes, whereas in reality their expression is controlled by a number of factors beyond the KSHV replication cycle. Some genes encoding proteins, such as viral interleukin 6 (vIL-6), that are induced during lytic replication are also induced entirely independently of lytic replication (25). Notch signaling has been demonstrated to induce a wide variety of KSHV nonstructural genes without lytic viral replication (23) (so-called class II genes [156]). KSHV has many different gene expression profiles that depend on virus replication status, cell and tissue type, immune signaling, and other factors—a complexity that is obscured by dichotomizing KSHV gene expression into only latent and lytic forms.

Organization and Features of the KSHV Genome

The KSHV genome was first sequenced from the virus-infected lymphoma cell line BC-1 2 years after its discovery (127, 153). Because of the extensive collinear homology between KSHV and the first sequenced rhadinovirus, herpesvirus saimiri, KSHV genes (or ORFs) are named according to their herpesvirus saimiri positional homologs (e.g., ORF4 to ORF75) if obvious gene similarity is present. Those genes unique to KSHV are given a K prefix as they occur starting from the left end of the genome (e.g., ORFs K1 to K15) (153). KSHV is unique among the HHVs in the extent of its extensive molecular piracy of genes from the host genome. These stolen genes include not only DNA replication genes found in other herpesviruses but also regulatory, cytokine, receptor, and immune signaling genes that contribute to KSHV-related pathogenesis.

The LUR is approximately 145 kb and possesses at least 84 viral genes thus far identified (Fig. 5). Structural (e.g., capsid) and lytic replication genes common to other herpesviruses are present in the KSHV genome and tend to be grouped together. These KSHV genes generally share the highest degree of homology to other herpesviral genes. Conservation of structural proteins leads to cross-reactivity with virion structural antigens of other viruses in serologic assays, although this problem can in part be overcome by identifying unique antigens on structural proteins through peptide mapping (138). The DNA polymerase (ORF9), KSHV thymidine kinase (ORF21), and phosphotransferase (ORF36) (14) are conserved with other herpesviruses and are targets for antiherpesviral drugs. KSHV has other DNA synthesis enzymes that are not found in most other herpesviruses, including dihydrofolate reductase (ORF2), ribonucleotide reductase, and thymidylate synthase (ORF70). The host genes are regulated by the retinoblastoma cell cycle checkpoint protein. KSHV probably uses these viral enzymes to overcome the G_1/S checkpoint during lytic replication or by inducing artificial S phase, which can allow viral DNA replication. These genes are also potential drug targets against lytic virus production.

While genes required for lytic replication are largely conserved with other herpesviruses, those genes expressed during latency are unique to KSHV. KSHV, for example, does not possess direct sequence homologs to any of the EBV latency genes, such as those for EBV nuclear antigens (EBNAs) and latent membrane proteins (LMPs). Despite these differences, KSHV and EBV tend to target the same regulatory cellular circuits. This is not surprising, since the

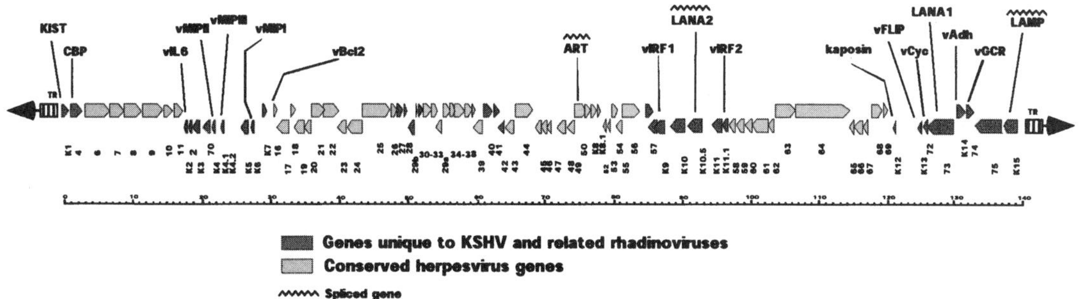

FIGURE 5 Genomic map of KSHV sequenced from the BC-1 KSHV-infected PEL cell line. The viral genome contains an ~145-kb LUR flanked on both sides by reiterated terminal repeat (TR) units of high GC content (>85%). Conserved herpesvirus gene blocks are interspersed with blocks containing genes unique to KSHV and other rhadinoviruses. These nonconserved regions contain numerous homologs to host cell genes involved in cell cycle regulation, apoptosis, and immune regulation.

viruses share similar environments, and face similar biological hurdles, during parts of their life cycles. In general, KSHV has pirated and modified cellular genes for use during its replication and survival, while EBV targets the same pathways using complex viral transcription-activating proteins. As an example, KSHV encodes an IL-6 homolog, whereas EBV LMP1 induces expression of cellular IL-6; many other parallel examples exist. Conserved and nonconserved genes are segregated into blocks of genes, which tend to be regulated together.

The KSHV-pirated genes express proteins that function similarly to host proteins but have modified regulation exploited by the virus (Table 1). Known homologs to regulatory genes include genes encoding a complement binding protein, vIL-6, viral macrophage inflammatory proteins (vMIPs; also called viral CC-chemokine ligands), vBCL-2, viral interferon regulatory factors (vIRF1, vIRF2, and LANA2), a viral FLICE-inhibitory protein (vFLIP), a viral cyclin (vCYC), a viral adhesion molecule (vOX2, or vAdh), and a viral G-protein-coupled receptor (vGCR; ORF74). Additional KSHV proteins, such as LANA1 (ORF73) and KIST (KSHV immunosignaling transducer; ORF K1), do not have known cellular homologs but have roles similar to those of oncoproteins found in other viruses (48, 95).

Finally, KSHV shares with other herpesviruses a repertoire of virus-encoded microRNAs (miRNAs) (141). These small (~22-bp), double-stranded RNAs are largely located on the right end of the genome between ORFs K12 and K13. KSHV miRNAs are generated by Drosha processing of alternative transcripts from the latency locus that arise by read-through of polyadenylation sites (12). Cellular targets for these miRNAs are an area of active investigation.

EPIDEMIOLOGY

KSHV-related diseases are a major unmet public health problem. Although the incidence of AIDS-associated KS declined 70 to 90% after the introduction of effective antiretroviral therapy, these drugs do not inhibit KSHV infection, and a second emergence of KS among persons with low HIV loads and high $CD4^+$ cell counts has been reported (110). Finally, although KSHV is poorly transmissible through transfusion, transfusion transmission can occur and may cause silent transmission and disease (40, 68).

Distribution and Geography

Unlike other HHVs, KSHV is an uncommon infection (~2 to 3%) of North American and northern European populations (139). Rates of infection are higher among Italian and other Mediterranean populations and highest in African populations (13, 54, 84). This correlates with the worldwide distribution of KS disease prior to the emergence of the AIDS epidemic (Table 2). Prior to the 1980s, KS was a rare tumor in the United States and England but occurred much more frequently in Italian, Greek, and other Mediterranean-basin populations. The highest rates of KS prior to the AIDS epidemic occurred in Central African countries.

Two ecological studies in Italy found close correlations between provincial KSHV infection rates in blood donors and historical rates of KS disease, with increasing rates of infection and disease occurring in a north-south gradient along the Italian peninsula (13, 180). Not all studies, however, find a close geographic correlation between infection rate and disease. Despite overall low infection rates in the Americas, very high KSHV infection rates are present among isolated South American indigenous populations (7), but not the general populations (140). Viral genotypes isolated from these Amerindian populations most closely match KSHV strains isolated in Asia, suggesting that the virus first migrated with humans to the Americas across the Bering Strait thousands of years ago (46).

Transmission

Sexual Transmission

In American and European populations, the groups at highest risk for KSHV infection are homosexual and bisexual men, in whom infection rates range from 30 to 60% (54, 84). While compelling evidence indicates that KSHV is sexually transmitted (Fig. 6), the specific behaviors resulting in KSHV transmission are disputed, and heterosexual transmission appears to be uncommon in these areas.

KSHV, however, is not appreciably shed into semen, and direct transmission through anal intercourse is unlikely. KSHV, like other herpesviruses, is asymptomatically shed from the oropharynx (17). A significant risk factor for virus transmission among homosexual men has been found to be deep kissing, although oral-penile contact and oral-anal contact are also significant risk factors for infection or seroconversion (43, 63). Since heterosexual couples also engage in kissing and oral-penile contact, the reasons why homosexual couples are much more susceptible to infection remain unclear. Use of saliva as a sexual lubricant for anal intercourse may also contribute to high infection rates. At present, it is not known whether HIV immunodeficiency enhances KSHV transmission.

Nonsexual Transmission

Explanations for the extremely high rates of KSHV and KS in sub-Saharan Africa are lacking. KSHV infection is common among presexually active African children, and evidence for sexual transmission among adults is scant. Areas of relatively high endemicity in Europe, including Italy, also show evidence for horizontal nonsexual transmission among children and possibly adults (181). Congenital and perinatal mother-to-child transmission is rare, but transmission from mothers to infants and children is common (104), presumably related to oropharyneal shedding and saliva contact.

Initial investigations of KS among AIDS patients found that persons infected with HIV through blood products had low rates of KS (6). This led to the assumption that the agent causing KS is not transfusion transmitted. However, case control studies demonstrate that the virus is detectable in approximately one-half of peripheral blood mononuclear cell (PBMC) samples from AIDS-KS patients using standard PCR techniques (121, 179), and the rate of virus detection may be dependent on the level of host immunosuppression (179).

Direct demonstration of blood-borne transmission has been found in both U.S. and African studies (40, 68, 111). Transfusion transmission is less efficient than for other viruses (~4% per infected transfusion) (68). Despite the low efficiency of blood-borne transmission, the large numbers of transfusions performed suggest that thousands of transmission events might take place in the United States alone

TABLE 1 Selected KSHV proteins and their known or putative functions

Protein[a]	Gene	Function(s)[b]
KIST	ORF K1	ITAM-mediated signaling, cell transformation
Complement binding protein	ORF4	Complement binding, immune signaling?
DNA synthesis and repair		
DNA polymerase	ORF9	Nucleotide synthesis and repair; cellular homologs under E2F transcriptional control
Dihydrofolate reductase	ORF2	
Thymidylate synthase	ORF70	
Thymidine kinase	ORF21	
Uracil DNA glucosidase	ORF46	
Polymerase processivity factor (PF-8)	ORF59	
Ribonucleotide reductase	ORF60, ORF61	
Structural proteins		
Scaffolding protein	ORF17.5	Assembly
Major capsid protein	ORF25	Major component of capsid hexamers and pentamers
TRI-2	ORF26	Triplex protein, location of KS330 representational difference analysis (RDA) fragment
SCIP	ORF65	Serologic antigen
MHC presentation inhibitors		
K3	ORF K3	Inhibit surface presentation of MHC I, inhibits T-cell costimulatory molecules (B7.2)
K5	ORF K5	
vIL-6	ORF K2	Secreted cytokine, B-cell proliferation, apoptosis inhibitor, angiogenesis
Viral chemokines		
vMIP-I (vMIP-1a)	ORF K6	Secreted CC chemokines, angiogenesis, Th2 chemotaxis, HIV coreceptor inhibition
vMIP-II (vMIP-1b)	ORF K4	
vMIP-III (BCK)	ORF K4.1	
vBCL-2	ORF16	Apoptosis inhibitor
Activator of replication and transcription (ART, RTA)	ORF50	Major lytic transactivator, homologous to EBV RTA transactivator
K8.1	ORF K8.1	Serologic antigen; glycoprotein analog to EBV gp350/220?
vIRF1	ORF K9	Cell transformation, interferon antagonist, anti-apoptotic factor/HAT inhibitor
LANA2	ORF K10.5	p53 inhibitor
vIRF2	ORF K11.1	PKR inhibition
Kaposins A, B, C, etc.	ORF K12 locus	Cell transformation, multiple transcribed and translated species having different expression patterns
vFLIP	ORF K13 (ORF71)	Inhibits Fas-dependent apoptosis; NF-κB inhibition
vCYC	ORF72	Directs CDK4/6 phosphorylation of pRB1 and histone H1
LANA1	LANA1	Serologic antigen, episomal binding protein, p53 and pRB1 inhibitor
vGCR	ORF74	IL-8-like receptor, constitutively activated receptor, induces VEGF and SAPK, cell transformation
vAdh (vOX-2)	ORF K14	N-CAM-like adhesion molecule
Latency-associated membrane protein	ORF K15	TRAF binding

[a] Italics indicate type I or constitutive expression patterns in PEL cells.

[b] ITAM, immunoreceptor tyrosine activation motif; HAT, histone acetyltransferase; VEGF, vascular endothelial growth factor; SAPK, stress-activated protein kinase; TRAF, tumor necrosis factor receptor-associated factors.

TABLE 2 Patterns of KSHV infection and KS prior to the AIDS epidemic

KS incidence	Region(s)	KSHV prevalence in the population (%)	Transmission	Risk groups
Low	North America, northern Europe, East Asia	0–5	Sexual, iatrogenic	Homosexual men, STD[a] clinic attendees, transplant recipients
Intermediate	Mediterranean, Middle Eastern countries, Caribbean	5–20	Sexual, iatrogenic, nonsexual	Homosexual men, STD clinic attendees, transplant recipients, older adults
High	Africa	>50	Nonsexual, sexual	Children, older adults, those of lower socioeconomic status

[a] STD, sexually transmitted disease.

each year. Far higher rates of transmission are likely to occur in settings where the virus has a higher prevalence.

Transplantation

KSHV transmission during transplantation presents the most immediate public health concern that is amenable to simple interventions. KS represents 3 to 8% of all posttransplant tumors and occurs in 0.1 to 0.5% of transplant patients in most settings, but it can be an even more common posttransplant neoplasm in countries with elevated KS rates in the general population (105, 144). Up to 5% of transplant patients developed KS posttransplantation in one Saudi Arabian registry study (144).

European studies demonstrate that this is principally due to reactivation of KSHV infection in the recipient. Approximately one-third of transplant KS patients are infected from the donated organ and develop KSHV-related diseases (101). The rate of disease among KSHV-positive transplant patients is strikingly high: between 25 and 68% of previously infected or newly infected patients develop KS (47, 147). Intriguingly, some KS tumors are derived from the donor rather than the recipient, suggesting that transmission of tumor cells rather than infectious virus contributes to transplantation KS. Transmission can occur after transplantation of any organ, including heart, bone, liver, and kidney, and all KSHV-related diseases, including KS, PEL, Castleman's disease, and bone marrow failure, have been reported in the transplant setting. In Europe and North America, few donors and recipients are likely to be found to be infected, but those that are are at extremely high risk for disease. The rates of mortality and graft loss are high among transplant KS patients (115), strongly arguing for primary screening.

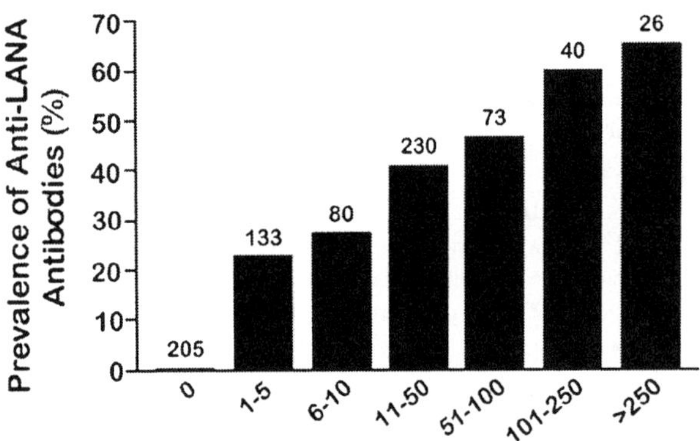

FIGURE 6 KSHV seroprevalence increases linearly with numbers of recent sex partners in this population-based sampling of homosexual and bisexual men (sera collected in 1984) from San Francisco, CA. This and related risk factor data suggest that KSHV is sexually transmitted, although the precise mechanism for transmission remains unclear. (Reprinted from reference 107 with permission of the Massachusetts Medical Society.)

African KS Epidemic

Prior to the AIDS epidemic, KS was the third most commonly reported tumor in some areas of Africa (Color Plate 32). With the onset of the AIDS epidemic, rates of KS have dramatically risen, and it is now the most commonly reported cancer in many sub-Saharan African countries. In Zimbabwe, for example, KS accounts for 31% of cancers (28), and in Uganda, it is the most common tumor in males and the second most common in females (behind cervical cancer) (176). Unlike in North America and Europe, men and women have similar KSHV infection rates in African countries (162). KS tumors, however, are more common in men, leading to speculation for a role of sex hormones in disease expression.

KS is virtually nonexistent among children from developed countries, but it is also one of the most common cancers among African children. Pediatric KS is fulminant disease that spreads lymphadenopathically, generally resulting in death within a year (193). As previously indicated, horizontal transmission appears to be the predominant means of infection (103). The ongoing epidemic of KS is a severe public health problem that is unchecked and unrecognized.

CLINICAL MANIFESTATIONS AND PATHOGENESIS

Primary Infection

Primary KSHV infection does not generally produce clinically important signs or symptoms, although transient fever might be associated with infection in children (80). Studies of AIDS patient cohorts show that KS can develop within weeks or months of primary infection, and in one case, an HIV-positive man developed transient angiolymphoid hyperplasia with microscopic foci of KS spindle cells immediately after infection (131). Among transplant patients infected by organ donation, KSHV-related diseases can erupt within 2 to 6 months of transplantation. This suggests that the incubation period for KS is primarily dependent on the state of immunosurveillance rather than length of time of infection. Among Dutch and American homosexual cohorts in which men are infected with both HIV and KSHV, those persons who were infected with KSHV first and HIV second tend to have a lower rate of developing KS (72, 149), implying that HIV-induced immune dysfunction impairs immunologic surveillance and control for KSHV.

Kaposi's Sarcoma

KS is a complex tumor characterized microscopically by a proliferation of spindle-shaped cells and irregular slit-like vascular channels. The spindle cells are probably derived from endothelial precursors, although immunophenotypic studies reveal ambiguous features that make precise identification of the progenitor cell elusive. The demarcation between infiltrating KS tumor cells and surrounding nontumor cells is often indistinct, particularly in early lesions of the skin. A common feature noted in KS lesions is the presence of an inflammatory infiltrate composed of lymphocytes and macrophages, suggesting an immune response against tumor-specific antigens.

KS often first appears on the skin (Fig. 7), particularly of the extremities, face, and genitalia, but it can disseminate to mucosal surfaces, lymphoid tissues, and viscera, especially in immunocompromised patients. Oral lesions on the gums, tongue, or palate are also frequent, and dentists may be the first clinicians to diagnose new-onset disease. KS skin lesions initially appear as bruised or discolored macules that progress to nodules and plaques, often with ulceration in late stages of disease. Advanced disease is also associated with edema and spread to surrounding lymph nodes. Visceral involvement is another manifestation of advanced KS. Gastrointestinal dissemination is frequently asymptomatic and can be difficult to diagnose due to submucosal infiltration of the tumor. Pulmonary involvement has a markedly worse prognosis than isolated skin or mucocutaneous disease and also may be difficult to distinguish radiologically from other opportunistic infections.

At initial presentation, KS lesions can be confused with other conditions or even simple bruises "that don't go away." Köbner phenomenon, where KS tumors appear at the site of an old scar, is not uncommon. The differential diagnosis, particular among HIV/AIDS patients, should include bacillary angiomatosis (due to *Bartonella*) and even skin manifestations of *Mycobacterium haemophilum*, but these conditions can be distinguished by site of lesion (mouth, nose, feet, or genitals) and risk factors (age, ethnicity, sexual orientation, history of HIV/AIDS, or history of local trauma) as well as appearance. KS tumors also present in combination with MCD in lymph nodes or with PELs in visceral cavities, resulting in a mixed tumor cell population and complex clinical presentation.

Pathological diagnosis is usually straightforward and can be confirmed by immunostaining for LANA1 protein (Fig. 8). Skin biopsies with precautions to prevent excess bleeding are used in most cases where lesions are readily accessible. Endoscopic examination is used for visceral disease.

All forms of KS (epidemic, endemic, classical, and iatrogenic) are KSHV positive and histologically indistinguishable and differ only in clinical or epidemiological characteristics. Classical KS is generally an indolent tumor occurring in elderly patients, particularly men of Mediterranean, Eastern European, or Middle Eastern ethnicity. No specific risk factors for classical KS have been identified, although country or region of birth (56, 62) and receipt of blood transfusions (5) may be associated with elevated dis-

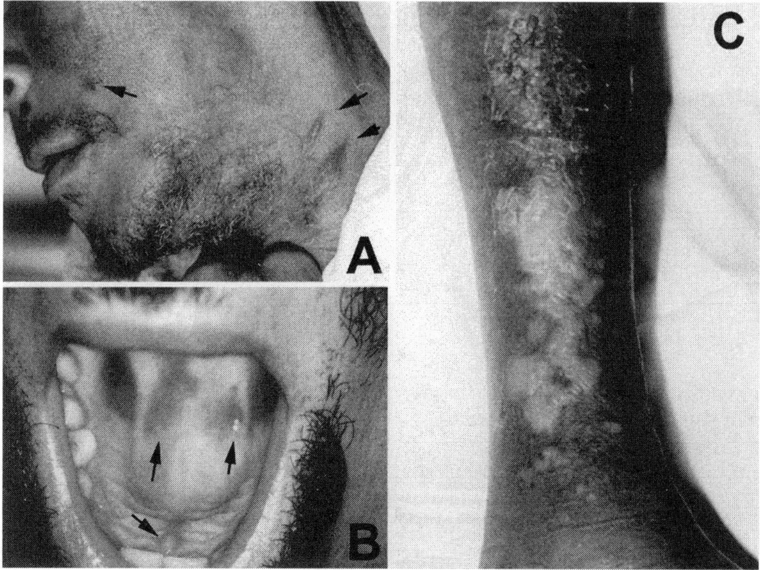

FIGURE 7 (A) KS on the face and neck of a patient with AIDS. These cutaneous lesions have a characteristic purple-red appearance. The neck lesions demonstrate the often-noted dermatomal distribution as well as the elliptical outline of cutaneous KS. (Courtesy of David Silvers, Columbia University College of Physicians and Surgeons, New York, NY.) (B) KS frequently involves mucosal surfaces. (C) A leg showing postradiation hyperpigmentation, ulceration, and nodular KS lesions that have recurred within the radiated area. (Panels B and C courtesy of Susan E. Krown, Memorial Sloan-Kettering Cancer Center, New York, NY.)

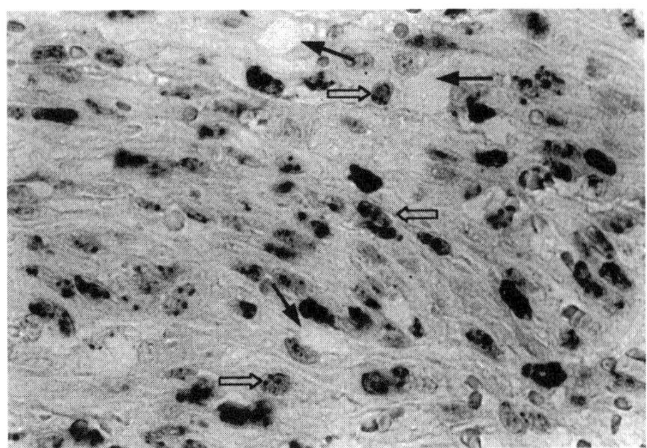

FIGURE 8 A photomicrograph of a KS tumor, immunostained for LANA1, infiltrating the dermis from a patient with AIDS-KS. All forms of KS (both HIV positive and HIV negative) have a similar histologic appearance. Vascular clefts (arrows) within the tumor are filled with red cells, most of which have been lost during tissue preparation. A mononuclear infiltrate in the tumor can be present, and cellular atypia or pleomorphism is generally uncommon in KS lesions. The characteristic speckled nuclear staining pattern (open arrows) for LANA1 can be seen in many of the cells.

ease risk. HIV-seronegative homosexual men also appear to be at increased risk for classical KS (49).

Endemic or African KS is similar to classical KS in having a male predominance, but it can be a progressive and rapidly fatal disease, especially in children. While the geographic pattern of occurrence in Africa overlaps with EBV-associated Burkitt's lymphoma, areas with high rates of KS and Burkitt's lymphoma are not identical (30). Endemic KS is not associated with specific immunodeficiency, although some patients may have diminished responses to skin test antigens (85).

AIDS-KS or epidemic KS is clinically aggressive, and visceral involvement is common. Male homosexual and bisexual AIDS patients are approximately 20 times more likely to present with KS at AIDS diagnosis than hemophilic AIDS patients (6), and cohort studies demonstrate that up to one-half of homosexual and bisexual men with AIDS develop KS over the course of their lifetime. The reported proportion of U.S. AIDS patients with KS as an initial AIDS-defining condition has declined since the beginning of the AIDS epidemic, perhaps due to changes in sexual practices (6) and the use of potent antiretroviral therapy.

KSHV DNA can be readily detected by in situ hybridization in nearly all tumor spindle cells of all epidemiological forms of KS (168). Probes commonly used for in situ hybridization are generally either PAN (polyadenylated nuclear RNA, ORF K7) or T0.7 (ORF K12), which are highly expressed small viral RNAs (170, 189). Most KS cells harboring the virus are in a virologically latent state in which few viral genes are active and infectious virus is not produced. Antibodies against LANA1 (ORF73) also are useful for immunopathological detection of virus in KS lesions (44). While vIL-6 is not found to be expressed in KS tumors in most studies (118), others do find a substantial proportion of tumors expressing this cytokine (15).

A small percentage of KS spindle cells (<1%) do undergo full lytic virus replication and export infectious virus. This minority lytic cell population may contribute to the pathology of KS through paracrine mechanisms or as a reservoir for persistent virus production. Consistent with this, transgenic mice expressing the vGCR (ORF74) under the control of an endothelial cell promoter develop angiogenic disease that strongly resembles KS (185). Since the vGCR is generally expressed only in the small percentage of cells undergoing active lytic replication, this suggests that the bulk of the tumor may be induced through paracrine mechanisms (86).

Primary Effusion Lymphomas

PELs possess a unique constellation of features that distinguishes them from other known lymphoproliferations (66). These lymphomas were first reported to occur in AIDS patients as body cavity-based lymphomas (87) but are now referred to as PELs. PEL usually presents as a localized pulmonary, cardiac, or abdominal effusion with tumor spread along serous membrane surfaces. The pleural cavity is the most common site of occurrence. Pulmonary or gastrointestinal KS may also generate local effusions, and mixed KS-PEL tumors should be considered in these cases. Usually there is no direct local tumor destruction or invasion into serous membranes, although spread to lymph nodes and lymphatics frequently occurs and circulating lymphoma cells can be isolated from the peripheral blood.

PELs are composed of post-germinal center, preterminally differentiated malignant B cells that do not usually express B-cell markers but can be identified as being of B-cell origin by clonal immunoglobulin chain rearrangements (1, 20, 51). They demonstrate morphological features that span those of large-cell immunoblastic lymphomas and anaplastic large-cell lymphomas, with abundant atypical mitosis, marked nuclear/cytoplasmic pleomorphism, and prominent nucleoli. These lymphomas consistently lack genetic alterations that have been associated with other lymphomas, including activation of the proto-oncogenes c-*myc*, *bcl-2*, and *ras* as well as mutations of p53 (1, 123).

PELs are all infected by KSHV at high copy number (50 to 150 viral genome copies/cell). The viral KSHV populations infecting a particular PEL are monoclonal by terminal repeat analysis, indicating that the lymphomas arise from single cells infected with the virus. Although PELs are defined primarily by their invariant association with KSHV, they have distinguishing clinical features as well. PEL cells have a marked tropism for serous surfaces and accumulate in fluid-filled visceral cavities. Malignant cells are largely confined to pleural, pericardial, and ascitic effusions; however, they can invade tissues underlying serous cavities as well to circulate in the bloodstream (8, 16).

The large majority of PELs are described as occurring in patients with compromised immune status, especially those with AIDS. Similar to KS, PELs demonstrate a strong association to an HIV transmission subgroup, and essentially all AIDS-related cases reported to date have been found in homosexual men. In these individuals, PELs respond poorly to therapy and are rapidly fatal, with a median survival of 2 to 3 months (1). Virtually all individuals with AIDS-related PEL are coinfected with clonal EBV. In contrast, PELs often have a much less aggressive course in HIV-seronegative patients, among whom they tend to occur in elderly persons. Both EBV-positive and EBV-negative PELs occur in HIV-negative patients (124).

Castleman's Disease

Castleman's disease, also known as angiofollicular lymphoid hyperplasia, is a rare, nonneoplastic, lymphoproliferative disorder related to excess IL-6-like activity. Histologically, Castleman's disease can be divided into three subtypes: hyaline-vascular, plasma cell, and mixed variants. Clinically, Castleman's disease occurs as solitary and multicentric forms (108). The majority of Castleman's disease is of the hyaline-vascular variant, which presents as solitary lymph node hyperplasia typically in the mediastinum or retroperitoneum. Other than isolated nodal enlargement, patients usually have no symptoms, and surgical excision of the involved lymph nodes is curative. In contrast, the plasma cell variant has an abundance of plasma cells and frequently multicentric or generalized presentation, and it is poorly responsive to treatment (50). Plasma cell variant MCD is associated with systemic symptoms, including fever, anemia, hypergammaglobulinemia, and hypoalbuminemia.

KSHV is associated with all subtypes of Castleman's disease and with the MCD variant in HIV-seronegative patients (57). HIV-seronegative patients who are KSHV infected tend to have a worse clinical prognosis; their disease is generally disseminated (multicentric) and complicated by type B symptoms, autoimmune hemolytic anemia, and polyclonal gammopathies. In one study, KSHV-infected MCD patients had an 80% mortality rate over an 8-month follow-up period (135). In contrast, although KSHV-negative disease is more frequently associated with subsequent non-Hodgkin's lymphoma than the KSHV-infected lesions, KSHV-negative Castleman's disease tends to be localized, affect younger persons, and be more readily treated by excision (135). KSHV-infected Castleman's tumors are frequently (25 to 50%) associated with intercurrent KS tumors that arise within lymph nodes affected by Castleman's disease.

In MCD, KSHV-infected cells have a peculiar and distinctive distribution. Immunohistochemical analysis shows that KSHV-infected cells comprise a minority population of B cells in the mantle zones, which surround germinal centers (44, 81, 135). Subsets of these cells have a centroblastic/immunoblastic morphology and demonstrate vIL-6 expression (135). This finding supports the notion that Castleman's disease is a syndrome of multiple etiologies involving aberrant IL-6 activity. Although Castleman's tumors infected with KSHV represent only a subset of all Castleman's lesions, this subset is the first recognized disorder that is likely to be caused by a virus-encoded cytokine.

Other Disorders Associated with KSHV

Less common KSHV-associated diseases include bone marrow failure (102) in the posttransplantation setting. While multiple myeloma, sarcoidosis, and primary pulmonary hypertension have been reported to be linked to KSHV infection, subsequent studies have failed to find any convincing evidence that the virus plays a role in these diseases in most patients.

Pathogenesis and KSHV Molecular Piracy

The specific mechanisms by which KSHV induces tumor formation remain incompletely defined. KSHV is a monoclonal infection in PELs, which are composed of fully transformed B cells (8, 78, 153). KS lesions, in contrast, are frequently oligoclonal or polyclonal but probably evolve into monoclonal lesions with disease progression (45, 153). The bulk of cells in Castleman's disease lesions, in further contrast, consist of hyperplastic, uninfected, untransformed cells. Only a fraction of cells, localized to the marginal zone of germinal centers, are infected with KSHV. Interestingly, while these infected cells are not monoclonal, they tend to show monotypic λ light-chain expression (41).

Many of the functions of the proteins encoded by the viral homologs of cellular genes appear to affect apoptosis and cell cycle regulation. For example, LANA1 is functionally similar to simian virus 40 T antigen in that it binds and inhibits both p53, which controls apoptotic signaling (48), and retinoblastoma protein (pRB1), which is responsible for cell cycle regulation (145). Other inhibitors of apoptosis include vBCL-2, which inhibits Bax pathway-mediated apoptosis (27, 157), and vIL-6, which acts as an autocrine factor for virus-infected PEL cells (25, 76). Evidence suggests that some proteins expressed during the lytic replication cycle, such as K-BZIP and vIRF1, also have p53 inhibitory functions (125, 134, 159) that may delay cell death during lytic replication so that capsid maturation is optimized.

Immune Evasion

KSHV possesses a number of proteins that target both adaptive and innate immunity. Many of these proteins are unique to KSHV, but like other viral functions, counterparts that achieve similar results subsequently have been found in other viruses. The KSHV vIRF1 molecule, for example, inhibits interferon-related transcription (52, 194) to prevent activation of an antiviral cell state. The ORF45 protein binds to and inactivates cellular IRF7, which acts upstream of the beta interferon promoter to dampen interferon activation, particularly during initial virus infection (192), a function also targeted during latency by the LANA2 protein (77). Similarly, vIRF2 and LANA2 proteins have been reported to antagonize PKR signaling, also preventing interferon activation (10, 122). The KSHV vIL-6 cytokine abrogates signaling from the beta interferon receptor (25), and the MIR1 and MIR2 proteins down-regulate expression of the gamma interferon receptor (97). It is evident that KSHV can target multiple sites in the interferon signaling response; most probably these proteins act in different combinations during different steps of the viral life cycle or in different cell types.

KSHV molecules target other components of the innate immune system as well. KIST (ORF K1 protein) possesses a functional immunoreceptor tyrosine activation motif and mimics an activated B-cell receptor (BCR) (91, 94) while down-modulating the host cell BCR (93). Together with ORF4 protein, a homolog to complement binding components of the BCR (165), these proteins may act as BCR signaling mimics to ensure survival of infected B cells. Immune signaling receptors may also be targeted by KSHV, although current evidence for this is weaker. While vFLIP was first described as a dominant-negative inhibitor of Fas signaling pathways activated during cell-mediated immune killing (173), evidence suggests that it has a more active role in inducing NF-κB signaling, which contributes to infected-cell survival and proliferation (26). NF-κB activation by vFLIP initiates multiple signaling pathways in infected cells that are presumed to be critical for survival of these cells, particularly infected B cells (64). This activity of vFLIP in endothelial cells probably accounts for their unusual spindle morphology in KS tumors (61, 109).

Adaptive immunity is also targeted by KSHV proteins to prevent efficient viral immune clearance. Proteins encoded by ORFs K3 and K5 blunt an adaptive cell-mediated immune response by down-regulating major histocompatibility complex class I (MHC I) molecules from the plasma membrane to prevent immune presentation of viral peptides (32, 70). This is achieved in a novel mechanism whereby K3 and K5 proteins act as E3 ligases to initiate ubiquitination of these membrane proteins, possibly at noncanonical cystine residues (11). Ubiquitination acts as an internalization for MHC I, resulting in its extraction from the plasma membrane and endosomal degradation. These proteins also play a role in inhibiting the cell surface presentation of costimulatory molecules required for T-cell receptor activation, such as B7.2 (69); CD1, involved in natural killer T-cell signaling (154); and the gamma-interferon receptor (97). Further, KSHV-secreted proteins, including vIL-6 and three virus-encoded chemokines, may help polarize anti-KSHV immune signaling toward an antibody-predominant Th2 response rather than a cell-mediated Th1 response (164, 169). Since KSHV is cell associated, antibody neutralization is unlikely to play a significant role in controlling virus infection.

LANA1 acts as a molecular tether between the host chromatin and the viral episome during latency and must be expressed for proper viral replication (3). Repeat regions in both EBNA1 and LANA1 inhibit their processing into antigenic peptides by retarding protein synthesis (which prevents rapid turnover of misfolded nascent proteins) and by inhibiting proteosomal turnover (89). This reduces opportunities for the host immune system to sample LANA1 peptides and prevents initiation of specific cytotoxic T lymphocyte immune responses against latently infected cells (188). Thus, during latency, KSHV protein expression is kept to minimal levels to avoid immune recognition, and those proteins that must be expressed to maintain the virus have evolved structural features to inhibit antigen presentation or to mimic host epitopes.

Cell Transformation and Proliferation

KSHV is primarily in a latent, unencapsidated and nontransmissible form in tumors. While a small percentage of tumor cells undergo productive virus replication at any one time, the bulk of tumor cells are noninfectious. The benefits to the virus from the virus-encoded "oncoproteins" can be divided into the two phases of the virus replication cycle (119). During lytic replication, these proteins prevent premature apoptosis and probably drive the infected cell into an S-phase-like state so that viral DNA can be rapidly replicated. The host cell is not an unwitting bystander to these changes and, in fact, actively initiates apoptosis and cell cycle arrest as an innate immune response to limit viral replication. DNA breaks and collapse of replication forks during the intense period of lytic viral DNA replication may constitute one trigger for this response (160). The cellular sensors for latent viral replication, if any, that require targeting by viral oncoproteins are less well described.

Cell cycle regulation is altered in infected cells by LANA1 interactions with pRB1 (145) as well as vCYC actions in inducing phosphorylation of pRB1 by partnering with CYC-dependent kinases (for a review, see references 116 and 175). The functions of vCYC appear to be very similar to those of the cellular class of D CYCs, although vCYC can also induce phosphorylation of H1 (59, 96). This suggests that vCYC may be active at stages of the cell cycle other than the G_1 checkpoint controlled by pRB1. Another KSHV protein, the vGCR, is mitogenic through its action as a constitutively active receptor acting on downstream mitogen-activated protein kinase and stress-activated protein kinase pathways (2).

To amplify its genome several hundred-fold during lytic virus replication, KSHV must prepare the cell environment to ensure proper nucleotide pools and replication enzyme availability. KSHV encodes many of the S-phase DNA synthesis enzymes required for its own replication. Several viral proteins, including the vGCR and vIL-6, have mitogenic activity that promotes cell cycle entry and may lay the cell cycle groundwork for genome replication. Surprisingly, some KSHV proteins, such as K-BZIP, also appear to arrest the cell in late G_1, as measured by chromatin content, by interacting with the CYC-dependent kinase CDK2 (71) and by activation of the CYC-dependent kinase inhibitor p21 (178). This is counterintuitive to the goal of generating an S-phase state for the infected cell and raises the interesting possibility that aberrant arrest may benefit viral DNA over cellular DNA replication. Mitogenic viral proteins may contribute to tumor cell proliferation if they act as paracrine factors on surrounding cells.

Disarming the G_1/S checkpoint activates cellular defenses to initiate apoptosis through p53. To counteract this, KSHV encodes a number of p53 pathway inhibitors so that the cell survives long enough for efficient virus maturation and egress. These include K-BZIP and vIRF1, which directly target p53 inhibition, and vBCL-2 and vIAP (viral inhibitor-of-apoptosis protein), which inhibit downstream mitochondrial apoptotic signaling. These proteins are expressed at high levels after KSHV enters lytic replication to prevent premature cell death. Several of these proteins are also expressed at low levels during virus latency, suggesting the possibility that they may also contribute to tumor cell survival.

Two of these proteins have additional novel features that may promote virus survival. Viral genome fragmentation, collapse of replication forks, and nucleotide misincorporation are likely to occur during virus replication, which can be expected to initiate DNA break responses. vIRF1 has been suggested to directly target the upstream signaling protein ATM (ataxia-telangectasia-mutated) to inhibit ATM signaling to p53 (160). In addition to apoptosis, autophagy contributes to tumor suppression and virus antigen presentation. KSHV vBCL-2 targets the autophagy control protein beclin, inhibiting this activity (137).

During latency, a similar but also different obstacle faces the virus. It is now apparent that a tricistronic cluster of proteins, together with a subset of miRNAs, are expressed constitutively during latency. These proteins include v-FLIP, which activates NF-κB and may inhibit Fas signaling; LANA1, which inhibits pRB1 and p53; and vCYC, which bypasses cellular CYC-dependent kinase inhibitors to phosphorylate pRB1. These proteins act in the same fashion as those which act during lytic replication to block apoptosis and to disarm the G_1/S checkpoint.

LABORATORY DIAGNOSIS

Diagnosis and Detection

Direct virus culture from patient specimens is not performed due to the technical limitations in primary isolation of KSHV in cell culture. PCR, however, has been used extensively as a research tool to detect viral DNA in tissues. While PCR has detected KSHV DNA sequences in nearly all (>95%) of the KS tumors examined to date, this technique is of limited use when examining PBMC, since only 1 in 50,000 to 100,000 cells are normally infected (121). Given the small amounts of circulating virus in infected individuals (including those with advanced KS), PBMC preparations are PCR positive for about one-half of patients with KS. Nested PCR, which is plagued by problems of contamination, is frequently required to detect the virus genome under these conditions.

Serologic Assays

Serologic assays have reasonable sensitivity and specificity in detecting KSHV infection (Table 3). No assays are currently approved for routine use in patient screening. This is due to the perceived lack of commercial viability for marketing KSHV assays rather than the technical specifications of the assays themselves. The most common assays use whole-cell antigen preparations from KSHV-infected PEL cell lines in an indirect immunofluorescence assay (IFA) format (120). These assays are divided into latent- or lytic-antigen assays depending on whether virus is induced into lytic replication through the use of tetradecanoyl phorbol acetate or another chemical agent. IFAs, which tend to be labor-intensive and require training, are generally being supplanted by enzyme-linked immunosorbent assay (ELISA)-based assays using recombinant antigens.

Latent-antigen IFAs detect antibodies directed against the ORF73-encoded LANA1 protein (83, 146). This highly charged nuclear phosphoprotein clusters in discrete nuclear speckles and migrates on immunoblots as a ca. 220-kDa doublet despite its predicted molecular mass of 150 kDa (53). Assays based on LANA1 IFA use unstimulated whole PEL cells, preferably adhered to glass slides using a cytospin technique, in which a characteristic nuclear speckling pattern of staining is present (54, 84). LANA1 positivity is usually determined at a 1:100 or 1:160 serum dilution, and extremely high antibody titers (>1:100,000) are not uncommon. This assay gives a 70 to 85% sensitivity rate in experienced hands and is generally highly specific. Generation of recombinant or peptide-mapped LANA epitopes tends to reduce assay sensitivity (132). In part, this can be overcome by use of baculovirus-prepared antigen, suggesting posttranslational modification of immunodominant LANA1 epitopes. Immunoblotting for LANA1 gives results similar to those of the whole-cell IFA, but extra effort is needed to efficiently transfer the antigen because of its apparent high molecular weight on gel electrophoresis (53).

Lytic-antigen IFAs generally have higher sensitivity than LANA assays, but lower specificity. PEL cells nonspecifically bind low-affinity human antibodies (54), and thus serum dilutions of less than 1:40 are likely to lead to a false-positive reaction. When appropriately counterstained, a diffuse cytoplasmic staining at a dilution of 1:40 or greater on lytic-antigen IFAs can have a sensitivity greater than 95%.

Given concerns about antigenic cross-reactivity in the lytic-antigen IFA, considerable effort has been put into development of recombinant lytic protein antigens. Most recombinant-antigen assays rely on two proteins, a viral glycoprotein, similar to EBV gp220/350, encoded by K8.1, and SCIP, encoded by ORF65 (22, 99, 161). Epitope mapping of both proteins has been performed, and peptide ELISAs have been developed which work well, particularly for the K8.1 peptide (138, 166). Some cross-reactivity of the amino terminus for KSHV ORF65 protein occurs with EBV-hyperimmune sera, but this can largely be avoided by using either a truncated C-terminal fragment or a synthetic peptide epitope.

Recombinant-antigen ELISA has distinct advantages in terms of cost, reproducibility, and ease of use. Individual sensitivities for these assays tend to be less than those of whole-cell IFAs, but combinations of recombinant-antigen assays (including a recombinant-LANA fragment assay) can be used to achieve >90% sensitivity (60). A combined three-antigen ELISA algorithm using K8.1 and ORF65 peptides together with recombinant LANA1 has been optimized to have ~93% sensitivity and 95% specificity (92). As in the diagnosis of other virus infections, recombinant-antigen ELISAs are often used for screening with immunoblot assay confirmation.

Antibody responses to KSHV tend to be rapid and persistent (Fig. 9). LANA1 antibodies often arise prior to ORF65 protein antibodies (particularly among HIV-infected persons), although exceptions to this are frequent (60, 131). Both LANA1 and ORF65 protein antibodies persist for years after infection and have stable titers throughout the asymptomatic period of infection (54, 60). Antibody titers may increase immediately prior to the onset of KS tumor formation, perhaps reflecting increased viremia concurrent with loss of immunologic control of the virus. However, the variability in absolute virus antibody titer in different individuals limits the usefulness of monitoring antibody titers as a means of predicting onset of disease.

For about 20% of HIV-positive persons, antibodies against LANA1 fail to develop at any time during the course of infection. In addition, seroreversion can occur during end-stage AIDS, even in persons with florid KS (53). In contrast, persons with HIV-negative KS tend to develop robust humoral immune responses. When HIV-negative KS patients are used as a "gold standard," the sensitivity of some assays may approach 100%, suggesting

TABLE 3 Serologic antigen assays for detecting KSHV infection

Antigen(s)	Gene	Sensitivity (%)	Specificity	Formats
LANA1	ORF73	~80	High	WB,[a] ELISA
K8.1A, K8.1B	K8.1	>90	Intermediate	WB, ELISA, peptide ELISA
SCIP	ORF65	~80	Intermediate	WB, ELISA
Whole cell (latent)		80	High	IFA, WB
Whole cell (lytic)		>95	Low	IFA, WB

[a] WB, Western blot.

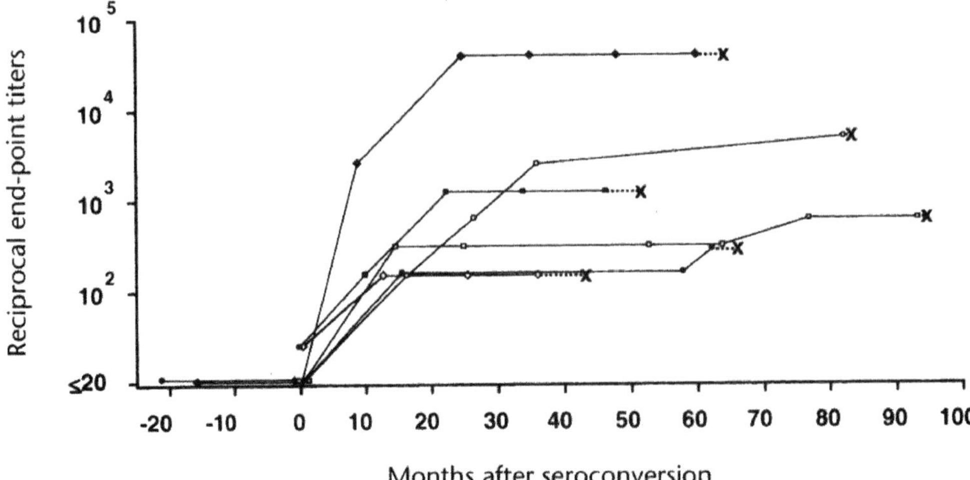

FIGURE 9 Antibody responses to KSHV infection are persistent for years after initial infection. This graph shows the reciprocal end-point titers for six men with AIDS who seroconverted to LANA1 IFA positivity at time zero. Antibody positivity remained stable for up to 8 years, until the patients developed KS (marked with an X). Note that anti-LANA1 titers are plotted on a log scale and in some patients can be positive at a dilution of 1:50,000 or greater. (Reprinted from reference 54 with permission of Macmillan Publishers Ltd.)

that assay performance may be affected by the types of populations for which it is used. This has been confirmed by studies showing loss of LANA reactivity, but not of reactivity with other KSHV antigens, for HIV patients with low $CD4^+$ cell counts (36).

PREVENTION

Since the exact modes of transmission are unknown, practical prevention measures have not been developed. Avoiding deep kissing and avoiding use of saliva as a sexual lubricant seem to be simple and reasonable recommendations to prevent oropharyngeal spread during sexual acitivity. Condom use is of unclear benefit for preventing KSHV transmission due to limited shedding in semen but should be encouraged to prevent other sexually transmitted infections. While it is unknown whether safe-sex practices have any practical effect on KSHV transmission, clinicians should counsel both HIV-seropositive and HIV-seronegative patients to engage in safe-sex practices to reduce the risk of acquiring opportunistic pathogens such as KSHV as well as limit the spread of HIV.

Screening guidelines for KSHV in the transplant setting have not yet been formally established. Assays to detect KSHV are not readily available to most clinicians, although they can be developed in-house by clinical laboratories with sufficient resources and expertise. Since rejection of otherwise healthy allografts from transplantation has critical clinical repercussions, only assays with high specificity (low false-positivity rates) should be considered for screening. At this time, elimination of KSHV-infected allografts from transplantation is not routinely practiced. Knowledge of the infection status of the donor and the recipient may allow the clinician either to consider antiviral prophylaxis or to at least monitor the transplant patient for early signs of KSHV-related disease.

Antibody screening for transplant patients, if available, should be strongly considered, particularly for patients in whom reduction in immunosuppressive therapy would have a fatal outcome (e.g., heart or liver transplant recipients). For these patients, if they are KSHV positive or received a transplant with a positive organ, careful follow-up, antiherpesvirus chemoprevention, and use of sirolimus can be considered.

There is no current development of a vaccine despite the established need in African and transplant populations. Unlike other herpesviruses, KSHV has been naturally lost from many populations and is poorly transmissible in others. This suggests that immunogenic vaccines may be capable of preventing infection and, if effective latent antigens are included, that therapeutic vaccines can be used once infection is established.

Chemoprevention

Chemoprevention is an important and underappreciated prevention possibility for persons at high risk for KS. In vitro assays suggest that cidofovir, foscarnet, and ganciclovir have higher specific activity against KSHV than acyclovir (14, 82, 114). A retrospective epidemiological study showed that AIDS patients receiving foscarnet for prevention and control of cytomegalovirus CMV retinitis have a lower incidence of KS occurrence (74). In a prospective, randomized clinical trial, AIDS patients receiving oral and intravenous ganciclovir (plus intraocular ganciclovir implants) had 75 and 93% reductions, respectively, in onset of new KS tumors compared to those receiving placebo (106). Similarly, foscarnet treatment used to prevent CMV retinitis can delay or prevent KS recurrence and spread among persons with established KS (151). Thus far, these drugs appear to have little activity once KS is established, but they may prevent emergence of new tumors.

TREATMENT OF KS

No specific antiviral therapy against KSHV has been developed to treat KS. KS is currently treated by surgical excision, intralesional or systemic chemotherapy, and localized irradiation. Localized tumors, particularly tumors in nonimmunosuppressed patients, can be excised or irradiated (up to 40 Gy over 20 fractions) with good outcome. KS is, however, a systemic viral disease, and local therapy does not prevent dissemination to other sites. Similarly, intralesional injection with vinblastine (0.2 mg/ml for 0.1 ml/cm^2 of tumor tissue) has a high partial response rate after single injection, but tumor regrowth is common. A wide range of chemotherapeutic agents either as single agents or in combination have moderate to good responses as palliative agents in AIDS-KS. KS is also responsive to systemic alpha interferon (1 to 50 MU/m^2), but whether this is due to antitumor, immunomodulatory, or antiviral activity remains to be explored.

Several novel therapies are being investigated (19). In contrast to KS, KSHV-positive MCD lesions have been reported to respond to ganciclovir treatment (18) as well as to rituximab (31, 129). In tissue culture cells, nutlin-3a, a reactivator of p53, prevents LANA1 interaction with p53 and MDM2 (155). This appears to specifically initiate apoptosis in KSHV-infected PEL cells. Switching immunosuppressive therapy to sirolimus, an mTOR (mammalian target of rapamycin) inhibitor and potential anticancer drug, has been reported to effectively control KS in a small series of transplant KS patients (167).

Among AIDS patients, the most effective control measure for KS is effective antiretroviral therapy. The rate of new KS diagnoses is markedly lower among persons on highly effective antiretroviral therapy (73, 75). Despite the efficacy of antiretroviral therapy, treatment has no apparent effect on long-term KSHV carriage, and as the AIDS population ages, there are worrisome reports of reemergence of KS among patients with low HIV loads and high CD4$^+$ cell counts (110).

REFERENCES

1. **Ansari, M. Q., D. B. Dawson, R. Nador, C. Rutherford, N. R. Schneider, M. J. Latimer, L. Picker, D. M. Knowles, and R. W. McKenna.** 1996. Primary body cavity-based AIDS-related lymphomas. *Am. J. Clin. Pathol.* **105:** 221–229.
2. **Bais, C., B. Santomasso, O. Coso, L. Arvanitakis, E. G. Raaka, J. S. Gutkind, A. S. Asch, E. Cesarman, M. C. Gershengorn, E. A. Mesri, and M. C. Gerhengorn.** 1998. G-protein-coupled receptor of Kaposi's sarcoma-associated herpesvirus is a viral oncogene and angiogenesis activator. *Nature* **391:**86–89.
3. **Ballestas, M. E., P. A. Chatis, and K. M. Kaye.** 1999. Efficient persistence of extrachromosomal KSHV DNA mediated by latency-associated nuclear antigen. *Science* **284:**641–644.
4. **Bechtel, J., A. Grundhoff, and D. Ganem.** 2005. RNAs in the virion of Kaposi's sarcoma-associated herpesvirus. *J. Virol.* **79:**10138–10146.
5. **Bendsoe, N., M. Dictor, J. Blomberg, S. Agren, and K. Merk.** 1990. Increased incidence of Kaposi sarcoma in Sweden before the AIDS epidemic. *Eur. J. Cancer* **26:** 699–702.
6. **Beral, V., T. A. Peterman, R. L. Berkelman, and H. W. Jaffe.** 1990. Kaposi's sarcoma among persons with AIDS: a sexually transmitted infection? *Lancet* **335:**123–128.
7. **Biggar, R. J., D. Whitby, V. Marshall, A. C. Linhares, and F. Black.** 2000. Human herpesvirus 8 in Brazilian Amerindians: a hyperendemic population with a new subtype. *J. Infect. Dis.* **181:**1562–1568.
8. **Boshoff, C., S. J. Gao, L. E. Healy, S. Matthews, A. J. Thomas, L. Coignet, R. A. Warnke, J. A. Strauchen, E. Matutes, O. W. Kamel, P. S. Moore, R. A. Weiss, and Y. Chang.** 1998. Establishing a KSHV+ cell line (BCP-1) from peripheral blood and characterizing its growth in Nod/SCID mice. *Blood* **91:**1671–1679.
9. **Boulanger, E., R. Duprez, E. Delabesse, J. Gabarre, E. Macintyre, and A. Gessain.** 2005. Mono/oligoclonal pattern of Kaposi sarcoma-associated herpesvirus (KSHV/HHV-8) episomes in primary effusion lymphoma cells. *Int. J. Cancer* **115:**511–518.
10. **Burysek, L., and P. M. Pitha.** 2001. Latently expressed human herpesvirus 8-encoded interferon regulatory factor 2 inhibits double-stranded RNA-activated protein kinase. *J. Virol.* **75:**2345–2352.
11. **Cadwell, K., and L. Coscoy.** 2005. Ubiquitination on nonlysine residues by a viral E3 ubiquitin ligase. *Science* **309:**127–130.
12. **Cai, X., and B. R. Cullen.** 2006. Transcriptional origin of Kaposi's sarcoma-associated herpesvirus microRNAs. *J. Virol.* **80:**2234–2242.
13. **Calabro, M. L., J. Sheldon, A. Favero, G. R. Simpson, J. R. Fiore, E. Gomes, G. Angarano, L. Chieco-Bianchi, and T. F. Schulz.** 1998. Seroprevalence of Kaposi's sarcoma-associated herpesvirus/human herpesvirus 8 in several regions of Italy. *J. Hum. Virol.* **1:**207–213.
14. **Cannon, J. S., F. Hamzeh, S. Moore, J. Nicholas, and R. F. Ambinder.** 1999. Human herpesvirus 8-encoded thymidine kinase and phosphotransferase homologues confer sensitivity to ganciclovir. *J. Virol.* **73:**4786–4793.
15. **Cannon, J. S., J. Nicholas, J. M. Orenstein, R. B. Mann, P. G. Murray, P. J. Browning, J. A. DiGiuseppe, E. Cesarman, G. S. Hayward, and R. F. Ambinder.** 1999. Heterogeneity of viral IL-6 expression in HHV-8-associated diseases. *J. Infect. Dis.* **180:**824–828.
16. **Carbone, A., A. Gloghini, E. Vaccher, V. Zagonel, C. Pastore, P. Dalla Palma, F. Branz, G. Saglio, R. Volpe, U. Tirelli, and G. Gaidano.** 1996. Kaposi's sarcoma-associated herpesvirus DNA sequences in AIDS-related and AIDS-unrelated lymphomatous effusions. *Br. J. Haematol.* **94:**533–543.
17. **Casper, C., E. Krantz, S. Selke, S. R. Kuntz, J. Wang, M. L. Huang, J. S. Pauk, L. Corey, and A. Wald.** 2007. Frequent and asymptomatic oropharyngeal shedding of human herpesvirus 8 among immunocompetent men. *J. Infect. Dis.* **195:**30–36.
18. **Casper, C., W. G. Nichols, M. L. Huang, L. Corey, and A. Wald.** 2004. Remission of HHV-8 and HIV-associated multicentric Castleman disease with ganciclovir treatment. *Blood* **103:**1632–1634.
19. **Casper, C., and A. Wald.** 2007. The use of antiviral drugs in the prevention and treatment of Kaposi sarcoma, multicentric Castleman disease and primary effusion lymphoma. *Curr. Top. Microbiol. Immunol.* **312:**289–307.
20. **Cesarman, E., Y. Chang, P. S. Moore, J. W. Said, and D. M. Knowles.** 1995. Kaposi's sarcoma-associated herpesvirus-like DNA sequences in AIDS-related body-cavity-based lymphomas. *N. Engl. J. Med.* **332:**1186–1191.
21. **Cesarman, E., P. S. Moore, P. H. Rao, G. Inghirami, D. M. Knowles, and Y. Chang.** 1995. In vitro establishment and characterization of two acquired immunodeficiency syndrome-related lymphoma cell lines (BC-1 and BC-2) containing Kaposi's sarcoma-associated herpesvirus-like (KSHV) DNA sequences. *Blood* **86:** 2708–2714.
22. **Chandran, B., C. Bloomer, S. R. Chan, L. Zhu, E. Goldstein, and R. Horvat.** 1998. Human herpesvirus-8 ORF

K8.1 gene encodes immunogenic glycoproteins generated by spliced transcripts. *Virology* **249:**140–149.

23. **Chang, H., D. P. Dittmer, S.-Y. Chul, Y. Hong, and J. U. Jung.** 2005. Role of Notch signal transduction in Kaposi's sarcoma-associated herpesvirus gene expression. *J. Virol.* **79:**14371–14382.
24. **Chang, Y., E. Cesarman, M. S. Pessin, F. Lee, J. Culpepper, D. M. Knowles, and P. S. Moore.** 1994. Identification of herpesvirus-like DNA sequences in AIDS-associated Kaposi's sarcoma. *Science* **265:**1865–1869.
25. **Chatterjee, M., J. Osborne, G. Bestetti, Y. Chang, and P. S. Moore.** 2002. Viral IL-6-induced cell proliferation and immune evasion of interferon activity. *Science* **298:** 1432–1435.
26. **Chaudhary, P. M., M. T. Eby, A. Jasmin, A. Kumar, L. Liu, and L. Hood.** 2000. Activation of the NF-kappaB pathway by caspase 8 and its homologs. *Oncogene* **19:** 4451–4460.
27. **Cheng, E. H., J. Nicholas, D. S. Bellows, G. S. Hayward, H. G. Guo, M. S. Reitz, and J. M. Hardwick.** 1997. A Bcl-2 homolog encoded by Kaposi sarcoma-associated virus, human herpesvirus 8, inhibits apoptosis but does not heterodimerize with Bax or Bak. *Proc. Natl. Acad. Sci. USA* **94:**690–694.
28. **Chokunonga, E., L. M. Levy, M. T. Bassett, B. G. Mauchaza, D. B. Thomas, and D. M. Parkin.** 2000. Cancer incidence in the African population of Harare, Zimbabwe: second results from the cancer registry 1993–1995. *Int. J. Cancer* **85:**54–59.
29. **Cohen, A., C. Brodie, and R. Sarid.** 2006. An essential role of ERK signalling in TPA-induced reactivation of Kaposi's sarcoma-associated herpesvirus. *J. Gen. Virol.* **87:** 795–802.
30. **Cook, P. J., and D. P. Burkitt.** 1971. Cancer in Africa. *Br. Med. Bull.* **27:**14–20.
31. **Corbellino, M., G. Bestetti, C. Scalamogna, S. Calattini, M. Galazzi, L. Meroni, D. Manganaro, M. Fasan, M. Moroni, M. Galli, and C. Parravicini.** 2001. Long-term remission of Kaposi sarcoma-associated herpesvirus-related multicentric Castleman disease with anti-CD20 monoclonal antibody therapy. *Blood* **98:**3473–3475.
32. **Coscoy, L., and D. Ganem.** 2000. Kaposi's sarcoma-associated herpesvirus encodes two proteins that block cell surface display of MHC class I chains by enhancing their endocytosis. *Proc. Natl. Acad. Sci. USA* **97:**8051–8056.
33. **Damania, B.** 2007. EBV and KSHV-related herpesviruses in nonhuman primates, p. 1093–1114. *In* A. Arvin, G. Campadelli-Fiume, E. Mocarski, P. S. Moore, B. Roizman, R. Whitley, and K. Yamanishi (ed.), *Human Herpesviruses: Biology, Therapy and Immunoprophylaxis*. Cambridge University Press, Cambridge, United Kingdom.
34. **Dedicoat, M., and R. Newton.** 2003. Review of the distribution of Kaposi's sarcoma-associated herpesvirus (KSHV) in Africa in relation to the incidence of Kaposi's sarcoma. *Br. J. Cancer* **88:**1–3.
35. **Deng, B., C. M. O'Connor, D. H. Kedes, and Z. H. Zhou.** 2007. Direct visualization of the putative portal in the Kaposi's sarcoma-associated herpesvirus capsid by cryoelectron tomography. *J. Virol.* **81:**3640–3644.
36. **de Souza, V. A., L. C. Pierrotti, L. M. Sumita, W. S. Freire, A. A. Segurado, and C. S. Pannuti.** 2007. Seroreactivity to Kaposi's sarcoma-associated herpesvirus (human herpesvirus 8) latent nuclear antigen in AIDS-associated Kaposi's sarcoma patients depends on $CD4^+$ T-cell count. *J. Med. Virol.* **79:**1562–1568.
37. **Desrosiers, R. C., V. G. Sasseville, S. C. Czajak, X. Zhang, K. G. Mansfield, A. Kaur, R. P. Johnson, A. A. Lackner, and J. U. Jung.** 1997. A herpesvirus of rhesus monkeys related to the human Kaposi sarcoma-associated herpesvirus. *J. Virol.* **71:**9764–9769.
38. **Deutsch, E., A. Cohen, G. Kazimirsky, S. Dovrat, H. Rubinfeld, C. Brodie, and R. Sarid.** 2004. Role of protein kinase C δ in reactivation of Kaposi's sarcoma-associated herpesvirus. *J. Virol.* **78:**10187–10192.
39. **Dittmer, D., M. Lagunoff, R. Renne, K. Staskus, A. Haase, and D. Ganem.** 1998. A cluster of latently expressed genes in Kaposi's sarcoma-associated herpesvirus. *J. Virol.* **72:**8309–8315.
40. **Dollard, S. C., K. E. Nelson, P. M. Ness, V. Stambolis, M. J. Kuehnert, P. E. Pellett, and M. J. Cannon.** 2005. Possible transmission of human herpesvirus-8 by blood transfusion in a historical United States cohort. *Transfusion* **45:**500–503.
41. **Du, M.-Q., H. Liu, T. C. Diss, H. Ye, R. A. Hamoudi, N. Dupin, V. Meignin, E. Oksenhendler, C. Boshoff, and P. G. Isaacson.** 2001. Kaposi sarcoma-associated herpesvirus infects monotypic (IgMλ) but polyclonal naive B cells in Castleman disease and associated lymphoproliferative disorders. *Blood* **97:**2130–2136.
42. **Duda, R. L., R. W. Hendrix, W. M. Huang, and J. F. Conway.** 2006. Shared architecture of bacteriophage SPO1 and herpesvirus capsids. *Curr. Biol.* **16:**R11–R13.
43. **Dukers, N. H., N. Renwick, M. Prins, R. B. Geskus, T. F. Schulz, G. J. Weverling, R. A. Coutinho, and J. Goudsmit.** 2000. Risk factors for human herpesvirus 8 seropositivity and seroconversion in a cohort of homosexual men. *Am. J. Epidemiol.* **151:**213–224.
44. **Dupin, N., C. Fisher, P. Kellam, S. Ariad, M. Tulliez, N. Franck, E. van Marck, D. Salmon, I. Gorin, J. P. Escande, R. A. Weiss, K. Alitalo, and C. Boshoff.** 1999. Distribution of human herpesvirus-8 latently infected cells in Kaposi's sarcoma, multicentric Castleman's disease, and primary effusion lymphoma. *Proc. Natl. Acad. Sci. USA* **96:**4546–4551.
45. **Duprez, R., V. Lacoste, J. Briere, P. Couppie, C. Frances, D. Sainte-Marie, E. Kassa-Kelembho, M. J. Lando, J. L. Essame Oyono, B. Nkegoum, O. Hbid, A. Mahe, C. Lebbe, P. Tortevoye, M. Huerre, and A. Gessain.** 2007. Evidence for a multiclonal origin of multicentric advanced lesions of Kaposi sarcoma. *J. Natl. Cancer Inst.* **99:**1086–1094.
46. **Fouchard, N., V. Lacoste, P. Couppie, M. Develoux, P. Mauclere, P. Michel, V. Herve, R. Pradinaud, G. Bestetti, M. Huerre, F. Tekaia, G. de The, and A. Gessain.** 2000. Detection and genetic polymorphism of human herpes virus type 8 in endemic or epidemic Kaposi's sarcoma from West and Central Africa, and South America. *Int. J. Cancer* **85:**166–170.
47. **Frances, C., C. Mouquet, A. G. Marcelin, S. Barete, R. Agher, D. Charron, H. Benalia, N. Dupin, J. C. Piette, M. O. Bitker, and V. Calvez.** 2000. Outcome of kidney transplant recipients with previous human herpesvirus-8 infection. *Transplantation* **69:**1776–1779.
48. **Friborg, J., Jr., W. Kong, M. O. Hottiger, and G. J. Nabel.** 1999. p53 inhibition by the LANA protein of KSHV protects against cell death. *Nature* **402:**889–894.
49. **Friedman-Kien, A. E., B. R. Saltzman, Y. Cao, M. S. Nestor, M. Mirabile, J. J. Li, and T. A. Peterman.** 1990. Kaposi's sarcoma in HIV-negative homosexual men. *Lancet* **335:**168–169.
50. **Frizzera, G., B. A. Peterson, E. D. Bayrd, and A. Goldman.** 1985. A systemic lymphoproliferative disorder with morphologic features of Castleman's disease: clinical findings and clinicopathologic correlations in 15 patients. *J. Clin. Oncol.* **3:**1202–1216.

51. **Gaidano, G., A. Gloghini, V. Gattei, M. F. Rossi, A. M. Cilia, C. Godeas, M. Degan, T. Perin, V. Canzonieri, D. Aldinucci, G. Saglio, A. Carbone, and A. Pinto.** 1997. Association of Kaposi's sarcoma-associated herpesvirus-positive primary effusion lymphoma with expression of the CD138/syndecan-1 antigen. *Blood* **90:**4894–4900.
52. **Gao, S.-J., C. Boshoff, S. Jayachandra, R. A. Weiss, Y. Chang, and P. S. Moore.** 1997. KSHV ORF K9 (vIRF) is an oncogene that inhibits the interferon signaling pathway. *Oncogene* **15:**1979–1986.
53. **Gao, S.-J., L. Kingsley, D. R. Hoover, T. J. Spira, C. R. Rinaldo, A. Saah, J. Phair, R. Detels, P. Parry, Y. Chang, and P. S. Moore.** 1996. Seroconversion to antibodies against Kaposi's sarcoma-associated herpesvirus-related latent nuclear antigens before the development of Kaposi's sarcoma. *N. Engl. J. Med.* **335:**233–241.
54. **Gao, S. J., L. Kingsley, M. Li, W. Zheng, C. Parravicini, J. Ziegler, R. Newton, C. R. Rinaldo, A. Saah, J. Phair, R. Detels, Y. Chang, and P. S. Moore.** 1996. KSHV antibodies among Americans, Italians and Ugandans with and without Kaposi's sarcoma. *Nat. Med.* **2:**925–928.
55. **Gao, S. J., Y. J. Zhang, J. H. Deng, C. S. Rabkin, O. Flore, and H. B. Jenson.** 1999. Molecular polymorphism of Kaposi's sarcoma-associated herpesvirus (human herpesvirus 8) latent nuclear antigen: evidence for a large repertoire of viral genotypes and dual infection with different viral genotypes. *J. Infect. Dis.* **180:**1466–1476. (Erratum, **180:**1756.)
56. **Geddes, M., S. Franceschi, D. Balzi, A. Arniani, L. Gafà, and R. Zanetti.** 1995. Birthplace and classic Kaposi's sarcoma in Italy. *J. Natl. Cancer Inst.* **87:**1015–1017.
57. **Gessain, A., A. Sudaka, J. Brière, N. Fouchard, M. A. Nicola, B. Rio, M. Arborio, X. Troussard, J. Audouin, J. Diebold, and G. de Thé.** 1996. Kaposi sarcoma-associated herpes-like virus (human herpesvirus type 8) DNA sequences in multicentric Castleman's disease: is there any relevant association in non-human immunodeficiency virus-infected patients? *Blood* **87:**414–416.
58. **Glaunsinger, B., and D. Ganem.** 2004. Highly selective escape from KSHV-mediated host mRNA shutoff and its implications for viral pathogenesis. *J. Exp. Med.* **200:**391–398.
59. **Godden-Kent, D., S. J. Talbot, C. Boshoff, Y. Chang, P. Moore, R. A. Weiss, and S. Mittnacht.** 1997. The cyclin encoded by Kaposi's sarcoma-associated herpesvirus stimulates cdk6 to phosphorylate the retinoblastoma protein and histone H1. *J. Virol.* **71:**4193–4198.
60. **Goudsmit, J., N. Renwick, N. H. Dukers, R. A. Coutinho, S. Heisterkamp, M. Bakker, T. F. Schulz, M. Cornelissen, and G. J. Weverling.** 2000. Human herpesvirus 8 infections in the Amsterdam Cohort Studies (1984–1997): analysis of seroconversions to ORF65 and ORF73. *Proc. Natl. Acad. Sci. USA* **97:**4838–4843.
61. **Grossmann, C., S. Podgrabinska, M. Skobe, and D. Ganem.** 2006. Activation of NF-κB by the latent vFLIP gene of Kaposi's sarcoma-associated herpesvirus is required for the spindle shape of virus-infected endothelial cells and contributes to their proinflammatory phenotype. *J. Virol.* **80:**7179–7185.
62. **Grulich, A. E., V. Beral, and A. J. Swerdlow.** 1992. Kaposi's sarcoma in England and Wales before the AIDS epidemic. *Br. J. Cancer* **66:**1135–1137.
63. **Grulich, A. E., J. M. Kaldor, O. Hendry, K. H. Luo, N. J. Bodsworth, and D. A. Cooper.** 1997. Risk of Kaposi's sarcoma and oroanal sexual contact. *Am. J. Epidemiol.* **145:**673–679.
64. **Guasparri, I., S. A. Keller, and E. Cesarman.** 2004. KSHV vFLIP is essential for the survival of infected lymphoma cells. *J. Exp. Med.* **199:**993–1003.
65. **Han, Z., and S. Swaminathan.** 2006. Kaposi's sarcoma-associated herpesvirus lytic gene ORF57 is essential for infectious virion production. *J. Virol.* **80:**5251–5260.
66. **Harris, N. L., E. S. Jaffe, J. Diebold, G. Flandrin, H. K. Muller-Hermelink, J. Vardiman, T. A. Lister, and C. D. Bloomfield.** 1999. World Health Organization classification of neoplastic diseases of the hematopoietic and lymphoid tissues: report of the Clinical Advisory Committee meeting-Airlie House, Virginia, November 1997. *J. Clin. Oncol.* **17:**3835–3849.
67. **Hayward, G. S., and J. C. Zong.** 2007. Modern evolutionary history of the human KSHV genome. *Curr. Top. Microbiol. Immunol.* **312:**1–42.
68. **Hladik, W., S. C. Dollard, J. Mermin, A. L. Fowlkes, R. Downing, M. M. Amin, F. Banage, E. Nzaro, P. Kataaha, T. J. Dondero, P. E. Pellett, and E. M. Lackritz.** 2006. Transmission of human herpesvirus 8 by blood transfusion. *N. Engl. J. Med.* **355:**1331–1338.
69. **Ishido, S., J. K. Choi, B. S. Lee, C. Wang, M. DeMaria, R. P. Johnson, G. B. Cohen, and J. U. Jung.** 2000. Inhibition of natural killer cell-mediated cytotoxicity by Kaposi's sarcoma-associated herpesvirus K5 protein. *Immunity* **13:**365–374.
70. **Ishido, S., C. Wang, B. S. Lee, G. B. Cohen, and J. U. Jung.** 2000. Downregulation of major histocompatibility complex class I molecules by Kaposi's sarcoma-associated herpesvirus K3 and K5 proteins. *J. Virol.* **74:**5300–5309.
71. **Izumiya, Y., S.-F. Lin, T. J. Ellison, A. M. Levy, G. L. Mayeur, C. Izumiya, and H.-J. Kung.** 2003. Cell cycle regulation by Kaposi's sarcoma-associated herpesvirus K-bZIP: direct interaction with cyclin-CDK2 and induction of G_1 growth arrest. *J. Virol.* **77:**9652–9661.
72. **Jacobson, L. P., F. J. Jenkins, G. Springer, A. Munoz, K. V. Shah, J. Phair, Z. Zhang, and H. Armenian.** 2000. Interaction of human immunodeficiency virus type 1 and human herpesvirus type 8 infections on the incidence of Kaposi's sarcoma. *J. Infect. Dis.* **181:**1940–1949.
73. **Jacobson, L. P., T. E. Yamashita, R. Detels, J. B. Margolick, J. S. Chmiel, L. A. Kingsley, S. Melnick, and A. Munoz.** 1999. Impact of potent antiretroviral therapy on the incidence of Kaposi's sarcoma and non-Hodgkin's lymphomas among HIV-1-infected individuals. Multicenter AIDS Cohort Study. *J. Acquir. Immune Defic. Syndr.* **21**(Suppl. 1)**:**S34–S41.
74. **Jones, J., T. Peterman, S. Chu, and H. Jaffe.** 1995. AIDS-associated Kaposi's sarcoma. *Science* **267:**1078–1079.
75. **Jones, J. L., D. L. Hanson, M. S. Dworkin, J. W. Ward, and H. W. Jaffe.** 1999. Effect of antiretroviral therapy on recent trends in selected cancers among HIV-infected persons. Adult/Adolescent Spectrum of HIV Disease Project Group. *J. Acquir. Immune Defic. Syndr.* **21**(Suppl. 1)**:**S11–S17.
76. **Jones, K. D., Y. Aoki, Y. Chang, P. S. Moore, R. Yarchoan, and G. Tosato.** 1999. Involvement of interleukin-10 (IL-10) and viral IL-6 in the spontaneous growth of Kaposi's sarcoma herpesvirus-associated infected primary effusion lymphoma cells. *Blood* **94:**2871–2879.
77. **Joo, C. H., Y. C. Shin, M. Gack, L. Wu, D. Levy, and J. U. Jung.** 2007. inhibition of interferon regulatory factor 7 (IRF7)-mediated interferon signal transduction by the Kaposi's sarcoma-associated herpesvirus viral IRF homolog vIRF3. *J. Virol.* **81:**8282–8292.
78. **Judde, J. G., V. Lacoste, J. Briere, E. Kassa-Kelembho, E. Clyti, P. Couppie, C. Buchrieser, M. Tulliez, J. Morvan, and A. Gessain.** 2000. Monoclonality or oligoclonality of human herpesvirus 8 terminal repeat sequences in Kaposi's sarcoma and other diseases. *J. Natl. Cancer Inst.* **92:**729–736.

79. **Kaposi, M.** 1872. Idiopathic multiple pigmented sarcoma of the skin. *Arch. Dermatol. Syphil.* **4:**265–273. (English translation in *CA Cancer J. Clin.* **32:** 342–347, 1982.)
80. **Kasolo, F. C., E. Mpabalwani, and U. A. Gompels.** 1997. Infection with AIDS-related herpesviruses in human immunodeficiency virus-negative infants and endemic childhood Kaposi's sarcoma in Africa. *J. Gen. Virol.* **78:**847–856.
81. **Katano, H., Y. Sato, T. Kurata, S. Mori, and T. Sata.** 2000. Expression and localization of human herpesvirus 8-encoded proteins in primary effusion lymphoma, Kaposi's sarcoma, and multicentric Castleman's disease. *Virology* **269:**335–344.
82. **Kedes, D. H., and D. Ganem.** 1997. Sensitivity of Kaposi's sarcoma-associated herpesvirus replication to antiviral drugs. Implications for potential therapy. *J. Clin. Investig.* **99:**2082–2086.
83. **Kedes, D. H., M. Lagunoff, R. Renne, and D. Ganem.** 1997. Identification of the gene encoding the major latency-associated nuclear antigen of the Kaposi's sarcoma-associated herpesvirus. *J. Clin. Investig.* **100:** 2606–2610.
84. **Kedes, D. H., E. Operskalski, M. Busch, R. Kohn, J. Flood, and D. Ganem.** 1996. The seroepidemiology of human herpesvirus 8 (Kaposi's sarcoma-associated herpesvirus): distribution of infection in KS risk groups and evidence for sexual transmission. *Nat. Med.* **2:**918–924.
85. **Kestens, L., M. Melbye, R. J. Biggar, W. J. Stevens, P. Piot, A. de Muynck, H. Taelman, M. de Feyter, L. Paluku, and P. L. Gigase.** 1985. Endemic Kaposi's sarcoma is not associated with immunodeficiency. *Int. J. Cancer* **36:**49–54.
86. **Kirshner, J. R., K. Staskus, A. Haase, M. Lagunoff, and D. Ganem.** 1999. Expression of the open reading frame 74 (G-protein-coupled receptor) gene of Kaposi's sarcoma (KS)-associated herpesvirus: implications for KS pathogenesis. *J. Virol.* **73:**6006–6014.
87. **Knowles, D. M., G. Inghirami, A. Ubriaco, and R. Dalla-Favera.** 1989. Molecular genetic analysis of three AIDS-associated neoplasms of uncertain lineage demonstrates their B-cell derivation and the possible pathogenetic role of Epstein-Barr virus. *Blood* **73:**792–799.
88. **Kudoh, A., M. Fujita, T. Kiyono, K. Kuzushima, Y. Sugaya, S. Izuta, Y. Nishiyama, and T. Tsurumi.** 2003. Reactivation of lytic replication from B cells latently infected with Epstein-Barr virus occurs with high S-phase cyclin-dependent kinase activity while inhibiting cellular DNA replication. *J. Virol.* **77:**851–861.
89. **Kwun, H. J., S. R. da Silva, I. Shah, N. Blake, P. S. Moore, and Y. Chang.** 2007. KSHV LANA1 mimics EBV EBNA1 immune evasion through central repeat domain effects on protein processing. *J. Virol.* **81:**8225–8235.
90. **Lacoste, V., P. Mauclere, G. Dubreuil, J. Lewis, M. C. Georges-Courbot, and A. Gessain.** 2001. A novel gamma 2-herpesvirus of the Rhadinovirus 2 lineage in chimpanzees. *Genome Res.* **11:**1511–1519.
91. **Lagunoff, M., R. Majeti, A. Weiss, and D. Ganem.** 1999. Deregulated signal transduction by the K1 gene product of Kaposi's sarcoma-associated herpesvirus. *Proc. Natl. Acad. Sci. USA* **96:**5704–5709.
92. **Laney, A. S., J. S. Peters, S. M. Manzi, L. A. Kingsley, Y. Chang, and P. S. Moore.** 2006. Use of a multiantigen detection algorithm for diagnosis of Kaposi's sarcoma-associated herpesvirus infection. *J. Clin. Microbiol.* **44:** 3734–3741.
93. **Lee, B. S., X. Alvarez, S. Ishido, A. A. Lackner, and J. U. Jung.** 2000. Inhibition of intracellular transport of B cell antigen receptor complexes by Kaposi's sarcoma-associated herpesvirus K1. *J. Exp. Med.* **192:**11–21.
94. **Lee, H., J. Guo, M. Li, J. K. Choi, M. DeMaria, M. Rosenzweig, and J. U. Jung.** 1998. Identification of an immunoreceptor tyrosine-based activation motif of K1 transforming protein of Kaposi's sarcoma-associated herpesvirus. *Mol. Cell. Biol.* **18:**5219–5228.
95. **Lee, H., R. Veazey, K. Williams, M. Li, J. Guo, F. Neipel, B. Fleckenstein, A. Lackner, R. C. Desrosiers, and J. U. Jung.** 1998. Deregulation of cell growth by the K1 gene of Kaposi's sarcoma-associated herpesvirus. *Nat. Med.* **4:**435–440.
96. **Li, M., H. Lee, D. W. Yoon, J. C. Albrecht, B. Fleckenstein, F. Neipel, and J. U. Jung.** 1997. Kaposi's sarcoma-associated herpesvirus encodes a functional cyclin. *J. Virol.* **71:**1984–1991.
97. **Li, Q., R. Means, S. Lang, and J. U. Jung.** 2007. Downregulation of gamma interferon receptor 1 by Kaposi's sarcoma-associated herpesvirus K3 and K5. *J. Virol.* **81:** 2117–2127.
98. **Liang, Y., J. Chang, S. J. Lynch, D. M. Lukac, and D. Ganem.** 2002. The lytic switch protein of KSHV activates gene expression via functional interaction with RBP-Jκ (CSL), the target of the Notch signaling pathway. *Genes Dev.* **16:**1977–1989.
99. **Lin, S. F., R. Sun, L. Heston, L. Gradoville, D. Shedd, K. Haglund, M. Rigsby, and G. Miller.** 1997. Identification, expression, and immunogenicity of Kaposi's sarcoma-associated herpesvirus-encoded small viral capsid antigen. *J. Virol.* **71:**3069–3076.
100. **Lukac, D. M., R. Renne, J. R. Kirshner, and D. Ganem.** 1998. Reactivation of Kaposi's sarcoma-associated herpesvirus infection from latency by expression of the ORF 50 transactivator, a homolog of the EBV R protein. *Virology* **252:**304–312.
101. **Luppi, M., P. Barozzi, G. Guaraldi, L. Ravazzini, V. Rasini, C. Spano, G. Riva, D. Vallerini, A. D. Pinna, and G. Torelli.** 2003. Human herpesvirus 8-associated diseases in solid-organ transplantation: importance of viral transmission from the donor. *Clin. Infect. Dis.* **37:** 606–607. (Author's reply, **37:**607.)
102. **Luppi, M., P. Barozzi, T. F. Schulz, G. Setti, K. Staskus, R. Trovato, F. Narni, A. Donelli, A. Maiorana, R. Marasca, S. Sandrini, G. Torelli, and J. Sheldon.** 2000. Bone marrow failure associated with human herpesvirus 8 infection after transplantation. *N. Engl. J. Med.* **343:**1378–1385.
103. **Lyall, E. G., G. S. Patton, J. Sheldon, C. Stainsby, J. Mullen, S. O'Shea, N. A. Smith, A. De Ruiter, M. O. McClure, and T. F. Schulz.** 1999. Evidence for horizontal and not vertical transmission of human herpesvirus 8 in children born to human immunodeficiency virus-infected mothers. *Pediatr. Infect. Dis. J.* **18:**795–799.
104. **Malope, B. I., R. M. Pfeiffer, G. Mbisa, L. Stein, E. M. Ratshikhopha, D. L. O'Connell, F. Sitas, P. MacPhail, and D. Whitby.** 2007. Transmission of Kaposi sarcoma-associated herpesvirus between mothers and children in a South African population. *J. Acquir. Immune. Defic. Syndr.* **44:**351–355.
105. **Margolius, L., M. Stein, D. Spencer, and W. R. Bezwoda.** 1994. Kaposi's sarcoma in renal transplant recipients. Experience at Johannesburg Hospital, 1966–1989. *S. Afr. Med. J.* **84:**16–17.
106. **Martin, D. F., B. D. Kuppermann, R. A. Wolitz, A. G. Palestine, H. Li, and C. A. Robinson.** 1999. Oral ganciclovir for patients with cytomegalovirus retinitis treated with a ganciclovir implant. *N. Engl. J. Med.* **340:**1063–1070.
107. **Martin, J. N., D. E. Ganem, D. H. Osmond, K. A. Page-Shafer, D. Macrae, and D. H. Kedes.** 1998. Sexual

transmission and the natural history of human herpesvirus 8 infection. *N. Engl. J. Med.* **338:**948–954.

108. **Maslovsky, I., L. Uriev, and G. Lugassy.** 2000. The heterogeneity of Castleman disease: report of five cases and review of the literature. *Am. J. Med. Sci.* **320:**292–295.
109. **Matta, H., R. M. Surabhi, J. Zhao, V. Punj, Q. Sun, S. Schamus, L. Mazzacurati, and P. M. Chaudhary.** 2007. Induction of spindle cell morphology in human vascular endothelial cells by human herpesvirus 8-encoded viral FLICE inhibitory protein K13. *Oncogene* **26:**1656–1660.
110. **Maurer, T., M. Ponte, and K. Leslie.** 2007. HIV-associated Kaposi's sarcoma with a high CD4 count and a low viral load. *N. Engl. J. Med.* **357:**1352–1353.
111. **Mbulaiteye, S. M., R. J. Biggar, P. M. Bakaki, R. M. Pfeiffer, D. Whitby, A. M. Owor, E. Katongole-Mbidde, J. J. Goedert, C. M. Ndugwa, and E. A. Engels.** 2003. Human herpesvirus 8 infection and transfusion history in children with sickle-cell disease in Uganda. *J. Natl. Cancer Inst.* **95:**1330–1335.
112. **Mbulaiteye, S. M., E. T. Katabira, H. Wabinga, D. M. Parkin, P. Virgo, R. Ochai, M. Workneh, A. Coutinho, and E. A. Engels.** 2006. Spectrum of cancers among HIV-infected persons in Africa: the Uganda AIDS-Cancer Registry Match Study. *Int. J. Cancer* **118:**985–990.
113. **McGeoch, D. J., D. Gatherer, and A. Dolan.** 2005. On phylogenetic relationships among major lineages of the Gammaherpesvirinae. *J. Gen. Virol.* **86:**307–316.
114. **Medveczky, M. M., E. Horvath, T. Lund, and P. G. Medveczky.** 1997. *In vitro* antiviral drug sensitivity of the Kaposi's sarcoma-associated herpesvirus. *AIDS* **11:** 1327–1332.
115. **Mendez, J. C., and C. V. Paya.** 2000. Kaposi's sarcoma and transplantation. *Herpes* **7:**18–23.
116. **Mittnacht, S., and C. Boshoff.** 2000. Viral cyclins. *Rev. Med. Virol.* **10:**175–184.
117. **Moore, P. S.** 2007. KSHV manipulation of the cell cycle and programmed cell death pathways, p. 540–558. *In* A. Arvin, G. Campadelli-Fiume, E. Mocarski, P. S. Moore, B. Roizman, R. Whitley, and K. Yamanishi (ed.), *Human Herpesviruses: Biology, Therapy and Immunoprophylaxis*. Cambridge University Press, Cambridge, United Kingdom.
118. **Moore, P. S., C. Boshoff, R. A. Weiss, and Y. Chang.** 1996. Molecular mimicry of human cytokine and cytokine response pathway genes by KSHV. *Science* **274:** 1739–1744.
119. **Moore, P. S., and Y. Chang.** 2003. Kaposi's sarcoma-associated herpesvirus immunoevasion and tumorigenesis: two sides of the same coin? *Annu. Rev. Microbiol.* **57:**609–639.
120. **Moore, P. S., S. J. Gao, G. Dominguez, E. Cesarman, O. Lungu, D. M. Knowles, R. Garber, P. E. Pellett, D. J. McGeoch, and Y. Chang.** 1996. Primary characterization of a herpesvirus agent associated with Kaposi's sarcoma. *J. Virol.* **70:**549–558. (Erratum, **70:**9083.)
121. **Moore, P. S., L. A. Kingsley, S. D. Holmberg, T. Spira, P. Gupta, D. R. Hoover, J. P. Parry, L. J. Conley, H. W. Jaffe, and Y. Chang.** 1996. Kaposi's sarcoma-associated herpesvirus infection prior to onset of Kaposi's sarcoma. *AIDS* **10:**175–180.
122. **Munoz-Fontela, C., L. Marcos-Villar, P. Gallego, J. Arroyo, M. Da Costa, K. M. Pomeranz, E. W. Lam, and C. Rivas.** 2007. Latent protein LANA2 from Kaposi's sarcoma-associated herpesvirus interacts with 14-3-3 proteins and inhibits FOXO3a transcription factor. *J. Virol.* **81:**1511–1516.
123. **Nador, R. G., E. Cesarman, A. Chadburn, D. B. Dawson, M. Q. Ansari, J. Sald, and D. M. Knowles.** 1996. Primary effusion lymphoma: a distinct clinicopathologic entity associated with the Kaposi's sarcoma-associated herpes virus. *Blood* **88:**645–656.
124. **Nador, R. G., E. Cesarman, D. M. Knowles, and J. W. Said.** 1995. Herpes-like DNA sequences in a body-cavity-based lymphoma in an HIV-negative patient. *N. Engl. J. Med.* **333:**943.
125. **Nakamura, H., M. Li, J. Zarycki, and J. U. Jung.** 2001. Inhibition of p53 tumor suppressor by viral interferon regulatory factor. *J. Virol.* **75:**7572–7582.
126. **Nealon, K., W. W. Newcomb, T. R. Pray, C. S. Craik, J. C. Brown, and D. H. Kedes.** 2001. Lytic replication of Kaposi's sarcoma-associated herpesvirus results in the formation of multiple capsid species: isolation and molecular characterization of A, B, and C capsids from a gammaherpesvirus. *J. Virol.* **75:**2866–2878.
127. **Neipel, F., J. C. Albrecht, and B. Fleckenstein.** 1997. Cell-homologous genes in the Kaposi's sarcoma-associated rhadinovirus human herpesvirus 8: determinants of its pathogenicity? *J. Virol.* **71:**4187–4192.
128. **Nekorchuk, M., Z. Han, T.-T. Hsieh, and S. Swaminathan.** 2007. Kaposi's sarcoma-associated herpesvirus ORF57 protein enhances mRNA accumulation independent of effects on nuclear RNA export. *J. Virol.* **81:** 9990–9998.
129. **Ocio, E. M., F. M. Sanchez-Guijo, M. Diez-Campelo, C. Castilla, O. J. Blanco, D. Caballero, and J. F. San Miguel.** 2005. Efficacy of rituximab in an aggressive form of multicentric Castleman disease associated with immune phenomena. *Am. J. Hematol.* **78:**302–305.
130. **Oettle, A. G.** 1962. Geographical and racial differences in the frequency of Kaposi's sarcoma as evidence of environmental or genetic causes. *Acta Unio Int. Contra Cancrum* **18:**330–363.
131. **Oksenhendler, E., D. Cazals-Hatem, T. F. Schulz, V. Barateau, L. Grollet, J. Sheldon, J. P. Clauvel, F. Sigaux, and F. Agbalika.** 1998. Transient angiolymphoid hyperplasia and Kaposi's sarcoma after primary infection with human herpesvirus 8 in a patient with human immunodeficiency virus infection. *N. Engl. J. Med.* **338:** 1585–1590.
132. **Olsen, S. J., R. Sarid, Y. Chang, and P. S. Moore.** 2000. Evaluation of the latency-associated nuclear antigen (ORF73) of Kaposi's sarcoma-associated herpesvirus by peptide mapping and bacterially expressed recombinant Western blot assay. *J. Infect. Dis.* **182:**306–310.
133. **Orenstein, J. M., S. Alkan, A. Blauvelt, K. T. Jeang, M. D. Weinstein, D. Ganem, and B. Herndier.** 1997. Visualization of human herpesvirus type 8 in Kaposi's sarcoma by light and transmission electron microscopy. *AIDS* **11:**F35–F45.
134. **Park, J., T. Seo, S. Hwang, D. Lee, Y. Gwack, and J. Choe.** 2000. The K-bZIP protein from Kaposi's sarcoma-associated herpesvirus interacts with p53 and represses its transcriptional activity. *J. Virol.* **74:**11977–11982.
135. **Parravicini, C., M. Corbellino, M. Paulli, U. Magrini, M. Lazzarino, P. S. Moore, and Y. Chang.** 1997. Expression of a virus-derived cytokine, KSHV vIL-6, in HIV-seronegative Castleman's disease. *Am. J. Pathol.* **151:**1517–1522.
136. **Parravicini, C., S. J. Olsen, M. Capra, F. Poli, G. Sirchia, S.-J. Gao, E. Berti, A. Nocera, E. Rossi, G. Bestetti, M. Pizzuto, M. Galli, M. Moroni, P. S. Moore, and M. Corbellino.** 1997. Risk of Kaposi's sarcoma-associated herpesvirus transmission from donor allografts among Italian posttransplant Kaposi's sarcoma patients. *Blood* **90:**2826–2829.

137. **Pattingre, S., A. Tassa, X. Qu, R. Garuti, X. H. Liang, N. Mizushima, M. Packer, M. D. Schneider, and B. Levine.** 2005. Bcl-2 antiapoptotic proteins inhibit Beclin 1-dependent autophagy. *Cell* **122:**927–939.
138. **Pau, C.-P., L. L. Lam, T. J. Spira, J. B. Black, J. A. Stewart, P. E. Pellett, and R. A. Respess.** 1998. Mapping and serodiagnostic application of a dominant epitope within the human herpesvirus 8 ORF 65-encoded protein. *J. Clin. Microbiol.* **36:**1574–1577.
139. **Pellett, P. E., D. J. Wright, E. A. Engels, D. V. Ablashi, S. C. Dollard, B. Forghani, S. A. Glynn, J. J. Goedert, F. J. Jenkins, T. H. Lee, F. Neipel, D. S. Todd, D. Whitby, G. J. Nemo, and M. P. Busch.** 2003. Multicenter comparison of serologic assays and estimation of human herpesvirus 8 seroprevalence among US blood donors. *Transfusion* **43:**1260–1268.
140. **Perez, C., M. Tous, S. Gallego, N. Zala, O. Rabinovich, S. Garbiero, M. J. Martinez, A. M. Cunha, S. Camino, A. Camara, S. C. Costa, M. Larrondo, V. Francalancia, F. Landreau, and M. A. Bartomioli.** 2004. Seroprevalence of human herpesvirus-8 in blood donors from different geographical regions of Argentina, Brazil, and Chile. *J. Med. Virol.* **72:**661–667.
141. **Pfeffer, S., A. Sewer, M. Lagos-Quintana, R. Sheridan, C. Sander, F. A. Grasser, L. F. van Dyk, C. K. Ho, S. Shuman, M. Chien, J. J. Russo, J. Ju, G. Randall, B. D. Lindenbach, C. M. Rice, V. Simon, D. D. Ho, M. Zavolan, and T. Tuschl.** 2005. Identification of microRNAs of the herpesvirus family. *Nat. Methods* **2:** 269–276.
142. **Poole, L. J., J. C. Zong, D. M. Ciufo, D. J. Alcendor, J. S. Cannon, R. Ambinder, J. M. Orenstein, M. S. Reitz, and G. S. Hayward.** 1999. Comparison of genetic variability at multiple loci across the genomes of the major subtypes of Kaposi's sarcoma-associated herpesvirus reveals evidence for recombination and for two distinct types of open reading frame K15 alleles at the right-hand end. *J. Virol.* **73:**6646–6660.
143. **Pozharskaya, V. P., L. L. Weakland, J. C. Zimring, L. T. Krug, E. R. Unger, A. Neisch, H. Joshi, N. Inoue, and M. K. Offermann.** 2004. Short duration of elevated vIRF-1 expression during lytic replication of human herpesvirus 8 limits its ability to block antiviral responses induced by alpha interferon in BCBL-1 cells. *J. Virol.* **78:**6621–6635.
144. **Qunibi, W., M. Akhtar, K. Sheth, H. E. Ginn, F. O. Al, E. B. DeVol, and S. Taher.** 1988. Kaposi's sarcoma: the most common tumor after renal transplantation in Saudi Arabia. *Am. J. Med.* **84:**225–232.
145. **Radkov, S. A., P. Kellam, and C. Boshoff.** 2000. The latent nuclear antigen of Kaposi sarcoma-associated herpesvirus targets the retinoblastoma-E2F pathway and with the oncogene Hras transforms primary rat cells. *Nat. Med.* **6:**1121–1127.
146. **Rainbow, L., G. M. Platt, G. R. Simpson, R. Sarid, S. J. Gao, H. Stoiber, C. S. Herrington, P. S. Moore, and T. F. Schulz.** 1997. The 222- to 234-kilodalton latent nuclear protein (LNA) of Kaposi's sarcoma-associated herpesvirus (human herpesvirus 8) is encoded by orf73 and is a component of the latency-associated nuclear antigen. *J. Virol.* **71:**5915–5921.
147. **Regamey, N., M. Tamm, M. Wernli, A. Witschi, G. Thiel, G. Cathomas, and P. Erb.** 1998. Transmission of human herpesvirus 8 infection from renal-transplant donors to recipients. *N. Engl. J. Med.* **339:**1358–1363.
148. **Renne, R., W. Zhong, B. Herndier, M. McGrath, N. Abbey, D. Kedes, and D. Ganem.** 1996. Lytic growth of Kaposi's sarcoma-associated herpesvirus (human herpesvirus 8) in culture. *Nat. Med.* **2:**342–346.
149. **Renwick, N., T. Halaby, G. J. Weverling, N. H. Dukers, G. R. Simpson, R. A. Coutinho, J. M. Lange, T. F. Schulz, and J. Goudsmit.** 1998. Seroconversion for human herpesvirus 8 during HIV infection is highly predictive of Kaposi's sarcoma. *AIDS* **12:**2481–2488.
150. **Rivas, C., A. E. Thlick, C. Parravicini, P. S. Moore, and Y. Chang.** 2001. Kaposi's sarcoma-associated herpesvirus LANA2 is a B-cell-specific latent viral protein that inhibits p53. *J. Virol.* **75:**429–438.
151. **Robles, R., D. Lugo, L. Gee, and M. A. Jacobson.** 1999. Effect of antiviral drugs used to treat cytomegalovirus end-organ disease on subsequent course of previously diagnosed Kaposi's sarcoma in patients with AIDS. *J. Acquir. Immune Defic. Syndr. Hum. Retrovirol.* **20:**34–38.
152. **Rose, T. M., K. B. Strand, E. R. Schultz, G. Schaefer, G. J. Rankin, M. E. Thouless, C. C. Tsai, and M. L. Bosch.** 1997. Identification of two homologs of the Kaposi's sarcoma-associated herpesvirus (human herpesvirus 8) in retroperitoneal fibromatosis of different macaque species. *J. Virol.* **71:**4138–4144.
153. **Russo, J. J., R. A. Bohenzky, M. C. Chien, J. Chen, M. Yan, D. Maddalena, J. P. Parry, D. Peruzzi, I. S. Edelman, Y. Chang, and P. S. Moore.** 1996. Nucleotide sequence of the Kaposi sarcoma-associated herpesvirus (HHV8). *Proc. Natl. Acad. Sci. USA* **93:**14862–14867.
154. **Sanchez, D. J., J. E. Gumperz, and D. Ganem.** 2005. Regulation of CD1d expression and function by a herpesvirus infection. *J. Clin. Investig.* **115:**1369–1378.
155. **Sarek, G., S. Kurki, J. Enback, G. Iotzova, J. Haas, P. Laakkonen, M. Laiho, and P. M. Ojala.** 2007. Reactivation of the p53 pathway as a treatment modality for KSHV-induced lymphomas. *J. Clin. Invest.* **117:**1019–1028.
156. **Sarid, R., O. Flore, R. A. Bohenzky, Y. Chang, and P. S. Moore.** 1998. Transcription mapping of the Kaposi's sarcoma-associated herpesvirus (human herpesvirus 8) genome in a body cavity-based lymphoma cell line (BC-1). *J. Virol.* **72:**1005–1012.
157. **Sarid, R., T. Sato, R. A. Bohenzky, J. J. Russo, and Y. Chang.** 1997. Kaposi's sarcoma-associated herpesvirus encodes a functional bcl-2 homologue. *Nat. Med.* **3:** 293–298.
158. **Sarid, R., J. S. Wiezorek, P. S. Moore, and Y. Chang.** 1999. Characterization and cell cycle regulation of the major Kaposi's sarcoma-associated herpesvirus (human herpesvirus 8) latent genes and their promoter. *J. Virol.* **73:**1438–1446.
159. **Seo, T., J. Park, D. Lee, S. G. Hwang, and J. Choe.** 2001. Viral interferon regulatory factor 1 of Kaposi's sarcoma-associated herpesvirus binds to p53 and represses p53-dependent transcription and apoptosis. *J. Virol.* **75:**6193–6198.
160. **Shin, Y. C., H. Nakamura, X. Liang, P. Feng, H. Chang, T. F. Kowalik, and J. U. Jung.** 2006. Inhibition of the ATM/p53 signal transduction pathway by Kaposi's sarcoma-associated herpesvirus interferon regulatory factor 1. *J. Virol.* **80:**2257–2266.
161. **Simpson, G. R., T. F. Schulz, D. Whitby, P. M. Cook, C. Boshoff, L. Rainbow, M. R. Howard, S. J. Gao, R. A. Bohenzky, P. Simmonds, C. Lee, A. de Ruiter, A. Hatzakis, R. S. Tedder, I. V. Weller, R. A. Weiss, and P. S. Moore.** 1996. Prevalence of Kaposi's sarcoma associated herpesvirus infection measured by antibodies to recombinant capsid protein and latent immunofluorescence antigen. *Lancet* **348:**1133–1138.
162. **Sitas, F., H. Carrara, V. Beral, R. Newton, G. Reeves, D. Bull, U. Jentsch, R. Pacella-Norman, D. Bourboulia, D. Whitby, C. Boshoff, R. Weiss, M. Patel, P. Ruff,**

W. R. Bezwoda, E. Retter, and M. Hale. 1999. Antibodies against human herpesvirus 8 in black South African patients with cancer. *N. Engl. J. Med.* **340:**1863–1871.

163. **Soulier, J., L. Grollet, E. Oksenhendler, P. Cacoub, D. Cazals-Hatem, P. Babinet, M.-F. d'Agay, J.-P. Clauvel, M. Raphael, L. Degos, and F. Sigaux.** 1995. Kaposi's sarcoma-associated herpesvirus-like DNA sequences in multicentric Castleman's disease. *Blood* **86:**1276–1280.
164. **Sozzani, S., W. Luini, G. Bianchi, P. Allavena, T. N. Wells, M. Napolitano, G. Bernardini, A. Vecchi, D. D'Ambrosio, D. Mazzeo, F. Sinigaglia, A. Santoni, E. Maggi, S. Romagnani, and A. Mantovani.** 1998. The viral chemokine macrophage inflammatory protein-II is a selective Th2 chemoattractant. *Blood* **92:**4036–4039.
165. **Spiller, O. B., L. Mark, C. E. Blue, D. G. Proctor, J. A. Aitken, A. M. Blom, and D. J. Blackbourn.** 2006. Dissecting the regions of virion-associated Kaposi's sarcoma-associated herpesvirus complement control protein required for complement regulation and cell binding. *J. Virol.* **80:**4068–4078.
166. **Spira, T. J., L. Lam, S. C. Dollard, Y. X. Meng, C. P. Pau, J. B. Black, D. Burns, B. Cooper, M. Hamid, J. Huong, K. Kite-Powell, and P. E. Pellett.** 2000. Comparison of serologic assays and PCR for diagnosis of human herpesvirus 8 infection. *J. Clin. Microbiol.* **38:**2174–2180.
167. **Stallone, G., A. Schena, B. Infante, S. Di Paolo, A. Loverre, G. Maggio, E. Ranieri, L. Gesualdo, F. P. Schena, and G. Grandaliano.** 2005. Sirolimus for Kaposi's sarcoma in renal-transplant recipients. *N. Engl. J. Med.* **352:**1317–1323.
168. **Staskus, K. A., W. Zhong, K. Gebhard, B. Herndier, H. Wang, R. Renne, J. Beneke, J. Pudney, D. J. Anderson, D. Ganem, and A. T. Haase.** 1997. Kaposi's sarcoma-associated herpesvirus gene expression in endothelial (spindle) tumor cells. *J. Virol.* **71:**715–719.
169. **Stine, J. T., C. Wood, M. Hill, A. Epp, C. J. Raport, V. L. Schweickart, Y. Endo, T. Sasaki, G. Simmons, C. Boshoff, P. Clapham, Y. Chang, P. Moore, P. W. Gray, and D. Chantry.** 2000. KSHV-encoded CC chemokine vMIP-III is a CCR4 agonist, stimulates angiogenesis, and selectively chemoattracts TH2 cells. *Blood* **95:**1151–1157.
170. **Sun, R., S.-F. Lin, L. Gradoville, and G. Miller.** 1996. Polyadenylated nuclear RNA encoded by Kaposi sarcoma-associated herpesvirus. *Proc. Natl. Acad. Sci. USA* **93:**11883–11888.
171. **Sun, R., S. F. Lin, L. Gradoville, Y. Yuan, F. Zhu, and G. Miller.** 1998. A viral gene that activates lytic cycle expression of Kaposi's sarcoma-associated herpesvirus. *Proc. Natl. Acad. Sci. USA* **95:**10866–10871.
172. **Sun, R., S. F. Lin, K. Staskus, L. Gradoville, E. Grogan, A. Haase, and G. Miller.** 1999. Kinetics of Kaposi's sarcoma-associated herpesvirus gene expression. *J. Virol.* **73:**2232–2242.
173. **Thome, M., P. Schneider, K. Hofman, H. Fickenscher, E. Meinl, F. Neipel, C. Mattmann, K. Burns, J.-L. Bodmer, M. Schröter, C. Scaffidl, P. H. Krammer, M. E. Peter, and J. Tschopp.** 1997. Viral FLICE-inhibitory proteins (FLIPs) prevent apoptosis induced by death receptors. *Nature* **386:**517–521.
174. **Trus, B. L., J. B. Heymann, K. Nealon, N. Cheng, W. W. Newcomb, J. C. Brown, D. H. Kedes, and A. C. Steven.** 2001. Capsid structure of Kaposi's sarcoma-associated herpesvirus, a gammaherpesvirus, compared to those of an alphaherpesvirus, herpes simplex virus type 1, and a betaherpesvirus, cytomegalovirus. *J. Virol.* **75:**2879–2890.
175. **Verschuren, E. W., N. Jones, and G. I. Evan.** 2004. The cell cycle and how it is steered by Kaposi's sarcoma-associated herpesvirus cyclin. *J. Gen. Virol.* **85:**1347–1361.
176. **Wabinga, H. R., D. M. Parkin, F. Wabwire-Mangen, and J. Mugerwa.** 1993. Cancer in Kampala, Uganda, in 1989–91: changes in incidence in the era of AIDS. *Int. J. Cancer* **54:**5–22.
177. **Walter, P. R., E. Philippe, C. Nguemby-Mbina, and A. Chamlian.** 1984. Kaposi's sarcoma: presence of herpes-type particles in a tumor specimen. *Hum. Pathol.* **15:**1145–1146.
178. **Wang, S. E., F. Y. Wu, M. Fujimuro, J. Zong, S. D. Hayward, and G. S. Hayward.** 2003. Role of CCAAT/enhancer-binding protein alpha (C/EBPalpha) in activation of the Kaposi's sarcoma-associated herpesvirus (KSHV) lytic-cycle replication-associated protein (RAP) promoter in cooperation with the KSHV replication and transcription activator (RTA) and RAP. *J. Virol.* **77:**600–623.
179. **Whitby, D., M. R. Howard, M. Tenant-Flowers, N. S. Brink, A. Copas, C. Boshoff, T. Hatzioannou, F. E. A. Suggett, D. M. Aldam, A. S. Denton, R. F. Miller, I. V. D. Weller, R. A. Weiss, R. S. Tedder, and T. F. Schulz.** 1995. Detection of Kaposi's sarcoma-associated herpesvirus (KSHV) in peripheral blood of HIV-infected individuals predicts progression to Kaposi's sarcoma. *Lancet* **364:**799–802.
180. **Whitby, D., M. Luppi, P. Barozzi, C. Boshoff, R. A. Weiss, and G. Torelli.** 1998. Human herpesvirus 8 seroprevalence in blood donors and lymphoma patients from different regions of Italy. *J. Natl. Cancer Inst.* **90:**395–397.
181. **Whitby, D., M. Luppi, C. Sabin, P. Barozzi, A. R. Di Biase, F. Balli, F. Cucci, R. A. Weiss, C. Boshoff, and G. Torelli.** 2000. Detection of antibodies to human herpesvirus 8 in Italian children: evidence for horizontal transmission. *Br. J. Cancer* **82:**702–704.
182. **Whitman, A. G., O. F. Dyson, P. J. Lambert, T. L. Oxendine, P. W. Ford, and S. M. Akula.** 2007. Changes occurring on the cell surface during KSHV reactivation. *J. Electron Microsc.* **56:**27–36.
183. **Wu, F. Y., Q. Q. Tang, H. Chen, C. ApRhys, C. Farrell, J. Chen, M. Fujimuro, M. D. Lane, and G. S. Hayward.** 2002. Lytic replication-associated protein (RAP) encoded by Kaposi sarcoma-associated herpesvirus causes $p21^{CIP-1}$-mediated G_1 cell cycle arrest through CCAAT/enhancer-binding protein-α. *Proc. Natl. Acad. Sci. USA* **99:**10683–10688.
184. **Wu, L., P. Lo, X. Yu, J. K. Stoops, B. Forghani, and Z. H. Zhou.** 2000. Three-dimensional structure of the human herpesvirus 8 capsid. *J. Virol.* **74:**9646–9654.
185. **Yang, B. T., S. C. Chen, M. W. Leach, D. Manfra, B. Homey, M. Wiekowski, L. Sullivan, C. H. Jenh, S. K. Narula, S. W. Chensue, and S. A. Lira.** 2000. Transgenic expression of the chemokine receptor encoded by human herpesvirus 8 induces an angioproliferative disease resembling Kaposi's sarcoma. *J. Exp. Med.* **191:**445–454.
186. **Yoo, S. M., F. C. Zhou, F. C. Ye, H. Y. Pan, and S. J. Gao.** 2005. Early and sustained expression of latent and host modulating genes in coordinated transcriptional program of KSHV productive primary infection of human primary endothelial cells. *Virology* **343:**47–64.
187. **Yu, F., J. N. Harada, H. J. Brown, H. Deng, M. J. Song, T. T. Wu, J. Kato-Stankiewicz, C. G. Nelson, J. Vieira, F. Tamanoi, S. K. Chanda, and R. Sun.** 2007. Systematic identification of cellular signals reactivating

Kaposi sarcoma-associated herpesvirus. *PLoS Pathog.* **3:** e44.

188. **Zaldumbide, A., M. Ossevoort, E. J. Wiertz, and R. C. Hoeben.** 2007. In cis inhibition of antigen processing by the latency-associated nuclear antigen I of Kaposi sarcoma herpes virus. *Mol. Immunol.* **44:**1352–1360.
189. **Zhong, W., and D. Ganem.** 1997. Characterization of ribonucleoprotein complexes containing an abundant polyadenylated nuclear RNA encoded by Kaposi's sarcoma-associated herpesvirus (human herpesvirus 8). *J. Virol.* **71:**1207–1212.
190. **Zhu, F. X., J. M. Chong, L. Wu, and Y. Yuan.** 2005. Virion proteins of Kaposi's sarcoma-associated herpesvirus. *J. Virol.* **79:**800–811.
191. **Zhu, F. X., T. Cusano, and Y. Yuan.** 1999. Identification of the immediate-early transcripts of Kaposi's sarcoma-associated herpesvirus. *J. Virol.* **73:**5556–5567.
192. **Zhu, F. X., X. Li, F. Zhou, S. J. Gao, and Y. Yuan.** 2006. Functional characterization of Kaposi's sarcoma-associated herpesvirus ORF45 by bacterial artificial chromosome-based mutagenesis. *J. Virol.* **80:**12187–12196.
193. **Ziegler, J. L., and E. Katongole-Mbidde.** 1996. Kaposi's sarcoma in childhood: an analysis of 100 cases from Uganda and relationship to HIV infection. *Int. J. Cancer* **65:**200–203.
194. **Zimring, J. C., S. Goodbourn, and M. K. Offermann.** 1998. Human herpesvirus 8 encodes an interferon regulatory factor (IRF) homolog that represses IRF-1-mediated transcription. *J. Virol.* **72:**701–707.
195. **Zong, J. C., D. M. Ciufo, D. J. Alcendor, X. Wan, J. Nicholas, P. J. Browning, P. L. Rady, S. K. Tyring, J. M. Orenstein, C. S. Rabkin, I. J. Su, K. F. Powell, M. Croxson, K. E. Foreman, B. J. Nickoloff, S. Alkan, and G. S. Hayward.** 1999. High-level variability in the ORF-K1 membrane protein gene at the left end of the Kaposi's sarcoma-associated herpesvirus genome defines four major virus subtypes and multiple variants or clades in different human populations. *J. Virol.* **73:**4156–4170.

Adenoviruses

OLLI RUUSKANEN, JORDAN P. METCALF, OLLI MEURMAN, AND GÖRAN AKUSJÄRVI

26

Adenoviruses were first isolated in 1953 from adenoids and tonsils surgically removed from children (54). Soon after the recovery of adenoviruses from patients with respiratory illness, their role as a major cause of febrile infections in young children and in army recruits was recognized. The illness was originally called acute respiratory disease, but the signs and symptoms are similar to those of other viral respiratory syndromes, which should replace the old nonspecific expression.

Adenoviruses are most closely linked with infections of the respiratory tract and conjunctivae and account for 5 to 8% of all pediatric respiratory infections. Adenoviruses are also an important cause of childhood diarrhea. They have also been implicated in aseptic meningitis, myocarditis, encephalitis, hepatitis, and hemorrhagic cystitis and are increasingly recognized as an important cause of morbidity and mortality in stem cell and solid-organ transplant recipients.

VIROLOGY

Classification

Adenoviruses are widespread in nature and have been isolated from a large number of species, including fish (*Ichtadenovirus*), amphibians (*Siadenovirus*), reptiles (*Atadenovirus*), and the two most-studied genera, those isolated from primates (*Mastadenovirus*) and birds (*Aviadenovirus*) (11). There is no common antigenic determinant that characterizes the whole family. However, all members of the *Adenoviridae* family have virus particles of similar sizes, structures, and polypeptide compositions.

The human adenoviruses comprise 51 distinct serotypes that are grouped into six subgroups (A to F) based on various immunologic, biological, and biochemical characteristics (Table 1) (120). Based on hemagglutination with rat and monkey red blood cells, human adenoviruses were originally classified into four subgroups. Since then, multiple additional criteria, such as oncogenic potential, DNA sequence homology, restriction endonuclease cleavage patterns, polypeptide composition, and immunologic characteristics, have been used to further subdivide the human adenoviruses into six subgroups; subgroup B is further divided into B1 and B2 based on tropism and restriction cleavage patterns (Table 1). Members within each subgroup are classified on the basis of immunologic differences. Antibodies directed against the two major capsid proteins, hexon and fiber, are the most important determinants in the classification of serotypes. The genetic relatedness of serotypes within each subgroup is high. Based on DNA-DNA hybridization, members of each subgroup generally share greater than 85% homology, whereas serotypes belonging to different subgroups are less than 20% homologous (120).

Virus Composition

Adenoviruses are nonenveloped icosahedral viruses (20 triangular surfaces and 12 vertices) with a diameter of 65 to 80 nm. The three-dimensional structure of the approximately 150×10^6-Da adenovirus particle has been determined by cryoelectron microscopy (cryo-EM) combined with three-dimensional image reconstruction (115). The crystallographic structure of the adenovirus type 2 hexon capsomer has been refined to 2.2-Å resolution.

Figure 1 summarizes the composition as well as the predicted location of the various viral polypeptides in the virion. The capsid consists of 252 major capsomers: 240 hexons form the facets of the icosahedron, and 12 pentons are located at the corners of the virus particle. The hexon capsomer is a trimer of the hexon polypeptide held tightly together by noncovalent interactions. The pentons consist of two distinct structural entities: the penton base, which anchors the pentons to the capsid, and the fiber, which forms an elongated structure protruding from the vertices. The fiber is a trimer of polypeptide IV, and the penton base is a pentamer of polypeptide III. Adenoviruses belonging to different subgroups have fibers of different lengths and flexibilities. The length difference of the fibers results from a difference in the number of repeat units in the shaft regions of the fiber polypeptides. The viral capsid consists of four additional protein components, polypeptides IIIa, VI, VIII, and IX (Fig. 1). Polypeptide VI is located underneath the peripentonal hexons, and polypeptide VIII is located under the facets; these proteins provide a link between the inside surface of the capsid and the viral DNA. Polypeptide IIIa has been proposed to span the capsid and link adjacent facets to the vertex regions, but recent data suggest that the electron density at the outside of the virus particle previously assigned to IIIa is, in fact, polypeptide IX, which functions as a glue protein

TABLE 1 Classification of human adenoviruses[a]

Subgroup	Serotype(s)	HA subgroup[b]	Production of tumors in animals	% GC	Tropism
	12, 18, 31	IV	High	47–49	Intestine
B1	3, 7, 16, 21, 50	I	Weak	50–52	Respiratory
B2	11, 14, 34, 35	I	Weak	50–52	Renal
C	1, 2, 5, 6	III	Low or none	57–59	Respiratory
D	8–10, 13, 15, 17, 19, 20, 22–30, 32, 33, 36–39, 42–49, 51	II	Low or none	57–60	Ocular and other
E	4	III	Low or none	57	Respiratory
F	40, 41	III	Low or none	57–59	Intestinal

[a] Adapted from reference 120.
[b] HA subgroups are classified as follows: I, complete agglutination of monkey erythrocytes; II, complete agglutination of rat erythrocytes; III, partial agglutination of rat erythrocytes; IV, no agglutination.

stabilizing hexon capsomers on the outside. The viral core consists of four proteins, polypeptides V, VII, X (μ), and terminal protein (TP). In contrast to most DNA viruses, adenovirus codes for its own basic histone-like proteins, V, VII, and μ, which complex to the viral DNA within the virion. In addition, the termini of the viral DNA are covalently linked to the TP, which functions as a protein primer during viral DNA replication. For a more extensive review on virus structure, see reference 115.

Viral Genome

The viral genome consists of a linear double-stranded DNA molecule with a length of approximately 30,000 to 38,000 bp. The entire nucleotide sequence has been established for a large number of human and animal adenovirus serotypes (see GenBank). The lytic cycle is divided into two distinct phases: an early phase preceding viral DNA replication and a late phase that follows DNA replication and is characterized by expression of the structural proteins of the viral capsid. The viral DNA encodes a total of nine different transcription units, six that are active early after infection (E1A, E1B E2A, E3, E4, and L1) and three that become activated at intermediate (pIX and IVa2) and late (major late transcription unit [MLTU]) times of infection (Fig. 2). All transcription units, except pIX and IVa2, generate a complex set of alternatively spliced mRNAs that codes for multiple proteins, many that have distinct biological activities (Table 2 and below) (58). In addition, adenoviruses encode at least one (but usually both) of the highly structured small RNAs, the so-called virus-associated (VA) RNAI and VA RNAII (86), that perform important functions during the lytic infection cycle by blocking activation of the interferon response and probably the RNA interference (RNAi) machinery (4).

Biology

The replication strategy of adenovirus is summarized in Fig. 3. The infection cycle takes approximately 30 h in tissue culture cells and results in the production of approximately 50,000 to 100,000 new virus particles per cell. Here we divide the infectious cycle into four stages: entry, early events, late events, and virus assembly.

Entry

Adenovirus binds with a high efficiency to receptors on the surface of the host cell through the knob region of the fiber. The cellular receptors mediating the initial binding of adenovirus to the cell surface have recently been identified for several serotypes. The best-studied adenovirus receptor is CAR (coxsackie and adenovirus receptor), an immunoglobulin superfamily member protein containing two immunoglobulin-like extracellular domains that is also used by coxsackie B virus for infection (12). CAR appears to be a preferred primary receptor used by serotypes belonging to all subgroups, except subgroup B. Subgroup B viruses use the complement regulatory protein CD46 for virus attachment (150). Several members of subgenus D have been shown to use sialic acid as a cellular receptor. Adenovirus infects many cell types efficiently in vitro, while adenovirus infection of ciliated epithelia of the lung in vivo is relatively inefficient. This inefficiency appears to result from the fact that CAR is expressed in the tight junctions and along the basolateral membrane and therefore is not readily available for virus attachment (140). Consequently, the initial infection may be mediated by other components, like coagulation factor IX, dipalmitoyl phosphatidylcholine, or lactorferrin (62), that function as bridging factors between adenovirus and the cell.

With the exception of the subgroup F viruses (types 40 and 41 [Table 1]), all sequenced adenovirus serotypes encode a penton base protein with an RGD peptide motif. The RGD peptide serves as an interaction motif mediating contact with several cellular $\alpha\beta$ integrin adhesion receptors, which function as the secondary receptor for virus attachment. In addition to the initially discovered $\alpha_v\beta_3$ and $\alpha_v\beta_5$ integrins, other RGD binding integrins have also been characterized (150). Penton base interaction with the integrins activates internalization of adenovirus through phosphatidylinositol 3 kinase signaling (78). The virus is taken up by clathrin-mediated endocytosis (90). The vertex capsomer, the penton, is lost in the acidic endosome (Fig. 3). At this step polypeptide VI is released from the interior of the virus capsid. Since polypeptide VI has membrane-lytic activity (144), this protein may have a specific role in helping the partially dismantled virus disrupt the endosome and escape into the cytoplasm. By a

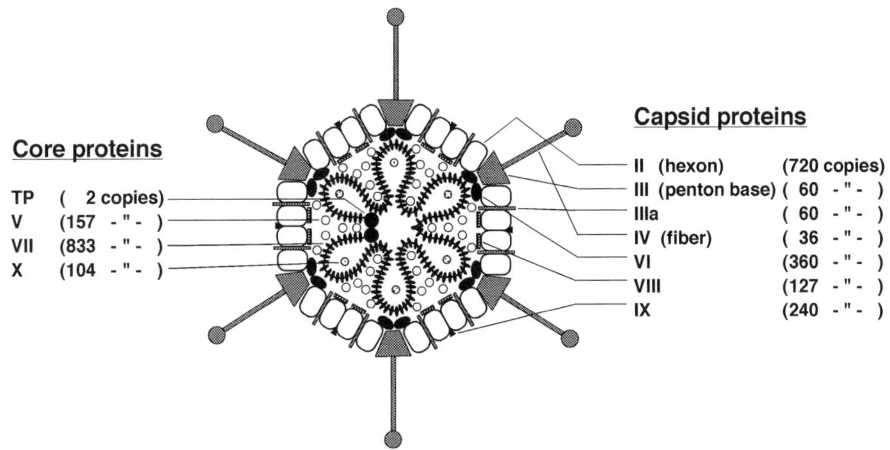

FIGURE 1 Schematic model illustrating the architecture of the adenovirus particle. The tentative location and copy number of polypeptides are indicated for the core and capsid proteins. (Adapted from reference 115 with permission.)

microtubule-dependent transport mechanism the virus is transported toward the nucleus, where it docks to a nuclear pore complex (132). Within 45 min of initial binding to the cell surface receptor, the viral DNA is injected into the cell nucleus. Viral entry is efficient, with 40% of the particles that bind to the cell surface delivering their DNA to the nucleus. Less than 5% of the incoming viruses end up degraded in lysosomes (51).

Early Events

Expression of the early viral mRNAs and proteins is temporally regulated during the infectious cycle. Thus, the first transcription unit to be activated is the E1A region, and transcripts from this region can be detected within 45 min after infection. The maximum rate of E1A transcription is then maintained for at least 16 h. The E1A proteins are essential for the initiation of the lytic infectious cycle since

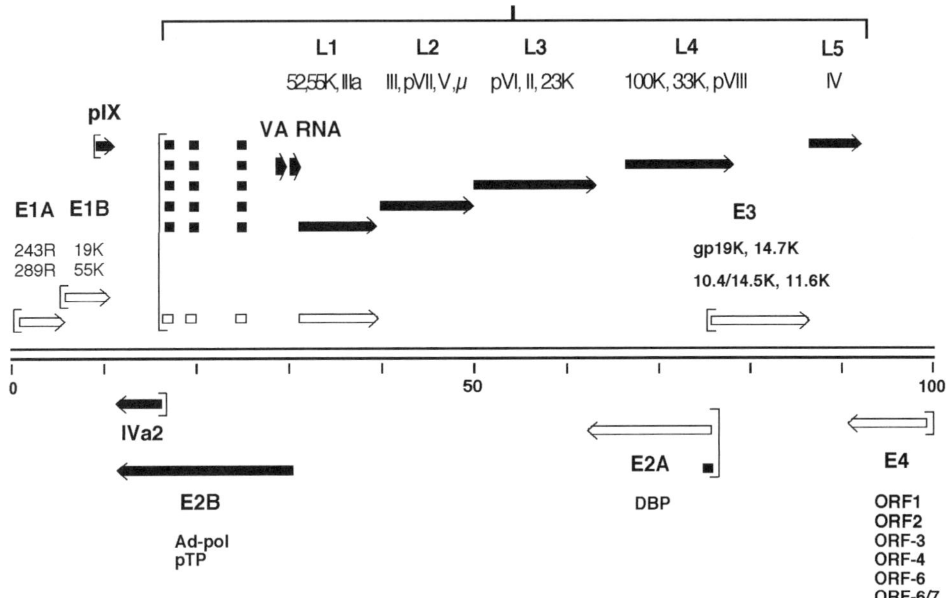

FIGURE 2 Adenovirus transcription map, here exemplified with human adenovirus type 2. Note that the alternatively sliced structures of individual mRNAs expressed from the different early and late units are not shown (see reference 120 for a detailed transcription map). White arrows indicate early transcription units, and black arrows indicate late transcription units. The functions of the nonstructural proteins expressed from respective transcription units are summarized in Table 2.

TABLE 2 Adenovirus early and late nonstructural proteins[a]

Protein	Function
Early	
E1A-289R	Major transcriptional activator protein encoded by the virus; regulates viral and some cellular promoters (13)
E1A-243R	Repressor of enhancer-dependent transcription and activator of some growth-regulated genes; activates cell cycling by displacing the pRb family of proteins from the E2F transcription factor (13)
E1B-19K	Homolog of the cellular BCL-2 protein; inhibits apoptosis by sequestering BAK and BAX (143)
E1B-55K	Inhibits the function of p53 (13); binds p53 and inactivates its transcription regulatory properties; forms a complex with the E4-ORF6 protein. This complex induces p53 ubiquitination and degradation and facilitates nuclear to cytoplasmic export of viral mRNAs late after infection (39)
E2A-DBP	Single-stranded DNA binding protein involved in viral DNA replication (136)
E2B-Ad-Pol	Adenovirus-encoded DNA polymerase (136)
E2B-pTP	Terminal precursor protein that functions as a protein primer for initiation of viral DNA replication (136)
E3-gp19K	Protects virus-infected cells against lysis by cytotoxic T cells by blocking major histocompatibility complex class I-restricted antigen presentation (79)
E3-14.7K	Inhibitor of TNF and TRAIL-induced apoptosis (79)
E3-10.4/14.5K	Receptor internalization and degradation complex; stimulates clearance of the Fas ligand and TRAIL receptors from the cell surface (79)
E3-11.6K	ADP; promotes virus release after completion of the infectious cycle (79)
E4-ORF3	Inhibits the MRN[b] DNA repair complex (128); inhibits the interferon-mediated antiviral response by disrupting the PML[c] oncogenic domain (134)
E4-ORF4	Binds to the B subunit of protein phosphatase 2A (14) and regulates a variety of activities in the cell, including transcription and RNA splicing; induces p53-independent apoptosis in transformed cells (65)
E4-ORF6	Forms a complex with the E1B-55K protein. This complex induces p53 ubiquitination and degradation and facilitates nuclear to cytoplasmic export of viral mRNAs late after infection (39)
E4-ORF6/7	Transcription factor inducing cooperative and stable binding of E2F to the E2 promoter (137)
Late	
L1-52,55K	Scaffolding protein in virus assembly; interacts with IVa2 and controls viral DNA encapsidation (100)
L3-23K	Viral protease that cleaves certain viral precursor proteins during virus maturation (142)
L4-100K	Required for hexon trimerization and nuclear transport; also enhances translation of tripartite-leader-containing mRNAs (26)
IVa2	Scaffolding protein and transcription factor augmenting major late promoter activity; binds to the viral packaging sequence and, together with the L1-52,55K protein, stimulates viral DNA encapsidation (100)
VA RNA	Two low-molecular-weight RNA polymerase III transcripts. VA RNAI is required for efficient translation late after infection. Protects virus-infected cells against the antiviral effect of interferon by preventing activation of the interferon-induced eIF2α kinase (86). Both VA RNAs suppress RNAi (4).

[a] For additional information, see reference 29a.
[b] MRN, Mre11-Rad50-NBS1.
[c] PML, promyelocytic leukemia protein.

they are key regulators of both viral and cellular transcription and necessary for efficient S-phase entry of the infected cell (14). Transcription from regions E1B, E3, and E4 begins around 1.5 h postinfection. Region E2 is the last early transcription unit to be activated, and RNA synthesis begins around 3 h postinfection. The central functions of the different early viral proteins in establishing a productive virus infection are summarized in Table 2.

Viral transcription units are reminiscent of bacterial operons in their organization. Genes with related biological functions are coordinately expressed. Thus, E1A codes for the viral proteins that regulate transcription, and E1B codes for proteins that protect the virus-infected cell from apoptotic death. Region E2 codes for the viral proteins that are directly involved in adenovirus DNA replication. Region E3 codes for proteins that counteract the host cell's antiviral defense mechanisms. Region E4 is slightly more complex and codes for proteins that regulate gene expression at the levels of transcription, RNA splicing, mRNA export, and protein stability. The major late transcription unit codes for the structural proteins of the virion. The VA RNAs function as decoy RNAs, subverting the activity

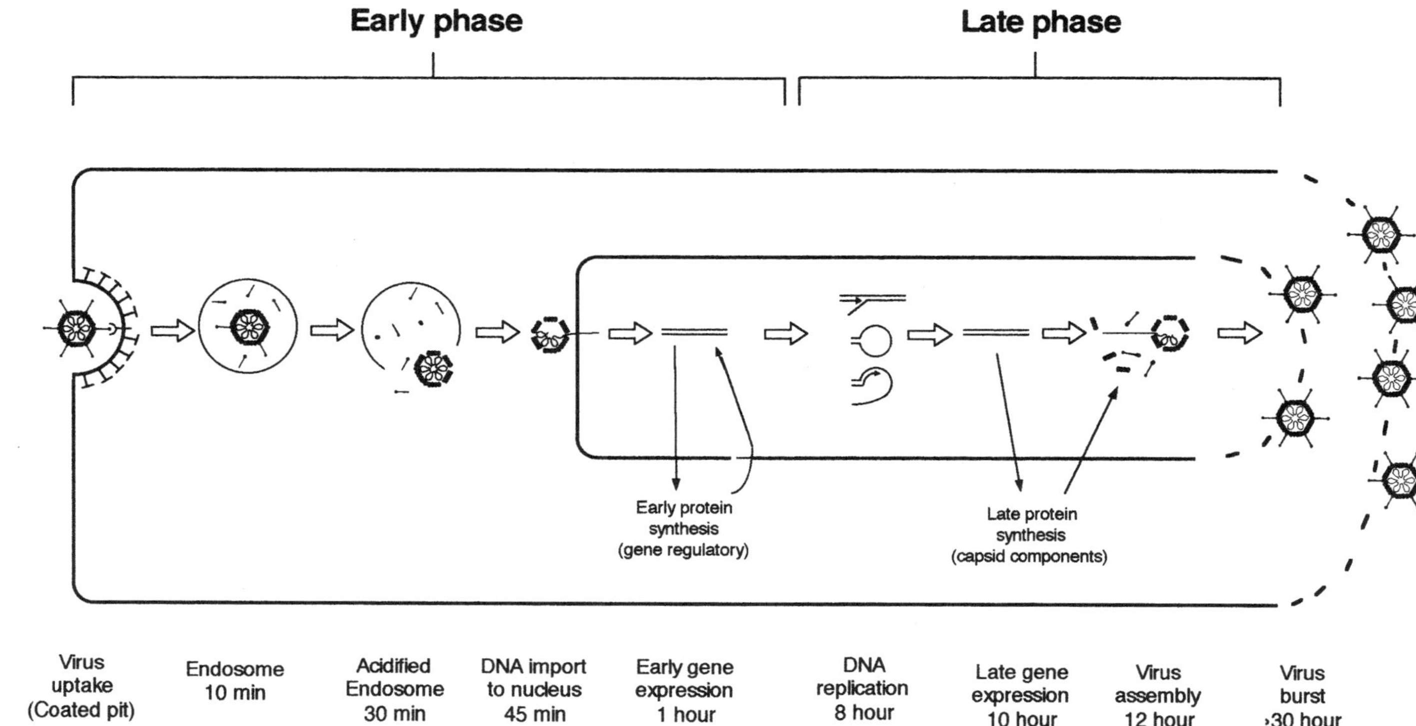

FIGURE 3 Diagram of adenovirus replication cycle. The approximate time scale for the different steps in the adenovirus life cycle is indicated at the bottom. See text for further details. For more extensive reviews, see references 51 and 120.

of cellular pathways that respond to double-stranded RNA.

LATE EVENTS

The late phase of the infectious cycle follows DNA replication, which begins around 8 h after infection. Adenoviruses use an unusual single-stranded DNA displacement strategy to replicate their DNA (120, 136). Initiation of viral DNA replication requires origin sequences that are located within the inverted terminal repeats at both ends of the chromosome. Replication initiates at either the left or right origin sequence and results in the displacement of the complementary strand as a single-stranded molecule (Fig. 3). Because of the inverted terminal repeat sequences, the displaced single-stranded DNA molecule can form partial duplex DNA structures that can be used to initiate DNA synthesis of the second strand. Initiation of adenovirus DNA replication occurs by a protein-priming mechanism in which the precursor terminal protein (pTP) covalently attached to the first nucleotide of the nascent strand functions as a primer for the virus-encoded DNA polymerase (Ad-Pol). Elongation is rapid and processive and also requires the viral single-stranded DNA binding protein. Only about 10% of viral DNA is incorporated into new virions.

Late after infection, transcription initiates predominantly at the so-called adenovirus major late promoter. Transcription from this promoter accounts for more than 30% of total RNA synthesis at late times of infection. This does not necessarily mean that the major late promoter is a strong promoter, since efficient transcription requires viral DNA replication, which amplifies the number of DNA templates available for transcription initiation (77). The major late transcription unit generates five families of late mRNAs with coterminal 3′ ends (L1 to L5 [Fig. 2]). Following selection of the poly(A) site, a complex set of mature mRNAs is generated by alternative RNA splicing (58). Most of the major late mRNAs encode structural proteins of the virion, whereas a few mRNAs encode proteins that are nonstructural and essential for replication (Table 2). Late during infection large amounts of the adenovirus VA RNAs (VA RNAI and VA RNAII) are synthesized. VA RNAI protects virus-infected cells against the antiviral effect of interferon by inhibiting the activity of the interferon-induced eIF2α-protein kinase (86). More recently, the VA RNAs have also been shown to suppress RNAi (4).

Late during infection, diminished cellular protein synthesis results in almost exclusive translation of late viral proteins. Mechanistically, this occurs by a selective transport of late viral mRNAs to the cytoplasm combined with an almost exclusive translation of mRNAs derived from the MLTU late after infection. The transcription of cellular genes is not inhibited, but nuclear to cytoplasmic transport of cellular mRNAs is strongly reduced in late virus-infected cells (9). Despite this inhibition of transport, viral mRNAs account for only 20% of the total cytoplasmic pool of mRNA. Nevertheless, more than 90% of total protein synthesis in late virus-infected cells is virus specific. Late adenovirus mRNAs possess the unique ability to be translated independently of the normal cap recognition process. Thus, inhibition of host protein synthesis has been shown to result from a virus-mediated block in cap-binding complex phosphorylation. The viral L4-100K protein has been shown to block association of the Mnk1 protein kinase, which is responsible for phosphorylation of the eIF4E component of the cap-binding complex (26). The tripartite leader, which is attached to all mRNAs derived from the MLTU, has been shown to be crucial for the cap-independent translation of viral mRNAs late after infection (26).

Virus Assembly

Most viral polypeptides are rapidly transported to the cell nucleus after synthesis. The very first step in virus assembly involves the formation of capsomers from monomeric polypeptide subunits: hexon, penton base, and fiber capsomers. The penton base and the fiber are then combined to form the penton, the vertex capsomer. Formation of the hexon capsomer requires the viral L4-100K protein, whereas fiber trimerization appears to be a spontaneous process. Structural components are made in huge excess in late virus-infected cells. Only 20% of hexon capsomers are incorporated into virions, and only 10% of viral DNA is encapsidated. Despite this inefficient process, around 100,000 virus particles are produced per infected cell (28).

During the assembly process, the first step is the formation of so-called empty capsids. These contain specific scaffolding proteins that are not found as stable polypeptides in mature virions and the structural proteins of the virion, except the core proteins, which come in at a later stage, together with the viral DNA. Empty capsids, which have a low density, mature into heavy intermediates by encapsidation of increasing amounts of the viral DNA. A *cis*-acting packaging element has been localized at the left end of the viral DNA, immediately downstream of the left inverted terminal repeat. This sequence element causes a preferential encapsidation of viral DNA into empty capsids beginning with the left end of the viral chromosome. The nonstructural virus-encoded IVa2 and L4-22K proteins bind to the packaging sequence (149). By a currently unclear mechanism, the L1-52,55K protein together with IVa2 and L4-22K facilitates encapsidation of the viral DNA into the empty capsids (100). After DNA encapsidation is completed, the young virions mature to fully infectious virions by proteolytic cleavage of five viral polypeptides that are made as precursor proteins (pIIIa, pV, pVI, pVII, and pTP). This proteolytic trimming is done by the L3-23K protease (142).

The infectious cycle is completed by the release of new virus particles from the infected cell. Two viral proteins have been suggested to promote viral escape by enhancing lysis of infected cells. The adenovirus death protein (ADP; also called E3-11.6K) is synthesized at very late stages of infection (>20 h postinfection) and promotes cell lysis. It may be the key factor that ensures efficient release of virus from infected cells (131). The virus-encoded E4-ORF4 protein has also been suggested to do the same by activating the apoptotic machinery at the very late stage of infection (84).

Host Range

Adenoviruses are generally species specific, so human adenoviruses preferentially infect humans. However, experimental infections have been established in rats, hamsters, rabbits, dogs, and swine. In most cases, virus production has been low and symptoms have been mild. In some cases, asymptomatic infections can lead to latency with prolonged persistence of the virus. In hamsters and other rodents, infections leading to tumorigenesis have been observed.

Inactivation by Chemical and Physical Agents

The sensitivities of different adenovirus serotypes to chemical biocides vary widely (117). Chloramine-T (*p*-toluenesulfonchloramide) at 5% for 15 min or at 0.6% for 30 min or 500 ppm of sodium hypochlorite for 10 min can be used to inactivate adenoviruses. Immersion in a water bath at 75°C for 30 s or 60°C for 2 min also kills the virus. Phenylmercuric borate, isopropyl alcohol, ether, cetrimide, and chlorhexidine gluconate do not inactivate adenoviruses.

EPIDEMIOLOGY

Adenovirus infections occur worldwide as endemic, epidemic, and sporadic infections. The most common adenovirus serotypes in clinical materials are the low-numbered respiratory types of subgenus C (1, 2, and 5) and subgenus B (3 and 7), as well as the gastroenteritis types 40 and 41. In the comprehensive World Health Organization (WHO) epidemiological study from 1967 to 1976, serotypes 2, 1, 7, 3, and 5 (in decreasing order) made up 90% of the 24,184 typed isolates (118). This study did not, however, include serotypes 40 and 41, which could not be isolated during that time. In a recent U.S. study from 2004 to 2006 with 2,237 adenovirus-positive specimens collected from 22 medical facilities, it was found that adenovirus types 3 (35%), 2 (24%), 1 (18%), and 5 (5%) were the most prevalent types. In children aged <7 years, types 1 and 2 were more prevalent than in older children (50). Recently, the emergence and spread of a virulent strain of adenovirus type 14 have been reported within the United States (22).

Each serotype consists of numerous genotypes, which can be differentiated by restriction enzyme analysis or sequencing (50). Within a serotype, especially in subgenus C, several genotypes circulate in parallel, but the prevailing genotypes change with time and show differences in geographic distribution. In hospital outbreaks, genotype analysis has been used to confirm the transmission pathways and similarities of strains. For stem cell transplant recipients, molecular typing can be used to discern whether a patient is having a reactivation of a latent adenovirus infection, a nosocomial infection, a community-acquired infection, or a donor-associated infection (50).

Incidence and Prevalence of Infection

Many adenovirus infections are subclinical. In large population-based respiratory "virus watch" studies, about 50% of persons from whom virus is isolated are asymptomatic (42, 43). However, some of these isolations are made during prolonged excretion of virus in stools after symptomatic infection. Thus, it is possible that the proportion of asymptomatic infections is smaller. Infection caused by gastroenteritis types 40 and 41 is often asymptomatic. In a study of gastroenteritis in Texas day care centers, 46% of such infections were asymptomatic.

Adenovirus infections induce the formation of neutralizing antibodies that are type specific and offer protection against reinfections caused by the same serotype. Protection is not complete, however, and reinfections may occur. In a Seattle, WA, virus watch study, reinfections were observed in 6% of seropositive family members (43); many of these were asymptomatic. In an adenovirus 3 outbreak in a boys' boarding school, previous infection provided 88% protection against reinfection. Similarly, previous neutralizing antibodies provided 87% protection in staff exposed to the index patient during a hospital epidemic caused by adenovirus 3a.

Of adenovirus serotypes causing respiratory infections, types 1, 2, 5, and 6 are mostly endemic, whereas 4, 7, 14, and 21 cause epidemics. Type 3 occurs both endemically and epidemically. Outbreaks have been described to occur in closed communities such as boarding schools and day care centers and among new military recruits (8). Community-wide epidemics also occur. The serotypes causing ocular infections (8, 19, and 37) are often endemic under the poor hygienic conditions of developing countries, but in Western countries, they occur mostly in epidemics which are sometimes nosocomial. The gastroenteritis serotypes 40 and 41 occur endemically throughout the world.

Rates of Age-Specific Attack

Adenovirus infections are most common between 6 months and 5 years of age but continue to occur throughout life. In the metropolitan New York virus watch study, the incidence of infection per 100 person-years was 40.8 in the age group 0 to 1 years, 33.6 between 2 and 4 years, 15.6 between 5 and 9 years, and 14.4 in the age group 10 years and older (42). These figures concur with seroepidemiological figures showing that about 33% of children have contracted at least one adenovirus infection by the age of 6 to 12 months and some have already contracted three or four adenovirus infections (Table 3).

The incidence of enteric adenovirus infections is from 4 to 7 per 100 person-years in young children (106). About half of preschool-age children have neutralizing antibodies against these serotypes.

The WHO epidemiological study indicates that serotypes 1, 2, and 5 are commonly contracted during the first years of life; serotypes 3 and 7 are contracted during school years; and some other types, such as 4, 8, and 19, are not contracted until adulthood (118).

Risk Factors and High-Risk Groups

Persons with impaired cell-mediated immunity have an increased risk of developing severe adenoviral infections. Severe and occasionally fatal disseminated infections have been observed in neonates, in patients with congenital im-

TABLE 3 Prevalence of serum neutralizing antibodies against adenoviruses in different age groups[a,b]

Age group	Total no. of serotypes neutralized						
	0	1	2	3	4	5	>6
6–12 mo	67[c]	14	14	2	2	0	0
1–3 yr	38	21	19	12	7	3	1
3–6 yr	8	21	20	20	14	7	10
6–9 yr	5	10	27	18	10	9	22
9–12 yr	5	8	12	15	22	12	26

[a] Data from reference 27. (Reprinted with permission of Cambridge University Press.)

[b] Sera tested against adenovirus serotypes 1 to 33.

[c] Percentage of children with neutralized antibodies against the number of serotypes indicated (27).

munodeficiency, and in recipients of hematopoietic stem cell transplants. Adenovirus infections are common in human immunodeficiency virus (HIV)-infected patients, but most of these infections are mild or asymptomatic.

Seasonality

Seasonal patterns depend on viral serotypes, population groups, and types of exposure (Fig. 4). Outbreaks of adenoviral respiratory disease are most common in winter and spring (19). Outbreaks of pharyngoconjunctival fever have been associated with swimming pools and occur most often in summer. Adenovirus gastroenteritis shows no distinct seasonal pattern (42, 118).

Transmission

Routes

Adenovirus infections are transmitted by direct contact, by small-droplet aerosols, by the fecal-oral route, and sometimes by water. The endemic adenoviruses of subgenus C (1, 2, and 5) causing childhood respiratory infections spread by direct contact via respiratory secretions or feces. Self-inoculation with fingers contaminated with infectious secretions is the most important route of transmission (118). For the epidemic types (especially 4 and 7), respiratory spread by contact and by aerosols is important (30, 108). Aerosol exposure, as measured by adenovirus DNA in ventilation filters, correlated with the number of hospitalizations during an outbreak caused by adenovirus 4 (30). In a military recruit setting, adenovirus was identified in the air and on the surfaces of pillows, lockers, and rifles (108). In such circumstances the route of transmission may affect the clinical picture. In volunteer studies, aerosolized adenovirus inhaled into the lungs caused lower respiratory disease more often than the same virus applied to the mouth, nasal mucosa, or intestine.

Serotypes causing pharyngoconjunctival fever and keratoconjunctivitis spread by contact through contaminated fingers or ophthalmologic instruments, and also by swimming pool water. The enteric serotypes 40 and 41 spread via the fecal-oral route.

Risk Factors

Close contact in crowded institutions and under low socioeconomic conditions increases the risk for adenovirus infections. Outbreaks have been described to occur in day care centers, schools, hospitals, shipyards, and military quarters. In households, about 50% of susceptible members will become infected after exposure (43). The risk increases with prolonged shedding of the virus. In one family study, 94% of the siblings and 56% of the parents had manifestations of acute illness during the follow-up after exposure; adenovirus disease was confirmed in 63 and 20% of these cases, respectively (111).

Variable attack rates have been observed in closed communities. In an epidemic caused by adenovirus type 3 in a boys' boarding school, the attack rate was 80% among susceptible persons without neutralizing antibodies, but about half of the infections were subclinical. On the other hand, in an outbreak caused by adenovirus 21 in an isolated Antarctic station, the infection rate was only 15%, although 89% of the personnel were susceptible (123).

Nosocomial Infections

Adenoviruses cause outbreaks of nosocomial respiratory infections. In one outbreak due to adenovirus type 3 in a pediatric long-term care facility, 56% of 63 residents developed adenoviral illness. Seventeen patients (49%) were admitted to intensive care units, and two died (60). An epidemic of adenovirus 7a infection in a neonatal nursery causing the death of two patients most likely spread from patient to staff and subsequently to other patients by infected staff (38).

Adenoviruses have caused several keratoconjunctivitis epidemics that have spread via contaminated fingers and improperly disinfected tonometers. One outbreak (141) comprised 110 nosocomial cases, and an attack rate of 17% was observed in another (66).

Duration of Infectiousness

Respiratory adenoviruses are excreted in nasopharyngeal secretions for 5 to 10 days and, especially types 1 and 2, in stool for weeks or months after initial infection. Inter-

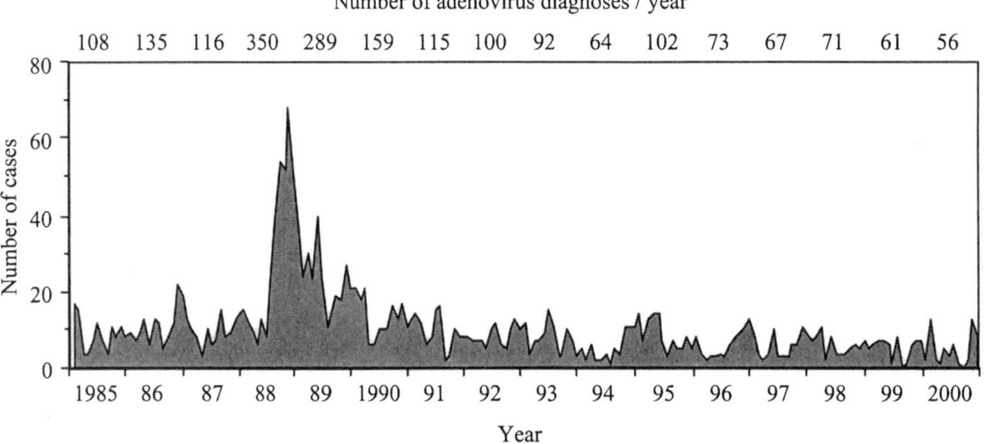

FIGURE 4 Monthly distribution of 1,958 adenovirus infections diagnosed by rapid antigen detection from nasopharyngeal aspirates at the Department of Virology, University of Turku, Turku, Finland, from 1985 to 2000. The peak in 1988 to 1989 was partly caused by a nationwide epidemic of adenovirus type 3.

mittent excretion lasting up to 906 days has been observed. Adenoviruses can remain viable for weeks under proper conditions on common surfaces. With gastroenteritis caused by adenoviruses 40 and 41, fecal excretion lasts 1 to 14 days (108).

PATHOGENESIS

Incubation Period

The incubation period for adenovirus infection, calculated from exposures to ill index patients or point sources, has been calculated to average 7 to 13 days, with a range from 2 to 21 days (67, 111).

Site of Infection

The primary site of replication of adenovirus is the epithelia of the organs involved. This includes the corneal epithelia, the epithelial lining of the upper and lower respiratory tract, and the urinary tract. In contrast, lymphocytes may be the site of chronic persistence of the virus in the nasopharynx. The virus may also persist in other tissues, as it can be detected by PCR in 10% of biopsy samples from patients with various forms of interstitial lung disease not thought to be related to adenovirus (70) and in 30% of normal duodenal biopsy samples (74).

Cultures of the appropriate site during active infection have a high positive yield. This includes cultures of nasopharyngeal swabs or aspirates, throat swabs or washes, conjunctival swabs or scrapings, bronchoalveolar lavage fluid, stool or rectal swabs, urine or urethral swabs, cervical swabs, cerebrospinal fluid, and tissue samples. In disseminated infection, adenovirus has also been cultured from solid organs, including the liver, spleen, kidneys, heart, and brain, and adenoviral DNA is detectable in the blood.

Pathology

Adenoviral pneumonia is characterized by a necrotizing bronchiolitis and alveolitis. The alveolar and bronchiolar cells are enlarged. Alveolar hyaline membranes may be prominent, and there may be extensive alveolar cellular debris. Characteristic cells with basophilic intranuclear inclusions with indistinct nuclear membranes known as "smudge" cells are usually seen (Fig. 5). Other epithelial cells with small eosinophilic nuclear inclusions, amphophilic nuclear inclusions, or basophilic inclusions with a clear halo may be seen. An interstitial and/or alveolar infiltrate is also present. The type of infiltrate may be neutrophilic, monocytic, or lymphocytic or mixed monocytic-lymphocytic (119, 127). The type of intranuclear inclusions and cellular character of infiltrate likely depend on the duration of infection prior to examination.

When there is hepatic involvement, fatty necrosis with neutrophilic infiltration or monocytic infiltration has been described, and amphophilic and basophilic intranuclear inclusions and smudge cells are seen (45, 92).

Adenoviral colitis occurs in the immunocompromised, particularly in patients with HIV or those who have undergone bone marrow transplantation. Pathological findings include characteristic adenovirus epithelial intranuclear inclusions and disorientation of the epithelia with a chronic inflammatory infiltrate, sometimes with focal mucosal necrosis (83, 146).

Encephalitis occurs rarely. Autopsy reveals perivascular mononuclear infiltrates, which have also been seen in patients with fatal, disseminated, adenoviral pneumonia with encephalitis (97).

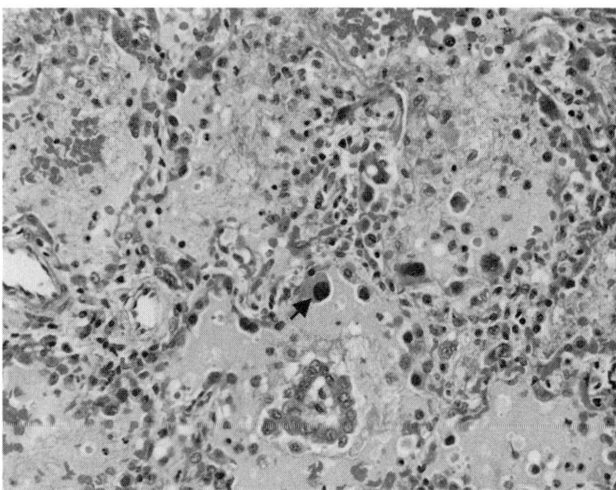

FIGURE 5 Pulmonary histopathology from a patient with a fatal case of adenoviral pneumonia. Characteristic epithelial smudge cells (arrow) show remarkedly enlarged nuclei containing inclusion bodies surrounded by thin rims of cytoplasm. Inclusion bodies are basophilic or amphophilic when stained with hemotoxylin and eosin. Unlike with herpesvirus infections, no syncytia or multinucleated giant cells are present.

Virus-Mediated Tissue Damage

Three mechanisms are likely responsible for the extensive tissue damage that occurs: (i) direct cytotoxicity due to viral replication or viral components, (ii) cytotoxicity due to the inflammatory cell infiltrate, and (iii) cytotoxicity due to effects related to cytokines stimulated by the virus.

Modulation of Cellular Functions by Adenovirus Replication

Adenovirus requires host cellular transcription factors to complete the replicative cycle. During this cycle the virus profoundly alters normal cellular function, presumably to create conditions that enhance replication. E1A proteins activate cell cycling through subdomain interactions with retinoblastoma protein and p300 (7, 104). Proapoptotic effects of E1A are counteracted by several adenovirus proteins, including E1B-55K, E4-ORF6, and E1B-19K (5, 81). These functions would be necessary to prolong function of host cells to promote viral replication. However, at late stages, viral proteins act to inhibit cellular processes and viability. E1B-55K together with the E4-ORF6 protein inhibits nuclear export of cellular mRNAs (52, 101). Host mRNA translation is also inhibited (56). Cellular integrity is disturbed through the action of an L3 viral protease on the cellular cytokeratin K18 (24). Furthermore, production of the E3-11.6K ADP induces cell death through caspase-dependent and non-caspase-dependent pathways (152).

Adenovirus structural proteins also interfere with cellular processes. Several of the adenovirus subtypes bind the receptor CAR. This binding disrupts cellular tight junctions and facilitates virus release (139). The penton base of adenovirus binds to cellular integrins and inhibits cell adhesion (6).

Adenovirus replication is not required for inflammation. Nonreplicating adenovirus vectors clearly cause significant tissue damage in mice, rats, nonhuman primates, and, unfortunately, humans. This damage likely comes from induction of proinflammatory cytokines and recruitment of inflammatory cells.

Innate Immune Cytokine Responses to Adenovirus

Much of the data regarding induction of cytokines by adenovirus are derived from animal data or from studies using nonreplicating adenovirus vectors. In a nonpermissive mouse model of intratracheal exposure to adenovirus, tumor necrosis factor alpha (TNF-α) and interleukin 6 (IL-6) mRNAs are induced in alveolar macrophages but not epithelial or endothelial cells (153). Intravenous infusion of a nonreplicating adenovirus vector in mice induced TNF-α, IL-6, and IL-12, with tissue macrophages and splenic dendritic cells and macrophages contributing to this response (151). Instillation of wild-type adenoviruses 3p and 7h, which cause pneumonia in humans, into a mouse induces the proinflammatory cytokines IL-1 β, TNF-α, gamma interferon, and IL-12 and the mouse IL-8 homologs MIP-2 and KC (64). When human monocytes and monocyte-derived macrophages were exposed to wild-type adenovirus type 2, TNF-α was induced in both cell types, but IL-1β was induced only in monocytes (69).

Exposure of human peripheral blood mononuclear cells to wild-type adenovirus type 7 induced interferon (not further specified) in culture. Alpha interferon levels were also elevated in two patients with adenovirus-induced hemolytic-uremic syndrome (16).

The source of adenovirus-induced cytokines and chemokines is likely not limited to dendritic cells and macrophages. IL-8 is also induced in epithelial cell cultures by adenovirus and adenovirus vectors and in a human lung slice model in which epithelial cells are the predominant cell type (17).

Induction of cytokines during active adenovirus infection in humans appears to be a marker of disease severity. Among 38 children with lower respiratory tract infections with adenovirus, TNF-α in serum was detected with a higher frequency in patients with severe disease or fatal outcome than in those with less severe disease, as was IL-6. IL-8 was detectable in serum in all groups of patients, and levels correlated with disease severity (91). The cytokine response is likely important in inflammation and cell injury, but it may also be important in limiting dissemination or severity of adenovirus illnesses. Although anti-TNF-α strategies may decrease inflammation induced by administration of adenovirus vectors to mice (10), this therapy may predispose humans to severe adenovirus infections (2).

Adaptive Immunity and Adenovirus

The adaptive immune response is important in preventing reinfection or, in the case of immunization, significant infection with adenovirus. Neutralizing and nonneutralizing antibodies to adenovirus are produced during infection. Serologic studies show a high rate of seroconversion. In children with acute adenovirus infection detected by antigen detection or seroconversion, immunoglobulin G (IgG) antibody increased in 77%, IgM increased in 48%, and IgA increased in 37%. IgM peaked at 10 to 20 days after the onset of illness and remained elevated for 2 months. IgA titers were variable, decreasing to undetectable levels in some patients and persisting for the duration of the study, 90 days, in others. In a similar study of infected military recruits, IgG levels increased in 89%, IgA levels increased in 77%, and IgM titers increased in 39%. IgA levels also increase in relevant secretions during adenovirus infections of the nasopharynx, conjunctiva, and intestine (94, 95).

The importance of T-cell responses to adenovirus infection is not well understood, but it is generally regarded that T cells play a role in limiting the severity of disease. For example, there is high morbidity and mortality associated with adenovirus infection of patients with transplants, hematologic malignancies, or AIDS. Many of these patients are infected by a serotype which usually causes only mild disease in immunocompetent patients. Furthermore, recovery of T-cell counts, decrease in T-cell suppression, or infusion of donor lymphocytes decreases viral shedding and the severity of the illness (138).

Both adenovirus-specific $CD4^+$ and $CD8^+$ T cells are present in healthy adults (40, 96). A role in containment of adenovirus infection has been proposed for both. Adenovirus-specific $CD4^+$ T-cell clones contain viral replication in infected cell lines and primary bronchial epithelial cells (53). Adenovirus-specific $CD8^+$ T-cell clones kill transformed lymphoblastoid cells expressing adenovirus hexon (130).

Adenovirus Persistence and Latency

The recognition of adenovirus persistence dates back to the discovery of the virus. Rowe and colleagues, while trying to develop cell lines from resected human adenoids, noted the development of cytopathic effect (CPE) in culture (107). This was attributed to infection of the cells with adenovirus, which was present in the original subjects in an asymptomatic persistent or latent state. In a similar fashion, viral shedding occurs for months to years after infection.

There are several adenovirus proteins that appear to play a role in evasion of the immune system. This was discovered when infection of cells with adenoviruses with mutations of these proteins increased the sensitivity of these cells to lysis by TNF exposure. These proteins in the E3 region, E3-10.4K, E3-14.5K, and E3-14.7K, act by downstream inhibition of TNF, either through phospholipase A2 or NF-κB (36). Another mechanism that may assist in immune evasion is displayed by E3-19K, which decreases expression of major histocompatibility complex class I molecules in adenovirus-infected cells. Also, adenovirus E1B-19K and E3 proteins counteract destruction of infected cells through inhibition of TNF-related apoptosis-inducing ligand (TRAIL), and E3 proteins also inhibit Fas ligand-induced apoptosis (36, 55).

These viral factors likely contribute to persistence of adenovirus in human tissues by preventing elimination of virus-infected cells. There has also been speculation that persistence, or true latency with integration of adenovirus genes, plays a role in the development of human illnesses. One study comparing lung tissue from patients with chronic obstructive pulmonary disease (COPD) to patients with similar smoking histories without the disease found that COPD patients had increased amounts of adenovirus E1A as revealed by PCR and increased detection of the E1A RNA by in situ hybridization (87). Follow-up studies by the same group showed that areas of increased E1A expression in alveolar epithelia correlated with cellular inflammation and severe emphysema (105). This issue has not been settled, however, as a recent study has shown a low incidence of E1A RNA expression and E1A DNA in patients with COPD (88).

One study of adenovirus persistence in children measured the presence of adenovirus capsid in bronchoalveolar lavage fluid from children with treatment-resistant asthma and found high rates of adenovirus detection in these children compared to children of similar age without asthma (82). This finding should be tempered by the fact that others have shown that steroid treatment of patients with interstitial lung disease increases the detection of adenovirus by PCR (70). In any case, these studies raise provocative questions about the possible role of persistent or latent adenovirus in the development of chronic respiratory diseases.

CLINICAL MANIFESTATIONS

Major Clinical Syndromes

Acute Respiratory Infection

Adenovirus infections most commonly occur in children between 6 months and 5 years of age and manifest as febrile upper respiratory tract infections. Most infections are mild and self-limited. Adenoviral infections cannot be distinguished from upper respiratory infections induced by other viruses (19, 20, 43). In one 12-month study, adenovirus was identified by PCR in 3% of 543 acute respiratory illnesses; the mean duration of adenovirus illness was 18.6 days. Interestingly, another virus was present in 60% of adenovirus-positive cases (72). Clinical findings for adenovirus infections consist of tonsillitis, pneumonia, acute otitis media, febrile convulsions, fever without focus of infections, and laryngitis (25, 112). High and persistent fever is common in children. In hospitalized children with adenovirus infection, the mean maximal temperature was 39.4°C, and the mean duration of fever was 5.4 days (range, 2 to 13 days) (112, 114).

About half of children with adenovirus infection have a marked leukocytosis (>15,000/mm^3), elevated erythrocyte sedimentation rate (>30 mm/h), and elevated serum C-reactive protein levels (>40 mg/liter), in contrast to most cases of influenza virus, parainfluenza virus, and respiratory syncytial virus-induced illnesses. Except for respiratory syncytial virus infections (which in up to 60% of the cases acute otitis media is found), the number of possible bacterial coinfections does not differ in different virus infections. The cause of the elevated laboratory values in adenovirus infections is unknown (99, 113).

Tonsillitis

Tonsillitis is a frequent clinical manifestation of adenovirus infection. One 1-year study of 110 children with acute febrile tonsillitis found that adenoviruses were the most common causative agent and accounted for 19% of cases (102). Adenoviruses and group A streptococci do not usually induce mixed infections in children. In adenoviral tonsillitis the exudates are most often thin and follicular or netlike but sometimes may have thick membranes (102, 114) (Color Plate 33). Neither white blood cell (WBC) count, serum C-reactive protein, nor erythrocyte sedimentation rate distinguishes bacterial from viral tonsillitis. Just over one-half of patients with both adenoviral and streptococcal tonsillitis have WBC counts of 15,000/mm^3 or above. Although age overlap occurs, adenoviral tonsillitis occurs most often in children less than 3 years of age, whereas beta-hemolytic streptococci induce tonsillopharyngitis in 5- to 17-year-old children. Adenovirus infection is a frequent cause of tonsillitis unresponsive to antibiotic therapy and requiring referral to a hospital (114).

Pneumonia

Approximately 10 to 20% of childhood pneumonias are attributed to adenoviruses. Pneumonia is a main diagnosis of 4 to 18% of hospitalized children identified with an adenovirus infection (63, 112, 137). Adenoviral pneumonia results primarily from infections with serotypes 7, 21, and 3. These types may also cause disseminated disease.

Adenoviral pneumonia cannot be clinically distinguished from other viral or bacterial pneumonias. Chest roentgenogram findings vary from diffuse to patchy interstitial infiltrates. Consolidation and pleural effusions have been described. Parahilar peribronchial infiltrates and atelectasis occur in most children with abnormal roentgenographic findings associated with adenovirus infection. Adenoviral pneumonia may be associated with disseminated infection involving the heart, liver, pancreas, kidneys, and central nervous system. The fatality rate can be as high as 30% (22, 145). Permanent lung damage after adenoviral pneumonia has been reported to occur in 27 to 65% of those who had adenovirus type 7 pneumonia. These changes include bronchiectasis, bronchiolitis obliterans, and unilateral hyperlucent lung (McLeod) syndrome. Many patients with normal chest roentgenograms have abnormal pulmonary function tests, often consistent with pulmonary obstruction (125). The young age of the child and measles are risk factors predisposing patients to chronic lung damage. Measles induces temporary suppression of cell-mediated immunity, which appears to predispose children to more severe adenovirus disease.

Adenoviral infection may mimic a bacterial infection and is a common cause of ineffective and unnecessary antibiotic treatment. High-grade and prolonged fever and common abnormal laboratory findings are the major reasons for antibiotic treatment in clinical practice (112, 114).

Pharyngoconjunctival Fever and Keratoconjunctivitis

Pharyngoconjunctival fever and keratoconjunctivitis are two well-described infections in the eye caused by adenoviruses. Pharyngoconjunctival fever occurs principally in children and is associated with types 3 and 7. Epidemic keratoconjunctivitis occurs mainly in adults and is usually caused by adenovirus types 8, 19, and 37 (41, 118). Recently, an outbreak induced by adenovirus type 22 was reported (32). In 99 children with acute conjunctivitis seen in a pediatric practice, *Haemophilus influenzae* (42%), adenoviruses (20%), and *Streptococcus pneumoniae* (12%) were the most common etiologic agents. Simultaneous infection with two pathogens was uncommon. The clinical features of conjunctivitis by the three different pathogens are summarized in Table 4. Eleven (65%) of the 17 children with both pharyngitis and conjunctivitis had adenovirus cultured from the conjunctiva (47).

Pharyngoconjunctival fever is often associated with preauricular adenopathy. Conjunctivitis is usually unilateral or asymmetric. In the early stage, adenoviral conjunctivitis cannot be distinguished clinically from bacterial, allergic, or other viral acute conjunctivitis. The duration of conjunctivitis is 1 to 2 weeks. Symptoms include watering, redness, discomfort, and photophobia. The

TABLE 4 Clinical features of conjunctivitis caused by three different pathogens[a]

Clinical feature	*H. influenzae* (n = 42)	*S. pneumoniae* (n = 12)	Adenoviruses (n = 20)
Mean age of patients (yr)	3.6	3.1	8.5
Bilateral disease (%)	74	50	35
Purulent exudate (%)	93	83	45
Concurrent otitis (%)	33	8	10
Concurrent pharyngitis (%)	5	8	55

[a] Modified from reference 47 with permission.

palpebral conjunctiva is hyperemic and contains diffuse infiltration and papillary or follicular hypertrophy. In severe cases, subconjunctival hemorrhages, chemosis, or pseudomembranes occur. Epidemics following swimming pool exposure have been described.

A large number of epidemics of adenoviral keratoconjunctivitis have been described. Outbreaks of keratoconjunctivitis typically occur in industrial plants, ophthalmology clinics, hospitals, nursing homes, camps, military bases, and child care centers. The virus is transmitted by the hands of medical personnel and by contaminated ophthalmic solutions and instruments. In industrial and military base outbreaks, spread may occur by the common use of bathrooms and inadequate hygiene. Adenoviruses can remain viable for several weeks on wash basins and hand towels. The illness is first characterized by conjunctivitis, chemosis, pain, photophobia, and lacrimation. A diffuse punctate epithelial keratitis occurs within 3 to 4 days. It may resolve within 2 weeks but can develop into focal subepithelial keratitis with pathognomonic corneal opacities. In rare cases, stromal infiltration may persist for months or even years. Fortunately, the illness is usually self-limited, and the patient's vision remains unaffected (41).

Enteric Infection

Adenoviruses are detected in 4 to 15% of stools from children with gastroenteritis in hospitals, outpatient clinics, and day care centers. In one study of 834 fecal specimens positive for viruses, rotavirus occurred in 56% of the specimens, adenovirus in 15%, minireovirus in 15%, astrovirus in 8%, calicivirus in 3%, and Norwalk-like virus in 2% (68). In another study conducted nearly 20 years later with 427 fecal specimens positive for viruses, rotavirus occurred in 58% of the specimens, norovirus in 31%, adenovirus in 7%, astrovirus in 3%, and human bocavirus in 2% (75). Of the adenoviruses detected in the feces, types 40 and 41 comprise 30 to 80%, respectively, in different studies. The other common adenovirus types found in the stools are 1, 2, 3, 5, 7, and 31. Adenoviral diarrhea is most common in children less than 2 years of age. By the age of 3 years, 30 to 100% of children have neutralizing antibodies to adenovirus types 40 and 41.

No special feature clinically differentiates adenoviral diarrhea from diarrheas induced by other viruses. The clinical profile of adenoviral diarrhea in children has been well characterized (61, 68, 148). The stools are usually watery and nonbloody, in contrast to bacterial diarrheas. Mucus is noted in 19 to 57% of cases. The maximum daily frequency of stools varies from 3 to 15. The mean duration of diarrhea is 3 to 11 days, often being significantly longer than rotavirus-induced diarrhea. In patients seeking care for diarrhea, the severity of adenoviral diarrhea has been similar to that of rotavirus infection, whereas in studies of outpatients, rotaviral disease seemed to be more severe than adenoviral disease (109). Type 41 adenovirus-induced diarrhea lasts longer than type 40-induced diarrhea (12.2 days, versus 8.6 days). Enteric adenoviruses seem to induce longer enteritis than nonenteric adenoviruses (133). Fever and vomiting in enteric adenovirus infections are common. Although adenoviral gastroenteritis is usually a mild disease, fatal cases in immunocompromised patients have been described. Transmission to family contacts seems to be rare.

Viral and bacterial copathogens in adenoviral diarrhea have been found in 13 to 18% of the cases, and other viruses were detected in respiratory specimens from 26% of 47 patients, when adenovirus was visualized in the fecal sample (21, 68).

Fever Syndromes

In 105 hospitalized patients with adenovirus infection, 17% had fever with no identifiable site of infection (112). In another study, adenovirus was cultured from 6% of 116 patients with fever without a localized cause (31). Samples for virus isolation, virus antigen detection, or PCR tests from the nasopharynx and feces should be included in the workup of febrile patients without focus of infection.

Virus infection is the most common cause of febrile convulsion and is detected in up to half of cases. Adenoviruses are the most common single etiologic agents and caused 13% of 144 cases in one study. In three patients, adenovirus was also detected from cerebrospinal fluid, suggesting that febrile convulsions may have been the sole manifestation of adenoviral central nervous system infection (103).

Hemorrhagic Cystitis

Adenovirus type 11 has been recovered from the urine of 19 to 91% of children with hemorrhagic cystitis. The disease occurs more often in boys than in girls. In addition to gross hematuria, the clinical manifestations included urgency, frequency, and fever. The duration of gross hematuria varies from 2 days to 2 weeks, and there are no changes in serum creatinine levels. Exfoliated bladder epithelial cells are found to contain adenoviral antigen by immunofluorescence.

Hemorrhagic cystitis associated with adenovirus type 11 has been described to occur following bone marrow and renal transplantations. Female gender, seropositivity for the antibody to adenovirus prior to bone marrow transplant (BMT), and acute graft-versus-host disease are significant risk factors. Studies from the United States reported adenovirus-associated hemorrhagic cystitis after BMT in only 0.3 to 1.0% of recipients (3, 121). In 22 cases of acute hemorrhagic cystitis due to adenovirus after renal transplantation, the disease was associated with gross hematuria, urinary frequency, burning urination, fever, and negative bacterial cultures. The symptoms lasted for 2 to 4 weeks, and serum creatinine increased in 17 of the 18 cases described. Most patients were treated with steroid pulse therapy, but the value of this therapy is unproven. Recently, intravesical instillation of cidofovir in the treatment of adenovirus-induced hemorrhagic cystitis was reported (35).

Infection in Military Recruits

Adenovirus infections are commonly recognized in military recruits. Physical and mental stress and crowding are considered major reasons for the susceptibility. The most common clinical manifestations in military recruits mimic those found in children: febrile illness associated with nasal congestion, sore throat, and cough. A large epidemic of keratoconjunctivitis with nearly 3,000 cases occurred at a U.S. military base in the Philippines, and this event led to recommendations for management of the epidemic (Table 5) (98). In one study of 108 young men with febrile tonsillitis in the military service, adenoviruses caused 31% of the cases, whereas group A streptococcal infections were detected in 38% (147). In 17% of cases of streptococcal tonsillitis, evidence of concurrent adenovirus infection was also found, in contrast to adenoviral tonsillitis in children (102).

Adenoviral pneumonia in military conscripts was originally classified as atypical pneumonia until the viral etiology was discovered. Clinically and radiologically it may resemble *Mycoplasma pneumoniae* pneumonia. Most often the illness is induced by adenovirus types 4 and 7, which are the types included in the oral live vaccine used successfully between 1971 and 1991 in the U.S. Army. As a result of vaccine unavailability, severe epidemics of adenovirus 4 infections affecting thousands of trainees have been reported, and adenovirus 4 is now responsible for nearly all diagnosed cases of adenovirus infections in U.S. military recruits (64). From 2002 to 2006, epidemiological studies using molecular diagnostic procedures revealed the emergence of adenovirus type 14 in U.S. military recruits, raising questions about the efficacy of the live type 4 and type 7 vaccines currently in field tests (15).

TABLE 5 Epidemic keratoconjunctivitis preventive measures[a]

General recommendations
- Wash hands thoroughly.
- Clean and sterilize instruments.
- Use unit doses of ophthalmic solutions.
- Examine "red eye" patients in a separate area.
- Educate staff about epidemic keratoconjunctivitis and other transmissible eye diseases.
- Avoid use of cloth towels in bathrooms.

Termination of an outbreak
- Observe above recommendations.
- Communicate the existence of an outbreak to all staff.
- Segregate patients by presence or absence of epidemic keratoconjunctivitis.
- Discard all open ophthalmic solutions.
- Remove infected personnel and patients from clinic for 2 wks.
- Determine the cause of the outbreak and mode of transmission.
- Educate patients about epidemic keratoconjunctivitis.
- Postpone elective procedures.
- Act with speed and decisiveness.

[a] Adapted from reference 41 with permission of Oxford University Press.

Infection in Newborn Infants

Newborn infants are susceptible to a disseminated form of adenovirus infection that is often fatal. Adenovirus outbreaks in neonatal intensive care units have been reported. Mothers often have viral symptoms preceding or shortly after delivery, and there may be prolonged rupture of membranes. The illness starts within 10 days of age with lethargy, fever or hypothermia, anorexia, apnea, hepatomegaly, bleeding, and progressive pneumonia. Conjunctivitis is not a common finding. Death occurred in 11 of 13 newborns. Adenovirus types 3, 7, 21, and 30 have been cultured most often from the lungs and liver (1).

Infection in Immunocompromised Patients

Adenovirus infections in immunosuppressed patients are often more persistent, severe, and associated with different types of adenoviruses than in healthy hosts. Severe adenovirus infections are being increasingly recognized in recipients of hematopoietic stem cell transplants (HSCT) (37, 59). One early study conducting weekly viral surveillance cultures from the throat and stools and, in adults, also from urine during the first 100 days after transplant in 201 BMT recipients over a 4-year period found that the incidence of adenovirus isolation was 31% for children and 14% for adults. Thirty-one percent of all adenovirus-positive patients had definite or probable adenoviral disease; these patients represented 6.5% of all patients. Other large studies of BMT patients in the 1980s in Seattle, WA, and in Baltimore, MD, described adenoviral disease in 5 and 40%, respectively; incidences of 3 to 12% have been reported in other studies. Children suffer adenovirus infections more often than adults and also develop them earlier after transplantation. Most adenovirus infections in children develop within 30 days after transplantation, whereas in adults infection usually develops more than 90 days after transplantation. The infection is thought to be secondary to reactivation of persistent or latent viruses or the transmission of latent virus via donor graft. In young children, infection may be acquired from a family contact or nosocomially (23).

The adenovirus types cultured from BMT recipients differ from those cultured from otherwise healthy subjects. Most often the disease has been caused by adenovirus belonging to subgroup B (types 11, 34, and 35) (121). In one study, 31 of 51 patients with adenovirus were also infected by herpes simplex virus, cytomegalovirus, or both (121). A definite diagnosis of adenoviral disease requires histopathological confirmation or virus detection from tissue. Adenoviral disease is considered probable if virus is detected from two or more body sites in association with compatible symptoms without any other identifiable cause (59).

The clinical manifestations of adenovirus infection in HSCT recipients include high fever, pneumonia, hemorrhagic cystitis, encephalitis, hepatitis, nephritis, and colitis. Adenovirus has been the major contributor to mortality in about one half of those with definite disease. Most of the fatal outcomes result from fulminant pneumonia, hepatic failure, nephritis, or colitis. Acute graft-versus-host disease, T-cell-depleted grafts, lymphocytopenia ($<300/mm^3$), and detection of adenovirus from multiple sites are clear risk factors for disease (23, 121). Routine viral cultures, PCR tests, or rapid detection of adenovirus antigen in nasopharyngeal mucus, feces, conjunctivae, and possibly from lung biopsy samples should be included in the etiologic workup of immunocompromised patients with suspected infection. Recently, weekly monitoring of blood samples for adenovirus DNA by real-time quantitative PCR has been shown to be useful in recognition of patients at risk for a potentially severe infection. Adenovirus DNA in blood has preceded the onset of clinical symptoms by 2 to 3 weeks. Increased or increasing viral loads are associated with an increased risk of death, and antiviral treatment should be considered (23, 33, 53, 59, 126).

Adenovirus was cultured from 10% of more than 500 liver transplant patients, with a median time of 26 days from transplantation, in one study. Urine was the most common site of adenovirus isolation, but the virus was also detected from WBCs of several children. Hepatitis was the most common invasive disease (29% of infections), and serotype 5 caused most cases of hepatitis. All patients had high fever lasting 6 to 44 days. In addition to elevated transaminase levels, the patients had characteristic histopathology in the liver consisting of adenoviral inclusions or microabscesses. Recently, adenovirus viremia was found to be relatively common in adult lung, liver, kidney, and heart transplant recipients, but most infections were asymptomatic, and screening for adenovirus DNA is not recommended in solid-organ transplant recipients (57, 59).

Adenovirus infections occur frequently in HIV-positive patients. The actuarial risk of adenovirus infection at 1 year in late-stage HIV disease was 31 to 38%. Infection occurred most often in the gastrointestinal tract, but half of the patients remained asymptomatic or minimally symptomatic.

Uncommon Clinical Manifestations

Adenoviruses have been isolated from the cerebrospinal fluid and brain of patients with meningoencephalitis. Often the patients have been neonates or immunocompromised persons with disseminated disease. In one adenovirus type 7 epidemic affecting 32 previously healthy children, 25% had meningoencephalitis and 10% died. All children also had respiratory symptoms, including pneumonia in six cases (124). In the California Encephalitis Project, adenovirus was found as a possible cause of encephalitis in about 1% of 1,570 patients studied (48).

Sensitive molecular techniques have suggested that adenoviruses may be causative agents of myocarditis. Adenovirus sequences were found by PCR in 39% of 38 myocardial samples from patients with suspected acute viral myocarditis, although 10 adenovirus-positive myocardial samples did not fulfill histopathological criteria for myocarditis (85). In a recent study, cardiac samples were obtained for PCR analysis from 624 patients with myocarditis and from 149 patients with dilated cardiomyopathy. Adenovirus was identified in 23 and 12% of the samples, respectively (18).

Adenovirus infections have been thought to induce mesenteric lymphadenopathy, which then could act as a mechanical lead point for the intussusception. In one study, 20% of 25 children with intussusception had nonenteric adenovirus in their stools, compared with 4% of 24 healthy controls (14). Adenoviruses have been detected in children with pertussis; and on the other hand, adenovirus infection may induce pertussis-like prolonged cough.

In one study, 15 adenovirus culture-positive men had urethritis and 3 adenovirus-positive women had vaginal discharge and genital ulcers or fissures. In all cases, adenoviruses were isolated from the urethra or cervix, findings which suggest that adenoviruses may be a sexually transmissible cause of genital ulcers and urethritis (129).

Bacterial Complications

Acute otitis media (AOM) occurs in 30 to 37% of children with adenovirus infection, and 3 to 10% of AOM patients have evidence of adenovirus infection. Adenovirus was found in 2% of 581 middle ear fluid samples from AOM patients (110).

Excluding in military conscripts, adenovirus-induced febrile tonsillitis is seldom associated with group A beta-hemolytic streptococci. However, approximately one-half of military conscripts with adenoviral pneumonia have concomitant bacterial infection. By contrast, bacterial coinfections have been very rare in adenoviral keratoconjunctivitis in active-duty military personnel. Serologic evidence of *Streptococcus pneumoniae*, nontypeable *Haemophilus influenzae*, *Moraxella catarrhalis*, and *Mycoplasma pneumoniae* infections was found in 47% of 19 children with adenoviral pneumonia (63). Except for blood culture and lung tissue culture, there are neither generally available nor accepted methods to detect bacterial coinfection in patients with viral respiratory tract infections.

LABORATORY DIAGNOSIS

The clinical picture of adenovirus infection is variable and commonly resembles that due to other microbes. Therefore, adenovirus infections can seldom be diagnosed on clinical grounds alone, and the laboratory is needed for specific diagnosis.

Virus Isolation

Specimen Types

Adenoviruses have been isolated from stool, throat swabs, nasopharyngeal aspirates, conjunctival swabs and scrapings, urine, cerebrospinal fluid, blood, and a variety of biopsy specimens. The optimal specimen type depends on the clinical picture and to some extent on the adenovirus serotype in question.

Most adenovirus infections involve viral excretion in stool, which makes it a practical specimen for detection. However, excretion of the respiratory serotypes in stool can continue for several months. Therefore, isolation from stool does not have the same diagnostic significance as isolation from the involved site, for example, respiratory tract or eye specimens.

Specimens should preferably be collected within a week after onset of illness. After that, in most cases the excretion of virus and the sensitivity of isolation will decrease. Swab and biopsy specimens should be collected in transport medium. Stool and cerebrospinal fluid specimens can be transported as such in clean containers. Adenoviruses are relatively stable. Shipment on ice (4°C) or frozen is preferable for maximum sensitivity, but most adenoviruses can be grown in specimens transported at room temperature.

Cell Culture

Adenoviruses are species specific, and isolation is best achieved in human cells, although cynomolgus monkey kidney cells can also be used. All adenovirus serotypes, except 40 and 41, grow well and produce CPE in a variety of human epithelial cells. The best sensitivity is achieved with human embryonic kidney cells, but because these are expensive and difficult to obtain, continuous cell lines are commonly used. Suitable continuous cell lines include A549, HeLa, HEp-2, KB, and MRC-5 strains.

Some strains of the enteric serotypes 40 and 41 will grow in these cell lines, but the best growth is achieved in Graham 239 cells (human embryonic kidney cells transformed by adenovirus 5 DNA). Because of strain variation in the growth pattern, sensitivity is increased by simultaneous inoculation of the specimens into two or three different cell lines.

Adenoviruses produce typical CPE, which often starts at the periphery of the monolayer. The cells become rounded, with characteristic refractile intranuclear inclusions. The appearance of CPE is relatively slow, especially in the continuous cell lines. For the best sensitivity, a 4-week incubation with blind passage is recommended. Virus isolation is still the "gold standard" of adenovirus diagnosis. In comparative studies concerning respiratory infection, isolation sensitivity has been 85 to 100%. Among healthy children, 2 to 8% have adenoviruses in their throat or fecal specimens, and fecal excretion particularly can persist for months. In general, however, adenovirus isolation can be considered diagnostically significant and indicative of an acute infection.

Isolated viruses can be identified as adenoviruses by various immunologic techniques, e.g., immunofluorescence, enzyme immunoassay (EIA), or latex agglutination. Serotyping of the isolates can be done by neutralization or, with some isolates, by hemagglutination inhibition. Reference antisera are available from American Type Culture Collection. PCR combined with restriction endonuclease analysis or sequencing has become an alternative to neutralization in isolate identification. A practical modification of cell culture is the shell vial assay, in which monolayers grown on coverslips are inoculated, using centrifugation to enhance the infection, and after 1 to 2 days of incubation are stained with monoclonal antibodies to the hexon protein. The sensitivities of different shell vial cultures are variable.

Antigen Detection

Monoclonal or polyclonal antibodies directed against the group-specific hexon antigen can be used for the direct detection of all adenoviruses in clinical specimens. Commercial monoclonal antibodies are available.

In respiratory and eye specimens, infected cells can be detected by immunofluorescence, whereas immunoassay methods (EIA and time-resolved fluoroimmunoassay) can be used to detect both cell-bound and free antigenic proteins. Nasopharyngeal aspirates are preferable specimens. The best sensitivity is obtained if the specimen is collected during the first 4 to 5 days after onset of illness, but some patients remain positive for 2 to 3 weeks. The sensitivity of the immunoassay methods has been 75 to 90% for children but considerably lower for adults. Immunofluorescence has a lower sensitivity than immunoassays. Commercial point-of-care tests for adenovirus are becoming more available. In one study, a rapid (10-min) immunochromatography kit showed 95% sensitivity compared to adenovirus isolation and 91% sensitivity compared to PCR as the standard (44). Point-of-care tests would be useful for clinicians, and more comparative studies with commercial tests are needed.

In fecal specimens, adenovirus antigens can be detected by immunoassays and by latex agglutination. Antigen detection is especially suitable, because the enteric serotypes 40 and 41 grow poorly in cell culture. In addition to group-specific immunoassays, immunoassays specific for the enteric serotypes have also been developed. The sensitivity of EIAs for enteric adenoviruses in stool has been 85 to 100%. EIAs have also been used to detect adenovirus antigens in conjunctival specimens. Compared to culture, EIA has shown a sensitivity of 70 to 80% when specimens were collected early in the course of illness.

Direct visualization by EM is also used to detect adenoviruses in stool, although it is impractical under most diagnostic circumstances. The characteristic morphology of adenoviruses makes them easy to identify by EM and allows a rapid diagnosis whenever the amount of viral particles in the specimen is large enough. Enteric adenoviruses occur in stools in considerably larger quantities than respiratory adenoviruses, and the sensitivity of EM is comparable to that of immunoassays. The enteric adenoviruses can be identified by the use of immuno-EM.

PCR Tests

Adenovirus DNA can be detected directly from respiratory specimens, plasma, conjunctivae, stools, urine, and genital specimens using PCR. As with many other respiratory viruses, PCR is more sensitive than conventional virus culture or virus antigen detection. In one study of 1,038 samples from children with respiratory illness, 101 of 130 specimens positive for adenovirus by PCR were negative by fluorescent-antibody testing (71). In another study of 181 respiratory samples from children, virus culture and direct immunofluorescence identified 7 positive samples, compared to 17 by real-time PCR (135).

Quantitative detection of adenovirus is helpful for clinical decisions (93). Since PCR may detect latent adenovirus in the respiratory, gastrointestinal, or urinary tract, a high adenovirus DNA load may be more often associated with active disease or more severe disease (33, 34, 122). In situ hybridization is a valuable method in pathogenesis studies, but it is rarely applicable in everyday diagnosis.

Serology

Acute adenovirus infection can be diagnosed by detecting significant increases in titer of antibody to the common hexon antigen by complement fixation or by EIA. The sensitivity of complement fixation is about 50 to 70%, and that of EIA is about 70 to 80%. In small children the responses are more attenuated than in older children and adults. IgM antibodies are detectable in 20 to 50% of infections, but the immune responses are often poor and difficult to interpret. Neutralization and hemagglutination inhibition tests are sensitive but measure serotype-specific antibodies, so these assays are not suitable for routine diagnosis.

PREVENTION

Isolation of patients with adenoviral illness has not been recommended routinely. Recent observations on detection of adenoviruses by PCR in the air and on surfaces (30, 108) suggest that proper cleaning, isolation of patients with suspected or confirmed cases of adenovirus infection, and restriction of new admissions may be essential in limiting the risk of nosocomial spread. Respiratory isolation with an airborne-infection isolation room (as droplet precautions may not be effective) should be considered when the patient is treated in the intensive care unit and for patients with severe adenovirus type 3, 7, or 14 infections.

Careful hand washing both before and after contact with the patient is recommended, but routine soap and water may not reliably remove adenovirus. A 60% ethanol hand gel reduced significantly the infectivity titer of adenoviruses on finger pads (116). Use of disposable gloves should be considered when examining a patient with suspected adenovirus infection. During epidemics, medical staff should be instructed not to rub their eyes or to do so only with a clean tissue or paper towel (41).

Hospital outbreaks have been controlled by grouping of patients into cohorts; use of gloves, gowns, and goggles; and exclusion of symptomatic staff from the unit. Dirty towels may be the source of infection in outbreaks, and disposable paper towels or hot-air blowers have been recommended. All staff should be taught the signs and symptoms of adenovirus infections, the potential for spread, and cleaning and sterilization techniques. Table 5 shows the preventive measures for epidemic keratoconjunctivitis.

Immunoprophylaxis

No data are available about the possible preventive efficacy of intravenous immunoglobulin or high-titer immunoglobulin products.

Safe and effective live oral adenovirus vaccines containing types 4 and 7 in enteric tablets were introduced in 1971. These adenovirus strains replicate in the intestine and induce type-specific neutralizing serum antibodies. The vaccine program dramatically reduced adenoviral disease rates, by 95 to 99%, and total respiratory disease rates, by 50 to 60%, in the U.S. Army, findings demonstrating the dominant role of adenovirus infections in military populations (Fig. 6). Due to the cessation of production by the sole manufacturer, no adenovirus vaccine has been available since 1999. It has been estimated that each year's loss of adenovirus vaccine will be responsible for 10,650 preventable infections and 820 hospitalizations among the estimated 213,000 active-duty and reserve trainees (89). Studies with new live type 4 and type 7 adenovirus vaccines are ongoing.

TREATMENT

At present there is no specific antiviral treatment of proven value for adenovirus infections. Ribavirin, ganciclovir, and cidofovir are variably active against adenoviruses in vitro and thus potentially effective for treatment. Ester prodrugs of cidofovir have oral bioavailablity and lower renal toxicity, but they are not yet in clinical use (76). Ribavirin shows in vitro inhibitory activity only for group C adenoviruses, and intravenous ribavirin has poor or no efficacy in the treatment of severe adenoviral disease (46, 73). Several case studies have reported evidence of clinical efficacy of cidofovir (a monophosphate nucleotide analog of cytosine) treatment (80). A recent summary of the literature described 130 patients, mostly HSCT recipients, who had been treated with cidofovir, 5 mg/kg of body weight, once per week for 1 week to 11 months. Renal toxicity (mostly mild proteinuria or mild elevation of the serum creatinine) was recorded in 13% of the cases. Of 20 patients with pneumonia, 9 (45%) survived. Thirty patients were treated with 1 mg/kg three times per week for 2 weeks to 8 months. Renal toxicity was recorded for 7 (29%) of 24 patients, and all 6 patients with pneumonia survived (29). In many centers, adenovirus DNA loads in plasma are monitored weekly in HSCT patients, and cidofovir treatment is started when adenovirus DNA is detected or increases progressively. In addition, patients often receive intravenous immunoglobulin, which has activity against a wide range of adenovirus serotypes, but its clinical efficacy is unknown. A decrease in the plasma virus load has been shown to predict a good clinical response. On the other hand, retrospective studies have shown that antiviral therapy may not be necessary for all children who develop adenovirus viremia after BMT. Systematic studies

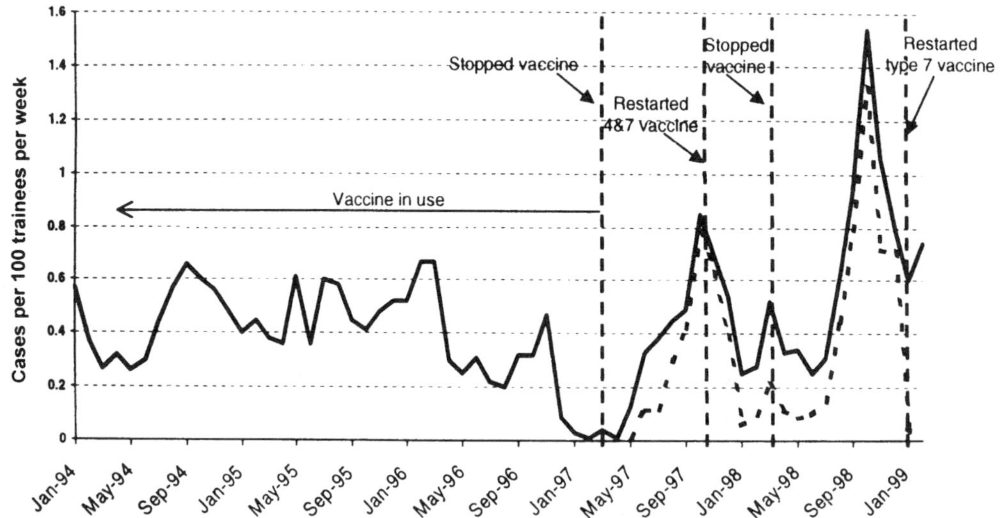

FIGURE 6 Use of adenovirus vaccines and febrile respiratory illness and adenovirus infection rates among U.S. Army trainees from 1994 to 1999. (Reprinted from reference 49 with permission.)

on the dose, safety, and virologic and clinical efficacy of intravenous cidofovir in adenovirus infections are needed.

REFERENCES

1. **Abzug, M. J., and M. J. Levin.** 1991. Neonatal adenovirus infection: four patients and review of the literature. *Pediatrics* **87:**890–896.
2. **Ahmad, N. M., K. M. Ahmad, and F. Younus.** 2007. Severe adenovirus pneumonia (AVP) following infliximab infusion for the treatment of Crohn's disease. *J. Infect.* **54:**e29–e32.
3. **Ambinder, R. F., W. Burns, M. Forman, P. Charache, R. Arthur, W. Beschorner, G. Santos, and R. Saral.** 1986. Hemorrhagic cystitis associated with adenovirus infection in bone marrow transplantation. *Arch. Intern. Med.* **146:**1400–1401.
4. **Andersson, M. G., P. C. Haasnoot, N. Xu, S. Berenjian, B. Berkhout, and G. Akusjarvi.** 2005. Suppression of RNA interference by adenovirus virus-associated RNA. *J. Virol.* **79:**9556–9565.
5. **Aoyagi, M., F. Higashino, M. Yasuda, A. Takahashi, Y. Sawada, Y. Totsuka, T. Kohgo, H. Sano, M. Kobayashi, and M. Shindoh.** 2003. Nuclear export of adenovirus E4orf6 protein is necessary for its ability to antagonize apoptotic activity of BH3-only proteins. *Oncogene* **22:**6919–6927.
6. **Bai, M., B. Harfe, and P. Freimuth.** 1993. Mutations that alter an Arg-Gly-Asp (RGD) sequence in the adenovirus type 2 penton base protein abolish its cell-rounding activity and delay virus reproduction in flat cells. *J. Virol.* **67:**5198–5205.
7. **Baluchamy, S., N. Sankar, A. Navaraj, E. Moran, and B. Thimmapaya.** 2007. Relationship between E1A binding to cellular proteins, c-myc activation and S-phase induction. *Oncogene* **26:**781–787.
8. **Barraza, E. M., S. L. Ludwig, J. C. Gaydos, and J. F. Brundage.** 1999. Reemergence of adenovirus type 4 acute respiratory disease in military trainees: report of an outbreak during a lapse in vaccination. *J. Infect. Dis.* **179:**1531–1533.
9. **Beltz, G. A., and S. J. Flint.** 1979. Inhibition of HeLa cell protein synthesis during adenovirus infection. Restriction of cellular messenger RNA sequences to the nucleus. *J. Mol. Biol.* **131:**353–373.
10. **Benihoud, K., S. Esselin, D. Descamps, B. Jullienne, B. Salone, P. Bobé, D. Bonardelle, E. Connault, P. Opolon, I. Saggio, and M. Perricaudet.** 2007. Respective roles of TNF-alpha and IL-6 in the immune response-elicited *[sic]* by adenovirus-mediated gene transfer in mice. *Gene Ther.* **14:**533–544.
11. **Benko, M., and B. Harrach.** 2003. Molecular evolution of adenoviruses. *Curr. Top. Microbiol. Immunol.* **272:**3–35.
12. **Bergelson, J. M., J. A. Cunningham, G. Droguett, E. A. Kurt-Jones, A. Krithivas, J. S. Hong, M. S. Horwitz, R. L. Crowell, and R. W. Finberg.** 1997. Isolation of a common receptor for coxsackie B viruses and adenoviruses 2 and 5. *Science* **275:**1320–1323.
13. **Berk, A. J.** 2005. Recent lessons in gene expression, cell cycle control, and cell biology from adenovirus. *Oncogene* **24:**7673–7685.
14. **Bhisitkul, D. M., K. M. Todd, and R. Listernick.** 1992. Adenovirus infection and childhood intussusception. *Am. J. Dis. Child.* **146:**1331–1333.
15. **Binn, L. N., J. L. Sanchez, and J. C. Gaydos.** 2007. Emergence of adenovirus type 14 in US military recruits—a new challenge. *J. Infect. Dis.* **196:**1436–1437.
16. **Blachar, Y., E. Leibovitz, and S. Levin.** 1990. The interferon system in two patients with hemolytic uremic syndrome associated with adenovirus infection. *Acta Paediatr. Scand.* **79:**108–109.
17. **Booth, J. L., K. M. Coggeshall, B. E. Gordon, and J. P. Metcalf.** 2004. Adenovirus type 7 induces interleukin-8 in a lung slice model and requires activation of Erk. *J. Virol.* **78:**4156–4164.
18. **Bowles, N. E., J. Ni, D. L. Kearney, M. Pauschinger, H. P. Schultheiss, R. McCarthy, J. Hare, J. T. Bricker, K. R. Bowles, and J. A. Towbin.** 2003. Detection of viruses in myocardial tissues by polymerase chain reaction. Evidence of adenovirus as a common cause of myocarditis in children and adults. *J. Am. Coll. Cardiol.* **42:**466–472.
19. **Brandt, C. D., H. W. Kim, B. C. Jeffries, G. Pyles, E. E. Christmas, J. L. Reid, R. M. Chanock, and R. H. Parrott.** 1972. Infections in 18,000 infants and children in a controlled study of respiratory tract disease. II. Variation in adenovirus infections by year and season. *Am. J. Epidemiol.* **95:**218–227.
20. **Brandt, C. D., H. W. Kim, A. J. Vargosko, B. C. Jeffries, J. O. Arrobio, B. Rindge, R. H. Parrott, and R. M. Chanock.** 1969. Infections in 18,000 infants and children in a controlled study of respiratory tract disease. I. Adenovirus pathogenicity in relation to serologic type and illness syndrome. *Am. J. Epidemiol.* **90:**484–500.
21. **Brandt, C. D., W. J. Rodriguez, H. W. Kim, J. O. Arrobio, B. C. Jeffries, and R. H. Parrott.** 1984. Rapid presumptive recognition of diarrhea-associated adenoviruses. *J. Clin. Microbiol.* **20:**1008–1009.
22. **Centers for Disease Control and Prevention.** 2007. Acute respiratory disease associated with adenovirus serotype 14—four states, 2006–2007. *Morb. Mortal. Wkly. Rep.* **56:**1181–1184.
23. **Chakrabarti, S., V. Mautner, H. Osman, K. E. Collingham, C. D. Fegan, P. E. Klapper, P. A. Moss, and D. W. Milligan.** 2002. Adenovirus infections following allogeneic stem cell transplantation: incidence and outcome in relation to graft manipulation, immunosuppression, and immune recovery. *Blood* **100:**1619–1627.
24. **Chen, P. H., D. A. Ornelles, and T. Shenk.** 1993. The adenovirus L3 23-kilodalton proteinase cleaves the amino-terminal head domain from cytokeratin 18 and disrupts the cytokeratin network of HeLa cells. *J. Virol.* **67:**3507–3514.
25. **Cheng, C. C., L. M. Huang, C. L. Kao, P. I. Lee, J. M. Chen, C. Y. Lu, C. Y. Lee, S. Y. Chang, and L. Y. Chang.** 2008. Molecular and clinical characteristics of adenoviral infections in Taiwanese children in 2004–2005. *Eur. J. Pediatr.* **167:**633–640.
26. **Cuesta, R., Q. Xi, and R. J. Schneider.** 2000. Adenovirus-specific translation by displacement of kinase Mnk1 from cap-initiation complex eIF4F. *EMBO J.* **19:**3465–3474.
27. **D'Ambrosio, E., N. Del Grosso, A. Chicca, and M. Midulla.** 1982. Neutralizing antibodies against 33 human adenoviruses in normal children in Rome. *J. Hyg.* **89:** 155–161.
28. **D'Halluin, J. C.** 1995. Virus assembly. *Curr. Top. Microbiol. Immunol.* **199**(Pt. 1)**:**47–66.
29. **Doan, M. L., G. B. Mallory, S. L. Kaplan, M. K. Dishop, M. G. Schecter, E. D. McKenzie, J. S. Heinle, and O. Elidemir.** 2007. Treatment of adenovirus pneumonia with cidofovir in pediatric lung transplant recipients. *J. Heart Lung Transplant.* **26:**883–889.

29a. **Doerfler, W., and P. Böhm (ed.).** 1995. *The Molecular Repertoire of Adenoviruses*, parts I, II, and III. Springer Verlag, Berlin, Germany.

30. **Echavarria, M., S. A. Kolavic, S. Cersovsky, F. Mitchell, J. L. Sanchez, C. Polyak, B. L. Innis, and L. N. Binn.** 2000. Detection of adenoviruses (AdV) in culture-negative environmental samples by PCR during an AdV-associated respiratory disease outbreak. *J. Clin. Microbiol.* **38:**2982–2984.
31. **Edwards, K. M., J. Thompson, J. Paolini, and P. F. Wright.** 1985. Adenovirus infections in young children. *Pediatrics* **76:**420–424.
32. **Engelmann, I., I. Madisch, H. Pommer, and A. Heim.** 2006. An outbreak of epidemic keratoconjunctivitis caused by a new intermediate adenovirus 22/H8 identified by molecular typing. *Clin. Infect. Dis.* **43:**e64–e66.
33. **Erard, V., M. L. Huang, J. Ferrenberg, L. Nguy, T. L. Stevens-Ayers, R. C. Hackman, L. Corey, and M. Boeckh.** 2007. Quantitative real-time polymerase chain reaction for detection of adenovirus after T cell-replete hematopoietic cell transplantation: viral load as a marker for invasive disease. *Clin. Infect. Dis.* **45:**958–965.
34. **Faix, D. J., H. S. Houng, J. C. Gaydos, S. K. Liu, J. T. Connors, X. Brown, L. V. Asher, D. W. Vaughn, and L. N. Binn.** 2004. Evaluation of a rapid quantitative diagnostic test for adenovirus type 4. *Clin. Infect. Dis.* **38:** 391–397.
35. **Fanourgiakis, P., A. Georgala, M. Vekemans, A. Triffet, J. M. De Bruyn, V. Duchateau, P. Martiat, E. De Clercq, R. Snoeck, E. Wollants, A. Rector, M. Van Ranst, and M. Aoun.** 2005. Intravesical instillation of cidofovir in the treatment of hemorrhagic cystitis caused by adenovirus type 11 in a bone marrow transplant recipient. *Clin. Infect. Dis.* **40:**199–201.
36. **Fessler, S. P., F. Delgado-Lopez, and M. S. Horwitz.** 2004. Mechanisms of E3 modulation of immune and inflammatory responses. *Curr. Top. Microbiol. Immunol.* **273:**113–135.
37. **Feuchtinger, T., P. Lang, and R. Handgretinger.** 2007. Adenovirus infection after allogeneic stem cell transplantation. *Leuk. Lymphoma* **48:**244–255.
38. **Finn, A., E. Anday, and G. H. Talbot.** 1988. An epidemic of adenovirus 7a infection in a neonatal nursery: course, morbidity, and management. *Infect. Control. Hosp. Epidemiol.* **9:**398–404.
39. **Flint, S. J., and R. A. Gonzalez.** 2003. Regulation of mRNA production by the adenoviral E1B 55-kDa and E4 Orf6 proteins. *Curr. Top. Microbiol. Immunol.* **272:**287–330.
40. **Flomenberg, P., V. Piaskowski, R. L. Truitt, and J. T. Casper.** 1996. Human adenovirus-specific $CD8^+$ T-cell responses are not inhibited by E3-19K in the presence of gamma interferon. *J. Virol.* **70:**6314–6322.
41. **Ford, E., K. E. Nelson, and D. Warren.** 1987. Epidemiology of epidemic keratoconjunctivitis. *Epidemiol. Rev.* **9:**244–261.
42. **Fox, J. P., C. D. Brandt, F. E. Wassermann, C. E. Hall, I. Spigland, A. Kogon, and L. R. Elveback.** 1969. The virus watch program: a continuing surveillance of viral infections in metropolitan New York families. VI. Observations of adenovirus infections: virus excretion patterns, antibody response, efficiency of surveillance, patterns of infections, and relation to illness. *Am. J. Epidemiol.* **89:** 25–50.
43. **Fox, J. P., C. E. Hall, and M. K. Cooney.** 1977. The Seattle Virus Watch. VII. Observations of adenovirus infections. *Am. J. Epidemiol.* **105:**362–386.
44. **Fujimoto, T., T. Okafuji, T. Okafuji, M. Ito, S. Nukuzuma, M. Chikahira, and O. Nishio.** 2004. Evaluation of a bedside immunochromatographic test for detection of adenovirus in respiratory samples, by comparison to virus isolation, PCR, and real-time PCR. *J. Clin. Microbiol.* **42:** 5489–5492.
45. **Garcia, A. G., M. E. Fonseca, M. de Bonis, H. I. Ramos, Z. P. Ferro, and J. P. Nascimento.** 1993. Morphological and virological studies in six autopsies of children with adenovirus pneumonia. *Mem. Inst. Oswaldo Cruz* **88:**141–147.
46. **Gavin, P. J., and B. Z. Katz.** 2002. Intravenous ribavirin treatment for severe adenovirus disease in immunocompromised children. *Pediatrics* **110:**e9.
47. **Gigliotti, F., W. T. Williams, F. G. Hayden, J. O. Hendley, J. Benjamin, M. Dickens, C. Gleason, V. A. Perriello, and J. Wood.** 1981. Etiology of acute conjunctivitis in children. *J. Pediatr.* **98:**531–536.
48. **Glaser, C. A., S. Honarmand, L. J. Anderson, D. P. Schnurr, B. Forghani, C. K. Cossen, F. L. Schuster, L. J. Christie, and J. H. Tureen.** 2006. Beyond viruses: clinical profiles and etiologies associated with encephalitis. *Clin. Infect. Dis.* **43:**1565–1577.
49. **Gray, G. C., P. R. Goswami, M. D. Malasig, A. W. Hawksworth, D. H. Trump, M. A. Ryan, and D. P. Schnurr for the Adenovirus Surveillance Group.** 2000. Adult adenovirus infections: loss of orphaned vaccines precipitates military respiratory disease epidemics. *Clin. Infect. Dis.* **31:**663–670.
50. **Gray, G. C., T. McCarthy, M. G. Lebeck, D. P. Schnurr, K. L. Russell, A. E. Kajon, M. L. Landry, D. S. Leland, G. A. Storch, C. C. Ginocchio, C. C. Robinson, G. J. Demmler, M. A. Saubolle, S. C. Kehl, R. Selvarangan, M. B. Miller, J. D. Chappell, D. M. Zerr, D. L. Kiska, D. C. Halstead, A. W. Capuano, S. F. Setterquist, M. L. Chorazy, J. D. Dawson, and D. D. Erdman.** 2007. Genotype prevalence and risk factors for severe clinical adenovirus infection, United States 2004–2006. *Clin. Infect. Dis.* **45:**1120–1131.
51. **Greber, U. F., M. Willetts, P. Webster, and A. Helenius.** 1993. Stepwise dismantling of adenovirus 2 during entry into cells. *Cell* **75:**477–486.
52. **Halbert, D. N., J. R. Cutt, and T. Shenk.** 1985. Adenovirus early region 4 encodes functions required for efficient DNA replication, late gene expression, and host cell shutoff. *J. Virol.* **56:** 250–257.
53. **Heemskerk, B., T. van Vreeswijk, L. A. Veltrop-Duits, C. C. Sombroek, K. Franken, R. M. Verhoosel, P. S. Hiemstra, D. van Leeuwen, M. E. Ressing, R. E. Toes, M. J. van Tol, and M. W. Schilham.** 2006. Adenovirus-specific $CD4^+$ T cell clones recognizing endogenous antigen inhibit viral replication in vitro through cognate interaction. *J. Immunol.* **177:**8851–8859.
54. **Hilleman, M. R., and J. H. Werner.** 1954. Recovery of new agent from patients with acute respiratory illness. *Proc. Soc. Exp. Biol. Med.* **85:**183–188.
55. **Hu, B., H. Zhu, S. Qiu, Y. Su, W. Ling, W. Xiao, and Y. Qi.** 2004. Enhanced TRAIL sensitivity by E1A expression in human cancer and normal cell lines: inhibition by adenovirus E1B19K and E3 proteins. *Biochem. Biophys. Res. Commun.* **325:**1153–1162.
56. **Huang, J. T., and R. J. Schneider.** 1991. Adenovirus inhibition of cellular protein synthesis involves inactivation of cap-binding protein. *Cell* **65:**271–280.
57. **Humar, A., K. Doucette, D. Kumar, X. L. Pang, D. Lien, K. Jackson, and J. Preiksaitis.** 2006. Assessment of adenovirus infection in adult lung transplant recipients using molecular surveillance. *J. Heart Lung Transplant.* **25:**1441–1446.
58. **Imperiale, M. J., G. Akusjärvi, and K. N. Leppard.** 1995. Post-transcriptional control of adenovirus gene expression. *Curr. Top. Microbiol. Immunol.* **199**(Pt. 2)**:**139–171.

59. **Ison, M. G.** 2006. Adenovirus infections in transplant recipients. *Clin. Infect. Dis.* **43:**331–339.
60. **James, L., M. O. Vernon, R. C. Jones, A. Stewart, X. Lu, L. M. Zollar, M. Chudoba, M. Westercamp, G. Alcasid, L. Duffee-Kerr, L. Wood, S. Boonlayangoor, C. Bethel, K. Ritger, C. Conover, D. D. Erdman, and S. I. Gerber.** 2007. Outbreak of human adenovirus type 3 infection in a pediatric long-term care facility—Illinois, 2005. *Clin. Infect. Dis.* **45:**416–420.
61. **Jarecki-Khan, K., S. R. Tzipori, and L. E. Unicomb.** 1993. Enteric adenovirus infection among infants with diarrhea in rural Bangladesh. *J. Clin. Microbiol.* **31:**484–489.
62. **Johansson, C., M. Jonsson, M. Marttila, D. Persson, X.-L. Fan, J. Skog, L. Frängsmyr, G. Wadell, and N. Arnberg.** 2007. Adenoviruses use lactoferrin as a bridge for CAR-independent binding to and infection of epithelial cells. *J. Virol.* **81:**954–963.
63. **Juven, T., J. Mertsola, M. Waris, M. Leinonen, O. Meurman, M. Roivainen, J. Eskola, P. Saikku, and O. Ruuskanen.** 2000. Etiology of community-acquired pneumonia in 254 hospitalized children. *Pediatr. Infect. Dis. J.* **19:**293–298.
64. **Kajon, A. E., A. P. Gigliotti, and K. S. Harrod.** 2003. Acute inflammatory response and remodeling of airway epithelium after subspecies B1 human adenovirus infection of the mouse lower respiratory tract. *J. Med. Virol.* **71:**233–244.
65. **Kleinberger, T.** 2000. Induction of apoptosis by adenovirus E4orf4 protein. *Apoptosis* **5:**211–215.
66. **Koo, D., B. Bouvier, M. Wesley, P. Courtright, and A. Reingold.** 1989. Epidemic keratoconjunctivitis in a university medical center ophthalmology clinic; need for re-evaluation of the design and disinfection of instruments. *Infect. Control Hosp. Epidemiol.* **10:**547–552.
67. **Kotloff, K. L., G. A. Losonsky, J. G. Morris, Jr., S. S. Wasserman, N. Singh-Naz, and M. M. Levine.** 1989. Enteric adenovirus infection and childhood diarrhea: an epidemiologic study in three clinical settings. *Pediatrics* **84:**219–225.
68. **Krajden, M., M. Brown, A. Petrasek, and P. J. Middleton.** 1990. Clinical features of adenovirus enteritis: a review of 127 cases. *Pediatr. Infect. Dis. J.* **9:**636–641.
69. **Kristoffersen, A. K., H. Sindre, Y. Mandi, H. Rollag, and M. Degre.** 1997. Effect of adenovirus 2 on cellular gene activation in blood-derived monocytes and macrophages. *APMIS* **105:**402–409.
70. **Kuwano, K., Y. Nomoto, R. Kunitake, N. Hagimoto, T. Matsuba, Y. Nakanishi, and N. Hara.** 1997. Detection of adenovirus E1A DNA in pulmonary fibrosis using nested polymerase chain reaction. *Eur. Respir. J.* **10:**1445–1449.
71. **Kuypers, J., N. Wright, J. Ferrenberg, M. L. Huang, A. Cent, L. Corey, and R. Morrow.** 2006. Comparison of real-time PCR assays with fluorescent-antibody assays for diagnosis of respiratory virus infections in children. *J. Clin. Microbiol.* **44:**2382–2388.
72. **Lambert, S. B., K. M. Allen, J. D. Druce, C. J. Birch, I. M. Mackay, J. B. Carlin, J. R. Carapetis, T. P. Sloots, M. D. Nissen, and T. M. Nolan.** 2007. Community epidemiology of human metapneumovirus, human coronavirus NL63, and other respiratory viruses in healthy preschool-aged children using parent-collected specimens. *Pediatrics* **120:**e929–e937.
73. **Lankester, A. C., B. Heemskerk, E. C. Claas, M. W. Schilham, M. F. Beersma, R. G. Bredius, M. J. van Tol, and A. C. Kroes.** 2004. Effect of ribavirin on the plasma viral DNA load in patients with disseminating adenovirus infection. *Clin. Infect. Dis.* **38:**1521–1525.
74. **Lawler, M., P. Humphries, C. O'Farrelly, H. Hoey, O. Sheils, M. Jeffers, D. S. O'Brian, and D. Kelleher.** 1994. Adenovirus 12 E1A gene detection by polymerase chain reaction in both the normal and coeliac duodenum. *Gut* **35:**1226–1232.
75. **Lee, J. I., J. Y. Chung, T. H. Han, M. O. Song, and E. S. Hwang.** 2007. Detection of human bocavirus in children hospitalized because of acute gastroenteritis. *J. Infect. Dis.* **196:**994–997.
76. **Lenaerts, L., and L. Naesens.** 2006. Antiviral therapy for adenovirus infections. *Antivir. Res.* **71:**172–180.
77. **Leong, K., and A. J. Berk.** 1986. Adenovirus early region 1A protein increases the number of template molecules transcribed in cell-free extracts. *Proc. Natl. Acad. Sci. USA* **83:**5844–5848.
78. **Li, E., D. Stupack, R. Klemke, D. A. Cheresh, and G. R. Nemerow.** 1998. Adenovirus endocytosis via α_v integrins requires phosphoinositide-3-OH kinase. *J. Virol.* **72:**2055–2061.
79. **Lichtenstein, D. L., and W. S. Wold.** 2004. Experimental infections of humans with wild-type adenoviruses and with replication-competent adenovirus vectors: replication, safety, and transmission. *Cancer Gene Ther.* **11:**819–829.
80. **Ljungman, P., P. Ribaud, M. Eyrich, S. Matthes-Martin, H. Einsele, M. Bleakley, M. Machaczka, M. Bierings, A. Bosi, N. Gratecos, C. Cordonnier, and Infectious Diseases Working Party of the European Group for Blood and Marrow Transplantation.** 2003. Cidofovir for adenovirus infections after allogeneic hematopoietic stem cell transplantation: a survey by the Infectious Diseases Working Party of the European Group for Blood and Marrow Transplantation. *Bone Marrow Transplant.* **31:**481–486.
81. **Lomonosova, E., T. Subramanian, and G. Chinnadurai.** 2005. Mitochondrial localization of p53 during adenovirus infection and regulation of its activity by E1B-19K. *Oncogene* **24:**6796–6808.
82. **Macek, V., J. Sorli, S. Kopriva, and J. Marin.** 1994. Persistent adenoviral infection and chronic airway obstruction in children. *Am. J. Respir. Crit. Care Med.* **150:**7–10.
83. **Maddox, A., N. Francis, J. Moss, C. Blanshard, and B. Gazzard.** 1992. Adenovirus infection of the large bowel in HIV positive patients. *J. Clin. Pathol.* **45:**684–688.
84. **Marcellus, R. C., J. N. Lavoie, D. Boivin, G. C. Shore, G. Ketner, and P. E. Branton.** 1998. The early region 4 orf4 protein of human adenovirus type 5 induces p53-independent cell death by apoptosis. *J. Virol.* **72:**7144–7153.
85. **Martin, A. B., S. Webber, F. J. Fricker, R. Jaffe, G. Demmler, D. Kearney, Y. H. Zhang, J. Bodurtha, B. Gelb, and J. Ni.** 1994. Acute myocarditis. Rapid diagnosis by PCR in children. *Circulation* **90:**330–339.
86. **Mathews, M. B.** 1995. Structure, function, and evolution of adenovirus virus-associated RNAs. *Curr. Top. Microbiol. Immunol.* **199**(Pt. 2)**:**173–187.
87. **Matsuse, T., S. Hayashi, K. Kuwano, H. Keunecke, W. A. Jefferies, and J. C. Hogg.** 1992. Latent adenoviral infection in the pathogenesis of chronic airways obstruction. *Am. Rev. Respir. Dis.* **146:**177–184.
88. **McManus, T. E., A. M. Marley, N. Baxter, S. N. Christie, J. S. Elborn, L. G. Heaney, P. V. Coyle, and J. C. Kidney.** 2007. Acute and latent adenovirus in COPD. *Respir. Med.* **101:**2084–2090.
89. **McNeill, K. M., R. M. Hendrix, J. L. Lindner, F. R. Benton, S. C. Monteith, M. A. Tuchs Cheres, G. C. Gray, and J. C. Gaydos.** 1999. Large, persistent epidemic of adenovirus type 4-associated acute respiratory disease in U.S. army trainees. *Emerg. Infect. Dis.* **5:**798–801.

90. **Meier, O., K. Boucke, S. V. Hammer, S. Keller, R. P. Stidwill, S. Hemmi, and U. F. Greber.** 2002. Adenovirus triggers macropinocytosis and endosomal leakage together with its clathrin-mediated uptake. *J. Cell Biol.* **158:**1119–1131.
91. **Mistchenko, A. S., R. A. Diez, A. L. Mariani, J. Robaldo, A. F. Maffey, G. Bayley-Bustamante, and S. Grinstein.** 1994. Cytokines in adenoviral disease in children: association of interleukin-6, interleukin-8, and tumor necrosis factor alpha levels with clinical outcome. *J. Pediatr.* **124:**714–720.
92. **Mistchenko, A. S., J. F. Robaldo, F. C. Rosman, E. R. Koch, and A. E. Kajon.** 1998. Fatal adenovirus infection associated with new genome type. *J. Med. Virol.* **54:**233–236.
93. **Miura-Ochiai, R., Y. Shimada, T. Konno, S. Yamazaki, K. Aoki, S. Ohno, E. Suzuki, and H. Ishiko.** 2007. Quantitative detection and rapid identification of human adenoviruses. *J. Clin. Microbiol.* **45:**958–967.
94. **Nishio, O., K. Sakae, Y. Ishihara, S. Isomura, and S. Inouye.** 1992. Adenovirus infection and specific secretory IgA responses in the intestine of infants. *Microbiol. Immunol.* **36:**623–631.
95. **Nordbo, S. A., T. Nesbakken, K. Skaug, and E. F. Rosenlund.** 1986. Detection of adenovirus-specific immunoglobulin A in tears from patients with keratoconjunctivitis. *Eur. J. Clin. Microbiol.* **5:**678–680.
96. **Olive, M., L. C. Eisenlohr, and P. Flomenberg.** 2001. Quantitative analysis of adenovirus-specific $CD4^+$ T-cell responses from healthy adults. *Viral Immunol.* **14:**403–413.
97. **Osamura, T., R. Mizuta, H. Yoshioka, and S. Fushiki.** 1993. Isolation of adenovirus type 11 from the brain of a neonate with pneumonia and encephalitis. *Eur. J. Pediatr.* **152:**496–499.
98. **Paparello, S. F., L. S. Rickman, H. N. Mesbahi, J. B. Ward, L. G. Siojo, and C. G. Hayes.** 1991. Epidemic keratoconjunctivitis at a U.S. military base: Republic of the Philippines. *Mil. Med.* **156:**256–259.
99. **Peltola, V., J. Mertsola, and O. Ruuskanen.** 2006. Comparison of total white blood cell count and serum C-reactive protein levels in confirmed bacterial and viral infections. *J. Pediatr.* **149:**721–724.
100. **Perez-Romero, P., K. E. Gustin, and M. J. Imperiale.** 2006. Dependence of the encapsidation function of the adenovirus L1 52/55-kilodalton protein on its ability to bind the packaging sequence. *J. Virol.* **80:**1965–1971.
101. **Pilder, S., M. Moore, J. Logan, and T. Shenk.** 1986. The adenovirus E1B-55K transforming polypeptide modulates transport or cytoplasmic stabilization of viral and host cell mRNAs. *Mol. Cell. Biol.* **6:**470–476.
102. **Putto, A.** 1987. Febrile exudative tonsillitis: viral or streptococcal? *Pediatrics* **80:**6–12.
103. **Rantala, H., M. Uhari, and H. Tuokko.** 1990. Viral infections and recurrences of febrile convulsions. *J. Pediatr.* **116:**195–199.
104. **Rasti, M., R. J. Grand, J. S. Mymryk, P. H. Gallimore, and A. S. Turnell.** 2005. Recruitment of CBP/p300, TATA-binding protein, and S8 to distinct regions at the N terminus of adenovirus E1A. *J. Virol.* **79:**5594–5605.
105. **Retamales, I., W. M. Elliott, B. Meshi, H. O. Coxson, P. D. Pare, F. C. Sciurba, R. M. Rogers, S. Hayashi, and J. C. Hogg.** 2001. Amplification of inflammation in emphysema and its association with latent adenoviral infection. *Am. J. Respir. Crit. Care Med.* **164:**469–473.
106. **Rodriguez, W. J., H. W. Kim, C. D. Brandt, R. H. Schwartz, M. K. Gardner, B. Jeffries, R. H. Parrott, R. A. Kaslow, J. I. Smith, and H. Takiff.** 1985. Fecal adenoviruses from a longitudinal study of families in metropolitan Washington, D.C.: laboratory, clinical, and epidemiologic observations. *J. Pediatr.* **107:**514–520.
107. **Rowe, W. P., R. J. Huebner, L. K. Gilmore, R. H. Parrot, and T. G. Ward.** 1953. Isolation of a cytopathogenic agent from human adenoids undergoing spontaneous degeneration in tissue culture. *Proc. Soc. Exp. Biol. Med.* **84:**570–573.
108. **Russell, K. L., M. P. Broderick, S. E. Franklin, L. B. Blyn, N. E. Freed, E. Moradi, D. J. Ecker, P. E. Kammerer, M. A. Osuna, A. E. Kajon, C. B. Morn, and M. A. Ryan.** 2006. Transmission dynamics and prospective environmental sampling of adenovirus in a military recruit setting. *J. Infect. Dis.* **194:**877–885.
109. **Ruuska, T., and T. Vesikari.** 1991. A prospective study of acute diarrhoea in Finnish children from birth to 2 1/2 years of age. *Acta Paediatr. Scand.* **80:**500–507.
110. **Ruuskanen, O., M. Arola, T. Heikkinen, and T. Ziegler.** 1991. Viruses in acute otitis media: increasing evidence for clinical significance. *Pediatr. Infect. Dis. J.* **10:** 425–427.
111. **Ruuskanen, O., J. Mertsola, and O. Meurman.** 1988. Adenovirus infection in families. *Arch. Dis. Child.* **63:** 1250–1253.
112. **Ruuskanen, O., O. Meurman, and H. Sarkkinen.** 1985. Adenoviral diseases in children: a study of 105 hospital cases. *Pediatrics* **76:**79–83.
113. **Ruuskanen, O., A. Putto, H. Sarkkinen, O. Meurman, and K. Irjala.** 1985. C-reactive protein in respiratory virus infections. *J. Pediatr.* **107:**97–100.
114. **Ruuskanen, O., H. Sarkkinen, O. Meurman, P. Hurme, T. Rossi, P. Halonen, and P. Hanninen.** 1984. Rapid diagnosis of adenoviral tonsillitis: a prospective clinical study. *J. Pediatr.* **104:**725–728.
115. **San Martin, C., and R. M. Burnett.** 2003. Structural studies on adenoviruses. *Curr. Top. Microbiol. Immunol.* **272:**57–94.
116. **Sattar, S. A., M. Abebe, A. J. Bueti, H. Jampani, J. Newman, and S. Hua.** 2000. Activity of an alcohol-based hand gel against human adeno-, rhino-, and rotaviruses using the fingerpad method. *Infect. Control Hosp. Epidemiol.* **21:**516–519.
117. **Sauerbrei, A., K. Sehr, A. Brandstadt, A. Heim, K. Reimer, and P. Wutzler.** 2004. Sensitivity of human adenoviruses to different groups of chemical biocides. *J. Hosp. Infect.* **57:**59–66.
118. **Schmitz, H., R. Wigand, and W. Heinrich.** 1983. Worldwide epidemiology of human adenovirus infections. *Am. J. Epidemiol.* **117:**455–466.
119. **Schonland, M., M. L. Strong, and A. Wesley.** 1976. Fatal adenovirus pneumonia: clinical and pathological features. *S. Afr. Med. J.* **50:**1748–1751.
120. **Shenk, T.** 1996. Adenoviridae: the viruses and their replication, p. 2111–2148. *In* B. N. Fields, D. M. Knipe, and P. M. Howley (ed.), *Fields Virology*, 3rd ed. Lippincott-Raven Publishers, Philadelphia, PA.
121. **Shields, A. F., R. C. Hackman, K. H. Fife, L. Corey, and J. D. Meyers.** 1985. Adenovirus infections in patients undergoing bone-marrow transplantation. *N. Engl. J. Med.* **312:**529–533.
122. **Shike, H., C. Shimizu, J. Kanegaye, J. L. Foley, and J. C. Burns.** 2005. Quantitation of adenovirus genome during acute infection in normal children. *Pediatr. Infect. Dis. J.* **24:**29–33.
123. **Shult, P. A., F. Polyak, E. C. Dick, D. M. Warshauer, L. A. King, and A. D. Mandel.** 1991. Adenovirus 21 infection in an isolated Antarctic station: transmission of the virus and susceptibility of the population. *Am. J. Epidemiol.* **133:**599–607.

124. **Similä, S., R. Jouppila, A. Salmi, and R. Pohjonen.** 1970. Encephalomeningitis in children associated with an adenovirus type 7 epidemic. *Acta Paediatr. Scand.* **59:** 310–316.
125. **Simila, S., O. Linna, P. Lanning, E. Heikkinen, and M. Ala-Houhala.** 1981. Chronic lung damage caused by adenovirus type 7: a ten-year follow-up study. *Chest* **80:** 127–131.
126. **Sivaprakasam, P., T. F. Carr, M. Coussons, T. Khalid, A. S. Bailey, M. Guiver, K. J. Mutton, A. J. Turner, J. D. Grainger, and R. F. Wynn.** 2007. Improved outcome from invasive adenovirus infection in pediatric patients after hemopoietic stem cell transplantation using intensive clinical surveillance and early intervention. *J. Pediatr. Hematol. Oncol.* **29:**81–85.
127. **Steen-Johnsen, J., I. Orstavik, and A. Attramadal.** 1969. Severe illnesses due to adenovirus type 7 in children. *Acta Paediatr. Scand.* **58:**157–163.
128. **Stracker, T. H., C. T. Carson, and M. D. Weitzman.** 2002. Adenovirus oncoproteins inactivate the Mre11-Rad50-NBS1 DNA repair complex. *Nature* **418:**348–352.
129. **Swenson, P. D., M. S. Lowens, C. L. Celum, and J. C. Hierholzer.** 1995. Adenovirus types 2, 8, and 37 associated with genital infections in patients attending a sexually transmitted disease clinic. *J. Clin. Microbiol.* **33:** 2728–2731.
130. **Tang, J., M. Olive, R. Pulmanausahakul, M. Schnell, N. Flomenberg, L. Eisenlohr, and P. Flomenberg.** 2006. Human $CD8^+$ cytotoxic T cell responses to adenovirus capsid proteins. *Virology* **350:**312–322.
131. **Tollefson, A. E., A. Scaria, T. W. Hermiston, J. S. Ryerse, L. J. Wold, and W. S. Wold.** 1996. The adenovirus death protein (E3-11.6K) is required at very late stages of infection for efficient cell lysis and release of adenovirus from infected cells. *J. Virol.* **70:**2296–2306.
132. **Trotman, L. C., N. Mosberger, M. Fornerod, R. P. Stidwill, and U. F. Greber.** 2001. Import of adenovirus DNA involves the nuclear pore complex receptor CAN/Nup214 and histone H1. *Nat. Cell Biol.* **3:**1092–1100.
133. **Uhnoo, I., G. Wadell, L. Svensson, and M. E. Johansson.** 1984. Importance of enteric adenoviruses 40 and 41 in acute gastroenteritis in infants and young children. *J. Clin. Microbiol.* **20:**365–372.
134. **Ullman, A. J., N. C. Reich, and P. Hearing.** 2007. Adenovirus E4 ORF3 protein inhibits the interferon-mediated antiviral response. *J. Virol.* **81:**4744–4752.
135. **van de Pol, A. C., A. M. van Loon, T. F. Wolfs, N. J. Jansen, M. Nijhuis, E. K. Breteler, R. Schuurman, and J. W. Rossen.** 2007. Increased detection of respiratory syncytial virus, influenza viruses, parainfluenza viruses, and adenoviruses with real-time PCR in samples from patients with respiratory symptoms. *J. Clin. Microbiol.* **45:**2260–2262.
136. **Van der Vliet, P. C.** 1995. Adenovirus DNA replication. *Curr. Top. Microbiol. Immunol.* **199**(Pt. 2)**:**1–30.
137. **Van Lierde, S., L. Corbeel, and E. Eggermont.** 1989. Clinical and laboratory findings in children with adenovirus infections. *Eur. J. Pediatr.* **148:**423–425.
138. **van Tol, M. J., E. C. Claas, B. Heemskerk, L. A. Veltrop-Duits, C. S. de Brouwer, T. van Vreeswijk, C. C. Sombroek, A. C. Kroes, M. F. Beersma, E. P. de Klerk, R. M. Egeler, A. C. Lankester, and M. W. Schilham.** 2005. Adenovirus infection in children after allogeneic stem cell transplantation: diagnosis, treatment and immunity. *Bone Marrow Transplant.* **35**(Suppl. 1)**:** S73–S76.
139. **Walters, R. W., P. Freimuth, T. O. Moninger, I. Ganske, J. Zabner, and M. J. Welsh.** 2002. Adenovirus fiber disrupts CAR-mediated intercellular adhesion allowing virus escape. *Cell* **110:**789–799.
140. **Walters, R. W., T. Grunst, J. M. Bergelson, R. W. Finberg, M. J. Welsh, and J. Zabner.** 1999. Basolateral localization of fiber receptors limits adenovirus infection from the apical surface of airway epithelia. *J. Biol. Chem.* **274:**10219–10226.
141. **Warren, D., K. E. Nelson, J. A. Farrar, E. Hurwitz, J. Hierholzer, E. Ford, and L. J. Anderson.** 1989. A large outbreak of epidemic keratoconjunctivitis: problems in controlling nosocomial spread. *J. Infect. Dis.* **160:**938–943.
142. **Weber, J. M.** 1995. Adenovirus endopeptidase and its role in virus infection. *Curr. Top. Microbiol. Immunol.* **199**(Pt. 1)**:**227–235.
143. **White, E.** 2001. Regulation of the cell cycle and apoptosis by the oncogenes of adenovirus. *Oncogene* **20:** 7836–7846.
144. **Wiethoff, C. M., H. Wodrich, L. Gerace, and G. R. Nemerow.** 2005. Adenovirus protein VI mediates membrane disruption following capsid disassembly. *J. Virol.* **79:**1992–2000.
145. **Wildin, S. R., T. Chonmaitree, and L. E. Swischuk.** 1988. Roentgenographic features of common pediatric viral respiratory tract infections. *Am. J. Dis. Child.* **142:** 43–46.
146. **Yan, Z., S. Nguyen, M. Poles, J. Melamed, and J. V. Scholes.** 1998. Adenovirus colitis in human immunodeficiency virus infection: an underdiagnosed entity. *Am. J. Surg. Pathol.* **22:**1101–1106.
147. **Ylikoski, J., and J. Karjalainen.** 1989. Acute tonsillitis in young men: etiological agents and their differentiation. *Scand. J. Infect. Dis.* **21:**169–174.
148. **Yolken, R. H., F. Lawrence, F. Leister, H. E. Takiff, and S. E. Strauss.** 1982. Gastroenteritis associated with enteric type adenovirus in hospitalized infants. *J. Pediatr.* **101:**21–26.
149. **Zhang, W., and M. J. Imperiale.** 2000. Interaction of the adenovirus IVa2 protein with viral packaging sequences. *J. Virol.* **74:**2687–2693.
150. **Zhang, Y., and J. M. Bergelson.** 2005. Adenovirus receptors. *J. Virol.* **79:**12125–12131.
151. **Zhang, Y., N. Chirmule, G. P. Gao, R. Qian, M. Croyle, B. Joshi, J. Tazelaar, and J. M. Wilson.** 2001. Acute cytokine response to systemic adenoviral vectors in mice is mediated by dendritic cells and macrophages. *Mol. Ther.* **3:**697–707.
152. **Zou, A., I. Atencio, W. M. Huang, M. Horn, and M. Ramachandra.** 2004. Overexpression of adenovirus E3-11.6K protein induces cell killing by both caspase-dependent and caspase-independent mechanisms. *Virology* **326:**240–249.
153. **Zsengeller, Z., K. Otake, S. A. Hossain, P. Y. Berclaz, and B. C. Trapnell.** 2000. Internalization of adenovirus by alveolar macrophages initiates early proinflammatory signaling during acute respiratory tract infection. *J. Virol.* **74:**9655–9667.

Polyomaviruses

JOHN E. GREENLEE AND FRANK J. O'NEILL

27

Polyomaviruses are widely distributed in humans and other animal species. The prototype member of the genus, polyomavirus of mice, was discovered in 1953 as an agent capable of producing tumors in its natural host (49). A second polyomavirus, murine K virus (now known as mouse pneumotropic virus [MPtV]), was discovered in 1952 and identified as a member of the papovavirus group in 1963 (55). An additional virus, the polyomavirus simian virus 40 (SV40), was discovered in 1960 as a contaminant of lots of rhesus monkey kidney cells used to prepare polio vaccine stocks (101). Infectious SV40 was subsequently detected in both the Salk and Sabin polio vaccines, as well as in adenovirus vaccines, and was inadvertently administered to millions of individuals worldwide (101). The virus became an object of intense experimental interest after it was shown to cause tumors in experimental animals (101). SV40 also became a favorite laboratory model for the molecular biological analysis of oncogenic cell transformation (54, 72, 101).

The first evidence that polyomaviruses might also be indigenous to humans came in 1965, when Zu Rhein et al. and Silverman and Rubinstein independently detected structures resembling polyomaviruses in brain material from patients with a fatal demyelinating disease, progressive multifocal leukoencephalopathy (PML) (45). Isolation of the agent was not achieved until 1971, when Padgett et al. recovered a previously unknown human polyomavirus, JC virus (JCV), by inoculation of brain material from a PML patient into primary cultures of human fetal glial cells (81). Since that time, JCV has been consistently recovered from PML brains and, more recently, has been associated with an encephalitis involving cerebellar granule cells.

In the same year in which JCV was isolated, a second human papovavirus, BK virus (BKV), was recovered from the urine of human renal transplant patients (38). BKV has since been repeatedly recovered from urine and also been associated with a number of urological conditions (52). Recently, additional polyomaviruses, Li, WU, and Merkel cell virus (MCV; also known as MCPyV), have been identified using molecular techniques in human samples.

JCV, BKV, and SV40 are also able to transform cells in tissue culture and to produce tumors in experimental animals. For this reason, there has been strong interest in the relationship of these agents to human cancer, but such an association has not been proven.

VIROLOGY

Classification

Polyomaviruses were initially considered a genus within the family *Papovaviridae*, which included papillomaviruses and polyomaviruses. In 2000, these agents, which are structurally and genetically unrelated, were reclassified as two separate families, *Papillomaviridae* and *Polyomaviridae*. Polyomaviruses have been isolated from a number of animal species (Table 1; Fig. 1) but have only been associated with clinical disease in mice, monkeys, humans, and birds.

Virus Structure and Composition

Polyomaviruses are unenveloped, 40- to 45-nm, icosahedral agents whose genomic material is comprised of supercoiled, circular, double-stranded DNA (Fig. 2) (54). JCV, BKV, and SV40 DNAs contain 5,130, 4,963, and 5,243 bp, respectively (54). The three agents exhibit extensive (69 to 75%) DNA homology. Sequences showing greatest divergence between these three agents lie in the regulatory region (RR), on the late side of the origin of replication (54). Both JCV and BKV differ from SV40 in that they are able to agglutinate human type O erythrocytes, as well as erythrocytes of several animal species.

Four major groups of BKV have been described. Group I comprises the prototype strain, Dunlop (DUN), as well as two other strains, MM and GS. Group II contains the SB strain, group III contains the AS strain, and group IV contains the MG and RF strains (54). GS and MM viruses have sequence differences around the replication origin (54). MGV and RFV, although antigenically similar to BKV, have a bipartite genome consisting of two complementing defective molecules, one having a deletion corresponding to the BKV early region and the other having a deletion corresponding to the BKV late region (82, 83).

Although the genomes of JCV, BKV, and SV40 yield only single serotypes of virus, extensive variation may occur in the RRs of each (54), resulting in multiple strains of each agent. Strains which are shed in urine and involved in transmission of infection are termed archetypal strains. Strains differing from the archetypal strain in their RRs are

TABLE 1 Major human and animal polyomaviruses[a]

Agent	Abbreviation	Species specificity	Major site(s) of persistent infection	Pathogenicity	
				Healthy hosts	Immunosuppressed hosts
Humans					
JC virus	JCV	High	Kidney (brain, PBMCs, possibly other organs)	Inapparent or mild	PML (cerebellar granule cell infection)
BK virus	BKV	High	Kidneys	Inapparent or mild	Cystitis, ureteral stenosis, nephritis
WU virus	WUV	Unknown	Unknown	Unknown	Unknown
LI virus	LIV	Unknown	Unknown	Unknown	Unknown
Merkel cell polyomavirus	MCV or MCPyV	Unknown	Unknown	Unknown	Isolated from cutaneous Merkel cell carcinoma tissue
Nonhuman primates					
Simian virus 40	SV40	High (rhesus macaques, cynomolgus monkeys, humans)	Kidney	Inapparent or mild	In monkeys: interstitial pneumonia; PML-like illness in simian AIDS
SA12 *or* baboon polyomavirus type 1	SA12	High	Kidney	Inapparent or mild	Unknown
Simian lymphotrophic polyomavirus	LPV	High	B lymphocytes	Inapparent or mild	Unknown
Baboon polyomavirus type 2		High	Kidney	Inapparent or mild	Unknown
Other mammals					
Polyomavirus (mice)	PyV	High	Kidney	Inapparent or mild	Inapparent or mild (tumor induction in neonatal animals)
Mouse pneumotropic virus (K virus)	MPtV; formerly KV	High	Kidney	Endothelial cells acutely; persistence in renal tubular epithelium	Fatal interstitial pneumonia (neonatal or immunosuppressed animals)
Hamster polyomavirus	HaPV	High	Kidney	Tichoepitheliomas, lymphomas	Lymphomas
Rabbit kidney vacuolating virus	RKV	Unknown	Kidney	Unknown	Unknown
Rat polyomavirus		High	?Kidney	Inapparent or mild	Sialoadenitis
Bovine polyomavirus	BPV	High	Kidney	Inapparent or mild	Unknown
Birds					
Avian polyomavirus	APV	Low (psittacine and other birds)	Kidney, small intestine	Lethal multiorgan involvement	Lethal multiorgan involvement
Goose hemorrhagic polyomavirus	GHPV	High	Kidney	Endothelial involvement with multiorgan hemorrhage	Endothelial involvement with multiorgan hemorrhage

[a] Adapted from reference 84.

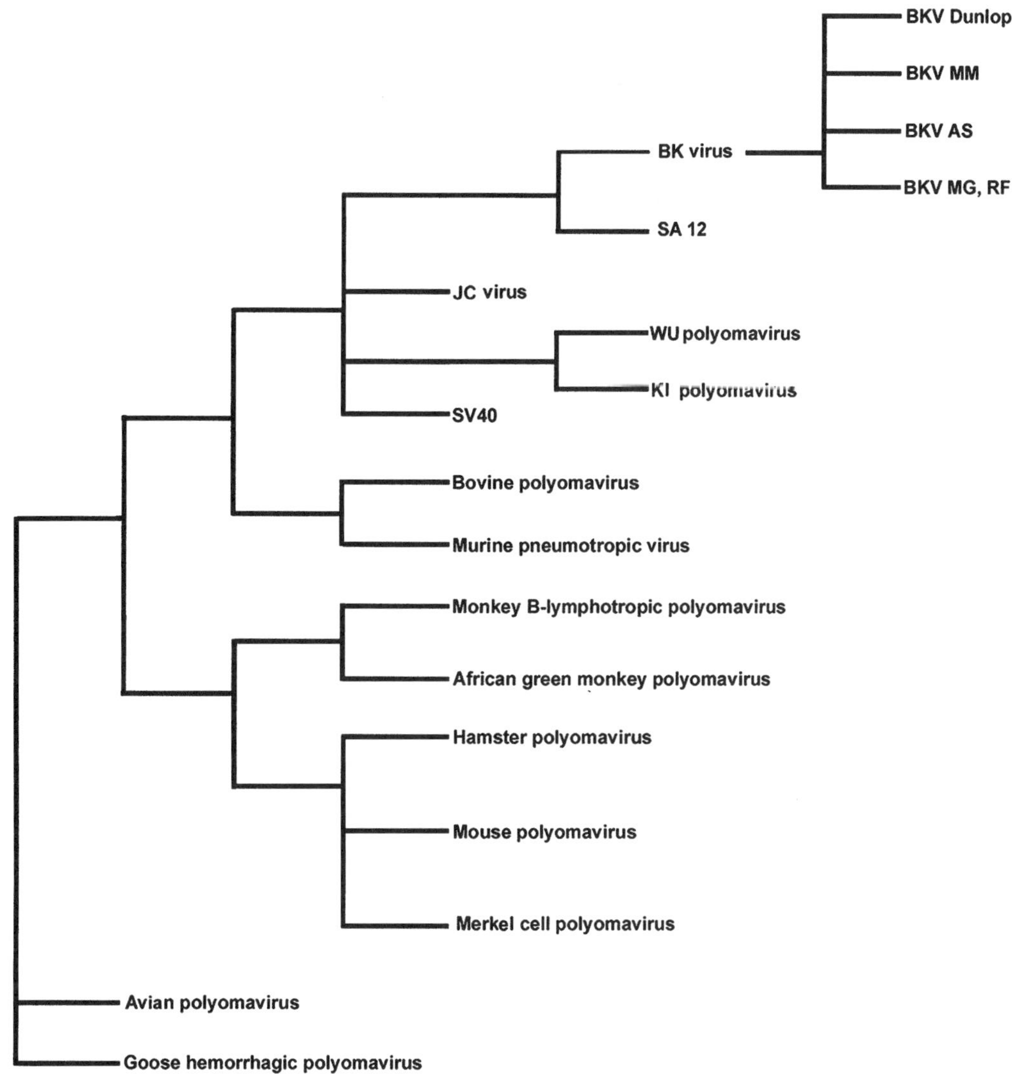

FIGURE 1 Taxonomic relationships of the major polyomaviruses.

termed variant or rearranged strains (119). As discussed below, variance from archetypal genomic sequences has been postulated to account for differences in the biological behavior of these agents, including host range, regulation of viral growth, and ability to cause disease.

Regulatory and Structural Proteins

Polyomaviruses encode two groups of viral proteins: early proteins, which control viral synthesis but are not components of the virion, and late proteins, which include the viral capsid (Table 2) (54). Early and late regions of the viral genome are separated at their 5′ termini by RR sequences of approximately 500 bp which contain a single replication origin (Fig. 3). The RR plays an important role in controlling early and late gene expression and also in initiating viral DNA replication.

The early proteins have been most thoroughly studied in the case of SV40. The roles of these proteins in SV40 synthesis are thought to apply to BKV and JCV as well. The most important early protein is large T antigen (T-Ag), a 708-amino-acid protein which is expressed predominantly in the cell nucleus but is also present at the cell membrane (Fig. 4) (54). T-Ag binds to the viral origin of replication as well as the RR and has multiple functions, many of which are accomplished by the ability of T-Ag to bind to and modulate the activity of cellular proteins. Functions of T-Ag include initiation of viral DNA replication and regulation of synthesis of both viral and cell proteins (Table 2). T-Ag is the only viral protein essential for viral DNA synthesis. T-Ag also interacts with multiple cellular proteins, including tumor suppressor proteins pRb, p107, p130, and p53. T-Ag plays an essential role in virus-induced cell transformation (54), and the presence of T-Ag in cells has been used as a marker for polyomavirus-induced cell transformation (Fig. 4 and 5). T-Ag also serves as a recognition site for T-cell-mediated cytotoxicity (110). Small t antigen (t-ag) is a histone-rich protein which shares its N terminus with T-Ag but has a unique C terminus. The functions of t-ag and of the late agnoprotein are outlined in Table 2 (54).

Three structural proteins comprise the viral capsid: Vp1, Vp2, and Vp3. Vp1 is a 45-kDa protein which makes up the major portion of the viral capsid and is the major protein involved in viral attachment to cells (54). Vp2 and

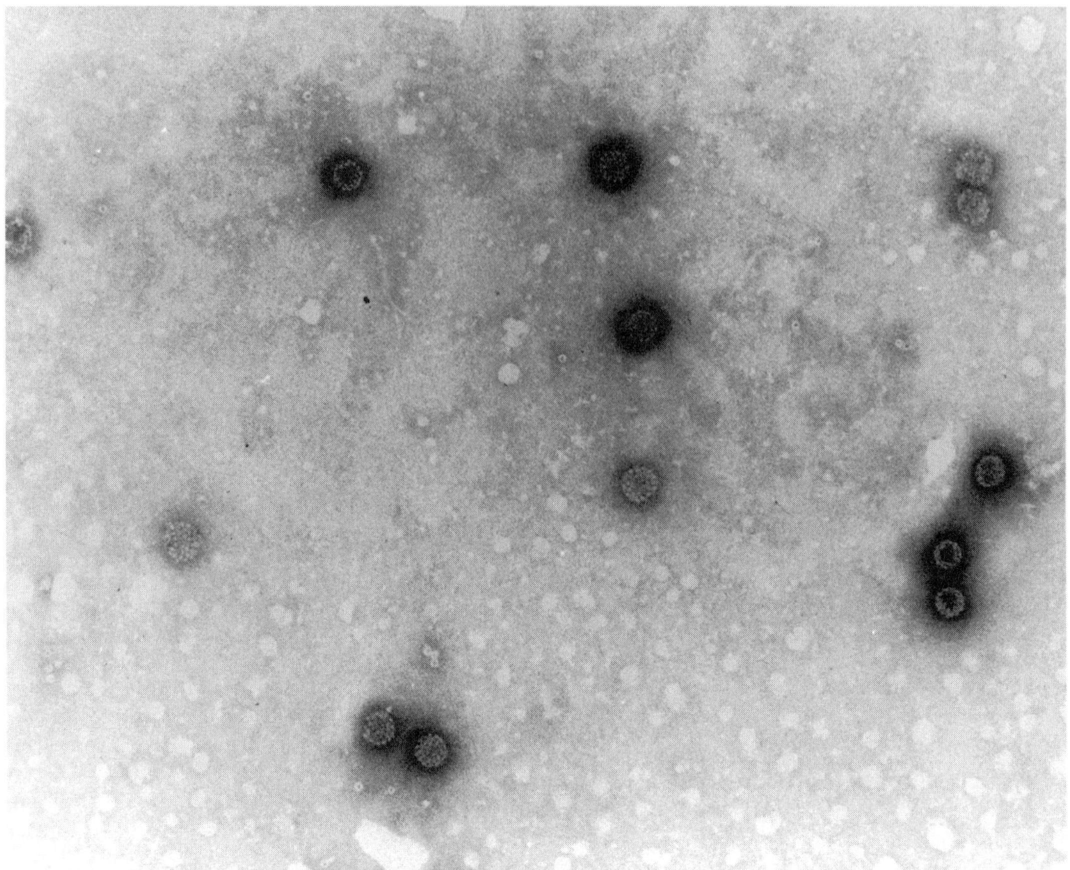

FIGURE 2 Electron micrograph of BKV extracted from human fetal kidney cells, concentrated by ultracentrifugation, and stained with 2% phosphotungstic acid, showing characteristic 42-nm particles.

Vp3 are minor constituents of the viral capsid. Extensive antigenic similarity exists between the T-Ags and t-ags of JCV BKV, and SV40. A lesser degree of antigenic cross-reactivity exists among intact JCV, BKV, and SV40 virions (45).

Biology

Virus Attachment and Entry into Cells

JCV and BKV infection can be blocked by pretreatment of cells with neuraminidase, suggesting that the receptors for these viruses contain sialic acid (54). Terminal alpha(2,6)-linked sialic acid is a crucial component of the JCV receptor (32). This moiety is present within the central nervous system (CNS) on the surface of oligodendrocytes and astrocytes but not cortical neurons, and it is also present on B lymphocytes, T lymphocytes, and cells within the kidneys and lungs (32). JCV also attaches to the 5HT2AR serotonin receptor present on cultured glial cells, and viral attachment can be blocked by monoclonal antibodies specific for this protein (34). Other receptors may also exist. JCV can infect cultured human brain microvascular endothelial cells without using the serotonin receptor (20). BKV attachment to cells has been less extensively studied than has JCV attachment. An N-linked glycoprotein containing alpha(2,3)-linked sialic acid appears to be a critical component of the cellular receptor for BKV (30). Addition of the gangliosides GD1b and GT1b to LNCaP cells, which are normally resistant to BKV infection, makes the cells susceptible to the virus (30, 65).

Internalization of JCV into susceptible cells differs from internalization of BKV or SV40. Internalization of JCV involves endocytosis of the virus within clathrin-coated pits, and transport of JCV to the cell nucleus involves microtubules and microfilaments (54). In contrast, BKV and SV40 enter cells by endocytosis into caveosomes and from there into the endoplasmic reticulum (54); virus-containing vesicles are then transported intracellularly to fuse with the outer membrane of the cell nucleus, releasing viral particles into perinuclear cisternae. Uncoating of JCV and BKV DNAs is thought to occur exclusively within the cell nucleus, although uncoating of SV40 may also begin within the endoplasmic reticulum (54).

Viral Replication

The steps of viral replication have been most clearly defined for SV40, with BKV and JCV being thought to replicate in a similar fashion. Viral transcription occurs in two stages, with early viral genes being transcribed off of one DNA strand in one direction and late viral genes being transcribed after the early genes and off the other strand in the opposite direction (54). The early promoter of SV40 is located near the replication origin and contains a TATA

TABLE 2 Functions of early and late polyomavirus-encoded proteins[a]

Function	Comment(s)
T-Ag functions	
Viral DNA replication	T-Ag forms a double hexamer and in the presence of ATP causes untwisting of the early viral DNA palindrome within the origin. Using its helicase activity, the complex unwinds the viral DNA bidirectionally. Cellular proteins, topoisomerase I, and DNA polymerase/primase are recruited to the replication origin to form a replication complex which is involved in the initiation of the replication of viral DNA molecules.
Activation of late viral gene expression	T-Ag effects an alteration of the cellular repressors which normally bind near the late promoter. This derepression, perhaps in combination with recruitment of transcription factors, activates late transcription. Alternatively, replicated viral DNAs appear in sufficient amounts to titrate the repressors.
Down-regulation of T-Ag expression	Two possible mechanisms for this down-regulation have been reported. (i) T-Ag activates expression of the late genes at the late promoter by helping to recruit transcription factors. Activation of the late promoter sequesters the transcription factors also required for the activation of the T-Ag promoter, causing its own down-regulation. (ii) In autoregulation, T-Ag binds to viral DNA at sites which block expression of the T-Ag gene.
Initiation and maintenance of cell transformation	When T-Ag binds to and/or inactivates tumor suppressors p53, Rb, and perhaps several others, the suppression or control of cell growth is then reversed and the cells become morphologically transformed and display several parameters of transformation. Also, the cells may form tumors in appropriate animals and can assume an immortal phenotype in culture. T-Ag may be required for immortalization of polyomavirus-transformed cells.
t-ag	
Leads to intracellular accumulations of viral DNA and viral replication; regulates PP2A	
Reverses the apoptotic effect of T-Ag	
Causes cell cycle progression; increases tumorgenicity of T-Ag-transformed cells	
Binds several cellular proteins, e.g., p300 and PP2A	
Induces telomerase and cellular AKT kinase activities	
Late (capsid) functions	
Vp1	Major capsid protein; involved in virus attachment to cell surface receptors
Vp2, Vp3	Minor capsid proteins
Agnoprotein	May serve a role in viral morphogenesis perhaps by retarding polymerization
	May help with intracellular migration of Vp1 to the perinuclear region and entry of Vp1 into the nucleus with consequent viral assembly
	Involved with late transcriptional regulation
	May play a role in cell-to-cell spread of virus

[a] Data from reference 54.

box, three GC-rich regions, and an enhancer region of 72-bp tandem repeats all contained within the RR (54). Archetypal SV40 strains isolated directly from simians usually contain only a single 72-bp enhancer element, whereas partial duplication of this region is characteristic of strains cultivated in vitro (77). The early GC-rich regions are bound by the Sp1 cellular transcription factor, and the enhancer region is believed to be bound to other transcription factors. Transcription is mediated by cellular RNA polymerase II, resulting first in the production of mRNAs encoding T-Ag and t-ag (54). During late transcription there is differential splicing to form the mRNAs encoding the agnoprotein, as well as Vp1, Vp2, and Vp3. Assembly of virions occurs in the cell nucleus, followed by release of viral particles during cell lysis (54).

Host Range

Polyomaviruses are extremely species specific. In general, neither JCV nor BKV causes productive infection in species other than humans. SV40 naturally infects rhesus and cynomolgus monkeys but was shown to produce limited infection in humans following exposure to contaminated vaccines (69). Inoculation of laboratory rodents (or, in the case of JCV or BKV, nonhuman primates) with JCV, BKV, or SV40 causes a variety of neoplasms, usually at or near the site of inoculation. The three agents usually do not cause systemic infection in nonhuman species, although in one study BKV was shown to cause systemic infection and interstitial nephritis in immunosuppressed cynomolgus monkeys (120). Species specificity and ability to infect specific cell populations are controlled by regulatory elements unique to each virus (54).

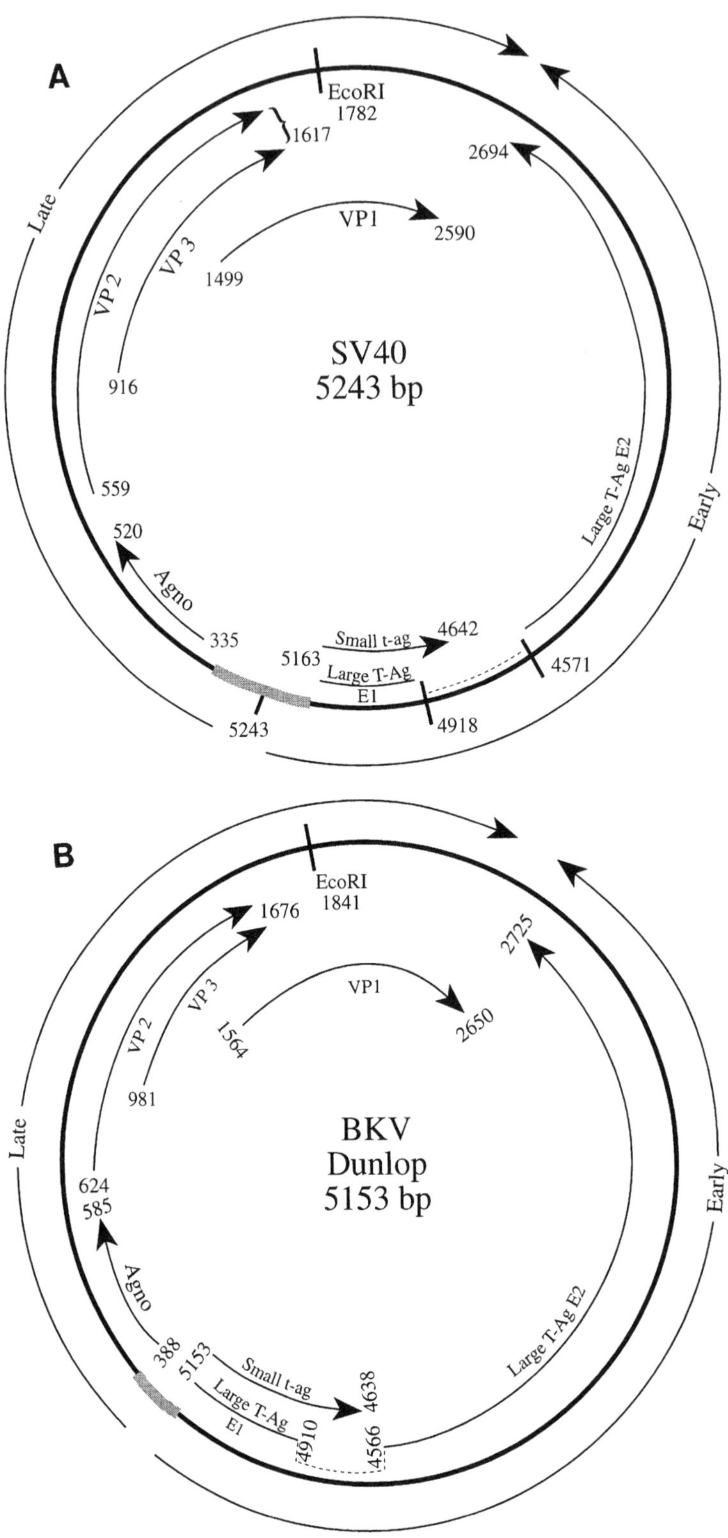

FIGURE 3 Viral gene transcription maps of SV40 (A), BKV (B), and JCV (C) DNAs. The checkerboard area on the thick solid line indicates the portion of the RR. The thin dashed line indicates intron sequences spliced out of large T-Ag. (Adapted from references 33 [A], 100 [B], and 4 [C].)

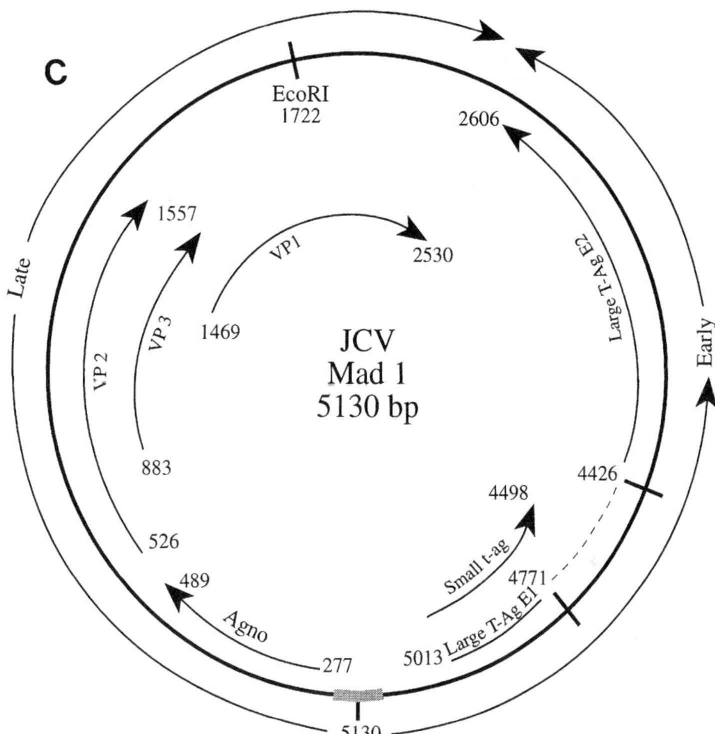

FIGURE 3 *(Continued)*

Growth in Cell Culture

JCV, BKV, and SV40 readily replicate in primary human fetal glial (PHFG) cells. Other than their ability to replicate in PHFG cells, however, the culture requirements of these three agents differ considerably (75). JCV was initially isolated in PHFG cells, and this culture system has been used most extensively in studies of the virus (81). Although several other cell culture systems have been developed, these have been less extensively employed (45). The archetypal strain of JCV has proven much more difficult to culture. Limited growth of the JCV archetype has been shown to occur in PHFG cells, and very slow growth of the virus also occurs in human embryonic kidney (HEK) and human endothelial cell cultures (78).

BKV grows most readily in human fibroblasts, early-passage primary cultures of HEK and PHFG cells. The virus also grows in simian BSC-1 cells and, to a limited extent, in simian Vero cells (37). SV40 can be isolated in cell lines derived from African green monkey kidney cells (BSC-1, CV-1, and Vero cells) and has also been propagated in several human tumor cell lines (75, 79). SV40 grows poorly in human fibroblasts, such as WI-38 cells, and even less efficiently in HEK cells (62, 63, 75, 79).

Interaction of Polyomaviruses with Glial Cell Cultures

The infections caused by SV40 and BKV in PHFG cultures differ significantly from that caused by JCV. Inoculation of PHFG cells with SV40 results in a progressive lytic infection of certain cell populations, resulting in high titers of infectious virus, and a transforming infection in others (Fig. 6) (77, 80). Inoculation of PHFG cultures with BKV produces an infection which is nearly identical to that seen with SV40, and serial passage of BKV-infected brain cultures resulted in the development of both persistently infected and transformed cell lines (Fig. 6) (80). In contrast, the Mad-1 strain of JCV causes a productive infection in PHFG cells which evolves over weeks. JCV infection in this culture system has a more limited cytopathic effect than does that produced by BKV or SV40 and in some studies has been described to involve spongioblasts or oligodendroblasts almost exclusively (Fig. 6) (80).

Cell Transformation by Polyomaviruses

In primary cell cultures or cell lines which are permissive, each polyomavirus replicates to generate progeny virus. Infection of cells which are nonpermissive for these viruses, however, does not result in viral replication. Instead, such cells usually express early but not late viral proteins, develop distinctive biological and biochemical properties such as the ability to grow from single cells or to grow in agar or serum-free media, and are considered transformed (76). Some, but not all, transformants become capable of indefinite serial passage and are considered immortal in culture. In general, cell transformation has required the use of cell culture systems derived from species other than those infected in nature by the virus. Most cell transformation studies involving SV40, BKV, and JCV have employed cultured rodent cells. However, BKV and SV40 have been shown to transform primary cultures of human diploid cells, including PHFG cells, HEK cells, and fibroblasts (75). Studies of chimeric SV40/BKV and SV40/JCV T-Ags demonstrated that three regions of SV40 T-Ag are required for immortalization of human cells: the N terminus, a central region containing the Rb-binding domain, and the C terminus (76). The mechanisms by which immortalization occurs are not well understood, however, and neither JCV nor BKV matches SV40 in its ability to im-

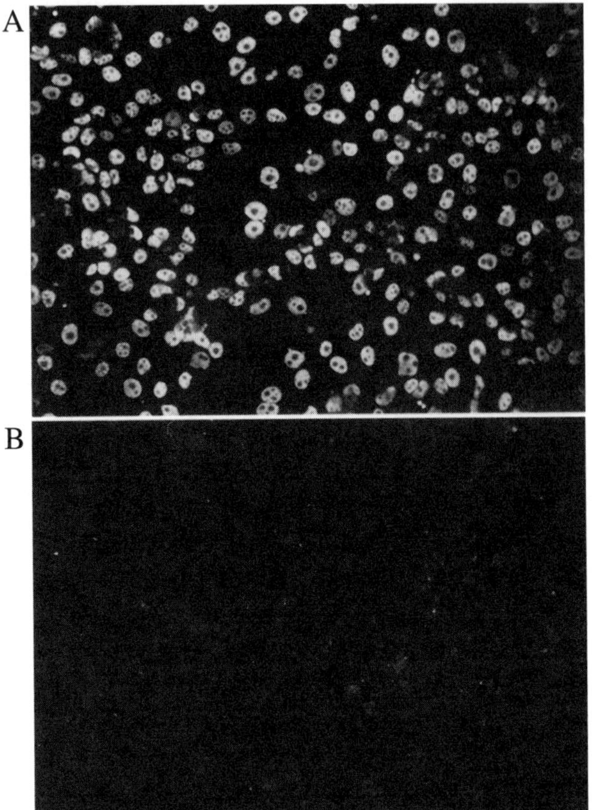

FIGURE 4 (A) Identification of SV40 T-Ag by immunofluorescence in transformed simian TC-7 kidney cells. Cells were grown in a monolayer and reacted with monoclonal antibodies PAb 416, PAb 108, and PAb 101 directed against T-Ag as described by O'Neill et al. (78a). (B) Naïve TC-7 cells (not containing T-Ag-encoding DNA sequences) reacted with monoclonal antibodies as in panel A (negative control).

mortalize human cells. The ability of these three viruses to produce tumors in animals is discussed below.

Inactivation by Chemical and Physical Agents

Polyomaviruses withstand prolonged drying at room temperature and are relatively resistant to heat. Because they lack a lipid envelope, they are unaffected by ether and other lipid solvents. The viruses can be inactivated by β-propiolactone, proteolytic digestion, formaldehyde, prolonged heating to above 50°C, and exposure to UV light. The ability of these agents to persist at room temperature can present significant risks of inadvertent contamination in laboratories in which these agents have been studied.

EPIDEMIOLOGY

JCV and BKV

JCV and BKV are ubiquitous in human populations. Acquisition of antibody to JCV and BKV begins in infancy (90, 102). The prevalence of antibody to JCV is 10% in children 5 years of age and rises to 76% by late adult life (102). Serologic evidence of infection by BKV is present in 37% of individuals by 5 years of age and 83% by adolescence; these rates fall to 53% in individuals over 50 years of age (102). Studies of geographically isolated populations indicate that BKV and JCV are worldwide in distribution (102). Antibodies to BKV and JCV have been detected in populations so isolated as to be without evidence of contact with measles and influenza viruses (102). The high prevalence of serum antibody response to JCV or BKV is not further increased in immunosuppressed patients, including those with human immunodeficiency virus (HIV) infection. This is in contrast to the prevalence of symptomatic infection with these agents. PML occurs essentially only in immunocompromised patients and is most prevalent in patients with AIDS. Similarly, although BKV is a ubiquitous agent, it is associated with significant human disease only in immunosuppressed patients, in particular in the setting of renal or other organ transplantation.

Recently Identified Human Polyomaviruses

Within the last 2 years, three additional polyomaviruses were identified through application of molecular screening techniques. Two of these, KI virus and WU virus, were detected by PCR screening of human respiratory secretions and stool samples (3, 9, 41). KI polyomavirus has been found in nasopharyngeal aspirates and stool samples but not in urine or blood. Sequencing studies of KI polyomavirus have shown it to be phylogenetically related to JCV, BKV, and SV40 in the early region but to have little homology in the late region. WU virus appears to be closely related to but distinct from KI virus. Both agents appear to be worldwide in distribution. The two viruses have been detected in essentially equal frequencies in patients with and without respiratory illness, and it is not yet known whether either agent is associated with human disease (74). In early 2008, a third polyomavirus, MCV, was iden-

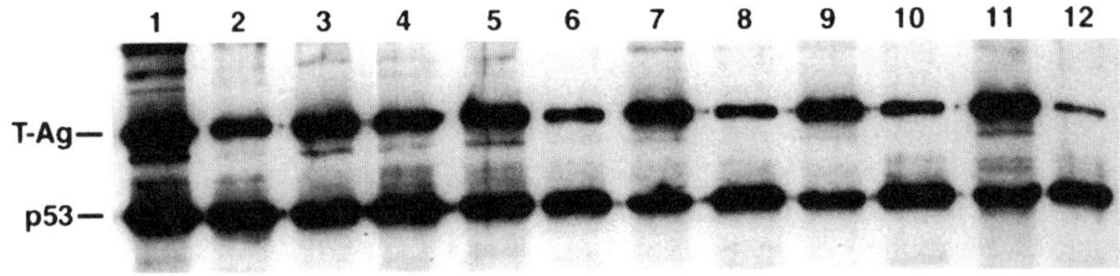

FIGURE 5 Western blot of SV40 T-Ag and p53 from transformed human cells. SV40 T-Ag was immunoprecipitated in even-numbered lanes and p53 was immunoprecipitated in odd-numbered lanes, and the immunoprecipitates were subjected to electrophoresis in agarose gels and analyzed by Western blotting using a cocktail of antibodies to T-Ag or p53 (95). The illustration shows that immunoprecipitation of either protein results in coprecipitation of the second protein.

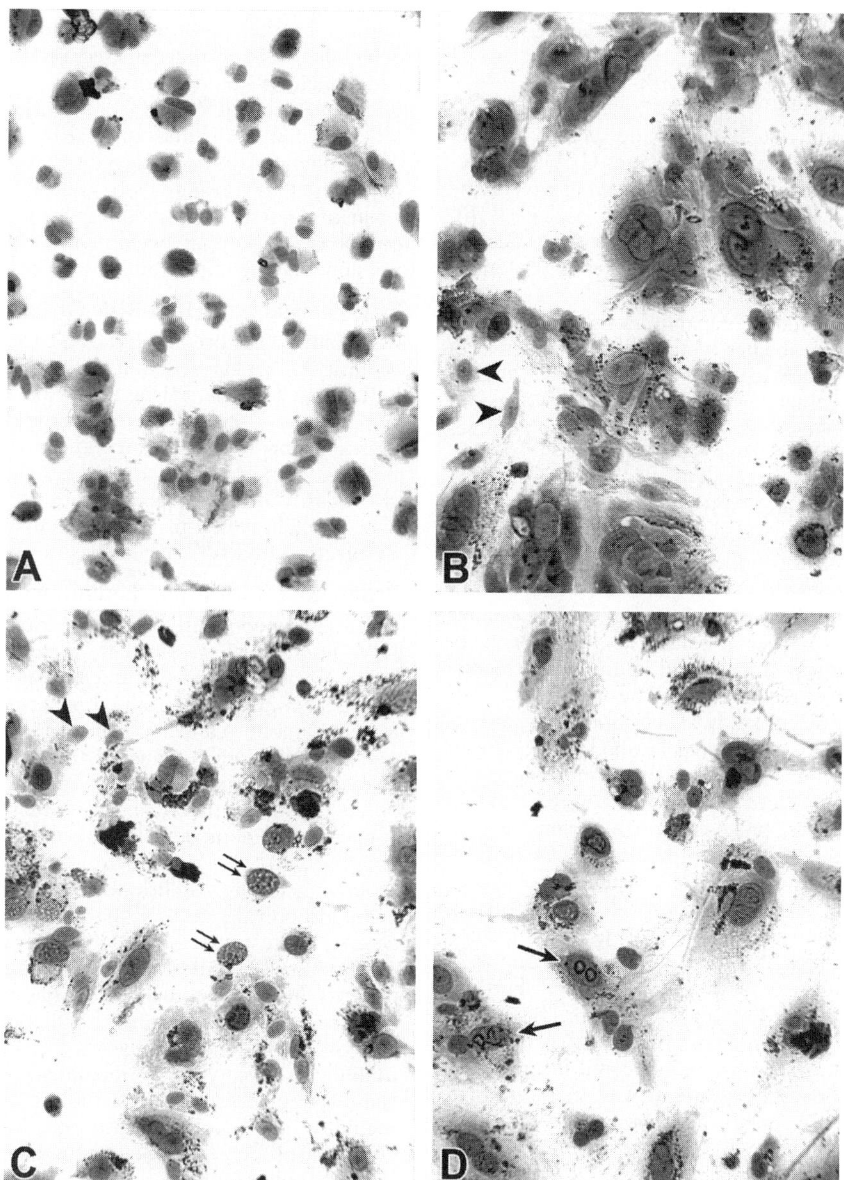

FIGURE 6 Interaction of JCV, BKV, and SV40 with primary cultures of human fetal brain or glial cells. Cells were infected with a 1/10 dilution of the Mad-1 strain of JCV or a 1/1,000 dilution of SV40 or BKV (~1 infectious unit per cell). Cells were transferred to 22-mm square glass coverslips after 2 weeks for the Mad-1-infected cells and immediately after inoculation for cultures infected with BKV or SV40. In JCV-infected cells, cytopathic effect did not appear until 3 to 4 weeks. In cultures infected with BKV or SV40, cytopathic effect became extensive within 8 to 10 days. (A) Uninfected human fetal brain cells containing relatively small, moderately stained nuclei. (B) Mad-1-infected human fetal brain cells with large nuclei and multinucleated cells. There were also occasional giant multinucleated cells that contained many nuclei (not shown) and also some cells with small nuclei, similar to those in uninfected cells (arrowheads in panels B and C). (C) SV40-infected cells, also with large, darkly staining nuclei. Some nuclei were reticulated or mottled (double arrows), but multinucleated cells were rare. (D) BKV-infected cells. Again, the nuclei were enlarged and intensely stained. Multinucleated cells were again rare. Some nuclei contained what appeared to be doughnut-shaped nucleoli (arrows). This was unique to BKV infection (Wright's stain; magnification, ×152).

tified in cutaneous Merkel cell carcinoma tissue using molecular methods, including digital transcriptome subtraction (36). None of these three viruses have yet been grown or characterized in tissue culture or studied in experimental animals.

SV40 as a Human Agent

Over 150 million individuals worldwide received SV40-contaminated polio or adenovirus vaccines (101). The frequency of antibody response to SV40 in groups receiving contaminated polio vaccines was as great as 24% (16). Early studies of children receiving contaminated vaccines demonstrated subclinical SV40 infection with prolonged fecal excretion of the virus (45). Up to 27% of personnel working for monkey export companies have been reported to have anti-SV40 antibodies, and serologic evidence of SV40 infection has been reported for 51 to 55% of laboratory workers in contact with monkeys or involved in preparation of monkey cells for tissue culture purposes (16). These data indicate that SV40 is capable of replication in human hosts.

Serologic, virologic, and PCR studies from a number of laboratories have also suggested the existence of a human agent closely related to or identical to SV40 (45). The existence of a human SV40-like agent has been controversial, however. Although a number of investigators have reported antibodies to SV40 in human sera, these have for the most part been at low titer, and many of the reports failed to exclude cross-reacting antibodies to JCV or BKV (19, 70, 104). One recent study of sera from 699 patients with and without cancer detected antibodies to JCV or BKV in both patient and control population groups (19). Although antibodies reactive with SV40 were found in 6.6% of serum samples, preabsorption experiments confirmed that these were actually antibodies to JCV or BKV which were cross-reactive with SV40. Attempts to amplify SV40 from urine of AIDS patients as well as from human sewage collected from widely dispersed areas in Europe and Africa have been unsuccessful despite the fact that JCV and BKV DNAs were readily detected (13, 103). Furthermore, although infectious JCV and BKV virions have been repeatedly recovered from human urine, this has not been the case with SV40, nor was SV40 detected in molecular studies of renal tissue from 19 patients with interstitial nephritis, although these studies did identify JCV and BKV (5). The existence of an SV40-like agent in humans thus remains unproven.

Transmission and Primary Infection

Neither JCV nor BKV has been consistently associated with symptomatic illness. For this reason the routes by which JCV and BKV infections are acquired in nature have not been defined, nor is the distribution of either agent during primary infection known. The most thorough data concerning polyomavirus transmission come from studies of nonhuman agents. Mouse polyomavirus has been reported to cause infection by respiratory spread (28). Infection with MPtV, the only polyomavirus for which detailed comparative studies of respiratory versus oral inoculation have been carried out, is acquired orally, with initial replication of the virus in intestinal endothelial cells (46). SV40 produced asymptomatic infection in volunteers after either oral or respiratory inoculation and was shown to cause transient viremia and prolonged viruria (16). JCV and BKV DNAs have been detected in human feces, suggesting that both viruses, like MPtV, may be transmitted by the oral route (12, 91, 113). Both JCV and BKV DNAs have been detected in human tonsils. However, PCR analysis of nasopharyngeal aspirates from 201 children requiring hospitalization for acute respiratory illnesses failed to detect JCV DNA and detected BKV DNA—but not infectious virus—in only 2 of the 201 patients (108). Neither JCV DNA nor BKV DNA was identified in saliva from 60 HIV-infected adults and 10 healthy adult controls (108). These data, in aggregate, suggest that while JCV and BKV may persist in tonsillar tissue, neither JCV nor BKV is a frequent cause of childhood respiratory infections and that nasopharynx, oropharyngeal tissues, and salivary glands do not appear to be important sites of primary infection (108).

Risk Factors and High-Risk Groups

Most individuals become infected with BKV and JCV, and acquisition or persistence of either agent is not known to be increased in the setting of impaired host immunity. In contrast, as discussed below, urinary excretion of both agents is increased under conditions of immunosuppression, and clinical disease due to either agent—PML in the case of JCV or nephropathy in the case of BKV—occurs almost exclusively in immunocompromised individuals. Reinfection by BKV or JCV has not been documented.

Progressive Multifocal Leukoencephalopathy

PML is an opportunistic demyelinating infection caused by JCV. The disease was initially identified in patients with hematologic malignancies and was later described to occur in other immunocompromised patients, including individuals undergoing cancer chemotherapy, patients immunosuppressed for organ transplantation or collagen vascular disease, and patients with protracted granulomatous disorders (including tuberculosis or sarcoidosis), patients with congenital immune deficiencies, and rare patients with celiac disease (45). Prior to the AIDS epidemic, PML was an extremely rare condition. In patients with AIDS, however, the prevalence of PML is greatly increased. In the absence of treatment with highly active antiretroviral therapy (HAART), PML is the cause of death in 4% of AIDS patients (45). Subclinical PML has been detected postmortem in AIDS patients who died of other conditions (45). Within the past few years, PML has occurred in rare individuals receiving monoclonal antibodies directed against specific components of the host immune response, including natalizumab, rituximab, and alemtuzumab (17, 56, 59, 61, 67, 112), as well as the broader-spectrum agent mycophenolate mofetil.

Association of BKV with Renal and Other Urological Diseases

BKV has been associated with hemorrhagic cystitis, ureteral infection in which BKV-infected cells may cause ureteral obstruction, urethritis, and interstitial nephritis (23, 90). Hemorrhagic cystitis has been described to occur in children, in whom the condition is thought to represent a complication of primary infection (90). More frequently, however, hemorrhagic cystitis, ureteral obstruction, and urethritis are associated with renal or bone marrow transplantation (54, 90).

Interstitial nephritis represents the major urological complication of BKV infection. Rarely, this is seen in children with immunodeficiency syndromes (25). More commonly, the condition is associated with renal or other organ transplantation (89, 90). BKV-associated nephropathy may involve 5% of renal transplant patients and when present is associated with graft failure in 60 to 70% of patients (51, 90). BKV-associated interstitial nephritis has been reported to occur in patients with AIDS, but the association with AIDS is much less strong than is the association with organ transplantation.

PATHOGENESIS

Animal Models of Human Polyomavirus Infection

Neither JCV nor BKV produces productive infection paralleling human infection in nonhuman species. Thus, much of the current knowledge about the biological behavior of polyomaviruses in their natural hosts comes from studies of nonhuman agents. SV40 produces renal involvement in its simian host, as do JCV and BKV in humans. In immunocompromised animals, SV40 has been associated with fatal interstitial pneumonia, renal tubular necrosis, meningoencephalitis, and a PML-like illness (45). Mouse polyomavirus produces a protracted, widely disseminated infection followed by a latent renal infection which can be reactivated by pregnancy (45).

The polyomavirus most extensively studied as a possible model for human infection is MPtV. In mice less than 6 days of age, MPtV produces an overwhelming infection of systemic and pulmonary vascular endothelial cells; death results from interstitial pneumonia (47). Older animals also develop widespread infection of vascular endothelial cells but survive acute infection. By 2 to 3 months following initial infection, viral nucleic acids, T-Ag, and V antigens can be detected in renal tubular epithelial cells, suggesting that viral persistence involves not actual latency but rather a chronic, low-level productive infection, similar to that now believed to occur in humans (48) (Fig. 7). Initial protection against lethal infection depends greatly on the ability of the host to mount a prompt antibody response. Cell-mediated immunity, although not essential for containment of acute infection, appears to be required for containment of persistent infection, and failure of T-lymphocyte function allows progression of infection by cell-to-cell spread (48).

Viral Persistence

Both JCV and BKV persist in renal tubular epithelial cells (54). JCV DNA sequences have also been identified in the lungs and spleens of PML patients (18) and in the kidneys, liver, and brain of a patient with non-AIDS immunodeficiency who did not have PML (14). Both archetypal and variant forms of JCV DNA have been detected in the brains of up to 33% of individuals without HIV infection or PML (35, 45, 117). These findings are of interest in that they suggest that JCV may persist in the brain and that PML might be a consequence of reactivated infection within the CNS.

Following initial detection of JCV DNA by in situ hybridization in B lymphocytes within the spleen and bone marrow of a patient with AIDS PML (53), a number of studies using PCR methods have detected JCV in peripheral blood mononuclear cells (PBMCs) or other leukocytes. This finding has been of considerable interest because infection of circulating blood leukocytes could provide a mechanism for viral entry into the brain. However, the role of these cells as sites of JCV persistence and replication remains uncertain (14, 29, 73, 87). Detection of JCV DNA sequences has been reported for PBMCs from 28.9% of 157 HIV-positive patients and from 16.5% of HIV-negative patients (29). However, JCV DNA sequences both for the noncoding region of the genome and for Vp1 were detected in only 0.9% of blood donors (26). In another study, DNA encoding JCV T-Ag was detected in blood from 31.8% of 60 AIDS patients but only in 2.3% of 88 immunologically normal blood donors (60). For the AIDS patients, mRNA sequences encoding JCV Vp1 were found in 38% of JCV DNA-positive urine samples but in blood from only one patient (60). Other investigators have also detected JCV DNA in T lymphocytes, monocytes, and polymorphonuclear leukocytes (105, 106). These studies confirm that JCV may infect B lymphocytes and that the frequency of infection may be increased by immunosuppression. However, the studies also suggest that blood leukocyte infection by JCV may be latent and that other leukocyte populations may also support viral persistence, making it uncertain to what extent these cells are involved in dissemination of viral infection. An unanswered question in studies of postmortem material is whether viral DNA detected in multiple organs is present in circulating lymphocytes rather than in organ parenchyma.

Detailed PCR studies of systemic BKV infection have not been reported, and although the virus persists in the

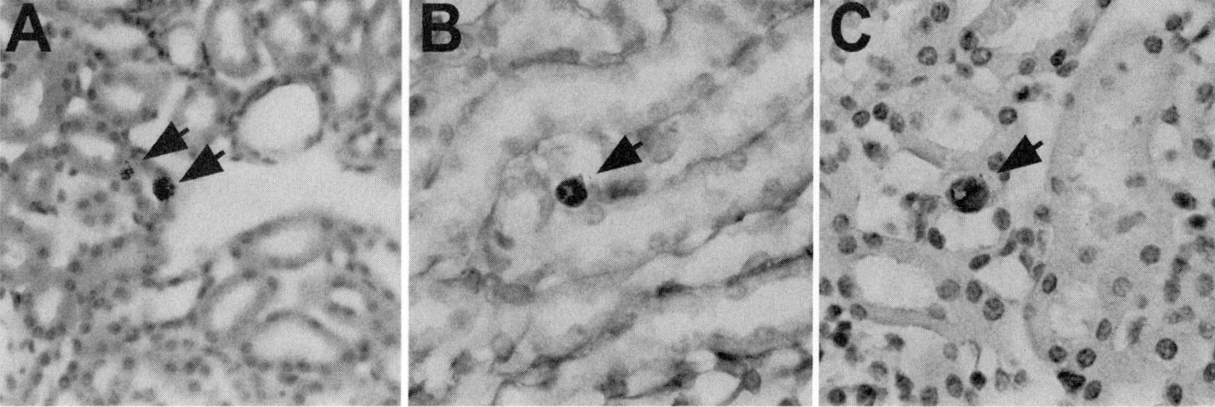

FIGURE 7 Polyomavirus persistence as a chronic productive infection, as shown in a kidney of a nonimmunosuppressed mouse 6 months after inoculation with murine pneumotropic (K) virus. Arrows indicate the presence of viral nucleic acids (A), T-Ag (B), and Vp1 antigen (C) indicative of viral replication in renal tubular epithelial cells.

kidneys, the distribution of BKV during persistent infection has not otherwise been defined (90). The virus has been detected in lymphocytes, and BKV DNA has been detected in the brains of a minority of individuals without HIV infection or PML (35, 90). The significance of these observations in terms of BKV persistence and reactivation is not known.

Reactivation of Persistent Infection

Reactivation of persistent infection by JCV or BKV has been largely defined in terms of urinary excretion of virus or viral DNA. Whether reactivated infection occurs in other sites such as the brain is unknown. Older studies based on serology, urinary cytology, and viral culture strongly associated reactivation or urinary excretion of JCV or BKV with immunosuppression. Serologic evidence for reactivation of BKV was detected in 22 to 44% of individuals undergoing renal transplantation or chemotherapy for malignant disease (90). Excretion of infectious BKV or virus-infected urothelial cells has been demonstrated for immunosuppressed patients, for diabetics, and during pregnancy (45, 90). Longitudinal studies of HIV-infected patients have documented urinary excretion of BKV for 37% of patients and JCV for 22% (57). Urinary excretion of either virus was more likely with patients with low CD4 counts or low β_2-microglobulin levels and did not correlate with serologic markers for either virus. Excretion of JCV did not appear to increase the likelihood of developing PML (57).

Recent studies using more sensitive PCR methods demonstrate that asymptomatic urinary excretion of JCV and BKV, unaccompanied by a rise in antibody titers, is common in healthy individuals (93, 121). Approximately 23% of healthy individuals excrete JCV DNA in their urine, with approximately 1.8% excreting BKV (93). In one study, urinary excretion of BKV DNA was 24% in children under 9 years of age, possibly reflecting excretion during primary infection. BKV DNA excretion fell to under 20% until age 30 and then gradually increased, reaching 44% by age 80 to 89 (121). Urinary excretion of JCV DNA was less than 10% in children 0 to 9 years of age and then steadily increased thereafter, reaching 75% by age 80 to 89 (121). Other studies have confirmed high rates of JCV DNA excretion in older individuals (88) and have indicated that urinary excretion of JCV DNA is continuous, whereas excretion of BKV DNA appears to be more sporadic (88). These data plus older studies would suggest that urinary excretion of JCV or BKV is ongoing in many individuals but that excretion of infectious virus is increased under conditions of immunosuppression. JCV DNAs recovered from nonimmunocompromised patients have been predominantly archetypal, whereas JCV strains recovered from immunocompromised patients may consist of both archetypal forms and rearranged variants (1, 119). Sequencing studies of BKV DNAs amplified from urine have detected both archetypal and rearranged forms of the virus (21).

Reactivation of Human Polyomavirus Infection during Pregnancy

Reactivation of BKV or JCV infection is a common event during pregnancy. A rise in antibody titers indicative of reactivated human polyomavirus infection or reinfection with these agents is found in approximately one-third of pregnant women (22). Significant rises in antibody titers occur most frequently at the end of the second trimester. Initially high antibody titers did not prevent reactivation of infection (22). Urinary excretion of JCV DNA and BKV DNA has been found to be increased in pregnant women versus healthy controls (111).

Whether reactivation of human polyomavirus infection during pregnancy might result in infection of the fetus is doubtful. Most serologic studies have failed to demonstrate evidence of congenital infection (42). One study reported detection of DNA encoding both BKV Vp1 and the BKV RR in brains and kidneys, as well as placentas of aborted fetuses (86). JCV DNA was not detected.

Immune Responses to JCV and BKV

Primary infection with JCV or BKV elicits both antibody- and T-cell-mediated immune responses (27, 54), with persistence of antibody throughout life. The respective roles of the B- and T-cell responses in control of acute infection are not known (27). However, impairment of the T-cell-mediated immune response results in increased urinary excretion of JCV or BKV despite continued high levels of circulating antibody, similar to the effect of immunosuppression on persistent MPtV infection in mice. Impaired T-cell function is almost invariably present in individuals developing PML or BKV-associated nephritis.

Pathogenesis of PML

PML almost always occurs in the setting of immunosuppression, involving both T-cell-mediated and antibody-mediated immune responses (45, 54). Studies of non-AIDS PML have demonstrated a general impairment of T-cell-mediated immunity, with selective impairment of the T-cell-mediated immune response specific for JCV (45). Many patients with non-AIDS PML have an impaired antibody response against the virus, as do patients with AIDS PML. Remission of PML following a reduction in immunosuppressive therapy in a renal transplantation patient was shown to be accompanied by a rise in titers of antibody to JCV in serum and the appearance of anti-JCV antibody in cerebrospinal fluid (CSF) (45). A similar rise in antibody has been observed during immune reconstitution in patients receiving HAART. In vitro studies of PBMC proliferation in response to purified JCV have demonstrated an absence of CD4 cell proliferation in PBMCs of patients with PML but not in controls. Nine of the 10 patients whose PML entered remission following HAART had positive responses, and restoration of JCV-specific CD4 T-cell responses was associated with JCV clearance from the CSF (40).

Despite the fact that most individuals are persistently infected with JCV, PML is an unusual event, even in AIDS. This discrepancy suggests that immunosuppression alone does not account for disease onset. The detection of JCV DNA in brains of immunologically normal patients suggests that PML might arise from reactivation of infection latent in the CNS (35, 45, 117). By the same token, the more frequent detection of JCV DNA in PBMCs from AIDS patients, with the caveats discussed above, could also provide a mechanism for viral entry into the brain. Pathological studies have documented a close association between AIDS PML lesions and HIV-infected T-cell/macrophage infiltrates, and large amounts of HIV antigens have been identified in some AIDS PML lesions (99). A direct facilitory role for HIV tat or other proteins has been suggested by studies in cell-free systems, but an actual effect of tat on JCV replication has not been proven (109).

Whether specific genetic susceptibility to JCV exists in patients developing PML is unknown.

An important question concerning the pathogenesis of PML has to do with the nature of the infectious virus. As noted above, archetypal JCV is at best rarely associated with PML, and most PML isolates have had RR duplications, deletions, or rearrangements. Although these genomic changes have been shown to alter the behavior of JCV in tissue culture, their role in causing PML has not been determined (78). JCV tropism for cerebellar granule cells, however, appears to correlate with a unique deletion in the region of the Vp1 gene corresponding to the C terminus (24), suggesting that the deletions or rearrangements seen in the genomes of PML-associated JCV strains may have pathogenic importance.

Recently, cases of PML have been described to occur in non-AIDS patients receiving the monoclonal antibody immunosuppressive agents natalizumab, rituximab, and alemtuzumab. Additional cases have recently been described in patients treated with mycophenolate mofetil, which affects both B cells and T cells. Natalizumab reacts with the $\alpha 4$ subunit of $\alpha 4\beta 1$ and $\alpha 4\beta 7$ integrins, which are expressed on the surface of all leukocytes except neutrophils (56, 61, 112). The agent is thought to inhibit migration of T lymphocytes and other PBMCs across vascular endothelial cells and could thus interfere with lymphocyte-mediated immune surveillance within the CNS. Rituximab targets $CD20^+$ B cells and could thus alter humoral immune surveillance. Alemtuzumab is directed against the CD52 glycoprotein expressed on the majority of B and T cells, monocytes, and natural killer cells and thus has a wide potential spectrum of action (67). The effects of each of these agents on JCV persistence and reactivation have not been defined. Here as well, however, only rare patients receiving these agents (in the case of natalizumab, only 3 of well over 17,000 patients) develop PML.

Pathology of PML

The pathological changes of PML may be present in the cerebrum, cerebellum, or brain stem (45, 92). The cerebral cortex and deep gray matter appear normal, but areas of retraction within the subcortical or deep white matter indicate myelin loss. Histopathological examination of PML lesions demonstrates loss of oligodendrocytes in demyelinated areas, and the remaining oligodendrocytes may have enlarged nuclei or contain actual intranuclear inclusions (45, 92). Astrocytes in and around PML lesions frequently develop hyperchromatic or multiple nuclei and mitotic figures (Fig. 8) (45, 92). JCV nucleic acids and early and late viral proteins are present within the nuclei of infected oligodendrocytes (45) (Fig. 9). Atypical astrocytes in PML contain viral nucleic acids but only occasionally express early or late viral proteins (45, 99). Electron microscopic examination of the brains of PML patients demonstrates crystalline arrays of viral particles within infected oligodendrocytes. Small numbers of viral particles can be found in occasional morphologically normal astrocytes but not within atypical astrocytes (45). Myelin breakdown and lipid-laden macrophages become evident as the disease progresses. In non-AIDS PML, extensive inflammation is unusual, although small numbers of lymphocytes may be seen around vessels and in demyelinated areas. Demyelination in AIDS PML is often more extensive than in non-AIDS cases (114), and brains may contain areas of actual necrosis (99, 114). Lymphocytic perivascular infiltrates are more evident (99, 114) and may at times be accompanied by parenchymal infiltrates which may include macrophages and multinucleated giant cells (114). Although atypical astrocytes have been considered a pathological hallmark

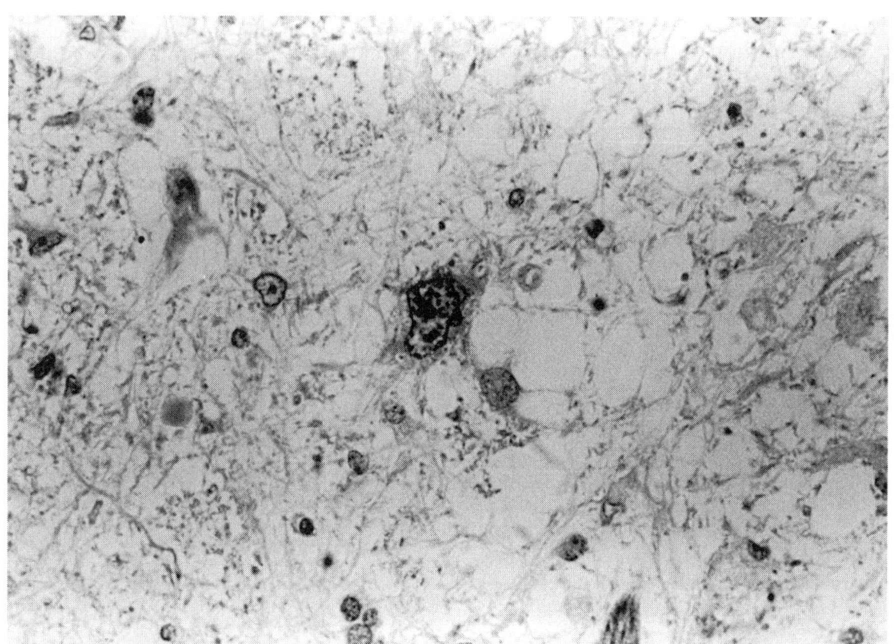

FIGURE 8 Section from edge of a PML lesion, stained for polyomavirus common structural antigen and labeled using immunoperoxidase techniques. There is extensive loss of myelin. Oligodendrocytes have enlarged nuclei that exhibit intense staining for common structural antigen. Giant astrocytes within the lesion remain unlabeled. Magnification, ×216.

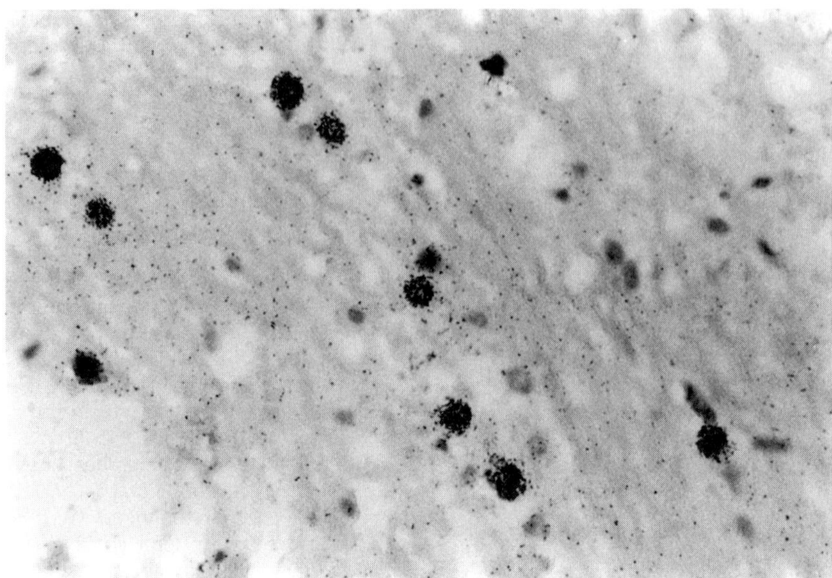

FIGURE 9 Section of PML-affected brain probed for JCV nuclei acids using in situ hybridization methods. Large numbers of exposed emulsion grains, indicative of specific hybridization, overlie nuclei of infected oligodendrocytes. Magnification, ×200.

for PML, these cells are often infrequent or absent in the brains of AIDS PML patients and may also be rare or absent in non-AIDS cases.

Pathogenesis of BKV-Associated Urinary Tract Disease

The major known site of BKV persistence is the renal tubular epithelium, and persistent infection of these cells, like that seen with JCV and with MPtV, appears to involve not a state of viral latency but rather ongoing productive infection at low level. The great majority of cases of symptomatic reactivated BKV infections have involved the kidneys, with a smaller number involving the ureter, bladder, or urethra, either by cell-to-cell spread within the kidneys or by infection of lower urinary tract structures by infected urine (90). Hemorrhagic cystitis has been reported during both presumed acute and chronic infection (90).

In children, hemorrhagic cystitis is thought to represent primary infection (90). More frequently, however, hemorrhagic cystitis, ureteral obstruction, and urethritis are associated with renal or bone marrow transplantation (54, 90). The conditions which predispose to BKV nephritis, like those which predispose to PML, are not fully understood. BKV viruria and viremia have been reported to occur in 26.5% of renal transplant patients and 25.5% of heart transplant patients, with BKV viremia occurring in 12.2 and 7% of these patients, respectively (71). In this study, elevation in serum creatinine was seen in both groups of patients. In this and other studies, actual development of nephritis correlated with renal transplantation, with use of mycophenylate mofetil in initial immunosuppression, and, in one study, with an absence of a detectable antibody response (43, 71, 90).

Pathology of BKV-Associated Urinary Tract Disease

The characteristic finding associated with BKV excretion (and occasionally JCV excretion) under conditions of immunosuppression is the excretion of cells containing intranuclear inclusions ("decoy cells"), which may be present in urine or in tissue samples. Decoy cell inclusions typically contain BKV virions, although cells infected by JCV may contain similar inclusions. In cases of ureteral stenosis, BKV-infected decoy cells may be numerous enough to cause luminal narrowing or actual occlusion (23). Characteristic pathological changes in the kidneys of individuals developing BKV-associated nephropathy include streaky fibrosis of the renal medulla as well as circumscribed areas of cortical scarring. Renal tubular epithelial cells may exhibit nuclear enlargement and at times intranuclear inclusions which contain BKV antigens and nucleic acids. Areas of infection exhibit peritubular infiltrates of mononuclear inflammatory cells (51, 90).

Association of Polyomavirus Infections with Human Neoplasia

SV40, BKV, and JCV are all capable of causing CNS tumors in experimental animals (45). For this reason there has been a long-standing interest in whether these agents might also cause tumors in humans. However, tumor production by any of these viruses usually requires conditions not easily found in nature, including use of large quantities of virus, inoculation of the agent into species other than its natural host, and inoculation under conditions of compromised immune status or into sites, such as the CNS, which are relatively sequestered from the host immune response. JCV, BKV, and, in particular, SV40 antigens or DNA have been detected by immunohistological or PCR methods in a number of human tumors, including choroid plexus papillomas and other brain tumors, mesotheliomas, colonic and esophageal tumors, and non-Hodgkin's lymphomas. Recently, much of this work has been called into question, in particular in the case of SV40. Studies employing improved PCR methods and more stringent controls have also failed to confirm most earlier reports identifying polyomavirus DNA in human tumors. The existence of a human SV40-like virus is at best uncertain, and studies of army veterans exposed to SV40 in contaminated adenovirus or poliovirus vaccines have not shown an increased incidence of cancer over time (94). Some SV40 isolates have been found, upon careful examination, to contain plasmid DNA sequences, indicating laboratory contamination (64). Other isolates have been shown to be 776-SV40, a widely used laboratory strain which has never been directly isolated from monkeys and which may also represent contamination rather than natural infection. Only one group of investigators has attempted to duplicate PCR isolation of polyomaviruses from the same tumor material in different laboratories (95). In this study, PCR analysis of the same 225 brain tumor samples was carried out in two geographically separated laboratories. JCV, BKV, or SV40 DNAs were detected in a small number of cases. However, neither laboratory could confirm the other laboratory's positive cases (95). At present, there is insufficient evidence to associate JCV, BKV, or SV40 with human neoplasia (95).

Recently, a previously unknown polyomavirus, MPV, has been identified in 8 of 10 human cutaneous Merkel cell carcinomas, tumors occurring predominantly in immunosuppressed older individuals (36). The agent was not detected in tissues from 84 tumor-negative controls but was detected in a lymph node metastasis from one tumor patient. In six of the eight positive samples, viral DNA was integrated into the host genome. These data, although of great interest, await confirmation by other investigators.

CLINICAL MANIFESTATIONS

Acute JCV or BKV infection is usually asymptomatic. One 13-year-old immunocompetent girl was reported to have undergone seroconversion to JCV positivity in association with chronic meningoencephalitis (10), and JCV DNA has been detected in CSF from an individual with meningitis in the setting of systemic lupus erythematosus (116). BKV has been isolated from urine of pediatric patients with both hemorrhagic and nonhemorrhagic cystitis. JCV and BKV DNAs were detected by PCR in 3.8 and 1.5% of 181 CSF samples from individuals with meningitis and encephalitis, respectively, but not in 20 CSF samples from control subjects (6). In none of these studies, however, was a causative role for either virus proven, and two of the positive samples (one positive for JCV and one positive for BKV) were also positive for *Mycobacterium tuberculosis*, suggesting a much more likely cause of the neurologic illnesses (6).

Progressive Multifocal Leukoencephalopathy

PML usually begins insidiously. Initial symptoms and signs suggest focal cerebral involvement: these may include alterations in personality, changes in intellect, focal weakness, difficulty with motor skills, or sensory loss (45, 92). Involvement of the dominant cerebral hemisphere may result in expressive or receptive dysphasia. Visual field abnormalities, including actual cortical blindness, occur in 50% of patients (45). Occasionally, PML begins with signs of brain stem or cerebellar involvement, with difficulty in phonation or swallowing, abnormalities of extraocular movements, or ataxia (45). Spinal cord involvement is rare and is virtually never symptomatic (8).

The course of PML is almost always remorselessly progressive. Initial symptoms are followed by the appearance of multifocal neurologic signs, increasing dementia, and eventual progression to a vegetative state. Most patients with non-AIDS PML die within 1 year, but death may occur within as little as 2 months, and cases have been reported with survival times of 8 to 10 years or longer (45). Survival in AIDS PML averages 4 months. Rarely, PML may stabilize or remit. Remission of non-AIDS PML has been reported spontaneously and following reduction of immunosuppressive medications (45). Remission of AIDS PML may also occasionally occur spontaneously or during antiretroviral treatment (45). HAART significantly increases overall survival in patients with AIDS PML but may not arrest progression in individual cases (118).

Clinical Diagnosis

PML should be considered in any immunocompromised patient, in particular with HIV infection, who develops progressive neurologic deficits involving multiple areas of the brain (45). Hematologic studies and blood chemistries are unhelpful in the diagnosis of PML. CSF is usually normal but may occasionally contain increased protein or, rarely, a lymphocytic pleocytosis (45).

The most useful screening study for PML is magnetic resonance imaging (45), which will show altered signal in subcortical and deep white matter on T2 and FLAIR images (Fig. 10). Some, but not all, PML lesions are enhanced with intravenous gadolinium. Computed tomography is less reliable, and changes consistent with demyelination may be absent on computed tomography despite clinically evident disease.

Several other infectious agents that may mimic PML clinically are common in immunosuppressed patients and, in particular, in AIDS patients. These include CNS invasion by *Toxoplasma gondii*, *Cryptococcus neoformans*, or *Mycobacterium tuberculosis*. These infections may occur

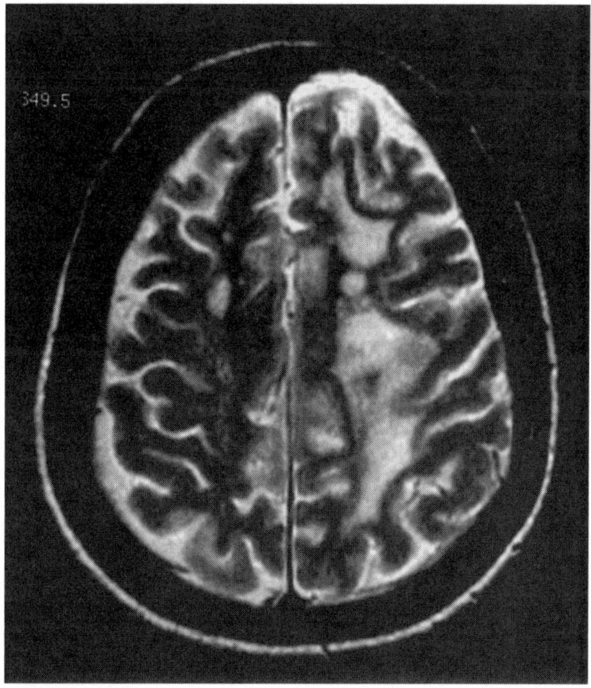

FIGURE 10 T2 weighted magnetic resonance image of a patient developing PML in the setting of AIDS. Multifocal areas of demyelination are seen as areas of increased signal, appearing white against the darker background. (Courtesy of Jay Tsuruda.)

together with or in the absence of PML. CNS lymphoma may also mimic PML, in particular in AIDS patients. Brain biopsy to rule out treatable conditions may thus be crucial where the diagnosis of PML is at all in question or where there is concern about other, coexisting conditions.

JCV Infection of Cerebellar Granule Neurons

JCV has traditionally been thought to produce an infection limited to cells of glial origin: oligodendrocytes and astrocytes. However, two cases have been reported in which JCV infected cerebellar granule neurons (31, 58). One of these patients had accompanying PML, whereas PML lesions were not detected in the second individual (58). Analysis of JCV DNA from the granule cells of the patient with coexisting PML revealed a unique deletion in the region of the Vp1 gene corresponding to the C terminus not present in JCV DNA present in the patient's white-matter lesions, suggesting that the deletion, with its accompanying frameshift, may have enabled the virus to infect granule cell neurons (24).

BKV Urinary Tract Infection

Urinary tract involvement by BKV may cause cystitis, ureteral obstruction, or interstitial nephritis. Cystitis due to BKV may be hemorrhagic or nonhemorrhagic, may occur during primary or reactivated infection, and may be occult or symptomatic. In transplant patients, hemorrhagic cystitis associated with BKV usually occurs well after organ transplantation and should be differentiated from that seen soon after transplantation, which is more commonly due to cyclophosphamide or other immunosuppressive agents (90). Ureteral stenosis may result in hydronephrosis. A diagnostic concern in such patients may be ureteral necrosis secondary to vascular compromise unrelated to viral infection.

The major complication of BKV infection is interstitial nephritis. Cases have been described to occur in rare children with severe immunodeficiency syndromes and in occasional patients with AIDS (90). However, the condition is more frequently seen following organ or stem cell transplantation and is seen in 4 to 8% of renal transplant patients (51, 90). In some cases, the condition may be accompanied by symptomatic cystitis or ureteral obstruction. More commonly, however, BKV-associated nephritis is clinically silent and is manifested in 40 to 60% of cases by progressive renal failure (51, 90). In renal transplant patients, the condition may be confused with graft rejection (51, 90). Limited data suggest that the likelihood of nephritis is increased in patients treated with tacrolimus or mycophenylate mofetil (90).

Other Conditions Associated with BKV Infection

In a handful of cases, all of them in profoundly immunocompromised patients, the virus has been reported to cause interstitial pneumonia (90). In one renal transplant patient, BKV was associated with a widespread infection of vascular endothelial cells resulting in muscle weakness, anasarca, and myocardial infarction (85). BKV has also been associated with cases of retinitis and of meningoencephalitis, but in none of these cases has there been clear proof that BKV was the causative agent (90).

LABORATORY DIAGNOSIS

JCV Infection and PML

PML was initially a pathological diagnosis, with diagnostic accuracy enhanced by immunohistochemistry for JCV antigens or in situ DNA hybridization methods. At present, the diagnostic study of choice for PML is PCR analysis of CSF for JCV DNA (96). PCR can also be used to supplement morphological studies of brain biopsy or autopsy material. In earlier studies, use of PCR analysis of CSF enabled specific diagnosis in 80 to 90% of cases (45). HAART has been shown to reduce viral load of JCV in CSF, however, and while CSF PCR remains a valuable diagnostic tool in this setting, the diagnostic yield in patients treated with HAART has been shown to be reduced to 57.5% (68). Tissue culture isolation is extremely cumbersome and essentially never used for diagnostic purposes.

BKV Infection

Urological infection by BKV can be diagnosed by identification of decoy cells in urine or by PCR. These plus detection of BKV viremia and viruria are of value in diagnosis of BKV nephritis. Decoy cells are found in 40 to 60% of transplant patients and have a predictive value of approximately 20% for the presence of nephritis (51). Viremia with over 7,000 copies of BKV DNA per ml has a predictive value of approximately 60% (51). Urinary excretion of over 100 times the number of copies per ml in plasma has a predictive value of 40%. Definitive diagnosis requires renal biopsy showing inflammatory changes with CD20-positive lymphocytic infiltrates and cells containing inclusions positive for BKV by immunohistological staining. Detection of BKV in renal tissue has a positive predictive value of 70%, whereas negative biopsy PCR makes the diagnosis unlikely (51).

Serologic Assays for JCV and BKV

Antibodies to JCV and BKV can be measured by hemagglutination inhibition or enzyme-linked immunosorbent assay methods. However, serologic tests for JCV or BKV are not usually useful, since most individuals have antibody, and immunosuppression may prevent a rise in antibody titer.

PREVENTION AND TREATMENT

Prevention

Measures to prevent JCV or BKV infection have not been developed, nor have consistently effective antiviral drugs been developed for either virus.

Treatment of PML

Cytosine arabinoside has been used anecdotally for many years to treat PML. Controlled studies of the agent have shown no benefit in HIV-infected individuals (50). However, in an uncontrolled study, neurologic stabilization or improvement was observed in 7 of 19 non-AIDS PML patients treated with intravenous cytosine arabinoside at 2 mg/kg of body weight for 5 days (2). Clinical improvement has been described for a number of AIDS and non-AIDS patients treated with the DNA synthesis inhibitor, cidofovir, including cases in which cidofovir was added to HAART or in which it was used with cytosine arabinoside (11, 39, 66, 97). Treatment was not beneficial in all cases, and controlled trials have not yet been reported. Camptothecin and topotecan have been used in individual cases of PML, but therapeutic efficacy has not been confirmed (7). The use of cytosine arabinoside, cidofovir, camptothecin, and topotecan may be accompanied by significant toxicity. Recently, based on the observation that JCV binds to the serotonin receptor, one study reported stabilization of disease and improvement in PML lesions following treatment with the serotonin reuptake inhibitor, mirtazapine (115). Additional treatment data for this agent have not been reported.

Over the past decade, it has become clear that the use of HAART in patients with AIDS PML improves survival in many patients and, over time, appears to have decreased the disease incidence (44, 107). However, AIDS patients may develop or have progression of PML while under treatment, and HAART is not effective in patients with non-AIDS PML. A complication of HAART in PML can be that of an immune reconstitution syndrome, in which recovery of immunocompetence is accompanied by severe inflammation at the site of PML lesions, with accompanying cerebral edema and a potentially fatal course. Treatment of this condition may require use of corticosteroids and reduction or temporary cessation of HAART (107).

Treatment of BKV Infection

Therapy for BKV infection, like that for PML, does not yet exist. In one recent prospective study, monitoring of viral load and preemptive withdrawal of immunosuppression were associated with resolution of BKV viremia and absence of BK nephritis (15). Treatment attempts have also included cidofovir, leflunomide (an immunosuppressive drug whose active metabolite, A77 1726, has antiviral activity), or a combination of both (51). There are no controlled studies to support the use of either agent (51), and cidofovir is nephrotoxic and is primarily excreted by the kidneys.

Portions of the work cited from our laboratories have been supported by the U.S. Department of Veterans Affairs.

REFERENCES

1. **Agostini, H. T., C. F. Ryschkewitsch, and G. L. Stoner.** 1998. Rearrangements of archetypal regulatory regions in JC virus genomes from urine. *Res. Virol.* **149:**163–170.
2. **Aksamit, A. J.** 2001. Treatment of non-AIDS progressive multifocal leukoencephalopathy with cytosine arabinoside. *J. Neurovirol.* **7:**386–390.
3. **Allander, T., K. Andreasson, S. Gupta, A. Bjerkner, G. Bogdanovic, M. A. Persson, T. Dalianis, T. Ramqvist, and B. Andersson.** 2007. Identification of a third human polyomavirus. *J. Virol.* **81:**4130–4136.
4. **Amirhaeri, S., F. Wohlrab, E. O. Major, and R. D. Wells.** 1988. Unusual DNA structure in the regulatory region of the human papovavirus JC virus. *J. Virol.* **62:** 922–931.
5. **Baksh, F. K., S. D. Finkelstein, P. A. Swalsky, G. L. Stoner, C. F. Ryschkewitsch, and P. Randhawa.** 2001. Molecular genotyping of BK and JC viruses in human polyomavirus-associated interstitial nephritis after renal transplantation. *Am. J. Kidney Dis.* **38:**354–365.
6. **Behzad-Behbahani, A., P. E. Klapper, P. J. Vallely, G. M. Cleator, and A. Bonington.** 2003. BKV-DNA and JCV-DNA in CSF of patients with suspected meningitis or encephalitis. *Infection* **31:**374–378.
7. **Berger, J. R.** 2000. Progressive multifocal leukoencephalopathy. *Curr. Treat. Options Neurol.* **2:**361–368.
8. **Bernal-Cano, F., J. T. Joseph, and I. J. Koralnik.** 2007. Spinal cord lesions of progressive multifocal leukoencephalopathy in an acquired immunodeficiency syndrome patient. *J. Neurovirol.* **13:**474–476.
9. **Bialasiewicz, S., D. M. Whiley, S. B. Lambert, D. Wang, M. D. Nissen, and T. P. Sloots.** 2007. A newly reported human polyomavirus, KI virus, is present in the respiratory tract of Australian children. *J. Clin. Virol.* **40:**15–18.
10. **Blake, K., D. Pillay, W. Knowles, D. W. Brown, P. D. Griffiths, and B. Taylor.** 1992. JC virus associated meningoencephalitis in an immunocompetent girl. *Arch. Dis. Child.* **67:**956–957.
11. **Blick, G., M. Whiteside, P. Griegor, U. Hopkins, T. Garton, and L. LaGravinese.** 1998. Successful resolution of progressive multifocal leukoencephalopathy after combination therapy with cidofovir and cytosine arabinoside. *Clin. Infect. Dis.* **26:**191–192.
12. **Bofill-Mas, S., M. Formiga-Cruz, P. Clemente-Casares, F. Calafell, and R. Girones.** 2001. Potential transmission of human polyomaviruses through the gastrointestinal tract after exposure to virions or viral DNA. *J. Virol.* **75:** 10290–10299.
13. **Bofill-Mas, S., S. Pina, and R. Girones.** 2000. Documenting the epidemiologic patterns of polyomaviruses in human populations by studying their presence in urban sewage. *Appl. Environ. Microbiol.* **66:**238–245.
14. **Bordin, G., R. Boldorini, R. Caldarelli Stefano, and E. Omodeo Zorini.** 1997. Systemic infection by JC virus in non-HIV induced immunodeficiency without progressive multifocal leukoencephalopathy. *Ann. Ital. Med. Int.* **12:** 35–38.
15. **Brennan, D. C., I. Agha, D. L. Bohl, M. A. Schnitzler, K. L. Hardinger, M. Lockwood, S. Torrence, R. Schuessler, T. Roby, M. Gaudreault-Keener, and G. A. Storch.** 2005. Incidence of BK with tacrolimus versus cyclosporine and impact of preemptive immunosuppression reduction. *Am. J. Transplant.* **5:**582–594.
16. **Butel, J. S., and J. A. Lednicky.** 1999. Cell and molecular biology of simian virus 40: implications for human infections and disease. *J. Natl. Cancer Inst.* **91:**119–134.
17. **Calabrese, L. H., E. S. Molloy, D. Huang, and R. M. Ransohoff.** 2007. Progressive multifocal leukoencephalopathy in rheumatic diseases: evolving clinical and pathologic patterns of disease. *Arthritis Rheum.* **56:**2116–2128.
18. **Caldarelli-Stefano, R., L. Vago, E. Omodeo-Zorini, M. Mediati, L. Losciale, M. Nebuloni, G. Costanzi, and P. Ferrante.** 1999. Detection and typing of JC virus in autopsy brains and extraneural organs of AIDS patients and non-immunocompromised individuals. *J. Neurovirol.* **5:** 125–133.
19. **Carter, J. J., M. M. Madeleine, G. C. Wipf, R. L. Garcea, P. A. Pipkin, P. D. Minor, and D. A. Galloway.** 2003. Lack of serologic evidence for prevalent simian virus 40 infection in humans. *J. Natl. Cancer Inst.* **95:**1522–1530.
20. **Chapagain, M. L., S. Verma, F. Mercier, R. Yanagihara, and V. R. Nerurkar.** 2007. Polyomavirus JC infects human brain microvascular endothelial cells independent of serotonin receptor 2A. *Virology* **20:**55–63.
21. **Chatterjee, M., T. B. Weyandt, and R. J. Frisque.** 2000. Identification of archetype and rearranged forms of BK virus in leukocytes from healthy individuals. *J. Med. Virol.* **60:**353–362.
22. **Coleman, D. V., S. D. Gardner, C. Mulholland, V. Fridiksdottir, A. A. Porter, R. Lilford, and H. Valdimarsson.** 1983. Human polyomaviruses in pregnancy. A model for the study of defense mechanisms to virus reactivation. *Clin. Exp. Immunol.* **53:**289–296.
23. **Coleman, D. V., E. F. D. MacKenzie, S. D. Gardner, J. M. Poulding, B. Amer, and W. J. I. Russell.** 1978. Human polyomavirus (BK) infection and ureteric stenosis in renal allograft recipients. *J. Clin. Pathol.* **31:**338–347.
24. **Dang, X., and I. J. Koralnik.** 2006. A granule cell neuron-associated JC virus variant has a unique deletion in the VP1 gene. *J. Gen. Virol.* **87:**2533–2537.

25. **de Silva, L. M., P. Bale, J. de Courcy, D. Brown, and W. Knowles.** 1995. Renal failure due to BK virus infection in an immunodeficient child. *J. Med. Virol.* **45:**192–196.
26. **Dolei, A., V. Pietropaolo, E. Gomes, C. Di Taranto, M. Ziccheddu, M. A. Spanu, C. Lavorino, M. Manca, and A. M. Degener.** 2000. Polyomavirus persistence in lymphocytes: prevalence in lymphocytes from blood donors and healthy personnel of a blood transfusion centre. *J. Gen. Virol.* **81:**1967–1973.
27. **Drummond, J. E., K. V. Shah, and A. D. Donnenberg.** 1985. Cell-mediated immune responses to BK virus in normal individuals. *J. Med. Virol.* **17:**237–247.
28. **Dubensky, T. W., and L. P. Villarreal.** 1984. The primary site of replication alters the eventual site of persistent infection by polyomavirus in mice. *J. Virol.* **50:**541–546.
29. **Dubois, V., H. Moret, M. E. Lafon, C. B. Janvresse, E. Dussaix, J. Icart, A. Karaterki, A. Ruffault, Y. Taoufik, C. Vignoli, and D. Ingrand.** 1998. Prevalence of JC virus viraemia in HIV-infected patients with or without neurological disorders: a prospective study. *J. Neurovirol.* **4:** 539–544.
30. **Dugan, A. S., S. Eash, and W. J. Atwood.** 2005. An N-linked glycoprotein with alpha(2,3)-linked sialic acid is a receptor for BK virus. *J. Virol.* **79:**14442–14445.
31. **Du Pasquier, R. A., S. Corey, D. H. Margolin, K. Williams, L. A. Pfister, U. De Girolami, J. J. MacKey, C. Wüthrich, J. T. Joseph, and I. J. Koralnik.** 2003. Productive infection of cerebellar granule cell neurons by JC virus in an HIV+ individual. *Neurology* **61:**775–782.
32. **Eash, S., R. Tavares, E. G. Stopa, S. H. Robbins, L. Brossay, and W. J. Atwood.** 2004. Differential distribution of the JC virus receptor-type sialic acid in normal human tissues. *Am. J. Pathol.* **164:**419–428.
33. **Eckhart, W.** 1990. Polyomavirinae and their replication, p. 1593–1607. *In* B. N. Fields, D. M. Knipe, R. M. Chanock, M. S. Hirsch, J. L. Melnick, T. P. Monath, and B. Roizman (ed.), *Fields Virology*, 2nd ed. Raven Press, New York, NY.
34. **Elphick, G. F., W. Querbes, J. A. Jordan, G. V. Gee, S. Eash, K. Manley, A. Dugan, M. Stanifer, A. Bhatnagar, W. K. Kroeze, B. L. Roth, and W. J. Atwood.** 2004. The human polyomavirus, JCV, uses serotonin receptors to infect cells. *Science* **19:**1380–1383.
35. **Elsner, C., and K. Dorries.** 1992. Evidence of human polyomavirus BK and JC infection in normal brain tissue. *Virology* **191:**72–80.
36. **Feng, H., M. Shuda, Y. Chang, and P. S. Moore.** 2008. Clonal integration of a polyomavirus in human Merkel cell carcinoma. *Science* **319:**1096–1100.
37. **Flaegstad, T., and T. Traavik.** 1987. BK virus in cell culture: infectivity quantitation and sequential expression of antigens detected by immunoperoxidase staining. *J. Virol. Methods* **16:**139–146.
38. **Gardner, S. D., D. M. Field, D. V. Coleman, and B. Hulme.** 1971. New human papovavirus isolated from urine after renal transplantation. *Lancet* **i:**1253–1257.
39. **Garvey, L., E. C. Thomson, and G. P. Taylor.** 2006. Progressive multifocal leukoencephalopathy: prolonged survival in patients treated with protease inhibitors and cidofovir: a case series. *AIDS* **20:**791–793.
40. **Gasnault, J., M. Kahraman, M. G. de Goër de Herve, D. Durali, J. F. Delfraissy, and Y. Taoufik.** 2003. Critical role of JC virus-specific CD4 T-cell responses in preventing progressive multifocal leukoencephalopathy. *AIDS* **17:**1443–1449.
41. **Gaynor, A. M., M. D. Nissen, D. M. Whiley, I. M. Mackay, S. B. Lambert, G. Wu, D. C. Brennan, G. A. Storch, T. P. Sloots, and D. Wang.** 2007. Identification of a novel polyomavirus from patients with acute respiratory tract infections. *PLoS Pathog.* **3:**e64.
42. **Gibson, P. E., A. M. Field, S. D. Gardner, and D. V. Coleman.** 1981. Occurrence of IgM antibodies against BK and JC polyomaviruses during pregnancy. *J. Clin. Pathol.* **34:**674–679.
43. **Ginevri, F., R. De Santis, P. Comoli, N. Pastorino, C. Rossi, G. Botti, I. Fontana, A. Nocera, M. Cardillo, M. R. Ciardi, F. Locatelli, R. Maccario, F. Perfumo, and A. Azzi.** 2003. Polyomavirus BK infection in pediatric kidney-allograft recipients: a single-center analysis of incidence, risk factors, and novel therapeutic approaches. *Transplantation* **75:**1266–1270.
44. **Giudici, B., B. Vaz, S. Bossolasco, S. Casari, A. M. Brambilla, W. Luke, A. Lazzarin, T. Weber, and P. Cinque.** 2000. Highly active antiretroviral therapy and progressive multifocal leukoencephalopathy: effects on cerebrospinal fluid markers of JC virus replication and immune response. *Clin. Infect. Dis.* **30:**95–99.
45. **Greenlee, J. E.** 1998. Progressive multifocal leukoencephalopathy, p. 399–430. *In* M. J. Aminoff and C. G. Goetz (ed.), *Handbook of Clinical Neurology*. Elsevier Science B. V., Amsterdam, The Netherlands.
46. **Greenlee, J. E.** 1979. Pathogenesis of K virus infection in newborn mice. *Infect. Immun.* **26:**705–713.
47. **Greenlee, J. E.** 1981. Effect of host age on experimental K virus infection in mice. *Infect. Immun.* **33:**297–303.
48. **Greenlee, J. E., R. C. Phelps, and W. G. Stroop.** 1991. The major site of murine K-papovavirus persistence and reactivation is the renal tubular epithelium. *Microb. Pathog.* **11:**237–247.
49. **Gross, L.** 1953. A filterable agent, recovered from Ak leukemic extracts, causing salivary gland carcinomas in C3H mice. *Proc. Soc. Exp. Biol. Med.* **83:**414–421.
50. **Hall, C. D., U. Dafni, D. Simpson, D. Clifford, P. E. Wetherill, B. Cohen, J. McArthur, H. Hollander, C. Yainnoutsos, E. Major, L. Millar, and J. Timpone for The AIDS Clinical Trials Group 243 Team.** 1998. Failure of cytarabine in progressive multifocal leukoencephalopathy associated with human immunodeficiency virus infection. *N. Engl. J. Med.* **338:**1345–1351.
51. **Hariharan, S.** 2006. BK virus nephritis after renal transplantation. *Kidney Int.* **69:**655–662.
52. **Hirsch, H. H., and J. Steiger.** 2003. Polyomavirus BK. *Lancet Infect. Dis.* **3:**611–623.
53. **Houff, S. A., E. O. Major, D. A. Katz, C. V. Kufta, J. L. Sever, S. Pittaluga, J. R. Roberts, J. Gitt, N. Saini, and W. Lux.** 1988. Involvement of JC virus-infected mononuclear cells from the bone marrow and spleen in the pathogenesis of progressive multifocal leukoencephalopathy. *N. Engl. J. Med.* **318:**301–305.
54. **Imperiale, M. J., and E. O. Major.** 2007. Polyomaviruses, p. 2263–2298. *In* D. M. Knipe, P. M. Howley, D. E. Griffin, R. A. Lamb, M. A. Martin, B. Roizman, and S. E. Straus (ed.), *Fields Virology*, 5th ed. Williams & Wilkins, Philadelphia, PA.
55. **Kilham, L., and H. W. Murphy.** 1953. A pneumotropic virus isolated from C3H mice carrying the Bittner milk agent. *Proc. Soc. Exp. Biol. Med.* **82:**133–137.
56. **Kleinschmidt-DeMasters, B. K., and K. L. Tyler.** 2005. Progressive multifocal leukoencephalopathy complicating treatment with natalizumab and interferon beta-1a for multiple sclerosis. *N. Engl. J. Med.* **353:**369–374.
57. **Knowles, W. A., D. Pillay, M. A. Johnson, J. F. Hand, and D. W. Brown.** 1999. Prevalence of long-term BK and JC excretion in HIV-infected adults and lack of correlation with serological markers. *J. Med. Virol.* **59:**474–479.
58. **Koralnik, I. J., C. Wuthrich, X. Dang, M. Rottnek, A. Gurtman, D. Simpson, and S. Morgello.** 2005. JC virus

granule cell neuronopathy: a novel clinical syndrome distinct from progressive multifocal leukoencephalopathy. *Ann. Neurol.* **57:**576–580.

59. **Kranick, S. M., E. M. Mowry, and M. R. Rosenfeld.** 2007. Progressive multifocal leukoencephalopathy after rituximab in a case of non-Hodgkin lymphoma. *Neurology* **69:**704–706.
60. **Lafon, M. E., H. Dutronc, V. Dubois, I. Pellegrin, P. Barbeau, J. M. Ragnaud, J. L. Pellegrin, and H. J. Fleury.** 1998. JC virus remains latent in peripheral blood B lymphocytes but replicates actively in urine from AIDS patients. *J. Infect. Dis.* **177:**1502–1505.
61. **Langer-Gould, A., S. W. Atlas, A. J. Green, A. W. Bollen, and D. Pelletier.** 2005. Progressive multifocal leukoencephalopathy in a patient treated with natalizumab. *N. Engl. J. Med.* **353:**375–381.
62. **Lebkowski, J. S., S. Clancy, and M. P. Calos.** 1985. Simian virus 40 replication in adenovirus-transformed human cells antagonizes gene expression. *Nature* **317:**169–171.
63. **Lewis, E. D., and J. L. Manley.** 1985. Repression of simian virus 40 early transcription by viral DNA replication in human 293 cells. *Nature* **317:**172–175.
64. **Lopez-Rios, F., P. B. Illei, V. Rusch, and M. Ladanyi.** 2004. Evidence against a role for SV40 infection in human mesotheliomas and high risk of false-positive PCR results owing to presence of SV40 sequences in common laboratory plasmids. *Lancet* **364:**1157–1166.
65. **Low, J. A., B. Magnuson, B. Tsai, and M. J. Imperiale.** 2006. Identification of gangliosides GD1b and GT1b as receptors for BK virus. *J. Virol.* **80:**1361–1366.
66. **Marra, C. M., N. Rajicic, D. E. Barker, B. A. Cohen, D. Clifford, M. J. Donovan Post, A. Ruiz, B. C. Bowen, M. L. Huang, J. Queen-Baker, J. Andersen, S. Kelly, and S. Shriver.** 2002. A pilot study of cidofovir for progressive multifocal leukoencephalopathy in AIDS. *AIDS* **16:**1791–1797.
67. **Martin, S. I., F. M. Marty, K. Fiumara, S. P. Treon, J. G. Gribben, and L. R. Baden.** 2006. Infectious complications associated with alemtuzumab use for lymphoproliferative disorders. *Clin. Infect. Dis.* **43:**16–24.
68. **Marzocchetti, A., S. Di Giambenedetto, A. Cingolani, A. Ammassari, R. Cauda, and A. De Luca.** 2005. Reduced rate of diagnostic positive detection of JC virus DNA in cerebrospinal fluid in cases of suspected progressive multifocal leukoencephalopathy in the era of potent antiretroviral therapy. *J. Clin. Microbiol.* **43:**4175–4177.
69. **Melnick, J. L., and S. Stinebaugh.** 1962. Excretion of vacuolating SV-40 virus (papova virus group) after ingestion as a contaminant of oral polio vaccine. *Proc. Soc. Exp. Biol. Med.* **109:**965–968.
70. **Minor, P., P. Pipkin, Z. Jarzebek, and W. Knowles.** 2003. Studies of neutralising antibodies to SV40 in human sera. *J. Med. Virol.* **70:**490–495.
71. **Munoz, P., M. Fogeda, E. Bouza, E. Verde, J. Palomo, and R. Banares.** 2005. Prevalence of BK virus replication among recipients of solid organ transplants. *Clin. Infect. Dis.* **41:**1720–1725.
72. **Mutti, L., M. Carbone, G. G. Giordano, and A. Giordano.** 1998. Simian virus 40 and human cancer. *Monaldi Arch. Chest Dis.* **53:**198–201.
73. **Newman, J. T., and R. J. Frisque.** 1997. Detection of archetype and rearranged variants of JC virus in multiple tissues from a pediatric PML patient. *J. Med. Virol.* **52:** 243–252.
74. **Norja, P., I. Ubillos, K. Templeton, and P. Simmonds.** 2007. No evidence for an association between infections with WU and KI polyomaviruses and respiratory disease. *J. Clin. Virol.* **40:**307–311.
75. **O'Neill, F. J., H. Carney, and Y. Hu.** 1998. Host range analysis of simian virus 40, BK virus and chimaeric SV40/BKV: relative expression of large T-antigen and Vp1 in infected and transformed cells. *Dev. Biol. Stand.* **94:**191–205.
76. **O'Neill, F. J., R. J. Frisque, X. Xu, Y. X. Hu, and H. Carney.** 1995. Immortalization of human cells by mutant and chimeric primate polyomavirus T-antigen genes. *Oncogene* **10:**1131–1139.
77. **O'Neill, F. J., J. E. Greenlee, and H. Carney.** 2003. The archetype enhancer of simian virus 40 DNA is duplicated during virus growth in human cells and rhesus monkey kidney cells but not in green monkey kidney cells. *Virology* **310:**173–182.
78. **O'Neill, F. J., J. E. Greenlee, K. Dorries, S. A. Clawson, and H. Carney.** 2003. Propagation of archetype and nonarchetype JC virus variants in human fetal brain cultures: demonstration of interference activity by archetype JC virus. *J. Neurovirol.* **9:**567–576.

78a. **O'Neill, F. J., Y. Hu, and H. C. Carney.** 1997. Identification of p53 unbound to T-antigen in human cells transformed by simian virus 40 T-antigen variants. *Oncogene* **14:**955–965.

79. **O'Neill, F. J., X. L. Xu, and T. H. Miller.** 1990. Host range determinant in the late region of SV40 and RF virus affecting growth in human cells. *Intervirology* **31:** 175–187.
80. **Oster-Granite, M. L., O. Narayan, R. T. Johnson, and R. M. Herndon.** 1978. Studies of cultured human and simian fetal brain cells. II. Infections with human (BK) and simian (SV40) papovaviruses. *Neuropathol. Appl. Neurobiol.* **4:**443–455.
81. **Padgett, B. L., D. L. Walker, G. M. Zu Rhein, and R. J. Eckroade.** 1971. Cultivation of a papova-like virus from human brain with progressive multifocal leukoencephalopathy. *Lancet* **i:**1257–1260.
82. **Pater, A., M. M. Pater, and G. di Mayorca.** 1980. The arrangement of the genome of the human papovavirus RF virus. *J. Virol.* **36:**480–487.
83. **Pater, M. M., A. Pater, and G. di Mayorca.** 1981. Genome analysis of MG virus, a human papovavirus. *J. Virol.* **39:**968–972.
84. **Perez-Losada, M., R. G. Christensen, D. A. McClellan, B. J. Adams, R. P. Viscidi, J. C. Demma, and K. A. Crandall.** 2006. Comparing phylogenetic codivergence between polyomaviruses and their hosts. *J. Virol.* **80:** 5663–5669.
85. **Petrogiannis-Haliotis, T., G. Sakoulas, J. Kirby, I. J. Koralnik, A. M. Dvorak, R. Monahan-Earley, P. C. De Girolami, U. De Girolami, M. Upton, E. O. Major, L.-A. Pfister, and J. T. Joseph.** 2001. BK-related polyomavirus vasculopathy in a renal-transplant recipient. *N. Engl. J. Med.* **345:**1250–1255.
86. **Pietropaolo, V., C. Di Taranto, A. M. Degener, L. Jin, L. Sinibaldi, A. Baiocchini, M. Melis, and N. Orsi.** 1998. Transplacental transmission of human polyomavirus BK. *J. Med. Virol.* **56:**372–376.
87. **Pietropaolo, V., D. Fioriti, P. Simeone, M. Videtta, C. Di Taranto, A. Arancio, N. Orsi, and A. M. Degener.** 2003. Detection and sequence analysis of human polyomaviruses DNA from autoptic samples of HIV-1 positive and negative subjects. *Int. J. Immunopathol. Pharmacol.* **16:**269–276.
88. **Polo, C., J. L. Perez, A. Mielnichuck, C. G. Fedele, J. Niubo, and A. Tenorio.** 2004. Prevalence and patterns of polyomavirus urinary excretion in immunocompetent adults and children. *Clin. Microbiol. Infect.* **10:**640–644.
89. **Randhawa, P., and D. C. Brennan.** 2006. BK virus infection in transplant recipients: an overview and update. *Am. J. Transplant.* **6:**2000–2005.

90. **Reploeg, M. D., G. A. Storch, and D. B. Clifford.** 2001. BK virus: a clinical review. *Clin. Infect. Dis.* **33:** 191–202.
91. **Ricciardiello, L., L. Laghi, P. Ramamirtham, C. L. Chang, D. K. Chang, A. E. Randolph, and C. R. Boland.** 2000. JC virus DNA sequences are frequently present in the human upper and lower gastrointestinal tract. *Gastroenterology* **119:**1228–1235.
92. **Richardson, E. P.** 1961. Progressive multifocal leukoencephalopathy. *N. Engl. J. Med.* **265:**815–823.
93. **Rodrigues, C., D. Pinto, and R. Medeiros.** 2007. Molecular epidemiology characterization of the urinary excretion of polyomavirus in healthy individuals from Portugal—a Southern European population. *J. Med. Virol.* **79:**1194–1198.
94. **Rollison, D. E., W. F. Page, H. Crawford, G. Gridley, S. Wacholder, J. Martin, R. Miller, and E. A. Engels.** 2004. Case-control study of cancer among US Army veterans exposed to simian virus 40-contaminated adenovirus vaccine. *Am. J. Epidemiol.* **160:**317–324.
95. **Rollison, D. E., U. Utaipat, C. Ryschkewitsch, J. Hou, P. Goldthwaite, R. Daniel, K. J. Helzlsouer, P. C. Burger, K. V. Shah, and E. O. Major.** 2005. Investigation of human brain tumors for the presence of polyomavirus genome sequences by two independent laboratories. *Int. J. Cancer* **113:**769–774.
96. **Romero, J. R., and D. W. Kimberlin.** 2003. Molecular diagnosis of viral infections of the central nervous system. *Clin. Lab. Med.* **23:**843–865, vi.
97. **Salmaggi, A., E. Maccagnano, A. Castagna, S. Zeni, F. Fantini, P. Cinque, and M. Savoiardo.** 2001. Reversal of CSF positivity for JC virus genome by cidofovir in a patient with systemic lupus erythematosus and progressive multifocal leukoencephalopathy. *Neurol. Sci.* **22:** 17–20.
98. **Samorei, I. W., M. Schmid, M. Pawlita, H. V. Vinters, K. Diebold, C. Mundt, and R. W. von Einsiedel.** 2000. High sensitivity detection of JC-virus DNA in postmortem brain tissue by in situ PCR. *J. Neurovirol.* **6:**61–74.
99. **Schmidbauer, M., H. Budka, and K. V. Shah.** 1990. Progressive multifocal leukoencephalopathy (PML) in AIDS and in the pre-AIDS era. A neuropathological comparison using immunocytochemistry and in situ DNA hybridization for virus detection. *Acta Neuropathol.* **80:**375–380.
100. **Seif, I., G. Khoury, and R. Dhar.** 1979. The genome of human papovavirus BKV. *Cell* **18:**963–977.
101. **Shah, K. V.** 2006. SV40 and human cancer: a review of recent data. *Int. J. Cancer* **120:**215–223.
102. **Shah, K. V.** 1996. Polyomaviruses, p. 2027–2043. *In* B. N. Fields, D. M. Knipe, and P. M. Howley (ed.), *Fields Virology*, 3rd ed. Lippincott-Raven Publishers, Philadelphia, PA.
103. **Shah, K. V., R. W. Daniel, H. D. Strickler, and J. J. Goedert.** 1997. Investigation of human urine for genomic sequences of the primate polyomaviruses simian virus 40, BK virus, and JC virus. *J. Infect. Dis.* **176:** 1618–1621.
104. **Shah, K. V., D. A. Galloway, W. A. Knowles, and R. P. Viscidi.** 2004. Simian virus 40 (SV40) and human cancer: a review of the serological data. *Rev. Med. Virol.* **14:** 231–239.
105. **Shimizu, N., A. Imamura, O. Daimaru, H. Mihara, Y. Kato, R. Kato, T. Oguri, M. Fukada, T. Yokochi, K. Yoshikawa, H. Komatsu, R. Ueda, and M. Nitta.** 1999. Distribution of JC virus DNA in peripheral blood lymphocytes of hematological disease cases. *Intern. Med.* **38:** 932–937.
106. **Smith, M. A., H. D. Strickler, M. Granovsky, G. Reaman, M. Linet, R. Daniel, and K. V. Shah.** 1999. Investigation of leukemia cells from children with common acute lymphoblastic leukemia for genomic sequences of the primate polyomaviruses JC virus, BK virus, and simian virus 40. *Med. Pediatr. Oncol.* **33:**441–443.
107. **Subsai, K., S. Kanoksri, C. Siwaporn, L. Helen, O. Kanokporn, and P. Wantana.** 2006. Neurological complications in AIDS patients receiving HAART: a 2-year retrospective study. *Eur. J. Neurol.* **13:**233–239.
108. **Sundsfjord, A., A. R. Spein, E. Lucht, T. Flaegstad, O. M. Seternes, and T. Traavik.** 1994. Detection of BK virus DNA in nasopharyngeal aspirates from children with respiratory infections but not in saliva from immunodeficient and immunocompetent adult patients. *J. Clin. Microbiol.* **32:**1390–1394.
109. **Tada, H., J. Rappaport, M. Lashgari, S. Amini, F. Wong-Staal, and K. Khalili.** 1990. Trans-activation of the JC virus late promoter by the tat protein of type 1 human immunodeficiency virus in glial cells. *Proc. Natl. Acad. Sci. USA* **87:**3479–3483.
110. **Tevethia, S. S.** 1990. Recognition of simian virus 40 T antigen by cytotoxic T lymphocytes. *Mol. Biol. Med.* **7:** 83–96.
111. **Tsai, R. T., M. Wang, W. C. Ou, Y. L. Lee, S. Y. Li, C. Y. Fung, Y. L. Huang, T. Y. Tzeng, Y. Chen, and D. Chang.** 1997. Incidence of JC viruria is higher than that of BK viruria in Taiwan. *J. Med. Virol.* **52:** 253–257.
112. **Van Assche, G., M. Van Ranst, R. Sciot, B. Dubois, S. Vermeire, M. Noman, J. Verbeeck, K. Geboes, W. Robberecht, and P. Rutgeerts.** 2005. Progressive multifocal leukoencephalopathy after natalizumab therapy for Crohn's disease. *N. Engl. J. Med.* **353:**362–368.
113. **Vanchiere, J. A., R. K. Nicome, J. M. Greer, G. J. Demmler, and J. S. Butel.** 2005. Frequent detection of polyomaviruses in stool samples from hospitalized children. *J. Infect. Dis.* **192:**658–664.
114. **Vazeux, R., M. Cumont, P. M. Girard, X. Nassif, P. Trotot, C. Marche, L. Matthiessen, C. Vedrenne, J. Mikol, and D. Henin.** 1990. Severe encephalitis resulting from coinfections with HIV and JC virus. *Neurology* **40:**944–948.
115. **Verma, S., K. Cikurel, I. J. Koralnik, S. Morgello, C. Cunningham-Rundles, Z. R. Weinstein, C. Bergmann, and D. M. Simpson.** 2007. Mirtazapine in progressive multifocal leukoencephalopathy associated with polycythemia vera. *J. Infect. Dis.* **196:**709–711.
116. **Viallard, J. F., E. Ellie, E. Lazaro, M. E. Lafon, and J. L. Pellegrin.** 2005. JC virus meningitis in a patient with systemic lupus erythematosus. *Lupus* **14:**964–966.
117. **White, F. A., III, M. Ishaq, G. L. Stoner, and R. J. Frisque.** 1992. JC virus DNA is present in many human brain samples from patients without progressive multifocal leukoencephalopathy. *J. Virol.* **66:**5726–5734.
118. **Wyen, C., C. Lehmann, G. Fätkenheuer, and C. Hoffmann.** 2005. AIDS-related progressive multifocal leukoencephalopathy in the era of HAART: report of two cases and review of the literature. *AIDS Patient Care STDS* **19:**486–494.
119. **Yogo, Y., T. Kitamura, C. Sugimoto, T. Ueki, Y. Aso, K. Hara, and F. Taguchi.** 1990. Isolation of a possible archetypal JC virus DNA sequence from nonimmunocompromised individuals. *J. Virol.* **64:**3139–3143.
120. **Zaragoza, C., R. M. Li, G. A. Fahle, S. H. Fischer, M. Raffeld, A. M. Lewis, Jr., and J. B. Kopp.** 2005. Squirrel monkeys support replication of BK virus more effi-

ciently than simian virus 40: an animal model for human BK virus infection. *J. Virol.* **79:**1320–1326.

121. **Zhong, S., H. Y. Zheng, M. Suzuki, Q. Chen, H. Ikegaya, N. Aoki, S. Usuku, N. Kobayashi, S. Nukuzuma, Y. Yasuda, N. Kuniyoshi, Y. Yogo, and T. Kitamura.** 2007. Age-related urinary excretion of BK polyomavirus by nonimmunocompromised individuals. *J. Clin. Microbiol.* **45:**193–198.

Papillomavirus

WILLIAM BONNEZ

28

Human papillomaviruses (HPVs) primarily infect the stratified squamous epithelia of humans. HPV was originally thought only to cause warts, but during the past 30 years, the great biological importance of these ubiquitous viruses has become recognized. HPVs are, in fact, responsible for a wide array of diseases, both benign and malignant. Hand and plantar warts, and external anogenital warts, also called condylomata acuminata, have been known since antiquity. However, over the past 130 years rarer diseases such as recurrent respiratory papillomatosis (laryngeal warts) and epidermodysplasia verruciformis have become recognized and were related to HPV infection in the late 1960s and early 1970s. In 1974 the role of HPV in cancer of the uterine cervix was first suspected. This oncogenic potential had already been established for the cottontail rabbit (Shope) papillomavirus in 1932 and for bovine papillomaviruses (BPV) starting in 1951. In the 1970s, analysis of HPV isolates led to the recognition of multiple HPV genotypes, and an association was also established between HPVs and squamous benign and preinvasive malignant lesions of the uterine cervix. These preinvasive malignant lesions, also called dysplasias, cervical intraepithelial neoplasias (CIN), or squamous intraepithelial neoplasias (SIL), are the precursors to invasive cervical carcinoma. As studies on the biology of HPVs progressed, it became clear that some of these viruses possessed genes capable of transforming and immortalizing cells in vitro. Subsequent epidemiological observations showed that some genital HPV types, the "low-risk" HPVs (e.g., types 6 and 11), were never or rarely associated with malignancies, whereas others, the "high-risk" HPVs (e.g., types 16 and 18), were linked. The use of PCR assays to diagnose HPV infection and prospective epidemiological studies have demonstrated that HPVs play a central role in the vast majority of cervical cancers. HPVs are also associated with many other cancers, with a causal link becoming increasingly established for squamous cell carcinomas (SCC) of the anus, vulva, vagina, penis, and oropharynx. In 2006 the first highly effective HPV vaccine directed at HPV type 6 (HPV-6), -11, -16, and -18 became available. A second, bivalent (HPV-16 and -18) vaccine was introduced in late 2007. These vaccines and their future expanded congeners hold the realistic promise of eradicating many of the HPV-related diseases.

VIROLOGY

Classification

HPVs have a supercoiled, single double-stranded circular DNA genome enclosed in an unenveloped, icosahedral capsid. These characteristics are shared by all the members of the *Papillomaviridae* family (see http://www.ncbi.nlm.nih.gov/ICTVdb/Ictv/index.htm). Papillomaviruses are widespread among higher vertebrates but are species specific. Because HPVs could not be grown for many years, and because sufficient quantities of most of them cannot be purified for direct biochemical and antigenic characterization, HPVs are classified by genotypes and not serotypes.

Genotypes

Papillomavirus genotypes are classified as distinct if their genomes have less than 90% homology in the DNA sequences of the L1 open reading frame (ORF), which encodes the major capsid protein. Subtypes have between 90 and 95% DNA homology, and variants have between 95 and 98% DNA homology. The *Papillomaviridae* family has 18 genera. HPVs belong to the *Alpha-*, *Beta-*, *Gamma-*, *Mu-*, and *Nupapillomavirus* genera. Although papillomaviruses share the same general genomic organization, some particularities characterize each genus. For example, the beta- and gammapapillomaviruses lack an E5 ORF. A genus may be further divided into species defined by a particular representative. For example, HPV-16, an alpha-papillomavirus, is the representative type of species 9, which also includes types 31, 33, 35, 52, and 67 (Fig. 1) (44). At the end of 2007, 107 HPV genotypes had been formally identified (Table 1). The number is continuously expanding, with over 300 types at various stages of characterization. There is an imperfect concordance between the phylogeny of the HPV types and their biology. All the betapapillomaviruses are associated with cutaneous lesions, with species 1 and 2 regrouping the epidermodysplasia verruciformis HPV types. The gamma-, mu-, and nupapillomaviruses are all associated with cutaneous lesions. Among the alphapapillomaviruses the situation is more complex. Species 1, 6, 7, 9, 10, 11, 13, 14, and 15 include only genital (mucosal) HPV types, while species 2 includes only cutaneous types, but species 3, 4, 5, and 8 include both cutaneous and genital types.

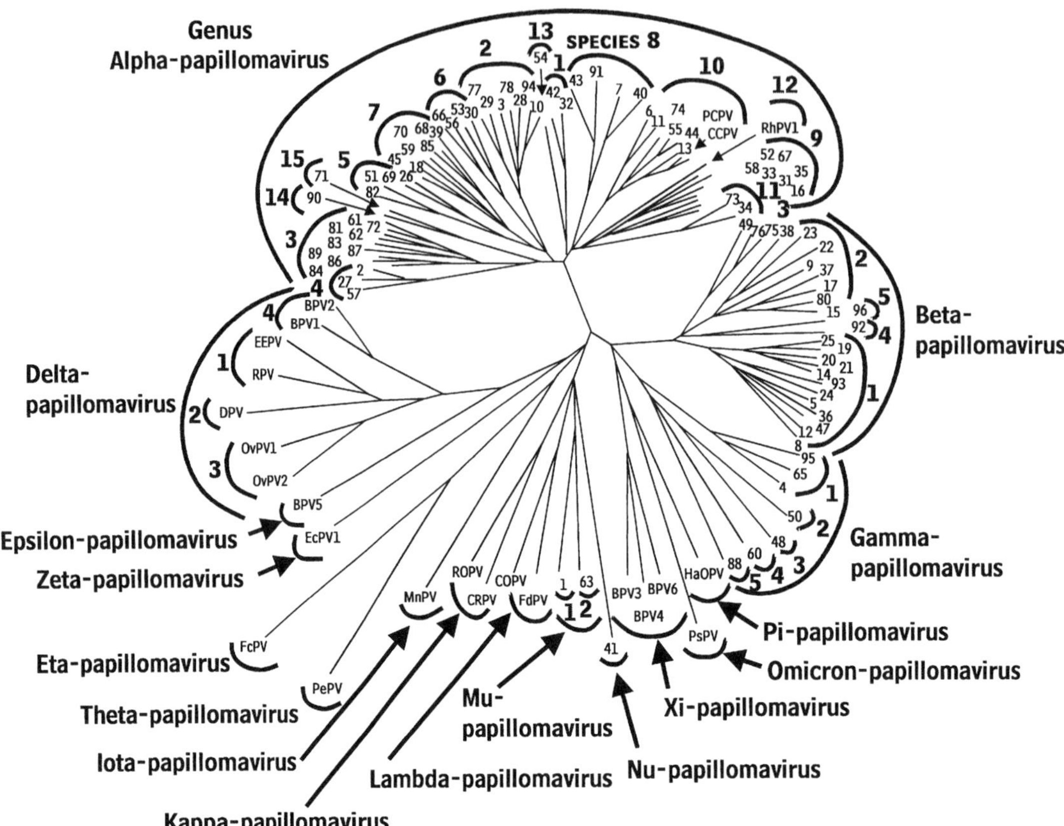

FIGURE 1 Phylogenetic tree of papillomaviruses. The tree was established on the basis of DNA sequence homology in the L1 ORF. Abbreviations: COPV, canine oral papillomavirus; CCPV, common chimpanzee papillomavirus; CRPV, cottontail rabbit papillomavirus; DPV, deer papillomavirus; EcPV, *Equus caballus* (horse) papillomavirus; EEPV, European elk papillomavirus; FdPV, *Felis domesticus* (cat) papillomavirus; FPV, *Fringilla coelebs* (chaffinch) papillomavirus; HaOPV, hamster oral papillomavirus; MnPV, *Mastomys natalensis* (rodent) papillomavirus; OvPV, ovine papillomavirus; PCPV, pygmy chimpanzee papillomavirus; PePV, *Psittacus erithacus timneh* (parrot) papillomavirus; PsPV, *Phocoena spinipinnis* (porpoise) papillomavirus; RhPV, rhesus monkey papillomavirus; ROPV, rabbit oral papillomavirus. (Tree slightly modified from reference 44 with permission of Elsevier.)

Serotypes

HPV virions induce humoral and cellular immune responses in animals and humans (51, 52). Antibodies react with major (L1) and minor (L2) proteins that constitute the viral capsid. Denatured papillomavirus virions exhibit a common antigen, not displayed during a natural infection, which has been used to generate a diagnostic antibody for immunocytochemistry. The DNA sequence encoding this common papillomavirus antigen has been mapped to a small region of the gene coding for the major capsid protein. Undenatured virions from different HPV types do not appear to share a common dominant antigen, even though the amino terminus of L2 contains epitopes shared broadly among papillomaviruses. Virus-like particles (VLPs) can be made by expressing the capsid genes, either for L1 alone or for L1 and L2 together. The study of papillomavirus L1 VLPs has shown that serotypes generally correspond to genotypes (122).

Composition

Papillomaviruses share the same structure, a naked, T = 7 icosahedral capsid containing a double-stranded, superhelicoidal, circular DNA molecule associated with cellular histone proteins H2a, H2b, H3, and H4. The capsid consists of 72 pentamers that are either pentavalent or hexavalent (Fig. 2). Each pentamer is composed of five major capsid proteins. The minor capsid protein is located in the center of the pentamer, possibly only in the pentavalent pentamers. Purified papillomavirus virions measure 55 to 60 nm in diameter (Fig. 2).

Genome

The viral genome is approximately 8,000 bp long (40 to 50% G+C content). The apparent molecular weight of 3×10^6 to 5×10^6 represents 10 to 13% of the virion's weight. Papillomavirus genomes share the same general organization (Fig. 3), which usually consists of eight ORFs, all located on the same strand. These have been designated as either early or late. The early ORFs (E1, E2, E4, E5, E6, and E7), originally numbered by diminishing size, code for nonstructural, regulatory proteins. The E3 ORF does not code for a protein, and different E8 ORFs have been identified only in kappa- and xipapillomaviruses—in the latter, E8 has the properties of E5. E5 is absent from the beta-

TABLE 1 HPV types and their disease associations[a]

Disease	HPV type(s)	
	Frequent association[b]	Less frequent association
Cutaneous		
Deep plantar warts	1, 2	4, 63
Common warts	2, 1, 4	26,[c] 27, 29, 41,[d] 57, 65, 77[d]
Common warts of meat, poultry, and fish handlers	7, 2	1, 3, 4, 10, 28
Flat warts	3, 10	27,[c] 38, 41,[d] 49,[c] 75, 76
Intermediate warts	10	26, 28
Epidermodysplasia verruciformis	5,[d] 8,[d] 9, 12, 14,[d] 15, 17[d]	19, 20[d,e] 21, 22, 23, 24, 25, 36, 37, 38, 47,[d] 50, 93
Anogenital or mucosal		
Condylomata acuminata	6, 11	42, 43, 44,[e] 45,[d] 51,[d] 54, 70
Intraepithelial neoplasia		
Unspecified		26,[d] 30,[d] 34,[e] 39,[d] 40, 53,[d] 57, 59,[d] 61, 62, 67, 68,[d] 69, 71, 81, 83
Low grade	6, 11	16,[d] 18,[d] 31,[d] 33,[d] 35,[d] 42, 43, 44,[e] 45,[d] 51,[d] 52,[d] 74[c]
High grade	16,[d] 18[d]	6, 11, 31,[d] 33,[d] 35,[d] 39,[d] 42, 44,[e] 45,[d] 51,[d] 52,[d] 56,[d] 58,[d] 66[d]
Bowen's disease	16[d]	31,[d] 34[e]
Bowenoid papulosis	16[d]	31,[d] 34,[e] 39,[d] 42, 45,[d] 67[d]
Cervical carcinoma	16,[d] 18[d]	31,[d] 33,[d] 35,[d] 39,[d] 45,[d] 51,[d] 52,[d] 56,[d] 58,[d] 59,[d] 66,[d] 67,[d] 68,[d] 73,[c,d] 82[d]
Recurrent respiratory papillomatosis	6, 11	
Miscellaneous		
Focal epithelial hyperplasia	13, 32	
Conjunctival papillomas and carcinomas	6, 11, 16[d]	18,[d] 33,[d] 45[d]
Others, cutaneous[f]		36, 37, 38,[d] 41,[d] 48,[c,d] 60, 72,[c] 80,[g] 88, 92, 93, 94, 95, 96, 107
Others, genital (mucosal)		30,[d] 84,[h] 85, 86,[d] 87, 89, 90, 91, 97, 101, 102, 103, 106

[a] I am grateful to Ola Forslund (Lund University, Malmö, Sweden) for sharing information. Most sequence information can be found in the GenBank and EMBL databases. The compendia *Human Papillomaviruses*, Los Alamos National Laboratory, Los Alamos, NM, are available on the Internet at http://hpv-web.lanl.gov/COMPENDIUM_PDF/. Data on HPV-78, -98, -99, -100, -104, and -105 are not currently available.

[b] The distinction between frequent and less frequent is arbitrary in many instances. Large descriptive statistics of HPV type distribution by disease are not available for all HPV types. Moreover, many HPV types have been looked for or identified only once or a few times.

[c] First recovered from immunosuppressed or HIV-infected patients.

[d] The malignant potential of this type is definite, probable (e.g., types 26, 53, 66, 68, 73, 82), or uncertain but possible because it has been isolated in one or a few lesions that were malignant (e.g., types 14, 17, 20, 38, and 47).

[e] HPV-46 was found to be a subtype of HPV-20, HPV-64 was found to be a subtype of HPV-34, and HPV-55 was found to be a subtype of HPV-44.

[f] Includes types isolated from a cystic plantar wart, oral cavity, kerathoanacanthoma, hand SCC, or malignant melanoma.

[g] Identified in normal skin.

[h] Identified in normal cervicovaginal cells.

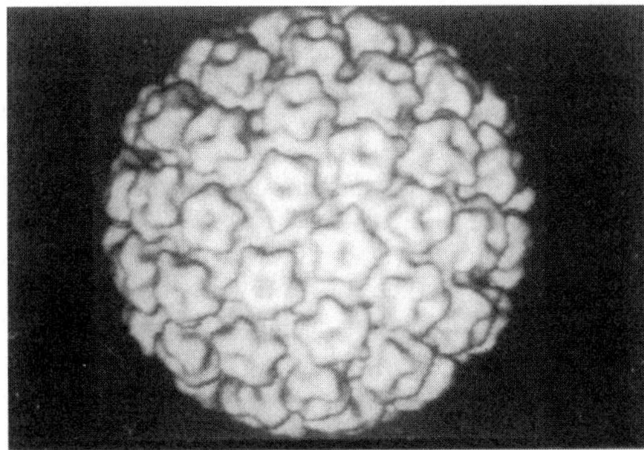

FIGURE 2 Structure of the papillomavirus virion. A cryo-electron micrograph of the HPV-1 capsid is shown (diameter, 60 nm). (Reprinted from reference 3a with permission.)

and gammapapillomaviruses, along with E4 from the etapapillomaviruses. E6 is absent from the xi- and theta-papillomaviruses, and E7 is absent from the omicronpapillomaviruses. The late ORFs (L1 and L2) code for the capsid proteins.

An important, typically 1-kb-long, noncoding region, referred to as the upstream regulatory region (URR) or long control region, lies between the early and late ORFs. The URR includes the origin of replication (*ori*), the E6/E7 gene promoter (promoter P97 of HPV-16), and the enhancer and silencers. The URR is thought to determine HPV tissue specificity. The function of the URR is governed by at least several of the internal transcriptional regulatory motifs (Fig. 4). These *cis*-acting elements bind to the various cellular and viral proteins that *trans*-regulate genomic function. At least four components are shared by the URRs of the papillomavirus types examined so far: (i)

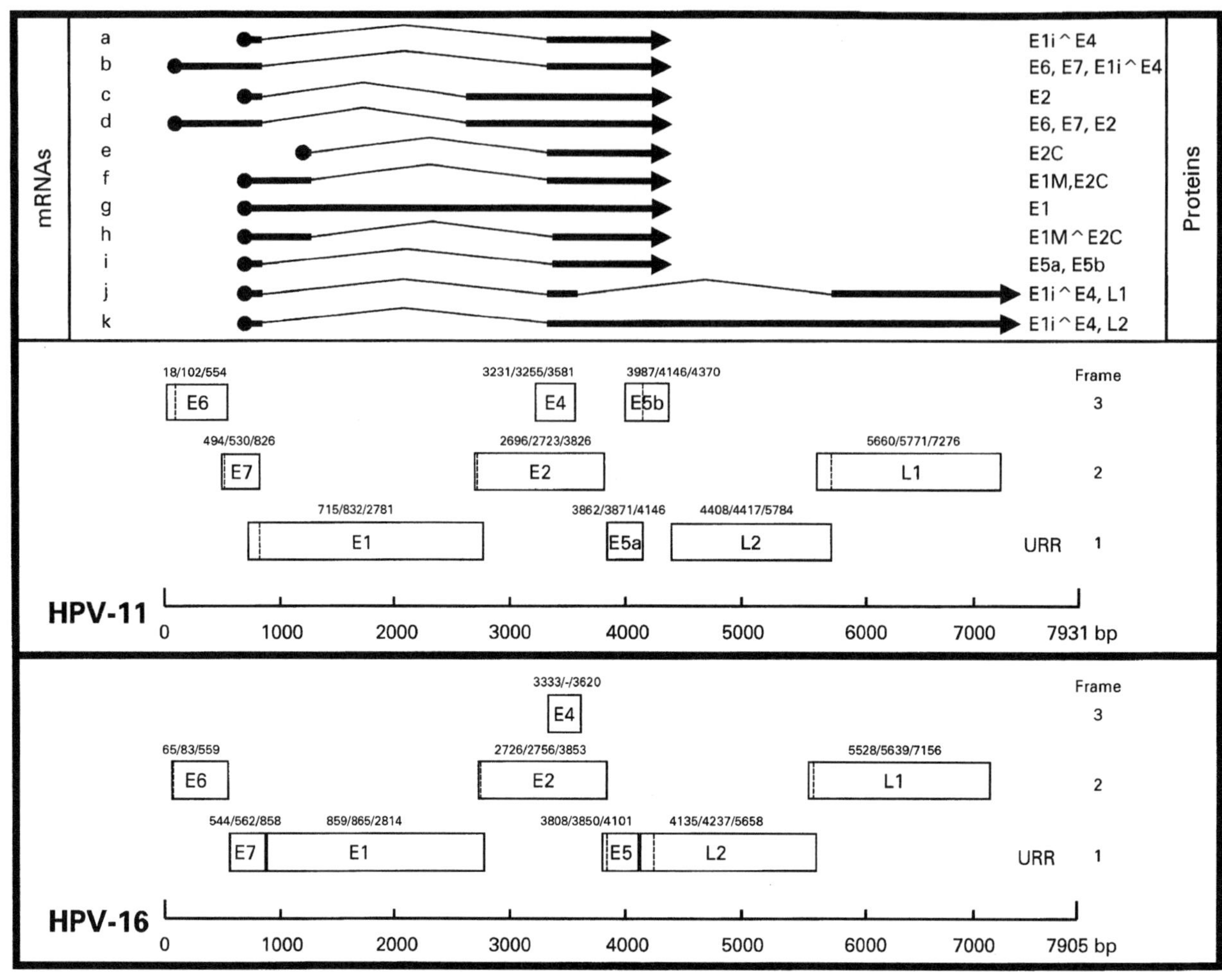

FIGURE 3 HPV genetic maps. (Bottom) linearized HPV-16 DNA map; (middle) linearized HPV-11 DNA map; (top) HPV-11 transcription map. By convention, the map origin of papillomaviruses is defined as the position homologous to the HpaI single restriction site of HPV-1. The open boxes correspond to the ORFs in the respective translation frames. The numbers above each ORF indicate the nucleotide position of the preceding stop codon (left solid vertical line) /start codon (dashed vertical line)/stop codon (right vertical line). Each HPV-11 mRNA is depicted with its cap site (solid circle), exons (thick line), introns (thin angled line), and poly(A) site (arrow). The putative corresponding proteins are indicated on the right of the mRNAs.

a polyadenylation signal for late mRNAs at the 5′ end, (ii) E2 protein binding sites, (iii) an E1 binding site associated with the origin of replication, and (iv) a TATA box in the E6 gene promoter. The molecular mechanisms of URR function and regulation are complex (166). Viral gene transcription results in an abundance of mRNA species due to complicated and multiple splicing patterns that reflect posttranscriptional regulation (166). These splicing patterns also differ among HPV types (Fig. 4). In addition, full or truncated ORFs may appear on different messages (e.g., E2 and E6). Some mRNAs are translated as fusion proteins (E1 and E4), whereas others are polycistronic (E6 and E7).

Proteins

Because of the multiple splicing patterns of viral gene expression, there are more protein products than ORFs. Table 2 summarizes the information on characterized proteins. L1 and L2 are structural proteins that form the capsid. L1 is called the major capsid protein because it represents 83% of the viral coat and has hemagglutinating activity. Experimentally, HPV L1 induces a strong and type-specific neutralizing antibody response (122). L2 is larger and dispensable in the formation of the capsid, but it appears to be important for both entry and egress of the viral genome and for encapsidation of the viral DNA. Experimentally, it also generates a weak but cross-specific neutralizing antibody response.

E1 and E2 proteins are involved in viral DNA replication (see "Biology" below) (67). E1 is the only viral protein with enzymatic activity as an ATPase that is part of the helicase function of E1. E1 also contributes to the maintenance of the viral episome and is often absent when the viral DNA is integrated. The E2 of HPV-16 possesses transcription regulatory properties and represses the activity of the E6/E7 promoter by binding to the E2 binding sites proximal to the E6 promoter (Fig. 4). In contrast, viral integration disrupts the E2 ORF and allows the free trans-

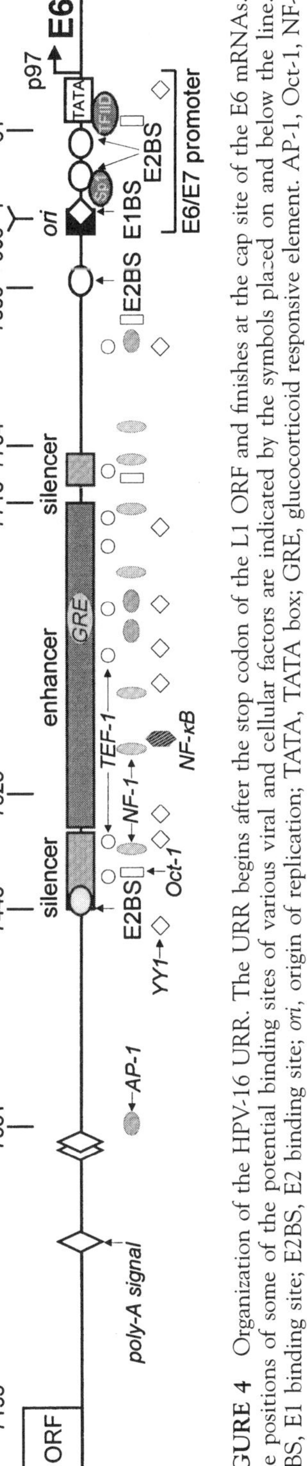

FIGURE 4 Organization of the HPV-16 URR. The URR begins after the stop codon of the L1 ORF and finishes at the cap site of the E6 mRNAs. The positions of some of the potential binding sites of various viral and cellular factors are indicated by the symbols placed on and below the line. E1BS, E1 binding site; E2BS, E2 binding site; *ori*, origin of replication; TATA, TATA box; GRE, glucocorticoid responsive element. AP-1, Oct-1, NF-1, NF-κB, Sp1, TEF-1, TFIID, and YY1 are cellular transcription factors.

activation of the E6/E7 promoter by several cellular transcription factors (159). The differential methylation of the E2 binding sites appears to be important in carcinogenesis.

Differential RNA splicing and proteolytic cleavage produce a variety of the most abundant cytoplasmic HPV protein, E4 (actually E1-E4 proteins, because they retain the first five amino acids of E1). With the exception of a conserved leucine-rich motif that appears to be important in the interaction with the cytokeratin networks, the E4 family of proteins shows substantial heterogeneity at the amino acid level among HPV types. Although the role of E4 remains to be defined, these proteins form a filamentous cytoplasmic network that colocalizes with the cytokeratin network of intermediate filaments in the lower epithelial layers (67). E4 proteins form solitary perinuclear structures in the more differentiated layers of the epidermis. Some of the speculated functions of E4 are the coordination of genome amplification, G_2-M arrest, and posttranscriptional gene regulation (67).

E5 is a small, membrane-bound protein that has weak transforming abilities in high-risk HPVs (67). However, it is unclear how this is accomplished because the protein is undetectable in tissues and the gene is often found to be deleted in cervical carcinomas. E5 interacts with cellular growth factor receptors, including the epidermal growth factor (EGF) receptor and, in the case of HPV-6, also with the erbB2 and platelet growth factor receptors (Fig. 5). Because it associates with an adaptin-like protein, E5 may interfere with the endocytosis and inactivation of these cell receptors. E5 also binds to the endosomal pore-forming protein, a 16-kDa protein with ATPase activity that participates in the endosomal proton pump. The resulting inhibition of endosome acidification increases the half-life of the EGF receptor. EGF activates the phosphokinase C pathway of signal transduction, which leads through the mitogen-activated protein (MAP) kinase activation pathway to the activation of the c-*jun* and c-*fos* oncogenes. c-Jun and c-Fos assemble in a heterodimer to form activation protein 1 (AP-1), which has potent transcriptional activity. c-*fos* is required for the malignant progression of skin tumors. It has been proposed that rather than acidifying the endosome, E5 acts by disturbing the protein trafficking from early to late endosomal structures. E5 may also activate the MAP kinase directly, and E5 can enhance endothelin-1-induced keratinocyte growth. E5 may also cause a decrease of expression of HLA-A and HLA-B molecules of the class I major histocompatibility complex, thus contributing to immune evasion. In addition, E5 suppresses cellular apoptosis and gap-junction communication between keratinocytes.

E6 and E7 are nuclear proteins that play a central role in malignant transformation (67, 133). Both proteins bind to a variety of cellular factors, with the highest affinity belonging to the E6 and E7 proteins of high-risk oncogenic HPVs, such as HPV-16 and -18. Thus, what follows mostly applies to E6 and E7 of the high-risk HPVs.

E6 is a zinc-binding protein that binds tightly to double-stranded DNA. In combination with the E6-associated protein (E6-AP), it associates with the p53 protein, prompting the accelerated degradation of p53 through the ubiquitin pathway. p53 is an important cell cycle regulator that is activated by DNA damage. Among its different functions (Fig. 6), p53 contributes to cell cycle arrest in G_1 phase. It transactivates the gene families *WAF1/CIP1* and *INK*, whose respective p21 and p16 proteins directly

TABLE 2 HPV proteins and their possible functions

Viral protein	Size (kDa)	Functions and properties[a]
E1	68–76	Participation in viral DNA replication Has a binding site in the URR and forms a hexameric ring around the DNA Forms a heterodimer with E2 Interacts with several of the cellular replicative proteins (DNA polymerase, primase complex, RP-A, etc.) Associates with histone H1 Binds to Ini1/hsSNF5, a chromatin remodeling complex that facilitates the access of transcription factors to DNA regulatory sequences Interacts with several cyclin/cyclin-dependent kinase complexes, especially cyclin E, leading to E1 phosphorylation, which is necessary for E1 nuclear localization DNA-dependent ATPase and helicase activities Maintenance of viral episomes Transcriptional repression (alone)/activation (with E2)
E2	40–58	Participation in DNA viral replication Has several binding sites in the URR. High-risk HPVs have four binding sites. Forms a heterodimer with E1 and dramatically increases the DNA-binding specificity of E1 Partitioning of viral episomes during cell replication by interacting with Brd4, a double bromodomain-containing chromatin adaptor protein Recruits histone acetyltransferases and may alter chromatin remodeling Viral transcription repression of E6/E7 at high level Viral transcription activation (E2 N terminus) at low level Cellular differentiation transcription regulation through interaction with the C/EBP transcription factors Interacts with L2 and may contribute to encapsidation of viral DNA Induces apoptosis (estrogen- and progesterone-dependent effect)
E4 (several) and E1-E4	10–17	Function unknown Bind to the cytokeratin filament network Are associated with the cornified cell envelope and may contribute to virion release ? Coordination of genome amplification ? Mitosis blockade ? Posttranscriptional gene regulation by binding to E4-DBP helicase
E5	10	? Malignant transformation Enhances growth factor receptor signal transduction Binds to and cooperates with cellular growth factor receptors (epithelial growth factor and platelet-derived growth factor) (HPV-6 but not HPV-16) Binds to Golgi's vacuolar ATPase 16-kDa protein (proton pump) and inhibits the acidification of endosomes and Golgi complex, which stabilize the epithelial growth factor receptor and platelet-derived growth factor, respectively Alternatively, E5 could interfere with protein trafficking from early to late endosomes Activates cellular oncogenes c-*jun* and c-*fos*, whose protein products form the AP-1 transcription factor (may be able to activate AP-1 directly) Can enhance endothelin-1-induced keratinocyte growth Might stimulate arachidonic acid metabolism independent of binding to platelet-derived growth factor Inhibits cell-to-cell communication through gap junctions Inhibits cell motility Immune evasion by inhibition of HLA-A and HLA-B cell surface antigens Apoptosis inhibition
E6	16–19	Inhibition of keratinocyte differentiation Binds to E6-AP, a calcium-binding protein and ubiquitin E3 ligase. Together they bind to and cause the degradation by ubiquitination of the tumor suppressor protein p53 and acceleration of its degradation by the ubiquitination pathway. This leads to the deactivation of the tumor suppressor gene *Notch1* and the activation of the oncogene *erb2* (HPV-16 and HPV-18) Leads in the same manner to the degradation of cell proliferation regulatory proteins Bak, multicopy maintenance protein 7, c-Myc, DLG Stimulation of malignant transformation By binding of E6 and E6-AP to PDZ domain proteins (DLG, MUPP1, MAGGI, and hScribble), leading to transformation by loss of cell polarization, cell signaling, and of cell-to-cell communication

(*Continued on next page*)

TABLE 2 *(Continued)*

Viral protein	Size (kDa)	Functions and properties
		Cellular immortalization
		By binding and degradation with E6-AP of the NFX cellular repressor of the hTERT (telomerase) promoter, thereby causing elongation and repair of chromosome telomeres
		Stimulation of cell proliferation
		Interacts with p300/CBP (transcription coactivator acetyltransferase), paxillin (focal adhesion protein), IRF-3 (transcription factor), E6TP1 (putative GAP protein), MUPP1 (putative DLG analog), Tyk2, and protein kinase N (high-risk HPVs)
		Interacts with Gps2, a protein that binds to p300/CBP (low- and high-risk HPVs)
		Inhibition of apoptosis
		By binding and degrading Bak, FADD, procaspase 8
		By reducing p53 levels
		Inhibition of the immune response (HPV-16 or -18)
		By binding to IRF-3
		By interacting with Tyk2 and interference with JAK-STAT activation of the IFN-α cascade
		By altering the expression and function of TLR-9
		By inhibiting the IL-8 and IP-10 induction of the IFN-γ response
		By down-regulating E-cadherin, which depletes the epidermis from Langerhans cells
		Cooperation with E7 to counteract the E7-induced increased level of p53
		Contributes to chromosome destabilization (high-risk HPVs)
		Enhances DNA integration and mutagenicity (high-risk HPVs)
		Binding to Bak, Gps2, E6-AP, and zylin (focal adhesion protein) (low-risk HPVs)
E6*	5–8	Has antiproliferative and antiviral replicative effects
		Inhibits E6-directed degradation of p53
E7	10–14	Stimulation of malignant transformation (high-risk HPVs) and cell proliferation (all HPVs)
		Interferes with pRB, a tumor suppressor gene product, and abrogates pRB's inhibitory effect on cell proliferation by releasing E2F, a family of transcription factors involved with the S phase of the cell cycle (high-risk HPVs)
		Interferes with the p107 and 130 proteins, pRB-like proteins that inhibit cell proliferation
		Inactivates the HDAC protein by binding first to the HDAC complex protein Mi-2β and causes increased levels of E2F. HDAC normally represses gene expression by facilitating chromatin condensation.
		Enhances DNA integration and mutagenicity
		Binds c-Jun and FOXM1c and activates the proliferation-associated transcription factors AP-1 and FOXM1c, respectively
		Inhibits cyclin-dependent kinase inhibitors $p21^{WAF1/CIP1}$ and $p27^{KIP1}$
		Activates cyclins E and A directly, by binding to cyclin E and histone 1 kinase, and indirectly, by activating the Cdc25A phosphatase
		Causes increased levels of $p16^{INK4A}$, an inhibitor of cyclin D1-CDK4 and cyclin D1-CDK6. But because the cell cycle is made resistant by E7 to the growth arrest that would otherwise ensue, $p16^{INK4A}$ has been used as a biomarker of potential malignancy
		Causes resistance to TGF-β, an inhibitor of keratinocyte growth
		Causes an increased level of p53 that is counteracted by E6
		Causes centriole amplification that results in aneuploidy
		Apoptosis modulation (estrogen- and progesterone-dependent effect)
		By interacting with p53 and binding to p600 (involved with anchorage-independent growth and cellular transformation)
		By interacting with the IκB kinase complex, leading to an increase in the precursor NF-κB proteins
		By inhibition of caspase 8
		Inhibition of the immune response (all HPVs)
		By binding and inhibiting IFN-α
		By binding and preventing the translocation to the nucleus of P48/IRF-9, which normally binds to the interferon-specific response element
		By binding and inactivating the IFN-γ-induced transcription factor IRF-1, thereby decreasing the expression of IFN-β, the transporter associated with antigen processing 1 (TAP1), and monocyte chemotactic protein 1
		By altering the expression and function of TLR-9
		Causes resistance to TNF produced by cytotoxic T cells

(Continued on next page)

TABLE 2 HPV proteins and their possible functions *(Continued)*

Viral protein	Size (kDa)	Functions and properties
		Other known and unknown functions Angiogenic properties Regulates the expression of the calcium-binding S100P protein and of the mitochondrial ADP/ATP carrier protein Interacts with the M2 pyruvate kinase, an enzyme of the carbohydrate metabolism
L1	54–58	Major capsid protein Assembles into pentamers and is sufficient to form VLPs Contains the dominant, type-specific, neutralizing epitope(s)
L2	63–78	Minor capsid protein Binds to DNA Facilitates the egress of the viral DNA from the endosome after entry Interacts with E2 Facilitates transport of L1 protein to the nucleus and localization to the POD nuclear domains ? Stabilizes capsid (stoichiometry unclear) N terminus contains minor, cross-reactive, neutralizing epitope(s)

[a] DLG, disk large; MUPP1, multiple PDZ protein1; IRF-3, interferon regulatory factor 3; TLR-9, Toll-like receptor 9; HDAC, histone deacetylase.

interact with a cyclin/cyclin-dependent kinase/proliferating cell nuclear antigen (PCNA) complex that is responsible for phosphorylating and inactivating the retinoblastoma (pRB) protein. The *Notch1* gene is induced; its protein is a determinant of keratinocyte differentiation and acts as a tumor suppressor protein. The net result is the arrest of the cell cycle in G_1 phase. Another function of p53 is the induction of apoptosis through the down-regulation of the *bcl2* gene and the activation of the *bax* gene. E6 interacts with various other cellular proteins (Table 1), including tumor suppressors (e.g., disk large [DLG], hScrib, and MAGI), transcription factors (e.g., c-Myc, p300/CBP, interferon regulatory factor 3, TBP, hADA3, p-CAF, and AMF-1), and proteins implicated in cell signaling and cell-to-cell communication (PSD-95/DLG/ZO–1–PDZ proteins, including multiple PDZ protein 1). E6 can cause cell immortalization by interacting with the promoter complex of the human telomerase (hTERT), a ribonucleoprotein enzyme that maintains the length of chromosomal telomeres, thus preventing cellular senescence. E6* proteins are truncated polypeptides resulting from splicing patterns present only in high-risk HPVs. They inhibit the E6-mediated degradation of p53 and have a negative regulatory effect on cellular and viral replication.

E7 is a zinc-binding protein whose amino terminus has homologies to adenovirus E1A and the large T antigen of polyomaviruses. E7 binds to and inactivates the hypophosphorylated pRB, a product of the tumor suppressor gene *Rb-1*. pRB associates with the transcription factor E2F and its associated protein, DP1 (differentiation-regulated transcription factor 1 protein). This results in the arrest of the cell cycle in G_1 phase. E7 protein can also bind to pRB-related proteins p107 and p130 (these three proteins are called the pRB pocket proteins) and through slightly different mechanisms (Fig. 6) cause the same overall effect, namely, the triggering of cell cycle progression. In addition, E7 inhibits inhibitors of the cyclin-dependent kinases ($p21^{WAF1/CIP1}$ and $p27^{KIP1}$). Like E6, E7 possesses some transcription regulatory activity (it stimulates the AP-1 transcription factor), and it is able to cooperate with v-*ras* in transforming primary rodent cells. Table 2 lists additional interactions of E7.

The transforming and immortalizing properties of the E6 and E7 genes have been demonstrated in various cell lines but also in transgenic animals, in which they induce carcinomas at the site of expression. Considerably less is known about the role of E6 and E7 of the low-risk HPVs.

Biology

Replication Strategy

Papillomavirus DNA replication appears to be governed by the state of differentiation of the keratinocytes in the squamous epithelium (Table 3). The first step is viral entry into the basal keratinocyte (144). Heparan sulfate and the glycosaminoglycans are strong candidates as cellular receptors for HPV. This initial binding seems to be followed by binding to a second receptor, an uncharacterized extracellular matrix component, possibly laminin, that leads to entry of the virus by a clathrin-coated pit mechanism into the endosome. A second trafficking pathway may be the Golgi apparatus, where furin, a membrane protease, could cleave L2 and release the viral DNA. The virus initiates its replication as an episome after entering a basal cell, generating a low number (less than 20 to 50) of copies per cell. Viral replication is dependent on the replicative machinery of the cell and is in part controlled by the transport of E1 in the nucleus, which is dependent on phosphorylation by cellular cyclin-dependent kinases. Viral DNA replication begins with displacement of the histones associated with the viral DNA and the unwinding of the supercoiled viral DNA (138). E1 binds to a receptor in the URR that incorporates the origin of replication. E2 contributes to the specificity of this binding and is then released. E1 has helicase and ATPase activities. In cooperation with E2, topoisomerase I, and replication protein A, E1 displaces the histones associated with the viral DNA and unwinds the DNA supercoiled conformation (Fig. 7). E1 subsequently forms a bidirectional replication fork complex with cellular proteins (polymerase α/primase, DNA polymerase δ/PCNA, replication factor C, topoisomerase II, and DNA ligase). HPV DNA replication progresses bidirectionally from the origin of replication. Viral DNA is then encapsidated in a process that involves its association with cellular histone proteins (H2a, H2b, H3, and H4). A

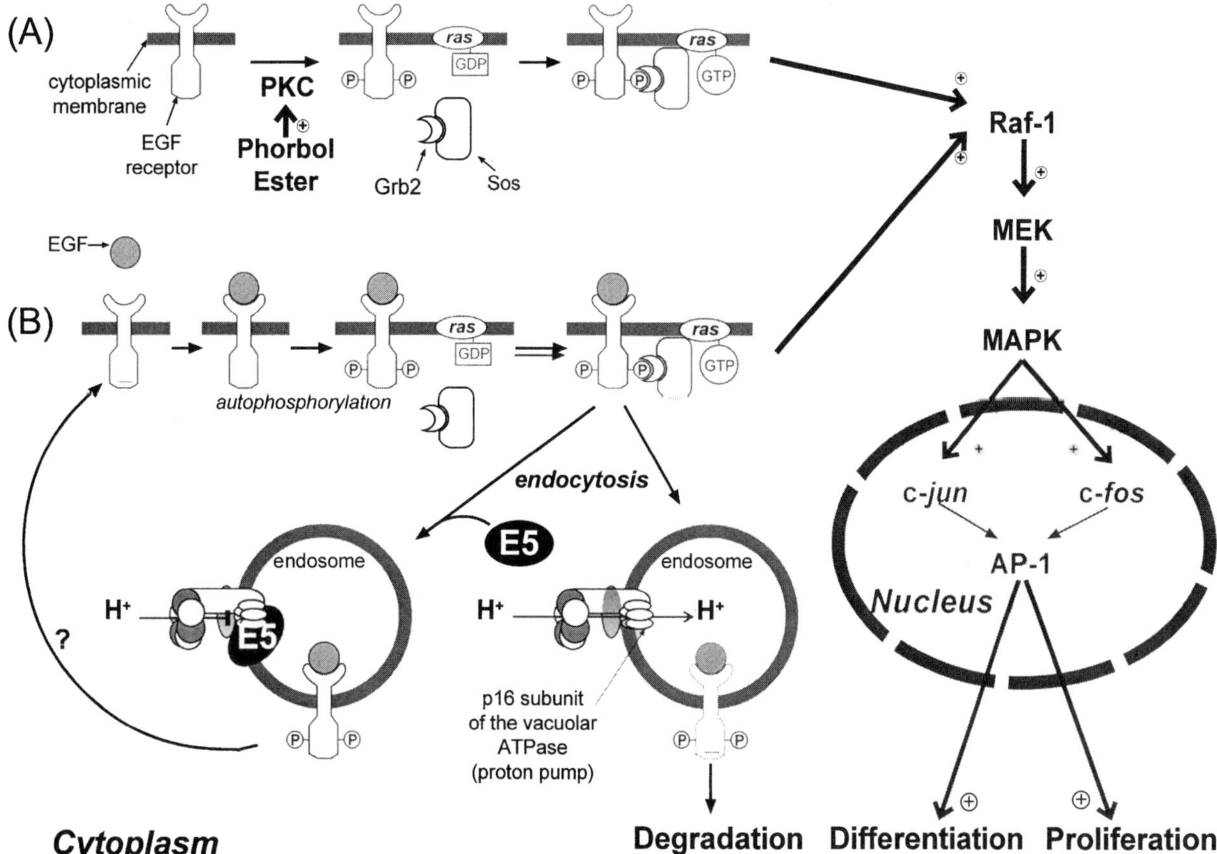

FIGURE 5 Epithelial growth factor (EGF) receptor, phorbol ester, and HPV E5 protein interactions. (A) Upon exposure to a phorbol ester, phosphokinase C (PKC) gets activated and phosphorylates the EGF receptor. This allows the binding of a complex of proteins, Grb2 and Sos, that are brought in contact with the cytoplasmic membrane. The Ras protein becomes activated by Sos after exchange of GDP for GTP. This is the trigger for the actuation of a cascade of protein kinases, Raf-1, MEK, MAPK, that ultimately induces the expression of the transcription factor AP-1, which is made up of two proto-oncoproteins, Fos and Jun. The net result is a stimulation of cell proliferation and differentiation. (B) Under physiological conditions, the EGF receptor is activated by the binding of its ligand, EGF. Autophosphorylation ensues, which precipitates the sequence of events detailed in panel A. Eventually, the process stops when the EGF receptor becomes internalized by endocytosis. As the endosome becomes acidic, the EGF receptor is degraded. The acidification of the endosome is dependent on a proton pump that includes a p16 protein subunit. Papillomavirus E5 inactivates the proton pump by binding to the p16 subunit. It is believed that the undegraded EGF receptor is then recycled to the cytoplasmic membrane. The overall effect is an increase of cellular differentiation and proliferation.

transient binding of L2 with E2 protein presumably guides the DNA into the aggregation of viral L1 and L2 proteins that eventually form the capsid. The release of viral particles is probably passive, resulting from the disintegration of the upper squamous epithelium, possibly facilitated by the E1-E4 protein. Desquamating cells are infectious.

Host Range

Papillomaviruses are widespread among higher vertebrates, but each type usually has a narrow species specificity, and HPVs infect only humans. BPV cause papillomas or fibropapillomas in cattle, but those BPV types producing fibropapillomas (BPV type 1 [BPV-1] and BPV-2) can induce, naturally or experimentally, fibromas and fibrosarcomas in a variety of mammals, such as horses (sarcoid), rabbits, and hamsters (30). The cottontail rabbit (Shope) papillomavirus causes skin papillomas in its natural hosts, the cottontail rabbit *(Sylvilagus floridanus)* and the jackrabbit *(Lepus californicus)*, but papillomas and carcinomas in its experimental host, the domestic rabbit *(Oryctolagus cuniculus)* (30). No animal papillomaviruses have been shown to infect humans.

Growth in Cell Culture and Animal Models

Infection with HPV virions or transfection with HPV DNA of keratinocyte monolayers results in transient replication of the viral DNA without visible cytopathic effect or production of virus. Tissue cultures derived from cutaneous warts or laryngeal papillomas have a normal morphological appearance and no viral gene expression. In

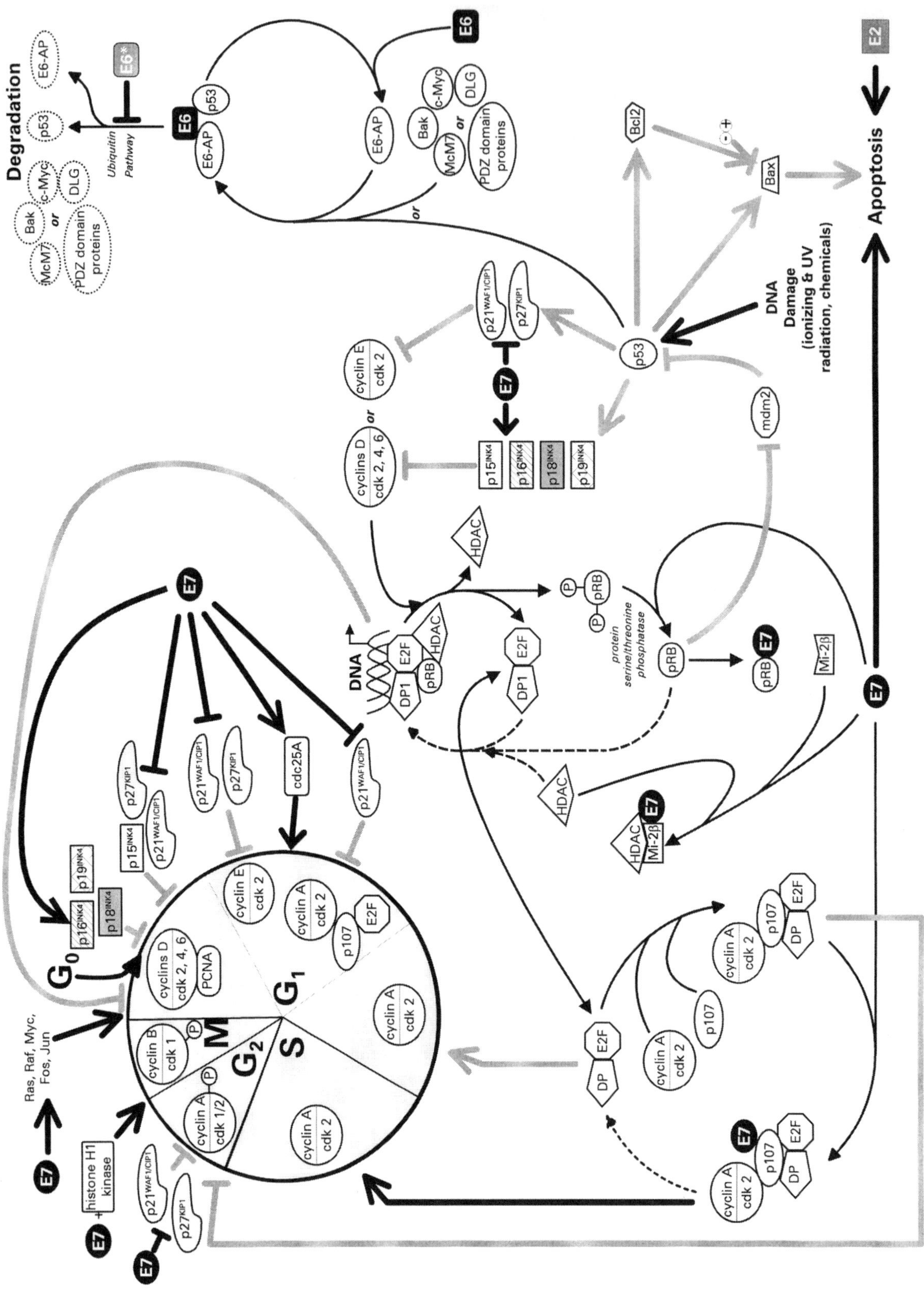
Degradation
Bak
c-Myc
DLG
McM7
or
PDZ domain proteins
p53
E6-AP
Ubiquitin Pathway
E6*
E6
E6-AP
p53
E6-AP
Bak
c-Myc
McM7
DLG
or
PDZ domain proteins
E6
or
cyclin E
cdk 2
cyclins D
cdk 2, 4, 6
or
$p21^{WAF1/CIP1}$
$p27^{KIP1}$
E7
$p15^{INK4}$
$p16^{INK4}$
$p18^{INK4}$
$p19^{INK4}$
p53
mdm2
Bcl2
Bax
Apoptosis
E2
DNA
Damage
(ionizing & UV radiation, chemicals)
E7
HDAC
DNA
DP1
E2F
pRB
HDAC
P
pRB
P
E2F
DP1
protein serine/threonine phosphatase
pRB
pRB
E7
Mi-2β
E7
HDAC
HDAC
Mi-2β
E7
$p27^{KIP1}$
$p15^{INK4}$
$p21^{WAF1/CIP1}$
$p21^{WAF1/CIP1}$
$p27^{KIP1}$
cdc25A
$p21^{WAF1/CIP1}$
$p16^{INK4}$
$p19^{INK4}$
$p18^{INK4}$
G_0
cyclins D
cdk 2, 4, 6
PCNA
cyclin E
cdk 2
cyclin A
cdk 2
p107
E2F
G_1
cyclin A
cdk 2
S
G_2
M
cyclin B
cdk 1
P
cyclin A
cdk 1/2
P
cyclin A
cdk 2
Ras, Raf, Myc, Fos, Jun
E7
E7
histone H1 kinase
$p21^{WAF1/CIP1}$
$p27^{KIP1}$
E7
DP
E2F
cyclin A
cdk 2
p107
cyclin A
cdk 2
p107
DP
E2F
cyclin A
cdk 2
p107
E7
DP
E2F

TABLE 3 Tissue differentiation and HPV markers of productive infection[a]

Tissue layer	DNA	RNA[b]				Virions
		E1, E2	E6, E7	E4, E5	L1, L2	
Stratum corneum	+++					++
Stratum granulosum	+++	++	+	++	+	++
Stratum spinosum						
High	+++	++	++	++	+	+
Low	++	++	++	+		
Stratum basale	+	+				

[a] Relative abundance, from low (+) to high (+++).

[b] In high-grade intraepithelial neoplasias, E6 and E7 mRNAs are usually more abundant than E4, E5, L1, and L2 mRNAs; the converse is true in low-grade lesions. The table applies mostly to anogenital HPVs.

contrast, cell lines from cervical carcinomas can exhibit a transformed phenotype and retain HPV DNA, such as HPV-16 (CaSki and SiHa) or HPV-18 (HeLa and C4-1). These cell lines carry HPV DNA in integrated form with a disruption of the early region of the viral genome and therefore lack a permissive infection. Permissive infections (infections yielding viral particles) have been established using immortalized, nonmalignant cell lines derived from CIN containing episomal HPV-16 (W12 cells) or HPV-31b (CIN 612 cells). This has been accomplished by induction of full epithelial differentiation by planting the cells either on the musculofascial layer of the flank of a nude (athymic) mouse (W12 cells) or on an organotypic "raft" culture system (CIN 612 cells) followed by stimulation with phorbol ester, an inducer of phosphokinase C and cell differentiation (Fig. 5). The raft system has undergone further refinements that only very recently have allowed the high multiplicity of infection that ensures the production and propagation of HPV infectious virions in vitro.

Immunodeficient mice (e.g., athymic or with severe combined immunodeficiency [SCID]) grafted orthotopically or heterotopically with HPV-infected human xenografts are otherwise the only means to reproduce the natural infectious cycle. They provide sustained propagation of HPV virions and duplicate the macroscopic, microscopic, and molecular features of natural lesions (13). These models demonstrated that HPV-6 and -11 induce condylomata acuminata and that HPV-16 induces intraepithelial neoplasias (18).

Inactivation by Physical and Chemical Agents

Little is known about their resistance to physical and chemical agents, but papillomaviruses appear to be hardy. Viral capsids resist treatment with ether, acid, and heat for 1 h at 50°C. Exposure to 100°C for 1 h is necessary to abolish HPV-11 gene expression in the SCID mouse xenograft model (21). Moreover, the heat generated during laser surgery or electrocoagulation produces a plume of smoke that contains HPV DNA and has been implicated in transmitting infection to health care workers. However, HPV is inactivated by autoclaving and 70% ethanol. Consequently, standard autoclaving procedures should be used to sterilize surgical instruments that are potentially contaminated with HPV, and the smoke released from vaporized HPV lesions should be evacuated.

EPIDEMIOLOGY

Distribution and Geography

HPV infections and diseases are widely distributed worldwide, although some geographic variations occur. For example, focal epithelial hyperplasia (Heck's disease), an oral disease related to HPV-13 and -32, mostly affects American Indians, Inuits, and South Africans (117). Geographic disparities in the prevalence of common warts can be seen within countries. The most comprehensive surveys of the worldwide distribution are those of cervical HPV infections and diseases (36, 43). In women with normal cervical cytology, HPV-16 is the dominant genotype worldwide, but there are exceptions in Eastern Africa, Japan, and Taiwan, where HPV-52 is more common than HPV-16. HPV-18, which is usually second worldwide, is replaced at that rank by HPV-58 in Western Africa and South America and by HPV-66 in southern Europe (43). Overall, in invasive cervical carcinomas, HPV-16 is the most common HPV type (53.5%), followed by HPV-18 (17.2%), HPV-45 (6.7%), HPV-31 (2.9%), HPV-33 (2.6), HPV-52 (2.3%), HPV-58 (2.2%), HPV-35 (1.4%), and others (36). Although the ranking rarely does change for HPV-16 and -18 according to location, in North America, HPV-31, -33, and -45 are, respectively, the third, fourth, and fifth most common HPVs, but in Asia, HPV-58, -33, and -53 occupy these ranks. The geographic variation is more striking when looking at the variants of HPV-16 with their North American, European, African, Asian, and Asian American lineages (164).

FIGURE 6 Model of the biological interactions of high-risk proteins with the cell cycle and apoptosis (see text for details). Symbols: ⊕, activation; ⊖, inhibition. Thick lines with open arrowheads (➔) indicate up-regulation; the same lines with a broken end denote down-regulation. Thick gray lines represent the regulations in normal cells, whereas the thick black lines show the regulations in HPV-infected cells; thin arrows (→) show direct interactions. Note that the symbols are not drawn proportional to the protein molecular weights and that the protein complex aggregations are not necessarily concomitant or involve the direct protein-to-protein contacts shown. DP, differentiation-regulated transcription factor polypeptide; HDAC, histone deacetylase; mdm2, murine double minute 2 protein; DLG, disk large.

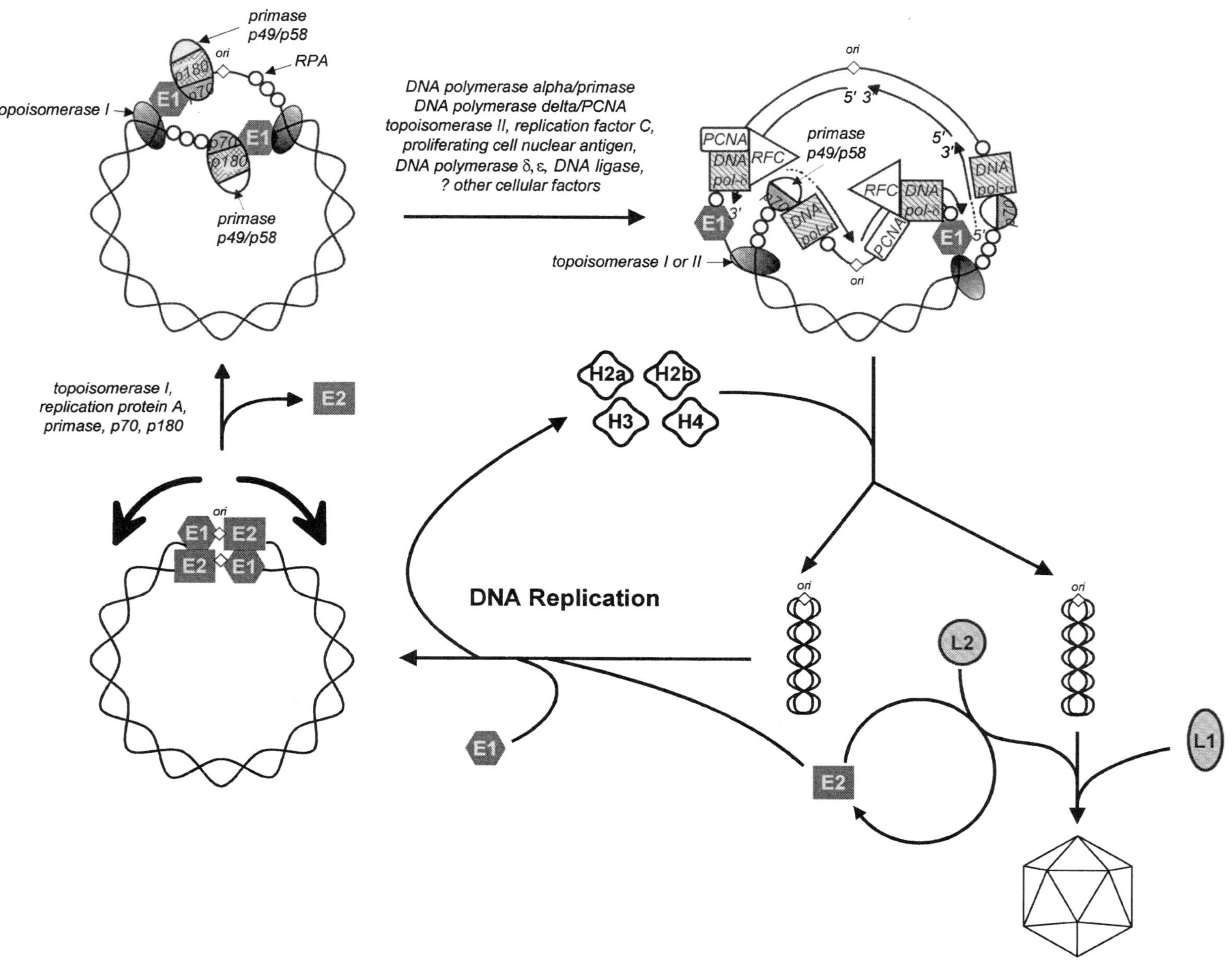

FIGURE 7 Model of HPV DNA replication and encapsidation.

Incidence and Prevalence of Infection

HPV infections are endemic. No epidemic patterns of HPV infection have been recognized. The moderate transmissibility, variable incubation period, latency, and spontaneous resolution of HPV infections ordinarily impede the recognition of HPV disease outbreaks.

Cutaneous Warts

Cutaneous HPV infections are extremely prevalent, with rates of 80% in immunocompetent hosts and 95% in immunocompromised patients (2). HPV DNA can be found on healthy skin and can still be present in half of the subjects when new samples are obtained from them 6 years later.

Cutaneous warts (common, plantar, and flat warts) are very common among the general population. Mostly a disease of school-age children, common (hand) warts represent about 70% of all cutaneous warts (80). The prevalence of common warts ranges from 0.8 to 22% (80). Plantar warts make up to a third of cutaneous warts and are found in a wider age group, primarily adolescents and young adults. Flat or juvenile warts constitute 4 to 8% of the cutaneous warts, with a peak prevalence among 10- to 12-year-olds (80). An increased incidence of plantar warts has been noted in the winter months.

Genital HPV Infections and Diseases

No seasonality is recognized generally in the acquisition of HPV infection or the expression of HPV diseases. In the U.S. female population, one study based on 3,262 sexually active women aged 18 to 25 (94) found that 26.9% of subjects were positive for a genital HPV, with 20% of the total sample being positive for a high-risk HPV. Remarkably, 62% of the infections were by multiple types, and 14.3% of women reporting only one lifetime sexual partner were positive. A second survey on a sample of 1,921 females aged 14 to 59 years (49) found that the overall prevalence of HPV DNA was 26.8%, with the majority represented by high-risk HPV infections, 15.2%. The peak rate was in the 14- to 19-year-old group (44.8%), followed by the 20- to 24-year-old group (17.4%). Here again, having only one lifetime sexual partner offered limited protection, as 11.5% of these women were positive. A meta-analysis of 78 studies of women with normal cytology indicated an overall worldwide HPV prevalence of 10.4%, with figures from as low as 8% for Asia to as high as 22% for Africa (28). Rates of HPV DNA prevalence on the male genitalia vary from 1.3 to 79%, with a majority of studies reporting rates of 20% and higher (47). In the United States, about 20 million people are estimated to be infected with genital HPVs, half of them aged between 15 and 24 years (153). About 6.2 million individuals contract a sexually transmitted HPV infection every year. It is estimated that 80% of the U.S. sexually active population will get a genital HPV infection in their lifetime.

Most infections are rapidly cleared, or at least become undetectable (148). In a prospective study of 331 18- to 35-year-old women who had HPV DNA-positive cervical samples, half had cleared the virus by 9 months (61). The median time to clearance was longer for high-risk types (9.8 months) than for low-risk types (4.3 months). By 14 months, only a tenth of the subjects were still positive. Typically, with repeated testing over time, only a minority of patients will be positive every time, while another subgroup will be consistently negative (69).

The incidence of anogenital warts is increasing. The number of initial visits for genital warts to physicians' offices in the United States increased from 222,000 in 2000 to 422,000 in 2006 (31). A similar increase was noted from the insurance claims of 5.9 million 15- to 59-year-old members enrolled in approximately 30 health plans in the United States (83). The rate of new genital warts rose from 117.8 claims per 100,000 person-years at risk in 1998 to 205.0 in 2001 (data were age standardized to the 2001 U.S. privately insured population). The highest rates were in the 10- to 29-year-old group. The NHANES survey indicates that in the United States, 5.6% of persons aged 18 to 59 years reported ever having genital warts, with a greater number of women (7.2%) than men (3.4%) (44a). A random survey of 69,147 women 18 to 45 years of age from the general population in Denmark, Iceland, Norway, and Sweden showed that 10.6% reported ever having had clinically diagnosed genital warts (81).

The prevalence of HPV infections in neonates and infants appears to be low (65). No more than 1% of babies have oral or genital HPV infections (131), and genital warts are highly unusual in children. Fifty percent to 75% of children with genital warts acquire them from sexual abuse, and 1 to 2% of sexually abused children have genital warts (65). Nevertheless, the presence of genital warts alone is not sufficient to establish a case of sexual abuse. Nonsexual transmission of anogenital warts appears to be possible. Family members of children with anogenital warts have been shown to have cutaneous warts that harbor HPV-6 (64). Conversely, the presence of HPV-1 or HPV-2, nongenital genotypes, in about 20% of genital warts recovered from prepubertal children suggests the existence of nongenital sources, such as autoinoculation or nonsexual contact, but does not necessarily exclude fondling (64). In young children (less than 2 years old), anogenital warts are more likely the result of vertical transmission, whereas horizontal, nongenital, or genital transmission is more likely in older children (11). Recommendations for the evaluation of children with genital warts suspected of sexual abuse are available (71).

The prevalence of cervical HPV disease is best measured by cervical cytology. Rates vary between 0.9 and 4.8% depending on the criteria and age and decrease after age 24 (84). In one study, 2.5% of cervical cytology samples had evidence of HPV-related cervical disease with low-grade SIL (LSIL) (1.97%), high-grade SIL (HSIL) (0.51%), SCC (0.026%), and adenocarcinomas (0.0046%) (141). In addition to these well-recognized entities are ambiguous cytological abnormalities that are as common. They are called atypical squamous cells (ASC), either of unknown significance (ASC-US) or which cannot exclude HSIL (ASC-H) (both subcategories used to be grouped as ASCUS).

An HPV infection is present in virtually all cervical cancers (SCC and adenocarcinomas) (105, 152). It is a necessary, if not sufficient, condition for the development of cervical cancer (128). In 2002, cervical cancer was worldwide the second most common cancer in women, with 493,000 new cases and 274,000 deaths (114). The burden is mostly in developing countries, where 83% of the cases occur. The highest incidences are observed in eastern Africa (42.7/100,000, age adjusted), southern Africa (38.2), Central America (30.6), and South America (28.6) (114). In the United States, according to 2007 estimates, cervical cancer is in decline; it ranks 14th in incidence (11,150 new cases) and 16th in mortality (3,670 deaths) among all female cancers (75). Cervical cancer is not the only cancer attributable to HPV. In 2002, worldwide and both sexes combined, 100% of the 492,800 cases of cervical cancers could be attributed to HPV, but so could 40% of the 26,300 cases of penile cancer, 40% of the 40,000 cases or vulvar or vaginal cancers, 90% of the 30,400 cases of anal cancers, 3% of the 274,300 cases of mouth cancers, and up to 70% of the 52,000 cases of oropharyngeal cancers (46, 113). Globally, these other cancers represent up to about 17% of all genital HPV-related cancers, and they represent a third in the developed world (113). These figures do not account for the premalignant conditions attributable to HPV.

Recurrent Respiratory Papillomatosis

The age of onset of recurrent respiratory papillomatosis has a bimodal distribution that includes young children and young adults, but not the elderly (42). In the United States, the estimated annual incidence rates are 4.3/100,000 in children less than 14 years of age and 1.8/100,000 in young adolescents (older than 15 years) and adults. The estimated prevalence rates for these two populations are 10.9/100,000 and 4.5/100,000, respectively.

Other HPV Diseases

Epidemiological data are lacking for other HPV diseases, such as the very rare epidermodysplasia verruciformis. Focal epithelial hyperplasia (Heck's disease) is also a relatively uncommon disease that is mostly found in children and adolescents (117).

Risk Factors

Cutaneous Warts

Use of heated swimming pools or communal baths is an activity that appears to promote the acquisition of plantar warts (76). In one controlled experiment, students who wore protective footwear during swimming were much less prone to developing plantar warts than those who did not. Nail biting is associated with the presence of periungual warts.

Some primary and secondary immunodeficiencies are risk factors for acquiring cutaneous warts. Patients with ataxia-telangiectasia, Wiskott-Aldrich syndrome, common variable immunodeficiency, or other various primary humoral and cellular defects may develop extensive verrucosis (5). An approximate 10-fold increase in prevalence of cutaneous warts has been noted in lymphoma patients, whereas a 4- to 12-fold increase has been reported for human immunodeficiency virus (HIV)-infected individuals. Organ transplant recipients are particularly susceptible to developing cutaneous warts or HPV-containing SCC in the sunlight-exposed areas of their body (87). Three years posttransplantation, between 25 and 42% of patients have cutaneous warts; this number rises to 92% after 5 years or more (87). In transplant patients the lifetime risk of developing SCC or basal cell carcinoma increases 100- or 10-fold, respectively (87). A great diversity of HPV types, mucosal, cutaneous, and epidermodysplasia verruciformis associated, as well as many potentially novel HPV types are found in these lesions, often in association (44).

People working with meat, poultry, or fish are uniquely prone to hand warts, up to one-half of whom are affected (92). Particularly intriguing is the predominance of HPV-7 in these lesions, since HPV-7 has rarely been found elsewhere, with the exception of oral lesions in immunosuppressed or immunodeficient patients. Associations between UV tanning beds and body warts and between cocaine snorting and nasal warts have also been reported.

Epidermodysplasia Verruciformis

Epidermodysplasia verruciformis is an autosomal recessive genodermatosis causing an abnormal susceptibility to betapapillomaviruses (72, 108). It results from the mutation of two adjacent genes, *EVER1/TMC6* and *EVER2/TMC8*, coding for transmembrane proteins in the endoplasmic reticulum.

Genital HPV Infection and Anogenital Warts

Sexual intercourse with a partner who has genital warts is a risk factor for the development of genital warts. About two-thirds of the sexual partners of persons with anogenital warts will develop the disease within 2 years (84, 107). The risk of developing genital warts is most strongly and directly linked to lifetime number of sexual partners (57, 84). Other markers of sexual behavior, such as sexually active years and number of regular partners, are additional risk factors. Markers of sexual behavior yet to be identified could be the confounding variables explaining inconsistent risk factors such as cigarette smoking, contraceptive use, prior sexually transmitted diseases, pregnancy, and alcohol consumption (57, 84). HIV infection increases the risk of genital warts (111).

Some of the same risk factors condition the presence of cervical HPV infection and disease. Age is a major risk factor for the acquisition of cervical infection, with a peak in the 14- to 19-year-old group (49). This is consistent with sexual transmission. Genital HPV infection is very uncommon in virgins, but when present it is likely the reflection of nonintromissive sexual play (158). Such activity, practiced by about a third of self-declared virgin adolescents, is not regarded by the subject as sexual intercourse but is conducive to the transmission of infectious agents, including HPV. The risk of infection rapidly decreases after age 30, but an unexplained second peak at older ages may occur (148). Sexual behavior reflected by an early age at sexual debut, higher number of lifetime sexual partners, and higher number of recent sexual partners is a risk factor (148). Lesbians are not free from these risk factors (97). The past and present sexual activity of the male partner is also important (68). Less consistent risk factors include the use of oral contraceptives, smoking, not using condoms, and some HLA polymorphisms (148). There may also be a protective effect from the consumption of fruits and vegetables, or from absorbing or having circulating levels of vitamins C and E, carotenoids, and xanthophylls (148). Other potential risk factors include multiparity, other sexually transmitted infections (herpes simplex virus and *Chlamydia trachomatis*), and cervical chronic inflammation. The risk factors may have different effects on low-risk and high-risk HPV infections and how they contribute to the progression from infection to premalignancy and to cancer (128, 148). In that regard, the most decisive factor is the HPV genotype (129). Different HPV types have different oncogenicities, generally derived from the phylogeny, and HPV-16 is very clearly the most oncogenic of all. Different variants of HPV-16 carry their own oncogenic profiles, with the African and Asian variants being more oncogenic than the European ones (164). Very similar risk factors for anogenital HPV infections have been implicated in males, including number of sexual partners, lack of condom use, smoking, and lack of circumcision (116).

Although they have been less studied, the risk factors related to sexual behavior, sexual partner history, and presence of high-risk oncogenic HPV DNA have been identified in the development of anal, penile, and vulvar or vaginal SCC (57). Anal receptive intercourse, in both men and women, is a risk factor for the acquisition of anal warts and preinvasive and invasive SCC (58). Because all genital HPVs share the same mode of transmission, it is not surprising that a history of anogenital warts carries an increased risk for the presence of all of these anogenital cancers (57).

Renal allograft recipients have a 10- to 100-fold increased risk of developing anogenital warts, intraepithelial neoplasias, and cancer, a risk that is proportional to the duration of immunosuppression (110). The risk probably extends to other allograft transplant recipients and has been observed in women treated with immunosuppressive agents for glomerulonephritis. Cervical and oral malignancies associated with HPV have also been observed in these populations (3, 87, 110). Patients with diabetes mellitus may be at risk for the development of condyloma acuminatum. However, diabetic women do not appear to have an increased risk of cervicovaginal infection during pregnancy.

The association between infections with HIV and anogenital HPV has been well documented (110). In HIV-seropositive women, depending on populations and methods of diagnosis, there is a 4- to 40-fold increase in the incidence and prevalence of condylomata acuminata and CIN compared to that in HIV-seronegative controls. This added risk is present even in HIV patients with a normal CD4 cell count, although it rises with lower CD4 counts or higher HIV viral load. HIV infection probably promotes the reactivation of HPV infection rather than new acquisition, since HIV-seropositive women shed HPV more persistently and in larger quantities than controls (68). The quantity and persistence of HPV DNA, as well as the presence of high-risk HPV types within lesions, are risk factors for the development of CIN. Anal intraepithelial neoplasias (AIN) are more common in HIV-positive men and women (110). Surprisingly, HPV has been found to be more prevalent in the anus (79%) than in the cervix (53%) in HIV-seropositive women (112). The same imbalance is found in the anus (43%) and cervix (24%) in HIV-seronegative women (112).

Contrary to expectations, the incidence of cervical cancer has not changed because of HIV-induced immunosuppression or because of highly active antiretroviral therapy (10). Whether anal cancer risk is increased by HIV-induced immunosuppression is unclear. Of the HPV-related malignancies, only penile cancer seems to be affected by the severity of immunosuppression (10, 53). These observations could suggest that the higher rates of HPV-associated cancers and precursor lesions in HIV subjects reflect in large part behavioral characteristics more than a deficient immune system.

Recurrent Respiratory Papillomatosis

The juvenile- and adult-onset variants of recurrent respiratory papillomatosis are usually linked to different risk factors (42). With the juvenile-onset form, the children are often firstborn and delivered vaginally by teenage mothers who have condyloma acuminatum. For the adult-onset form of the disease, patients report a higher number of lifetime sexual partners and a higher frequency of oral sex than controls. The disease is very rare among siblings. Recurrent respiratory papillomatosis has not been reported to occur in transplant recipients or HIV-infected individuals.

Association between HPV and Cancer

On the basis of biological and epidemiological arguments, it is now accepted that HPV infection is a necessary condition for the development of preinvasive and invasive cervical cancer (128). The epidemiological evidence can be summarized as follows: (i) HPV DNA is consistently present in virtually all CIN, SCC, or adenocarcinoma specimens, and specific genotypes (mostly 16 and 18), so-called high risk, are responsible for this association (36); (ii) the presence of HPV-16 antibodies is associated with cervical cancer (51); (iii) the prevalence of the high-risk HPV types increases relative to the low-risk types as the grade of the preinvasive cancer worsens (36); (iv) the strength of the association between HPV and preinvasive or invasive cervical cancers, as measured by the relative risk, ranges in most studies from 20 to 70, which is larger than the magnitude of the association between lung cancer and smoking (57); (v) no other risk factors for preinvasive and invasive cancers approach the strength and consistency of HPV infection (57); (vi) persistent but not transient exposure to high-risk HPV leads to cervical disease progression, which suggests that the cancer risk disappears with exposure cessation (148); and finally, (vii) HPV infection precedes the development of preinvasive cancer (128).

Although the evidence is less developed than for the cervix, high-risk HPVs are implicated in the development of SCC at sites other than the cervix (57, 113). It is estimated that about 40% of penile, vulvar, and vaginal cancers and 90% of anal cancers are attributable to HPV. In the case of the penile, vulvar, and vaginal cancers, the percentage attributed to HPV is not higher because among those cancers, only the basaloid and bowenoid histologic variants are related to HPV.

In the nasal and sinus cavities, four of five exophytic papillomas and only a third of the inverted (Schneiderian) papillomas contain HPV, usually HPV-6 or HPV-11 (25). There is mounting evidence that HPV plays a role in some of the SCC of the mouth, sinonasal tract, and larynx (147). Strong evidence has now emerged to impute up to 70% of oropharyngeal cancers to oncogenic HPVs, mostly HPV-16 (46). These HPV-related cancers tend to occur in younger subjects and are associated with sexual behavior markers of young age at intercourse, number of lifetime sexual partners, history of genital warts, performance of oral sex, and number of oral sex partners. Limited or conflicting evidence exists for an association between HPV infection and SCC of the esophagus (146), lung (145), and conjunctiva (79).

Non-melanoma skin cancers (NMSCs) include mostly SCC and basal cell carcinomas. Actinic keratoses represent the precursor lesion for SCC. HPV infection is present in 33 to 99% of NMSCs and precursors in immunosuppressed patients and in 21 to 100% of immunocompetent patients (139). A wide assortment of cutaneous and anogenital HPV types are detected in these NMSCs. However, the great majority of the genotypes are related to epidermodysplasia verruciformis. The clear oncogenic potential of a subset of these HPVs may, along with UV light, contribute to the development of NMSCs and precursor lesions. However, a causal link with HPV is difficult to prove for several reasons: (i) the high number of HPV types, including most of the novel ones, that are isolated from these lesions is perplexing; (ii) the HPV types found vary from patient to patient but also from lesion to lesion, and multiple infections are common; (iii) these HPVs are found in the normal skin (and in a small number of melanomas) of 33 to 73% of tested subjects; (iv) they are typically present at low copy numbers; (v) they are often at the surface of the epithelium rather than within; and (vi) the oncogenicity of epidermodysplasia verruciformis-associated HPVs is poorly understood and so far cannot be explained by any consistent molecular mechanisms (139).

Reinfections

HPV-associated diseases can recur, and relapses are well documented. How often these events represent reinfection versus relapse of a previous subclinical or clinical infection is often impossible to determine. Laryngeal and genital HPV infections can remain latent and subsequently relapse either at the site of the former lesion or in the normal-appearing skin surrounding the ablated lesion (95). Five types of observations would suggest that relapses are more common than reinfections. First, attempts to treat the male sexual partners of women with genital HPV lesions have had no effect on the treatment failure rate in the females (120). Second, studies of HPV types present in the lesions of both sexual partners show only partial concordance either at the genotype or subtype level (28, 70). Epidemiological studies suggest that in males but not in females, a history of genital warts in the previous 5 years in the sexual partner does not predict anogenital wart recurrence. Third, the frequent presence of HPV-6 or HPV-11 DNA in the plucked pubic or perianal hairs of patients with condyloma acuminatum indicates a potential viral reservoir for relapse (22). Fourth, with the use of ever more sensitive and specific HPV PCR assays, it is possible to demonstrate that infections that appear to be transient are in fact persistent (159; D. R. Brown, personal communication). Fifth, therapeutically induced immunosuppression in solid-organ transplantation leads to an increase of HPV infections and diseases (see "Risk factors" above). Although this could be the result of increased susceptibility to HPV, infection relapse is a more likely explanation.

Transmission

Routes

The epidemiology of plantar warts suggests an indirect mode of transmission, for example, through fomites present in communal baths or swimming pools (76). The virus probably enters the epidermis directly, because special footwear is protective. Direct natural or experimental transmission is possible (125); so is autoinoculation from genital lesions. Because epidermodysplasia verruciformis is so rare, until recently it was unclear where the viral natural reservoir was. It is now evident that these HPV types are widely spread at low levels in the population, in normal skin or in actinic keratoses and NMSCs (139).

Several observations strongly support sexual transmission of condyloma acuminatum and other anogenital HPV infections (35, 84). The peak incidence of condyloma acuminatum occurs between ages 20 and 25 years, which follows the onset of sexual activity. The presence of condyloma acuminatum and a history of sexually transmitted diseases are associated. The risk for HPV infection increases with the number of sexual partners, and sexual partners share in part the same HPV infections or diseases. Sexual activity appears to precede the development of anogenital warts (6). Similarly, the association between anal warts and anal intercourse also indicates a direct route of transmission through sexual contact (28, 106). The concordance of HPV-16 variants between partners is another argument for the sexual transmission of HPV (28).

As discussed above, young children can acquire anogenital HPV infections by nonsexual routes, like in utero and perinatal exposure, nonsexual direct contact, and autoinoculation. However, the importance of alternate routes of transmission is probably negligible. Even the very low rate of HPV infection in virgin women does not exclude all forms of sexual activity. Although HPV DNA can be recovered from the underwear of women with anogenital warts or on surgical instruments used for gynecologic examination, a role for fomites in the transmission of anogenital HPV has not been demonstrated, but it is reasonable to assume that sex toys could be such a vehicle.

The mode of transmission of respiratory papillomatosis has not been directly established. In its juvenile-onset form, the disease could be acquired by vaginal delivery through an HPV-infected birth canal, whereas the adult form of the disease might result from oral sex (42). Nevertheless, respiratory papillomatosis can be present at birth or after cesarean delivery, indicating possible in utero transmission (42). Transmission among family members is very rare (42).

Risk Factors

The risk of transmission after direct or indirect contact with cutaneous warts is probably low and may be mitigated by the presence of cofactors such as the immunity of the recipient and the nature and duration of the contact (73). Plantar warts tend to appear on weight-bearing areas, which suggests that microscopic injury to the skin fosters viral entry. Shaving, finger sucking, or nail biting may favor the extension of lesions and cause a Koebner phenomenon (125). In vitro observations suggest that the wound repair epithelium is more susceptible to an active infection. However, manual workers other than meat packers, abattoir workers, or fish handlers do not appear to be prone to the development of warts, and trauma was not found to be a risk factor in meat handlers. Perhaps moisture and warmth are additional risk factors (76).

The risk of developing condyloma acuminatum or acquiring anogenital HPV infection after one sexual contact with an affected individual is unknown but is presumably low. However, as expected, repetitive contact increases the risk. In a study of 603 female college students negative for HPV DNA at baseline, resampling every 4 months with a cervicovaginal lavage found a cumulative prevalence of 29% at 1 year, 32% at 2 years, 48% at 3 years, and 54% at 4 years (158). In a study of 18- to 20-year-old male students sampled at 4-month intervals at different sites (glans, shaft, scrotum, urine, and under the fingernails), the cumulative incidence of any genital HPV infection was

62% after 2 years (115). About two-thirds of sexual partners of individuals with anogenital warts will develop warts within 2 years (107). Genital warts appear in areas, such as the vulvar fourchette, that are more likely to be traumatized during intercourse; microabrasions or lacerations are also thought to play a role in HPV transmission.

Limited evidence suggests that macroscopic lesions are more contagious than microscopic ones. In one study of women with HPV infection, 67% of 42 male consorts of women with visible condylomata acuminata developed clinical or subclinical lesions, compared to 46% of 39 partners of women with subclinical lesions (82). Transmission of condyloma acuminatum by household contact is probably very rare in the absence of sexual contact or abuse.

The risk of acquiring recurrent respiratory papillomatosis following vaginal delivery from a woman with anogenital warts has been estimated to range between 1:80 and 1:500 (42). Firstborn babies carry more risk than babies of subsequent births, presumably because of longer delivery (42). Furthermore, viral load has been shown to condition the risk of HPV-16 transmission from mother to child. Oral sex appears to be a risk factor for the adult-onset form of the disease.

Oropharyngeal cancers tend to occur in younger subjects and are associated with sexual behavior markers of young age at intercourse, number of lifetime sexual partners, history of genital warts, performance of oral sex, and number of oral sex partners (46).

Nosocomial Infection

Cryoprobes have been responsible for transmission of warts from patient to patient, thus making sprays preferable for cryotherapy. Electrocautery and laser therapy present a unique risk for the operator because HPV DNA can be recovered from the smoke generated from the procedure. The surgeon's mucosal membranes, as well as the operating room, may become contaminated. Laser surgeons appear to have a higher prevalence of hand and nasopharyngeal warts. These observations have led to the use of smoke evacuation systems, and to wearing gowns, gloves, and goggles during the procedure.

Duration of Infectivity

The duration of infectivity is unknown. Patients with anogenital warts of long duration may be less infectious than those with a shorter disease history (107).

PATHOGENESIS IN HUMANS

The duration of incubation for HPV diseases is poorly known. For cutaneous warts, experimental inoculation leads to the development of lesions within 3 to 4 months, on average, but as early as 6 weeks or as late as 2 years (125). Similar incubation periods have been observed in natural-history studies with sexual partners of patients with condyloma acuminatum for whom the date of exposure could be estimated (6, 107). In a study of 51 female university students with an incident cervical HPV-6 or -11 infection, 51% developed genital warts within a median of 2.9 months (157). Among 603 subjects monitored over a 36-month period after an incident HPV infection, 47 and 29% of the students developed LSIL of the cervix and vagina, respectively (157). The median times for lesion clearance were 5.5 and 4.7 months, respectively. When limited to HPV-16 and -18 infections, the cumulative incidences for CIN 2 and CIN 3 were 20 and 7%, respectively.

Virus Replication

HPVs infect the squamous keratinized (skin) and nonkeratinized (mucosa) stratified epithelia. The mucosae of the mouth, upper airways, vagina, cervix, and anal canal are major targets, but HPV has been found in other locations as well, such as the conjunctiva, lacrimal sac, nasal passages, bronchi, esophagus, cervical glandular tissue, and bladder (25, 79, 113, 145, 146). Epithelia next to a squamo-columnar junction (sinuses, larynx, anus, and cervix) are particularly vulnerable. In the case of the uterine cervix, by a process called squamous metaplasia triggered by hormonal and pH changes, this squamo-columnar junction recedes toward the os, the glandular epithelium being replaced by squamous epithelium. The area traveled by this slowly moving junction is called the transformation zone and is the site where cervical cancer is found. HPV DNA has been found in prostatic tissue and semen, although conflicting reports exist on the prevalence and biological significance of this association. Metastases of HPV-induced lesions also contain HPV DNA. However, whereas BPV can infect lymphocytes and metastasize, similar evidence with HPV remains controversial.

The duration of HPV infections and diseases is highly variable, ranging from weeks to years. Lesion regression is not random. The regression of treated lesions may be accompanied by the regression of the untreated lesions, a phenomenon consistent with a host response (136). Several histologic events accompany the spontaneous regression of warts (136). Spongiosis of the basal cells occurs and a lymphomonocytic infiltrate develops in the dermis and lower epidermis. Necrosis and apoptosis are present in the epidermis; the dermis exhibits focal thrombosis and hemorrhages. The lymphocytic infiltrate is primarily T cells, with CD4 cells predominating. The lymphocytes display the isomorphs $CD45RA^+$ and $CD45RO^+$, indicating the presence of naïve and memory cells, respectively. Lymphocytes, Langerhans cells, and keratinocytes are immunologically activated; they display HLA-DR and ICAM-1 molecules. In addition, the lymphocytes exhibit high-affinity interleukin 2 (IL-2) receptors (CD25). These histologic changes are consistent with a delayed-type hypersensitivity reaction. An increase in natural killer (NK) cell activity has also been associated with resolution of CIN 1. Thus, the cellular immune system appears to be important in HPV disease regression.

Latency and Cancer

HPV can be recovered not only from skin and mucosal lesions but also from the normal surrounding tissues, where lesions usually relapse (95). Remarkably, HPV-6 or -11 DNA is found in a third to a half of the hair follicles plucked from the pubic and perianal area of patients with condylomata acuminata (22). The vast majority of HPV infections are latent (22, 84, 139). Probably less than a third of anogenital infections are symptomatic (84). Many of the cervical HPV infections are transient, especially in younger women, and usually contain a low copy number of HPV DNA (69). Transient expression is more common during the luteal phase than during the follicular phase of menstruation. Whereas an infection with a high-risk HPV is associated with a risk of developing CIN that appears to be specific of each genotype, the effect of viral load on persistence and disease progression is more complex than previously appreciated, and the relevance of multiple concomitant HPV infections is largely unknown (133, 159). The issue of persistence itself is fraught with methodological difficulties, including the frequency of sampling and the detection sensitivity of the HPV DNA assay used (159). Therefore, it is unclear if the body is capable of truly clearing an HPV infection and how often, or if the virus persists in a latent state, undetected and producing no viral particles (128, 159). We also do not know the viral and cellular factors that induce, maintain, or abrogate latency (45, 128). Anecdotally, the initiation of an oral contraceptive treatment has been associated with a flare-up of genital warts.

The oncogenic properties of several animal papillomaviruses, such as BPV and cottontail rabbit papillomavirus, were experimentally demonstrated long ago (30). A cancer precursor can be produced by infecting human foreskin with HPV-16 prior to grafting in SCID mice (18).The anogenital HPV types most capable of immortalizing and transforming cells in vitro are those associated with cervical cancer. Different viral genes, notably E6 and E7 from high-risk types, have transforming, immortalization, and oncogenic potential, especially in combination, when introduced into cell lines or transgenic animals. These genes interfere with cell cycle regulation and apoptosis (see "Virology" above) (Table 2).

HPV-induced malignant transformation seems to result from a complex series of events that are independent of viral particle production. Integration of HPV DNA into the host genome appears to be associated with the progression from high-grade CIN to cancer. Integration occurs in the majority of invasive cervical carcinomas but is rare in benign and premalignant lesions; however, this may be an underestimation (159, 167). Integrated and episomal forms may coexist in the same cells. Possible sites of viral integration in the host genome may exist on a variety of chromosomes and in proximity to cellular oncogenes. The site of integration in the viral genome is typically restricted between the 3′ end of E1 and the 5′ end of E2, resulting in disruption, deletion, or inactivation of the E2 ORF. These changes appear to disrupt the viral and cellular regulatory controls of viral gene expression mediated by the E2 proteins (67, 133, 159, 166, 167). Integration may also disrupt the E1, E4, E5, L1, and L2 ORFs, but the E6 and E7 ORFs are typically spared. Viral integration does not appear to be necessary for progression to malignancy, given that up to a quarter of invasive cervical cancers contain only viral episomes (159). In addition, on the rare occasions when low-risk oncogenic HPVs such as HPV-6 and -11 have been associated with squamous cell cancers, the viral genome undergoes deletions, mutations, and amplifications in the URR but remains episomal. DNA sequence heterogeneity exists within each genotype, and molecular variants have different oncogenic potentials (164).

Although the E6 and E7 genes are necessary for immortalization and malignant transformation, they are not sufficient. Hybrid clones from the fusion of cell lines containing HPV-16 do not necessarily retain their malignant phenotype, as would be expected if this phenotype was solely dependent on the presence of the viral genes (167). Therefore, internal cellular and molecular mechanisms so far mostly unidentified are often capable of keeping the oncogenic process in check. However, one internal signal that has been identified is the CDKN2A gene, which codes for the $p16^{INK4A}$ protein. Its role is to inhibit the cell cycle by inactivating cyclin D1-CDK4 or cyclin D1-CDK6 complexes, thus down-regulating cyclin E. Methylation, mutation, or deletion of CDKN2A is necessary for E6 to regain its immortalizing effects. E7 by itself increases $p16^{INK4A}$ levels, which makes this protein a potentially useful biomarker of malignancy, but it also circumvents the inhibiting effect $p16^{INK4A}$ would have by stimulating the downstream cyclins A and E (Fig. 6). External signals also contribute to the down-regulation of the transcription and oncogenesis of the high-risk HPVs. These cytokines include tumor necrosis factor alpha, alpha interferon (IFN-α), IFN-β, IFN-γ, retinoic acid, and tumor growth factor β (TGF-β) (67, 133, 167). Some potential mechanisms have been identified. The transcription complex AP-1 is a heterodimer made of c-Jun and c-Fos (Fig. 5) or c-Jun and Fra I. Only c-Jun and c-Fos can bind and participate in the activation of the HPV E6/E7 promoter. Tumor necrosis factor alpha and retinoic acid induce the Fra I gene, thus favoring the formation of the c-Jun–Fra I complex, the net effect being a down-regulation of the HPV promoter.

Other endogenous factors associated with malignant transformation have been identified. Cellular oncogenes (e.g., c-*myc* and c-*ras*) may be activated by the nearby integration of viral DNA into the host chromosome. This is significant because the E7 gene can cooperate with activated *ras* to induce transformation in primary rodent cells.

Methylation has emerged as an important epigenetic mechanism of carcinogenesis control by causing the inactivation of viral and cellular genes and their regulatory sequences (159). The promoter region of several tumor suppressor genes can be inactivated by aberrant methylation of the GpC islands. E7 is thought to be able to stimulate the transcription of some DNA methylases, causing methylation of the pRB pocket proteins and inhibition of E2F-regulated transcription.

Various cytogenetic abnormalities have been observed in cervical carcinomas, such as alterations of chromosome 1 and allelic losses on the short arm of chromosome 3 or 17 or the long arm of chromosome 11. This loss of heterozygosity may eventually lead to the disappearance of suppressor genes; for example, *p53* is located on 17p. E6 and E7 genes can induce chromosomal abnormalities in vitro. Chromosome markers have been used to study the cellular clonality of cervical lesions. Low-grade lesions are typically polyclonal, while high-grade lesions seem to be oligoclonal, or monoclonal if concomitant with an invasive cancer. Invasive cancers are monoclonal.

Genetic host factors appear to be important in the development of cervical cancer. For example, the family-attributable risk of cervical cancer is higher in full sisters than in adopted or half sisters of women with cervical cancer. One case control study examining the association of HLA class A, B, C, DRB1, and DQB1 allele combinations in cervical SCC found several effects, all less than twofold in magnitude (90). The HLA class I alleles A*0301, B*4402, and Cw*0501 conferred an increased risk, and B*1501 conferred a decreased risk. The combination of HLA class II alleles DRB1*1101 and DQB1*0301 decreased the risk, while the combination of DRB1*1302 and DQB1*02 increased the risk. In high-order interaction effects, most of the combinations containing B*4402 or DQB1*0301 were associated with an increased risk. Of interest, the combination B*4402-DRB1*1101-DQB1*0301 increased the risk of cancer 10-fold. All these associations were also observed in cervical adenocarcinoma and vulvar squamous cell cancer.

Numerous exogenous factors play a putative role in HPV-related and malignant transformation, including UV and X-ray radiations, smoking tobacco, steroid hormones, *Chlamydia*, and viruses like HIV, herpes simplex virus, and Epstein-Barr virus. However, much remains to be learned about their contributions and mechanisms of action.

Histopathology

Epidermal basal cells are arranged around a central, putative basal stem cell, in groups of approximately 10. These groups define the base of the epidermal proliferative unit. One may speculate that HPV needs to infect the basal stem cell to become established. Two different HPV types can infect the same cell. As the putative basal cell divides, the viral genome replicates. Some viral copies are transmitted to the daughter cell that is eventually thrust upward to form a parabasal cell. As they ascend toward the surface of the epithelium, the keratinocytes stop dividing but continue to differentiate (Fig. 8). Differentiation is a process associated with the expression of different keratins. Viral replication is independent of cellular replication and may continue as the keratinocytes reach the upper layers of the stratum spinosum. However, to replicate, the virus has to activate and appropriate the cell molecular replicative machinery. The viral particles are shed with the desquamating cells of the stratum corneum.

The typical histologic features of benign cutaneous HPV disease include thickening of the stratum spinosum (acanthosis), stratum granulosum (parakeratosis), and stratum corneum (hyperkeratosis) (Fig. 8). The persistence of nuclei in the stratum corneum is also a feature of parakeratosis. The presence of koilocytes (koilocytosis) (from the Greek *koilos*, cave) is strongly indicative of HPV infection. The koilocyte is an enlarged keratinocyte that develops in the upper layers of the stratum spinosum and in the stratum granulosum. It is recognized by a clear halo that surrounds a central nucleus, shriveled and shrunken on tissue sections and enlarged on cytologic smears (Fig. 9). The cell may be binucleated or the nucleus may be bilobar. The cytoarchitecture of the lesion is papillomatous, with fronds of epidermis extending toward both the dermis and the surface. A combination of the same histologic characteristics can be found in the mucosal epithelia infected by HPV. Because such epithelia are not keratinized, hyperkeratosis is not a frequent or prominent feature. In an inverted papilloma, the papillomatosis is frank but strictly limited to the dermis, thus giving a flat lesion. HPV type also contributes to variations in the histology of lesions. Figures 10 and 11 illustrate the histology of different types of warts.

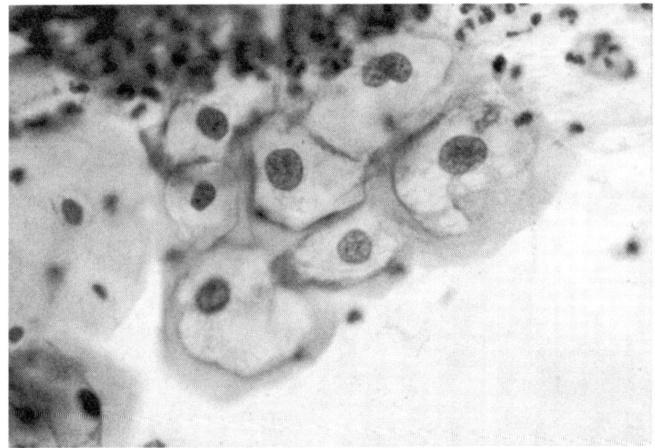

FIGURE 9 Pap smear demonstrating koilocytic atypia. In contrast to the histologic specimen, by cytology koilocytes have one or two relatively large, smooth, oval nuclei, surrounded by a very large halo of amorphous substance. (Courtesy of Clara E. Mesonero, Cape Cod Hospital, Cape Cod, MA.)

HPV infection of the cervical squamous epithelium can result in a range of histopathological entities for which different classification schemes have been designed (Fig. 12). This evolution reflects the many fine points of the surgical pathology diagnosis and the debates that surround them. What follows is only a crude description of the squamous epithelial changes.

Cervical flat condylomas are benign lesions characterized by the presence of koilocytes. The abnormal proliferation of the basal layer is one of the features that defines intraepithelial neoplasia. These lesions, which are preinvasive cancers, are graded according to the extent of basal-type cell proliferation. Proliferation up to the lower third of the epithelium is mild dysplasia or CIN 1, up to the

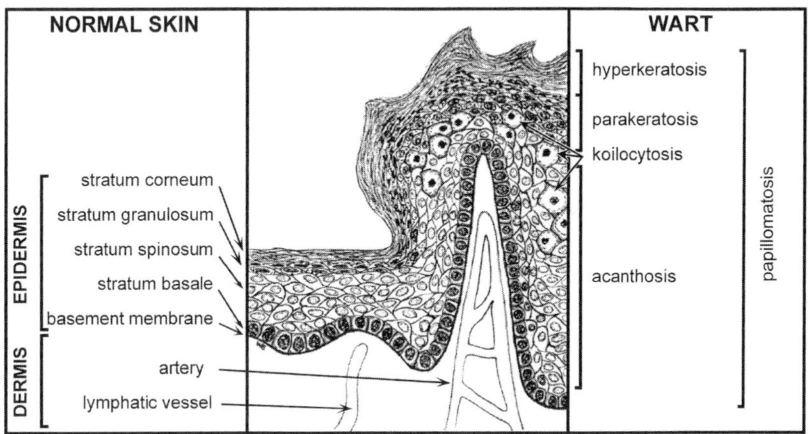

FIGURE 8 Drawing of the histologic features of normal skin and of a wart.

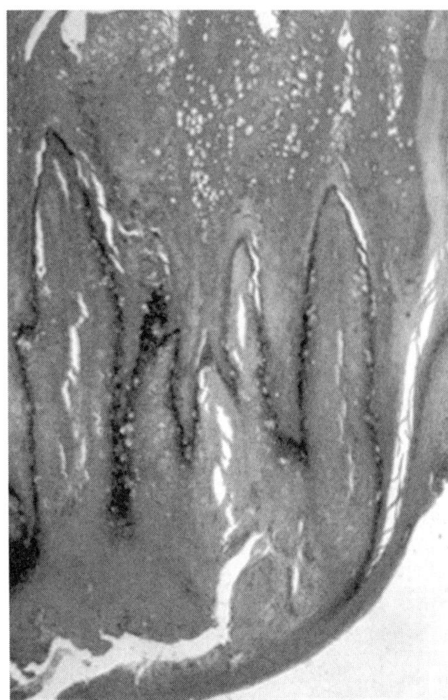

FIGURE 10 Histology of a cutaneous wart (hemalun-eosin stain; low-power view). The darkly stained layer is the stratum granulosum. Koilocytes are profuse and disrupt the stratum granulosum. The persistence of nuclei in the stratum corneum is a feature of parakeratosis. Note the thick stratum corneum. (Courtesy of Clara E. Mesonero, Cape Cod Hospital, Cape Cod, MA.)

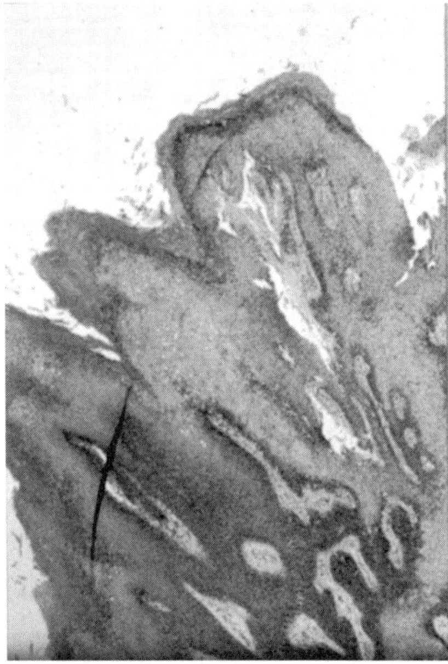

FIGURE 11 Histology of condyloma acuminatum (hemalun-eosin stain; high-power view). The figure demonstrates many koilocytes in the stratum spinosum. Koilocytes are relatively large cells with a shrunken, irregular nucleus surrounded by a halo. (Courtesy of Clara E. Mesonero, Cape Cod Hospital, Cape Cod, MA.)

upper two-thirds is moderate dysplasia or CIN 2, and up to the full epithelium is severe dysplasia/carcinoma in situ (CIS), or CIN 3. In CIS the full epithelium is abnormal. The local breach of the basal membrane by the epithelial cells characterizes an invasive SCC. The other features of this abnormal cellular proliferation are more prominent as the severity of the lesion increases. They include an enlarged cell nucleus/cytoplasm ratio, coarse granularity of the nucleus, numerous and abnormal mitotic figures, and some abnormal and necrosed cells (atypia defines these abnormal or atypical cellular changes). Koilocytosis may be absent, particularly in the higher grades, which otherwise display anisocytosis. The cytological equivalents of cervical condyloma and CIN are LSIL for cervical condyloma and CIN 1 and HSIL for CIN 2 or 3 (Fig. 12). As a parallel, some pathologists now use the terminology of low-grade CIN (L-CIN) and high-grade CIN (H-CIN) for histology.

From a normal-appearing cervix to CIS there is a graded risk of progression toward invasive cancer (102). This gradient can be superimposed on a gradient of increased prevalence of high-risk HPV types (Fig. 12) (36, 132). Although it would seem that lesions slowly progress through each stage of CIN before becoming invasive, a rapid progression can occur without recognition of the intermediate stage, and progression from a normal cervix to H-CIN can occur in as little as 2 years (128).

Immune Responses

The immunology of HPV infections is poorly understood (51, 52, 108, 137). The frequency, severity, and persistence of HPV infections and diseases in immunocompromised patients have long indicated that immunity, cell-mediated immunity in particular, contributes to the development and resolution of HPV infections. Although various and mostly nonspecific, immunologic alterations have been reported to occur in patients with HPV infections, few have been associated with specific genetic alterations. The model for this is epidermodysplasia verruciformis, a genodermatosis associated with inactivating mutations in two genes, *EVER1/TMC6* and *EVER2/TMC8*, that code for transporter proteins in the endoplasmic reticulum (108). A mutation in the CXCR4 chemokine receptor gene has been found in patients with the WHIM (warts, hypogammaglobulinemia, infections, and myelokathexis) syndrome (108). Cutaneous papillomatosis has been described to occur in patients with SCID due to defective either γc cytokine receptor subunit or Janus kinase 3 (JAK-3) (108). HPV-16 E6 and E7 may abrogate the expression and function of Toll-like receptor 9.

There is a cytokine and chemokine response to HPV-associated cell proliferation that promotes leukocyte trafficking and angiogenesis. The molecules include tumor necrosis factor alpha; monocyte chemotactic protein 1 (MCP-1); chemokine CCL27; vascular endothelial cell growth factor; IFN-α, -β, and -γ; IL-5 and -8; IFN-γ-inducible protein 10 (IP-10 [CXCL10]); retinoic acid; and TGF-β (67, 133, 167). Some of these responses are consistent with the notable mononuclear cell infiltrate present in the dermis and epidermis during wart or condyloma regression. These cells allow the development of a local and systemic specific immune response. The respective roles in antigen presentation of the Langerhans cells, which are the epidermal professional antigen-presenting cells, and the keratinocytes, which upon immunologic activation can

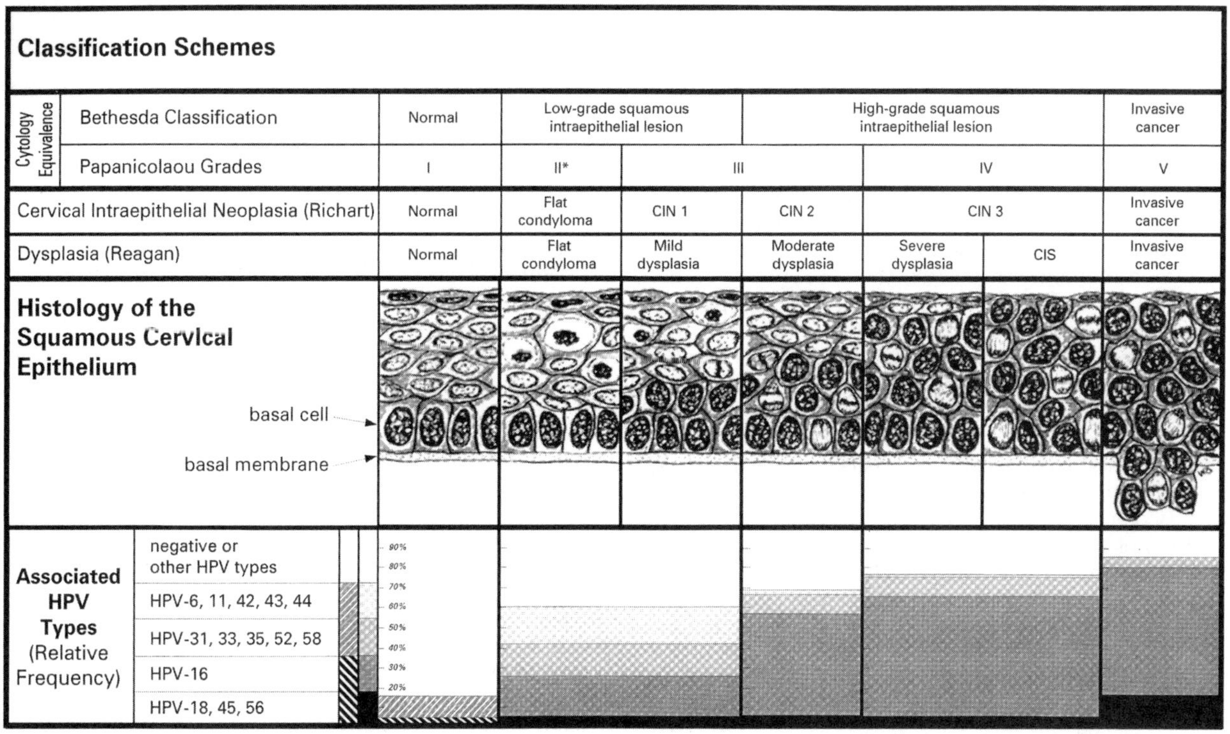

Classification Schemes

Cytology Equivalence: Bethesda Classification	Normal	Low-grade squamous intraepithelial lesion		High-grade squamous intraepithelial lesion			Invasive cancer
Cytology Equivalence: Papanicolaou Grades	I	II*	III		IV		V
Cervical Intraepithelial Neoplasia (Richart)	Normal	Flat condyloma	CIN 1	CIN 2	CIN 3		Invasive cancer
Dysplasia (Reagan)	Normal	Flat condyloma	Mild dysplasia	Moderate dysplasia	Severe dysplasia	CIS	Invasive cancer

Histology of the Squamous Cervical Epithelium

basal cell

basal membrane

Associated HPV Types (Relative Frequency)

negative or other HPV types

HPV-6, 11, 42, 43, 44

HPV-31, 33, 35, 52, 58

HPV-16

HPV-18, 45, 56

FIGURE 12 Diagrammatic representation of the nomenclature, histologic features, and distribution of associated HPV types in HPV-related cervical lesions. The dysplasia and the CIN classifications are primarily histologic classifications that are also used for cytology, whereas the Bethesda classification is designed mainly for cytology (see text for details). *, This category in the Pap classification also included atypical squamous cells of the Bethesda classification.

also behave as antigen-presenting cells, are unclear. However, the density of Langerhans cells is generally decreased in nonregressing warts, which may be related to the downregulation of E-cadherin by E6. It is also likely that the major histocompatibility complex has a role in the immunologic control of HPV infection (90). What governs the persistence, progression, or regression of HPV infection and disease is largely unknown. Humoral and cellular immune responses develop but are incompletely effective and changing. As already discussed, HPV E5, E6, and E7 proteins interact at several levels in the immune response to suppress it (78). Furthermore, general immune responsiveness appears to be blunted in older women with HPV infection compared to age-matched controls (60).

The humoral response to the early viral proteins is typically modest or absent in most patients. Patients with invasive cervical cancer are the most significant exception; approximately half of them develop antibodies to HPV-16 E6 and E7 peptides or fusion proteins. Otherwise, the most consistent and strongest immune response in patients infected with HPV is to the L1 protein in the native conformation it assumes in virions or recombinant VLPs (51, 123). These L1 antibodies can be neutralizing, but this requires them to be of high titer, which is rarely the case, as the HPV VLP vaccine studies have shown (34, 85). The immune response to native L1 is typically type specific (122).

HPV L1 VLP-based enzyme immunoassays usually lack high enough sensitivity (50 to 70%) to be useful clinically. However, they are specific and detect an immunoglobulin G (immunoglobulin A to a lesser extent) immune response that decreases only a little over time. Hence, they measure HPV exposure. This makes them excellent seroepidemiological tools that have complemented and supported the results obtained by HPV DNA detection, itself a measure of present infection (51).

Lymphoproliferative responses to different HPV proteins can be detected in some patients with HPV infections, especially those with cervical preinvasive cancers. The most consistent and strongest of these responses are against E6 and E7 (51, 52). The same proteins are also the targets of a cytotoxic T-cell response (51, 52). NK cell cytotoxicity against HPV-infected keratinocytes is present in epidermodysplasia verruciformis and CIN (108). The precise nature and role of these responses in disease persistence and resolution largely remain to be established and explained in the context of the immunogenetic factors that govern HPV disease (51, 52, 90, 108, 137).

CLINICAL MANIFESTATIONS

Cutaneous Warts

Three major types of cutaneous warts are recognized: deep plantar warts, common warts, and flat or plane warts (73).

Deep plantar warts (verrucae plantaris), also termed myrmecias (from Greek, ant hill), are usually solitary lesions preferentially located on the weight-bearing surfaces of the foot. These deeply set and painful lesions can be 2 mm to 1 cm in diameter. They interrupt the ordered pattern of surrounding rete ridges and look like a circular, disorganized bundle of keratotic fibers, sometimes containing dark speckles, surrounded by a slightly raised keratotic ring. The black dots represent thrombosed capillaries (Color Plate 34). Occasionally, the lesion is completely covered by the keratotic ring and can take on the appearance of a corn or callus. Tenderness and the appearance of punctate, thrombosed capillaries after paring the horny layer with a scalpel are features distinguishing a deep plantar wart from a callus or a fibrokeratoma. Occasionally, myrmecias can develop on the palms of the hands.

Common warts (verrucae vulgaris) are usually multiple, well-circumscribed, exophytic, hyperkeratotic, round papules with a coarse surface ranging in size from 1 mm to 1 cm (Color Plate 35). They are normally found on the dorsum of the hand, between the fingers, and around the nail bed. They can also grow under the nail bed, causing nail loss (onycholysis). Mosaic warts are a variant of common warts and may be found on several areas of the foot, including the sole, the knuckles, and around the toenails (Color Plate 36). They appear as multiple, confluent, shallow, slightly raised, keratotic lesions. These painless lesions coalesce and may cover several square centimeters. Filiform warts are common warts usually located on the face, particularly the lips, nares, or eyelids. They are thin, fleshy projections, usually 1 to 3 mm in diameter and a few millimeters long. Cutaneous horns are an uncommon presentation of common warts and may be confused with keratoacanthoma, basal carcinomas, SCC, actinic keratoses, or seborrheic keratoses. The warts of meat handlers busually resemble typical common warts (92). Common warts may be confused with nevi, seborrheic keratoses, acrochordons (skin tags), molluscum contagiosum, keratoacanthomas, lichen planus, lichen nitidus, syringomas, dermofibromas, or SCC. In the healthy host, malignant transformation of common warts into Bowen's disease, verrucous carcinoma, or SCC is a rare event and may be related to the presence of high-risk oncogenic HPV types in the lesions (130).

Most cutaneous warts are asymptomatic. Bleeding and pain, particularly with deep plantar warts, may occur in pressure areas. The natural history of cutaneous warts is poorly defined. In children, the rates of spontaneous resolution after 1 and 5 years of follow-up are 50 and 90%, respectively (100). Individual deep plantar and common warts spontaneously take about 1 month to disappear. They either blacken, become inflamed, or involute. In any given patient, two-thirds of the warts that resolve spontaneously will do so within the first 2 months.

Plane or flat warts (verrucae planae) present as multiple, flat, small, asymmetric, smooth papules with a pink to tan color. They are found mostly on the face (especially the chin and eyelids), neck, and hands of children. Taller lesions are sometimes called intermediate warts. Lichen planus and freckles may be confused with flat warts. Reddening, swelling, and itching of lesions announce simultaneous flat wart regression, a process that lasts 2 to 7 weeks.

In immunocompromised patients, HPV-associated lesions may take on appearances other than that of common warts, such as warty keratoses (Color Plate 37), or epidermodysplasia verruciformis-like plaques distributed in the sun-exposed areas (dorsum of the hands, face, scalp, and neck). In these patients, malignant or benign lesions such as SCC, basal cell carcinomas, Bowen's disease, keratoacanthoma, or actinic keratoses can contain HPV (139).

Epidermodysplasia Verruciformis

Epidermodysplasia verruciformis is characterized by the appearance of flat wart-like lesions, red to brown plaques (Color Plate 38), or pityriasis versicolor-like lesions over the face, the torso, and the extensor surfaces of the extremities, usually during the first decade (72, 108). Over 20 different HPV types have been isolated from epidermodysplasia verruciformis lesions (Table 1), often coexisting in the same patient. HPV-3 is uniquely associated with lesions resembling large flat warts. The prevalence of plantar and common warts appears to be increased in these patients. In about half the patients, beginning before the age of 30 years and extending over the following decades, lesions in sun-exposed areas, primarily those associated with HPV-5, -8, or -47, undergo premalignant and malignant changes. They form papillomas, seborrheic keratoses, and SCC. The malignancies remain locally invasive and slow growing, unless they have been exposed to local irradiation. Biopsy is useful in the diagnosis and management of epidermodysplasia verruciformis.

Anogenital HPV Diseases

The full evaluation of a patient with potential anogenital HPV disease should include a history that reviews symptoms, particularly those pertaining to emotional well-being, sexual intercourse, urination, and defecation. Duration of symptoms and treatment received should be asked along with age at first intercourse, number of past and current sexual partners, sexual practices, and use of barrier methods of contraception. The patient's history of other sexually transmitted diseases (STD) (including HIV infection) and treatments should be recorded, as should the histories of anogenital warts, intraepithelial neoplasias, and cancers in the sexual partners. The physical examination should be done aided, if necessary, by the application of 3 to 5% acetic acid (white vinegar) and the use of a colposcope (a biomicroscope offering several magnifications, ranging typically from ×6 to ×40, and a long focal length) or a powerful magnifying glass. The female internal genitalia should be examined with a speculum. A Pap smear may be obtained at that time (160). A diagram displaying the anatomic location of the lesions will facilitate evaluation and monitoring. A digital rectal examination completes the examination in immunocompromised patients (HIV patients and transplant recipients) and men who have sex with men. Immunocompromised women should have a pelvic examination.

External Genitalia and Anus

Condylomata acuminata (singular, condyloma acuminatum; from the Greek *kondylōma*, knuckle, knob, and Latin *acumen*, sharp point), also known as anogenital warts or venereal warts, are slightly hyperkeratotic, firm, exophytic papules that are flesh colored to dark gray and are either sessile or attached by a broad short peduncle (Color Plate 39). On the skin, small lesions tend to be smooth, round papules with an accentuation of the skin ridges. Larger skin lesions or mucosal lesions are more cornified and may have an irregular, jagged, mulberry-like or pointed surface contour. Sizes usually vary from a millimeter to 2 cm, but can reach several square centimeters, particularly when several lesions coalesce like cobblestones to form a plaque. Individual lesions are devoid of hair.

In men, the predominant location of lesions is the penile shaft in circumcised individuals and the preputial cavity otherwise (35, 107). One percent to 25% of patients will have urethral warts that are usually located between the meatus and the fossa navicularis (107). Warts rarely extend beyond the distal first 3 cm, and involvement of the proximal urethra and bladder is exceptional. Meatal eversion or the use of an otoscope or pediatric nasal speculum facilitates the inspection of meatal warts. Although perianal warts can occur in heterosexual men, they are much more common in homosexual men (106). The scrotum, perineum, groin, and pubic area are rarely affected.

In women, the great majority of lesions are found over the posterior introitus, including the fourchette, spreading toward the labia minora and majora and clitoris. In decreasing order of frequency, the perineum, vagina, anus, cervix, and urethra represent less than 25% of the usually affected sites (35, 107). Young girls with anogenital warts should have a careful examination of the anus and genitals, and according to the findings or age of the patient, proper referrals have to be made (71).

For both sexes, anoscopic examination is recommended if there is a history of receptive anal intercourse, if perianal warts are present, or if the patient has anal symptoms. Because lesions rarely extend beyond the pectinate line, sigmoidoscopy is not ordinarily performed. An oral examination is indicated for the presence of associated oral warts.

Itching, burning, even pain and tenderness are the most common symptoms of condylomata acuminata (35). Yet approximately three-quarters of patients are asymptomatic (35). Nonetheless, the disease has a significant psychosexual impact on about half of the patients before or after treatment. During pregnancy or immunosuppression, warts may increase in number or size and may obstruct the birth canal. The natural history of condyloma acuminatum is poorly defined, but 10 to 20% of patients will experience a spontaneous remission within 3 to 4 months of presentation to a physician. Genital warts disappear spontaneously by involution.

Diagnosis

Molluscum contagiosum is the disease most frequently mistaken for condyloma acuminatum. Lesions of molluscum contagiosum are usually small, circular, well-defined, dome-shaped, sessile papules. They are flesh to wax colored, not pigmented, with a smooth or dotted surface containing a central depression from which a cheesy material can be extruded. Their anatomic distribution helps the differential diagnosis because they predominate over the pubis and can extend to the trunk. Condyloma latum of syphilis is a relatively large, smooth, sessile, moist, flat-topped lesion that is few in number. The medical history and serology help with the diagnosis. Nodular scabies appears as red, scaly or crusted, deeply set nodules accompanied by an intense pruritus, particularly at night. The differential diagnosis includes other dermatologic conditions. Hidradenoma papilliferum, encountered on the keratinized vulva, resembles a large wart. Acrochordons (skin tags) are soft, skin-colored tumors. Epidermoid cysts and angiokeratomas can be found on the scrotum. Lichen planus, lichen sclerosus et atrophicus, lichen nitidus, or syringomas manifest as small and plane lesions that may be difficult to recognize. Small penile warts in the corona glandis may be very difficult to distinguish from a normal anatomic variant called hirsutoid papillomatosis (pearly coronal papules, papillae corona glandis). Whether the sometimes painful papillae that may be present on the vulvar introitus represent the female equivalent of hirsutoid papillomatosis or are lesions caused by HPV (i.e., vulvar papillomatosis) has been controversial. In both sexes, one may encounter sessile papules or macules that have a brown to slate blue pigmentation (Color Plate 40). These lesions are particularly important to recognize because they may represent benign condylomas infected with HPV-6 or -11 (41), nevi, seborrheic keratoses, or intraepithelial neoplasias infected with HPV-16 or -18 (41). The poor correlation between appearance and histology or HPV type argues for the biopsy of these lesions. Biopsy should also be considered if lesions are large, bleed, appear in plaques, or are in unusual locations. There should be a lower threshold to biopsy immunosuppressed or immunodeficient patients.

The use of the colposcope in conjunction with soaking the genitalia for 3 to 5 min with 3 to 5% acetic acid prior to examination has allowed better recognition of subclinical HPV lesions, which are more often than macroscopic lesions associated with high-risk HPV infections (143). Subclinical lesions appear mostly as small acetowhite papules. In surveys of male partners of patients with condyloma acuminatum, from one-third to more than two-thirds of the detectable lesions are seen only with the aid of the colposcope, and a smaller percentage is seen by acetowhitening alone (143). On the vulva, HPV infection may produce white patches that are enhanced or exposed after application of acetic acid. In some surveys, over 80% of women with or exposed to condyloma acuminatum were found to have subclinical infections. The clinical significance of acetowhite lesions is presently unknown, in part because acetowhitening lacks specificity and possibly sensitivity for diagnosis of HPV infection on the external genitalia (155). Anecdotal evidence suggests that acetowhite lesions may also be caused by menstruation or recent coitus. Subclinical lesions are usually transient, and diagnosis and treatment of asymptomatic subclinical diseases are not recommended (143, 160). Furthermore, dermatitis, folliculitis, candidiasis, psoriasis, lichen sclerosus et atrophicus, lichen simplex chronicus, and trauma can produce the same symptoms of pain, discomfort, and itching in the absence of visible lesions. The distinct entity of vulvar vestibulitis, also called focal vulvitis, does not appear to be related to HPV infection.

Vagina and Cervix

Vaginal warts manifest as either spiked condylomas, white, keratinized nodosities centered on a capillary loop, or flat condylomas (107). The latter may be confused with the occasional normal anatomic variant of micropapillary projections that are located over the distal third of the vagina, and extend over the introitus (vulvar papillomatosis).

Cervical warts are found in less than 10% of women with genital warts (107). Three variants are recognized: the flat condyloma (Color Plate 41), and the rarer exophytic and inverted (endophytic) condylomas. These lesions are also acetowhite, and colposcopic examination facilitates their identification (Color Plate 42). Because colposcopy is not entirely reliable, several biopsies of suspicious-looking areas are usually required for evaluation. Nevertheless, in the developing world, simple naked-eye visual inspection aided by acetic acid is able to contribute effectively to the prevention of cervical cancer. This screening can be further improved when followed by HPV DNA testing.

Preinvasive and Invasive Malignant Lesions

The clinical appearance of HPV-related preinvasive and invasive malignant cervical lesions is defined by colposcopic criteria that attempt to match histopathology (Color Plates 41 and 42) (55). Most of the lesions of CIN and SCC develop in the transitional zone. Usually not accessible to visual inspection, the glandular epithelium is vulnerable to HPV infections, especially by HPV-18, which may cause adenocarcinoma (36).

Depending on histologic grade, CIN lesions may regress, persist, or progress at various rates. According to a recent meta-analysis, the risks of progression over 2 years to HSIL from ASCUS and LSIL are 7 and 21%, respectively (102). Over 2 years, the risks of progression to invasive cancer are low, 0.25% for ASCUS, 0.15% for LSIL, and 1.4% for HSIL. In contrast, the rates of regression to normal cytology or histology are high, 68% for ASCUS, 47% for LSIL, and 35% for HSIL, and independent of duration of follow-up.

Intraepithelial neoplasias at the anogenital sites are often referred to by the acronyms of PIN (penile intraepithelial neoplasia), VIN (vulvar intraepithelial neoplasia), VAIN (vaginal intraepithelial neoplasia), and AIN. Intraepithelial neoplasias can coexist in different anatomic locations, thus reflecting the multicentric nature of the disease. Clinically, these lesions may present on the skin as pigmented papules, leukoplakia, or red macules (41). Bowenoid papulosis is a distinct clinicopathological entity made of the multicentric aggregation of pigmented papules, ranging from dark red to dark blue, with the histologic features of an intraepithelial neoplasia and the cytoarchitecture of a condyloma (Color Plate 40). It may evolve into Bowen's disease, which is a carcinoma in situ that presents as a red to brown, flat, scaly plaque with an irregular surface but well-demarcated borders. On the glans penis, Bowen's disease is known as erythroplasia of Queyrat. High-risk HPVs are typically associated with these premalignant conditions. Adequate natural history data on intraepithelial neoplasias of the external genitalia are nonexistent. Like CIN, VAIN and early vaginal cancer are best recognized with the colposcope, after the application of acetic acid; biopsy is necessary to establish a diagnosis.

On the external genitalia, warts may exceptionally evolve into verrucous carcinoma, a slow-growing, large, locally invasive SCC (130). Some authors distinguish Buschke-Loewenstein tumor (also called condylomatous carcinoma or giant condyloma) from what others consider to be a less aggressive form of verrucous carcinoma (Color Plate 43) (130). Buschke-Loewenstein tumors look like large condylomas with a locally invasive behavior.

Recurrent Respiratory Papillomatosis

An altered cry in infants or hoarseness of voice in older individuals is the presenting clinical manifestation of recurrent respiratory papillomatosis (42). Stridor or respiratory distress may also be present. The disease is recognized by laryngoscopic examination. The lesions are fungating and smooth (Color Plate 44), and are encountered specifically where the ciliated and squamous epithelia are juxtaposed. The lesions are also found along the tract of tracheostomies. The severity of the disease is inversely related to the age of onset; thus, tracheostomy is required in 14% of children but in 6% of adults. Extralaryngeal spread is also more common in children (31%) than in adults (16%). Lesion growth and extension toward the lung compromise the respiratory tract, and frequent surgical treatment may be needed to prevent asphyxiation. About one in five patients requires more than 40 lifetime operations. Most lesions contain HPV-6 or -11. HPV-11-containing lesions might be more aggressive. Despite the low oncogenic risk usually associated with these genotypes in other anatomic locations, in less than 10% of individuals malignant transformation can occur, resulting in verrucous carcinomas or SCC, especially if the lesions were previously treated with irradiation. Disease extension to the lung or the aerodigestive tract carries a risk of malignant transformation as high as 85%. Unexpectedly, recurrent respiratory papillomatosis appears to be rare in the HIV-infected population.

Miscellaneous

The different HPV-related lesions of the oral cavity are clinically similar but can be differentiated by histology (15, 117). The most common are oral squamous cell papillomas (or squamous papillomas). A closely related entity differentiated on histology is oral condylomata acuminata. These two types of lesions are caused by the same HPV types, mostly HPV-6, -11, and -16. Verrucae vulgaris lesions are less common and are caused by cutaneous HPVs, such as HPV-2, -4, and -57. HPV DNA, particularly HPV-16 DNA, can be found in various oral intraepithelial neoplasias, verrucous carcinomas, and SCC, as well as in proliferative verrucous leukoplakia (117). Focal epithelial hyperplasia (Heck's disease) manifests as multiple, asymptomatic, 1- to 5-mm, soft, sessile papules distributed preferentially on the lower lip but also on the buccal mucosa, lower lip, tongue, and gums (117). The lesions usually disappear over time. Oral hairy leukoplakia is a condition found in HIV-infected patients and is caused by Epstein-Barr virus infection, although coinfection with HPV does occur (117). HPV infection may cause papillomas and malignant tumors of the conjunctiva (79). An intriguing and strong association exists between HPV-5 and psoriasis skin lesions (108).

LABORATORY DIAGNOSIS

The role of the laboratory includes not only confirming the clinical diagnosis by histology or screening precursor and malignant lesions in the cervix by cytology but also detecting HPV DNA in cervical samples to aid in the screening and prevention of cervical cancer. Table 4 details some of the characteristics of the diagnostic methods that are currently used for anogenital HPV infections. A practical method for HPV isolation by in vitro culture is not yet available.

Cytology and Colposcopy

Cytology has been applied to the diagnosis of HPV infections of the penis, vulva, and anus, but cervical cytology,

TABLE 4 Diagnostic methods for anogenital HPV infection[a]

HPV diagnostic method (name of FDA-approved diagnostic kit)	Tested material or subject	HPV type determination	Availability to the clinician	Relevance for patient management	Sensitivity	Specificity
Clinical examination (cervix not included)						
With naked eye	Patient	No	+++++	+++++	+	++
And with acetic acid application	Patient	No	+++++	++	++	+
And examination with colposcope	Patient	No	+++	+++	++	++
Colposcopy	Patient	No	+++	+++++	+++	++
Cervicography	Patient	No	+	+++++	+++	+/++
Cytology						
Cervical	Swabbing, washing	No	+++++	+++++	++	++
Noncervical	Swabbing	No	++[b]	?+++[c]	++	++
Histology						
Light microscopy	Tissue	No	+++++	+++	++	+++
Electron microscopy	Tissue	No	+	+	+	++++
Immunocytochemistry	Swabbing, washing, tissue	No	++	++	++	++++
Nucleic acid hybridization						
Tissue in situ	Tissue	Possible	+	?	++	++++
Hybrid capture (Hybrid Capture II System)	Swabbing, washing, tissue	Possible[d]	+++	+++	++++	++++
PCR assay	Swabbing, washing, tissue	Possible	+	?	+++++	+++/+++++
Serology	Serum	Yes	+	+	++	+++

[a] + to +++++, from the lowest to the highest magnitude.
[b] This rating takes into account the fact that the technique needs to be associated with high-resolution anoscopy.
[c] In HIV patients and in men who have sex with men.
[d] The commercial kit distinguishes only between low-risk (types 6, 11, 42, 43, and 44) and high-risk (types 16, 18, 31, 33, 35, 39, 45, 51, 52, 56, 58, 59, and 68) HPV types.

in the form of the Papanicolaou (Pap) smear, remains the most extensively used. Cells can be collected by washings, but swabbing or scraping is standard. The optimal method of collection combines the use of the Ayre spatula to scrape the exocervix and the Cytobrush to sample the endocervix (98). The Cervex-Brush ("broom"), which is designed to sample both areas simultaneously, does not perform as well in traditional cytology (98). The sample can be placed directly on a glass slide and fixed (traditional cytology). A newer, now common, alternate approach is to place the sample (ThinPrep; Cytyc Corp.) or the head of the broom (SurePath [formerly AutoCyte]; TriPath Imaging, Inc.) in a liquid fixative (66, 126). The cells are dispersed and are either gathered on a filter and transferred to the glass slide (ThinPrep) or centrifuged on a gradient, with the suspended cells allowed to sediment on the glass slide (SurePath). Both liquid-based preparation technologies appear to offer performance characteristics at least equal to those of traditional cytology (66, 126). Their higher cost and longer processing time are offset by the ability to test the cervical sample for HPV DNA.

Koilocytes and dyskeratocytes (small, very keratinized squamous cells with orange cytoplasm and nucleus atypia) are hallmarks of cervical HPV infection (Fig. 9). However, atypical squamous metaplasia and, to a lesser degree, dyskeratosis correlate independently with the presence of HPV infection by PCR better than koilocytosis. Cytology is at least 10 times less sensitive than PCR for the diagnosis of HPV infection and should not be used for such a purpose (see "Epidemiology" above).

Over the years different classification schemes which remain in use throughout the world, have been applied to the Pap smear (Fig. 12). The shortcomings of these classification schemes led to a consensus effort in the United States to develop a more rigorous approach to Pap smear and cervical cancer screening. The result, initially proposed in 1988 and revised in 1992 and 2001, is known as the Bethesda system (http://www.bethesda2001.cancer.gov) (8, 135). The Bethesda system has three main components: a judgment on the adequacy of the specimen, a categorization of the smear with a codified descriptive diagnosis, and a set of guidelines for management and follow-up. Squamous cell abnormalities fall into four categories: (i) atypical squamous cells (a) of undetermined significance (ASC-US) or (b) for which HSIL cannot be excluded (ASC-H), (ii) LSIL, (iii) HSIL, and (iv) SCC. In a nationwide survey in the United States, 2.8% of Pap smears were categorized as atypical squamous cells, 1.97% as LSIL, 0.51% as HSIL, 0.026% as SCC, and 0.0046% as adenocarcinoma (141).

The performance characteristics of the Pap smear are difficult to determine accurately. A recent systematic review estimated that the sensitivity ranges from 30 to 87% and the specificity ranges from 86 to 100% (66). It is clearly an imperfect tool for the diagnosis of preinvasive and invasive cervical cancer, but it is still a preferred screening test because it is easy to obtain and has a low cost, and with periodic repetitions the chance of missing invasive cancer diminishes. A development in cervical cytological screening has been the use of computer-aided diagnosis systems to attempt to increase speed, accuracy, and reproducibility while keeping the cost down (66). Automated screening can be implemented for initial screening (triage) (66), thus diminishing technologist workload considerably. The AutoPap Primary Screening System (TriPath) has been approved for this purpose by the Food and Drug Administration (FDA). An alternate use of automated screening is quality control rescreening. This is a response to the obligation that American laboratories have to rescreen 10% of their negative smears. The AutoPap 300 QC Screener and the PAPNET systems are FDA approved for quality control rescreening (66).

Abnormal cervical cytology is usually supplemented by colposcopy for two purposes: the visual diagnostic of the lesion and selection of a biopsy site for further histologic identification (55). After applying 5% acetic acid, the cervix is examined with a colposcope. The application of an iodine solution (Lugol solution) may be included in the examination (Schiller test). Various scoring schemes have been developed to try to differentiate between typical condylomas, low-grade and high-grade intraepithelial neoplasia, and cancer. They rely to various degrees on color, shape of lesion margins or surface contours, appearance of the vessels (punctation and mosaicism), and iodine staining (Color Plates 41 and 42) (55). A troublesome shortcoming of colposcopy is that like all visually based interpretive diagnostic methods, it suffers from limited accuracy compared to histology, as well as poor intra- and interobserver agreement, particularly when contiguous diagnostic categories are concerned (4, 103). However, it is an indispensable tool for identifying the biopsy sites.

The colposcopic technique has been applied to the screening of patients at risk of anal cancer. The scoring system developed for the cervix is as effective for the anus in allowing discrimination between L-CIN and H-CIN.

Cervicography is a derivative of colposcopy and colpophotography (55). A picture of the cervix obtained with a special camera is sent for review by an expert. The system is patented, and National Testing Laboratories, in St. Louis, MO, is the worldwide licensee. The interpretation of colpophotographs suffers, like colposcopy, from poor intra- and interobserver agreement (4, 161). Cervicography, because it is cheaper than colposcopy, has been proposed as a screening tool to complement the Pap smear. It is more sensitive than cervical cytology but not as sensitive as colposcopy. Cervicography does not replace colposcopy, and its place in the process of screening cervical cancers and its precursors remains to be established.

New technologies in development for the detection of cervical preinvasive and invasive cancers include (i) speculoscopy, a visual inspection of the cervix after the application of acetic acid and of a chemical light source; (ii) the Polarprobe, an optoelectronic instrument that in contact with the cervix emits electrical impulses and light pulses at various frequencies and wavelengths and measures the tissue response; and (iii) fluorescence spectroscopy in which a fiberoptic probe applied on the cervix emits a laser light and the fluorescence of the tissue is recorded (161). In low-resource settings, in the absence of cytological screening and colposcopy, the simple technique of direct visual inspection of the cervix with the naked eye followed by immediate treatment, if indicated, has proved advantageous (128, 161).

Histology

Histology is the "gold standard" for confirming diagnosis of HPV disease and is the most important among the laboratory resources available to the clinician. However, sampling error, sample size, and fixation artifacts can all contribute to an inconclusive diagnosis. Histology is not an appropriate tool for the diagnosis of HPV infection because it selects only small areas for biopsy, and most HPV infections are asymptomatic (28, 49, 94, 95).

Histologic criteria allow the diagnosis of the different HPV diseases (Fig. 10 and 11). They are neither absolute nor easy to define, and subjectivity and experience contribute to differences in interpretation. Interobserver variability is a substantial limitation that affects histology and cytology equally. Even among well-trained pathologists, interobserver agreement on cervical biopsies is only moderate, and it is worst for CIN 2 (128). The clinical identity of a lesion cannot always be established from the histology. For example, whereas anogenital warts, flat warts, and myrmecias are easily recognized and differentiated as such, other cutaneous warts might be more difficult to identify.

Transmission electron microscopy is of little use in the diagnosis of HPV lesions, but it may reveal the presence of intranuclear viral particles that are typically organized in crystalline arrays or pseudoarrays. HPV intranuclear particles have been noted in histologically or colposcopically normal cervical samples.

Immunocytochemistry

Denaturation of papillomavirus virions by boiling and mercaptoethanol treatment uncovers an antigen that is shared among papillomaviruses. Antibodies to the common papillomavirus or genus-specific antigen are commercially available (DAKO antibody; Accurate Chemical and Scientific Corp., Westbury, NY) and have been used for the immunocytochemical diagnosis of HPV infection (Fig. 13). The sensitivity of this test is limited and varies with lesion type. The common papillomavirus antigen has been found in 68% of common warts, 58% of plantar warts, about 50% of anogenital and oral warts and laryngeal papillomas, about 40% of CIN 1, 20% of CIN 2, 8% of conjunctival papillomas, and 5% of cases of bowenoid papillomatosis. The reasons for this low and variable sensitivity are unknown but may be related to sampling, HPV type, relative abundance, or periodic expression of L1 protein. The specificity of the assay in the diagnosis of condylomata acuminata appears to be excellent compared to that of in situ hybridization.

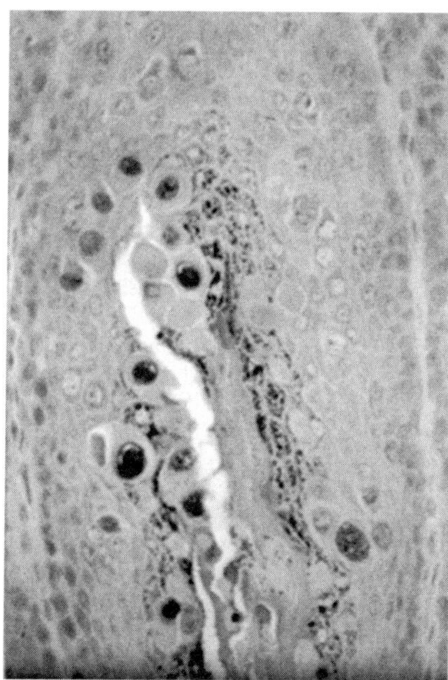

FIGURE 13 Immunocytochemistry of condyloma acuminatum with an antibody directed against the common papillomavirus antigen (high-power view). Several intense nuclear signals are visible. (Courtesy of Clara E. Mesonero, Cape Cod Hospital, Cape Cod, MA.)

Nucleic Acid Detection Assays

In situ hybridization is a method that is applicable to the visualization of HPV nucleic acids under the microscope in cells or tissues, typically a paraffin-embedded tissue section. Probes can be sense or antisense. Antisense probes offer the advantage of binding to both viral DNA and mRNAs, and either of these targets can be selected by denaturing and pretreating with RNase or not (149). The advantages of in situ hybridization include the ability to type the infecting HPV, to detect cellular double infections, to distinguish integrated (speckled nuclear signal) from episomal (diffuse nuclear signal) infections, and to relate infection to associated histopathological features. Different commercial tests have been developed, but none are approved by the FDA.

The hybrid capture system is an FDA-approved proprietary assay based on liquid hybridization, now in its second generation (Hybrid Capture II; Digene Diagnostics, Inc.) (29). Cells or DNA extracted from tissue is added to an alkaline reaction mixture that denatures the DNA. Two pools of RNA probes are added in parallel. Pool A contains probes for low-risk HPV types (types 6, 11, 42, 43, and 44), whereas pool B contains probes for high-risk HPV types (types 16, 18, 31, 33, 35, 39, 45, 51, 52, 56, 58, 59, and 68). However, the American College of Obstetricians and Gynecologists and the American Society for Colposcopy and Cervical Pathology recommend testing with the high-risk probes only (29). The mixtures are added to microtiter plates coated with antibodies that immobilize RNA/DNA hybrids. An alkaline phosphatase-conjugated antibody directed to RNA/DNA hybrids is reacted, and all unbound antibody is enzymatically degraded. The immobilized complex is detected with a sensitive chemoluminescent substrate to the alkaline phosphatase. The assay is rapid and quantitative, which may be useful for prognosis but does not give a type-specific diagnosis, only that the sample contains a low-risk or a high-risk HPV. It also does not detect any of genotypes 26, 53, 66, 73, and 82, altogether present in about 1% of cervical cancers (29). The technique is directly applicable to aliquots of the samples collected for liquid-based cytology. Compared to PCR, it has the advantages of ease of use, simplicity, and not being susceptible to sample cross-contamination. Although the Hybrid Capture II assay is overall slightly less sensitive than PCR, it is more sensitive for patients with LSIL and has a better positive predictive value.

PCR diagnosis offers the highest sensitivity for the detection of HPV DNA (104). It also permits typing. A variety of methods have been described, and among the commercial assays developed, none has been FDA approved to date (29, 104). They are based on the use of either general (also called consensus or generic) primers or a mixture of primers (degenerate primer system). Typing can be done by retesting the sample with type-specific primers or by applying type-specific probes to the amplicon. The cost and the need to enforce strict measures to prevent contamination and false-positive results are the main limitations of PCR, which is otherwise the leading investigational tool for HPV diagnosis.

Serologic Assays

There are no serologic assays satisfactory for the clinical diagnosis of HPV infection. The most consistently sensitive assays are VLP-based enzyme-linked immunosorbent assays used chiefly for the diagnosis of HPV-6, -11, -16, and -18 infections (14, 51, 124). They cannot identify much more than half to two-thirds of infected subjects if they are to retain a high specificity. These assays and their derivatives, like the Luminex bead technology, are investigational, and they have been useful for epidemiological surveys and the assessment of the immune response following immunization.

PREVENTION

General

No specific environmental precautions have been developed for the control of HPV infections. However, surgical instruments in contact with areas potentially infected by HPV should be properly sterilized according to standard procedures developed for viruses. Disposable materials should not be reused. Contaminated surfaces can be disinfected with household bleach (5.25% sodium hypochlorite) diluted 1:10 in water.

Some is known of the value of barrier methods in preventing the dissemination of HPV infections and diseases, but wart dressings while swimming have been useful for the prevention of plantar warts. There is now strong evidence that condoms are effective in reducing the transmission of genital HPV. In a randomized study of 125 couples of women with CIN and their male sexual partners, there was a greater rate of CIN (1.5-fold) and HPV DNA clearance (5.7-fold) in the women from the couples assigned to condom use. Similarly, there was a higher (1.9-fold) rate of clearance of HPV-associated flat lesions in the males, and the clearance effect of condoms in males was seen only in the couples with concordant HPV types (12). In a prospective study of 82 college-aged, initially virgin women, 100% consistent condom use, as opposed to 5% or less use, was associated with a statistically significant (threefold) decreased risk of cervical, vulvar, and vaginal HPV infection (156). Although the protective effect of condoms is modest, their use can be recommended in nascent sexual relationships or after treatment of one sexual partner for HPV disease.

Smoke evacuation systems should be used during electrosurgery or laser surgery. Protective garments, including goggles, mask, gloves, and gown, are recommended.

Patients with epidermodysplasia verruciformis and immunodeficient or immunosuppressed patients with cutaneous lesions should avoid UV light exposure to minimize the risk of malignant conversion.

There are no validated isolation procedures of HPV-infected individuals. There is no evidence that school activities should be restricted for children with recurrent respiratory papillomatosis.

Passive Immunoprophylaxis

Although the potential efficacy of passive immunoprophylaxis using hyperimmune globulins raised against VLPs has been demonstrated with experimental animal papillomavirus infections, no data are available for HPV infections (23).

Chemoprophylaxis

It is possible to prevent the relapse of anogenital warts with either podofilox or 5-fluorouracil (5-FU) (see "Treatment" below), but effective chemoprophylaxis against new HPV infection is not yet available in clinical practice. Carrageenan, a readily available polysaccharide already included in some vaginal lubricants, has shown excellent microbicidal activity in vitro and in an animal model (121). Clinical studies are ongoing. In contrast, the spermicide nonoxynol 9 has been shown to potentiate HPV transmission (121).

Active Immunization

The most dramatic change in the field of papillomaviruses has been the commercial release in June 2006 of the first prophylactic vaccine against HPV. This vaccine, Gardasil (Merck), is quadrivalent and directed at HPV-6, -11, -16, and -18. HPV-6 and -11 account for about 90% of genital warts, while HPV-16 and -18 are found in about 90% of cervical cancers. A similar vaccine, but limited to HPV-16 and -18, Cervarix (GlaxoSmithKline), became available in some countries in early 2007 but might not be available in the United States before 2009. These two vaccines are based on VLPs produced by the expression in yeast cells (Gardasil) or insect cells (Cervarix) of the L1 gene. The major capsid protein reassembles spontaneously into a noninfectious capsid devoid of viral DNA but identical morphologically and immunologically to the native virion. The key property of HPV virions and VLPs is to induce neutralizing antibodies that were shown to protect against a viral challenge by HPV or animal papillomaviruses (23, 123, 124).

The clinical indications of Gardasil are supported by a series of clinical trials (14). In a pivotal randomized controlled trial, a monovalent HPV-16 VLP vaccine was shown at 1.5 years of follow-up to completely prevent persistent cervical HPV-16 infection compared to adjuvant (aluminum hydroxyphosphate sulfate) alone. Phase III trials, involving a total of 17,000 females, aged 16 to 26 years, who were seronegative and HPV DNA negative for the vaccine types, have shown that Gardasil is 99% effective in preventing CIN 2 or 3 and adenocarcinoma in situ (AIS) caused by HPV-16 or -18 at 3 years of follow-up. The results published so far with Cervarix are quite comparable. Gardasil was also 100% effective preventing, at 3 years of follow-up, any grades of CIN, AIS, VIN 1, VAIN 1, and external genital warts caused by HPV-6, -11, -16, or -18 and VIN 2 or 3 and VAIN 2 or 3 caused by HPV-16 or -18. In the intention-to-treat analysis, including subjects who did not receive the full immunization series or who had an abnormal Pap smear at entry, the efficacy was 82 to 98%. When women who were seropositive or HPV DNA positive for the vaccine types at enrollment were added, the vaccine efficacy dropped to 44% for CIN 2 or 3 and AIS and to 76% for genital warts. With longer follow-up, more subjects are likely to reach a disease end point in the control group than in the vaccine group, thus further increasing the vaccine efficacy. Nevertheless, these results clearly show that vaccination has the greatest benefits if given before the onset of sexual activity and acquisition of an HPV infection. Vaccination in 9- to 15-year-old boys and girls induced a neutralizing immune response, which was used as the end point for vaccine approval for this age group. Actually, this immune response is inversely proportional to age and superior in titer to the response generated in older girls and women. Evidence for the vaccine's excellent clinical efficacy has now been demonstrated in women up to 45 years of age.

Gardasil is approved in the United States for the prevention in women of cervical cancer, AIS, CIN, VIN 2 and 3, VAIN 2 and 3, and genital warts. The vaccine is given by intramuscular injections in a three-dose regimen (day 0 and months 2 and 6). Pregnancy is a contraindication. The Advisory Committee on Immunization Practices has issued guidelines for vaccine administration, recommending the vaccination of 11- to 12-year-old girls, with a catch-up vaccination for 13- to 18-year-old girls. The vaccine can be given from 9 to 26 years of age (96). The vaccine has shown great safety. The only significant adverse reactions from the immunization series have been pain at the injection site (85%) and swelling (26%). Fever was reported with 13.5% of the vaccine immunizations, compared to 10.2% with the placebo. Importantly, vaccination does not alter any of the cervical screening recommendations. The cost of the vaccine in the United States is about $120 per dose, but this does not include the costs for storage and delivery.

Remaining questions about the vaccine (14) include the true efficacy in preventing cervical cancer, the impact on the rate of abnormal Pap smears, whether a booster will be necessary (not at least for 5 years), the efficacy in boys and men, and the efficacy against other HPV diseases caused by the types included in the current vaccine and more multivalent vaccines in development.

Prevention of Perinatal and Congenital Infection

Delivery by cesarean section in pregnant women with condyloma acuminatum is not indicated for the prevention of disease transmission to the baby (42). There is no consensus on the use of cesarean section for the delivery of babies whose mothers have had a child with recurrent respiratory papillomatosis.

Prevention of Anogenital Malignancies

There are several guidelines available for the screening of cervical cancer (31, 127, 150, 160). They have been summarized in Table 5. Consensus guidelines were updated in 2006 and published in late 2007 to help the health care provider through the proper management of cytological abnormalities and CIN (162, 163). They, along with the corresponding algorithms (http://www.asccp.org/pdfs/consensus/algorithms_hist_07.pdf), can be downloaded from the American Society for Colposcopy and Cervical Pathology website (http://www.asccp.org/consensus.shtml). Important points are that initial follow-up rather than intervention is recommended for adolescents with ASC or CIN 1 regardless of colposcopy results, or with CIN 2 or 3 and negative colposcopy. Observation is also recommended for young women with CIN 2 or 3 and normal colposcopy. Less intensive evaluation is recommended during pregnancy as well. Recommendations have also been introduced for the management of glandular abnormalities. Another major change is the increased role of HPV DNA testing for the triaging of women with low-grade Pap smear abnormalities as well as for the follow-up of some women. Evidence has been developed for the use of high-risk HPV DNA testing in the management of the following situations (38): (i) ASC-US or ASC-H, regardless of the patient's age; (ii) management of LSIL in older women (especially after the age of 40 years, regardless of menopausal status); (iii) the follow-up after colposcopy of women with ASC-US, ASC-H, or LSIL; and (iv) the observation of women after treatment.

Screening strategies for anal cancer based on anal cytology have been proposed (109). The procedure, which can be self-administered, consists of the introduction into the anal canal, more than 2 cm from the anus, of a Dacron swab moistened with saline or water, or of a cervical Cytobrush. The collected material is processed like a conventional or liquid-based Pap smear. A cost-effectiveness analysis of cytological screening every 2 or 3 years in homosexual and bisexual men indicated cost savings and life expectancy benefits similar to those of other preventive health measures such as cervical cytology. Nevertheless, anal cytology is not yet recommended, except in New York State, as a standard practice in these populations (101, 109). The reasons for this reluctance include (i) the poor to moderate inter- and intraobserver reliability of the interpretation of anal cytology and histology; (ii) the absence of clinically validated screening strategies adapted to the various populations at risk; (iii) the limited understanding of the natural evolution of anal HSIL, which are also prone to recur after treatment (32); (iv) the absence of standardized medical and surgical treatment guidelines, as well as the absence of corroborative comparative studies; (v) the lack of evidence that this type of screening has an impact on the prevention of anal cancer; and (vi) the insufficient number of physicians trained in how to evaluate, biopsy, and treat a cytology-positive patient with anoscopy under magnified optics (high-resolution anoscopy).

TREATMENT

A consistently effective and safe treatment for HPV infections is not available. Present therapeutic options are directed at eradicating the disease, not the infection, by destroying the lesions with physical or chemical means or by stimulating an inflammatory or immune response. A majority of these treatments have been developed empirically, but few have been thoroughly tested, and none is completely satisfactory.

This section reviews the most commonly used and best-evaluated forms of treatment for HPV diseases. Additional information on these and other approaches can be found in several sources (3, 9, 16, 26, 42, 86, 88, 89, 134, 160). Tables 6 to 8 summarize information regarding the effectiveness in treatment of cutaneous warts and condylomata acuminata of several of the therapies discussed below. The current HPV VLP vaccine has not shown any therapeutic effect.

Chemical Methods

Acids

Salicylic acid alone, or in combination with lactic acid (SAL), has been used for the topical treatment of cutaneous warts (88, 89). This is a keratolytic agent, but the exact mode of action is unknown. Salicylic acid-based compounds are useful for self-treatment of cutaneous warts. They are well tolerated, although there can be hypersen-

TABLE 5 Summary of cervical cancer screening guidelines[a]

Parameter	Organization	Guideline
When to begin Pap test screening?	USPSTF, ACS, ACOG	Approximately 3 yr after a woman begins having sexual intercourse, but no later than age 21 yr
How often?	USPSTF	Every 3 yr (regardless of the cervical cytology technique used)
	ACS	(i) At initiation of screening Annually with conventional cytology *or* Every 2 yr using liquid-based cytology (ii) At or after age 30, women who have had three consecutive, technically satisfactory normal/negative cytology results may be screened every 2–3 yr *unless* (a) They have a history of in utero DES[b] exposure (b) They are HIV positive (c) They are immunocompromised by organ transplantation, chemotherapy, or chronic corticosteroid treatment
	ACOG	(i) Annually after initiation of screening (regardless of the cervical cytology technique used) (ii) At or after age 30, women who have had three consecutive, technically satisfactory normal/negative cytology results may be screened every 2–3 yr *unless* (a) They have a history of CIN 2 or 3 and have not had after treatment at least three consecutive negative cervical (or vaginal if posthysterectomy) cytology screening results (b) They have a history of in utero DES exposure (c) They are HIV positive (d) They are immunocompromised by organ transplantation, chemotherapy, or chronic corticosteroid treatment
When to discontinue screening?	USPSTF	At age 65 in women who have had normal results previously and who are not otherwise at high risk for cervical cancer
	ACS	At age 70 or older in women with an intact cervix and who have had three or more documented, consecutive, technically satisfactory, normal/negative cervical cytology tests and no abnormal/positive cytology tests within the 10-yr period prior to age 70 Exceptions (a) Women who have not been previously screened (b) Women for whom information about previous screening is unavailable (c) Women for whom past screening is unlikely (d) Women with a history of cervical cancer or in utero exposure to DES (e) Women who are immunocompromised (e.g., due to organ transplantation, HIV infection, chemotherapy, or chronic corticosteroid treatment) (f) Women who have tested positive for HPV DNA
ACOG	No age recommendation	
Screening after hysterectomy	USPSTF, ACS, ACOG	Not necessary if (total) hysterectomy was for benign disease
Screening with HPV DNA testing (Hybrid Capture II test for high-risk HPV)	USPSTF	Not recommended
	ACS and ACOG	Can be used with cytology, only at age 30 or older, and if both tests are negative, they should not be repeated more frequently than every 3 yr

(Continued on next page)

TABLE 5 *(Continued)*

Parameter	Organization	Guideline
Additional guidelines	ACS	(i) Regular health care visits, including gynecologic care (including pelvic examination) and STD screening and prevention, should be done. (ii) Counseling and education related to HPV infection are critical if HPV DNA testing is done.
	ACOG	(i) Yearly testing using cytology alone remains an acceptable screening plan. (ii) Annual examinations, including pelvic examination, are still recommended.
	CDC	(i) Women who have external genital warts do not need to have Pap tests more frequently than women who do not have warts, unless otherwise indicated. (ii) For HIV-infected women a cervical cytology should be obtained twice in the first year after diagnosis of HIV infection and, if the results are normal, annually thereafter.

[a] ACS, American Cancer Society (127) (http://caonline.amcancersoc.org/cgi/content/short/52/6/342); USPSTF, U.S. Preventive Services Task Force (150) (http://www.ahrq.gov/clinic/3rduspstf/cervicalcan/cervcanrr.htm, http://www.ahrq.gov/clinic/uspstf/uspscerv.htm); ACOG, American College of Obstetrics and Gynecology (1); CDC, Centers for Disease Control and Prevention (160) (http://www.cdc.gov/std/treatment/).
[b] DES, diethylstilbestrol.

sitivity reactions to colophony, a component of the collodion base often used in salicylic acid preparations.

Bichloroacetic acid and trichloroacetic acid (TCA) are keratolytic, cauterizing agents favored by gynecologists for the treatment of genital warts on the moist areas (26, 88). They cannot be applied on large areas, and their application is painful. Adverse reactions, including ulceration and scabbing, are more common than with cryotherapy. Monochloracetic acid in combination with 60% salicylic acid has been more effective than placebo (83%, versus 54%) for the treatment of plantar warts.

Fixatives

A 3% formaldehyde solution or 10% glutaraldehyde solution or gel is effective for the treatment of plantar warts, but sensitization to these compounds can occur. In addition, formaldehyde may cause painful skin fissures.

Antimitotics, Antimetabolites, and Cytotoxic, Blistering, and Cauterizing Agents

Antimitotics and antimetabolites take advantage of the increased cellular replication in wart tissues. Podophyllin is extracted from the rhizome of *Podophyllum peltatum* or the more potent *Podophyllum emodi* (26, 88, 134). It is usually prepared as a benzoin tincture, 25% podophyllum (USP). Podophyllotoxin, a lignan, is the molecule most responsible for the antiwart and toxic activities of podophyllin. It is available as a purified compound, podofilox. Podophyllin and podofilox act by preventing microtubule polymerization, thus disrupting the mitotic spindle. Podophyllin may also damage HPV DNA. These preparations have been most extensively used for the treatment of condyloma acuminatum. Local adverse reactions (pain, erythema, tenderness, erosions, and ulcerations) result from the intense acute inflammation and necrosis following topical application. The podofilox solution might be worse in that respect than the cream formulation or podophyllin (26). Care should be exercised not to paint the healthy skin or to leave the medication on for more than 24 h. Podophyllin should be applied by a health practitioner and no more than once a week. Podofilox (solution or gel) is better tolerated and can be applied by the patient (9). Its efficacy, which is variable and modest, has been confirmed in several randomized studies (9, 26). Systemic adverse reactions include sensitization to benzoin or guaiacum wood. Ingestion or extensive application of these compounds has been responsible for gastroenteric, neurologic, hematologic, and renal toxicities that may be fatal (9, 26). Podophyllin or podofilox should not be used during pregnancy. Treatment is contraindicated if the wart area is greater than 10 cm^2.

5-FU, a pyrimidine analog, prevents the synthesis of DNA, and to a minor degree that of RNA, by blocking the methylation of thymidylic acid (26, 88, 134) and is used in a variety of regimens as a 5% cream for the treatment of anogenital warts. Sensitization dermatitis and ulcerations occur infrequently but can be severe. 5-FU has been associated with hematologic abnormalities, such as bone marrow suppression and vaginal adenomatosis or carcinoma. The use of 5-FU is contraindicated during pregnancy. Another pyrimidine antagonist, 5-iodo-2′-deoxyuridine, or idoxuridine, has been used topically for condylomata acuminata, with up to an 80% complete response rate.

Bleomycin is a glycopeptidic mixture that causes breaks in single- and double-stranded DNA. This cytotoxic agent has been well studied for the intralesional treatment of cutaneous warts, particularly periungual warts (88, 89, 134). At the recommended doses (<5 mg), no systemic toxicities have been reported. Most patients experience pain that can be severe. Administration of a local anesthetic or the addition of lidocaine to bleomycin helps control pain. Intralesional administration imposes a limit to the number of lesions to be treated. As a result, alternate modes of delivery, such as bifurcated needle puncture, dermography (tattooing machine), and medicated topical dressing, have been proposed. Bleomycin should not be used in children, pregnant women, or patients with peripheral vascular disease.

Estradiol and 16-α-hydroxyestrone are estrogenic compounds that stimulate the growth of experimental human

TABLE 6 Some common treatment modalities for cutaneous warts

Agent (U.S. commercial preparation)	Usual formulation and regimen[a]	Wart type[b]	Complete response rate[c] (%)
Salicylic acid (17%)-lactic acid-collodion, 1:1:4 (e.g., Duofilm, Occlusal-HP, Wart-Off)	Daily for up to 12 wk	HW	67
		Single PW	84
		MW	50
Fixatives			
Formaldehyde, 3%	Daily (bedtime)	PW	94
Glutaraldehyde	Daily	MW	47
Podophyllin (Podocon-25 or Podofin)	15% Podophyllin, qd	Single PW	81
5-FU (Effudex cream, 5%)	2% 5-FU in propylene glycol, qd	MW	47
	5% 5-FU in DMSO, qd	MW	53
Bleomycin	1-mg/ml solution, 0.1–0.2 ml/wart	HW	~70
	Intralesional, once, 0.7% solution	MW	~50
Retinoids	0.05% Tretinoin cream	CW	85
	Etretinate, orally	CW	84
Cantharidin (Cantharone,Verr-Canth)	Topical, once	CW	87
Silver nitrate stick	qd or every 3 days	CW	43
Cryotherapy	Every 3 wk, up to 6 times	CW	41–45
		HW	~75
		PW	29–50
Electrosurgery	Once	PW	65
CO_2 laser surgery	Once	CW	32
		Periungual	71
		PW	50–90

[a] qd, once a day; DMSO, dimethyl sulfoxide.
[b] CW, cutaneous warts; HW, hand warts; PW, plantar warts; MW, mosaic warts.
[c] These rates are derived from available studies (88, 89). Because of great dissimilarities between the studies and the usual absence of controls, these rates are not necessarily comparable and they are provided for indication only.

TABLE 7 Common treatment modalities for anogenital warts

Agent (U.S. commercial preparation)	Usual formulation and regimen[a]	Complete response rate[b] (%)	Relapse rate[b] (%)
Podophyllin (Podocon-25 or Podofin; 15-ml bottle)	25% in benzoin solution; qwk up to six times	35–51	60–85
Podofilox (Condylox; 3.5-ml bottle or 3.5-g tube)	0.5% Solution or gel; self-applied; bid 3 days/wk, ≤4 wk	57–72[c]	32–50
Imiquimod (Aldara; box of 12 single-use 250-mg packets)	5% Cream; self-applied, tiw, qod hs, ≤16 wk	56	13
Kunecatechins (Veregen; 15-g tube)	15% Ointment; self-applied, tid, ≤16 wk	57	
TCA (Tri-Chlor; 15-ml bottle)	50–90% Solution; qwk up to six times	64–83	55
5-FU (Effudex cream; 25-g tube)	5% Cream; highly variable regimens	43–58	
Cryotherapy	Liquid-nitrogen spray; one or two cycles qwk up to six times	64–76	19–40
Cold-blade surgery	Scissor excision	87–94	20–31
Electrosurgery	Variable techniques (e.g., electrocoagulation, electrocautery, and fulguration)	58–94	22
CO_2 laser surgery	Variable techniques	93–99	49–65[d]
Intralesional IFN-α2b or n3 (Intron A, Alferon N)	1 MU; tiw for 3–8 wks; from one to all lesions injected	40–52	18–37

[a] qwk, once a week; bid, twice a day; tid, thrice a day; qod, every other day; hs, at night; tiw, thrice weekly; MU, million units.
[b] These numbers represent the 95% confidence limits, whenever appropriate, derived from results of the selected studies (9, 16, 17, 26).
[c] Results given for the solution formulation.
[d] Based on randomized comparative studies.

TABLE 8 Suggested approaches to the treatment of warts

Type of wart or lesion	Treatment options[a]
Plantar and hand warts	First line Salicylic acid-based paints (H) Cryotherapy (O) Second line Formaldehyde (H) Glutaraldehyde (H) Silver nitrate stick (H) Cantharidin (O) Bleomycin (especially periungual warts) (O) Third line Electrosurgery (O) Laser surgery (O) Contact immunotherapy (O)
Flat warts	First line No treatment Second line Cryotherapy Electrocautery Retinoids Contact immunotherapy
Epidermodysplasia verruciformis lesions	Benign-appearing lesion Observation or treatment; sun protection measures Preinvasive or invasive malignant lesion Surgical excision Cryotherapy Laser surgery
Condylomata acuminata	First line Imiquimod (H) Podofilox (H) Cryotherapy[b] (O) TCA (O) Podophyllin[b] (O) Scissor excision (O) (if few and small lesions) Second line Electrosurgery (O) Laser surgery (O) Intralesional interferon (O)
Anal warts	Cryotherapy TCA Cold-blade surgery Infrared coagulator Electrosurgery Laser surgery
Vaginal warts	Cryotherapy (liquid nitrogen spray, not a cryoprobe) TCA Laser surgery
Cervical warts	Electrosurgery (LEEP) Cryotherapy Laser surgery
Intraepithelial neoplasia of the external genitalia	Laser surgery Cryotherapy (penis) Cold-blade surgery Imiquimod
AIN	Infrared coagulator TCA Imiquimod Cryotherapy Podophyllin Electrosurgery Cold-blade surgery
VAIN	Laser surgery
CIN	Electrosurgery (LEEP) Cryotherapy Laser surgery
Recurrent respiratory papillomatosis	Primary therapy Microsurgery with microdebrider CO_2 laser surgery Photodynamic (laser) therapy Cold-blade surgery Adjuvant therapy Intralesional cidofovir Interferon Photodynamic (laser) therapy I3C
Oral warts (papillomas, verrucae, condylomata)	Cold-blade excision Cryotherapy Podophyllin
Focal epithelial hyperplasia	No treatment

[a] H, home treatment; O, office-based treatment. The reader may also consult several published guidelines or reviews mentioned in the text (3, 9, 16, 26, 42, 86, 88, 89, 134, 160).
[b] Recommended for intrameatal warts.

papillomas. Indole-3-carbinole (I3C), a molecule abundant in cruciferous vegetables (e.g., cabbage and broccoli), has an inhibitory effect by increasing the 2-hydroxylation of estradiol, thus favoring the formation of 2-hydroxyestrone instead of 16-α-hydoxyestrone (42). I3C (Indoplex) is a popular dietary supplement in the management of recurrent respiratory papillomatosis. While one study of oral I3C for the treatment of CIN 2 or 3 has shown promising results, the use of this supplement for the treatment of recurrent respiratory papillomatosis has been submitted to only an open-label, noncomparative trial (16, 42).

Retinoids impede epidermal growth and differentiation. A 0.05% tretinoin cream gave more than twice the rate of complete response that placebo did in patients with plantar warts (88). Uncontrolled trials have also indicated a beneficial effect of systemic retinoids for the treatment of plantar and common warts (88). Retinoids are teratogenic.

Cantharidin is a compound extracted from the blister beetle, *Cantharis vesicatoria* (Spanish fly) (88). Its topical application causes acantholysis. Excellent responses have been documented for the treatment of cutaneous warts. The blistering is painful, but it is usually well tolerated and does not cause scars. Care should be exercised not to apply cantharidin on healthy skin or near mucosal membranes, especially the conjunctiva. It is not recommended for use during pregnancy. Systemic absorption of cantharidin causes severe toxicities.

Silver nitrate sticks are chemical cauterizers that have been applied to cutaneous warts (88). Three applications at 3-day intervals on common warts gave a fourfold increase in complete response over placebo. Occasional hyperpigmentation is reported.

Allergic Sensitization

Sensitization with 1-nitro-2,4-dinitrochlorobenzene, followed by application of the compound on the lesions, has been used for the treatment of recalcitrant cutaneous and genital warts (27). Complete response rates of about 80 to 100% have been reported in uncontrolled studies. The occurrence of severe allergic reactions has led to a decline in use. More recently, other sensitizing agents, 2,3-diphenylcyclopropenone (diphencyprone), squaric acid dibutyl ester, and 10% masoprocol cream (Actinex), have been advocated for their greater safety (27).

Interferons, Immunomodulators, Antivirals, and Others

Interferons have been extensively evaluated in the treatment of condyloma acuminatum, but they have also been used to treat other HPV diseases (26, 88). Intralesional administration is more effective than parenteral administration. Although the initial experience with topical interferons was negative, more recent studies suggest superiority to either placebo or podofilox for the treatment of external genital or intravaginal warts (26). Topical interferon formulations are not available in the United States. Systemic interferon has little effect on HPV DNA copy number in vivo (19). Experience with the pegylated formulations of interferon is lacking. The common side effects of interferon are well known, and their intensity is in part related to dose (see chapter 11). Interferons are very costly and contraindicated during pregnancy.

Imiquimod, an imidazoquinoline, is an inducer of IFN-α and other cytokines that is available as a 5% cream (Aldara) for the treatment of condyloma acuminatum (26, 33, 88). An attractive feature of this immunotherapy is that it is patient applied. In the pivotal study, patients were randomized to topical treatment with imiquimod at 5 or 1% or vehicle cream, thrice a week, every other night for up to 16 weeks, with a 12-week follow-up for those free of lesions (33). The complete response rates were 50, 21, and 11%, respectively, and the corresponding recurrence rates were 13, 0, and 10%, respectively. The 5% preparation was significantly more effective than the others combined. Side effects of imiquimod are local and include itching and burning sensations, as well as erythema, erosion, and swelling. Women respond approximately twice as well as men, but higher rates of disease eradication, as well as of local side effects, can be obtained with daily application (50). Imiquimod has been used for the treatment of cutaneous warts, Bowen disease, and bowenoid papulosis (33). It is superior to placebo for the treatment of VIN (150a).

Cimetidine has immunomodulatory properties in addition to its H_2-blocking effect. Although advocated for the treatment of cutaneous warts (26, 88), its was ineffective in controlled studies.

Two nucleic acid analogs have shown some degree of effectiveness in HPV infections. Ribavirin, a nucleoside analog with known activity against RNA viruses, was found to have some efficacy in a cottontail rabbit papillomavirus animal model, as well as an encouraging effect in a few pilot studies on recurrent respiratory papillomatosis (42). Cidofovir [(S)-1-(3-hydroxy-2-phosphonylmethoxypropyl) cytosine (HPMPC); Vistide], a nucleotide analog effective against cytomegalovirus and other herpesvirus infections, has been found to be effective in a variety of conditions caused by HPV when delivered either intralesionally or topically (26, 88, 134). They include condyloma acuminatum, recurrent respiratory papillomatosis, aerodigestive tumors, VIN, CIN, and cutaneous and oral warts (134). These results, except for condyloma acuminatum, are all based on uncontrolled, nonrandomized studies. Cidofovir is a potential carcinogen in humans.

Veregen is 15% ointment of kunecatechins that was approved in October 2006 by the FDA but has not yet been launched on the U.S. market. This botanical is made from a partially purified fraction of a water extract of green tea (*Camellia sinensis*) leaves. It contains more than 55% epigallocatechin gallate and other catechins. The mechanism of action is unknown, but it is possibly antiviral. The product is self-applied three times a day on the lesions until complete disappearance, but for not more than 16 weeks. It has been approved on the basis of two still-unpublished phase III clinical trials that enrolled about 1,000 immunocompetent patients with genital warts (http://www.fda.gov/cder/foi/label/2006/021902lbl.pdf). The complete clearance rates by week 16 were 57.2% for Veregen-treated patients and 33.7% for vehicle-treated patients (147a). As with imiquimod, results were better in females than males. Erythema, itching, burning, pain or discomfort, and erosion or ulceration were, in order of frequency, the most common adverse effects; they were noted in at least about half of the patients. The drug is contraindicated during pregnancy. The potential drawbacks of this new medication are the frequency of application—no compliance data are available—and its red color, which may stain undergarments.

Physical Methods

Curettage and Cold-Blade Excision

Curettage is used for the removal of cutaneous warts but has not been rigorously evaluated. Its main drawback is the formation of scars that are sometimes painful. Excision of anogenital warts with scissors has been used with good success (20). Scarring is also a complication but is minimal (20). Local anesthesia is required with either technique.

Cold-blade conization of the cervix has long been the standard mode of biopsy and treatment for CIN. It is now being replaced by electrosurgical techniques. The development of microresectors, small instruments that resemble biopsy forceps, has facilitated the resection of laryngeal papillomas.

Electrosurgery

Electrosurgery encompasses various techniques in which tissue ablation is the result of electric current. Depending on the wave form of the current, its voltage and amperage, and the number (one or two) and contact of the electrodes with the tissue, the methods are called electrocautery, electrodessication, electrofulguration, electrocoagulation, and electrosection. It is unknown which method is best, but scarring is a notable side effect with all. Because scars tend to be painful, electrosurgery should be discouraged for plantar warts (26, 62). Electrofulguration is useful for the treatment of facial warts, and electrocoagulation and electrodessication are appropriate for the treatment of condyloma acuminatum. A topical anesthetic containing prilocaine and lidocaine (EMLA cream) provides good pain control for the removal of condylomata acuminata.

Large loop excision of the transitional zone (LLETZ), also known under the more general descriptor of loop electrosurgical excision procedure (LEEP), is an electrosurgical procedure that has largely replaced cold-blade conization of the cervix in the management of CIN (118, 162, 163). It requires local anesthesia. It has been associated with higher rates of preterm deliveries.

Cryotherapy and Heat Therapy

Cryotherapy, or treatment by cold, relies on three types of cryogenics: carbonic ice (boiling temperature, −78.5°C), nitrous oxide (−89.5°C), and liquid nitrogen (−196°C) (74). The treatment is delivered by a cryogenic pencil, a cotton swab, a cryoprobe, or a spray. Cryogenic pencils have been responsible for wart transmission, making liquid nitrogen spray the preferred method of delivery. The aim is to produce an ice ball around the lesion in the form of a frozen halo extending 1 to 2 mm beyond the margins. Some advocate a second freezing immediately after the lesion thaws, which may be advantageous for the treatment of plantar warts if not hand warts. Freezing is accompanied by a brief stinging pain. Mild discomfort or pain may reappear after tissue thawing. Scarring is infrequent and usually minimal (19). The procedure is well tolerated by the vast majority of patients (19). Cryotherapy is widely used for the treatment of most HPV diseases, including CIN (62, 142). It is also the procedure of choice for pregnant patients.

Heat has been used to a lesser extent than cold to treat HPV diseases. In one study, an infrared coagulator was effective in completely eradicating condyloma acuminatum in 82% of patients (7). This technique is also becoming attractive for the treatment of AIN, including high grade, because of good clearance and control rates of the disease (63). Cold coagulation requires a 100°C probe to be in contact with the lesion for 20 s. This technique has been applied to the treatment of CIN, with success rates exceeding 93% in some uncontrolled experiments. Anecdotal but dramatic improvements have been reported after either immersion of cutaneous warts in a 45 to 50°C water bath for up to 75 min or application of a radiofrequency heat generator for 30 to 60 s (140). In a controlled experiment, 86% of 29 treated warts disappeared, compared to 41% of 17 control warts (140).

Laser Therapy

Lasers deliver high-energy, monochromatic, collimated light. The CO_2 laser has been the laser of choice for the treatment of HPV diseases, but the pulsed-dye, argon, and KTP lasers have also been used (26, 44, 99, 165). The energy of its infrared light (λ = 10,600 nm) is well absorbed by the intracellular water, which is then vaporized. Varying the width of the beam controls the energy density of the light delivered, which can be used for cutting (narrow beam) or superficial vaporization (broad beam) (119). One can reduce the energy of a broad beam so that the tissue is coagulated rather than vaporized, a technique called brushing. An additional variable is how the light is emitted: continuously, pulsed, or superpulsed, the last being favored. The determination of proper laser techniques has been largely empirical. The great variation in the techniques used may account for differences in outcomes (26, 99, 119). Because of the pain generated and the need for the patient's cooperation, laser ablation usually requires local or general anesthesia. A lidocaine/prilocaine cream (EMLA cream) is an effective solution for local anesthesia of the external genitalia. Postoperative pain, bleeding, swelling, and scarring occur in up to a quarter of the patients treated. The high cost of the procedure is an additional drawback. Laser therapy is a suitable option for the treatment of vulvar warts during pregnancy.

Photodynamic laser therapy is an evolving and successful approach for the treatment of cutaneous warts, genital HPV diseases, and recurrent respiratory papillomatosis (42, 89). The concept is to deliver a photosensitizing agent to the lesion, either topically (5-aminolevulinic acid) or systemically [e.g., *meso*-tetra (*m*-hydroxyphenyl)porphyrin (*m*-THPP) or 5-aminolevulinic acid]. Exposure of the tumor to intense light of the proper wavelength activates the compound and selectively destroys the tissue.

Occlusive Therapy

The therapeutic application on the wart of an occlusive dressing with duct tape has received a lot of popular attention, especially after the positive results of a randomized clinical trial (56). This trial had limitations with blinding and follow-up, and two subsequent trials failed to replicate these results (40, 154).

Therapeutic Vaccines

Many efforts are ongoing to develop a therapeutic vaccine, with E6 and E7 usually being the targets, using approaches as diverse as chimeric VLPs, peptides, proteins, viral or bacterial vectors, and nucleic acids and cell-based or prime-boost strategies (24, 77). The few successes have been modest and have not been validated with phase III clinical trials. ZYC101a, for example, is a plasmid DNA coding for HPV-16 E7 HLA-A-2-restricted sequences and HPV-18 E6 and E7 sequences encapsulated in biodegradable microparticles (59). It was administered intramuscularly to women with CIN2 or 3 in a phase II study. The two different dosages tried were associated with CIN regression at conization compared to placebo, but only in women younger than 25 years. HspE7 is a fusion protein of the heat shock protein 65 of bacillus Calmette-Guérin with an HPV-16 E7 sequence. This vaccine has been used with encouraging, if modest, results in uncontrolled phase II studies of AIN, recurrent respiratory papillomatosis, and CIN (42, 77).

Suggestion, Hypnosis, and Homeopathy

The idea that cutaneous warts respond to suggestion is widely disseminated, but randomized, controlled studies have failed to provide convincing evidence of a suggestion effect (88). Hypnosis was found by some investigators to be superior to suggestion, but it appears that the results are inconsistent and the methodologies are defective (54, 88). Homeopathy has so far failed to show superiority to placebo for the treatment of either plantar or cutaneous warts (89).

Management and Treatment Approaches

Our incomplete knowledge of the natural history of HPV diseases and of the comparative effectiveness and tolerance of the available therapies has unfortunately resulted in a wide variety of management options whose relative merits are often difficult to ascertain. Table 8 offers some guidelines, and the following section addresses more specific points of management.

Cutaneous Warts

Health practitioners probably treat only a minority of cutaneous warts. In most patients the lesions cause little inconvenience and resolve spontaneously, making treatment unjustified. None of the comparative trials available has shown differences in effectiveness between SAL paint, cryotherapy, and glutaraldehyde for the treatment of common warts (89). A combination of SAL paint and cryotherapy does not give cure rates that are substantially different from those of either treatment alone. Paring of plantar warts prior to topical treatment increases the effectiveness of the treatment. This can be done by the patient using a pumice stone, or by the practitioner with a scalpel blade. SAL paints and fixatives can be applied by the patient and should be the first line of treatment. It is important to remember that no treatment is highly successful; the complete response rate is about 60 to 70% at 3 months (89). It is therefore important to avoid the production of scars.

Epidermodysplasia verruciformis lesions should be monitored for premalignant and malignant transformation, as well as protected from sun exposure (93). Excisional surgery, cryotherapy, or laser surgery can be used for the management of the lesions (93). Grafting may be necessary to cover extensive skin defects, and artificial skin has been used successfully to that effect.

Anogenital Lesions

Condyloma Acuminatum

Treatment for condyloma acuminatum is aimed at improving cosmesis and psychological well-being, relieving symptoms, or freeing an obstructed birth canal. We do not know the impact of treatment on HPV infection transmission, on the rare development of an HPV-related malignancy, or on the acquisition of recurrent respiratory papillomatosis in the newborn (6, 107). Presently, treatment should not seek to eradicate HPV infection or subclinical infection; such attempts have failed and caused high rates of morbidity (120). Therefore, treatment is not appropriate for every patient. The benefits should be weighed against adverse effects and costs associated with therapy and against the possibility of spontaneous resolution, which occurs within 3 to 4 months in approximately 10 to 20% of patients. With the possible exception of long disease duration, there are no strong or reliable indicators of disease refractoriness to treatment (19). Warts appearing at new sites (recurrence) or during treatment can be treated with the same therapy. Warts appearing at previously treated sites (relapse) may benefit from a different therapy.

There is no evidence that evaluating and treating the male partner has an impact on HPV infection, CIN risk, or disease relapse in the treated woman (120, 160). However, no comparable data exist regarding the female partner of the male patient. At present, partner evaluation is not necessary for the management of the patient, but it may be appropriate in order to address specific STD transmission risks, education, and counseling (160). Condom use can be beneficial in couples in which at least one of the partners has HPV disease (12).

Podophyllin is inferior to podofilox, excisional surgery, electrosurgery, and cryotherapy (26, 31, 142, 160). Although podofilox is more effective than podophyllin, both drugs are associated with high recurrence rates. Podofilox is superior to a vehicle only in preventing recurrences when used prophylactically after treatment. Cryotherapy and TCA application appear to be therapeutically equivalent, and cryotherapy is not significantly different from electrosurgery (142). Intralesional interferon treatment has been found to be more effective than placebo, but most studies have failed to show similar superiority with parenteral interferon. When used in combination, interferon treatment adds little to the efficacy of cryotherapy or laser therapy, but it does enhance the effect of podophyllin (19).

Podofilox is an attractive form of treatment because it is administered by the patient. Imiquimod is also self-administered and is probably more effective overall. However, a complete response may take up to 16 weeks of treatment, and men fare significantly less well than women (50). The simplest and most effective office-based treatment modalities are cryotherapy and TCA application. Podophyllin is less effective, and electrosurgery requires both equipment and skills. Surgical excision with scissors is well suited to the treatment of lesions that are small in size and number. Urethral warts can be treated with podophyllin or cryotherapy (160). Interferon treatment or laser surgery should not be first-line choices because of their high cost. For recalcitrant lesions, intralesional interferon is useful for small numbers of lesions and laser surgery is useful for numerous ones.

Cryotherapy, TCA application, electrosurgery, cold-blade excision, and laser surgery are all appropriate for the treatment of condyloma acuminatum in the pregnant patient. Anogenital warts in immunocompromised patients respond relatively poorly to treatment (17). Intralesional interferon is ineffective in HIV-seropositive patients, but imiquimod has been beneficial in a very modest way on the partial clearance of lesions or on decreasing the recurrence rate (17, 37). Since the aim is often to control the disease rather than to eradicate it, one should choose approaches that minimize the potential side effects of cumulative treatments.

No intervention, either as a primary approach or because of previous treatment failures, may be necessary in the absence of changing lesions, intraepithelial neoplasia, or carcinoma, provided proper follow-up and evaluation (e.g., yearly) are done.

Internal Warts and Intraepithelial Neoplasias

The evaluation and management of intraepithelial neoplasias and internal warts should be left to experienced practitioners. Guidelines have been established for the cervix (162, 163). The scarcity of rigorous comparative studies makes it difficult to evaluate the respective merits of several proposed therapies for these conditions. This is compounded in some instances by the complete absence of adequate natural history data.

The most common treatments include cryotherapy (cryoprobes should not be used for vaginal warts due to the risk of perforation), surgical cold-blade excision for intra-anal warts, and laser surgery. 5-FU for therapy or recurrence prophylaxis for vaginal warts has fallen out of favor because of the often severe adverse effects, including ulcerations. TCA application and interferon with or without electrosurgery are among additional options for the treatment of vaginal or cervical warts.

VIN were traditionally treated by vulvectomy, whose mutilating outcome can be palliated by simultaneous grafting (skinning vulvectomy). In expert hands, laser therapy offers better cosmetic results. Treatment with a 5-FU cream is poorly tolerated when applied daily, but a less intensive regimen is effective for prophylaxis. The topical application of 2 g of 5% 5-FU cream twice a week for 6 months resulted in a twofold reduction in the rate of CIN relapse compared to no treatment in HIV-positive women who had undergone CIN 3 treatment by ablative methods (91). Like its vulvar counterpart, PIN has been treated with radiotherapy, cold-blade surgery, cryotherapy, and, more recently, laser surgery (151). In treating VAIN, radiotherapy has been largely replaced by laser surgery. 5-FU cream regimens have also been used. Surgical excision, cryotherapy, TCA, electrosurgery, and podophyllin have all been used but not compared for the treatment of anal intraepithelial neoplasia (17, 86). Electrosurgery (LEEP), laser surgery, and cryotherapy are the three major options available for treatment of CIN (39, 99, 118). These techniques have largely supplanted cold-knife conization, particularly LEEP, which is speedy and technically less demanding. Overall, they appear to be quite comparable in effectiveness, and choice is dictated by equipment availability and lesion size and location (39, 99).

Patient Education

The public is largely uninformed about genital HPV disease, and the information is complex; thus, education is a necessary part of the practitioner-patient interaction. The diagnosis of genital HPV disease is emotionally charged, and education is also an opportunity to engage the trust of the patient so that optimal care can be offered. For patients and health professionals, abundant high-quality and current information materials (including in Spanish) about HPV are easily available on the World Wide Web from the Centers for Disease Control and Prevention (CDC) (http://www.cdc.gov/std/hpv/default.htm). The American Social Health Association (http://www.ashastd.org) also offers excellent resources for patients, including links to support groups. The two organizations operate the same hotline at 1-800-227-8922 (Monday through Friday from 9:00 a.m. to 8:00 p.m., eastern standard time).

Recurrent Respiratory Papillomatosis

Although numerous therapeutic options have been considered for the treatment of recurrent respiratory papillomatosis, the microdebrider device is now favored by most American surgeons instead of the CO_2 laser or cold-steel surgery (42). Photodynamic laser therapy will probably gain acceptance due to early encouraging results. Because many patients require scores of procedures during a lifetime, selection of a skilled operator is essential to minimize long-term side effects. Tracheostomy should be avoided since the surgical site often becomes involved with the disease, which may also spread further down the respiratory tree. Radiotherapy of recurrent respiratory papillomatosis has been associated with malignant transformation and is contraindicated. Parenteral interferon is used as an adjuvant therapy. A randomized, controlled trial of IFN-α-n3 proved disappointing because the benefits of treatment appeared limited to the first 6 months. A subsequent trial with lymphoblastoid IFN-α-n1 was more encouraging and indicated that about one-fourth of the treated patients benefit from a long-lasting response. Adjuvant treatment with intralesional cidofovir has now replaced oral ribavirin, but convincing evidence for either treatment is lacking (42). Most patients will have tried I3C (Indoplex). Patients and families may find support and information at the Recurrent Respiratory Papillomatosis Foundation (http://www.rrpf.org), the International RRP ISA Center (http://www.rrpwebsite.org; P.O. Box 30821, Seattle, WA 98113-0821), or the American Laryngeal Papilloma Foundation (http://www.alpf.org) (c/o William Lazar, P.O. Box 6108, Spring Hill, FL 34611; telephone and fax, 352-684-7191).

Oral Warts

Surgical excision, cryotherapy, and podophyllin application are among the therapeutic choices for the management of oral warts (3). Focal epithelial hyperplasia usually does not require treatment because of its self-limited evolution.

REFERENCES

1. **American College of Obstetricians and Gynecologists.** 2003. ACOG practice bulletin. Cervical cytology screening. No. 45, August 2003. *Int. J. Gynaecol. Obstet.* **83:** 237–247.
2. **Antonsson, A., O. Forslund, H. Ekberg, G. Sterner, and B. Göran Hansson.** 2000. The ubiquity and impressive genomic diversity of human skin papillomaviruses suggest a commensalic nature of these viruses. *J. Virol.* **74:**11636–11641.
3. **Baccaglini, L., J. C. Atkinson, L. L. Patton, M. Glick, G. Ficarra, and D. E. Peterson.** 2007. Management of oral lesions in HIV-positive patients. *Oral Surg. Oral Med. Oral Pathol. Oral Radiol. Endod.* **103**(Suppl.)**:**S50e1–S50e23.

3a. **Baker, T. S., W. W. Newcomb, N. H. Olson, L. M. Cowsert, and J. C. Brown.** 1991. Structures of bovine and human papillomaviruses. Analysis by cryoelectron microscopy and three-dimensional image reconstruction. *Biophys. J.* **60:**1445–1456.

4. **Ballagh, S.** 2004. Factors affecting the reproducibility and validity of colposcopy for product development: review of current literature. *J. Acquir. Immune Defic. Syndr.* **37**(Suppl. 3)**:**S152–S155.
5. **Barnett, N., H. Mak, and J. A. Winkelstein.** 1983. Extensive verrucosis in primary immunodeficiency diseases. *Arch. Dermatol.* **119:**5–7.
6. **Barrett, T. J., J. D. Silbar, and J. P. McGinley.** 1954. Genital warts—a venereal disease. *JAMA* **154:**333–334.
7. **Bekassy, Z., and L. Weström.** 1987. Infrared coagulation in the treatment of condyloma acuminata in the female genital tract. *Sex. Transm. Dis.* **14:**209–212.
8. **Berek, J. S.** 2003. Simplification of the new Bethesda 2001 classification system. *Am. J. Obstet. Gynecol.* **188:** S2–S5; discussion, S6–S7.
9. **Beutner, K. R., D. J. Wiley, J. M. Douglas, S. K. Tyring, K. Fife, K. Trofatter, and K. M. Stone.** 1998. Genital warts and their treatment. *Clin. Infect. Dis.* **28:**S37–S56.
10. **Biggar, R. J., A. K. Chaturvedi, J. J. Goedert, and E. A. Engels.** 2007. AIDS-related cancer and severity of immunosuppression in persons with AIDS. *J. Natl. Cancer Inst.* **99:**962–972.
11. **Bingham, E. A.** 1994. Significance of anogenital warts in children. *Br. J. Hosp. Med.* **53:**469–472.

12. **Bleeker, M. C., J. Berkhof, C. J. Hogewoning, F. J. Voorhorst, A. J. van den Brule, T. M. Starink, P. J. Snijders, and C. J. Meijer.** 2005. HPV type concordance in sexual couples determines the effect of condoms on regression of flat penile lesions. *Br. J. Cancer* **92:**1388–1392.
13. **Bonnez, W.** 2005. The HPV xenograft severe combined immunodeficiency mouse model. *Methods Mol. Med.* **119:** 203–216.
14. **Bonnez, W.** 2007. Human papillomavirus vaccine—recent results and future developments. *Curr. Opin. Pharmacol.* **7:**1–8.
15. **Bonnez, W.** 2002. Issues with HIV and oral human papillomavirus infections. *AIDS Reader* **12:**174–176.
16. **Bonnez, W.** 2002. Papillomaviruses, p. 1349–1374. *In* V. L. Yu, R. Weber, and D. Raoult (ed.), *Antimicrobial Therapy and Vaccines*, 2nd ed., vol. 1. *Microbes*. Apple Tree Productions, LLC, New York, NY.
17. **Bonnez, W.** 2008. Sexually transmitted human papillomavirus infection, p. 953–980. *In* R. Dolin, H. Masur, and M. Saag (ed.), *AIDS Therapy*, 3rd ed. W. B. Saunders, Philadelphia, PA.
18. **Bonnez, W., C. DaRin, C. Borkhuis, K. de Mesy Jensen, R. C. Reichman, and R. C. Rose.** 1998. Isolation and propagation of human papillomavirus type 16 in human xenografts implanted in the severe combined immunodeficiency mouse. *J. Virol.* **72:**5256–5261.
19. **Bonnez, W., D. Oakes, A. Bailey-Farchione, A. Choi, D. Hallahan, P. Pappas, M. Halloway, L. Corey, G. Barnum, A. Dunne, M. H. Stoler, L. M. Demeter, and R. C. Reichman.** 1995. A randomized, double-blind, placebo-controlled trial of systemically administered alpha-, beta-, or gamma-interferon in combination with cryotherapy for the treatment of condyloma acuminatum. *J. Infect. Dis.* **171:**1081–1089.
20. **Bonnez, W., D. Oakes, A. Choi, S. J. D'Arcy, P. G. Pappas, L. Corey, M. H. Stoler, L. M. Demeter, and R. C. Reichman.** 1996. Therapeutic efficacy and complications of excisional biopsy of condyloma acuminatum. *Sex. Transm. Dis.* **23:**273–276.
21. **Bonnez, W., R. C. Rose, C. Borkhuis, C. Da Rin, and R. C. Reichman.** 1994. Evaluation of the temperature sensitivity of human papillomavirus (HPV) type 11 using the human xenograft severe combined immunodeficiency (SCID) mouse model. *J. Clin. Microbiol.* **32:**1575–1577.
22. **Boxman, I. L. A., A. Hogewoning, L. H. C. Mulder, J. N. Bouwes Bawinck, and J. ter Schegget.** 1999. Detection of human papillomavirus types 6 and 11 in pubic and perianal hair from patients with genital warts. *J. Clin. Microbiol.* **37:**2270–2273.
23. **Breitburd, F., and P. Coursaget.** 1999. Human papillomavirus vaccines. *Semin. Cancer Biol.* **9:**431–444.
24. **Brinkman, J. A., S. H. Hughes, P. Stone, A. S. Caffrey, L. I. Muderspach, L. D. Roman, J. S. Weber, and W. M. Kast.** 2007. Therapeutic vaccination for HPV induced cervical cancers. *Dis. Markers* **23:**337–352.
25. **Buchwald, C., and B. Norrild.** 1997. Human papillomavirus in sinonasal papillomas and in normal mucosa. *Papillomavirus Rep.* **8:**99–104.
26. **Buck, H. W., Jr.** 2007. Warts (genital). *BMJ Clin. Evidence* **12:**1–20.
27. **Buckley, D. A., and A. W. Du Vivier.** 2001. The therapeutic use of topical contact sensitizers in benign dermatoses. *Br. J. Dermatol.* **145:**385–405.
28. **Burchell, A. N., R. L. Winer, S. de Sanjosé, and E. L. Franco.** 2006. Chapter 6. Epidemiology and transmission dynamics of genital HPV infection. *Vaccine* **24**(Suppl. 3)**:** S52–S61.
29. **Burd, E. M.** 2007. Human papillomavirus detection and utility of testing. *Clin. Microbiol. Newsl.* **29:**159–167.
30. **Campo, M. S.** 2002. Animal models of papillomavirus pathogenesis. *Virus Res.* **89:**249–261.
31. **Centers for Disease Control and Prevention.** 2007. *Sexually Transmitted Disease Surveillance, 2006*. Centers for Disease Control and Prevention, Atlanta, GA.
32. **Chang, G. J., J. M. Berry, N. Jay, J. M. Palefsky, and M. L. Welton.** 2002. Surgical treatment of high-grade anal squamous intraepithelial lesions: a prospective study. *Dis. Colon Rectum* **45:**453–458.
33. **Chang, Y. C., V. Madkan, R. Cook-Norris, K. Sra, and S. Tyring.** 2005. Current and potential uses of imiquimod. *South. Med. J.* **98:**913–920.
34. **Christensen, N. D., J. W. Kreider, K. V. Shah, and R. F. Rando.** 1992. Detection of human serum antibodies that neutralize infectious human papillomavirus type 11 virions. *J. Gen. Virol.* **73:**1261–1267.
35. **Chuang, T.-Y., H. O. Perry, L. T. Kurland, and D. M. Ilstrup.** 1984. Condyloma acuminatum in Rochester, Minn, 1950–1978. I. Epidemiology and clinical features. *Arch. Dermatol.* **120:**469–475.
36. **Clifford, G., S. Franceschi, M. Diaz, N. Munoz, and L. L. Villa.** 2006. Chapter 3. HPV type-distribution in women with and without cervical neoplastic diseases. *Vaccine* **24**(Suppl. 3)**:**S26–S34.
37. **Conant, M. A.** 2000. Immunomodulatory therapy in the management of viral infections in patients with HIV infection. *J. Am. Acad. Dermatol.* **43:**S27–S30.
38. **Cox, J. T.** 2006. Human papillomavirus testing in primary cervical screening and abnormal Papanicolaou management. *Obstet. Gynecol. Surv.* **61:**S15–S25.
39. **Cox, J. T.** 1999. Management of cervical intraepithelial neoplasia. *Lancet* **353:**857–859.
40. **de Haen, M., M. G. Spigt, C. J. van Uden, P. van Neer, F. J. Feron, and A. Knottnerus.** 2006. Efficacy of duct tape vs placebo in the treatment of verruca vulgaris (warts) in primary school children. *Arch. Pediatr. Adolesc. Med.* **160:**1121–1125.
41. **Demeter, L. M., M. H. Stoler, W. Bonnez, P. Pappas, L. Corey, J. Strussenberg, and R. C. Reichman.** 1993. Penile intraepithelial neoplasia: clinical presentation and an analysis of the physical state of human papillomavirus DNA. *J. Infect. Dis.* **168:**38–46.
42. **Derkay, C. S., and D. H. Darrow.** 2006. Recurrent respiratory papillomatosis. *Ann. Otol. Rhinol. Laryngol.* **115:** 1–11.
43. **de Sanjose, S., M. Diaz, X. Castellsague, G. Clifford, L. Bruni, N. Munoz, and F. X. Bosch.** 2007. Worldwide prevalence and genotype distribution of cervical human papillomavirus DNA in women with normal cytology: a meta-analysis. *Lancet Infect. Dis.* **7:**453–459.
44. **de Villiers, E. M., C. Fauquet, T. R. Broker, H. U. Bernard, and H. zur Hausen.** 2004. Classification of papillomaviruses. *Virology* **324:**17–27.
44a. **Dinh, T. H., M. Sternberg, E. F. Dunne, and L. E. Markowitz.** 2008. Genital warts among 18- to 59-year-olds in the United States, national health and nutrition examination survey, 1999–2004. *Sex. Transm. Dis.* **35:**357–360.
45. **Doorbar, J.** 2005. The papillomavirus life cycle. *J. Clin. Virol.* 32(Suppl. 1)**:**S7–S15.
46. **D'Souza, G., A. R. Kreimer, R. Viscidi, M. Pawlita, C. Fakhry, W. M. Koch, W. H. Westra, and M. L. Gillison.** 2007. Case-control study of human papillomavirus and oropharyngeal cancer. *N. Engl. J. Med.* **356:**1944–1956.
47. **Dunne, E. F., C. M. Nielson, K. M. Stone, L. E. Markowitz, and A. R. Giuliano.** 2006. Prevalence of HPV infection among men: a systematic review of the literature. *J. Infect. Dis.* **194:**1044–1057.

48. Reference deleted.
49. **Dunne, E. F., E. R. Unger, M. Sternberg, G. McQuillan, D. C. Swan, S. S. Patel, and L. E. Markowitz.** 2007. Prevalence of HPV infection among females in the United States. *JAMA* **297:**81381–81389.
50. **Edwards, L.** 2000. Imiquimod in clinical practice. *J. Am. Acad. Dermatol.* **43:**S12–S17.
51. **Egelkrout, E. M., and D. A. Galloway.** 2007. The humoral immune response to human papillomavirus, p. 277–312. *In* R. L. Garcea and D. DiMaio (ed.), *The Papillomaviruses*. Springer, New York, NY.
52. **Eiben Lyons, G., M. I. Nishimura, and W. M. Kast.** 2007. Cell-mediated immune responses to human papillomavirus, p. 313–335. *In* R. L. Garcea and D. DiMaio (ed.), *The Papillomaviruses*. Springer, New York, NY.
53. **Engels, E. A., R. M. Pfeiffer, J. J. Goedert, P. Virgo, T. S. McNeel, S. M. Scoppa, and R. J. Biggar.** 2006. Trends in cancer risk among people with AIDS in the United States 1980–2002. *AIDS* **20:**1645–1654.
54. **Erwin, D. M.** 1992. Hypnotherapy for warts (verruca vulgaris): 41 consecutive cases with 33 cures. *Am. J. Clin. Hypn.* **35:**1–10.
55. **Farley, J., J. W. McBroom, and C. M. Zahn.** 2005. Current techniques for the evaluation of abnormal cervical cytology. *Clin. Obstet. Gynecol.* **48:**133–146.
56. **Focht, D. R., III, C. Spicer, and M. P. Fairchok.** 2002. The efficacy of duct tape vs cryotherapy in the treatment of verruca vulgaris (the common wart). *Arch. Pediatr. Adolesc. Med.* **156:**971–974.
57. **Franco, E. L.** 1996. Epidemiology of anogenital warts and cancer. *Obstet. Gynecol. Clin. N. Am.* **23:**597–623.
58. **Frisch, M., B. Glimelius, A. J. van den Brule, J. Wohlfahrt, C. J. Meijer, J. M. Walboomers, S. Goldman, C. Svensson, H. O. Adami, and M. Melbye.** 1997. Sexually transmitted infection as a cause of anal cancer. *N. Engl. J. Med.* **337:**1350–1358.
59. **Garcia, F., K. U. Petry, L. Muderspach, M. A. Gold, P. Braly, C. P. Crum, M. Magill, M. Silverman, R. G. Urban, M. L. Hedley, and K. J. Beach.** 2004. ZYC101a for treatment of high-grade cervical intraepithelial neoplasia: a randomized controlled trial. *Obstet. Gynecol.* **103:**317–326.
60. **Garcia-Pineres, A. J., A. Hildesheim, R. Herrero, M. Trivett, M. Williams, I. Atmetlla, M. Ramirez, M. Villegas, M. Schiffman, A. C. Rodriguez, R. D. Burk, M. Hildesheim, E. Freer, J. Bonilla, C. Bratti, J. A. Berzofsky, and L. A. Pinto.** 2006. Persistent human papillomavirus infection is associated with a generalized decrease in immune responsiveness in older women. *Cancer Res.* **66:**11070–11076.
61. **Giuliano, A. R., R. Harris, R. L. Sedjo, S. Baldwin, D. Roe, M. R. Papenfuss, M. Abrahamsen, P. Inserra, S. Olvera, and K. Hatch.** 2002. Incidence, prevalence, and clearance of type-specific human papillomavirus infections: The Young Women's Health Study. *J. Infect. Dis.* **186:**462–469.
62. **Glover, M. G.** 1990. Plantar warts. *Foot Ankle* **11:**172–178.
63. **Goldstone, S. E., A. Z. Kawalek, and J. W. Huyett.** 2005. Infrared coagulator: a useful tool for treating anal squamous intraepithelial lesions. *Dis. Colon Rectum* **48:**1042–1054.
64. **Gutman, L. T., M. E. Herman-Giddens, and W. C. Phelps.** 1993. Transmission of human genital papillomavirus disease: comparison of data from adults and children. *Pediatrics* **91:**31–38.
65. **Hammerschlag, M. R.** 1998. Sexually transmitted diseases in sexually abused children: medical and legal implications. *Sex. Transm. Dis.* **74:**167–174.
66. **Hartmann, K. E., K. Nanda, S. Hall, and E. Myers.** 2001. Technologic advances for evaluation of cervical cytology: is newer better? *Obstet. Gynecol. Surv.* **56:**765–774.
67. **Hebner, C. M., and L. A. Laimins.** 2006. Human papillomaviruses: basic mechanisms of pathogenesis and oncogenicity. *Rev. Med. Virol.* **16:**83–97.
68. **Ho, G. Y., R. Bierman, L. Beardsley, C. J. Chang, and R. D. Burk.** 1998. Natural history of cervicovaginal papillomavirus infection in young women. *N. Engl. J. Med.* **338:**423–428.
69. **Ho, G. Y. F., R. D. Burk, S. Klein, A. S. Kadish, C. J. Chang, P. Palan, J. Basu, R. Tachezy, R. Lewis, and S. Romney.** 1995. Persistent genital human papillomavirus infection as a risk factor for persistent cervical dysplasia. *J. Natl. Cancer Inst.* **87:**1365–1371.
70. **Ho, L., S.-K. Tay, S.-Y. Chan, and H.-U. Bernard.** 1993. Sequence variants of human papillomavirus type 16 from couples suggest sexual transmission with low infectivity and polyclonality in genital neoplasia. *J. Infect. Dis.* **168:**803–809.
71. **Hornor, G.** 2004. Ano-genital warts in children: sexual abuse or not? *J. Pediatr. Health Care* **18:**165–170.
72. **Jablonska, S., and S. Majewski.** 1994. Epidermodysplasia verruciformis: immunological and clinical aspects. *Curr. Top. Microbiol. Immunol.* **186:**157–175.
73. **Jablonska, S., S. Majewski, S. Obalek, and G. Orth.** 1997. Cutaneous warts. *Clin. Dermatol.* **15:**309–319.
74. **Jackson, A. D.** 1999. Cryosurgery: a guide for GPs. *Practitioner* **243:**131–136.
75. **Jemal, A., R. Siegel, E. Ward, T. Murray, J. Xu, and M. J. Thun.** 2007. Cancer statistics, 2007. *CA Cancer J. Clin.* **57:**43–66.
76. **Johnson, L. W.** 1995. Communal showers and the risk of plantar warts. *J. Fam. Pract.* **40:**136–138.
77. **Kadish, A. S., and M. H. Einstein.** 2005. Vaccine strategies for human papillomavirus-associated cancers. *Curr. Opin. Oncol.* **17:**456–461.
78. **Kanodia, S., L. M. Fahey, and W. M. Kast.** 2007. Mechanisms used by human papillomaviruses to escape the host immune response. *Curr. Cancer Drug Targets* **7:**79–89.
79. **Kiire, C. A., and B. Dhillon.** 2006. The aetiology and associations of conjunctival intraepithelial neoplasia. *Br. J. Ophthalmol.* **90:**109–113.
80. **Kilkenny, M., K. Merlin, R. Young, and R. Marks.** 1998. The prevalence of common skin conditions in Australian school students. 1. Common, plane and plantar viral warts. *Br. J. Dermatol.* **138:**840–845.
81. **Kjaer, S. K., T. N. Tran, P. Sparen, L. Tryggvadottir, C. Munk, E. Dasbach, K. L. Liaw, J. Nygard, and M. Nygard.** 2007. The burden of genital warts: a study of nearly 70,000 women from the general female population in the 4 Nordic countries. *J. Infect. Dis.* **196:**1447–1454.
82. **Kokelj, F., E. Baraggino, G. Stinco, and U. Wiesenfeld.** 1993. Study of the partners of women with human papillomavirus infection. *Int. J. Dermatol.* **32:**661–663.
83. **Koshiol, J. E., S. A. Laurent, and J. M. Pimenta.** 2004. Rate and predictors of new genital warts claims and genital warts-related healthcare utilization among privately insured patients in the United States. *Sex. Transm. Dis.* **31:**748–752.
84. **Koutsky, L.** 1997. Epidemiology of genital human papillomavirus infection. *Am. J. Med.* **102:**3–8.
85. **Koutsky, L. A.** 2007. Quadrivalent vaccine against human papillomavirus to prevent high-grade cervical lesions. *N. Engl. J. Med.* **356:**1915–1927.
86. **Lacey, C. J.** 2005. Therapy for genital human papillomavirus-related disease. *J. Clin. Virol.* **32**(Suppl. 1)**:**S82–S90.
87. **Leigh, I. M., J. A. Buchanan, C. A. Harwood, R. Cerio, and A. Storey.** 1999. Role of human papillomaviruses in

cutaneous and oral manifestations of immunosuppression. *J. Acquir. Immune Defic. Syndr.* **21**:S49–S57.

88. **Lipke, M. M.** 2006. An armamentarium of wart treatments. *Clin. Med. Res.* **4**:273–293.
89. **Luk, N. M., and Y. M. Tang.** 2007. Warts (nongenital). *BMJ Clin. Evidence* **12**:1–18.
90. **Madeleine, M. M., L. G. Johnson, A. G. Smith, J. A. Hansen, B. B. Nisperos, S. Li, L. P. Zhao, J. R. Daling, S. M. Schwartz, and D. A. Galloway.** 2008. Comprehensive analysis of HLA-A, HLA-B, HLA-C, HLA-DRB1, and HLA-DQB1 loci and squamous cell cervical cancer risk. *Cancer Res.* **68**:3532–3539.
91. **Maiman, M., D. H. Watts, J. Andersen, P. Clax, M. Merino, and M. A. Kendall.** 1999. Vaginal 5-fluorouracil for high-grade cervical dysplasia in human immunodeficiency virus infection: a randomized trial. *Obstet. Gynecol.* **94**:954–961.
92. **Maitland, N. J., M. Keefe, A. al-Ghamdi, and D. Coggon.** 1995. Human papillomavirus type 7 and the butcher's wart. *Papillomavirus Rep.* **6**:33–37.
93. **Majewski, S., and S. Jablonska.** 1995. Epidermodysplasia verruciformis as a model of human papillomavirus-induced genetic cancer of the skin. *Arch. Dermatol.* **131**: 1312–1318.
94. **Manhart, L. E., K. K. Holmes, L. A. Koutsky, T. R. Wood, D. L. Kenney, Q. Feng, and N. B. Kiviat.** 2006. Human papillomavirus infection among sexually active young women in the United States: implications for developing a vaccination strategy. *Sex. Transm. Dis.* **33**: 502–508.
95. **Maran, A., C. A. Amella, T. P. Di Lorenzo, K. J. Auborn, L. B. Taichman, and B. M. Steinberg.** 1995. Human papillomavirus type 11 transcripts are present at low abundance in latently infected respiratory tissues. *Virology* **212**:285–294.
96. **Markowitz, L. E., E. F. Dunne, M. Saraiya, H. W. Lawson, H. Chesson, and E. R. Unger for the Centers for Disease Control and Prevention and Advisory Committee on Immunization Practices.** 2007. Quadrivalent human papillomavirus vaccine: recommendations of the Advisory Committee on Immunization Practices (ACIP). *Morb. Mortal. Wkly Rep.* **56**:1–24.
97. **Marrazzo, J. M., L. A. Koutsky, N. B. Kiviat, J. M. Kuypers, and K. Stine.** 2001. Papanicolaou test screening and prevalence of genital human papillomavirus among women who have sex with women. *Am. J. Public Health* **91**:947–952.
98. **Martin-Hirsch, P., R. Lilford, G. Jarvis, and H. C. Kitchener.** 1999. Efficacy of cervical-smear collection devices: a systematic review and meta-analysis. *Lancet* **354**:1763–1770.
99. **Martin-Hirsch, P. L., E. Paraskevaidis, and H. Kitchener.** 2000. Surgery for cervical intraepithelial neoplasia. *Cochrane Database of Systematic Reviews* CD001318.
100. **Massing, A. M., and W. L. Epstein.** 1963. Natural history of warts. A two year study. *Arch. Dermatol.* **87**:306–310.
101. **Masur, H., J. E. Kaplan, and K. K. Holmes.** 2002. Guidelines for preventing opportunistic infections among HIV-infected persons—2002. Recommendations of the U.S. Public Health Service and the Infectious Diseases Society of America. *Ann. Intern. Med.* **137**: 435–478.
102. **Melnikow, J., J. Nuovo, A. R. Willan, B. K. Chan, and L. P. Howell.** 1998. Natural history of cervical squamous intraepithelial lesions: a meta-analysis. *Obstet. Gynecol.* **92**:727–735.
103. **Mitchell, M. F., D. Schottenfeld, G. Tortolero-Luna, S. B. Cantor, and R. Richards-Kortum.** 1998. Colposcopy for the diagnosis of squamous intraepithelial lesions: a meta-analysis. *Obstet. Gynecol.* **91**:626–631.
104. **Molijn, A., B. Kleter, W. Quint, and L. J. van Doorn.** 2005. Molecular diagnosis of human papillomavirus (HPV) infections. *J. Clin. Virol.* **32**(Suppl. 1):S43–S51.
105. **Munoz, N., F. X. Bosch, X. Castellsague, M. Diaz, S. de Sanjose, D. Hammouda, K. V. Shah, and C. J. Meijer.** 2004. Against which human papillomavirus types shall we vaccinate and screen? The international perspective. *Int. J. Cancer* **111**:278–285.
106. **Oriel, J. D.** 1971. Anal warts and anal coitus. *Br. J. Vener. Dis.* **47**:373–376.
107. **Oriel, J. D.** 1971. Natural history of genital warts. *Br. J. Vener. Dis.* **47**:1–13.
108. **Orth, G.** 2006. Genetics of epidermodysplasia verruciformis: insights into host defense against papillomaviruses. *Semin. Immunol.* **18**:362–374.
109. **Palefsky, J. M.** 2000. Anal squamous intraepithelial lesions in human immunodeficiency virus-positive men and women. *Semin. Oncol.* **27**:471–479.
110. **Palefsky, J. M., M. L. Gillison, and H. D. Strickler.** 2006. Chapter 16. HPV vaccines in immunocompromised women and men. *Vaccine* **24**(Suppl. 3):S140–S146.
111. **Palefsky, J. M., E. A. Holly, M. L. Ralston, S. P. Arthur, N. Jay, J. M. Berry, M. M. DaCosta, R. Botts, and T. M. Darragh.** 1998. Anal squamous intraepithelial lesions in HIV-positive and HIV-negative homosexual and bisexual men: prevalence and risk factors. *J. Acquir. Immune Defic. Syndr. Hum. Retrovirol.* **17**:320–326.
112. **Palefsky, J. M., E. A. Holly, M. L. Ralston, M. Da Costa, and R. M. Greenblatt.** 2001. Prevalence and risk factors for anal human papillomavirus infection in human immunodeficiency virus (HIV)-positive and high risk HIV-negative women. *J. Infect. Dis.* **183**:383–391.
113. **Parkin, D. M., and F. Bray.** 2006. Chapter 2. The burden of HPV-related cancers. *Vaccine* **24**(Suppl. 3):S11–S25.
114. **Parkin, D. M., F. Bray, J. Ferlay, and P. Pisani.** 2005. Global cancer statistics, 2002. *CA Cancer J. Clin.* **55**: 74–108.
115. **Partridge, J. M., J. P. Hughes, Q. Feng, R. L. Winer, B. A. Weaver, L.-F. Xi, M. E. Stern, S.-K. Lee, S. F. O'Reilly, S. E. Hawes, N. B. Kiviat, and L. A. Koutsky.** 2007. Genital human papillomavirus infection in men: incidence and risk factors in a cohort of university students. *J. Infect. Dis.* **196**:1128–1136.
116. **Partridge, J. M., and L. A. Koutsky.** 2006. Genital human papillomavirus infection in men. *Lancet Infect. Dis.* **6**:21–31.
117. **Praetorius, F.** 1997. HPV-associated diseases of oral mucosa. *Clin. Dermatol.* **15**:399–413.
118. **Prendiville, W.** 1995. Large loop excision of the transformation zone. *Clin. Obstet. Gynecol.* **38**:622–639.
119. **Reid, R.** 1991. Physical and surgical principles of laser surgery in the lower genital tract. *Obstet. Gynecol. Clin. N. Am.* **18**:429–474.
120. **Riva, J. M., T. V. Sedlacek, M. F. Cunnane, and C. E. Mangan.** 1989. Extended carbon dioxide laser vaporization in the treatment of subclinical papillomavirus infection of the lower genital tract. *Obstet. Gynecol.* **73**: 25–30.
121. **Roberts, J. N., C. B. Buck, C. D. Thompson, R. Kines, M. Bernardo, P. L. Choyke, D. R. Lowy, and J. T. Schiller.** 2007. Genital transmission of HPV in a mouse model is potentiated by nonoxynol-9 and inhibited by carrageenan. *Nat. Med.* **13**:857–861.
122. **Rose, R. C., W. Bonnez, C. Da Rin, D. J. McCance, and R. C. Reichman.** 1994. Serological differentiation

of human papillomavirus types 11, 16 and 18 using recombinant virus-like particles. *J. Gen. Virol.* **75:**2445–2449.

123. **Rose, R. C., W. Bonnez, R. C. Reichman, and R. L. Garcea.** 1993. Expression of human papillomavirus type 11 L1 protein in insect cells: in vivo and in vitro assembly of viruslike particles. *J. Virol.* **67:**1936–1944.
124. **Rose, R. C., R. C. Reichman, and W. Bonnez.** 1994. Human papillomavirus type 11 (HPV-11) recombinant virus-like particles (VLPs) induce the formation of neutralizing antibodies and detect HPV-specific antibodies in human sera. *J. Gen. Virol.* **75:**2075–2079.
125. **Rowson, K. E. K., and B. W. J. Mahy.** 1967. Human papova (wart) virus. *Bacteriol. Rev.* **31:**110–131.
126. **Saslow, D., P. E. Castle, J. T. Cox, D. D. Davey, M. H. Einstein, D. G. Ferris, S. J. Goldie, D. M. Harper, W. Kinney, A. B. Moscicki, K. L. Noller, C. M. Wheeler, T. Ades, K. S. Andrews, M. K. Doroshenk, K. G. Kahn, C. Schmidt, O. Shafey, R. A. Smith, E. E. Partridge, Gynecologic Cancer Advisory Group, and F. Garcia.** 2007. American Cancer Society Guideline for human papillomavirus (HPV) vaccine use to prevent cervical cancer and its precursors. *CA Cancer J. Clin.* **57:**7–28.
127. **Saslow, D., C. D. Runowicz, D. Solomon, A. B. Moscicki, R. A. Smith, H. J. Eyre, and C. Cohen.** 2002. American Cancer Society guideline for the early detection of cervical neoplasia and cancer. *CA Cancer J. Clin.* **52:**342–362.
128. **Schiffman, M., P. E. Castle, J. Jeronimo, A. C. Rodriguez, and S. Wacholder.** 2007. Human papillomavirus and cervical cancer. *Lancet* **370:**890–907.
129. **Schiffman, M., R. Herrero, R. Desalle, A. Hildesheim, S. Wacholder, A. C. Rodriguez, M. C. Bratti, M. E. Sherman, J. Morales, D. Guillen, M. Alfaro, M. Hutchinson, T. C. Wright, D. Solomon, Z. Chen, J. Schussler, P. E. Castle, and R. D. Burk.** 2005. The carcinogenicity of human papillomavirus types reflects viral evolution. *Virology* **337:**76–84.
130. **Schwartz, R. A.** 1995. Verrucous carcinoma of the skin and mucosa. *J. Am. Acad. Dermatol.* **32:**1–21.
131. **Smith, E. M., J. M. Ritchie, J. Yankowitz, D. Wang, L. P. Turek, and T. H. Haugen.** 2004. HPV prevalence and concordance in the cervix and oral cavity of pregnant women. *Infect. Dis. Obstet. Gynecol.* **12:**45–56.
132. **Smith, J. S., L. Lindsay, B. Hoots, J. Keys, S. Franceschi, R. Winer, and G. M. Clifford.** 2007. Human papillomavirus type distribution in invasive cervical cancer and high-grade cervical lesions: a meta-analysis update. *Int. J. Cancer* **121:**621–632.
133. **Snijders, P. J., R. D. Steenbergen, D. A. Heideman, and C. J. Meijer.** 2006. HPV-mediated cervical carcinogenesis: concepts and clinical implications. *J. Pathol.* **208:**152–164.
134. **Snoeck, R.** 2006. Papillomavirus and treatment. *Antivir. Res.* **71:**181–191.
135. **Solomon, D., D. Davey, R. Kurman, A. Moriarty, D. O'Connor, M. Prey, S. Raab, M. Sherman, D. Wilbur, T. Wright, Jr., and N. Young.** 2002. The 2001 Bethesda System: terminology for reporting results of cervical cytology. *JAMA* **287:**2114–2119.
136. **Stanley, M.** 2006. Immune responses to human papillomavirus. *Vaccine* **24**(Suppl. 1)**:**S16–S22.
137. **Stanley, M. A., M. R. Pett, and N. Coleman.** 2007. HPV: from infection to cancer. *Biochem. Soc. Trans.* **35:** 1456–1460.
138. **Stenlund, A.** 2007. DNA replication of papillomaviruses, p. 145–174. *In* R. L. Garcea and D. DiMaio (ed.), *The Papillomaviruses*. Springer, New York, NY.
139. **Sterling, J. C.** 2005. Human papillomaviruses and skin cancer. *J. Clin. Virol.* **32**(Suppl. 1)**:**S67–S71.
140. **Stern, P., and N. Levine.** 1992. Controlled localized heat therapy in cutaneous warts. *Arch. Dermatol.* **128:** 945–948.
141. **Stoler, M. H.** 2000. Advances in cervical screening technology. *Mod. Pathol.* **13:**275–284.
142. **Stone, K. M., T. M. Becker, A. Hadgu, and S. J. Kraus.** 1990. Treatment of external genital warts: a randomised clinical trial comparing podophyllin, cryotherapy, and electrodessication. *Genitourin. Med.* **66:**16–19.
143. **Strand, A., and E. Rylander.** 1998. Human papillomavirus. Subclinical and atypical manifestations. *Dermatol. Clin.* **16:**817–822.
144. **Streeck, R. E., H.-C. Selinka, and M. Sapp.** 2007. Viral entry and receptors, p. 89–107. *In* R. L. Garcea and D. DiMaio (ed.), *The Papillomaviruses*. Springer, New York, NY.
145. **Syrjanen, K. J.** 2002. HPV infections and lung cancer. *J. Clin. Pathol.* **55:**885–891.
146. **Syrjanen, K. J.** 2002. HPV infections and oesophageal cancer. *J. Clin. Pathol.* **55:**721–728.
147. **Syrjanen, S.** 2005. Human papillomavirus (HPV) in head and neck cancer. *J. Clin. Virol.* **32**(Suppl. 1)**:**S59–S66.
147a. **Tatti, S., J. M. Swinehart, C. Thielert, H. Tawfik, A. Mescheder, and K. R. Beutner.** 2008. Sinecatechins, a defined green tea extract, in the treatment of external anogenital warts: a randomized controlled trial. *Obstet. Gynecol.* **111:**1371–1379.
148. **Trottier, H., and E. L. Franco.** 2006. The epidemiology of genital human papillomavirus infection. *Vaccine* **24**(Suppl. 1)**:**S1–S15.
149. **Unger, E. R.** 2000. In situ diagnosis of human papillomaviruses. *Clin. Lab. Med.* **20:**289–301.
150. **U.S. Preventive Services Task Force.** January 2003, posting date. Screening for Cervical Cancer. AHRQ publication no. 03-515A, January 2003. Agency for Healthcare Research and Quality, Rockville, MD.
150a. **van Seters, M., M. van Beurden, F. J. ten Kate, I. Beckmann, P. C. Ewing, M. J. Eijkemans, M. J. Kagie, C. J. Meijer, N. K. Aaronson, A. Kleinjan, C. Heijmans-Antonissen, F. J. Zijlstra, M. P. Burger, and T. J. Helmerhorst**. 2008. Treatment of vulvar intraepithelial neoplasia with topical imiquimod. *N. Engl. J. Med.* **358:** 1465–1473.
151. **von Krogh, G., and S. Horenblas.** 2000. The management and prevention of premalignant penile lesions. *Scand. J. Urol. Nephrol.* **34:**220–229.
152. **Walboomers, J. M., M. V. Jacobs, M. M. Manos, F. X. Bosch, J. A. Kummer, K. V. Shah, P. J. Snijders, J. Peto, C. J. Meijer, and N. Munoz.** 1999. Human papillomavirus is a necessary cause of invasive cervical cancer worldwide. *J. Pathol.* **189:**12–19.
153. **Weinstock, H., S. Berman, and W. Cates, Jr.** 2004. Sexually transmitted diseases among American youth: incidence and prevalence estimates, 2000. *Perspect. Sex. Reprod. Health* **36:**6–10.
154. **Wenner, R., S. K. Askari, P. M. Cham, D. A. Kedrowski, A. Liu, and E. M. Warshaw.** 2007. Duct tape for the treatment of common warts in adults: a double-blind randomized controlled trial. *Arch. Dermatol.* **143:** 309–313.
155. **Wikström, A., M.-A. Hedblad, B. Johansson, M. Kalantari, S. Syrjänen, M. Lindberg, and G. von Krogh.** 1992. The acetic acid test in evaluation of subclinical genital papillomavirus infection: a comparative study on penoscopy, histopathology, virology and scanning electron microscopy findings. *Genitourin. Med.* **68:**90–99.

156. **Winer, R. L., J. P. Hughes, Q. Feng, S. O'Reilly, N. B. Kiviat, K. K. Holmes, and L. A. Koutsky.** 2006. Condom use and the risk of genital human papillomavirus infection in young women. *N. Engl. J. Med.* **354:**2645–2654.
157. **Winer, R. L., N. B. Kiviat, J. P. Hughes, D. E. Adam, S. K. Lee, J. M. Kuypers, and L. A. Koutsky.** 2005. Development and duration of human papillomavirus lesions, after initial infection. *J. Infect. Dis.* **191:**731–738.
158. **Winer, R. L., S. K. Lee, J. P. Hughes, D. E. Adam, N. B. Kiviat, and L. A. Koutsky.** 2003. Genital human papillomavirus infection: incidence and risk factors in a cohort of female university students. *Am. J. Epidemiol.* **157:**218–226.
159. **Woodman, C. B., S. I. Collins, and L. S. Young.** 2007. The natural history of cervical HPV infection: unresolved issues. *Nat. Rev. Cancer* **7:**11–22.
160. **Workowski, K. A., and S. M. Berman.** 2006. Sexually transmitted diseases treatment guidelines, 2006. *Morb. Mortal. Wkly. Rep. Recomm. Rep.* **55:**1–94.
161. **Wright, T. C., Jr.** 2003. Chapter 10. Cervical cancer screening using visualization techniques. *J. Natl. Cancer Inst. Monogr.* **31:**66–71.
162. **Wright, T. C., Jr., L. S. Massad, C. J. Dunton, M. Spitzer, E. J. Wilkinson, and D. Solomon.** 2007. 2006 consensus guidelines for the management of women with abnormal cervical cancer screening tests. *Am. J. Obstet. Gynecol.* **197:**346–355.
163. **Wright, T. C., Jr., L. S. Massad, C. J. Dunton, M. Spitzer, E. J. Wilkinson, and D. Solomon.** 2007. 2006 consensus guidelines for the management of women with cervical intraepithelial neoplasia or adenocarcinoma in situ. *Am. J. Obstet. Gynecol.* **197:**340–345.
164. **Xi, L. F., L. A. Koutsky, A. Hildesheim, D. A. Galloway, C. M. Wheeler, R. L. Winer, J. Ho, and N. B. Kiviat.** 2007. Risk for high-grade cervical intraepithelial neoplasia associated with variants of human papillomavirus types 16 and 18. *Cancer Epidemiol. Biomarkers Prev.* **16:**4–10.
165. **Zeitouni, N. C., S. Shieh, and A. R. Oseroff.** 2001. Laser and photodynamic therapy in the management of cutaneous malignancies. *Clin. Dermatol.* **19:**328–338.
166. **Zheng, Z. M., and C. C. Baker.** 2006. Papillomavirus genome structure, expression, and post-transcriptional regulation. *Frontiers Biosci.* **11:**2286–2302.
167. **zur Hausen, H.** 2002. Papillomaviruses and cancer: from basic studies to clinical application. *Nat. Rev. Cancer* **2:** 342–350.

Human Parvoviruses

LARRY J. ANDERSON AND DEAN D. ERDMAN

29

Parvoviruses have been isolated from a wide range of animals, including chickens, geese, cats, dogs, mice, mink, pigs, and raccoons. These viruses tend to be species specific and can cause a variety of serious diseases in their host species (137). The first parvoviruses isolated from humans were adeno-associated parvoviruses, which have not yet been associated with disease in humans. Until recently, the only parvovirus associated with human disease was human parvovirus B19, which was fortuitously identified in 1975 during an evaluation of tests for hepatitis B virus antigens (32). Parvovirus B19 has been associated with erythema infectiosum, transient aplastic crisis, chronic anemia in patients with abnormal immune systems, and hydrops fetalis and has been purported to be associated with a number of other conditions (151). Two additional parvoviruses have recently been detected in humans by molecular screening for new sequences (3, 69). One, human bocavirus (HBoV), has been associated with acute respiratory illness, and the other, PARV4, has yet to be associated with human disease.

VIROLOGY

Classification and Serotypes

Parvoviridae are small, nonenveloped, single-stranded DNA viruses that infect a variety of animals, usually in a species-specific fashion. The family *Parvoviridae* is divided into two subfamilies: the *Densovirinae*, which infect insects, and the *Parvovirinae*, which infect vertebrates. The members of the *Parvovirinae* that infect humans are the focus of this chapter. The subfamily *Parvovirinae* is divided into five genera: *Parvovirus*, *Erythrovirus*, *Dependovirus*, *Amdovirus*, and *Bocavirus* (137). The parvoviruses known to infect humans include B19 parvovirus in the genus *Erythrovirus*, adeno-associated viruses (AAVs) in the genus *Dependovirus*, HBoV in the genus *Bocavirus*, and PARV4 and PARV5, not yet placed into a genus (Fig. 1).

AAVs require coinfection with another virus, usually an adenovirus or herpesvirus, to replicate. AAVs can establish a latent infection by integrating into the host cell genome or in an extrachromosomal state. The ability of AAV DNA to integrate into the human genome in a site-specific manner on chromosome 19 has made them a candidate vector for gene therapy (see chapter 16) (145). Latent AAV can be rescued by infection with a helper virus or in vitro by stressing the cell with UV or ionizing radiation. Members of the other genera in the subfamily *Parvovirinae* do not require a helper virus for productive infection but do require actively dividing cells.

Multiple genotypes of AAV have been detected in humans using PCR-based assays, with many newer types being discovered recently (50). B19 parvovirus has one serotype but three genotypes, 1 to 3. Among these, genotype 1 is presently most commonly detected in the majority of studies. Genotype 2 has been infrequently detected since the 1960s, and genotype 3 has been infrequently detected with the exception of a study in Ghana (37). The three genotypes appear to have similar biological and antigenic properties. To date, sequence studies of HBoV isolates have identified two genotypes (76). Sequence studies of PARV4 and PARV5 isolates have also identified two genotypes, one related to PARV4 and the other related to PARV5 (49).

Composition

Parvoviruses are icosahedral particles between 20 and 25 nm in diameter containing 60 copies of the structural proteins (Fig. 2). B19 capsids contain two proteins, termed VP1 and VP2, whereas AAV capsids contain three proteins, designated VP1 to VP3. X-ray crystallography has been used to determine the structure for a number of parvoviruses, including minute virus of mice; AAV 2, 4, and 5; and B19 parvovirus (72, 73, 112). For some parvoviruses, the location of amino acids associated with cell receptor and antibody binding sites have been determined.

The encapsidated single-stranded DNA genome varies from 4 to 6 kb in size and contains negative-stranded DNA or a combination of negative and positive strands of various proportions. AAV and B19 and presumably PARV4 and PARV5 virions contain equal numbers of positive- and negative-sense DNA strands, while this ratio has not yet been determined for HBoV (49, 137). Parvovirus DNA contains palindromic sequences at each end that form terminal hairpin structures. These hairpin structures permit self-priming and are essential for replication. Parvovirus genomes contain two major open reading frames; one encodes nonstructural (NS) proteins in the left half of the genome, and the other encodes structural capsid proteins in the right half of the genome. Some parvoviruses, in-

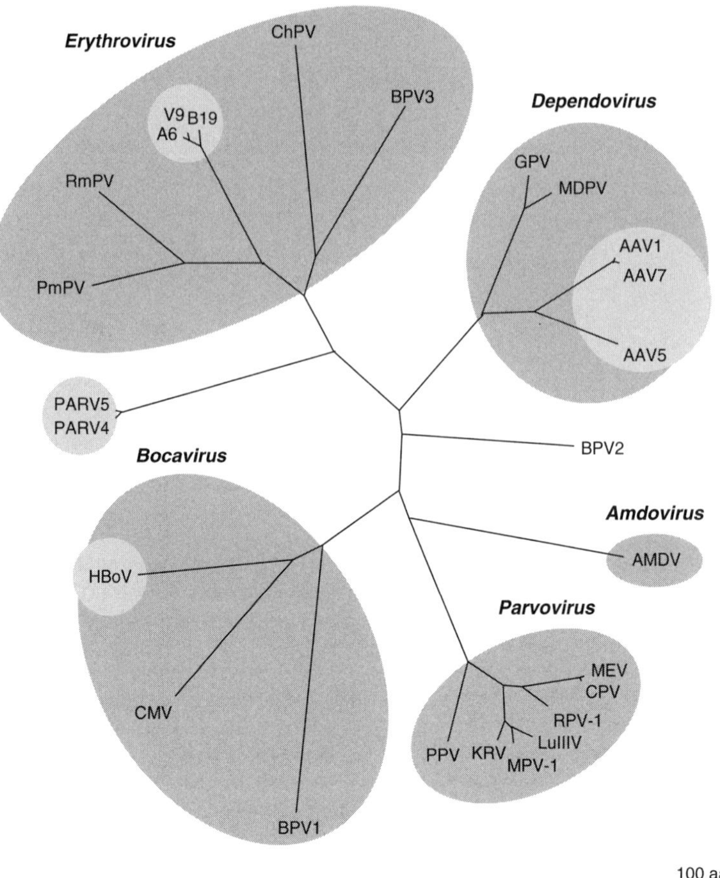

FIGURE 1 Phylogenetic relationships between NS genes of selected members of the subfamily *Parvovirinae*. Shown is an estimated-maximum-parsimony tree generated with PAUP* software showing clustering of different parvovirus genera and ungrouped parvoviruses. The parvoviruses that infect humans are indicated with lighter gray shading. aa, amino acids; AAV, adeno-associated virus; CMV, canine minute virus; BPV, bovine parvovirus; PPV, porcine parvovirus; KRV, Kilham rat virus; MPV, mouse parvovirus; LuIIIV, LuIII virus; RPV, rat parvovirus; CPV, canine parvovirus; MEV, mink enteritis virus; AMDV, Aleutian mink disease virus; MDPV, muscovy duck parvovirus; GPV, goose parvovirus; ChPV, chipmunk parvovirus; RmPV, rhesus macaque parvovirus; PmPV, pig-tailed macaque parvovirus. B19, V9, and A6 are human parvovirus B19 strains; PARV4 and PARV5 are human parvovirus strains.

cluding HBoV, have additional minor open reading frames (3).

Multiple mRNA species are produced by splicing mechanisms. For example, the B19 genome encodes nine mRNA species from a single promoter (Fig. 3) (109). These nine mRNAs translate at least five proteins: VP1, VP2, and at least three NS proteins (Table 1) (90, 108, 134). The NS proteins play a key role in production of infectious virus, probably by regulating transcription, participating in replication, and assisting in encapsidation of virion DNA (98). The NS proteins can be toxic to cells, and this toxicity may contribute to cytopathology during infection. AAV has three promoters, and HBoV has three promoter-like sequences (3, 137).

VP2 or VP3 is the major component of the virion. In the case of B19 parvovirus, VP2 comprises about 95% of the virion and VP1 comprises 5% (111). The VP2 proteins expressed in a Chinese hamster ovary cell line or in a baculovirus system will self-assemble into empty capsids. VP1 can be incorporated into VP2 empty capsids, but it does not self-assemble unless its unique amino terminus is truncated (147). VP1 contains the VP2 sequences plus an additional 227 amino acids at its amino terminus. Empty capsids that include both VP1 and VP2 elicit neutralizing antibodies, while those containing only VP2 do not (70). Most parvoviruses, including AAV, B19 parvovirus, HBoV, and PARV4 and PARV5, have a calcium-dependent phospholipase A2 (PLA2) in the unique region of the VP1 protein (33). PLA2 is presumed to facilitate infection in cells by altering membranes of virion containing endosomes.

Biology

Replication of parvoviruses requires cellular functions expressed only during the S phase of cell division and thus requires actively dividing cells.

Receptors

B19 parvovirus attaches to the cell surface through globoside or P antigen (20), is endocytosed, and migrates to

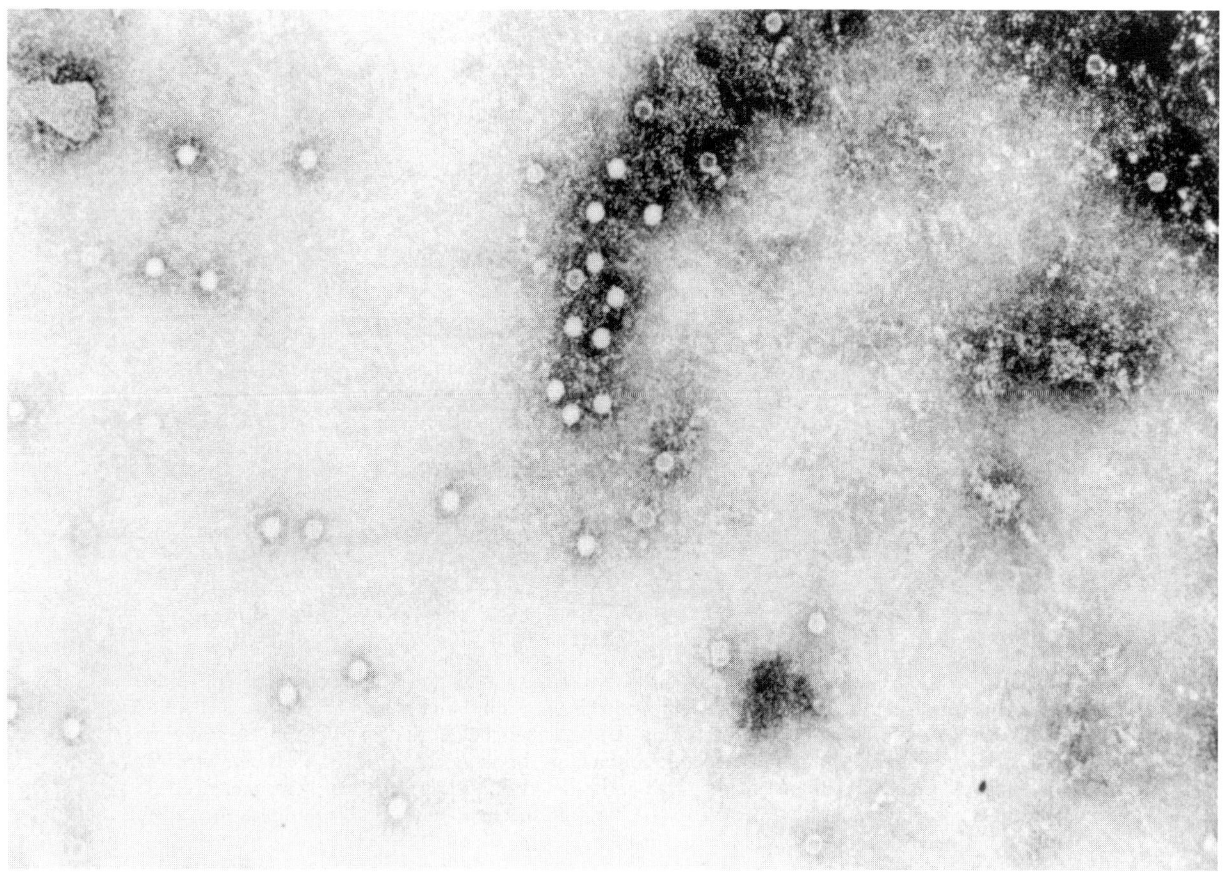

FIGURE 2 Electron micrograph of B19 empty particles in a serum specimen from a patient with transient aplastic crisis. Magnification, ×170,000. (Courtesy of G. William Gary, CDC, Atlanta, GA.)

the nucleus. $\alpha 5\beta 1$ integrin acts as a coreceptor for infection, and its presence appears to explain some tissue specificity of B19 infection (146). Ku80 autoantigen has also been reported to be a coreceptor for B19 parvovirus (102).

A variety of receptors have been identified for other parvoviruses, including transferrin receptors for some members of genus parvovirus and heparin sulfate proteoglycan, human fibroblast growth factor receptor 1, and integrin for AAVs (33). However, the receptors for bocavirus and PARV4 and PARV5 have not yet been identified.

Replication Strategy

Transcription of mRNA and replication of virion DNA occur in the nucleus. Replication of virion DNA is initiated at the terminal hairpins and produces dimer and dimer duplex intermediate forms, which are cleaved to form single-stranded virion DNA (Fig. 4) (110). Plus- and minus-sense single-stranded virion DNA strands are encapsidated with equal frequencies, and the resultant virions are released through cell lysis.

Host Range

Erythroid precursor cells appear to be the primary cells and bone marrow appears to be the primary tissue for B19 parvovirus replication (99). Extramedullary hematopoiesis makes fetal liver an important site of fetal infection in utero (101). Erythroid cells with marginated chromatin and nuclear inclusions (Fig. 5) are typical of B19 parvovirus infection and are found during active infection in the bone marrow as giant pronormoblasts and in blood and other tissues in the fetus (5).

During infection in humans, B19 parvovirus has also been detected in nonerythroid tissues and cells (e.g., myocardial cells, epidermal cells, granulocyte precursors, megakaryocytes, and macrophages), but it is not known if the virus replicates in these nonerythroid cells. Studies have demonstrated the presence of B19-like particles or B19 DNA in fetal myocardial cells and macrophages of infected fetuses (106, 116), B19 antigen and parvovirus-like particles in endothelial cells from erythematous skin lesions from a patient with B19 infection (135), and B19-like particles and B19 antigen in granulocytic precursor cells or large, bizarre granulocytes from patients with B19-associated pancytopenia (77).

Less is known about the tissue tropism of other parvoviruses. AAV has been most often detected in specimens from the genital tract but has also been detected in muscle and a variety of other tissues (47, 50, 63). HBoV has been most often detected in respiratory specimens but also from stool specimens and serum (91). PARV4 and PARV5 have been detected in serum and blood specimens from otherwise healthy individuals and from autopsy bone marrow and lymphoid tissue specimens from human immunodeficiency virus-infected persons (49, 94).

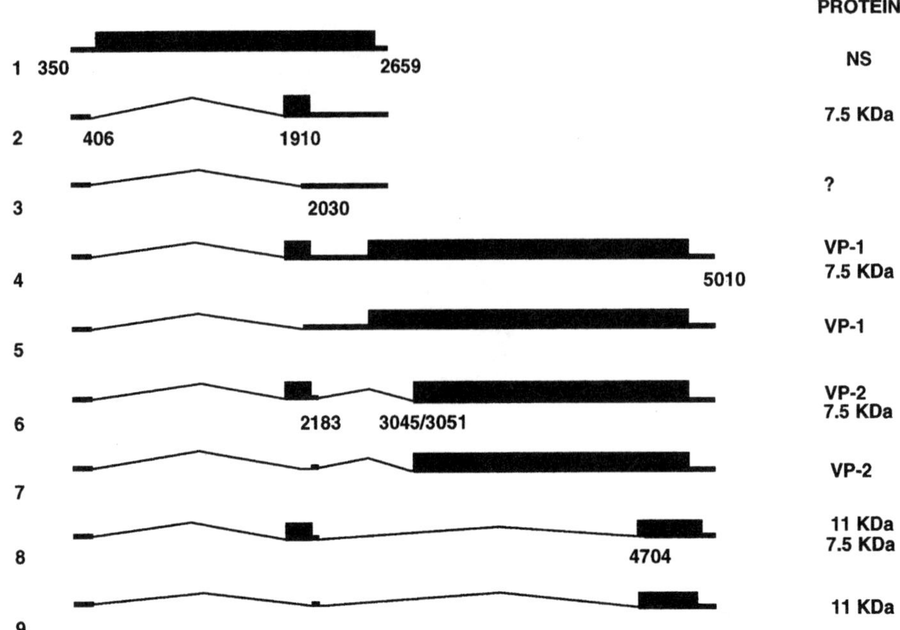

FIGURE 3 Schematic of B19 mRNA produced in erythroid progenitor cells. The thin line represents introns, and the thick line represents the nontranslated portion of exons. The solid boxes represent translated portions of exons. The numbers below the line indicate the start or end of the respective exon. All mRNAs are initiated at the same promoter (P6). The NS protein (first mRNA) is encoded in one reading frame; the 7.5-kDa, VP1, and VP2 proteins are encoded in a second reading frame (−1 relative to the NS protein); and the 11.0-kDa protein is encoded in the third reading frame. (Based on data from references 90 and 109.)

Growth in Cell Culture

Productive B19 parvovirus infection in vitro was first accomplished in late erythroid precursor cells present in bone marrow explant culture systems (101, 110). Subsequently, several human leukemic cell lines, including UT-7, MB-02, JK-1, and KU812, have been shown to support low levels of B19 replication (97). Erythropoietin either is necessary for or markedly increases B19 replication in these cell culture systems. In one study, hypoxia improved B19 parvovirus replication in KU812 cells (23).

With the appropriate helper virus, AAVs can replicate in a variety of tissue culture systems (15). If a helper virus is not present, AAV integrates into the host cell genomic DNA in a site-specific fashion. When cells containing integrated AAV are infected with helper virus or subjected to certain chemical or physical treatments, AAV genes are expressed, the integrated DNA is released, and virions are produced. No tissue culture system has yet been shown to support HBoV or PARV4 or PARV5 replication.

TABLE 1 Proteins of human parvovirus B19

Protein	Size (kDa)	No. of amino acids	Function
NS protein	77	671	Replication
VP1	83	781	Virus capsid
VP2	58	554	Virus capsid
7.5 kDa	7.5	72	Unknown
11 kDa	11	94	Unknown

B19 has not been shown to replicate in animals, and no animal parvoviruses have been shown to replicate in humans, with the exception of simian parvoviruses. Serologic tests have suggested that exposed animal handlers may have been infected with one of the simian erythroviruses (21). Infection of other erythroviruses in their respective host species has been proposed as a model for B19 parvovirus disease (57, 107).

Inactivation by Physical and Chemical Agents

Nonenveloped viruses, such as parvoviruses, are stable under ordinary environmental conditions and more difficult to inactivate on environmental surfaces. The choice and concentration of the inactivating agent, inactivation time, and presence of organic material all impact the effectiveness of inactivation. The effectiveness of surface inactivation also varies by the virus, but detergent- and phenolic acid-based products do not inactivate nonenveloped viruses. Solutions with 5,000 ppm of free chlorine (e.g., 1/10 dilution of household bleach) and 70% aqueous alcohol solutions inactivate some nonenveloped viruses, and 2% glutaraldehyde solutions inactivate most nonenveloped viruses (126). Inactivation of blood or blood products is problematic. Infection in persons receiving heat-treated clotting factor concentrates indicates that the virus can withstand dry-heat treatment at 80°C for as long as 72 h or at 100°C for 30 min (125). Based on in vitro studies, the B19 parvovirus is more sensitive to liquid heat treatment, and the level of sensitivity depends on the composition of the solution (60).

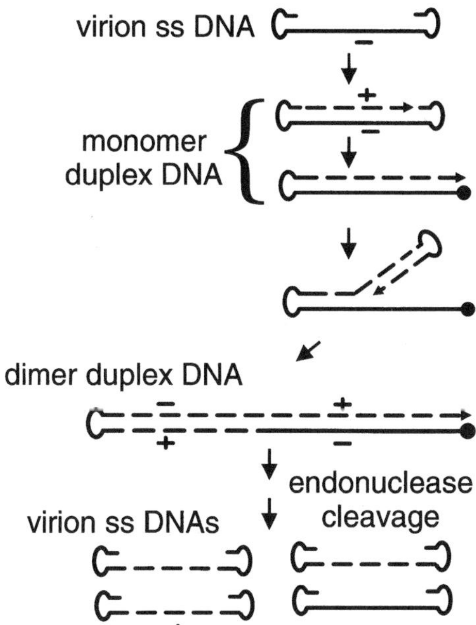

FIGURE 4 Schematic of replication of B19 virion DNA. Replication is initiated at the 3′-terminal hairpin by host DNA polymerases and proceeds to form monomer duplex DNA and then dimer duplex DNA. The dimer duplex DNA is cleaved by cellular endonucleases into positive- and negative-sense single-stranded DNAs (ssDNAs), which are packaged with equal frequencies into B19 virions. (Reprinted from reference 110 with permission of the American Association for the Advancement of Science.)

EPIDEMIOLOGY

Distribution

B19 parvovirus infection is common throughout the world, although the percentage of persons positive for immunoglobulin G (IgG) antibody as a measure of past infection varies by location and timing of the last B19 epidemic (30, 67, 144). AAVs, bocavirus, and PARV4 and PARV5 have been detected in multiple locations globally.

Incidence and Prevalence

In most communities, the prevalence of B19 parvovirus antibody increases from 2 to 15% among children 1 to 5 years of age to 20 to 40% among children 6 to 9 years of age and to 35 to 60% among children 11 to 19 years of age (30, 74, 144). Antibody prevalence continues to increase with age, reaching 75 to 90% among persons over 50 years of age in several studies (Fig. 6). The greatest rate of increase in IgG positivity occurs in school-age children, consistent with the observation that erythema infectiosum, the most commonly recognized manifestation of B19 infection, is most often diagnosed in this age group.

Subclinical infection is common, and most adults with B19 IgG antibody will not give a history suggestive of a B19-associated illness. In outbreaks of B19 infection, 50% or more of infected persons may be asymptomatic or report a nonrash illness (29, 115, 149).

B19 infections are most often noted as outbreaks of erythema infectiosum in schools. Outbreaks in the United States usually occur in the winter and spring and often continue for months or until school recesses for the summer (29, 54). During school outbreaks, 25 to 50% of students have been reported to have clinical or serologic evidence of infection. Staff in schools are also commonly infected (25, 54, 140); 20% of susceptible staff developed infection during one outbreak. Infections also occur endemically when no outbreak activity is noted in the community. Since recurrences of erythema infectiosum or transient aplastic crisis are rare, it is assumed that past infection, as indicated by the presence of B19 IgG antibodies, confers long-term protection from disease. Experimental inoculation of one patient with low levels of B19 IgG antibody led to an asymptomatic infection, indicating that past infection may not always prevent reinfection (8).

AAV and HBoV infections are common. In one study, nearly 90% of children had serologic evidence of HBoV (39). The majority of AAV data are for AAV 2, for which 50% or more of persons 10 to 19 years of age have antibodies (42). Less is known about timing and extent of infection with PARV4 and PARV5.

Seasonality

In temperate climates in the northern hemisphere, B19 parvovirus outbreaks most often occur during the late winter and spring. These outbreaks are cyclical, with increased B19 transmission occurring every 4 to 10 years in a given community (74, 105).

Seasonal patterns of PARV4 and PARV5 infections are not known, and those for HBoV are yet to be clearly defined. Depending on the study, HBoV has most often been reported to occur during the fall and winter months (76, 83, 94) and less often with no clear seasonality (13, 48) or a spring peak in activity (9).

Transmission

The primary route of source of B19 parvovirus is likely the respiratory tract; i.e., B19 DNA can be found in respiratory secretions (8, 29, 115). The virus has also been demonstrated in urine and blood specimens from patients during the acute phase of infection and by PCR in the blood for up to months after acute infection (8, 29, 87, 115). In the community, infection probably occurs through the respiratory tract after exposures through close contact, droplets, and/or fomites. B19 DNA has been detected on surfaces in a room where a B19-infected abortus was delivered (35). In volunteer studies, infection occurred in four of five exposed persons after intranasal inoculation (8). Transmission also occurs percutaneously, including after transfusion of contaminated blood or blood from an infected mother to her fetus, and after tattooing (125, 131). Vertical transmission from mother to fetus has been reported to occur in 25 to 50% of infants of mothers infected during pregnancy (78, 119).

The risk of B19 parvovirus transmission from a single unit of blood is low, with levels $\geq 10^5$ IU of B19 DNA present per ml in 1/500 to 1/10,000 units in one study (127a). The risk has been high after receipt of many types of multiunit blood products. B19 DNA has been detected in 25 to 100% of products such as albumin and factor VIII concentrates, which may contain components from 5,000 or more units, and infection has often been associated with receipt of these products. The small size of the B19 virion and the resistance of the virus to inactivation have made it difficult to remove or inactivate during the preparation of these products. Screening units for B19 DNA can decrease the frequency and level of B19 in blood products (17, 53).

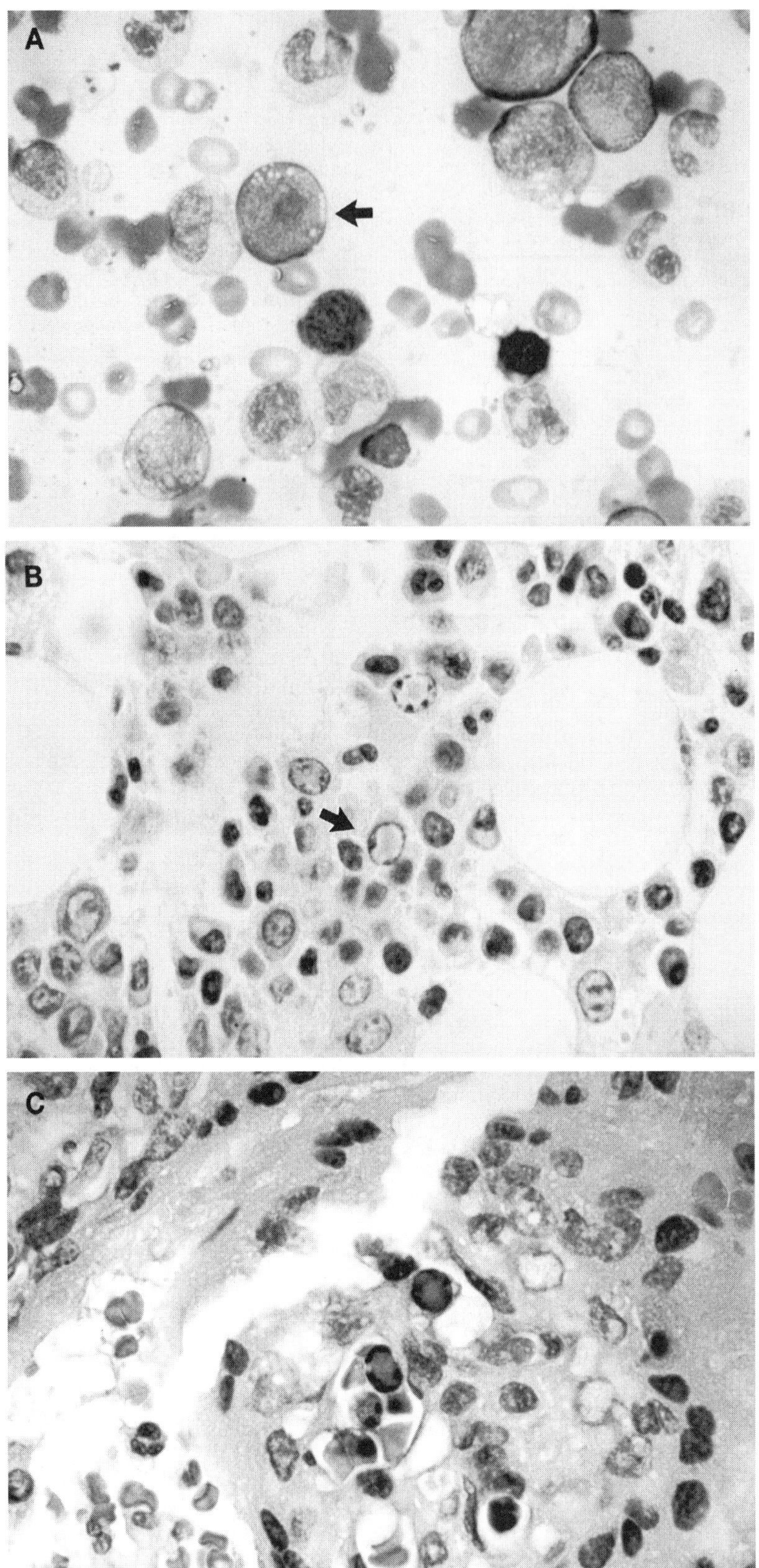

FIGURE 5 (A) Wright-Giemsa stain of a bone marrow aspirate from a patient with B19 infection. Note the giant pronormoblasts (arrow) with multiple vacuoles in the darkly stained (basophilic) cytoplasm, high nucleus-to-cytoplasm ratio, and prominent nucleoli. (B) Hematoxylin and eosin stain of bone marrow biopsy section from a patient with B19 infection. Note the prominent nuclear inclusions, marginated chromatin, and high nucleus-to-cytoplasm ratio in erythroid precursor cells (arrow). (C) Hematoxylin and eosin stain of placental tissue from a fetus that died with B19 infection. Note the ground-glass-appearing nuclear inclusions and marginated chromatin in erythroid precursor cells within fetal vessels. Magnifications, ×625. (All panels courtesy of Sherif R. Zaki, CDC, Atlanta, GA.)

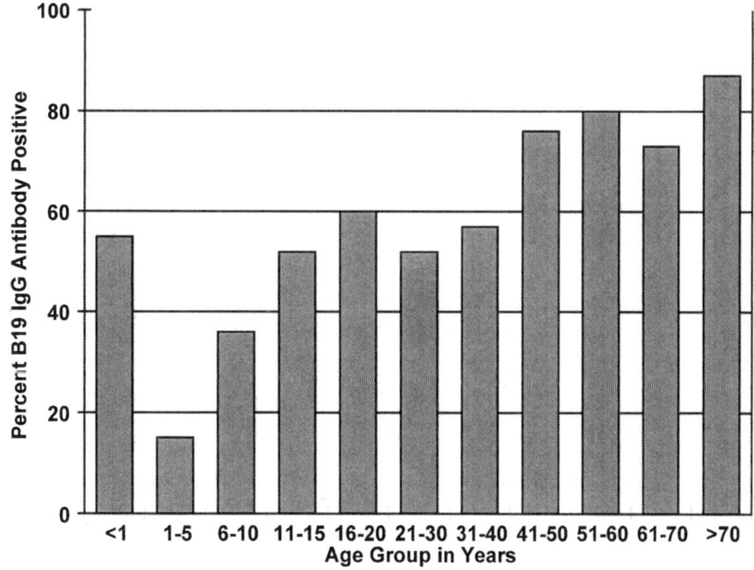

FIGURE 6 Rates of B19 IgG antibody positivity by age. (Adapted from reference 30.)

B19 parvovirus is transmitted efficiently in households, with about 50% of susceptible exposed household members becoming infected, while in schools and child care centers, about 20% of susceptible staff may be infected (29, 54, 115, 140). In pregnant women living in communities with outbreaks of B19 disease, infection rates among susceptible persons have ranged from 4 to 14%. Risk factors for infection include working as a teacher or child care worker or having children at home (25, 67, 140).

Nosocomial transmission of B19 among staff and patients has been reported with infection rates as high as 50%, but it is often difficult to differentiate hospital-acquired from community-acquired infection in such outbreaks (35, 51, 103, 129). Nosocomial transmission can, however, occur, and standard precautions are recommended for all B19-infected patients and droplet precautions are recommended for those most likely to have high-titer infection, i.e., those with chronic B19 infection and those with transient aplastic crisis (52). Those with chronic infection are considered infectious until the infection has been cured; those with transient aplastic crisis are considered infectious up to 5 days after onset of illness; and those with erythema infectiosum are most likely to be infectious before, but not after, onset of their illness.

The routes of transmission for AAV, HBoV, and PARV4 and PARV5 are not well understood. The presence of HBoV in feces and respiratory secretions suggests two sources of virus for its transmission.

PATHOGENESIS IN HUMANS

The course of disease for erythema infectiosum, the most common manifestation of B19 parvovirus infection, suggests that it is immune mediated in part. The estimated incubation period to onset of rash has usually been between 1 and 2 weeks but sometimes as long as 3 weeks (4). In experimental infection in humans, the first symptoms of fever, malaise, and myalgia occurred 1 to 2 weeks after inoculation of the virus. These symptoms developed during viremia and were accompanied by a reticulocytopenia, a drop in hemoglobin, and moderate but clinically insignificant lymphopenia, thrombocytopenia, and neutropenia (8). The viremia and reticulocytopenia resolved by days 11 to 16 as volunteers mounted an antibody response; the rash or arthralgias were noted at 15 to 17 days after inoculation (Fig. 7).

During the viremia, the bone marrow has a marked decrease in the number of erythroid cells but a relatively normal number of myeloid cells. The arrest of hematopoiesis during viremia is consistent with the expected impact of a lytic infection of red cell precursor cells. On the other hand, the fact that onset of rash and/or arthritic symptoms occurs coincident with the host antibody response and decreasing levels of viremia suggests that the host immune response is important to the pathogenesis of these symptoms. The occurrence of rash in an immunocompromised patient after treatment with immune globulin and again after the patient mounted an antibody response suggests that anti-B19 antibody is important to the pathogenesis of the rash (82). B19-antibody immune complexes could explain these findings. Immune complexes have been detected in sera of experimentally infected adults by an immune adherence assay (8) and in sera of 31 of 38 B19-infected patients by a C1q binding assay (51). The finding of B19 antigens and viral particles in vascular endothelial cells from B19-associated rash lesions suggests that infection of these cells might also contribute to the pathogenesis of the rash (135).

The pathogenesis of B19-associated arthritis is less clear. B19 parvovirus DNA has been detected by PCR assays in synovial tissue from the joints of patients with B19-associated arthritis and other types of arthritis and from control patients (64, 113, 133). However, there is no evidence that B19 replicates in synovial tissue. In B19-associated arthritis, it is possible that virally expressed proteins are cytotoxic to cells; e.g., NS2 contributes to joint inflammation. The PLA2 activity in VP1 can activate synoviocytes, induce mediators of inflammation, and, possibly, participate in B19-associated arthritis (88).

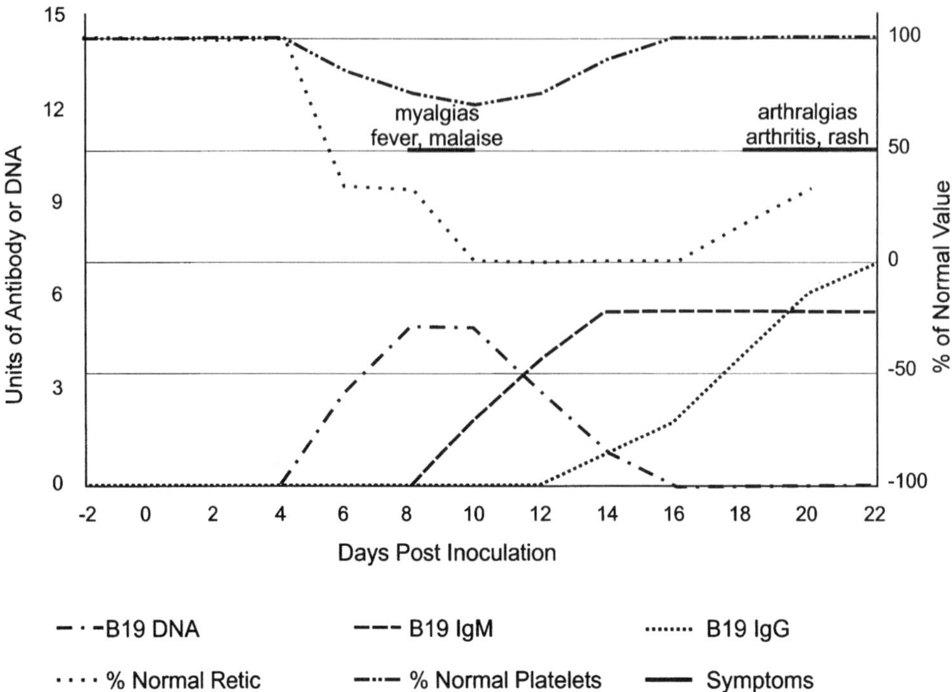

FIGURE 7 Schematic of clinical and laboratory findings during the course of B19 infection in adult volunteers. Note the drop in reticulocyte (Retic) and platelet counts and the presence of symptoms (fever, myalgias, and malaise) associated with peak viremia (days 6 to 12). During this period, there is also a transient drop in neutrophil and lymphocyte counts. Associated with the drop in reticulocyte counts, there is a progressive drop in hemoglobin levels to about 90% of normal by days 14 to 16. The timing of the drop in hemoglobin levels corresponds to the time of anemia in patients with transient aplastic crisis. Note the second period of symptoms (rash, arthritis, and arthralgias) on days 18 to ≥22. This second period of illness corresponds to symptoms of erythema infectiosum. (Data from reference 8.)

Virus Replication Patterns

As noted above, B19-associated anemia correlates with viremia and is presumed to be related to the cytopathic effect of the virus on hematopoietic precursor cells. In immunocompetent persons, the immune response controls the infection within 7 to 10 days and before a significant anemia develops. In persons with borderline compensated hemoglobin levels, even a short cessation of red cell production can produce a self-limited but serious anemia, i.e., transient aplastic crisis. A variety of conditions, including sickle cell disease, hereditary spherocytosis, thalassemia, and acquired hemolytic anemias, have been associated with transient aplastic crisis.

Some patients with compromised immunity due to human immunodeficiency virus infection, malignancies, chemotherapy, or organ transplantation are unable to control B19 parvovirus replication and develop a chronic lytic infection of red cell precursors and an associated chronic reticulocytopenic anemia (19, 36, 80, 151). Patients with chronic infection usually respond to treatment with intravenous immune globulin (IVIG) with a prompt reticulocytosis and clearing of viremia. Chronic infection with anemia has also been rarely noted in patients with presumed normal immune systems (19, 36, 80, 151). Detection of B19 parvovirus in blood, bone marrow, synovial tissue, and liver in adults without evidence of recent infection (i.e., presumably from infection many years earlier) complicates the task of linking B19 parvovirus to disease based on its detection in these tissues (64, 86, 113).

The fetus is susceptible to severe B19 anemia because it has a need for increased red cell production and an immature immune system that is not always able to control the infection (151). B19-associated myocarditis may also contribute to fetal disease. Transplacentally transferred maternal antibodies presumably provide some protection to the fetus during the later stages of pregnancy.

Although the primary cell type for productive B19 infection is erythroid precursor cells, a number of other cells have P antigen and may be susceptible to infection (20). For example, endothelial cells, myocardial cells, cells in the placenta, fetal liver cells, and megakaryocytes have P antigen and, in some instances, have been positive for B19 DNA or antigens (116, 117, 135, 148). In vitro, macrophage infection has been facilitated by the presence of antibody, presumably through Fc receptor-mediated phagocytosis of virus-antibody complexes (100). This may be the mechanism by which phagocytic cells in the bone marrow and synovial tissue become infected.

Immune Response

An IgM antibody response begins 10 to 14 days after infection, and an IgG response begins shortly thereafter (8) (Fig. 7). This antibody response correlates with clearing infection. B19 IgG antibodies persist long term and presumably confer protection from disease. The ability of IVIG to control and sometimes cure chronic infection in the immunodeficient patient clearly demonstrates the importance of antibodies in B19 immunity (36, 80). Various assays have been used to characterize the antibody response to B19. Some of these assays have identified differences in the types of antibody seen early from those seen later after an acute infection. For example, antibodies against linear epitopes on the VP2 protein are present during the acute phase and then lost in the late convalescent phase, whereas VP1 linear and conformational epitopes are present during both the acute and the convalescent phases of infection (92, 132). An antibody response to the NS protein has also been detected later in the course of the illness (~6 weeks after onset of illness) and has been associated with chronic symptomatic infection in some, but not all, studies (61, 68, 152). Neutralizing antibodies can also be detected, and epitopes associated with neutralization activity have been identified on both the VP1 unique and the VP1/VP2 shared regions of the structural proteins. There is very limited information on the cellular immune response to B19 infection (71, 151).

There is little information on the immune response to natural infection with the other parvoviruses other than the data on antibodies against AAV and HBoV noted above and studies of AAV gene therapy (27).

CLINICAL MANIFESTATIONS OF B19 PARVOVIRUS

Asymptomatic Infection

Asymptomatic infection, or atypical illness, is probably the most common manifestation of B19 infection. Investigations of B19-infected persons in outbreaks (29, 140, 149) found that as many as 50% reported no rash and 25% reported no symptoms.

Erythema Infectiosum

Erythema infectiosum, or fifth disease, is the most commonly recognized clinical manifestation of B19 parvovirus infection. It is a mild rash illness manifested by a malar erythematous rash (slapped cheek) (Color Plate 15) and reticulated or lacelike rash on the trunk and extremities (4). B19 infection has also been associated with other types of rashes, including morbilliform, confluent, vesicular, and purpuric patterns. Erythema infectiosum is most commonly diagnosed in school-age children. The child is usually afebrile but may experience a mild systemic illness 1 to 4 days before the onset of rash. These systemic symptoms presumably correspond to the time of viremia noted in infected volunteers. Various nonrash symptoms have been noted in some patients, including headache, sore throat, coryza, pruritus, gastrointestinal symptoms, and arthralgias and/or arthritis. In most patients, symptoms resolve over the course of a few weeks, but in some, they last months and, rarely, even years. A typical feature of erythema infectiosum is the recrudescence of rash after a variety of nonspecific stimuli, such as change in temperature, exposure to sunlight, or emotional stress.

Patients with erythema infectiosum usually do not undergo laboratory evaluation, but they may have reticulocytopenia and clinically insignificant anemia, lymphopenia, neutropenia, and thrombocytopenia before and possibly at the onset of rash.

Transient Aplastic Crisis

Transient aplastic crisis is the best-understood manifestation of infection. The lytic infection of red cell precursors leads to cessation of hematopoiesis, which in persons with a poorly compensated hematopoietic system, like those with sickle cell disease, may develop a severe, self-limited reticulocytopenic anemia, i.e., transient aplastic crisis. Patients present with symptoms of a severe anemia, i.e., pallor, weakness, and lethargy (124, 130), and sometimes also with nonspecific systemic symptoms and, infrequently, a rash. During the acute phase of the illness, patients have no reticulocytes and may have a drop in hemoglobin levels of 30% or more. The bone marrow has a hypoplastic or aplastic erythroid and normal myeloid series. About 7 to 10 days after onset of illness and coincident with development of an antibody response, reticulocytosis develops and the hemoglobin begins to return to preinfection levels.

B19 Infection in Immunodeficient Patients

B19 infection in immunodeficient patients is a potentially life-threatening illness that can be treated with IVIG. Some patients with deficient immune systems develop a chronic B19 infection and associated chronic, severe reticulocytopenic anemia (19, 36). These patients often respond to IVIG with a brisk reticulocytosis and resolution of B19-associated anemia. In some patients, the infection may resolve completely, whereas in others, viremia and anemia may recur, resulting in the need for additional treatment with IVIG.

Hydrops Fetalis

Hydrops fetalis is a potential complication of B19 infection during pregnancy, and this possibility can generate considerable concern in the pregnant woman and her family. The B19 parvovirus-infected fetus may not be able to control infection and may develop a severe reticulocytopenic anemia leading to high-output congestive heart failure, hydrops, and sometimes death (46, 139). Maternal infection in the second half of pregnancy appears to present less risk to the fetus, possibly because transplacental transfer of maternal antibody may occur and protect the fetus. B19 can also infect fetal myocardial cells, which may contribute to cardiac dysfunction and heart failure (116, 151). Although most fetuses that survive B19 infection are normal at delivery, one study of fetuses requiring intrauterine transfusions found evidence of developmental delay in some infected children at 6 months to 8 years of age (104).

Approximately 30 to 50% (78, 119) of maternal B19 parvovirus infections lead to fetal infection, and 2 to 10% lead to fetal death (41, 67, 78, 119). B19 infection has also been detected in approximately 5 to 20% of autopsy cases of nonimmune hydrops (41, 43). Although case reports have suggested that B19 might be teratogenic, most studies of children born to women infected with B19 during pregnancy have not demonstrated an increased risk of birth defects (41, 67, 121). If B19 causes birth defects, it is likely an uncommon occurrence.

Arthralgias and Arthritis

Arthralgias and arthritis associated with B19 infection have been described for children and adults but most commonly for adult females (41, 67, 78, 119). This condition usually manifests as a symmetrical peripheral polyarthropathy commonly involving the hands, wrists, knees, and feet, although any joint can be affected. Joint symptoms may develop with or without other symptoms and before, during, or after rash onset and include tenderness and swelling. Symptoms usually resolve over the course of a few weeks but can persist for months and, rarely, for years. It is not a destructive arthritis. As with the rash of erythema infectiosum, joint symptoms can recur after a variety of stimuli.

The predisposition of B19 parvovirus infection to cause joint disease has led to studies of B19 in patients with rheumatoid arthritis. While some have suggested higher frequencies of B19 antibody or DNA in patients with chronic arthritis (including rheumatoid arthritis), these findings have been inconsistent, and a link between B19 and chronic arthritis has not been proven (127, 151). B19 parvovirus does not appear to be an important cause of rheumatoid arthritis, although B19-associated arthritis may sometimes be confused with early chronic arthritis, including rheumatoid arthritis.

Other Disease Associations

Other disease associations have been reported but not established for B19 parvovirus infection. The list of possible B19-associated conditions includes a wide range of cardiovascular, skin, endocrine, hematologic, hepatic, neurologic, ocular, renal, respiratory, and rheumatic disorders (138, 151). Some of the purported associations are simply coincidental occurrences of a common infection and the disease. Others are probably instances in which B19 is one of several causes of the disease, and some represent instances in which false-positive laboratory results led to a spurious association. False-positive results for B19 IgM antibody assays can be a substantial problem. The exquisite sensitivity of PCR makes even low levels of specimen contamination an ongoing concern in interpreting positive results.

Hepatitis has been noted during acute B19 infection, and B19 DNA has been detected in the liver and serum of patients with acute hepatitis, but an etiologic link between B19 and hepatic injury has not been demonstrated (148).

Glomerulonephritis may occur following B19-associated transient aplastic crisis in patients with sickle cell disease and in otherwise healthy patients with B19 infection (65, 136). B19 infection has been reported in association with conjunctivitis (150) and acute pneumonia (16, 18). Some diseases associated with decreased numbers of platelets and white cells may be caused by B19 infection (8). B19 infection has been detected in patients with a wide range of rashes, including morbilliform, vesicular, and confluent ones, in addition to the slapped cheek and reticular, lace-like rash on the trunk and extremities characteristic of erythema infectiosum. Other dermatologic illnesses reported with B19 infection include papular purpuric "gloves and socks" syndrome and papular acrodermatitis of childhood, Gianotti-Crosti syndrome, and livedo reticularis (24, 34, 58).

Case reports of vascular purpura were the first vasculitis-like findings associated with B19 infection (95). However, reports of B19 infection being assocated with other vasculitides, including Henoch-Schönlein purpura, Wegener's granulomatosis, polyarteritis nodosa, and Kawasaki disease, have not been substantiated (151).

B19 parvovirus infection has been associated uncommonly with various neurologic abnormalities, including peripheral neuropathies, meningitis, and encephalopathy. B19 DNA has been detected in cerebrospinal fluid from several patients with meningitis during acute B19 infection (12, 84), and B19 antigens and DNA have been detected in fetal brain tissue (66). These findings suggest that B19 infection may occasionally lead to neurologic disease.

Whether B19 parvovirus infection may cause acute or chronic myocarditis is unresolved, except in the fetus. B19 probably can cause myocarditis in the fetus (98).

Clinical Illness Associated with Other Parvovirus Infections

AAVs and PARV4 and PARV5 have not yet been linked to human disease. HBoV has been detected typically in 1 to 10% of respiratory specimens from children and adults with acute respiratory illnesses (2, 13, 48, 76, 83, 89, 93, 120). The illness in HboV-positive patients is indistinguishable from that caused by other respiratory viruses and includes upper respiratory tract illness and the range of lower respiratory tract syndromes like pneumonia, bronchitis, and bronchiolitis. Detection of HBoV in healthy controls is uncommon, so infection appears to be associated with acute respiratory illness in younger children (2, 48, 76, 93). The role the virus plays in the illness, however, is confounded by detection of coinfecting viruses in up to 90% of specimens (2, 48, 62, 118). HBoV has also been detected in 1 to 9% of stool specimens from children hospitalized with acute gastroenteritis (but is not yet linked to gastroenteritis) (83, 85, 142) and in blood (2, 48).

LABORATORY DIAGNOSIS

Serologic, antigen detection, and nucleic acid detection assays have been used to detect B19 parvovirus infection. Acute infection in the healthy patient is most often demonstrated by detecting serum B19 IgM antibodies, and past infection is demonstrated by detecting B19 IgG antibodies. Antibody assays are not reliable for diagnosing chronic infection in immunocompromised patients, in whom detection of B19 DNA by PCR or probe hybridization assays is required.

Detection of AAV, HboV, and PARV4 and PARV5 has been primarily accomplished with PCR-based assays. Past infection has been determined using a variety of serologic assays for IgG antibodies.

Virus Isolation

Although erythroid precursor cells derived from human bone marrow, peripheral blood, and several continuous cell lines with erythroid precursor-like features support B19 infection, they do so inefficiently, and isolation has not been used to detect infection (97). Isolation studies have been used to evaluate inactivation methods for blood or plasma products (60).

Antigen Detection

Enzyme and radioimmunoassays have been developed for B19 parvovirus antigens, but they lack sufficient sensitivity to reliably diagnose acute infection. Immunohistochemical techniques have proven useful for detecting B19 antigens in various tissues and cells, most commonly in fetal tissues and bone marrow specimens (5).

Nucleic Acid Detection

Nucleic acid detection has become a key part of B19 parvovirus diagnostics for both detecting infection and screening blood products. Probe hybridization assays used in the past are being replaced by PCR assays, especially real-time PCR assays, which have the advantages of both high sensitivity and decreased risk of template contamination (17, 114).

PCR assays have been developed using a variety of primers and methods. Both the sensitivity and specificity of PCR can vary among assays and laboratories (14). The most sensitive PCR assays use a second amplification step (nested PCR) or a sensitive method to detect the PCR product, e.g., dot blot hybridization, Southern blot, or enzyme immunoassays (40, 43, 87). Very sensitive PCR assays have been used to detect B19 DNA in chronic infections and to extend the time during acute infection when DNA can be detected. For example, with probe hybridization assays, B19 DNA is usually not detected at onset of rash in patients with erythema infectiosum, while it is often detected at and within a month of onset of rash with PCR assays. Since the clinical significance of low levels of B19 DNA is not always clear and PCR assays are subject to false-positive results, a positive PCR result must be interpreted carefully and in the context of appropriate clinical and laboratory controls.

In situ hybridization studies have been successfully used to detect infection in patients as well as determine which cells and tissues are infected (5).

The majority of recent studies of AAVs and studies of PARV4 and PARV5 and HBoV have been based on a variety of PCR assays to detect the viral DNA (50, 93).

Antibody Assays

B19 IgM antibody assays have been the key to diagnosing most infections. The initial assays used a capture antibody format as an enzyme immunoassay or radioimmunoassay. The assays proved sensitive and specific for detecting IgM antibodies in patients with erythema infectiosum and transient aplastic crisis and have been considered the standard against which other assays are compared (6, 7, 31). The best antigen for these assays is empty capsids made from VP2 or VP2 plus VP1 proteins expressed in vitro (45, 70). Expressed proteins that do not form empty capsids may not include all the epitopes needed to detect a response in all patients.

IgM antibody develops within 10 to 12 days after infection and is present in over 90% of patients with erythema infectiosum at onset of rash and in about 80% of patients with transient aplastic crisis at the time of presentation (6, 7, 31). IgM positivity increases to over 90% in patients with transient aplastic crisis by 3 to 7 days after presentation. The IgM response begins to wane the second month after infection but may remain positive for 6 months or more.

Indirect IgM antibody assays have been used but tend to be both less sensitive and less specific than the IgM capture format (22, 128). The capture assay method eliminates competition from IgG antibodies, which can lead to false-negative results, and decreases the risk of rheumatoid factor or nonspecific sticking of IgM antibodies, which can lead to false-positive results. Other serologic indicators of acute or active B19 infection include low avidity (56) and the presence of antibodies against linear VP2 epitopes (10, 92).

IgG antibodies appear a few days after IgM antibodies and persist long term. Unlike the IgM antibody assays, the IgG indirect format should be as good as or better than the capture format.

A variety of serologic assays have been used to detect AAVs in a serotype-specific fashion (42). A serologic assay for HBoV has recently been described based on cloned expressed capsid proteins forming empty capsids (39).

Prevention

As noted above, B19 parvovirus and HBoV are probably most often transmitted via respiratory secretions through close contact, contact with contaminated fomites, and possibly through droplet aerosol transmission. Attention to good hygienic practices, such as hand washing and not sharing food or drinks, may be effective in reducing the spread of B19 and, though not yet studied, can be recommended to control spread during outbreaks.

Nosocomial transmission has been reported after exposure to patients with transient aplastic crisis but should not be a risk after exposure to patients with erythema infectiosum. By the time the rash of erythema infectiosum is noted, the patient no longer has high-titer viremia and has low levels of or no virus in respiratory secretions (7, 151). Patients with transient aplastic crisis are probably a risk for transmitting B19 as long as a week after onset of illness. The risk for transmission from immunodeficient patients is poorly understood but may be prolonged. Patients with transient aplastic crisis should be placed on droplet isolation precautions for 7 days, and immunodeficient patients with chronic infection should be placed on droplet precautions for the duration of their hospitalization (52). No vaccine or chemoprophylaxis is available for B19 infection. A vaccine made from empty capsids is, however, being developed and evaluated (11).

Community outbreaks of B19 disease, usually manifested as erythema infectiosum in schools, often raise concern about infection in persons at risk for complications, especially pregnant women. The risk of fetal death from an exposure can be defined by the following equation: rate of fetal death from an exposure = rate of susceptibility to B19 × expected rate of infection from the exposure × rate of fetal death with infection (26). Depending on the community and antibody assay, between 40 and 60% of women in their childbearing years will test positive for B19 IgG antibodies and presumably not be susceptible to infection. Infection occurs in about 50% of susceptible persons during household exposure to a patient with erythema infectiosum or transient aplastic crisis (29, 115), in about 20% of susceptible staff working in a school during an outbreak of erythema infectiosum (54), in about 6% of susceptible residents of a community during one B19 outbreak (25), and in about 1 to 3% of women with no specific exposure during a year or a pregnancy (38, 67, 79, 141). The risk of fetal death with maternal infection is between 2 and 10% (28, 59, 67, 96, 119). Thus, the risk of fetal death in pregnancy can be estimated to be between 0.4 and 3.0% after exposure to B19 in the household and between 0.16 and 1.2% after exposures associated with working in a school or child care setting with a B19 disease outbreak. Persons should be informed of potential exposures to B19, and efforts to decrease the risk of exposures (e.g., avoiding the workplace or school environment) should be made on an individual basis after consultation with family members, health care providers, public health officials, and employers or school officials (26).

TREATMENT

Although most B19 parvovirus illnesses, including erythema infectiosum, are mild and require no treatment, several complications require treatment. B19-associated arthralgias or arthritis may benefit from nonsteroidal, anti-inflammatory medications. Patients with transient aplastic crisis often require hospitalization and transfusion therapy until the immune response controls the infection 1 to 10 days after presentation. In one study of 62 patients with sickle cell disease who developed transient aplastic crisis, 54 (87%) required blood transfusions (55). The death of one patient before transfusion therapy highlights the importance of prompt evaluation and treatment of patients with transient aplastic crisis (130). Patients with chronic infection and associated anemia (most but not all such patients will have compromised immune systems) should be treated with IVIG. Commercial IVIG at a dosage of 400 mg/kg of body weight for 5 or 10 days or at a dosage of 1 g/kg for 3 days has been used successfully (80, 81). Patients can be monitored with hemoglobin and reticulocyte count, and if they develop a reticulocytopenic anemia and recurrent B19 viremia, then retreatment with IVIG is indicated. IVIG treatment has not been shown to be effective for treatment of nonanemia manifestations of chronic infection (123).

Management and treatment of the fetus of a B19-infected pregnant woman are problematic. Some studies have advocated monitoring the fetus with ultrasound to look for evidence of hydrops and treating hydropic fetuses with intrauterine blood transfusion. However, since the fetus can survive and be normal without treatment and intrauterine blood transfusion can cause fetal death, this approach to managing the hydropic fetus needs to be considered carefully. Intrauterine blood transfusion may be beneficial to an affected fetus, but the efficacy of this treatment has not been proven to date (44, 46, 75, 143). In one study, 9 of 12 fetuses treated with intrauterine blood transfusions, compared to 13 of 26 untreated ones, survived and were normal at delivery (44); analysis indicated a significant difference after adjusting for severity of ultrasound findings and gestational age. Although most B19-infected transfused fetuses that survive are normal, one study of 24 transfused hydropic fetuses reported that some suffered long-term complications (104), which included delayed psychomotor development in 5 of the 16 survivors (severe in 2). The available data suggest that intrauterine blood transfusions may be helpful and should be considered in the management of some fetuses with B19-associated disease. Unfortunately, the data do not clearly indicate when the benefits of this procedure outweigh the risks.

REFERENCES

1. **Ager, E. A., T. D. Y. Chin, and J. D. Poland.** 1966. Epidemic erythema infectiosum. *N. Engl. J. Med.* **275:** 1326–1331.
2. **Allander, T., T. Jartti, S. Gupta, H. G. Niesters, P. Lehtinen, R. Osterback, T. Vuorinen, M. Waris, A. Bjerkner, A. Tiveljung-Lindell, B. G. van den Hoogen, T. Hyypia, and O. Ruuskanen.** 2007. Human bocavirus and acute wheezing in children. *Clin. Infect. Dis.* **44:**904–910.
3. **Allander, T., M. T. Tammi, M. Eriksson, A. Bjerkner, A. Tiveljung-Lindell, and B. Andersson.** 2005. Cloning of a human parvovirus by molecular screening of respiratory tract samples. *Proc. Natl. Acad. Sci. USA* **102:** 12891–12896.
4. **Anderson, L. J.** 1987. Role of parvovirus B19 in human disease. *Pediatr. Infect. Dis. J.* **6:**711–718.
5. **Anderson, L. J., T. J. Torok, and S. R. Zaki.** 1998. Human parvovirus B19, p. 3.0–3.20. *In* C. M. Wilfert (ed.), *Pediatric Infectious Diseases*. Current Medicine, Inc., and Churchill Livingstone, Philadelphia, PA.
6. **Anderson, L. J., C. Tsou, R. A. Parker, T. L. Chorba, H. Wulff, P. Tattersall, and P. P. Mortimer.** 1986. Detection of antibodies and antigens of human parvovirus B19 by enzyme-linked immunosorbent assay. *J. Clin. Microbiol.* **24:**522–526.
7. **Anderson, M. J., L. R. Davis, S. E. Jones, and J. R. Pattison.** 1982. The development and use of an antibody capture radioimmunoassay for specific IgM to a human parvovirus-like agent. *J. Hyg.* **88:**309–324.
8. **Anderson, M. J., P. G. Higgins, L. R. Davis, J. S. Willman, S. E. Jones, I. M. Kidd, J. R. Pattison, and D. A. J. Tyrrell.** 1985. Experimental parvoviral infection in humans. *J. Infect. Dis.* **152:**257–265.
9. **Arnold, J. C., K. K. Singh, S. A. Spector, and M. H. Sawyer.** 2006. Human bocavirus: prevalence and clinical spectrum at a children's hospital. *Clin. Infect. Dis.* **43:** 283–288.
10. **Azzi, A., E. Manaresi, K. Zakrzewska, R. DeSantis, M. Musiani, and M. Zerbini.** 2004. Antibody response to B19 parvovirus VP1 and VP2 linear epitopes in patients with haemophilic arthritis. *J. Med. Virol.* **72:**679–682.
11. **Ballou, W. R., J. L. Reed, W. Noble, N. S. Young, and S. Koenig.** 2003. Safety and immunogenicity of a recombinant parvovirus B19 vaccine formulated with MF59C.1. *J. Infect. Dis.* **187:**675–678.
12. **Barah, F., P. J. Vallely, M. L. Chiswick, G. M. Cleator, and J. R. Kerr.** 2001. Association of human parvovirus B19 infection with acute meningoencephalitis. *Lancet* **358:**729–730.
13. **Bastien, N., N. Chui, J. L. Robinson, B. E. Lee, K. Dust, L. Hart, and Y. Li.** 2007. Detection of human bocavirus in Canadian children in a 1-year study. *J. Clin. Microbiol.* **45:**610–613.
14. **Baylis, S. A., N. Shah, and P. D. Minor.** 2004. Evaluation of different assays for the detection of parvovirus B19 DNA in human plasma. *J. Virol. Methods* **121:**7–16.
15. **Berns, K., and C. R. Parrish.** 2006. *Parvoviridae*, p. 2437–2477. *In* D. M. Knipe, P. M. Howley, D. E. Griffin, R. A. Lamb, M. A. Martin, B. Roizman, and S. E. Straus (ed.), *Fields Virology*, 5th ed., vol. 2. Lippincott Williams & Wilkins, Philadelphia, PA.
16. **Beske, F., S. Modrow, J. Sorensen, H. Schmidt, S. Kriener, R. Allwinn, T. Klingebiel, D. Schwabe, and T. Lehrnbecher.** 2007. Parvovirus B19 pneumonia in a child undergoing allogeneic hematopoietic stem cell transplantation. *Bone Marrow Transplant.* **40:**89–91.
17. **Bonvicini, F., G. Gallinella, G. A. Gentilomi, S. Ambretti, M. Musiani, and M. Zerbini.** 2006. Prevention of iatrogenic transmission of B19 infection: different approaches to detect, remove or inactivate virus contamination. *Clin. Lab.* **52:**263–268.
18. **Bousvaros, A., R. Sundel, G. M. Thorne, K. McIntosh, M. Cohen, D. D. Erdman, A. Perez-Atayde, T. H. Finkel, and A. A. Colin.** 1998. Parvovirus B19-associated interstitial lung disease, hepatitis, and myositis. *Pediatr. Pulmonol.* **26:**365–369.
19. **Brown, K. E.** 1997. Human parvovirus B19 epidemiology and clinical manifestations. *Monogr. Virol.* **20:**42–60.
20. **Brown, K. E., S. M. Anderson, and N. S. Young.** 1993. Erythrocyte P antigen: cellular receptor for B19 parvovirus. *Science* **262:**114–117.
21. **Brown, K. E., Z. Liu, G. Gallinella, S. Wong, I. P. Mills, and M. G. O'Sullivan.** 2004. Simian parvovirus infection: a potential zoonosis. *J. Infect. Dis.* **190:**1900–1907.
22. **Bruu, A.-L., and S. A. Nordbo.** 1995. Evaluation of five commercial tests for detection of immunoglobulin M an-

tibodies to human parvovirus B19. *J. Clin. Microbiol.* **33:**1363–1365.

23. **Caillet-Fauquet, P., M. L. Draps, M. Di Giambattista, Y. de Launoit, and R. Laub.** 2004. Hypoxia enables B19 erythrovirus to yield abundant infectious progeny in a pluripotent erythroid cell line. *J. Virol. Methods* **121:**145–153.
24. **Carrascosa, J., M. Just, M. Ribera, and C. Ferrandiz.** 1998. Papular acrodermatitis of childhood related to poxvirus and parvovirus B19 infection. *Cutis* **61:**265–267.
25. **Cartter, M. L., T. A. Farley, S. Rosengren, D. L. Quinn, S. M. Gillespie, G. W. Gary, and J. L. Hadler.** 1991. Occupational risk factors for infection with parvovirus B19 among pregnant women. *J. Infect. Dis.* **163:**282–285.
26. **Centers for Disease Control.** 1989. Risks associated with human parvovirus B19 infection. *Morb. Mortal. Wkly. Rep.* **38:**81–88, 93–97.
27. **Chen, J., Q. Wu, P. Yang, H. C. Hsu, and J. D. Mountz.** 2006. Determination of specific CD4 and CD8 T cell epitopes after AAV2- and AAV8-hF.IX gene therapy. *Mol. Ther.* **13:**260–269.
28. **Chisaka, H., K. Ito, H. Niikura, J. Sugawara, T. Takano, T. Murakami, Y. Terada, K. Okamura, H. Shiroishi, K. Sugamura, and N. Yaegashi.** 2006. Clinical manifestations and outcomes of parvovirus B19 infection during pregnancy in Japan. *Tohoku J. Exp. Med.* **209:**277–283.
29. **Chorba, T., P. Coccia, R. C. Holman, T. Tattersall, L. J. Anderson, J. Sudman, N. S. Young, E. Kurczynski, U. M. Saarinen, R. Moir, D. N. Lawrence, J. M. Jason, and B. Evatt.** 1986. The role of parvovirus B19 in aplastic crisis and erythema infectiosum (fifth disease). *J. Infect. Dis.* **154:**383–393.
30. **Cohen, B. J., and M. M. Buckley.** 1988. The prevalence of antibody to human parvovirus B19 in England and Wales. *J. Med. Microbiol.* **25:**151–153.
31. **Cohen, B. J., P. P. Mortimer, and M. S. Pereira.** 1983. Diagnostic assays with monoclonal antibodies for the human serum parvovirus-like virus (SPLV). *J. Hyg.* **91:**113–130.
32. **Cossart, Y. E., A. M. Field, B. Cant, and D. Widdows.** 1975. Parvovirus-like particles in human sera. *Lancet* **i:**72–73.
33. **Cotmore, S. F., and P. Tattersall.** 2007. Parvoviral host range and cell entry mechanisms. *Adv. Virus Res.* **70:**183–232.
34. **Dereure, O., B. Montes, and J. J. Guilhou.** 1995. Acute generalized livedo reticularis with myasthenialike syndrome revealing parvovirus B19 primary infection. *Arch. Dermatol.* **131:**744–745.
35. **Dowell, S. F., T. J. Torok, J. A. Thorp, J. Hedrick, D. D. Erdman, S. R. Zaki, C. J. Hinkle, W. L. Bayer, and L. J. Anderson.** 1995. Parvovirus B19 infection in hospital workers: community or hospital acquisition? *J. Infect. Dis.* **172:**1076–1079.
36. **Eid, A. J., R. A. Brown, R. Patel, and R. R. Razonable.** 2006. Parvovirus B19 infection after transplantation: a review of 98 cases. *Clin. Infect. Dis.* **43:**40–48.
37. **Ekman, A., K. Hokynar, L. Kakkola, K. Kantola, L. Hedman, H. Bonden, M. Gessner, C. Aberham, P. Norja, S. Miettinen, K. Hedman, and M. Soderlund-Venermo.** 2007. Biological and immunological relations among human parvovirus B19 genotypes 1 to 3. *J. Virol.* **81:**6927–6935.
38. **Enders, M., A. Weidner, and G. Enders.** 2007. Current epidemiological aspects of human parvovirus B19 infection during pregnancy and childhood in the western part of Germany. *Epidemiol. Infect.* **135:**563–569.
39. **Endo, R., N. Ishiguro, H. Kikuta, S. Teramoto, R. Shirkoohi, X. Ma, T. Ebihara, H. Ishiko, and T. Ariga.** 2007. Seroepidemiology of human bocavirus in Hokkaido Prefecture, Japan. *J. Clin. Microbiol.* **45:**3218–3223.
40. **Erdman, D. D., J. Usher, C. Tsou, E. O. Caul, G. W. Gary, S. Kajigaya, N. S. Young, and L. J. Anderson.** 1991. Human parvovirus B19 specific IgG, IgA, and IgM antibodies and DNA in serum specimens from persons with erythema infectiosum. *J. Med. Virol.* **35:**110–115.
41. **Ergaz, Z., and A. Ornoy.** 2006. Parvovirus B19 in pregnancy. *Reprod. Toxicol.* **21:**421–435.
42. **Erles, K., P. Sebokova, and J. R. Schlehofer.** 1999. Update on the prevalence of serum antibodies (IgG and IgM) to adeno-associated virus (AAV). *J. Med. Virol.* **59:**406–411.
43. **Essary, L., C. Vnencak-Jones, S. Manning, S. Olson, and J. Johnson.** 1998. Frequency of parvovirus B19 infection in nonimmune hydrops fetalis and utility of three diagnostic methods. *Hum. Pathol.* **29:**696–701.
44. **Fairley, C. K., J. S. Smoleniec, O. E. Caul, and E. Miller.** 1995. Observational study of effect of intrauterine transfusions on outcome of fetal hydrops after parvovirus B19. *Lancet* **346:**1335–1337.
45. **Ferguson, M., and A. Heath.** 2004. Report of a collaborative study to calibrate the Second International Standard for parvovirus B19 antibody. *Biologicals* **32:**207–212.
46. **Forestier, F., J.-D. Tissot, Y. Vial, F. Daffos, D. Fernand, and P. Hohlfeld.** 1999. Haematological parameters of parvovirus B19 infection in 13 fetuses with hydrops foetalis. *Br. J. Haematol.* **104:**925–927.
47. **Friedman-Einat, M., Z. Grossman, F. Mileguir, Z. Smetana, M. Ashkenazi, G. Barkai, N. Varsano, E. Glick, and E. Mendelson.** 1997. Detection of adeno-associated virus type 2 sequences in the human genital tract. *J. Clin. Microbiol.* **35:**71–78.
48. **Fry, A. M., X. Lu, M. Chittaganpitch, T. Peret, J. Fischer, S. F. Dowell, L. J. Anderson, D. Erdman, and S. J. Olsen.** 2007. Human bocavirus: a novel parvovirus epidemiologically associated with pneumonia requiring hospitalization in Thailand. *J. Infect. Dis.* **195:**1038–1045.
49. **Fryer, J. F., E. Delwart, F. Bernardin, P. W. Tuke, V. V. Lukashov, and S. A. Baylis.** 2007. Analysis of two human parvovirus PARV4 genotypes identified in human plasma for fractionation. *J. Gen. Virol.* **88:**2162–2167.
50. **Gao, G., L. H. Vandenberghe, M. R. Alvira, Y. Lu, R. Calcedo, X. Zhou, and J. M. Wilson.** 2004. Clades of adeno-associated viruses are widely disseminated in human tissues. *J. Virol.* **78:**6381–6388.
51. **Garcia-Tapia, A. M., C. F.-M. del Alamo, J. A. Giron, J. Mira, F. de la Rubia, A. Martinez-Rodriguez, M. V. Martin-Reina, R. Lopez-Caparrox, R. Caliz, M. S. Caballero, and A. Bascunana.** 1996. Spectrum of parvovirus B19 infection: analysis of an outbreak of 43 cases in Cadiz, Spain. *Clin. Infect. Dis.* **21:**1424–1430.
52. **Garner, J. S., and The Hospital Infection Control Practices Advisory Committee.** 1996. Guideline for isolation precautions in hospitals, 2nd ed., part 2. Rationale and recommendations. *Infect. Control Hosp. Epidemiol.* **17:**53–80.
53. **Geng, Y., C. G. Wu, S. P. Bhattacharyya, D. Tan, Z. P. Guo, and M. Y. Yu.** 2007. Parvovirus B19 DNA in Factor VIII concentrates: effects of manufacturing procedures and B19 screening by nucleic acid testing. *Transfusion* **47:**883–889.
54. **Gillespie, S. M., M. L. Cartter, S. Asch, J. B. Rokos, G. W. Gary, C. J. Tsou, D. B. Hall, L. J. Anderson, and E. S. Hurwitz.** 1990. Occupational risk of human parvovirus B19 infection for school and day-care personnel

during an outbreak of erythema infectiosum. *JAMA* **263:** 2061–2065.

55. **Goldstein, A. R., M. J. Anderson, and G. R. Serjeant.** 1987. Parvovirus associated aplastic crisis in homozygous sickle cell disease. *Arch. Dis. Child.* **62:**585–588.
56. **Gray, J. J., B. J. Cohen, and U. Desselberger.** 1993. Detection of human parvovirus B19-specific IgM and IgG antibodies using a recombinant viral VP1 antigen expressed in insect cells and estimation of the time of infection by testing for antibody avidity. *J. Virol. Methods* **44:**11–24.
57. **Green, S. W., I. Malkovska, M. G. O'Sullivan, and K. E. Brown.** 2000. Rhesus and pig-tailed macaque parvoviruses: identification of two new members of the Erythrovirus genus in monkeys. *Virology* **269:**105–112.
58. **Harel, L., I. Straussberg, A. Zeharia, D. Praiss, and J. Amir.** 2002. Papular purpuric rash due to parvovirus B19 with distribution on the distal extremities and the face. *Clin. Infect. Dis.* **35:**1558–1561.
59. **Harger, J., S. Adler, W. Koch, and G. Harger.** 1998. Prospective evaluation of 618 pregnant women exposed to parvovirus B19: risks and symptoms. *Obstet. Gynecol.* **91:**413–420.
60. **Hattori, S., M. Yunoki, M. Tsujikawa, T. Urayama, Y. Tachibana, I. Yamamoto, S. Yamamoto, and K. Ikuta.** 2007. Variability of parvovirus B19 to inactivation by liquid heating in plasma products. *Vox Sang.* **92:**121–124.
61. **Hemauer, A., A. Gigler, K. Searle, K. Beckenlehner, U. Raab, K. Broliden, H. Wolf, G. Enders, and S. Modrow.** 1999. Seroprevalence of parvovirus B19 NS1-specific IgG in B19-infected and uninfected individuals and in infected pregnant women. *J. Med. Virol.* **60:**48–55.
62. **Hindiyeh, M. Y., N. Keller, M. Mandelboim, D. Ram, J. Rubinov, L. Regev, V. Levy, S. Orzitzer, H. Shaharabani, R. Azar, E. Mendelson, and Z. Grossman.** 2008. High rate of human bocavirus and adenovirus coinfection in hospitalized Israeli children. *J. Clin. Microbiol.* **46:**334–337.
63. **Hobbs, J. A.** 2006. Detection of adeno-associated virus 2 and parvovirus B19 in the human dorsolateral prefrontal cortex. *J. Neurovirol.* **12:**190–199.
64. **Hokynar, K., J. Brunstein, M. Soderlund-Venermo, O. Kiviluoto, E. K. Partio, Y. Konttinen, and K. Hedman.** 2000. Integrity and full coding sequence of B19 virus DNA persisting in human synovial tissue. *J. Gen. Virol.* **81:**1017–1025.
65. **Ieiri, N., O. Hotta, and Y. Taguma.** 2005. Characteristics of acute glomerulonephritis associated with human parvovirus B19 infection. *Clin. Nephrol.* **64:**249–257.
66. **Isumi, H., T. Nunoue, A. Nishida, and S. Takashima.** 1999. Fetal brain infection with human parvovirus B19. *Pediatr. Neurol.* **21:**661–663.
67. **Jensen, I., P. Thorsen, B. Jeune, B. Moller, and B. Vestergaard.** 2000. An epidemic of parvovirus B19 in a population of 3,596 pregnant women: a study of sociodemographic and medical risk factors. *Br. J. Obstet. Gynaecol.* **107:**637–643.
68. **Jones, L., D. D. Erdman, and L. Anderson.** 1999. Prevalence of antibodies to human parvovirus B19 nonstructural protein (NS1) in persons with varied clinical outcomes following B19 infection. *J. Infect. Dis.* **180:** 500–504.
69. **Jones, M. S., A. Kapoor, V. V. Lukashov, P. Simmonds, F. Hecht, and E. Delwart.** 2005. New DNA viruses identified in patients with acute viral infection syndrome. *J. Virol.* **79:**8230–8236.
70. **Kajigaya, S., H. Fujii, A. Field, S. Anderson, S. Rosenfeld, L. J. Anderson, T. Shimada, and N. S. Young.** 1991. Self-assembled B19 parvovirus capsids, produced in a baculovirus system, are antigenically and immunogenically similar to native virions. *Proc. Natl. Acad. Sci. USA* **88:**4646–4650.
71. **Kajigaya, S., and M. Momeoda.** 1997. Immune response to B19 infection. *Monogr. Virol.* **20:**120–136.
72. **Kaufmann, B., A. Lopez-Bueno, M. G. Mateu, P. R. Chipman, C. D. Nelson, C. R. Parrish, J. M. Almendral, and M. G. Rossmann.** 2007. Minute virus of mice, a parvovirus, in complex with the Fab fragment of a neutralizing monoclonal antibody. *J. Virol.* **81:**9851–9858.
73. **Kaufmann, B., A. A. Simpson, and M. G. Rossmann.** 2004. The structure of human parvovirus B19. *Proc. Natl. Acad. Sci. USA* **101:**11628–11633.
74. **Kelly, H., D. Siebert, R. Hammond, J. Leydon, P. Kiely, and W. Maskill.** 2000. The age-specific prevalence of human parvovirus immunity in Victoria, Australia compared with other parts of the world. *Epidemiol. Infect.* **124:**449–457.
75. **Kempe, A., B. Rosing, C. Berg, D. Kamil, A. Heep, U. Gembruch, and A. Geipel.** 2007. First-trimester treatment of fetal anemia secondary to parvovirus B19 infection. *Ultrasound Obstet. Gynecol.* **29:**226–228.
76. **Kesebir, D., M. Vazquez, C. Weibel, E. D. Shapiro, D. Ferguson, M. L. Landry, and J. S. Kahn.** 2006. Human bocavirus infection in young children in the United States: molecular epidemiological profile and clinical characteristics of a newly emerging respiratory virus. *J. Infect. Dis.* **194:**1276–1282.
77. **Kobayashi, S., A. Maruta, T. Yamamoto, N. Katayama, R. Higuchi, Y. Sakano, H. Fujita, H. Koharazawa, N. Tomita, J. Taguchi, F. Kodama, Y. Nakamura, and A. Shimizu.** 1998. Human parvovirus B19 capsid antigen in granulocytes in parvovirus-B19-induced pancytopenia after bone marrow transplantation. *Acta Haematol.* **100:** 195–199.
78. **Koch, W., J. Harger, B. Barnstein, and S. Adler.** 1998. Serologic and virologic evidence for frequent intrauterine transmission of human parvovirus B19 with a primary maternal infection during pregnancy. *Pediatr. Infect. Dis. J.* **17:**489–494.
79. **Koch, W. C., and S. P. Adler.** 1989. Human parvovirus B19 infections in women of childbearing age and within families. *Pediatr. Infect. Dis. J.* **8:**83–87.
80. **Koduri, P., R. Kumapley, J. Valladares, and C. Teter.** 1999. Chronic pure red cell aplasia caused by parvovirus B19 in AIDS: use of intravenous immunoglobulin—a report of eight patients. *Am. J. Hematol.* **61:**16–20.
81. **Kurtzman, G., N. Frickhofen, J. Kimball, D. W. Jenkins, A. W. Nienhuis, and N. S. Young.** 1989. Pure red-cell aplasia of ten years' duration due to persistent parvovirus B19 infection and its cure with immunoglobulin therapy. *N. Engl. J. Med.* **321:**519–523.
82. **Kurtzman, G. J., B. Cohen, P. Meyers, A. Amunullah, and N. S. Young.** 1988. Persistent B19 parvovirus infection as a cause of severe chronic anaemia in children with acute lymphocytic leukaemia. *Lancet* **ii:**1159–1162.
83. **Lau, S. K., C. C. Yip, T. L. Que, R. A. Lee, R. K. Au-Yeung, B. Zhou, L. Y. So, Y. L. Lau, K. H. Chan, P. C. Woo, and K. Y. Yuen.** 2007. Clinical and molecular epidemiology of human bocavirus in respiratory and fecal samples from children in Hong Kong. *J. Infect. Dis.* **196:** 986–993.
84. **Laurenz, M., B. Winkelmann, J. Roigas, M. Zimmering, U. Querfeld, and D. Müller.** 2006. Severe parvovirus B19 encephalitis after renal transplantation. *Pediatr. Transplant.* **10:**978–981.
85. **Lee, J. I., J. Y. Chung, T. H. Han, M. O. Song, and E. S. Hwang.** 2007. Detection of human bocavirus in

children hospitalized because of acute gastroenteritis. *J. Infect. Dis.* **196:**994–997.

86. **Lefrere, J. J., A. Servant-Delmas, D. Candotti, M. Mariotti, I. Thomas, Y. Brossard, F. Lefrere, R. Girot, J. P. Allain, and S. Laperche.** 2005. Persistent B19 infection in immunocompetent individuals: implications for transfusion safety. *Blood* **106:**2890–2895.
87. **Lindblom, A., A. Isa, O. Norbeck, S. Wolf, B. Johansson, K. Broliden, and T. Tolfvenstam.** 2005. Slow clearance of human parvovirus B19 viremia following acute infection. *Clin. Infect. Dis.* **41:**1201–1203.
88. **Lu, J., N. Zhi, S. Wong, and K. E. Brown.** 2006. Activation of synoviocytes by the secreted phospholipase A2 motif in the VP1-unique region of parvovirus B19 minor capsid protein. *J. Infect. Dis.* **193:**582–590.
89. **Lu, X., M. Chittaganpitch, S. J. Olsen, I. M. Mackay, T. P. Sloots, A. M. Fry, and D. D. Erdman.** 2006. Real-time PCR assays for detection of bocavirus in human specimens. *J. Clin. Microbiol.* **44:**3231–3235.
90. **Luo, W., and C. R. Astell.** 1993. A novel protein encoded by small RNAs of parvovirus B19. *Virology* **195:** 448–455.
91. **Mackay, I. M.** 2007. Human bocavirus: multisystem detection raises questions about infection. *J. Infect. Dis.* **196:**968–970.
92. **Manaresi, E., G. Gallinella, M. Zerbini, S. Venturoli, G. Gentilomi, and M. Musiami.** 1999. IgG immune response to B19 parvovirus VP1 and VP2 linear epitopes by immunoblot assay. *J. Med. Virol.* **57:**174–178.
93. **Manning, A., V. Russell, K. Eastick, G. H. Leadbetter, N. Hallam, K. Templeton, and P. Simmonds.** 2006. Epidemiological profile and clinical associations of human bocavirus and other human parvoviruses. *J. Infect. Dis.* **194:**1283–1290.
94. **Manning, A., S. J. Willey, J. E. Bell, and P. Simmonds.** 2007. Comparison of tissue distribution, persistence, and molecular epidemiology of parvovirus B19 and novel human parvoviruses PARV4 and human bocavirus. *J. Infect. Dis.* **195:**1345–1352.
95. **McNeely, M., J. Friedman, and E. Pope.** 2005. Generalized petechial eruption induced by parvovirus B19 infection. *J. Am. Acad. Dermatol.* **52:**S109–S113.
96. **Miller, E., C. Fairley, B. J. Cohen, and C. Seng.** 1998. Immediate and long term outcome of human parvovirus B19 infection during pregnancy. *Br. J. Obstet. Gynaecol.* **105:**174–178.
97. **Miyagawa, E., T. Yoshida, H. Takahashi, K. Yamaguchi, T. Nagano, Y. Kiriyama, K. Okochi, and H. Sato.** 1999. Infection of the erythroid cell line, KU812ep6 with human parvovirus B19 and its application to titration of B19 infectivity. *J. Virol. Methods* **83:**45–54.
98. **Modrow, S.** 2006. Parvovirus B19: the causative agent of dilated cardiomyopathy or a harmless passenger of the human myocard? *Ernst Schering Res. Found. Workshop* **2006:**63–82.
99. **Morey, A. L., D. J. P. Ferguson, K. O. Leslie, D. J. Taatjes, and K. A. Fleming.** 1993. Intracellular localization of parvovirus B19 nucleic acid at the ultrastructural level by in situ hybridization with digoxigenin-labelled probes. *Histochem. J.* **25:**421–429.
100. **Morey, A. L., G. Patou, S. Myint, and K. Fleming.** 1992. In vitro culture for the detection of infectious human parvovirus B19 and B19-specific antibodies using foetal haematopoietic precursor cells. *J. Gen. Virol.* **73:** 3313–3317.
101. **Morey, A. L., H. J. Porter, J. W. Keeling, and K. A. Fleming.** 1992. Non-isotopic in situ hybridisation and immunophenotyping of infected cells in the investigation of human fetal parvovirus infection. *J. Clin. Pathol.* **45:**673–678.
102. **Munakata, Y., T. Saito-Ito, K. Kumura-Ishii, J. Huang, T. Kodera, T. Ishii, Y. Hirabayashi, Y. Koyanagi, and T. Sasaki.** 2005. Ku80 autoantigen as a cellular coreceptor for human parvovirus B19 infection. *Blood* **106:** 3449–3456.
103. **Myamoto, K., M. Ogami, Y. Takahashi, T. Mori, S. Akimoto, H. Terashita, and T. Terashita.** 2000. Outbreak of human parvovirus B19 in hospital workers. *J. Hosp. Infect.* **45:**238–241.
104. **Nagel, H. T., T. R. de Haan, F. P. Vandenbussche, D. Oepkes, and F. J. Walther.** 2007. Long-term outcome after fetal transfusion for hydrops associated with parvovirus B19 infection. *Obstet. Gynecol.* **109:**42–47.
105. **Naides, S. J.** 1988. Erythema infectiosum (fifth disease) occurrence in Iowa. *Am. J. Public Health* **78:**1230–1231.
106. **Naides, S. J., and C. P. Weiner.** 1989. Antenatal diagnosis and palliative treatment of non-immune hydrops fetalis secondary to fetal parvovirus B19 infection. *Prenatal Diagn.* **9:**105–114.
107. **O'Sullivan, M. G., D. K. Anderson, J. A. Goodrich, H. Tulli, S. W. Green, N. S. Young, and K. E. Brown.** 1997. Experimental infection of cynomolgus monkeys with simian parvovirus. *J. Virol.* **71:**4517–4521.
108. **Ozawa, K., J. Ayub, and N. Young.** 1988. Functional mapping of the genome of the B19 (human) parvovirus by in vitro translation after negative hybrid selection. *J. Virol.* **62:**2508–2511.
109. **Ozawa, K., J. Ayub, H. Yu-Shu, G. Kurtzman, T. Shimada, and N. Young.** 1987. Novel transcription map for the B19 (human) pathogenic parvovirus. *J. Virol.* **61:** 2395–2406.
110. **Ozawa, K., G. Kurtzman, and N. Young.** 1986. Replication of the B19 parvovirus in human bone marrow cell cultures. *Science* **233:**883–886.
111. **Ozawa, K., and N. Young.** 1987. Characterization of capsid and noncapsid proteins of B19 parvovirus propagated in human erythroid bone marrow cell cultures. *J. Virol.* **61:**2627–2630.
112. **Padron, E., V. Bowman, N. Kaludov, L. Govindasamy, H. Levy, P. Nick, R. McKenna, N. Muzyczka, J. A. Chiorini, T. S. Baker, and M. Agbandje-McKenna.** 2005. Structure of adeno-associated virus type 4. *J. Virol.* **79:**5047–5058.
113. **Peterlana, D., A. Puccetti, R. Beri, M. Ricci, S. Simeoni, L. Borgato, L. Scilanga, S. Ceru, R. Corrocher, and C. Lunardi.** 2003. The presence of parvovirus B19 VP and NS1 genes in the synovium is not correlated with rheumatoid arthritis. *J. Rheumatol.* **30:**1907–1910.
114. **Peterlana, D., A. Puccetti, R. Corrocher, and C. Lunardi.** 2006. Serologic and molecular detection of human parvovirus B19 infection. *Clin. Chim. Acta* **372:** 14–23.
115. **Plummer, F. A., G. W. Hammond, K. Forward, L. Sekla, L. M. Thompson, S. E. Jones, I. M. Kidd, and M. J. Anderson.** 1985. An erythema infectiosum-like illness caused by human parvovirus infection. *N. Engl. J. Med.* **313:**74–79.
116. **Porter, H. J., T. Y. Khong, M. F. Evans, V. T.-W. Chan, and K. A. Fleming.** 1988. Parvovirus as a cause of hydrops fetalis: detection by in situ DNA hybridisation. *J. Clin. Pathol.* **41:**381–383.
117. **Porter, H. J., A. M. Quantrill, and K. A. Fleming.** 1988. B19 parvovirus infection of myocardial cells. *Lancet* **i:**535–536.
118. **Pozo, F., M. L. Garcia-Garcia, C. Calvo, I. Cuesta, P. Perez-Brena, and I. Casas.** 2007. High incidence of hu-

man bocavirus infection in children in Spain. *J. Clin. Virol.* **40:**224–228.

119. **Public Health Laboratory Service Working Party on Fifth Disease.** 1990. Prospective study of human parvovirus (B19) infection in pregnancy. *Br. Med. J.* **300:** 1166–1170.

120. **Qu, X. W., Z. J. Duan, Z. Y. Qi, Z. P. Xie, H. C. Gao, W. P. Liu, C. P. Huang, F. W. Peng, L. S. Zheng, and Y. D. Hou.** 2007. Human bocavirus infection, People's Republic of China. *Emerg. Infect. Dis.* **13:**165–168.

121. **Rodis, J. F., C. Rodner, A. A. Hansen, A. F. Borgida, I. Deoliveira, and S. S. Rosengren.** 1998. Long-term outcome of children following maternal human parvovirus B19 infection. *Obstet. Gynecol.* **91:**125–128.

122. **Ros, C., M. Gerber, and C. Kempf.** 2006. Conformational changes in the VP1-unique region of native human parvovirus B19 lead to exposure of internal sequences that play a role in virus neutralization and infectivity. *J. Virol.* **80:**12017–12024.

123. **Saag, K. G., C. A. True, and S. J. Naides.** 1993. Intravenous immunoglobulin treatment of chronic parvovirus B19 arthropathy. *Arthritis Rheum.* **36**(Suppl.)**:**S67.

124. **Saarinen, U. A., T. L. Chorba, P. Tattersall, N. S. Young, L. J. Anderson, E. Palmer, and P. F. Coccia.** 1986. Human parvovirus B19-induced epidemic red cell aplasia in patients with hereditary hemolytic anemia. *Blood* **67:**1411–1417.

125. **Santagostino, E., P. Mannucci, A. Gringeri, A. Azzi, M. Morfini, R. Musso, R. Santoro, and M. Schiavoni.** 1997. Transmission of parvovirus B19 by coagulation factor concentrates exposed to 100°C heat after lyophilization. *Transfusion* **37:**517–522.

126. **Sattar, S. A., V. S. Springthorpe, Y. Karim, and P. Loro.** 1989. Chemical disinfection of non-porous inanimate surfaces experimentally contaminated with four human pathogenic viruses. *Epidemiol. Infect.* **102:**493–505.

127. **Schmid, S., W. Bossart, B. A. Michel, and P. Bruhlmann.** 2007. Outcome of patients with arthritis and parvovirus B19 DNA in synovial membranes. *Rheumatol. Int.* **27:**747–751.

127a. **Schmidt, M., A. Themann, C. Drexler, M. Bayer, G. Lanzer, E. Menichetti, S. Lechner, D. Wessin, B. Prokoph, J. P. Allain, E. Seifried, and M. K. Hourfar.** 2007. Blood donor screening for parvovirus B19 in Germany and Austria. *Transfusion* **47:**1775–1782.

128. **Schwarz, T. F., G. Jager, and S. Gilch.** 1997. Comparison of seven commercial tests for the detection of parvovirus B19-specific IgM. *Zentbl. Bakteriol.* **285:**525–530.

129. **Seng, C., P. Watkins, D. Morse, S. P. Barrett, M. Zambon, N. Andrews, M. Atkins, S. Hall, Y. K. Lau, and B. J. Cohen.** 1994. Parvovirus B19 outbreak on an adult ward. *Epidemiol. Infect.* **113:**345–353.

130. **Serjeant, G. R., G. E. Serjeant, P. W. Thomas, M. J. Anderson, G. Patou, and J. R. Pattison.** 1993. Human parvovirus infection in homozygous sickle cell disease. *Lancet* **341:**1237–1240.

131. **Shneerson, J. M., P. P. Mortimer, and E. M. Vandervelde.** 1980. Febrile illness due to a parvovirus. *Br. Med. J.* **1:**1580.

132. **Soderlund, M., C. S. Brown, W. J. M. Spaan, L. Hedman, and K. Hedman.** 1995. Epitope type-specific IgG responses to capsid proteins VP1 and VP2 of human parvovirus B19. *J. Infect. Dis.* **172:**1431–1436.

133. **Soderlund, M., R. von Essen, J. Haapasarri, U. Kiistala, O. Kiviluoto, and K. Hedman.** 1997. Persistence of parvovirus B19 DNA in synovial membranes of young patients with and without chronic arthropathy. *Lancet* **349:**1063–1065.

134. **St. Amand, J., and C. R. Astell.** 1993. Identification and characterization of a family of 11-kDa proteins encoded by the human parvovirus B19. *Virology* **192:**121–131.

135. **Takahashi, M., M. Ito, F. Sakamoto, N. Shimizu, T. Furukawa, M. Takahashi, and Y. Matsunaga.** 1995. Human parvovirus B19 infection: immunohistochemical and electron microscopic studies of skin lesions. *J. Cutan. Pathol.* **22:**168–172.

136. **Takeda, S., C. Takaeda, E. Takazakura, and J. Haratake.** 2001. Renal involvement induced by human parvovirus B19 infection. *Nephron* **89:**280–285.

137. **Tattersall, P., M. Bergoin, M. E. Bloom, K. E. Brown, R. M. Linden, N. Muzyczka, C. R. Parrish, and P. Tijssen.** 2005. *Parvoviridae*, p. 353–369. *In* C. M. Fauquet, M. A. Mayo, J. Maniloff, U. Desselberger, and L. A. Ball (ed.), *Virus Taxonomy: VIIIth Report of the International Committee on Taxonomy of Viruses*. Elsevier Academic Press, London, England.

138. **Torok, T. J.** 1997. Unusual clinical manifestations reported in patients with parvovirus B19 infection. *Monogr. Virol.* **20:**61–92.

139. **Torok, T. J., Q.-Y. Wang, G. W. Gary, C.-F. Yang, T. M. Finch, and L. J. Anderson.** 1992. Prenatal diagnosis of intrauterine infection with parvovirus B19 by the polymerase chain reaction technique. *Clin. Infect. Dis.* **14:**149–155.

140. **Tuckerman, J. G., T. Brown, and B. J. Cohen.** 1986. Erythema infectiosum in a village primary school: clinical and virological studies. *J. R. Coll. Gen. Practitioners* **36:**267–270.

141. **van Gessel, P. H., M. A. Gaytant, A. C. Vossen, J. M. Galama, N. T. Ursem, E. A. Steegers, and H. I. Wildschut.** 2006. Incidence of parvovirus B19 infection among an unselected population of pregnant women in the Netherlands: a prospective study. *Eur. J. Obstet. Gynecol. Reprod. Biol.* **128:**46–49.

142. **Vicente, D., G. Cilla, M. Montes, E. G. Perez-Yarza, and E. Perez-Trallero.** 2007. Human bocavirus, a respiratory and enteric virus. *Emerg. Infect. Dis.* **13:**636–637.

143. **von Kaisenberg, C. S., and W. Jonat.** 2001. Fetal parvovirus B19 infection. *Ultrasound Obstet. Gynecol.* **18:** 280–288.

144. **Vyse, A. J., N. J. Andrews, L. M. Hesketh, and R. Pebody.** 2007. The burden of parvovirus B19 infection in women of childbearing age in England and Wales. *Epidemiol. Infect.* **135:**1354–1362.

145. **Warrington, K. H., Jr., and R. W. Herzog.** 2006. Treatment of human disease by adeno-associated viral gene transfer. *Hum. Genet.* **119:**571–603.

146. **Weigel-Kelley, K. A., M. C. Yoder, and A. Srivastava.** 2003. $\alpha5\beta1$ integrin as a cellular coreceptor for human parvovirus B19: requirement of functional activation of $\beta1$ integrin for viral entry. *Blood* **102:**3927–3933.

147. **Wong, S., M. Momoeda, A. Field, S. Kajigaya, and N. S. Young.** 1994. Formation of empty B19 parvovirus capsids by the truncated minor capsid protein. *J. Virol.* **68:**4690–4694.

148. **Wong, S., N. S. Young, and K. E. Brown.** 2003. Prevalence of parvovirus B19 in liver tissue: no association with fulminant hepatitis or hepatitis-associated aplastic anemia. *J. Infect. Dis.* **187:**1581–1586.

149. **Woolf, A. D., G. V. Campion, A. Chishick, S. Wise, B. J. Cohen, P. T. Klouda, O. Caul, and P. A. Dieppe.** 1989. Clinical manifestations of human parvovirus B19 in adults. *Arch. Intern. Med.* **149:**1153–1156.

150. **Yoshida, M., and T. Tezuka.** 1994. Conjunctivitis caused by human parvovirus B19 infection. *Ophthalmologica* **208:**161–162.
151. **Young, N. S., and K. E. Brown.** 2004. Parvovirus B19. *N. Engl. J. Med.* **350:**586–597.
152. **Zakrzewska, K., A. Azzi, E. De Biasi, P. Radossi, R. De Santis, P. G. Davoli, and G. Tagariello.** 2001. Persistence of parvovirus B19 DNA in synovium of patients with haemophilic arthritis. *J. Med. Virol.* **65:**402–407.

TT Virus

PETER SIMMONDS

30

TT virus (TTV) and its relatives are small nonenveloped viruses with circular single-stranded DNA genomes. They frequently or ubiquitously infect humans and a range of other mammalian species. Infections are characterized by their lifelong persistence and their great genetic variability. Despite the original claimed association between TTV infection and hepatitis in humans when TTV was first discovered, in 1997, no evidence convincingly links infections with TTV or related viruses to clinical disease.

VIROLOGY

Discovery

TTV was identified in the plasma of an individual who developed non-A-E hepatitis after blood transfusion, using representational different analysis (RDA). RDA provided the method for the specific amplification of nucleic acid sequences present in plasma of an individual (initials, T. T.) during the period of his acute hepatitis but which were absent before transfusion (47). The cloning of the newly christened TT virus provided nucleotide sequences that allowed the development of methods for its detection by PCR. The original PCR method used primers from the N22 region (a part of the gene encoding the TTV structural protein; see "Composition" below) and was used to investigate other cases of posttransfusion hepatitis and other liver diseases of unexplained etiology (see "Pathogenesis and Clinical Manifestations" below).

The cloning of the N22 region allowed the sequence of the rest of the TTV genome to be determined and its genome organization to be characterized (43, 53). The genome was shown to be comprised of single-stranded DNA with coding sequences on the antigenomic strand. The length of the genome of the originally described (prototype) isolate of TTV (TA278) is 3,853 bases, forming a covalently closed circle (43). This genomic configuration is most similar to that of the animal virus chicken anemia virus (CAV), with some similarities in its arrangement of coding sequences (see "Classification" below).

In the years following the discovery of TTV, further highly divergent groups of TTV-like viruses have been found in humans, in nonhuman primates, and in a variety of other mammalian species. Independently, a virus also with a claimed association with posttransfusion and other forms of hepatitis was discovered by RDA. This virus was described as SEN V (75), but it has now become apparent that it represents a different genotype of TTV (see "Genetic Variability" below). More divergent human viruses include TTV-like minivirus (TTMV), which was accidentally discovered by PCR of human plasma samples using TTV-specific primers that matched homologous sequences in TTMV but generated a noticeably shorter amplicon than expected for TTV (72). Its overall genome length was additionally much shorter than that of TTV (approximately 2.8 kb). More recently, further TTV-like variants were cloned from a plasma sample of an individual at high risk for human immunodeficiency virus infection (24). These variants were initially described as small anellovirus types 1 and 2 (SAV-1 and -2) because their genome lengths were shorter than those of TTV and TTMV. Recent findings indicate that the originally published SAV-1 and SAV-2 sequences may have been incomplete (46); their finally determined sizes of 3.2 kb suggested to the authors the alternative designation TTV-like midivirus (TTMDV).

Using highly conserved primers from the untranslated region (UTR), a variety of TTV-like viruses have subsequently been found to be circulating in nonhuman primates, such as chimpanzees, African monkeys, macaques, New World primates (49, 77), and the tupaia (50), as well as a variety of domestic animals (pig, cat, and dog [8, 55]).

Classification

The classification of TTV and other small DNA viruses with single-stranded circular DNA genomes has recently been revised (7). TTV and its human virus relatives, TTMDV and TTMV, are now classified in a newly designated genus, *Anellovirus*, a term referring to the ring (Latin: anello)-like configuration of its genome. This is an "orphan" genus currently unassigned to any virus family. Tentatively included in the *Anellovirus* genus are related viruses found in nonhuman primates and other mammalian species. Although the genome organization of TTV and its relatives shows similarities to that of CAV, the latter virus remains classified as the type member of the *Gyrovirus* genus within the virus family *Circoviridae*.

However, the circovirus family includes a variety of avian and mammalian small DNA viruses such as the highly pathogenic pig virus porcine circovirus (in the genus *Circovirus*), but none of these show any resemblance to CAV (or TTV and its relatives) in genome organization, coding strategy, protein composition, capsid structure (11), or presumed mechanism of replication. The current classification is likely to be revised in the future.

Genetic Variability

TTV is characterized by extreme genetic diversity (Fig. 1). This has led to considerable problems in classification and the development of methods for screening, genetic characterization, and genotype identification. The situation is made more complex by the discovery of TTMV and TTMDV, which contain their own sets of genotypes and genetic groups, and by the existence of a wide range of homologs of TTV and TTMV in nonhuman primates, as well as even more divergent viruses in other mammalian species (Fig. 1) (2, 8, 10, 40, 49, 51, 77, 83). Although the phylogenetic tree in Fig. 1 is based on the majority of publicly available complete genome sequences of TTV and related viruses, it likely depicts only a small subset of TTV-like variants in nature. The most conserved region of the genome between genetic variants of human and animal TTV-like viruses is the UTR (Fig. 2). PCR using primers from this region can amplify each of the five main genetic groups of human TTV, as well as TTMV, TTMDV variants, and primate TTV-like viruses.

Among nonhuman primates, TTV variants are species specific; for example, chimpanzees harbor a range of TTV genotypes distinct from those infecting humans, although the genotypes themselves fall into three of the five main genetic groups of TTV (Fig. 1). TTV sequences from primates more distantly related to humans, such as macaques and the New World tamarins and owl monkeys, are in-

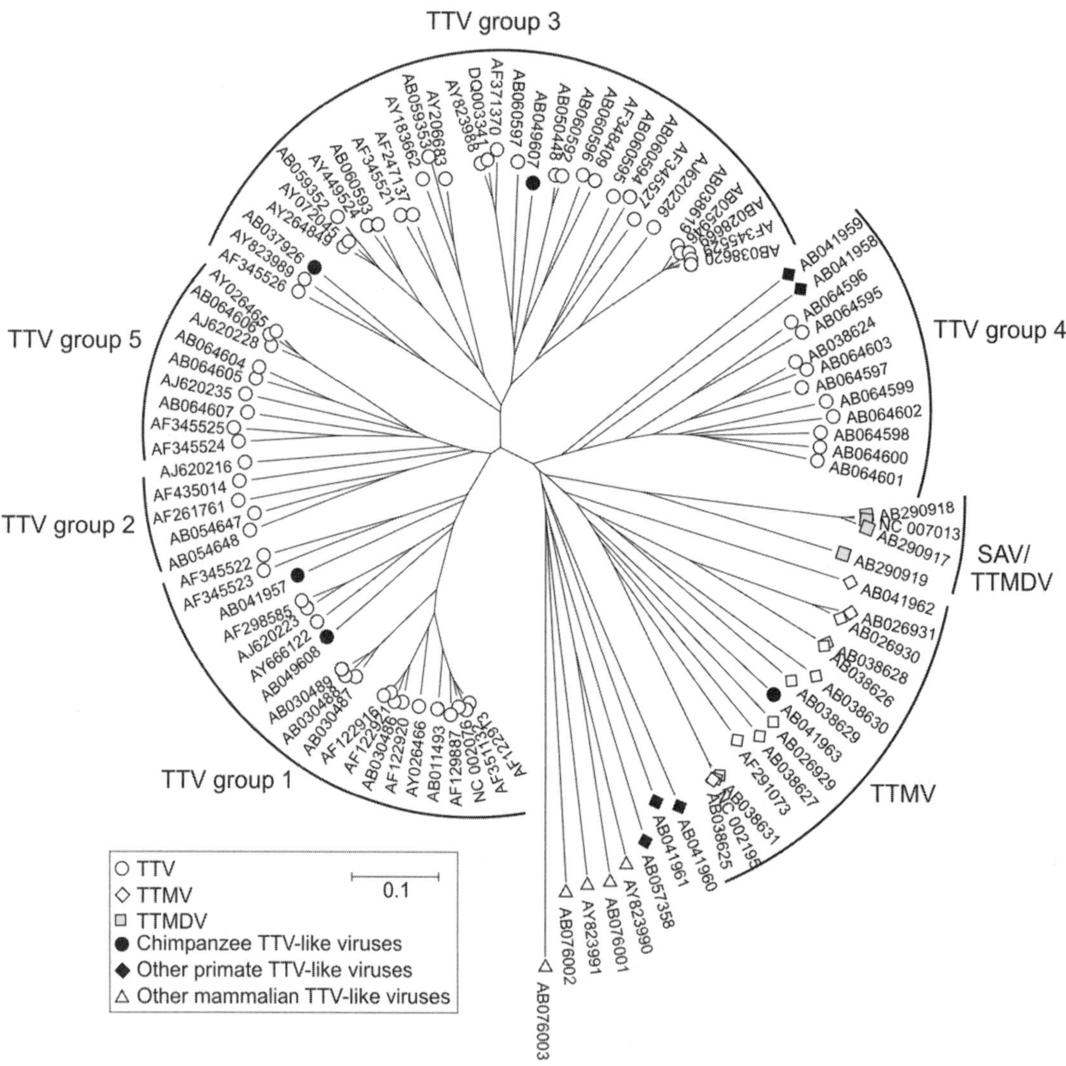

FIGURE 1 Sequence diversity in the ORF1 protein-coding sequence of TTV and related viruses. An alignment of ORF1 coding sequences between positions 211 and 862 (numbered from the start of the reading frame of the TA278 [NC_002076] reference sequence) was created using ClustalW, and a neighbor-joining phylogenetic tree was constructed from amino acid distances. Sequences from nonhuman primates, such as the chimpanzee, were frequently interspersed within the human-derived TTV and TTMV variants, while those from nonprimate mammalian species (pig, cat, and dog) were the most divergent.

		71	TATA box		Conserved region	160
TTV Grp. 1	NC_002076	GGGTCTACGTCCTC	ATATAA	GTAACTG	CACTTCCGAATGGCTGAGTTT	TCCACGCCCGTCCGCAG--CGGTGAAGCCA-----CGGAGGGAG-ATCTC
Grp. 2	AB050448	.TC.TAT.CG....	......	.....A.	....	..T..............--...CAGCA...-----.......T.-...C.
Grp. 3	AB054647	.............G	......	AGCG...	....	.................--...CAGC....-----.......T.-...C.
Grp. 4	AB064599	T.TC..C.CA.TGA	......	.C...A.	.GG.GA......TA.......	.TTC.............--..AG..C..G.G----..C..C...CGG.CG
Grp. 5	AB064605	.T...........A	......	A.G.G.A	....	ATGCT..........G.--A.AG..-....C----G.C..A..C--..CG
TTMV	NC_002195	..AGACT.CA.ACT	......	TA....A	....	ATGC....A.A.G.AGACTG.AGC.GTT..-----------CT.-..TA.
	AB038627	..AGT..ACAAACT	......	C.....A	....	ATGC....A.A.GAAGACAG.A.C.CTT..-----------.T.-.CTC.
	AB041962	...G.C.ACAAACT	......	CC..G.A	....	ATGC....A.A.G.AGACGG.A.C.CTT..-----------.T.-.CTC.
TTMDV SAV1	NC_007013	.A.A..CTTAAACT	......	CC..G..	GGG.GG...............	A..C...TA.A.G.TGCAGG.ACCGGAT.GAGCGCA.CGA....-G..C.
SAV2	AY622909	.A.A..TTAAAACT	......	CC..G..	GGG.GG...............	A..C...TA.A.G.TGCAGG.ACCGGAT.GAGCGCA.CGA....-G..C.
Macaque	AB041958	CCCGTCG.CAT..G	...A..	....G..	...A.T...............	ATACT.T...G......GT.....G..GAGC----GAC..TA.CG.C.C.
Macaque	AB041959	...GAA.A.GG.CA	......	.CCGGA.	....	.T.C.C.GA.A.GCAG.CGA..ACG.A..GCGCAG.CTG.T...TGA.CT
Tamarin	AB041960	ATTGGACGAAAACT	......	AG...C.	GGG.GA...............	A.TC....G.GTGTAG.AGAC.--CGA..GG-------.....AGG.AT
Owl monkey	AB041961	CTT.TCGG.AGAGG	......	.C..G..	....GA...............	A..GT...G.GGA....CGTCTGCCGAG.GG-------..C...GCG.GA
Tupaia	AB057358	ACA.AA.A...AC.	...AGT	AA..TGC	AGG.....G............	ATGC....A.CGGT...AG.CA.C.GA...C---------------G...
Pig	AB076001	TCCCACTAAAGTGA	......	..G.G..	..G..................	ATGC....A.CGGTAGA------C.GA--.C---------------.G..
Pig	AY823990	TCCCACGAAAG.GA	......	...GG..	AGG..................	ATGC....A.CGGTAGA------C.GA--.C---------------.G..
Cat	AB076003	...A.ACA.GGGGT	......	....G.A	....GA...............	A.TG..T.A.C.G.ACT-GGT.AC.G.A.GTGCGAAC.GA..T.AG.AGT
Dog	AB076002	C.CCT.T.CA.TCT	....CT	TGCG...	..G..................	ATGCT...G.GGTCGGACAGC.--C---.GA-------...CG--CG.GT
CAV	NC_001427	.C.CAAG.C..TCT	.....T	TG.G.GC	ACA.A...GTC...A.TAGG.	ATACGCAAG.CGGT.C.GGT..ATGCA.GG-------..AC.GCGGA.AA

		161	Conserved region	250
TTV Grp. 1	NC_002076	CG-CGTCCCGAGGGCGGGTGCCGAAG-----GTGAGTTTACACACCG-A	AGTCAAGGGGCAATTCGGGC	TCGGGACTGGCCGGGCTAT-GGGCAAGGC
Grp. 2	AB050448	..-.....................G..-----...............-C	....	...................-.........
Grp. 3	AB054647	..-.....................G..-----...............-C	....	...................-.........
Grp. 4	AB064599	A.-..A....T.......A......-----...............-C	....	...................-.......A.
Grp. 5	AB064605	AA-..C..................G..-----...............-C	....	................CCC-.........
TTMV	NC_002195	A.G.TGA..A.................-----......GA.AC.....-.	....	.A..TCAGTCTG.C.GA.C-.......AA
	AB038627	A.G.TGA..A.................-----......GA.AC.....-.	....	.A..TCAGTCTG.C.GA.C-.......AA
	AB041962	A.G.TGAA.TT.......A.......-----......GA.AC.....-T	....T...............	.A.TTCAGTCTG.C.GA.C-.......AA
TTMDV SAV1	NC_007013	..G.TG....T.......A...CG..-----......GA.AC.....-.	G...T...............	.A...CAGTCTA.C.GA.C-.......AA
SAV2	AY622909	A.G.TG...AT.......A...CG..-----......GA.AC.....-.	G...T...............	.A...CAGTCTA.C.GA.C-.......AA
Macaque	AB041958	A.A.CAG..CT.............G..-----................-C	....	A--..G.........ATCT.......TG
Macaque	AB041959	..G.CG....T...............C---G.GAG......C.C.GC-G	....	AA...CGGTCT....GACC-.........
Tamarin	AB041960	.CG.AG....T.......AC...C..AGCATTCCGAA-GGT.TG.G.CG	C..GT...............	A....CTCCCGG.C.GACC-........T
Owl monkey	AB041961	.CGA.CGA.T-.......A....GGAA-CATCC..AG--GT.TGTG.-.	C...T...............	AG.A.CACCCGGC.CAAC--........
Tupaia	AB057358	T.A..AG.T.--...........G..G---CTGTGCCGCG...TG.CGG	...........CT.......	AGC.AGAGTCTG.C.GA.C-....CTAA.
Pig	AB076001	TAG..A-.T.--...........G..G---AT------CC..G.T.CGG	...........CTA......	AG.A.CAGCTGA.C.GA---....CTACA
Pig	AY823990	TAG..A-.T.--...........G..G---AT------CC.TG.T.CGG	...........CTA......	AG.A.CAGCTAG.C.GA---....CTATG
Cat	AB076003	.ATG.AA.TAG.A...C.G..G.GT.C---C.GAG.CC.GG.GG...-G	...........TTA......	GAT.CGACC.G.T.A.----...TGG.C.
Dog	AB076002	GCGA.G....-.............GACTCCT.C.GAGCAG.GAGAG.CG	....	AA...C.ACCGT.CAGC---.......AT
CAV	NC_001427	.CGGCCG.T.G....A.TGAATCGGCG-----------------.TTAG	CCGAG........CCT....	-.CA.CGGA....C..A--G.......TA

FIGURE 2 Alignment of nucleotide sequences from the UTR of TTV and related human viruses (upper box) and homologs in other primates and mammalian species and the avian virus CAV (lower box). Highly conserved regions are boxed, including the putative TATA box at position 85 in the prototype TTV sequence, TA278 (NC_002076). Periods indicate sequence identity with prototype TTV sequence; dashes indicate gaps introduced to preserve alignment of homologous nucleotide sites.

creasingly divergent from TTV variants infecting humans (Fig. 1) (49). TTMV infection has been detected in chimpanzees (50, 77), again with genotypes distinct from but interspersed with human genotypes. A complication of primate studies is the cross-species transmission of TTV genotypes; for example, it is known that human TTV variants can infect chimpanzees and macaques (3, 76). Cross-species transmission may occur in captivity or through the administration of human plasma-derived blood products containing infectious TTV or related viruses that frequently occurs in experimental animals. In the future, samples should ideally be collected from animals in the wild to investigate further their species specificity.

Composition

TTV is a nonenveloped small virus with a diameter, as measured by electronmicroscopy, of 30 to 32 nm. Its density in plasma on sucrose gradients ranged from 1.31 to 1.34 g/cm^3, although this value was slightly higher for TTV virions excreted in feces (1.34 to 1.35 g/cm^3) (21). TTV purified from plasma of infected individuals was found to be frequently immune complexed with immunoglobulin G (21). The virion is likely composed of copies of only a single viral protein. TTV and related viruses are stable in the environment. For example, infectious TTV can be recovered from human feces (32), a finding that suggests that environmental sources of TTV may exist in contaminated water supplies, as documented for enteroviruses and caliciviruses. Consistent with these conclusions, the related CAV shows considerable resistance to a number of virus inactivation methods (82). The temperature required to reduce or eliminate infectivity is well above those used for plasma product inactivation (84).

The genomes of TTV and related viruses contain several open reading frames (ORFs) that code for several putative viral proteins from either spliced or unspliced mRNA transcripts (Fig. 3). The antigenomic sequence of TTV ranges from 3,750 to 3,900 bases in length, in which a total of four gene sequences can be consistently identified among the different genetic groups. The largest ORF (ORF1) potentially encodes a protein of 770 amino acids in the TTV prototype strain, TA278, while homologous proteins in prototype strains of related TTMV and TTMDV human viruses are shorter, at 673 and 663 amino acids (Fig. 3). The ORF1 product is likely to form the nucleocapsid, with perhaps the amino terminus being responsible for binding, encapsidation, and nuclear targeting of genomic DNA.

The translation of other ORFs requires splicing of viral mRNAs. Three main species of mRNA of 2.8, 1.2, and 1.0 kb have been detected after in vitro transfection of TTV DNA (27) and in bone marrow and liver tissues in vivo (52). These mRNAs share common 5′ and 3′ ends (Fig. 3); for the large transcript, splicing removed an intron between positions 185 and 277, leaving the entire coding sequence of ORF1. For the shorter mRNA of 1.3 kb, splicing removed the sequence between positions 771 and 2374 to join the coding sequence ORF2 with that of ORF4. The 1.0-kb transcript was generated by the removal of an intron from position 771 to position 2564 or 2567 to join ORF2 to ORF5. Each transcript can be translated from an initiating methionine at position 354 or 581; thus, a total of six distinct proteins can be expressed during replication (64). TTMV and TTMDV show the same arrangement of open reading as TTV, and it is therefore likely that nonstructural proteins comparable to those from ORF2/ORF4 and ORF2/ORF5 would be produced, as well as the structural protein from ORF1.

The UTR of the TTV genome contains conserved promoter sites, a TATA box, and cap sites consistent with the transcription of mRNAs from position 98 and termination around the polyadenylation signal at position 3073. The region contains a number of transcription promoters and regulatory elements responsible for transcriptional control (26). Although the nucleotide sequences of the UTRs of TTV and related viruses are distinct, there are some restricted regions of sequence identity or close sequence similarity interspersed with more variable regions (Fig. 2). This includes regions of clear sequence homology with more divergent sequences from macaques and New World primate species, with TTV-like viruses infecting other mammals and remarkably even in the otherwise dissimilar UTR of CAV. Apart from the TATA box, the functional constraints that have retained this sequence similarity are uncertain.

Replication

TTV and TTMV are likely to replicate in the nucleus of the infected cell, using host polymerases. The replication of small DNA viruses such as the parvoviruses is cell cycle dependent, and their replication is confined to rapidly dividing cells, such as those in the bone marrow, the gut, and fetal tissue. It is unknown whether the replication of TTV and TTMV is restricted in a similar way, or whether they encode proteins with transforming activity, perhaps corresponding to the T antigens of the polyomaviruses, that drive cells into division.

TTV can be cultured in the laboratory through inoculation of plasma-derived virus onto Chang liver cells (15) or stimulated peripheral blood mononuclear cells (34, 38). However, in contrast to the relative ease of culture of CAV and circoviruses, TTV replication in vitro occurs at low levels and serial passage has not been reported. In vivo, high levels of TTV DNA have been detected in the liver, peripheral blood mononuclear cells, bone marrow, and other tissues (23, 34, 56, 57, 63, 74). Double-stranded, presumed replicative intermediates of DNA have been detected in liver and bone marrow (56, 57). There is currently no evidence for a directly cytopathic or immunopathogenic effect of TTV replication in vivo, although the limited replication of TTV achieved in Chang cells in vitro was associated with detectable cytopathogenic changes (15). Replication in the respiratory tract was suggested by the detection of high levels of TTV DNA in respiratory secretions (14, 17, 18, 35).

EPIDEMIOLOGY

Distribution and Geography

TTV and the related viruses TTMDV and TTMV are widely distributed in human populations throughout the

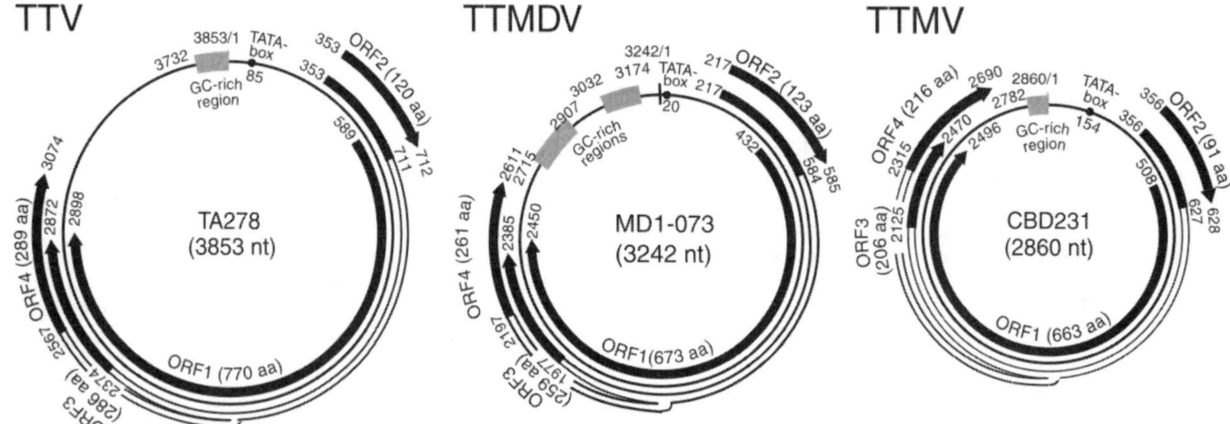

FIGURE 3 Genome organization of TTV, TTMV, and TTMDV showing the arrangement of genes on the antigenomic strand. Closed arrows represent the principal ORFs in each virus; thin lines between ORFs represent introns in the viral mRNAs. aa, amino acids; nt, nucleotides. (Reproduced with kind permission from reference 46.)

world. The original surveys used detection methods based on primers that amplified the variable N22 region, so sequences similar to the prototype strain (TA278, genotype 1) are vastly overrepresented in the database of published sequences. Using primers based on the conserved sequences in the UTR (Fig. 2), >80% frequencies of viremia with TTV and/or related viruses have been found in every population studied (1, 6, 20, 36, 68, 71). Through the use of primers specific for individual genotypes or genogroups of TTV, or those that differentiate TTV from TTMV sequences, high frequencies of coinfection with multiple variants of TTV have been described. In recent surveys (5, 33), 84 to 89% of study populations (generally healthy adults) were viremic for TTV or TTMV, with coinfections of TTV and TTMV in 41% and frequencies of coinfection with multiple genotypes of TTV or TTMV of 40 to 70%. Infection with TTV-like viruses in pigs was similarly highly prevalent (66 to 84% [8, 39, 40]).

Because of the near ubiquity of TTV and related viruses, the large number of genogroups and genotypes, and the difficulty in detecting coinfections, it is premature to conclude anything from previous investigations of possible geographic or risk group associations of genetic variants of these viruses.

Transmission

The detection of >80% frequencies of viremia in adult populations indicates a considerable incidence of infection early in life. Although limited by the use of N22 primers, most of the original studies have demonstrated that infection with TTV occurs in the perinatal period; samples collected at birth are generally PCR negative, with a rapidly rising prevalence of infection over the subsequent months (12, 13, 28, 69, 70). However, there are also conflicting reports of detection of TTV DNA in cord blood, implying in utero infection (42, 66). Using semiconserved primers from the UTR, my group found all samples collected around the time of birth to be PCR negative, while the frequency of viremia in children aged 6 to 12 months was 75% and stabilized at that level over the subsequent 5 years (68). During close follow-up of a newborn child (4), high levels of TTV DNA were detected in saliva from days 4 to 9 after birth, a period that coincided with a mild rhinitis. The TTV variant infecting the neonate was genetically identical to that present in maternal saliva in the neonatal period. Although anecdotal, these findings are consistent with findings of other studies indicating rapid acquisition of TTV infections around the time of birth. As described above, TTV is present at high concentrations in saliva (14, 17, 18), and it may therefore be transmissible by kissing or other close contact between a child and his or her parents or siblings.

There are likely other sources of TTV infection. TTV is present in peripheral blood and has been demonstrated to be transmissible by parenteral routes such as blood transfusion (47). However, this route is probably insignificant compared to the rapid acquisition of TTV in the perinatal period. Infectious TTV can be recovered from feces, providing an additional potential source of oral transmission (32). The likely great stability of TTV may lead to general environmental contamination.

PATHOGENESIS AND CLINICAL MANIFESTATIONS

Pathology

Infection with TTV and related viruses is characterized by persistent lifelong viremia in humans and nonhuman primates, with circulating levels typically ranging from 10^4 to 10^6 DNA copies/ml (20, 62). Levels of viremia reflect the balance between virus production and clearance from the circulation by the immune-complex formation and destruction of virus-infected cells; it has been estimated that a production rate of $>10^{10}$ virions per day is required to maintain observed levels of viremia (37).

The sites of replication of TTV in vivo responsible for this high level of virus production are uncertain. Initial investigations concentrated on the liver, given its originally described association with posttransfusion hepatitis. By in situ hybridization and/or quantitative PCR, evidence for replication of TTV in the liver has been documented (44, 48, 65), corroborated by the detection of double-stranded replicative intermediates in this tissue (57) and high levels of TTV excreted in bile (32, 45, 81). The latter may be the main source of TTV in the gastrointestinal tract and its excretion in feces. Despite the evidence for hepatic replication of TTV, there is no evidence for cytopathology or specific inflammatory changes associated with replication, or (despite earlier claims [78]) for its involvement in hepatocellular carcinoma or other malignant changes (41).

The replication of TTV is not restricted to the liver. High viral loads, double-stranded replicative forms of TTV DNA, and mRNA transcripts have been detected in bone marrow (16, 29, 52, 56), spleen (22), and other lymphoid tissue (25). TTV DNA is frequently detectable in peripheral blood mononuclear cells (3, 31, 54, 58). In these lymphoid cells, TTV shows a very broad tropism, as viral DNA can be detected in T and B lymphocytes, monocytes, and NK cells (34, 54, 74, 85). TTV tropism extends to granulocytes and other polymorphonuclear cells (34, 74). Bone marrow is the major site of replication of the related CAV, and the TTV findings may reflect a broader dependence of circoviruses for replication in rapidly dividing cells. No specific pathology has been attributed to the replication of TTV in bone marrow or lymphoid tissue.

Immune Responses

TTV infection is likely to be acquired around the time of birth (see "Transmission" above), and this may lead to substantial immune tolerance, as described for other viruses such as hepatitis B virus. Immunopathological changes such as inflammation and lymphocyte infiltration are not observed in tissues where TTV replication occurs (see "Pathology" above). The hypothesis that TTV and related viruses escape immunologic detection is supported by the persistent nature of infection and the presence of multiple circulating genetic variants in plasma (see "Genetic Variability" above) that may represent repeated rounds of reinfection. However, antibody reactivity to whole virions (80) or recombinant proteins expressed from ORF1 (19, 59) is frequently found in viremic and nonviremic individuals, and virions purified from plasma are often complexed with immunoglobulin G (21). Despite this, there is no evidence at present for an association with or presence of TTV in immune-complex deposition diseases such as glomerulonephritis.

Higher frequencies of TTV viremia and higher viral loads have been found among immunosuppressed individuals and in those with other intercurrent illnesses, indicating a potential role of the immune system in controlling TTV replication (9, 67, 79, 85). TTV might thus act as an opportunistic pathogen in certain immunodeficiency states, analogous to the behavior of human cytomegalovirus in AIDS, although it remains unclear what role the immune system plays in the natural course of TTV infection. Of great theoretical interest are the mechanisms of immune evasion that have evolved in TTV to establish persistent infection in immunocompetent individuals.

Disease Associations

As infection with TTV and/or related viruses is (almost) universally present in human populations, it is unlikely that these viruses are pathogenic per se. Numerous studies on the frequency of viremia detectable by PCR using N22 primers have been carried out, and they have provided no evidence for associations with any form of hepatitis (posttransfusion, chronic idiopathic, acute, or fulminant), despite the detection of virus replication in the liver. It is possible that certain genotypes of TTV may be specifically pathogenic, but there is currently no evidence to support this hypothesis.

More recent investigations have concentrated on potential roles of TTV and related viruses in childhood respiratory disease; high levels of TTV DNA are found in respiratory secretions and saliva (14, 17, 18, 35), and the respiratory tract may thus be a major site of TTV replication. Infection with TTV coincided with a mild rhinitis in a neonate (4), and children hospitalized with acute respiratory disease or with bronchiectasis showed higher TTV viral loads than controls (35, 36, 61). Higher TTV viral loads were associated with impairment of lung function among asthmatic children, although frequencies of detection and viral loads were comparable to those of children without asthma (60).

High levels of TTV replication in bone marrow have been suggested as being responsible for an otherwise unexplained case of aplastic anemia (29). Interestingly, infection of chickens with the related CAV is associated with anemia and lymphopenia that are generally only clinically apparent in association with other viral coinfections, such as with Marek's disease virus. It is unknown whether infections with other viruses have an equivalent effect on TTV infection in humans, but investigating the association of TTV and related viruses with such hematologic abnormalities may be a fruitful area of research in the future. In common with other small DNA viruses such as parvoviruses and circoviruses, TTV is not known to be associated with tumorigenesis or malignant transformation of cells, although it has been suggested that infections with TTV-like viruses may be associated with chromosomal translocations and childhood leukemia (30).

LABORATORY DIAGNOSIS

PCR is the principal method used for the detection of TTV DNA in clinical specimens. Methods that use heminested or fully nested primers are capable of extremely high sensitivity and specificity. The UTR of TTV is much more conserved than the coding region and therefore more appropriate as a target sequence for PCR (73). PCR based on primers from regions around the transcription start site (Fig. 2) indicated that frequencies of TTV and TTMV infections were close to universal, not only in humans but also in a range of nonhuman primates (see "Distribution and Geography" above).

Because of the great genetic variability of TTV and TTMV, it has not been possible to date to develop effective genotyping assays for either virus. To attempt to do so would be premature, as it is unlikely that the full genetic diversity of TTV and related viruses has been documented. For the foreseeable future, genotype identification of TTV will have to remain based on nucleotide sequencing of the N22 region and the UTR.

PREVENTION AND TREATMENT

As infection with TTV and/or related viruses is universal, measures to prevent transmission are unwarranted. Similarly, there is no current indication to treat individuals infected with TTV.

REFERENCES

1. **Abe, K., T. Inami, K. Asano, C. Miyoshi, N. Masaki, S. Hayashi, K. Ishikawa, Y. Takebe, K. M. Win, A. R. El-Zayadi, K. H. Han, and D. Y. Zhang.** 1999. TT virus infection is widespread in the general populations from different geographic regions. *J. Clin. Microbiol.* **37:**2703–2705.
2. **Abe, K., T. Inami, K. Ishikawa, S. Nakamura, and S. Goto.** 2000. TT virus infection in nonhuman primates and characterization of the viral genome: identification of simian TT virus isolates. *J. Virol.* **74:**1549–1553.
3. **Barril, G., J. M. Lopez-Alcorocho, A. Bajo, N. Ortiz-Movilla, J. A. Sanchez-Tomero, J. Bartolome, R. Selgas, and V. Carreno.** 2000. Prevalence of TT virus in serum and peripheral mononuclear cells from a CAPD population. *Perit. Dial. Int.* **20:**65–68.
4. **Biagini, P., R. N. Charrel, P. de Micco, and X. de Lamballerie.** 2003. Association of TT virus primary infection with rhinitis in a newborn. *Clin. Infect. Dis.* **36:**128–129.
5. **Biagini, P., P. Gallian, J. F. Cantaloube, H. Attoui, P. de Micco, and X. de Lamballerie.** 2006. Distribution and genetic analysis of TTV and TTMV major phylogenetic groups in French blood donors. *J. Med. Virol.* **78:**298–304.
6. **Biagini, P., P. Gallian, M. Touinssi, J. F. Cantaloube, J. P. Zapitelli, X. de Lamballerie, and P. de Micco.** 2000. High prevalence of TT virus infection in French blood donors revealed by the use of three PCR systems. *Transfusion* **40:**590–595.
7. **Biagini, P., D. Todd, M. Bendinelli, S. Hino, A. Mankertz, S. Mishiro, C. Niel, H. Okamoto, S. Raidal, B. W. Ritchie, and C. G. Teo.** 2004. Anellovirus, p. 335–341. *In* C. M. Fauquet, M. A. Mayo, J. Maniloff, U. Desselberger, and L. A. Ball (ed.), *Virus Taxonomy: Eighth Report of the International Committee on Taxonomy of Viruses.* Elsevier/Academic Press, London, United Kingdom.
8. **Bigarre, L., V. Beven, C. de Boisseson, B. Grasland, N. Rose, P. Biagini, and A. Jestin.** 2005. Pig anelloviruses are highly prevalent in swine herds in France. *J. Gen. Virol.* **86:**631–635.
9. **Christensen, J. K., J. Eugen-Olsen, M. Srensen, H. Ullum, S. B. Gjedde, B. K. Pedersen, J. O. Nielsen, and K. Krogsgaard.** 2000. Prevalence and prognostic significance of infection with TT virus in patients infected with human immunodeficiency virus. *J. Infect. Dis.* **181:**1796–1799.
10. **Cong, M. E., B. Nichols, X. G. Dou, J. E. Spelbring, K. Krawczynski, H. A. Fields, and Y. E. Khudyakov.** 2000. Related TT viruses in chimpanzees. *Virology* **274:** 343–355.
11. **Crowther, R. A., J. A. Berriman, W. L. Curran, G. M. Allan, and D. Todd.** 2003. Comparison of the structures of three circoviruses: *Chicken Anemia Virus, Porcine Cir-*

covirus Type 2, and *Beak and Feather Disease Virus*. *J. Virol.* **77:**13036–13041.

12. **Davidson, F., D. MacDonald, J. L. K. Mokili, L. E. Prescott, S. Graham, and P. Simmonds.** 1999. Early acquisition of TT virus (TTV) in an area endemic for TTV infection. *J. Infect. Dis.* **179:**1070–1076.
13. **de Martino, M., M. Moriondo, C. Azzari, M. Resti, L. Galli, and A. Vierucci.** 2000. TT virus infection in human immunodeficiency virus type 1 infected mothers and their infants. *J. Med. Virol.* **61:**347–351.
14. **Deng, X., H. Terunuma, R. Handema, M. Sakamoto, T. Kitamura, M. Ito, and Y. Akahane.** 2000. Higher prevalence and viral load of TT virus in saliva than in the corresponding serum: another possible transmission route and replication site of TT virus. *J. Med. Virol.* **62:**531–537.
15. **Desai, M., R. Pal, R. Deshmukh, and D. Banker.** 2005. Replication of TT virus in hepatocyte and leucocyte cell lines. *J. Med. Virol.* **77:**136–143.
16. **Fanci, R., R. De Santis, K. Zakrzewska, C. Paci, and A. Azzi.** 2004. Presence of TT virus DNA in bone marrow cells from hematologic patients. *New Microbiol.* **27:** 113–117.
17. **Gallian, P., P. Biagini, S. Zhong, M. Touinssi, W. Yeo, J. F. Cantaloube, H. Attoui, P. de Micco, P. J. Johnson, and X. de Lamballerie.** 2000. TT virus: a study of molecular epidemiology and transmission of genotypes 1, 2 and 3. *J. Clin. Virol.* **17:**43–49.
18. **Goto, K., K. Sugiyama, T. Ando, F. Mizutani, K. Terabe, K. Tanaka, M. Nishiyama, and Y. Wada.** 2000. Detection rates of TT virus DNA in serum of umbilical cord blood, breast milk and saliva. *Tohoku J. Exp. Med.* **191:**203–207.
19. **Handa, A., B. Dickstein, N. S. Young, and K. E. Brown.** 2000. Prevalence of the newly described human circovirus, TTV, in United States blood donors. *Transfusion* **40:** 245–251.
20. **Hu, Y. W., M. I. Al Moslih, M. T. Al Ali, S. R. Khameneh, H. Perkins, F. Diaz-Mitoma, J. N. Roy, S. Uzicanin, and E. G. Brown.** 2005. Molecular detection method for all known genotypes of TT virus (TTV) and TTV-like viruses in thalassemia patients and healthy individuals. *J. Clin. Microbiol.* **43:**3747–3754.
21. **Itoh, Y., M. Takahashi, M. Fukuda, T. Shibayama, T. Ishikawa, F. Tsuda, T. Tanaka, T. Nishizawa, and H. Okamoto.** 2000. Visualization of TT virus particles recovered from the sera and feces of infected humans. *Biochem. Biophys. Res. Commun.* **279:**718–724.
22. **Jelcic, I., A. Hotz-Wagenblatt, A. Hunziker, H. H. Zur, and E. M. de Villiers.** 2004. Isolation of multiple TT virus genotypes from spleen biopsy tissue from a Hodgkin's disease patient: genome reorganization and diversity in the hypervariable region. *J. Virol.* **78:**7498–7507.
23. **Jiang, X. J., K. X. Luo, and H. T. He.** 2000. Intrahepatic transfusion-transmitted virus detected by in situ hybridization in patients with liver diseases. *J. Viral Hepatitis* **7:** 292–296.
24. **Jones, M. S., A. Kapoor, V. V. Lukashov, P. Simmonds, F. Hecht, and E. Delwart.** 2005. New DNA viruses identified in patients with acute viral infection syndrome. *J. Virol.* **79:**8230–8236.
25. **Kakkola, L., N. Kaipio, K. Hokynar, P. Puolakkainen, P. S. Mattila, A. Kokkola, E. K. Partio, A. M. Eis-Hubinger, M. Soderlund-Venermo, and K. Hedman.** 2004. Genoprevalence in human tissues of TT-virus genotype 6. *Arch. Virol.* **149:**1095–1106.
26. **Kamada, K., T. Kamahora, P. Kabat, and S. Hino.** 2004. Transcriptional regulation of TT virus: promoter and enhancer regions in the 1.2-kb noncoding region. *Virology* **321:**341–348.
27. **Kamahora, T., S. Hino, and H. Miyata.** 2000. Three spliced mRNAs of TT virus transcribed from a plasmid containing the entire genome in COS1 cells. *J. Virol.* **74:** 9980–9986.
28. **Kazi, A., H. Miyata, K. Kurokawa, M. A. Khan, T. Kamahora, S. Katamine, and S. Hino.** 2000. High frequency of postnatal transmission of TT virus in infancy. *Arch. Virol.* **145:**535–540.
29. **Kikuchi, K., H. Miyakawa, K. Abe, M. Kako, K. Katayama, S. Fukushi, and S. Mishiro.** 2000. Indirect evidence of TTV replication in bone marrow cells, but not in hepatocytes, of a subacute hepatitis/aplastic anemia patient. *J. Med. Virol.* **61:**165–170.
30. **Leppik, L., K. Gunst, M. Lehtinen, J. Dillner, K. Streker, and E.-M. de Villiers.** 2007. In vivo and in vitro intragenomic rearrangement of TT viruses. *J. Virol.* **81:** 9346–9356. [Epub ahead of print.]
31. **Lopez-Alcorocho, J. M., L. F. Mariscal, S. De Lucas, E. Rodriguez-Inigo, M. Casqueiro, I. Castillo, J. Bartolome, M. Herrero, M. L. Manzano, M. Pardo, and V. Carreno.** 2000. Presence of TTV DNA in serum, liver and peripheral blood mononuclear cells from patients with chronic hepatitis. *J. Viral Hepatitis* **7:**440–447.
32. **Luo, K., W. Liang, H. He, S. Yang, Y. Wang, H. Xiao, D. Liu, and L. Zhang.** 2000. Experimental infection of nonenveloped DNA virus (TTV) in rhesus monkey. *J. Med. Virol.* **61:**159–164.
33. **Maggi, F., E. Andreoli, L. Lanini, C. Fornai, M. Vatteroni, M. Pistello, S. Presciuttini, and M. Bendinelli.** 2005. Relationships between total plasma load of torquetenovirus (TTV) and TTV genogroups carried. *J. Clin. Microbiol.* **43:**4807–4810.
34. **Maggi, F., C. Fornai, L. Zaccaro, A. Morrica, M. L. Vatteroni, P. Isola, S. Marchi, A. Ricchiuti, M. Pistello, and M. Bendinelli.** 2001. TT virus (TTV) loads associated with different peripheral blood cell types and evidence for TTV replication in activated mononuclear cells. *J. Med. Virol.* **64:**190–194.
35. **Maggi, F., M. Pifferi, C. Fornai, E. Andreoli, E. Tempestini, M. Vatteroni, S. Presciuttini, S. Marchi, A. Pietrobelli, A. Boner, M. Pistello, and M. Bendinelli.** 2003. TT virus in the nasal secretions of children with acute respiratory diseases: relations to viremia and disease severity. *J. Virol.* **77:**2418–2425.
36. **Maggi, F., M. Pifferi, E. Tempestini, C. Fornai, L. Lanini, E. Andreoli, M. Vatteroni, S. Presciuttini, A. Pietrobelli, A. Boner, M. Pistello, and M. Bendinelli.** 2003. TT virus loads and lymphocyte subpopulations in children with acute respiratory diseases. *J. Virol.* **77:**9081–9083.
37. **Maggi, F., M. Pistello, M. Vatteroni, S. Presciuttini, S. Marchi, P. Isola, C. Fornai, S. Fagnani, E. Andreoli, G. Antonelli, and M. Bendinelli.** 2001. Dynamics of persistent TT virus infection, as determined in patients treated with alpha interferon for concomitant hepatitis C virus infection. *J. Virol.* **75:**11999–12004.
38. **Mariscal, L. F., J. M. Lopez-Alcorocho, E. Rodriguez-Inigo, N. Ortiz-Movilla, S. De Lucas, J. Bartolome, and V. Carreno.** 2002. TT virus replicates in stimulated but not in nonstimulated peripheral blood mononuclear cells. *Virology* **301:**121–129.
39. **Martinez, L., T. Kekarainen, M. Sibila, F. Ruiz-Fons, D. Vidal, C. Gortázar, and J. Segalés.** 2006. Torque teno virus (TTV) is highly prevalent in the European wild boar (Sus scrofa). *Vet. Microbiol.* **118:**223–229.
40. **McKeown, N. E., M. Fenaux, P. G. Halbur, and X. J. Meng.** 2004. Molecular characterization of porcine TT virus, an orphan virus, in pigs from six different countries. *Vet. Microbiol.* **104:**113–117.

41. **Michitaka, K., and M. Onji.** 2003. Causes of non-B, non-C hepatocellular carcinoma: is TTV a causative agent? *Intern. Med.* **42:**1157–1158.
42. **Morrica, A., F. Maggi, M. L. Vatteroni, C. Fornai, M. Pistello, P. Ciccorossi, E. Grassi, A. Gennazzani, and M. Bendinelli.** 2000. TT virus: evidence for transplacental transmission. *J. Infect. Dis.* **181:**803–804.
43. **Mushahwar, I. K., J. C. Erker, A. S. Muerhoff, T. P. Leary, J. N. Simons, L. G. Birkenmeyer, M. L. Chalmers, T. J. Pilot-Matias, and S. M. Dexai.** 1999. Molecular and biophysical characterization of TT virus: evidence for a new virus family infecting humans. *Proc. Natl. Acad. Sci. USA* **96:**3177–3182.
44. **Nakagawa, H., H. Shimomura, T. Hasui, H. Tsuji, and T. Tsuji.** 1994. Quantitative detection of hepatitis C virus genome in liver tissue and circulation by competitive reverse transcription polymerase chain reaction. *Dig. Dis. Sci.* **39:**225–233.
45. **Nakagawa, N., J. Ikoma, T. Ishihara, N. Yasui-Kawamura, N. Fujita, M. Iwasa, M. Kaito, S. Watanabe, and Y. Adachi.** 2000. Biliary excretion of TT virus (TTV). *J. Med. Virol.* **61:**462–467.
46. **Ninomiya, M., T. Nishizawa, M. Takahashi, F. R. Lorenzo, T. Shimosegawa, and H. Okamoto.** 2007. Identification and genomic characterization of a novel human torque teno virus of 3.2 kb. *J. Gen. Virol.* **88:**1939–1944.
47. **Nishizawa, T., H. Okamoto, K. Konishi, H. Yoshizawa, Y. Miyakawa, and M. Mayumi.** 1997. A novel DNA virus (TTV) associated with elevated transaminase levels in posttransfusion hepatitis of unknown aetiology. *Biochem. Biophys. Res. Commun.* **241:**92–97.
48. **Ohbayashi, H., Y. Tanaka, S. Ohoka, R. Chinzei, S. Kakinuma, M. Goto, M. Watanabe, F. Marumo, and C. Sato.** 2001. TT virus is shown in the liver by in situ hybridization with a PCR-generated probe from the serum TTV-DNA. *J. Gastroenterol. Hepatol.* **16:**424–428.
49. **Okamoto, H., M. Fukuda, A. Tawara, T. Nishizawa, Y. Itoh, I. Hayasaka, F. Tsuda, T. Tanaka, Y. Miyakawa, and M. Mayumi.** 2000. Species-specific TT viruses and cross-species infection in nonhuman primates. *J. Virol.* **74:**1132–1139.
50. **Okamoto, H., T. Nishizawa, M. Takahashi, A. Tawara, Y. Peng, J. Kishimoto, and Y. Wang.** 2001. Genomic and evolutionary characterization of TT virus (TTV) in tupaias and comparison with species-specific TTVs in humans and non-human primates. *J. Gen. Virol.* **82:**2041–2050.
51. **Okamoto, H., T. Nishizawa, A. Tawara, Y. Peng, M. Takahashi, J. Kishimoto, T. Tanaka, Y. Miyakawa, and M. Mayumi.** 2000. Species-specific TT viruses in humans and nonhuman primates and their phylogenetic relatedness. *Virology* **277:**368–378.
52. **Okamoto, H., T. Nishizawa, A. Tawara, M. Takahashi, J. Kishimoto, T. Sai, and Y. Sugai.** 2000. TT virus mRNAs detected in the bone marrow cells from an infected individual. *Biochem. Biophys. Res. Commun.* **279:**700–707.
53. **Okamoto, H., T. Nishizawa, and M. Ukita.** 1999. A novel unenveloped DNA virus (TT Virus) associated with acute and chronic non-A to G hepatitis. *Intervirology* **42:**196–204.
54. **Okamoto, H., M. Takahashi, N. Kato, M. Fukuda, A. Tawara, S. Fukuda, T. Tanaka, Y. Miyakawa, and M. Mayumi.** 2000. Sequestration of TT virus of restricted genotypes in peripheral blood mononuclear cells. *J. Virol.* **74:**10236–10239.
55. **Okamoto, H., M. Takahashi, T. Nishizawa, A. Tawara, K. Fukai, U. Muramatsu, Y. Naito, and A. Yoshikawa.** 2002. Genomic characterization of TT viruses (TTVs) in pigs, cats and dogs and their relatedness with species-specific TTVs in primates and tupaias. *J. Gen. Virol.* **83:**1291–1297.
56. **Okamoto, H., M. Takahashi, T. Nishizawa, A. Tawara, Y. Sugai, T. Sai, T. Tanaka, and F. Tsuda.** 2000. Replicative forms of TT virus DNA in bone marrow cells. *Biochem. Biophys. Res. Commun.* **270:**657–662.
57. **Okamoto, H., M. Ukita, T. Nishizawa, J. Kishimoto, Y. Hoshi, H. Mizuo, T. Tanaka, Y. Miyakawa, and M. Mayumi.** 2000. Circular double-stranded forms of TT virus DNA in the liver. *J. Virol.* **74:**5161–5167.
58. **Okamura, A., M. Yoshioka, M. Kubota, H. Kikuta, H. Ishiko, and K. Kobayashi.** 1999. Detection of a novel DNA virus (TTV) sequence in peripheral blood mononuclear cells. *J. Med. Virol.* **58:**174–177.
59. **Ott, C., L. Duret, I. Chemin, C. Trépo, B. Mandrand, and F. Komurian-Pradel.** 2000. Use of a TT virus ORF1 recombinant protein to detect anti-TT virus antibodies in human sera. *J. Gen. Virol.* **81**(Pt. 12)**:**2949–2958.
60. **Pifferi, M., F. Maggi, E. Andreoli, L. Lanini, E. D. Marco, C. Fornai, M. L. Vatteroni, M. Pistello, V. Ragazzo, P. Macchia, A. Boner, and M. Bendinelli.** 2005. Associations between nasal torquetenovirus load and spirometric indices in children with asthma. *J. Infect. Dis.* **192:**1141–1148.
61. **Pifferi, M., F. Maggi, D. Caramella, E. De Marco, E. Andreoli, S. Meschi, P. Macchia, M. Bendinelli, and A. L. Boner.** 2006. High torquetenovirus loads are correlated with bronchiectasis and peripheral airflow limitation in children. *Pediatr. Infect. Dis. J.* **25:**804–808.
62. **Pistello, M., A. Morrica, F. Maggi, M. L. Vatteroni, G. Freer, C. Fornai, F. Casula, S. Marchi, P. Ciccorossi, P. Rovero, and M. Bendinelli.** 2001. TT virus levels in the plasma of infected individuals with different hepatic and extrahepatic pathology. *J. Med. Virol.* **63:**189–195.
63. **Pollicino, T., G. Raffa, G. Squadrito, L. Costantino, I. Cacciola, S. Brancatelli, C. Alafaci, M. G. Florio, and G. Raimondo.** 2003. TT virus has a ubiquitous diffusion in human body tissues: analyses of paired serum and tissue samples. *J. Viral Hepatitis* **10:**95–102.
64. **Qiu, J., L. Kakkola, F. Cheng, C. Ye, M. Soderlund-Venermo, K. Hedman, and D. J. Pintel.** 2005. Human circovirus TT virus genotype 6 expresses six proteins following transfection of a full-length clone. *J. Virol.* **79:**6505–6510.
65. **Rodriguez-Inigo, E., M. Casqueiro, J. Bartolome, N. Ortiz-Movilla, J. M. Lopez-Alcorocho, M. Herrero, F. Manzarbeitia, H. Oliva, and V. Carreno.** 2000. Detection of TT virus DNA in liver biopsies by in situ hybridization. *Am. J. Pathol.* **156:**1227–1234.
66. **Saback, F. L., S. A. Gomes, V. S. de Paula, R. R. S. da Silva, L. L. Lewis-Ximenez, and C. Niel.** 1999. Age-specific prevalence and transmission of TT virus. *J. Med. Virol.* **59:**318–322.
67. **Shibayama, T., G. Masuda, A. Ajisawa, M. Takahashi, T. Nishizawa, F. Tsuda, and H. Okamoto.** 2001. Inverse relationship between the titre of TT virus DNA and the CD4 cell count in patients infected with HIV. *AIDS* **15:**563–570.
68. **Simmonds, P., L. E. Prescott, C. Logue, F. Davidson, A. E. Thomas, and C. A. Ludlam.** 1999. TT virus—part of the normal human flora? *J. Infect. Dis.* **180:**1748–1750.
69. **Sugiyama, K., K. Goto, T. Ando, F. Mizutani, K. Terabe, Y. Kawabe, and Y. Wada.** 1999. Route of TT virus infection in children. *J. Med. Virol.* **59:**204–207.
70. **Sugiyama, K., K. Goto, T. Ando, F. Mizutani, K. Terabe, and T. Yokoyama.** 2001. Highly diverse TTV population in infants and their mothers. *Virus Res.* **73:**183–188.

71. **Takahashi, K., H. Hoshino, Y. Ohta, N. Yoshida, and S. Mishiro.** 1998. Very high prevalence of TT virus (TTV) infection in general population of Japan revealed by a new set of PCR primers. *Hepatol. Res.* **12:**233–239.
72. **Takahashi, K., Y. Iwasa, M. Hijikata, and S. Mishiro.** 2000. Identification of a new human DNA virus (TTV-like mini virus, TLMV) intermediately related to TT virus and chicken anemia virus. *Arch. Virol.* **145:**979–993.
73. **Takahashi, K., Y. Ohta, and S. Mishiro.** 1998. Partial 2.4 kb sequences of TT virus (TTV) genome from 8 Japanese isolates: diagnostic and phylogenetic implications. *Hepatol. Res.* **12:**111–120.
74. **Takahashi, M., S. Asabe, Y. Gotanda, J. Kishimoto, F. Tsuda, and H. Okamoto.** 2002. TT virus is distributed in various leukocyte subpopulations at distinct levels, with the highest viral load in granulocytes. *Biochem. Biophys. Res. Commun.* **290:**242–248.
75. **Tanaka, Y., D. Primi, R. Y. Wang, T. Umemura, A. E. Yeo, M. Mizokami, H. J. Alter, and J. W. Shih.** 2001. Genomic and molecular evolutionary analysis of a newly identified infectious agent (SEN virus) and its relationship to the TT virus family. *J. Infect. Dis.* **183:**359–367.
76. **Tawara, A., Y. Akahane, M. Takahashi, T. Nishizawa, T. Ishikawa, and H. Okamoto.** 2000. Transmission of human TT virus of genotype 1a to chimpanzees with fecal supernatant or serum from patients with acute TTV infection. *Biochem. Biophys. Res. Commun.* **278:**470–476.
77. **Thom, K., C. Morrison, J. C. Lewis, and P. Simmonds.** 2003. Distribution of TT virus (TTV), TTV-like minivirus, and related viruses in humans and nonhuman primates. *Virology* **306:**324–333.
78. **Tokita, H., S. Murai, H. Kamitsukasa, M. Yagura, H. Harada, M. Takahashi, and H. Okamoto.** 2002. High TT virus load as an independent factor associated with the occurrence of hepatocellular carcinoma among patients with hepatitis C virus-related chronic liver disease. *J. Med. Virol.* **67:**501–509.
79. **Touinssi, M., P. Gallian, P. Biagini, H. Attoui, B. Vialettes, Y. Berland, C. Tamalet, C. Dhiver, I. Ravaux, P. de Micco, and X. de Lamballerie.** 2001. TT virus infection: prevalence of elevated viraemia and arguments for the immune control of viral load. *J. Clin. Virol.* **21:**135–141.
80. **Tsuda, F., H. Okamoto, M. Ukita, T. Tanaka, Y. Akahane, K. Konishi, H. Yoshizawa, Y. Miyakawa, and M. Mayumi.** 1999. Determination of antibodies to TT virus (TTV) and application to blood donors and patients with post-transfusion non-A to G hepatitis in Japan. *J. Virol. Methods* **77:**199–206.
81. **Ukita, M., H. Okamoto, N. Kato, Y. Miyakawa, and M. Mayumi.** 1999. Excretion into bile of a novel unenveloped DNA virus (TT virus) associated with acute and chronic non-A-G hepatitis. *J. Infect. Dis.* **179:**1245–1248.
82. **Urlings, H. A., G. F. de Boer, D. J. van Roozelaar, and G. Koch.** 1993. Inactivation of chicken anaemia virus in chickens by heating and fermentation. *Vet. Q.* **15:**85–88.
83. **Verschoor, E. J., S. Langenhuijzen, and J. L. Heeney.** 1999. TT viruses (TTV) of non-human primates and their relationship to the human TTV genotypes. *J. Gen. Virol.* **80:**2491–2499.
84. **Welch, J., C. Bienek, E. Gomperts, and P. Simmonds.** 2006. Resistance of porcine circovirus and chicken anemia virus to virus inactivation procedures used for blood products. *Transfusion* **46:**1951–1958.
85. **Zhong, S., W. Yeo, M. Tang, C. Liu, X. R. Lin, W. M. Ho, P. Hui, and P. J. Johnson.** 2002. Frequent detection of the replicative form of TT virus DNA in peripheral blood mononuclear cells and bone marrow cells in cancer patients. *J. Med. Virol.* **66:**428–434.

Hepatitis B Virus

ALEXANDER J. V. THOMPSON, SALLY J. BELL, AND STEPHEN A. LOCARNINI

31

It has been almost 40 years since the discovery of the hepatitis B virus (HBV), and yet the diseases it causes (hepatitis, liver failure, and hepatocellular carcinoma [HCC]) remain major public health challenges. In spite of the development of an effective vaccine and its implementation through the 1980s, there is still a huge burden of liver disease due to chronic hepatitis B (CHB). Worldwide, over 400 million people have CHB, with the majority being in the Asia-Pacific region, and there are at least one million deaths each year as a direct consequence of infection. The main public health strategy to control hepatitis B for the last 20 years has been primary prevention through vaccination, and excellent progress has been made. However, in order to reduce the complications of CHB, which include the development of cirrhosis with hepatic decompensation and HCC for the at-risk population, an additional strategy is clearly required. The World Heath Organization (WHO) has termed this strategy chemoprevention, which is the use of antiviral agents to control HBV replication and thereby block the development of the complications that make HBV infection the 10th leading cause of death worldwide. The success of highly active antiretroviral therapy (HAART) for the treatment of patients with human immunodeficiency virus (HIV) infection is based on the use of multiple drugs which have different sites of action. For CHB, the licensed therapies include only two classes: interferon (IFN) and the nucleos(t)ide analogs (NA). How these new therapeutics will be used and what type of therapeutics will be needed in the future for the successful implementation of chemoprevention require urgent attention. The goal of chemoprevention for CHB must be to improve the quality and the outcomes of care for patients with CHB.

VIROLOGY

Classification

HBV is the prototype member of the family *Hepadnaviridae*. *Hepadnaviridae* are divided into the orthohepadnaviruses of mammals and avihepadnaviruses of birds (Table 1). The focus of this chapter is human HBV. HBV is an enveloped, 3.2-kb double-stranded DNA virus which may be classified into eight major genotypes (A to H) based on a nucleotide diversity of 8% or more (Table 2) (145).

Virus Structure: Virion and Subviral Particles

Three types of virus-associated particles are typically present in the blood of HBV-infected persons. The virus is spherical, with a diameter of 42 nm. Negative-staining electron microscopy usually reveals a double-shelled structure for the virus (Fig. 1A). The outer shell or envelope is formed by HBV surface antigen (HBsAg) proteins, while the inner shell, with a diameter of 27 to 32 nm, is the viral nucleocapsid or hepatitis B core antigen (HBcAg). The viral nucleocapsid encloses the viral DNA and virion DNA polymerase (Pol). As well as virions, the sera of viremic patients contain large numbers of two types of noninfectious particles: spherical particles 17 to 25 nm in diameter and filamentous forms 20 nm in diameter with a variable length. Both types of subviral particles are composed of HBsAg.

Genome Organization and Viral Proteins

The genome of HBV is a circular, partially double-stranded relaxed circular (rc) DNA molecule (104). The two linear DNA strands are held in a circular configuration by a 226-bp cohesive overlap between the 5′ ends of the two DNA strands that contain 11-nucleotide (nt) direct repeats called DR1 and DR2 (57). All known complete HBV genomes are gapped and circular (Fig. 1B), comprising between 3,181 and 3,221 bases depending on the genotype (Table 2). The minus strand is not a closed circle and has a nick near the 5′ end of the plus strand. The viral Pol is covalently bound to the 5′ end of the minus strand. The 5′ end of the plus strand contains an 18-base-long oligoribonucleotide, which is capped in the same manner as mRNA (189). The 3′ end of the plus strand is not at a fixed position, so most viral genomes contain a single-stranded gap region of variable length ranging from 20 to 80% of the genomic length that can be filled in by the viral DNA Pol.

The HBV genetic information is found on the minus-strand DNA in four open reading frames (ORFs), the longest of which encodes the viral Pol (Pol ORF). The envelope ORF (pre-S1, pre-S2, and S) is located within the Pol ORF, while the precore/core and the X ORFs overlap partially with it. The ORFs overlap in a frameshifted

TABLE 1 Taxonomy of *Hepadnaviridae*[a]

Virus genus and host	Virus
Orthohepadnavirus	
Human	Hepatitis B virus
Chimpanzee	Chimpanzee hepatitis B virus
White-handed gibbon	Gibbon hepatitis B virus
Orangutan	Orangutan hepatitis B virus
Gorilla	Gorilla hepatitis B virus
Woolly monkey	Woolly monkey hepatitis B virus
Woodchuck	Woodchuck hepatitis virus
Ground squirrel	Ground squirrel hepatitis virus
Arctic squirrel	Arctic squirrel hepatitis virus
Avihepadnavirus	
Pekin duck	Duck hepatitis B virus
Grey teal	Grey teal hepatitis B virus
Heron	Heron hepatitis B virus
Maned duck	Maned duck hepatitis B virus
Ross's goose	Ross's goose hepatitis virus
Snow goose	Snow goose hepatitis B virus
"White stork"	Stork hepatitis B virus
Grey crowned crane	Crane hepatitis B virus

[a] Adapted from reference 145.

manner such that the minus-strand DNA is read one and a half times. The transcriptional template of the virus is the covalently closed circular DNA (cccDNA) which exists in the cell nucleus as a viral minichromosome. From this template four major RNA species, the 3.5-, 2.4-, 2.1-, and 0.7-kb viral RNA transcripts, are transcribed. The enhancer II/basal core, large surface antigen (pre-S1), major surface antigen (S), and enhancer I/X gene promoters direct the expression of these four transcripts, respectively (57) (Fig. 2A).

Pol ORF

The Pol gene is the longest ORF, spanning almost 80% of the genome and overlapping the other three ORFs. The Pol is translated from pregenomic RNA (pgRNA) (Fig. 2A). The 834 to 845 codons found in the Pol ORF have sequence homology to reverse transcriptases (57), and most parts of the ORF are essential for viral replication. The 90-kDa product of the Pol ORF is a multifunctional protein that has at least four domains (Fig. 2B) (57). The N-terminal domain contains the terminal protein that is covalently linked to the 5′ end of the minus strand of virion DNA. This part of Pol ORF is necessary for priming of minus-strand synthesis. An intervening domain with no specific recognized function is referred to as the spacer or tether region. The third domain contains the RNA- and DNA-dependent DNA polymerase activities, that is, the reverse transcriptase. The C-terminal domain contains RNase H activity that cleaves the RNA in the RNA-DNA hybrids during reverse transcription.

The terminal protein's role in protein priming of reverse transcription includes the provision of the substrate tyrosine at amino acid 63 of the HBV Pol for the formation of the covalent bond between the enzyme and the first nucleotide (G) of the minus-strand DNA (201). The DNA Pol domain contains the amino acid motif YMDD, which is essential for reverse transcriptase activity (147) (Fig. 2B). The RNase H domain, besides degrading the RNA template, also plays a role in viral RNA packaging, in optimizing priming of minus-strand DNA synthesis, and in elongation of the minus-strand viral DNA.

The Pol contains at least two T-cell epitopes within its catalytic domains at amino acid residues 107 to 115 and 227 to 235 (33). Changes in these epitopes have been related to successful IFN-α therapy and viral clearance during acute infection.

Precore/Core ORF

The precore/core ORF encodes the core protein P21, which is the major polypeptide of the nucleocapsid and expresses the HBcAg. The HBc protein is 183, 185, or 195 amino acids long, depending on the genotype of the virus (Table 2). The core ORF is preceded by a short, upstream, in-phase ORF called the precore region, from which the soluble HBV ecore antigen (HBeAg) is made (57).

HBc Protein

The HBc protein has two distinct domains: amino acid residues 1 to 144 are required for the assembly of the 32-nm nucleocapsid, while the arginine-rich C-terminal

TABLE 2 Overview of the eight genotypes of HBV

Genotype	Genome length (nt)	Frequency of mutation[a]		Global distribution
		PC	BCP	
A	3,221	Uncommon	Common	Western Europe, United States, Central Africa, India
B	3,215	Common	Common	Japan, Taiwan, Indonesia, China, United States
Bj	3,215	Common	Uncommon	Japan
Ba	3,215	Common	Uncommon	China, Taiwan, Indonesia, Vietnam
C	3,215	Common	Common	East Asia, Taiwan, Korea, China, United States, Japan, Polynesia
D	3,182	Common	Common	Mediterranean region, India, United States
E	3,212	ND	ND	West Africa
F	3,215	Uncommon	ND	Central and South America, Polynesia
G	3,248	Very common	ND	United States, Europe
H	3,215	ND	ND	Central and South America

[a] PC, precore mutations such as G1896A; BCP, basal core promoter mutations such as A1762T and G1764A; very common, most isolates; common, up to 50% of isolates; uncommon, less than 10% of isolates; ND, not described.

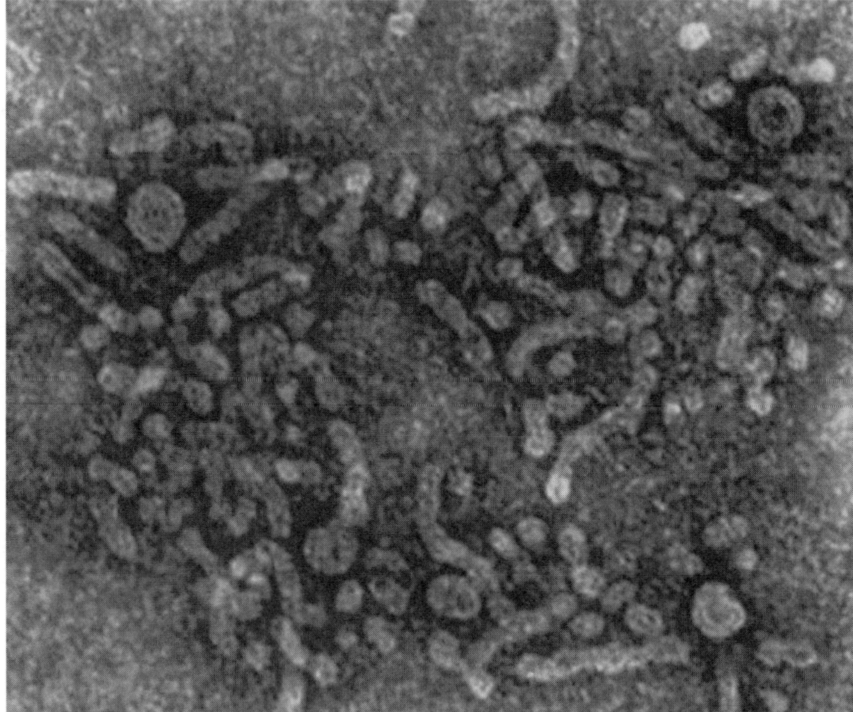

B

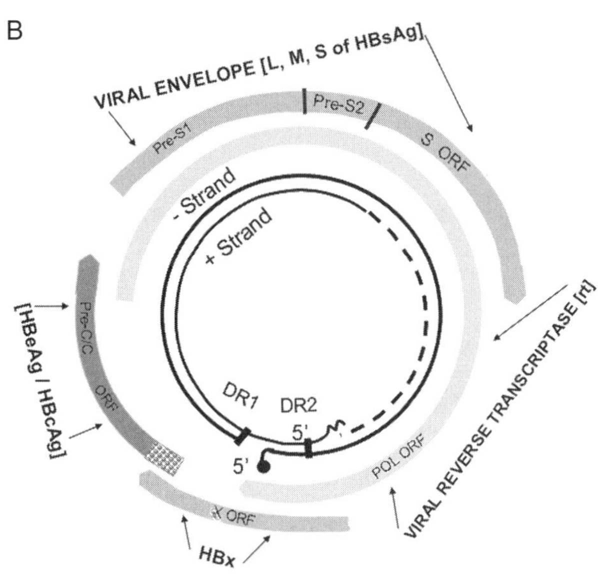

FIGURE 1 (A) Electron micrograph of the various forms found in the blood of HBV-infected persons. The 42-nm virions, both full and empty, can be seen. Within the empty particles, the 27- to 32-nm core structure can be visualized. The excess 22-nm subviral particles and filamentous forms of HBsAg are also present. (B) The circular double-stranded DNA genome of HBV showing the four main ORFs. The minus (−) and plus (+) DNA strands are marked. The HBV Pol and capped mRNA oligomer at the 5′ end of the minus and plus strands, respectively, as well as DR1 and DR2 are shown. The space between DR1 and DR2 is the "cohesive overlap region." The plus strand is typically incomplete.

residues from around residue 140 onward form a protamine-like domain that mediates nucleic acid binding and is involved in viral encapsidation and DNA replication (57). This arginine-rich region contains four clusters and includes a potential nuclear localization sequence. The core protein contains many hydrophilic and charged amino acids, and when expressed, it becomes phosphorylated (75). Phosphorylation of serines 170 to 172 between arginine cluster 3 and 4 appears to block nucleic acid binding and may possibly negatively regulate nuclear localization of the core protein (75). The HBc protein is also translated from pgRNA (Fig. 2A) and carries the HBcAg epitopes.

HBe Protein

HBeAg is the soluble secretory form of the HBc protein and is classified as an accessory protein of the virus. The precore sequence is upstream of the core sequence, and translation initiating from the precore initiation codon produces the precore protein, which contains the entire core protein sequence plus an additional 29 amino acids at the N-terminal end (P25) (57). The precore protein is translated from the precore mRNA (Fig. 2A). The first 19 amino acids of the precore protein form a secretion signal that allows the translocation of the precore protein into the lumen of the endoplasmic reticulum (ER). These 19 amino acids are cleaved off by a host cell signal peptidase,

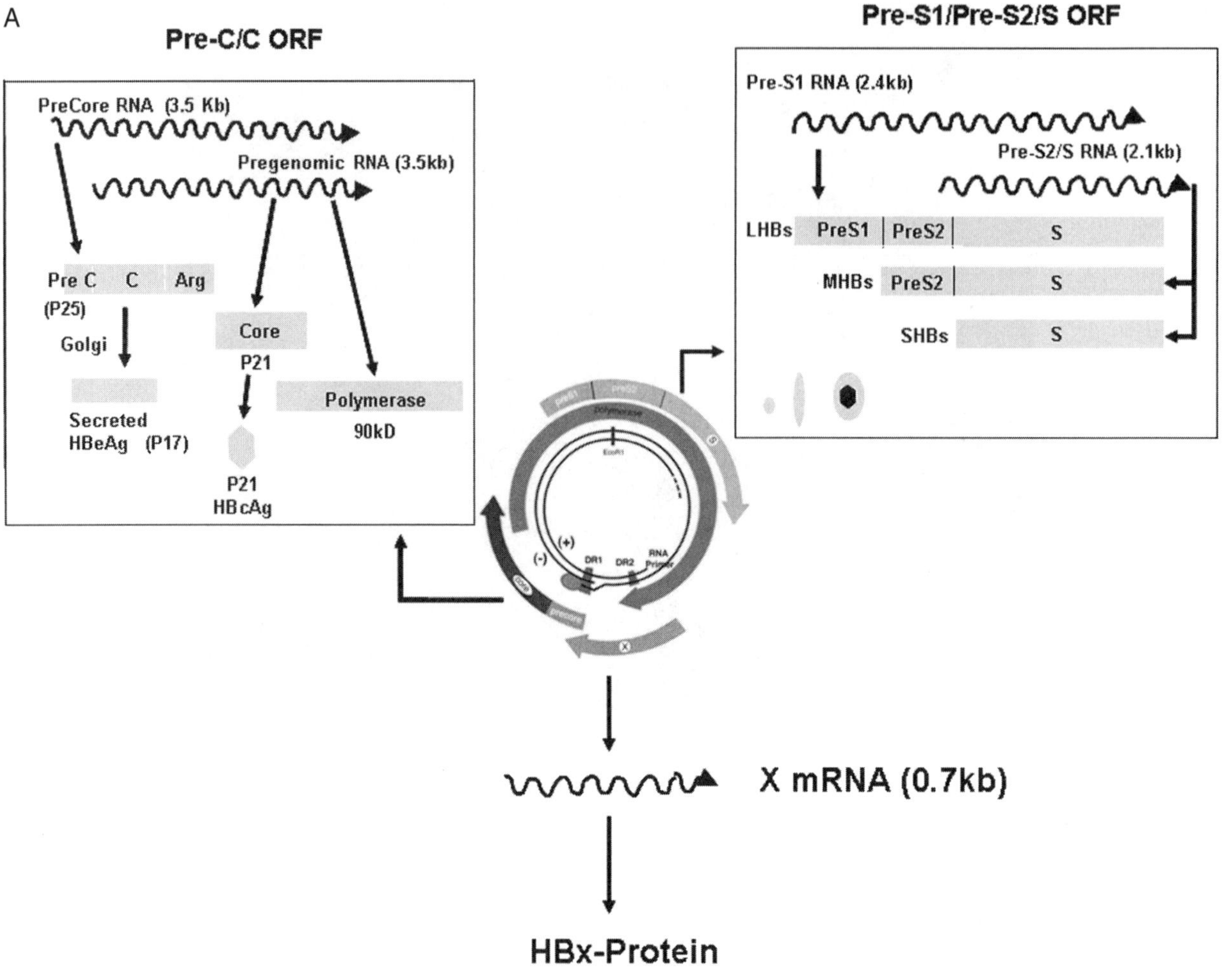

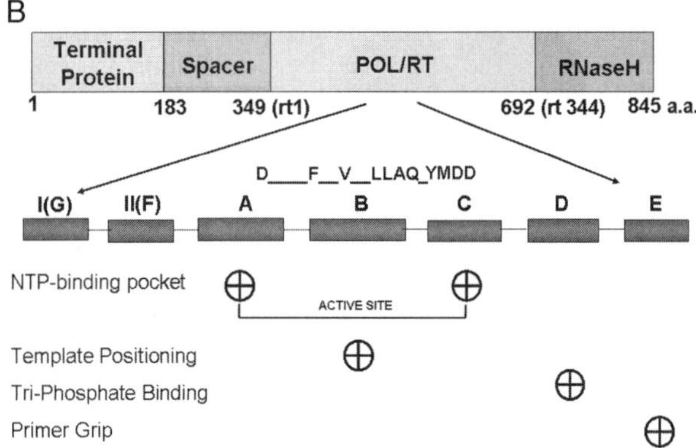

FIGURE 2 (A) Biosynthesis of the precore/core, Pol, envelope, and X proteins from the various HBV transcripts. The two major genomic 3.5-kb transcripts are the larger precore mRNA from which the precore protein (HBeAg) is made and the smaller pgmRNA that encodes the core and Pol and is the template for reverse transcription. The single 2.4-kb RNA makes LHBs, while the various 2.1-kb mRNAs translate MHBs and SHBs. The HBx protein is translated from the 0.7-kb mRNA. (B) Functional domains of the Pol-reverse transcriptase of HBV. (C) HBV DNA genome showing the overlapping ORFs and, in particular, how the Pol-envelope overlap can affect each of the proteins during the emergence of NA drug resistance.

leaving the precore protein derivative P22. P22 is then secreted through the ER and Golgi apparatus and further modified by C-terminal cleavage of up to 34 amino acids, resulting in the secretion of a heterogeneous population of proteins of approximately 17 kDa, serologically defined as HBeAg (57) (Fig. 3). Thus, HBe protein differs in almost all aspects from HBc protein, although the primary sequences of these two molecules are almost identical. Some of the HBe protein does not reach the ER lumen and is not cleaved at all. The P25 HBe protein also expresses a nuclear transport signal (75). Thus, HBe proteins of variable lengths are found in practically all compartments of the cell as well as being secreted.

The HBe protein is essential for the establishment of persistent infection. Mutants of HBV without a functional precore sequence and HBe protein are found commonly during chronic infection. High levels of secreted HBe protein are found in the tolerant phase of chronic infection and are associated with very high viral loads and near-normal liver histology. Elimination of HBeAg is usually accompanied by hepatitic flares produced as a consequence of heightened immunoreactivity to virus-infected hepato-

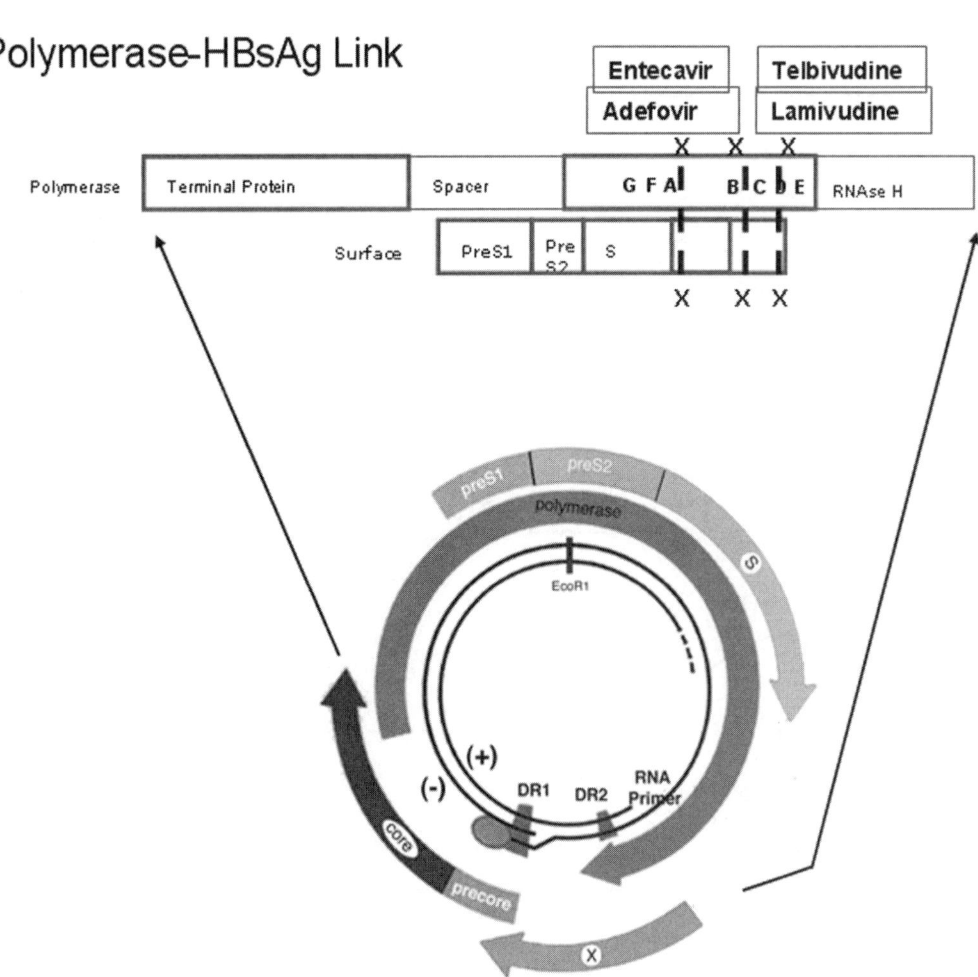

FIGURE 2 *(Continued)*

cytes. The viral load drops significantly during these flares, presumably as a consequence of the antiviral activity of the host's immune response. An HBeAg-negative mutant of the woodchuck HBV is infectious for newborn woodchucks but is unable to establish persistent infection (30). Similar scenarios have been described for HBV, suggesting that the HBe protein may act to suppress the immune elimination of HBV-infected hepatocytes. It certainly can function as a tolerogen in vivo (120).

HBeAg has at least two B-cell epitopes, one of which is linear (HBe1) and the other of which is conformational (HBe2). The HBe1 and HBe2 epitopes have been mapped to core amino acid residues 85 and 138, respectively, and two immunodominant core epitopes (HBc) are localized between residues 74 and 83 (HBc1), colinear with HBe1, and to residues 107 to 118 (HBc2). Not surprisingly, HBcAg and HBeAg are highly cross-reactive at the T-cell level (33). Two cytotoxic T-lymphocyte (CTL) epitopes of HBc can be mapped to residues 18 to 27 (human leukocyte antigen A2 [HLA-A2] restricted) and residues 141 to 151 (HLA-A31 and HLA-Aw69 restricted). Core peptides 91 to 110 and 111 to 125 are potential HLA-A2-restricted CTL epitopes. Three T-helper cell epitopes have been found on the core protein, at amino acid residues 1 to 20, 50 to 69, and 117 to 131 (33).

Pre-S/S ORF

HBsAg contains small (SHBs), medium (MHBs), and large (LHBs) proteins, all of which exist in two forms differing in the extent of glycosylation (Fig. 2A). N-linked glycosylation and glucosidase processing are necessary for virion, but not subviral particle, secretion (75). The filaments consist of the same ratio of surface proteins as the virion envelope.

SHBs

The SHBs domain is 226 amino acids long and is the most abundant protein in all three HBV-associated particles. SHBs is found in glycosylated and nonglycosylated forms. It contains a high number of cysteine residues that are cross-linked with each other, forming a conformational loop that is the major antigenic determinant of HBsAg, the "a" determinant (22). The a determinant is present on all known HBsAg isolates and has the subdeterminants "d" or "y" and "w" or "r." Determinant d has a lysine at position 122, and y is represented by an arginine; likewise, determinant w has a lysine at position 160 and r is an arginine (127). These antigenic subtypes are able to elicit cross-protecting anti-HBs following immunization. The a determinant has been renamed the major hydrophilic re-

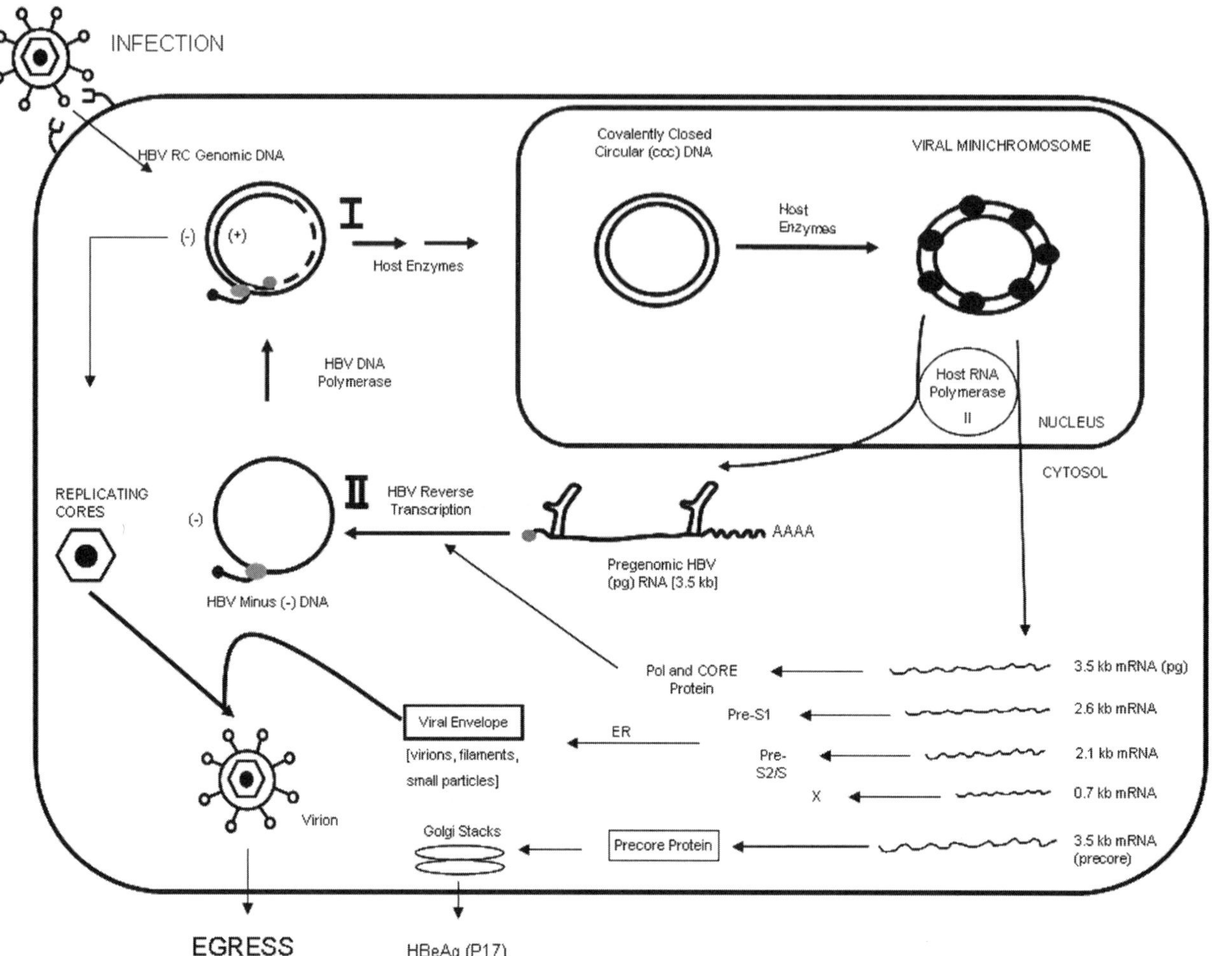

FIGURE 3 Replication cycle of HBV. Following attachment, penetration, and uncoating, the viral nucleocapsid is released into the cytosol and transported to the nuclear pore. The genomic DNA is delivered into the nucleus, where it is converted into cccDNA and the viral minichromosome is generated. Transcription of the viral minichromosome produces the genomic and subgenomic HBV mRNA transcripts. Translation of the pgRNA in the cytosol produces the core and Pol proteins, and in association with HSP60 all are selectively packaged into a replication complex. Within the nucleocapsid, reverse transcription begins. The envelope proteins (pre-S1, pre-S2, and S) are translated at the rough ER and then bud into the lumen of the intermediate compartment. Approximately 50% of the pre-S1-enriched ER membrane areas envelope core particles. The HBV virions, small particles, and tubules are then secreted into the extracellular space by the constitutive pathway. The nucleocapsids can also be transported to the nucleus via an intracellular conversion pathway, increasing the copy number of cccDNA molecules.

gion, spanning amino acids 99 to 160, and is considered the major neutralization domain for anti-HBs.

MHBs

The MHBs pre-S2 domain is a minor component of the virion or HBs particle and consists of the S domain and a 55-amino-acid N-terminal extension (57). It is either singly or doubly glycosylated but is not essential for virus assembly and release. The immunogenic epitopes are not conformationally dependent, as is the case for SHBs.

The central part of the pre-S2 domain carries the major antigenic epitope, and the region between amino acids 3 and 16 has the ability to bind polymerized human serum albumin (75). The significance of this binding is unknown. MHBs is considerably more immunogenic than SHBs at the B-cell level (122), and pre-S2-containing HBs particles generated from animal cell lines have been used in some countries as a prophylactic vaccine (169).

LHBs

LHBs contains a further N-terminal extension to the M protein of 108 or 119 amino acids (depending on the subtype or genotype [Table 2]) and is more prevalent than MHBs in virions and filaments but less prevalent in HBs spheres. Thus, LHBs contains three domains, pre-S1, pre-S2, and S, and is glycosylated. In the mature virions and HBs particles, the pre-S domains are exposed on the particle surface and both the S domains and parts of the pre-

S2 sequence are covered by the pre-S1 sequence of LHBs (75). In contrast to MHBs, LHBs is essential for infection and viral morphogenesis. The N-terminal end of the pre-S domain is myristylated, a function that is not required for virion formation and release but is essential for virion infectivity (18).

LHBs has important antigenic sites for both B and T cells that appear to play critical roles in recovery from viral infection or protection from infection (121). The major immunogenic epitopes within the pre-S1 coding region are at amino acids 27 to 35, 72 to 78, and 95 to 107. LHBs is also highly immunogenic at the T-cell level in humans, at residues 21 to 48 as well as 81 to 108.

X ORF

The X ORF encodes a polypeptide 154 amino acids in length (HBx) with a molecular mass of 17 kDa (Fig. 2A). This is the second accessory protein of HBV and is conserved in a similar form across all the mammalian hepadnaviruses. The expression of full-length HBx protein is dispensable for virus production in vitro but is a critical component of the infectivity process in vivo (200). HBx behaves as a transcriptional transactivator of a number of viral and cellular gene promoters through direct interaction with transcription factors such as the RPB5 subunit of RNA polymerase II, TATA-binding protein, and ATB and is also involved in the activation of signal transduction pathways, such as the Ras/Raf/mitogen-activated protein kinase cascade (75).

Another important effect of HBx protein is its potential as a cofactor in HBV-mediated carcinogenesis (79). The mechanism(s) whereby HBx contributes to the development of HCC is unknown, although the HBx-associated transactivation activity may lead to alterations in cellular gene expression that contribute to transformation (143). This is supported by the finding that HBx binds to and inactivates the transcription factor and tumor suppressor p53 (170, 179). HBx has also been shown to deregulate cell cycle checkpoints and abrogate p53-dependent apoptosis (180). Finally, the 26S proteasome complex is another functionally important target of HBx, suppressing viral antigen presentation and evading immune elimination (69).

Viral Replication Cycle

Replication of HBV revolves around two key processes:

- Generation of HBV cccDNA from genomic RC DNA and its subsequent processing by host enzymes to produce viral RNA
- Reverse transcription of the pgRNA within the viral nucleocapsid to form RC DNA, completing the cycle (Fig. 3). Earlier and later events are described below in the context of these two processes. The detailed molecular biology of HBV replication has been presented recently (8) and is not repeated here.

Early Events: Attachment, Penetration, and Uncoating

The first stage of infection is attachment to a susceptible hepatocyte and penetration of HBV into the cell cytoplasm following the binding of the HBV envelope to its specific cellular receptor and/or coreceptor. The cellular protein complex forming the receptor for HBV is still to be identified. Similarly, subsequent events such as penetration and uncoating are also unclear, but it is likely that a process of receptor-mediated endocytosis, and not membrane fusion, is responsible for the delivery of viral nucleocapsids into the cytoplasm.

Key Step One: Conversion of Genomic RC DNA into cccDNA and Transcription of the Viral Minichromosome

Intracellular viral nucleocapsids are transported to the nuclear membrane, where they uncoat (138). The genomic RC DNA is released into the nucleus and then converted into cccDNA using host cell enzymes, resulting in the formation of the viral minichromosome, the major template of HBV that is used for the transcription of all the viral mRNAs (12, 123) (Fig. 3).

Two classes of transcript are synthesized from the HBV minichromosome: genomic length and subgenomic length (57). Both classes contain heterogeneous transcripts that are of positive orientation, are capped at the 5′ end, and are polyadenylated at the 3′ end. The subgenomic transcripts function exclusively as mRNAs for translation of the envelope (pre-S1, pre-S2, and S proteins) and X proteins. The two genomic transcripts are longer than genomic length and contain the precore, core, and Pol ORF. The precore/core mRNA is not used for reverse transcription and functions in translation of the precore protein, which is processed and then secreted as HBeAg (57). The pgRNA is multifunctional, serving as the template for reverse transcription into the viral (minus) DNA strand and for translation of HBcAg as well as HBV Pol. The viral envelope, the small particles, and filaments are synthesized and assembled at the ER membranes and then bud into its lumen. The HBc protein is synthesized in the cytosol and assembled independently of the enveloped proteins (57, 75).

Key Step Two: HBV Genomic Replication via Reverse Transcription

HBV genomic replication is initiated with packaging of the pgRNA and the viral Pol/reverse transcriptase (HBV Pol) into subviral core particles, forming replication complexes. Reverse transcription occurs within the HBV nucleocapsid. As the HBV Pol is being translated off the pgRNA molecule, the N-terminal region (terminal protein) binds to a unique RNA stem-loop structure, known as epsilon (ε), at the 5′ end of the pgRNA (3) (Fig. 4). This RNA structure also acts as a packaging signal around which core dimers assemble into nucleocapsids. The HBV Pol undergoes a conformational change which results in enzymatic activation, with the terminal protein domain priming DNA synthesis (201). This Pol-oligonucleotide complex is then translocated to the complementary sequences of a direct repeat (DR1) region located at the 3′ end of the pgRNA. From here, minus-strand DNA synthesis continues until it reaches the 5′ end of the pgRNA molecule (189), generating a terminal redundancy of 8 or 9 nt. While reverse transcription is proceeding, the pgRNA is degraded by the RNase H activity of the HBV Pol, except for the 5′ capped terminal 18 nt that contains the DR1 sequence (57). This fragment includes a 6-nt homology to the DR sequence. The 18-nt capped RNA structure is then translocated to a second DR sequence (DR2) on the 5′ end of the newly made minus DNA strand, where it acts as a primer for plus-strand synthesis, using the minus strand as a template (Fig. 3) (189).

Synthesis of the plus DNA strand proceeds from the RNA primer to the 5′ end of the minus DNA strand (189).

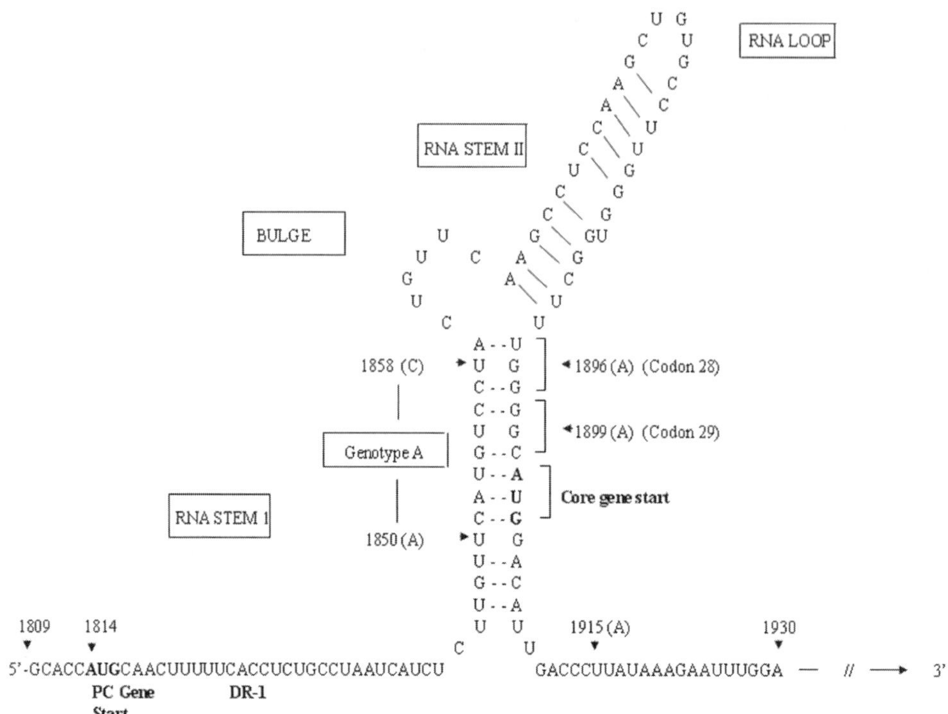

FIGURE 4 Diagrammatic representation of the epsilon (ε) stem-loop structure of HBV. This is a highly conserved structure within the eight genotypes of HBV. The positions of base changes for genotype A-2 (Ae) are shown, as are the common translational precore mutations of G1896A (precore stop codon: UAG) and G1899A.

The short terminal redundancy of the minus DNA strand permits the transfer of the 3′ end of the growing short plus strand from the protein-linked 5′ end to the 3′ end of the minus strand, thereby circularizing the genome and allowing continuation of DNA synthesis, generating the genomic RC DNA molecule with the HBV Pol covalently attached to the 5′ end of the minus DNA strand (Fig. 3). Synthesis of the plus-strand DNA continues until it reaches about 50 to 70% of the length of the minus strand.

Viral Assembly and Release

The assembly of nucleocapsids containing genomic RC DNA occurs in the cytosol, and these are selectively enveloped prior to exiting the cell. Immature nucleocapsids containing pgRNA are incompetent for envelopment, which can occur only after initiation of reverse transcription (57). Minus-strand DNA synthesis appears to be coupled to phosphorylation of the nucleocapsid, which is required for envelopment to occur. A further bias exists in favor of the export of genomes that have completed minus-strand DNA synthesis and at least started plus-strand synthesis (57). Correct assembly of replicating cores with the viral envelopes requires a critical relative molar ratio of pre-S1 to S. Insufficient S or excessive pre-S1 production results in abnormal assembly and release (57).

GENOTYPES

There are currently eight recognized genotypes of HBV, designated A to H, that vary by 8% or more at the nucleotide level over the entire genome (75, 156). These genotypes show a distinct geographic distribution (Table 2). As genotype designation is now based on the entire genomic sequence, it is a more reliable classification than the previously used serologic subtype nomenclature (*adw*, *adr*, *ayw*, and *ayn*), which is based on the immunoreactivity of particular antibodies to a limited number of amino acids in the envelope protein. HBV genotypes have unique insertions or deletions. For example, HBV genotype A varies from the other genotypes by an insertion of 6 nt at the portion of the core gene corresponding to the C terminus (145). HBV genotype D has a 33-nt deletion at the portion of the pre-S1 region corresponding to the N terminus. HBV genotypes E and G have a 3-nt deletion also in the portion of the pre-S1 region corresponding to the N terminus. HBV genotype G also has a 36-nt insertion in the portion of the core gene corresponding to the N terminus (75), and the precore/core region has two translational stop codons at positions 2 and 28 and so causes HBeAg-negative disease. Subgenotypes have recently been described for a number of these genotypes (A, B, C, and F). Recombination between two HBV genotypes, generating even more diversity, has also been reported for genotypes B and C and genotypes A and D (145).

Important pathogenic and therapeutic differences appear to exist among HBV genotypes. Differences of intra- and extracellular expression of viral DNA and antigens between genotypes have been observed in vitro, with HBV DNA levels in cell lysates being highest for genotype C, followed by genotypes B and D, findings suggesting differential replication activity (158). Clinical studies have found that in Taiwan, genotype C is associated with more severe liver disease than genotype B, while in Western countries, genotype A has a more favorable prognosis than genotype D (24, 49, 78). An association between genotype F HBV and increased risk of HCC has been observed in Alaska Native people (99). Response to antiviral therapy may also be influenced by genotype. Patients infected with genotype A appear to respond better to IFN therapy than those infected with genotype D, while patients infected with genotype B may respond better than those infected with genotype C (53). Similarly, there may be genotype-specific differences in response to NA therapy. However, current management and treatment guidelines do not recommend a role for genotype determination.

VARIANT VIRUSES

The replication strategy of HBV is essentially error prone. This poor fidelity results from the lack of a proofreading or editing mechanism for the HBV Pol, with the consequent potential for every nucleotide in the genome to be replaced daily (58). Although mutations can occur randomly along the HBV genome, the overlapping ORFs constrain the evolution rate, limiting the number and location of viable mutations. Despite this, many variants exist within a host at any given time; HBV therefore exists as a quasispecies, defined as a mixture of genetic variants evolved from a single inoculum. The predominant virus is selected as the fittest variant present following this random mutation process, in the face of various selective pressures. Three forms of variant HBV that occur commonly in clinical practice are discussed below.

Mutations Affecting HBeAg and HBcAg

Precore and basal core promoter (BCP) variants are defective for HBeAg production, typically emerge after HBeAg seroconversion, and are the most common cause of HBeAg-negative CHB. BCP variants affect the BCP and typically involve the double mutation of A1762T plus G1764A. This results in a transcriptional reduction of the precore mRNA (70), with a significant decrease in HBeAg levels. This pattern of mutation is found in genotype A-infected individuals as the major cause of HBeAg loss (70) and typically in association with the precore mutations in the other viral genotypes (Table 1) (4). Importantly, these BCP mutations do not affect the transcription of HBV pgRNA or the translation of the core protein or Polymerase. By removing the inhibitory effect of the precore protein on HBV replication, the BCP mutations appear to enhance viral replication by suppressing precore mRNA relative to pgRNA (70) and have been associated with an increase in viral load.

The second group of mutants includes HBV mutants with a translational stop codon mutation at nt 1896 (codon 28: TGG; tryptophan) of the precore gene. The single base substitution (G to A) at nt 1896 gives rise to a translational stop codon (TGG to TAG; TAG = stop codon) in the second last codon (codon 28) of the precore gene located within the ε structure of pgRNA. nt G1896 forms a base pair with nt 1858 at the base of the stem-loop. In HBV genotypes B, D, E, and G and some strains of genotype C, nt 1858 is a thymidine (Table 2). Thus, the stop codon mutation created by G1896A (T-A) stabilizes the ε structure. In contrast, the precore stop codon mutation is rarely detected in HBV genotype A and F strains and some strains of HBV genotype C, as the nucleotide at position 1858 is a cytidine (C), maintaining the preferred Watson-Crick (G-C) base-pairing. Other mutations have been found within the precore transcript that block HBeAg production, including abolition of the initiation codon methionine residue (4).

Envelope Gene Mutations

Envelope mutants may be selected by hepatitis B immunoglobulin (HBIG) therapy in the posttransplantation setting or by vaccines following prophylactic immunization. Viral genomes that cannot synthesize pre-S1 and pre-S2 proteins have been found to occur frequently and may be the dominant virus population in patients with CHB (61). The pre-S1 mutants are associated with intracellular retention of the viral envelope proteins and the classical histologic appearance of ground-glass hepatocytes. The pre-S2 region overlaps the spacer region of the Pol, which is not essential for enzyme activity; thus, both envelope mutants replicate in their infected host, but with differing histopathological sequelae.

The licensed hepatitis B vaccine contains the major HBsAg. The subsequent anti-HBs response to the major hydrophilic region of HBsAg located from residues 99 to 170 induces protective immunity. Mutations within this epitope have been selected during prophylactic vaccination (22) and following treatment of liver transplant recipients with HBIG prophylaxis (21). Most vaccine HBIG escape isolates have a mutation from glycine to arginine at residue 145 of HBsAg (sG145R) or aspartate to alanine at residue 144 (sD144A). The sG145R mutation has been associated with vaccine failure (22) and has been shown to be transmitted and cause disease. Other important mutations have been found at a major histocompatibility complex class I-restricted T-cell epitope in HBsAg between codons 28 and 51.

Pol Mutations

Antiviral-agent-resistant Pol mutants emerge in the setting of NA therapy and are responsible for virologic breakthrough and treatment failure (Fig. 5). They are discussed in more detail below.

LABORATORY DIAGNOSIS

HBV infection is usually diagnosed using specific serologic assays (also see chapter 5). During the course of infection, the viral proteins HBsAg, HBcAg, and HBeAg stimulate

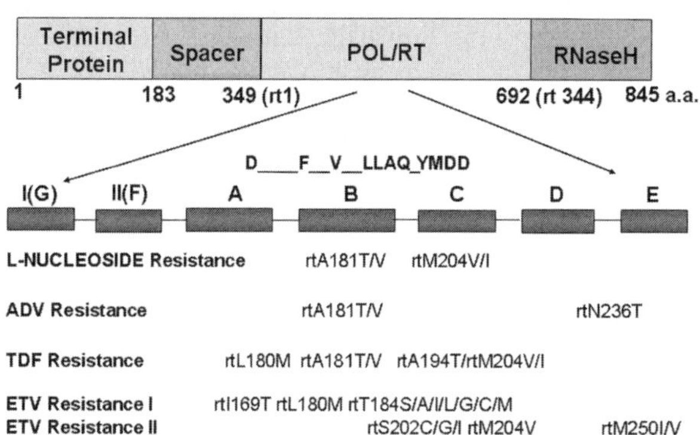

FIGURE 5 Location of the primary mutations associated with LMV and LdT resistance as well as ADV, TDF, and ETV resistance, in the major catalytic domains of the HBV Pol gene. a.a., amino acids.

the immune system to produce the corresponding antibodies anti-HBs, anti-HBc, and anti-HBe. The assays for serum HBsAg and its resultant antibody are critical because the persistence of HBsAg for longer than 6 months defines chronic infection and the presence of anti-HBs indicates immunity from vaccination or disease resolution. Beyond diagnosis, novel quantitative assays for HBeAg and HBsAg and ultrasensitive assays for anti-HBe and anti-HBs are providing new insight into the dynamics of humoral immunity in the setting of CHB. The quantification of HBV DNA has recently become a primary tool in the management of CHB. Data are emerging on the relationship between the magnitude of HBV DNA load and the relative risk of developing liver disease (27, 71). Consequently, HBV DNA now plays a central role in defining antiviral treatment eligibility and efficacy. The development of resistance can also be identified by an increase in the level of HBV DNA, generally considered to be a $>1\text{-}\log_{10}$ increase from nadir for a compliant patient in two consecutive serum samples taken 1 month apart (102). Recent advances in molecular diagnostics allow analysis of intrahepatic HBV replicative intermediates, such that comparison of the peripheral serum compartment to the liver compartment is possible.

Serologic Markers of HBV Infection

Acute Hepatitis B (AHB)

Of the viral markers associated with acute infection (Table 3), HBsAg is typically the first to become detectable (15). It appears early, usually 6 to 12 weeks after exposure, and is present before the onset of symptoms. HBeAg appears soon after HBsAg and has been shown to be a useful marker of replication activity and infectivity. As the antigen titers peak, the serum alanine aminotransferase (ALT) levels begin to rise and symptoms first become apparent. Antibodies to the antigens begin to appear during this symptomatic phase, which is consistent with hepatitis B being essentially an immunomediated disease. The first antibody raised is directed against the core antigen and is of the immunoglobulin M (IgM) class, anti-HBc IgM (15). In combination with the presence of HBsAg, anti-HBc IgM is the best indicator of acute infection. Anti-HBc IgM peaks in early convalescence before gradually declining over 3 to 12 months, irrespective of whether the disease becomes self-limiting or progresses to chronic disease. As the anti-HBc IgM titer falls, a corresponding increase in titer of anti-HBc IgG occurs, which typically remains detectable for life (15). Anti-HBe is detected either concurrently with or soon after the appearance of anti-HBc IgM, and its appearance is associated with the rapid clearance of HBeAg. The seroconversion of HBeAg to anti-HBe coincides with a dramatic increase in ALT, probably because of antibodies causing the immune lysis of infected cells. Often anti-HBe will persist for years, but in the absence of any active viral replication, the titer declines. Finally, anti-HBs, the antibody to HBsAg, appears, although it may not be detectable for 3 to 6 months. Anti-HBs is the neutralizing antibody and is recognized as a marker of disease resolution. In some patients, there may be a window period when HBsAg cannot be detected and anti-HBs has not yet appeared; however, anti-HBc IgM is usually found at this time. Anti-HBs is also the marker for confirming successful vaccination. Anti-HBs should be the only HBV antibody found after immunization (Table 3) and provides protective immunity.

The use of DNA amplification techniques, such as PCR, allows detection of HBV DNA in the serum a few weeks after infection, but there is little advantage over the newer, more sensitive HBsAg detection assays (11). HBV DNA assays may occasionally help to identify HBV as the etiology of liver disease in HBsAg-negative patients; this occurs in the rare patient with fulminant HBV infection who has cleared HBsAg by the time of presentation.

CHB

The persistence of high levels of HBsAg for >6 months following acute hepatitis indicates the establishment of chronic infection (14). The serologic profile correlates with acute infection, but as the levels of ALT and anti-HBc IgM decline, HBsAg remains. In the early stages of chronic infection, ongoing replication can be identified by the presence of HBsAg, HBeAg, and HBV DNA. The antibody response consists mostly of anti-HBc IgG, measured as total anti-HBc, with minimal contribution from anti-HBc IgM. HBeAg titers may decline over time, with eventual seroconversion of HBeAg to anti-HBe. This seroconversion occurs at a rate of up to 5 to 20% per year in adults and is often accompanied by a flare in disease activity, known as the seroconversion illness. A number of abortive flares of active hepatitis may occur over several years before final anti-HBe seroconversion. In most cases, the loss of HBeAg is associated with a decrease in circulating levels of HBV DNA (which may become undetectable), normalization of ALT levels, and a significant clinical improvement despite the lasting presence of HBsAg. However, HBV DNA may remain detectable and disease progress as HBeAg-negative CH-B.

HBV Viral Load Assays

Previous obstacles to the widespread use of HBV DNA testing have been the lack of quality-controlled reagents, lack of standardization between assays, and limitations in sensitivity. New commercial assays with wider dynamic ranges and lower limits of detection are now available and a WHO international standard for HBV DNA has been

TABLE 3 Profile of serologic markers for HBV infection

Marker	Incubation period	Acute hepatitis	Recovery period	Immunity	Vaccine immunity	Chronic infection
HBsAg	±	+	±	−	−	+
Anti-HBs	−	−	−	+	+	−
HBeAg	±	−	−	−	−	±
Anti-HBe	−	+	+	+	−	±
Anti-HBc IgM	−	±	−	−	−	−
Anti-HBc total	−	±	+	+	−	+

established, allowing for comparisons of assay results expressed as international units per milliliter (Table 4) (144). HBV DNA detection and quantification offer several advantages other than being an adjunct to serologic testing. HBV viral load is now recognized to be a key prognostic marker and an important parameter for determining eligibility for antiviral therapy. Serial viral load measurements are now the standard of care for monitoring patients on therapy, both for efficacy and for the development of antiviral resistance.

HBV DNA nucleic acid tests employ either signal or target amplification technologies, and each has its respective advantages and disadvantages (Table 4) (132). Generally, signal amplification assays are less sensitive than target amplification assays; however, they are more suitable for testing large sample numbers because there is no requirement to purify HBV DNA from plasma or serum. Another advantage is that they do not require the strict measures to limit contamination from amplified DNA. The target amplification assays offer excellent sensitivity, and because of this, they should be the test of choice in the evaluation of new antiviral agents or drug combinations. They may be less suited to laboratories where a high throughput is required, as not all target amplification assays are compatible with semiautomated extraction instruments.

Novel Diagnostic Tests

Assays for Intrahepatic HBV Replicative Intermediates

HBV cccDNA provides a difficult obstacle for both immune clearance and antiviral therapy to overcome. The level of serum HBV DNA may not reflect what is taking place in the liver. For example, as HBV replication does not employ a semiconservative mechanism, any NA-based therapy can only indirectly affect the preexisting cccDNA template. Quantification of the various intrahepatic HBV replicative forms, in particular the HBV cccDNA, total intrahepatic HBV DNA (RC DNA), and pgRNA, has therefore been used to gain further insights into the natural history of HBV infection as well as for evaluating the efficacy of specific antiviral therapy.

Patients with HBeAg-negative CHB have lower levels of cccDNA than their HBeAg-positive counterparts (85, 185, 191). Virion productivity, defined as the ratio of RC DNA to cccDNA, is reduced in HBeAg-negative CHB (Fig. 6). This reduced replicative activity has been associated with lower levels of pgRNA, implying transcriptional down-regulation. In the context of antiviral therapy, preliminary data suggest that the pretreatment cccDNA level may predict antiviral response and that a significant decline of cccDNA to low end-of-treatment levels may predict durable off-treatment viral suppression, indicating clearance of infected cells (185, 191).

Quantitative HBeAg and HBsAg Assays

One of the drawbacks to measuring the intrahepatic HBV intermediates is the requirement to use liver tissue. Some studies have found a correlation between the levels of circulating HBsAg and the levels of intrahepatic HBV cccDNA. This has led to renewed interest in the development of sensitive quantitative assays for HBsAg as well as HBeAg.

Quantitative HBsAg assays. HBsAg titers correlate with intrahepatic cccDNA and serum HBV DNA in the different phases of disease (38). HBsAg titer has been observed to decline with cccDNA on treatment (185, 191). Quantitative HBsAg titer may therefore be a useful surrogate marker for cccDNA and have clinical utility in predicting treatment response in both HBeAg-positive and -negative patients. A number of enzyme-linked immunosorbent assays for quantitative HBsAg titer are commercially available and offer a less invasive alternative to the measurement of intrahepatic HBV DNA replicative forms.

Quantitative HBeAg assays. HBeAg seroconversion is an established therapeutic end point for the management of HBeAg-positive CHB. A low HBeAg titer pretreatment and a rapid decline of HBeAg titer on therapy both predict for HBeAg seroconversion during treatment with pegylated IFN-α (PEG) and NA (54, 131). Conversely, the failure of HBeAg to fall on treatment predicts nonresponse. The predictive power of HBeAg titer appears greater than for HBV viral load (54). Rising HBeAg titer has also been shown to predict lamivudine (LMV) resistance before virologic breakthrough (131).

Ultrasensitive Immunoassays for Anti-HBs and Anti-HBe

The presence of large amounts of HBsAg and HBeAg in the serum may affect the ability to detect circulating

TABLE 4 Properties of HBV viral load assays[a]

Assay	LLQ	ULQ	Conversion factor (IU > copies)
Target amplification			
COBAS HBV MONITOR (Roche Diagnostics)	2×10^2 copies/ml	2×10^5 copies/ml	Not applicable[b]
COBAS TaqMan HBV (Roche Diagnostics)	3×10^1 IU/ml	1.1×10^8 IU/ml	5.82
RealArt HBV PCR (QIAGEN)	2×10^1 IU/ml	2×10^8 IU/ml	6
RealTime HBV PCR (Abbott Molecular)	1×10^1 IU/ml	1×10^9 IU/ml	3.41
Signal amplification			
HBV Hybrid Capture II (Digene)	1.4×10^5 copies/ml	1.7×10^9 copies/ml	Not applicable[b]
VERSANT HBV DNA 3.0 (Siemens Medical Solutions)	3.5×10^2 IU/ml	1.8×10^7 IU/ml	5.7

[a] LLQ, lower limit of quantification; ULQ, upper limit of quantification.

[b] Assay was developed before the establishment of the WHO international standard. Note that some assays can detect smaller amounts of HBV DNA, but this is outside the linear quantification range.

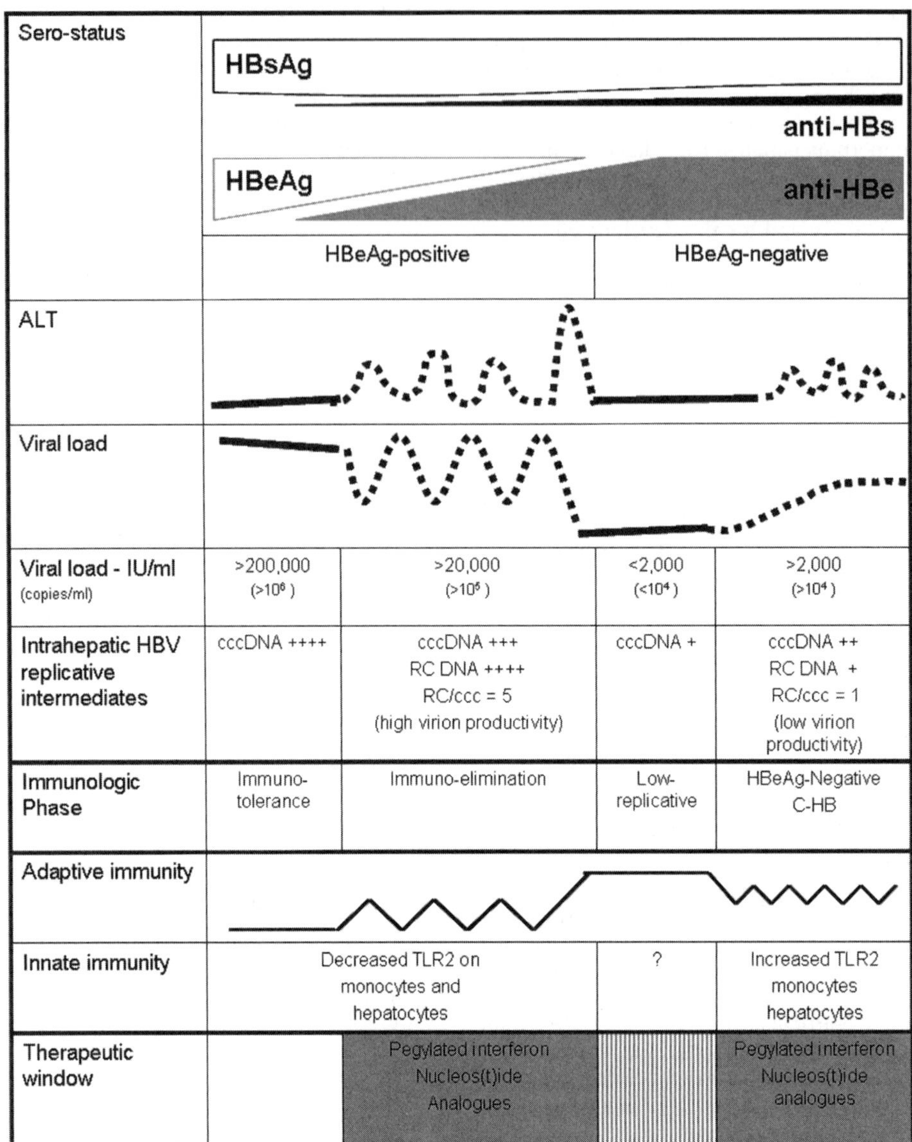

Sero-status
HBsAg
anti-HBs
HBeAg
anti-HBe
HBeAg-positive
HBeAg-negative
ALT
Viral load
Viral load - IU/ml (copies/ml)
>200,000 (>10⁶)
>20,000 (>10⁵)
<2,000 (<10⁴)
>2,000 (>10⁴)
Intrahepatic HBV replicative intermediates
cccDNA ++++
cccDNA +++ RC DNA ++++ RC/ccc = 5 (high virion productivity)
cccDNA +
cccDNA ++ RC DNA + RC/ccc = 1 (low virion productivity)
Immunologic Phase
Immuno-tolerance
Immuno-elimination
Low-replicative
HBeAg-Negative C-HB
Adaptive immunity
Innate immunity
Decreased TLR2 on monocytes and hepatocytes
?
Increased TLR2 monocytes hepatocytes
Therapeutic window
Pegylated interferon Nucleos(t)ide Analogues
Pegylated interferon Nucleos(t)ide analogues

FIGURE 6 Natural history of CHB, showing relationships between serology, biochemistry, molecular virology (serum and liver compartment), and immunologic parameters of the innate and adaptive arms. (Adapted from reference 103.)

antibodies and may obscure the onset of seroconversion. The available qualitative commercial assays usually detect anti-HBs and anti-HBe antibodies only after the respective antigens have been cleared from the serum. More sensitive immunoassays detect antibody in the presence of excess serum antigen (111) and may identify serologic responses in the context of active viral replication. For example, all patients with "active" CHB and the majority of patients with immunotolerant CHB demonstrate ongoing humoral immune responses, including anti-HBe and anti-surface antibody (anti-HBs) production (112). In fact, anti-HBe may appear years before the actual loss of HBeAg or onset of liver injury. Similarly, anti-HBs may coexist with virions and subviral HBsAg particles for many years before viral clearance and loss of HBsAg. The concept of a relatively nonoverlapping seroconversion from HBeAg-positive to anti-HBe-positive status during CHB may need amendment (Fig. 6).

PATHOGENESIS

HBV is not normally cytopathic, and the liver inflammation and disease that complicate infection are thought to be immunomediated (Fig. 7). Experimental study of the immunopathogenesis of HBV has been limited by a lack of available animal models and in vitro cell lines permissive for HBV infection. HBV can infect chimpanzees but typically causes a self-limiting acute hepatitis, different in severity and outcome from human disease. Although important data have been obtained, this work is resource intensive and not widely accessible. Other animal models include the infection of ducks and woodchucks with their

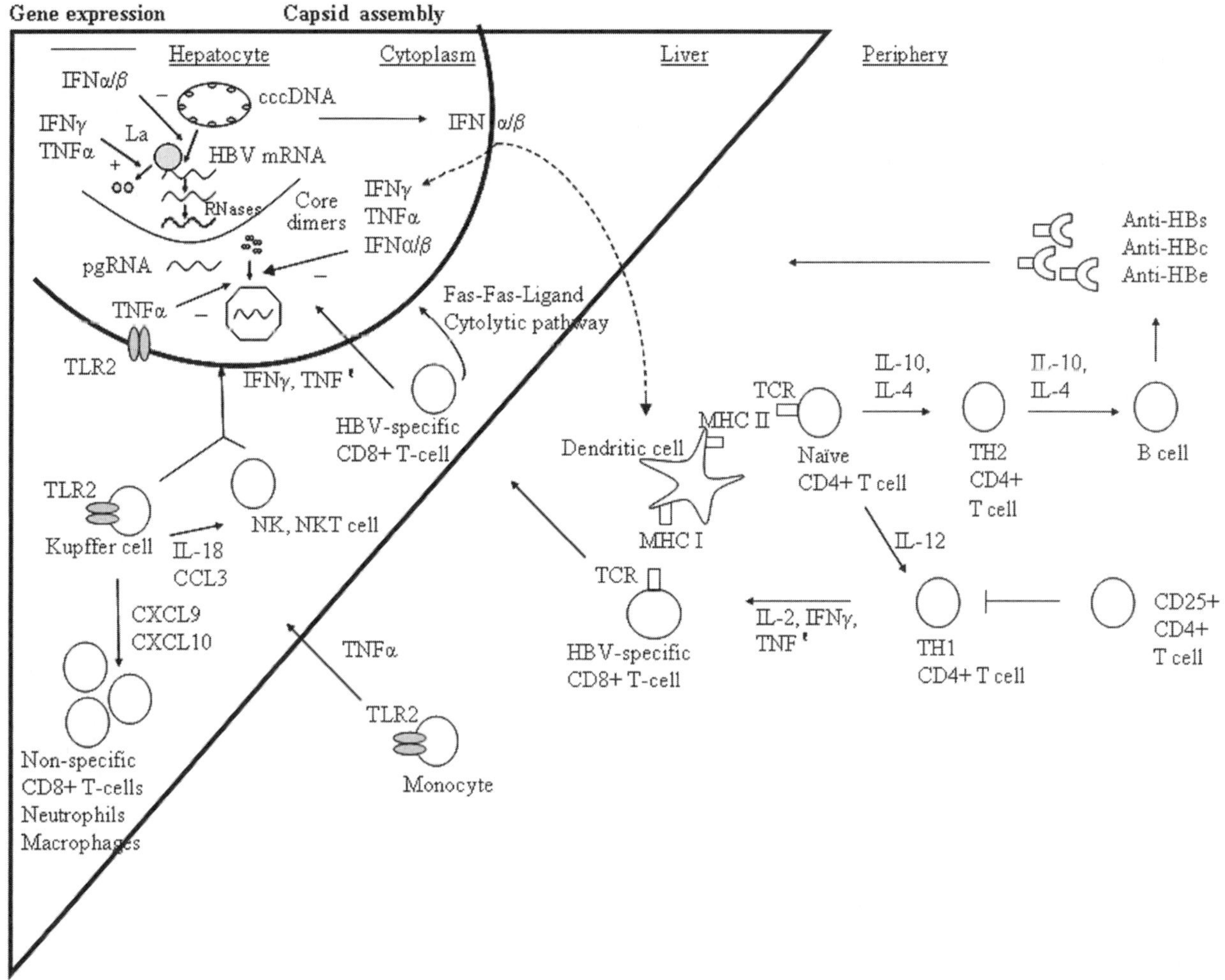

FIGURE 7 The host immune response directed against HBV requires coordinated action of both innate immunity and cellular and humoral adaptive immunity, to affect both noncytolytic and cytolytic activity. The pathways of noncytolytic clearance are highlighted (see text). The key cytokines involved are IFN-γ, TNF-α, and IFN-α/β. IFN-γ and TNF-α, secreted by antigen-specific CTL or by the antigen-nonspecific macrophages and T cells that they activate, abolish HBV gene expression and replication in the livers of transgenic mice without killing the hepatocytes. These cytokines activate two independent virocidal pathways. The first pathway eliminates HBV nucleocapsid particles and their cargo of replicating viral genomes, by preventing capsid assembly in a proteasome- and kinase-dependent manner. The second pathway destabilizes the viral RNA by an SSB/La-dependent mechanism. IFN-γ and TNF-α induce proteolytic cleavage of the La autoantigen, which normally protects several HBV RNA endoribonuclease cleavage sites from cellular RNases. Type I IFN (IFN-α/β) also inhibits HBV replication at a posttranscriptional level. IFN-β has been shown to activate hepatocellular mechanisms that prevent the formation of replication-competent HBV capsids. The molecular mechanism(s) that mediates this inhibition has not yet been defined; type I IFN-inducible genes with known antiviral activity, including those for double-stranded RNA-dependent protein kinase and interferon regulatory factor 1, have been implicated. Type I IFNs have also been shown to inhibit transcription of HBV RNAs in some models.

respective HBVs. Transgenic mouse models have allowed for a better understanding of the role of cytokines and noncytolytic viral clearance in the pathogenesis of HBV.

Acute HBV

In contrast to HCV, HBV does not start to replicate efficiently immediately postinoculation (188). Instead, experimental data from animal models and humans show that a lag period of 4 to 7 weeks is observed before HBV DNA and HBV antigens become detectable in the serum or liver. The explanation for this lag phase remains unclear. There is evidence to support a role for innate immune control during this period, via NK/NK T-cell activation and Toll-like receptor (TLR) signaling (72, 74, 176). However, a recent study of acute HBV infection in chimpanzees that analyzed the activation of hepatic cellular genes longitudinally by gene array (187) found that no genes were activated during the lag phase, despite a strong adaptive immune response and then clearing of the HBV in all animals, suggesting that HBV might be a stealth virus that evades early innate immunity.

Once HBV DNA becomes detectable, replication increases exponentially to peak at levels of $>10^{12}$ copies/ml in serum (186). In adult-acquired acute HBV infection, in which the host is able to control the virus, viral replication then declines, preceding the onset of clinical hepatitis (184). In acutely infected chimpanzees, a similar rapid drop in viral replication occurs before any detectable cellular infiltration or liver injury has occurred (60). This phenomenon is explained by the process of noncytolytic clearance, involving cytokine-mediated inhibition of HBV replication without the direct destruction of infected cells. The cells that mediate these early antiviral effects have not yet been identified in human infection, but studies from both the chimpanzee and transgenic mouse models have shown that HBV-specific $CD8^+$ cytotoxic T lymphocytes (CTLs) are important. In the chimpanzee model, monoclonal antibody-mediated depletion of $CD8^+$ T cells at the peak of viremia delays viral clearance until virus-specific T cells return to the liver (162). HBsAg-specific $CD8^+$ T cells, adoptively transferred to HBV transgenic mice, recognize their cognate antigen, lyse a small number of local hepatocytes, and, concurrently, produce cytokines that down-regulate HBV replication throughout the liver (116). A key role for the cytokines IFN-γ, TNF-α, and IFN-α/β has been identified (188) (Fig. 7). HBV-specific CTLs are therefore thought to be the most important effector cells involved in HBV clearance.

The disappearance of most of the HBV DNA from blood and liver is followed by the development of clinically apparent hepatitis, with peak ALT levels and maximal $CD4^+$ and $CD8^+$ T-cell responses in the blood (60, 162). Massive chemokine-mediated recruitment of intrahepatic inflammatory cells occurs, including HBV-specific and nonspecific T cells ("bystander lymphocytes"), neutrophils, NK cells, and monocytes/macrophages (184). Much of the hepatocellular damage occurring during acute hepatitis, therefore, results from secondary, non-antigen-specific inflammatory responses set in motion by the earlier HBV-specific CTL response. This combination of cytolytic and noncytolytic mechanisms serves to prevent infection of new hepatocytes and clear infected hepatocytes.

Humoral responses are also important in controlling HBV replication. HBV clearance is associated with the production of anti-HBs antibodies, and sera with high levels of anti-HBs can control or prevent HBV infection. The pathogenetic role of antibody directed against the nonenvelope proteins is not clear. Anti-HBe does not have virus-neutralizing activity; however, protection of chimpanzees against infection with HBV by passive administration of anti-HBc/HBe antibodies has been observed, suggesting a possible but undefined role for anti-HBe (153).

The integrated activation of the cellular and humoral arms of the adaptive immune response is therefore required for clearance of acute HBV infection; HBV-specific antibodies, together with HBV-specific memory T cells, then provide protective immunity against future infections.

Chronic HBV

The mechanisms of HBV persistence are not fully understood but are likely multifactorial, including characteristics of the host immune response (both developmental and genetic), strategies of HBV-specific immunosuppression, and the persistence of stable forms of the HBV genome such as cccDNA.

The likelihood of viral clearance depends on the age and immune status of the individual. Persistent infection is more likely to occur following vertical transmission or after horizontal transmission to children or immunocompromised adults. The single most important predictor of persistence is therefore the maturity of the host immune system at the time of infection, and the majority of the world's chronic HBV infections occur in areas of endemicity where infection occurs between the neonatal period and 5 years of age.

HBV displays a number of strategies to achieve persistence. In individuals with CHB, the HBV-specific $CD4^+$ and $CD8^+$ T-cell responses are significantly diminished relative to those in individuals with resolved infection, in both frequency and function. This relative collapse of virus-specific adaptive immunity appears to be regulated by the quantity of HBV replication present (Fig. 6). In animal models of chronic viral infection, the sustained presence of viral antigens may lead to a progressive functional decline in virus-specific CTL responses and ultimately T-cell deletion. Similarly, the frequency and function of both intrahepatic and peripheral HBV-specific T cells are inversely proportional to the level of HBV DNA in CHB (183). The effect of HBV infection on other components of the immune system remains unclear, but HBV-induced dendritic cell dysfunction or up-regulation of $CD25^+$ $CD4^+$ regulatory T cells might be relevant to persistence.

HBV produces a number of viral proteins that may promote chronicity. HBeAg, the secreted form of the viral nucleocapsid, is not required for infection or replication, yet it is absolutely required for the establishment of chronicity. Viral mutants defective for HBeAg production may cause acute, even fulminant, hepatitis but not de novo CHB (it should be noted, however, that these variants emerge to become the dominant virus during the natural history of established CHB, in the HBeAg-negative phase of disease; this always occurs in the context of a prior HBeAg-positive phase [Fig. 6]). The tolerizing effect of HBeAg in mouse models has been well characterized (119) and likely contributes to the poor core-specific T-cell responses that occur in patients with HBeAg-positive CHB. A second role for HBeAg in immune evasion has been identified: TLR2 expression and function have been observed to be down-regulated on peripheral monocytes, Kupffer cells, and hepatocytes from patients with HBeAg-positive disease, whereas HBeAg-negative CHB was associated with the up-regulation of TLR2 (176). A relationship between HBeAg and TLR2 may therefore contribute to persistence of infection, and the innate immune system may regulate adaptive immunity in CHB.

Viral particles consisting of HBsAg are produced far in excess of infectious virions during the life cycle of HBV. These particles are not infectious but are thought to act as a decoy for HBV-specific humoral immunity and also promote a state of low T-cell response and T-cell deletion.

EPIDEMIOLOGY

There are approximately 2 billion people who have been infected with HBV worldwide, most of whom live in Asia. This number includes both persons who have cleared the virus and more than 400 million who remain chronically infected.

Acute Hepatitis B

The introduction of the HBV vaccine has had a dramatic impact on the reported incidence of AHB. In the United States, the reported rate of acute HBV infection has declined since 1990, falling from 8.5 per 100,000 population to 1.8 per 100,000 population in 2005, the lowest rate ever recorded (182). Symptomatic AHB remains primarily a disease of adulthood; in the same survey the highest rates of AHB occurred among persons aged 25 to 44 years (3.6/100,000), and the lowest rates occurred among persons aged <15 years (0.03/100,000). The most common risk factors were sexual exposure (sexual contact with a person known to have HBV infection, multiple sex partners, and men having sex with men) and injection drug use. Similar trends have been seen in other countries, including Italy and Egypt, where the frequency of acute HBV infection as a cause of symptomatic hepatitis decreased from 43.4% in 1983 to 28.5% in 2002, following the introduction of childhood immunization in 1991 (199).

Chronic Hepatitis B

A total of 400 million people have been estimated to have CHB (126). Among infected patients, 15 to 40% develop serious liver disease, resulting in up to 1.2 million deaths per year. HBV infection is the 10th leading cause of death worldwide (88).

Chronic HBV infection is endemic in Southeast Asia, China, sub-Saharan Africa, Micronesia, and Polynesia and among the indigenous populations of Alaska, northern Canada, Greenland, Australia, and New Zealand (Fig. 8). In these high-prevalence regions, more than 7% of the population is chronically infected (prevalence has been reported as up to 10 to 20% [114]). Patterns of infection vary considerably from country to country, city to city, and even village to village and can change with time. Most infections are acquired early in childhood, and the risk of chronicity is inversely related to age at infection (see below) (62). Approximately 45% of the global population lives in an area of high prevalence (88). Moderate prevalence rates, of 2 to 7%, are seen in the southern regions of Eastern and Central Europe, the Amazon Basin, the Middle East, and the Indian subcontinent (Fig. 8) (113). Low-prevalence regions include much of North America, the United Kingdom, and northern Europe, where the incidence of chronic HBV infection is less than 2%. In these countries, HBV is seen predominantly in immigrants from countries with high prevalence and in their unvaccinated offspring, as well as in specific groups with percutaneous and sexual risk factors (see below).

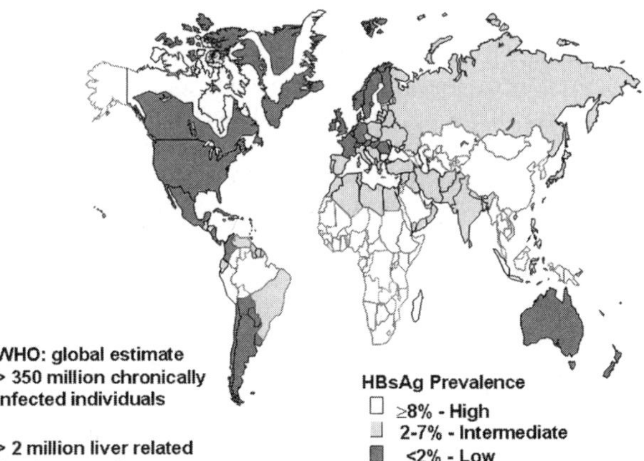

FIGURE 8 Global prevalence of HBsAg. The WHO clarifies areas as being of high, medium, or low endemicity for HBV if the prevalence rate of HBsAg is >8, 2 to 7, or <2%, respectively.

Transmission

HBV can be detected in serum, urine, saliva, nasopharyngeal secretions, urine, tears, vaginal secretions, menstrual blood, and semen (88). The virus can therefore be transmitted by perinatal, percutaneous, or sexual exposure or via close person-to-person contact in the presence of open cuts and sores (a common transmission method in children). The most common method of transmission is perinatal infection (154).

The mode of transmission of HBV infection varies geographically. In high-prevalence areas such as Southeast Asia and China, perinatal and early childhood horizontal transmissions are most common, resulting in high levels of chronicity (95% with perinatal infection and 30% with infection before 5 years of age). Perinatal transmission is likely to occur at birth or in the neonatal period. Given the efficacy of neonatal vaccination, in utero infection is probably uncommon. The primary determinants of vertical transmission are HBeAg status and HBV DNA level. The transmission rate in HBeAg-positive women is 90% without vaccination, compared to 32% for HBeAg-negative women (155).

In low-prevalence areas, sexual and percutaneous spread (primarily injection drug use) is also seen. In this setting, HBV infection typically manifests as adult-acquired acute hepatitis (see below). Progression to chronic hepatitis is rare in immunocompetent adults, occurring in <1% of individuals (150). Patients already infected with HIV or immunosuppressed for other reasons are at increased risk of chronicity after AHB (13).

Uncommon Modes of Transmission

Transfusion-related hepatitis B is now uncommon in countries where blood is obtained from unpaid donors screened for HBsAg and anti-HBc, with an estimated risk in the United States of 1/63,000 (148). Nosocomial HBV transmission still occurs despite the availability of vaccination and postexposure prophylaxis, although HBV infection in health care workers (HCW) has declined dramatically in countries with HCW vaccination programs (107). The most common route is patient to patient or patient to HCW via needlestick injuries (from syringes or suture needles) or scalpel. Nurses, dialysis staff, surgeons, dentists, and their assistants are at highest risk. Incomplete vaccination of staff, failure to apply universal precautions, and incorrect needle disposal technique are the most common reasons for transmission. Knowledge of a patient's infectious status does not prevent exposure. HBV DNA levels are the best marker of infectivity. Transmission from any organ donation from HBsAg-positive donors is well recognized, and all donations are screened for HBsAg. Anti-HBc-positive liver donors can also transmit infection. This is less common in renal and other transplants (178).

CLINICAL MANIFESTATIONS

Acute Hepatitis B

The incubation period of AHB varies from 1 to 4 months postinfection. Clinical presentation varies from asymptomatic infection in two-thirds of patients to icteric hepatitis and, rarely, fulminant liver failure (see chapter 5). A serum sickness-like illness, characterized by fever, arthralgias, and rash, may develop in the prodromal period, followed by constitutional symptoms, anorexia, nausea, jaundice, and right upper quadrant discomfort. Clinical symptoms coincide with biochemical abnormalities. The biochemical diagnosis of acute hepatitis is characterized by elevations in the concentration of serum ALT and bilirubin. ALT values in AHB are usually greater than 500 IU/ml, with ALT being higher than aspartate transaminase. Elevations in bilirubin are usually modest, 5 to 10 mg/dl (85 to 170 μmol/liter). The symptoms and jaundice generally disappear after 1 to 3 months, although fatigue may persist in some patients even after normalization of liver function tests.

The most serious complication of AHB is fulminant hepatic failure (FHF). This is unusual, occurring in <0.5% of patients, and is defined as the onset of hepatic encephalopathy within 8 weeks of the development of jaundice. The risk of FHF may be higher in patients acutely infected with BCP or precore variants, coinfected with other hepatitis viruses, or with underlying liver disease. The development of coagulopathy (marked by an international normalized ratio [INR] of >1.6) should raise concern about the risk of development of FHF and warrants consultation with a liver transplant center, as the prognosis is poor.

Chronic Hepatitis B

Most cases of CHB occur in endemic populations as the result of perinatal or early childhood horizontal transmission. The natural course of disease is determined by the interplay between virus replication and the host immune response, and it may be divided into a number of phases: (i) the immune tolerance phase, (ii) the immune elimination phase, (iii) the low or nonreplicative phase, and (iv) HBeAg-negative CHB (Fig. 6).

The immune tolerance phase is characterized by high levels of viral replication, with serum HBV viral load up to 10^{12} copies/ml and detectable HBeAg, but no evidence of active liver disease as manifested by lack of symptoms, normal serum ALT measurement, and minimal changes on liver biopsy. The quasispecies is dominated by a single dominant variant, and HBV-specific T-cell responses are weak or undetectable (183). The immune tolerance phase usually lasts 10 to 30 years, during which there is a very low rate of spontaneous HBeAg clearance, reported at only 15% after 20 years of infection (105).

Transition from the immune tolerance to the immune elimination phase typically occurs during the second and third decades of life. This transition is marked by increased HBV-specific T-cell immunity, falling HBV DNA titers, increased serum ALT, and necroinflammatory histologic changes. Immune pressure drives an increase in viral quasispecies diversity. The immune elimination phase may last for years, during which time disease activity fluctuates and progressive liver damage accumulates. The most important factor influencing prognosis appears to be prolonged viral replication at levels of $>10^4$ copies/ml (see below). In a small percentage of patients, severe ALT flares result in hepatic decompensation and, rarely, death from hepatic failure. HBeAg seroconversion is used as the serologic marker of the end of the immune elimination phase and correlates with a significant drop in viral load, often to undetectable levels, and histologic arrest or improvement. HBV is not cleared from the liver, however, and the nuclear cccDNA reservoir persists. Spontaneous HBeAg clearance increases to an annual rate of 10 to 20% during the immune elimination phase (105).

Patients in the low or nonreplicative phase are HbeAg negative and anti-HBe positive. An arbitrary threshold below which HBV replication is not thought to be clinically significant has been set at $>10^4$ copies/ml (106). In some patients serum HBV DNA is no longer detectable, even when tested by sensitive PCR assays. Liver disease remits as evidenced by normal serum ALT concentrations and resolution of necroinflammation in liver biopsies. HBV-specific T-cell reactivity is high and thought to maintain viral suppression (108). The remaining HBV quasispecies is a diverse population, with positive selection of viral variants defective for HBeAg production that are able to persist, but at the cost of reduced-replication phenotype (95, 177). The annual rate of delayed clearance of HBsAg has been estimated to be 0.5 to 2% in Western patients and much lower (0.1 to 0.8%) in Asian countries (1, 92). HBsAg seroconversion is regarded as a "cure" and is associated with a good prognosis. It is unlikely that HBV DNA is ever completely cleared from the liver, however, and a small risk of reactivation persists in settings of potent immunosuppression like allogeneic bone marrow transplantation or HIV infection.

A percentage of patients continue to have moderate levels of HBV replication and active liver disease (elevated serum ALT and chronic inflammation on liver biopsies) but remain HBeAg negative. This typically occurs following the emergence of variants of HBV that are phenotypically HBeAg negative and genotypically include precore or BCP mutants. It remains unclear whether this occurs as a smooth transition from the HBeAg-positive immune elimination phase or as reactivation from the low or nonreplicative phase.

In adult-acquired CHB the immune tolerance phase is typically absent, with disease progressing immediately to the immune elimination phase. Some of these patients will be immunosuppressed, and in this setting the disease course may be more aggressive. This has been clearly documented in the setting of HIV coinfection, which confers an increased risk of cirrhosis and liver-related morbidity (164). In immunocompetent adults, however, a higher rate of spontaneous and treatment-induced HBsAg seroconversion and lower rates of progression to cirrhosis occur.

Complications of CHB

The major complications of CHB are cirrhosis, hepatic decompensation, and HCC. Extrahepatic manifestations can also occur (see below). Between 15 and 40% of individuals with CHB will develop liver sequelae during their lifetime, with the highest risk in men (6, 7). CHB has a variable natural history, and accurately predicting prognosis in an individual patient is difficult. Studies to identify the characteristics of patients at risk have been limited by the long duration of follow-up required. However, more recently a key role has been identified for a viral load of $>10^4$ copies/ml (>2,000 IU/ml), over the age of 30 years, as a risk factor for clinical progression to cirrhosis and HCC (27, 71).

Cirrhosis

The current challenge in CHB is to identify patients at risk for progressive liver disease, so that therapy may be offered early to alter the natural history. The major risk factors for progression to cirrhosis are viral load, the presence of fibrosis on liver biopsy, and elevated serum ALT. Other factors which influence progression to cirrhosis include viral genotype; coinfection with other viruses, such as HCV, HDV, and HIV; and alcohol consumption (195).

In patients with CHB, the strongest independent predictor of progression to cirrhosis is HBV viral load. In a prospective study of 3,582 community-based HBsAg-positive Taiwanese aged greater than 30 years, the risk of cirrhosis increased as baseline viral load increased (71) and a critical threshold of viral load of 10^4 DNA copies/ml (2,000 IU/ml) was identified (Fig. 9). The effect of viral load was independent of age, sex, cigarette smoking, alcohol consumption, HBeAg status, and alanine transaminase level. The annual incidence of cirrhosis was 0.9%, lower than the reported rate of 2 to 7% observed in tertiary referral center populations (47, 68, 94). A second large prospective study, conducted in mainland China (28), has confirmed this central role for viral load in prognostication (71). Whether these data can be extrapolated to younger patients, particularly those still in the immunotolerant phase of disease, or to HBsAg carriers in Western countries with adult-acquired HBV infection, remains unclear.

Elevated serum ALT, especially frequent ALT flares, has been shown to be a risk factor for progressive disease (64). Mild elevations of serum ALT also predict for poor outcome, however, and it is likely that only a persistently low-normal serum ALT (<0.5 times the upper limit of normal [ULN]) is reassuring (198). Liver biopsy remains a useful clinical tool, and histology has prognostic significance. The probability of evolution to cirrhosis is increased in patients with moderate to severe inflammatory changes (47, 94) or advanced fibrosis (130).

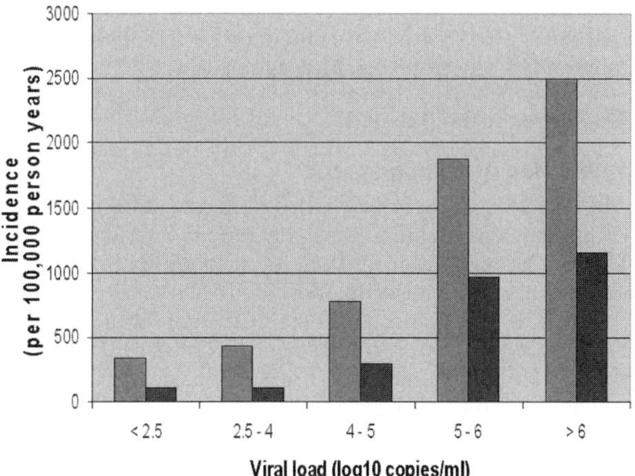

FIGURE 9 HBV DNA level predicts the risk of cirrhosis (light gray bars) and HCC (dark gray bars). Elevated serum HBV DNA level (>10^4 copies/ml) is a strong predictor of risk for both cirrhosis and HCC. (Adapted from references 27 and 71.)

Viral factors have been shown to have an influence on the risk of disease progression. In Asian countries, where genotypes B and C predominate, more rapid and frequent progression to cirrhosis has been noted in patients with genotype C disease (34, 159). Much of this risk is explained by the observation that the age of HBeAg seroconversion is greater in genotype C than in genotype B patients, confirming the critical role of prolonged viremia. Genotype D has been associated with more advanced disease than genotype A in Western populations (9, 46, 50). There are no natural history studies that compare all four of the major genotypes. In addition to genotype, a pathogenic role has been proposed for the common viral mutants associated with HBeAg-negative CHB. HBeAg-negative disease has been associated with severe and progressive disease; a significant proportion of patients have been found to have established cirrhosis on liver biopsy (35, 97). The BCP mutation has been identified as a risk factor for cirrhosis (48). The role of the precore variant, the most common variant associated with HBeAg-negative disease, remains unclear.

Hepatic Decompensation

Decompensated liver disease develops as a complication of cirrhosis. The estimated 5-year risk of progression to decompensation is 20 to 23% (141). Risk factors for decompensation include persistent viremia, age, and markers of impaired synthetic function (including low albumin, low platelets, high bilirubin, and ascites) (93). Once decompensation occurs, the estimated 5-year survival rate is 14 to 35%, compared to 80 to 85% for compensated patients. The advent of NA therapy has had a dramatic impact on this natural history, again confirming the critical role viral replication plays in disease progression (see below).

HCC

Seropositivity for HBsAg is one of the most important risk factors for the development of HCC. The relative risk of developing HCC if HBsAg positive varies from 7-fold in Japan to 60- to 98-fold in Taiwan, likely proportional to the respective population-attributable risks of 10 and 94% (27). More important for clinical practice is risk stratification for individual patients with CHB.

Viral load has a profound impact on the risk of development of HCC in CHB patients (Fig. 9) (27). A biological gradient of risk according to a single measurement of serum HBV DNA level has been defined in a large prospective Taiwanese cohort. The cumulative incidence of HCC over 13 years of follow-up varied from 1.3 to 14.9% for HBV DNA levels of <300 and >10^6 copies/ml (<60 and >200,000 IU/ml), respectively. Individuals were at highest risk if the viral load was persistently >10^5 copies/ml (>20,000 IU/ml). Conversely, a significant reduction in HCC risk was observed in those who had a high entry at baseline but in whom viral load was significantly reduced at follow-up. HBV DNA level remained an independent predictor of HCC even after adjusting for known covariates, including sex, age, cigarette smoking, alcohol consumption, HBeAg status, serum ALT level, and the presence of cirrhosis at baseline. The importance of HBV viral load in hepatic carcinogenesis was further emphasized by the finding that LMV therapy for patients with advanced fibrosis or cirrhosis reduces the risk of HCC (93).

A number of Asian studies have identified viral factors that are associated with the development of HCC. Genotype C is associated with increased risk compared to genotype B (77, 197), likely secondary to the prolonged high-level viremia that occurs with genotype C infection. BCP mutations have been linked to hepatic carcinogenesis (76). BCP mutations are more common in genotype C disease; again, the common factor is likely to be the degree and duration of viremia. More recently, genotype F disease has been associated with the development of HCC among Alaska Native people (99).

Extrahepatic Manifestations

HBV infection is associated with several extrahepatic manifestations which are thought to be mediated by circulating immunocomplexes (67). These include the serum sickness-like prodrome of acute HBV infection, polyarteritis nodosa, HBV-associated glomerulonephritis (GN), mixed essential cryoglobulinemia, and neurologic manifestations.

A serum sickness-like prodrome precedes clinical hepatitis by 1 to 6 weeks in 10 to 30% of those acquiring acute HBV infection. Also known as the "arthritis-dermatitis" syndrome, it is characterized by a symmetrical generalized inflammatory arthritis, typically involving the small joints of the hands and feet, which may be indistinguishable from acute rheumatoid arthritis. The joint lesions are nondestructive, however. Skin manifestations are variable, occurring in more than 50% at the time of, or shortly after, the joint symptoms. Lesions described include maculopapular, petechial, or purpuric rash; palpable purpura; Henoch-Schönlein-type purpura; erythema multiforme; toxic erythema; lichenoid dermatitis; and urticaria. Fever is common. Renal involvement with proteinuria or hematuria is much less common. Angioneurotic edema may rarely occur.

Polyarteritis nodosa is a rare but serious complication of HBV infection. The syndrome normally presents within 4 months of the clinical onset of HBV infection, with abdominal pain due to arteritis of medium-sized vessels causing ischemia of the intestine and gallbladder. The finding of microaneurysms of blood vessels in the renal, hepatic, or mesenteric circulations on angiography is virtually pathognomonic. Tissue biopsy of affected organs revealing inflammation of the medium-sized arteries confirms the diagnosis. Treatment involves antiviral therapy, immunosuppression, and plasma exchange. The prognosis is poor without treatment, with a mortality rate of up to 50%.

GN is more commonly associated with CHB. A number of patterns of glomerular injury have been described, including membranoproliferative GN, membranous GN, and, rarely, mesangial proliferative GN. In children the disease is usually self-limited; however, progression to renal failure has been described to occur in adults. The association of HBV infection with mixed essential cryoglobulinemia is controversial. Rare cases have been reported; however, the majority of cases are now recognized to be associated with HCV infection (51).

Other manifestations of HBV-related vasculitis include mononeuritis multiplex and polyneuropathy. Guillain-Barré syndrome has been reported. Associations with polymyalgia rheumatica, polymyositis, and HLA-B27-positive ankylosing spondylitis have also been reported, although a causative link remains controversial.

LOW-LEVEL (OCCULT) HBV INFECTION

Occult HBV infection is defined by the presence of detectable HBV DNA in a patient in whom HBsAg is not measurable. In a small number of these patients, viral variants may be identified that produce an antigenically modified HBs protein not detectable using commercial HBsAg assays, or carrying mutations that inhibit pre-S/S gene expression (139). However, in most cases the occult status does not seem to result from genomic heterogeneity. Rather, the occult expression results from strong suppression of viral gene expression. Most of these patients have very low levels of HBV DNA in the serum (typically 10^2 to 10^3 copies/ml), accounting for the failure to detect HBsAg. The epidemiology of occult HBV remains poorly defined. It remains rare in the Western world. It appears to be more common in areas of endemicity, in the setting of coinfection with HCV and HIV, in patients with a history of injection drug use, in hemophiliacs, and in patients on hemodialysis (139). There is increasing evidence that occult HBV is relevant clinically. Carriers of occult HBV may be a source of HBV transmission in the case of blood donation. There is a risk of viral reactivation in patients who are immunosuppressed. Although there are no prospective data, there is evidence to suggest an association between occult HBV and progressive liver fibrosis and HCC (139).

MANAGEMENT OF HBV INFECTION

■ Acute Hepatitis B

In immunocompetent adults, AHB is a spontaneously resolving infection in the majority of cases. Antiviral therapy is not generally indicated. However, there has been some interest in whether NA therapy would benefit patients with severe AHB. The use of LMV in German patients presenting to a transplant center with severe AHB, defined by an INR of >2.0, was found to improve the mortality rate compared to a historical control (166). In contrast, a recent randomized controlled trial in India failed to demonstrate a benefit of LMV therapy in severe AHB defined by two of three criteria: hepatic encephalopathy; serum bilirubin of ≥10.0 mg/dl (171 μmol/liter); and an INR of ≥1.6 (81). No patients in this study required liver transplantation, and it is likely that the patients represented a "less severe" population than in the German cohort. Despite the negative findings of this well-conducted study, therefore, a trial of NA therapy may be reasonable in fulminant HBV with profound coagulopathy.

■ Chronic Hepatitis B

Principles of Management

The aim of treatment for CHB is the prevention of clinical complications, including decompensated liver disease and HCC. The prevention of these clinical end points may be achieved by durable suppression of HBV replication (106). As clinical end points may take years to eventuate, a sustained virologic response has been adopted as the goal of therapy in both clinical trials and day-to-day practice. Virologic response has been recently defined as a decrease in serum HBV DNA to levels undetectable by sensitive PCR assays, with loss of HBeAg in patients who were initially HBeAg positive. In HBeAg-positive CHB, HBeAg seroconversion has been shown to correlate with sustained viral suppression and clinical benefit and is therefore an end point for therapy (125). There is no clear end point for therapy in the setting of HBeAg-negative CHB, as relapse is common on treatment cessation (106).

Indications for Therapy

Candidates for antiviral therapy fall into three groups: patients with HBeAg-positive CHB, patients with HBeAg-negative CHB, and patients with advanced fibrosis/cirrhosis (who may be either HBeAg positive or negative). The clinical utility of this approach is based on the expected differences in the duration of therapy that will be required for these groups.

HBeAg-Positive CHB

The clearly defined clinical end point for therapy in HBeAg-positive CHB is HBeAg seroconversion. Therefore, a trial of therapy should be offered to all patients with active disease, defined by a viral load of $>10^5$ copies/ml and either a raised ALT of >2 times the ULN or moderate to severe inflammation on liver biopsy. In patients with an ALT of <2 times the ULN in the presence of viral replication, the decision of whether to commence therapy is influenced by the severity of both inflammation and fibrosis on liver biopsy. Most professional bodies would recommend a trial of observation for 3 to 6 months to allow for spontaneous seroconversion prior to initiating therapy (44, 91, 106). The options for therapy include IFN-based therapy or one of the approved NA (Table 5).

HBeAg-Negative CHB

There is no agreed upon end point of therapy for patients with HBeAg-negative CHB. A sustained virologic response may be achieved in a small percentage of patients using IFN-based therapy; however, most patients require prolonged therapy with an NA. Treatment decisions must weigh the risk of future clinical complications against the long-term costs and risk of antiviral resistance. Liver biopsy is useful in decision making, as the presence of significant fibrosis should trigger consideration of therapy. Treatment is reasonable for patients with a viral load of $>10^4$ copies/ml and evidence of moderate to severe inflammation or significant fibrosis (106). For patients with mild fibrosis and inflammation but ongoing replication, there are no data to determine whether the risk of long-term antiviral resistance outweighs the benefit of initial viral suppression (Table 4).

Cirrhosis

Sustained viral suppression improves clinical outcomes in the setting of CHB and advanced liver disease (93). Long-term NA therapy would normally be recommended. It is critical that these patients be monitored closely both for initial virologic response and subsequently for the development of antiviral resistance to allow institution of salvage therapy before the serum ALT becomes elevated. Patients with compensated cirrhosis and HBeAg-positive CHB can be considered for PEG with close monitoring for hepatitis flare and long-term monitoring for virologic relapse (19). Patients with decompensated liver disease should not receive IFN-based therapy because of the risk of hepatitis flare; rather, long-term NA therapy and referral to a transplant center are indicated.

Antiviral Therapy

There are two strategies of therapy currently available for the management of CHB: (i) NA and (ii) standard IFN-α (sIFN-α) or PEG.

NA

The development of safe and efficacious orally available antiviral NA has advanced the treatment of CHB significantly during the past 10 years (Table 5). The recognition that sustained viral suppression with NA reduced hepatic necroinflammatory activity and reversed fibrosis (including cirrhosis) has led to the current focus on the importance of viral load in pathogenesis, as well as fundamentally altering the understanding of hepatic fibrogenesis (41). The first NA, LMV, a synthetic deoxycytidine analog with an unnatural L conformation, gained approval from the U.S. Food and Drug Administration (FDA) for treatment of CHB in 1996. Telbivudine (LdT), another L-nucleoside, has also been recently approved for the treatment of CHB. The related L-nucleoside emtricitabine (FTC) has similar anti-HBV efficacy but is only licensed for use for HIV. Adefovir dipivoxil (ADV), a prodrug for the acyclic dAMP analog adefovir, gained approval in 2002, and clinical trials of structurally similar tenofovir disoproxil fumarate (TDF), which is currently used to treat HIV infection, are under way. The most potent anti-HBV drug discovered to date is the deoxyguanosine analog entecavir (ETV) (149), which has recently been approved by the FDA for first-line use against HBV. Clevudine and LB80380 were in phase III trials in 2008.

The advantages of NA are ease of administration, rapid viral suppression, and lack of side effects. The major disadvantages are the requirement for prolonged therapy in the majority of patients, the development of resistance to single agents, and the paucity of data surrounding the use of these agents during conception and pregnancy. The latter is especially important for younger patients during their fertile years. The description of these agents and their pharmacology is summarized in chapter 12.

LMV

LMV, the (−) enantiomer of 2′,3′dideoxy-3′-thiacytidine, is a cytosine NA. It was the first NA licensed for use in the treatment of CHB. In HBeAg-positive patients, 48 weeks of treatment with LMV results in a mean decline of serum HBV DNA of 4 to 5 $\log_{10}$ copies/ml, and HBeAg seroconversion occurs in 16 to 18% (Table 5) (106). The rate of HBeAg seroconversion increases with prolonged duration of therapy, up to 50% by 5 years. Viral suppression is associated with histologic improvement and reversal of fibrosis. Pretreatment ALT is the strongest predictor of response—seroconversion is greatest in patients with baseline ALT greater than five times the ULN in clinical trials. Seroconversion is unlikely if the baseline ALT is less than twice the ULN (32).

LMV-induced HBeAg seroconversion is regarded as an end point for therapy in HBeAg-positive patients. Following treatment withdrawal, HBeAg seroconversion is durable in 50 to 80% of patients in clinical trials. Factors that have been identified to increase durability include longer duration of consolidation therapy, younger age, lower DNA level at the time of treatment withdrawal, and genotype B versus genotype C. It is therefore recommended that therapy be continued for at least 6 months after seroconversion. The significance of virologic factors in determining LMV response remains controversial, although it may be relevant in the development of LMV resistance (31).

LMV is also effective in HBeAg-negative patients. Several studies have demonstrated that 1 year of therapy will suppress HBV DNA to levels undetectable in 60 to 70%

TABLE 5 Responses to approved antiviral therapies among treatment-naïve patients with HBeAg-positive and HBeAg-negative CHB[a]

Parameter	Patient HBeAg status	sIFN-α, 5 MU daily or 10 MU TIW,[b] 12–24 wks (%)	Control	LMV, 100 mg daily, 48–52 wks (%)	Placebo	ADV, 10 mg daily, 48 wks (%)	Placebo	ETV, 0.5 mg daily, 48 wks (%)	LdT, 600 mg daily, 52 wks (%)	PEG, 180 μg weekly, 48 wks (%)	PEG + LMV, 180 μg weekly + 100 mg daily, 48 wks (%)
Loss of serum DNA[c]	Positive	37	17	40–44	16	21	0	67	60	25	69
	Negative	60–70	10–20	60–73	NA[d]	51	0	90	88	63	87
Loss of HBeAg	Positive	33	12	17–32	6–11	24	11	22	26	30/34[e]	27/28[e]
HBeAg seroconversion	Positive	Difference of 18%		16–21	4–6	12	6	21	22	27/32[e]	24/27[e]
Loss of HBsAg	Positive	7.80	1.80	<1	0	0	0	2	0	3	3
Normalization of ALT	Positive	Difference of 23%		41–75	7–24	48	16	68	77	39	46
	Negative	60–70	10–20	60–79	NA	72	29	78	74	38	49
Histologic improvement	Positive	NA	NA	49–56	23–25	53	25	72	65	38	41
	Negative	NA	NA	60–66	NA	64	33	70	67	48	38
Durability of response	Positive	80–90		50–80		90		69	80	NA	NA
	Negative	10–20		<10		5		NA	NA	20	20
Clinical benefit[f]											
Increase in Child-Pugh score				3.40	8.80						
HCC				3.90	7.40						

[a] Adapted from reference 106.
[b] MU TIW, million (10^6) units three times per week.
[c] DNA assays of variable sensitivity.
[d] NA, not available.
[e] Values are for 48 and 72 weeks, i.e., at end of treatment and 24 weeks posttreatment.
[f] Comparison of long-term LMV therapy in the setting of advanced fibrosis or cirrhosis; study terminated at 32.4 months owing to a significant difference between treatment groups in the number of end points reached.

of patients using sensitive PCR assays (Table 5). This is unlikely to reflect increased potency compared to HBeAg-positive cohorts, but rather a lower baseline viral load. Despite effective viral suppression, 90% of patients relapse when treatment is stopped. Long-term therapy is therefore required for sustained viral suppression. Unfortunately, prolonged therapy is complicated by the progressive development of LMV resistance (see below).

The one prospective, double-blind, randomized, placebo-controlled trial of LMV therapy with a clinical end point included 651 Asian patients with evidence of active viral replication and bridging fibrosis or cirrhosis on liver biopsy (134). A statistically significant reduction in overall disease progression (defined by an increase in Child-Turcotte-Pugh score, hepatic decompensation, or new-onset HCC) and HCC development was observed in comparing LMV therapy to placebo. Patients with decompensated cirrhosis also benefit from LMV, which may delay or even obviate liver transplantation (175). Clinical improvement occurs over 3 to 6 months; unfortunately, in this group, the risk of HCC persists. LMV can therefore improve clinical outcome in patients with advanced liver disease. Prospective data on clinical outcomes in patients with less advanced disease are lacking, although retrospective analyses suggest that clinical outcome is improved in patients maintaining viral suppression after starting therapy with LMV (128).

LMV therapy is very well tolerated in general. There is now considerable worldwide experience with LMV, which has been used in both HBV and HIV infections for over a decade. Various mild adverse events have been reported for patients receiving LMV, but all were observed to occur at the same frequency among controls (43).

Despite these encouraging results, the use of LMV has been complicated by the frequent emergence of drug resistance (see below). The development of newer antiviral drugs with improved resistance profiles has meant that LMV monotherapy is no longer recommended for treatment-naïve patients. For economic reasons, however, it is likely that widespread use will continue in the developing world.

ADV

ADV is the orally bioavailable prodrug of adefovir, an analog of AMP. Similar to other NA, it inhibits HBV DNA Pol by acting as a chain terminator, inhibiting both the reverse transcriptase and DNA Pol. The degree of HBV suppression achieved is less than that with LMV therapy, with a mean viral load decline of 3 to 3.5 $\log_{10}$ copies/ml after 1 year of treatment (Table 5) (134). Furthermore, approximately 30% of NA-naïve patients will be primary nonresponders (defined as having a <1-$\log_{10}$ drop in viral load by 6 months of treatment) (42). The ADV dosage approved for clinical use was limited to 10 mg per day by the 8% risk of nephrotoxicity observed at the higher dosage of 30 mg daily. Suboptimal dosage may therefore contribute to the primary nonresponse rate (43).

HBeAg seroconversion appears to be durable and similar to that observed with LMV therapy. ADV is also effective in the management of HBeAg-negative CHB. Although the relapse rate is very high in HBeAg-negative CHB if therapy is stopped after 48 weeks (92%) (65), it may be possible to withdraw therapy in patients after long-term viral suppression. In a cohort of 33 patients who maintained virologic suppression on ADV for a median of 4 to 5 years, 67% maintained biochemical remission to a median follow-up of 18 months. Although all experienced virologic relapse, VR, HBV DNA levels remained relatively low (similar to the inactive HBsAg carrier state, <50,000 copies/ml), and in most cases, they declined over time. Persistent biochemical relapse and reinstitution of ADV was required in only 3% (63).

The risk of ADV nephrotoxicity and the observed primary nonresponse rate make ADV less suitable as a therapy for patients with advanced liver disease, either compensated or decompensated. No trials have evaluated ADV as primary therapy in this clinical context. "Add-on" ADV has been shown to be effective as salvage therapy in decompensated CHB complicated by LMV resistance (146).

Although less potent as an antiviral agent compared to LMV, ADV offers the benefit of a much reduced incidence of drug resistance; furthermore, the resistance profile differs greatly from that of LMV, and cross-resistance has not been observed. ADV has activity against both wild-type and LMV-resistant HBV in vitro and clinically.

ETV

ETV is an analog of 2′-deoxyguanosine. It inhibits HBV replication at three different steps: (i) the priming of HBV DNA Pol, (ii) the reverse transcription of minus-strand DNA, and (iii) the synthesis of plus-strand HBV DNA. ETV is more potent than LMV or ADV, reducing HBV DNA by 6 to 7 $\log_{10}$ copies/ml after 48 weeks of treatment (134).

ETV was compared to LMV in the phase III registration trial for the management of HBeAg-positive CHB (26). At week 48, ETV was associated with superior rates of DNA undetectability, normalization of ALT, and histologic improvement (Table 5). HBeAg seroconversion rates were similar. Limited data are available on the durability of ETV-associated HBeAg seroconversion, but of patients who stopped treatment at 48 weeks, 70% remained HBeAg negative through 96 weeks (26, 59). In the setting of HBeAg-negative CHB, ETV was again associated with improved rates of undetectable HBV DNA, normalization of ALT, and histologic improvement compared to LMV. Data on the durability of response are lacking, but experience with other NA would suggest that most patients would relapse if therapy were stopped after 1 year (106). Few published data are available on the safety and efficacy of ETV in decompensated cirrhosis. Studies are ongoing.

ETV is very well tolerated, and clinical trials have found a safety profile similar to that of LMV. Preclinical studies in rats treated with doses 3 to 40 times the maximal human dose found an increased risk of tumors in the lungs, brain, and liver. Similar events have not been observed in humans (45), in whom no difference in the incidence of any neoplasm has been observed with the use of ETV compared to LMV.

ETV resistance is rare in NA-naïve patients and emerges slowly, as discussed below (36). ETV therefore offers the benefit of potent antiviral effect combined with a favorable resistance profile. Of the currently available agents, it is recommended as the first-line NA monotherapy for NA-naïve patients with compensated liver disease.

LdT

LdT is an L-nucleoside with a potent anti-HBV effect. Forty-eight weeks of therapy will reduce HBV viral load by 6 $\log_{10}$ copies/ml. In clinical trials, LdT has been shown to be more potent than LMV in suppressing HBV (Table 5) (83). However, the rate of HBeAg loss observed was similar to that obtained with LMV. Despite the potent antiviral effect, LdT is also associated with a high rate of resistance, and LdT-resistant mutants are cross-resistant to LMV (see below). For this reason, LdT monotherapy is likely to have a limited role in the treatment of HBV infection.

TDF

TDF is structurally similar to ADV. TDF and ADV are equipotent in vitro, but because TDF is associated with less nephrotoxicity, the clinical trial dose was 30 times greater (300 mg per day). This explains the much greater potency seen in studies (reductions in viral load of 6 to 7 $\log_{10}$ copies/ml) (134). TDF has activity against both HIV and HBV. It is currently approved as monotherapy and combination therapy (with FTC) for the management of HIV and HIV-HBV coinfection. TDF-FTC combination therapy is currently recommended as first-line therapy for HBV infection in the setting of HIV infection (66). It is not yet approved for the management of HBV monoinfection, though TDF-FTC combination therapy holds the promise of potent viral suppression and a high barrier to resistance. As discussed below, TDF is effective for the management of both LMV and ADV resistance. Although generally well tolerated, TDF therapy may rarely be associated with Fanconi syndrome and renal insufficiency (174).

FTC

FTC (5′-fluorothiacytidine) is a fluorinated cytosine analog that is structurally similar to LMV. It inhibits both HBV DNA Pol and HIV reverse transcriptase. Clinical studies show that 48 weeks of FTC reduced HBV DNA by 3 to 4 $\log_{10}$ copies/ml and significantly improved liver histology (96). However, despite virologic, biochemical, and histologic improvement, this study of 248 patients (63% HBeAg positive) failed to show any benefit in HBeAg seroconversion compared to placebo—12% in the two groups (96). Furthermore, mutants with FTC resistance mutations in the YMDD motif (rtM204V) were detected in 13% of patients at 48 weeks, mutants which are cross-resistant to LMV.

FTC monotherapy is unlikely to have an important role in the management of HBV given the frequency of drug resistance and the issue of cross-resistance to LMV. It does hold promise in combination with TDF for NA-naïve monoinfected patients.

Combination Therapy

The challenge in the use of long-term NA therapy is reducing the rate of resistance. Although combination therapy has been shown to prevent antiviral resistance in HIV, the promise of combination therapy is yet to be fulfilled in CHB. The limited data available to date are disappointing. Although several combination studies in cohorts of NA-naïve patients have demonstrated that the rate of LMV resistance can be reduced when used in combination with either PEG or a second NA, combination therapy has not yet been shown to reduce the rate of resistance to antiviral compounds that have a low rate of resistance. This may be due to the relatively short-term follow-up, as well as the choice of NA which have been shown to be cross-resistant (e.g., LMV and LdT). With appropriate drug selection, combination therapy will likely become standard therapy for CHB in the future.

As discussed below, the use of add-on ADV combination therapy has been shown to be superior to sequential monotherapy following the development of LMV resistance (140). This treatment strategy has been shown to limit secondary ADV resistance.

NA Resistance

Drug resistance is important because it is associated with the loss of virologic, biochemical, and, eventually, histologic therapeutic gain. In the setting of advanced liver disease, resistance may lead to hepatitis flares, hepatic decompensation, and death (93).

Virologic breakthrough is defined as a >1 $\log_{10}$ increase in serum HBV DNA from nadir, in two consecutive samples taken 1 month apart, in a patient who had an initial virologic response (102, 106). Virologic breakthrough is usually followed by biochemical breakthrough, with its associated risks of flare and decompensation. However, virologic breakthrough may occur months and sometimes years before biochemical breakthrough; hence, early detection is possible prior to the development of clinical complications. This is particularly important in the setting of advanced liver disease.

LMV and Other L-NA Resistance

Antiviral resistance to LMV has been mapped to the YMDD locus in the catalytic domain (C domain) of HBV Pol (157). The mutations within the reverse transcriptase gene that have been selected during LMV therapy are designated rtM204I/V/S (domain C) plus or minus rtL180M (domain B) (157), with mutations in other regions of the HBV Pol being detected (Fig. 5). For other L-nucleosides such as LdT, the B-domain (rtA181T/V) and C-domain (rtM204I) changes are most important for the development of resistance (Fig. 5).

LMV resistance increases progressively during treatment at rates between 14 and 32% annually, exceeding 70% after 48 months of treatment (82). Factors that increase the risk of development of resistance include high pretherapy serum HBV DNA and ALT levels and incomplete suppression of viral replication (82). LMV resistance does not confer cross-resistance to ADV.

Mutations that confer LMV resistance decrease in vitro sensitivity to LMV by 100-fold to 1,000-fold. The rtM204I substitution has been detected in isolation, but rtM204V and rtM204S are found only in association with other changes in the B or A domain (39). Four major patterns of resistance can be identified: (i) rtM204I, (ii) rtL180M plus rtM204V, (iii) rtL180M plus rtM204I, and (iv) rtV173L plus rtL180M plus rtM204V. The molecular mechanism of LMV resistance is steric hindrance caused by the β-branched side group of the valine or isoleucine colliding with the oxathiolane ring of LMV in the deoxynucleoside triphosphate binding site (5).

Management of LMV resistance

ADV. ADV is effective in the management of LMV-resistant variants. While early treatment responses have been shown to be equivalent in patients with compensated liver disease who are treated with ADV monotherapy (switch) and those treated with combination LMV-ADV (add-on), it is now clear that the risk of ADV resistance is increased in the setting of monotherapy. Rates of genotypic resistance as high as 18% have been reported after 48 weeks of ADV monotherapy, compared to 0% in NA-naïve patients (89). The optimal strategy for the use of ADV therapy in the setting of LMV resistance is therefore to add on (versus switching to) ADV (140). ADV should be added on early, at the time of genotypic versus phenotypic resistance, when the viral load remains <200,000 IU/ml (<10^6 copies/ml), to promote virologic response (84, 140).

ETV. In studies with follow-up limited to 48 weeks, ETV monotherapy at a dosage of 1 mg per day appeared to be effective for the management of LMV resistance (higher than the 0.5 mg per day recommended for NA-naïve patients) (151). However, concern has been raised about ETV as a therapeutic strategy for LMV resistance following the recognition that the M204V and M204I LMV mutations are required as the first "hit" in the two-hit process producing ETV resistance (see below) (160). De novo combination ETV-LMV therapy has not been investigated, but it is not recommended for this reason (106).

TDF. TDF is effective for the management of LMV-resistant HBV; it results in a significant reduction in serum HBV DNA levels (171). It is more effective than ADV as a primary salvage therapy, and it is also effective as secondary therapy following inadequate response to ADV salvage (172).

ADV Resistance

Resistance to ADV was initially associated with mutations in the B (rtA181T/V) and D (N236T) domains of the enzyme (Fig. 5) (2). HBV resistance to ADV occurs less frequently (around 2% after 2 years, 4% after 3 years, and 18% after 4 years) than resistance to LMV. These ADV-associated mutations in HBV Pol result in only a modest (three- to eightfold) increase in 50% inhibitory concentration and partial cross-resistance to TDF, probably because the molecular mechanisms of resistance are similar, with indirect perturbation of the triphosphate binding site between the A and D domains (5). The rtN236T mutation does not significantly affect sensitivity to LMV (2), but the rtA181T/V mutation results in partial cross-resistance to LMV.

Although published data are limited, in vitro resistance profiles suggest that treatment options for ADV resistance include LMV, ETV, and TDF (101). LMV should be added on, especially in patients with a history of LMV resistance, which has been reported to reemerge rapidly following the reintroduction of LMV monotherapy (55). Although the mutations result in partial cross-resistance with TDF in vitro, limited clinical experience suggests that the higher relative dose of TDF allows effective salvage therapy for ADV resistance (168).

ETV Resistance

Resistance to ETV has been observed in patients who were also LMV resistant (160). Mutations in the viral Pol associated with the emergence of ETV resistance were mapped to the B domain (rtI169T or rtS184G and rtL180M), C domain (rtS202I and rtM204V), and E domain (rtM250V) of HBV Pol (Fig. 5). In the absence of the LMV mutations, rtM250V causes a ninefold increase in the 50% inhibitory concentration, while the double mutation rtT184G plus rtS202I has no effect (160, 181). The molecular mechanism of resistance for the rtM250V change is the alteration of the binding interaction between the DNA primer strand and DNA template strand with the incoming deoxynucleoside triphosphate (181). The mechanism for rtT184G plus rtS202I is an allosteric change with altered geometry of the nucleotide binding pocket and DNA template binding of the Pol near the YMDD site (181). ETV-resistant mutants are susceptible to ADV in vitro, but few data are available on the efficacy of ADV as salvage therapy for patients with ETV-resistant disease.

LdT Resistance

LdT selects for mutations in the YMDD motif, although to date mainly rtM204I mutations have been observed (83). LdT-resistant mutants are therefore cross-resistant to LMV. The rate of resistance observed with LdT therapy is lower than for LMV; however, it is substantial and increases exponentially after the first year of therapy. The rates of genotypic resistance observed at 1 and 2 years of therapy were 4.4 and 2.7% and 21.6 and 8.6% in HBeAg-positive and -negative patients, respectively (compared to 9.1 and 9.8% and 35 and 21.9% for LMV) (106).

Multidrug Resistance

Recently, multidrug-resistant HBV has been reported for patients who received sequential treatment with NA monotherapies (160, 194). The development of multidrug resistance will almost certainly have implications for the efficacy of rescue therapy, as in the case of multidrug-resistant HIV. Successive evolution of different patterns of resistance mutations has been reported during long-term LMV monotherapy. The isolates of HBV with these initial mutations appear to be associated with decreased replication fitness compared with that of wild-type HBV; however, additional mutations that can restore replication fitness are frequently detected as treatment is continued.

Pol-HBsAg Mutations

The Pol gene overlaps the envelope gene (Fig. 2C), and changes in the HBV Pol selected during antiviral resistance can cause concomitant changes to the overlapping reading frame of the envelope. Thus, the major resistance mutations associated with LMV, ADV, ETV, and LdT failure also have the potential to alter the C-terminal region of HBsAg. For example, changes associated with LMV and ETV resistance, such as rtM204V, result in a change at sI195M in the surface antigen, while the rtM204I change, which is associated with LMV and LdT resistance, is linked to three possible changes: sW196S, sW196L, or a termination codon. To date, only one published study has examined the effect of the main LMV resistance mutations on the altered antigenicity of HBsAg (167). One of the common HBV quasispecies selected during LMV treatment is rtV173L plus rtL180M plus rtM204V, which results in changes in HBsAg: sE164D plus sI195M. Approximately 10% of monoinfected individuals carry this "triple Pol mutant" (40). In binding assays, HBsAg expressing these LMV resistance-associated residues had reduced anti-HBs binding. This reduction was similar to that of the classical vaccine escape mutant, sG145R.

The ADV resistance mutation rtN236T does not affect the envelope gene and overlaps with the stop codon at the end of the envelope gene. The rtA181T mutation selected by ADV and/or LMV results in a stop codon mutation, sW172stop. The ADV resistance mutation at rtA181V results in the sL173F change. HBV with mutations that result in a stop codon in the envelope gene such as those for LMV and ADV would be present in association with a low percentage of the wild type to enable viral assembly and release.

The ETV resistance-associated changes of rtI169T, rtS184G, and rtS202I also affect HBsAg and result in sF161L, sL/V176G, and sV194F mutations. rtM250V is located after the end of HBsAg. sF161L is located within the region that was defined as the a determinant or major hydrophilic region, which includes amino acids 90 to 170 of HBsAg (20). This region is a highly conformational epitope, characterized by multiple disulfide bonds formed from sets of cysteines at residues 107 and 138, 137 and 149, and 139 and 147 (20). Since distal substitutions such as sE164D significantly affect anti-HBs binding (167), the influence of other changes to HBsAg driven by NA resistance, such as sF161L, needs further investigation in order to determine the effect on the envelope structure and subsequent anti-HBs binding. The HBsAg change linked to rtM204V has already been covered.

Although evidence for the spread of transmission of antiviral-resistant HBV is limited, there has been a report of the transmission of LMV-resistant HBV to an HIV patient undergoing LMV as part of antiretroviral therapy (161). In addition, HBV strains bearing LMV resistance mutations were also found in a cohort of dialysis patients with occult HBV (10). Therefore, it is important to recognize that both primary and compensatory antiviral-resistant mutations may result in associated changes to the viral envelope that could have substantial public health relevance.

Conclusions

Resistance will remain an important issue in the management of patients with CHB because long-term—probably lifelong—therapy with NA will be required in the majority of patients. One of the important lessons learned from the HIV paradigm is that resistance will occur if viral replication is present during treatment, as occurs with existing monotherapy regimens (142). The introduction of combination therapy seems clear for proper management of patients with CHB because combination therapy not only reduces the viral load and quasispecies pool but also has the great advantage of reducing the risk of selecting resistance, especially if differing resistance mutation profiles of the various antiviral agents are used. Another strong argument for combination is that because of the overlap between the Pol and S genes, the selection of drug-resistant HBV may have important clinical, diagnostic, and public health implications. Envelope changes in HBV have been detected with LMV, ADV, ETV, and LdT usage. The significance of these changes warrants further investigation to determine what effect these changes have on the natural history of drug-resistant HBV and its possible transmissibility in the hepatitis B-vaccinated community at large.

IFN-α

IFNs have antiviral, antiproliferative, and immunomodulatory effects. Standard IFN-α (sIFN-α) has been shown to be effective in suppressing HBV replication and was the first treatment approved for chronic HBV infection in most countries. More recently, PEG has been licensed for the management of CHB. The attachment of polyethylene glycol to a protein (pegylation) reduces its rate of absorption following subcutaneous injection, reduces renal and cellular clearance, and decreases the immunogenicity of the protein. All of these effects tend to enhance the half-life of the pegylated versus the native protein. This allows PEG to be administered once weekly yet maintain a more sustained viral suppression between doses. One phase II clinical study has suggested that the efficacy of PEG is similar to or slightly superior to that of sIFN-α (37). PEG has largely replaced sIFN-α in clinical practice because of the more convenient dosing schedule. The advantages of IFN use include the finite course of treatment and the durability of HBeAg seroconversion. The disadvantages are the side effect profile and, in HBeAg-negative disease, the lack of durable viral suppression.

sIFN-α

sIFN-α was one of the first therapies investigated for CHB. The literature dates back over two decades; however, large prospective randomized controlled trials are scarce. A meta-analysis of 15 randomized controlled trials using sIFN-α for the treatment of HBeAg-positive disease concluded that viral suppression, normalization of ALT, and HBeAg seroconversion (33 versus 12%) were significantly more common than in untreated controls if patients received sIFN-α for 3 to 6 months and were monitored for 6 to 12 months (Table 5). The most important predictors of HBeAg seroconversion were an ALT level greater than twice the ULN and a low level of HBV DNA (16). In long-term follow-up studies, the durability of sIFN-α-induced HBeAg seroconversion has been reported to be 80 to 90% at 4 to 8 years (106). In contrast to NA therapy, IFN-based therapy may lead to HBsAg seroconversion. Treatment-related HBsAg loss has been reported for 7.8% of sIFN-α-treated patients, compared to 1.8% of controls ($P = 0.001$) (190). Studies in North America and Europe have reported delayed HBsAg seroconversion in 12 to 65% within 5 years of HBeAg loss (although this was not observed in the Asian studies, likely reflecting the higher prevalence of genotype A adult-acquired disease in the West [80]).

Clinical outcome studies comparing responders and nonresponders have found that HBeAg seroconversion predicted better long-term survival and survival free of hepatic decompensation (125, 173). These data are mostly from long-term follow-up studies. There has been only one prospective randomized controlled trial comparing clinical outcome following sIFN-α with placebo (98). This Taiwanese study found treated patients to have a lower incidence of HCC (1.5 versus 12%; $P = 0.04$) and an improved survival rate (98 versus 57%; $P = 0.02$) after a median 8-year follow-up.

sIFN-α also has an antiviral effect in the setting of HBeAg-negative CHB; however, relapse posttherapy is frequent, with sustained response rates of only 15 to 30% (109, 129). Of long-term responders, however, up to 20% clear HBsAg by 5 years, and the risk of progression to cirrhosis, HCC, and liver-related death is reduced (17, 109, 129). Retreatment may lead to sustained response in a further 20 to 30% of patients (109).

The use of sIFN-α in the setting of cirrhosis is limited by the risk of hepatitis flare, which may precipitate hepatic decompensation. Approximately 20 to 40% of HBeAg-positive patients develop a flare of their ALT during treatment. In compensated cirrhosis the risk appears to be small, and less than 1% of cirrhotic patients included in HBeAg-positive cohorts developed hepatic decompensation (135). Treatment response was comparable to that of precirrhotic patients. However, sIFN-α offers little virologic benefit once liver disease progresses to Child-Pugh class B or C, and sIFN-α is complicated by significant toxicity and exacerbations of liver disease, even at low doses (133). IFN is therefore contraindicated in this setting, and NA provide a safe and effective alternative.

sIFN-α therapy is associated with multiple adverse effects. Common symptoms include an initial flu-like illness, anorexia, weight loss, fatigue, mild alopecia, and skin rashes. Emotional lability is common—anxiety, irritability, depression, and even suicidal tendencies have been described. IFN is myelosuppressive, although profound neutropenia and thrombocytopenia are uncommon. Regular monitoring of blood counts is required during therapy. Autoimmune disease has been described, most commonly hyper- or hypothyroidism. Retinal changes and impaired vision occur rarely. IFN therapy of CHB is accompanied by a hepatitis flare in 30 to 40% of patients. Although this is considered to be a marker of treatment response, indicating an increased likelihood of HBeAg seroconversion, it may precipitate hepatic decompensation, especially in the setting of cirrhosis.

PEG

There is evidence to support the use of PEG in both HBeAg-positive and -negative CHB. In HBeAg-positive CHB, a number of trials have compared the efficacy of PEG monotherapy to both LMV monotherapy and PEG-LMV combination therapy. In the phase III registration trial, 48 weeks of pegylated IFN-α2a at a dosage of 180 μg/week was compared to the combination of pegylated IFN-α2a plus LMV at 100 mg daily or LMV monotherapy (86). The primary end point was HBeAg seroconversion 24 weeks posttreatment. At the end of treatment, combination therapy had achieved the most profound viral suppression. The rates of HBeAg seroconversion were similar between treatment arms. However, the HBeAg seroconversion rate was significantly higher in the two groups that received PEG therapy at 24 weeks posttreatment (Table 5), suggesting that clinical benefit may continue to increase after treatment is stopped. Furthermore, 16 patients receiving PEG (1.5%) experienced HBsAg seroconversion, compared with no patients in the LMV monotherapy group (P = 0.001). The authors concluded that PEG was superior to LMV in inducing HBeAg seroconversion and that combination therapy did not offer any benefit (86).

A number of factors predict response to PEG in HBeAg-positive patients. HBeAg seroconversion is more likely in the setting of an ALT level greater than twice the ULN, a high histologic activity index, a low HBV DNA level, and genotype A or B versus C or D HBV (73). HBsAg seroconversion may be more likely in the setting of genotype A disease, occurring in 14% after 52 weeks of therapy (53).

Only one study has used PEG for the treatment of HBeAg-negative CHB (110). The study also compared PEG alone or in combination with LMV to LMV monotherapy. The sustained viral responses, defined as undetectable HBV DNA (<400 copies/ml) and normal ALT, were 15 and 16% in the groups that received PEG, versus 6% in the LMV monotherapy group (P = 0.007 and P = 0.003, respectively). Although virologic suppression was improved relative to that obtained with 48 weeks of LMV, most patients therefore relapsed on treatment cessation.

The limitation of all studies that have compared PEG to LMV is that the LMV and PEG were stopped simultaneously (in HBeAg-positive patients, before the majority had achieved HBeAg seroconversion) (86, 110). Primary end points were defined at 24 weeks posttreatment. In clinical practice, LMV would be continued until a clinical end point was achieved. Virologic relapse is otherwise almost universal. The efficacy of PEG in patients with LMV-resistant YMDD mutations has not been well studied. In a series of 16 such patients (the largest cohort reported), only 2 patients seroconverted and achieved sustained virologic suppression and biochemical normalization (90).

Like sIFN-α, PEG should be used with caution in patients with advanced liver disease, as a treatment-induced flare might precipitate hepatic decompensation. Although there are no data specifically addressing the use of PEG in cirrhotic patients, it is reasonable to extrapolate from the experience with sIFN-α. Treatment of patients with compensated cirrhosis would therefore be reasonable. In the two phase III trials, approximately 15 to 25% of the HBeAg-positive and -negative cohorts had advanced fibrosis or cirrhosis on liver biopsy, respectively, and no instances of hepatic decompensation were recorded. PEG should not be used for patients with Child-Pugh class B or C cirrhosis.

The two IFN preparations have similar side effect profiles (see above). The convenience of once-weekly dosing has meant that PEG is now the more widely used form of IFN, but there are few convincing data that it offers superior efficacy or improved side effect profile.

Tα-1

Thymosin-α-1 (Tα-1) is a synthetic thymic extract. Thymosin derivatives regulate multiple aspects of T-cell function. Tα-1 is approved for the treatment of HBV in several countries, mainly in Asia. Treatment is usually well tolerated, but antiviral efficacy remains controversial, with a number of smaller clinical trials finding conflicting results (23). A meta-analysis published in 2001 that included a total of 353 patients from five controlled trials concluded that patients treated with Tα-1 were significantly more likely than controls to have a virologic response, defined as a loss of HBV DNA and HBeAg (23). The maximal rate of response was not seen until 12 months after discontinuing therapy. Although Tα-1 is well tolerated, data on its clinical efficacy therefore require confirmation.

Novel Antiviral Strategies

Novel antiviral strategies include the following.

1. TLR ligands. In the transgenic HBV mouse model, TLR3, -4, -5, -7, and -9 ligands exerted an indirect antiviral effect via induction of type I IFN (72). The TLR2 ligand Pam-2-Cys has been shown to have direct antiviral efficacy in a cell culture model of HBV replication (165).
2. Selective targeting of antiviral drugs to the liver. Two approaches have been taken. The first has involved conjugation of antiviral agents to ligands that are selectively taken up by the liver; the second has involved the creation of prodrugs that require activation in the liver.
3. RNA interference. Gene expression can be silenced with small inhibitory RNA and short hairpin RNA. These short strands of double-stranded RNA contain sequence

homologous to the gene of interest. Together they are recruited into the cytoplasmic-RNA-induced silencing complex. This natural cellular mechanism then cleaves the target mRNA and inhibits protein expression. In vitro and animal studies have suggested a potential therapeutic role for these molecules, assuming that delivery is feasible (115, 196).

4. Vaccine-based HBV-specific immunomodulatory therapy. Therapeutic vaccine approaches have included highly immunogenic S and pre-S antigen vaccines, DNA vaccines, and T-cell vaccines. The ex vivo culture and priming of human dendritic cells with viral antigens, followed by autologous transfusion, are being explored as a form of immunotherapy.

HIV AND HBV COINFECTION

CHB affects nearly 10% of HIV-infected patients. HIV impacts directly on the outcome of HBV infection, complicating its natural history, diagnosis, and management. In the setting of HIV and HBV coinfection, levels of serum HBV DNA tend to be higher and spontaneous HBeAg seroconversion occurs at a lower rate. For reasons that remain unclear, liver damage, especially fibrosis, progresses at a higher rate than in HBV monoinfection, despite hepatic necroinflammation typically being less severe. With improved control of HIV disease with HAART, liver disease has emerged as one of the leading causes of death in patients with HIV (164).

Therefore, all patients with HIV should be screened for HBV infection. It is recommended that testing for both anti-HBc and HBsAg be performed, as patients with HIV can have occult HBV. Similarly, all HBV patients should undergo HIV testing (106).

Anti-HBV therapy should be considered for all HIV-HBV-coinfected patients with evidence of liver disease, irrespective of the CD4 cell count (163). In coinfected patients not requiring HAART, HBV therapy should be based on agents that do not target HIV. ETV, previously recommended as first-line therapy in this situation, is now recognized to have anti-HIV activity and is associated with the accumulation of HIV type 1 variants with the LMV resistance mutation M184V (118). Therapeutic options therefore include ADV (10 mg) or PEG. Although LdT does not target HIV, its use as monotherapy is not recommended because of the risk of selection of the M204I mutation in the YMDD motif.

In contrast, in patients with CD4 counts of less than 350 cells/μl, the use of agents with dual anti-HIV and anti-HBV activity should be considered. These include LMV (or FTC) and TDF, ideally as combination therapy. HBV resistance is more common in the setting of coinfection, and combination therapy will prevent or delay the development of antiviral resistance. Combination therapy may also limit the risk of immune reconstitution disease resulting in serious hepatic flare and precipitating liver decompensation, a particular risk for patients presenting with advanced HIV infection and reduced functional hepatic reserve due to HBV-related cirrhosis.

The hepatitis B vaccine should be given to all HIV-positive persons who are negative for HBV seromarkers. The vaccine should be given when CD4 cell counts are $\geq$200/μl, as response is poor below this level. Persons with CD4 counts below 200 μl should receive HAART first, deferring HBV vaccine until CD4 counts rise above 200/μl.

PREVENTION

Effective strategies for the prevention of HBV infection include (i) the avoidance of high-risk behavior and the prevention of exposure to blood or bodily fluids, (ii) active immunization with the hepatitis B vaccine, and (iii) active-passive immunization with vaccine and HBIG after a suspected high-risk exposure.

The global HIV epidemic has led to widespread education campaigns directed at decreasing the transmission of blood-borne viruses, including HBV, HCV, and HIV. Changes in sexual practice, the increased use of condoms, and needle exchange programs all appear to have reduced the incidence of HBV infection. The screening of blood and blood products has led to a dramatic decline in transfusion-acquired HBV infection. The improved disposal of needles and other sharp objects in the hospital setting, as well as the advent of new devices designed to decrease inadvertent needlestick injury, has reduced occupational exposures. Unfortunately, such primary preventive measures are likely to be less effective in countries with high prevalence of disease, where perinatal or early horizontal infection is common. In these areas, immunoprophylaxis, both passive and active, is the most effective strategy.

The WHO has recommended that all countries provide universal HBV vaccination programs for infants and adolescents, with appropriate catch-up programs. In addition, persons at high risk should be targeted (including persons at occupational risk, institutionalized persons, dialysis patients, recipients of blood products, household members and sexual partners of CHB patients, travelers to areas of endemicity, persons who have more than one sexual partner in a 6-month period, men who have sex with men, injection drug users, and prisoners) (137). Prevaccination testing is useful only in adults from areas of endemicity, to identify those who are either infected or immune and therefore do not require vaccination. It is not cost-effective in low-prevalence areas.

HBV Vaccines

Effective hepatitis B vaccines have been available since 1981. Multiple formulations are now licensed, either as a monovalent vaccine or in fixed combination with other vaccines (including hepatitis A, *Haemophilus influenzae* type B, diphtheria, tetanus, pertussis, and poliomyelitis). All currently licensed hepatitis B vaccines are now recombinant proteins made by incorporating the SHBs gene of HBV into the yeast expression vector *Saccharomyces cerevisiae*, to generate recombinant HBsAg. They therefore contain the S epitope (the major antigenic determinant, or the a determinant) but not the pre-S1 or pre-S2 epitope. Plasma-derived vaccines are no longer used. Third-generation recombinant vaccines containing two or three surface epitopes (S, pre-S2, and/or pre-S1) have been generated from animal cell lines and have been used in some countries as prophylactic vaccines. These may provide enhanced immunogenicity and therefore be potentially applicable in nonresponders to the standard vaccine (169, 192).

Currently licensed vaccines are very effective at eliciting protective humoral immunity directed against HBsAg (137). The standard vaccination schedule consists of three doses of vaccine, given intramuscularly, at 10 to 20 μg in adults and 5 to 10 μg in children. The second dose is given 1 month after the first dose, and the third is given 6 months after the first dose. It is not necessary to restart the series if there have been prolonged intervals between doses. The complete vaccine series elicits protective antibody levels in >95% of infants, children, and adolescents (137). The efficacy of the vaccine is almost 100% in immunocompetent people who develop antibody levels of >10 IU/ml. The response declines with increasing age beyond 30 years; protection falls to 90% by the age of 40 years, and by 60 years protective antibody levels are achieved in only 65 to 75%. Other risk factors for nonresponse include obesity and immunodeficiency.

Postvaccination testing is recommended only in the following groups: infants born to HBV-infected mothers, the immunocompromised (including HIV-infected and dialysis patients), HCW and other persons at occupational risk of exposure, and sexual partners of HBV-infected persons. Nonresponse is defined as the failure to mount an anti-HBs response of >10 IU/ml 1 to 6 months after the third dose of vaccine. In nonresponders, 25 to 50% of immunocompetent adults will respond to one additional dose of vaccine. For individuals who remain seronegative after this booster dose, a second series (three additional doses) of the double-dose vaccine should be given; 50 to 60% will seroconvert (136). Those remaining seronegative are likely to be true nonresponders.

The duration of protection is at least 15 years (117, 124). Even if anti-HBs titers decline to become undetectable, an amnestic response appears to persist, providing protective immunity. A small number of high-risk individuals in whom protective antibody titers have been lost have been reported to develop markers of HBV infection (anti-HBc). However, in most the infections were asymptomatic and detected by regular blood monitoring in the setting of clinical trials. Routine testing postvaccination, and routine booster vaccination, is therefore not recommended. Additional information is still needed to establish the need for a booster beyond 15 years after immunization in those who are at high risk for exposure (e.g., HCW). Boosters may be considered to provide reassurance of protective immunity in these special groups (52).

The hepatitis B vaccine appears to be very safe. Anaphylaxis is rare and the only serious adverse effect that has been documented. There are no data to support a link with demyelinating disorders, Guillain-Barré syndrome, autoimmune disorders (including systemic lupus erythematosus), chronic fatigue syndrome, sudden infant death syndrome, or other disorders (137).

Passive immunization with HBIG will provide temporary immunity against HBV infection in those who are not immune. The most common indication for use is for postexposure prophylaxis (see below). It is also used to prevent HBV recurrence after liver transplantation in HBsAg-positive recipients.

Postexposure Prophylaxis

Postexposure prophylaxis is the standard of care for all nonvaccinated individuals exposed to infectious blood or bodily fluids, including infants born to HBsAg-positive mothers, and following percutaneous (e.g., needlestick), mucosal, or sexual exposure to HBV. This consists of the first dose of HBV vaccination within 12 h followed by second and third doses at 1 and 6 months, respectively. HBIG should be administered with the first dose of vaccine and can be repeated at 1 month if there has been previous nonresponse to the vaccine. Vaccinated individuals with documented responses do not require prophylaxis.

Impact of Vaccination on Transmission

Active-passive vaccination was shown to prevent >95% of perinatal transmissions in the mid-1980s (100). Taiwan was the first country to introduce universal neonatal vaccination, in 1986. Since the program began, the prevalence of HBsAg in children under 5 years of age has decreased from 9.3% in 1984 to 1.3% in 1994. This suggests not only protection of those vaccinated but also prevention of horizontal transmission. The incidence of both fulminant hepatitis (29) and HCC in children has declined sharply (25) (Fig. 10). According to the WHO, as of March 2000, 116 countries had included hepatitis B vaccine in their national programs, including most countries in eastern and Southeast Asia, the Pacific Islands, Australia, North and South America, Western Europe, and the Middle East. However, many low-income countries in sub-Saharan Africa, the Indian subcontinent, and the Newly Independent States do not use the vaccine. The price of the hepatitis B vaccine has been one of the main obstacles to its introduction in many of these countries.

IMMUNOSUPPRESSION AND REACTIVATION

Immunosuppression is a special situation in which antiviral therapy is indicated for HBV. Reactivation of HBV replication with increase in ALT levels has been reported for 20 to 50% of HBsAg-positive patients undergoing immunosuppression or cancer chemotherapy (193). Case reports document reactivation following intra-arterial chemoembolization for HCC, rituximab therapy for lymphoma, anti-TNF therapies for inflammatory bowel disease or rheumatoid arthritis, and HIV infection (193). Although most cases are asymptomatic, icteric flares, hepatic decompensation, and death have all been reported. Patients with high pretreatment viral load, defined by HBeAg positivity or HBV DNA at >60,000 IU/ml, are at higher risk of reactivation. The degree of immunosuppression is also im-

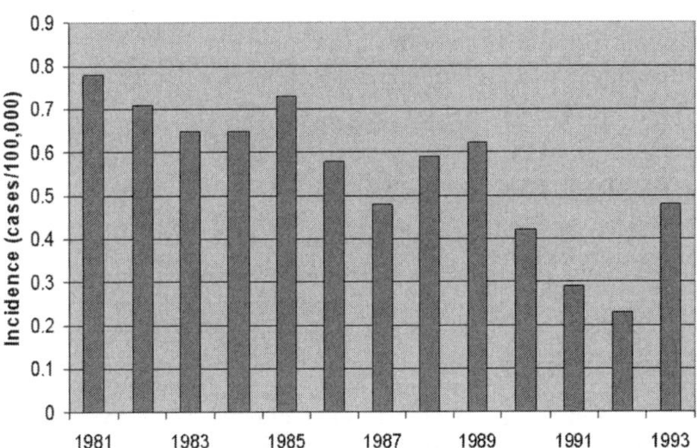

FIGURE 10 Impact of universal vaccination on the incidence of HCC in Taiwan. A universal vaccination program was implemented in Taiwan in July 1984. Subsequently, the incidence of HCC was found to decline ($P < 0.01$ for the comparison of values before July 1990 with those after July 1990). (Adapted from reference 25.)

portant. Corticosteroids and anthracyclines have both been linked to reactivation, particularly when included in the intensive combination chemotherapy used with bone marrow transplantation. The monoclonal antibody rituximab appears to be associated with a particular risk of severe hepatitis flare (193).

Prophylactic therapy with LMV has been shown to reduce the rate of HBV reactivation, severity of associated hepatitis, and mortality (87, 193). HBsAg-positive patients with baseline viral loads of less than 10^4 copies/ml should be commenced on LMV at the onset of immunosuppression. Recommendations for the duration of maintenance therapy vary from 6 weeks to 6 months (106, 193). Patients with baseline HBV DNA levels of $>10^4$ copies/ml should continue antiviral therapy until a therapeutic end point is reached, as viral relapse after withdrawal of LMV has been reported. In this setting, where therapy may be prolonged, an alternate NA such as ETV may be more appropriate.

HBsAg-negative, anti-HBc- or anti-HBs-positive patients remain at risk of reactivation of HBV when profoundly immunosuppressed. Reactivation is infrequent, however, and few data support therapy in this situation (193). It may be reasonable to monitor such patients closely and to initiate treatment when the serum HBV DNA level becomes detectable or when a hepatitis flare is diagnosed. Prophylactic LMV therapy is reasonable in the setting of rituximab therapy, as case reports of fatal hepatic flares in HBsAg-negative patients have been described.

LIVER TRANSPLANTATION FOR CHB

Liver transplantation for HBV infection in the 1980s was associated with rapid recurrence with poor outcomes despite HBIG (152). With the advent of the NA in combination with high-dose HBIG to prevent graft reinfection, transplantation with viral control became possible, although HBIG was expensive and not readily available worldwide, and disease progression associated with drug resistance was common. Low-dose HBIG plus LMV provides safe and effective prophylaxis at a significantly lower cost (56). Subsequently, the use of single agents with lower resistance rates or combination therapy has delayed or prevented resistance, and liver transplant outcomes for CHB are now equivalent to those with other liver diseases, with a 5-year survival rate of 75%. Viral control can result in a dramatic improvement in liver function in the pretransplant patient such that transplantation for decompensation is no longer required for some patients.

REFERENCES

1. **Alward, W. L., B. J. McMahon, D. B. Hall, W. L. Heyward, D. P. Francis, and T. R. Bender.** 1985. The long-term serological course of asymptomatic hepatitis B virus carriers and the development of primary hepatocellular carcinoma. *J. Infect. Dis.* **151:**604–609.
2. **Angus, P., R. Vaughan, S. Xiong, H. Yang, W. Delaney, C. Gibbs, C. Brosgart, D. Colledge, R. Edwards, A. Ayres, A. Bartholomeusz, and S. Locarnini.** 2003. Resistance to adefovir dipivoxil therapy associated with the selection of a novel mutation in the HBV polymerase. *Gastroenterology* **125:**292–297.
3. **Bartenschlager, R., and H. Schaller.** 1992. Hepadnaviral assembly is initiated by polymerase binding to the encapsidation signal in the viral RNA genome. *EMBO J.* **11:** 3413–3420.
4. **Bartholomeusz, A., and S. Schaefer.** 2004. Hepatitis B virus genotypes: comparison of genotyping methods. *Rev. Med. Virol.* **14:**3–16.
5. **Bartholomeusz, A., B. G. Tehan, and D. K. Chalmers.** 2004. Comparisons of the HBV and HIV polymerase, and antiviral resistance mutations. *Antivir. Ther.* **9:**149–160.
6. **Beasley, R. P.** 1988. Hepatitis B virus. The major etiology of hepatocellular carcinoma. *Cancer* **61:**1942–1956.
7. **Beasley, R. P., C. C. Lin, C. S. Chien, C. J. Chen, and L. Y. Hwang.** 1982. Geographic distribution of HBsAg carriers in China. *Hepatology* **2:**553–556.
8. **Beck, J., and M. Nassal.** 2007. Hepatitis B virus replication. *World J Gastroenterol.* **13:**48–64.
9. **Bell, S. J., A. Lau, A. Thompson, K. J. Watson, B. Demediuk, G. Shaw, R. Y. Chen, A. Ayres, L. Yuen, A. Bartholomeusz, S. A. Locarnini, and P. V. Desmond.** 2005. Chronic hepatitis B: recommendations for therapy based on the natural history of disease in Australian patients. *J. Clin. Virol.* **32:**122–127.
10. **Besisik, F., C. Karaca, F. Akyuz, S. Horosanli, D. Onel, S. Badur, M. S. Sever, A. Danalioglu, K. Demir, S. Kaymakoglu, Y. Cakaloglu, and A. Okten.** 2003. Occult HBV infection and YMDD variants in hemodialysis patients with chronic HCV infection. *J. Hepatol.* **38:**506–510.
11. **Biswas, R., E. Tabor, C. C. Hsia, D. J. Wright, M. E. Laycock, E. W. Fiebig, L. Peddada, R. Smith, G. B. Schreiber, J. S. Epstein, G. J. Nemo, and M. P. Busch.** 2003. Comparative sensitivity of HBV NATs and HBsAg assays for detection of acute HBV infection. *Transfusion* **43:**788–798.
12. **Bock, C. T., P. Schranz, C. H. Schroder, and H. Zentgraf.** 1994. Hepatitis B virus genome is organized into nucleosomes in the nucleus of the infected cell. *Virus Genes* **8:**215–229.
13. **Bodsworth, N., B. Donovan, and B. N. Nightingale.** 1989. The effect of concurrent human immunodeficiency virus infection on chronic hepatitis B: a study of 150 homosexual men. *J. Infect. Dis.* **160:**577–582.
14. **Bowden, S.** 2002. *Laboratory Diagnosis of Hepatitis B Infection.* International Medical Press, London, United Kingdom.
15. **Bowden, S.** 2006. Serological and molecular diagnosis. *Semin. Liver Dis.* **26:**97–103.
16. **Brook, M. G., P. Karayiannis, and H. C. Thomas.** 1989. Which patients with chronic hepatitis B virus infection will respond to alpha-interferon therapy? A statistical analysis of predictive factors. *Hepatology* **10:**761–763.
17. **Brunetto, M. R., F. Oliveri, B. Coco, G. Leandro, P. Colombatto, J. M. Gorin, and F. Bonino.** 2002. Outcome of anti-HBe positive chronic hepatitis B in alpha-interferon treated and untreated patients: a long term cohort study. *J. Hepatol.* **36:**263–270.
18. **Bruss, V., J. Hagelstein, E. Gerhardt, and P. R. Galle.** 1996. Myristylation of the large surface protein is required for hepatitis B virus in vitro infectivity. *Virology* **218:**396–399.
19. **Buster, E. H., B. E. Hansen, M. Buti, J. Delwaide, C. Niederau, P. P. Michielsen, R. Flisiak, P. E. Zondervan, S. W. Schalm, and H. L. Janssen.** 2007. Peginterferon alpha-2b is safe and effective in HBeAg-positive chronic hepatitis B patients with advanced fibrosis. *Hepatology* **46:** 388–394.
20. **Carman, W. F.** 1997. The clinical significance of surface antigen variants of hepatitis B virus. *J. Viral. Hepat.* **4**(Suppl. 1)**:**11–20.
21. **Carman, W. F., C. Trautwein, F. J. van Deursen, K. Colman, E. Dornan, G. McIntyre, J. Waters, V. Kliem, R. Muller, H. C. Thomas, and M. P. Manns.** 1996. Hep-

atitis B virus envelope variation after transplantation with and without hepatitis B immune globulin prophylaxis. *Hepatology* **24:**489–493.

22. **Carman, W. F., A. R. Zanetti, P. Karayiannis, J. Waters, G. Manzillo, E. Tanzi, A. J. Zuckerman, and H. C. Thomas.** 1990. Vaccine-induced escape mutant of hepatitis B virus. *Lancet* **336:**325–329.
23. **Chan, H. L., J. L. Tang, W. Tam, and J. J. Sung.** 2001. The efficacy of thymosin in the treatment of chronic hepatitis B virus infection: a meta-analysis. *Aliment. Pharmacol. Ther.* **15:**1899–1905.
24. **Chan, H. L., S. W. Tsang, M. L. Wong, C. H. Tse, N. W. Leung, F. K. Chan, and J. J. Sung.** 2002. Genotype B hepatitis B virus is associated with severe icteric flare-up of chronic hepatitis B virus infection in Hong Kong. *Am. J. Gastroenterol.* **97:**2629–2633.
25. **Chang, M.-H., C.-J. Chen, M.-S. Lai, H.-M. Hsu, T.-C. Wu, M.-S. Kong, D.-C. Liang, W.-Y. Shau, and D.-S. Chen for the Taiwan Childhood Hepatoma Study Group.** 1997. Universal hepatitis B vaccination in Taiwan and the incidence of hepatocellular carcinoma in children. *N. Engl. J. Med.* **336:**1855–1859.
26. **Chang, T. T., R. G. Gish, R. de Man, A. Gadano, J. Sollano, Y. C. Chao, A. S. Lok, K. H. Han, Z. Goodman, J. Zhu, A. Cross, D. DeHertogh, R. Wilber, R. Colonno, and D. Apelian.** 2006. A comparison of entecavir and lamivudine for HBeAg-positive chronic hepatitis B. *N. Engl. J. Med.* **354:**1001–1010.
27. **Chen, C. J., H. I. Yang, J. Su, C. L. Jen, S. L. You, S. N. Lu, G. T. Huang, and U. H. Iloeje.** 2006. Risk of hepatocellular carcinoma across a biological gradient of serum hepatitis B virus DNA level. *JAMA* **295:**65–73.
28. **Chen, G., W. Lin, F. Shen, U. H. Iloeje, W. T. London, and A. A. Evans.** 2006. Past HBV viral load as predictor of mortality and morbidity from HCC and chronic liver disease in a prospective study. *Am. J. Gastroenterol.* **101:** 1797–1803.
29. **Chen, H. L., C. J. Chang, M. S. Kong, F. C. Huang, H. C. Lee, C. C. Lin, C. C. Liu, I. H. Lee, T. C. Wu, S. F. Wu, Y. H. Ni, H. Y. Hsu, D. S. Chen, and M. H. Chang.** 2004. Pediatric fulminant hepatic failure in endemic areas of hepatitis B infection: 15 years after universal hepatitis B vaccination. *Hepatology* **39:**58–63.
30. **Chen, H. S., M. C. Kew, W. E. Hornbuckle, B. C. Tennant, P. J. Cote, J. L. Gerin, R. H. Purcell, and R. H. Miller.** 1992. The precore gene of the woodchuck hepatitis virus genome is not essential for viral replication in the natural host. *J. Virol.* **66:**5682–5684.
31. **Chen, R. Y., R. Edwards, T. Shaw, D. Colledge, W. E. Delaney IV, H. Isom, S. Bowden, P. Desmond, and S. A. Locarnini.** 2003. Effect of the G1896A precore mutation on drug sensitivity and replication yield of lamivudine-resistant HBV in vitro. *Hepatology* **37:**27–35.
32. **Chien, R.-N., Y.-F. Liaw, and M. Atkins for the Asian Hepatitis Lamivudine Trial Group.** 1999. Pretherapy alanine transaminase level as a determinant for hepatitis B e antigen seroconversion during lamivudine therapy in patients with chronic hepatitis B. *Hepatology* **30:**770–774.
33. **Chisari, F. V., and C. Ferrari.** 1995. Hepatitis B virus immunopathogenesis. *Annu. Rev. Immunol.* **13:**29–60.
34. **Chu, C. J., M. Hussain, and A. S. Lok.** 2002. Hepatitis B virus genotype B is associated with earlier HBeAg seroconversion compared with hepatitis B virus genotype C. *Gastroenterology* **122:**1756–1762.
35. **Chu, C. J., E. B. Keeffe, S. H. Han, R. P. Perrillo, A. D. Min, C. Soldevila-Pico, W. Carey, R. S. Brown, Jr., V. A. Luketic, N. Terrault, and A. S. Lok.** 2003. Prevalence of HBV precore/core promoter variants in the United States. *Hepatology* **38:**619–628.
36. **Colonno, R. J., R. Rose, C. J. Baldick, S. Levine, K. Pokornowski, C. F. Yu, A. Walsh, J. Fang, M. Hsu, C. Mazzucco, B. Eggers, S. Zhang, M. Plym, K. Klesczewski, and D. J. Tenney.** 2006. Entecavir resistance is rare in nucleoside naive patients with hepatitis B. *Hepatology* **44:**1656–1665.
37. **Cooksley, G.** 2003. The treatment of hepatitis B e antigen-positive chronic hepatitis B with pegylated interferon. *J. Hepatol.* **39**(Suppl. 1)**:**S143–S145.
38. **Deguchi, M., N. Yamashita, M. Kagita, S. Asari, Y. Iwatani, T. Tsuchida, K. Iinuma, and I. K. Mushahwar.** 2004. Quantitation of hepatitis B surface antigen by an automated chemiluminescent microparticle immunoassay. *J. Virol. Methods* **115:**217–222.
39. **Delaney, W. E., IV, S. Locarnini, and T. Shaw.** 2001. Resistance of hepatitis B virus to antiviral drugs: current aspects and directions for future investigation. *Antivir. Chem. Chemother.* **12:**1–35.
40. **Delaney, W. E., IV, H. Yang, C. E. Westland, K. Das, E. Arnold, C. S. Gibbs, M. D. Miller, and S. Xiong.** 2003. The hepatitis B virus polymerase mutation rtV173L is selected during lamivudine therapy and enhances viral replication in vitro. *J. Virol.* **77:**11833–11841.
41. **Dienstag, J. L., R. D. Goldin, E. J. Heathcote, H. W. Hann, M. Woessner, S. L. Stephenson, S. Gardner, D. F. Gray, and E. R. Schiff.** 2003. Histological outcome during long-term lamivudine therapy. *Gastroenterology* **124:** 105–117.
42. **Durantel, D., S. Carrouee-Durantel, B. Werle-Lapostolle, M. N. Brunelle, C. Pichoud, C. Trepo, and F. Zoulim.** 2004. A new strategy for studying in vitro the drug susceptibility of clinical isolates of human hepatitis B virus. *Hepatology* **40:**855–864.
43. **Durantel, S., B. Werle, D. Durantel, C. Pichoud, G. Currie, S. Xiong, C. Brosgart, C. Trepo, and F. Zoulim.** 2004. Different profiles of response to adefovir dipivoxil and factors that may influence response in patients with chronic hepatitis B. *Hepatology* **40:**654A.
44. **Elsevier.** 2003. Proceedings of the European Association for the Study of the Liver (EASL) International Consensus Conference on Hepatitis B. September 14–16, 2002. Geneva, Switzerland. *J. Hepatol.* **39**(Suppl. 1)**:**S1–S235.
45. **Entecavir Review Team.** Briefing document for NDA 21-797, and NDA 21-798, ETV oral solution 0.05 mg/ml. http://www.fda.gov/ohrms/dockets/ac/05/briefing/2005-4094B1_02_FDA-Background-Memo.pdf.
46. **Fattovich, G., L. Brollo, A. Alberti, P. Pontisso, G. Giustina, and G. Realdi.** 1988. Long-term follow-up of anti-HBe-positive chronic active hepatitis B. *Hepatology* **8:**1651–1654.
47. **Fattovich, G., L. Brollo, G. Giustina, F. Noventa, P. Pontisso, A. Alberti, G. Realdi, and A. Ruol.** 1991. Natural history and prognostic factors for chronic hepatitis type B. *Gut* **32:**294–298.
48. **Fattovich, G., G. Giustina, S. W. Schalm, S. Hadziyannis, J. Sanchez-Tapias, P. Almasio, E. Christensen, K. Krogsgaard, F. Degos, M. Carneiro de Moura, et al., for The EUROHEP Study Group on Hepatitis B Virus and Cirrhosis.** 1995. Occurrence of hepatocellular carcinoma and decompensation in western European patients with cirrhosis type B. *Hepatology* **21:**77–82.
49. **Feld, J., J. Y. Lee, and S. Locarnini.** 2003. New targets and possible new therapeutic approaches in the chemotherapy of chronic hepatitis B. *Hepatology* **38:**545–553.
50. **Feld, J. J., and E. J. Heathcote.** 2006. Hepatitis B e antigen-positive chronic hepatitis B: natural history and treatment. *Semin. Liver Dis.* **26:**116–129.
51. **Ferri, C., M. Sebastiani, D. Giuggioli, M. Cazzato, G. Longombardo, A. Antonelli, R. Puccini, C. Michelassi,**

and A. L. Zignego. 2004. Mixed cryoglobulinemia: demographic, clinical, and serologic features and survival in 231 patients. *Semin. Arthritis Rheum.* **33:**355–374.

52. **Fitzsimons, D., G. Francois, A. Hall, B. McMahon, A. Meheus, A. Zanetti, B. Duval, W. Jilg, W. O. Bocher, S. N. Lu, U. Akarca, D. Lavanchy, S. Goldstein, J. Banatvala, and P. V. Damme.** 2005. Long-term efficacy of hepatitis B vaccine, booster policy, and impact of hepatitis B virus mutants. *Vaccine* **23:**4158–4166.
53. **Flink, H. J., M. van Zonneveld, B. E. Hansen, R. A. de Man, S. W. Schalm, and H. L. A. Janssen for the HBV 99-01 Study Group.** 2006. Treatment with Peg-interferon α-2b for HBeAg-positive chronic hepatitis B: HBsAg loss is associated with HBV genotype. *Am. J. Gastroenterol.* **101:**297–303.
54. **Fried, M., Y.-F. Liaw, and K. Luo.** 2005. Role of baseline and on-treatment quantitative HBeAg levels in predicting response to Peginterferon alfa-2a (40kD) (Pegasys) monotherapy in a large, multinational trial of patients with chronic hepatitis B. *Hepatology* **42:**268A.
55. **Fung, S. K., P. Andreone, S. H. Han, K. Rajender Reddy, A. Regev, E. B. Keeffe, M. Hussain, C. Cursaro, P. Richtmyer, J. A. Marrero, and A. S. Lok.** 2005. Adefovir-resistant hepatitis B can be associated with viral rebound and hepatic decompensation. *J. Hepatol.* **43:**937–943.
56. **Gane, E. J., P. W. Angus, S. Strasser, D. H. Crawford, J. Ring, G. P. Jeffrey, and G. W. McCaughan.** 2007. Lamivudine plus low-dose hepatitis B immunoglobulin to prevent recurrent hepatitis B following liver transplantation. *Gastroenterology* **132:**931–937.
57. **Ganem, D., and R. Schneider.** 2001. Hepadnaviridae: the viruses and their replication, p. 2923–2970. *In* D. M. Knipe, P. M. Howley, D. E. Griffin, R. A. Lamb, M. A. Martin, B. Roizman, and S. E. Straus (ed.), *Fields Virology*, 4th ed., vol. 2. Lippincott Williams & Wilkins, Philadelphia, PA.
58. **Girones, R., and R. H. Miller.** 1989. Mutation rate of the hepadnavirus genome. *Virology* **170:**595–597.
59. **Gish, R., T. T. Chang, R. de Man, A. Gadano, J. Sollano, K. H. Han, A. Lok, J. Zhu, and L. Fernandes.** 2005. Entecavir results in substantial virologic and biochemical improvement through 96 weeks of treatment in HBeAg(+) chronic hepatitis B patients (Study ETV-022). *Hepatology* **42:**267A.
60. **Guidotti, L. G., R. Rochford, J. Chung, M. Shapiro, R. Purcell, and F. V. Chisari.** 1999. Viral clearance without destruction of infected cells during acute HBV infection. *Science* **284:**825–829.
61. **Günther, S., L. Fischer, I. Pult, M. Sterneck, and H. Will.** 1999. Naturally occurring variants of hepatitis B virus. *Adv. Virus Res.* **52:**25–137.
62. **Gust, I. D.** 1996. Epidemiology of hepatitis B infection in the Western Pacific and South East Asia. *Gut* **38**(Suppl. 2)**:**S18–S23.
63. **Hadziyannis, S., I. Sevastianos, I. Rapt, and N. Tassopoulos.** 2006. Sustained biochemical and virological remission after discontinuation of 4 to 5 years of adefovir dipivoxil (ADV) treatment in HBeAg-negative chronic hepatitis B. *Hepatology* **44:**231A.
64. **Hadziyannis, S. J., and G. V. Papatheodoridis.** 2006. Hepatitis B e antigen-negative chronic hepatitis B: natural history and treatment. *Semin. Liver Dis.* **26:**130–141.
65. **Hadziyannis, S. J., N. C. Tassopoulos, E. J. Heathcote, T. T. Chang, G. Kitis, M. Rizzetto, P. Marcellin, S. G. Lim, Z. Goodman, J. Ma, S. Arterburn, S. Xiong, G. Currie, and C. L. Brosgart.** 2005. Long-term therapy with adefovir dipivoxil for HBeAg-negative chronic hepatitis B. *N. Engl. J. Med.* **352:**2673–2681.
66. **Hammer, S. M., M. S. Saag, M. Schechter, J. S. Montaner, R. T. Schooley, D. M. Jacobsen, M. A. Thompson, C. C. Carpenter, M. A. Fischl, B. G. Gazzard, J. M. Gatell, M. S. Hirsch, D. A. Katzenstein, D. D. Richman, S. Vella, P. G. Yeni, and P. A. Volberding.** 2006. Treatment for adult HIV infection: 2006 recommendations of the International AIDS Society—USA panel. *Top. HIV Med.* **14:**827–843.
67. **Han, S. H.** 2004. Extrahepatic manifestations of chronic hepatitis B. *Clin. Liver Dis.* **8:**403–418.
68. **Hsu, Y. S., R. N. Chien, C. T. Yeh, I. S. Sheen, H. Y. Chiou, C. M. Chu, and Y. F. Liaw.** 2002. Long-term outcome after spontaneous HBeAg seroconversion in patients with chronic hepatitis B. *Hepatology* **35:**1522–1527.
69. **Hu, Z., Z. Zhang, E. Doo, O. Coux, A. L. Goldberg, and T. J. Liang.** 1999. Hepatitis B virus X protein is both a substrate and a potential inhibitor of the proteasome complex. *J. Virol.* **73:**7231–7240.
70. **Hunt, C. M., J. M. McGill, M. I. Allen, and L. D. Condreay.** 2000. Clinical relevance of hepatitis B viral mutations. *Hepatology* **31:**1037–1044.
71. **Iloeje, U. H., H. I. Yang, J. Su, C. L. Jen, S. L. You, and C. J. Chen.** 2006. Predicting cirrhosis risk based on the level of circulating hepatitis B viral load. *Gastroenterology* **130:**678–686.
72. **Isogawa, M., M. D. Robek, Y. Furuichi, and F. V. Chisari.** 2005. Toll-like receptor signaling inhibits hepatitis B virus replication in vivo. *J. Virol.* **79:**7269–7272.
73. **Janssen, H. L., and G. K. Lau.** 2005. Chronic hepatitis B: HBeAg seroconversion after pegylated interferon and nucleos(t)ide analogs. *Hepatology* **42:**1459. (Author's reply, **42:**1459–1460.)
74. **Kakimi, K., L. G. Guidotti, Y. Koezuka, and F. V. Chisari.** 2000. Natural killer T cell activation inhibits hepatitis B virus replication in vivo. *J. Exp. Med.* **192:**921–930.
75. **Kann, M.** 1998. Hepadnaviridae: structure and molecular virology, p. 77–105. *In* A. J. Zuckerman and H. C. Thomas (ed.), *Viral Hepatitis*, 2nd ed. Churchill Livingstone, New York, NY.
76. **Kao, J. H., and D. S. Chen.** 2003. Clinical relevance of hepatitis B virus genotypes Ba and Bj in Taiwan. *Gastroenterology* **125:**1916–1917. (Author's reply, **125:**1917–1918.)
77. **Kao, J. H., P. J. Chen, M. Y. Lai, and D. S. Chen.** 2000. Hepatitis B genotypes correlate with clinical outcomes in patients with chronic hepatitis B. *Gastroenterology* **118:**554–559.
78. **Kao, J. H., P. J. Chen, M. Y. Lai, and D. S. Chen.** 2004. Hepatitis B virus genotypes and spontaneous hepatitis B e antigen seroconversion in Taiwanese hepatitis B carriers. *J. Med. Virol.* **72:**363–369.
79. **Koike, K., T. Tsutsumi, H. Fujie, Y. Shintani, and M. Kyoji.** 2002. Molecular mechanism of viral hepatocarcinogenesis. *Oncology* **62**(Suppl. 1)**:**29–37.
80. **Krogsgaard, K., the Long-Term Follow-up Investigator Group, Executive Team on Anti-Viral Treatment.** 1998. The long-term effect of treatment with interferon-α2a in chronic hepatitis B. *J. Viral Hepat.* **5:**389–397.
81. **Kumar, M., S. Satapathy, R. Monga, K. Das, S. Hissar, C. Pande, B. C. Sharma, and S. K. Sarin.** 2007. A randomized controlled trial of lamivudine to treat acute hepatitis B. *Hepatology* **45:**97–101.
82. **Lai, C. L., J. Dienstag, E. Schiff, N. W. Leung, M. Atkins, C. Hunt, N. Brown, M. Woessner, R. Boehme, and L. Condreay.** 2003. Prevalence and clinical correlates of YMDD variants during lamivudine therapy for patients with chronic hepatitis B. *Clin. Infect. Dis.* **36:**687–696.

83. **Lai, C. L., N. Leung, E. K. Teo, M. Tong, F. Wong, H. W. Hann, S. Han, T. Poynard, M. Myers, G. Chao, D. Lloyd, and N. A. Brown.** 2005. A 1-year trial of telbivudine, lamivudine, and the combination in patients with hepatitis B e antigen-positive chronic hepatitis B. *Gastroenterology* **129:**528–536.
84. **Lampertico, P., M. Vigano, E. Manenti, M. Iavarone, G. Lunghi, and M. Colombo.** 2005. Adefovir rapidly suppresses hepatitis B in HBeAg-negative patients developing genotypic resistance to lamivudine. *Hepatology* **42:**1414–1419.
85. **Laras, A., J. Koskinas, E. Dimou, A. Kostamena, and S. J. Hadziyannis.** 2006. Intrahepatic levels and replicative activity of covalently closed circular hepatitis B virus DNA in chronically infected patients. *Hepatology* **44:**694–702.
86. **Lau, G. K., T. Piratvisuth, K. X. Luo, P. Marcellin, S. Thongsawat, G. Cooksley, E. Gane, M. W. Fried, W. C. Chow, S. W. Paik, W. Y. Chang, T. Berg, R. Flisiak, P. McCloud, and N. Pluck.** 2005. Peginterferon alfa-2a, lamivudine, and the combination for HBeAg-positive chronic hepatitis B. *N. Engl. J. Med.* **352:**2682–2695.
87. **Lau, G. K., H. H. Yiu, D. Y. Fong, H. C. Cheng, W. Y. Au, L. S. Lai, M. Cheung, H. Y. Zhang, A. Lie, R. Ngan, and R. Liang.** 2003. Early is superior to deferred preemptive lamivudine therapy for hepatitis B patients undergoing chemotherapy. *Gastroenterology* **125:**1742–1749.
88. **Lavanchy, D.** 2004. Hepatitis B virus epidemiology, disease burden, treatment, and current and emerging prevention and control measures. *J. Viral. Hepat.* **11:**97–107.
89. **Lee, Y. S., D. J. Suh, Y. S. Lim, S. W. Jung, K. M. Kim, H. C. Lee, Y. H. Chung, W. Yoo, and S. O. Kim.** 2006. Increased risk of adefovir resistance in patients with lamivudine-resistant chronic hepatitis B after 48 weeks of adefovir dipivoxil monotherapy. *Hepatology* **43:**1385–1391.
90. **Leemans, W. F., H. J. Flink, H. L. Janssen, H. G. Niesters, S. W. Schalm, and R. A. de Man.** 2006. The effect of pegylated interferon-alpha on the treatment of lamivudine resistant chronic HBeAg positive hepatitis B virus infection. *J. Hepatol.* **44:**507–511.
91. **Liaw, Y. F., N. Leung, R. Guan, G. K. Lau, I. Merican, G. McCaughan, E. Gane, J. H. Kao, and M. Omata.** 2005. Asian-Pacific consensus statement on the management of chronic hepatitis B: a 2005 update. *Liver Int.* **25:**472–489.
92. **Liaw, Y. F., I. S. Sheen, T. J. Chen, C. M. Chu, and C. C. Pao.** 1991. Incidence, determinants and significance of delayed clearance of serum HBsAg in chronic hepatitis B virus infection: a prospective study. *Hepatology* **13:**627–631.
93. **Liaw, Y. F., J. J. Sung, W. C. Chow, G. Farrell, C. Z. Lee, H. Yuen, T. Tanwandee, Q. M. Tao, K. Shue, O. N. Keene, J. S. Dixon, D. F. Gray, and J. Sabbat.** 2004. Lamivudine for patients with chronic hepatitis B and advanced liver disease. *N. Engl. J. Med.* **351:**1521–1531.
94. **Liaw, Y. F., D. I. Tai, C. M. Chu, and T. J. Chen.** 1988. The development of cirrhosis in patients with chronic type B hepatitis: a prospective study. *Hepatology* **8:**493–496.
95. **Lim, S. G., Y. Cheng, S. Guindon, B. L. Seet, L. Y. Lee, P. Hu, S. Wasser, F. J. Peter, T. Tan, M. Goode, and A. G. Rodrigo.** 2007. Viral quasi-species evolution during hepatitis B e antigen seroconversion. *Gastroenterology* **133:**951–958.
96. **Lim, S. G., T. M. Ng, N. Kung, Z. Krastev, M. Volfova, P. Husa, S. S. Lee, S. Chan, M. L. Shiffman, M. K. Washington, A. Rigney, J. Anderson, E. Mondou, A. Snow, J. Sorbel, R. Guan, and F. Rousseau.** 2006. A double-blind placebo-controlled study of emtricitabine in chronic hepatitis B. *Arch. Intern. Med.* **166:**49–56.
97. **Lin, C. L., L. Y. Liao, C. S. Wang, P. J. Chen, M. Y. Lai, D. S. Chen, and J. H. Kao.** 2005. Basal core-promoter mutant of hepatitis B virus and progression of liver disease in hepatitis B e antigen-negative chronic hepatitis B. *Liver Int.* **25:**564–570.
98. **Lin, S. M., I. S. Sheen, R. N. Chien, C. M. Chu, and Y. F. Liaw.** 1999. Long-term beneficial effect of interferon therapy in patients with chronic hepatitis B virus infection. *Hepatology* **29:**971–975.
99. **Livingston, S. E., J. P. Simonetti, B. J. McMahon, L. R. Bulkow, K. J. Hurlburt, C. E. Homan, M. M. Snowball, H. H. Cagle, J. L. Williams, and V. P. Chulanov.** 2007. Hepatitis B virus genotypes in Alaska Native people with hepatocellular carcinoma: preponderance of genotype F. *J. Infect. Dis.* **195:**5–11.
100. **Lo, K. J., Y. T. Tsai, S. D. Lee, T. C. Wu, J. Y. Wang, G. H. Chen, C. L. Yeh, B. N. Chiang, S. H. Yeh, A. Goudeau, P. Coursaget, and M. Tong.** 1985. Immunoprophylaxis of infection with hepatitis B virus in infants born to hepatitis B surface antigen-positive carrier mothers. *J. Infect. Dis.* **152:**817–822.
101. **Locarnini, S.** 2005. Molecular virology and the development of resistant mutants: implications for therapy. *Semin. Liver Dis.* **25**(Suppl. 1):9–19.
102. **Locarnini, S., A. Hatzakis, J. Heathcote, E. B. Keeffe, T. J. Liang, D. Mutimer, J. M. Pawlotsky, and F. Zoulim.** 2004. Management of antiviral resistance in patients with chronic hepatitis B. *Antivir. Ther.* **9:**679–693.
103. **Lok, A. S.** 2002. Chronic hepatitis B. *N. Engl. J. Med.* **346:**1682–1683.
104. **Lok, A. S., U. Akarca, and S. Greene.** 1994. Mutations in the pre-core region of hepatitis B virus serve to enhance the stability of the secondary structure of the pre-genome encapsidation signal. *Proc. Natl. Acad. Sci. USA* **91:**4077–4081.
105. **Lok, A. S., C. L. Lai, P. C. Wu, E. K. Leung, and T. S. Lam.** 1987. Spontaneous hepatitis B e antigen to antibody seroconversion and reversion in Chinese patients with chronic hepatitis B virus infection. *Gastroenterology* **92:**1839–1843.
106. **Lok, A. S., and B. J. McMahon.** 2007. Chronic hepatitis B. *Hepatology* **45:**507–539.
107. **Mahoney, F. J., K. Stewart, H. Hu, P. Coleman, and M. J. Alter.** 1997. Progress toward the elimination of hepatitis B virus transmission among health care workers in the United States. *Arch. Intern. Med.* **157:**2601–2605.
108. **Maini, M. K., C. Boni, C. K. Lee, J. R. Larrubia, S. Reignat, G. S. Ogg, A. S. King, J. Herberg, R. Gilson, A. Alisa, R. Williams, D. Vergani, N. V. Naoumov, C. Ferrari, and A. Bertoletti.** 2000. The role of virus-specific CD8(+) cells in liver damage and viral control during persistent hepatitis B virus infection. *J. Exp. Med.* **191:**1269–1280.
109. **Manesis, E. K., and S. J. Hadziyannis.** 2001. Interferon alpha treatment and retreatment of hepatitis B e antigen-negative chronic hepatitis B. *Gastroenterology* **121:**101–109.
110. **Marcellin, P., G. K. Lau, F. Bonino, P. Farci, S. Hadziyannis, R. Jin, Z. M. Lu, T. Piratvisuth, G. Germanidis, C. Yurdaydin, M. Diago, S. Gurel, M. Y. Lai, P. Button, and N. Pluck.** 2004. Peginterferon alfa-2a alone, lamivudine alone, and the two in combination in

patients with HBeAg-negative chronic hepatitis B. *N. Engl. J. Med.* **351:**1206–1217.

111. **Maruyama, T., S. Iino, K. Koike, K. Yasuda, and D. R. Milich.** 1993. Serology of acute exacerbation in chronic hepatitis B virus infection. *Gastroenterology* **105:**1141–1151.
112. **Maruyama, T., A. McLachlan, S. Iino, K. Koike, K. Kurokawa, and D. R. Milich.** 1993. The serology of chronic hepatitis B infection revisited. *J. Clin. Investig.* **91:**2586–2595.
113. **Mast, E. E., M. J. Alter, and H. S. Margolis.** 1999. Strategies to prevent and control hepatitis B and C virus infections: a global perspective. *Vaccine* **17:**1730–1733.
114. **Maynard, J. E.** 1990. Hepatitis B: global importance and need for control. *Vaccine* **8**(Suppl. 1):S18–S20; discussion, S21–S23.
115. **McCaffrey, A. P., H. Nakai, K. Pandey, Z. Huang, F. H. Salazar, H. Xu, S. F. Wieland, P. L. Marion, and M. A. Kay.** 2003. Inhibition of hepatitis B virus in mice by RNA interference. *Nat. Biotechnol.* **21:**639–644.
116. **McClary, H., R. Koch, F. V. Chisari, and L. G. Guidotti.** 2000. Relative sensitivity of hepatitis B virus and other hepatotropic viruses to the antiviral effects of cytokines. *J. Virol.* **74:**2255–2264.
117. **McMahon, B. J., D. L. Bruden, K. M. Petersen, L. R. Bulkow, A. J. Parkinson, O. Nainan, M. Khristova, C. Zanis, H. Peters, and H. S. Margolis.** 2005. Antibody levels and protection after hepatitis B vaccination: results of a 15-year follow-up. *Ann. Intern. Med.* **142:**333–341.
118. **McMahon, M. A., B. L. Jilek, T. P. Brennan, L. Shen, Y. Zhou, M. Wind-Rotolo, S. Xing, S. Bhat, B. Hale, R. Hegarty, C. R. Chong, J. O. Liu, R. F. Siliciano, and C. L. Thio.** 2007. The HBV drug entecavir—effects on HIV-1 replication and resistance. *N. Engl. J. Med.* **356:**2614–2621.
119. **Milich, D., and T. J. Liang.** 2003. Exploring the biological basis of hepatitis B e antigen in hepatitis B virus infection. *Hepatology* **38:**1075–1086.
120. **Milich, D. R., J. E. Jones, J. L. Hughes, J. Price, A. K. Raney, and A. McLachlan.** 1990. Is a function of the secreted hepatitis B e antigen to induce immunologic tolerance in utero? *Proc. Natl. Acad. Sci. USA* **87:**6599–6603.
121. **Milich, D. R., A. McLachlan, F. V. Chisari, S. B. Kent, and G. B. Thorton.** 1986. Immune response to the pre-S(1) region of the hepatitis B surface antigen (HBsAg): a pre-S(1)-specific T cell response can bypass nonresponsiveness to the pre-S(2) and S regions of HBsAg. *J. Immunol.* **137:**315–322.
122. **Milich, D. R., G. B. Thornton, A. R. Neurath, S. B. Kent, M. L. Michel, P. Tiollais, and F. V. Chisari.** 1985. Enhanced immunogenicity of the pre-S region of hepatitis B surface antigen. *Science* **228:**1195–1199.
123. **Newbold, J. E., H. Xin, M. Tencza, G. Sherman, J. Dean, S. Bowden, and S. Locarnini.** 1995. The covalently closed duplex form of the hepadnavirus genome exists in situ as a heterogeneous population of viral minichromosomes. *J. Virol.* **69:**3350–3357.
124. **Ni, Y. H., L. M. Huang, M. H. Chang, C. J. Yen, C. Y. Lu, S. L. You, J. H. Kao, Y. C. Lin, H. L. Chen, H. Y. Hsu, and D. S. Chen.** 2007. Two decades of universal hepatitis B vaccination in Taiwan: impact and implication for future strategies. *Gastroenterology* **132:**1287–1293.
125. **Niederau, C., T. Heintges, S. Lange, G. Goldmann, C. M. Niederau, L. Mohr, and D. Haussinger.** 1996. Long-term follow-up of HBeAg-positive patients treated with interferon alfa for chronic hepatitis B. *N. Engl. J. Med.* **334:**1422–1427.
126. **Ocama, P., C. K. Opio, and W. M. Lee.** 2005. Hepatitis B virus infection: current status. *Am. J. Med.* **118:**1413.
127. **Okamoto, H., F. Tsuda, Y. Akahane, Y. Sugai, M. Yoshiba, K. Moriyama, T. Tanaka, Y. Miyakawa, and M. Mayumi.** 1994. Hepatitis B virus with mutations in the core promoter for an e antigen-negative phenotype in carriers with antibody to e antigen. *J. Virol.* **68:**8102–8110.
128. **Papatheodoridis, G. V., E. Dimou, K. Dimakopoulos, S. Manolakopoulos, I. Rapti, G. Kitis, D. Tzourmakliotis, E. Manesis, and S. J. Hadziyannis.** 2005. Outcome of hepatitis B e antigen-negative chronic hepatitis B on long-term nucleos(t)ide analog therapy starting with lamivudine. *Hepatology* **42:**121–129.
129. **Papatheodoridis, G. V., E. Manesis, and S. J. Hadziyannis.** 2001. The long-term outcome of interferon-alpha treated and untreated patients with HBeAg-negative chronic hepatitis B. *J. Hepatol.* **34:**306–313.
130. **Park, B. K., Y. N. Park, S. H. Ahn, K. S. Lee, C. Y. Chon, Y. M. Moon, C. Park, and K. H. Han.** 2007. Long-term outcome of chronic hepatitis B based on histological grade and stage. *J. Gastroenterol. Hepatol.* **22:** 383–388.
131. **Park, N. H., J. W. Shin, J. H. Park, S. J. Bang, D. H. Kim, and K. R. Joo.** 2005. Monitoring of HBeAg levels may help to predict the outcomes of lamivudine therapy for HBeAg positive chronic hepatitis B. *J. Viral. Hepat.* **12:**216–221.
132. **Pawlotsky, J. M.** 2002. Molecular diagnosis of viral hepatitis. *Gastroenterology* **122:**1554–1568.
133. **Perrillo, R., C. Tamburro, F. Regenstein, L. Balart, H. Bodenheimer, M. Silva, E. Schiff, C. Bodicky, B. Miller, C. Denham, C. Brodeur, K. Roach, and J. Albrecht.** 1995. Low-dose, titratable interferon alfa in decompensated liver disease caused by chronic infection with hepatitis B virus. *Gastroenterology* **109:**908–916.
134. **Perrillo, R. P.** 2005. Current treatment of chronic hepatitis B: benefits and limitations. *Semin. Liver Dis.* **25**(Suppl. 1):20–28.
135. **Perrillo, R. P., E. R. Schiff, G. L. Davis, H. C. Bodenheimer, Jr., K. Lindsay, J. Payne, J. L. Dienstag, C. O'Brien, C. Tamburro, I. M. Jacobson, R. Sampliner, D. Feit, J. Lefkowitch, M. Kuhns, C. Meschievitz, B. Sanghvi, J. Albrecht, A. Gibes, and The Hepatitis Interventional Therapy Group.** 1990. A randomized, controlled trial of interferon alfa-2b alone and after prednisone withdrawal for the treatment of chronic hepatitis B. *N. Engl. J. Med.* **323:**295–301.
136. **Poland, G. A.** 1998. Hepatitis B immunization in health care workers. Dealing with vaccine nonresponse. *Am. J. Prev. Med.* **15:**73–77.
137. **Poland, G. A., and R. M. Jacobson.** 2004. Clinical practice: prevention of hepatitis B with the hepatitis B vaccine. *N. Engl. J. Med.* **351:**2832–2838.
138. **Rabe, B., A. Vlachou, N. Pante, A. Helenius, and M. Kann.** 2003. Nuclear import of hepatitis B virus capsids and release of the viral genome. *Proc. Natl. Acad. Sci. USA* **100:**9849–9854.
139. **Raimondo, G., T. Pollicino, I. Cacciola, and G. Squadrito.** 2007. Occult hepatitis B virus infection. *J. Hepatol.* **46:**160–170.
140. **Rapti, I., E. Dimou, P. Mitsoula, and S. J. Hadziyannis.** 2007. Adding-on versus switching-to adefovir therapy in lamivudine-resistant HBeAg-negative chronic hepatitis B. *Hepatology* **45:**307–313.

141. **Realdi, G., G. Fattovich, S. Hadziyannis, S. W. Schalm, P. Almasio, J. Sanchez-Tapias, E. Christensen, G. Giustina, and F. Noventa for The Investigators of the European Concerted Action on Viral Hepatitis (EUROHEP).** 1994. Survival and prognostic factors in 366 patients with compensated cirrhosis type B: a multicenter study. *J. Hepatol.* **21:**656–666.
142. **Richman, D. D.** 2000. The impact of drug resistance on the effectiveness of chemotherapy for chronic hepatitis B. *Hepatology* **32:**866–867.
143. **Rossner, M. T.** 1992. Review: hepatitis B virus X-gene product: a promiscuous transcriptional activator. *J. Med. Virol.* **36:**101–117.
144. **Saldanha, J., W. Gerlich, N. Lelie, P. Dawson, K. Heermann, and A. Heath.** 2001. An international collaborative study to establish a World Health Organization international standard for hepatitis B virus DNA nucleic acid amplification techniques. *Vox Sang.* **80:**63–71.
145. **Schaefer, S.** 2007. Hepatitis B virus taxonomy and hepatitis B virus genotypes. *World J. Gastroenterol.* **13:**14–21.
146. **Schiff, E., C.-L. Lai, S. Hadziyannis, P. Neuhaus, N. Terrault, M. Colombo, H. Tillmann, D. Samuel, S. Zeuzem, J.-P. Villeneuve, S. Arterburn, K. Borroto-Esoda, C. Brosgart, and S. Chuck for the Adefovir Dipivoxil Study 435 International Investigators Group.** 2007. Adefovir dipivoxil for wait-listed and post-liver transplantation patients with lamivudine-resistant hepatitis B: final long-term results. *Liver Transplant.* **13:**349–360.
147. **Schlicht, H., R. Bartenschlager, and H. Schaller.** 1991. Biosynthesis and enzymatic functions of the hepadnaviral reverse transcriptase, p. 171–180. *In* A. McLachlan (ed.), *Molecular Biology of the Hepatitis B Viruses.* CRC Press, Boca Raton, FL.
148. **Schreiber, G. B., M. P. Busch, S. H. Kleinman, and J. J. Korelitz for The Retrovirus Epidemiology Donor Study.** 1996. The risk of transfusion-transmitted viral infections. *N. Engl. J. Med.* **334:**1685–1690.
149. **Shaw, T., and S. Locarnini.** 2004. Entecavir for the treatment of chronic hepatitis B. *Expert Rev. Anti-Infect. Ther.* **2:**853–871.
150. **Sherlock, S.** 1987. The natural history of hepatitis B. *Postgrad. Med. J.* **63**(Suppl. 2)**:**7–11.
151. **Sherman, M., C. Yurdaydin, J. Sollano, M. Silva, Y. F. Liaw, J. Cianciara, A. Boron-Kaczmarska, P. Martin, Z. Goodman, R. Colonno, A. Cross, G. Denisky, B. Kreter, and R. Hindes.** 2006. Entecavir for treatment of lamivudine-refractory, HBeAg-positive chronic hepatitis B. *Gastroenterology* **130:**2039–2049.
152. **Starzl, T. E., A. J. Demetris, and D. Van Thiel.** 1989. Liver transplantation (1). *N. Engl. J. Med.* **321:**1014–1022.
153. **Stephan, W., A. M. Prince, and B. Brotman.** 1984. Modulation of hepatitis B infection by intravenous application of an immunoglobulin preparation that contains antibodies to hepatitis B e and core antigens but not to hepatitis B surface antigen. *J. Virol.* **51:**420–424.
154. **Stevens, C. E., R. P. Beasley, J. Tsui, and W. C. Lee.** 1975. Vertical transmission of hepatitis B antigen in Taiwan. *N. Engl. J. Med.* **292:**771–774.
155. **Stevens, C. E., P. T. Toy, M. J. Tong, P. E. Taylor, G. N. Vyas, P. V. Nair, M. Gudavalli, and S. Krugman.** 1985. Perinatal hepatitis B virus transmission in the United States. Prevention by passive-active immunization. *JAMA* **253:**1740–1745.
156. **Stuyver, L., S. De Gendt, C. Van Geyt, F. Zoulim, M. Fried, R. F. Schinazi, and R. Rossau.** 2000. A new genotype of hepatitis B virus: complete genome and phylogenetic relatedness. *J. Gen. Virol.* **81:**67–74.
157. **Stuyver, L. J., S. A. Locarnini, A. Lok, D. D. Richman, W. F. Carman, J. L. Dienstag, and R. F. Schinazi.** 2001. Nomenclature for antiviral-resistant human hepatitis B virus mutations in the polymerase region. *Hepatology* **33:**751–757.
158. **Sugiyama, M., Y. Tanaka, T. Kato, E. Orito, K. Ito, S. K. Acharya, R. G. Gish, A. Kramvis, T. Shimada, N. Izumi, M. Kaito, Y. Miyakawa, and M. Mizokami.** 2006. Influence of hepatitis B virus genotypes on the intra- and extracellular expression of viral DNA and antigens. *Hepatology* **44:**915–924.
159. **Sumi, H., O. Yokosuka, N. Seki, M. Arai, F. Imazeki, T. Kurihara, T. Kanda, K. Fukai, M. Kato, and H. Saisho.** 2003. Influence of hepatitis B virus genotypes on the progression of chronic type B liver disease. *Hepatology* **37:**19–26.
160. **Tenney, D. J., S. M. Levine, R. E. Rose, A. W. Walsh, S. P. Weinheimer, L. Discotto, M. Plym, K. Pokornowski, C. F. Yu, P. Angus, A. Ayres, A. Bartholomeusz, W. Sievert, G. Thompson, N. Warner, S. Locarnini, and R. J. Colonno.** 2004. Clinical emergence of entecavir-resistant hepatitis B virus requires additional substitutions in virus already resistant to lamivudine. *Antimicrob. Agents Chemother.* **48:**3498–3507.
161. **Thibault, V., C. Aubron-Olivier, H. Agut, and C. Katlama.** 2002. Primary infection with a lamivudine-resistant hepatitis B virus. *AIDS* **16:**131–133.
162. **Thimme, R., S. Wieland, C. Steiger, J. Ghrayeb, K. A. Reimann, R. H. Purcell, and F. V. Chisari.** 2003. $CD8^+$ T cells mediate viral clearance and disease pathogenesis during acute hepatitis B virus infection. *J. Virol.* **77:**68–76.
163. **Thio, C. L., and S. Locarnini.** 2007. Treatment of HIV/HBV coinfection: clinical and virologic issues. *AIDS Rev.* **9:**40–53.
164. **Thio, C. L., E. C. Seaberg, R. Skolasky, Jr., J. Phair, B. Visscher, A. Munoz, and D. L. Thomas.** 2002. HIV-1, hepatitis B virus, and risk of liver-related mortality in the Multicenter Cohort Study (MACS). *Lancet* **360:**1921–1926.
165. **Thompson, A. J. V., D. S. Preiss, X. Chen, P. Revill, P. Desmond, K. Visvanathan, and S. A. Locarnini.** 2006. Hepatocyte interleukin-1 receptor and toll-like receptor signalling: effects on HBV replication in vitro. *Hepatology* **44:**537A.
166. **Tillmann, H. L., J. Hadem, L. Leifeld, K. Zachou, A. Canbay, C. Eisenbach, I. Graziadei, J. Encke, H. Schmidt, W. Vogel, A. Schneider, U. Spengler, G. Gerken, G. N. Dalekos, H. Wedemeyer, and M. P. Manns.** 2006. Safety and efficacy of lamivudine in patients with severe acute or fulminant hepatitis B, a multicenter experience. *J. Viral Hepat.* **13:**256–263.
167. **Torresi, J., L. Earnest-Silveira, G. Deliyannis, K. Edgtton, H. Zhuang, S. A. Locarnini, J. Fyfe, T. Sozzi, and D. C. Jackson.** 2002. Reduced antigenicity of the hepatitis B virus HBsAg protein arising as a consequence of sequence changes in the overlapping polymerase gene that are selected by lamivudine therapy. *Virology* **293:**305–313.
168. **Trojan, J., M. Stuermer, G. Teuber, A. Berger, and D. Faust.** 2007. Treatment of patients with lamivudine-resistant and adefovir dipivoxil-resistant chronic hepatitis B virus infection: is tenofovir the answer? *Gut* **56:**436–437. (Author's reply, **56:**437.)
169. **Tron, F., F. Degos, C. Brechot, A. M. Courouce, A. Goudeau, F. N. Marie, P. Adamowicz, P. Saliou, A. Laplanche, J. P. Benhamou, and M. Girard.** 1989. Ran-

domized dose range study of a recombinant hepatitis B vaccine produced in mammalian cells and containing the S and PreS2 sequences. *J. Infect. Dis.* **160:**199–204.

170. **Truant, R., J. Antunovic, J. Greenblatt, C. Prives, and J. A. Cromlish.** 1995. Direct interaction of the hepatitis B virus HBx protein with p53 leads to inhibition by HBx of p53 response element-directed transactivation. *J. Virol.* **69:**1851–1859.
171. **Van Bommel, F., A. Schernick, U. Hopf, and T. Berg.** 2003. Tenofovir disoproxil fumarate exhibits strong antiviral effect in a patient with lamivudine-resistant severe hepatitis B reactivation. *Gastroenterology* **124:**586–587.
172. **van Bommel, F., B. Zollner, C. Sarrazin, U. Spengler, D. Huppe, B. Moller, H. H. Feucht, B. Wiedenmann, and T. Berg.** 2006. Tenofovir for patients with lamivudine-resistant hepatitis B virus (HBV) infection and high HBV DNA level during adefovir therapy. *Hepatology* **44:**318–325.
173. **van Zonneveld, M., P. Honkoop, B. E. Hansen, H. G. Niesters, S. D. Murad, R. A. de Man, S. W. Schalm, and H. L. Janssen.** 2004. Long-term follow-up of alpha-interferon treatment of patients with chronic hepatitis B. *Hepatology* **39:**804–810.
174. **Verhelst, D., M. Monge, J. L. Meynard, B. Fouqueray, B. Mougenot, P. M. Girard, P. Ronco, and J. Rossert.** 2002. Fanconi syndrome and renal failure induced by tenofovir: a first case report. *Am. J. Kidney Dis.* **40:**1331–1333.
175. **Villeneuve, J. P., L. D. Condreay, B. Willems, G. Pomier-Layrargues, D. Fenyves, M. Bilodeau, R. Leduc, K. Peltekian, F. Wong, M. Margulies, and E. J. Heathcote.** 2000. Lamivudine treatment for decompensated cirrhosis resulting from chronic hepatitis B. *Hepatology* **31:**207–210.
176. **Visvanathan, K., N. A. Skinner, A. J. Thompson, S. M. Riordan, V. Sozzi, R. Edwards, S. Rodgers, J. Kurtovic, J. Chang, S. Lewin, P. Desmond, and S. Locarnini.** 2007. Regulation of Toll-like receptor-2 expression in chronic hepatitis B by the precore protein. *Hepatology* **45:**102–110.
177. **Volz, T., M. Lutgehetmann, P. Wachtler, A. Jacob, A. Quaas, J. M. Murray, M. Dandri, and J. Petersen.** 2007. Impaired intrahepatic hepatitis B virus productivity contributes to low viremia in most HBeAg-negative patients. *Gastroenterology* **133:**843–852.
178. **Wachs, M. E., W. J. Amend, N. L. Ascher, P. N. Bretan, J. Emond, J. R. Lake, J. S. Melzer, J. P. Roberts, S. J. Tomlanovich, F. Vincenti, and P. Stock.** 1995. The risk of transmission of hepatitis B from HBsAg(−), HBcAb(+), HBIgM(−) organ donors. *Transplantation* **59:**230–234.
179. **Wang, X. W., K. Forrester, H. Yeh, M. A. Feitelson, J. R. Gu, and C. C. Harris.** 1994. Hepatitis B virus X protein inhibits p53 sequence-specific DNA binding, transcriptional activity, and association with transcription factor ERCC3. *Proc. Natl. Acad. Sci. USA* **91:**2230–2234.
180. **Wang, X. W., M. K. Gibson, W. Vermeulen, H. Yeh, K. Forrester, H. W. Sturzbecher, J. H. Hoeijmakers, and C. C. Harris.** 1995. Abrogation of p53-induced apoptosis by the hepatitis B virus X gene. *Cancer Res.* **55:**6012–6016.
181. **Warner, N., S. Locarnini, and D. Colledge.** 2004. Molecular modeling of entecavir resistant mutations in the hepatitis B polymerase selected during therapy. *Hepatology* **40:**245A.
182. **Wasley, A., J. T. Miller, and L. Finelli.** 2007. Surveillance for acute viral hepatitis—United States, 2005. *Morb. Mortal. Wkly. Rep. Surveill. Summ.* **56:**1–24.
183. **Webster, G. J., S. Reignat, D. Brown, G. S. Ogg, L. Jones, S. L. Seneviratne, R. Williams, G. Dusheiko, and A. Bertoletti.** 2004. Longitudinal analysis of $CD8^+$ T cells specific for structural and nonstructural hepatitis B virus proteins in patients with chronic hepatitis B: implications for immunotherapy. *J. Virol.* **78:**5707–5719.
184. **Webster, G. J., S. Reignat, M. K. Maini, S. A. Whalley, G. S. Ogg, A. King, D. Brown, P. L. Amlot, R. Williams, D. Vergani, G. M. Dusheiko, and A. Bertoletti.** 2000. Incubation phase of acute hepatitis B in man: dynamic of cellular immune mechanisms. *Hepatology* **32:**1117–1124.
185. **Werle-Lapostolle, B., S. Bowden, S. Locarnini, K. Wursthorn, J. Petersen, G. Lau, C. Trepo, P. Marcellin, Z. Goodman, W. E. Delaney IV, S. Xiong, C. L. Brosgart, S. S. Chen, C. S. Gibbs, and F. Zoulim.** 2004. Persistence of cccDNA during the natural history of chronic hepatitis B and decline during adefovir dipivoxil therapy. *Gastroenterology* **126:**1750–1758.
186. **Whalley, S. A., J. M. Murray, D. Brown, G. J. Webster, V. C. Emery, G. M. Dusheiko, and A. S. Perelson.** 2001. Kinetics of acute hepatitis B virus infection in humans. *J. Exp. Med.* **193:**847–854.
187. **Wieland, S., R. Thimme, R. H. Purcell, and F. V. Chisari.** 2004. Genomic analysis of the host response to hepatitis B virus infection. *Proc. Natl. Acad. Sci. USA* **101:**6669–6674.
188. **Wieland, S. F., and F. V. Chisari.** 2005. Stealth and cunning: hepatitis B and hepatitis C viruses. *J. Virol.* **79:**9369–9380.
189. **Will, H., W. Reiser, T. Weimer, E. Pfaff, M. Buscher, R. Sprengel, R. Cattaneo, and H. Schaller.** 1987. Replication strategy of human hepatitis B virus. *J. Virol.* **61:**904–911.
190. **Wong, D. K., A. M. Cheung, K. O'Rourke, C. D. Naylor, A. S. Detsky, and J. Heathcote.** 1993. Effect of alpha-interferon treatment in patients with hepatitis B e antigen-positive chronic hepatitis B. A meta-analysis. *Ann. Intern. Med.* **119:**312–323.
191. **Wursthorn, K., M. Lutgehetmann, M. Dandri, T. Volz, P. Buggisch, B. Zollner, T. Longerich, P. Schirmacher, F. Metzler, M. Zankel, C. Fischer, G. Currie, C. Brosgart, and J. Petersen.** 2006. Peginterferon alpha-2b plus adefovir induce strong cccDNA decline and HBsAg reduction in patients with chronic hepatitis B. *Hepatology* **44:**675–684.
192. **Yap, I., and S. H. Chan.** 1996. A new pre-S containing recombinant hepatitis B vaccine and its effect on non-responders: a preliminary observation. *Ann. Acad. Med. Singap.* **25:**120–122.
193. **Yeo, W., and P. J. Johnson.** 2006. Diagnosis, prevention and management of hepatitis B virus reactivation during anticancer therapy. *Hepatology* **43:**209–220.
194. **Yim, H. J., M. Hussain, Y. Liu, S. N. Wong, S. K. Fung, and A. S. Lok.** 2006. Evolution of multi-drug resistant hepatitis B virus during sequential therapy. *Hepatology* **44:**703–712.
195. **Yim, H. J., and A. S. Lok.** 2006. Natural history of chronic hepatitis B virus infection: what we knew in 1981 and what we know in 2005. *Hepatology* **43:**S173–S181.
196. **Ying, R. S., C. Zhu, X. G. Fan, N. Li, X. F. Tian, H. B. Liu, and B. X. Zhang.** 2007. Hepatitis B virus is inhibited by RNA interference in cell culture and in mice. *Antivir. Res.* **73:**24–30.
197. **Yu, M. W., S. H. Yeh, P. J. Chen, Y. F. Liaw, C. L. Lin, C. J. Liu, W. L. Shih, J. H. Kao, D. S. Chen, and**

C. J. Chen. 2005. Hepatitis B virus genotype and DNA level and hepatocellular carcinoma: a prospective study in men. *J. Natl. Cancer Inst.* **97:**265–272.

198. **Yuen, M. F., H. J. Yuan, D. K. Wong, J. C. Yuen, W. M. Wong, A. O. Chan, B. C. Wong, K. C. Lai, and C. L. Lai.** 2005. Prognostic determinants for chronic hepatitis B in Asians: therapeutic implications. *Gut* **54:** 1610–1614.
199. **Zakaria, S., R. Fouad, O. Shaker, S. Zaki, A. Hashem, S. S. El-Kamary, and G. Esmat.** 2007. Changing patterns of acute viral hepatitis at a major urban referral center in Egypt. *Clin. Infect. Dis.* **44:**e30–e36.
200. **Zoulim, F., J. Saputelli, and C. Seeger.** 1994. Woodchuck hepatitis virus X protein is required for viral infection in vivo. *J. Virol.* **68:**2026–2030.
201. **Zoulim, F., and C. Seeger.** 1994. Reverse transcription in hepatitis B viruses is primed by a tyrosine residue of the polymerase. *J. Virol.* **68:**6–13.

Human Lymphotropic Viruses: HTLV-1 and HTLV-2

WILLIAM A. BLATTNER AND MANHATTAN E. CHARURAT

32

The discovery of the first human retrovirus, human T-cell lymphotropic virus type 1 (HTLV-1), in 1979 ushered in a new age of medical virology (137). The long-standing search for a human homolog to cancer-causing retroviruses in animals, first discovered at the beginning of the 20th century, ended at a time when most researchers had abandoned the quest and focused instead on virus-transforming genes that occur as oncogenes in human tumors. HTLV-2 was identified 3 years later, in 1982 (78). By using techniques that led to the isolation of these viruses, human immunodeficiency virus type 1 (HIV-1) was isolated in 1983 (6) and was shown to be the cause of AIDS in 1984 (46, 150). These initial breakthroughs were followed by the molecular characterization of the human genera of the family *Retroviridae: Deltaretrovirus* (formerly termed *Oncornavirus*; HTLV) and *Lentivirus* (HIV). The association of HTLV-1 with adult T-cell leukemia/lymphoma (ATL) and HTLV-1-associated myelopathy/tropical spastic paraparesis (HAM/TSP), as well as other diseases, was established by clinical epidemiological studies (13, 24, 51, 78), whereas links of HTLV-2 to diseases are less certain (1a). In 2005, HTLV-3 was discovered in Central Africa (175). A single isolate termed HTLV-4 has also been sequenced (21). Clinical disease associations have yet to be recognized for these new viruses, which have closely related nonhuman primate homologs (105).

VIROLOGY

Classification

Within the taxa of DNA and RNA reverse-transcribing viruses, the HTLVs, along with bovine leukemia virus, are classified within the genus *Deltaretrovirus* in the family *Retroviridae* (47). HTLV-1 and HTLV-2 are RNA viruses that contain a diploid genome that replicates through a DNA intermediary able to integrate into the host T-lymphocyte genome as a provirus. The integration process is essential to the ability of this class of virus to cause lifelong infection, evade immune clearance, and produce diseases of long latency such as leukemia/lymphoma. The high degree of sequence stability of the viral genome—despite hundreds of thousands of years of evolution—arose because HTLV-1 favors viral expansion through proliferation of proviral DNA-harboring cells rather than infection of new cells by cell-free virions like HIV (3). Therefore, the replicative machinery of the cell, rather than the error-prone viral reverse transcriptase, is responsible for maintaining viral genomic stability. The phylogeny of the HTLVs has become more complex as systematic studies of nonhuman primates and humans residing in Central Africa have been carried out. A close relationship exists between the human and simian versions of these viruses. Figure 1 shows the phylogenetic relationship between the simian and human versions of the primate T-lymphotropic viruses. HTLV-3 is genetically equidistant (approximately 62% homology) from HTLV-1 and HTLV-2, which in turn are approximately 60% homologous (156). HTLV-4 has only been reported for a handful of individuals from west central Africa (175) (see "Molecular Epidemiology of HTLV-1, -2, and -3" below).

Composition of the Virus

The HTLV-1 virion is approximately 100 nm in diameter, with a thin electron-dense outer envelope and an electron-dense, roughly spherical core. The total provirus genome consists of 9,032 nucleotides, with identical sequences termed long terminal repeats (LTRs) at the 5′ and 3′ ends of the genome, which contain regulatory elements called Tax-responsive elements that control virus expression and virion production (Fig. 2). The newly discovered HTLV-3 has only two Tax-responsive elements in its LTR, while both HTLV-1 and -2 have three. In the absence of the third Tax-responsive element, HTLV-3 contains a unique activator upstream of the 21-bp repeat elements, protein-1 transcription factor, to compensate for this function (20).

The major structural and regulatory proteins of HTLV-1 are summarized in Table 1. HTLV-1 shares with other replication-competent retroviruses the three main genomic regions of *gag* (group-specific antigen), *pol* (protease/polymerase/integrase), and *env* (envelope). Production of the Gag proteins occurs as a result of the translation of the full-length mRNA, which yields a large precursor polypeptide that is subsequently cleaved by the virally encoded protease. For the Pol proteins, production depends on translation made possible when the stop codon of the *gag* gene is bypassed, leading to a large polypeptide including Gag- and Pol-related proteins, which are subsequently cleaved into functional proteins by the viral protease. Production of the Env surface and transmembrane proteins

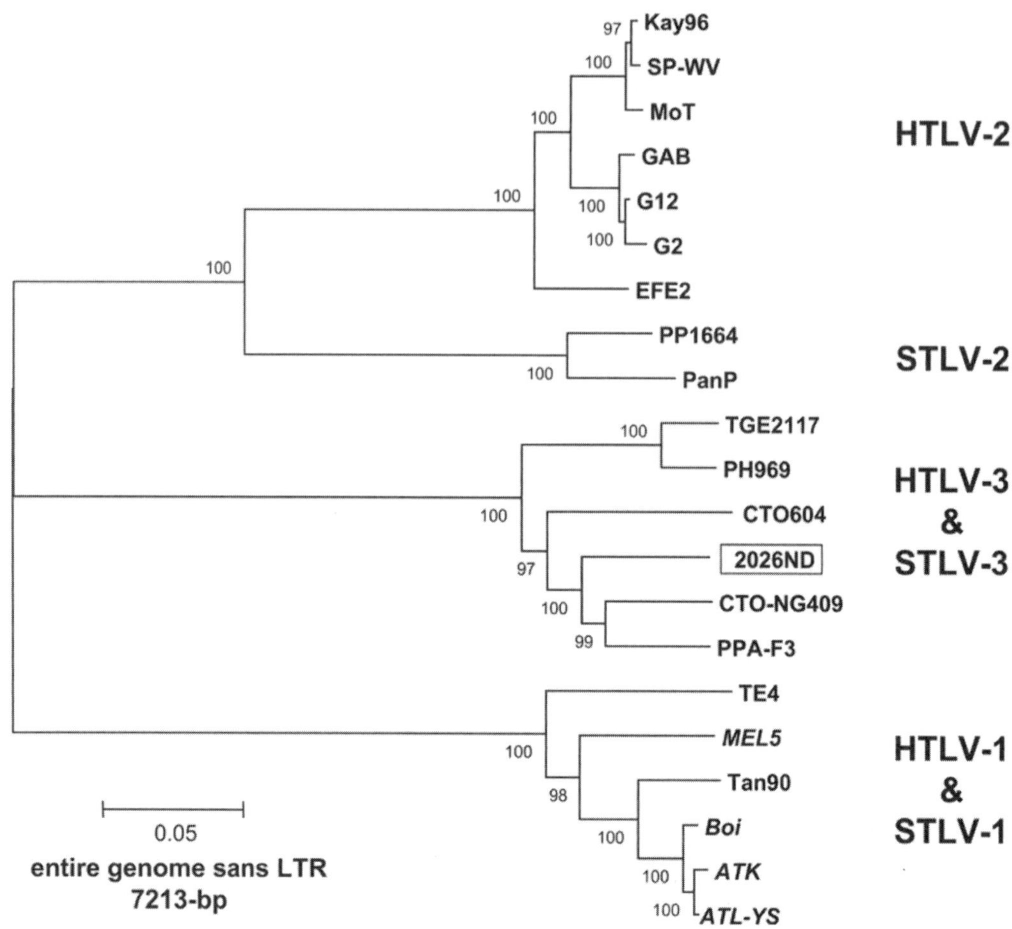

FIGURE 1 Phylogenetic relationship of HTLV-1, -2, and -3. Each type varies by approximately 60% from each other. STLV, simian T-lymphotropic virus. (Reprinted from reference 156 with permission.)

involves translation of spliced mRNA (Fig. 3), which results in an envelope precursor that is cleaved into the subunits. The precursor proteins have characteristic molecular weights (MWs) that can be detected immunologically by Western blot analysis (Table 1). The Gag proteins function as structural proteins of the matrix, capsid, and nucleocapsid. The *pol* gene encodes several enzymes: a protease that cleaves Gag and Gag-Pol polypeptides into proteins of the mature virion, a reverse transcriptase that generates a double-stranded DNA from the RNA genome, and an integrase that integrates viral DNA into the host cell chromosomes. The *env* gene encodes the major components of the viral coat: the surface glycoprotein (gp46; MW, 46,000) and the transmembrane glycoprotein (gp21; MW, 21,000).

Unlike other vertebrate leukemia viruses, the deltaretroviruses have an additional region called pX that contains four open reading frames (ORFs). pX ORFs III and IV code for two transcription-regulatory proteins, the Tax and Rex proteins, whose functions are involved in regulation of virus expression. pX ORFs I and II encode other accessory and regulatory genes whose functions involve cell cycle regulation. Tax is responsible for enhanced transcription of viral and cellular gene products and is essential for transformation of human T lymphocytes (147); Rex (regulator of expression of virion proteins for HTLV) stabilizes viral mRNA and modulates the splicing and transport from the nucleus of viral RNA (87). As shown in Fig. 3, two overlapping reading frames are involved in the expression of both of these gene products, translated from a doubly spliced mRNA employing the initiation codon from *env* and the remaining sequences from the pX region. HIV-1 employs a similar strategy for expressing Tat and Rev proteins, which perform regulatory functions similar to those of Tax and Rex of HTLV-1. pX ORF I, also produced by this double-splicing mechanism, codes for a hydrophobic 12-kDa protein, $p12^{I}$; pX ORF II results in the production of two nuclear proteins, $p13^{II}$ and $p30^{II}$ (92). Recently, an antisense RNA from the negative strand of the pX region has been discovered, which codes for the HTLV-1 bZip protein (HBZ) that down-regulates viral transcription (50). The roles of these pX gene products and accessory gene products in disease pathogenesis are described in Table 1.

Biology

The replication strategy of the HTLVs involves a replication cycle typical of all members of the *Retroviridae* family (Fig. 3), whereby the RNA genome undergoes reverse transcription into a DNA provirus that integrates into the host

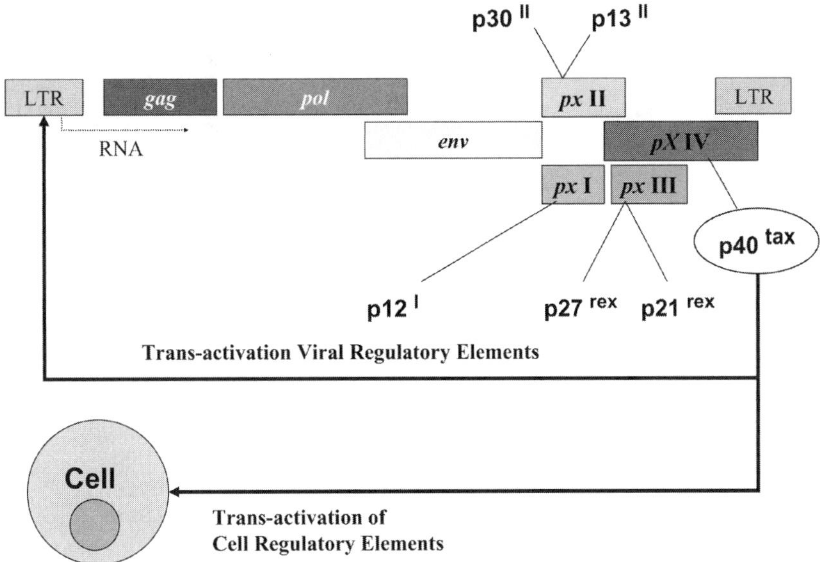

FIGURE 2 Genomic structure of HTLV-1. The LTR is organized into three regions: (i) US, R, and U3, which house the polyadenylation site; (ii) *rev* (response element); and (iii) the 21-bp enhancer *trans*-activating response elements. The last two elements are involved in controlling virus expression. Shown are the *gag* gene (group-specific antigen), whose products form the skeleton of the virion (matrix, capsid, nucleocapsid, and nucleic acid binding protein); the *pol/pro* gene (the gene for reverse transcriptase, integrase, and protease), the *env* gene (the envelope gene), the *tax* gene (the *trans*-activator gene), and the *rex* gene (the viral regulatory gene involved in promoting genomic RNA production). (Courtesy of Robert C. Gallo.)

genome. Subsequently, new virions are produced via this integrated DNA template under the regulation of viral regulatory genes. In HeLa cells, integration does not specifically target transcription units (e.g., CpG islands) and transcription start sites like with some other retroviruses. Instead, integration site preference correlates with the sequence and structure of virus-encoded integrase, which is consistent with the hypothesis that integrase is the major determinant of retroviral integration site selection (36).

Receptors

HTLV-1 preferentially infects CD4 T-helper cells, whereas HTLV-2 has a preferential tropism for the CD8 cell type. Additionally, HTLV-1 infects a wide range of cells in vitro, including endothelial cells, fibroblasts, and CD8 T cells (but at a lower frequency based on studies of T cells from patients with HAM/TSP [126]). HTLV-1 is transmitted through a viral synapse and enters target cells via interaction with the glucose transporter GLUT1. The discovery of GLUT1 as the major receptor for HTLV-1 derived from careful molecular analysis of the extracellular surface component of the gp41 HTLV-1 envelope that mapped the surface glycoprotein binding domain to the first 160 residues of the HTLV-1 and -2 envelopes (108). The discovery of GLUT1 helps explain why many animal species and cell types can be infected either experimentally (mice, rats, rabbits, and New World primate species) or naturally (Old World primates), because GLUT1 is widely distributed in mammalian cells. CD8 cells are rich in GLUT1 compared to CD4 cells, so the cellular tropism of HTLV-1 must be explained by additional factors.

Recently, it has been discovered that heparan sulfate proteoglycans are required for efficient entry of HTLV-1 (75). High levels of heparan sulfate proteoglycans are found on activated primary CD4 T cells compared to CD8 T cells. Conversely, CD8 T cells, the primary target of HTLV-2, express GLUT1 at dramatically higher levels than CD4 T cells, thus explaining the preference of HTLV-2 for CD8 cells. HTLV-2 surface glycoprotein binding and viral entry are markedly higher for CD8 T cells, while HTLV-1 surface glycoprotein binding and viral entry are higher on CD4 T cells rich in heparan sulfate proteoglycans. Infection of CD4 cells by HTLV-2 can be increased if CD4 cells are made to overexpress GLUT1, whereas HTLV-1 infection of CD8 cells can be increased by using transfection to increase heparan sulfate proteoglycan expression on CD8 cells (75). Studies employing chimeric HTLV-1 and -2 viruses in which envelope sequences are swapped demonstrate that cellular tropism is determined by type-specific envelope mapping to the C-terminal portion of gp21, indicating that *env* is a major viral determinant for HTLV T-cell tropism (176). Additionally, neuropilin-1, the receptor for semaphorin-3A and VEGF-A165 and a member of the immune synapse, is a physical and functional partner of HTLV-1 Env proteins in HTLV-1 cell entry (54). Thus, both cellular and viral envelope factors account for the complex tropism of the HTLVs.

HTLV is preferentially transmitted via direct contact between infected and targeted cells through a structure referred to as the virologic synapse, which is formed between the envelope glycoprotein of the virus and a cellular binding partner (16). It is hypothesized that early during infection, most new HTLV-1-infected cells are produced by cell-to-cell synapse, resulting in a polyclonal infection of both CD4 and CD8 T cells. This model is consistent with epidemiological data suggesting that cell-free biological flu-

TABLE 1 Major structural and regulatory proteins of HTLV-1

Viral gene	Gene product[a]	Function
LTR		Regulation of viral gene expression, integration of provirus into host genetic material, and regulation of virion production
gag	p15	Nucleocapsid is a small basic protein found in the virion in association with the genome RNA characterized with zinc finger motifs associated with nucleic acid binding
gag	p19	Matrix protein forms a close linkage to the internal surface of the viral envelope via myristic acid
gag	p24	Capsid protein forms the major internal structural feature of the core shell of the virion
gag	p53	Precursor protein for other Gag proteins
pol	Integrase	Integrates viral DNA into the host cell chromosomes
pol	Reverse transcriptase (95 kDa)	Reverse transcriptase generates a double-stranded DNA from the RNA genome
pro	Protease (p14)	Cleaves Gag and Gag-Pol polypeptides into proteins of the mature virion
env	gp46	Envelope surface glycoprotein attached to surface lipid bilayer involved in virion binding to target cell
env	p21e	Envelope transmembrane protein
px IV	Tax (p40)	Transactivator for enhanced transcription of viral and cellular gene products
px III	Rex (p27/p21)	Regulator of expression of virion proteins for HTLV stabilizes viral mRNAs and modulates the splicing and transport from the nucleus of viral RNA
px I	ORF I ($p12^{I}$)	Activation of STAT5 and interference with MHC class I trafficking; down-modulation of ICAM-1 and -2 and reduced adherence of NK cells
px II	ORF II ($p30^{II}$, $p13^{II}$)	Inhibition of acetyltransferase activity of P/CAF on histones and stabilization of p53; alters cell cycle G_2 regulation of T lymphocytes
px minus strand	HBZ	Leucine zipper protein inhibits CREB-2 binding to the viral LTR promoter, reducing viral replication; down-modulates Tax effects on bZIP transcription factors. HBZ mRNA directly contributes to the proliferation of T cells.

[a] MWs: matrix membrane-associated protein, 19,000 (p19; can be chemically cross-linked to the lipid bilayer of the external envelope); internal core shell protein, 24,000 (p24); external, highly glycosolated envelope, 46,000; transmembrane, 21,000 (43).

ids do not transmit HTLV-1. In later stages of infection, when equilibrium between viral replication and immune response is established, HTLV-1 mainly multiplies through mitosis of the host cells (162).

Replication

Once viral attachment takes place, fusion of the virion with the cell membrane results in uncoating of the diploid RNA genome of the virus (Fig. 3). The virally encoded RNA-dependent DNA polymerase (reverse transcriptase) complexed to the genomic RNA of the virus transcribes viral RNA into double-stranded DNA. This double-stranded viral cDNA is transported to the nucleus as a ribonucleoprotein complex that includes the p24 capsid protein as well as integrase and reverse transcriptase. There the cDNA, through a complex process mediated by the viral integrase, is inserted into the host genome. The genomic integration of HTLV-1 establishes a lifelong infection and is integral to both the virus replication cycle and amplification through expansion of HTLV-infected host cells (162).

Elements in the viral LTR (Fig. 2) are essential to integration and replication; they form the sites for covalent attachment of the provirus to cellular DNA and provide important regulatory components for transcription. Additional key regulatory elements of HTLV are *tax*, which activates transcription of the viral genome, and *rex*, which modulates the processing of the viral RNA expressing unspliced forms of the viral mRNA. The recently discovered HBZ leucine zipper protein encoded by the antisense pX gene inhibits CREB-2 binding to the viral promoter, thus modulating the viral replicating impact of Tax (50). When the DNA provirus is expressed (transcribed by a cellular RNA polymerase), viral genomic RNA, mRNA, and subsequently viral proteins are made by the cell. Under the influence of Rex, which stabilizes viral mRNA and regulates its splicing and transport, new genomic RNA is assembled at the cell membrane and packaged for release (budding). During the budding process, the envelope incorporates some of the cell's lipid bilayer, producing an infectious virion of about 100 nm (Fig. 3).

EPIDEMIOLOGY

Molecular Epidemiology of HTLV-1, -2, and -3

The four recognized HTLVs are closely related to simian counterparts and are approximately 60% homologous with each other (Fig. 1). Based on sequencing data, HTLV-1 is composed of three types—termed Cosmopolitan, Melanesian (Papua New Guinea, Melanesia, and Australian aborigines), and Central African—with up to 10% sequence

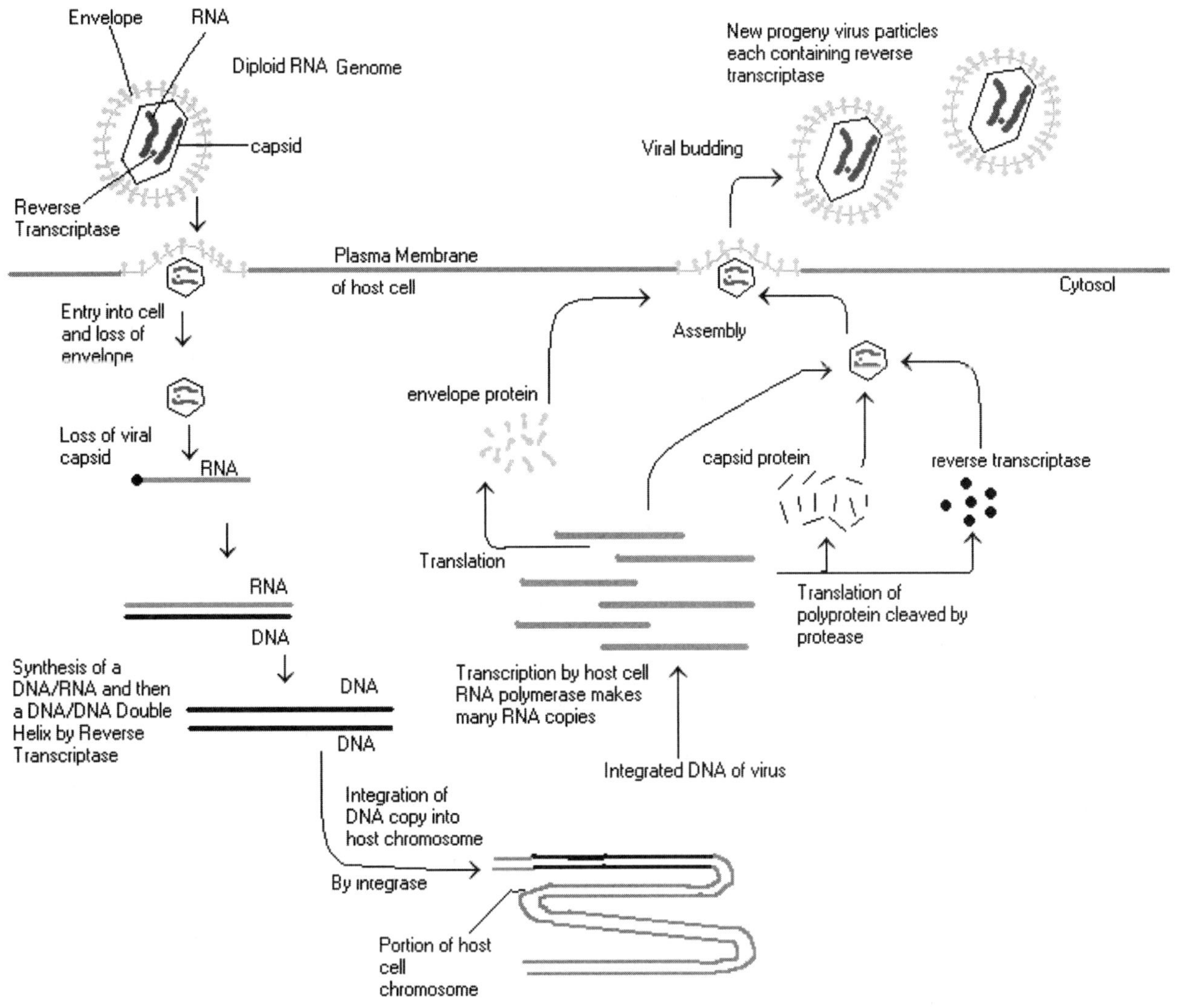

FIGURE 3 Replication cycle of HTLV-1. Virus infection involves initial binding to the surface of the target CD4 cell, uncoating, and release of viral genetic material. Virally encoded reverse transcriptase creates a DNA copy that is integrated into the host genome under the influence of viral integrase. Viral replication involves the production of both genomic RNA and polyproteins that are cleaved by the viral protease, resulting in virion assembly at the cell surface. See the text for details. (Adapted from reference 1 with permission of the publisher.)

variation (53). It is postulated that these lineages arose from separate interspecies transmissions from simians to humans (167). The Cosmopolitan strain has the widest distribution worldwide and consists of four subtypes that vary by 1 to 3%. Subtype A (Transcontinental) occurs in Japan, the Caribbean, Colombia, Chile, and India; subtype B (Japanese) is found in Japan and India; subtype C (West African) is found in the Caribbean and Africa, brought to the Caribbean through the slave trade (168); and subtype D (North African) was first identified among Mashhadi Jews.

HTLV-2 consists of four types—A, B, C, and D—that are geographically distributed throughout the Americas and in West Africa. Prevalence ranges from 1 to 3% on average but is as high as 20% in some Native American populations and is above 50% in some drug user cohorts (11). Both HTLV-2 types A and B are found in West Africa and Cameroon. Between these subtypes, sequence differences of 2 to 4% are observed (90). In contrast to HTLV-1, HTLV-2 appears to originate from a common human ancestor virus that emerged from only one simian-to-human transmission (3). There are no epidemiological data to suggest that disease incidence or subtype is impacted by viral type for either HTLV-1 or HTLV-2.

The new variant viruses, HTLV-3 and -4, have been detected only in Central Africa. For the regions of HTLV-3 that have been sequenced, there is an overall 60% nucleotide homology between HTLV-1, -2, and -3 (3, 20, 156). The full-length sequence of HTLV-3 suggests that it shares structural features that could make a pathogenic virus similar to HTLV-1, but no disease association has been made (156).

No serotypes for either HTLV-1 or HTLV-2 correspond to these genetically defined types. Serologically, there is significant cross-reactivity between HTLV-1 and -2, reflecting their approximate 65% sequence homology. There are limited data on seroreactivity for HTLV-3. The strongest antibody response to the major antigens of HTLV-1 and -2 occurs to the major capsid antigen p24, whereas p19, the matrix protein, which has approximately 50% homology, is less cross-reactive and previously served as a means of distinguishing HTLV-1 from HTLV-2.

Distribution

HTLV-1

HTLV-1 is widely disseminated (Fig. 4). Between 15 million and 25 million people are estimated worldwide to harbor HTLV-1 infection. Over the lifetime of the infected carriers, 3 to 5% will develop an aggressive T-cell malignancy ATL and another 2 to 3% will experience chronic inflammatory diseases, mainly HAM/TSP (52). In some areas of endemicity, over 70% of all lymphoid malignancies are attributable to HTLV-1 exposure (32). The incidence of HAM/TSP among carriers is approximately half that of ATL, with the remainder of nonmalignant disease accounted for by a variety of conditions detailed below.

Japan and the Pacific

The distributions of both HTLV-1 and -2 vary by geographic region, race, ethnicity, and risk factors. Endemic clusters of HTLV-1 seropositivity or infection are present in southern Japan, the islands of the Ryukyu Chain (including Okinawa), and some isolated villages in the north of Japan among aboriginal Ainu populations; most of the seropositive persons in northern Japan are immigrants from areas in the south where infections are endemic (119). Rates of infection among persons older than 40 years exceed 15% in these areas. China, Taiwan, Korea, and Vietnam are largely free of infection; the high rates (>15%) in Melanesia are attributed to the Melanesian virus type (169).

The Caribbean and Americas

Another major endemic focus of HTLV-1 infection occurs in the Caribbean, where rates of seropositivity in Jamaica, Trinidad and Tobago, Martinique, Barbados, St. Lucia, Haiti, and the Dominican Republic range between 5 and 14% (15, 107). In Trinidad and Tobago, seropositivity (5 to 14%) is restricted almost exclusively to persons of African descent, even though individuals of Indo-Asian ethnic background have shared a common environment for over a century (7). In Jamaica, different rates of seropositivity occur in different regions, with the highest rates (10%) observed in the lowland, high-rainfall areas (107). Seropositivity is found more frequently in persons of lower socioeconomic class and those who lack formal education (15). Men and women attending clinics for sexually transmitted diseases (STDs) have the highest rate of seropositivity (>15%) (122). The rate in blood donors is lower (1 to 5%) (109).

Foci of seropositivity are also present in South and Central America, including Brazil (>15% in Bahia), Colombia, Venezuela, Guyana, Surinam, Panama, and Honduras (5 to 14%). With the exception of some foci among Native Americans, HTLV-1 is rare in the rest of Central and North America (22). In Chile, identified pockets of HTLV-1 in persons of non-African descent raise the possibility of a trans-Pacific viral passage. A study of DNA from pre-Columbian mummies has confirmed that the molecular characteristics of this Chilean virus are closely related to the virus from Japan (100).

In the United States, large-scale screening of blood supplies has documented rates of HTLV-1 or -2 of 0.43 per 1,000; approximately half of the positive results are associated with HTLV-2 infection (95). In a significant proportion of HTLV-1-positive cases, the donor either has links to an area of endemic infection or has a history of risk-related behaviors, such as injecting drugs (95). Persons of African ancestry have higher rates of seropositivity (143). Similarly, migrant populations from Okinawa to Hawaii, from the Caribbean to the United States, and from the Caribbean to the United Kingdom are at risk of HTLV positivity, as are those who experience exposure through sexual contact or blood transfusion in areas where the virus is endemic (14, 66).

Africa

In most African countries, the actual HTLV-1 prevalence cannot be estimated because of a lack of information and the potential for cross-reactivity with related HTLVs (see above) in the area (155). Limited data from the Ivory Coast, Ghana, Nigeria, Zaire, Kenya, and Tanzania document that more than 5% of the general population is infected (35).

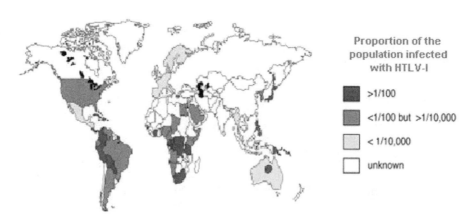

FIGURE 4 HTLV-1 infection clusters with high rates in selected geographic areas.

The Middle East and Europe

Surveys in the Middle East have been largely negative, with the exception of Iranian Jews from northeastern Iran (Mashhad) and emigrants from that area now residing in Israel and New York (40). Surveys in southern India and Indonesia have identified some HTLV-1-positive cases; in the Seychelles in the Indian Ocean, HTLV-1 is highly endemic (>15%).

In Europe, occasional infections are detected among migrants from areas of endemic infection. In the most western European countries, HTLV-1 is still uncommon in the general population. The infection has been reported to occur in specific groups in addition to the immigrants from areas of endemicity, including sex workers and injection drug users (138).

HTLV-2

HTLV-2 has a more restricted distribution than HTLV-1 and occurs primarily in the Americas and parts of Africa. A major reservoir is among injection drug users in the United States and southern Europe, with rates ranging from 10 to 15% and higher (11). Amerindians residing in North, Central, and South America have various rates of positivity for HTLV-2 (5 to 30%). Pockets of infection are present among the Seminoles in southern Florida and the Pueblo and Navajo in New Mexico but not among various tribes in Alaska. In Central America, the Guaymi Indians residing in northeastern Panama near the Costa Rican border have high seropositivity rates (>15%), but this does not hold true for the Guaymi living in southwestern Panama (142).

Incidence and Prevalence of Infection

HTLV-1

HTLV-1 seroprevalence is characterized by an age-dependent rise that is observed in diverse geographic areas. For example, the patterns of infection in Jamaica and Okinawa, Japan, are similar (Fig. 5). The prevalence rate among children of both sexes is low (approximately 1%), and the male-to-female ratio is 1. During adolescence, coincident with the onset of sexual activity, the prevalence begins to rise and a divergence in infection rates between males and females emerges, with female rates exceeding male rates by up to 50%. This trend continues into adulthood, with male rates plateauing by the age of 40 years but female rates continuing to rise to a peak at about the age of 60 years. The reason for this female excess is thought to be the more efficient transmission from males to females than from females to males. Part of this age-dependent rise, at least in Japan, has been attributed to a "cohort effect," in which declining rates of infection in younger birth cohorts give the appearance of rising rates in older birth cohorts (118). This pattern is observed in follow-up studies of Japanese emigrants to Hawaii, for whom rates of infection decline in successive generations (66). Possible explanations for this declining intergenerational prevalence include changes in standard of living, improved nutrition, changes in breast-feeding patterns, elimination of many coincident infectious diseases, and declines in other STDs. Nevertheless, older Japanese couples discordant for HTLV-1 show evidence of ongoing male-to-female and female-to-male transmission. There is no evidence to support the concept that reactivation of immunosilent infection in seronegative persons accounts for this age-dependent rise. However, there are isolated instances of ATL patients who lack HTLV-1 antibodies and are positive for a replication-defective virus as demonstrated by PCR (58, 89).

HTLV-2

HTLV-2 also exhibits a characteristic age-dependent rise in seropositivity. Among populations of Amerindians in areas of endemic infection, a curve similar to that of HTLV-1 seropositivity occurs, but with no gender differences at any age (106). Among injection drug users, the sharing of eye dropper injection equipment—a common practice before the wide availability of disposable syringes—is linked to unusually high rates of seropositivity in

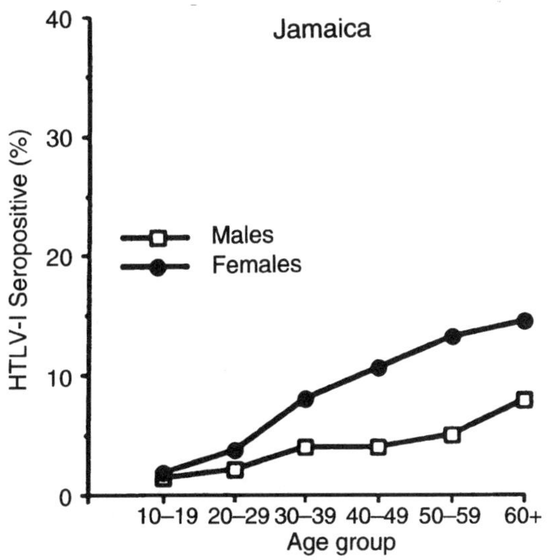

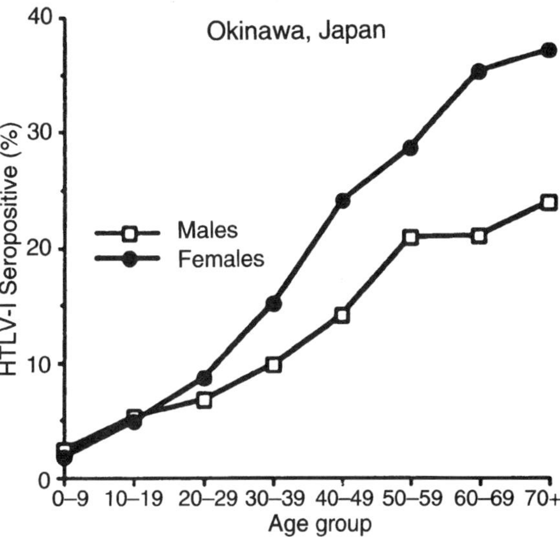

FIGURE 5 Age-specific seroprevalence of HTLV-1 in Jamaica and Okinawa, Japan. There is a characteristic pattern of higher rates in females than in males, with an age-dependent increase in seroprevalence and a plateauing in males at age 50 years but an increase in females. (Reprinted from references 76 and 123 with permission of the publisher.)

older groups and may explain why rates are significantly higher than those reported for younger injection drug users. There is no evidence of a virus-positive, antibody-negative state.

Associated Diseases

ATL

In areas of endemicity such as southern Japan and the Caribbean Islands, the annual incidence of virus-associated leukemia is approximately 3/100,000 per year and may account for one-half of all adult lymphoid malignancies (136). ATL occurs in 1 per 1,000 carriers per year, resulting in 2,500 to 3,000 cases per year worldwide (113). ATL rarely occurs in the pediatric age group, but cases in 5- and 6-year-old children have been reported (141). Most ATL cases occur between the late 30s and late 50s (Fig. 6) rather than in the older age groups, which is typical of B-cell lymphomas in developed countries. Before the age of 50 years, HTLV-1 is the major single cause of lymphoma in areas of endemic infection. Compared to Japan, where the peak occurrence is between 50 and 60 years of age, cases in the West Indies and Brazil among persons of African descent peak approximately a decade earlier; immigrants from these regions to areas where infection is not endemic sustain this differential in the age-specific incidence (15). The male-to-female ratio for ATL cases is approximately 1, which contrasts with the excess of infections among females in adulthood. The decline in attributable risk for ATL after age 50 argues that early-life exposure to HTLV-1 contributes substantially to subsequent risk of lymphoid malignancy with a latency of decades.

HAM/TSP

The lifetime incidence of HAM/TSP in HTLV-1 carriers is estimated to be less than 5% (range of 0.3 to 4%). The disease geographically clusters in regions of HTLV-1 endemicity. For example, disease incidence is higher in Jamaica, where the virus is endemic, than in Japan. HAM/TSP appears to have a much shorter latency than ATL, and blood transfusion is a major risk factor for HAM/TSP but not for ATL. The incidence of HAM/TSP has been estimated at approximately half that of ATL, but cases are more prevalent because of the long survival associated with this chronic degenerative neurologic condition.

Females are approximately twice as likely to be affected; markers of sexual transmission have been associated with disease in females (102). Cases tend to peak in the 30- to 50-year age group, but cases have been reported for children as young as 3 years of age. HAM/TSP is considered uncommon in children, although case reports have increased in recent years (2, 139). In a report of seven children with infective dermatitis and HAM/TSP, the progression of neurologic symptoms was remarkably rapid (139).

The pattern of occurrence, linking blood transfusions and markers of sexual transmission, suggests that both peri- and postnatal and adult sexually acquired infections are linked to disease risk.

Transmission

Table 2 summarizes the routes, modes, and cofactors associated with HTLV-1 and -2 transmission. The routes of transmission are better characterized for HTLV-1 because injection drug use accounts for the majority of HTLV-2 infections in the United States and there are few studies among noninjection drug user cohorts. Data on HTLV-3 are not available in the absence of a reliable serologic tool for distinguishing viral subtype.

Routes

Mother-to-Child Transmission

Mother-to-child transmission of HTLV-1 is the principal means of childhood infection. Maternal transmission

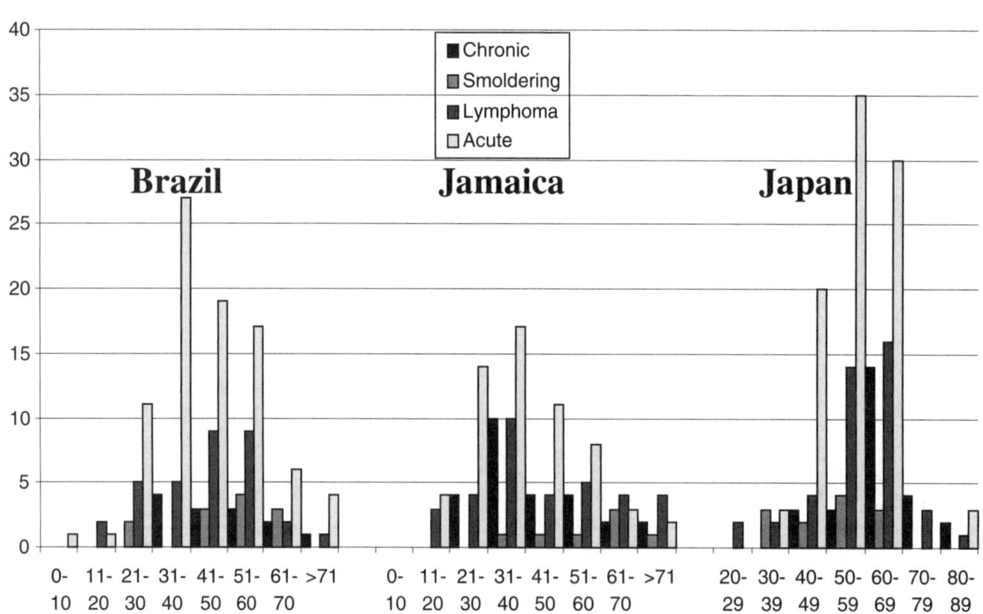

FIGURE 6 Age distribution of ATL patients. Compared here are the age-specific prevalences of ATL in patients from Japan, Brazil, and the Caribbean. Age is given on the *x* axis, and the number of cases is given on the *y* axis. (Courtesy of Barry Haralad and Maria Pombo-Oliveira.)

TABLE 2 Transmission of HTLV-1 and HTLV-2

Mode of transmission or cofactor	HTLV-1	HTLV-2
Mode of transmission		
Mother to infant		
Transplacental	Low efficiency	Not known
Breast milk	High efficiency	Probable but not quantified
Sexual		
Male to female	Most efficient	Yes but not quantified
Female to male	Efficient	Yes but not quantified
Male to male	Efficient	Not known
Parenteral		
Blood transfusion	Very efficient	Very efficient
Intravenous drug use	Efficient	More efficient
Cofactors		
Elevated virus load		
Mother to infant	Yes	Not known
Heterosexual	Yes	Not known
Ulcerative genital lesions	Yes	Not known
Cellular transfusion products	Yes	Yes
Sharing of needles and paraphernalia	Yes	Yes

accounts for approximately 2 to 5% of HTLV-1 infections, and such early-life infections are associated with the greatest risk of ATL. The risk of infection in children of seropositive mothers correlates with the provirus load in breast milk, the concordance of human leukocyte antigen (HLA) class I type between mother and child, and the duration of breast-feeding (12, 99). Among children who received prolonged breast-feeding, the rate of infection ranged between 15 and 25% (174).

In Japanese intervention trials, breast-feeding accounts for most occurrences of perinatal transmission. Although 20% of breast-fed infants seroconvert to HTLV-1 only 1 to 2% of bottle-fed infants of HTLV-1-positive mothers become infected (65). Children usually seroconvert in the first 2 years of life; the rates remain stable until the early teenage years, when new infections occur via sexual transmission. Maternal antibodies, present during the first 6 months of the child's life, appear to provide some protection for children exposed through breast milk, and infection rates increase as maternal antibody levels decline (173).

The viral load of the mother, as measured by antibody titer and viral antigen level, is the best predictor of the risk of mother-to-infant transmission (173), with the risk of transmission found to increase from 4.7/1,000 person-months when the provirus load in breast milk was <0.18% to 28.7/1,000 person-months when it was >1.5% (99). The presence of antibody to the Tax antigen and antibodies to certain envelope epitopes is associated with enhanced transmission. These antibodies are a surrogate for elevated maternal viral load, the major risk factor for transmission (173).

Limited studies of mother-to-child transmission of HTLV-2 infection have been performed to date. The detection of HTLV-2 in breast milk, the 1 to 2% prevalence rate among preadolescent Guaymi Indians (a noninjecting drug use cohort from Panama at high risk for HTLV-2), and finding that seropositive children had seropositive mothers support this route of infection (170).

Sexual Transmission

HTLV-1 is present in genital secretions of infected individuals and can be transmitted through sexual intercourse. Sexual transmission of HTLV-1 occurs more efficiently from males to females than from females to males (94). Numerous studies of married or stable heterosexual couples show a significant excess of couples concordant for HTLV-1 infection. Based on a cohort of discordant couples followed for 10 years in which 27.3% of the initially seronegative women converted to antibody-positive status and 6.7% of the initially seronegative men seroconverted, the incidence rate of male-to-female transmission is found to be 4.2 times higher than that of female-to-male transmission (148).

Markers of sexual activity, such as increased number of sexual partners and contact with female prostitutes, are associated with HTLV-1 transmission. STDs, such as syphilis and genital ulcer disease, are also linked to increased transmission, but female-to-male transmission can occur in the absence of detectable cofactors, as reported among U.S. Marine Corps veterans married to Okinawan women (19). Among homosexual men in Trinidad, the percentage of infected persons increased with the number of lifetime partners (8). The duration of a steady sexual relationship with a seropositive partner is also associated with seroconversion. Elevated HTLV-1 load, as measured by antibody titer or quantitative PCR, correlates with heightened risk of sexual transmission (157). The presence of anti-Tax antibody (perhaps a measure of in vitro proliferation) has also been associated with transmission (27).

Sexual transmission of HTLV-2 has been difficult to study because of the frequency of coincidental injection drug abuse among study populations (e.g., drug-addicted female prostitutes) (81). Among Amerindian populations, sexual transmission of HTLV-2 was documented in cross-sectional studies showing high concordance rates for seropositivity in couples (96).

Parenteral Transmission

Parenteral transmission by transfusion, transplantation, or drug injection is another means of acquiring infection. Although the probability of acquiring infection through transfusion has been significantly decreased through blood donor screening, transfusion of contaminated cellular components can result in seroconversion in more than 40% of recipients (109). Among U.S. blood donors who are confirmed to be HTLV positive, approximately half are HTLV-1 positive and half are HTLV-2 positive. Their major risk factors for infection are injection drug use, having been born in an area where the virus is endemic, and sexual contact with a person with this profile. Characteristics of the donor such as elevated antibody titer (a surrogate for viral load) are not associated with increased risk of transmission. The use of immunosuppressive drugs such as corticosteroids by the recipients of blood components may heighten susceptibility by blunting the cellular immune response to HTLV-1 following exposure. Transmission of HTLV-2 has been well documented for 50% of the recipients of known units of positive blood (37).

HTLV has been considered a contraindication to organ donation, but according to the United Network for Organ Sharing database, the prevalences of HTLV-1 and -2 infections in organ donors are 0.027 and 0.064%, respectively. No reports of HTLV-related diseases in the recipients were reported in one cohort at 1 year posttransplantation (152). The current standard of care involves antibody screening of donors and, if needed because of indeterminant Western blot results, molecular screening (see below) is also performed, an algorithm that has eliminated transplant-associated transmission.

Parenteral drug abuse has been associated with transmission of HTLV-1 and -2, but most HTLV-positive drug abusers are HTLV-2 infected. This suggests a difference in the transmission efficiencies of the two viruses among drug abusers (95). Risk factors for seroconversion include sharing of drug paraphernalia and blood exposure, which was more common before the wide availability of disposable syringes.

Environmental and Socioeconomic Cofactors

There is no evidence for seasonal variation in HTLV infection. Given the relative inefficiency of HTLV-1 transmission and its association with lymphoid cells, vector transmission is not thought to occur (107). The association of HTLV-1 with markers of lower socioeconomic status, such as poor housing, hygiene, and nutrition, remains unexplained.

Other means of transmission are rare. One case of a health care worker who seroconverted to HTLV-1 after experiencing a "microtransfusion" when a syringe loaded with blood punctured his foot (83), as well as transmission of HTLV-2 to a laboratory worker caused by a needlestick injury when she was re-capping a syringe after collecting material for an arterial blood gas analysis (114), are the only reported instances of nosocomial infection to date. Casual contact does not seem to be sufficient for transmission.

PATHOGENESIS

HTLV-1 is associated with two categories of disease: (i) an aggressive CD4 T-cell leukemia/lymphoma called ATL and (ii) a series of virus- and immune-mediated diseases, most prominently a form of chronic inflammatory neurologic disease, HAM/TSP, which is associated with demyelination of the long motor neurons of the spinal cord. In the case of ATL, HTLV-1 is monoclonally integrated into the leukemic cells, whereas in HAM/TSP, neurologic damage appears to result from overexpression of virus and altered immune response. At the center of disease pathogenesis are the gene products of the pX reading frame (*pX* I to *pX* IV in Fig. 2 and Table 1), which not only are engaged in promoting viral replication but also impact cellular functions that favor viral replication. The most important of these viral gene products coded for by pX IV is the p40 Tax viral regulatory protein, which, like its counterpart Tat from HIV-1, plays an important role in promoting viral growth and disease pathogenesis. Both Tax and Tat promote *trans*-acting, transcriptional activation of the LTR, but the effect of Tax on disease pathogenesis appears to be mediated via transactivation of a variety of cellular growth (transcription) factors and bioactive cytokines, interruption of cell cycle regulatory factors resulting in interruption of cell cycle arrest, blocking of normal apoptotic pathways, and interference with DNA repair (Fig. 7). However, Tax expression is not necessary for maintenance of the malignant genotype because, in most ATL cases, Tax is not expressed. In contrast, overexpression of Tax is prominent in the inflammatory and autoimmune diseases linked to HTLV. The additional accessory proteins coded for by the pX region also play a role in pathogenesis.

Incubation Period

The incubation period between infection and disease onset ranges from months to years. Blood transfusion-associated cases of HAM/TSP have developed within a few months of transmission. For ATL, the incubation period appears to be years to decades. For infective dermatitis, a childhood immunodeficiency condition, disease occurs within the first few months of life following infection at birth or via breast milk transmission.

Viral and Host Factors

Tax Modulation of Transcription Factors

Tax protein is responsible for the transactivation of virus transcription not only via *tax*-responsive elements of the viral LTR (Fig. 2) but also through action on a series of cellular transcription factors, including nuclear factor κB (NF-κB), activator protein-1 (AP-1), cyclic AMP response element binding proteins/activating transcription factors (CREB/ATF), serum response factor (SRF), and nuclear factor of activated T cells (NFAT) (Fig. 8). The impact on NF-κB involves not only direct effects on activation but also ubiquitization of the IκB kinase, which turns off the down-modulator of NF-κB activity (61). Tax1 but not Tax2 interacts with NF-κB2/p100 and activates it by inducing the cleavage of p100 into the active transcription factor p52. Activation of NF-κB2/p100 and Tax1 binding to the PDZ domain binding motif (lacking in HTLV-2) are both responsible for the augmented transforming activity of Tax1, which is thought to be crucial to HTLV-1 leukemogenesis (64). A PDZ motif is also present in the C terminus of the HTLV-3 Tax protein, like that in HTLV-1, which is important for cellular signal transduction and transformation; thus, yet-to-be-discovered disease associations with HTLV-3 might be predicted to include lymphoproliferative malignancy (156).

Tax-Induced Transduction of Signaling Molecules in Cellular Proliferation

An important strategy employed by HTLV in promoting T-cell growth involves direct transduction of a series of key signaling molecules (Fig. 8). Tax by transactivation stimulates the gene expression of receptors and their ligands, thus setting up an autocrine stimulatory process that di-

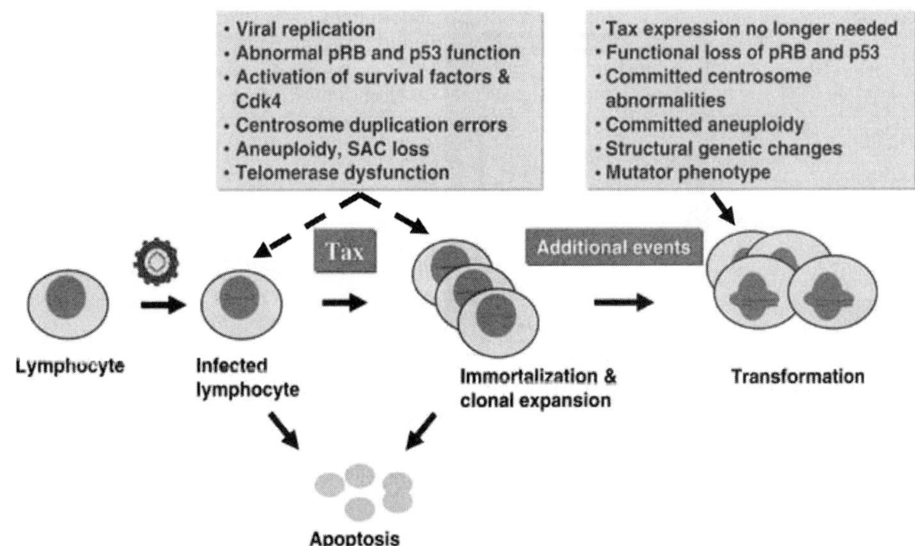

FIGURE 7 HTLV lymphomagenesis: progression of T lymphocytes from immortalization and clonal expansion to transformation. Various changes in the cell during the different stages are listed in the shaded boxes. As shown, virus-infected cells can also go into apoptosis. (Reprinted from reference 56 with permission of Macmillan Publishers Ltd.)

rectly activates transcriptional activation. The first such autocrine loop was recognized for interleukin 2 (IL-2) and the IL-2 receptor (IL-2R).

In addition to transactivation of the pathways detailed above, Tax activates the proto-oncogenes c-*fos* and c-*erg*, as well as the gene for granulocyte-macrophage colony-stimulating factor, an array of early response genes, the human lymphotoxin gene, and parathyroid hormone-related protein gene, while it transrepresses the β-polymerase gene. Overproduction of gamma interferon via this pathway has been implicated in promoting the chronic inflammation that characterizes diseases such as HAM/TSP. In addition to the interaction of Tax with nuclear regulatory elements (e.g., the NF-κB pathway), Tax also operates cytoplasmically through the induction of nuclear translocation of active transcriptional factors, but not via pathways typical of other oncoviral proteins that target tumor suppressor genes (182).

Tax Effects on the Cell Cycle

Tax also has effects on regulators of the cell cycle (Fig. 8). Cyclin D2, required for G_1 cell progression, is a target for up-regulation by Tax. In vitro experiments confirmed that exogenous Tax causes a significant shift of cells from G_0/G_1 to S and G_2/M phases of the cell cycle (101). Tax also induces IL-2 and IL-2R in an autocrine fashion, which also might contribute to the up-regulation of cyclin D2 through its promoter. Thus, Tax up-regulates uncontrolled cell proliferation that promotes the potential for oncogenic transformation and unregulated immune control.

Tax and Tumor Suppressors

Tax stimulates cell growth by directly binding to tumor suppressor genes such as p53, Rb, and human homolog of *Drosophila* discs large (hDLG) (56). p53, a DNA-binding transcription factor that guards against cellular DNA damage and transformation, is inactivated by Tax (120) by competing with it for binding the p300/CBP transcriptional coactivator and/or through an NF-κB/RelA(p65) pathway to perturb p53 function. Tax blocks the ability of p53 to activate DNA repair proteins and to hold the cell at a cycle checkpoint (G_1/S) so that repair cannot be made. As noted below, Tax also blocks apoptosis pathways, so damaged cells do not die but rather persist, which can result in lymphomagenesis (56). Tax causes hyperphosphorylation of the tumor suppressor protein Rb through direct binding of Cdk4, thus supporting cell proliferation and possibly also contributing to its degradation. One of the proteins bound by Tax is hDLG, a human homolog of the *Drosophila* disks large PDZ-containing tumor suppressor that binds Tax1 and is correlated with cellular transformation in vitro. Comparison between HTLV-1 and -2 Tax proteins revealed that the reduced ability of Tax2 to transform cells correlated with a loss of the C-terminal component that binds to the PDZ domain (38).

Tax Modulation of Apoptosis

Tax functions as an oncoprotein both to induce proliferation by mechanisms summarized above and to trigger cellular apoptosis. For example, the Fas (CD95)/FasL pathway and IL-1β-converting enzyme appear to be mediators of the Tax apoptotic effect (29). Tax represses transcription of the Bax gene, the product of which accelerates apoptosis (18). Tax also supports antiapoptotic activity by activating NF-κB (84) and CREB to transactivate BCL2 with inhibition of apoptosis (117), as well as by direct transcriptional transactivation of cellular regulators of apoptosis (130, 164). The choice between proliferation and death is likely influenced by cellular environment, cell background, and whether the cell's tumor suppressor functions have been defeated (56). Another strategy involves Tax making HTLV-infected cells resistant to various physical, chemical, and biological inducers of apoptosis, which may contribute to the risk of malignant transformation because such cells survive with damaged DNA following environmental carcinogenic exposures (79).

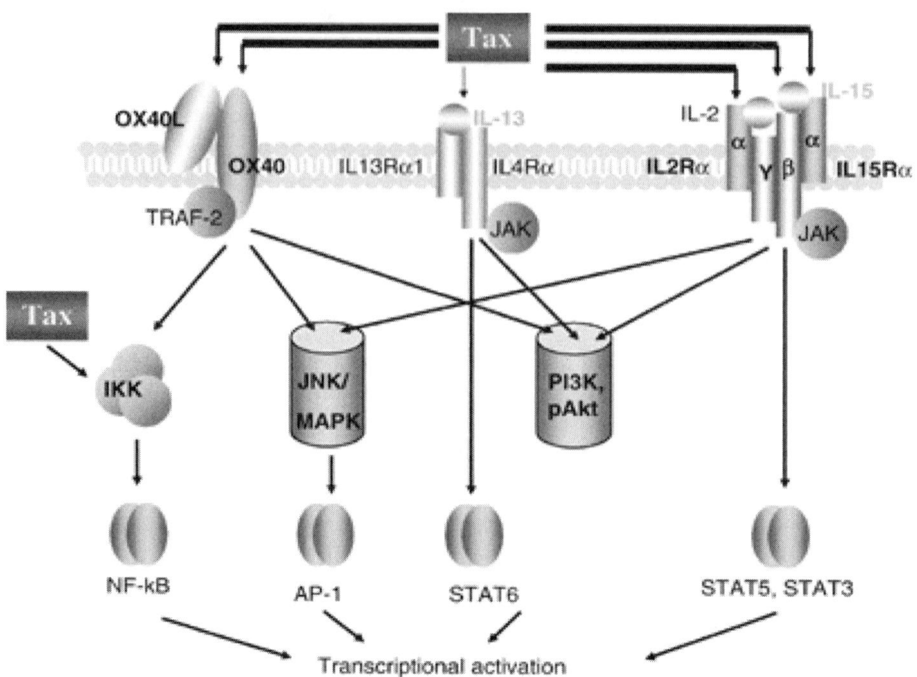

FIGURE 8 Cytoplasmic signaling of Tax-stimulated regulatory proteins. Tax by transactivation stimulates the gene expression of receptors OX40, IL-2Rα, and IL-15Rα1 and ligands OX40L, IL-13, and IL-15. IL-15, which is a close relative of IL-2 that shares a common backbone, is also up-regulated, as are the separate IL-4/IL-13R and IL-13 ligand and OX40 receptor and OX40 ligand. The activation of both ligand and receptor for OX40, a member of the tumor necrosis factor family, suggests that costimulatory signals delivered from OX40 contribute to a transformed phenotype. Receptor ligand binding results in the activation of growth- and survival-controlling signaling cascades and activation of transcription factors employing the Janus tyrosine kinase (JAK3) signal transducer of activated T cells (STAT5a and STAT5b) pathway to enter the nucleus and stimulate target gene transcription. Tax also stimulates transforming growth factor β1 to protect infected cells from cytotoxicity but employs transcription factors Smad 3 and Smad 4 to repress transforming growth factor β1, thus modulating this effect to the advantage of HTLV-induced cell proliferation. (Reprinted from reference 56 with permission of Macmillan Publishers Ltd.)

Tax DNA Repair and Aneuploidy

In addition to its negative impacts on p53's DNA repair function, Tax also induces structural DNA damage and alters chromosomal stability, resulting in harm to the cell's genomic integrity on the path to malignant transformation (Fig. 7). DNA polymerase β is down-regulated by Tax, affecting both base excision repair (72) and nucleotide excision repair (80). The telomerase reverse transcriptase (TERT) gene is inhibited by Tax, which also contributes to chromosomal instability, resulting in telomere shortening and eventual senescence through competition by Tax for the MYC binding site in the TERT promoter (74, 82). The high frequency of aneuploidy observed in ATL appears to result from Tax directly binding to mitotic arrest deficiency protein 1 (MAD1) and disturbing segregation of chromosomes during mitosis (74). Additionally, Tax also induces defective mitotic spindle assembly checkpoint function (82) and causes abnormal amplification of cellular centrosomes, which causes chromosomal missegregation (56).

As noted above, Tax also inactivates p53 and Rb, which are essential to repair at the G_1 tetraploid/polyploid checkpoint (161). Given the high frequency of aneuploidy in ATL, the transition from oligoclonal expansion to malignant transformation is brought about by the impact of Tax on chromosomal stability (56).

Effects of pX I and II Proteins

pX I produces $p12^I$, which activates NFAT, localizes in the endoplasmic reticulum and *cis*-Golgi apparatus, and elevates cytoplasmic calcium, which precedes T-cell activation and is essential for establishing persistent infection. In addition, $p12^I$ targets cellular pathways involved in T-cell proliferation through the STAT5 pathway, thus contributing, along with Tax, to T-cell activation. $p12^I$ also interferes with trafficking of the heavy chain of major histocompatibility complex (MHC) class I to the surface of T cells, thus contributing to persistence of infected cells by blocking immune recognition. $p13^{II}$ localizes to the mitochondria. $p30^{II}$ localizes to the nucleolus, stabilizes p53, and abrogates p53 suppressor cell function (43), as well as the function of other cell cycle regulators (33). The interaction between $p30^{II}$ and Rex appears to govern the switch between virus latency and replication (153).

Immune Responses

In the face of prodigious mechanisms for expansion of viral infection, a robust and targeted cell-mediated immune response is mounted to control viral infection. In most cases, this response is effective given the relatively infrequent occurrence of disease among carriers, but at times the immune response may contribute to disease occurrence.

Viral Load

Until molecular amplification tools became available, it was assumed that HTLV-1 had a low rate of expression because levels of plasma-associated virus were undetectable and the variation in sequence diversity around the world was minimal. HIV-1, in contrast, was shown to have a very high rate of virus production and high levels of plasma-associated virus, rapid turnover, and a highly mutable genome responding to strong selective pressures from the immune system. However, the proviral load of HTLV-1 is remarkably high compared with that of other retroviruses (127). Quantitative PCR shows that the median proviral load among healthy carriers involves between 0.1 and 1.0% of peripheral blood cells (30). In patients with HAM/TSP, between 5 and 10% of peripheral blood cells are infected, and in some cases 30% of peripheral blood cells harbor the virus. Careful molecular analysis of HTLV-1 in various disease states has indicated that HTLV-1 infection is largely an oligoclonal rather than a polyclonal expansion. These observations are consistent with the hypothesis that most HTLV-1 replication and expansion occur via proliferation of infected cells containing integrated provirus rather than through infection by free virions. As a consequence, discussed below, cell-mediated immune responses are key for controlling viral infection.

Humoral Immune Responses

Antibodies to the various antigens of HTLV-1 occur at high levels in carriers and among patients with ATL and HAM/TSP. During primary HTLV infection, the first specific antibodies to emerge are directed against the Gag proteins. Over several weeks to months, anti-Env antibodies appear and about 50% of infected individuals develop detectable antibodies to p40 Tax protein (27). Antibody titers vary from patient to patient, are significantly higher in patients with HAM/TSP and among those at risk for this disease, and correlate with the proviral burden (30, 173). This may explain the paradoxical finding of high antibody titers among women who transmit HTLV-1 to their infants through prolonged breast-feeding (174). The explanation for this paradox is that transplacental maternal antibodies appear to protect the infant from infection in the first months of life, but subsequently the infant becomes infected via maternal virus transmitted via breast milk, most likely by cell-associated infection. Other than this apparent protection afforded the baby through passive antibody transfer from an infected mother at birth, few data suggest that humoral immune responses play a role in protection from disease. The high titers observed in patients with HAM/TSP and ATL seem to reflect immune responses in the context of high viral burden observed in these conditions rather than as a direct correlate of disease risk.

Cell-Mediated Immunity

Cytotoxic T lymphocytes (CTL) targeted at viral antigens expressed on infected cells play an essential role in the regulation of viral expression. Among chronic carriers, infected individuals mount a strong cell-mediated immune response to the virus, and up to 1% of CD8-positive CTL can recognize at least one epitope of HTLV. Freshly isolated cells have substantial expression of activation markers, indicating that these cells have recently encountered the Tax antigen (59, 69, 135).

Host Virus Immune Response

A proposed model of this viral interaction with the host cell-mediated immune response is shown in Fig. 9.

HAM/TSP

In the case of HAM/TSP, there is an imbalance in immune response manifested by an overexpression of Tax, high levels of Tax-specific CTL, and excessive elevation of HTLV viral load. For instance, CXCL10/IP-10, a T-helper type 1 (Th1)-associated chemokine, has been found to be significantly elevated in the cerebrospinal fluid (CSF) of HAM /TSP patients compared to healthy controls (129). Other cytokines in the Th1 pathway such as transcription factors T-beta, GATA-3, IL-12Rβ2, and suppressors of cytokine signaling are also markedly elevated in HAM/TSP patients (57). The role for CD8-mediated cell killing as the primary means of viral suppression may explain the epidemiological observation that recipients of infected blood products who are also receiving exogenous immunosuppressive medications are more susceptible to HTLV-1 infection, due to the host's inability to clear initial virus infection (109). CD4 CD25 T-cell subsets, the target of HTLV-1 infection (Fig. 9), stimulate and expand HTLV-I Tax-specific CD8 T cells, which may play an important role in the pathogenesis of HTLV-1-associated neurologic disease (179). The finding that Tax1A is more frequent in HAM/TSP than Tax1B may point to a viral motif in Tax1A that contributes to pathogenesis. Such a mechanism is consistent with the hypothesis that there is molecular mimicry between a viral and cellular antigen. This hypothesis is supported by the finding that HAM/TSP patients make antibodies to heterogeneous nuclear ribonuclear protein A1 (hnRNP A1), a neuron-specific autoantigen (97). Monoclonal antibodies to Tax cross-reacted with hnRNP A1 show molecular mimicry between the two proteins and provide a pathogenic basis for autoimmune neurologic disease. Additionally, the finding that there are oligoclonal immunoglobulin bands in the CSF of HAM/TSP patients that react to HTLV-1 antigens supports this hypothesis (69).

Host Immunogenetic Factors

An association between class I HLA haplotypes and protection against HAM/TSP suggests that carriers of certain antigen-presenting motifs augment the efficient control of HTLV-1-containing cells. Thus, carriers of the HLA-A*02 haplotype are less prone to developing HAM/TSP. Non-HLA-A*02-positive carriers may be at increased risk of HAM/TSP because of an impaired cell-mediated immune response against HTLV-infected cells, resulting in overexpression of HTLV (4, 73). Additionally, HLA-DRB1*0101 doubles the odds of HAM/TSP in the absence of the protective effect of HLA-A*02 (73). These data suggest that deficient immune recognition of Tax epitopes blunts a robust cell-mediated immune response.

Impact of CD8 Lymphotropism of HTLV-2

In contrast to the predominant CD4 lymphotropism of HTLV-1, HTLV-2 provirus in vivo is integrated at the

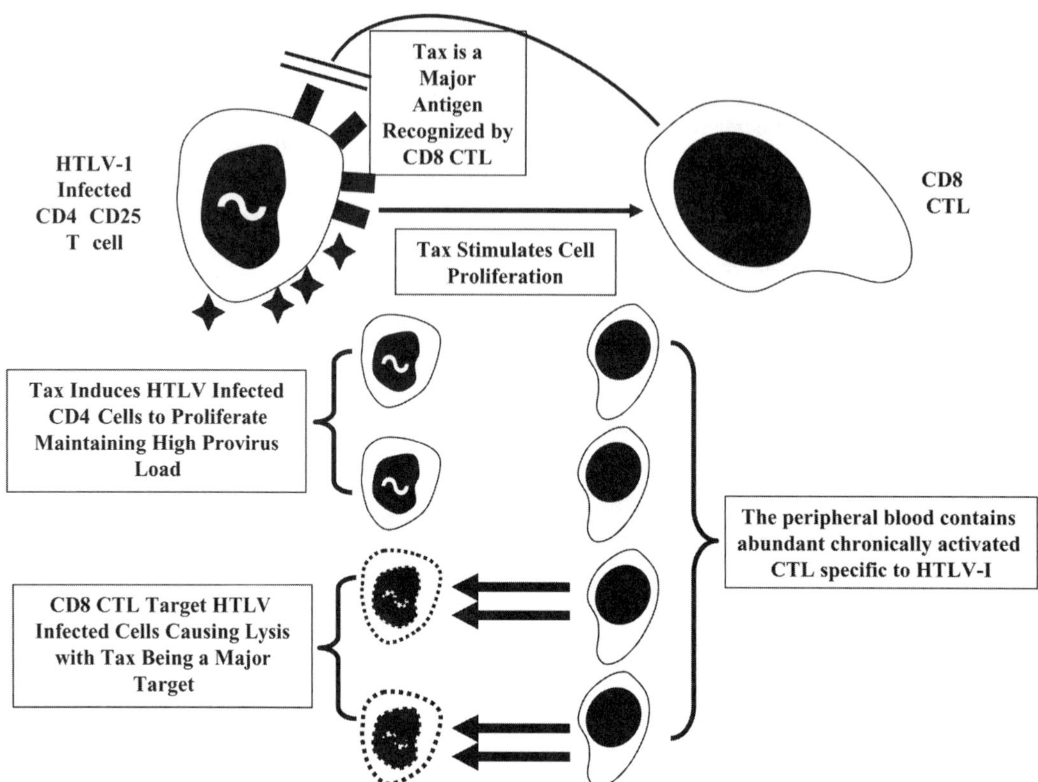

FIGURE 9 Model of CD8 CTL-mediated control of HTLV-1 infection. HTLV-1 infects CD4 T lymphocytes, with expansion of infection primarily via cell replication. As HTLV-1-specific antigens, particularly Tax, are expressed, a robust CD8 CTL response is generated that results in killing of CD4-infected cells. The inability of some persons to control HTLV-1 expansion is thought to contribute to disease pathogenesis. In this model, the dynamic equilibrium between viral replication and immune destruction is mediated through Tax overexpression, causing CD4 target cell proliferation and a robust cell-mediated response to the antigen in particular, thereby leading to CTL-mediated lysis of these HTLV-1-infected CD4 cells (59, 70, 71, 135). As a consequence of ongoing Tax proliferation, there is a cell-associated expansion of HTLV-1 genome-containing CD4 cells and a compensatory expansion of CD8 CTL. As the number of CD4 cells containing the HTLV-1 genome expands, HTLV-1 antigens are expressed on the cell surface and become targets for CD8-mediated cytotoxic killing. (Reprinted from reference 3b with permission of the publisher.)

highest levels into CD8 lymphocytes but may also be demonstrated in CD4 cells (93). A delayed hypersensitivity response is normal among HTLV-2-infected individuals, suggesting intact cell-mediated or Th1-type immunity (125). Although subtle differences may exist, the overall distribution of lymphocyte subsets is not perturbed in persons with HTLV-2 (88, 140). However, total immunoglobulin G levels are higher in HTLV-2-infected persons (146), and HTLV-2 may induce expression of gamma interferon, granulocyte macrophage colony-stimulating factor, and other cytokines (17, 98). Although HTLV-2 provirus has also been demonstrated in macrophages (183), whether such infection influences macrophage regulation or function to a clinically notable degree is not known. More intensive diagnostic evaluation and follow-up of HTLV-2-infected individuals is needed to confirm the relationship between HTLV-2 and recurrent pneumonia or asthma, and other diseases.

Natural History of Associated Diseases

ATL

Following initial infection, there is a proliferation of infected cells that is down-modulated by CTL immune responses. No acute infection syndrome has been identified. Oligoclonal infection of mainly CD4 postthymic T cells manifests within months, and the infected cells resemble transformed, but not malignant, cells (157). In some instances, monoclonal infection of T cells is observed. Such oligoclonal and monoclonal expansions have been noted to appear and sometimes disappear spontaneously. Thus, for ATL, the net effect of Tax and other ORF products is that the normal checks to transition between cell cycle phases are abrogated (Fig. 7), thus contributing to the potential for heightened mutation. Genetic damage that would normally be repaired accumulates, apoptotic cell death does not occur, and Tax induces aneuploidy directly—all in the path to malignancy. Subsequently, T cells can accumulate DNA mutations, resulting in transformation and monoclonal outgrowth of a truly malignant cell. At the stage of malignancy, the *tax* gene is silent and Tax is no longer expressed, as transformation of the malignant cell is complete.

HAM/TSP

The pathogenesis of HAM/TSP appears to involve dysregulation of immune function. This condition and other diseases with "autoimmune" manifestations of HTLV-1, coupled with the inability to down-regulate HTLV-1 expression, appear to result from a failure of the cell-mediated immune response in HAM/TSP among carriers at risk. In the case of HAM/TSP, the major pathological manifestations appear to result from collateral damage to neurologic tissues as part of a cell-mediated immune assault on abundant CD4 HTLV-1-containing cells that infiltrate the central nervous system (CNS) (60). Elevated levels of lymphokines such as IL-6, tumor necrosis factor beta (TNF-β), and IL-2 are found in the CSF. However, attempts to document the presence of HTLV-1 in demyelinated lesions have not demonstrated a direct role for the virus in the target cell.

It is possible that HTLV-1 induces an autoimmune-like process through molecular mimicry or by indirect effects on immune function. Autoantibodies against nuclear and perinuclear human brain proteins cross-reacting with different HTLV-1 epitopes have been found in the sera of HAM/TSP patients (49). Virus loads are high in HAM/TSP, suggesting a deficiency in the ability of the host to control viral proliferation. Furthermore, the pattern of oligoclonal expansion observed in healthy carriers is amplified in HAM/TSP. Up to one in five peripheral blood cells is infected with a high proportion of CD8-positive CTL targeting HTLV-1. Immunogenetic factors are associated with disease and possibly overexpression of the virus (154).

The finding of HTLV-1 in CD8 cells and the coincidence of CD8 cells in spinal cord lesions raise the possibility that these cells may contribute to induction of local spinal cord damage. Alternatively, because CTL against HTLV-1 account for a significant percentage of such lymphocytes, the pathogenesis of demyelination has been hypothesized to result from collateral damage due to local overproduction of harmful cytokines secreted by these cells. Thus, the tissue damage in the CNS in patients with HAM/TSP may be caused by lymphocytes chronically activated by the HTLV-1 Tax protein, which cause secretion of harmful cytokines and metalloproteinases in the local environment (4, 10). The CD4 CD25 T-cell population is the main reservoir for HTLV-1 in HAM/TSP patients (181).

Other HTLV-Associated Conditions

For other HTLV-1-associated autoimmune diseases such as uveitis and arthritis, HTLV-1-infected cells at the site of pathological changes and lymphokine and cytokine overexpression may account for the local pathological manifestations (67). Such a model of acute tissue damage is consistent with the short latency for HAM/TSP.

CLINICAL MANIFESTATIONS

Acute seroconversion is associated with no clinical syndrome: the time from infection to seroconversion can vary from 1 to 2 months, as seen with transfusion cases. The time from seroconversion to disease can vary from 18 weeks with HAM/TSP to many decades with ATL. As summarized in Table 3, there are a wide range of clinical conditions linked to HTLV-1, some of which result from virally induced cell transformation, as in ATL, while others appear to result from the indirect effects of virus-induced immunologic perturbation.

ATL

Before the discovery and isolation of HTLV-1, ATL was characterized as an aggressive leukemia/lymphoma of mature T lymphocytes, with varied clinical manifestations: generalized lymphadenopathy, visceral involvement, hypercalcemia, cutaneous skin involvement, lytic bone lesions, and leukemia cells with pleotrophic features. Almost all patients with ATL present with lymphadenopathy and 50% have hepatosplenomegaly (160).

The Lymphoma Study Group in Japan has classified ATL into four clinical types based on clinical features and cell morphology: acute, chronic, smoldering, and lymphoma/leukemia types (178). Figure 10 shows the characteristic morphological features of the leukemia cells and examples of the cutaneous manifestations that may be the first indication of disease. The prototypic acute ATL is distinguished by increased numbers of leukemic T cells with characteristic pleomorphic morphology (Fig. 10A), skin lesions (Fig. 10D), systemic lymphadenopathy, hepatosplenomegaly, and metabolic disorders, especially hypercalcemia.

Chronic ATL (Fig. 10B) resembles chronic T-lymphocytic leukemia; cells have a characteristic cleaved morphology called buttock cells, the white blood cell count is increased, and skin lesions are evident. Some patients manifest mild lymphadenopathy and hepatosplenomegaly, and the serum lactate dehydrogenase level is sometimes elevated. Hypercalcemia and hyperbilirubinemia are not characteristic of this type of ATL.

Smoldering ATL (Fig. 10C) may clinically resemble mycosis fungoides/Sézary syndrome, with cutaneous involvement manifesting as erythema or as infiltrative plaques or tumors (Fig. 10D), and Pautrier's microabscesses characteristic of mycosis fungoides may be observed. This

TABLE 3 HTLV-associated diseases[a]

Disease	HTLV-1	HTLV-2
Childhood		
Infective dermatitis	++++	No
Persistent lymphadenopathy	++	No
Adult		
ATL	+++	No
HTLV-associated myelopathy	++++	+++
Infective dermatitis	+++	No
Polymyositis	++	Unknown
Uveitis	+++	Unknown
HTLV-associated arthritis	+++	Unknown
Sjögren syndrome	+++	Unknown
Strongyloidiasis	++	Unknown
Pulmonary infiltrative pneumonitis	++	Unknown
Invasive cervical cancer	+	Unknown
Small cell carcinoma of lung	+	Unknown

[a] ++++, very strong evidence; +++, strong evidence; ++, possible association; +, weak association; no, evidence does not support association; unknown, no data to support association or lack of association.

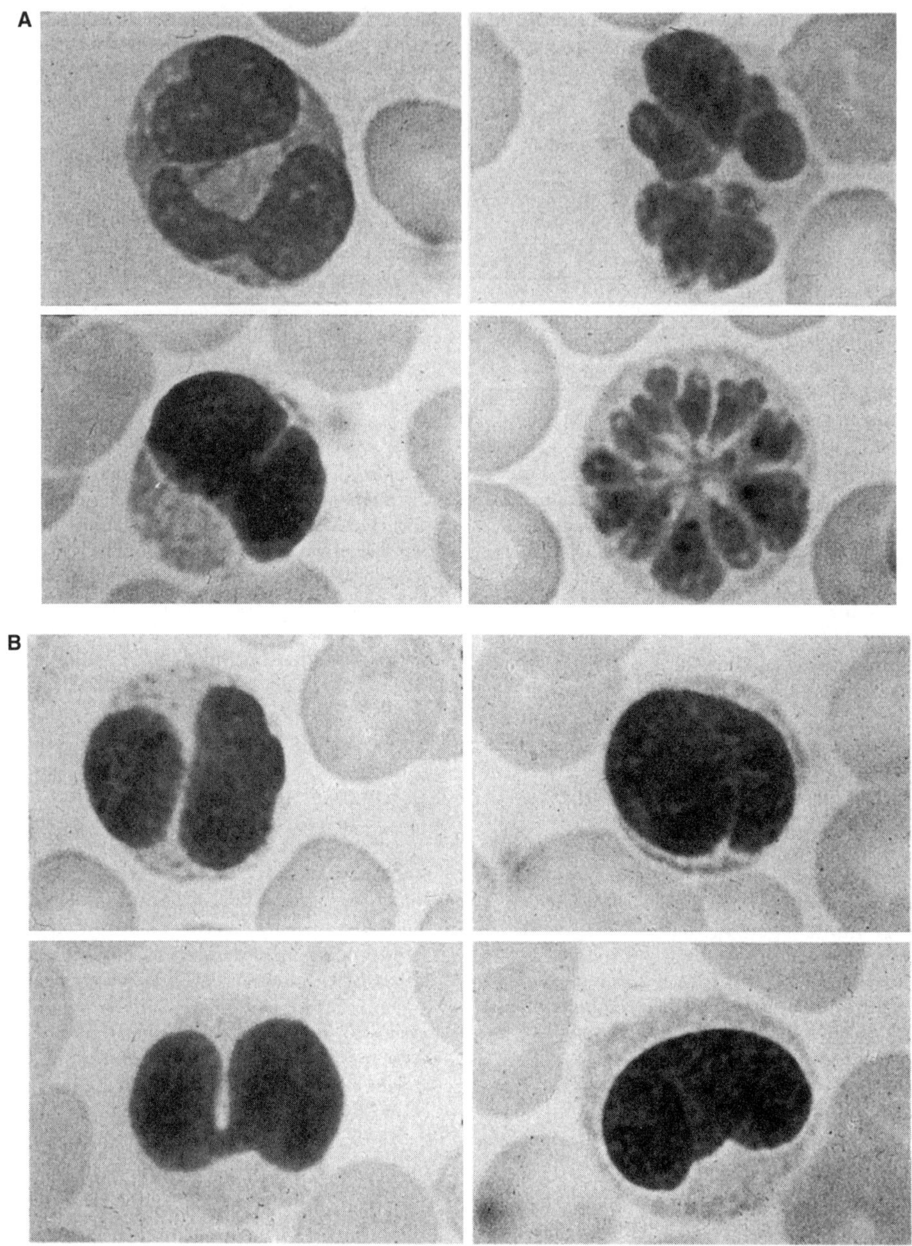

FIGURE 10 Photomicrographs of typical peripheral blood leukemic cells from patients with acute ATL (A), chronic ATL (B), and smoldering ATL (C) and cutaneous manifestations (D). Details of the features are discussed in the text. (Panels A, B, and C are reprinted from reference 178 and panel D is reprinted from reference 177 with permission of the publisher.)

was the case in the first patient from whom the virus was isolated in the United States by Gallo and colleagues (48).

In patients with chronic or smoldering ATL, a long prodrome of symptoms or signs is usually noted before transformation to an acute ATL. Sometimes ATL manifests as a non-Hodgkin's T-cell lymphoma with no other clinical features of ATL except monoclonal integration of HTLV-1 in the proviral DNA of the tumor cells. These cases are termed lymphoma-type ATL and are indistinguishable from peripheral T-cell lymphomas.

Between 50 and 60% of ATL patients have the acute type, 20% have the chronic and lymphoma type, and 5% have the smoldering type. Most patients with the acute and lymphoma types die within 6 months of diagnosis in the absence of therapy (Fig. 11), particularly if hypercalcemia is a presenting sign. In general, the smoldering type is the least aggressive; patients with the chronic type have a relatively poor prognosis, with death occurring within a few years of diagnosis. The cause of death is usually an explosive growth of tumor cells, hypercalcemia, bacterial sepsis, and other infections observed in patients with immunodeficiency.

Opportunistic infections are often present and contribute to a rapid progression to death in patients with acute

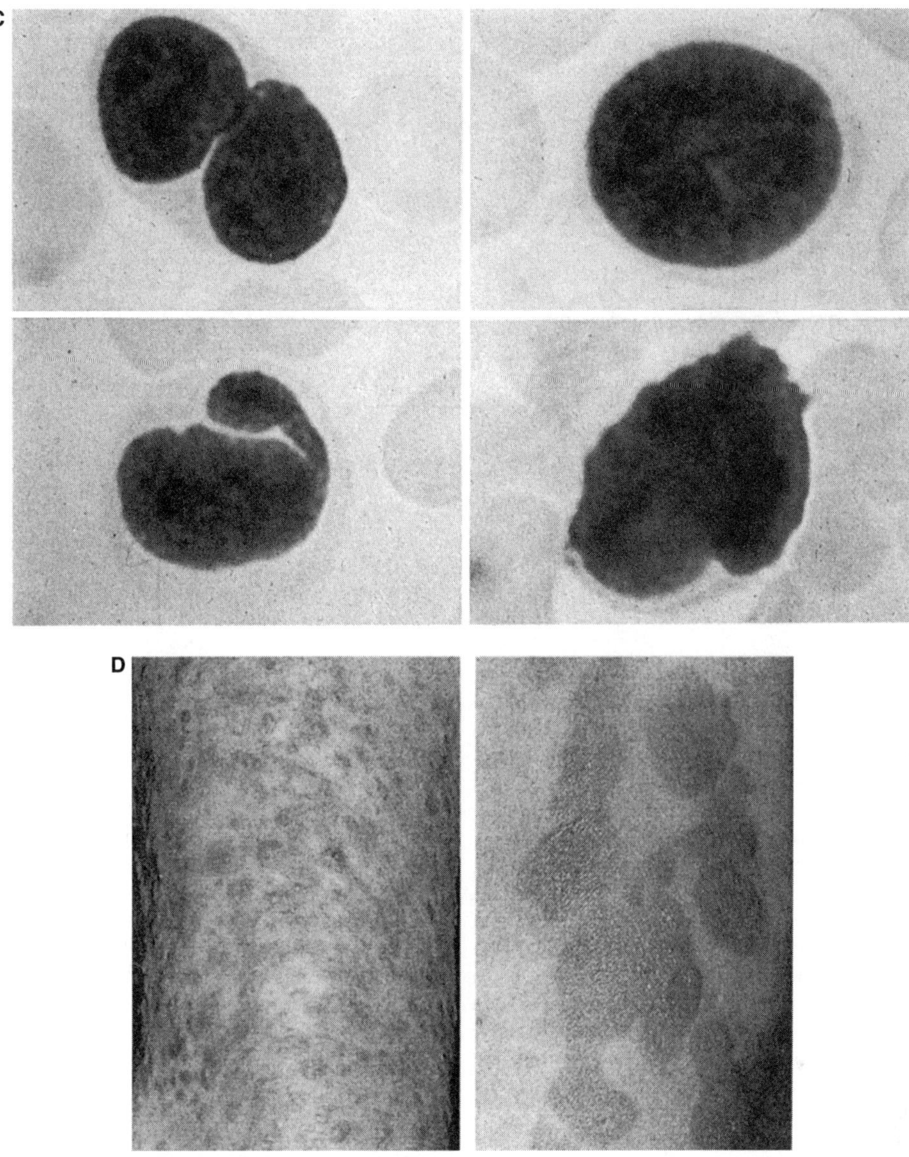

FIGURE 10 *(Continued)*

and lymphoma-type ATL. Immunocompromise is not due to the type of immune ablation observed for HIV-1, even though CD4 cells are infected by HTLV-1; rather, the immunodeficiency is associated with rapidly proliferating malignancy, and the pattern of opportunistic infections is typical for those reported for patients with aggressive non-Hodgkin's lymphomas.

The diagnosis of ATL is based on testing serum for HTLV-1 antibodies in patients with the characteristic features of T-cell malignancy. Proviral HTLV-1 can also be detected in the blood leukemia cells or in biopsy specimens from the patient, but such studies require a laboratory with specialized expertise. In some cases of ATL in patients from high-risk areas with typical clinical features, antibody is absent but a defective integrated virus with a retained *tax* function can be detected with sophisticated molecular probes (89).

Other Cancers

HTLV-1 has been associated with isolated cases of other malignancies. In one case of small cell cancer of the lung, viral sequences were monoclonally integrated into the tumor cells (112). There is a statistically increased prevalence of HTLV-1 antibodies in patients with invasive carcinoma of the cervix, but this could result from shared sexual risk factors rather than a direct effect of HTLV-1 in carcinogenesis. Japanese patients with a variety of malignancies show elevated rates of HTLV-1 infections compared with healthy populations, but biases such as blood transfusion might have influenced the association.

HAM/TSP

The onset of HAM/TSP is often subtle, and the florid clinical picture is not usually seen at first presentation. A single symptom or physical sign may be the only evidence

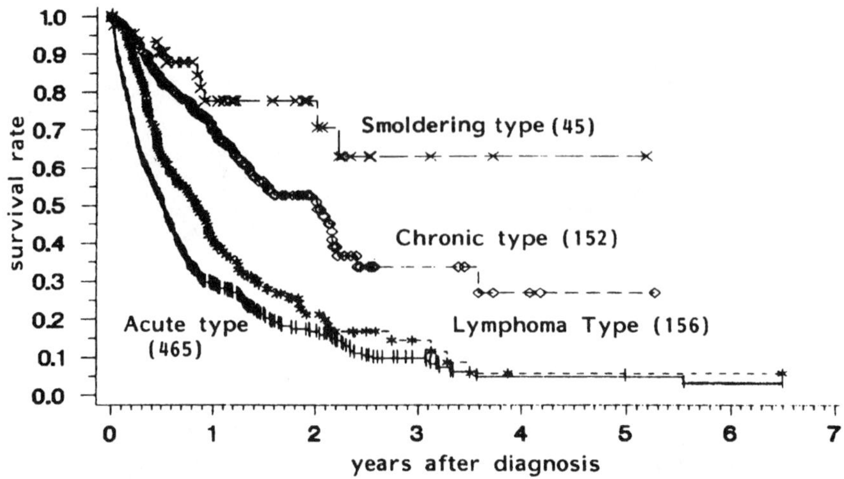

FIGURE 11 Survival patterns of patients with different ATL subtypes after polychemotherapy. Patients with acute and lymphoma-type ATL have the poorest prognosis after chemotherapy (see the text). (Reprinted from reference 165 with permission of the publisher.)

of early HAM/TSP. Symptoms often begin with a stiff gait, progressing (usually slowly) to increasing spasticity and lower-extremity weakness, back pain, urinary incontinence, and impotence in men. Patients may complain of sensory symptoms such as tingling, pins and needles, and burning. Vibration sense is frequently impaired. Hyperreflexia of lower limbs, often with clonus and Babinski's sign, may be detected. Hyperreflexia of upper limbs, as well as positive Hoffmann's and Tromner's signs, are also frequent. Exaggerated jaw jerk is seen in some patients, and ataxia sometimes develops. Magnetic resonance imaging sometimes detects isolated lesions of the CNS (86). The syndrome is significantly different from classic multiple sclerosis. HAM/TSP follows a slow course without the waxing and waning of symptoms characteristic of multiple sclerosis and without the changes in affect or the multiple magnetic resonance imaging abnormalities.

HAM/TSP patients characteristically have HTLV-1 antibodies or antigens in the blood and CSF. Detection of provirus load in CSF is associated with HAM/TSP (180). CSF may show mild lymphocytic pleocytosis; lobulated lymphocytes with morphological similarity to ATL cells may also be present in the blood and CSF. Mild to moderate increases in protein levels may be observed in the CSF, and oligoclonal bonds with specific reactivity to HTLV-1 antigens are detected (69).

The diagnosis of HAM/TSP is suspected in unexplained CNS disease with loss of pyramidal tract functions and is confirmed by a positive result when testing sera for HTLV-1 antibodies. The definite diagnosis of HAM/TSP requires demonstration of HTLV-1 infection and the exclusion of other causes of myelopathy, such as spinal cord compression, paraneoplastic syndromes, parasitic myelopathy, vitamin B_{12} and folate deficiency, multiple sclerosis, and amyotrophic lateral sclerosis, among others. A modified model is proposed for diagnosing HAM/TSP with levels of ascertainment as definite, probable, and possible, according to myelopathic symptoms, serologic findings, and/or detection of HTLV-I DNA and exclusion of other disorders (34).

The link of HTLV-2 with HAM/TSP is now well established, although the case attack rate appears to be less than that for HTLV-1 carriers, including an ongoing prospective follow-up of a U.S. transfusion cohort (134). Some of the HTLV-2-positive cases had features reminiscent of the ataxic form of HAM/TSP found in Jamaica. Patients have oligoclonal bands in the CSF reminiscent of what is observed for HTLV-1-positive patients with specific reactivity for virus-specific antigens: an indirect mechanism of pathogenesis like that seen in HTLV-1-induced perturbation of immune function has been hypothesized. The demyelinating lesions from these patients show infiltration with CD8 cells, and only rarely is an HTLV-2-positive cell observed in lesions.

Other Syndromes

In areas where the virus is endemic, skeletal muscle polymyositis is associated with HTLV-1 seropositivity; these cases are indistinguishable from the polymyositis seen in areas where HTLV-1 is not endemic. A large-joint polyarthropathy has been reported in Japan among elderly patients (67). A distinguishing feature of these cases is the presence of HTLV-1-producing cells in the synovial infiltrate. Another disease associated with HTLV-1 is uveitis. Patients with HTLV-1-positive uveitis complain of blurred, foggy vision or ocular floaters with an acute or subacute onset. Visual acuity is moderately affected. The most characteristic findings are vitreous opacities associated with mild iritis and mild retinal vasculitis. The clinical course is slowly progressive or persistent unless the condition is treated with corticosteroids. More than 90% of cases recur within 3 years, with a mean interval between episodes of 16 months (128).

Although there is no proven etiologic link, a few individuals from Japan with HTLV-1 infection have presented with CD4 cell decline and AIDS-like opportunistic infection in the absence of HIV infection or other predisposing underlying malignancy such as ATL (158). Strongyloidiasis refractory to treatment has also been reported to occur in HTLV-1 carriers (151). Among older adults, HTLV-1 carriers have decreased skin test response to recall antigens (172). HTLV-1 has also been associated with Sjögren syndrome (42). An increased prevalence of HTLV-1 among tuberculosis patients and a high prevalence of tuberculosis among HTLV-1-infected individuals exist (110). Additionally, HTLV-1 carriers have a reduced delayed-type hypersensitivity response to *Mycobacterium tuberculosis* purified protein derivative (111). These data are consistent with the concept that HTLV-1 is associated with some forms of subtle immune perturbation.

The association of infective dermatitis syndrome with HTLV-1 infection in children in Jamaica (91) appears to be an immunodeficiency syndrome induced by HTLV-1 and represents the first childhood HTLV-1 syndrome. These patients are born to HTLV-1-positive mothers and experience a syndrome of failure to thrive. They are prone to refractory generalized eczema with exudates and crusting on the scalp, ear, eyelid margins, paranasal skin, neck, axilla, and groin. Recurrent bacterial superinfections with beta-hemolytic streptococci, *Staphylococcus aureus*, or both are frequent but can be suppressed by chronic antibiotic therapy (133). This syndrome usually emerges in the first few years after birth and can persist into adulthood. Infrequent cases emerging in adolescence suggest that induction of disease can occur following exposure of young adults. Some affected individuals go on to develop ATL or HAM/TSP.

Whether coinfection with HTLV-1 and HIV-1 results in a more rapid progression to AIDS is controversial. Given the effect of HTLV-1 Tax on cellular proliferation, a number of in vitro studies document accelerated killing of HIV-1-infected cells that might predict an influence of HTLV infection on HIV-1-related AIDS progression. Several epidemiological studies suggest that HTLV-1 infection can promote HIV-1 replication and accelerate the clinical progression to AIDS, but other studies have not confirmed this observation (23).

HTLV-2 Disease Associations

The original isolations of HTLV-2 came from patients diagnosed with T-cell hairy cell leukemia. In one of these cases, the tumor involved B cells, while the HTLV-2 was in the T cells (144). Several cases of large granulocytic cell leukemia (a non-T-cell malignancy with a similar pattern) have also been reported (78, 145). It is possible that these leukemias are the same entity. Systematic surveys have not identified a clear association of this type of lymphoid malignancy with HTLV-2, suggesting that these patients may be coincidentally infected (41). In addition to an increased risk of HAM/TSP with HTLV-2 infection (described above), HTLV-2-positive drug users also show an excess of asthma-related deaths and an increased frequency of skin and soft tissue infections (116).

HTLV-2-infected individuals may show increased incidences of acute bronchitis, bladder or kidney infection, arthritis, and asthma, and a higher incidence of pneumonia than HTLV-seronegative individuals (124). The biological basis for a putative increased susceptibility to certain infections in humans with chronic HTLV-2 infection is not well described.

LABORATORY DIAGNOSIS

Virus Isolation

Isolation of HTLV by culture is used only in the context of research studies to characterize the viral sequence and study disease pathogenesis and is not a routine diagnostic procedure. The technique employs cocultivation of patient cells with human peripheral blood mononuclear cells that have been stimulated in vitro with mitogens (e.g., phytohemagglutinin) and growth factors (e.g., IL-2). When peripheral blood from patients with ATL is cultured, the virus-positive cell that emerges has a normal karyotype and the tumor cells themselves do not grow.

Another method of virus detection is the antigen capture assay. Because HTLV-1 is so strongly cell associated, plasma antigenemia is not present at detectable levels. Antigen assays are used for detection of virus antigen in the supernatant of short-term cell cultures.

Nucleic Acid Detection

PCR assays previously employed in the research setting to confirm HTLV infection, distinguish HTLV type, and quantify the level of virus under various clinical conditions (62) are now available commercially to clinicians in practice. Refinements of the PCR assay resulted in a highly sensitive and reproducible detection system with limits of detection at 10 molecules of DNA in 1 mg of human DNA (about 1 infected cell in 100,000 peripheral blood mononuclear cells) (127). Provirus load is the most frequently used marker for prognosis and disease progression in infected patients. With some modification, the technique is also used in real time to detect viral RNA in different infected cells. This helps to identify actively replicating virus to evaluate viral gene expression and to correlate transcript levels to key stages of the virus life cycle and, ultimately, pathogenesis. Commercial molecular detection is increasingly being applied in the clinical setting, for example, to distinguish a false-positive antibody test or to confirm infection in the context of transplantation. For research applications, flow-based systems have allowed the detection of cell-specific viral antigen expression, usually Gag or Tax specific in subsets of T lymphocytes (59).

Serologic Assays

The primary test for HTLV-1 or -2 infection is detection of virus-specific antibody by a variety of techniques. Because HTLV infection is chronic, almost all HTLV-1 antibody-positive patients are also virus positive. Samples are first screened by one of several assays using whole-virus lysates, sometimes enriched with recombinant antigens. The most widely used assay for detection of HTLV-1 in the United States is the enzyme-linked immunosorbent assay (ELISA) technique, using whole disrupted virus. In Japan, a particle agglutination assay is used. These assays are highly sensitive and specific for virus infection (104). The ELISAs for HTLV-1 and -2 are cross-reactive. Virus subtype is distinguished by Western blot technology, which uses a combination of whole virus and recombinantly produced peptides. This assay is used to confirm that an ELISA sample is truly positive and to distinguish between HTLV-1 and HTLV-2 types (25). The criterion for Western blot confirmation is the presence of antibody to the p24 *gag* gene product and one of the HTLV-1 *env* gene products, p21e (transmembrane), gp46 (external envelope), or gp61 (whole envelope). Sera with no reactivity to viral protein bands are considered negative; sera with partial reactivity are called indeterminate. Because the virus is highly cell associated, additional tests are sometimes needed to demonstrate antibody to the *env*-encoded components of the virus. Additional approaches, such as the line immunoassay, are gaining popularity because they identify the virus type without the need for confirmation by Western blotting (171). Confirmation by immunofluorescence assay is often used for the particle agglutination assay in Japan. Titer determination to allow quantification of antibody is possible with modifications to the ELISA and particle agglutination assay.

Cellular Assays

In the research setting, detection of cellular immune responses to HTLV-1 involves standard CTL assays using chromium release by either leukemic cells or transformed cells treated with HTLV-1 peptides or infected with recombinant virus. More recently, flow cytometry-based assays adapting tetramer technology have provided a much more precise measure of cell-specific CTL quantities. In these assays, peripheral blood mononuclear cells can be directly quantitated by the ability of MHC class I-restricted tetramers to bind Tax peptides (59).

PREVENTION

Infection Control Measures

Transmission of HTLV is mediated by live cells, not via cell-free body fluids. For this reason, HTLV-1 is not an easily transmitted virus. Universal precautions like those recommended for HIV-1 are applicable for viral inactivation and protection from potentially infectious blood or bodily secretions. Guidelines for prevention and counseling have been developed for HTLV-1 and HTLV-2 by a Centers for Disease Control and Prevention working group (26). Standard prevention approaches address each of the major avenues of transmission and are similar for both viruses: screen blood, eliminate breast-feeding by known infected mothers (or, where not feasible, limit breast-feeding to the first 6 months of life), and advise use of condoms by discordant couples.

The value of blood donor screening has been well documented in Japan, where up to 15% of HTLV-1 infections have been eliminated (28). In areas where the infection is not endemic, such as the United States, the cost-effectiveness of screening has been questioned, but because of the risk of HAM/TSP in the transfusion setting, all blood bank units in the United States are screened. Because HTLV-1 is transmitted only in blood units containing cells and not in plasma, plasma donations are not screened for HTLV-1.

Pregnant women who are HTLV-1 positive should not breast-feed their infants. However, in developing countries, where safe alternatives to breast-feeding may not be available, limiting breast-feeding to the first 6 months may afford some protection via maternal antibodies (174).

The use of condoms is recommended for couples who are discordant for HTLV infection. Given the relatively low frequency of sexual transmission for each sexual encounter, couples who desire a pregnancy could plan to have unprotected sex during periods of maximal fertility. Such decisions require careful discussion between the physician and patient, and there are no absolute guidelines in this particular area.

Counseling of seropositive patients involves a clear discussion of the distinction of HTLV from HIV. In addition, the HTLV type should be defined by serologic methods, and the distinctions in disease associations of the two virus types should be emphasized.

On a population level, prevention measures that have been developed for HIV infection also are applicable to HTLV. Because in areas where the virus is endemic the populations at risk for HIV are also at risk for HTLV-1 (e.g., persons at risk for STDs, persons with high rates of partner exchange, and commercial sex workers), HIV prevention guidelines will also benefit those at risk for HTLV-1. Therefore, prevention measures that promote condom use, treatment of STDs, and decrease of high-risk exposures will also prevent HTLV-1 infection. Nosocomial infection has been reported in only two instances (83, 114), suggesting that HTLV-1 is unlikely to be transmitted in this setting. There is no therapy for HTLV-1 infection and thus no chemoprophylaxis. Passive immunoprophylaxis is hypothetically effective, as noted below, in animal studies, but it has no practical clinical application given the low risk for transmission except through sexual, breast-feeding, and transfusion exposure, where other prevention methods are more applicable.

Vaccines

While vaccines against HTLV-1 are feasible, there has been no impetus to develop or market an HTLV-1 vaccine because of the low rate of disease. This decision is based on the observation that while the incidence of disease is not dissimilar to the estimated incidence of hepatocellular carcinoma in hepatitis B virus antigen carriers, there is no acute morbidity for HTLV-1 comparable to hepatitis B virus-induced acute hepatitis.

Experimentally, vaccines containing whole virus and recombinant HTLV-1 envelope antigens successfully prevent HTLV-1 infection in monkey and rabbit models (44, 85). Protection is correlated with the presence of neutralizing antibodies, indicating that humoral immunity can be an effective barrier against infection, even when the challenge is cell associated. The HTLV-1 envelope is relatively highly conserved, and neutralizing antibody appears to protect against challenge with even major strain variants, consistent with the conclusion that a single serotype will protect against all variants (103). Therefore, a synthetic vaccine against one HTLV-1 isolate could protect against other HTLV-1 isolates. A vaccine that induces cell-mediated immune responses in nonhuman-primate studies has also been shown to be effective (5).

TREATMENT

Unlike for HIV-1, there is no proven antiviral therapy for HTLV-1. Hypothetically, some drugs that target HIV-1 reverse transcriptase might have effects against HTLV-1, as shown by in vitro studies showing inhibition of viral growth. However, therapeutic effects have not been systematically evaluated in clinical trials, although anecdotal reports suggest some antitumor effects (see below). Furthermore, the exact way in which HTLV-1 contributes to disease pathogenesis has not been clearly defined. In ATL, the role of active viral replication is far from clear because the tumor cell harbors many oncogenic mutations in cell regulatory genes, which may not be reversible by treating the virus. HAM/TSP, with its high viral load and substantial cell-mediated immune response to HTLV-1, would appear to be a better candidate for antiviral treatment, but therapy that targets the immune response itself or a combination of antiviral and immunomodulator therapies may afford an equally attractive avenue for experimental treatment. The opportunity exists to investigate the impact of antiviral therapy on persons coinfected with HTLV-1 or

-2 and HIV-1, and studies are needed to determine if, for example, the viral load of HTLV-1 or -2 is modulated by anti-HIV-1 therapy. However, one report indicated that a high viral load of HTLV-2 protected against HIV-1 disease progression. The mechanism appears to involve heightened production of C-C chemokines in response to HTLV-2 infection, blocking HIV-1 infection (31). Further systematic study of this relationship is warranted.

The major diseases caused by HTLV-1 infection are chronic diseases of the hematopoietic and neurologic system, which have proved refractory to most conventional and experimental chemotherapeutic regimens. Consequently, individuals with such diseases have a poor prognosis.

ATL

Despite advances in support and development of novel treatment agents, the prognosis for patients with ATL remains poor. While response rates, even for the poorest risk categories, are over 50% and complete remissions are achieved in 20%, these responses are short-lived, with relapses within weeks to months (143). Therapeutic approaches tested over the past two decades have employed a variety of approaches, with modest improvements in response, but more recent strategies offer greater hope (68, 115). With a 70% 5-year survival rate with no therapy and because of complicating infections caused by bone marrow suppression, patients with chronic and smoldering ATL are not treated or are given prednisone with or without cyclophosphamide. The acute and lymphoma types of ATL are aggressive high-grade lymphomas with a generally poor prognosis and historically at best have 20% remission rates with a variety of traditional chemotherapy approaches, but remissions are short-lived and the mortality rate is high.

Significant prognostic factors include poor performance status at diagnosis, age over 40 years, extensive disease, hypercalcemia, and a high serum lactate dehydrogenase level. Approximately 13 to 15% of patients with such aggressive cases experience a long-term survival (over 2 years), which has been associated with several factors: complete remission, longer time to remission, and total doxorubicin dose. Relapses in these long-term survivors often occurred in the CNS and proved refractory to subsequent therapy.

Experimental approaches that use monoclonal antibodies to IL-2R linked with cell toxins selectively targeted to the leukemic cells are being tested, with some evidence of at least partial responses (165). In phase I trials, use of a combination of antiretrovirals and interferon has been reported to induce remission in some cases (39, 55), which are unexplained because the regimen does not cause direct cytotoxic killing of the leukemia cells and does not directly counteract virus-specific pathways of leukemogenesis (10).

Combinations of doxorubicin and etoposide have resulted in complete remission rates of 40% (166). The current focus of therapy is the use of allogeneic hematopoietic stem cell transplantation for patients with ATL (45), in which all evaluable patients entered complete remission, with a median survival time of 9.6 months and an estimated 3-year survival of 45.3%, relapse-free survival of 33.8%, and disease relapse of 39.3%. One transplant patient showed reappearance of cells harboring the integration of HTLV-1 previously observed in his leukemia cells, but the patient continues in clinical remission, suggesting a possible reversion to the preleukemic carrier state (159). Additionally, some patients achieved a second complete remission, including by reduction or cessation of immunosuppression, suggesting a graft-versus-ATL effect (45).

A study of arsenic trioxide demonstrated responses in patients failing prior chemotherapy but involved a high level of toxicity (63). Newer agents like proteasome inhibitors, retinoids, and angiogenesis inhibitors, as well as cellular immunotherapy, are being evaluated (9, 121).

HAM/TSP

Treatment of HAM/TSP with corticosteroids benefits some patients, particularly when given early in the clinical course or in those with rapidly progressive disease. Treatment with danazol, an androgenic steroid, has reversed urinary and fecal incontinence in some patients, but not the spastic limb disease or the underlying neurologic deficit. Experimental studies with some therapies currently being implemented for multiple sclerosis may be of value because the mechanism of immune pathogenesis may be shared between the two diseases (131).

Treatment with alpha interferon has shown to be of short-term benefit and appears to decrease provirus load (149). Beta 1a interferon also has been reported to reduce the HTLV-1 mRNA load, but the provirus load remained unchanged and there was only a slight improvement in motor function (132).

Given the emerging picture of disease pathogenesis with an inability to control high viral expression, therapy with antiviral drugs would appear to be a promising avenue for research. The combination of two nucleoside analogs, zidovudine and lamivudine, has been evaluated in 16 patients with HAM/TSP (163), but after a year of follow-up, no significant changes in provirus load and no clinical improvements were observed. These studies will be dependent on identifying agents that target cell-associated virus with sufficient specificity to block the HTLV-1 reverse transcriptase and other virus-specific targets.

REFERENCES

1. **Alberts, B., D. Bray, A. Johnson, J. Lewis, M. Raff, K. Roberst, and P. Walter.** 1998. *Essential Cell Biology: an Introduction to the Molecular Biology of the Cell.* Garland Science Publishing, New York, NY.

1a. **Araujo, A., and W. W. Hall.** 2004. Human T-lymphotropic virus type II and neurological disease. *Ann. Neurol.* **56:**10–19.

2. **Araujo, A. P., L. M. Fontenelle, P. A. Padua, H. S. Maia Filho, and Q. Araujo Ade.** 2002. Juvenile human T lymphotropic virus type 1-associated myelopathy. *Clin. Infect. Dis.* **35:**201–204.

3. **Azran, I., Y. Schavinsky-Khrapunsky, E. Priel, M. Huleihel, and M. Aboud.** 2004. Implications of the evolution pattern of human T-cell leukemia retroviruses on their pathogenic virulence. *Int. J. Mol. Med.* **14:**909–915.

3a. **Bangham, C. R.** 2000. The immune response to HTLV-I. *Curr. Opin. Immunol.* **12:**397–402.

3b. **Bangham, C. R. M.** 2000. HTLV-I infections. *J. Clin. Pathol.* **53:**581–586.

4. **Bangham, C. R. M., A. G. Kermode, and S. E. Hall.** 1996. The cytotoxic T-lymphocyte response to HTLV-I: the main determinant of disease? *Semin. Virol.* **7:**41–48.

5. **Barouch, D. H., Z. Y. Yang, W. P. Kong, B. Korioth-Schmitz, S. M. Sumida, D. M. Truitt, M. G. Kishko, J. C. Arthur, A. Miura, J. R. Mascola, N. L. Letvin, and G. J. Nabel.** 2005. A human T-cell leukemia virus

type 1 regulatory element enhances the immunogenicity of human immunodeficiency virus type 1 DNA vaccines in mice and nonhuman primates. *J. Virol.* **79:**8828–8834.

6. **Barre-Sinoussi, F., J.-C. Chermann, F. Rey, M. T. Nugeyre, S. Chamaret, J. Gruest, C. Dauguet, C. Axler-Blin, F. Vezinet-Brun, C. Rouzioux, W. Rozenbaum, and L. Montagnier.** 1983. Isolation of a T-lymphotropic retrovirus from a patient at risk for acquired immune deficiency syndrome (AIDS). *Science* **220:**868–871.
7. **Bartholomew, C., W. Charles, C. Saxinger, W. Blattner, M. Robert-Guroff, C. Raju, P. Ratan, W. Ince, D. Quamina, and K. Basdeo-Maharaj.** 1985. Racial and other characteristics of human T cell leukemia/lymphoma (HTLV-I) and AIDS (HTLV-III) in Trinidad. *Br. Med. J.* **290:**1243–1246.
8. **Bartholomew, C., W. C. Saxinger, J. W. Clark, M. Gail, A. Dudgeon, B. Mahabir, B. Hull-Drysdale, F. Cleghorn, R. C. Gallo, and W. A. Blattner.** 1987. Transmission of HTLV-I and HIV among homosexual men in Trinidad. *JAMA* **257:**2604–2608.
9. **Bazarbachi, A., D. Ghez, Y. Lepelletier, R. Nasr, H. de The, M. E. El-Sabban, and O. Hermine.** 2004. New therapeutic approaches for adult T-cell leukaemia. *Lancet Oncol.* **5:**664–672.
10. **Bazarbachi, A., R. Nasr, M. E. El-Sabban, A. Mahe, R. Mahieux, A. Gessain, N. Darwiche, G. Dbaibo, J. Kersual, Y. Zermati, L. Dianoux, M. K. Chelbi-Alix, H. de The, and O. Hermine.** 2000. Evidence against a direct cytotoxic effect of alpha interferon and zidovudine in HTLV-I associated adult T cell leukemia/lymphoma. *Leukemia* **14:**716–721.
11. **Biggar, R. J., Z. Buskell-Bales, P. N. Yakshe, D. Caussy, G. Gridley, and L. Seeff.** 1991. Antibody to human retroviruses among drug users in three east coast American cities, 1972–1976. *J. Infect. Dis.* **163:**57–63.
12. **Biggar, R. J., J. Ng, N. Kim, M. Hisada, H. C. Li, B. Cranston, B. Hanchard, and E. M. Maloney.** 2006. Human leukocyte antigen concordance and the transmission risk via breast-feeding of human T cell lymphotropic virus type I. *J. Infect. Dis.* **193:**277–282.
13. **Blattner, W. A., V. S. Kalynaraman, M. Robert-Guroff, T. A. Lister, D. A. Galton, P. S. Sarin, M. H. Crawford, D. Catovsky, M. Greaves, and R. C. Gallo.** 1982. The human type-C retrovirus, HTLV, in Blacks from the Caribbean region, and relationship to adult T-cell leukemia/lymphoma. *Int. J. Cancer* **30:**257–264.
14. **Blattner, W. A., A. Nomura, J. W. Clark, G. Y. Ho, Y. Nakao, R. Gallo, and M. Robert-Guroff.** 1986. Modes of transmission and evidence for viral latency from studies of human T-cell lymphotrophic virus type I in Japanese migrant populations in Hawaii. *Proc. Natl. Acad. Sci. USA* **83:**4895–4898.
15. **Blattner, W. A., C. Saxinger, D. Riedel, B. Hull, G. Taylor, F. Cleghorn, R. Gallo, B. Blumberg, and C. Bartholomew.** 1990. A study of HTLV-I and its associated risk factors in Trinidad and Tobago. *J. Acquir. Immune Defic. Syndr.* **3:**1102–1108.
16. **Blot, V., L. Delamarre, F. Perugi, D. Pham, S. Bénichou, R. Benarous, T. Hanada, A. H. Chishti, M. C. Dokhélar, and C. Pique.** 2004. Human Dlg protein binds to the envelope glycoproteins of human T-cell leukemia virus type 1 and regulates envelope mediated cell-cell fusion in T lymphocytes. *J. Cell Sci.* **117:**3983–3993.
17. **Bovolenta, C., E. Pilotti, M. Mauri, M. Turci, P. Ciancianaini, P. Fisicaro, U. Bertazzoni, G. Poli, and C. Casoli.** 2002. Human T-cell leukemia virus type 2 induces survival and proliferation of CD34(+) TF-1 cells through activation of STAT1 and STAT5 by secretion of interferon-gamma and granulocyte macrophage-colony-stimulating factor. *Blood* **99:**224–231.
18. **Brauweiler, A., J. E. Gerrus, J. C. Reed, and J. K. Nyborg.** 1997. Repression of bax gene expression by the HTLV-1 Tax protein: implications for suppression of apoptosis in virally infected cells. *Virology* **231:**135–140.
19. **Brodine, S. K., K. C. Hyams, C. A. Molgaard, S. I. Ito, R. J. Thomas, C. R. Roberts, A. L. Golbeck, E. C. Oldfield III, and W. A. Blattner.** 1995. The risk of human T cell leukemia virus and viral hepatitis infection among US Marines stationed in Okinawa, Japan. *J. Infect. Dis.* **171:**693–696.
20. **Calattini, S., S. A. Chevalier, R. Duprez, P. Afonso, A. Froment, A. Gessain, and R. Mahieux.** 2006. Human T-cell lymphotropic virus type 3: complete nucleotide sequence and characterization of the human Tax3 protein. *J. Virol.* **80:**9876–9888.
21. **Calattini, S., S. A. Chevalier, R. Duprez, S. Bassot, A. Froment, R. Mahieux, and A. Gessain.** 2005. Discovery of a new human T-cell lymphotropic virus (HTLV-3) in Central Africa. *Retrovirology* **2:**30.
22. **Carneiro-Proietti, A. B., B. C. Catalan-Soares, C. M. Castro-Costa, E. L. Murphy, E. C. Sabino, M. Hisada, B. Galvão-Castro, L. C. Alcantara, C. Remondegui, K. Verdonck, and F. A. Proietti.** 2006. HTLV in the Americas: challenges and perspectives. *Rev. Panam. Salud Publica* **19:**44–53.
23. **Casoli, C., E. Pilotti, and U. Bertazzoni.** 2007. Molecular and cellular interactions of HIV-1/HTLV coinfection and impact on AIDS progression. *AIDS Rev.* **9:**140–149.
24. **Catovsky, D., M. F. Greaves, M. Rose, D. A. Galton, A. W. Goolden, D. R. McCluskey, J. M. White, I. Lampert, G. Bourikas, R. Ireland, A. I. Brownell, J. M. Bridges, W. A. Blattner, and R. C. Gallo.** 1982. Adult T-cell lymphoma-leukaemia in Blacks from the West Indies. *Lancet* **i:**639–643.
25. **Centers for Disease Control.** 1992. Update: serologic testing for human T-lymphotrophic virus type 1—United States. *Morb. Mortal. Wkly. Rep.* **41:**259.
26. **Centers for Disease Control and Prevention and the U.S.P.H.S. Working Group.** 1993. Guidelines for counseling persons infected with human T-lymphotropic virus type I (HTLV-I) and type II (HTLV-II). *Ann. Intern. Med.* **118:**448–454.
27. **Chen, Y. M., A. Okayama, T. H. Lee, N. Tachibana, N. Mueller, and M. Essex.** 1991. Sexual transmission of human T-cell leukemia virus type I associated with the presence of anti-Tax antibody. *Proc. Natl. Acad. Sci. USA* **88:**1182–1186.
28. **Chiyoda, S., K. Kinoshita, S. Egawa, J. Inoue, K. Watanabe, and M. Ifuku.** 2001. Decline in the positive rate of human T-lymphotropic virus type-1 (HTLV-1) antibodies among blood donors in Nagasaki. *Intern. Med.* **40:**14–17.
29. **Chlichlia, K., M. Busslinger, M. E. Peter, H. Walczak, P. H. Krammer, V. Schirrmacher, and K. Khazaie.** 1997. ICE-proteases mediate HTLV-I Tax-induced apoptotic T-cell death. *Oncogene* **14:**2265–2272.
30. **Cho, I., M. Sugimoto, S. Mita, M. Tokunaga, F. Imamura, and M. Ando.** 1995. In vivo proviral burden and viral RNA expression in T cell subsets of patients with human T lymphotropic virus type-1-associated myelopathy/tropical spastic paraparesis. *Am. J. Trop. Med. Hyg.* **53:**412–418.
31. **Ciancianaini, P., G. Magnani, E. Barchi, D. Padrini, T. Zauli, S. Ghezzi, C. Grosso, C. Casoli, and U. Bertazzoni.** 2001. Serological and clinical follow-up of an Italian IVDU cohort of HTLV-II/HIV-1 co-infected patients. Ev-

idence of direct relationship between CD4 count and HTLV-II proviral load. *AIDS Res. Hum. Retrovir.* **17:**S70.
32. **Cleghorn, F. R., A. Manns, R. Falk, P. Hartge, B. Hanchard, N. Jack, E. Williams, E. Jaffe, F. White, C. Bartholomew, et al.** 1995. Effect of human T-lymphotropic virus type I infection on non-Hodgkin's lymphoma incidence. *J. Natl. Cancer Inst.* **87:**1009–1014.
33. **Datta, A., L. Silverman, A. J. Phipps, H. Hiraragi, L. Ratner, and M. D. Lairmore.** 2007. Human T-lymphotropic virus type-1 p30 alters cell cycle G2 regulation of T lymphocytes to enhance cell survival. *Retrovirology* **4:**49.
34. **De Castro-Costa, C. M., A. Q. Araujo, M. M. Barreto, O. M. Takayanagui, M. P. Sohler, E. L. da Silva, S. M. de Paula, R. Ishak, J. G. Ribas, L. C. Rovirosa, H. Carton, E. Gotuzzo, W. W. Hall, S. Montano, E. L. Murphy, J. Oger, C. Remondegui, and G. P. Taylor.** 2006. Proposal for diagnostic criteria of tropical spastic paraparesis /HTLV-I-associated myelopathy (TSP/HAM). *AIDS Res. Hum. Retrovir.* **22:**931–935.
35. **Delaporte, E., M. Peeters, J. P. Durand, A. Dupont, D. Schrijvers, L. Bedjabaga, C. Honore, S. Ossari, A. Trebucq, R. Josse, and M. Merlin.** 1989. Seroepidemiological survey of HTLV-I infection among randomized populations of western central African countries. *J. Acquir. Immune Defic. Syndr.* **2:**410–413.
36. **Derse, D., B. Crise, Y. Li, G. Princler, N. Lum, C. Stewart, C. F. McGrath, S. H. Hughes, D. J. Munroe, and X. Wu.** 2007. Human T-cell leukemia virus type 1 integration target sites in the human genome: comparison with those of other retroviruses. *J. Virol.* **81:**6731–6741.
37. **Donegan, E., M. P. Busch, J. A. Galleshaw, G. M. Shaw, and J. W. Mosley for The Transfusion Safety Study Group.** 1990. Transfusion of blood components from a donor with human T-lymphotropic virus type II (HTLV-II) infection. *Ann. Intern. Med.* **113:**555–556.
38. **Endo, K., A. Hirata, K. Iwai, M. Sakurai, M. Fukushi, M. Oie, M. Higuchi, W. W. Hall, F. Gejyo, and M. Fujii.** 2002. Human T-cell leukemia virus type 2 (HTLV-2) Tax protein transforms a rat fibroblast cell line but less efficiently than HTLV-1 Tax. *J. Virol.* **76:**2648–2653.
39. **Ezaki, K., M. Hirano, R. Ohno, K. Yamada, K. Naito, Y. Hirota, S. Shirakawa, and K. Kimura.** 1991. A combination trial of human lymphoblastoid interferon and bestrabucil (KM2210) for adult T-cell leukemia-lymphoma. *Cancer* **68:**695–698.
40. **Farid, R., M. Etemadi, H. Baradaran, and B. Nikkin.** 1993. Seroepidemiology and virology of HTLV-I in the city of Mashhad, northeastern Iran. *Serodiagn. Immunother. Infect. Dis.* **5:**251.
41. **Feuer, G., and P. L. Green.** 2005. Comparative biology of human T-cell lymphotropic virus type 1 (HTLV-1) and HTLV-2. *Oncogene* **24:**5996–6004.
42. **Fox, R. I., M. Stern, and P. Michelson.** 2000. Update in Sjogren syndrome. *Curr. Opin. Rheumatol.* **12:**391–398.
43. **Franchini, G.** 2001. HTLV and immortalization/transformation: current concepts and clinical relevance. *AIDS Res. Hum. Retrovir.* **17:**S5.
44. **Frangione-Beebe, M., B. Albrecht, N. Dakappagari, R. T. Rose, C. L. Brooks, S. P. Schwendeman, M. D. Lairmore, and P. T. Kaumaya.** 2000. Enhanced immunogenicity of a conformational epitope of human T-lymphotropic virus type 1 using a novel chimeric peptide. *Vaccine* **19:**1068–1081.
45. **Fukushima, T., Y. Miyazaki, S. Honda, F. Kawano, Y. Moriuchi, M. Masuda, R. Tanosaki, A. Utsunomiya, N. Uike, S. Yoshida, J. Okamura, and M. Tomonaga.** 2005. Allogeneic hematopoietic stem cell transplantation provides sustained long-term survival for patients with adult T-cell leukemia/lymphoma. *Leukemia* **19:**829–834.
46. **Gallo, R., S. Z. Salahuddin, M. Popovic, G. Shearer, M. Kaplan, B. F. Haynes, T. J. Palker, R. R. Redfield, J. Oleske, B. Safai, F. White, P. Foster, and P. D. Markham.** 1984. Frequent detection and isolation of cytopathic retroviruses (HTLV-III) from patients with AIDS and at risk for AIDS. *Science* **224:**500–503.
47. **Gallo, R., F. Wong-Staal, L. Montagnier, W. A. Haseltine, and M. Yoshida.** 1988. HIV/HTLV gene nomenclature. *Nature* **333:**504.
48. **Gallo, R. C., P. S. Sarin, E. P. Gelmann, M. Robert-Guroff, E. Richardson, V. S. Kalynaraman, D. Mann, G. D. Sidhu, R. E. Stahl, S. Zolla-Pazner, J. Leibowitch, and M. Popovic.** 1983. Isolation of human T-cell leukemia virus in acquired immune deficiency syndrome (AIDS). *Science* **220:**865–867.
49. **Garcia-Vallejo, F., M. C. Dominguez, and O. Tamayo.** 2005. Autoimmunity and molecular mimicry in tropical spastic paraparesis/human T-lymphotropic virus-associated myelopathy. *Braz. J. Med. Biol. Res.* **38:**241–250.
50. **Gaudray, G., F. Gachon, J. Basbous, M. Biard-Piechaczyk, C. Devaux, and J. M. Mesnard.** 2002. The complementary strand of the human T-cell leukemia virus type 1 RNA genome encodes a bZIP transcription factor that down-regulates viral transcription. *J. Virol.* **76:**12813–12822.
51. **Gessain, A., F. Barin, J. C. Vernant, O. Gout, L. Maurs, A. Calender, and G. De The.** 1985. Antibodies to human T-lymphotropic virus type-I in patients with tropical spastic paraparesis. *Lancet* **ii:**407–410.
52. **Gessain, A., and R. Mahieux.** 2000. A virus called HTLV-1. Epidemiological aspects. *Presse Med.* **29:**2233–2239. (In French.)
53. **Gessain, A., R. Yanagihara, G. Franchini, R. M. Garruto, C. L. Jenkins, A. B. Ajdukiewicz, R. C. Gallo, and D. C. Gajdusek.** 1991. Highly divergent molecular variants of human T-lymphotropic virus type I from isolated populations in Papua New Guinea and the Solomon Islands. *Proc. Natl. Acad. Sci. USA* **88:**7694–7698.
54. **Ghez, D., Y. Lepelletier, S. Lambert, J.-M. Fourneau, V. Blot, S. Janvier, B. Arnulf, P. M. van Endert, N. Heveker, C. Pique, and O. Hermine.** 2006. Neuropilin-1 is involved in human T-cell lymphotropic virus type 1 entry. *J. Virol.* **80:**6844–6854.
55. **Gill, P. S., W. Harrington, M. H. Kaplan, R. C. Ribeiro, J. M. Bennett, H. A. Liebman, M. Bernstein-Singer, B. M. Espina, L. Cabral, S. Allen, S. Kornblau, M. C. Pike, and A. M. Levine.** 1995. Treatment of adult T-cell leukemia-lymphoma with a combination of interferon alfa and zidovudine. *N. Engl. J. Med.* **332:**1744–1748.
56. **Grassmann, R., M. Aboud, and K. T. Jeang.** 2005. Molecular mechanisms of cellular transformation by HTLV-1 Tax. *Oncogene* **24:**5976–5985.
57. **Guerreiro, J. B., S. B. Santos, D. J. Morgan, A. F. Porto, A. L. Muniz, J. Lotto, A. L. Teixeira, Jr., M. M. Teixeira, and E. M. Carvalho.** 2006. Levels of serum chemokines discriminate clinical myelopathy associated with human T lymphotropic virus type 1 (HTLV-1)/tropical spastic paraparesis (HAM/TSP) disease from HTLV-1 carrier state. *Clin. Exp. Immunol.* **145:**296–301.
58. **Hall, W. W., C. R. Liu, O. Schneewind, H. Takahashi, M. H. Kaplan, G. Roupe, and A. Vahlne.** 1991. Deleted HTLV-I provirus in blood and cutaneous lesions of patients with mycosis fungoides. *Science* **253:**317–320.
59. **Hanon, E., S. Hall, G. P. Taylor, M. Saito, R. Davis, Y. Tanaka, K. Usuku, M. Osame, J. N. Weber, and C. R. Bangham.** 2000. Abundant Tax protein expression in

CD4+ T cells infected with human T-cell lymphotropic virus type I (HTLV-I) is prevented by cytotoxic T lymphocytes. *Blood* **95:**1386–1392.
60. **Hanon, E., J. C. Stinchcombe, M. Saito, B. E. Asquith, G. P. Taylor, Y. Tanaka, J. N. Weber, G. M. Griffiths, and C. R. Bangham.** 2000. Fratricide among CD8(+) T lymphocytes naturally infected with human T cell lymphotropic virus type I. *Immunity* **13:**657–664.
61. **Harhaj, N. S., S. C. Sun, and E. W. Harhaj.** 2007. Activation of NF-κB by the human T cell leukemia virus type I Tax oncoprotein is associated with ubiquitin-dependent relocalization of IκB kinase. *J. Biol. Chem.* **282:**4185–4192.
62. **Heneine, W., R. F. Khabbaz, R. B. Lal, and J. E. Kaplan.** 1992. Sensitive and specific polymerase chain reaction assays for diagnosis of human T-cell lymphotropic virus type I (HTLV-I) and HTLV-II infections in HTLV-I/II-seropositive individuals. *J. Clin. Microbiol.* **30:**1605–1607.
63. **Hermine, O., H. Dombret, J. Poupon, B. Arnulf, F. Lefrere, P. Rousselot, G. Damaj, R. Delarue, J. P. Fermand, J. C. Brouet, L. Degos, B. Varet, H. de The, and A. Bazarbachi.** 2004. Phase II trial of arsenic trioxide and alpha interferon in patients with relapsed/refractory adult T-cell leukemia/lymphoma. *Hematol. J.* **5:**130–134.
64. **Higuchi, M., C. Tsubata, R. Kondo, S. Yoshida, M. Takahashi, M. Oie, Y. Tanaka, R. Mahieux, M. Matsuoka, and M. Fujii.** 2007. Cooperation of NF-κB2/p100 activation and the PDZ domain binding motif signal in human T-cell leukemia virus type 1 (HTLV-1) Tax1 but not HTLV-2 Tax2 is crucial for interleukin-2-independent growth transformation of a T-cell line. *J. Virol.* **81:**11900–11907.
65. **Hino, S., S. Katamine, K. Kawase, T. Miyamoto, H. Doi, Y. Tsuji, and T. Yamabe.** 1994. Intervention of maternal transmission of HTLV-1 in Nagasaki, Japan. *Leukemia* **8**(Suppl. 1)**:**S68–S70.
66. **Ho, G. Y., A. M. Nomura, K. Nelson, H. Lee, B. F. Polk, and W. A. Blattner.** 1991. Declining seroprevalence and transmission of HTLV-I in Japanese families who immigrated to Hawaii. *Am. J. Epidemiol.* **134:**981–987.
67. **Ijichi, S., T. Matsuda, I. Maruyama, T. Izumihara, K. Kojima, T. Niimura, Y. Maruyama, S. Sonoda, A. Yoshida, and M. Osame.** 1990. Arthritis in a human T lymphotropic virus type I (HTLV-I) carrier. *Ann. Rheum. Dis.* **49:**718–721.
68. **Ishitsuka, K., and K. Takamura.** 10 December 2007. Treatment of adult T-cell leukemia/lymphoma: past, present, and future. *Eur. J. Haematol.* **80:**185–196. [Epub ahead of print.]
69. **Jacobson, S., A. Gupta, D. Mattson, E. Mingioli, and D. E. McFarlin.** 1990. Immunological studies in tropical spastic paraparesis. *Ann. Neurol.* **27:**149–156.
70. **Jacobson, S., J. S. Reuben, R. D. Streilein, and T. J. Palker.** 1991. Induction of CD4+, human T lymphotropic virus type-1-specific cytotoxic T lymphocytes from patients with HAM/TSP. Recognition of an immunogenic region of the gp46 envelope glycoprotein of human T lymphotropic virus type-1. *J. Immunol.* **146:**1155–1162.
71. **Jacobson, S., H. Shida, D. E. McFarlin, A. S. Fauci, and S. Koenig.** 1990. Circulating CD8+ cytotoxic T lymphocytes specific for HTLV-I pX in patients with HTLV-I associated neurological disease. *Nature* **348:**245–248.
72. **Jeang, K. T., S. G. Widen, O. J. Semmes IV, and S. H. Wilson.** 1990. HTLV-I trans-activator protein, tax, is a trans-repressor of the human beta-polymerase gene. *Science* **247:**1082–1084.
73. **Jeffery, K. J., K. Usuku, S. E. Hall, W. Matsumoto, G. P. Taylor, J. Procter, M. Bunce, G. S. Ogg, K. I. Welsh, J. N. Weber, A. L. Lloyd, M. A. Nowak, M. Nagai, D. Kodama, S. Izumo, M. Osame, and C. R. Bangham.** 1999. HLA alleles determine human T-lymphotropic virus-I (HTLV-I) proviral load and the risk of HTLV-I-associated myelopathy. *Proc. Natl. Acad. Sci. USA* **96:**3848–3853.
74. **Jin, D. Y., F. Spencer, and K. T. Jeang.** 1998. Human T cell leukemia virus type 1 oncoprotein Tax targets the human mitotic checkpoint protein MAD1. *Cell* **93:**81–91.
75. **Jones, K. S., K. Fugo, C. Petrow-Sadowski, Y. Huang, D. C. Bertolette, I. Lisinski, S. W. Cushman, S. Jacobson, and F. W. Ruscetti.** 2006. Human T-cell leukemia virus type 1 (HTLV-1) and HTLV-2 use different receptor complexes to enter T cells. *J. Virol.* **80:**8291–8302.
76. **Kajiyama, W., S. Kashiwagi, H. Nomura, H. Ikematsu, J. Hayashi, and W. Ikematsu.** 1986. Seroepidemiologic study of antibody to adult T-cell leukemia virus in Okinawa, Japan. *Am. J. Epidemiol.* **123:**41–47.
77. Reference deleted.
78. **Kalynaraman, V. S., M. G. Sarngadharan, M. Robert-Guroff, I. Miyoshi, D. Golde, and R. C. Gallo.** 1982. A new subtype of human T-cell leukemia virus (HTLV-II) associated with a T-cell variant of hairy cell leukemia. *Science* **218:**571–573.
79. **Kao, S. Y., F. J. Lemoine, and S. J. Marriott.** 2000. HTLV-1 Tax protein sensitizes cells to apoptotic cell death induced by DNA-damaging agents. *Oncogene* **19:**2240–2248.
80. **Kao, S. Y., F. J. Lemoine, and S. J. Marriott.** 2000. Suppression of DNA repair by human T cell leukemia virus type 1 Tax is rescued by a functional p53 signaling pathway. *J. Biol. Chem.* **275:**35926–35931.
81. **Kaplan, J. E., R. F. Khabbaz, E. L. Murphy, S. Hermansen, C. Roberts, R. Lal, W. Heneine, D. Wright, L. Matijas, R. Thomson, D. Rudolph, W. M. Switzer, S. Kleinman, M. Busch, and G. B. Schreiber for The Retrovirus Epidemiology Donor Study Group.** 1996. Male-to-female transmission of human T-cell lymphotropic virus types I and II: association with viral load. *J. Acquir. Immune Defic. Syndr. Hum. Retrovirol.* **12:**193–201.
82. **Kasai, T., Y. Iwanaga, H. Iha, and K. T. Jeang.** 2002. Prevalent loss of mitotic spindle checkpoint in adult T-cell leukemia confers resistance to microtubule inhibitors. *J. Biol. Chem.* **277:**5187–5193.
83. **Kataoka, R., N. Takehara, Y. Iwahara, T. Sawada, Y. Ohtsuki, Y. Dawei, H. Hoshino, and I. Miyoshi.** 1990. Transmission of HTLV-I by blood transfusion and its prevention by passive immunization in rabbits. *Blood* **76:**1657–1661.
84. **Kawakami, A., T. Nakashima, H. Sakai, S. Urayama, S. Yamasaki, A. Hida, M. Tsuboi, H. Nakamura, H. Ida, K. Migita, Y. Kawabe, and K. Eguchi.** 1999. Inhibition of caspase cascade by HTLV-I Tax through induction of NF-κB nuclear translocation. *Blood* **94:**3847–3854.
85. **Kazanji, M., J. Tartaglia, G. Franchini, B. de Thoisy, A. Talarmin, H. Contamin, A. Gessain, and G. de Thé.** 2001. Immunogenicity and protective efficacy of recombinant human T-cell leukemia/lymphoma virus type 1 NYVAC and naked DNA vaccine candidates in squirrel monkeys *(Saimiri sciureus)*. *J. Virol.* **75:**5939–5948.
86. **Kitajima, M., Y. Korogi, Y. Shigematsu, L. Liang, M. Matsuoka, T. Yamamoto, M. Jhono, K. Eto, and M. Takahashi.** 2002. Central nervous system lesions in adult T-cell leukaemia: MRI and pathology. *Neuroradiology* **44:**559–567.

87. **Kiyokawa, T., M. Seiki, S. Iwashita, K. Imagawa, F. Shimizu, and M. Yoshida.** 1985. p27x-III and p21x-III, proteins encoded by the pX sequence of human T-cell leukemia virus type I. *Proc. Natl. Acad. Sci. USA* **82:** 8359–8363.
88. **Klimas, N. G., J. B. Page, R. Patarca, D. Chitwood, R. Morgan, and M. A. Fletcher.** 1993. Effects of retroviral infections on immune function in African-American intravenous drug users. *AIDS* **7:**331–335.
89. **Korber, B., A. Okayama, R. Donnelly, N. Tachibana, and M. Essex.** 1991. Polymerase chain reaction analysis of defective human T-cell leukemia virus type I proviral genomes in leukemic cells of patients with adult T-cell leukemia. *J. Virol.* **65:**5471–5476.
90. **Kubo, T., S. W. Zhu, S. Ijichi, H. Takahashi, and W. W. Hall.** 1994. Molecular characterization of human T-cell leukemia virus, type II (HTLV-II). *AIDS Res. Hum. Retrovir.* **10:**465.
91. **LaGrenade, L., B. Hanchard, V. Fletcher, B. Cranston, and W. Blattner.** 1990. Infective dermatitis of Jamaican children: a marker for HTLV-I infection. *Lancet* **336:** 1345–1347.
92. **Lairmore, M. D., B. Albrecht, C. D'Souza, J. W. Nisbet, W. Ding, J. T. Bartoe, P. L. Green, and W. Zhang.** 2000. In vitro and in vivo functional analysis of human T cell lymphotropic virus type 1 pX open reading frames I and II. *AIDS Res. Hum. Retrovir.* **16:**1757–1764.
93. **Lal, R. B., S. M. Owen, D. L. Rudolph, C. Dawson, and H. Prince.** 1995. In vivo cellular tropism of human T-lymphotropic virus type II is not restricted to CD8+ cells. *Virology* **210:**441–447.
94. **Larsen, O., S. Andersson, Z. da Silva, K. Hedegaard, A. Sandstrom, A. Naucler, F. Dias, M. Melbye, and P. Aaby.** 2000. Prevalences of HTLV-1 infection and associated risk determinants in an urban population in Guinea-Bissau, West Africa. *J. Acquir. Immune Defic. Syndr.* **25:**157–163.
95. **Lee, H. H., P. Swanson, J. D. Rosenblatt, I. S. Chen, W. C. Sherwood, D. E. Smith, G. E. Tegtmeier, L. P. Fernando, C. T. Fang, M. Osame, and S. H. Kleinman.** 1991. Relative prevalence and risk factors of HTLV-I and HTLV-II infection in US blood donors. *Lancet* **337:** 1435–1439.
96. **Leon-Ponte, M., O. Noya, N. Bianco, and G. Echeverria de Perez.** 1996. Highly endemic human T-lymphotropic virus type II (HTLV-II) infection in a Venezuelan Guahibo Amerindian group. *J. Acquir. Immune Defic. Syndr. Hum. Retrovirol.* **13:**281–286.
97. **Levin, M. C., S. M. Lee, Y. Morcos, J. Brady, and J. Stuart.** 2002. Cross-reactivity between immunodominant human T lymphotropic virus type I Tax and neurons: implications for molecular mimicry. *J. Infect. Dis.* **186:**1514–1517.
98. **Lewis, M. J., V. W. Gautier, X. P. Wang, M. H. Kaplan, and W. W. Hall.** 2000. Spontaneous production of C-C chemokines by individuals infected with human T lymphotropic virus type II (HTLV-II) alone and HTLV-II/HIV-1 coinfected individuals. *J. Immunol.* **165:**4127–4132.
99. **Li, H. C., R. J. Biggar, W. J. Miley, E. M. Maloney, B. Cranston, B. Hanchard, and M. Hisada.** 2004. Provirus load in breast milk and risk of mother-to-child transmission of human T lymphotropic virus type I. *J. Infect. Dis.* **190:**1275–1278.
100. **Li, H. C., T. Fujiyoshi, H. Lou, S. Yashiki, S. Sonoda, L. Cartier, L. Nunez, I. Munoz, S. Horai, and K. Tajima.** 1999. The presence of ancient human T-cell lymphotropic virus type I provirus DNA in an Andean mummy. *Nat. Med.* **5:**1428–1432.
101. **Liang, M. H., T. Geisbert, Y. Yao, S. H. Hinrichs, and C. Z. Giam.** 2002. Human T-lymphotropic virus type 1 oncoprotein Tax promotes S-phase entry but blocks mitosis. *J. Virol.* **76:**4022–4033.
102. **Lima, M. A., R. C. Harab, D. Schor, M. J. Andrada-Serpa, and A. Q. Araújo.** 2007. Subacute progression of human T-lymphotropic virus type I-associated myelopathy/tropical spastic paraparesis. *J. Neurovirol.* **13:**468–473.
103. **Lynch, M. P., and P. T. Kaumaya.** 2006. Advances in HTLV-1 peptide vaccines and therapeutics. *Curr. Protein Pept. Sci.* **7:**137–145.
104. **Madeleine, M. M., S. Z. Wiktor, J. J. Goedert, A. Manns, P. H. Levine, R. J. Biggar, and W. A. Blattner.** 1993. HTLV-I and HTLV-II world-wide distribution: reanalysis of 4,832 immunoblot results. *Int. J. Cancer* **54:** 255–260.
105. **Mahieux, R., and A. Gessain.** 2005. New human retroviruses: HTLV-3 and HTLV-4. *Med. Trop.* **65:**525–528. (In French.)
106. **Maloney, E. M., R. J. Biggar, J. V. Neel, M. E. Taylor, B. H. Hahn, G. M. Shaw, and W. A. Blattner.** 1992. Endemic human T cell lymphotropic virus type II infection among isolated Brazilian Amerindians. *J. Infect. Dis.* **166:**100–107.
107. **Maloney, E. M., E. L. Murphy, J. P. Figueroa, W. N. Gibbs, B. Cranston, B. Hanchard, M. Holding-Cobham, K. Malley, and W. A. Blattner.** 1991. Human T-lymphotropic virus type I (HTLV-I) seroprevalence in Jamaica. II. Geographic and ecologic determinants. *Am. J. Epidemiol.* **133:**1125–1134.
108. **Manel, N., N. Taylor, S. Kinet, F. J. Kim, L. Swainson, M. Lavanya, J. L. Battini, and M. Sitbon.** 2004. HTLV envelopes and their receptor GLUT1, the ubiquitous glucose transporter: a new vision on HTLV infection? *Front. Biosci.* **9:**3218–3241.
109. **Manns, A., R. J. Wilks, E. L. Murphy, G. Haynes, J. P. Figueroa, M. Barnett, B. Hanchard, and W. A. Blattner.** 1992. A prospective study of transmission by transfusion of HTLV-I and risk factors associated with seroconversion. *Int. J. Cancer* **51:**886–891.
110. **Marinho, J., B. Galvao-Castro, L. C. Rodrigues, and M. L. Barreto.** 2005. Increased risk of tuberculosis with human T-lymphotropic virus-1 infection: a case-control study. *J. Acquir. Immune Defic. Syndr.* **40:**625–628.
111. **Marsh, B. J.** 1996. Infectious complications of human T cell leukemia/lymphoma virus type I infection. *Clin. Infect. Dis.* **23:**138–145.
112. **Matsuzaki, H., H. Hata, N. Asou, M. Yoshida, F. Matsuno, M. Takeya, K. Yamaguchi, I. Sanada, and K. Takatsuki.** 1992. Human T-cell leukemia virus-1-positive cell line established from a patient with small cell lung cancer. *Jpn. J. Cancer Res.* **83:**450–457.
113. **Matutes, E.** 2007. Adult T-cell leukaemia/lymphoma. *J. Clin. Pathol.* **60:**1373–1377.
114. **Menna-Barreto, M.** 2006. HTLV-II transmission to a health care worker. *Am. J. Infect. Control* **34:**158–160.
115. **Moarbess, G., H. El-Hajj, Y. Kfoury, M. E. El-Sabban, Y. Lepelletier, O. Hermine, C. Deleuze-Masquefa, P. A. Bonnet, and A. Bazarbachi.** 2008. EAPB0203, a member of the imidazoquinoxaline family, inhibits growth and induces caspase dependent apoptosis in T cell lymphomas and HTLV-I associated adult T-cell leukemia/lymphoma. *Blood* **111:**3770–3777.
116. **Modahl, L. E., K. C. Young, K. F. Varney, H. Khayam-Bashi, and E. L. Murphy.** 1995. Injection drug users seropositive for human T-lymphotropic virus type II (HTLV-II) are at increased risk for pneumonia. *J. Acquir. Immune Defic. Synd. Hum. Retrovirol.* **10:**260.

117. **Mori, N., M. Morishita, T. Tsukazaki, C. Z. Giam, A. Kumatori, Y. Tanaka, and N. Yamamoto.** 2001. Human T-cell leukemia virus type I oncoprotein Tax represses Smad-dependent transforming growth factor beta signaling through interaction with CREB-binding protein/p300. *Blood* **97:**2137–2144.

118. **Morofuji-Hirata, M., W. Kajiyama, K. Nakashima, A. Noguchi, J. Hayashi, and S. Kashiwagi.** 1993. Prevalence of antibody to human T-cell lymphotropic virus type I in Okinawa, Japan, after an interval of 9 years. *Am. J. Epidemiol.* **137:**43–48.

119. **Mueller, N., N. Tachibana, S. O. Stuver, A. Okayama, J. Ishizaki, E. Shishime, K. Murai, S. Shioiri, and K. Tsuda.** 1990. Epidemiologic perspectives of HTLV-I, p. 281–294. *In* W. A. Blattner (ed.), *Human Retrovirology: HTLV.* Lippincott-Raven, Philadelphia, PA.

120. **Mulloy, J. C., T. Kislyakova, A. Cereseto, L. Casareto, A. LoMonico, J. Fullen, M. V. Lorenzi, A. Cara, C. Nicot, C.-Z. Giam, and G. Franchini.** 1998. Human T-cell lymphotropic/leukemia virus type 1 Tax abrogates p53–induced cell cycle arrest and apoptosis through its CREB/ATF functional domain. *J. Virol.* **72:**8852–8860.

121. **Murata, K., and Y. Yamada.** 2007. The state of the art in the pathogenesis of ATL and new potential targets associated with HTLV-1 and ATL. *Int. Rev. Immunol.* **26:**249–268.

122. **Murphy, E. L., J. P. Figueroa, W. N. Gibbs, A. Brathwaite, M. Holding-Cobham, D. Waters, B. Cranston, B. Hanchard, and W. A. Blattner.** 1989. Sexual transmission of human T-lymphotropic virus type I (HTLV-I). *Ann. Intern. Med.* **111:**555–560.

123. **Murphy, E. L., J. P. Figueroa, W. N. Gibbs, M. Holding-Cobham, B. Cranston, K. Malley, A. J. Bodner, S. S. Alexander, and W. A. Blattner.** 1991. Human T-lymphotropic virus type I (HTLV-I) seroprevalence in Jamaica. I. Demographic determinants. *Am. J. Epidemiol.* **133:**1114–1124.

124. **Murphy, E. L., B. Wang, R. A. Sacher, J. Fridey, J. W. Smith, C. C. Nass, B. Newman, H. E. Ownby, G. Garratty, S. T. Hutching, and G. B. Schreiber.** 2004. Respiratory and urinary tract infections, arthritis, and asthma associated with HTLV-I and HTLV-II infection. *Emerg. Infect. Dis.* **10:**109–116.

125. **Murphy, E. L., Y. Wu, H. E. Ownby, J. W. Smith, R. K. Ruedy, R. A. Thomson, D. I. Ameti, D. J. Wright, and G. J. Nemo.** 2001. Delayed hypersensitivity skin testing to mumps and Candida albicans antigens is normal in middle-aged HTLV-I- and-II-infected U.S. cohorts. *AIDS Res. Hum. Retrovir.* **17:**1273–1277.

126. **Nagai, M., M. B. Brennan, J. A. Sakai, C. A. Mora, and S. Jacobson.** 2001. CD8+ T cells are an in vivo reservoir for HTLV-I. *Blood* **98:**1858–1861.

127. **Nagai, M., K. Usuku, W. Matsumoto, D. Kodama, N. Takenouchi, T. Moritoyo, S. Hashiguchi, M. Ichinose, C. R. Bangham, S. Izumo, and M. Osame.** 1998. Analysis of HTLV-I proviral load in 202 HAM/TSP patients and 243 asymptomatic HTLV-I carriers: high proviral load strongly predisposes to HAM/TSP. *J. Neurovirol.* **4:** 586–593.

128. **Nakao, K., N. Ohba, M. Nakagawa, and M. Osame.** 1999. Clinical course of HTLV-I-associated uveitis. *Jpn. J. Ophthalmol.* **43:**404–409.

129. **Narikawa, K., K. Fujihara, T. Misu, J. Feng, J. Fujimori, I. Nakashima, I. Miyazawa, H. Sato, S. Sato, and Y. Itoyama.** 2005. CSF-chemokines in HTLV-I-associated myelopathy: CXCL10 up-regulation and therapeutic effect of interferon-alpha. *J. Neuroimmunol.* **159:** 177–182.

130. **Nicot, C., R. Opavsky, R. Mahieux, J. M. Johnson, J. N. Brady, L. Wolff, and G. Franchini.** 2000. Tax oncoprotein trans-represses endogenous B-myb promoter activity in human T cells. *AIDS Res. Hum. Retrovir.* **16:** 1629–1632.

131. **Oger, J.** 2007. HTLV-1 infection and the viral etiology of multiple sclerosis. *J. Neurol. Sci.* **262:**100–104.

132. **Oh, U., Y. Yamano, C. A. Mora, J. Ohayon, F. Bagnato, J. A. Butman, J. Dambrosia, T. P. Leist, H. McFarland, and S. Jacobson.** 2005. Interferon-beta1a therapy in human T-lymphotropic virus type I-associated neurologic disease. *Ann. Neurol.* **57:**526–534.

133. **Oliveira Mde, F., C. Brites, N. Ferraz, P. Magalhaes, F. Almeida, and A. Bittencourt.** 2005. Infective dermatitis associated with the human T cell lymphotropic virus type I in Salvador, Bahia, Brazil. *Clin. Infect. Dis.* **40:** e90–e96.

134. **Orland, J. R., J. Engstrom, J. Fridey, R. A. Sacher, J. W. Smith, C. Nass, G. Garratty, B. Newman, D. Smith, B. Wang, K. Loughlin, and E. L. Murphy for the HTLV Outcomes Study.** 2003. Prevalence and clinical features of HTLV neurologic disease in the HTLV Outcomes Study. *Neurology* **61:**1588–1594.

135. **Parker, C. E., S. Daenke, S. Nightingale, and C. R. Bangham.** 1992. Activated, HTLV-1-specific cytotoxic T-lymphocytes are found in healthy seropositives as well as in patients with tropical spastic paraparesis. *Virology* **188:**628–636.

136. **Parkin, D. M.** 2006. The global health burden of infection-associated cancers in the year 2002. *Int. J. Cancer* **118:**3030–3044.

137. **Poiesz, B. J., F. W. Ruscetti, A. F. Gazdar, P. A. Bunn, J. D. Minna, and R. C. Gallo.** 1980. Detection and isolation of type C retrovirus particles from fresh and cultured lymphocytes of a patient with cutaneous T-cell lymphoma. *Proc. Natl. Acad. Sci. USA* **77:**7415–7419.

138. **Price, J., B. A. Cant, J. A. Barbara, and R. S. Tedder.** 2001. Human T-cell leukaemia/lymphoma virus risk may be enhanced in some selected donor populations. *Vox. Sang.* **80:**148–150.

139. **Primo, J. R., C. Brites, F. Oliveira Mde, O. Moreno-Carvalho, M. Machado, and A. L. Bittencourt.** 2005. Infective dermatitis and human T cell lymphotropic virus type 1-associated myelopathy/tropical spastic paraparesis in childhood and adolescence. *Clin. Infect. Dis.* **41:**535–541.

140. **Prince, H. E., E. R. Jensen, and J. York.** 1992. Lymphocyte subsets in HTLV-II-infected former blood donors: relationship to spontaneous lymphocyte proliferation. *Clin. Immunol. Immunopathol.* **65:**201–206.

141. **Proietti, F. A., A. B. Carneiro-Proiletti, B. C. Catalan-Soares, and E. L. Murphy.** 2005. Global epidemiology of HTLV-I infection and associated diseases. *Oncogene* **24:**6058–6068.

142. **Reeves, W. C., J. R. Cutler, F. Gracia, J. E. Kaplan, L. Castillo, T. M. Hartley, M. M. Brenes, M. Larreategui, S. de Loo de Lao, C. Archbold, et al.** 1990. Human T cell lymphotropic virus infection in Guaymi Indians from Panama. *Am. J. Trop. Med. Hyg.* **43:**410–418.

143. **Roberts, C. R., D. R. Fipps, J. F. Brundage, S. E. Wright, M. Goldenbaum, S. S. Alexander, and D. S. Burke.** 1992. Prevalence of human T-lymphotropic virus in civilian applicants for the United States Armed Forces. *Am. J. Public Health* **82:**70–73.

144. **Rosenblatt, J. D., J. V. Giorgi, D. W. Golde, J. B. Ezra, A. Wu, C. D. Winberg, J. Glaspy, W. Wachsman, and I. S. Chen.** 1988. Integrated human T-cell leukemia virus II genome in CD8 + T cells from a patient with

"atypical" hairy cell leukemia: evidence for distinct T and B cell lymphoproliferative disorders. *Blood* **71:**363–369.

145. **Rosenblatt, J. D., D. W. Golde, W. Wachsman, J. V. Giorgi, A. Jacobs, G. M. Schmidt, S. Quan, J. C. Gasson, and I. S. Chen.** 1986. A second isolate of HTLV-II associated with atypical hairy-cell leukemia. *N. Engl. J. Med.* **315:**372–377.
146. **Rosenblatt, J. D., S. Plaeger-Marshall, J. V. Giorgi, P. Swanson, I. S. Chen, E. Chin, H. J. Wang, M. Canavaggio, M. A. Hausner, and A. C. Black.** 1990. A clinical, hematologic, and immunologic analysis of 21 HTLV-II-infected intravenous drug users. *Blood* **76:**409–417.
147. **Ross, T. M., S. M. Pettiford, and P. L. Green.** 1996. The tax gene of human T-cell leukemia virus type 2 is essential for transformation of human T lymphocytes. *J. Virol.* **70:**5194–5202.
148. **Roucoux, D. F., B. Wang, D. Smith, C. C. Nass, J. Smith, S. T. Hutching, B. Newman, T. H. Lee, D. M. Chafets, and E. L. Murphy.** 2005. A prospective study of sexual transmission of human T lymphotropic virus (HTLV)-I and HTLV-II. *J. Infect. Dis.* **191:**1490–1497.
149. **Saito, M., M. Nakagawa, S. Kaseda, T. Matsuzaki, M. Jonosono, N. Eiraku, R. Kubota, N. Takenouchi, M. Nagai, Y. Furukawa, K. Usuku, S. Izumo, and M. Osame.** 2004. Decreased human T lymphotropic virus type I (HTLV-I) provirus load and alteration in T cell phenotype after interferon-alpha therapy for HTLV-I-associated myelopathy/tropical spastic paraparesis. *J. Infect. Dis.* **189:**29–40.
150. **Sarngadharan, M. G., A. L. DeVico, L. Bruch, J. Schüpbach, and R. C. Gallo.** 1984. HTLV-III: the etiologic agent of AIDS. *Princess Takamatsu Symp.* **15:**301–308.
151. **Satoh, M., and A. Kokaze.** 2004. Treatment strategies in controlling strongyloidiasis. *Expert Opin. Pharmacother.* **5:**2293–2301.
152. **Shames, B. D., A. M. D'Alessandro, and H. W. Sollinger.** 2002. Human T-cell lymphotrophic virus infection in organ donors: a need to reassess policy? *Am. J. Transplant.* **2:**658–663.
153. **Sinha-Datta, U., A. Datta, S. Ghorbel, M. D. Dodon, and C. Nicot.** 2007. Human T-cell lymphotrophic virus type I rex and p30 interactions govern the switch between virus latency and replication. *J. Biol. Chem.* **282:** 14608–14615.
154. **Sonoda, S.** 1990. Genetic and immunologic determinants of HTLV-I associated diseases, p. 315. *In* W. A. Blattner (ed.), *Human Retrovirology: HTLV.* Lippincott-Raven, Philadelphia, PA.
155. **Switzer, W. M., I. Hewlett, L. Aaron, N. D. Wolfe, D. S. Burke, and W. Heneine.** 2006. Serologic testing for human T-lymphotropic virus-3 and -4. *Transfusion* **46:**1647–1648.
156. **Switzer, W. M., S. H. Qari, N. D. Wolfe, D. S. Burke, T. M. Folks, and W. Heneine.** 2006. Ancient origin and molecular features of the novel human T-lymphotropic virus type 3 revealed by complete genome analysis. *J. Virol.* **80:**7424–7438.
157. **Tachibana, N., A. Okayama, S. Ishihara, S. Shioiri, K. Murai, K. Tsuda, N. Goya, Y. Matsuo, M. Essex, S. Stuver, and N. Mueller.** 1992. High HTLV-I proviral DNA level associated with abnormal lymphocytes in peripheral blood from asymptomatic carriers. *Int. J. Cancer* **51:**593–595.
158. **Taguchi, H., and I. Miyoshi.** 1989. Immune suppression in HTLV-I carriers: a predictive sign of adult T-cell leukemia. *Acta Med. Okayama* **43:**317–321.
159. **Tajima, K., R. Amakawa, K. Uehira, N. Matsumoto, T. Shimizu, Y. Miyazaki, M. Fujimoto, Y. Kishimoto, and S. Fukuhara.** 2000. Adult T-cell leukemia successfully treated with allogeneic bone marrow transplantation. *Int. J. Hematol.* **71:**290–293.
160. **Takatsuki, K.** 2005. Discovery of adult T-cell leukemia. *Retrovirology* **2:**16.
161. **Takemoto, S., R. Trovato, A. Cereseto, C. Nicot, T. Kislyakova, L. Casareto, T. Waldmann, G. Torelli, and G. Franchini.** 2000. p53 stabilization and functional impairment in the absence of genetic mutation or the alteration of the p14(ARF)-MDM2 loop in ex vivo and cultured adult T-cell leukemia/lymphoma cells. *Blood* **95:**3939–3944.
162. **Tanaka, G., A. Okayama, T. Watanabe, S. Aizawa, S. Stuver, N. Mueller, C. C. Hsieh, and H. Tsubouchi.** 2005. The clonal expansion of human T lymphotropic virus type 1-infected T cells: a comparison between seroconverters and long-term carriers. *J. Infect. Dis.* **191:** 1140–1147.
163. **Taylor, G. P., P. Goon, Y. Furukawa, H. Green, A. Barfield, A. Mosley, H. Nose, A. Babiker, P. Rudge, K. Usuku, M. Osame, C. R. Bangham, and J. N. Weber.** 2006. Zidovudine plus lamivudine in human T-lymphotropic virus type-I-associated myelopathy: a randomised trial. *Retrovirology* **3:**63.
164. **Tsukahara, T., M. Kannagi, T. Ohashi, H. Kato, M. Arai, G. Nunez, Y. Iwanaga, N. Yamamoto, K. Ohtani, M. Nakamura, and M. Fujii.** 1999. Induction of Bcl-x_L expression by human T-cell leukemia virus type 1 Tax through NF-κB in apoptosis-resistant T-cell tranfectants with Tax. *J. Virol.* **73:**7981–7987.
165. **Tsukasaki, K., S. Ikeda, K. Murata, T. Maeda, S. Atogami, H. Sohda, S. Momita, T. Jubashi, Y. Yamada, M. Mine, et al.** 1993. Characteristics of chemotherapy-induced clinical remission in long survivors with aggressive adult T-cell leukemia/lymphoma. *Leukocyte Res.* **17:**157–166.
166. **Tsukasaki, K., K. Tobinai, M. Shimoyama, M. Kozuru, N. Uike, Y. Yamada, M. Tomonaga, K. Araki, M. Kasai, K. Takatsuki, M. Tara, C. Mikuni, and T. Hotta.** 2003. Deoxycoformycin-containing combination chemotherapy for adult T-cell leukemia-lymphoma: Japan Clinical Oncology Group Study (JCOG9109). *Int. J. Hematol.* **77:**164–170.
167. **Vandamme, A. M., M. Salemi, and J. Desmyter.** 1998. The simian origins of the pathogenic human T-cell lymphotropic virus type I. *Trends Microbiol.* **6:**477–483.
168. **Van Dooren, S., M. Salemi, and A. M. Vandamme.** 2001. Dating the origin of the African human T-cell lymphotropic virus type-i (HTLV-I) subtypes. *Mol. Biol. Evol.* **18:**661–671.
169. **Vidal, A. U., A. Gessain, M. Yoshida, F. Tekaia, B. Garin, B. Guillemain, T. Schulz, R. Farid, and G. De The.** 1994. Phylogenetic classification of human T cell leukaemia/lymphoma virus type I genotypes in five major molecular and geographical subtypes. *J. Gen. Virol.* **75:**3655–3666.
170. **Vitek, C. R., F. I. Gracia, R. Giusti, K. Fukuda, D. B. Green, L. C. Castillo, B. Armien, R. F. Khabbaz, P. H. Levine, J. E. Kaplan, and W. A. Blattner.** 1995. Evidence for sexual and mother-to-child transmission of human T lymphotropic virus type II among Guaymi Indians, Panama. *J. Infect. Dis.* **171:**1022–1026.
171. **Wattel, E., M. Cavrois, A. Gessain, and S. Wain-Hobson.** 1996. Clonal expansion of infected cells: a way of life for HTLV-I. *J. Acquir. Immune Defic. Syndr. Hum. Retrovirol.* **13**(Suppl. 1)**:**S92–S99.

172. **Welles, S. L., N. Tachibana, A. Okayama, S. Shioiri, S. Ishihara, K. Murai, and N. E. Mueller.** 1994. Decreased reactivity to PPD among HTLV-I carriers in relation to virus and hematologic status. *Int. J. Cancer* **56:** 337–340.

173. **Wiktor, S. Z., E. J. Pate, E. L. Murphy, T. J. Palker, E. Champegnie, A. Ramlal, B. Cranston, B. Hanchard, and W. A. Blattner.** 1993. Mother-to-child transmission of human T-cell lymphotropic virus type I (HTLV-I) in Jamaica: association with antibodies to envelope glycoprotein (gp46) epitopes. *J. Acquir. Immune Defic. Syndr.* **6:**1162–1167.

174. **Wiktor, S. Z., E. J. Pate, P. S. Rosenberg, M. Barnett, P. Palmer, D. Medeiros, E. M. Maloney, and W. A. Blattner.** 1997. Mother-to-child transmission of human T-cell lymphotropic virus type I associated with prolonged breast-feeding. *J. Hum. Virol.* **1:**37–44.

175. **Wolfe, N. D., W. Heneine, J. K. Carr, A. D. Garcia, V. Shanmugam, U. Tamoufe, J. N. Torimiro, A. T. Prosser, M. Lebreton, E. Mpoudi-Ngole, F. E. McCutchan, D. L. Birx, T. M. Folks, D. S. Burke, and W. M. Switzer.** 2005. Emergence of unique primate T-lymphotropic viruses among central African bushmeat hunters. *Proc. Natl. Acad. Sci. USA* **102:**7994–7999.

176. **Xie, L., and P. L. Green.** 2005. Envelope is a major viral determinant of the distinct in vitro cellular transformation tropism of human T-cell leukemia virus type 1 (HTLV-1) and HTLV-2. *J. Virol.* **79:**14536–14545.

177. **Yamaguchi, K., T. Kiyokawa, G. Futami, T. Ishii, and K. Takatsui.** 1990. Pathogenesis of adult T-cell leukemia from clinical pathologic features, p. 163. *In* W. A. Blattner (ed.), *Human Retrovirology: HTLV.* Lippincott-Raven, Philadelphia, PA.

178. **Yamaguchi, K., M. Shimoyama, and K. Takatsuki.** 1990. *Adult T-Cell Leukemia and HTLV-1 Related Diseases.* Eisai, Tokyo, Japan.

179. **Yamano, Y., C. J. Cohen, N. Takenouchi, K. Yao. U. Tomaru, H. C. Li, Y. Reiter, and S. Jacobson.** 2004. Increased expression of human T lymphocyte virus type I (HTLV-1) Tax 11-19 peptide–human histocompatibility leukocyte antigen A*201 complexes on $CD4^+$ $CD25^+$ T cells detected by peptide-specific, major histocompatibility complex-restricted antibodies in patients with HTLV-I-associated neurologic disease. *J. Exp. Med.* **199:**1367–1377.

180. **Yamano, Y., M. Nagai, M. Brennan, C. A. Mora, S. S. Soldan, U. Tomaru, N. Takenouchi, S. Izumo, M. Osame, and S. Jacobson.** 2002. Correlation of human T-cell lymphotropic virus type 1 (HTLV-1) mRNA with proviral DNA load, virus-specific CD8(+) T cells, and disease severity in HTLV-1-associated myelopathy (HAM/TSP). *Blood* **99:**88–94.

181. **Yamano, Y., N. Takenouchi, H. C. Li, U. Tomaru, K. Yao, C. W. Grant, D. A. Maric, and S. Jacobson.** 2005. Virus-induced dysfunction of CD4+CD25+ T cells in patients with HTLV-I-associated neuroimmunological disease. *J. Clin. Investig.* **115:**1361–1368.

182. **Yoshida, M.** 2001. Multiple viral strategies of HTLV-1 for dysregulation of cell growth control. *Annu. Rev. Immunol.* **19:**475–496.

183. **Zehender, G., L. Meroni, S. Varchetta, C. De Maddalena, B. Cavalli, M. Gianotto, A. B. Bosisio, C. Colasante, G. Rizzardini, M. Moroni, and M. Galli.** 1998. Human T-lymphotropic virus type 2 (HTLV-2) provirus in circulating cells of the monocyte/macrophage lineage in patients dually infected with human immunodeficiency virus type 1 and HTLV-2 and having predominantly sensory polyneuropathy. *J. Virol.* **72:**7664–7668.

Human Immunodeficiency Virus

JOHN C. GUATELLI, ROBERT F. SILICIANO, DANIEL R. KURITZKES, AND DOUGLAS D. RICHMAN

33

Human immunodeficiency virus (HIV), the etiologic agent of AIDS, is estimated to have infected over 60 million people (353; http://www.unaids.org/en/hiv_data/default.asp). Over 95% of these infections have occurred among young adults in the developing world. The AIDS pandemic is now the fourth leading cause of mortality worldwide, and approximately 33 million people are currently living with HIV infection (353). Infection with HIV type 1 (HIV-1) is prevalent throughout the world and is characterized by a progressive deterioration of the immune system that is almost uniformly fatal if untreated.

Although the first known human case of HIV infection dates to 1959 (392), AIDS was first recognized as a clinical entity in 1981. The syndrome was identified by clusters of unusual diseases including Kaposi's sarcoma and *Pneumocystis jiroveci* pneumonia in young homosexual men (136, 224, 325). These patients were noted to have immunodeficiency due to depletion of CD4$^+$ helper T cells. AIDS cases were subsequently found in intravenous drug users, hemophiliacs, and infants born to mothers with AIDS, suggesting that AIDS was caused by a blood-borne as well as sexually transmitted pathogen. In 1983, HIV-1 was isolated (19), and this novel human retrovirus was proposed as the cause of AIDS. Within several years an antibody test was developed to detect infection, the nucleotide sequence of the genome of HIV-1 was determined (244, 289, 308, 363), and the first antiretroviral drug—the nucleoside analog zidovudine—was shown to have activity in vitro and in patients (238, 382). Since then, enormous progress in both basic and clinical research has provided the tools to suppress viral replication to a degree sufficient to prevent or reverse the immunologic and clinical sequelae of HIV infection. Nevertheless, neither curative therapy for this disease nor a vaccine able to stop its spread is available.

The HIV strains arose from cross-species transmission of nonhuman primate lentiviruses (150). Evidence for cross-species transmission became apparent in 1985, when studies of West African prostitutes revealed the presence of antibodies that were more highly reactive with proteins of simian immunodeficiency virus (SIV) than with those of HIV-1 (17). This observation led to the discovery of HIV-2 (33), a virus more closely related genetically to the SIVs than to HIV-1. SIVsm, isolated from sooty mangabeys (*Cercocebus atys*), is very closely related to HIV-2 strains isolated from West African people, and the sooty mangabey appears to be the source of HIV-2 infection in humans. In contrast, the source of HIV-1 appears to be the chimpanzee subspecies *Pan troglodytes troglodytes*, in which SIVcpz strains are endemic (126, 182). Presumably, SIVcpz has been introduced into the human population from *P. t. troglodytes* on three occasions to yield the major HIV-1 groups: main (M), outlier (O), and non-M, non-O (N), although the gorilla subspecies *Gorilla gorilla gorilla* may have been an intermediate reservoir during the transmission of group O viruses from chimpanzees to humans (357). The natural range of *P. t. troglodytes* is West Equatorial Africa, an area in which the three genetically distinct HIV-1 groups are endemic.

VIROLOGY

Classification

HIV-1 and HIV-2 are enveloped RNA viruses belonging to the family *Retroviridae*. These viruses reverse transcribe their genomes to form double-stranded DNA, which integrates into the genomic DNA of the host. HIV-1, HIV-2, and the SIVs are members of the *Lentivirus* genus. Viruses in this genus are characterized by cytopathicity in vitro, lack of oncogenicity, the establishment of chronic infections, and relatively low rates of pathogenesis. SIV has been found in at least 26 species of nonhuman African primates, including African green monkeys (SIVagm) and sooty mangabeys (SIVsm) (150). In their natural hosts these viruses are generally not pathogenic. However, introduction of African SIVsm or SIVagm into Asian rhesus macaques results in an AIDS-like illness, similar to that caused by HIV infection in humans (201).

Genotypes, Serotypes, and Antigenicity

Among the three genetic groups of HIV-1 (M, O, and N), group M viruses dominate the pandemic. This group is further divided into genetic subtypes or clades (A through D, F through H, J, and K) based on nucleotide sequence relatedness (Fig. 1); subtype C is the most prevalent worldwide. Many viral isolates appear to be recombinants containing sequences from more than one subtype. These are designated CRF (for "circulating recombinant form") (298). For example, the former subtype E is thought to be a recombinant between subtypes A and E, and its current

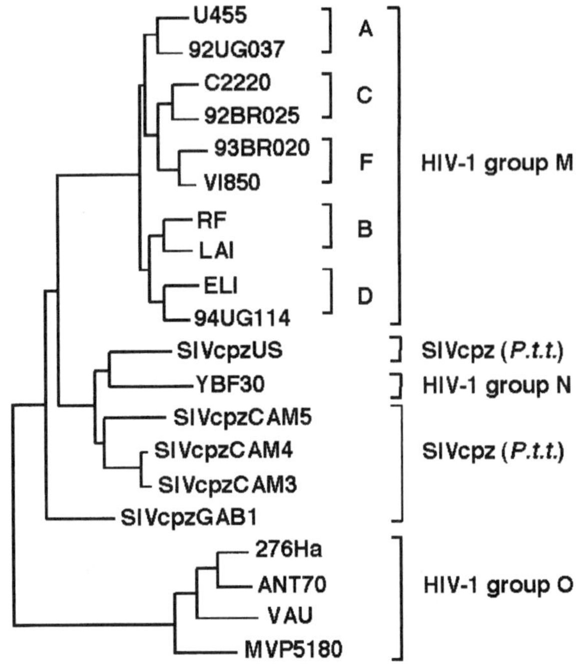

FIGURE 1 Evolutionary relationships between members of the HIV-1 and SIVcpz lineages, based on the phylogenetic analysis of Env protein sequences. The three genetic groups of HIV-1 (M, N, and O) are indicated by brackets on the right, as are related groups of SIVcpz strains from *P. t. troglodytes*, the apparent nonhuman primate source of HIV-1 strains. Five subtypes within group M are also indicated. The scale bar indicates 0.1 amino acid replacement per site. (Modified from reference 150 with permission of the American Association for the Advancement of Science.)

designation is CRF01-AE. Numerous unique recombinant forms (URF), detected in individuals and resulting from coinfection with two subtypes, have not been recognized to undergo sustained transmission like CRFs. Mosaic viruses that contain parts resembling four or more subtypes are given the suffix cpx (for "complex"); for example, the former subtype I has been given the designation CRF04-cpx to indicate that it is a complex circulating recombinant form. The current designations of specific HIV-1 strains as CRFs versus parental subtypes are subject to change, since putative evolutionary relationships can be confounded by sampling history and high rates of recombination (1). Both humoral and cellular immune responses to each of the proteins of HIV have been detected. Antibody reactivity to multiple proteins forms the basis for the confirmatory Western blot assay. The primary structural proteins, Gag and Env, elicit the greatest antibody responses, which form the basis for the diagnostic enzyme-linked immunosorbent assay (EIA). Neutralizing antibodies are directed to the envelope glycoproteins, gp120 and gp41, which are exposed on the surfaces of infected cells and virions. However, there are no clearly defined HIV-1 serotypes. HIV-1 Env is composed of a surface domain (gp120) and a transmembrane domain (gp41), which are noncovalently associated and form trimeric spikes (Fig. 2). The peptide sequence of gp120 contains conserved (C) and variable (V) regions.

Several features of this protein render the virus relatively resistant to humoral immunity (193, 380). Regions of gp120 that are involved in binding interactions with cellular molecules required for infectivity are conserved but are poorly accessible to antibodies. For example, the binding site for CD4, the primary cellular receptor for the primate immunodeficiency viruses, is recessed and surrounded by variable, glycosylated regions (Fig. 2). In addition, the surface of gp120 is heavily glycosylated. This glycosylation reduces the antigenicity of Env, presumably by allowing the molecule to appear to the immune system as "self." Extensive glycosylation also provides a "shield" that appears to protect virions from neutralizing antibodies. Similarly, the binding site for the chemokine receptors, the so-called coreceptors for these viruses, is masked by the variable loops V2 and V3 (Fig. 2) (297).

Antibodies to gp120 become detectable in the sera of HIV-infected individuals within 2 to 3 weeks after infection (243). However, these early antibodies are not neutralizing. They appear to recognize the interactive regions of gp120 and gp41, which, although immunogenic, are not exposed in the assembled trimeric glycoprotein complex (380). Subsequently, antibodies appear that may recognize the V3 or V2 loops and are neutralizing but usually restricted in activity to the infecting strain. Such antibodies appear to drive the selection of escape variants, so that patient serum can neutralize previous but not contemporaneous autologous isolates (296). Finally, antibodies appear that have more broadly neutralizing activity against a variety of isolates. Many of these interfere with the binding interaction between gp120 and CD4. These antibodies recognize discontinuous epitopes, the key residues of which are located within the binding pocket for CD4 on gp120 (the so-called CD4BS epitopes [Fig. 2]). Other broadly neutralizing antibodies recognize epitopes that are near conserved structures involved in coreceptor binding (the so-called CD4i epitopes [Fig. 2]). An unusual neutralization epitope is distant from the receptor binding sites on the outer domain of gp120. This epitope (2G12 [Fig. 2]) is carbohydrate based and is formed by a conserved cluster of oligomannoses (42). Lastly, broadly cross-reactive neutralization epitopes are located in the membrane-proximal region of the ectodomain of gp41 (262).

Composition of Virus

Virion Morphology, Structure, Size, and Genomic Organization

By electron microscopy, the HIV-1 virion measures approximately 100 to 150 nm in diameter (Fig. 3). Mature viral particles are characterized by an electron-dense conical core. The core is surrounded by a lipid envelope that is acquired as the virion buds from the infected cell. The virion core contains two copies of single-stranded positive-sense genomic RNA, each of which encodes the complete viral repertoire of structural, enzymatic, and regulatory proteins. The HIV genome is approximately 10 kb in length and is organized similarly to that of other retroviruses (Fig. 4). The sequence is flanked by the two long terminal repeats (LTRs). The 5′ LTR contains the enhancer/promoter sequences for viral transcription, and the 3′ LTR contains the polyadenylation signal. From 5′ to 3′ the viral genome contains the *gag* gene, which encodes the virion structural components; the *pol* gene, which encodes the viral en-

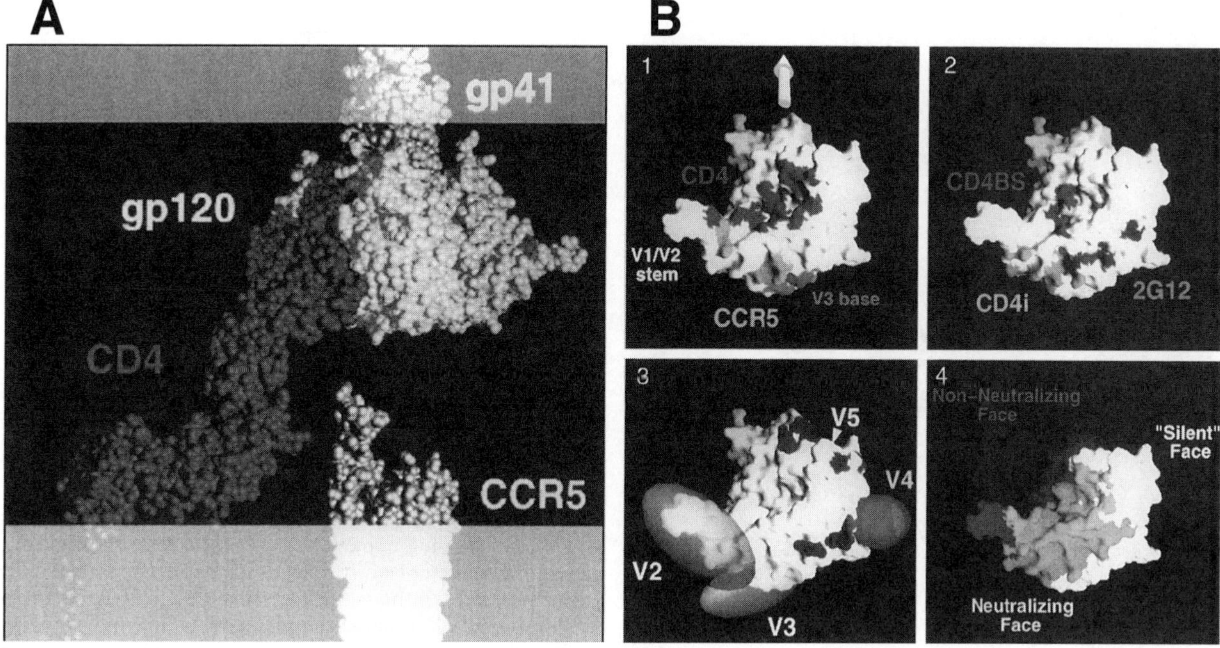

FIGURE 2 (A) Structural representation of the envelope glycoprotein complex of HIV-1 interacting with the cellular receptor molecules CD4 and CCR5. The shaded area at the top represents the viral lipid envelope; that at the bottom represents the cellular plasma membrane. The surface subunit gp120 and the transmembrane subunit gp41 of HIV Env form a trimeric complex. The variable loops of the gp120 are not shown and would extend over the outer surface of the complex. (B) Structural representation of the gp120 surface, emphasizing the relationships among the binding sites for CD4 and CCR5, the location of neutralization epitopes, and the protection from antibody responses afforded by the variable loops and by glycosylation. (Panel 1) Surface of the core of gp120, missing most of the major variable loops (V1, V2, V3, and V4). The arrow points to the viral membrane. The interaction sites for CCR5 are lightly shaded; those for CD4 are more darkly shaded. (Panel 2) Conserved neutralization epitopes are indicated: the CD4BS epitopes are darkly shaded, the CD4i epitopes are lightly shaded, and the 2G12 epitope is darkly shaded and toward the right; see the text for definition. (Panel 3) Protection from antibody responses is provided by the V2 and V3 loops, as well as by N-linked glycosylation (sites are shaded). (Panel 4) The neutralizing face of gp120 (light shading) includes the binding sites for CD4 and CCR5; the nonneutralizing face (dark shading) includes the region that interacts with gp41; and the silent face (white) is minimally immunogenic due to glycosylation. (Modified from reference 380a with permission of the American Association for the Advancement of Science.)

zymes; and the *env* gene, which encodes the envelope glycoproteins. The primate immunodeficiency viral genomes contain six additional genes: *vif*, *vpr*, *tat*, *rev*, *nef*, and either *vpx* (in HIV-2 and SIV) or *vpu* (in HIV-1) (Fig. 4 and Table 1) (97). The products of these genes function via interactions with host cell proteins to optimize viral replication by a variety of mechanisms discussed below.

Major Structural and Regulatory Proteins

The major structural and core proteins of HIV are synthesized from *gag* as a large, myristoylated precursor protein (pr55) that is subsequently cleaved by the viral proteinase to yield the matrix (MA; p17), capsid (CA; p24), and nucleocapsid (NC; p7) proteins (158, 234). The matrix protein is a peripheral membrane protein located along the inner leaflet of the viral lipid envelope, where it directs the incorporation of the envelope glycoproteins (Env) into the forming virion (88). The MA protein is also found in the virion core; it may participate in the transport of the viral preintegration complex to the nucleus after reverse transcription is completed (36). The capsid protein (p24) assembles to form the conical core of the virion. The core structure follows the principles of a fullerene cone composed primarily of a curved array of hexameric CA subunits, with the inclusion of several pentameric subunits to allow closure of the cone (203). The nucleocapsid protein (p7) is an RNA binding protein required for packaging of the genomic RNA into the virion (134). Several smaller cleavage products, p1, p2, and p6, are also generated from the p55 precursor. The p6 protein contains the so-called late or L domain required for viral budding; it mediates the incorporation of the viral accessory protein Vpr into virions (3).

The viral enzymes are also produced by proteolytic cleavage from a large precursor molecule. During translation, a ribosomal frameshift occasionally occurs between the *gag* and *pol* open reading frames, resulting in the synthesis of a *gag-pol* precursor protein (pr170) (170). The ratio of Gag-Pol to Gag produced is approximately 1:20. Subsequent cleavage of pr170 yields the Gag protein prod-

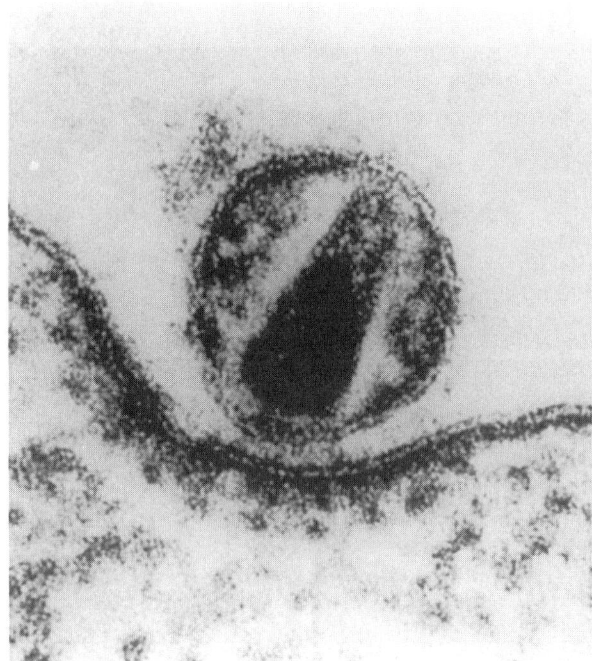

FIGURE 3 Electron micrograph of an HIV-1 virion budding from an infected cell. The viral glycoprotein complexes are barely discernible on the surface of the virion membrane. The electron-dense material just beneath the viral lipid bilayer corresponds to the MA (p17) protein. The conical virion core is composed of the CA (p24) protein. Also within the core are the NC (p7) protein which binds the genomic RNA, the p6 protein required for budding, the accessory protein Vpr, the RT, the IN, and two copies of the genomic RNA. The accessory protein Nef is also virion-associated. (Micrograph courtesy of H. Gelderbloom.)

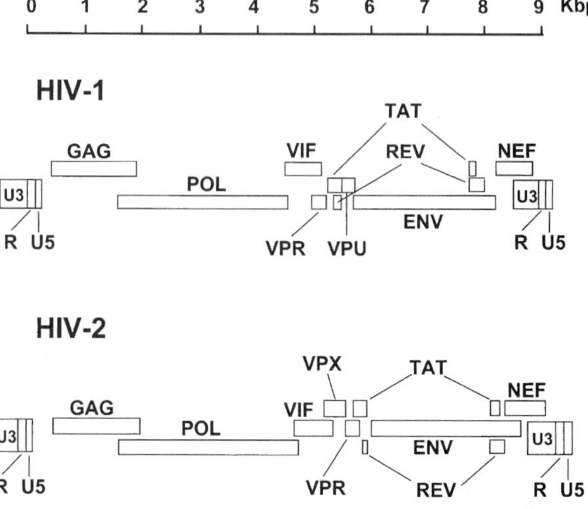

FIGURE 4 Genomic organization of HIV-1 and HIV-2. The viral open reading frames are shown; the roles of their gene products are described in the text and in Table 1. The open reading frames of the *tat* and *rev* genes are interrupted by an intron. The LTRs found at each end of the fully reverse-transcribed viral DNA are composed of U3, R, and U5 regions; the definitions of their boundaries are described in the text. The major genetic differences between these viruses are the lack of the Vpu open reading frame and the presence of the Vpx open reading frame in HIV-2; these features render HIV-2 more similar to most SIVs than to HIV-1.

ucts and the retroviral enzymes protease (p11), reverse transcriptase (RT)/RNase H (p66/p51), and integrase (p32). The aspartyl protease (p11) cleaves the structural and enzymatic proteins from the large polyprotein precursors. This enzyme is a symmetric dimer that is activated by dimerization during virion assembly (170, 177). Pharmacologic inhibition of the viral protease results in the formation of noninfectious particles. The RT enzyme is a heterodimer with 66- and 51-kDa subunits. This enzyme provides both the RT activity, which allows RNA-dependent DNA polymerization, and the RNase H activity, which allows the specific degradation of RNA present in RNA-DNA heteroduplexes. The RNase H domain is present only in the larger of the two subunits (76). The integrase mediates insertion of the viral DNA into that of the chromosome of the host cell (106). To accomplish this, integrase comprises two activities: a DNA-cleaving activity, which cuts the host DNA and processes the ends of the HIV-DNA, and a DNA strand transfer activity, which covalently attaches the viral DNA to that of the host, most frequently in transcriptionally active open reading frames.

The protein product of the *env* gene is synthesized in the endoplasmic reticulum as an 88-kDa polypeptide (373). This protein undergoes glycosylation in the endoplasmic reticulum and Golgi. The resulting molecule, gp160, contains N-linked, high-mannose sugars that account for approximately half of the final molecular mass of 160 kDa. Much of the newly synthesized gp160 is retained in intracellular compartments and eventually degraded; however, a fraction is cleaved by cellular serine proteases such as furin to generate the transmembrane (gp41) and surface (gp120) subunits (373). This cleavage event is required for viral infectivity, because it allows subsequent exposure of a sequence within the ectodomain of gp41 that mediates fusion of the virion and target cell membranes (228). Following proteolytic cleavage, gp120 remains noncovalently associated with gp41 on the cell surface. The complex is incorporated into the envelope of budding virions via an interaction between the cytoplasmic domain of gp41 and the p17 matrix protein (88). The envelope glycoproteins are arranged as trimers in a spike-and-knob configuration (Fig. 2). Recent analyses suggest that as few as 8 to 14 Env trimers may be incorporated per virion (54, 391).

The primate immunodeficiency viruses encode several nonenzymatic and nonstructural gene products (97). Two of these genes, *tat* and *rev*, are essential for viral replication. Tat is a 14-kDa *trans*-activating protein that markedly enhances the rate of transcription from the 5′ LTR by recruiting cellular factors that enhance the processivity of the cellular RNA polymerase II complex (10, 195, 245). Tat recruits a cyclin-dependent protein kinase complex (Cdk9 plus cyclin T) to a structured region near the 5′ end of the primary viral transcript (the *trans*-acting responsive region) (367, 381). Cdk9 hyperphosphorylates the C-terminal domain of RNA polymerase II, allowing efficient elongation of the nascent viral mRNA (263). In the absence of Tat, viral transcription is essentially stalled just after initiation.

The 18-kDa Rev protein mediates the transport of singly spliced and unspliced viral RNAs from the nucleus to

TABLE 1 HIV genes and gene products

Gene	Protein	Size	Function
Structural			
gag	Matrix (MA)	p17	Structural protein (recruits envelope glycoprotein)
	Capsid (CA)	p24	Structural protein (forms conical core)
	Nucleocapsid (NC)	p7	Binds viral RNA to encapsidate genome
	p6	p6	Budding
pol	Protease (PR)	p12	Viral enzyme: cleavage of polyprotein precursors
	Reverse transcriptase (RT)	p66/p51	Viral enzyme: reverse transcription and RNase H activities
	Integrase (IN)	p32	Viral enzyme: integration of viral cDNA into host chromosomes
env	Surface glycoprotein (SU)	gp120	Viral envelope glycoprotein: receptor binding
	Transmembrane (TM)	gp41	Viral envelope glycoprotein: fusion
Regulatory			
tat	Tat	p14	Transactivates viral transcription
rev	Rev	p19	Transports unspliced mRNA to cytoplasm
vif	Vif	p24	Promotes virion infectivity by degrading the cellular cytidine deaminases APOBEC3F and APOBEC3G
nef	Nef	p27	Down-regulates class I MHC and CD4; enhances viral infectivity; facilitates T-cell activation
vpu[a]	Vpu	p16	Promotes release of viral particles; induces degradation of CD4
vpr	Vpr	p15	Arrests cell cycle in G_2; facilitates nuclear entry of the preintegration complex and viral replication in macrophages
vpx[a]	Vpx	p14	Facilitates nuclear entry of the preintegration complex and viral replication in macrophages

[a] *vpu* is found almost exclusively in HIV-1; *vpx* is found only in HIV-2 and SIV.

the cytoplasm. These RNAs encode the HIV-1 structural and enzymatic proteins and include the viral genomic RNA (219). Rev directly links these viral RNAs to a specific nuclear export pathway. The N-terminal region of Rev contains a basic domain that binds a structured region in the RNA (the Rev response element [RRE], which overlaps the coding sequence of the gp41), while the C-terminal region contains a prototypical, leucine-rich, nuclear export signal that binds to the nuclear export protein CRM1, also known as exportin 1 (116, 220, 369). In the absence of Rev activity, viral mRNAs are inefficiently exported from the nucleus, and as a consequence of prolonged nuclear retention, they undergo extensive splicing to yield subgenomic mRNAs encoding only a subset of viral proteins that includes Tat, Rev, and Nef.

The other nonenzymatic and nonstructural genes of HIV-1 and HIV-2 (*vif, vpr, vpx, vpu,* and *nef*) are not essential for viral replication under certain conditions in vitro and consequently have been termed "accessory genes." Nevertheless, these genes are highly conserved among isolates of primate lentiviruses, and their importance for viral replication and pathogenicity in vivo has been documented by using the macaque/SIV and SHIV animal models of AIDS (84, 183). The critical roles of these genes have also been confirmed by the use of physiologic culture systems, in particular primary cultures of T lymphocytes and macrophages (123, 154, 331). The accessory gene products appear to function by mediating interactions with cellular proteins or pathways. With the current exception of Nef, the function of each of these gene products involves the modulation of specific cellular ubiquitin ligases that control protein expression at the level of proteosomal degradation (81). In the cases of Vif and Vpu, specific cellular proteins that are deleterious to viral replication are targeted for degradation.

The 23-kDa Vif protein targets the cellular cytidine deaminases APOBEC3F and APOBEC3G for degradation by the proteasome (323). In the absence of Vif, these proteins are incorporated into virions, where they deaminate cytosine residues in the minus strand of the forming viral cDNA. The resulting uracil residues lead to inactivating hypermutation (G-to-A transitions in the plus strand) (153). Consequently, Vif is required for the production of infectious virions (339) and for viral replication in primary cultures of T lymphocytes (123). Cells of certain immortalized lines allow the replication of Vif-negative virus (hence the "accessory gene" designation), simply because they lack APOBEC3F and APOBEC3G (322). These cytidine deaminases may play a role in an innate cellular defense against both exogenous retroviruses and endogenous retroelements (99).

The 14-kDa HIV-1 Vpr protein appears to have two distinct functions. First, the expression of Vpr arrests cells in the G_2 phase of the cell cycle (302). This has two known consequences: the yield of progeny virions is increased due to enhanced viral transcription during the prolonged G_2 phase (302), and apoptosis (programmed cell death) is induced (8). Transcriptional activation by Vpr may occur immediately after infection (169), because Vpr is incorporated into virion cores by direct association with the p6 *gag* gene product (190). Second, Vpr is required for efficient viral replication in macrophages (154). Vpr is a component of the viral preintegration complex, which forms after virion entry and contains the viral cDNA and integrase (236). Vpr appears to contribute to the transport of the preintegration complex into the nucleus, particularly in nondividing cells such as macrophages where the complex must cross an intact nuclear envelope (286). The two functions of HIV-1 Vpr are divided between two gene products in SIV and HIV-2. In these viruses, Vpr causes G_2 arrest and Vpx allows efficient nuclear transport of the preintegration complex and viral replication in macrophages; both Vpr and Vpx are virion-associated proteins (115). Vpr (and probably Vpx) interacts with and probably modulates the activity of a specific ubiquitin ligase that is involved in the regulation of cellular DNA replication and the response to host cell DNA damage (81, 199). Presumably by stimulating the degradation of a currently unidentified cellular protein(s), Vpr activates a cellular sensor of replication stress (the ataxia telangiectasia-mutated and Rad3-related protein), blocking entry of the cell into M phase and ultimately leading to cell death by apoptosis (8).

The 16-kDa Vpu protein is an integral membrane protein encoded by HIV-1 but not by HIV-2 or SIV (340). Vpu enhances the release of virions from infected cells (188), apparently by inhibiting the endocytosis of Gag and by counteracting an unidentified cellular factor that tethers nascent virions to the plasma membrane (250). The virion release function of Vpu maps to the transmembrane domain of the protein, which forms an ion channel reminiscent of the M2 protein of influenza A virus (102, 314). Vpu also induces the rapid degradation of CD4 by linking it while still in the endoplasmic reticulum to the proteosomal degradation machinery via the cellular protein β-TrCP (374); this function maps to the cytoplasmic domain of Vpu, which interacts with both CD4 and β-TrCP. Vpu and Env are translated from bicistronic mRNAs, suggesting that the coordinated expression of these two genes is important (318). By degrading CD4 during virus production, Vpu prevents an inhibitory effect of the viral receptor on the infectivity of progeny virions that would otherwise occur due to the interaction of Env and CD4 (202).

The 27-kDa Nef protein modulates both cellular signal transduction and membrane trafficking. Nef is a peripheral membrane protein that contains two well-defined protein interaction motifs: an SH3 binding domain and a dileucine-based protein-sorting motif (73, 146, 307). HIV-1 Nef facilitates T-cell activation, and it activates specific signaling pathways (212). These effects may enhance viral transcription and stimulate the production of cytokines such as interleukin-2. Nef also affects membrane trafficking by interacting with cellular proteins that coat transport vesicles (21, 196). The consequences of this include the down-regulation of CD4 and class I major histocompatibility complex (MHC) from the cell surface (127, 316). The down-regulation of class I MHC provides escape from immune surveillance by enabling infected cells to avoid destruction by cytotoxic T lymphocytes (CTL) (65). Nef is a virion-associated protein, and it enhances the infectivity of virions by an incompletely described mechanism (270). Patients infected with naturally occurring Nef mutants of HIV-1 and macaque monkeys infected experimentally with Nef mutants of SIV experience attenuated rates of disease progression, indicating that this protein is required for high viral burdens and maximal pathogenesis (80, 183). On the other hand, most SIV and HIV-2 Nef proteins, but not HIV-1 Nef, are able to down-regulate the T-cell receptor (CD3), and this effect has been hypothesized to account for the ability of SIVs to sustain nonpathogenic infection in their natural hosts, presumably by reducing the chronic activation of the immune system typical of pathogenic lentiviral infections (311).

Biology

Replication Strategy

The entire replication cycle of HIV-1 (Fig. 5), from the binding of virions to target cells to the release of infectious progeny, is completed in approximately 24 h in vitro and in vivo (186, 278). Replication is initiated by attachment of the virus to a target cell through the interaction of the viral envelope glycoprotein, gp120, with the cellular receptor molecule, CD4 (75, 216, 230). The binding of gp120 to CD4 induces conformational changes in gp120, which enable binding to the cellular coreceptor molecules (379). The two major coreceptor molecules for HIV-1 are CXCR4 and CCR5 (4, 58, 108). These molecules are transmembrane proteins that function in the host as receptors for chemoattractant cytokines (chemokines). The natural ligand for CXCR4 is the stromal cell-derived factor 1 (SDF-1), and the natural ligands for CCR5 are the β-chemokines CCL3, CCL4, and CCL5 (formerly known as MIP-1α, MIP-1β, and RANTES, respectively). Binding of gp120 to these coreceptors is obligatory for the fusion of virus with the host cell, and natural as well as synthetic ligands for these molecules can block the infectivity of HIV-1. Some primary isolates of HIV-1 can utilize either CXCR4 or CCR5 as a coreceptor for entry, but many can utilize only CCR5. Binding of gp120 to the coreceptors allows exposure of a fusogenic motif in the amino-terminal ectodomain of gp41; this leads to fusion of the lipid bilayer of the virion with that of the host cell (27). The fusion-competent core of the gp41 forms a six-helix bundle analogous in structure to the low-pH (fusion-competent) conformation of the influenza A virus hemagglutinin (51). Formation of this so-called hairpin conformation is required for the viral and cellular membranes to reach sufficient proximity to fuse. Entry of HIV into the cell occurs primarily at the plasma membrane and does not require internalization of the virus into cellular endosomes. Consequently, the entry of HIV-1 is acid independent and is not blocked by weak bases or drugs that inhibit acidification of the endo-lysosomal system (217).

Synthesis of the viral cDNA can begin in cell-free virions (386), but it is completed in the target cell cytoplasm within so-called reverse transcription complexes that travel toward the cell nucleus along microtubules (229). The syn-

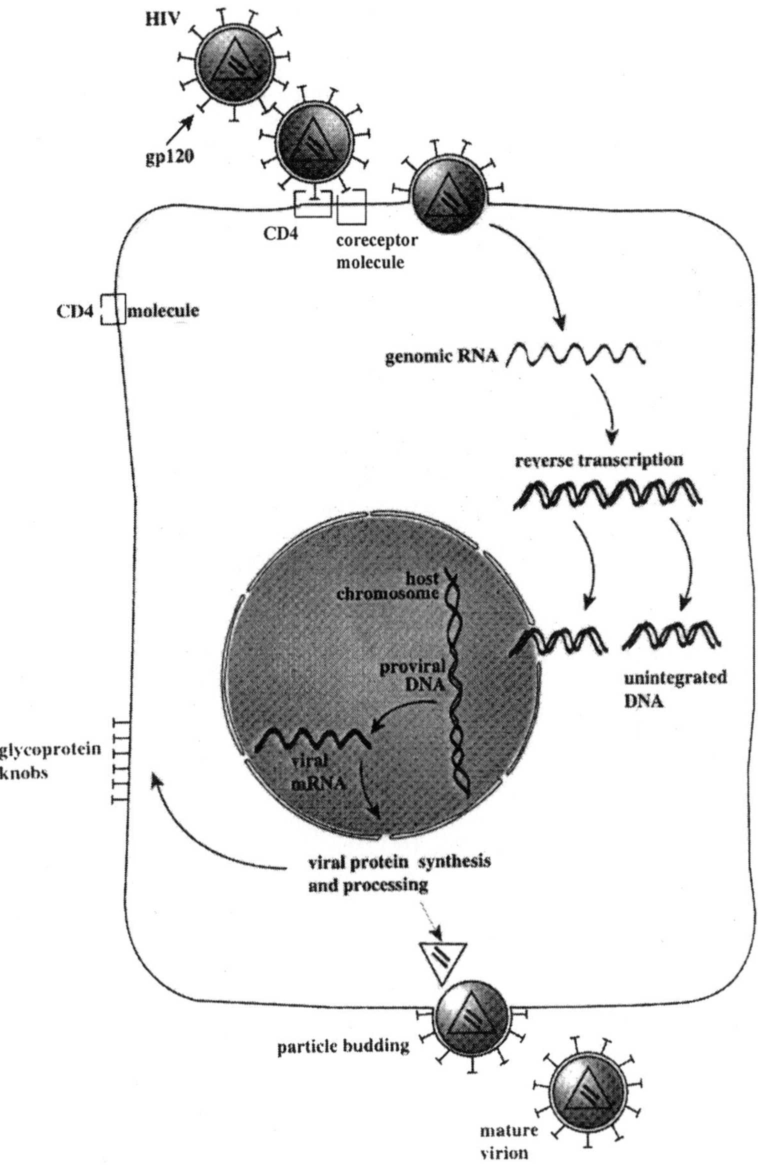

FIGURE 5 Replication cycle of HIV.

thesis of the viral cDNA is discontinuous. The RT synthesizes the first complementary strand of DNA (the minus strand) by using the viral genomic RNA as a template and a host tRNA-Lys as a primer. The tRNA primer binding site defines the 3′ end of the U5 region of the LTR. Viral RNase H degrades the original RNA template. The RT then synthesizes the second strand of DNA (the plus strand), beginning at two polypurine tracks: one defines the 5′ end of the U3 region of the LTR, and the other is located near the center of the genome (53, 378). Strand-switching events that utilize sequence complementarity at each end of the viral RNA occur during the synthesis of both minus- and plus-strand DNAs, generating the U3-R-U5 direct repeats (the LTRs) at each end of the complete, double-stranded cDNA. These strand transfer events lead to the utilization of both copies of the virion-associated genomic RNA as templates during reverse transcription, so that genetic recombination occurs when the two copies are dissimilar in sequence (384). Such recombination generates genetic variants following coinfection of the same target cell with genetically distinct viruses.

The reverse-transcribed viral genome remains associated with several viral proteins as the preintegration complex. This nucleoprotein complex can be viewed as an uncoated virion core that lacks the major capsid protein p24 but contains the viral matrix protein (p17), Vpr, integrase, and RT in addition to the viral cDNA (36, 107, 236). Transport of the preintegration complex into the nucleus is facilitated by protein sequences within the various subunits. These include the matrix protein, Vpr, and the integrase itself. A "flap" structure within the middle of the viral plus-strand cDNA, which is formed during the process of reverse transcription, also contributes to efficient nuclear import (385). After translocation to the nucleus, the double-stranded linear DNA is integrated into the host cell chromosome by the virally encoded integrase in concert with host cell DNA repair enzymes to form the provirus (41, 105). Covalently closed DNA circles with either one or two LTR junctions are also formed by host enzymes in the nucleus, but these forms are dead-end products that cannot integrate into the target cell DNA. Integration requires the cellular coactivator protein p75/LEDGF (209), which tethers the viral integrase enzyme to the host cell chromatin. This mechanism probably provides at least part of the basis for the preferential integration of HIV into genes that are transcriptionally active (313). Chromosomal integration is required for viral replication. Integration also yields the form of the viral genome responsible for establishing a permanent, latent reservoir in the host.

The activation of HIV transcription and gene expression from the integrated provirus is dependent on the activity of both cellular and viral factors. The virion-associated protein Vpr is a weak transactivator of transcription and may stimulate the initial expression of viral RNAs (169). Specific sites within the 5′ LTR are recognized by cellular transcription factors including NF-κB, AP-1, SP1, and NFAT, several of which are induced during the activation of T cells (130). Transcription is initiated from a single site in the viral 5′ LTR, the 5′ boundary of the R region. The activity of the HIV promoter is repressed by chromatin structure; chromatin remodeling induced by histone acetylation can relieve this repression and activate transcription (359). The primary transcript is alternatively spliced to generate over 30 species of viral mRNAs. The early viral transcripts are extensively spliced to form a group of mRNAs that are 1.8 to 2.0 kb in size and which encode the proteins Tat, Rev, and Nef (317). Tat markedly increases the level of viral transcription by recruiting cellular factors to the nascent RNAs, facilitating their elongation as discussed above. Once Rev is synthesized, the incompletely spliced (approximately 5-kb) and unspliced (9-kb) viral mRNAs are exported from the nucleus (168). These RNAs encode the accessory gene products Vif, Vpr, and Vpu; all the structural and enzymatic proteins; and genomic RNA. Thus, Rev mediates a transition from early-gene expression (Tat, Rev, and Nef) to late-gene expression (Gag, Pol, Env, Vif, Vpr, and Vpu) about 6 to 8 h after infection in vitro (186).

The assembly of virions occurs primarily at the plasma membrane. The Gag and Gag-Pol precursor polyproteins are synthesized in the cytoplasm and associate with the plasma membrane via N-terminal myristolation and binding to specific membrane lipids (264). Dimerization of Gag precursor activates the viral protease, which cleaves the precursor proteins to generate the individual structural and enzymatic polypeptides described above. In contrast to Gag, the Env glycoproteins are synthesized in association with cellular membranes. Env is then recruited into the forming virion at the plasma membrane by association of the cytoplasmic domain of gp41 with p17 MA. The capsid protein p24 forms the core structure, and the nucleocapsid protein p7 binds the genomic RNA. The Gag polyprotein is sufficient for virion assembly and budding. Budding requires a specific domain (the L-domain) in the p6 region of Gag, which binds endosomal proteins involved in the biogenesis of multivesicular bodies (MVBs) (336, 362). MVBs are late endosomal structures that contain internal vesicles, and the viral budding process is topologically similar to the formation of the vesicles within MVBs. How the virus utilizes this cellular machinery for budding while avoiding degradation in late endosomes and lysosomes is unknown. Virion assembly occurs selectively at the basal-lateral surfaces of polarized epithelial cells, at the uropod of T cells, and at regions of cell-cell contact that are enriched in cellular transmembrane proteins termed tetraspanins (83, 176). HIV-1, like measles virus and influenza virus, buds from specialized regions of the plasma membrane that are enriched in cholesterol and glycolipids (so-called lipid rafts) (254). Presumably, this modified lipid composition facilitates budding and/or fusion of the virions with target cells. In addition to the virally encoded proteins, virions of HIV-1 incorporate a number of cellular proteins, including major histocompatibility antigens (9), adhesion molecules such as ICAM-1 (117), cyclophilin A (213), and a large number of cytoskeletal and endosomal proteins (55). The roles of these incorporated cellular proteins for the virus are not clear.

Host Range, Tropism, and Cytopathic Effect

The natural host range of HIV-1 and HIV-2 is restricted to humans, although chimpanzees have been infected with HIV-1 under experimental conditions (121, 249) and cynomologous monkeys and rhesus macaques have been infected with HIV-2 (89, 287). Unlike infection in humans, HIV-1 is generally nonpathogenic in chimpanzees and virus replication declines over time. Studies of the molecular determinants of the host range of primate lentiviruses have revealed novel, innate intracellular defense mechanisms that restrict infection. In particular, the inability of Old World monkey cells to support infection with HIV-1 is due to the expression of a specific form of the protein TRIM5α, which targets the capsid protein of incoming virions to inhibit viral replication by an incompletely understood mechanism (341).

The primary cellular targets for HIV-1 infection in vivo are $CD4^+$ T lymphocytes and macrophages. In vitro, most isolates of HIV-1 replicate efficiently in primary cultures of $CD4^+$ T cells while only a subset are capable of replication in immortalized $CD4^+$ T-cell lines. This cellular tropism is the result of the selective interaction of Env glycoproteins with specific coreceptor molecules (387). For example, many primary isolates (derived from patients by minimal passage in primary cultures of T cells) utilize CCR5 exclusively and fail to grow in T-cell lines, which typically express CXCR4 but not CCR5. Other primary isolates utilize both CCR5 and CXCR4, and consequently these isolates grow in both primary cells and T-cell lines. Exclusive use of CXCR4 is a feature found in occasional clones from later-stage patients and laboratory strains of HIV-1 that have been adapted by extensive passage using CXCR4-expressing immortalized T cells. HIV-1 also replicates in vitro in monocyte-derived macrophages. Macrophage-tropic isolates utilize CCR5 as the cellular coreceptor. The basis of macrophage tropism remains incompletely understood, because although these cells express CXCR4, they are not permissive for the replication of viruses that use only this coreceptor. Within Env, the principal determinants of specific coreceptor usage and macrophage tropism map to the V3 loop, but other regions of gp120 can also mediate CXCR4 usage (261, 371). HIV can also enter dendritic cells (DC) and Langerhans' cells via the interaction between gp120 and C-type lectins on the cell surface. Although these professional antigen-presenting cells do not support robust productive infection, they can retain infectious virions and transmit them to $CD4^+$ T cells (104, 131). This so-called transinfection may be an important part of the mechanism of transmission of HIV at mucosal surfaces and of its initial spread to regional lymphoid tissue.

In vitro, the fusion of infected and uninfected cells leads to a cytopathic effect characterized by the formation of multinucleated giant cells (syncytia). The formation of syncytia begins with cell clustering, followed by cell-cell fusion and ballooning of cell membranes (Fig. 6). Not all primary isolates of HIV-1 induce syncytia in immortalized T-cell lines in vitro. Frequently, isolates derived early in the course of infection are non-syncytium-inducing (NSI) whereas isolates from later stage patients often have a syncytium-inducing (SI) phenotype (28, 346). The NSI phenotype is the result of exclusive use of CCR5 by the Env of the isolate, while the SI phenotype is the result of the additional ability to use CXCR4, allowing viral growth in T-cell lines. In longitudinal analyses of patient isolates, the acquisition of tropism for cells expressing only CXCR4 is associated with a more rapid decline in $CD4^+$ T-cell numbers and clinical progression of disease (67, 293). Use of CXCR4 as a coreceptor may be viewed as a marker for expanded tropism, potentially explaining the association of this phenotype with more rapidly progressive disease.

Inactivation by Physical and Chemical Agents

HIV is sensitive to a variety of chemical agents including glutaraldehyde, hypochlorite, quaternary ammonium compounds, phenolics, ethanol, and iodine (92). Cell-free virus is inactivated most readily; infectivity is decreased by at least 10^6-fold after 1 min of exposure of cell-free virus to 0.5% glutaraldehyde or 35% ethanol. Cell-associated virus is less susceptible to inactivation; exposure of cell-associated virus to 35% ethanol for 5 min is inadequate, but exposure to 75% ethanol for 1 min is sufficient. Cell-associated virus suspended in blood is the most resistant to inactivation; glutaraldehyde (0.5%), hypochlorite (25,000 ppm), and 75% ethanol are effective after 1 min, but quaternary ammonium compounds and phenolics are ineffective even after 10 min.

HIV is also sensitive to UV light (92). As in the case of chemical inactivation, cell-associated virus and virus in blood are more resistant to inactivation by UV light. A 10-min exposure of cell-free virus to UV light in a typical biosafety cabinet is sufficient for inactivation, but 30 min is required to inactivate cell-associated virus, and even 60 min fails to inactivate cell-associated virus suspended in blood.

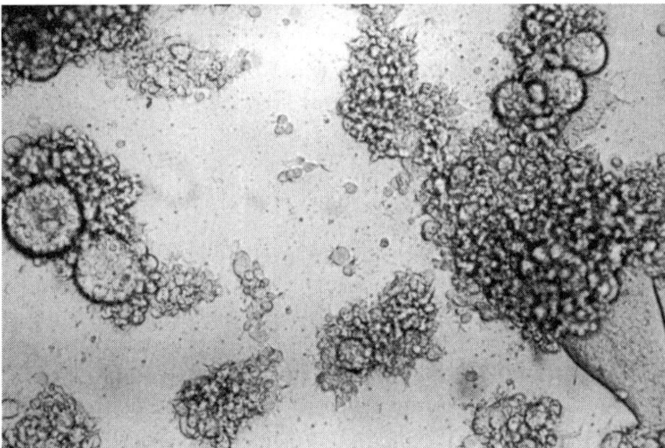

FIGURE 6 Formation of syncytia during replication of HIV-1 in a culture of T lymphoblastoid cells. In immortalized T-cell lines, the interaction of the viral glycoprotein complex with the cellular receptors CD4 and CXCR4 allows cell-cell fusion and the formation of multinucleated giant cells.

EPIDEMIOLOGY

Distribution and Geography

The AIDS pandemic can be viewed as a composite of multiple epidemics, each occurring in specific geographic regions and populations. While HIV-2 has remained largely confined to West Africa, HIV-1 has spread throughout the world. Group M viruses are responsible for the vast majority of HIV-1 infections. Viruses belonging to the distinct subtypes or clades within group M have been isolated in geographically distinct regions of the world. In the United States, Europe, and Australia, the prevalence of subtype B illustrates a founder effect in which one or several viral variants were introduced and then disseminated through the population (133). Subtype B is found only rarely in Africa. Instead, subtype A predominates in West Africa, subtypes A and D predominate in East Africa, and subtype C predominates in southern Africa. Variants of HIV-1 appear to quickly expand to become the major subtype when introduced into a specific population or geographic area. For example, in Thailand, subtype B viruses predominated among intravenous drug users in Bangkok while CRF-01AE (formerly designated subtype E) recombinant viruses spread throughout the country by heterosexual contact (370).

The distribution of HIV-1 subtypes is complex and uneven and probably reflects a stochastic dissemination. Multiple subtypes cocirculate within areas of central Africa, Southeast Asia, and South America. In regions where different subtypes are prevalent, recombination between subtypes is apparent (299). The incidence of coinfection and subsequent recombination may be high in areas such as Africa and Southeast Asia where multiple subtypes of HIV-1 are known to circulate simultaneously. For example, in Camaroon, mixed infections were observed in approximately 10% of cases and included coinfection with two subtypes within group M, coinfection with M and O viruses, and even coinfection with HIV-1 and HIV-2 (343). Recombination events between all of the HIV-1 subtypes belonging to group M have been detected, as has recombination between group M and group O viruses (344).

Incidence and Prevalence of Infection

According to World Health Organization estimates, approximately 30 million persons are estimated to have died while 33 million are living with HIV infection or AIDS. A total of 2.5 million new cases were estimated to have occurred globally during the year 2006. Approximately 95% of all HIV infections have occurred in the developing world and among young and middle-aged adults.

The prevalence and incidence rates of HIV infection vary considerably in different regions of the world and reflect the progress of local epidemics fueled by distinct modes of transmission, socioeconomic environments, and behavioral factors (79). Sub-Saharan Africa accounts for over 60% of the current cases of HIV infection and for 75% of the world's HIV-infected women and children, although it contains only 10% of the world's population. The overall prevalence of disease in adults between 15 and 49 years of age in sub-Saharan Africa is approximately 6%, and many countries in this region have prevalences of over

10%. Although the prevalence of infection has stabilized in some regions of Africa, this reflects approximately equal rates of incidence and mortality. Africa continues to account for the majority of new cases in the world. Asia accounts for over 20% of the world's cases of HIV-1 infection, with over 6 million cases as of 2006. The majority of these have occurred in India. Latin America accounts for over 4% of the world's cases of HIV infection, with 1.6 million cases. Although the prevalence among adults in Europe is less than 1%, regions in Eastern Europe have experienced recent marked increases in prevalence, attributable to high rates of injection drug use. Eastern Europe and Central Asia now account for 1.6 million cases. North America accounts for approximately 4% of the world's cases of HIV infection.

Transmission

Transmission of HIV occurs through direct contact with infected body fluids, including blood and blood products (166), semen (166), vaginal and cervical secretions (361), amniotic fluid (246), and breast milk (348). Despite detection of HIV-1 nucleic acids in saliva and tears (120, 141), there have been no documented cases of transmission via these body fluids. Transmission most commonly occurs during sexual contact, with the transfer of semen, genital secretions, or blood from an infected individual to the uninfected partner. Unprotected receptive anal intercourse, with associated mucosal trauma, carries the highest risk of sexual transmission. In the majority of instances, transmission from male to female and from female to male takes place during vaginal intercourse, although cases have occurred after fellatio. Sexual transmission is facilitated by the presence of underlying sexually transmitted diseases including chancroid, herpes genitalis, and syphilis, which disrupt the integrity of the skin or mucosal linings (140, 332).

Transmission is also more likely when the source partner is acutely infected and the concentration of virus in genital secretions is highest (31). The exact mechanism of sexual transmission is unclear. The form of the transmitted inoculum may be cell-associated virus or cell-free virions. How HIV breaches the mucosal barrier is also uncertain; the possibilities include facilitation at areas of disruption in the mucosa as noted above, transcytosis of virions through epithelial cells with release into the lamina propria, and uptake of virions into Langerhans' cells with transinfection of T cells as discussed above.

Infection also occurs through direct inoculation of infected blood, transfusion of infected blood products, transplantation of infected tissues, and the reuse of contaminated needles. The risk of HIV-1 transmission following occupational percutaneous exposure to infected blood via a contaminated needle is approximately 0.3% (132, 157). The likelihood of transmission is influenced by many factors including the type of needle (hollow versus solid bore), the depth of penetration, the volume of the inoculum, and the amount of infectious virus in the inoculum.

The third primary mode of transmission of HIV-1 is from an infected mother to her child during pregnancy, delivery, or breast-feeding. The risk of maternal-fetal transmission is 13 to 40% (100), but this can be significantly reduced by prophylatic treatment of the mother and the newborn with antiretrovirals (66). Unfortunately, the beneficial effects of perinatal prophylaxis with antiretroviral therapy can be lost by subsequent infection of the infant during breast-feeding.

Patterns of Transmission

The primary modes of transmission vary in different regions. The mode of transmission in sub-Saharan Africa is heterosexual in 90% of cases; almost 60% of the HIV-positive individuals in this region are women. This region also accounts for 87% of the world's total number of HIV-infected children, in whom infection is acquired perinatally.

The pattern of spread of HIV in South and Southeast Asia is exemplified by the epidemic in Thailand, which began among injection drug users and sex workers and then spread into the general population. Prevalences reached a peak of 10% among military recruits and 6.4% in prenatal clinics by 1993 to 1994, but they have declined subsequently due to control measures such as condom use in commercial sex establishments (79). Heterosexual transmission plays a major role in the epidemics in Southeast Asia, as evidenced by the fact that 25% of the infected adults are women. In Latin America, the initial epidemic primarily involved men having sex with men. However, injection drug use and heterosexual transmission have become significant modes of spread in this region.

The dramatic recent rise in incidence rates in Eastern Europe and Central Asia has been fueled by injection drug use and has occurred primarily among men in the Ukraine and other countries of the former Soviet Union (129). Eastern Europe has also been the site of nosocomial outbreaks of HIV infection caused by improper reuse of medical equipment. In Western and Northern Europe, the initial epidemic involved men having sex with men. More recently, the incidence of infection in other populations has increased, with heterosexual contact and injection drug use accounting for an increasing number of cases.

In the United States, the prevalence of AIDS remains greatest among homosexual and bisexual men. Between 2001 and 2004 the proportion of new AIDS cases in African-Americans and Hispanics increased to 50 and 20% of the total number of cases in the United States, respectively. The proportion of new cases attributed to heterosexual transmission in the United States increased markedly from 4% in 1985 to 34% by 2004. Heterosexual transmission in the United States has been strongly associated with sexual contact with an injection drug user. The proportion of women infected with HIV in the United States has also increased markedly since the beginning of the epidemic, from 7% of cases in the early 1980s to 27% in 2004. Despite these increases in HIV infection among U.S. women, the incidence of infection among infants declined dramatically from 907 cases in 1992 to fewer than 100 by 2003; this decline was attributable to the treatment of infected women, prenatal screening, and peripartum chemoprophylaxis.

PATHOGENESIS

Incubation Period

In classic virologic terms, the incubation period is the interval between acquisition of the infection and onset of the illness. For HIV-1 infection, the term is problematic in the sense that a symptomatic illness, called primary HIV-1 infection, develops in some infected individuals within 1 to 4 weeks after exposure whereas clinical immunodeficiency (AIDS) typically appears after a prolonged asymptomatic period measured in years following primary infection. During this time, active viral replication and critical pathophysiologic changes occur. Patients with advanced HIV-1 infection show numerous immunologic abnormalities, the most prominent of which are severe quantitative and qualitative defects in the CD4$^+$ T-lymphocyte compartment. Much of the decline in CD4$^+$ T-cell counts occurs during the asymptomatic period between initial infection and the development of clinically apparent immunodeficiency. In adults, the average length of this asymptomatic period is 10 years. Opportunistic infections by organisms that do not cause disease in immunocompetent individuals herald the development of AIDS. These infections usually do not occur until the CD4$^+$ T-cell count has dropped from the normal levels of 600 to 1,000 cells/μl to below 200 cells/μl. The degree of loss of CD4$^+$ T cells is an excellent predictor of progression to AIDS, and a CD4$^+$ T-cell count below 200 cells/μl is now considered to be an AIDS-defining condition. Susceptibility to particular opportunistic infections appears in a predictable way, such that some infections appear as the CD4 count falls below 200 cells/μl (*Pneumocystis* pneumonia) while other infections are seen only in patients whose CD4 counts have fallen to below 100 cells/μl (*Mycobacterium avium* complex infection) or 50 cells/μl (cytomegalovirus retinitis). These findings suggest that the loss of CD4$^+$ T cells is central to the development of clinical immunodeficiency. Therefore, understanding the mechanism of CD4 depletion is the central problem in AIDS pathogenesis.

Patterns of Virus Replication

Organ and Cell Specificity

Although in untreated individuals virus is detected in the blood throughout the course of HIV-1 infection, most evidence suggests that virus replication occurs predominantly in the peripheral lymphoid organs, especially the spleen, lymph nodes, and gut-associated lymphoid tissue (272, 360). However, HIV-1 virions can infect CD4$^+$ cells in any tissue. Target cells include not only mature CD4$^+$ T cells in lymphoid tissues but also developing T cells in the thymus and the ubiquitous tissue macrophages, which express small amounts of CD4. Fusion and entry occur if appropriate coreceptors are expressed. However, the course of subsequent events in the virus life cycle depends on the cell type (CD4$^+$ T cell versus macrophage) and the state of activation of the cell.

CD4$^+$ T Lymphocytes

The cellular dynamics of infection of CD4$^+$ T lymphocytes by HIV-1 are illustrated in Fig. 7. CD4$^+$ T cells are heterogeneous with respect to activation state (resting versus activated) and previous antigen exposure (naïve versus

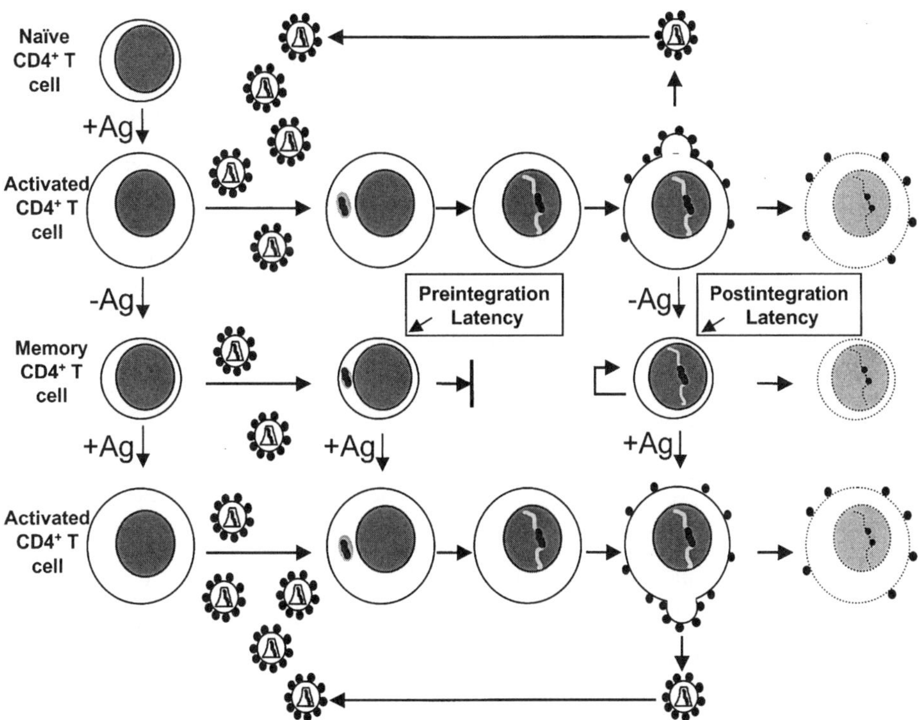

FIGURE 7 Cellular dynamics of HIV-1 infection of CD4$^+$ T cells. Successive steps in the life cycle of the virus are indicated by horizontal arrows. Transitions between resting (small) and activated (large) CD4$^+$ T cells are illustrated by vertical arrows. HIV-1 can infect resting and activated CD4$^+$ T cells, but integration of the reverse-transcribed HIV-1 provirus, which is necessary for virus production, occurs only in antigen-activated T cells. Productive infection requires antigen (Ag)-driven activation of recently infected resting CD4$^+$ cells or infection of antigen-activated CD4$^+$ T cells. Productively infected cells generally die within a few days from cytopathic effects of the infection, but some survive long enough to go back to a resting state, thereby establishing a stable latent reservoir.

memory), and HIV-1 pathogenesis must be considered in the context of this heterogeneity. Normally, the majority of mature CD4$^+$ T lymphocytes are in a resting G_0 state. These resting T cells are among the most quiescent cells in the body and are simply waiting to encounter antigen. About half are memory cells, which have previously responded to some antigen, while the remainder are naïve T cells.

The frequently transmitted CCR5-tropic (R5) forms of HIV-1 can bind to and fuse with activated CD4$^+$ T cells and a small subset of resting memory CD4$^+$ T cells (281). CXCR4-tropic (X4) viruses can enter essentially all CD4$^+$ T cells due to the broad expression of CXCR4 in CD4$^+$ T cells. Although reverse transcription can occur in both resting and activated T cells, the process is slow in resting T cells and there are blocks at a subsequent step in the virus life cycle such that resting CD4$^+$ T cells probably do not become productively infected without some form of activating stimulus. For example, the host cytidine deaminase APOBEC3G and other members of this family of proteins appear to play a significant role in restricting productive infection of resting CD4$^+$ T cells, monocytes, and most dendritic cells (DC) (57, 276, 284). In addition, in resting CD4$^+$ T cells, entry of the preintegration complex containing the reverse-transcribed HIV-1 DNA into the nucleus may not occur (35). Thus, in resting T cells, reverse-transcribed HIV-1 genomes reside in the cytoplasm for a finite period (days to weeks) before the preintegration complex becomes nonfunctional. If the T cell is activated by antigen before the preintegration complex becomes nonfunctional, the subsequent replicative steps can occur. In this sense, resting T cells carrying unintegrated HIV-1 DNA represent a latent reservoir for the virus, a condition known as preintegration latency (37). In untreated asymptomatic HIV-1-infected individuals, most of the viral DNA present in resting CD4$^+$ T cells is in this unintegrated form (26, 59). Because transcription of unintegrated viral DNA in the cytoplasm cannot occur, latently infected cells carrying this form of viral DNA presumably escape detection by immunologic mechanisms.

Following encounter with antigen, resting CD4$^+$ T cells undergo blast transformation and enter a state in which they are highly susceptible to productive infection by HIV-1. In activated T cells, APOBEC3G is sequestered in an inactive form and there is no block to nuclear import. Thus, the infection progresses rapidly to integration, viral gene expression, and virus production. Gene expression from the HIV-1 LTR is dependent on host transcription factors such as NF-κB that are up-regulated in activated T cells (247). This adaptation allows HIV-1 gene expression and virus production to be dramatically increased in activated CD4$^+$ T cells and largely shut off in resting CD4$^+$ T cells.

From this point, there are several possible fates for infected cells (Fig. 7). In vitro studies have shown that HIV-1 infection can be highly cytopathic for activated CD4$^+$ T cells and can induce cell killing by mechanisms that are described below. Some of these cells can also be destroyed by immunologic mechanisms including HIV-1-specific CTL. As a result of these mechanisms, the half-life of productively infected CD4$^+$ T cells is relatively short, generally <1 day. However, some of the productively infected CD4$^+$ T cells escape both the viral cytopathic effects and immunologic effector mechanisms and revert to a resting memory state carrying integrated provirus (61). This is a reflection of the normal physiology of T-cell activation; a fraction of the T cells that respond to any given antigen survive and enter the long-lived pool of memory T cells. In a resting state, these memory CD4$^+$ T cells are likely to have little or no virus gene expression and are thus unrecognized by the immune system. Because the viral DNA is in an integrated state in these cells, it is highly stable. These cells therefore provide a long-term, stable latent reservoir for the virus, a phenomenon termed postintegration latency (59, 61). On subsequent exposure to antigen, these cells become activated and release infectious virus. Thus, as emphasized in Fig. 7, antigen plays a critical role in driving CD4$^+$ T cells into states in which they are susceptible to productive infection by HIV-1 and subsequent destruction by viral cytopathic effects or immune mechanisms.

Macrophages

The cellular dynamics of HIV-1 infection are different in macrophages and CD4$^+$ T cells. HIV-1 can replicate in macrophages (164, 255), although integration and replication can occur only in dividing cells for most retroviruses. Specific amino acid sequences in the HIV-1 Gag, Vpr, and integrase (IN) proteins and even a portion of the reverse-transcribed HIV-1 DNA all participate in targeting the viral preintegration complex for nuclear import, permitting integration and replication in nondividing cells such as macrophages (34, 154). Infection is not cytopathic in macrophages, and in vitro studies suggest that infected macrophages can continue to produce virus for long periods (164, 255). Infected macrophages may thus serve as a reservoir of virus in vivo. Virus production by macrophages is particularly apparent late in the course of disease when few CD4$^+$ T cells remain and in the setting of opportunistic infections (265).

Time Course of the Infection

The natural history of HIV-1 infection may be divided into three phases (Fig. 8). During the initial phase, known as primary or acute HIV-1 infection, virus present in the infecting inoculum replicates in the host, producing a viremia that spreads the virus throughout the body. Viremia is eventually reduced by the emergence of a vigorous antiviral immune response. These events occur during the first several weeks following exposure to HIV-1. Primary HIV-1 infection has been studied most carefully for the 50 to 70% of individuals who develop constitutional symptoms. In these individuals, a transient illness resembling infectious mononucleosis appears 2 to 3 weeks after exposure (see below). During the acute illness, levels of genomic HIV-1 RNA in the plasma (a reflection of the free-virion concentration) are usually higher than 10^6 copies/ml and can be as high as 10^8 copies/ml. Antibodies to HIV-1 are initially absent, and seroconversion usually occurs within a few weeks after onset of the acute illness.

As the immune response to HIV-1 develops, there is a dramatic reduction in the level of viremia. Typically, viremia falls to a lower plateau level (the "set point"). Set point values for plasma HIV-1 RNA levels are usually between 10^3 and 10^5 copies/ml. The CD4$^+$ T-cell count is typically reduced during symptomatic primary HIV-1 infection, reflecting both virus-induced CD4$^+$ T-cell depletion and sequestration of circulating CD4$^+$ T cells in lymphoid organs. After the acute illness resolves, peripheral CD4$^+$ T-cell counts generally rise again, but usually not to preinfection levels.

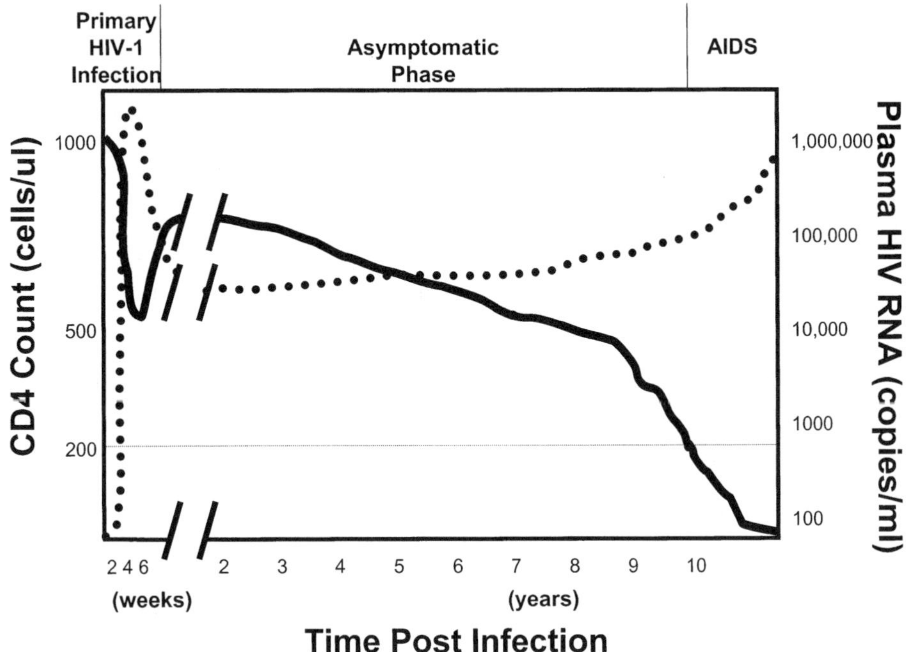

FIGURE 8 The three stages of disease in a hypothetical case of HIV-1 infection. Solid line, CD4 count; broken line, plasma HIV RNA.

During acute infection, there is rapid and dramatic depletion of $CD4^+$ T cells from the gut-associated lymphoid tissue (225, 327, 360). This early CD4 depletion in the gut is much more pronounced than CD4 depletion in other organs. The early loss of $CD4^+$ T cells from the gastrointestinal mucosa allows translocation of microbial products, which cause immune system activation, which in turn contributes to CD4 depletion (30).

Primary HIV-1 infection provides clues regarding the importance of various immune effector mechanisms in controlling HIV-1 infection. Virus-specific CTL appear early and probably represent a critical host factor in the control of acute HIV-1 infection (191). In rhesus monkeys depleted of $CD8^+$ T cells, the viremia of primary SIV infection is not brought under control and the animals progress quickly to AIDS (312). Thus, is it very likely that through the lysis of infected cells and perhaps also through the release of chemokines such as MIP-1α (CCL3), MIP-1β (CCL4), and RANTES (CCL5) that inhibit HIV-1 entry, CTL help to reduce the level of circulating virus to the lower levels that are characteristic of the asymptomatic phase of infection.

The second phase of HIV-1 infection is the long asymptomatic period between primary infection and the development of clinical immunodeficiency. The most important and characteristic pathophysiologic feature of the asymptomatic phase of HIV-1 infection is the gradual loss of $CD4^+$ T cells. Although the asymptomatic phase may represent a phase of clinical latency, the virus replicates continuously during this period. As primary infection resolves, plasma virus levels fall to a relatively stable steady-state level which is different in different patients and which determines the rate of disease progression (233). The higher the set point of the plasma HIV-1 RNA level (often referred to as the viral load), the more rapidly the patient loses $CD4^+$ T cells and progresses to AIDS. The plasma HIV-1 RNA level and the CD4 count are both used in making decisions about when to initiate therapy. The plasma HIV-1 RNA level determines how rapidly CD4 cells will be lost, and the CD4 count reflects the degree of impairment of immunologic function and the risk of opportunistic infections.

There is tremendous variation in the length of the asymptomatic period in different infected individuals. Some individuals progress to AIDS within 2 years of infection, whereas others, termed long-term nonprogressors (LTNP), have lived with HIV-1 infection for over 20 years without experiencing significant $CD4^+$ T-cell depletion. Many individuals in this category eventually do progress to AIDS in the absence of treatment. Nevertheless, a subset of LTNP, termed elite controllers, actually have no measurable viremia in the absence of treatment (364). Many of these individuals harbor forms of HIV-1 that appear to be replication competent, but it appears that the virus is held in check by immunologic mechanisms (25). These individuals frequently carry the class I MHC allele HLA B*5701, suggesting a role for CTL (235). It is likely that both virologic and host immunologic factors (discussed below) play a role in limiting HIV-1 replication and disease progression in elite controllers and LTNP. Some LTNP are infected with strains of HIV-1 that are defective in accessory genes such as *nef* (78). Polymorphisms in structural and regulatory regions of other chemokine receptors or chemokine genes have subtle but significant effects on the rate of disease progression (156, 258).

Viral loads are on the average lower in women than in men in the first 5 years after infection, although rates of disease progression are similar to those observed in men (334). Rates of disease progression may be influenced by environmental factors, particularly other concurrent infections. Although a direct relationship between rate of progression and concurrent infections has not yet been clearly established, the activation of CD4$^+$ T cells in response to other infections provides the virus with an increased number of target cells, allowing transient spikes in viremia, which can also be observed after immunizations with recall antigens (333).

Another important factor in disease progression is the evolution of viral variants with mutations in the envelope protein leading to a change in the pattern of chemokine receptor utilization. In many infected individuals, mutations in *env* lead to a change in the pattern of chemokine receptor utilization from CCR5 to CXCR4. These so-called X4 viruses have a potentially wider host cell range due to the broader distribution of CXCR4 and have been associated in some studies with higher replication rates and higher cytopathic potential. The appearance of X4 viruses is temporally associated with more rapid CD4$^+$ T-cell decline (321). The rate of disease progression is thus influenced by the characteristics of the infecting virus, host genetic factors influencing virus entry and antiviral immune responses, and possibly environmental factors related to immune system activation.

Factors in Disease Progression

Although rates of progression differ, the fundamental relationship between viral load and the rate of CD4$^+$ T-cell loss remains a central feature of AIDS pathogenesis, indicating that viral replication is the driving force for CD4 depletion. However, the exact mechanisms are still uncertain. Although HIV-1 is cytopathic for T cells in vitro, it is unclear whether the fraction of cells infected is high enough to account for the depletion of the entire CD4$^+$ T-cell compartment as a consequence of direct infection. At any given time, only a small fraction of CD4$^+$ T cells are productively infected. Thus, it is likely that additional mechanisms contribute to CD4$^+$ T-cell depletion. These include alterations in lymphoid tissue microenvironments and chronic immune activation.

Histopathologic Changes

During the asymptomatic phase of the infection, there are important changes in the structure and function of the peripheral lymphoid organs, best defined in studies of lymph nodes (272). Early in the asymptomatic period, the lymph nodes show characteristics of immune activation. Scattered productively infected CD4$^+$ T cells are seen throughout the lymph nodes. The B-cell areas of the lymph nodes show a pattern of follicular hyperplasia indicative of intense B-cell stimulation. Virus particles are readily detected in the germinal centers, where they are found associated with the network of follicular DC (FDC). These cells express Fc receptors and three types of complement receptors (CR1, CR2, and CR3) and as a result are capable of binding antigens that have bound antibody or activated complement. FDC may serve as filters that trap virus particles and thereby lower the level of infectious virus in the circulation. FDC are not susceptible to HIV infection; however, they play an important role in the activation of B lymphocytes in response to antigen. During the asymptomatic phase of HIV-1 infection, there is progressive disruption of the normal architecture of the lymph nodes, with loss of the FDC network and follicular involution (272). The loss of FDC may be in part responsible for the abnormal B-cell function observed in HIV-1-infected individuals. In contrast to FDC, blood-derived DC, which play an important role in the presentation of antigens to T cells, can bind virus and transmit the virus to the CD4$^+$ T cells with which they interact during the course of an immune response (43). Following stimulation with inflammatory cytokines, immature tissue DC migrate to the lymph nodes where they present antigens taken up in the tissues to T cells in the lymph nodes. DC may carry virions bound via DC-SIGN to the nodes where they mediate infection of CD4$^+$ T cells (131).

Viral Dynamics

Analysis of changes in the level of viral RNA following initiation of therapy with potent inhibitors of HIV-1 RT or protease (PR) has provided a striking picture of the very dynamic nature of the infection (114) (Fig. 9). Both types of drugs have the effect of blocking the new rounds of infection of susceptible cells without inhibiting the release of virions by cells that are already infected. Following the initiation of therapy, plasma virus levels drop by approximately 2 log units within less than 2 weeks, indicating that the half-life of virus in plasma is very short (now estimated to be on the order of minutes) and that the half-life of most productively infected cells is also very short (<1 day) (163, 367). Thus, most of the plasma virus is produced by cells that have only recently become infected. Continuous new rounds of viral replication sustain the infection. Most current evidence favors the view that the short-lived, productively infected cells responsible for most of the virus production are activated CD4$^+$ T cells (389).

Because the rates of clearance and decay are largely independent of the stage of disease and other factors, the level of viral RNA in the plasma reflects the rate of virus production. Because the half-life of free virus particles is extremely short, the steady-state level of viral RNA genomes in the blood reflects very recent virus production (278). The magnitude of the first phase of decay indicates that infected cells with longer half-lives such as chronically infected macrophages make a relatively minor contribution to plasma viremia in untreated individuals.

After the rapid initial phase of decay, there is a second, slower phase of decay, reflecting either the clearance of virions that have accumulated in the germinal centers or lymphoid organs or the decay of a longer-lived population of virus-producing cells (277), perhaps infected macrophages or infected CD4$^+$ T cells that are in a lower state of activation (389). The second phase of decay reduces plasma virus levels down to below the limit of detection of current assays (50 copies of HIV-1 RNA/ml of plasma). The rapid drop in viremia initially raised hopes that eradication of the infection with antiretroviral therapy might be possible (277). However, resting memory CD4$^+$ T cells in the postintegration state of latency (Fig. 7) persist even in patients who have responded well to highly active antiretroviral therapy (HAART) and have had no detectable free virus in the blood for several years (62, 113, 376). These cells appear to represent the major barrier to curing the infection with antiretroviral drugs (112). The reservoir of resting memory CD4$^+$ T cells with integrated HIV-1 DNA is established early in primary infection (60) and shows minimal decay in infected adults (112) and children (279). There are currently two hypotheses to explain the extraordinary stability of the latent reservoir. The first is that the stability is simply a reflection of the fact that the virus has taken up residence in memory T cells, cells which by nature survive for prolonged periods. In this sense, the mechanism of HIV-1 persistence resembles that of Epstein-Barr virus, which establishes latent infection in memory B

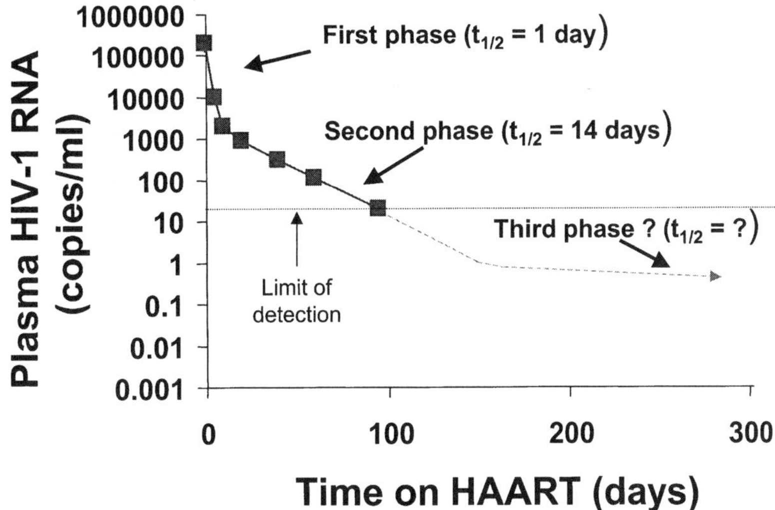

FIGURE 9 Hypothetical plot of plasma virus in a patient who is taking an effective regimen of drugs that block infection of new cells. The plasma virus level drops rapidly in the first 2 weeks of treatment, reflecting the short half-life of the virus in plasma and the short half-life of most of the productively infected cells. These cells appear to be activated $CD4^+$ T cells. The decline in plasma virus level shows a second, slower phase, which is due to turnover of cells infected before initiation of therapy. These may be persistently infected macrophages or $CD4^+$ T cells that are in a lower state of activation. Alternatively, this RNA could represent the clearance of virions that had accumulated in the germinal centers of lymphoid tissue. The second phase brings the viral load down to below the limit of detection, but the virus persists in reservoirs, including an extremely stable reservoir of latent virus in resting memory $CD4^+$ T cells.

cells. A distinct but not mutually exclusive hypothesis is that the reservoir is continually reseeded by a low level of viral replication that may continue even in patients whose plasma virus levels are below the limit of detection (90, 122, 288, 383, 388). Even in patients who have suppression of viremia to below the limit of detection of ultrasensitive clinical assays (50 copies of HIV-1 RNA/ml), free virus particles are continuously present (90). Recent studies suggest that a new steady-state level of viremia is reached in patients receiving HAART, with average values of ~3 copies/ml (218). While all patients receiving HAART are continuously viremic, direct analysis of this residual viremia does not provide evidence for viral evolution (184, 252), and it is possible that the residual viremia simply reflects release of virus from latently infected cells that become activated or from other stable reservoirs rather than reflecting ongoing replication (15). If this is the case, the use of even more intensive drug regimens will not accelerate the intrinsic decay rate of the latent reservoir.

T-Cell Dynamics and Mechanisms of CD4 Depletion

In infected individuals, the rate of $CD4^+$ T-cell loss exceeds the rate at which $CD4^+$ T cells are produced through thymic differentiation and clonal expansion of peripheral $CD4^+$ T cells. $CD4^+$ T cells may be lost through a number of potential mechanisms, some operative for noninfected cells. In addition, the possibility that the production of $CD4^+$ T cells is decreased in HIV-1 infection needs consideration. Pathologic examination of thymuses from AIDS patients suggests that HIV-1 infection accelerates the thymic involution that normally occurs with age. The decline in naïve $CD4^+$ and $CD8^+$ T-cell numbers in the peripheral blood of infected individuals has been interpreted as indicating a defect in thymopoeisis in HIV-1 infection (301). Unfortunately, it is difficult to measure directly the rate at which new T cells are produced in the thymus. To monitor ongoing thymic production of new T cells, studies have quantitated T-cell receptor excision circles (TRECs) produced as a by-product of the VDJ recombination reactions that occur in the thymus as new T cells are generated (91). These DNA circles are stable in cells after the gene rearrangements that produce functional T-cell receptors occur. Lower than normal TREC levels in peripheral blood $CD4^+$ and $CD8^+$ T cells have been observed in some HIV-1-infected adults, with partial reversal on treatment. Interpretation of TREC measurements is complicated by the fact that TRECs can be diluted out by proliferation of mature T cells. However, careful analysis of TRECs generated by rearrangement of the α and β chains of the T-cell receptor has provided convincing evidence for a defect in thymocyte proliferation in HIV-1-infected individuals (85).

Most evidence suggests that accelerated $CD4^+$ T-cell loss is a critical factor in $CD4^+$ T-cell depletion. Under some experimental conditions, HIV-1 infection of susceptible cell types in vitro results in death of the infected cell. Syncytia or multinucleated giant cells may form by the fusion of infected cells expressing Env and noninfected cells expressing CD4 (329). Inclusion of noninfected $CD4^+$ T cells in short-lived syncytia provides a potential mechanism for $CD4^+$ T-cell depletion. The extent to which syncytium formation contributes to $CD4^+$ T-cell depletion in vivo is unclear.

In addition, under some conditions, HIV-1-infected T cells appear to die from the infection independent of any cell-cell fusion events (44, 345). Most potential mechanisms for HIV-1-induced single-cell killing involve the Env glycoprotein, which is poorly tolerated by many cell types. The fusogenic properties of the Env protein are an important determinant of the intrinsic toxicity of this protein for host cells (44). Other HIV-1 proteins including Nef, Vif, and Vpr have also been implicated in the death of infected cells (306, 335).

Another potential mechanism for the loss of $CD4^+$ T cells in HIV-1 infection involves the destruction of such cells by components of the immune system, particularly $CD8^+$ CTL. As discussed below, the natural immune response to HIV-1 infection includes a strong $CD8^+$ CTL response, and it is quite likely that $CD8^+$ CTL mediate the destruction of infected cells in vivo. The destruction of productively infected cells by CTL is beneficial to the host because it leads to a more rapid cessation of virus production from cells that are destined to die.

In HIV-1 infection, several interesting reactions can potentially cause the loss of $CD4^+$ T cells that are not infected. HIV-1 infection is associated with high levels of immune activation, and activated T cells are susceptible to apoptosis (198). Interestingly, in situ studies of lymph nodes from HIV-1-infected children and SIV-infected rhesus monkeys have shown that cells undergoing programmed cell death are distinct from cells productively infected with virus, supporting the notion that indirect cell-killing mechanisms may contribute to $CD4^+$ T-cell depletion (111). Rates of T-cell proliferation are increased severalfold, and steady-state considerations suggest that this increased rate of $CD4^+$ T-cell proliferation must be more than balanced by an increased rate of destruction of T cells in the periphery (155, 241). The proximal cause of the immune hyperactivation seen in untreated HIV-1 infection remains unclear. One theory suggests that microbial translocation from the gastrointestinal tract contributes to the activation.

In addition to the quantitative depletion of $CD4^+$ T cells that occurs during the course of HIV-1 infection, there are qualitative defects in the function of the surviving $CD4^+$ T cells. Infection with HIV-1 results in dramatic effects on B-lymphocyte function. While normal absolute numbers of circulating B cells are found in HIV-1-infected individuals, circulating levels of immunoglobulins are high, reflecting polyclonal B-cell activation, but antibody responses to specific immunogens are very poor, particularly in patients with AIDS. Part of the B-cell defect may be intrinsic and not simply a consequence of defects in $CD4^+$ T-cell help. However, the precise mechanisms remain obscure.

Immune Responses

Immunodeficiency develops in HIV-1-infected individuals despite the presence of readily detectable B- and T-lymphocyte responses to HIV-1. Virtually all infected individuals develop antibody responses to several of the protein products of the HIV-1 genome. Even more striking is the finding that most infected individuals also have very high levels of virus-specific CTL. On the other hand, $CD4^+$ T-cell responses are generally reduced. Current research is focused on understanding which elements of the immune response are the most important in controlling viral replication and why the response as a whole is not more effective in eliminating the virus.

Antibody Responses

All infected individuals make a readily measurable antibody response to HIV-1. Only antibodies to the extracellular portion of the Env glycoprotein can neutralize the virus. In general, levels of neutralizing antibodies are low even when high levels of antibodies to HIV-1 Env glycoproteins are present, indicating that many anti-Env antibodies are not neutralizing. When neutralizing antibodies do arise, the virus can escape through the accumulation of mutations in the *env* gene. Of the protein products of the HIV-1 genome, the Env glycoprotein gp120 shows by far the greatest sequence variability. Neutralization-resistant variants have been obtained in vitro in infected cultures maintained in the presence of neutralizing antibody and arise readily when HIV-1 infection of human T cells is maintained in immunodeficient SCID mice (285). Antibodies present in patient sera can neutralize autologous virus isolates obtained at earlier time points but generally cannot neutralize the contemporaneous isolate (368). This appears to reflect the rapid and continuous evolution of the ectodomain of Env in the face of a neutralizing-antibody response (119). B-cell depletion studies in the SIV model have provided evidence that neutralizing antibodies do contribute to the control of viral replication during chronic infection.

Antibodies to gp120 become detectable in the sera of HIV-infected individuals within 2 to 3 weeks after infection (243). However, these early antibodies are not neutralizing. They appear to be directed against disassembled envelope glycoproteins, and they recognize the interactive regions of gp120 and gp41, which, although immunogenic, are not exposed in the assembled trimeric glycoprotein complex (380). Subsequently, antibodies appear that are neutralizing but are usually restricted in activity to the infecting strain (296). Finally, antibodies appear that have more broadly neutralizing activity against a variety of isolates but in relatively low titers. Many of these interfere with the binding interaction between gp120 and CD4. Such antibodies recognize discontinuous epitopes, the key residues of which are located within the binding pocket for CD4 on gp120 (the so-called CD4BS epitopes). Other broadly neutralizing antibodies recognize epitopes that are near conserved structures involved in coreceptor binding (the so-called CD4i epitopes).

CTL Responses

HIV-1-specific $CD8^+$ CTL are readily detected in healthy seropositive individuals and are sometimes detected in patients with AIDS (135, 365). As discussed above, CTL appear early in response to acute HIV-1 infection and help to control the high-level viremia characteristic of this stage of infection by lysing productively infected cells. CTL may also control viral replication through the release of chemokines (64). Vigorous HIV-1-specific CTL responses are observed in many long-term survivors of HIV-1 infection (152). The frequency of HIV-1-specific CTL appears to decline as the clinical and immunologic status of the patient deteriorates. In the SIV system, $CD8^+$ T cells help to control viremia in both acute and chronic infection (174, 312). The MHC genotype influences the rate of disease progression (179), and particular class I MHC alleles have been associated with slower disease progression, probably as a result of the capacity of the relevant alleles to present conserved epitopes in HIV-1 proteins to CTL. As mentioned above, certain MHC class I alleles are overrepresented in patients who control viremia without antiretroviral drugs. The breadth of the CTL response is also important, and perhaps as a consequence, heterogeneity at the class I loci is also associated with slower disease progression (46).

The HIV-1-specific CTL response can lead to the evolution of escape mutants. Mutations affecting recognition by HIV-1-specific CTL accelerate AIDS pathogenesis (6, 137). Viral escape from CTL responses can involve mutations that diminish viral fitness, as evidenced by reversion of the mutations on transmission of the virus to a new host with a different HLA genotype (200). While mutational escape provides one mechanism by which HIV-1 persists in the face of an ongoing CTL response, the functional capacity of HIV-1-specific CTL is compromised in patients with progressive disease. HIV-1-specific CTL express the inhibitory receptor PD-1 which is associated with clonal exhaustion (77, 280, 350). CTL carry out other functions including the production of cytokines. The maintenance of "polyfunctional" CTL has been associated with slower disease progression (23).

Helper T-Cell Responses

The one component of the immune response to HIV-1 that is not readily demonstrable in most infected people is the helper T-cell response to HIV-1 proteins. It appears that HIV-1-specific $CD4^+$ T cells are inactivated early in the course of the infection. They can be readily detected only in the rare individuals in whom the disease does not progress (LTNP). Treatment of infected individuals with antiretroviral therapy early in primary HIV-1 infection facilitates the development of this HIV-1-specific immune response.

To recapitulate, vigorous B- and $CD8^+$ T-cell responses to HIV-1 have been demonstrated in infected individuals. Although such responses ultimately fail to control the infection, they may delay the onset of symptomatic disease for years. Two principal mechanisms allow HIV-1 to evade host immune responses, sequence variability and latency. The ability of the virus to evade these responses through these mechanisms, coupled with the progressive virus-induced destruction of the $CD4^+$ T-cell compartment, eventually leads to immunodeficiency.

Central Nervous System Disease

Neurologic problems are common in HIV-1-infected persons (226). In addition to opportunistic infections and malignancies affecting the central nervous system (CNS), there is a unique dementia syndrome, HIV-associated dementia (HAD), that appears to result from direct effects of HIV-1 on the CNS. HAD appears late in the course of disease, roughly coincident with the development of clinical immunodeficiency, and is an AIDS-defining condition.

The pathogenesis of HAD is complex and poorly understood. As is the case with HIV-1-induced immunodeficiency, the pathogenesis of HAD involves complex interactions between various types of infected and uninfected cells in the CNS. HIV-1 probably gains access to the CNS from the bloodstream, which means that it requires a mechanism for crossing the blood-brain barrier. This may occur either by direct infection of capillary endothelial cells (95) or, more likely, by ingress of infected monocytes/macrophages (147). This "Trojan horse" mechanism resembles the mechanism by which other lentiviruses gain access to the CNS. Although CNS disease does not become apparent until late in the course of infection, entry of HIV-1 into the CNS may occur very early. Studies using an artificial blood-brain barrier demonstrated that up-regulation of adhesion molecules and proinflammatory cytokines is critical for transendothelial migration. Heightened trafficking may occur with peripheral activation of monocytes in late-stage HIV-1 infection, which is generally when HAD occurs. Proinflammatory cytokines such as tumor necrosis factor alpha (TNF-α) may also alter the permeability of the blood-brain barrier to free virus (109).

The principal cellular target cells for HIV-1 replication in the CNS are brain macrophages and microglial cells (192). Both cell types are derived from peripheral blood monocytes and are presumed to undergo gradual turnover. In some cases, syncytia composed of numerous infected macrophages and microglial cells can be observed in the vicinity of blood vessels in the CNS. No convincing evidence exists for the presence of HIV-1 DNA in neurons, endothelial cells, or oligodendrocytes (342). Progress in our understanding of the extent of infection within the CNS has been hampered by the obvious difficulty in obtaining tissue and by uncertainties with regard to the relationship between the level of virus in the cerebrospinal fluid and that in the brain parenchyma. In an animal model of AIDS dementia (394), SIV-infected cells were not detected in the CNS in monkeys during the asymptomatic stage of the infection (290) but were present following progression to AIDS (290, 394).

Certain strains of HIV-1 may have an increased propensity to invade (neurotropism) and cause damage in (neurovirulence) the nervous system. The development of HAD is not universal in advanced AIDS, suggesting that there may be viral as well as host genetic determinants of heightened risk. Indeed, distinct strains of HIV-1 isolated from both peripheral blood and the nervous system of the same individual can have different biological characteristics and cellular tropisms. Brain isolates tend to be more macrophage-tropic with specifically conserved regions in a portion of the envelope, the V3 domain (56, 128). These observations suggest that infection with a "neurotropic and neurovirulent" strain might lead to clinically significant CNS involvement (221, 283).

How viral infection of brain macrophages and microglial cells leads to CNS dysfunction is still unclear. The simplest hypothesis is that infected cells release soluble products that damage other cells in the CNS. The list of potential mediators is long (192) and includes viral proteins such as gp120, Tat, and Nef, as well as inflammatory mediators such as TNF-α, NO, and prostaglandins. A major problem is that most of these potential neurotoxins have been implicated based on in vitro cell culture studies or correlative in vivo studies.

Concern exists that the virus might persist in the CNS and produce disease even in treated patients who had no detectable virus in plasma, in part because of the limited CNS penetration by certain protease inhibitors. Other important factors include the active efflux of antiretroviral drugs through transporters including P-glycoprotein (185). While case reports alerted clinicians to this possibility, describing patients who had undetectable or low plasma HIV RNA levels yet significantly higher CSF HIV RNA levels, there have been relatively few clinical examples of "CNS escape." In fact, significant reductions in the incidence rates of HAD have been noted since 1996 (32). HAART regimens can actually improve neuropsychological performance and radiological abnormalities in those with HAD (110). Turnover of infected microglial cells over the course of weeks to months may result in replacement by uninfected monocytes from the blood. Thus, as is the case with HIV-1-induced immune deficiency, HAD appears to be driven by active viral replication.

CLINICAL MANIFESTATIONS

The cardinal manifestation of HIV-1 infection is the progressive loss of CD4$^+$ T lymphocytes. The resulting defect in cellular immunity leads to development of the opportunistic infections and malignancies that characterize AIDS. In addition, certain organ-specific syndromes may be caused directly by the virus itself. A comprehensive discussion of the myriad complications of HIV-1 infection is beyond the scope of this chapter. Instead, an overview of the major clinical manifestations is presented. The reader is referred to the many excellent textbooks of infectious diseases and AIDS medicine for more detailed discussions of specific syndromes and opportunistic pathogens.

Major Clinical Syndromes

Primary Infection

Symptomatic primary infection with HIV-1 occurs in approximately 30 to 70% of infected individuals (349). Symptoms begin around 14 days after exposure, and peak virus titers occur a week later (206). The most frequently described symptoms include fever, pharyngitis, headache, arthralgias, myalgias, and malaise (Table 2). A nonpruritic maculopapular rash on the face and trunk is also commonly observed. Generalized lymphadenopathy is a frequent finding. Mucocutaneous ulceration occurs and helps to differentiate primary HIV-1 infection from other viral syndromes. Oral candidiasis is frequently noted, and invasive esophageal candidiasis is well documented (349). Other gastrointestinal symptoms can include nausea, vomiting, and diarrhea. Aseptic meningoencephalitis is the most common neurologic manifestation of primary HIV-1 infection. Acute peripheral neuropathy, myelopathy, and mononeuritis multiplex are less frequently observed (349). In the majority of patients, symptoms resolve within a month. Persistence of symptoms beyond 8 to 12 weeks, along with a severely depressed CD4$^+$ lymphocyte count, may be clues to unusually rapid progression of HIV-1 disease.

The virologic and immunologic aspects of primary HIV-1 infection are discussed elsewhere in this chapter (see "Pathogenesis" above). The principal laboratory abnormality is a decrease in the absolute CD4$^+$ lymphocyte count. In most patients there is also an increase in the number of reactive CD8$^+$ T lymphocytes. Hematologic abnormalities are uncommon except for mild thrombocytosis. Serum aspartate transaminase and alkaline phosphatase levels may be mildly elevated, but clinical hepatitis is an infrequent finding (349).

Progression to AIDS

In most patients, a prolonged asymptomatic period follows the resolution of primary infection. In the absence of antiretroviral therapy, the median time from acquisition of HIV-1 infection to AIDS is approximately 8 to 10 years. Use of the term "clinical latency" to describe this interval is misleading, given the presence of continuous virus replication and CD4$^+$ lymphocyte depletion. On average, there is a loss of 30 to 60 CD4$^+$ cells/μl per year, although in many patients CD4$^+$ lymphocyte counts may remain stable for several years before rapidly declining. Progression to AIDS within 1 to 2 years of primary HIV-1 infection occurs in fewer than 5% of patients. Rapid progression often follows severe primary infection and may be associated with transmission of syncytium-inducing (CXCR4-utilizing) variants of HIV-1 (256).

In many patients, fatigue and lymphadenopathy continue to occur during the otherwise asymptomatic phase of HIV-1 infection. The occurrence of minor clinical events, such as oral hairy leukoplakia (secondary to Epstein-Barr virus), oral or vaginal candidiasis, herpes zoster, and a variety of other dermatologic disorders, may be an early sign of progression. Worsening fatigue, night sweats, and weight loss become more common with advancing disease. The risk of serious, potentially life-threatening opportunistic infections increases significantly at CD4$^+$ cell counts below 200/μl. For this reason, a CD4 count of less than 200/μl was selected as a diagnostic criterion of AIDS according to the 1993 revised Centers for Disease Control and Prevention (CDC) case definition (49).

TABLE 2 Frequency of signs and symptoms in patients with acute HIV-1 infection

Sign or symptom	Frequency (%) reported in reference:			
	187 (n = 31)	74 (n = 40)	356[a] (n = 74)	310[b] (n = 41)
Fever	87	88	80	~95
Lethargy and/or fatigue	26	NA[c]	67	~90
Myalgia	42	60	63	~60
Rash	68	58	53	~30
Headache	39	55	51	~55
Sore throat and/or pharyngitis	48	43	51	~70
Lymphadenopathy	6	38	43	~50
Arthralgia	29	28	26	NA
Diarrhea	32	NA	32	~45
Night sweats	NA	50	NA	~45
Oral ulcers	13	8	30	NA

[a] Group 3 from reference 356.
[b] Estimated from Fig. 1 in reference 310.
[c] NA, not available.

Systemic Manifestations

Infection with HIV produces a variety of clinical manifestations affecting nearly every organ system. Improvement of most of these manifestations following the institution of potent antiretroviral therapy strongly implicates HIV replication or immune activation in their pathogenesis.

The majority of HIV-infected individuals experience some form of dermatologic disorder during the course of their disease. Pruritus and xerosis are frequent symptoms in patients with early infection. A variety of noninfectious inflammatory conditions are commonly observed, including seborrheic dermatitis, papular pruritic eruption, and eosinophilic folliculitis (69).

Neurologic manifestations of HIV infection include disorders of the CNS and peripheral nervous system, opportunistic infections, malignancies, vascular complications, and myopathies. The most frequently recognized "primary" neurologic manifestation of HIV infection is HAD (or the AIDS dementia complex), which occurs in up to 27% of patients with late-stage HIV disease (326). This syndrome involves progressive cognitive, motor, and behavioral deficits that usually begin in patients with moderately advanced HIV disease ($CD4^+$ cell counts below $200/\mu l$). Computed tomography or magnetic resonance imaging studies of the brain usually show evidence of cortical atrophy, ventricular enlargement, and diffuse white matter abnormalities. Rapid clinical improvement in the response to treatment argues for a central role of HIV in the pathogenesis of AIDS dementia (324).

Disorders of the peripheral nervous system can be classified as distal symmetric polyneuropathy, toxic neuropathy, inflammatory demyelinating polyneuropathy, progressive polyradiculopathy, and mononeuropathy multiplex (326). Up to 35% of patients with HIV infection develop signs or symptoms of distal symmetric polyneuropathy in later stages of disease (328). Symptoms begin as burning pain and numbness in the feet and may progress to the point that ambulation becomes impossible. Subjective complaints of distal polyneuropathy may precede objective findings on neurologic examination by several months. In more advanced cases there is diminished vibratory sensation and loss of ankle reflexes. Toxic neuropathy due to treatment with the dideoxynucleoside analogs (ddI, ddC, d4T) is indistinguishable from the distal symmetric polyneuropathy related to HIV infection but usually is reversible on early withdrawal of the responsible agent. Inflammatory demyelinating polyneuropathy is characterized by progressive weakness and areflexia resembling that of Guillain-Barré syndrome. This form of neuropathy, along with mononeuropathy multiplex, may occur during primary HIV-1 infection and is thought to have an autoimmune basis (326).

Nonspecific interstitial pneumonitis and lymphocytic interstitial pneumonitis have been associated with HIV infection. It is not known whether interstitial pneumonitis is a primary consequence of HIV infection in the lungs or is due to secondary immunologic mechanisms activated by HIV. The occurrence of lymphocytic interstitial pneumonitis is most frequent in infants with perinatally acquired HIV (see below). Clinical signs and symptoms of interstitial lung disease are similar to those in HIV-uninfected patients. Histologic features include lymphocytic or mononuclear cell infiltration and the absence of known pulmonary pathogens (237).

Disorders of the digestive tract are an important cause of morbidity in patients with HIV infection. Oral pathology attributable to HIV infection includes xerostomia, recurrent aphthous stomatitis, and gingivitis. Giant aphthous ulcers of the esophagus also occur, but they are less common than aphthous stomatitis. Diarrheal illness is common and usually can be attributed to infection with specific enteric pathogens. Although cases of chronic diarrhea in the absence of intestinal pathogens were thought initially to represent an AIDS enteropathy, most such cases are now thought to represent unrecognized infection with *Cryptosporidium*, microsporidia, or *M. avium* complex. Extensive HIV-1 infection occurs in gut-associated lymphoid tissue, so that a direct contribution of HIV-1 to intestinal dysfunction remains a possibility (352).

Endocrine dysfunction and metabolic disorders are well described as complications of HIV infection. Hypogonadism with loss of libido and testicular atrophy are common findings. It is uncertain whether the primary abnormality is at the level of the hypothalamus or the testis. Fertility is decreased and the rate of fetal loss is increased, particularly among women with advanced stages of disease (304). HIV-associated abnormalities of thyroid function are unusual. Similarly, pancreatic and adrenal insufficiency usually result from drug toxicity or opportunistic infections rather than from HIV infection per se.

Wasting syndrome in HIV infection is defined as the unintentional loss of >10% of body weight. When accompanied by constitutional symptoms for longer than 30 days, wasting in the absence of opportunistic infection or malignancy is sufficient to make a diagnosis of AIDS (49). In the developing world, the high prevalence of HIV-associated wasting has given AIDS the appellation "slim disease." In developing countries, some degree of HIV-associated wasting occurs in nearly one-third of otherwise asymptomatic patients (in the absence of effective antiretroviral therapy) and in 60 to 90% of patients with AIDS (319). As in starvation and cancer, death from wasting in AIDS occurs at 66% of ideal body weight (143).

Multiple mechanisms contribute to the pathophysiology of AIDS wasting syndrome. Unlike starvation, wasting in AIDS is often the result of loss of body cell mass rather than of adipose fat. Inadequate caloric intake and inappropriate nutrient utilization are important factors leading to the depletion of lean body mass. Anorexia due to intercurrent opportunistic infection or the side effects of medication, and malabsorption due to diarrhea can contribute to malnutrition. Although elevated serum triglyceride levels are commonly observed in patients with AIDS, the level of hypertriglyceridemia is not correlated with the extent of weight loss. Cytokine-induced changes in lipid metabolism may contribute to this finding, but the role of specific cytokines, such as TNF-α, interleukin-1, and alpha interferon, remains controversial. It has been suggested that an increase in resting energy expenditure (the basal metabolic rate) accounts for the weight loss in AIDS, but total energy expenditure is reduced during episodes of weight loss (215). Weight loss is accelerated during episodes of intercurrent opportunistic infections due to diminished caloric intake. Nevertheless, the difficulty in reversing the loss of lean body mass with nutritional support alone speaks to an underlying metabolic disorder in some patients with AIDS.

Anemia and neutropenia are the most frequently encountered hematologic disorders in HIV-infected individuals. Although a large number of drugs used in the treatment of HIV infection and its complications can cause bone marrow suppression, HIV infection per se is clearly associated with anemia and neutropenia, particularly in late-stage disease. Anemia and neutropenia have been noted in 4 and 11%, respectively, of untreated patients with AIDS (294). The anemia associated with HIV infection is normochromic and normocytic. Laboratory tests of iron status reveal a pattern suggestive of the anemia of chronic disease. Although the hypergammaglobulinemia associated with HIV infection may lead to a positive Coombs' test in 20% of patients, other evidence in support of hemolysis as a cause of anemia in HIV infection is rare (2). Similarly, antigranulocyte antibodies detected in many HIV-infected patients do not appear to play a major role in the development of HIV-associated neutropenia. Progenitor cells for myeloid, erythroid, and megakaryocyte lineages from HIV-infected individuals have a reduced capacity for growth in vitro. It is not known whether diminished growth capacity in vitro is due to HIV infection of $CD34^+$ progenitor cells or is the result of abnormal patterns of cytokine secretion. Despite evidence that $CD34^+$ cells can be infected with HIV-1 under certain conditions in vitro, these cells do not seem to harbor HIV-1 in vivo.

In contrast to anemia and neutropenia, thrombocytopenia in HIV infection is usually due to immune-mediated destruction of platelets. Platelet-associated antibodies are detected in the majority of patients with HIV-associated thrombocytopenia, and examination of the bone marrow reveals increased numbers of megakaryocytes, suggesting peripheral destruction of platelets. The incidence and severity of immune thrombocytopenia appear to increase with diminishing $CD4^+$ T-cell count. Some degree of thrombocytopenia is present in 5 to 10% of patients at earlier stages of HIV disease and in up to 30% of patients with AIDS (2).

A variety of rheumatologic syndromes have been detected in HIV-infected individuals, including Reiter's syndrome, psoriatic arthritis, polymyositis, vasculitis, and sicca syndrome (181). Inappropriate immune activation and polyclonal B-cell activation leading to hypergammaglobulinemia and autoantibody production are implicated in the pathogenesis of these HIV-associated syndromes, but precise pathogenetic mechanisms have not been defined.

HIV infection is also associated with a rapidly progressive form of glomerulosclerosis (HIV-associated nephropathy), leading to nephrotic-range proteinuria and renal insufficiency. The incidence of HIV-associated nephropathy is highest among African-Americans and injection drug users. Renal biopsy reveals collapsing focal segmental sclerosis of involved glomeruli, as well as tubulointerstitial changes accompanied by an interstitial mononuclear cell infiltrate and the presence of HIV-1 RNA in tubular epithelial cells and glomerular podocytes (375). Control of viral replication by effective antiretroviral therapy has been associated with resolution of histologic changes. Despite reductions in HIV-1 levels in the kidneys, persistence of viral RNA transcripts suggests that the kidneys may serve as a reservoir for HIV-1 infection.

Complications

Opportunistic infections. The incidence and severity of opportunistic infections increase as cellular immunity wanes during the course of HIV-1 infection. The widespread use of potent antiretroviral therapy and effective chemoprophylaxis has markedly reduced the incidence of opportunistic infections in HIV-infected patients in the developed world. However, because of limited access or avoidance of care, patients continue to present late in the course of HIV disease with active opportunistic infections.

The $CD4^+$ T-cell count is the most useful marker for predicting the immediate risk of developing a particular opportunistic infection. Such complications are rare in patients with CD4 counts above 500 cells/μl. As the CD4 count drops below 500 cells/μl, patients may begin to experience oral candidiasis, pneumococcal infections, and a host of cutaneous disorders including recurrent reactivation of herpes simplex virus and varicella-zoster virus infections, dermatophyte infections, pityariasis, and onychomycosis. The risk of more serious opportunistic infections such as *Pneumocystis* pneumonia, *Candida* esophagitis, reactivation of latent histoplasmosis and other systemic fungal infections, *Toxoplasma* encephalitis, and cryptococcal meningitis increases significantly as the CD4 count falls below 200 cells/μl. At CD4 counts under 50/μl, patients are at increased risk for the occurrence of disseminated infection with M. *avium* complex, reactivation of cytomegalovirus infection, cryptosporidiosis, and progressive multifocal leukoencephalopathy due to JC virus infection.

Infection with HIV-1 significantly increases the risk of pulmonary and extrapulmonary tuberculosis. The HIV-1 pandemic has contributed to a 5- to 10-fold increase in the incidence of tuberculosis in resource-poor countries, where more than 80% of patients newly diagnosed with tuberculosis are coinfected with HIV (71). In contrast to other opportunistic infections, the risk of tuberculosis is increased even in patients with well-preserved CD4 counts. A study of South African gold miners found that the incidence of tuberculosis doubled within the first year of HIV infection (330). Numerous other opportunistic infections have been catalogued in patients with advanced HIV disease but are beyond the scope of this chapter.

Oncologic complications. The oncologic manifestations of HIV infection arise as opportunistic malignancies in the setting of severe immune deficiency. Non-Hodgkin's lymphoma (often associated with high-level Epstein-Barr virus replication), Kaposi's sarcoma (associated with human herpesvirus 8 infection) (52), and cervical cancer (due to oncogenic serotypes of human papillomavirus) are recognized as AIDS-defining cancers when they occur in HIV-infected patients. Other malignancies, including Hodgkin's disease, anorectal carcinoma, liver cancer, and stomach cancer, also occur more often among HIV-infected patients than in the general population (142). By contrast, rates of common epithelial malignancies such as breast, prostate, and colorectal cancer are not increased.

HIV-1 Infection in Children

In the absence of preventive antiretroviral therapy, 15 to 30% of children born to HIV-infected mothers acquire HIV infection through mother-to-child transmission (24, 305). The course of HIV-1 infection is accelerated in children with vertically acquired HIV-1 compared to that in HIV-infected adults. Because of the lymphocytosis of infancy, the absolute $CD4^+$ lymphocyte count may not accurately reflect functional immune status and must be adjusted for age. Without potent antiretroviral therapy, approximately 20% of infected infants develop AIDS in the first year of life and 28% die before 5 years of age (101). In the developed world, the 5-year survival rate for children who develop signs of HIV infection within the first 5 months of life is 45%, compared to 74% for children with a later onset of disease (125). In poor countries, the 2-year mortality of HIV-infected children exceeds 50% (253). Lymphadenopathy, splenomegaly, and hepatomegaly are the most common signs of HIV infection in the first year of life. Growth failure and developmental delay are manifestations of HIV infection in children. Progressive encephalopathy is found in approximately 15% of infected children (320). Another unique manifestation is lymphoid interstitial pneumonitis, which occurs in 30 to 40% of children with HIV infection (320). Abnormalities in immunoglobulin synthesis predispose to recurrent pyogenic infections with organisms that are common causes of infection in young children, such as *Streptococcus pneumoniae*, *Haemophilus influenzae*, *Staphylococcus aureus*, and *Salmonella* spp. The most frequently encountered opportunistic infections in children are *Pneumocystis* pneumonia, *Candida* esophagitis, disseminated cytomegalovirus infection, cryptosporidiosis, and disseminated *M. avium* complex infection (320).

Clinical Diagnosis

Prior to the discovery of HIV-1, AIDS was defined in part by the occurrence of opportunistic infections suggestive of immunodeficiency in patients not receiving immunosuppressive therapy and without a history of congenital immunodeficiency. This definition remains useful in helping to identify patients with advanced HIV-1 disease. Thus, the occurrence of opportunistic infections such as *Pneumocystis* pneumonia, *Candida* esophagitis, cryptococcal meningitis, toxoplasmosis, or chronic ulcerative herpes simplex in the absence of a known cause of immunodeficiency should raise the possibility of HIV-1 infection. Recurrent or disseminated zoster, pneumococcal infection in a young adult, oral or recurrent vulgovaginal candidiasis, disseminated papillomavirus infection, persistent fever, night sweats, lymphadenopathy, weight loss, and chronic diarrhea all may be evidence of infection with HIV-1. Similarly, a diagnosis of HIV-1 infection should be considered for patients with unexplained lymphopenia, anemia, or neutropenia and in those with idiopathic thrombocytopenia. In such cases, information should be sought from the patient to determine if he or she is at risk for HIV infection (e.g., men who have sex with men, current or prior injection drug use, female sexual partners of bisexual men or injection drug users, a history of unprotected sex with a new or unknown partner, or a history of transfusion or occupational exposure).

A difficult challenge is to identify and diagnose individuals at risk for HIV-1 infection during the asymptomatic stages of illness. Early diagnosis is essential to provide appropriate counseling and advice regarding modification of behaviors that may spread the virus to other individuals, as well as to institute antiretroviral therapy prior to immune depletion. For this reason, the CDC recommends that HIV testing be performed as part of routine medical care at least once in all persons aged 13 to 64 years and annually in those at high risk of HIV infection (29). The presence of another sexually transmitted disease, infection with hepatitis B or C viruses, or active tuberculosis should prompt testing for HIV-1 infection.

The clinical diagnosis of primary HIV infection is particularly challenging due to the relatively nonspecific nature of the presenting signs and symptoms (Table 2), which may be confused with other viral infections including adenovirus or enterovirus infection, influenza, or mononucleosis. This difficulty is further confounded by the observation that patients with acute HIV infection who seek medical attention usually do so in a primary-care or emergency room setting, where clinicians may be less attuned to the possibility of primary HIV infection. In one study, approximately 1% of heterophile-negative sera from patients tested to exclude acute mononucleosis were found to have high titers of HIV-1 RNA but to give negative results on HIV antibody testing, suggesting acute infection (303).

LABORATORY DIAGNOSIS

A diagnosis of infection with HIV can be made by virologic, serologic, or molecular biological tests. For the majority of patients with clinical symptoms suggestive of HIV infection and for those at high risk for HIV infection, diagnosis is straightforward. The broad application of HIV diagnostic tests to persons at low or zero risk of acquiring HIV infection, however, requires an understanding of the performance characteristics of these assays.

Virus Isolation

HIV-1 can be cultured from plasma or peripheral blood mononuclear cells (PBMC) of infected individuals. A positive culture provides direct evidence of HIV-1 infection, but virus culture is rarely necessary to establish a diagnosis. The overall sensitivity of PBMC culture is 95% or more in patients with $CD4^+$ cell counts below 500/μl, but sensitivity is lower in patients with higher CD4 counts. Virus isolation is now limited to research purposes.

Antigen Detection Assays

The presence of circulating HIV-1 capsid (p24) antigen can be detected by antigen capture EIA. Because high titers of p24 antigen are present in the sera of acutely infected individuals during the interval prior to seroconversion, p24 antigen detection can be used to diagnose primary HIV-1 infection. In one study, the sensitivity and specificity of the p24 antigen assay were 88.6 and 100%, respectively (74). After seroconversion, p24 antigen is complexed with p24 antibodies and becomes undetectable in the majority of infected individuals. For this reason, p24 antigen assays are not useful diagnostic tests in asymptomatic individuals at risk for HIV-1 infection.

Serum p24 antigen becomes detectable again in 30 to 70% of patients during the course of HIV-1 infection and is associated with an increased risk of clinical progression (5, 103). The sensitivity of p24 assays can be improved by pretreatment of serum samples to dissociate antigen-antibody complexes. Heat denaturation of plasma, coupled with tyramide signal amplification, has been reported to make p24 antigen detection as sensitive as detection of viral RNA by PCR (315).

Nucleic Acid Detection

Qualitative Assays for Proviral HIV-1 DNA

Evidence for HIV-1 infection can be established by demonstrating the presence of proviral DNA in PBMC. Assays for detecting proviral DNA employ PCR to amplify con-

TABLE 3 Characteristics of assays for quantification of plasma HIV-1 RNA

Assay	Range (no. of copies/ml)
Ultrasensitive RT-PCR (HIV-1 Monitor 1.5)	50–75,000
bDNA[a] (Versant 3.0)	80–8,000,000
NASBA[b] (NucliSens QT)	50–500,000
Real-time PCR	
RealTime HIV-1 assay	40–10,000,000
Cobas TaqMan HIV-1 test	48–10,000,000

[a] bDNA, branched DNA assay.
[b] NASBA, nucleic acid and sequence-based amplification.

served sequences in the HIV-1 *gag* or *pol* gene, coupled to a detection step based on hybridization of a labeled oligonucleotide probe specific for the amplified gene sequences. With carefully standardized procedures and rigorous quality assurance and quality control, experienced laboratories can achieve 100% sensitivity and specificity. Scrupulous attention to guard against contamination from the carryover of PCR products is essential to prevent false-positive results.

Despite the excellent performance of these assays in proficency panels, the sensitivity of HIV-1 DNA PCR assays in clinical practice is only 96 to 99%. As with virus culture and p24 antigen detection, sensitivity is lower in individuals with higher CD4$^+$ cell counts due to the lower titer of circulating infected PBMC. The greatest potential clinical utility of HIV-1 DNA PCR assays is in the early diagnosis of HIV-1 infection in neonates (see below). Clinical applications of these tests in adults are relatively limited, but occasionally DNA PCR testing may be helpful in resolving indeterminate Western blot results for high-risk individuals.

Assays for Quantifying HIV-1 RNA in Plasma

Quantitative assay of HIV-1 RNA levels in plasma is used to monitor the course of disease and the response to antiretroviral therapy in patients already known to be HIV-1 infected. Several assays based on different methodologies have been approved by the Food and Drug Administration for clinical use.

Despite methodological differences, results of the commercially available quantitative HIV-1 RNA assays are highly correlated (Table 3) (204). The assays have a lower limit of quantification of approximately 40 to 80 copies/ml. The assay range can be extended by using larger volumes of plasma and pelleting virion particles prior to RNA extraction, but the precision with which plasma HIV-1 RNA can be quantified diminishes substantially at titers below 200 copies/ml. Serial testing of clinically stable patients not receiving antiretroviral therapy (or receiving a stable failing regimen) has shown the relative stability of plasma HIV-1 RNA levels over the short term (weeks to months), with a biological variation of approximately 0.3 to 0.4 $\log_{10}$ copies/ml (20). Thus, changes of greater than 0.5 to 0.7 $\log_{10}$ (three- to fivefold) are likely to reflect significant changes in HIV-1 replication. These assays are specific for HIV-1 belonging to group M and do not reliably detect HIV-1 group O or HIV-2.

Clinical Utility of Plasma HIV-1 RNA Monitoring

Numerous studies have demonstrated the correlation of plasma HIV-1 RNA levels with stage of disease. Patients with AIDS or symptomatic HIV infection have significantly higher titers of plasma HIV-1 RNA than do those with asymptomatic infection, although the HIV-1 RNA level and CD4$^+$ T-cell count are weakly correlated. Individuals with plasma HIV-1 RNA levels of >100,000 copies/ml within 6 months of seroconversion are 10 times more likely to progress to AIDS within 5 years than patients with lower levels of plasma HIV-1 RNA (231). Although plasma HIV-1 RNA levels are strong predictors of the risk of disease progression, they are weak predictors of the rate of CD4 count decline (Table 4) (300). This seeming paradox may be explained by the large variance observed in CD4 slopes and the weak association between CD4 slope and risk of disease progression (232).

In the absence of treatment, plasma HIV-1 RNA levels may provide prognostic information in late stages of disease (214) and in children with perinatally acquired HIV-1 infection (269). However, some studies suggest that the CD4 count is a better predictor of disease progression than is the plasma HIV-1 RNA level in patients with very low CD4 counts (below 50 cells/μl) (72).

The dynamic response of plasma HIV-1 RNA to treatment makes it possible to assess the effectiveness of antiviral therapy within a matter of weeks. A decrease in the plasma HIV-1 RNA level confers a significant reduction in

TABLE 4 Association of plasma HIV-1 RNA level with decline in CD4$^+$ T-cell count and risk of AIDS and death[a]

Plasma HIV-1 RNA level from bDNA assay (copies/ml)	Change in CD4$^+$ T-cell count/yr (cells/μl)	% who progressed to AIDS within 6 yr	% who died from AIDS within 6 yr
<500	−36.3	5.4	0.9
501–3,000	−44.8	16.6	6.3
3,001–10,000	−55.2	31.7	18.1
10,001–30,000	−64.8	55.2	34.9
>30,000	−76.5	80.0	69.5

[a] Adapted from reference 233.

the risk of disease progression, independent of the baseline plasma HIV-1 RNA level and CD4 count and independent of the increase in CD4 count due to treatment (223). Much of the benefit of antiretroviral therapy can be attributed to the effect on plasma HIV-1 RNA levels. A 0.3-$\log_{10}$ (2-fold) reduction in plasma HIV-1 RNA levels confers a 30% reduction in the risk of progression to AIDS or death (68); a 1-$\log_{10}$ (10-fold) reduction reduces the risk of disease progression by approximately two-thirds (180). Although initial studies suggested that HIV-1 RNA was a more significant predictor of the response to antiretroviral therapy than was the change in CD4 count, subsequent studies have made clear the prognostic importance of improvement in both markers (138, 162).

Sample Collection

Blood for plasma HIV-1 RNA testing should be collected into tubes containing EDTA as an anticoagulant, and the plasma should be separated and stored frozen at −70°C until used in testing. Studies show that HIV-1 RNA is stable for up to 48 h at room temperature in the presence of EDTA, but samples ideally should be processed within 6 h after collection. Events leading to immune activation, such as vaccination or acute infectious illness, can transiently raise the plasma HIV-1 RNA level (333). Therefore, plasma HIV-1 RNA testing should not be performed within 4 weeks of an intercurrent infection or immunization. Because of differences between assay formats and commercial laboratories, the same laboratory should be used for serial tests on samples from an individual patient.

Current treatment guidelines recommend obtaining a plasma HIV-1 RNA level as part of the initial patient evaluation. Virus load testing also should be performed immediately before and within 2 to 8 weeks after initiating treatment, to assess the initial response to a regimen. A decline in the plasma HIV-1 RNA level of approximately 2.0 $\log_{10}$ is expected for treatment-naïve patients within 8 weeks of starting an initial antiretroviral regimen, and the plasma virus level should become undetectable (below 50 copies/ml) by 16 weeks. However, more than 24 weeks may be required for plasma virus titers to fall below the limit of detection in patients with high pretreatment levels of viremia (above 100,000 copies/ml). Declines of 1 $\log_{10}$ or more within 8 weeks should be expected following a change in regimen due to treatment failure. Subsequently, plasma HIV-1 RNA levels should be obtained every 3 to 4 months to monitor the success of antiretroviral therapy.

Plasma HIV-1 RNA Assays for Diagnosing Primary HIV-1 Infection

Quantitative plasma HIV-1 RNA assays are frequently used for diagnosing primary HIV-1 infection, although they are not approved for this purpose. These assays are highly sensitive (100%), but occasional false-positive tests result in a specificity of only 97.4% (74). Because of the potential social and legal ramifications of a false-positive HIV-1 test, additional testing (e.g., serial EIA and Western blots) should be performed to clarify a patient's HIV infection status. However, HIV-1 RNA levels are lower than 10,000 copies/ml in nearly all false-positive assays but exceed 100,000 copies/ml in the great majority of patients with primary HIV-1 infection. Thus, plasma HIV-1 RNA testing should be considered in cases in which a history of recent exposure and symptoms consistent with acute HIV-1 infection provide a high index of suspicion. A qualitative HIV-1 RNA assay approved for HIV-1 diagnosis (Aptima HIV-1 [Gen-Probe]) may prove useful but has not been extensively evaluated in this setting.

Nucleic acid amplification tests also are used to screen donated blood to exclude the presence of HIV-1 (and hepatitis C virus) infection. To maximize efficiency, samples from many donors are pooled and individual samples are tested only if the pool tests positive. Of 12.6 million donations that were p24-antigen negative and seronegative, 4 were found to be positive by nucleic acid amplification testing (1/3,150,000) (338).

Serologic Assays

In most cases, infection is diagnosed by demonstrating the presence of antibodies specific for HIV-1 or HIV-2. The mean time to seroconversion in patients with acute HIV-1 infection is approximately 25 days (40, 205). Antibodies to HIV become detectable within 6 to 12 weeks of infection in the majority of infected individuals and within 6 months in virtually all patients (124, 165). Serologic diagnosis is a two-stage process: sera that give a positive reaction by an initial antibody screening assay (EIA, chemiluminometric, or rapid immunoassay) are retested to exclude the possibility of clerical or laboratory error; repeatedly reactive sera are then tested by a confirmatory assay to verify that reactive antibodies are directed against HIV antigens. Assays have been developed for detection of HIV antibodies in serum, whole blood, saliva, urine, and dried blood collected on filter paper.

HIV EIA

Antigens for HIV-1 or HIV-2 EIA are prepared from lysates of HIV-infected human T-cell lines, recombinant HIV proteins produced in bacterial or yeast expression systems, or chemically synthesized oligopeptides. Biological false-positive reactions may occur in assays that use viral lysates as a source of HIV-1 antigen ("first-generation" HIV-1 EIAs) due to reactivity of antibodies directed against human leukocyte antigen (HLA) proteins that are expressed by lymphoid cell lines used to prepare viral lysates. Such antibodies are commonly found in multiparous women who are exposed to foreign HLA proteins on fetal cells and in multiply transfused individuals. Second-generation assays that use recombinant or synthetic HIV-1 antigens circumvent the problem of HLA antibodies, but cross-reactivity to contaminating bacterial or yeast proteins can be an alternative cause of false-positive reactions. Assays based on recombinant or synthetic envelope antigens may fail to detect antibodies to the highly divergent HIV-1 subtypes from groups N and O (211, 309).

In a comparison of commercial HIV-1 EIA kits using serum from individuals with documented HIV-1 infection, sensitivities ranged from 98.1 to 100%. The specificity of these assays in populations with a low prevalence of HIV-1 infection ranges from 99.6 to 100.0%. The American Red Cross Blood Services report an overall specificity of 99.8% when HIV-1 EIAs are used to screen donated blood (366). Comparable sensitivities and specificities were reported in a comprehensive evaluation of HIV-1 EIA kits using sera from European, African, and South American subjects (358).

False-negative HIV-1 EIAs usually are the result of absent or low levels of HIV-specific immunoglobulin G (IgG) in the weeks following primary infection. Whereas first- and second-generation HIV-1 EIAs detect primarily

IgG antibodies, antigen sandwich EIAs (third-generation assays) can detect all classes of antibodies to HIV-1. Third-generation EIAs have greater sensitivity in detecting HIV-1 antibodies in the early stages of infection, and their use significantly shortens the time to seroconversion. The lower reactivity of sera from newly HIV-1-infected patients can be turned to clinical advantage in the diagnosis of recent seroconversion. Third-generation EIAs can be made less sensitive ("detuned") so that the time to seroconversion is increased by approximately 4 months (173). Patients infected within 5 to 6 months of testing are reactive on the sensitive EIA but nonreactive on the less sensitive EIA. A two-step algorithm using a sensitive and a less sensitive EIA testing strategy correctly identified 95% of recent seroconverters in a large retrospective study (173). This strategy may be helpful in identifying patients for clinical studies of early HIV-1 infection and for estimating the incidence of HIV-1 infection.

In addition to the standard HIV EIA, rapid diagnostic tests based on red cell or particle agglutination as well as dot blot assays have been developed. The simplicity and wide range of operating temperature for some of these rapid tests make them particularly well suited for point-of-care testing. Field testing of a rapid test approved for detection of HIV-1 and HIV-2 antibodies in whole blood, plasma, and oral fluids (OraQuick Advance [OraSure Technologies]) found a sensitivity of 99.7% in whole blood and 99.1% in oral fluid, with specificities of 99.9 and 99.6%, respectively (82). However, the occurrence of 16 false-positive reactions in one study resulted in a specificity of only 99.0%. For this reason, a positive result by a rapid HIV antibody test should be verified by a confirmatory assay such as a Western blot.

Western Blots

Even with a specificity of 99.8%, the predictive value of a positive assay is unacceptably low (about 70%) when applied to low-risk populations (47). Assuming a prevalence of 0.5% for HIV-1 infection in the U.S. population, two false-positive results would occur for every five infected individuals identified. For this reason, a confirmatory test is essential to exclude false-positive results. (Confirmatory tests are not routinely run on samples that test negative by a screening assay.) The confirmatory test most commonly used in the United States is the Western blot. Antibodies against the major HIV-1 proteins (Gag, Pol, and Env) can be identified by Western blot testing. Antibodies against the Gag proteins (p17, p24, and p55) appear earliest in the course of HIV-1 infection but decrease in titer with progression of HIV-1 disease, whereas antibodies to Env (gp160 or gp120/gp41) usually persist even in advanced stages of HIV-1 disease. Coordinate use of the HIV-1 EIA and Western blot results in a specificity approaching 100%. In a study of military recruits from U.S. counties with a low prevalence of HIV-1 infection, only 1 of 135,187 samples tested gave a false-positive result (38).

Criteria for interpretation of HIV-1 Western blots have been developed by several groups, but no uniform standard has been adopted (38, 48). The most widely recognized criteria are as follows: (i) American Red Cross, at least one band from each structural gene product (*gag*, *pol*, and *env*); (ii) CDC and Association of State and Territorial Public Health Directors, any two of p24, gp41, or gp120/160; (iii) Consortium for Retrovirus Serology Standardization, p24 or p31 and one of gp41 or gp120/160; and (iv) World Health Organization, reactivity to two envelope glycoproteins.

Interpretation of HIV-1 Serologic Tests

Sera that give a positive reaction in a screening assay on more than one occasion are termed "repeatedly reactive." Sera that react on only one occasion are not considered to represent true positives and are reported as negative or unreactive. If the results of a repeatedly reactive screening assay are confirmed by a positive Western blot result, a diagnosis of HIV-1 infection can be made. A negative Western blot result with a serum sample that is repeatedly reactive by HIV-1 EIA suggests a false-positive EIA result. However, a repeatedly reactive EIA and negative or partly reactive Western blot could be evidence of recently acquired HIV-1 infection in the appropriate setting and should be followed by repeat testing in a few weeks. Because of the "window" period between initial infection with HIV-1 and seroconversion, a negative EIA result firmly excludes the possibility of infection only in individuals who have not engaged in high-risk behavior or whose last possible exposure to HIV-1 was 6 months or more prior to testing.

On occasion, sera that are repeatedly reactive by HIV-1 EIA will yield an atypical pattern on Western blot in which one or two bands characteristic of HIV-1 are identified, which is fewer than the number of bands required to meet criteria for a positive blot. Interpretation of these results depends on the clinical situation. For persons with a history of exposure to HIV-1 or at high risk for HIV-1 infection, an indeterminate Western blot result may be evidence of recent HIV-1 infection, particularly if antibodies directed against Gag proteins are present. In such cases, evolution of a fully positive Western blot can usually be demonstrated within 6 months (38, 171). If the clinical suspicion for HIV infection is high and the Western blot remains indeterminate, testing with an EIA and Western blot specific for HIV-2 is recommended (see below) (38, 260). In some states, an alternative confirmatory test (e.g., indirect immunofluorescence assay) is used to resolve indeterminate results. Qualitative PCR tests for HIV-1 RNA or proviral DNA may also be useful in this situation (see above).

Persons at low risk for HIV-1 infection (e.g., those identified incidentally as a result of blood donation) with persistently indeterminate HIV-1 Western blot results are most probably uninfected (38, 171). Long-term follow-up of such individuals has failed to uncover other evidence of HIV-1 infection by virus culture, PCR, or clinical progression in the majority of such cases (38, 171). Cross-reacting antibodies responsible for repeatedly reactive HIV-1 EIA and persistent indeterminate Western blots have been associated with rheumatoid arthritis, systemic lupus erythematosus, polyclonal gammopathy, and antibodies to HLA DR.

Serologic Diagnosis of HIV-2

The combination HIV-1/HIV-2 antigen sandwich EIAs commonly used by blood banks screen simultaneously for HIV-1 and HIV-2 antibodies. The sensitivity of a third-generation HIV-1/HIV-2 combination EIA tested against a panel of European, Central African, and West African sera was found to be 99.7% for detection of HIV-1 and 99.5% for detection of HIV-2 (14). Because of the very low prevalence of HIV-2 infection in the United States, the CDC does not recommend routine testing for HIV-2 other than in blood banks. Persons for whom HIV-2 testing should be considered include immigrants from countries where HIV-2 is endemic, those with sex partners known to be infected with HIV-2, those who have received blood transfusions in countries in which HIV-2 is endemic, those who have shared needles with an HIV-2-infected individual or an individual from a country where HIV-2 is endemic, and children of women with known HIV-2 infection or who are at risk for HIV-2 infection (259).

Diagnosis of HIV-1 Infection in Neonates and Infants

Placental transfer of HIV-1 IgG antibodies from infected mothers to their fetuses poses special challenges to the early diagnosis of HIV-1 in infants and neonates. All infants born of HIV-1-infected mothers are initially HIV-1 seropositive, but in the absence of antiretroviral therapy only 15 to 30% of these infants are themselves infected with HIV-1 (24, 305). Titers of maternal IgG decay over 12 to 15 months. Persistence of HIV-1 antibodies beyond 15 months is therefore considered diagnostic of infection in the infant. Infection with HIV-1 can reasonably be excluded by two or more negative HIV-1 serologic tests performed at least 1 month apart for infants older than 6 months of age.

Early identification of infected infants is essential to maximize the potential benefits of antiretroviral and prophylactic therapies while minimizing the exposure of uninfected infants to the potential toxicities of these therapies. Consequently, the diagnosis of HIV-1 infection in infants depends on virologic assays (e.g., virus culture or DNA or RNA PCR). Current guidelines recommend testing infants born to HIV-infected mothers at age 48 h, at age 1 to 2 months, and at age 3 to 6 months. A positive test suggests the possibility of HIV-1 infection and should be confirmed by a second test as soon as possible. DNA PCR testing is positive in approximately 40% of infected children by age 48 h and in 93% of infected children by age 14 days (93). Virus culture has similar sensitivity and specificity to those of DNA PCR tests. Plasma HIV-1 RNA testing detected infection in significantly more infected infants at birth and at 6 weeks of age than did either HIV-1 culture or DNA PCR (194). Serum p24 antigen assays are less sensitive than other virologic assays for diagnosis of HIV-1 infection in infants, and they have a high false-positive rate when used for infants younger than 1 month (251).

HIV-1 Drug Resistance Testing

HIV-1 resistance to antiretroviral agents can be assessed by genotypic and phenotypic assays (160, 161). Advances in molecular diagnostic techniques have made these tests routinely available to clinicians. Genotypic assays determine the sequence of PR or RT coding regions of the *pol* gene, whereas phenotypic assays determine the susceptibility of a patient's virus to specific drugs in an infected cell culture system. The two kinds of assays provide complementary information. Each approach has distinct advantages and disadvantages, and the two types of assays share certain limitations.

Resistance assays for HIV-1 depend on initial amplification of the coding sequences of selected HIV genes targeted by drugs from plasma viral RNA by reverse transcription followed by PCR. For genotypic analysis, the amplicons are then subjected to automated DNA sequencing, probed by hybridization-based assays, or tested by point mutation assay. Automated sequencing provides the most comprehensive data regarding genotypic changes associated with drug resistance. Phenotypic tests are performed by generating recombinant viruses or pseudoviruses, using sequences from patient samples together with a molecular clone of HIV-1 with the gene of interest deleted. The resulting recombinant viruses (or pseudoviruses) have a common genetic backbone but express PR, RT, IN, or Env from the patient's virus. This approach eliminates many of the problems associated with older assays performed with primary virus isolates in PBMC, which had considerable interassay variation.

A limitation shared by currently available drug resistance assays is their relative insensitivity to the presence of minority species in the virus population. Resistant variants of HIV-1 generally are not detected by most genotypic and phenotypic assays until they constitute more than 20 to 30% of the quasispecies. In addition, technical limitations in the RT-PCR step required to amplify viral sequences from plasma HIV-1 RNA make it difficult to obtain reliable results when the plasma HIV-1 RNA level is <1,000 copies/ml.

Genotypic assays have the relative advantage of being faster and easier to perform, resulting in shorter turnaround times and lower cost than phenotypic assays. In addition, sentinel mutations may be detectable by genotypic assay before a shift in drug susceptibility becomes apparent. A major limitation of genotypic assays is the difficulty in predicting the consequences of mutational interactions on phenotype. Likewise, the extent of cross-resistance among drugs within a class (e.g., PR inhibitors) can be difficult to predict on the basis of genotype alone. The Stanford University HIV Drug Resistance Database (http://hivdb.stanford.edu/) offers useful guidance and a variety of tools for the interpretation of genotypic resistance tests.

Phenotypic assays have the advantage of providing susceptibility data in a format that is familiar to most clinicians (i.e., 50% inhibitory concentration or fold resistance), as well as the capacity to determine drug susceptibility, even if the genetic basis of resistance to a particular drug is uncertain, and the net effect of different mutations on drug susceptibility and cross-resistance. A disadvantage of phenotypic assays is their more limited availability (only a few laboratories offer HIV-1 drug susceptibility testing as a diagnostic service) and higher cost compared to genotypic assays.

Numerous retrospective studies have demonstrated the correlation between genotype or phenotype at the time of regimen switch and the subsequent virologic response to salvage therapy. One meta-analysis showed that the risk of virologic failure was reduced by 30 to 50% for each drug in the salvage regimen to which the virus was susceptible, as predicted by the resistance test employed (80). In randomized trials (94), selection of a salvage regimen with the assistance of resistance testing resulted in significantly greater decreases in the level of plasma HIV-1 RNA or a greater proportion of patients achieving a plasma HIV-1 RNA level below the limit of detection, although follow-up in most studies was brief.

Resistance testing is recommended to help guide the choice of new regimens after treatment failure and for pregnant women (159). In addition, resistance testing should be performed prior to initiating therapy in treatment-naïve patients, particularly in areas with a high prevalence of drug resistance in recently transmitted viruses. Testing is also advisable for patients with primary HIV infection, but treatment should not be delayed while awaiting results. Because resistant variants can be replaced by wild-type virus within weeks of discontinuing treatment, resistance testing is most accurate when the sample is obtained while the patient is still taking the failing antiretroviral regimen. If high-level resistance to a drug is detected, that drug is unlikely to be useful in a treatment regimen. Failure to detect resistance to a previously used drug does not necessarily imply activity of that drug, however, for reasons cited above. Because sample mix-ups and PCR contamination can lead to reporting of erroneous results, clinicians should not hesitate to repeat a resistance test if the results are markedly discordant with the treatment history or results of viral load and CD4 testing.

PREVENTION

General

The frightening image of AIDS as a lethal plague sweeping across the globe without prospect of control belies the fact that the mechanisms and risks of transmission are clearly defined. High titers of HIV are found in two bodily fluids, blood and semen. Exchange of these fluids and contact with female genital secretions, in which the virus is more difficult to quantify, account for most infections. By excluding blood donors at risk of infection and by testing blood products for HIV, transmission by this route can be virtually eliminated.

The major causes of transmission of HIV, sexual intercourse and injection drug use, represent two extremely strong biological drives. Transmission can be significantly diminished, if not avoided, by monogamous sex with a known uninfected partner, use of barrier contraceptives, and not sharing drug paraphernalia. Many individuals have successfully modified their risk behaviors to prevent infection. For example, in the San Francisco homosexual men's cohort, HIV spread early and rapidly between 1978 and 1984. When the mechanism of its transmission was recognized and behavior changed as a result, new infections in this cohort diminished remarkably (197). Unfortunately, a new generation of young men who have sex with men are often ignoring these stark lessons, and transmission continues; these men also contribute significantly to transmission in developing countries (355). Educational programs regarding condom use appear to have dampened rates of transmission in some locales. Needle exchange programs to reduce sharing of contaminated paraphernalia by intravenous drug users reduces HIV transmission, but in many places in the United States, former Soviet Republics, and Southeast Asia, socioeconomic, political, or religious considerations thwart implementation of this intervention (178).

A very high priority is the development of a vaginal microbicide effective against HIV (96). Ideally the microbicide would be active against other sexually transmitted infections as well, since they increase transmission rates of HIV by producing mucosal ulceration and local inflammation (140). In many cultural and social situations, women who have limited choice regarding sexual encounters could utilize an effective microbicide prophylactically without the need for a partner's consent. Unfortunately, the similarity between the retroviral envelope and the host cell membrane provides a challenge to identification of inactivating agents with selective activity. In phase 3 trials, the topical microbicides nonoxydal-9 and cellulose sulfate both increased transmission of HIV, presumably by disrupting the integrity of the natural mucosal barrier (354), while Carraguard fared no better than placebo. Consequently, the design of a promising candidate has remained elusive.

With the inadequacy of behavioral interventions, microbicides, and vaccines to impact transmission, preexposure prophylaxis emerged as a prevention strategy (208, 275). Proven efficacy in animal models and the simplicity of taking pills without the need for informing others make preexposure prophylaxis appealing. The risks are false sense of security, disinhibition, drug toxicity, and drug resistance. Off-label use among men who have sex with men occurs commonly. Randomized controlled trials are currently lacking, and several were aborted because of political and regulatory snafus (www.prepwatch.org/).

Three randomized trials of uninfected men have shown a 50 to 60% protective effect of circumcision against heterosexually acquired HIV (13, 16, 139). This intervention is less effective than condom use but does not require adherence with each sex act. No data have yet been generated on the protection of women or men who have sex with men. The increased incidence of transmission associated with genital herpes motivated a randomized controlled trial of the use of valacyclovir to reduce transmission (395), but results from this trial were discouraging.

Efforts to empower individuals at risk for HIV infection to understand and implement risk reduction remain a high priority worldwide in the absence of an effective vaccine. Such practices may dampen the rates of transmission; however, widespread implementation of behavioral modification is an unrealistic expectation.

Passive Immunoprophylaxis

Studies of the administration of passive antibody either to prevent transmission or to impact ongoing infection have yet to provide evidence of benefit. One critical challenge is the difficulty in eliciting potent broadly neutralizing antibody by natural infection or most vaccines. The administration of monoclonal antibodies or polyclonal sera that provide neutralizing activity against the challenge virus can confer protection from infection in both murine and rhesus macaque models (39, 257, 354). The administration of a mixture of three neutralizing monoclonal antibodies delayed the reemergence of detectable viremia in several subjects after their suppressive antiretroviral regimen was withdrawn (351). The viruses that emerged were neutralization escape mutants to monoclonal antibody 2G12, indicating that the selective pressure conferred by that antibody contributed to the delayed emergence of replicating virus. Additional trials of passive administration of mixtures of neutralizing monoclonal antibodies are in progress.

Active Immunization

The AIDS pandemic can be controlled only by an effective vaccine, but the challenges are substantial (Table 5) (248). Ideally, a vaccine would induce sustained high levels of both broadly cross-reactive neutralizing antibodies and CD8 CTL responses (86). Studies of macaques have indicated protective value of neutralizing antibody (257). However, neutralizing-antibody responses to infection are of low titer and restricted cross-reactivity in humans, and most antibodies to the HIV envelope exhibit poor neu-

TABLE 5 Obstacles to an effective vaccine for HIV

1. The immune responses conferring protection and mediating viral clearance and the viral antigens that elicit these responses are not defined.
2. HIV displays great antigenic diversity among individuals.
3. HIV mutates readily to generate escape mutants and genetic diversity within individuals.
4. Mucosal immunity may be needed.
5. Enhancing antibodies exist.
6. The viral genome integrates into the host cell chromosome.
7. The major target organ of HIV is the immune system.
8. No inexpensive, simple animal models exist.
9. The elicitation of a sustained, high-level, broadly reactive virus-specific CTL response with a safe immunogen is without precedent.
10. The most effective viral vaccine vectors are subject to preexisting anti-vector immunity and elicit immunity that compromises reuse.
11. High-titer broadly reactive neutralizing antibody responses do not occur within a year in any subject or over many years in most subjects with natural infection.
12. No immunogen has been designed that elicits neutralizing antibody that is high titer or not strain specific.

tralizing activity. Neutralizing antibody develops within 2 to 3 months after infection; however, this antibody is strain specific, and more broadly reactive neutralizing antibody responses develop only over years and only in a subset of individuals (296). Neutralizing-antibody responses to candidate vaccines have been weak and restricted to laboratory-adapted strains rather than primary isolates (39). Modified envelope protein preparations have not yet been designed that elicit neutralizing antibody to heterologous strains. Thus, although neutralizing antibody comprises the basis of most protective viral vaccines (274), new basic insights are needed to elicit protective humoral responses to HIV infection.

Extensive efforts have been employed to induce HIV-specific CTL (248, 296). Historically this has been done using live, attenuated virus to express viral antigen in the context of autologous HLA-restricted presentation of epitopes. The use of live, attenuated HIV has been complicated by concerns about the balance between attenuation and immunogenicity (175, 296) which may be unpredictable and highly variable in the outbred human population. Efforts to induce CTL have thus focused on the expression of HIV antigens either with "naked" DNA or with viral or bacterial vectors. Virtually every available vector has been studied as a candidate, but the most extensive studies with primate and human trials have included poxviruses (vaccinia and avian) and adenoviruses (see chapter 16). The literature is replete with negative or borderline levels of protection. Substantial CTL responses after DNA priming with adenovirus or poxvirus boosting or after sequential vector immunizations have resulted in reductions in the HIV RNA "set point" and rates of progression in rhesus macaque models of SIV or SHIV infection (7, 18). However, the first large trial of an adenovirus type 5 vector expressing *gag*, *pol*, and *nef* (Merck) was discontinued before completion because of discouraging results.

Postexposure Prophylaxis

Occupational Exposure

Approximately 1 in 300 health care providers becomes infected with HIV after percutaneous exposure with a needle used on a seropositive patient (50, 132). With the inoculum size in such transmissions probably representing close to one human infectious dose, prompt administration of chemoprophylaxis may be beneficial. Because of the low rate of transmission, controlled randomized trials are not feasible and decisions must be based on judgment, retrospective studies, and animal models. A retrospective analysis of the use of zidovudine for postexposure prophylaxis of health care workers after percutaneous exposure to infected blood suggested an 80% reduction in the risk of seroconversion (50). Extrapolation from other applications of chemoprophylaxis for infections would argue that the earlier the administration and the more potent the regimen, the greater the likelihood that the prophylaxis will work. Because most HIV-infected patients in hospital and clinic situations have been treated with antiretrovirals and thus may harbor drug-resistant virus, guidelines for significant exposure to blood from such patients recommend prophylaxis with multiple drugs. U.S. Public Health Service Guidelines have been recently disseminated with background information and recommendations (271).

Prevention of needlestick transmission is best accomplished by prevention of needlesticks. This requires care and attention by health care workers during injection and phlebotomy procedures, use of gloves, proper disposal of sharp instruments, and use of needles with guards and other devices designed to minimize risk.

The issue of risk to patients from infected providers has raised much controversy. The mechanism of transmission in one outbreak associated with a Florida dentist remains unexplained (63). Nevertheless, routine health care provided by HIV-infected providers poses no measurable risk of transmission.

Sexual Exposure

Considerations similar to those for health care providers apply to postexposure prophylaxis following sexual exposure due to rape, broken condom, or unprotected consensual sex. The decision regarding implementation and regimen requires judgment (http://www.cdc.gov/hiv/resources/guidelines/index.htm#prophylaxis). Postexposure prophylaxis following unprotected consensual sex is not being investigated as intensively as is preexposure prophylaxis.

Maternal-Fetal Transmission

Maternal-fetal transmission represents a special situation: 2.3 million children worldwide were living with HIV infection at the end of 2006, with 1,000 newly infected children daily, half of whom will die by their second birthday if they are not treated (353). Maternal-fetal transmission occurs antepartum by transplacental transmission, during delivery, and via breast-feeding (372). From 13 to 40% of HIV-infected pregnant women transmit infection to their newborn infants (372). Perinatal administration of the relatively impotent antiviral ZDV to treatment-naïve pregnant women with more than 200 CD4 cells/μl of blood and to their newborns reduced transmission from 25.5 to 8.3% (66). More recent studies indicate that the protection is conferred primarily as postexposure prophylaxis in the newborn (172). Perinatal antiretroviral treatment represents an extremely cost-effective measure because life-threatening infection is prevented by a short duration of treatment, thus providing a strong impetus for routine testing of all pregnant women globally to permit the preventive benefit of this intervention and to provide longitudinal care for both mother and infant (372).

The cost-effectiveness of single-dose nevirapine prophylaxis, which is associated with a 50% reduced risk of mother-to-infant transmission, has prompted extensive implementation of programs, primarily in sub-Saharan Africa. However, several concerns remain to be addressed, and regimens with improved efficacy are urgently needed. Selection for nevirapine resistance in mother and child is frequent and compromises first-line treatment regimens in the developing world (210). Transmisssion from breast-feeding results in infection of a proportion of those protected perinatally by prophylaxis. Although exclusive bottle-feeding reduces the risk of HIV transmission, this gain is offset in developing countries by increases in infant mortality from diarrheal and respiratory infections (70, 347). A healthy mother is important for the welfare and survival of the newborn. Each of these concerns would be addressed if the mother received effective antiretroviral treatment at diagnosis of pregnancy.

Full suppression of plasma HIV RNA by potent combination therapy during pregnancy has resulted in no observed transmissions and, importantly, no discernible toxicity to the newborns. Rates of maternal-fetal transmission do not exceed 1% in women receiving antiviral therapy and perinatal prophylaxis (87). The residual infections probably represented antenatal infection in mothers with residual virus replication.

TREATMENT

The improvement in AIDS mortality statistics reflects drug usage in Western Europe and the Americas (Fig. 10) (239, 268). Opportunistic disease has been reversed and prevented. Health care costs have diminished. Many ill and disabled patients have returned to normal and functional lifestyles. This dramatic impact does come with costs—the expense, inconvenience, and toxicity of antiretroviral therapy. These costs and the benefits of treatment create a tension in the decision-making process regarding when to initiate therapy.

As described above, the clinical manifestations of HIV disease are primarily opportunistic consequences of the progressive destruction of the immune system by the persistent replication of HIV. Some manifestations, including dementia, wasting, thrombocytopenia, and neuropathy, can be the direct consequences of HIV infection and are often directly responsive to antiretroviral therapy. Most symptoms, however, result from opportunistic infections and malignancies. Specific prophylactic strategies and treatments for these AIDS-related conditions and other important management issues of patients with HIV infection, including nutrition, psychological counseling, social management, and treatment of addiction, are beyond the scope of this chapter. Moreover, the field changes so rapidly that practice is often based on information not yet in the peer-reviewed literature. Treatment guidelines (151) provide recent expert consensus summaries regarding important treatment issues such as appropriate regimens, timing of initiation and switching, and HIV drug resistance testing. These are updated approximately annually; however, the changing practice of experts may often precede the publication of these consensus guidelines. Consequently this chapter, rather than providing an obsolete and inadequate manual for chemotherapy, summarizes the pathogenetic principles and challenges of the treatment of HIV infection itself. The antiretroviral drugs, including their mechanisms of action, pharmacology, and toxicities, are summarized in chapter 11.

Virologic and Immunologic Principles Underlying Antiretroviral Chemotherapy

The primary goal in the management of the HIV-infected patient treated with antiviral therapy should be to achieve prolonged suppression of viral replication. While a small subset of individuals, for reasons attributable to the genetic composition of the virus or immunologic responses, may survive for years to decades without an increase in viral burden (45, 273), HIV infection in most individuals leads to increasing levels of HIV, decline in $CD4^+$ T-cell numbers, and death.

As discussed above (see "Pathogenesis"), the turnover of virus particles in the body is tremendous, clearance of virus from the plasma is rapid (minutes to hours), and the clearance rate constant varies little among individuals and different stages of disease. The steady-state levels of HIV RNA in the blood are thus determined by the rate of virus production. These rates of production are a function of the number of infected lymphocytes in the lymphoid tissue (148, 149). The rate of decline of CD4 lymphocytes is thus directly related to the steady-state level of plasma HIV RNA. The higher the RNA levels, the faster the loss of CD4 cells and the shorter the duration of HIV infection before death (233). Since the CD4 count determines the risk of disease and death, and the level of HIV RNA determines the rate of CD4 cell decline, these values are routinely used clinically to assess clinical status and urgency to initiate chemotherapy (151).

When potent combination therapy is effectively administered, levels of HIV RNA in plasma and infected cells in lymphoid tissue rapidly decrease (Fig. 9 and 11a). The clearance dynamics of HIV with treatment are discussed above (see "Pathogenesis"). Failure to reduce plasma HIV RNA levels to below the limit of detection of 50 copies/ml with the currently available assays indicates inadequate suppression and a risk for the outgrowth of resistant virus. For patients sustaining suppression below this level of 50 copies/ml (Fig. 11b), many will sustain steady-state levels of 1 to 50 copies HIV RNA/ml, which is not associated with clinical progression or viral evolution. The relative contributions of smoldering replication, release of virions from activated latently infected cells, and persistently infected long-lived cells have not been well delineated (90, 121, 389).

Compartments and Reservoirs

The treatment of HIV is complicated by the existence of tissue compartments and cellular reservoirs. Although there is trafficking between the blood and CNS, much virus in the CNS evolves independently (56, 98, 337, 377). Similar observations have been made for virus in semen (266, 282, 393). Drug penetration into these compartments differs from penetration into the circulation and lymphoid tissue and varies with each drug. Latently infected CD4 lymphocytes represent a small fraction of in-

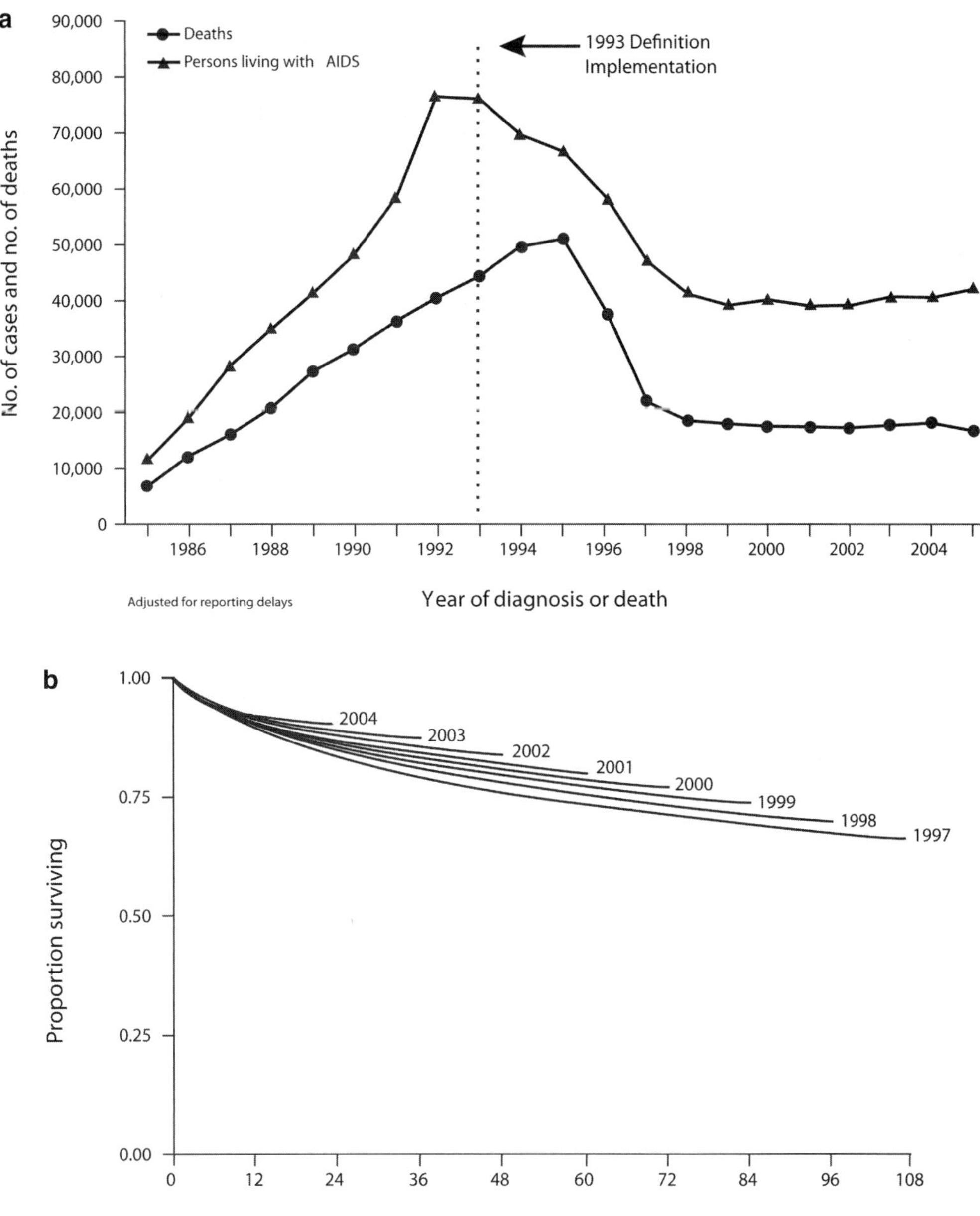

FIGURE 10 (a) Estimated number of AIDS cases and deaths of adults and adolescents with AIDS in the United States and dependent areas during the period from 1985 to 2005. The number of deaths is adjusted for reporting delays. (b) Estimated proportion of persons surviving with AIDS in the United States and dependent areas by year of diagnosis. With new infections continuing unabated and with survival increasing as a result of improving treatment, one consequence is the progressive accumulaton of persons living with HIV infection. (Both figures adapted from the CDC [http://www.cdc.gov/hiv/].)

fected cells during active infection, but, like immunologic memory, they persist for life (112). Such cells survive, archiving virus that can be drug resistant and can reemerge and propagate after the withdrawal of chemotherapy.

Immunologic Restoration with Antiretroviral Therapy

The immunologic consequences of suppressing virus replication are dramatic (Fig. 11c). The increase in CD4 lymphocyte numbers has two phases. In the first month or two the increase is often large (20 to 100 cells/μl of blood) (11, 22, 144, 267). The magnitude is proportional to the steady-state HIV RNA levels, which drive the level of generalized activation of the immune system. The normal distribution of lymphocytes is 2% in the circulation and 98% in the lymphoid tissues. With the immune activation of HIV infection, the distribution shifts to 1% and 99% (148, 390). Therapy largely corrects this shift and results in re-

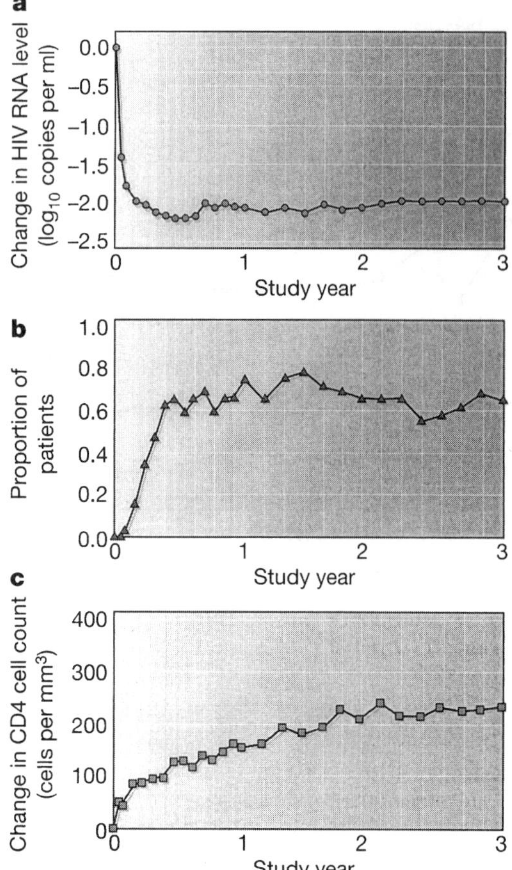

FIGURE 11 Three-year treatment with indinavir, zidovudine, and lamivudine. (a) Median changes in serum HIV RNA level (Amplicor assay with quantification limit of 500 copies/ml) from baseline. (b) Proportions of patients with serum HIV RNA levels lower than 50 copies/ml (ultradirect assay). (c) Median changes in CD4 cell count from baseline. The number of contributing patients in each trial and at each time point was between 30 and 33. Details regarding the study and analyses are published in reference 145. (Adapted from reference 292 with permission.)

distribution of mostly CD45RO$^+$ memory T cells from the lymphoid tissue back to the circulation (267, 390). Production of new cells, mostly of the CD45RA-naïve phenotype, is generated both by restored thymic mass and function, which is age related, and by peripheral proliferation (91, 227).

However, it is the restoration of immune function that has transformed the natural history of AIDS. Both CD4$^+$ and CD8$^+$ T-cell responses to recall antigens are regenerated (11, 189). Persistent opportunistic infections are often resolved. Occasionally subclinical chronic infections with *M. avium* complex or cytomegalovirus, for example, are manifested when a restored immune response produces a local inflammatory reaction (118). Patient care has been transformed by the ability to withdraw prophylactic or suppressive chemotherapy for *Pneumocystis*, *Toxoplasma*, cytomegalovirus, *M. avium* complex, *Leishmania*, *Cryptococcus*, and *Candida* infections, which had previously been lifelong commitments (240).

Antiviral Resistance in Antiretroviral Chemotherapy

Antiretroviral drugs select for the emergence of drug-resistant viral variants. These mutations and their impact on phenotype and treatment have been reviewed in detail for each of the classes of antiretroviral drugs (159, 161), but it is important to note that the speed, magnitude, and clinical impact of the emergence of resistance differ among antiretrovirals. The likelihood that resistant mutants will emerge is a function of at least four factors: (i) the viral mutation frequency, (ii) the intrinsic mutability of the viral target site with respect to a specific antiviral, (iii) the selective pressure of the antiviral drug, and (iv) the magnitude and rate of virus replication.

For single-stranded RNA viruses, whose genomic replication lacks a proofreading mechanism, the mutation frequencies are approximately 10^{-5} per nucleotide per replication cycle or approximately 1 mutation for every progeny genome (167, 222). Some mutations at a single nucleotide result in greater than 100-fold reductions in susceptibility, for example, to lamivudine or nonnucleoside RT inhibitors (161). For many nucleosides and PR inhibitors, high-level resistance requires the cumulative acquisition of multiple mutations.

With regard to the selective pressure of the antiviral drug, one definition of an antiviral drug is a compound that confers sufficient selective pressure on virus replication to select for drug-resistant mutants. With increasing drug exposure, the selective pressure on the replicating virus population increases to promote the more rapid emergence of drug-resistant mutants. For example, higher doses of AZT or of ritonavir monotherapy tend to select for drug-resistant virus more readily than do lower doses (242, 295). Increasing selective pressure for resistant mutants increases the likelihood of such mutants arising as long as significant levels of virus replication persist (Fig. 12). As antiviral drug activity increases still more, the amount of virus replication diminishes to the point where the likelihood of emergence of resistance begins to diminish, as is being seen with potent PR inhibitors, and becomes nil when virus replication is completely inhibited. The ultimate goal of chemother-

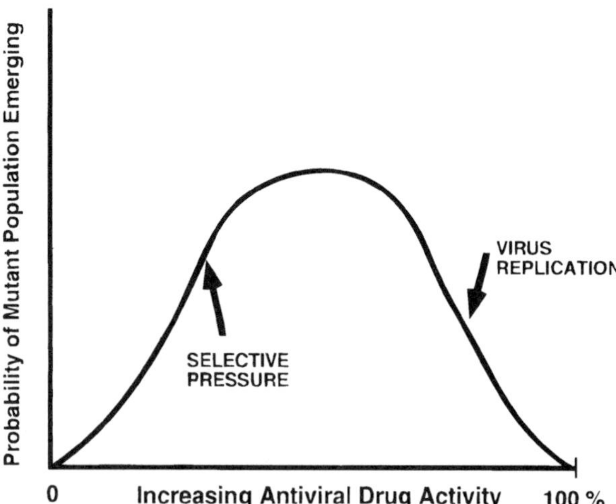

FIGURE 12 Hypothetical impact of antiviral drug activity on the probability of the emergence of drug resistance. (Reprinted from reference 291.)

TABLE 6 Approved antiretroviral drugs[a]

Drug	Yr approved by FDA	Major toxicities
Nucleoside and nucleotide RT inhibitors		
Zidovudine (AZT)	1987	Anemia, neutropenia, nausea, headache, insomnia, myalgia and weakness, elevated serum lactate level, steatohepatitis, ?fat redistribution
Didanosine (ddI)	1991	Peripheral neuropathy, pancreatitis, sicca syndrome
Zalcitabine (ddC)[c]	1992	Peripheral neuropathy
Stavudine (d4T)	1994	Peripheral neuropathy, elevated liver function tests, elevated serum lactate, steatohepatitis, ?fat redistribution
Lamivudine (3TC)	1995	
Abacavir (ABC)	1998	Nausea, anorexia, abdominal pain, hypersensitivity reactions
Tenofovir (TDF)[b]	2001	Fanconi syndrome
Emtricitabine (FTC)	2003	
Nonnucleoside RT inhibitors		
Nevirapine	1996	Rash, hepatitis
Delavirdine[c]	1997	Rash, hepatitis, nausea, diarrhea
Efavirenz	1998	Altered dreams, confusion, dizziness, rash; teratogenicity in primates
Etravirine	2007	Rash, nausea
Protease inhibitors[d]		
Saquinavir[e]	1995	Diarrhea, abdominal pain, nausea
Indinavir[e]	1996	Nausea, abdominal discomfort, nephrolithiasis, dry skin and nail changes, indirect hyperbilirubinemia
Ritonavir	1996	Circumoral parathesia, altered taste, diarrhea, weakness, nausea
Nelfinavir	1997	Diarrhea, nausea, weakness, abdominal pain
Fosamprenavir[e,f]	1999	Rash, nausea, diarrhea
Lopinavir[e]	2000	Diarrhea, fatigue, nausea, stomach discomfort
Atazanavir	2003	Hyperbilirubinemia
Tipranavir	2005	Rash, hepatitis
Darunavir	2006	Rash, nausea, diarrhea
Entry inhibitors		
Enfuvirtide	2003	Injection site reactions
Maraviroc	2007	
Integrase inhibitor		
Raltegravir	2007	

[a] Refer to chapter 11 for a detailed discussion.
[b] Technically, tenofovir is a nucleotide.
[c] No longer marketed.
[d] All approved protease inhibitors, with the exception of atazanavir, can produce elevated cholesterol and triglycerides, insulin resistance, and fat redistribution to various degrees.
[e] Often or usually used with low-dose ritonavir for pharmacological enhancement.
[f] Approved as amprenavir in 1999 and replaced by fosamprenavir in 2003.

apy of HIV is to thus identify drug regimens that completely inhibit virus replication.

The magnitude and rate of replication of the virus population have major consequences for the likelihood of emergence of resistant mutants. Approximately 10 billion (10^{10}) HIV-1 virions are generated daily (278), and approximately 1 mutation is generated for each new genome of 9,200 nucleotides (222). Thus, genomes with each possible mutation as well as many with double mutations should be generated daily. Incompletely suppressed viral replication with drug regimens sufficient to exert selective pressure drives the evolution and fixation of drug-resistant virus at a rate Darwin himself never imagined. Moreover, drug-resistant virus is readily archived in latently infected cells to confound treatment modifications for the remainder of the patient's life (113, 376).

Impact of Resistance on Treatment

As resistance mutations accumulate, drug susceptibility diminishes, progressively reducing the potency of components of combination antiretroviral regimens. Continued replication in the presence of drug selects for even greater levels of resistance to each administered drug and progressive cross-resistance to drugs of the same class. Thus, impotent regimens, suboptimal adherence, pharmacologic hurdles, and ineffectively treated compartments permit the emergence of resistant virus; its emergence drives a vicious cycle of treatment failure and yet more difficult treatment challenges. Regimens for patients failing to respond to treatment with resistant virus are constrained by more limited options but must still contend with the same obstacles of adherence, pharmacology, and tolerability that challenged the first regimen.

Resistant virus in genital secretions, blood, or milk can be transmitted during sex, needle sharing, childbirth, or nursing (206). Rates of transmission of drug-resistant virus appear to be increasing, with up to 20% of primary infections being due to drug-resistant virus strains, many of which exhibit resistance to multiple classes of drug (206, 207). Such patients are more likely to fail their first treatment regimen.

Resistance Testing To Manage Patients

The accumulation of drug resistance due to treatment failure and transmission raises challenges to the effective treatment of individuals and to public health that have resulted from widespread antibiotic resistance. As discussed above, the use of drug resistance testing has been incorporated into standard HIV care (160, 161). Drug resistance assays can help determine which drugs will not work, thereby diminishing cost, toxicity, and inconvenience, and which drugs are most likely to be effective.

Antiretroviral Drugs

As of 2008, 22 antiretroviral drugs had been approved for use in the United States (Table 6) and several more were in various stages of clinical development. Although any function in a genetically efficient organism is a candidate for an inhibitory drug, the currently approved drugs are directed against RT, PR, IN, and viral entry, with the RT inhibitors being classified as nucleosides or nonnucleosides. They are described in detail in chapter 11.

The use of these drugs in the management of HIV-infected patients has developed into a remarkably complex specialty. These drugs must be used in various combinations of three or more drugs for optimal efficacy. Each drug has a complicated pharmacology that often interacts with other components of the regimen or with nonantiretroviral drugs. Treatment success is related to rigorous adherence. Initial regimens have become increasingly tolerable and convenient with many regimens involving once-daily administration. Regimens for persons who have experienced treatment failure become increasingly complex and are attended by higher rates of undesirable side effects.

New Antiretroviral Drugs

Drug candidates continue to be discovered and developed to obtain greater potency, activity against drug-resistant virus, diminished pharmacologic interactions with other drugs, and lower toxicity. Compounds designed against new targets should not be affected by resistance in PR or RT. Moreover, they may have unique attributes regarding both antiviral activity and toxicity.

The correlation of risk of progression with certain class I HLA haplotypes and with the breadth and magnitude of cell-mediated immune responses has prompted interest in therapeutic immunization to enhance these beneficial responses. This approach in general has been aimed at delivering immunogens while the immune system is fully protected by potent antiretroviral chemotherapy and then ascertaining whether a benefit can be discerned after withdrawal of therapy. Of concern, an effective prophylactic vaccine has yet to be identified, the concept of therapeutic vaccination has yet to be proven by example, exposure to autologous HIV antigens using numerous strategic treatment interruption approaches has consistently shown no benefit, and to date therapeutic immunization trials have shown either no benefit or worse (12).

REFERENCES

1. **Abecasis, A. B., P. Lemey, N. Vidal, T. de Oliveira, M. Peeters, R. Camacho, B. Shapiro, A. Rambaut, and A. M. Vandamme.** 2007. Recombination confounds the early evolutionary history of human immunodeficiency virus type 1: subtype g is a circulating recombinant form. *J. Virol.* **81:**8543–8551.
2. **Aboulafia, D. M., and R. T. Mitsuyasu.** 1991. Hematologic abnormalities in AIDS. *Hematol. Oncol. Clin. North. Am.* **5:**195–214.
3. **Accola, M. A., B. Strack, and H. G. Gottlinger.** 2000. Efficient particle production by minimal Gag constructs which retain the carboxy-terminal domain of human immunodeficiency virus type 1 capsid-p2 and a late assembly domain. *J. Virol.* **74:**5395–5402.
4. **Alkhatib, G., C. Combadiere, C. C. Broder, Y. Feng, P. E. Kennedy, P. M. Murphy, and E. A. Berger.** 1996. CC CKR5: a RANTES, MIP-1α, MIP-1β receptor as a fusion cofactor for macrophage-tropic HIV-1. *Science* **272:**1955–1958.
5. **Allain, J. P., Y. Laurian, D. A. Paul, F. Verroust, M. Leuther, C. Gazengel, D. Senn, M. J. Larrieu, and C. Bosser.** 1987. Long-term evaluation of HIV antigen and antibodies to p24 and gp41 in patients with hemophilia. Potential clinical importance. *N. Engl. J. Med.* **317:**1114–1121.
6. **Allen, T. M., D. H. O'Connor, P. Jing, J. L. Dzuris, B. R. Mothe, T. U. Vogel, E. Dunphy, M. E. Liebl, C. Emerson, N. Wilson, K. J. Kunstman, X. Wang, D. B. Allison, A. L. Hughes, R. C. Desrosiers, J. D. Altman, S. M. Wolinsky, A. Sette, and D. I. Watkins.** 2000. Tat-specific cytotoxic T lymphocytes select for SIV escape

variants during resolution of primary viraemia. *Nature* **407:**386–390.

7. **Amara, R. R., F. Villinger, J. D. Altman, S. L. Lydy, S. P. O'Neil, S. I. Staprans, D. C. Montefiori, Y. Xu, J. G. Herndon, L. S. Wyatt, M. A. Candido, N. L. Kozyr, P. L. Earl, J. M. Smith, H. L. Ma, B. D. Grimm, M. L. Hulsey, J. Miller, H. M. McClure, J. M. McNicholl, B. Moss, and H. L. Robinson.** 2001. Control of a mucosal challenge and prevention of AIDS by a multiprotein DNA/MVA vaccine. *Science* **292:**69–74.
8. **Andersen, J. L., J. L. DeHart, E. S. Zimmerman, O. Ardon, B. Kim, G. Jacquot, S. Benichou, and V. Planelles.** 2006. HIV-1 Vpr-induced apoptosis is cell cycle dependent and requires Bax but not ANT. *PLoS Pathog.* **2:**e127.
9. **Arthur, L. O., J. W. Bess, Jr., R. C. Sowder, R. E. Benveniste, D. L. Mann, J. C. Chermann, and L. E. Henderson.** 1992. Cellular proteins bound to immunodeficiency viruses: implications for pathogenesis and vaccines. *Science* **258:**1935–1938.
10. **Arya, S. K., C. Guo, S. F. Josephs, and F. Wong-Staal.** 1985. Trans-activator gene of human T-lymphotropic virus type III (HTLV-III). *Science* **229:**69–73.
11. **Autran, B., G. Carcelain, T. S. Li, C. Blanc, D. Mathez, R. Tubiana, C. Katlama, P. Debre, and J. Leibowitch.** 1997. Positive effects of combined antiretroviral therapy on $CD4^+$ T cell homeostasis and function in advanced HIV disease. *Science* **277:**112–116.
12. **Autran, B., D. Costagliola, R. Murphy, N. Wincker, B. Clotet, J. Gatell, R. Tubiana, S. Staszewski, B. Walker, C. Katlama, and the ORVACS Study Group.** 2007. *Abstr. 14th Conf. Retroviruses Oppor. Infect.*, abstr. 126LB.
13. **Auvert, B., D. Taljaard, E. Lagarde, J. Sobngwi-Tambekou, R. Sitta, and A. Puren.** 2005. Randomized, controlled intervention trial of male circumcision for reduction of HIV infection risk: the ANRS 1265 Trial. *PLoS Med.* **2:**e298.
14. **Ayres, L., F. Avillez, A. Garcia-Benito, F. Deinhardt, L. Gurtler, F. Denis, G. Leonard, S. Ranger, P. Grob, and H. Joller-Jemelka.** 1990. Multicenter evaluation of a new recombinant enzyme immunoassay for the combined detection of antibody to HIV-1 and HIV-2. *AIDS* **4:**131–138.
15. **Bailey, J. R., A. R. Sedaghat, T. Kieffer, T. Brennan, P. K. Lee, M. Wind-Rotolo, C. M. Haggerty, A. R. Kamireddi, Y. Liu, J. Lee, D. Persaud, J. E. Gallant, J. Cofrancesco, Jr., T. C. Quinn, C. O. Wilke, S. C. Ray, J. D. Siliciano, R. E. Nettles, and R. F. Siliciano.** 2006. Residual human immunodeficiency virus type 1 viremia in some patients on antiretroviral therapy is dominated by a small number of invariant clones rarely found in circulating $CD4^+$ T cells. *J. Virol.* **80:**6441–6457.
16. **Bailey, R. C., S. Moses, C. B. Parker, K. Agot, I. Maclean, J. N. Krieger, C. F. Williams, R. T. Campbell, and J. O. Ndinya-Achola.** 2007. Male circumcision for HIV prevention in young men in Kisumu, Kenya: a randomised controlled trial. *Lancet* **369:**643–656.
17. **Barin, F., S. M'Boup, F. Denis, P. Kanki, J. S. Allan, T. H. Lee, and M. Essex.** 1985. Serological evidence for virus related to simian T-lymphotropic retrovirus III in residents of west Africa. *Lancet* **ii:**1387–1389.
18. **Barouch, D. H., S. Santra, J. E. Schmitz, M. J. Kuroda, T. M. Fu, W. Wagner, M. Bilska, A. Craiu, X. X. Zheng, G. R. Krivulka, K. Beaudry, M. A. Lifton, C. E. Nickerson, W. L. Trigona, K. Punt, D. C. Freed, L. Guan, S. Dubey, D. Casimiro, A. Simon, M. E. Davies, M. Chastain, T. B. Strom, R. S. Gelman, D. C. Montefiori, M. G. Lewis, E. A. Emini, J. W. Shiver, and N. L. Letvin.** 2000. Control of viremia and prevention of clinical AIDS in rhesus monkeys by cytokine-augmented DNA vaccination. *Science* **290:**486–492.
19. **Barré-Sinoussi, F., J. C. Chermann, F. Rey, M. T. Nugeyre, S. Chamaret, J. Gruest, C. Dauguet, C. Axler-Blin, F. Vezinet-Brun, C. Rouzioux, W. Rozenbaum, and L. Montagnier.** 1983. Isolation of a T-lymphotropic retrovirus from a patient at risk for acquired immune deficiency syndrome (AIDS). *Science* **220:**868–871.
20. **Bartlett, J. A., R. DeMasi, D. Dawson, and A. Hill.** 1998. Variability in repeated consecutive measurements of plasma human immunodeficiency virus RNA in persons receiving stable nucleoside reverse transcriptase inhibitor therapy or no treatment. *J. Infect. Dis.* **178:**1803–1805.
21. **Benichou, S., M. Bomsel, M. Bodeus, H. Durand, M. Doute, F. Letourneur, J. Camonis, and R. Benarous.** 1994. Physical interaction of the HIV-1 Nef protein with beta-COP, a component of non-clathrin-coated vesicles essential for membrane traffic. *J. Biol. Chem.* **269:**30073–30076.
22. **Bennett, K. K., V. G. DeGruttola, I. C. Marschner, D. V. Havlir, and D. D. Richman.** 2002. Baseline predictors of CD4 T-lymphocyte recovery with combination antiretroviral therapy. *J. Acquir. Immune. Defic. Syndr.* **31:**20–26.
23. **Betts, M. R., M. C. Nason, S. M. West, S. C. De Rosa, S. A. Migueles, J. Abraham, M. M. Lederman, J. M. Benito, P. A. Goepfert, M. Connors, M. Roederer, and R. A. Koup.** 2006. HIV nonprogressors preferentially maintain highly functional HIV-specific $CD8^+$ T cells. *Blood* **107:**4781–4789.
24. **Blanche, S., C. Rouzioux, M. L. Moscato, F. Veber, M. J. Mayaux, C. Jacomet, J. Tricoire, A. Deville, M. Vial, and G. Firtion for the HIV Infection in Newborns French Collaborative Study Group.** 1989. A prospective study of infants born to women seropositive for human immunodeficiency virus type 1. *N. Engl. J. Med.* **320:**1643–1648.
25. **Blankson, J. N., J. R. Bailey, S. Thayil, H. C. Yang, K. Lassen, J. Lai, S. K. Gandhi, J. D. Siliciano, T. M. Williams, and R. F. Siliciano.** 2007. Isolation and characterization of replication-competent human immunodeficiency virus type 1 from a subset of elite suppressors. *J. Virol.* **81:**2508–2518.
26. **Blankson, J. N., D. Finzi, T. C. Pierson, B. P. Sabundayo, K. Chadwick, J. B. Margolick, T. C. Quinn, and R. F. Siliciano.** 2000. Biphasic decay of latently infected $CD4^+$ T cells in acute human immunodeficiency virus type 1 infection. *J. Infect. Dis.* **182:**1636–1642.
27. **Bosch, M. L., P. L. Earl, K. Fargnoli, S. Picciafuoco, F. Giombini, F. Wong-Staal, and G. Franchini.** 1989. Identification of the fusion peptide of primate immunodeficiency viruses. *Science* **244:**694–697.
28. **Bozzette, S. A., J. A. McCutchan, S. A. Spector, B. Wright, and D. D. Richman.** 1993. A cross-sectional comparison of persons with syncytium- and non-syncytium-inducing human immunodeficiency virus. *J. Infect. Dis.* **168:**1374–1379.
29. **Branson, B. M., H. H. Handsfield, M. A. Lampe, R. S. Janssen, A. W. Taylor, S. B. Lyss, and J. E. Clark.** 2006. Revised recommendations for HIV testing of adults, adolescents, and pregnant women in health-care settings. *Morb. Mortal. Wkly. Rep. Recomm. Rep.* **55:**1–17.
30. **Brenchley, J. M., D. A. Price, T. W. Schacker, T. E. Asher, G. Silvestri, S. Rao, Z. Kazzaz, E. Bornstein, O. Lambotte, D. Altmann, B. R. Blazar, B. Rodriguez, L. Teixeira-Johnson, A. Landay, J. N. Martin, F. M. Hecht, L. J. Picker, M. M. Lederman, S. G. Deeks, and D. C. Douek.** 2006. Microbial translocation is a cause of sys-

temic immune activation in chronic HIV infection. *Nat. Med.* **12:**1365–1371.

31. **Brenner, B. G., M. Roger, J. P. Routy, D. Moisi, M. Ntemgwa, C. Matte, J. G. Baril, R. Thomas, D. Rouleau, J. Bruneau, R. LeBlanc, M. Legault, C. Tremblay, H. Charest, and M. A. Wainberg.** 2007. High rates of forward transmission events after acute/early HIV-1 infection. *J. Infect. Dis.* **195:**951–959.
32. **Brodt, H. R., B. S. Kamps, P. Gute, B. Knupp, S. Staszewski, and E. B. Helm.** 1997. Changing incidence of AIDS-defining illnesses in the era of antiretroviral combination therapy. *AIDS* **11:**1731–1738.
33. **Brun-Vezinet, F., M. A. Rey, C. Katlama, P. M. Girard, D. Roulot, P. Yeni, L. Lenoble, F. Clavel, M. Alizon, and S. Gadelle.** 1987. Lymphadenopathy-associated virus type 2 in AIDS and AIDS-related complex. Clinical and virological features in four patients. *Lancet* **i:**128–132.
34. **Bukrinsky, M. I., S. Haggerty, M. P. Dempsey, N. Sharova, A. Adzhubel, L. Spitz, P. Lewis, D. Goldfarb, M. Emerman, and M. Stevenson.** 1993. A nuclear localization signal within HIV-1 matrix protein that governs infection of non-dividing cells. *Nature* **365:**666–669.
35. **Bukrinsky, M. I., N. Sharova, M. P. Dempsey, T. L. Stanwick, A. G. Bukrinskaya, S. Haggerty, and M. Stevenson.** 1992. Active nuclear import of human immunodeficiency virus type 1 preintegration complexes. *Proc. Natl. Acad. Sci. USA* **89:**6580–6584.
36. **Bukrinsky, M. I., N. Sharova, T. L. McDonald, T. Pushkarskaya, W. G. Tarpley, and M. Stevenson.** 1993. Association of integrase, matrix, and reverse transcriptase antigens of human immunodeficiency virus type 1 with viral nucleic acids following acute infection. *Proc. Natl. Acad. Sci. USA* **90:**6125–6129.
37. **Bukrinsky, M. I., T. L. Stanwick, M. P. Dempsey, and M. Stevenson.** 1991. Quiescent T lymphocytes as an inducible virus reservoir in HIV-1 infection. *Science* **254:** 423–427.
38. **Burke, D. S., J. F. Brundage, R. R. Redfield, J. J. Damato, C. A. Schable, P. Putman, R. Visintine, and H. I. Kim.** 1988. Measurement of the false positive rate in a screening program for human immunodeficiency virus infections. *N. Engl. J. Med.* **319:**961–964.
39. **Burton, D. R.** 1997. A vaccine for HIV type 1: the antibody perspective. *Proc. Natl. Acad. Sci. USA* **94:**10018–10023.
40. **Busch, M. P., L. L. Lee, G. A. Satten, D. R. Henrard, H. Farzadegan, K. E. Nelson, S. Read, R. Y. Dodd, and L. R. Petersen.** 1995. Time course of detection of viral and serologic markers preceding human immunodeficiency virus type 1 seroconversion: implications for screening of blood and tissue donors. *Transfusion* (Paris) **35:**91–97.
41. **Bushman, F. D., T. Fujiwara, and R. Craigie.** 1990. Retroviral DNA integration directed by HIV integration protein in vitro. *Science* **249:**1555–1558.
42. **Calarese, D. A., H. K. Lee, C. Y. Huang, M. D. Best, R. D. Astronomo, R. L. Stanfield, H. Katinger, D. R. Burton, C. H. Wong, and I. A. Wilson.** 2005. Dissection of the carbohydrate specificity of the broadly neutralizing anti-HIV-1 antibody 2G12. *Proc. Natl. Acad. Sci. USA* **102:**13372–13377.
43. **Cameron, P. U., P. S. Freudenthal, J. M. Barker, S. Gezelter, K. Inaba, and R. M. Steinman.** 1992. Dendritic cells exposed to human immunodeficiency virus type-1 transmit a vigorous cytopathic infection to $CD4^+$ T cells. *Science* **257:**383–387.
44. **Cao, J., I. W. Park, A. Cooper, and J. Sodroski.** 1996. Molecular determinants of acute single-cell lysis by human immunodeficiency virus type 1. *J. Virol.* **70:**1340–1354.
45. **Cao, Y., L. Qin, L. Zhang, J. Safrit, and D. D. Ho.** 1995. Virologic and immunologic characterization of long-term survivors of human immunodeficiency virus type 1 infection. *N. Engl. J. Med.* **332:**201–208.
46. **Carrington, M., G. W. Nelson, M. P. Martin, T. Kissner, D. Vlahov, J. J. Goedert, R. Kaslow, S. Buchbinder, K. Hoots, and S. J. O'Brien.** 1999. HLA and HIV-1: heterozygote advantage and B*35-Cw*04 disadvantage. *Science* **283:**1748–1752.
47. **Centers for Disease Control and Prevention.** 1988. Update: serologic testing for antibody to human immunodeficiency virus. *Morb. Mortal. Wkly. Rep.* **36:**833–845.
48. **Centers for Disease Control and Prevention.** 1989. Interpretation and use of the Western blot assay for serodiagnosis of human immunodeficiency virus type 1 infections. *Morb. Mortal. Wkly. Rep.* **38:**1–7.
49. **Centers for Disease Control and Prevention.** 1992. 1993 revised classification system for HIV infection and expanded surveillance case definition for AIDS among adolescents and adults. *Morb. Mortal. Wkly. Rep.* **41:**1–19.
50. **Centers for Disease Control and Prevention.** 2001. Updated U.S. Public Health Service guidelines for the management of occupational exposures to HBV, HCV, and HIV and recommendations for postexposure prophylaxis. *Morb. Mortal. Wkly. Rep.* **50:**1–52.
51. **Chan, D. C., D. Fass, J. M. Berger, and P. S. Kim.** 1997. Core structure of gp41 from the HIV envelope glycoprotein. *Cell* **89:**263–273.
52. **Chang, Y., E. Cesarman, M. S. Pessin, F. Lee, J. Culpepper, D. M. Knowles, and P. S. Moore.** 1994. Identification of herpesvirus-like DNA sequences in AIDS-associated Kaposi's sarcoma. *Science* **266:**1865–1869.
53. **Charneau, P., M. Alizon, and F. Clavel.** 1992. A second origin of DNA plus-strand synthesis is required for optimal human immunodeficiency virus replication. *J. Virol.* **66:**2814–2820.
54. **Chertova, E., J. J. Bess, Jr., B. J. Crise, R. C. Sowder II, T. M. Schaden, J. M. Hilburn, J. A. Hoxie, R. E. Benveniste, J. D. Lifson, L. E. Henderson, and L. O. Arthur.** 2002. Envelope glycoprotein incorporation, not shedding of surface envelope glycoprotein (gp120/SU), is the primary determinant of SU content of purified human immunodeficiency virus type 1 and simian immunodeficiency virus. *J. Virol.* **76:**5315–5325.
55. **Chertova, E., O. Chertov, L. V. Coren, J. D. Roser, C. M. Trubey, J. W. Bess, Jr., R. C. Sowder II, E. Barsov, B. L. Hood, R. J. Fisher, K. Nagashima, T. P. Conrads, T. D. Veenstra, J. D. Lifson, and D. E. Ott.** 2006. Proteomic and biochemical analysis of purified human immunodeficiency virus type 1 produced from infected monocyte-derived macrophages. *J. Virol.* **80:**9039–9052.
56. **Chesebro, B., K. Wehrly, J. Nishio, and S. Perryman.** 1992. Macrophage-tropic human immunodeficiency virus isolates from different patients exhibit unusual V3 envelope sequence homogeneity in comparison with T-cell-tropic isolates: definition of critical amino acids involved in cell tropism. *J. Virol.* **66:**6547–6554.
57. **Chiu, Y. L., V. B. Soros, J. F. Kreisberg, K. Stopak, W. Yonemoto, and W. C. Greene.** 2005. Cellular APOBEC3G restricts HIV-1 infection in resting $CD4^+$ T cells. *Nature* **435:**108–114.
58. **Choe, H., M. Farzan, Y. Sun, N. Sullivan, B. Rollins, P. D. Ponath, L. Wu, C. R. Mackay, G. LaRosa, W. Newman, N. Gerard, C. Gerard, and J. Sodroski.** 1996. The beta-chemokine receptors CCR3 and CCR5 facili-

tate infection by primary HIV-1 isolates. *Cell* **85:**1135–1148.

59. **Chun, T. W., L. Carruth, D. Finzi, X. Shen, J. A. DiGiuseppe, H. Taylor, M. Hermankova, K. Chadwick, J. Margolick, T. C. Quinn, Y. H. Kuo, R. Brookmeyer, M. A. Zeiger, P. Barditch-Crovo, and R. F. Siliciano.** 1997. Quantification of latent tissue reservoirs and total body viral load in HIV-1 infection. *Nature* **387:**183–188.
60. **Chun, T. W., D. Engel, M. M. Berrey, T. Shea, L. Corey, and A. S. Fauci.** 1998. Early establishment of a pool of latently infected, resting $CD4^+$ T cells during primary HIV-1 infection. *Proc. Natl. Acad. Sci. USA* **95:**8869–8873.
61. **Chun, T. W., D. Finzi, J. Margolick, K. Chadwick, D. Schwartz, and R. F. Siliciano.** 1995. In vivo fate of HIV-1-infected T cells: quantitative analysis of the transition to stable latency. *Nat. Med.* **1:**1284–1290.
62. **Chun, T. W., L. Stuyver, S. B. Mizell, L. A. Ehler, J. A. Mican, M. Baseler, A. L. Lloyd, M. A. Nowak, and A. S. Fauci.** 1997. Presence of an inducible HIV-1 latent reservoir during highly active antiretroviral therapy. *Proc. Natl. Acad. Sci. USA* **94:**13193–13197.
63. **Ciesielski, C. A., D. W. Marianos, G. Schochetman, J. J. Witte, and H. W. Jaffe.** 1994. The 1990 Florida dental investigation. The press and the science. *Ann. Intern. Med.* **121:**886–888.
64. **Cocchi, F., A. L. DeVico, A. Garzino-Demo, S. K. Arya, R. C. Gallo, and P. Lusso.** 1995. Identification of RANTES, MIP-1α, and MIP-1β as the major HIV-suppressive factors produced by $CD8^+$ T cells. *Science* **270:**1811–1815.
65. **Collins, K. L., B. K. Chen, S. A. Kalams, B. D. Walker, and D. Baltimore.** 1998. HIV-1 Nef protein protects infected primary cells against killing by cytotoxic T lymphocytes. *Nature* **391:**397–401.
66. **Connor, E. M., R. S. Sperling, R. Gelber, P. Kiselev, G. Scott, M. J. O'Sullivan, R. VanDyke, M. Bey, W. Shearer, and R. L. Jacobson for the Pediatric AIDS Clinical Trials Group Protocol 076 Study Group.** 1994. Reduction of maternal-infant transmission of human immunodeficiency virus type 1 with zidovudine treatment. *N. Engl. J. Med.* **331:**1173–1180.
67. **Connor, R. I., H. Mohri, Y. Cao, and D. D. Ho.** 1993. Increased viral burden and cytopathicity correlate temporally with $CD4^+$ T-lymphocyte decline and clinical progression in human immunodeficiency virus type 1-infected individuals. *J. Virol.* **67:**1772–1777.
68. **Coombs, R. W., S. L. Welles, C. Hooper, P. S. Reichelderfer, R. T. D'Aquila, A. J. Japour, V. A. Johnson, D. R. Kuritzkes, D. D. Richman, S. Kwok, J. Todd, J. B. Jackson, V. DeGruttola, C. S. Crumpacker, and J. Kahn for the AIDS Clinical Trials Group (ACTG) 116B/117 Study Team and the ACTG Virology Committee Resistance and HIV-1 RNA Working Groups.** 1996. Association of plasma human immunodeficiency virus type 1 RNA level with risk of clinical progression in patients with advanced infection. *J. Infect. Dis.* **174:**704–712.
69. **Coopman, S. A., R. A. Johnson, R. Platt, and R. S. Stern.** 1993. Cutaneous disease and drug reactions in HIV infection. *N. Engl. J. Med.* **328:**1670–1674.
70. **Coovadia, H. M., N. C. Rollins, R. M. Bland, K. Little, A. Coutsoudis, M. L. Bennish, and M. L. Newell.** 2007. Mother-to-child transmission of HIV-1 infection during exclusive breastfeeding in the first 6 months of life: an intervention cohort study. *Lancet* **369:**1107–1116.
71. **Corbett, E. L., B. Marston, G. J. Churchyard, and K. M. De Cock.** 2006. Tuberculosis in sub-Saharan Africa: opportunities, challenges, and change in the era of antiretroviral treatment. *Lancet* **367:**926–937.
72. **Cozzi Lepri A., T. L. Katzenstein, H. Ullum, A. N. Phillips, P. Skinhoj, J. Gerstoft, and B. K. Pedersen.** 1998. The relative prognostic value of plasma HIV RNA levels and CD4 lymphocyte counts in advanced HIV infection. *AIDS* **12:**1639–1643.
73. **Craig, H. M., M. W. Pandori, and J. C. Guatelli.** 1998. Interaction of HIV-1 Nef with the cellular dileucine-based sorting pathway is required for CD4 down-regulation and optimal viral infectivity. *Proc. Natl. Acad. Sci. USA* **95:**11229–11234.
74. **Daar, E. S., S. Little, J. Pitt, J. Santangelo, P. Ho, N. Harawa, P. Kerndt, J. V. Glorgi, J. Bai, P. Gaut, D. D. Richman, S. Mandel, and S. Nichols for the Los Angeles County Primary HIV Infection Recruitment Network.** 2001. Diagnosis of primary HIV-1 infection. *Ann. Intern. Med.* **134:**25–29.
75. **Dalgleish, A. G., P. C. Beverley, P. R. Clapham, D. H. Crawford, M. F. Greaves, and R. A. Weiss.** 1984. The CD4 (T4) antigen is an essential component of the receptor for the AIDS retrovirus. *Nature* **312:**763–767.
76. **Davies, J. F., Z. Hostomska, Z. Hostomsky, S. R. Jordan, and D. A. Matthews.** 1991. Crystal structure of the ribonuclease H domain of HIV-1 reverse transcriptase. *Science* **252:**88–95.
77. **Day, C. L., D. E. Kaufmann, P. Kiepiela, J. A. Brown, E. S. Moodley, S. Reddy, E. W. Mackey, J. D. Miller, A. J. Leslie, C. DePierres, Z. Mncube, J. Duraiswamy, B. Zhu, Q. Eichbaum, M. Altfeld, E. J. Wherry, H. M. Coovadia, P. J. Goulder, P. Klenerman, R. Ahmed, G. J. Freeman, and B. D. Walker.** 2006. PD-1 expression on HIV-specific T cells is associated with T-cell exhaustion and disease progression. *Nature* **443:**350–354.
78. **Deacon, N. J., A. Tsykin, A. Solomon, K. Smith, M. Ludford-Menting, D. J. Hooker, D. A. McPhee, A. L. Greenway, A. Ellett, C. Chatfield, V. A. Lawson, S. Crowe, A. Maerz, S. Sonza, J. Learmont, J. S. Sullivan, A. Cunningham, D. Dwyer, D. Dowton, and J. Mills.** 1995. Genomic structure of an attenuated quasi species of HIV-1 from a blood transfusion donor and recipients. *Science* **270:**988–991.
79. **De Cock, K. M., and H. A. Weiss.** 2000. The global epidemiology of AIDS. *Trop. Med. Int. Health* **5:**A3–A9.
80. **De Gruttola, V., L. Dix, R. D'Aquila, D. Holder, A. Phillips, M. Ait-Khaled, J. Baxter, P. Clevenbergh, S. Hammer, R. Harrigan, D. Katzenstein, R. Lanier, M. Miller, M. Para, S. Yerly, A. Zolopa, J. Murray, A. Patick, V. Miller, S. Castillo, L. Pedneault, and J. Mellors.** 2000. The relation between baseline HIV drug resistance and response to antiretroviral therapy: re-analysis of retrospective and prospective studies using a standardized data analysis plan. *Antiviral Ther.* **5:**41–48.
81. **DeHart, J. L., E. S. Zimmerman, O. Ardon, C. M. Monteiro-Filho, E. R. Arganaraz, and V. Planelles.** 2007. HIV-1 Vpr activates the G2 checkpoint through manipulation of the ubiquitin proteasome system. *Virol. J.* **4:**57.
82. **Delaney, K. P., B. M. Branson, A. Uniyal, P. R. Kerndt, P. A. Keenan, K. Jafa, A. D. Gardner, D. J. Jamieson, and M. Bulterys.** 2006. Performance of an oral fluid rapid HIV-1/2 test: experience from four CDC studies. *AIDS* **20:**1655–1660.
83. **Deschambeault, J., J. P. Lalonde, G. Cervantes-Acosta, R. Lodge, E. A. Cohen, and G. Lemay.** 1999. Polarized human immunodeficiency virus budding in lymphocytes involves a tyrosine-based signal and favors cell-to-cell viral transmission. *J. Virol.* **73:**5010–5017.
84. **Desrosiers, R. C., J. D. Lifson, J. S. Gibbs, S. C. Czajak, A. Y. Howe, L. O. Arthur, and R. P. Johnson.** 1998.

Identification of highly attenuated mutants of simian immunodeficiency virus. *J. Virol.* **72:**1431–1437.

85. **Dion, M. L., J. F. Poulin, R. Bordi, M. Sylvestre, R. Corsini, N. Kettaf, A. Dalloul, M. R. Boulassel, P. Debre, J. P. Routy, Z. Grossman, R. P. Sekaly, and R. Cheynier.** 2004. HIV infection rapidly induces and maintains a substantial suppression of thymocyte proliferation. *Immunity* **21:**757–768.
86. **Dittmer, U., D. M. Brooks, and K. J. Hasenkrug.** 1999. Requirement for multiple lymphocyte subsets in protection by a live attenuated vaccine against retroviral infection. *Nat. Med.* **5:**189–193.
87. **Dorenbaum, A.** 2001. *Abstr. 8th Conf. Retroviruses Oppor. Infect.*, abstr. LB7.
88. **Dorfman, T., F. Mammano, W. A. Haseltine, and H. G. Gottlinger.** 1994. Role of the matrix protein in the virion association of the human immunodeficiency virus type 1 envelope glycoprotein. *J. Virol.* **68:**1689–1696.
89. **Dormant, D., J. Livartowski, S. Chararet, D. Guetard, D. Henin, R. Levagueresse, P. F. van de Moortelle, B. Larke, P. Gourmelon, R. Vazeaux, H. Metivier, J. Flageat, L. Court, J. J. Hauw, and L. Montagnier.** 1989. HIV-2 in rhesus monkeys: serological, virological, and clinical results. *Intervirology* **30:**59–65.
90. **Dornadula, G., H. Zhang, B. VanUitert, J. Stern, L. Livornese, Jr., M. J. Ingerman, J. Witek, R. J. Kedanis, J. Natkin, J. DeSimone, and R. J. Pomerantz.** 1999. Residual HIV-1 RNA in blood plasma of patients taking suppressive highly active antiretroviral therapy. *JAMA* **282:**1627–1632.
91. **Douek, D. C., R. D. McFarland, P. H. Keiser, E. A. Gage, J. M. Massey, B. F. Haynes, M. A. Polis, A. T. Haase, M. B. Feinberg, J. L. Sullivan, B. D. Jamieson, J. A. Zack, L. J. Picker, and R. A. Koup.** 1998. Changes in thymic function with age and during the treatment of HIV infection. *Nature* **396:**690–695.
92. **Druce, J. D., D. Jardine, S. A. Locarnini, and C. J. Birch.** 1995. Susceptibility of HIV to inactivation by disinfectants and ultraviolet light. *J. Hosp. Infect.* **30:**167–180.
93. **Dunn, D. T., C. D. Brandt, A. Krivine, S. A. Cassol, P. Roques, W. Borkowsky, A. De Rossi, E. Denamur, A. Ehrnst, and C. Loveday.** 1995. The sensitivity of HIV-1 DNA polymerase chain reaction in the neonatal period and the relative contributions of intra-uterine and intra-partum transmission. *AIDS* **9:**F7–F11.
94. **Durant, J., P. Clevenbergh, P. Halfon, P. Delgiudice, S. Porsin, P. Simonet, N. Montagne, C. A. Boucher, J. M. Schapiro, and P. Dellamonica.** 1999. Drug-resistance genotyping in HIV-1 therapy: the VIRADAPT randomised controlled trial. *Lancet* **353:**2195–2199.
95. **Edinger, A. L., J. L. Mankowski, B. J. Doranz, B. J. Margulies, B. Lee, J. Rucker, M. Sharron, T. L. Hoffman, J. F. Berson, M. C. Zink, V. M. Hirsch, J. E. Clements, and R. W. Doms.** 1997. CD4-independent, CCR5-dependent infection of brain capillary endothelial cells by a neurovirulent simian immunodeficiency virus strain. *Proc. Natl. Acad. Sci. USA* **94:**14742–14747.
96. **Elias, C. J., and L. L. Heise.** 1994. Challenges for the development of female-controlled vaginal microbicides. *AIDS* **8:**1–9.
97. **Emerman, M., and M. H. Malim.** 1998. HIV-1 regulatory/accessory genes: keys to unraveling viral and host cell biology. *Science* **280:**1880–1884.
98. **Epstein, L. G., C. Kuiken, B. M. Blumberg, S. Hartman, L. R. Sharer, M. Clement, and J. Goudsmit.** 1991. HIV-1 V3 domain variation in brain and spleen of children with AIDS: tissue-specific evolution within host-determined quasispecies. *Virology* **180:**583–590.
99. **Esnault, C., O. Heidmann, F. Delebecque, M. Dewannieux, D. Ribet, A. J. Hance, T. Heidmann, and O. Schwartz.** 2005. APOBEC3G cytidine deaminase inhibits retrotransposition of endogenous retroviruses. *Nature* **433:**430–433.
100. **European Collaborative Study.** 1991. Children born to women with HIV-1 infection: natural history and risk of transmission. *Lancet* **337:**253–260.
101. **European Collaborative Study.** 1994. Natural history of vertically acquired human immunodeficiency virus-1 infection. *Pediatrics* **94:**815–819.
102. **Ewart, G. D., T. Sutherland, P. W. Gage, and G. B. Cox.** 1996. The Vpu protein of human immunodeficiency virus type 1 forms cation-selective ion channels. *J. Virol.* **70:**7108–7115.
103. **Fahey, J. L., J. M. Taylor, R. Detels, B. Hofmann, R. Melmed, P. Nishanian, and J. V. Giorgi.** 1990. The prognostic value of cellular and serologic markers in infection with human immunodeficiency virus type 1. *N. Engl. J. Med.* **322:**166–172.
104. **Fahrbach, K. M., S. M. Barry, S. Ayehunie, S. Lamore, M. Klausner, and T. J. Hope.** 2007. Activated CD34-derived Langerhans cells mediate transinfection with human immunodeficiency virus. *J. Virol.* **81:**6858–6868.
105. **Farnet, C. M., and F. D. Bushman.** 1997. HIV-1 cDNA integration: requirement of HMG I(Y) protein for function of preintegration complexes in vitro. *Cell* **88:**483–492.
106. **Farnet, C. M., and F. D. Bushman.** 1996. HIV cDNA integration: molecular biology and inhibitor development. *AIDS* **10**(Suppl. A)**:**S3–S11.
107. **Farnet, C. M., and W. A. Haseltine.** 1991. Determination of viral proteins present in the human immunodeficiency virus type 1 preintegration complex. *J. Virol.* **65:**1910–1915.
108. **Feng, Y., C. C. Broder, P. E. Kennedy, and E. A. Berger.** 1996. HIV-1 entry cofactor: functional cDNA cloning of a seven-transmembrane, G protein-coupled receptor. *Science* **272:**872–877.
109. **Fiala, M., D. J. Looney, M. Stins, D. D. Way, L. Zhang, X. Gan, F. Chiappelli, E. S. Schweitzer, P. Shapshak, M. Weinand, M. C. Graves, M. Witte, and K. S. Kim.** 1997. TNF-α opens a paracellular route for HIV-1 invasion across the blood-brain barrier. *Mol. Med.* **3:**553–564.
110. **Filippi, C. G., G. Sze, S. J. Farber, M. Shahmanesh, and P. A. Selwyn.** 1998. Regression of HIV encephalopathy and basal ganglia signal intensity abnormality at MR imaging in patients with AIDS after the initiation of protease inhibitor therapy. *Radiology* **206:**491–498.
111. **Finkel, T. H., G. Tudor-Williams, N. K. Banda, M. F. Cotton, T. Curiel, C. Monks, T. W. Baba, R. M. Ruprecht, and A. Kupfer.** 1995. Apoptosis occurs predominantly in bystander cells and not in productively infected cells of HIV- and SIV-infected lymph nodes. *Nat. Med.* **1:**129–134.
112. **Finzi, D., J. Blankson, J. D. Siliciano, J. B. Margolick, K. Chadwick, T. Pierson, K. Smith, J. Lisziewicz, F. Lori, C. Flexner, T. C. Quinn, R. E. Chaisson, E. Rosenberg, B. Walker, S. Gange, J. Gallant, and R. F. Siliciano.** 1999. Latent infection of $CD4^+$ T cells provides a mechanism for lifelong persistence of HIV-1, even in patients on effective combination therapy. *Nat. Med.* **5:**512–517.
113. **Finzi, D., M. Hermankova, T. Pierson, L. M. Carruth, C. Buck, R. E. Chaisson, T. C. Quinn, K. Chadwick, J. Margolick, R. Brookmeyer, J. Gallant, M. Markowitz, D. D. Ho, D. D. Richman, and R. F. Siliciano.** 1997. Identification of a reservoir for HIV-1 in patients

on highly active antiretroviral therapy. *Science* **278:** 1295–1300.

114. **Finzi, D., and R. F. Siliciano.** 1998. Viral dynamics in HIV-1 infection. *Cell* **93:**665–671.

115. **Fletcher, T. M., III, B. Brichacek, N. Sharova, M. A. Newman, G. Stivahtis, P. M. Sharp, M. Emerman, B. H. Hahn, and M. Stevenson.** 1996. Nuclear import and cell cycle arrest functions of the HIV-1 Vpr protein are encoded by two separate genes in HIV-2/SIV(SM). *EMBO J.* **15:**6155–6165.

116. **Fornerod, M., M. Ohno, M. Yoshida, and I. W. Mattaj.** 1997. CRM1 is an export receptor for leucine-rich nuclear export signals. *Cell* **90:**1051–1060.

117. **Fortin, J. F., R. Cantin, G. Lamontagne, and M. Tremblay.** 1997. Host-derived ICAM-1 glycoproteins incorporated on human immunodeficiency virus type 1 are biologically active and enhance viral infectivity. *J. Virol.* **71:**3588–3596.

118. **French, M. A., P. Price, and S. F. Stone.** 2004. Immune restoration disease after antiretroviral therapy. *AIDS* **18:** 1615–1627.

119. **Frost, S. D., T. Wrin, D. M. Smith, S. L. Kosakovsky Pond, Y. Liu, E. Paxinos, C. Chappey, J. Galovich, J. Beauchaine, C. J. Petropoulos, S. J. Little, and D. D. Richman.** 2005. Neutralizing antibody responses drive the evolution of human immunodeficiency virus type 1 envelope during recent HIV infection. *Proc. Natl. Acad. Sci. USA* **102:**18514–18519.

120. **Fujikawa, L. S., S. Z. Salahuddin, A. G. Palestine, H. Masur, R. B. Nussenblatt, and R. C. Gallo.** 1985. Isolation of human T-lymphotropic virus type III from the tears of a patient with the acquired immunodeficiency syndrome. *Lancet* **ii:**529–530.

121. **Fultz, P. N., H. M. McClure, R. B. Swenson, C. R. McGrath, A. Brodie, J. P. Getchell, F. C. Jensen, D. C. Anderson, J. R. Broderson, and D. P. Francis.** 1986. Persistent infection of chimpanzees with human T-lymphotropic virus type III/lymphadenopathy-associated virus: a potential model for acquired immunodeficiency syndrome. *J. Virol.* **58:**116–124.

122. **Furtado, M. R., D. S. Callaway, J. P. Phair, K. J. Kunstman, J. L. Stanton, C. A. Macken, A. S. Perelson, and S. M. Wolinsky.** 1999. Persistence of HIV-1 transcription in peripheral-blood mononuclear cells in patients receiving potent antiretroviral therapy. *N. Engl. J. Med.* **340:**1614–1622.

123. **Gabuzda, D. H., K. Lawrence, E. Langhoff, E. Terwilliger, T. Dorfman, W. A. Haseltine, and J. Sodroski.** 1992. Role of vif in replication of human immunodeficiency virus type 1 in $CD4^+$ T lymphocytes. *J. Virol.* **66:** 6489–6495.

124. **Gaines, H., M. von Sydow, A. Sonnerborg, J. Albert, J. Czajkowski, P. O. Pehrson, F. Chiodi, L. Moberg, E. M. Fenyo, and B. Asjo.** 1987. Antibody response in primary human immunodeficiency virus infection. *Lancet* **i:**1249–1253.

125. **Galli, L., M. de Martino, P. A. Tovo, C. Gabiano, M. Zappa, C. Giaquinto, S. Tulisso, A. Vierucci, M. Guerra, and P. Marchisio for the Italian Register for HIV Infection in Children.** 1995. Onset of clinical signs in children with HIV-1 perinatal infection. *AIDS* **9:**455–461.

126. **Gao, F., E. Bailes, D. L. Robertson, Y. Chen, C. M. Rodenburg, S. F. Michael, L. B. Cummins, L. O. Arthur, M. Peeters, G. M. Shaw, P. M. Sharp, and B. H. Hahn.** 1999. Origin of HIV-1 in the chimpanzee *Pan troglodytes troglodytes*. *Nature* **397:**436–441.

127. **Garcia, J. V., and A. D. Miller.** 1991. Serine phosphorylation-independent downregulation of cell-surface CD4 by nef. *Nature* **350:**508–511.

128. **Gartner, S., P. Markovits, D. M. Markovitz, M. H. Kaplan, R. C. Gallo, and M. Popovic.** 1986. The role of mononuclear phagocytes in HTLV-III/LAV infection. *Science* **233:**215–219.

129. **Gayle, H.** 2000. An overview of the global HIV/AIDS epidemic, with a focus on the United States. *AIDS* **14**(Suppl. 2):S8–S17.

130. **Gaynor, R.** 1992. Cellular transcription factors involved in the regulation of HIV-1 gene expression. *AIDS* **6:** 347–363.

131. **Geijtenbeek, T. B., D. S. Kwon, R. Torensma, S. J. van Vliet, G. C. van Duijnhoven, J. Middel, I. L. Cornelissen, H. S. Nottet, V. N. KewalRamani, D. R. Littman, C. G. Figdor, and Y. van Kooyk.** 2000. DC-SIGN, a dendritic cell-specific HIV-1-binding protein that enhances trans-infection of T cells. *Cell* **100:**587–597.

132. **Gerberding, J. L., C. E. Bryant-LeBlanc, K. Nelson, A. R. Moss, D. Osmond, H. F. Chambers, J. R. Carlson, W. L. Drew, J. A. Levy, and M. A. Sande.** 1987. Risk of transmitting the human immunodeficiency virus, cytomegalovirus, and hepatitis B virus to health care workers exposed to patients with AIDS and AIDS-related conditions. *J. Infect. Dis.* **156:**1–8.

133. **Gilbert, M. T., A. Rambaut, G. Wlasiuk, T. J. Spira, A. E. Pitchenik, and M. Worobey.** 2007. The emergence of HIV/AIDS in the Americas and beyond. *Proc. Natl. Acad. Sci. USA* **104:**18566–18570.

134. **Gorelick, R. J., S. M. Nigida, Jr., J. W. Bess, Jr., L. O. Arthur, L. E. Henderson, and A. Rein.** 1990. Noninfectious human immunodeficiency virus type 1 mutants deficient in genomic RNA. *J. Virol.* **64:**3207–3211.

135. **Gotch, F. M., D. F. Nixon, N. Alp, A. J. McMichael, and L. K. Borysiewicz.** 1990. High frequency of memory and effector gag specific cytotoxic T lymphocytes in HIV seropositive individuals. *Int. Immunol.* **2:**707–712.

136. **Gottlieb, M. S., R. Schroff, H. M. Schanker, J. D. Weisman, P. T. Fan, R. A. Wolf, and A. Saxon.** 1981. *Pneumocystis carinii* pneumonia and mucosal candidiasis in previously healthy homosexual men: evidence of a new acquired cellular immunodeficiency. *N. Engl. J. Med.* **305:**1425–1431.

137. **Goulder, P. J., C. Brander, Y. Tang, C. Tremblay, R. A. Colbert, M. M. Addo, E. S. Rosenberg, T. Nguyen, R. Allen, A. Trocha, M. Altfeld, S. He, M. Bunce, R. Funkhouser, S. I. Pelton, S. K. Burchett, K. McIntosh, B. T. Korber, and B. D. Walker.** 2001. Evolution and transmission of stable CTL escape mutations in HIV infection. *Nature* **412:**334–338.

138. **Grabar, S., M. Le, V. C. Goujard, C. Leport, M. D. Kazatchkine, D. Costagliola, and L. Weiss.** 2000. Clinical outcome of patients with HIV-1 infection according to immunologic and virologic response after 6 months of highly active antiretroviral therapy. *Ann. Intern. Med.* **133:**401–410.

139. **Gray, R. H., G. Kigozi, D. Serwadda, F. Makumbi, S. Watya, F. Nalugoda, N. Kiwanuka, L. H. Moulton, M. A. Chaudhary, M. Z. Chen, N. K. Sewankambo, F. Wabwire-Mangen, M. C. Bacon, C. F. Williams, P. Opendi, S. J. Reynolds, O. Laeyendecker, T. C. Quinn, and M. J. Wawer.** 2007. Male circumcision for HIV prevention in men in Rakai, Uganda: a randomised trial. *Lancet* **369:**657–666.

140. **Greenblatt, R. M., S. A. Lukehart, F. A. Plummer, T. C. Quinn, C. W. Critchlow, R. L. Ashley, L. J. D'Costa, J. O. Ndinya-Achola, L. Corey, and A. R. Ronald.** 1988. Genital ulceration as a risk factor for human immunodeficiency virus infection. *AIDS* **2:**47–50.

141. **Groopman, J. E., S. Z. Salahuddin, M. G. Sarngadharan, P. D. Markham, M. Gonda, A. Sliski, and R. C.**

Gallo. 1984. HTLV-III in saliva of people with AIDS-related complex and healthy homosexual men at risk for AIDS. *Science* **226:**447–449.

142. **Grulich, A. E., M. T. van Leeuwen, M. O. Falster, and C. M. Vajdic.** 2007. Incidence of cancers in people with HIV/AIDS compared with immunosuppressed transplant recipients: a meta-analysis. *Lancet* **370:**59–67.
143. **Grunfeld, C., and D. P. Kotler.** 1992. Wasting in the acquired immunodeficiency syndrome. *Semin. Liver Dis.* **12:**175–187.
144. **Gulick, R. M., J. W. Mellors, D. Havlir, J. J. Eron, C. Gonzalez, D. McMahon, D. D. Richman, F. T. Valentine, L. Jonas, A. Meibohm, E. A. Emini, and J. A. Chodakewitz.** 1997. Treatment with indinavir, zidovudine, and lamivudine in adults with human immunodeficiency virus infection and prior antiretroviral therapy. *N. Engl. J. Med.* **337:**734–739.
145. Reference deleted.
146. **Guy, B., M. P. Kieny, Y. Riviere, P. C. Le, K. Dott, M. Girard, L. Montagnier, and J. P. Lecocq.** 1987. HIV F/3′ orf encodes a phosphorylated GTP-binding protein resembling an oncogene product. *Nature* **330:**266–269.
147. **Haase, A. T.** 1986. Pathogenesis of lentivirus infections. *Nature* **322:**130–136.
148. **Haase, A. T.** 1999. Population biology of HIV-1 infection: viral and $CD4^+$ T cell demographics and dynamics in lymphatic tissues. *Annu. Rev. Immunol.* **17:**625–656.
149. **Haase, A. T., K. Henry, M. Zupancic, G. Sedgewick, R. A. Faust, H. Melroe, W. Cavert, K. Gebhard, K. Staskus, Z. Q. Zhang, P. J. Dailey, H. H. Balfour, Jr., A. Erice, and A. S. Perelson.** 1996. Quantitative image analysis of HIV-1 infection in lymphoid tissue. *Science* **274:**985–989.
150. **Hahn, B. H., G. M. Shaw, K. M. De Cock, and P. M. Sharp.** 2000. AIDS as a zoonosis: scientific and public health implications. *Science* **287:**607–614.
151. **Hammer, S. M., M. S. Saag, M. Schechter, J. S. Montaner, R. T. Schooley, D. M. Jacobsen, M. A. Thompson, C. C. Carpenter, M. A. Fischl, B. G. Gazzard, J. M. Gatell, M. S. Hirsch, D. A. Katzenstein, D. D. Richman, S. Vella, P. G. Yeni, and P. A. Volberding.** 2006. Treatment for adult HIV infection: 2006 recommendations of the International AIDS Society—USA panel. *JAMA* **296:**827–843.
152. **Harrer, T., E. Harrer, S. A. Kalams, T. Elbeik, S. I. Staprans, M. B. Feinberg, Y. Cao, D. D. Ho, T. Yilma, A. M. Caliendo, R. P. Johnson, S. P. Buchbinder, and B. D. Walker.** 1996. Strong cytotoxic T cell and weak neutralizing antibody responses in a subset of persons with stable nonprogressing HIV type 1 infection. *AIDS Res. Hum. Retroviruses* **12:**585–592.
153. **Harris, R. S., K. N. Bishop, A. M. Sheehy, H. M. Craig, S. K. Petersen-Mahrt, I. N. Watt, M. S. Neuberger, and M. H. Malim.** 2003. DNA deamination mediates innate immunity to retroviral infection. *Cell* **113:** 803–809.
154. **Heinzinger, N. K., M. I. Bukinsky, S. A. Haggerty, A. M. Ragland, V. Kewalramani, M. A. Lee, H. E. Gendelman, L. Ratner, M. Stevenson, and M. Emerman.** 1994. The Vpr protein of human immunodeficiency virus type 1 influences nuclear localization of viral nucleic acids in nondividing host cells. *Proc. Natl. Acad. Sci. USA* **91:**7311–7315.
155. **Hellerstein, M., M. B. Hanley, D. Cesar, S. Siler, C. Papageorgopoulos, E. Wieder, D. Schmidt, R. Hoh, R. Neese, D. Macallan, S. Deeks, and J. M. McCune.** 1999. Directly measured kinetics of circulating T lymphocytes in normal and HIV-1-infected humans. *Nat. Med.* **5:**83–89.
156. **Hendel, H., N. Henon, H. Lebuanec, A. Lachgar, H. Poncelet, S. Caillat-Zucman, C. A. Winkler, M. W. Smith, L. Kenefic, S. O'Brien, W. Lu, J. M. Andrieu, D. Zagury, F. Schachter, J. Rappaport, and J. F. Zagury.** 1998. Distinctive effects of CCR5, CCR2, and SDF1 genetic polymorphisms in AIDS progression. *J. Acquir. Immune. Defic. Syndr. Hum. Retrovirol.* **19:**381–386.
157. **Henderson, D. K., B. J. Fahey, M. Willy, J. M. Schmitt, K. Carey, D. E. Koziol, H. C. Lane, J. Fedio, and A. J. Saah.** 1990. Risk for occupational transmission of human immunodeficiency virus type 1 (HIV-1) associated with clinical exposures. A prospective evaluation. *Ann. Intern. Med.* **113:**740–746.
158. **Henderson, L. E., M. A. Bowers, R. C. Sowder, S. A. Serabyn, D. G. Johnson, J. W. Bess, Jr., L. O. Arthur, D. K. Bryant, and C. Fenselau.** 1992. Gag proteins of the highly replicative MN strain of human immunodeficiency virus type 1: posttranslational modifications, proteolytic processings, and complete amino acid sequences. *J. Virol.* **66:**1856–1865.
159. **Hirsch, M. S., F. Brun-Vezinet, B. Clotet, B. Conway, D. R. Kuritzkes, R. T. D'Aquila, L. M. Demeter, S. M. Hammer, V. A. Johnson, C. Loveday, J. W. Mellors, D. M. Jacobsen, and D. D. Richman.** 2003. Antiretroviral drug resistance testing in adults infected with human immunodeficiency virus type 1: 2003 recommendations of an International AIDS Society—USA Panel. *Clin. Infect. Dis.* **37:**113–128.
160. **Hirsch, M. S., F. Brun-Vezinet, R. T. D'Aquila, S. M. Hammer, V. A. Johnson, D. R. Kuritzkes, C. Loveday, J. W. Mellors, B. Clotet, B. Conway, L. M. Demeter, S. Vella, D. M. Jacobsen, and D. D. Richman.** 2000. Antiretroviral drug resistance testing in adult HIV-1 infection: recommendations of an International AIDS Society—USA Panel. *JAMA* **283:**2417–2426.
161. **Hirsch, M. S., B. Conway, R. T. D'Aquila, V. A. Johnson, F. Brun-Vezinet, B. Clotet, L. M. Demeter, S. M. Hammer, D. M. Jacobsen, D. R. Kuritzkes, C. Loveday, J. W. Mellors, S. Vella, and D. D. Richman for the International AIDS Society—USA Panel.** 1998. Antiretroviral drug resistance testing in adults with HIV infection: implications for clinical management. *JAMA* **279:**1984–1991.
162. **HIV Surrogate Marker Collaborative Group.** 2000. Human immunodeficiency virus type 1 RNA level and CD4 count as prognostic markers and surrogate end points: a meta-analysis. *AIDS Res. Hum. Retroviruses* **16:** 1123–1133.
163. **Ho, D. D., A. U. Neumann, A. S. Perelson, W. Chen, J. M. Leonard, and M. Markowitz.** 1995. Rapid turnover of plasma virions and CD4 lymphocytes in HIV-1 infection. *Nature* **373:**123–126.
164. **Ho, D. D., T. R. Rota, and M. S. Hirsch.** 1986. Infection of monocyte/macrophages by human T lymphotropic virus type III. *J. Clin. Investig.* **77:**1712–1715.
165. **Ho, D. D., M. G. Sarngadharan, L. Resnick, F. Dimarzoveronese, T. R. Rota, and M. S. Hirsch.** 1985. Primary human T-lymphotropic virus type III infection. *Ann. Intern. Med.* **103:**880–883.
166. **Ho, D. D., R. T. Schooley, T. R. Rota, J. C. Kaplan, T. Flynn, S. Z. Salahuddin, M. A. Gonda, and M. S. Hirsch.** 1984. HTLV-III in the semen and blood of a healthy homosexual man. *Science* **226:**451–453.
167. **Holland, J. J., J. C. De La Torre, and D. A. Steinhauer.** 1992. RNA virus populations as quasispecies. *Curr. Top. Microbiol. Immunol.* **176:**1–20.
168. **Hope, T., and R. J. Pomerantz.** 1995. The human immunodeficiency virus type 1 Rev protein: a pivotal pro-

tein in the viral life cycle. *Curr. Top. Microbiol. Immunol.* **193:**91–105.

169. **Hrimech, M., X. J. Yao, F. Bachand, N. Rougeau, and E. A. Cohen.** 1999. Human immunodeficiency virus type 1 (HIV-1) Vpr functions as an immediate-early protein during HIV-1 infection. *J. Virol.* **73:**4101–4109.
170. **Jacks, T., M. D. Power, F. R. Masiarz, P. A. Luciw, P. J. Barr, and H. E. Varmus.** 1988. Characterization of ribosomal frameshifting in HIV-1 gag-pol expression. *Nature* **331:**280–283.
171. **Jackson, J. B.** 1992. Human immunodeficiency virus (HIV)-indeterminate western blots and latent HIV infection. *Transfusion* (Paris) **32:**497–499.
172. **Jackson, J. B., P. Musoke, T. Fleming, L. A. Guay, D. Bagenda, M. Allen, C. Nakabiito, J. Sherman, P. Bakaki, M. Owor, C. Ducar, M. Deseyve, A. Mwatha, L. Emel, C. Duefield, M. Mirochnick, M. G. Fowler, L. Mofenson, P. Miotti, M. Gigliotti, D. Bray, and F. Mmiro.** 2003. Intrapartum and neonatal single-dose nevirapine compared with zidovudine for prevention of mother-to-child transmission of HIV-1 in Kampala, Uganda: 18-month follow-up of the HIVNET 012 randomised trial. *Lancet* **362:**859–868.
173. **Janssen, R. S., G. A. Satten, S. L. Stramer, B. D. Rawal, T. R. O'Brien, B. J. Weiblen, F. M. Hecht, N. Jack, F. R. Cleghorn, J. O. Kahn, M. A. Chesney, and M. P. Busch.** 1998. New testing strategy to detect early HIV-1 infection for use in incidence estimates and for clinical and prevention purposes. *JAMA* **280:**42–48.
174. **Jin, X., D. E. Bauer, S. E. Tuttleton, S. Lewin, A. Gettie, J. Blanchard, C. E. Irwin, J. T. Safrit, J. Mittler, L. Weinberger, L. G. Kostrikis, L. Zhang, A. S. Perelson, and D. D. Ho.** 1999. Dramatic rise in plasma viremia after $CD8^+$ T cell depletion in simian immunodeficiency virus-infected macaques. *J. Exp. Med.* **189:**991–998.
175. **Johnson, R. P., J. D. Lifson, S. C. Czajak, K. S. Cole, K. H. Manson, R. Glickman, J. Yang, D. C. Montefiori, R. Montelaro, M. S. Wyand, and R. C. Desrosiers.** 1999. Highly attenuated vaccine strains of simian immunodeficiency virus protect against vaginal challenge: inverse relationship of degree of protection with level of attenuation. *J. Virol.* **73:**4952–4961.
176. **Jolly, C. and Q. J. Sattentau.** 2007. Human immunodeficiency virus type 1 assembly, budding, and cell-cell spread in T cells take place in tetraspanin-enriched plasma membrane domains. *J. Virol.* **81:**7873–7884.
177. **Kaplan, A. H., M. Manchester, and R. Swanstrom.** 1994. The activity of the protease of human immunodeficiency virus type 1 is initiated at the membrane of infected cells before the release of viral proteins and is required for release to occur with maximum efficiency. *J. Virol.* **68:**6782–6786.
178. **Kaplan, E. H.** 1995. Economic analysis of needle exchange. *AIDS* **9:**1113–1119.
179. **Kaslow, R. A., and J. M. McNicholl.** 1999. Genetic determinants of HIV-1 infection and its manifestations. *Proc. Assoc. Am. Physicians* **111:**299–307.
180. **Katzenstein, D. A., S. M. Hammer, M. D. Hughes, H. Gundacker, J. B. Jackson, S. Fiscus, S. Rasheed, T. Elbeik, R. Reichman, A. Japour, T. C. Merigan, and M. S. Hirsch for the AIDS Clinical Trials Group Study 175 Virology Study Team.** 1996. The relation of virologic and immunologic markers to clinical outcomes after nucleoside therapy in HIV-infected adults with 200 to 500 CD4 cells per cubic millimeter. *N. Engl. J. Med.* **335:**1091–1098.
181. **Kaye, B. R.** 1989. Rheumatologic manifestations of infection with human immunodeficiency virus (HIV). *Ann. Intern. Med.* **111:**158–167.
182. **Keele, B. F., F. Van Heuverswyn, Y. Li, E. Bailes, J. Takehisa, M. L. Santiago, F. Bibollet-Ruche, Y. Chen, L. V. Wain, F. Liegeois, S. Loul, E. M. Ngole, Y. Bienvenue, E. Delaporte, J. F. Brookfield, P. M. Sharp, G. M. Shaw, M. Peeters, and B. H. Hahn.** 2006. Chimpanzee reservoirs of pandemic and nonpandemic HIV-1. *Science* **313:**523–526.
183. **Kestler, H. W., III, D. J. Ringler, K. Mori, D. L. Panicali, P. K. Sehgal, M. D. Daniel, and R. C. Desrosiers.** 1991. Importance of the nef gene for maintenance of high virus loads and for development of AIDS. *Cell* **65:**651–662.
184. **Kieffer, T. L., M. M. Finucane, R. E. Nettles, T. C. Quinn, K. W. Broman, S. C. Ray, D. Persaud, and R. F. Siliciano.** 2004. Genotypic analysis of HIV-1 drug resistance at the limit of detection: virus production without evolution in treated adults with undetectable HIV loads. *J. Infect. Dis.* **189:**1452–1465.
185. **Kim, R. B., M. F. Fromm, C. Wandel, B. Leake, A. J. Wood, D. M. Roden, and G. R. Wilkinson.** 1998. The drug transporter P-glycoprotein limits oral absorption and brain entry of HIV-1 protease inhibitors. *J. Clin. Investig.* **101:**289–294.
186. **Kim, S. Y., R. Byrn, J. Groopman, and D. Baltimore.** 1989. Temporal aspects of DNA and RNA synthesis during human immunodeficiency virus infection: evidence for differential gene expression. *J. Virol.* **63:**3708–3713.
187. **Kinloch-de Loes, S., B. J. Hirschel, B. Hoen, D. A. Cooper, B. Tindall, A. Carr, J. H. Saurat, N. Clumeck, A. Lazzarin, and L. Mathiesen.** 1995. A controlled trial of zidovudine in primary human immunodeficiency virus infection. *N. Engl. J. Med.* **333:**408–413.
188. **Klimkait, T., K. Strebel, M. D. Hoggan, M. A. Martin, and J. M. Orenstein.** 1990. The human immunodeficiency virus type 1-specific protein vpu is required for efficient virus maturation and release. *J. Virol.* **64:**621–629.
189. **Komanduri, K. V., M. N. Viswanathan, E. D. Wieder, D. K. Schmidt, B. M. Bredt, M. A. Jacobson, and J. M. McCune.** 1998. Restoration of cytomegalovirus-specific $CD4^+$ T-lymphocyte responses after ganciclovir and highly active antiretroviral therapy in individuals infected with HIV-1. *Nat. Med.* **4:**953–956.
190. **Kondo, E., and H. G. Gottlinger.** 1996. A conserved LXXLF sequence is the major determinant in p6gag required for the incorporation of human immunodeficiency virus type 1 Vpr. *J. Virol.* **70:**159–164.
191. **Koup, R. A., J. T. Safrit, Y. Cao, C. A. Andrews, G. McLeod, W. Borkowsky, C. Farthing, and D. D. Ho.** 1994. Temporal association of cellular immune responses with the initial control of viremia in primary human immunodeficiency virus type 1 syndrome. *J. Virol.* **68:**4650–4655.
192. **Krebs, F. C., H. Ross, J. McAllister, and B. Wigdahl.** 2000. HIV-1-associated central nervous system dysfunction. *Adv. Pharmacol.* **49:**315–385.
193. **Kwong, P. D., R. Wyatt, J. Robinson, R. W. Sweet, J. Sodroski, and W. A. Hendrickson.** 1998. Structure of an HIV gp120 envelope glycoprotein in complex with the CD4 receptor and a neutralizing human antibody. *Nature* **393:**648–659.
194. **Lambert, J. S., D. R. Harris, E. R. Stiehm, J. Moye, Jr., M. G. Fowler, W. A. Meyer III, J. Bethel, and L. M. Mofenson.** 2003. Performance characteristics of HIV-1 culture and HIV-1 DNA and RNA amplification assays for early diagnosis of perinatal HIV-1 infection. *J. Acquir. Immune. Defic. Syndr.* **34:**512–519.
195. **Laspia, M. F., A. P. Rice, and M. B. Mathews.** 1989. HIV-1 Tat protein increases transcriptional initiation and stabilizes elongation. *Cell* **59:**283–292.

196. **LeGall, S., L. Erdtmann, S. Benichou, C. Berlioz-Torrent, L. Liu, R. Benarous, J. M. Heard, and O. Schwartz.** 1998. Nef interacts with the mu subunit of clathrin adaptor complexes and reveals a cryptic sorting signal in MHC I molecules. *Immunity* **8:**483–495.
197. **Lemp, G. F., S. F. Payne, G. W. Rutherford, N. A. Hessol, W. Winkelstein, Jr., J. A. Wiley, A. R. Moss, R. E. Chaisson, R. T. Chen, and D. W. Feigal, Jr.** 1990. Projections of AIDS morbidity and mortality in San Francisco. *JAMA* **263:**1497–1501.
198. **Lenardo, M., K. M. Chan, F. Hornung, H. McFarland, R. Siegel, J. Wang, and L. Zheng.** 1999. Mature T lymphocyte apoptosis—immune regulation in a dynamic and unpredictable antigenic environment. *Annu. Rev. Immunol.* **17:**221–253.
199. **Le Rouzic E., N. Belaidouni, E. Estrabaud, M. Morel, J. C. Rain, C. Transy, and F. Margottin-Goguet.** 2007. HIV1 Vpr arrests the cell cycle by recruiting DCAF1/VprBP, a receptor of the Cul4-DDB1 ubiquitin ligase. *Cell Cycle* **6:**182–188.
200. **Leslie, A. J., K. J. Pfafferott, P. Chetty, R. Draenert, M. M. Addo, M. Feeney, Y. Tang, E. C. Holmes, T. Allen, J. G. Prado, M. Altfeld, C. Brander, C. Dixon, D. Ramduth, P. Jeena, S. A. Thomas, A. St. John, T. A. Roach, B. Kupfer, G. Luzzi, A. Edwards, G. Taylor, H. Lyall, G. Tudor-Williams, V. Novelli, J. Martinez-Picado, P. Kiepiela, B. D. Walker, and P. J. Goulder.** 2004. HIV evolution: CTL escape mutation and reversion after transmission. *Nat. Med.* **10:**282–289.
201. **Letvin, N. L., M. D. Daniel, P. K. Sehgal, R. C. Desrosiers, R. D. Hunt, L. M. Waldron, J. J. MacKey, D. K. Schmidt, L. V. Chalifoux, and N. W. King.** 1985. Induction of AIDS-like disease in macaque monkeys with T-cell tropic retrovirus STLV-III. *Science* **230:**71–73.
202. **Levesque, K., Y. S. Zhao, and E. A. Cohen.** 2003. Vpu exerts a positive effect on HIV-1 infectivity by downmodulating CD4 receptor molecules at the surface of HIV-1-producing cells. *J. Biol. Chem.* **278:**28346–28353.
203. **Li, S., C. P. Hill, W. I. Sundquist, and J. T. Finch.** 2000. Image reconstructions of helical assemblies of the HIV-1 CA protein. *Nature* **407:**409–413.
204. **Lin, H. J., L. Pedneault, and F. B. Hollinger.** 1998. Intra-assay performance characteristics of five assays for quantification of human immunodeficiency virus type 1 RNA in plasma. *J. Clin. Microbiol.* **36:**835–839.
205. **Ling, A. E., K. E. Robbins, T. M. Brown, V. Dunmire, S. Y. Thoe, S. Y. Wong, Y. S. Leo, D. Teo, J. Gallarda, B. Phelps, M. E. Chamberland, M. P. Busch, T. M. Folks, and M. L. Kalish.** 2000. Failure of routine HIV-1 tests in a case involving transmission with preseroconversion blood components during the infectious window period. *JAMA* **284:**210–214.
206. **Little, S. J.** 2000. Transmission and prevalence of HIV resistance among treatment-naive subjects. *Antiviral Ther.* **5:**33–40.
207. **Little, S. J., S. Holte, J. P. Routy, E. S. Daar, M. Markowitz, A. C. Collier, R. A. Koup, J. W. Mellors, E. Connick, B. Conway, M. Kilby, L. Wang, J. M. Whitcomb, N. S. Hellmann, and D. D. Richman.** 2002. Antiretroviral-drug resistance among patients recently infected with HIV. *N. Engl. J. Med.* **347:**385–394.
208. **Liu, A. Y., R. M. Grant, and S. P. Buchbinder.** 2006. Preexposure prophylaxis for HIV: unproven promise and potential pitfalls. *JAMA* **296:**863–865.
209. **Llano, M., D. T. Saenz, A. Meehan, P. Wongthida, M. Peretz, W. H. Walker, W. Teo, and E. M. Poeschla.** 2006. An essential role for LEDGF/p75 in HIV integration. *Science* **314:**461–464.
210. **Lockman, S., R. L. Shapiro, L. M. Smeaton, C. Wester, I. Thior, L. Stevens, F. Chand, J. Makhema, C. Moffat, A. Asmelash, P. Ndase, P. Arimi, E. van Widenfelt, L. Mazhani, V. Novitsky, S. Lagakos, and M. Essex.** 2007. Response to antiretroviral therapy after a single, peripartum dose of nevirapine. *N. Engl. J. Med.* **356:**135–147.
211. **Loussert-Ajaka, I., T. D. Ly, M. L. Chaix, D. Ingrand, S. Saragosti, A. M. Courouce, F. Brun-Vezinet, and F. Simon.** 1994. HIV-1/HIV-2 seronegativity in HIV-1 subtype O infected patients. *Lancet* **343:**1393–1394.
212. **Lu, X., X. Wu, A. Plemenitas, H. Yu, E. T. Sawai, A. Abo, and B. M. Peterlin.** 1996. CDC42 and Rac1 are implicated in the activation of the Nef-associated kinase and replication of HIV-1. *Curr. Biol.* **6:**1677–1684.
213. **Luban, J., K. L. Bossolt, E. K. Franke, G. V. Kalpana, and S. P. Goff.** 1993. Human immunodeficiency virus type 1 Gag protein binds to cyclophilins A and B. *Cell* **73:**1067–1078.
214. **Lyles, R. H., C. Chu, J. W. Mellors, J. B. Margolick, R. Detels, J. V. Giorgi, Q. Al-Shboul, and J. P. Phair.** 1999. Prognostic value of plasma HIV RNA in the natural history of *Pneumocystis carinii* pneumonia, cytomegalovirus and *Mycobacterium avium* complex. Multicenter AIDS Cohort Study. *AIDS* **13:**341–349.
215. **Macallan, D. C., C. Noble, C. Baldwin, S. A. Jebb, A. M. Prentice, W. A. Coward, M. B. Sawyer, T. J. McManus, and G. E. Griffin.** 1995. Energy expenditure and wasting in human immunodeficiency virus infection. *N. Engl. J. Med.* **333:**83–88.
216. **Maddon, P. J., A. G. Dalgleish, J. S. McDougal, P. R. Clapham, R. A. Weiss, and R. Axel.** 1986. The T4 gene encodes the AIDS virus receptor and is expressed in the immune system and the brain. *Cell* **47:**333–348.
217. **Maddon, P. J., J. S. McDougal, P. R. Clapham, A. G. Dalgleish, S. Jamal, R. A. Weiss, and R. Axel.** 1988. HIV infection does not require endocytosis of its receptor, CD4. *Cell* **54:**865–874.
218. **Maldarelli, F., S. Palmer, M. S. King, A. Wiegand, M. A. Polis, J. Mican, J. A. Kovacs, R. T. Davey, D. Rock-Kress, R. Dewar, S. Liu, J. A. Metcalf, C. Rehm, S. C. Brun, G. J. Hanna, D. J. Kempf, J. M. Coffin, and J. W. Mellors.** 2007. ART suppresses plasma HIV-1 RNA to a stable set point predicted by pretherapy viremia. *PLoS Pathog.* **3:**e46.
219. **Malim, M. H., J. Hauber, S. Y. Le, J. V. Maizel, and B. R. Cullen.** 1989. The HIV-1 rev trans-activator acts through a structured target sequence to activate nuclear export of unspliced viral mRNA. *Nature* **338:**254–257.
220. **Malim, M. H., D. F. McCarn, L. S. Tiley, and B. R. Cullen.** 1991. Mutational definition of the human immunodeficiency virus type 1 Rev activation domain. *J. Virol.* **65:**4248–4254.
221. **Mankowski, J. L., M. T. Flaherty, J. P. Spelman, D. A. Hauer, P. J. Didier, A. M. Amedee, M. Murphey-Corb, L. M. Kirstein, A. Munoz, J. E. Clements, and M. C. Zink.** 1997. Pathogenesis of simian immunodeficiency virus encephalitis: viral determinants of neurovirulence. *J. Virol.* **71:**6055–6060.
222. **Mansky, L. M., and H. M. Temin.** 1995. Lower in vivo mutation rate of human immunodeficiency virus type 1 than that predicted from the fidelity of purified reverse transcriptase. *J. Virol.* **69:**5087–5094.
223. **Marschner, I. C., A. C. Collier, R. W. Coombs, R. T. D'Aquila, V. DeGruttola, M. A. Fischl, S. M. Hammer, M. D. Hughes, V. A. Johnson, D. A. Katzenstein, D. D. Richman, L. M. Smeaton, S. A. Spector, and

M. S. Saag. 1998. Use of changes in plasma levels of human immunodeficiency virus type 1 RNA to assess the clinical benefit of antiretroviral therapy. *J. Infect. Dis.* **177:**40–47.

224. **Masur, H., M. A. Michelis, J. B. Greene, I. Onorato, R. A. Stouwe, R. S. Holzman, G. Wormser, L. Brettman, M. Lange, H. W. Murray, and S. Cunningham-Rundles.** 1981. An outbreak of community-acquired *Pneumocystis carinii* pneumonia: initial manifestation of cellular immune dysfunction. *N. Engl. J. Med.* **305:** 1431–1438.
225. **Mattapallil, J. J., D. C. Douek, B. Hill, Y. Nishimura, M. Martin, and M. Roederer.** 2005. Massive infection and loss of memory CD4$^+$ T cells in multiple tissues during acute SIV infection. *Nature* **434:**1093–1097.
226. **McArthur, J. C., N. Sacktor, and O. Selnes.** 1999. Human immunodeficiency virus-associated dementia. *Semin. Neurol.* **19:**129–150.
227. **McCune, J. M., R. Loftus, D. K. Schmidt, P. Carroll, D. Webster, L. B. Swor-Yim, I. R. Francis, B. H. Gross, and R. M. Grant.** 1998. High prevalence of thymic tissue in adults with human immunodeficiency virus-1 infection. *J. Clin. Investig.* **101:**2301–2308.
228. **McCune, J. M., L. B. Rabin, M. B. Feinberg, M. Lieberman, J. C. Kosek, G. R. Reyes, and I. L. Weissman.** 1988. Endoproteolytic cleavage of gp160 is required for the activation of human immunodeficiency virus. *Cell* **53:**55–67.
229. **McDonald, D., M. A. Vodicka, G. Lucero, T. M. Svitkina, G. G. Borisy, M. Emerman, and T. J. Hope.** 2002. Visualization of the intracellular behavior of HIV in living cells. *J. Cell Biol.* **159:**441–452.
230. **McDougal, J. S., M. S. Kennedy, J. M. Sligh, S. P. Cort, A. Mawle, and J. K. Nicholson.** 1986. Binding of HTLV-III/LAV to T4$^+$ T cells by a complex of the 110K viral protein and the T4 molecule. *Science* **231:**382–385.
231. **Mellors, J. W., L. A. Kingsley, C. R. Rinaldo, Jr., J. A. Todd, B. S. Hoo, R. P. Kokka, and P. Gupta.** 1995. Quantitation of HIV-1 RNA in plasma predicts outcome after seroconversion. *Ann. Intern. Med.* **122:**573–579.
232. **Mellors, J. W., J. B. Margolick, J. P. Phair, C. R. Rinaldo, R. Detels, L. P. Jacobson, and A. Munoz.** 2007. Prognostic value of HIV-1 RNA, CD4 cell count, and CD4 cell count slope for progression to AIDS and death in untreated HIV-1 infection. *JAMA* **297:**2349–2350.
233. **Mellors, J. W., A. Munoz, J. V. Giorgi, J. B. Margolick, C. J. Tassoni, P. Gupta, L. A. Kingsley, J. A. Todd, A. J. Saah, R. Detels, J. P. Phair, and C. R. Rinaldo, Jr.** 1997. Plasma viral load and CD4$^+$ lymphocytes as prognostic markers of HIV-1 infection. *Ann. Intern. Med.* **126:**946–954.
234. **Mervis, R. J., N. Ahmad, E. P. Lillehoj, M. G. Raum, F. H. Salazar, H. W. Chan, and S. Venkatesan.** 1988. The *gag* gene products of human immunodeficiency virus type 1: alignment within the *gag* open reading frame, identification of posttranslational modifications, and evidence for alternative *gag* precursors. *J. Virol.* **62:**3993–4002.
235. **Migueles, S. A., M. S. Sabbaghian, W. L. Shupert, M. P. Bettinotti, F. M. Marincola, L. Martino, C. W. Hallahan, S. M. Selig, D. Schwartz, J. Sullivan, and M. Connors.** 2000. HLA B*5701 is highly associated with restriction of virus replication in a subgroup of HIV-infected long term nonprogressors. *Proc. Natl. Acad. Sci. USA* **97:**2709–2714.
236. **Miller, M. D., C. M. Farnet, and F. D. Bushman.** 1997. Human immunodeficiency virus type 1 preintegration complexes: studies of organization and composition. *J. Virol.* **71:**5382–5390.
237. **Mitchell, D. M., and R. F. Miller.** 1995. AIDS and the lung: update 1995. 2. New developments in the pulmonary diseases affecting HIV infected individuals. *Thorax* **50:**294–302.
238. **Mitsuya, H., K. J. Weinhold, P. A. Furman, M. H. St. Clair, S. N. Lehrman, R. C. Gallo, D. Bolognesi, D. W. Barry, and S. Broder.** 1985. 3′-Azido-3′-deoxythymidine (BW A509U): an antiviral agent that inhibits the infectivity and cytopathic effect of human T-lymphotropic virus type III/lymphadenopathy-associated virus in vitro. *Proc. Natl. Acad. Sci. USA* **82:** 7096–7100.
239. **Mocroft, A., B. Ledergerber, C. Katlama, O. Kirk, P. Reiss, M. A. d'Arminio, B. Knysz, M. Dietrich, A. N. Phillips, and J. D. Lundgren.** 2003. Decline in the AIDS and death rates in the EuroSIDA study: an observational study. *Lancet* **362:**22–29.
240. **Mofenson, L. M., J. Oleske, L. Serchuck, D. R. Van, and C. Wilfert.** 2005. Treating opportunistic infections among HIV-exposed and infected children: recommendations from CDC, the National Institutes of Health, and the Infectious Diseases Society of America. *Clin. Infect. Dis.* **40**(Suppl. 1)**:**S1–S84.
241. **Mohri, H., A. S. Perelson, K. Tung, R. M. Ribeiro, B. Ramratnam, M. Markowitz, R. Kost, A. Hurley, L. Weinberger, D. Cesar, M. K. Hellerstein, and D. D. Ho.** 2001. Increased turnover of T lymphocytes in HIV-1 infection and its reduction by antiretroviral therapy. *J. Exp. Med.* **194:**1277–1287.
242. **Molla, A., M. Korneyeva, Q. Gao, S. Vasavanonda, P. J. Schipper, H. M. Mo, M. Markowitz, T. Chernyavskiy, P. Niu, N. Lyons, A. Hsu, G. R. Granneman, D. D. Ho, C. A. Boucher, J. M. Leonard, D. W. Norbeck, and D. J. Kempf.** 1996. Ordered accumulation of mutations in HIV protease confers resistance to ritonavir. *Nat. Med.* **2:**760–766.
243. **Moore, J. P., Y. Cao, D. D. Ho, and R. A. Koup.** 1994. Development of the anti-gp120 antibody response during seroconversion to human immunodeficiency virus type 1. *J. Virol.* **68:**5142–5155.
244. **Muesing, M. A., D. H. Smith, C. D. Cabradilla, C. V. Benton, L. A. Lasky, and D. J. Capon.** 1985. Nucleic acid structure and expression of the human AIDS/lymphadenopathy retrovirus. *Nature* **313:**450–458.
245. **Muesing, M. A., D. H. Smith, and D. J. Capon.** 1987. Regulation of mRNA accumulation by a human immunodeficiency virus trans-activator protein. *Cell* **48:** 691–701.
246. **Mundy, D. C., R. F. Schinazi, A. R. Gerber, A. J. Nahmias, and H. W. Randall, Jr.** 1987. Human immunodeficiency virus isolated from amniotic fluid. *Lancet* **ii:** 459–460.
247. **Nabel, G., and D. Baltimore.** 1987. An inducible transcription factor activates expression of human immunodeficiency virus in T cells. *Nature* **326:**711–713.
248. **Nabel, G. J.** 2001. Challenges and opportunities for development of an AIDS vaccine. *Nature* **410:**1002–1007.
249. **Nara, P. L., W. G. Robey, L. O. Arthur, D. M. Asher, A. V. Wolff, C. J. Gibbs, Jr., D. C. Gajdusek, and P. J. Fischinger.** 1987. Persistent infection of chimpanzees with human immunodeficiency virus: serological responses and properties of reisolated viruses. *J. Virol.* **61:** 3173–3180.
250. **Neil, S. J., S. W. Eastman, N. Jouvenet, and P. D. Bieniasz.** 2006. HIV-1 Vpu promotes release and prevents endocytosis of nascent retrovirus particles from the plasma membrane. *PLoS Pathog.* **2:**e39.
251. **Nesheim, S., F. Lee, M. L. Kalish, C. Y. Ou, M. Sawyer, S. Clark, L. Meadows, V. Grimes, R. J. Simonds,**

and A. Nahmias. 1997. Diagnosis of perinatal human immunodeficiency virus infection by polymerase chain reaction and p24 antigen detection after immune complex dissociation in an urban community hospital. *J. Infect. Dis.* **175:**1333–1336.

252. **Nettles, R. E., T. L. Kieffer, P. Kwon, D. Monie, Y. Han, T. Parsons, J. Cofrancesco, Jr., J. E. Gallant, T. C. Quinn, B. Jackson, C. Flexner, K. Carson, S. Ray, D. Persaud, and R. F. Siliciano.** 2005. Intermittent HIV-1 viremia (Blips) and drug resistance in patients receiving HAART. *JAMA* **293:**817–829.

253. **Newell, M. L., H. Coovadia, M. Cortina-Borja, N. Rollins, P. Gaillard, and F. Dabis.** 2004. Mortality of infected and uninfected infants born to HIV-infected mothers in Africa: a pooled analysis. *Lancet* **364:**1236–1243.

254. **Nguyen, D. H., and J. E. Hildreth.** 2000. Evidence for budding of human immunodeficiency virus type 1 selectively from glycolipid-enriched membrane lipid rafts. *J. Virol.* **74:**3264–3272.

255. **Nicholson, J. K., G. D. Cross, C. S. Callaway, and J. S. McDougal.** 1986. In vitro infection of human monocytes with human T lymphotropic virus type III/lymphadenopathy-associated virus (HTLV-III/LAV). *J. Immunol.* **137:**323–329.

256. **Nielsen, C., C. Pedersen, J. D. Lundgren, and J. Gerstoft.** 1993. Biological properties of HIV isolates in primary HIV infection: consequences for the subsequent course of infection. *AIDS* **7:**1035–1040.

257. **Nishimura, Y., T. Igarashi, N. Haigwood, R. Sadjadpour, R. J. Plishka, A. Buckler-White, R. Shibata, and M. A. Martin.** 2002. Determination of a statistically valid neutralization titer in plasma that confers protection against simian-human immunodeficiency virus challenge following passive transfer of high-titered neutralizing antibodies. *J. Virol.* **76:**2123–2130.

258. **O'Brien, S. J., and J. P. Moore.** 2000. The effect of genetic variation in chemokines and their receptors on HIV transmission and progression to AIDS. *Immunol. Rev.* **177:**99–111.

259. **O'Brien, T. R., J. R. George, J. S. Epstein, S. D. Holmberg, and G. Schochetman.** 1992. Testing for antibodies to human immunodeficiency virus type 2 in the United States. *Morb. Mortal. Wkly. Rep.* **41:**1–9.

260. **O'Brien, T. R., J. R. George, and S. D. Holmberg.** 1992. Human immunodeficiency virus type 2 infection in the United States. Epidemiology, diagnosis, and public health implications. *JAMA* **267:**2775–2779.

261. **O'Brien, W. A., Y. Koyanagi, A. Namazie, J. Q. Zhao, A. Diagne, K. Idler, J. A. Zack, and I. S. Chen.** 1990. HIV-1 tropism for mononuclear phagocytes can be determined by regions of gp120 outside the CD4-binding domain. *Nature* **348:**69–73.

262. **Ofek, G., M. Tang, A. Sambor, H. Katinger, J. R. Mascola, R. Wyatt, and P. D. Kwong.** 2004. Structure and mechanistic analysis of the anti-human immunodeficiency virus type 1 antibody 2F5 in complex with its gp41 epitope. *J. Virol.* **78:**10724–10737.

263. **Okamoto, H., C. T. Sheline, J. L. Corden, K. A. Jones, and B. M. Peterlin.** 1996. Trans-activation by human immunodeficiency virus Tat protein requires the C-terminal domain of RNA polymerase II. *Proc. Natl. Acad. Sci. USA* **93:**11575–11579.

264. **Ono, A., S. D. Ablan, S. J. Lockett, K. Nagashima, and E. O. Freed.** 2004. Phosphatidylinositol (4,5) bisphosphate regulates HIV-1 Gag targeting to the plasma membrane. *Proc. Natl. Acad. Sci. USA* **101:**14889–14894.

265. **Orenstein, J. M., C. Fox, and S. M. Wahl.** 1997. Macrophages as a source of HIV during opportunistic infections. *Science* **276:**1857–1861.

266. **Overbaugh, J., R. J. Anderson, J. O. Ndinya-Achola, and J. K. Kreiss.** 1996. Distinct but related human immunodeficiency virus type 1 variant populations in genital secretions and blood. *AIDS Res. Hum. Retroviruses* **12:**107–115.

267. **Pakker, N. G., D. W. Notermans, R. J. de Boer, M. T. Roos, F. de Wolf, A. Hill, J. M. Leonard, S. A. Danner, F. Miedema, and P. T. Schellekens.** 1998. Biphasic kinetics of peripheral blood T cells after triple combination therapy in HIV-1 infection: a composite of redistribution and proliferation. *Nat. Med.* **4:**208–214.

268. **Palella, F. J., Jr., K. M. Delaney, A. C. Moorman, M. O. Loveless, J. Fuhrer, G. A. Satten, D. J. Aschman, and S. D. Holmberg for the HIV Outpatient Study Investigators.** 1998. Declining morbidity and mortality among patients with advanced human immunodeficiency virus infection. *N. Engl. J. Med.* **338:**853–860.

269. **Palumbo, P. E., C. Raskino, S. Fiscus, S. Pahwa, T. Schutzbank, S. A. Spector, C. J. Baker, and J. A. Englund.** 1999. Virologic and immunologic response to nucleoside reverse-transcriptase inhibitor therapy among human immunodeficiency virus-infected infants and children. *J. Infect. Dis.* **179:**576–583.

270. **Pandori, M. W., N. J. Fitch, H. M. Craig, D. D. Richman, C. A. Spina, and J. C. Guatelli.** 1996. Producer-cell modification of human immunodeficiency virus type 1: Nef is a virion protein. *J. Virol.* **70:**4283–4290.

271. **Panlilio, A. L., D. M. Cardo, L. A. Grohskopf, W. Heneine, and C. S. Ross.** 2005. Updated U.S. Public Health Service guidelines for the management of occupational exposures to HIV and recommendations for postexposure prophylaxis. *Morb. Mortal. Wkly. Rep. Recomm. Rep.* **54:**1–17.

272. **Pantaleo, G., C. Graziosi, J. F. Demarest, L. Butini, M. Montroni, C. H. Fox, J. M. Orenstein, D. P. Kotler, and A. S. Fauci.** 1993. HIV infection is active and progressive in lymphoid tissue during the clinically latent stage of disease. *Nature* **362:**355–358.

273. **Pantaleo, G., S. Menzo, M. Vaccarezza, C. Graziosi, O. J. Cohen, J. F. Demarest, D. Montefiori, J. M. Orenstein, C. Fox, and L. K. Schrager.** 1995. Studies in subjects with long-term nonprogressive human immunodeficiency virus infection. *N. Engl. J. Med.* **332:**209–216.

274. **Parren, P. W., and D. R. Burton.** 2001. The antiviral activity of antibodies in vitro and in vivo. *Adv. Immunol.* **77:**195–262.

275. **Paxton, L. A., T. Hope, and H. W. Jaffe.** 2007. Pre-exposure prophylaxis for HIV infection: what if it works? *Lancet* **370:**89–93.

276. **Peng, G., T. Greenwell-Wild, S. Nares, W. Jin, K. J. Lei, Z. G. Rangel, P. J. Munson, and S. M. Wahl.** 2007. Myeloid differentiation and susceptibility to HIV-1 are linked to APOBEC3 expression. *Blood* **110:**393–400.

277. **Perelson, A. S., P. Essunger, Y. Cao, M. Vesanen, A. Hurley, K. Saksela, M. Markowitz, and D. D. Ho.** 1997. Decay characteristics of HIV-1-infected compartments during combination therapy. *Nature* **387:**188–191.

278. **Perelson, A. S., A. U. Neumann, M. Markowitz, J. M. Leonard, and D. D. Ho.** 1996. HIV-1 dynamics in vivo: virion clearance rate, infected cell life-span, and viral generation time. *Science* **271:**1582–1586.

279. **Persaud, D., T. Pierson, C. Ruff, D. Finzi, K. R. Chadwick, J. B. Margolick, A. Ruff, N. Hutton, S. Ray,**

and R. F. Siliciano. 2000. A stable latent reservoir for HIV-1 in resting CD4+ T lymphocytes in infected children. *J. Clin. Investig.* **105:**995–1003.

280. **Petrovas, C., J. P. Casazza, J. M. Brenchley, D. A. Price, E. Gostick, W. C. Adams, M. L. Precopio, T. Schacker, M. Roederer, D. C. Douek, and R. A. Koup.** 2006. PD-1 is a regulator of virus-specific CD8+ T cell survival in HIV infection. *J. Exp. Med.* **203:**2281–2292.
281. **Pierson, T., T. L. Hoffman, J. Blankson, D. Finzi, K. Chadwick, J. B. Margolick, C. Buck, J. D. Siliciano, R. W. Doms, and R. F. Siliciano.** 2000. Characterization of chemokine receptor utilization of viruses in the latent reservoir for human immunodeficiency virus type 1. *J. Virol.* **74:**7824–7833.
282. **Pillai, S. K., B. Good, S. K. Pond, J. K. Wong, M. C. Strain, D. D. Richman, and D. M. Smith.** 2005. Semen-specific genetic characteristics of human immunodeficiency virus type 1 env. *J. Virol.* **79:**1734–1742.
283. **Pillai, S. K., S. L. Pond, Y. Liu, B. M. Good, M. C. Strain, R. J. Ellis, S. Letendre, D. M. Smith, H. F. Gunthard, I. Grant, T. D. Marcotte, J. A. McCutchan, D. D. Richman, and J. K. Wong.** 2006. Genetic attributes of cerebrospinal fluid-derived HIV-1 env. *Brain* **129:**1872–1883.
284. **Pion, M., A. Granelli-Piperno, B. Mangeat, R. Stalder, R. Correa, R. M. Steinman, and V. Piguet.** 2006. APOBEC3G/3F mediates intrinsic resistance of monocyte-derived dendritic cells to HIV-1 infection. *J. Exp. Med.* **203:**2887–2893.
285. **Poignard, P., R. Sabbe, G. R. Picchio, M. Wang, R. J. Gulizia, H. Katinger, P. W. Parren, D. E. Mosier, and D. R. Burton.** 1999. Neutralizing antibodies have limited effects on the control of established HIV-1 infection in vivo. *Immunity* **10:**431–438.
286. **Popov, S., M. Rexach, G. Zybarth, N. Reiling, M. A. Lee, L. Ratner, C. M. Lane, M. S. Moore, G. Blobel, and M. Bukrinsky.** 1998. Viral protein R regulates nuclear import of the HIV-1 pre-integration complex. *EMBO J.* **17:**909–917.
287. **Putkonen, P., B. Bottiger, K. Warstedt, R. Thorstensson, J. Albert, and G. Biberfeld.** 1989. Experimental infection of cynomolgus monkeys *(Macaca fascicularis)* with HIV-2. *J. Acquir. Immune Defic. Syndr.* **2:**366–373.
288. **Ramratnam, B., J. E. Mittler, L. Zhang, D. Boden, A. Hurley, F. Fang, C. A. Macken, A. S. Perelson, M. Markowitz, and D. D. Ho.** 2000. The decay of the latent reservoir of replication-competent HIV-1 is inversely correlated with the extent of residual viral replication during prolonged anti-retroviral therapy. *Nat. Med.* **6:**82–85.
289. **Ratner, L., W. A. Haseltine, R. Patarca, K. J. Livak, B. Starcich, S. F. Josephs, E. R. Doran, J. A. Rafalski, E. A. Whitehorn, K. Baumeister, L. Ivanoff, S. R. Petteway, Jr., M. L. Pearson, J. A. Lautenberger, T. S. Papas, J. Ghrayeb, N. T. Chang, R. C. Gallo, and F. Wong-Staal.** 1985. Complete nucleotide sequence of the AIDS virus, HTLV-III. *Nature* **316:**277–284.
290. **Reinhart, T. A., M. J. Rogan, D. Huddleston, D. M. Rausch, L. E. Eiden, and A. T. Haase.** 1997. Simian immunodeficiency virus burden in tissues and cellular compartments during clinical latency and AIDS. *J. Infect. Dis.* **176:**1198–1208.
291. **Richman, D. D.** 1996. The implications of drug resistance for strategies of combination antiviral chemotherapy. *Antiviral Res.* **29:**31–33.
292. **Richman, D. D.** 2001. HIV chemotherapy. *Nature* **410:** 995–1001.
293. **Richman, D. D., and S. A. Bozzette.** 1994. The impact of the syncytium-inducing phenotype of human immunodeficiency virus on disease progression. *J. Infect. Dis.* **169:**968–974.
294. **Richman, D. D., M. A. Fischl, M. H. Grieco, M. S. Gottlieb, P. A. Volberding, O. L. Laskin, J. M. Leedom, J. E. Groopman, D. Mildvan, M. S. Hirsch, G. G. Jackson, D. T. Durack, S. Nusinoff-Lehrman, and the AZT Collaborative Working Group.** 1987. The toxicity of azidothymidine (AZT) in the treatment of patients with AIDS and AIDS-related complex. A double-blind, placebo-controlled trial. *N. Engl. J. Med.* **317:**192–197.
295. **Richman, D. D., J. M. Grimes, and S. W. Lagakos.** 1990. Effect of stage of disease and drug dose on zidovudine susceptibilities of isolates of human immunodeficiency virus. *J. Acquir. Immune Defic. Syndr.* **3:**743–746.
296. **Richman, D. D., T. Wrin, S. J. Little, and C. J. Petropoulos.** 2003. Rapid evolution of the neutralizing antibody response to HIV type 1 infection. *Proc. Natl. Acad. Sci. USA* **100:**4144–4149.
297. **Rizzuto, C. D., R. Wyatt, N. Hernandez-Ramos, Y. Sun, P. D. Kwong, W. A. Hendrickson, and J. Sodroski.** 1998. A conserved HIV gp120 glycoprotein structure involved in chemokine receptor binding. *Science* **280:**1949–1953.
298. **Robertson, D. L., J. P. Anderson, J. A. Bradac, J. K. Carr, B. Foley, R. K. Funkhouser, F. Gao, B. H. Hahn, M. L. Kalish, C. Kuiken, G. H. Learn, T. Leitner, F. McCutchan, S. Osmanov, M. Peeters, D. Pieniazek, M. Salminen, P. M. Sharp, S. Wolinsky, and B. Korber.** 2000. HIV-1 nomenclature proposal. *Science* **288:**55–56.
299. **Robertson, D. L., P. M. Sharp, F. E. McCutchan, and B. H. Hahn.** 1995. Recombination in HIV-1. *Nature* **374:**124–126.
300. **Rodriguez, B., A. K. Sethi, V. K. Cheruvu, W. Mackay, R. J. Bosch, M. Kitahata, S. L. Boswell, W. C. Mathews, D. R. Bangsberg, J. Martin, C. C. Whalen, S. Sieg, S. Yadavalli, S. G. Deeks, and M. M. Lederman.** 2006. Predictive value of plasma HIV RNA level on rate of CD4 T-cell decline in untreated HIV infection. *JAMA* **296:**1498–1506.
301. **Roederer, M., J. G. Dubs, M. T. Anderson, P. A. Raju, L. A. Herzenberg, and L. A. Herzenberg.** 1995. CD8 naive T cell counts decrease progressively in HIV-infected adults. *J. Clin. Investig.* **95:**2061–2066.
302. **Rogel, M. E., L. I. Wu, and M. Emerman.** 1995. The human immunodeficiency virus type 1 *vpr* gene prevents cell proliferation during chronic infection. *J. Virol.* **69:** 882–888.
303. **Rosenberg, E. S., A. M. Caliendo, and B. D. Walker.** 1999. Acute HIV infection among patients tested for mononucleosis. *N. Engl. J. Med.* **340:**969.
304. **Ross, A., L. Van der Paal, R. Lubega, B. N. Mayanja, L. A. Shafer, and J. Whitworth.** 2004. HIV-1 disease progression and fertility: the incidence of recognized pregnancy and pregnancy outcome in Uganda. *AIDS* **18:** 799–804.
305. **Ryder, R. W., W. Nsa, S. E. Hassig, F. Behets, M. Rayfield, B. Ekungola, A. M. Nelson, U. Mulenda, H. Francis, K. Mwandagalirwa, et al.** 1989. Perinatal transmission of the human immunodeficiency virus type 1 to infants of seropositive women in Zaire. *N. Engl. J. Med.* **320:**1637–1642.
306. **Sakai, K., J. Dimas, and M. J. Lenardo.** 2006. The Vif and Vpr accessory proteins independently cause HIV-1-induced T cell cytopathicity and cell cycle arrest. *Proc. Natl. Acad. Sci. USA* **103:**3369–3374.
307. **Saksela, K., G. Cheng, and D. Baltimore.** 1995. Proline-rich (PxxP) motifs in HIV-1 Nef bind to SH3 domains of a subset of Src kinases and are required for

the enhanced growth of Nef+ viruses but not for downregulation of CD4. *EMBO J.* **14:**484–491.

308. **Sanchez-Pescador, R., M. D. Power, P. J. Barr, K. S. Steimer, M. M. Stempien, S. L. Brown-Shimer, W. W. Gee, A. Renard, A. Randolph, and J. A. Levy.** 1985. Nucleotide sequence and expression of an AIDS-associated retrovirus (ARV-2). *Science* **227:**484–492.
309. **Schable, C., L. Zekeng, C. P. Pau, D. Hu, L. Kaptue, L. Gurtler, T. Dondero, J. M. Tsague, G. Schochetman, H. Jaffe, et al.** 1994. Sensitivity of United States HIV antibody tests for detection of HIV-1 group O infections. *Lancet* **344:**1333–1334.
310. **Schacker, T., A. C. Collier, J. Hughes, T. Shea, and L. Corey.** 1996. Clinical and epidemiologic features of primary HIV infection. *Ann. Intern. Med.* **125:**257–264.
311. **Schindler, M., J. Munch, O. Kutsch, H. Li, M. L. Santiago, F. Bibollet-Ruche, M. C. Muller-Trutwin, F. J. Novembre, M. Peeters, V. Courgnaud, E. Bailes, P. Roques, D. L. Sodora, G. Silvestri, P. M. Sharp, B. H. Hahn, and F. Kirchhoff.** 2006. Nef-mediated suppression of T cell activation was lost in a lentiviral lineage that gave rise to HIV-1. *Cell* **125:**1055–1067.
312. **Schmitz, J. E., M. J. Kuroda, S. Santra, V. G. Sasseville, M. A. Simon, M. A. Lifton, P. Racz, K. Tenner-Racz, M. Dalesandro, B. J. Scallon, J. Ghrayeb, M. A. Forman, D. C. Montefiori, E. P. Rieber, N. L. Letvin, and K. A. Reimann.** 1999. Control of viremia in simian immunodeficiency virus infection by $CD8^+$ lymphocytes. *Science* **283:**857–860.
313. **Schroder, A. R., P. Shinn, H. Chen, C. Berry, J. R. Ecker, and F. Bushman.** 2002. HIV-1 integration in the human genome favors active genes and local hotspots. *Cell* **110:**521–529.
314. **Schubert, U., S. Bour, A. V. Ferrer-Montiel, M. Montal, F. Maldarell, and K. Strebel.** 1996. The two biological activities of human immunodeficiency virus type 1 Vpu protein involve two separable structural domains. *J. Virol.* **70:**809–819.
315. **Schupbach, J., M. Flepp, D. Pontelli, Z. Tomasik, R. Luthy, and J. Boni.** 1996. Heat-mediated immune complex dissociation and enzyme-linked immunosorbent assay signal amplification render p24 antigen detection in plasma as sensitive as HIV-1 RNA detection by polymerase chain reaction. *AIDS* **10:**1085–1090.
316. **Schwartz, O., V. Marechal, G. S. Le, F. Lemonnier, and J. M. Heard.** 1996. Endocytosis of major histocompatibility complex class I molecules is induced by the HIV-1 Nef protein. *Nat. Med.* **2:**338–342.
317. **Schwartz, S., B. K. Felber, D. M. Benko, E. M. Fenyo, and G. N. Pavlakis.** 1990. Cloning and functional analysis of multiply spliced mRNA species of human immunodeficiency virus type 1. *J. Virol.* **64:**2519–2529.
318. **Schwartz, S., B. K. Felber, E. M. Fenyo, and G. N. Pavlakis.** 1990. Env and Vpu proteins of human immunodeficiency virus type 1 are produced from multiple bicistronic mRNAs. *J. Virol.* **64:**5448–5456.
319. **Schwenk, A., B. Buger, D. Wessel, H. Stutzer, D. Ziegenhagen, V. Diehl, and M. Schrappe.** 1993. Clinical risk factors for malnutrition in HIV-1-infected patients. *AIDS* **7:**1213–1219.
320. **Scott, G. B.** 1991. HIV infection in children: clinical features and management. *J. Acquir. Immune Defic. Syndr.* **4:**109–115.
321. **Shankarappa, R., J. B. Margolick, S. J. Gange, A. G. Rodrigo, D. Upchurch, H. Farzadegan, P. Gupta, C. R. Rinaldo, G. H. Learn, X. He, X. L. Huang, and J. I. Mullins.** 1999. Consistent viral evolutionary changes associated with the progression of human immunodeficiency virus type 1 infection. *J. Virol.* **73:**10489–10502.
322. **Sheehy, A. M., N. C. Gaddis, J. D. Choi, and M. H. Malim.** 2002. Isolation of a human gene that inhibits HIV-1 infection and is suppressed by the viral Vif protein. *Nature* **418:**646–650.
323. **Sheehy, A. M., N. C. Gaddis, and M. H. Malim.** 2003. The antiretroviral enzyme APOBEC3G is degraded by the proteasome in response to HIV-1 Vif. *Nat. Med.* **9:** 1404–1407.
324. **Sidtis, J. J., C. Gatsonis, R. W. Price, E. J. Singer, A. C. Collier, D. D. Richman, M. S. Hirsch, F. W. Schaerf, M. A. Fischl, and K. Kieburtz for the AIDS Clinical Trials Group.** 1993. Zidovudine treatment of the AIDS dementia complex: results of a placebo-controlled trial. *Ann. Neurol.* **33:**343–349.
325. **Siegal, F. P., C. Lopez, F. S. Hammer, A. E. Brown, S. J. Kornfeld, J. Gold, J. Hassett, S. Z. Hirschman, C. Cunningham-Rundles, B. R. Adelsberg, D. M. Parham, M. Siegal, S. Cunningham-Rundles, and D. Armstrong.** 1981. Severe acquired immunodeficiency in male homosexuals manifested by chronic perianal ulcerative herpes simplex lesions. *N. Engl. J. Med.* **305:** 1439–1444.
326. **Simpson, D. M., and M. Tagliati.** 1994. Neurologic manifestations of HIV infection. *Ann. Intern. Med.* **121:** 769–785.
327. **Smit-McBride, Z., J. J. Mattapallil, M. McChesney, D. Ferrick, and S. Dandekar.** 1998. Gastrointestinal T lymphocytes retain high potential for cytokine responses but have severe $CD4^+$ T-cell depletion at all stages of simian immunodeficiency virus infection compared to peripheral lymphocytes. *J. Virol.* **72:**6646–6656.
328. **So, Y. T., D. M. Holtzman, D. I. Abrams, and R. K. Olney.** 1988. Peripheral neuropathy associated with acquired immunodeficiency syndrome. Prevalence and clinical features from a population-based survey. *Arch. Neurol.* **45:**945–948.
329. **Sodroski, J., W. C. Goh, C. Rosen, K. Campbell, and W. A. Haseltine.** 1986. Role of the HTLV-III/LAV envelope in syncytium formation and cytopathicity. *Nature* **322:**470–474.
330. **Sonnenberg, P., J. R. Glynn, K. Fielding, J. Murray, P. Godfrey-Faussett, and S. Shearer.** 2005. How soon after infection with HIV does the risk of tuberculosis start to increase? A retrospective cohort study in South African gold miners. *J. Infect. Dis.* **191:**150–158.
331. **Spina, C. A., T. J. Kwoh, M. Y. Chowers, J. C. Guatelli, and D. D. Richman.** 1994. The importance of nef in the induction of human immunodeficiency virus type 1 replication from primary quiescent CD4 lymphocytes. *J. Exp. Med.* **179:**115–123.
332. **Stamm, W. E., H. H. Handsfield, A. M. Rompalo, R. L. Ashley, P. L. Roberts, and L. Corey.** 1988. The association between genital ulcer disease and acquisition of HIV infection in homosexual men. *JAMA* **260:**1429–1433.
333. **Stanley, S. K., M. A. Ostrowski, J. S. Justement, K. Gantt, S. Hedayati, M. Mannix, K. Roche, D. J. Schwartzentruber, C. H. Fox, and A. S. Fauci.** 1996. Effect of immunization with a common recall antigen on viral expression in patients infected with human immunodeficiency virus type 1. *N. Engl. J. Med.* **334:** 1222–1230.
334. **Sterling, T. R., D. Vlahov, J. Astemborski, D. R. Hoover, J. B. Margolick, and T. C. Quinn.** 2001. Initial plasma HIV-1 RNA levels and progression to AIDS in women and men. *N. Engl. J. Med.* **344:**720–725.
335. **Stewart, S. A., B. Poon, J. B. Jowett, and I. S. Chen.** 1997. Human immunodeficiency virus type 1 Vpr in-

duces apoptosis following cell cycle arrest. *J. Virol.* **71:** 5579–5592.

336. **Strack, B., A. Calistri, S. Craig, E. Popova, and H. G. Gottlinger.** 2003. AIP1/ALIX is a binding partner for HIV-1 p6 and EIAV p9 functioning in virus budding. *Cell* **114:**689–699.

337. **Strain, M. C., S. Letendre, S. K. Pillai, T. Russell, C. C. Ignacio, H. F. Gunthard, B. Good, D. M. Smith, S. M. Wolinsky, M. Furtado, J. Marquie-Beck, J. Durelle, I. Grant, D. D. Richman, T. Marcotte, J. A. McCutchan, R. J. Ellis, and J. K. Wong.** 2005. Genetic composition of human immunodeficiency virus type 1 in cerebrospinal fluid and blood without treatment and during failing antiretroviral therapy. *J. Virol.* **79:**1772–1788.

338. **Stramer, S. L., S. Caglioti, and D. M. Strong.** 2000. NAT of the United States and Canadian blood supply. *Transfusion* (Paris). **40:**1165–1168.

339. **Strebel, K., D. Daugherty, K. Clouse, D. Cohen, T. Folks, and M. A. Martin.** 1987. The HIV 'A' (sor) gene product is essential for virus infectivity. *Nature* **328:**728–730.

340. **Strebel, K., T. Klimkait, and M. A. Martin.** 1988. A novel gene of HIV-1, *vpu*, and its 16-kilodalton product. *Science* **241:**1221–1223.

341. **Stremlau, M., C. M. Owens, M. J. Perron, M. Kiessling, P. Autissier, and J. Sodroski.** 2004. The cytoplasmic body component TRIM5α restricts HIV-1 infection in Old World monkeys. *Nature* **427:**848–853.

342. **Takahashi, K., S. L. Wesselingh, D. E. Griffin, J. C. McArthur, R. T. Johnson, and J. D. Glass.** 1996. Localization of HIV-1 in human brain using polymerase chain reaction/in situ hybridization and immunocytochemistry. *Ann. Neurol.* **39:**705–711.

343. **Takehisa, J., L. Zekeng, E. Ido, I. Mboudjeka, H. Moriyama, T. Miura, M. Yamashita, L. G. Gurtler, M. Hayami, and L. Kaptue.** 1998. Various types of HIV mixed infections in Cameroon. *Virology* **245:**1–10.

344. **Takehisa, J., L. Zekeng, E. Ido, Y. Yamaguchi-Kabata, I. Mboudjeka, Y. Harada, T. Miura, L. Kaptu, and M. Hayami.** 1999. Human immunodeficiency virus type 1 intergroup (M/O) recombination in Cameroon. *J. Virol.* **73:**6810–6820.

345. **Terai, C., R. S. Kornbluth, C. D. Pauza, D. D. Richman, and D. A. Carson.** 1991. Apoptosis as a mechanism of cell death in cultured T lymphoblasts acutely infected with HIV-1. *J. Clin. Investig.* **87:**1710–1715.

346. **Tersmette, M., R. E. de Goede, B. J. Al, I. N. Winkel, R. A. Gruters, H. T. Cuypers, H. G. Huisman, and F. Miedema.** 1988. Differential syncytium-inducing capacity of human immunodeficiency virus isolates: frequent detection of syncytium-inducing isolates in patients with acquired immunodeficiency syndrome (AIDS) and AIDS-related complex. *J. Virol.* **62:**2026–2032.

347. **Thior, I., S. Lockman, L. M. Smeaton, R. L. Shapiro, C. Wester, S. J. Heymann, P. B. Gilbert, L. Stevens, T. Peter, S. Kim, E. van Widenfelt, C. Moffat, P. Ndase, P. Arimi, P. Kebaabetswe, P. Mazonde, J. Makhema, K. McIntosh, V. Novitsky, T. H. Lee, R. Marlink, S. Lagakos, and M. Essex.** 2006. Breastfeeding plus infant zidovudine prophylaxis for 6 months vs formula feeding plus infant zidovudine for 1 month to reduce mother-to-child HIV transmission in Botswana: a randomized trial: the Mashi Study. *JAMA* **296:**794–805.

348. **Thiry, L., S. Sprecher-Goldberger, T. Jonckheer, J. Levy, P. Van de Perre, P. Henrivaux, J. Cogniaux-LeClerc, and N. Clumeck.** 1985. Isolation of AIDS virus from cell-free breast milk of three healthy virus carriers. *Lancet* **ii:**891–892.

349. **Tindall, B., and D. A. Cooper.** 1991. Primary HIV infection: host responses and intervention strategies. *AIDS* **5:**1–14.

350. **Trautmann, L., L. Janbazian, N. Chomont, E. A. Said, S. Gimmig, B. Bessette, M. R. Boulassel, E. Delwart, H. Sepulveda, R. S. Balderas, J. P. Routy, E. K. Haddad, and R. P. Sekaly.** 2006. Upregulation of PD-1 expression on HIV-specific $CD8^+$ T cells leads to reversible immune dysfunction. *Nat. Med.* **12:**1198–1202.

351. **Trkola, A., H. Kuster, P. Rusert, B. Joos, M. Fischer, C. Leemann, A. Manrique, M. Huber, M. Rehr, A. Oxenius, R. Weber, G. Stiegler, B. Vcelar, H. Katinger, L. Aceto, and H. F. Gunthard.** 2005. Delay of HIV-1 rebound after cessation of antiretroviral therapy through passive transfer of human neutralizing antibodies. *Nat. Med.* **11:**615–622.

352. **Ullrich, R., M. Zeitz, W. Heise, M. L'age, G. Hoffken, and E. O. Riecken.** 1989. Small intestinal structure and function in patients infected with human immunodeficiency virus (HIV): evidence for HIV-induced enteropathy. *Ann. Intern. Med.* **111:**15–21.

353. **United Nations Programme on HIV/AIDS and World Health Organization.** December 2007, posting date. *AIDS Epidemic Update, 2007.* Joint United Nations Programme on HIV/AIDS and World Health Organization, Geneva, Switzerland. http://data.unaids.org/pub/EPISlides/2007/2007_epiudate_en.pdf.

354. **van Damme, L.** 2000. *Abstr. XIII Int. AIDS Conf.*, abstr. PL04.

355. **van Griensven, F.** 2007. Men who have sex with men and their HIV epidemics in Africa. *AIDS* **21:**1361–1362.

356. **Vanhems, P., J. Hughes, A. C. Collier, J. Vizzard, L. Perrin, D. A. Cooper, B. Hirschel, and L. Corey.** 2000. Comparison of clinical features, CD4 and CD8 responses among patients with acute HIV-1 infection from Geneva, Seattle and Sydney. *AIDS* **14:**375–381.

357. **Van Heuverswyn F., Y. Li, C. Neel, E. Bailes, B. F. Keele, W. Liu, S. Loul, C. Butel, F. Liegeois, Y. Bienvenue, E. M. Ngolle, P. M. Sharp, G. M. Shaw, E. Delaporte, B. H. Hahn, and M. Peeters.** 2006. Human immunodeficiency viruses: SIV infection in wild gorillas. *Nature* **444:**164.

358. **Van Kerckhoven, I., G. Vercauteren, P. Piot, and G. van der Groen.** 1991. Comparative evaluation of 36 commercial assays for detecting antibodies to HIV. *Bull. W. H. O.* **69:**753–760.

359. **Van Lint, C., S. Emiliani, M. Ott, and E. Verdin.** 1996. Transcriptional activation and chromatin remodeling of the HIV-1 promoter in response to histone acetylation. *EMBO J.* **15:**1112–1120.

360. **Veazey, R. S., M. DeMaria, L. V. Chalifoux, D. E. Shvetz, D. R. Pauley, H. L. Knight, M. Rosenzweig, R. P. Johnson, R. C. Desrosiers, and A. A. Lackner.** 1998. Gastrointestinal tract as a major site of $CD4^+$ T cell depletion and viral replication in SIV infection. *Science* **280:**427–431.

361. **Vogt, M. W., D. J. Witt, D. E. Craven, R. Byington, D. F. Crawford, R. T. Schooley, and M. S. Hirsch.** 1986. Isolation of HTLV-III/LAV from cervical secretions of women at risk for AIDS. *Lancet* **i:**525–527.

362. **von Schwedler, U. K., M. Stuchell, B. Muller, D. M. Ward, H. Y. Chung, E. Morita, H. E. Wang, T. Davis, G. P. He, D. M. Cimbora, A. Scott, H. G. Krausslich, J. Kaplan, S. G. Morham, and W. I. Sundquist.** 2003. The protein network of HIV budding. *Cell* **114:**701–713.

363. **Wain-Hobson, S., P. Sonigo, O. Danos, S. Cole, and M. Alizon.** 1985. Nucleotide sequence of the AIDS virus, LAV. *Cell* **40:**9–17.

364. **Walker, B. D.** 2007. Elite control of HIV infection: implications for vaccines and treatment. *Top. HIV Med.* **15:**134–136.
365. **Walker, B. D., S. Chakrabarti, B. Moss, T. J. Paradis, T. Flynn, A. G. Durno, R. S. Blumberg, J. C. Kaplan, M. S. Hirsch, and R. T. Schooley.** 1987. HIV-specific cytotoxic T lymphocytes in seropositive individuals. *Nature* **328:**345–348.
366. **Ward, J. W., A. J. Grindon, P. M. Feorino, C. Schable, M. Parvin, and J. R. Allen.** 1986. Laboratory and epidemiologic evaluation of an enzyme immunoassay for antibodies to HTLV-III. *JAMA* **256:**357–361.
367. **Wei, P., M. E. Garber, S. M. Fang, W. H. Fischer, and K. A. Jones.** 1998. A novel CDK9-associated C-type cyclin interacts directly with HIV-1 Tat and mediates its high-affinity, loop-specific binding to TAR RNA. *Cell* **92:**451–462.
368. **Wei, X., J. M. Decker, S. Wang, H. Hui, J. C. Kappes, X. Wu, J. F. Salazar-Gonzalez, M. G. Salazar, J. M. Kilby, M. S. Saag, N. L. Komarova, M. A. Nowak, B. H. Hahn, P. D. Kwong, and G. M. Shaw.** 2003. Antibody neutralization and escape by HIV-1. *Nature* **422:**307–312.
369. **Wen, W., J. L. Meinkoth, R. Y. Tsien, and S. S. Taylor.** 1995. Identification of a signal for rapid export of proteins from the nucleus. *Cell* **82:**463–473.
370. **Weniger, B. G., Y. Takebe, C. Y. Ou, and S. Yamazaki.** 1994. The molecular epidemiology of HIV in Asia. *AIDS* **8**(Suppl. 2)**:**S13–S28.
371. **Westervelt, P., D. B. Trowbridge, L. G. Epstein, B. M. Blumberg, Y. Li, B. H. Hahn, G. M. Shaw, R. W. Price, and L. Ratner.** 1992. Macrophage tropism determinants of human immunodeficiency virus type 1 in vivo. *J. Virol.* **66:**2577–2582.
372. **Wilfert, C. M.** 2001. Prevention of mother-to-child transmission of HIV-1. *Antiviral Ther.* **6:**161–177.
373. **Willey, R. L., J. S. Bonifacino, B. J. Potts, M. A. Martin, and R. D. Klausner.** 1988. Biosynthesis, cleavage, and degradation of the human immunodeficiency virus 1 envelope glycoprotein gp160. *Proc. Natl. Acad. Sci. USA* **85:**9580–9584.
374. **Willey, R. L., F. Maldarelli, M. A. Martin, and K. Strebel.** 1992. Human immunodeficiency virus type 1 Vpu protein induces rapid degradation of CD4. *J. Virol.* **66:** 7193–7200.
375. **Winston, J. A., L. A. Bruggeman, M. D. Ross, J. Jacobson, L. Ross, V. D. D'Agati, P. E. Klotman, and M. E. Klotman.** 2001. Nephropathy and establishment of a renal reservoir of HIV type 1 during primary infection. *N. Engl. J. Med.* **344:**1979–1984.
376. **Wong, J. K., M. Hezareh, H. F. Gunthard, D. V. Havlir, C. C. Ignacio, C. A. Spina, and D. D. Richman.** 1997. Recovery of replication-competent HIV despite prolonged suppression of plasma viremia. *Science* **278:** 1291–1295.
377. **Wong, J. K., C. C. Ignacio, F. Torriani, D. Havlir, N. J. Fitch, and D. D. Richman.** 1997. In vivo compartmentalization of human immunodeficiency virus: evidence from the examination of *pol* sequences from autopsy tissues. *J. Virol.* **71:**2059–2071.
378. **Wu, A. M., and R. C. Gallo.** 1975. Reverse transcriptase. *Crit. Rev. Biochem.* **3:**289–347.
379. **Wu, L., N. P. Gerard, R. Wyatt, H. Choe, C. Parolin, N. Ruffing, A. Borsetti, A. A. Cardoso, E. Desjardin, W. Newman, C. Gerard, and J. Sodroski.** 1996. CD4-induced interaction of primary HIV-1 gp120 glycoproteins with the chemokine receptor CCR-5. *Nature* **384:** 179–183.
380. **Wyatt, R., P. D. Kwong, E. Desjardins, R. W. Sweet, J. Robinson, W. A. Hendrickson, and J. G. Sodroski.** 1998. The antigenic structure of the HIV gp120 envelope glycoprotein. *Nature* **393:**705–711.
380a. **Wyatt, R., and J. Sodroski.** 1998. The HIV-1 envelope glycoproteins: fusogens, antigens, and immunogens. *Science* **280:**1881–1888.
381. **Yang, X., M. O. Gold, D. N. Tang, D. E. Lewis, E. Guilar-Cordova, A. P. Rice, and C. H. Herrmann.** 1997. TAK, an HIV Tat-associated kinase, is a member of the cyclin-dependent family of protein kinases and is induced by activation of peripheral blood lymphocytes and differentiation of promonocytic cell lines. *Proc. Natl. Acad. Sci. USA* **94:**12331–12336.
382. **Yarchoan, R., R. W. Klecker, K. J. Weinhold, P. D. Markham, H. K. Lyerly, D. T. Durack, E. Gelmann, S. N. Lehrman, R. M. Blum, and D. W. Barry.** 1986. Administration of 3′-azido-3′-deoxythymidine, an inhibitor of HTLV-III/LAV replication, to patients with AIDS or AIDS-related complex. *Lancet* **i:**575–580.
383. **Yerly, S., L. Kaiser, T. V. Perneger, R. W. Cone, M. Opravil, J. P. Chave, H. Furrer, B. Hirschel, and L. Perrin.** 2000. Time of initiation of antiretroviral therapy: impact on HIV-1 viraemia. The Swiss HIV Cohort Study. *AIDS* **14:**243–249.
384. **Yu, H., A. E. Jetzt, Y. Ron, B. D. Preston, and J. P. Dougherty.** 1998. The nature of human immunodeficiency virus type 1 strand transfers. *J. Biol. Chem.* **273:** 28384–28391.
385. **Zennou, V., C. Petit, D. Guetard, U. Nerhbass, L. Montagnier, and P. Charneau.** 2000. HIV-1 genome nuclear import is mediated by a central DNA flap. *Cell* **101:**173–185.
386. **Zhang, H., G. Dornadula, and R. J. Pomerantz.** 1998. Natural endogenous reverse transcription of HIV-1. *J. Reprod. Immunol.* **41:**255–260.
387. **Zhang, L., T. He, Y. Huang, Z. Chen, Y. Guo, S. Wu, K. J. Kunstman, R. C. Brown, J. P. Phair, A. U. Neumann, D. D. Ho, and S. M. Wolinsky.** 1998. Chemokine coreceptor usage by diverse primary isolates of human immunodeficiency virus type 1. *J. Virol.* **72:** 9307–9312.
388. **Zhang, L., B. Ramratnam, K. Tenner-Racz, Y. He, M. Vesanen, S. Lewin, A. Talal, P. Racz, A. S. Perelson, B. T. Korber, M. Markowitz, and D. D. Ho.** 1999. Quantifying residual HIV-1 replication in patients receiving combination antiretroviral therapy. *N. Engl. J. Med.* **340:**1605–1613.
389. **Zhang, Z., T. Schuler, M. Zupancic, S. Wietgrefe, K. A. Staskus, K. A. Reimann, T. A. Reinhart, M. Rogan, W. Cavert, C. J. Miller, R. S. Veazey, D. Notermans, S. Little, S. A. Danner, D. D. Richman, D. Havlir, J. Wong, H. L. Jordan, T. W. Schacker, P. Racz, K. Tenner-Racz, N. L. Letvin, S. Wolinsky, and A. T. Haase.** 1999. Sexual transmission and propagation of SIV and HIV in resting and activated $CD4^+$ T cells. *Science* **286:**1353–1357.
390. **Zhang, Z. Q., D. W. Notermans, G. Sedgewick, W. Cavert, S. Wietgrefe, M. Zupancic, K. Gebhard, K. Henry, L. Boies, Z. Chen, M. Jenkins, R. Mills, H. McDade, C. Goodwin, C. M. Schuwirth, S. A. Danner, and A. T. Haase.** 1998. Kinetics of $CD4^+$ T cell repopulation of lymphoid tissues after treatment of HIV-1 infection. *Proc. Natl. Acad. Sci. USA* **95:**1154–1159.
391. **Zhu, P., E. Chertova, J. Bess, Jr., J. D. Lifson, L. O. Arthur, J. Liu, K. A. Taylor, and K. H. Roux.** 2003. Electron tomography analysis of envelope glycoprotein trimers on HIV and simian immunodeficiency virus virions. *Proc. Natl. Acad. Sci. USA* **100:**15812–15817.

392. **Zhu, T., B. T. Korber, A. J. Nahmias, E. Hooper, P. M. Sharp, and D. D. Ho.** 1998. An African HIV-1 sequence from 1959 and implications for the origin of the epidemic. *Nature* **391:**594–597.
393. **Zhu, T., N. Wang, A. Carr, D. S. Nam, R. Moor-Jankowski, D. A. Cooper, and D. D. Ho.** 1996. Genetic characterization of human immunodeficiency virus type 1 in blood and genital secretions: evidence for viral compartmentalization and selection during sexual transmission. *J. Virol.* **70:**3098–3107.
394. **Zink, M. C., J. P. Spelman, R. B. Robinson, and J. E. Clements.** 1998. SIV infection of macaques—modeling the progression to AIDS dementia. *J. Neurovirol.* **4:**249–259.
395. **Zuckerman, R. A., A. Lucchetti, W. L. Whittington, J. Sanchez, R. W. Coombs, R. Zuniga, A. S. Magaret, A. Wald, L. Corey, and C. Celum.** 2007. Herpes simplex virus (HSV) suppression with valacyclovir reduces rectal and blood plasma HIV-1 levels in HIV-1/HSV-2-seropositive men: a randomized, double-blind, placebo-controlled crossover trial. *J. Infect. Dis.* **196:**1500–1508.

Colorado Tick Fever Virus and Other Arthropod-Borne *Reoviridae*

STEVEN YUKL AND JOSEPH K. WONG

34

The earliest accounts of what was most likely Colorado tick fever emerged in the middle of the 19th century from settlers and mountaineers in the Rocky Mountains who termed it, along with other febrile illnesses, "mountain fever." By the time the rickettsial disease Rocky Mountain spotted fever (RMSF) was identified as a distinct entity in the first decade of the 20th century, cases of RMSF without rash were also being described, and some of these cases were likely Colorado tick fever (19, 30, 31, 88, 97). In 1930, Becker described the clinical manifestations and gave them the name Colorado tick fever (10). The clinical features and epidemiology were further characterized by Topping in 1940 (94). In 1944, Florio and colleagues reported the experimental transmission of the disease to animals and adult volunteers, thus establishing the (viral) etiology (41).

The development of viral cultures in chicken embryos and mice by Koprowski and Cox in the 1940s (56) and subsequent refinements in viral isolation and molecular biology permitted further description of Colorado tick fever virus (CTFV). Much is now known about its ecological niche and life cycle in vertebrate and invertebrate hosts as well as the epidemiology, pathogenesis, and clinical course of infection in humans (13, 17, 18, 25, 31, 32). A growing body of genetic sequence information has helped to delineate the relationship between CTFV and related viruses (3, 4, 6, 63).

VIROLOGY

Classification

Three genera of arthropod-transmitted viral agents of medical importance have been identified within the family *Reoviridae: Orbivirus, Coltivirus*, and the new genus *Seadornavirus* (Southeast Asian dodeca-RNA virus). Although all were previously included in the same genus (*Orbivirus*), recognition of the fundamental difference in their genome structure (10 double-stranded RNA [dsRNA] segments in orbiviruses, versus 12 dsRNA segments in coltiviruses and seadornaviruses) and other genetic attributes have prompted the current classification (43, 49–51, 54, 76). Species designations of members of each genus have been based on analysis of electropherotypes, RNA cross-hybridization assays, RNA sequence analysis, serologic reactivity, and the ability to reassort and produce viable progeny in coinfection experiments (63).

CTFV is the type species of the genus *Coltivirus* (after Colorado tick fever). A number of other coltiviruses have been isolated and partially characterized and identified to species level. Eyach virus (EYAV) has been isolated from *Ixodes ricinus* and *Ixodes ventalloi* ticks in central Europe (22, 82). In a serologic survey of patients with meningoencephalitis and polyradiculitis in the former Czechoslovakia, 10 and 20% (respectively) had demonstrable antibody to EYAV, but a definite causal relationship remains to be proven (62). A coltivirus isolated from *Lepus californicus* hares in an area of northern California (outside the territory of *Dermacentor andersoni*) has been designated S6-14-03 virus (58, 76). Although this isolate has not been proven to cause human disease, it has been postulated to be responsible for Colorado tick fever-like human infection in California (98). A coltivirus dubbed Salmon River tick fever virus was isolated from a patient in Idaho with an illness similar to Colorado tick fever (71, 98). Whether this represents an antigenic variant of CTFV or a unique virus remains to be determined. CTFV, EYAV, and S6-14-03 have been fully or partially sequenced. Nucleotide sequence homologies among CTFVs range from 90 to 100% for conserved segments such as genome segment 12, while homologies between CTFV and EYAV isolates range from 53 to 58% in this segment. These viruses constitute the *Coltivirus* genus (3, 4, 6).

Previously grouped within the genus *Coltivirus*, the *Seadornavirus* genus comprises a distinct group of arthropod-borne agents in East Asia (4, 6, 63) (Fig. 1). The current taxonomy recognizes three distinct species: (i) the type species, Banna virus (BAV); (ii) Kadipiro virus; and (iii) Liao Ning virus. The pathogenic potential of these viruses in humans remains to be determined, although associations of BAV infection with febrile illnesses and encephalitis are convincing. Seadornaviruses are serologically distinct from CTFV and EYAV, have a lower G+C content than coltiviruses (37 to 39%, versus 48 to 52%), and show genetic distances in the RNA-dependent RNA polymerase of more than 90% compared to coltiviruses. Phylogenetic reconstructions based on sequences from the RNA-dependent RNA polymerase suggest that seadornaviruses are more closely related to rotaviruses than to other members of the *Reoviridae*. Furthermore, structural studies demonstrate

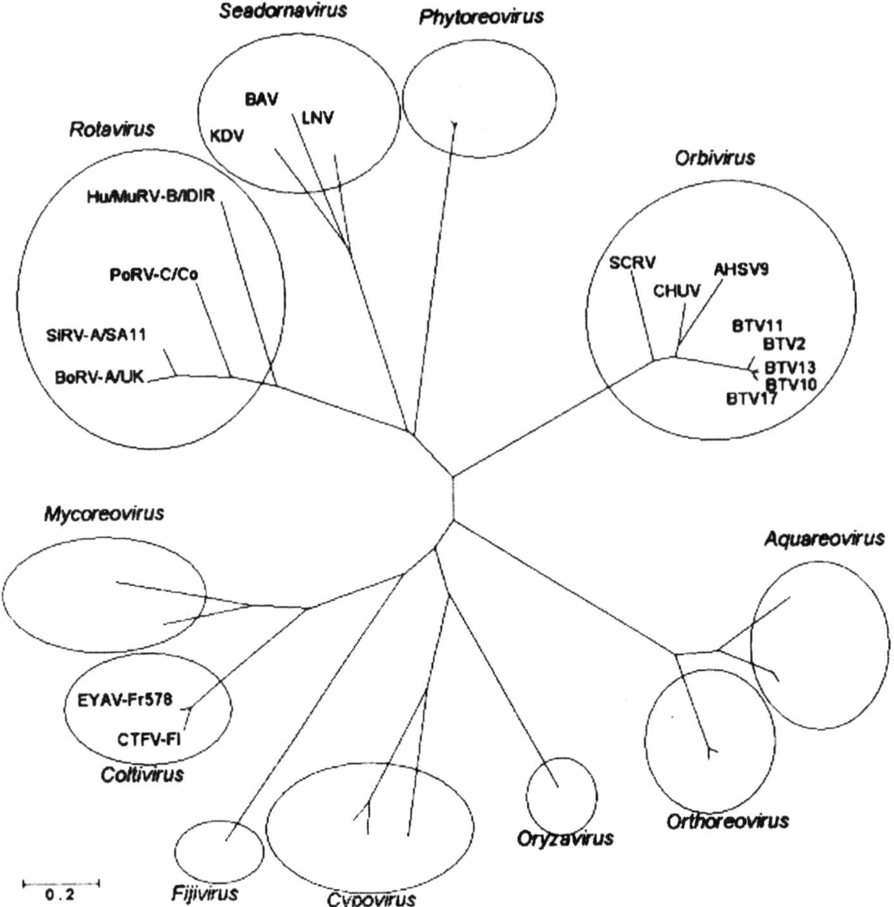

FIGURE 1 Phylogenetic relationship between members of *Coltivirus*, *Seadornavirus*, and *Orbivirus* with other *Reoviridae*, based on analysis of partial polymerase sequence. Each forms a distinct sequence cluster. Seadornaviruses appear to be most closely related to rotaviruses. KDV, Kadipiro virus; LNV, Liao Ning virus; SCRV, St. Croix River virus; AHSV, African horse sickness virus; CHUV, Chuzan virus; BTV, bluetongue virus; BoRV, bovine rotavirus; SiRV, simian rotavirus; PoRV, porcine rotavirus; Hu/MuRV, human/murine rotavirus. (Reprinted from reference 7 with permission.)

similarities between BAV proteins and those of rotavirus. The BAV outer capsid viral protein 9 (VP9) has homology to the rotavirus receptor binding protein VP8, and there are additional similarities between BAV VP10 and the VP5 domain of rotavirus VP4 (70).

At present, there are 21 recognized orbiviral species comprising over 200 identified serotypes, as well as a number of as-yet-unclassified viruses (50, 63). The best-studied members of the genus *Orbivirus* are a number of veterinary pathogens, including bluetongue virus and African horse sickness virus, but several other groups within the genus (including Changuinola, Kemerovo, Lebombo, and Orungo) appear to be capable of infecting humans and causing disease. In the southwestern United States, orbiviral infection with an agent(s) related to the Kemerovo-Lipovnik serogroup of the Great Island virus species or the Sixgun City virus (Chenuda virus species) is suspected to be the cause of an acute febrile illness characterized by myalgia, abdominal pain, vomiting, and pancytopenia (63, 97, 98). It seems quite likely that additional members of the *Coltivirus* and *Seadornavirus* genera will be identified in the future (71).

Composition and Biology

CTFV particles consist of nonenveloped double capsid structures with icosahedral symmetry and an outer capsid diameter of approximately 80 nm. The capsid is smoother than that of orbivirus particles, with less prominent surface projections (Fig. 2). BAV has a structure more similar to that of rotaviruses, with protein fibers extending from the surface (70). Though CTFV does not acquire an envelope, electron microscopic (EM) studies frequently demonstrate association of viral particles with membrane (74–76, 78).

The genome of all members of the *Reoviridae* consists of segmented dsRNA. Orbiviruses contain 10 segments, rotaviruses contain 11 segments, and coltiviruses and seadornaviruses contain 12 segments ranging in approximate molecular mass from 0.24×10^6 to 2.53×10^6 (approximately 0.35 to 3.7 kbp). The 29-kB genome of CTFV is the longest of any genome in *Reoviridae* characterized to date (3), while *Seadornavirus* genomes average 21 kB. If the genetic organization conforms to that of the other *Reoviridae*, each segment should encode a monocistronic message and gene product (46, 54, 55, 76, 83). However, genome segment 9 of CTFV produces two different pro-

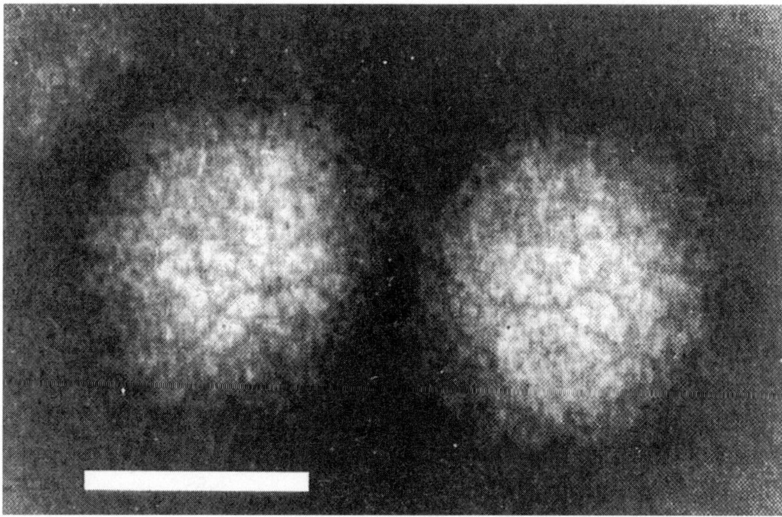

FIGURE 2 Negative-contrast electron micrograph of CTFV virions. The bar represents 50 nm. (Reprinted from reference 76 with permission of Elsevier.)

teins through the use of a functionally "leaky" stop codon, allowing translation of both a truncated protein (VP9, a structural protein) and a longer, read-through protein (VP9′) (67).

Comparatively more is known about the gene products of orbiviruses and seadornaviruses than of CTFV. BAV (the prototype seadornavirus) has seven structural proteins. VP4 and VP9 form the outer capsid, while VP1, VP2, VP3, VP8, and VP10 form an inner core with a smoother surface (70). VP9 is involved in binding to the cell surface and may play a role in internalization (65). VP3 has guanyltransferase activity (69).

As stated above, less is known about the gene products of CTFV. VP1 of CTFV has sequence homology to and includes signature motifs characteristic of the RNA-dependent RNA polymerases of other reoviruses (3). Putative functions of other CTFV genes and their orbiviral homologs have been described previously (Table 1).

The natural segmentation of the genome of *Reoviridae* allows reassortment, as has been shown to occur by comparative studies of CTFV isolates acquired from the same location at different times. The adaptive advantage of this ability to reassort presumably outweighs the inherent cost of maintaining this segmented organization, both by permitting the generation of a larger number of potentially advantageous variants (positive selection) and by allowing salvage of portions of genomes that have suffered deleterious mutations owing to the inherent infidelity of RNA genome replication (purifying selection) (21).

Some genetic variability has also been demonstrated by differential polyacrylamide gel electrophoresis mobility of some of the RNA segments from different isolates obtained simultaneously from one location (15). Antigenic variation of CTFV is demonstrable by serum cross-neutralization studies (53). However, there is relative conservation of CTFV sequences based on RNA-RNA hybridization under conditions that allow hybridization with as low as 74% homology (12). A more complete understanding of the degree and role of genetic heterogeneity in the biology of CTFV awaits thorough characterization of individual gene products and comparative sequence data.

Of note, recent studies on bluetongue virus have shown that the endocytic pathway is important to viral entry of orbiviruses and that completion of the infectious cycle necessitates exposure to relatively low pH conditions (42). It is not known whether coltiviruses and seadornaviruses share similar entry requirements, but the observed similarities between the receptor binding proteins of BAV and bluetongue virus suggest that this may be the case (70).

Orbiviruses, coltiviruses, and seadornaviruses are all rendered noninfectious at a pH of 3. Unlike the orbiviruses, coltiviruses are relatively sensitive to treatment with deoxycholate, although with rare exception, members of each genus are relatively resistant to ether and other solvents (76, 96).

EPIDEMIOLOGY AND ECOLOGY

The geographic distribution of Colorado tick fever, which is defined by the distribution of the arthropod and vertebrate hosts for CTFV, consists of mountainous and highland areas at altitudes between 4,000 and 10,000 ft (1,000 to 2,500 m) in the western United States and southwestern Canada (Fig. 3) (32, 97). Because reporting of cases is not required, the several hundred cases reported annually likely underestimate the true annual incidence by a factor of 10 or more (25, 71, 88). As an example, the recent declassification of Colorado tick fever as a reportable disease in Colorado has resulted in an apparent but misleading decline in disease incidence in that state (http://www.cdphe.state.co.us/dc/zoonosis.asp) (J. Poppy, personal communication, 2001).

Cases occur between March and October, with 90% of cases occurring between May and September (Fig. 4) (32, 45). This seasonal distribution probably reflects the heightened numbers and activity of the arthropod vector *Dermacentor andersoni* (wood tick) and its natural vertebrate hosts (including the golden-mantled ground squirrel, Columbian ground squirrel, yellow pine chipmunk, and least chipmunk), as well as the greater exposure of human hosts participating in occupational and recreational activities during the summer months. Ticks are particularly numer-

TABLE 1 Coding organization of *Coltivirus*, *Seadornavirus*, and *Orbivirus* segments[a,b]

Coltivirus		Function	Seadornavirus		Orbivirus (BTV)	Function
CTFV	EYAV		BAV	KAV		
VP1	VP1	**RNA-dependent RNA polymerase**	VP1	VP1	VP1	**RNA-dependent RNA polymerase**
VP2	VP2	**Capping enzyme—guanylyltransferase**	VP3	VP3	VP4	**Capping enzyme—guanylyltransferase**
VP3	VP3	**RNA replication factor**			VP3	(Core)
VP4	VP4	*Unknown*/(outer coat)	VP4	VP4	VP2,VP5	(Outer capsid)
VP5	VP5	*Unknown*/(NS)	VP5	VP6		
VP6	VP7	**Nucleotide binding, NTPase**	VP6, VP2	VP5, VP2	VP6	(Inner core, binds ssRNA, dsRNA)
VP7	VP6	*RNA replication factor* (NS)	VP11	VP12		
VP8	VP8	*Unknown* (core)	VP8	VP9	VP7	(Core)
VP9	VP9	*Structural and NS* (core)	VP10	VP10	VP8	(Core)
VP10	VP10	**Kinase**	VP7	VP7	NS1	(NS, tubules)
VP11	VP11	*Unknown* (cell attachment)	VP9	VP11	NS2	(NS, binds ssRNA)
VP12	VP12	*RNA replication factor* (dsRNA binding)	VP12	VP8	NS3	(Virus budding)

[a] Adapted from references 7 and 83a.
[b] Coltivirus functions shared by homologous segment of *Seadornavirus* and/or *Orbivirus* are listed in bold type. When the putative function of a segment from *Coltivirus* does not coincide with the function in *Seadornavirus*, the function in *Coltivirus* is italicized and the function in *Seadornavirus* is in parentheses. Functions of *Coltivirus* and *Seadornavirus* genetic segments are shown in column 3; *Orbivirus* genetic segments are shown in column 7. KAV, Kadipiro virus; BTV, bluetongue virus; NS, nonstructural; ssRNA, single-stranded RNA.

ous in grassy and low-brush areas, on south-facing slopes, and near streams (29, 32, 97).

The preponderance of males between the ages of 15 and 40 among reported cases of Colorado tick fever does not stem from increased susceptibility but, rather, reflects the greater likelihood of exposure of this population to the vector carrying CTFV. There is no difference in likelihood of infection based on age or sex in populations when normalized for exposure (31, 45).

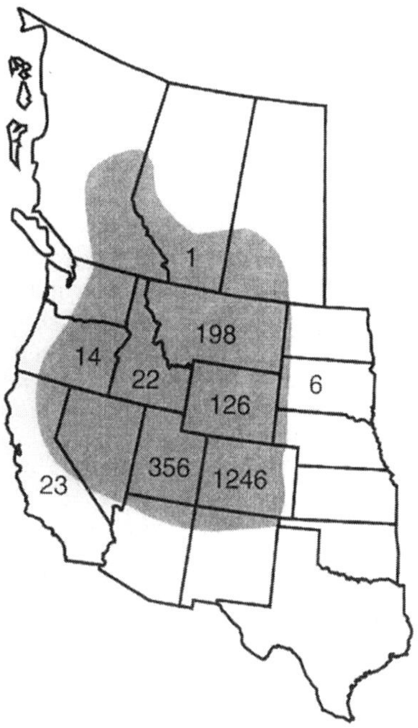

FIGURE 3 Distribution of *Dermacentor andersoni* ticks (shaded area) and numbers of cases of Colorado tick fever from 1990 to 1996. (Modified from reference 98 with permission of Elsevier.)

Although CTFV has been isolated from several tick species, *D. andersoni* has been the only species demonstrated to transmit disease to humans (31). However, it has been postulated that *Dermacentor variabilis* may transmit CTFV or the Colorado tick fever-related virus (S6-14-03) in regions of California that lie outside the area of distribution of *D. andersoni* (98). The life span of *D. andersoni* has been reported to be as long as 3 years, and once this species is infected, it remains so for life. Acquisition of infection can occur in the larval, nymphal, or adult stage with transstadial persistence, but transovarial transmission does not occur. Hence, passage of CTFV between generations of ticks requires an intermediate reservoir provided by the small mammalian hosts. These natural mammalian hosts develop subclinical infections followed by persistent viremia lasting weeks to months. Hibernating animals appear to sustain viremia for longer periods; this may be one mechanism that allows CTFV to survive the winter and to initiate a new cycle of infection when fed upon by larval and nymphal ticks in the spring and summer. The virus titer in an infected adult tick of 10^2 to 10^5 mouse 50% lethal doses/ml (homogenized tissue) can be maintained for up to a year. Transmission to humans or animals occurs by transfer of virus in saliva during feeding. Mature adult ticks prefer blood meals from large animals such as deer, elk, porcupines, and, occasionally, humans (25, 31, 71, 97). Human-to-human transmission can occur during the viremic phase of illness, and there has been at least one documented case of transfusion-related Colorado tick fever (81).

PATHOGENESIS

Organ and Cellular Pathology

EM studies of cultured cells following infection reveal viral particles in association with granular matrices within the

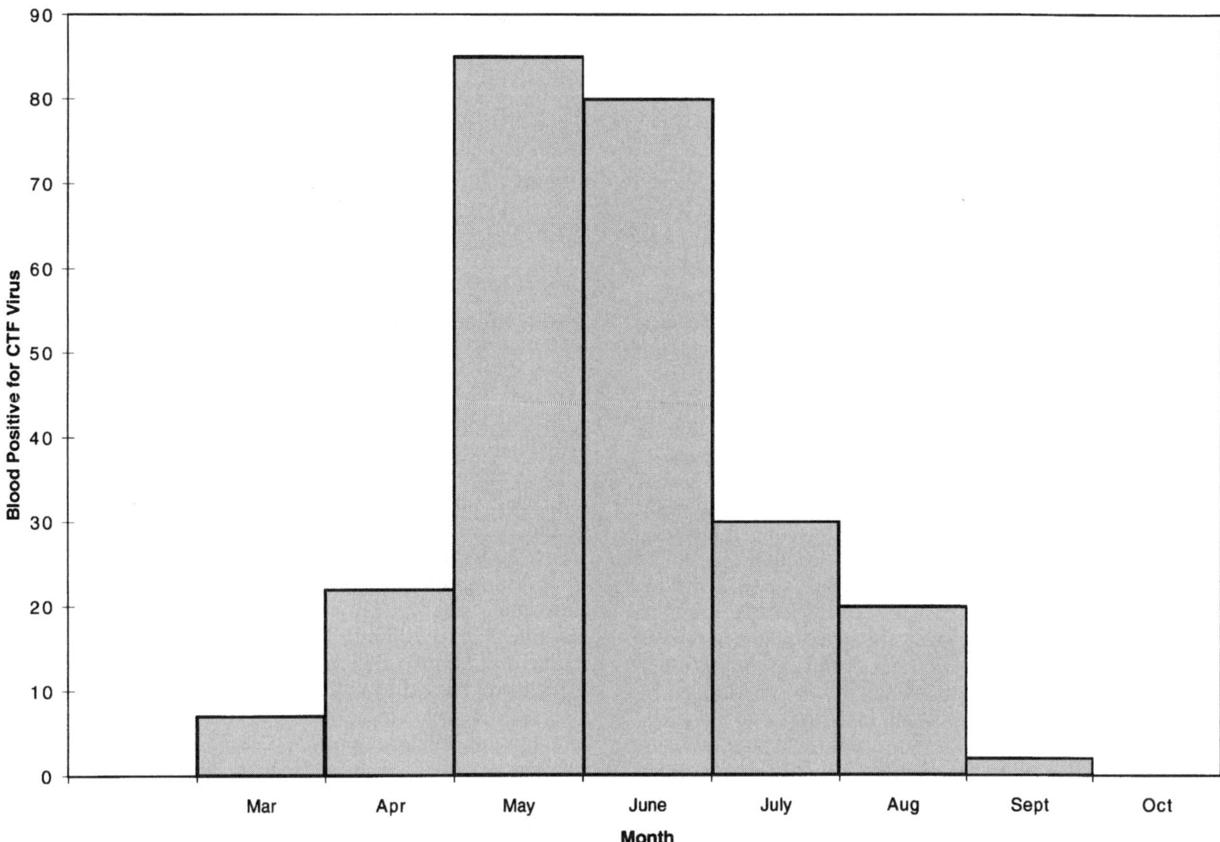

FIGURE 4 Frequency distribution, by month, of confirmed illness due to CTFV in Colorado during 1973 and 1974. (Modified from reference 45 with permission.)

cytoplasm. Filamentous arrays are also seen lying in parallel bundles, both in the cytoplasm and in the nucleus (nuclear filaments are not seen with other reovirus infections). In late stages of infection, the matrices become larger and viral particles become more numerous, but the viral particles are still contained within cells. There is no evidence for release of virus until cells undergo dissolution. EM of neurons infected in vivo fail to demonstrate a comparable cytopathic effect (7, 74, 75, 78).

The tropism of CTFV for hematopoietic cells is demonstrated by the ability to detect viral antigen within erythrocytes by various methods (virus isolation, histochemical staining, fluorescent-antibody [FA] staining, and EM) long after the acute phase of infection (13, 35, 45, 77). Since CTFV antigens are intracellular and not found on the erythrocyte surface, the virus may be shielded from immune clearance by neutralizing antibody throughout the natural life span of the erythrocyte. CTFV is able to infect and replicate within human hematopoietic progenitor cell lines, thus providing not only an explanation for the intraerythrocytic persistence but also a possible explanation for the frequently encountered leukopenia and thrombocytopenia (79). This pathology could be either due to a direct cytopathic effect on infected stem cells as they differentiate toward these cell lineages or a consequence of host immune clearance of those infected cells capable of displaying viral antigen. In patients infected with CTFV, mononuclear cells are also less able to produce colony-stimulating factors, and a circulating inhibitory factor (possibly lactoferrins or interferon) can be demonstrated in patient sera (1).

Only three deaths have been attributed to Colorado tick fever, all in children. Autopsies of two patients, both of whom died from bleeding diatheses, reported purpura and cutaneous petechiae. Hyaline membrane disease, encephalitis, and swollen endothelial cells were described to occur in a 4-year-old boy. A 10-year-old girl had disseminated intravascular coagulation with focal necrosis involving the brain, liver, spleen, heart, and intestinal tract (26, 30). Studies on suckling mice and hamsters have disclosed similar histopathological findings (47, 64).

Immune Response

High levels of alpha interferon can be detected in a majority of Colorado tick fever patients during the first 10 days of infection. These levels appear to correlate with fever but not with other clinical parameters (2). One-third of patients develop detectable neutralizing antibody titers within 10 days of onset of symptoms. By 30 days, more than 90% are antibody positive, but nearly half of all patients continue to have detectable viremia by either indirect FA assay or viral culture (presumably due to intraerythrocytic persistence) (45). It is not known whether other immune mechanisms are involved in viral clearance.

Convalescence is accompanied by lasting immunity against reinfection. Only a single case has been reported of a patient experiencing either relapse or reinfection a year after her initial infection. Interestingly, the second episode was accompanied by loss of previously demonstrated neutralizing antibody titers (45). Experimental rechallenge of immune subjects with CTFV failed to produce clinical disease (with the exception of several hours of headache in some of the subjects) (41).

CLINICAL MANIFESTATIONS

Individuals with Colorado tick fever typically have a history of tick attachment or exposure (>90%) and residence or travel within areas of endemicity. Following an incubation period of 3 to 5 days (range, 1 to 14 days), fever is noted along with malaise, headache, myalgias, and gastrointestinal upset (Table 2). In approximately half of all cases a characteristic "saddleback" fever pattern is seen. This consists of 2 to 3 days of fever, followed by an afebrile period of up to several days, followed by return of fever for 2 to 3 days. Rarely, this can be followed by yet another febrile period. Thereafter, most patients recover without sequelae, although some have reported prolonged lassitude lasting weeks to months. It is likely that mild or subclinical infection occurs but has been underrepresented in the literature (30, 31, 45).

Physical examination during the acute phase of disease can reveal altered sensorium, neck stiffness, photophobia, mild conjunctivitis, and, occasionally, lymphadenopathy and splenomegaly. Rash is seen in a minority of cases. When present, it appears as faint, fine macules or maculopapules on the trunk or, at times, the extremities (45). Hemorrhagic diatheses with attendant petechiae, particularly in those under age 10, have been attributed to thrombocytopenia and, in at least one case report, to frank disseminated intravascular coagulation (DIC) (26, 30). Central nervous system (CNS) involvement can range from self-limited meningitis to encephalitis with coma and death (2, 88). Other reported complications have included hepatitis, epididymo-orchitis, pericarditis, myocarditis, and pneumonitis (28, 36, 48, 61, 81). Rare deaths have been attributed to bleeding or CNS complications (26, 30, 88).

There have been occasional reports of Colorado tick fever acquired by women during pregnancy, including one case of abortion 2 weeks after infection, one case of multiple congenital abnormalities in a mother infected in the first trimester (Colorado tick fever was thought not to be causal), and a case of apparent perinatal transmission with self-limited disease in the neonate (13, 30). No published reports describe the course of Colorado tick fever in human immunodeficiency virus-infected or other immunocompromised hosts, although one clinical review reports that immunocompromised individuals may be at risk for more severe disease (14).

Laboratory Findings

The most characteristic routine laboratory feature is a moderate leukopenia, of 2,000 to 4,000 leukocytes/mm^3 or less, with a relative lymphocytosis (approximately 60% of patients). Other findings can include a "left shift" (at times with the appearance of metamyelocytes and even myelocytes) and toxic granulation. Thrombocytopenia can occur with or without DIC. Anemia (usually mild) may be present, but hemolysis is not a typical feature in the absence of DIC. There can be mild elevations of hepatic transaminases and creatine phosphokinase (25, 31, 45, 55, 71).

Mild to moderate cerebrospinal fluid (CSF) pleocytosis can occur, usually with a lymphocyte predominance (typical range, 0 to 500 mm^3), although there is a single case report of Colorado tick fever meningoencephalitis with a CSF leukocyte count of 1,578 and 89% neutrophils. CSF glucose has ranged from 40 mg/dl to normal and CSF protein has ranged from normal to 170 mg/dl in Colorado tick fever patients with meningoencephalitis (28, 38).

Differential Diagnosis

Consideration of a diagnosis of Colorado tick fever must depend largely on epidemiological features. Because ticks can transmit a number of other infectious diseases, the differential diagnosis includes tularemia, RMSF, ehrlichiosis, Lyme disease, and tick-borne relapsing fever. Although the vectors for relapsing fever (*Ornithodoros* spp.), ehrlichiosis (*Dermacentor variabilis*, *Amblyomma* spp., and *Ixodes* spp.) and Lyme disease (*Ixodes* spp.) are different from the principal vector transmitting CTFV to humans, this distinction is often not made by patients or health care providers (32, 87, 97). Colorado tick fever must also be distinguished

TABLE 2 Symptom frequency in 320 patients suspected of having Colorado tick fever in Colorado for the years 1973 and 1974[a]

Symptom	% Positive for CTFV (n = 222)	% Negative for CTFV (n = 98)
Fever	97	97
Headache	88	87
Myalgia	79	74
Lethargy	61	63
Abdominal pain[b]	21	33
Vomiting	24	24
Stiff neck	18	26
Sore throat[c]	19	34
Diarrhea	5	8
Skin rash	5	16
Bleeding	0	2
Petechiae	1	5
Vertigo	5	0

[a] Modified from reference 45 with permission.
[b] Differences statistically significant ($P < 0.05$).
[c] Differences statistically significant ($P < 0.01$).

from a number of other viral diseases, in particular those caused by the enteroviruses (because of the similar seasonal association). Distinguishing Colorado tick fever from RMSF can be difficult early in the course of disease. However, the typical improvement after 2 to 3 days, the possible appearance of the relapsing-fever pattern, the relative leukopenia, and the failure of the rash to evolve to a purpuric/petechial nature (as is seen with the vasculitic process of RMSF) would all point away from the diagnosis of RMSF (19, 25, 31, 32, 71, 87, 97).

The distributions of human monocytotropic ehrlichiosis (HME), caused by *Ehrlichia chaffeensis*, and human granulocytic ehrlichiosis (HGE), caused by *Ehrlichia phagocytophila*, overlap only marginally with that of Colorado tick fever (27, 40, 44). *E. chaffeensis* is concentrated in the southeastern and south central United States, with sporadic cases reported from the Rocky Mountain and western states, consistent with the distribution of *Amblyomma americanum* (the Lone Star tick) in the southeast and south central United States and *Dermacentor variabilis* in the western United States (37, 101). HGE has been predominantly described in the upper Midwest (Minnesota and Wisconsin), Northeast (New York and Massachusetts), and, more recently, northern California, conforming to the geographic distribution of the *Ixodes* tick vectors (8, 9, 20, 91, 101). Nevertheless, it seems prudent that these two tick-borne "emerging" diseases should remain in the differential diagnosis of suspected Colorado tick fever patients, especially those with severe disease. In particular, the cytopenias seen with HGE and severe cases of HME might be confused with that of Colorado tick fever.

LABORATORY DIAGNOSIS

Specific diagnosis of CTFV can be made by (i) viral isolation, (ii) demonstration of viral antigens, (iii) serology, or (iv) PCR-based detection of viral nucleic acids. Although CTFV can be cultured directly (in Vero or BHK-21 cells), the most sensitive method of isolation is intracerebral or intraperitoneal inoculation of blood clot suspensions or erythrocytes into suckling mice. The mice sicken and die 4 to 8 days after inoculation. Specific isolation is confirmed by FA staining of smears of mouse brain or blood or by cell culture. The blood clot intended for virus isolation should be stored refrigerated but not frozen. Typically, such procedures are available only through reference laboratories. When available, a source tick can be retained for species identification and virus isolation.

A more rapid, albeit less sensitive (60 to 70% compared with culture), approach to specific diagnosis is by direct immunofluorescence staining of blood smears for the presence of viral antigen (25, 31, 32, 55, 71, 97). Though diagnostic yield by either isolation or direct demonstration of antigen is greatest during the acute phase of disease, viremia is at times detectable well into the period of convalescence (45). Nearly 50% of patients are culture positive after 4 weeks and 5 to 17% are culture positive up to 12 weeks after onset of clinical symptoms. Antigen is detectable in erythrocytes by direct FA assay in nearly 10% of patients as long as 20 weeks after onset of symptoms. There is no apparent relationship between the persistence of viremia and the duration of symptoms.

Paired acute- and convalescent-phase sera can be assayed for antibody titer in a variety of ways, including complement fixation (CF), indirect FA assay, enzyme-linked immunosorbent assay (ELISA), and an assay for neutralizing antibody measuring plaque reduction. CF antibodies may appear relatively late, whereas neutralizing antibodies are typically detectable from 14 to 21 days after onset of symptoms. Immunoglobulin M detectable by ELISA appears at about or slightly before neutralizing antibody but declines abruptly after 6 weeks (25, 31–34, 55, 71, 97). A recent ELISA for immunoglobulin M using synthetic antigens and a separate Western blot analysis may be more sensitive than earlier ELISA systems for diagnosis but will require validation (5). Different ELISAs are also available for EYAV (using VP6) and BAV (using VP9) (66, 68).

Molecular diagnosis based on reverse transcription-PCR (RT-PCR) of RNA isolated from cell-free plasma or erythrocytes has been investigated for Colorado tick fever (5, 52). These methods appear to be comparable to or slightly more sensitive than viral isolation in the first week following infection but have the important advantage of providing rapid results and do not require the highly specialized reagents needed for virus isolation and identification. They should be superior to serologic assays for diagnosis in acute infection. However, these methods have only been applied to a limited number of viral isolates and retrospectively collected clinical samples and have not been prospectively tested except on experimentally infected animals (5). Furthermore, assays vary in sensitivity depending on virus strain, presumably due to sequence variation (52), although recent RT-PCR assays appear to be capable of detecting a single genome and are at least 10 times more sensitive than standard plaque assays (5, 57). The utility and validity of these assays should increase when more complete sequence data become available from additional clinical viral isolates, permitting further assay refinement. Such approaches that permit early diagnosis are needed because the most important diagnostic and therapeutic decisions are faced during acute infection, when clinical distinction from RMSF and other potentially more serious tick-borne diseases is most challenging. Microarrays that have been developed to simultaneously screen for multiple viral pathogens currently include probes for *Coltivirus* and *Seadornavirus* (102).

PREVENTION

Individuals should be educated and encouraged to take preventive measures when outdoors in areas of endemicity during the late spring and summer months. Wearing long-sleeved shirts and light-colored clothing, frequent self-inspection for ticks, and use of repellents such as DEET (*N*,*N*-diethyl-*m*-toluamide) or permethrin (only for treatment of clothing or bedding) should be advised (31, 32, 55, 97).

Patients recovering from Colorado tick fever should not donate blood for a period of at least 6 months because of the intraerythrocytic persistence of virus.

In the 1960s, a Colorado tick fever vaccine was developed using formalinized infected murine brain extracts. This vaccine elicits a neutralizing antibody response, but because of the modest morbidity of natural infection, the vaccination program has since been abandoned (92).

TREATMENT

The typical, uncomplicated case of Colorado tick fever requires no specific therapy. Reassurance, analgesics, and an-

TABLE 3 Orbiviruses that naturally infect humans[a]

Characteristic	Changuinola virus	Kemerovo virus[b]	Oklahoma tick fever virus[c]	Lebombo virus	Orungo virus
Geographic distribution	Panama	Russia and Eastern Europe	Oklahoma and Texas	Nigeria and South Africa	Western and central Africa
Insect vectors	Phlebotamine flies	*Ixodes* ticks	Ticks (presumed)	*Aedes* and *Mansonia* mosquitoes	*Aedes*, *Anopheles*, and *Culex* mosquitoes
Reported clinical syndromes	Self-limited febrile illness in one adult	Fever, encephalitis, ?polyradiculitis	Fever, pancytopenia	Fever in one child	Fever, headache, myalgias, nausea, and vomiting (diarrhea, flaccid paralysis, seizures, normal routine CSF parameters in one child)
Specific diagnosis[d]	Rise in serologic titer; viral isolation in i.c.[e]-inoculated suckling mice, plaques in Vero and LLC-MK2 cell cultures	Rise in serologic titer; viral isolation in i.c.-inoculated newborn mice, hamsters, chicken embryos; plaques in primary chicken embryo, Vero, and BHK-21 cell cultures	Rise in serologic titer; viral isolation yet to be successful	Rise in serologic titer; viral isolation in i.c.-inoculated suckling mice, plaques in Vero and LLC-MK2 cell cultures	Rise in serologic titers; viral isolation in i.c.-inoculated suckling and weanling mice, plaques in Vero and BHK-21 cell cultures

[a] Data from references 22, 24, 46, 63, 84, 97, and 100.
[b] The Kemerovo serogroup includes Kemerovo, Tribec, and Lipovnik viruses as well as 33 other serotypes that are not known to be pathogenic for humans.
[c] Serologically related to the Kemerovo serogroup of Great Island virus and the Sixgun City serotype of Chenuda virus.
[d] Reagents to assay for various combinations of CF antibodies, neutralizing antibodies, and indirect FA assay are available at only a limited number of reference laboratories. Suspected cases can be referred to Division of Vector-Borne Infectious Diseases, CDC, Fort Collins, CO; R. Shope, University of Texas, Medical Branch, Galveston; or U.S. Army Medical Research Institute for Infectious Diseases, Ft. Detrick, MD.
[e] i.c., intracerebrally.

tipyretics can be given, with the caveat that aspirin and other nonsteroidal anti-inflammatory drugs with antiplatelet activities should be avoided (particularly in children) because of the occurrence of thrombocytopenia (25, 31, 32, 45, 55, 71).

In vitro activity against CTFV has been demonstrated for ribavirin, 3-deazaguanine, and, to a lesser extent, 3-deazauridine (MICs of 3.2, 3.2, and 32 μg/ml, respectively, in MA-104 cells and MICs of 32, 3.2, and 10 to 100 μg/ml, respectively, in Vero cells). In mice inoculated intracerebrally with CTFV, intracerebral or intraperitoneal ribavirin triacetate (but not ribavirin) reduced the mortality rate, while intracerebral 3-deazaguanine increased the mean survival time (84, 85). However, no experience with humans has been published. At present, no specific antiviral therapy exists for Colorado tick fever.

SEADORNAVIRUSES

BAV (23, 59) was first isolated from the CSF and blood of patients with febrile syndromes and encephalitis (98, 103) as well as from mosquitoes (23, 86, 98) in southern and western China in 1987. Numerous additional isolates have since been reported from patients in China and Indonesia. Insect vectors for BAV include *Anopheles*, *Aedes*, and *Culex* mosquitoes. Viral sequences with similarity to BAV have also been found in cattle and pigs (90), suggesting a potential role for livestock as an animal reservoir. BAV is currently classified as a pathogen requiring biosafety level 3 laboratory containment and is the only species of the genus to be isolated from humans (7). BAV is endemic in areas of tropical and subtropical Asia that overlap with Japanese encephalitis virus and dengue virus, so it is likely that infection with BAV may be underestimated. Indeed, recent retrospective surveys of serum from Chinese patients with suspected Japanese encephalitis and other encephalitic syndromes suggest BAV infection in 8 to 12%. No specific treatment exists for BAV infection.

Kadipiro virus and Liao Ning virus are serologically distinct seadornaviruses that have also been obtained from mosquitoes in Indonesia and China (23, 86, 98). Sequence comparisons of the viral polymerase gene show homology ranging from 24 to 42%. However, these viruses have not been isolated from humans. Liao Ning virus is the only species of *Seadornavirus* that is able to replicate in a variety of mammalian cell lines and is also able to establish pathogenic infection in adult mice (11). A serologic assay for antibody to VP9 antigen (the outer coat protein) of BAV has been developed, as have RT-PCR assays for BAV and Kadipiro virus.

ORBIVIRUSES AND HUMAN DISEASE

The name *Orbivirus* derives from the appearance of virus particles as large, doughnut-shaped capsomeres by negative-contrast EM (orbi from Latin *orbis*, meaning "ring"). Though the most-studied orbiviruses are agents of veterinary import, a number of serogroups within the genus cause human disease (55, 76). They are predominantly transmitted by arthropod vectors (ticks, gnats, midges, and mosquitoes).

Changuinola virus was first isolated from a man in Panama experiencing a self-limited febrile illness. Serologic surveys in the area verify human exposure, but the frequency of clinical disease is unknown. The virus can be isolated from phlebotamine flies (55, 95). The Kemerovo serogroup includes at least three tick-borne serotypes (Kemerovo, Tribec, and Lipovnik) of the *Great Island virus* genus that have been implicated as agents causing febrile illness and CNS infection in Russia and eastern Europe (24, 55, 60, 62). Serologic evidence of infection with a virus related to Lipovnik and Sixgun City viruses (a serotype of the Chenuda virus) was found in several patients from Texas and Oklahoma who were hospitalized with febrile illnesses associated with tick exposure and various degrees of transient leukopenia, thrombocytopenia, and anemia. The etiologic agent(s) has not been successfully isolated (97, 99). The clinical syndrome has been given the name Oklahoma tick fever. Orungo virus has a wide geographic distribution in western and central Africa (55, 93). The principal vector is *Aedes* mosquitoes (though it is also isolated from *Anopheles* and *Culex*). The epidemiology of infection with Orungo virus therefore parallels that of yellow fever, and serologic surveys done during outbreaks of yellow fever demonstrate a high incidence of apparent coinfection with Orungo virus (72). In these studies, the contribution of Orungo virus to clinical illness was thought (understandably) to be small relative to that of yellow fever virus, but Orungo virus has been incriminated in febrile syndromes independent of yellow fever (38), and in at least one case it has been associated with CNS complications (39, 55). Lebombo virus has been isolated from a febrile Nigerian child and from *Aedes* and *Mansonia* mosquitoes in Nigeria and South Africa (55, 73). Lebombo and Orungo viruses are distinct serologically and by RNA-RNA hybridization and genetic reassortment studies (16).

Over several years in the 1980s, four laboratory workers in a South African veterinary vaccine packaging plant were apparently infected with neurotropic attenuated strains of African horse sickness virus (89, 100). Three of the four cases included fronto-temporal encephalitis, and all four had evidence of uveochorioretinitis. The diagnosis was made based on specific serologic studies (CF, enzyme immunoassay, and neutralizing antibody) and the serologic exclusion of a battery of other viral and nonviral entities, including herpes simplex virus (though two of the four received 10-day courses of acyclovir) and Rift Valley fever virus. Several other laboratory workers demonstrated antibody to African horse sickness virus without overt clinical symptoms. The mode of acquisition was thought to be inhalation of lyophilized virus in laboratory accidents. Despite episodic outbreaks of African horse sickness virus and bluetongue virus around the world, natural human infection has not been reported.

Table 3 summarizes some of the clinical aspects of these naturally acquired human orbiviral diseases. As with coltiviruses and seadornaviruses, we are likely to encounter many more orbiviruses that have the capacity to cause human disease.

REFERENCES

1. **Andersen, R. D., M. A. Entringer, and W. A. Robinson.** 1985. Virus-induced leukopenia: Colorado tick fever as a human model. *J. Infect. Dis.* **151:**449–453.
2. **Ater, J. L., J. C. Overall, Jr., T. J. Yeh, R. T. O'Brien, and A. Bailey.** 1985. Circulating interferon and clinical symptoms in Colorado tick fever. *J. Infect. Dis.* **151:**966–968.

3. **Attoui, H., F. Billoir, P. Biagini, J. F. Cantaloube, R. de Chesse, P. de Micco, and X. de Lamballerie.** 2000. Sequence determination and analysis of the full-length genome of Colorado tick fever virus, the type species of genus *Coltivirus* (family *Reoviridae*). *Biochem. Biophys. Res. Commun.* **273:**1121–1125.
4. **Attoui, H., F. Billoir, P. Biagini, P. de Micco, and X. de Lamballerie.** 2000. Complete sequence determination and genetic analysis of Banna virus and Kadipiro virus: proposal for assignment to a new genus *(Seadornavirus)* within the family *Reoviridae*. *J. Gen. Virol.* **81**(Pt. 6)**:** 1507–1515.
5. **Attoui, H., F. Billoir, J. M. Bruey, P. de Micco, and X. de Lamballerie.** 1998. Serologic and molecular diagnosis of Colorado tick fever viral infections. *Am. J. Trop. Med. Hyg.* **59:**763–768.
6. **Attoui, H., R. N. Charrel, F. Billoir, J. F. Cantaloube, P. de Micco, and X. de Lamballerie.** 1998. Comparative sequence analysis of American, European and Asian isolates of viruses in the genus Coltivirus. *J. Gen. Virol.* **79**(Pt. 10)**:**2481–2489.
7. **Attoui, H., F. Mohd Jaffar, P. de Micco, and X. de Lamballerie.** 2005. Coltiviruses and Seadornaviruses in North America, Europe, and Asia. *Emerg. Infect. Dis.* **11:**1673–1679.
8. **Bakken, J. S., J. S. Dumler, S. M. Chen, M. R. Eckman, L. L. Van Etta, and D. H. Walker.** 1994. Human granulocytic ehrlichiosis in the upper Midwest United States. A new species emerging? *JAMA* **272:**212–218.
9. **Bakken, J. S., J. Krueth, C. Wilson-Nordskog, R. L. Tilden, K. Asanovich, and J. S. Dumler.** 1996. Clinical and laboratory characteristics of human granulocytic ehrlichiosis. *JAMA* **275:**199–205.
10. **Becker, F. E.** 1930. Tick borne infections in Colorado. *Colo. Med.* **27:**87–95.
11. **Billoir, F., H. Attoui, S. Simon, P. Gallian, P. deMicco, and X. de Lamballerie.** 1999. Molecular diagnosis of group B coltivirus infections. *J. Virol. Methods* **81:**39–45.
12. **Bodkin, D. K., and D. L. Knudson.** 1987. Genetic relatedness of Colorado tick fever virus isolates by RNA-RNA blot hybridization. *J. Gen. Virol.* **68**(Pt. 4)**:**1199–1204.
13. **Bowen, G. S.** 1988. Colorado tick fever, p. 159–176. *In* T. P. Monath (ed.), *The Arboviruses: Ecology and Epidemiology*. CRC Press, Boca Raton, FL.
14. **Bratton, R., and G. Corey.** 2005. Tick-borne disease. *Am. Family Physician* **71:**2323–2330.
15. **Brown, S. E., B. R. Miller, R. G. McLean, and D. L. Knudson.** 1989. Co-circulation of multiple Colorado tick fever virus genotypes. *Am. J. Trop. Med. Hyg.* **40:**94–101.
16. **Brown, S. E., H. G. Morrison, N. Karabatsos, and D. L. Knudson.** 1991. Genetic relatedness of two new Orbivirus serogroups: Orungo and Lebombo. *J. Gen. Virol.* **72**(Pt. 5)**:**1065–1072.
17. **Burgdorfer, W.** 1959. Colorado tick fever. The behavior of Colorado tick fever virus in the porcupine. *J. Infect. Dis.* **104:**101–104.
18. **Burgdorfer, W.** 1960. Colorado tick fever. The behavior of Colorado tick fever virus in rodents. *J. Infect. Dis.* **107:** 384–388.
19. **Calisher, C. H.** 1994. Medically important arboviruses of the United States and Canada. *Clin. Microbiol. Rev.* **7:** 89–116.
20. **Centers for Disease Control and Prevention.** 1995. Human granulocytic ehrlichiosis—New York, 1995. *Morb. Mortal. Wkly. Rep.* **44:**593–595.
21. **Chao, L.** 1994. Evolution of genetic exchange in RNA viruses, p. 233–250. *In* S. S. Morse (ed.), *The Evolutionary Biology of Viruses*. Raven Press, Ltd., New York, NY.
22. **Chastel, C., A. J. Main, A. Couatarmanac'h, G. Le Lay, D. L. Knudson, M. C. Quillien, and J. C. Beaucournu.** 1984. Isolation of Eyach virus (*Reoviridae*, Colorado tick fever group) from Ixodes ricinus and I. ventalloi ticks in France. *Arch. Virol.* **82:**161–171.
23. **Chen, B. Q., and S. J. Tao.** 1996. Arbovirus survey in China in recent ten years. *Chin. Med. J.* **109:**13–15.
24. **Chumakov, M. P., L. G. Karpovich, E. S. Sarmanova, G. I. Sergeeva, M. B. Bychkova, V. O. Tapupere, H. Libikova, V. Mayer, J. Rehacek, O. Kozuch, and E. Ernek.** 1963. Report on the isolation from *Ixodes persulcatus* ticks and from patients in western Siberia of a virus differing from the agent of tick-borne encephalitis. *Acta Virol.* **7:**82–83.
25. **Craven, R. B.** 1991. Orbiviruses and other reoviruses, p. 713–718. *In* R. B. Belshe (ed.), *Textbook of Human Virology*. Mosby-Year Book, Inc., St. Louis, MO.
26. **Dawson, D. L., and T. M. Vernon.** 1972. Colorado tick fever—Colorado. *Morb. Mortal. Wkly. Rep.* **21:**374.
27. **Dawson, J. E., C. K. Warner, S. Standaert, and J. G. Olson.** 1996. The interface between research and the diagnosis of an emerging tick-borne disease, human ehrlichiosis due to Ehrlichia chaffeensis. *Arch. Intern. Med* **156:** 137–142.
28. **Draughn, D. E., O. F. Sieber, Jr., and J. H. Umlauf, Jr.** 1965. Colorado tick fever encephalitis. *Clin. Pediatr.* **4:** 626–628.
29. **Eklund, C. M., G. M. Kohls, and W. L. Jellison.** 1958. Isolation of Colorado tick fever virus from rodents in Colorado. *Science* **128:**413.
30. **Eklund, C. M., G. M. Kohls, W. L. Jellison, W. Burgdorfer, K. C. Kennedy, and L. Thomas.** 1959. The clinical and ecological aspects of Colorado tick fever, p. 197–203. *In Proc. 6th Int. Conf. Trop. Med. Malaria*, vol. 5. Instituto de Medicinia Tropical, Lisbon, Portugal.
31. **Emmons, R. W.** 1981. Colorado tick fever, p. 113–124. *In* J. H. Steele (ed.), *CRC Handbook on Zoonoses*. CRC Press, Boca Raton, FL.
32. **Emmons, R. W.** 1988. Ecology of Colorado tick fever. *Annu. Rev. Microbiol.* **42:**49–64.
33. **Emmons, R. W., D. V. Dondero, V. Devlin, and E. H. Lennette.** 1969. Serologic diagnosis of Colorado tick fever. A comparison of complement-fixation, immunofluorescence, and plaque-reduction methods. *Am. J. Trop. Med. Hyg.* **18:**796–802.
34. **Emmons, R. W., and E. H. Lennette.** 1966. Immunofluorescent staining in the laboratory diagnosis of Colorado tick fever. *J. Lab. Clin. Med.* **68:**923–929.
35. **Emmons, R. W., L. S. Oshiro, H. N. Johnson, and E. H. Lennette.** 1972. Intra-erythrocytic location of Colorado tick fever virus. *J. Gen. Virol.* **17:**185–195.
36. **Emmons, R. W., and H. I. Schade.** 1972. Colorado tick fever simulating acute myocardial infarction. *JAMA* **222:** 87–88.
37. **Eng, T. R., J. R. Harkess, D. B. Fishbein, J. E. Dawson, C. N. Greene, M. A. Redus, and F. T. Satalowich.** 1990. Epidemiologic, clinical, and laboratory findings of human ehrlichiosis in the United States, 1988. *JAMA* **264:**2251–2258.
38. **Fabiyi, A., O. Tomori, and M. S. el Bayoumi.** 1975. Epidemics of a febrile illness associated with UgMP 359 virus in Nigeria. *West Afr. Med. J. Niger. Med. Dent. Pract.* **23:**9–11.
39. **Familusi, J. B., D. L. Moore, A. K. Fomufod, and O. R. Causey.** 1972. Virus isolates from children with febrile convulsions in Nigeria. A correlation study of clinical and laboratory observations. *Clin. Pediatr.* **11:**272–276.
40. **Fishbein, D. B., J. E. Dawson, and L. E. Robinson.** 1994. Human ehrlichiosis in the United States, 1985 to 1990. *Ann. Intern. Med.* **120:**736–743.

41. **Florio, L., M. Stewart, and E. R. Mugrage.** 1944. The experimental transmission of Colorado tick fever. *J. Exp. Med.* **80:**165–187.
42. **Forzan, M., M. Marsch, and P. Roy.** 2007. Bluetongue virus entry into cells. *J. Virol.* **81:**4819–4827.
43. **Francki, R. I. B., C. M. Fauquet, D. L. Knudson, and F. Brown.** 1991. Classification and nomenclature of viruses. *Arch. Virol. Suppl.* **2:**186.
44. **Goodman, J. L., C. Nelson, B. Vitale, J. E. Madigan, J. S. Dumler, T. J. Kurtti, and U. G. Munderloh.** 1996. Direct cultivation of the causative agent of human granulocytic ehrlichiosis. *N. Engl. J. Med.* **334:**209–215.
45. **Goodpasture, H. C., J. D. Poland, D. B. Francy, G. S. Bowen, and K. A. Horn.** 1978. Colorado tick fever: clinical, epidemiologic, and laboratory aspects of 228 cases in Colorado in 1973–1974. *Ann. Intern. Med.* **88:**303–310.
46. **Green, I. J.** 1970. Evidence for the double-stranded nature of the RNA of Colorado tick fever virus, an ungrouped arbovirus. *Virology* **40:**1056–1059.
47. **Hadlow, W. J.** 1957. Histopathologic changes in suckling mice infected with the virus of Colorado tick fever. *J. Infect. Dis.* **101:**158–167.
48. **Hierholzer, W. J., and D. W. Barry.** 1971. Colorado tick fever pericarditis. *JAMA* **217:**825.
49. **ICTVdB Management.** 2006. 00.060.0.04.001. Colorado tick fever virus. *In* C. Büchen-Osmond (ed.), *ICTVdB—The Universal Virus Database*, version 4. Columbia University, New York, NY. http://www.ncbi.nlm.nih.gov/ICTVdb/ICTVdB/.
50. **ICTVdB Management.** 2006. 00.060.0.02. Orbivirus. *In* C. Büchen-Osmond (ed.), *ICTVdB—The Universal Virus Database*, version 4. Columbia University, New York, NY. http://www.ncbi.nlm.nih.gov/ICTVdb/ICTVdB/.
51. **ICTVdB Management.** 2006. 00.060.0.10. Seadornavirus. *In* C. Büchen-Osmond (ed.), *ICTVdB—The Universal Virus Database*, version 4. Columbia University, New York, NY. http://www.ncbi.nlm.nih.gov/ICTVdb/ICTVdB/.
52. **Johnson, A. J., N. Karabatsos, and R. S. Lanciotti.** 1997. Detection of Colorado tick fever virus by using reverse transcriptase PCR and application of the technique in laboratory diagnosis. *J. Clin. Microbiol.* **35:**1203–1208.
53. **Karabatsos, N., J. D. Poland, R. W. Emmons, J. H. Mathews, C. H. Calisher, and K. L. Wolff.** 1987. Antigenic variants of Colorado tick fever virus. *J. Gen. Virol.* **68**(Pt. 5)**:**1463–1469.
54. **Knudson, D. L.** 1981. Genome of Colorado tick fever virus. *Virology* **112:**361–364.
55. **Knudson, D. L., and T. P. Monath.** 1990. Orbiviruses, p. 1405–1433. *In* B. N. Fields and D. M. Knipe (ed.), *Virology*. Raven Press, Ltd., New York, NY.
56. **Koprowski, H., and H. R. Cox.** 1946. Adaptation of Colorado tick fever virus to mice and developing chick embryo. *Proc. Soc. Exp. Biol. Med.* **62:**320–322.
57. **Lambert, A. J., O. Kosoy, J. O. Velez, B. J. Russell, and R. S. Lanciotti.** 2007. Detection of Colorado tick fever viral RNA in acute human serum samples by a quantitative RT-PCR assay. *J. Virol. Meth.* **140:**43–48.
58. **Lane, R. S., R. W. Emmons, V. Devlin, D. V. Dondero, and B. C. Nelson.** 1982. Survey for evidence of Colorado tick fever virus outside of the known endemic area in California. *Am. J. Trop. Med. Hyg.* **31:**837–843.
59. **Li, Q. P., S. C. Hsiah, C. Zhie, L. Ma, B. L. Ah, Y. O. Lin, S. B. Wu, Y. J. Zhang, E. K. Yah, C. Wang, L. M. Se, G. D. Yan, Y. Ho, Z. J. Zhao, B. C. Chen, P.-T. Shu, and J. M. Zuo.** 1992. First isolations of 8 strains of new orbivirus (BANNA) from patients with innominate fever in Xinjiang. *Endem. Dis. Bull.* **7:**77–81.
60. **Libikova, H., F. Heinz, D. Ujhazyova, and D. Stunzner.** 1978. Orbiviruses of the Kemerovo complex and neurological diseases. *Med. Microbiol. Immunol.* **166:**255–263.
61. **Loge, R. V.** 1985. Acute hepatitis associated with Colorado tick fever. *West. J. Med.* **142:**91–92.
62. **Malkova, D., J. Holubova, J. M. Kolman, Z. Marhoul, F. Hanzal, H. Kulkova, K. Markvart, and L. Simkova.** 1980. Antibodies against some arboviruses in persons with various neuropathies. *Acta Virol.* **24:**298.
63. **Mertens, P. P. C., R. Duncan, H. Attoui, and T. S. Dermody.** 2005. *Reoviridae*, p. 447–454. *In* C. M. Fauquet, M. A. Mayo, J. Maniloff, U. Desselberger, and L. A. Ball (ed.), *Virus Taxonomy: Classification and Nomenclature of Viruses. Eighth Report of the International Committee on Taxonomy of Viruses.* Elsevier/Academic Press, San Deigo, CA.
64. **Miller, J. K., V. N. Tompkins, and J. C. Sieracki.** 1961. Pathology of Colorado tick fever in experimental animals. *Arch. Pathol.* **72:**149–157.
65. **Mohd Jaafar, F., H. Attoui, M. W. Bahar, C. Siebold, G. Sutton, P. P. Mertens, P. De Micco, D. I. Stuart, J. M. Grimes, and X. De Lamballerie.** 2005. The structure and function of the outer coat protein VP9 of Banna virus. *Structure* **13:**17–28.
66. **Mohd Jaafar, F., H. Attoui, P. De Micco, and X. De Lamballerie.** 2004. Recombinant VP6-based enzyme-linked immunosorbent assay for detection of immunoglobulin G antibodies to Eyach virus (genus Coltivirus). *J. Clin. Virol.* **30:**248–253.
67. **Mohd Jaafar, F., H. Attoui, P. De Micco, and X. De Lamballerie.** 2004. Termination and read-through proteins encoded by genome segment 9 of Colorado tick fever virus. *J. Gen. Virol.* **85**(Pt. 8)**:**2237–2244.
68. **Mohd Jaafar, F., H. Attoui, P. Gallian, I. Isahak, K. T. Wong, S. K. Cheong, V. S. Nadarajah, J. F. Cantaloube, P. Biagini, P. De Micco, and X. De Lamballerie.** 2004. Recombinant VP9-based enzyme-linked immunosorbent assay for detection of immunoglobulin G antibodies to Banna virus (genus *Seadornavirus*). *J. Virol. Methods* **116:**55–61.
69. **Mohd Jaafar, F., H. Attoui, P. P. Mertens, P. de Micco, and X. de Lamballerie.** 2005. Identification and functional analysis of VP3, the guanyltransferase of Banna virus (genus *Seadornavirus*, family *Reoviridae*). *J. Gen. Virol.* **86**(Pt. 4)**:**1141–1146.
70. **Mohd Jaafar, F., H. Attoui, P. P. C. Mertens, P. deMicco, and X. de Lamballerie.** 2005. Structural organization of an encephalitic human isolate of Banna virus (genus *Seadornavirus*, family *Reoviridae*). *J. Gen. Virol.* **86:**1147–1157.
71. **Monath, T. P.** 1995. Colorado tick fever, p. 1446–1447. *In* G. L. Mandell, J. E. Bennett, and R. Dolin (ed.), *Principles and Practice of Infectious Diseases*, 4th ed. Churchill Livingstone, New York, NY.
72. **Monath, T. P., R. B. Craven, A. Adjukiewicz, M. Germain, D. B. Francy, L. Ferrara, E. M. Samba, H. N'Jie, K. Cham, S. A. Fitzgerald, P. H. Crippen, D. I. Simpson, E. T. Bowen, A. Fabiyi, and J. J. Salaun.** 1980. Yellow fever in the Gambia, 1978–1979: epidemiologic aspects with observations on the occurrence of orungo virus infections. *Am. J. Trop. Med. Hyg.* **29:**912–928.
73. **Moore, D. L., O. R. Causey, D. E. Carey, S. Reddy, A. R. Cooke, F. M. Akinkugbe, T. S. David-West, and G. E. Kemp.** 1975. Arthropod-borne viral infections of man in Nigeria, 1964–1970. *Ann. Trop. Med. Parasitol.* **69:**49–64.
74. **Murphy, F. A., E. C. Borden, R. E. Shope, and A. Harrison.** 1971. Physicochemical and morphological relationships of some arthropod-borne viruses to bluetongue

virus—a new taxonomic group. Electron microscopic studies. *J. Gen. Virol.* **13:**273–288.

75. **Murphy, F. A., P. H. Coleman, A. K. Harrison, and G. W. Gary, Jr.** 1968. Colorado tick fever virus: an electron microscopic study. *Virology* **35:**28–40.
76. **Murphy, F. A., C. M. Fauquet, D. H. L. Bishop, S. A. Ghabrial, A. W. Jarvis, G. P. Martelli, M. A. Mayo, and M. D. Summers** (ed.). 1995. *Virus Taxonomy: Classification and Nomenclature of Viruses. Sixth Report of the International Committee on Taxonomy of Viruses.* Springer-Verlag, Vienna, Austria.
77. **Oshiro, L. S., D. V. Dondero, R. W. Emmons, and E. H. Lennette.** 1978. The development of Colorado tick fever virus within cells of the haemopoietic system. *J. Gen. Virol.* **39:**73–79.
78. **Oshiro, L. S., and R. W. Emmons.** 1968. Electron microscopic observations of Colorado tick fever virus in BHK 21 and KB cells. *J. Gen. Virol.* **3:**279–280.
79. **Philipp, C. S., C. Callaway, M. C. Chu, G. H. Huang, T. P. Monath, D. Trent, and B. L. Evatt.** 1993. Replication of Colorado tick fever virus within human hematopoietic progenitor cells. *J. Virol.* **67:**2389–2395.
80. Reference deleted.
81. **Randall, W. H., J. Simmons, E. A. Caspter, and R. N. Philip.** 1975. Transmission of Colorado tick fever virus by blood transfusion—Montana. *Morb. Mortal. Wkly. Rep.* **24:**422–427.
82. **Rehse-Kupper, B., J. Casals, E. Rehse, and R. Ackermann.** 1976. Eyach—an arthropod-borne virus related to Colorado tick fever virus in the Federal Republic of Germany. *Acta Virol.* **20:**339–342.
83. **Roy, P.** 1993. Dissecting the assembly of orbiviruses. *Trends Microbiol.* **1:**299–305.

83a.**Roy, P.** 1996. Orbivirus structure and assembly. *Virology* **216:**1–11. (Erratum, **218:**296.)

84. **Smee, D. F., J. L. Morris, D. L. Barnard, and A. Van Aerschot.** 1992. Selective inhibition of arthropod-borne and arenaviruses in vitro by 3′-fluoro-3′-deoxyadenosine. *Antivir. Res.* **18:**151–162.
85. **Smee, D. F., R. W. Sidwell, S. M. Clark, B. B. Barnett, and R. S. Spendlove.** 1981. Inhibition of bluetongue and Colorado tick fever orbiviruses by selected antiviral substances. *Antimicrob. Agents Chemother.* **20:**533–538.
86. **Song, L., B. Chen, and Z. Zhao.** 1995. Isolation and identification of new members of coltivirus from mosquitoes collected in China. *Chin. J. Virol.* **9:**7–10. (Abstract in English.)
87. **Spach, D. H., W. C. Liles, G. L. Campbell, R. E. Quick, D. E. Anderson, Jr., and T. R. Fritsche.** 1993. Tick-borne diseases in the United States. *N. Engl. J. Med.* **329:** 936–947.
88. **Spruance, S. L., and A. Bailey.** 1973. Colorado tick fever. A review of 115 laboratory confirmed cases. *Arch. Intern. Med.* **131:**288–293.
89. **Swanepoel, R., B. J. Erasmus, R. Williams, and M. B. Taylor.** 1992. Encephalitis and chorioretinitis associated with neurotropic African horsesickness virus infection in laboratory workers. Part III. Virological and serological investigations. *S. Afr. Med. J.* **81:**458–461.
90. **Tao, S. J., and B. Q. Chen.** 2005. Studies of Coltivirus in China. *Chin. Med. J. (Engl. Ed.)* **118:**581–586.
91. **Telford, S. R., III, T. J. Lepore, P. Snow, C. K. Warner, and J. E. Dawson.** 1995. Human granulocytic ehrlichiosis in Massachusetts. *Ann. Intern. Med.* **123:**277–279.
92. **Thomas, L. A., R. N. Philip, E. Patzer, and E. Casper.** 1967. Long duration of neutralizing-antibody response after immunization of man with a formalinized Colorado tick fever vaccine. *Am. J. Trop. Med. Hyg.* **16:**60–62.
93. **Tomori, O., and A. Fabiyi.** 1976. Neutralizing antibodies to Orungo virus in man and animals in Nigeria. *Trop. Geogr. Med.* **28:**233–238.
94. **Topping, H. N.** 1940. Colorado tick fever. *Public Health Rep.* **55:**2224–2237.
95. **Travassos da Rosa, A. P., R. B. Tesh, F. P. Pinheiro, J. F. Travassos da Rosa, P. H. Peralta, and D. L. Knudson.** 1984. Characterization of the Changuinola serogroup viruses *(Reoviridae: Orbivirus)*. *Intervirology* **21:**38–49.
96. **Trent, D. W., and L. V. Scott.** 1966. Colorado tick fever virus in cell culture. II. Physical and chemical properties. *J. Bacteriol.* **91:**1282–1288.
97. **Tsai, T. F.** 1991. Arboviral infections in the United States. *Infect. Dis. Clin. N. Am.* **5:**73–102.
98. **Tsai, T. F.** 2005. Coltiviruses and Seadornaviruses (Colorado tick fever), p. 1900–1901. *In* G. L. Mandell, J. E. Bennett, and R. Dolin (ed.), *Principles and Practice of Infectious Diseases.* Churchill Livingstone, Philadelphia, PA.
99. **Tsai, T. F.** 2005. Orthoreoviruses and Orbiviruses, p. 1899–1900. *In* G. L. Mandell, J. E. Bennett, and R. Dolin (ed.), *Principles and Practice of Infectious Diseases,* 6th ed. Churchill Livingstone, Philadelphia, PA.
100. **van der Meyden, C. H., B. J. Erasmus, R. Swanepoel, and O. W. Prozesky.** 1992. Encephalitis and chorioretinitis associated with neurotropic African horsesickness virus infection in laboratory workers. Part I. Clinical and neurological observations. *S. Afr. Med. J.* **81:**451–454.
101. **Walker, D. H., and S. J. Dumler.** 2000. Ehrlichia chaffeensis (human monocytotropic ehrlichiosis), Ehrlichia phagocytophila (human granulocytotropic ehrlichiosis), and other Ehrlichia, p. 2057–2064. *In* G. L. Mandell, J. E. Bennett, and R. Dolin (ed.), *Principles and Practice of Infectious Diseases,* 5th ed. Churchill Livingstone, Philadelphia, PA.
102. **Wang, D., A. Urisman, Y. T. Liu, M. Springer, T. G. Ksiazek, D. D. Erdman, E. R. Mardis, M. Hickenbotham, V. Magrini, J. Eldred, J. P. Latreille, R. K. Wilson, D. Ganem, and J. L. DeRisi.** 2003. Viral discovery and sequence recovery using DNA microarrays. *PLoS Biol.* **1**(2):E2.
103. **Zhao, Z., Y. Huang, and Y. Zhou.** 1994. Isolation of a kind of new virus from patients with viral encephalitis in Beijing. *Chin. J. Virol.* **8:**297–299. (Abstract in English.)

Rotaviruses

MANUEL A. FRANCO AND HARRY B. GREENBERG

35

Upper respiratory tract infections and acute infectious diarrhea are two of the most frequent diseases of young children. During the 1960s and early 1970s, numerous unsuccessful attempts were made to grow the viral agents responsible for acute infectious diarrhea of children. The etiologic agent of epizootic diarrhea of infant mice was identified by electron microscopy (EM) in 1963 (2). Nonetheless, it was not until the discovery of the virus responsible for calf scours by EM in 1969 by Mebus et al. (91), and of the human Norwalk virus by Kapikian et al. (73) in 1972, that the methodology for identification of the viruses responsible for severe diarrhea in children was established. Using EM, Bishop et al. (15) identified the first human rotavirus in an intestinal biopsy sample from a child with diarrhea. At roughly the same time, other groups used immuno EM to identify the enteric caliciviruses and astroviruses, which were also difficult to grow in vitro, as additional causes of acute infectious diarrhea in children. Quickly, the virus causing epizootic diarrhea of infant mice and the calf scours virus were found to be related to the human rotavirus, grouped in the genus *Rotavirus*, and identified as one of the most important pathogens of acute diarrhea in both children and the young of many animals (43).

Rotaviruses are responsible for 29 to 45% of all hospitalizations due to diarrhea worldwide, and it has been estimated that they cause the death of approximately 1,600 children daily (106) (Fig. 1). Probably because efficient and widespread accesses to rehydration and other supportive measures are generally available, rotaviruses are not responsible for a substantial number of deaths in developed countries. Nonetheless, rotavirus is still a very important public health problem, responsible for a large number of hospitalizations. For example, in the United States rotaviruses are the most common enteric pathogens identified in children under 5 years and cause approximately 60,000 hospitalizations and 37 deaths annually (46).

VIROLOGY

Classification

Rotaviruses belong to the *Reoviridae* family of icosahedral, nonenveloped, segmented double-stranded RNA (dsRNA) viruses. Rotaviruses are classified into groups (A through E) depending on the presence of cross-reactive epitopes primarily located on the internal structural protein VP6. Group A rotaviruses are the most frequent pathogens of humans, and groups D through E have been found only in nonhuman animals. Unless otherwise stated, we refer only to group A rotaviruses in this chapter. Group B rotaviruses are sporadic pathogens of animals and were implicated in several large outbreaks of severe acute adult diarrhea in China in the 1980s and, less frequently, in the 1990s. More recently, they have been identified in children and adults with diarrhea in Asia (8). Group C rotaviruses are primarily veterinary pathogens but have been reported to be sporadically associated with diarrhea in children. Seroprevalence of antibodies for these rotaviruses is relatively high in humans, specially those living in rural areas, suggesting transmission from animals to humans (65). Despite occasional studies implicating the importance of group B or C rotaviruses in humans, group A rotaviruses continue to be by far the most frequently identified pathogens.

Group A rotaviruses have been serologically classified into subgroups depending on the presence of epitopes localized on the major internal capsid protein on the virion, VP6 (43). Four subgroup specificities have been defined: subgroup I (most animal and a few human strains), subgroup II (most human and a few animal strains), subgroups I and II, and neither subgroup I nor subgroup II; only rare human strains belong to the last two categories. The subgroup classification was useful in early epidemiological studies but is less commonly utilized today.

Antibodies that neutralize rotavirus in vitro are used to further classify the virus into serotypes. The two outer viral capsid proteins (VP7 and VP4), which induce neutralizing antibodies, segregate independently, and thus a binary serotyping classification system has been developed, much like for influenza virus. Antibodies against VP7 define the G (glycosylated protein) serotypes, and antibodies against VP4 define the P (protease-sensitive protein) serotypes. Historically, hyperimmune serum and, later, monoclonal antibodies (MAbs) against distinct rotavirus strains were used to classify viral serotypes. Because antibodies against VP7 generally predominate in hyperimmune sera and serotype-specific MAbs to neutralizing epitopes on VP7 are easy to isolate, the classification of G serotypes has been extensive and clear-cut. More recently, the G protein has been characterized based on its sequence analysis (geno-

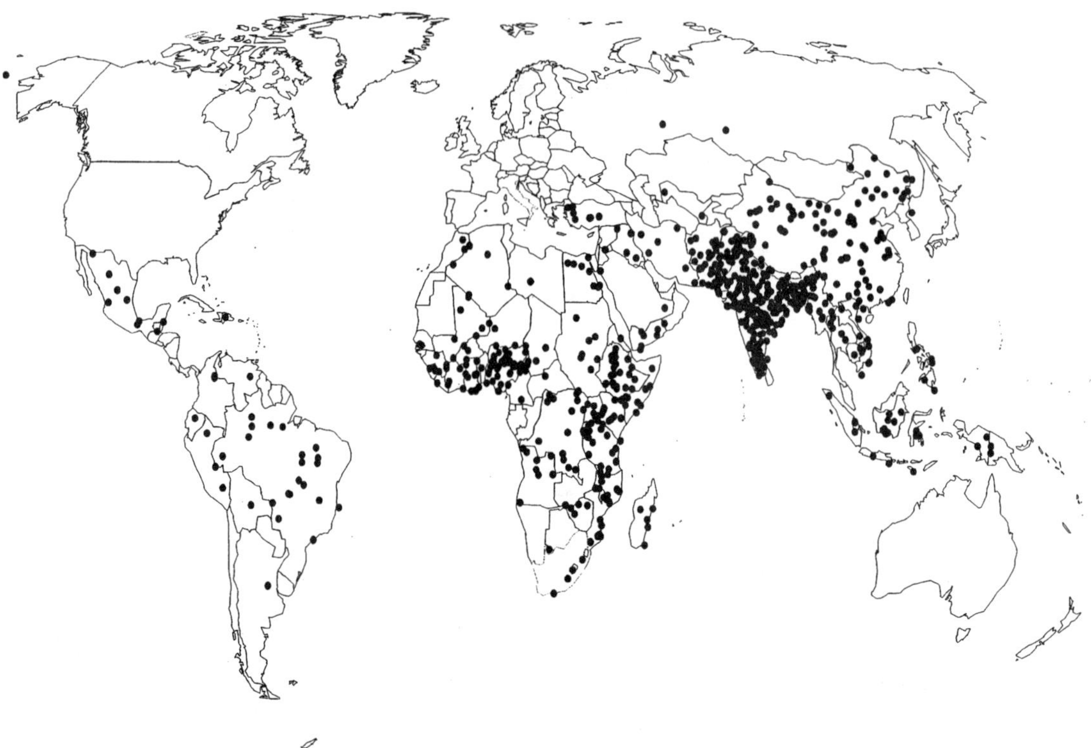

FIGURE 1 Estimated global distribution of deaths due to rotavirus. Each dot represents 1,000 deaths attributed to rotavirus per year at the indicated location. The total world death toll is approximately 600,000 children per year. (Figure courtesy of R. Glass; adapted from reference 53 with permission.)

type), and this classification correlates well with traditional serologic designations. In contrast, to obtain good P serotyping reagents, it has been necessary to raise polyclonal antibodies against the different recombinant VP4 proteins (129), and these reagents have not been widely available. For this reason, many more distinct types of VP4 have been identified by comparison of gene sequence (genotype) than by serology. A significant, but not absolute, correlation has been found between P serotypes and P genotypes. For example, the most common human P serotypes, 1A and 1B, correspond to genotypes 8 and 4, respectively, but genotypes 2 and 3 can both correspond to P serotype 5B (43). For these reasons, a dual system for classification of rotaviruses according to their VP4 genotype and serotype is in use.

Using this nomenclature, the P serotype (if available) is followed by the genotype in square brackets. For example, the Wa strain of human rotavirus is designated P1A[8], G1. Of the 15 G serotypes and 26 P genotypes described, 10 and 11, respectively, have been isolated from humans (128). Human rotavirus strains belonging to the G1, G3, G4, and G9 serotypes are preferentially associated with P[8], while G2 serotype strains are most frequently associated with the P[4] genotype. Worldwide, five G serotypes (G1 to G4 and G9) and three P genotypes (P[4], P[6], and P[8]) account for most human rotavirus infections (128).

Composition of Virus

Virion Morphology

Rotaviruses, as determined by conventional EM (which does not permit clear identification of the spike protein), are 70-nm particles that have a multilayered icosahedral structure. The viral particle forms three concentric layers of proteins: the core comprises VP1, VP2, and VP3 and the genome (Color Plate 45); the intermediate layer is formed by VP6, the most abundant viral protein; and the external layer comprises VP7 and VP4. In vitro treatment of a complete infectious virus, or triple-layered particles (TLPs), with calcium chelating agents removes the outer viral capsid (VP4 and VP7), producing double-layered, noninfectious particles (DLPs). Pioneering structural studies of rotavirus using cryo-EM (112, 155) obtained detailed functional and structural information about these relatively large and complex viruses (Color Plate 45). The 60 spike structures that protrude from the surface of the viral particle are formed by trimers of VP4 that interact at their base with both the outer-layer (VP7) and middle-layer (VP6) proteins (40, 43). The structural changes of VP4, which probably occur during penetration, recall those of enveloped virus fusion proteins (40).

The particle has three types of aqueous channels that connect the central core, containing the genome, with the viral surface. These channels have been classified depending on their location, relative to the icosahedral symmetry, into three types (I, II, and III), and are thought to be important in the entry of metabolites required for RNA transcription (112). The exit of nascent mRNA from the DLP occurs via type I channels. Viral transcription may occur simultaneously from each of the 12 type I channels in the viral particle. Approximately one-fourth of the viral RNA is organized in an ordered dodecahedral structure localized near a VP1 (the viral polymerase)-VP3 complex at the base of the type I channels (112). The continuous translocation of nascent mRNA through the capsid is critical for efficient mRNA elongation, and blockage of that translocation causes premature termination of transcription (80).

Viral Genome

Rotavirus contains 11 segments of dsRNA that range in size from 0.6 to 3.3 kbp, with a total genomic size of approximately 18 kb. These segments are numbered according to their size, from the largest (segment 1) to the smallest (segment 11) (43). With the exceptions of segments 9 and 11 (which are biscistronic in at least some viral strains), each RNA segment contains a single open reading frame (ORF), with relatively short 5′ and 3′-terminal conserved noncoding regions. These conserved noncoding terminal sequences differ among group A, B, and C rotaviruses, and this could be one of the factors that restricts reassortment between rotaviruses of different groups. Positive strands of the dsRNA are capped at their 5′ ends but do not possess a polyadenylation tract at their 3′ ends (108).

The genome of rotavirus is highly diverse. In decreasing order of relative importance, three primary sources for this diversity have been proposed: point mutations, reassortment, and rearrangement of the viral genome (108). In vitro studies have revealed a mutation rate of $<5 \times 10^{-5}$ mutations per nucleotide per viral replication. This rate of mutation suggests that the average rotavirus genome differs from its parental genome by at least one mutation. Reassortment of gene segments occurs at a relatively high frequency during mixed infections with two or more rotaviruses, both in vitro and in vivo. In humans, the capacity for rotaviruses to reassort influences the generation of serotypic diversity less dramatically than for influenza virus, although reassortment clearly occurs, especially in less developed countries (50, 128).

Rearrangements (concatemerization, partial gene duplications, and deletions) of the viral genome have been observed, especially with rotavirus recovered from chronically infected immunodeficient children (153). Rotavirus with rearranged genomes can also be obtained in vitro following multiple passages at a high multiplicity of infection. To date, gene rearrangements have exclusively involved the nonstructural proteins and VP6 (108).

Viral Structural and Nonstructural Proteins

In addition to six structural proteins (designated VP followed by a number), rotaviruses encode six nonstructural proteins (designated NSP followed by a number). The gene coding assignments for these proteins were initially established with prototypic rotavirus strains, like the simian SA11 strain, that were easily cultured in vitro (Table 1).

VP1 binds the 3′ end of the viral RNA, but its transcriptase is not active unless it is associated with VP2 (108). Virus-like particles (VLPs) formed by the VP1-VP2 complex are the minimal combination that supports RNA replication (108). Strategies aimed at developing agents with the capacity to specifically block the viral polymerase could be useful in the control of rotavirus infection.

VP2 binds dsRNA and dsDNA and assembles in the cytoplasm of infected cells in core-like particles 45 nm in diameter (43). The role of VP2 in the assembly of VP1 and VP3 and in replicase activity appears to be primarily structural (108). The results of replicase assays performed with mutant VP2 containing a deletion in its RNA-binding domain suggest that the essential role of VP2 in replication is linked to the protein's ability to bind the mRNA template for minus-strand synthesis (108).

VP3 is found at the vertices of the inner core. In addition to the RNA polymerase activity, viral cores have been shown to contain a nonspecific guanylyltransferase activity that caps viral and nonviral mRNAs in vitro (24). This viral guanylyltransferase activity and a methyltransferase activity have both been assigned to VP3, making this protein a multifunctional capping enzyme (24).

VP4 trimers form the spike protein on the virion surface (43). Based on structural data showing that VP4 interacts with both VP7 and VP6, it has been proposed that the assembly of VP4 on the virion precedes that of VP7, but this hypothesis has been challenged by other data (see "Replication strategy" below). VP4 has been shown to be the viral attachment protein, both in vivo and in vitro, and to be a determinant of viral growth in vitro and a virulence factor in vivo (43). Trypsin treatment of rotavirus cleaves VP4 into VP8 (amino-terminal) and VP5 proteins and greatly enhances viral infectivity in vitro (43).

VP8* contains most of the sequence variation in VP4 and determines the viral P genotype (43). Antibodies against VP8* neutralize the virus by inhibiting viral attachment. VP8* has been shown to be responsible for the binding of sialic acid and for the hemagglutinating activity present in many animal strains but absent in most human rotavirus strains. Structural analysis of the VP8* protein shows that it belongs to the galectin family of lectins expressed in enterocytes (94).

VP5* has been shown to function as a rotavirus attachment protein that does not require cell surface sialic acid residues to mediate viral infectivity (82). In addition, VP5* is a specific membrane-permeabilizing protein which is likely to play a role in cellular entry (55). The membrane permeabilization induced by VP5* is size selective, which suggests that the role of VP5* in the rotavirus entry process may be to expose TLPs to low Ca^{2+} which uncoats the virus, rather than to mediate the detergent-like lysis of early endosomal membranes (43).

VP6 is the major structural protein of the inner viral capsid (middle viral layer). VP6 is the most immunogenic viral protein and carries group- and subgroup-specific epitopes. Coexpression of VP2 from group A rotavirus and VP6 from group C rotavirus leads to the formation of chimeric DLPs (43). Thus, the VP6 domains necessary for binding to VP2 are conserved in different rotavirus serogroups and are necessary for DLP formation. Although not required for in vitro replicase activity, VP6 is required for transcriptase activity, but its exact role in this function is not known (13).

VP7 can be coded by gene segment 7, 8, or 9, depending on the viral strain (43). It is the major constituent of the outer rotavirus layer, and the target of type-specific, as well as heterotypic, neutralizing antibodies. Three major antigenic regions (regions A, B, and C) have been identified on VP7 using murine MAbs. These regions can be the target of both cross-reactive and serotype-specific antibodies (43). VP7 is a glycoprotein with three potential sites for N glycosylation which are used variably, depending on the viral strain. Glycosylation of VP7 can influence its antigenicity. The retention of VP7 in the endoplasmic re-

TABLE 1 dsRNA segments and encoded proteins of simian rotavirus SA11[a]

dsRNA segment (size [bp])	Protein designation and protein structure/function[b]	Protein size (no. of aa[c]) and mol mass (kDa)	No. of protein copies/ particle	Protein location	Function
1 (3,302)	VP1 (Pol)	1,088 (125.005)	<25	Inner capsid at 5-fold axis	RNA-dependent RNA polymerase; ssRNA[d] binding; part of minimal replication complex; forms a transcription complex with VP3
2 (2,690)	VP2 (T1)	880 (102.431)	180	Inner capsid shell	Inner capsid structural protein; non-sequence-specific RNA-binding activity; myristoylated; part of minimal replication complex
3 (2,591)	VP3 (cap)	835 (98.120)	<25	Inner capsid at 5-fold axis	Guanylyltransferase; methyltransferase; basic protein; part of virion transcription complex
4 (2,362)	VP4	776 (86.782)	120	Outer capsid spike	Trimers form outer capsid spike, P-type neutralization antigen, hemagglutinin, and cell attachment protein; involved in virulence. Cleavage by trypsin into VP5* and VP8* enhances infectivity.
	VP5*	529 *247–776 (60.000)			VP5* permeabilizes membranes.
	VP8*	247 *1–247 (28.000)			VP8* hemagglutinin; highly variable and determines P genotypes
5 (1,611)	NSP1	495 (58.654)	0	Nonstructural	Associates with cytoskeleton; extensive sequence diversity between strains; two conserved cysteine-rich zinc finger motifs; RNA binding; has a role in suppressing the host IFN-α response; nonessential in vitro in some strains; has role in host range restriction
6 (1,356)	VP6 (T13)	397 (44.816)	780	Middle capsid	Major virion protein; structural protein; homotrimeric structure; subgroup antigen; myristoylated; hydrophobic; required for transcription
7 (1,049)	NSP3	315 (34.600)	0	Nonstructural	Homodimer; specifically binds 3′ end of rotavirus mRNA; binds eIF4G1; involved in translational regulation
8 (1,059)	NSP2 (Vip)	317 (36.700)	0	Nonstructural: in viroplasms	Nonspecific ssRNA binding; accumulates in viroplasm; involved in viroplasm formation and NTPase and helicase activity; homomultimer (4–8 subunits); binds NSP5 and VP1; regulates NSP5 autophosphorylation
9 (1,062)	VP7	326 (37.368)	780	Virion surface glycoprotein	Outer capsid structural glycoprotein; G-type neutralization antigen, N-linked high mannose glycosylation and trimming, rough ER

(Continued on next page)

TABLE 1 *(Continued)*

dsRNA segment (size [bp])	Protein designation and protein structure/function[b]	Protein size (no. of aa[c]) and mol mass (kDa)	No. of protein copies/particle	Protein location	Function
10 (751)	NSP4	175 (20.290)	0	Nonstructural	Enterotoxin, receptor for budding of DLPs through ER membrane, N-linked high mannose glycosylation; uncleaved signal sequence; rough ER transmembrane glycoprotein; putative, Ca^{2+}/Sr^{2+} binding site; modulates intracellular calcium levels and RNA replication; secreted cleavage product
11 (667)	NSP5	198 (21.725)	0	Nonstructural: present in viral inclusion bodies	Interacts with NSP2 and NSP6; homomultimerizes; O-linked glycosylation; (hyper-)phosphorylated; autocatalytic kinase activity; binds ssRNA; component of viroplasm; essential for viral replication
	NSP6	92 (11.012)	0	Nonstructural	Product of second out-of-frame ORF; interacts with NSP5; localizes to viroplasm

[a] Adapted with permission from an annotated table by Eric Mossel, Frank Ramig, and Mary Estes that appears in http://www.iah.bbsrc.ac.uk/dsRNA_virus_proteins/Rotavirus.htm.

[b] Protein structure/function: Pol, RNA polymerase; T1, inner virus structural protein with T = 1 symmetry; Cap, capping enzyme; T13, inner virus structural protein with T = 13 symmetry; Vip, viral inclusion body or viroplasm matrix protein. Other species of rotavirus within the genus may have proteins with differences in sizes.

[c] aa, amino acids.

[d] ssRNA, single-stranded RNA.

ticulum (ER) is mediated by a signal peptide sequence, as well as other unique residues of the protein (43).

The amino acid sequence of NSP1 is the most highly variable of all the rotavirus proteins. NSP1 has been reported to bind zinc and RNA and has been implicated in host range restriction in the mouse model (43). NSP1 appears to be dispensable for growth in cell culture. Recent studies indicate that NSP1 functions as an E3 ubiquitin ligase that promotes degradation of IRF3 and IRF7, and inhibits the cellular type I interferon (IFN) response in vitro after rotavirus infection (9).

NSP2 interacts with NSP5, has a helicase activity, and is present at a high concentration in the viroplasm, where viral replication takes place. It has been proposed that NSP2 functions as a molecular motor, catalyzing the packaging of viral mRNA into core-like replication intermediates, through the energy derived from its NTPase activity (108).

NSP3 is a sequence-specific RNA binding protein that binds the nonpolyadenylated 3′ end of the rotavirus mRNAs (111). NSP3 also interacts with the cellular translation initiation factor eIF4GI and competes with cellular poly(A) binding protein (111). It has been postulated that the competition between NSP3 and poly(A) binding protein for eIF4G is responsible for the shutoff of host cell translation and the enhancement of translation of viral mRNA (111). In agreement with this hypothesis, mutation of the RNA NSP3 binding sites decreases protein translation (108). However, it remains to be clarified why small interfering RNA for NSP3, which restores cellular protein synthesis, does not decrease the synthesis of viral proteins (95).

The capacity of NSP4 to bind both DLPs and VP4 probably plays an important role in viral morphogenesis. NSP4 is the intracellular receptor that permits DLPs to enter the ER and is a key player in intracellular calcium regulation during rotavirus infection (43). NSP4 was the first putative viral enterotoxin described (7): NSP4, or an active NSP4-derived peptide, induces diarrhea in neonatal mice through the activation of an age- and Ca^{2+}-dependent plasma membrane anion channel distinct from the cystic fibrosis transmembrane regulator (CFTR) (96). Recently, NSP4 has been shown to traffic to caveolae a specific subset of rafts at the plasma membrane (43). In the porcine model, the NSP4 gene is associated with virulence of a human rotavirus (62). The role of NSP4 in inducing diarrhea in humans remains to be determined (43).

NSP5, a product of gene segment 11, is a phosphoprotein with putative autocatalytic kinase activity and is present in infected cells as various isoforms (108). The isoforms vary according to different patterns of O-linked glycosylation. In infected cells NSP5 forms oligomers which are localized to the viroplasm and associated with NSP2, suggesting that it plays a role in viral replication (108).

NSP6 is the product of the second ORF of segment 11. It interacts with NSP5 and might have a regulatory role in the self-association of NSP5 and thus in viral replication (108).

Biology

Replication Strategy

Viral replication is understood mainly from in vitro studies. The process of viral attachment and entry is mediated by multiple interactions between rotavirus and the cell surface, and it varies for different rotavirus strains (Fig. 2) (82). For some nonhuman animal strains a first binding step between VP8* and sialic acid seems to be important for cell attachment. For many human and some animal strains which do not require sialic acid for binding, an initial binding to the ganglioside GM1a may be the first step in entry. As a second step for sialic acid-dependent strains, and as a first or second step for sialic acid-independent strains, a protein-protein interaction has been identified in the viral attachment cascade: the $\alpha 2\beta 1$ integrin (via an interaction with VP4) and the $\alpha 4\beta 1$ integrin (probably via an interaction with VP7) have been shown to function as cellular receptors for SA11 rotavirus, a sialic acid-dependent rotavirus (31, 82). Biochemical studies showing the involvement of N-glycoproteins, glycolipids, and cholesterol in rotavirus infection suggest that the integrins mentioned above, other integrins, and other proteins involved in the attachment and entry process are likely to form part of lipid microdomains (rafts) in the cell membrane. The presence of correct combinations of several distinct molecules on the lipid rafts, and not any single molecule functioning as the receptor, may determine the susceptibility of a given cell to rotavirus (82). Rotaviruses have been proposed to enter cells by endocytosis and by direct plasma membrane penetration. Both VP4 and VP7 have been shown to permeabilize membranes, suggesting that these proteins are involved in viral penetration (82). The permeabilization of membranes by VP4 depends on a hydrophobic domain on VP5* and is size selective (41). Entry probably occurs by the endocytic route, in which the size-selective membrane permeabilization induced by VP5* permits the exit of Ca^{2+} from the putative viral endosome (41). Due to the low Ca^{2+} concentration in the endosome, the viral particle would then lose VP7. The free VP7 and VP4 could, in turn, have a detergent-like effect on early endosomal membranes, permitting the access of DLPs (free of VP4 and VP7) to the cytoplasm (43).

In the cytoplasm, the DLPs gain transcriptase activity, which had been restricted by the presence of VP4 and VP7, and begin to synthesize viral mRNAs. The mRNAs produced by the transcriptase are exact copies of each genome segment, with a 5′-terminal cap 1 structure and without a 3′-terminal poly(A). The viral mRNAs are then translated, giving rise to the structural and nonstructural proteins necessary to complete the viral replication cycle. Preferential translation of viral proteins is favored by the shutoff of host protein synthesis mediated by NSP3 (111). Viral proteins accumulate in the cytoplasm in electron-dense regions called viroplasms, where the viral genome is replicated and the assembly of progeny DLPs takes place (108). A hypothetical initial stage in viral assembly involves the assortment of single-stranded positive RNA strands corresponding to each of the 11 gene segments. How this occurs is one of the critical mysteries of rotavirus

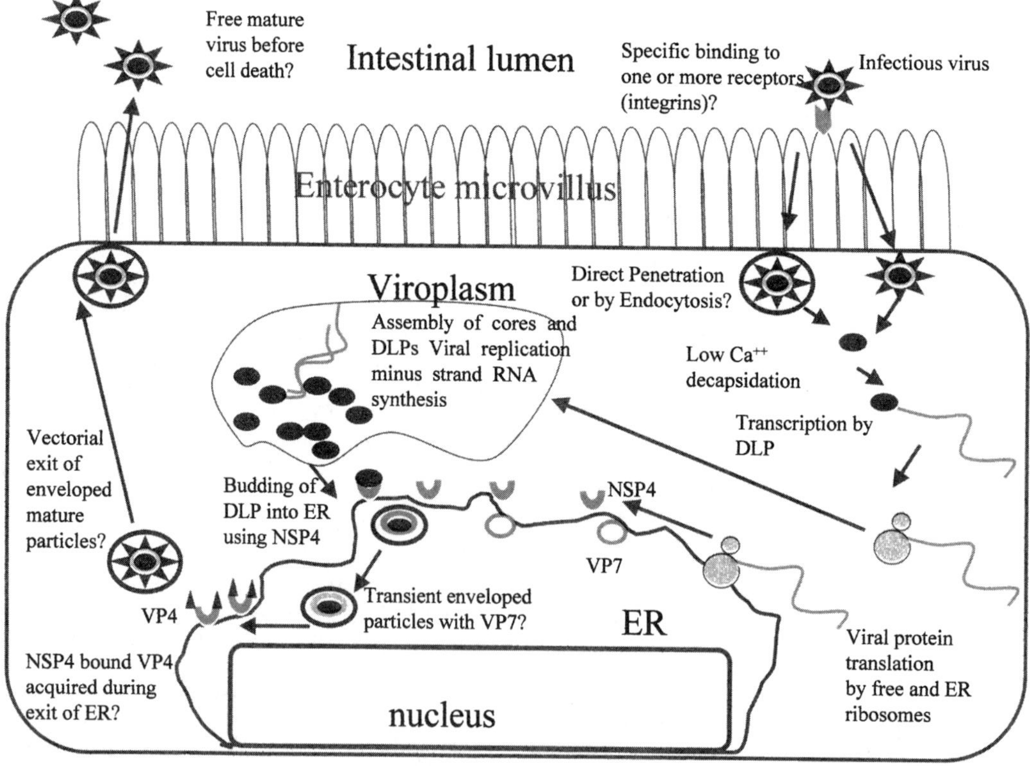

FIGURE 2 Schematic representation of the rotavirus replication cycle in intestinal polarized epithelial cells. For references, see "Replication strategy." As indicated by the question marks, many aspects of this cycle remain uncertain.

replication. The process is not random, because rotaviruses with a particle-to-PFU ratio of less than 5 have been described. The viral polymerase can carry out dsRNA synthesis only when capsid protein is available to package its newly made product. For this reason, free dsRNA does not accumulate in cells and does not trigger dsRNA-dependent IFN signaling (108). A viral intermediate particle that consists of VP1, VP2, VP3, and probably all the nonstructural proteins, except NSP4, is the simplest structure with replicase activity that can be isolated from infected cells, and its formation is postulated to follow gene assortment (108). Most probably, this complex then acquires VP6 and during this process the nonstructural proteins are lost. Subsequently, the DLPs, via VP6, interact with NSP4, which has been synthesized by ER ribosomes (5). This interaction leads to budding of the DLPs into the ER lumen. In this organelle the DLPs acquire a transient lipid membrane. In a very poorly understood mechanism (probably related to the high Ca^{2+} levels of the ER), the viral particles acquire VP7 that is initially present in the ER membrane. When and how the viral particles acquire VP4 and lose the transient enveloping membrane is not known. The exit of the mature TLP from the ER and the cell has not been completely elucidated, and two mechanisms have been proposed (25). In the polarized Caco-2 cell line (derived from a human colon adenocarcinoma), rotavirus is initially released from the apical pole of the cells via a raft-dependent pathway, before cell lysis occurs (25). This mechanism could help explain the lack of substantial histopathology associated with viral shedding that has been observed in some studies of infected animals (25). Alternatively, the virus can exit the cell after cell lysis. The mechanism of cell death induced by rotavirus (before or after viral exit) is not well known; current models in vitro and in vivo in mice suggest that it is dependent of cell apoptosis (19, 23).

The efficient dissemination of rotaviruses to the environment is ensured because they are shed in the feces at a very high concentration (10^{11} particles per g) and are very resistant to degradation at ambient temperature. For example, infectious porcine rotavirus can be recovered after 32 months if stool samples were maintained at approximately 10°C (114).

Host Range

Although animal and human group A rotaviruses can reassort in vitro and in several cases human rotaviruses have been found that have genes of animal rotavirus origin (90), significant species restriction of rotavirus replication exists. This restriction formed the basis for the development of Jennerian rotavirus vaccines (see "Prevention" below). In general, rotavirus from one species has not proven capable of efficiently spreading and maintaining itself in another species. However, interspecies primary transmission and reassortment in vivo are not rare events in certain areas of the world (50). In India, rotaviruses recovered from neonates and children commonly have a P8[11] VP4 type, which is the predominate P type found in buffaloes and cattle (50). G5 rotaviruses that are probably reassortants with porcine rotavirus are endemic in certain areas of Brazil (50). In Malawi, the current predominant rotavirus strains are G8. The similarity of the VP7 gene sequence of the prototype G8 strain isolated in Malawi to that of bovine serotype G8 rotavirus suggests that they may represent human/bovine reassortant viruses (50).

Growth in Cell Culture

Although initially growth of human rotavirus in vitro was very difficult, the discovery that trypsin treatment enhanced viral yield led to the cultivation of most isolates. Biochemical studies of rotavirus gene expression and function have been performed in both the MA104 (monkey kidney) and Caco-2 (human colon cancer) epithelial cell lines (32).

Infectious cDNAs have been derived from most pathogenic human RNA viruses, but transfection of purified rotavirus RNA or cDNA into permissive tissue culture cells has not yet yielded infectious virus. Very recently, the first reverse-genetics method to create rotaviruses with cDNA-derived genes has been described, but this method requires helper virus and appears to be quite inefficient (78). However, recent demonstrations that both reoviruses and orbiviruses are amenable to efficient reverse-genetics manipulation offer promise that the same methodologies will shortly be available for rotaviruses (20, 76). An alternative approach that has recently been used to study the function of individual viral genes involves inhibition of specific RNAs with small interfering RNA (43).

EPIDEMIOLOGY

Distribution

Rotavirus infections occur worldwide, and throughout the world most children develop antirotavirus antibodies by the age of 2 years. Thus, the incidences of rotavirus infection are the same in developed and developing countries, implying that improvements in sanitation and hygiene will not effectively control rotavirus infection. Even in developed countries with good sanitation, the burden of rotavirus disease is very substantial. In the United States, an effective universal rotavirus immunization program would be estimated to prevent 13 deaths, 44,000 hospitalizations, 137,000 emergency department visits, 256,000 office visits, and 1,100,000 episodes of diarrhea requiring only home care for children <5 years of age (151). Group B rotavirus has been associated with recent sporadic cases of diarrhea in adults and children in India, suggesting that it has the potential to reemerge as an important pathogen (8). In a prospective study of diarrhea in adults in Sweden, rotaviruses were found in 3% of patients, and in 35% of these group C rotavirus was detected, suggesting that this virus could be a more common cause of diarrhea in adults than previously realized (102).

Incidence and Prevalence of Infection

The estimated incidence of rotavirus-induced diarrhea varies depending on the method used for detection. The incidence in developing countries determined by prospective studies has varied between 0.07 and 0.8 episode per child per year (128). Compared with diarrhea caused by other microorganisms, diarrhea caused by rotavirus is generally more severe and is more frequently associated with dehydration. Because of the significant association with dehydration, the proportion of children with rotavirus-induced diarrhea depends on the epidemiological settings under study. Rotavirus infections account for a low percentage (8%) of all cases of community-acquired diarrhea, 28% of outpatient or clinic visit-associated diarrhea, and 39% of hospitalizations for diarrhea among young children (106).

The incidence of various rotavirus serotypes varies by geographic location and time. While P1A[8]G1 strains account for more than 70% of rotavirus infections in North America, Europe, and Australia, these viruses represent only about 30% of the infections in South America and Asia and 23% in Africa (128). These variable frequencies could be due to differences in sanitary and climate conditions, or to closer contact of individuals with animal rotaviruses in areas with more rotavirus diversity, or both (128). Not withstanding these differences, approximately 90 and 65% of human rotavirus strains circulating worldwide share some epitopes on VP4 and VP7, respectively, the two proteins that are the target of protective antibodies.

Most epidemiological studies up to the early 1990s showed a predominance of G1 to G4 strains, but since then P[8]G9 and P[6]G9 strains have begun to emerge worldwide, and they currently account for 4.1% of all isolates in recent studies (128). In The Netherlands, a major outbreak of diarrhea in neonates due to a P[6]G9 virus was postulated to be casually associated with a lack of protective maternal antibodies (152). G9 viruses have also been associated with more severe gastroenteritis (GE) in Latin America (81). However, the appearance of a P[6]G9 virus in Philadelphia, PA, did not cause especially severe disease or significantly displace previously extant serotypes (26). More recently, in several countries worldwide, but specifically in India, a high prevalence of G12 viruses has been detected, suggesting that this serotype may be the next emerging rotavirus strain (113). Thus, although rotaviruses with limited serologic variability predominate worldwide, unusual serotypes currently circulate and can arise sporadically in both developed and developing countries, but especially in the latter (128).

Subclinical Infections

Approximately 50% of all rotavirus infections appear to be asymptomatic (140). The percentage of asymptomatic infections increases during the second, third, and subsequent infections, presumably due to the development of both homo- and heterotypic immunity.

Epidemic Patterns and Seasonality

In the temperate zones of the world (mostly developed countries), rotaviral infection occurs primarily during epidemic peaks in the cooler months of the year (27). This pattern is not seen in countries within 10° of the equator, where infection occurs in an endemic fashion year-round (27). No clear explanation is available for the rotavirus winter epidemic peaks: higher airborne transmission (27), higher stability of rotavirus with low relative humidity, and indoor crowding have all been proposed. However, a clear association between lower relative humidity and development of rotavirus infections has not been found in all settings (43).

In the United States, a yearly wave of rotaviral illness spreads across the country, originating in the southwest in November and ending in the northeast in March (136). A convincing explanation for this interesting observation has not been found. A similar phenomenon has been seen in Europe, where an annual rotavirus epidemic starts in Spain, usually in December, followed by France in February and ending in Northern Europe in England and Wales in February or March, and The Netherlands and Finland in March (79).

Age-Specific Attack Rates

The peak incidence of rotaviral illness in children in developing countries is between 6 and 11 months of age. In contrast, in developed countries, like the United States and Canada, the highest rates occur during the second year of life. This difference between developed and developing countries has been proposed to be due to the seasonal pattern of rotavirus infection in developed countries. A child born just after the rotavirus season in a developed country would have almost a year before being exposed to the next rotavirus season, whereas children born in a tropical country where rotavirus is endemic are exposed throughout the year. While rotaviral infection is frequently asymptomatic in neonates (14, 75, 144), first infections after 3 months of age are more likely to be symptomatic. Strains isolated from neonates have been reported to have a particular P type, and also specific differences in their VP7 and NSP4 genes, compared with pathogenic strains of similar serotype (75). However, it is likely the newborn host, rather than the viral strain, that is primarily responsible for the avirulent phenotype of rotavirus infection seen in newborns (144). The relative resistance to rotavirus illness in infants less than 3 months old may be due to antibodies acquired by placental transfer from the mother (144). Rotaviral disease of adults is seen occasionally in the elderly, especially in persons who take care of sick children. In families, almost 50% of the caretakers of children with rotavirus-induced diarrhea become infected with rotavirus, and 50% of these infections are accompanied by mild symptoms (120). In challenge studies of adults with virulent rotavirus, low levels of preexisting serum antibody are associated with symptoms (146).

Risk Factors and High-Risk Groups

Malnutrition, with its probable associated immunodeficiency, has been linked to severe dehydrating rotavirus disease (35). In developed countries, low-birth-weight and premature infants appear to be at greater risk for hospitalization with rotavirus-induced GE (100). Interestingly, human immunodeficiency virus (34) has not proven to be a substantial risk factor for rotavirus illness, whereas severe combined immunodeficiency diseases have (52). In the United States, while breast-feeding was found to be modestly protective, low-birth-weight infants, children in child care, those covered by Medicaid or without insurance, and children having another child in the household had an increased risk of rotavirus-associated hospitalization (37). Being a child of African-American descent (46), maternal age, and having a mother with less than a high school education may also increase risk of rotavirus-associated hospitalization (37). Thus, socioeconomic factors seem to increase the risk for hospitalization with rotavirus-induced GE (37).

Reinfections

Prospective study shows that rotavirus reinfections are very common. One study found that 96, 69, 42, 22, and 13% of children were reinfected 1, 2, 3, 4, and 5 times, respectively (140). The severity of disease rapidly decreased after the first infection, and remarkably, no child experienced moderate or severe disease after the second reinfection.

Transmission

Rotaviruses are usually transmitted by the fecal-oral route, but some limited indirect evidence suggests that they could also be transmitted by the respiratory route (43). Nasal shedding of an attenuated, but not a virulent, human rotavirus was seen in a pig model, suggesting that this route of transmission might depend on the viral strain (6). The origin of a rotavirus that infects a child who is not in contact with other children is not clear, but such infection could be due to subclinical infection in household adults (43). Although rotaviruses have been detected in both treated and untreated sewage water, waterborne outbreaks are probably rare due to the relative instability of rotavirus at high relative humidity (43). Food-borne outbreaks are also rare, although it has been reported that oyster and mussel samples can be heavily contaminated by rotavirus (43).

The duration of viral excretion in infected children, as determined both by enzyme-linked immunosorbent assay (ELISA) and a sensitive PCR method, ranges from 4 to 57 days after onset of diarrhea (118). Viral excretion stops in 10 days in about 43% of children and within 20 days in 70% of children. Extended excretion (mainly following initial infection) is detected for 25 to 57 days in the remaining 30% of children.

Institutions, like day care centers, with high concentrations of young children have an increased risk of developing outbreaks of rotavirus disease. Moist surfaces, including the telephone, water fountains, and water play tables, are common sources of rotavirus contamination in day care centers (43). Rotavirus infection occurs frequently in neonatal nurseries, and although most of these infections are asymptomatic, some are not (152). Nosocomial rotavirus infections, especially in newborn nurseries, are often caused by a single strain that differs from strains circulating concurrently outside of the hospital (39, 43).

PATHOGENESIS IN HUMANS

Incubation Period

In studies of experimental infection of adult volunteers, the incubation period for rotavirus is generally less than 48 h. This very short incubation period, which permits substantial viral replication before the amplification of a memory immune response, may be one of the factors that explains the multiple reinfections that occur with rotavirus (48).

Patterns of Virus Replication

An important study from an immunologic point of view showed that in cattle, rotaviruses penetrate but do not replicate in the intestinal M cells that cover Peyer's patches, an observation suggesting that rotaviruses can come in contact with the immune system by means of these cells (135). Until recently, it was thought that in immunocompetent children, rotavirus infection was restricted to the mature enterocytes on the tips of the small intestinal villi (43); recent studies in both healthy humans and animals have established that most rotavirus infections are associated with viral antigenemia (16), RNAemia (116), and some level of viremia (17) during the initial phase of rotavirus-induced diarrhea. In mice, the level and location of extraintestinal replication vary among rotavirus strains, and initial steps of viral replication seem to occur in several leukocyte subsets (44). However, the clinical relevance of the findings of extraintestinal spread and replication is still unclear, and in children and in animals the great bulk of rotavirus replication occurs in the mature villus tip cells of the small bowel (Fig. 3). Immunostaining with antibodies against nonstructural proteins in liver and kidney autopsy samples from severely immunodeficient children with chronic rotavirus infection suggests that extraintestinal viral replication occurs under these circumstances (52).

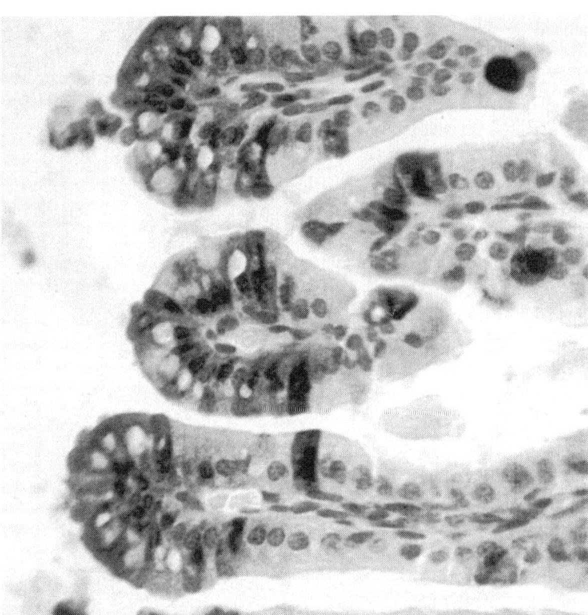

FIGURE 3 Cross section of the small bowel villi from a rotavirus-infected mouse; the sample was immunostained for rotavirus antigen. Note the growth of rotavirus restricted to the mature villus tip cells of the small bowel.

Factors in Disease Production

The pathological changes in the intestines of children infected with rotavirus include shortening and atrophy of the villi, mononuclear infiltration in the lamina propia, and distended cisternae of the ER (43). However, a direct relationship between the extent of histopathological changes and disease severity has not been demonstrated. For example, in a study of intestinal biopsy samples from children with rotavirus-induced diarrhea, 95% of 40 patients did not have prominent histopathological changes despite their symptoms (77). In the mouse model, rotavirus disease is associated with very modest histopathological findings, suggesting that the mechanism or mechanisms for the induction of rotavirus-induced diarrhea could be similar in mice and humans. In all species examined to date, the bulk of rotavirus infection appears to be restricted to the mature villus tip cells of the small bowel (Fig. 3), while low levels of viremia and extraintestinal replication in other organs probably take place. Using a semiquantitative PCR assay, a direct correlation was found between the levels of viral RNA in stool and the severity of diarrhea (72), but this observation needs to be confirmed.

Studies of the physiological basis of rotavirus-induced diarrhea in humans and in several animal models have yielded diverse and sometimes contradictory findings (43). In the pig model, rotavirus infection is associated with decreased intestinal lactase content, increased fecal lactose loss, and an increased fecal osmotic gap (43). These findings are consistent with the hypothesis that malabsorption of carbohydrates causes an osmotic diarrhea during rotaviral infection. In humans, a lactase deficiency has also been associated with rotavirus-induced GE (103). The most common explanation for the malabsorption and lactase deficiency associated with rotavirus-induced diarrhea is the direct destruction of the enterocyte during viral replication. An alternative explanation, which would be more in accord with the cases of rotavirus disease not associated with substantial histopathological findings, is that rotavirus affects the turnover of microvillar membrane disaccharidases (43). In support of this theory, rotavirus reduces sucrase-isomaltase expression and activity in human intestinal epithelial tumor cell lines by perturbing protein targeting and the organization of the microvillar cytoskeleton, before apparent cell destruction occurs (25). In children, rotavirus-induced diarrhea causes increased mucosal permeability, as measured by the lactulose-mannitol intestinal permeability test (103). A possible explanation for these in vivo findings is suggested by in vitro experiments that show that rotavirus induces structural and functional alterations in tight junctions of polarized intestinal Caco-2 cell monolayers, without alterations in cell and monolayer integrity (25).

There are other potential causes of rotavirus-induced diarrhea. The heterologous SA11 recombinant NSP4 and a synthetic peptide derived from it induce an age-dependent secretory diarrhea in mice (7). NSP4 is thus the first identified viral enterotoxin (7). In these studies, mouse pups born to dams immunized with the NSP4-derived peptide were partially protected from the diarrhea induced by heterologous rotavirus. The homologous mouse NSP4 has also been shown to induce diarrhea in mice. Since CFTR knockout mice, which do not respond to any known intestinal secretagogues, experience homologous rotavirus-induced diarrhea and NSP4 and the NSP4-derived peptide also induce diarrhea in these mice, NSP4 may mediate its effect through a novel secretory (non-CFTR-dependent) pathway or by another nonsecretory mechanism (43). In addition, rotavirus infection may induce intestinal fluid and electrolyte secretion by activation of the enteric nervous system in the intestinal wall (84), but further studies need to be performed to establish the relative importance of this mechanism. The fact that children with rotavirus-induced GE can be successfully treated with acetorphan, an enkephalinase inhibitor that acts on the enteric nervous system, supports a role for this mechanism in rotavirus-induced diarrhea (127). The three mechanisms (malabsorption, NSP4, and enteric nervous system) proposed to explain rotavirus-induced diarrhea could play different relative roles depending upon the animal species analyzed and, for a given species, could be operating together, with the relative importance of each mechanism varying depending upon the stage of infection. Determining the relative importance of each mechanism in human rotavirus-induced diarrhea would help in developing vaccine strategies or strategies to treat rotavirus-induced diarrhea.

Immune Responses

Although symptomatic reinfection with rotaviruses seems to be frequent, the severity and number of rotavirus infections diminish with the age of the child, and severe infections seem to be primarily limited to the initial infection (48). This pattern of infection strongly suggests that a protective immune response against rotavirus develops after primary infection, but that the generation of complete immunity requires multiple infections (29). Chronic rotavirus infection, prolonged symptoms, and extraintestinal infection in children with severe combined T and/or B immunodeficiencies (52, 153) also argue for an important role of adaptive immune responses to rotavirus. Some, but not all, strains of T- and B-cell-immunodeficient mice become chronically infected with murine rotavirus (48).

Innate Immunity

Studies with mice have shown that rotaviruses are inactivated in the stomachs of adult but not newborn mice (12), which suggests that the development of gastric acid and pepsin secretion may be an important factor in host defense against rotavirus. Interleukin 1, IFN-α, and IFN-γ cytokines can induce a dose-dependent resistance to rotavirus infection in vitro (11). Certain cytokines (interleukin 10, IFN-γ, and IFN-α) and chemokines are produced in the intestines of mice (122) and in the serum of children (70) after rotavirus infection, suggesting that innate intestinal immunity may play a role in modulating infection. The relative importance of IFN-α in innate immunity to rotavirus has been highlighted recently by the fact that NSP1 inhibits IFN-α responses (9). These and/or other innate mechanisms may explain the observation that some, but not all, mouse strains with combined T- and B-cell deficiency clear rotavirus infection successfully (48). A passive innate mechanism that has been associated with an antirotavirus effect is the presence of the lactadherin glycoprotein in human milk. This protein binds to rotavirus and inhibits its replication in vitro (99). Lactadherin levels in maternal milk are significantly higher in asymptomatic than symptomatic children with rotavirus infection, suggesting that this glycoprotein, rather than immunoglobulin A (IgA), could be mediating the antiviral effect of maternal milk.

Specific Humoral and Cell-Mediated Immune Responses

Because rotavirus replication is primarily restricted to enterocytes in vivo, the immune responses against rotavirus originate in, and exhibit their effector function directly at, the intestinal mucosa. Hence, rotaviruses can serve as an excellent model for the study of basic aspects of intestinal immunity. Such studies in neonatal and adult mice have shown that intestinal T-cell and neutralizing antibody responses are relatively weak in neonatal mice after homologous rotavirus infection (4, 67, 138). Nevertheless, protection from reinfection is primarily mediated by antibodies, but T cells can also play a role. Moreover, the presence of the integrin $\alpha 4\beta 7$ (the intestinal homing receptor) has been shown to be required by B cells, but not $CD8^+$ T cells, for the migration of the lymphocytes to the intestine to provide immunity to rotavirus (48). The migration of the B cells to the intestine also depends on the presence of the CCR9 and CCR10 chemokine receptors (45). However, immune responses of humans may differ substantially from those in animals. For example, while mice develop a primary lifelong protective intestinal IgA response against rotavirus, humans do not and are reinfected multiple times.

A rotavirus-specific IgA coproantibody response occurs in 70 to 84% of children after a symptomatic infection (48). This IgA response has been reported to peak from 1 to 4 weeks after infection and then to decrease rapidly (29, 89). The relatively short duration of human intestinal antiviral IgA is probably one of the factors that contribute to multiple reinfections with rotavirus. The ratio of salivary virus-specific IgA1 to IgA2 in very young children is higher than the ratio in adults, suggesting that the response in children is qualitatively different (more sensitive to intestinal proteases, for example) from that of adults (49). During the acute phase of infection, IgM serum antibodies predominate, being subsequently replaced by IgG and, to a lesser extent, IgA (58). The IgG serum response is longer lasting than salivary or fecal IgA (30, 48). During acute infection, rotavirus-specific serum IgA has been shown to be directed principally against VP2 and VP6 and to broaden to include other structural and nonstructural proteins in the convalescent phase (71). Secondary infections will generally boost the fecal IgA response, and in many, but not all, children, they induce protective fecal antirotavirus IgA levels (29). Studies of human neutralizing antibody responses against rotavirus have shown that upon first exposures to rotavirus, children develop higher homotypic than heterotypic antibody levels (48). However, as the number of rotavirus infections increases, children develop more heterotypic antibodies. Recent studies with human MAbs suggest that the fine specificity of human neutralizing antibodies may differ from those of the most extensively studied animal neutralizing antibodies (60, 94).

In older children without documented recent rotavirus infection who underwent surgery for diverse causes, the presence of blood circulating rotavirus-specific antibody-secreting cells (ASC) correlated with intestinal ASC (21). Thus, the measurement of blood ASC may be a good surrogate marker for intestinal antiviral responses. More recently, human rotavirus-specific B cells have been characterized in detail, for both mice and naturally infected and vaccinated children, by flow cytometry (69, 121). Interestingly, a significant fraction of naïve human B cells bind rotavirus VP6 (107), and the VH1-46 gene is a dominant gene used by these cells (150).

The rotavirus-specific T-cell immune response in both children and adults has been studied by lymphoproliferation (104) and, more recently, by flow cytometry (68). The frequency of rotavirus-specific T cells in children with acute rotavirus infection is relatively low, at least in comparison to several chronic viral infections (68). This finding may be related to recent studies that suggest that children with acute rotavirus infection have circulating T-cell lymphopenia (145). More studies of the T-cell response to rotavirus, specially those that identify the epitopes recognized by the T cells, are needed to clarify the role of cellular immune responses to rotavirus in humans.

Correlates of Immune Protection

Studies in animal models and humans have shown that local intestinal antibody is probably the primary protective effector mechanism against rotavirus (48). In mice, other mechanisms, like $CD8^+$ T cells induced by natural infection, can also mediate a modest level of protection (48).

Protective humoral immune responses in several, but not all, animal models are associated with the presence of neutralizing antibodies directed at VP4 and/or VP7 (48). In mice, nonneutralizing antibodies directed against VP6 have also been shown to be able to protect (22). Since these VP6 antibodies were not active when present on the luminal side of the intestinal tract, they appear to mediate intracellular viral inactivation during transcytosis through the enterocyte (22, 28). In addition, as mentioned previously, suckling pups nursed by dams vaccinated with an NSP4-derived peptide are partially protected from heterologous rotavirus-induced diarrhea (7). In pigs (the only animal model in which protection from disease and not viral infection is measured), vaccination with VLPs composed of VP2 and VP6 did not induce protection against challenge with a human rotavirus, despite the presence of a substantial intestinal antibody response, while protection with VLPs composed of VP2 and VP6 is induced in mice (48). In addition, in the pig model, NSP4 antibodies do not correlate with protection (156). Unlike pigs, neonatal mice are moderately well protected against rotavirus after vaccination with adjuvant intranasal recombinant VP6, a vaccine that specifically requires the induction of $CD4^+$ T cells (138). Adult mice are better protected by this vaccine than neonatal mice (138). Thus, immunity may vary according to the immunogen, the animal species, the age of the animal at vaccination, and the route of immunization (48, 138).

In studies performed in day care centers and orphanages, where antibodies to rotavirus were measured very shortly before a rotavirus outbreak, intestinal and/or serum antibody levels correlated with protection against rotavirus reinfection (48). Rotavirus-specific antibodies (stool IgA in particular) have also been correlated with protection in some studies (29), but not in others, involving naturally infected as well as vaccinated children (48). In general, serum antibody levels have correlated better with protection following natural infection than following vaccination (48, 141). At present, we do not have a precise and reliable marker for vaccine-induced protection. This absence has been an impediment to the development of new rotavirus vaccines, since the only way of determining whether a vaccine is effective is in field efficacy trials. Both serum neutralizing antibodies and serum and stool G-type-specific antibodies correlated with protection in studies carried out in an orphanage and day care center (89). Nonetheless, neutralizing antibodies did not correlate with protection in other settings (48). Likewise, in vaccine studies, some investigators, but not others, found a correlation between the presence of neutralizing antibodies and protection (48). Younger children develop lower levels of neutralizing antibodies to the Rotarix vaccine (see below), and the frequency of children who develop these antibodies is significantly lower than the level of protection induced by the vaccine (147). Thus, although neutralizing antibodies seem to play a role in protection, it is possible that antibodies against other proteins (VP6 and/or NSP4) or other mechanisms also play a role in immunity.

The role of maternal antibodies acquired transplacentally and through milk has been studied in several animal models of rotavirus infection (101). In the pig model, antibodies acquired transplacentally (simulated by the passive transfer of serum from rotavirus-infected animals) or by colostrum reduced the severity of primary rotavirus disease (101). These antibodies also inhibited the development of an effective mucosal immune response, and animals that received these antibodies were more susceptible to viral reinfection than the ones that did not receive the antibodies (101). The relative importance of transplacentally acquired versus breast-feeding-acquired antibodies in protection against rotaviruses in children is not clear. It has been postulated that the relative resistance of newborns to rotavirus-induced diarrhea is due to transplacentally acquired antibodies (144). Children breast-fed with milk that contains antirotavirus neutralizing antibodies develop diarrhea at a rate similar to non-breast-fed children, or those breast-fed with milk that did not have the antibodies (54). In contrast, breast-feeding may slightly decrease vaccine take rates, indicating a modest antirotavirus effect (54). Breast-fed children and non-breast-fed children develop both symptomatic and asymptomatic rotavirus infections to the same extent (99). The concentration of lactadherin but not rotavirus-specific secretory milk IgA is higher in the breast milk of mothers of children with asymptomatic infection than in that of mothers of children with rotavirus-induced diarrhea. Thus, breast-feeding probably confers limited protection against rotavirus, but this effect is apparently minor compared to the effect breast-feeding has against several bacterially induced diarrheas.

Correlates of Disease Resolution

In animal models, the mechanisms that mediate disease resolution are multiple and probably redundant. In mice, $CD8^+$ T cells are probably the first acquired immune mechanism that mediates rotavirus clearance (48), but in their absence, antibody or other mechanisms can perform this function. The mechanisms responsible for disease and infection resolution in humans have not been studied.

CLINICAL MANIFESTATIONS

Major Clinical Syndromes

The primary clinical syndrome caused by rotavirus infection is acute GE. Typically, rotavirus-induced diarrhea is watery, lasts for approximately 5 days, is preceded by the sudden onset of vomiting (typically lasting 1 to 2 days), and is frequently accompanied by several days of fever (37.9°C or greater) and dehydration (137). Respiratory symptoms, while common in children with rotavirus infection, have not been specifically linked to this virus, although in the mouse model the virus appears to replicate at low levels in the lungs (44). The vomiting associated with rotavirus disease has been correlated with the increased levels of serum IFN-α in acutely infected children (36). Since the maximal temperature and duration of fever were not correlated with levels of serum IFN-α, it is probable that other endogenous inflammatory mediators are responsible. Severe diarrhea in a child under the age of 3 years during the cool months of the year, in a country with a temperate climate, strongly suggests the diagnosis of rotavirus. Nonetheless, the clinical characteristics of rotavirus illness are not distinct enough to permit diagnosis based solely on physical exam and history, and laboratory confirmation is necessary for a definitive diagnosis, although such diagnosis is seldom needed for therapeutic purposes in children with mild to moderate GE.

Laboratory abnormalities in children with rotavirus infection are related to vomiting and dehydration (high urine specific gravity and electrolyte alterations) and should be investigated depending on their severity. The presence of reducing sugars in stool should alert the clinician to probable lactose intolerance (59). Occult blood and fecal leukocytes are found infrequently (less than 16 and 39%, respectively) in rotavirus-infected children, but these findings are present at higher frequencies in children with bacterial infections and may redirect the differential diagnosis (63). Overtly bloody stools, prolonged diarrhea, leukocytosis, and a raised erythrocyte sedimentation rate suggest a bacterial etiology and are rarely associated with rotavirus infection (137). One recent study requiring confirmation found that up to 20% of children with rotavirus-induced GE had elevated alanine aminotransferase and aspartate aminotransferase, suggesting that some hepatic involvement may occur during infection (134).

Rotavirus infection can cause severe and prolonged disease in children with severe combined primary immunodeficiencies, some of whom shed virus chronically and develop antigenemia and dissemination of infection (52). Severe rotavirus disease can be a particular threat to severely immunosuppressed pediatric bone marrow and liver transplant recipients (47). The role of rotavirus-induced disease in immunosuppressed adults with human immunodeficiency virus and in adult transplant patients (34, 139) is less important.

Complications

Rotaviruses are not a major cause of prolonged diarrhea. However, diarrhea of rotavirus origin, especially in developing countries, can be the initiating factor for malnutrition, with its accompanying immunodeficiency, which in turn makes the child susceptible to other infectious diseases (88). Thus, the effects of rotavirus disease may not be limited to the morbidity and mortality associated per se with an episode of acute diarrhea. Most (but not all) studies have not found an association between natural rotavirus infection and intussusception (98, 117). In mice, rotavirus enhances lipopolysaccharide-induced intussusception (149). Moreover, natural rotavirus infection in children thickens the intestinal wall and enlarges mesenteric lymph nodes (10), suggesting a potential mechanism by which infection could promote intussusception. Studies aimed at clarifying this potential association are of great relevance, because RotaShield (Wyeth/Lederle), the first licensed rotavirus vaccine, was withdrawn from the market because of its temporal association with very rare cases of intestinal intussusception. These cases mostly occurred in the first week after administration of the first vaccine dose (97). Although studies have failed to identify the reasons why RotaShield induced intussusception, it is important to note (see "Prevention" below) that this complication occurred mostly (80%) in children older than 3 months of age (132). A relationship between rotavirus infection and the development of diabetes has been proposed but is not supported by recent experiments in mice and children (86), and further studies are needed to clarify this issue. A possible association between group C rotavirus and the development of biliary atresia has been supported by some studies (119) but not other studies (18). However, in rodents certain strains of heterologous simian group A rotavirus induce biliary atresia (85). This disease is autoimmune in nature, since adoptive transfer of T cells from mice with rotavirus-induced biliary atresia into naïve syngeneic severe combined immunodeficient recipient mice resulted in bile duct-specific inflammation, in the absence of detectable virus. Preliminary evidence requiring confirmation associates rotavirus infection with celiac disease (157). Seizures have been reported in association with rotavirus infection and in association with mild GE due to other viruses (1). The casual relationship between rotavirus and seizures has been supported by the detection of rotavirus in some cerebrospinal fluid samples by PCR (1). Electrolyte abnormalities and fever associated with infection could also explain some of the seizures, and a firm conclusion concerning the mechanism of seizures cannot be drawn at present. Many other rare complications have been associated with rotavirus infection, but due to the high frequency of rotavirus infections, these associations probably occurred by chance.

LABORATORY DIAGNOSIS

Virus Isolation

Cell Culture

At present, cultivation of human group A rotavirus is relatively straightforward but a time-consuming and labor-intensive task. In contrast, very few group B and C rotaviruses have been grown in vitro. The best results for growing group A human rotavirus are obtained using fecal samples (rectal swabs are less efficient) (43). With pretreatment of virus with trypsin (5 to 10 μg/ml) and subsequent incorporation of trypsin (0.5 to 1 μg/ml) in the medium of infected MA104 cells in roller tubes, 75% of human rotaviruses can be grown in vitro (43). Primary simian kidney cells (148) and intestinally derived cell lines, like the human colon adenocarcinoma cell line Caco-2 (33), are probably superior to MA104 cells for primary isolation of rotavirus.

Antigen Detection

The first method available for making the diagnosis of rotavirus infection was electron microscopy. Although this method has generally been replaced by the more readily available solid-phase immunoassays, it can still be of use, for example, for detecting non-group A rotavirus and mixed infections with other enteric viruses. Commercially available ELISA kits are more sensitive than latex agglutination tests for detecting rotavirus in stool samples and are probably the most commonly used system for making the diagnosis of rotavirus infection (51). The commercial ELISA kits available can have a sensitivity and specificity of up to 98 and 100%, respectively. Among the ELISAs, those that employ specimen-specific negative controls (preimmune sera as capture antibodies) are superior in minimizing false-positive reactions (51). ELISAs that use G and P serotype-specific MAbs are also available to type the most frequent rotavirus strains that infect humans.

Nucleic Acid Detection

In the early rotavirus studies, the characteristic migration patterns of genomic dsRNA during polyacrylamide gel electrophoresis were used as an important laboratory and epidemiological tool. This method of differentiating rotavirus strains is called electropherotyping. Although this method is still useful to differentiate rotaviruses of group A from rotaviruses of other groups, the different electropherotypes among group A strains do not correspond to specific serotypes and are of limited value (43).

Reverse transcriptase PCR amplification of rotavirus nucleic acid from stool specimens is the most sensitive way to detect group A, B, and C rotaviruses (3, 56). With this method, in a case control study, up to 29% of asymptomatic children less than 1 year of age were found to be positive for rotavirus (3). This observation needs confirmation or refutation, since high rates of apparent infection in asymptomatic children have never been observed using ELISA or EM diagnostic assays. If these findings are correct, they suggest that symptomatic children must shed much more PCR-positive material than asymptomatic children. In agreement with this conclusion, a correlation has been observed between the severity of rotavirus-induced diarrhea and the quantity of RNA shed (72). G (66) and P (87) genotyping by PCR is more sensitive and specific than solid-phase immunoassays based on serotype-specific MAbs. Future developments in rotavirus nucleic acid detection will probably involve quantitative real-time PCR assays (92), and microarray assays to simultaneously detect multiple rotavirus variants (61).

Serologic Assays

Detection of rotavirus-specific serum and stool antibodies is generally performed by ELISA, and the use of these ELISAs is restricted to epidemiological and vaccine studies. The most sensitive and rapid serologic test to make the diagnosis of primary rotavirus infection relies on the detection of virus-specific IgM in serum (58). However, children without rotavirus-induced diarrhea can have low levels of this antibody. A fourfold increase in convalescent-phase over acute-phase serum IgA and/or IgG titers can also be used to diagnose primary infections. An increase in IgA titer in convalescent-phase stool samples is a more sensitive marker of rotavirus reinfection than seroconversion (30). However, measurement of coproantibodies in breast-fed children is complicated by their presence at various levels in maternal milk. Measurement of rotavirus neutralizing antibodies is commonly performed by plaque reduction or focus reduction assay (147). Serotype-specific responses to defined VP7 or VP4 epitopes can be measured by traditional competition immunoassay (130).

PREVENTION

General

Standard precautions are adequate, and strict isolation of rotavirus-infected patients is not necessary to avoid spread of nosocomial rotavirus infections (38). The risk of nosocomial infection is not increased by room contact with a rotavirus-infected patient or by the sharing of attending personnel. Precaution should be exercised in disinfection of surfaces thought to be contaminated with rotavirus, since rotaviruses have been shown to be highly resistant to many commonly used disinfectants (43). A spray composed of 0.1% *o*-phenylphenol and 79% ethanol is highly effective at decontaminating surfaces (43). These measures combined with careful hand washing will limit the spread of rotavirus infection in hospitals or other institutional settings. Nonetheless, the fact that the incidences of rotavirus infection are similar in developed and less developed countries suggests that these measures will not replace the need for an effective vaccine.

Passive Immunoprophylaxis

The feasibility of passively protecting newborns by immunizing mothers with rotavirus vaccine has been demonstrated in animal models and human trials in which oral vaccination of mothers increased milk antibodies (110); however, the efficacy of this strategy in humans has not been evaluated.

Active Immunization

Because animal and human rotaviruses share antigens capable of inducing protective immunity (154), Jennerian vaccines (vaccination of humans with a host range-restricted and hence attenuated rotavirus of animal origin) have been the most extensively tested rotavirus vaccines.

Based on evidence that indicated that protection against rotavirus depended on serotype G-specific antibodies (57), a quadrivalent vaccine with the four most common human G serotypes was made by combining a rhesus rotavirus (serotype 3) and three monoreassortants of this virus that possessed the gene encoding VP7 of human rotavirus serotypes 1, 2, and 4. This vaccine was shown to prevent 49, 80, and 100% of all episodes, of severe episodes, and of dehydrating diarrhea episodes, respectively. The quadrivalent rhesus vaccine (RotaShield) was licensed for use in the United States but then withdrawn from the market because of its association with intussusception (97). RotaShield appears to trigger an increase in the number of intussusceptions within the first week following vaccination. However, the impact of this vaccine on the total attributable risk of intussusception is quite small and age dependent (124). Nonetheless, given the reported strength of the temporal association, it seems unlikely that this vaccine will ever be reconsidered for widespread use.

Two new orally administered, live attenuated rotavirus vaccines have been recently licensed for use in many countries worldwide. The vaccine produced by Merck (RotaTeq) contains five monoreassortants of a bovine virus with G1, G2, G3, G4, and P1A[8] human rotavirus genes and is given in a three-dose schedule (143). The vaccine produced by GlaxoSmithKline (Rotarix) is an attenuated human G1P1A[8] virus given in a two-dose schedule (125). In trials that involved over 60,000 infants, both of these vaccines were shown to be safe and to provide protection against any and severe rotavirus-induced diarrhea of more than 70 and 98%, respectively. Importantly, both vaccines reduced the rates of all GE-related hospitalizations of any cause by more than 40% (4). Despite these encouraging results, and the fact that Rotarix has been shown to work in malnourished children from Venezuela (109), it is still undetermined if these vaccines will work effectively in very poor developing countries in Africa and Asia, in which children can be malnourished and atypical rotavirus strains may frequently circulate. Moreover, the intussusception associated with RotaShield was predominantly seen in children older than 3 months of age, but the children studied in the large safety evaluations of the two new vaccines were predominately 2 months of age. Thus, the safety of the new rotavirus vaccines in children of more than 3 months of age has not been well established, and the development of third-generation vaccines may be desirable (4). The Advisory Committee on Immunization Practices, as endorsed by the American Academy of Pediatrics (AAP) (105), recommends routine immunization of infants with three doses of RotaTeq, administered orally at 2, 4, and 6 months of age. The first dose should be administered between 6 and 12 weeks of age; immunization should not be initiated for infants older than 12 weeks of age. Subsequent doses should be administered at 4- to 10-week intervals, and all three doses of vaccine should be administered by 32 weeks of age. Both Rotarix and RotaTeq can be coadministered with other childhood vaccines.

In addition to the newly licensed vaccines, several other live oral vaccines are being evaluated or in use (4). The Lanzhou lamb rotavirus strain, which was developed in China, has been in use in that country since 2000; however, controlled clinical trial data supporting its efficacy and safety have not been published in the English literature. A bovine reassortant vaccine developed in the United States by the National Institutes of Health has been shown to provide high levels of protection, and in a new approach to vaccine development, this vaccine was licensed to seven companies in three developing countries where it is currently under development and evaluation. Based on the observation that neonatal rotavirus infection protects against severe rotavirus-induced GE later in life (14), two vaccines derived from neonatal rotavirus strains (the Indian 116E and the Australian RV3 P[6]G3) are also under evaluation. As a strategy to lower the risk of intussusception, some investigators are proposing neonatal administration of live oral vaccines, since such complications are very rare at this age (142). Also, to try to minimize this and other potential complications, strategies for future rotavirus vaccines include several nonlive vaccines, like recombinant viral antigens (VP6), rotavirus VLPs, DNA vaccination with selected rotavirus genes, and vaccination with synthetic peptides (48).

TREATMENT

Since rotavirus disease spontaneously resolves in a few days to 1 or 2 weeks without treatment, therapy is aimed at preventing dehydration, which is the main serious complication. The standard hydration solution used is one recommended by the World Health Organization. It was derived from the formula initially developed to treat secretory cholera-induced diarrhea and thus has a high sodium concentration and an osmolarity of 331 mmol/liter. Rehydration formulas with reduced osmolarity (224 mmol/liter) have been suggested to be superior to this formulation in treatment of children with non-cholera-induced diarrhea, especially the subset of patients with most severe persistent disease (42, 64, 115). Rice-based rehydration solutions have been shown to have little advantage over the standard World Health Organization formula, which contains glucose (93). If oral rehydration fails, or if the patient is severely dehydrated or in shock, intravenous fluids must be administered (74). A CDC committee endorsed by the AAP has elaborated detailed recommendations for oral rehydration and treatment of GE in children (74).

Several studies have indicated that passive oral immunotherapy can shorten the duration of rotavirus infection in animals and humans. The rationale for this type of treatment has been studied while treating immunocompromised children with chronic rotavirus-induced diarrhea (83). Treatment with antirotavirus immunoglobulin of bovine colostral origin was shown to reduce the daily and total stool output and stool frequency and to accelerate viral clearance in children with rotavirus-induced diarrhea. It is not clear, however, whether this strategy will be economically feasible or logistically practical. Administration of some strains of lactobacilli (the bacteria present in yogurt) to children with rotavirus-induced diarrhea stimulated a stronger immune response to rotavirus and shortened the duration of diarrhea in some, but not all, studies (126, 133). The CDC committee declined to recommend the use of lactobacilli because their efficacy had not been fully evaluated, although these bacteria were considered to be safe (74). This committee also did not recommend loperamide, anticholinergic agents, bismuth subsalicylate, or adsorbents for the symptomatic treatment of diarrhea in children 1 month to 5 years of age. Because of the associated side effects, like ileus, the use of opiates and atropine is contraindicated for treatment of children with diarrhea.

Several other compounds, like racecadotril (127) (an enkephalinase inhibitor with antisecretory and antidiarrheal actions) and nitazoxanide (123), have, in limited clinical studies, been shown to be safe and effective against rotavirus-induced diarrhea, but more data are required before these drugs can be recommended. Zinc supplementation is effective at preventing and treating diarrhea in children of developing countries, but its use in developed countries needs further evaluation (74).

Early refeeding after rehydration of children with diarrhea is recommended (74). A meta-analysis found that this practice does not prolong diarrhea and that it may reduce the duration of diarrhea by approximately 0.5 day (74). Recommended foods include complex carbohydrates (rice, wheat, potatoes, bread, and cereals), lean meats, yogurt, fruits, and vegetables. Fatty foods and foods high in simple sugars (including juices and soft drinks) should be avoided. The AAP initially recommended gradual reintroduction of milk-based formulas or cow's milk in the management of acute diarrhea, beginning with diluted milk mixtures. Based on several studies (59), this recommendation has changed, and at present the recommendation is that children with diarrhea can receive a regular age-appropriate diet, including undiluted milk, but with active clinical monitoring to identify the few children who develop malabsorption and lactose intolerance (74). Lactose intolerance should be suspected if diarrheal disease severity worsens 3 to 4 days after the onset of diarrhea and for those who are passing significant amounts of reducing sugars in their stool (59). In Thai and other Asian children with genetically determined low lactase levels, a lactose-free diet seems to be better for recovery from rotavirus infection (131).

REFERENCES

1. **Abe, T., M. Kobayashi, K. Araki, H. Kodama, Y. Fujita, T. Shinozaki, and H. Ushijima.** 2001. Infantile convulsions with mild gastroenteritis. *Brain Dev* **22:**301–306.
2. **Adams, W. R., and L. M. Kraft.** 1963. Epizootic diarrhea of infant mice: identification of the etiologic agent. *Science* **141:**359–360.
3. **Amar, C. F., C. L. East, J. Gray, M. Iturriza-Gomara, E. A. Maclure, and J. McLauchlin.** 2007. Detection by PCR of eight groups of enteric pathogens in 4,627 faecal samples: re-examination of the English case-control Infectious Intestinal Disease Study (1993–1996). *Eur. J. Clin. Microbiol. Infect. Dis.* **26:**311–323.
4. **Angel, J., M. A. Franco, and H. B. Greenberg.** 2007. Rotavirus vaccines: recent developments and future considerations. *Nat. Rev. Microbiol.* **5:**529–539.
5. **Au, K. S., N. M. Mattion, and M. K. Estes.** 1993. A subviral particle binding domain on the rotavirus nonstructural glycoprotein NS28. *Virology* **194:**665–673.
6. **Azevedo, M. S., L. Yuan, K. I. Jeong, A. Gonzalez, T. V. Nguyen, S. Pouly, M. Gochnauer, W. Zhang, A. Azevedo, and L. J. Saif.** 2005. Viremia and nasal and rectal shedding of rotavirus in gnotobiotic pigs inoculated with Wa human rotavirus. *J. Virol.* **79:**5428–5436.
7. **Ball, J. M., P. Tian, C. Q.-Y. Zeng, A. P. Morris, and M. K. Estes.** 1996. Age-dependent diarrhea induced by a rotaviral nonstructural glycoprotein. *Science* **272:**101–104.
8. **Barman, P., S. Ghosh, S. Samajdar, U. Mitra, P. Dutta, S. K. Bhattacharya, T. Krishnan, N. Kobayashi, and T. N. Naik.** 2006. RT-PCR based diagnosis revealed importance of human group B rotavirus infection in childhood diarrhoea. *J. Clin. Virol.* **36:**222–227.
9. **Barro, M., and J. T. Patton.** 2007. Rotavirus NSP1 inhibits expression of type I interferon by antagonizing the function of interferon regulatory factors IRF3, IRF5, and IRF7. *J. Virol.* **81:**4473–4481.
10. **Bass, D., E. Cordoba, C. Dekker, A. Schuind, and C. Cassady.** 2004. Intestinal imaging of children with acute rotavirus gastroenteritis. *J. Pediatr. Gastroenterol. Nutr.* **39:**270–274.
11. **Bass, D. M.** 1997. Interferon gamma and interleukin 1, but not interferon alfa, inhibit rotavirus entry into human intestinal cell lines. *Gastroenterology* **113:**81–89.
12. **Bass, D. M., R. Baylor, R. Broom, and H. B. Greenberg.** 1992. Molecular basis of age-dependent gastric inactivation of rhesus rotavirus in the mouse. *J. Clin. Investig.* **89:**1741–1745.
13. **Bican, P., J. Cohen, A. Charpilienne, and R. Scherrer.** 1982. Purification and characterization of bovine rotavirus cores. *J. Virol.* **43:**1113–1117.
14. **Bishop, R. F., G. L. Barnes, E. Cipriani, and J. S. Lund.** 1983. Clinical immunity after neonatal rotavirus infection. A prospective longitudinal study in young children. *N. Engl. J. Med.* **309:**72–76.
15. **Bishop, R. F., G. P. Davidson, I. H. Holmes, and B. J. Ruck.** 1973. Virus particles in epithelial cells of duodenal mucosa from children with acute non-bacterial gastroenteritis. *Lancet* **ii:**1281–1283.
16. **Blutt, S. E., C. D. Kirkwood, V. Parreno, K. L. Warfield, M. Ciarlet, M. K. Estes, K. Bok, R. F. Bishop, and M. E. Conner.** 2003. Rotavirus antigenaemia and viraemia: a common event? *Lancet* **362:**1445–1449.
17. **Blutt, S. E., D. O. Matson, S. E. Crawford, M. A. Staat, P. Azimi, B. L. Bennett, P. A. Piedra, and M. E. Conner.** 2007. Rotavirus antigenemia in children is associated with viremia. *PLoS Med.* **4:**e121.
18. **Bobo, L., C. Ojeh, D. Chiu, A. Machado, P. Colombani, and K. Schwarz.** 1997. Lack of evidence for rotavirus by polymerase chain reaction/enzyme immunoassay of hepatobiliary samples from children with biliary atresia. *Pediatr. Res.* **41:**229–234.
19. **Boshuizen, J. A., J. H. Reimerink, A. M. Korteland-van Male, V. J. van Ham, M. P. Koopmans, H. A. Buller, J. Dekker, and A. W. Einerhand.** 2003. Changes in small intestinal homeostasis, morphology, and gene expression during rotavirus infection of infant mice. *J. Virol.* **77:**13005–13016.
20. **Boyce, M., and P. Roy.** 2007. Recovery of infectious bluetongue virus from RNA. *J. Virol.* **81:**2179–2186.
21. **Brown, K. A., J. A. Kriss, C. A. Moser, W. J. Wenner, and P. A. Offit.** 2000. Circulating rotavirus-specific antibody-secreting cells (ASCs) predict the presence of rotavirus-specific ASCs in the human small intestinal lamina propria. *J. Infect. Dis.* **182:**1039–1043.
22. **Burns, J. W., P. M. Siadat, A. A. Krishnaney, and H. B. Greenberg.** 1996. Protective effect of rotavirus VP6-specific IgA monoclonal antibodies that lack neutralizing activity. *Science* **272:**104–107.
23. **Chaibi, C., J. Cotte-Laffitte, C. Sandre, A. Esclatine, A. L. Servin, A. M. Quero, and M. Geniteau-Legendre.** 2005. Rotavirus induces apoptosis in fully differentiated human intestinal Caco-2 cells. *Virology* **332:**480–490.
24. **Chen, D., C. L. Luongo, M. L. Nibert, and J. T. Patton.** 1999. Rotavirus open cores catalyze 5′-capping and methylation of exogenous RNA: evidence that VP3 is a methyltransferase. *Virology* **265:**120–130.
25. **Chwetzoff, S., and G. Trugnan.** 2006. Rotavirus assembly: an alternative model that utilizes an atypical trafficking pathway. *Curr. Top. Microbiol. Immunol* **309:**245–261.

26. **Clark, H. F., D. A. Lawley, A. Schaffer, J. M. Patacsil, A. E. Marcello, R. I. Glass, V. Jain, and J. Gentsch.** 2004. Assessment of the epidemic potential of a new strain of rotavirus associated with the novel G9 serotype which caused an outbreak in the United States for the first time in the 1995–1996 season. *J. Clin. Microbiol.* **42:** 1434–1438.
27. **Cook, S. M., R. I. Glass, C. W. LeBaron, and M. S. Ho.** 1990. Global seasonality of rotavirus infections. *Bull. W. H. O.* **68:**171–177.
28. **Corthesy, B., Y. Benureau, C. Perrier, C. Fourgeux, N. Parez, H. Greenberg, and I. Schwartz-Cornil.** 2006. Rotavirus anti-VP6 secretory immunoglobulin A contributes to protection via intracellular neutralization but not via immune exclusion. *J. Virol.* **80:**10692–10699.
29. **Coulson, B. S., K. Grimwood, I. L. Hudson, G. L. Barnes, and R. F. Bishop.** 1992. Role of coproantibody in clinical protection of children during reinfection with rotavirus. *J. Clin. Microbiol.* **30:**1678–1684.
30. **Coulson, B. S., K. Grimwood, P. J. Masendycz, J. S. Lund, N. Mermelstein, R. F. Bishop, and G. L. Barnes.** 1990. Comparison of rotavirus immunoglobulin A coproconversion with other indices of rotavirus infection in a longitudinal study in childhood. *J. Clin. Microbiol.* **28:** 1367–1374.
31. **Coulson, B. S., S. L. Londrigan, and D. J. Lee.** 1997. Rotavirus contains integrin ligand sequences and a disintegrin-like domain that are implicated in virus entry into cells. *Proc. Natl. Acad. Sci. USA* **94:**5389–5394.
32. **Cuadras, M. A., D. A. Feigelstock, S. An, and H. B. Greenberg.** 2002. Gene expression pattern in Caco-2 cells following rotavirus infection. *J. Virol.* **76:**4467–4482.
33. **Cumino, A. C., M. O. Giordano, L. C. Martinez, S. I. Medeot, J. V. Pavan, S. Yudowsky, M. B. Isa, A. R. Depetris, and S. V. Nates.** 1998. Culture amplification in human colon adenocarcinoma cell line (CaCo-2) combined with an ELISA as a supplementary assay for accurate diagnosis of rotavirus. *J. Virol. Methods* **76:**81–85.
34. **Cunliffe, N. A., J. S. Gondwe, C. D. Kirkwood, S. M. Graham, N. M. Nhlane, B. D. Thindwa, W. Dove, R. L. Broadhead, M. E. Molyneux, and C. A. Hart.** 2001. Effect of concomitant HIV infection on presentation and outcome of rotavirus gastroenteritis in Malawian children. *Lancet* **358:**550–555.
35. **Dagan, R., Y. Bar-David, B. Sarov, M. Katz, I. Kassis, D. Greenberg, R. I. Glass, C. Z. Margolis, and I. Sarov.** 1990. Rotavirus diarrhea in Jewish and Bedouin children in the Negev region of Israel: epidemiology, clinical aspects and possible role of malnutrition in severity of illness. *Pediatr. Infect. Dis. J.* **9:**314–321.
36. **De Boissieu, D., P. Lebon, J. Badoual, Y. Bompard, and C. Dupont.** 1993. Rotavirus induces alpha-interferon release in children with gastroenteritis. *J. Pediatr. Gastroenterol. Nutr.* **16:**29–32.
37. **Dennehy, P. H., M. M. Cortese, R. E. Begue, J. L. Jaeger, N. E. Roberts, R. Zhang, P. Rhodes, J. Gentsch, R. Ward, D. I. Bernstein, C. Vitek, J. S. Bresee, and M. A. Staat.** 2006. A case-control study to determine risk factors for hospitalization for rotavirus gastroenteritis in U.S. children. *Pediatr. Infect. Dis. J.* **25:**1123–1131.
38. **Dennehy, P. H., and G. Peter.** 1985. Risk factors associated with nosocomial rotavirus infection. *Am. J. Dis. Child.* **139:**935–939.
39. **Desikan, P., J. D. Daniel, C. N. Kamalarathnam, and M. M. Mathan.** 1996. Molecular epidemiology of nosocomial rotavirus infection. *J. Diarrhoeal Dis. Res.* **14:**12–15.
40. **Dormitzer, P. R., E. B. Nason, B. V. Prasad, and S. C. Harrison.** 2004. Structural rearrangements in the membrane penetration protein of a non-enveloped virus. *Nature* **430:**1053–1058.
41. **Dowling, W., E. Denisova, R. LaMonica, and E. R. Mackow.** 2000. Selective membrane permeabilization by the rotavirus VP5* protein is abrogated by mutations in an internal hydrophobic domain. *J. Virol.* **74:**6368–6376.
42. **Dutta, P., U. Mitra, S. Dutta, B. Manna, M. K. Chatterjee, A. De, and S. K. Bhattacharya.** 2000. Hypoosmolar oral rehydration salts solution in dehydrating persistent diarrhoea in children: double-blind, randomized, controlled clinical trial. *Acta Paediatr.* **89:**411–416.
43. **Estes, M. K., and A. Z. Kapikian.** 2007. Rotaviruses, p. 1917–1974. *In* D. M. Knipe, P. M. Howley, D. E. Griffin, R. A. Lamb, M. A. Martin, B. Roizman, and S. E. Straus (ed.), *Fields Virology*, 5th ed., vol. 2. Lippincott Williams & Wilkins, Philadelphia, PA.
44. **Fenaux, M., M. A. Cuadras, N. Feng, M. Jaimes, and H. B. Greenberg.** 2006. Extraintestinal spread and replication of a homologous EC rotavirus strain and a heterologous rhesus rotavirus in BALB/c mice. *J. Virol.* **80:** 5219–5232.
45. **Feng, N., M. C. Jaimes, N. H. Lazarus, D. Monak, C. Zhang, E. C. Butcher, and H. B. Greenberg.** 2006. Redundant role of chemokines CCL25/TECK and CCL28/MEC in IgA+ plasmablast recruitment to the intestinal lamina propria after rotavirus infection. *J. Immunol.* **176:** 5749–5759.
46. **Fischer, T. K., C. Viboud, U. Parashar, M. Malek, C. Steiner, R. Glass, and L. Simonsen.** 2007. Hospitalizations and deaths from diarrhea and rotavirus among children <5 years of age in the United States, 1993–2003. *J. Infect. Dis.* **195:**1117–1125.
47. **Fitts, S. W., M. Green, J. Reyes, B. Nour, A. G. Tzakis, and S. A. Kocoshis.** 1995. Clinical features of nosocomial rotavirus infection in pediatric liver transplant recipients. *Clin. Transplant.* **9:**201–204.
48. **Franco, M. A., J. Angel, and H. B. Greenberg.** 2006. Immunity and correlates of protection for rotavirus vaccines. *Vaccine* **24:**2718–2731.
49. **Friedman, M. G., N. Entin, R. Zedaka, and R. Dagan.** 1996. Subclasses of IgA antibodies in serum and saliva samples of newborns and infants immunized against rotavirus. *Clin. Exp. Immunol.* **103:**206–211.
50. **Gentsch, J. R., A. R. Laird, B. Bielfelt, D. D. Griffin, K. Banyai, M. Ramachandran, V. Jain, N. A. Cunliffe, O. Nakagomi, C. D. Kirkwood, T. K. Fischer, U. D. Parashar, J. S. Bresee, B. Jiang, and R. I. Glass.** 2005. Serotype diversity and reassortment between human and animal rotavirus strains: implications for rotavirus vaccine programs. *J. Infect. Dis.* **192**(Suppl. 1)**:**S146–S159.
51. **Gilchrist, M. J., T. S. Bretl, K. Moultney, D. R. Knowlton, and R. L. Ward.** 1987. Comparison of seven kits for detection of rotavirus in fecal specimens with a sensitive, specific enzyme immunoassay. *Diagn. Microbiol. Infect. Dis.* **8:**221–228.
52. **Gilger, M. A., D. O. Matson, M. E. Conner, H. M. Rosenblatt, M. J. Finegold, and M. K. Estes.** 1992. Extraintestinal rotavirus infections in children with immunodeficiency. *J. Pediatr.* **120:**912–917.
53. **Glass, R. I., J. S. Bresee, U. Parashar, M. Miller, and J. R. Gentsch.** 1997. Rotavirus vaccines at the threshold. *Nat, Med,* **3:**1324–1325.
54. **Glass, R. I., D. J. Ing, B. J. Stoll, and R. T. Ing.** 1991. Immune response to rotavirus vaccines among breast-fed and nonbreast-fed children. *Adv. Exp. Med. Biol.* **310:** 249–254.

55. **Golantsova, N. E., E. E. Gorbunova, and E. R. Mackow.** 2004. Discrete domains within the rotavirus VP5* direct peripheral membrane association and membrane permeability. *J. Virol.* **78:**2037–2044.
56. **Gouvea, V., R. I. Glass, P. Woods, K. Taniguchi, H. F. Clark, B. Forrester, and Z. Y. Fang.** 1990. Polymerase chain reaction amplification and typing of rotavirus nucleic acid from stool specimens. *J. Clin. Microbiol.* **28:** 276–282.
57. **Green, K. Y., K. Taniguchi, E. R. Mackow, and A. Z. Kapikian.** 1990. Homotypic and heterotypic epitope-specific antibody responses in adult and infant rotavirus vaccinees: implications for vaccine development. *J. Infect. Dis* **161:**667–679.
58. **Grimwood, K., J. C. Lund, B. S. Coulson, I. L. Hudson, R. F. Bishop, and G. L. Barnes.** 1988. Comparison of serum and mucosal antibody responses following severe acute rotavirus gastroenteritis in young children. *J. Clin. Microbiol.* **26:**732–738.
59. **Haffejee, I. E.** 1990. Cow's milk-based formula, human milk, and soya feeds in acute infantile diarrhea: a therapeutic trial. *J. Pediatr. Gastroenterol. Nutr.* **10:**193–198.
60. **Higo-Moriguchi, K., Y. Akahori, Y. Iba, Y. Kurosawa, and K. Taniguchi.** 2004. Isolation of human monoclonal antibodies that neutralize human rotavirus. *J. Virol.* **78:** 3325–3332.
61. **Honma, S., V. Chizhikov, N. Santos, M. Tatsumi, M. D. Timenetsky, A. C. Linhares, J. D. Mascarenhas, H. Ushijima, G. E. Armah, J. R. Gentsch, and Y. Hoshino.** 2007. Development and validation of DNA microarray for genotyping group A rotavirus VP4 (P[4], P[6], P[8], P[9], and P[14]) and VP7 (G1 to G6, G8 to G10, and G12) genes. *J. Clin. Microbiol.* **45:**2641–2648.
62. **Hoshino, Y., L. J. Saif, S. Y. Kang, M. M. Sereno, W. K. Chen, and A. Z. Kapikian.** 1995. Identification of group A rotavirus genes associated with virulence of a porcine rotavirus and host range restriction of a human rotavirus in the gnotobiotic piglet model. *Virology* **209:**274–280.
63. **Huicho, L., D. Sanchez, M. Contreras, M. Paredes, H. Murga, L. Chinchay, and G. Guevara.** 1993. Occult blood and fecal leukocytes as screening tests in childhood infectious diarrhea: an old problem revisited. *Pediatr. Infect. Dis. J.* **12:**474–477.
64. **International Study Group on Reduced-Osmolarity ORS Solutions.** 1995. Multicentre evaluation of reduced-osmolarity oral rehydration solution. *Lancet* **345:**282–285.
65. **Iturriza-Gomara, M., I. Clarke, U. Desselberger, D. Brown, D. Thomas, and J. Gray.** 2004. Seroepidemiology of group C rotavirus infection in England and Wales. *Eur. J. Epidemiol.* **19:**589–595.
66. **Iturriza-Gomara, M., J. Green, D. W. Brown, U. Desselberger, and J. J. Gray.** 1999. Comparison of specific and random priming in the reverse transcriptase polymerase chain reaction for genotyping group A rotaviruses. *J. Virol. Methods* **78:**93–103.
67. **Jaimes, M. C., N. Feng, and H. B. Greenberg.** 2005. Characterization of homologous and heterologous rotavirus-specific T-cell responses in infant and adult mice. *J. Virol.* **79:**4568–4579.
68. **Jaimes, M. C., O. L. Rojas, A. M. González, I. Cajiao, A. Charpilienne, P. Pothier, E. Kohli, H. B. Greenberg, M. A. Franco, and J. Angel.** 2002. Frequencies of virus-specific $CD4^+$ and $CD8^+$ T lymphocytes secreting gamma interferon after acute natural rotavirus infection in children and adults. *J. Virol.* **76:**4741–4749.
69. **Jaimes, M. C., O. L. Rojas, E. J. Kunkel, N. H. Lazarus, D. Soler, E. C. Butcher, D. Bass, J. Angel, M. A. Franco, and H. B. Greenberg.** 2004. Maturation and trafficking markers on rotavirus-specific B cells during acute infection and convalescence in children. *J. Virol.* **78:** 10967–10976.
70. **Jiang, B., L. Snipes-Magaldi, P. Dennehy, H. Keyserling, R. C. Holman, J. Bresee, J. Gentsch, and R. I. Glass.** 2003. Cytokines as mediators for or effectors against rotavirus disease in children. *Clin. Diagn. Lab. Immunol.* **10:** 995–1001.
71. **Johansen, K., L. Granqvist, K. Karlen, G. Stintzing, I. Uhnoo, and L. Svensson.** 1994. Serum IgA immune response to individual rotavirus polypeptides in young children with rotavirus infection. *Arch. Virol.* **138:**247–259.
72. **Kang, G., M. Iturriza-Gomara, J. G. Wheeler, P. Crystal, B. Monica, S. Ramani, B. Primrose, P. D. Moses, C. I. Gallimore, D. W. Brown, and J. Gray.** 2004. Quantitation of group A rotavirus by real-time reverse-transcription-polymerase chain reaction: correlation with clinical severity in children in South India. *J. Med. Virol.* **73:**118–122.
73. **Kapikian, A. Z., R. G. Wyatt, R. Dolin, T. S. Thornhill, A. R. Kalica, and R. M. Chanock.** 1972. Visualization by immune electron microscopy of a 27-nm particle associated with acute infectious nonbacterial gastroenteritis. *J. Virol.* **10:**1075–1081.
74. **King, C. K., R. Glass, J. S. Bresee, and C. Duggan.** 2003. Managing acute gastroenteritis among children: oral rehydration, maintenance, and nutritional therapy. *Morb. Mortal. Wkly. Rep. Recomm. Rep.* **52:**1–16.
75. **Kirkwood, C. D., B. S. Coulson, and R. F. Bishop.** 1996. G3P2 rotaviruses causing diarrhoeal disease in neonates differ in VP4, VP7 and NSP4 sequence from G3P2 strains causing asymptomatic neonatal infection. *Arch. Virol.* **141:**1661–1676.
76. **Kobayashi, T., A. A. R. Antar, K. W. Boehme, P. Danthi, E. A. Eby, K. M. Guglielmi, G. H. Holm, E. M. Johnson, M. S. Magninnis, S. Naik, W. B. Skelton, D. J. Wetzel, G. J. Wilson, J. D. Chappell, and T. S. Dermody.** 2007. A plasmid-based reverse genetics system for animal double-stranded RNA viruses. *Cell Host Microbe* **1:**147–157.
77. **Kohler, T., U. Erben, H. Wiedersberg, and N. Bannert.** 1990. Histological findings of the small intestinal mucosa in rotavirus infections in infants and young children. *Kinderaerztl. Prax.* **58:**323–327. (In German.)
78. **Komoto, S., J. Sasaki, and K. Taniguchi.** 2006. Reverse genetics system for introduction of site-specific mutations into the double-stranded RNA genome of infectious rotavirus. *Proc. Natl. Acad. Sci. USA* **103:**4646–4651.
79. **Koopmans, M., and D. Brown.** 1999. Seasonality and diversity of group A rotaviruses in Europe. *Acta Paediatr. Suppl.* **88:**14–19.
80. **Lawton, J. A., M. K. Estes, and B. V. Prasad.** 1999. Comparative structural analysis of transcriptionally competent and incompetent rotavirus-antibody complexes. *Proc. Natl. Acad. Sci. USA* **96:**5428–5433.
81. **Linhares, A. C., T. Verstraeten, J. Wolleswinkel-van den Bosch, R. Clemens, and T. Breuer.** 2006. Rotavirus serotype G9 is associated with more-severe disease in Latin America. *Clin. Infect. Dis.* **43:**312–314.
82. **Lopez, S., and C. F. Arias.** 2006. Early steps in rotavirus cell entry. *Curr. Top. Microbiol. Immunol.* **309:**39–66.
83. **Losonsky, G. A., J. P. Johnson, J. A. Winkelstein, and R. H. Yolken.** 1985. Oral administration of human serum immunoglobulin in immunodeficient patients with viral gastroenteritis. A pharmacokinetic and functional analysis. *J. Clin. Investig.* **76:**2362–2367.
84. **Lundgren, O., A. T. Peregrin, K. Persson, S. Kordasti, I. Uhnoo, and L. Svensson.** 2000. Role of the enteric

nervous system in the fluid and electrolyte secretion of rotavirus diarrhea. *Science* **287**:491–495.

85. **Mack, C. L., R. M. Tucker, B. R. Lu, R. J. Sokol, A. P. Fontenot, Y. Ueno, and R. G. Gill.** 2006. Cellular and humoral autoimmunity directed at bile duct epithelia in murine biliary atresia. *Hepatology* **44**:1231–1239.
86. **Makela, M., V. Oling, J. Marttila, M. Waris, M. Knip, O. Simell, and J. Ilonen.** 2006. Rotavirus-specific T cell responses and cytokine mRNA expression in children with diabetes-associated autoantibodies and type 1 diabetes. *Clin. Exp. Immunol.* **145**:261–270.
87. **Masendycz, P. J., E. A. Palombo, R. J. Gorrell, and R. F. Bishop.** 1997. Comparison of enzyme immunoassay, PCR, and type-specific cDNA probe techniques for identification of group A rotavirus gene 4 types (P types). *J. Clin. Microbiol.* **35**:3104–3108.
88. **Mata, L., A. Simhon, J. J. Urrutia, and R. A. Kronmal.** 1983. Natural history of rotavirus infection in the children of Santa Maria Cauque. *Prog. Food Nutr. Sci.* **7**:167–177.
89. **Matson, D. O., M. L. O'Ryan, I. Herrera, L. K. Pickering, and M. K. Estes.** 1993. Fecal antibody responses to symptomatic and asymptomatic rotavirus infections. *J. Infect. Dis.* **167**:577–583.
90. **Matthijnssens, J., M. Rahman, V. Martella, Y. Xuelei, S. De Vos, K. De Leener, M. Ciarlet, C. Buonavoglia, and M. Van Ranst.** 2006. Full genomic analysis of human rotavirus strain B4106 and lapine rotavirus strain 30/96 provides evidence for interspecies transmission. *J. Virol.* **80**:3801–3810.
91. **Mebus, C. A., N. R. Underdahl, M. B. Rhodes, and M. J. Twiehaus.** 1969. Calf diarrhea (scours): reproduced with a virus from a field outbreak. *Univ. Nebraska Res. Bull.* **233**:1–16.
92. **Min, B. S., Y. J. Noh, J. H. Shin, S. Y. Baek, K. I. Min, S. R. Ryu, B. G. Kim, M. K. Park, S. E. Choi, E. H. Yang, S. N. Park, S. J. Hur, and B. Y. Ahn.** 2006. Assessment of the quantitative real-time polymerase chain reaction using a cDNA standard for human group A rotavirus. *J. Virol. Methods* **137**:280–286.
93. **Molina, S., C. Vettorazzi, J. M. Peerson, N. W. Solomons, and K. H. Brown.** 1995. Clinical trial of glucose-oral rehydration solution (ORS), rice dextrin-ORS, and rice flour-ORS for the management of children with acute diarrhea and mild or moderate dehydration. *Pediatrics* **95**:191–197.
94. **Monnier, N., K. Higo-Moriguchi, Z. Y. Sun, B. V. Prasad, K. Taniguchi, and P. R. Dormitzer.** 2006. High-resolution molecular and antigen structure of the VP8* core of a sialic acid-independent human rotavirus strain. *J. Virol.* **80**:1513–1523.
95. **Montero, H., C. F. Arias, and S. Lopez.** 2006. Rotavirus nonstructural protein NSP3 is not required for viral protein synthesis. *J. Virol.* **80**:9031–9038.
96. **Morris, A. P., J. K. Scott, J. M. Ball, C. Q. Zeng, W. K. O'Neal, and M. K. Estes.** 1999. NSP4 elicits age-dependent diarrhea and Ca(2+) mediated I(−) influx into intestinal crypts of CF mice. *Am. J. Physiol.* **277**:G431–G444.
97. **Murphy, B. R., D. M. Morens, L. Simonsen, R. M. Chanock, J. R. La Montagne, and A. Z. Kapikian.** 2 April 2003. Reappraisal of the association of intussusception with the licensed live rotavirus vaccine challenges initial conclusions. *J. Infect. Dis.* **187**:1301–1308. [Epub ahead of print.]
98. **Nakagomi, T.** 2000. Rotavirus infection and intussusception: A view from retrospect. *Microbiol. Immunol.* **44**:619–628.
99. **Newburg, D. S., J. A. Peterson, G. M. Ruiz-Palacios, D. O. Matson, A. L. Morrow, J. Shults, M. L. Guerrero, P. Chaturvedi, S. O. Newburg, C. D. Scallan, M. R. Taylor, R. L. Ceriani, and L. K. Pickering.** 1998. Role of human-milk lactadherin in protection against symptomatic rotavirus infection. *Lancet* **351**:1160–1164.
100. **Newman, R. D., J. Grupp-Phelan, D. K. Shay, and R. L. Davis.** 1999. Perinatal risk factors for infant hospitalization with viral gastroenteritis. *Pediatrics* **103**:E3.
101. **Nguyen, T. V., L. Yuan, M. S. Azevedo, K. I. Jeong, A. M. Gonzalez, C. Iosef, K. Lovgren-Bengtsson, B. Morein, P. Lewis, and L. J. Saif.** 2006. High titers of circulating maternal antibodies suppress effector and memory B-cell responses induced by an attenuated rotavirus priming and rotavirus-like particle-immunostimulating complex boosting vaccine regimen. *Clin. Vaccine Immunol.* **13**:475–485.
102. **Nilsson, M., B. Svenungsson, K. O. Hedlund, I. Uhnoo, A. Lagergren, T. Akre, and L. Svensson.** 2000. Incidence and genetic diversity of group C rotavirus among adults. *J. Infect. Dis.* **182**:678–684.
103. **Noone, C., I. S. Menzies, J. E. Banatvala, and J. W. Scopes.** 1986. Intestinal permeability and lactose hydrolysis in human rotaviral gastroenteritis assessed simultaneously by non-invasive differential sugar permeation. *Eur. J. Clin. Investig.* **16**:217–225.
104. **Offit, P. A., E. J. Hoffenberg, N. Santos, and V. Gouvea.** 1993. Rotavirus-specific humoral and cellular immune response after primary, symptomatic infection. *J. Infect. Dis.* **167**:1436–1440.
105. **Parashar, U. D., J. P. Alexander, and R. I. Glass.** 2006. Prevention of rotavirus gastroenteritis among infants and children. Recommendations of the Advisory Committee on Immunization Practices (ACIP). *Morb. Mortal. Wkly. Rep. Recomm. Rep.* **55**:1–13.
106. **Parashar, U. D., C. J. Gibson, J. S. Bresse, and R. I. Glass.** 2006. Rotavirus and severe childhood diarrhea. *Emerg. Infect. Dis.* **12**:304–306.
107. **Parez, N., A. Garbarg-Chenon, C. Fourgeux, F. Le Deist, A. Servant-Delmas, A. Charpilienne, J. Cohen, and I. Schwartz-Cornil.** 2004. The VP6 protein of rotavirus interacts with a large fraction of human naive B cells via surface immunoglobulins. *J. Virol.* **78**:12489–12496.
108. **Patton, J. T., L. S. Silvestri, M. A. Tortorici, R. Vasquez-Del Carpio, and Z. F. Taraporewala.** 2006. Rotavirus genome replication and morphogenesis: role of the viroplasm. *Curr. Top. Microbiol. Immunol.* **309**:169–187.
109. **Perez-Schael, I., B. Salinas, M. Tomat, A. C. Linhares, M. L. Guerrero, G. M. Ruiz-Palacios, A. Bouckenooghe, and J. P. Yarzabal.** 2007. Efficacy of the human rotavirus vaccine RIX4414 in malnourished children. *J. Infect. Dis.* **196**:537–540.
110. **Pickering, L. K., A. L. Morrow, I. Herrera, M. O'Ryan, M. K. Estes, S. E. Guilliams, L. Jackson, C. S. Carter, and D. O. Matson.** 1995. Effect of maternal rotavirus immunization on milk and serum antibody titers. *J. Infect. Dis.* **172**:723–728.
111. **Piron, M., T. Delaunay, J. Grosclaude, and D. Poncet.** 1999. Identification of the RNA-binding, dimerization, and eIF4GI-binding domains of rotavirus nonstructural protein NSP3. *J. Virol.* **73**:5411–5421.
112. **Prasad, B. V., R. Rothnagel, C. Q. Zeng, J. Jakana, J. A. Lawton, W. Chiu, and M. K. Estes.** 1996. Visualization of ordered genomic RNA and localization of transcriptional complexes in rotavirus. *Nature* **382**:471–473.
113. **Rahman, M., J. Matthijnssens, X. Yang, T. Delbeke, I. Arijs, K. Taniguchi, M. Iturriza-Gomara, N. Iftekha-**

ruddin, T. Azim, and M. Van Ranst. 2007. Evolutionary history and global spread of the emerging g12 human rotaviruses. *J. Virol.* **81:**2382–2390.

114. **Ramos, A. P., C. C. Stefanelli, R. E. Linhares, B. G. de Brito, N. Santos, V. Gouvea, R. de Cassia Lima, and C. Nozawa.** 2000. The stability of porcine rotavirus in feces. *Vet. Microbiol.* **71:**1–8.
115. **Rautanen, T., S. Kurki, and T. Vesikari.** 1997. Randomised double blind study of hypotonic oral rehydration solution in diarrhoea. *Arch. Dis. Child.* **76:**272–274.
116. **Ray, P., M. Fenaux, S. Sharma, J. Malik, S. Subodh, S. Bhatnagar, H. Greenberg, R. I. Glass, J. Gentsch, and M. K. Bhan.** 2006. Quantitative evaluation of rotaviral antigenemia in children with acute rotaviral diarrhea. *J. Infect. Dis.* **194:**588–593.
117. **Rennels, M. B., U. D. Parashar, R. C. Holman, C. T. Le, H. G. Chang, and R. I. Glass.** 1998. Lack of an apparent association between intussusception and wild or vaccine rotavirus infection. *Pediatr. Infect. Dis. J.* **17:** 924–925.
118. **Richardson, S., K. Grimwood, R. Gorrell, E. Palombo, G. Barnes, and R. Bishop.** 1998. Extended excretion of rotavirus after severe diarrhoea in young children. *Lancet* **351:**1844–1848.
119. **Riepenhoff-Talty, M., V. Gouvea, M. J. Evans, L. Svensson, E. Hoffenberg, R. J. Sokol, I. Uhnoo, S. J. Greenberg, K. Schakel, G. Zhaori, J. Fitzgerald, S. Chong, M. el-Yousef, A. Nemeth, M. Brown, D. Piccoli, J. Hyams, D. Ruffin, and T. Rossi.** 1996. Detection of group C rotavirus in infants with extrahepatic biliary atresia. *J. Infect. Dis.* **174:**8–15.
120. **Rodriguez, W. J., H. W. Kim, C. D. Brandt, R. H. Schwartz, M. K. Gardner, B. Jeffries, R. H. Parrott, R. A. Kaslow, J. I. Smith, and A. Z. Kapikian.** 1987. Longitudinal study of rotavirus infection and gastroenteritis in families served by a pediatric medical practice: clinical and epidemiologic observations. *Pediatr. Infect. Dis. J.* **6:**170–176.
121. **Rojas, O. L., L. Caicedo, C. Guzman, L. S. Rodriguez, J. Castaneda, L. Uribe, Y. Andrade, R. Pinzon, C. F. Narvaez, J. M. Lozano, B. De Vos, M. A. Franco, and J. Angel.** 2007. Evaluation of circulating intestinally committed memory B cells in children vaccinated with attenuated human rotavirus vaccine. *Viral Immunol.* **20:** 300–311.
122. **Rollo, E. E., K. P. Kumar, N. C. Reich, J. Cohen, J. Angel, H. B. Greenberg, R. Sheth, J. Anderson, B. Oh, S. J. Hempson, E. R. Mackow, and R. D. Shaw.** 1999. The epithelial cell response to rotavirus infection. *J. Immunol.* **163:**4442–4452.
123. **Rossignol, J. F., M. Abu-Zekry, A. Hussein, and M. G. Santoro.** 2006. Effect of nitazoxanide for treatment of severe rotavirus diarrhoea: randomised double-blind placebo-controlled trial. *Lancet* **368:**124–129.
124. **Rothman, K. J., Y. Young-Xu, and F. Arellano.** 2006. Age dependence of the relation between reassortant rotavirus vaccine (RotaShield) and intussusception. *J. Infect. Dis.* **193:**898. (Author reply **193:**898–899.)
125. **Ruiz-Palacios, G. M., I. Perez-Schael, F. R. Velazquez, H. Abate, T. Breuer, S. C. Clemens, B. Cheuvart, F. Espinoza, P. Gillard, B. L. Innis, Y. Cervantes, A. C. Linhares, P. Lopez, M. Macias-Parra, E. Ortega-Barria, V. Richardson, D. M. Rivera-Medina, L. Rivera, B. Salinas, N. Pavia-Ruz, J. Salmeron, R. Ruttimann, J. C. Tinoco, P. Rubio, E. Nunez, M. L. Guerrero, J. P. Yarzabal, S. Damaso, N. Tornieporth, X. Saez-Llorens, R. F. Vergara, T. Vesikari, A. Bouckenooghe, R. Clemens, B. De Vos, and M. O'Ryan.** 2006. Safety and efficacy of an attenuated vaccine against severe rotavirus gastroenteritis. *N. Engl. J. Med.* **354:**11–22.
126. **Salazar-Lindo, E., P. Miranda-Langschwager, M. Campos-Sanchez, E. Chea-Woo, and R. B. Sack.** 2004. Lactobacillus casei strain GG in the treatment of infants with acute watery diarrhea: a randomized, double-blind, placebo controlled clinical trial [ISRCTN67363048]. *BMC Pediatr* **4:**18.
127. **Salazar-Lindo, E., J. Santisteban-Ponce, E. Chea-Woo, and M. Gutierrez.** 2000. Racecadotril in the treatment of acute watery diarrhea in children. *N. Engl. J. Med.* **343:**463–467.
128. **Santos, N., and Y. Hoshino.** 2005. Global distribution of rotavirus serotypes/genotypes and its implication for the development and implementation of an effective rotavirus vaccine. *Rev. Med. Virol.* **15:**29–56.
129. **Sereno, M. M., and M. I. Gorziglia.** 1994. The outer capsid protein VP4 of murine rotavirus strain Eb represents a tentative new P type. *Virology* **199:**500–504.
130. **Shaw, R. D., K. J. Fong, G. A. Losonsky, M. M. Levine, Y. Maldonado, R. Yolken, J. Flores, A. Z. Kapikian, P. T. Vo, and H. B. Greenberg.** 1987. Epitope-specific immune responses to rotavirus vaccination. *Gastroenterology* **93:**941–950.
131. **Simakachorn, N., Y. Tongpenyai, O. Tongtan, and W. Varavithya.** 2004. Randomized, double-blind clinical trial of a lactose-free and a lactose-containing formula in dietary management of acute childhood diarrhea. *J. Med. Assoc. Thail.* **87:**641–649.
132. **Simonsen, L., C. Viboud, A. Elixhauser, R. J. Taylor, and A. Z. Kapikian.** 2005. More on RotaShield and intussusception: the role of age at the time of vaccination. *J. Infect. Dis.* **192**(Suppl. 1)**:**S36–S43.
133. **Szymanski, H., J. Pejcz, M. Jawien, A. Chmielarczyk, M. Strus, and P. B. Heczko.** 2006. Treatment of acute infectious diarrhoea in infants and children with a mixture of three Lactobacillus rhamnosus strains—a randomized, double-blind, placebo-controlled trial. *Aliment. Pharmacol. Ther.* **23:**247–253.
134. **Teitelbaum, J. E., and R. Daghistani.** 12 April 2007. Rotavirus causes hepatic transaminase elevation. *Dig. Dis. Sci.* **52:**3396–3398.
135. **Torres Medina, A.** 1984. Effect of rotavirus and/or Escherichia coli infection on the aggregated lymphoid follicles in the small intestine of neonatal gnotobiotic calves. *Am. J. Vet. Res.* **45:**652–660.
136. **Turcios, R. M., A. T. Curns, R. C. Holman, I. Pandya-Smith, A. LaMonte, J. S. Bresee, and R. I. Glass.** 2006. Temporal and geographic trends of rotavirus activity in the United States, 1997–2004. *Pediatr. Infect. Dis. J.* **25:** 451–454.
137. **Uhnoo, I., S. E. Olding, and A. Kreuger.** 1986. Clinical features of acute gastroenteritis associated with rotavirus, enteric adenoviruses, and bacteria. *Arch. Dis. Child.* **61:** 732–738.
138. **VanCott, J. L., A. E. Prada, M. M. McNeal, S. C. Stone, M. Basu, B. Huffer, Jr., K. L. Smiley, M. Shao, J. A. Bean, J. D. Clements, A. H. Choi, and R. L. Ward.** 2006. Mice develop effective but delayed protective immune responses when immunized as neonates either intranasally with nonliving VP6/LT(R192G) or orally with live rhesus rotavirus vaccine candidates. *J. Virol.* **80:**4949–4961.
139. **van Kraaij, M. G., A. W. Dekker, L. F. Verdonck, A. M. van Loon, J. Vinje, M. P. Koopmans, and M. Rozenberg-Arska.** 2000. Infectious gastro-enteritis: an uncommon cause of diarrhoea in adult allogeneic and autologous stem cell transplant recipients. *Bone Marrow Transplant.* **26:**299–303.

140. **Velázques, F. R., D. O. Matson, J. J. Calva, L. Guerrero, A. L. Morrow, S. Carter-Campell, R. I. Glass, M. K. Estes, L. K. Pickering, and G. M. Ruiz-Palacios.** 1996. Rotavirus infection in infants as protection against subsequent infections. *N. Engl. J. Med.* **335:**1022–1028.
141. **Velazquez, F. R., D. O. Matson, M. L. Guerrero, J. Shults, J. J. Calva, A. L. Morrow, R. I. Glass, L. K. Pickering, and G. M. Ruiz-Palacios.** 2000. Serum antibody as a marker of protection against natural rotavirus infection and disease. *J. Infect. Dis.* **182:**1602–1609.
142. **Vesikari, T., A. Karvonen, B. D. Forrest, Y. Hoshino, R. M. Chanock, and A. Z. Kapikian.** 2006. Neonatal administration of rhesus rotavirus tetravalent vaccine. *Pediatr. Infect. Dis. J.* **25:**118–122.
143. **Vesikari, T., D. O. Matson, P. Dennehy, P. Van Damme, M. Santosham, Z. Rodriguez, M. J. Dallas, J. F. Heyse, M. G. Goveia, S. B. Black, H. R. Shinefield, C. D. Christie, S. Ylitalo, R. F. Itzler, M. L. Coia, M. T. Onorato, B. A. Adeyi, G. S. Marshall, L. Gothefors, D. Campens, A. Karvonen, J. P. Watt, K. L. O'Brien, M. J. DiNubile, H. F. Clark, J. W. Boslego, P. A. Offit, and P. M. Heaton.** 2006. Safety and efficacy of a pentavalent human-bovine (WC3) reassortant rotavirus vaccine. *N. Engl. J. Med.* **354:**23–33.
144. **Vial, P. A., K. L. Kotloff, and G. A. Losonsky.** 1988. Molecular epidemiology of rotavirus infection in a room for convalescing newborns. *J. Infect. Dis.* **157:**668–673.
145. **Wang, Y., P. H. Dennehy, H. L. Keyserling, K. Tang, J. R. Gentsch, R. I. Glass, and B. Jiang.** 2007. Rotavirus infection alters peripheral T-cell homeostasis in children with acute diarrhea. *J. Virol.* **81:**3904–3912.
146. **Ward, R. L., D. I. Bernstein, R. Shukla, E. C. Young, J. R. Sherwood, M. M. McNeal, M. C. Walker, and G. M. Schiff.** 1989. Effects of antibody to rotavirus on protection of adults challenged with a human rotavirus. *J. Infect. Dis.* **159:**79–88.
147. **Ward, R. L., C. D. Kirkwood, D. S. Sander, V. E. Smith, M. Shao, J. A. Bean, D. A. Sack, and A. D. Bernstein.** 2006. Reductions in cross-neutralizing antibody responses in infants after attenuation of the human rotavirus vaccine candidate 89-12. *J. Infect. Dis.* **194:**1729–1736.
148. **Ward, R. L., D. R. Knowlton, and M. J. Pierce.** 1984. Efficiency of human rotavirus propagation in cell culture. *J. Clin. Microbiol.* **19:**748–753.
149. **Warfield, K. L., S. E. Blutt, S. E. Crawford, G. Kang, and M. E. Conner.** 2006. Rotavirus infection enhances lipopolysaccharide-induced intussusception in a mouse model. *J. Virol.* **80:**12377–12386.
150. **Weitkamp, J. H., N. L. Kallewaard, A. L. Bowen, B. J. Lafleur, H. B. Greenberg, and J. E. Crowe, Jr.** 2005. VH1-46 is the dominant immunoglobulin heavy chain gene segment in rotavirus-specific memory B cells expressing the intestinal homing receptor alpha4beta7. *J. Immunol.* **174:**3454–3460.
151. **Widdowson, M. A., M. I. Meltzer, X. Zhang, J. S. Bresee, U. D. Parashar, and R. I. Glass.** 2007. Cost-effectiveness and potential impact of rotavirus vaccination in the United States. *Pediatrics* **119:**684–697.
152. **Widdowson, M. A., G. J. van Doornum, W. H. van der Poel, A. S. de Boer, U. Mahdi, and M. Koopmans.** 2000. Emerging group-A rotavirus and a nosocomial outbreak of diarrhoea. *Lancet* **356:**1161–1162. (Letter.)
153. **Wood, D. J., T. J. David, I. L. Chrystie, and B. Totterdell.** 1988. Chronic enteric virus infection in two T-cell immunodeficient children. *J. Med. Virol.* **24:**435–444.
154. **Wyatt, R. G., C. A. Mebus, R. H. Yolken, A. R. Kalica, H. D. James, Jr., A. Z. Kapikian, and R. M. Chanock.** 1979. Rotaviral immunity in gnotobiotic calves: heterologous resistance to human virus induced by bovine virus. *Science* **203:**548–550.
155. **Yeager, M., J. A. Berriman, T. S. Baker, and A. R. Bellamy.** 1994. Three-dimensional structure of the rotavirus haemagglutinin VP4 by cryo-electron microscopy and difference map analysis. *EMBO J.* **13:**1011–1018.
156. **Yuan, L., S. Honma, S. Ishida, X. Y. Yan, A. Z. Kapikian, and Y. Hoshino.** 2004. Species-specific but not genotype-specific primary and secondary isotype-specific NSP4 antibody responses in gnotobiotic calves and piglets infected with homologous host bovine (NSP4[A]) or porcine (NSP4[B]) rotavirus. *Virology* **330:**92–104.
157. **Zanoni, G., R. Navone, C. Lunardi, G. Tridente, C. Bason, S. Sivori, R. Beri, M. Dolcino, E. Valletta, R. Corrocher, and A. Puccetti.** 2006. In celiac disease, a subset of autoantibodies against transglutaminase binds toll-like receptor 4 and induces activation of monocytes. *PLoS Med.* **3:**e358.

Respiratory Syncytial Virus, Human Metapneumovirus, and Parainfluenza Viruses

JOHN V. WILLIAMS, PEDRO A. PIEDRA, AND JANET A. ENGLUND

36

Respiratory syncytial virus (RSV), human metapneumovirus (hMPV), and the parainfluenza viruses (PIVs) are the most important causes of lower respiratory tract illnesses in infants and children. RSV was first isolated from chimpanzees with coryza in 1956 (174) but was soon shown to be the major cause of bronchiolitis and pneumonia in infants (18). RSV was named after the cell fusion that is characteristic of its growth in some continuous tissue culture cell lines. PIV types 1, 2, and 3 were first recovered in 1956 (35, 37) and were recognized as the major causes of croup, or laryngotracheobronchitis, in children. PIV types 4A and 4B have been recovered from adults and children with upper respiratory illnesses but are difficult to isolate in the tissue cultures usually employed in virus diagnostic laboratories (228). hMPV was first discovered in The Netherlands in 2001 (229) and soon thereafter was documented to be an important cause of lower respiratory tract illness in children worldwide. These three viruses cause frequent reinfections in older children and adults that are generally mild in healthy persons but may cause serious disease in immunocompromised patients or patients with underlying cardiopulmonary diseases.

VIROLOGY

Classification

RSV, PIV, and hMPV belong to the *Paramyxoviridae* family. RSV is a member of the genus *Pneumovirus*, hMPV is a member of the genus *Metapneumovirus*, and the PIVs are members of the genus *Paramyxovirus*. A number of related animal paramyxoviruses are important pathogens (Table 1; see also chapter 39). RSV is comprised of two heterotypic strains of viruses that are antigenically distinct, classified as subgroups A and B (177). The major difference between these subgroups is the antigenic properties of the G surface glycoprotein protein (81). The fusion (F) surface glycoprotein remains antigenically conserved between the RSV subgroups (Table 2) (81). The two RSV surface glycoproteins evoke antibody responses that are important for conferring protection against life-threatening RSV illness. In addition, strain differences exist within the RSV A and B subgroups.

In contrast to RSV, PIVs have no clinically significant antigenic variants within each of the five strains (1, 2, 3, 4A, and 4B) recognized (121). Immune responses to the two PIV surface glycoproteins, hemagglutinin-neuraminidase (HN) and F, also appear to correlate with protection against infection.

Several hMPV genes, including the F, G, and P genes, have been used for subtyping, and phylogenetic analyses of these sequences have defined two major genetic subgroups of hMPV, A and B, each with two minor subgroups (161, 230). The two major hMPV groups (A and B) show significant genetic variability in the G gene and relative conservation in the F gene. F protein induces neutralizing antibodies and appears to be the major protective antigen.

Structure

The virions are pleomorphic and range in diameter from 150 to 300 nm (42). Shapes can vary from almost spherical to filamentous. Large filamentous forms are often noninfectious because they may lack a nucleocapsid. All of these viruses have an envelope consisting of spike-like glycoproteins (peplomers) and a lipid bilayer derived from the host cell. The main elements of their structures are illustrated in Fig. 1. The lipid-containing envelope is lined by a matrix (M) protein that surrounds the helical nucleocapsid. The diameter of the nucleocapsid of PIV is 18 nm, while that of RSV is slightly smaller, at 12 to 15 nm. The genomes are single-stranded RNA with negative sense but vary in size. The RSV genome consists of 15.2×10^3 nucleotides, the PIV genome consists of 15.5×10^3 nucleotides, and the hMPV genome consists of 13.3×10^3 nucleotides. The organization of the genome differs for the three viruses (Fig. 2). Eleven proteins are encoded by the RSV genome, two of which are nonstructural. hMPV encodes nine proteins analogous to those of RSV, but NS1 and NS2 are lacking in hMPV. The gene order of hMPV differs from that of RSV. PIVs have at least six structural proteins and one or more nonstructural proteins. The nucleocapsid comprises the RNA bound to the nucleoprotein, with clumps of the small phosphoproteins and large L proteins that have RNA-dependent RNA polymerase activity.

The compositions and major proteins of RSV, the PIVs, and hMPV are compared in Table 2. RSV, PIV, and hMPV all have an F protein in the envelope, but each has a distinct second large surface glycoprotein. PIV has an HN protein that has hemagglutinating and neuraminidase ac-

TABLE 1 Animal viruses related to human respiratory paramyxoviruses

Human strain	Related animal strain[a]	Animal host(s)	Disease
PIV type 1	Sendai virus	Rodents	Pneumonia
PIV type 2	Simian virus 5	Dogs	Canine croup
PIV type 3	Bovine PIV type 3	Cattle	Shipping fever
RSV	Bovine/ovine RSV	Cattle, sheep	Shipping fever
hMPV	Avian metapneumovirus (formerly turkey rhinotracheitis virus)	Turkeys, chickens	Swollen head syndrome

[a] Sendai virus of rats is closely related to PIV type 1; simian virus 5, a cause of canine croup, is related to PIV type 2. Bovine PIV type 3 contributes to the economically important shipping fever complex of cattle and is closely related to human PIV type 3.

tivities, while RSV and hMPV have a large glycoprotein, designated the G protein, that is important for attachment (predicted for hMPV) but lacks hemagglutinating and neuraminidase activities. RSV has a highly conserved short hydrophobic (SH) protein in the envelope whose function remains undefined.

Replication

Infection is initiated by attachment of the virion to a susceptible cell by the HN or G protein (150). The F protein must be cleaved by cellular proteolytic enzymes to become activated and fusion capable. The cleaved F proteins (F1 and F2) act to fuse the host cell membrane to the virus lipid envelope to allow the nucleocapsid to enter the cytoplasm. RSV and PIV replicate solely in the cytoplasm, with no requirements for nuclear processing. The virion polymerases (P+C and L) transcribe the negative-strand RNA to mRNA for production of the viral proteins (Fig. 3). The negative-strand RNA also serves as a template for synthesis of the genomic intermediate positive-strand RNA. The virion-complementary RNA is then copied into progeny negative-strand RNA. The virion is assembled with the progeny negative-strand RNA and structural virus proteins and then released by budding from the host cell membrane.

Host Range

Human RSV infects nonhuman primates, including chimpanzees, as well as rodents, including cotton rats and mice. Disease manifestations due to RSV in primates and cotton rats have similarities to human disease. RSV infection in mice is generally characterized by more general symptoms such as weight loss and fur ruffling, with minimal pulmonary symptoms despite histopathological changes in the lungs. Closely related RSV viruses causing symptomatic disease are found in cattle and sheep (31). Counterparts of the human PIVs are found in animals (Table 1).

Both RSV and PIV can be propagated in many different continuous and primary cell lines, including HEp-2, human embryonic lung diploid fibroblasts, and monkey kidney cells. PIV type 3 infection of certain continuous cell lines produces syncytia; the other PIVs are less likely to produce syncytia. PIV type 4 in particular is characterized by the lack of syncytium production.

hMPV is capable of infecting hamsters, cotton rats, mice, and nonhuman primates under experimental conditions (146, 250). The only other virus in the *Metapneumovirus* genus is avian metapneumovirus (formerly turkey rhinotracheitis virus), which is an important pathogen of commercial poultry. While an initial report indicated that hMPV did not replicate in experimentally inoculated chickens and turkeys (229), another group recently reported that turkeys inoculated intranasally with hMPV developed rhinitis associated with hMPV RNA detection by reverse transcriptase PCR (RT-PCR) but without confirmed productive hMPV replication (232). hMPV was initially recovered in tertiary monkey kidney cells but has been cultivated in a number of other cell types, most commonly LLC-MK2.

TABLE 2 Proteins of RSV, hMPV, and PIV[a]

RSV		hMPV		PIV	
Gene	Protein	Gene	Protein	Gene	Protein
F	Fusion	F	Fusion	F	Fusion
G	Attachment	G	Attachment	HN	Hemagglutinin-neuraminidase
M	Matrix	M	Matrix	M	Matrix
N	Nucleoprotein	N	Nucleoprotein	NP	Nucleoprotein
P	Phosphoprotein	P	Phosphoprotein	P+C	Polymerase complex
L	Large polymerase complex	L	Large (RNA polymerase)	L	Large polymerase complex
SH	Short hydrophobic	SH	Short hydrophobic		
M2-1	Nonstructural	M2-1	Nonstructural		
M2-2	Nonstructural	M2-2	Nonstructural		
NS1	Nonstructural				
NS2	Nonstructural				

[a] Data from references 41a and 42.

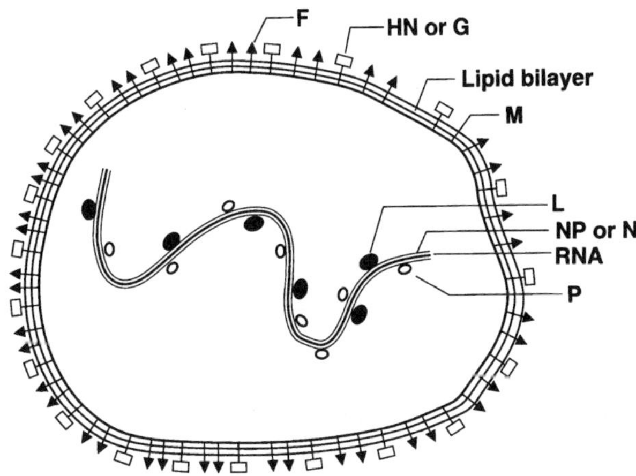

FIGURE 1 Schematic presentation of the structure of viruses of the family *Paramyxoviridae*, including PIVs and RSV. L, large protein of the polymerase complex; NP or N, nucleoprotein; P, phosphoprotein. HN is an attachment protein for PIV, and G protein is an attachment protein for RSV.

Stability

Because of their lipid-containing envelopes, these respiratory viruses are sensitive to ether and other lipid solvents. RSV and the PIVs differ in their lability; RSV is relatively unstable, and isolation in tissue culture is enhanced by immediate inoculation into sensitive tissue cultures without freezing the specimen. By contrast, the PIVs are relatively stable and remain viable in a virus stabilizing medium for up to 5 days at 4°C (14).

EPIDEMIOLOGY

Geographic Distribution

RSV, PIV, and hMPV are recognized as causes of upper and lower respiratory tract disease across all age groups worldwide. These ubiquitous respiratory pathogens are an especially important cause of disease in young children. In particular, RSV infection in infants is associated with high rates of morbidity and mortality (212, 215). Importantly, respiratory diseases remain the most significant cause of mortality in young children worldwide, with an estimated 3 million to 4 million children under 5 years of age dying annually (178).

Age-Specific Infection Rates

Infections with all three viruses are common during early childhood (88, 92). Approximately two-thirds of infants are infected with RSV and PIV type 3 during the first year of life (Table 3). Infants and young children are also commonly infected with hMPV, although the mean age of infection is approximately 6 months older. Most primary infections in children occur during the first 2 years of life and are symptomatic; RSV infections are more likely to involve the lower respiratory tract, and PIV type 3 infections are more likely to produce illnesses limited to the upper respiratory tract (Table 4). Virtually all children are infected with RSV by 2 years of age and with hMPV by 5 years of age. Infections with PIV types 1 and 2 occur at a lower rate; by the age of 5 years, 74 and 59% of children have been infected with types 1 and 2, respectively (90).

Severe disease due to RSV infection in children without underlying chronic conditions is most common in infants younger than 6 months of age. After primary infection, the incidence of RSV lower respiratory tract infection falls with increasing age (92, 118) until late adulthood, when increasing rates are again noted in the elderly (67). Immunity induced by primary infection has a limited effect on illness associated with the first reinfection, but the severity of illness is significantly reduced by the third RSV infection (92). Repeated infections in children and adults occur frequently, indicating that protection against reinfection is incomplete (92).

Hospitalization of children for hMPV infection occurs primarily in the first year of life, although many studies report that the peak age of hospitalization for hMPV is

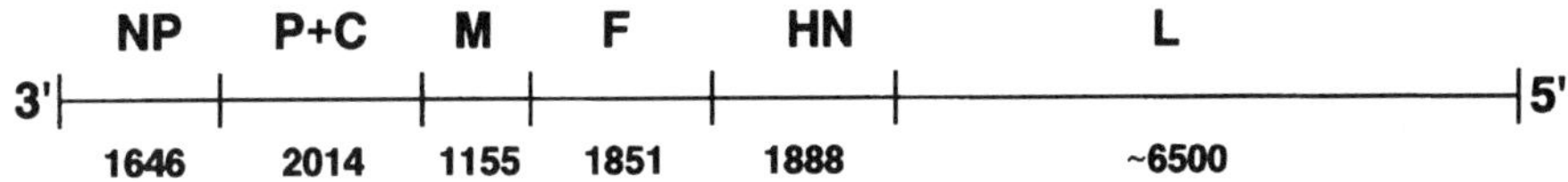

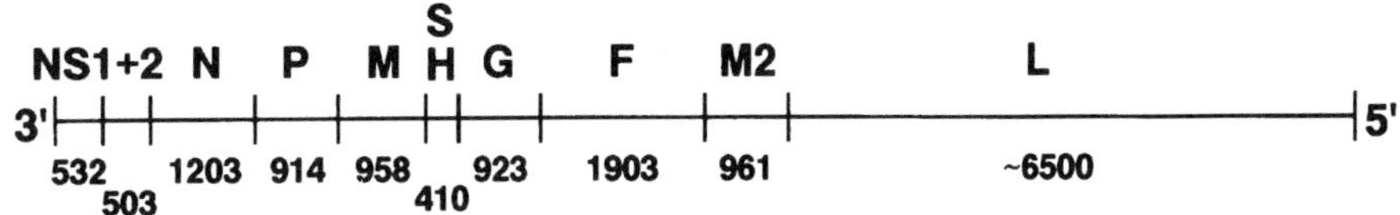

FIGURE 2 Schematic presentation of the genomes of PIV type 3 and RSV. Abbreviations: NP, nucleoprotein; P+C, small proteins of the polymerase complex; M, matrix; F, fusion; HN, hemagglutinin-neuraminidase; L, large protein of the polymerase complex; NS, nonstructural proteins; N, nucleoprotein; P, phosphoprotein; SH, strongly hydrophobic protein; G, attachment protein; M2, small envelope protein. (Data from references 41a and 42.)

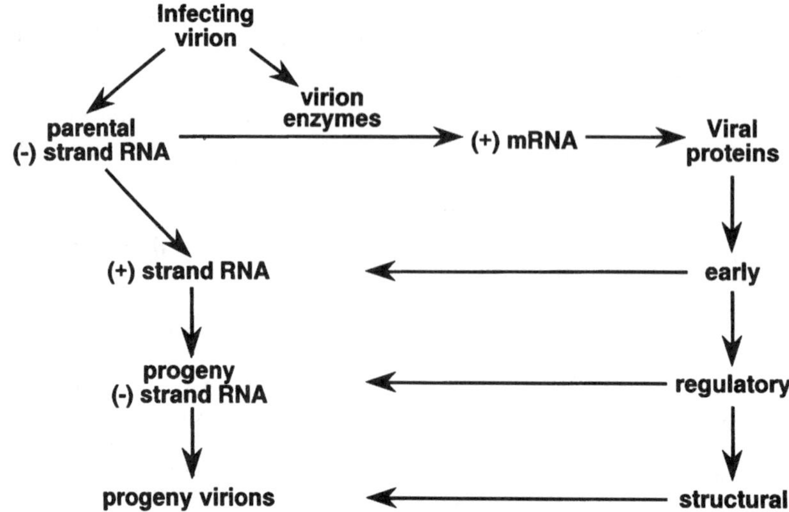

FIGURE 3 Schematic presentation of the replication strategy of viruses of the family *Paramyxoviridae*. (−), negative sense; (+), positive sense. (Data from reference 150.)

from 6 to 12 months of age and thus later than the peak age of hospitalization for RSV (24). For PIVs, lower respiratory tract infection occurs most frequently in children younger than 4 years of age (88). Repeated infection is common but usually results in upper respiratory infection or inapparent infection (88). Immunity elicited after infection appears to be very important in reducing the severity of disease following reinfection.

Reinfection

Reinfections with these viruses are common. Overall, 76 and 67% of children are reinfected with RSV and PIV type 3, respectively, during the second year of life (Table 5). Only 3% of children <5 years of age develop lower tract disease with PIV type 3 reinfection, compared to 11% who have lower tract disease with RSV. Reinfections with these viruses also cause a sizable proportion of upper respiratory illnesses in healthy older children and adults. RSV and PIV reinfections are common causes of hospitalization of adult patients with chronic lung conditions like asthma and chronic obstructive pulmonary disease (67, 89). RSV can cause serious lower respiratory tract infection among immunocompromised adults (142), residents of chronic care facilities, and the elderly who live in the community (68, 70). The clinical presentation of disease and morbidity and mortality caused by RSV in the noninstitutionalized elderly population are similar to those observed with influenza A infection (68). Two to nine percent of pneumonia hospitalizations and deaths in older adults are due to RSV (113). hMPV also causes reinfections in both children and adults (246, 252).

Clinical Attack Rates

RSV, PIV, and hMPV are the most important causes of lower respiratory tract disease in children (50, 202, 209). Almost 30% of infants have a medically attended illness, usually diagnosed as bronchiolitis or pneumonia, in the first year of life due to RSV (253). RSV-related hospitalization rates for lower respiratory tract diseases are similar in developed and developing countries (185). At least 2% of all infants are hospitalized with RSV disease, with the peak occurrence in the second month of life (210). Infants from low-income households and many Native American or aboriginal populations have a much higher risk of hospitalization than those from upper- and middle-income groups (89). The frequency of RSV lower tract disease decreases gradually during the preschool years. The frequency of primary and repeat hMPV infection has not been well characterized, although it appears that rates of clinical hMPV disease are lower than that of RSV. PIV type 3 infects children at an early age, but these infections are much less likely to involve the lower respiratory tract.

TABLE 3 RSV and PIV type 3 infection rates in children younger than 5 years[a]

Age (mo)	RSV		PIV type 3	
	Total no. of children	No. (%) infected	Total no. of children	No. (%) infected
0–12	125	86 (68.8)	121	81 (66.9)
13–24	92	76 (82.6)	90	61 (67.8)
25–36	65	30 (46.2)	63	23 (36.5)
37–48	39	13 (33.3)	39	13 (33.3)
49–60	24	12 (50.0)	24	4 (16.7)
Total	345	217 (62.8)	337	182 (54.0)

[a] Data from references 88 and 92.

TABLE 4 Primary infection rate for RSV and PIV type 3 in children younger than 3 years[a]

Age (mo)	RSV			PIV type 3		
	Total no. of children	No. (%) infected	No. (%) with LRD[b]	Total no. of children	No. (%) infected	No. (%) with LRD[b]
0–12	125	85 (68.0)	27 (21.6)	121	75 (62.0)	13 (10.7)
13–24	34	33 (97.1)	2 (5.9)	37	30 (81.1)	8 (21.6)
25–36	1	1 (100)	0	3	2 (66.7)	0
Total	160	119 (74.4)	29 (18.1)	161	107 (66.5)	21 (13.0)

[a] Data from references 88 and 92.
[b] LRD, lower respiratory tract disease.

Lower respiratory tract disease due to PIV types 1 and 2 has its highest incidence between 6 and 18 months of age. The total impact of the three PIVs combined, as reflected by admissions to the hospital, is about the same as that of RSV. The PIVs have lower rates than RSV in infants but higher rates than RSV in the 1- to 4-year age group (90).

The economic impact of acute RSV infection alone in the United States is considerable. The total annual cost of hospitalization has more than doubled those previously estimated, because recent rates of bronchiolitis hospitalization have increased substantially (210). Using 2002 data for an estimated 149,000 children hospitalized with bronchiolitis, total annual hospitalization costs in the United States were approximately $543 million (193).

Epidemic Occurrence

In temperate climates, RSV produces annual epidemics that are characterized by bronchiolitis in infants; RSV outbreaks are less clearly delineated in tropical areas, where year-round infection is reported (86). RSV subgroup A infections usually predominate, but sometimes RSV subgroup B infections are more prevalent, and in certain settings, subgroup B may alternate with subgroup A (36, 177).

Different lineages of hMPV frequently circulate in a community during the same winter season, although one subgroup may predominate in a given year (93, 163, 252). Viruses from each subgroup appear to be capable of causing severe lower respiratory tract disease; different subgroups have not been convincingly associated with varying severity of disease.

PIV type 1 causes croup epidemics every other year (88). PIV type 2 infections usually follow the same pattern as PIV type 1, but the manifestations of PIV type 2 infections are milder. PIV type 3 is the least predictable; infections occur in an endemic pattern most of the time but outbreaks do occur, usually in the spring.

Outbreaks of infections with these respiratory viruses are common in closed populations of young children, especially in pediatric hospital wards or large day care centers (78). Epidemic RSV disease in nursing homes (69) and homes for adolescents with developmental disabilities (160) has also been described.

Epidemics of RSV or PIV can be recognized by clinical syndrome, for example, seasonal outbreaks of bronchiolitis in infants in the autumn and winter months or croup epidemics due to PIV types 1 and 2 in slightly older infants and toddlers in the autumn. PIV type 3 outbreaks tend to occur in late winter or springtime. hMPV generally follows the RSV season in the late winter or early spring. Many upper respiratory illnesses that occur in older children and adults during these periods are caused by reinfections with these viruses.

Seasonality

Distinct seasonal patterns of infections occur for these agents in the temperate zones (86, 88). Seasonality differs in other climate areas: in tropical and subtropical areas, disease may be endemic year-round or increased during distinct seasons, such as rainy seasons. In Alaska, RSV and hMPV are detected during most months of the year. RSV commonly produces epidemics in midwinter, particularly in large urban centers, but some variations have been observed. For example, in the southern United States, the RSV season generally begins earlier than in other regions of the United States. Epidemics that alternate between large midwinter epidemics followed by small early spring outbreaks in the following season have been reported from some countries. PIV type 1 has a unique pattern of occurrence, with epidemics that occur every other year in the autumn. Since 1973, both PIV types 1 and 2 have been epidemic in the autumn of odd-numbered years. PIV type 3 infections have occurred in late winter or early spring or

TABLE 5 Reinfection rates for RSV and PIV type 3 in children 1 to 5 years of age[a]

Age (mo)	RSV			PIV type 3		
	Total no. of children	No. (%) infected	No. (%) with LRD[b]	Total no. of children	No. (%) infected	No. (%) with LRD[b]
13–24	58	44 (75.9)	11 (19.0)	55	37 (67.3)	2 (4)
25–36	64	29 (45.3)	7 (10.9)	62	21 (33.9)	2 (3)
37–48	39	13 (33.3)	3 (7.7)	39	13 (33.3)	1 (3)
49–60	24	12 (50.0)	0	24	4 (16.7)	0
Total	185	98 (53.0)	21 (11.4)	180	75 (41.7)	5 (3)

[a] Data from references 88 and 92.
[b] LRD, lower respiratory tract disease.

during months when PIV types 1 and 2 are not prevalent. PIV type 4 appears to be more common during autumn and winter (227). Outbreaks of RSV and PIVs are less predictable in the tropics; most studies have shown increased prevalence in the rainy season (34).

Transmission

Most evidence indicates that these viruses are transmitted by respiratory secretions through direct contact or via fomites (100) or by large-droplet spread (98). RSV has been recovered from environmental surfaces in infected patients' rooms for up to 6 h (101). Entry likely occurs through contact with the nasal mucosa or eyes, in contrast to the less permissive oral route (103). Transmission by small-particle aerosols of RSV has not been proven, and if it occurs, it is an infrequent route. Clinical observations suggest that PIVs and hMPV are transmitted similarly to RSV (105). Although PIV types 1 and 3 have been recovered from air samples collected in the vicinity of infected patients (173), direct contact and transmission via fomites are likely to be more important. The high initial and subsequent infection rates suggest that these viruses spread readily, that reinfected persons may be infectious, and that relatively small inocula are necessary to infect.

Nosocomial infections are common with RSV, hMPV, and PIV type 3 (155, 213) and can involve health care workers and patients as both sources and transmitters of disease. Spread of RSV can be limited in these settings by adherence to strict hand washing procedures and cohorting of infected and exposed individuals (80). Use of gloves, masks, and goggles in the hospital setting will also limit spread (79). A preschool or school-age sibling is the most likely introducer of RSV and PIVs into the family, with approximately half of family members becoming infected once the virus is introduced (43). On average, the time between primary and secondary infections in family members is 5 to 6 days.

Virus Shedding Patterns

Infants and young children shed RSV for a mean of 9 days, while immunocompetent adults generally shed for less than 4 days. Infants may excrete RSV for over 3 weeks after onset of illness, and prolonged excretion for weeks to months may occur in immunocompromised hosts. In hospitalized infants with lower respiratory tract infection, nearly all infected infants shed RSV during the first 7 days of hospitalization, and the majority still shed virus at the time of discharge from the hospital (102). A few critically ill infants may continue to shed for up to 27 days. Infants with lower respiratory tract disease shed RSV for a longer period than those with an upper respiratory illness. High viral titers, 10^5 to 10^7 PFU/ml, can often be found in secretions from the upper and lower respiratory tract in young children (63, 102). Substantially lower viral quantities are found in the upper respiratory tract of immunocompetent or immunocompromised adults (63). Decline in viral titer is not consistently observed in infants until days 3 to 6 of hospitalization, although they may already be improving clinically by that time.

The duration of viral shedding for PIVs is approximately a week, although this is variable and dependent on age, number of prior infections, and severity of infection (105). PIV type 3 may be excreted for up to 4 weeks, and 17% of specimens from infected children are positive during the third week after onset of illness (76). Some children may excrete PIV as early as 6 days before the onset of illness. The persistent shedding of virus from young children facilitates the spread of infection. Prolonged PIV type 3 shedding may occur in children with primary infection and adults with underlying chronic lung disease (76, 95). Prolonged viral shedding (mean, 4 weeks) occurs in children and adults with compromised immune function due to malignancy, organ transplantation, congenital and acquired immunodeficiency, and prolonged steroid treatment (95). Even longer shedding of parainfluenza viruses and persistent shedding in asymptomatic patients have been noted using more sensitive molecular detection methods, especially for immunocompromised patients (191). Impairment of T-cell function appears to be the common denominator in children with prolonged shedding due to RSV, hMPV, and PIVs (108, 143).

PATHOGENESIS

Organ Specificity

In the immunocompetent host, RSV, hMPV, and PIV replication is restricted to the respiratory epithelium. Viremia or isolation of PIV type 3 from cerebrospinal fluid has been reported rarely. All these viruses spread primarily from cell to cell in the upper respiratory tract and at times progress to the lower respiratory tract. The inoculum size is an important variable for achieving RSV and PIV infections in adults and possibly infants and children (131, 237).

Histopathology

The pulmonary histopathology of bronchiolitis has been described primarily from infants and young children who have succumbed acutely from RSV infection (2, 55). Limited data are available for PIVs, although the histopathology appears to be similar to that of RSV (55, 129). The earliest lesion to develop within 24 h of onset is necrosis of the bronchiolar epithelium with denudation of the ciliated epithelial cells. This is followed by migration of lymphocytes into affected tissues, resulting in peribronchiolar infiltration (Fig. 4). The submucosal and adventitial tissues become edematous, accompanied by increased secretions from mucus-producing cells. Plugs consisting of mucus, cellular debris, fibrin strands, and DNA-like materials occlude the smaller bronchioles. Fatal RSV infection has been characterized by viral antigen detected primarily in cellular debris obstructing the lumen of the small airways and in multinucleated cells lining the bronchiolar lumen, near absence of CD8-positive lymphocytes and natural killer cells, and increased expression of apoptosis markers (241). The major pathological features are air trapping with distension of some segments or obstruction with alveolar collapse. Polymorphonuclear cells are absent, except for cells in the exudate of large airways. Histologic recovery is slow, beginning with regeneration of the basal epithelial layer within 3 to 4 days and exuberant regeneration of the ciliated epithelial cells starting at the end of the second week (2). The plugs of cellular debris are eventually resorbed (Fig. 5).

Interstitial inflammation with mononuclear cell infiltration is the rule in RSV and PIV pneumonia (Fig. 6) (55, 147). The epithelial cells are flattened, with loss of cilia. The subepithelial tissues of bronchiolar and interalveolar walls are thickened due to mononuclear cell infiltration. Subsequently, significant epithelial necrosis, an intense mononuclear inflammatory response extending from the smaller bronchioles into alveoli, hyaline membrane for-

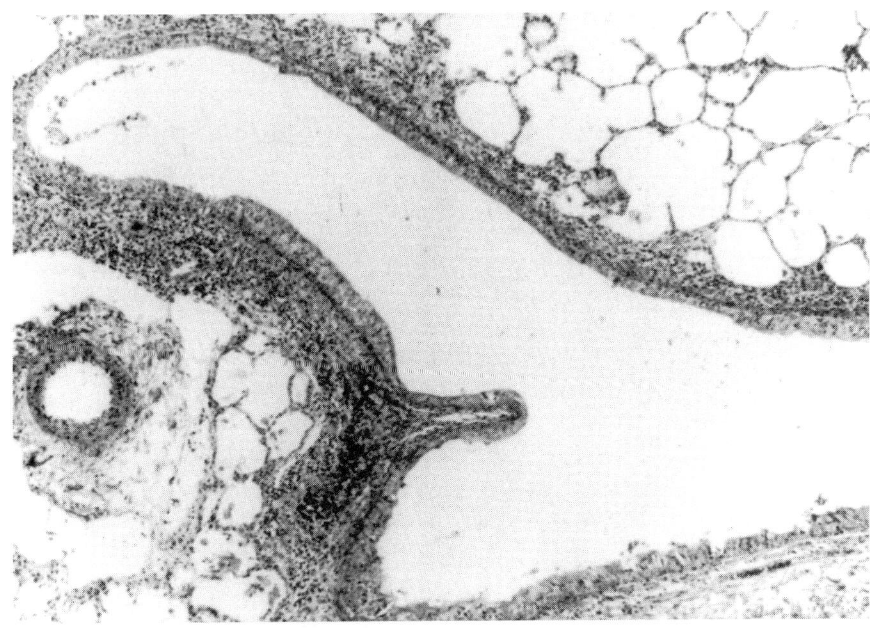

FIGURE 4 Characteristic histopathological changes of the airways of an infant with bronchiolitis due to RSV infection. Note the peribronchial mononuclear cell inflammation, relatively normal alveoli, and focal ulceration on top with regenerative epithelial changes. Hematoxylin and eosin stain; magnification, ×45.

mation in alveolar spaces, and edema of interalveolar walls may occur. Histologic differences observed between bronchiolitis and pneumonia may represent a continuum of disease possibly related to the size of the viral inoculum, with higher concentrations of virus resulting in pneumonia (147).

hMPV has been detected only in respiratory tract specimens, suggesting that its replication is limited to respiratory epithelia. In lung transplant recipients infected with hMPV, both acute and organizing lung injury occur, with diffuse alveolar damage and cytoplasmic inclusion bodies (219). Bronchoalveolar lavage fluid from immunocom-

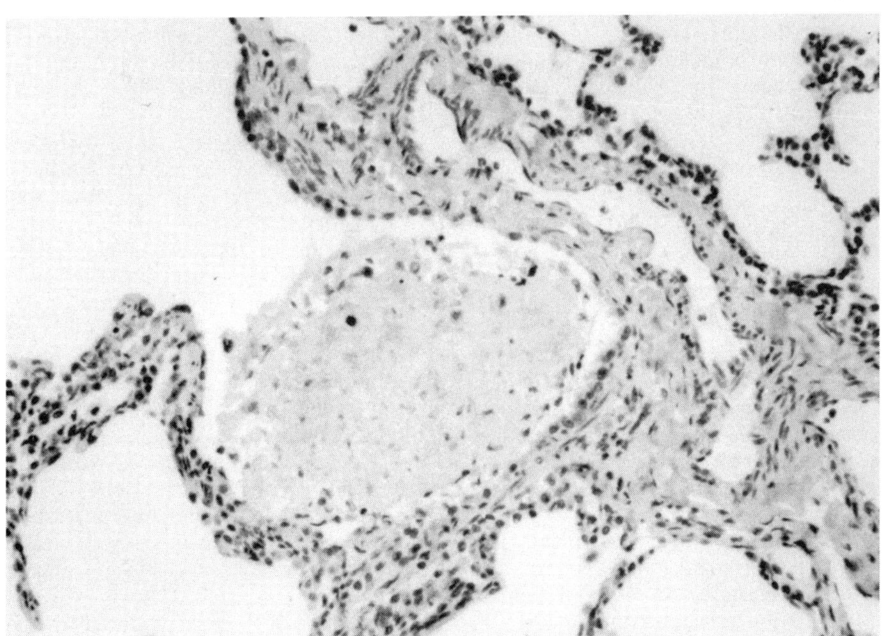

FIGURE 5 Histopathological features of resolving RSV bronchiolitis in an infant. Note the plug of mucus and cellular debris in a terminal respiratory bronchus. Hematoxylin and eosin stain; magnification, ×144.

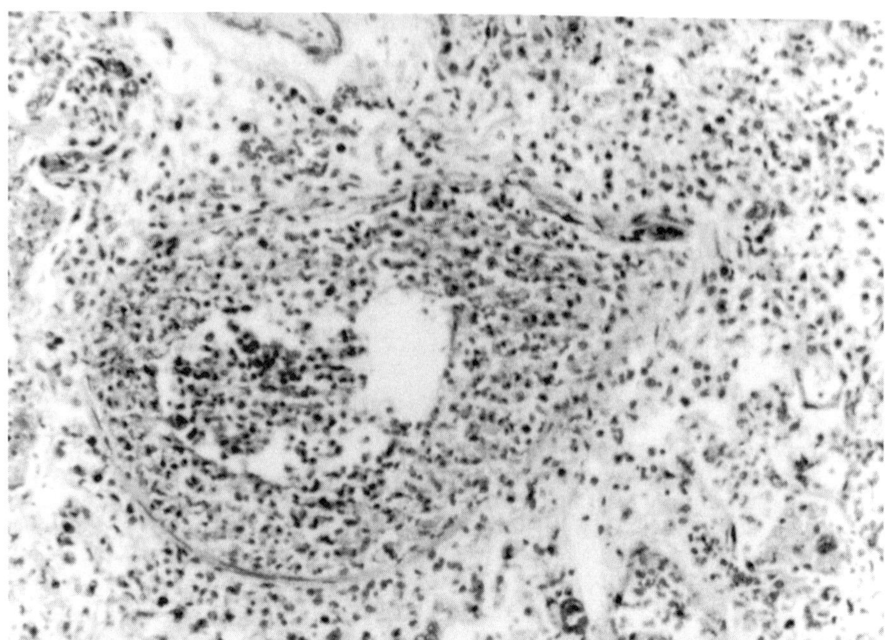

FIGURE 6 Histopathology in an infant with congenital immunodeficiency and RSV pneumonia. Note the plugging of a terminal bronchus by cellular debris and parenchymal infiltration with necrosis. Hematoxylin and eosin stain; magnification, ×72.

promised patients contains sloughed, degenerated epithelial cells with eosinophilic cytoplasmic inclusions, multinucleated giant cells, and histiocytes (231). Because available histopathological evidence comes from lung biopsy and bronchoalveolar lavage specimens from patients with underlying immunodeficiencies or malignancies, these findings may not reflect what occurs in otherwise healthy humans. The pathological features of hMPV infection in mice, cotton rats, and macaques include disruption of respiratory epithelial architecture, sloughing of epithelial cells, loss of ciliation, and inflammatory infiltrates (4, 146, 250). Histopathological changes or evidence of infection was not detected in any other tissues. In macaques and cotton rats, viral antigen is localized almost exclusively at the apical surface of ciliated respiratory epithelial cells.

IMMUNE RESPONSES

Innate Response: Cytokines and Inflammatory Mediators

Upon virus infection of the respiratory epithelium, the innate immune response is the first line of host defense. The mannan-binding lectin, surfactant proteins, and other collectins act as opsonins with activity against RSV and likely hMPV and PIVs. Signaling receptors such as Toll-like receptor 4, which recognizes the F protein of RSV, can activate the NF-κB signaling pathway, inducing expression of cytokines and costimulatory molecules. Gene polymorphisms of the pattern recognition receptors (Toll-like receptor 4 and surfactant protein D) and of downstream-induced antiviral molecules (interleukin 4 [IL-4], IL-8, IL-10, and tumor necrosis factor alpha [TNF-α]) and other innate immune genes have been associated with severe RSV infection (29, 66, 127). Cytokine production is depressed in infants and children compared with adults and may account for their less-than-optimal immune response (159).

Interferon plays an important role in promoting early recovery from viral diseases. RSV infection is notable for little or no local interferon production (104). The host interferon response to RSV is suppressed by RSV nonstructural proteins NS1 and NS2. Detectable levels of interferon have been found in 30% of children with PIV infection and may be associated with diminished shedding of the virus (104). The P/C gene of PIV type 1 inhibits the interferon response by inhibiting interferon regulatory factor 3 activation and subsequent interferon production (149).

The clinical significance of the cytokine profiles associated with severity of RSV and other respiratory viruses is slowly emerging. Although it was thought that the inflammatory response generated against RSV contributed substantially to the development of respiratory disease, more recent data suggest that a robust early inflammatory response is critical in the control of viral replication and of respiratory disease (19, 149, 241). Each respiratory virus has a unique cytokine profile even though the clinical presentations of disease may be identical (19, 149, 241).

IL-2 and gamma interferon (IFN-γ) are the predominant RSV-stimulated cytokine responses of memory T cells from young children exposed to one RSV season, older children with one or more prior RSV infections, and adults (11, 166). Some children also develop an increase in IL-5 mRNA. RSV-specific memory T cells appear to have a dominant Th1 response and are similar for different age groups.

TNF-α and IL-8 are produced by RSV-infected human alveolar macrophages. These cytokines attract neutrophils and macrophages to the site of infection (16). IL-8 is also produced by RSV-infected human epithelial cells in vitro (15, 16). IL-6, a promoter of mucosal B lymphocytes and immunoglobulin A (IgA) production, and TNF-α are detected in the nasal secretions and tracheal aspirates of the majority of infants and young children with acute primary RSV infection, although peak concentrations are not correlated with the peak of mucosal RSV-specific IgA responses (164). Higher plasma IL-8 levels have been detected in RSV-infected infants who require mechanical ventilation than in nonventilated infants (22). IL-6, IL-8, and IL-10 have been inversely correlated with duration of oxygen support (19), and a similar inverse correlation has been observed between the duration of mechanical ventilation and the production of IL-12 in RSV-infected infants (23). A robust inflammatory response may be protective against more severe disease, and IL-12 may play a critical role in the development of an RSV-specific immune response during recovery of the infection.

The respiratory epithelium plays a role in modulating the inflammatory response to RSV. Macrophage inflammatory protein 1α (MIP-1α), IL-8, and RANTES have been detected in lower airway secretions of RSV-infected children (114a). Through the release of MIP-1α and RANTES, epithelial cells may augment the recruitment and activation of monocytes, basophils, and eosinophils (207).

Various mediators of inflammation, in particular degranulation products of mucosal mast cells and eosinophils, have been associated with severity of involvement in bronchiolitis. Histamine and leukotrienes C4, D4, and E4 are the major mast cell mediators responsible for constriction of smooth muscle, increased mucus production, and increased vascular permeability. In infants with RSV and PIV type 3 bronchiolitis, elevated levels of histamine, leukotriene C4, and eosinophilic cationic protein have been detected during the acute phase of the disease and have been associated with wheezing and hypoxemia in RSV-infected infants (84, 204, 233, 240).

Data on human innate immune responses to hMPV are limited. Increased levels of IL-8 and decreased levels of RANTES have been reported to be present in nasal secretions of hMPV-infected children compared with levels from RSV-infected children (128). Children infected with hMPV appear to have significantly lower levels of IL-1β, IL-6, IL-8, IL-12, and TNF-α than do RSV- or influenza virus-infected infants (149). hMPV infection of human dendritic cells (DCs) ex vivo (97) induces production of TNF-α, IL-6 in myeloid DCs, and IFN-α in both myeloid and plasmacytoid DCs.

Humoral, Cell-Mediated, Mucosal Immune Responses

Humoral immune responses in infants hospitalized following primary RSV infection consist of virus-specific IgM antibodies that may persist up to 10 weeks after the illness and virus-specific IgG and IgA antibodies that are produced within the second week, peak by 3 to 4 weeks, and decline to low or nondetectable levels by the following RSV season. Reinfection with RSV results in a rapid increase in all three classes of antibody. Age-specific and preexisting-virus-specific maternal antibodies appear to influence the development of serum antibodies to the F and G surface glycoproteins and serum neutralizing antibodies in infants undergoing primary RSV infection (180). Older infants are able to develop a more appropriate protein-specific and functionally active neutralizing antibody response after primary RSV infection. The avidity of the antibody in response to primary infection, however, appears to be low regardless of age (172). Primary infection with RSV subgroup A virus elicits antibodies that cross-react with subgroup B virus (175). In contrast, primary subgroup B infection induces cross-reactive antibodies to subgroup A virus less efficiently. The IgG responses to F and G surface glycoproteins after primary RSV infection are predominantly of the IgG1 subclass and, less frequently, the IgG3 subclass, a finding consistent with the protein domain bearing the dominant antigenic sites (234). In contrast, adults respond to the heavily glycosylated G protein with IgG1 and IgG2 subclass antibodies, while a dominant IgG1 subclass response to the less glycosylated F protein occurs (235).

Antibodies directed to the G protein most likely neutralize the virus by preventing attachment of virus to cells, while antibodies directed to the F surface glycoprotein neutralize the virus by preventing virus-cell fusion and inhibiting cell-to-cell spread (17, 225). Other effector mechanisms mediated by IgG1 and IgG3, like complement-enhanced neutralization and antibody-dependent cell cytotoxicity, help clear virus and virus-infected cells. Since RSV infection is restricted to the mucosa, the antibodies present in the lower and upper respiratory tract are important for disease prevention. In adults, IgG1 and IgG2 concentrations in serum and the terminal airways are similar (171).

Cellular immune responses are thought to play an important role in clearing RSV and PIV infections and preventing lethal disease. Immunocompetent infants infected with RSV, hMPV, or PIVs stop shedding virus within 21 days following infection, but persons with deficient cellular immunity may shed virus for months (114) and progress to fatal infection (60, 108, 242).

The role of the cytotoxic T lymphocytes in RSV, hMPV, and PIV lung disease in humans has not been fully elucidated. RSV-specific cytotoxic T-cell responses occur in a minority of infants with RSV bronchiolitis, with the highest responses occurring in children with mild lung disease (126). Infants who develop RSV-specific cytotoxic T-cell responses after RSV lower respiratory tract illness in the first year of life appear to be less likely to develop a lower respiratory tract illness in the second year of life (166). A direct correlation has been observed between RSV-specific CD8 cytotoxic activity and RSV-induced IFN-γ and inversely with IL-4 (166). In adults, RSV-specific cytotoxic T cells recognize the N (nucleoprotein) protein, the SH proteins, the F protein, the M protein, and, poorly, the M2 protein but not the G protein (13, 39). In elderly adults, development of severe RSV infection may be due to low numbers of RSV-specific CD8 memory T cells that maintain effector function (49). RSV-specific cytotoxic T cells appear to be important for recovery from infection, and their maintenance is critical for the control of subsequent RSV infections.

Secretory antibodies found in the nasal secretions consist of IgA, IgM, IgG, and IgE classes and are directed to at least the major surface glycoproteins of these viruses (168, 181). Younger infants have a lower rate and magnitude of IgG and IgA secretory antibody responses to RSV than older infants. With primary infection, secretory IgG and IgM antibodies peak between 8 to 13 days, while secretory IgA peaks between 14 to 28 days after onset of illness. After 2 months, infants have low or nondetectable levels of virus-specific secretory antibodies to all three immunoglobulin classes. Primary infections with PIVs result in low, transient virus-specific IgA responses in secretions (238).

The production of virus-specific IgE antibody has been associated with disease severity (239, 240). During primary RSV and PIV infections, secretory virus-specific IgE antibody has been detected primarily in infants with bronchiolitis. Virus-IgE complexes may induce mast cells to release mediators that are responsible for smooth muscle constriction, increased mucus production, and vascular permeability.

Correlates of Immune Protection

Infants with high levels of maternally acquired RSV- and PIV type 3-specific antibodies are better protected against lower respiratory tract illness than those with lower levels (88, 92). The level of neutralizing antibody in cord blood directly correlates with the age at which primary RSV infection occurs and is inversely related to the severity of illness. The risk of reinfection in children and adults is also inversely related to the level of serum neutralizing antibodies (88, 92). In children and adults, a minimum protective level of serum neutralizing antibody is associated with a 3.5-fold-lower likelihood of RSV-associated hospitalization (197). Other humoral correlates of immunity against RSV and PIV infections are IgG antibodies directed to the F surface glycoprotein and to the homologous G (HN for PIV) surface glycoprotein of the infecting virus strain (91, 137). However, even in the presence of high levels of virus-specific antibodies, primary infection and reinfection can occur (88, 92). Serum neutralizing antibody is a good correlate of immunity against RSV disease of the lower respiratory tract but not of the upper respiratory tract. For PIVs, serum antibodies to both HN and F proteins confer protection (203).

CLINICAL MANIFESTATIONS

Respiratory Syncytial Virus

Any respiratory virus may be associated with a wide spectrum of illness severity ranging from inapparent infection or mild afebrile upper respiratory illness to severe and fulminating pneumonia. However, RSV and PIVs produce distinct clinical syndromes that are hallmarks of infection with these viruses.

Children

The signal illness for RSV in infants is bronchiolitis manifested by expiratory wheezing, air trapping, nasal flaring, subcostal retractions, and, sometimes, cyanosis (Table 6). Conversely, RSV is the most common virus associated with bronchiolitis, detected in approximately 70% of children with bronchiolitis during the peak season (215). Fever is not a prominent finding in infants with RSV infection; approximately 50% of infants presenting to the hospital with RSV disease will have moderate or greater elevations in temperature. RSV pneumonia is common with primary infection, and infants may have signs and symptoms of both clinical conditions simultaneously. The clinical presentation may depend on the proportion of the small airways partially occluded by the inflammatory process. This results in expiratory wheezing and air trapping, whereas subsegmental atelectasis results from complete occlusion of the small airways. Radiographic findings depend upon the same factors. Partial occlusion of the bronchioles results in hyperaeration and flattening of the diaphragm (Fig. 7). Complete occlusion results in atelectasis that may be lobar, usually involving the right middle or right upper lobe (Fig. 8).

TABLE 6 Clinical manifestations of RSV and hMPV infection at various ages

Infants
Bronchiolitis
Pneumonia
Croup
Asthma exacerbation
Upper respiratory tract infection
Otitis media
Older children and adults
Upper respiratory tract infection
Croup
Laryngitis
Bronchitis
Asthma exacerbation
Pneumonia (elderly)
Chronic obstructive pulmonary disease exacerbation (elderly)

Hypoxia is a common finding in infants with lower respiratory tract disease (125). The arterial blood PO_2 is often less than 60 mm Hg, and the oxygen saturation may be below 90%. Apnea has been documented to occur in about 20% of hospitalized young infants with RSV illness (10), and apnea may be the presenting sign of RSV in premature babies or infants less than 3 months of age. Oxygen saturation is lower on average in infants with apnea, even if other signs of severe disease like subcostal retractions are absent. Infants with apnea tend to be younger, to be born before 37 weeks' gestation, and to have a history of apnea of prematurity. Some deaths in infants who die unexpectedly at home may be a result of RSV infection accompanied by apnea. Interstitial pneumonitis is not commonly recognized with RSV infection, but cases are overrepresented in autopsy series (55). Therefore, the recognition of interstitial involvement should alert the caregiver to the need for repeat clinical assessment and measurement of oxygen saturation.

Otitis media is a frequent complication of RSV infection in children, with rates up to 60% in some studies. RSV has been detected alone, but it is commonly detected with bacteria in middle ear fluid samples (186). Severity decreases with age and following repeated infections, such that mild upper respiratory tract disease characterized by rhinorrhea, hoarseness, sore throat, and sinusitis is more typical of RSV infection in school-age children (86, 107).

Adults

The common clinical presentation of RSV infection in otherwise healthy adults is similar to that reported for older children. Initial symptoms commonly include upper respiratory tract disease complaints like nasal congestion, cough, sore throat or hoarseness, earache, and low-grade fever (Table 6). Adults may have minimal or no symptoms and still have RSV isolated from secretory specimens, or they may be symptomatic, with sore throat, bronchitis, and even wheezing. In elderly persons, clinical symptoms with RSV infection are often indistinguishable from influenza

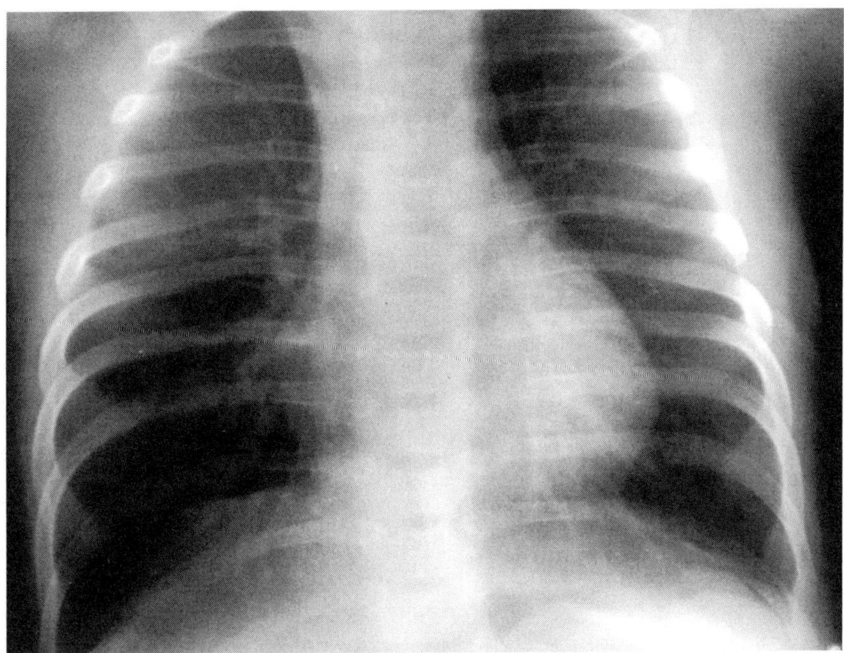

FIGURE 7 Chest radiograph of an infant with bronchiolitis due to RSV. Peribronchial thickening with hyperaeration and flattened diaphragms bilaterally are evident. (Reprinted from reference 139 with permission of Elsevier.)

virus infection, with the possible exception of a lower frequency of high-grade fever (70). In adults with underlying pulmonary disease, RSV infection may commonly manifest as increased dyspnea with or without hypoxia, and it may be accompanied by cough, fever, nasal congestion, and wheezing (67). The last two findings occur more frequently with RSV than with influenza virus infection (70). Clinical findings of RSV in adults are generally nonspecific, and definitive diagnosis requires laboratory testing.

PIV

The signal illness for PIV in children is croup, or laryngotracheobronchitis. Croup is manifested by fever, hoarseness, and a barking cough in a child usually between 6 and 18 months of age. Severe narrowing of the subglottic area of the trachea may progress to cause inspiratory stridor (Fig. 9). Observation in the hospital may be required for children with severe stridor, so that the airway can be secured. PIV type 1 is the major cause of croup (51). PIV type 2 also is associated with croup, usually during the season that PIV type 1 is active. PIV type 3 is a cause of sporadic croup and also is associated with bronchiolitis and pneumonia in young infants but with much less frequency than that observed with RSV (Fig. 10). PIV type 4 disease has been less well described; PIV type 4 disease can manifest as bronchiolitis, paroxysmal cough, or upper respiratory tract disease (153).

PIV disease in adults commonly manifests as a relatively nonspecific upper respiratory tract illness, with rhinorrhea, nasal congestion, and hoarseness commonly noted. Reinfection with PIV is a common cause of serious morbidity in adults with chronic lung disease (89).

Human Metapneumovirus

hMPV has been associated with a variety of respiratory symptoms and diagnoses. Children with hMPV infection typically present with upper respiratory symptoms like rhinorrhea, cough, and fever (Tables 6 and 7). Conjunctivitis, vomiting, diarrhea, and rash are occasionally reported but are not prominent in most studies. The lower respiratory tract syndromes most frequently associated with hMPV are bronchiolitis, croup, pneumonia, and asthma exacerbation. These illnesses are neither clinically nor radiographically distinct from the same clinical syndromes caused by other common respiratory viruses (Fig. 11). Reinfections with hMPV are more likely to be limited to the upper respiratory tract in otherwise healthy children (247, 252). hMPV is associated with a substantial proportion of acute otitis media (AOM) in children, and viral RNA has been detected in middle ear fluid from patients with AOM (208, 251).

A causal relationship between hMPV infection and asthma development or exacerbations is currently unproven. One study of outpatient children did not find an association between hMPV and asthma exacerbations (201), while another found a highly significant association between hMPV and the diagnosis of acute asthma exacerbation (247). hMPV infection has been detected in up to 60% (71) of children hospitalized for wheezing or adults hospitalized for asthma exacerbations (246, 249). One study reporting a strong association between infantile hMPV bronchiolitis and asthma at age 5 years (82) requires confirmation, in part because of the difficulty of making the diagnosis of asthma during infancy, when acute wheezing frequently is associated with viral infections. hMPV is rarely detected in asymptomatic children (247).

Infections in Immunocompromised Patients

Immunocompromised children and adults are vulnerable to severe RSV, PIV, and hMPV infections (64, 108, 142). RSV and PIV infections are especially devastating for infants with severe combined immunodeficiency syndrome

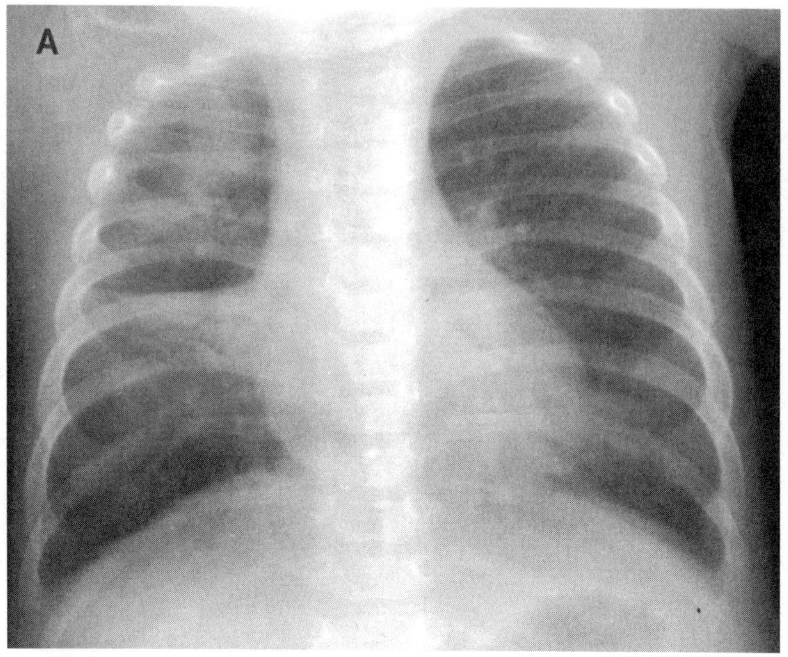

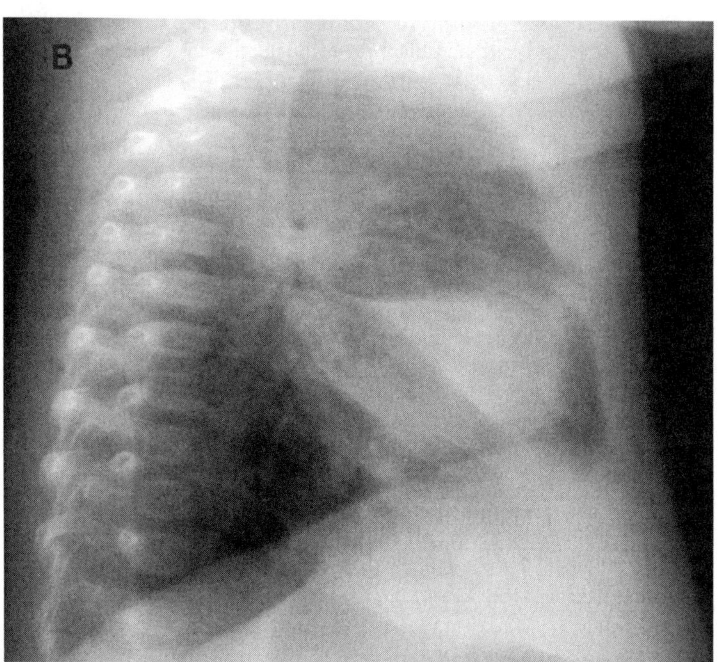

FIGURE 8 Posterior-anterior (A) and lateral (B) chest radiographs of an infant with bronchiolitis and pneumonia due to RSV. Bilateral perihilar and peribronchial infiltrations and partial or segmental atelectasis of the right middle and right upper lobes are evident. (Reprinted from reference 139 with permission of Elsevier.)

(SCID) (77, 129), in whom persistent viral shedding and the development of progressive pneumonia occur. Children or adults who acquire RSV or hMPV during or shortly after chemotherapy for malignancy also may have severe, life-threatening disease (60, 64). Children with human immunodeficiency virus (HIV) infection have a higher rate of pneumonia, decreased likelihood of wheezing, prolonged viral carriage with intermittent disease, and increased morbidity following infection by one of these viruses. Although the clinical course is generally not fulminant in HIV-positive patients when good supportive care and antiretroviral therapy are available (130, 143), the overall mortality of these patients in developing countries is substantial, with reported rates ranging from 10 to 65% (162).

Hematopoietic stem cell transplant (HCT) recipients of all ages may have a more fulminant course following RSV or PIV infection, particularly if the infection occurs around the time of transplantation (123, 190, 242). Adults with

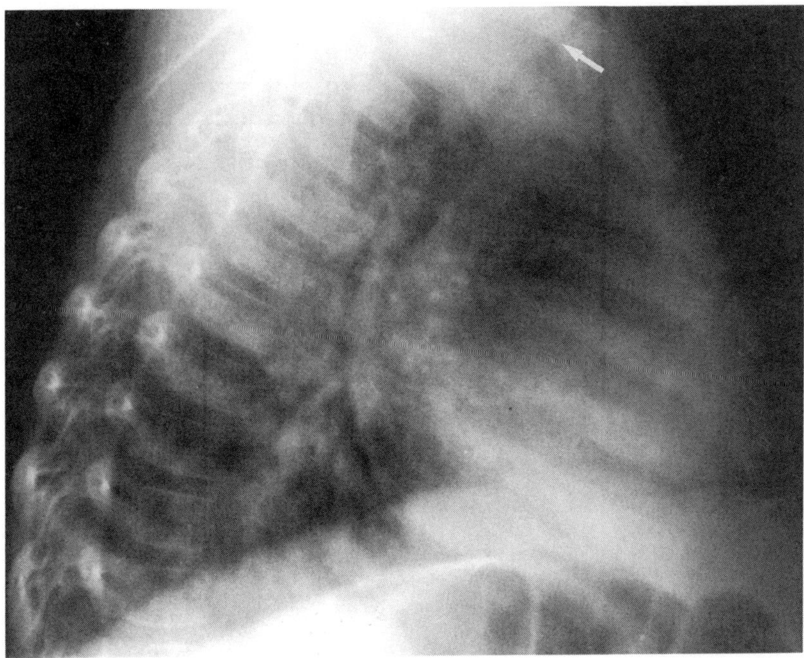

FIGURE 9 Chest radiograph of a child with croup due to PIV type 1. Peribronchial thickening, scattered infiltrates, and marked narrowing of the superior portion of the trachea (arrow) are evident.

leukemia (45), those with profound chemotherapy-induced myelosuppression (45, 245), and solid-organ transplant recipients, particularly lung and pediatric heart recipients, are also at risk of fatal outcome. Initial clinical symptoms related to RSV infection in these patients are similar to those in immunocompetent persons and variably include low-grade fever, cough, rhinorrhea, nasal congestion, and sore throat. In immunocompromised adults with RSV infection, other common clinical findings include sinusitis, otitis media or otalgia, nausea, and tachypnea. Upper res-

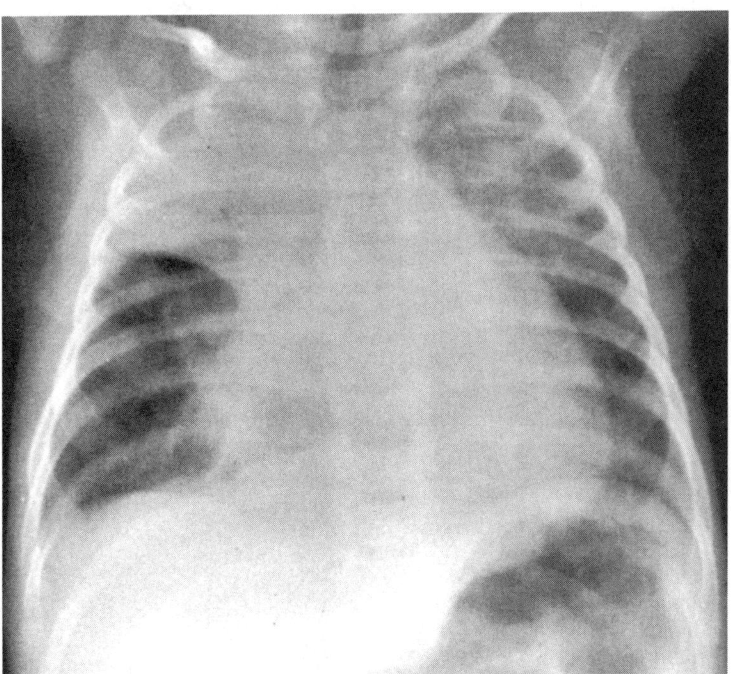

FIGURE 10 Chest radiograph of an infant with pneumonia due to PIV type 3. Right upper lobe atelectasis and multilobar infiltrates are evident.

TABLE 7 Clinical features of hMPV infection in children

Feature	Value in indicated reference[a]					
	52a	66a	178a	192	247	252
No. of hMPV-infected patients	50	53	26	19	49	118
Fever (%)	44	77	73	100	52	54
Rhinorrhea (%)	90	64	77	38	88	82
Cough (%)	90	68	92	90	90	66
Wheezing (%)	56	51	—	28	52	NA
Vomiting (%)	36	—	—	—	10	20
Diarrhea (%)	14	—	—	6	17	14
Rash (%)	—	—	—	12	4	3
Abnormal chest radiograph		56	85	68	50	NA
Bronchiolitis (%)	48	—	23	9	59	NA
Pneumonia (%)	34	—	23	38	8	NA
Croup (%)		—	—	—	18	NA
Asthma (%)		—	27	19	14	NA
AOM (%)		—	15	12	37	50

[a] —, not reported; NA, not applicable. References 52a, 66a, 178a, and 192 include only hospitalized children. Reference 247 includes only children with lower respiratory illness. Reference 252 includes only children with upper respiratory illness.

piratory tract disease may progress to lower respiratory tract disease over the next week or two, with the likelihood of disease progression probably related to the patient's underlying immune status. Risk factors for disease progression include lack of engraftment, decreased lymphocyte count, and older age at time of transplantation (184). Evidence of pulmonary infiltrates on chest radiograph may be delayed or absent for patients with severe neutropenia. Chest computed tomography or magnetic resonance imaging may be useful to document the extent of lower tract disease, although findings are frequently nonspecific. Over 1 or 2 weeks, lower respiratory tract involvement may become

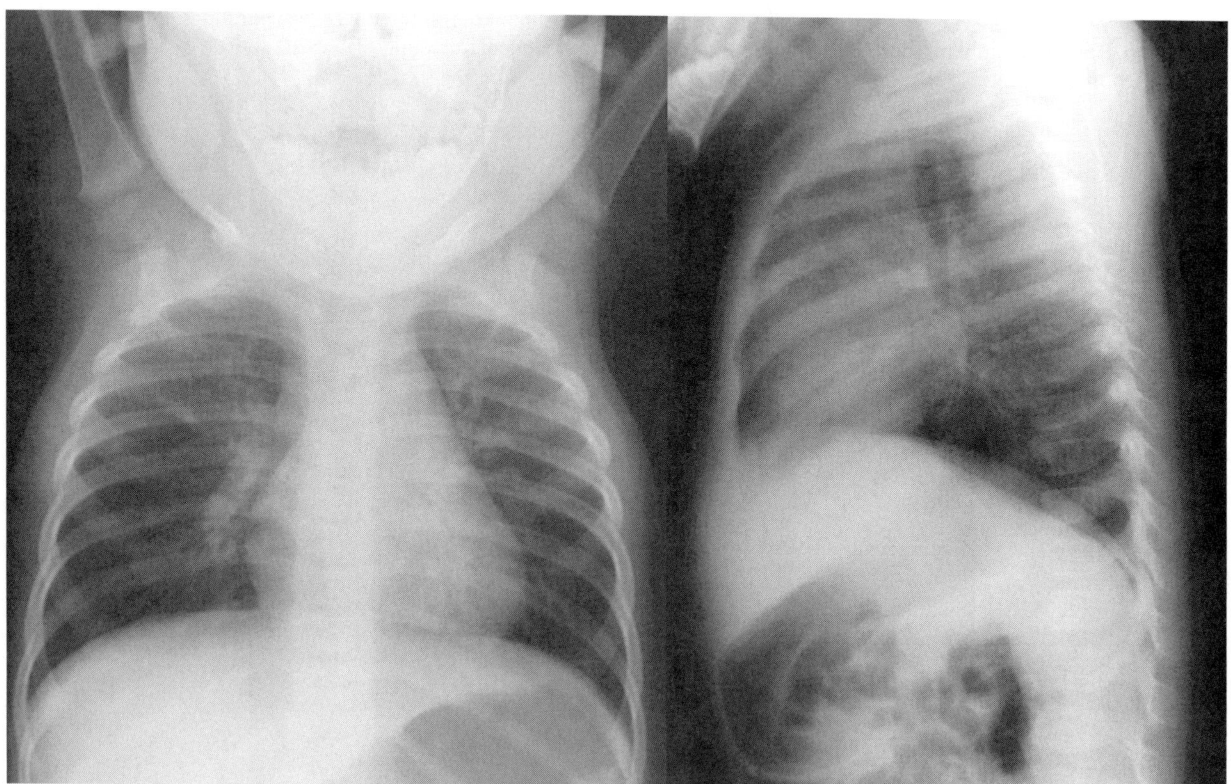

FIGURE 11 Chest radiographs of a 6-month-old infant with bronchiolitis due to hMPV. Peribronchial thickening and hyperinflation are evident.

evident as confirmed by increasing respiratory distress, worsening hypoxia, and, frequently, the need for assisted ventilation. Recovery following assisted ventilation for RSV pneumonia is possible but remains uncommon despite advances in life support.

Many immunocompromised adults with PIV infection first present with symptoms of mild upper respiratory tract disease, but in contrast to RSV, influenza virus, and hMPV infections, detection of PIV in asymptomatic HCT recipients is relatively common (191). In contrast to the case with RSV infection, less than half of PIV-infected patients have a fever. In severely immunocompromised patients, such as allogeneic HCT recipients less than 100 days post-transplantation, PIV infection may progress to lower respiratory tract disease (158). These patients generally have cough, tachypnea, hypoxia, and infiltrates on chest radiographs. Progressive pulmonary disease may require ventilatory support. Concomitant infections with other viruses or fungi or severe graft-versus-host disease is relatively common in adult patients with PIV pneumonitis (158, 183).

hMPV also causes severe infections in immunocompromised hosts. Fatal infection attributed to hMPV has been reported to occur in cancer patients, and hMPV may be a relatively common cause of acute respiratory infection in children and adults with malignancy and HCTs or organ transplants (27, 152, 248). Asymptomatic hMPV infection in HCT recipients was described in one study, but all other reports note severe disease due to hMPV in immunocompromised hosts. Further long-term prospective studies are needed to characterize fully the extent and severity of disease due to hMPV in immunocompromised hosts.

Complications

AOM is the most common complication of RSV and PIV infection (119). The virus infection causes dysfunction of the eustachian tube, resulting in negative pressure in the middle ear. Normal clearance mechanisms for bacteria that reside in the nasopharynx are disrupted, and purulent middle ear infection may result. Acute sinusitis may develop by the same pathogenetic process.

Bacterial pneumonia may complicate lower tract infections due to these viruses, although the risk following RSV infections is very low, as determined by studies of hospitalized children in the United States and Europe (73, 109). Superinfections with pneumococci and staphylococci are more common after PIV infections (139). Outbreaks of bacterial tracheitis have been reported in conjunction with PIV type 1 epidemics (56).

The relationship between the development of reactive-airway disease and RSV infections is intriguing (87, 222). Children with RSV bronchiolitis in infancy have a high risk of recurrent wheezing illness during the first decade of life. Longitudinal studies of pulmonary mechanics after RSV bronchiolitis have shown persistent abnormalities. The use of prophylaxis in infants with palivizumab, a monoclonal antibody to prevent RSV hospitalization, was recently associated with a lower incidence of physician-diagnosed asthma and recurrent wheezing in the subsequent 2 years of life (212). Additional intervention trials will be needed to clarify the causality of early virus infection and childhood asthma. RSV and PIV infections are associated frequently with exacerbations of reactive-airway disease in older children and adults, and prevention of these infections in this high-risk group could significantly reduce morbidity (89).

Clinical Diagnosis

The clinical presentation of an acute respiratory illness at the time of community outbreaks of RSV or PIV may allow a reasonable estimate of the viral etiology in young children. For instance, an infant with severe bronchiolitis accompanied by hypoxia who presents in midwinter during an RSV epidemic is likely to be infected with RSV, and similarly, a child with croup in the autumn is likely to have PIV type 1. Epidemiological and clinical features, including age, season, and clinical findings, are helpful in determining the etiology of disease, particularly during relatively discrete winter outbreaks. However, differentiating RSV from hMPV in an individual child with bronchiolitis is not possible, and conversely, wheezing is often unrelated to RSV or hMPV infection. Because clinical care in young children is generally supportive in nature, routine viral screening for all children with bronchiolitis is not currently recommended (6). The nonspecific manifestations of infection by these viruses in very young and older children and adults with underlying diseases such as immunodeficiency, or those who are hospitalized for respiratory symptoms, therefore require laboratory methods for etiologic diagnosis.

The differential diagnosis of croup due to PIV infection includes upper airway obstruction due to foreign bodies or bacterial epiglottitis, an entity less commonly seen since the decline of *Haemophilus influenzae* type b infections.

LABORATORY DIAGNOSIS

Sample Type and Handling

The diagnosis of respiratory viral infections is critically dependent on the type and quality of the clinical specimen and proper handling of the specimen prior to laboratory studies (107). Adequate clinical specimens are needed to avoid false-negative diagnoses. The preferred specimen type for the diagnosis of RSV, hMPV, and PIV in infants and young children is a nasal wash (99, 120) or aspirate (3). This specimen is obtained from the young infant by holding the infant upright or at a 45° angle, and, using either a bulb syringe or a soft plastic catheter attached to suction, instilling and rapidly withdrawing a small amount of normal saline (1 to 3 ml/nostril). The amount of RSV present in nasal wash specimens from young children is very high, ranging from 10^3 to 10^8 PFU/ml (63, 106), or 10^3 to 10^{11} genome copies/ml by RT-PCR (mean, 7.6 $\log_{10}$) (148).

An adequate clinical specimen can be verified by the identification of epithelial cells on microscopic examination of the fluid or examination of a cell pellet following centrifugation. In general, nasopharyngeal swabs are not as sensitive or reliable as nasal washes or aspirates for the diagnosis of RSV and PIV (99, 167). Specimens from adults are less sensitive than those from children due to decreased viral load. Other clinical specimens which have proven useful for the detection of RSV, PIV, and hMPV in patients of all ages include endotracheal aspirates collected from intubated patients (188), bronchoalveolar lavage fluid (60, 64), nasal mucosal epithelium collected by scraping, and lung tissue obtained by biopsy or at autopsy (60, 64, 244).

RSV is very labile and requires special handling (107, 188). Clinical specimens collected for culture should be transported on ice and inoculated onto sensitive cell culture lines quickly. Loss of infectivity occurs after 1 h at 37°C; complete loss of viability occurs with slow freezing at −20°C followed by thawing (20). Specimens should be inoculated into culture within 4 h of collection, and those that are not immediately processed should be flash frozen using alcohol and dry-ice baths (107). hMPV appears to be similarly labile, but PIVs are more stable and can be maintained in a viral transport medium for up to 5 days at 4°C (14). The recovery of PIV and RSV following freezing can be enhanced by the addition of sucrose or glycerol to the holding medium (111).

Virus Isolation

Heteroploid cell lines like HEp-2 or Vero cells are used in many laboratories for the culture of RSV, but other, less permissive cell types that may be used include human embryonic lung diploid fibroblasts, primary monkey kidney cells, and human amniotic or kidney cell lines. Mixed cell cultures, containing two or more cell lines, have also been utilized with or without centrifugation to enhance respiratory virus detection (182). Primary isolation of RSV in cell culture generally takes 3 to 5 days, although viral antigen may be detected in cellular cytoplasm within 10 h of inoculation (144). RSV is identified by a characteristic syncytial pattern formed by the infected cells (Fig. 12). The sensitivity of various cell lines for RSV must be monitored, however, because the ability of cells to form the characteristic syncytia associated with RSV may change over time (188).

For PIV isolation, primary monkey kidney cells and continuous monkey kidney cell lines like LLC-MK2, with trypsin added in the medium, are equally sensitive, although the latter is less expensive (75). Infection of cell lines with PIV is generally detected by hemadsorption, typically using guinea pig erythrocytes. Infection can generally be detected within 5 to 14 days, and hemadsorbing viruses can be characterized by hemadsorption inhibition, hemagglutination inhibition (HI), or immunofluorescence (IF) (176). PIV type 3 can produce a recognizable cytopathic effect in continuous cell lines, which can be adapted as an end point in neutralization assays (176), but cytopathic effect is generally not detected with other PIV types. PIV type 4 has an even more restricted host range in cell culture, growing mainly in LLC-MK2 cells without syncytium formation and typical cytopathic effect, except for the appearance of round cells that progress to destruction of cell monolayers (227).

The use of trypsin in addition to sensitive cell lines such as LLC-MK2 cells is required for the growth of hMPV in culture. In contrast to the rapid cytopathic effect induced by RSV, the cytopathic effect caused by hMPV consisting of cell rounding and syncytia (Fig. 13) generally is not seen for several weeks after inoculation, and it may not even be detectable until after blind passage.

Although cell culture continues to be valuable in detecting other viruses, providing isolates for subtyping or further analysis, and avoiding incorrect diagnosis, the use of virus isolation is decreasing due to its expense, its demands for technologist time, and the improved sensitivity of molecular detection methods.

Antigen Detection

Fluorescein-labeled antibody detection methods for RSV or PIV antigens have been reliably used to detect infection with RSV and PIVs for many years; adaptation of these methods to detect hMPV is now also possible. The rapid diagnosis of RSV and PIVs using direct or indirect IF

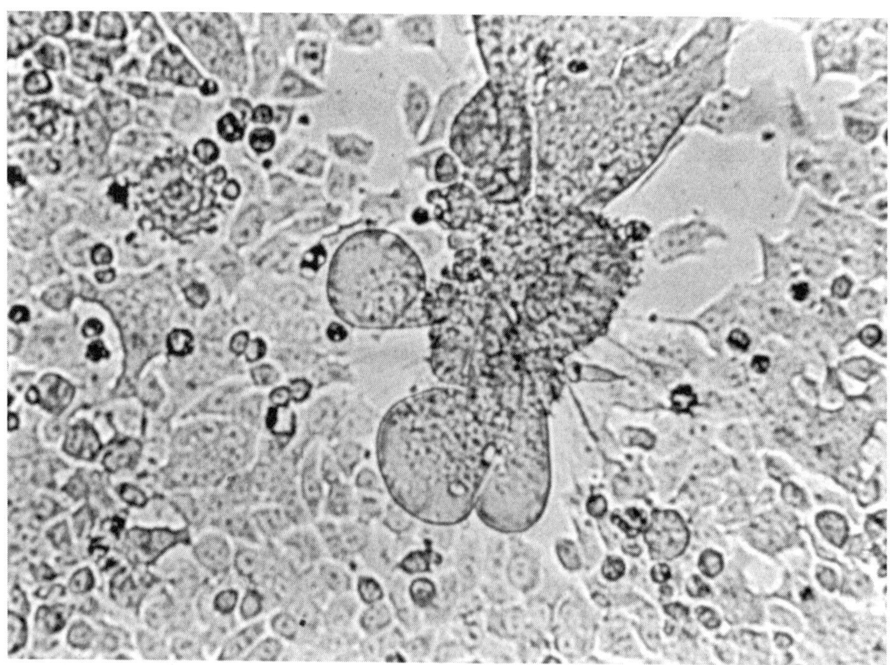

FIGURE 12 Cytopathic effect of RSV in cell culture on a continuous human epithelial cell line (HEp-2 cells) after 1 week of incubation. Large syncytial cells are evident, with ballooning and coalescence of RSV-infected cells.

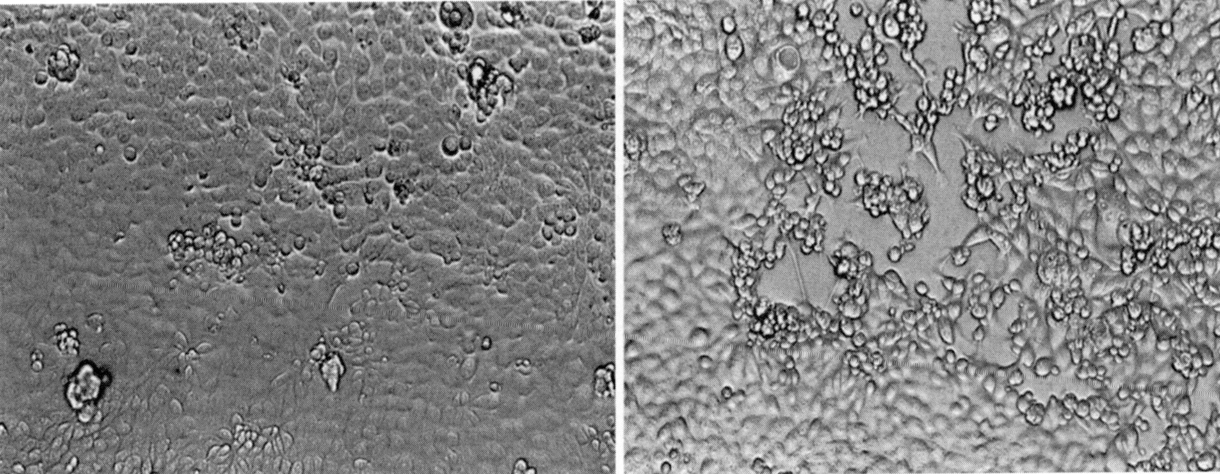

FIGURE 13 (Left) Cytopathic effect of hMPV in cell culture on a continuous monkey kidney epithelial cell line (LLC-MK2 cells) after 14 days of incubation. (Right) Rounding up and detachment of cells are evident, with developing syncytia.

methods has become more widely utilized with the advent of commercially available specific reagents (138, 141, 224). Advantages of IF methods include the direct examination of a clinical specimen for epithelial cells (permitting quality control for the submitted specimen), rapid results, low cost, and elimination of the need to test large numbers of specimens at one time. Of note, detection in any specimen by indirect IF is more sensitive than detection by antigen detection kits. The use of shell vials permits amplification of virus in the clinical specimen, increases the sensitivity of isolation, and permits earlier diagnosis than routine cell culture (165). The IF method depends on the experience of the laboratory technician with specialized equipment, and it may not be suitable for large-scale testing. Furthermore, incorrect or indeterminate results may occur with specimens with thick mucus or cellular debris or the use of nonspecific antibody reagents (165). There is no commercially available rapid antigen detection test for hMPV, although hMPV-specific monoclonal antibodies are now commercially available.

The availability of sensitive and specific enzyme-linked immunosorbent assay (ELISA) kits for the detection of RSV antigen in clinical specimens provides a rapid, reliable, and relatively inexpensive diagnostic test. Similar antigen detection tests are not available for PIVs or hMPV. Such RSV tests are widely utilized because of the demand by clinicians for rapid diagnosis. Currently available IF and ELISA reagents for RSV in pediatric specimens have sensitivities and specificities ranging from 80 to 95% (36, 53). Antigen detection tests with nasopharyngeal specimens obtained from adult patients have much lower sensitivity, most likely because of the substantially lower viral titer (often <100 PFU of RSV/ml in immunocompromised adults) (63).

In general, ELISA kits do not require expensive equipment or highly skilled personnel, take only 15 to 20 min from start to finish, are suitable for single specimens or batch testing of many specimens, and are inexpensive compared to cell culture. The cost per test, excluding technician time, averages less than $20. Although licensed for use with nasal wash specimens from pediatric patients, the tests have been demonstrated to be specific (although not always sensitive) with other secretions, including bronchoalveolar lavage or endotracheal tube aspirates. Disadvantages of rapid antigen test kits include absence of evaluation of the quality of the clinical sample and potential false positives when samples with blood or mucus are tested. Such kits, and particularly simplified kits which are waived by the Clinical Laboratory Improvement Amendments, have also been successfully used in clinics, at the bedside, and by nonlaboratory personnel (224).

Nucleic Acid Detection

Amplification methods to detect RSV or PIV genomes directly in respiratory secretions have not been widely used in the clinical setting due to the effectiveness of less expensive and more rapid antigen detection methods utilizing IF or ELISA. In the research setting, RT-PCR has been used for the subtyping of RSV (218) and for the identification of RSV in clinical specimens like respiratory secretions (189) or middle ear fluid (86). A more sensitive assay utilized in the analysis of genetic variability of RSV uses amplified cDNAs with secondary restriction fragment analysis (218).

By contrast, hMPV studies have relied on nucleic acid amplification techniques for detection. In general, reliable diagnosis of hMPV currently depends on molecular techniques based on standard or real-time RT-PCR assays. Several different RT-PCR methods appear to be quite sensitive, although they are labor-intensive and time-consuming (44, 148).

Use of multiple simultaneous PCRs in clinical samples may be useful when PIVs and RSV are cocirculating (72). Ribonuclease protection assays have been developed which permit the recognition of extensive variability in the RNA encoding the G glycoprotein region of RSV, resulting in a sensitive method to determine genomic diversity in outbreak settings (217). PCR sequencing assays have been applied to the molecular epidemiology of PIV infection by analyzing a portion of the PIV type 3 F protein gene (133).

Antibody Assays

Acute- and convalescent-phase sera are generally required for the serologic diagnosis of RSV or PIV. A fourfold increase in antibody after at least 2 weeks, and preferably 3 to 4 weeks, or the appearance of specific IgM antibody is required for serologic confirmation of infection. Antibody assays have been more useful in epidemiological studies and retrospective diagnosis due to the time interval before convalescent-phase sera can be collected. Furthermore, young infants may not generate a reliable response to RSV or may have antibody responses obscured by maternal antibody. Immunocompromised patients or older persons who have had repeated infections may not demonstrate rises in antibody titer (107).

Complement-fixing (CF) antibody titers for RSV and PIV are specific but lack sensitivity (36) and may therefore underestimate disease prevalence. Antibody to RSV may be more sensitively measured by ELISA, neutralization, indirect IF, and plaque reduction (with or without complement enhancement) assays (188, 198, 211). RSV antibodies measured by the microneutralization test correlate best with protection from RSV disease in an animal model (258). Other RSV antibody assays of investigational interest include ELISA detection of antibody to specific viral proteins (33), determination of specific anti-F-protein antibody (198), capture immunoassays using monoclonal antibodies (65), radioimmunoprecipitation assays (226), and Western blot analysis (195). Analysis by Western blotting permits the quantitative and qualitative measurement of the repertoire of various RSV antibodies to specific RSV proteins and can differentiate immune responses to natural infection from those obtained by immunization with a purified RSV protein (195).

Antibody to PIV in serum and respiratory secretions can be measured by CF, neutralization, or HI techniques (38, 176). The serologic tests have been adapted to microtiter methods, enabling serodiagnosis with small quantities of sera. As with RSV, the detection of CF antibodies may be insensitive in detecting infection. When only CF or HI antibodies to PIV are measured in clinical studies, careful interpretation of the results is required because heterologous cross-reactions are frequent among the paramyxovirus group, including mumps virus (176).

Serologic evidence of previous hMPV infection has been determined by measuring virus-neutralizing antibodies in plaque reduction assays (229) and by ELISA methods based on recombinant hMPV proteins (157).

PREVENTION

The international health impact and economic burden attributed to RSV, PIV, and hMPV contribute to the urgency of developing safe and effective vaccines against these pathogens (46, 185). Progress has been slow (57), in part because of the serious adverse experience observed with the use of the formalin-inactivated RSV (FI-RSV) vaccine in young children (140), the early failures with live attenuated virus vaccines, and the ineffective immune response elicited by primary RSV infection. The identification of serum neutralizing antibody as a correlate of protection against serious RSV infection has been an important advance in this field. New methods of increasing neutralizing activity in serum by active and passive immunization are being actively investigated, with the ultimate goal being the prevention of RSV and PIV morbidity in selected groups.

Management of Nosocomial Outbreaks

RSV and PIVs are common causes of nosocomial infections contributing to significant morbidity and mortality in pediatric wards (83, 108, 170). hMPV probably causes nosocomial outbreaks but is likely underrecognized due to lack of available diagnostic tests. Nosocomial RSV infections in adults with leukemia and bone marrow transplants are associated with a high mortality rate (114, 244). Nosocomial outbreaks characteristically occur from multiple introductions of community RSV strains (217). For prevention of nosocomial transmission, contact isolation precautions are effective as long as compliance with the policy is maintained among personnel (154). Patients known or suspected to be infected with RSV should be kept in contact isolation and isolated or cohorted until symptoms have resolved and repeated diagnostic tests for RSV are negative (32). A single negative viral culture following a positive one is insufficient to remove isolation precautions.

Hospital personnel commonly play a role in the transmission of RSV to susceptible patients. Hand washing before and after contact with a patient should limit the transmission of RSV, but hand washing is frequently neglected (54). The use of masks and goggles can decrease nosocomial infections in hospitalized children and medical personnel by preventing viral infection of personnel, who then transmit virus to susceptible children (1, 79). Strict compliance with glove and gown isolation precautions can also significantly reduce nosocomial RSV infections (80, 154). Such strict measures are appropriate in high-risk settings like pediatric intensive care units or bone marrow transplant settings. Restriction of visitors, and particularly young children, in hospital wards at high risk for RSV infection may be necessary during community epidemic periods. Continued compliance through the respiratory virus season by all members of the health care team is critical to any successful infection control policy. The Committee on Infectious Diseases of the American Academy of Pediatrics has provided guidelines for the prevention of nosocomial infections attributed to RSV and PIVs, as illustrated in Table 8 (5a).

Prophylaxis

Passive Immunoprophylaxis

Virus-specific neutralizing antibodies correlate with immunity against severe lower respiratory tract RSV infections. Protection against RSV replication occurs primarily in the lower respiratory tract, with only a limited reduction

TABLE 8 Control measures for the prevention of nosocomial RSV, PIV, and hMPV infections

Institute contact isolation precautions (strict adherence).
Pay strict attention to good hand washing and/or use of gloves.
Wear a gown to prevent exposure of clothing to contaminated secretions.
Screen subjects for RSV and PIV infections.
Cohort infected patients.
Exclude visitors with respiratory infections.
Prevent staff with respiratory illness from caring for susceptible patients.
Consider the use of eye-nose goggles when caring for subjects at high risk for severe viral infections.

in viral replication of the upper respiratory tract. Prophylactic monthly intravenous infusion of a human immune globulin pool enriched for RSV neutralizing antibodies (RSVIG) in high-risk children with prematurity, bronchopulmonary dysplasia, and congenital heart disease at a high dose (750 mg/kg of body weight) protected against lower respiratory tract RSV disease and hospitalization for RSV disease even though the number of RSV infections was not significantly reduced (94). The RSVIG product Respigam is no longer manufactured.

A chimeric human-mouse monoclonal antibody specific for the F protein of RSV, palivizumab (Synagis), has been approved for use in high-risk children since 1998. The administration of 15 mg of palivizumab per kg intramuscularly at 4-week intervals during the RSV season has been shown to be safe and effective in preventing serious RSV illness and hospitalization in preterm children, children with chronic lung disease, and children with hemodynamically significant heart disease (7, 125). The drug is supplied in single-dose vials containing 100 mg of lyophilized product. Motavizumab, the next-generation RSV F protein monoclonal antibody, has been demonstrated to be more effective than palivizumab in preventing medically attended lower respiratory tract illness and is undergoing clinical evaluation as of this writing (256).

Guidelines issued by the American Academy of Pediatrics recommend that prophylaxis with palivizumab be considered for infants and children younger than 2 years of age who have chronic lung disease that requires medical therapy within the 6 months prior to the anticipated start of the RSV season or who have hemodynamically significant heart disease (7). Infants born at 32 weeks of gestation or earlier who do not have chronic lung disease are also considered good candidates for palivizumab. Infants born at 28 weeks of gestation or earlier are recommended to receive prophylaxis during their first RSV season, whenever it occurs during their first 12 months of life. Infants born at 29 to 32 weeks of gestation are candidates for prophylaxis if they are 6 months of age or younger at the start of the RSV season. Palivizumab was efficacious and licensed for use in infants without lung disease who are born at 32 to 35 weeks of gestation, but because this group includes such a large number of infants and because of the high cost of palivizumab, palivizumab is recommended only if two or more risk factors for severe RSV disease are present. Risk factors may include child care attendance, school-age siblings, congenital abnormalities of the airways, severe neuromuscular disease, and environmental air pollutants. Exposure to tobacco smoke is considered a modifiable risk factor that can be controlled by the family, and thus it is not considered by the American Academy of Pediatrics as one of the risk factors for prophylaxis, although few parents are able to stop smoking during the period infants are most vulnerable to severe RSV disease. Passive immunoprophylaxis against PIV and hMPV infection has not been studied in children.

Active Immunization

In the 1960s, field studies were conducted with FI-RSV and PIV vaccines (40, 140). The FI-RSV vaccine was a crude RSV-monkey kidney cell harvest precipitated with a very high concentration of alum and concentrated 100-fold. The PIV vaccine was prepared similarly, although some lots were grown in embryonated eggs. In all four studies, some children, usually less than 2 years of age, who received the RSV vaccine experienced more severe respiratory disease on subsequent infection with RSV. Enhanced disease was not observed in the PIV vaccinees. RSV vaccinees had a nearly 8-fold-increased risk of pneumonia and a 16-fold-increased risk of hospitalization compared to the controls (140). The enhanced respiratory disease that was described to occur in children <2 years of age appeared to be similar to the naturally occurring disease in infants <6 months of age who are hospitalized with RSV bronchiolitis or pneumonia. Importantly, many young children who received the vaccine did not have an adverse outcome when infected with RSV, suggesting that variables other than the RSV vaccine may have been required for the development of vaccine-enhanced disease. The pathogenesis of vaccine-enhanced disease remains poorly defined. Advances in the development of new RSV vaccines have been hampered by the inability to identify the immune mechanism responsible for vaccine-enhanced disease.

Other RSV and PIV vaccines that have been developed and tested in animal or human models include animal-derived vaccines, adenovirus vector vaccines, subunit protein vaccines, live attenuated vaccine candidates derived from multiple passages selecting for temperature sensitivity, and genetic recombinant vaccines (Table 9). Purified F protein vaccines prepared from the F protein of RSV subgroup A (A2 strain) have been shown to be safe, immunogenic, and possibly protective against disease in RSV-seropositive children (187, 194, 196). This vaccine is undergoing evaluation in the elderly. Other candidate RSV protein vaccines, such as FG chimeric and BBG2Na vaccines, consisting of a conserved G protein fragment fused to the albumin binding domain of streptococcal G protein, have failed to progress in clinical studies. PIV type 3 subunit vaccines with proven efficacy in animal models have not been evaluated in clinical human trials for safety, immunogenicity, or efficacy (5).

Live attenuated vaccines could potentially circumvent the issues related to the enhanced disease of inactivated RSV vaccine and also take advantage of mucosal immunity. However, developing an attenuated, genetically stable, nontransmissible, and immunogenic live RSV vaccine for use in infants has proven difficult (57). Early attenuated cold-adapted temperature-sensitive phenotypes were found to require further attenuation by chemical mutagenesis (124, 200). Studies of genetically characterized live attenuated, temperature-sensitive RSV vaccines (134, 255) have been carried out with infants down to 2 months of age (134). None of the infants and young children who received the live attenuated RSV vaccines developed enhanced disease on subsequent exposure to RSV (254).

Inactivated and live attenuated PIV vaccines have been studied (Table 9). A live attenuated bovine PIV type 3 vaccine has been tested in infants, children, and adults (135, 136, 255) with good safety and immunogenicity. Evaluation of cold-adapted, live attenuated PIV type 3 vaccine in children has paralleled that of the live attenuated RSV vaccine (135, 255). The live attenuated bovine PIV type 3 vaccine is also being studied as a vaccine vector for the expression of the surface glycoproteins of human PIV and/or hMPV (110, 221).

Live attenuated hMPV vaccines are under development using reverse-genetics approaches. A recombinant chimeric bovine/human PIV vaccine that expressed hMPV F protein was immunogenic and protective against challenge

TABLE 9 RSV, PIV, and hMPV vaccine candidates

Virus	Type of vaccine	Population(s) evaluated	Result(s)	Reference(s)
RSV	Formalin inactivated	Young children	Enhanced disease	140
	Live attenuated: cpts-248/404 (cold passage, temperature sensitive) and recombinant live attenuated rA2cp248/404/1030 SH	Chimpanzees, adults, and seropositive and seronegative children	Immunogenic but insufficiently attenuated in young seronegative children	134, 254, 255
	Purified fusion protein vaccine (PFP-1, PFP-2, PFP-3)	Adults, children, children with cystic fibrosis, pregnant women, postpartum women	Immunogenic and safe in seropositive children and adults; passive transfer of antibody from immunized women to babies; no longer manufactured	187, 194, 196
	Polypeptides to G protein (BB2GNa)	Healthy young adults	Safe and immunogenic	199
PIV	Formalin inactivated	Young children	Safe, immunogenic, not effective	40
	Bovine origin PIV-3	Chimpanzees, adults, children	Safe, immunogenic, no longer being developed	135
	Cold-adapted, live attenuated	Chimpanzees, adults, young children, and infants	Safe in preliminary studies; no longer manufactured	132
	Chimeric virus—PIV type 3 backbone with PIV type 1 genes for HN and F proteins	Not evaluated in animals	No data	221
hMPV	Chimeric virus—hMPV F protein in bovine PIV type 3 backbone	Hamsters, cotton rats, and African green monkeys	Safe, immunogenic, and protective in animal models	47, 220

with hMPV in hamsters (220). Recombinant F protein subunit vaccines for hMPV have been demonstrated to be effective in rodents (47, 122).

Maternal Immunization

RSV-specific serum neutralizing antibodies are efficiently transferred from the mother to the newborn (52, 91). High levels of neutralizing antibodies acquired transplacentally by the neonate protect against lower respiratory tract disease during the first several months of life, but the decline of virus-specific immunity provided by maternal antibodies closely mirrors the half-life of IgG1, the principal IgG subclass antibody to RSV F and G glycoproteins that is transplacentally transferred in preterm and term neonates (52).

One strategy to protect infants younger than 6 months of age from RSV disease is to augment maternal antibody by administration of an RSV vaccine to the mother during pregnancy (59, 61). In studies of pregnant and postpartum women (58, 179), the purified F protein vaccine was nonreactogenic and immunogenic. Many of the postpartum women had ≥4-fold rises in their serum neutralizing antibody titers, and antibody levels in babies born to immunized women were higher than in control infants at birth and at 2 and 6 months of age. However, development of RSV F subunit vaccines has been suspended by pharmaceutical companies.

TREATMENT

Supportive Treatment

Previously healthy children and immunocompetent healthy adults who are infected with RSV generally require supportive treatment only. Antibiotic treatment is usually not necessary except as adjunct treatment for AOM or sinusitis (73, 109). The potential hypoxemia, apnea, and poor oral intake resulting from infection in young infants require close medical management, and hospitalization, generally for 1 to 3 days, may be required for children less than 1 year of age. Intravenous fluid replacement and oxygen therapy may be necessary. Secondary bacterial pneumonia is uncommon (109). Because the hypoxemia is related to unequal ventilation-to-perfusion ratios, infants will generally respond to inspired-oxygen concentrations of 40 or lower (107). Corticosteroid therapy is not effective in the treatment of acute RSV disease and does not benefit pulmonary function during convalescence in young infants (48, 156). Thus, systemic or inhaled steroids are not generally recommended for the treatment of RSV disease. In general, the use of systemic theophylline or other bronchodilators is not recommended. Bronchodilator therapy in younger infants appears to be less beneficial than in older children, and systemic bronchodilators like theophylline appear to carry more risk than nebulized ones. Because some children with lower respiratory tract disease may respond to aerosolized bronchodilators, a closely monitored trial of aerosol bronchodilator therapy, like salbutamol, may be warranted in infants over the age of 6 months (107). The prolonged or continuous use of these therapies in the very young infant can be potentially dangerous.

Supportive management in the care of lower respiratory tract disease due to RSV in the older child or high-risk adult may include oxygen therapy, close attention to fluid and electrolyte balance, and often aerosolized bronchodilators. In patients with underlying pulmonary or heart disease, recovery from the effects of RSV infection may take weeks to months.

Treatment of croup, the most common clinical presentation of PIV infection, generally consists of reassurance of the family and providing advice regarding the need for medical attention. Treatment of a crouping child in a mist tent has not been shown to be of benefit and is no longer recommended (25, 151). Systemic glucocorticoid therapy, including intramuscular dexamethasone, oral prednisolone, and nebulized budesonide (145, 223), is efficacious in mild to moderate and severe croup in the young child. The decision to use and the route of administration—oral, injected, or aerosolized—should be based on the clinical assessment of the child, ease of administration, cost, and duration of use. Epinephrine is used for symptomatic relief in patients with moderate to severe symptoms, but because the benefits of racemic epinephrine are short-lived, such patients must be observed carefully after therapy to be sure that their clinical condition does not deteriorate after the effects of epinephrine have diminished. Children with airway obstruction or signs of hypoxia require admission to an intensive care setting for close monitoring. They may benefit from treatment with intravenous dexamethasone; children with severe disease may require intubation. Antibiotic therapy is generally not beneficial except in cases of secondary bacterial infection, as suggested by persistent high fevers or purulent material noted at endotracheal intubation. Lower respiratory tract infections due to PIV in young children or immunocompromised hosts may require hospitalization and adjunct therapy, including intravenous fluids and oxygen support.

The majority of children infected with hMPV can be managed at home with supportive care. For infants and children who require hospitalization, therapy is supportive, including supplementary oxygen and intravenous hydration. Bronchodilators and corticosteroids have been used empirically, but there are no controlled trials of these medications for hMPV and no data to support or refute efficacy.

Management of Severe Disease

Infants with respiratory failure require mechanical ventilation and may require pressor support. Severe RSV disease in very young infants can result in life-threatening damage to the lungs and secondary end organ failure affecting the cardiac, renal, and hepatic systems. The use of other ventilatory support modalities, like high-frequency ventilation, mixtures of gases such as helium and oxygen or nitrous oxide, or extracorporeal membrane oxygenation (ECMO) to permit healing of the lung has been reported, with some success. Prolonged supportive therapy (for days to several weeks) with extracorporeal membrane oxygenation may be required for RSV infection (216).

Upper respiratory tract disease due to RSV in immunocompromised hosts (64) may progress to severe lower respiratory tract disease requiring ventilatory support. Underlying immunosuppression, high inspired-oxygen concentrations, and the accompanying barotrauma may result in pulmonary hemorrhage, adult respiratory distress syndrome, or both. The presence of pneumonia and associated respiratory failure in severely immunocompromised patients generally culminates in multiorgan system failure, with mortality rates in intubated patients approaching 80 to 90% (64, 114, 244). Supportive care in these immunocompromised patients includes fluid and nutritional support, as well as aggressive therapy for secondary fungal, bacterial, or viral infections. Antiviral therapy is frequently utilized (discussed below).

PIV infection with lower respiratory tract disease in immunosuppressed patients, particularly very young patients or those in the immediate posttransplantation period, may result in a similar clinical picture (12, 242), although the overall mortality rate does not appear to be as high as with RSV (230). Supportive and management measures are similar to those used for RSV disease.

Antiviral Treatment

Ribavirin, a synthetic guanosine nucleoside, has been licensed for the treatment of RSV respiratory disease in children since 1986 and for the treatment of RSV disease in mechanically ventilated patients since 1993. Ribavirin is the only approved drug for lower respiratory tract disease due to RSV (9), but concerns regarding efficacy in children, cost, and drug administration issues have resulted in minimal current use of the drug, except in immunocompromised patients (8). Ribavirin is administered by a small-particle aerosol from a solution containing the drug at a concentration of 20 mg/ml of sterile water via aerosol for 2 to 20 h per day. Aerosol administration results in high levels of ribavirin in the secretions, with levels exceeding 1,000 μM and little systemic absorption.

The therapeutic use of ribavirin in children infected with RSV remains controversial (30, 236). Potential benefits of ribavirin therapy include the inhibition of RSV-specific IgE production in nasal secretions, which has been associated with the development of wheezing and hypoxemia (206), and possibly improved pulmonary mechanics in ribavirin-treated infants (212). While studies have demonstrated efficacy in terms of decreasing clinical severity of disease and improvement in oxygenation (106, 169, 214), many are limited by the small numbers of patients studied, differences in enrollment criteria and clinical scoring systems, and type of placebo used. The 1996 American Academy of Pediatrics guidelines for ribavirin use state that "ribavirin treatment may be considered for the following patients hospitalized with RSV lower respiratory tract disease" (8), specifically for infants at high risk for severe or complicated RSV infection.

The duration of therapy in immunocompromised hosts with serious lower respiratory tract disease is generally longer than the 5 days utilized in immunocompetent children. Delayed antiviral treatment of RSV infections in markedly immunocompromised patients, like bone marrow transplant recipients who receive antiviral therapy only after the initiation of mechanical ventilation, is not generally successful (243). Initiation of antiviral therapy at the stage of upper respiratory tract disease may decrease viral load and possibly reduce the risk of respiratory failure (21,

85). Intermittent therapy utilizing higher drug concentrations (60 mg of ribavirin/ml of water) administered over 2 h three times daily to provide the same total amount of drug compared favorably with standard ribavirin therapy in one small clinical trial in children and in an uncontrolled trial in immunocompromised adults (85). This delivery method may improve patient access, improve compliance with therapy, and decrease environmental release of drug (62). A small randomized trial comparing short intermittent ribavirin in HCT patients with RSV upper respiratory tract disease demonstrated good tolerability and a trend of decreasing viral load over time compared to no treatment (21).

The potential environmental release of ribavirin has caused concern in hospital personnel because of the potential teratogenicity of ribavirin in the rodent model (28). Exposure is contraindicated in pregnant women because of its teratogenic potential. Ribavirin has been detected in the erythrocytes of some health care workers (115, 205). Administration of ribavirin via a ventilator, using a high-dose, short-duration method of drug delivery (62), or with a vacuum-exhausted treatment hood (26) results in minimal or no detectable ribavirin in the rooms of treated children.

Systemic immunotherapy (117), combined immunotherapy and ribavirin (96, 243), and aerosolized immunotherapy have been used for treating RSV disease. Standard intravenous immunoglobulin and RSVIG have not been found to be efficacious in the treatment of established RSV disease in hospitalized infants. High titers of RSV-specific antibody in different forms, including monoclonal humanized murine antibody and recombinant human monoclonal antibody Fab fragments, have been shown to be effective therapeutically when introduced directly into the lungs of RSV-infected mice (56) or cotton rats (258), leading to speculation that treatment of RSV disease could be carried out by antibody fractions administered by aerosol therapy. Controlled therapeutic trials with RSVIG and palivizumab have not shown clinical benefit in hospitalized infants. The combination of high-titer RSVIG and ribavirin has been associated with therapeutic success in uncontrolled studies in severely immunocompromised adults with RSV disease. Studies are now under way evaluating the treatment effects of higher-potency RSV monoclonal antibodies (motavizumab) in pediatric patients.

Other antiviral agents that have been evaluated include parenteral IFN-α (41). The side effects of interferon and the lack of clinical benefits make it unlikely that this therapy, as currently applied, will be utilized for the treatment of childhood RSV infections. Other promising antiviral compounds include novel fusion inhibitors, small RNA-inhibitory molecules, and high-titer monoclonal antibody preparations.

There is no licensed antiviral therapy for the treatment of PIV infections. Ribavirin has effects against PIV in cell culture and has been used for the treatment of lower respiratory tract disease in immunocompromised hosts (242). Case reports documenting decreased viral load and clinical improvement in three children with severe combined immunodeficiency following multiple treatments with aerosolized ribavirin therapy have been published (99). Ribavirin has also been utilized in bone marrow transplant recipients with upper and lower respiratory tract infection with PIV, without apparent benefit (183, 242). Intravenous ribavirin administered by intermittent dosing or constant infusion has been used in individual patients for the treatment of serious PIV infections (116). Controlled studies of ribavirin treatment of croup or other PIV infections have not been reported.

Antiviral therapy for the treatment of severe hMPV disease has not been studied in humans. One animal study suggested benefit with ribavirin and corticosteroid treatment of experimentally infected mice (112). Both ribavirin and polyclonal human immunoglobulin possessed in vitro virus-inhibiting activity against hMPV equivalent to their activity against RSV (257). There are no published animal or human data for these interventions.

REFERENCES

1. **Agah, R., J. D. Cherry, A. Garakian, and M. Chapin.** 1987. Respiratory syncytial virus (RSV) infection rate in personnel caring for children with RSV infections. Routine isolation procedure vs routine procedure supplemented by use of masks and goggles. *Am. J. Dis. Child.* **141:**695–697.
2. **Aherne, W., T. Bird, S. Court, P. S. Gardner, and J. McQuillin.** 1970. Pathological changes in virus infection of the lower respiratory tract in children. *J. Clin. Pathol.* **23:**7–18.
3. **Ahluwalia, G., J. Embree, P. McNicol, B. Law, and G. W. Hammond.** 1987. Comparison of nasopharyngeal aspirate and nasopharyngeal swab specimens for respiratory syncytial virus diagnosis by cell culture, indirect immunofluorescence assay, and enzyme-linked immunosorbent assay. *J. Clin. Microbiol.* **25:**763–767.
4. **Alvarez, R., K. S. Harrod, W. J. Shieh, S. Zaki, and R. A. Tripp.** 2004. Human metapneumovirus persists in BALB/c mice despite the presence of neutralizing antibodies. *J. Virol.* **78:**14003–14011.
5. **Ambrose, C., P. R. Wyde, M. Ewasyshyn, A. Bonneau, B. Caplan, H. Meyer, and M. Klein.** 1991. Evaluation of the immunogenicity and protective efficacy of a candidate parainfluenza virus type 3 subunit vaccine in cotton rats. *Vaccine* **9:**505–511.

5a. **American Academy of Pediatrics.** 1994. Parainfluenza virus infections, p. 341. *In* G. Peter (ed.), *Red Book: Report of the Committee on Infectious Diseases*. American Academy of Pediatrics, Elk Grove Village, IL.

6. **American Academy of Pediatrics.** 2006. Diagnosis and management of bronchiolitis. *Pediatrics* **118:**1774–1793.
7. **American Academy of Pediatrics Committee on Infectious Diseases.** 1998. Prevention of respiratory syncytial virus infections. *Pediatrics* **102:**1211–1216.
8. **American Academy of Pediatrics Committee on Infectious Diseases.** 1996. Reassessment of the indications for ribavirin therapy in respiratory syncytial virus infections. *Pediatrics* **97:**137.
9. **American Academy of Pediatrics Committee on Infectious Diseases.** 1993. Use of ribavirin in the treatment of respiratory syncytial virus infection. *Pediatrics* **92:**501.
10. **Anas, N., C. Boettrich, C. B. Hall, and J. G. Brooks.** 1982. The association of apnea and respiratory syncytial virus infection in infants. *J. Pediatr.* **101:**65–68.
11. **Anderson, L., C. Tsou, C. Potter, H. L. Keyserling, T. F. Smith, G. Ananaba, and C. R. Bangham.** 1994. Cytokine response to respiratory syncytial virus stimulation of human peripheral blood mononuclear cells. *J. Infect. Dis.* **170:**1201–1208.
12. **Apalsch, A. M., M. Green, J. Ledesma-Medina, B. Nour, and E. R. Wald.** 1995. Parainfluenza and influenza

virus infections in pediatric organ transplant recipients. *Clin. Infect. Dis.* **20:**394–399.

13. **Bangham, C. R., P. J. Openshaw, L. A. Ball, A. M. King, G. W. Wertz, and B. A. Askonas.** 1986. Human and murine cytotoxic T cells specific to respiratory syncytial virus recognize the viral nucleoprotein (N), but not the major glycoprotein (G), expressed by vaccinia virus recombinants. *J. Immunol.* **137:**3973–3977.
14. **Baxter, B. D., R. B. Couch, S. B. Greenberg, and J. A. Kasel.** 1977. Maintenance of viability and comparison of identification methods for influenza and other respiratory viruses of humans. *J. Clin. Microbiol.* **6:**19–22.
15. **Becker, S., H. Koren, and D. Henke.** 1993. Interleukin-8 expression in normal nasal epithelium and its modulation by infection with respiratory syncytial virus and cytokines tumor necrosis factor, interleukin-1 and interleukin-6. *Am. J. Respir. Cell Mol. Biol.* **8:**20–27.
16. **Becker, S., J. Quay, and J. Soukup.** 1991. Cytokine (tumor necrosis factor, IL-6 and IL-8) production by respiratory syncytial virus-infected human alveolar macrophages. *J. Immunol.* **147:**4307–4312.
17. **Beeler, J. A., and K. van Wyke Coelingh.** 1989. Neutralization epitopes of the F glycoprotein of respiratory syncytial virus: effect of mutation upon fusion function. *J. Virol.* **63:**2941–2950.
18. **Beem, M., F. H. Wright, D. Hamre, M. Clements, M. Wilson, S. Hall, and E. Tierny.** 1960. Association of the chimpanzee coryza agent with acute respiratory disease in children. *N. Engl. J. Med.* **263:**523.
19. **Bennett, B. L., R. P. Garofalo, S. G. Cron, Y. M. Hosakote, R. L. Atmar, C. G. Macias, and P. A. Piedra.** 2007. Immunopathogenesis of respiratory syncytial virus bronchiolitis. *J. Infect. Dis.* **195:**1532–1540.
20. **Berthaume, L., J. Poncas, and V. Pavilanis.** 1974. Comparative structure, morphogenesis, and biological characteristics of the respiratory syncytial (RS) and pneumonia virus of mice. *Arch. Gesamte Virusforsch.* **45:**39–51.
21. **Boeckh, M., J. Englund, Y. Li, C. Miller, A. Cross, H. Fernandez, J. Kuypers, H. Kim, J. Gnann, and R. Whitley.** 2007. Randomized controlled multicenter trial of aerosolized ribavirin for respiratory syncytial virus upper respiratory tract infection in hematopoietic cell transplant recipients. *Clin. Infect. Dis.* **44:**245–249.
22. **Bont, L., C. Heijnen, A. Kavelaars, W. van Aaldern, F. Brus, J. Draaisma, S. Geelen, and H. van Vught.** 1999. Peripheral blood cytokine responses and disease severity in respiratory syncytial virus bronchiolitis. *Eur. Respir. J.* **14:**144–149.
23. **Bont, L., A. Kavelaars, C. Heijnen, H. van Vught, and J. L. Kimpen.** 2000. Monocyte interleukin-12 production is inversely related to duration of respiratory failure in respiratory syncytial virus bronchiolitis. *J. Infect. Dis.* **181:**1772–1775.
24. **Bosis, S., S. Esposito, H. G. Niesters, P. Crovari, A. D. Osterhaus, and N. Principi.** 2005. Impact of human metapneumovirus in childhood: comparison with respiratory syncytial virus and influenza viruses. *J. Med. Virol.* **75:**101–104.
25. **Bourchier, D., K. P. Dawson, and D. M. Ferguson.** 1984. Humidification in viral croup: a controlled trial. *Aust. Paediatr.* **20:**289–291.
26. **Bradley, J.** 1990. Environmental exposure to ribavirin aerosol. *Pediatr. Infect. Dis. J.* **9:**595–598.
27. **Cane, P. A., B. G. van den Hoogen, S. Chakrabarti, C. D. Fegan, and A. D. Osterhaus.** 2003. Human metapneumovirus in a haematopoietic stem cell transplant recipient with fatal lower respiratory tract disease. *Bone Marrow Transplant.* **31:**309–310.
28. **Canonico, M., M. Kende, and J. W. Huggins.** 1984. Toxicology and pharmacology of ribavirin in experimental animals, p. 65. *In* R. Smith, V. Knight, and J. Smith (ed.), *Clinical Applications of Ribavirin*. Academic Press, New York, NY.
29. **Capasso, M., R. A. Avvisati, C. Piscopo, N. Laforgia, F. Raimondi, F. de Angelis, and A. Iolascon.** 2007. Cytokine gene polymorphisms in Italian preterm infants: association between interleukin-10 −1082 G/A polymorphism and respiratory distress syndrome. *Pediatr. Res.* **61:**313–317.
30. **Carmack, M., and C. G. Prober.** 1992. Respiratory syncytial virus and ribavirin quo vad. *Infect. Agents Dis.* **1:** 99–107.
31. **Cash, P., W. H. Wunner, and C. R. Pringle.** 1977. A comparison of the polypeptides of human and bovine respiratory syncytial viruses and murine pneumonia virus. *Virology* **82:**369–379.
32. **Centers for Disease Control and Prevention, Infectious Disease Society of America, and American Society of Blood and Marrow Transplantation.** 2000. Guidelines for preventing opportunistic infections among hematopoietic stem cell transplant recipients. *Morb. Mortal. Wkly. Rep. Recomm. Rep.* **49:**1–128, CE1–CE7.
33. **Cevenini, R., M. Donati, S. Bertini, A. Moroni, and V. Sambri.** 1986. Capture-ELISA for sera IgM antibody to respiratory syncytial virus. *J. Hyg. Camb.* **97:**5111.
34. **Chan, P. K., R. Y. Sung, K. S. Fung, M. Hui, K. W. Chik, F. A. Adeyemi-Doro, and A. F. Cheng.** 1999. Epidemiology of respiratory syncytial virus infection among paediatric patients in Hong Kong: seasonality and disease impact. *Epidemiol. Infect.* **123:**257–262.
35. **Chanock, R. M.** 1956. Association of a new type of cytopathogenic myxovirus with infantile croup. *J. Exp. Med.* **104:**555–576.
36. **Chanock, R. M., H. Kim, A. Vargosko, A. Deleva, K. M. Johnson, C. Cumming, and R. H. Parrott.** 1961. Respiratory syncytial virus: virus recovery and other observations during 1960 outbreak of bronchiolitis, pneumonia, and minor respiratory diseases in children. *JAMA* **176:**647–653.
37. **Chanock, R. M., R. H. Parrott, K. Cook, B. E. Andrews, J. A. Bella, T Reichelderfer, A. Z. Kapikian, F. M. Mastrota, and R. J. Huebner.** 1958. Newly recognized myxoviruses from children with respiratory disease. *N. Engl. J. Med.* **258:**207–213.
38. **Chanock, R. M., D. C. Wong, R. J. Huebner, and J. A. Bell.** 1960. Serologic response in individuals infected with parainfluenza viruses. *Am. J. Public Health* **50:**1858–1865.
39. **Cherrie, A. H., K. Anderson, G. W. Wertz, and P. J. M. Openshaw.** 1992. Human cytotoxic T cells stimulated by antigen on dendritic cells recognize the N, SH, F, M, 22K, and 1b proteins of respiratory syncytial virus. *J. Virol.* **66:** 2102–2110.
40. **Chin, J., R. L. Magoffin, L. A. Shearer, J. H. Schieble, and E. H. Lennette.** 1969. Field evaluation of a respiratory syncytial virus vaccine and a trivalent parainfluenzavirus vaccine in a pediatric population. *Am. J. Epidemiol.* **89:**449–463.
41. **Chipps, B., W. Sullivan, and J. Portnoy.** 1993. Alpha-2A-interferon for treatment of bronchiolitis caused by respiratory syncytial virus. *Pediatr. Infect. Dis. J.* **12:**653–658.

41a. **Collins, P. L., R. M. Chanock, and K. McIntosh.** 1996. Parainfluenza viruses, p. 1205. *In* B. N. Fields, D. M. Knipe, and P. M. Howley (ed.), *Fields Virology*, 3rd ed. Lippincott-Raven Publishers, Philadelphia, PA.

42. **Collins, P. L., K. McIntosh, and R. M. Chanock.** 1996. Respiratory syncytial virus, p. 1313. *In* B. N. Fields, D. M.

Knipe, and P. M. Howley (ed.), *Fields Virology*, 3rd ed. Lippincott-Raven Publishers, Philadelphia, PA.

43. **Cooney, M. K., J. P. Fox, and C. E. Hall.** 1975. The Seattle Virus Watch. VI. Observations of infections with an illness due to influenza, mumps and respiratory syncytial viruses and *Mycoplasma pneumoniae*. *Am. J. Epidemiol.* **101:**532–551.
44. **Cote, S., Y. Abed, and G. Boivin.** 2003. Comparative evaluation of real-time PCR assays for detection of the human metapneumovirus. *J. Clin. Microbiol.* **41:**3631–3635.
45. **Couch, R. B., J. A. Englund, and E. Whimbey.** 1997. Respiratory viral infections in immunocompetent and immunocompromised persons. *Am. J. Med.* **102:**2–9; discussion, 25–26.
46. **Crowe, J. E., Jr.** 1995. Current approaches to the development of vaccines against disease caused by respiratory syncytial virus (RSV) and parainfluenza virus (PIV). A meeting report of the WHO Programme for Vaccine Development. *Vaccine* **13:**415–521.
47. **Cseke, G., D. W. Wright, S. J. Tollefson, J. E. Johnson, J. E. Crowe, Jr., and J. V. Williams.** 2007. Human metapneumovirus fusion protein vaccines that are immunogenic and protective in cotton rats. *J. Virol.* **81:** 698–707.
48. **Dabbous, I. A., J. S. Tkachyk, and S. J. Stamm.** 1966. A double blind study on the effects of corticosteroids in the treatment of bronchiolitis. *Pediatrics* **37:**477–484.
49. **de Bree, G., J. Heidema, E. van Leeuwen, G. van Bleek, R. Jonkers, H. Jansen, R. van Lier, and T. Out.** 2005. Respiratory syncytial virus-specific CD8+ memory T cell responses in elderly persons. *J. Infect. Dis.* **191:**1710–1718.
50. **Denny, F. W., and W. A. Clyde, Jr.** 1986. Acute lower respiratory tract infections in nonhospitalized children. *J. Pediatr.* **108:**635–646.
51. **Denny, F. W., T. F. Murphy, W. A. Clyde, Jr., A. Collier, M. LaPoint, and F. W. Henderson.** 1983. Croup: an 11 year study in a pediatric practice. *Pediatrics* **71:**871–876.
52. **de Sierra, T. M., M. L. Kumar, T. E. Wasser, B. R. Murphy, and E. K. Subbarao.** 1993. Respiratory syncytial virus-specific immunoglobulins in preterm infants. *J. Pediatr.* **122:**787–791.

52a. **Dollner, H., K. Risnes, A. Radtke, and S. A. Nordbo.** 2004. An outbreak of human metapneumovirus infection in Norwegian children. *Pediatr. Infect. Dis. J.* **23:**436–440.

53. **Dominguez, E. A., L. H. Taber, and R. B. Couch.** 1993. Comparison of rapid diagnostic techniques for respiratory syncytial and influenza A virus respiratory infections in young children. *J. Clin. Microbiol.* **31:**2286–2290.
54. **Donowitz, L. G.** 1987. Handwashing technique in a pediatric intensive care unit. *Am. J. Dis. Child.* **141:**683.
55. **Downham, M. A. P. S., P. S. Gardner, J. McQuillin, and J. Ferris.** 1975. Role of respiratory viruses in childhood mortality. *Br. Med. J.* **1:**235–239.
56. **Edwards, K. M., C. Dundon, and W. A. Altemeier.** 1983. Bacterial tracheitis as a complication of croup. *Pediatr. Infect. Dis. J.* **2:**390–391.
57. **Englund, J.** 2005. In search of a vaccine for respiratory syncytial virus: the saga continues. *J. Infect. Dis.* **191:** 1036–1039.
58. **Englund, J., W. P. Glezen, and P. A. Piedra.** 1998. Maternal immunization against viral disease. *Vaccine* **16:** 1456–1463.
59. **Englund, J. A., and W. P. Glezen.** 1991. Maternal immunization for the prevention of infection in early infancy. *Semin. Pediatr. Infect. Dis.* **2:**225–231.
60. **Englund, J. A., M. Boeckh, J. Kuypers, W. G. Nichols, R. C. Hackman, R. A. Morrow, D. N. Fredricks, and L. Corey.** 2006. Brief communication: fatal human metapneumovirus infection in stem-cell transplant recipients. *Ann. Intern. Med.* **144:**344–349.
61. **Englund, J. A., I. N. Mbawuike, H. Hammill, M. C. Holleman, B. D. Baxter, and W. P. Glezen.** 1993. Maternal immunization with influenza or tetanus toxoid vaccine for passive antibody protection in young infants. *J. Infect. Dis.* **168:**647–656.
62. **Englund, J. A., P. A. Piedra, Y. M. Ahn, B. E. Gilbert, and P. Hiatt.** 1994. High-dose, short-duration ribavirin aerosol therapy compared with standard ribavirin therapy in children with suspected respiratory syncytial virus infection. *J. Pediatr.* **125:**635–641.
63. **Englund, J. A., P. A. Piedra, A. Jewell, K. Patel, B. B. Baxter, and E. Whimbey.** 1996. Rapid diagnosis of respiratory syncytial virus infections in immunocompromised adults. *J. Clin. Microbiol.* **34:**1649–1653.
64. **Englund, J. A., C. J. Sullivan, M. C. Jordan, L. P. Dehner, G. M. Vercellotti, and H. H. Balfour, Jr.** 1988. Respiratory syncytial virus infection in immunocompromised adults. *Ann. Intern. Med.* **109:**203–208.
65. **Erdman, D. D., and L. J. Anderson.** 1990. Monoclonal antibody-based capture enzyme immunoassays for specific immunoglobulin G (IgG), IgA, and IgM antibodies to respiratory syncytial virus. *J. Clin. Microbiol.* **28:**2744–2749.
66. **Ermers, M., B. Hoebee, H. Hodemaekers, T. Kimman, J. Kimpen, and L. Bont.** 2003. IL-13 genetic polymorphism identifies children with late wheezing after respiratory syncytial virus infection. *J. Allergy Clin. Immunol.* **119:**1086–1091.

66a. **Esper, F., R. A. Martinello, D. Boucher, C. Weibel, D. Ferguson, M. L. Landry, and J. S. Kahn.** 2004. A 1-year experience with human metapneumovirus in children aged <5 years. *J. Infect. Dis.* **189:**1388–1396.

67. **Falsey, A. R.** 2007. Respiratory syncytial virus infection in adults. *Semin. Respir. Crit. Care Med.* **28:**171–181.
68. **Falsey, A. R., C. Cunningham, W. Barker, R. Kouides, J. Yuen, M. E. Menegus, and L. Weiner.** 1995. Respiratory syncytial virus and influenza infections in the hospitalized elderly. *J. Infect. Dis.* **172:**389–394.
69. **Falsey, A. R., and E. E. Walsh.** 1992. Humoral immunity to respiratory syncytial virus infection in the elderly. *J. Med. Virol.* **36:**39–43.
70. **Falsey, A. R., and E. E. Walsh.** 2000. Respiratory syncytial virus infection in adults. *Clin. Microbiol. Rev.* **13:** 371–384.
71. **Falsey, A. R., and E. E. Walsh.** 2006. Viral pneumonia in older adults. *Clin. Infect. Dis.* **42:**518–524.
72. **Fan, J., K. J. Henrickson, and L. L. Savatski.** 1998. Rapid simultaneous diagnosis of infections with respiratory syncytial viruses A and B, influenza viruses A and B, and human parainfluenza virus types 1, 2, and 3 by multiplex quantitative reverse transcription-polymerase chain reaction-enzyme hybridization assay (Hexaplex). *Clin. Infect. Dis.* **26:**1397–1402.
73. **Field, C. M. B., J. H. Connolly, G. Murtagh, L. Weiner, C. Bonville, and R. F. Betts.** 1966. Antibiotic treatment of epidemic bronchiolitis—a double blind trial. *Br. Med. J.* **1:**83.
74. **Fishaut, M., D. Tubergen, and K. McIntosh.** 1980. Cellular response to respiratory viruses with particular reference to children with disorders of cell-mediated immunity. *J. Pediatr.* **96:**179–186.
75. **Frank, A. L., R. B. Couch, C. A. Griffis, and B. D. Baxter.** 1979. Comparison of different tissue cultures for

isolation and quantitation of influenza and parainfluenza viruses. *J. Clin. Microbiol.* **10:**32–36.

76. **Frank, A. L., L. H. Taber, C. R. Wells, J. M. Wells, W. P. Glezen, and A. Paredes.** 1981. Patterns of shedding of myxoviruses and paramyxoviruses in children. *J. Infect. Dis.* **144:**433.
77. **Frank, J. A., Jr., R. W. Warren, J. A. Tucker, J. Zeller, and C. M. Wilfert.** 1983. Disseminated parainfluenza infection in a child with severe combined immunodeficiency. *Am. J. Dis. Child.* **137:**1172–1174.
78. **Frank, A. L., and W. P. Glezen.** 1990. Respiratory tract infections in children in day care. *Semin. Pediatr. Infect. Dis.* **1:**234–244.
79. **Gala, C. L., C. B. Hall, K. C. Schnabel, P. H. Pincus, P. Blossom, S. W. Hildreth, R. F. Betts, and R. G. Douglas, Jr.** 1986. The use of eye-nose goggles to control nosocomial respiratory syncytial virus infection. *JAMA* **256:**2706–2708.
80. **Garcia, R., I. Raad, D. Abi-Said, G. Bodey, R. Champlin, J. Tarrand, L. A. Hill, J. Umphrey, J. Neumann, J. Englund, and E. Whimbey.** 1997. Nosocomial respiratory syncytial virus infections: prevention and control in bone marrow transplant patients. *Infect. Control Hosp. Epidemiol.* **18:**412–416.
81. **Garcia-Barreno, B., C. Palomo, C. Penas, T. Delgado, P. Perez-Brena, and J. A. Melero.** 1989. Marked differences in the antigenic structure of human respiratory syncytial virus F and G glycoproteins. *J. Virol.* **63:**925–932.
82. **Garcia-Garcia, M. L., C. Calvo, I. Casas, T. Bracamonte, A. Rellan, F. Gozalo, T. Tenorio, and P. Perez-Brena.** 2007. Human metapneumovirus bronchiolitis in infancy is an important risk factor for asthma at age 5. *Pediatr. Pulmonol.* **42:**458–464.
83. **Gardner, P. S., S. D. Court, J. T. Brocklebank, M. A. Downham, and D. Weightman.** 1973. Virus cross-infection in paediatric wards. *Br. Med. J.* **2:**571–575.
84. **Garofalo, R., J. L. Kimpen, R. C. Welliver, and P. L. Ogra.** 1992. Eosinophil degranulation in the respiratory tract during naturally acquired respiratory syncytial virus infection. *J. Pediatr.* **120:**28–32.
85. **Ghosh, S., R. E. Champlin, J. Englund, S. A. Giralt, K. Rolston, I. Raad, K. Jacobson, J. Neumann, C. Ippoliti, S. Mallik, and E. Whimbey.** 2000. Respiratory syncytial virus upper respiratory tract illnesses in adult blood and marrow transplant recipients: combination therapy with aerosolized ribavirin and intravenous immunoglobulin. *Bone Marrow Transplant.* **25:**751–755.
86. **Glezen, P., and F. W. Denny.** 1973. Epidemiology of acute lower respiratory disease in children. *N. Engl. J. Med.* **288:**498–505.
87. **Glezen, W. P.** 1984. Reactive airway disorders in children. Role of respiratory virus infections. *Clin. Chest Med.* **5:**635–643.
88. **Glezen, W. P., A. L. Frank, L. H. Taber, and J. A. Kasel.** 1984. Parainfluenza virus type 3: seasonality and risk of infection and reinfection in young children. *J. Infect. Dis.* **150:**851–857.
89. **Glezen, W. P., S. B. Greenberg, R. L. Atmar, P. A. Piedra, and R. B. Couch.** 2000. Impact of respiratory virus infections on persons with chronic underlying conditions. *JAMA* **283:**499–505.
90. **Glezen, W. P., F. A. Loda, and F. W. Denny.** 1997. Parainfluenza viruses, p. 551–567. *In* A. S. Evans and R. A. Kaslow (ed.), *Viral Infections in Humans*, vol. 3. Plenum Medical Books, New York, NY.
91. **Glezen, W. P., A. Paredes, J. E. Allison, L. H. Taber, and A. L. Frank.** 1981. Risk of respiratory syncytial virus infection for infants from low-income families in relationship to age, sex, ethnic group, and maternal antibody level. *J. Pediatr.* **98:**708–715.
92. **Glezen, W. P., L. H. Taber, A. L. Frank, and J. A. Kasel.** 1986. Risk of primary infection and reinfection with respiratory syncytial virus. *Am. J. Dis. Child.* **140:**543–546.
93. **Gray, G. C., A. W. Capuano, S. F. Setterquist, D. D. Erdman, N. D. Nobbs, Y. Abed, G. V. Doern, S. E. Starks, and G. Boivin.** 2006. Multi-year study of human metapneumovirus infection at a large US Midwestern Medical Referral Center. *J. Clin. Virol.* **37:**269–276.
94. **Groothuis, J. R., E. A. Simoes, M. J. Levin, C. B. Hall, C. E. Long, W. J. Rodriguez, J. Arrobio, H. C. Meissner, D. R. Fulton, R. C. Welliver, D. A. Tristram, G. R. Siber, G. A. Prince, M. Van Raden, and V. G. Hemming for The Respiratory Syncytial Virus Immune Globulin Study Group.** 1993. Prophylactic administration of respiratory syncytial virus immune globulin to high-risk infants and young children. *N. Engl. J. Med.* **329:**1524–1530.
95. **Gross, P. A., R. H. Green, and M. G. Curnen.** 1973. Persistent infection with parainfluenza type 3 virus in man. *Am. Rev. Respir. Dis.* **108:**894–898.
96. **Gruber, W. C., S. Z. Wilson, B. J. Throop, and P. R. Wyde.** 1987. Immunoglobulin administration and ribavirin therapy: efficacy in respiratory syncytial virus infection of the cotton rat. *Pediatr. Res.* **21:**270–274.
97. **Guerrero-Plata, A., A. Casola, G. Suarez, X. Yu, L. Spetch, M. E. Peeples, and R. P. Garofalo.** 2006. Differential response of dendritic cells to human metapneumovirus and respiratory syncytial virus. *Am. J. Respir. Cell Mol. Biol.* **34:**320–329.
98. **Hall, C. B.** 2007. The spread of influenza and other respiratory viruses: complexities and conjectures. *Clin. Infect. Dis.* **45:**353–359.
99. **Hall, C. B., and R. G. Douglas, Jr.** 1975. Clinically useful method for the isolation of respiratory syncytial virus. *J. Infect. Dis.* **131:**1–5.
100. **Hall, C. B., and R. G. Douglas, Jr.** 1981. Modes of transmission of respiratory syncytial virus. *J. Pediatr.* **99:**100–103.
101. **Hall, C. B., R. G. Douglas, Jr., and J. M. Geiman.** 1980. Possible transmission by fomites of respiratory syncytial virus. *J. Infect. Dis.* **141:**98–102.
102. **Hall, C. B., R. G. Douglas, Jr., and J. M. Geiman.** 1975. Quantitative shedding patterns of respiratory syncytial virus in infants. *J. Infect. Dis.* **132:**151–156.
103. **Hall, C. B., R. G. Douglas, Jr., K. C. Schnabel, and J. M. Geiman.** 1981. Infectivity of respiratory syncytial virus by various routes of inoculation. *Infect. Immun.* **33:**779–783.
104. **Hall, C. B., R. G. Douglas, Jr., R. L. Simons, and J. M. Geiman.** 1978. Interferon production in children with respiratory syncytial, influenza, and parainfluenza virus infections. *J. Pediatr.* **93:**28–32.
105. **Hall, C. B., J. M. Geiman, B. B. Breese, and R. G. Douglas, Jr.** 1977. Parainfluenza viral infections in children: correlation of shedding with clinical manifestations. *J. Pediatr.* **91:**194–198.
106. **Hall, C. B., J. McBride, D. M. Galagan, S. W. Hildreth, and K. C. Schnabel.** 1985. Ribavirin treatment of respiratory syncytial virus infection in infants with underlying cardiopulmonary disease. *JAMA* **254:**3047–3051.
107. **Hall, C. B., and C. A. McCarthy.** 2005. Respiratory syncytial virus, p. 2008–2026. *In* G. L. Mandell, J. E. Bennett, and R. Dolin (ed.), *Principles and Practice of Infectious Diseases*, 6th ed. Churchill Livingstone, Inc., New York, NY.

108. **Hall, C. B., K. R. Powell, N. E. MacDonald, C. L. Gala, M. E. Menegus, S. C. Suffin, and H. J. Cohen.** 1986. Respiratory syncytial viral infection in children with compromised immune function. *N. Engl. J. Med.* **315:**77–81.
109. **Hall, C. B., K. R. Powell, K. C. Schnabel, C. L. Gala, and P. H. Pincus.** 1988. Risk of secondary bacterial infection in infants hospitalized with respiratory syncytial viral infection. *J. Pediatr.* **113:**266–271.
110. **Haller, A. A., T. Miller, M. Mitiku, and K. Coelingh.** 2000. Expression of the surface glycoproteins of human parainfluenza virus type 3 by bovine parainfluenza virus type 3, a novel attenuated virus vaccine vector. *J. Virol.* **74:**11626–11635.
111. **Hambling, M. H.** 1964. Survival of the respiratory syncytial virus during storage under various conditions. *Br. J. Exp. Pathol.* **45:**647–655.
112. **Hamelin, M. E., G. A. Prince, and G. Boivin.** 2006. Effect of ribavirin and glucocorticoid treatment in a mouse model of human metapneumovirus infection. *Antimicrob. Agents Chemother.* **50:**774–777.
113. **Han, L. L., J. P. Alexander, and L. J. Anderson.** 1999. Respiratory syncytial virus pneumonia among the elderly: an assessment of disease burden. *J. Infect. Dis.* **179:**25–30.
114. **Harrington, R. D., T. M. Hooton, R. C. Hackman, G. A. Storch, B. Osborne, C. A. Gleaves, A. Benson, and J. D. Meyers.** 1992. An outbreak of respiratory syncytial virus in a bone marrow transplant center. *J. Infect. Dis.* **165:**987–993.
114a. **Harrison, A. M. C., C. A. Bonville, H. F. Rosenberg, and J. B. Domachowske.** 1999. Respiratory syncytial virus-induced chemokine expression in the lower airways: eosinophil recruitment and degranulation. *Am. J. Respir. Crit. Care Med.* **159:**1918–1924.
115. **Harrison, R., J. Bellows, and D. Rempel.** 1988. Assessing exposures of health care personnel to aerosols of ribavirin. *Morb. Mortal. Wkly. Rep.* **37:**560–563.
116. **Hayden, F. G., C. A. Sable, J. D. Connor, and J. Lane.** 1996. Intravenous ribavirin by constant infusion for serious influenza and parainfluenzavirus infection. *Antivir. Ther.* **1:**51–56.
117. **Hemming, V. G., W. Rodriguez, H. W. Kim, C. D. Brandt, R. H. Parrott, B. Burch, G. A. Prince, P. A. Baron, R. J. Fink, and G. Reaman.** 1987. Intravenous immunoglobulin treatment of respiratory syncytial virus infections in infants and young children. *Antimicrob. Agents Chemother.* **31:**1882–1886.
118. **Henderson, F. W., A. M. Collier, W. A. Clyde, Jr., and F. W. Denny.** 1979. Respiratory-syncytial-virus infections, reinfections and immunity. A prospective, longitudinal study in young children. *N. Engl. J. Med.* **300:** 530–534.
119. **Henderson, F. W., A. M. Collier, M. A. Sanyal, J. M. Watkins, D. L. Fairclough, W. A. Clyde, Jr., and F. W. Denny.** 1982. A longitudinal study of respiratory viruses and bacteria in the etiology of acute otitis media with effusion. *N. Engl. J. Med.* **306:**1377–1383.
120. **Henrickson, K.** 1995. Parainfluenza viruses, p. 1489–1496. *In* G. Mandell, R. Dolin, and J. E. Bennett (ed.), *Principles and Practice of Infectious Diseases,* 4th ed. Churchill Livingstone, New York, NY.
121. **Henrickson, K. J., and L. L. Savatski.** 1992. Genetic variation and evolution of human parainfluenza virus type 1 hemagglutinin neuraminidase: analysis of 12 clinical isolates. *J. Infect. Dis.* **166:**995–1005.
122. **Herfst, S., M. de Graaf, E. Scharauwen, N. Ulbrandt, A. Barnes, K. Senthil, A. Osterhaus, R. Fouchier, and B. van den Hoogen.** 2007. Immunization of Syrian golden hamsters with F subunit vaccine of human metapneumovirus induces protection against challenge with homologous or heterologous strains. *J. Gen. Virol.* **88:**2702–2709.
123. **Hertz, M. I., J. A. Englund, D. Snover, P. B. Bitterman, and P. B. McGlave.** 1989. Respiratory syncytial virus-induced acute lung injury in adult patients with bone marrow transplants: a clinical approach and review of the literature. *Medicine* (Baltimore) **68:**269–281.
124. **Hsu, K. H., J. E. Crowe, Jr., M. D. Lubeck, A. R. Davis, P. P. Hung, R. M. Chanock, and B. R. Murphy.** 1995. Isolation and characterization of a highly attenuated respiratory syncytial virus (RSV) vaccine candidate by mutagenesis of the incompletely attenuated RSV A2 ts-1 NG-1 mutant virus. *Vaccine* **13:**509–515.
125. **The IMpact-RSV Study Group.** 1998. Palivizumab, a humanized respiratory syncytial virus monoclonal antibody, reduces hospitalization from respiratory syncytial virus infection in high-risk infants. *Pediatrics* **102:**531–537.
126. **Isaacs, D., C. R. Bangham, and A. J. McMichael.** 1987. Cell-mediated cytotoxic response to respiratory syncytial virus in infants with bronchiolitis. *Lancet* **ii:**769–771.
127. **Janssen, R., L. Bont, C. L. Siezen, H. M. Hodemaekers, M. J. Ermers, G. Doornbos, R. van't Slot, C. Wijmenga, J. J. Goeman, J. L. Kimpen, H. C. van Houwelingen, T. G. Kimman, and B. Hoebee.** 2007. Genetic susceptibility to respiratory syncytial virus bronchiolitis is predominantly associated with innate immune genes. *J. Infect. Dis.* **196:**826–834.
128. **Jartti, T., B. van den Hoogen, R. P. Garofalo, A. D. Osterhaus, and O. Ruuskanen.** 2002. Metapneumovirus and acute wheezing in children. *Lancet* **360:**1393–1394.
129. **Jarvis, W. R., P. J. Middleton, and E. W. Gelfand.** 1979. Parainfluenza pneumonia in severe combined immunodeficiency disease. *J. Pediatr.* **94:**423–425.
130. **Josephs, S., H. W. Kim, C. D. Brandt, and R. H. Parrott.** 1988. Parainfluenza 3 virus and other common respiratory pathogens in children with human immunodeficiency virus infection. *Pediatr. Infect. Dis. J.* **7:** 207–209.
131. **Kapikian, A. Z., R. M. Chanock, T. E. Reichelderfer, T. G. Ward, R. J. Huebner, and J. A. Bell.** 1961. Inoculation of human volunteers with parainfluenza virus type 3. *JAMA* **178:**537.
132. **Karron, R. A., R. B. Belshe, P. F. Wright, B. Thumar, B. Burns, F. Newman, J. C. Cannon, J. Thompson, T. Tsai, M. Paschalis, S. L. Wu, Y. Mitcho, J. Hackell, B. R. Murphy, and J. M. Tatem.** 2003. A live human parainfluenza type 3 virus vaccine is attenuated and immunogenic in young infants. *Pediatr. Infect. Dis. J.* **22:** 394–405.
133. **Karron, R. A., K. L. O'Brien, J. L. Froehlich, and V. A. Brown.** 1993. Molecular epidemiology of a parainfluenza type 3 virus outbreak on a pediatric ward. *J. Infect. Dis.* **167:**1441–1445.
134. **Karron, R. A., P. F. Wright, R. B. Belshe, B. Thumar, R. Casey, F. Newman, F. P. Polack, V. B. Randolph, A. Deatly, J. Hackell, W. Gruber, B. R. Murphy, and P. L. Collins.** 2005. Identification of a recombinant live attenuated respiratory syncytial virus vaccine candidate that is highly attenuated in infants. *J. Infect. Dis.* **191:** 1093–1104.
135. **Karron, R. A., P. F. Wright, S. L. Hall, M. Makhene, J. Thompson, B. A. Burns, S. Tollefson, M. C. Steinhoff, M. H. Wilson, and D. O. Harris.** 1995. A live attenuated bovine parainfluenza virus type 3 vaccine is safe, infectious, immunogenic, and phenotypically stable in infants and children. *J. Infect. Dis.* **171:**1107–1114.

136. **Karron, R. A., P. F. Wright, F. K. Newman, M. Makhene, J. Thompson, R. Samorodin, M. H. Wilson, E. L. Anderson, M. L. Clements, and B. R. Murphy.** 1995. A live human parainfluenza type 3 virus vaccine is attenuated and immunogenic in healthy infants and children. *J. Infect. Dis.* **172:**1445–1450.
137. **Kasel, J. A., E. E. Walsh, A. L. Frank, B. D. Baxter, L. H. Taber, and W. P. Glezen.** 1987. Relation of serum antibody to glycoproteins of respiratory syncytial virus with immunity to infection in children. *Viral Immunol.* **1:**199–205.
138. **Kellogg, J. A.** 1991. Culture vs direct antigen assays for detection of microbial pathogens from lower respiratory tract specimens suspected of containing the respiratory syncytial virus. *Arch. Pathol. Lab. Med.* **115:**451–458.
139. **Khamapirad, T., and W. P. Glezen.** 1987. Clinical and radiographic assessment of acute lower respiratory tract disease in infants and children. *Semin. Respir. Infect.* **2:** 130–144.
140. **Kim, H. W., J. G. Canchola, C. D. Brandt, G. Pyles, R. M. Chanock, K. Jensen, and R. H. Parrott.** 1969. Respiratory syncytial virus disease in infants despite prior administration of antigenic inactivated vaccine. *Am. J. Epidemiol.* **89:**422–434.
141. **Kim, H. W., R. G. Wyatt, B. F. Fernie, C. D. Brandt, J. O. Arrobio, B. C. Jeffries, and R. H. Parrott.** 1983. Respiratory syncytial virus detection by immunofluorescence in nasal secretions with monoclonal antibodies against selected surface and internal proteins. *J. Clin. Microbiol.* **18:**1399–1404.
142. **Kim, Y. J., M. Boeckh, and J. A. Englund.** 2007. Community respiratory virus infections in immunocompromised patients: hematopoietic stem cell and solid organ transplant recipients, and individuals with human immunodeficiency virus infection. *Semin. Respir. Crit. Care Med.* **28:**222–242.
143. **King, J. C., Jr., A. R. Burke, J. D. Clemens, P. Nair, J. J. Farley, P. E. Vink, S. R. Batlas, M. Rao, and J. P. Johnson.** 1993. Respiratory syncytial virus illnesses in human immunodeficiency virus- and noninfected children. *Pediatr. Infect. Dis. J.* **12:**733–739.
144. **Kisch, A. L., K. M. Johnson, and R. M. Chanock.** 1962. Immunofluorescence with respiratory syncytial virus. *Virology* **16:**177–189.
145. **Klassen, T. P., M. E. Feldman, L. K. Watters, T. Sutcliffe, and P. C. Rowe.** 1994. Nebulized budesonide for children with mild-to-moderate croup. *N. Engl. J. Med.* **331:**285–289.
146. **Kuiken, T., B. G. van den Hoogen, D. A. van Riel, J. D. Laman, G. van Amerongen, L. Sprong, R. A. Fouchier, and A. D. Osterhaus.** 2004. Experimental human metapneumovirus infection of cynomolgus macaques (Macaca fascicularis) results in virus replication in ciliated epithelial cells and pneumocytes with associated lesions throughout the respiratory tract. *Am. J. Pathol.* **164:**1893–1900.
147. **Kurlandsky, L. E., G. French, P. M. Webb, and D. D. Porter.** 1988. Fatal respiratory syncytial virus pneumonitis in a previously healthy child. *Am. Rev. Respir. Dis.* **138:**468–472.
148. **Kuypers, J., N. Wright, J. Ferrenberg, M. L. Huang, A. Cent, L. Corey, and R. Morrow.** 2006. Comparison of real-time PCR assays with fluorescent-antibody assays for diagnosis of respiratory virus infections in children. *J. Clin. Microbiol.* **44:**2382–2388.
149. **Laham, F. R., V. Israele, J. M. Casellas, A. M. Garcia, C. M. Lac Prugent, S. J. Hoffman, D. Hauer, B. Thumar, M. I. Name, A. Pascual, N. Taratutto, M. T. Ishida, M. Balduzzi, M. Maccarone, S. Jackli, R. Passarino, R. A. Gaivironsky, R. A. Karron, N. R. Polack, and F. P. Polack.** 2004. Differential production of inflammatory cytokines in primary infection with human metapneumovirus and with other common respiratory viruses of infancy. *J. Infect. Dis.* **189:**2047–2056.
150. **Lamb, R. A., and D. Kolakofsky.** 1996. Paramyxoviridae and their replication, p. 1177. *In* B. N. Fields, D. M. Knipe, and P. M. Howley (ed.), *Fields Virology*, 3rd ed. Lippincott-Raven Publishers, Philadelphia, PA.
151. **Landau, L. I., and G. C. Geelhoed.** 1994. Aerosolized steroids for croup. *N. Engl. J. Med.* **331:**322–323.
152. **Larcher, C., C. Geltner, H. Fischer, D. Nachbaur, L. C. Muller, and H. P. Huemer.** 2005. Human metapneumovirus infection in lung transplant recipients: clinical presentation and epidemiology. *J. Heart Lung Transplant.* **24:**1891–1901.
153. **Lau, S. K. P., W.-K. To, P. W. T. Tse, A. K. H. Chan, P. C. Y. Woo, H.-W. Tsoi, A. F. Y. Leung, K. S. M. Li, P. K. S. Chan, W. W. L. Lim, R. W. H. Yung, K.-H. Chan, and K.-Y. Yuen.** 2005. Human parainfluenza virus 4 outbreak and the role of diagnostic tests. *J. Clin. Microbiol.* **43:**4515–4521.
154. **Leclair, J. M., J. Freeman, B. F. Sullivan, C. M. Crowley, and D. A. Goldmann.** 1987. Prevention of nosocomial respiratory syncytial virus infections through compliance with glove and gown isolation precautions. *N. Engl. J. Med.* **317:**329–334.
155. **Lee, N., P. K. Chan, I. T. Yu, K. K. Tsoi, G. Lui, J. J. Sung, and C. S. Cockram.** 2007. Co-circulation of human metapneumovirus and SARS-associated coronavirus during a major nosocomial SARS outbreak in Hong Kong. *J. Clin. Virol.* **40:**333–337.
156. **Leer, J. A., Jr., J. L. Green, E. M. Heimlich, J. S. Hyde, H. L. Moffet, G. A. Young, and B. A. Barron.** 1969. Corticosteroid treatment in bronchiolitis. A controlled, collaborative study in 297 infants and children. *Am. J. Dis. Child.* **117:**495–503.
157. **Leung, J., F. Esper, C. Weibel, and J. S. Kahn.** 2005. Seroepidemiology of human metapneumovirus (hMPV) on the basis of a novel enzyme-linked immunosorbent assay utilizing hMPV fusion protein expressed in recombinant vesicular stomatitis virus. *J. Clin. Microbiol.* **43:** 1213–1219.
158. **Lewis, V. A., R. Champlin, J. Englund, R. Couch, J. M. Goodrich, K. Rolston, D. Przepiorka, N. Q. Mirza, H. M. Yousuf, M. Luna, G. P. Bodey, and E. Whimbey.** 1996. Respiratory disease due to parainfluenza virus in adult bone marrow transplant recipients. *Clin. Infect. Dis.* **23:**1033–1037.
159. **Lilic, D., A. J. Cant, M. Abinun, J. E. Calvert, and G. P. Spickett.** 1997. Cytokine production differs in children and adults. *Pediatr. Res.* **42:**237–240.
160. **Louie, J. K., D. P. Schnurr, C. Y. Pan, D. Kiang, C. Carter, S. Tougaw, J. Ventura, A. Norman, V. Belmusto, J. Rosenberg, and G. Trochet.** 2007. A summer outbreak of human metapneumovirus infection in a long-term-care facility. *J. Infect. Dis.* **196:**705–708.
161. **Mackay, I. M., S. Bialasiewicz, Z. Waliuzzaman, G. R. Chidlow, D. C. Fegredo, S. Laingam, P. Adamson, G. B. Harnett, W. Rawlinson, M. D. Nissen, and T. P. Sloots.** 2004. Use of the P gene to genotype human metapneumovirus identifies 4 viral subtypes. *J. Infect. Dis.* **190:**1913–1918.
162. **Madhi, S. A., H. Ludewick, Y. Abed, K. P. Klugman, and G. Boivin.** 2003. Human metapneumovirus-associated lower respiratory tract infections among hospitalized human immunodeficiency virus type 1 (HIV-1)-infected and HIV-1-uninfected African infants. *Clin. Infect. Dis.* **37:**1705–1710.

163. **Madhi, S. A., H. Ludewick, L. Kuwanda, N. van Niekerk, C. Cutland, and K. P. Klugman.** 2007. Seasonality, incidence, and repeat human metapneumovirus lower respiratory tract infections in an area with a high prevalence of human immunodeficiency virus type-1 infection. *Pediatr. Infect. Dis. J.* **26:**693–699.
164. **Matsuda, K., H. Tsutsumi, Y. Okamoto, and C. Chiba.** 1995. Development of interleukin 6 and tumor necrosis factor alpha activity in nasopharyngeal secretions of infants and children during infection with respiratory syncytial virus. *Clin. Diagn. Lab. Immunol.* **2:**322–324.
165. **Matthey, S., D. Nicholson, S. Ruhs, B. Alden, M. Knock, K. Schultz, and A. Schmuecker.** 1992. Rapid detection of respiratory viruses by shell vial culture and direct staining by using pooled and individual monoclonal antibodies. *J. Clin. Microbiol.* **30:**540–544.
166. **Mbawuike, I. N., K. Fujihashi, S. DiFabio, S. Kawabata, J. R. McGhee, R. B. Couch, and H. Kiyono.** 1999. Human interleukin-12 enhances interferon-gamma-producing influenza-specific memory CD8+ cytotoxic T lymphocytes. *J. Infect. Dis.* **180:**1477–1486.
167. **McIntosh, K., R. M. Hendry, M. L. Fahnestock, and L. T. Pierik.** 1982. Enzyme-linked immunosorbent assay for detection of respiratory syncytial virus infection: application to clinical samples. *J. Clin. Microbiol.* **16:**329–333.
168. **McIntosh, K., H. B. Masters, I. Orr, R. K. Chao, and R. M. Barkin.** 1978. The immunologic response to infection with respiratory syncytial virus in infants. *J. Infect. Dis.* **138:**24–32.
169. **Meert, K. L., A. P. Sarnaik, M. J. Gelmini, and M. W. Lieh-Lai.** 1994. Aerosolized ribavirin in mechanically ventilated children with respiratory syncytial virus lower respiratory tract disease: a prospective, double-blind, randomized trial. *Crit. Care Med.* **22:**566–572.
170. **Meissner, H. C., S. A. Murray, M. A. Kiernan, D. R. Snydman, and K. McIntosh.** 1984. A simultaneous outbreak of respiratory syncytial virus and parainfluenza virus type 3 in a newborn nursery. *J. Pediatr.* **104:**680–684.
171. **Merrill, W. W., G. P. Naegel, J. J. Olchowski, and H. Y. Reynolds.** 1985. Immunoglobulin G subclass proteins in serum and lavage fluid of normal subjects. Quantitation and comparison with immunoglobulins A and E. *Am. Rev. Respir. Dis.* **131:**584–587.
172. **Meurman, O., M. Waris, and K. Hedman.** 1992. Immunoglobulin G antibody avidity in patients with respiratory syncytial virus infection. *J. Clin. Microbiol.* **30:** 1479–1484.
173. **Miller, W. S., and M. S. Artenstein.** 1967. Aerosol stability of three acute respiratory disease viruses. *Proc. Soc. Exp. Biol. Med.* **125:**222–227.
174. **Morris, J. A., R. E. Blount, Jr., and R. E. Savage.** 1956. Recovery of cytopathogenic agent from chimpanzees with coryza. *Proc. Soc. Exp. Biol. Med.* **92:**544–549.
175. **Muelenaer, P. M., F. W. Henderson, V. G. Hemming, E. E. Walsh, L. J. Anderson, G. A. Prince, and B. R. Murphy.** 1991. Group-specific serum antibody responses in children with primary and recurrent respiratory syncytial virus infections. *J. Infect. Dis.* **164:**15–21.
176. **Mufson, M. A.** 1989. Parainfluenza viruses, mumps virus, and New Castle disease virus, p. 669. *In* E. Lennette and N. J. Schmitt (ed.), *Diagnostic Procedures for Viral, Rickettsial and Chlamydial Infections*, 6th ed. American Public Health Association, Washington, DC.
177. **Mufson, M. A., C. Orvell, B. Rafnar, and E. Norrby.** 1985. Two distinct subtypes of human respiratory syncytial virus. *J. Gen. Virol.* **66**(Pt. 10)**:**2111–2124.
178. **Mulholland, K.** 2007. Childhood pneumonia mortality—a permanent global emergency. *Lancet* **370:**285–289.
178a. **Mullins, J. A., D. D. Erdman, G. A. Weinberg, K. Edwards, C. B. Hall, F. J. Walker, M. Iwane, and L. J. Anderson.** 2004. Human metapneumovirus infection among children hospitalized with acute respiratory illness. *Emerg. Infect. Dis.* **10:**700–705.
179. **Munoz, F. M., P. A. Piedra, and W. P. Glezen.** 2003. Safety and immunogenicity of respiratory syncytial virus purified fusion protein-2 vaccine in pregnant women. *Vaccine* **21:**3465–3467.
180. **Murphy, B. R., D. W. Alling, M. H. Snyder, E. E. Walsh, G. A. Prince, R. M. Chanock, V. G. Hemming, W. J. Rodriguez, H. W. Kim, and B. S. Graham.** 1986. Effect of age and preexisting antibody on serum antibody response of infants and children to the F and G glycoproteins during respiratory syncytial virus infection. *J. Clin. Microbiol.* **24:**894–898.
181. **Murphy, B. R., B. S. Graham, G. A. Prince, E. E. Walsh, R. M. Chanock, D. T. Karzon, and P. F. Wright.** 1986. Serum and nasal-wash immunoglobulin G and A antibody response of infants and children to respiratory syncytial virus F and G glycoproteins following primary infection. *J. Clin. Microbiol.* **23:**1009–1014.
182. **Navarro-Marí, J. M., S. Sanbonmatsu-Gámez, M. Pérez-Ruiz, and M. De La Rosa-Fraile.** 1999. Rapid detection of respiratory viruses by shell vial assay using simultaneous culture of HEp-2, LLC-MK2, and MDCK cells in a single vial. *J. Clin. Microbiol.* **37:**2346–2347.
183. **Nichols, W. G., L. Corey, T. Gooley, C. Davis, and M. Boeckh.** 2001. Parainfluenza virus infections after hematopoietic stem cell transplantation: risk factors, response to antiviral therapy, and effect on transplant outcome. *Blood* **98:**573–578.
184. **Nichols, W. G., T. Gooley, and M. Boeckh.** 2001. Community-acquired respiratory syncytial virus and parainfluenza virus infections after hematopoietic stem cell transplantation: the Fred Hutchinson Cancer Research Center experience. *Biol. Blood Marrow Transplant.* **7**(Suppl.)**:**11S–15S.
185. **Nokes, D. J., E. A. Okiro, M. Ngama, R. Ochola, L. J. White, P. D. Scott, M. English, P. A. Cane, and G. F. Medley.** 2008. Respiratory syncytial virus infection and disease in infants and young children observed from birth in Kilifi District, Kenya. *Clin. Infect. Dis.* **46:**50–57.
186. **Okamoto, Y., K. Kudo, K. Shirotori, M. Nakazawa, E. Ito, K. Togawa, J. A. Patel, and P. L. Ogra.** 1992. Detection of genomic sequences of respiratory syncytial virus in otitis media with effusion in children. *Ann. Otol. Rhinol. Laryngol. Suppl.* **157:**7–10.
187. **Paradiso, P. R., S. W. Hildreth, D. A. Hogerman, D. J. Speelman, E. B. Lewin, J. Oren, and D. H. Smith.** 1994. Safety and immunogenicity of a subunit respiratory syncytial virus vaccine in children 24 to 48 months old. *Pediatr. Infect. Dis. J.* **13:**792–798.
188. **Parrott, R. H., H. Kim, and C. D. Brandt.** 1979. Respiratory syncytial virus, p. 695. *In* E. Lennette and N. J. Schmitt (ed.), *Diagnostic Procedures for Viral, Rickettsial and Chlamydial Infections*, 5th ed. American Public Health Association, Washington, DC.
189. **Paton, A. W., J. C. Paton, A. J. Lawrence, P. N. Goldwater, and R. J. Harris.** 1992. Rapid detection of respiratory syncytial virus in nasopharyngeal aspirates by reverse transcription and polymerase chain reaction amplification. *J. Clin. Microbiol.* **30:**901–904.
190. **Peck, A. J., L. Corey, and M. Boeckh.** 2004. Pretransplantation respiratory syncytial virus infection: impact of

a strategy to delay transplantation. *Clin. Infect. Dis.* **39:** 673–680.

191. **Peck, A. J., J. A. Englund, J. Kuypers, K. A. Guthrie, L. Corey, R. Morrow, R. C. Hackman, A. Cent, and M. Boeckh.** 2007. Respiratory virus infection among hematopoietic cell transplant recipients: evidence for asymptomatic parainfluenza virus infection. *Blood* **110:** 1681–1688.
192. **Peiris, J. S., W. H. Tang, K. H. Chan, P. L. Khong, Y. Guan, Y. L. Lau, and S. S. Chiu.** 2003. Children with respiratory disease associated with metapneumovirus in Hong Kong. *Emerg. Infect. Dis.* **9:**628–633.
193. **Pelletier, A. J., J. M. Mansbach, and C. A. Camargo, Jr.** 2006. Direct medical costs of bronchiolitis hospitalizations in the United States. *Pediatrics* **118:**2418–2423.
194. **Piedra, P. A., S. G. Cron, A. Jewell, N. Hamblett, R. McBride, M. A. Palacio, R. Ginsberg, C. M. Oermann, and P. W. Hiatt.** 2003. Immunogenicity of a new purified fusion protein vaccine to respiratory syncytial virus: a multi-center trial in children with cystic fibrosis. *Vaccine* **21:**2448.
195. **Piedra, P. A., W. P. Glezen, J. A. Kasel, R. C. Welliver, A. M. Jewel, Y. Rayford, D. A. Hogerman, S. W. Hildreth, and P. R. Paradiso.** 1995. Safety and immunogenicity of the PFP vaccine against respiratory syncytial virus (RSV): the Western blot assay aids in distinguishing immune responses of the PFP vaccine from RSV infection. *Vaccine* **13:**1095–1101.
196. **Piedra, P. A., S. Grace, A. Jewell, S. Spinelli, D. Bunting, D. A. Hogerman, F. Malinoski, and P. W. Hiatt.** 1996. Purified fusion protein vaccine protects against lower respiratory tract illness during respiratory syncytial virus season in children with cystic fibrosis. *Pediatr. Infect. Dis. J.* **15:**23.
197. **Piedra, P. A., A. M. Jewell, S. G. Cron, R. L. Atmar, and W. P. Glezen.** 2003. Correlates of immunity to respiratory syncytial virus (RSV) associated-hospitalization: establishment of minimum protective threshold levels of serum neutralizing antibodies. *Vaccine* **21:**3479–3482.
198. **Piedra, P. A., P. R. Wyde, W. L. Castleman, M. W. Ambrose, A. M. Jewell, D. J. Speelman, and S. W. Hildreth.** 1993. Enhanced pulmonary pathology associated with the use of formalin-inactivated respiratory syncytial virus vaccine in cotton rats is not a unique viral phenomenon. *Vaccine* **11:**1415–1423.
199. **Power, U. F., T. N. Nguyen, E. Rietveld, R. L. de Swart, J. Groen, A. D. Osterhaus, R. de Groot, N. Corvaia, A. Beck, N. Bouveret-Le-Cam, and J. Y. Bonnefoy.** 2001. Safety and immunogenicity of a novel recombinant subunit respiratory syncytial virus vaccine (BBG2Na) in healthy young adults. *J. Infect. Dis.* **184:** 1456–1460.
200. **Randolph, V. B., M. Kandis, P. Stemler-Higgins, M. S. Kennelly, Y. M. McMullen, D. J. Speelman, and C. Weeks-Levy.** 1994. Attenuated temperature-sensitive respiratory syncytial virus mutants generated by cold adaptation. *Virus Res.* **33:**241–259.
201. **Rawlinson, W. D., Z. Waliuzzaman, I. W. Carter, Y. C. Belessis, K. M. Gilbert, and J. R. Morton.** 2003. Asthma exacerbations in children associated with rhinovirus but not human metapneumovirus infection. *J. Infect. Dis.* **187:**1314–1318.
202. **Ray, C. G., C. J. Holberg, L. L. Minnich, Z. M. Shehab, A. L. Wright, and L. M. Taussig for The Group Health Medical Associates.** 1993. Acute lower respiratory illnesses during the first three years of life: potential roles for various etiologic agents. *Pediatr. Infect. Dis. J.* **12:**10–14.
203. **Ray, R., Y. Matsuoka, T. L. Burnett, B. J. Glaze, and R. W. Compans.** 1990. Human parainfluenza virus induces a type-specific protective immune response. *J. Infect. Dis.* **162:**746–749.
204. **Renzi, P. M., J. P. Turgeon, J. P. Yang, S. P. Drblik, J. E. Marcotte, L. Pedneault, and S. Spier.** 1997. Cellular immunity is activated and a TH-2 response is associated with early wheezing in infants after bronchiolitis. *J. Pediatr.* **130:**584–593.
205. **Rodriguez, W. J., R. H. Bui, J. D. Connor, H. W. Kim, C. D. Brandt, R. H. Parrott, B. Burch, and J. Mace.** 1987. Environmental exposure of primary care personnel to ribavirin aerosol when supervising treatment of infants with respiratory syncytial virus infections. *Antimicrob. Agents Chemother.* **31:**1143–1146.
206. **Rosner, I. K., R. C. Welliver, P. J. Edelson, K. Geraci-Ciardullo, and M. Sun.** 1987. Effect of ribavirin therapy on respiratory syncytial virus-specific IgE and IgA responses after infection. *J. Infect. Dis.* **155:**1043–1047.
207. **Saito, T., R. W. Deskin, A. Casola, H. Haeberle, B. Olszewska, P. B. Ernst, R. Alam, P. L. Ogra, and R. Garofalo.** 1997. Respiratory syncytial virus induces selective production of the chemokine RANTES by upper airway epithelial cells. *J. Infect. Dis.* **175:**497–504.
208. **Schildgen, O., and A. Simon.** 2005. Induction of acute otitis media by human metapneumovirus. *Pediatr. Infect. Dis. J.* **24:**1126.
209. **Selwyn, B. J., for the Coordinated Data Group of BOSTID Researchers.** 1990. The epidemiology of acute respiratory tract infection in young children: comparison of findings from several developing countries. *Rev. Infect. Dis.* **12**(Suppl. 8)**:**S870–S888.
210. **Shay, D. K., R. C. Holman, R. D. Newman, L. L. Liu, J. W. Stout, and L. J. Anderson.** 1999. Bronchiolitis-associated hospitalizations among US children, 1980–1996. *JAMA* **282:**1440–1446.
211. **Siber, G. R., J. Leszcynski, V. Pena-Cruz, C. Ferren-Gardner, R. Anderson, V. G. Hemming, E. E. Walsh, J. Burns, K. McIntosh, and R. Gonin.** 1992. Protective activity of a human respiratory syncytial virus immune globulin prepared from donors screened by microneutralization assay. *J. Infect. Dis.* **165:**456–463.
212. **Simoes, E. A.** 1999. Respiratory syncytial virus infection. *Lancet* **354:**847–852.
213. **Simon, A., A. Müller, K. Khurana, S. Engelhart, M. Exner, O. Schildgen, A. M. Eis-Hübinger, W. Kamin, T. Schaible, K. Wadas, R. A. Ammann, A. Wilkesmann, and DSM RSV Paed Study Group.** 14 September 2007. Nosocomial infection: a risk factor for a complicated course in children with respiratory syncytial virus infection—results from a prospective multicenter German surveillance study. *Int. J. Hyg. Environ. Health* doi:10.1016/j.ijheh.2007.07.020.
214. **Smith, D. W., L. R. Frankel, L. H. Mathers, A. T. Tang, R. L. Ariagno, and C. G. Prober.** 1991. A controlled trial of aerosolized ribavirin in infants receiving mechanical ventilation for severe respiratory syncytial virus infection. *N. Engl. J. Med.* **325:**24–29.
215. **Smyth, R. L., and P. J. Openshaw.** 2006. Bronchiolitis. *Lancet* **368:**312–322.
216. **Steinhorn, R. H., and T. P. Green.** 1990. Use of extracorporeal membrane oxygenation in the treatment of respiratory syncytial virus bronchiolitis: the national experience, 1983 to 1988. *J. Pediatr.* **116:**338–342.
217. **Storch, G. A., C. B. Hall, L. J. Anderson, C. S. Park, and D. E. Dohner.** 1993. Antigenic and nucleic acid analysis of nosocomial isolates of respiratory syncytial virus. *J. Infect. Dis.* **167:**562–566.

218. **Sullender, W. M., L. Sun, and L. J. Anderson.** 1993. Analysis of respiratory syncytial virus genetic variability with amplified cDNAs. *J. Clin. Microbiol.* **31:**1224–1231.
219. **Sumino, K. C., E. Agapov, R. A. Pierce, E. P. Trulock, J. D. Pfeifer, J. H. Ritter, M. Gaudreault-Keener, G. A. Storch, and M. J. Holtzman.** 2005. Detection of severe human metapneumovirus infection by real-time polymerase chain reaction and histopathological assessment. *J. Infect. Dis.* **192:**1052–1060.
220. **Tang, R. S., K. Mahmood, M. Macphail, J. M. Guzzetta, A. A. Haller, H. Liu, J. Kaur, H. A. Lawlor, E. A. Stillman, J. H. Schickli, R. A. Fouchier, A. D. Osterhaus, and R. R. Spaete.** 2005. A host-range restricted parainfluenza virus type 3 (PIV3) expressing the human metapneumovirus (hMPV) fusion protein elicits protective immunity in African green monkeys. *Vaccine* **23:**1657–1667.
221. **Tao, T., A. P. Durbin, S. S. Whitehead, F. Davoodi, P. L. Collins, and B. R. Murphy.** 1998. Recovery of a fully viable chimeric human parainfluenza virus (PIV) type 3 in which the hemagglutinin-neuraminidase and fusion glycoproteins have been replaced by those of PIV type 1. *J. Virol.* **72:**2955–2961.
222. **Taussig, L. M., A. L. Wright, C. J. Holberg, M. Halonen, W. J. Morgan, and F. D. Martinez.** 2003. Tucson Children's Respiratory Study: 1980 to present. *J. Allergy Clin. Immunol.* **111:**661–675; quiz, 676.
223. **Tibballs, J., F. A. Shann, and L. I. Landau.** 1992. Placebo-controlled trial of prednisolone in children intubated for croup. *Lancet* **340:**745–748.
224. **Todd, S. J., L. Minnich, and J. L. Waner.** 1995. Comparison of rapid immunofluorescence procedure with TestPack RSV and Directigen FLU-A for diagnosis of respiratory syncytial virus and influenza A virus. *J. Clin. Microbiol.* **33:**1650–1651.
225. **Tristram, D. A., R. C. Welliver, C. K. Mohar, D. A. Hogerman, S. W. Hildreth, and P. Paradiso.** 1993. Immunogenicity and safety of respiratory syncytial virus subunit vaccine in seropositive children 18–36 months old. *J. Infect. Dis.* **167:**191–195.
226. **Tsutsumi, H., T. Honjo, K. Nagai, Y. Chiba, S. Chiba, and S. Tsugawa.** 1989. Immunoglobulin A antibody response to respiratory syncytial virus structural proteins in colostrum and milk. *J. Clin. Microbiol.* **27:**1949–1951.
227. **Vachon, M. L., N. Dionne, E. Leblanc, D. Moisan, M. G. Bergeron, and G. Boivin.** 2006. Human parainfluenza type 4 infections, Canada. *Emerg. Infect. Dis.* **12:** 1755–1758.
228. **Vainionpaa, R., and T. Hyypia.** 1994. Biology of parainfluenza viruses. *Clin. Microbiol. Rev.* **7:**265–275.
229. **van den Hoogen, B. G., J. C. de Jong, J. Groen, T. Kuiken, R. de Groot, R. A. Fouchier, and A. D. Osterhaus.** 2001. A newly discovered human pneumovirus isolated from young children with respiratory tract disease. *Nat. Med.* **7:**719–724.
230. **van den Hoogen, B. G., S. Herfst, L. Sprong, P. A. Cane, E. Forleo-Neto, R. L. de Swart, A. D. Osterhaus, and R. A. Fouchier.** 2004. Antigenic and genetic variability of human metapneumoviruses. *Emerg. Infect. Dis.* **10:**658–666.
231. **Vargas, S. O., H. P. Kozakewich, A. R. Perez-Atayde, and A. J. McAdam.** 2004. Pathology of human metapneumovirus infection: insights into the pathogenesis of a newly identified respiratory virus. *Pediatr. Dev. Pathol.* **7:**478–486; discussion, 421.
232. **Velayudhan, B. T., K. V. Nagaraja, A. J. Thachil, D. P. Shaw, G. C. Gray, and D. A. Halvorson.** 2006. Human metapneumovirus in turkey poults. *Emerg. Infect. Dis.* **12:**1853–1859.
233. **Volovitz, B., H. Faden, and P. L. Ogra.** 1988. Release of leukotriene C4 in respiratory tract during acute viral infection. *J. Pediatr.* **112:**218–222.
234. **Wagner, D. K., B. S. Graham, P. F. Wright, E. E. Walsh, H. W. Kim, C. B. Reimer, D. L. Nelson, R. M. Chanock, and B. R. Murphy.** 1986. Serum immunoglobulin G antibody subclass responses to respiratory syncytial virus F and G glycoproteins after primary infection. *J. Clin. Microbiol.* **24:**304–306.
235. **Wagner, D. K., D. L. Nelson, E. E. Walsh, C. B. Reimer, F. W. Henderson, and B. R. Murphy.** 1987. Differential immunoglobulin G subclass antibody titers to respiratory syncytial virus F and G glycoproteins in adults. *J. Clin. Microbiol.* **25:**748–750.
236. **Wald, E. R., B. Dashefsky, and M. Green.** 1988. In re ribavirin: a case of premature adjudication? *J. Pediatr.* **112:**154–158.
237. **Watt, P. J., B. S. Robinson, C. R. Pringle, and D. A. Tyrrell.** 1990. Determinants of susceptibility to challenge and the antibody response of adult volunteers given experimental respiratory syncytial virus vaccines. *Vaccine* **8:**231–236.
238. **Welliver, R., D. T. Wong, T. S. Choi, and P. L. Ogra.** 1982. Natural history of parainfluenza virus infection in childhood. *J. Pediatr.* **101:**180–187.
239. **Welliver, R. C., D. T. Wong, E. Middleton, Jr., M. Sun, N. McCarthy, and P. L. Ogra.** 1982. Role of parainfluenza virus-specific IgE in pathogenesis of croup and wheezing subsequent to infection. *J. Pediatr.* **101:**889–896.
240. **Welliver, R. C., D. T. Wong, M. Sun, E. Middleton, Jr., R. S. Vaughan, and P. L. Ogra.** 1981. The development of respiratory syncytial virus-specific IgE and the release of histamine in nasopharyngeal secretions after infection. *N. Engl. J. Med.* **305:**841–846.
241. **Welliver, T. P., R. P. Garofalo, Y. Hosakote, K. H. Hintz, L. Avendano, K. Sanchez, L. Velozo, H. Jafri, S. Chavez-Bueno, P. L. Ogra, L. McKinney, J. L. Reed, and R. C. Welliver, Sr.** 2007. Severe human lower respiratory tract illness caused by respiratory syncytial virus and influenza virus is characterized by the absence of pulmonary cytotoxic lymphocyte responses. *J. Infect. Dis.* **195:**1126–1136.
242. **Wendt, C. H., D. J. Weisdorf, M. C. Jordan, H. H. Balfour, Jr., and M. I. Hertz.** 1992. Parainfluenza virus respiratory infection after bone marrow transplantation. *N. Engl. J. Med.* **326:**921–926.
243. **Whimbey, E., R. E. Champlin, and J. A. Englund.** 1995. Combination therapy with aerosolized ribavirin and intravenous immunoglobulin for respiratory syncytial virus disease in adult bone marrow transplant recipients. *Bone Marrow Transplant.* **16:**393–399.
244. **Whimbey, E., R. B. Couch, J. A. Englund, M. Andreef, J. M. Goodrich, I. I. Raad, V. Lewis, N. Mirza, M. A. Luna, and B. Baxter.** 1995. Respiratory syncytial virus pneumonia in hospitalized adult patients with leukemia. *Clin. Infect. Dis.* **21:**376–379.
245. **Whimbey, E., J. A. Englund, and R. B. Couch.** 1997. Community respiratory virus infections in immunocompromised patients with cancer. *Am. J. Med.* **102:**10–18; discussion, 25–26.
246. **Williams, J. V., J. E. Crowe, Jr., R. Enriquez, P. Minton, R. S. Peebles, Jr., R. G. Hamilton, S. Higgins, M. Griffin, and T. V. Hartert.** 2005. Human metapneumovirus infection plays an etiologic role in acute asthma exacerbations requiring hospitalization in adults. *J. Infect. Dis.* **192:**1149–1153.

247. **Williams, J. V., P. A. Harris, S. J. Tollefson, L. L. Halburnt-Rush, J. M. Pingsterhaus, K. M. Edwards, P. F. Wright, and J. E. Crowe, Jr.** 2004. Human metapneumovirus and lower respiratory tract disease in otherwise healthy infants and children. *N. Engl. J. Med.* **350:**443–450.
248. **Williams, J. V., R. Martino, N. Rabella, M. Otegui, R. Parody, J. M. Heck, and J. E. Crowe, Jr.** 2005. A prospective study comparing human metapneumovirus with other respiratory viruses in adults with hematologic malignancies and respiratory tract infections. *J. Infect. Dis.* **192:**1061–1065.
249. **Williams, J. V., S. J. Tollefson, P. W. Heymann, H. T. Carper, J. Patrie, and J. E. Crowe.** 2005. Human metapneumovirus infection in children hospitalized for wheezing. *J. Allergy Clin. Immunol.* **115:**1311–1312.
250. **Williams, J. V., S. J. Tollefson, J. E. Johnson, and J. E. Crowe, Jr.** 2005. The cotton rat *(Sigmodon hispidus)* is a permissive small animal model of human metapneumovirus infection, pathogenesis, and protective immunity. *J. Virol.* **79:**10944–10951.
251. **Williams, J. V., S. J. Tollefson, S. Nair, and T. Chonmaitree.** 2006. Association of human metapneumovirus with acute otitis media. *Int. J. Pediatr. Otorhinolaryngol.* **70:**1189–1193.
252. **Williams, J. V., C. K. Wang, C. F. Yang, S. J. Tollefson, F. S. House, J. M. Heck, M. Chu, J. B. Brown, L. D. Lintao, J. D. Quinto, D. Chu, R. R. Spaete, K. M. Edwards, P. F. Wright, and J. E. Crowe, Jr.** 2006. The role of human metapneumovirus in upper respiratory tract infections in children: a 20-year experience. *J. Infect. Dis.* **193:**387–395.
253. **Wright, A. L., L. M. Taussig, C. G. Ray, H. R. Harrison, and C. J. Holberg.** 1989. The Tucson Children's Respiratory Study. II. Lower respiratory tract illness in the first year of life. *Am. J. Epidemiol.* **129:**1232–1246.
254. **Wright, P. F., R. A. Karron, R. B. Belshe, J. R. Shi, V. B. Randolph, P. L. Collins, A. F. O'Shea, W. C. Gruber, and B. R. Murphy.** 2007. The absence of enhanced disease with wild type respiratory syncytial virus infection occurring after receipt of live, attenuated, respiratory syncytial virus vaccines. *Vaccine* **25:**7372–7378.
255. **Wright, P. F., R. A. Karron, R. B. Belshe, J. Thompson, J. E. Crowe, Jr., T. G. Boyce, L. L. Halburnt, G. W. Reed, S. S. Whitehead, E. L. Anderson, A. E. Wittek, R. Casey, M. Eichelberger, B. Thumar, V. B. Randolph, S. A. Udem, R. M. Chanock, and B. R. Murphy.** 2000. Evaluation of a live, cold-passaged, temperature-sensitive, respiratory syncytial virus vaccine candidate in infancy. *J. Infect. Dis.* **182:**1331–1342.
256. **Wu, H., D. S. Pfarr, S. Johnson, Y. A. Brewah, R. M. Woods, N. K. Patel, W. I. White, J. F. Young, and P. A. Kiener.** 2007. Development of motavizumab, an ultra-potent antibody for the prevention of respiratory syncytial virus infection in the upper and lower respiratory tract. *J. Mol. Biol.* **368:**652–665.
257. **Wyde, P. R., S. N. Chetty, A. M. Jewell, G. Boivin, and P. A. Piedra.** 2003. Comparison of the inhibition of human metapneumovirus and respiratory syncytial virus by ribavirin and immune serum globulin in vitro. *Antivir. Res.* **60:**51–59.
258. **Wyde, P. R., D. K. Moore, T. Hepburn, C. L. Silverman, T. G. Porter, M. Gross, G. Taylor, S. G. Demuth, and S. B. Dillon.** 1995. Evaluation of the protective efficacy of reshaped human monoclonal antibody RSHZ19 against respiratory syncytial virus in cotton rats. *Pediatr. Res.* **38:**543–550.

Color Insert

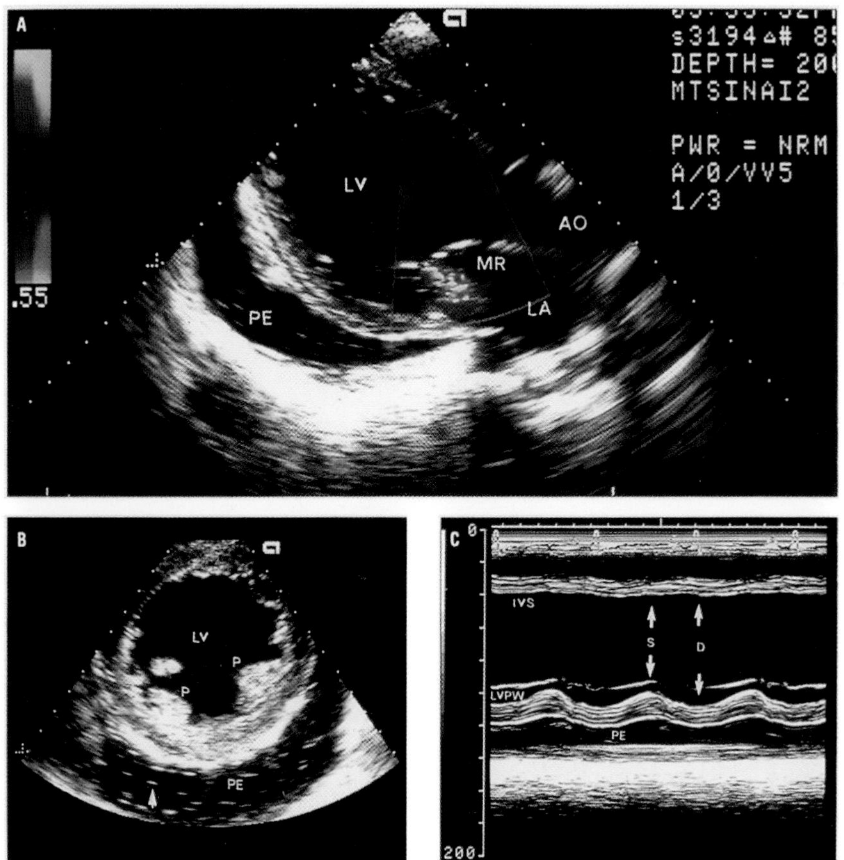

COLOR PLATE 1

COLOR PLATE 1 (Chapter 7) Echocardiographic features of myocarditis. (A) Two-dimensional parasternal long-axis view demonstrating LV dilation and a pericardial effusion (PE). Color Doppler interrogation provides evidence of mitral regurgitation. (B) Parasternal long-axis view demonstrating LV dilation and normal papillary muscles (P). (C) M mode demonstrating systolic dysfunction with flattened interventricular septal motion (IVS), fair LV posterior wall excursion (LVPW), LV dilation with increased LV end-diastolic dimension (D), and reduced systolic function (S) and PE.

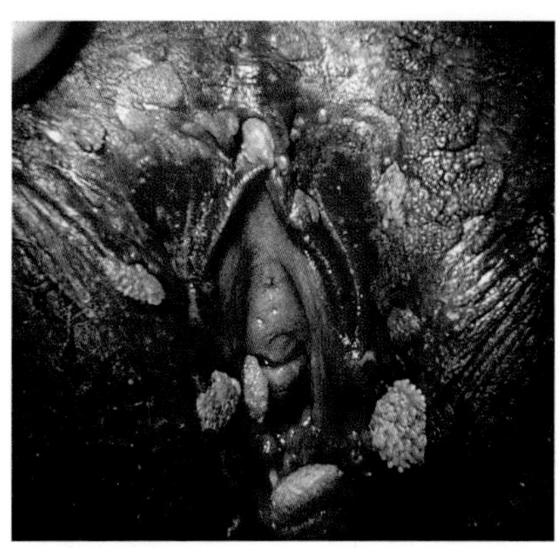
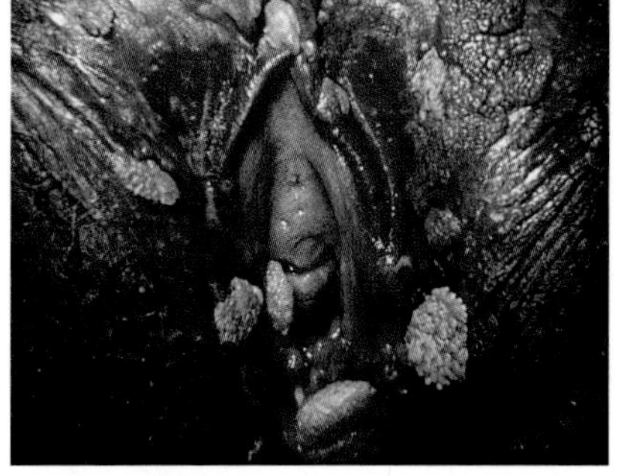

COLOR PLATE 2

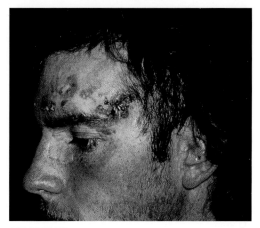

COLOR PLATE 3

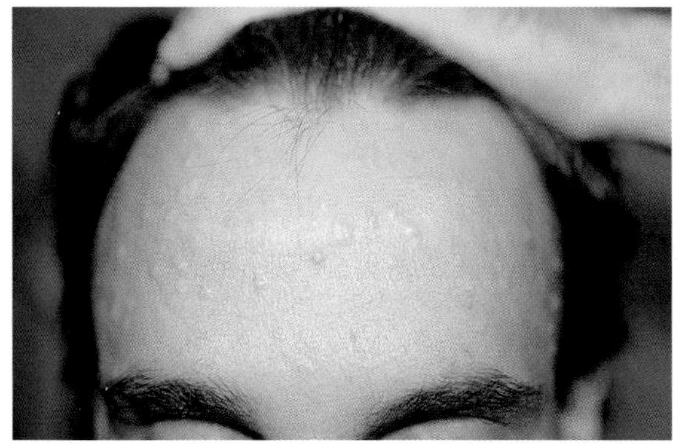

COLOR PLATE 4

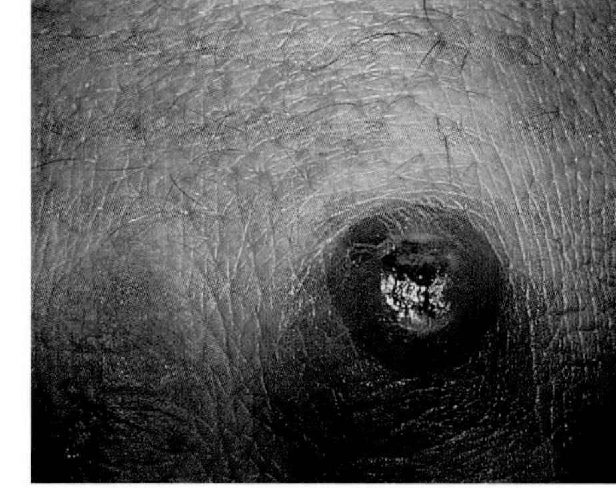

COLOR PLATE 5

COLOR PLATE 2 (Chapter 8) Condyloma acuminatum associated with HPV-6.

COLOR PLATE 3 (Chapter 8) Multiple primary squamous cell carcinomas associated with HPV-8 on the forehead of a man with EV.

COLOR PLATE 4 (Chapter 8) Disseminated molluscum contagiosum in an AIDS patient.

COLOR PLATE 5 (Chapter 8) Nodular stage of orf on the hand of a shepherd from Mexico.

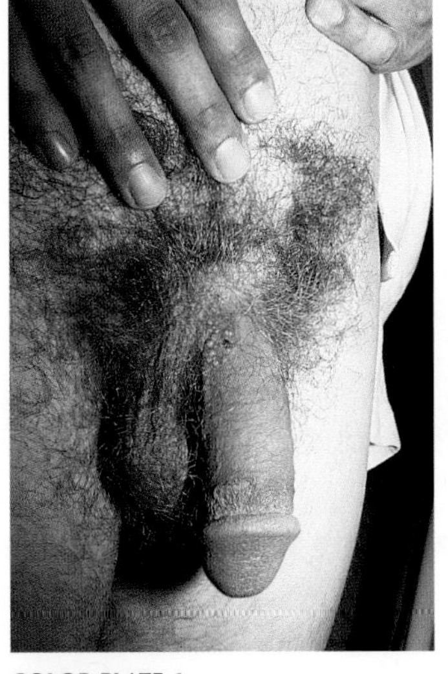

COLOR PLATE 6

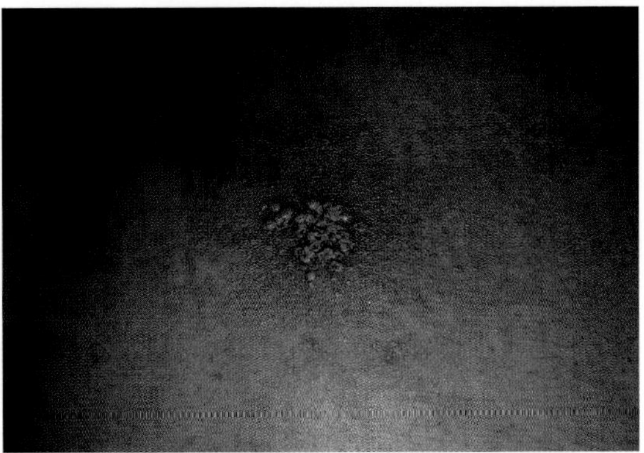

COLOR PLATE 7

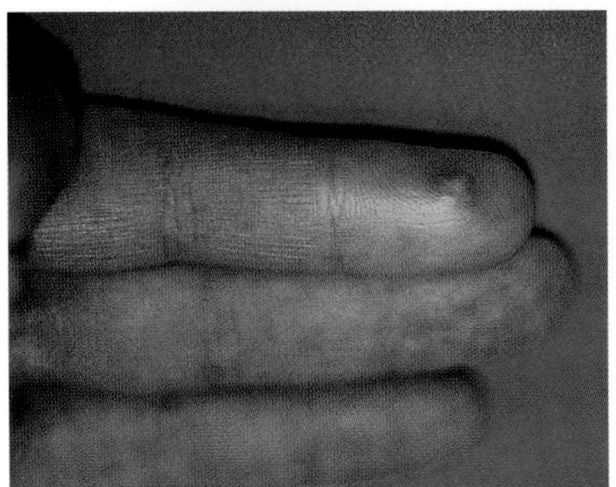

COLOR PLATE 8

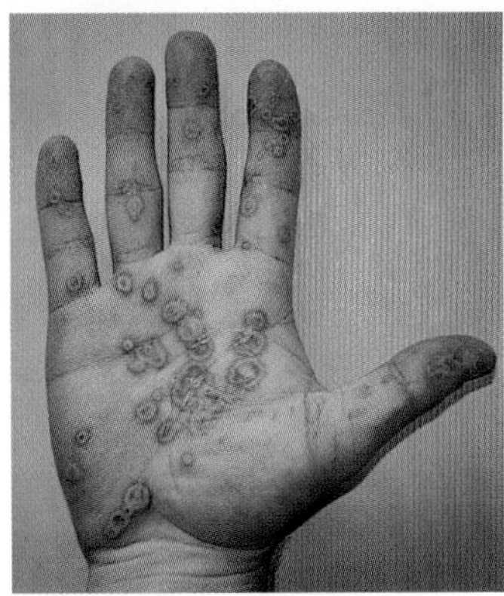

COLOR PLATE 9

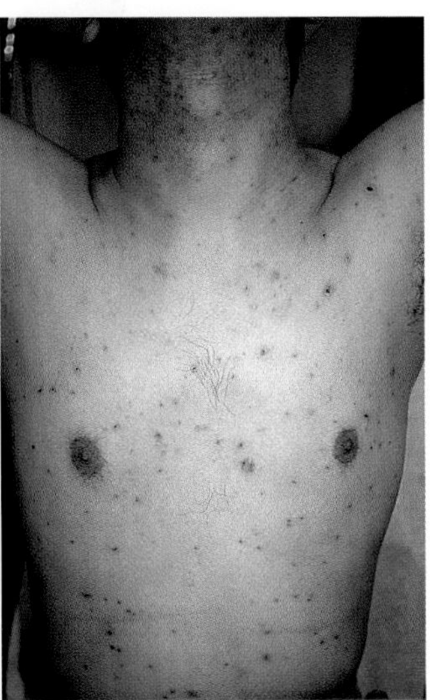

COLOR PLATE 10

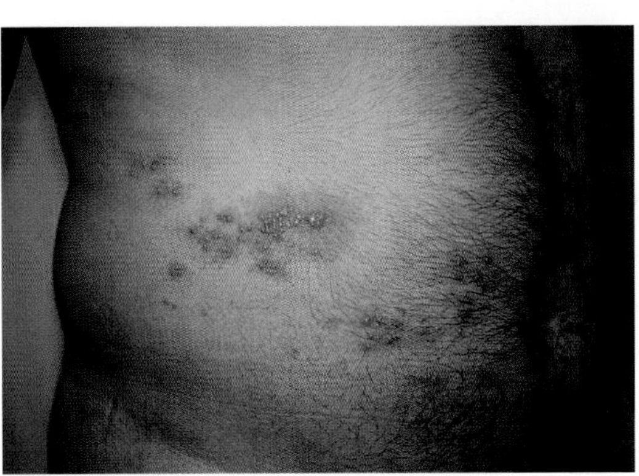

COLOR PLATE 11

COLOR PLATE 6 (Chapter 8) First-episode genital herpes (due to HSV-2) in a man who gave a history of always using condoms during sex.

COLOR PLATE 7 (Chapter 8) Recurrent HSV-2 infection of the buttock.

COLOR PLATE 8 (Chapter 8) Herpes whitlow due to HSV-2 in a health care worker following a puncture wound from a needle used to culture genital herpes.

COLOR PLATE 9 (Chapter 8) Erythema multiforme following an outbreak of herpes labialis.

COLOR PLATE 10 (Chapter 8) Primary varicella in an adult Japanese man.

COLOR PLATE 11 (Chapter 8) Thoracic herpes zoster in an otherwise healthy man.

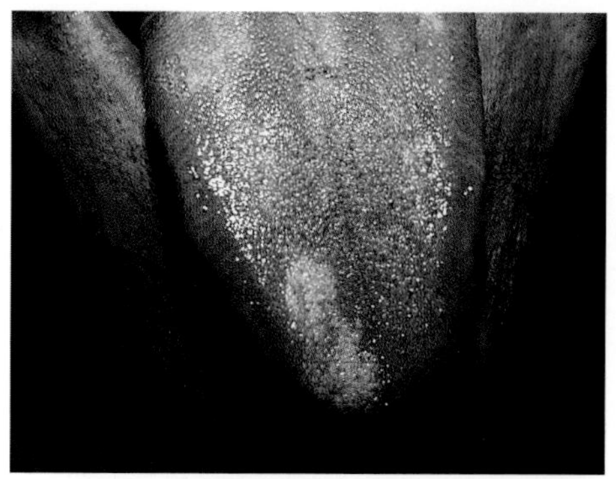

COLOR PLATE 12

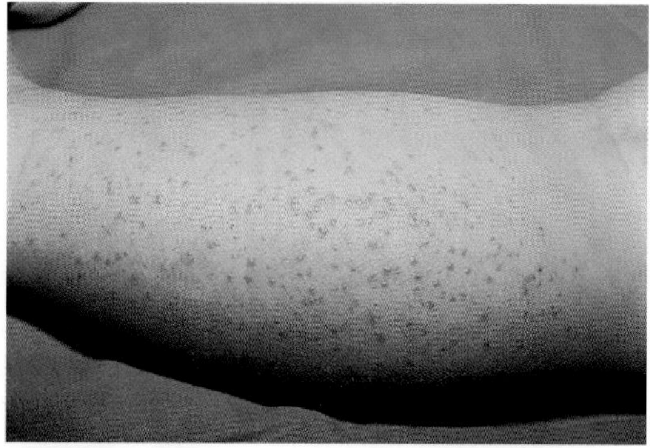

COLOR PLATE 13

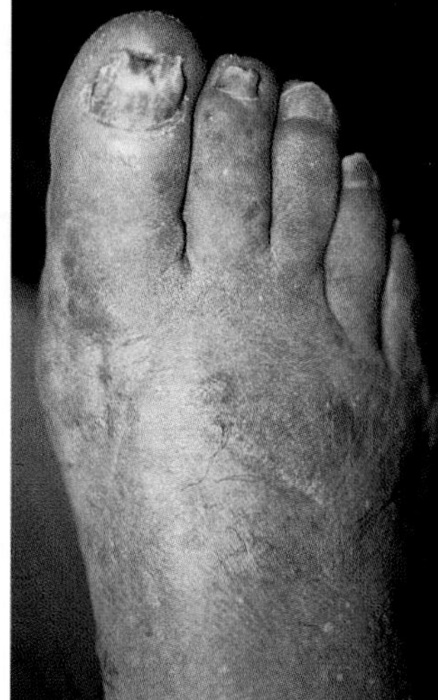

COLOR PLATE 14

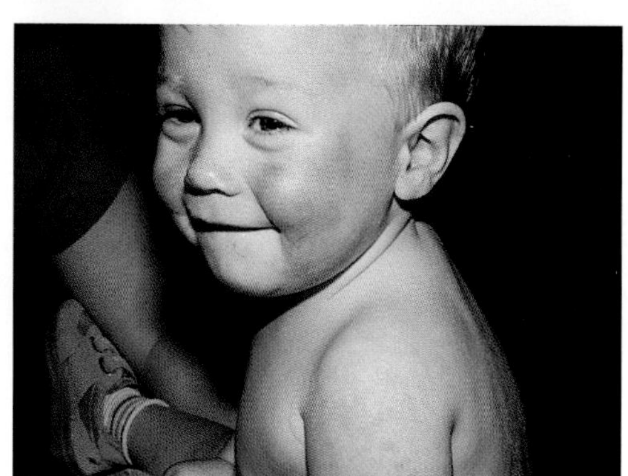

COLOR PLATE 15

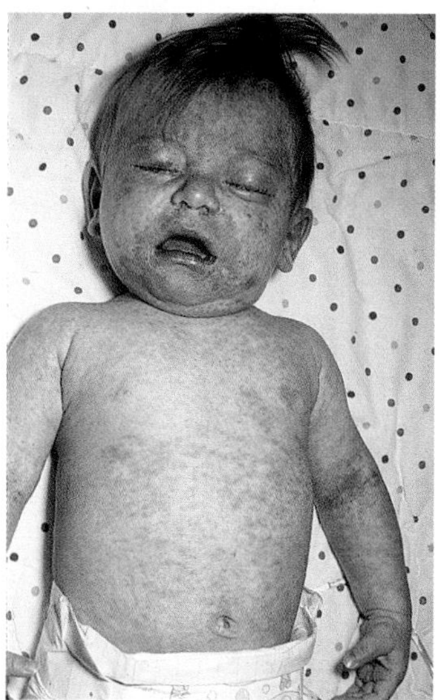

COLOR PLATE 16

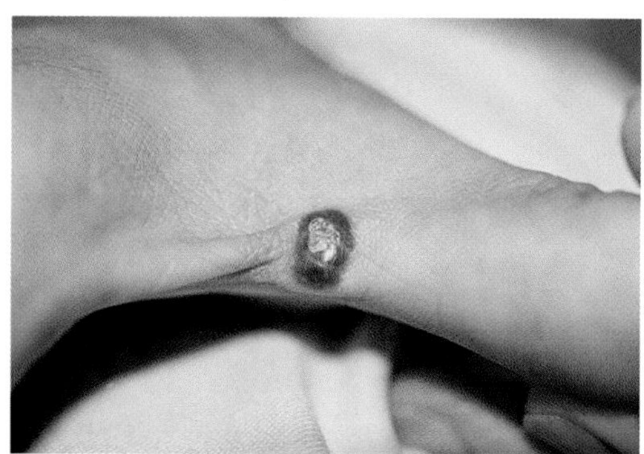

COLOR PLATE 17

COLOR PLATE 12 (Chapter 8)	Oral hairy leukoplakia associated with EBV in an AIDS patient.
COLOR PLATE 13 (Chapter 8)	Papules of Gianotti-Crosti syndrome associated with EBV.
COLOR PLATE 14 (Chapter 8)	Kaposi's sarcoma associated with HHV-8 in an HIV-negative elderly Italian man.
COLOR PLATE 15 (Chapter 8)	Erythema infectiosum (fifth disease) associated with parvovirus B19.
COLOR PLATE 16 (Chapter 8)	Measles in an infant.
COLOR PLATE 17 (Chapter 8)	Bacillary angiomatosis associated with *Bartonella quintana* in an HIV-positive man.

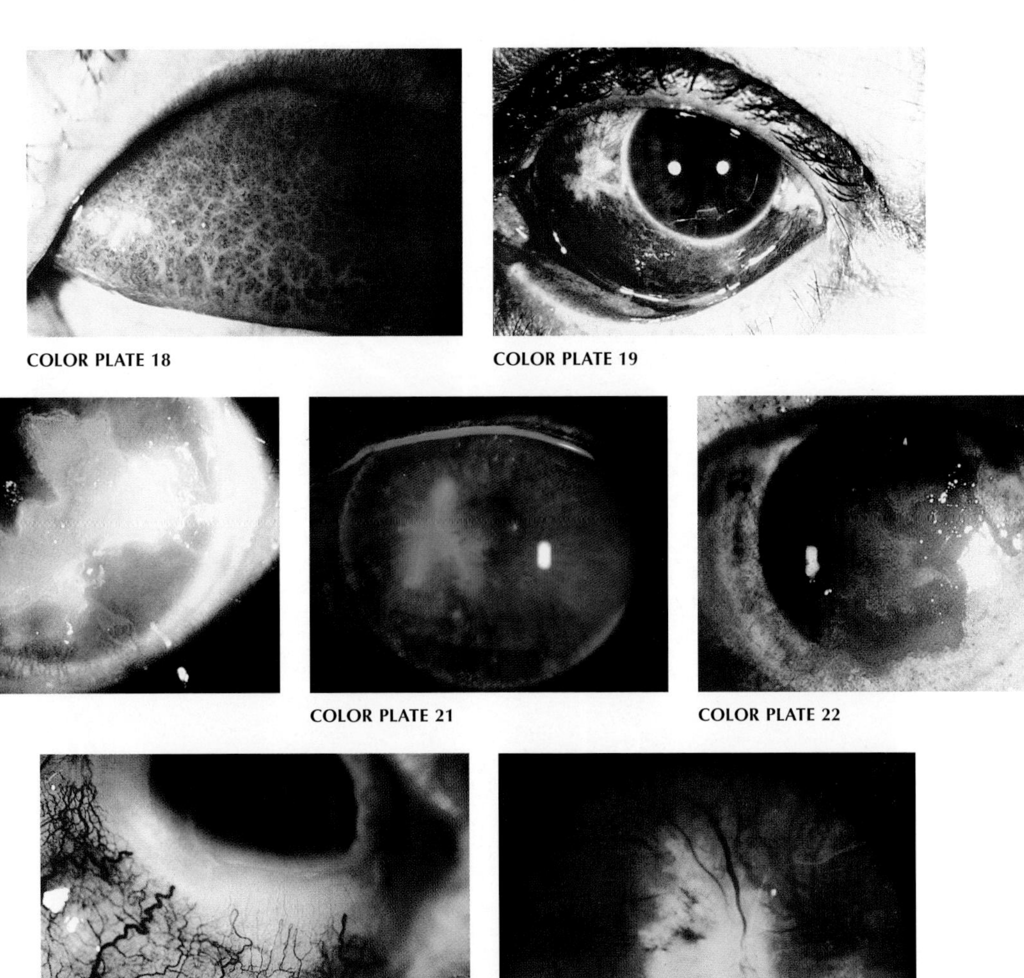

COLOR PLATE 18

COLOR PLATE 19

COLOR PLATE 20

COLOR PLATE 21

COLOR PLATE 22

COLOR PLATE 23

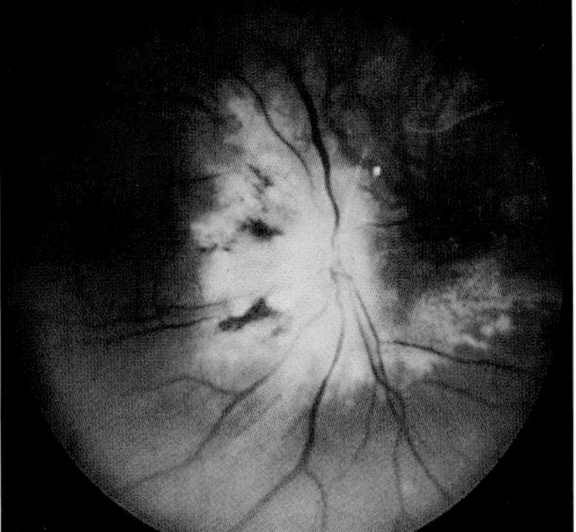

COLOR PLATE 24

COLOR PLATE 18 (Chapter 10) Intense papillary response in the superior conjunctival tarsal plate due to adenovirus infection. (Reprinted from N. K. Ragge and D. L. Easty, ed., *Immediate Eye Care*, Mosby Year Book, Inc., Philadelphia, PA, 1991, with permission of Elsevier.)

COLOR PLATE 19 (Chapter 10) Acute hemorrhagic conjunctivitis. (Courtesy of P. Asbell. Reprinted from N. K. Ragge and D. L. Easty, ed., *Immediate Eye Care*, Mosby Year Book, Inc., Philadelphia, PA, 1991, with permission of Elsevier.)

COLOR PLATE 20 (Chapter 10) Large ameboid corneal ulcer in a malnourished child with measles. (Courtesy of J. Stanford Smith. Reprinted from N. K. Ragge and D. L. Easty, ed., *Immediate Eye Care*, Mosby Year Book, Inc., Philadelphia, PA, 1991, with permission of Elsevier.)

COLOR PLATE 21 (Chapter 10) Dendritic corneal ulceration demonstrated using fluorescein and illuminated in cobalt blue light.

COLOR PLATE 22 (Chapter 10) Ameboid corneal ulceration occurring as a result of locally induced immunosuppression by steroids. Both Rose Bengal and fluorescein stains were used.

COLOR PLATE 23 (Chapter 10) Diffuse scleritis secondary to herpes zoster. Note the dusky red color due to the injection of the scleral, episcleral, and conjunctival vascular beds.

COLOR PLATE 24 (Chapter 10) CMV optic neuritis. Note the clear view indicative of little vitreous inflammation. (Courtesy of S. Lightman.)

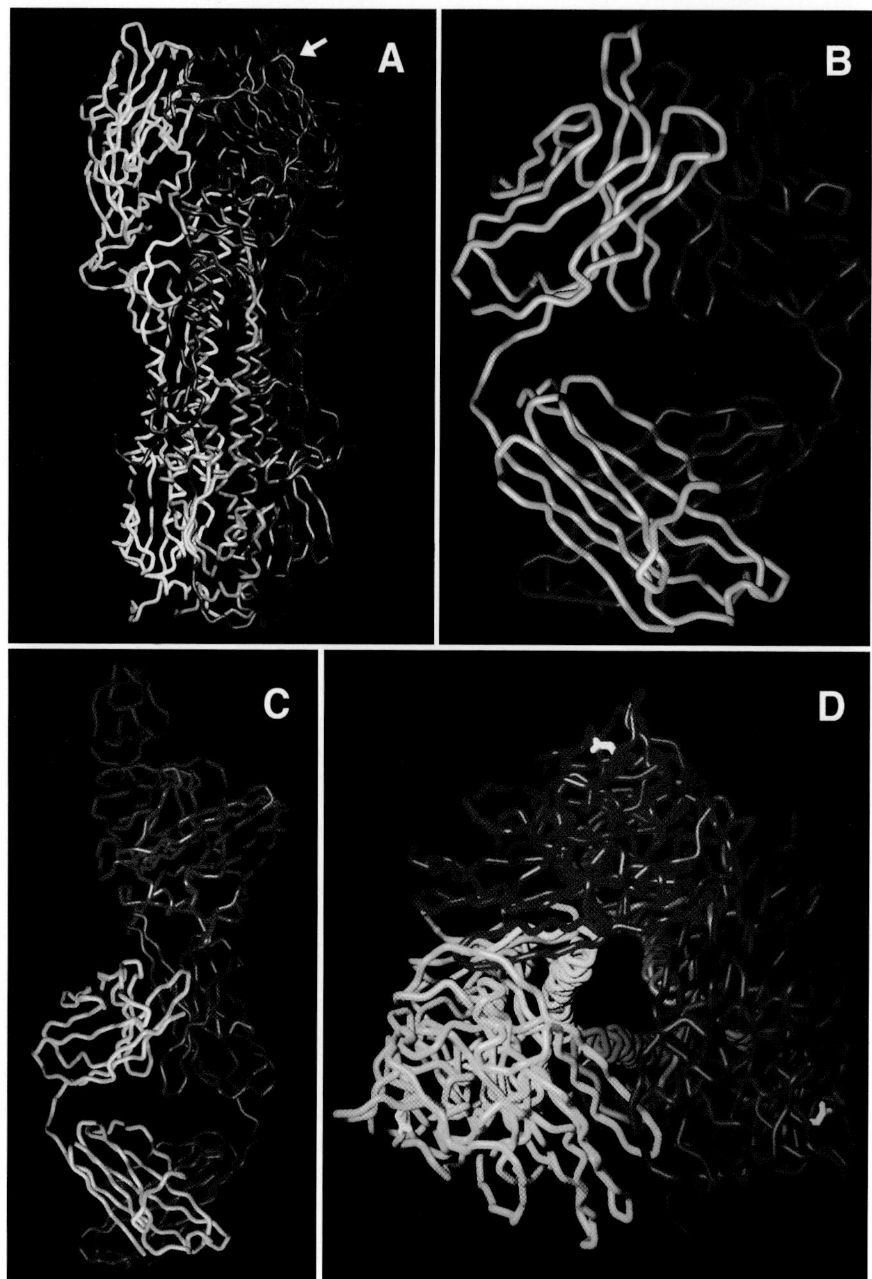

COLOR PLATE 25

COLOR PLATE 25 (Chapter 14) Three-dimensional structure of the interaction of influenza virus HA with a neutralizing antibody. (A) α-Carbon backbone structure of a water-soluble influenza virus HA released from viral membranes by protease digestion, as determined by X-ray crystallography (57, 58). Individual subunits of the trimeric structure are colored red, blue, and yellow. The molecule is oriented such that the sialic acid binding pockets are at the top and the region that connects with the membrane anchor domain is toward the bottom. (B) α-Carbon backbone structure of the variable domain of an anti-HA MAb. The heavy and light chains, respectively, are dark and light blue. The molecule is oriented with the antigen-binding region toward the top. (C) Interaction of HA with the variable region of an anti-HA MAb (3). Antibody colors are the same as in panel B; HA is in red. The region of the HA bound by the MAb is located in panel A by the arrow. (D) Top view of HA trimers, looking toward the membrane surface. The side chain of the single modified residue in an antigenic MAb escape variant (selected by a different antibody than those shown in panel C or D) is in white. Note the exposed location. Comparison of variant and wild-type structures revealed only minimal conformational alterations: the new side chain simply replaces its predecessor.

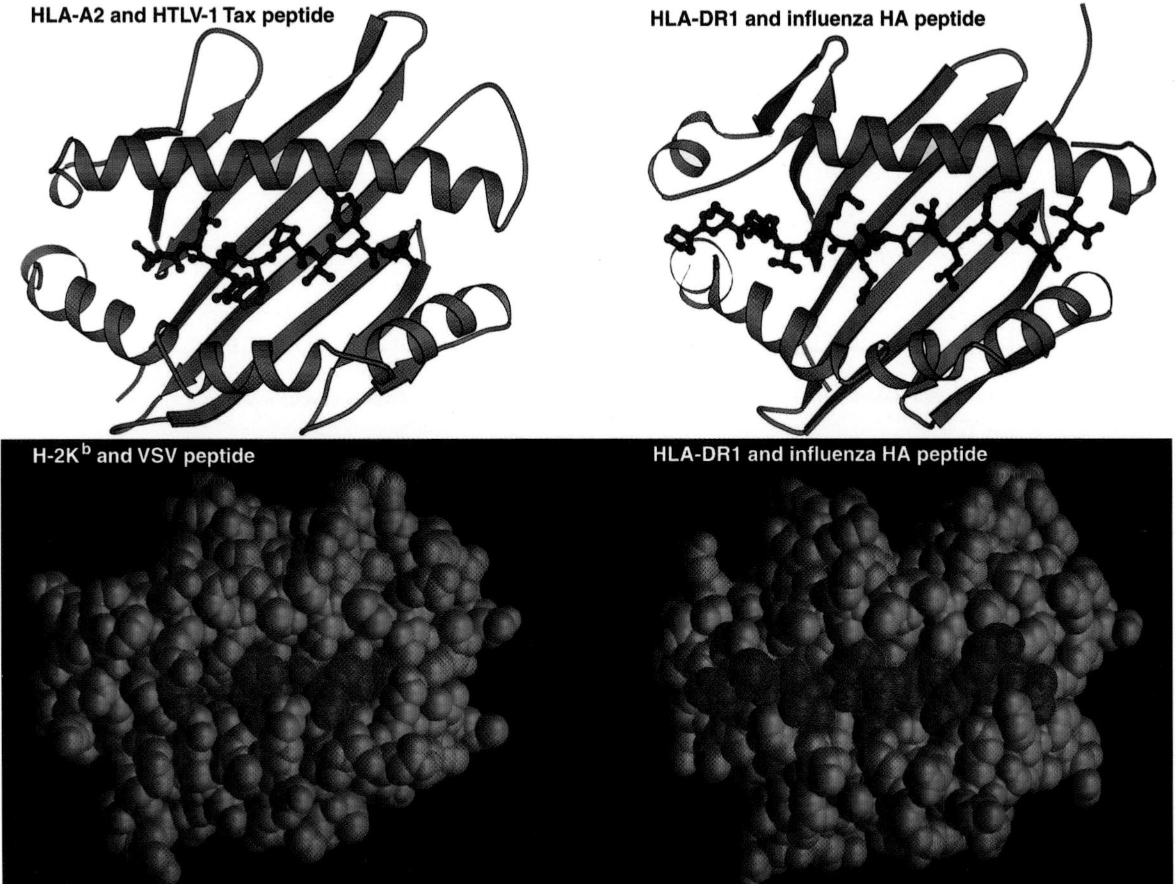

COLOR PLATE 26

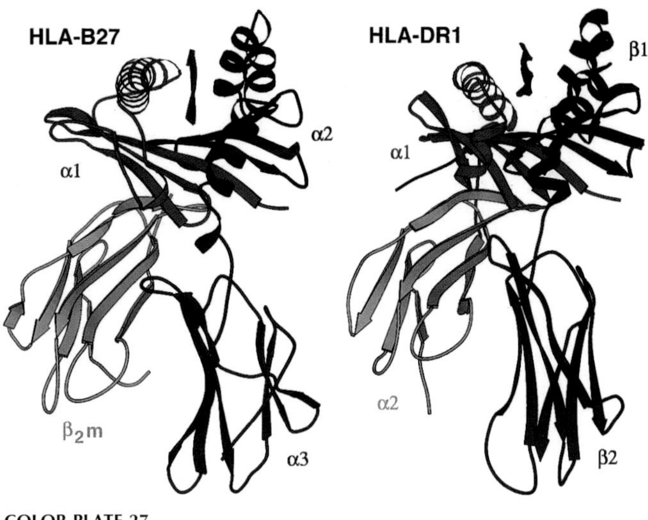

COLOR PLATE 27

COLOR PLATE 26 (Chapter 14) Three-dimensional structure of MHC class I and class II molecules. Shown is the structure of the α-carbon backbone of class I (left) and class II (right) molecules (48) bearing antigenic peptides (short red ribbon) in the groove, as determined by X-ray crystallography of water-soluble molecules released from the cell surface by protease digestion. The molecule is oriented with the top toward the TCR.

COLOR PLATE 27 (Chapter 14) Three-dimensional structure of MHC molecules bearing antigenic peptides. Ribbon α-carbon backbone (top) and space-filling main- and side-chain (bottom) representations of class I (9, 46) (left) and class II (right) molecules bearing antigenic peptides from viral proteins. The view is from the perspective of a TCR.

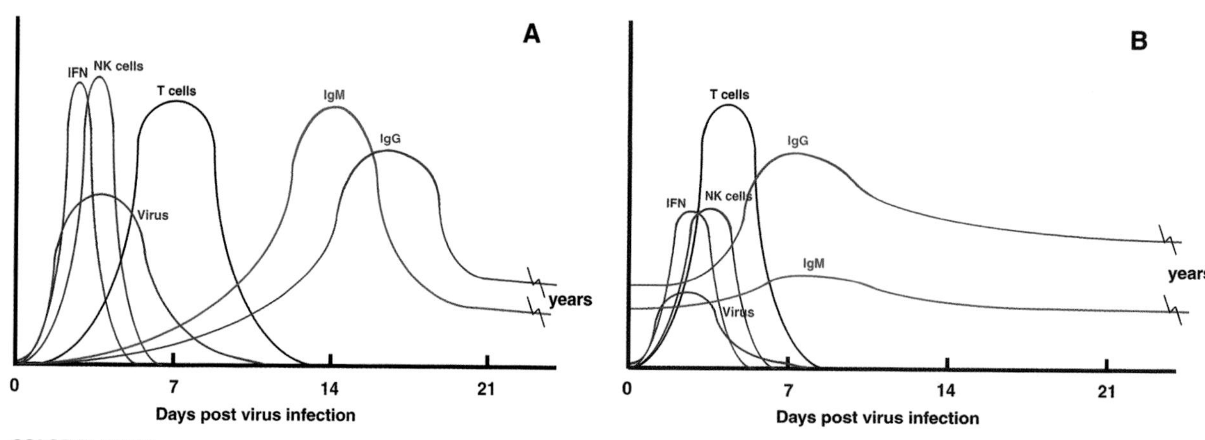

COLOR PLATE 28

COLOR PLATE 28 (Chapter 14) Time course of an idealized antiviral immune response. (A) Response to a primary viral infection. All values are in arbitrary activity units, except the magnitude of serum Ig responses, which is expressed in relative amounts of protein. Since IgG antibodies are of higher affinity than IgM antibodies, the IgG response will have a much greater biological effect on viral replication. "T cells" represents the aggregate activities of T_{CD4^+} and T_{CD8^+}. (B) Response to a secondary viral infection. Note that the presence of preexisting antibodies limits (or sometimes completely prevents) the replication of viruses serologically cross-reactive to those previously encountered. The presence of a cross-reactive antigen triggers a rapid increase in IgG antibodies. T-cell responses occur more rapidly but may not include T_{CD8^+} if viral replication is greatly limited. The reduction in IFN and NK cell activity merely reflects the decreased number of virus-infected cells.

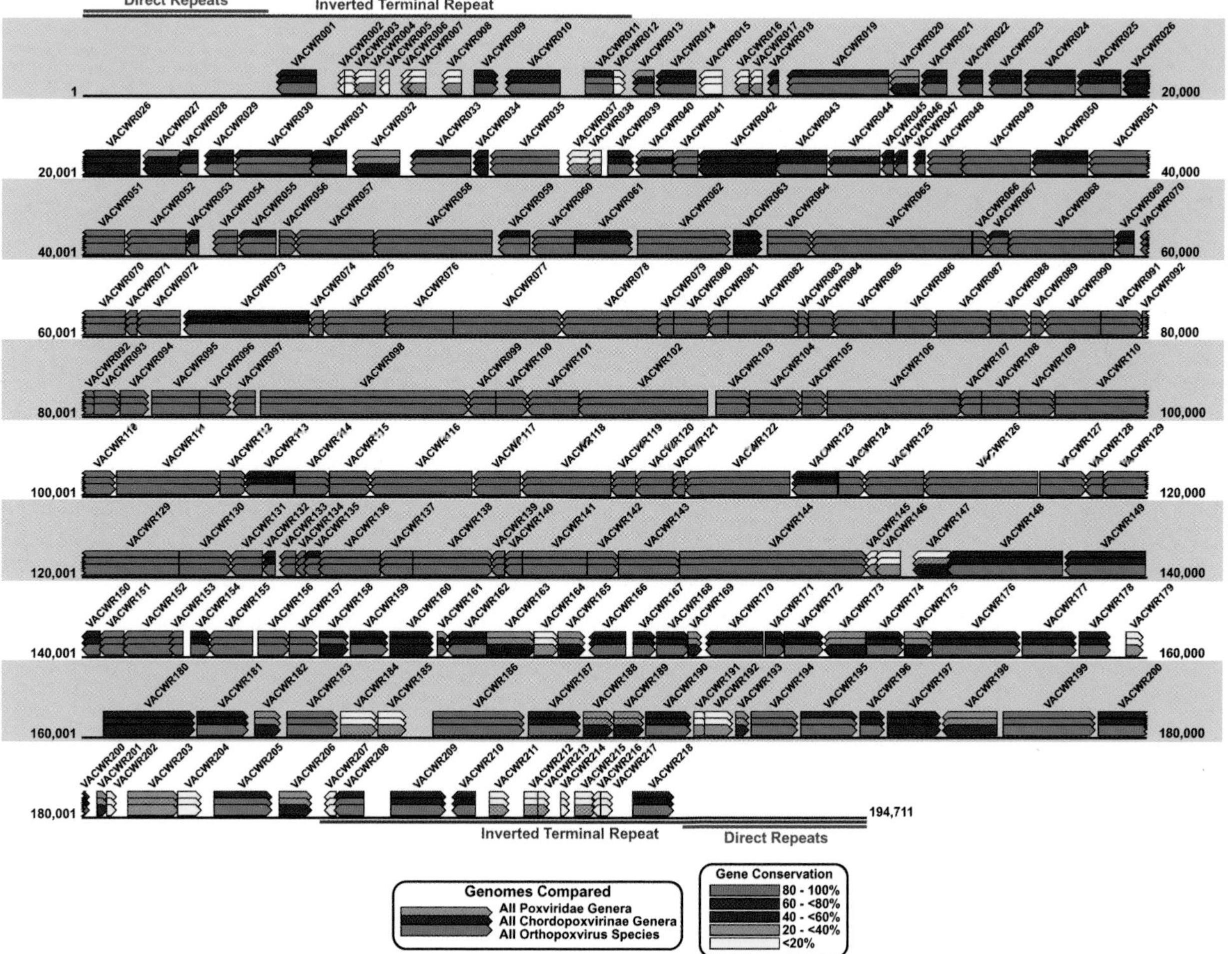

COLOR PLATE 29

COLOR PLATE 29 (Chapter 18) Schematic representation of the genome of the WR strain of VACV. The genome is a linear double-stranded molecule with terminal hairpins, inverted terminal repeats, and a series of direct repeats within the inverted repeats. Each overlapping bar indicates gene conservation between the WR strain and all poxviruses, vertebrate poxviruses, and orthopoxviruses. The bars are color coded according to the percentage of gene conservation across the indicated taxa. (Reprinted from reference 15 with permission.)

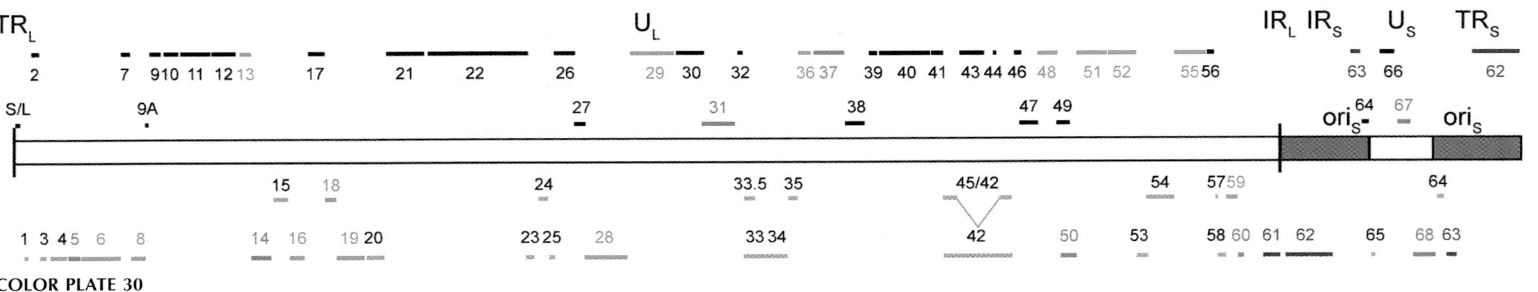

COLOR PLATE 30

COLOR PLATE 30 (Chapter 21) The V2V genome. The 125-kbp linear double-stranded DNA consists of a long unique segment (U_L) of approximately 100 kbp that is flanked by terminal and internal repeats of 88 bp (TR_L and IR_L) and a short unique sequence (U_S) of approximately 5.4 kbp that is bounded by repeated sequences (TR_S and IR_S) of 6.8 kbp. There are two origins (ori_S) for DNA replication in the repeats that bound the U_S. ORFs are to scale and are identified by number; genes containing ORFs below the genome are transcribed from right to left, while those above the genome are transcribed from left to right. Red is used for the ORFs for IE genes, green is used for glycoproteins, and blue is used for DNA synthesis and nucleotide metabolism. ORFs 62, 63, and 64 are present in two copies, as they are fully contained within the repeats flanking the U_S.

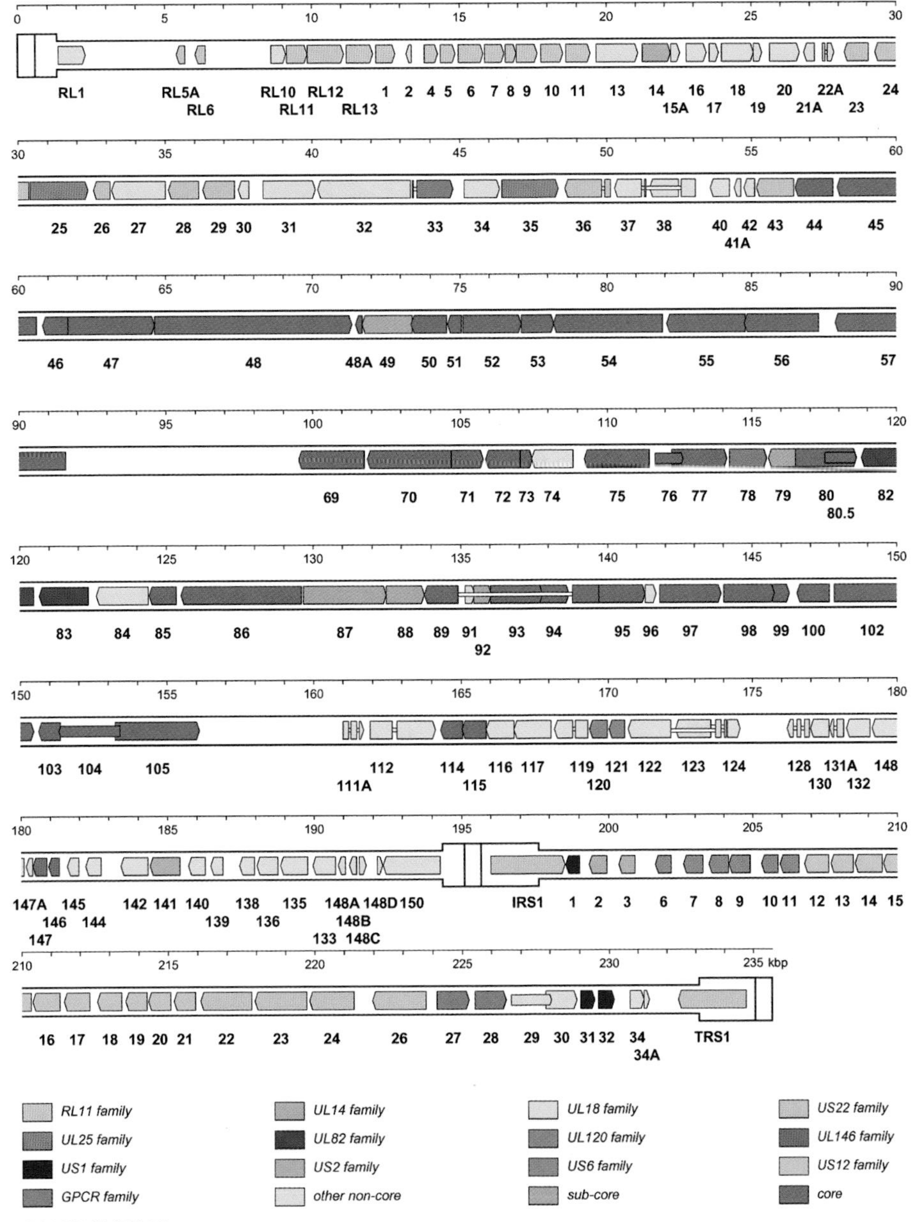

COLOR PLATE 31 (Chapter 22) Consensus genetic map of wild-type HCMV based on the Merlin genome. RL and RS (which contain the *a* sequence as a direct repeat at the genome termini and as an inverted repeat internally) are shown in a thicker format than UL and US. Protein-coding regions are indicated by colored arrows grouped according to the key, with gene nomenclature below. Introns are shown as narrow white bars. Genes corresponding to those in AD169 RL and RS are given their full nomenclature, but the UL and US prefixes have been omitted from UL1-UL150 (12 to 194 kbp) and US1-US34A (199 to 231 kbp). Colors differentiate between genes on the basis of conservation across the *Alpha-*, *Beta-*, and *Gammaherpesvirinae* (core genes) or between the *Beta-* and *Gammaherpesvirinae* (subcore genes), with subsets of the remaining noncore genes grouped into gene families. GPCR, G-protein-coupled receptor. (Reprinted from reference 46 with permission.)

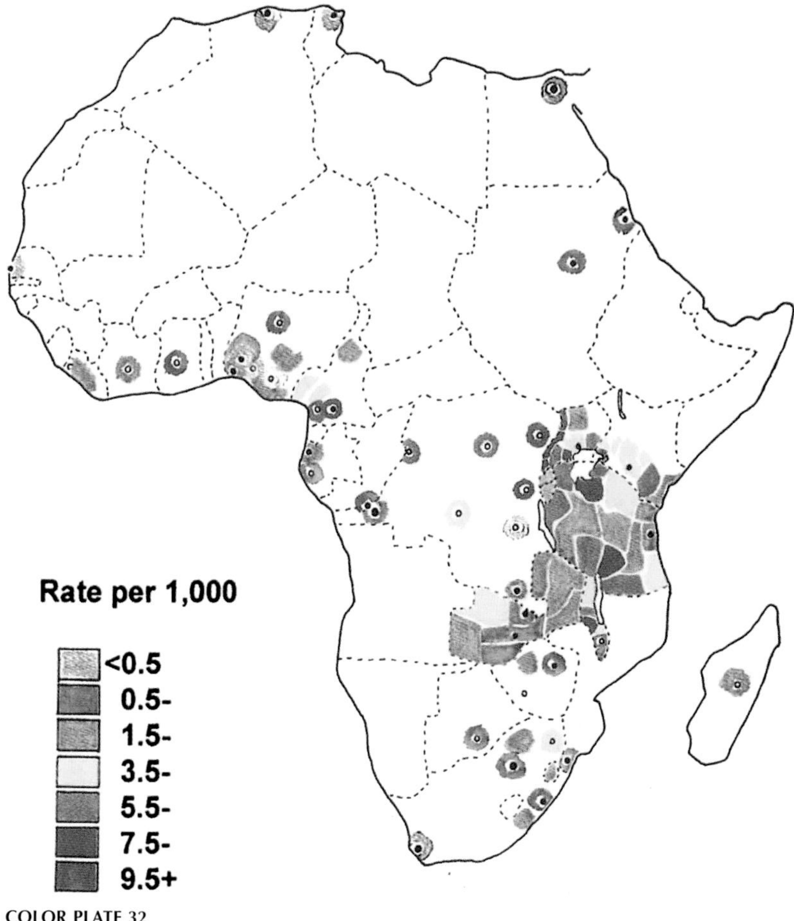

COLOR PLATE 32

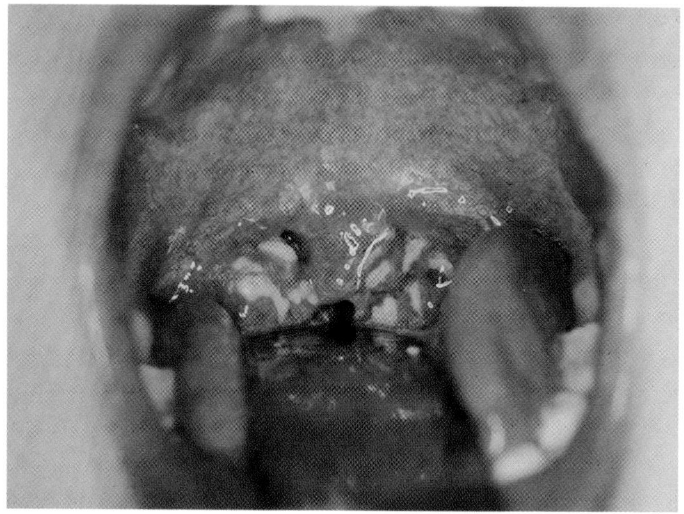

COLOR PLATE 33

COLOR PLATE 32 (Chapter 25) Map of KS prevalence throughout Africa prior to the AIDS epidemic. This map was constructed from surveys performed by Denis Burkitt, who first described Burkitt's lymphoma. It is evident that KS was hyperendemic throughout this continent. With the onset of the AIDS epidemic, a second epidemic of KSHV-related cancer has occurred, and KS is the most commonly reported cancer in most sub-Saharan African countries.

COLOR PLATE 33 (Chapter 26) Adenoviral tonsillitis in a 3-year-old child. Note the follicular exudates. (Reprinted from reference 114 with permission.)

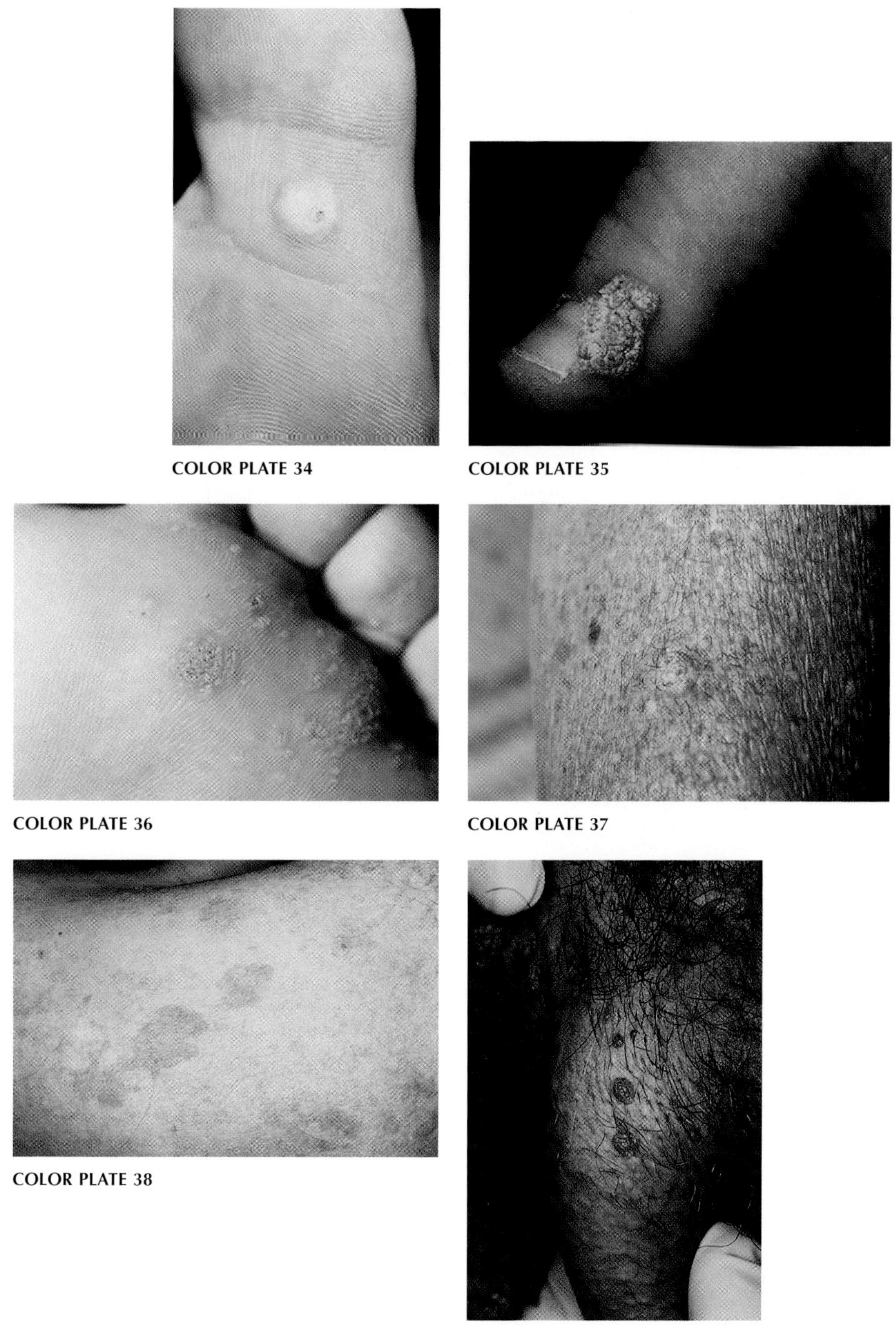

COLOR PLATE 34

COLOR PLATE 35

COLOR PLATE 36

COLOR PLATE 37

COLOR PLATE 38

COLOR PLATE 39

COLOR PLATE 34 (Chapter 28) Plantar wart, myrmecia. (Courtesy of Mark H. Goldgeier, University of Rochester.)

COLOR PLATE 35 (Chapter 28) Common wart. (Courtesy of Mark H. Goldgeier, University of Rochester.)

COLOR PLATE 36 (Chapter 28) Plantar wart, mosaic wart. (Courtesy of Mark H. Goldgeier, University of Rochester.)

COLOR PLATE 37 (Chapter 28) Warty keratosis on the forearm of a transplant recipient. (Courtesy of Anthony A. Gaspari, University of Maryland.)

COLOR PLATE 38 (Chapter 28) Epidermodysplasia verruciformis, pityriasis-like plaques caused by HPV. (Courtesy of Eliott J. Androphy, University of Massachusetts.)

COLOR PLATE 39 (Chapter 28) Condylomata acuminata of the penis. Lesions are at different stages of development.

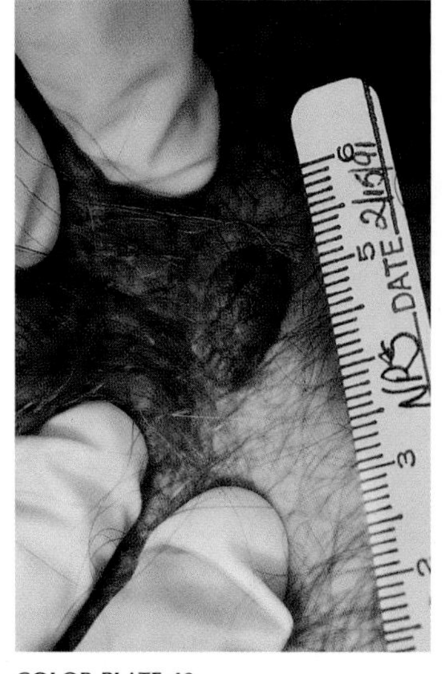

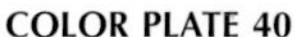

COLOR PLATE 40

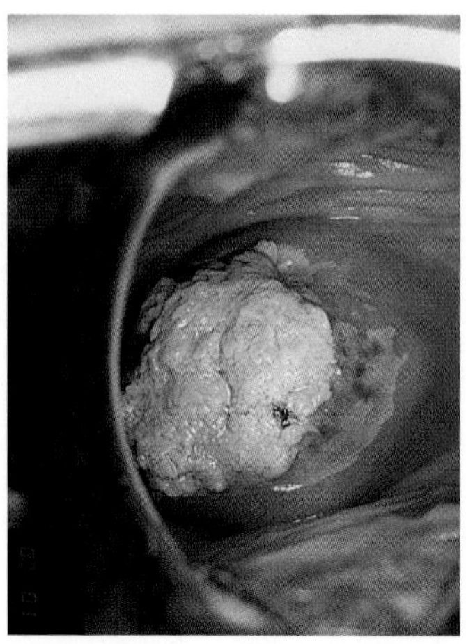

COLOR PLATE 41

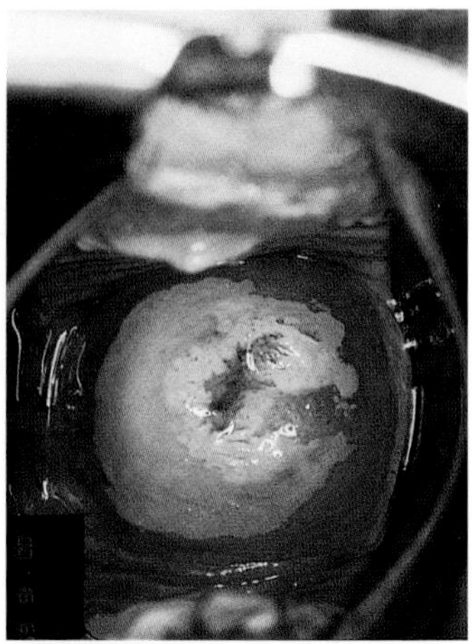

COLOR PLATE 42

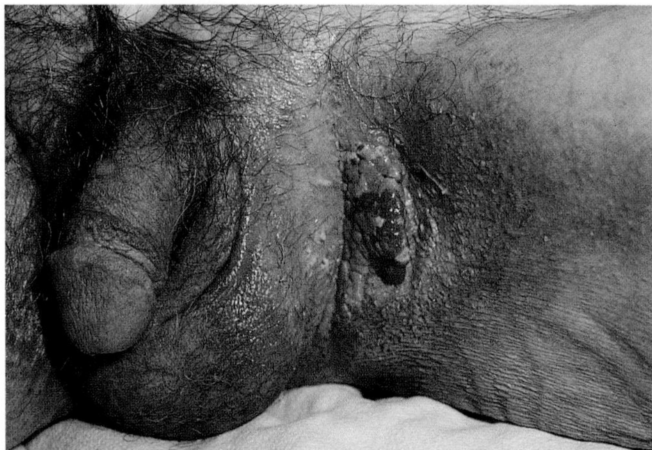

COLOR PLATE 43

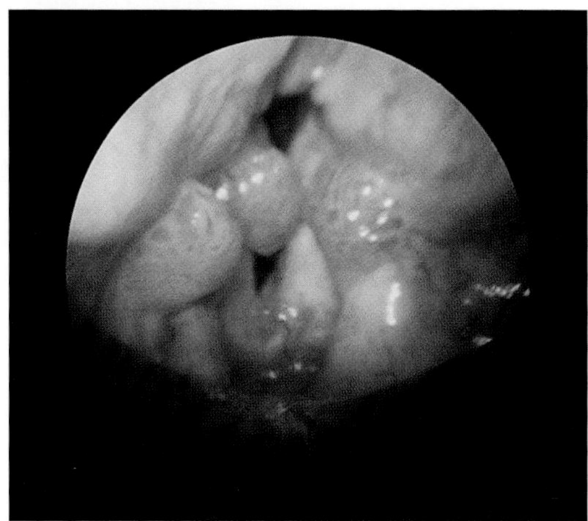

COLOR PLATE 44

COLOR PLATE 40 (Chapter 28) Large pigmented condyloma acuminatum of the inguinal fold. The clinical appearance is also consistent with bowenoid papillomatosis.

COLOR PLATE 41 (Chapter 28) Colpophotograph showing a well-developed cervical condyloma adjacent to a flat, pale acetowhite area (upper quadrants of the cervix) with jagged borders and satellite lesions, consistent with a low-grade HPV infection. (Courtesy of Richard C. Cherkis, University of Rochester.)

COLOR PLATE 42 (Chapter 28) Colpophotograph demonstrating different grades of HPV cervical disease. Centered around the cervical os is an acetowhite area with an internal gray-white demarcation and a few punctate vessels suggestive of a moderate-grade lesion. This lesion is surrounded, mostly in the lower quadrants, by a fainter acetowhite area, with straight margins and no vessels suggestive of a lower-grade HPV lesion. (Courtesy of Richard C. Cherkis, University of Rochester.)

COLOR PLATE 43 (Chapter 28) Buschke-Loewenstein tumor of the inguinal fold.

COLOR PLATE 44 (Chapter 28) Laryngeal papilloma narrowing the airway. (Courtesy of Haskins K. Kashima, Johns Hopkins University.)

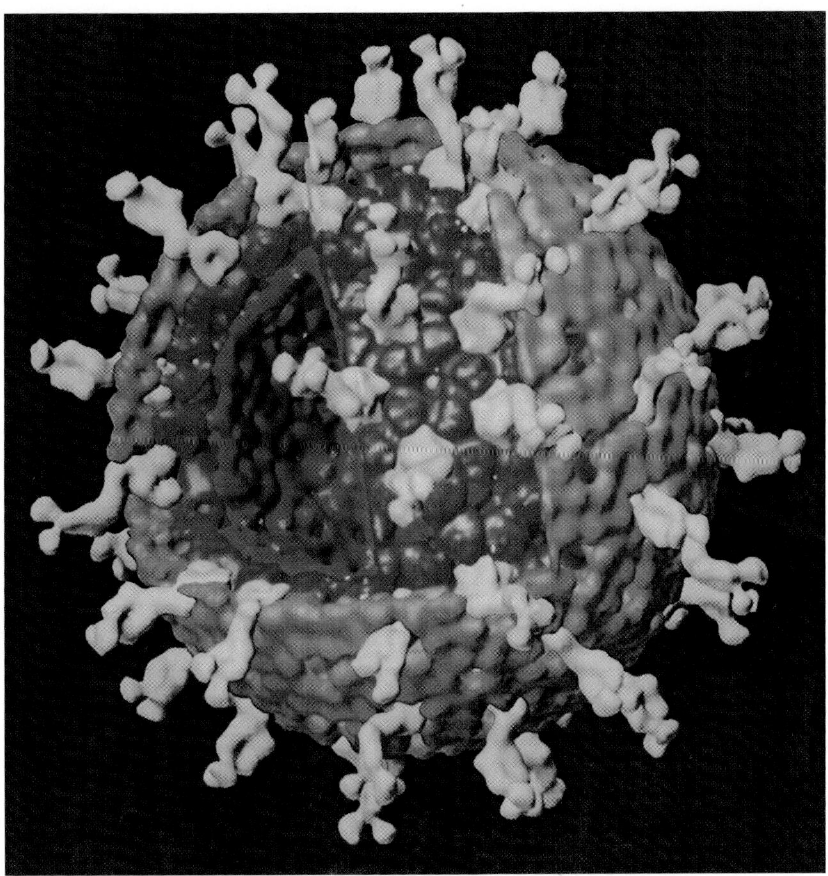

COLOR PLATE 45

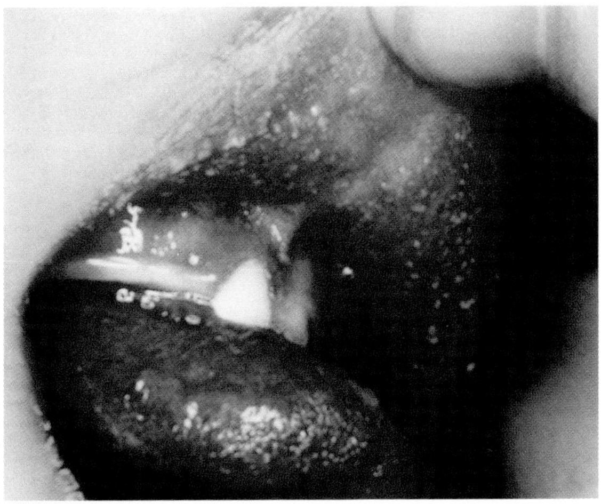

COLOR PLATE 46

COLOR PLATE 45 (Chapter 35) Computer image reconstruction of a rotavirus TLP based on cryoelectron microscopy. The diameter of the viral particle, including the spikes, is 1,000 Å. Both the outer and inner capsids are constructed with a T = 131 (levo) icosahedral lattice symmetry. VP4 (the spike protein) and VP7 compose the outer viral layer; in the cutaway, the middle layer is composed of VP6, and inside this layer can be seen the core (that surrounds VP1 and VP3 and the viral RNA) formed by VP2. (Image courtesy of Mark Yeager, reproduced with permission from reference 155.)

COLOR PLATE 46 (Chapter 37) Koplik's spots on the oral mucosa of a child with measles seen just after the appearance of the rash. The erythematous mucosa is peppered with numerous tiny bluish-white elevations. (Courtesy of the late Saul Krugman.)

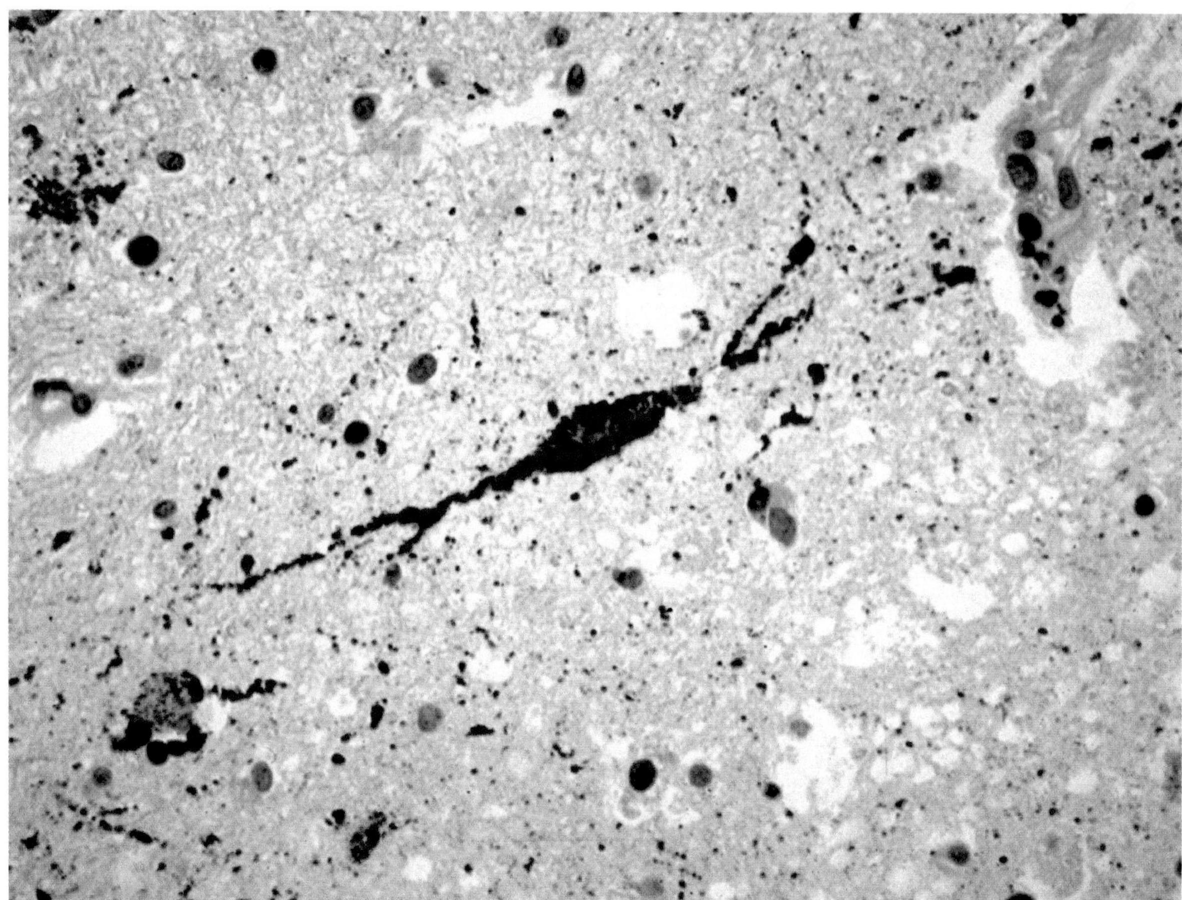

COLOR PLATE 47

COLOR PLATE 47 (Chapter 39) NiV infection in the brain of a person for whom the infection was fatal. Viral antigens are present in neurons and neuronal processes. Immunoalkaline phosphatase staining, naphthol fast red substrate with light hematoxylin counterstain; original magnification, ×100. (Photomicrograph courtesy of S. R. Zaki and W. J. Shieh.)

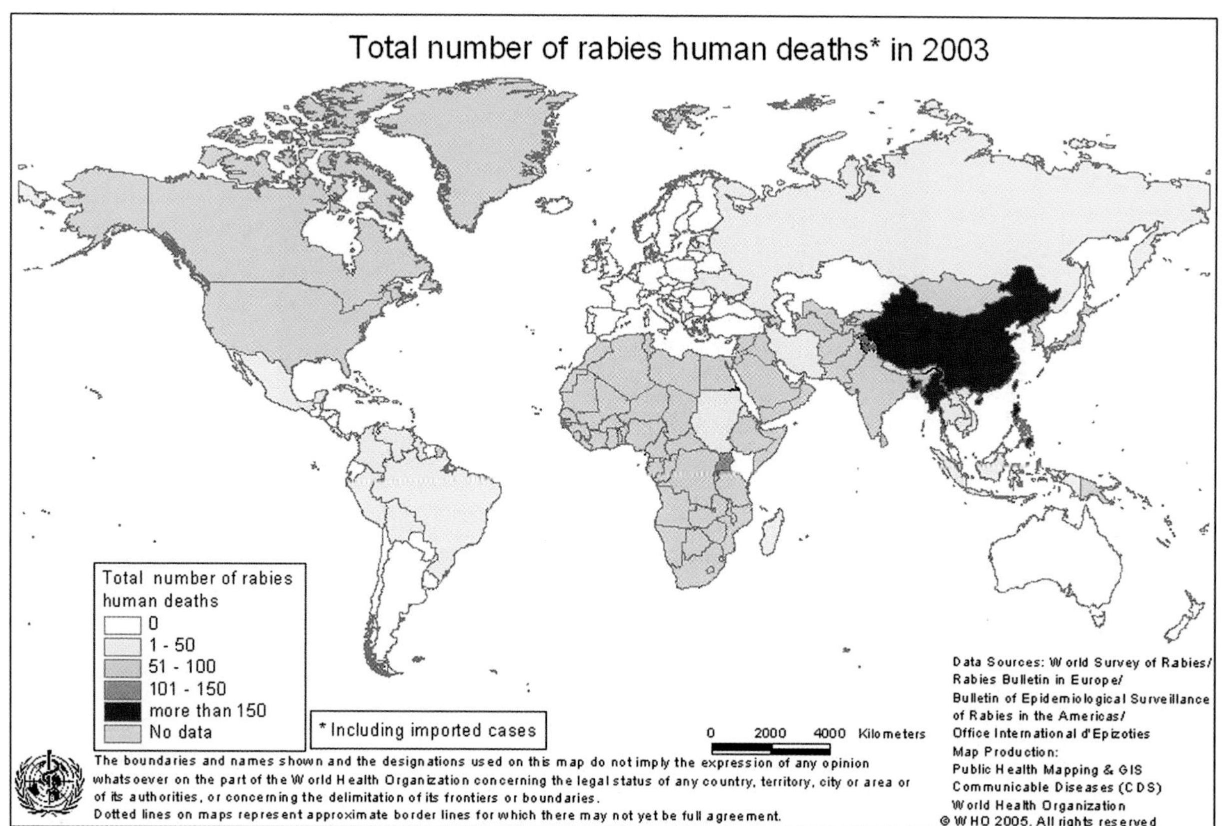

COLOR PLATE 48

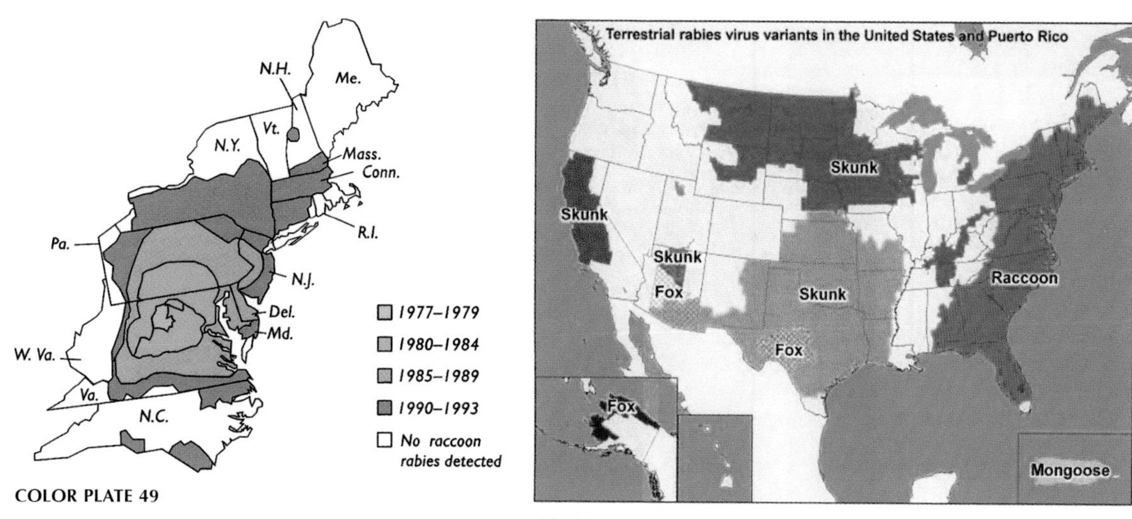

COLOR PLATE 49

COLOR PLATE 50

COLOR PLATE 48 (Chapter 40) Map of human rabies deaths in 2003. (Source: World Health Organization [http://gamapserver.who.int/mapLibrary/app/searchResults.aspx].)

COLOR PLATE 49 (Chapter 40) Concentric spread of raccoon rabies in the eastern United States between 1977 and 1993. (Reprinted from reference 31a with permission.)

COLOR PLATE 50 (Chapter 40) Distribution of terrestrial rabies strains in the United States in 2006. (Reprinted from reference 16.)

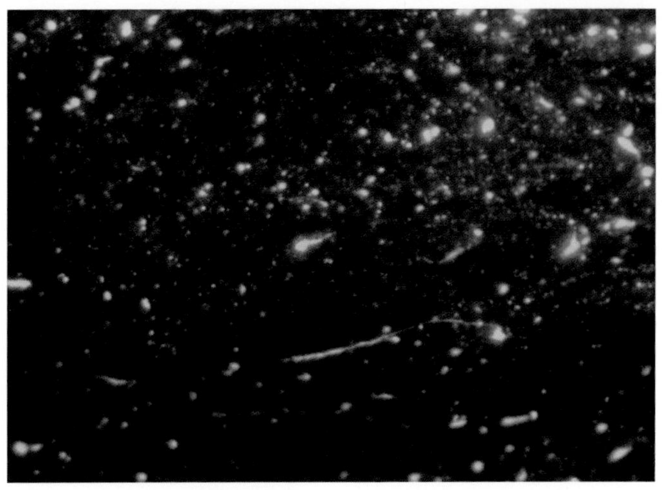

COLOR PLATE 51

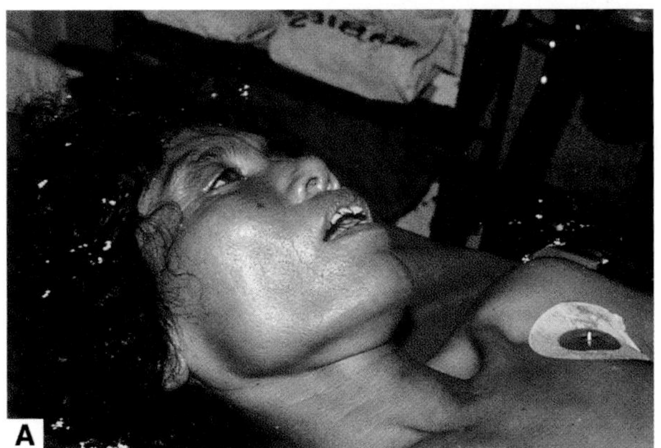

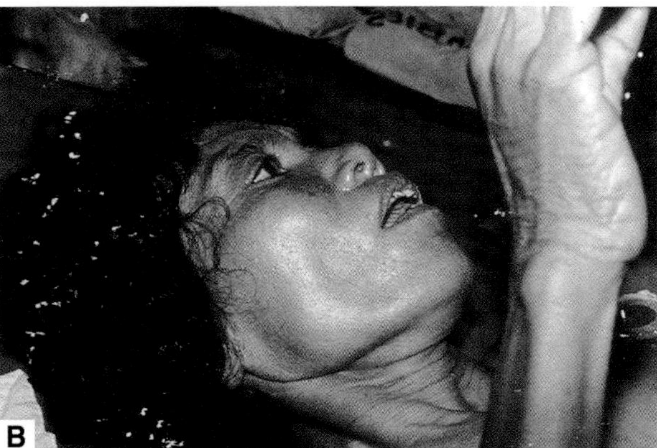

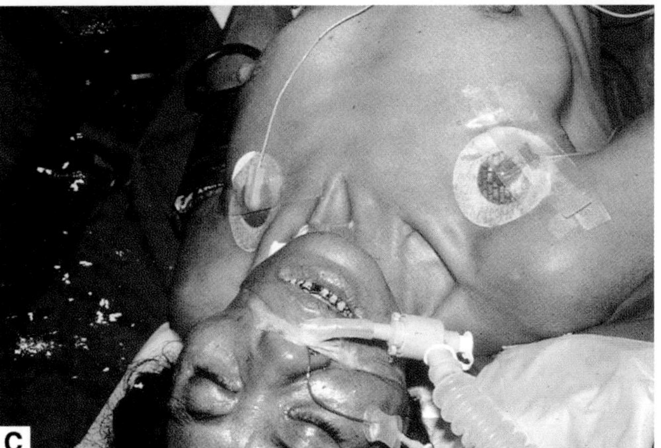

COLOR PLATE 52

COLOR PLATE 51 (Chapter 40) Immunofluorescence staining of rabies antigen in brain tissue.

COLOR PLATE 52 (Chapter 40) Clinical features of furious rabies. (A) The grimace and stare which accompany the pharyngeal spasms of hydrophobia. (B) Aerophobia provoked by air movement across the patient's face. (C) Inspiratory spasm. (Reprinted from reference 78a with permission of *Current Medicine*.)

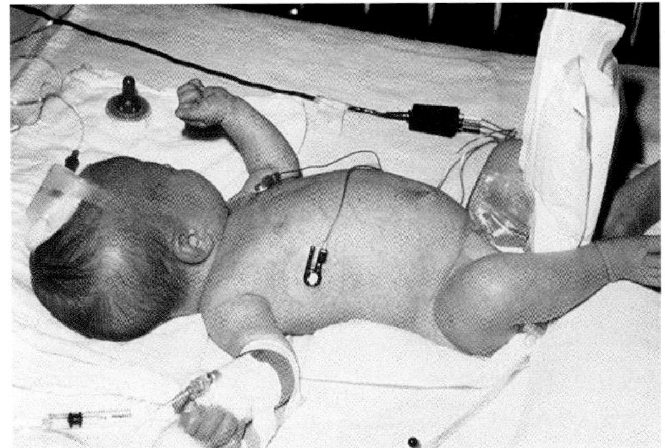

COLOR PLATE 53

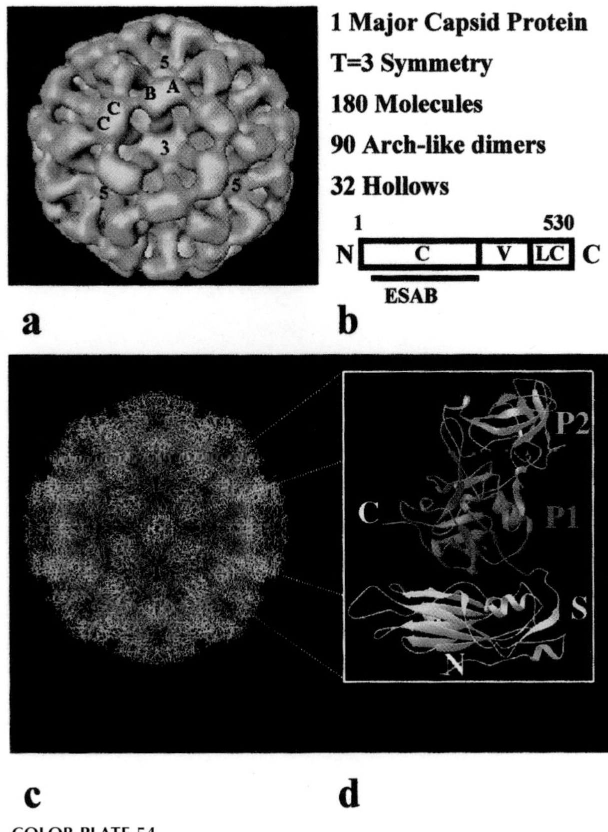

COLOR PLATE 54

COLOR PLATE 53 (Chapter 45) Newborn with overwhelming sepsis due to echovirus 11. Note typical EV exanthem. This child's illness began within the first week of life and ended with her death due to hepatic failure at approximately 1 month of age.

COLOR PLATE 54 (Chapter 48) Structure of Norwalk virus (NV) particles. (a) Surface representation of the three-dimensional surface structure of recombinant NV (rNV) particles viewed along the icosahedral threefold axis. This structure was determined by image processing of the rNV particles shown in Fig. 1C. The rNV particles have a distinct architecture, and they exhibit T=3 icosahedral symmetry; the twofold, threefold, and fivefold axes of symmetry are shown. Cup-like depressions are evident at the threefold and fivefold axes. The capsid structure is made up of 90 arch-like dimers of a single protein that form two types of capsomers; A/B capsomers (n = 60) surround the three- and fivefold axes of symmetry, and C/C capsomers (n = 30) are located at the twofold axes of symmetry. (b) Summary of the properties of the single protein that makes up the NV capsid structure. A linear schematic of the three domains (C, conserved; V, variable; LC, less conserved) in the single capsid protein and a region predicted to fold into an eight-stranded antiparallel beta-barrel is shown. (c) X-ray crystallographic structure of rNV capsid at 3.4-Å resolution, as viewed along the icosahedral twofold axis. Only backbone atoms of the 180 subunits are depicted, and the structure is depth cued, with deeper blue at lower radii and lighter blue at higher radii. (d) Ribbon presentation of the C subunit of rNV capsid protein. The N-terminal arm, S domain, and P1 and P2 subdomains are colored in green, yellow, red, and blue, respectively. The N and C termini of the capsid protein are indicated. The C terminus faces a hollow, the N terminus faces the interior of the capsid, and the P2 subdomain faces the exterior of the capsid. (Panels a, c, and d kindly provided by B. V. V. Prasad; modified from references 105a and 106 with permission.)

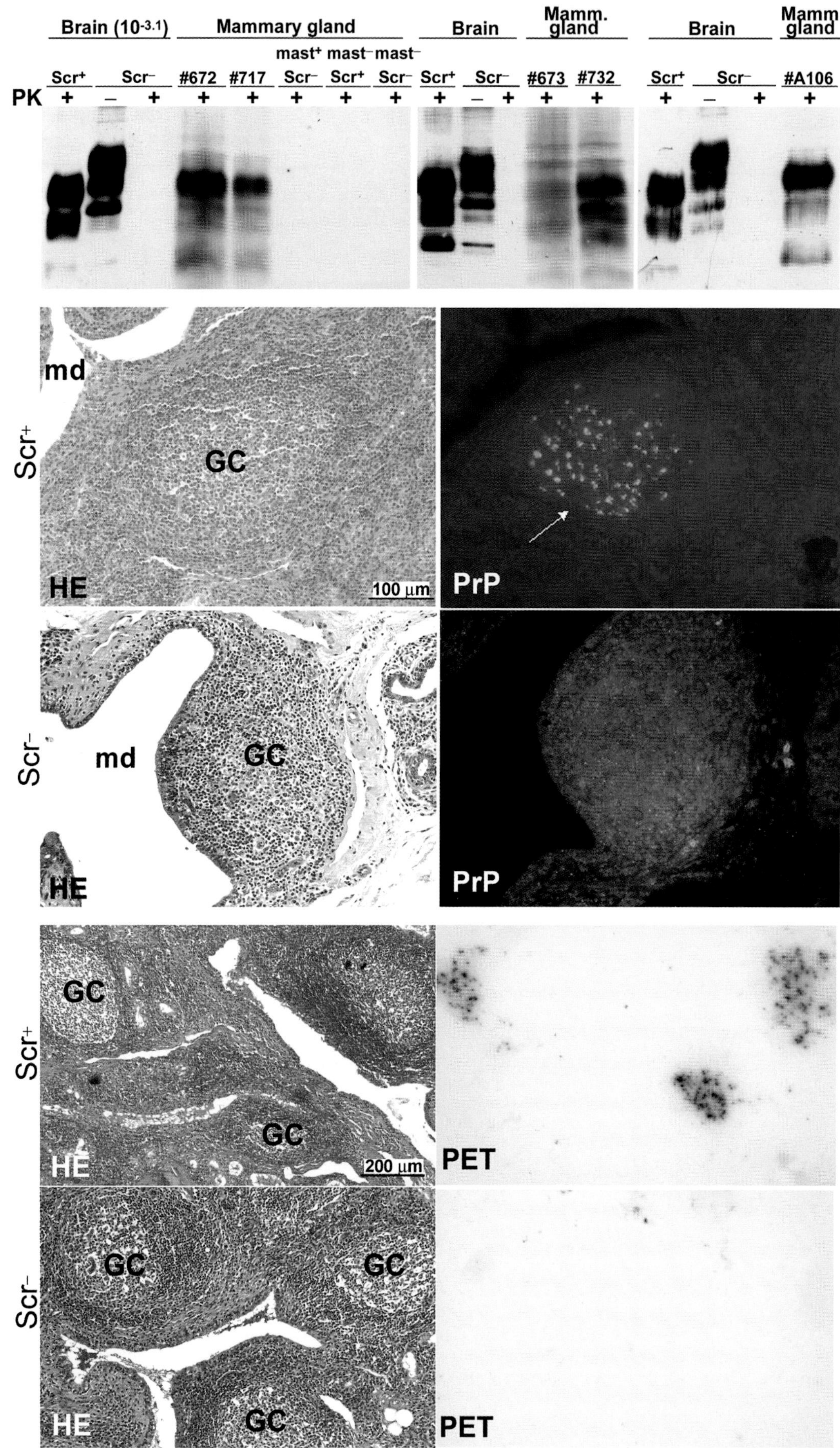

Brain (10-3.1)
Mammary gland
Brain
Mamm. gland
Brain
Mamm. gland
mast+ mast− mast−
Scr+
Scr−
#672
#717
Scr−
Scr+
Scr−
Scr+
Scr−
#673
#732
Scr+
Scr−
#A106
PK
md
GC
Scr+
HE
100 μm
PrP
Scr−
md
GC
HE
PrP
GC
Scr+
GC
HE
200 μm
PET
GC
GC
Scr−
HE
GC
PET

COLOR PLATE 55 (Chapter 57) Inflamed mammary glands of scrapie-infected sheep accumulate PrP^{Sc}. (Top) Western blots with a PrP-specific antibody. Lanes 1 to 3, 9 to 11, and 14 to 16 from left: native and PK-digested brain homogenates (diluted 1,400-fold) from a scrapie-infected (Scr^+) and a scrapie-free (Scr^-) sheep. Lanes 6 to 8: mammary glands from an Scr^- sheep with follicular mastitis ($mast^+$), an Scr^+ sheep from a flock with neither visna/maedi virus seropositivity nor mastitis ($mast^-$), and an Scr^- $mast^-$ sheep. Each one of five Scr^+ $mast^+$ sheep displayed mammary PrP^{Sc} (lanes 4, 5, 12, 13, and 17). Non-scrapie-infected brain and mammary gland extracts showed no PrP^{Sc} upon PK digestion (lanes 3, 6 to 8, 11, and 16). (Middle) Mammary gland micrographs from visna/maedi virus-seropositive Scr^+ $mast^+$ sheep and from Scr^- $mast^+$ sheep. Lymphoid follicles are adjacent to milk ducts (md). Immunofluorescence stains reveal abundant PrP deposits within mammary lymphoid follicles (arrow) from Scr^+ but not from Scr^- sheep. GC, germinal center (the area including FDCs). (Bottom) PK-treated paraffin-embedded tissue (PET) blots of mammary gland sections reveal punctate PrP^{Sc} deposits colocalizing with lymphoid follicles in Scr^+ $mast^+$ but not in Scr^- $mast^+$ sheep. HE, hematoxylin and eosin.

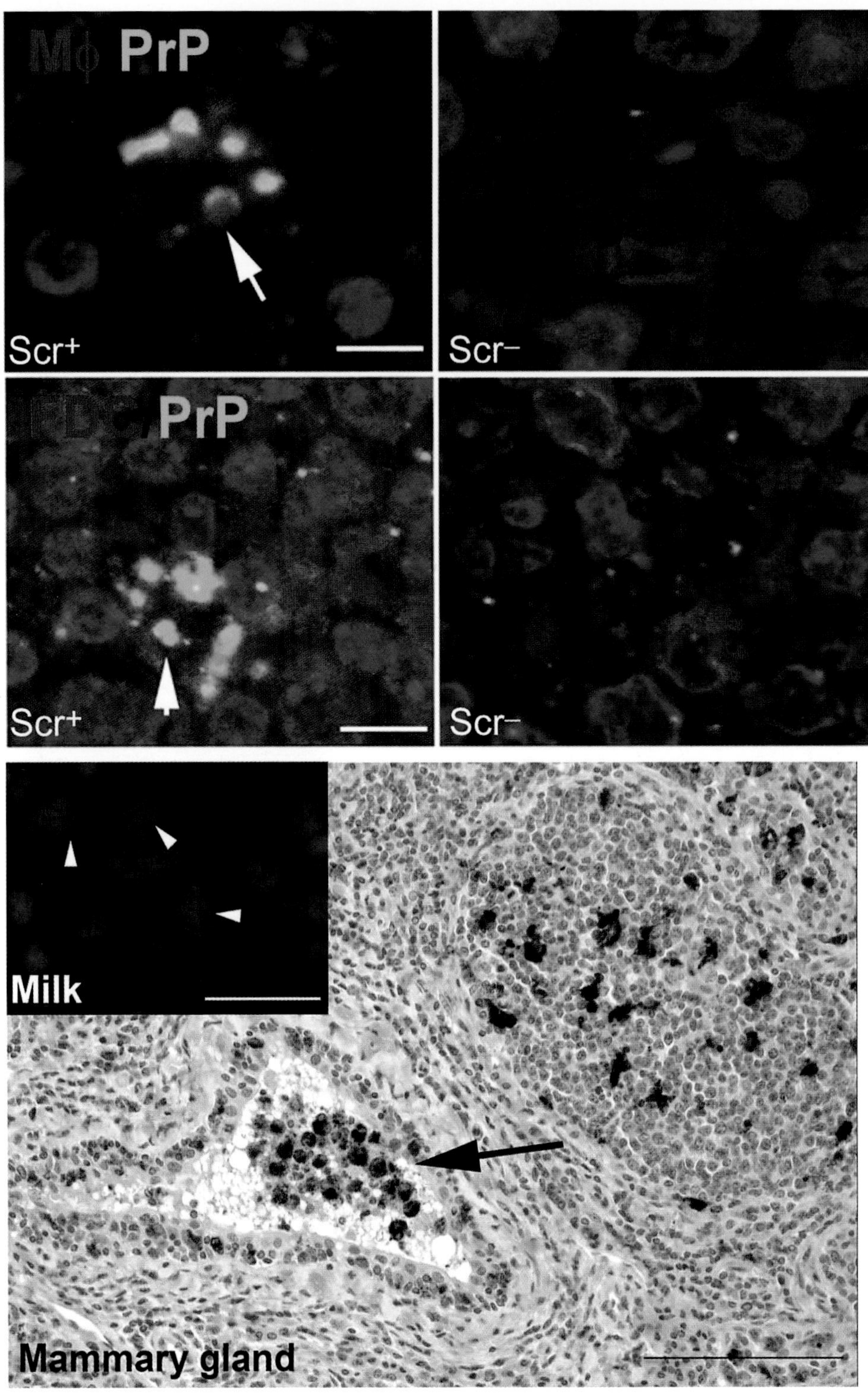

COLOR PLATE 56

COLOR PLATE 56 (Chapter 57) Mammary PrP^{Sc} localizes to macrophages and FDCs. (Top) Mammary gland from a sheep with coincident mastitis, visna/maedi virus seropositivity, and scrapie (sample no. 732). Shown are confocal laser scanning micrographs of lymphoid follicles immunostained for PrP (green), macrophages (Mϕ, red) or FDCs (red), and nuclear DNA (blue). PrP^{Sc} associates with $CD68^+$ Mϕ and FDCs in scrapie-positive (Scr^+, arrows) but not in scrapie-free (Scr^-) sheep. Bars = 6.3 μm (top) and 7.5 μm (bottom). (Bottom) $CD68^+$ macrophages (arrow) and degenerating leukocytes within milk ducts and in adjacent lymphoid follicles of an inflamed mammary gland, as well as in milk sediment (inset, arrowheads). Bars = 100 μm (mammary gland) and 20 μm (milk cells).

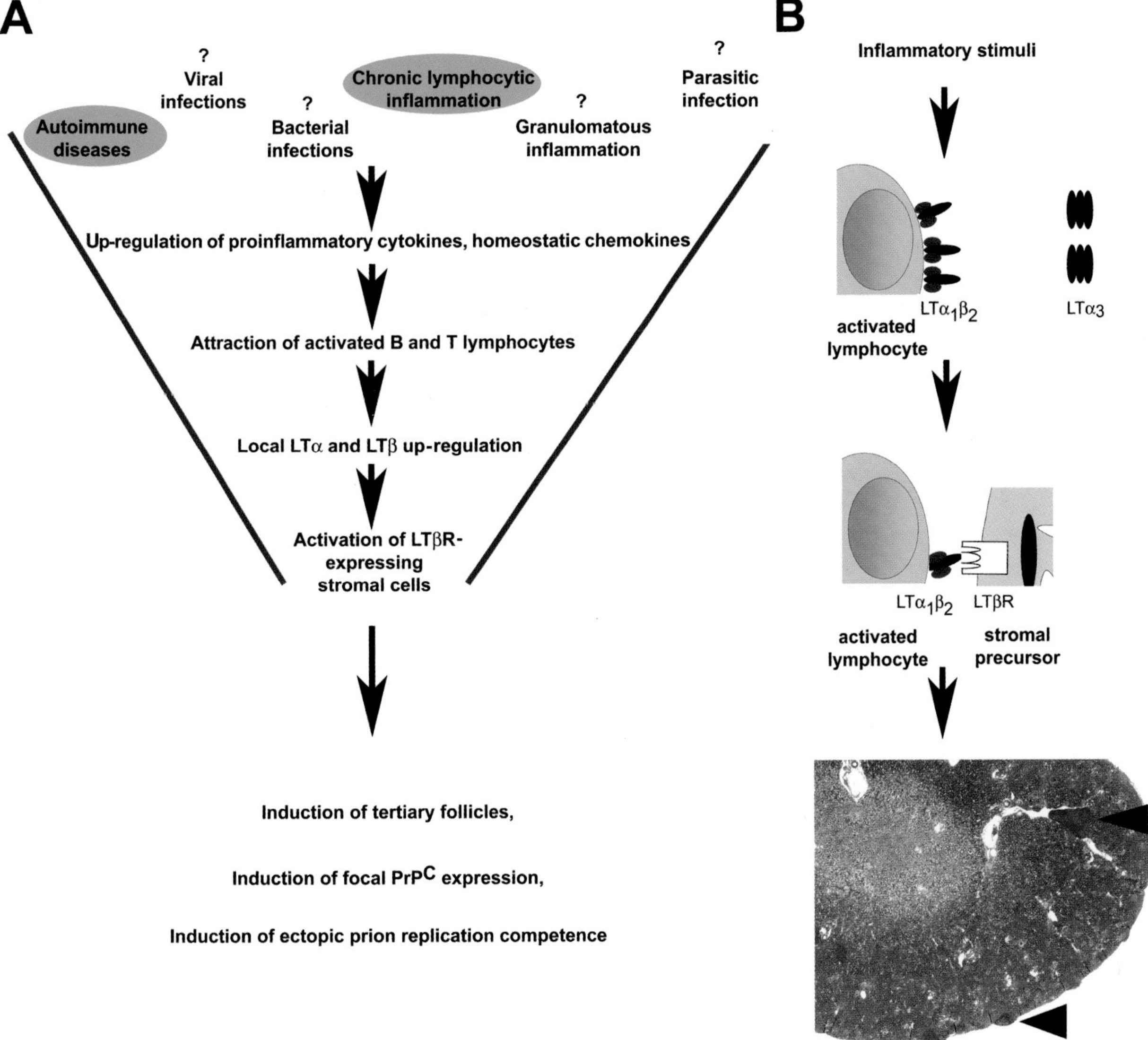

COLOR PLATE 57

COLOR PLATE 57 (Chapter 57) Induction of tertiary follicles and prion replication competence in nonlymphoid organs. (A) Hypothetical hierarchical cascade inducing the generation of tertiary follicles in nonlymphoid organs, and possibly giving rise to ectopic prion replication competence. Autoimmune diseases as well as chronic lymphocytic inflammations have been demonstrated to induce prion replication competence in nonlymphoid organs (green), whereas others have not been investigated yet (question marks). (B) Schematic drawing of the events that contribute to the generation of tertiary follicles upon an inflammatory stimulus that has attracted and activated lymphocytes and induced up-regulation of LTs. LTβR$^+$ stromal precursor cells will be activated upon binding to LTs (LTα_3 or LT$\alpha_1\beta_2$) provided by lymphocytes, leading to the expression of homeostatic chemokines and further LTs, generating a positive-feedback loop that leads to the formation of tertiary follicles containing FDCs and other cells of the immune system.

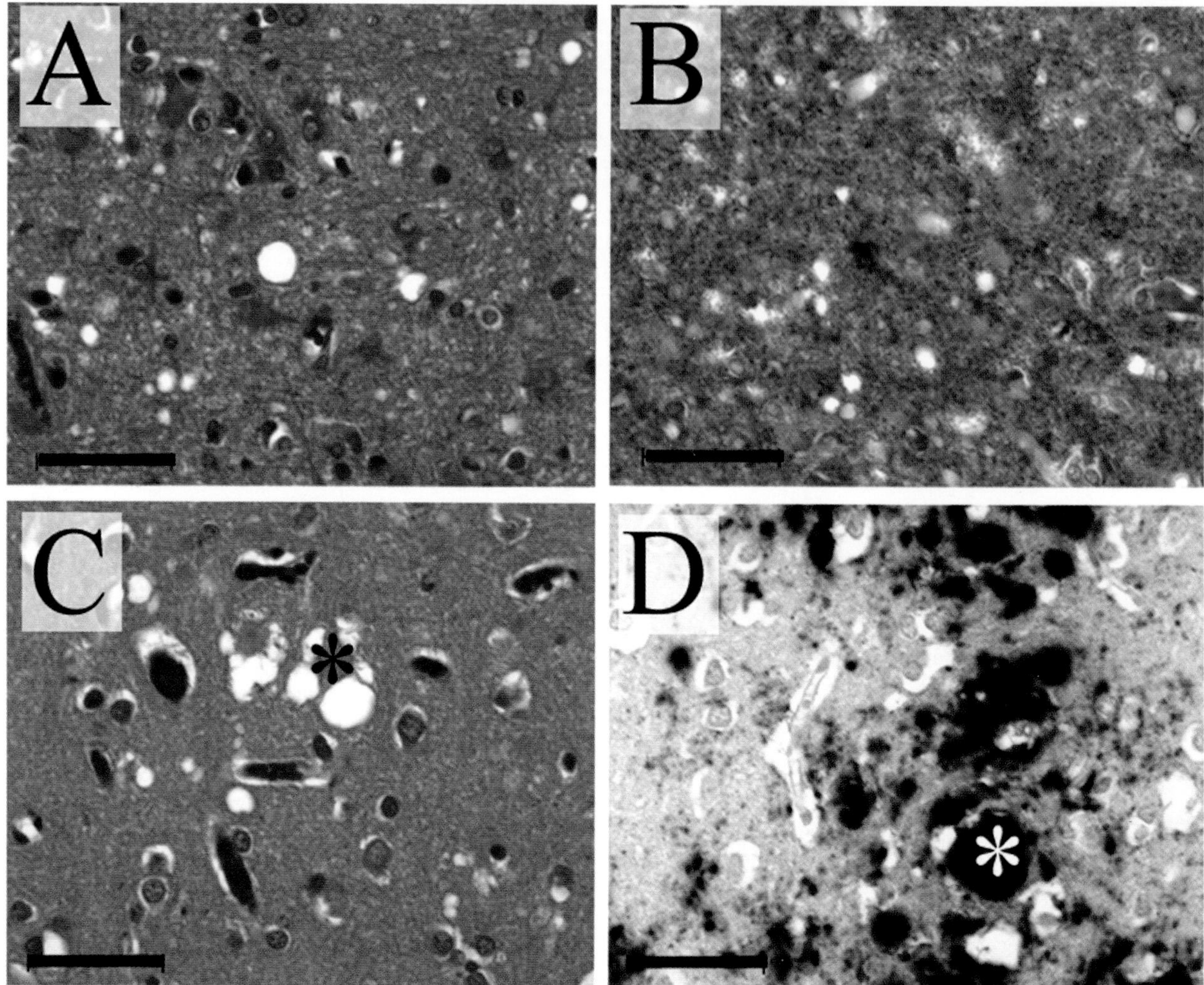

COLOR PLATE 58

COLOR PLATE 58 (Chapter 57) Histologic features of prion diseases. CNS parenchyma of sCJD (A and B) and vCJD (C and D) showing astrogliosis and widespread spongiform changes. PrP depositions are synaptic (A and B) and in the form of florid plaques (asterisks [C and D]). Panels A and C are standard hematoxylin-eosin stains; panels B and D are immunohistochemical stainings for PrP. Bars = 50 μm.

Measles Virus

WILLIAM J. MOSS AND DIANE E. GRIFFIN

37

Measles is a highly contagious disease caused by infection with measles virus (MV) and characterized by a prodromal illness of fever, cough, coryza, and conjunctivitis followed by the appearance of a generalized maculopapular rash. Measles is one of the most important infectious diseases of humans and has caused millions of deaths since its emergence thousands of years ago. MV most closely resembles rinderpest virus, a pathogen of cattle, and probably evolved as a zoonotic infection in communities where cattle and humans lived in close proximity. MV is thought to have become established in humans about 5,000 to 10,000 years ago when populations achieved sufficient size in Middle Eastern river valley civilizations to maintain virus transmission.

Abu Becr, an Arab physician also known as Rhazes, is generally credited with distinguishing smallpox from measles in the 9th century. He dated the first description of measles to the 6th century. However, epidemics identified as measles were not recorded until the 11th and 12th centuries, and measles was first mentioned as a childhood disease in 1224. The name "morbilli" was derived from the Italian meaning "little diseases" to distinguish it from plague, "il morbo." Thomas Sydenham's description of an outbreak of measles in London in 1670 provided an accurate clinical picture of the disease, called attention to its increased severity in adults, and recorded the danger of pulmonary complications. Sanvages in 1763 defined morbilli as measles but called it rubeola, leading to confusion with rubella.

Introduction of MV into previously unexposed populations has been associated with high mortality. Thousands died as a result of European exploration of the New World, largely due to the introduction of diseases such as smallpox and measles into native Amerindian populations. The high mortality from these diseases facilitated the European conquest of the Americas (87).

Many of the basic principles of measles epidemiology and infection were elucidated by Peter Panum, a Danish physician who was sent to the Faroe Islands in 1846 during a large measles epidemic (110). Panum deduced the highly contagious nature of the disease, the 14-day incubation period, and the lifelong immunity following infection and postulated a respiratory route of transmission.

In the mid-18th century, Francis Home, a Scottish physician, attempted to immunize children by inoculating their scarified skin with blood taken from infected individuals shortly after the rash appeared (35). Of the 12 inoculated children, 10 developed mild measles after a short incubation period of only 8 to 10 days. Home's work was regarded with skepticism until 1905, when Hektoen demonstrated the transmission of measles by transfer of blood from patients in the acute stage to susceptible volunteers. The viral etiology of measles was confirmed when Goldberger and Anderson reproduced the disease in monkeys inoculated with filtered respiratory tract secretions from patients with measles. MV first was isolated from the blood and propagated in tissue culture in 1954 by John Enders and Thomas Peebles (38); their viruses included an isolate from a child named David Edmonston. The development of the widely used live attenuated vaccines, derived from the Edmonston MV strain, soon followed.

VIROLOGY

Classification

MV is a member of the genus *Morbillivirus* within the family *Paramyxoviridae*. Other members of the genus include canine distemper virus, affecting dogs and other mammalian carnivores; rinderpest virus, affecting domestic cattle and swine; peste des petits ruminants virus, affecting sheep and goats; phocine distemper virus, causing epizootic disease in seals; and porpoise and dolphin morbilliviruses, causing epizootic disease in porpoises and dolphins. Morbilliviruses differ from other paramyxoviruses in lacking neuraminidase activity and in the formation of intranuclear inclusion bodies as a distinctive feature of their cytopathology.

Serotypes

There is only one serotype of MV, and recovery from measles confers lifelong immunity to disease. Although antigenic changes have been detected in the hemagglutinin (H) surface protein, these variations have not reduced the protective immunity induced by wild-type MV infection or measles vaccines. MV remains a monotypic virus, probably because of functional constraints on the amino acid sequence and tertiary structure of the MV surface proteins (48).

Genetic and Antigenic Variation

Estimates of MV mutation rates range from 10^{-4} to 10^{-3} per nucleotide per year (83). Despite the high degree of genetic variation expected of a single-stranded RNA virus, analyses of H, fusion (F), nucleoprotein (N), and phosphoprotein (P) gene sequences have shown that MVs isolated during the 1950s and 1960s, including vaccine strains, were remarkably homogeneous. Despite diverse geographic origins and different attenuation methods, these strains differed in sequence by no more than 0.5 to 0.6% at the nucleotide level.

Sequence analyses of the N, H, P, and matrix (M) genes of more recent wild-type MVs have demonstrated some genetic variability relative to vaccine strains and wild-type viruses isolated in the 1950s and 1960s. Genetic characterization of wild-type MVs is based on sequence analysis of the genes coding for the N and H proteins. One of the most variable regions of the MV genome is the 450-nucleotide sequence at the carboxy terminal of the N protein, with up to 12% variability between wild-type viruses. The World Health Organization recognizes 8 clades of MV (designated A through H) and 23 genotypes (145). New genotypes will probably be identified with improved surveillance and molecular characterization. As measles control efforts intensify, molecular surveillance of circulating MV strains can be used to document interruption of MV transmission and to identify the source and transmission pathways of MV outbreaks (121).

These genetic changes have been accompanied by minor antigenic changes in the corresponding H, N, and M proteins of some wild-type MV isolates (132). Serum specimens from vaccinated persons and from persons naturally infected during the 1950s and 1960s have comparable neutralization titers to vaccine viruses and to recently isolated wild-type MVs, although sera from persons infected in the 1990s have higher neutralization titers to the homologous wild-type virus (132). As an example of how genetic changes have not significantly altered important antigenic epitopes, MV isolates from a genotype circulating in the People's Republic of China during 1993 and 1994 differed from other wild-type viruses by as much as 6.9% in the H gene and 7.0% in the N gene but did not differ significantly from other wild-type viruses in their anti-H monoclonal antibody-binding patterns and were neutralized by human postvaccination antiserum (148). Thus, neutralizing epitopes on the H protein are highly conserved among MVs. Many centuries of selective pressure exerted by naturally acquired immunity, and more recently by vaccine-induced immunity, have not resulted in the selection of new antigenic types.

Composition of the Virus

Virion Morphology

Measles virions are spherical, enveloped particles with a helical nucleocapsid and are morphologically indistinguishable from the virions of other paramyxoviruses (Fig. 1). The virion diameter averages 150 nm and varies between 100 and 250 nm. The envelope, a lipid bilayer derived from the plasma membrane of the infected host cell, carries surface projections composed of two transmembrane glycoproteins, the H and F proteins. On the inner surface of the envelope is the M protein, which interacts with the nucleocapsid and cytoplasmic tails of the H and F transmembrane glycoproteins to play a key role in virus maturation (Fig. 2). The helical nucleocapsid is packed within the envelope in the form of a symmetrical coil consisting of about 2,500 copies of the N protein bound to the genomic RNA, together with a relatively small number of copies of the P protein and the large polymerase protein (L).

Genome

The MV genome consists of linear, single-stranded, nonsegmented RNA of negative polarity and contains about 16,000 nucleotides (Fig. 2), although the number of nucleotides varies between virus strains and even between viruses of the same strain with different passage histories. The genome begins at the 3′ end with a 53-nucleotide leader sequence that shows a high degree of complementarity to the extragenic 40-nucleotide trailer sequence at the 5′ end of the genome, theoretically allowing the formation of a stable panhandle structure. It is likely that these regions contain sequences that promote encapsidation of the nascent RNA by N protein and binding sites for the viral RNA polymerase. After the leader sequence are six consecutive nonoverlapping genes that encode the N, P, M, F, H, and L proteins (Fig. 2). The P gene encodes two additional nonstructural proteins, C and V. The intergenic regions consist of a single trinucleotide, GAA, with a single variation between the H and L genes. In addition, there is an untranslated GC-rich region of about 1,000 nucleotides at the M-F gene boundary that spans the 5′ end of the M gene and the 3′ end of the F gene.

Structural and Regulatory Proteins

Six MV gene products are structural proteins (Table 1). Three proteins, N, P, and L, are complexed with viral RNA to form the nucleocapsid, and three proteins, M, H, and F, participate in the formation of the virus envelope. There is a transcriptional gradient from N to L for the mRNAs that encode these proteins, and this determines their relative abundance. The N mRNA is the first transcribed from the genome and thus is the most abundant. When expressed from a recombinant vaccinia virus or a plasmid containing only the N gene, N is an insoluble protein that migrates to the nucleus, where it self-assembles into helical nucleocapsid-like structures. When coexpressed with the P protein in MV-infected cells, N is retained in the cytoplasm as a soluble N-P complex. N binds both to RNA and to P and is required for transcription and replication. The N protein surrounds genomic and antigenomic RNAs that possess the leader sequence to form nucleocapsid structures, which are the templates for both mRNA transcription and RNA replication. The conserved N-terminal portion of the protein is required for self-assembly into nucleocapsids and for RNA binding (77). The C-terminal 125 residues are more variable, and this domain belongs to a family of proteins with intrinsically disordered regions, structurally similar to the acidic activation domains of cellular transcription factors (84). Sequence differences in the variable C terminus of N provide the basis for the identification of different MV genotypes, and this portion of the N protein contains a major T-cell epitope.

The P protein is a polymerase cofactor activated by phosphorylation that forms tetramers and links L to N to form the replicase complex. The P protein modulates the assembly of functional MV nucleocapsids after binding to individual molecules of N protein in the cytoplasm to form a soluble N-P complex that is required for RNA encapsi-

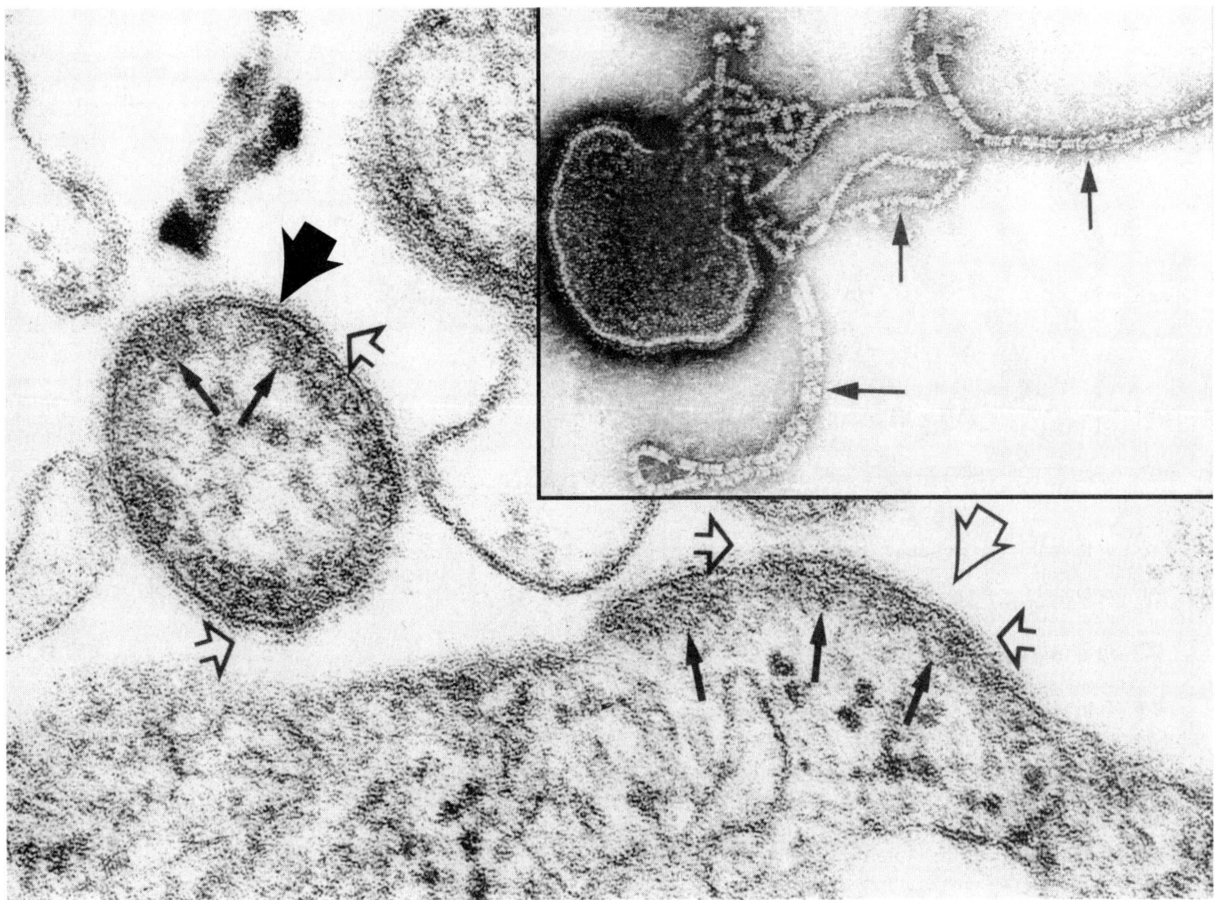

FIGURE 1 MV growing in cell culture. An extracellular virion (large solid arrow) is coated with glycoprotein spikes (small open arrows), with the viral nucleocapsid (small solid arrows) positioned beneath the envelope. An infected cell has a region on the membrane (large open arrow) with viral glycoprotein spikes and subjacent viral nucleocapsids that is a site of MV maturation and budding. Free paramyxovirus nucleocapsids (small solid arrows) from a disrupted viron are shown in the inset. (Courtesy of Cynthia Goldsmith, William Bellini, and Erskine Palmer of the Centers for Disease Control and Prevention, Atlanta, GA.)

dation. P also binds to the L protein to form an L-P complex that is involved in mRNA transcription and genome replication. The P gene of MV, like that of many members of the *Paramyxoviridae* family, encodes nonstructural proteins in addition to P. C is a basic protein translated using an initiator methionine codon in an overlapping reading frame. V shares the initiator methionine and the amino-terminal 231 amino acids of the P protein, but a nontemplated guanosine residue is added through RNA editing that shifts the reading frame to produce a different C terminus that is cysteine rich and has zinc-binding properties. Neither C nor V is necessary for MV replication in vitro, but both interact with cellular proteins to down-regulate the response to infection, particularly the production of alpha and beta interferons (IFN-α and IFN-β) (17, 97).

The L protein interacts with the P protein to form the MV RNA-dependent RNA polymerase. Although P is required for polymerase activity, the L protein, which contains six regions that are highly conserved among the RNA polymerases of minus-strand RNA viruses, appears to contain the catalytic activities.

H is the receptor-binding protein and an important determinant of cellular tropism. It is a type II transmembrane glycoprotein on the surface of infected cells and of virions, and it is present as a disulfide-linked homodimer which self-associates to form tetramers. H has a 34-amino-acid cytoplasmic tail preceding a single hydrophobic transmembrane region and a large C-terminal ectodomain with a propeller-like structure and 13 strongly conserved cysteines. The primary function of H is to bind to MV receptors on the surface of host cells (139). The H protein is also responsible for the ability of measles virions to agglutinate simian erythrocytes by binding to a simian homolog of human CD46. Antibodies that block hemagglutination generally also neutralize virus infectivity. A second essential function of H is to interact with the F protein to mediate fusion of the virion envelope with the host cell membrane and entry of the nucleocapsid into the cell (139).

F is a highly conserved type I transmembrane glycoprotein, synthesized as an inactive precursor, F_0, which is subsequently processed to the active disulfide-linked F_1 and F_2

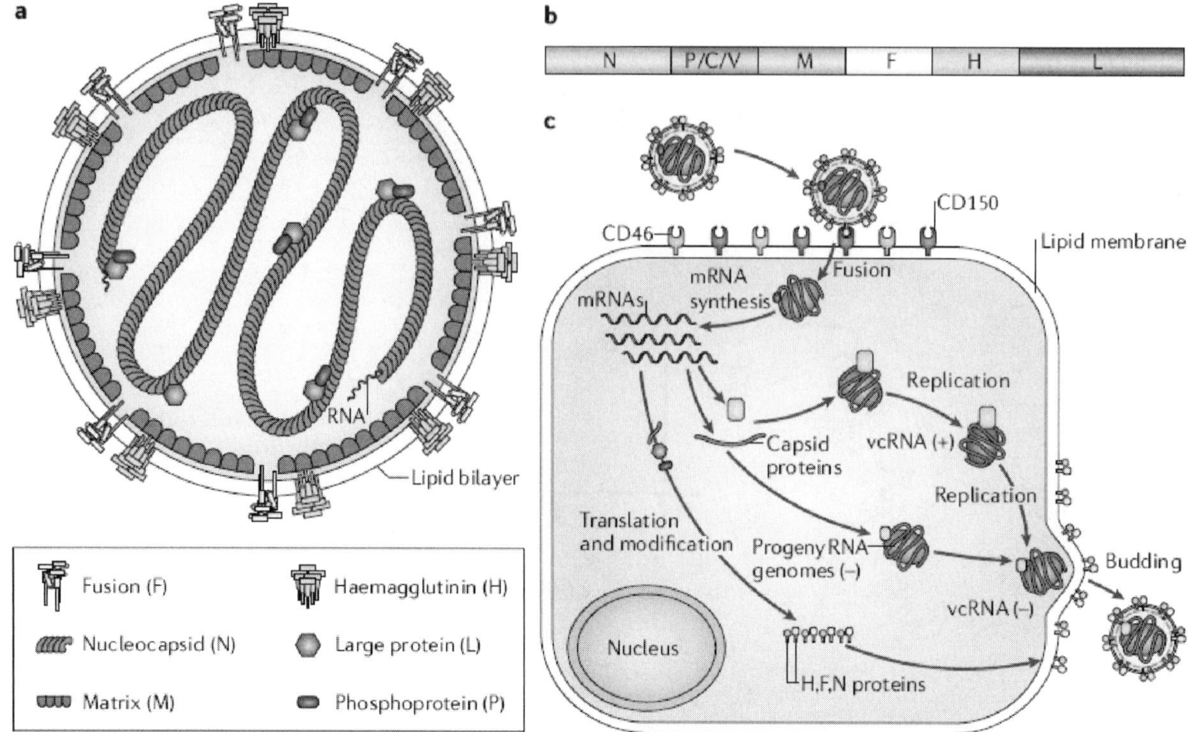

FIGURE 2 MV structure, genome, and replication cycle. (a) MV is a spherical, nonsegmented, single-stranded, negative-sense RNA virus. Of the six structural proteins, the phosphoprotein P, large protein L, and nucleoprotein N form the nucleocapsid that encloses the viral RNA. The hemagglutinin protein H, fusion protein F, and matrix protein M, together with lipids from the host cell membrane, form the viral envelope. (b) The MV RNA genome is composed of approximately 16,000 nucleotides encoding eight proteins, two of which (V and C) are nonstructural proteins alternatively translated from the P gene. (c) The H protein interacts with F to mediate attachment and fusion of the viral envelope with the host cell membrane through specific receptors (CD46 and CD150), enabling viral entry into the cell. The remaining MV proteins are involved in viral replication. The P protein regulates transcription, replication, and assembly of nucleocapsids. The M protein is critical for viral assembly. (From reference 90 with permission of the publisher.)

that cooperate with H for fusion and entry. After synthesis and glycosylation in the endoplasmic reticulum, F_0 is transported to the Golgi, where it is cleaved by furin into F_1 and F_2 (Table 1). The F_1 subunit, derived from the carboxy terminus of F_0, is anchored in the viral envelope and has a cytoplasmic tail, the terminal 14 amino acids of which are highly conserved among morbilliviruses. At its amino terminus there is a 25-amino-acid hydrophobic region, the fusion peptide, which interacts with the host cell membrane to induce fusion and is highly conserved among paramyxovirus fusion proteins. Fully processed active $F_{1,2}$ proteins are found as trimers or tetramers, forming the F peplomers on the surface of infected cells and virions. The function of F is to trigger fusion of the viral envelope with the host cell membrane. Expression of F alone is not sufficient to induce fusion. The interaction of H with the cellular receptor brings the fusion peptide region of the F_1 subunit into a position permitting it to initiate fusion. Synthetic peptide analogs of the fusion peptide inhibit both cell fusion and virus penetration but do not prevent virus attachment.

The M protein, a basic protein with several conserved hydrophilic domains, is the second most abundant viral protein and forms a continuous layer on the inner surface of the envelope. It interacts with progeny nucleocapsids and with the cytoplasmic tails of the F and H proteins to mediate virion maturation. Binding of M to nucleocapsids inhibits transcription of MV mRNA.

Biology

Receptors

Two cellular receptors for MV have been identified: membrane cofactor protein (MCP) or CD46 (29, 99) and signaling lymphocyte activation molecule (SLAM) or CD150 (133). CD46 is a widely distributed human complement regulatory protein expressed on all nucleated cells. It acts as a cofactor for the proteolytic inactivation of C3b/C4b by factor I but also induces proliferation and differentiation of regulatory T cells (79). SLAM is an important costimulatory molecule expressed on cells of the immune system (149). The cytoplasmic domain has tyrosines and SH-2 domain-binding regions that constitute an immunoreceptor tyrosine-based switch motif that binds small SH-2 domain adaptor proteins important for cell signaling. Both vaccine and wild-type strains of MV can use SLAM

TABLE 1 Major structural and regulatory proteins of MV[a]

MV protein	No. of amino acids	Location within: Infected cell	Location within: Virion	Function and special features
Nucleoprotein (N)	525	Cytoplasm	Nucleocapsid	Most abundant of viral proteins. Closely associated with full-length and positive-sense RNA in forming nucleocapsids.
Phosphoprotein (P)	507	Cytoplasm	Nucleocapsid	More abundant in infected cells than in virions. Regulation of transcription and replication. Complex formation with N and L.
C	186	Cytoplasm and nucleus	Not present	Read from the same transcript as P gene, but in different reading frame. Regulates transcription and sensitivity to antiviral effects of alpha and beta interferon.
V	298	Cytoplasm	Not present	Read from an "edited" transcript of P gene. Regulates transcription and sensitivity to antiviral effects of alpha and beta interferon.
Matrix (M)	335	Inner leaflet of plasma membrane; cytoplasm in persistent infections	Inner surface of membrane	Virion assembly and budding.
Fusion (F)	553	Endoplasmic reticulum, Golgi, and plasma membrane	Type I transmembrane surface protein	Glycosylated. Membrane fusion, virus entry, and hemolysis activity in conjunction with H. Active form cleaved from F_0 to F_1 and F_2.
Hemagglutinin (H)	617	Endoplasmic reticulum, Golgi, and plasma membrane	Type II transmembrane surface protein	Glycosylated. Receptor binding. Hemagglutination activity. Disulfide-linked dimer.
Large (L)	2,213	Cytoplasm	Nucleocapsid	Catalytic component of viral polymerase. Least abundant protein. RNA transcription and replication. Complex formed with P.

[a] Adapted from reference 54a with permission of the publisher.

as a receptor. Vaccine strains tend to use CD46 efficiently, whereas wild-type strains often do not. The receptor-binding regions for CD46 and SLAM on H are contiguous or overlapping, and most H proteins can bind both receptors; however, affinity and efficiency of entry differ. In general, binding affinity for SLAM is higher than for CD46, and differences in the efficiency of receptor usage may involve interactions with F.

MV probably uses at least one additional receptor. The distributions of SLAM and CD46 in tissues do not account for the tropism and sites of MV replication in acute infections, where epithelial and endothelial cells, as well as cells of the immune system, are infected, or in chronic infections, where cells of the central nervous system (CNS) are important targets for infection. In addition, several in vitro studies have shown that infection can occur independently of either CD46 or SLAM (66). Receptors used by attenuated vaccine strains adapted to growth in cells from nonsusceptible hosts probably represent an additional category of MV receptors that have not been identified.

Replication

Infection is initiated when the MV H protein on the virion envelope attaches to the extracellular domain of CD46 or CD150. The fusion peptide at the amino terminus of the F_1 subunit, which is physically associated with H, initiates fusion of the envelope with the cell membrane, resulting in entry of the viral nucleocapsid into the cell cytoplasm. The virion RNA-dependent RNA polymerase is then activated and begins transcribing monocistronic mRNAs from the nucleocapsid template.

Transcription occurs sequentially following the gene order. The polymerase terminates synthesis at the end of each gene following polyadenylation and reinitiates at the consensus sequence of the next gene without transcribing the intergenic nucleotides. The viral mRNAs are capped and methylated at the 5′ end and polyadenylated at the 3′ end. The poly(A) tails are synthesized by a slippage or stuttering mechanism in which the polymerase reiteratively copies the sequence of four to seven U's at the end of the gene (70). The polymerase sometimes fails to reinitiate and detaches from the nucleocapsid, resulting in the mRNA abundance gradient (70).

The envelope glycoproteins, H and F, are synthesized and glycosylated in the endoplasmic reticulum, further processed in the Golgi, and transported to the cytoplasmic membrane as oligomers to form the H and F peplomers. The other MV proteins accumulate in the cytoplasm. The availability of N appears to regulate the transition from mRNA transcription to RNA replication because the synthesis of genome length positive- and negative-sense RNAs is coupled to their concomitant encapsidation by N. To initiate encapsidation, the RNA polymerase catalyzes the sequence-specific binding of N from soluble N-P complexes to nascent leader RNA, releasing P protein. The continuing encapsidation by N, which is coupled to further RNA synthesis, masks the consensus signals at each gene boundary, preventing termination and RNA processing and yielding the full-length nucleocapsid. Positive- and negative-sense RNAs are encapsidated, but the majority of the nucleocapsids contain negative-sense viral RNA. A small number of P-L polymerase complexes associate with each of the nucleocapsids.

M proteins associate with the inner surface of the cytoplasmic membrane, with the cytoplasmic tails of H and F, and with each other, excluding cellular membrane proteins from patches of cytoplasmic membrane destined for virion budding. M also binds to newly synthesized nucleocapsids, bringing them into association with these modified areas of cell membrane. Measles virions are produced by budding, and cellular proteins are also required. Progeny nucleocapsids attach to growing actin filaments. The vectorial growth of the actin filament transports the nucleocapsid from the cytoplasm to the plasma membrane, initiating the budding process.

Host Range

Because of the specificity of the host receptors and the high infectivity of MV, humans are the only natural host for MV. Nonhuman primates can be infected experimentally with MV and develop an illness similar to measles in humans, thus serving as models for measles pathogenesis and for the evaluation of vaccines. However, native populations of nonhuman primates are not of sufficient size to maintain MV transmission in the wild. Rodent-adapted strains of MV have been developed by repeated intracerebral passage of virus in newborn animals. Although these strains do not produce an acute disease resembling measles in humans, they also are used as models of MV pathogenesis.

Growth in Cell Culture

Primary cultures of human and monkey kidney cells have traditionally been used for isolating MV. Problems with supply and the potential contamination of primary monkey cells with simian viruses led to the use of continuous monkey kidney cell lines (e.g., Vero cells) for MV isolation and propagation. However, a derivative (B95-a) of the Epstein-Barr virus-transformed marmoset B-lymphocyte cell line B95-8 has greater sensitivity than Vero cells for the isolation of wild-type strains of MV (81). After serial passage in cultures of primary human or monkey kidney cells, MV isolates can be successfully propagated in a wide variety of human and simian cell types and adapted to grow in chicken embryo fibroblasts, an adaptation important for the development of measles vaccines.

The incorporation of MV H and F proteins into the cytoplasmic membranes of infected cells causes them to fuse with adjacent infected and uninfected cells. Consequently, replication of wild-type MV in permissive cells results in characteristic cytopathic effects that include the formation of multinucleated giant cells, as well as the production of eosinophilic intranuclear and intracytoplasmic inclusion bodies. Eosinophilic Cowdry type A intranuclear inclusion bodies are characteristic of morbillivirus infection. The intranuclear inclusion bodies are composed of helical nucleocapsids that appear smooth by electron microscopy and contain only the N protein. In contrast, intracytoplasmic inclusions are composed of helical nucleocapsids that appear "fuzzy" by electron microscopy and contain P and M proteins in addition to N.

Inactivation of MV by Physical and Chemical Agents

MV is inactivated by lipid solvents, such as ether or acetone, and by detergents. It is also acid labile, losing infectivity below pH 4.5, and is inactivated by proteolytic enzymes, by drying on surfaces, and by exposure to sunlight. It is thermolabile, with a half-life at 37°C of 2 h, and is completely inactivated by exposure to 56°C for 30 min. MV may retain infectivity for a week at 0°C and can be stored for long periods at −70°C. It can be freeze-dried, and lyophilized virus is stable for prolonged periods at refrigerator temperature (0°C to 8°C), a characteristic important for the storage and transportation of live attenuated measles vaccines.

EPIDEMIOLOGY

Deaths from measles are due largely to an increased susceptibility to secondary bacterial and viral infections, attributed to a prolonged state of immune suppression. The disease burden caused by measles has decreased over the past decades because of a number of factors. Measles mortality declined in developed countries in association with economic development, improved nutritional status, and supportive care, particularly antibiotic therapy for secondary bacterial pneumonia. The introduction of measles vaccines beginning in the 1960s led to substantial reductions in measles incidence, morbidity, and mortality in both developed and developing countries. Remarkable progress in reducing measles incidence and mortality has been, and continues to be, made in resource-poor countries as a consequence of increasing measles vaccine coverage, provision of a second opportunity for measles vaccination through supplementary immunization activities (SIA), and efforts by the World Health Organization, the United Nations Children's Fund, and their partners to target countries for accelerated and sustained measles mortality reduction. Specifically, this targeted strategy aims to achieve greater than 90% measles vaccination coverage in every district and to ensure that all children receive a second opportunity for measles immunization (147).

In 2003, the World Health Assembly endorsed a resolution urging member countries to reduce the number of deaths attributed to measles by 50% by the end of 2005 compared with 1999 estimates. This target was met. Overall global measles mortality in 2005 was estimated to be 345,000 deaths (uncertainty bounds, 247,000 and 458,000 deaths), a 60% decrease from 1999 (140). This achievement attests to the enormous public health significance of measles vaccination. The new goal is to reduce global measles deaths by 90% by 2010 compared to the estimated number in 2000. To achieve this goal, continued progress needs to be made in delivering measles vaccines to the world's children. Overall global measles mortality in 2006 was estimated to be 242,000 deaths (uncertainty bounds, 173,000 and 325,000 deaths) (146). The largest decrease in measles mortality was in Africa, where measles mortality decreased 91% from 2000 to 2006. Despite this enormous progress, measles remains a leading vaccine-preventable cause of childhood mortality worldwide, particularly in sub-Saharan Africa and Asia, and continues to cause outbreaks in communities with low vaccination coverage rates in industrialized nations.

Geographic Distribution

Measles occurs throughout the world, wherever MV is circulating or introduced into susceptible populations. Most measles cases currently occur in sub-Saharan Africa and Asia. Small isolated populations, such as island populations, cannot sustain MV transmission and require the importation of MV for outbreaks to occur. Sustained indigenous MV transmission has been eliminated in many regions including the Americas. In the United States, the number of measles cases had declined 99.9% by 2006 since the introduction of measles vaccine (122). However, outbreaks in unvaccinated, susceptible populations within the United States continue to occur through importation of MV (111). Persons in the United States who do not receive measles vaccine because of philosophical or religious exemption are at particular risk of measles (43).

Incidence and Prevalence of Infection

MV is one of the most highly contagious infectious pathogens, and measles outbreaks can occur in populations in which fewer than 10% of persons are susceptible. Chains of transmission commonly occur among household contacts, school-age children, and health care workers. The contagiousness of MV is best expressed by the basic reproductive number R_0, which represents the average number of secondary cases that arise if an infectious agent is introduced into a completely susceptible population. In the 1951 measles epidemic in Greenland, the index patient attended a community dance which resulted in an R_0 of 200 (20). In more typical settings, the estimated R_0 for MV is 12 to 18, compared to only 5 to 7 for smallpox virus and 2 to 3 for severe acute respiratory syndrome coronavirus. The high infectivity of MV implies that a high level of population immunity is required to interrupt MV transmission.

There are no latent or epidemiologically significant persistent MV infections and no animal reservoirs. Thus, MV can be maintained in human populations only via an unbroken chain of acute infections, requiring a continuous supply of susceptible individuals. Newborns become susceptible to measles when passively acquired maternal antibody is lost, and they are the main source of new susceptible individuals. For births to provide a sufficient number of susceptible persons to maintain MV transmission, a population size of 300,000 to 500,000 persons with 5,000 to 10,000 births per year is required (13). In smaller populations, episodic outbreaks are dependent on the importation of MV by infected individuals.

Prior to the introduction of measles vaccine, more than 130 million cases of measles and 7 million to 8 million deaths occurred globally each year, and almost everyone was infected during childhood or adolescence. In the United States, the prevalence of antibodies to MV in 18-year-old persons exceeded 98% and the incidence of measles, as in almost every other country, was equal to the number of surviving newborns. The widespread use of live attenuated measles vaccines significantly reduced the incidence of measles and lowered measles morbidity and mortality; indigenous MV transmission has been eliminated in many regions.

Subclinical Infections

MV infections in nonimmune individuals are almost always symptomatic. Subclinical measles is defined as a fourfold rise in MV-specific immunoglobulin G (IgG) antibody titer following exposure to wild-type MV in an asymptomatic individual. Subclinical infection may be important in boosting protective antibody levels in children with waning immunity (138). Whether partially immune individuals with subclinical infection can sustain MV transmission is unknown. However, MV has been isolated from a naturally immune, asymptomatically reinfected individual (135), and acquisition from a person with subclinical infection was implicated in one investigation (143).

Epidemic Patterns

When measles is endemic, its incidence has a typical temporal pattern characterized by yearly seasonal epidemics superimposed on longer epidemic cycles of 2 to 5 years or more. In temperate climates, annual measles outbreaks typically occur in the late winter and early spring. These annual outbreaks are likely to be the result of social networks facilitating transmission (e.g., congregation of children at school) and environmental factors favoring the viability and transmission of MV (44). Measles cases continue to occur during the interepidemic period in large populations but at low incidence. The longer cycles occurring every several years result from the accumulation of susceptible persons over successive birth cohorts and the subsequent decline in the number of susceptible individuals following an outbreak. The interval between epidemics is shorter in populations with high birth rates because the number of susceptible individuals reaches the epidemic threshold more quickly. Measles vaccination programs that achieve coverage rates in excess of 80% extend the interepidemic period to 4 to 8 years by reducing the number of susceptible individuals.

Age-Specific Attack Rates

Secondary attack rates in susceptible household and institutional contacts generally exceed 90%. The average age at MV infection depends on the rate of contact with infected persons, the rate of decline of protective maternal antibodies, and the vaccine coverage rate. Infants in the first few months of life are protected by passively acquired maternal antibodies, and measles is rare in this age group. In densely populated urban settings with low vaccination coverage rates, measles is a disease of young children. The cumulative distribution can reach 50% by 1 year of age, with a significant proportion of children acquiring MV infection before the age of 9 months, the age of routine vaccination in many countries. As measles vaccine coverage increases or population density decreases, the age distribution shifts toward older children. In such situations, measles cases predominate in school-age children. Infants and younger children, although susceptible if not protected by immunization, are not exposed to MV at a rate sufficient to cause a large disease burden in this age group. As vaccination coverage increases further, the age distribution of cases may be shifted into adolescence and young adulthood, as seen in measles outbreaks in the United States and the Americas (25, 72), necessitating targeted measles vaccination programs for these older age groups.

Infants in the first months of life are protected against measles by maternally acquired IgG antibodies. An active transport mechanism in the placenta is responsible for the transfer of IgG antibodies from the maternal circulation to the fetus, starting at about 28 weeks' gestation and continuing until birth. Three factors determine the degree and duration of protection in the newborn: (i) the level of maternal antimeasles antibodies, (ii) the efficiency of placental transfer, and (iii) the rate of catabolism in the child. Although providing passive immunity to young infants, maternally acquired antibodies can interfere with the immune responses to the attenuated measles vaccine by inhibiting replication of vaccine virus (3). In general, maternally acquired antibodies are no longer present in the majority of children by 9 months of age (16), the time of routine measles vaccination in many countries. Women with vaccine-induced immunity tend to have lower anti-MV antibody levels than women with naturally acquired immunity, and their children may be susceptible to measles at an earlier age. The half-life of antimeasles antibodies has been estimated to be 48 days in the United States and Finland but is shorter in some developing countries. Infants born to human immunodeficiency virus (HIV)-infected women may have lower levels of protective maternal antibodies independent of their own HIV infection status and may thus be susceptible to measles at a younger age (127).

Reinfection

Wild-type MV infection induces lifelong immunity to disease, and reinfection is not required to maintain this protective immunity. On reexposure, immune individuals may be reinfected and support limited virus replication, as evidenced by increases in their preexisting levels of humoral and cellular immunity to MV. Such reinfections are almost always asymptomatic and rarely result in transmission of MV to susceptible contacts (see "Subclinical infections" above).

Seasonality

In temperate climates the incidence of measles peaks in late winter and early spring and reaches a nadir in late summer and early autumn. Where widespread immunization has reduced MV transmission, the temporal distribution of cases is determined by importations of MV and outbreaks may occur at any time.

Transmission

MV is transmitted primarily by respiratory droplets over short distances and, less commonly, by small-particle aerosols that remain suspended in the air for long periods. The symptoms induced during the prodrome, particularly sneezing and coughing, enhance transmission. Airborne transmission appears to be important in certain settings, including schools, physicians' offices, hospitals, and enclosed public gathering places (33). Direct contact with infected secretions can transmit MV, but the virus does not survive long on fomites and is inactivated by heat and UV radiation. Transmission across the placenta can occur when measles occurs during pregnancy, but congenital measles is uncommon.

Duration of Infectiousness

Persons with measles are infectious for several days before and after the onset of rash, when levels of MV in blood and body fluids are highest and when the symptoms of cough, coryza, and sneezing are most severe. The fact that MV is contagious prior to the onset of recognizable disease hinders the effectiveness of quarantine measures. MV can be isolated from the urine as late as 1 week after rash onset. MV shedding is prolonged in children with impaired cell-mediated immunity. Giant cells were detected in nasal secretions for up to 28 days after the onset of rash in malnourished Kenyan children with severe measles (125), and MV antigen was detected for up to 13 days after rash onset in malnourished Nigerian children (30). Prolonged presence of MV RNA has been associated with HIV infection (114) and congenital measles (96). However, whether detection of MV by these methods indicates prolonged contagiousness is unclear.

Risk Factors for Transmission

The risk of MV transmission is increased by more frequent, prolonged, and intimate contact between susceptible persons and infectious persons. The risk of transmission is substantially greater if contact occurs when the infectious person is in the late prodromal stage with more pronounced coryza, cough, and sneezing than later when these symptoms have abated. Patterns of air circulation may determine the risk of transmission when airborne transmission is involved. The risk of transmission can be >90% when infected and susceptible children share the same household. In day care centers and schools, the risk of transmission often exceeds 50%.

Nosocomial Transmission

Medical settings are well-recognized sites of MV transmission. Patients may present to health care facilities during the prodrome when the diagnosis is not obvious, although the patients are infectious and likely to infect susceptible contacts. Health care workers can acquire measles from infected patients and transmit MV to others. Nosocomial transmission can be reduced by maintaining a high index of clinical suspicion, using appropriate isolation precautions when measles is suspected, administering measles vaccine to susceptible patients and health care workers, and documenting immunity to measles (i.e., receipt of two doses of measles vaccine or detection of antibodies to MV) in health care workers.

Morbidity and Mortality

Measles case fatality proportions vary, depending on the average age of infection, nutritional and immunologic status of the population, measles vaccine coverage, and access to health care. In developed countries, fewer than 1 in 1,000 children with measles die. In areas of endemic infection in sub-Saharan Africa, the measles case fatality proportion may be 5% or higher. Measles is a major cause of child deaths in refugee camps and in internally displaced populations. Measles case fatality proportions in children during humanitarian emergencies, such as refugees, have been as high as 20 to 30% (124).

The measles case fatality proportion is highest at the extremes of age. Exposure to an index patient within the household may result in more severe disease, perhaps because of transmission of a larger inoculum of virus (1). Vaccinated children, should they develop disease after exposure, have less severe disease and significantly lower mortality rates. Vaccination programs, by increasing the average age of infection, shift the burden of disease out of the age group with the highest case fatality rate (infancy), further reducing measles mortality.

Measles and malnutrition have important bidirectional interactions. Measles is more severe in malnourished children. Children with severe malnutrition, such as those with marasmus or kwashiorkor, are at particular risk of death following measles. Measles, in turn, can exacerbate malnutrition by decreasing intake (particularly in children with mouth ulcers), increasing metabolic demands, and enhancing gastrointestinal loss of nutrients as a consequence of a protein-losing enteropathy. Measles in persons with vitamin A deficiency leads to severe keratitis, corneal scarring, and blindness (128).

Measles mortality may be higher in girls than boys (51), although older historical data and recent surveillance data from the United States do not support this conclusion (115). Supporting the hypothesis of biological differences in the response to MV was the observation that girls were more likely than boys to have delayed mortality following receipt of high-titer measles vaccine (see below) (63). The underlying mechanisms are likely to be differences in immune responses to MV between girls and boys, although no cogent explanation has been developed.

In regions of high HIV prevalence and crowding, such as urban centers in sub-Saharan Africa, HIV-infected children may play a role in sustaining MV transmission (89). Children born to HIV-infected mothers have lower levels of passively acquired maternal antibodies and are thus susceptible to measles at an earlier age than children born to uninfected mothers (91, 127). Protective antibody levels wane within 2 to 3 years in vaccinated HIV-infected children (94). Children with defective cell-mediated immunity can develop measles without the characteristic rash (89). Finally, HIV-infected children have prolonged shedding of MV RNA (114), potentially increasing the period of infectivity. Counteracting the increased susceptibility of HIV-infected children to measles is the high mortality rate of HIV-infected children, particularly in sub-Saharan Africa, such that these children do not live long enough to build up a sizable pool of susceptible children (67). This may change with increased access to antiretroviral therapy.

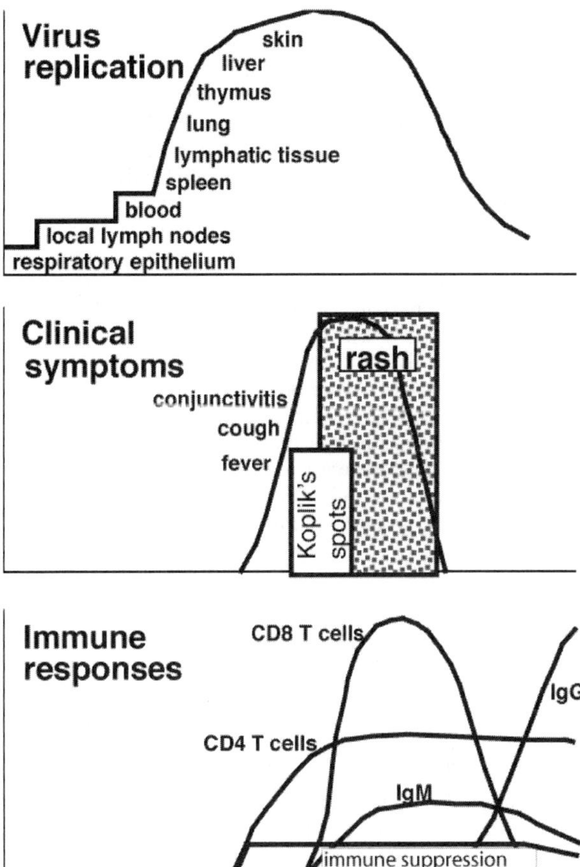

FIGURE 3 Basic pathogenesis of MV infection. Panels summarize features of the pathogenesis of MV infection. (Top) Spread of the virus from the initial site of infection in the respiratory epithelia to the skin. Sites of infection are overlaid with virus titer. (Middle) Appearance of clinical signs and symptoms in relation to viral replication and the immune responses. (Bottom) Immune responses to measles virus. The clinical manifestations arise coincident with the onset of the immune response. (From reference 54b with permission of the publisher.)

PATHOGENESIS IN HUMANS

Incubation Period

The incubation period for measles, i.e., the time from infection to clinical disease, is approximately 10 days to the onset of fever and 14 days to the onset of rash. The incubation period may be shorter in infants or following a large inoculum of virus and may be longer (up to 3 weeks) in adults.

Virus Replication

Infection is initiated when MV reaches epithelial cells in the respiratory tract, oropharynx, or conjunctivae (Fig. 3). The lower respiratory tract is more susceptible than the nasopharynx, which is more susceptible than the oral mucosa. Direct observations pertaining to the early multiplication of MV in humans are lacking, but experimental studies with monkeys and experimental and histopathologic observations of humans suggest that during the first 2 to 4 days after infection MV proliferates locally in the respiratory mucosa and spreads, perhaps within infected pulmonary macrophages and dendritic cells, to draining lymph nodes, where further replication occurs. MV infection of macrophages increases the expression of LFA-1, an integrin that promotes adherence to endothelial cells and transendothelial migration into surrounding tissues (71).

Virus then enters the bloodstream in infected leukocytes, primarily monocytes (42), producing the primary viremia that disseminates infection to sites throughout the reticuloendothelial system. When MV is administered parenterally, bypassing the usual respiratory route, the incubation period is shortened by 2 to 4 days, suggesting that during natural measles the virus is initially confined to tissues at the portal of entry for this period. Lymphoid tissues throughout the body, including tonsils, adenoids, submucosal lymphoid tissue in the respiratory and gastrointestinal tracts, lymph nodes, thymus, spleen, appendix, and Peyer's patches, become major sites of virus replication. Although clinically inapparent, MV replication at these sites is evidenced by lymphoid hyperplasia and the formation of multinucleated giant cells. In the thymus, MV infection of epithelial cells leads to apoptosis of uninfected thymocytes and a decrease in the size of the thymic cortex.

Further replication results in a secondary viremia that begins 5 to 7 days after infection and disseminates MV to tissues throughout the body, including the skin, conjunctivae, CNS, oropharynx, respiratory mucosa, lungs, genital mucosa, kidneys, gastrointestinal tract, and liver (Fig. 3). Replication of MV in these target organs, together with the host immune response, is responsible for the prodromal signs and symptoms that occur 8 to 12 days after infection and mark the end of the incubation period. The prodromal signs and symptoms reflect involvement of epithelial surfaces in the oropharynx, respiratory tract, gastrointestinal tract, and conjunctivae. During this secondary viremia, virus is again carried within infected monocytes and lymphocytes, more than 5% of which may be infected.

Infection of vascular endothelial cells plays a central role in measles pathogenesis. Infection of the endothelial cells of small vessels in the lamina propria and dermis during the secondary viremia precedes infection of the overlying epithelium, and inflammatory changes in and around these vessels are an integral part of the local pathology and characteristic rash.

Pathology

The most striking and consistent pathological feature of MV infection is the formation of multinucleated giant cells that result from the fusion of infected cells with infected and uninfected neighboring cells (Fig. 4). Endothelial cells of small vessels show evidence of MV infection, including inclusion bodies, MV antigens, or MV RNA, during the prodrome and the first days of rash. This is accompanied by vascular dilatation, perivascular infiltration with mononuclear cells, and increased vascular permeability. Changes in the skin, conjunctivae, and mucous membranes of the respiratory and gastrointestinal tracts are secondary to changes in the underlying small blood vessels. MV antigen and RNA also have been detected in perifollicular histiocytes in lymph nodes and spleen, in epithelial cells of Hassall's corpuscles in the thymus, in biliary duct epithelial cells in the liver, in the epithelium of submucosal glands in the respiratory and gastrointestinal tracts, and in the cells lining hair follicles and sweat glands in the skin.

The rash and Koplik's spots of measles have similar pathogenesis and histopathology (Fig. 4). The initial event is infection of endothelial cells in superficial vessels in the dermis. The earliest histopathological changes are mild hyperemia, edema, and lymphocytic infiltration of the dermis, with swelling and proliferation of endothelial cells in capillaries, precapillary vessels, and small veins. MV antigens and viral nucleocapsids can be detected in these endothelial cells on the day before and on the first day of the rash (80). Infection of the overlying epidermis is due to the spread of virus from the infected vascular endothelial cells in the subjacent dermis and by infiltration of infected leukocytes. This leads to the formation of epithelial giant cells containing eosinophilic intracytoplasmic and intranuclear inclusion bodies. A lymphohistocytic infiltrate accumulates around the dilated dermal vessels, and the infected epithelial cells become necrotic. By the third day, this process results in the formation of a vesicle under the stratum corneum that undergoes desiccation and desquamation. In the mucous membranes of the mouth, the necrotic epithelial cells of Koplik's spots slough, leaving a tiny shallow ulcer.

During the secondary viremia, infection of capillary endothelial cells throughout the respiratory tract produces

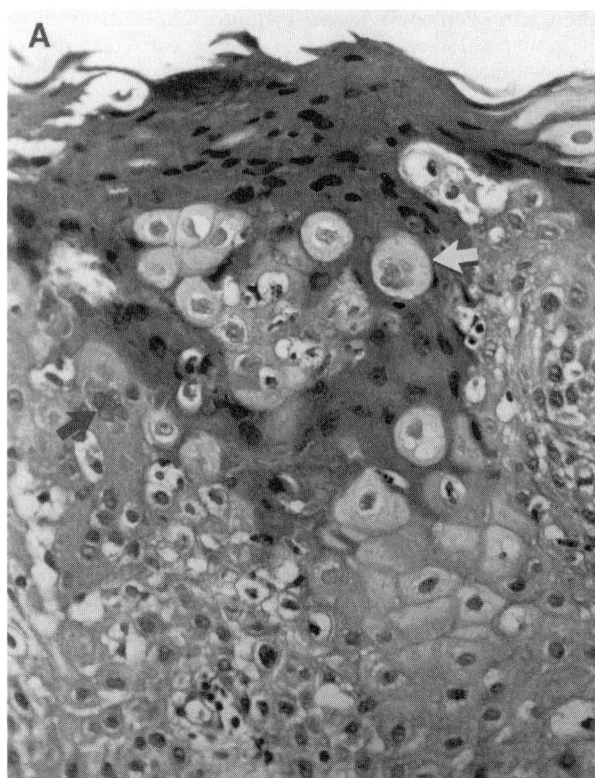

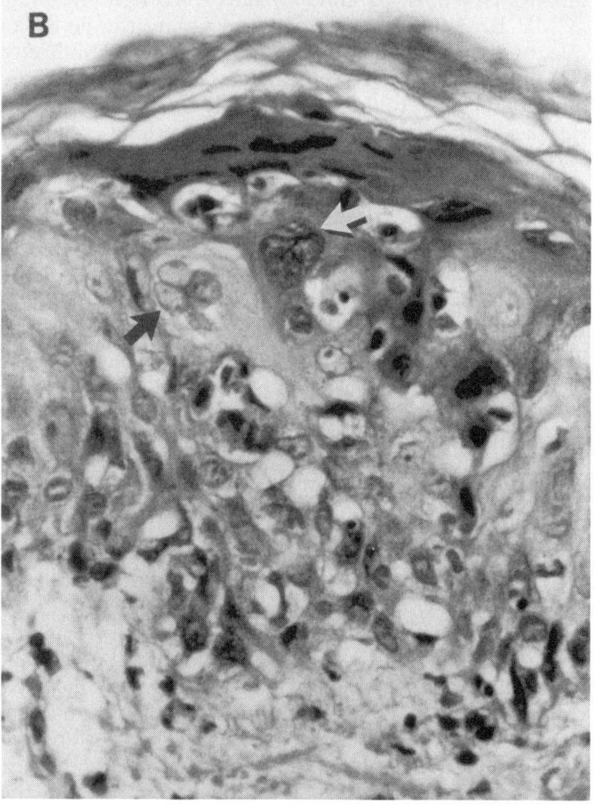

FIGURE 4 Histopathology of Koplik's spots (A) and the skin rash (B) of measles. The epidermal changes in both are characterized by multinucleated giant cells (arrows), focal parakeratosis, dyskeratosis and spongiosis, intracellular edema, and a sparse lymphocytic infiltrate. (Courtesy of D. W. R. Suringa, Tampa, FL.)

foci of peribroncheolar inflammation, dilated submucosal vessels, perivascular and interstitial mononuclear cell infiltrates, and epithelial hyperplasia. Epithelial giant cells develop in the mucosa from the trachea to the alveoli, and some are shed into the lumen. This pathological process is well developed by the onset of the prodrome and accounts for the cough and coryza. The damage caused to the respiratory tract by MV infection also predisposes to secondary bacterial infections. In the normal host, virus replication and giant-cell formation cease within 2 or 3 days after the onset of the rash, and measles giant cells disappear from the respiratory tract shortly thereafter.

Immune Responses

MV-specific immune responses are essential for recovery from measles and for the establishment of long-term immunity to disease, but they also play a role in the pathogenesis of measles and its complications. Immune responses to MV are first apparent during the prodrome and are well developed by the onset of rash. Marked activation of the immune system is manifested by T- and B-cell activation, spontaneous proliferation of peripheral blood mononuclear cells, and increased levels of cytokines and soluble cell surface proteins in the circulation (92) (Fig. 3). Immune suppression, evidenced by impaired delayed-type hypersensitivity skin test responses to recall antigens and reduced humoral and cellular immune responses to new antigens, occurs at the same time and increases susceptibility to secondary viral and bacterial infections (92). Immune activation and suppression persist for many weeks after recovery from measles.

Innate Immune Responses

Nonspecific immune responses contribute to the control of MV replication during the incubation period. MV infection of some types of cells in vitro induces the production of IFN-α and IFN-β, but IFN induction by wild-type strains is generally less efficient than by vaccine strains (100). Increased levels of IFN and IFN-induced proteins are detectable in blood after measles immunization, but elevated levels of biologically active IFN in plasma have not been documented during natural infection (61). MV shuts down IFN production by plasmacytoid dendritic cells but stimulates IFN production by myeloid dendritic cells in vitro (150). Induction of IFN mRNA and protein synthesis may occur at the cell surface through signaling initiated by interaction of the virus with CD46 or Toll-like receptor 2 (TLR-2) or after virus has entered the cell (134).

Humoral Immune Responses

The onset of clinically apparent disease coincides with the appearance of MV-specific adaptive humoral and cellular immune responses (Fig. 3). Antibodies to MV are first detectable within several days after rash onset (14). The isotype of MV-specific antibody is initially IgM; this is followed by a switch to IgG3 and then, in the memory phase, to IgG1 and IgG4 (14). IgM antibodies generally decline to undetectable levels within 6 to 8 weeks. IgG titers rise rapidly, peak within 3 to 4 weeks, and then gradually decline, but they generally persist for life. IgG is initially of low avidity, but the avidity increases steadily over several months. IgG1 is efficiently transported across the placenta, and levels of antibody to MV are often higher in the newborn than in the mother. The role of mucosal immunity to MV is unclear. IgA, IgM, and IgG antibodies to MV are found in secretions, and sampling of saliva has provided a noninvasive method for determining immune status (15).

The most abundant and most rapidly produced antibody is to N. Because of the abundance of anti-N antibody, the absence of this antibody is a reliable indicator of seronegativity. The M protein elicits only small amounts of antibody, except in atypical measles. Antibodies to H are the primary antibodies measured by tests based on neutralization of virus infectivity (27). Human convalescent-phase sera show reactivity to linear epitopes, as well as to epitopes dependent on conformation and glycosylation. Major conformational epitopes have been localized to H regions between amino acids 368 to 396 and in the SLAM-binding region (40). These epitopes were predicted to form part of the exposed surfaces on top of the molecule, and elucidation of the crystal structure of H confirms that the highly conserved binding sites and neutralizing epitopes are positioned in an exposed region of the protein, unshielded from N-linked sugars (22, 65). Antibodies to F contribute to virus neutralization, probably by preventing fusion of the virus membrane with the cell membrane at the time of virus entry (118).

Antibody can protect from MV infection and may contribute to recovery from infection. Antibody is sufficient for protection because infants are protected by maternal antibody, and passive transfer of immune serum can modify or interfere with measles vaccination and can partially protect children from measles after exposure. The best correlate of protection from infection is the level of neutralizing antibody. In infants, the level of maternal antibody correlates with failure of the humoral response to vaccination (3). In outbreaks, antibody levels correlate with protection from disease, with a plaque reduction neutralizing titer of 120 mIU/ml generally considered to be the level needed for protection from disease and 1,000 mIU/ml being the level for protection from infection (19).

IgG antibodies to MV persist for decades and provide lifelong protection (4). Reexposure may boost antibody titers but is not required for long-term immunity. Immunologic memory is evidenced by continued synthesis of antibodies to MV and by persistence of MV-specific T cells. There is no evidence for the persistence of infectious or latent MV, but MV antigens may persist for prolonged periods in follicular dendritic cells in the absence of virus replication. The extensive replication of MV in lymphoid tissues during the acute phase of measles may maximize the input of MV antigens to these cells, contributing to the persistence of MV-specific antibody production (54).

Contributions of antibody to virus clearance are less clear. Failure to mount an adequate antibody response carries a poor prognosis, and levels of antibody-dependent cellular cytotoxicity correlate with clearance of the cell-associated viremia (47). Antibody binding to infected cells alters intracellular virus replication and may contribute to control of infection (49). However, transient depletion of B cells does not affect virus clearance in infected monkeys (112). Children with congenital agammaglobulinemia, who produce no detectable antibody to the virus, recover from MV infection (52). Such evidence indicates that cell-mediated immunity, rather than antibody, is the essential component for MV clearance.

Cellular Immune Responses

A vigorous $CD8^+$ T-cell response occurs during MV infection (Fig. 3). MV-specific and proliferating $CD8^+$ T cells with evidence of clonal expansion are detectable in blood at the time of the rash and in bronchoalveolar lavage fluid during pneumonitis (73). IFN-γ, soluble CD8, and β_2-microglobulin levels are increased in plasma (59, 62) and CD8$^+$ T-cell memory is established after infection (73, 74, 98). Depletion of CD8$^+$ T cells in infected monkeys impairs the control of virus replication (113). MV antigens that induce CD8$^+$ T cells include the N, P, H, and F proteins (73), although H contains the majority of epitopes recognized by HLA-A2-positive humans (103).

CD4$^+$ T cells are also activated in response to MV infection. CD4$^+$ T cells proliferate during the rash, and the concentration of soluble CD4 in plasma is elevated during acute disease and remains so for several weeks after recovery (57). MV-specific T-cell proliferation and the production of cytokines are stimulated during measles, and CD4$^+$ T-cell memory is established after recovery.

MV-specific T cells are responsible for production of a variety of cytokines and soluble factors during disease and recovery. Levels of IFN-γ, neopterin (a product of IFN-γ-activated macrophages), and soluble interleukin-2 receptor in plasma rise during the prodrome, prior to appearance of the rash (59, 60). This is followed by increases in IL-2 levels at the time of the rash. As the rash fades, IL-4, IL-10, and IL-13 levels increase, and elevation of the levels of these cytokines persists in some individuals for weeks (62, 93). This pattern of cytokine production suggests early activation of CD8$^+$ (IFN-γ) and type 1 CD4$^+$ (IFN-γ and IL-2) T cells during the rash followed by activation of type 2 CD4$^+$ T cells (IL-4 and IL-13) and then regulatory T cells (IL-10) during recovery (58).

The cellular immune response is necessary for development of the characteristic measles rash. Biopsies show infiltration of CD4$^+$ and CD8$^+$ T cells and macrophages into areas of virus replication (113). Individuals with deficiencies in cellular immunity may develop measles without a rash (37, 86).

MV-Induced Immunosuppression

The intense immune responses induced by MV infection are paradoxically associated with depressed responses to unrelated (non-MV) antigens, and they last for several weeks to months beyond resolution of the acute illness. This state of immune suppression enhances susceptibility to secondary bacterial and viral infections that cause pneumonia and diarrhea and is responsible for much measles-related morbidity and mortality. Delayed-type hypersensitivity responses to recall antigens, such as tuberculin, are suppressed (131) and cellular and humoral responses to new antigens are impaired following MV infection. Reactivation of tuberculosis and remission of autoimmune diseases have been described after measles and are attributed to this state of immune suppression.

Abnormalities of both the innate and adaptive immune responses following MV infection have been described (Fig. 5) (92). Transient lymphopenia (a reduction in the number of lymphocytes in the blood), with a reduction in both CD4$^+$ and CD8$^+$ T-lymphocyte counts, occurs in children following MV infection (123). Functional abnormalities of immune cells are also detected, including decreased lymphocyte proliferative responses (69). Dendritic cells, major antigen-presenting cells, mature poorly, lose the ability to stimulate proliferative responses in lymphocytes, and undergo cell death when infected with MV in vitro. The dominant type 2 cytokine response in children recovering from measles can inhibit type 1 responses and increase susceptibility to intracellular pathogens (55, 57). The production of IL-12, important for the generation of type 1 immune responses, decreases following binding of the CD46 receptor (78) and is low for several weeks in children with measles (7). This diminished ability to produce IL-12 could result in a limited type 1 immune response to other pathogens. A role for immunomodulatory cytokines in the immune suppression following measles is

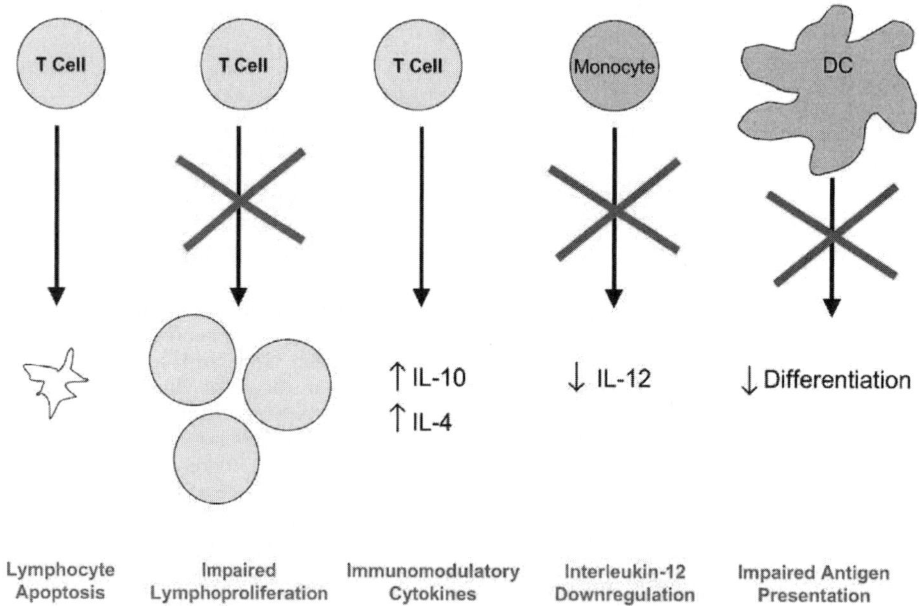

FIGURE 5 Potential mechanisms of immune suppression following MV infection. (From reference 92 with permission of the publisher.)

supported by the finding of elevated levels of IL-10 in plasma from children with measles; this cytokine is capable of inhibiting immune responses (93).

CLINICAL MANIFESTATIONS

Typical Measles

The prodromal phase of measles begins with fever, malaise, and anorexia followed by coryza, conjunctivitis, and cough. The catarrhal symptoms increase in intensity, as does the fever, reaching a peak at the height of the skin eruption on about the fifth day. Coryza can be intense, with a profuse mucopurulent nasal discharge. The cough can be severe, with a brassy, barking quality. Sore throat, eye pain, headache, and myalgia can occur, especially in adolescents and adults. Ocular findings include palpebral conjunctivitis with lacrimation, edema of the lids, photophobia, and punctate keratitis visible on slit lamp examination or with fluorescein staining.

Two to three days before the onset of the rash, Koplik's spots, the pathognomonic enanthem of measles, appear as small (1-mm) white lesions on the buccal mucosa, allowing the astute clinician to diagnose measles prior to the onset of rash (Fig. 6; Color Plate 46). Initially, only a few are present opposite the second molars, but they can spread to coat the entire buccal mucosa. Usually by the third day of rash the lesions slough, the erythema fades, and the mucosal membranes regain their normal appearance. Koplik's spots may not be recognized unless the buccal mucosa is examined carefully, and they may also be seen on the conjunctivae and other mucosal surfaces, including the gastrointestinal tract.

The intense inflammation of lymphoid tissues during the prodrome can result in generalized lymphadenopathy and mild splenomegaly, with posterior auricular, cervical, and occipital lymph nodes typically becoming enlarged. Lymphoid inflammation is also responsible for the most frequent abdominal complication of measles, acute nonsuppurative appendicitis, which can develop prior to the rash.

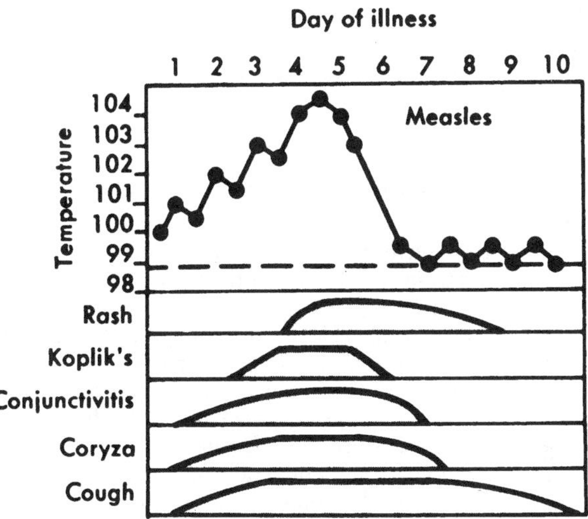

FIGURE 6 Schematic diagram of the clinical course of a typical case of measles. (From reference 82a with permission of Elsevier.)

The rash begins 3 or 4 days after the onset of prodromal symptoms. The earliest lesions, consisting of 3- to 4-mm dull-red blanching maculopapules, appear behind the ears, on the forehead at the hairline, and on the upper part of the neck. The rash then spreads downward over the face, neck, upper extremities, and trunk and continues downward until it reaches the feet by the third day. The rash is most profuse in the areas first affected. The lesions on the face and neck tend to become confluent, producing a blotchy appearance characteristic of measles (Fig. 7), whereas those on the abdomen and limbs tend to be more discrete. In severe cases, the rash may be associated with edema, especially of the face. The rash begins to fade by the third day in the order of its appearance, so that the rash may be fading on the face by the time it appears on the legs. The fading rash can leave a brownish discoloration of the skin, probably the result of capillary hemorrhage, which resolves during the next 10 days with fine desquamation that usually spares the hands and feet. In fair-skinned children the rash may become purpuric. This type of eruption is not related to severe hemorrhagic measles or the thrombocytopenic purpura that occasionally occurs after the rash has disappeared. Malnourished children and children infected with HIV may have a more severe, desquamating rash at the end of the acute illness.

In uncomplicated measles, fever reaches a peak of 39 to 40°C at the height of the skin eruption, with rapid defervescence on the third or fourth day of rash (Fig. 6).

Tracheobronchitis and peribronchial interstitial pneumonitis are common features of uncomplicated measles. Pulmonary infiltrates may be seen on chest radiographs taken during the acute phase of measles. The illness typically reaches its climax between the second and third days of rash. The temperature then falls rapidly over the following 24 to 48 h, the coryza and conjunctivitis clear, and the cough decreases in severity, although it may persist for a week or more. Most children in developed countries recover fully within a few days. Persistence or recurrence of fever beyond the third day of rash usually indicates a secondary bacterial infection.

Although uncommon in children, hepatic dysfunction has been frequently documented in adults with measles (82). These abnormalities are generally subclinical and self-limited. Myositis, evidenced by myalgia and elevated levels of creatine phosphokinase, is observed in 30 to 40% of adolescents and adults during the acute phase of measles, and one-third have hypocalcemia (141).

Modified Measles

Modified measles occurs in partially immunized persons, including persons given immune globulin following exposure to measles and infants with residual maternal antibody. Modified measles is usually a mild version of measles, although the incubation period may be prolonged, lasting up to 21 days. The prodrome is shortened or absent, fever is reduced, Koplik's spots are fewer, the rash is short-lived and markedly attenuated, and complications are extremely rare. Patients with modified measles rarely transmit MV to others.

Atypical Measles

A severe atypical measles syndrome was observed in recipients of formalin-inactivated measles vaccine (FIMV) who were subsequently exposed to wild-type MV (50). An estimated 600,000 to 900,000 children were immunized with FIMV between 1963 and 1967. After exposure to wild-type

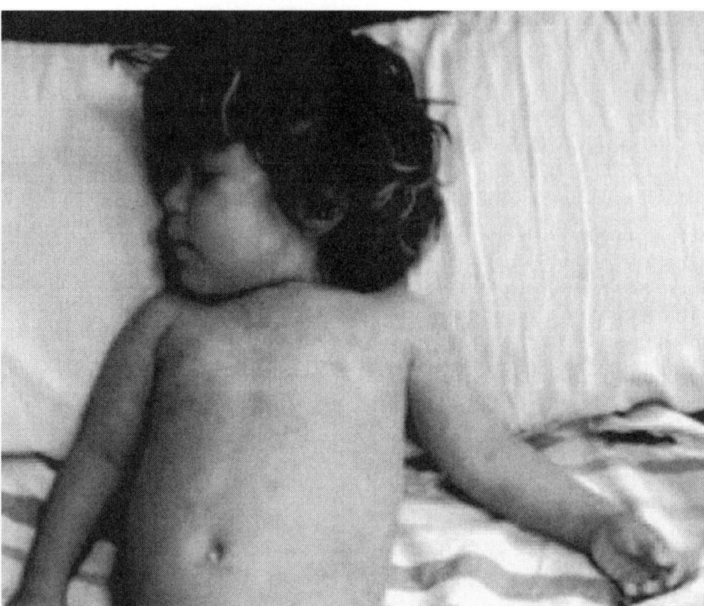

FIGURE 7 Measles rash. Note the characteristic blotchy appearance. (From reference 90 with permission of the publisher.)

MV, vaccinated individuals were at risk of developing high fever, headache, myalgia, abdominal pain, anorexia, nonproductive cough, and dyspnea followed by an atypical rash that began on the palms and soles and spread centripetally to the proximal extremities and trunk, sparing the face. The rash was initially erythematous and maculopapular but frequently progressed to vesicular, petechial, or purpuric lesions. Most patients had pneumonitis with interstitial infiltrates and segmental pulmonary consolidation, and many had pleural effusions, hilar adenopathy, and nodular parenchymal lesions. Hepatocellular enzyme levels were often markedly elevated, and some patients have had evidence of myositis and disseminated intravascular coagulation. Cases of atypical measles were reported many years after administration of FIMV, but the clinical characteristics in adults were more variable than those in children. Despite its severity, atypical measles was self-limited, although pulmonary abnormalities persisted.

In rhesus macaques, the FIMV induces a poor cytotoxic T-cell response and antibody that does not undergo affinity maturation (116, 117). Low-avidity antibody can neutralize in vitro infection with viruses that use CD46 as a receptor, as routinely measured by plaque reduction neutralizing titer assays with Vero cells, but cannot neutralize infection with wild-type viruses that primarily use CD150 (117). This difference in neutralization properties may be due to the higher-affinity interaction between MV and CD150 than between MV and CD46. Subsequent infection with MV induces an anamnestic antibody response, but the antibody produced is also of low avidity and cannot neutralize wild-type virus. This leads to the formation of complexes of nonneutralizing antibody and MV, resulting in immune complex deposition, vasculitis, and pneumonitis in rhesus macaques (116, 117). The exact nature of the defect in immune priming exhibited by FIMV has not yet been identified.

Measles during Pregnancy and the Neonatal Period

Morbidity and mortality are increased in pregnant women with measles, due to an increased risk of MV pneumonia during the third trimester and peripartum period. Measles during pregnancy has not been associated with congenital abnormalities in the fetus but is associated with an increased incidence of premature delivery and spontaneous abortion (8). Congenital measles, in which the rash is present at birth or appears during the first 10 days of life, varies from a mild illness to a rapidly fatal disease. In the absence of immunoglobulin prophylaxis, the overall mortality is about 30%. Mortality is higher in premature infants than in term infants; it is also higher in infants who fail to develop rash (8). Postnatally acquired measles in the neonate is rare because passively acquired maternal antibodies result in protection of most newborns. In the absence of protective maternal antibodies, however, measles in neonates is often severe.

Measles in Immunocompromised Patients

Children and adults with deficient cell-mediated immunity may develop severe, progressive, and frequently fatal MV infection, often in the absence of the typical rash and characteristic prodrome. The most frequent manifestation is giant-cell pneumonia (Hecht pneumonia), characterized by increasing respiratory insufficiency, progressive interstitial pneumonia with multinucleated giant cells throughout the tracheobronchial and alveolar epithelium (Fig. 8), the presence of measles giant cells in pulmonary and nasopharyngeal secretions, and a chest radiograph showing diffuse interstitial and alveolar infiltrates resembling adult respiratory distress syndrome (76, 89). The case fatality rate for MV pneumonia has been estimated to be about 70% in oncology patients and about 40% in HIV-infected patients (76).

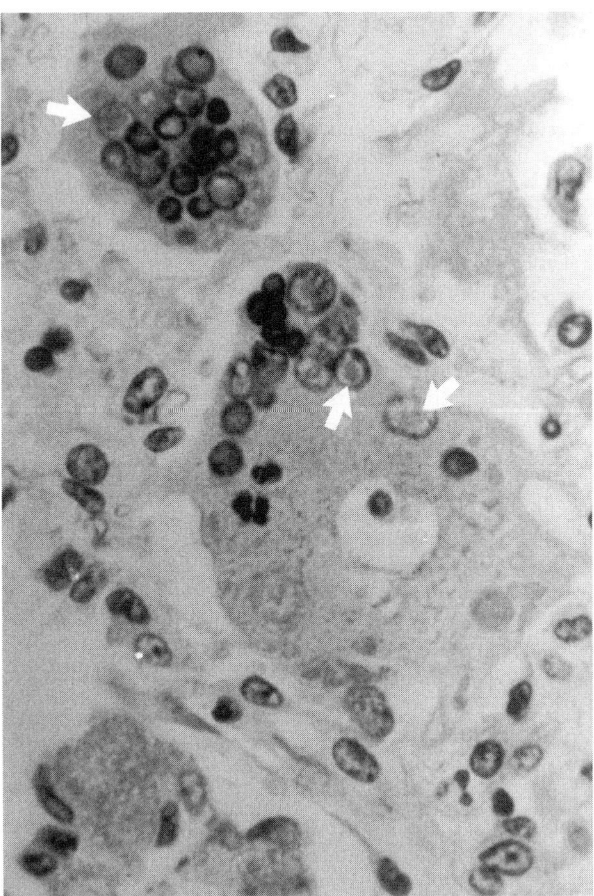

FIGURE 8 Measles giant-cell pneumonia. Two multinucleated epithelial giant cells are visible in alveolar spaces in the lung of an immunosuppressed child who died of giant cell pneumonia. Eosinophilic Cowdry type A inclusion bodies are visible in many nuclei (arrows). (From reference 37 with permission of the Massachusetts Medical Society.)

The other frequent manifestation of progressive MV infection in immunocompromised patients is measles inclusion body encephalitis (MIBE). MIBE may accompany or follow giant cell pneumonia, but more often occurs as the sole clinical manifestation months after MV infection (95). The disease usually presents with refractory focal myoclonic seizures and altered mental status and progresses to generalized seizures, coma, and death. Mortality exceeds 85%. Patients with MIBE are frequently afebrile and have normal cerebrospinal fluid (CSF) and head computed tomography and magnetic resonance imaging scans. Electroencephalograms are abnormal but nonspecific. Progression is often rapid, with the majority of deaths occurring within 6 to 8 weeks of onset. Survivors have severe neurologic sequelae. At autopsy or biopsy, the brain shows gliosis and focal necrosis, lymphocytic perivascular cuffing, and eosinophilic intranuclear and intracytoplasmic inclusions in glial cells and neurons. MV antigens are detectable by immunofluorescent staining, and MV RNA can be detected by reverse transcriptase PCR (RT-PCR). Live attenuated measles vaccine may also cause MIBE in severely immunodeficient infants (12).

Measles is severe in malnourished children, frequently resulting in secondary infections causing pneumonia and diarrhea; its case fatality rate exceeds 10%. Many factors are likely to contribute to the increased morbidity and mortality, including early age at infection, rapid loss of maternal antibody, vitamin A deficiency, and prior or concurrent infection with other pathogens. However, depressed cell-mediated immune responses secondary to malnutrition probably contribute significantly to the high risk of morbidity and mortality.

Complications

In developed countries, about 10% of measles cases are associated with complications, although the rate exceeded 20% during the 1989 to 1990 measles epidemic in the United States, primarily because of the high proportion of cases in adolescents and adults (18). The most common complications are otitis media (5 to 9%), diarrhea (5 to 9%), pneumonia (1 to 7%), and encephalitis (0.1%). Pneumonia is more common in young children, while encephalitis is more common in adolescents and adults. In developing countries, measles is a devastating disease with complication rates as high as 80% in many epidemics, and case fatality rates may exceed 10%. Diarrhea and pneumonia are frequently fatal. Keratitis in children with vitamin A deficiency can lead to corneal ulceration and blindness, and secondary bacterial infections cause otitis media, osteomyelitis, and other pyogenic complications.

Respiratory Tract Complications

The most frequent complications of measles involve the respiratory tract. Coryza, mild laryngitis, and tracheobronchitis with cough are almost invariably present in uncomplicated measles. Only when they are unusually severe or prolonged are they considered complications. Pneumonia is the most frequent life-threatening complication of measles (32) and may present clinically as bronchiolitis in infants or as bronchopneumonia or lobar pneumonia in infants and older children. Although the incidence in developed countries is less than 10%, pneumonia accounts for more than 60% of measles-associated deaths. In children, pneumonia is usually caused by secondary bacterial infection and occurs predominantly in those younger than 5 years. Common bacterial pathogens are *Streptococcus pneumoniae*, *Haemophilus influenzae* type b, and *Staphylococcus aureus*. Secondary bacterial pneumonia should be suspected in any child with measles who develops respiratory distress in association with persistence or recurrence of fever.

Symptomatic pneumonia is observed in 5 to 15% of immunocompetent adults with measles. In contrast to pneumonia in children, pneumonia in adults is more commonly caused by MV itself rather than a secondary bacterial infection. Respiratory distress and hypoxemia develop in parallel with the rash, and there is evidence of prolonged and extensive MV replication, including high and persistent fever, persistent rash, persistent viremia, and laboratory evidence of hepatitis and myositis (82). Pneumonia caused by bacterial superinfection develops later, usually 5 to 10 days after onset of the rash. Typically, deteriorating clinical and pulmonary status, high fever, elevated white blood cell count, and purulent sputum develop in a patient whose rash is resolving. In patients with MV pneumonia, chest radiographs reveal bilateral diffuse reticulonodular interstitial infiltrates. Segmental pulmonary consolidation, parenchymal nodules, hilar adenopathy, and pleural effusions are rarely observed except in atypical measles. Measles pneumonia is frequently a severe illness in healthy young adults, but fatalities are rare.

Otitis media is usually signaled by increasing irritability and ear pulling in infants or earache in older children, together with persistence or recurrence of fever. In severe cases, the first sign of otitis media may be spontaneous perforation of the tympanic membrane, with a purulent discharge from the middle ear. The incidence of otitis media is increased in infants.

Laryngotracheobronchitis (croup) due to MV occurs in up to 20% of children with measles who are younger than 2 years; it should be suspected when a child with measles develops inspiratory stridor, progressive hoarseness, a barking cough, and suprasternal retraction. Increased restlessness, dyspnea, anxiety, and tachycardia suggest increasing airway obstruction (obstructive laryngitis), which may require tracheostomy. Bronchiolitis may also complicate measles in infants and children younger than 2 years and is clinically indistinguishable from bronchiolitis caused by respiratory syncytial virus. Sinusitis occurs in 2 to 4% of patients with measles, primarily in adolescents and adults, and has been observed in 25% of young adults hospitalized with pneumonia.

Neurologic Complications

Uncomplicated measles is frequently accompanied by CSF pleocytosis and electroencephalographic abnormalities, but there is no evidence that the parenchyma of the brain is directly infected. Infection of vascular endothelial cells is a central feature of the pathogenesis of uncomplicated measles, and vascular endothelial cells in the brain are not spared (41). MV infection of vascular endothelial cells in the CNS provides a route of entry for virus into the brain parenchyma in the rare patients who develop MIBE. The neurologic complications of measles are listed in Table 2.

Acute Postinfectious Measles Encephalomyelitis

Acute postinfectious measles encephalomyelitis is the most common neurologic complication of measles. It is rare in children younger than 2 years but occurs in about 1 in 1,000 cases of measles in older children and somewhat more frequently in adults (75). Onset is usually during the first week after onset of the rash, but this complication occasionally develops during the prodrome or shortly after the rash has cleared. Onset is typically abrupt, starting with irritability, headache, vomiting, and confusion and progressing rapidly to obtundation and coma. These manifestations are frequently accompanied by seizures and by recurrence or accentuation of fever. Some patients develop other focal neurologic signs, including cerebellar ataxia, myelitis, optic neuritis, and retinopathy. There are usually signs of meningeal irritation, and the CSF shows a mild lymphocytic pleocytosis and a moderately elevated protein concentration. Mortality is 10 to 20%, and the majority of survivors have neurologic sequelae. Acute postinfectious measles encephalomyelitis appears to be an autoimmune disease. The neuropathology is similar to that of experimental allergic encephalomyelitis, with lymphocytic perivascular cuffing and periveinular demyelination (75). Neither MV RNA nor viral antigens have been detected in the brain, and there is no intrathecal synthesis of MV-specific antibody. However, antibodies to myelin basic protein are present in the CSF. The pathogenesis is unclear, but possibilities include altered presentation of myelin antigens, activation and expansion of autoreactive lymphocytes as a result of the immune activation and dysregulation, and molecular mimicry. There appear to be regions of homology between MV proteins and myelin basic protein, but neither cross-reactive antibodies nor cross-reactive T cells have been identified.

Subacute Sclerosing Panencephalitis

A second form of measles encephalitis, subacute sclerosing panencephalitis (SSPE), is a rare delayed complication of measles that occurs in approximately 1 in 10,000 cases (11). Typically, SSPE presents in children 6 to 8 years after measles that occurred in early childhood, generally prior to the age of 2 years (64). The onset is insidious, with symptoms of progressive loss of cortical function developing over months. In the early stages, subtle personality changes and deteriorating intellectual capacity are often manifested by declining school performance. There may also be awkwardness and stumbling. Later, myoclonic jerks develop, accompanied by characteristic electroencephalographic changes consisting of stereotyped periodic high-amplitude slow-wave complexes (Rodermacker complexes). Patients subsequently develop ataxia, progressive mental deterioration, and extrapyramidal dyskinesias, including choreoathetosis and dystonic posturing. Progressive loss of vision is caused by chorioretinitis, optic atrophy, or cortical blindness. Disease progression is variable, and periods of remission are common, but in most cases death occurs within 1 to 3 years of onset.

TABLE 2 Neurologic complications of measles[a]

Disease	Host	Typical age of measles	MV in brain	Incidence	Pathology	Time course
Acute postinfectious measles encephalitis	Normal	>2 years	No	1:1,000 cases	Demyelination and perivascular inflammation	Monophasic course over weeks
Subacute sclerosing panencephalitis (SSPE)	Normal	<2 years	Yes	1:10,000 cases	Inclusion bodies and inflammation	Progressive course over years
Measles inclusion body encephalitis (MIBE)	Immune suppressed	Any	Yes	Unknown	Inclusion bodies in neurons and glial cells	Progressive course over months

[a] Adapted from reference 54b with permission of the publisher.

Pathologic examination reveals diffuse encephalitis involving both white and gray matter with lymphocytic perivascular cuffing, diffuse lymphocytic infiltration, extensive microglial proliferation, and patchy demyelination. Neurons and glial cells contain typical MV nuclear and cytoplasmic inclusion bodies that are composed of MV nucleocapsids, antigens, and RNA. Although large amounts of viral RNA and N and P protein are present in nucleocapsids, synthesis of one or more of the MV envelope proteins is markedly reduced or absent or the protein is functionally defective, resulting in deficient virion assembly and budding (130). Infectious MV and multinucleated giant cells are not present. The defective MVs in the brains of SSPE patients have multiple mutations throughout the genome, especially hypermutations within the M gene and alterations in the H and F genes (68).

Patients with SSPE have exceptionally high titers of antibody to MV in their serum and CSF. Synthesis of antibody to MV by plasma cells in the CNS results in elevated levels of immunoglobulin in the CSF; much of the immunoglobulin is MV specific. Because this antibody to MV is of limited heterogeneity, electrophoretic analysis of the CSF reveals oligoclonal bands (88).

The pathogenesis of SSPE is unclear, but sequence analysis of MV RNA from various parts of the brain suggests that MV in the CNS is clonal. Neurons and glial cells are not fully permissive for MV and, when infected, downregulate MV transcription and also increase the 3′-5′ transcription gradient, resulting in a marked reduction in the synthesis of envelope glycoproteins. The infected cells produce MV nucleocapsids and defective interfering particles but little or no infectious virus. Antibodies to MV may contribute to this process by further inhibiting transcription of MV mRNA in the infected cells and by removing MV proteins from the cell membrane. The result is the establishment of a persistent infection that can slowly progress by cell-to-cell spread within the brain. Immune lysis of cells expressing even small amounts of MV envelope proteins may limit progression of the infection and could account for the prolonged latent period of SSPE.

Measles Inclusion Body Encephalitis

The third form of measles encephalitis, MIBE, is a progressive, generally fatal MV infection of the brain that occurs in immunocompromised patients. MIBE is described above (see "Measles in Immunocompromised Patients").

Gastrointestinal Complications

MV infection of epithelial surfaces and lymphoid tissues throughout the gastrointestinal tract is responsible for the nausea, vomiting, diarrhea, and diffuse abdominal pain observed in 30 to 60% of children and adults with measles, as well as for rare cases of nonsuppurative appendicitis. Involvement of the liver is reflected by laboratory evidence of hepatitis in the majority of adults with measles but rarely by symptomatic hepatitis or jaundice (82). In developed countries, these manifestations are self-limited and generally resolve as the rash disappears. In developing countries, severe and persistent diarrhea occurs in 20 to 70% of children with measles and is frequently associated with secondary bacterial or protozoal infection (53). In this setting, diarrhea aggravates preexisting malnutrition and vitamin A deficiency and results in significant morbidity and mortality.

Cardiovascular Complications

Electrocardiographic evidence of myocarditis and pericarditis, including prolongation of the P-R interval, ST segment abnormalities and T wave inversions, can be detected in 15 to 30% of children and adults during the acute phase of measles (45). These abnormalities may be associated with MV infection of vascular endothelial cells but are transient and rarely result in symptomatic disease. Prolongation of the Q-T interval may also be observed, presumably related to the transient hypocalcemia that can occur during the acute phase of measles.

Ocular Complications

Conjunctivitis and punctate keratitis are features of uncomplicated measles and resolve as the rash disappears. In malnourished children with vitamin A deficiency, these lesions frequently progress to corneal ulceration, which may be complicated by secondary bacterial infection. Consequently, measles is an important cause of childhood blindness in developing countries where malnutrition is prevalent.

Other Complications

Mild to moderate thrombocytopenia is common during the acute phase of uncomplicated measles but is asymptomatic and transient, resolving soon after the rash disappears. Rarely, thrombocytopenic purpura develops several weeks after uncomplicated measles. This complication resembles idiopathic thrombocytopenic purpura and has an excellent prognosis.

Severe hemorrhagic measles (black measles) is an extremely rare form characterized by the sudden onset of high fever, seizures, delirium, respiratory distress, and a confluent hemorrhagic eruption in the skin and mucous membranes. Bleeding from the nose, mouth, gastrointestinal tract, and genitourinary tract are frequently severe and uncontrollable, and mortality is high. The pathogenesis appears to involve disseminated intravascular coagulopathy associated with extensive MV infection of the vascular endothelium.

Tuberculosis may be exacerbated or reactivated by measles, presumably because of the prolonged suppression of cell-mediated immunity induced by MV infection (131). This has not been seen to occur after live attenuated MV vaccine, although suppression of tuberculin skin test reactivity and in vitro lymphoproliferative responses occur after measles vaccination.

There are conflicting and inconclusive data suggesting that persistent MV infection causes or contributes to the development of chronic diseases of unknown etiology, including multiple sclerosis, Paget's disease, inflammatory bowel disease, and otosclerosis (115). However, no causal association has been established between MV or measles vaccines and these conditions.

Clinical Diagnosis

Measles is readily diagnosed on clinical grounds. Koplik's spots are especially helpful because they appear early and are pathognomonic for measles. The clinical diagnosis is more difficult during the prodrome and when the illness and rash are attenuated by passively acquired MV antibodies or prior immunization or when the rash is absent in immunocompromised patients and severely malnourished children. It is also more difficult in regions where the incidence of measles is low because other pathogens are responsible for the majority of measles-like illnesses (fever and rash). The Centers for Disease Control and Prevention case definition for measles requires (i) a generalized maculopapular rash of at least 3 days' duration; (ii) fever of at least 38.3°C (101°F); and (iii) either cough, coryza, or conjunctivitis. While the Centers for Disease Control and Prevention case definition has a sensitivity of at least 90%, its specificity is only about 25% in the absence of endemic and epidemic measles.

The differential diagnosis of measles includes a number of conditions associated with fever and rash: rubella, enterovirus infections, drug eruptions and other allergic rashes, scarlet fever, meningococcemia, roseola infantum caused by human herpesvirus 6, erythema infectiosum caused by parvovirus B19, and dengue virus infection. Other diseases that may cause maculopapular rashes resembling measles include toxic shock syndrome, infectious mononucleosis caused by Epstein-Barr virus, toxoplasmosis, and Kawasaki's disease.

LABORATORY DIAGNOSIS

Virus Isolation

Measles can be diagnosed by isolating virus in cell culture from respiratory secretions, nasopharyngeal and conjunctival swabs, peripheral blood mononuclear cells, and urine. Spin amplification (shell vial) assays, with fluorescent-antibody staining for MV antigens, can improve the speed and sensitivity of culture diagnosis. Nevertheless, virus isolation remains technically difficult and unavailable in most clinical settings.

Cytologic Diagnosis and Antigen Detection

Direct detection of giant cells in respiratory secretions or urine, on accessible epithelial surfaces such as the pharynx, nasal mucosa, buccal mucosa, or conjunctiva, or in tissue obtained by biopsy, provides a rapid and practical means of diagnosis. Characteristic multinucleated giant cells containing eosinophilic intranuclear and intracytoplasmic inclusion bodies are ordinarily present during the prodrome and for the first 2 or 3 days of the rash. Multinucleated giant cells with eosinophilic intranuclear inclusion bodies are also produced by herpes simplex and varicella-zoster virus infections. Detection of MV antigens by immunofluorescent or immunoenzyme staining increases sensitivity and specificity. These techniques can detect MV antigens later in the disease, when infectious virus can no longer be isolated. Polyclonal sera and monoclonal antibodies are both effective, but antibodies to the MV N protein are most useful because this viral protein is the most abundant antigen.

Nucleic Acid Detection

Detection of MV RNA by RT-PCR amplification of RNA extracted from clinical specimens or tissue can be accomplished using primers targeted to highly conserved regions of the MV N, H, or F genes. These techniques provide an extremely sensitive and specific means of diagnosis and are especially useful in CNS infections, where infectious virus cannot be readily isolated, and in immunocompromised patients, who may not be capable of antibody responses. RT-PCR assays can be applied to specimens obtained under field conditions and, when combined with nucleotide sequencing, permit the precise identification and characterization of MV genotypes for molecular epidemiologic studies.

Serologic Diagnosis

Serologic testing has been the mainstay of the laboratory diagnosis of measles. A fourfold or greater increase in MV-specific IgG antibody levels between acute- and convalescent-phase sera or the detection of MV-specific IgM or low-avidity IgG antibodies in a single specimen of serum or saliva is considered diagnostic for acute MV infection. The presence of IgG antibody to MV in a single serum specimen is evidence of prior infection or immunization. In primary infection in the normal host, detectable antibodies to MV generally appear in the serum within 1 to 3 days of rash onset and reach peak levels in 2 to 4 weeks. Because some patients have already had a substantial rise in antibody titer if the initial serum sample is obtained 4 days or more after rash onset, acute-phase serum should be obtained as soon as possible after the onset of symptoms. Convalescent-phase serum should be obtained 2 to 4 weeks later, although an interval of 7 days is often sufficient to demonstrate a rising antibody level. MV-specific IgM antibodies may not be detectable by some currently available assays until 4 to 5 days or more after rash onset, and MV-specific IgM antibodies usually fall to undetectable levels within 4 to 8 weeks of rash onset (10).

A number of methods are available for measuring the levels of antibodies to MV. Neutralization tests are sensitive and specific, the results are highly correlated with immunity to infection, and they provide the most clinically relevant measure of response to immunization (21). However, they require propagation of MV in cell culture and are thus expensive, laborious, and not widely available. The hemagglutination inhibition (HI) test was the most widely used means of serologic diagnosis until the introduction of enzyme immunoassays (EIA). HI test results correlate well with those of conventional neutralization tests, and the presence of HI antibody is indicative of immunity to measles. The complement fixation test is less sensitive than HI or neutralization tests and is more difficult to perform; it is now used only rarely. EIA use antigens prepared from MV-infected cells or recombinant MV proteins and can detect both IgM and IgG antibodies. Sensitive EIA can detect MV-specific IgM antibodies in patients with secondary immune responses to MV, albeit at lower IgM-to-IgG ratios than observed in patients with primary immune responses. Thus, the presence of IgM antibody is not necessarily indicative of primary MV infection. Recent MV infection can also be distinguished from past infection by the presence of low-avidity antibody and IgG3 (34).

PREVENTION

General

Environmental measures, including disinfection, have little impact on the spread of MV because the virus is highly labile and fomites do not play a significant role in transmission. Quarantine is generally futile because exposure often occurs during the prodrome and before the diagnosis is made. Respiratory isolation is indicated for all hospitalized patients with measles until 5 days after onset of the rash. Immunocompromised patients with measles may continue to shed virus and should be isolated for the duration of their illness. Susceptible medical personnel exposed to measles should be relieved from patient contact from days 5 to 21 after exposure, regardless of whether they receive postexposure immunization with vaccine or immune globulin (IG). Personnel who become ill should be relieved from patient contact until 5 days after onset of rash.

Passive Immunoprophylaxis

IG can prevent or modify measles in susceptible persons, but administration of attenuated measles vaccine is the preferred intervention. Live attenuated measles vaccine may provide some protection to immunocompetent persons if administered within 72 h of exposure and has the advantage of inducing long-term immunity. Administration of IG to immunocompetent persons within 72 h of exposure usually prevents MV infection and almost always prevents clinical measles. Even if administered up to 6 days after exposure, IG prevents or modifies the disease. Prophylaxis with IG is recommended for susceptible household and nosocomial contacts who are at risk of developing severe measles, particularly children younger than 1 year, immunocompromised persons (including HIV-infected persons previously immunized with live attenuated measles vaccine), and pregnant women. Except for premature infants, children younger than 6 months are usually partially or completely protected by passively acquired maternal antibody. If measles is diagnosed in a mother, all unimmunized children in the household should receive IG. The recommended dose of IG is 0.25 ml/kg of body weight given intramuscularly; immunocompromised persons should receive 0.5 ml/kg. The maximum total dose is 15 ml. Intravenous IG (IVIG) contains antibodies to MV, and the usual dose of 100 to 400 mg/kg should provide adequate prophylaxis for measles exposures occurring as long as 3 weeks or more after IVIG administration.

In countries where the use of measles vaccine has been widespread for decades, most adults are immune as a consequence of vaccination rather than natural infection, and the reduction in indigenous MV transmission has eliminated the immunologic "boosting" associated with reexposure. Consequently, levels of antibody to MV in adults are considerably lower than they were when wild-type MV infection was prevalent, resulting in lower titers of passively acquired maternal antibody to MV in newborns (85) and lower titers of antibody to MV in current lots of IG (39).

Susceptible persons who receive postexposure prophylaxis with IG should be immunized with live attenuated measles vaccine (if it is not contraindicated). Measles vaccine should be given 5 months after IG if the dose was 0.25 mg/kg (standard dose) or 6 months after IG if the dose was 0.5 mg/kg (for immunocompromised persons).

Active Immunization

The process of adaptation of MV grown in nonsusceptible hosts, such as the chicken embryo and canine and bovine kidney cells, led successfully to the development of live attenuated vaccine (LAV) strains. The first live attenuated measles vaccine was developed by passage of the Edmonston strain of MV in chicken embryo fibroblasts to produce the Edmonston B virus (Fig. 9) (36). Licensed in 1963, this vaccine was protective but also induced fever and rash in a large proportion of immunized children. Reactions were reduced when immunoglobulin that contained antibodies to MV was given at the time of vaccination.

More extensive passage of the Edmonston B virus in chicken embryo fibroblasts produced the more attenuated Schwarz vaccine that was licensed in 1965 and currently serves as the standard measles vaccine in much of the

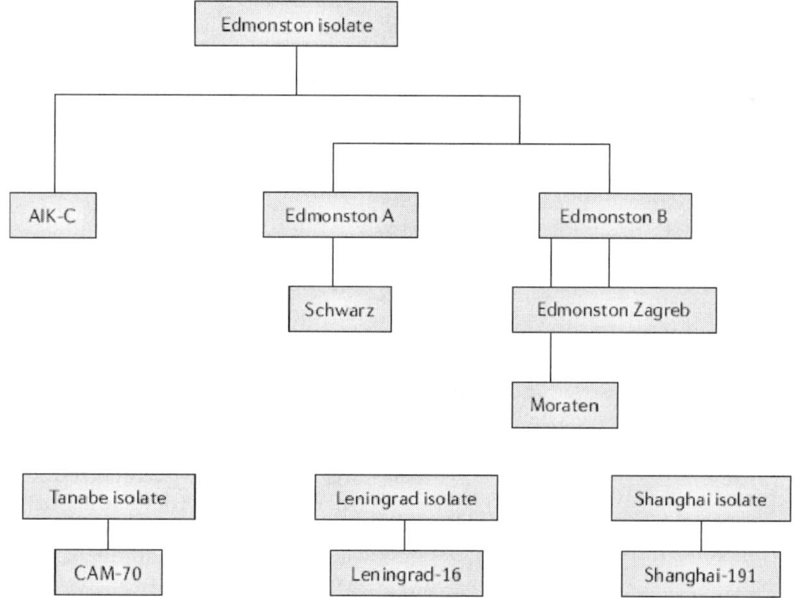

FIGURE 9 Measles vaccines. Most attenuated measles vaccines were developed from the Edmonston strain of MV. The Edmonston B vaccine was the first licensed measles vaccine but was associated with a high frequency of fever and rash. The further attenuated Schwarz and Edmonston-Zagreb vaccines are widely used throughout the world. The Moraten vaccine is the only measles vaccine used in the United States. (From reference 22a with permission of the publisher.)

world (Fig. 9). The Moraten strain (licensed in 1968) used in the United States is closely related to the Schwarz strain (Fig. 9) (120). Other Edmonston-derived vaccine strains (e.g., Zagreb, AIK-C) and attenuated strains developed independently (e.g., CAM, Leningrad-16, and Shanghai-191) are also successful vaccines. Few antigenic differences have been described among MV vaccine strains (all genotype A) regardless of the geographic origin of the parent virus. However, the Edmonston-Zagreb vaccine is produced in human diploid cells rather than chicken embryo fibroblasts and may be more reactogenic and immunogenic in young infants and when delivered by the aerosol route (23).

The lyophilized LAV is relatively stable, but the reconstituted vaccine rapidly loses infectivity. LAV is inactivated by light and heat, and after reconstitution it loses about half of its potency at 20°C and almost all potency at 37°C within an hour. Therefore, a cold chain must be maintained prior to and after reconstitution. LAVs replicate less efficiently than wild-type MV but induce both neutralizing antibody and cellular immune responses qualitatively similar to that induced by natural disease, although antibody titers are lower (105). Antibodies first appear 12 to 15 days after vaccination and peak at 1 to 3 months. In many countries, LAV is combined with other live attenuated virus vaccines such as those for mumps, rubella (MMR), and varicella (MMRV).

Administration

The recommended age of vaccination varies from 6 to 15 months. This age varies regionally and is a balance between the optimum age for seroconversion and the probability of acquiring measles before that age. In areas where measles remains prevalent, measles vaccination is routinely performed at 9 months, whereas in areas with little measles, vaccination is often at 12 to 15 months. During epidemics and in HIV-1-infected infants in developing countries, vaccination at 6 months with a second dose at 9 months is recommended.

LAV is administered subcutaneously or intramuscularly. However, there is substantial interest in alternate routes of delivery that would not require needles and syringes. Neither oral nor intranasal administration is effective, but respiratory delivery may be more promising. There are several ongoing efforts to evaluate aerosol delivery of aqueous and dry-powder forms of LAV. Aerosol administration was advocated by Albert Sabin in the early 1980s, is highly effective in boosting preexisting antibody titers, and may hold promise for use in older children. Respiratory routes of vaccination have also been advocated as a means of lowering the age of immunization. However, the primary immune response to aerosolized measles vaccine is weaker than it is to subcutaneous administration of the same vaccine (142). The reasons for this are not known but may be related to dose or efficiency of delivery and infection.

It is generally accepted that the proportions of children who develop protective levels of antibody are approximately 85% at 9 months of age and 95% at 12 months of age (24), although these proportions vary by vaccine strain and host characteristics (144). Genetic background affects the likelihood of seroconversion and antibody titers (28, 106). Common childhood illnesses at the time of vaccination may also reduce immune responses, although this is not frequent and should not be a reason for withholding vaccination (126). Any potential decrease in seroconversion must be balanced against the loss of the opportunity for vaccination and the consequent risk of the child acquiring measles. Similar compromises must be considered with respect to immunizing individuals infected with HIV. Overall, measles vaccine has been well tolerated and immunogenic in HIV-infected children and adults, although antibody levels may wane (94). Because of the potential severity of wild-type MV infection in HIV-infected individuals (89), LAV is recommended for routine administration to HIV-infected infants except those who are severely immunocompromised (144). LAV is also contraindicated in individuals with other severe deficiencies of cellular immunity because of the possibility of disease due to progressive pulmonary or CNS infection.

The dose of MV routinely used for immunization is between 10^3 and 10^4 PFU. When 10- to 100-fold-higher doses were used, seroconversion in younger infants improved, and in 1990 the Expanded Programme on Immunization (EPI) recommended use of the high-titer Edmonston-Zagreb vaccine at 6 months of age in countries where measles before the age of 9 months was a significant cause of death. However, subsequent follow-up of children receiving high-titer vaccines in countries with high childhood mortality showed an increased mortality in girls over the subsequent 2 to 3 years, and this recommendation was withdrawn (63). Mortality was not due to measles but, rather, to a relative increase in the deaths due to other infections. The pathogenesis of delayed increased mortality after the high-titer vaccine is not understood but occurred primarily in those who developed a rash after vaccination and may be related to long-term suppression of immune responses similar to that induced by measles or alteration of immune responses associated with a change in the sequence of delivery of vaccines (2).

The duration of vaccine-induced immunity is variable. Secondary vaccine failure rates have been estimated to be approximately 5% at 10 to 15 years after immunization but are probably lower when vaccination is given after 12 months of age (5). Waning antibody levels occur within 2 to 3 years of measles vaccination of HIV-infected children in the absence of antiretroviral therapy (94). However, decreasing antibody titers do not necessarily imply a complete loss of protective immunity because a secondary immune response usually develops after reexposure to MV, with a rapid rise in antibody titers without overt clinical disease (107).

Vaccine Side Effects

Standard doses of currently licensed measles vaccines are safe in immunocompetent children and adults. Fever to 39.4°C (103°F) occurs in 5 to 15% of seronegative vaccine recipients and can induce seizures in children predisposed to febrile seizures; 2 to 5% of vaccine recipients develop transient rash. Encephalitis or encephalopathy occurs in fewer than 1 in 10^6 vaccinees, an incidence lower than that reported for encephalitis or encephalopathy of unknown etiology. LAV is not a recognized cause of SSPE, which has declined in incidence in parallel with the vaccine-induced decline in the incidence of measles. Mild transient thrombocytopenia has been reported, with an incidence of approximately 1 in 10^6 vaccine recipients (9).

Although assumed to be rare, the risk of disease caused by attenuated measles vaccine virus in HIV-infected persons is unknown. The only documented case of fatal disease induced by measles vaccine virus in an HIV-infected person was in a 20-year-old man who died with MV giant-cell pneumonitis 15 months after receiving his second dose of measles vaccine (6). He had a very low $CD4^+$ T-lymphocyte count but no HIV-related symptoms at the time of vaccination. Fatal disseminated infection with measles vaccine virus has been found rarely in persons with other impairments of immune function, and MIBE caused by vaccine virus was reported to have occurred in a child with an uncharacterized immune deficiency (12).

As with wild-type MV infection, measles vaccine is associated with immunosuppression. However, this immune suppression is less pronounced than after wild-type MV infection and resolves within weeks after vaccination (102). Manifestations include decreased lymphoproliferative responses to mitogens and antigens, altered patterns of cytokine production, and suppression of delayed-type hypersensitivity skin test responses. Tuberculin skin test reactivity may be abrogated for 4 to 6 weeks after immunization, but unlike wild-type MV infection, measles vaccine does not exacerbate tuberculosis.

Much public attention has focused on a purported association between MMR vaccine and autism following publication of a report in 1998 hypothesizing that MMR vaccine may cause a syndrome of autism and intestinal inflammation (137). The events that followed, and the public concern over the safety of MMR vaccine, led to diminished vaccine coverage in the United Kingdom and provide important lessons in the misinterpretation of epidemiologic evidence and the communication of scientific results to the public (101). The publication that incited the concern was a case series describing 12 children with a regressive developmental disorder and chronic enterocolitis. Nine of the children had autism. Onset of the developmental delay was associated by the parents with MMR vaccination in eight children. This simple temporal association was misinterpreted and misrepresented as a possible causal relationship, first by the lead author of the study and then by the media and public. Subsequently, several comprehensive reviews and additional epidemiological studies rejected evidence of a causal relationship between MMR vaccination and autism (26).

Contraindications

Contraindications to measles vaccination include pregnancy; anaphylactic allergy to eggs, gelatin, or neomycin; severe immune suppression associated with HIV infection defined as a percentage of $CD4^+$ T-lymphocytes of <15%; other conditions associated with severe impairment of cellular immunity; and recent administration of IG, IVIG, or other IG-containing products.

Investigational Measles Vaccines

A new measles vaccine would be advantageous if it could be used in infants younger than 6 months. This would both close the "window of susceptibility" between decay of maternal antibody and vaccination and facilitate delivery by allowing measles vaccine to be given at the same time as other World Health Organization EPI vaccines. Additional motivations for development of a new vaccine would be to increase thermostability, to avoid the use of needles and syringes for delivery, and to provide a vaccine that would be safe for use in immunocompromised individuals (56). A number of experimental vaccines have been developed, and vaccination with individual MV proteins expressed in plants, in viral or bacterial vectors, or as DNA, peptides, or proteins has been explored by using animal models. Delivery of viral genes into host cells for processing and antigen presentation without the need for virus infection, along with thermostability, inexpensive manufacture, and the potential for mucosal administration, makes DNA vaccines an attractive possibility for development. Studies of vaccination of juvenile macaques indicated that DNA vaccines could protect from measles and did not predispose to atypical measles. However, studies of infant macaques have shown induction of lower levels of antibody, particularly in the face of maternal antibody, and limited protection from challenge (119). Therefore, DNA vaccines will have to be improved if further development is contemplated.

In addition to DNA vaccines, several viruses and bacteria have been used to express MV proteins and tested as experimental vaccines. Sindbis virus-based alphavirus replicon particle vaccines expressing MV H induced high-titer, dose-dependent, MV-neutralizing antibody after a single vaccination in mice. Vaccination of juvenile rhesus macaques with a single dose, and infant macaques with two doses, induced sustained levels of high-titer MV-neutralizing antibody and IFN-γ-producing memory T cells. Most monkeys were protected from disease, but not from viremia, when challenged 18 months later (109). Recombinant bacille Calmette-Guérin, the mycobacterium used for neonatal immunization against tuberculosis, has been engineered to express the MV N protein and used to immunize infant rhesus macaques.

Measles Vaccination Strategies

Different goals for measles control have been established, necessitating different vaccination strategies. Three broad goals can be defined: mortality reduction, regional elimination, and global eradication.

Mortality Reduction

Mortality reduction, the least demanding of the three goals, calls for a reduction in measles mortality from a predetermined level through reductions in incidence, case fatality, or both. Although a reduction in case fatality using appropriate case management is an important component, measles mortality reduction is achieved largely through a reduction in incidence. To reduce incidence, measles vaccine is administered as a single dose through routine immunization services in child health clinics, with the optimal age of immunization determined by the transmission intensity and rate of decline in the levels of maternal antibodies. If vaccination coverage is sufficiently high, substantial reductions in incidence and mortality occur, the interepidemic period lengthens, and the age distribution shifts toward older children, further contributing to a reduction in case fatality.

Regional Elimination

Measles elimination is the interruption of MV transmission within a defined geographic area, such as a country, continent, or region. Small outbreaks of primary and secondary cases may still occur following importation from outside the region, but sustained transmission does not occur. Because of the high infectivity of MV and the fact that not all persons develop protective immunity following vaccination, a single dose of measles vaccine does not achieve a sufficient level of population immunity to eliminate measles. A second opportunity for measles immunization is necessary to eliminate measles by providing protective immunity to children who failed to respond to the first dose and to those who were not previously vaccinated. Two broad strategies to administer the second dose have been used. In countries with sufficient infrastructure, the second dose of measles vaccine is administered through routine immunization services, typically prior to the start of school (4 to 6 years of age). High coverage can be ensured by school entry requirements. A second approach, first developed by the Pan American Health Organization (PAHO) for South and Central America (108), involves mass immunization campaigns (called supplementary immunization activities [SIA]) to deliver the second dose of measles vaccine. This strategy was very successful in eliminating measles in South and Central America and has resulted in a marked reduction in measles incidence and mortality in parts of sub-Saharan Africa (104).

The PAHO strategy consists of four subprograms: catch-up, keep-up, follow-up, and mop-up. The catch-up phase is a one-time, mass immunization campaign that targets all children within a broad age group regardless of whether they have previously had wild-type MV infection or measles vaccination. The goal is to rapidly achieve a high level of population immunity and interrupt MV transmission. These campaigns are conducted over a short period, usually several weeks, and during a low-transmission season. Under the PAHO strategy, children aged 9 months to 14 years were targeted for vaccination. In many countries, this is a substantial proportion of the total population. The appropriate target age range depends on the age distribution of measles seropositivity. In regions where measles is endemic, the majority of older children are likely to be immune. Nevertheless, seroprevalence studies usually are not conducted prior to catch-up campaigns, and this broad age range first adopted by PAHO has been widely used in sub-Saharan Africa and Asia. These campaigns require large investments of financial resources and personnel; extensive logistical planning to transport and store vaccines, maintain cold chains, and dispose of syringes and needles; and community mobilization to ensure participation. But if successful, SIA are cost-effective and can abruptly interrupt MV transmission, with dramatic declines in incidence and mortality.

Keep-up refers to the need to maintain greater than 90% routine measles vaccine coverage through improved access to measles vaccination and a reduction in missed opportunities (e.g., because of false contraindications to vaccination). Follow-up refers to periodic mass campaigns to prevent the accumulation of susceptible children. Follow-up campaigns typically target children 1 to 4 years of age, a narrower age group than targeted in catch-up campaigns. Follow-up campaigns should be conducted when the estimated number of susceptible children reaches the size of one birth cohort, generally every 3 to 5 years after the catch-up campaign. Mop-up campaigns target difficult-to-reach children in sites of measles outbreaks or low vaccine coverage. Difficult-to-reach children include those living on the street or in areas of conflict.

Global Eradication

The possibility of measles eradication has been discussed for almost 40 years (129). Serious discussion of measles eradication began in the late 1960s, when smallpox eradication was nearing completion and the effective, long-term immunity induced by measles vaccine became apparent. MV meets many of the biological criteria for disease eradication (90). MV has no nonhuman reservoir and is accurately diagnosed, and measles vaccination is a highly effective intervention. Although MV displays sufficient genetic variability to conduct molecular epidemiologic analyses, the antigenic epitopes against which protective antibodies develop have remained stable. Where MV differs from smallpox virus and poliovirus is that it is more highly infectious, necessitating much higher levels of population immunity to interrupt transmission.

The vaccination strategy necessary for measles eradication is not different from that of regional elimination; the only difference is that the target population is global. The success of measles elimination in large geographic regions suggests that measles eradication is possible. Two doses of measles vaccine, administered through routine immunization services or via SIA, would need to be administered to the children of the world. Many believe this to be a realistic and morally imperative goal, but as polio eradication efforts have shown, the endgame may be full of challenges.

TREATMENT

Symptomatic and Supportive Therapy

Treatment of uncomplicated measles is symptomatic and includes bed rest, hydration, and antipyretics. Secondary bacterial infections are a major cause of morbidity and mortality following measles (32), and effective case management involves prompt treatment with antibiotics. Various strategies have been used to guide antibiotic therapy in children with measles. Antibiotics are indicated for children with measles who have clinical evidence of bacterial infection, including pneumonia, otitis media, skin infection, eye infection, or severe mouth ulcers. *S. pneumoniae* and *H. influenzae* type B are the most common causes of bacterial pneumonia following measles, and antibiotic therapy should be directed against these pathogens. Vaccines against these pathogens lower the incidence of secondary bacterial infections. Whether all children with measles, or all hospitalized children with measles, should be given prophylactic antibiotics remains controversial. Limited evidence suggests that antibiotics administered as prophylaxis to all children presenting with measles may reduce the incidence of pneumonia but not mortality (32). The potential benefits of antibiotic prophylaxis need to be weighed against the risks of accelerating antibiotic resistance.

Vitamin A

Vitamin A is effective for the treatment of measles, and its administration has resulted in marked reductions in morbidity and mortality in hospitalized children with measles. The World Health Organization recommends administration of two daily doses of 200,000 IU of vitamin A to all children 12 months of age or older with measles. Lower doses (100,000 IU) are recommended for children younger than 12 months. Overall, this regimen results in a 64% reduction in the risk of mortality (31). Pneumonia-specific mortality is reduced, and the impact is greatest in children younger than 2 years (31). The mechanisms by which vitamin A reduces measles morbidity and mortality are not known, but these effects are probably mediated through beneficial effects on epithelial cells and host immune responses.

While vitamin A deficiency is not a recognized problem in the United States, many American children with measles have low serum vitamin A levels, and these children experience increased morbidity following measles. The Committee on Infectious Diseases of the American Academy of Pediatrics recommends that the administration of two consecutive daily doses of vitamin A (200,000 IU orally for children 1 year and older; 100,000 IU for children 6 months to 1 year of age) be considered for children 6 to 24 months of age hospitalized for measles and its complications, as well as for children with measles older than 6 months who have immunodeficiency, ophthalmologic evidence of vitamin A deficiency, impaired intestinal absorption, or moderate to severe malnutrition or are recent immigrants from areas where high measles-related mortality rates have been observed.

Prophylactic administration of vitamin A also reduces measles mortality. Vitamin A has been widely distributed through polio and measles SIA as well as through routine child health services. Vitamin A supplementation of apparently healthy children has resulted in a 39% reduction in measles-associated mortality (136).

Antiviral Therapy

There is no antiviral therapy of proven efficacy for measles. Ribavirin inhibits MV replication in cell culture and has been reported to reduce the severity of measles in children and adults (46). Anecdotal reports have described previously healthy, pregnant, and immunocompromised patients with measles pneumonia and immunocompromised patients with subacute MIBE who recovered following treatment with aerosolized and/or intravenous ribavirin (76, 95). However, the clinical benefits of ribavirin treatment have yet to be clearly demonstrated.

Numerous therapeutic agents have been used to treat SSPE, including IFN, ribavirin, amantadine, isoprinosine, inoseplex, and levamasole. Experience has been anecdotal, and any benefits have been transient at best.

REFERENCES

1. **Aaby, P., J. Bukh, I. M. Lisse, and A. J. Smits.** 1984. Overcrowding and intensive exposure as determinants of measles mortality. *Am. J. Epidemiol.* **120:**49–63.
2. **Aaby, P., H. Jensen, B. Samb, B. Cisse, M. Sodemann, M. Jakobsen, A. Poulsen, A. Rodrigues, I. M. Lisse, F. Simondon, and H. Whittle.** 2003. Differences in female-male mortality after high-titre measles vaccine and association with subsequent vaccination with diphtheria-tetanus-pertussis and inactivated poliovirus: reanalysis of West African studies. *Lancet* **361:**2183–2188.
3. **Albrecht, P., F. A. Ennis, E. J. Saltzman, and S. Krugman.** 1977. Persistence of maternal antibody in infants beyond 12 months: mechanism of measles vaccine failure. *J. Pediatr.* **91:**715–718.
4. **Amanna, I. J., N. E. Carlson, and M. K. Slifka.** 2007. Duration of humoral immunity to common viral and vaccine antigens. *N. Engl. J. Med.* **357:**1903–1915.
5. **Anders, J. F., R. M. Jacobson, G. A. Poland, S. J. Jacobsen, and P. C. Wollan.** 1996. Secondary failure rates of measles vaccines: a metaanalysis of published studies. *Pediatr. Infect. Dis. J.* **15:**62–66.
6. **Angel, J. B., P. Walpita, R. A. Lerch, M. S. Sidhu, M. Masuredar, R. A. DeLellis, J. T. Noble, D. R. Snydman, and S. A. Udem.** 1998. Vaccine-associated measles pneumonitis in an adult with AIDS. *Ann. Intern. Med.* **129:**104–106.
7. **Atabani, S. F., A. A. Byrnes, A. Jaye, I. M. Kidd, A. F. Magnusen, H. Whittle, and C. L. Karp.** 2001. Natural measles causes prolonged suppression of interleukin-12 production. *J. Infect. Dis.* **184:**1–9.
8. **Atmar, R. L., J. A. Englund, and H. Hammill.** 1992. Complications of measles during pregnancy. *Clin. Infect. Dis.* **14:**217–226.
9. **Beeler, J., F. Varricchio, and R. Wise.** 1996. Thrombocytopenia after immunization with measles vaccines: review of the vaccine adverse events reporting system (1990 to 1994). *Pediatr. Infect. Dis. J.* **15:**88–90.
10. **Bellini, W. J., and R. F. Helfand.** 2003. The challenges and strategies for laboratory diagnosis of measles in an international setting. *J. Infect. Dis.* **187**(Suppl. 1)**:**S283–S290.
11. **Bellini, W. J., J. S. Rota, L. E. Lowe, R. S. Katz, P. R. Dyken, S. R. Zaki, W. J. Shieh, and P. A. Rota.** 2005. Subacute sclerosing panencephalitis: more cases of this fatal disease are prevented by measles immunization than was previously recognized. *J. Infect. Dis.* **192:**1686–1693.
12. **Bitnun, A., P. Shannon, A. Durward, P. A. Rota, W. J. Bellini, C. Graham, E. Wang, E. L. Ford-Jones, P. Cox, L. Becker, M. Fearon, M. Petric, and R. Tellier.** 1999. Measles inclusion-body encephalitis caused by the vaccine strain of measles virus. *Clin. Infect. Dis.* **29:**855–861.
13. **Black, F. L.** 1966. Measles endemicity in insular populations: critical community size and its evolutionary implication. *J. Theor. Biol.* **11:**207–211.
14. **Bouche, F. B., O. T. Ertl, and C. P. Muller.** 2002. Neutralizing B cell response in measles. *Viral Immunol.* **15:**451–471.
15. **Brown, D. W., M. E. Ramsay, A. F. Richards, and E. Miller.** 1994. Salivary diagnosis of measles: a study of notified cases in the United Kingdom, 1991–3. *Br. Med. J.* **308:**1015–1017.
16. **Caceres, V. M., P. M. Strebel, and R. W. Sutter.** 2000. Factors determining prevalence of maternal antibody to measles virus throughout infancy: a review. *Clin. Infect. Dis.* **31:**110–119.
17. **Caignard, G., M. Guerbois, J. L. Labernardiere, Y. Jacob, L. M. Jones, F. Wild, F. Tangy, and P. O. Vidalain.** 2007. Measles virus V protein blocks Jak1-mediated phosphorylation of STAT1 to escape IFN-alpha/beta signaling. *Virology* **368:**351–362.
18. **Centers for Disease Control.** 1991. Measles—United States, 1990. *Morb. Mortal. Wkly. Rep.* **40:**369–372.
19. **Chen, R. T., L. E. Markowitz, P. Albrecht, J. A. Stewart, L. M. Mofenson, S. R. Preblud, and W. A. Orenstein.** 1990. Measles antibody: reevaluation of protective titers. *J. Infect. Dis.* **162:**1036–1042.
20. **Christensen, P. E., H. Schmidt, H. O. Bang, V. Andersen, B. Jordal, and O. Jensen.** 1953. An epidemic of measles in southern Greenland, 1951. Measles in virgin soil. II. The epidemic proper. *Acta Med. Scand.* **144:**430–449.
21. **Cohen, B. J., S. Audet, N. Andrews, and J. Beeler.** 2007. Plaque reduction neutralization test for measles antibodies: description of a standardised laboratory method for use in immunogenicity studies of aerosol vaccination. *Vaccine* **26:**59–66.
22. **Colf, L. A., Z. S. Juo, and K. C. Garcia.** 2007. Structure of the measles virus hemagglutinin. *Nat. Struct. Mol. Biol.* **14:**1227–1228.

22a. **Cutts, F. T.** 1993. The immunological basis for immunization series module 7: measles. Document WHO/EPI/GEN/93.17. World Health Organization, Geneva, Switzerland.

23. **Cutts, F. T., C. J. Clements, and J. V. Bennett.** 1997. Alternative routes of measles immunization: a review. *Biologicals* **25:**323–338.
24. **Cutts, F. T., M. Grabowsky, and L. E. Markowitz.** 1995. The effect of dose and strain of live attenuated measles vaccines on serological responses in young infants. *Biologicals* **23:**95–106.
25. **de Quadros, C. A., B. S. Hersh, A. C. Nogueira, P. A. Carrasco, and C. M. da Silveira.** 1998. Measles eradication: experience in the Americas. *Bull. W. H. O.* **76**(Suppl. 2)**:**47–52.
26. **DeStefano, F. and W. W. Thompson.** 2004. MMR vaccine and autism: an update of the scientific evidence. *Expert Rev. Vaccines* **3:**19–22.
27. **de Swart, R. L., S. Yuksel, and A. D. Osterhaus.** 2005. Relative contributions of measles virus hemagglutinin- and fusion protein-specific serum antibodies to virus neutralization. *J. Virol.* **79:**11547–11551.
28. **Dhiman, N., I. G. Ovsyannikova, J. M. Cunningham, R. A. Vierkant, R. B. Kennedy, V. S. Pankratz, G. A. Poland, and R. M. Jacobson.** 2007. Associations between measles vaccine immunity and single-nucleotide polymorphisms in cytokine and cytokine receptor genes. *J. Infect. Dis.* **195:**21–29.
29. **Dorig, R. E., A. Marcil, A. Chopra, and C. D. Richardson.** 1993. The human CD46 molecule is a receptor for measles virus (Edmonston strain). *Cell* **75:**295–305.
30. **Dossetor, J., H. C. Whittle, and B. M. Greenwood.** 1977. Persistent measles infection in malnourished children. *Br. Med. J.* **1:**1633–1635.
31. **D'Souza, R. M. and R. D'Souza.** 2002. Vitamin A for the treatment of children with measles—a systematic review. *J. Trop. Pediatr.* **48:**323–327.
32. **Duke, T., and C. S. Mgone.** 2003. Measles: not just another viral exanthem. *Lancet* **361:**763–773.
33. **Ehresmann, K. R., C. W. Hedberg, M. B. Grimm, C. A. Norton, K. L. MacDonald, and M. T. Osterholm.** 1995. An outbreak of measles at an international sporting event with airborne transmission in a domed stadium. *J. Infect. Dis.* **171:**679–683.
34. **El Mubarak, H. S., S. A. Ibrahim, H. W. Vos, M. M. Mukhtar, O. A. Mustafa, T. F. Wild, A. D. Osterhaus, and R. L. de Swart.** 2004. Measles virus protein-specific IgM, IgA, and IgG subclass responses during the acute and convalescent phase of infection. *J. Med. Virol.* **72:**290–298.
35. **Enders, J. F.** 1964. Francis Home and his experimental approach to medicine. *Bull. Hist. Med.* **38:**101–112.
36. **Enders, J. F., S. L. Katz, and A. Holloway.** 1962. Development of attenuated measles-virus vaccines. *Am. J. Dis. Child.* **103:**335–340.
37. **Enders, J. F., K. McCarthy, A. Mitus, and W. J. Cheatham.** 1959. Isolation of measles virus at autopsy in cases of giant-cell pneumonia without rash. *N. Engl. J. Med.* **261:**875–881.
38. **Enders, J. F. and T. C. Peebles.** 1954. Propagation in tissue cultures of cytopathic agents from patients with measles. *Proc. Soc. Exp. Biol. Med.* **86:**277–286.
39. **Endo, A., H. Izumi, M. Miyashita, K. Taniguchi, O. Okubo, and K. Harada.** 2001. Current efficacy of postexposure prophylaxis against measles with immunoglobulin. *J. Pediatr.* **138:**926–928.
40. **Ertl, O. T., D. C. Wenz, F. B. Bouche, G. A. Berbers, and C. P. Muller.** 2003. Immunodominant domains of the measles virus hemagglutinin protein eliciting a neutralizing human B cell response. *Arch. Virol.* **148:**2195–2206.
41. **Esolen, L. M., K. Takahashi, R. T. Johnson, A. Vaisberg, T. R. Moench, S. L. Wesselingh, and D. E. Griffin.** 1995. Brain endothelial cell infection in children with acute fatal measles. *J. Clin. Investig.* **96:**2478–2481.
42. **Esolen, L. M., B. J. Ward, T. R. Moench, and D. E. Griffin.** 1993. Infection of monocytes during measles. *J. Infect. Dis.* **168:**47–52.
43. **Feikin, D. R., D. C. Lezotte, R. F. Hamman, D. A. Salmon, R. T. Chen, and R. E. Hoffman.** 2000. Individual and community risks of measles and pertussis associated with personal exemptions to immunization. *JAMA* **284:**3145–3150.
44. **Fine, P. E., and J. A. Clarkson.** 1982. Measles in England and Wales—I. An analysis of factors underlying seasonal patterns. *Int. J. Epidemiol.* **11:**5–14.
45. **Finkel, H. E.** 1964. Measles myocarditis. *Am. Heart J.* **67:**679–683.
46. **Forni, A. L., N. W. Schluger, and R. B. Roberts.** 1994. Severe measles pneumonitis in adults: evaluation of clinical characteristics and therapy with intravenous ribavirin. *Clin. Infect. Dis.* **19:**454–462.
47. **Forthal, D. N., G. Landucci, A. Habis, M. Zartarian, and J. Katz.** 1994. Measles virus-specific functional antibody responses and viremia during acute measles. *J. Infect. Dis.* **169:**1377–1380.
48. **Frank, S. A., and R. M. Bush.** 2007. Barriers to antigenic escape by pathogens: trade-off between reproductive rate and antigenic mutability. *BMC Evol. Biol.* **7:**229.
49. **Fujinami, R. S., and M. B. Oldstone.** 1979. Antiviral antibody reacting on the plasma membrane alters measles virus expression inside the cell. *Nature* **279:**529–530.
50. **Fulginiti, V. A., J. J. Eller, A. W. Downie, and C. H. Kempe.** 1967. Altered reactivity to measles virus: atypical measles in children previously immunized with inactivated measles virus vaccines. *JAMA* **202:**1075.
51. **Garenne, M.** 1994. Sex differences in measles mortality: a world review. *Int. J. Epidemiol.* **23:**632–642.
52. **Good, R. A., and S. J. Zak.** 1956. Disturbances in gamma globulin synthesis as "experiments of nature." *Pediatrics* **18:**109–149.
53. **Greenberg, B. L., R. B. Sack, E. Salazar-Lindo, E. Budge, M. Gutierrez, M. Campos, A. Visberg, R. Leon-Barua, A. Yi, and D. Maurutia.** 1991. Measles-associated diarrhea in hospitalized children in Lima, Peru: pathogenic agents and impact on growth. *J. Infect. Dis.* **163:** 495–502.
54. **Griffin, D. E.** 1995. Immune responses during measles virus infection. *Curr. Top. Microbiol. Immunol.* **191:**117–134.
54a. **Griffin, D. E.** 2001. Measles virus. *In* D. M. Knipe and P. M. Howley (ed.), *Fields Virology*, 4th ed. Lippincott Williams & Wilkins, Philadelphia, PA.
54b. **Griffin, D. E.** 2007. Measles virus, p. 1551–1585. *In* D. M. Knipe and P. M. Howley (ed.), *Fields Virology*, 5th ed. Lippincott Williams & Wilkins, Philadelphia, PA.
55. **Griffin, D. E., S. J. Cooper, R. L. Hirsch, R. T. Johnson, I. L. Soriano, S. Roedenbeck, and A. Vaisberg.** 1985. Changes in plasma IgE levels during complicated and uncomplicated measles virus infections. *J. Allergy Clin. Immunol.* **76:**206–213.
56. **Griffin, D. E., C. H. Pan, and W. J. Moss.** 2008. Measles vaccines. *Front. Biosci.* **13:**1352–1370.
57. **Griffin, D. E., and B. J. Ward.** 1993. Differential CD4 T cell activation in measles. *J. Infect. Dis.* **168:**275–281.
58. **Griffin, D. E., B. J. Ward, and L. M. Esolen.** 1994. Pathogenesis of measles virus infection: an hypothesis for altered immune responses. *J. Infect. Dis.* **170**(Suppl. 1)**:** S24–S31.
59. **Griffin, D. E., B. J. Ward, E. Jauregui, R. T. Johnson, and A. Vaisberg.** 1989. Immune activation in measles. *N. Engl. J. Med.* **320:**1667–1672.

60. **Griffin, D. E., B. J. Ward, E. Jauregui, R. T. Johnson, and A. Vaisberg.** 1990. Immune activation during measles: interferon-γ and neopterin in plasma and cerebrospinal fluid in complicated and uncomplicated disease. *J. Infect. Dis.* **161:**449–453.
61. **Griffin, D. E., B. J. Ward, E. Jauregui, R. T. Johnson, and A. Vaisberg.** 1990. Natural killer cell activity during measles. *Clin. Exp. Immunol.* **81:**218–224.
62. **Griffin, D. E., B. J. Ward, E. Jauregui, R. T. Johnson, and A. Vaisberg.** 1992. Immune activation during measles: β_2-microglobulin in plasma and cerebrospinal fluid in complicated and uncomplicated disease. *J. Infect. Dis.* **166:**1170–1173.
63. **Halsey, N. A.** 1993. Increased mortality after high-titre measles vaccines: too much of a good thing. *Pediatr. Infect. Dis. J.* **12:**462–465.
64. **Halsey, N. A., J. F. Modlin, J. T. Jabbour, L. Dubey, D. L. Eddins, and D. D. Ludwig.** 1980. Risk factors in subacute sclerosing panencephalitis: a case-control study. *Am. J. Epidemiol.* **111:**415–424.
65. **Hashiguchi, T., M. Kajikawa, N. Maita, M. Takeda, K. Kuroki, K. Sasaki, D. Kohda, Y. Yanagi, and K. Maenaka.** 2007. Crystal structure of measles virus hemagglutinin provides insight into effective vaccines. *Proc. Natl. Acad. Sci. USA* **104:**19535–19540.
66. **Hashimoto, K., N. Ono, H. Tatsuo, H. Minagawa, M. Takeda, K. Takeuchi, and Y. Yanagi.** 2002. SLAM (CD150)-independent measles virus entry as revealed by recombinant virus expressing green fluorescent protein. *J. Virol.* **76:**6743–6749.
67. **Helfand, R. F., W. J. Moss, R. Harpaz, S. Scott, and F. Cutts.** 2005. Evaluating the impact of the HIV pandemic on measles control and elimination. *Bull. W. H. O.* **83:** 329–337.
68. **Hirano, A., A. H. Wang, A. F. Gombart, and T. C. Wong.** 1992. The matrix proteins of neurovirulent subacute sclerosing panencephalitis virus and its acute measles virus progenitor are functionally different. *Proc. Natl. Acad. Sci. USA* **89:**8745–8749.
69. **Hirsch, R. L., D. E. Griffin, R. T. Johnson, S. J. Cooper, I. Lindo de Soriano, S. Roedenbeck, and A. Vaisberg.** 1984. Cellular immune responses during complicated and uncomplicated measles virus infections of man. *Clin. Immunol. Immunopathol.* **31:**1–12.
70. **Horikami, S. M., and S. A. Moyer.** 1995. Structure, transcription, and replication of measles virus. *Curr. Top. Microbiol. Immunol.* **191:**35–50.
71. **Hummel, K. B., W. J. Bellini, and M. K. Offermann.** 1998. Strain-specific differences in LFA-1 induction on measles virus-infected monocytes and adhesion and viral transmission to endothelial cells. *J. Virol.* **72:**8403–8407.
72. **Hutchins, S., L. Markowitz, W. Atkinson, E. Swint, and S. Hadler.** 1996. Measles outbreaks in the United States, 1987 through 1990. *Pediatr. Infect. Dis. J.* **15:**31–38.
73. **Jaye, A., A. F. Magnusen, A. D. Sadiq, T. Corrah, and H. C. Whittle.** 1998. *Ex vivo* analysis of cytotoxic T lymphocytes to measles antigens during infection and after vaccination in Gambian children. *J. Clin. Investig.* **102:** 1969–1977.
74. **Jaye, A., A. F. Magnusen, and H. C. Whittle.** 1998. Human leukocyte antigen class I- and class II-restricted cytotoxic T lymphocyte responses to measles antigens in immune adults. *J. Infect. Dis.* **177:**1282–1289.
75. **Johnson, R. T., D. E. Griffin, R. L. Hirsch, J. S. Wolinsky, S. Roedenbeck, I. Lindo de Soriano, and A. Vaisberg.** 1984. Measles encephalomyelitis—clinical and immunologic studies. *N. Engl. J. Med.* **310:**137–141.
76. **Kaplan, L. J., R. S. Daum, M. Smaron, and C. A. McCarthy.** 1992. Severe measles in immunocompromised patients. *JAMA* **267:**1237–1241.
77. **Karlin, D., S. Longhi, and B. Canard.** 2002. Substitution of two residues in the measles virus nucleoprotein results in an impaired self-association. *Virology* **302:**420–432.
78. **Karp, C. L., M. Wysocka, L. M. Wahl, J. M. Ahearn, P. J. Cuomo, B. Sherry, G. Trinchieri, and D. E. Griffin.** 1996. Mechanism of suppression of cell-mediated immunity by measles virus. *Science* **273:**228–231.
79. **Kemper, C., A. C. Chan, J. M. Green, K. A. Brett, K. M. Murphy, and J. P. Atkinson.** 2003. Activation of human $CD4^+$ cells with CD3 and CD46 induces a T-regulatory cell 1 phenotype. *Nature* **421:**388–392.
80. **Kimura, A., K. Tosaka, and T. Nakao.** 1975. Measles rash. I. Light and electron microscopic study of skin eruptions. *Arch.Virol.* **47:**295–307.
81. **Kobune, F., H. Sakata, and A. Sugiura.** 1990. Marmoset lymphoblastoid cells as a sensitive host for isolation of measles virus. *J. Virol.* **64:**700–705.
82. **Krause, P. J., J. D. Cherry, J. Seda-Tous, J. G. Champion, M. Strassburg, C. Sullivan, M. J. Spencer, Y. J. Bryson, R. C. Welliver, and K. M. Boyer.** 1979. Epidemic measles in young adults. Clinical, epidemiologic, and serologic studies. *Ann. Intern. Med.* **90:**873–876.

82a. **Krugman, S., S. L. Katz, and A. A. Gershon.** 1985. Measles, p. 152. *Infectious Diseases of Children.* C. V. Mosby, St. Louis, MO.

83. **Kuhne, M., D. W. Brown, and L. Jin.** 2006. Genetic variability of measles virus in acute and persistent infections. *Infect. Genet. Evol.* **6:**269–276.
84. **Longhi, S., V. Receveur-Brechot, D. Karlin, K. Johansson, H. Darbon, D. Bhella, R. Yeo, S. Finet, and B. Canard.** 2003. The C-terminal domain of the measles virus nucleoprotein is intrinsically disordered and folds upon binding to the C-terminal moiety of the phosphoprotein. *J. Biol. Chem.* **278:**18638–18648.
85. **Maldonado, Y. A., E. C. Lawrence, R. DeHovitz, H. Hartzell, and P. Albrecht.** 1995. Early loss of passive measles antibody in infants of mothers with vaccine-induced immunity. *Pediatrics* **96:**447–450.
86. **Markowitz, L. E., F. W. Chandler, E. O. Roldan, M. J. Saldana, K. C. Roach, S. S. Hutchins, S. R. Preblud, C. D. Mitchell, and G. B. Scott.** 1988. Fatal measles pneumonia without rash in a child with AIDS. *J. Infect. Dis.* **158:**480–483.
87. **McNeill, W. H.** 1976. *Plagues and Peoples.* Penguin, London, United Kingdom.
88. **Metz, H., M. Gregoriou, and P. Sandifer.** 1964. Subacute sclerosing pan-encephalitis. A review of 17 cases with special reference to clinical diagnostic criteria. *Arch. Dis. Child.* **39:**554–557.
89. **Moss, W. J., F. Cutts, and D. E. Griffin.** 1999. Implications of the human immunodeficiency virus epidemic for control and eradication of measles. *Clin. Infect. Dis.* **29:**106–112.
90. **Moss, W. J., and D. E. Griffin.** 2006. Global measles elimination. *Nat. Rev. Microbiol.* **4:**900–908.
91. **Moss, W. J., M. Monze, J. J. Ryon, T. C. Quinn, D. E. Griffin, and F. Cutts.** 2002. Prospective study of measles in hospitalized human immunodeficiency virus (HIV)-infected and HIV-uninfected children in Zambia. *Clin. Infect. Dis.* **35:**189–196.
92. **Moss, W. J., M. O. Ota, and D. E. Griffin.** 2004. Measles: immune suppression and immune responses. *Int. J. Biochem. Cell Biol.* **36:**1380–1385.
93. **Moss, W. J., J. J. Ryon, M. Monze, and D. E. Griffin.** 2002. Differential regulation of interleukin (IL)-4, IL-5, and IL-10 during measles in Zambian children. *J. Infect. Dis.* **186:**879–887.
94. **Moss, W. J., S. Scott, N. Mugala, Z. Ndhlovu, J. A. Beeler, S. A. Audet, M. Ngala, S. Mwangala, C.**

Nkonga-Mwangilwa, J. J. Ryon, M. Monze, F. Kasolo, T. C. Quinn, S. Cousens, D. E. Griffin, and F. T. Cutts. 2007. Immunogenicity of standard-titer measles vaccine in HIV-1-infected and uninfected Zambian children: an observational study. *J. Infect. Dis.* **196:**347–355.

95. **Mustafa, M. M., S. D. Weitman, N. J. Winick, W. J. Bellini, C. F. Timmons, and J. D. Siegel.** 1993. Subacute measles encephalitis in the young immunocompromised host: report of two cases diagnosed by polymerase chain reaction and treated with ribavirin and review of the literature. *Clin. Infect. Dis.* **16:**654–660.

96. **Nakata, Y., T. Nakayama, Y. Ide, R. Kizu, G. Koinuma, and M. Bamba.** 2002. Measles virus genome detected up to four months in a case of congenital measles. *Acta Paediatr.* **91:**1263–1265.

97. **Nakatsu, Y., M. Takeda, S. Ohno, R. Koga, and Y. Yanagi.** 2006. Translational inhibition and increased interferon induction in cells infected with C protein-deficient measles virus. *J. Virol.* **80:**11861–11867.

98. **Nanan, R., C. Carstens, and H. W. Kreth.** 1995. Demonstration of virus-specific $CD8^+$ memory T cells in measles-seropositive individuals by in vitro peptide stimulation. *Clin. Exp. Immunol.* **102:**40–45.

99. **Naniche, D., G. Varior-Krishnan, F. Cervoni, T. F. Wild, B. Rossi, C. Rabourdin-Combe, and D. Gerlier.** 1993. Human membrane cofactor protein (CD46) acts as a cellular receptor for measles virus. *J. Virol.* **67:**6025–6032.

100. **Naniche, D., A. Yeh, D. Eto, M. Manchester, R. M. Friedman, and M. B. A. Oldstone.** 2000. Evasion of host defenses by measles virus: wild-type measles virus infection interferes with induction of alpha/beta interferon production. *J. Virol.* **74:**7478–7484.

101. **Offit, P. A., and S. E. Coffin.** 2003. Communicating science to the public: MMR vaccine and autism. *Vaccine* **22:**1–6.

102. **Okada, H., T. A. Sato, A. Katayama, K. Higuchi, K. Shichijo, T. Tsuchiya, N. Takayama, Y. Takeuchi, T. Abe, N. Okabe, and M. Tashiro.** 2001. Comparative analysis of host responses related to immunosuppression between measles patients and vaccine recipients with live attenuated measles vaccines. *Arch. Virol.* **146:**859–874.

103. **Ota, M. O., Z. Ndhlovu, S. Oh, S. Piyasirisilp, J. A. Berzofsky, W. J. Moss, and D. E. Griffin.** 2007. Hemagglutinin protein is a primary target of the measles virus-specific HLA-A2-restricted $CD8^+$ T cell response during measles and after vaccination. *J. Infect. Dis.* **195:** 1799–1807.

104. **Otten, M., R. Kezaala, A. Fall, B. Masresha, R. Martin, L. Cairns, R. Eggers, R. Biellik, M. Grabowsky, P. Strebel, J. M. Okwo-Bele, and D. Nshimirimana.** 2005. Public-health impact of accelerated measles control in the WHO African Region 2000–03. *Lancet* **366:**832–839.

105. **Ovsyannikova, I. G., N. Dhiman, R. M. Jacobson, R. A. Vierkant, and G. A. Poland.** 2003. Frequency of measles virus-specific $CD4^+$ and $CD8^+$ T cells in subjects seronegative or highly seropositive for measles vaccine. *Clin. Diagn. Lab. Immunol.* **10:**411–416.

106. **Ovsyannikova, I. G., V. S. Pankratz, R. A. Vierkant, R. M. Jacobson, and G. A. Poland.** 2006. Human leukocyte antigen haplotypes in the genetic control of immune response to measles-mumps-rubella vaccine. *J. Infect. Dis.* **193:**655–663.

107. **Ozanne, G., and M. A. d'Halewyn.** 1992. Secondary immune response in a vaccinated population during a large measles epidemic. *J. Clin. Microbiol.* **30:**1778–1782.

108. **Pan American Health Organization.** 1999. *Measles Eradication. Field Guide*. Pan American Health Organization, Washington, DC.

109. **Pan, C. H., A. Valsamakis, T. Colella, N. Nair, R. J. Adams, F. P. Polack, C. E. Greer, S. Perri, J. M. Polo, and D. E. Griffin.** 2005. Inaugural Article. Modulation of disease, T cell responses, and measles virus clearance in monkeys vaccinated with H-encoding alphavirus replicon particles. *Proc. Natl. Acad. Sci. USA* **102:** 11581–11588.

110. **Panum, P.** 1938. Observations made during the epidemic of measles on the Faroe Islands in the year 1846. *Med Classics* **3:**829–886.

111. **Parker, A. A., W. Staggs, G. H. Dayan, I. R. Ortega-Sanchez, P. A. Rota, L. Lowe, P. Boardman, R. Teclaw, C. Graves, and C. W. LeBaron.** 2006. Implications of a 2005 measles outbreak in Indiana for sustained elimination of measles in the United States. *N. Engl. J. Med.* **355:**447–455.

112. **Permar, S. R., S. A. Klumpp, K. G. Mansfield, A. A. Carville, D. A. Gorgone, M. A. Lifton, J. E. Schmitz, K. A. Reimann, F. P. Polack, D. E. Griffin, and N. L. Letvin.** 2004. Limited contribution of humoral immunity to the clearance of measles viremia in rhesus monkeys. *J. Infect. Dis.* **190:**998–1005.

113. **Permar, S. R., S. A. Klumpp, K. G. Mansfield, W. K. Kim, D. A. Gorgone, M. A. Lifton, K. C. Williams, J. E. Schmitz, K. A. Reimann, M. K. Axthelm, F. P. Polack, D. E. Griffin, and N. L. Letvin.** 2003. Role of $CD8^+$ lymphocytes in control and clearance of measles virus infection of rhesus monkeys. *J. Virol.* **77:**4396–4400.

114. **Permar, S. R., W. J. Moss, J. J. Ryon, M. Monze, F. Cutts, T. C. Quinn, and D. E. Griffin.** 2001. Prolonged measles virus shedding in human immunodeficiency virus-infected children, detected by reverse transcriptase-polymerase chain reaction. *J. Infect. Dis.* **183:**532–538.

115. **Perry, R. T., and N. A. Halsey.** 2004. The clinical significance of measles: a review. *J. Infect. Dis.* **189**(Suppl. 1)**:**S4–S16.

116. **Polack, F. P., P. G. Auwaerter, S. H. Lee, H. C. Nousari, A. Valsamakis, K. M. Leiferman, A. Diwan, R. J. Adams, and D. E. Griffin.** 1999. Production of atypical measles in rhesus macaques: evidence for disease mediated by immune complex formation and eosinophils in the presence of fusion-inhibiting antibody. *Nat. Med.* **5:** 629–634.

117. **Polack, F. P., S. J. Hoffman, G. Crujeiras, and D. E. Griffin.** 2003. A role for nonprotective complement-fixing antibodies with low avidity for measles virus in atypical measles. *Nat. Med.* **9:**1209–1213.

118. **Polack, F. P., S. H. Lee, S. Permar, E. Manyara, H. G. Nousari, Y. Jeng, F. Mustafa, A. Valsamakis, R. J. Adams, H. L. Robinson, and D. E. Griffin.** 2000. Successful DNA immunization against measles: neutralizing antibody against either the hemagglutinin or fusion glycoprotein protects rhesus macaques without evidence of atypical measles. *Nat. Med.* **6:**776–781.

119. **Premenko-Lanier, M., G. Hodge, P. Rota, A. Tamin, W. Bellini, and M. McChesney.** 2006. Maternal antibody inhibits both cellular and humoral immunity in response to measles vaccination at birth. *Virology* **350:** 429–432.

120. **Rota, J. S., Z. D. Wang, P. A. Rota, and W. J. Bellini.** 1994. Comparison of sequences of the H, F, and N coding genes of measles virus vaccine strains. *Virus Res.* **31:** 317–330.

121. **Rota, P. A., J. S. Rota, S. B. Redd, M. J. Papania, and W. J. Bellini.** 2004. Genetic analysis of measles viruses

isolated in the United States between 1989 and 2001: absence of an endemic genotype since 1994. *J. Infect. Dis.* **189**(Suppl. 1):S160–S164.

122. **Roush, S. W., T. V. Murphy, and the Vaccine-Preventable Disease Table Working Group.** 2007. Historical comparisons of morbidity and mortality for vaccine-preventable diseases in the United States. *JAMA* **298:**2155–2163.
123. **Ryon, J. J., W. J. Moss, M. Monze, and D. E. Griffin.** 2002. Functional and phenotypic changes in circulating lymphocytes from hospitalized Zambian children with measles. *Clin. Diagn. Lab. Immunol.* **9:**994–1003.
124. **Salama, P., F. Assefa, L. Talley, P. Spiegel, A. van Der Veen, and C. A. Gotway.** 2001. Malnutrition, measles, mortality, and the humanitarian response during a famine in Ethiopia. *JAMA* **286:**563–571.
125. **Scheifele, D. W., and C. E. Forbes.** 1972. Prolonged giant cell excretion in severe African measles. *Pediatrics* **50:**867–872.
126. **Scott, S., F. T. Cutts, and B. Nyandu.** 1999. Mild illness at or after measles vaccination does not reduce seroresponse in young children. *Vaccine* **17:**837–843.
127. **Scott, S., W. J. Moss, S. Cousens, J. A. Beeler, S. A. Audet, N. Mugala, T. C. Quinn, D. E. Griffin, and F. T. Cutts.** 2007. The influence of HIV-1 exposure and infection on levels of passively acquired antibodies to measles virus in Zambian infants. *Clin. Infect. Dis.* **45:**1417–1424.
128. **Semba, R. D., and M. W. Bloem.** 2004. Measles blindness. *Surv. Ophthalmol.* **49:**243–255.
129. **Sencer, D. J., H. B. Dull, and A. D. Langmuir.** 1967. Epidemiologic basis for eradication of measles in 1967. *Public Health Rep.* **82:**253–256.
130. **Sidhu, M. S., J. Crowley, A. Lowenthal, D. Karcher, J. Menonna, S. Cook, S. Udem, and P. Dowling.** 1994. Defective measles virus in human subacute sclerosing panencephalitis brain. *Virology* **202:**631–641.
131. **Tamashiro, V. G., H. H. Perez, and D. E. Griffin.** 1987. Prospective study of the magnitude and duration of changes in tuberculin reactivity during uncomplicated and complicated measles. *Pediatr. Infect. Dis. J.* **6:**451–454.
132. **Tamin, A., P. A. Rota, Z. D. Wang, J. L. Heath, L. J. Anderson, and W. J. Bellini.** 1994. Antigenic analysis of current wild type and vaccine strains of measles virus. *J. Infect. Dis.* **170:**795–801.
133. **Tatsuo, H., N. Ono, K. Tanaka, and Y. Yanagi.** 2000. SLAM (CDw150) is a cellular receptor for measles virus. *Nature* **406:**893–897.
134. **ten Oever, B. R., M. J. Servant, N. Grandvaux, R. Lin, and J. Hiscott.** 2002. Recognition of the measles virus nucleocapsid as a mechanism of IRF-3 activation. *J. Virol.* **76:**3659–3669.
135. **Vardas, E., and S. Kreis.** 1999. Isolation of measles virus from a naturally-immune asymptomatically re-infected individual. *J. Clin. Virol.* **13:**173–179.
136. **Villamor, E., and W. W. Fawzi.** 2000. Vitamin A supplementation: implications for morbidity and mortality in children. *J. Infect. Dis.* **182**(Suppl. 1)**:**S122–S133.
137. **Wakefield, A. J., S. H. Murch, A. Anthony, J. Linnell, D. M. Casson, M. Malik, M. Berelowitz, A. P. Dhillon, M. A. Thomson, P. Harvey, A. Valentine, S. E. Davies, and J. A. Walker-Smith.** 1998. Ileal-lymphoid-nodular hyperplasia, non-specific colitis, and pervasive developmental disorder in children. *Lancet* **351:**637–641.
138. **Whittle, H. C., P. Aaby, B. Samb, H. Jensen, J. Bennett, and F. Simondon.** 1999. Effect of subclinical infection on maintaining immunity against measles in vaccinated children in West Africa. *Lancet* **353:**98–101.
139. **Wild, T. F., and R. Buckland.** 1995. Functional aspects of envelope-associated measles virus proteins. *Curr. Top. Microbiol. Immunol.* **191:**51–64.
140. **Wolfson, L. J., P. M. Strebel, M. Gacic-Dobo, E. J. Hoekstra, J. W. McFarland, and B. S. Hersh.** 2007. Has the 2005 measles mortality reduction goal been achieved? A natural history modelling study. *Lancet* **369:**191–200.
141. **Wong, R. D., and M. B. Goetz.** 1993. Clinical and laboratory features of measles in hospitalized adults. *Am. J. Med.* **95:**377–383.
142. **Wong-Chew, R. M., R. Islas-Romero, M. L. Garcia-Garcia, J. A. Beeler, S. Audet, J. I. Santos-Preciado, H. Gans, L. Lew-Yasukawa, Y. A. Maldonado, A. M. Arvin, and J. L. Valdespino-Gomez.** 2006. Immunogenicity of aerosol measles vaccine given as the primary measles immunization to nine-month-old Mexican children. *Vaccine* **24:**683–690.
143. **World Health Organization.** 2000. Strategies for reducing global measles mortality. *Wkly. Epidemiol. Rec.* **75:**411–416.
144. **World Health Organization.** 2004. Measles vaccines. *Wkly. Epidemiol. Rec.* **79:**130–142.
145. **World Health Organization.** 2006. Global distribution of measles and rubella genotypes—update. *Wkly. Epidemiol. Rec.* **81:**474–479.
146. **World Health Organization.** 2007. Progress in global measles control and mortality reduction, 2000–2006. *Wkly. Epidemiol. Rec.* **82:**418–424.
147. **World Health Organization and United Nations Children's Fund.** 2001. *Measles Mortality Reduction and Regional Elimination Strategic Plan 2001–2005*. World Health Organization, Geneva, Switzerland.
148. **Xu, W., A. Tamin, J. S. Rota, L. Zhang, W. J. Bellini, and P. A. Rota.** 1998. New genetic group of measles virus isolated in the People's Republic of China. *Virus Res.* **54:**147–156.
149. **Yanagi, Y., N. Ono, H. Tatsuo, K. Hashimoto, and H. Minagawa.** 2002. Measles virus receptor SLAM (CD150). *Virology* **299:**155–161.
150. **Zilliox, M. J., G. Parmigiani, and D. E. Griffin.** 2006. Gene expression patterns in dendritic cells infected with measles virus compared with other pathogens. *Proc. Natl. Acad. Sci. USA* **103:**3363–3368.

Mumps Virus

JOHN W. GNANN, JR.

38

Mumps virus, a member of the family *Paramyxoviridae*, causes a distinctive and generally benign systemic infection that is clinically characterized by fever and parotitis. In older literature, mumps is often termed "epidemic parotitis." In unvaccinated populations, mumps is most common among school-age children, but it has become an uncommon disease in countries where comprehensive childhood immunization programs have been established.

VIROLOGY

Classification

Mumps virus is classified as a member of the order *Mononegavirales* (viruses with nonsegmented, negative-sense, single-stranded RNA genomes), family *Paramyxoviridae*, subfamily *Paramyxovirinae*, and genus *Rubulavirus*. In general, members of the family *Paramyxoviridae* possess nonsegmented RNA genomes, bind to neuraminic acid receptors on host cells, replicate in the cytoplasm, are inactivated by ether, and cause respiratory infections in humans.

Serologic testing with hemagglutination inhibition or neutralization assays has identified only one serotype of mumps virus, although minor antigenic differences among mumps virus isolates can be detected using panels of glycoprotein-specific monoclonal antibodies (118). Infection can be efficiently prevented by vaccination with a single strain of mumps virus. Mumps virus shares some serologic cross-reactivity with other paramyxoviruses, especially parainfluenza viruses, which can complicate interpretation of serodiagnostic assays (63).

Composition

Mumps virus virions are markedly pleomorphic, irregularly spherical particles that range from 50 to 300 nm in diameter (average, about 200 nm). An outer envelope encloses a helically coiled ribonucleocapsid core. The envelope is about 10 nm thick and is composed of three layers: glycoprotein spikes which project 10 to 15 nm from the outer surface of the envelope, a lipid bilayer acquired from the host cell as the virus buds from the cytoplasmic membrane, and an inner structural matrix (M) protein (Fig. 1).

Genome

The mumps virus genome is a linear molecule of single-stranded, negative-sense RNA that contains approximately 15.3 kb and encodes seven major and several minor proteins (47). All of the mumps virus genes have been sequenced (38), and the genome is organized as follows: 3′-NP-V/P-M-F-SH-HN-L-5′ (Fig. 2). The three proteins associated with the ribonucleoprotein complex are the nucleocapsid protein (NP), the phosphoprotein (P), and the large (L) protein. The envelope contains M and two surface glycoproteins that mediate hemagglutinin-neuraminidase (HN) and fusion (F) activities. The small hydrophobic (SH) protein is membrane associated (124).

Viral Proteins

The nucleocapsid protein is the major viral structural protein and tightly encloses the genomic RNA (126). Complement-fixing antibody recognizes NP as the "S antigen." P is also associated with the nucleocapsid (141). The L protein, a high-molecular-weight polypeptide present in small amounts, functions in conjunction with P in the transcriptase complex as an RNA-dependent RNA polymerase (103). Full-length transcription of the V/P gene yields the V protein (also known as NS1), while RNA editing during the transcription of V/P produces P as well as the nonstructural I protein (also known as NS2) (40). The V protein is thought to block host antiviral responses by inhibiting the interferon signal transduction pathway (5, 79). The function of the I protein is not known.

The M protein is a nonglycosylated membrane-associated protein (39). The function of the M protein is to link the ribonucleocapsid with the host cell membrane and to position newly assembled nucleocapsids under the appropriate region of the host cell membrane prior to viral budding. HN is an N-glycosolated protein bound to the membrane via a hydrophobic domain near its amino terminus (137). This transmembrane molecule carries both hemagglutination and neuraminidase activities in the same domain of the protein, with functions activated by protein conformational changes (125). HN is responsible for binding of mumps virus to sialic acid receptors on the host cell membrane. In addition, HN works in concert with the

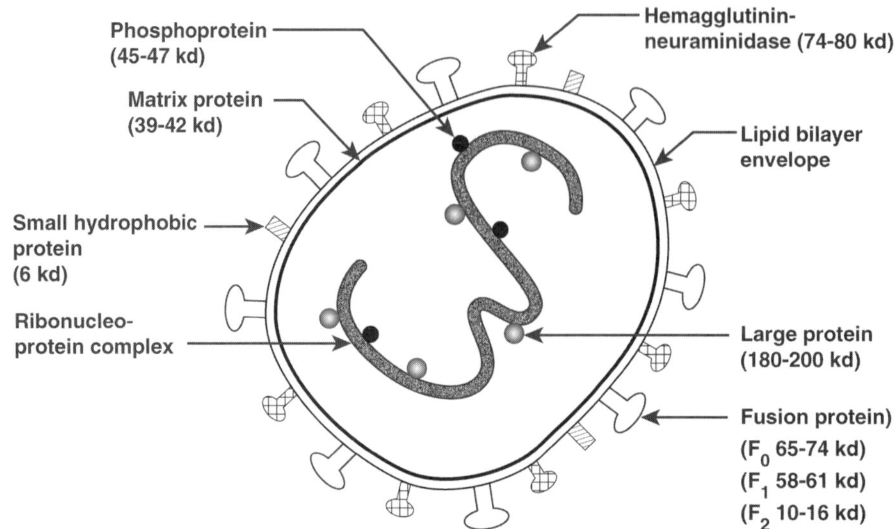

FIGURE 1 Structure of the mumps virus virion. Molecular masses of viral proteins as measured by gel electrophoresis are shown in parentheses. (Data from reference 47.)

F protein to mediate both virus-to-cell and cell-to-cell membrane fusion (125, 127). Antibody directed against HN is neutralizing and inhibits viral infectivity. In complement fixation (CF) assays, HN is the "V antigen."

The F protein is an N-glycosylated molecule anchored into the envelope by a sequence of hydrophobic amino acids near the carboxyl terminus (39). Penetration of the viral nucleocapsid into the target cell does not occur if fusion activity is inhibited. In addition, antibody directed against the F protein blocks hemolytic activity of mumps virus. The fusion molecule is expressed as a precursor protein (F_0) that is cleaved by a cellular protease to its active form, which consists of two disulfide-linked glycoproteins (F_1 and F_2) (98). After attachment, fusion is initiated when a hydrophobic sequence near the amino terminus of F_1 interacts with the lipid bilayer of the host cell membrane (128).

The function of the membrane-associated SH protein has not been fully defined (123). However, recent studies employing reverse transcriptase PCR (RT-PCR) methodology have demonstrated 12 distinct viral genotypes (tentatively designated A to L) based on the sequence of the SH gene (65). These molecular tools will allow more precise studies of mumps transmission and epidemiology (64, 99, 105). Genetic characterization of SH is also a useful tool for distinguishing wild-type and vaccine strains of mumps virus (1).

Specific changes in mumps virus gene sequences may modulate viral neurovirulence (83, 89, 110, 114). In the suckling hamster model, mumps virus strains vary significantly in their degree of neurotropism, possibly due to differences in the HN surface glycoprotein (87).

Biology

Penetration of mumps virus virions into target cells begins with binding of the HN surface glycoprotein to sialic acid-containing receptors on the cell surface. Fusion of the viral and cellular membranes allows the viral nucleocapsid to enter the cytoplasm of the host cell, where mumps virus replication is initiated. The nucleocapsid-associated protein is complexed in the virion with genomic RNA to form the ribonucleocapsid, which serves as a template for RNA synthesis. Replication is initiated by the binding of the RNA-dependent RNA polymerase, a complex of P and the L protein, to the ribonucleocapsid. The input genomic RNA is transcribed into mRNAs that are 5′ capped and 3′ polyadenylated (Fig. 3). RNA synthesis begins at the 3′ end of the genome and proceeds sequentially by a stop-start mechanism in which transcription is terminated and reinitiated at each gene junction. This results in a gradient

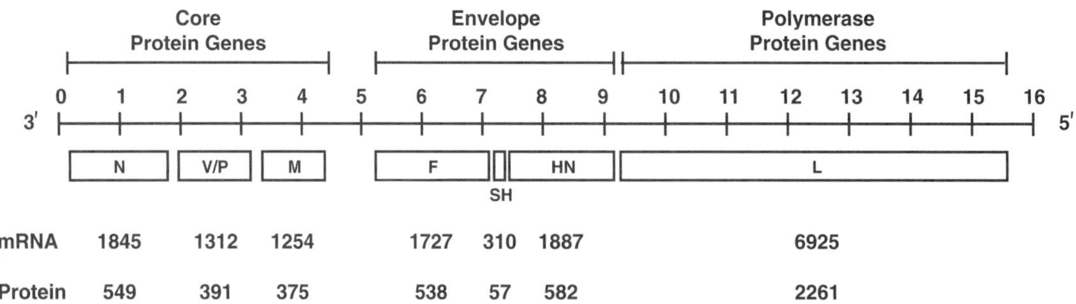

FIGURE 2 Genome organization of mumps virus. Number of nucleotides in mRNA and amino acid residues in corresponding protein are shown below map. (Data from reference 109.)

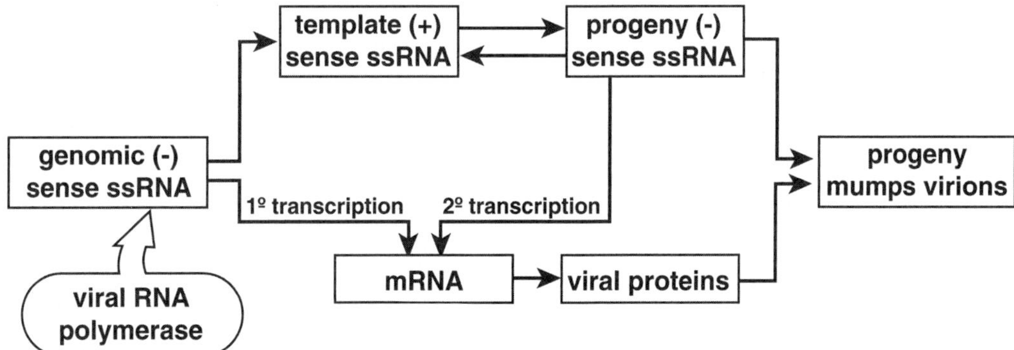

FIGURE 3 Replication strategy of mumps virus.

of mRNA synthesis, with fewer copies of downstream mRNAs due to the occasional failure of the RNA polymerase to properly reinitiate at the next gene junction. Following primary transcription and translation of viral proteins, RNA synthesis proceeds with production of replicative intermediates (positive-sense RNA) and subsequently progeny negative-sense RNAs. The switch from producing monocistronic mRNAs to synthesis of full-length RNA species is controlled by intracellular concentrations of nucleocapsid protein. The nascent full-length negative-sense RNA strands may serve as templates for replication or as templates for secondary transcription, or they may be packaged into progeny virions. The newly assembled nucleocapsids are actively transported from the cytoplasm to the plasma membrane of the host cell. Under the direction of the M protein, viral nucleocapsids are aligned along the inner surface of the cellular membrane beneath the newly synthesized viral glycoproteins. The progeny virions are released from the cell by budding, incorporating a portion of the cellular cytoplasmic membrane into the envelope.

Host Range

Although humans are the only known natural host for mumps virus, mumps virus infection can be experimentally induced in a variety of mammalian species. Suckling hamsters have proven to be a useful model for investigations of mumps virus neuropathology.

Cell Growth

Mumps virus can be propagated in many mammalian cell lines, including Vero, primary rhesus monkey kidney, human embryonic kidney, BSC-1, and HeLa cells, as well as embryonated hens' eggs. In vitro cytopathic effects generally appear within 3 to 6 days after inoculation and may be either fusing or nonfusing, depending on the virus strain and cell lines involved. The classic cytopathic effect is cell-to-cell fusion producing giant multinucleated syncytia. Other cytopathic changes that may be observed include cell pyknosis and lysis, eosinophilic intracytoplasmic inclusions, and spindle formation. The degree of neurovirulence of a mumps virus strain cannot be predicted by in vitro cytopathology.

Stability and Inactivation

Mumps virus will retain infectivity at 4°C for several hours (longer in protein-stabilized media) and at −70°C for years. Mumps virus can be inactivated by treatment with formalin, ether or other organic solvents, detergents, UV irradiation, or heating to 56°C.

EPIDEMIOLOGY

Incidence and Prevalence of Mumps Virus Infection

Mumps has a worldwide distribution and, in susceptible urban populations, is a disease of school-age children (4). Over 50% of mumps cases occur in children between 5 and 9 years of age. In unvaccinated populations, 92% of children have antibodies against mumps virus by age 15. Infection is commonly acquired at school, with secondary spread to susceptible family members. Mumps is rare in children under 1 year of age, presumably due to the protective effect of passively acquired maternal antibody. Mumps is generally a benign disease; the case fatality ratio from 1962 to 1971 was 1.6 to 3.8 per 10,000 cases (which is likely an overestimation, due to reporting bias), with most deaths resulting from encephalitis. Prior to the release of the mumps vaccine in the United States in 1967, mumps was an endemic disease, with annual peak activity occurring between January and May. Localized epidemics of mumps in closed populations (isolated communities, boarding schools, military units, etc.) were also well recognized.

United States

The largest number of mumps cases reported in the United States occurred in 1941, when the incidence was 250 cases per 100,000 population (30). When the mumps vaccine first entered clinical usage in 1968, the incidence of mumps was 76 cases per 100,000 population. Mumps vaccine was recommended for routine use in the United States in 1977. In 1985, only 2,982 cases of mumps were reported (1.1 cases per 100,000 population), which is a 98% reduction from the 185,691 cases reported in 1967 (24). Between 1985 and 1987, the incidence of mumps in the United States increased fivefold, to 5.2 cases per 100,000 population (23, 30). More than one-third of the cases reported during this interval occurred in adolescents, reflecting the failure to adequately vaccinate this cohort of children during the 1970s (121, 139). Since 1987, the incidence of mumps in the United States has steadily declined, and only 231 cases were reported in 2003, the lowest total ever recorded (29, 60). In 1989, the Centers for Disease Control Advisory Committee on Immunization Practices issued a recommendation that all children receive a second dose of the measles-mumps-rubella (MMR) vaccine, which has reduced the problem of primary vaccine failure (28).

A series of outbreaks in the United States and Canada in 2005–2006 reemphasized the potential for mumps virus to cause localized epidemics even in highly vaccinated populations (34, 68). In 2006, a total of 6,584 cases of mumps were reported, with a national incidence of 2.2 cases per 100,000 population (34). The U.S. outbreak was centered in the Midwest and peaked in April 2006; 34% of the cases occurred in Iowa. The highest age-specific rate was in persons aged 18 to 24 years (median age, 22 years), many of whom were college students (26). Among the Iowa patients, 7% were unvaccinated, 14% had received 1 dose of MMR, 49% had received ≥2 doses of MMR vaccine, and 30% had unknown vaccine status. While some cases can be attributed to failure to vaccinate, most represented primary (insufficient initial immune response) or secondary (waning immune response) vaccine failure (20, 106). This suggests the need for a mumps vaccine with a longer duration of protection or modification in vaccination policy, perhaps focusing on young adults (31, 34).

Lifelong immunity follows natural infection. Adult patients with apparent symptomatic mumps virus reinfection have been reported, but diagnoses were made serologically and not by viral isolation; serologic cross-reactivity with other paramyxoviruses cannot be excluded (53).

PATHOGENESIS

Transmission and Viral Replication

Mumps is highly contagious. Humans can be experimentally infected by inoculation of mumps virus onto the nasal or buccal mucosa, suggesting that natural infection results from airborne spread of droplets of respiratory secretions from infected to susceptible individuals. Humans are most contagious near the time of onset of parotitis. Mumps virus can be isolated from saliva from 5 to 6 days before to 5 days after the onset of clinical symptoms, indicating that an infected person is potentially able to transmit mumps for a period of about 10 days. The mean incubation period from exposure to onset of clinical symptoms is 18 days. During the incubation period, a primary round of viral replication takes place in epithelial cells of the nasal mucosa or upper respiratory tract, followed by spread of virus to regional lymph nodes. This is followed by a transient plasma viremia (possibly via infected T lymphocytes), resulting in dissemination of mumps virus to glandular and neural tissues. Positive cultures from blood are uncommon. The viremic phase is terminated by the onset of the humoral immune response. Mumps virus can be isolated from saliva from nearly all patients with acute mumps parotitis.

Mumps virus also replicates in the kidney, involving epithelial cells of the distal tubules and renal collecting system. Virus can be recovered from up to 72% of urine samples collected during the first 5 days of clinical illness; viruria may persist for up to 2 weeks (132). Mild renal function abnormalities are common in patients with mumps, but permanent impairment of renal function is rare (132).

CNS

Central nervous system (CNS) involvement in mumps is very common, although it is usually asymptomatic (10). The proposed pathogenesis involves spread of virus (or infected mononuclear cells) across the endothelium of the choroid plexus and replication in the choroidal epithelial cells, with release of virions into the cerebrospinal fluid (CSF). CSF collected during the early phases of mumps meningoencephalitis will yield mumps virus in 30 to 50% of cases (96).

Mumps virus can establish persistent infection in neuronal cell lines (86) and chronic CNS infection in animal models, but it does not routinely cause chronic infections in humans. In patients with mumps meningitis, the persistence of leukocytes and oligoclonal mumps-specific immunoglobulins in the CSF for months after the acute infection suggests the possibility of ongoing antigenic stimulation from chronic mumps virus CNS infection (133). A few anecdotal case reports of chronic mumps encephalitis have appeared (54, 62), but sufficient data do not exist to confirm a role for mumps virus as a cause of chronic CNS infection in humans.

Histopathology

Since mumps is rarely a fatal illness, few pathological descriptions from autopsy series are available. Most observations of mumps pathology have been derived from patients who died with acute mumps encephalitis (16). Mumps parotitis is characterized by diffuse periductal and interstitial edema with infiltration by lymphocytes and monocytes. The ductal epithelial cells degenerate and the ductal lumen becomes occluded with neutrophils and necrotic debris, but the glandular cells are generally not involved.

The brains of patients who died with mumps encephalitis have exhibited variable neuropathological findings (16, 21). Reported abnormalities have included diffuse cerebral edema, meningeal infiltration with mononuclear leukocytes, perivascular cuffing with mononuclear cells, proliferation of glial cells, focal neuronal destruction, and localized demyelinization. Histologic changes indicate direct viral cytopathic effect, as well as changes (e.g., demyelinization) that suggest an autoimmune postinfectious encephalopathy. In the suckling hamster model, mumps virus CNS infection is associated with the development of stenosis of the sylvian aqueduct and with granular ependymitis (57). These findings suggest a possible (but unproven) linkage between mumps CNS infections and aqueductal stenosis in children (3).

Orchitis is a common complication of mumps in men. Virus replicates in cells of the seminiferous tubules, resulting in infiltration by leukocytes and hemorrhagic interstitial edema. Swelling within the closed space bounded by the tunica albuginea causes severe pain and can produce vascular insufficiency and areas of infarction. Severe cases of mumps orchitis can result in atrophy of the germinal epithelium with scarring and fibrosis.

Immune Responses

The relative contributions of the humoral and cell-mediated immune responses to viral clearance during mumps have not been precisely established. Mumps-specific immunoglobulin M (IgM) is detectable within 10 to 12 days after initiation of infection and usually falls to undetectable levels after 6 months (102). Mumps-specific secretory IgA appears in saliva within 5 days of disease onset and correlates with the termination of viral shedding. The antimumps IgG response is detectable by enzyme-linked immunosorbent assay (ELISA) during the first week of the acute infection and by CF assay by day 10 to 14.

IgG titers peak at about 3 to 4 weeks after the onset of infection and persist for decades. Antibodies directed against HN (and possibly the F protein) have viral neutralizing activity (61).

Infection with mumps virus also induces a specific cell-mediated immune response. Peripheral lymphocytes that proliferate when stimulated with mumps virus S and V antigens in an in vitro blastogenesis assay as well as HLA-restricted cytotoxic T lymphocytes (CTLs) can be detected in peripheral blood following natural infection or immunization. Lymphocytes isolated from the CSF of patients with mumps meningitis will proliferate when stimulated with mumps virus antigens and demonstrate cytotoxicity to autologous mumps virus-infected target cells. Recruitment of CTLs into the CNS in patients with mumps may play a role in the immunopathological changes observed in human brains after fatal mumps encephalitis (74).

Elevated levels of cytokines and immunoglobulins can be measured in CSF from patients with mumps meningitis. CSF interferon levels decline within a week in patients with self-limited mumps meningitis but remain elevated in the CSF of those patients who have more severe CNS involvement or persistent CSF pleocytosis (91). Intrathecal production of mumps-specific IgG and IgM is a common feature of mumps meningitis in children, although there is no apparent correlation between the severity of clinical meningoencephalitis and titers of mumps-specific immunoglobulins in the CSF (44).

A delayed hypersensitivity response to intradermally injected mumps virus antigen develops about 3 to 12 weeks after the clinical illness. While used as a "control" antigen for tuberculin skin testing, the mumps skin test is not a reliable indicator of mumps immune status.

CLINICAL MANIFESTATIONS

Clinical Syndromes

Following an incubation period of about 18 days (range, 14 to 28 days), symptomatic mumps begins with a short, nonspecific prodromal phase characterized by fever, malaise, headache, and anorexia. Young children may initially complain of ear pain. Patients then develop the characteristic salivary gland pain and swelling (Table 1). In some case series, <50% of patients with acute mumps virus infections have developed classic disease with parotitis. Symptomatic parotitis is most common among children aged 2 to 9 years. Up to 50% of mumps virus infections may be associated with nonspecific or respiratory symptoms, and 15 to 20% are asymptomatic (43). Over 90% of unvaccinated adults with no history of mumps are found to be seropositive when tested for mumps antibody, indicating prior subclinical infection.

TABLE 1 Clinical manifestations of mumps

Common
- Salivary gland enlargement (especially parotitis)
- "Aseptic" meningitis
- Epididymo-orchitis (postpubertal males)

Uncommon
- Hearing loss
- Encephalitis
- Oophoritis (postpubertal females)
- Mastitis (postpubertal females)
- Pancreatitis
- Polyarthritis
- Myocarditis
- Thyroiditis
- Hepatitis
- Thrombocytopenia
- Ocular involvement
- Nephritis

Parotid glands are most commonly involved, although other salivary glands may be enlarged in 10% of cases. Involvement of the submandibular glands may mimic anterior cervical adenopathy. Sublingual gland involvement is least frequent and may be associated with tongue swelling. Involvement of other salivary glands without parotitis is rare. Parotitis may initially be unilateral, with swelling of the contralateral gland occurring 2 to 3 days later; bilateral parotitis eventually develops in 75 to 90% of patients with symptomatic salivary gland involvement. Presternal pitting edema occurs in about 5% of patients and may be secondary to lymphatic obstruction caused by enlarged salivary glands (2). Painful parotid gland swelling progresses over 2 or 3 days, lifting the ear lobe outward and obscuring the angle of the mandible (which helps distinguish parotitis from cervical adenopathy). The orifice of Stensen's duct is often erythematous and edematous. Patients complain of trismus, difficulty chewing, and difficulty speaking. Drinking citrus juice may exacerbate the parotid pain. Fever (up to 40°C) and parotid enlargement peak on the third day of illness, followed by defervescence and resolution of parotid pain and swelling within about 1 week. Long-term sequelae of parotitis are uncommon, although sialectasis and recurrent sialadenitis have been reported.

Results of routine laboratory studies of patients with mumps are generally nonspecific. The peripheral leukocyte count is mildly elevated (10,000 to 12,000 cells/mm^3), with a mild lymphocytosis (30 to 40% lymphocytes). Approximately 30% of mumps patients will have an elevated serum amylase, reflecting inflammation of the salivary glands or pancreas (9); these can be distinguished by isoenzyme analysis or by pancreatic lipase determination.

CNS

CNS involvement is the most common extrasalivary manifestation of mumps and occurs with sufficient frequency (10 to 30% of mumps cases) that it should be considered a part of the natural history and not a complication (10, 50). For reasons that remain unexplained, mumps CNS disease is three to four times more likely to occur among male children than among females (21, 75, 84). The spectrum of CNS diseases associated with mumps ranges from mild aseptic meningitis, which is very common, to fulminant and potentially fatal encephalitis, which is very rare, occurring in less than 0.1% of cases of acute mumps (75, 84). CSF pleocytosis is present in 40 to 60% of patients with acute mumps, although only 10 to 30% of mumps patients will have clinical evidence of meningeal irritation. That is, half of the mumps patients demonstrated to have CSF pleocytosis will not have CNS symptoms (10, 21).

CNS symptoms usually appear about 5 days after the onset of parotitis, although development of CNS findings before or simultaneously with parotitis is well recognized (8, 75, 84). Mumps CNS disease can also occur in patients without clinical evidence of parotitis; indeed, 40 to 50% of patients with symptomatic mumps meningitis have no evidence of salivary gland enlargement. The diagnosis of mumps cannot be excluded in a patient with meningoencephalitis simply because the patient does not have clinically apparent salivary gland involvement.

Mumps CNS infection manifests as high fever, vomiting, and headache that lasts for 48 to 96 h (8, 100, 112) (Table 2). The majority of mumps patients with CNS involvement will have signs of meningeal irritation but no evidence of cortical dysfunction. Defervescence is accompanied by overall clinical recovery, and the total duration of illness in uncomplicated cases is 7 to 10 days. Mumps meningitis is a benign disease with essentially no risk of mortality or long-term morbidity.

The onset of seizures, an altered level of consciousness, or focal neurologic abnormalities in a patient with mumps are indicative of encephalitis (75, 84). The mortality rate for patients with mumps encephalitis is less than 1.5%, and permanent sequelae are rare. Even among patients who are profoundly encephalopathic, the probability of complete recovery is high; sustained seizures and focal neurologic deficits may indicate a less favorable prognosis (75).

CSF pleocytosis (>5 leukocytes/mm^3) occurs in 40 to 60% of patients with mumps parotitis and is a prominent feature of patients with mumps meningoencephalitis (6) (Table 3). Mumps virus can be isolated from about 33% of CSF specimens in which there is pleocytosis. Lumbar puncture in patients with mumps meningoencephalitis usually reveals a normal opening pressure and an elevated leukocyte count of 200 to 600 cells/mm^3 (ranging up to 2,000 cells/mm^3) that is >80% lymphocytes (21, 84, 140). About 50% of patients will have a moderately elevated CSF protein, and 10 to 20% will have moderate hypoglycorrhachia (CSF glucose, 20 to 40 mg/dl) (66, 140). Depressed CSF glucose is an unusual finding in viral meningitis and has been reported most often with mumps virus, lymphocytic choriomeningitis virus, and herpes simplex virus infections. CSF pleocytosis often persists for weeks after resolution of clinical mumps disease (9). There is no definite correlation between the magnitude of the CSF abnormalities and the clinical course, although one study reported that higher CSF protein and lower CSF glucose levels were associated with longer durations of hospitalization (69, 84).

Numerous neurologic complications have been described in association with mumps encephalitis, including behavioral disturbances and personality changes (19, 75), seizure disorders (112), cranial nerve palsies (especially facial and ocular palsies) (14), muscular weakness (including hemiparesis), ataxia (75, 88), myelitis (11, 134), Guillain-Barré syndrome (36), and hydrocephalus (51, 131, 135).

TABLE 2 Initial clinical findings in patients with CNS mumps virus infection[a]

Sign or symptom	% of patients
Fever	95
Vomiting	75
Headache	70
Neck stiffness	70
Parotitis	50
Lethargy	40
Abdominal pain	15
Seizures	15

[a] Compiled from 248 cases (8, 84, 96, 100). Modified from reference 50 with permission.

TABLE 3 Initial CSF findings in patients with CNS mumps virus infection[a]

Finding	Mean	Typical range
Leukocyte count (cells/mm^3)	450	100–1,000
Leukocyte differential (% lymphocytes)	90	70–100
Protein (mg/dl)	65	30–150
Glucose (mg/dl)	55	30–70

[a] Compiled from 116 cases (73, 112, 115, 140). Modified from reference 50 with permission.

Electroencephalograms recorded from patients with acute mumps encephalitis characteristically show moderate to severe slowing without spikes or lateralizing signs. Modern imaging techniques (computed tomography, magnetic resonance imaging, etc.) have not been systematically evaluated as diagnostic tools for patients with mumps CNS infection (93).

Special Populations

Maternal mumps virus infection during the first trimester of pregnancy may result in an increased frequency of spontaneous abortion; infection during the second or third trimester is generally uncomplicated. Fetal wastage occurs as a result of infection of the placenta and/or fetus during the early viremic phase. Villous necrosis with intracytoplasmic inclusion bodies in decidual cells have been seen in placentas from spontaneous abortions following maternal mumps (48). In addition, mumps virus has been isolated from fetal tissue following a spontaneous first-trimester abortion that occurred during acute maternal mumps (80). A possible association between mumps occurring during the first trimester and low birth weight has been described. There is no clear connection between mumps occurring during pregnancy and congenital defects (119). Mumps virus is known to be excreted in breast milk, but perinatal mumps virus infection is extremely rare.

Mumps virus has not usually been shown to cause severe or prolonged infections in patients with congenital or acquired immunodeficiency syndromes.

Complications

Gonadal involvement can occur in both men and women with mumps (92). Epididymo-orchitis is rare in prepubertal boys with mumps but occurs in 25 to 38% of men (13, 90). Orchitis is usually unilateral; bilateral involvement occurs in 17 to 38% of cases. Orchitis typically develops within 4 to 10 days after the onset of parotitis, although orchitis can develop prior to or even in the absence of parotitis (22, 41). Patients with mumps orchitis present with severe testicular pain and swelling accompanied by high fever (39 to 41°C), nausea, vomiting, and headache. Physical examination demonstrates warmth and erythema of the scrotum with marked tenderness of the testicle, which may be swollen to three or four times its normal size. Epididymitis is also present in 85% of cases (12, 138). The testicular swelling and constitutional symptoms resolve within 5 to 7 days, although residual testicular tenderness persists for several weeks in up to 20% of patients. Testicular atrophy may follow orchitis in 35 to 50% of cases, but impotence or sterility is uncommon even among patients with bilateral orchitis. A proposed association between mumps-related testicular atrophy and subsequent testicular malignancy appears to be unlikely (37).

Oophoritis occurs in 5% of postpubertal women with mumps. Women with mumps oophoritis typically report fever, nausea, vomiting, and adnexal pain. Sequelae are uncommon, although impaired fertility and premature menopause following mumps can occur. Fifteen percent of postpubertal women with mumps complain of breast swelling and tenderness consistent with mastitis.

Mumps-associated pancreatitis manifests as fever, nausea, vomiting, and epigastric pain. Some epidemiological data suggested an association between mumps pancreatitis and juvenile diabetes mellitus; however, the dramatic decline in the incidence of mumps has not been mirrored by a corresponding decline in the occurrence of juvenile-onset diabetes mellitus.

Migratory polyarthritis (or, less frequently, monarticular arthritis) has been observed in mumps patients (52, 56). The pathogenesis of mumps-related arthritis is uncertain; virus has not been isolated from joint fluid, and there is no evidence of immune complex deposition. The arthritis may involve large and small joints and usually begins 10 to 14 days after the onset of parotitis. The joint symptoms may last 4 to 6 weeks but usually resolve with no permanent joint damage.

Symptomatic mumps myocarditis is rare, although electrocardiographic changes have been reported to occur in 3 to 15% of patients (6). The most common electrocardiographic abnormalities are prolongation of the PR interval, flattening or inversion of T waves, and depression of ST segments. Rare cases of inflammatory myocarditis with lymphocytic infiltration in patients with mumps have been described. A proposed linkage of mumps with pediatric endocardial fibroelastosis remains unproven (101).

Sensorineural hearing loss is a well-recognized complication of mumps that occurs with a frequency of 0.5 to 5.0 episodes/100,000 mumps cases (70, 71, 95). In one series collected among military personnel, transient high-frequency hearing loss occurred in 4.4% of cases (136). The onset of deafness may be either gradual or abrupt and may be accompanied by vertigo. Hearing changes result from direct damage to the cochlea by the mumps virus and may be either transient or permanent (55).

Other infrequent complications of mumps include thyroiditis, hepatitis, nephritis (67), and thrombocytopenia. Rare ocular complications of mumps include iritis, keratitis, and central retinal vein occlusion (45, 104). A mumps virus-associated hemophagocytic syndrome has been described (59).

Clinical Diagnosis

The presentation of a febrile child with parotitis strongly suggests the diagnosis of mumps, particularly if the individual is known to be susceptible and has been exposed to mumps during the preceding 2 to 3 weeks. However, the etiology of aseptic meningitis may not be apparent if there is no concomitant salivary gland enlargement. Mumps meningoencephalitis has been confused with nonparalytic poliomyelitis, particularly when mumps cases occur during the summer. The CSF pleocytosis is generally higher in mumps and the nuchal rigidity and fever resolve more quickly than in poliomyelitis (21). To further complicate the diagnosis, mumps encephalitis can occasionally be associated with local muscle weakness that clinically resembles poliomyelitis. Since mumps and poliomyelitis are both becoming rare diseases in industrialized nations, the presentation of fever, meningoencephalitis, and focal motor weakness requires specific laboratory testing to establish the diagnosis.

A variety of other infectious and noninfectious disorders can cause parotid enlargement that may be confused with mumps (97). Other viruses (including parainfluenza virus, coxsackievirus, adenovirus, Epstein-Barr virus, human herpesvirus 6, and influenza A virus) can cause fever and parotid gland enlargement (32). Accurate diagnosis requires viral culture or specific serologic testing. Parotid gland enlargement has also been described to occur in patients with AIDS, especially children (15, 120). Bacterial parotitis (usually caused by *Staphylococcus aureus* or gram-negative bacilli) is most often unilateral and occurs in debilitated patients with poor oral intake, postoperative patients, and premature infants. Physical examination reveals erythematous skin overlying a hard, warm, and very tender parotid gland. Parotid massage expresses pus from Stensen's duct. Tumors, cysts, and duct obstruction due to salivary stones can also result in unilateral parotid swelling.

Drugs and systemic illness can result in parotid swelling which is typically bilateral and nontender. Medications associated with salivary gland enlargement include iodides, phenothiazines, phenylbutazone, and thiouracil. Chronic diseases in which parotitis can appear include cirrhosis, diabetes mellitus, malnutrition, chronic renal failure, sarcoidosis (uveoparotid fever), tuberculosis, lymphoma, amyloidosis, and Sjögren syndrome.

LABORATORY DIAGNOSIS

Virus Isolation and Nucleic Acid Amplification

The clinical diagnosis is accurate and reliable in most cases of mumps. However, atypical clinical presentations (e.g., meningitis or orchitis without parotitis) may require laboratory confirmation. Virus culture is the definitive diagnostic test, although it may not be routinely available. Mumps virus can be isolated from saliva from virtually all patients with acute mumps parotitis from 2 to 3 days before until 4 to 5 days after the onset of symptoms. Most diagnostic laboratories isolate mumps virus on primary rhesus monkey kidney cells or on human embryonic kidney cells. Hemagglutinin molecules on the surface of mumps virus-infected cells will bind guinea pig erythrocytes. Confirmation of a clinical isolate as mumps virus has traditionally been performed by a hemadsorption inhibition assay in which mumps-specific antiserum is used to block the adherence of erythrocytes to mumps virus-infected cells. This technique has been replaced by immunofluorescence methods with polyclonal or monoclonal anti-mumps virus antibodies to positively identify mumps virus in tissue culture.

A nested RT-PCR assay for detection of mumps RNA in CSF has been described (108). Although clinical experience with this assay is currently limited, RT-PCR is likely to become the diagnostic method of choice for mumps virus CNS infection (17, 76, 78, 129).

Serologic Assays

Humoral immune responses to mumps virus infection or immunization can be measured by a variety of techniques, all of which are limited to some extent by inherent antigenic cross-reactivity between mumps virus and other paramyxoviruses (63). Serologic assays are designed to detect a fourfold increase in mumps-specific IgG between acute-phase (collected at the time of clinical disease) and convalescent-phase (collected 2 to 4 weeks later) serum specimens. Detection of neutralizing antibody, which appears during the convalescent phase of mumps and persists for years, is a reliable but technically demanding assay (107). The hemagglutination inhibition assay is simple and sensitive, but reagents are not routinely commercially available. The CF assay was widely used in the past but has now been replaced by sensitive and specific ELISAs (85, 102). ELISA has the advantages of simplicity and ability to measure either IgG or IgM. Demonstration of high-titer mumps-specific IgM in the acute-phase specimen is indicative of recent infection (77). An IgM response is detectable by the fifth day of clinical illness, peaks at 1 week, and persists for at least 6 weeks (49). Measurement of IgM for diagnosis of acute mumps has the additional advantage of low (or absent) cross-reactivity with parainfluenza viruses (130).

As measured by the CF assay, anti-V (HN) antibodies peak at about 2 to 4 weeks after infection and persist for years, while anti-S (NP) antibodies decline over several months to undetectable levels. In the past, CF was used to distinguish between current or recent infection (high anti-S) and remote infection (low/absent anti-S, high anti-V), but CF has been replaced by more specific and sensitive serologic assays (46). ELISA is routinely used to determine mumps immune status, although the labor-intensive plaque reduction neutralization assay is more sensitive and specific (85, 94).

PREVENTION

Children with mumps are usually isolated for about 1 week after the appearance of parotitis, although this practice is of dubious benefit to classmates since the virus is known to be shed in respiratory secretions for several days prior to the onset of clinical symptoms.

Mumps can be efficiently prevented by use of an effective vaccine containing live attenuated virus. A formalin-inactivated mumps virus vaccine has also been developed, but the duration of protection may be shorter, so the killed-virus vaccine is less widely used. The vaccine currently used in the United States contains the Jeryl-Lynn B strain of live mumps virus that was attenuated by serial passage in embryonated hens' eggs and chicken embryo cell cultures. The mumps vaccine is a component of the MMR vaccine and is given by subcutaneous injection in two doses. The Advisory Committee on Immunization Practices recommends that the first dose of MMR vaccine be given at 12 to 15 months of age and the second dose given at 4 to 6 years of age (28). Neutralizing antibody appears within 2 weeks of immunization. Recent studies from Finland showed that 74% of vaccinees had detectable mumps antibody 15 years after the second MMR vaccine dose (31). Early studies concluded that a single immunization provided protective immunity to 97% of recipients (58). However, studies conducted during mumps virus outbreaks in the 1980s indicated an efficacy rate of 75 to 91% following a single dose (122, 139). The two-dose MMR vaccination schedule was adopted in the United States in 1989 in response to increased rates of measles but also effectively addressed the problem of primary mumps vaccine failure seen with a single dose (24). Most states now require presumptive evidence of mumps immunity (either two doses of vaccine, physician-documented disease, or laboratory-demonstrated seropositivity) before children are allowed to enroll in school. Health care workers without evidence of mumps immunity should also be immunized (27). A quadrivalent vaccine (MMR plus varicella vaccine) has recently been approved for use in the United States (111).

The Jeryl-Lynn B-based vaccine is safe, well tolerated, and cost-effective (142). In healthy children, immunization causes no symptoms, and virus cannot be isolated from blood, urine, or saliva. Administration of MMR vaccine is contraindicated in pregnant women, in persons who have received immunoglobulin therapy within the preceding 3 months (which might limit immune responses to the vaccine), or in persons who are significantly immunocompromised. Asymptomatic human immunodeficiency virus-infected children should receive mumps immunization (7). Mumps vaccine is produced in chicken embryo cell cultures and may contain trace amounts of egg protein and neomycin, so immunization is not recommended for any person with a history of severe allergic reactions to those substances. Egg-allergic children can be safely immunized by following a desensitization protocol (72, 82). Anaphylactic reactions to MMR or mumps vaccine are extremely rare (25). Other strains of live attenuated mumps vaccine (including Urabe AM9 and Leningrad-3) have been associated with higher rates of vaccine-associated aseptic meningitis and are no longer widely used (18, 35). In some countries, the Urabe mumps vaccine strain was replaced by the highly attenuated Rubini strain, which provides unacceptably low levels of clinical protection (106, 117). A rat-based neurovirulence assay has been developed to assess the safety of candidate mumps vaccine viruses (113).

Mumps vaccine can be safely administered to an individual of unknown immune status, although vaccine given to a susceptible person following exposure to mumps may not provide protection (33). This circumstance most often arises when an individual with no history of mumps is exposed to a patient with active infection. Mumps immune globulin is of no proven value in this setting and is not commercially available. The immune status of the exposed individual can be rapidly determined by ELISA, although it is generally safe to assume that adults born in the United States before 1957 have been naturally infected and are immune (24).

TREATMENT

Therapy of patients with uncomplicated mumps consists of conservative measures to provide symptomatic relief, such as analgesics, antipyretics, rest, and hydration. There is currently no established role for corticosteroids, antiviral chemotherapy, or passive immunotherapy in mumps. Case reports and small series have claimed that administration of $\alpha 2$ interferon is beneficial in men with mumps orchitis, but this therapy has not been adequately studied in a controlled fashion (42, 116). Symptomatic measures to alleviate the pain and swelling of mumps orchitis include bed rest, scrotal support, opioid analgesics, and application of ice packs. Surgical decompression was frequently performed in the past for mumps orchitis but is no longer recommended (81).

Patients with mumps and clinical evidence of encephalitis (e.g., altered mental status, seizures, or focal neurologic findings) should be hospitalized for observation.

Supportive care for patients with mumps meningoencephalitis includes bed rest, fever control, hydration, antiemetics, and anticonvulsants as required. Lumbar puncture may temporarily relieve the headache in some patients with mumps meningitis. Corticosteroids have been used in the treatment of mumps encephalitis (112) and orchitis, but there are no data from controlled studies to support this approach, and corticosteroid use is not routinely recommended.

REFERENCES

1. **Afzal, M. A., J. Buchanan, J. A. Dias, M. Cordeiro, M. L. Bentley, C. A. Shorrock, and P. D. Minor.** 1997. RT-PCR based diagnosis and molecular characterisation of mumps viruses derived from clinical specimens collected during the 1996 mumps outbreak in Portugal. *J. Med. Virol.* **52:**349–353.
2. **Alhaj, S., I. Ozyylmaz, G. Altun, and H. Cam.** 2007. Eyelid, facial and presternal edema in mumps. *Pediatr. Infect. Dis. J.* **26:**661.
3. **Alp, H., H. Tan, Z. Orbak, and H. Keskin.** 2005. Acute hydrocephalus caused by mumps meningoencephalitis. *Pediatr. Infect. Dis. J.* **24:**657–658.
4. **Anderson, R. M., J. A. Crombie, and B. T. Grenfell.** 1987. The epidemiology of mumps in the UK: a preliminary study of virus transmission, herd immunity and the potential impact of immunization. *Epidemiol. Infect.* **99:** 65–84.
5. **Andrejeva, J., K. S. Childs, D. F. Young, T. S. Carlos, N. Stock, S. Goodbourn, and R. E. Randall.** 2004. The V proteins of paramyxoviruses bind the IFN-inducible RNA helicase, mda-5, and inhibit its activation of the IFN-beta promoter. *Proc. Natl. Acad. Sci. USA* **101:** 17264–17269.
6. **Arita, M., Y. Ueno, and Y. Masuyama.** 1981. Complete heart block in mumps myocarditis. *Br. Heart J.* **46:**342–344.
7. **Aurpibul, L., T. Puthanakit, T. Sirisanthana, and V. Sirisanthana.** 2007. Response to measles, mumps, and rubella revaccination in HIV-infected children with immune recovery after highly active antiretroviral therapy. *Clin. Infect. Dis.* **45:**637–642.
8. **Azimi, P. H., H. G. Cramblett, and R. E. Hayers.** 1969. Mumps meningoencephalitis in children. *JAMA* **207:** 509–512.
9. **Azimi, P. H., S. Shaban, M. D. Hilty, and R. E. Haynes.** 1975. Mumps meningoencephalitis: prolonged abnormality of cerebrospinal fluid. *JAMA* **234:**1161–1162.
10. **Bang, H. O., and J. Bang.** 1943. Involvement of the central nervous system in mumps. *Acta Med. Scand.* **113:** 487–505.
11. **Bansal, R., J. Kalita, U. K. Misra, and J. Kishore.** 1998. Myelitis: a rare presentation of mumps. *Pediatr. Neurosurg.* **28:**204–206.
12. **Başekim, C. C., E. Kizilkaya, Z. Pekkafali, K. V. Baykal, and A. F. Karsli.** 2000. Mumps epididymo-orchitis: sonography and color Doppler sonographic findings. *Abdom. Imaging* **25:**322–325.
13. **Beard, C. M., R. C. Benson, P. P. Kelalis, L. R. Eveback, and L. T. Kurland.** 1977. The incidence and outcome of mumps orchitis in Rochester, Minnesota, 1935–1974. *Mayo Clin. Proc.* **52:**3–7.
14. **Beardwell, A.** 1969. Facial palsy due to the mumps virus. *Br. J. Clin. Pract.* **23:**37–38.
15. **Bern, C., H. Barucha, and P. S. Patil.** 1992. Parotid disease and human immunodeficiency virus infection in Zambia. *Br. J. Surg.* **79:**768–770.
16. **Bistrian, B., C. A. Phillips, and I. S. Kaye.** 1972. Fatal mumps meningoencephalitis. *JAMA* **222:**478–479.
17. **Boddicker, J. D., P. A. Rota, T. Kreman, A. Wangeman, L. Lowe, K. B. Hummel, R. Thompson, W. J. Bellini, M. Pentella, and L. E. Desjardin.** 2007. Real-time reverse transcription-PCR assay for detection of mumps virus RNA in clinical specimens. *J. Clin. Microbiol.* **45:**2902–2908.
18. **Bonnet, M. C., A. Dutta, C. Weinberger, and S. A. Plotkin.** 2006. Mumps vaccine virus strains and aseptic meningitis. *Vaccine* **24:**7037–7045.
19. **Brown, E. H., and W. H. Dunnett.** 1974. A retrospective survey of the complications of mumps. *J. R. Coll. Gen. Practitioners* **24:**552–556.
20. **Brunnell, P. A.** 2006. Mumps outbreak 2006: evaluating vaccine efficacy complicated by disease's characteristics. *Infect. Dis. Child.* **196:**24–26.
21. **Bruyn, H. B., H. M. Sexton, and H. D. Brainend.** 1957. Mumps meningoencephalitis: a clinical review of 119 cases with one death. *Calif. Med.* **86:**153–160.
22. **Casella, R., B. Leibundgut, K. Lehmann, and T. C. Gasser.** 1997. Mumps orchitis: report of a mini-epidemic. *J. Urol.* **158:**2158–2161.
23. **Centers for Disease Control.** 1989. Mumps—United States, 1985–1988. *Morb. Mortal. Wkly. Rep.* **38:**101–105.
24. **Centers for Disease Control and Advisory Committee on Immunization Practices.** 1989. Mumps prevention. *Morb. Mortal. Wkly. Rep.* **38:**388–400.
25. **Centers for Disease Control and Prevention.** 1996. Update: vaccine side effects, adverse reactions, contraindications, and precautions. Recommendations of the Advisory Committee on Immunization Practices (ACIP). *Morb. Mortal. Wkly. Rep. Recomm. Rep.* **45:**1–35.
26. **Centers for Disease Control and Prevention.** 2006. Brief report: update: mumps activity—United States, January 1–October 7, 2006. *Morb. Mortal. Wkly. Rep.* **55:**1152–1153.
27. **Centers for Disease Control and Prevention.** 2006. Notice to readers: updated recommendations of the Advisory Committee on Immunization Practices (ACIP) for the control and elimination of mumps. *Morb. Mortal. Wkly. Rep.* **55:**629–630.
28. **Centers for Disease Control and Prevention.** 2007. Recommended immunization schedules for persons aged 0–18 years—United States, 2007. *Morb. Mortal. Wkly. Rep.* **55:**Q1–Q4.
29. **Centers for Disease Control and Prevention.** 1995. Mumps surveillance—United States, 1988–1993. *Morb. Mortal. Wkly. Rep.* **44**(SS-3)**:**1–14.
30. **Cochi, S. L., S. R. Preblud, and W. A. Orenstein.** 1988. Perspectives on the relative resurgence of mumps in the United States. *Am. J. Dis. Child.* **142:**499–507.
31. **Davidkin, I., S. Jokinen, M. Broman, P. Leinikki, and H. Peltola.** 2008. Persistence of measles, mumps, and rubella antibodies in an MMR-vaccinated cohort: a 20-year follow-up. *J. Infect. Dis.* **197:**950–956.
32. **Davidkin, I., S. Jokinen, A. Paananen, P. Leinikki, and H. Peltola.** 2005. Etiology of mumps-like illnesses in children and adolescents vaccinated for measles, mumps, and rubella. *J. Infect. Dis.* **191:**719–723.
33. **Davidson, W. L., E. B. Buynak, M. B. Leagus, J. E. Whitman, and M. R. Hilleman.** 1967. Vaccination of adults with live attenuated mumps virus vaccine. *JAMA* **201:**995–998.
34. **Dayan, G. H., P. Quinlisk, A. A. Parker, A. E. Barskey, M. L. Harris, J. M. Hill Schwartz, K. Hunt, C. G. Filey, D. P. Leschinsky, A. L. O'Keefe, and J. Clayton.** 2008.

Recent resurgence of mumps in the United States. *N. Engl. J. Med.* **358:**1580–1589.

35. **Dourado, I., S. Cunha, M. G. Teixeira, C. P. Farrington, A. Melo, R. Lucena, and M. L. Barreto.** 2000. Outbreak of aseptic meningitis associated with mass vaccination with a Urabe-containing measles-mumps-rubella vaccine: implications for immunization programs. *Am. J. Epidemiol.* **151:**524–530.
36. **Duncan, S., R. G. Will, and J. Catnach.** 1990. Mumps and Guillian-Barré syndrome. *J. Neurol. Neurosurg. Psychiatry* **53:**709. (Letter.)
37. **Ehrengut, W., and M. Schwartau.** 1977. Mumps orchitis and testicular tumours. *Br. Med. J.* **2:**191.
38. **Elango, N., T. Varsanyi, J. Kövamees, and E. Norrby.** 1988. Molecular cloning and characterization of six genes, determination of gene order and intergenic sequences and leader sequence of mumps virus. *J. Gen. Virol.* **69:**2893–2900.
39. **Elliott, G. D., M. A. Afzal, S. J. Martin, and B. K. Rima.** 1989. Nucleotide sequence of the matrix, fusion and putative SH protein genes of mumps virus and their deduced amino acid sequences. *Virus Res.* **12:**61–75.
40. **Elliott, G. D., R. P. Yeo, M. A. Afzal, E. J. B. Simpson, J. A. Curran, and B. K. Rima.** 1990. Strain variable editing during transcription of the P gene of mumps virus may lead to the generation of non-structural proteins NS1 (V) and NS2. *J. Gen. Virol.* **71:**1555–1560.
41. **Emerson, C., W. W. Dinsmore, and S. P. Quah.** 2007. Are we missing mumps epididymo-orchitis? *Int. J. STD AIDS* **18:**341–342.
42. **Erpenbach, K. H.** 1991. Systemic treatment with interferon-alpha 2B: an effective method to prevent sterility after bilateral mumps orchitis. *J. Urol.* **146:**54–56.
43. **Falk, W. A., K. Buchan, M. Dow, J. Z. Garson, E. Hill, M. Nosal, M. Tarrant, R. C. Westbury, and F. M. White.** 1989. The epidemiology of mumps in southern Alberta 1980–1982. *Am. J. Epidemiol.* **130:**736–749.
44. **Forsberg, P., A. Fryden, H. Link, and C. Orvell.** 1986. Viral IgM and IgG antibody synthesis within the central nervous system in mumps meningitis. *Acta Neurol. Scand.* **73:**372–380.
45. **Foster, R. E., C. Y. Lowder, D. M. Meisler, G. S. Kosmorsky, and B. Baetz-Greenwalt.** 1990. Mumps neuroretinitis in an adolescent. *Am. J. Ophthalmol.* **110:**91–92.
46. **Freeman, R., and M. H. Hambling.** 1980. Serologic studies on 40 cases of mumps virus infection. *J. Clin. Pathol.* **33:**28–32.
47. **Galinski, M. S., and S. L. Wechsler.** 1991. The molecular biology of the paramyxovirus genus, p. 41–82. *In* D. W. Kingbury (ed.), *The Paramyxoviruses*. Plenum Press, New York, NY.
48. **Garcia, A. G., J. M. Pereira, N. Vidigal, Y. Y. Lokato, C. S. Pegado, and J. P. Branco.** 1980. Intrauterine infection with mumps virus. *Obstet. Gynecol.* **56:**756–759.
49. **Glikmann, G., M. Pedersen, and C. H. Mordhorst.** 1986. Detection of specific immunoglobulin M to mumps virus in serum and cerebrospinal fluid samples from patients with acute mumps infection, using an antibody capture enzyme immunoassay. *Acta Pathol. Microbiol. Immunol. Scand.* **94:**145–156.
50. **Gnann, J. W.** 1994. Mumps virus, p. 555–562. *In* R. R. McKendall and W. G. Stroop (ed.), *Handbook of Neurovirology*. Marcel Dekker Inc., New York, NY.
51. **Gonzalez-Gil, J., M. T. Zarrabeitia, E. Altuzarra, I. Sanchez-Molina, and R. Calvet.** 2000. Hydrocephalus: a fatal late consequence of mumps encephalitis. *J. Forensic Sci.* **45:**204–207.
52. **Gordon, S. C., and C. B. Lauter.** 1984. Mumps arthritis: a review of the literature. *Rev. Infect. Dis.* **6:**338–343.
53. **Gut, J. P., C. Lablache, S. Behr, and A. Kirn.** 1995. Symptomatic mumps virus reinfections. *J. Med. Virol.* **45:**17–23.
54. **Haginoya, K., K. Ike, K. Iinuma, T. Yagi, K. Kon, H. Yokoyama, and Y. Numazaki.** 1995. Chronic progressive mumps virus encephalitis in a child. *Lancet* **346:**50.
55. **Hall, R., and H. Richards.** 1987. Hearing loss due to mumps. *Arch. Dis. Child.* **62:**189–191.
56. **Harel, L., J. Amir, O. Reish, A. H. Cohen, I. Varsano, and N. Varsano.** 1990. Mumps arthritis in children. *Pediatr. Infect. Dis. J.* **9:**928–929.
57. **Herndon, R. M., R. T. Johnson, L. E. Davis, and L. R. Descalzi.** 1974. Ependymitis in mumps virus meningitis. Electron microscopical studies of cerebrospinal fluid. *Arch. Neurol.* **30:**475–479.
58. **Hilleman, M. R., E. B. Buynak, R. E. Weibel, and J. Stokes.** 1968. Live, attenuated mumps-virus vaccine. *N. Engl. J. Med.* **278:**227–232.
59. **Hiraiwa, K., K. Obara, and A. Sato.** 2005. Mumps virus-associated hemophagocytic syndrome. *Emerg. Infect. Dis.* **11:**343.
60. **Hopkins, R. S., R. A. Jajosky, P. A. Hall, D. A. Adams, F. J. Connor, P. Sharp, W. J. Anderson, R. F. Fagan, J. J. Aponte, D. A. Nitschke, C. A. Worsham, N. Adekoya, and M. H. Chang.** 2005. Summary of notifiable diseases—United States, 2003. *Morb. Mortal. Wkly. Rep.* **52:**1–85.
61. **Houard, S., T. M. Varsanyi, F. Milican, E. Norrby, and A. Bollen.** 1995. Protection of hamsters against experimental mumps virus (MuV) infection by antibodies raised against the MuV surface glycoproteins expressed from recombinant vaccinia virus vectors. *J. Gen. Virol.* **76**(Pt. 2):421–423.
62. **Ito, M., T. Go, T. Okuno, and H. Mikawa.** 1991. Chronic mumps virus encephalitis. *Pediatr. Neurol.* **7:**467–470.
63. **Ito, Y., M. Tsurudome, M. Hishiyama, and A. Yamada.** 1987. Immunological interrelationships among human and non-human paramyxoviruses revealed by immunoprecipitation. *J. Gen. Virol.* **68:**1289–1297.
64. **Jin, L., D. W. Brown, P. A. Litton, and J. M. White.** 2004. Genetic diversity of mumps virus in oral fluid specimens: application to mumps epidemiological study. *J. Infect. Dis.* **189:**1001–1008.
65. **Jin, L., B. Rima, D. Brown, C. Orvell, T. Tecle, M. Afzal, K. Uchida, T. Nakayama, J. W. Song, C. Kang, P. A. Rota, W. Xu, and D. Featherstone.** 2005. Proposal for genetic characterisation of wild-type mumps strains: preliminary standardisation of the nomenclature. *Arch. Virol.* **150:**1903–1909.
66. **Johnstone, J. A., C. A. C. Ross, and M. Dunn.** 1972. Meningitis and encephalitis associated with mumps infection. *Arch. Dis. Child.* **47:**647–651.
67. **Kabakus, N., H. Aydinoglu, S. A. Bakkaloglu, and H. Yekeler.** 1999. Mumps interstitial nephritis: a case report. *Pediatr. Nephrol.* **13:**930–931.
68. **Kancherla, V. S., and I. C. Hanson.** 2006. Mumps resurgence in the United States. *J. Allergy Clin. Immunol.* **118:**938–941.
69. **Kanra, G., P. Isik, A. Kara, A. B. Cengiz, G. Secmeer, and M. Ceyhan.** 2004. Complementary findings in clinical and epidemiologic features of mumps and mumps meningoencephalitis in children without mumps vaccination. *Pediatr. Int.* **46:**663–668.
70. **Kanra, G., A. Kara, A. B. Cengiz, P. Isik, M. Ceyhan, and A. Atas.** 2002. Mumps meningoencephalitis effect on hearing. *Pediatr. Infect. Dis. J.* **21:**1167–1169.
71. **Kayan, A.** 1990. Bilateral sensorineural hearing loss due to mumps. *Br. J. Clin. Pathol.* **44:**757–759.

72. **Khakoo, G. A., and G. Lack.** 2000. Recommendations for using MMR vaccine in children allergic to eggs. *BMJ* **320:**929–932.
73. **Kilham, L., J. Levens, and J. Enders.** 1949. Nonparalytic poliomyelitis and mumps meningoencephalitis. *JAMA* **140:**934–936.
74. **Kimura, H., Y. Ando, M. Shibata, T. Abe, and T. Morishima.** 1993. T-cell receptor V alpha region usage in the cerebrospinal fluid of patients with mumps meningitis. *J. Med. Virol.* **41:**306–311.
75. **Koskiniemi, M., M. Donner, and O. Pettay.** 1983. Clinical appearance and outcome in mumps encephalitis in children. *Acta Paediatr. Scand.* **72:**603–609.
76. **Krause, C. H., K. Eastick, and M. M. Ogilvie.** 2006. Real-time PCR for mumps diagnosis on clinical specimens—comparison with results of conventional methods of virus detection and nested PCR. *J. Clin. Virol.* **37:**184–189.
77. **Krause, C. H., P. J. Molyneaux, D. O. Ho-Yen, P. McIntyre, W. F. Carman, and K. E. Templeton.** 2007. Comparison of mumps-IgM ELISAs in acute infection. *J. Clin. Virol.* **38:**153–156.
78. **Kubar, A., M. Yapar, B. Besirbellioglu, I. Y. Avci, and C. Guney.** 2004. Rapid and quantitative detection of mumps virus RNA by one-step real-time RT-PCR. *Diagn. Microbiol. Infect. Dis.* **49:**83–88.
79. **Kubota, T., N. Yokosawa, S. Yokota, N. Fujii, M. Tashiro, and A. Kato.** 2005. Mumps virus V protein antagonizes interferon without the complete degradation of STAT1. *J. Virol.* **79:**4451–4459.
80. **Kurtz, J. B., A. H. Tomlinson, and J. Pearson.** 1982. Mumps virus isolated from a fetus. *Br. Med. J.* **284:**471.
81. **Lane, T. M., and J. Hines.** 2006. The management of mumps orchitis. *BJU Int.* **97:**1–2.
82. **Lavi, S., B. Zimmerman, G. Koren, and R. Gold.** 1990. Administration of measles, mumps, and rubella virus vaccine (live) to egg allergic children. *JAMA* **263:**269–271.
83. **Lemon, K., B. K. Rima, S. McQuaid, I. V. Allen, and W. P. Duprex.** 2007. The F gene of rodent brain-adapted mumps virus is a major determinant of neurovirulence. *J. Virol.* **81:**8293–8302.
84. **Levitt, L. P., T. A. Rich, S. W. Kindle, A. L. Lewis, E. H. Gates, and J. O. Bond.** 1970. Central nervous system mumps. *Neurology* **20:**829–834.
85. **Linde, G. A., M. Granstrom, and C. Örvell.** 1987. Immunoglobulin class and immunoglobulin G subclass enzyme-linked immunosorbent assays compared with microneutralization assay for serodiagnosis of mumps infection and determination of immunity. *J. Clin. Microbiol.* **25:**1653–1658.
86. **Löve, A., T. Andersson, E. Norrby, and K. Kristenssan.** 1987. Mumps virus infection of dissociated rodent spinal ganglion in vitro. Expression and disappearance of viral structural protein in neurons. *J. Gen. Virol.* **68:**1755–1759.
87. **Löve, A., R. Rydbeck, K. Kristensson, C. Örvell, and E. Norrby.** 1985. Hemagglutinin-neuraminidase glycoprotein as a determinant of pathogenicity in mumps virus hamster encephalitis: analysis of mutants selected with monoclonal antibodies. *J. Virol.* **53:**67–74.
88. **Majda-Stanislawska, E.** 2000. Mumps cerebellitis. *Eur. Neurol.* **43:**117.
89. **Malik, T., C. Wolbert, J. Mauldin, C. Sauder, K. M. Carbone, and S. A. Rubin.** 2007. Functional consequences of attenuating mutations in the haemagglutinin neuraminidase, fusion and polymerase proteins of a wild-type mumps virus strain. *J. Gen. Virol.* **88:**2533–2541.
90. **Manson, A. L.** 1990. Mumps orchitis. *Urology* **36:**355–358.
91. **Martin, R., A. Vallbracht, and H. W. Kreth.** 1991. Interferon-gamma secretion by in vivo activated cytotoxic T lymphocytes from the blood and cerebrospinal fluid during mumps meningitis. *J. Neuroimmunol.* **33:**191–198.
92. **Masarani, M., H. Wazait, and M. Dinneen.** 2006. Mumps orchitis. *J. R. Soc. Med.* **99:**573–575.
93. **Matsukuma, E., Z. Kato, K. Orii, T. Asano, K. Orii, E. Matsui, H. Kaneko, and N. Kondo.** 2008. Acute mumps cerebellitis with abnormal findings in MRI diffusion-weighted images. *Eur. J. Pediatr.* **167:**829–830.
94. **Mauldin, J., K. Carbone, H. Hsu, R. Yolken, and S. Rubin.** 2005. Mumps virus-specific antibody titers from pre-vaccine era sera: comparison of the plaque reduction neutralization assay and enzyme immunoassays. *J. Clin. Microbiol.* **43:**4847–4851.
95. **McKenna, M. J.** 1997. Measles, mumps, and sensorineural hearing loss. *Ann. N. Y. Acad. Sci.* **830:**291–298.
96. **McLean, D. M., S. J. Walker, and G. A. McNaughton.** 1964. Mumps meningoencephalitis, Toronto 1963. *Can. Med. Assoc. J.* **90:**458–462.
97. **McQuone, S. J.** 1999. Acute viral and bacterial infections of the salivary glands. *Otolaryngol. Clin. N. Am.* **32:**793–811.
98. **Merz, D. C., A. C. Server, M. N. Waxham, and J. S. Wolinsky.** 1983. Biosynthesis of mumps virus F glycoprotein: nonfusing strains efficiently cleave the F glycoprotein precursor. *J. Gen. Virol.* **64:**1457–1467.
99. **Muhlemann, K.** 2004. The molecular epidemiology of mumps virus. *Infect. Genet. Evol.* **4:**215–219.
100. **Murray, H. G. S., C. M. B. Field, and W. J. McLeod.** 1960. Mumps meningo-encephalitis. *Br. Med. J.* **1:**1850–1853.
101. **Ni, J., N. E. Bowles, Y. H. Kim, G. Demmler, D. Kearney, J. T. Bricker, and J. A. Towbin.** 1997. Viral infection of the myocardium in endocardial fibroelastosis. Molecular evidence for the role of mumps virus as an etiologic agent. *Circulation* **95:**133–139.
102. **Nigro, G., F. Nanni, and M. Midulla.** 1986. Determination of vaccine-induced and naturally acquired class-specific antibodies by two indirect ELISAs. *J. Virol. Methods* **13:**91–106.
103. **Okazaki, K., K. Tanabayashi, K. Takeuchi, M. Hishiyama, K. Okazaki, and A. Yamada.** 1992. Molecular cloning and sequence analysis of the mumps virus gene encoding the L protein and the trailer sequence. *Virology* **188:**926–930.
104. **Onal, S., and E. Toker.** 2005. A rare ocular complication of mumps: kerato-uveitis. *Ocul. Immunol. Inflamm.* **13:**395–397.
105. **Palacios, G., O. Jabado, D. Cisterna, F. de Ory, N. Renwick, J. E. Echevarria, A. Castellanos, M. Mosquera, M. C. Freire, R. H. Campos, and W. I. Lipkin.** 2005. Molecular identification of mumps virus genotypes from clinical samples: standardized method of analysis. *J. Clin. Microbiol.* **43:**1869–1878.
106. **Peltola, H., P. S. Kulkarni, S. V. Kapre, M. Paunio, S. S. Jadhav, and R. M. Dhere.** 2007. Mumps outbreaks in Canada and the United States: time for new thinking on mumps vaccines. *Clin. Infect. Dis.* **45:**459–466.
107. **Pipkin, P. A., M. A. Afzal, A. B. Heath, and P. D. Minor.** 1999. Assay of humoral immunity to mumps virus. *J. Virol. Methods* **79:**219–225.
108. **Poggio, G. P., C. Rodriguez, D. Cisterna, M. C. Freire, and J. Cello.** 2000. Nested PCR for rapid detection of mumps virus in cerebrospinal fluid from patients with neurological diseases. *J. Clin. Microbiol.* **38:**274–278.
109. **Pringle, C. R.** 1991. The genetics of paramyxoviruses, p. 1–39. *In* D. W. Kingbury (ed.), *The Paramyxoviruses*. Plenum Press, New York, NY.

110. **Rafiefard, F., B. Johansson, T. Tecle, and C. Orvell.** 2005. Characterization of mumps virus strains with varying neurovirulence. *Scand. J. Infect. Dis.* **37:**330–337.
111. **Reisinger, K. S., M. L. Brown, J. Xu, B. J. Sullivan, G. S. Marshall, B. Nauert, D. O. Matson, P. E. Silas, F. Schodel, J. O. Gress, and B. J. Kuter.** 2006. A combination measles, mumps, rubella, and varicella vaccine (ProQuad) given to 4- to 6-year-old healthy children vaccinated previously with M-M-RII and Varivax. *Pediatrics* **117:**265–272.
112. **Ritter, B. S.** 1958. Mumps meningoencephalitis. *J. Pediatr.* **52:**424–432.
113. **Rubin, S. A., M. A. Afzal, C. L. Powell, M. L. Bentley, G. R. Auda, R. E. Taffs, and K. M. Carbone.** 2005. The rat-based neurovirulence safety test for the assessment of mumps virus neurovirulence in humans: an international collaborative study. *J. Infect. Dis.* **191:**1123–1128.
114. **Rubin, S. A., G. Amexis, M. Pletnikov, Z. Li, J. Vanderzanden, J. Mauldin, C. Sauder, T. Malik, K. Chumakov, and K. M. Carbone.** 2003. Changes in mumps virus gene sequence associated with variability in neurovirulent phenotype. *J. Virol.* **77:**11616–11624.
115. **Russell, R. R., and J. C. Donald.** 1958. The neurological complications of mumps. *Br. Med. J.* **2:**27–30.
116. **Rüther, U., S. Stilz, E. Röhl, C. Nunnensiek, J. Rassweiler, U. Dörr, and P. Jipp.** 1995. Successful interferon-alpha 2a therapy for a patient with acute mumps orchitis. *Eur. Urol.* **27:**174–176.
117. **Schlegel, M., J. J. Osterwalder, R. L. Galeazzi, and P. L. Vernazza.** 1999. Comparative efficacy of three mumps vaccines during disease outbreak in Eastern Switzerland: cohort study. *BMJ* **319:**352.
118. **Server, A. C., D. C. Merz, M. N. Waxham, and J. S. Wolinsky.** 1982. Differentiation of mumps virus strains with monoclonal antibody to the HN glycoprotein. *Infect. Immun.* **35:**179–186.
119. **Siegel, M. S.** 1973. Congenital malformations following chickenpox, measles, mumps, and hepatitis. Results of a cohort study. *JAMA* **226:**1521.
120. **Soberman, N., J. C. Leonidas, W. E. Berdon, V. Bonagura, J. O. Haller, M. Posher, and L. Mandel.** 1991. Parotid enlargement in children seropositive for human immunodeficiency virus: imaging findings. *Am. J. Roentgenol.* **157:**553–556.
121. **Sosin, D. M., S. L. Cochi, R. A. Gunn, C. E. Jennings, and S. R. Preblud.** 1989. Changing epidemiology of mumps and its impact on university campuses. *Pediatrics* **84:**779–784.
122. **Sullivan, K. M., T. J. Halpin, J. S. Marks, and R. Kim-Farley.** 1985. Effectiveness of mumps vaccine in a school outbreak. *Am. J. Dis. Child.* **139:**909–912.
123. **Takeuchi, K., K. Tanabayashi, M. Hishiyama, and A. Yamada.** 1996. The mumps virus SH protein is a membrane protein and not essential for virus growth. *Virology* **225:**156–162.
124. **Takeuchi, K., K. Tanabayashi, M. Hishiyama, A. Yamada, and A. Sigiura.** 1991. Variations of nucleotide sequences and transcription of the SH gene among mumps virus strains. *Virology* **181:**364–366.
125. **Takimoto, T., G. L. Taylor, H. C. Connaris, S. J. Crennell, and A. Portner.** 2002. Role of the hemagglutinin-neuraminidase protein in the mechanism of paramyxovirus-cell membrane fusion. *J. Virol.* **76:**13028–13033.
126. **Tanabayashi, K., K. Takeuchi, M. Hishiyama, A. Yamada, M. Tsurudome, Y. Ho, and A. Sugiura.** 1990. Nucleotide sequence of the leader and nucleocapsid protein gene of mumps virus and epitope mapping with the *in vitro* expressed nucleocapsid protein. *Virology* **177:** 124–130.
127. **Tanabayashi, K., K. Takeuchi, K. Okazaki, M. Hishiyama, and A. Yamada.** 1992. Expression of mumps virus glycoproteins in mammalian cells from cloned cDNAs: both F and HN proteins are required for cell fusion. *Virology* **187:**801–804.
128. **Tanabayashi, K., K. Takeuchi, K. Okazaki, M. Hishiyama, and A. Yamada.** 1993. Identification of an amino acid that defines the fusogenicity of mumps virus. *J. Virol.* **67:**2928–2931.
129. **Uchida, K., M. Shinohara, S. Shimada, Y. Segawa, R. Doi, A. Gotoh, and R. Hondo.** 2005. Rapid and sensitive detection of mumps virus RNA directly from clinical samples by real-time PCR. *J. Med. Virol.* **75:**470–474.
130. **Ukkonen, P., O. Vaisanen, and K. Penttinen.** 1980. Enzyme-linked immunosorbent assay for mumps and parainfluenza type 1 immunoglobulin G and immunoglobulin M antibodies. *J. Clin. Microbiol.* **11:**319–323.
131. **Uno, M., T. Takano, T. Yamano, and M. Shimada.** 1997. Age-dependent susceptibility in mumps-associated hydrocephalus: neuropathologic features and brain barriers. *Acta Neuropathol.* **94:**207–215.
132. **Utz, J. P., V. N. Houk, and D. W. Alling.** 1964. Clinical and laboratory studies of mumps. IV. Viruria and abnormal renal function. *N. Engl. J. Med.* **270:**1283–1286.
133. **Vandvik, B., E. Norrby, J. Steen-Johnsen, and K. Stensvold.** 1978. Mumps meningitis: prolonged pleocytosis and occurrence of mumps virus-specific oligoclonal IgG in the cerebrospinal fluid. *Eur. Neurol.* **17:**13–22.
134. **Venketasubramanian, N.** 1997. Transverse myelitis following mumps in an adult—a case report with MRI correlation. *Acta Neurol. Scand.* **96:**328–331.
135. **Viola, L., A. Chiaretti, M. Castorina, L. Tortorolo, M. Piastra, A. Villani, P. Valentini, and G. Polidori.** 1998. Acute hydrocephalus as a consequence of mumps meningoencephalitis. *Pediatr. Emerg. Care* **14:**212–214.
136. **Vuori, M., E. A. Lahikainen, and T. Peltonen.** 1962. Perceptive deafness in connection with mumps. *Acta Otolaryngol.* **55:**231.
137. **Waxham, M. N., J. Aronowski, A. C. Server, J. S. Wolinsky, J. A. Smith, and H. M. Goodman.** 1988. Sequence determination of the mumps virus HN gene. *Virology* **164:**318–325.
138. **Wharton, I. P., A. H. Chaudhry, and M. E. French.** 2006. A case of mumps epididymitis. *Lancet* **367:**702.
139. **Wharton, M., S. L. Cochi, R. H. Hutcheson, J. M. Bistowish, and W. Schaffner.** 1988. A large outbreak of mumps in the postvaccine era. *J. Infect. Dis.* **158:**1253–1260.
140. **Wilfert, C. M.** 1969. Mumps meningoencephalitis with low cerebrospinal fluid glucose, prolonged pleocytosis and elevation of protein. *N. Engl. J. Med.* **280:**855–859.
141. **Yamada, A., K. Takeuchi, K. Tamabayashi, M. Hishiyama, Y. Takahashi, and A. Sigiura.** 1990. Differentiation of the mumps vaccine strains from the wild viruses by the nucleotide sequences of the P gene. *Vaccine* **8:** 553–557.
142. **Zhou, F., S. Reef, M. Massoudi, M. J. Papania, H. R. Yusuf, B. Bardenheier, L. Zimmerman, and M. M. McCauley.** 2004. An economic analysis of the current universal 2-dose measles-mumps-rubella vaccination program in the United States. *J. Infect. Dis.* **189**(Suppl. 1)**:**S131–S145.

Zoonotic Paramyxoviruses

PAUL A. ROTA, THOMAS G. KSIAZEK, AND WILLIAM J. BELLINI

39

This chapter focuses on recently emergent paramyxoviruses that are associated with zoonotic disease, Hendra virus (HeV) (68, 69), Nipah virus (NiV) (16), and Menangle virus (MeV) (6). These viruses, which have emerged over the last 14 years, are potential threats to agriculture as well as clinically relevant to humans (Table 1). In particular, HeV and NiV have caused fatal diseases in animals and humans, and outbreaks of NiV continue to occur almost annually. Molecular biological studies have made substantial contributions to the characterization of recently emergent zoonotic paramyxoviruses. Sequencing studies provided an accurate picture of the relative taxonomic position of these viruses, and molecular techniques were used to provide rapid diagnostic capabilities. In the case of outbreaks of NiV in Malaysia, Bangladesh, and India, molecular biological data quickly identified the etiologic agent present, and reverse transcriptase PCR (RT-PCR) and serologic assays were used to rapidly confirm NiV infections in humans and animals (11, 16, 40, 41).

There has been only one report of human illness due to MeV (80, 81), and one study has detected an antibody response to Tioman virus (TiV) (19) in humans (117, 118). It is interesting that all of these viruses share a common reservoir in large fruit bats *(Pteropus)*, also known as flying foxes (37). Because of their clear potential to cause severe disease in humans and animals, NiV and HeV have been designated class C select agents and have been the focus of intense study since their emergence (38).

VIROLOGY

Classification

HeV was originally named equine morbillivirus because initial sequencing studies and morphological studies conducted following its emergence in 1994 led to the conclusion that HeV was most closely related to the morbilliviruses (68). However, subsequent studies showed that HeV is neither a morbillivirus nor an equine virus. Analysis of the sequences of the entire genomes of both HeV and NiV has since provided convincing evidence that these viruses are members of a novel genus, *Henipavirus*, within the subfamily *Paramyxovirinae* (Fig. 1) (57). HeV and NiV are related viruses that share 68 to 92% amino acid identity in their protein coding regions and 40 to 67% nucleotide homology in the untranslated regions of their genomes (39, 40). Among the other four genera within the *Paramyxovirinae*, the henipaviruses are more closely related to the respiroviruses and morbilliviruses than to the rubulaviruses and avulaviruses.

The recent genetic characterization of a number of novel paramyxoviruses has substantially increased our appreciation of the diversity within this viral family (6, 16, 19, 27, 50, 68, 80). In several cases, these viruses demonstrated a departure from the restricted host range that has been the norm for most members of the *Paramyxoviridae*. For example, viruses closely related to the morbillivirus canine distemper virus were associated with disease outbreaks in harbor seals (74), striped dolphins (24), and Serengeti lions (88).

Genome Structure and Gene Function

The single-stranded, negative-sense RNA genomes of NiV and HeV have the same gene order, 3′ N-P-M-F-G-L 5′ (individual proteins are discussed below), as the respiroviruses and the morbilliviruses (Fig. 2), and HeV and NiV retain a number of genetic features found in viruses throughout the subfamily (39, 40). Though most studies have shown that HeV and NiV share many genetic, biological, and biochemical features with other paramyxoviruses, the henipaviruses have several distinguishing genetic and biochemical features.

The genomes of HeV and NiV are 18,234 and 18,246 nucleotides in length, which, until the recent characterization of Beilong and J viruses (48, 54), made them the largest genomes among the paramyxoviruses. In contrast, the average genome size for the other members of the *Paramyxovirinae* is approximately 15,500 nucleotides. The larger size of the HeV and NiV genomes is mostly due to the unusually large sizes of the open reading frame for the phosphoprotein (P protein) gene and the large 3′ untranslated regions of several of the genes (40). The functional significance of the large 3′ untranslated regions has not been explored. The "rule of six" states that the total length of the genomic RNA of viruses within the subfamily *Paramyxovirinae* must be evenly divisible by six in order for the viruses to replicate (8). The sizes of the genomes of both HeV and NiV are evenly divisible by six, suggesting that like other members of the *Paramyxovirinae*, the henipaviruses adhere to the rule of six. It was also interesting

TABLE 1 Characteristics of zoonotic paramyxovirus infections of humans

Virus	Year identified	Presumed reservoir	Nonhuman species infected		Total no. of reported incidents in humans			Clinical disease in humans
			Natural	Experimental	Outbreaks	Cases	Deaths	
HeV	1994	Fruit bats	Horses	Horses, cats, guinea pigs	6	3	2	Influenza-like illness, pneumonia, encephalitis
MeV	1997	Fruit bats	Pigs	NA[b]	1	2	0	Febrile, rash illness
NiV	1999	Fruit bats	Pigs, cats, dogs, horses	Pigs, cats, hamsters, fruit bats, guinea pigs	7[a]	387[a]	191[a]	Pneumonia, encephalitis

[a] Includes one outbreak in Malaysia and Singapore (16), one outbreak in India (11), and five outbreaks in Bangladesh, 2001 to 2005 (25); not all cases were confirmed by laboratory testing.
[b] NA, not applicable.

to observe that for HeV and NiV the differences in entire genome sizes as well as the sizes of the individual genes are evenly divisible by six (40), and studies with a minigenome replication assay confirmed that NiV and HeV conform to the rule of six (36).

The complete nucleotide sequence of a horse isolate of HeV was completed in 2000 (105, 106) and since that time, only a few other HeV isolates have been sequenced; these have been found to be virtually identical (35, 43). The complete genomic sequences of the NiV strains associated with the outbreaks in Malaysia in 1999 (NiV-M) and Bangladesh in 2004 (NiV-B) have been determined (41). The genome of NiV-B is six nucleotides longer than that of NiV-M, the prototype strain of NiV, and two nucleotides shorter than that of HeV. The additional six nucleotides map to the 5′ untranslated region of the fusion (F) protein gene. The gene order and sizes of all the open reading frames except V are conserved between NiV-B and

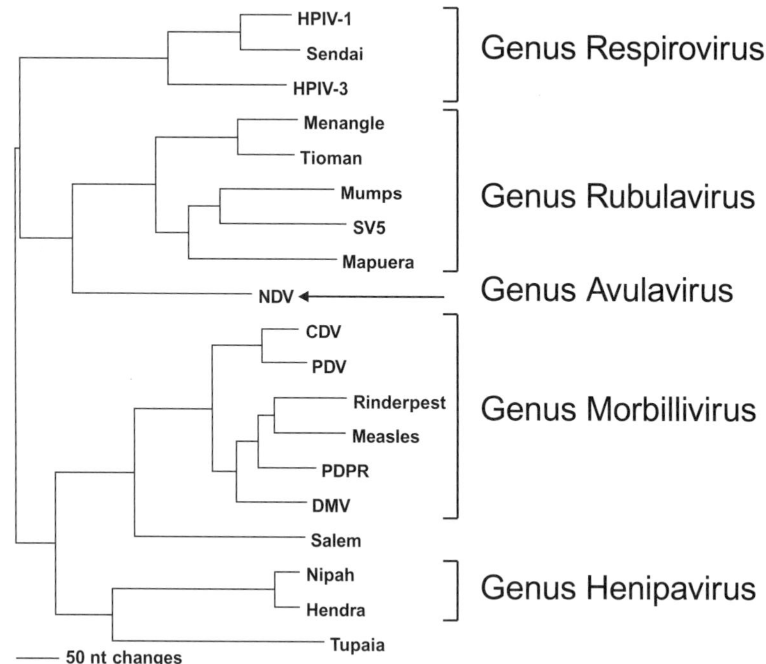

FIGURE 1 Phylogenetic analysis of the sequences of the open reading frame of the N protein gene from viruses in the subfamily *Paramyxovirinae*. The genus name is at the right. The scale, representing the number of nucleotide (nt) changes, is shown at the bottom left. Accession numbers are as follows: canine distemper virus (CDV), AF014953; dolphin morbillivirus (DMV), X75961; HeV, AF017149; human parainfluenza virus 1 (HPIV-1), D01070; human parainfluenza virus 3 (HPIV-3), D10025; Mapuera virus, X85128; MeV, AF326114; mumps virus, D86172; measles virus, K01711; Newcastle disease virus (NDV), AF064091; NiV, AF212302; peste-des-petits-ruminants virus (PDPR), X74443; phocid distemper virus (PDV), X75717; rinderpest virus, X68311; Salem virus, AF237881; Sendai virus, X00087; simian virus 5 (SV5), M81442; TiV, AF298895; and Tupaia virus, AF079780.

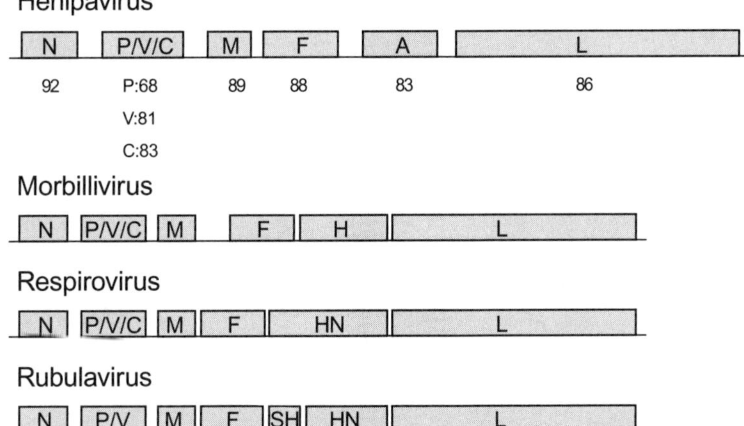

FIGURE 2 Schematic representation of the genomes of viruses in the subfamily *Paramyxovirinae*. Genomes are single-stranded, negative-sense RNA shown in the 3′-to-5′ (left-to-right) orientation. Gray boxes indicate protein coding regions, and solid lines indicate noncoding regions. Numbers under the protein coding regions on the henipavirus genome indicate the percent amino acid identity between HeV and NiV for the indicated protein. Abbreviations for the structural genes are as follows: N, nucleoprotein; P, phosphoprotein; M, matrix protein; F, fusion protein; A, attachment protein; H, hemagglutinin protein; HN, hemagglutinin-neuraminidase; L, polymerase. The schematic genome for rubulaviruses is that of mumps virus and shows the position of the gene for the small hydrophobic protein (SH).

NiV-M. The overall nucleotide homology between the genomes of NiV-B and NiV-M is 91.8%; the predicted amino acid homologies between the proteins expressed by NiV-M and NiV-B are all greater than 92% (41).

Although NiV strains show a high level of sequence conservation, the degree of sequence variation among strains appears to be related to their geographic distribution. The nucleoprotein (N protein) gene sequence of a bat isolate of NiV from Cambodia is more closely related to the sequence of NiV-M than to the sequence of NiV-B, while sequences obtained from samples from an outbreak in India were more closely related to NiV-B (11).

The genomes of paramyxoviruses contain a number of conserved *cis*-acting signals that regulate gene expression and replication. The *cis*-acting signals on the genomes of HeV and NiV, including the gene start sites, gene stop sites, RNA editing sites, genomic termini, and intergenic sequences, are nearly identical between these viruses and are very closely related to the corresponding sequences within the genomes of respiroviruses and morbilliviruses (39, 40, 104–107). However, HeV and NiV are the only paramyxoviruses in which the intergenic sequence, CTT, is conserved at every gene junction (40, 106). The development of minigenome replication assays and reverse-genetics systems for HeV and NiV (28, 36, 120) will permit more detailed functional studies of how the control regions on the genomes of HeV and NiV compare to those of other paramyxoviruses. For example, a recent study used a minigenome replication assay to show that the antigenomic promoter of NiV is bipartite as in other paramyxoviruses. However, fine-mapping studies identified some differences in the internal control elements (104).

Proteins

The P protein is an essential component of the replication complex for all paramyxoviruses, including HeV and NiV. The P protein of NiV contains binding domains for the N protein at both its amino and carboxyl termini (12). The coding strategy for the P protein gene of the henipaviruses is similar to that found in the respiroviruses and morbilliviruses. In each case, a faithful transcript of the P protein gene codes for the P protein, while the transcript encoding the V protein is produced by RNA editing. RNA editing refers to the insertion of nontemplated guanosine (G) nucleotides into the mRNA of the P protein gene to permit access to additional open reading frames (98). The V proteins of the respiroviruses, morbilliviruses, and henipaviruses share the same amino terminus as their respective P proteins, which, at the editing site, are joined to a unique, carboxyl-terminal cysteine-rich domain encoded by an open reading frame that is unique to V (Fig. 3). The P protein genes of the henipaviruses also code for a C protein, which is produced by ribosomal choice from an overlapping reading frame located near the 5′ terminus of the P protein gene mRNA. As in the case of the morbilliviruses, the translational start site for the C protein of HeV and NiV is located downstream of the start codon for the P/V protein (39, 105). The P protein genes of HeV and NiV also have the capacity to code for a protein that is analogous to the W protein described for Sendai virus (100). W protein is produced by the addition of two nontemplated G's at the RNA editing site. The W proteins of HeV and NiV have not been detected in infected cells, though their function has been studied using transient expression of cloned copies of the gene. The P protein gene of HeV, but not NiV, also contains another short open reading frame that codes for a protein with unknown function designated SB. While a similar coding region has been located in the P protein cistrons of vesicular stomatitis virus and Marburg virus, expression of SB has not been demonstrated for HeV (105).

As for other paramyxoviruses, the C, V, and W proteins of NiV and HeV function as virulence factors that interfere with the innate immune system. NiV C, V, and W proteins

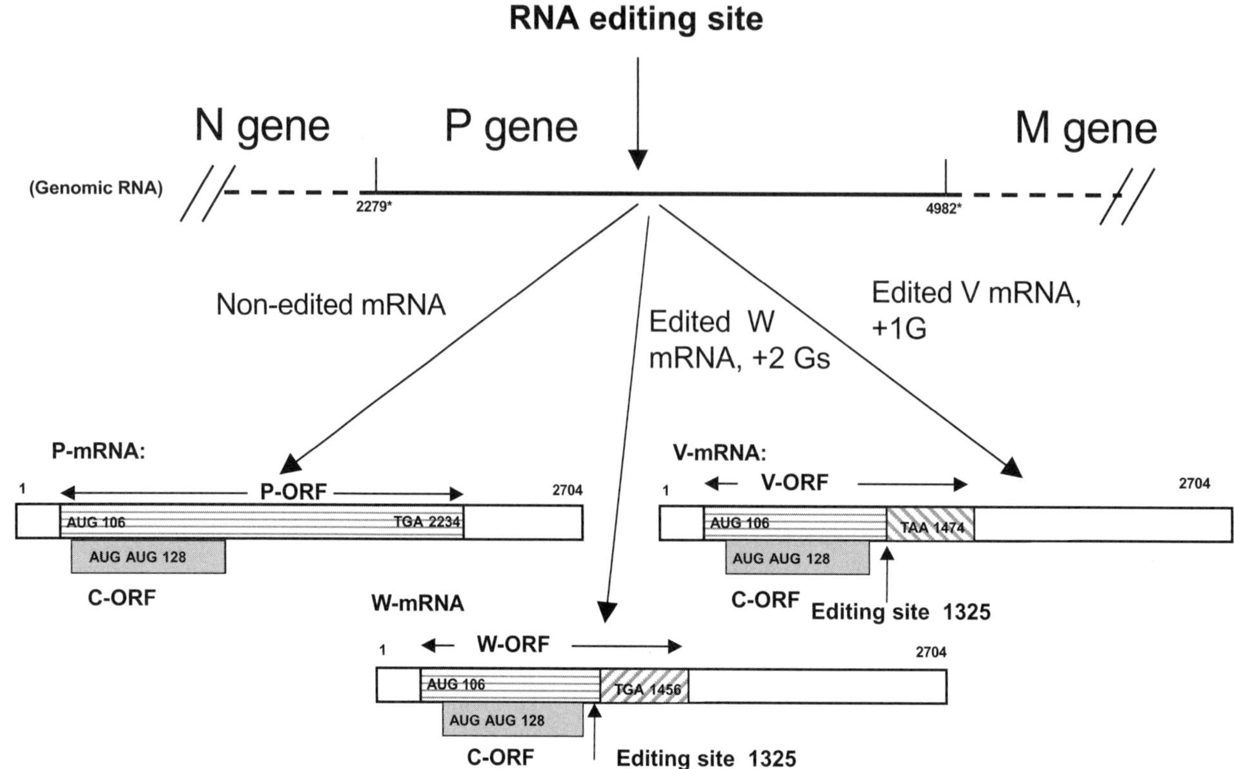

FIGURE 3 Schematic representation of the coding strategy found in the P protein gene of NiV. The predicted P protein mRNA is 2,704 nucleotides in length (nucleotides with asterisks indicate the location of the P protein gene sequence within the sequence with GenBank accession no. AF212302). The P protein is encoded by a faithful transcript of the viral genomic RNA from an opening reading frame beginning at nucleotide 106 of the mRNA. The RNA editing site is indicated by the vertical arrow. The addition of a nontemplated G nucleotide at the RNA editing site (nucleotide 1325) allows access to a different reading frame (−1 relative to P). The V protein contains the amino-terminal domain of the P protein (horizontal lines) joined to the cysteine-rich domain that is unique to the V protein (diagonal lines). The addition of two nontemplated G nucleotides at the RNA editing site produces the mRNA for the W protein in which the amino-terminal domain of P is joined to carboxyl-terminal domain unique for W (diagonal lines). The C protein (gray box) is expressed from an opening reading frame (ORF) that begins at nucleotide 128 (or 131) and overlaps P in the +1 frame.

can rescue growth of interferon (IFN)-sensitive viruses, and cells expressing both V and W of NiV block activation of an IFN-inducible promoter in primate cells (78). The V protein sequesters STAT1 and STAT2 in high-molecular-weight complexes, preventing both nuclear transportation and activation (86, 87), while W protein has been shown to sequester STAT1 in the nucleus (95, 96). The P protein also inhibits the nuclear translocation of STAT1 (95). The V and W proteins also block virus activation of the IFN-β promoter and of an IFN regulatory factor 3-responsive, IFN-stimulated promoter (95). The ability to block IFN signaling has been mapped to a single amino acid on the NiV V protein (33).

The genes coding for the RNA-dependent RNA polymerase (L protein) of HeV and NiV have a linear domain structure that is conserved in all of the *Mononegavirales* (82). In domain III, all of the negative-strand RNA viruses have a predicted catalytic site with the amino acid sequence GDNQ. The sequence QDNE is found only in HeV, NiV, and Tupaia paramyxovirus (40, 99, 106). However, substitution of the E for Q did not affect the function of the L protein of NiV in a minigenome replication assay (56). As for the other paramyxoviruses, the N, P, and L proteins are necessary and sufficient for transcription and genome replication (36).

HeV and NiV have two virion membrane glycoproteins, the F protein and the attachment protein (G), which perform the same functions as the membrane glycoproteins of the morbilliviruses and respiroviruses. As with the other paramyxoviruses, both the G and F proteins of HeV and NiV are required for cell fusion, and heterotypic mixtures of the G and F proteins of HeV and NiV are also fusion competent (5, 97).

The F proteins of *Paramyxovirinae* are type I membrane glycoproteins that facilitate the viral entry process by mediating fusion of the virion membrane with the plasma membrane of the host cell. F proteins are synthesized as inactive precursors, F_0, that are converted to biologically active subunits, F_1 and F_2, following proteolytic cleavage by a host cell protease. The F peptide, located at the amino terminus of the F_1 protein, is highly conserved within the *Paramyxovirinae* (52). The F peptides of HeV and NiV are related to the F proteins of other paramyxoviruses, with the exception that HeV and NiV have leucine at the first position, while almost all of the other viruses have phenylalanine (39). However, substitution of phenylalanine for leucine in the F_1 subunit of NiV does not affect its ability to form syncytia (64).

Among the paramyxoviruses, the carboxyl terminus of the F_2 protein subunit contains either single basic or multiple basic amino acids that comprise the cleavage site between F_1 and F_2. F proteins with multiple basic amino acids (e.g., those of morbilliviruses) are cleaved by furin-like protease during exocytosis from the host cell. F proteins of viruses with a single basic amino acid (e.g., those of respiroviruses) are cleaved at the cell surface by trypsin-like proteases. These viruses usually require the addition of exogenous trypsin to replicate in cell culture. While HeV and NiV have a single basic residue at the cleavage site, both produce productive infections in a variety of cell lines in the absence of exogenous trypsin. In addition, the cleavage site of the F proteins of NiV and HeV do not contain a furin-like protease consensus sequence (R-X-R/K-R) found in most morbilliviruses, rubulaviruses, and pneumoviruses (51, 52), and in fact, the basic amino acids do not appear to be required for cleavage (64). Cleavage of the F protein of NiV and HeV occurs by a novel mechanism involving clathrin-mediated endocytosis via a tyrosine-dependent signal on the cytoplasmic tail (59, 60, 101). The F proteins of both HeV and NiV require the endosomal protease cathepsin L for proteolytic processing (76). N-glycans of the F protein of NiV are required for proper proteolytic processing, and these glycans may modulate access to neutralization epitopes (1, 65).

As for other paramyxoviruses, the NiV surface glycoproteins are the primary targets for neutralizing antibodies (22, 31, 97). Recombinant vaccinia viruses expressing NiV F and G proteins elicit neutralizing antibodies against NiV and protect Syrian hamsters and pigs against lethal NiV challenge (31, 97, 110). Antibodies to F or G protein also provided passive protection in the hamster challenge model (30, 31).

Biology

The replication strategies of the henipaviruses and MeV conform to those of other *Paramyxovirinae;* likewise, these enveloped, negative-sense RNA viruses are vulnerable to the same physical and chemical inactivating agents as those viruses (50; see also chapter 36). MeV, NiV, and HeV were initially isolated in Vero cells, and in vitro studies have shown that NiV and HeV have an impressively broad host cell range (5), which is well correlated to what has been observed in natural and experimental infections.

Attachment and Receptors

The attachment proteins of the *Paramyxoviridae* are type II membrane glycoproteins and are responsible for binding to receptors on host cells (50, 51). Unlike many other paramyxoviruses, neither of the henipaviruses has been shown to have erythrocyte binding or neuraminidase activities. The attachment proteins of the henipaviruses are most closely related to the hemagglutinin-neuraminidases of the respiroviruses (122). The conservation of most of the structurally important amino acids suggests that the attachment proteins of HeV and NiV would have structures that are very similar to the structure proposed for the attachment proteins of other paramyxoviruses (52). EphrinB2, the membrane-bound ligand for the EphB class of receptor tyrosine kinases, specifically binds to the attachment (G) glycoproteins of henipaviruses and is a functional receptor for HeV and NiV (4, 70). While ephrinB3 has also been shown to be a functional receptor for both viruses, the binding of NiV to ephrinB3 is much more efficient than the binding of HeV (70–72), and the G protein of NiV has distinct binding regions for ephrinB2 and ephrinB3 (71). EphrinB3 but not ephrinB2 is expressed in the brain stem, so the difference in the abilities of HeV and NiV to bind to these cellular receptors is consistent with the neuroinvasiveness of NiV (70–72). NiV infection does not appear to down-regulate cell surface expression of ephrinB2 or ephrinB3 (91).

MeV and TiV

The sequences of the complete genomes of the antigenically related MeV and TiV clearly showed that both MeV and TiV are members of the rubulaviruses (6, 7, 20). Like other members of the genus, these viruses lack the gene for the small hydrophobic protein, which is found in mumps virus and simian virus 5. The coding strategy for the P protein genes is also the same as that found in the other rubulaviruses. The unedited transcript codes for the V protein, while a two-G insertion at the RNA editing site produces the transcript coding for the P protein. MeV lacks detectable neuraminidase and erythrocyte binding activity (79), and the hemagglutinin-neuraminidases of MeV and TiV lack the hexapeptide, NRKSCS, that is proposed to be essential for neuraminidase activity (6). Compared to the other rubulaviruses, TiV and MeV also have some unique genetic features in their RNA start sites and intergenic regions (19, 20).

PATHOGENESIS

The development or characterization of animal models to study henipavirus infections is critical for understanding their pathogenesis and for development of therapeutics or vaccines. Both cats and golden hamsters have been used as small-animal models, and both develop fatal disease after challenge with NiV. In cats, virus is mostly present in the respiratory epithelium, while hamsters develop neurologic disease (30, 31, 67). NiV in pigs causes a febrile respiratory illness with or without neurologic signs (61, 63, 109). Infection of fruit bats with NiV did produce clinical signs; some of the bats seroconverted with intermittent excretion of low levels of virus (62). The pathogenesis and immune responses of human infections are described below for each virus.

Hendra Virus

Epidemiology

Distribution and Geography

There have been six outbreaks of HeV among horses recognized between 1994 and 2006. All have occurred in Queensland, Australia, and three have involved spillover to humans. The first incident occurred in September 1994 at a stable in Hendra, a suburb of Brisbane. An outbreak of acute respiratory disease resulted in 14 horse deaths (68, 69, 93). Approximately 1 week after exposure to the index horse case, a pregnant mare recently moved to the stable, a stable hand, and a horse trainer developed an influenza-like illness. The stable hand recovered completely after 6 weeks, but the horse trainer died on the seventh day of illness.

The second incident, in October 1995, involved the death in Brisbane of a farmer from Mackay (75). The patient lived on a horse stud and often assisted a veterinary surgeon during treatment of horses. In August 1994, the patient developed meningitis shortly after he cared for, and assisted in the autopsies of, two horses that died, one from acute respiratory distress and the other from rapid-onset neurologic symptoms. Both horses were retrospectively diagnosed with HeV (42). The patient recovered completely and remained symptom free for 13 months before his fatal illness, which is believed to have resulted from reactivation of virus that entered a latent phase following the initial disease.

Transmission

Despite the potential for HeV to infect a wide variety of animals under experimental conditions (111, 112), horses appear to be the primary source of human HeV infection. Each of the HeV-infected persons reported extensive contact with horses. In the first incident, both infected persons had close contact with a dying mare, particularly the horse trainer with fatal disease, who had abrasions on his hands and arms and was exposed to nasal discharge while trying to feed the incapacitated horse (93). The infected farmer from Mackay in the second incident cared for sick horses and assisted in their autopsies without using gloves, masks, or protective eyewear (75). No evidence of infection was found in 22 other persons who reported feeding or nursing sick horses or participating in their autopsies or in more than 110 other persons associated with, or living near, the affected stables (58, 93). These data indicate that transmission of infection from horses to humans is not very efficient and requires very close contact. Laboratory experiments suggest that the urine and saliva from infected horses are important in disease transmission (111), whereas respiratory spread is less likely. Human-to-human transmission of HeV has not been documented, either among domestic contacts or among health care workers (58, 93).

Reservoir

No epidemiological connection could be found between the first two HeV incidents, which occurred within 1 month of each other at locations 1,100 km apart. No evidence of HeV infection was found among horses, other farm animals, or more than 40 species of wildlife in Queensland (89, 108). However, HeV antibodies were detected in several fruit bat species in Queensland, and the virus isolated from a fruit bat was indistinguishable from that isolated from horses and humans (34, 35, 119). These findings suggest that fruit bats, which have the capacity to travel long distances, may have been the link between the two incidents and may also be the natural reservoir for HeV. This hypothesis is supported by the observation that natural or experimental infection of fruit bats is largely subclinical (111, 112). It is postulated that transmission to horses may occur through the ingestion of pasture recently contaminated by the urine or infected fetal tissue of fruit bats (26, 34).

Pathogenesis in Humans

The incubation period of acute disease is approximately 5 to 7 days. The pathology of these infections and factors in disease production are incompletely characterized because of the small number of cases. The autopsy of the horse trainer who died in the first HeV incident showed a severe interstitial pneumonia. Both lungs were congested, hemorrhagic, and edematous. Histologic examination showed focal necrotizing alveolitis, with giant cells, syncytium formation, and viral inclusions. Postmortem lung, liver, kidney, and spleen samples were inoculated in cell culture, resulting in the appearance of prominent syncytia in cultures inoculated with kidney material (68, 93). The findings at autopsy of the farmer from Mackay, who died more than 1 year after initial infection with HeV, were quite different (75). A leptomeningitis with lymphocyte and plasma cell infiltration was prominent, with discrete foci of necrosis in the neocortex, basal ganglia, brain stem, and cerebellum. Multinucleate endothelial cells were observed in the brain, liver, spleen, and lungs. Immunohistochemical (IHC) studies showed the presence of viral antigen in the cytoplasm of some cells, but most frequently scattered throughout the neuropil, although virus could not be isolated from the brain.

These findings suggest that following initial infection with the virus, possibly through the oral/respiratory route or through direct inoculation of cutaneous abrasions with infectious secretions, viremia develops, resulting in spread to various organs, including the central nervous system. The pathogenesis of recurrence of fatal disease in the farmer from Mackay is unclear. The antibody profile during the fatal illness was indicative of an anamnestic response to viral antigens (75). This patient had abundant immunoglobulin M (IgM) antibody suggestive of a reinfection, but no exposure to horses was documented prior to the recurrence. The failure to isolate virus from this patient's brain supports speculation that the pathogenesis may be similar to that of subacute sclerosing panencephalitis, as both diseases are caused by paramyxoviruses and are characterized by recurrence of fatal neurologic disease following complete recovery from an initial infection. However, the pathological findings and rapid course of this disease are strikingly different from those of subacute sclerosing panencephalitis.

Clinical Manifestations

The two patients in the first HeV incident had abrupt onset of an influenza-like illness, characterized by myalgia, headaches, lethargy, and vertigo (68, 69). One patient remained lethargic for 6 weeks but fully recovered. The other patient developed nausea and vomiting on the fourth day of illness and deteriorated rapidly in the next 2 days, requiring admission to an intensive care unit and mechanical ventilation. He died on the seventh day of illness. The fatal patient in the first HeV incident showed thrombocytopenia; increased levels of creatine phosphokinase, lactic dehydrogenase, aspartate aminotransferase, alanine aminotransferase, and glutamyltransferase; and features of dehydration and acidosis (68). Chest radiographs showed diffuse alveolar shadowing. No laboratory abnormalities were detected in the patient who survived.

Unlike the first two patients, the affected farmer in the second HeV incident primarily had neurologic manifestations (75). He initially presented with features of meningitis, including headache, drowsiness, vomiting, and neck stiffness. Thirteen months following complete recovery, the patient presented again with a 2-week history of irritable mood and lower back pain, three episodes of focal seizures of the right arm, and an episode of generalized tonic-clonic seizures. In the following week, he continued to have a low-grade fever and focal and generalized seizures. By day 7, he developed dense right hemiplegia, signs of brain stem involvement, and depressed consciousness, requiring intubation. The patient remained unconscious and febrile until he died 25 days after admission. Cerebrospinal fluid (CSF) examination showed an elevated protein level, normal glucose level, and mononuclear pleocytosis. Magnetic resonance imaging (MRI) of the brain showed multifocal cortical lesions sparing the subcortical white matter that became more pronounced and widespread prior to death.

Nipah Virus

Epidemiology

Distribution and Geography

The first known human infections with NiV occurred during an outbreak of severe encephalitis in 1998 to 1999, during which 265 patients (40% fatal) with viral encephalitis and 11 patients (1 fatal) with laboratory-confirmed NiV disease were reported in peninsular Malaysia and Singapore, respectively (9, 10, 16). This outbreak began in October 1998 in Malaysia near the city of Ipoh and then spread southward in conjunction with the movement of pigs, resulting in three other clusters of human disease in Malaysia. The largest, accounting for approximately 85% of all cases of outbreak-associated encephalitis, occurred in the Bukit Pelandok area of Negeri Sembilan state, a region with extensive pig farming activities. In Singapore, abattoir workers who slaughtered pigs imported from outbreak-affected areas in Malaysia were exclusively affected (14, 79). Adult males of Chinese or Indian ethnicity, who were primarily involved in pig farming activities, accounted for more than three-fourths of the cases. Infections were also documented among abattoir workers (14, 79), veterinary personnel, and military personnel involved in pig culling activities to control the outbreak. Since this outbreak, human cases of NiV encephalitis have occurred in several small outbreaks in India, in 2001 (11), and Bangladesh, from 2001 through 2007 (2, 46, 113–116; Centers for Disease Control and Prevention [CDC] and ICDRB, unpublished data).

The sequence analysis of different strains of NiV has also provided some information about the transmission patterns of the virus. Molecular biological data suggest that there were at least two introductions of NiV into pigs prior to the outbreak in 1999. Only one of these variants was associated with the explosive spread within pig farms and subsequent transmission to humans, suggesting that a single spillover from the reservoir triggered the outbreak. In contrast, the sequence heterogeneity observed between samples obtained from the outbreak in Bangladesh in 2004 suggests multiple spillovers between the reservoir and humans (41).

Transmission

Direct, close contact with pigs is the primary source of human NiV infection (63, 78). Activities involving close contact with pigs (e.g., medicating sick pigs and assisting in birthing) were associated with the greatest risk of human infection (77). In pigs, extensive infection of the upper and lower airways is seen with evidence of tracheitis and bronchial and interstitial pneumonia, and a harsh, nonproductive cough is a prominent clinical feature (16, 44). Vasculitis of small vessels in the kidney is also seen (16, 44), and viral antigen is detected by IHC studies as focal staining in renal tubular epithelium. Therefore, exposure to respiratory secretions and possibly the urine of infectious pigs likely results in transmission of virus among pigs and to humans. In experimental studies, transmission among pigs occurs through both oral and in-contact exposure (44).

Serologic studies demonstrate evidence of infection among other species of animals, including dogs and cats (16, 44), on and near farms with NiV-infected pigs. Because NiV can be found by IHC staining in renal glomeruli of infected dogs and cats and virus can be isolated from the urine of experimentally infected cats, virus may be transmitted by exposure to the urine of these two species. It is unclear whether humans are at risk from exposure to infected animals other than pigs, but this possibility cannot be excluded, because some patients reported no direct contact with pigs and others reported contact with dogs that died of unknown causes (29, 77).

Although NiV is excreted in respiratory secretions and urine of patients (18), one survey of health care workers demonstrated no evidence of human-to-human transmission (66). This finding may be the result of standard universal precautions practiced by the health care workers, although no special precautions were used in the initial period of the outbreak before the identification of NiV. Alternatively, the lack of transmission may be related to the lower viral load in respiratory secretions and urine of humans compared with pigs, as suggested by IHC studies of necropsy tissue (16).

In Bangladesh pigs may not have acted as intermediate hosts of the virus, and transmission directly from bats or from fruits or commodities contaminated by bats may have resulted in the primary infections in the small outbreaks occurring there (3, 55). Transmission from patients to relatives or caregivers in contact with patients during the course of disease was strongly implicated in at least some of the cases in Bangladesh and perhaps in India (3, 11, 32). This may be related to care in settings in which standard precautions are not the usual practice and in which infection control is not at the standard that was used in the intensive care setting in Malaysia during the 1998–1999 NiV outbreak.

Reservoir

Knowing the similarities between NiV and HeV, surveillance for the natural reservoir for NiV focused on bats. Neutralizing antibodies to NiV were found in a total of 21 bats belonging to four fruit bat species and one insectivorous bat species in peninsular Malaysia (119). Attempts to detect the virus in sera from bats using both cell culture and amplification of RNA were unsuccessful. Bat colonies were noted proximal to pig farms near the city of Ipoh, where the outbreak in pigs was first noticed, supporting the hypothesis that transmission from bats to pigs initiated the outbreak and that bats could be the natural reservoir (119).

Evidence of henipaviruses in several species of the genus *Pteropus* has suggested that the geographic range of the henipaviruses is significant and ranges from African coastal islands to the Western Pacific Islands (Fig. 4), including

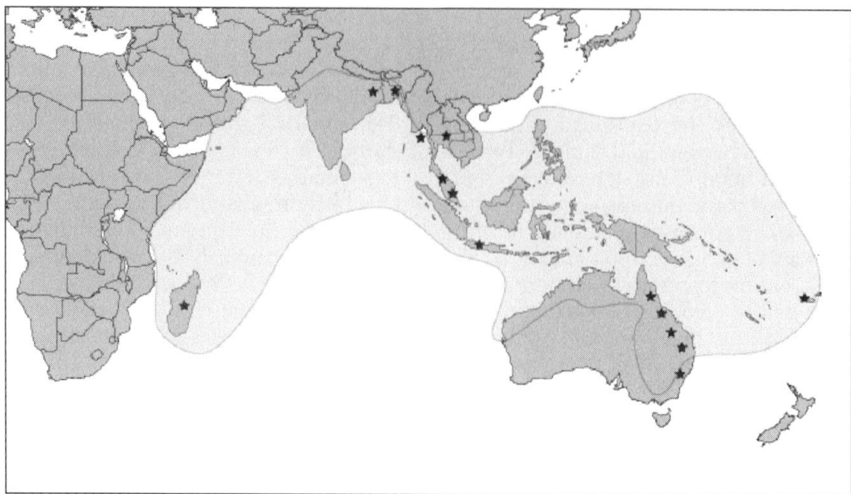

FIGURE 4 Range of the genus *Pteropus* (shaded area) and locations where henipaviruses have been described (stars) to occur in the local *Pteropus* species.

American Samoa, Thailand, Cambodia, Indonesia, Bangladesh, and Madagascar (2, 47, 73, 85, 94, 102, 103; CDC, unpublished). These findings primarily implicate species within the genus *Pteropus*, suggesting that this genus shares a coevolutionary relationship with the *Henipavirus* genus. This, in turn, may suggest that yet other members of the genus *Pteropus* may also harbor henipaviruses.

Pathogenesis in Humans

The exact incubation period of NiV disease is not known. For 94 patients (77), the period between the last contact with pigs and onset of illness ranged from several days to 2 months, and it was 2 weeks or less for 92% of patients.

Histopathology

A multiorgan vasculitis associated with infection of endothelial cells is the hallmark pathological feature of Nipah disease (29). Occasionally, multinucleate giant cells characteristic of paramyxovirus infections are observed in the affected vascular endothelium. Infection is most pronounced in the central nervous system, where a diffuse vasculitis characterized by segmental endothelial cell damage, mural necrosis, karyorrhexis, and infiltration with polymorphonuclear leukocytes and mononuclear cells is noted (Color Plate 47). The lesions are primarily seen in the cerebral cortex and brain stem, with extension to parenchymal tissue, where extensive areas of rarefaction necrosis are seen. Eosinophilic, mainly intracytoplasmic, viral inclusions with a "melted-tallow" appearance are seen in the affected neurons and parenchymal cells. IHC studies with NiV antigen show intense staining of endothelial and parenchymal cells. Evidence of endothelial infection and vasculitis is also seen in other organs, including the lungs, heart, spleen, and kidneys. NiV has been isolated from CSF, tracheal secretions, throat and nasal swabs, and urine specimens from patients (29, 77).

The widespread distribution of vasculitis throughout the central nervous system and, to a lesser extent, in other organs and the isolation of virus from a variety of clinical specimens suggest that following initial infection with the virus, possibly through the respiratory tract or direct inoculation of cutaneous abrasions with infectious secretions, viremia develops, resulting in systemic spread. Involvement of the uncus of the temporal lobe in some patients has led to speculation that virus may be spread along the olfactory tract to the uncus following inhalation and local replication (90), as in the case of herpes simplex encephalitis. The nonspecific neurologic manifestations of Nipah disease probably reflect widespread vasculitis, but the distinctive features, such as segmental myoclonus and brain stem dysfunction, indicate a predilection of the virus for certain neurons.

Immune Responses

Limited data are available on the immune response to NiV infection and correlates of immune protection and disease resolution. A serum IgM response has been demonstrated shortly after onset of illness, with 50% of patients being antibody positive on the first day of illness and 100% being antibody positive by the third day (84). Persistence of an IgM antibody response was demonstrated for 95% of 37 patients in serum obtained a mean of 83 days after onset of illness. An IgG antibody response is seen in 10 to 29% of patients in the first 10 days of illness and in 100% of patients after days 17 to 18 of illness.

The presence of IgM antibody appears to reduce the rate of isolation of virus from throat and respiratory secretions (18). The presence of antibody in the serum or CSF, however, does not appear to influence the rate of isolation of virus from CSF (17), suggesting that humoral immunity plays a minor role in recovery from neurologic disease.

Clinical Manifestations

The onset of NiV disease is abrupt, usually with the development of fever. Often, patients deteriorate rapidly, requiring hospitalization 3 to 4 days after onset of symptoms. Severe encephalitis is the most prominent clinical manifestation. Fever (97%), headache (65%), dizziness (36%), vomiting (27%), and reduced level of consciousness (21%) are the most common features at presentation (29). Several other features of neurologic involvement, particularly signs of brain stem dysfunction, are noted in patients during the course of illness (Table 2). The disease in 3 of the 11 patients in Singapore presented as an atypical pneu-

TABLE 2 Neurologic features in patients with laboratory-confirmed NiV disease, Malaysia, 1998 to 1999[a]

Feature	% of patients (n = 94)
Absent or reduced reflexes	56
Abnormal pupils	52
Tachycardia (heart rate > 120/min)	39
Hypertension (blood pressure > 160/90 mm Hg)	38
Abnormal doll's-eye reflex	38
Segmental myoclonus	32
Meningism	28
Seizures	23
Nystagmus	16
Cerebellar signs	9
Bilateral ptosis	4

[a] Adapted from reference 29 with permission of the Massachusetts Medical Society.

monia, with fever and infiltrates on chest radiography (79). One of these three patients later developed features of encephalitis. The disparity in clinical presentation (i.e., greater prevalence of respiratory symptoms) and outcome (i.e., lower fatality rate) of patients in Singapore compared with those in Malaysia likely reflects more sensitive case finding due to increased awareness in the at-risk population.

NiV disease was fatal in up to one-third of hospitalized patients in Malaysia. The following are all associated with a poor prognosis: older age; evidence of brain stem involvement; the presence of segmental myoclonus, seizures, or areflexia; elevated hepatic enzyme levels or low platelet counts; and isolation of virus from the CSF (17, 29).

Laboratory Abnormalities

Thrombocytopenia (30%), leukopenia (11%), and elevated levels of alanine aminotransferase (33%) and aspartate transaminase (42%) are the most common hematologic abnormalities (29). CSF studies are frequently abnormal, with elevated white blood cell counts and/or protein levels (29, 79), but the presence of abnormal CSF findings does not correlate with severity of disease (17).

Computed tomography scans of the brain are generally unremarkable. On MRI, small, discrete lesions measuring 2 to 7 mm are seen in the subcortical and deep white matter of the cerebral hemispheres during both the acute and late phases of illness (29, 79, 90). These lesions possibly represent focal areas of ischemia and infarction resulting from the vasculitis. The pattern and extent of brain involvement on MRI do not appear to correlate with specific clinical features, severity of coma, or outcome of disease (63). Electroencephalography (EEG) shows the following abnormalities: diffuse slow waves with focal sharp waves; continuous, diffuse, irregular slow waves; and intermittent, diffuse slow waves (29, 90). Focal EEG abnormalities occur primarily in the temporal lobes.

Complications

Residual neurologic deficits, including a vegetative state, cognitive impairments, and cerebellar disabilities, occur in 10 to 15% of patients (29, 79, 90). Recurrence of neurologic dysfunction is seen in some patients, including neurologic relapse with seizures and/or cognitive impairment or focal signs such as isolated cranial nerve dysfunction. Findings at autopsy of a patient who died of encephalitis that developed 10 weeks following an initial asymptomatic infection showed evidence of neuronal death, neuronophagia, parenchymal inflammation, and perivascular cuffing, suggestive of a primary viral encephalitis rather than a vasculitis or infarction (90). MRI showed patchy areas of confluent cortical involvement, mainly in the cerebral hemispheres. The distinctive pathology and the MRI features of patients with relapse suggest that the pathogenesis may differ from that of acute Nipah encephalitis.

In a recent study (92), delayed progression to neurologic illness following Nipah fever was not observed, but persistent fatigue and functional impairment were frequent. Neurologic sequelae were frequent following Nipah encephalitis. Neurologic dysfunction may persist for years after acute infection, and new neurologic dysfunction may develop after acute illness. Survivors of NiV infection may experience substantial long-term neurologic and functional morbidity.

Clinical Diagnosis

Encephalitis can be diagnosed by the presence of fever, headache, reduced level of consciousness, and focal neurologic signs, as well as abnormalities on CSF examination and EEG studies. Clues to the Nipah virus etiology are provided by the history of contact with pigs, particularly in the context of an outbreak; the presence of segmental myoclonus; and MRI findings of small, discrete lesions in the subcortical and deep white matter of the cerebral hemispheres. MRI findings are particularly useful in distinguishing encephalitis caused by NiV from that caused by Japanese encephalitis virus, the most common arboviral encephalitis worldwide and which is endemic in China, India, and other parts of Southeast Asia, and by herpes simplex virus, the most common sporadic form of encephalitis worldwide.

Menangle Virus

Epidemiology

Distribution and Geography

From mid-April to early September 1997, at a piggery in New South Wales, Australia, a decline was noticed in the farrowing rate of sows, associated with an increase in the proportion of malformed, mummified, and stillborn piglets, with occasional abortions (80, 81). Affected piglets had craniofacial and spinal abnormalities and degeneration of the brain and spinal cord. A new paramyxovirus, MeV, was isolated from the brain, heart, and lung specimens of several affected piglets. No disease was seen in postnatal pigs of any age, but a high proportion of serum specimens (>95%) collected from these animals contained high titers of antibodies that neutralized the virus. Evidence of infection with MeV was also detected in porcine sera from two other associated piggeries that received weaned pigs from the affected piggery, but not in sera from several other piggeries throughout Australia (49).

A serologic survey on persons who came into contact with the affected piglets (13) detected a high titer of neutralizing antibodies in two workers, one at the affected piggery and one at an associated piggery. Both workers had an influenza-like illness concomitant with the outbreak in pigs, and no alternative cause was identified despite serologic testing. Thus, the illness was attributed to MeV infection.

Transmission

Close contact with infected piglets appears to be the primary mode of transmission of MeV to humans. The worker reported splashes of amniotic fluid and blood to the face and the frequent occurrence of minor wounds on his hands and forearms (13). The other worker performed autopsies on pigs without gloves or protective eyewear. Of note, a large breeding colony of fruit bats roosted within 200 m of the affected piggery, and sera from several bats had antibodies that neutralized MeV (80). In addition, antibodies were found in sera collected in 1996, before the outbreak, and from a colony of fruit bats 24 km from the piggery. All other sera collected from a variety of wild and domestic animals (e.g., cattle, sheep, birds, rodents, feral cats, and a dog) in the vicinity of the affected piggery tested seronegative for the virus. Thus, fruit bats are likely the primary reservoirs of MeV.

Clinical Manifestations

The two affected workers had similar illnesses, characterized by abrupt onset of fever, malaise, chills, drenching sweats, and severe headache (13). On the fourth day of illness, both developed a spotty, red, nonpruritic rash. Bilateral hypochondrial tenderness was present in one patient, and an abdominal ultrasound conducted 2 months after the illness showed splenomegaly and liver size at the upper limit of normal. Both patients recovered after approximately 10 days of illness.

LABORATORY DIAGNOSIS

Virus Isolation

Traditional techniques of virus isolation in cell culture, electron microscopy, enzyme-linked immunosorbent assay-based serology, neutralization assays, and IHC techniques have been employed in the diagnosis of the zoonotic paramyxoviruses (16, 23, 45, 80). Vero cell culture supports the growth of HeV, NiV, and MeV. Both HeV and NiV were first identified as syncytium-forming agents in Vero cell cultures, and electron microscopic studies revealed the presence of typical paramyxovirus "herringbone" nucleocapsid structures (16, 17). NiV has been successfully isolated from human specimens, including nasal and throat swabs as well as urine and CSF (29). The kidneys have been the only human source of HeV isolation from humans (68). In contrast, MeV has not been isolated from human specimens, but virus isolations from the tissues of stillborn piglets were readily obtained (80).

NiV and HeV are internationally classified as biosafety level or biosecurity level 4 (BSL-4) agents; thus, clinical specimens suspected to be infected with these agents must be handled with caution. Propagation of viruses from clinical specimens known to be infected with henipaviruses is not recommended without appropriate containment facilities. The CDC, Atlanta, GA, and the Australian Animal Health Laboratory, Geelong, Australia, have adopted the approach that primary virus isolation from specimens of outbreaks not already proven to be henipaviruses take place at BSL-3. However, if the results of cell culture suggest the presence of these agents, cultures should be transferred to BSL-4 to conform to biosafety guidelines (23).

Antigen and RNA Detection

IHC is an excellent technique for the detection of the zoonotic paramyxoviruses (16, 23, 42, 45) in the absence of BSL-4 facilities. Tissue specimens can be formalin fixed with minimal risk to the laboratory workers. Convalescent-phase human serum was initially used for antigen detection in the investigations of the first HeV outbreak, but subsequently, a wide variety of immunologic reagents became available from the Australian Animal Health Laboratory and CDC, including polyvalent and monoclonal antibodies to both HeV and NiV. HeV and NiV are genetically closely related (16, 39); thus, the investigation of more current NiV outbreaks benefited greatly from the availability of immunologic reagents made to HeV. To date, there are no commercially available antigen detection systems.

Diagnostic specimens from suspected cases can be disrupted in chaotropic salts in preparation for RNA extraction and RT-PCR. The addition of the chaotropic agent (guanidinium isothiocyanate) almost immediately abrogates paramyxovirus infectivity, and it minimizes human exposure to the infected tissues. RT-PCRs with conserved primer pairs (or families of degenerative primers) flanking the P protein gene editing region (16, 98) of the *Paramyxovirinae* subfamily results in the amplification of approximately 140 nucleotides of sequence spanning the P protein gene editing site. This strategy worked extremely well in the investigation of the NiV outbreak in Malaysia and Singapore and was instrumental in the rapid characterization of this new viral agent as related to, but different from, HeV (6). This method can be used in conjunction with fresh or formalin-fixed tissues from a variety of sources, including brain, lung, and kidney as well as CSF, for the detection of viral sequences.

Serology

Enzyme-linked immunosorbent assays using both indirect and antibody capture formats have been configured for the detection of IgM and IgG antibodies to HeV and NiV (23). The necessity of these simple serologic assays for detection of acute disease and epidemiological surveillance studies is unquestioned. However, viral antigen preparation for the henipaviruses is expensive and must take place in a BSL-4 facility. While sufficient quantities were prepared and made available for the diagnostic needs of the HeV and NiV outbreaks, alternative approaches to viral antigen production from virus-infected cells are currently being explored. One alternative is the expression of individual viral proteins following the incorporation of the viral genes in baculovirus expression or similar expression systems. Serum neutralization of HeV and NiV infection of Vero cell monolayer cultures is currently performed at BSL-4. These tests are very specific and have been used in conjunction with enzyme immunoassays and radioimmunoprecipitation assays to confirm acute infection and previous exposure to the viruses. In addition, the neutralization assay has been used to detect neutralizing antibody to HeV and NiV in animal serum specimens, particularly bat serum, in attempts to identify possible reservoirs of these agents (23, 119, 121).

PREVENTION

No passive immunoprophylaxis, antiviral chemoprophylaxis, or vaccine is currently available for henipavirus infections. The principal means of preventing human infections are early recognition of animal disease and use of precautions to avoid exposure. Since interruption of transmission to horses or pigs from the natural reservoir of these viruses, presumably fruit bats, is difficult, early identification of infected animals and use of appropriate personal protective measures to prevent transmission are keys to reducing the risk to humans. For example, persons handling horses in areas in which HeV may be endemic should be educated regarding the features of disease in horses and should use appropriate protective equipment (e.g., gloves, gowns, and face visors). Similarly, pig farmers in areas in which NiV may be endemic should be educated regarding the features of Nipah encephalitis in pigs and to report any unusual disease. Since transmission is possible without close contact with pigs, exposure to potentially infected animals should be completely avoided, if possible. Persons handling pigs or their excreta should wear protective equipment such as gloves, masks, gowns, and face visors.

Nipah Virus

Infection in piggeries with NiV or MeV can be eradicated through a combination of quarantine, segregation, and culling. During the outbreak in Malaysia, a national swine testing and surveillance program was initiated in which a sample of adult sows from pig farms was tested for antibody to NiV. Farms with antibody-positive animals were considered infected, and pigs from these farms were culled. A similar program to identify infected farms by testing pigs entering abattoirs is also being developed.

During community outbreaks, additional control measures may be required, including the restriction of movement of animals between farms, the culling of pigs from infected farms, and the temporary closure of abattoirs that slaughter pigs from farms in outbreak-affected areas. Recent data suggest that disinfection of fruit and boiling of palm sap, potentially contaminated by bats, might also be warranted in areas where repeated NiV outbreaks have occurred (3, 54).

In areas where large populations of fruit bats of the genus *Pteropus* congregate or frequent fruit or other agricultural products, means of reducing exposure of persons to potentially contaminated plants, areas, and products and means of disinfection of fruits or commodities before consumption should be considered.

Person-to-person transmission of NiV appears to have occurred in Bangladesh and perhaps in India (3, 11, 32). Therefore, it is likely that there is some risk for human-to-human transmission, since viral antigen is detected in human kidney and respiratory tract tissues and virus has been isolated from human urine and respiratory secretion specimens (16, 18). Given the potential severity of illness, those in contact with patients, including health care workers, should use standard and droplet precautions (e.g., strict attention to good hand washing practices, wearing a mask, and wearing gloves) during contact with secretions, excretions, and body fluids of patients.

TREATMENT

Symptomatic therapy includes the use of antipyretic and antiepileptic drugs and mechanical ventilatory support for severely ill patients. Because of the histopathological features of vasculitis-induced thrombosis, aspirin and pentoxifylline were used empirically in some NiV patients (29).

No specific antiviral therapy for infection by henipaviruses has been proven effective to date. One HeV patient recovered completely without any specific treatment, and neither patient with fatal disease received antiviral therapy. In vitro ribavirin is inhibitory for HeV at a concentration of 10 to 50 μg/ml, and the drug also crosses the blood-brain barrier, with a mean CSF/plasma ratio of 0.7 (15, 21). In Malaysia, ribavirin was administered either orally or intravenously to 140 patients with suspected Nipah encephalitis; 54 patients who were managed prior to the availability of ribavirin or refused treatment were selected as controls (15). Of the 140 patients who received ribavirin, 128 received it orally (2 g on day 1, 1.2 g three times daily on days 2 to 4, 1.2 g twice daily on days 5 and 6, and 0.6 g twice daily for another 1 to 4 days), whereas 12 received ribavirin intravenously (loading dose of 30 mg/kg of body weight, followed by 16 mg/kg every 6 h for 4 days and 8 mg/kg every 8 h for 3 days). A total of 45 (32%) of the 140 treated patients died, compared with 29 (54%) of the 54 controls, representing a 40% decline in the mortality rate in the treated group. Because a small number of patients received intravenous ribavirin, its effectiveness could not be adequately compared with that of oral ribavirin.

Despite the absence of any known published information on the in vitro effect of acyclovir on NiV infection or replication, acyclovir was empirically administered to all nine patients with encephalitis in Singapore. While only one of these patients died, several deteriorated before recovering, so the influence of acyclovir therapy on the course of disease is unknown.

Humanized monoclonal antibodies directed against the G protein are very efficient at neutralizing NiV (123, 124). Galectin-1, an endogenous lectin secreted by a variety of cell types, has pleiotropic immunomodulatory functions and also appears to have antiviral effects against NiV (53). A peptide based on the heptad repeats of the hPIV3 F protein was also able to inhibit HeV infection (83). A novel minigenome assay based on polymerase 1-driven transcription has been used to screen a library of small molecules to identify potential lead compounds for further study (28).

REFERENCES

1. **Aguilar, H. C., K. A. Matreyek, C. M. Filone, S. T. Hashimi, E. L. Levroney, O. A. Negrete, A. Bertolotti-Ciarlet, D. Y. Choi, I. McHardy, J. A. Fulcher, S. V. Su, M. C. Wolf, L. Kohatsu, L. G. Baum, and B. Lee.** 2006. N-glycans on Nipah virus fusion protein protect against neutralization but reduce membrane fusion and viral entry. *J. Virol.* **80:**4878–4889.
2. **Anonymous.** 2003. Outbreaks of encephalitis due to Nipah/Hendra-like viruses, western Bangladesh. *Health Sci. Bull.* (English) **1:**1–6.
3. **Anonymous.** 2004. Person-to-person transmission of Nipah virus during outbreak in Faridpur District, 2004. *Health Sci. Bull.* **2:**5–9.
4. **Bonaparte, M. I., A. S. Dimitrov, K. N. Bossart, G. Crameri, B. A. Mungall, K. A. Bishop, V. Choudhry, D. S. Dimitrov, L. F. Wang, B. T. Eaton, and C. C. Broder.** 2005. Ephrin-B2 ligand is a functional receptor for Hendra virus and Nipah virus. *Proc. Natl. Acad. Sci. USA* **102:**10652–10657.
5. **Bossart, K. N., L. F. Wang, M. N. Flora, K. B. Chua, S. K. Lam, B. T. Eaton, and C. C. Broder.** 2002. Membrane fusion tropism and heterotypic functional activities of the Nipah virus and Hendra virus envelope glycoproteins. *J. Virol.* **76:**11186–11198.

6. **Bowden, T. R., M. Westenberg, L. F. Wang, B. T. Eaton, and D. B. Boyle.** 2001. Molecular characterization of Menangle virus, a novel paramyxovirus which infects pigs, fruit bats and humans. *Virology* **283:**358–373.
7. **Bowden, T. R., and D. B. Boyle.** 2005. Completion of the full-length genome sequence of Menangle virus: characterization of the polymerase gene and genomic 5′ trailer region. *Arch. Virol.* **150:**2125–2137.
8. **Calain, P., and L. Roux.** 1993. The rule of six, a basic feature for efficient replication of Sendai virus defective interfering RNA. *J. Virol.* **67:**4822–4830.
9. **Centers for Disease Control and Prevention.** 1999. Outbreak of Hendra-like virus—Malaysia and Singapore, 1998–1999. *Morb. Mortal. Wkly. Rep.* **48:**265–269. (Erratum, **48:**339.)
10. **Centers for Disease Control and Prevention.** 1999. Update: outbreak of Nipah virus—Malaysia and Singapore, 1999. *Morb. Mortal. Wkly. Rep.* **48:**335–337.
11. **Chadha, M. S., J. A. Comer, L. Lowe, P. A. Rota, P. E. Rollin, W. J. Bellini, T. G. Ksiazek, and A. Mishra.** 2006. Nipah virus-associated encephalitis outbreak, Siliguri, India. *Emerg. Infect. Dis.* **12:**235–240.
12. **Chan, Y. P., C. L. Koh, S. K. Lam, and L. F. Wang.** 2004. Mapping of domains responsible for nucleocapsid protein-phosphoprotein interaction of Henipaviruses. *J. Gen. Virol.* **85:**1675–1684.
13. **Chant, K., R. Chan, M. Smith, D. E. Dwyer, and P. Kirkland for The NSW Expert Group.** 1998. Probable human infection with a newly described virus in the family Paramyxoviridae. *Emerg. Infect. Dis.* **4:**273–275.
14. **Chew, M. H., P. M. Arguin, D. K. Shay, R. T. Goh, P. E. Rollin, W. J. Shieh, S. R. Zaki, P. A. Rota, A. E. Ling, T. G. Ksiazek, S. K. Chew, and L. J. Anderson.** 2000. Risk factors for Nipah virus infection among abattoir workers in Singapore. *J. Infect. Dis.* **181:**1760–1763.
15. **Chong, H. T., A. Kamarulzaman, C. T. Tan, K. J. Goh, T. Thayaparan, S. R. Kunjapan, N. K. Chew, K. B. Chua, and S. K. Lam.** 2001. Treatment of acute Nipah encephalitis with ribavirin. *Ann. Neurol.* **49:**810–813.
16. **Chua, K. B., W. J. Bellini, P. A. Rota, B. H. Harcourt, A. Tamin, S. K. Lam, T. G. Ksiazek, P. E. Rollin, S. R. Zaki, W. J. Shieh, C. S. Goldsmith, J. T. Roehrig, B. Eaton, A. R. Gould, H. Field, P. Daniel, A. E. Ling, C. J. Peters, L. J. Anderson, and B. W. J. Mahy.** 2000. Nipah virus: a recently emergent deadly paramyxovirus. *Science* **288:**1432–1435.
17. **Chua, K. B., S. K. Lam, C. T. Tan, P. S. Hooi, K. J. Goh, N. K. Chew, K. S. Tan, A. Kamarulzaman, and K. T. Wong.** 2000. High mortality in Nipah encephalitis is associated with presence of virus in cerebrospinal fluid. *Ann. Neurol.* **48:**802–805.
18. **Chua, K. B., S. K. Lam, K. J. Goh, P. S. Hooi, T. G. Ksiazek, A. Kamarulzaman, J. Olson, and C. T. Tan.** 2001. The presence of Nipah virus in respiratory secretions and urine of patients during an outbreak of Nipah virus encephalitis in Malaysia. *J. Infect.* **42:**40–44.
19. **Chua, K. B., L. F. Wang, S. K. Lam, G. Crameri, M. Yu, T. Wise, D. Boyle, A. D. Hyatt, and B. T. Eaton.** 2001. Tioman virus, a novel paramyxovirus isolated from fruit bats in Malaysia. *Virology* **283:**215–229.
20. **Chua, K. B., L. F. Wang, S. K. Lam, and B. T. Eaton.** 2002. Full length genome sequence of Tioman virus, a novel paramyxovirus in the genus Rubulavirus isolated from fruit bats in Malaysia. *Arch. Virol.* **147:**1323–1348.
21. **Connor, E., S. Morrison, J. Lane, J. Oleske, R. L. Sonke, and J. Connor.** 1993. Safety, tolerance, and pharmacokinetics of systemic ribavirin in children with human immunodeficiency virus infection. *Antimicrob. Agents Chemother.* **37:**532–539.
22. **Crameri, G., L. F. Wang, C. Morrissy, J. White, and B. T. Eaton.** 2002. A rapid immune plaque assay for the detection of Hendra and Nipah viruses and anti-virus antibodies. *J. Virol. Methods* **99:**41–51.
23. **Daniels, P., T. Ksiasek, and B. T. Eaton.** 2001. Laboratory diagnosis of Nipah and Hendra virus infections. *Microbes Infect.* **3:**289–295.
24. **Domingo, M., J. Visa, M. Pumarola, A. J. Marco, L. Ferrer, R. Rabanal, and S. Kennedy.** 1992. Pathologic and immunocytochemical studies of morbillivirus infection in striped dolphins *(Stenella coeruleoalba)*. *Vet. Pathol.* **29:**1–10.
25. **Epstein, J. H., H. E. Field, S. Luby, J. R. Pulliam, and P. Daszak.** 2006. Nipah virus: impact, origins, and causes of emergence. *Curr. Infect. Dis. Rep.* **8:**59–65.
26. **Field, H. E., P. C. Barratt, R. J. Hughes, J. Shield, and N. D. Sullivan.** 2000. A fatal case of Hendra virus infection in a horse in north Queensland: clinical and epidemiological features. *Aust. Vet. J.* **78:**279–280.
27. **Franke, J., S. Essbauer, W. Ahne, and S. Blahak.** 2001. Identification and molecular characterization of 18 Paramyxoviruses isolated from snakes. *Virus Res.* **80:**67–74.
28. **Freiberg, A., L. K. Dolores, S. Enterlein, and R. Flick.** 2008. Establishment and characterization of plasmid-driven minigenome rescue systems for Nipah virus: RNA polymerase I- and T7-catalyzed generation of functional paramyxoviral RNA. *Virology* **370:**33–44.
29. **Goh, K. J., C. T. Tan, N. K. Chew, P. S. Tan, A. Kamarulzaman, S. A. Sarji, K. T. Wong, B. J. Abdullah, K. B. Chua, and S. K. Lam.** 2000. Clinical features of Nipah virus encephalitis among pig farmers in Malaysia. *N. Engl. J. Med.* **342:**1229–1235.
30. **Guillaume, V., H. Contamin, P. Loth, M. C. Georges-Courbot, A. Lefeuvre, P. Marianneau, K. B. Chua, S. K. Lam, R. Buckland, V. Deubel, and T. F. Wild.** 2004. Nipah virus: vaccination and passive protection studies in a hamster model. *J. Virol.* **78:**834–840.
31. **Guillaume, V., H. Contamin, P. Loth, I. Grosjean, M. C. Courbot, V. Deubel, R. Buckland, and T. F. Wild.** 2006. Antibody prophylaxis and therapy against Nipah virus infection in hamsters. *J. Virol.* **80:**1972–1978.
32. **Gurley, E. S., J. M. Montgomery, M. J. Hossain M. R. Islam, M. A. R. Molla, S. M. Shamsuzzaman, K. Akram, K. Zaman, N. Asgari, J. A. Comer, A. K. Azad, P. E. Rollin, T. G. Ksiazek, and R. F. Breiman.** 2007. Risk of nosocomial transmission of Nipah virus in a Bangladesh hospital. *Infect. Control Hosp. Epidemiol.* **28:**740–742.
33. **Hagmaier, K., N. Stock, S. Goodbourn, L. F. Wang, and R. Randall.** 2006. A single amino acid substitution in the V protein of Nipah virus alters its ability to block interferon signaling in cells from different species. *J. Gen. Virol.* **87:**3649–3653.
34. **Halpin, K., P. L. Young, H. Field, and J. S. Mackenzie.** 1999. Newly discovered viruses of flying foxes. *Vet. Microbiol.* **68:**83–87.
35. **Halpin, K., P. L. Young, H. E. Field, and J. S. Mackenzie.** 2000. Isolation of Hendra virus from pteropid bats: a natural reservoir of Hendra virus. *J. Gen. Virol.* **81:**1927–1932.
36. **Halpin, K., B. Bankamp, B. H. Harcourt, W. J. Bellini, and P. A. Rota.** 2004. Nipah virus conforms to the rule of six in a minigenome replication assay. *J. Gen. Virol.* **85:**701–707.
37. **Halpin, K., A. D. Hyatt, R. K. Plowright, J. H. Epstein, P. Daszak, H. E. Field, L. Wang, and P. W. Daniels.** 2007. Emerging viruses: coming in on a wrinkled wing and a prayer. *Clin. Infect. Dis.* **44:**711–717.

38. **Halpin, K., and B. A. Mungall.** 2007. Recent progress in henipavirus research. *Comp. Immunol. Microbiol. Infect. Dis.* **30:**287–307.
39. **Harcourt, B. H., A. Tamin, T. G. Ksiazek, P. E. Rollin, L. J. Anderson, W. J. Bellini, and P. A. Rota.** 2000. Molecular characterization of Nipah virus, a newly emergent paramyxovirus. *Virology* **271:**334–349.
40. **Harcourt, B. H., A. Tamin, K. Halpin, T. G. Ksiazek, P. E. Rollin, L. J. Anderson, W. J. Bellini, and P. A. Rota.** 2001. Molecular characterization of polymerase gene and genomic termini of Nipah virus. *Virology* **287:** 192–201.
41. **Harcourt, B. H., L. Lowe, A. Tamin, X. Liu, B. Bankamp, N. Bowden, P. E. Rollin, J. A. Comer, T. G. Ksiazek, M. J. Hossain, E. S. Gurley, R. F. Breiman, W. J. Bellini, and P. A. Rota.** 2005. Genetic characterization of Nipah virus, Bangladesh, 2004. *Emerg. Infect. Dis.* **11:**1594–1597.
42. **Hooper, P. T., A. R. Gould, G. M. Russell, J. A. Kattenbelt, and G. Mitchell.** 1996. The retrospective diagnosis of a second outbreak of equine morbillivirus infection. *Aust. Vet. J.* **74:**244–245.
43. **Hooper, P. T., A. R. Gould, A. D. Hyatt, M. A. Braun, J. A. Kattenbelt, S. G. Hengstberger, and H. A. Westbury.** 2000. Identification and molecular characterization of Hendra virus in a horse in Queensland. *Aust. Vet. J.* **78:**281–282.
44. **Hooper, P. T., and M. M. Williamson.** 2000. Hendra and Nipah virus infections. *Vet. Clin. N. Am. Equine Pract.* **16:**597–603, xi.
45. **Hooper, P. T., G. M. Russell, P. W. Selleck, R. A. Lunt, C. J. Morrissy, M. A. Braun, and M. M. Williamson.** 1999. Immunohistochemistry in the identification of a number of new diseases in Australia. *Vet. Microbiol.* **68:** 89–93.
46. **Hsu, V. P., M. J. Hossain, U. D. Parashar, M. M. Ali, T. G. Ksiazek, I. Kuzmin, M. Niezgoda, C. Rupprecht, J. Breese, and R. F. Breiman.** 2004. Nipah virus encephalitis reemergence, Bangladesh. *Emerg. Infect. Dis.* **10:** 2082–2087.
47. **Iehlé, C., G. Razafitrimo, J. Razainirina, N. Andriaholinirina, S. M. Goodman, C. Faure, M.-C. Georges-Courbot, D. Rousset, and J.-M. Reynes.** 2007. Henipavirus and Tioman virus antibodies in pteropodid bats, Madagascar. *Emerg. Infect. Dis.* **13:**159–161.
48. **Jack, P. J. M., D. B. Boyle, B. T. Eaton, and L.-F. Wang.** 2005. The complete genome sequence of J virus reveals a unique genome structure in the family *Paramyxoviridae*. *J. Virol.* **79:**10690–10700.
49. **Kirkland, P. D., R. J. Love, A. W. Philbey, A. D. Ross, R. J. Davis, and K. G. Hart.** 2001. Epidemiology and control of Menangle virus in pigs. *Aust. Vet. J.* **79:**199–206.
50. **Lamb, R. A., and D. Kolakofsky.** 1996. *Paramyxoviridae:* The viruses and their replication, p. 1177–1202. *In* B. N. Fields, D. M Knipe, and P. M. Howley (ed.), *Fields Virology*, 3rd ed. Lippincott-Raven Publishers, Philadelphia, PA.
51. **Lamb, R. A., and T. S. Jardetzky.** 2007. Structural basis of viral invasion: lessons from paramyxovirus F. *Curr. Opin. Struct. Biol.* **17:**427–436.
52. **Langedijk, J. P. M., F. J. Daus, and J. T. van Oirschot.** 1997. Sequence and structure alignment of *Paramyxoviridae* attachment proteins and discovery of enzymatic activity for a morbillivirus hemagglutinin. *J. Virol.* **71:**6155–6167.
53. **Levroney, E. L., H. C. Aguilar, J. A. Fulcher, L. Kohatsu, K. E. Pace, M. Pang, K. B. Gurney, L. G. Baum, and B. Lee.** 2005. Novel innate immune functions for galectin-1: galectin-1 inhibits cell fusion by Nipah virus envelope glycoproteins and augments dendritic cell secretion of proinflammatory cytokines. *J. Immunol.* **175:**413–420.
54. **Li, Z., M. Yu, H. Zhang, D. E. Magoffin, P. J. Jack, A. Hyatt, H. Y. Wang, and L. F. Wang.** 2006. Beilong virus, a novel paramyxovirus with the largest genome of non-segmented negative-stranded RNA viruses. *Virology* **346:** 219–228.
55. **Luby, S. P., M. Rahman, M. J. Hossain, L. S. Blum, M. M. Husain, E. Gurley, R. Khan, B.-N. Ahmed, S. Rahman, N. Nahar, E. Kenah, J. A. Comer, and T. G. Ksiazek.** 2006. Foodborne transmission of Nipah virus, Bangladesh. *Emerg. Infect. Dis.* **12:**1888–1894.
56. **Magoffin, D. E., K. Halpin, P. A. Rota, and L. F. Wang.** 2007. Effects of single amino acid substitutions at the E residue in the conserved GDNE motif of the Nipah virus polymerase (L) protein. *Arch. Virol.* **152:**827–832.
57. **Mayo, M. A., and M. H. van Regenmortel.** 2000. ICTV and the Virology Division News. *Arch. Virol.* **145:**1985–1988.
58. **McCormack, J. G., A. M. Allworth, L. A. Selvey, and P. W. Selleck.** 1999. Transmissibility from horses to humans of a novel paramyxovirus, equine morbillivirus (EMV). *J. Infect.* **38:**22–23.
59. **Meulendyke, K. A., M. A. Wurth, R. O. McCann, and R. E. Dutch.** 2005. Endocytosis plays a critical role in proteolytic processing of the Hendra virus fusion protein. *J. Virol.* **79:**12643–12649.
60. **Michalski, W. P., G. Crameri, L. F. Wang, B. J. Shiell, and B. Eaton.** 2000. The cleavage activation and sites of glycosylation in fusion protein of Hendra virus. *Virus Res.* **69:**83–93.
61. **Middleton, D. J., H. A. Westbury, C. J. Morrissy, B. M. van der Heide, G. M. Russell, M. A. Braun, and A. D. Hyatt.** 2002. Experimental Nipah virus infection in pigs and cats. *J. Comp. Pathol.* **126:**124–136.
62. **Middleton, D. J., C. J. Morrissy, B. M. van der Heide, G. M. Russell, M. A. Braun, H. A. Westbury, K. Halpin, and P. W. Daniels.** 2007. Experimental Nipah virus infection in pteropid bats (Pteropus poliocephalus). *J. Comp. Pathol.* **136:**266–272.
63. **Mohd Nor, M. N., C. H. Gan, and B. L. Ong.** 2000. Nipah virus infection of pigs in peninsular Malaysia. *Rev. Sci. Tech. Off. Int. Epizoot.* **19:**160–165.
64. **Moll, M., S. Diederich, H. D. Klenk, M. Czub, and A. Maisner.** 2004. Ubiquitous activation of the Nipah virus fusion protein does not require a basic amino acid at the cleavage site. *J. Virol.* **78:**9705–9712.
65. **Moll, M., A. Kaufmann, and A. Maisner.** 2004. Influence of N-glycans on processing and biological activity of the Nipah virus fusion protein. *J. Virol.* **78:**7274–7278.
66. **Mounts, A. W., H. Kaur, U. D. Parashar, T. G. Ksiazek, D. Cannon, J. T. Arokiasamy, L. J. Anderson, M. S. Lye, and the Nipah Virus Nosocomial Study Group.** 2001. A cohort study of health care workers to assess nosocomial transmissibility of Nipah virus, Malaysia, 1999. *J. Infect. Dis.* **183:**810–813.
67. **Mungall, B. A., D. Middleton, G. Crameri, J. Bingham, K. Halpin, G. Russell, D. Green, J. McEachern, L. I. Pritchard, B. T. Eaton, L. F. Wang, K. N. Bossart, and C. C. Broder.** 2006. Feline model of acute Nipah virus infection and protection with a soluble glycoprotein-based subunit vaccine. *J. Virol.* **80:**12293–12302.
68. **Murray, K., P. Selleck, P. Hooper, A. Hyatt, A. Gould, L. Gleeson, H. Westbury, L. Hiley, L. Selvey, B. Rodwell, and P. Ketterer.** 1995. A morbillivirus that caused fatal disease in horses and humans. *Science* **268:**94–97.

69. **Murray, K., R. Rogers, L. Selvey, P. Selleck, A. Hyatt, A. Gould, L. Gleeson, P. Hooper, and H. Westbury.** 1995. A novel morbillivirus pneumonia of horses and its transmission to humans. *Emerg. Infect. Dis.* **1:**31–33.
70. **Negrete, O. A., E. L. Levroney, H. C. Aguilar, A. Bertolotti-Ciarlet, R. Nazarian, S. Tajyar, and B. Lee.** 2005. EphrinB2 is the entry receptor for Nipah virus, an emergent deadly paramyxovirus. *Nature* **436:**401–405.
71. **Negrete, O. A., M. C. Wolf, H. C. Aguilar, S. Enterlein, W. Wang, E. Muhlberger, S. V. Su, A. Bertolotti-Ciarlet, R. Flick, and B. Lee.** 2006. Two key residues in ephrinB3 are critical for its use as an alternative receptor for Nipah virus. *PLoS Pathog.* **2**(2)**:**e7.
72. **Negrete, O. A., D. Chu, H. C. Aguilar, and B. Lee.** 2007. Single amino acid changes in the Nipah and Hendra virus attachment glycoproteins distinguish ephrinB2 from ephrinB3 usage. *J. Virol.* **81:**10804–10814.
73. **Olson, J. G., C. Rupprecht, P. E. Rollin, U. S. An, M. Niezgoda, T. Clemins, J. Walston, and T. G. Ksiazek.** 2002. Antibodies to Nipah-like virus in bats *(Pteropus lylei)*, Cambodia. *Emerg. Infect. Dis.* **8:**987–988.
74. **Osterhaus, A. D. M. E., and E. J. Vedder.** 1988. Identification of virus causing recent seal deaths. *Nature* **335:** 20.
75. **O'Sullivan, J. D., A. M. Allworth, D. L. Paterson, T. M. Snow, R. Boots, L. J. Gleeson, A. R. Gould, A. D. Hyatt, and J. Bradfield.** 1997. Fatal encephalitis due to novel paramyxovirus transmitted from horses. *Lancet* **349:**93–95.
76. **Pager, C. T., and R. E. Dutch.** 2005. Cathepsin L is involved in proteolytic processing of the Hendra virus fusion protein. *J. Virol.* **79:**12714–12720.
77. **Parashar, U. D., L. M. Sunn, F. Ong, A. W. Mounts, M. T. Arif, T. G. Ksiazek, M. A. Kamaluddin, A. N. Mustafa, H. Kaur, L. M. Ding, G. Othman, H. M. Radzi, P. T. Kitsutani, P. C. Stockton, J. Arokiasamy, H. E. Gary, Jr., and L. J. Anderson.** 2000. Case-control study of risk factors for human infection with a new zoonotic paramyxovirus, Nipah virus, during a 1998–1999 outbreak of severe encephalitis in Malaysia. *J. Infect. Dis.* **181:**1755–1759.
78. **Park, M.-S., M. L. Shaw, J. Muñoz-Jordan, J. F. Cros, T. Nakaya, N. Bouvier, P. Palese, A. García-Sastre, and C. F. Basler.** 2003. Newcastle disease virus (NDV)-based assay demonstrates interferon-antagonist activity for the NDV V protein and the Nipah virus V, W, and C proteins. *J. Virol.* **77:**1501–1511.
79. **Paton, N. I., Y. S. Leo, S. R. Zaki, A. P. Auchus, K. E. Lee, A. E. Ling, S. K. Chew, B. Ang, P. E. Rollin, T. Umapathi, I. Sng, C. C. Lee, E. Lim, and T. G. Ksiazek.** 1999. Outbreak of Nipah-virus infection among abattoir workers in Singapore. *Lancet* **354:**1253–1256.
80. **Philbey, A. W., P. D. Kirkland, A. D. Ross, R. J. Davis, A. B. Gleeson, R. J. Love, P. W. Daniels, A. R. Gould, and A. R. Hyatt.** 1998. An apparently new virus (family Paramyxoviridae) infectious for pigs, humans and fruit bats. *Emerg. Infect. Dis.* **4:**269–271.
81. **Philbey, A. W., A. D. Ross, P. D. Kirkland, and R. J. Love.** 2007. Skeletal and neurological malformations in pigs congenitally infected with Menangle virus. *Aust. Vet. J.* **85:**134–140.
82. **Poch, O., B. M. Blumberg, L. Bougueleret, and N. Tordo.** 1990. Sequence comparison of five polymerases (L proteins) of unsegmented negative-strand RNA viruses: theoretical assignment of functional domains. *J. Gen. Virol.* **71:**1153–1162.
83. **Porotto, M., P. Carta, Y. Deng, G. E. Kellogg, M. Whitt, M. Lu, B. A. Mungall, and A. Moscona.** 2007. Molecular determinants of antiviral potency of paramyxovirus entry inhibitors. *J. Virol.* **81:**10567–10574.
84. **Ramasundrum, V., C. T. Tan, K. B. Chua, H. T. Chong, K. J. Goh, N. K. Chew, K. S. Tan, T. Thayaparan, S. R. Kunjapan, V. Petharunam, Y. L. Loh, T. G. Ksiazek, and S. K. Lam.** 2000. Kinetics of IgM and IgG seroconversion in Nipah virus infection. *Neurol. J. Southeast Asia* **5:**23–28.
85. **Reynes, J. M., D. Counor, S. Ong, C. Faure, V. Seng, S. Molia, J. Walston, M. C. Georges-Courbot, V. Deubel, and J. L. Sarthou.** 2005. Nipah virus in Lyle's flying foxes, Cambodia. *Emerg. Infect. Dis.* **11:**1042–1047.
86. **Rodriguez, J. J., J. P. Parisien, and C. M. Horvath.** 2002. Nipah virus V protein evades alpha and gamma interferons by preventing STAT1 and STAT2 activation and nuclear accumulation. *J. Virol.* **76:**11476–11483.
87. **Rodriguez, J. J., L. F. Wang, and C. M. Horvath.** 2003. Hendra virus V protein inhibits interferon signaling by preventing STAT1 and STAT2 nuclear accumulation. *J. Virol.* **77:**11842–11845.
88. **Roelke-Parker, M. E., L. Munson, C. Packer, R. Kock, S. Cleaveland, M. Carpenter, S. J. O'Brien, A. Pospischil, R. Hofmann-Lehmann, and H. Lutz.** 1996. A canine distemper virus epidemic in Serengeti lions (Panthera leo). *Nature* **379:**441–445. (Erratum, **381:** 172.)
89. **Rogers, R. J., I. C. Douglas, F. C. Baldock, R. J. Glanville, K. T. Seppanen, L. J. Gleeson, P. N. Selleck, and K. J. Dunn.** 1996. Investigation of a second focus of equine morbillivirus infection in coastal Queensland. *Aust. Vet. J.* **74:**243–244.
90. **Sarji, S. A., B. J. Abdullah, K. J. Goh, C. T. Tan, and R. T. Wong.** 2000. MR imaging features of Nipah encephalitis. *Am. J. Roentgenol.* **175:**437–442.
91. **Sawatsky, B., A. Grolla, N. Kuzenko, H. Weingartl, and M. Czub.** 2007. Inhibition of henipavirus infection by Nipah virus attachment glycoprotein occurs without cell-surface downregulation of ephrin-B2 or ephrin-B3. *J. Gen. Virol.* **88:**582–591.
92. **Sejvar, J. J., J. Hossain, S. K. Saha, E. S. Gurley, S. Banu, J. D. Hamadani, M. A. Faiz, F. M. Siddiqui, O. D. Mohammad, A. H. Mollah, R. Uddin, R. Alam, R. Rahman, C. T. Tan, W. Bellini, P. Rota, R. F. Breiman, and S. P. Luby.** 2007. Long-term neurological and functional outcome in Nipah virus infection. *Ann. Neurol.* **62:**235–242.
93. **Selvey, L. A., R. M. Wells, J. G. McCormack, A. J. Ansford, K. Murray, R. J. Rogers, P. S. Lavercombe, P. Selleck, and J. W. Sheridan.** 1995. Infection of humans and horses by a newly described morbillivirus. *Med. J. Aust.* **162:**642–645.
94. **Sendow, I., H. E. Field, J. Curran, Darminto, C. Morrissy, G. Meehan, T. Buick, and P. Daniels.** 2005. Henipavirus in *Pteropus vampyrus* bats, Indonesia. *Emerg. Infect. Dis.* **12:**711–712.
95. **Shaw, M. L., A. Garcia-Sastre, P. Palese, and C. F. Basler.** 2004. Nipah virus V and W proteins have a common STAT1-binding domain yet inhibit STAT1 activation from the cytoplasmic and nuclear compartments, respectively. *J. Virol.* **78:**5633–5641.
96. **Shaw, M. L., W. B. Cardenas, D. Zamarin, P. Palese, and C. F. Basler.** 2005. Nuclear localization of the Nipah virus W protein allows for inhibition of both virus- and Toll-like receptor 3-triggered signaling pathways. *J. Virol.* **79:**6078–6088.
97. **Tamin, A., B. H. Harcourt, T. G. Ksiazek, P. E. Rollin, W. J. Bellini, and P. A. Rota.** 2002. Functional properties of the fusion and attachment glycoproteins of Nipah virus. *Virology* **296:**190–200.

98. **Thomas, S. M., R. A. Lamb, and R. G. Paterson.** 1988. Two mRNAs that differ by two non-templated nucleotides encode the amino coterminal proteins P and V of the paramyxovirus SV5. *Cell* **54:**891–902.
99. **Tidona, C. A., H. W. Kurz, H. R. Gelderblom, and G. Darai.** 1999. Isolation and molecular characterization of a novel cytopathogenic paramyxovirus from tree shrews. *Virology* **258:**425–434.
100. **Vidal, S., J. Curran, and D. Kolakofsky.** 1990. Editing of the Sendai virus P/C mRNA by G insertion occurs during mRNA synthesis via a virus-encoded activity. *J. Virol.* **64:**239–246.
101. **Vogt, C., M. Eickmann, S. Diederich, M. Moll, and A. Maisner.** 2005. Endocytosis of the Nipah virus glycoproteins. *J. Virol.* **79:**3865–3872.
102. **Wacharapluesadee, S., B. Lumlertdacha, K. Boongird, S. Wanghongsa, L. Chanhome, P. Rollin, P. Stockton, C. E. Rupprecht, T. G. Ksiazek, and T. Hemachudha.** 2005. Bat Nipah virus, Thailand. *Emerg. Infect. Dis.* **11:** 1949–1951.
103. **Wacharapluesadee, S., and T. Hemachudha.** 2007. Duplex nested RT-PCR for detection of Nipah virus RNA from urine specimens of bats. *J. Virol. Methods* **141:**97–101.
104. **Walpita, P., and C. J. Peters.** 2007. Cis-acting elements in the antigenomic promoter of Nipah virus. *J. Gen. Virol.* **88:**2542–2551.
105. **Wang, L.-F., W. P. Michalski, M. Yu, L. I. Pritchard, G. Crameri, B. Shiell, and B. T. Eaton.** 1998. A novel P/V/C gene in a new member of the *Paramyxoviridae* family, which causes lethal infection in humans, horses, and other animals. *J. Virol.* **72:**1482–1490.
106. **Wang, L.-F., M. Yu, E. Hansson, L. I. Pritchard, B. Shiell, W. P. Michalski, and B. T. Eaton.** 2000. The exceptionally large genome of Hendra virus: support for creation of a new genus within the family *Paramyxoviridae*. *J. Virol.* **74:**9972–9979.
107. **Wang, L. F., B. H. Harcourt, M. Yu, A. Tamin, P. A. Rota, W. J. Bellini, and B. T. Eaton.** 2001. Molecular biology of Hendra and Nipah viruses. *Microbes Infect.* **3:** 279–296.
108. **Ward, M. P., F. Black, A. J. Childs, F. C. Baldock, W. R. Webster, B. J. Rodwell, and S. L. Brouwer.** 1996. Negative findings from serological studies of equine morbillivirus in the Queensland horse population. *Aust. Vet. J.* **74:**241–243.
109. **Weingartl, H., S. Czub, J. Copps, Y. Berhane, D. Middleton, P. Marszal, J. Gren, G. Smith, S. Ganske, L. Manning, and M. Czub.** 2005. Invasion of the central nervous system in a porcine host by Nipah virus. *J. Virol.* **79:**528–534.
110. **Weingartl, H. M., Y. Berhane, J. L. Caswell, S. Loosmore, J. C. Audonnet, J. A. Roth, and M. Czub.** 2006. Recombinant Nipah virus vaccines protect pigs against challenge. *J. Virol.* **80:**7929–7938.
111. **Williamson, M. M., P. T. Hooper, P. W. Selleck, L. J. Gleeson, P. W. Daniels, H. A. Westbury, and P. K. Murray.** 1998. Transmission studies of Hendra virus (equine morbillivirus) in fruit bats, horses and cats. *Aust. Vet. J.* **76:**813–818.
112. **Williamson, M. M., P. T. Hooper, P. W. Selleck, H. A. Westbury, and R. F. Slocombe.** 2000. Experimental Hendra virus infection in pregnant guinea-pigs and fruit bats (Pteropus poliocephalus). *J. Comp. Pathol.* **122:** 201–207.
113. **World Health Organization.** September 2001. Nipah virus. Fact sheet no. 262. http://www.who.int/mediacentre/factsheets/fs262/en/print.html.
114. **World Health Organization.** 2004. Nipah virus outbreak(s) in Bangladesh, January–April 2004. *Wkly. Epidemiol. Rec.* **79:**168–171.
115. **World Health Organization.** 12 February 2004. Nipah-like virus in Bangladesh. http://www.who.int/csr/don/2004_02_12/en/print.html.
116. **World Health Organization.** 26 February 2004. Nipah-like virus in Bangladesh—update. http://www.who.int/csr/don/2004_02_26/en/print.html.
117. **Yaiw, K. C., J. Bingham, G. Crameri, B. Mungall, A. Hyatt, M. Yu, B. Eaton, D. Shamala, L. F. Wang, and K. T. Wong.** 3 October 2007. Tioman virus, a paramyxovirus of bat origin, causes mild disease in pigs and has a predilection for lymphoid tissues. *J. Virol.* doi:101128/JVI.01660-07. (Subsequently published, *J. Virol.* **82:** 565–568, 2008.) Oct. 3. Epub.
118. **Yaiw, K. C., G. Crameri, L. Wang, H. T. Chong, K. B. Chua, C. T. Tan, K. J. Goh, D. Shamala, and K. T. Wong.** 2007. Serological evidence of possible human infection with Tioman virus, a newly described paramyxovirus of bat origin. *J. Infect. Dis.* **196:**884–886.
119. **Yob, J. M., H. Field, A. M. Rashidi, C. Morrissy, B. van der Heide, P. A. Rota, A. Adzhar, J. White, P. Daniels, A. Jamaluddin, and T. G. Ksiazek.** 2000. Nipah virus infection in bats (order Chiroptera) in peninsular Malaysia. *Emerg. Infect. Dis.* **7:**439–441.
120. **Yoneda, M., V. Guillaume, F. Ikeda, Y. Sakuma, H. Sato, T. F. Wild, and C. Kai.** 2006. Establishment of a Nipah virus rescue system. *Proc. Natl. Acad. Sci. USA* **103:**16508–16513.
121. **Young, P. L., K. Halpin, P. W. Selleck, H. Field, J. L. Gravel, M. A. Kelly, and J. S. Mackenzie.** 1996. Serologic evidence for the presence in Pteropus bats of a paramyxovirus related to equine morbillivirus. *Emerg. Infect. Dis.* **2:**239–240.
122. **Yu, M., E. Hansson, J. P. Langedijk, B. T. Eaton, and L. F. Wang.** 1998. The attachment protein of Hendra virus has high structural similarity but limited primary sequence homology compared with viruses in the genus paramyxovirus. *Virology* **251:**227–233.
123. **Zhu, Z., A. S. Dimitrov, K. N. Bossart, G. Crameri, K. A. Bishop, V. Choudhry, B. A. Mungall, Y. R. Feng, A. Choudhary, M. Y. Zhang, Y. Feng, L. F. Wang, X. Xiao, B. T. Eaton, C. C. Broder, and D. S. Dimitrov.** 2006. Potent neutralization of Hendra and Nipah viruses by human monoclonal antibodies. *J. Virol.* **80:**891–899.
124. **Zhu, Z., A. S. Dimitrov, S. Chakraborti, D. Dimitrova, X. Xiao, C. C. Broder, and D. S. Dimitrov.** 2006. Development of human monoclonal antibodies against diseases caused by emerging and biodefense-related viruses. *Expert Rev. Anti-Infect. Ther.* **4:**57–66.

Rhabdoviruses

THOMAS P. BLECK AND CHARLES E. RUPPRECHT

40

Rabies is a viral disease producing an almost uniformly fatal encephalitis in humans and other mammals. This disease has been present throughout recorded history and literature and likely predates the evolution of humanity. The thought of rabies produces both loathing and fascination. Rabies virus stands apart as the most uniformly fatal of all viruses and remains one of the most common viral causes of mortality in the developing world.

Rabies exposure also has profound worldwide medical and economic implications (175), with as many as four million people receiving postexposure prophylaxis to prevent rabies (116). Although current vaccine technology allows the production of safe agents for postexposure prophylaxis, the expense involved often leads to the use of older, more dangerous vaccines in the developing world, with their attendant risk of catastrophic neurologic complications.

Rabies was the Latin word for madness, derived from *rabere*, meaning "to rave." It is related to the Sanskrit word *rabhas*, meaning "violence." The Greek word for rabies, *lyssa*, also meant "madness" and is the source of the taxonomic name of the viral genus *(Lyssavirus)*. Baer reports that the Babylon Eshnuna code probably contains the first surviving mention of rabies, dating back to the 23rd century BC (11). This disorder played a role in Greek mythology; in Homer's *Iliad*, Hector is compared to a mad dog, and the author evokes rabies when he uses the dog star Sirius to represent malignant influences on human health. Democritus provided the first clear description of animal rabies in about 500 BC.

Wound cauterization was the preferred treatment in the writings of Celsus in the first century AD and remained the only real treatment until Pasteur introduced immunization in 1885. St. Hubert, a medieval European healing saint, was pictured with a large key which was heated and used for cauterization. Maimonides recommended thorough wound cleansing, suction, cautery, and rest in the 12th century (11). Wound cautery remained part of official recommendations for the management of bites from rabid animals into the middle of the 20th century (11). Another attempt at treatment in classical times, which has remained a part of popular culture even though its original use has long been forgotten, was placement of some of the hair of the dog that bit the patient into the wound (66).

The time of the introduction of rabies into the western hemisphere remains a subject of debate. There is folkloric evidence of a disease of foxes resembling rabies among the native peoples of the Pacific Northwest, which was transmitted to both dogs and humans (15). Bats were thought to spread the disease among cattle and humans in Central America in the early 16th century (12). The first clear description of rabies in the New World emerged from what is now California in 1703 (153). Epizootics of canine and fox rabies have occurred in the northern and eastern United States since the 18th century, in part reflecting the importation of foxes for hunting (142).

The diagnosis of rabies remained a clinical one until 1903, when the Italian physician Adelchi Negri described the cytoplasmic inclusions which bear his name (125). Negri initially thought that this inclusion body was part of the life cycle of a parasite (126). This remained the only pathological marker for rabies until the introduction of fluorescent-antibody techniques in 1958 (72).

Vesicular stomatitis virus was identified in 1925 (79). It is of significant veterinary importance, producing a febrile vesicular eruption in cattle and horses. Human disease was thought to occur only incidentally after contact with infected animals. More recently, epidemics of encephalitis primarily affecting children have been caused by Chandipura virus, a member of the vesiculoviruses group (156). Much of the basic virology of the rhabdoviruses has been elucidated by studies of vesiculoviruses.

VIROLOGY

Classification

The *Rhabdoviridae* is a group of over 200 negatively stranded RNA viruses and consists of seven genera, four of which infect animals (*Lyssavirus*, *Vesiculovirus*, *Ephemerovirus*, and *Novirhabdovirus;* the last is confined to fish), and the plant rhabdovirus groups (78). The type species of *Lyssavirus* is rabies virus (serotype 1) (142), that of *Vesiculovirus* is VSV, that of *Ephemerovirus* is bovine ephemeral fever virus, and that of *Novirhabdovirus* is hirame rhabdovirus. Rabies is enzootic, and sometimes epizootic, in a variety of mammalian species, including wild and domestic Canidae (e.g., dogs, foxes, and coyotes), Mephitidae (e.g., skunks, badgers, and martens), Viverridae (e.g., mongooses, civets, and genets), and Procyonidae (e.g., raccoons and their allies) and the Chiroptera (both insectivorous and hematophagous bats). A patient who died from raccoon rabies was recently described (35a). The six other members of the *Lyssavirus* genus rarely cause human disease (Table 1). In addition, four putative members of the *Lyssavirus* genus have recently been isolated from bats (Irkut virus, isolated from *Murina leucogaster*, Siberia; Aravan virus, *Myotis blythi*, Kyrgyzstan; Khujand virus, *Myotis mystacinus*, Tajikistan; and West Caucasian virus, *Miniopterus schreibersi*, Russia) (104a).

Vesiculoviruses share many of the virologic characteristics of the lyssaviruses. They infect a large number of animal and insect species; humans occasionally are infected by contact with animals, typically via respiratory secretions (138). Seven vesiculoviruses are known to occasionally infect humans (Table 2) (18); there are many other vesiculoviruses, however.

Composition

The rabies virus, in common with the other lyssaviruses, is bullet shaped, with an average length of 180 nm (range, 130 to 200 nm) and an average diameter of 75 nm (60 to 110 nm) (181). The complete virus consists of a helical nucleocapsid with between 30 and 35 coils; unwound, its length is between 4.2 and 4.6 μm (151). The nucleocapsid is enclosed in a lipoprotein envelope which is 7.5 to 10 nm thick; from this envelope, glycoprotein (G protein) spikes project out another 10 nm (50). These spikes cover the surface of the virus except for a portion of the blunt end.

TABLE 1 Members of the *Lyssavirus* genus[a]

Virus	Serotype	Reservoir	Comments	Cross-protection with rabies vaccine
Rabies virus	1	Found worldwide except for a few island nations, Australia, and Antarctica. The vast majority of human cases occur in areas of uncontrolled domestic dog rabies.		Not applicable
Lagos bat virus	2	Probably enzootic in fruit bats. At least 10 cases have been identified, including 3 in domestic animals, in Nigeria, South Africa, Zimbabwe, the Central African Republic, Senegal, and Ethiopia. No reported human cases.	First isolated in 1956 from brains of Nigerian fruit bats. Some cases were initially diagnosed as rabies but displayed weak immunofluorescence and were later distinguished by monoclonal antibody or nucleotide sequence analysis.	Marginal
Mokola virus	3	Probably an insectivore or rodent species. Cases have been identified in Nigeria, South Africa, Cameroon, Zimbabwe, the Central African Republic, and Ethiopia. At least 19 known cases, including 11 in domestic animals and 2 in humans.	First isolated from shrews in Nigeria in 1968	None
Duvenhage virus	4	Probably insectivorous bats. Cases have been identified in South Africa, Zimbabwe, and Senegal. Four cases known, including one human death. No cases in domestic animals.	First identified in 1970 in a man with a rabies-like encephalitis in South Africa (virus named after the patient). Negri bodies were present, but immunofluorescent stains were negative.	Marginal
European bat lyssavirus 1	5	European insectivorous bats (probably *Eptesicus serotinus*). Over 400 bat cases, one confirmed human death, and another suspected. No known domestic animal cases.	Suspected as early as 1954 but not identified until 1985. Almost all cases are in the common European house bat.	Marginal
European bat lyssavirus 2	6	European insectivorous bats (probably *Myotis dasycneme*). Five known cases, including one human death. No known domestic animal cases.	First identified in a Swiss bat biologist who died in Finland	Marginal
Australian bat lyssavirus	7	Fruit bats, flying foxes, insectivorous bats	Originally called Ballina virus after the site of its discovery	

[a] Adapted from reference 142.

TABLE 2 Vesiculoviruses reported to cause human infection[a]

Type of vesiculovirus	Area(s) of endemicity	Reported clinical illness
VSV—New Jersey	Southeastern United States to northern South America	Influenza-like
VSV—Indiana	Central America and northern South America	Influenza-like
VSV—Alagoas	Colombia and Brazil	Unknown
Calchaqui virus	Argentina	Unknown
Piry virus	Brazil	Influenza-like
Chandipura virus	India	Influenza-like; encephalitis
Isfahan virus	Iran	Unknown

[a] From reference 153a.

The rabies viral genome is a nonsegmented, single negatively stranded RNA molecule with a molecular mass of 4.6×10^6 Da and contains a sequence of 11,932 nucleotides (158). Rabies virus RNA contains five genes; starting from the 3′ end, they are named N, P (formerly NS or M_1), M (or M_2), G, and L (Table 3) (139). The N nucleoprotein binds to the RNA and may be involved in control of replication of viral RNA in rhabdoviruses. It is a potential immunogen (74) and is also useful for molecular epidemiological studies of the virus (91). In VSV, an analogous rhabdovirus, it is required to switch from the transcription of gene products from the RNA to the production of a full-length positively stranded RNA, which then serves as a template for new negatively stranded RNA production for the formation of new nucleocapsids (22). The P phosphoprotein appears to control the L protein, which is the RNA-dependent RNA polymerase used in the replication of negatively stranded RNA viruses (108, 159). The M, or matrix, protein is located between the nucleocapsid and lipoprotein envelope (43) and is responsible for the assembly and budding of bullet-shaped particles, in concert with the G protein (115).

The G protein is involved in cellular reception and is the only antigen that induces virus-neutralizing antibodies; variability in the sequence of this protein appears to be responsible for the serotypic differences among lyssaviruses (140). Mutations at position 333 (producing substitution of glutamine or isoleucine for arginine) cause loss of virulence (147). This arginine residue appears to be essential for G protein-mediated fusion of the viral envelope with neurons (120). Molecular modifications of the G protein can increase its antigenicity (128) and may aid in the search for better vaccines (119). A recent attempt at taxonomic revision based on the G protein divides some lyssaviruses into two phylogroups: group I (rabies virus, European bat virus, Duvenhage virus, and Australian bat virus) and group II (Lagos bat virus and Mokola virus) (9). Lagos bat virus demonstrates considerable genetic diversity (49).

Replication Strategy

Although the neuronal receptor which mediates viral attachment has not yet been determined, it is likely to be a ganglioside (100). One important binding site for the virus is the nicotinic acetylcholine receptor (see "Pathogenesis" below), but it is probably not the only one. Once bound to the receptor, the virus is probably internalized by receptor-mediated endocytosis. This forms a coated pit, which then fuses with a lysosome, "whose enzymes set the nucleocapsid free to be discharged then into the cytosol" (73). The molecular events which result in viral envelope membrane fusion with the host neuronal endosome remain to be defined. Viral reproduction occurs in areas of the cell rich in ribosomes. The genome is transcribed into five mRNAs for production of the viral proteins described above, and then a full-length positively stranded RNA is produced as the template for the progeny viral genome (54). The viral envelope forms from host cisternal membranes, into which the G and M proteins are inserted (121). Both the G and M proteins influence pathogenicity, exerting control over replication and spread between cells (136). The envelope includes small amounts of some host proteins (108). In natural infections, the virus appears to accumulate in cytoplasmic cisterns, from which it is re-

TABLE 3 Rhabdoviral genes and their products

Gene	Synonym(s)	Size of product (kDa)	Function(s)
N (nucleocapsid)		50	
P (phosphorylated protein)	M_1, NS	40	Originally thought to encode a nonstructural protein but now known to produce a structural protein which is phosphorylated by kinases in the host cell and joins with L
M (matrix)	M_2	26	
G (glycoprotein)		65	Attachment to host cell receptors
L (large)		160–190	RNA-dependent RNA polymerase; required for transcription of the negatively stranded viral RNA. Appears to form a complex with P.

leased either by fusion of the cisternal membrane with the cell membrane or upon dissolution of the cell (73). Altered regulation of host genes may also be involved in the replication and spread of the virus (135).

The virus does not tolerate extremes of pH (below 3 or above 11) and can be inactivated by UV light, sunlight, or desiccation. It can also be inactivated by exposure to formalin, phenol, ether, trypsin, β-propiolactone, and most detergents.

EPIDEMIOLOGY

Rabies is currently distributed worldwide except for Antarctica and a few island nations. In 2005 (the last year for which global data are available), 112 nations reported the presence of rabies, and 50 reported its absence (180). Animals and humans dying in Australia from Australian bat virus encephalitis have the typical neuropathological changes of rabies (89, 144, 152), and the disease appears to be preventable by standard rabies vaccines (160).

The epidemiology of human rabies primarily reflects that of animal rabies in the community (162). For example, in developing areas where canine rabies remains common, most cases of human rabies result from dog bites. Conversely, human rabies in regions where dogs are vaccinated most commonly stems from exposure to rabid wild animals.

In 2005, the World Health Organization (WHO) estimated that 55,000 humans die annually from rabies (see also Color Plate 48) (178). In Africa and Asia, the vast majority of cases (more than 85%) are diagnosed on clinical grounds alone, and the source of exposure is not reported for more than half of the cases. An estimated four million persons receive postexposure prophylaxis annually, with the vast majority of persons being treated with vaccine types carrying a risk of neurologic complications (8).

In the United States, one to seven cases have been reported annually for the past decade; in 2006, three were reported. In countries with a very low prevalence, such as the United States, an increasing percentage of cases are imported, occur after very long incubation periods, or lack a known source of exposure. In the United States, the exposure sources of human rabies cases have changed from predominantly domestic animals (1945 to 1965) to bats in recent years. A recent review found that 34% of reported cases of bat rabies virus infections in humans involved no history of bat contact (51).

Animal Rabies

Cases of animal rabies throughout the world can be separated into two groups. In the developing world, rabies is predominantly a problem of domestic animals, with a smaller contribution from wild animals. In the more developed nations, animal control procedures have largely eliminated rabies from domestic animals, and wild animals are the major group affected. Throughout the world, the percentages of animal rabies cases diagnosed by laboratory methods range from 63% in Asia to 97% in Europe. In the United States, the prevalence of animal rabies has been increasing during the past two decades (Fig. 1).

A new outbreak of raccoon rabies in the United States began in 1977 near the Virginia-West Virginia border, and in the ensuing two decades the outbreak has expanded to involve most of the eastern states. Over 20,000 cases of raccoon rabies have been reported, with several thousand secondary cases in dogs and other animals (143). In the state of New York alone, the number of humans receiving postexposure prophylaxis increased from 84 in 1989 to over 1,000 in 1992, at a cost of nearly $1,000 per patient treated (31). The median cost per patient in Massachusetts was $2,376 in 1995, with estimates of the total cost to the state as high as $6.4 million (104). Rabies had been in-

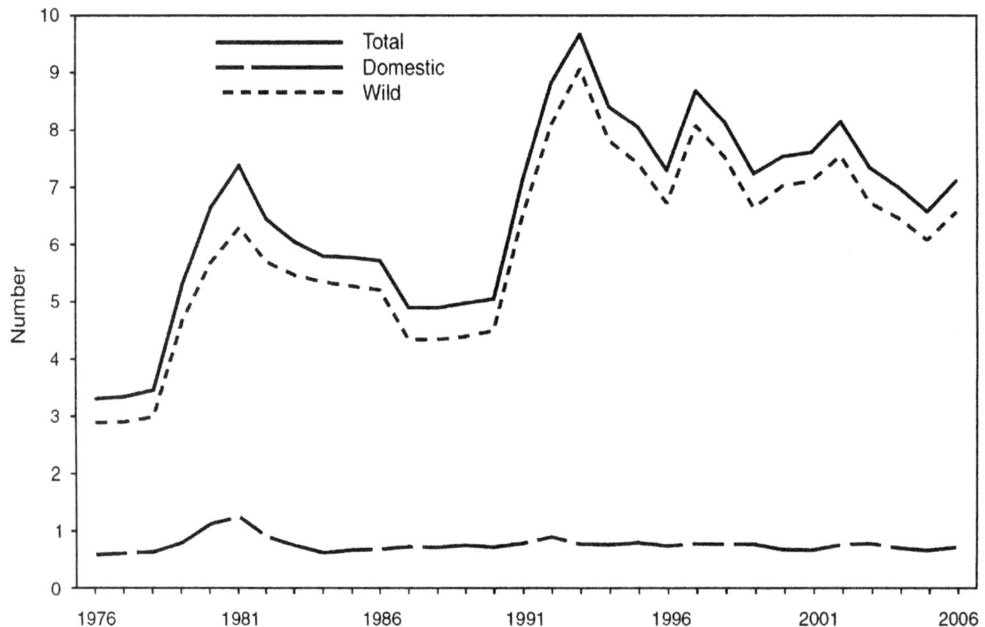

FIGURE 1 Reported cases of animal rabies in the United States by year through 2006. Data are from the National Center for Zoonotic, Vector-Borne, and Enteric Diseases. Numbers on the y axis are in thousands. (Source: CDC Annual Summaries of Notifiable Diseases.)

creasing among previously rarely affected species in other parts of the United States, such as coyotes (41), but this species is now free of the disease as a consequence of oral rabies vaccination. The likelihood that humans will unknowingly transport rabid animals during the incubation phase, thereby allowing the disease access to previously unaffected populations, appears to be increasing (34). Color Plate 49 depicts the concentric spread of raccoon rabies in the eastern United States between 1977 and 1993.

Bat rabies appears to be the most rapidly increasing source of human infections in the United States (103). This determination is possible in part due to the generation of nucleotide sequences for cases of rabies in which the source of exposure is unknown. The distribution of terrestrial wild animal species frequently infected with rabies virus is shown in Color Plate 50 (16). The epizoology of bat rabies is complex, involving not only typical reservoirs (e.g., the common big brown bat, *Eptesicus fuscus*) but also previously rarely affected bat species (e.g., the silver-haired bat, *Lasionycteris noctivagans*) (38). Eighteen of the 26 human rabies cases known to have been contracted from bats in the United States since 1980 involve silver-haired bat rabies virus (33). The mode of transmission of rabies in many current cases is uncertain but probably involves bites, and the molecular epidemiological evidence reinforces the importance of avoiding contact with downed bats or other wildlife (32, 145).

PATHOGENESIS

The pathogenesis of rabies virus infection was elucidated in an exquisite series of studies by Murphy and others (121). The process involves centripedal spread of the virus via peripheral nerves to the central nervous system (CNS), proliferation of the virus within the CNS, and centrifugal spread via peripheral nerves to many tissues. Following introduction through a break in the skin, through mucosal surfaces, or through the respiratory tract, rabies virus replicates within peripheral neurons, but it is not usually found in peripheral glial cells. Its appearance in dorsal root ganglion cells within 60 to 72 h of inoculation, and prior to its appearance in spinal cord neuronal cell bodies, confirms its transport within sensory neurons. The virus may also replicate in muscle cells, and in so doing, it may also infect the specialized muscle cells of the muscle spindle. It then infects the nerve innervating the spindle and moves centrally through the axons of these neurons as described above.

Subsequent studies have suggested that another major site of neuronal invasion is the neuromuscular junction. In experimental models, active rabies virus colocalizes with cholinesterase-positive binding sites 1 h after intramuscular or subcutaneous injection (169). Inactivation of the virus prevents this binding. Pretreatment with α-bungarotoxin or D-tubocurarine to block nicotinic acetylcholine receptors inhibits viral attachment (106). A partial amino acid sequence homology exists between rabies virus G protein and the sequences of several snake neurotoxins which bind specifically to the nicotinic acetylcholine receptor (107). Thus, it appears that the virus can enter both motor and sensory nerves.

In contrast to experimental infections, natural rabies virus infection may require a period of local viral replication, presumably to increase the inoculum, before nervous system infection can occur. During this period, the administration of antirabies immunoglobulin and the development of antirabies immunity by active immunization are able to prevent spread of the virus into the nervous system and are thereby able to prevent clinical disease. Once the virus has entered peripheral nerves, current therapeutic techniques may not prevent its subsequent replication and spread. However, current research holds the promise of antibody delivery across the blood-brain barrier, which may allow more effective later treatments (52).

Once the virus invades peripheral nerve cells, it quickly moves to the central processes of these neurons. It appears to move via retrograde axoplasmic flow (30, 161), in contrast to herpes simplex virus and tetanus toxin, which make use of microtubular transport systems (20). After reaching the spinal cord, the virus rapidly spreads throughout the CNS. In so doing, it appears to follow the established patterns of synaptic connectivity (164). Electron micrographic studies indicate that in animal models, virtually every neuron is infected (121). Recent data indicate that CNS glial cells as well as neurons can be infected (92).

After CNS infection is established, the virus spreads out to the rest of the body via the peripheral nerves. Many tissues become infected. Besides direct viral replication in the salivary glands, the high concentration of virus in saliva results from viral shedding from sensory nerve endings in the oral mucosa (121).

The mechanisms by which rabies virus produces such severe CNS dysfunction are obscure, since in many cases the pathological evidence of neuronal necrosis is minimal or absent (see below). Interference with neurotransmission (36), including the cholinergic systems mentioned above, and with endogenous opioid systems (102) have been invoked, and the almost 30-fold increase in local nitric oxide production (88) may be a clue to the discovery of an excitotoxic mechanism. There is an inverse relationship between the concentration of G protein produced and the pathogenicity of different viral strains, and there is a monotonic relationship between pathogenicity and the induction of apoptosis (118, 136). The host cytokine response is also important in the development of clinical rabies (28). In point of fact, however, we do not understand why this disease is almost invariably fatal.

Pathology

The gross appearance of the brain at autopsy is usually unremarkable (60), except for the vascular congestion which frequently occurs in patients dying after prolonged mechanical ventilation. The microscopic CNS pathology of rabies is classically described as an encephalitis with Negri bodies. However, as noted in Table 4, not all autopsy specimens show the perivascular lymphocytic cuffing and necrosis which characterize encephalitis, and some cases appear histologically as meningitis (55).

Negri bodies are usually concentrated in the hippocampal pyramidal cells and, slightly less frequently, in cortical neurons (Fig. 2A) and cerebellar Purkinje cells (Fig. 2B) (60). These cytoplasmic inclusions are round or oval, between 1 and 7 μm across, and usually eosinophilic. Immunofluorescence staining (Color Plate 51) and ultrastructural analyses confirm that these inclusions contain rabies viral nucleocapsids (48). The lyssa body, which is acidophilic, has been demonstrated to be ultrastructurally identical to the Negri body (154).

TABLE 4 Histologic markers of rabies[a]

Histology	% of cases with marker	Mean duration of illness before death (days)
Encephalitis with Negri bodies	56.3	72.7
Negri bodies only	14.6	66.5
Vascular congestion only	12.5	38.2
Encephalitis only	8.3	Not stated
Encephalitis and equivocal inclusions	8.3	41.5
Meningitis	6.3	Not stated

[a] Data from reference 55.

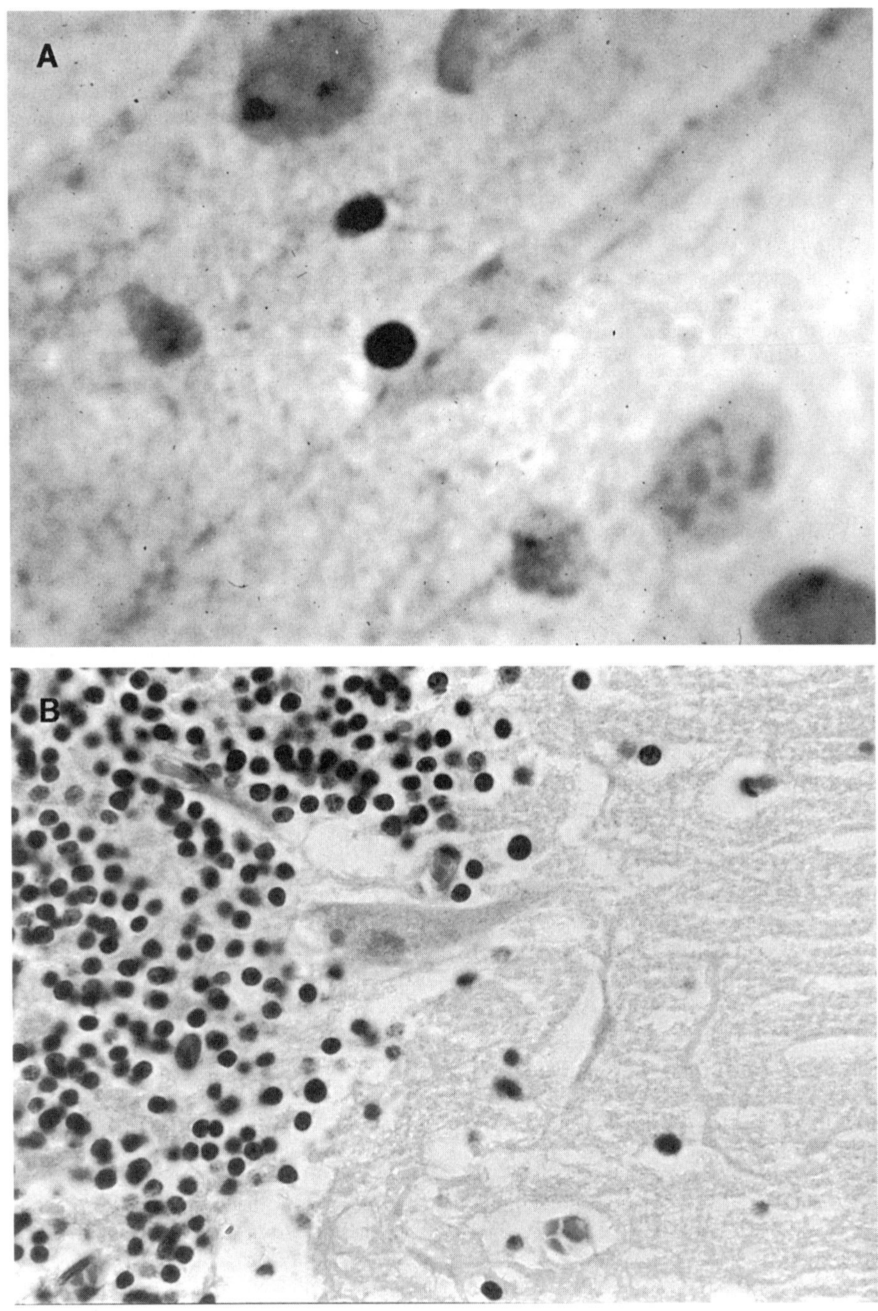

FIGURE 2 Negri bodies. (A) Negri body in a pyramidal neuron; (B) Negri body in a cerebellar Purkinje cell.

Paralytic rabies appears to have the majority of its pathology in the spinal cord, with severe inflammation and neuronal destruction (39). The brain stem is involved to a lesser extent than the spinal cord. A minority of these patients has Negri bodies in the cortex. Segmental demyelination occurs in the peripheral nerves in these patients, which is of particular interest in view of the resemblance of paralytic rabies to acute inflammatory polyneuropathy (Guillain-Barré syndrome).

The systemic pathology of rabies is most remarkable for the presence of myocarditis in a large number of cases (42). The etiology of this cardiac disorder is uncertain, but it resembles the myocarditis which occurs in hypercatecholaminergic states such as pheochromocytoma, subarachnoid hemorrhage, and tetanus (20). However, the presence of Negri bodies in the hearts of some patients suggests a more direct role for the virus in the genesis of this condition (65). Detection of atrial ganglioneuritis suggests that the virus reaches the myocardium via centrifugal spread from the nervous system (117). Other autopsy findings usually reflect the complications encountered with aggressive support through the course of a critical illness, such as upper gastrointestinal tract bleeding.

Immune Responses

The human immune response to natural rabies virus infection is insufficient to prevent disease. Some investigators have speculated that this is a consequence of an insufficient antigenic load (4); this contention has been disputed by others (84). Viral replication at an immunologically "privileged" site may also impair the host response. Rabies virus is capable of producing immunosuppression (174), and only a minority of unvaccinated rabies patients develops a measurable antibody response (99). However, patients who develop a cellular immune response to the virus tend to have the encephalitic (furious) form of the disease rather than the paralytic form, and they die faster than those who do not mount such a response as determined by a lymphocyte proliferation assay (83). Some investigators believe that interleukin 1 production in the CNS during rabies virus infection may be sufficient to explain the immunosuppressive effect of the virus (80).

In experimental infection, rabies virus may be able to persist in some macrophages, from which it may later emerge from its persistent state to produce disease (137). This may help to explain the very long incubation periods occasionally reported between exposure and death. Alternatively, the virus may persist in neurons until activation.

CLINICAL MANIFESTATIONS

Human Rabies

Transmission

Several variables affect the risk of rabies and the rate of clinical disease development after exposure to a rabid animal (172). The viral inoculum appears to play an important role; in clinical practice, this is most commonly reflected in the extent of exposure to the saliva of a rabid animal (Table 5). Exposures in which saliva prominently contaminates a wound, as in a bite on exposed skin, are more likely to produce rabies than a bite through thick clothing, which removes most of the saliva from the animal's teeth. Multiple bites are more likely to transmit the disease than a single bite. The location of the bite also exerts an important influence on the likelihood of developing rabies; bites on the face are more strongly associated with the disease than those on the extremities. Salivary contamination of a wound can also result in viral transfer, as can exposure of mucous membranes or (rarely) the respiratory tract to aerosolized virus (44).

The factors responsible for the difference in disease incidence after otherwise similar bites on different parts of the body remain to be elucidated. One possibility is that multiple severe bites to the face occur more commonly in cases in which the animal is more severely infected.

Human-to-human transmission has been documented in cases of organ and corneal transplants from unsuspected infected donors (85). In 2004, two separate instances of such transmission occurred. In the United States, four patients (recipients of kidneys, a liver, and a blood vessel) died of rabies between 7 and 23 days after transplantation (27). A recipient of a lung died rapidly of respiratory failure and did not develop rabies. Later that year, three of six organ recipients in Germany died following transplantation (81). The reasons why the other recipients did not develop rabies are unknown. In an unrelated transplant, one patient who received a cornea was quickly managed with standard postexposure prophylaxis plus interferon and did not develop rabies (155).

TABLE 5 Approximate mortality rates in nonvaccinated patients after exposure to rabid dogs[a]

Location of exposure	Type	Extent	Mortality rate (%)
Face	Bite	Multiple, deep	60
Head (other than face)	Bite	Multiple, deep	50
Face	Bite	Single	30
Fingers or hand	Bite	Severe	15
Face	Bite	Multiple, superficial	10
Hand	Bite	Multiple, superficial	5
Trunk or legs	Scratch	Superficial	3
Exposed skin	Bleeding	Superficial wound	2
Skin covered by clothing	Wound	Superficial	0.5
Recent wound	Contamination by saliva		0.1
Wounds more than 24 h old	Contamination by saliva		0.0

[a] Data from reference 172.

Incubation

The reported incubation period for rabies varies from a few days to over 19 years, although 75% of patients become ill in the first 90 days after exposure (Table 6).

Prodromal Symptoms

The initial symptoms of rabies are usually those associated with other systemic viral infections, such as fever, headache, malaise, and disorders of the upper respiratory and gastrointestinal tracts (4). Neurologic complaints during this period include subtle changes in personality and cognition (so-called "mental status") and paresthesias or pain at or near the exposure site. Because of the nonspecific nature of these complaints, rabies is seldom considered early in the differential diagnosis of these patients. In one series, this diagnosis was considered in only 3 of 21 patients on their first visit to a physician, despite a compatible exposure history in many of the patients (174). This prodromal period lasts on average about 4 days, but up to 10 days may elapse before more specific symptoms and signs supervene (18).

Myoedema may be present in the prodromal stage and persists throughout the course of the disease (87). This finding appears as mounding of a part of the muscle struck with a percussion hammer, which then flattens and disappears over a few seconds. The sensitivity and specificity of this finding are unknown.

Established Neurologic Disease

Human rabies virus infections are typically divided into two forms: furious and paralytic (or dumb). The furious form includes patients whose symptoms are dominated by encephalitis and thus present with the hydrophobia, delirium, and agitation which form the common concept of rabies. About 20% of patients present with the paralytic form and have little clinical evidence of cerebral cortical involvement until late in their course. Occasional patients run a course intermediate between the two forms. As noted above, the pathological distinction between the two forms is primarily quantitative, with the spinal cord and brain stem bearing the brunt of the illness in the paralytic form. The pathogenetic distinction between the two types of rabies is unclear; it does not appear to be based on virologic or antigenic differences (110). No host factors accounting for this difference have yet been defined.

In either form, the course of symptomatic rabies usually lasts between 2 and 14 days before coma supervenes. Death follows an average of 18 days after the onset of symptoms, but the range is quite broad (4). Older reports of intensive support suggested that critical care could prolong survival by about 50% (70); more recent studies have not shown further improvement in this regard (79).

Furious Rabies

Hydrophobia is the symptom most identified with furious rabies. William Gowers (77) provides a seminal description of hydrophobia and its sequelae:

> ... some discomfort about the throat, an occasional sense of choking, or a little difficulty in swallowing liquids.... The attempt to drink occasions some spasm in the pharynx, which increases in the course of a few hours, and spreads to the muscles of respiration, causing a short, quick inspiration, a "catch in the breath...." This increases in severity to a strong inspiratory effort, in which the extraordinary muscles of respiration, sternomastoid, scaleni, etc., and even the facial muscles, take part; the shoulders are raised, and the angles of the mouth drawn outwards. As the intensity of the spasm increases, so does the readiness with which it is excited. It may be caused by the mere contact of water with the lips, and a state of cutaneous hyperæsthesia develops, so that various impressions, such as a draught of air, which normally excite a respiratory effort, bring on the spasm. The mere movement of air caused by raising the bedclothes may be sufficient. The patient is often unable to swallow the saliva, which is usually abundant and viscid, so that it hangs about the mouth and is expelled with difficulty.... Vomiting is common.... The attacks of spasm are very distressing to the patient; the mental state which they occasion increases the readiness with which they are produced; and in some cases the mere sight of water of the sound of dropping water will cause an attack. It may even be excited by visual impressions which cause a similar sensation, as the reflection from a looking glass, or even a strong light. The sufferer's horror and dread of these excitants become intense. Thus the disturbance in the act of swallowing liquids, which constitutes ... the first symptom and keynote of the disease, spreads, on the one hand, to mental disturbance, and on the other to ex-

TABLE 6 Durations of different stages of rabies[a]

Stage	Type (% of cases)	Duration (% of cases)	Associated findings
Incubation period		Under 30 days (25) 30–90 days (50) 90 days–1 yr (20) More than 1 yr (5)	None
Prodrome and early symptoms		2–10 days	Paresthesias or pain at the wound site, fever, malaise, anorexia, nausea, and vomiting
Acute neurologic disease	Furious rabies (80)	2–7 days	Hallucinations, bizarre behavior, anxiety, agitation, biting, hydrophobia, autonomic dysfunction, syndrome of inappropriate antidiuretic hormone
	Paralytic rabies (20)	2–7 days	Ascending flaccid paralysis
Coma death[b]		0–14 days	

[a] Data from reference 65.
[b] Rare recoveries have been reported.

tensive muscular spasm. In each of these directions further symptoms develop. The spasm, at first confined to the muscles of deglutition and respiration, spreads to the other muscles of the body, and the paroxysms, at first respiratory, afterwards become general, and assume a convulsive character, although still excited by the same causes. The convulsions may consist of general muscular rigidity, sometimes tetanoid in character, with actual opisthotonus.... Actual delusions occasionally supervene, and there may even be wild delirium. The mental derangement is most intense during the paroxysms of spasms, and the frenzied patient may spit his saliva at those about him, and often attempts to bite them with his teeth, making occasional strange sounds in his throat which have been thought to resemble the barking of a dog

Hydrophobia appears to represent an exaggerated irritant reflex of the respiratory tract, possibly as a consequence of involvement of the nucleus ambiguus (166). This finding and other signs of rabies are illustrated in Color Plate 52.

Other findings of furious rabies include episodic hyperactivity, seizures, and aerophobia. Hyperventilation is frequently present during this period. With the onset of coma, evidence of pituitary dysfunction, especially disordered water balance (either inappropriate antidiuresis or diabetes insipidus), frequently develops. Hyperventilation gives way to ventilatory dysfunction, including forms of periodic and ataxic respiration (166), and eventually apnea supervenes. Cardiac arrhythmias, predominantly supraventricular tachycardias and bradycardias (70), are common and may be a consequence of either brain stem dysfunction or myocarditis (37). Autonomic dysfunction is common and may include pupillary dilation, anisocoria, piloerection, markedly increased salivation and sweating, and, rarely, priapism (84). The last finding may include spontaneous ejaculation as well as erections and may be the presenting symptom of rabies (58).

With the exception of some rare cases, patients entering coma generally die within 1 to 2 weeks despite maximal supportive care. Furious rabies patients who receive maximal intensive care support and survive for a longer-than-expected period appear to pass in the paralytic phase prior to death (71).

Although cerebral edema has been described to occur in patients with rabies, it is probably a consequence of hypoxia rather than a manifestation of the infection itself (65).

Paralytic (Dumb) Rabies

In contrast to patients with furious rabies, those with paralytic rabies lack hydrophobia, aerophobia, hyperactivity, and seizures. Their initial findings may suggest an ascending paralysis, resembling acute inflammatory polyneuropathy (Guillain-Barré syndrome), or a symmetric tetraparesis. In some cases, weakness is more severe in the extremity through which the virus was introduced. Meningeal signs (headache and neck stiffness) may be prominent despite the normal sensorium. As the disease progresses, the patient with paralytic rabies becomes confused and then progressively declines into coma.

Nonneurologic Findings

In addition to the cardiac arrhythmias mentioned above, the systemic complications of rabies are similar to those in other critically ill patients. Although the virus may disseminate to many organs, pathological proof of its role in nonneurologic organ dysfunction is lacking. As the disease progresses, hypoxemia may develop; its cause is uncertain, but it is frequently attributed to atelectasis, aspiration pneumonia, or congestive heart failure secondary to myocarditis. Hypotension is probably a consequence of volume depletion but may also reflect brain stem involvement. A variety of gastrointestinal disturbances have been reported in addition to bleeding, including vomiting, diarrhea, and ileus (14). Vomiting may be sufficiently severe to produce Boerhaave syndrome (127). In patients who avoid or survive these complications, death is usually due to rabies myocarditis, with cardiac arrhythmia or congestive heart failure as mechanisms (165).

Animal Rabies

A complete description of the behavioral effects of rabies in all of the species which may be infected is beyond the scope of this text. WHO studies have established a crude ranking of rabies susceptibility, which is summarized in Table 7, but this was accomplished using fixed (i.e., laboratory strain) rabies virus rather than the variants associated with reservoir hosts (113).

Rabies in dogs and cats has phases and types similar to those of the human disease. In dogs, the prodromal phase is frequently characterized by subtle behavioral change. Most dogs then enter an excitative (furious) phase, during which they are agitated and restless and may bite without provocation. Paralysis of the laryngeal musculature produces a characteristic high-pitched bark (62). In the paralytic (dumb) phase, the animal displays a "dropped jaw" as a consequence of masseter weakness. However, up to 24% of experimentally infected dogs in one study died without showing any signs of illness and yet were pathologically demonstrated to be rabid (61). The incubation period in dogs may be as long as 8.5 months (157). However, more recent studies suggest that the incubation period depends on the inoculum and strain involved; experiments designed to simulate natural infection suggest an incubation period of 7 to 125 days (61). Other exper-

TABLE 7 Susceptibilities of various animal species to rabies[a]

Very high	High	Moderate	Low
Wolves	Hamsters	Dogs	Opossums
Foxes	Skunks	Primates	
Coyotes	Raccoons		
Kangaroo rats	Domestic cats		
Cotton rats	Rabbits		
Jackals	Bats		
Voles	Cattle		

[a] Data from reference 179.

imental studies suggest that up to 20% of infected dogs may recover from rabies without treatment (62).

Cats exhibit a 2- to 3-day prodromal phase, characterized by subtle behavioral changes, slight fever, pupillary dilation, and impaired corneal reflexes. Most rabid cats then enter a furious phase, during which they frequently scratch or bite without provocation. During this 2- to 4-day period, tremor, incoordination, and hypersalivation are common. A paralytic phase then ensues, during which convulsions may also develop. Death follows in most animals in a few days. Rare experimental cases of a more chronic form of rabies in cats have been reported (26).

A description of the behavioral changes of wild animals is contained in Baer's text (10).

Diagnosis of Human Rabies

The diagnosis of rabies poses little difficulty in a nonimmunized patient presenting with hydrophobia after a bite by a known rabid animal. While this situation sadly remains common in many parts of the world, the presentation of rabies in areas where domestic animals are immunized is very seldom this straightforward. As the disease becomes rarer, physicians and patients are less apt to consider the diagnosis. Furthermore, an increasingly large percentage of cases in the United States are not associated with a known exposure to a potentially rabid animal.

During the incubation period, no diagnostic studies in the patient are useful; recognition of an exposure to a potentially rabid animal should prompt prophylactic treatment as outlined below. When symptoms begin, standard laboratory testing does not help to distinguish rabies reliably from other encephalitides. In one study, the cerebrospinal fluid (CSF) was classically abnormal in a minority of patients, revealing a lymphocytic pleocytosis (5 to 30 cells/μl), a normal glucose, and a modest protein elevation (less than 100 mg/dl) (85). However, the majority of recent human cases has abnormal CSF; the reason for this change is unknown. Computed tomographic scans, although rarely reported, are typically normal (90) unless hypoxia has intervened. In rare cases, there may be nonspecific hypodensity of the basal ganglia (8). Minimal experience with magnetic resonance imaging suggests that areas of brain involvement with rabies exhibit high T2 signal intensity and enhancement of T1 signal after gadolinium administration (132). Several patients have had lesions in the region of the hypothalamus (Fig. 3) (19). In the transplant-related cases, patients developed large areas of abnormal T2 signal, but the extent to which this was a consequence of immunosuppression is uncertain (27).

The cornerstones of diagnosing rabies in humans are skin biopsy, detection of virus in saliva, and serology on serum and CSF. Direct immunofluorescent-antibody staining (DFA) of a skin biopsy sample obtained from the nape of the neck, above the hairline, remains a standard diagnostic test for human rabies (24). The virus tends to localize in the nerves innervating hair follicles. During the first week of symptoms, about 50% of samples reveal rabies virus, with an increasing percentage thereafter (21). Reverse transcriptase (RT-PCR) is sometimes used as a diagnostic procedure in suspected rabies, especially in human cases (46). This test can be performed on CSF or on tissue, but it is most useful for humans when performed on saliva. The CSF does not appear to yield a positive PCR result until CNS tissue sloughs into the CSF. The RT-PCR assay, followed by genetic sequencing, allows more specific determination of the geographic and host species origins of a particular rabies virus (6, 123). It can be successfully performed on decomposed brain material (171), with which older techniques failed (1). The older corneal impression test (183) is no longer in common use.

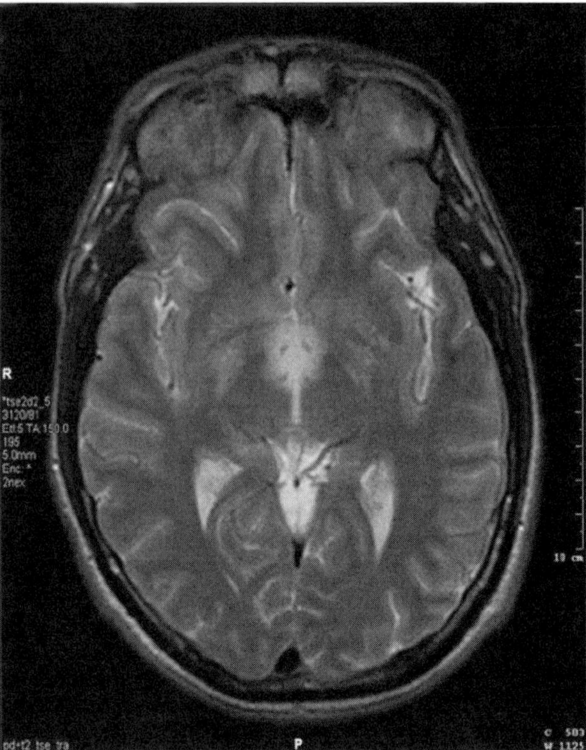

FIGURE 3 T2-weighted magnetic resonance image from a patient with rabies. (Reprinted from reference 19 with permission of Elsevier.)

In the developing world, equipment and reagents for these tests are often not available. A recently developed technique, the direct rapid immunohistochemical test, performs as well as DFA and can be performed with a light microscope (56).

The rapid fluorescent focus inhibition test (RFFIT) is a serologic test for neutralizing antirabies antibody most commonly performed in the United States (150). Among patients who have received neither postexposure prophylaxis nor immunologic therapies, serum antibody is detectable in a small number by day 6 of clinical illness, in 50% by day 8, and usually in 100% by day 15. Any levels in CSF are diagnostically valuable; this is true even for patients who have received postexposure prophylaxis. CSF may also be examined for the presence of specific oligoclonal bands not found in the serum as a method of confirming CNS infection (3).

A bisynchronous periodic electroencephalographic (EEG) pattern was described for a 17-year-old patient with rabies confirmed at autopsy (101), but the sensitivity and specificity of this finding are uncertain. Periodic EEG activity is much more common in herpes simplex encephalitis (HSE); this diagnosis should be strongly considered in any encephalitic patient, although HSE more typically produces unilateral or independent bilateral periodic discharges. Others have reported desynchronization or slowing of the EEG (68). Conflicting experimental studies suggest that in mice, the EEG may slow or remain unchanged until the animal nears death, but sleep architecture becomes disrupted quite early (75, 76). This has not been studied in humans but might be of some diagnostic value.

Differential Diagnosis

When considering the possibility of furious rabies, the major differential diagnostic consideration is that of another viral encephalitis. In the absence of a known exposure to a rabid animal, and in cases where hydrophobia and hyperactivity are not prominent, there is little clinical information to distinguish among these possibilities (173). Since the CSF and EEG findings in rabies occasionally mimic those of HSE, some patients will receive empirical therapy with acyclovir while awaiting a more secure diagnosis (e.g., PCR for herpes simplex virus DNA in the CSF). While there are no data currently available concerning this approach, anecdotal information regarding the use of adenine arabinoside in rabies suggests that it had no effect on the course of the disease (85).

Tetanus is occasionally confused with rabies, because opisthotonic posturing may be seen in either (20). However, the other symptoms of rabies, such as hydrophobia, are not part of tetanus, and the CSF and EEG are normal in tetanus patients unless they have suffered hypoxic injury. The spasms of rabies may lack the marked stimulus sensitivity of tetanus, and patients with rabies lack the persistent rigidity of tetanus patients. Strychnine poisoning should also be considered in the differential diagnosis and may require elimination by laboratory testing.

Paralytic rabies may be confused with acute inflammatory polyneuropathy, transverse myelitis, or poliomyelitis. Electromyographic studies may be useful in the distinction of rabies from polyneuropathy. In transverse myelitis, the complaint of an aching pain at the level of the lesion may by helpful, as may the finding of a high T2 signal lesion in the spinal cord in some cases. A sensory level is characteristic of transverse myelitis, whereas sensory function is typically normal in rabies patients (84). Although a high fever often precedes the weakness of poliomyelitis, the resolution of fever with the onset of neurologic findings may be a useful clue favoring this diagnosis over rabies. A history of poliomyelitis immunization may help to resolve the issue.

The sometimes prolonged incubation period of rabies recalls another group of diseases, the slow infections of the CNS caused by conventional viruses (e.g., progressive multifocal leukoencephalopathy) (98). However, rabies requires neither a defect in host immunity nor a mutation in the virus to produce disease, thus distinguishing it from the agents in this group. The spongiform changes in brain tissue (25) resemble those of another group of slow infections, the prion diseases (17). The need for careful distinction between these infections has been heightened by the emergence of bovine spongiform encephalopathy, with which rabies may be confused (67).

Although CNS reactions to the rabies vaccines available in more developed countries are exceptionally rare, patients receiving older vaccine forms containing myelin determinants occasionally develop acute disseminated encephalomyelitis (ADEM; also called postvaccinal encephalomyelitis; see "Prophylaxis" below). ADEM is a syndrome with many known precipitants in addition to rabies vaccine, and it also occurs cryptogenically. Symptomatically, ADEM resembles a more typical encephalitis or occasionally presents as a mass lesion resembling a brain abscess. ADEM typically begins 10 to 14 days after vaccine exposure, which would constitute an unusually brief incubation period for rabies. In the absence of viral isolation, a high RFFIT titer in spinal fluid is evidence for rabies rather than ADEM, even in patients who have been immunized (167, 168). ADEM produces high-T2 lesions visible by magnetic resonance imaging (122). This may also occur in patients experiencing postvaccinal myelitis (148).

Patients exposed to a potentially rabid animal may develop a psychological reaction termed rabies hysteria (63). These patients may refuse to attempt to drink water, in contrast to the patient with rabies who, at least initially, makes the attempt but is halted by pharyngeal spasms. Patients with rabies hysteria may have read extensively about the disease and appear to manifest other findings of the condition.

PREVENTION

Rabies vaccination for both prevention and postexposure prophylaxis was developed in the latter part of the 19th century, initially by Galtier and shortly thereafter by Pasteur (133).

Prophylaxis

While the control of animal rabies is clearly central to the prevention of human rabies, only a few nations have succeeded in eliminating the risk of rabies, and these must usually maintain quarantine procedures lest the disease reappear. Therefore, procedures for prophylaxis before exposure (for domestic animals and selected humans) and postexposure prophylaxis for humans remain essential for the prevention of clinical rabies. The law requires prophylaxis for cats and dogs in many countries; in the United States, the use of 1-, 3-, or 4-year vaccines is permitted (124). Vaccination should be performed by, or under the direction of, a licensed veterinarian; failure to properly administer the vaccine can lead to a lack of immunity, with tragic results (45). Some vaccines may lack potency, and measurement of animal seroconversion rates may be considered to augment control in developing countries (59). Immunization of livestock is also recommended in areas of increasing rabies prevalence.

Vaccination of wild animals can be an effective veterinary public health measure (146). The use of vaccines which are effective after ingestion (e.g., in bait) allows vaccination of free-ranging animals (113, 141). An intensive 4-year campaign in Belgium eliminated rabies from the fox population (23). This approach may also be effective in dogs. A similar campaign appears to have eliminated rabies from red foxes in parts of Canada (111).

Veterinary vaccines prepared in continuous cell lines cost about $0.50 per dose in the United States. In contrast, Semple-type human vaccines cost about $5 for a course; Vero cell vaccine in France costs about $160 per course, and human diploid cell vaccine (HDCV) in the United States costs more than $500 per course (131).

Preexposure prophylaxis is confined to people with a relatively high risk of rabies exposure, such as veterinarians, laboratory workers using rabies virus, cavers, and people planning a visit of more than 30 days to countries where the prevalence of rabies in dogs is high. Current recommendations for international travelers are available from http://www.cdc.gov/diseases/rabies.html. A series of three intramuscular (or intradermal, if using a vaccine prepared for this route) injections over a 3-week course is sufficient; antibody response determination is not required for healthy hosts. Serology every 2 to 3 years is usually recommended for individuals frequently at risk of exposure, with a routine booster dose administered only as needed. An adequate antibody response is generally considered to be complete neutralization at the 1:5 level by RFFIT, or the 0.5-IU/ml concentration suggested by the WHO.

One study suggests that if a person previously vaccinated by the intradermal route is exposed to rabies, a booster injection may not provide a rapid anamnestic response for at least several days (96). However, in this circumstance rabies immune globulin is not required; no vaccinated person exposed to rabies has been known to succumb to rabies if a booster vaccine was given on days 0 and 3.

Postexposure Prophylaxis

The cornerstone of rabies prevention is good wound care, which can reduce the risk of rabies by up to 90% (47). The wound should be washed thoroughly with a 20% soap solution, which is as effective as the formerly recommended quaternary ammonium compounds (5). Following wound care, the clinician must decide whether to institute passive and active immunization (94). Prompt consultation with public health officials is advised, since this decision is based on the current incidence of rabies in the animal species involved in the exposure (112). The most recent report of the Advisory Committee on Immunization Practices is also an important source of information (35). A recent decision analysis model may also be useful in deciding who should receive prophylaxis (29).

In general, a healthy dog or cat in a country of low prevalence which has bitten (or otherwise transferred saliva to) a human is observed for 10 days. If its behavior remains normal, the patient need not receive postexposure prophylaxis beyond proper wound care. If the animal's behavior changes, it should undergo immediate pathological examination for evidence of rabies virus infection. If infection is confirmed, there is adequate time to institute postexposure prophylaxis. Wild-mammal exposure, especially if the animal exhibits uncharacteristic behavior, warrants postexposure prophylaxis in most circumstances. If the animal is available for pathological examination, and DFA of the brain does not indicate the presence of rabies virus, postexposure prophylaxis may be discontinued.

Postexposure prophylaxis appears to be safe in pregnancy; it should not be withheld when an indication exists (40).

Rabies immune globulin is available in human (HRIG) and equine (pooled antiserum of equine origin [ARS] and purified antirabies serum of equine origin [ERIG]) forms. These immunoglobulins are purified from the sera of donors who are hyperimmunized with rabies vaccine. Immunoglobulin should be routinely administered. HRIG is given in a dose of 20 IU/kg of body weight, with as much of the dose as possible injected in the vicinity of the wound and the remainder injected intramuscularly. The dose of ERIG is 40 IU/kg. The recent development of a hybridoma line secreting human monoclonal antibodies to several different rabies virus antigens (53) holds promise for the eventual production and global availability of HRIG without the need for hyperimmunized donors.

Failure to infiltrate wounds with rabies immune globulin and surgical closure of wounds prior to immune globulin infiltration have been associated with the development of rabies in patients despite otherwise proper postexposure prophylaxis (176).

Many different forms of rabies vaccine have been produced since Pasteur's original success in 1885. In some developing nations, vaccine prepared from virus grown in adult animal nerve tissue (Semple vaccine) is still employed, but it carries a risk of central and peripheral neurologic complications in the range of 1 in 200 to 1 in 1,600 vaccinees (18). Several cases of Guillain-Barré syndrome have been reported as a complication of its use (163). Its efficacy is uncertain. Although neurologic and inflammatory reactions are often assumed to be a consequence of an immune reaction to myelin basic protein in the vaccine, only a minority of patients appears to develop antibody against this constituent of myelin (86). Suckling-mouse brain vaccine is effective and safer, with a neurologic complication rate of approximating 1 in 8,000. DNA vaccines are another approach that, if proven effective, would eliminate the risk of these reactions (130). Production of vaccine in sheep CNS, a common method of Semple-type vaccine production, also carries the theoretical risk of transmitting the scrapie prion (7).

The currently employed human vaccines in the United States include HDCV and purified chicken embryo vaccine (PCEC). These vaccines are remarkably safe and immunogenic. Local reactions (pain, swelling, and induration) may be common, but systemic complaints (fever, headache, malaise, nausea, abdominal pain, and adenopathy) occur in a minority of patients. Serious reactions have been exceedingly rare, with Guillain-Barré syndrome reported to occur in a few patients (13) and a chimpanzee (2). To report a vaccine reaction, call the appropriate company: for persons receiving HDCV, contact Sanofi Pasteur (1-800-VACCINE [822-2463]; http://www.vaccineplace.com/products/), and for PCEC, contact Novartis Vaccines and Diagnostics (1-800-244-7668; http://www.rabavert.com).

Corticosteroids should not be given to patients experiencing a vaccine reaction, since they interfere with the development of immunity, unless that reaction is life threatening. Immunocompromised patients may not respond adequately to vaccination and should undergo measurement of antibody titers 2 to 4 weeks after immunization to ensure adequate immunization. Some have suggested that patients infected with human immunodeficiency virus may need larger doses of vaccine, but the dosing of vaccine in all immunocompromised patients remains controversial (69, 97).

In other countries, other postexposure treatment (PET) vaccines (e.g., vaccines grown in chicken embryos or Vero cell cultures) (82) and regimens are often employed. Consultation with the rabies officer of the state health department may be helpful for the management of patients in whom postexposure prophylaxis has been initiated with a vaccine not approved for use in the United States.

The usual dose of HDCV or rabies vaccine, adsorbed, for postexposure prophylaxis is 1.0 ml intramuscularly on the day of exposure (or as soon as possible thereafter), repeated on days 3, 7, 14, and 28. Other schedules are available; physicians not familiar with their use should consult local public health authorities and review the most recent

WHO and CDC recommendations (35). The various immunogenicities of different regimens, and their interaction with the response to immunoglobulin (108), raise the possibility of treatment failure if the recommendations are not carefully followed (105). If possible, the vaccine should be administered in the deltoid muscle. Gluteal injections, which may miss the muscle, have been associated with some vaccine failures. In small children, it may be given in the lateral thigh. The vaccine must not be given in the same region as the immunoglobulin. Intradermal vaccine administration (0.1 ml) was previously only recommended for preexposure prophylaxis, but in 1996 the WHO recommended it as an alternative for PET. Patients who have been previously vaccinated receive 1.0 ml intramuscularly on days 0 and 3 only, without rabies immune globulin.

A single case of a transient false-positive enzyme-linked immunosorbent assay result for human immunodeficiency virus after HDCV immunization was reported in 1994 (129). Subsequent screening of samples from 50 patients recently immunized against rabies revealed no similar cases (134), but in view of a similar phenomenon with other vaccines, physicians administering rabies vaccines should be aware of this possibility.

The limited extent of cross-protection among different lyssaviruses, and the possibility that antigenic differences in lyssaviruses from different locales may impair vaccine efficacy, should prompt future efforts to produce a vaccine effective against all lyssavirus variants. The nucleic acid vaccine approach is also promising (182). Further research in these areas may produce a stable, inexpensive vaccine which could lead to very simple, safe, and effective prophylaxis and PET.

Personnel caring for rabies patients should practice standard universal and respiratory precautions. In addition, they should receive a preexposure immunization sequence (see above) and maintain a serum antirabies antibody titer of 0.5 IU/ml (57). Exposures to potentially contaminated secretions or tissues should lead to standard postexposure prophylaxis.

TREATMENT

There is no established, specific treatment for rabies once symptoms have begun. Despite excellent intensive care, almost all patients succumb to the disease or its complications within a few weeks of onset. The three patients in the 1970s who survived, two of whom made apparently complete recoveries (18, 172), represent very unusual occurrences. Each of these patients had some history of vaccination prior to the onset of illness, and it seems likely that this treatment modified their course. Another case with partial recovery was reported in 1994 for a child who received rabies vaccine without immunoglobulin (24). Based upon these experiences, one might consider beginning postexposure prophylaxis (including HRIG) in previously untreated patients when the diagnosis of rabies is made, but there have been no survivors reported with this approach, and it is not recommended.

Supportive therapy for rabies patients includes endotracheal intubation, sedation, mechanical ventilation, fluid and electrolyte replacement, nutritional support, and management of intercurrent illnesses and complications. The details of intensive care for these patients have been discussed elsewhere (145). However, none of the patients in that series survived more than 17 days despite aggressive antirabies and symptomatic treatment.

Trials of many agents have been undertaken in clinical rabies, including interferons, interferon-inducing agents, ribavirin, and cytosine arabinoside, without beneficial effects (57). In 2003, a working group reviewed the potential treatments for human rabies and proposed a management schema for consideration if one were to attempt treatment (93). The use of rabies vaccine, rabies immunoglobulin, monoclonal antibodies, ribavirin, alpha interferon, and ketamine was proposed. In addition to its antiexcitotoxic properties, ketamine inhibits rabies viral replication in tissue culture (109). Whether excitotoxicity is important in the pathogenesis of neuronal damage in rabies is uncertain; apoptosis may be more important (170).

The longstanding contention that symptomatic rabies patients who had not received at least partial PET always died was challenged in 2004 by the survival and eventual complete recovery of such a patient (177). A 15-year-old girl developed encephalitis 1 month after contact with a silver-haired bat; she did not receive any PET. At the time of her presentation, samples of serum and CSF already contained antibodies against rabies virus, so she was not treated with either vaccine or immunoglobulin. Her physicians administered ketamine, midazolam, ribavirin, and amantadine. She was hospitalized for 76 days, and when discharged from the hospital she had substantial neurologic dysfunction. However, over the ensuing 2 years she has recovered and was able to attend college.

The components of her treatment that allowed recovery remain debated (95), and subsequent attempts at treatment have not been successful (114). Nevertheless, her recovery points to the possibility of future triumphs over rabies. Given that the vast majority of cases occur in areas that are too poor to provide critical care services on a large scale, prevention and PET must remain the cornerstones of our approach to management of this disease.

REFERENCES

1. **Albas, A., C. I. Ferrari, L. H. da Silva, F. Bernardi, and F. H. Ito.** 1999. Influence of canine brain decomposition on laboratory diagnosis of rabies. *Rev. Soc. Bras. Med. Trop.* **32:**19–22.
2. **Alford, P. L., and W. C. Satterfield.** 1995. Paralytic illness resembling inflammatory polyradiculoneuropathy in a chimpanzee. *J. Am. Vet. Med. Assoc.* **207:**83–85.
3. **Alvarez, L., R. Fajardo, E. Lopez, R. Pedroza, T. Hemachudha, N. Kamolvarin, G. Cortes, and G. M. Baer.** 1994. Partial recovery from rabies in a nine-year-old boy. *Pediatr. Infect. Dis. J.* **13:**1154–1155.
4. **Anderson, L. J., K. G. Nicholson, R. V. Tauxe, and W. G. Winkler.** 1984. Human rabies in the United States, 1960 to 1979: epidemiology, diagnosis, and prevention. *Ann. Intern. Med.* **100:**728–735.
5. **Anderson, L. J., and W. G. Winkler.** 1979. Aqueous quaternary ammonium compounds and rabies treatment. *J. Infect. Dis.* **139:**494–495.
6. **Arai, Y. T., K. Yamada, Y. Kameoka, T. Horimoto, K. Yamamoto, S. Yabe, M. Nakayama, and M. Tashiro.** 1997. Nucleoprotein gene analysis of fixed and street rabies virus variants using RT-PCR. *Arch. Virol.* **142:**1787–1796.
7. **Arya, S. C.** 1994. Transmissible spongiform encephalopathies and sheep-brain derived rabies vaccines. *Biologicals* **22:**73. (Letter.)

8. **Awasthi, M., H. Parmar, T. Patankar, and M. Castillo.** 2001. Imaging findings in rabies encephalitis. *Am. J. Neuroradiol.* **22:**677–680.
9. **Badrane, H., C. Bahloul, P. Perrin, and N. Tordo.** 2001. Evidence of two *Lyssavirus* phylogroups with distinct pathogenicity and immunogenicity. *J. Virol.* **75:**3268–3276.
10. **Baer, G. M. (ed.).** 1991. *The Natural History of Rabies*, 2nd ed. CRC Press, Boca Raton, FL.
11. **Baer, G. M.** 1994. Rabies—an historical perspective. *Infect. Agents Dis.* **3:**168–180.
12. **Baer, G. M.** 1991. Vampire bat and bovine paralytic rabies, p. 389–403. *In* G. M. Baer (ed.), *The Natural History of Rabies*, 2nd ed. CRC Press, Boca Raton, FL.
13. **Bernard, K. W., P. W. Smith, F. J. Kader, and M. J. Moran.** 1982. Neuroparalytic illness and human diploid cell rabies vaccine. *JAMA* **248:**3136–3138.
14. **Bhatt, D. R., M. A. W. Hattwick, R. Gerdson, R. W. Emmons, and H. N. Johnson.** 1974. Human rabies: diagnosis, complications, and prognosis. *Am. J. Dis. Child.* **127:**862–869.
15. **Blancou, J., M. F. A. Aubert, and M. Artois.** 1991. Fox rabies, p. 257–290. *In* G. M. Baer (ed.), *The Natural History of Rabies*, 2nd ed. CRC Press, Boca Raton, FL.
16. **Blanton, J. D., C. A. Hanlon, and C. E. Rupprecht.** 2007. Rabies surveillance in the United States during 2006. *J. Am. Vet. Med. Assoc.* **231:**540–556.
17. **Bleck, T. P., and S. R. Alston.** 1995. Prion diseases, p. 11.1–11.16. *In* T. P. Bleck (ed.), *Atlas of Infectious Diseases*, vol. III. *Central Nervous System and Eye Infections*. (Series editor, G. L. Mandell.) Livingstone, New York, NY.
18. **Bleck, T. P., and C. E. Rupprecht.** 2000. Rabies, p. 1811–1820. *In* G. L. Mandell, J. E. Bennett, and R. Dolin (ed.), *Principles and Practice of Infectious Diseases*, 5th ed. Churchill Livingstone, New York, NY.
19. **Bleck, T. P., and C. E. Rupprecht.** 2005. Rhabdoviruses, p. 2047–2056. *In* G. L. Mandell, J. E. Bennett, and R. Dolin (ed.), *Principles and Practice of Infectious Diseases*, 6th ed. Churchill Livingstone, New York, NY.
20. **Bleck, T. P., and J. S. Brauner.** 2004. Tetanus, p. 625–648. *In* W. M. Scheld, R. J. Whitley, and C. M. Marra (ed.), *Infections of the Central Nervous System*, 3rd ed. Lippincott Williams & Wilkins, New York, NY.
21. **Blenden, D. C., W. Creech, and M. J. Torres-Anjel.** 1986. Use of immunofluorescence examination to detect rabies virus in the skin of humans with clinical encephalitis. *J. Infect. Dis.* **154:**698–701.
22. **Blumberg, B. M., C. Giorgi, and D. Kolakofsky.** 1983. N protein of vesicular stomatitis virus selectively encapsidates leader RNA in vitro. *Cell* **32:**559–567.
23. **Brochier, B., D. Boulanger, F. Costy, and P.-P. Pastoret.** 1994. Toward rabies elimination in Belgium by fox vaccination using a vaccinia-rabies glycoprotein recombinant virus. *Vaccine* **12:**1368–1371.
24. **Bryceson, A. D., B. M. Greenwood, D. A. Warrell, N. M. Davidson, H. M. Pope, J. H. Lawrie, H. J. Barnes, W. E. Bailie, and G. E. Wilcox.** 1975. Demonstration during life of rabies antigen in humans. *J. Infect. Dis.* **131:**71–74.
25. **Bundza, A., and K. M. Charlton.** 1988. Comparison of spongiform lesions in experimental scrapie and rabies in skunks. *Acta Neuropathol.* **3:**275–280.
26. **Bunn, T. O.** 1991. Cat rabies, p. 380–387. *In* G. M. Baer (ed.), *The Natural History of Rabies*, 2nd ed. CRC Press, Boca Raton, FL.
27. **Burton, E. C., D. K. Burns, M. J. Opatowsky, W. H. El-Feky, B. Fischbach, L. Melton, E. Sanchez, H. Randall, D. L. Watkins, J. Chang, and G. Klintmalm.** 2005. Rabies encephalomyelitis: clinical, neuroradiological, and pathological findings in 4 transplant recipients. *Arch. Neurol.* **62:**873–882.
28. **Camelo, S., M. Lafage, and M. Lafon.** 2000. Absence of the p55 Kd TNF-alpha receptor promotes survival in rabies virus acute encephalitis. *J. Neurovirol.* **6:**507–518.
29. **Cantor, S. B., R. D. Clover, and R. F. Thompson.** 1994. A decision-analytic approach to postexposure rabies prophylaxis. *Am. J. Public. Health* **84:**1144–1148.
30. **Ceccaldi, P. E., J. P. Gillet, and H. Tsiang.** 1989. Inhibition of the transport of rabies virus in the central nervous system. *J. Neuropathol. Exp. Neurol.* **48:**620–630.
31. **Centers for Disease Control.** 1992. Extension of the raccoon rabies epizootic—United States, 1992. *Morb. Mortal. Wkly. Rep.* **41:**661–664.
31a. **Centers for Disease Control and Prevention.** 1994. Raccoon rabies epizootic—United States, 1993. *Morb. Mortal. Wkly. Rep.* **43:**269–273.
32. **Centers for Disease Control and Prevention.** 1995. Human rabies—Alabama, Tennessee, and Texas, 1994. *Morb. Mortal. Wkly. Rep.* **44:**269–272.
33. **Centers for Disease Control and Prevention.** 1996. Human rabies—Connecticut, 1995. *Morb. Mortal. Wkly. Rep.* **45:**207–209.
34. **Centers for Disease Control and Prevention.** 1995. Translocation of coyote rabies—Florida, 1994. *Morb. Mortal. Wkly. Rep.* **44:**580–587.
35. **Centers for Disease Control and Prevention.** 1999. Human rabies prevention—United States, 1999: recommendations of the Advisory Committee on Immunization Practices (ACIP). *Morb. Mortal. Wkly. Rep.* **48**(RR-1)**:** 1–41.
35a. **Centers for Disease Control and Prevention.** 2003. First human death associated with raccoon rabies—Virginia, 2003. *Morb. Mortal. Wkly. Rep. 2003;* **52:**1102–1103.
36. **Charlton, K. M.** 1994. The pathogenesis of rabies and other lyssaviral infections: recent studies, p. 95–119. *In* C. E. Rupprecht, B. Dietzschold, and H. Koprowski (ed.), *Lyssaviruses*. Springer-Verlag, Berlin, Germany.
37. **Cheetham, H. D., J. Hart, N. F. Coghill, and B. Fox.** 1970. Rabies with myocarditis. Two cases in England. *Lancet* **i:**921–922.
38. **Childs, J. E., C. V. Trimarchi, and J. W. Krebs.** 1994. The epidemiology of bat rabies in New York State, 1988–92. *Epidemiol. Infect.* **113:**501–511.
39. **Chopra, J. S., A. K. Banerjee, J. M. K. Murthy, and S. R. Pal.** 1980. Paralytic rabies: a clinicopathologic study. *Brain* **103:**789–802.
40. **Chutivongse, S., H. Wilde, M. Benjavongkulchai, P. Chomchey, and S. Punthawong.** 1995. Postexposure rabies vaccination during pregnancy: effect on 202 women and their infants. *Clin. Infect. Dis.* **20:**818–820.
41. **Clark, K. A., S. U. Neill, J. S. Smith, P. J. Wilson, V. W. Whadford, and G. W. McKirihan.** 1994. Epizootic canine rabies transmitted by coyotes in south Texas. *J. Am. Vet. Med. Assn.* **204:**536–540.
42. **Cohen, S. L., S. Gardner, C. Lanyi, J. R. McDonald, H. Ree, P. A. Southorn and A. W. Woodruff.** 1976. A case of rabies in man: some problems of diagnosis and management. *Br. Med. J.* **1:**1041–1042.
43. **Coll, J. M.** 1995. The glycoprotein G of rhabdoviruses. *Arch. Virol.* **140:**827–851.
44. **Constantine, D. G.** 1967. *Rabies Transmission by Air in Bat Caves*. U.S. Public Health Service, Washington, DC.
45. **Conti, L. A., G. Tucker, and S. Heston.** 1994. Rabies in a dog vaccinated by its owner. *J. Am. Vet. Med. Assoc.* **205:**1250. (Letter.)
46. **Crepin, P., L. Audry, Y. Rotivel, A. Gacoin, C. Caroff, and H. Bourhy.** 1998. Intravitam diagnosis of human ra-

bies by PCR using saliva and cerebrospinal fluid. *J. Clin. Microbiol.* **36:**1117–1121.

47. **Dean, D. J.** 1963. Pathogenesis and prophylaxis of rabies in man. *N. Y. State J. Med.* **63:**3507–3513.
48. **De Brito, T., M. D. Araujo, and A. Tiriba.** 1973. Ultrastructure of the Negri body in human rabies. *J. Neurol. Sci.* **20:**363–372.
49. **Delmas, O., E. C. Holmes, C. Talbi, F. Larrous, L. Dacheux, C. Bouchier, and H. Bourhy.** 2008. Genomic diversity and evolution of the lyssaviruses. *PLoS ONE* **3:** e2057.
50. **de Mattos, C. A., C. C. de Mattos, and C. E. Rupprecht.** 2001. Rhabdoviruses, p. 1245–1277. *In* B. N. Fields, D. M. Knipe, and P. M. Howley (ed.), *Fields Virology*, 4th ed. Lippincott Williams & Wilkins, Philadelphia, PA.
51. **De Serres, G, F. Dallaire, M. Côte, and D. M. Skowronski.** 2008. Bat rabies in the United States and Canada from 1950 through 2007: human cases with and without bat contact. *Clin. Infect. Dis.* **46:**1329–1337.
52. **Dietzschold, B.** 1993. Antibody-mediated clearance of viruses from the mammalian central nervous system. *Trends Microbiol.* **1:**63–66.
53. **Dorfman, N., B. Dietschold, W. Kajiyama, Z. F. Fu, H. Koprowski, and A. L. Notkins.** 1994. Development of human monoclonal antibodies to rabies. *Hybridoma* **13:** 397–402.
54. **Dubois-Dalcq, M., K. V. Holmes, and B. Rentier.** 1984. Assembly of rhabdoviridae, p. 21–43. *In* M. Dubois-Dalcq, K. V. Holmes, B. Rentier, B. Dietzschold, and H. Koprowski (ed.), *Assembly of Enveloped RNA Viruses*. Springer-Verlag, Vienna, Austria.
55. **Dupont, J. R., and K. M. Earle.** 1965. Human rabies encephalitis. A study of forty-nine fatal cases with a review of the literature. *Neurology* **15:**1023–1034.
56. **Dürr, S., S. Naïssengar, R. Mindekem, C. Diguimbye, M. Niezgoda, I. Kuzmin, C. E. Rupprecht, and J. Zinsstag.** 2008. Rabies diagnosis for developing countries. *PLoS Negl. Trop. Dis.* **2:**e206.
57. **Dutta, J. K., and T. K. Dutta.** 1994. Treatment of clinical rabies in man: drug therapy and other measures. *Clin. Pharmacol. Ther.* **32:**594–597.
58. **Dutta, J. K.** 1994. Rabies presenting with priapism. *J. Assoc. Physicians India* **42:**430. (Letter.)
59. **Eng, T. R., D. B. Fishbein, H. E. Talamante, M. Fekadu, G. F. Chavez, F. J. Muro, and G. M. Baer.** 1994. Immunogenicity of rabies vaccines used during an urban epizootic of rabies in Mexico. *Vaccine* **12:**1259–1306.
60. **Esiri, M. M., and P. G. E. Kennedy.** 1992. Virus diseases, p. 335–399. *In* J. H. Adams, and L. W. Duchen (ed.), *Greenfield's Neuropathology*. Oxford University Press, New York, NY.
61. **Fekadu, M., F. W. Chandler, and A. K. Harrison.** 1982. Pathogenesis of rabies in dogs inoculated with an Ethiopian rabies virus strain. Immunofluorescence, histologic and ultrastructural studies of the central nervous system. *Arch. Virol.* **71:**109–126.
62. **Fekadu, M.** 1991. Canine rabies, p. 367–378. *In* G. M. Baer (ed.), *The Natural History of Rabies*, 2nd ed. CRC Press, Boca Raton, FL.

62a. **Fine, S. M.** 2005. Vesicular stomatitis virus and related viruses, p. 2044–2047. *In* G. L. Mandell, J. E. Bennett, and R. Dolin (ed.), *Principles and Practice of Infectious Diseases*, 6th ed. Churchill Livingstone, New York, NY.

63. **Fishbain, D. A., S. Barsky, and M. Goldberg.** 1992. Monosymptomatic hypochondriacal psychosis: belief of contracting rabies. *Int. J. Psychiatry Med.* **22:**3–9.
64. Reference deleted.
65. **Fishbein, D. B.** 1991. Rabies in humans, p. 519–549. *In* G. M. Baer (ed.), *The Natural History of Rabies*, 2nd ed. CRC Press, Boca Raton, FL.
66. **Fleming, G.** 1872. *Rabies and hydrophobia*, p. 7. Chapman and Hall, London, England.
67. **Foley, G. L., and J. F. Zachary.** 1995. Rabies-induced spongiform change and encephalitis in a heifer. *Vet. Pathol.* **32:**309–311.
68. **Gastaut, H., and G. Miletto.** 1955. Interprétation physiopathogénetique de la rage furieuse. *Rev. Neurol.* **92:**1–25.
69. **Gibbons, R. V., and C. E. Rupprecht.** 2001. Postexposure rabies prophylaxis in immunocompromised patients. *JAMA* **285:**1574–1575.
70. **Gode, G. R., A. V. Raju, T. S. Jayalakshmi, H. L. Kaul, and N. K. Bhide.** 1976. Intensive care in rabies therapy: clinical observations. *Lancet* **ii:**6–8.
71. **Gode, G. R., R. Saksena, R. K. Batra, P K. Kalia, and N. K. Bhide.** 1988. Treatment of 54 clinically diagnosed rabies patients with two survivals. *Indian J. Med. Res.* **88:** 564–566.
72. **Goldwasser, R. A., and R. E. Kissling.** 1958. Fluorescent antibody staining of street and fixed rabies virus antigens. *Proc. Soc. Exp. Biol. Med.* **98:**219–223.
73. **Gosztonyi, G.** 1994. Reproduction of lyssaviruses: ultrastructural composition of lyssaviruses and functional aspects of pathogenesis, p. 43–68. *In* C. E. Rupprecht, B. Dietzschold, and H. Koprowski (ed.), Lyssaviruses. Springer-Verlag, Berlin, Germany.
74. **Goto, H., N. Minimoto, H. Ito, T. R. Luo, M. Sugiyama, T. Kinjo, and A. Kawai.** 1995. Expression of the nucleoprotein of rabies virus in Escherichia coli and mapping of antigenic sites. *Arch. Virol.* **140:**1061–1074.
75. **Gourmelon, P., D. Briet, D. Clarençon, L. Court, and H. Tsiang.** 1991. Sleep alterations in experimental street rabies virus infection occur in the absence of major EEG abnormalities. *Brain Res.* **554:**159–165.
76. **Gourmelon, P., D. Briet, L. Court, and H. Tsiang.** 1986. Electrophysiological and sleep alterations in experimental mouse rabies. *Brain Res.* **398:**128–140.
77. **Gowers, W. R.** 1888. *A Manual of Diseases of the Nervous System*, p. 1237–1254. P. Blakiston & Co., Philadelphia, PA.
78. **Gubala, A. J., D. F. Proll, R. T. Barnard, C. J. Cowled, S. G. Crameri, A. D. Hyatt, and D. B. Boyle.** 2008. Genomic characterisation of Wongabel virus reveals novel genes within the Rhabdoviridae. *Virology* **376:**13–23.

78a. **Hanley, D. F., J. D. Glass, J. C. McArthur, and R. T. Johnson.** 1995. Viral encephalitis and related conditions, p. 3.24–3.28. *In* T. P. Bleck (ed.), *Atlas of Infectious Diseases*, vol. III. *Central Nervous System and Eye Infections*. (Series editor, G. L. Mandell.) Churchill Livingstone, Inc., New York, NY.

79. **Hansom, R. P.** 1952. The natural history of vesicular stomatitis. *Bacteriol. Rev.* **16:**179–204.
80. **Haour, F., C. Marquette, E. Ban, M. Crumeyrolle-Arias, W. Rostene, H. Tsiang, and G. Fillion.** 1995. Receptors for interleukin-1 in the central nervous system and neuroendocrine systems. *Ann. Endocrinol.* **56:**173–179.
81. **Hellenbrand, W., C. Meyer, G. Rasch, I. Steffens, and A. Ammon.** 2005. Cases of rabies in Germany following organ transplantation. *Euro. Surveill.* **10:**E0502.
82. **Hemachuda, T., E. Mitrabhakdi, H. Wilde, A. Vejabhuti, S. Siripataravanit, and D. Kingnate.** 1999. Additional reports of failure to respond to treatment after rabies exposure in Thailand. *Clin. Infect. Dis.* **28:**143–144.
83. **Hemachuda, T., P. Phanuphak, and B. Sriwanthana.** 1988. Immunologic study of human encephalitic and paralytic rabies. A preliminary study of 16 patients. *Am. J. Med.* **84:**673–677.

84. **Hemachuda, T.** 1994. Human rabies: clinical aspects, pathogenesis, and potential therapy, p. 121–143. *In* C. E. Rupprecht, B. Dietzschold, and H. Koprowski (ed.), *Lyssaviruses*. Springer-Verlag, Berlin, Germany.
85. **Hemachuda, T.** 1989. Rabies. *Handb. Clin. Neurol.* **56:** 383–404.
86. **Hemachudha, T., D. E. Griffin, R. T. Johnson, and J. J. Giffels.** 1988. Immunologic studies of patients with chronic encephalitis induced by post-exposure Semple rabies vaccine. *Neurology* **38:**42–44.
87. **Hemachudha, T., K. Phanthumchinda, P. Phanuphak, and S. Manatsathit.** 1987. Myoedema as a clinical sign in paralytic rabies. *Lancet* **i:**1210.
88. **Hooper, D. C., S. T. Ohnishi, R. Kean, Y. Numagami, B. Dietzschold, and H. Koprowski.** 1995. Local nitric oxide production in viral and autoimmune diseases of the central nervous system. *Proc. Natl. Acad. Sci. USA* **92:**5312–5316.
89. **Hooper, P. T., G. C. Fraxer, R. A. Foster, and G. J. Storie.** 1999. Histopathology and immunohistochemistry of bats infected by Australian bat lyssavirus. *Aust. Vet. J.* **77:**595–599.
90. **Houff, S. A., R. C. Burton, R. W. Wilson, T. E. Henson, W. T. London, G. M. Baer, L. J. Anderson, W. G. Winkler, D. L. Madden, and J. L. Sever.** 1979. Human-to-human transmission of rabies virus by corneal transplant. *N. Engl. J. Med.* **300:**603–604.
91. **Ito, N., M. Sugiyama, K. Oraveerakul, P. Piyaviriyakul, B. Lumlertdacha, Y. T. Arai, Y. Tamura, Y. Mori, and N. Minamoto.** 1999. Molecular epidemiology of rabies in Thailand. *Microbiol. Immunol.* **43:**551–559.
92. **Jackson, A. C., C. C. Phelan, and J. P. Rossiter.** 2000. Infection of Bergmann glia in the cerebellum of a skunk experimentally infected with street rabies virus. *Can. J. Vet. Res.* **64:**226–228.
93. **Jackson, A. C., M. J. Warrell, C. E. Rupprecht, W. H. Wunner, T. P. Bleck, and H. Wilde.** 2003. Management of rabies in humans. *Clin. Infect. Dis.* **36:**60–63.
94. **Jackson, A. C.** 2000. Rabies. *Curr. Treatment Options Neurol.* **2:**369–373.
95. **Jackson, A. C.** 2005. Recovery from rabies. *N. Engl. J. Med.* **352:**2549–2550.
96. **Jaijaroensup, W., S. Limusanno, P. Khawplod, K. Serikul, P. Chomchay, W. Kaewchompoo, T. Tantawichien, and H. Wilde.** 1999. Immunogenicity of rabies postexposure booster injections in subjects who had previously received intradermal preexposure vaccination. *J. Travel Med.* **6:**234–237.
97. **Jaijaroensup, W., T. Tantawichien, P. Khawplod, S. Tepsumethanon, and H. Wilde.** 1999. Postexposure rabies vaccination in patients infected with human immunodeficiency virus. *Clin. Infect. Dis.* **28:**913–914.
98. **Johnson, R. T.** 1994. Slow infections of the central nervous system caused by conventional viruses. *Ann. N. Y. Acad. Sci.* **724:**6–13.
99. **Kasempimolporn, S., T. Hemachuda, P. Khawplod, and S. Manatsathit.** 1991. Human immune response to rabies nucleocapsid and glycoprotein antigens. *Clin. Exp. Immunol.* **84:**195–199.
100. **Kawai, A., and K. Morimoto.** 1994. Functional aspects of lyssavirus proteins, p. 27–42. *In* C. E. Rupprecht, B. Dietzschold, and H. Koprowski (ed.), *Lyssaviruses*. Springer-Verlag, Berlin, Germany.
101. **Komsuoglu, S. S., F. Dora, and O. Kalabay.** 1981. Periodic EEG activity in human rabies encephalitis. *J. Neurol. Neurosurg. Psychiatry* **44:**264–265.
102. **Koschel, K., and P. Munzel.** 1984. Inhibition of opiate receptor-mediated signal transmission by rabies virus in persistently infected NG-108-15 mouse neuroblastoma–rat glioma hybrid cells. *Proc. Natl. Acad. Sci. USA* **81:**950–954.
103. **Krebs, J. W., C. E. Rupprecht, and J. E. Childs.** 2000. Rabies surveillance in the United States during 1999. *J. Am. Vet. Med. Assoc.* **217:**1799–1811.
104. **Kreindel, S. M., M. McGuill, M. Meltzer, C. Rupprecht, and A. DeMaria Jr.** 1998. The cost of rabies postexposure prophylaxis: one state's experience. *Public Health Rep* **113:**247–251.
104a. **Kuzmin, I. V., X. Wu, N. Tordo, and C. E. Rupprecht.** 2008. Complete genomes of Aravan, Khujand, Irkut, and West Caucasian bat viruses, with special attention to the polymerase gene and non-coding regions. *Virus Res.* **136:** 81–90.
105. **Lang, J., G. H. Simanjuntak, S. Soerjosembodo, and C. Koesharyono.** 1998. Suppressant effect of human or equine rabies immunoglobulins on the immunogenicity of postexposure rabies vaccination under the 2-1-1 regimen: a field trial in Indonesia. MAS054 Clinical Investigator Group. *Bull. W. H. O.* **76:**491–495.
106. **Lentz, T. L., T. G. Burrage, A. L. Smith, J. Crick, and G. H. Tignor.** 1982. Is the acetylcholine receptor a rabies virus receptor? *Science* **215:**182–184.
107. **Lentz, T. L., P. T. Wilson, E. Hawrot, and D. W. Speicher.** 1984. Amino acid sequence similarity between rabies virus glycoprotein and snake venom curaremimetic neurotoxins. *Science* **226:**847–848.
108. **Levy, J. A., H. Fraenkel-Conrat, and R. A. Owens.** 1994. *Virology*, p. 77–85. Prentice Hall, Englewood Cliffs, NJ.
109. **Lockhart, B. P., N. Tordo, and H. Tsiang.** 1992. Inhibition of rabies virus transcription in rat cortical neurons with the dissociative anesthetic ketamine. *Antimicrob. Agents Chemother.* **36:**1750–1755.
110. **Lopez, A., P. Miranda, E. Tejada, and D. B. Fishbein.** 1992. Outbreak of human rabies in the Peruvian jungle. *Lancet* **339:**408–411.
111. **MacInnes, C. D., S. M. Smith, R. R. Tinline, N. R. Ayers, P. Bachmann, D. G. Ball, L. A. Calder, S. J. Crosgrey, C. Fielding, P. Hauschildt, J. M. Honig, D. H. Johnston, K. F. Lawson, C. P. Nunan, M. A. Pedde, B. Pond, R. B. Stewart, and D. R. Voigt.** 2001. Elimination of rabies from red foxes in eastern Ontario. *J. Wildl. Dis.* **37:**119–132.
112. **Mann, J. M., M. J. Burkhart, and O. J. Rollag.** 1980. Anti-rabies treatment in New Mexico: impact of a comprehensive consultations-biologics system. *Am. J. Public Health* **70:**128–132.
113. **Matter, H. C., H. Kharmachi, N. Haddad, S. Ben Youseff, C. Sghaier, R. Ben Khelifa, J. Jemli, L. Mirabet, F. X. Meslin, and A. I.Wandeler.** 1995. Test of three bait types for oral immunization of dogs against rabies in Tunisia. *Am. J. Trop. Med. Hyg.* **52:**489–495.
114. **McDermid, R. C., L. Saxinger, B. Lee, J. Johnstone, R. T. Gibney, M. Johnson, and S. M. Bagshaw.** 2008. Human rabies encephalitis following bat exposure: failure of therapeutic coma. *Can. Med. Assoc. J.* **178:**557–561.
115. **Mebatsion, T., F. Weiland, and K. K. Conzelmann.** 1999. Matrix protein of rabies virus is responsible for the assembly and budding of bullet-shaped particles and interacts with the transmembrane spike glycoprotein G. *J. Virol.* **73:**242–250.
116. **Meslin, F.-X., D. B. Fishbein, and H. C. Matter.** 1994. Rationale and prospects for rabies elimination in developing countries, p. 1–26. *In* C. E. Rupprecht, B. Dietzschold, and H. Koprowski (ed.), *Lyssaviruses*. Springer-Verlag, Berlin, Germany.

117. **Metze, K., and W. Feiden.** 1991. Rabies virus ribonucleoprotein in the heart. *N. Engl. J. Med.* **324:**1814–1815.
118. **Morimoto, K., D. C. Hooper, S. Spitsin, H. Koprowski, and B. Dietzschold.** 1999. Pathogenicity of different rabies virus variants inversely correlates with apoptosis and rabies virus glycoprotein expression in infected primary neuron cultures. *J. Virol.* **73:**510–518.
119. **Morimoto, K., J. P. McGettigan, H. D. Foley, D. C. Hooper, B. Dietzschold, and M. J. Schnell.** 2001. Genetic engineering of live rabies vaccine. *Vaccine* **19:** 3543–3551.
120. **Morimoto, K., Y.-J. Ni, and A. Kawai.** 1992. Syncytium formation is induced in the murine neuroblastoma cell cultures which produce pathogenic G proteins of the rabies virus. *Virology* **189:**203–216.
121. **Murphy, F. A., S. P. Bauer, A. K. Harrison, and W. C. Winn.** 1973. Comparative pathogenesis of rabies and rabies-like viruses. Infection of the central nervous system and centrifugal spread to peripheral tissues. *Lab. Investig.* **29:**1–16.
122. **Murthy, J. M.** 1998. MRI in acute disseminated encephalomyelitis following Semple antirabies vaccine. *Neuroradiology* **40:**420–423.
123. **Nadin-Davis, S. A.** 1998. Polymerase chain reaction protocols for rabies virus discrimination. *J. Virol. Methods* **75:**1–8.
124. **National Association of State Public Health Veterinarians, Inc. (NASPHV) and Centers for Disease Control and Prevention (CDC).** 2008. Compendium of animal rabies prevention and control, 2008: National Association of State Public Health Veterinarians, Inc. (NASPHV). *Morb. Mortal. Wkly. Rep. Recomm. Rep.* **57**(RR-2)**:**1–9.
125. **Negri, A.** 1903. Zur Aetiologie der Tollwuth. Die Diagnose der Tollwuth auf Grund der neuen Befunde. *Z. Hyg. Infectionskr.* **44:**519–540.
126. **Negri, A.** 1909. Uber die Morphologie und den Entwicklungszyklus des Parasiten der Tollwut (Neurorcytes Hydrophobiae Calkins). *Z. Hyg. Infektionskr.* **43:** 507–526.
127. **Oon, C. T.** 2000. Boerhaave's syndrome (ruptured oesophagus) in a case of rabies. *Singap. Med. J.* **41:**83–85.
128. **Otvos, L., G. R. Krivulka, L. Urge, G. I. Szendrei, L. Nagy, Z. Q. Xiang, and H. C. J. Ertl.** 1995. Comparison of the effects of amino acid substitutions and beta-*N*- vs. alpha-*O*-glycosylation on the T-cell stimulatory activity and conformation of an epitope on the rabies virus glycoprotein. *Biochim. Biophys. Acta* **1267:**55–64.
129. **Pearlman, E., and S. Ballas.** 1994. False-positive human immunodeficiency virus screening test related to rabies vaccination. *Arch. Pathol. Lab. Med.* **118:**805–806.
130. **Perrin, P., Y. Jacob, and N. Tordo.** 2000. DNA-based immunization against Lyssaviruses. *Intervirology* **43:**302–311.
131. **Petricciani, J. C.** 1993. Ongoing tragedy of rabies. *Lancet* **342:**1067–1068.
132. **Pleasure, S. J., and N. J. Fischbein.** 2000. Correlation of clinical and neuroimaging findings in a case of rabies encephalitis. *Arch. Neurol.* **57:**1765–1769.
133. **Plotkin, S. A., and H. Koprowski.** 1994. Rabies vaccine, p. 649–670. *In* S. A. Plotkin, and E. A. Mortimer (ed.), *Vaccines*, 2nd ed. W. B. Saunders, Philadelphia, PA.
134. **Plotkin, S. A., E. Loupi, and C. Blondeau.** 1995. False-positive positive human immunodeficiency virus screening test related to rabies vaccination. *Arch. Pathol. Lab. Med.* **119:**679. (Letter.)
135. **Prosniak, M., D. C. Hooper, B. Dietzschold, and H. Koprowski.** 2001. Effect of rabies virus infection on gene expression in mouse brain. *Proc. Natl. Acad. Sci. USA* **98:**2758–2763.
136. **Pulmanausahakul, R., J. Li, M. J. Schnell, and B. Dietzschold.** 2008. The glycoprotein and the matrix protein of rabies virus affect pathogenicity by regulating viral replication and facilitating cell-to-cell spread. *J. Virol.* **82:**2330–2338.
137. **Ray, N. B., L. C. Ewalt, and D. L. Lodmell.** 1995. Rabies virus replication in primary murine bone marrow macrophages and in human and murine macrophage-like cell lines: implications for viral persistence. *J. Virol.* **69:** 764–772.
138. **Reif, J. S., P. A. Webb, T. P. Monath, J. K. Emerson, J. D. Poland, G. E. Kemp, and G. Cholas.** 1987. Epizootic vesicular stomatitis in Colorado, 1982: infection in occupational risk groups. *Am. J. Trop. Med. Hyg.* **36:** 177–182.
139. **Rose, J. K., and M. A. Whitt.** 2001. Rhabdoviruses: the viruses and their replication, p. 1221–1244. *In* B. N. Fields, D. M. Knipe, and P. M. Howley (ed.), *Fields Virology*, 4th ed. Lippincott Williams & Wilkins, Philadelphia, PA.
140. **Rupprecht, C. E., B. Dietzschold, W. H. Wunner, and H. Koprowski.** 1991. Antigenic relationships of lyssaviruses, p. 69–100. *In* G. M. Baer (ed.), *The Natural History of Rabies*, 2nd ed. CRC Press, Boca Raton, FL.
141. **Rupprecht, C. E., C. A. Hanlon, M. Niezgoda, J. R. Buchanan, D. Diehl, and H. Koprowski.** 1993. Recombinant rabies vaccines: efficacy assessment in free-ranging animals. *Onderstepoort J. Vet. Res.* **60:**463–468.
142. **Rupprecht, C. E., J. S. Smith, M. Fekadu, and J. E. Childs.** 1995. The ascension of wildlife rabies: a cause for public health concern or intervention? *Emerg. Infect. Dis.* **1:**107–114.
143. **Rupprecht, C. E., and J. S. Smith.** 1994. Raccoon rabies: the re-emergence of an epizootic in a densely populated area. *Semin. Virol.* **5:**155–164.
144. **Samaratunga, H., J. W. Searle, and N. Hudson.** 1998. Non-rabies Lyssavirus human encephalitis from fruit bats: Australian bat Lyssavirus (pteropid Lyssavirus) infection. *Neuropathol. Appl. Neurobiol.* **24:**331–335.
145. **Schmida, T. O.** 1995. Resurgence of rabies. *Arch. Pediatr. Adolesc. Med.* **149:**1043.
146. **Schneider, L. G.** 1995. Rabies virus vaccines. *Dev. Biol. Stand.* **84:**49–54.
147. **Seif, I., P. Coulon, P. E. Rollin, and A. Flamand.** 1985. Rabies virulence: effect on pathogenicity and sequence characterization of rabies virus mutations affecting antigenic site III of the glycoprotein. *J. Virol.* **53:**926–934.
148. **Shah, H., T. Patankar, S. Prasad, and B. Vakil.** 1999. Post-vaccinal diffuse myelitis: magnetic resonance imaging features. *J. Assoc. Physicians India* **47:**929–930.
149. Reference deleted.
150. **Smith, J. S., P. A. Yager, and G. M. Baer.** 1973. A rapid reproducible test for determining rabies neutralizing antibody. *Bull. W. H. O.* **48:**535–541.
151. **Sokol, F., H. D. Schlumberger, T. K. Wiktor, H. Koprowski, and K. Hummeler.** 1969. Biochemical and biophysical studies on the nucleocapsid and on the RNA of rabies virus. *Virology* **38:**651–665.
152. **Speare, R., L. Skerratt, R. Foster, L. Berger, P. Hooper, R. Lunt, D. Blair, D. Hansman, M. Goulet, and S. Cooper.** 1997. Australian bat lyssavirus infection in three fruit bats from north Queensland. *Commun. Dis. Intell.* **21:**117–120.
153. **Steele, J. H., and P. J. Fernandez.** 1991. History of rabies and global aspects, p. 1–24. *In* G. M. Baer (ed.),

The Natural History of Rabies, 2nd ed. CRC Press, Boca Raton, FL.

153a. **Stoeckle, M.** 1990. Vesicular stomatitis virus and related viruses, p. 1289–1291. *In* G. L. Mandell, R. G. Douglas, Jr., and J. E. Bennett (ed.), *Principles and Practice of Infectious Disease*, 3rd ed. Churchill Livingstone, New York, NY.

154. **Sung, J. H., M. Hayano, A. R. Mastri, and T. Okagaki.** 1976. A case of human rabies and ultrastructure of the Negri body. *J. Neuropathol. Exp. Neurol.* **35:**541–559.

155. **Sureau, P., D. Portnoi, D. Rollin, C. Lapresle, C. Lapresle, and A. Chaouhi-Berbich.** 1981. Prevention de la transmission inter-humaine de la rage greffe de cornee. *C. R. Seances Acad. Sci.* **293:**689–692.

156. **Tandale, B. V., S. S. Tikute, V. A. Arankalle, P. S. Sathe, M. V. Joshi, S. N. Ranadive, P. C. Kanojia, D. Eshwarachary, M. Kumarswamy, and A. C. Mishra.** 2008. Chandipura virus: a major cause of acute encephalitis in children in North Telangana, Andhra Pradesh, India. *J. Med. Virol.* **80:**118–124.

157. **Tierkel, E. S., H. Koprowski, J. Black, and R. H. Gorrie.** 1949. Preliminary observations in the comparative prophylactic vaccination of dogs against rabies with living virus vaccines and phenolized vaccine. *J. Am. Vet. Res.* **10:**361–376.

158. **Tordo, N., O. Poch, A. Ermine, G. Keith, and F. Rougeon.** 1988. Completion of the rabies virus genome sequence determination: highly conserved domains among the L (polymerase) proteins of unsegmented negative-strand RNA viruses. *Virology* **165:**565–576.

159. **Tordo, N., O. Poch, A. Ermine, G. Keith, and F. Rougeon.** 1986. Walking along the rabies genome: is the large G-L intergenic region a remnant gene? *Proc. Natl. Acad. Sci. USA* **83:**3914–3918.

160. **Torvaldsen, S., and T. Watson.** 1998. Rabies prophylaxis in Western Australia: the impact of Australian bat lyssavirus. *Commun. Dis. Intell.* **22:**149–152.

161. **Tsiang, H.** 1992. Pathogenesis of rabies virus infection of the nervous system. *Adv. Virus Res.* **42:**375–412.

162. **Turner, G. S.** 1976. A review of the world epidemiology of rabies. *Trans. R. Soc. Trop. Med. Hyg.* **70:**175–178.

163. **Udawat, H., H. R. Chaudhary, R. K. Goyal, V. K. Chaudhary, and R. Mathur.** 2001. Guillain-Barre syndrome following antirabies Semple vaccine—a report of six cases. *J. Assoc. Physicians India* **49:**384–385.

164. **Ugolini, G.** 1995. Specificity of rabies virus as a transneuronal tracer of motor networks: transfer from hypoglossal motoneurons to connected second-order and higher order central nervous system cell groups. *J. Comp. Neurol.* **356:**457–480.

165. **Warrell, D. A., N. M. Davidson, H. M. Pope, W. E. Bailie, J. H. Lawrie, L. D. Ormerod, A. Kertesz, and P. Lewis.** 1976. Pathophysiologic studies in human rabies. *Am. J. Med.* **60:**180–190.

166. **Warrell, D. A.** 1976. The clinical picture of rabies in man. *Trans. R. Soc. Trop. Med. Hyg.* **701:**188–195.

167. **Warrell, M. J., S. Looareesuwan, S. Manatsathit, N. J. White, P. Phuapradit, A. Vejjajiva, C. H. Hoke, D. S. Burke, and D. A. Warrell.** 1988. Rapid diagnosis of rabies and post-vaccinal encephalitides. *Clin. Exp. Immunol.* **71:**229–234.

168. **Warrell, M. J.** 2008. Emerging aspects of rabies infection: with a special emphasis on children. *Curr. Opin. Infect. Dis.* **21:**251–257.

169. **Watson, H. D., G. H. Tignor, and A. L. Smith.** 1981. Entry of rabies virus into the peripheral nerves of mice. *J. Gen. Virol.* **56:**371–382.

170. **Weli, S. C., C. A. Scott, C. A. Ward, and A. C. Jackson.** 2006. Rabies virus infection of primary neuronal cultures and adult mice: failure to demonstrate evidence of excitotoxicity. *J. Virol.* **80:**10270–10273.

171. **Whitby, J. E., P. Johnstone, and C. Sillero-Zubiri.** 1997. Rabies virus in the decomposed brain of an Ethiopian wolf detected by nested reverse transcription-polymerase chain reaction. *J. Wildl. Dis.* **33:**912–915.

172. **Whitley, R. J., and M. Middlebrooks.** 1991. Rabies, p. 127–144. *In* W. M. Scheld, R. J. Whitley, and D. T. Durack (ed.), *Infections of the Central Nervous System*. Raven Press, New York, NY.

173. **Whitley, R. J.** 1990. Viral encephalitis. *N. Engl. J. Med.* **323:**242–250.

174. **Wiktor, T. J., P. C. Doherty, and H. Koprowski.** 1977. Suppression of cell mediated immunity by street rabies virus. *J. Exp. Med.* **145:**1617–1622.

175. **Wilde, H., P. Tipkong, and P. Khawplod.** 1999. Economic issues in postexposure rabies treatment. *J. Travel Med.* **6:**238–242.

176. **Wilde, H., S. Sirikawin, A. Sabcharoen, D. Kingate, T. Tantawichien, P. A. Harischandra, N. Chaiyabutr, D. G. de Silva, L. Fernando, J. B. Liyanage, and V. Sitprija.** 1996. Failure of postexposure treatment of rabies in children. *Clin. Infect. Dis.* **22:**228–232.

177. **Willoughby, R. E., Jr., K. S. Tieves, G. M. Hoffman, N. S. Ghanayem, C. M. Amlie-Lefond, M. J. Schwabe, M. J. Chusid, and C. E. Rupprecht.** 2005. Survival after treatment of rabies with induction of coma. *N. Engl. J. Med.* **352:**2508–2514.

178. **World Health Organization.** 2005. *WHO Expert Consultation on Rabies: First Report*. World Health Organization, Geneva, Switzerland.

179. **World Health Organization.** 1973. *Sixth Report of the Expert Committee on Rabies*. Technical report series 523. World Health Organization, Geneva, Switzerland.

180. **World Health Organization.** 2001. *World Survey of Rabies N° 34 for the year 1998*. World Health Organization, Geneva, Switzerland. http://whqlibdoc.who.int/hq/1996/WHO_EMC_ZOO_96.3.pdf.

181. **Wunner, W. H.** 1991. The chemical composition and molecular structure of rabies viruses, p. 31–67. *In* G. M. Baer (ed.), *The Natural History of Rabies*, 2nd ed. CRC Press, Boca Raton, FL.

182. **Xiang, Z. Q., S. L. Spitalnik, J. Cheng, J. Erikson, B. Wojczyk, and H. C. J. Ertl.** 1995. Immune responses to nucleic acid vaccines to rabies virus. *Virology* **209:**569–579.

183. **Zaidman, G. W., and A. Billingsley.** 1998. Corneal impression test for the diagnosis of acute rabies encephalitis. *Ophthalmology* **105:**249–251.

Filoviruses

MIKE BRAY

41

The two genera of filoviruses, *Marburgvirus* and *Ebolavirus*, are certainly the most virulent, and are possibly the most mysterious, of the viral pathogens that afflict humans. They cause severe hemorrhagic fever in humans and nonhuman primates that resembles fulminant septic shock. In a series of epidemics in central Africa that have involved as many as 450 patients, case fatality rates have ranged from 50 to 90% (Fig. 1, Table 1). The frequency of outbreaks has been increasing over the past decade. At the time of this writing, Marburg hemorrhagic fever has been detected among miners in a remote area of Uganda, and international teams are responding to a large Ebola virus epidemic in the Democratic Republic of the Congo (DRC). Filoviruses also cause lethal disease in wild primates. The spread of the Zaire species of Ebola virus has been especially devastating, killing thousands of gorillas and chimpanzees in the Gabon/Republic of the Congo region during the past decade. Like other agents of hemorrhagic fever, Marburg and Ebola viruses are presumably maintained through cyclic transmission in an animal reservoir, but despite 40 years of investigation, the maintenance host(s) has still not been identified. Certain bat species are prime suspects as the source of infection for both humans and wild primates, but no virus has yet been isolated from these animals.

The virulence of the filoviruses for primates is truly remarkable. In the most thoroughly studied animal model of lethal hemorrhagic fever, the injection of a small dose of Ebola Zaire or Marburg virus into a cynomolgus macaque results within a few days in the onset of fever and prostration, followed by the development of disseminated intravascular coagulation (DIC) and increased vascular permeability, leading to hemorrhagic phenomena, a fall in blood pressure, shock, multiorgan failure, and death by the end of the week. This inexorably progressive disease is now known to result from a catastrophic failure of innate antiviral defenses, in which proinflammatory mediators released from infected macrophages are responsible for the major features of illness.

Fortunately for residents of central Africa and the rest of humanity, filoviral hemorrhagic fever is not very contagious. Person-to-person transmission occurs almost exclusively through direct contact with virus-containing body fluids, and there is no evidence of spread by insect vectors or the respiratory route. Once recognized, an outbreak can therefore be brought to an end through case tracking and the rigorous enforcement of standard barrier nursing measures. Considerable progress has been made in developing vaccines that solidly protect nonhuman primates against both Ebola and Marburg viruses, including one that prevents disease when inoculated soon after virus challenge. If approved for human use, these could be of major benefit in protecting members of international response teams, local doctors and nurses, and persons exposed to virus during an epidemic. Some types of experimental therapy have also prevented death in filovirus-infected monkeys when initiated early in the incubation period, and these may eventually prove valuable for postexposure prophylaxis in humans.

VIROLOGY

Because of the lack of any approved vaccines or antiviral drugs, Marburg and Ebola viruses are classified as category A agents of bioterrorism, which can be studied only in high-containment (biosafety level 4 [BSL-4]) laboratories.

Phylogenetic Classification

The family *Filoviridae* is part of the order of single-stranded, negative-sense RNA viruses, the *Mononegavirales*. The scientific name derives from the Latin word *filum* (thread), reflecting the agents' unique filamentous morphology (Fig. 2A). The family contains two genera, *Marburgvirus* and *Ebolavirus*, which are virtually identical in genomic structure but differ extensively in nucleotide sequence. The genus *Ebolavirus* contains four species, with shared and unique epitopes: Zaire, Sudan, Côte d'Ivoire, and Reston. The various Marburg virus isolates show some sequence divergence, but only one species, Lake Victoria, is recognized. The cellular replication mechanisms of Ebola and Marburg viruses are identical except for the makeup of the replication complex and production of the surface glycoprotein (GP), as described below. Because the major antigens of the two viral genera do not induce cross-reactive immune responses, vaccines that protect animals against one are inactive against the other.

Composition of Virus

Virion Morphology

Filoviral virions are long, pencil-like structures that measure 80 nm in diameter but can range in length from 800

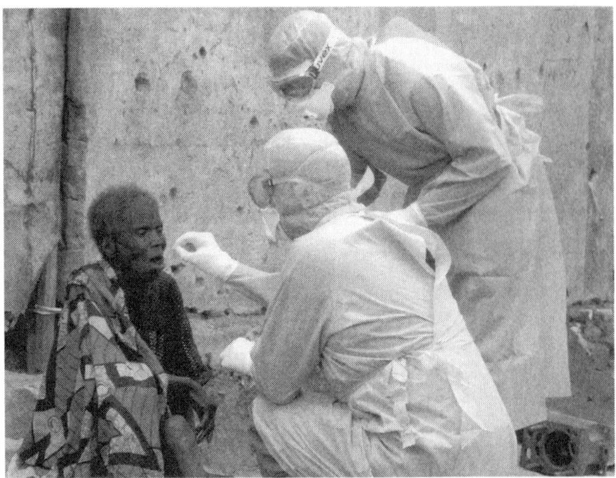

FIGURE 1 Members of an outbreak response team collect a saliva sample for testing by RT-PCR during the epidemic of Marburg hemorrhagic fever in Uige, Angola, in 2005. Saliva testing can accurately identify patients with full-blown filoviral hemorrhagic fever, but it is less sensitive than blood testing for detecting cases early in the disease course. (Courtesy of Steve Jones, Arthur Marx, and Ute Stroher, Public Health Agency of Canada.)

to more than 10,000 nm. Individual particles appear straight, branched, or U shaped when viewed by electron microscopy (Fig. 2A). The outer surface of the virion is made up of a lipid bilayer derived from the host cell, in which trimeric spikes of the virion GP are embedded (Fig. 3A) (26). The central core is made up of a helical nucleocapsid, consisting of the genome and its encapsidating proteins, nucleoprotein (NP), VP35, and VP30 (66). The nucleocapsid is linked to the inner surface of the envelope by a major matrix protein, VP40, and a minor protein, VP24. The RNA-dependent RNA polymerase, or L protein, is also carried within the virion.

Genome Length and Composition

The filoviruses have the longest genomes of the *Mononegavirales*, averaging just over 19 kb. The 3′ and 5′ ends contain conserved, complementary sequences, which presumably play a role in the initiation of transcription and genome replication (59). The order of the seven genes resembles that in the rhabdoviruses and paramyxoviruses (Fig. 3B). Most genes possess long noncoding regions at their 3′ and 5′ ends. A conserved UAAUU transcriptional signal is present at the 5′ end of start sites and the 3′ end of stop sites; in some instances, more commonly in Ebola than in Marburg virus, the signal is enclosed within short

TABLE 1 Known cases and epidemics of filoviral hemorrhagic fever[a]

Virus	Yr	Location	Source of infection	Mode of spread	No. of cases	CFR[b] (%)
Marburg	1967	Europe	Imported monkeys	Laboratory, hospital	31	23
	1975	South Africa	Unknown	Direct contact	3	33
	1980	Kenya	Unknown		2	50
	1987	Kenya	Unknown		1	100
	1998	DRC	Unknown	Repeated introductions	154	83
	2004	Angola	Unknown	Hospital, direct contact	374	88
	2007	Uganda	Unknown		4	?
Ebola Zaire	1976	Zaire	Unknown	Hospital	318	88
	1977	Zaire	Unknown		1	100
	1994	Gabon	Unknown	Hospital/healer	49	65
	1995	DRC	Unknown	Hospital	317	77
	1996	Gabon	Dead chimp	Nonhospital contact	37	57
	1996	Gabon	Unknown	Nonhospital contact	60	75
	1996	South Africa	Doctor infected in Gabon	Hospital contact	2	50
	2001	Gabon		Direct contact	65	82
	2001	Republic of the Congo	Unknown	Direct contact	57	75
	2002	Republic of the Congo	Unknown	Direct contact	143	89
	2003	Republic of the Congo	Unknown	Direct contact	35	83
	2007	DRC	Unknown	Unknown	26	?
Ebola Sudan	1976	Sudan	Unknown	Hospital	284	53
	1979	Sudan	Unknown	Hospital	34	65
	2000	Uganda	Unknown	Hospital	425	53
	2004	Sudan	Unknown	Unknown	17	41
Ebola Côte d'Ivoire	1994	Côte d'Ivoire	Dead chimp		1	0
Ebola Reston	1989	Virginia	Imported macaques	Unknown	—*[c]	
	1990	Pennsylvania	Imported macaques	Unknown	—*	
	1992	Italy	Imported macaques	Unknown	—*	
	1996	Texas	Imported macaques	Unknown	—*	

[a] A few instances of laboratory-acquired infection are not included. As this volume went to press, few data were available on the 2007 Uganda and DRC outbreaks.

[b] CFR, case fatality rate.

[c] *, in episodes of Ebola Reston virus infection, quarantined macaques developed fatal hemorrhagic fever, but none of the people exposed to them became ill.

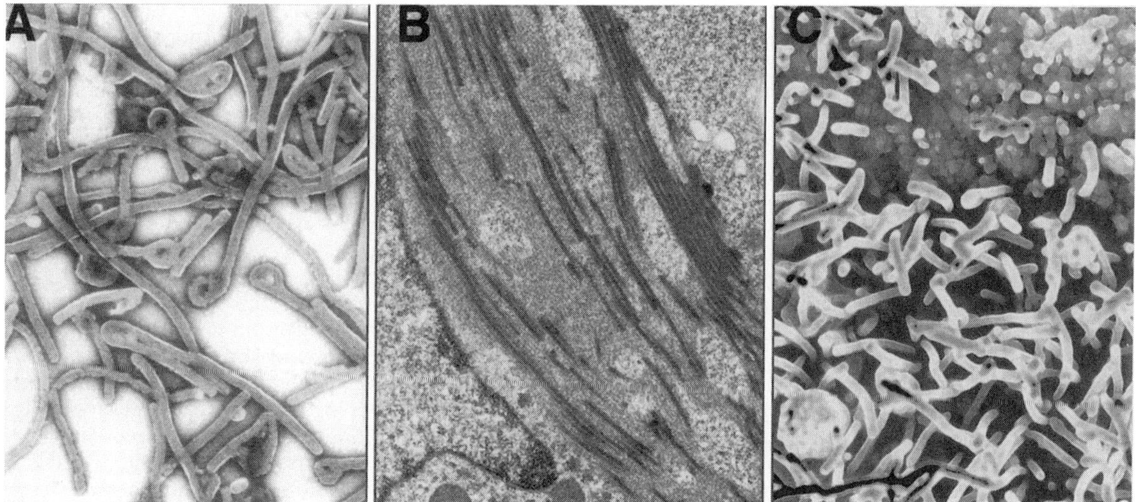

FIGURE 2 (A) Negative-contrast electron micrograph of Ebola Zaire virus virions, concentrated by centrifugation from a Vero cell supernatant and dried onto a grid (magnification, ×17,000); (B) transmission electron micrograph of nucleocapsids in a cytoplasmic inclusion body in an infected hepatocyte; (C) scanning electron micrograph of Ebola Zaire virus virions budding from the surface of an infected primary human umbilical vein endothelial cell. (Courtesy of Tom Geisbert, USAMRIID.)

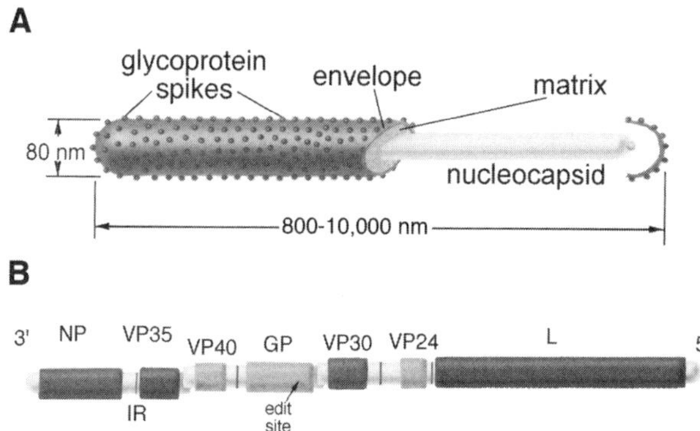

FIGURE 3 (A) Diagram of a filovirus virion, showing the single-stranded negative-sense RNA genome with its associated nucleocapsid proteins, enveloped in a lipid bilayer bearing GP spikes. The NP and VP30 bind to virion RNA to make up the nucleocapsid, and VP35 and the polymerase (L protein) join them in forming a replication complex. Matrix proteins VP24 and VP40 link the nucleocapsid to GP embedded in the lipid membrane bilayer. (B) Schematic representation of the genomes of Marburg and Ebola viruses. The seven genes encoding viral structural proteins are drawn roughly to scale; coding regions are shaded. Most genes are separated by intergenic regions (IR), but some overlap in short sequences containing a conserved transcriptional signal. Indicated for Ebola virus is the "editing site" at which transcription of the GP gene generates either a full-length membrane-anchored GP or a nonstructural sGP, depending upon whether the polymerase does or does not add a single uncoded adenosine.

gene overlaps. Transcription of each gene terminates at a series of five or six U's, where repeated copying results in addition of a long poly(A) tail.

Major Structural and Regulatory Proteins

GP

The surface of filoviral virions bears a single type of GP that is responsible for interactions with host cells and is the primary target for neutralizing antibodies. The Marburg virus GP is expressed from a single open reading frame. In contrast, all Ebola virus species encode their surface GPs in two contiguous reading frames offset by a single nucleotide (26). The major product, encoded by the upstream reading frame, is a C-terminally truncated version of GP that lacks a hydrophobic membrane anchor and is secreted from infected cells (sGP). Full-length protein is expressed only when the RNA polymerase "stutters" while transcribing a series of seven U's at a so-called "editing site" and inserts an additional adenosine. Such a site is absent from the Marburg virus GP gene.

Both sGP and the full-length molecule undergo extensive N- and O-linked glycosylation in the Golgi apparatus and are cleaved by a furin-like enzyme into two segments that remain linked by a disulfide bond. The final membrane-bound product, designated $GP_{1,2}$, is composed of a 140-kDa GP_1 that is responsible for receptor binding and a 26-kDa membrane-anchored GP_2 containing a hydrophobic stretch of amino acids that fuses with the host cell membrane (38, 45). $GP_{1,2}$ molecules aggregate into homotrimers on the virion surface. Studies of GP processing and function have been aided by the generation of nonpathogenic pseudotyped viruses, usually a retrovirus in which the native GP gene has been replaced by that of Ebola or Marburg virus (95).

Because large amounts of sGP are released into the plasma of humans and animals infected with Ebola virus, it has been speculated that the protein contributes in some way to disease severity, perhaps by acting as a "decoy" that binds large amounts of antibody. The argument is weakened, however, by the fact that Marburg virus causes an essentially identical disease but lacks an equivalent protein. The actual physiological role (if any) of sGP in the maintenance and transmission of Ebola virus can be determined only through studies of viral replication in its reservoir host.

Matrix Proteins

The major filoviral matrix protein, VP40, the most abundant protein in the virion, is the driving force behind the assembly and release of new viral particles from infected cells. Expression of VP40 alone from transfected plasmids results in the budding and release of virus-like particles from the cell surface that closely resemble infectious virions; production is increased when GP is also present (7, 38, 45, 57, 70). Like homologous proteins of other viruses, VP40 has evolved to resemble host cell proteins by acquiring a "late domain" sequence that is recognized by elements of the cellular vesicular protein-sorting machinery, particularly Tsg101 and the ubiquitin ligase Nedd4, permitting interactions with microtubules that carry it to the cell membrane (45). Once it has arrived, VP40 associates with cholesterol-rich lipid rafts, which serve as organizing centers for virion formation (2, 7). Interaction of the hydrophobic C terminus of VP40 with the lipid bilayer apparently enables the N-terminal portions of adjacent molecules to oligomerize, initiating the process of virion assembly (45). VP24, which is also hydrophobic and membrane associated, may help link VP40 and GP to the ribonucleoprotein (RNP) core.

Nucleocapsid

The filoviral nucleocapsid is a tubular structure 50 nm in diameter, with a central axial channel (Fig. 3A). Its principal component is the NP, an approximately 100-kDa phosphoprotein whose hydrophobic N-terminal segment binds to genomic RNA. Expression of NP alone in plasmid-transfected cells results in the formation and cytoplasmic accumulation of empty helical tubes, indicating that NP serves as the backbone of the nucleocapsid. When VP24 and VP35 are coexpressed, structures form that are indistinguishable from nucleocapsids seen in virus-infected cells (66). In the presence of VP40, the nucleocapsids move to the inner surface the cell membrane, demonstrating the critical role of that protein in assembling the structures required for virion budding. VP30, a minor component of the nucleocapsid, is a phosphoprotein with an N-terminal cluster of basic amino acids that bind to RNA.

Biology

Replication Strategy

Marburg and Ebola viruses can replicate in a wide range of human cells, including macrophages, dendritic cells, hepatocytes, adrenal cortical cells, and fibroblasts, causing extensive necrosis that contributes significantly to the severity of illness. The ability of the filoviruses to enter a broad variety of cell types suggests that they do not employ a specific receptor (although several candidates have been nominated over the past decade, none has held up under further examination). Instead, the mannose-rich oligosaccharides on the Ebola and Marburg virus surface GPs are able to bind to widely distributed cell surface C-type lectins, including DC-SIGN. Virions then enter coated pits and are enveloped by endocytic vesicles. Acidification of the internalized vesicle leads to a conformational change in GP_2, exposing hydrophobic amino acids that carry out membrane fusion, resulting in the release of virion contents into the cytoplasm (26).

Transcription of viral genes is performed in the case of Marburg virus by a replication complex consisting of NP, VP35, and the L protein, while that of Ebola virus also includes VP30 (62). Transcription begins at the 3′ end of the genome, producing a leader RNA and seven polyadenylated mRNAs. Production of virion proteins continues until the accumulation of a gene product, probably NP or VP30, triggers the synthesis of complementary copies of the viral genome ("antigenomes") that serve as templates for genome replication. As new genomes form, they become encapsidated by NP and other proteins to produce nucleocapsids, which form parallel aggregates in eosinophilic cytoplasmic inclusion bodies (Fig. 2B and 4B). Meanwhile, new $GP_{1,2}$ molecules emerging from the Golgi apparatus migrate to lipid rafts, where association with VP40 and nucleocapsids causes assembly and extrusion of new virions (Fig. 2C) (38).

Studies of filoviral assembly and budding have been aided markedly by the expression of combinations of proteins in plasmid-transfected cells (38, 66). Similarly, the activity of the replication complex has been examined using noninfectious in vitro reconstitution systems, in which a "minigenome" (a strand of RNA in which a negative-sense reporter gene is flanked by filoviral 3′ leader and 5′ trailer sequences) is expressed within cells into which plasmids encoding filoviral proteins have also been transfected (62). The same approach has been used to generate infectious virus, in this case by expressing all seven filoviral proteins from transfected plasmids and providing an antigenome template through intracellular transcription by T7 polymerase (64, 86). This reverse-genetics strategy has been used to generate modified viruses with defined sequences that are providing definitive answers to a number of important questions, including the identification of determinants of viral virulence (86).

Host Range and Natural Reservoir

Marburg virus and all species of Ebola virus cause severe disease in all types of nonhuman primates so far tested, but other animals are less susceptible to infection. At the time of the 1967 outbreak in Germany, guinea pigs were found to develop a mild febrile illness after inoculation of patient specimens, and the passage of virus from animal to animal soon resulted in the acquisition of lethal virulence. Ebola Zaire and Ebola Sudan viruses have since been adapted to guinea pigs in similar fashion.

Mice are much more resistant to filoviruses. Newborn animals can be lethally infected, but susceptibility is lost by the second week of life, probably as a result of maturation of type I interferon responses. However, Ebola Zaire virus from the 1976 outbreak was adapted through sequential passage in progressively older suckling mice, leading to the isolation of a variant that is uniformly lethal for adult mice when inoculated intraperitoneally (12). This "mouse-

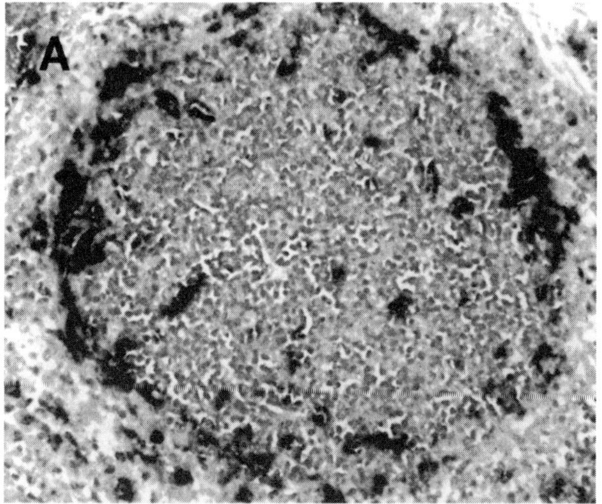

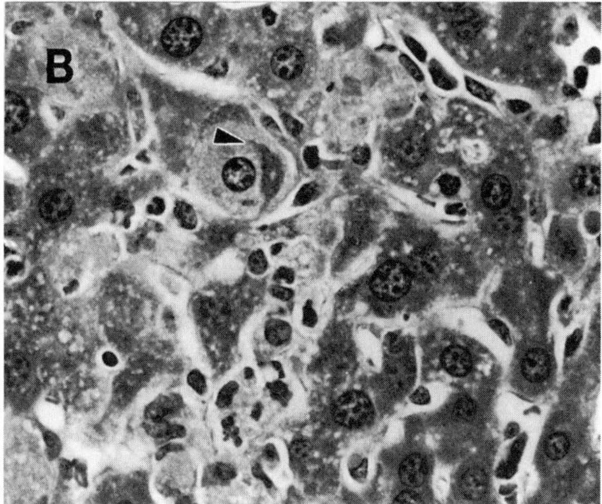

FIGURE 4 (A) In situ hybridization of viral RNA in marginal-zone macrophages of the spleen of a mouse, day 3 after infection with mouse-adapted Ebola Zaire virus. (Courtesy of Tammy Gibb, USAMRIID.) (B) Multifocal necrosis in the liver of a mouse 4 days after infection with the same virus. Some infected hepatocytes contain large acidophilic viral inclusions (arrowhead). (Courtesy of Kelly Davis, USAMRIID.)

adapted virus" differs from its wild-type precursor at five nucleotides that result in amino acid changes, but only those in NP and VP24 are required for virulence in mice (22). The variant is more effective than wild-type virus at suppressing murine type I interferon responses, but it appears to be attenuated for primates (13).

As noted above, the natural reservoirs of the filoviruses have not been identified. Both Marburg and Ebola viruses have been recovered from wild African primates, but it is clear that those animals cannot serve as maintenance hosts, because their populations are too small to support the spread of a rapidly lethal disease. Instead, it appears likely that the filoviruses persist through continuous transmission in one or more species of small animals that are widely distributed in central Africa (72).

Because a number of single cases and epidemics have been associated with exposure to bats, these animals have long been the leading candidate for the natural reservoir. Following the 1995 Kikwit, DRC, outbreak of Ebola hemorrhagic fever, it was demonstrated that inoculation of the causative agent produced persistent viremia in the absence of any apparent illness in several species of fruit and insectivorous bats, while other animals were resistant to infection (85). A small percentage of fruit bats captured in Gabon and Republic of the Congo have tested positive for immunoglobulin G (IgG) antibodies to Ebola virus, and tissues from some have given a positive signal by nested reverse transcription-PCR (RT-PCR), but virus has not been recovered (54). However, the percentages of positive animals were roughly the same at sites where epidemics had occurred and in a region where Ebola hemorrhagic fever had never been reported (73). Similarly, some fruit bats of the species *Rousettus aegyptiacus* collected in Gabon were found to be positive both for Marburg virus sequences by RT-PCR and for anti-Marburg virus IgG, but neither infectious virus nor viral antigen could be detected in PCR-positive tissues (88). As Marburg hemorrhagic fever has never been seen in Gabon, the relationship between these findings and the occurrence of human disease is unclear.

Growth in Cell Culture

Filoviruses replicate to high titers in many types of cultured cells, including Vero monkey kidney cells, human umbilical vein endothelial cells, and primary human macrophages. Plaque assays for virus titration based on uptake of the vital dye, neutral red, have been developed in the Vero E6 cell line. Ebola Zaire and some isolates of Marburg virus cause cell death through necrosis, while the Sudan, Reston, and Côte d'Ivoire strains of Ebola virus are less cytopathic. Syncytium formation is not observed.

Inactivation by Physical and Chemical Agents

Filoviruses are quite stable in aqueous suspensions. The titers of Ebola Zaire virus in growth medium remained nearly constant for several days at 37°C, for weeks at room temperature, and for months at 4°C (M. Bray, unpublished data), suggesting that virus in body fluids or other materials would remain infectious for similar periods. The agents also withstand repeated cycles of freezing and thawing.

Filoviruses can be inactivated by gamma irradiation, heating at 60°C for 30 min, or treatment with bleach, formaldehyde, or phenolic or quaternary ammonium disinfectants. In outbreak settings, the solution used most commonly to disinfect personal protective equipment is bleach diluted in water to a concentration of 0.1% active chlorine. More concentrated solutions are employed to inactivate virus in contaminated bedding and other materials that are known to contain virus. Guidelines are provided in publications available through the websites of the CDC Special Pathogens Branch (http://www.cdc.gov/ncidod/dvrd/spb/) and Médecins Sans Frontières (http://www.msf.org).

EPIDEMIOLOGY

Except for the 1967 outbreak in Germany and Yugoslavia and a few accidental laboratory infections, filoviral hemorrhagic fever has been seen only in Africa. The disease has presumably occurred sporadically among local residents for millennia, as single cases or small clusters of infection. Large outbreaks apparently only began to occur in the second half of the 20th century, as an unintended consequence of the construction of clinics and hospitals, which in the absence of proper infection control have served as amplifying centers for the rapid spread of disease.

Distribution and Geography

Outbreaks have occurred at widely separated sites over a region of Africa extending roughly 10° to either side of the equator (Table 1). They have not been associated with any one type of vegetation pattern or topography. The proposal that the filoviruses are maintained in ubiquitous species of flying animals (bats) may elucidate why outbreaks occur at widely dispersed sites, but it does little to explain their rarity.

Incidence and Prevalence of Infection

Table 1 lists all known naturally occurring cases of Marburg and Ebola hemorrhagic fever. The bulk of current evidence indicates that Marburg virus and the Zaire and Sudan subtypes of Ebola always cause severe disease in humans. Although immunofluorescence assays performed during the 1980s reported prevalences of antifilovirus antibodies exceeding 20% in some countries in central Africa, suggesting the widespread occurrence of mild illness or asymptomatic infection, those results are now attributed to a lack of assay specificity. More recent studies using enzyme-linked immunosorbent assay (ELISA) in the aftermath of the Kikwit and other epidemics indicate that unrecognized infection, if it occurs, is a rare phenomenon (17, 51).

The only direct evidence that some humans might be able to resist filovirus infection came in a single report from Gabon, based on the detection of proinflammatory cytokines and specific antibody responses in a small number of family caregivers during an outbreak in 1996 (53). This phenomenon has not been reported from any of the numerous epidemics that have occurred since that time.

Epidemic Patterns

Epidemics have occurred in three distinct patterns. In the majority of outbreaks, a chain of person-to-person transmission begins when one or a few people become ill after exposure to the as-yet-unidentified reservoir host. At some point, one of these sick individuals is admitted to a medical facility lacking basic infection control practices, resulting in the spread of virus to nurses and doctors, to other patients on the ward, and to their family caregivers. In Yambuku, the reuse of contaminated syringes resulted in a massive wave of simultaneous cases (97). In Kikwit, by contrast, the initial spread of virus to the members of an operating team, probably in blood droplets aerosolized during surgery, was followed by multiple chains of person-to-person transmission (49).

The second pattern, which characterized both the original outbreaks of Marburg hemorrhagic fever in Europe and recent Ebola virus epidemics in the border region of Gabon and Republic of the Congo, is a point-source outbreak that begins when multiple individuals come into contact with an infected nonhuman primate. In 1967, this occurred in vaccine laboratories, but more recent exposures in Africa have resulted from the butchering and consumption of infected chimpanzees and gorillas (56). The third epidemic pattern, which has been seen only in the Durba/Watsa, DRC, outbreak of Marburg hemorrhagic fever, is characterized by multiple independent introductions of virus into a community, resulting in the repeated occurrence of primary infections (6).

Marburg Hemorrhagic Fever

The first known outbreak of filoviral hemorrhagic fever occurred in 1967, when monkeys were imported from Uganda to Marburg and Frankfurt, Germany, and to Belgrade, Yugoslavia, as a source of primary kidney cells for polio vaccine production. Although the animals appeared well on arrival, 25 people who tended them or processed their tissues developed a severe hemorrhagic disease (60). Six doctors and nurses who treated the first wave of patients became infected; 7 of the 31 total cases were fatal. Subsequent serologic studies revealed one case of illness that was recognized during the outbreak, but there was no evidence of asymptomatic or subclinical infection. Follow-up studies in Uganda failed to reveal the source of the virus.

With the exception of a few accidental laboratory infections, all known cases of filoviral hemorrhagic fever since 1967 have occurred in Africa. Between 1967 and 1998, only six Marburg virus infections were detected. The first was in a hitchhiker who arrived in South Africa from Rhodesia in 1975; infection also spread to a traveling companion and to a nurse where the two were treated (28). Cases also occurred in 1980 and 1987 in persons who had visited a cave in western Kenya inhabited by large numbers of bats. Studies of captured and sentinel animals in the cave failed to isolate virus.

The first known epidemic of Marburg hemorrhagic fever in Africa was detected in 1998 among men illegally mining for gold in abandoned, bat-infested mines in the Durba/Watsa area of eastern DRC (5). Local clinic records revealed that four similar outbreaks of a severe hemorrhagic illness had occurred in the same area since 1983. Sequence analysis indicated that in contrast to all other known filovirus epidemics, a number of distinct strains of virus had been introduced on separate occasions into the affected community; only a small percentage of the more than 150 cases were the result of person-to-person transmission (6). These observations suggest that infection among the miners resulted from repeated exposure to the virus-containing excreta of a mixed population of bats, but this hypothesis remains unproven. A cluster of new cases of Marburg hemorrhagic fever identified in Uganda in mid-2007 also occurred in miners exposed to bats. Testing of captured animals is currently being performed.

As if to demonstrate the unpredictability of filoviral hemorrhagic fever, the largest Marburg virus epidemic to date occurred in 2005 in Angola, many hundreds of miles from any previously recognized infection (Fig. 1, Table 1). An initial chain of transmission went unrecognized until the virus was introduced into the pediatric ward of Uige provincial hospital, causing a wave of lethal illness among the young patients, possibly through the use of contaminated transfusion equipment. The epidemic then spread to nurses, doctors, and family caregivers and into the surrounding community. An isolation ward was established at the hospital through the efforts of local and international health workers, but only a few infected persons were willing to enter it, necessitating the development of a new containment strategy based on home isolation (47, 76).

Ebola Hemorrhagic Fever

Ebola Zaire Virus

In June 1976, an explosive outbreak of hemorrhagic fever occurred in a small missionary hospital in Yambuku, close to the Ebola River in northern Zaire (the present DRC) (97). The disease was apparently introduced by one of the dozens of sick persons who arrived each morning for treatment, which typically consisted of injections given with syringes that were reused after being rinsed in a pan of water. Within days, nearly 100 people were ill, and the epidemic was further amplified when doctors, nurses, and family members caring for the horde of dying patients also became infected. Many victims were young women attending a prenatal clinic and their children; all who had been infected by contaminated syringes died. The outbreak ended when everyone fled the facility and the remaining patients underwent traditional quarantine in their home villages.

The Zaire subtype of Ebola virus was not seen again for almost 20 years, until another hospital-based epidemic occurred in 1995 in Kikwit, DRC. An initial chain of person-to-person transmission went unrecognized for several months, until an individual with abdominal pain and bloody diarrhea underwent surgery at a Kikwit hospital, spreading infection to the entire operating team. Once the outbreak had been recognized, a combined local and international effort employed a combination of case tracking, quarantine of patient contacts, creation of an isolation ward, and rigorous enforcement of barrier nursing procedures to bring it to a halt (49). The 244 dead included 80 medical workers. Retrospective analysis found that only those persons who had touched patients, been contaminated by their body fluids, or prepared cadavers for burial were at risk of disease (21). The causative agent of the Kikwit outbreak proved to be almost identical in sequence to the agent which caused the 1976 epidemic (80). Such a high degree of sequence preservation over almost 20 years suggests that filoviruses undergo relatively few replication cycles in their unknown natural reservoir. A new Ebola Zaire virus outbreak began in central DRC in mid-2007; its epidemiology has not yet been determined.

After 1995, the epicenter of Ebola Zaire virus infection shifted from the DRC to the border region of Gabon and Republic of the Congo, where the agent has caused die-offs among gorillas and chimpanzees that have occasionally spilled over into human populations when infected animals were consumed as "bush meat" (55). In the first such episode to reach the attention of the medical research community, a point source outbreak occurred when 18 people butchered, cooked, and ate a dead chimp found in the forest (35). Viruses from this and two other outbreaks in Gabon in the late 1990s showed a high degree of homology with the agent from Kikwit, providing further evidence of the genetic stability of filoviruses across central Africa.

The bush meat trade has presumably been responsible for the series of epidemics that have continued to occur since 2000 in the Gabon/Republic of the Congo region (Table 1). Most have begun in logging camps and among hunters living deep in the forest. In several instances, treatment by local healers has abetted the spread of infection. Efforts have been initiated to warn villagers of the danger posed by sick animals.

Ebola Sudan Virus

A few months after the first known outbreak of Ebola hemorrhagic fever took place in Zaire, a second large epidemic occurred far to the north in Sudan. The first cases were seen among workers in a cloth factory in Nzara, but once they had been taken for treatment to the regional hospital in Maridi, the virus spread to medical staff and family members (96). The presence of a large colony of insectivorous bats in the factory roof suggested that those animals had been the source of infection. The same viral subtype caused much smaller outbreaks in the Maridi area in 1979 and in 2004.

The largest epidemic of filoviral hemorrhagic fever to date took place in the Gulu district of Uganda in 2000 (98). An initial chain of person-to-person transmission went unrecognized until student nurses in the local hospital began to develop a severe hemorrhagic illness. Nearly 4 months was required for a combined local and international response to bring the epidemic to an end. The establishment of a small clinical laboratory made it possible to collect and process blood specimens from patients. Because of the approximately 50% case fatality rate, the data have been especially useful in identifying biological markers predictive of survival or death (41, 81, 82).

Ebola Côte d'Ivoire Virus

In 1994, ethologists tracking a troop of chimpanzees in the Tai Forest of Côte d'Ivoire noted the disappearance of a number of animals. When a freshly dead chimp was discovered, one of the scientists performed a necropsy, and 6 days later she became severely ill (27). Ebola hemorrhagic fever was eventually diagnosed, but the patient recovered, and no secondary transmission occurred. As well as revealing the existence of a new subtype of Ebola virus more than 1,000 miles from any previously known human infection, this event provided further evidence of the threat posed by the filoviruses to wild primates. Follow-up studies in the Tai forest have failed to identify a viral reservoir.

Ebola Reston Virus

Ebola virus made its Western Hemisphere debut in 1989, when cynomolgus macaques imported from the Philippines to a quarantine facility in Reston, VA, developed a severe hemorrhagic illness, and electron microscopic examination of specimens unexpectedly revealed a filovirus (43). Monkeys throughout the facility soon began to fall ill, and it was decided to kill them all and decontaminate the building. An investigation at the supplier's holding compound in the Philippines revealed ongoing transmission of virus among the captive primates, but the source of infection could not be determined (61). Similar outbreaks occurred over the following 6 years in quarantine units in Pennsylvania, Texas, and Italy that had received macaques from the same source, but they stopped once the supplier had ceased operations.

Sequencing of the Reston agent showed that it was a distinct subtype of Ebola virus, suggesting that it might have been transferred from Africa to the Philippines through European exploration or trade. Although highly pathogenic for laboratory primates, Ebola Reston virus is measurably less virulent than the Zaire and Sudan subtypes. A striking feature of the Reston outbreak was the absence of illness in veterinary personnel who were exposed to sick animals without wearing protective equipment. Several were later found to have developed antibodies to Ebola virus antigens, suggesting that they had undergone asymptomatic infection (19). These limited data have been widely accepted as evidence that the Reston virus is not pathogenic for humans, but it seems more prudent to conclude that the threat to humans is not known.

Age-Specific Attack Rates

Even though children are fully susceptible to filoviral infection, the vast majority of patients in outbreaks have been adults. This skewed age distribution indicates that unlike malaria and some other tropical diseases that predominantly afflict children, Ebola and Marburg hemorrhagic fever are not transmitted by mosquitoes or other arthropods. Epidemiological studies have also shown that these diseases rarely spread to all members of a family, ruling out respiratory transmission (21). Outbreaks would obviously be far more difficult to contain if the filoviruses were transmitted by either of these routes.

The predominance of adult cases has a simple explanation: primary infections result from direct contact with the reservoir host or with sick or dead nonhuman primates, while secondary transmission takes place chiefly during hands-on care of patients or preparation of a cadaver for burial. All of these activities are far more likely to be carried out by adults than by children. The exception, of course, is the passive acquisition of infection that can occur through the use of contaminated medical equipment.

Risk Factors and High-Risk Groups

Risk factors for filoviral hemorrhagic fever differ for primary and secondary infections. Because primary cases arise through contact with wild animals, hunters and those who butcher and cook their quarry are at greatest risk of infection. As noted above, consumption of bats or exposure to their excretions has been proposed as the source of infection in a number of single cases and epidemics of both Ebola and Marburg hemorrhagic fever, but this remains unproven. By contrast, transmission of virus from nonhuman primates took place in the 1967 Marburg outbreak, for the single case in Côte d'Ivoire, and in the repeated epidemics that have occurred in the Gabon/Republic of the Congo region since the mid-1990s (27, 55, 56, 60). Laboratory investigators are also at risk of primary infection through accidental needlesticks or other types of exposure.

Secondary Marburg or Ebola viral infection takes place when medical personnel or family members caring for patients become contaminated with virus-containing body fluids. Most such cases have occurred when patients with unrecognized filoviral hemorrhagic fever were treated in central African medical facilities lacking basic infection control procedures. Local and expatriate nurses and doctors have played the tragic role of "sentinels" in several large hospital-based outbreaks. The lack of protective measures such as rubber gloves and routine hand washing in such settings can be explained in part by the fact that the most common febrile syndromes in the region, such as malaria and yellow fever, are not transmitted through direct contact.

Transmission

Routes

Because filoviruses disseminate rapidly to macrophages and dendritic cells in every tissue, all body fluids of patients should be expected to contain virus. Skin contact, not normally thought of as a route of transmission for systemic viral infections, poses a major risk in filoviral hemorrhagic fever, because sweat glands are sites of active viral replication (Fig. 5). Infection could be acquired by touching a patient, whether living or deceased, followed by transfer of virus from the hands to the mouth or eyes (99). Only trained individuals wearing protective clothing should prepare cadavers for burial.

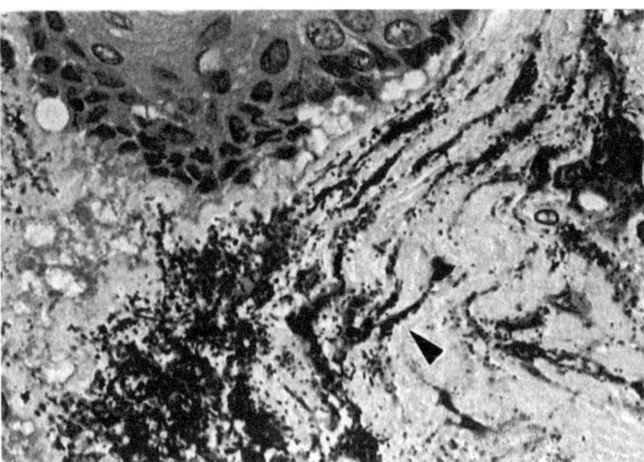

FIGURE 5 Immunoperoxidase-stained skin biopsy sample from a fatal case of Ebola Zaire virus infection in the 1995 Kikwit outbreak. Viral antigen is seen in fibroblasts and endothelial cells, outlining small vessels (arrowhead). (Courtesy of Sherif Zaki, CDC.)

Just as filoviruses spread to macrophages and dendritic cells in all tissues, disease can also be initiated by introducing virus into any part of the body. Mucous membranes contain especially large numbers of these sentinel cells, making them particularly vulnerable. Laboratory primates have been lethally infected by dropping a small amount of virus suspension into the mouth or eye. Aerosols generated during medical or laboratory procedures are also a potential source of infection. For example, spraying from high-pressure hoses during routine cleanup of animal waste may have played a role in the rapid spread of virus among macaques during the Reston incident. Paradoxically, even though virus is present in the saliva and pulmonary secretions of patients with Ebola or Marburg hemorrhagic fever, epidemiological studies have shown that person-to-person transmission by the airborne route is rare. Nevertheless, all personnel involved in patient care must use respiratory protection to avoid even a low risk of infection.

Basic infection control measures for use in epidemics of filoviral hemorrhagic fever, including hand washing, the use of protective clothing, gloves, goggles, and masks, proper handling of specimens, and disinfection and disposal of infectious wastes, are described in a joint CDC-WHO publication available through their websites. These measures are based on the same principles of universal precautions that are followed in all modern hospitals to prevent the spread of infection.

Nosocomial Infection

The occurrence of large hospital-based epidemics of filoviral hemorrhagic fever in central Africa illustrates the potentially catastrophic consequences of bringing large numbers of sick people into close proximity in the absence of basic infection control regimens. By contrast, the admission of unrecognized Ebola or Marburg hemorrhagic fever patients to hospitals with better hygienic practices has resulted in few secondary infections. Thus, even though the doctors and nurses who cared for patients in the 1967 Marburg hemorrhagic fever outbreak knew nothing about the disease they were treating, only six became infected, and no tertiary transmission occurred (60). Similarly, the admission of a Marburg virus-infected traveler to a South African hospital in 1975 led to only a single secondary case (28). Two decades later, a Gabonese physician with unrecognized Ebola hemorrhagic fever was treated without special precautions in South Africa, but only one member of the nursing staff became infected (27). Similarly, treatment of a researcher with undiagnosed Ebola virus infection in Switzerland did not result in secondary transmission (75). The fact that minimal transmission occurred in the absence of special precautions suggests that such basic measures as the use of gloves and hand washing are the most important factors in preventing the spread of infection.

Duration of Infectiousness

Virus disappears from the blood as the illness resolves, but some may remain for weeks to months in "immunologically privileged" sites. Both Marburg and Ebola viruses have been recovered from the anterior chamber of the eye and from semen 2 to 3 months into the convalescent period. Following the 1967 Marburg outbreak, a patient who had recovered sufficiently to leave the hospital infected his wife, apparently through sexual intercourse (60). After the 1995 Kikwit outbreak, some vaginal, rectal, and conjunctival swabs from one female patient were positive by RT-PCR at day 33, and virus was recovered from the semen of a male patient 82 days after disease onset (77).

PATHOGENESIS IN HUMANS

The fulminant course and high mortality rate of Ebola and Marburg hemorrhagic fever result from a combination of factors:

- The ability of filoviruses to suppress type I interferon responses and spread rapidly to macrophages, dendritic cells, and other cell types
- The extensive tissue damage caused by necrosis of infected cells
- The physiological effects of high levels of proinflammatory mediators released from infected macrophages
- Severe impairment of adaptive immune responses, through necrosis of infected dendritic cells and massive "bystander" apoptosis of lymphocytes

Hemorrhagic phenomena may occur, but bleeding is rarely the cause of death.

Patterns of Virus Replication

Like all microbes, filoviruses are confronted by macrophages and dendritic cells at their site of entry, but in contrast to most organisms, they are able to use these "sentinel cells" as their principal site of replication (Fig. 6). Suppression of type I interferon responses by two viral proteins, VP24 and VP35, may play an important role in the ability of the filoviruses to overcome these primary barriers to infection (3, 74). Infected macrophages migrate to local lymph nodes, while free virions released into the lymph or bloodstream disseminate to fixed macrophages in the liver, spleen, and other tissues, from which infection then spreads to hepatocytes, adrenal cortical cells, fibroblasts, and other cell types (Fig. 4). Even though lymphocytes remain uninfected, massive numbers undergo apoptosis during the course of illness, as seen in septic shock (30, 71). In Ebola virus-infected primates, this consists of the early loss of NK cells, followed by $CD8^+$ and $CD4^+$ T cells; similar changes occur in mice (10).

The increased vascular permeability seen in filoviral hemorrhagic fever was at one time assumed to result from direct infection and injury of the endothelial lining of blood vessels, but studies with nonhuman primates have found no evidence of viral replication in these cells until late in the disease course (34). Because this acquired susceptibility to infection may reflect changes in endothelial function induced by the presence in the plasma of high levels of vasoactive mediators, it may be seen as a result rather than a cause of illness. Altered vascular function may be viewed as a physiological response that is beneficial in the case of a localized infectious process but catastrophic when it occurs throughout the organism (11). Its etiology in filoviral hemorrhagic fever appears to be similar to that in septic shock.

Characteristic Histopathological Changes

Pathological changes in the tissues of filovirus-infected humans and animals can be divided into those caused directly by viral replication and those produced indirectly through host responses to infection (Fig. 6) (59). Among the former, the most prominent abnormality is the necrosis of virus-infected macrophages and dendritic cells in lymph nodes, thymus, spleen, liver, and other lymphoid organs that severely disrupts their normal architecture (Fig. 4). Dissemination to parenchymal cells in the liver, adrenal glands, and other tissues also causes extensive injury. In the liver, virus spreads from Kupffer cells to hepatocytes, producing innumerable small foci of necrosis (Fig. 4B). Infected cells contain eosinophilic viral inclusion bodies consisting of masses of viral nucleocapsids. Hepatic damage is particularly prominent in macaques infected with Marburg virus from the 2005 Angola epidemic (29).

Histopathological changes that result indirectly from filoviral infection can be separated into two categories. The first consists of manifestations of DIC. In laboratory primates, the expression of cell surface tissue factor causes macrophages to become encased in fibrin, most prominently in the spleen and other lymphoid tissues (34). Fibrin deposits are also seen in glomeruli and proximal tubules of the kidneys. For unknown reasons, such changes are rare or absent in lethally infected rodents (36). The development of DIC also leads to perivascular and interstitial hemorrhage, most prominently in the bladder and in the lining of the gastrointestinal tract.

The second type of indirect injury is the death of large numbers of uninfected lymphocytes in germinal centers of lymph nodes and lymphoid follicles of the spleen and thymus (10, 30, 96). Massive lymphocytolysis is a nonspecific accompaniment of septic shock and other types of severe infection, induced by proapoptotic mediators and the disruption of normal physiological mechanisms that regulate the size of lymphocyte populations (71). In combination with the destruction of dendritic cells and other antigen-presenting cells, lymphocyte apoptosis may prevent generation of the adaptive immune responses needed to contain and eliminate viral infection.

Immune Responses

Nonspecific Responses: Cytokines and Other Proinflammatory Mediators

The major signs and symptoms of filoviral hemorrhagic fever are produced indirectly, through the physiological

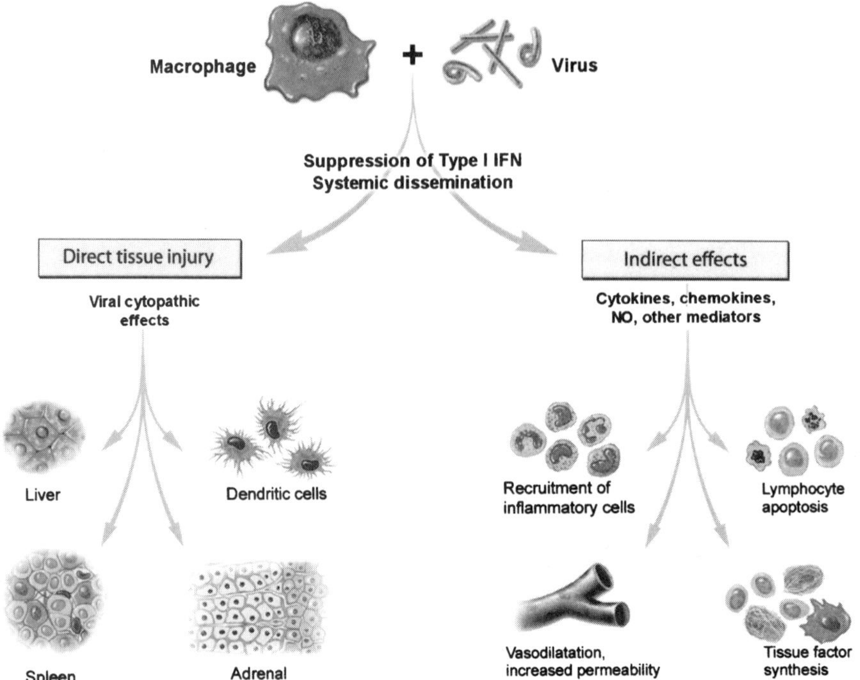

FIGURE 6 Pathogenetic mechanisms of filoviral hemorrhagic fever, based on data from human cases and studies of lethal infection of rodents and nonhuman primates. Macrophages are the primary site of viral replication. Suppression of type I interferon responses permits rapid dissemination from the initial site of infection to macrophages and dendritic cells in the spleen, lymph nodes, and other lymphoid tissues and to hepatocytes and parenchymal cells of other organs, resulting in extensive necrosis. At the same time, the release of proinflammatory cytokines, chemokines, nitric oxide, and other mediators and the production of cell surface tissue factor by infected macrophages cause a diffuse increase in vascular permeability and DIC, producing a systemic inflammatory syndrome resembling septic shock. Lymphocytes remain uninfected but undergo programmed cell death, apparently brought about through the proapoptoptic effects of inflammatory mediators and a loss of normal support signals from infected dendritic cells. The massive loss of lymphocytes and dendritic cells creates a state of "immune paralysis" in the terminal phase of illness.

effects of substances produced by infected monocytes, macrophages, and dendritic cells. Cultured human macrophages infected with Ebola Zaire virus release the proinflammatory cytokines and chemokines tumor necrosis factor alpha (TNF-α), interleukin 6 (IL-6), macrophage inflammatory protein 1α (MIP-1α), MIP-1β, alpha interferon (IFN-α), and RANTES into the growth medium (40). The same mediators, plus IFN-β, IFN-γ, IL-18, and the potent vasodilator nitric oxide (NO), are present in the plasma of Ebola virus-infected nonhuman primates, and high levels of proinflammatory cytokines have also been detected in serum samples from acutely ill patients in African outbreaks (40, 81, 90). Nitric oxide levels are especially high in fatal cases. In infected macaques treated with rNAPc2 (see below), concentrations of IL-6 and MIP-1α in plasma correlated inversely with the response to therapy (31). Although TNF-α has long been considered a critical component of the damaging host response in filoviral hemorrhagic fever, a study comparing fatal and nonfatal cases in the Gulu outbreak found that IL-6, IL-8, IL-10, and MIP-1β were markedly elevated in patients who died from infection, but TNF-α was not significantly increased (41).

The principal significance of the release of proinflammatory cytokines from filovirus-infected macrophages and dendritic cells is their role in bringing about circulatory failure, the basic cause of death in filoviral hemorrhagic fever. Those mediators are probably no different from those produced during any localized inflammatory process, such as viral pharyngitis or an infected wound. In such settings, cytokines, chemokines, and other products help to eliminate infection by enhancing local blood flow, increasing endothelial permeability, and inducing the expression of endothelial cell surface adhesion and procoagulant molecules, so as to bring about the entry of antibodies, complement, granulocytes, and other immune cells into the affected area. In filoviral hemorrhagic fever, by contrast, changes in vascular function take place everywhere at once, causing a diffuse "leak" of water, salts, and small proteins from the plasma into the tissues that results in hemoconcentration and circulatory collapse. The effects of mediators released from filovirus-infected macrophages on endothelial cell function have been demonstrated in cell culture experiments, which indicate that tyrosine phosphorylation of platelet endothelial cell adhesion molecule

1 may play a critical role in decreased endothelial barrier function (9, 24).

The expression of cell surface tissue factor by infected macrophages also plays a critical role in producing the hemorrhagic fever syndrome by triggering the extrinsic coagulation pathway (33). The release into the plasma of innumerable membrane microparticles from infected cells appears to be of special importance in the induction of DIC. Because tissue factor production begins with the first infected macrophage, coagulopathy can be detected early in the disease course. D-Dimers are the first disease marker detected in the plasma of infected macaques, and they are extremely elevated in the plasma of patients dying from Ebola hemorrhagic fever (33, 78).

Specific Immune Responses

Little is known about the development of specific immune responses over the course of filoviral hemorrhagic fever. All current animal models involve rapidly progressive, uniformly lethal infection, in which no antibody response or evidence of cell-mediated immunity is detected before death. Data from African epidemics have been limited to the measurement of virus-specific IgM and IgG responses (see below). Cell-mediated immunity must also play a critical role in eliminating virus-infected cells, but data on its evolution during the course of illness are still lacking.

Correlates of Disease Resolution

Studies performed during the Kikwit epidemic showed that most fatally infected patients had persistent high-level viremia in the absence of a detectable antibody response. In contrast, those patients who survived developed virus-specific IgM and IgG responses, generally during the second week of illness (50). Similar observations were made during the Gulu outbreak (89). These observations are consistent with our current understanding of pathogenesis, in which a massive loss of dendritic cells, the principal antigen-presenting cells of the body, and lymphocytes, the effectors of a specific immune response, takes place over the course of illness. The few patients who survive are those who manage to mobilize an early adaptive immune response before excessive destruction of dendritic cells and lymphocytes has occurred. As discussed below, this concept is leading to the development of novel postexposure interventions based on the use of fast-acting vaccines to generate protective immune responses (20, 25).

The roughly 50% survival rate in the large outbreak of Sudan Ebola virus hemorrhagic fever made it possible to examine whether human genetic variation might influence the outcome of infection (82). Sequence-based HLA-B typing of isolated leukocytes showed that alleles B*67 and B*15 were linked to a fatal outcome, while B*07 and B*14 were more common in survivors. Mouse studies have also shown marked differences in immune responses to Ebola virus proteins, depending on genotype (93).

CLINICAL MANIFESTATIONS

Clinical Syndrome

Marburg virus and the Sudan, Zaire, and Côte d'Ivoire subtypes of Ebola virus cause similar diseases in humans (18, 23, 27, 28, 60, 75). After an incubation period averaging 5 to 7 days, illness begins with the abrupt onset of fever, weakness, muscle pain, and headache. Patients frequently develop diarrhea, nausea, vomiting, and abdominal pain; such signs have sometimes been so severe as to bring about inappropriate surgical intervention. Other findings include bilateral conjunctival injection, pharyngitis, and the development of a macropapular rash, which usually begins on the flanks during the first week of illness and then spreads to cover all of the body except for the face. It may be difficult to recognize in dark-skinned individuals.

Despite the syndrome's name, severe bleeding is not a common finding in filoviral hemorrhagic fever. Less than half of patients in the Kikwit epidemic showed significant hemorrhagic manifestations; when present, they usually took the form of petechiae, ecchymoses, conjunctival hemorrhages, and failure of venipuncture sites to clot (18). Major hemorrhage is associated almost exclusively with fatal cases and usually involves the gastrointestinal tract. As the disease progresses, the combination of systemic vascular leakage and limited fluid intake results in worsening circulatory failure, with multiorgan dysfunction, anuria, obtundation, coma, and a terminal fall in body temperature. Death usually occurs 6 to 9 days after the onset of symptoms.

For the small percentage of individuals who survive Marburg or Ebola hemorrhagic fever, full recovery takes weeks to months. Convalescent patients may be amnestic for the period of illness. They often display a striking degree of weakness and weight loss, and appetite may be only slowly regained. Hair loss and sloughing of skin often occur several weeks after the end of the acute illness, presumably as a result of the spread of virus to the dermis, resulting in necrosis of infected hair follicles (Fig. 7). Migratory arthralgias, principally involving the large joints, may persist for months.

Laboratory Abnormalities

Changes in standard laboratory tests in filoviral hemorrhagic fever resemble those seen in sepsis and other severe infections (13, 23, 27, 28, 78). Alterations in total blood cell count include an early increase in total granulocytes, with numerous immature forms, reflecting the role of chemokines in mobilizing cells from the bone marrow. The apoptotic death of lymphocytes results in some degree of lymphopenia, while DIC is marked by a falling platelet count, circulating fibrin degradation products, and pro-

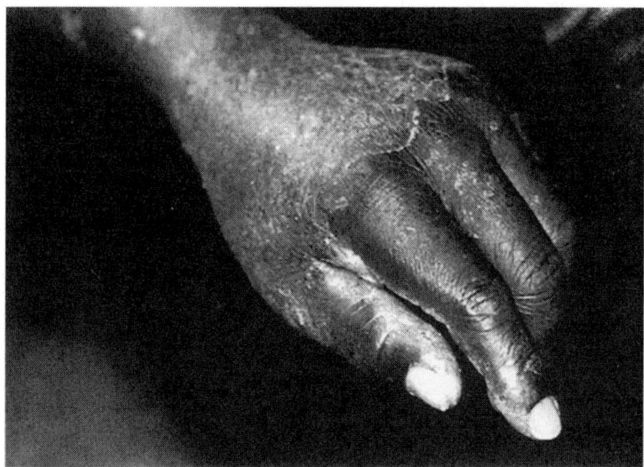

FIGURE 7 Extensive desquamation of the forearm and hand of an Ebola Sudan virus survivor, 3 weeks after disease onset, Gulu, Uganda, 2000. (Courtesy of Dan Bausch, Tulane University.)

longed coagulation times (59). Viral infection of the liver results in elevated levels of aspartate aminotransferase and alanine aminotransferase; alkaline phosphatase and bilirubin levels remain normal or are only moderately elevated (13, 78). Increased vascular permeability and decreased plasma volume are reflected in a rise in hemoglobin concentration and hematocrit and a fall in the albumin concentration. Blood urea nitrogen and creatinine increase as circulatory failure reduces organ perfusion.

Studies from the Gulu outbreak showed that elevated levels of liver enzymes (aspartate and alanine aminotransferases), amylase, blood urea nitrogen, and creatinine, with a reduced level of albumin, were predictive of a fatal outcome (78). All patients showed elevated levels of D-dimers early in the disease course, but they were especially high in fatal cases.

Clinical Diagnosis

Because the signs and symptoms of filoviral hemorrhagic fever and accompanying changes on standard laboratory tests reflect nonspecific host responses, the disease may easily be mistaken for any of a variety of severe infectious processes. In central Africa, these may include other types of viral hemorrhagic fever, such as Lassa, Crimean-Congo, or yellow fever, or more common illnesses such as malaria or typhoid fever (46). Once an outbreak is recognized, however, filoviral infection becomes easier to identify, because sick individuals can be linked to a known chain of transmission.

Outside the setting of an epidemic, a high index of suspicion would be required for a doctor to consider the diagnosis of filoviral hemorrhagic fever when examining an acutely ill patient. If the person has recently returned from an area where outbreaks have occurred in the past, the physician should keep in mind the extreme rarity of filoviral infections, relative to other endemic diseases in central Africa, to avoid making an overly hasty diagnosis. A number of sick people who have arrived in Europe or North America from that region and were suspected to be suffering from Marburg or Ebola hemorrhagic fever have proven on diagnostic workup to have malaria or another treatable illness.

LABORATORY DIAGNOSIS

Because virus isolation cannot be performed under the typical conditions of an outbreak in central Africa, field diagnostic tests are based on the detection of viral RNA or antigens or a specific antibody response. A variety of specimens, including urine and saliva, can be used for testing, but because all symptomatic patients are viremic, blood is considered the best sample. In recent outbreaks, efforts to reduce the risk posed by hypodermic needles have led to the use of saliva as an initial diagnostic specimen (Fig. 1) (47). Given an appropriate history of contact with a confirmed patient, a positive result on a saliva swab can be considered diagnostic of filoviral infection, but a negative test does not rule it out and should be followed up by analysis of a blood sample. A diagnosis of Ebola or Marburg hemorrhagic fever can also be made postmortem, through immunohistopathological study of a formalin-fixed skin biopsy sample (99).

Whenever Marburg or Ebola hemorrhagic fever is considered a possible diagnosis, all specimens must be handled using appropriate safety precautions. In the setting of an African epidemic, all personnel who collect or process patient material should wear gloves, a gown, and a mask and employ eye protection, preferably a clear face shield (Fig. 1) (4). Once removed from the outbreak site, samples should be manipulated only within a BSL-4 containment laboratory. In the United States, specific diagnostic tests can be performed by the Special Pathogens Branch, CDC, Atlanta, GA (404-639-1115; http://www.cdc.gov), or by the U.S. Army Medical Research Institute of Infectious Diseases (USAMRIID), Fort Detrick, Frederick, MD (301-619-2772; http://www.usamriid.army.mil).

Virus Isolation

Filovirus isolation through growth in cell culture is the "gold standard" for diagnosis. Because such testing cannot be performed in the setting of African epidemics, confirmation of the identity of the causative agent requires that patient samples be kept cold and shipped to a BSL-4 laboratory. Vero cells (especially the E6 clone) are most widely used to isolate and quantitate virus from clinical samples.

Antigen Detection

Viral antigens in body fluids of humans and animals can be detected and measured by an antigen capture ELISA, which has been validated for experimentally infected nonhuman primates and employed in several African epidemics (50, 89). Testing can be performed using gamma-irradiated material. Serially diluted samples are added to wells of a 96-well plate coated with monoclonal antibodies against filoviral antigens. After incubation, the wells are rinsed, and retained antigens are revealed by adding enzyme-linked antibodies and performing a color reaction. This method allows rapid detection and monitoring of illness but may fail to detect small quantities of virus; a negative result therefore does not rule out infection.

A simpler method for antigen detection that has recently been tested under field conditions is an immunofiltration-based modification of ELISA in which polyethylene filter elements inside a small plastic column are coated with a monoclonal antibody to Ebola virus VP40 (58). After a sample of diluted serum or urine is passed through the column, it is rinsed, peroxidase-conjugated anti-VP40 antibody is added, and a color reaction is performed. A quantitative readout can be obtained using a small battery-powered device. Columns can be prepared ahead of time and stored refrigerated or dried.

Nucleic Acid Detection

RT-PCR assays were first used to diagnose Ebola hemorrhagic fever in the Kikwit epidemic, and they have since been employed in Gulu, Uganda, and during the Angola epidemic of Marburg hemorrhagic fever (89). In contrast to antigen detection methods, a generator is needed to power the thermocycler. Testing can be performed outside of biocontainment using samples denatured by treatment with guanidinium isothiocyanate. RT-PCR has been found to be more sensitive than antigen-based tests for rapid diagnosis; in the Gulu epidemic, the technique identified infected patients 24 to 48 h earlier than an ELISA method (81, 89). Batch methods permit testing many samples at one time (87). The quantitation of circulating virus has prognostic significance, as fatally infected patients in Gulu had 100-fold-higher mean circulating viral titers than those who survived.

Two new approaches to specific detection of filoviral nucleic acid have recently been described. The first is based on RT-PCR, using primers conjugated to tags of differing molecular weights, followed by decoupling of the tags from the DNA product and their identification by mass spectrometry (68). The other is a panmicrobial chip-based assay containing probes for filoviral sequences, which has proven capable of discriminating a case of malaria from Marburg hemorrhagic fever under laboratory conditions (69). Neither has yet been assessed in the setting of a disease outbreak.

Serologic Assays

The detection of filovirus-specific antibodies in serum has been used both to diagnose patients during outbreaks and to assess the prevalence of exposure to filoviruses among various population groups. During the Kikwit outbreak, the presence of Ebola virus-specific IgM or IgG in plasma was found to be an important prognostic marker, as it was detected in all patients who survived infection but in few who died (50). IgM disappeared from the serum of survivors during convalescence, but specific IgG could still be detected 2 years later. IgM capture assays can therefore be used to diagnose acute illness, while IgG testing identifies persons who have recovered from filoviral infection.

Serosurveys carried out in central Africa during the 1980s made use of immunofluorescence assays in which a monolayer of inactivated virus-infected cells served as the substrate. The test proved to be nonspecific, producing a high background level of positivity wherever it was employed—a result that has sometimes been mistakenly interpreted as demonstrating that infection by nonpathogenic filoviruses occurs frequently throughout central Africa. Immunofluorescence assays have since been abandoned in favor of IgG ELISA for population screening, but even this more specific test has given a positive signal in up to 6% of serum samples from persons outside of Africa (8). To be meaningful, any method used for large serosurveys must be proven to be specific by including a large number of control samples from groups outside the region of interest.

PREVENTION

General

Naturally occurring primary cases of filoviral hemorrhagic fever result from contact with infected nonhuman primates or the as-yet-unidentified reservoir host. In regions of the Republic of the Congo where filoviral hemorrhagic fever is endemic, educational efforts have been initiated to warn local residents of the danger posed by gorillas, chimpanzees, and other animals found sick or dead in the forest. Because the few nonhuman primates imported from central Africa undergo prolonged quarantine before being transferred to laboratories, they do not pose a risk to researchers. Prevention of secondary infection requires measures to block any contact with virus-containing body fluids. As early as the first Ebola virus epidemics, it was recognized that strict barrier nursing with respiratory protection and the careful disposal of contaminated excretions could prevent the spread of infection.

Passive Immunoprophylaxis

Attempts to model passive immunoprophylaxis in animals have given positive results in rodents but have failed in nonhuman primates. Immune plasma or whole blood has been given to patients with filoviral hemorrhagic fever on a number of occasions (see below) but has rarely been used in an effort to prevent illness. The most experience has been obtained in Russia, where immunoglobulin from goats or horses hyperimmunized with Ebola Zaire virus is approved for treating accidental infections in laboratory workers (52). The equine immunoglobulin protected baboons and guinea pigs when administered shortly after Ebola virus challenge, but it caused only a brief delay of death in mice and macaques (44). These products have been administered to several allegedly exposed individuals, who did not become ill, but it is not clear that any of them was actually infected. In the only reported case of an actual Ebola virus infection in a Russian laboratory worker, injection of 12 ml of equine immunoglobulin a few hours after an accidental needlestick did not prevent a fatal outcome (1).

Although mice were solidly protected when homologous immune serum was administered before or after exposure to mouse-adapted Ebola virus, rhesus macaques that received transfusions of whole blood from immune animals soon after Ebola Zaire virus challenge showed no change in the lethal disease course (37, 42). Monoclonal antibodies against Ebola virus have also proven beneficial for pre- and postexposure prophylaxis in mice and guinea pigs, but none has protected a primate. Interestingly, some antibodies targeting epitopes on the viral GP were highly protective in mice but produced no measurable effect in plaque reduction assays, suggesting that they acted through antibody-dependent cytotoxicity (94). A human monoclonal antibody produced by phage display, using mRNA from survivors of the 1995 Ebola Zaire virus outbreak, protected guinea pigs but showed no benefit in nonhuman primates (67).

Active Immunization

Several types of vaccines have been developed that protect nonhuman primates against an otherwise uniformly lethal Marburg or Ebola virus challenge, suggesting that they would also be effective in humans. The first successful approach used a prime-boost strategy, in which three injections of DNA encoding the NP and GP of Ebola Zaire virus were followed by a single inoculation of a replication-defective recombinant adenovirus encoding the same antigens (84). Subsequent testing showed that the adenovirus was effective when given alone, inducing protective immunity in as little as 1 week (83). These approaches elicit strong cell-mediated and humoral immune responses; both are believed to be necessary to achieve solid protection in primates. The DNA vaccine has proven safe in phase I testing, and the adenovirus is currently being evaluated. If approved for human use, prime-boost vaccination could provide long-term protection to lab workers and members of international teams who frequently respond to hemorrhagic fever outbreaks, while the single-shot product could be administered during an epidemic to protect local health care workers and others at risk of infection.

An even more rapidly acting vaccine has also been developed in the form of a recombinant, attenuated vesicular stomatitis virus (VSV) encoding the GP of Ebola or Marburg virus (48). A single injection induces solid resistance in nonhuman primates to subsequent challenge with the corresponding pathogen. Each vaccine was also active when given by the nasal or oral route, potentially facilitating large-scale use in epidemics. Remarkably, the VSV vaccines also protected macaques when administered after virus challenge. In an experiment that simulated a laboratory accident, the VSV-Marburg virus chimera prevented disease when inoculated 30 min after an injection of Marburg virus, while injection of the Ebola virus vaccine after Ebola Zaire virus challenge protected 50% of animals (20, 25). If approved for human use, such fast-acting products could be employed both as conventional vaccines and as "drugs" to treat persons who have been exposed to a filovirus but have not yet become ill.

Two other approaches to preexposure immunization have also protected laboratory primates and might find application in disease outbreaks. A live recombinant Ebola virus vaccine based on parainfluenza virus type 3 was effective when given by the intranasal route (16). A preparation of noninfectious Ebola virus-like particles also protected laboratory primates, though a series of doses was required (91).

Postexposure Prophylaxis

Several types of treatment have prevented the death of laboratory primates when initiated soon after Marburg or Ebola virus challenge, suggesting that they would be beneficial for postexposure prophylaxis in humans. These treatments aim to induce the rapid development of antigen-specific responses, slow or halt pathogen replication, or block the development of damaging host responses.

The most effective treatments yet devised are the single-shot live, chimeric VSV vaccines described in the previous section. Because the outer surface of the vaccine virions is coated with the GP of Marburg or Ebola virus, they replicate within the same cell types as targeted by the corresponding pathogen, initiating immune responses specific for the filoviral GP. The VSV vaccines protect only against the filovirus whose GP they encode, indicating that protection is based not on nonspecific antiviral mechanisms, such as IFN-α, but on the rapid development of an antigen-specific response (20, 25).

No licensed antiviral drug, including the nucleoside analog ribavirin, inhibits the replication of Marburg or Ebola virus. A few experimental compounds and some licensed preparations of type I interferon have protected rodents but not nonhuman primates (15). Attention has recently turned to antisense oligonucleotides and small interfering RNA molecules, which are being evaluated as therapies for a wide range of diseases. In a preliminary evaluation, phosphorodiamidate morpholino oligomers targeting predicted sequences in the mRNA of three Ebola virus genes prevented the death of most rhesus macaques when therapy was begun before viral challenge (92). Treatment with small interfering RNA targeting Ebola virus has been successful in guinea pigs, but results for nonhuman primates have not yet been reported (32). Because future therapies may use enhanced delivery systems and combinations of molecules targeting multiple genes, it seems reasonable to expect improvements in efficacy.

Improved understanding of the role of host responses in the pathogenesis of filoviral hemorrhagic fever is also identifying new targets for intervention. The first such effort focused on preventing the initiation of DIC by blocking the binding of tissue factor to factor VIIa, using recombinant nematode anticoagulant protein C2 (rNAPC2), an anticoagulant in advanced human trials for unrelated applications (31). When nine macaques were given daily injections of rNAPC2, beginning on the day of or the day after virus challenge, most showed a marked reduction in coagulopathy. Unexpectedly, treatment also resulted in a striking decrease in peak circulating levels of IL-6 and MCP-1 and a 100-fold drop in the peak level of viremia in the three animals that survived infection. When macaques infected with the highly pathogenic Marburg Angola virus were treated with the same drug, a delay in death was seen in five of six animals, and one survived (29). The unexpectedly broad effect of blocking a single host response has revealed an interlocking connection among viral replication, coagulation, and inflammation.

Based on its pathophysiology, filoviral hemorrhagic fever can be considered a variant of septic shock, suggesting that patients might benefit from treatments now in use for sepsis (14). The potential fruitfulness of this approach is shown by a recent experiment based on the observations that gram-negative bacterial sepsis and Ebola hemorrhagic fever are both characterized by a significant fall in the plasma protein C level over the course of illness and that recombinant human activated protein C has reduced the mortality from sepsis in large clinical trials. Its administration to a group of 11 Ebola virus-infected macaques by constant intravenous infusion resulted in a significant prolongation of the mean time to death and the survival of 2 animals (39).

Management of Outbreaks

Beginning with the 1995 Kikwit epidemic, large outbreaks of filoviral hemorrhagic fever in central Africa have been managed through a combined effort of local and national health workers and international response teams, in which the WHO, CDC, Public Health Agency of Canada, and Médecins Sans Frontières have been the principal participants. In principle, the task they face in halting an epidemic is quite straightforward. Because person-to-person transmission occurs almost exclusively through direct physical contact with body fluids of patients, it can be prevented by establishing a case definition; finding, isolating, and treating everyone who meets that definition; and monitoring all those with whom they have been in close contact. Case recognition is facilitated by rapid diagnostic methods; as patients are identified, they are gathered into a single treatment facility, so as to favor isolation measures. Once the last patient has died or recovered and the last person at risk of disease has remained healthy for two to three times the average incubation period, the epidemic is over.

In practice, outbreak control is far more challenging. Recent experience has shown that the arrival in an African village of aid workers clad from head to foot in protective gear, and their efforts to have patients transferred to a frightening isolation ward (from which no one may have emerged alive), can cause sick persons to hide or flee and the general populace to resist the team's efforts (4, 76). In the recent Angola epidemic, only a small percentage of persons who met the case definition were willing to enter an isolation unit established at the province hospital, necessitating a new strategy of home-based treatment by family members provided with protective gear. No more than the most basic symptomatic care was possible under such conditions (47).

Such a reaction by the local population may be unavoidable so long as a diagnosis of filoviral hemorrhagic fever is equivalent to a death sentence (4). The lack of any specific therapy, combined with the risk faced by doctors and nurses attempting to care for patients, makes the development of effective treatment a formidable challenge. It is hoped that progress in vaccine development will soon make it safe for health workers to perform medical care, as well as provide an additional means of limiting the spread of infection. Even the ability to provide all patients with intravenous fluid replacement would represent major progress. Looking further ahead, the introduction of specific therapy will require approved protocols and the creation of a mobile logistical base and laboratory sufficient to support a clinical trial. Whatever form prophylaxis and therapy may take in the future, it is clear that effective management of a filovirus epidemic will require close collaboration between the response team and the affected community.

TREATMENT

Symptomatic

Patients with Marburg or Ebola hemorrhagic fever suffer fever, muscle and bone pain, and gastrointestinal disturbances as a result of massive systemic cytokine release, and the shift of water from plasma into the tissues causes thirst, weakness, and other symptoms. Analgesics, antipyretics, and fluid replacement help to relieve their suffering.

Specific Therapy

There is no specific treatment for Marburg or Ebola hemorrhagic fever. Patients in the original Marburg virus outbreak were treated with a variety of antibiotics, platelets, clotting factors, electrolyte solutions, albumin, and corticosteroids, without clear evidence of benefit (60). Since then, human convalescent-phase serum has been administered on several occasions to patients with filoviral hemorrhagic fever, but its efficacy has never been proven. One individual accidentally infected with Ebola Sudan virus in the laboratory survived after receiving convalescent-phase serum and IFN-α, but it is not clear that either treatment affected the disease course (23). Similarly, the two reported patients who were accidentally infected in Russian containment laboratories received many types of interventions, including dialysis and massive plasma replacement. The person infected with Ebola Zaire virus died, but the other, infected with Marburg virus, survived (1, 65).

The only attempt that has been made to introduce a specific form of therapy during an African outbreak occurred toward the end of the 1995 Kikwit epidemic, when eight hospitalized patients were transfused with whole blood from convalescent individuals, and all but one of them survived (63). Although the results appeared to be very encouraging, retrospective analysis of the epidemic showed that the seven "responders" would very likely have survived without any form of treatment, because by the time they were transfused they had already lived a mean of 11 days after the onset of illness (79). When this approach was later duplicated in the laboratory by giving whole blood from immune macaques to Ebola Zaire virus-infected animals, no benefit was observed (42).

CONCLUSION

The past decade has seen remarkable progress in filovirus research. The pathogenesis of lethal Ebola and Marburg hemorrhagic fever is now well understood, and a number of vaccines and forms of postexposure prophylaxis have been developed that are protective in nonhuman primates, suggesting that they will also benefit humans. At the same time, the frequency of epidemics in central Africa has continued to increase, and case fatality rates remain as high as they were in the 1970s. The unexpected emergence of Marburg virus in Angola and Uganda has made it clear that no country in the region is safe from the filovirus threat.

The continuing failure to reduce the toll of illness and death from filoviral hemorrhagic fever means that we must now begin to translate progress in the laboratory to success in the field. Delivering safe and effective vaccines and therapies to the sites of Marburg and Ebola virus outbreaks is a challenging undertaking that will require extensive collaboration among scientists, clinicians, and public health officials in the industrialized nations where the majority of research is performed and their counterparts in the countries where epidemics take place. The road will be long and difficult, but the alternative—failure to make use of our new capabilities—is unacceptable. Only by combining our best scientific skills with our best moral impulses can we humans gain the upper hand over these frightening diseases.

REFERENCES

1. **Akinfeeva, A., O. Aksionova, I. Vasilevich, A. Gin'ko, K. Zar'kov, N. Zybavichene, L. Katkova, O. Kuzovlev, V. Kuzubov, L. Lokteva, and E. Ryabchikova.** 2005. A case of Ebola hemorrhagic fever. *Infektsionnie Bolezni* **3:** 85–88.
2. **Aman, M. J., C. M. Bosio, R. G. Panchal, J. C. Burnett, A. Schmaljohn, and S. Bavari.** 2003. Molecular mechanisms of filovirus cellular trafficking. *Microbes Infect.* **5:** 639–649.
3. **Basler, C. F., A. Mikulasova, L. Martinez-Sobrido, J. Paragas, E. Muhlberger, M. Bray, H. D. Klenk, P. Palese, and A. Garcia-Sastre.** 2003. The Ebola virus VP35 protein inhibits activation of interferon regulatory factor 3. *J. Virol.* **77:**7945–7956.
4. **Bausch, D., H. Feldmann, T. Geisbert, M. Bray, A. Sprecher, P. Boumandouki, P. Rollin, and C. Roth.** 2007. Filovirus outbreaks: time to refocus on the patient. *J. Infect. Dis.* **196** (Suppl. 2):S136–S141.
5. **Bausch, D. G., M. Borchert, T. Grein, C. Roth, R. Swanepoel, M. L. Libande, A. Talarmin, E. Bertherat, J. J. Muyembe-Tamfum, B. Tugume, R. Colebunders, K. M. Konde, P. Pirad, L. L. Olinda, G. R. Rodier, P. Campbell, O. Tomori, T. G. Ksiazek, and P. E. Rollin.** 2003. Risk factors for Marburg hemorrhagic fever, Democratic Republic of the Congo. *Emerg. Infect. Dis.* **9:** 1531–1537.
6. **Bausch, D. G., S. T. Nichol, J. J. Muyembe-Tamfum, M. Borchert, P. E. Rollin, H. Sleurs, P. Campbell, F. K. Tshioko, C. Roth, R. Colebunders, P. Pirard, S. Mardel, L. A. Olinda, H. Zeller, A. Tshomba, A. Kulidri, M. L. Libande, S. Mulangu, P. Formenty, T. Grein, H. Leirs, L. Braack, T. Ksiazek, S. Zaki, M. D. Bowen, S. B. Smit, P. A. Leman, F. J. Burt, A. Kemp, and R. Swanepoel.** 2006. Marburg hemorrhagic fever associated with multiple genetic lineages of virus. *N. Engl. J. Med.* **355:** 909–919.
7. **Bavari, S., C. M. Bosio, E. Wiegand, G. Ruthel, A. B. Will, T. W. Geisbert, M. Hevey, C. Schmaljohn, A. Schmaljohn, and M. J. Aman.** 2002. Lipid raft microdomains: a gateway for compartmentalized trafficking of Ebola and Marburg viruses. *J. Exp. Med.* **195:**593–602.

8. **Becker, S., H. Feldmann, C. Will, and W. Slenczka.** 1992. Evidence for occurrence of filovirus antibodies in humans and imported monkeys: do subclinical filovirus infections occur worldwide? *Med. Microbiol. Immunol.* **181:**43–55.
9. **Bockeler, M., U. Stroher, J. Seebach, T. Afanasieva, N. Suttorp, H. Feldmann, and H. J. Schnittler.** 2007. Breakdown of para-endothelial barrier function in Marburg virus infection is associated with early tyrosine phosphorylation of PECAM-1. *J. Infect. Dis.* **196**(Suppl. 2)**:**S337–S346.
10. **Bradfute, S., D. Braun, J. Shamblin, J. Geisbert, J. Paragas, L. Hensley, and T. Geisbert.** 2007. Lymphocyte death in a mouse model of Ebola virus infection. *J. Infect. Dis.* **196**(Suppl. 2)**:**S296–S304.
11. **Bray, M.** 2005. Pathogenesis of viral hemorrhagic fever. *Curr. Opin. Immunol.* **17:**399–403.
12. **Bray, M., K. Davis, T. Geisbert, C. Schmaljohn, and J. Huggins.** 1998. A mouse model for evaluation of prophylaxis and therapy of Ebola hemorrhagic fever. *J. Infect. Dis.* **178:**651–661.
13. **Bray, M., S. Hatfill, L. Hensley, and J. W. Huggins.** 2001. Haematological, biochemical and coagulation changes in mice, guinea-pigs and monkeys infected with a mouse-adapted variant of Ebola Zaire virus. *J. Comp. Pathol.* **125:**243–253.
14. **Bray, M., and S. Mahanty.** 2003. Ebola hemorrhagic fever and septic shock. *J. Infect. Dis.* **188:**1613–1617.
15. **Bray, M., and J. Paragas.** 2002. Experimental therapy of filovirus infections. *Antiviral Res.* **54:**1–17.
16. **Bukreyev, A., P. E. Rollin, M. K. Tate, L. Yang, S. R. Zaki, W. J. Shieh, B. R. Murphy, P. L. Collins, and A. Sanchez.** 2007. Successful topical respiratory tract immunization of primates against Ebola virus. *J. Virol.* **81:** 6379–6388.
17. **Busico, K. M., K. L. Marshall, T. G. Ksiazek, T. H. Roels, Y. Fleerackers, H. Feldmann, A. S. Khan, and C. J. Peters.** 1999. Prevalence of IgG antibodies to Ebola virus in individuals during an Ebola outbreak, Democratic Republic of the Congo, 1995. *J. Infect. Dis.* **179**(Suppl. 1)**:**S102–S107.
18. **Bwaka, M. A., M. J. Bonnet, P. Calain, R. Colebunders, A. De Roo, Y. Guimard, K. R. Katwiki, K. Kibadi, M. A. Kipasa, K. J. Kuvula, B. B. Mapanda, M. Massamba, K. D. Mupapa, J. J. Muyembe-Tamfum, E. Ndaberey, C. J. Peters, P. E. Rollin, and E. Van den Enden.** 1999. Ebola hemorrhagic fever in Kikwit, Democratic Republic of the Congo: clinical observations in 103 patients. *J. Infect. Dis.* **179**(Suppl. 1)**:**S1–S7.
19. **Centers for Disease Control.** 1990. Update: filovirus infection among persons with occupational exposure to nonhuman primates. *Morb. Mortal. Wkly. Rep.* **39:**266.
20. **Daddario-DiCaprio, K. M., T. W. Geisbert, U. Stroher, J. B. Geisbert, A. Grolla, E. A. Fritz, L. Fernando, E. Kagan, P. B. Jahrling, L. E. Hensley, S. M. Jones, and H. Feldmann.** 2006. Postexposure protection against Marburg haemorrhagic fever with recombinant vesicular stomatitis virus vectors in non-human primates: an efficacy assessment. *Lancet* **367:**1399–1404.
21. **Dowell, S. F., R. Mukunu, T. G. Ksiazek, A. S. Khan, P. E. Rollin, and C. J. Peters for the Commission de Lutte contre les Epidémies à Kikwit.** 1999. Transmission of Ebola hemorrhagic fever: a study of risk factors in family members, Kikwit, Democratic Republic of the Congo, 1995. *J. Infect. Dis.* **179**(Suppl. 1)**:**S87–S91.
22. **Ebihara, H., A. Takada, D. Kobasa, S. Jones, G. Neumann, S. Theriault, M. Bray, H. Feldmann, and Y. Kawaoka.** 2006. Molecular determinants of Ebola virus virulence in mice. *PLoS Pathog.* **2:**e73.
23. **Emond, R. T., B. Evans, E. T. Bowen, and G. Lloyd.** 1977. A case of Ebola virus infection. *Br. Med. J.* **2:**541–544.
24. **Feldmann, H., H. Bugany, F. Mahner, H. D. Klenk, D. Drenckhahn, and H. J. Schnittler.** 1996. Filovirus-induced endothelial leakage triggered by infected monocytes/macrophages. *J. Virol.* **70:**2208–2214.
25. **Feldmann, H., S. M. Jones, K. M. Daddario-Dicaprio, J. B. Geisbert, U. Stroher, A. Grolla, M. Bray, E. A. Fritz, L. Fernando, F. Feldmann, L. E. Hensley, and T. W. Geisbert.** 2007. Effective post-exposure treatment of Ebola infection. *PLoS Pathog.* **3:**e2.
26. **Feldmann, H., V. E. Volchkov, V. A. Volchkova, and H. D. Klenk.** 1999. The glycoproteins of Marburg and Ebola virus and their potential roles in pathogenesis. *Arch. Virol. Suppl.* **15:**159–169.
27. **Formenty, P., C. Hatz, B. Le Guenno, A. Stoll, P. Rogenmoser, and A. Widmer.** 1999. Human infection due to Ebola virus, subtype Cote d'Ivoire: clinical and biologic presentation. *J. Infect. Dis.* **179**(Suppl. 1)**:**S48–S53.
28. **Gear, J. S., G. A. Cassel, A. J. Gear, B. Trappler, L. Clausen, A. M. Meyers, M. C. Kew, T. H. Bothwell, R. Sher, G. B. Miller, J. Schneider, H. J. Koornhof, E. D. Gomperts, M. Isaacson, and J. H. Gear.** 1975. Outbreak of Marburg virus disease in Johannesburg. *Br. Med. J.* **4:** 489–493.
29. **Geisbert, T., K. Daddario-DiCaprio, J. Geisbert, E. Fritz, H. Young, P. Formenty, T. Larsen, and L. Hensley.** 2007. Marburg (Angola) virus infection of rhesus monkeys: pathogenesis and treatment with recombinant nematode anticoagulant protein c2. *J. Infect. Dis.* **196** (Suppl. 2)**:**S372–S381.
30. **Geisbert, T. W., L. E. Hensley, T. R. Gibb, K. E. Steele, N. K. Jaax, and P. B. Jahrling.** 2000. Apoptosis induced in vitro and in vivo during infection by Ebola and Marburg viruses. *Lab. Investig.* **80:**171–186.
31. **Geisbert, T. W., L. E. Hensley, P. B. Jahrling, T. Larsen, J. B. Geisbert, J. Paragas, H. A. Young, T. M. Fredeking, W. E. Rote, and G. P. Vlasuk.** 2003. Treatment of Ebola virus infection with a recombinant inhibitor of factor VIIa/tissue factor: a study in rhesus monkeys. *Lancet* **362:**1953–1958.
32. **Geisbert, T. W., L. E. Hensley, E. Kagan, E. Z. Yu, J. B. Geisbert, K. Daddario-Dicaprio, E. A. Fritz, P. B. Jahrling, K. McClintock, J. R. Phelps, A. C. Lee, A. Judge, L. B. Jeffs, and I. Maclachlan.** 2006. Postexposure protection of guinea pigs against a lethal Ebola virus challenge is conferred by RNA interference. *J. Infect. Dis.* **193:**1650–1657.
33. **Geisbert, T. W., H. A. Young, P. B. Jahrling, K. J. Davis, E. Kagan, and L. E. Hensley.** 2003. Mechanisms underlying coagulation abnormalities in Ebola hemorrhagic fever: overexpression of tissue factor in primate monocytes/macrophages is a key event. *J. Infect. Dis.* **188:**1618–1629.
34. **Geisbert, T. W., H. A. Young, P. B. Jahrling, K. J. Davis, T. Larsen, E. Kagan, and L. E. Hensley.** 2003. Pathogenesis of Ebola hemorrhagic fever in primate models: evidence that hemorrhage is not a direct effect of virus-induced cytolysis of endothelial cells. *Am. J. Pathol.* **163:** 2371–2382.
35. **Georges-Courbot, M. C., C. Y. Lu, J. Lansoud-Soukate, E. Leroy, and S. Baize.** 1997. Isolation and partial molecular characterisation of a strain of Ebola virus during a recent epidemic of viral haemorrhagic fever in Gabon. *Lancet* **349:**181.
36. **Gibb, T. R., M. Bray, T. W. Geisbert, K. E. Steele, W. M. Kell, K. J. Davis, and N. K. Jaax.** 2001. Patho-

genesis of experimental Ebola Zaire virus infection in BALB/c mice. *J. Comp. Pathol.* **125:**233–242.

37. **Gupta, M., S. Mahanty, M. Bray, R. Ahmed, and P. E. Rollin.** 2001. Passive transfer of antibodies protects immunocompetent and immunodeficient mice against lethal Ebola virus infection without complete inhibition of viral replication. *J. Virol.* **75:**4649–4654.
38. **Hartlieb, B., and W. Weissenhorn.** 2006. Filovirus assembly and budding. *Virology* **344:**64–70.
39. **Hensley, L., E. Stevens, S. Yan, J. Geisbert, W. Macias, T. Larsen, K. Daddario-DiCaprio, G. Cassell, P. Jahrling, and T. Geisbert.** 2007. Recombinant human activated protein C for the postexposure treatment of Ebola hemorrhagic fever. *J. Infect. Dis.* **196**(Suppl. 2)**:**S390–S399.
40. **Hensley, L. E., H. A. Young, P. B. Jahrling, and T. W. Geisbert.** 2002. Proinflammatory response during Ebola virus infection of primate models: possible involvement of the tumor necrosis factor receptor superfamily. *Immunol. Lett.* **80:**169–179.
41. **Hutchinson, K., and P. Rollin.** 2007. Cytokine and chemokine expression in humans infected with Ebola Sudan virus. *J. Infect. Dis.* **196**(Suppl. 2)**:**S357–S363.
42. **Jahrling, P., J. Geisbert, J. Swearengen, T. Larsen, and T. Geisbert.** 2007. Ebola hemorrhagic fever: evaluation of passive immunotherapy in nonhuman primates. *J. Infect. Dis.* **196**(Suppl. 2)**:**S400–S403.
43. **Jahrling, P. B., T. W. Geisbert, D. W. Dalgard, E. D. Johnson, T. G. Ksiazek, W. C. Hall, and C. J. Peters.** 1990. Preliminary report: isolation of Ebola virus from monkeys imported to USA. *Lancet* **335:**502–505.
44. **Jahrling, P. B., T. W. Geisbert, J. B. Geisbert, J. R. Swearengen, M. Bray, N. K. Jaax, J. W. Huggins, J. W. LeDuc, and C. J. Peters.** 1999. Evaluation of immune globulin and recombinant interferon-alpha2b for treatment of experimental Ebola virus infections. *J. Infect. Dis.* **179**(Suppl. 1)**:**S224–S234.
45. **Jasenosky, L. D., and Y. Kawaoka.** 2004. Filovirus budding. *Virus Res.* **106:**181–188.
46. **Jeffs, B.** 2006. A clinical guide to viral haemorrhagic fevers: Ebola, Marburg and Lassa. *Trop. Dr.* **36:**1–4.
47. **Jeffs, B., M. Iscla, I. Grovas, C. Dorion, M. H. Bengi, P. N. Folo, P. Roddy, O. de la Rosa, D. Weatherill, P. P. Palma, O. Bernal, J. Rodriguez-Martinez, B. Barcelo, D. Pou, and M. Borchert.** 2007. The MSF intervention in the Uige Marburg Epidemic 2005—lessons learnt in Uige Provincial Hospital. *J. Infect. Dis.* **196**(Suppl. 2)**:**S154–S161.
48. **Jones, S. M., H. Feldmann, U. Stroher, J. B. Geisbert, L. Fernando, A. Grolla, H. D. Klenk, N. J. Sullivan, V. E. Volchkov, E. A. Fritz, K. M. Daddario, L. E. Hensley, P. B. Jahrling, and T. W. Geisbert.** 2005. Live attenuated recombinant vaccine protects nonhuman primates against Ebola and Marburg viruses. *Nat. Med.* **11:**786–790.
49. **Khan, A. S., F. K. Tshioko, D. L. Heymann, B. Le Guenno, P. Nabeth, B. Kerstiens, Y. Fleerackers, P. H. Kilmarx, G. R. Rodier, O. Nkuku, P. E. Rollin, A. Sanchez, S. R. Zaki, R. Swanepoel, O. Tomori, S. T. Nichol, C. J. Peters, J. J. Muyembe-Tamfum, and T. G. Ksiazek for the Commission de Lutte contre les Epidémies à Kikwit.** 1999. The reemergence of Ebola hemorrhagic fever, Democratic Republic of the Congo, 1995. *J. Infect. Dis.* **179**(Suppl. 1)**:**S76–S86.
50. **Ksiazek, T. G., P. E. Rollin, A. J. Williams, D. S. Bressler, M. L. Martin, R. Swanepoel, F. J. Burt, P. A. Leman, A. S. Khan, A. K. Rowe, R. Mukunu, A. Sanchez, and C. J. Peters.** 1999. Clinical virology of Ebola hemorrhagic fever (EHF): virus, virus antigen, and IgG and IgM antibody findings among EHF patients in Kikwit, Democratic Republic of the Congo, 1995. *J. Infect. Dis.* **179**(Suppl. 1)**:**S177–S187.
51. **Ksiazek, T. G., C. P. West, P. E. Rollin, P. B. Jahrling, and C. J. Peters.** 1999. ELISA for the detection of antibodies to Ebola viruses. *J. Infect. Dis.* **179**(Suppl. 1)**:** S192–S198.
52. **Kudoyarova-Zubavichene, N. M., N. N. Sergeyev, A. A. Chepurnov, and S. V. Netesov.** 1999. Preparation and use of hyperimmune serum for prophylaxis and therapy of Ebola virus infections. *J. Infect. Dis.* **179**(Suppl. 1)**:**S218–S223.
53. **Leroy, E. M., S. Baize, V. E. Volchkov, S. P. Fisher-Hoch, M. C. Georges-Courbot, J. Lansoud-Soukate, M. Capron, P. Debre, J. B. McCormick, and A. J. Georges.** 2000. Human asymptomatic Ebola infection and strong inflammatory response. *Lancet* **355:**2210–2215.
54. **Leroy, E. M., B. Kumulungui, X. Pourrut, P. Rouquet, A. Hassanin, P. Yaba, A. Delicat, J. T. Paweska, J. P. Gonzalez, and R. Swanepoel.** 2005. Fruit bats as reservoirs of Ebola virus. *Nature* **438:**575–576.
55. **Leroy, E. M., P. Rouquet, P. Formenty, S. Souquiere, A. Kilbourne, J. M. Froment, M. Bermejo, S. Smit, W. Karesh, R. Swanepoel, S. R. Zaki, and P. E. Rollin.** 2004. Multiple Ebola virus transmission events and rapid decline of central African wildlife. *Science* **303:**387–390.
56. **Leroy, E. M., S. Souquiere, P. Rouquet, and D. Drevet.** 2002. Re-emergence of Ebola haemorrhagic fever in Gabon. *Lancet* **359:**712.
57. **Licata, J. M., R. F. Johnson, Z. Han, and R. N. Harty.** 2004. Contribution of Ebola virus glycoprotein, nucleoprotein, and VP24 to budding of VP40 virus-like particles. *J. Virol.* **78:**7344–7351.
58. **Lucht, A., P. Formenty, H. Feldmann, M. Gotz, E. Leroy, P. Bataboukila, A. Grolla, F. Feldmann, T. Wittmann, P. Campbell, C. Atsangandoko, P. Boumandouki, E. Finke, P. Miethe, S. Becker, and R. Grunow.** 2007. Development of an immunofiltration-based antigen detection assay for rapid diagnosis of Ebola virus infections. *J. Infect. Dis.* **196**(Suppl. 2)**:**S184–S192.
59. **Mahanty, S., and M. Bray.** 2004. Pathogenesis of filoviral haemorrhagic fevers. *Lancet Infect. Dis.* **4:**487–498.
60. **Martini, G. A.** 1969. Marburg agent disease in man. *Trans. R. Soc. Trop. Med. Hyg.* **63:**295–302.
61. **Miranda, M. E., T. G. Ksiazek, T. J. Retuya, A. S. Khan, A. Sanchez, C. F. Fulhorst, P. E. Rollin, A. B. Calaor, D. L. Manalo, M. C. Roces, M. M. Dayrit, and C. J. Peters.** 1999. Epidemiology of Ebola (subtype Reston) virus in the Philippines, 1996. *J. Infect. Dis.* **179** (Suppl. 1)**:**S115–S119.
62. **Muhlberger, E., M. Weik, V. E. Volchkov, H. D. Klenk, and S. Becker.** 1999. Comparison of the transcription and replication strategies of Marburg virus and Ebola virus by using artificial replication systems. *J. Virol.* **73:**2333–2342.
63. **Mupapa, K., M. Massamba, K. Kibadi, K. Kuvula, A. Bwaka, M. Kipasa, R. Colebunders, and J. J. Muyembe-Tamfum for the International Scientific and Technical Committee.** 1999. Treatment of Ebola hemorrhagic fever with blood transfusions from convalescent patients. *J. Infect. Dis.* **179**(Suppl. 1)**:**S18–S23.
64. **Neumann, G., H. Feldmann, S. Watanabe, I. Lukashevich, and Y. Kawaoka.** 2002. Reverse genetics demonstrates that proteolytic processing of the Ebola virus glycoprotein is not essential for replication in cell culture. *J. Virol.* **76:**406–410.
65. **Nikiforov, V. V., I. Turovskii Iu, P. P. Kalinin, L. A. Akinfeeva, L. R. Katkova, V. S. Barmin, E. I. Riabchikova, N. I. Popkova, A. M. Shestopalov, V. P. Nazarov,**

et al. 1994. A case of a laboratory infection with Marburg fever. *Zh. Mikrobiol. Epidemiol. Immunobiol.*:104–106. (In Russian.)

66. **Noda, T., H. Ebihara, Y. Muramoto, K. Fujii, A. Takada, H. Sagara, J. H. Kim, H. Kida, H. Feldmann, and Y. Kawaoka.** 2006. Assembly and budding of Ebola virus. *PLoS Pathog.* **2**:e99.
67. **Oswald, W. B., T. W. Geisbert, K. J. Davis, J. B. Geisbert, N. J. Sullivan, P. B. Jahrling, P. W. Parren, and D. R. Burton.** 2007. Neutralizing antibody fails to impact the course of Ebola virus infection in monkeys. *PLoS Pathog.* **3**:e9.
68. **Palacios, G., T. Briese, V. Kapoor, O. Jabado, Z. Liu, M. Venter, J. Zhai, N. Renwick, A. Grolla, T. W. Geisbert, C. Drosten, J. Towner, J. Ju, J. Paweska, S. T. Nichol, R. Swanepoel, H. Feldmann, P. B. Jahrling, and W. I. Lipkin.** 2006. MassTag polymerase chain reaction for differential diagnosis of viral hemorrhagic fever. *Emerg. Infect. Dis.* **12**:692–695.
69. **Palacios, G., P. L. Quan, O. J. Jabado, S. Conlan, D. L. Hirschberg, Y. Liu, J. Zhai, N. Renwick, J. Hui, H. Hegyi, A. Grolla, J. E. Strong, J. S. Towner, T. W. Geisbert, P. B. Jahrling, C. Buchen-Osmond, H. Ellerbrok, M. P. Sanchez-Seco, Y. Lussier, P. Formenty, M. S. Nichol, H. Feldmann, T. Briese, and W. I. Lipkin.** 2007. Panmicrobial oligonucleotide array for diagnosis of infectious diseases. *Emerg. Infect. Dis.* **13**:73–81.
70. **Panchal, R. G., G. Ruthel, T. A. Kenny, G. H. Kallstrom, D. Lane, S. S. Badie, L. Li, S. Bavari, and M. J. Aman.** 2003. In vivo oligomerization and raft localization of Ebola virus protein VP40 during vesicular budding. *Proc. Natl. Acad. Sci. USA* **100**:15936–15941.
71. **Parrino, J., R. Hotchkiss, and M. Bray.** 2007. Prevention of immune cell apoptosis as potential therapeutic strategy for severe infections. *Emerg. Infect. Dis.* **13**:191–198.
72. **Peterson, A. T., D. S. Carroll, J. N. Mills, and K. M. Johnson.** 2004. Potential mammalian filovirus reservoirs. *Emerg. Infect. Dis.* **10**:2073–2081.
73. **Pourrut, X., A. Delicat, P. Rollin, T. Ksiazek, J. Gonzalez, and E. Leroy.** 2007. Spatial and temporal patterns of Zaire Ebolavirus antibody prevalence in the possible reservoir bat species. *J. Infect. Dis.* **196**(Suppl. 2):S176–S183.
74. **Reid, S. P., L. W. Leung, A. L. Hartman, O. Martinez, M. L. Shaw, C. Carbonnelle, V. E. Volchkov, S. T. Nichol, and C. F. Basler.** 2006. Ebola virus VP24 binds karyopherin $\alpha 1$ and blocks STAT1 nuclear accumulation. *J. Virol.* **80**:5156–5167.
75. **Richards, G. A., S. Murphy, R. Jobson, M. Mer, C. Zinman, R. Taylor, R. Swanepoel, A. Duse, G. Sharp, I. C. De La Rey, and C. Kassianides.** 2000. Unexpected Ebola virus in a tertiary setting: clinical and epidemiologic aspects. *Crit. Care Med.* **28**:240–244.
76. **Roddy, P., D. Weatherill, B. Jeffs, Z. Abaakouk, P. N. Folo, M. H. Bengi, C. Dorion, P. Rodriguez, P. P. Palma, O. de la Rosa, L. Villa, I. Grovas, and M. Borchert.** 2007. The Médecins Sans Frontières intervention in the Marburg epidemic Uige/Angola, 2005—II: lessons learnt in the community. *J. Infect. Dis.* **196**(Suppl. 2):S162–S167.
77. **Rodriguez, L. L., A. De Roo, Y. Guimard, S. G. Trappier, A. Sanchez, D. Bressler, A. J. Williams, A. K. Rowe, J. Bertolli, A. S. Khan, T. G. Ksiazek, C. J. Peters, and S. T. Nichol.** 1999. Persistence and genetic stability of Ebola virus during the outbreak in Kikwit, Democratic Republic of the Congo, 1995. *J. Infect. Dis.* **179**(Suppl. 1):S170–S176.
78. **Rollin, P., D. Bausch, and A. Sanchez.** 2007. Blood chemistry measurements and D-dimer levels associated with fatal and nonfatal outcomes of Ebola virus (Sudan) disease in humans. *J. Infect. Dis.* **196**(Suppl. 2):S364–S371.
79. **Sadek, R. F., A. S. Khan, G. Stevens, C. J. Peters, and T. G. Ksiazek.** 1999. Ebola hemorrhagic fever, Democratic Republic of the Congo, 1995: determinants of survival. *J. Infect. Dis.* **179**(Suppl. 1):S24–S27.
80. **Sanchez, A., T. G. Ksiazek, P. E. Rollin, M. E. Miranda, S. G. Trappier, A. S. Khan, C. J. Peters, and S. T. Nichol.** 1999. Detection and molecular characterization of Ebola viruses causing disease in human and nonhuman primates. *J. Infect. Dis.* **179**(Suppl. 1):S164–S169.
81. **Sanchez, A., M. Lukwiya, D. Bausch, S. Mahanty, A. J. Sanchez, K. D. Wagoner, and P. E. Rollin.** 2004. Analysis of human peripheral blood samples from fatal and nonfatal cases of Ebola (Sudan) hemorrhagic fever: cellular responses, virus load, and nitric oxide levels. *J. Virol.* **78**:10370–10377.
82. **Sanchez, A., K. Wagoner, and P. Rollin.** 2007. Sequence-based HLA-B typing of patients infected with Ebola virus (Uganda 2000): identification of alleles associated with fatal and nonfatal disease. *J. Infect. Dis.* **196**(Suppl. 2):S329–S336.
83. **Sullivan, N. J., T. W. Geisbert, J. B. Geisbert, L. Xu, Z. Y. Yang, M. Roederer, R. A. Koup, P. B. Jahrling, and G. J. Nabel.** 2003. Accelerated vaccination for Ebola virus haemorrhagic fever in non-human primates. *Nature* **424**:681–684.
84. **Sullivan, N. J., A. Sanchez, P. E. Rollin, Z. Y. Yang, and G. J. Nabel.** 2000. Development of a preventive vaccine for Ebola virus infection in primates. *Nature* **408**: 605–609.
85. **Swanepoel, R., P. A. Leman, F. J. Burt, N. A. Zachariades, L. E. Braack, T. G. Ksiazek, P. E. Rollin, S. R. Zaki, and C. J. Peters.** 1996. Experimental inoculation of plants and animals with Ebola virus. *Emerg. Infect. Dis.* **2**:321–325.
86. **Theriault, S., A. Groseth, H. Artsob, and H. Feldmann.** 2005. The role of reverse genetics systems in determining filovirus pathogenicity. *Arch. Virol. Suppl.* **2005**:157–177.
87. **Towner, J., T. Sealy, T. Ksiazek, and S. Nichol.** 2007. High-throughput molecular detection of hemorrhagic fever virus threats with applications for outbreak settings. *J. Infect. Dis.* **196**(Suppl. 2):S205–S212.
88. **Towner, J. S., X. Pourrut, C. G. Albariño, C. N. Nkogue, B. H. Bird, G. Grard, T. G. Ksiazek, J.-P. Gonzalez, S. T. Nichol, and E. M. Leroy.** 2007. Marburg virus infection detected in a common African bat. *PLoS ONE* **2**:e764.
89. **Towner, J. S., P. E. Rollin, D. G. Bausch, A. Sanchez, S. M. Crary, M. Vincent, W. F. Lee, C. F. Spiropoulou, T. G. Ksiazek, M. Lukwiya, F. Kaducu, R. Downing, and S. T. Nichol.** 2004. Rapid diagnosis of Ebola hemorrhagic fever by reverse transcription-PCR in an outbreak setting and assessment of patient viral load as a predictor of outcome. *J. Virol.* **78**:4330–4341.
90. **Villinger, F., P. E. Rollin, S. S. Brar, N. F. Chikkala, J. Winter, J. B. Sundstrom, S. R. Zaki, R. Swanepoel, A. A. Ansari, and C. J. Peters.** 1999. Markedly elevated levels of interferon (IFN)-gamma, IFN-alpha, interleukin (IL)-2, IL-10, and tumor necrosis factor-alpha associated with fatal Ebola virus infection. *J. Infect. Dis.* **179**(Suppl. 1):S188–S191.
91. **Warfield, K. L., D. L. Swenson, G. G. Olinger, W. V. Kalina, M. J. Aman, and S. Bavari.** 2007. Ebola virus-like particle vaccine protects nonhuman primates against

lethal Ebola virus challenge. *J. Infect. Dis.* **196**(Suppl. 2): S430–S437.

92. **Warfield, K. L., D. L. Swenson, G. G. Olinger, D. K. Nichols, W. D. Pratt, R. Blouch, D. A. Stein, M. J. Aman, P. L. Iversen, and S. Bavari.** 2006. Gene-specific countermeasures against Ebola virus based on antisense phosphorodiamidate morpholino oligomers. *PLoS Pathog.* **2:**e1.
93. **Wilson, J. A., M. Bray, R. Bakken, and M. K. Hart.** 2001. Vaccine potential of Ebola virus VP24, VP30, VP35, and VP40 proteins. *Virology* **286:**384–390.
94. **Wilson, J. A., M. Hevey, R. Bakken, S. Guest, M. Bray, A. L. Schmaljohn, and M. K. Hart.** 2000. Epitopes involved in antibody-mediated protection from Ebola virus. *Science* **287:**1664–1666.
95. **Wool-Lewis, R. J., and P. Bates.** 1998. Characterization of Ebola virus entry by using pseudotyped viruses: identification of receptor-deficient cell lines. *J. Virol.* **72:** 3155–3160.
96. **World Health Organization.** 1978. Ebola haemorrhagic fever in Sudan, 1976. *Bull. W. H. O.* **56:**247–270.
97. **World Health Organization.** 1978. Ebola haemorrhagic fever in Zaire, 1976. *Bull. W. H. O.* **56:**271–293.
98. **World Health Organization.** 2001. Outbreak of Ebola hemorrhagic fever, Uganda, August 2000–January 2001. *Wkly. Epidemiol. Rec.* **76:**41–48.
99. **Zaki, S. R., W. J. Shieh, P. W. Greer, C. S. Goldsmith, T. Ferebee, J. Katshitshi, F. K. Tshioko, M. A. Bwaka, R. Swanepoel, P. Calain, A. S. Khan, E. Lloyd, P. E. Rollin, T. G. Ksiazek, and C. J. Peters for the Commission de Lutte contre les Epidémies à Kikwit.** 1999. A novel immunohistochemical assay for the detection of Ebola virus in skin: implications for diagnosis, spread, and surveillance of Ebola hemorrhagic fever. *J. Infect. Dis.* **179**(Suppl. 1)**:**S36–S47.

Influenza Virus

FREDERICK G. HAYDEN AND PETER PALESE

42

"If influenza is a riddle wrapped in mystery inside an enigma, then the viral genes are the riddle, the variable surface antigens for which they code are the mystery, and the course and cause of epidemics the ultimate enigma."
E. Kilbourne, 1980

Influenza viruses are unique among the viruses with regard to their antigenic variability, seasonality, and impact on the general population. They can cause explosive outbreaks of febrile respiratory illness across all age groups and often substantial mortality, particularly in aged and chronically ill persons. Epidemics resembling influenza have been recorded since antiquity. The plague of Athens in 430 to 427 BC, described by Thucydides, has been postulated to be due to epidemic influenza complicated by toxigenic staphylococcal disease (74). The greatest effects of influenza are seen when novel strains to which most persons are susceptible cause worldwide outbreaks, or pandemics. The most profound of these in modern times was the 1918 pandemic that claimed at least 40 million lives worldwide (66). Recently, sequencing of RNA fragments from tissue samples taken from 1918 pandemic victims enabled reconstruction of the extinct 1918 virus and study of its virulence in animal models (149, 157).

Influenza virus was first isolated from chickens with fowl plague in 1901. Swine influenza virus, possibly transmitted to swine from humans during the 1918 pandemic, was isolated initially in 1931, and the first human influenza A virus was recovered in 1933 (Fig. 1). Recognition of antigenic variation, growth in embryonated eggs, and the ability of virus to agglutinate erythrocytes followed shortly. These discoveries provided reliable means of virus isolation and serologic testing. Influenza B and C viruses were first isolated in 1940 and 1947, respectively. During the 1940s, crude inactivated vaccines were introduced, and these were followed by more purified, less reactogenic ones. In 1948, the World Health Organization (WHO) established an influenza surveillance program to monitor global activity and to facilitate strain selection for vaccines.

Among the first antiviral agents, amantadine and rimantadine were shown to have prophylactic and therapeutic activities for influenza A in the mid-1960s, and the neuraminidase (NA) inhibitors followed in the late 1990s. Despite the availability of improved vaccines and antivirals, seasonal influenza remains an important public health problem. The annual burden of interpandemic influenza in the United States has averaged approximately 20 million respiratory illnesses, over 200,000 hospitalizations, and 36,000 deaths in recent years (152).

VIROLOGY

Classification

Influenza A, B, and C viruses belong to the family *Orthomyxoviridae*, which is characterized by a segmented, negative-strand RNA genome (121). The influenza A and B virus types each carry eight different RNA segments, while the influenza C virus genome has only seven. Infections by strains of all three influenza types (genera) can be associated with classical influenza symptoms in humans. The fourth genus of the *Orthomyxoviridae* consists of the Thogoto viruses. Its members, Dhori and Thogoto viruses, are tick-borne agents which possess six and seven RNA segments, respectively, but are not recognized as human pathogens. The fifth orthomyxovirus genus is made up of the isaviruses (infectious salmon anemia virus).

The influenza A, B, and C virus types were defined originally by the observation that antisera made against the core proteins of a specific strain cross-reacted in complement fixation (CF) assays only with those belonging to the same type and not with those of another type. Sequencing studies have confirmed this classification scheme, showing that genes coding for the matrix protein (M1) or the nucleoprotein (NP) of strains belonging to one type are more closely related to each other than to the corresponding genes of strains from different influenza virus types; however, nucleotide sequence comparisons indicate that all influenza virus types share a common ancestor (121).

Subtypes occur only among the influenza A viruses. The extent of serologic cross-reactivity for the surface glycoproteins, the hemagglutinin (HA) and the NA, was previously used to differentiate them; more recently, sequencing of the corresponding genes has been used to differentiate them. Based on sequence analysis, 16 distinct HA and 9 distinct NA subtypes are now recognized in animal influenza viruses, but only 3 HA subtypes (H1, H2, and H3) and 2 NA subtypes (N1 and N2) are known to have caused extensive outbreaks in humans (Fig. 1). Virus strains are named on the basis of type, location of isolation, serial

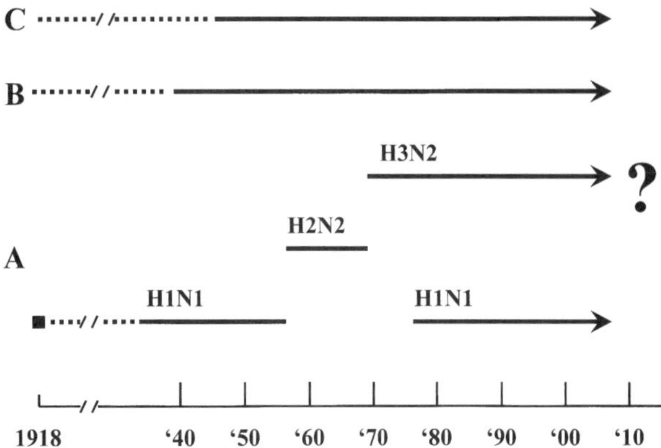

FIGURE 1 Circulation of human influenza A, B, and C viruses. Solid lines indicate that strains have been isolated and characterized. Three different influenza A virus HA subtypes (H1, H2, and H3) and two NA subtypes (N1 and N2) were identified in humans during the 20th century. The RNA genome of the extinct pandemic 1918 virus has been sequenced from RNA fragments in formalin-fixed and frozen tissue samples from 1918 victims following RT-PCR (149). The virus was then reconstructed in the laboratory by reverse genetics (solid square) (157).

number from that location, year of isolation, and, in the case of influenza A viruses, the subtypes of the HA and NA antigens [e.g., A/Brisbane/10/2006 (H3N2)].

Composition

Influenza viruses are spherical lipid-containing viruses with a diameter of approximately 120 nm (Fig. 2A). Filamentous forms of the virus can also be observed with electron microscopy, appear to be infectious, and are postulated to be predominant particles during productive infection in the lungs. The activities and functions of the viral structural and nonstructural (NS) proteins are summarized in Table 1. The virus surface is covered by HA and NA glycoprotein spikes, the structures of which have been resolved by X-ray diffraction (21, 162). A small number of molecules of the M2 protein are also found in the membrane of the virus particle. Below the lipid membrane is a layer of the M1 protein surrounding the ribonucleoprotein (RNP) core. This core consists of the eight RNA segments which are associated with one to several copies of the viral polymerase complex (PB1, PB2, and PA) proteins and are covered by viral NP molecules.

Surface Proteins

The HA is a trimeric rod-shaped spike with a hydrophobic carboxy terminus anchored in the viral envelope and the hydrophilic end projecting outward from the virus. The exposed portion contains the antigenic domains and binding sites for sialic acid (*N*-acetylneuraminic acid) residues in receptors of host cells or erythrocytes (Fig. 2B). The HA facilitates both attachment of the virus to host cell receptors and penetration of the virus. Posttranslational proteolytic cleavage into HA1 and HA2 by a serine protease is essential for infectivity. Certain avian HAs (H5 and H7) contain extra basic amino acids in the HA cleavage site, which allow for activation by cellular proteases (e.g., furin) widely distributed in tissues and result in systemic replication in birds and sometimes mammalian hosts (60). These so-called highly pathogenic avian influenza (HPAI) viruses have caused multiple outbreaks in poultry and, recently, sporadic disease in humans (Table 2). The HA2 portion appears to be responsible for fusion of the virus envelope and cell membrane, whereas the HA1 portion contains the binding sites for host cell receptors, as well as at least four major antigenic domains. The overall configuration of the HA and its functions are conserved during virus evolution, but frequent amino acid substitutions occur in the antigenic sites. Antibodies to HA neutralize viral infectivity; antibodies to HA2 do not prevent infection but reduce viral replication in animal models.

NA is a mushroom-shaped tetramer that is anchored in the lipid envelope at its amino terminus (20). It cleaves terminal sialic acid residues from various glycoconjugates and plays an essential role in release of virus from infected cells and spread within the respiratory tract. By removing sialic acid residues from the virion envelope and cell surface and from mucins present in respiratory tract secretions, the NA activity (receptor-destroying enzyme [RDE]) prevents aggregation of viral particles and may enable penetration of virus through respiratory secretions (121). One strain, A/WSN/33(HlN1), possesses an NA capable of binding plasminogen, which in turn causes HA cleavage activation and increased virulence. Anti-NA antibodies and NA enzyme inhibitors prevent release of virus from infected cells. A balance of HA and NA activities is essential for efficient virus replication.

The M2 protein, present only in influenza A viruses, appears on the surface of infected cells and is also incorporated into virions as a third integral membrane protein. The ion channel activity of M2 plays a role in uncoating of virus in endosomes and possibly in regulation of virus assembly. Antibody to M2 is associated with reduced viral replication and heterosubtypic protection in animals (34). M2 is the viral target of amantadine and rimantadine. The BM2 protein of influenza B viruses is possibly the homolog of the M2 protein of the A viruses. In addition to HA, NA, and BM2 proteins, the influenza B viruses have a fourth protein (NB) inserted into their lipid membrane.

The single glycoprotein of influenza C virus encompasses receptor-binding, membrane-fusing, and receptor-destroying activities. It is directed against 9-*O*-acetyl-*N*-acetylneuraminic acid, a receptor different from *N*-acetylneuraminic acid, which is recognized by influenza A and B viruses (121).

Genome

Influenza A and B viruses each possess eight different RNA segments that can code for 11 different proteins (Fig. 3A). Influenza C viruses lack an NA gene and thus have only seven RNA segments that code for at least nine different polypeptides. In nature, a reassortment of gene segments after coinfection of cells by human and animal influenza A viruses may be responsible for the emergence of new pandemic strains (see below and Fig. 4). However, reassortment of genes among viruses belonging to different influenza virus types has not been observed. Apparently, the proteins of different virus types have evolved sufficiently to preclude replication of intertypic reassortants. In addition, recombination is a very rare event. Homologous recombination between corresponding RNA segments of different influenza viruses has not been observed, in contrast to the high frequency of recombination observed among the genomes of positive-sense RNA viruses, like

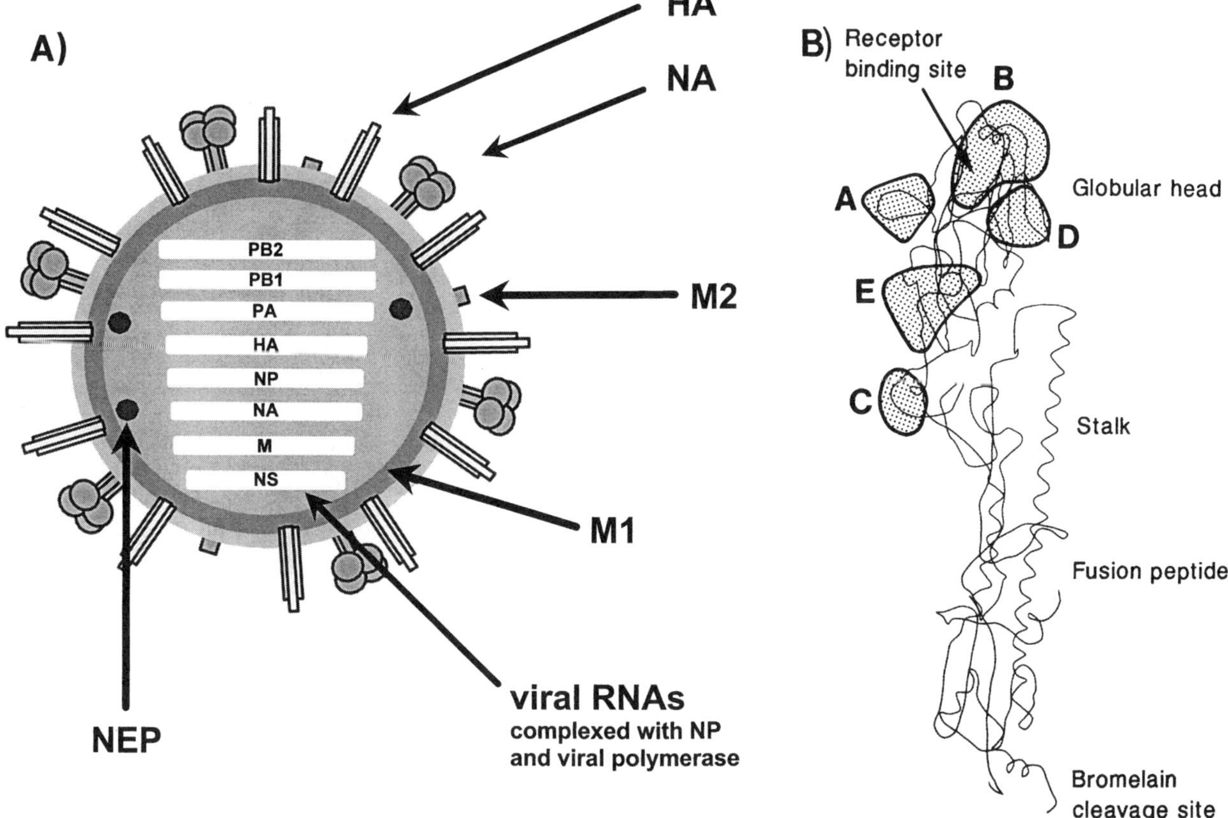

FIGURE 2 (A) Schematic diagram of an influenza A virus. HA, NA, and M2 are transmembrane proteins anchored in the lipid membrane of the virus. Inside the lipid membrane is a layer of the M1 protein. The RNP core consists of the different RNA segments which are covered by NP molecules. In addition, they carry an RNA-dependent RNA polymerase complex (P proteins). The RNA segments possess a panhandle-fork-corkscrew structure which appears to be stabilized by base pairing between the 3′ and 5′ ends of the RNAs. NEP is also part of the viral core structure. (B) Schematic depiction of influenza virus HA. Antigenic changes cluster into five highly variable regions (A to E) surrounding the receptor-binding pocket. The latter is too small to allow ingress of antibody and remains conserved. See Color Plate 25 depicting the interaction of neutralizing antibody with HA. (Panel B courtesy of Robert Webster, St. Jude Children's Hospital, Memphis, TN.)

TABLE 1 Influenza A virus RNA segments and proteins

RNA segment	Protein	Protein size (amino acids)	Functional activity(ies)
1	PB2	759	Cap binding, endonuclease
2	PB1	757	RNA polymerase
	PB1-F2	87	Proapoptotic acivity
3	PA	716	RNA polymerase subunit, proteolysis
4	HA	~560	Attachment to receptors, fusion of membranes
5	NP	498	Structural component of RNP, nuclear import of RNA
6	NA	~450	NA/sialidase activity, release of virus
7	M1	252	Structural protein, nuclear export of RNA, viral budding
	M2	96	Ion channel
8	NS1	~230	Interferon antagonist, possible role in viral gene expression
	NEP (NS2)	121	Nuclear export factor

TABLE 2 Recent examples of human illness due to infection by avian influenza viruses[a]

Yr	Location	Influenza A subtype	No. of laboratory-confirmed human illnesses	Primary syndrome/comment
1996	United Kingdom	H7N7 (LP)	1	Conjunctivitis
1997	Hong Kong SAR	H5N1 (HP)	18	Pneumonia; six deaths
1999	Hong Kong SAR	H9N2 (LP)	2	ILI
2002	Virginia	H7N2 (LP)	1	ILI
2003	China, Hong Kong SAR	H5N1 (HP)	2	ARI; one death plus one other ARI death in a family member
2003	The Netherlands	H7N7 (HP)	89	Conjunctivitis (78 cases), ILI ± conjunctivitis (7 cases), other (4 cases); 1 fatal pneumonia. Limited human-human transmission likely.
2003	Hong Kong SAR	H9N2 (LP)	1	ILI
2003	New York	H7N2 (LP)	1	ARI in immunocompromised host
2004	Egypt	H10N7 (LP)	2	ILI
2004	Canada	H7N3 (LP) H7N3 (HP)	1 1	Conjunctivitis
2004–present[b]	Asia, Middle East, eastern Europe, Africa	H5N1 (HP)	>350[b]	Pneumonia, ARDS; mortality rate, approximately 63%. Limited, nonsustained human-human transmission to date[b]
2007	United Kingdom	H7N2 (LP)	4	ILI, conjunctivitis
2007	Hong Kong SAR	H9N2 (LP)	1	ARI

[a] Abbreviations: LP, low chicken pathogenicity; HP, high chicken pathogenicity; ILI, influenza-like illness; ARI, acute respiratory illness (not specified).
[b] Consult the WHO and CDC websites for updated information.

polioviruses, and retroviruses. Occasionally, nonhomologous recombination (mostly with cellular RNA) possibly resulting from a "jumping" polymerase has been observed in influenza virus RNAs; this recombination may have accounted for emergence of an HPAI virus in several instances (122). Influenza A virus isolates obtained during a single outbreak are variable in genetic sequence. This genetic heterogeneity provides a basis for evolutionary adaptation and the ability of the virus to cope with selective immunologic and drug pressures.

The complete genomes of the influenza A, B, and C viruses have been sequenced. Influenza A viruses code for approximately 13,600 nucleotides (nt) (73), influenza B viruses for 14,600 nt, and influenza C viruses for approximately 12,900 nt (168). A genomic map of an influenza A virus is shown in Fig. 3. Each RNA codes for a different protein, with the two smallest RNA segments each transcribing an additional spliced mRNA.

Biology

Replication Strategy

Influenza A and B viruses adsorb to receptors on the cell surface which contain sialic acid (121) (Fig. 5). It is not known whether the natural receptors are glycolipids carrying sialic acids or whether specific carbohydrate-containing membrane proteins are the major target for the initial binding. Human influenza viruses preferentially attach to sialic acid with an $\alpha(2,6)$ linkage to galactose-containing oligosaccharides, whereas avian and equine viruses prefer $\alpha(2,3)$ linkages. Influenza C virus binds to 9-*O*-acetyl-*N*-acetylneuraminic acid-bearing receptors. After internalization into endosomes, the cleaved HA undergoes an acid pH-triggered conformational change into a fusogenic form. This event facilitates the fusion of the viral and endosomal membranes. The ion channel in the viral membrane comprised of M2 polypeptides is also activated by the acid pH in the endosomes. This process results in an influx of protons into the virion interior, which probably loosens the M1 protein from the RNP core and ultimately facilitates RNP release into the cytoplasm (uncoating). The RNA of the incoming virus particle (vRNA) remains associated with viral protein throughout the uncoating process and enters the nucleus as RNP through the nuclear pore complex (116).

Following uncoating of the virus and transportation of the RNP into the nucleus, transcription and replication of the viral genome take place in the nucleus. The incoming viral RNP is the template for the viral RNA-dependent RNA polymerase, which produces two different species of viral RNA: (i) an mRNA that derives its first 9 to 15 nt from host mRNA, is capped at the 5′ end, and carries a poly(A) tail lacking the 3′ 15 to 16 nt of the template RNA, and (ii) a full-length complementary copy (cRNA) of the template RNA. This cRNA itself becomes a template for the amplification of viral RNAs, leading to additional copies of vRNA (Fig. 6). The minimal promoter sequences of the vRNA and the cRNA molecules appear to be the highly conserved 3′ sequences. In addition, the 5′ sequences of the templates are part of the transcription-replication complex (50) (Fig. 6). Both the vRNA- and the cRNA-RNP templates appear to have panhandle-fork-corkscrew structures (36, 38).

mRNA synthesis is regulated, but control of the switch from transcription (mRNA synthesis) to replication (amplification of vRNA) is not well understood. Although the different vRNA molecules appear to be equimolar in the virus and in infected cells, the mRNAs of the HA, M, NP, and NS genes are much more abundant than those of the

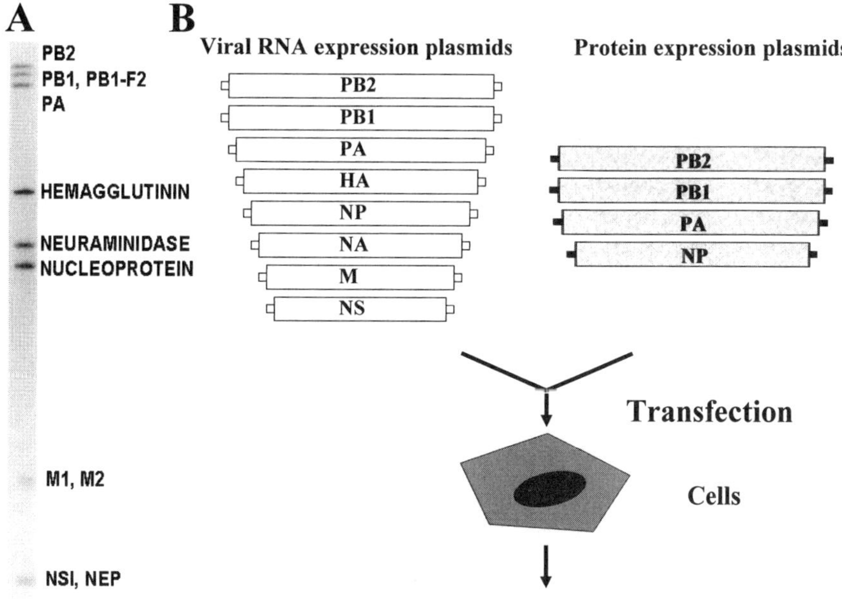

FIGURE 3 (A) Genetic map of influenza A/PR/8/34 (H1N1) virus. Purified RNAs were separated on a polyacrylamide gel; assignment of genes coding for one or two viral proteins is indicated. (B) Plasmid-only rescue of infectious influenza virus. Twelve plasmids are introduced into mammalian cells: four plasmids lead to expression of the viral proteins required for viral RNA replication (PA, PB1, PB2, and NP), and eight plasmids express precise copies of the eight viral RNA segments (PA, PB1, PB2, HA, NP, NA, M, and NS). The resulting viral RNAs are replicated and transcribed by the reconstituted influenza virus RNA-dependent RNA polymerase. Recombinant infectious influenza virus is generated 48 to 72 h after transfection of cells (37, 107). Recently, several improvements of the plasmid-only rescue for influenza A viruses have been introduced (119). Also, reverse-genetics systems for influenza B and C viruses have been successfully developed (23, 59, 63, 99).

three polymerase (P) genes or of the NA gene. Also, mRNA synthesis is down-regulated altogether late in the replication cycle, while vRNA synthesis continues. Finally, protein expression is affected by several additional mechanisms: (i) for the M and NS genes, partial splicing of their mRNAs leads to the expression of two viral proteins from each of these RNA segments; (ii) coupled stop-start translation of tandem cistrons gives rise to two proteins, the M and the BM2 proteins, from the M segment of influenza B viruses; and (iii) ribosomal initiation from AUG codons located in different reading frames on the PB1 gene of influenza A viruses and on the NA gene of influenza B viruses leads to the expression of two additional proteins, PB1-F2 and NB, respectively (in addition to the PB1 and NA proteins of the corresponding RNAs) (19, 121).

Assembly and packaging of RNAs into infectious viruses involve several cellular compartments. The viral P proteins and the NP have specific nuclear localization signals, so they can travel into the nucleus, where they associate with viral RNAs to form RNPs. The nuclear export of these RNPs likewise requires a unique mechanism and depends critically on the presence of the M1 protein and nuclear export protein (NEP) (88, 117). M1 binds to viral RNPs in the nucleus and promotes their export by interacting with NEP, which possesses a nuclear export signal and the ability to interact with M1 (1, 117). The virus-induced Raf/MEK/ERK signal cascade is essential for efficient replication, and blockade of this pathway slows viral RNP export and reduces viral titers.

Following the export of the RNPs into the cytoplasm, they assemble at the cytoplasmic membrane under patches of the viral glycoproteins HA and NA. M1 plays a critical role in the assembly and budding of infectious virus. Virus particles bud from the cytoplasmic membrane, while the NA clears the virus and the cell membrane of sialic acids to prevent virus-virus aggregation and virus-cell surface retention, respectively. Once the virus particle is outside the cell, the NA may further help to remove sialic acids from mucous substances in the respiratory tract, thus allowing the virus to reach other epithelial cells.

The packaging of vRNAs into influenza virus particles most likely involves a specific packaging mechanism: the 3′ and 5′ noncoding regions of the vRNA segments contain *cis*-acting signals which are required for packaging the vRNAs into virus particles. In addition, sequences in the coding regions of the influenza A virus RNAs contribute to the efficient packaging of just the eight different segments in virus particles (39, 87). Thus, the available evidence points away from a random packaging model, although the precise mechanism by which the packaging of a full complement of just eight RNAs occurs remains to be elucidated.

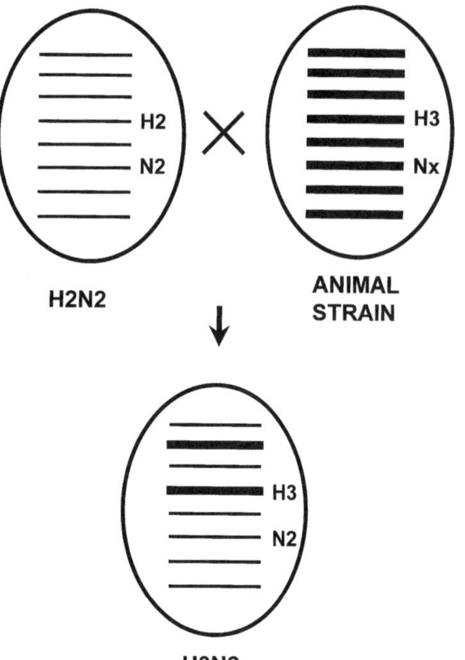

FIGURE 4 Reassortment of influenza A viruses leading to a new pandemic strain. Coinfection of the same cell with a human H2N2 (thin lines) virus and an animal (avian) strain with an H3 HA (thick lines) results in reassortment. The H3N2 virus responsible for the pandemic in 1968 is postulated to derive its PB1 and H3 genes (thick lines) from the animal strain and its remaining six RNAs, including the N2 gene, from the H2N2 parent (thin lines) (105).

Genetic Engineering of Influenza Viruses

The genome of negative-sense RNA viruses is not infectious, and thus transfection of cDNA-derived influenza virus RNAs does not result in the formation of infectious virus particles. However, systems have been developed which allow the in vitro reconstitution of biologically active RNP from synthetic RNAs and purified viral proteins. Transfection of synthetic RNPs into helper virus-infected cells allowed the rescue of transfectant viruses which contain one or more genetically engineered segments (42). Recently, new helper virus-free systems for producing recombinant influenza A viruses have been developed (37, 107) (Fig. 3B). Plasmids are transfected into cells, and infectious virus can be generated within 48 to 72 h. In these plasmid-only systems, the vRNAs, as well as the viral RNA polymerase, are generated from the transfected plasmids. Improvements in this technology now make it easy to do structure-function analysis of individual viral proteins and have opened the way for the construction of improved influenza virus vaccines and influenza virus vectors (119). Reverse-genetics systems have also been successfully developed for influenza B and C viruses (23, 59, 63).

Host Range

Type A influenza viruses have a broad host range (60, 115). Wild avian species, particularly ducks and other aquatic waterfowl, are the primary reservoir and harbor all known 16 HA and 9 NA subtypes. Other principal natural hosts of influenza A viruses are humans, swine, and horses. Outbreaks have also been documented for other species, including marine mammals (whales and seals), mink, dogs, and ruminants (e.g., reindeer). In avian species, influenza viruses replicate in both the respiratory and gastrointestinal tracts, and there can be shedding of high quantities of virus

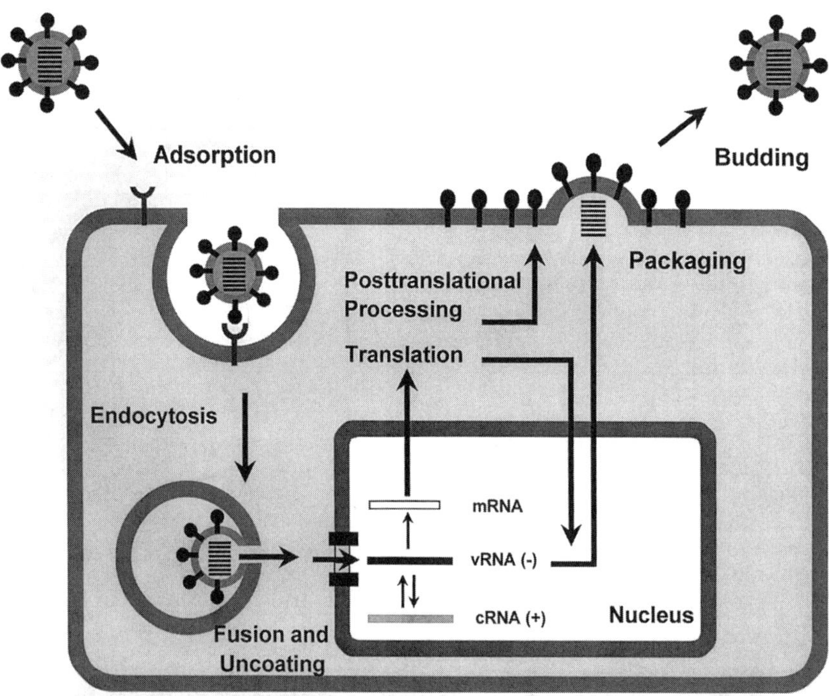

FIGURE 5 Replication of influenza virus. For a description of different replication steps, see the text.

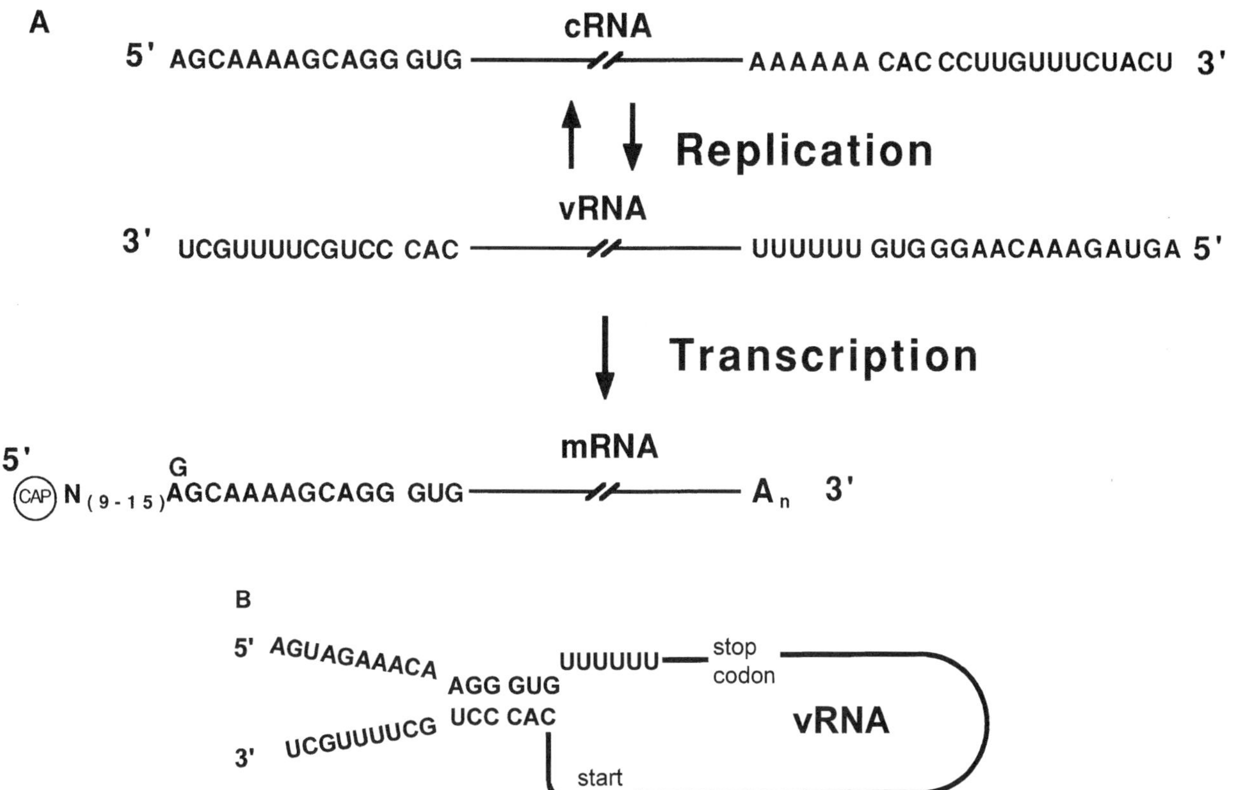

FIGURE 6 Transcription and replication of influenza virus RNAs. (A) The 3′-terminal 15 nt and the 5′-terminal 22 nt of an NS gene (vRNA) are shown. The 3′-terminal 12 nt and the 5′-terminal 13 nt are highly conserved among influenza virus RNAs. The six U's at the 5′ end are part of the polyadenylation signal. Transcription leads to a polyadenylated mRNA which is primed by short capped RNA molecules derived from nascent cellular transcripts and terminates at the stretch of six U's near the 5′ end of the incoming vRNA. Full-length cRNAs are copied from vRNAs and are then used as templates for the generation of new vRNA molecules. All RNAs are shown as linear molecules. (B) The vRNA is represented here by a panhandle-fork structure. The 3′ and 5′ ends are postulated to base pair, but it is not known which RNA structure (panhandle-fork-corkscrew) is the predominant one in vivo.

in the feces. Infectious virus is readily recovered from cold lakes and other water sources frequented by birds. In contrast to the progressive changes of human viruses, avian viruses generally show little antigenic variation within the same subtype, although the rapid evolution and antigenic variation of HPAI A (H5N1) viruses is an exception (143, 161). Thus, aquatic birds represent an enormous migratory reservoir of influenza A virus genes that can be potentially incorporated into influenza viruses transmitted to other species.

The fact that influenza A viruses populate nonhuman species has important consequences for the epidemiology of the virus. First, reassortment among human and nonhuman influenza A viruses may lead to new pandemic viruses (see Fig. 4 and below). Second, the presence of an animal reservoir will enable the virus to continue to circulate outside the human population, so eradication of human influenza A by immunization of humans is unlikely. Influenza B and C viruses are primarily pathogens of humans, but influenza B virus may infect seals, dogs, cats, and possibly swine. However, widespread animal-to-animal or human-to-animal transmission of influenza B viruses has not been identified to date. Influenza C viruses have been isolated from swine.

Full explanations do not exist currently for the host range characteristics of the different influenza viruses. The virulence and host range of influenza viruses relate to the surface glycoproteins, as well as to other viral proteins (121). Experimental infection has been accomplished in a variety of species, including hamsters, cotton rats, guinea pigs, horses, and nonhuman primates, but mice, ferrets, chickens, and swine are most commonly used. Pigs can be experimentally infected with avian influenza viruses representing nearly all HA subtypes. Ferrets can be infected with nonadapted human influenza viruses and serve as a useful model for studying viral virulence and transmission (85, 157). Recently, a transmission model for influenza viruses was developed using guinea pigs (81).

Growth in Cell Culture

Traditionally, influenza viruses have been grown in embryonated chicken eggs, both for laboratory purposes and for vaccine production. Primary cell cultures, including African green and rhesus monkey, hamster, bovine, or chicken kidney cells and established cell lines like Madin-Darby canine kidney (MDCK) and mink lung epithelial cells, can be used to replicate influenza viruses (126). Propagation in nonprimary cell lines lacking the protease needed for HA cleavage requires the addition of trypsin in serum-free medium. Although plaque assays provide a more accurate and sensitive quantitation of infectious virus, hemagglutination by chicken or human erythrocytes remains a frequently used tool to identify and measure the replication of influenza viruses in eggs and cell culture. Future influenza vaccine manufacturing will rely increasingly on the growth of virus in cell culture to avoid the cumbersome use of embryonated eggs, and various cell systems are being developed or already used for vaccine virus production (e.g., MDCK, Per.C6, and Vero).

Inactivation by Physical and Chemical Agents

Influenza virus proteins and RNAs can be readily inactivated by ionizing radiation, high (>9) or low (<5) pH, and temperatures above 50°C. The stability of the virus depends on the surrounding medium, its protein concentration, and its ionic strength. Influenza viruses are enveloped viruses and thus are susceptible to all agents which affect membranes, including ionic and nonionic detergents, chlorination, and organic solvents (25). At 4°C in phosphate-buffered saline solution containing physiological protein (albumin) concentrations, influenza viruses are stable for months. On the other hand, drying of viral suspensions inactivates the virus in less than 12 h on porous environmental surfaces and in 24 to 48 h on nonporous environmental surfaces (4, 10). The virus can remain infectious for 24 h or more after aerosolization under conditions of low (25%) or high (80%) relative humidity but is less stable under conditions of intermediate (50%) relative humidity (137).

EPIDEMIOLOGY

Influenza viruses have a worldwide distribution and cause outbreaks with variable intensities annually. Rapid onset and dissemination of infection are characteristic features of epidemic influenza. These relate to a short incubation period, which averages 2 days and ranges from 1 to 5 days, and high concentrations of virus in respiratory secretions during the initial phase of illness. Influenza surveillance information is available through the Centers for Disease Control and Prevention (CDC) website (http://www.cdc.gov/ncidod/diseases/flu/weekly/htm).

Transmission

Influenza viruses spread from person to person by airborne droplets expelled during coughing, sneezing, or speaking. The relative contributions to transmission of droplet, short-distance small-particle aerosols, and hand contamination self-inoculation routes of exposure are currently uncertain (11). Zoonotic influenza virus infections (discussed below; Table 2) are also spread by these routes through direct and indirect exposures and perhaps rarely by gastrointestinal infection. For human viruses, the human infectious dose is estimated to be 1 to 5 50% tissue culture infectious doses following experimental small-particle (1 to 5 μm) aerosol exposure. Aerosol dissemination has been shown to occur in ferrets and guinea pigs (81, 82) and implicated in outbreaks, where clinical attack rates may exceed 70% after common-source exposure in confined spaces (134). Influenza virus RNA is readily detected on fomites (10), and virus retains infectiousness longer on hard, nonporous surfaces, in low humidity, and at cooler temperatures (4, 81), but the importance of transmission via fomites is unclear. One hypothesis, that epidemic spread involves long-range atmospheric transmission of aerosolized influenza virus, remains unconfirmed. The biological, environmental, and social factors that contribute to influenza seasonality are complex and incompletely understood (80).

Antigenic Change

The changing antigenicity of influenza viruses enables continued circulation in human populations and makes their behavior unpredictable (44). Relatively minor changes, called antigenic drift, result from stepwise point mutations in the gene segment coding for the HA or NA. Sequential amino acid changes in antigenically important regions accumulate over a period of years. In the case of influenza A virus, these result from the selective pressure of increasing levels of population immunity and lead to the emergence of epidemiologically important drift variants every 2 to 3 years. Amino acid substitutions in HA and NA have been observed at rates of approximately 0.5 to 1% per year over a two-decade period. Changes occur predominantly in the HA1 peptide and are distributed over the surface of the molecule, as well as clustering into five hypervariable regions (Fig. 2B; see Color Plate 25). Viral lineages undergoing the greatest number of mutations in a restricted number of rapidly evolving HA1 codons appear to be the progenitors of future epidemic strains (14). Drift strains of epidemiological importance usually have mutations in two or more of the antigenic sites of the HA and arise when such mutations lead to substantial antigenic change (72). Such variants have reduced susceptibility to preexisting immunity in the population and are able to spread because of larger numbers of susceptible individuals and a higher likelihood of causing symptomatic infections. Antigenic variation has occurred more rapidly in H3 than H1 viruses and is less pronounced in influenza B and C viruses. Multiple evolutionary lines of influenza B or C viruses may cocirculate. Viruses representing two influenza B virus lineages, designated B/Victoria/2/87 and B/Yamagata/16/88, have circulated in various proportions in recent years. Seasonal influenza viruses undergo frequent reassortment that contributes to their evolution and genetic diversity. New antigenic variants of public health concern are usually identified by monospecific antisera raised in animals, typically ferrets, and by convalescent-phase sera from persons immunized with vaccines containing previous strains.

For influenza A viruses, marked changes in HA with or without change in NA, called antigenic shift, are due to the acquisition of new gene segments. This may occur during genetic reassortment in cells dually infected by a human and an animal virus (Fig. 4) or possibly by direct interspecies transmission (60). When such viruses are introduced into a population that has no preexisting immunity, they can lead to the generation of pandemics.

Pandemic Influenza

Over the past 300 years, at least six pandemics of influenza have probably occurred, including three well-characterized ones in the 20th century (128). These have appeared at irregular intervals and been notable for high illness rates in all susceptible age groups, particularly in young persons, and usually for significant increases in mortality rates (Table 3). Pandemics have spread globally over 6- to 9-

TABLE 3 Influenza A virus pandemics and other important influenza events during the past century

Yr(s) of appearance	Duration of circulation (yr)	Virus subtype	Common designation	Estimated mortality in the United States	Comment
1889	?28	H3N?[a]		High	Estimated mortality of 270,000–360,000 in Europe
1918	39	H1N1	Spanish, swine	548,000	Ancestor likely avian
1957	11	H2N2	Asian	86,000	Avian reassortant
1968	Ongoing	H3N2	Hong Kong	34,000	Avian reassortant
1976	<1	H1N1	Swine	1 death	Outbreak limited to one U.S. military base
1977	Ongoing	H1N1	Russian	Negligible	Reappearance of earlier circulating virus
1997, 2003	Ongoing in poultry	H5N1	Avian, bird, or chicken	Not applicable	First proven avian-human transmission

[a] The subtype designation of this virus is uncertain but is proposed on the basis of retrospective serologic studies of elderly adults who were living at the times of the pandemic (30).

month periods. Because they spread at the pace of human traffic and often irrespective of season, future pandemics are likely to disseminate more rapidly, in part because of air travel patterns (32). Second and sometimes third waves of infection separated by several months may occur. At least two of the 20th-century pandemic strains appeared to have emerged from China.

Cumulative illness rates have often exceeded 50% in the general population during successive waves of a pandemic. Older adults usually experience lower illness frequency, perhaps related to prior experience with related viruses, but the case fatality ratios are usually highest in the very young and elderly. However, the 1918 pandemic caused an increase in mortality in young adults up to the age of 30. The relatively low rate of mortality of people older than 30 years of age is compatible with the idea that an H1 virus circulated in the human population before 1889 and resulted in partial protection against the 1918 virus in the older segment of the population (120). During the 1918 pandemic, >30-fold differences in population mortality occurred across countries and about 4-fold differences occurred within countries, including the United States (101). In the era encompassing virus isolation, pandemics in 1957 and to a lesser extent in 1968 also caused increases in mortality compared to interpandemic periods (Table 3). In each of the 20th-century pandemics, large portions of the excess influenza-related deaths (>99% in 1918, 36% in 1957, and 48% in 1968) occurred in those aged <65 years, followed by smaller proportions over the subsequent decade (140). In contrast, disease due to the reappearance of an H1N1 subtype virus in 1977, after a 20-year hiatus since circulation of essentially the same strain, principally affected those younger than 25 years and caused negligible excess mortality.

Serologic studies with elderly individuals suggest that viruses with HA of the H3 subtype caused pandemic disease in the late 19th century (Table 2) (30). The origin of these pandemic strains and the mechanisms for apparent recycling of strains in the human population remain unresolved issues. Explanations include dormancy in a frozen state, which appears to be likely for the 1977 H1N1 strain; interspecies transmission and adaptation of an animal influenza virus to become infectious and pathogenic for humans; and, more commonly, reassortment of genes between animal and human influenza viruses. Analysis of the 1957 pandemic strain found that this H2N2 subtype virus resulted from acquisition of three new gene segments (HA, NA, and PB1) of avian origin by the previously circulating human H1N1 strain. Similarly, the 1968 pandemic H3N2 virus acquired two new genes (HA and PB1) from an avian virus closely related to viruses isolated from ducks in Asia in 1963 (165) (Fig. 4).

Changes in the receptor specificity of the avian influenza virus HA appear to be a key factor in generation of viruses that are capable of sustained human transmission, and the HAs of all pandemic viruses characterized to date bind to human-like α2,6-sialylated glycans. One or two amino acid changes can alter receptor binding patterns of the 1918 virus HA and reduce transmissibility among ferrets without altering replication or lethality, although the predictive value of this model for human transmission is uncertain, and one 1918 virus HA from a fatal case shows dual α2,3 and α2,6 binding (158). Avian H5N1 viruses transmit inefficiently or not at all among ferrets and have failed to show sustained human-to-human transmission, despite several H5N1 HAs showing mutations associated with dual α2,3 and α2,6 binding (167). However, an H5N1 virus engineered to bind preferentially to α2,6 receptors also was not transmitted among ferrets, and changes in multiple genes are likely necessary to generate a pandemic virus (85).

Although avian viruses cannot usually directly infect humans, swine can be infected by both human and avian viruses and may serve as an intermediate host needed for reassortment of these viruses, the so-called "mixing vessel," or as the species in which avian viruses can adapt to a mammalian host. Avian-human reassortment and avian-like influenza A viruses with limited zoonotic spread to humans have been identified in swine (103). However, the pig has not been positively identified as the intermediate host for any of the known pandemic strains. The origin of the genes of the 1918 pandemic strain remains unknown, but it is likely that some of the genes were derived from avian influenza viruses (149, 157).

The concept of China and Southeast Asia as the site of origin or epicenter of new pandemic viruses is supported by the presence of high concentrations and cohabitation of domestic avian species (especially ducks), swine, and humans. The avian reservoir provides a mechanism for maintaining the virus while not circulating in humans and a source for the introduction of influenza virus subtypes into humans. For example, avian viruses which contain an antigenically conserved H2 HA similar to that of the 1957 pandemic strain continue to circulate in birds and were recently identified in swine (84). H1N1 viruses, derived from that responsible for the 1918 pandemic, continue to circulate in domestic swine and occasionally cause human infections (103).

Epidemic Influenza

Seasonality

Influenza activities of various intensities occur annually in temperate areas, most often during the winter or early spring months (44) (Fig. 7). The distinct seasonality of epidemic influenza appears to be related to reintroduction of virus each season, behavioral factors influencing exposure (e.g., school and indoor crowding), factors affecting viral survival in the environment (e.g., low temperature and relative humidity), and/or host determinants influenced by seasonal changes (80, 81). Antigenic and genetic analyses indicate that H3N2 epidemics in temperate regions are seeded from an area of continuous virus circulation with temporally overlapping epidemics in East-Southeast Asia and not from persistent circulation of virus in temperate areas during the summer months (133a).

The onset of influenza activity ranges from October to April in the northern hemisphere but usually peaks between December and March. Influenza typically peaks between May and August in the southern hemisphere. Activity may occur year-round in the tropics, but seasonal variation with epidemics, more often during high-rainfall periods, is evident. Summertime outbreaks may occur on cruise ships and among large groups of land-based travelers, especially when new antigenic variants have emerged elsewhere. Consequently, an influenza diagnosis should be considered during the summer in those with febrile respiratory illness who have recently traveled in the tropics, in the southern hemisphere, or with international groups.

In a given community or region, outbreaks due to a particular virus usually peak in about 3 weeks and are of short duration (6 to 10 weeks). Successive or overlapping waves of infection by different influenza A subtypes and influenza B virus may cause prolonged influenza activity. Influenza B viruses cause widespread epidemics every 3 to 4 years, but cocirculation of two or three influenza viruses

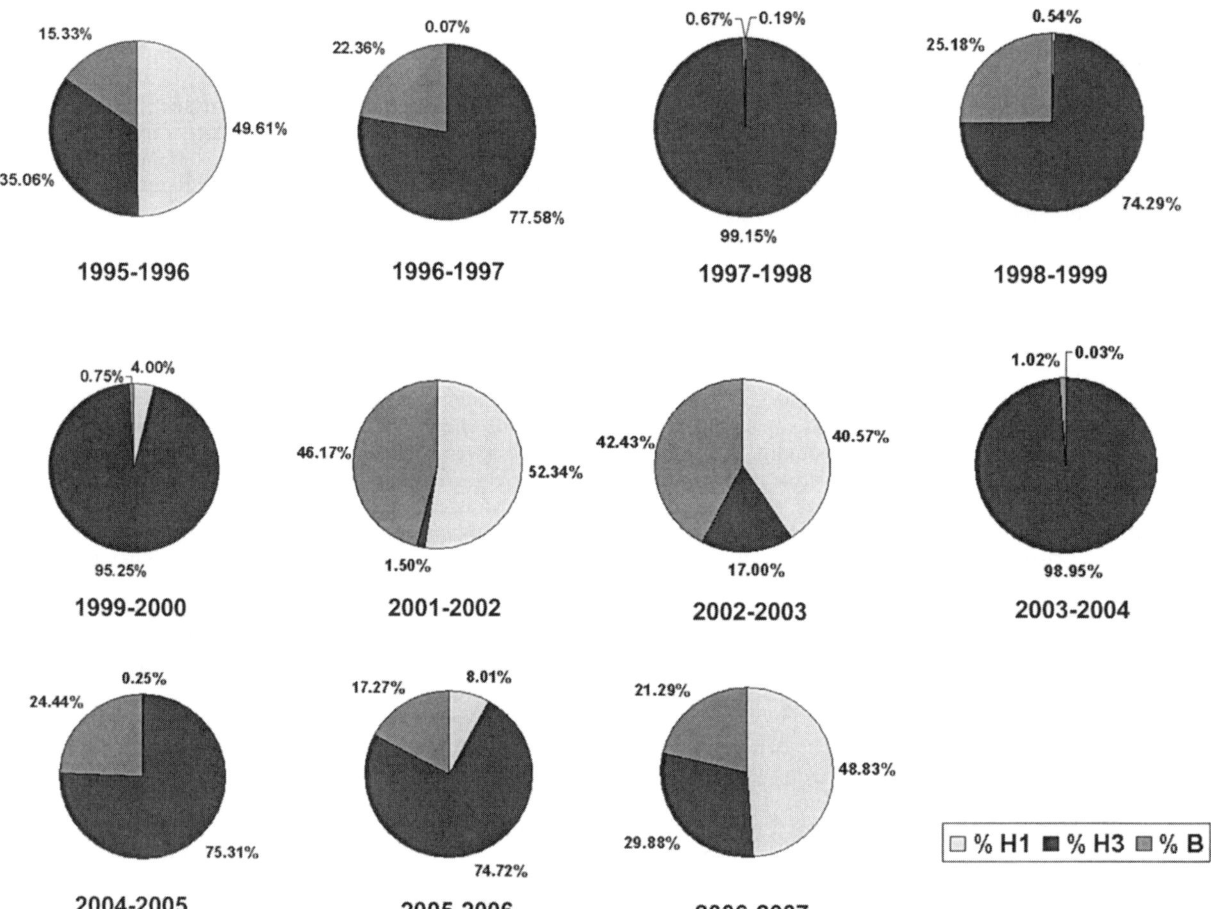

FIGURE 7 Influenza activity in the United States, 1995 to 2007, based on isolates reported to the Influenza Branch, CDC. Influenza activity has occurred each year during this interpandemic period, often with mixtures of influenza A subtypes and/or B viruses. (Figure kindly provided by Lynnette Brammer and Joe Bresee, Influenza Division, CDC.)

(H3, H1, and B) may occur within a single season. The isolation of an antigenically drifted virus late in the spring months during a limited outbreak (herald wave) may foreshadow an epidemic in the next season.

Community Impact

School-age children play a central role in the dissemination of influenza in the community and spread virus to their younger siblings and parents in the household. Increased school absenteeism is an early epidemiological marker of epidemic influenza, and school closings may blunt outbreaks. Epidemic attack rates up to 60 to 75% have been described to occur in schoolchildren. Epidemics are also marked by increases in visits to primary-care physicians and emergency rooms for febrile respiratory illness, workplace absenteeism, and subsequently hospitalizations for pneumonia. The overall incidence of influenza is highest in school-age children and adolescents and declines with increasing age, such that attack rates are about fourfold lower in people over age 60 than in those age groups. Influenza is the single most common cause of medically attended acute respiratory illness. Up to one-half of influenza A H3N2 subtype or B illnesses lead to physician contact. Approximately 5 to 15% of teens or adults and 25% of children <5 years old seek medical care for acute respiratory disease during epidemics (44). Influenza virus has been associated with 15 to 25% of all respiratory illnesses seen by physicians and up to 40% of those seen in patients over the age of 15 years.

The impact of influenza varies considerably with age, underlying condition, and the epidemic strain (153). In the United States, increases in pneumonia and influenza hospitalizations range from 16,000 to over 220,000 per epidemic, less than one-half of which involve adults 65 years of age or older (152). Admissions for exacerbations of chronic respiratory diseases and cardiovascular disease, particularly congestive heart failure, also increase. The peak of hospitalizations lags about 1 week after the peak of influenza activity. Hospitalization rates for all influenza-related complications are about 1 to 3 per 1,000 persons and are highest in those aged less than 1 year or over 64 years, among whom approximately 3 to 6 per 1,000 are hospitalized annually (44). Among children, hospitalization rates are highest in those <6 months of age and decline through 6 years of age. A (H3N2) subtype epidemics are associated with two- to threefold increases in pneumonia rates and two- to fivefold increases in hospitalization rates for adults with high-risk medical conditions. Diabetic persons experience increased hospitalizations and mortality due to ketoacidosis and pneumonia during influenza epidemics. However, most adults but less than one-half of children requiring hospitalization for respiratory disease have a previously recognized underlying medical condition (127). Contemporary strains of the H3N2 subtype of influenza A virus typically cause the most severe illness and highest hospitalization rates and those of the H1N1 subtype of influenza usually cause the lowest, with influenza B epidemics intermediate in severity.

Mortality

The overall case fatality rate is low, generally 0.01% or less, but influenza epidemics are often associated with mortality rates well in excess of those observed during comparable time periods in the absence of influenza outbreaks. Annual influenza-associated mortality averaged about 34,000 (8,000 to 68,000) per epidemic in the United States between 1979 and 2001 (140, 152). Mortality rates are highest in infants, the elderly, and those with underlying cardiopulmonary disease. About 90% of deaths occur in those ≥65 years of age, and the mortality rates in those over 65 years old are over 50-fold higher than in younger persons and are especially high in those aged 85 years and above. A hereditary predisposition to influenza-related death has been postulated, particularly in association with the 1918 pandemic and recently with subtype A (H5N1) infections, but the possible mechanisms have not been elucidated.

Most mortality is attributable principally to lower respiratory complications or cardiovascular disease. Pneumonia and influenza deaths account for only about one-quarter of all excess deaths, but they serve as important markers of influenza activity (Fig. 8). Up to two-thirds of the excess deaths are related to cardiovascular disease. Excess mortality due to pneumonia and influenza-related deaths in the United States occurs particularly in association with H3N2 subtype epidemics (Fig. 8). Increases in mortality rates generally lag several weeks behind the peak of influenza activity and persist for approximately 6 weeks afterwards.

Influenza C

Influenza C virus infection is worldwide in distribution and generally nonseasonal but may cause prolonged community outbreaks (89, 90). Symptomatic infections usually occur between 1 and 4 years of age, but influenza C virus usually represents <1% of viruses from children with respiratory illness (89, 90). Most children ≥6 years and adults are seropositive. Influenza C virus has been associated with outbreaks in closed populations, including those in children's homes and the military.

Nosocomial Infections

Influenza A and, less often, B viruses are important causes of nosocomial outbreaks involving hospital wards, intensive care units, nursing homes, and other closed populations (134). Because of the short incubation period of influenza and its efficient transmission, rapid dissemination of virus can lead to explosive outbreaks in such populations. Outbreaks are typically brief, lasting from 1 to 3 weeks. Clinical attack rates among groups of institutionalized adults range from 10 to 60%, with substantial ward-to-ward variation. Up to 10% of influenza cases in hospitalized adults are nosocomially acquired. Nosocomial influenza is usually associated with 4 to 5 days of fever and 1 week or more of illness. Lower respiratory tract complications develop in one-third or more of affected adults. Mortality rates range widely (0 to 30%). Health care personnel are often involved during the course of both community and hospital outbreaks of influenza. Secondary infections in health care workers are common (20 to 50% attack rates) and can lead to absenteeism and disruption of services. Infected workers can initiate or perpetuate outbreaks by transmitting infection to susceptible patients, and health care provider immunization has been associated with reduced influenza-associated illness and mortality in chronic-care facilities (57).

Nursing home residents are disproportionately impacted by influenza because of higher frequencies of underlying disease, decreased vaccine responsiveness, and greater likelihood of influenza exposure, due to residence in semi-

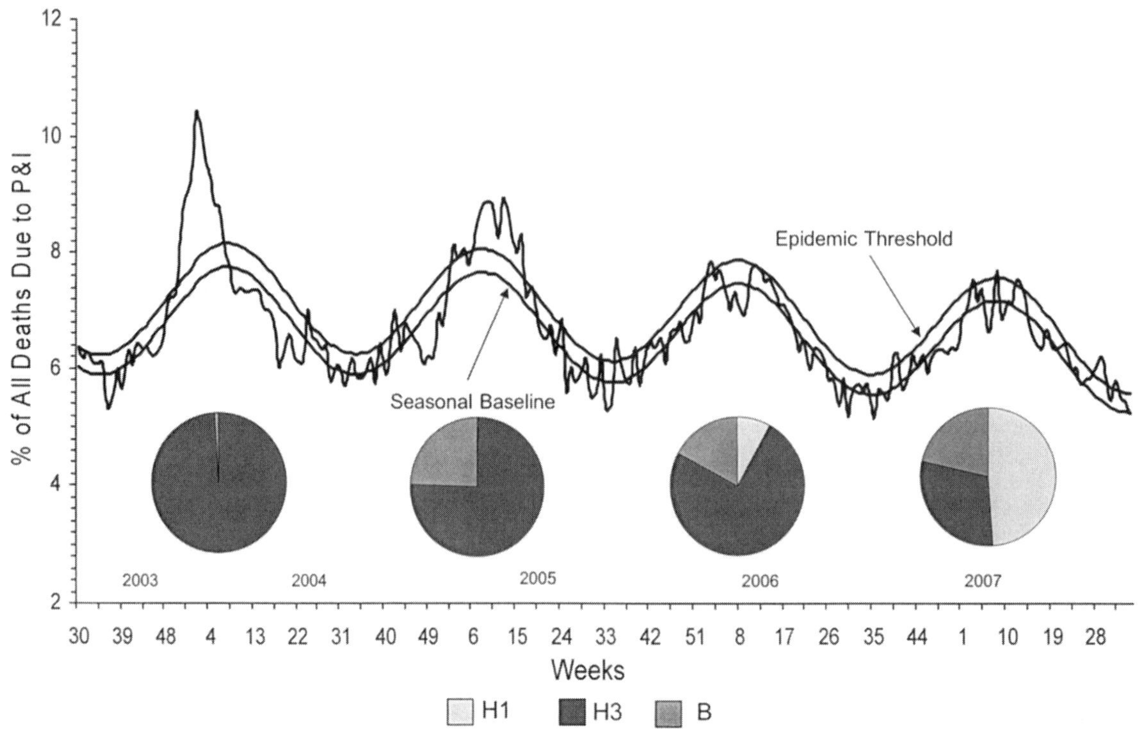

FIGURE 8 Pneumonia and influenza (P&I) deaths presented as a percentage of total deaths in the United States, 2002 to 2007. Total deaths and those attributed to pneumonia and influenza deaths are reported weekly from 122 cities in the United States to the CDC. Excess mortality above the epidemic threshold has been seen particularly in association with influenza A (H3N2) subtype activity. (Figure kindly provided by Lynnette Brammer and Joe Bresee, Influenza Division, CDC.)

closed facilities, compared to elderly persons in the community. Nursing home outbreaks are more likely in larger homes and in those with lower immunization rates, but outbreaks have occurred despite immunization rates exceeding 90% and sometimes out of season during the summer months. Nosocomial influenza should be considered in hospitalized or nursing home patients with unexplained febrile illness or respiratory deterioration, especially during periods of influenza activity in the community or if multiple cases occur.

Zoonotic Infections

Animal influenza viruses cause occasional zoonotic infections of humans. Such events are usually associated with inefficient human-to-human spread but create the conditions for the potential emergence of an animal-human reassortment virus. Transmission of H1N1 subtype virus from swine is most frequently implicated, including the Fort Dix outbreak in 1976 and sporadic fatal pneumonic disease, particularly in pregnant or immunocompromised persons (103). Reassortant H3N2 swine viruses with genes of avian, human, and swine viral origin have recently caused sporadic human illnesses (103). The recent detection of H2N3 subtype virus in swine raises concern about potential for human infection (84). Serologic evidence of infection by multiple subtypes of avian viruses is present in Chinese agricultural workers, and experimental human infection has developed after intranasal exposure to H4, H6, and H10 subtype viruses (5, 165).

H5N1 Virus

In 1997, direct interspecies transmission of an avian influenza A H5N1 subtype virus led to severe illness and six deaths among 18 recognized cases in Hong Kong (Table 2) (145). This experience established that avian influenza viruses could cause human infections without adaptation in an intermediate host and despite differences in receptor specificity. The virus possessed a polybasic amino acid HA cleavage site characteristic of HPAI viruses and was uniquely lethal in animals without adaptation. The virulent H5N1 subtype appeared to arise as a reassortant of avian influenza viruses, likely including a goose H5N1 subtype virus and possibly a quail H9N2 subtype virus, which provided multiple internal genes (79). Subsequent reassortment events and genetic changes led to further outbreaks in birds in Hong Kong, fatalities in one family visiting Fujian Province in 2003, and then major poultry outbreaks and associated human cases in Thailand, Vietnam, and Cambodia starting in 2003 to 2004 (http://www.who.int/csr/disease/avian_influenza/ai_timeline/en/index.html) (161). The emergence of a dominant Z genotype was associated with spread of virus across Asia to Europe, the Middle East, and Africa (161). Poultry trade practices, live-poultry markets, duck abundance, and rice cropping intensity are contributory to the persistence of the virus, which is currently entrenched in several countries. The virus has continued to evolve, with 10 lineages now recognized, 4 of which (clades 0, 1, 2, and 7) have caused fatal human illness (166). Progenitors of the clade 1 and 2 viruses appear to have come from southern China.

The epizootic in birds has resulted in loss through illness or culling of over 200 million poultry, predominantly chickens and ducks, but relatively few human cases to date despite numerous exposures (166). Episodes of nonsustained person-to-person transmission to household and health care contacts have been recognized uncommonly; subclinical human infections have been rare to date (166). One explanation for the rare event of a chicken-to-human transmission is that only large amounts of virus lead to infection (and disease) in humans, but the host factors that might contribute to susceptibility are poorly understood.

Other Avian Viruses

Purulent conjunctivitis due to H7N7 subtype influenza virus has followed exposure to infected seals or laboratory materials (Table 2). In 2000, a large outbreak of HPAI H7N7 virus in poultry in Holland and Belgium was associated with scores of human illnesses, principally conjunctivitis but also influenza-like illness and one fatal pneumonia in a veterinarian, and evidence of human-to-human transmission (98). Sporadic human infections by other H7 viruses, sometimes without apparent symptoms and detected serologically, have been reported in Canada, Italy, and the United States. H9N2 subtype viruses continue to circulate in domestic poultry and swine, likely facilitated by aerosol transmission, and have caused human infections in China.

PATHOGENESIS

Viral Replication

The initial site of infection is the respiratory tract mucosa (44, 165) and is mediated by HA binding to sialylated glycans on epithelial cells (165). The α2,6-linked receptors preferred by human viruses are present in both the upper and lower respiratory tract, particularly tracheobronchial epithelium and type 1 pneumocytes, whereas the α2,3-linked receptors preferred by avian viruses are present in the distal bronchioles, type 2 pneumocytes, and alveolar macrophages (159). These distribution patterns may explain in part the high frequency of tracheobronchitis in seasonal influenza and of viral pneumonia and the relative paucity of upper respiratory manifestations in avian H5N1 infection. In volunteers experimentally infected with a human virus, approximately 10- to 100-fold-smaller viral inocula are needed to initiate infection after small-particle aerosol exposure of the lower respiratory tract than after intranasal inoculation of the upper respiratory tract. Intervention studies with intranasal or inhaled delivery of antivirals like zanamivir (118) indicate that infection by human influenza viruses is initiated most commonly in the pharynx or tracheobronchial tree.

The duration of virus shedding in respiratory secretions is generally 3 to 6 days during uncomplicated influenza in adults and older children. Hospitalized adults may shed infectious virus for a week or longer after illness onset (76). Longer periods of shedding (1 to 3 weeks) are commonly seen in infants and children and in those experiencing H5N1 illness (26, 27, 166). In H5N1 disease, viral levels are higher in tracheal aspirates than in the upper respiratory tract and higher in the throat than in the nose. Prolonged virus shedding (weeks to months) has been described to occur in patients with immunodeficiency, including advanced human immunodeficiency virus (HIV) disease (95). Influenza does not appear to be unusually protracted in patients with hypo- or agammaglobulinemia. In uncomplicated influenza, virus shedding begins about 1 day before onset of illness and titers in nasal washings peak within several days at 10^4 to 10^7 50% tissue culture infectious doses per ml (55). Fever and the severity of illness correlate temporally with the quantity of virus detectable in respiratory secretions. Influenza viremia or invasion of extrapulmonary tissues has been documented only rarely in seasonal influenza. Virus has been recovered from the heart, liver, spleen, kidneys, adrenals, muscles, and meninges, and in children with encephalopathy, viral RNA has been detected in cerebrospinal fluid (CSF). Viremia, gastrointestinal infection, and extrapulmonary dissemination, sometimes including the central nervous system (CNS), occur in some HPAI H5N1-infected patients, and detection of H5N1 viral RNA in blood or feces is associated with a worse prognosis (26, 48, 166).

Pathological Changes

In apparently uncomplicated influenza, bronchial histopathology shows degeneration of respiratory epithelial cells with loss of ciliated tufts and desquamation; pseudometaplastic changes of the epithelium; and edema, hyperemia, and mononuclear cell infiltrates in the lamina propria (97). In fatal influenza viral pneumonia, the gross pathological findings include hemorrhagic, airless lungs and severe tracheobronchitis (110). The pathological features are necrotizing tracheobronchitis and bronchiolitis with loss of ciliated epithelium, fibrin exudation, and inflammatory cell infiltration; hyaline membrane formation; intra-alveolar and intrabronchiolar hemorrhage; and interstitial edema, hemorrhage, and mononuclear cell infiltration (Fig. 9) (97). Later changes include diffuse alveolar damage, lymphohistiocytic alveolitis, metaplastic epithelial regeneration, and sometimes extensive fibrosis. Influenza virus antigens have been demonstrated in virtually all cells of the respiratory tract, and virus has been recovered from pulmonary tissues as late as 3 weeks after illness onset in fatal cases and sometimes later in steroid-treated H5N1 disease (48). Both direct cytopathic effects (CPE) and virally induced apoptosis contribute to the pathological changes. Exuberant local and systemic cytokine and chemokine responses associated with H5N1 disease have been postulated to cause inflammation and cellular infiltration in the lungs and other organs. The severity of pneumonitis relates to cell-mediated immune responses and can be enhanced by transfer of certain types of T lymphocytes in murine models, but the extent to which immunopathological host responses contribute to disease has not been determined for humans.

Patients with fatal cases of influenza often show pathological changes in other organs. Diffuse congestion and generalized swelling of the brain and myocardial inflammation with edema, interstitial hemorrhage, myocyte necrosis, and lymphocytic infiltration have been found in one-third or more of autopsies. The few autopsies of patients with fatal H5N1 have also shown lymphocyte depletion, hemophagocytosis, and hepatitis (110).

Pathogenesis of Symptoms

Direct viral involvement of the upper and lower respiratory tract accounts for much of the illness associated with influenza, particularly the high frequency of cough and

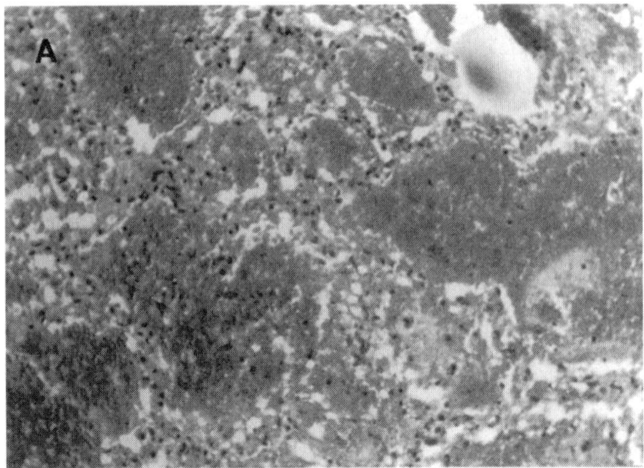

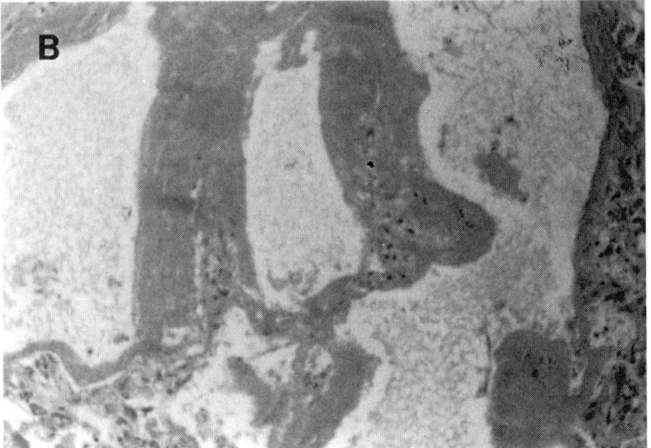

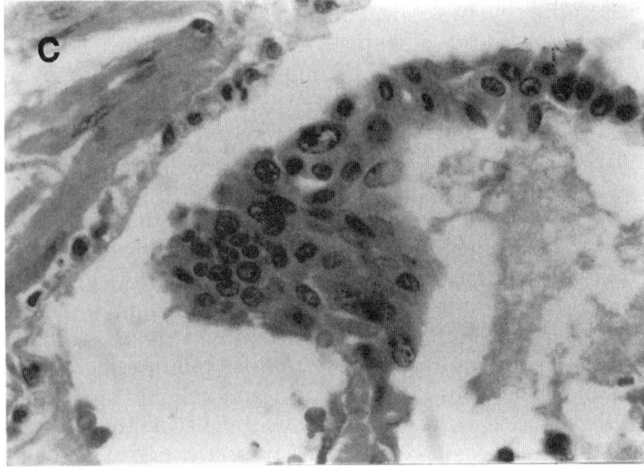

FIGURE 9 Photomicrographs of lung tissue from patients with primary influenza A viral pneumonia. Histologic sections were stained with hematoxylin and eosin and were viewed at an original magnification of approximately ×125. (A) Intra-alveolar hemorrhage with erythrocytes and exudate filling alveoli; (B) extensive hyaline membrane formation; (C) early regenerative phase with a metaplastic epithelium. (Figure kindly provided by Phillip Feldman, Department of Pathology, University of Virginia.)

tracheal irritation. Even in apparently uncomplicated influenza, bronchoscopy shows tracheobronchial inflammation, and pulmonary function abnormalities persist for weeks to months after infection (155). Pulmonary function studies have detected restrictive and obstructive ventilatory defects, abnormal gas exchange with increased alveolar-arterial oxygen gradients, decreased carbon monoxide diffusing capacity, and airway hyperreactivity.

The cause of the marked constitutional symptoms during influenza relates in part to elaboration of proinflammatory cytokines and chemokines. Various mediators, including alpha interferon (IFN-α), IFN-γ, tumor necrosis factor alpha (TNF-α), and interleukins (interleukin 1 [IL-1], -2, -4, -5, -6, -10, and -12), are expressed in the respiratory tracts of experimentally infected animals. Levels of TNF-α and the chemokine macrophage inflammatory protein 2 (MIP-2) in bronchoalveolar lavage fluid correlate with the extent of pulmonary inflammation, and administration of anti-TNF or anti-MIP-2 antibody improves survival rates in mice. MIP-1α-deficient mice have reduced influenza-induced pulmonary inflammation but also delayed viral clearance. In murine models of H5N1 infection, mice with knockouts of IL-6, MIP-1α, or TNF-α or its receptors or those treated with glucocorticoids have mortality rates comparable to those of wild-type mice; mice without IL-1 receptors show increased mortality rates (135).

In vitro infection of human respiratory epithelial cells results in elaboration of IL-6, -8, -11; TNF-α; RANTES; and other mediators. IFN-α, IFN-γ, IL-6, TNF-α, IL-8, IL-1b, IL-10, MCP-10, and MIP-1α and -1β levels in nasal lavage samples and IL-6 and TNF-α levels in blood also increase during experimental human influenza (55). Early increases in nasal IFN-α, IFN-γ, and IL-6 correlate with viral titers and illness measures. Interferon levels increase in respiratory secretions and blood during uncomplicated human influenza. Interferon concentrations peak about 1 day after the peak of virus shedding and fall in temporal association with decreases in viral replication. In natural human influenza, levels of IL-6, IFN-α, IFN-γ, TNF-α, and IL-10 in the nose and blood are increased early; IL-6 levels correlate with illness measures, and nasal IFN-γ levels correlate with decreases in viral titers (67). Hypercytokinemia of proinflammatory and Th1 cytokines occurs in patients hospitalized with serious human influenza, in whom elevated plasma IL-6 levels correlate with prolonged hospitalization (75), and is especially marked in H5N1 patients, in whom the highest cytokine levels are found in those with fatal illness (26).

The mechanisms of cytokine induction are incompletely defined, but viral replication appears to drive these responses. Upper respiratory tract viral loads in patients hospitalized with either seasonal influenza or H5N1 infection correlate with plasma cytokine and chemokine levels (26, 75). Influenza HA activates cellular transcription factor NF-κB binding and transactivation of target genes encoding certain cytokines, cellular adhesion molecules, and other acute-phase proteins. Viral NA can also stimulate TNF and IL-1 production by monocytes and activate latent transforming growth factor β. Virus-associated double-stranded RNA interacting with Toll-like receptors 3 and 7 and with the helicase retinoic acid-inducible gene (RIG-I) appear to play an important role in initiating acute-phase responses and inducing cytokine elaboration during acute influenza (160).

Viral Pathogenicity

Virulence is a multigenic characteristic and does not relate to a specific subtype. The H1N1 pandemic of 1918 was especially severe, perhaps related to the greater pneumotropism of the virus. Unlike a conventional human virus, the 1918 virus causes a lethal pneumonia with sustained viral replication in experimentally infected macaques and a dysregulated immune response characterized by deficient interferon responses early and prolonged proinflammatory responses (71). The polymerase genes from the 1918 influenza virus are required for full pathogenicity in animals (149, 157), and one mutation in PB1-F2 (Asp66Ser) is associated with increased replication of this and other influenza A viruses in mice. In humans, infections by H3N2 subtype viruses cause pulmonary function changes which have not been commonly found during recent H1N1 subtype infections. Certain pandemics have been more virulent during the second wave of infection. Although it has been postulated that the virus undergoes adaptation to its human host, specific alterations have not been identified.

Pathogenicity and cell tropism of influenza viruses relate in part to the HA cleavability by particular host cell enzymes (60). One lethal avian influenza virus has been linked to an HA mutation associated with loss of a glycosylation site and enhanced HA cleavability. Serine proteases, presumably derived from host epithelial cells, cleave the HA precursor molecule into HA1 and HA2 to render human influenza viruses infectious. Protease activity present in human nasal secretions, common house dust mites, and importantly, proteases produced by some bacteria, including *Staphylococcus aureus*, can enhance viral replication. Certain bacterial enzymes like streptokinase can proteolytically activate plasmin to cleave HA. Host range restriction, replication kinetics, and virulence are also influenced by multiple other genes. For example, the multifunctional NS1 protein counteracts the double-stranded-RNA-activated protein kinase and other antiviral responses induced by interferon (41), limits the induction of IFN-β, interacts with the cellular protein nucleolin, and also interacts via its C terminus with PDZ-binding proteins to modulate viral pathogenicity (63a). Apoptosis appears to be an important mechanism for inducing cell death by influenza viruses and is mediated by several viral proteins, including NA and NS1. The extent of viral NA expression influences virulence in animal models of influenza and predicts lethality from secondary pneumococcal infection (124). The unique virulence of HPAI H5N1 viruses appears to be multifactorial, including high HA cleavability, high replication competence related to its polymerase complex (especially the PB2 protein for certain strains), and ability to subvert host innate immune responses (106, 123).

Various factors contribute to the increased risk of bacterial infections following influenza. Infection damages the bronchial epithelium and disrupts mucociliary clearance, promotes pharyngeal colonization by bacterial pathogens by increasing adherence to epithelial cells, and depresses the chemotaxis and bactericidal activity of alveolar macrophages and polymorphonuclear leukocytes (PMNs). Viral NA activity can expose cellular receptors that enhance binding by pneumococci and result in lethal viral-bacterial interactions in murine models (124). The production of nitric oxide, which exerts antiviral effects, is depressed in influenza virus-infected macrophages. Rapid onset of reduced intracellular killing and lysozyme secretion occurs with in vitro infection of PMNs. Decreased PMN chemotaxis, intracellular killing, and other functional changes have been linked to altered signal transduction steps, including binding of G proteins. Purified viral NP inhibits PMN chemotaxis and superoxide production. Depressed mitogen-stimulated blastogenic responses also develop early in illness and are accompanied by cutaneous anergy. Lymphopenia with decreases in both T- and B-cell counts and normal CD4/CD8 ratios occurs early during acute infection. Decreased mitogenic responses may persist for 4 weeks after infection. Some H5N1 viruses show high resistance to antiviral cytokines and the ability to infect and kill monocyte-derived or blood myeloid dendritic cells in vitro.

Immune Responses

Recovery from infection and protection against reinfection are associated with specific host immune responses (44, 100). The observation that the 1977 H1N1 reemergence rarely affected persons who had been infected with essentially the same virus over 20 years earlier indicates that immunity to reinfection and illness caused by homotypic virus is durable. Serologic evidence of reinfection by the same or closely related strains is common, especially in closed populations, but reinfections are usually subclinical in adults. The first lifetime influenza A virus infection results in immune memory for the subtype to which the strain belongs, such that subsequent infections or immunizations reinforce the antibody response to the first virus. This phenomenon has been termed "original antigenic sin." Previously infected persons may produce cross-reacting antibodies to the subtype causing initial infection, as well as strain-specific antibodies to previously encountered related viruses.

General

Nonspecific host factors may contribute to protection or early response to infection. Various lectins, including mucins in nasal secretions, surfactant proteins, and serum mannose-binding lectin, directly inhibit influenza viruses through binding to their surface glycoproteins, as well as promote uptake by phagocytic cells (150). Neutrophil-derived α-defensins inhibit influenza virus replication in vitro, possibly by interfering with protein kinase C activation (136). The pattern of HA glycosylation influences viral opsonization and complement-mediated lysis of infected cells. Human bronchoalveolar lavage fluids also inhibit HA activity. Nasal interferon levels peak early and correlate directly with viral titers. Failure of endogenous interferon responses has been described to occur in patients with severe influenza viral pneumonia and also in a macaque model of infection by the 1918 virus (71). Type I interferons cause Mx protein expression that leads to species-specific cellular resistance to influenza virus infection (160). Other nonspecific immune responses include increased natural killer (NK) cell activity and detectable but low levels of interferon in serum during the first few days of infection. NK cell activity correlates directly with degree of illness and virus shedding in experimental human influenza. Apoptosis-dependent phagocytosis by macrophages of virus-infected cells may contribute to elimination of virus.

Humoral Immunity

Following primary infection in children, serum hemagglutination inhibition (HAI) and anti-NA antibodies develop within 10 days and persist for years (165). The principal neutralizing antibody responses are strain-specific serum immunoglobulin M (IgM) and IgG antibodies and nasal

IgA antibodies directed against HA. Virus-specific serum IgM, IgG, and IgA antibodies are present in adults within the first week after illness onset (132). Serum HAI titers gradually decrease over the first 6 months but may be boosted by infection with related viruses; IgA responses remain detectable for several months. Otherwise healthy persons infected with avian A (H5N1) virus show serum neutralizing antibody responses with kinetics similar to those following primary infection in children with human influenza A viruses.

Protection against infection and illness by the homologous virus correlates directly with levels of neutralizing IgA in nasal secretions and of serum IgG-neutralizing or HAI antibodies (100). Serum HAI antibody titers of 1:32 to 1:40 and above generally correlate with protection against illness due to the homotypic strain in immunocompetent persons (24), but protective titers vary widely with virus strain, age, and probably general immune status. Antibodies in either serum or nasal secretions confer resistance regardless of subclass if present in sufficient titer. Heterosubtypic humoral immunity, as assessed by HAI titers, provides no significant protection against infection. Nonneutralizing antibodies, which increase phagocytosis of opsonized viruses by Fc receptor-bearing cells, occur following primary infection and may contribute to viral clearance by macrophages. In addition, subtype-specific antibodies which mediate cell lysis by complement binding or by antibody-dependent cellular cytotoxicity develop after infection or immunization. Antibody to M2 protein also inhibits virus replication, perhaps through one of these mechanisms.

Cell-Mediated Immunity

Influenza virus infection elicits cell-mediated immune responses that are detectable before the appearance of humoral responses (94). Virus-specific lymphocyte blastogenic responses, T-lymphocyte cellular cytotoxicity, and cutaneous delayed-type hypersensitivity are detectable within 6 days after infection. Animal and limited human studies indicate that these responses, particularly cytotoxic T lymphocytes (CTLs), play a role in termination of virus replication and recovery from infection. CTL responses require several days for induction but may modify the risk of illness or complications. Human CTLs are generally type specific but cross-reactive for cells infected by different influenza A virus subtypes, major histocompatibility complex class I restricted, and $CD8^+$ T cell mediated (43). Specific clones are directed at epitopes on internal (NP, M protein, or polymerase) or surface glycoproteins. Heterosubtypic CTL responses recognize mainly NP and M protein. Human $CD8^+$ and $CD4^+$ CTLs recognize epitopes of animal influenza viruses (64), and nonexposed healthy adults possess H5N1-reactive $CD4^+$ T cells directed against M protein, NP, NA, and also HA (133). Mutations in CTL epitopes may abrogate major histocompatibility complex class I presentation and allow escape from immune recognition (130). CTL activity correlates with more rapid viral clearance in experimentally infected seronegative adults. Granzyme B elaboration in virus-stimulated peripheral blood mononuclear cell cultures of CTL activity appears to be lower in immunized elderly adults who develop influenza than those who do not. The half-life of influenza CTL memory has been estimated to be 4 years.

CLINICAL MANIFESTATIONS

Influenza causes illness in the majority of those infected, although depending on prior immunity, up to one-half of serologically proven infections in adults may be subclinical. Infection may result in a range of clinical syndromes, including common cold, pharyngitis, tracheobronchitis, and, in children, bronchiolitis or croup.

Influenza Syndrome

Classic influenza presents abruptly with prominent systemic symptoms, including fever, malaise, headache, and myalgia, and with respiratory symptoms of cough and often sore throat (70, 112). Fever may be quite high and may be continuous or intermittent, especially if antipyretics are used. Pharyngeal and conjunctival injection, minor cervical adenopathy, and clear nasal discharge are common, but physical findings are generally nonspecific. Fever and systemic complaints usually abate by 3 to 5 days in adults, but respiratory complaints increase, with dry cough, substernal burning, and nasal congestion. Slight neutrophilia and lymphopenia occur early, followed by neutropenia. Influenza is associated with elevations of acute-phase proteins, serum amyloid A, and C-reactive protein, especially in hospitalized elderly persons. Acute influenza impairs psychomotor performance and lengthens reaction times.

Recovery is often slow; cough and malaise commonly persist for 2 to 4 weeks. Apparently uncomplicated influenza is often associated with prolonged abnormalities in gas exchange and pulmonary mechanics indicative of small-airway dysfunction (155). These may contribute to the asthenia and decreased exercise tolerance reported by patients during convalescence. The frequency and severity of clinically apparent influenza are greater in smokers. Allergic patients also experience increased severity of acute symptoms, bronchospastic exacerbations, and prolonged convalescence. Premorbid psychological status correlates with prolonged convalescence. Severity also relates to virus type; H3N2 subtype infections are associated with higher frequencies of lower respiratory symptoms, pulmonary function changes, and physician visits than H1N1 subtype infections.

Influenza C virus has been associated with 3.5% of common colds in adults and may cause febrile bronchitis and influenza-like illnesses, as well as a range of syndromes, including febrile coryza, bronchiolitis, and pneumonia, in children (90). Rhinorrhea and cough are the most commonly recognized symptoms and may last several weeks.

The diagnosis of influenza is often based on clinical and epidemiological grounds in the context of a known outbreak. In adults presenting with both fever and cough during community outbreaks, a suspected influenza diagnosis has been confirmed virologically in up to 80% (15, 96). The absence of fever, cough, or nasal congestion decreases the likelihood of influenza. However, clinical diagnosis often lacks accuracy, especially in children below the age of 5 years or when influenza prevalence is low, since the acute respiratory symptoms of influenza mimic those of other viral infections, including those due to respiratory syncytial virus, parainfluenza virus, and adenoviruses.

Specific Populations

Infants and Children

Influenza virus infection occurs in about one-third of infants during the first year of life and is associated with increased severity because of their lack of immunity and their small-caliber airways. Maternally derived antibodies provide some protection in infants, although hospitalization rates are highest in children younger than 6 months and progressively decrease thereafter (109). Approximately 40% of initial infections in young children are subclinical or cause afebrile upper respiratory tract illness (45). About 90% of symptomatic patients have fever, cough, and rhinitis, up to 40% have emesis or diarrhea, and 25% or more have otitis media or lower respiratory tract disease (127). Pneumonia develops in about 5 to 15% of young children. Underlying conditions, like bronchopulmonary dysplasia and congenital heart or neurologic disease, are present in a minority. In adolescents, otitis media, usually resolving without antibiotics, and pneumonia complicate about 5% of cases. More than 1% of infections in the pediatric population result in hospitalization (109). Influenza A and B virus infections have been associated with 68 and 36%, respectively, of croup admissions and 36 and 11%, respectively, of all pediatric hospitalizations for respiratory illness during epidemic periods.

Influenza is underrecognized in infants and young children (127). Unexplained fever or suspected sepsis, bronchiolitis, croup, vomiting, diarrhea, and neurologic manifestations, including apnea, seizures in up to 36%, and meningitis-like presentations, lead to hospitalization. Abdominal pain can mimic acute appendicitis. Myositis, usually manifested as calf tenderness and pain impeding ambulation for hours to several days, occurs in about 20% of influenza B virus-infected children. Myositis and gastrointestinal symptoms are associated more frequently with influenza B than with influenza A virus infections. The latter can lead to obliterative bronchiolitis and chronic pulmonary disease in infants. Acute influenza encephalopathy in children aged 1 to 6 years is manifested by sudden onset of fever, seizures, rapidly progressive coma, and often death. Less common findings include thalamic necrosis, increased CSF protein or pleocytosis, and the presence of viral RNA in the CSF. Abnormal transaminases without the hyperammonemia or hypoglycemia typical of Reye's syndrome may occur. The incidence of Reye's syndrome in children with influenza, estimated to be less than 1 case per 10^5, has markedly decreased in temporal association with the reduced use of salicylates.

Pregnancy

Approximately 5 to 10% of pregnant women have serologic evidence of influenza virus infection. Excess mortality during pregnancy, primarily due to overwhelming pulmonary disease, has been documented during pandemics and sporadically during epidemics (70, 128a). In the 1957 pandemic, up to 10% of influenza deaths were among pregnant women in New York City. Increased risks of complications and hospitalization (two- to fourfold) occur with increasing stage of pregnancy in women with seasonal influenza, especially in those with comorbidity (29). The third trimester of pregnancy and early puerperium appear to be periods of increased risk for severe disease and viral pneumonia. Maternal infection has been associated with preterm delivery, fetal distress, and cesarean delivery. Reported associations with teratogenic effects or an increased risk of childhood leukemia, schizophrenia (1957 pandemic), or Parkinson's disease remain to be proven (128a). Transplacental spread of virus has been documented rarely. H5N1 disease is associated with high mortality rates, fetal loss, and transplacental dissemination of virus (48). Administration of inactivated vaccine is considered safe during any stage of pregnancy.

Elderly

Viral shedding and illness duration may be more prolonged in elderly adults. Aged mice show defects in cellular immunity and cytokine responses that correlate with delayed viral clearance. Elderly patients with influenza may not complain of typical systemic symptoms. Lassitude, lethargy, confusion, anorexia, decreased activity level, cough, and low-grade fever may be the primary findings (70, 112). Presentation with complications such as bacterial pneumonia or exacerbations of underlying asthma, chronic obstructive pulmonary disease, or congestive heart failure also occurs. The elderly may experience myalgia and/or muscle weakness profound enough to impair ambulation in association with high creatine phosphokinase levels.

Immunocompromised Hosts

The course of influenza in HIV-infected patients and other immunocompromised hosts may be more prolonged, and viral shedding for months has been observed in those with advanced immunodeficiency. An increased frequency of cardiopulmonary complications and hospitalizations occurs in HIV-infected persons, and persons with AIDS experience excess pneumonia and influenza-related mortality during epidemics (78). Influenza in HIV-infected children has been associated with an eightfold-increased risk of hospitalization for lower respiratory illness.

Influenza virus infections in oncology patients have been associated with variable prolongation of clinical course, increased hospitalizations, and interruption of chemotherapy. Acute-leukemia patients with chemotherapy-induced neutropenia have high risks of pneumonia and death following influenza (52). Chronically immunosuppressed transplant patients are at increased risk for influenza complications, including severe pneumonia, bacterial superinfection, and, in children, neurologic abnormalities. Most transplant patients have self-limited infections, but fever may be prolonged and hospitalization frequent. Up to 50% of bone marrow transplant recipients develop lower respiratory tract disease, and up to 20% die without antiviral therapy, with the highest risk during the period of aplasia (52). Infection in transplant patients has been linked with rejection, graft loss, and possibly hemolytic-uremic syndrome.

Complications

Influenza complications are common and may be manifested in the upper (otitis media and sinusitis) or lower (bronchitis, croup, and pneumonia) respiratory tract, as exacerbations of preexisting chronic diseases (asthma, chronic obstructive pulmonary disease, cystic fibrosis, and congestive heart failure) or, less often, systemically. The most common complications are bronchitis in adults, which occurs in up to 20% of patients seeking care, and otitis media in children. Influenza is linked to approximately 10% of community-acquired pneumonias in adults (68). In patients with reactive-airway or chronic obstructive pulmonary disease, influenza is an important cause of exacerbations, and most illnesses are associated with spirometric deteriorations, usually lasting less than 3 months (155). Exacerbations of asthma, with FEV_1 (forced expiratory volume in 1 s) decreases lasting 2 to 9 days, occur in most cases of clinically apparent influenza. In patients with cystic fibrosis, influenza virus infections are associated with increased hospitalizations and disease progression, including decreases in spirometry.

Viral Pneumonia

Influenza A virus can cause severe primary viral pneumonia in those with underlying conditions and previously healthy adults (68, 155). Approximately 15 to 20% of young adults with influenza developed pneumonia in 1918, with associated fatality rates of 30% or higher; bacterial pathogens were detected from the lungs or blood in a majority of fatal cases (12). During the 1957 pandemic, approximately 30% of persons with fatal cases had influenza viral pneumonitis or tracheobronchitis without coexistent bacterial infection. Mild forms of viral pneumonia with patchy radiographic infiltrates are more common, particularly in children, than severe primary influenza viral pneumonia. The latter occurs in 2 to 18% of adults hospitalized with pneumonia during epidemic periods. Over 90% of cases have been linked to influenza A virus infection, and most recognized cases occur in those over the age of 40 years. Various risk factors, including underlying cardiopulmonary disease, rheumatic heart disease (particularly mitral stenosis), malignancy, organ transplantation, corticosteroid or cytotoxic therapy, pregnancy, and possibly HIV infection, have been identified. However, nearly 40% of cases occur in those with no recognized underlying disease.

Patients present with a preceding influenza syndrome, followed by increasing cough, tachypnea, and dyspnea, typical of acute respiratory distress syndrome (ARDS). The interval from onset of illness to disabling pulmonary symptoms is variable (<1 to 20 days), but most patients deteriorate within 1 to 4 days. Sputum production occurs in about one-half, and hemoptysis occurs in about one-third. Sputum Gram smear may show abundant PMNs without significant numbers of bacteria. The illness progresses over 1 to 4 days to cause severe respiratory failure. Chest radiographs are nonspecific but typically show bilateral, diffuse mid-lung and lower-lung infiltrates (Fig. 10). Presentation as Goodpasture's syndrome or a syndrome mimicking pulmonary embolism has been described. Advanced techniques of assisted ventilation have improved the outlook in severe cases, but fatality rates average about 50%. A correlation between clinical and radiographic improvement, which initially occurs within 2 to 3 weeks, has been observed in survivors. Bronchiolitis obliterans with organizing pneumonia, pulmonary fibrosis, and chronic functional impairment may develop in survivors.

Progressive pneumonia with development of ARDS and often multiorgan failure occur in the majority of patients with sporadic H5N1 disease (166). The median times from illness onset to presentation for care and to death are about 4 and 9 days, respectively.

Secondary Pneumonia

Secondary bacterial pneumonias account for about 25% of influenza-associated deaths in interpandemic periods and were found in 70% of patients with life-threatening pneumonia during the 1957 and 1968 pandemics (124). Reappearance of fever, increased respiratory symptoms, or cough productive of purulent sputum suggests the possibility of superimposed bacterial infection (138), but presentation with bacterial or mixed viral-bacterial pneumonia without a biphasic illness also occurs. Fungal infections, particularly *Aspergillus* infections, have been rarely reported in association with cutaneous anergy and lymphocytopenia. The most common bacterial pathogen complicating influenza is *Streptococcus pneumoniae*, but *S. aureus* accounts for 12 to 25% or more of secondary bacterial infections, and *Haemophilus influenzae* is common (12, 138). Group A beta-hemolytic streptococci, gram-negative bacilli, and *Neisseria meningitidis* infections are also seen. Severe pneumococcal pneumonia including empyema and lung abscess has been associated with influenza in previously healthy children. During the 1957 pandemic, *S. aureus* suprainfection was the most common cause of fatal respiratory tract disease related to influenza and was associated with mortality rates of 28 to 48% irrespective of age or prior disease. Certain strains of *S. aureus* and other bacteria secrete proteases that enhance the infectivity of influenza viruses through HA cleavage and induce severe combined viral-bacterial pneumonia in animals. Severe and often fatal cases of community-acquired, methicillin-resistant *S. aureus* pneumonia associated with influenza are being increasingly seen in both children and adults (49). No association between preceding influenza and the occurrence of *Mycoplasma pneumoniae* or *Legionella pneumophila* infections has been found.

Nonpulmonary Complications

Other recognized but rare (<1% of cases) complications include a range of CNS syndromes (encephalitis or encephalopathy, meningitis, transverse myelitis, and polyneuritis), acute parotitis, myocarditis and pericarditis, acute myositis, rhabdomyolysis with myoglobinuria and acute renal failure, disseminated intravascular coagulopathy, arthritis, and Stevens-Johnson syndrome (70, 112). Creatine phosphokinase elevations may be as high as 10,000 IU/ml in influenza-associated rhabdomyolysis, which very rarely causes compartment syndromes. Subclinical electrocardiogram changes, including T-wave inversions, and associated echocardiographic abnormalities lasting usually 2 weeks or less occur in up to 15% of patients with apparently uncomplicated influenza. Severe cardiac involvement, rarely associated with recovery of virus from the myocardium or blood, has manifested as acute heart failure, pericardial tamponade or effusion, and fatal arrhythmia. Hepatic decompensation may occur in those with preexisting liver disease.

Acute CNS manifestations include seizures, coma without focal signs, delirium, extensor spasm, and increased intracranial pressure. Both an acute encephalopathy, which occurs at the height of illness and may be fatal, and a postinfectious encephalitis occur. Virus has been rarely isolated from the CSF or brain, although CNS dissemination has been documented in H5N1 disease (27). Postinfluenzal encephalitis begins 1 to 3 weeks after the illness and is ascribed to an autoimmune process with demyelination and vasculopathy. Patients develop fever and decreased consciousness or coma, in association with lymphocytic pleocytosis and diffuse slowing on electroencephalograms. Encephalopathic symptoms resolve in 2 to 25 days. Focal encephalitis also occurs. Influenza has been linked to delayed-onset encephalitis lethargica and postencephalitic parkinsonism.

Toxic shock syndrome may follow within 1 week of onset of influenza and has been linked to either respiratory tract colonization or infections, including sinusitis, pneumonia, or enterocolitis, with toxigenic *S. aureus* strains or group A streptococci. Influenza outbreaks are associated with an increased risk of invasive meningococcal disease, possibly related to virus-induced mucosal damage or immunosuppression. Cases usually occur within 2 weeks following influenza. Both influenza A and B virus infections

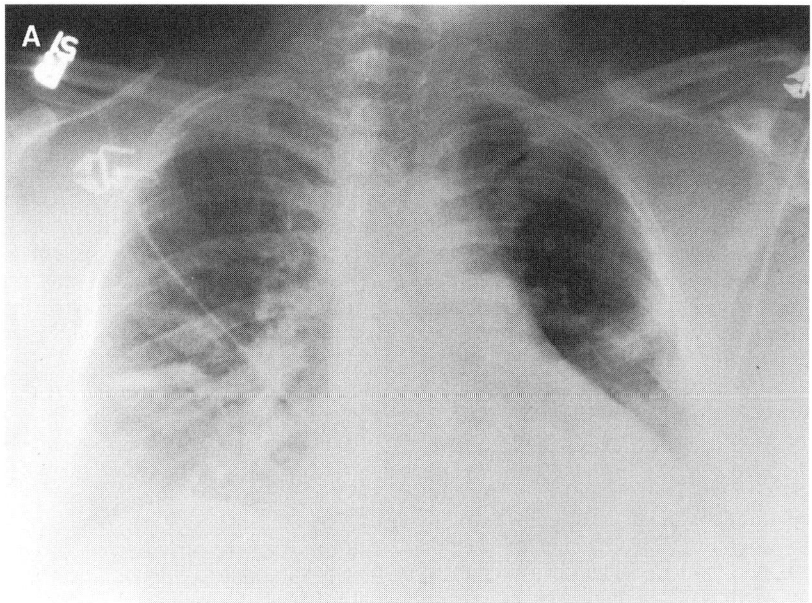

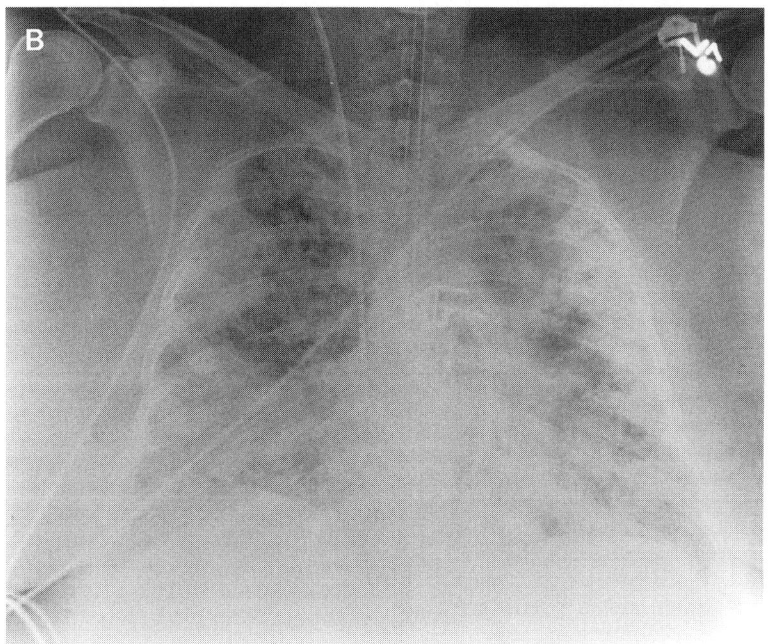

FIGURE 10 Sequential chest radiographs from a 30-year-old nonimmunocompromised female with acute influenza A virus pneumonia. (A) Her symptoms began 1 day before first radiograph, which shows right middle and bilateral lower lobe infiltrates. Her respiratory status deteriorated rapidly and she required mechanical ventilation but survived. (B) The second radiograph, taken approximately 24 h after admission, shows diffuse infiltrates.

have been associated with theophylline toxicity related to decreased clearance.

LABORATORY DIAGNOSIS

Virus Isolation

Influenza viruses can be readily isolated early in illness from a variety of respiratory specimens, including nose and throat swabs, nasal aspirates or washes, sputum, and tracheal aspirates. Throat swabs or washings contain lower virus concentrations and are usually less sensitive than nasal samples, except in sporadic A (H5N1) disease, in which the converse holds (26). Combined nose and throat swabs are a reasonable sample for upper respiratory tract sampling. If possible, tracheal aspirates or bronchial washings are advisable for seriously ill patients with lower respiratory disease, including that due to A (H5N1). Because freezing, especially in standard −20°C freezers, of specimens may cause greater loss of infectivity than short-term storage at

4°C, refrigerated samples should be transported for processing within 1 to 4 days. Freezing at or below −70°C preserves infectivity.

Embryonated hen's eggs are a practical isolation system but are less sensitive than cell culture for many contemporary human influenza viruses (126). Primary rhesus or cynomolgus monkey kidney cell cultures are sensitive for most strains. Several continuous epithelial cell lines, particularly MDCK and the rhesus monkey kidney-derived LLC-MK2, are useful for primary isolation in conjunction with incorporation of trypsin into serum-free medium to effect proteolytic activation of HA. Because of its relative temperature stability, 1-tosylamide-3-phenylethylchloromethyl ketone-treated trypsin (TPCK trypsin) is recommended. MDCK cells are comparable to primary rhesus monkey kidney cells in sensitivity for most influenza virus strains. MDCK cells that are stably transfected to overexpress α2,6-linked sialic acid receptors appear to be useful for both in vitro susceptibility testing and isolation of virus from clinical specimens (51). Other cell types (e.g., Vero, mink lung, and MRC-5 human embryonic lung cells) will support primary isolation if trypsin is used. Isolation may be facilitated by incubation at 33°C, rolling cell culture tubes, and centrifugation of the sample onto cell monolayers. Laboratory cross-contamination sometimes causes false-positive isolation results.

The CPE, particularly of influenza A viruses, is nonspecific and may be absent or difficult to detect. Over 50% of cultures show CPE within 3 days of inoculation, and over 90% shown CPE within 5 days. Virus replication is usually detected in cell culture by hemadsorption with guinea pig, turkey, or chicken erythrocytes performed at fixed times after inoculation or when CPE is noted. Because of changes in receptor specificity since 1993, use of chicken erythrocytes is not advised for detection of human strains. Blind hemadsorption of monolayers is positive in over 85% of samples at 2 days and nearly 100% of samples at 3 days after inoculation. For detection of avian influenza viruses or HAI antibody testing, avian or horse erythrocytes are used, since these predominantly express α2,3-linked sialic acid receptors.

Identification of isolates can be done by HAI testing using antisera to current strains and appropriate types of erythrocytes or by immunofluorescence (IF) or enzyme immunoassays (EIAs) using type- or subtype-specific antisera. Nucleic acid amplification tests with selected primers and probes or sequence analysis of HA and NA genes can also provide rapid typing. Rapid detection of influenza virus antigen can also be accomplished by EIA or IF testing of monolayers.

Centrifugation of samples onto MDCK monolayers in shell vials or plates combined with antigen detection has a sensitivity of about 80% (range, 56 to 100%) at 1 or 2 days. Shell vial monolayers of mink lung or rhesus monkey kidney cells may provide greater sensitivity. A commercial mixture of mink lung and A549 cells in shell vials is useful for detection of influenza and other respiratory viruses.

Primary isolation of influenza C virus has been accomplished in embryonated hen's eggs and a human malignant melanoma cell line (HMV-II) or sometimes MDCK cells, in which hemadsorption is positive with chicken but not guinea pig erythrocytes (90).

Antigen Detection

Direct detection of influenza viral antigens in respiratory secretions can be performed within about 1 to 4 h and has been accomplished with IF, EIA, radioimmunoassay, and time-resolved fluoroimmunoassay. Monoclonal antibodies directed against type-specific NP or other epitopes overcome the variable antigenicity of the surface glycoproteins and generally perform more accurately than polyclonal antisera. Direct and indirect IF microscopy of respiratory epithelial cells with commercially available monoclonal antibodies is rapid and has a sensitivity greater than those of point-of-care (POC) antigen tests (126). Noncommercial monoclonal antibodies specific for particular HAs are also available. Nasopharyngeal aspirates usually have higher cellular content and are superior to swabs; cytocentrifugation may enhance sensitivity.

Multiple commercial EIAs for rapid ($\leq$30 min) laboratory or POC diagnosis are available (http://www.cdc.gov/flu/professionals/diagnosis/rapidlab.htm#table). Sensitivity depends on sample type and quality, duration of illness, patient age, and perhaps influenza virus type. Median sensitivities and specificities are approximately 70 to 75% and 90 to 95%, respectively, compared to virus culture. Assay sensitivities are higher for children (~70 to 90%) than adults (~40 to 70%), in part because of higher viral levels. Nasopharyngeal aspirates and washes have higher yields than swabs; throat swabs or gargles are relatively insensitive. Lower clinical sensitivity has been reported in influenza B virus infections than in influenza A virus infections, and very low clinical sensitivity has been found in patients with A (H5N1) (166). Mucoid samples like sputa or tracheal aspirates cause false-positive or -negative reactions in some assays. POC test results should be interpreted with caution outside of the influenza season and confirmed by other methods.

NA Detection

A commercial assay that detects the specific enzymatic activity of influenza A and B viruses through the use of a substrate linked to a cleavable chromogenic marker is available for rapid diagnosis. The reported sensitivity ranges from 65 to 88% (126), although one study of pediatric nasal lavage samples found lower sensitivity than for an EIA for influenza A (113).

Nucleic Acid Detection

Reverse transcription-PCR (RT-PCR) has been used in detecting influenza A and B virus RNA in clinical samples. The sensitivity is approximately 90% compared to cell culture isolation, but RT-PCR can detect noninfectious virus and often has higher overall yield. The performance time is slower than for rapid antigen detection methods. Multiplex primer combinations are capable of distinguishing between types and subtypes in a single amplification. Two commercial multiplex RT-PCR assays (xTAG, Luminex; proFLU+, Prodesse) were approved in 2008 in the United States. Nucleic acid amplification tests with selected primers or combined with restriction enzyme analysis can detect influenza A viruses harboring M2 gene mutations associated with resistance to amantadine and rimantadine or selected NA mutations associated with resistance to oseltamivir, differentiate between the genes of vaccine-like strains and circulating ones, and provide data about HA genetic drift. Sensitive multiplex real-time PCR assays provide rapid (<5-h) quantitative detection of influenza A and B virus RNA, and in combination with shell vial can also provide isolates for analysis (125).

Serology

Serologic studies are not useful for rapid diagnosis of influenza, since most cases are reinfections and paired acute- and convalescent-phase sera are usually needed. Commonly used systems include CF, HAI, and enzyme-linked immunosorbent assay. Less commonly employed tests include neutralization (Nt) or microneutralization, single radial hemolysis, radial immunodiffusion, passive hemagglutination, and NA inhibition. The CF test utilizes type-specific internal antigens (NP), and unlike the HAI test, it is not influenced by the antigenic variability of the circulating strain or by the presence of serum inhibitors. However, CF is less sensitive than HAI or enzyme-linked immunosorbent assay and detects a rise in no more than 70% of infections. HAI titers reflect subtype- and strain-specific antibodies directed to HA. HAI testing requires inactivation of nonspecific inhibitors in the sample, and its sensitivity depends on the antigenic variant employed. Sensitivity is enhanced by antigen preparation in cell culture and, particularly for influenza B virus, ether treatment of antigen. Because anamnestic responses frequently occur, inclusion of antigens that resemble circulating strains and those of past prevalent strains increases diagnostic yield. Fourfold-or-greater rises occur in 80% or more of infections. The Nt test is the most specific of the conventional assays, correlates best with protective immunity, and is the current serologic method of choice in A (H5N1) infections. However, it is more labor-intensive and, for H5N1 diagnosis, requires use of biosafety level 3-enhanced conditions. Detection of HAI antibodies to H5 with horse erythrocytes or by Nt testing with pseudotyped virus expressing H5 HA may overcome this problem (151). Antibody detection by EIA is more sensitive than other assays and can be used to measure HA-specific responses or particular antibody types.

PREVENTION

Inactivated influenza vaccines were initially introduced in the 1940s but were impure, reactogenic, and variably potent. Less reactogenic whole-virus vaccines became available nearly four decades ago and were followed during the 1970s by purified split and subvirion preparations. Currently, use of inactivated influenza vaccine is the most important measure for reducing influenza virus-related morbidity and mortality (Table 4).

The effectiveness of various nonpharmaceutical interventions like social distancing, hand hygiene, cough etiquette, and masking in influenza prevention has received increased attention in the context of both seasonal influenza and pandemic preparedness (17). The value of hand hygiene for preventing influenza transmission remains to be rigorously proven, and in health care settings, the possible incremental value of using respirators compared with surgical or procedure masks remains uncertain. Timely implementation of multiple public health responses, including combinations of school closures, cancellation of mass gatherings, isolation, and voluntary quarantine, that were taken in some cities during the 1918 pandemic appears to have reduced its community impact, although the value of any individual intervention cannot be dissected in these retrospective studies (86). Holiday periods are associated with reduced seasonal influenza rates, and prolonged school closures are predicted to reduce peak attack rates and cumulative numbers of cases in children and adults (16). Such interventions are being contemplated as part of a community mitigation strategy in the face of a pandemic associated with high mortality (17).

Inactivated Vaccines

Current vaccines are formalin-inactivated whole-virus, detergent-disrupted or chemically disrupted split-virus (subvirion), or purified surface antigen preparations (35, 40). Antigens for inactivated vaccines are mass produced in embryonated chicken eggs by use of high-yield reassortant viruses that express the HA and NA of circulating strains. Residual egg proteins can rarely cause immediate hypersensitivity reactions in those with egg allergy and possibly contribute to other adverse effects. The HA content of vaccines is standardized (minimum of 15 μg per antigen for adults) (Table 5). The composition of influenza vaccines is determined semiannually on the basis of the antigenicity of circulating influenza viruses through the WHO's Global Influenza Surveillance Network (http://www.who.int/csr/disease/influenza/surveillance/en/). Recent seasonal vaccines contain antigens of two influenza A virus subtypes (H3N2 and H1N1) and of one influenza B virus. The waning of vaccine-induced immunity over time necessitates annual reimmunization, even if the vaccine antigens are unchanged. Annual guidelines for immunization are published by the CDC (35).

Immunogenicity

Inactivated vaccine is highly immunogenic in young adults but less so in the elderly, infants, and persons with chronic illness or immunosuppression, including those with HIV disease, solid-organ and bone marrow transplant recipients, and those receiving cancer chemotherapy. Immunogenicity is also lower in those with high preexisting antibody levels. Protection against illness correlates with the levels of serum HAI antibodies. In addition, parenteral immunization may stimulate limited mucosal antibody production and CTL responses (40). In primed healthy adults, immunization results in presumably protective levels of serum HAI antibody in >85% for the homologous strain. Because 60% or less of unprimed children respond, two doses of vaccine at least 1 month apart are required. Protective HAI antibody responses usually occur in responding adults, including those with cardiopulmonary disease, within 10 days. The duration of protection following immunization is uncertain but may last up to 2 to 3 years against homotypic virus.

Age-related declines in serologic and CTL memory responses to vaccine occur with advancing age, and failure of vaccine boosting occurs more commonly in the elderly (142). A second dose of vaccine at 1 or 3 months does not boost serum HAI titer responses in healthy, elderly persons (91), but vaccine containing fourfold-higher antigen content (60 μg of HA) appears to improve immunogenicity (22). An MF-59 adjuvanted vaccine available in Europe appears to be more immunogenic in the elderly. The degree of infirmity, rather than increasing age by itself, is a critical determinant of decreased vaccine responsiveness. T-cell responses may be better correlates of vaccine protection than antibody levels in the elderly (92). While later booster doses do not appear to increase protection in the frail elderly, a second dose may improve immunogenicity in certain high-risk groups (e.g., liver transplant or chemotherapy recipients).

TABLE 4 Target groups for influenza immunization[a,b]

Patients at increased risk for influenza-related complications
- Persons 50 yr and older[c]
- Children aged 6 mo to 18 yr[d]
- Women who will be pregnant during influenza season
- Persons with chronic cardiovascular (excluding hypertension), pulmonary (including asthma), renal, hepatic, hematologic, or metabolic disorders (including diabetes mellitus) or immunosuppression (including that due to HIV infection)
- Patients with neuromuscular conditions that compromise respiratory function or handling of secretions (including cognitive dysfunction, seizure disorder, or spinal cord injury)
- Residents of nursing homes and other long-term care facilities housing persons with chronic medical conditions
- Children and teenagers (6 mo–18 yr) who are receiving long-term aspirin therapy (risk for Reye's syndrome after influenza infection)

Close contacts of high-risk patients
- Physicians, nurses, and other health care personnel, volunteers and trainees in health care settings
- Employees of nursing homes and long-term care facilities
- Household contacts (including children) and caregivers (visiting nurses and home health aides) of persons at higher risk of complications, including children <5 yr old (especially contacts of infants <6 mo old) and adults >50 yr old

Providers of essential community services

Persons in settings with increased risk of exposure (e.g., those in student dormitories)

Other groups
- Nonimmunized travelers to areas where influenza may be circulating before travel (i) with large organized groups at any time of year, (ii) to the tropics, or (iii) to the southern hemisphere (April–September)

Anyone wishing to reduce risk of influenza (including school-age children)

[a] Based in part on Recommendations of the Advisory Committee on Immunization Practices, 2007 (35).

[b] When delays in vaccine availability are anticipated, available vaccine should be targeted preferentially to persons at increased risk of influenza complications and to health care workers. The optimal time for administration to high-risk individuals is October to November in the northern hemisphere.

[c] Immunization is recommended for persons aged 50 to 64 years in part because this age cohort has an increased prevalence of persons with high-risk conditions.

[d] Children aged 6 months to 8 years who have not been immunized against influenza before should receive two doses of vaccine the first year they are immunized, with the second dose administered ≥4 weeks after the first and if possible before the influenza season. Trivalent inactivated influenza vaccine is FDA approved for children 6 months and older, whereas LAIV is approved currently for those aged 2 to 49 years. If only one dose of vaccine (either trivalent inactivated influenza vaccine or LAIV) was administered in the initial season, two doses are recommended for the second season of immunization.

Efficacy

Vaccine efficacy in preventing clinical influenza relates to both host immune responses and the antigenic relatedness between the epidemic virus and vaccine strain. The efficacy of inactivated vaccines in preventing illness has ranged widely but is generally 60 to 90% in healthy children and adults. The higher levels of efficacy are seen when the antigenic match between the vaccine and circulating strains is good. Immunization of working adults reduces absenteeism and physician visits due to respiratory illness by about 30 to 60% during epidemic periods and may be cost saving. Immunization of children reduces the risk of influenza-related otitis media and the likelihood of illness in nonimmunized household contacts. Mass immunization of children also appears to lessen the impact of the epidemic in the community; wide-scale immunization of school-age children in Japan was temporally associated with reduced respiratory and overall mortality in older adults (129). Among ambulatory older adults in the community, immunization provides about 50 to 60% protection against influenza, is cost saving, and reduces hospitalizations and hospital deaths for pneumonia and other respiratory conditions, as well as mortality from cardiovascular conditions and all causes, by approximately 30 to 50% during outbreaks (111). However, the magnitude of influenza immunization's effect on overall mortality in the elderly is debated (141).

In nursing home residents, protective efficacy against influenzal illness ranges widely and averages only 20 to 45%. However, immunization reduces influenza-related hospitalizations and pneumonia by 50 to 60% and mortality by 65 to 80% in such persons. High nursing home immunization rates (≥80% of residents) may indirectly confer protection against outbreaks by increasing levels of herd immunity.

Populations targeted for immunization include both those at increased risk for influenza-related complications and persons who are in close contact with high-risk indi-

TABLE 5 Comparison of seasonal inactivated vaccines and LAIV[a]

Parameter	Inactivated vaccine	LAIV	Comment
Route of administration	Intramuscular injection	Intranasal spray	Deltoid for adults and older children; anterolateral thigh for infants and young children
No. of strains	Trivalent	Trivalent	Currently A (H1N1), A (H3N2), and B
Vaccine	Chemically disrupted virus or purified surface antigens	Live virus	Inactivated whole-virus vaccines under development for nonseasonal viruses
Dose strength	15 μg of HA/antigen	~10^7 infectious doses/virus	
Dose	0.25–0.5 ml	0.2 ml	Smaller volume of TIV[b] for children aged 6–35 mo
Production	Eggs	Eggs	Growth cell cultures under study and approved for TIV in some countries
FDA approval	Persons aged ≥6 mo	Healthy persons aged 2–49 yr	Only TIV approved for use in those with underlying medical conditions or pregnancy (see Table 5)
Frequency	Annual	Annual	4-wk interval between for children receiving vaccine for first time and requiring two doses
Shipment and storage	2–8°C	2–8°C	Do not place in freezer.
Packaging	Prefilled syringes, single-use and multiuse vials	Prefilled, single-use sprayer	Thimerosal-free TIV formulations available from some manufacturers

[a] Adapted from reference 35.
[b] TIV, trivalent inactivated influenza vaccine.

viduals and at risk of transmitting infection to them, particularly health care workers (Table 4). Health care worker immunization probably reduces the risk of nosocomial transmission and associated consequences (57). Foreign travelers, particularly elderly or high-risk persons, should be immunized before travel to the tropics during any time of the year or during April to September if travel is to the southern hemisphere. Pregnant women and HIV-infected persons are important risk groups. In addition, immunization is appropriate for anyone who wishes to reduce his or her risk of acquiring influenza.

Reactogenicity

Injection may cause local redness and induration for 1 or 2 days in up to one-third of vaccinees. Fever and constitutional symptoms beginning 6 to 12 h after vaccination and lasting for several days occur in 1 to 5% of adult recipients and more often in young children. Elderly subjects tend to have lower rates of local and systemic reactions. Because of the potential for causing febrile reactions, only split-virus or surface antigen vaccine should be used for seasonal immunization in children. Severe allergic reactions, including anaphylaxis, are rare and usually secondary to egg protein hypersensitivity, so the vaccine should be used with caution in patients who have documented allergies to eggs or egg products. Desensitization regimens have been described for such patients. A temporal association between immunization and Guillain-Barré syndrome (GBS) development within 6 weeks was found during the 1977 swine influenza immunization program, during which approximately 430 GBS cases occurred among 41 million vaccinees, a rate estimated to be sevenfold higher than expected. Whether influenza vaccines in certain seasons may be associated with a low risk of GBS (1 per 10^6) in older vaccinees is unresolved. Reported associations of influenza immunization with exacerbations of asthma, systemic vasculitis, recurrent GBS, adverse ocular effects, or pericarditis remain unproven; asthma exacerbations are not associated with inactivated vaccine. No important changes in drug metabolism have occurred with current vaccines. Pneumococcal and influenza vaccines can be given at the same time at different sites without increased side effects.

Special Populations

In HIV-infected persons, advanced disease is associated with low antibody responses, which are not augmented by a booster dose or doubled HA antigen content. Those with CD4 counts of $<100/mm^3$ rarely show antibody rises, but immunization appears to be protective in those with CD4 counts of $>200/mm^3$ despite diminished HAI responses. Influenza immunization may be followed 1 to 4 weeks later by transient increases in plasma virus titers in some recipients, but the clinical significance of such changes is doubtful, and no long-term effects on CD4 counts or clinical progression have been recognized (148).

Those with hematologic malignancy, including myeloma, often have reduced responsiveness to vaccine. Oncology patients manifest HAI antibody responses less often when they are immunized concurrently with or shortly after chemotherapy compared to immunization between courses of chemotherapy. If immunization is required during chemotherapy, a two-dose schedule of vaccination separated by 3 to 5 weeks has been suggested, since this significantly increases the antibody responses in lymphoma patients. For children with malignancy, immunization at least 1 month off chemotherapy and when the peripheral leukocyte count exceeds 1,000 improves immunogenicity.

Immunization is generally safe in solid-organ transplantation, but many recipients of such transplants, including heart, lung, and liver transplants, have deficient HAI responses. Immunization within the first 6 to 12 months following bone marrow transplantation is ineffective, but responsiveness gradually returns by 2 years in most patients. A booster dose 1 month after the initial one does not generally improve response rates but may in some transplant patients. Antiviral chemoprophylaxis (discussed below) offers an alternative or supplemental means of protection.

The H5 HA appears to be a weak human immunogen, and two doses of nonadjuvanted, inactivated split vaccine with a high HA antigen content (45 to 90 μg) are needed for immunogenicity in the majority of healthy adults and children (146, 154). Alum adjuvants do not improve immunogenicity much, but proprietary oil-in-water adjuvants (e.g., MF-59 and AS03) provide substantial HA antigen sparing and cross-clade immunogenicity (9, 77). Whole-virus A (H5N1) vaccines also appear to reduce antigen requirements and give broader immunogenicity.

Live Attenuated Vaccines

Intranasally administered live attenuated influenza virus vaccines (LAIV) have been used extensively in the former Soviet Union and were licensed for commercial use in the United States in 2003. Cold-adapted, temperature-sensitive, attenuated donor viruses (A/Ann/6/60/H2N2 and B/Ann Arbor/1/66), which are able to grow at 25°C but are restricted at 39°C, have been used to make reassortants containing six internal genes from donor virus and two genes encoding the HA and NA from wild-type strains (Table 5) (13). Several gene segments contribute to the attenuation/temperature sensitivity phenotype of the live attenuated influenza A (with mutations in PB1, PB2, and NP) and influenza B (with mutations in PA, NP, and M1) virus vaccines (58, 65). These reassortant viruses are well tolerated, genetically stable, rarely transmissible to contacts, and immunogenic following intranasal administration in seronegative children and adults. Serum antibody responses are lower in adults than following administration of inactivated vaccines. They appear to be safe in those with underlying pulmonary disease or HIV infection (CD4 count, >200 cells/mm^3) but are licensed for use in the United States only in healthy persons aged 2 to 49 years (Table 5). Intranasal LAIV may be associated with coryza (5 to 30%), sore throat (10%), and, in children, transient febrile reactions (5%) or decreased activity level typically on the second or third day after inoculation. An increased frequency of medically significant wheezing episodes has been found in children less than 2 years of age (8). Detection of LAIV virus lasts up to 1 week in adults and up to 3 weeks in very young children. Transmission of vaccine virus may sometimes occur among young children. Transmission of vaccine virus from adults has not been documented to date, but health care workers and others who receive LAIV should avoid contact with highly immunocompromised persons (e.g., stem cell transplant recipients in protected environments) for 1 week after immunization.

Immune responses to multivalent LAIV are influenced by preexisting immunity, the infectivity of each vaccine virus, and interference among vaccine viruses. The 50% infectious doses are about 10- to 100-fold lower for seronegative infants than adults, but interference among vaccine strains reduces responses in seronegative children. Although single doses are often immunogenic (7), two doses appear to be necessary to confer multistrain protection in young children. Potential advantages of *ca* vaccines include ease of administration (nose drops or coarse spray), induction of local secretory antibody, protection against drift variants, and possibly induction of heterosubtypic CTL responses.

The efficacy of trivalent LAIV is superior to that of inactivated vaccine in healthy children aged 6 to 59 months, including protection against antigenically drifted strains (8), but is comparable or somewhat lower in adults ≤65 years old (114). In children, LAIV is highly protective (efficacy, >90%) against influenza A and B illness and associated complications, including otitis media (7). Effectiveness against drift variant illness has been observed in children and working adults, but LAIV is less immunogenic in elderly adults. Compared to inactivated vaccine alone, combined administration of inactivated and intranasal LAIV may have given greater protection against influenza in elderly nursing home residents although not in ambulatory patients with chronic obstructive pulmonary disease. The intranasal replication and associated immunogenicity of A (H5N1) LAIV have been low to date.

Other Vaccines

Various approaches have been undertaken to improve the immunogenicity of inactivated vaccines, especially in elderly adults, and to develop alternative methods of production that avoid growth in chicken eggs. Mammalian cell substrates (e.g., Vero or MDCK cells) are being developed or already approved in some countries. Purified recombinant uncleaved HA, expressed in insect cells, shows dose-related immunogenicity and protection in young and older adults (156). Virosome vaccines that incorporate viral glycoproteins into unilamellar liposomes appear to be more immunogenic than standard inactivated vaccines after injection and are available in several European countries. One intranasal virosomal vaccine with the heat-labile toxin of *Escherichia coli* as an adjuvant was associated with Bell's palsy (102). Virus-like particle vaccines that contain HA, NA, and M proteins are in development. Adjuvants added to inactivated vaccines can increase immunogenicity as well as local and sometimes systemic reactogenicity in humans. Coadministration of certain immunomodulators (e.g., IL-2 or thymosin) at the time of immunization may enhance responses in older adults.

An influenza vaccine approach based on generating immune responses to conserved antigens might enable a broader spectrum of coverage and possibly reduce the impact of a new pandemic strain (146). An M2 protein-hepatitis B core protein conjugate vaccine is protective in mice, apparently through an antibody-mediated mechanism (104, 146). NA vaccines do not prevent infection but moderate illness severity. The supplementation of conventional inactivated vaccine with purified NA has been proposed to broaden heterovariant immunity. Approaches to stimulate CTL responses include various adjuvants, antigen-lipid conjugates, and injection of cDNA. In animals, administration of influenza vaccine antigens in liposomes, immune-stimulating complexes, or combined with diphtheria-tetanus-whole-cell pertussis vaccine or with cholera toxin B subunit enhances antibody responses and protection against experimental infection. Intramuscular injection of DNA encoding the influenza A virus NP in mice results in the generation of specific CTLs and Th1-type, cytokine-secreting CD4 lymphocytes that mediate heterosubtypic immunity. Polynucleotide vaccines expressing HA or adenovirus-vectored HA are protective in animals when given by injection or topical application to the respiratory tract.

Reverse genetics has been used to modify the HA of HPAI viruses to allow growth in eggs and other substrates under biosafety level 2 conditions (146). The rational design of attenuated influenza viruses for use as vaccines involves the introduction of *ts* attenuating mutations into cDNAs of different genes and rescue of viruses bearing the mutant genes. Such genetically engineered viruses are highly attenuated and protect mice against subsequent challenge with wild-type virus (144). Influenza virus mutants with truncated NS1 proteins have also been proposed as vaccine candidates, as they are highly attenuated and induce a self-adjuvant immune response by virtue of their enhanced activity to induce an interferon response in infected cells (3).

Antiviral Chemoprophylaxis

Amantadine and rimantadine are effective for prophylaxis and treatment of influenza A virus infections due to susceptible strains (53), but neither is effective for influenza B, and most recently circulating subtype A (H3N2) and some subtype A (H1N1) viruses show resistance (28). These agents share antiviral spectra, mechanisms of action, and cross-susceptibility or -resistance to influenza A viruses. Inhaled zanamivir and oral oseltamivir, which are NA inhibitors, are effective for prophylaxis for both influenza A and B virus infections (54, 56). Zanamivir and oseltamivir selectively inhibit the NA activities of a wide range of strains, including amantadine- and rimantadine-resistant influenza A viruses and all nine influenza A NA subtypes circulating in nature. Oseltamivir and inhaled zanamivir are approved in the United States and many countries for prophylaxis (Table 6). Oseltamivir has been stockpiled by the WHO for possible use in mass targeted chemoprophylaxis for containing emergence of a pandemic virus (33).

Efficacy

Prophylactic oral amantadine and rimantadine are 70 to 90% effective in preventing illness caused by susceptible strains of influenza A virus (53, 56). Efficacy has been shown in healthy adults and children and for nosocomial infection, household transmission, and pandemic influenza. Lower doses of rimantadine or amantadine (100 mg/day) appear to be effective for prophylaxis in young adults. Rimantadine prophylaxis in school-age children markedly decreases their risk of influenza A illness and also reduces the risk of influenza virus infection in their family contacts.

The efficacy of oseltamivir at 75 mg once daily for 6 weeks for seasonal prophylaxis is approximately 84% in unimmunized working adults and 89% in immunized nursing home residents. When used for postexposure prophylaxis in family contacts, 7 to 10 days of once-daily oseltamivir provides 73 to 89% protection (54, 56). Inhaled zanamivir at 10 mg once daily is also highly protective against influenza under similar circumstances. In one nursing home-based trial, zanamivir prophylaxis was more effective than oral rimantadine in protecting against influenza, in part because of the frequent failure of rimantadine prophylaxis due to drug-resistant strains (47).

Seasonal prophylaxis is an alternative or adjunct to immunization when the epidemic strain differs antigenically to a significant extent from the vaccine strain or when high-risk patients have a contraindication or are expected to mount an inadequate response to immunization. Combined use of vaccine and chemoprophylaxis offers the highest level of protection for high-risk patients. Protection requires drug administration for the duration of the epidemic, generally 6 to 10 weeks. Drug recipients may experience subclinical infection, which usually confers protection against infection by the same strain.

Because antiviral chemoprophylaxis does not interfere with the immune response to inactivated vaccine, they can be administered concurrently. However, concurrent use of any anti-influenza antiviral drug might interfere with the immunogenicity of LAIV. If influenza has already occurred in the community, prophylaxis can be given to unimmunized high-risk persons for 2 weeks beginning at the time of immunization. Short-term postexposure prophylaxis with rimantadine or amantadine for 10 days appears to be effective in protecting family contacts when circulating strains are susceptible, but concurrent treatment of ill children may lead to rapid selection and spread of drug-resistant virus to contacts receiving prophylaxis (53). In contrast, use of inhaled zanamivir or oral oseltamivir for both treatment of ill index cases and prophylaxis of healthy contacts is protective and usually not associated with resistance emergence (54, 56).

Tolerability

At usual doses in healthy adults (200 mg/day), amantadine is associated with more frequent minor adverse drug reactions, including nervousness, anxiety, insomnia, and difficulty concentrating, than rimantadine. Most complaints develop within a week of dosing but often resolve over time or promptly upon cessation. Higher amantadine doses are frequently associated with adverse effects and decreased psychomotor performance. More severe effects include stupor, delirium, confusion, hallucinations, and seizures. Risk factors, particularly in elderly patients, include impaired renal function (serum creatinine, >1.0 mg/dl), lower body mass (weight, <50 kg), female gender (which is associated with lower renal clearance of amantadine), coadministration of drugs that impair amantadine excretion (e.g., triamterene, trimethoprim, and possibly thiazides) or potentiate its CNS effects (e.g., anticholinergics and psychotropics), and preexisting seizure disorders.

Adults aged 65 years or older require only one-half of the body weight-adjusted dose of amantadine to achieve drug concentrations in plasma similar to those observed in young adults; doses of ≤100 mg per day are advisable in order to reduce the risk of toxicity. Dose reductions are also indicated in those with recognized renal disease or in persons with active seizure disorder (Table 6). Rimantadine

TABLE 6 Suggested dose regimens for antiviral administration in seasonal influenza[a]

Drug	Regimen
Amantadine	Children 1–9 yr of age: 5.0 mg/kg of body wt/day (up to 150 mg/day) in two divided doses
	Children ≥10 yr and adults <64 yr who have normal renal function: 100 mg twice daily
	Adults ≥65 yr: 100 mg once daily[a,b]
	Prophylaxis: same as treatment dose
	Dose reduction: creatinine clearance <60–80 ml/min or serum creatinine >1.0 mg/dl
Rimantadine[c]	Children 1–9 yr of age: 5 mg/kg/day (up to 150 mg/day)
	Children ≥10 yr and adults ≤64 yr: 200 mg once daily or 100 mg twice daily
	Adults ≥65 yr: 100 mg once daily
	Prophylaxis: same as treatment dose
	Dose reduction: severe hepatic dysfunction or creatinine clearance <10–20 ml/min
Zanamivir	Children ≥5 yr[d] and adults: 10 mg by oral inhalation (two inhalations) twice daily
	Prophylaxis[d]: 10 mg by oral inhalation (one inhalation) once daily
Oseltamivir	Children 1–12 yr: 30 mg for ≤15 kg, 45 mg for >15–23 kg, 60 mg for >23–40 kg twice daily
	Children ≥13 yr or weighing >40 kg and adults: 75 mg twice daily
	Prophylaxis in children ≥13 yr and adults: 75 mg once daily
	Prophylaxis in children 1–12 yr: 30 mg for ≤15 kg, 45 mg for >15–23 kg, 60 mg for >23–40 kg once daily
	Dose reduction: creatinine clearance <30 ml/min

[a] Dosing based in part on Recommendations of the Advisory Committee on Immunization Practices, 2007 (35). Amantadine and rimantadine are not recommended for use at present because of the high frequency of resistance in seasonal influenza A (H3N2), as well as some A (H1N1), viruses. The suggested duration of treatment is 5 days. Oseltamivir is currently the recommended treatment for H5N1 infections, for which twofold-higher doses, more prolonged treatment (10 days), and, where viruses are susceptible, combined administration with amantadine are considerations (163). The suggested duration of prophylaxis depends on epidemiological circumstances, e.g., 7 to 10 days for postcontact prophylaxis in households, 2 weeks or longer in health care facility outbreaks, and 4 to 6 weeks for protection of high-risk persons in community outbreaks.

[b] Further reductions are indicated for renal dysfunction or low weight (≤50 kg). Some authorities suggest a dosage of 1.4 mg/kg/day.

[c] Rimantadine has been approved by the FDA for the prevention and treatment of influenza A virus infection in adults and for prevention in children; it has not been approved for treatment in children.

[d] Approved by the FDA for treatment for those aged 7 years and above and for 10-day prophylaxis for those aged 5 years and above.

dose reductions are indicated for marked hepatic or renal insufficiency or in the elderly.

The dosing of zanamivir or oseltamivir does not need adjustment in the elderly. In patients with advanced renal insufficiency (creatinine clearance, <30 ml/min), the dose of oseltamivir should be reduced by half. Oseltamivir chemoprophylaxis is associated with gastrointestinal upset (nausea and emesis) in <5% of recipients and perhaps headache in elderly persons. Inhaled zanamivir is generally well tolerated when used for prophylaxis. The breath-activated proprietary Diskhaler device for delivery of inhaled zanamivir requires a cooperative patient who can effectively inspire. Compliance has generally been excellent, but certain groups (children <5 years old, persons with cognitive impairment, and very frail or hospitalized elderly persons) are not able to use it reliably.

Management of Nosocomial Outbreaks

Prevention of outbreaks in institutional populations requires an established plan that includes preapproved vaccine and medication orders; preseason immunization of residents and staff members; surveillance for influenza during the season; and, in the event of an outbreak, use of appropriate isolation techniques, immunization of residents and staff who have not received vaccine, and possibly antiviral chemoprophylaxis. A surveillance system is needed for detection of influenza-like illness in the facility and confirmation of viral etiology. Rapid antigen testing and institution of outbreak control measures increase the proportion of preventable cases compared to the delay associated with waiting for culture reports. Chemoprophylaxis both for patients, irrespective of immunization status, and for staff is indicated for outbreak control. Administration for 2 weeks or until new cases have ceased to occur for at least 1 week appears to be adequate in most nursing home outbreaks.

The choice of antiviral agent depends on multiple considerations, including circulating virus, tolerance, resistance, and cost. The dose of amantadine suggested for prophylaxis in nursing home residents aged ≥65 years (100 mg/day) has been associated with adverse effects in 22 to 47% of recipients, with excess falls, and with cessation of therapy in 7 to 37% because of side effects (69). The differences in risk of adverse drug reactions and less complex dose adjustment for renal impairment favor rimantadine over amantadine, when circulating influenza A virus strains are susceptible (69). NA inhibitors should be used for influenza B, mixed outbreaks of influenza A and B, when circulating influenza A strains are likely resistant to M2 inhibitors, or when influenza A cases continue to occur despite use of an M2 inhibitor.

When possible, isolation of infected patients, especially respiratory isolation in negative-pressure ventilated rooms in the hospital setting, is desirable. In the context of nursing home outbreaks, suggested guidelines (46) include confinement of ill residents to their rooms for at least 72 h; restriction of movement of nonill residents to other parts of the facility and consideration for confinement to their rooms, if an outbreak with high attack rates or severe illness is occurring; decentralization or postponement of activities which could expose large numbers of nonill residents to influenza; restriction from work of employees with influenza-like illness; minimizing work assignments of staff to multiple units of the facility; restricting visits by persons with respiratory illness; and discouraging visits to residents with illness.

TREATMENT

Symptomatic treatment of influenza commonly involves antipyretic-analgesic drugs, particularly acetaminophen or nonsteroidal anti-inflammatory agents, for relief of fever, aches, and other systemic symptoms. Aspirin should be avoided in children because of its association with Reye's syndrome. Antitussives are often needed for relief of cough. Antibiotics have not been shown to benefit the course or reduce the likelihood of complications and should be used for proven or presumed bacterial complications.

In those with lower-airway disease, correction of hypoxemia and treatment of bronchospasm are important. Ventilatory support with positive airway pressures can be lifesaving in patients with influenza viral pneumonia; extracorporeal membrane oxygenation has been used in some cases. The value of corticosteroids to treat bronchiolitis obliterans with organizing pneumonia or the fibroproliferative phase of ARDS associated with viral pneumonia is uncertain. In subtype A (H5N1) pneumonia, corticosteroids are not recommended, and higher doses may be associated with increased mortality (163, 166).

Amantadine and Rimantadine

In uncomplicated influenza A due to susceptible strains, early treatment (within ≤48 h of illness onset) with amantadine or rimantadine reduces viral replication and the duration of fever, symptoms, and functional disability by about 1 to 2 days in previously healthy adults (Table 6). Treatment is associated with more rapid improvement in peripheral airway dysfunction but not airway hyperreactivity. Whether treatment reduces the risk of influenza-related complications or provides therapeutic benefit in established complications or severe influenza in hospitalized patients is unknown. High-dose oral amantadine (400 to 550 mg per day) has been used in influenza viral pneumonia with uncertain benefit.

In children, rimantadine treatment has been associated with lower symptom burden and viral titers during the first 2 days of treatment than with acetaminophen but also with more prolonged shedding of virus and emergence of resistance. Early antiviral treatment in children may reduce viral antigen exposure and delay the development of specific immune responses. Rimantadine is not currently approved for therapy of influenza in children in the United States.

M2 inhibitor resistance due to a Ser31Asn mutation has become widespread globally among circulating strains of subtype A (H3N2) (28). Resistance is present in subtype A (H1N1) viruses variably, as well as in all clade 1 and some clade 2 A (H5N1) viruses. Consequently, the use of M2 inhibitors is generally not recommended at present. Influenza A viruses cross-resistant to amantadine and rimantadine have been recovered from patients as early as 2 to 3 days after the start of treatment and from about 30% of outpatient children and adults treated for influenza (53). Most immunocompromised patients who shed virus for more than 3 days while on treatment shed resistant variants (31). While immunocompetent patients recover promptly despite resistance emergence, prolonged shedding of resistant variants and illness have been observed in immunocompromised patients. Apparent transmission of resistant virus has caused failures of drug prophylaxis in family contacts and during nursing home outbreaks. Resistant variants appear to be pathogenic and can cause typical disabling influenzal illness.

Oseltamivir and Zanamivir

Inhaled zanamivir treatment provides 1- to 2.5-day reductions in time to alleviation of illness and return to usual activities compared to placebo in adults and children ≥5 years old, including those with mild to moderate underlying airway disease (54, 56). Zanamivir appears to be more effective than oseltamivir in treating influenza B virus infections in children (147). Zanamivir treatment reduces the frequency of antibiotic prescriptions for lower respiratory complications by about 40% (54). Among older adults, including those developing influenza despite immunization, inhaled zanamivir treatment appears to have therapeutic effects and tolerance similar to those in younger adults. Its therapeutic value in treating viral pneumonia or other lower respiratory tract disease due to influenza is unproven. Inhaled zanamivir reduces pharyngeal but not nasal viral recovery. Inhaled zanamivir is generally well tolerated during therapeutic use, although rare cases of bronchospasm and exacerbations of underlying airway disease, sometimes fatal, have been reported.

Early oseltamivir treatment of previously healthy adults reduces the time to illness alleviation by approximately 1 to 1.5 days, time to resumption of usual activities by 2 to 3 days, and frequency of secondary complications leading to antibiotic prescriptions by approximately 50%. Oseltamivir treatment of children aged 1 to 12 years with acute influenza reduces illness duration by 1.5 days and the frequency of complications, particularly otitis media, leading to antibiotic prescriptions (54, 56). Therapeutic use of NA inhibitors does not interfere with the serum antibody response to acute influenza. About 10 to 15% of treated persons experience nausea or emesis with oseltamivir. Gastrointestinal upset is usually not dose-limiting, typically occurs after the first doses, and can be reduced by ingesting the drug with food.

Oseltamivir therapy appears to reduce the risk of progression to pneumonia in highly immunocompromised hosts with influenza (18) and to reduce the risk of death in hospitalized patients (93). Oseltamivir treatment is associated with lower mortality in A (H5N1) disease, although progressive illness, sometimes related to resistance emergence, occurs (27, 166). Combinations of M2 and NA inhibitors show enhanced antiviral activity under experimental conditions, including against A (H5N1) disease (61), and have been used in cases of presumed influenza A viral pneumonia.

The efficacy and safety of these drugs in pregnancy have not been established, but no teratogenicity has been found in animal studies. Both zanamivir and oseltamivir carboxylate distribute across the placenta and into breast milk in animals. Given the potential teratogenicity of the M2 inhibitors, the NA inhibitors would be preferred for influenza treatment; the lower systemic exposure of inhaled zanamivir is a consideration in this decision.

Resistance has occurred uncommonly with both agents during clinical use (2), but oseltamivir resistance has been found recently in community isolates (108, 164). Oseltamivir-resistant variants have been recovered from immunocompetent outpatient adults (~1%), outpatient children (~4%), inpatient children (~18%), and subtype A (H5N1)-infected persons (~25%) during or immediately after treatment (2, 27). These variants possess amino acid substitutions (primarily Arg292Lys or Glu119Lys in N2 and His274Tyr in N1) in the NA; most oseltamivir-resistant variants retain susceptibility to zanamivir. Prolonged replication with resistant variants, sometimes with dual resistance to M2 inhibitors, has been recognized in immunocompromised hosts (62). Transmission of oseltamivir-resistant variants has been observed in families and in the community (108), and recently, oseltamivir-resistant H1N1 viruses with a His274Tyr mutation in N1 have appeared among community isolates in multiple countries (164), so careful monitoring of susceptibility patterns is necessary to guide antiviral choices (http://www.who.int/csr/disease/influenza/h1n1_table/en/index.html).

Investigational Agents

Antivirals

A number of anti-influenza compounds have been described, but few have undergone clinical testing (118). No parenteral antiviral is currently approved for influenza management in seriously ill patients. Intravenous zanamivir is highly active in experimental human influenza. Peramivir, an NA inhibitor with a prolonged duration of activity in animal models (169) and long plasma half-life in humans, is currently being studied for its activity when administered by intramuscular (outpatient) and intravenous (inpatient) routes. Inhaled NA inhibitors with a prolonged duration of antiviral action in animals are in clinical development. Monoclonal antibodies show activity in animal models of subtype A (H5N1) disease, and a retrospective analysis suggested that therapeutic use of convalescent-phase blood products in pneumonia patients in 1918 reduced mortality (83). Serotherapy with convalescent-phase plasma has been used in individual H5N1 patients.

Ribavirin is a nucleoside analog active in vitro against both influenza A and B viruses. If initiated early after symptom onset, aerosol ribavirin variably reduces illness in adults with uncomplicated influenza, but it was associated with no important clinical benefits in young children hospitalized with influenza (131). Aerosolized, oral, and intravenous forms of ribavirin have been used to treat individual patients with influenza pneumonia or other severe complications, including influenza myocarditis and subtype A (H5N1) illness. Combinations of ribavirin and oseltamivir show enhanced activity in a murine model of subtype A (H5N1) disease. However, ribavirin remains an investigational agent of unproven efficacy in influenza. A polymerase inhibitor, designated T-705, that is active against all three influenza types, including subtype A (H5N1) virus and some other RNA viruses in animal models (139), has good oral bioavailability in humans and is undergoing clinical study. A topically applied sialidase construct, designated DAS181, that cleaves receptors recognized by influenza viruses is active in animal models, including one due to subtype A (H5N1) infection (6), and is entering clinical development.

Intranasal recombinant IFN-α2 provided partial protection against illness in experimental human influenza when volunteers were infected by nasal inoculation, but it is ineffective in preventing natural influenza. Aerosolized interferon provides only limited protection in murine models of influenza. Various combinations of antivirals (e.g., M2 inhibitor with ribavirin, NA inhibitor, or interferon or NA inhibitor with polymerase inhibitor) show enhanced antiviral activity in preclinical studies, including H5N1 infections (61), and may eventually provide a strategy for treating severe infections in humans (118).

Other Modalities

Studies with animal models suggest that surfactant deficiency, due to alveolar cell destruction and exudate, may play a role in the development of respiratory failure in influenza pneumonia. Exogenous replacement is associated with improved gas exchange and pulmonary mechanics in experimental animal influenza in some studies but not others. Generation of reactive oxygen species by phagocytes may contribute to pulmonary damage, and administration of the xanthine oxidase inhibitor allopurinol or a free radical scavenger superoxide dismutase is associated with improved survival in experimentally infected animals. Vitamin E supplementation of influenza virus-infected aged mice improves survival and levels of Th1 cytokines and NK cell activity. Some agents with immunomodulator activity, like gemfibrozil, show activity in experimental animal models of influenza, but the usefulness of such interventions remains to be established in human influenza.

REFERENCES

1. **Akarsu, H., W. P. Burmeister, C. Petosa, I. Petit, C. W. Muller, R. W. Ruigrok, and F. Baudin.** 2003. Crystal structure of the M1 protein-binding domain of the influenza A virus nuclear export protein (NEP/NS2). *EMBO J.* **22:**4646–4655.
2. **Aoki, F. Y., G. Boivin, and N. Roberts.** 2007. Influenza virus susceptibility and resistance to oseltamivir. *Antivir. Ther.* **12**(4 Pt. B)**:**603–616.
3. **Baskin, C. R., H. Bielefeldt-Ohmann, A. Garcia-Sastre, T. M. Tumpey, N. Van Hoeven, V. S. Carter, M. J. Thomas, S. Proll, A. Solorzano, R. Billharz, J. L. Fornek, S. Thomas, C. H. Chen, E. A. Clark, K. Murali-Krishna, and M. G. Katze.** 2007. Functional genomic and serological analysis of the protective immune response resulting from vaccination of macaques with an NS1-truncated influenza virus. *J. Virol.* **81:**11817–11827.
4. **Bean, B., B. M. Moore, B. Sterner, L. R. Peterson, D. N. Gerding, and H. H. Balfour, Jr.** 1982. Survival of influenza viruses on environmental surfaces. *J. Infect. Dis.* **146:**47–51.

5. **Beare, A. S., and R. G. Webster.** 1991. Replication of avian influenza viruses in humans. *Arch. Virol.* **119:**37–42.
6. **Belser, J. A., X. Lu, K. Szretter, X. Jin, L. M. Aschenbrenner, S. Lee, S. Hawley, D. H. Kim, M. P. Malakhov, M. Yu, F. Fang, and J. M. Katz.** 2007. DAS181, a novel sialidase fusion protein, protects mice from lethal avian influenza H5N1 virus infection. *J. Infect. Dis.* **196:**1493–1499.
7. **Belshe, R., P. Mendelman, J. J. Treanor, J. King, W. C. Gruber, P. A. Piedra, D. I. Bernstein, F. G. Hayden, K. Kotloff, K. Zangwill, D. Iacuzio, and M. Wolff.** 1998. Efficacy of a trivalent live attenuated intranasal influenza vaccine in children. *N. Engl. J. Med.* **338:**1405–1412.
8. **Belshe, R. B., K. M. Edwards, T. Vesikari, S. V. Black, R. E. Walker, M. Hultquist, G. Kemble, and E. M. Connor for the CAIV-T Comparative Efficacy Study Group.** 2007. Live attenuated versus inactivated influenza vaccine in infants and young children. *N. Engl. J. Med.* **356:**685–696.
9. **Bernstein, D. I., K. M. Edwards, C. L. Dekker, R. Belshe, H. K. B. Talbot, I. L. Graham, D. L. Noah, F. He, and H. Hill.** 2008. Effects of adjuvants on the safety and immunogenicity of an avian influenza H5N1 vaccine in adults. *J. Infect. Dis.* **197:**1–9.
10. **Boone, S. A., and C. P. Gerba.** 2005. The occurrence of influenza A virus on household and day care center fomites. *J. Infect.* **51:**103–109.
11. **Brankston, G., L. Gitterman, Z. Hirji, C. Lemieux, and M. Gardam.** 2007. Transmission of influenza A in human beings. *Lancet Infect. Dis.* **7:**257–265.
12. **Brundage, J. F.** 2006. Interactions between influenza and bacterial respiratory pathogens: implications for pandemic preparedness. *Lancet Infect. Dis.* **6:**303–312.
13. **Buonagurio, D. A., T. M. Bechert, C. F. Yang, L. Shutyak, G. A. D'Arco, Y. Kazachkov, H. P. Wang, E. A. Rojas, R. E. O'Neill, R. R. Spaete, K. L. Coelingh, T. J. Zamb, M. S. Sidhu, and S. A. Udem.** 2006. Genetic stability of live, cold-adapted influenza virus components of the FluMist(R)/CAIV-T vaccine throughout the manufacturing process. *Vaccine* **24:**2151–2160.
14. **Bush, R. M., C. A. Bender, K. Subbarao, N. J. Cox, and W. M. Fitch.** 1999. Predicting the evolution of human influenza A. *Science* **286:**1921–1925.
15. **Call, S. A., M. A. Vollenweider, C. A. Hornung, D. L. Simel, and W. P. McKinney.** 2005. Does this patient have influenza? *JAMA* **293:**987–997.
16. **Cauchemez, S., A. J. Valleron, P. Y. Boelle, A. Flahault, and N. M. Ferguson.** 2008. Estimating the impact of school closure on influenza transmission from sentinel data. *Nature* **452:**750–754.
17. **Centers for Disease Control and Prevention.** 2007. Interim pre-pandemic planning guidance: community strategy for pandemic influenza mitigation in the United States—easy, targeted, layered use of nonpharmaceutical interventions. http://www.pandemicflu.gov/plan/community/community_mitigation.pdf.
18. **Chemaly, R. F., H. A. Torres, E. A. Aguilera, G. Mattiuzzi, M. Cabanillas, H. Kantarjian, V. Gonzalez, A. Safdar, and I. I. Raad.** 2007. Neuraminidase inhibitors improve outcome of patients with leukemia and influenza: an observational study. *Clin. Infect. Dis.* **44:**964–967.
19. **Chen, W., P. A. Calvo, D. Malide, J. Gibbs, U. Schubert, I. Bacik, S. Basta, R. O'Neill, J. Schickli, P. Palese, P. Henklein, J. R. Bennink, and J. W. Yewdell.** 2001. A novel influenza A virus mitochondrial protein that induces cell death. *Nat. Med.* **7:**1306–1312.
20. **Colman, P. M.** 1989. Influenza virus neuraminidase: enzyme and antigen, p. 175–218. *In* R. M. Krug (ed.), *The Influenza Viruses*. Plenum Press, New York, NY.
21. **Colman, P. M., J. N. Varghese, and W. G. Laver.** 1983. Structure of the catalytic and antigenic sites in influenza virus neuraminidase. *Nature* **303:**41–44.
22. **Couch, R. B., P. Winokur, R. Brady, R. Belshe, W. H. Chen, T. R. Cate, B. Sigurdardottir, A. Hoeper, I. L. Graham, R. Edelman, F. He, D. Nino, J. Capellan, and F. L. Ruben.** 2007. Safety and immunogenicity of a high dosage trivalent influenza vaccine among elderly subjects. *Vaccine* **25:**7656–7663.
23. **Crescenzo-Chaigne, B., and S. van der Werf.** 2007. Rescue of influenza C virus from recombinant DNA. *J. Virol.* **81:**11282–11289.
24. **Davies, J. R., and E. A. Grilli.** 1989. Natural or vaccine-induced antibody as a predictor of immunity in the face of natural challenge with influenza viruses. *Epidemiol. Infect.* **102:**325–333.
25. **De Benedictis, P., M. S. Beato, and I. Capua.** 2007. Inactivation of avian influenza viruses by chemical agents and physical conditions: a review. *Zoonoses Public Health* **54:**51–68.
26. **de Jong, M. D., C. P. Simmons, T. T. Thanh, V. M. Hien, G. J. Smith, T. N. Chau, D. M. Hoang, N. V. Chau, T. H. Khanh, V. C. Dong, P. T. Qui, B. V. Cam, D. Q. Ha, Y. Guan, J. S. Peiris, N. T. Chinh, T. T. Hien, and J. Farrar.** 2006. Fatal outcome of human influenza A (H5N1) is associated with high viral load and hypercytokinemia. *Nat. Med.* **12:**1203–1207.
27. **de Jong, M. D., T. T. Thanh, T. H. Khanh, V. M. Hien, G. J. D. Smith, N. V. Chau, B. V. Cam, P. T. Qui, D. Q. Ha, Y. Guan, J. S. M. Peiris, T. T. Hien, and J. Farrar.** 2005. Oseltamivir resistance during treatment of influenza A (H5N1) infection. *N. Engl. J. Med.* **353:**2667–2672.
28. **Deyde, V. M., X. Xu, R. A. Bright, M. Shaw, C. Smith, Y. Zhang, Y. Shu, L. Gubareva, N. Cox, and A. I. Klimov.** 2008. Surveillance of resistance to adamantanes among influenza A(H3N2) and A(H1N1) viruses isolated worldwide. *J.Infect. Dis.* **196:**249–257.
29. **Dodds, L., S. A. McNeil, D. B. Fell, V. M. Allen, A. Coombs, J. Scott, and N. MacDonald.** 2007. Impact of influenza exposure on rates of hospital admissions and physician visits because of respiratory illness among pregnant women. *Can. Med. Assoc. J.* **176:**463–468.
30. **Dowdle, W. R.** 1999. Influenza A virus recycling revisited. *Bull. W. H. O.* **77:**820–828.
31. **Englund, J. A., R. E. Champlin, P. R. Wyde, H. Kantarjian, R. L. Atmar, J. J. Tarrand, H. Yousuf, H. Regnery, A. I. Klimov, N. Cox, and E. Whimbey.** 1998. Common emergence of amantadine and rimantadine resistant influenza A viruses in symptomatic immunocompromised adults. *Clin. Infect. Dis.* **26:**1418–1424.
32. **Epstein, J. M., D. M. Goedecke, F. Yu, R. J. Morris, D. K. Wagener, and G. V. Bobashev.** 2007. Controlling pandemic flu: the value of international air travel restrictions. *PLoS ONE* **2**(5)**:**e401.
33. **Ferguson, N. M., D. A. T. Cummings, S. Cauchemez, C. Fraser, S. Riley, A. Meeyai, S. Iamsirithaworn, and D. S. Burke.** 2005. Strategies for containing an emerging influenza pandemic in Southeast Asia. *Nature* **437:**209–214.
34. **Fiers, W., M. De Filette, A. Birkett, S. Neirynck, and W. Min Jou.** 2004. A "universal" human influenza A vaccine. *Virus Res.* **103**(1–2)**:**173–176.
35. **Fiore, A. E., D. K. Shay, P. Haber, J. Iskander, T. M. Uyeki, G. Mootrey, J. S. Bresee, and N. Cox for the Centers for Disease Control and Prevention.** 2007. Prevention and control of influenza. Recommendations of the Advisory Committee on Immunization Practices (ACIP), 2007. *Morb. Mortal. Wkly. Rep.* **56**(RR-6)**:**1–54.

36. **Flick, R., and G. Hobom.** 1999. Interaction of influenza virus polymerase with viral RNA in the 'corkscrew' conformation. *J. Gen. Virol.* **80**(Pt. 10)**:**2565–2572.
37. **Fodor, E., L. Devenish, O. G. Engelhardt, P. Palese, G. G. Brownlee, and A. Garcia-Sastre.** 1999. Rescue of influenza A virus from recombinant DNA. *J. Virol.* **73:** 9679–9682.
38. **Fodor, E., D. C. Pritlove, and G. G. Brownlee.** 1995. Characterization of the RNA-fork model of virion RNA in the initiation of transcription in influenza A virus. *J. Virol.* **69:**4012–4019.
39. **Fujii, K., Y. Fujii, T. Noda, Y. Muramoto, T. Watanabe, A. Takada, H. Goto, T. Horimoto, and Y. Kawaoka.** 2005. Importance of both the coding and the segment-specific noncoding regions of the influenza A virus NS segment for its efficient incorporation into virions. *J. Virol.* **79:**3766–3774.
40. **Fukuda, K., R. A. Levandowski, C. B. Bridges, and N. J. Cox.** 2004. Inactivated influenza vaccine, p. 339–370. *In* S. A. Plotkin, and W. A. Orenstein (ed.), *Vaccines*. Elsevier, Philadelphia, PA.
41. **Garcia-Sastre, A.** 2006. Antiviral response in pandemic influenza viruses. *Emerg. Infect. Dis.* **12:**44–47.
42. **Garcia-Sastre, A., and P. Palese.** 1993. Genetic manipulation of negative-strand RNA virus genomes. *Annu. Rev. Microbiol.* **47:**765–790.
43. **Gianfrani, C., C. Oseroff, J. Sidney, R. W. Chesnut, and A. Sette.** 2000. Human memory CTL response specific for influenza A virus is broad and multispecific. *Hum. Immunol.* **61:**438–452.
44. **Glezen, W. P., and R. B. Couch.** 1997. Influenza viruses, p. 473–505. *In* A. S. Evans and R. A. Kaslow (ed.), *Viral Infections of Humans*. Plenum Medical Book Company, New York, NY.
45. **Glezen, W. P., L. H. Taber, A. L. Frank, W. C. Gruber, and P. A. Piedra.** 1997. Influenza virus infections in infants. *Pediatr. Infect. Dis. J.* **16:**1065–1068.
46. **Gomolin, I. H., H. B. Leib, N. H. Arden, and F. T. Sherman.** 1995. Control of influenza outbreaks in the nursing home: guidelines for diagnosis and management. *J. Am. Geriatr. Soc.* **43:**71–74.
47. **Gravenstein, S. M. M. C., P. M. Drinka, D. M. Osterweil, M. M. Schilling, P. R. Krause, M. M. Elliott, P. P. Shult, A. M. Ambrozaitis, R. M. Kandel, E. M. Binder, J. M. Hammond, J. M. McElhaney, N. P. Flack, J. P. Daly, and O. M. Keene.** 2005. Inhaled zanamivir versus rimantadine for the control of influenza in a highly vaccinated long-term care population. *J. Am. Med. Directors Assoc.* **6:**359–366.
48. **Gu, J., Z. Xie, Z. Gao, J. Liu, C. Korteweg, J. Ye, L. T. Lau, J. Lu, Z. Gao, B. Zhang, M. A. McNutt, M. Lu, V. M. Anderson, E. Gong, A. C. H. Yu, and W. I. Lipkin.** 2007. H5N1 infection of the respiratory tract and beyond: a molecular pathology study. *Lancet* **370:**1137–1145.
49. **Hageman, J. C., T. M. Uyeki, J. S. Francis, D. B. Jernigan, J. G. Wheeler, C. B. Bridges, S. J. Barenkamp, D. M. Sievert, A. Srinivasan, M. C. Doherty, L. K. McDougal, G. E. Killgore, U. A. Lopatin, R. Coffman, J. K. MacDonald, S. K. McAllister, G. E. Fosheim, J. B. Patel, and L. C. McDonald.** 2006. Severe community-acquired pneumonia due to Staphylococcus aureus, 2003–04 influenza season. *Emerg. Infect. Dis.* **12:**894–899.
50. **Hagen, M., T. D. Chung, J. A. Butcher, and M. Krystal.** 1994. Recombinant influenza virus polymerase: requirement of both 5′ and 3′ viral ends for endonuclease activity. *J. Virol.* **68:**1509–1515.
51. **Hatakeyama, S., Y. Sakai-Tagawa, M. Kiso, H. Goto, C. Kawakami, K. Mitamura, N. Sugaya, Y. Suzuki, and Y. Kawaoka.** 2005. Enhanced expression of an α2,6-linked sialic acid on MDCK cells improves isolation of human influenza viruses and evaluation of their sensitivity to a neuraminidase inhibitor. *J. Clin. Microbiol.* **43:**4139–4146.
52. **Hayden, F. G.** 1997. Prevention and treatment of influenza in immunocompromised patients. *Am. J. Med.* **102**(3A)**:**55–60.
53. **Hayden, F. G., and F. Y. Aoki.** 2005. Amantadine, rimantadine, and related agents, p. 705–729. *In* V. L. Yu, G. Edwards, P. S. McKinnon, C. Peloquin, and G. D. Morse (ed.), *Antimicrobial Therapy and Vaccines*. ESun Technologies, LLC, Pittsburgh, PA.
54. **Hayden, F. G., and F. Y. Aoki.** 2005. Influenza neuraminidase inhibitors, p. 773–789. *In* V. L. Yu, G. Edwards, P. S. McKinnon, C. Peloquin, and G. D. Morse (ed.), *Antimicrobial Therapy and Vaccines*. ESun Technologies, LLC, Pittsburgh, PA.
55. **Hayden, F. G., R. S. Fritz, M. Lobo, G. Alvord, W. Strober, and S. E. Straus.** 1998. Local and systemic cytokine responses during experimental human influenza A virus infection. *J. Clin. Investig.* **101:**643–649.
56. **Hayden, F. G., and A. T. Pavia.** 2006. Antiviral management of seasonal and pandemic influenza. *J. Infect. Dis.* **194**(S2)**:**S119–S126.
57. **Hayward, A. C., R. Harling, S. Wetten, A. M. Johnson, S. Munro, J. Smedley, S. Murad, and J. M. Watson.** 2006. Effectiveness of an influenza vaccine programme for care home staff to prevent death, morbidity, and health service use among residents: cluster randomised controlled trial. *Br. Med. J.* **333:**1241–1247.
58. **Hoffmann, E., K. Mahmood, Z. Chen, C.-F. Yang, J. Spaete, H. B. Greenberg, M. L. Herlocher, H. Jin, and G. Kemble.** 2005. Multiple gene segments control the temperature sensitivity and attenuation phenotypes of *ca* B/Ann Arbor/1/66. *J. Virol.* **79:**11014–11021.
59. **Hoffmann, E., K. Mahmood, C. F. Yang, R. G. Webster, H. B. Greenberg, and G. Kemble.** 2002. Rescue of influenza B virus from eight plasmids. *Proc. Natl. Acad. Sci. USA* **99:**11411–11416.
60. **Horimoto, T., and Y. Kawaoka.** 2005. Influenza: lessons from past pandemics, warnings from current incidents. *Nat. Rev. Microbiol.* **3:**591–600.
61. **Ilyushina, N. A., E. Hoffmann, R. Solomon, R. G. Webster, and E. A. Govorkova.** 2007. Amantadine-oseltamivir combination therapy for H5N1 influenza virus infection in mice. *Antivir. Ther.* **12:**363–370.
62. **Ison, M. G., L. V. Gubareva, R. L. Atmar, J. Treanor, and F. G. Hayden.** 2006. Recovery of drug-resistant influenza virus from immunocompromised patients: a case series. *J. Infect. Dis.* **193:**760–764.
63. **Jackson, D., A. Cadman, T. Zurcher, and W. S. Barclay.** 2002. A reverse genetics approach for recovery of recombinant influenza B viruses entirely from cDNA. *J. Virol.* **76:**11744–11747.
63a. **Jackson, D., H. J. Hossain, D. Hickman, D. R. Perez, and R. A. Lamb.** 2008. A new influenza virus virulence determinant: the NS1 protein four C-terminal residues modulate pathogenicity. *Proc. Natl. Acad. Sci. USA* **105:** 4381–4386.
64. **Jameson, J., J. Cruz, M. Terajima, and F. A. Ennis.** 1999. Human CD8+ and CD4+ T lymphocyte memory to influenza A viruses of swine and avian species. *J. Immunol.* **162:**7578–7583.
65. **Jin, H., B. Lu, H. Zhou, C. Ma, J. Zhao, C. F. Yang, G. Kemble, and H. Greenberg.** 2003. Multiple amino acid residues confer temperature sensitivity to human influenza virus vaccine strains (Flumist) derived from cold-adapted A/Ann Arbor/6/60. *Virology* **306:**18–24.

66. **Johnson, N. P., and J. Mueller.** 2002. Updating the accounts: global mortality of the 1918–1920 "Spanish" influenza pandemic. *Bull. Hist. Med.* **76:**105–115.
67. **Kaiser, L., R. S. Fritz, S. E. Straus, L. Gubareva, and F. G. Hayden.** 2001. Symptom pathogenesis during acute influenza: interleukin-6 and other cytokine responses. *J. Med. Virol.* **64:**262–268.
68. **Kaiser, L., and F. G. Hayden.** 1999. Hospitalizing influenza in adults. *Curr. Clin. Top. Infect. Dis.* **19:**112–134.
69. **Keyser, L. A., M. Karl, A. N. Nafziger, and J. S. Bertino. Jr.** 2000. Comparison of central nervous system adverse effects of amantadine and rimantadine used as sequential prophylaxis of influenza A in elderly nursing home patients. *Arch. Intern. Med.* **160:**1485–1488.
70. **Kilbourne, E. D.** 1987. *Influenza*. Plenum Medical Book Company, New York, NY.
71. **Kobasa, D., S. M. Jones, K. Shinya, J. C. Kash, J. Copps, H. Ebihara, Y. Hatta, J. Hyun Kim, P. Halfmann, M. Hatta, F. Feldmann, J. B. Alimonti, L. Fernando, Y. Li, M. G. Katze, H. Feldmann, and Y. Kawaoka.** 2007. Aberrant innate immune response in lethal infection of macaques with the 1918 influenza virus. *Nature* **445:**319–323.
72. **Koelle, K., S. Cobey, B. Grenfell, and M. Pascual.** 2006. Epochal evolution shapes the phylodynamics of interpandemic influenza A (H3N2) in humans. *Science* **314:**1898–1903.
73. **Lamb, R. A.** 1983. The influenza virus RNA segments and their encoded proteins, p. 21. *In* P. Palese and D. W. Kingsbury (ed.), *Genetics of Influenza Viruses*. Springer-Verlag, New York, NY.
74. **Langmuir, A. D., T. D. Worthen, J. Solomon, C. G. Ray, and E. Petersen.** 1985. The Thucydides syndrome. A new hypothesis for the cause of the plague of Athens. *N. Engl. J. Med.* **313:**1027–1030.
75. **Lee, N., C. K. Wong, P. K. S. Chan, S. W. M. Lun, G. Lui, B. Wong, D. S. C. Hui, C. W. K. Lam, C. S. Cockram, K. W. Choi, A. C. M. Yeung, J. W. Tang, and J. J. Y. Sung.** 2007. Hypercytokinemia and hyperactivation of phospho-p38 mitogen-activated protein kinase in severe human influenza A virus infection. *Clin. Infect. Dis.* **45:**723–731.
76. **Leekha, S., N. Zitterkopf, M. J. Espy, T. F. Smith, R. L. Thompson, and P. Sampathkumar.** 2007. Duration of influenza a virus shedding in hospitalized patients and implications for infection control. *Infect. Control Hosp. Epidemiol.* **28:**1071–1076.
77. **Leroux-Roels, I., A. Borkowski, T. Vanwolleghem, M. Drame, F. Clement, E. Hons, J. M. Devaster, and G. Leroux-Roels.** 2007. Antigen sparing and cross-reactive immunity with an adjuvanted rH5N1 prototype pandemic influenza vaccine: a randomised controlled trial. *Lancet* **370:**580–589.
78. **Lin, J. C., and K. L. Nichol.** 2001. Excess mortality due to pneumonia or influenza during influenza seasons among persons with acquired immunodeficiency syndrome. *Arch. Intern. Med.* **161:**441–446.
79. **Lin, Y. P., M. Shaw, V. Gregory, K. Cameron, W. Lim, A. Klimov, K. Subbarao, Y. Guan, S. Krauss, K. Shortridge, R. Webster, N. Cox, and A. Hay.** 2000. Avian-to-human transmission of H9N2 subtype influenza A viruses: relationship between H9N2 and H5N1 human isolates. *Proc. Natl. Acad. Sci. USA* **97:**9654–9658.
80. **Lofgren, E., N. H. Fefferman, Y. N. Naumov, J. Gorski, and E. N. Naumova.** 2007. Influenza seasonality: underlying causes and modeling theories. *J. Virol.* **81:**5429–5436.
81. **Lowen, A. C., S. Mubareka, J. Steel, and P. Palese.** 2007. Influenza virus transmission is dependent on relative humidity and temperature. *PloS Pathog.* **3:**1470–1476.
82. **Lowen, A. C., S. Mubareka, T. M. Tumpey, A. Garcia-Sastre, and P. Palese.** 2006. The guinea pig as a transmission model for human influenza viruses. *Proc. Natl. Acad. Sci. USA* **103:**9988–9992.
83. **Luke, T. C., E. M. Kilbane, J. L. Jackson, and S. L. Hoffman.** 2006. Meta-analysis: convalescent blood products for Spanish influenza pneumonia: a future H5N1 treatment? *Ann. Intern. Med.* **145:**599–609.
84. **Ma, W., A. L. Vincent, M. R. Gramer, C. B. Brockwell, K. M. Lager, B. H. Janke, P. C. Gauger, D. P. Patnayak, R. J. Webby, and J. A. Richt.** 2007. Identification of H2N3 influenza A viruses from swine in the United States. *Proc. Natl. Acad. Sci. USA* **104:**20949–20954.
85. **Maines, T. R., L. M. Chen, Y. Matsuoka, H. Chen, T. Rowe, J. Ortin, A. Falcon, N. T. Hien, L. Q. Mai, E. R. Sedyaningsih, S. Harun, T. M. Tumpey, R. O. Donis, N. J. Cox, K. Subbarao, and J. M. Katz.** 2006. Lack of transmission of H5N1 avian-human reassortant influenza viruses in a ferret model. *Proc. Natl. Acad. Sci. USA* **103:**12121–12126.
86. **Markel, H., H. B. Lipman, J. A. Navarro, A. Sloan, J. R. Michalsen, A. M. Stern, and M. S. Cetron.** 2007. Nonpharmaceutical interventions implemented by US cities during the 1918–1919 influenza pandemic. *JAMA* **298:**644–654.
87. **Marsh, G. A., R. Hatami, and P. Palese.** 2007. Specific residues of the influenza A virus hemagglutinin viral RNA are important for efficient packaging into budding virions. *J. Virol.* **81:**9727–9736.
88. **Martin, K., and A. Helenius.** 1991. Nuclear transport of influenza virus ribonucleoproteins: the viral matrix protein (M1) promotes export and inhibits import. *Cell* **67:**117–130.
89. **Matsuzaki, Y., C. Abiko, K. Mizuta, K. Sugawara, E. Takashita, Y. Muraki, H. Suzuki, M. Mikawa, S. Shimada, K. Sato, M. Kuzuya, S. Takao, K. Wakatsuki, T. Itagaki, S. Hongo, and H. Nishimura.** 2007. A nationwide epidemic of influenza c virus infection in Japan in 2004. *J. Clin. Microbiol.* **45:**783–788.
90. **Matsuzaki, Y., N. Katsushima, Y. Nagai, M. Shoji, T. Itagaki, M. Sakamoto, S. Kitaoka, K. Mizuta, and H. Nishimura.** 2006. Clinical features of influenza C virus infection in children. *J. Infect. Dis.* **193:**1229–1235.
91. **McElhaney, J. E., J. W. Hooton, N. Hooton, and R. C. Bleackley.** 2005. Comparison of single versus booster dose of influenza vaccination on humoral and cellular immune responses in older adults. *Vaccine* **23:**3294–3300.
92. **McElhaney, J. E., D. Xie, W. D. Hager, M. B. Barry, Y. Wang, A. Kleppinger, C. Ewen, K. P. Kane, and R. C. Bleackley.** 2006. T cell responses are better correlates of vaccine protection in the elderly. *J. Immunol.* **176:**6333–6339.
93. **McGeer, A., K. Green, A. Plevneshi, A. Shigayeva, N. Siddiqi, J. Raboud, and D. Low.** 2007. Antiviral therapy and outcomes of influenza requiring hospitalization in Ontario, Canada. *Clin. Infect. Dis.* **45:**1568–1575.
94. **McMichael, A.** 1994. Cytotoxic T lymphocytes specific for influenza virus. *Curr. Top. Microbiol. Immunol.* **189:**75–91.
95. **McMinn, P., A. Carrello, C. Cole, D. Baker, and A. Hampson.** 1999. Antigenic drift of influenza A (H3N2) virus in a persistently infected immunocompromised host is similar to that occurring in the community. *Clin. Infect. Dis.* **29:**456–458.
96. **Monto, A. S., S. Gravenstein, M. Elliott, M. Colopy, and J. Schweinle.** 2000. Clinical signs and symptoms predicting influenza infection. *Arch. Intern. Med.* **160:**3243–3247.

97. **Mulder, J., and J. E. Hers.** 1972. *Influenza*. Wolters-Noordhoof, Groningen, The Netherlands.
98. **Munster, V. J., E. de Witt, D. van Riel, W. E. Beyer, G. F. Rimmelzwaan, A. D. Osterhaus, T. Kuiken, and R. A. Fouchier.** 2007. The molecular basis of the pathogenicity of the Dutch highly pathogenic human influenza A H7N7 viruses. *J. Infect. Dis.* **196:**258–265.
99. **Muraki, Y., T. Murata, E. Takashita, Y. Matsuzaki, K. Sugawara, and S. Hongo.** 2007. A mutation on influenza C virus M1 protein affects virion morphology by altering the membrane affinity of the protein. *J. Virol.* **81:**8766–8773.
100. **Murphy, B. R., and M. L. Clements.** 1989. The systemic and mucosal immune response of humans to influenza A virus. *Curr. Top. Microbiol. Immunol.* **146:** 107–116.
101. **Murray, C. J., A. D. Lopez, B. Chin, D. Feehan, and K. H. Hill.** 2006. Estimation of potential global pandemic influenza mortality on the basis of vital registry data from the 1918–20 pandemic: a quantitative analysis. *Lancet* **368:**2211–2218.
102. **Mutsch, M., W. Zhou, P. Rhodes, M. Bopp, R. T. Chen, T. Linder, C. Spyr, and R. Steffen.** 2004. Use of the inactivated intranasal influenza vaccine and the risk of Bell's palsy in Switzerland. *N. Engl. J. Med.* **350:**896–903.
103. **Myers, K. P., C. W. Olsen, and G. C. Gray.** 2007. Cases of swine influenza in humans: a review of the literature. *Clin. Infect. Dis.* **44:**1084–1088.
104. **Neirynck, S., T. Deroo, X. Saelens, P. Vanlandschoot, W. M. Jou, and W. Fiers.** 1999. A universal influenza A vaccine based on the extracellular domain of the M2 protein. *Nat. Med.* **5:**1157–1163.
105. **Neumann, G., and Y. Kawaoka.** 2006. Host range restriction and pathogenicity in the context of influenza pandemic. *Emerg. Infect. Dis.* **12:**881–886.
106. **Neumann, G., K. Shinya, and Y. Kawaoka.** 2007. Molecular pathogenesis of H5N1 influenza virus infections. *Antivir. Ther.* **12**(4 Pt. B)**:**617–626.
107. **Neumann, G., T. Watanabe, H. Ito, S. Watanabe, H. Goto, P. Gao, M. Hughes, D. R. Perez, R. Donis, E. Hoffmann, G. Hobom, and Y. Kawaoka.** 1999. Generation of influenza A viruses entirely from cloned cDNAs. *Proc. Natl. Acad. Sci. USA* **96:**9345–9350.
108. **Neuraminidase Inhibitor Susceptibility Network.** 2007. Monitoring of neuraminidase inhibitor resistance among clinical influenza virus isolates in Japan during the 2003–2006 influenza seasons. *Wkly. Epidemiol. Rec.* **82:**149–150.
109. **Neuzil, K. M., B. G. Mellen, P. F. Wright, E. F. Mitchel, Jr., and M. R. Griffin.** 2000. The effect of influenza on hospitalizations, outpatient visits, and courses of antibiotics in children. *N. Engl. J. Med.* **342:**225–231.
110. **Ng, W. F., K. F. To, W. W. L. Lam, T. K. Ng, and K. C. Lee.** 2006. The comparative pathology of severe acute respiratory syndrome and avian influenza A subtype H5N1—a review. *Hum. Pathol.* **37:**381–390.
111. **Nichol, K. L., J. D. Nordin, D. B. Nelson, J. P. Mullooly, and E. Hak.** 2007. Effectiveness of influenza vaccine in the community-dwelling elderly. *N. Engl. J. Med.* **357:**1373–1381.
112. **Nicholson, K. G.** 1998. Human influenza, p. 219–264. *In* K. G. Nicholson, R. G. Webster, and A. J. Hay (ed.), *Textbook of Influenza*. Blackwell Science Ltd., Oxford, United Kingdom.
113. **Noyola, D. E., B. Clark, F. T. O'Donnell, R. L. Atmar, J. Greer, and G. J. Demmler.** 2000. Comparison of a new neuraminidase detection assay with an enzyme immunoassay, immunofluorescence, and culture for rapid detection of influenza A and B viruses in nasal wash specimens. *J. Clin. Microbiol.* **38:**1161–1165.
114. **Ohmit, S. E., J. C. Victor, J. R. Rotthoff, E. R. Teich, R. K. Truscon, L. L. Baum, B. Rangarajan, D. W. Newton, M. L. Boulton, and A. S. Monto.** 2006. Prevention of antigenically drifted influenza by inactivated and live attenuated vaccines. *N. Engl. J. Med.* **355:** 2513–2522.
115. **Olsen, B., V. J. Munster, A. Wallensten, J. Waldenstrom, A. D. M. E. Osterhaus, and R. A. M. Fouchier.** 2006. Global patterns of influenza A virus in wild birds. *Science* **312:**384–388.
116. **O'Neill, R. E., R. Jaskunas, G. Blobel, P. Palese, and J. Moroianu.** 1995. Nuclear import of influenza virus RNA can be mediated by viral nucleoprotein and transport factors required for protein import. *J. Biol. Chem.* **270:**22701–22704.
117. **O'Neill, R. E., J. Talon, and P. Palese.** 1998. The influenza virus NEP (NS2 protein) mediates the nuclear export of viral ribonucleoproteins. *EMBO J.* **17:**288–296.
118. **Ong, A. K., and F. G. Hayden.** 2007. John F. Enders Lecture 2006: antivirals for influenza. *J. Infect. Dis.* **196:** 181–190.
119. **Ozawa, M., H. Goto, T. Horimoto, and Y. Kawaoka.** 2007. An adenovirus vector-mediated reverse genetics system for influenza A virus generation. *J. Virol.* **81:** 9556–9559.
120. **Palese, P.** 2004. Influenza: old and new threats. *Nat. Med.* **10**(12 Suppl.)**:**S82–S87.
121. **Palese, P., and M. Shaw.** 2007. *Orthomyxoviridae:* the viruses and their replication, p. 1647–1689. *In* D. M. Knipe, P. M. Howley, D. E. Griffin, R. A. Lamb, M. A. Martin, B. Roizman, and S. E. Straus (ed.), *Fields Virology*, 5th ed. Lippencott Williams & Wilkins, Philadelphia, PA.
122. **Pasick, J., K. Handel, J. Robinson, J. Copps, D. Ridd, K. Hills, H. Kehler, C. Cottam-Birt, J. Neufeld, Y. Berhane, and S. Czub.** 2005. Intersegmental recombination between the haemagglutinin and matrix genes was responsible for the emergence of a highly pathogenic H7N3 avian influenza virus in British Columbia. *J. Gen. Virol.* **86:**727–731.
123. **Peiris, J. S. M., M. D. de Jong, and Y. Guan.** 2007. Avian influenza virus (H5N1): a threat to human health. *Clin. Microbiol. Rev.* **20:**243–267.
124. **Peltola, V. T., K. G. Murti, and J. A. McCullers.** 2005. Influenza virus neuraminidase contributes to secondary bacterial pneumonia. *J. Infect. Dis.* **192:**249–257.
125. **Perez-Ruiz, M., R. Yeste, M. J. Ruiz-Perez, A. Ruiz-Bravo, M. de la Rosa-Fraile, and J. M. Navarro-Mari.** 2007. Testing of diagnostic methods for detection of influenza virus for optimal performance in the context of an influenza surveillance network. *J. Clin. Microbiol.* **45:** 3109–3110.
126. **Petric, M., L. Comanor, and C. A. Petti.** 2006. Role of the laboratory in diagnosis of influenza during seasonal epidemics and potential pandemics. *J. Infect. Dis.* **194**(Suppl. 2)**:**S98–S110.
127. **Poehling, K. A., K. M. Edwards, G. A. Weinberg, P. Szilagyi, M. A. Staat, M. K. Iwane, C. B. Bridges, C. G. Grijalva, Y. Zhu, D. I. Bernstein, G. Herrera, D. Erdman, C. B. Hall, R. Seither, and M. R. Griffin for the New Vaccine Surveillance Network.** 2006. The underrecognized burden of influenza in young children. *N. Engl. J. Med.* **355:**31–40.
128. **Potter, C. W.** 1998. Chronicle of influenza pandemics, p. 3–18. *In* K. G. Nicholson, R. G. Webster, and A. J.

Hay (ed.), *Textbook of Influenza*. Blackwell Science Ltd., Oxford, United Kingdom.

128a. **Rasmussen, S. A., D. J. Jamieson, and J. S. Bresee.** 2008. Pandemic influenza and pregnant women. *Emerg. Infect. Dis.* **14:**95–100.

129. **Reichert, T. A., N. Sugaya, D. S. Fedson, W. P. Glezen, L. Simonsen, and M. Tashiro.** 2001. The Japanese experience with vaccinating schoolchildren against influenza. *N. Engl. J. Med.* **344:**889–896.

130. **Rimmelzwaan, G. F., A. C. Boon, J. T. Voeten, E. G. Berkhoff, R. A. Fouchier, and A. D. Osterhaus.** 2004. Sequence variation in the influenza A virus nucleoprotein associated with escape from cytotoxic T lymphocytes. *Virus Res.* **103**(1–2)**:**97–100.

131. **Rodriguez, W. J., C. B. Hall, R. Welliver, E. A. Simoes, M. E. Ryan, H. Stutman, G. Johnson, R. Van Dyke, J. R. Groothuis, J. Arrobio, K. Schabel, H. W. Kim, R. H. Parrott, and P. Pincus.** 1994. Efficacy and safety of aerosolized ribavirin in young children hospitalized with influenza: a double-blind, multicenter, placebo-controlled trial. *J. Pediatr.* **125:**129–135.

132. **Rothbarth, P. H., J. Groen, A. M. Bohnen, R. de Groot, and A. D. Osterhaus.** 1999. Influenza virus serology—a comparative study. *J. Virol. Methods* **78**(1–2)**:** 163–169.

133. **Roti, M., J. Yang, D. Berger, L. Huston, E. A. James, and W. W. Kwok.** 2008. Healthy human subjects have CD4+ T cells directed against H5N1 influenza virus. *J. Immunol.* **180:**1758–1768.

133a. **Russell, C. A., T. C. Jones, I. G. Barr, N. J. Cox, R. J. Garten, V. Gregory, I. D. Gust, A. W. Hampson, A. J. Hay, A. C. Hurt, J. C. de Jong, A. Kelso, A. I. Klimov, T. Kageyama, N. Komadina, A. S. Lapedes, Y. P. Lin, A. Mosterin, M. Obuchi, T. Odagiri, A. D. M. E. Osterhaus, G. F. Rimmelzwaan, M. W. Shaw, E. Skepner, K. Stohr, M. Tashiro, R. A. M. Fouchier, and D. J. Smith.** 2008. The global circulation of seasonal influenza A (H3N2) viruses. *Science* **320:**340–346.

134. **Salgado, C. D., B. M. Farr, K. K. Hall, and F. G. Hayden.** 2002. Influenza in the acute hospital setting. *Lancet Infect. Dis.* **2:**145–155.

135. **Salomon, R., E. Hoffmann, and R. G. Webster.** 2007. Inhibition of the cytokine response does not protect against lethal H5N1 influenza infection. *Proc. Natl. Acad. Sci. USA* **104:**12479–12481.

136. **Salvatore, M., A. Garcia-Sastre, P. Ruchala, R. I. Lehrer, T. Chang, and M. E. Klotman.** 2007. α-Defensin inhibits influenza virus replication by cell-mediated mechanism(s). *J. Infect. Dis.* **196:**835–843.

137. **Schaffer, F. L., M. E. Soergel, and D. C. Straube.** 1976. Survival of airborne influenza virus: effects of propagating host, relative humidity, and composition of spray fluids. *Arch. Virol.* **51:**263–273.

138. **Schwarzmann, S. W., J. L. Adler, R. J. Sullivan, and W. M. Marine.** 1971. Bacterial pneumonia during the Hong Kong influenza epidemic of 1968–1969. *Arch. Intern. Med.* **127:**1037–1041.

139. **Sidwell, R. W., D. L. Barnard, C. W. Day, D. F. Smee, K. W. Bailey, M. H. Wong, J. D. Morrey, and Y. Furuta.** 2007. Efficacy of orally administered T-705 on lethal avian influenza A (H5N1) virus infections in mice. *Antimicrob. Agents Chemother.* **51:**845–851.

140. **Simonsen, L., M. J. Clarke, L. B. Schonberger, N. Arden, N. J. Cox, and K. Fukuda.** 1998. Pandemic versus epidemic influenza mortality: a pattern of changing age distribution. *J. Infect. Dis.* **178:**53–60.

141. **Simonsen, L., R. J. Taylor, C. Viboud, M. A. Miller, and L. A. Jackson.** 2007. Mortality benefits of influenza vaccination in elderly people: an ongoing controversy. *Lancet Infect. Dis.* **7:**658–666.

142. **Skowronski, D., S. A. Tweed, and G. De Serres.** 2008. Rapid decline of influenza vaccine-induced antibody in the elderly: is it real, or is it relevant? *J. Infect. Dis.* **197:** 490–502.

143. **Smith, G. J. D., X. H. Fan, J. Wang, K. S. Li, K. Qin, J. X. Zhang, D. Vijaykrishna, C. L. Cheung, K. Huang, J. M. Rayner, J. S. M. Peiris, H. Chen, R. G. Webster, and Y. Guan.** 2006. Emergence and predominance of an H5N1 influenza variant in China. *Proc. Natl. Acad. Sci. USA* **103:**16936–16941.

144. **Stech, J., H. Garn, M. Wegmann, R. Wagner, and H. D. Klenk.** 2005. A new approach to an influenza live vaccine: modification of the cleavage site of hemagglutinin. *Nat. Med.* **11:**683–689.

145. **Subbarao, K., I. Klimov, J. Katz, H. Regnery, W. Lim, H. Hall, M. Perdue, D. Swayne, C. Bender, J. Huang, M. Hemphill, T. Rowe, M. Shaw, X. Xu, K. Fukuda, and N. Cox.** 1998. Characterization of an avian influenza A(H5N1) virus isolated from a child with a fatal respiratory illness. *Science* **279:**393–396.

146. **Subbarao, K., and T. Joseph.** 2007. Scientific barriers to developing vaccines against avian influenza viruses. *Nat. Rev. Immunol.* **7:**267–278.

147. **Sugaya, N., K. Mitamura, M. Yamazaki, D. Tamura, M. Ichikawa, K. Kimura, C. Kawakami, M. Kiso, M. Ito, S. Hatakeyama, and Y. Kawaoka.** 2007. Lower clinical effectiveness of oseltamivir against influenza B contrasted with influenza A infection in children. *Clin. Infect. Dis.* **44:**197–202.

148. **Sullivan, P. S., D. L. Hanson, M. S. Dworkin, J. L. Jones, J. W. Ward, and the Adult and Adolescent Spectrum of HIV Disease Investigators.** 2000. Effect of influenza vaccination on disease progression among HIV-infected persons. *AIDS* **14:**2781–2785.

149. **Taubenberger, J. K., A. H. Reid, R. M. Lourens, R. Wang, G. Jin, and T. G. Fanning.** 2005. Characterization of the 1918 influenza virus polymerase genes. *Nature* **437:**889–893.

150. **Tecle, T., M. R. White, E. C. Crouch, and K. L. Hartshorn.** 2007. Inhibition of influenza viral neuraminidase activity by collectins. *Arch. Virol.* **152:**1731–1742.

151. **Temperton, N. J., K. Hoschler, D. Major, C. Nicolson, R. Manvell, V. M. Hien, D. Q. Ha, M. de Jong, M. Zambon, Y. Takeuchi, and R. A. Weiss.** 2007. A sensitive retroviral pseudotype assay for influenza H5N1-neutralizing antibodies. *Influenza Other Respir. Viruses* **1:** 105–112.

152. **Thompson, W. W., D. K. Shay, E. Weintraub, L. Brammer, C. B. Bridges, N. J. Cox, and K. Fukuda.** 2004. Influenza-associated hospitalizations in the United States. *JAMA* **292:**1333–1340.

153. **Thompson, W. W., L. Comanor, and D. K. Shay.** 2006. Epidemiology of seasonal influenza: use of surveillance data and statistical models to estimate the burden of disease. *J. Infect. Dis.* **194**(Suppl. 2)**:**S82–S91.

154. **Treanor, J. J., J. D. Campbell, K. M. Zangwill, T. Rowe, and M. Wolff.** 2006. Safety and immunogenicity of an inactivated subvirion influenza A (H5N1) vaccine. *N. Engl. J. Med.* **354:**1343–1351.

155. **Treanor, J. J., and F. G. Hayden.** 2005. Viral infections, p. 867–919. *In* J. F. Murray and J. A. Nadel (ed.), *Textbook of Respiratory Medicine*. W. B. Saunders Company, Philadelphia, PA.

156. **Treanor, J. J., G. M. Schiff, F. G. Hayden, R. C. Brady, C. M. Hay, A. L. Meyer, J. Holden-Wiltse, H. Liang, A. Gilbert, and M. Cox.** 2007. Safety and immunogenicity of a baculovirus-expressed hemagglutinin influenza

vaccine: a randomized controlled trial. *JAMA* **297:** 1577–1582.

157. **Tumpey, T. M., C. F. Basler, P. V. Aguilar, H. Zeng, A. Solorzano, D. E. Swayne, N. J. Cox, J. M. Katz, J. K. Taubenberger, P. Palese, and A. Garcia-Sastre.** 2005. Characterization of the reconstructed 1918 Spanish influenza pandemic virus. *Science* **310:**77–80.
158. **Tumpey, T. M., T. R. Maines, N. Van Hoeven, L. Glaser, A. Solorzano, C. Pappas, N. J. Cox, D. E. Swayne, P. Palese, J. M. Katz, and A. Garcia-Sastre.** 2007. A two-amino acid change in the hemagglutinin of the 1918 influenza virus abolishes transmission. *Science* **315:** 655–659.
159. **van Riel, D., V. J. Munster, E. de Wit, G. F. Rimmelzwaan, R. A. M. Fouchier, A. D. M. E. Osterhaus, and T. Kuiken.** 2007. Human and avian influenza viruses target different cells in the lower respiratory tract of humans and other mammals. *Am. J. Pathol.* **171:** 1215–1223.
160. **Wang, J. P., E. A. Kurt-Jones, and R. W. Finberg.** 2007. Innate immunity to respiratory viruses. *Cell. Microbiol.* **9:**1641–1646.
161. **Webster, R. G., and E. A. Govorkova.** 2006. H5N1 influenza—continuing evolution and spread. *N. Engl. J. Med.* **355:**2174–2177.
162. **Wiley, D. C., and J. J. Skehel.** 1987. The structure and function of the hemagglutinin membrane glycoprotein of influenza virus. *Annu. Rev. Biochem.* **56:**365–394.
163. **World Health Organization.** 2007. Clinical management of human infection with avian influenza A (H5N1) virus. http://www.who.int/csr/disease/avian_influenza/guidelines/ClinicalManagement07.pdf.
164. **World Health Organization.** 2008. WHO/ECDC frequently asked questions for oseltamivir resistance. http://www.who.int/csr/disease/influenza/oseltamivir_faqs/en/print.html.
165. **Wright, P., G. Neumann, and Y. Kawaoka.** 2007. Orthomyxoviruses, p. 1691–1740. *In* D. M. Knipe, P. M. Howley, D. E. Griffin, R. A. Lamb, M. A. Martin, B. Roizman, and S. E. Straus (ed.), *Fields Virology*, 5th ed. Lippincott Williams & Wilkins, Philadelphia, PA.
166. **Writing Committee of the Second World Health Organization Consultation on Clinical Aspects of Human Infection with Avian Influenza A (H5N1) Virus.** 2008. Update on avian influenza A (H5N1) virus infection in humans. *N. Engl. J. Med.* **358:**261–273.
167. **Yamada, S., Y. Suzuki, T. Suzuki, M. Q. Le, C. A. Nidom, Y. Sakai-Tagawa, Y. Muramoto, M. Ito, M. Kiso, T. Horimoto, K. Shinya, T. Sawada, M. Kiso, T. Usui, T. Murata, Y. Lin, A. Hay, L. F. Haire, D. J. Stevens, R. J. Russell, S. J. Gamblin, J. J. Skehel, and Y. Kawaoka.** 2006. Haemagglutinin mutations responsible for the binding of H5N1 influenza A viruses to human-type receptors. *Nature* **444:**378–382.
168. **Yamashita, M., M. Krystal, and P. Palese.** 1989. Comparison of the three large polymerase proteins of influenza A, B, and C viruses. *Virology* **171:**458–466.
169. **Yun, N. E., N. S. Linde, M. A. Zacks, I. G. Barr, A. C. Hurt, J. N. Smith, N. Dziuba, M. R. Holbrook, L. Zhang, J. M. Kilpatrick, C. S. Arnold, and S. Paessler.** 2008. Injectable peramivir mitigates disease and promotes survival in ferrets and mice infected with the highly virulent influenza virus, A/Vietnam/1203/04 (H5N1). *Virology* **374:**198–209.

Bunyaviridae: Bunyaviruses, Phleboviruses, Nairoviruses, and Hantaviruses

GREGORY J. MERTZ

43

The family *Bunyaviridae* is the largest family of animal viruses and includes many viruses that are known human pathogens. The clinical diseases produced in humans range from acute febrile illnesses, such as sandfly fever, to more distinct clinical syndromes such as California encephalitis (CE), Rift Valley fever (RVF), Crimean-Congo hemorrhagic fever (CCHF), hemorrhagic fever with renal syndrome (HFRS), and the recently recognized hantavirus cardiopulmonary syndrome (HCPS), which is also referred to in the literature as hantavirus pulmonary syndrome. Sandfly fever, RVF, and HFRS are common. Although most of the remaining diseases probably cause no more than a few hundred cases each year, some are associated with a high mortality rate (particularly CCHF and HCPS), and two (CE and HCPS) are endemic in North America.

VIROLOGY

Classification

The family *Bunyaviridae* includes more than 300 viruses and is divided into five genera: *Bunyavirus*, *Phlebovirus*, *Nairovirus*, *Hantavirus*, and *Tospovirus* (14). All genera except the tospoviruses, which are plant viruses, infect vertebrate hosts and include human pathogens.

Representative groups and complexes for the bunyaviruses, phleboviruses, and nairoviruses, including major human pathogens, are shown in Table 1. In general, the genotypes are determined by molecular features, including conserved nucleotide sequences, genomic size, and genomic organization, whereas groups within each genus are determined primarily by serologic methods (14, 61). Within the larger genera, viruses may be classified into groups and complexes.

Antibodies are directed against a nucleocapsid protein (NP) and two major envelope glycoproteins. The nucleocapsid protein is usually more conserved within a genus than the glycoproteins. Serologic tests that are solely or primarily directed against nucleocapsid protein antigens tend to be sensitive but exhibit significant cross-reactivity, whereas assays that are directed solely or primarily against glycoprotein antigens tend to be useful in distinguishing between closely related viruses (14, 61).

Virion Structure, Genome Composition, and Major Proteins

Bunyaviruses are enveloped viruses about 100 nm in diameter (80 to 120 nm) with 5- to 10-nm glycoprotein spikes projecting from the envelope (Fig. 1) (9, 41, 158). The viruses are generally spherical but may be oval and elongated. The envelope surrounds a tripartite core containing the short (S), medium (M), and long (L) genome segments of single-stranded RNA with negative polarity (Fig. 1).

The lengths of the genomic segments vary among the genera, ranging from 6.3 to 12 kb for the L segment, 3.5 to 6 kb for the M segment, and 1 to 2.2 kb for the S segment. The range within each genus is much more restricted. For hantaviruses, segment lengths range from 6.5 to 7.0 kb for the L segment, 3.6 to 3.7 kb for the M segment, and 1.6 to 2.1 kb for the S segment.

Four major structural proteins are encoded by the three segments, and nonstructural proteins are encoded by some, but not all, viruses within the family. RNA-dependent RNA polymerase (RDRP; L protein) is encoded by the L segment, and nucleoprotein is encoded by the S segment. Glycoproteins (G1 and G2, or G_N and G_C for CCHFV) are encoded by the M segment (Fig. 1). Many of the structural proteins for the major viruses in the family have been sequenced (8, 28, 82, 101, 150), and successful reverse-genetics systems have recently been described for CCHF virus and Andes virus (ANDV) (49, 100).

REPLICATION STRATEGIES

There is considerable diversity in the replication strategies within the family, although all members of the family replicate in the cytoplasm and mature in the Golgi apparatus (Fig. 1) (9, 41, 89, 117, 158). Attachment and entry are mediated by one or both of the glycoproteins (Fig. 1, event 1). For phleboviruses, entry into cells is by endocytosis, a mechanism that may be shared by other members of the family. *Bunyaviridae* can fuse cells at acid pH, and conformational changes in G1 have been described for the *Bunyavirus* genus. Thus, for members of the family, entry and uncoating may occur through a common mechanism of entry by endocytosis followed by uncoating and release of the three nucleocapsids into the cytoplasm following fusion

TABLE 1 *Bunyaviridae*: genera, subgroups, and selected viruses that are human pathogens, excluding hantaviruses

Genus	Serogroup or complex	Geographic location of human pathogens	Selected human pathogens
Bunyavirus	California	North America, Europe	CE, La Crosse, Jamestown Canyon, and Tahyna viruses
	Simbu	South America	Oropouche virus
	Anopheles A	South America	Tacaiuma virus
	Bunyamwera	Africa, South America	Bunyamwera, Fort Sherman, Shokwe, and Xingu viruses
	Group C	North and South America	Apue, Itaqui, Madrid, and Oriboca viruses
Nairovirus	CCHF	Africa, Asia, Europe	CCHF and Dugbe viruses
	NSD	Africa, Asia	NSD virus
Phlebovirus	Sandfly fever group	North and South America, Africa, Europe, Asia	Alenquer, Punta Toro, RVF, sandfly fever Naples, Toscana, Chagres, and sandfly fever Sicilian viruses

of the viral envelope and endosomal membrane at acid pH (Fig. 1, event 2).

After uncoating, primary transcription of negative-strand viral RNA (vRNA) to mRNA is believed to involve vRNA, host primers, and the viral polymerase (RDRP) (Fig. 1, event 4). Transcription is followed by translation and by phosphorylation of the M segment-encoded proteins (Fig. 1, event 6). This is followed by genome replication, usually through synthesis of a full-length positive-strand cRNA that serves as a replicative intermediate, followed by synthesis of negative-strand vRNA (Fig. 1, events 3 and 5). These events are then followed by continued translation and RNA replication.

Replication of the S segment in the *Phlebovirus* and *Tospovirus* genomes is accomplished via an ambisense coding strategy. The NS protein is encoded in the 5′ half of the S segment, the N protein is encoded in the 3′ half of the segment, and the proteins are translated from separate mRNAs (not shown). Genetic reassortment has been demonstrated both in cell culture and in vivo in arthropod vectors between members of the same serogroup in the genus *Bunyavirus* but not between members of different serogroups in the same genus.

A key point in genome replication is the switch from transcription of genomic RNA (Fig. 1, event 3) to production of the positive-strand cRNA that serves as the replicative intermediate (Fig. 1, event 3). This is also a key component in the transcription and replication strategies of other negative-strand viruses such as vesicular stomatitis virus, influenza virus, and rhabdovirus. For vesicular stomatitis virus, the switch appears to be regulated by the nucleoprotein, and a similar mechanism may exist for members of the family *Bunyaviridae*.

These events are followed by terminal glycosylation of the glycoproteins, assembly of viral particles by budding into Golgi vesicles, transport of the cytoplasmic vesicles to the cell surface, fusion of the cytoplasmic vesicles with the plasma membrane, and release of virions through exocytosis (Fig. 1, events 7 to 11). In other negative-strand RNA viruses such as *Rhabdoviridae*, *Orthomyxoviridae*, and *Paramyxoviridae*, a viral matrix protein bridges the gap between envelope proteins and the nucleocapsids during assembly. *Bunyaviridae* lack a matrix protein. Thus, there may be direct transmembrane recognition between viral glycoproteins that accumulate on the luminal side and the ribonucleoprotein structures (nucleocapsids) that accumulate on the cytoplasmic side of vesicular membranes. In addition to morphogenesis in the Golgi apparatus that occurs in all members of the family, other mechanisms have been described. One member of the genus *Phlebovirus*, RVF virus, can bud at the surface of rat hepatocytes as well as into the Golgi cisternae.

Host Range, Growth in Cell Culture, and Inactivation

Members of the *Bunyavirus*, *Phlebovirus*, and *Nairovirus* genera infect both vertebrates and arthropods. Given the large number of viruses in the family, it is not surprising that the overall range of natural vertebrate hosts is broad, including rodents, lagomorphs, deer, birds, and sheep and other domestic animals (14, 61). However, for a particular virus the range varies from broad to very limited, the latter being particularly true of hantaviruses. Although "spill-over" may occur between small rodent species in nature and although rats, mice, and rabbits can be infected in the laboratory, each hantavirus tends to have a very restricted host range in nature (Table 2). The limited host range and similar phylogenetic relationships among hantaviruses and among the rodent hosts have led to the suggestion that hantaviruses may have coevolved with their rodent hosts. Recent evidence also suggests remote divergence of a clade of insectivore-borne hantaviruses (36). Although many members of the latter clade have recently been identified in soricids (shrews), none have been clearly associated with human disease. Humans are not believed to be a natural reservoir for any members of the family *Bunyaviridae*, but human infections, some of substantial medical importance, occur by members of each genus except the *Tospovirus* genus.

The range of arthropod hosts tends to be more limited within each genus and to be even more limited for groups or individual viruses within each genus (Table 3). With only a few exceptions, members of the genus *Bunyavirus* infect only mosquitoes. Most phleboviruses infect sand flies, but RVF virus can infect a wide range of arthropods and appears to be transmitted primarily by mosquitoes. The arthropod host range for nairoviruses appears to be largely limited to ticks, particularly those in the genus *Hyalomma* (83, 189).

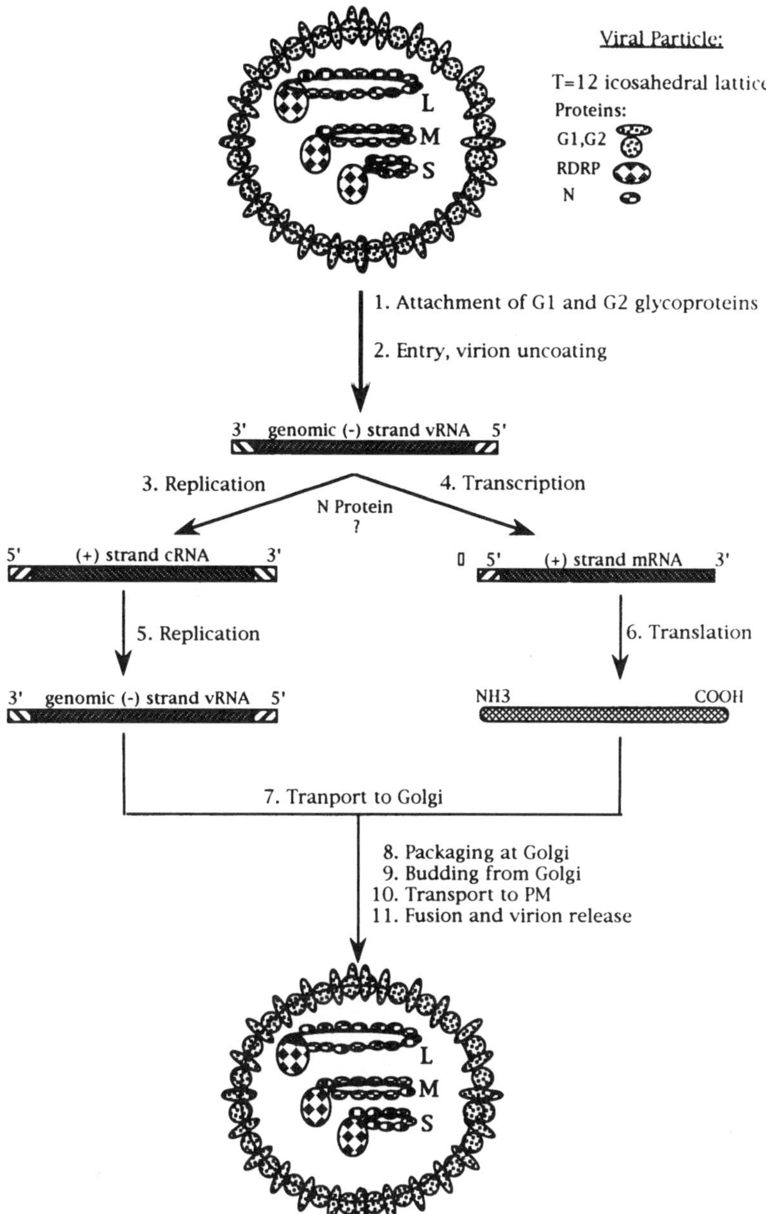

FIGURE 1 Model for replication of *Bunyaviridae*. The principal steps in replication are as follows: 1, attachment, in which G1 and/or G2 proteins bind to an unidentified receptor; 2, entry and uncoating, probably mediated by fusion; 3, replication, cRNA synthesis from vRNA genome; 4, transcription, mRNA synthesis from vRNA genome; 5, replication, vRNA synthesis from the cRNA template; 6, translation, L and M mRNA translation on free ribosomes and M translation on rough endoplasmic reticulum; 7, transport, movement of L, M, and S genomes into the Golgi complex and RDRP and N proteins; 8, packaging, assembly of genomic RNAs and proteins at the Golgi apparatus; 9 and 10, budding and transport, in which Golgi vesicles carry virions to the plasma membrane (PM); 11, fusion and virion release. (Courtesy of C. Jonsson, Department of Molecular Biology, Southern Research Institute.)

Most bunyaviruses replicate in BHK-21 or Vero E6 cells, are cytolytic, and plaque well. Although hantaviruses can be grown in Vero E6 cells, they are fastidious and are generally not cytopathic. Viral antigen can be detected by fluorescent antibody or other techniques, and plaque reduction assays are also possible with Vero E6 cells. Bunyaviruses in the *Bunyavirus* genus have been shown to cause persistent, noncytopathic infections in mosquito cell cultures. Suckling mice may also be used for isolation of many members of the family. Like other enveloped viruses, bunyaviruses are sensitive to acid pH, detergents, formalin, heat, and lipid solvents.

TABLE 2 Hantavirus species recognized to date[a]

Virus	Abbreviation	Synonym	Host(s)	Distribution of host	Disease
Hantaan	HTN		*A. agrarius*	Central and East Asia, Central and Eastern Europe	HFRS
Seoul	SEO		*R. norvegicus*, *Rattus rattus*	Worldwide; commensal rat hosts	HFRS, mild
Dobrava/Belgrade	DOB	BEL	*A. flavicollis*	Asia Minor, Europe, Palestine	HFRS
Saaremaa	SAA		*A. agrarius*	Central and Eastern Europe	HFRS, mild
Puumala	PUU		*C. glareolus*	Russia, Europe, Asia Minor	HFRS/NE
Sin Nombre	SN	Four Corners	*P. maniculatus*	Throughout United States, western Canada	HCPS
Black Creek Canal	BCC		*S. hispidus*	Southeastern United States to Peru	HCPS
New York	NY	NY-1	*P. leucopus*	Northeastern United States, southeastern Canada	HCPS
Bayou	BAY		*O. palustris*	Southeastern United States, Kansas to New Jersey	HCPS
Andes[b]	AND		*O. longicaudatus*	Southern Chile, Argentina	HCPS
Laguna Negra	LN		*C. laucha*	Paraguay, Bolivia	HCPS
Choclo			*O. fulvenscens*	Panama	HCPS, mild
Thottapalayam	TPM		*Sigmodon murinus*	Africa, India, Southeast Asia	Unknown
Tula	TUL		*Microtus arvalis*	Russia, Europe, Asia Minor	Unknown
Thai	THAI		*Bandicota indica*	Southeast Asia, India	Unknown
Khabarovsk			*Microtus fortis*	East Asia	
Prospect Hill	PH		*M. pennsylvanicus*	Northern and eastern United States, Canada, Alaska	Unknown
Bloodland Lake	BLLL	PVV	*M. ochrogaster*	Midwestern and eastern United States, southern Canada	Unknown
Isla Vista	Isla	CMMV	*M. californicus*	California, Oregon, Mexico	Unknown
El Moro Canyon	ELMC	HMV-1	*R. megalotis*	Western United States, Mexico, southwestern Canada	Unknown
Rio Segundo	RIOS	HMV-2	*R. mexicanus?*	Mexico, Costa Rica, Ecuador	Unknown
Rio Mamoré	RM		*O. microtis*	Bolivia, Brazil, Paraguay, Peru	Unknown
Calabazo			*Z. brivicauda*	Panama	Unknown

[a] Only those that are well characterized and clearly differentiated from previously characterized species are listed. (Courtesy of B. Hjelle.)
[b] Possibly synonymous with variant forms Bermejo, Oran, and Lechiguanas.

TABLE 3 Natural vertebrate hosts, vectors, and mechanisms of transmission for representative bunyaviruses that are human pathogens

Genus and virus	Vertebrate hosts	Vector(s)	Transmission
Bunyavirus			
La Crosse virus	Woodland rodents	*Aedes triseriatus*	Insect bite
Bunyamwera virus	Rodents, lagomorphs	*Aedes* species	Insect bite
Nairovirus			
CCHF virus	Herbivores, lagomorphs	*Hyalomma* ticks	Insect bites, infected animal tissues, person to person
Phlebovirus			
RVF virus	Sheep and other domestic animals	Mosquitoes	Insect bite, contact with blood or tissue of animals
Sandfly fever virus	Unknown	*Phlebotomus* species	Insect bite
Hantavirus	Rodents (persistent)	None	Aerosolized rodent excreta, person to person (Andes)

EPIDEMIOLOGY

General Principles

For members of the *Bunyavirus*, *Phlebovirus*, and *Nairovirus* genera, the infection is arthropod borne, although RVF may also be acquired by direct contact with infected animal carcasses or blood. Person-to-person transmission may also occur with CCHF virus and with ANDV infections, including nosocomial transmission of CCHF virus through contact with infected blood and person-to-person transmission of ANDV within households and other close contacts in Chile and Argentina. For most bunyaviruses, the period of viremia in the vertebrate host is brief, suggesting that infection in vertebrates is generally more important for amplification than for viral perpetuation. In contrast, infection in the insect is persistent. For several viruses in these genera, virus perpetuation can be maintained solely in the insect host for prolonged periods through both transovarial and horizontal transmission. For example, La Crosse virus survives over the winter in mosquito eggs, and RVF virus can survive in mosquito eggs for years during drought.

In contrast to the genera described above, hantaviruses have no arthropod vector, although infection and transovarial transmission in gamasid mites have been described (84). Virus perpetuation and amplification occur largely within a single rodent species that becomes chronically infected (Table 2). Infected rodents appear to be asymptomatic, but Puumala virus impairs overwinter survival in bank voles, and Sin Nombre virus (SNV)-infected juvenile but not adult deer mice have shorter survival than uninfected mice (34). There is also evidence that SNV-infected adult male deer mice and Seoul virus-infected male rats are more aggressive than uninfected adult males (70). There is no evidence for vertical transmission, and most evidence points to horizontal transmission following weaning and clearance of protective maternal antibodies (93). Virus is chronically shed in rodent excreta, and humans appear to acquire infection from aerosols from infected rodent excreta. The viability of virus in rodent excreta is not known, but Puumala virus remains viable for at least 12 days at room temperature (94). Finally, laboratory infections have been documented with many members of the family. In most cases, aerosol transmission has been the probable mode of transmission, but direct transmission of hantaviruses from contact with infected animals may also occur. Particular care, including biosafety level 4 (BSL-4) containment for some applications, should be taken with agents that carry a high risk of mortality, such as CCHF virus and the hantaviruses that cause HCPS.

CE Serogroup Viruses (*Bunyavirus* Genus)

The virus type or subtype, geographic location, and primary mosquito vector and vertebrate host or hosts for CE serogroup viruses that cause human infection are shown in Table 4. The group is named for the first virus isolated in this group, CE virus, which was isolated from humans with encephalitis in Kern County, CA, in 1943. Since then, however, this virus has not been associated with human disease, and La Crosse virus, first identified in 1960 from a fatal case of encephalitis, has accounted for most reported cases of CE (107). The majority of cases are reported from Ohio, Wisconsin, Minnesota, Illinois, Iowa, and Indiana, but cases have been reported in most states adjacent to or east of the Mississippi River and are reported sporadically in western states.

CE is endemic in the Midwest. From 1963 to 1981, the rate of reported cases remained relatively constant at about

TABLE 4 CE serogroup viruses

Virus	Geographic location(s)	Vector(s)	Hosts	Human infection
CE virus	Western United States, Canada	*Aedes melanimon*, *Aedes dorsalis*	Rodents, rabbits	Very rare
La Crosse virus	Midwestern and eastern United States	*A. triseriatus*	Chipmunk, squirrels	Endemic
Tahyna virus	Europe	*Aedes vexans*, *Culiseta annulata*	Domestic animals, rabbits	Endemic
Jamestown Canyon virus	North America	*Aedes* spp., *C. inornata*	White-tailed deer?	Uncommon

75 cases per year. Most cases occur between July and September in children, particularly boys, between the ages of 6 months and 16 years of age, with a peak incidence in children between the ages of 4 and 10 years. Most infections appear to be subclinical or to result in a viral syndrome without encephalitis. One survey in Minnesota estimated that 1 encephalitis case occurred for every 26 childhood La Crosse virus infections, while a large serosurvey in Indiana suggested that there might be more than 1,000 infections for every reported case of encephalitis in children less than 16 years old. Serosurveys show that acquisition of La Crosse virus infection continues throughout life, with about 20% of the population seropositive in areas of endemicity by the age of 60 years; presumably, adults who acquire infection are at little risk of developing encephalitis.

The primary vector is the mosquito *Aedes triseriatus*. The female *A. triseriatus* is a daytime feeder that breeds in rainwater in tree holes or other small containers, including discarded tires, thereby allowing breeding and disease transmission in areas distant from the mosquito's usual forest habitat. The virus can be maintained over winter by transovarial transmission where eggs deposited in the fall can survive the winter and hatch in the spring (188). There is some evidence that infected female mosquitoes may hibernate during the winter and lay eggs in the spring. At that point, virus can be amplified through infecting small mammals, particularly chipmunks and squirrels, and through horizontal transmission through mating with male mosquitoes. Humans are infected through bites from chronically infected female mosquitoes. As with other infections in this genus, infections in the mosquito are chronic, whereas viremia in the primary vertebrate hosts and in humans is limited.

Another CE serogroup virus, Jamestown Canyon virus, is widely distributed in North America and may be amplified in the white-tailed deer. It is transmitted by *Culiseta inornata* and *Aedes* species. In contrast to La Crosse virus, Jamestown Canyon virus more commonly causes encephalitis in adults than in children.

Hantaviruses

HCPS

HCPS was first recognized in May 1993 following a cluster of unexplained deaths in young adults in the rural Four Corners area of northwestern New Mexico and northeastern Arizona (17, 37, 71). SNV, a previously unrecognized hantavirus associated with the deer mouse, *Peromyscus maniculatus*, was found to be the virus responsible for most cases of HCPS, and specific serologic tests and tests for nucleic acid detection (reverse transcriptase PCR [RT-PCR]) were quickly developed (26, 37, 40, 46, 71–74, 77, 88, 136, 138, 152, 171). Cases have been reported in 31 states in the continental United States, including most states west of the Mississippi, and cases were diagnosed retrospectively from as early as 1959 (51, 137, 192).

Although SNV remains by far the most important pathogen in the United States and Canada, a limited number of HCPS cases in the United States have occurred outside the range of the deer mouse (Fig. 2) and are caused by distinct species. These include Black Creek Canal virus from the cotton rat, *Sigmodon hispidus*, in Florida (145, 146), New York virus (NYV) from *Peromyscus leucopus* (white-footed mouse) in the northeastern United States (78, 79, 169), and Bayou virus from rice rats (*Oryzomys palustris*) in Louisiana and Texas (133, 179). NYV is closely associated with SNV, whereas Black Creek Canal virus and Bayou virus are more closely associated with ANDV.

HCPS has also now been reported in Argentina, Canada, Bolivia, Brazil, Chile, Panama, Paraguay, and Uruguay. ANDV, which is carried by *Oligoryzomys longicaudatus*, causes severe HCPS along the southern Andes Mountains in central and southern Argentina and Chile. ANDV is of particular concern because of strong evidence for person-to-person transmission (47, 143, 191). Laguna Negra virus (host, *Calomys laucha*) is a recognized pathogen in Paraguay and Bolivia, and Juquitiba virus is a pathogen in Brazil. In Panama, Choclo virus was identified in patients and in the host, *Oligoryzomys fulvescens*, in an outbreak that began in January 2000 (187).

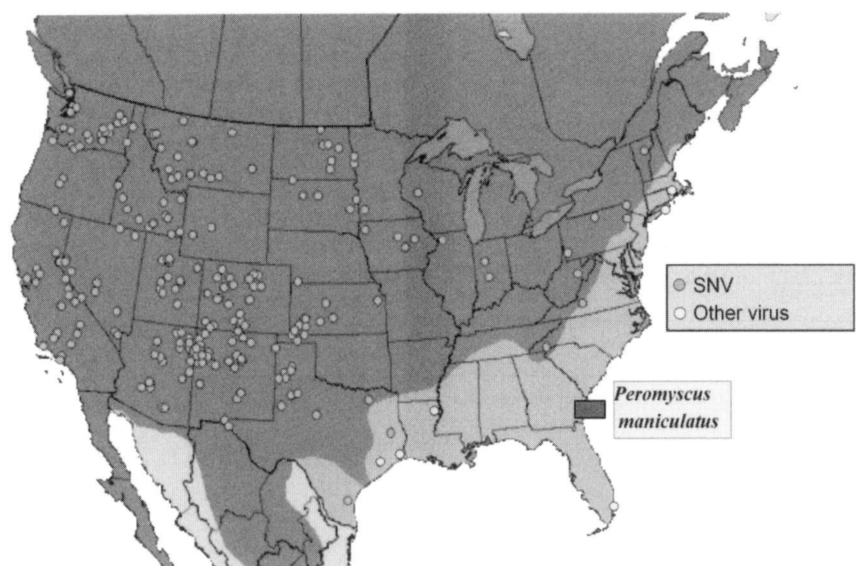

FIGURE 2 Distribution of *Peromyscus maniculatus* and location of hantavirus pulmonary syndrome cases as of 9 May 2006. The total number of cases was 438 in 30 states. (From the CDC.)

In addition to the viruses implicated in HCPS, hantaviruses that have been identified in New World rodents include Rio Mamore virus, amplified by RT-PCR from *Oligoryzomys microtus* collected in Bolivia in 1985; Calabazo virus (host, *Zygodontomys brevicauda*) in Panama (187); Prospect Hill virus in the meadow vole, *Microtus pennsylvanicus;* Isla Vista virus in the California vole, *Microtus californicus;* Bloodland Lake virus in the prairie vole, *Microtus ochrogaster;* El Moro Canyon virus in the western harvest mouse, *Reithrodontomys megalotis;* and Rio Segundo virus from *Reithrodontomys mexicanus* (75, 76, 80, 170, 180).

Current evidence suggests that subclinical infections with SNV and ANDV are uncommon. Although a small number of individuals without a history of HCPS, including mammalogists and persons living in rural areas of the Four Corners region of New Mexico and Arizona, have been found to have hantavirus antibodies, it is not clear whether these individuals have been infected with a pathogenic virus such as SNV. Surveys of hundreds of individuals presenting to health care facilities in the Four Corners region and equal numbers of national park workers and others presumed to have high-risk occupations have failed to identify seropositive persons (4, 17, 200).

Seroprevalence rates of 3 to 30% have been reported in some areas in Central and South America. Rates as high as 12% have been reported in some high-risk areas in Chile when testing was done by the Centers for Disease Control and Prevention (CDC) EIA using standard cutoff values, whereas seroprevalence rates were much lower (3%) and there was intertest agreement when samples were tested by the strip immunoblot assay and by neutralizing antibody testing and a higher cutoff was used for the EIA (P. Vial, personal communication). Seroprevalence rates exceeding 30% have been reported in Panama, where Choclo virus causes a mild form of HCPS with a low case fatality rate and where a high proportion of seropositive individuals have no history of HCPS (3). Although subclinical infections with SNV and ANDV may be rare, mild, symptomatic infections are probably underreported for all hantaviruses that cause HCPS. A number of persons have been identified in New Mexico, Chile, and elsewhere that have been hospitalized for only a few days and required low-flow, supplemental oxygen for only a brief period, and cases have been identified retrospectively that have not involved hospitalization. As of March 2007, 465 cases of HCPS had been reported in the United States, and 64 cases had been reported in Canada through December 2006. In the United States and Canada, there is a male predominance (64%), and the mean age is 38 years (range, 11 to 69 years) in the United States and 42 years in Canada (5). The overall case fatality rate among reported cases is 35% in the United States and 32% in Canada. Cases occur year-round, but most occur in the spring and summer.

Most persons with HCPS lived in rural areas or had occupations or recent activities that involved exposure to rural areas (4, 27, 200). In case-controlled studies of HCPS patients and near and far household controls, risk factors for HCPS included seeing increased numbers of small rodents in the home, cleaning food storage areas in the home, cleaning feed storage areas, and cleaning animal sheds (27, 200). Of note, risk factors almost always include indoor exposure (81).

Risk factors for person-to-person transmission of ANDV infection include close contact with the index case before or shortly after the onset of symptoms rather than following development of the cardiopulmonary phase, when patients typically present for hospital admission (47, 105, 123). In a prospective study of 476 household contacts of index cases with HCPS in Chile, the risk of HCPS was 17.6% in sex partners, versus 1.2% in other household contacts ($P < 0.001$), and 32.6% of 96 HCPS cases occurred in household clusters with two or more cases in the household (47).

Despite the evidence for person-to-person transmission with ANDV, particularly in close household contacts, and some person-to-person transmission in the 1996 outbreak in Argentina that suggested nosocomial transmission, nosocomial transmission of ANDV has not been clearly documented (15, 191). Similarly, a prospective study among health care workers who cared for substantial numbers of HCPS patients in 1993 showed no evidence of nosocomial transmission despite the fact that isolation was often not employed early in the epidemic.

Among U.S. patients, 78% were white, 19% were Native American, 14% were Hispanic, and 2% were black. The relative overrepresentation of Native Americans among all cases reflects the racial distribution in the rural Four Corners area, where SNV infection has been most common. In Chile, where 522 cases were reported through May 2007 and a median of 64 cases were reported annually between 2001 and 2006, the case fatality rate was 38%. The mean age (32 years) is lower than in the United States, in part because ANDV causes disease in young children, whereas SNV does not. Through the end of 2006, 841 cases were reported in Argentina (60), and similar numbers of cases have also been reported in Brazil. Both the number of cases and the numbers of deaths from HCPS in South America exceed the numbers of cases and deaths in the United States and Canada by a factor of at least 3.

HFRS

HFRS associated with Hantaan virus and *Apodemus agrarius* (striped field mouse) is distributed throughout the Far East, particularly in China and Korea, eastern Russia, and the Balkans (Table 2) (14, 29, 108–110, 124, 156, 157, 195). Another severe form of HFRS associated with Dobrava virus and *Apodemus flavicollis* (yellow-necked field mouse) occurs in the Balkans. Saaremaa virus, carried by *A. agrarius*, causes mild HFRS and occurs in eastern and central Europe. Another mild form of HFRS associated with Seoul virus (SEO) and *Rattus norvegicus* (brown rat) occurs worldwide (14, 25, 57, 58, 106, 108, 109, 111, 114, 195). The mildest form of HFRS, nephropathia epidemica (NE), is caused by Puumala virus, which is carried by *Clethrionomys glareolus* (red bank vole); NE occurs throughout Scandinavia, western Russia, and Europe (10, 108, 109, 140, 141, 143, 197). Although infection with the hantaviruses causing HFRS occurs in all age groups, infection and disease peak in adults 15 to 40 years of age; like HCPS, HFRS is uncommon in children (24, 147, 196). There may be 150,000 cases of HFRS per year, with the majority in Asia (183). In a study in two villages in an agricultural district in China, the ratio of subclinical to clinical hantavirus infections was 5.4:1 based on cross-sectional data, versus 14:1 based on prospective data, and clinical infections were more likely to be caused by Hantaan than by Seoul virus. Among rodents trapped in the area, most Hantaan virus infections were found in field-trapped A. *agrarius*, whereas most Seoul virus infections were found in *Rattus norvegicus* trapped in homes (147).

Human infections with Hantaan virus occur throughout the year but peak in November and December following peaks in rodent density and rodent reproductive activity. A smaller peak occurs in May through July in China and Korea, but Seoul virus may be the primary cause of the spring/summer peak. Human infections with Hantaan virus occur primarily in adults in rural areas. Some studies report a preponderance of Hantaan virus infections in men (2:1), but rates among men and women may be equal in areas where agricultural work is performed near the home or where crops are stored near homes during winter months (24, 147, 196). In the latter case, the field mice may be likely to invade homes and food storage areas. Specific occupational groups, including farmers, forest workers, and field soldiers, have been shown to be at higher risk, as have those who perform activities such as harvesting and those who sleep in straw huts (196).

Seoul virus infection appeared to account for approximately 20% of infections and <5% of cases of HFRS in rural China, but Seoul virus appears to cause most urban outbreaks. Large outbreaks have been described in Osaka, Japan; Seoul, Korea; and seaports in China. However, limited outbreaks have been described to occur in seaports throughout the world.

Puumala virus-associated HFRS (NE) primarily occurs among farmers and others living in rural areas (31, 64, 141, 160). Human infections occur throughout the year. In Scandinavian countries, where more than a thousand cases occur annually, most cases occur in the fall and early winter, when bank voles infest barns and homes (184). In temperate Europe, cases are less frequent, and peaks every 3 to 4 years appear to be related to mast years, when an abundance of oak and beech seeds leads to increased rodent populations (184). Seroprevalence in the population in Sweden ranges from about 2% in areas of nonendemicity to approximately 10 to 15% in areas of endemicity (160). The male-to-female ratio ranges from almost 2:1 to almost 5:1. The peak ages for Puumala infection and disease are similar to those for Seoul and Hantaan virus infections, and fewer than 5% of persons with NE are <15 years of age. There are approximately 100 hospitalizations a year in Sweden, and serosurveys in Sweden suggest that there are 10 to 20 infections for every hospitalized case (160).

As indicated above, humans acquire hantavirus infections by aerosol transmission from inhalation of infected rodent excreta, including urine, droppings, and saliva (108, 109, 182). There is no evidence of human-to-human transmission of the viruses that cause HFRS, including nosocomial transmission in hospitals. Seroconversions and clinical infections have occurred among animal handlers and persons visiting laboratories housing small rodents, and, rarely, following bites and dissection of infected animals and among persons working with hantaviruses in cell culture (116, 182). Despite a search for an ectoparasite as a potential vector, including demonstration of infection and transovarial transmission in gamasid mites (84), there is no conclusive evidence linking an ectoparasite vector with any hantavirus infection in humans.

Phleboviruses

RVF

RVF is endemic in sub-Saharan Africa, but major outbreaks occurred outside sub-Saharan Africa in Egypt in 1977 and 1993, in Yemen in 2000, in Saudi Arabia in 2000–2001, and in Kenya in 2007 (2, 19, 120, 127). Epizootics, particularly in sheep and cattle, and epidemics may result from periods of high rainfall as well as factors such as introduction of irrigation projects. Routes of transmission for RVF virus include transmission by insect vectors for epizootics and for most human infections, aerosol transmission in laboratories, and aerosol transmission and, perhaps, transmission from direct contact from necropsy or slaughter of infected animals (21, 61, 127). The virus has been isolated from several genera of mosquitoes and from sand flies, suggesting that multiple insect vectors may be important in maintaining epizootic disease. There is evidence that in the absence of epizootic disease, the virus can be maintained for years during drought through transovarial transmission (particularly in *Aedes mcintoshi*), persistence of infected viable mosquito eggs in soil, and reemergence of infection after rainfall and hatching of the infected eggs (61, 115). Amplification in sheep, cattle, and goats would appear to be more important than transmission between mosquitoes. The infection has a mortality rate of 10 to 30% in sheep, cattle, and goats and is associated with abortion and almost 100% mortality in pregnant animals.

Persons at risk include persons in rural, agricultural areas where an epidemic or epizootic is recognized, persons with exposure to areas where deaths and abortions are occurring in livestock (particularly if they perform necropsy), and persons with exposures in laboratories or abattoirs. Although adult men are at the highest risk, presumably through agricultural activities, disease occurs in all age groups and in both sexes. In an analysis of an outbreak of RVF in Kenya in 1997–1998, contact with sheep body fluids and sheltering livestock in one's home were significantly associated with infection (193). Infection may result in asymptomatic infection, mild disease, or severe disease with substantial morbidity and mortality (193).

Although humans can be infected from bites of mosquitoes and other arthropod vectors, contact with viremic animals, particularly livestock, appears to be the most common mode of acquisition. This is supported by multivariate analyses of risk factors for infection, which include contact with sheep body fluids and sheltering livestock in the home, as well as by relatively low rates of infection in young children (20, 193).

Sandfly Fever Viruses

Phlebotomus fever viruses are found in both hemispheres (14, 61). Sicilian and Naples viruses, transmitted by *Phlebotomus papatasi*, continue to cause human disease in the Balkans, the Middle East, northern Africa, and Southwest Asia, but infection now appears to be uncommon in Italy following eradication efforts with dichlorodiphenyltrichloroethane. Residual spraying of walls in homes was particularly successful, since the vectors feed primarily at night within buildings and tend to rest on building walls, but sand flies may penetrate mosquito netting. Most human infections occur in late spring, summer, and early fall. Epidemics have been described, particularly during wartime, including epidemics in Italy during the Second World War (148). The flight range of the sand fly is limited, so attack rates may vary considerably during epidemics. Toscana virus, which is transmitted by *Phlebotomus perniciosus*, is a continued cause of sporadic human disease in central Italy.

The viruses are presumably amplified in wildlife vertebrate hosts, but these have not been identified. Transstadial transmission and transovarial transmission in sand flies have been demonstrated and are probably the primary mechanisms of perpetuation, particularly in the desert (42, 176).

New World phleboviruses, including Chagres, Punta Toro, and Alenquer viruses, have been isolated during sporadic febrile illnesses from humans in Panama and Brazil who work or live in jungle areas. No epidemics have been identified, and the sand fly vectors appear to be limited to forests.

Nairoviruses

There are at least 34 viruses in the genus *Nairovirus*, all of which are tick borne, which have been classified in seven serogroups (44, 50, 121). These serogroups include the CCHF group, which includes the human pathogens CCHF virus and Hazara virus, and the Nairobi sheep disease (NSD) group, which includes the human pathogens NSD virus and Ganjam virus. Ganjam virus, which has been isolated from ticks collected from goats in India and has been associated with febrile illness in humans in India, appears to be an Asian variant of NSD virus (121). Dugbe virus infection was described for a patient who suffered from a febrile illness with prolonged thrombocytopenia in South Africa (13).

CCHF

CCHF virus is distributed over the geographic range of *Hyalomma* ticks, which includes Africa, Eastern Europe, the Middle East, and Asia through the western provinces of China (Fig. 3) (44, 61, 83, 172). There is little evidence for subclinical infection, and most humans in areas of endemicity are seronegative. CCHF is usually an uncommon, sporadic illness.

Infection occurs through tick bites or by direct contact with infected animals or humans or their tissues. Cows, sheep, goats, hares, and other herbivores have all been implicated in transmission and amplification of CCHF virus. While birds are not susceptible to CCHF virus infection, many *Hyalomma* species feed on birds, thereby allowing the migrating birds to play an important role in disseminating CCHF virus-infected ticks. Antibody to CCHF virus was found in 28% of cattle sera and 78% of cattle herds tested in South Africa and in 45% of cattle sera and 94% of herds tested in Zimbabwe (172). CCHF appears to be maintained both by transovarial and transstadial cycles in ticks and by a tick-vertebrate cycle. In temperate climates, peak transmission generally occurs in the spring and summer, when populations of ticks and their vertebrate hosts peak.

The risk of infection in humans after a bite from a CCHF virus-infected tick is not known but is presumed to be high. Secondary cases have occurred both in laboratory workers and in hospital workers with direct contact with patients, blood, and respiratory secretions, and tertiary cases have also been described among family contacts of health care workers with CCHF (12, 48, 162). There are multiple reports of nosocomial transmission, including one in which infection occurred in 8.7% of health care workers exposed to blood and in 33% of those with a needlestick injury (44, 183). Viremia is highest during the first 3 days of illness and may persist through the second week (163).

PATHOGENESIS IN HUMANS

CE Serogroup Viruses

The incubation period is approximately 3 to 7 days based on exposure histories and the incubation period in exper-

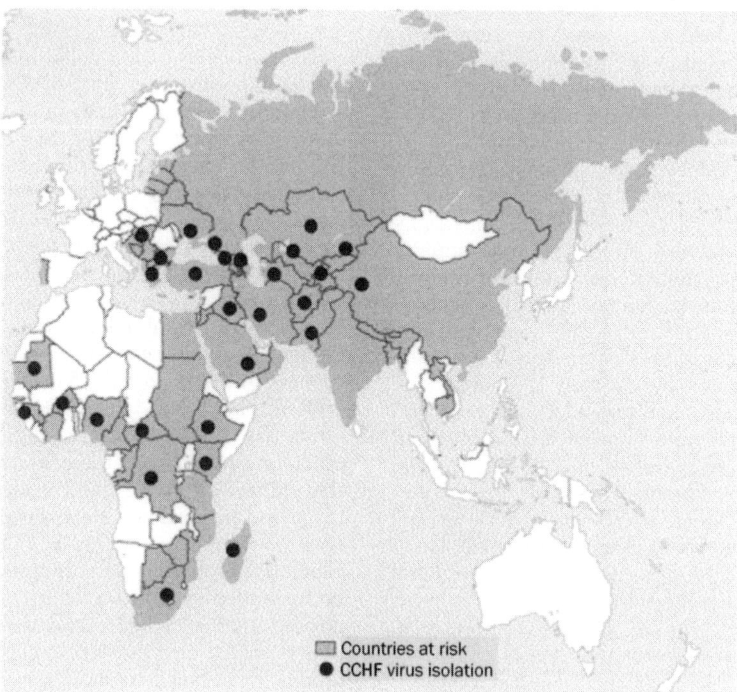

FIGURE 3 Worldwide distribution of CCHF virus. (Reprinted from reference 44 with permission of Elsevier.)

imental animals. Virus has only rarely been isolated from brain tissue of persons dying from encephalitis, and virus has not been recovered from blood, cerebrospinal fluid (CSF), or throat or rectal swabs (177). The few reported autopsies and a brain biopsy showed cerebral edema, mild leptomeningitis, glial nodules, perivascular cuffing, and rare, focal necrosis distributed in cortical gray matter of the temporal, parietal, and frontal lobes; basal nuclei; midbrain; and pons (6, 92, 177).

Antibodies against G1 neutralize virus, block fusion, and inhibit hemagglutination and presumably are important in virus clearance, recovery from infection, and prevention of reinfection. Passive administration of neutralizing antibody has been shown to protect experimental animals, and development of specific immune responses is correlated with recovery from illness in humans and with clearance of viremia in animals (39, 42).

Hantaviruses

The incubation period between rodent contact and onset of symptoms is usually difficult to determine, since the period of potential exposure may be prolonged. A small study of persons with NE suggested that the median was about 4 weeks, with a range of 1 to 8 weeks (159, 160). For the more severe forms of HFRS, the average incubation period has been estimated to be 21 days, with a range of 4 days to 6 weeks (97, 112, 196). Information on the incubation period for HCPS is also limited, but the median incubation period was 18 days, with a range of 10 to 34 days, in a small series of 11 patients with ANDV-associated HCPS in Chile in whom the potential period of exposure was limited to 48 h or less (186).

In persons who die from HFRS and HCPS, hantaviral antigens are widely distributed in organs, as demonstrated by immunohistochemical stains (87, 199). In HCPS, tissues from the lungs, kidneys, heart, spleen, pancreas, lymph nodes, adipose tissue, skeletal muscle, intestine, adrenal gland, and brain are stained; in contrast, only rare sinusoidal lining cells are stained in the liver (199). Viral antigens are seen primarily within capillary endothelial cells but are rarely detected in large veins or arteries. In HCPS, the most intense staining is found in pulmonary capillary endothelial cells. In the kidney, immunostaining is seen in interstitial capillaries in the medulla and cortex and in glomerular endothelial cells. In contrast, for persons dying of HFRS, immunohistochemical staining is most intense in tissues from the kidney. Immunohistochemical staining in tubular epithelial cells is prominent in HFRS but rare in HCPS.

In electron microscopic studies of autopsy tissue from HCPS patients, infrequent hantavirus inclusions have been observed in pulmonary capillary endothelial cells, and more rarely, virions averaging 58 nm have been observed in pulmonary capillary endothelial cells and interstitial macrophages (142, 199). Hantaviruses have been infrequently recovered from humans, so the duration of viremia and viral excretion has not been clearly determined. However, SNV RNA was uniformly detected in peripheral blood mononuclear cells (PBMC) by RT-PCR from persons hospitalized with HCPS, was detected intermittently in specimens collected 16 to 23 days after onset of symptoms, and was not detected in later specimens (74). In contrast, SNV RNA was detected by RT-PCR in only one of three bronchoalveolar lavage samples from patients in whom SNV RNA was easily detected in PBMC.

In autopsied patients with HFRS, capillary engorgement and focal hemorrhages were widely distributed in the kidneys, and there was hemorrhagic necrosis of the renal medulla (118). Retroperitoneal edema was present in persons who died of shock early in the course of illness. Widespread hemorrhages with or without hemorrhagic necrosis were described for the subepicardium and epicardium of the right atrium, anterior pituitary, meninges and subarachnoid space, pancreas, and skin. Hemorrhage and necrosis were most marked in the right atrium in patients who died early in the shock phase, whereas hemorrhagic necrosis of the anterior pituitary was most prominent in patients who survived the shock phase and died during the oliguric or diuretic phase (see "Clinical Manifestations" below). Although pulmonary edema has been described to occur in HFRS, most cases of fatal pulmonary edema described in the literature from the Korean War occurred during the oliguric and diuretic phases rather than the shock phase (11, 86, 98, 118). Pulmonary interstitial infiltrates also appeared to be much less prominent in HFRS than in HCPS (86, 118, 142, 199). In both HFRS and HCPS, there were infiltrates of large, atypical mononuclear cells in the spleen, lymph nodes, and hepatic portal triads. Renal biopsies of patients with NE have shown interstitial edema and hemorrhage, tubular degenerative changes, and glomerular inflammatory infiltrates, and changes consistent with acute tubular necrosis may persist for several months (11). In a series of 13 autopsies of patients with HCPS performed at the University of New Mexico (UNM), all had large, bilateral pleural effusions and large, rubbery, edematous lungs with an average combined weight of 1,920 g (two times the normal weight) (142). Splenomegaly was found in 5 of 12, and gastric mucosal hemorrhage was found in 3 of 13. Histologically, the lungs showed intra-alveolar and septal edema, interstitial infiltrates with mononuclear cells (primarily T lymphocytes, with a CD4/CD8 ratio of about 2:1 and macrophage/monocytic cells), and sparse to moderate hyaline membranes (142). Large immunoblasts, primarily activated $CD8^+$ cells, were found in pleural fluid and peripheral blood (Fig. 4) (128, 142). In contrast to findings in patients with adult respiratory distress syndrome, the type I alveolar lining cells were intact and type II lining cells were not activated; hyaline membranes were composed primarily of fibrin, and neutrophils and cellular debris were uncommon (Fig. 5). In contrast to the findings in HFRS, gross and histologic findings in patients with HCPS were normal for the brain, pituitary gland, heart, kidneys, adrenal gland, pancreas, and skin, and no patient had retroperitoneal edema (142). Of note, however, a group from Brazil recently reported pathological evidence of myocarditis in patients who died from HCPS (149).

Both HCPS and HFRS are thought to be capillary leak syndromes. Differences between the two syndromes include different primary target organs (the lungs in HCPS and the kidneys in HFRS) and a lack of widespread hemorrhage and hemorrhagic necrosis in HCPS despite the presence of thrombocytopenia in both syndromes. Although capillary endothelial cells are infected with hantaviruses in both syndromes and the degree of hantavirus infection is greatest in the capillary endothelial cells in the primary target organ, electron microscopic studies in both syndromes have failed to show any evidence of capillary endothelial cell necrosis or cytotoxicity. Thus, it has been postulated that T cells, cytokines, or other immune-mediated factors may act to create gaps between virus-

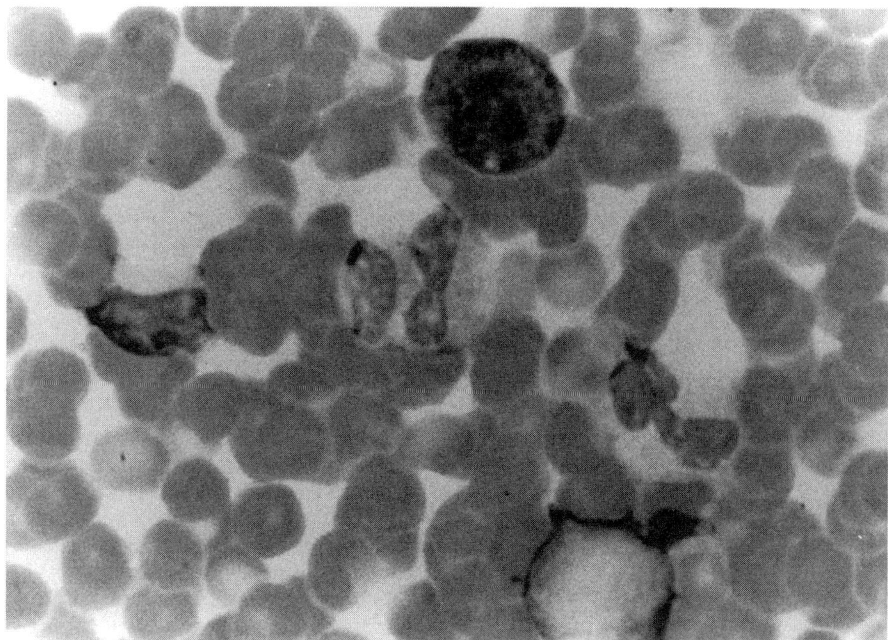

FIGURE 4 Peripheral blood smear from a patient with the cardiopulmonary stage of HCPS. Note the immunoblast with basophilic cytoplasm, prominent nucleolus, and high nuclear-to-cytoplasmic ratio. Also note immature neutrophils. (Courtesy of R. Fedderson.)

infected endothelial cells (128). In both syndromes, antihantavirus antibodies are invariably present at the onset of clinical involvement of the primary target organ. In HCPS, elevated levels in plasma of interleukin 2 (IL-2) and its receptors, gamma interferon, IL-6, and soluble receptors for tumor necrosis factor (TNF) suggest marked cytokine activation, and the same is suggested by increased levels of soluble IL-2 receptor, TNF, and kallikrein-kinins and by gamma interferon expression in HFRS. Circulating immune complexes, activation of the complement path-

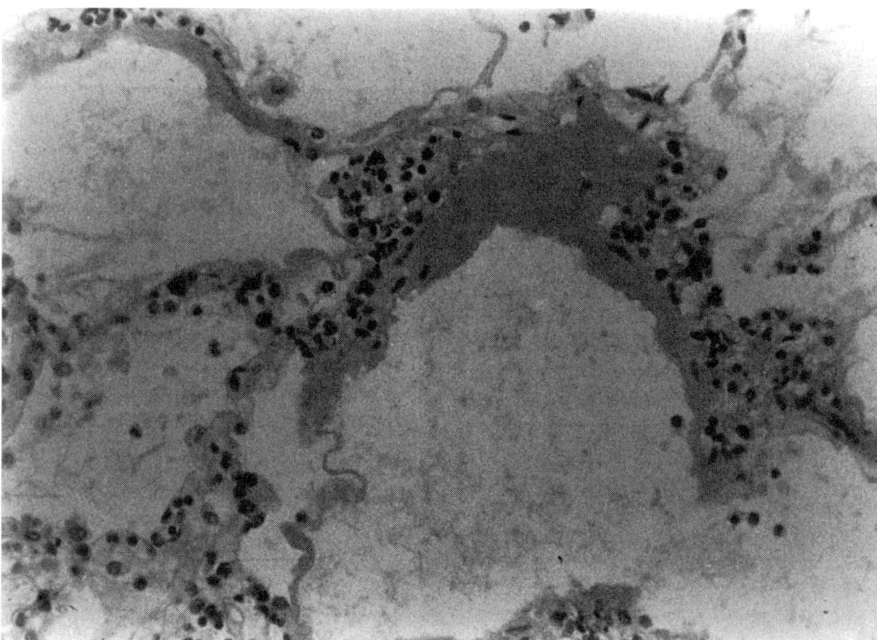

FIGURE 5 Pulmonary histology in a patient who died from HCPS. Note the intra-alveolar and septal edema, interstitial infiltrates with mononuclear cells, and sparse hyaline membrane. In contrast to patients with acute respiratory distress syndrome, the hyaline membranes are largely devoid of inflammatory cells and cellular debris. (Courtesy of K. Nolte.)

way, and deposition of immunoglobulins and complement in both the glomerular basement membrane and tubules are present in HFRS but not HCPS (128).

The role of viremia in the pathogenesis of HFRS and HCPS is not known, but there is emerging evidence that viremia with ANDV routinely precedes the onset of symptoms and development of antihantavirus antibodies in HCPS by periods of up to 15 days. High levels of vRNA can be detected by quantitative RT-PCR in patients with SNV-associated HCPS at the time of hospital admission, and there is a significant association between high viral load at admission and severe disease (134, 174, 194).

Virus isolation from humans with HFRS is difficult (65, 74, 91, 133, 145, 195), and there has been only one successful isolation from a human with HCPS. In that case, ANDV was isolated from the serum of a 10-year-old, seronegative Chilean boy 2 days before he developed fever and 6 days before he died from HCPS (52). Furthermore, in a recent prospective study of household contacts of index patients with HCPS in Chile, ANDV RNA was detected by RT-PCR in peripheral blood cells 5 to 15 days before the onset of symptoms or detection of antihantavirus antibodies in four household contacts who subsequently developed HCPS (47).

Early development of high titers of neutralizing antibody to SNV is associated with mild HCPS. Patients with severe or fatal acute SNV infection have significantly lower neutralizing antibody titers on the day of hospital admission than do patients with mild disease (7).

β_3 integrins mediate cellular entry of pathogenic hantaviruses (Hantaan, Seoul, and Puumala viruses, SNV, and NYV) but do not mediate the entry of Prospect Hill virus, a virus not associated with human disease, in human umbilical vein endothelial cells or in Vero E6 cells (53, 119). β_3 integrins are present on platelets, endothelial cells, and macrophages and are also known to regulate vascular permeability and platelet function.

Humoral and cell-mediated immune responses appear to persist for decades, and recurrent episodes of HFRS or HCPS have not been reported. Thus, it is presumed that infection leads to lifelong protection from repeat infection. Immune but not nonimmune spleen cells protected mice challenged with Hantaan virus, and protection was abolished after depletion of T cells but not after depletion of B cells (134).

Phleboviruses

RVF

The incubation period ranges from 2 to 6 days (21, 61, 127). Viremia occurs in domestic animals and in humans during the acute illness. In humans, the duration of the acute illness usually ranges from 2 to 5 days. In animals, target organs include the liver and brain, and in sheep, death usually results from hepatic necrosis. Deaths in humans most commonly occur among the small number who develop a hemorrhagic fever, shock, and liver necrosis during the acute episode, and virus can be detected or isolated from postmortem blood or liver samples (21, 61, 126, 127, 138, 139). In contrast, virus cannot be isolated from persons with the late clinical complications (encephalitis, retinitis, and uveitis). The time course, lack of viremia, and presence of virus-specific antibodies all suggest that these late complications may be immune mediated. Animal models for both the acute hepatic necrosis and the late encephalitis are available.

Sandfly Fever

In human volunteers, the incubation period ranges from 2 to 6 days (148). Infected humans are viremic during the acute febrile illness, and Toscana virus has been isolated from CSF of patients with aseptic meningitis (38). No deaths have been reported. Neutralizing antibodies persist after infection, and immunity is probably lifelong.

Nairoviruses

CCHF

The incubation period ranges from 3 to 6 days in nosocomial transmission, whereas the range after exposures to animals or ticks is 2 to 12 days (12, 17, 21, 172). Viremia is present during the illness, and titers are highest during the first 3 days of illness (163). In a series from South Africa from 1981 to 1987, 15 of 50 patients died between days 5 and 14 of illness (173).

The pathogenesis of CCHF is less well understood than for many of the other hemorrhagic fevers, in part due to the lack of an appropriate animal model. However, there is good evidence that disseminated intravascular coagulation (DIC) is present, particularly in the more severe cases (173). Fatal infections are also heralded by markedly elevated serum aspartate aminotransferase, alanine aminotransferase, and creatine kinase levels and, terminally, by elevated bilirubin, creatinine, and blood urea nitrogen. Clinically, multiple organ failure precedes death, with involvement of the brain, liver, kidneys, lungs, and heart. Hemophagocytosis, which may be associated with high levels of Th1 cytokines, has been reported in severe CCHF, and levels of the proinflammatory cytokines IL-6 and TNF alpha and DIC scores are higher in patients with fatal CCHF than in those with nonfatal CCHF (45, 96). Finally, a CCHF virus glycoprotein precursor is cleaved to generate a novel glycoprotein that is similar to an Ebola virus domain associated with increased vascular permeability and development of hemorrhages (151).

At autopsy, edema and focal hemorrhage and necrosis are present in multiple organs, including the liver and brain. Although focal hepatic necrosis is most common, massive hepatic necrosis has also been described (173). Focal hemorrhage and necrosis may be found in the brain, and herniation may occur. Renal lesions are characterized by focal, tubular necrosis.

Clinical recovery is temporally associated with resolution of viremia and with the appearance of specific immunoglobulin G (IgG) and IgM antibodies, generally between days 7 and 9 of illness. In contrast, endogenous antibody production was demonstrated in only 2 of 15 patients who died of CCHF (165). There is little information regarding the role of cell-mediated immune responses or the role of nonspecific defenses such as natural killer cells or cytokines.

CLINICAL MANIFESTATIONS

CE Serogroup Viruses (*Bunyavirus* Genus)

At the onset of the illness, patients typically have fever (100%); headache (~75%); and malaise, nausea, and vomiting (50 to 65%) (6, 30, 32, 69). Within 1 to 3 days this is accompanied by meningeal signs (~60%) and lethargy, with total resolution within 7 to 8 days. In the most severe form, fever and headache may begin abruptly, with progression to seizures in 12 to 24 h. Overall, approximately half of patients develop seizures, including some with status epilepticus. Approximately 10% develop coma. Most of the remainder develop disorientation or altered consciousness, but aseptic meningitis without altered consciousness is also described. Less commonly, hemiparesis, tremor, aphasia, ataxia, dysarthria, abnormal reflexes, and chorea have been reported. The case fatality rate is 1% or less, and the total duration of the illness rarely exceeds 10 to 14 days. Most persons recover without any obvious residua. However, persistent focal neurologic findings or learning difficulties have each been reported for about 2% of patients, and emotional lability is reported to persist in about 10%. Epilepsy persists in about 20% of those who experience seizures during the acute episode, and most persons tested within the first 5 years after an acute episode have an abnormal electroencephalogram (62).

Most children with CE have a peripheral white blood cell (WBC) count between 10,000 and 20,000 (median, ~16,000), but normal counts and counts as high as 30,000 have been reported (6, 30, 69). The CSF is almost always abnormal at some point during the acute illness. The CSF glucose is normal and the protein concentration is usually normal, but in about 30% of patients the latter is minimally elevated (range, 40 to 100 mg/dl). The CSF WBC count is elevated (median, ~100; range, 0 to 600 cells/mm^3) in at least 90% of cases, with a predominance of mononuclear cells in 60 to 85% of patients reported in three series.

In the age group at greatest risk for CE, the most common illnesses in the differential diagnosis include herpes simplex virus encephalitis, mumps meningitis or encephalitis, or enteroviral meningoencephalitis (6). Mumps and enteroviral infections tend to occur during community-wide epidemics. Parotitis would be diagnostic of mumps and rash would suggest enteroviral infection, although rash is rarely reported in CE. Focal central nervous system (CNS) findings, seizures, stupor, or coma would suggest CE or herpes simplex virus encephalitis. An absence of exposure to a rural, wooded area in the previous 2 weeks, occurrence outside the months of June through September, or illness in a child less than 1 year or greater than 15 years of age would suggest a diagnosis other than CE. Bacterial meningitis might be suggested in the 30% of patients with a predominance of leukocytes in the CSF, but the clinical course, normal glucose, and negative Gram stain and cultures would rule out bacterial meningitis (6).

Hantaviruses

HCPS

The illness typically begins with a febrile prodromal phase characterized by fever and myalgia; the latter is often prominent (Fig. 6) (103). Headache, backache, abdominal pain, diarrhea, nausea, and vomiting may also be present, particularly after the first 24 to 48 h. As with HFRS, fever and abdominal pain may dominate the clinical presentation, suggesting acute appendicitis or another cause of an acute surgical abdomen (Table 5). The febrile phase, which usually lasts 3 to 4 days but may last 10 to 12 days, is followed by the sudden onset of noncardiogenic pulmonary edema and, in some cases, by shock (17, 37, 71).

The cardiopulmonary or shock phase is heralded by the abrupt onset of cough and shortness of breath, which may be accompanied by dizziness. Pulmonary edema develops rapidly, usually over 12 h or less. All hospitalized patients have become hypoxic during this stage, and nearly all have required supplemental oxygen. Approximately 75% of cases require mechanical ventilation, and mortality is approximately 50% in those who require intubation. Monitoring with a flow-directed pulmonary artery catheter typically shows normal pulmonary wedge pressure (PWP), decreased cardiac index (CI), and elevated systemic vascular resistance (SVR) (Table 6). These parameters are helpful in clinically differentiating HCPS from septic shock. In the latter, the CI is typically elevated and the SVR is depressed.

Among hospitalized patients, death is usually preceded by the abrupt onset of a profound lactic acidosis and cardiogenic shock and by pulseless electrical activity despite the ability to maintain adequate oxygenation. Death may occur within hours of the first pulmonary symptoms, with deaths being uncommon after approximately 48 h of intubation. A lactate level of ≥4 mmol/liter, marked hemoconcentration, a CI of ≤2.2, and persistent hypotension are all indicators of a poor prognosis. Among hospitalized patients, death almost always results from shock with very low cardiac output and from cardiac arrhythmias. Death rarely occurs from respiratory failure provided that mechanical ventilation is available. Consequently, this chapter and many recent publications use the term hantavirus cardiopulmonary syndrome (HCPS) rather than hantavirus pulmonary syndrome to call attention to the important role of shock and arrhythmia in serious and fatal HCPS.

After 2 to 4 days, recovery is heralded by the onset of the diuretic phase. Clinical improvement is often rapid, allowing many patients to be extubated within 12 to 24 h after the onset of diuresis. Supplemental oxygen may be required for several days following extubation. The diuretic phase is typically followed by a convalescent phase that may last up to several months and is characterized by weakness and fatigue, but limited long-term follow-up studies suggest that patients recover fully without any residual abnormalities.

Ketai et al. reviewed chest radiographic findings in 16 patients with HCPS (99). Chest radiographs are usually normal during the prodromal, febrile phase and may be normal at the onset of pulmonary symptoms, but radiographic abnormalities invariably appear shortly after the onset of pulmonary symptoms (99). Early findings include radiological signs of bilateral interstitial edema, including Kerley B lines, hilar indistinctness, and peribronchial cuffing. Within 48 h (often within 2 or 3 h), radiographic signs of bilateral air space disease developed in 11 (69%), including all who required mechanical ventilation or died (Fig. 7).

The platelet count begins to drop shortly after the onset of fever (Fig. 6) (103). Although complete blood counts have been performed for only a few patients during the febrile prodrome, isolated thrombocytopenia was usually present in samples obtained 24 to 48 h before the onset of the shock phase. In the shock phase, characteristic hematologic abnormalities included thrombocytopenia, increased WBC counts with immature granulocytes, ≥10% immunoblasts, and elevation of lactate dehydrogenase. Patients with severe disease also exhibited hemoconcentration, hypoalbuminemia, and lactic acidosis. The immunoblasts are characterized by basophilic cytoplasm (occasionally with coarse granules), prominent nucleoli,

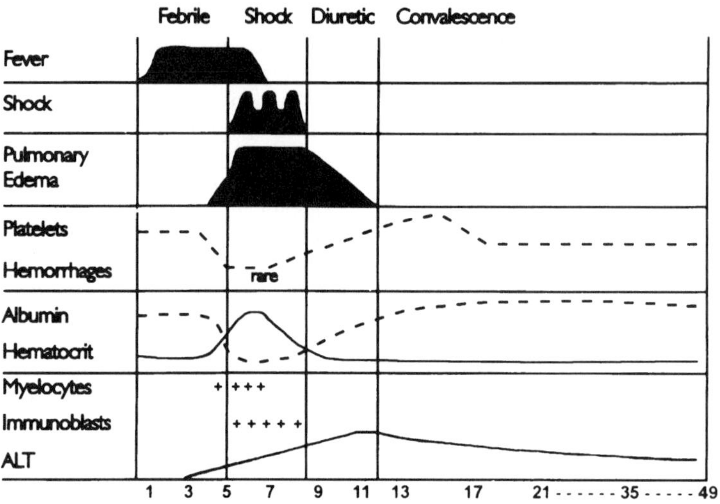

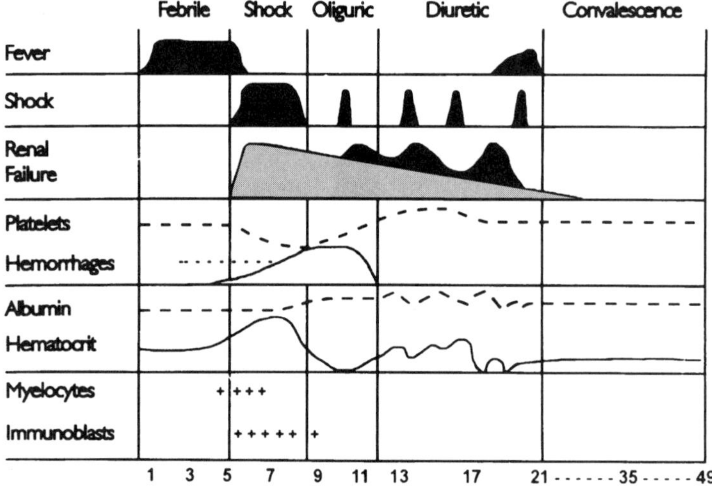

FIGURE 6 Clinical course and typical laboratory findings in severe HCPS and severe HFRS. (Reprinted from reference 103 with permission.)

and a high nuclear-to-cytoplasmic ratio (Fig. 4). Elevations in aspartate aminotransferase typically occur after the onset of the cardiopulmonary or shock phase and peak early in the convalescent phase (Fig. 6).

Pending definitive serologic studies, a clinical diagnosis can be established for patients in the shock or cardiopulmonary phase of HCPS through examination of the peripheral smear and by measurement of the CI, PWP, and SVR with a flow-directed pulmonary artery catheter (23, 102, 130). The differential diagnosis is broad but should include pneumonia, sepsis, endocarditis, and septic shock. Pending definitive diagnosis, antibiotic coverage should be provided to cover the most likely clinical syndromes. At UNM, we routinely cover for pathogens such as *Neisseria meningitidis*, *Streptococcus pneumoniae*, *Yersinia pestis*, and *Francisella tularensis* unless a specific pathogen or syndrome is suspected. Although SNV and other hantaviruses have not been transmitted nosocomially, isolation should be considered until the diagnosis is established or until infection with agents such as *N. meningitidis* or *Y. pestis* has been ruled out.

Clinical decisions regarding patient care such as transfer to a tertiary-care facility and institution of extracorporeal membrane oxygenation (ECMO) must often be made before the results of serologic testing are available (Fig. 8) (130). Fortunately, an initial clinical diagnosis of HCPS can be made with a high degree of confidence for patients who are in the cardiopulmonary phase based on the clinical presentation and a review of the peripheral blood smear. In a recent blinded analysis of patients with a febrile prodrome followed by pulmonary edema, the presence of four or more of the following findings had a sensitivity of 96% and specificity of 99% for diagnosis of HCPS (102). The five findings were thrombocytopenia, myelocytosis,

TABLE 5 Clinical and laboratory features of Hantaan virus-associated HFRS and HCPS

Abnormality	HFRS	HCPS
Prodrome with fever and myalgias	Present	Present
Facial flushing	Common early	Absent
Petechiae	Common late in prodrome	Absent in SNV infection, often present in ANDV infection
Conjunctival injection	Common early	Absent
Pulmonary edema	Uncommon except in oliguria	Present during cardiopulmonary stage
Proteinuria	Present with onset late in prodrome	Uncommon
Hemorrhage	GI,[a] CNS, and right atrial hemorrhage seen in severe cases and patients who died	Rare in SNV infection; clinical bleeding (from venipuncture sites, pulmonary hemorrhage) more common with ANDV
Renal failure/azotemia	Common	Uncommon/mild
Hemoconcentration	Uncommon except with shock	Present in 50% of patients
Thrombocytopenia	Present early	Present early
Nonproductive cough and shortness of breath	Uncommon	Present at onset of cardiopulmonary stage
Shock	Uncommon	Common during cardiopulmonary stage
Hypotension	Common	Very common

[a] GI, gastrointestinal.

lack of significant toxic granulation in neutrophils, hemoconcentration, and more than 10% lymphocytes with immunoblastic morphological features.

Unfortunately, it is very difficult to differentiate patients who are in the febrile, prodromal phase of HCPS from patients with other febrile illnesses based on clinical criteria or on routine laboratory findings. The diagnosis should be considered for persons who present with fever and moderate to severe myalgia, particularly if the person has had recent rural exposure or a recent high-risk exposure such as cleaning food or feed storage areas, catching mice, agricultural work, or increased numbers of mice in the home. Whenever practical, a complete blood count, including a platelet count, should be obtained. In the setting described above, the presence of thrombocytopenia should trigger both serologic testing for hantavirus and consideration of referral to a center with critical care capabilities. The differential diagnosis of fever and thrombocytopenia is broad. For patients with rural exposure in North America, the differential diagnosis would vary by region and the type of exposure but could include plague, tularemia, leptospirosis, ehrlichiosis, Colorado tick fever, relapsing fever, or spotless Rocky Mountain spotted fever.

HFRS

The clinical severity of HFRS varies according to the virus type. Hantaan-associated HFRS, also called Korean and epidemic hemorrhagic fever, has been divided into five stages: febrile, hypotensive, oliguric, diuretic, and convalescent (Fig. 6). Not all patients with Hantaan-associated HFRS have all five stages, and the stages appear to be somewhat less useful in understanding the clinical course of HFRS caused by the other viruses (11, 54, 161, 181).

Hantaan-Associated HFRS

In Hantaan-associated HFRS, illness begins with the onset of fever, which is universal and lasts from 3 to 7 days (11, 54, 161, 181). Symptoms such as malaise, myalgias, and headache are common, as are findings of flushing of the face and neck in conjunction with periorbital edema and conjunctival injection or hemorrhage (Table 5). After several days, the symptoms may worsen and be accompanied by nausea, vomiting, abdominal pain, and lower back pain, and petechiae may be found, particularly on the head, neck, trunk, and palate. As in the case of HCPS, patients at this stage have undergone an exploratory lap-

TABLE 6 Hemodynamic summary at clinical nadir of eight HCPS patients with shock[a]

Characteristic	HCPS (mean ± SEM)	Normal (range)
CI (liters/min/m^2)	2.1 ± 0.33	2.5–4.2
PWP (mm Hg)	15.6 ± 2.6	8–10
SVR (dyne·s·cm^{-5}/m^2)	2,114 ± 258	1,700–2,500
Pulmonary artery mean (mm Hg)	29.7 ± 3.5	8–20
Stroke volume index (ml/beat/m^2)	17.9 ± 3.5	33–47

[a] The clinical nadir is defined by the lowest value of the stroke volume index. All patients were receiving vasoactive or inotropic drugs at the time of measurement and had received volume resuscitation. (Reprinted from reference 68 with permission.)

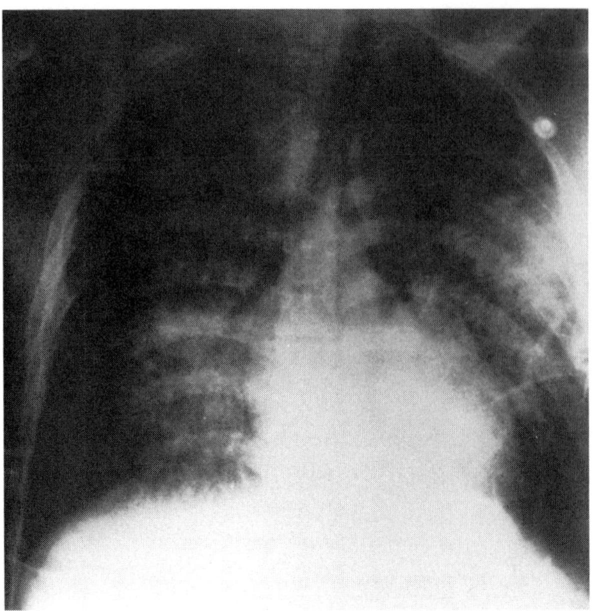

FIGURE 7 Bilateral pulmonary edema in a patient with the cardiopulmonary stage of HCPS. (Courtesy of L. Ketai.)

arotomy because the presentation is mistaken for an acute surgical abdomen. Laboratory findings include a normal or slightly elevated WBC and decreasing platelet count. Proteinuria is present, gradually increases during this phase, and persists through the oliguric phase.

Coincident with or shortly before resolution of the fever, some patients develop hypotension and shock. Mild degrees of hypotension may develop in up to 50% of patients, whereas shock develops in 10 to 15%. In patients with shock, the WBC is markedly elevated, with a left shift and immature forms, and there is marked thrombocytopenia and hemoconcentration. Patients at this stage may exhibit more widespread petechiae and bleeding, and DIC is usually present. One-third of deaths among patients who died during the Korean War and both deaths in a more recent series occurred during this stage (11, 54, 161). In the remainder, the hypotensive phase resolves after a period of several hours to 2 or 3 days.

During the second half of the first week of the illness, oliguric renal failure develops in up to 60 to 70% of patients. If present initially, hypotension and elevations in the hematocrit resolve during the oliguric phase, but hypervolemia with pulmonary edema, neurologic complications, and increased bleeding may occur. Dialysis may be required, particularly in patients with pulmonary edema.

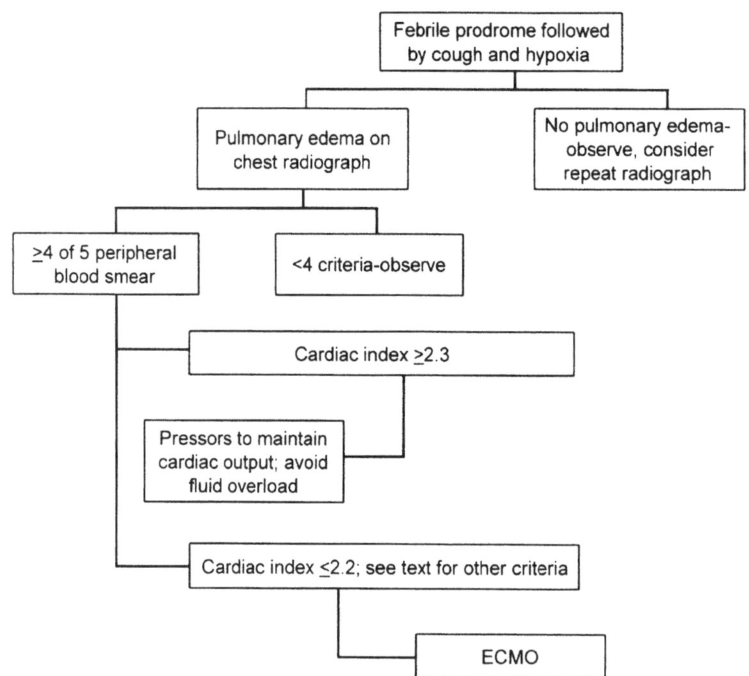

FIGURE 8 Flow diagram for the management of patients suspected of having HCPS in the cardiopulmonary stage pending IgG and IgM antihantavirus antibody results. Potential exposure at any time during the 6 weeks before the onset of symptoms includes living in or visiting any area, usually rural, where a rodent reservoir of a pathogenic hantavirus may be present or close contact with a person with HCPS who could have acquired ANDV infection. (Reprinted from reference 130 with permission.)

In a recent series, oliguric renal failure was present for a mean of 8 days (range, 3 to 17 days) (11). Deaths may occur secondary to pulmonary edema, electrolyte disturbances, shock, and CNS and other hemorrhages.

The diuretic phase begins about the middle of the second week of illness. Patients who have had mild disease generally recover quickly during this phase, but more severely ill patients are at risk of death from intravascular volume depletion, electrolyte disturbances, and secondary infection. This stage may be brief in patients with mild disease or may gradually resolve over several weeks in those with more severe disease; in a recent series, the mean duration was 6 days (range, 2 to 12 days) (11). The diuretic phase may be followed by a prolonged convalescent phase.

The risk of death during the Korean War was about 15%, whereas more recent reports suggest that the risk of death is 5 to 7%. During the Korean War, deaths were equally distributed among the hypotensive, oliguric, and diuretic phases (54, 160), whereas both deaths (7% mortality) occurred from shock on days 4 and 6 in a recent series of 26 patients treated at three U.S. military hospitals between 1981 and 1986 (11). Among the 24 survivors, 4 of 5 who developed pulmonary edema during the oliguric phase required hemodialysis, suggesting that the risk of death during the oliguric and diuretic phases may have been reduced by critical-care treatment and hemodialysis.

HFRS from Seoul, Saaremaa, and Dobrava Viruses

Seoul-associated HFRS is less severe and has less distinct phases, and overall mortality is estimated at less than 1%. Hemorrhagic manifestations appear to be less common, whereas abdominal pain, hepatomegaly, and hepatic dysfunction may be more common. Serologic evidence of hantavirus infection was found in 6.5% of patients with end-stage renal disease due to hypertension in Baltimore, MD (55, 56). These data suggest that a hantavirus may cause hypertension and end-stage renal disease but need to be confirmed by other groups and with prospective studies. Although the serologic data suggest that the antibodies react most strongly to Seoul virus, hantaviral RNA should be examined to determine whether the syndrome is caused by Seoul or a closely related virus. Saaremaa virus is also reported to cause a mild form of HFRS. Dobrava virus, in contrast, causes a severe form of HFRS with a mortality rate of 9 to 12%, hypotension in almost 50%, and oliguric renal failure requiring dialysis in 30 to 47% (184). Hemorrhage or hemorrhagic complications are reported for 9 to 26%, and shock is reported for 21 to 28% (184).

NE

NE is the mildest form of HFRS, with a mortality estimated to be about 0.2% in recent series (159, 160, 184). The syndrome begins with a fever that typically lasts between 2 and 9 days. Within 1 to 2 days of the onset of fever, most patients also develop headache, malaise, and backache. Abdominal pain has been reported for most patients, and as with other hantavirus infections, this presentation may mistakenly suggest an acute surgical abdomen. Shock is very rare. Petechiae and DIC were reported for 1 and 5% of patients in one series, but epistaxis was reported for 28% of patients in the same series (159, 160). Proteinuria (almost 100%), elevated creatinine (almost 100%) (with peaks of 2 to 10 mg/dl), and oliguria (~50% of cases) typically begin at about the third or fourth day of illness and last only a few days (184). This phase is followed by a diuretic phase that lasts for a week to 10 days. Rarely, patients with NE have also been reported to have encephalitis, Guillain-Barré syndrome, and disseminated encephalomyelitis as well as acute perimyocarditis (184). CSF examination is usually normal but may show slight elevations in protein and WBCs. Blurred vision due to myopia that may be caused by ciliary body and lens edema has been reported in about 10% of cases. The mean duration of hospitalization ranged from 8 to 22 days in three Scandinavian series, and the median time of missed work ranges from 36 to 48 days (160).

Phleboviruses

RVF

After an incubation period of 2 to 6 days, most patients with RVF develop a benign febrile illness with fever, myalgia, and malaise (21, 104, 115, 126, 127, 166, 168). Symptoms typically resolve in 2 to 5 days but may be followed by a prolonged convalescent period. In approximately 1 to 3% of patients, petechiae, gastrointestinal bleeding, jaundice, and shock may develop. The overall mortality of RVF has been estimated to be 1% or less (20). Among hospitalized patients with confirmed RVF, however, both mortality and complications have been reported at much higher frequencies. Among 165 patients hospitalized at one hospital in Saudi Arabia in 2000, hepatocellular failure occurred in 75%, acute renal failure occurred in 41%, and hemorrhagic complications occurred in 19%. Hepatorenal failure, shock, and severe anemia were major factors associated with death among the 56 patients who died (34%).

Mortality is also much higher than 1% in case series, probably because of underreporting of mild cases. In an analysis of 834 reported cases of RVF in Saudi Arabia in 2000–2001, of which 81% were laboratory confirmed, the overall mortality rate was 13.9%. Bleeding, neurologic manifestations, and jaundice were independently associated with increased mortality rates, and patients with leukopenia had lower mortality rates than patients with normal or increased leukocyte counts (120). Similarly, a case fatality rate of 29% was reported among 404 probable or confirmed cases of RVF in Kenya between November 2006 and January 2007 (20).

Patients with encephalitis often have a biphasic illness, with onset of headache, nuchal rigidity, confusion, hallucinations, coma, or focal neurologic findings 1 to 4 weeks after onset of RVF. Death may result. Patients with decreased visual acuity may have findings of retinitis with hemorrhages, exudates, and edema or of uveitis (166).

Ocular complications of RVF have long been recognized as serious but relatively uncommon (166). However, in a cross-sectional study of 30 hospitalized patients and 113 outpatients in Saudi Arabia, 212 eyes were affected, including 165 eyes in 113 outpatients and 47 eyes in 30 inpatients, with an interval of 4 to 15 days (mean, 8.8 days) between onset of symptoms of RVF and onset of visual symptoms (1). Macular or paramacular retinitis was identified in all affected eyes, ranging from retinal hemorrhage to optic disk edema and retinal vasculitis. Transient anterior uveitis was present in 31%. Visual acuity was less than 20/200 in 80%, and vision remained the same in 72% and deteriorated in 15% of affected eyes over time. Permanent visual loss was associated with macular and perimacular scarring, vascular occlusion, and optic atrophy.

Sandfly Fever

Most infections with sandfly fever viruses appear to result in clinical disease, but mild or subclinical infections may be more common in children. After an incubation period of 2 to 6 days, the patient develops a febrile illness that lasts 2 to 4 days (148). Toscana virus has been shown to cause aseptic meningitis in Italy and Portugal (38), but high seroprevalence rates in central Italy suggest that most persons infected with this virus have either subclinical infection or a clinical syndrome other than aseptic meningitis (39). No deaths have been reported with these viruses.

Nairoviruses

CCHF

The illness typically begins as an acute febrile illness with fever, chills, myalgia, headache, and nausea, with or without abdominal pain and emesis (12, 165, 172, 173). During this stage, patients are often flushed and have injected conjunctivae or chemosis. After 3 to 6 days of illness, often after a brief period of clinical improvement, most patients develop hemorrhagic manifestations (Fig. 9) (44). These may be limited to petechiae over the trunk and limbs or may involve large ecchymoses. Epistaxis, hematemesis, melena, and hematuria are common during this phase. Both hepatomegaly (20 to 40% of cases) and splenomegaly (14 to 23%) may be present (44). Patients may be somnolent, and dizziness and mild meningeal signs are common. Beginning at about the fifth day of illness, the most severely ill patients develop disseminated intravascular coagulation. Some series have emphasized hepatorenal failure, bradycardia, and hypotension in fatal cases, but these were not reported in recent series in Turkey (44).

Patients who survive have rapid lysis of fever and hemorrhagic manifestations that may be followed by a convalescent stage characterized by persistent fatigue. Poor prognostic indicators include overt DIC; hematemesis, melena, and somnolence: aspartate aminotransferase and alanine aminotransferase levels of >700 and >900 IU/liter, respectively; platelet counts below 20,000; and low platelet counts (below 50,000 cells/ml) that fail to increase over the first few days of hospitalization (44).

The case fatality rate has averaged about 30% but has ranged from 10% to more than 64% (44); the case fatality rate may be greater in nosocomial cases. The proportion of subclinical infections is not known, but one model suggested that CCHF developed in 20% of infected persons (59).

Clinical laboratory abnormalities are helpful in suggesting the diagnosis, and marked elevations in hepatic transaminases, thrombocytopenia, and findings consistent with severe DIC during the first few days of illness are of prognostic value. Leukopenia is usually present from the onset of illness in nonfatal cases, whereas granulocytosis is often present during the first week in fatal infections. Thrombocytopenia is uniformly present early in the course of the illness in fatal cases and appears to be universally present by the end of the first week of illness. DIC occurs in both fatal and nonfatal infections, but abnormal activated partial thromboplastin times, thrombin times, and fibrin degradation products occur earlier and are more abnormal in fatal than in nonfatal cases (173).

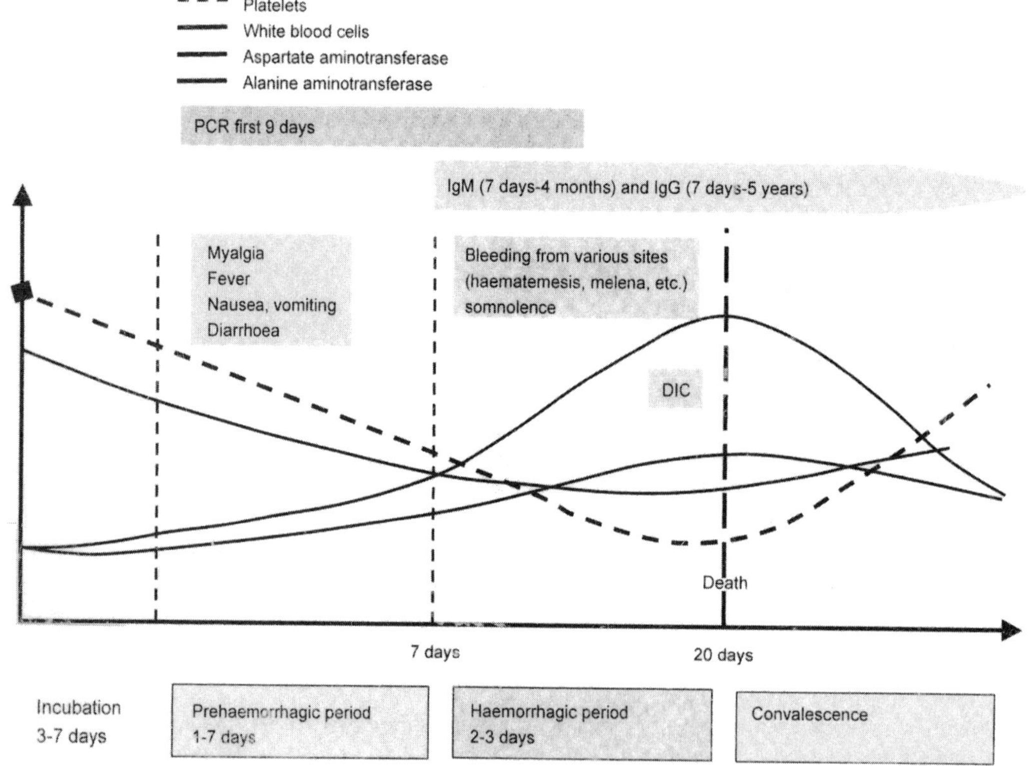

FIGURE 9 Clinical and laboratory course of CCHF. (Reprinted from reference 44 with permission of Elsevier.)

Prior to the development of hemorrhagic manifestations, the differential diagnosis would include any cause of febrile illness. Many patients will have an occupational or rural exposure history. Depending on the patient's location and recent travel history, the differential diagnosis could include leptospirosis, brucellosis, septicemic plague, malaria, tularemia, tick typhus, RVF or sandfly fever. Once hemorrhagic manifestations develop, the differential diagnosis should include other hemorrhagic fevers (see chapters 41, 44, and 52) that are known to be present in the region. These may include Kyasanur Forest disease, Omsk hemorrhagic fever, HFRS, Lassa fever, yellow fever, Ebola or Marburg virus infection, and dengue hemorrhagic fever or dengue shock syndrome. If nosocomial transmission occurs following an index case with an undiagnosed hemorrhagic fever, the differential diagnosis would be limited to known, regional causes of hemorrhagic fever and to agents that are known to be transmitted nosocomially. The latter include CCHF virus, Lassa fever virus, Marburg virus, and the Ebola viruses.

LABORATORY DIAGNOSIS

CE Serogroup Viruses

Although CE serogroup viruses cause productive, cytotoxic infections and replicate in many cell lines, including Vero and BHK-21 cells, repeated attempts to grow virus from throat swabs, blood, CSF, and stool have been unsuccessful. The diagnosis is usually established by serologic methods, including neutralization, hemagglutination inhibition (HI), complement fixation (CF), and enzyme-linked immunosorbent assay (ELISA) (6, 30, 32, 69, 107). Most patients are seropositive by IgM ELISA at the onset of illness. The neutralization assay is positive for most patients by the end of the first week of illness, and neutralizing antibody appears to persist for life. HI antibodies appear with neutralizing antibodies but are not as persistent, and CF antibodies appear only after 2 to 3 weeks of illness and are absent within a year (Fig. 10) (6).

Hantaviruses

In contrast to most other bunyaviruses, hantaviruses are fastidious in cell culture. They can only be grown in a few types of cells, particularly Vero E6 cells, and in experimental infections in rodents such as suckling or adult mice. Hantaan, Seoul, Puumala, Prospect Hill, and SNV (SNV and Convict Creek isolates) were originally recovered from their usual rodent hosts, albeit with some difficulty (40, 61, 110, 111, 114, 140, 152). As was already mentioned in the section on pathogenesis in humans, direct virus isolation in humans with HFRS and HCPS is difficult (52). In addition, virus isolation requires BSL-3 facilities, and the ANDV/hamster model for HCPS requires BSL-4 animal facilities (33). Since faster, safer laboratory methods are available for laboratory confirmation of hantavirus infection in humans, virus isolation is rarely attempted outside the research setting.

HCPS

As in the case of HFRS, specific IgG and IgM antibodies have been almost uniformly present in the first serum sam-

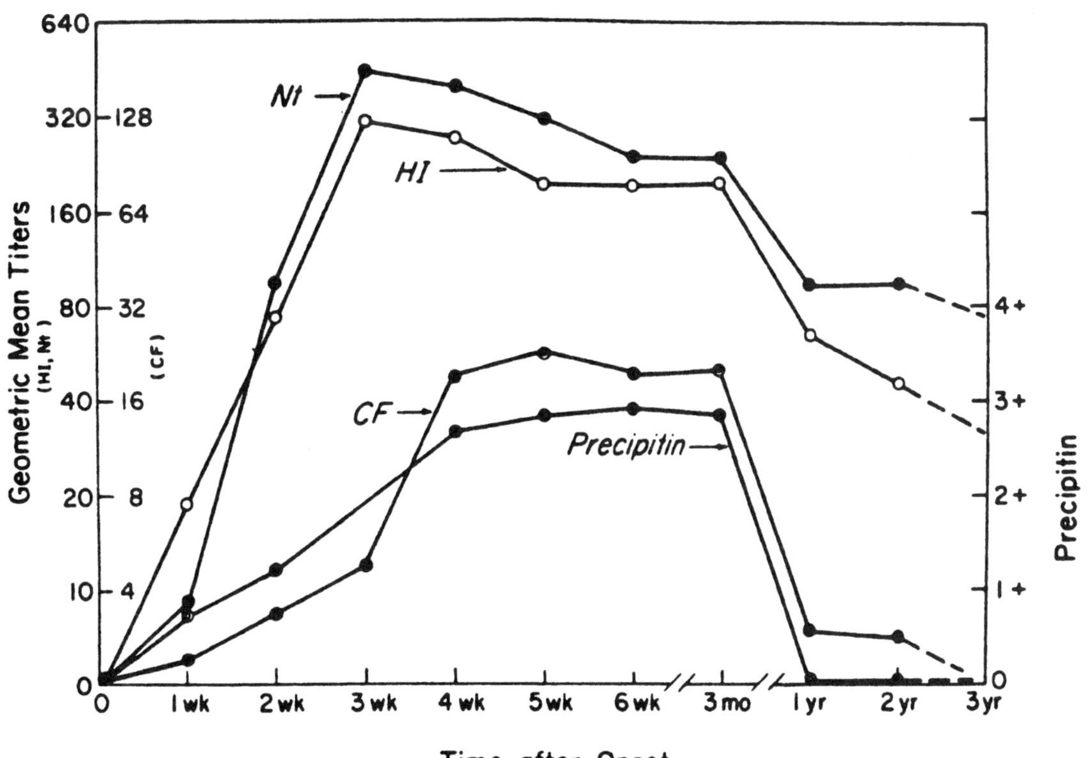

FIGURE 10 Serologic results in 66 patients with CE. The geometric means are plotted for neutralizing (Nt), HI, and CF titers, and the arithmetic means are plotted for precipitin antibodies. (Reprinted from reference 6 with permission.)

ples tested (71, 77, 88). Most available serum samples have been obtained shortly after the onset of the cardiopulmonary stage of HCPS, but testing of limited numbers of serum samples obtained early in the febrile prodrome has also detected specific IgG and IgM antibodies. Available serologic tests include ELISA, neutralization, HI, and Western and strip immunoblot assays.

In the United States, serologic testing to date has used ELISA and Western and strip immunoblot assays. The CDC has developed an IgG ELISA and an IgM capture ELISA based on recombinant N proteins of SNV that is available in many state laboratories. Investigators at UNM first developed a Western immunoblot assay for IgG and IgM antibodies to recombinant N protein and G1 protein, which was followed by development of an IgG and IgM strip immunoblot assay employing recombinant affinity-purified SNV N and G1 antigens (Fig. 11) (7, 77). Using Western immunoblotting, the dominant humoral epitopes of the N protein and G1 proteins of SNV were mapped, thereby allowing increased specificity. N protein is highly immunogenic and tends to be cross-reactive among hantaviruses. Inclusion of the N protein enhances the sensitivity of an assay, and cross-reactivity may be useful as in the case when one is performing serologic screening for a previously unrecognized hantavirus. However, it is difficult to differentiate among hantavirus species using the N protein.

In the Western immunoblot format, the first 59 amino acid residues of SNV N protein contain almost all the antigenic activity of the 428-amino-acid protein, and the dominant linear epitope of SNV G1 protein is confined to a variable region at residues 58 to 88 (73, 88). The latter elicits little or no cross-reactivity among hantaviruses but is conserved among SNV from different regions. Alternative methods that are useful in the serologic differentiation of hantavirus species include the neutralization and HI assays.

Viral RNA can be readily detected by RT-PCR in PBMC in persons with acute SNV or ANDV infection. Postmortem, hantavirus infection can be documented with serologic studies or by examination of tissue (particularly lung tissue) by RT-PCR or by immunohistochemical studies using monoclonal antibodies. RT-PCR is helpful in determining the hantavirus species and has proven useful in molecular epidemiological studies.

HFRS

In eastern Asia, infection with Hantaan and Seoul hantaviruses is usually diagnosed serologically with immunofluorescence assay (IFA), ELISA, or bead agglutination formats, and IgM antibody is determined by IgM capture ELISA. Similarly, NE is commonly diagnosed by detection of IgG antibodies to Puumala virus by IFA, ELISA, or radioimmunoassay RIA, and specific IgM antibody is determined by IgM capture ELISA (31, 64, 160, 184). As in the case of HCPS, IgM antibodies are almost invariably present at or within days of the onset of symptoms. However, in contrast to HCPS, where viral RNA can easily be detected in PBMC during the acute illness, viral RNA is detectable from blood or serum by RT-PCR in less than two-thirds of patients with acute Dobrava or Puumala virus infection (184).

Phleboviruses

RVF Virus

Virus isolation is simple provided that blood is obtained during the acute illness (21, 115, 126, 127, 139, 168). Sensitive isolation systems include Vero or AP61 mosquito cells, intracranially inoculated suckling mice, or intraperitoneally inoculated adult mice or hamsters. The virus grows easily in many cell lines, is cytopathic, and plaques easily. Serologic diagnosis may be accomplished with a single convalescent-phase serum sample using IgM capture ELISA (or less reliably by IgM IFA) or with comparison of acute- and convalescent-phase sera by neutralization, HI, IFA, or ELISA. Both antigen capture ELISA and nucleic acid hybridization techniques have also been used in place of viral isolation during the acute illness; both appear to be somewhat less sensitive than virus isolation (139). Neither virus isolation nor antigen or nucleic acid detection is helpful in patients with late complications such as encephalitis or ocular complications, but a presumptive diagnosis can be established based on rising serum IgG titers

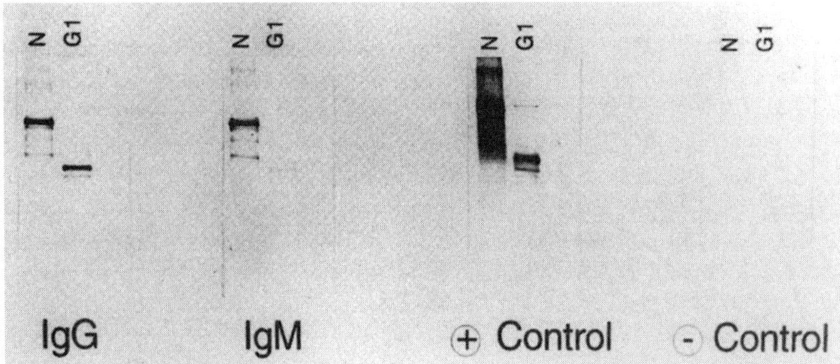

FIGURE 11 SNV recombinant Western blot assay for HCPS. Each panel is a replicate Western blot that contains SNV N (N) and SNV G1 (G1) proteins in separate lanes. The first two panels were reacted with serum from a patient with a clinical syndrome consistent with HCPS. Separate blots were used to detect IgG antibodies (first panel) and IgM antibodies (second panel). The serum sample was found to contain strong IgG and IgM reactivities to SNV N, strong IgG reactivity to SNV G1, and weak IgM reactivity to SNV G1. This pattern is typically seen for patients presenting with acute HCPS. Positive and negative serum samples, respectively, were tested with the blots shown in the last two panels. (Reprinted from reference 77 with permission.)

and through detection of specific IgM in serum and, occasionally, in CSF.

Sandfly Fever Viruses

Virus isolation is easily achieved from blood obtained during the 3-day fever; the viruses replicate well, are cytotoxic, and form plaques in Vero cells (42, 115, 148, 175, 176). Serologic diagnosis can be performed with IgM IFA or, preferably, by IgM capture ELISA shortly after resolution of the fever or by serology on paired sera using techniques such as ELISA, HI, or plaque reduction neutralization.

Nairoviruses

CCHF Virus

CCHF virus can be easily isolated from blood during the acute illness, particularly during the first 3 days, when virus titers are greatest (12, 163, 165, 172, 173). After intracranial inoculation of suckling mice, the mice die in 4 to 8 days, and the diagnosis can be established by CF or fluorescent-antibody testing of brains. Primary isolation can also be performed in cell culture and confirmed by detection of viral antigen by fluorescent-antibody testing once a cytopathic effect is seen. Comparison of primary isolation by intracerebral inoculation of suckling mice and cell culture inoculation of CER or Vero E6 cells suggests that the former is somewhat more sensitive (164). Virus isolation should be attempted only in BSL-4 facilities.

The method of choice for rapid viral diagnosis is real-time RT-PCR, which is highly sensitive and specific (35). An antigen capture ELISA, which is less sensitive, in one series detected antigen in most fatal cases and in approximately half of nonfatal cases (164).

Serodiagnosis can be made using acute- and convalescent-phase titers or by detection of IgM antibody in early convalescence. Serologic assays are usually negative during the first week of illness and for persons who die from CCHF. In order of decreasing sensitivity, the assays that were most sensitive in testing of a series of 35 survivors of CCHF (165) were ELISA, reversed passive HI, IFA, fluorescent-focus reduction, CF, and immunodiffusion. IgG antibodies became detectable by IFA on days 7 to 9 in the 35 survivors; IgM antibody was present in 1 patient on day 5 and was usually present 1 day before or after the first detection of IgG antibody. A neutralization test is available but appears to be more useful for screening sera for neutralizing activity than for routine diagnostic use.

PREVENTION

CE Serogroup Viruses

Infection with CE serogroup viruses may be prevented by use of insect repellents and by mosquito control through insecticide spraying and through control of breeding sites. Some communities have attempted removal of discarded tires and other artificial breeding sites, but control of natural breeding sites such as tree holes in woodlands is probably impractical.

Isolation of infected persons is not necessary. There is no known role for passive immunoprophylaxis or antiviral chemoprophylaxis. No vaccine is available, although immunization of mice with a vaccinia virus recombinant that expresses La Crosse virus glycoproteins protects mice from lethal challenge (63).

Hantaviruses

General guidelines for prevention of infection with hantaviruses include efforts to seal sites of potential rodent entry into homes and peridomestic buildings (particularly storage sheds), careful attention to preventing rodent access to food, and discouraging rodent nesting by eliminating potential nesting sites around the home and workplace. Detailed guidelines for cleaning up rodent-infested areas and for working with potentially infected rodents have been published (18, 131). There is no known role for passive immunoprophylaxis or antiviral chemoprophylaxis, but animal models using Hantaan virus suggest that antiviral chemoprophylaxis with intravenous ribavirin would probably offer some protection from clinical infection. In addition, passive administration of anti-ANDV neutralizing antibody 4 or 5 days after ANDV infection was protective in the Syrian hamster model (33).

Candidate recombinant Hantaan virus vaccines, including a vaccinia virus recombinant vaccine and a baculovirus-expressed subunit vaccine, have been developed at USAMRIID (153, 154). Vaccines with both G1 and G2 of Hantaan virus can elicit neutralizing antibody responses and provide partial protection from challenge in hamsters, and administration of baculovirus-expressed N protein also prevented virus expression in hamsters. However, these vaccines have been dropped from development, since the vaccinia virus recombinant vaccines were poorly immunogenic in humans, and the baculovirus products did not produce sufficient quantities of purified antigen (155). Investigational strategies include DNA vaccination for pathogenic hantaviruses, including Hantaan virus and ADNV (33).

Formalin-inactivated tissue culture-derived Hantaan and Seoul virus vaccines have been developed in Asia. A formalin-inactivated mouse brain-derived Hantaan virus vaccine has been licensed and widely used in Korea since 1990 (113). The vaccine is immunogenic and well tolerated, but rigorously performed, controlled efficacy trials have not been reported. In China, formalin-inactivated Hantaan virus vaccines have been prepared in Mongolian gerbil kidney cells or golden hamster kidney cells (198). These vaccines appear to be immunogenic, and field trials suggest efficacy. However, neither of the vaccines has been tested in randomized, placebo-controlled trials. A bivalent vaccine with inactivated Hantaan and Seoul viruses has also been developed in China (198). The bivalent vaccine appears to be immunogenic, but efficacy trials have not been reported.

Phleboviruses

RVF Virus

As one mode of transmission of RVF virus is via mosquito bites, the risk of infection could presumably be reduced by careful use of mosquito repellents, particularly during periods of high rainfall and high mosquito density, when the risk of epizootics is most marked. The risk of direct transmission from animals during handling, slaughter, autopsy, or disposal is also greatest during epizootics, and particular care should be taken at this time. The presence of an epizootic should be suspected in the setting of unexplained deaths of lambs and sheep and abortions in ewes in an area that is known to be at risk for RVF (127).

No special precautions are indicated when caring for infected persons or when handling blood or other tissues beyond those routinely used to prevent nosocomial transmission of blood-borne infections. However, extreme care should be taken in working with the virus. Furthermore, when the differential diagnosis could involve diseases such as CCHF, Lassa fever, or Ebola virus infection, which have substantial risk of nosocomial transmission, strict isolation would be indicated until RVF is diagnosed or the patient recovers. Parenteral ribavirin therapy was effective in preventing or significantly reducing the level of viremia in a rhesus monkey model, and alpha or purified human leukocyte interferon therapy was effective in the same model (132, 144, 167). Passive antibody and interferon inducers are also effective in animal models. No human trials have been reported for prevention or treatment of RVF, and there are no current guidelines for passive immunoprophylaxis or antiviral chemoprophylaxis of RVF.

A formalin-inactivated, cell culture-derived vaccine is available that is immunogenic and appears to be protective (95, 97, 125). Neutralizing antibody develops in almost all vaccinees after administration of vaccine on days 0, 7, and 28; an annual booster vaccination is required to maintain adequate neutralizing antibody levels. Although unlicensed, the vaccine should be considered for persons with a high risk of infection, such as some laboratory and veterinary workers in areas of endemicity and persons who work with the virus in research laboratories. Both inactivated and attenuated vaccines have been tested for the ability to prevent infection in sheep, cattle, goats, and other animals both to prevent epizootics and economic loss and to prevent human infections. Control measures in a recent outbreak in Kenya included a ban on slaughter of livestock, closure of livestock markets, and vaccination of animals with a live, attenuated vaccine (20).

Sandfly Fever Viruses

Infection with sandfly fever virus can best be avoided by use of insect repellents containing DEET. No special isolation requirements are necessary for persons with sandfly fever. There is no known role for passive immunoprophylaxis or active immunization to prevent sandfly fever. Although oral treatment with 1,200 mg of ribavirin per day prevented viremia and clinical manifestations in volunteers inoculated with Sicilian sandfly fever virus, this approach has not been evaluated during a natural epidemic (J. Huggins, personal communication). This model may suggest a role for short-term, oral prophylactic therapy with ribavirin for other, more serious bunyavirus infections. However, the significant potential for adverse effects with long-term oral ribavirin therapy at this dosage and the benign course of sandfly fever would argue against the routine use of ribavirin for this indication.

Nairoviruses

CCHF Virus

The risk of tick bites can be reduced by use of permethrin-impregnated clothing, by frequent inspection for the presence of ticks, and by gentle removal of ticks (without crushing the tick) if tick bites occur (135). Repellents such as DEET are relatively ineffective against ticks, but application of acaracides to domestic animals may be helpful. In light of the numerous examples of secondary, nosocomial transmission to health care workers, some with tertiary transmission to their families, strict isolation should be followed when caring for a patient with known or suspected CCHF. Recommendations for veterinarians, abattoir workers, and others who may acquire CCHF from direct contact are less clear, but presumably they would include avoidance of contact with blood and body tissues, particularly with animals that appear sick.

A formalin-inactivated suckling mouse brain-derived vaccine has been evaluated for immunogenicity in humans but appears to elicit only very low neutralizing antibody titers. There are no controlled data regarding antiviral chemoprophylaxis, but limited in vitro and animal data suggest that oral or intravenous chemoprophylaxis with ribavirin might be effective. In a nosocomial outbreak of CCHF at Tygerberg Hospital in Cape Town, South Africa, six of nine persons with needlestick exposure were given prophylactic ribavirin. One of the six treated persons developed a mild clinical disease, and the remainder remained clinically well and seronegative (16, 183). While this limited experience does not prove efficacy, this approach might be considered following a high-risk exposure in the laboratory or in a health care setting. Close follow-up for 14 days with administration of ribavirin if fever develops is another strategy (44).

TREATMENT

CE Serogroup Viruses

Treatment of CE is supportive. Seizures should be managed with analeptics, and cerebral edema, if present, should be managed initially with glycerol or mannitol.

Hantaviruses

HCPS

Principles of critical-care management for patients with the cardiopulmonary syndrome include oxygen delivery with intubation and ventilatory support as necessary (67). Because of the high potential for rapid clinical deterioration, whenever feasible, patients should be transferred to a facility with sophisticated critical-care facilities, ideally including the availability of ECMO. Monitoring of CI, PWP, and SVR with a flow-directed pulmonary artery catheter should be performed whenever possible. Inotropic support and vasopressors should be employed rather than fluids whenever possible to reduce the likelihood of worsening pulmonary edema.

Open-label intravenous ribavirin was available for persons with suspected HCPS from 8 June 1993 until 1 September 1994 through a CDC-sponsored protocol. Therapy was considered justified because it had reduced mortality in hantavirus-associated HFRS in a controlled trial and because all previously tested hantaviruses had been sensitive to ribavirin in vitro (85, 90). Subsequently, similar in vitro results were obtained with the hantavirus isolated from *Peromyscus maniculatus* (J. Huggins and S. Ruyo, personal communication). A total of 140 persons suspected of having HCPS were enrolled. HCPS was confirmed in 30; 5 died prior to receipt of the loading dose (22). Among the 64 patients in the United States, death occurred in 14 (47%) of 30 patients enrolled for ribavirin therapy, compared to 17 (50%) of 34 who were not enrolled for treatment. Ribavirin-associated toxicity included reversible anemia in 71% of recipients; 19% required transfusions (22). Adverse events that were less clearly related to ribavirin therapy included pancreatitis and hyperamylasemia, which were documented in 8% of patients.

A subsequent, Collaborative Antiviral Study Group-sponsored, prospective, placebo-controlled trial of intravenous ribavirin for suspected HCPS in the United States and Canada failed to reach its target accrual and was closed based on a futility analysis (129). However, there were no trends suggesting efficacy in patients enrolled during the cardiopulmonary phase, and the investigators were unable to enroll subjects in the febrile prodrome. The median time to progression to death or initiation of ECMO was 24 h or less in both treatment groups, suggesting that there is a very limited window of opportunity for intervention short of ECMO once patients present in the cardiopulmonary phase (Fig. 12) (129).

ECMO has been used at the UNM Health Sciences Center in patients who fit criteria that were associated with almost 100% mortality in a retrospective analysis of patients cared for at UNM. Of these 42 managed with ECMO, 27 (65%) survived to hospital discharge, including 22 (76%) of the last 29 treated patients (M. Crowley, personal communication). Criteria for ECMO include a CI of less than 2.3 l/min per m^2, or a ratio of arterial oxygen tension to fractional inspired oxygen (PaO_2/FIO_2) of less than 50, and a lack of response to conventional (non-ECMO) support (Fig. 8; 130).

HFRS

Management of HFRS should include monitoring for shock, hypotension, renal failure, and hemorrhage. Whenever possible, both critical-care facilities and hemodialysis should be readily available. Comparison of case fatality rates before and after the availability of hemodialysis and critical care suggests that mortality rates have been significantly reduced by the availability of the latter (11, 54, 161, 181). During the Korean War, the risk of death was about 15%, whereas more recent reports suggest that the risk of death is 5 to 7%. Furthermore, during the Korean War, deaths were equally distributed among the hypotensive, oliguric, and diuretic phases (54, 161). In contrast, among 26 patients treated at three U.S. military hospitals between 1981 and 1986, both deaths (7% mortality) occurred from shock on days 4 and 6. Among the 24 survivors, 4 of 5 who developed pulmonary edema during the oliguric phase required hemodialysis, suggesting that the risk of death during the oliguric and diuretic phases may have been reduced by critical-care treatment and hemodialysis (11).

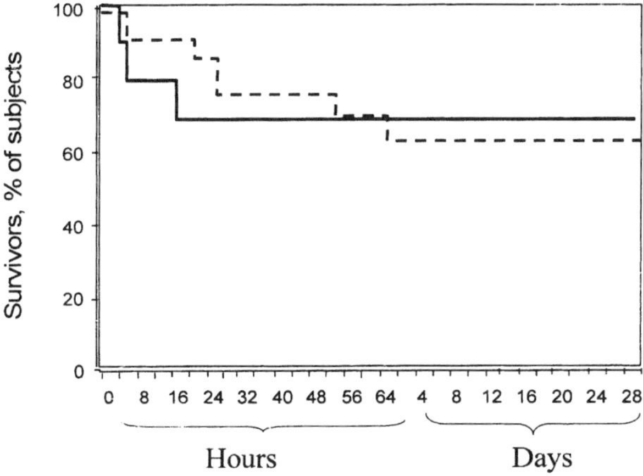

FIGURE 12 Survival without ECMO among ribavirin recipients versus placebo recipients in a trial of intravenous ribavirin therapy for HCPS. Solid line, ribavirin recipients (n = 10); broken line, placebo recipients (n = 13). (Reprinted from reference 129 with permission.)

A prospective, placebo-controlled trial of intravenous ribavirin was carried out in patients with serologically confirmed hantavirus-associated HFRS in the People's Republic of China (85). Nonpregnant patients 14 years of age or older with fever and proteinuria and with a significant exposure history or the presence of hantavirus-specific IgM antibodies were eligible for enrollment unless they had symptoms for more than 6 days, advanced renal failure, coma, or shock refractory to fluid replacement. Patients who received ribavirin received a loading dose of 33 mg/kg of body weight followed by 16 mg/kg every 6 h for 4 days and 8 mg/kg every 8 h for 3 days. Of 242 patients with serologically confirmed hantavirus-associated HFRS who were included in the efficacy analysis, there was a sevenfold decrease in the risk of mortality among ribavirin-treated patients (P = 0.01 [Fig. 13]) after adjustment for baseline estimators of mortality (85). Ribavirin therapy also significantly reduced the risk of developing oliguria or hemorrhage. The primary adverse effect of therapy was hemolytic anemia that resolved after discontinuation of therapy. The proportions of patients with severe anemia (hematocrit below 20) were similar in the two treatment groups. Development of severe anemia was gradual in the ribavirin-treated patients, whereas placebo-treated patients with severe anemia tended to develop acute drops in hematocrit secondary to gastrointestinal or urinary tract hemorrhage.

A similar placebo-controlled trial, also conducted in the People's Republic of China, evaluated the efficacy of treatment with alpha interferon at a dose of 10^7 U per day. Although the risk of hemorrhage was reduced with treatment, treatment with interferon did not reduce mortality (66).

Phleboviruses

RVF Virus

There is no specific therapy for RVF, for the hemorrhagic complications or for the late complications of encephalitis and retinitis. The experimental models described in the section on prevention suggest that early treatment with ribavirin, alpha or human leukocyte interferon, or passive neutralizing antibody might reduce the risk of complications, but no trials have been performed in humans. Steroids have been used in patients with retinal vasculitis and encephalitis, without apparent benefit.

Sandfly Fever Viruses

No specific therapy is available. Although prophylactic therapy with oral ribavirin successfully prevented sandfly fever in experimentally infected volunteers, it seems unlikely that initiation of ribavirin therapy after the onset of fever would have a significant impact on this benign, 2- to 4-day illness.

Nairoviruses

CCHF Virus

Aggressive, supportive therapy, preferably in a setting with critical-care capabilities, is essential for patients with this serious hemorrhagic fever. Hemorrhage can lead to large requirements for blood replacement, with attendant com-

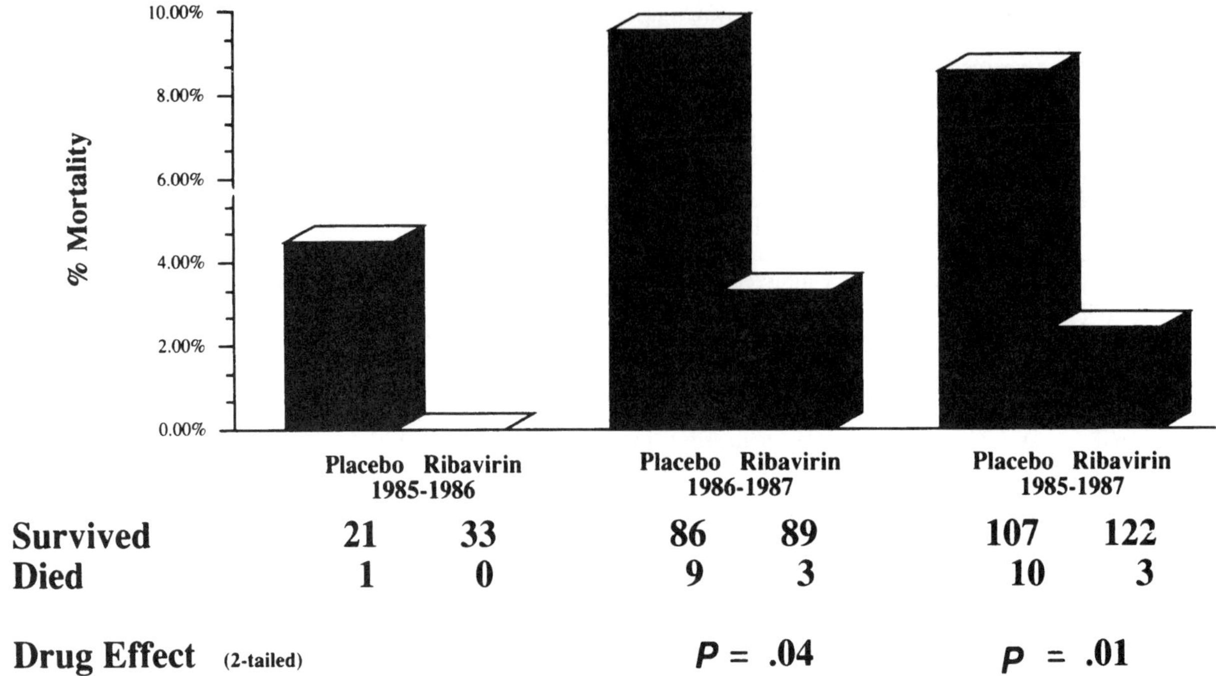

FIGURE 13 Effect of ribavirin or placebo therapy on patients with serologically confirmed HFRS. Top, percent mortality by enrollment date. Bottom, survival and death by study year. From the drug effect model the odds of death in controls were estimated as seven times greater than in the ribavirin group (95% confidence interval, 1.2 to 39.9). Baseline covariates in the logistic regression model were total serum protein and aspartate aminotransferase. (Reprinted from reference 85 with permission of The University of Chicago Press.)

plications. Replacement of platelets and coagulation factors with fresh frozen plasma may be indicated, and shock and less severe intravascular volume disturbances may necessitate invasive monitoring (24).

There is no proven, specific antiviral therapy for CCHF in humans. Ribavirin is active in vitro and in an infant mouse model of CCHF (178, 190). No controlled trials of ribavirin have been reported for humans, but several series have documented low mortality rates in persons with CCHF treated with ribavirin compared with historical controls. Among three health care workers given oral ribavirin 1 g four times a day for 4 days followed by 500 mg four times a day for 6 days (oral therapy was chosen because intravenous ribavirin was not available) within 1 to 4 days after the onset of fever, each patient became afebrile within 48 h of initiation of therapy (48). In another study of eight patients with severe CCHF treated with oral ribavirin at dosages of 4 g/day for 4 days and 2.4 g/day for 6 days, all survived (43). More recently, 88.9% of 69 patients survived who had confirmed CCHF and received oral ribavirin, reportedly at the dosages reported below for intravenous ribavirin (122). If intravenous ribavirin is available, the recommended regimen is a 30-mg/kg loading dose (maximum, 2 g) followed by 15 mg/kg (maximum, 1g) every 6 h for 4 days followed by 7.5 mg/kg (maximum, 500 mg) every 8 h for 6 days (44, 50, 129). One study reported that intravenous administration of specific immunoglobulin for CCHF virus hastened recovery and reduced mortality in patients treated in Bulgaria, but the study was uncontrolled (185).

REFERENCES

1. **Al-Hazmi, A., A. A. Al-Rajhi, E. B. Abboud, E. A. Ayoola, M. Al-Hazmi, R. Saadi, and N. Ahmed.** 2005. Ocular complications of Rift Valley fever outbreak in Saudi Arabia. *Ophthalmology* **112:**313–318.
2. **Al-Hazmi, M., E. Ayobanji Ayoola, M. Abdurahman, S. Banzal, J. Ashraf, A. El-Bushra, A. Hazmi, M. Abdullah, H. Abbo, A. Elamin, E.-T. Al-Sammani, M. Gadour, C. Menon, M. Hamza, I. Rahim, M. Hafez, M. Jambavalikar, H. Arishi, and A. Aqeel.** 2003. Epidemic Rift Valley fever in Saudi Arabia: a clinical study of severe illness in humans. *Clin. Infect. Dis.* **36:**245–252.
3. **Armien, B., J. M. Pascale, V. Bayard, C. Munoz, I. Mosca, G. Guerrero, A. Armien, E. Quiroz, C. Castillo, Y. Zaldivar, F. Gracia, B. Hjelle, and F. Koster.** 2004. High seroprevalence of hantavirus infection on the Aquero Peninsula of Panama. *Am. J. Trop. Med. Hyg.* **70:** 682–687.
4. **Armstrong, L. R., S. R. Zaki, M. J. Goldoft, R. L. Todd, A. S. Khan, R. F. Khabbaz, T. G. Ksiazek, and C. J. Peters.** 1995. Hantavirus cardiopulmonary syndrome associated with entering or cleaning rarely used, rodent-infested structures. *J. Infect. Dis.* **172:**1166.
5. **Artsorb, H., M. Drebot, R. Lindsay, D. Safronetz, D. Dick, and H. Feldman.** 2007. Hantavirus Pulmonary Syndrome in Canada 1989–2006, p. 89. *Abstr. VII Int. Conf. HFRS, HPS and Hantavirus*, Buenos Aires, Argentina, 13 to 15 June.
6. **Balfour, H. H., R. A. Siem, H. Bauer, and P. G. Quie.** 1973. California arbovirus (La Crosse) infections. I. Clinical and laboratory findings in 66 children with meningoencephalitis. *Pediatrics* **52:**680–691.

7. **Bharadwaj, M., R. Nofchissey, D. Goade, F. Koster, and B. Hjelle.** 2000. Humoral immune responses in the hantavirus cardiopulmonary syndrome. *J. Infect. Dis.* **182:**43–48.
8. **Bird, B. H., M. L. Khristova, P. E. Rollin, T. G. Ksiazek, and S. T. Nichol.** 2007. Complete genome analysis of 33 ecologically and biologically diverse Rift Valley fever virus strains reveals widespread virus movement and low genetic diversity due to recent common ancestry. *J. Virol.* **81:**2805–2816.
9. **Bouloy, M.** 1991. *Bunyaviridae:* genome organization and replication strategies. *Adv. Virus Res.* **40:**235–275.
10. **Brummer-Korvenkontio, M., A. Vaheri, T. Hovi, C. H. von Bonsdorff, J. Vuorimies, T. Manni, K. Penttinen, N. Oker-Blom, and J. Lahdevirta.** 1980. Nephropathia epidemica: detection of antigen in bank voles and serologic diagnosis of human infection. *J. Infect. Dis.* **41:**131–134.
11. **Bruno, P., L. H. Hassell, J. Brown, W. Tanner, and A. Lau.** 1990. The protean manifestations of hemorrhagic fever with renal syndrome. A retrospective review of 26 cases from Korea. *Ann. Intern. Med.* **113:**385–391.
12. **Burney, M. I., A. Ghafoor, M. Saleen, P. A. Webb, and J. Casals.** 1980. Nosocomial outbreak of viral hemorrhagic fever caused by Crimean hemorrhagic fever-Congo virus in Pakistan, January 1976. *Am. J. Trop. Med. Hyg.* **29:**941–947.
13. **Burt, F. J., D. C. Spencer, P. A. Leman, B. Patterson, and R. Swanepoel.** 1996. Investigation of tick-borne viruses as pathogens of humans in South Africa and evidence of Dugbe virus infection in a patient with prolonged thrombocytopenia. *Epidemiol. Infect.* **116:**353–361.
14. **Calisher, C. H.** 2001. History, classification and taxonomy of viruses in the family *Bunyaviridae*, p. 1–17. *In* R. M. Eliott (ed.), *The* Bunyaviridae. Plenum Press, New York, N.Y.
15. **Castillo, C., E. Villagra, L. Sanhueza, M. Ferres, J. Mardones, and G. J. Mertz.** 2004. Prevalence of antibodies to hantavirus among family and healthcare worker contacts of persons with hantavirus cardiopulmonary syndrome in Chile: lack of evidence for nosocomial transmission of Andes virus to healthcare workers in Chile. *Am. J. Trop. Med. Hyg.* **70:**302–304.
16. **Centers for Disease Control.** 1983. Management of patients with suspected viral hemorrhagic fever. *Morb. Mortal. Wkly. Rep.* **37:**S2.
17. **Centers for Disease Control and Prevention.** 1993. Outbreak of acute illness—southwestern United States, 1993. *Morb. Mortal. Wkly. Rep.* **42:**421.
18. **Centers for Disease Control and Prevention.** 1993. Hantavirus infection—southwestern United States: interim recommendations for risk reduction. *Morb. Mortal. Wkly. Rep.* **42**(RR-11)**:**1–13.
19. **Centers for Disease Control and Prevention.** 2000. Outbreak of Rift Valley fever—Yemen, August–October 2000. *Morb. Mortal. Wkly. Rep.* **49:**1065–1066.
20. **Centers for Disease Control and Prevention.** 2007. Rift Valley fever outbreak—Kenya, November 2006–January 2007. *Morb. Mortal. Wkly. Rep.* **56:**73–76.
21. **Chambers, P., and R. Swanepoel.** 1980. Rift Valley fever in abattoir workers. *Centr. Afr. J. Med.* **26:**122–126.
22. **Chapman, L. E., G. J. Mertz, C. J. Peters, H. M. Jolson, A. S. Khan, T. G. Ksiazek, F. T. Koster, K. F. Baum, P. E. Rollin, A. T. Pavia, R. C. Holman, J. C. Christenson, P. J. Rubin, R. E. Behrman, L. J. Bell, G. L. Simpson, and R. F. Sadek.** 1999. Intravenous ribavirin for hantavirus pulmonary syndrome: safety and tolerance during one year of open label experience. *Antiviral Ther.* **4:**211–219.
23. **Chapman, L. E., B. A. Ellis, F. T. Koster, M. Sotir, T. G. Ksiazek, G. J. Mertz, P. E. Rollin, K. F. Baum, A. T. Pavia, J. C. Christenson, P. J. Rubin, H. M. Jolson, R. E. Behrman, A. S. Khan, L. J. Wilson Bell, G. L. Simpson, J. Hawk, R. C. Holman, C. J. Peters, and the Ribavirin Study Group.** 2002. Discriminators between hantavirus-infected and uninfected persons enrolled in a trial of intravenous ribavirin for presumptive hantavirus pulmonary syndrome. *Clin. Infect. Dis.* **34:**293–304.
24. **Chen, H. X., F. X. Qiu, B. J. Dong, S. Z. Ji, Y. T. Li, Y. Wang, H. M. Wang, G. F. Zuo, X. X. Tao, and S. Y. Gao.** 1986. Epidemiologic studies on hemorrhagic fever with renal syndrome in China. *J. Infect. Dis.* **154:**394–398
25. **Childs, J. E., G. W. Korch, G. E. Glass, J. W. LeDuc, and K. V. Shah.** 1987. Epizootiology of hantavirus infections in Baltimore: isolation of a virus from Norway rats, and characteristics of infected rat populations. *Am. J. Epidemiol.* **126:**55–68.
26. **Childs, J. E., T. G. Ksiazek, C. F. Spiropoulou, J. W. Krebs, S. Morzunov, G. O. Maupin, K. L. Gage, P. E. Rollin, J. Sarisky, R. E. Enscore, J. K. Frey, C. J. Peters, and S. T. Nichol.** 1994. Serologic and genetic identification of *Peromyscus maniculatus* as the primary rodent reservoir for a new hantavirus in the southwestern United States. *J. Infect. Dis.* **169:**1271–1280.
27. **Childs, J. E., J. W. Krebs, T. G. Ksiazek, G. O. Maupin, K. L. Gage, P. E. Rollin, P. S. Zeitz, J. Sarisky, R. E. Enscore, J. C. Butler, J. E. Creek, G. E. Glass, and C. J. Peters.** 1995. A household-based, case-control study of environmental factors associated with hantavirus cardiopulmonary syndrome in the southwestern United States. *Am. J. Trop. Med. Hyg.* **52:**393–397.
28. **Chizhikov, V. E., C. F. Spiropoulou, S. P. Morzunov, M. C. Monroe, C. J. Peters, and S. T. Nichol.** 1995. Complete genetic characterization and analysis of isolation of Sin Nombre virus. *J. Virol.* **69:**8132–8136.
29. **Chu, Y. K., C. Rossi, J. W. Leduc, H. W. Lee, C. S. Schmaljohn, and J. M. Dalrymple.** 1994. Serological relationships among viruses in the *Hantavirus* genus, family Bunyaviridae. *Virology* **198:**196–204.
30. **Chun, R. W. M., W. H. Thompson, J. D. Grabow, and C. G. Matthews.** 1968. California arbovirus encephalitis in children. *Neurology* **18:**369–375.
31. **Clement, J., P. McKenna, P. Colson, P. Damoiseaux, C. Penalba, P. Halin, and D. Lombart.** 1994. Hantavirus epidemic in Europe, 1993. *Lancet* **343:**114.
32. **Cramblett, H. G., H. Stegmiller, and C. Spencer.** 1966. California encephalitis infections in children. *JAMA* **198:**108–112.
33. **Custer, D. M., E. Thompson, C. S. Schmaljohn, T. G. Ksiazek, and J. W. Hooper.** 2003. Active and passive vaccination against hantavirus pulmonary syndrome with Andes virus M genome segment-based DNA vaccine. *J. Virol.* **77:**9894–9905.
34. **Douglass, R. J., T. Wilson, W. J. Semmens, S. N. Zanto, C. W. Bond, R. C. Van Horn, and J. N. Mills.** 2001. Longitudinal studies of Sin Nombre virus in deer mouse-dominated ecosystems of Montana. *Am. J. Trop. Med. Hyg.* **65:**33–41.
35. **Drosten, C., S. Göttig, S. Schilling, M. Asper, M. Panning, H. Schmitz, and S. Günther.** 2002. Rapid detection and quantification of RNA of Ebola and Marburg viruses, Lassa virus, Crimean-Congo hemorrhagic fever virus, Rift Valley fever virus, dengue virus, and yellow fever virus by real-time reverse transcription-PCR. *J. Clin. Microbiol.* **40:**2323–2330.

36. **Dubey, S., N. Salamin, S. D. Ohdachi, P. Barriere, and P. Vogel.** 2007. Molecular phylogenetics of shrews (Mammalia: Soricidae) reveal timing of transcontinental colonizations. *Mol. Phylogenet. Evol.* **44:**126–137.
37. **Duchin, J. S., F. T. Koster, C. J. Peters, G. L. Simpson, B. Tempest, S. R. Zaki, T. G. Ksiazek, P. E. Rollin, S. Nichol, E. T. Umland, R. L. Moolenaar, S. E. Reef, K. B. Nolte, M. M. Gallaher, J. C. Butler, and R. F. Breiman for the Hantavirus Study Group.** 1994. Hantavirus cardiopulmonary syndrome: a clinical description of 17 patients with a newly recognized disease. *N. Engl. J. Med.* **330:**949–955.
38. **Ehrnst, A., C. J. Peters, B. Niklasson, A. Svedmyr, and B. Holmgren.** 1985. Neurovirulent Toscana virus (a sandfly fever virus) in a Swedish man after a visit to Portugal. *Lancet* **i:**1212–1213.
39. **Eitrem, R., M. Stylianou, and B. Niklasson.** 1991. High prevalence rates of antibody to three sandfly fever viruses (Sicilian, Naples, and Toscana) among Cypriots. *Epidemiol. Infect.* **107:**685–691.
40. **Elliott, L. H., T. G. Ksaizek, P. E. Rollin, C. F. Spiropoulou, S. Morzunov, M. Monroe, C. S. Goldsmith, C. D. Humphrey, S. R. Zaki, J. W. Krebs, G. Maupin, K. Gage, J. E. Childs, S. T. Nichol, and C. J. Peters.** 1994. Isolation of the causative agent of hantavirus cardiopulmonary syndrome. *Am. J. Trop. Med. Hyg.* **51:**102–108.
41. **Elliott, R. M.** 1990. Molecular biology of the *Bunyaviridae*. *J. Gen. Virol.* **71:**501–522.
42. **Endris, R. G., R. B. Tesh, and D. G. Young.** 1983. Transovarial transmission of Rio Grande virus (Bunyaviridae: Phlebovirus) by the sand fly, *Lutzomyia anthophora*. *Am. J. Trop. Med. Hyg.* **32:**862–864.
43. **Ergonul, O., A. Celikbas, B. Dokuzoguz, S. Eren, N. Baykam, and H. Esener.** 2004. Characteristics of patients with Crimean Congo hemorrhagic fever in a recent outbreak in Turkey and impact of oral ribarivin therapy. *Clin. Infect. Dis.* **39:**284–287.
44. **Ergonul, O.** 2006. Crimean-Congo hemorrhagic fever. *Lancet Infect. Dis.* **6:**203–214.
45. **Ergonul, O., S. Tuncbilek, N. Baykam, A. Celikbas, and B. Dokunzoguz.** 2006. Evaluation of serum levels of interleukin (IL)-6, IL-10, and tumor necrosis factor-alpha in patients with Crimean-Congo hemorrhagic fever. *J. Infect. Dis.* **193:**941–944.
46. **Feldmann, H., A. Sanchez, S. Morzunov, C. F. Spiropoulou, P. E. Rollin, T. G. Ksiazek, C. J. Peters, and S. T. Nichol.** 1993. Utilization of autopsy RNA for the synthesis of the nucleocapsid antigen of a newly recognized virus associated with hantavirus cardiopulmonary syndrome. *Virus Res.* **30:**351–367.
47. **Ferrés, M., P. Vial, C. Marco, L. Yañez, P. Godoy, C. Castillo, B. Hjelle, I. Delgado, S.-J. Lee, and G. J. Mertz for the Andes Virus Household Contacts Study Group.** 2007. Prospective evaluation of household contacts of persons with hantavirus cardiopulmonary syndrome in Chile. *J. Infect. Dis.* **195:**1563–1571.
48. **Fisher-Hoch, S. P., J. A. Khan, S. Rehman, S. Mirza, M. Khurshid, and J. B. McCormick.** 1995. Crimean-Congo haemorrhagic fever treated with ribavirin. *Lancet* **346:**472–475.
49. **Flick, R., K. Flick, H. Feldmann, and F. Elgh.** 2003. Reverse genetics for Crimean-Congo hemorrhagic fever virus. *J. Virol.* **77:**5997–6006.
50. **Flick, R., and C. A. Whitehouse.** 2005. Crimean-Congo hemorrrhagic fever virus. *Curr. Mol. Med.* **5:**753–760.
51. **Frampton, J. W., S. Lanser, C. R. Nichols, and P. J. Ettestad.** 1995. Sin Nombre virus infection in 1959. *Lancet* **346:**781–782.
52. **Galeno, H., J. Mora, E. Villagra, J. Fernandez, R. Hernandez, G. J. Mertz, and E. Ramirez.** 2002. First human isolate of hantavirus (Andes virus) in the Americas. *Emerg. Infect. Dis.* **8:**657–661.
53. **Gavrilovskaya, I. N., M. Shepley, R. Shaw, M. H. Ginsberg, and E. R. Mackow.** 1998. β_3 integrins mediate cellular entry of hantaviruses that cause respiratory failure. *Proc. Natl. Acad. Sci. USA* **95:**7074–7079.
54. **Giles, R. B., J. A. Sheedy, C. N. Ekman, H. F. Froeb, C. C. Conley, J. L. Stockard, D. W. Cugell, J. W. Vester, R. K. Kiyasu, G. Entwisle, and R. H. Yoe.** 1954. The sequelae of epidemic hemorrhagic fever with a note on causes of death. *Am. J. Med.* **16:**629–638.
55. **Glass, G. E., A. J. Watson, J. W. LeDuc, G. D. Kelen, T. C. Quinn, and J. E. Childs.** 1993. Infection with a ratborne hantavirus in U.S. residents is consistently associated with hypertensive renal disease. *J. Infect. Dis.* **167:**614–620.
56. **Glass, G. E., A. J. Watson, J. W. LeDuc, and J. E. Childs.** 1994. Domestic cases of hemorrhagic fever with renal syndrome in the United States. *Nephron* **68:**48–51.
57. **Gligic, A., M. Frusic, M. Obradovic, R. Stojanovic, D. Hlaca, C. J. Gibbs, R. Yanagihara, C. H. Calisher, and D. C. Gajdusek.** 1989. Hemorrhagic fever with renal syndrome in Yugoslavia: antigenic characterization of hantaviruses isolated from *Apodemus flavicollis* and *Clethrionomys glareolus*. *Am. J. Trop. Med. Hyg.* **41:**109–115.
58. **Gligic, A., N. Dimkovic, S. Y. Yiao, G. J. Buckle, D. Jovanovic, D. Velimirovic, R. Stojanovic, M. Obradovic, G. Diglisic, J. Micic, D. M. Asher, J. W. LeDuc, R. Yanagihara, and D. C. Gajdusek.** 1992. Belgrade virus: a new hantavirus causing severe hemorrhagic fever with renal syndrome in Yugoslavia. *J. Infect. Dis.* **166:**113–120.
59. **Goldfarb, L. G., M. P. Chumakov, A. A. Myskin, V. F. Kondratenko, and O. Y. Reznikov.** 1980. An epidemiological model of Crimean hemorrhagic fever. *Am. J. Trop. Med. Hyg.* **29:**260–264.
60. **Gonzalez Capri, S., M. Elder, M. L. Cacace, J. Cortes, M. Romero Bruno, M. I. Farace, and P. J. Padula.** 2007. Hantavirus pulmonary syndrome in Argentina, 1995–2006, abstr. S1-03, p. 22. *Abstr. VII Int. Conf. HFRS, HPS and Hantavirus*, Buenos Aires, Argentina 13 to 15 June.
61. **Gonzalez-Scarano, F., and N. Nathanson.** 1996. *Bunyaviridae*, p. 1473–1504. *In* B. N. Fields, D. M. Knipe, P. M. Howley, R. M. Chanock, J. L. Melnick, T. P. Monath, B. Roizman, and S. E. Straus (ed.), *Fields Virology*, 3rd ed., vol. 1. Lippincott-Raven, Philadelphia, PA.
62. **Grabow, J. D., C. G. Matthews, R. W. M. Chun, and W. H. Thompson.** 1969. The electroencephalogram and clinical sequelae of California arbovirus encephalitis. *Neurology* **19:**394–404.
63. **Griot, C., A. Pekosz, D. Lukac, S. S. Scherer, K. Stillmock, D. Schmeidler, M. J. Endres, F. Gonzalez-Scarano, and N. Nathanson.** 1993. Polygenic control of neuroinvasiveness in California serogroup bunyaviruses. *J. Virol.* **67:**3861–3867.
64. **Groen, J., M. N. Gerding, J. G. Jordans, J. P. Clement, J. H. Nieuwenhuijs, and A. D. Osterhaus.** 1995. Hantavirus infections in the Netherlands: epidemiology and disease. *Epidemiol. Infect.* **114:**373–383.
65. **Gu, X. S., Z. B. Song, Z. W. Jin, G. R. Meng, C. A. Zhang, D. Y. Yan, T. Gu, S. Q. Yang, J. R. He, F. J. Luo, Z. Q. You, Q. Su, J. K. Zhang, and L. T. Peng.** 1990. Isolation of a strain of Hantaan virus from peritoneal exudate cells of a patient with hemorrhagic fever with renal syndrome. *Chin. Med. J.* **103:**455–459.
66. **Gui, X. E., M. Ho, M. S. Cohen, Q. L. Wang, H. P. Huang, and Q. X. Xie.** 1987. Hemorrhagic fever with

renal syndrome: treatment with recombinant alpha interferon. *J. Infect. Dis.* **155:**1047–1051.

67. **Hallin, G. W., S. Q. Simpson, R. E. Crowell, D. S. James, F. T. Koster, G. J. Mertz, and H. Levy.** 1996. Cardiopulmonary manifestations of the hantavirus cardiopulmonary syndrome. *Crit. Care Med.* **24:**252–258.
68. **Hallin, G. W., and S. Q. Simpson.** 1996. Hantavirus cardiopulmonary syndrome. *PCCU* **11:**5.
69. **Hilty, M. D., R. E. Haynes, P. H. Azimi, and H. G. Cramblett.** 1972. California encephalitis in children. *Am. J. Dis. Child.* **124:**530–533.
70. **Hinson, E. R., S. M. Shone, M. C. Zink, G. E. Glass, and S. L. Klein.** 2004. Wounding: the primary mode of Seoul virus transmission among male Norway rats. *Am. J. Trop. Med. Hyg.* **70:**310 317.
71. **Hjelle, B., S. Jenison, G. Mertz, F. Koster, and K. Foucar.** 1994. Emergence of hantaviral disease in the southwestern United States. *West. J. Med.* **161:**467–473.
72. **Hjelle, B., S. Jenison, N. Torrez-Martinez, T. Yamada, K. Nolte, R. Zumwalt, K. MacInnes, and G. Myers.** 1994. A novel hantavirus associated with an outbreak of fatal respiratory disease in the southwestern United States: evolutionary relationships to known hantaviruses. *J. Virol.* **68:**592–596.
73. **Hjelle, B., F. Chavez-Giles, N. Torrez-Martinez, T. Yamada, J. Sarisky, M. Ascher, and S. Jenison.** 1994. Dominant glycoprotein epitope of Four Corners hantavirus is conserved across a wide geographical area. *J. Gen. Virol.* **75:**2881–2888.
74. **Hjelle, B., C. F. Spiropoulou, N. Torrez-Martinez, S. Morzunov, C. J. Peters, and S. T. Nichol.** 1994. Detection of Muerto Canyon virus RNA in peripheral blood mononuclear cells from patients with hantavirus cardiopulmonary syndrome. *J. Infect. Dis.* **170:**1013–1017.
75. **Hjelle, B., F. Chavez-Giles, N. Torrez-Martinez, T. Yates, J. Sarisky, J. Webb, and M. Ascher.** 1994. Genetic identification of a novel hantavirus of the harvest mouse *Reithrodontomys megalotis*. *J. Virol.* **68:**6751–6754.
76. **Hjelle, B., B. Anderson, N. Torrez-Martinez, W. Song, W. L. Gannon, and T. L. Yates.** 1995. Prevalence and geographic genetic variation of hantaviruses of New World harvest mice *(Reithrodontomys)*: identification of a divergent genotype from a Costa Rican *Reithrodontomys mexicanus*. *Virology* **207:**452–459.
77. **Hjelle, B., S. Jenison, D. E. Goade, W. B. Green, R. M. Feddersen, and A. A. Scott.** 1995. Hantaviruses: clinical, microbiologic and epidemiologic aspects. *Crit. Rev. Clin. Lab. Sci.* **32:**469–508.
78. **Hjelle, B., J. Krolikowski, N. Torrez-Martinez, F. Chavez-Giles, C. Vanner, and E. Laposata.** 1995. Phylogenetically distinct hantavirus implicated in a case of hantavirus cardiopulmonary syndrome in the northeastern United States. *J. Med. Virol.* **46:**21–27.
79. **Hjelle, B., S. W. Lee, W. Song, N. Torrez-Martinez, J. W. Song, R. Yanagihara, I. Gavrilovskaya, and E. R. Mackow.** 1995. Molecular linkage of hantavirus cardiopulmonary syndrome to the white-footed mouse, *Peromyscus leucopus*: genetic characterization of the M genome of New York virus. *J. Virol.* **69:**8137–8141.
80. **Hjelle, B., N. Torrez-Martinez, and F. T. Koster.** 1996. Hantavirus cardiopulmonary syndrome-related virus from Bolivia. *Lancet* **347:**57.
81. **Hjelle, B., and G. E. Glass.** 2000. Outbreak of hantavirus infection in the Four Corners region of the United States in the wake of the 1997–1998 El Nino-southern oscillation. *J. Infect. Dis.* **181:**1569–1573.
82. **Honig, J. E., J. C. Osborne, and S. T. Nichol.** 2004. Crimean-Congo hemorrhagic fever virus genome L RNA segment and encoded protein. *Virology* **321:**29–35.
83. **Hoogstraal, H.** 1979. The epidemiology of tick-borne Crimean-Congo hemorrhagic fever in Asia, Europe, and Africa. *J. Med. Entomol.* **15:**307–417.
84. **Houck, M. A., H. Qin, and H. R. Roberts.** 2001. Hantavirus transmission: potential role of ectoparasites. *Vector Borne Zoonotic Dis.* **1:**75–79.
85. **Huggins, J. W., C. M. Hsiang, T. M. Cosgriff, M. Y. Guang, J. I. Smith, Z. O. Wu, J. W. LeDuc, Z. M. Zheng, J. M. Meegan, Q. N. Wang, D. O. Oland, X. E. Gui, P. H. Gibbs, G. H. Yuan, and T. M. Zhang.** 1991. Prospective, double-blind, concurrent, placebo-controlled clinical trial of intravenous ribavirin therapy of hemorrhagic fever with renal syndrome. *J. Infect. Dis.* **164:** 1119–1127.
86. **Hullinghorst, R. L., and A. Steer.** 1953. Pathology of epidemic hemorrhagic fever. *Ann. Intern. Med.* **38:**77–101.
87. **Hung, T., J. Y. Zhou, Y. M. Tang, T. X. Zhao, L. J. Baek, and H. W. Lee.** 1992. Identification of Hantaan virus-related structures in kidneys of cadavers with haemorrhagic fever with renal syndrome. *Arch. Virol.* **122:** 187–199.
88. **Jenison, S., T. Yamada, C. Morris, B. Anderson, N. Torrez-Martinez, N. Keller, and B. Hjelle.** 1994. Characterization of human antibody responses to Four Corners hantavirus infections among patients with hantavirus cardiopulmonary syndrome. *J. Virol.* **68:**3000–3006.
89. **Jin, H., and R. M. Elliot.** 1991. Expression of functional Bunyamwera virus L protein by recombinant vaccinia viruses. *J. Virol.* **65:**4182–4189.
90. **Johnson, K. M.** 1993. Ribavirin treatment of arenavirus, hantavirus, pneumo-virus and paramyxovirus disease: topical and systemic therapy, p. 229. *In* J. Mills and L. Corey (ed.), *Antiviral Chemotherapy: New Directions for Clinical Application and Research,* vol. 3. PTR Prentice Hall, Englewood Cliffs, NJ.
91. **Juto, P., F. Elgh, C. Ahlm, O. A. Alexeyev, K. Edlund, A. Lundkvist, and G. Wadell.** 1997. The first human isolate of Puumala virus in Scandinavia as cultured from phytohemagglutinin stimulated leucocytes. *J. Med. Virol.* **53:**150–156.
92. **Kalfayan, B.** 1983. Pathology of La Crosse virus infection in humans, p. 179. *In* C. H. Calisher and W. H. Thompson (ed.), *California Serogroup Viruses*. A. R. Liss, New York, NY.
93. **Kallio, E. R., A. Poikonen, A. Vaheri, O. Vapalahti, H. Henttonen, E. Koskela, and T. Mappes.** 2006. Maternal antibodies postpone hantavirus infection and enhance individual breeding success. *Proc. R. Soc. Biol. Sci. Ser. B* **273:**2771–2776.
94. **Kallio, E. R., J. Klingström, E. Gustafsson, T. Manni, A. Vaheri, H. Henttonen, O. Vapalahti, and Å Lundkvist.** 2006. Prolonged survival of Puumala hantavirus outside the host: evidence for indirect transmission via the environment. *J. Gen. Virol.* **87:**2127–2134.
95. **Kark, J. D., Y. Aynor, and C. J. Peters.** 1982. A Rift Valley fever vaccine trial. I. Side effects and serologic response over a six-month follow-up. *Am. J. Epidemiol.* **116:**808–820.
96. **Karti, S. S., Z. Odabasi, V. Korten, M. Yilmaz, M. Sonmez, R. Caylan, E. Akdogan, N. Eren, I. Koksal, E. Ovali, B. R. Erickson, M. J. Vincent, S. T. Nichol, J. A. Comer, P. E. Rollin, and T. G. Ksiazek.** 2004. Crimean-Congo hemorrhagic fever in Turkey. *Emerg. Infect. Dis.* **19:**1379–1384.
97. **Kawamata, J., T. Yamanouchi, K. Dohmae, H. Miyamoto, M. Takahaski, K. Yamanishi, T. Kurata, and H. W. Lee.** 1987. Control of laboratory acquired hem-

orrhagic fever with renal syndrome (HFRS) in Japan. *Lab. Anim. Sci.* **37:**431–436.
98. **Kessler, W. H.** 1953. Gross anatomic features found in 27 autopsies of epidemic hemorrhagic fever. *Ann. Intern. Med.* **38:**73–76.
99. **Ketai, L. H., M. R. Williamson, R. J. Telepak, H. Levy, F. T. Koster, K. B. Nolte, and S. E. Allen.** 1994. Hantavirus pulmonary syndrome: radiographic findings in 16 patients. *Radiology* **191:**665–668.
100. **Khaiboullina, S., A. Rizvanov, D. Bourdreaux, G. P. Morzunov, and S. St. Jeor.** 2007. Reconstruction of a recombinant hantavirus from plasmids encoding all three viral segments, abstr. S501, p. 62. *Abstr. VII Int. Conf. HFRS, HPS and Hantavirus*, Buenos Aires, Argentina 13 to 15 June.
101. **Kinsella, E., S. G. Martin, A. Grolla, M. Czub, H. Feldmann, and R. Flick.** 2004. Sequence determination of the Crimean-Congo hemorrhagic fever virus L segment. *Virology* **321:**23–28.
102. **Koster, F. T., K. Foucar, B. Hjelle, A. Scott, Y. Y. Chong, R. Larson, and M. McCabe.** 2001. Presumptive diagnosis of hantavirus cardiopulmonary syndrome by routine complete blood count and blood smear review. *Am. J. Clin. Pathol.* **116:**665–672.
103. **Koster, F. T. and S. Jenison.** 1996. The hantaviruses, p. 2140–2147. *In* S. L. Gorbach, J. G. Bartlett, and N. R. Blacklow (ed.), *Infectious Diseases*, 2nd ed. The W. B. Saunders Company, Philadelphia, PA.
104. **Laughlin, L., J. M. Meegan, L. H. Strausbaugh, D. M. Morens, and R. H. Watten.** 1979. Epidemic Rift Valley fever in Egypt: observations on the spectrum of human illness. *Trans. R. Soc. Trop. Med. Hyg.* **73:**630–633.
105. **Lázaro, M. E., G. E. Cantoni, L. M. Claanni, A. J. Resa, E. R. Herrero, M. A. Iacono, D. A. Enria, and S. M. González Cappa.** 2007. Clusters of hantavirus infection, southern Argentina. *Emerg. Infect. Dis.* **13:**104–110.
106. **LeDuc, J. W., G. A. Smith, J. E. Childs, F. P. Pinheiro, J. I. Maiztegui, B. Niklasson, A. Antoniades, D. M. Robinson, M. Khin, K. F. Shortridge, M. T. Woosler, M. R. Elwell, P. L. T. Illbery, D. Koech, E. S. T. Rosa, and L. Rosen.** 1986. Global survey of antibody to Hantaan-related viruses among peridomestic rodents. *Bull. W.H.O.* **64:**139–144.
107. **LeDuc, J. W.** 1987. Epidemiology and ecology of the California serogroup viruses. *Am. J. Trop. Med. Hyg.* **37:** 60S–68S.
108. **Leduc, J. W.** 1989. Epidemiology of hemorrhagic fever viruses. *Rev. Infect. Dis.* **11:**S730–S735.
109. **LeDuc, J. W., J. E. Childs, G. E. Glass, and A. J. Watson.** 1993. Hantaan (Korean hemorrhagic fever) and related rodent zoonoses, p. 149–158. *In* S. S. Morse (ed.), *Emerging Viruses*. Oxford University Press, New York, NY.
110. **Lee, H. W., P. W. Lee, and K. M. Johnson.** 1978. Isolation of the etiologic agent of Korean hemorrhagic fever. *J. Infect. Dis.* **137:**298–308.
111. **Lee, H. W., L. J. Baek, and I. M. Johnson.** 1982. Isolation of Hantaan virus, the etiologic agent of Korean hemorrhagic fever, from wild urban rats. *J. Infect. Dis.* **146:**638–644.
112. **Lee, H. W., and K. M. Johnson.** 1982. Laboratory-acquired infections with Hantaan virus, the etiologic agent of Korean hemorrhagic fever. *J. Infect. Dis.* **146:** 645–651.
113. **Lee, H. W., Y. K. Chu, Y. D. Woo, C. N. An, H. Kim, E. Tkachenko, and A. Gligic.** 1999. Vaccines against hemorrhagic fever with renal syndrome, p. 147–156. *In* J. F. Saluzzo and B. Dodet (ed.), *Factors in the Emergence and Control of Rodent-Borne Viral Diseases*. Elsevier, New York, NY.
114. **Lee, P. W., H. L. Amyx, D. C. Gajdusek, R. T. Yanagihara, D. Goldgaber, and C. J. Gibbs.** 1982. New haemorrhagic fever with renal syndrome-related virus in indigenous wild rodents in United States. *Lancet* **ii:**1405.
115. **Linthicum, K., F. G. Davies, A. Kairo, and C. L. Bailey.** 1985. Rift Valley fever virus (family Bunyaviridae, genus Phlebovirus). Isolations from Diptera collected during an inter-epizootic period in Kenya. *J. Hyg. Camb.* **95:**197–203.
116. **Lloyd, G., E. T. W. Bowen, N. Jones, and A. Pendry.** 1984. HFRS outbreak associated with laboratory rats in UK. *Lancet* **i:**1175–1176.
117. **Lopez, N., R. Muller, C. Prehaude, and M. Bouloy.** 1995. The L protein of Rift Valley fever virus can rescue viral ribonucleoproteins and transcribe genome-like RNA molecules. *J. Virol.* **69:**3972–3979.
118. **Lukes, K. J.** 1954. The pathology of thirty-nine fatal cases of epidemic hemorrhagic fever. *Am. J. Med.* **16:** 639–650.
119. **Mackow, E. R., M. H. Ginsberg, and I. N. Gavrilovskaya.** 1999. β_3 integrins mediate cellular entry of pathogenic hantaviruses, p. 113–123. *In* J. F. Saluzzo and B. Dodet (ed.), *Factors in the Emergence and Control of Rodent-Borne Viral Diseases*. Elsevier, New York, NY.
120. **Madani, T. A., Y. Y. Al-Mazrou, M. H. Al-Jeffri, A. Mishkhas, A. M. Al-Rabeah, A. M. Turkistani, M. O. Al-Sayed, A. A. Abodahish, A. S. Khan, T. G. Ksiazek, and O. Shobokshi.** 2004. Rift Valley fever epidemic in Saudi Arabia: epidemiological, clinical and laboratory characteristics. *Clin. Infect. Dis.* **37:**1084–1092.
121. **Marczinke, B. I., and S. T. Nichol.** 2002. Nairobi sheep disease virus, an important tick-borne pathogen of sheep and goats in Africa, is also present in Asia. *Virology* **303:** 146–151.
122. **Mardani, M., M. Keshtkar Jahromi, K. Holakouie Naieni, and M. Zeinali.** 2003. The efficacy of oral ribavirin in the treatment of Crimean-Congo hemorrhagic fever in Iran. *Clin. Infect. Dis.* **36:**1613–1618.
123. **Martinez, V. P., C. Bellomo, J. San Juan, D. Pinna, R. Forlenza, M. Elder, and P. Padula.** 2005. Person-to-person transmission of Andes virus. *Emerg. Infect. Dis.* **11:**1848–1853.
124. **McCormick, J. B., D. R. Sasso, E. L. Palmer, and M. P. Kiley.** 1981. Morphological identification of the agent of Korean hemorrhagic fever (Hantaan virus) as a member of the Bunyaviridae. *Lancet* **i:**765–768.
125. **Meadors, G. F., III, P. H. Gibbs, and C. J. Peters.** 1986. Evaluation of a new Rift Valley fever vaccine: safety and immunogenicity trials. *Vaccine* **4:**179–184.
126. **Meegan, J., and R. E. Shope.** 1981. Emerging concepts on Rift Valley fever. *Perspect. Virol.* **11:**267.
127. **Meegan, J. M.** 1979. The Rift Valley fever epizootic in Egypt 1977–78. 1. Description of the epizootic and virological studies. *Trans. R. Soc. Trop. Med. Hyg.* **73:** 618–623.
128. **Mertz, G. J., B. L. Hjelle, T. M. Williams, and F. T. Koster.** 1999. Host responses in the hantavirus cardiopulmonary syndrome, p. 133–137. *In* J. F. Saluzzo and B. Dodet (ed.), *Factors in the Emergence and Control of Rodent-Borne Viral Diseases*. Elsevier, New York, NY.
129. **Mertz, G. J., L. Miedzinski, D. Goade, A. T. Pavia, B. Hjelle, C. O. Hansbarger, H. Levy, F. T. Koster, K. Baum, A. Lindemulder, W. Wang, L. Riser, H. Fernandez, and R. J. Whitley for the Collaborative Antiviral Study Group.** 2004. Placebo-controlled, double-blind trial of intravenous ribavirin for hantavirus

cardiopulmonary syndrome in North America. *Clin. Infect. Dis.* **39:**1307–1313.

130. **Mertz, G. J., B. Hjelle, M. Crowley, G. Iwamoto, V. Tomicic, and P. Vial.** 2006. Diagnosis and treatment of New World hantavirus infections. *Curr. Opin. Infect. Dis.* **19:**437–442.
131. **Mills, J. N., T. L. Yates, J. E. Childs, R. R. Parmenter, T. G. Ksiazek, P. E. Rollis, and C. J. Peters.** 1995. Guidelines for working with rodents potentially infected with hantavirus. *J. Mammal.* **76:**716–722.
132. **Morrill, J. C., G. B. Jennings, T. Cosgriff, P. H. Gibbs, and C. J. Peters.** 1989. Prevention of Rift Valley fever in rhesus monkeys with interferon-alpha. *Rev. Infect. Dis* **11:**S815–S825.
133. **Morzunov, S. P., H. Feldmann, C. F. Spiropoulou, V. A. Semenova, P. E. Rollin, T. G. Ksiazek, C. J. Peters, and S. T. Nichol.** 1995. A newly recognized virus associated with a fatal case of hantavirus cardiopulmonary syndrome in Louisiana. *J. Virol.* **69:**1980–1983.
134. **Nakamura, T., R. Yanagihara, C. J. Gibbs, and D. C. Gajdusek.** 1985. Immune spleen cell-mediated protection against fatal Hantaan virus infection in infant mice. *J. Infect. Dis.* **151:**691–697.
135. **Needham, G. R.** 1985. Evaluation of five popular methods for tick removal. *Pediatrics* **75:**997–1002.
136. **Nerurkar, V. R., K. J. Song, D. C. Gajdusek, and R. Yanagihara.** 1993. Genetically distinct hantavirus in deer mice. *Lancet* **342:**1058–1059.
137. **Nerurkar, V. R., J. W. Song, K. J. Song, J. W. Nagle, B. Hjelle, S. Jenison, and R. Yanagihara.** 1994. Genetic evidence for a hantavirus enzootic in deer mice *(Peromyscus maniculatus)* a decade before the recognition of hantaviral pulmonary syndrome. *Virology* **204:**563–568.
138. **Nichol, S. T., C. F. Spiropoulou, S. Morzunov, P. E. Rollin, T. G. Ksiazek, H. Feldmann, A. Sanchez, J. Childs, S. Zaki, and C. J. Peters.** 1993. Genetic identification of a novel hantavirus associated with an outbreak of acute respiratory illness in the southwestern United States. *Science* **262:**914–917.
139. **Niklasson, B., M. Grandien, C. J. Peters, and T. P. Gargan II.** 1983. Detection of Rift Valley fever virus antigen by enzyme-linked immunoabsorbent assay. *J. Clin. Microbiol.* **17:**1026–1031.
140. **Niklasson, B., and J. W. LeDuc.** 1984. Isolation of the nephropathia epidemica agent in Sweden. *Lancet* **i:** 1012–1013.
141. **Niklasson, B., B. Hornfeldt, M. Mullaart, B. Settergren, E. Tkachenko, Y. A. Myasnikov, E. V. Ryltceva, E. Leschinskaya, A. Malkin, and T. Dzagurova.** 1993. An epidemiologic study of hemorrhagic fever with renal syndrome in Bashkirtostan (Russia) and Sweden. *Am. J. Trop. Med. Hyg.* **48:**670–675.
142. **Nolte, K. B., R. M. Fedderson, K. Foucar, S. R. Zaki, F. T. Koster, D. Madar, T. L. Merlin, P. J. McFeeley, E. T. Umland, and R. E. Zumwalt.** 1995. Hantavirus cardiopulmonary syndrome in the United States: a pathological description of a disease caused by a new agent. *Hum. Pathol.* **26:**110–120.
143. **Padula, P. J., A. Edelstein, S. D. Miguel, N. M. Lopez, C. M. Rossi, and R. D. Rabinovich.** 1998. Hantavirus pulmonary syndrome outbreak in Argentina: molecular evidence for person-to-person transmission of Andes virus. *Virology* **241:**323–330.
144. **Peters, C. J., J. A. Reynolds, T. W. Sloane, D. E. Jones, and E. L. Stephen.** 1986. Prophylaxis of Rift Valley fever with antiviral drugs, immune serum, an interferon inducer, and a macrophage activator. *Antiviral Res.* **6:**285–297.
145. **Ravkov, E. V., P. E. Rollin, T. G. Ksiazek, C. J. Peters, and S. T. Nichol.** 1995. Genetic and serologic analysis of Black Creek Canal virus and its association with human disease and *Sigmodon hispidus* infection. *Virology* **210:**482–489.
146. **Rollin, P. E., T. G. Ksiazek, L. H. Elliott, E. V. Ravkov, M. L. Martin, S. Morzunov, W. Livingstone, M. Monroe, G. Glass, S. Ruo, A. S. Khan, J. E. Childs, S. T. Nichol, and C. J. Peters.** 1995. Isolation of Black Creek Canal virus, a new hantavirus from *Sigmodon hispidus* in Florida. *J. Med. Virol.* **46:**35–39.
147. **Ruo, S. L., Y. L. Li, Z. Tong, Q. R. Ma, Z. L. Liu, Y. W. Tang, K. L. Ye, J. B. McCormick, S. P. Fisher-Hoch, and Z. Y. Xu.** 1994. Retrospective and prospective studies of hemorrhagic fever with renal syndrome in rural China. *J. Infect. Dis.* **170:**527–534.
148. **Sabin, A., C. B. Philip, and J. R. Paul.** 1944. Phlebotomus (pappataci or sandfly fever): a disease of military importance. Summary of existing knowledge and preliminary report of original investigations. *JAMA* **125:**603–606.
149. **Saggioro, F. P., M. A. Rossi, M. I. S. Duarte, C. C. S. Martin, V. A. F. Alves, M. L. Moreli, L. T. M. Figueiredo, J. E. Moreira, A. A. Borges, and L. Neder.** 2007. Hantavirus infection induces a typical myocarditis that may be responsible for myocardial depression and shock in hantavirus pulmonary syndrome. *J. Infect. Dis.* **195:**1541–1549.
150. **Sanchez, A. J., M. J. Vincent, and S. T. Nichol.** 2002. Characterization of the glycoproteins of Crimean-Congo hemorrhagic fever virus. *J. Virol.* **76:**7263–7275.
151. **Sanchez, A. J., M. J. Vincent, B. R. Erickson, and S. T. Nichol.** 2006. Crimean-Congo hemorrhagic fever virus glycoprotein precursor is cleaved by furin-like and SKI-1 proteases to generate a novel 38-kilodalton glycoprotein. *J. Virol.* **80:**514–525.
152. **Schmaljohn, A. L., D. Li, D. L. Negley, D. S. Bressler, M. J. Turell, G. W. Korch, M. S. Ascher, and C. S. Schmaljohn.** 1995. Isolation and initial characterization of a newfound hantavirus from California. *Virology* **206:** 963–972.
153. **Schmaljohn, C., Y. K. Chu, A. L. Schmaljohn, and J. M. Dalrymple.** 1990. Antigenic subunits of Hantaan virus expressed by baculovirus and vaccinia virus recombinants. *J. Virol.* **64:**3162–3170.
154. **Schmaljohn, C., S. E. Hasty, and J. M. Dalrymple.** 1992. Preparation of candidate vaccinia-vectored vaccine for haemorrhagic fever with renal syndrome. *Vaccine* **10:**10–13.
155. **Schmaljohn, C., K. Kamrud, and J. Hooper.** 1999. Recombinant DNA vaccines for hantaviruses, p. 163–173. *In* J. F. Saluzzo and B. Dodet (ed.), *Factors in the Emergence and Control of Rodent-Borne Viral Diseases*. Elsevier, New York, NY.
156. **Schmaljohn, C. S., and J. M. Dalrymple.** 1983. Analysis of Hantaan virus RNA: evidence for a new genus of Bunyaviridae. *Virology* **131:**482–491.
157. **Schmaljohn, C. S., S. E. Hasty, J. M. Dalrymple, J. W. LeDuc, H. W. Lee, C. H. von Bonsdorff, M. Brummer-Korvenkontio, A. Vaheri, T. F. Tsai, H. L. Regnery, D. Goldgaber, and P. W. Lee.** 1985. Antigenic and genetic properties of viruses linked to hemorrhagic fever with renal syndrome. *Science* **227:**1041–1044.
158. **Schmaljohn, C. S.** 1996. *Bunyaviridae:* the viruses and their replication, p. 1447. *In* B. N. Fields, D. M. Knipe, P. M. Howley, R. M. Chanock, J. L. Melnick, T. P. Monath, B. Roizman, and S. E. Straus (ed.), *Fields Virology*, 3rd ed., vol. 1. Lippincott-Raven, Philadelphia, PA.

159. **Settergren, B., P. Juto, B. Trollfors, G. Wadell, and S. R. Norrby.** 1989. Clinical characteristics of nephropathia epidemica in Sweden: prospective study of 74 cases. *Rev. Infect. Dis.* **11:**921–927.
160. **Settergren, B.** 1991. Nephropathia epidemica (hemorrhagic fever with renal syndrome) in Scandinavia. *Rev. Infect. Dis.* **13:**736–744.
161. **Sheedy, J. A., H. R. Froeb, H. A. Batson, C. C. Conley, J. P. Murphy, R. B. Hunter, D. W. Cugell, R. B. Giles, S. C. Bershadsky, J. W. Vester, and R. H. Yoe.** 1954. The clinical course of epidemic hemorrhagic fever. *Am. J. Med.* **16:**619–628.
162. **Shepherd, A. J., R. Swanepoel, S. P. Shepherd, P. A. Leman, N. K. Blackburn, and A. F. Hallett.** 1985. A nosocomial outbreak of Crimean-Congo hemorrhagic fever at Tygerberg Hospital. Part V. Virological and serological observations. *S. Afr. Med. J.* **68:**733–736.
163. **Shepherd, A. J., R. Swanepoel, P. A. Leman, and S. P. Shepherd.** 1986. Comparison of methods for isolation and titration of Crimean-Congo hemorrhagic fever virus. *J. Clin. Microbiol.* **24:**654–656.
164. **Shepherd, A. J., R. Swanepoel, and D. E. Gill.** 1988. Evaluation of enzyme-linked immunosorbent assay and reversed passive hemagglutination for detection of Crimean-Congo hemorrhagic fever virus. *J. Clin. Microbiol.* **26:**347–353.
165. **Shepherd, A. J., R. Swanepoel, and P. A. Leman.** 1989. Antibody response in Crimean-Congo hemorrhagic fever. *Rev. Infect. Dis.* **11:**S801–S806.
166. **Siam, A., J. M. Meegan, and K. F. Gharbawi.** 1980. Rift Valley fever ocular manifestations: observations during the 1977 epidemic in Egypt. *Br. J. Ophthalmol.* **64:** 366–374.
167. **Sidwell, R. W., J. H. Huffman, B. B. Barnett, and D. Y. Pfat.** 1988. In vitro and in vivo phlebovirus inhibition by ribavirin. *Antimicrob. Agents Chemother.* **32:** 331–336.
168. **Smithburn, K. C., A. F. Mahaffy, A. J. Haddow, S. F. Kitchen, and J. F. Smith.** 1949. Rift Valley fever. Accidental infections among laboratory workers. *J. Immunol.* **62:**213–227.
169. **Song, J. W., L. J. Baek, D. C. Gajdusek, R. Yanagihara, I. Gavrilovskaya, B. J. Luft, E. R. Mackow, and B. Hjelle.** 1994. Isolation of pathogenic hantavirus from white footed mouse *(Peromyscus leucopus)*. *Lancet* **344:** 1637.
170. **Song, W., N. Torrez-Martinez, W. Irwin, F. J. Harrison, R. Davis, M. Ascher, M. Jay, and B. Hjelle.** 1995. Isla Vista virus: a genetically novel hantavirus of the California vole *Microtus californicus*. *J. Gen. Virol.* **76:** 3195–3199.
171. **Spiropoulou, C. F., S. Morzunov, H. Feldmann, A. Sanchez, C. J. Peters, and S. T. Nichol.** 1994. Genome structure and variability of a virus causing hantavirus cardiopulmonary syndrome. *Virology* **200:**715–723.
172. **Swanepoel, R., A. J. Shepherd, P. A. Leman, S. P. Shepherd, G. M. McGillivray, M. J. Erasmus, L. A. Searle, and D. E. Gill.** 1987. Epidemiologic and clinical features of Crimean-Congo hemorrhagic fever in southern Africa. *Am. J. Trop. Med. Hyg.* **36:**120–132.
173. **Swanepoel, R., D. E. Gill, A. J. Shepherd, P. A. Leman, J. H. Mynhardt, and S. Harvey.** 1989. The clinical pathology of Crimean-Congo hemorrhagic fever. *Rev. Infect. Dis.* **11:**S794–S800.
174. **Terajima, M., J. D. Hendershoot, H. Kariwa, F. T. Koster, B. Hjelle, D. Goade, M. C. DeFronzo, and F. A. Ennis.** 1999. High levels of viremia in patients with the hantavirus pulmonary syndrome. *J. Infect. Dis.* **180:** 2030–2034.
175. **Tesh, R., B. N. Chaniotis, P. H. Peralta, and K. M. Johnson.** 1974. Ecology of viruses isolated from Panamanian sandflies. *Am. J. Trop. Med. Hyg.* **23:**258–269.
176. **Tesh, R. B., and B. N. Chaniotis.** 1975. Transovarial transmission of viruses by phlebotomine sandflies. *Ann. N. Y. Acad. Sci.* **266:**125–134.
177. **Thompson, W. H., B. Kalfayan, and R. O. Aslow.** 1965. Isolation of California encephalitis group virus from a fatal human illness. *Am. J. Epidemiol.* **81:**245–253.
178. **Tignor, G. H., and C. A. Hanham.** 1993. Ribavirin efficacy in an in vivo model of Crimean-Congo hemorrhagic fever virus (CCHF) infection. *Antiviral Res.* **22:** 309–325.
179. **Torrez-Martinez, N., and B. Hjelle.** 1995. Enzootic of Bayou hantavirus in rice rats *(Oryzomys palustris)* in 1983. *Lancet* **346:**780–781.
180. **Torrez-Martinez, N., W. Song, and B. Hjelle.** 1995. Nucleotide sequence analysis of the M genomic segment of El Moro Canyon hantavirus: antigenic distinction from Four Corners hantavirus. *Virology* **211:**336–338.
181. **Tsai, T. F.** 1987. Hemorrhagic fever with renal syndrome: clinical aspects. *Lab. Anim. Sci.* **37:**419–427.
182. **Tsai, T. F.** 1987. Hemorrhagic fever with renal syndrome: mode of transmission to humans. *Lab. Anim. Sci.* **37:**428–430.
183. **Van de Wal, B. W., J. R. Joubert, P. H.Van Eeden, and J. B. King.** 1985. A nosocomial outbreak of Crimean-Congo hemorrhagic fever at Tygerberg Hospital. Part IV. Preventive and prophylactic measures. *S. Afr. Med. J.* **68:**729–732.
184. **Vapalahti, O., J. Mustonen, Å. Lundkvist, H. Henttonen, A. Plyusnin, and A. Vaheri.** 2003. Hantavirus infections in Europe. *Lancet Infect. Dis.* **3:**653–661.
185. **Vassilenko, S. M., T. L. Vassilev, L. G. Bozadjiev, I. L. Bineva, and G. Z. Kazarov.** 1990. Specific intravenous immunoglobulin for Crimean-Congo haemorrhagic fever. *Lancet* **335:**791–792.
186. **Vial, P. A., F. Valdivieso, G. Mertz, C. Castillo, E. Belmar, I. Delgado, M. Tapia, and M. Ferrés.** 2006. Incubation period of hantavirus cardiopulmonary syndrome. *Emerg. Infect. Dis.* **12:**1271–1273.
187. **Vincent, M. J., E. Quiroz, F. Gracia, A. J. Sanchez, T. G. Ksiazek, P. T. Kitsutani, L. A. Ruedas, D. S. Tinnin, L. Caceres, A. Garcia, P. E. Rollin, J. N. Mills, C. J. Peters, and S. T. Nichol.** 2000. Hantavirus pulmonary syndrome in Panama: identification of novel hantaviruses and their likely reservoirs. *Virology* **277:**14–19.
188. **Watts, D. M., W. H. Thompson, T. M. Yuill, G. R. DeFoliart, and R. P. Hanson.** 1974. Overwintering of La Crosse virus in *Aedes triseriatus*. *Am. J. Trop. Med. Hyg.* **23:**694–700.
189. **Watts, D. M., T. G. Ksiazek, K. J. Linthicum, and H. Hoogstral.** 1988. Crimean-Congo hemorrhagic fever, p. 177–260. *In* T. P. Monath (ed.), *The Arboviruses: Epidemiology and Ecology*, vol. 2. CRC Press, Boca Raton, FL.
190. **Watts, D. M., M. A. Ussery, D. Nash, and C. J. Peters.** 1989. Inhibition of Crimean-Congo hemorrhagic fever viral infectivity yields in vitro by ribavirin. *Am. J. Trop. Med. Hyg.* **41:**581–585.
191. **Wells, R. M., S. Sosa Estani, Z. E. Yadon, D. Enria, P. Padula, N. Pini, J. N. Mills, C. J. Peters, and E. L. Segura for the Hantavirus Pulmonary Syndrome Study Group for Patagonia.** 1997. An unusual hantavirus outbreak in southern Argentina: person-to-person transmission? *Emerg. Infect. Dis.* **3:**171–174.

192. **Wilson, C., B. Hjelle, and S. Jenison.** 1994. A probable case of hantavirus cardiopulmonary syndrome that occurred in New Mexico in 1975. *Ann. Intern. Med.* **120:** 813–817.
193. **Woods, C. W., A. M. Karpati, T. Grein, N. McCarthy, P. Gaturuku, E. Muichiri, L. Dunster, A. Henderson, A. S. Khan, R. Swanepoel, I. Bonmarin, L. Martin, P. Mann, B. L. Smoak, M. Ryan, T. G. Ksiazek, R. R. Arthur, A. Ndikuyeze, N. N. Agata, C. J. Peters, and the World Health Organization Hemorrhagic Fever Task Force.** 2002. An outbreak of Rift Valley fever in northeastern Kenya, 1997–98. *Emerg. Infect. Dis.* **8:**138–144.
194. **Xiao, R., S. Yang, F. Koster, C. Ye, C. Stidley, and B. Hjelle.** 2006. Sin Nombre viral RNA in patients with hantavirus cardiopulmonary syndrome. *J. Infect. Dis.* **194:**1403–1409.
195. **Xiao, S. Y., J. W. LeDuc, Y. K. Chu, and C. S. Schmaljohn.** 1994. Phylogenetic analysis of virus isolates of the genus Hantavirus, family Bunyaviridae. *Virology* **198:** 205–217.
196. **Xu, Z. Y., C. S. Guo, Y. L. Wu, X. W. Zhang, and K. Liu.** 1985. Epidemiologic studies of hemorrhagic fever with renal syndrome. Analysis of risk factors and mode of transmission. *J. Infect. Dis.* **152:**137–144.
197. **Yanagihara, R., D. Goldgaber, P. W. Lee, H. L. Amyx, D. C. Gajdusek, C. J. Gibb, and A. Svedmyr.** 1984. Propagation of nephropathia epidemica virus in cell culture. *Lancet* **i:**1013.
198. **Yongxin, Y., Z. Zhiyong, S. Zhihui, and D. Guanmu.** 1999. Inactivated cell-culture hantavirus vaccine developed in China, p. 157–161. *In* J. F. Saluzzo and B. Dodet (ed.), *Factors in the Emergence and Control of Rodent-Borne Viral Diseases*. Elsevier, New York, NY.
199. **Zaki, S. R., P. W. Greer, L. M. Coffield, C. S. Goldsmith, K. B. Nolte, K. Foucar, R. M. Feddersen, R. E. Zumwalt, G. L. Miller, A. S. Khan, P. E. Rollin, K. G. Ksiazek, S. T. Nichols, B. W. J. Mahy, and C. J. Peters.** 1995. Hantavirus cardiopulmonary syndrome. Pathogenesis of an emerging infectious disease. *Am. J. Pathol.* **146:**552–579.
200. **Zeitz, P. S., J. C. Butler, J. E. Cheek, M. C. Samuel, J. E. Childs, L. A. Shands, R. E. Turner, R. E. Voorhees, J. Sarisky, P. E. Rollin, T. G. Ksiazek, L. Chapman, S. E. Reef, K. K. Komatsu, C. Dalton, J. W. Krebs, G. O. Maupin, K. Gage, C. M. Sewell, R. F. Breiman, and C. J. Peters.** 1995. A case-control study of hantavirus cardiopulmonary syndrome during an outbreak in the southwestern United States. *J. Infect. Dis.* **171:**864–870.

Arenaviruses

C. J. PETERS

44

Arenaviruses are negative-stranded RNA viruses that cause chronic infections of rodents and zoonotically acquired diseases in humans (Table 1). The prototype arenavirus is lymphocytic choriomeningitis virus (LCMV), which has the common house mouse as its host and was the first recognized cause of aseptic meningitis in humans (7, 129). This virus has continued to be a human pathogen from wild mice in the United States but has also had a major role in elucidating our concepts of viral immunopathology and of T-cell function through experiments with laboratory strains of virus and inbred mice (160). Other arenaviruses known from South America and Africa are common causes of the viral hemorrhagic fever (HF) syndrome in the areas in which they occur naturally (Table 2). The first of these was Argentine HF, first recognized by its characteristic clinical syndrome and caused by Junin virus. After the virus was isolated in 1958, the virus and the disease were extensively studied by the Argentine medical establishment; they form the basis for much of our knowledge of the pathogenesis of the South American HFs. All the arenaviruses are aerosol infectious and through that property have caused many laboratory infections and deaths. Therefore, they also pose significant bioterrorism or biowarfare threats.

VIROLOGY

Serotypic and Genotypic Variation

The family *Arenaviridae* was first proposed because of similarities in the electron microscopic appearance of the viruses, virion density and RNA composition, the common thread of having rodent hosts, and their serologic relationships. Arenaviruses fall into two serologic groups. LCMV, Lassa virus, and other African arenaviruses compose the Old World arenaviruses (Fig. 1), and the viruses from North and South America are referred to as the New World, American, or Tacaribe arenavirus serologic complex (Fig. 2). These distinctions also identify evolutionary relationships, since the Old World viruses are maintained in nature by chronic infections of Old World rodents *(Rodentia; Muridae; Murinae)*, whereas the New World serologic complex has been associated only with rodents native to the Americas *(Rodentia; Muridae; Sigmodontinae)*. The latter species were formerly referred to as cricetine rodents but now are more properly called sigmodontine rodents (23, 129).

Genetic analysis segregates arenaviruses into the same two groups as do serologic tests (18, 61). Old World viruses form one major grouping, and each virus is identifiable, with the virus species named on the basis of geography, reservoir host, and serology (Fig. 3) (71, 89). New World, or Tacaribe complex, viruses similarly form the same genetic species by phylogenetic analysis as identified by consideration of serology and host rodent species (Fig. 4) (18). Indeed, the different New World viruses form three subgroups which mirror serologic cross-reactivity based on fluorescent-antibody testing with polyclonal and monoclonal antibodies.

Arenavirus genetic sequences are relatively conserved within the family, but even the relatively similar nucleocapsid (N) and G2 proteins of different arenaviruses differ by at least 15 to 20% in their deduced amino acid sequences (61). Sequence variation can be extreme within a single virus species (57, 157). Monoclonal antibodies identify a conserved 5-amino-acid motif in G2 which reacts with many polyclonal antisera and a monoclonal antibody. The segmented genome has the potential for reassortment. Reassortment and, occasionally, recombination in distant times have been suggested as one cause of evolutionary diversity (61). Intratypic reassortants have been prepared, and their phenotypic analysis has yielded variable results. The only intertypic reassortant reported is between Lassa and Mopeia viruses and is attenuated for guinea pigs and nonhuman primates.

Composition

Arenavirus genomes comprise two ambisense RNA molecules. They are composed of an approximately 3.4-kb S segment and a 7.2-kb L segment (23). The S segment codes for the N protein in the negative, antimessage sense at the 3′ end and the glycoprotein precursor (GPC) in the positive, message sense at the 5′ end. The L segment codes for the L protein (a putative polymerase) in the negative sense at the 3′ end and the Z protein (putative zinc binding protein) in the positive sense at the 5′ end. The Z protein (11 kDa) interacts with L through its RING domain and may have a role in regulating translation (77). It is also important in budding through its myristolated form and may even form particles by itself when expressed

TABLE 1 Arenaviruses, their hosts, and their geographic distribution

Virus (abbreviation)	Host(s)	Geographic distribution
Old World arenaviruses		
Lymphocytic choriomeningitis virus (LCMV)	*Mus domesticus, Mus musculus*	Europe, Americas, Australia, ?Asia
Lassa virus (LASV)	*Mastomys natalensis*	West Africa, particularly Sierra Leone, Liberia, Guinea, and Nigeria
Mopeia virus (MOPV)	*Mastomys natalensis* s.l.	Mozambique
Mobala virus (MOBV)	*Praomys jacksoni*	Central African Republic
Ippy virus (IPPYV)	*Arvicanthis* spp.	Central African Republic
New World or Tacaribe complex arenaviruses		
Tacaribe virus (TCRV)	*Artibeus* bat?	Trinidad
Tamiami virus (TAMV)	*Sigmodon hispidus*	United States (Florida)
Whitewater Arroyo virus (WWAV)	*Neotoma* spp.	United States (western states)
Bear Canyon virus (BCNV)	*Peromyscus californicus*	United States (western states)
Guanarito virus (GUAV)	*Zygodontomys brevicauda*	Venezuela, Portuguesa State
Pirital virus (PIRV)	*Sigmodon alstoni*	Venezuela
Pichinde virus (PICV)	*Oryxomys albigularis*	Colombia
Amapari virus (AMAV)	*Oryzomys goeldi*	Brazil (Ampa Territory)
Cupixi virus (CPXV)	*Neacomys guianae*	Brazil
Flexal virus (FLEV)	*Oryzomys* spp.	Brazil (Para State)
Sabia virus (SABV)	Unknown	Brazil (São Paulo State)
Allpaahuayo virus (ALLV)	*Oecomys bicolor*	Peru
Parana virus (PARV)	*Oryzomys buccinatus*	Paraguay (Misiones Province)
Machupo virus (MACV)	*Calomys callosus*	Bolivia (Beni Department)
Latino virus (LATV)	*Calomys callosus*	Bolivia (Beni Department)
Chapare virus (CHAV)	Unknown	Bolivia (Cochabamba Department)
Junin virus (JUNV)	*Calomys musculinus*	Argentina (pampas)
Oliveros virus (OLVV)	*Bolomys obscurus*	Argentina (pampas)

in cells; it interacts directly with GPC for this function (25, 45, 152). The GPC polyprotein is posttranslationally cleaved by a specific cellular protease (92) to G1 (44-kDa) and G2 (35-kDa) glycoproteins which form the virion spike that interacts with viral receptors and neutralizing antibodies. α-Dystroglycan is a major receptor for LCMV and Lassa and clade C New World viruses, although some LCMV strains can enter without participation of α-dystroglycan (148). The pathogenic New World arenaviruses fall within clade B and utilize the transferrin receptor as a receptor. Cleavage occurs in the Golgi region and requires prior glycosylation of GPC. The N protein (65 kDa) is an internal RNA binding protein. Virions contain all five proteins (Fig. 5).

Virus particles are approximately 100 nm in diameter, with a range of 60 to 300 nm. In section they often contain granular particles that are host ribosomes, giving rise to the name "arena," meaning "sandy" (Fig. 5). The role of the host cell ribosomes which are encapsulated in budding virions is not known, although they are not obligatory for subsequent viral infectivity. The RNA is within the lipid envelope complexed to the N protein and is circularized via the terminal nucleotides, which are conserved throughout the family at the 3′ end and in complementary form at the 5′ end of each segment. The surface exhibits peplomers consisting of a tetrameric complex with a G2 stalk inserted into the membrane and a G1 globular head bound by ionic interactions. Virions are formed by budding from the cell surface. In productively infected cells, electron-dense material thought to be nucleocapsids accumulates below the plasma membrane in the region of viral buds.

Biology

Replication Strategy

After uncoating in the endosomal compartment of the cell, the S RNA segment is of template polarity for production of mRNA for translation to N protein, but the viral polymerase must transcribe the genomic RNA to permit message formation for GPC (Fig. 6). Similar considerations apply to the L RNA segment, which directly serves as the template for the production of L protein mRNA; L protein is also believed to be present in virions. The mRNAs contain small amounts of nontemplated bases and are capped, possibly through "cap-snatching" mechanisms such as are used by bunyaviruses. This may relate to the sensitivity of both *Bunyaviridae* and *Arenaviridae* to ribavirin. The regulation of viral genomic replication, mRNA metabolism, and protein synthesis is not understood. The intergenic regions contain relatively stable stem-loop structures, and translation termination codons are found on either side and within the stems, providing a mechanism for independent regulation of each gene. In chronically infected cells, mRNA levels fall markedly, as does glycoprotein expression, but abundant nucleocapsids persist in the cytoplasm (147).

Phenotypic Characteristics

Phenotypic variation among strains is considerable, but the genotypic or biological basis has never been investigated. Low-passage Junin strains vary greatly in their pathogenicity for guinea pigs, and there is some suggestion that they may mimic the two principal human syndromes (hemorrhagic or neurologic) in macaques (127). The pathogenic-

TABLE 2 Arenaviruses pathogenic for humans

Virus	Geography	Ecology	Disease	Clinical description
LCMV	Europe, the Americas, perhaps elsewhere	Rural areas, particularly in the fall, when rodents enter houses; urban areas with rodent infestation	LCM	Usually recognized as aseptic meningitis; more severe CNS disease uncommon. Febrile illness with thrombocytopenia and leukopenia but lacking neurologic involvement is probably common but rarely diagnosed. Fulminant Lassa fever-like disease is seen rarely but is particularly likely in the immunosuppressed.
Lassa virus	West Africa	Villages, farms, diamond mines where *Mastomys* is common	Lassa fever	Severe systemic illness, increased vascular permeability, shock; severe cases are often associated with bleeding and encephalopathy
Junin virus	Argentine pampas	Agricultural zones, particularly along fence lines	Argentine HF	Classical viral HF; similar to Lassa fever, except that thrombocytopenia, florid bleeding, and neurologic manifestations are much more common
Machupo	Beni region of Bolivia	Cleared lands, particularly when crops are planted; villages invaded by rodents	Bolivian HF	Similar to Argentine HF
Guanarito	Portuguesa State, Venezuela	Cleared small-hold agricultural settlements and villages	Venezuelan HF	Similar to Argentine HF
Sabia	São Paulo State, Brazil	Suburban areas of small town?		Probably similar to Argentine HF. One of three known cases involved prominent hepatic necrosis; one was treated early with ribavirin, with apparent success.
Chapare	Cochabamba, Bolivia	Rural area or small town?		Typical arenaviral HF; only one case known

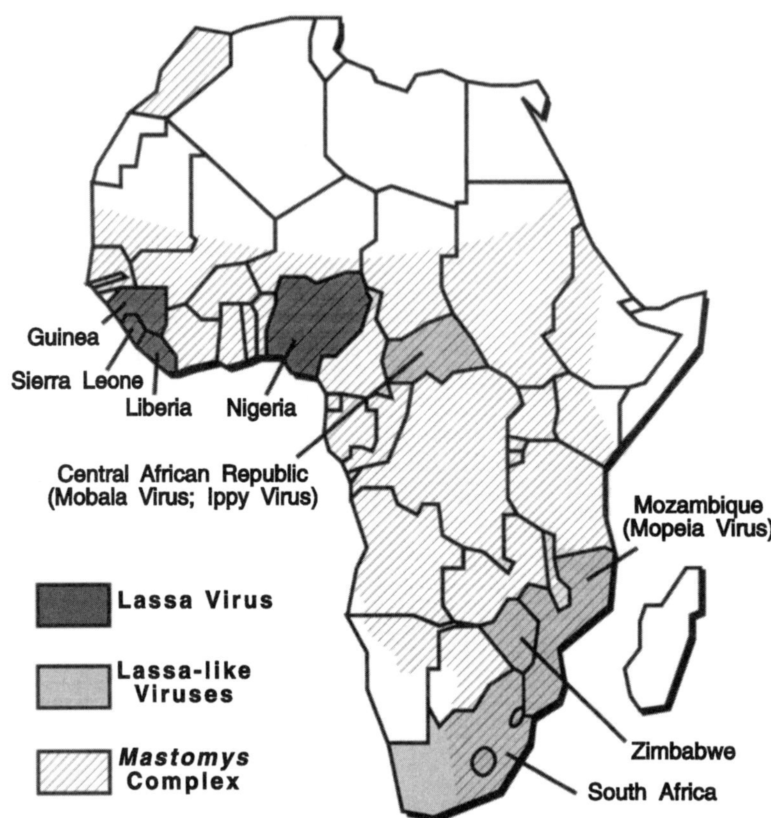

FIGURE 1 Old World arenaviruses and distribution of the genus *Mastomys* on the African continent. Lassa fever is a clinical problem in Sierra Leone, Liberia, Guinea, and Nigeria. Other arenaviruses are shown with their countries of isolation. It is not known if they are pathogenic for humans, but at least some are thought not to be so on the basis of reduced virulence for nonhuman primates. There are several other viruses from *Mastomys* and other species that have been isolated from antibody-positive rodent species in South Africa and are being characterized (R. Swanepoel, personal communication). LCMV has not been convincingly demonstrated on the African continent but may well exist in port cities and other areas where *M. musculus* has been introduced. (Prepared by A. Sanchez.)

ity of Lassa virus isolates for guinea pigs also parallels the severity of human disease in the patient. LCMV strains from hamster epidemics show less lethality and more chronic infection in experimental hamster infections than highly lethal laboratory strains such as WE or the extremely attenuated mouse neuroadapted strain ARM (60). As in many other arenavirus systems, the host genotype is critical in determining hamster susceptibility to a given LCMV strain. Arenaviruses have also been adapted to increase their virulence for selected experimental hosts by passage (127). The best-studied example of adaptation by arenaviruses is the work with variants of LCMV that can be isolated from different organs of neonatally infected mice. Macrophage-tropic viruses are capable of suppressing the cytotoxic T-lymphocyte response and result in chronic viremic infections of adult laboratory mice (2). Viruses isolated from the brains of mice infected with the same parental virus pool differ in one amino acid in the L and one in the G protein and give rise to the expected immunizing infections.

Host Range

Arenaviruses grow well in most mammalian cell lines, including endothelial cells, and infect most mammals (6, 90, 129). Generally, the interaction between arenaviruses and cells produces little or no cytopathic effect. Occasional combinations, particularly Vero cells, which are often used in diagnosis and assay of arenaviruses, produce rounding and detachment of affected cells and subsequent cell death. Carrier cultures are readily established with cyclic production of infectious virus. Infected cells from these cultures may contain large quantities of N protein but minimal GPC. There is evidence for the presence of defective interfering particles in cell cultures and some animal systems, but they have not been shown to have a major role in animal infections, with occasional exceptions (130, 148, 158).

Inactivation

Like most lipid-enveloped viruses, arenaviruses quickly lose infectivity after treatment with detergents or common disinfectants. They are also inactivated by low or high pH. Stability may be surprisingly high in protein-containing solutions around neutral pH. Heating for 60 min at 56 to 60°C reduces infectivity. Inactivation in serum while preserving other protein activity (viral antigen, antibody, or serum enzymes) can be achieved in several ways, including

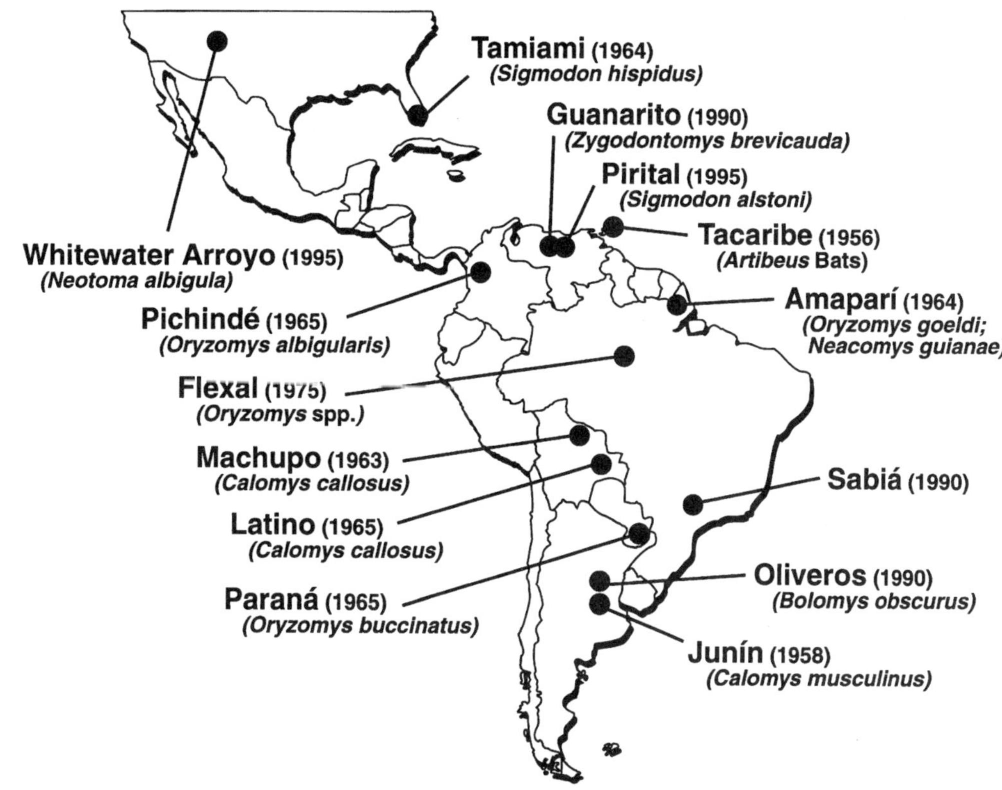

FIGURE 2 New World arenaviruses in the Americas. Circles denote the places of isolation and the approximate areas of known distribution. (Prepared by A. Sanchez.)

irradiation with a high-intensity ^{60}Co source in the frozen state (109).

EPIDEMIOLOGY

The distribution of an arenavirus is determined by the range of its host rodent and the pattern of infection within the rodent reservoir. Each arenavirus is associated with a single reservoir rodent (Table 1) (28), with the apparent exception of Tacaribe virus, known only from *Artibeus* bats in Trinidad. Guanarito virus was thought to have dual rodent reservoirs in Venezuela, but subsequent studies showed two different viral species (56). The rodent species specificity of arenaviruses is demonstrated by studies in agricultural areas of the Argentine pampas. Junin virus (the causative agent of Argentine HF) has *Calomys musculinus* as its reservoir. In contrast, infection is uncommon and chronic infection unknown in any of the seven other rodent species living in the same fields, with the possible exception of the related *Calomys laucha* (106, 107, 134, 135). At least two other arenavirus species circulate simultaneously with their specific reservoirs, Oliveros virus from *Bolomys obscurus*, a native South American rodent, and LCMV, brought to the New World with the introduction of its natural reservoir, *Mus musculus* (4).

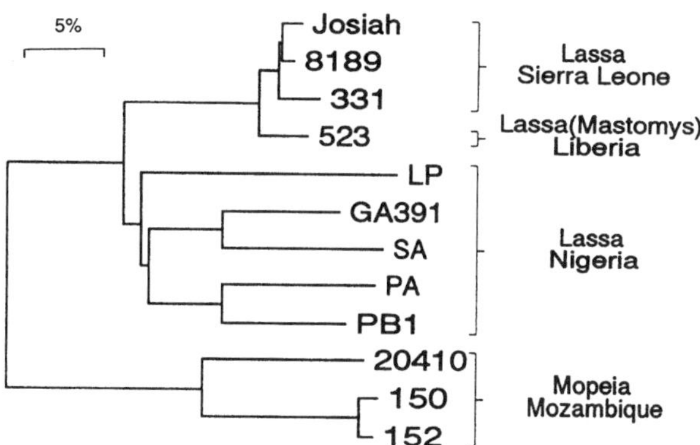

FIGURE 3 Phylogenetic relationships of the Old World arenaviruses. The tree is based on nucleotide sequences from the conserved region of the S RNA segment. Note that the geographically distant Lassa virus strains from Nigeria differ from those in Sierra Leone and Liberia. 20410 is the prototype Mopeia virus strain from Mozambique. (Prepared by J. C. S. Clegg.)

Chronic infection of the reservoir rodent species serves to maintain the continuity of virus transmission in nature, and humans are only incidental hosts. For some viruses, such as LCMV and Lassa virus, there is a tightly linked vertical mechanism of transmission. Chronic viremic infection in the mother leads to congenital infection and chronic viremia in the offspring. For other virus-host combinations there is a pattern of chronic viremia and/or chronic virus shedding which may occur even if infection is not neonatal but which nevertheless leads to virus perpetuation (28, 106).

Each reservoir host has its own ecology and habitat preferences; fluctuations of rodent populations and dynamics of virus circulation determine where the zones of risk occur.

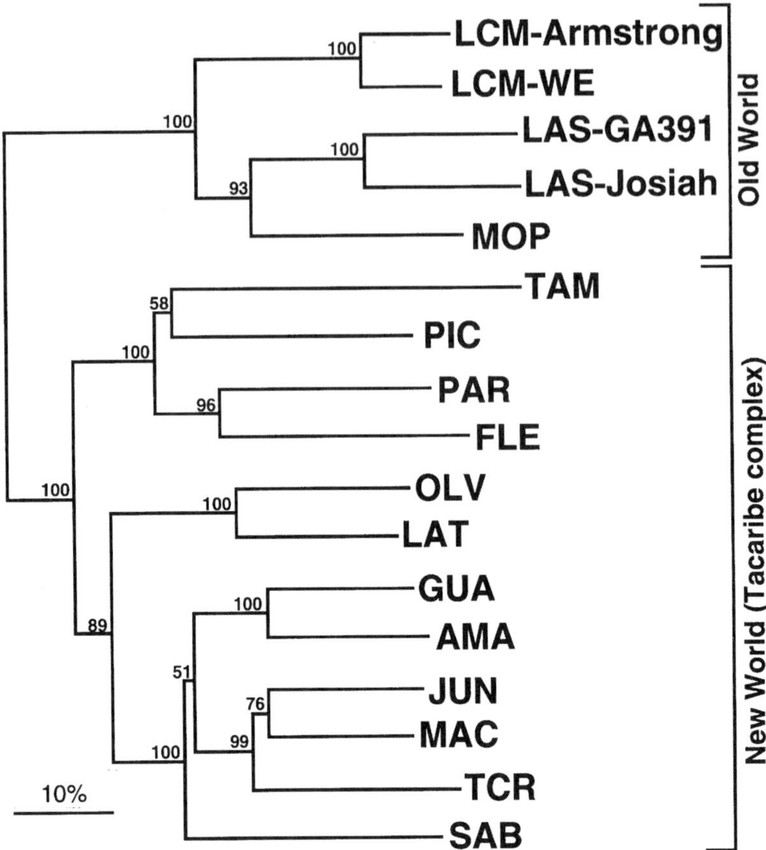

FIGURE 4 Phylogenetic relationships of the New World, or Tacaribe complex, arenaviruses and their relation to the Old World viruses. The tree is based on the nucleotide 613 to 649 region of the N protein gene constructed by the method of Fitch and Margoliash. Branch lengths are proportional to distance, with twofold weighting of transversions. The scale bar indicates 10% difference, and numbers indicate the percentage of 1,000 bootstrap replicates supporting interior nodes. See Table 1 for abbreviations. (Prepared by M. Bowen and S. Nichol.)

Transmission to Humans

The exact mechanisms of human infection are unknown. Arenaviruses are infectious via small-particle aerosols, and this route has been clearly implicated in human infections in the field and in the laboratory (10, 28, 34, 81, 150). Contamination of mucous membranes, contact with broken skin, and ingestion may be alternate routes of infection. Although plausible, there is no direct evidence for these possibilities. Intimate spousal contact has been associated with conjugal transmission of Lassa, Junin, and Machupo viruses (21, 43). Nosocomial spread of the HF viruses has occurred on occasion.

As with any viremic infection, transfusion or transplantation of organs could infect recipients. The reports of 13 infections derived from four donors between 2003 and early 2008 have emphasized that viremia and/or residual virus in internal organs may be much more common than previously suspected. The immunosuppressed recipients would be much more likely to be identified because of the severe disease that results than infected transfusion recipients who might only have febrile illness or aseptic meningitis (27a, 120, 125). One donor was suspected to have been infected by a pet hamster, and this was subsequently proven by tracing the virus back to a facility selling hamsters to pet stores and showing the identity by sequence analysis (5). Two donors had died from cerebral hemorrhages and one had died in a motorcycle accident. It is not completely certain whether they were symptomatic with LCMV infection at the time of death or whether the virus was transmitted by blood or actual infection of the transplanted organs.

Laboratory infections with arenaviruses have been quite common, and several have been fatal. Transmission may be associated with infected laboratory animals, virus propagation, or necropsy. Infections may occur without any overt incident, suggesting aerosol transmission, or may follow an obvious accident such as a cut or spill (10, 24, 90, 129, 143).

Lymphocytic Choriomeningitis Virus

LCMV is found wherever either of the two closely related species of the common house mouse (*Mus musculus* and *Mus domesticus*) are known to occur and possibly elsewhere as well. This geographic distribution includes Europe, the Americas, Australia, and Japan (4, 15, 90, 123).

The prevalence of infection in mouse populations is highly variable, and the factors underlying these geographic differences are unknown. In addition, infection in

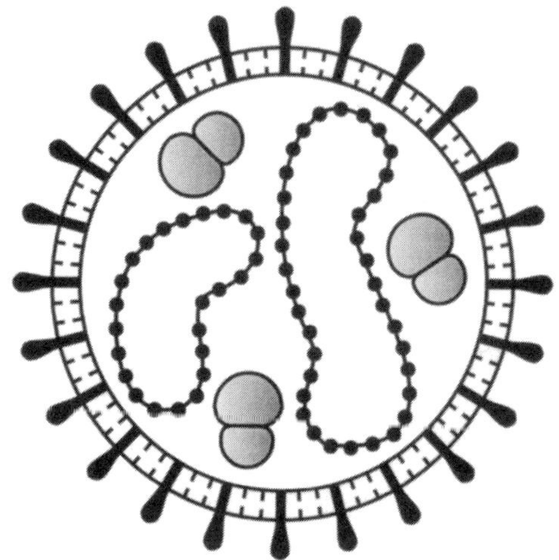

FIGURE 5 Diagram of an arenavirus virion. The typical diameter is around 100 nm, and the shape is pleomorphic but basically spherical. The envelope is composed of tetrameric complexes of G2 anchored in the lipid bilayer and attached to G1 by ionic forces; they are visible as peplomers. N proteins are thought to be circularized. The L protein and Z protein are both associated with virions, but their localization is unknown. (Prepared by A. Sanchez.)

a given area may be focal over distances of a few meters, reflecting the population structure and home range of *Mus* (28, 90, 139). Human infection with LCMV often occurs in rural areas, although considerable numbers of infected mice have been detected in urban environments. Human infection has been shown to be more common in areas of high infection prevalence in *Mus* species. Antibody studies in the United States and elsewhere usually find a prevalence of previous LCMV exposure of 1 to 9% in humans, although some samples are virtually nil (4, 29). In the greater metropolitan area of Birmingham, AL, no LCMV seropositivity has been found in persons under 30 years of age, although about 5% of persons in older age groups were positive (122). It is not known if these cross-sectional results represent a lesser risk in younger age groups compared to older persons or a decrease in recent years in the prevalence of murine infection, infectivity of mice, or human contact with mice.

Surprisingly few systematic data exist on the contribution of LCMV to human disease because of the infrequent application of specific diagnostic tests. LCMV was responsible for 8 to 11% of cases of febrile central nervous system (CNS) disease in studies carried out between 1941 and 1958 on patients principally drawn from a military referral hospital in Washington, DC (1, 105, 121). Occasional infections have also been detected from testing of sera submitted for atypical pneumonia serology. Human LCMV infections have autumn-winter predominance, involve all age groups, and generally occur sporadically. Antibodies have been found in 2 to 10% of several human populations, including those in Washington, DC; Baltimore, MD; Birmingham, AL (122); and some rural areas of Argentina and Germany (4).

Hamster colonies may also become infected with LCMV and provide the exception to the rule that infection of noncarrier rodents is not a major factor in transmission of arenaviruses (37, 62, 132). Crowding and viruria are major risk factors at work in colonies. Hamster-based epidemics have occurred in laboratory workers and pet owners, leading to hundreds of cases in Germany and the United States. Infections in hamster colonies and hamster-related human cases continue to be reported occasionally (5, 51, 87, 114, 131).

Most human infections are undoubtedly the result of exposure to naturally infected wild mice, but the possibility of infection from laboratory mice exists as well. Better-quality commercial laboratory mouse colonies are protected against entry of wild mice and are routinely tested for LCMV contamination, but occasional infections continue to occur in spite of precautions and monitoring (145). The prolonged excretion of LCMV by athymic mice infected as adults can lead to an increased risk from these

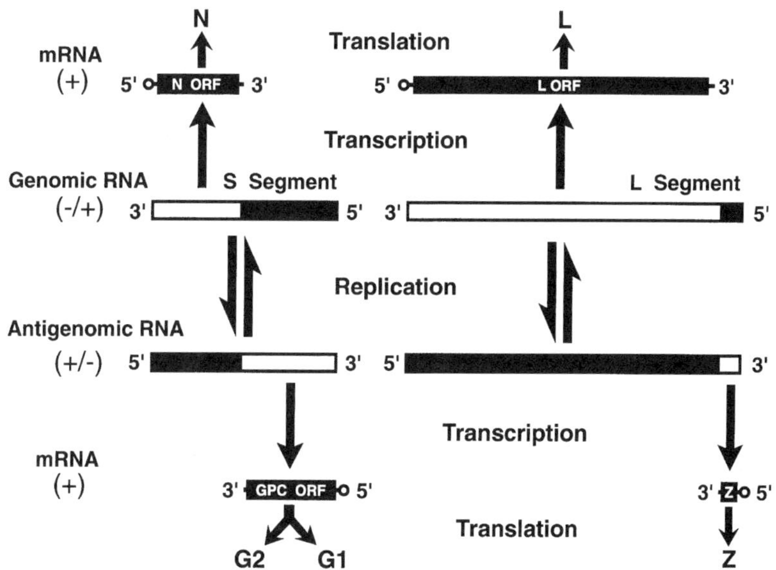

FIGURE 6 Replication strategy. See text for details. (Prepared by A. Sanchez.)

rodents if persons are exposed to virus in production or by use of contaminated materials in experiments (44). Procuring rodents from unmonitored and, particularly, unprotected breeding sources may result in virus contamination. The increasing use of rodents as pets and as food for pet reptiles in the United States makes further epidemics likely, since most of these colonies are not monitored.

Lassa Virus

In 1969, a severe systemic disease was transmitted from a nurse infected in the town of Lassa, Nigeria, to a nurse caring for her in Jos, Nigeria, and finally to a third nurse who was evacuated to the United States and who was the only survivor (54). Lassa virus was isolated from these patients with Lassa fever (24) and from the virologist after he was infected in the laboratory. Since the initial discovery of the virus, several nosocomial infections have been discovered and numerous exported cases have been documented.

Longitudinal field studies demonstrate that Lassa fever is an endemic disease in west Africa and is quite common (55, 104, 111). Indeed, it is thought that Lassa virus infects tens to hundreds of thousands of humans annually and causes hundreds to thousands of deaths. Unfortunately, there are insufficient surveillance data to provide precise estimates, and it is not possible to map the exact geographic range of Lassa virus. Disease is known primarily from Sierra Leone, Liberia, and Guinea and from the noncontiguous country of Nigeria (Fig. 1).

Lassa virus was first isolated in Sierra Leone from rodents of the genus *Mastomys natalensis*. *Mastomys* is a complex genus, and it now appears that the major reservoir is indeed *M. natalensis* as molecularly identified (50, 88, 105). These rodents are prolific and numerous in savannas and altered forests of west, central, and eastern Africa; in Sierra Leone, up to 14% of *Mastomys* rodents are infected in some villages (104). Human infection presumably occurs within houses, as the rodents live in close contact with humans and in peridomestic settings, particularly when these rodents are sought for food. Infection and disease are common in all age groups and both sexes, and there are more cases in the January-May dry season (104, 110, 111, 139). This may be related to the greater aerosol stability of the virus in lower relative humidity, the increase in *Mastomys* populations that follows the rainy season, or the habits of the infected rodents in the dry season (51, 151). With the war setting in Sierra Leone, there have been epidemics of Lassa fever related to the many conditions that accompany strife (16).

Person-to-person transmission of Lassa virus is believed to be common in the village setting, and small household epidemics have been observed (76). Nosocomial transmission occurs. One particularly dramatic episode in Nigeria, attributed to aerosols generated by a critically ill patient with prominent cough, resulted in 16 secondary cases with 12 deaths (26). Generally, however, there is minimal risk in the African hospital setting based on Sierra Leone studies (64).

Junin Virus

Junin virus occurs in a defined area of the Argentine pampas, where it was discovered in 1958 (Fig. 3). The very characteristic clinical disease of Argentine HF has allowed surveillance with addition of laboratory confirmation over the last two decades. Most remarkably, the area of endemicity has expanded from a zone of 16,000 km^2 centered around the town of Junin to subsume 120,000 km^2 containing more than a million inhabitants. Areas that have historically been active have experienced a decrease in incidence. This widening of the disease zone is not associated with obvious differences in agricultural practices, and the rodent reservoir has existed throughout the area for decades. Rodent infection rates measured in 1988 to 1989 paralleled the observed incidence of human disease in different geographic areas, suggesting that the underlying process involves a change in rodent-virus relationships leading to increased human exposure, but the nature of this change is unknown (107).

Over the years, the number of Argentine HF cases has varied from hundreds to a few thousand annually. Recently, vaccination of high-risk target populations has resulted in a marked decrease in human disease cases to fewer than 100/year, although the infected rodent vectors are still found in abundance. The most heavily affected group is adult men who work in agricultural occupations. Most human infections occur in the autumn, when rodents are most numerous, their infection rates are highest, and harvest activities take place. *C. musculinus* rodents have a predilection for linear habitats such as fence lines, making those areas particularly dangerous (106). Interestingly, in former years workers who harvested corn often slept in the fields and were severely impacted, but mechanization has not eliminated the disease. Drivers of machinery are infected by aerosols, sometimes from rodents that are macerated by mechanical harvesters.

Machupo Virus

Between 1959 and 1962, scattered cases of an unknown disease described as "black typhus" were reported from a remote area of Bolivia, the Beni Department (Fig. 3). Then epidemics in small towns began and led to the isolation of a virus named for the nearby Machupo River, which drains into the Amazon system. Machupo virus causes a chronic infection of a rodent that thrives in cleared areas, particularly planted fields, in the jungles of the Beni and causes sporadic infections of humans, mainly adult men. The rodent sometimes invades houses within small towns and causes epidemics with infection of men, women, and children. The best known such epidemic involved San Joaquin, Bolivia, with a population of about 3,000. Before the disease was controlled by trapping the numerous *Calomys callosus* rodents living in houses in the town, 637 cases with 113 deaths had occurred over a 2-year period (73). Since then, trapping teams led by immune Bolivian HF survivors have kept the towns free of rodents, and few cases have been reported. In 1971, a dramatic nosocomial outbreak occurred (124), and again in 1994, three sporadic cases were noted, with one of these leading to dissemination of fatal infection to six family members.

Guanarito Virus

In 1989, HF cases in the municipality of Guanarito and the state of Portuguesa in Venezuela were noted (Fig. 3). Virus isolation in mammalian cells and suckling mice revealed an arenavirus named Guanarito virus (137). Rodent trapping studies revealed extensive arenavirus infection in two common grassland rodent species, *Sigmodon alstoni* and *Zygodontomys brevicauda*. *S. alstoni* rodents had a high rate of virus isolation with low antibody prevalence, suggesting the type of chronic, viremic infection often seen with arenaviruses, and that species was proposed as the reservoir. It was subsequently found that the presumptive identifications of the virus and antibodies on the basis of fluorescent-antibody tests were mistaken and that there were actually two species of arenavirus present: Guanarito virus, which causes a chronic viremic infection of *Z. brevicauda*, and another distinct virus (Pirital virus is the proposed name) present in *S. alstoni* (157). The human epidemiology, pathogenicity, and geographic ranges of the two viruses are currently under study. The prototype Guanarito virus was isolated from a person with HF.

From 1989 to 1991, there were 104 cases of Venezuelan HF with 26 deaths. Subsequently there have been only a handful of cases. The emergence of the disease is thought to be related to the clearing of forested areas for small farms and ranches, with incursions of savanna rodent species into the fields and near houses. The details of exposure are unknown, but both sexes and all ages are affected, with the highest rates in adult males (137).

Sabia Virus

Sabia virus was isolated from a young woman dying in 1990 in São Paulo, Brazil, after she visited a nearby small town (Fig. 3). The virus was not identified as an arenavirus until 1992, when the laboratory technician working with the virus developed a moderate case of viral HF. During the further characterization of the virus, another laboratory infection occurred in the United States and was apparently aborted by ribavirin treatment (10). The reservoir and epidemiology of Sabia virus are unknown.

Chapare Virus

Little is known about Chapare virus except that the only known patient acquired it in a rural area near Cochabamba, Bolivia, outside the zone of endemicity for Machupo virus (38). The typical HF was fatal. It seems to be phylogenetically most closely related to Sabia virus.

PATHOGENESIS

Arenaviruses enter the human body through either inhalation or other routes and, based on animal model studies and human necropsy material, are presumed to replicate in the draining thoracic lymph node before producing a viremia (34, 81, 150). This viremia results in widespread infection, initially prominently involving macrophages but also spreading to other cell types throughout the body, particularly in the later stages. The duration of viremia is around 7 to 12 days in South American HFs but may be up to 3 weeks in Lassa fever; this long duration is important in giving an adequate window for chemotherapy or passive antibody to succeed.

Involvement of the CNS varies among arenavirus infections. In LCMV and Lassa virus infections, isolation has been made from cerebrospinal fluid (CSF) and/or brain in some cases with neurologic involvement. Neurologic manifestations are very common in Argentine and Bolivian HFs. The ready neuroinvasiveness of Junin and Machupo viruses in nonhuman primates and the serologic findings in the late neurologic syndrome seen in human Junin virus infections treated with passive antibodies suggest that Junin and Machupo viruses gain access to the human CNS in spite of the fact that no isolations have been made from the brain or CSF.

A recurring question with the arenaviral HFs is how the virus causes disease. The histologic lesions observed do not usually provide an obvious cause of death. Findings at necropsy are often composed of petechial and mucosal hemorrhages, vascular dilatation and congestion, and small foci of necrosis in organs such as the liver, adrenals, and kidneys, with a mild or absent inflammatory response (155). In the case of LCMV aseptic meningitis, the disease is likely to be due to the cellular immune response against the virus (see below); however, the HFs appear to have different modes of pathogenesis (123, 127).

Patients with HF present with fever and myalgia and later develop increased vascular permeability, hypotension, and shock. It is believed that the extensive macrophage and lymphoreticular infection is the basis for local and systemic release of physiologically active soluble mediators leading to many of the abnormalities observed (123). Tumor necrosis factor alpha and alpha/beta interferon are among the candidates for such mediators; both are present in sera from Argentine HF patients in high concentrations, and their levels correlate with mortality (63, 94). In animal models, leukotrienes, platelet-activating factor, and endorphins appear to contribute (127). Whether the infection per se results in mediator release or whether the immune response also participates is unknown; however, immunosuppression exacerbates rather than ameliorates the effects of Junin virus infection in the guinea pig model of HF (80). Immune complexes, disseminated intravascular coagulation, and complement activation by other means appear to have no important role in arenaviral HF (35, 127, 155).

Arenaviruses may exert cytopathic effects, but it is also common to observe large areas of immunohistochemical evidence of infection in a tissue with little overt necrosis (127). Thus, another candidate mechanism for arenavirus-induced disease is through functional effects of the viruses that are not associated with overt evidence of cellular damage. There are now several examples of chronic infections of laboratory rodents in which arenaviruses affect critical enzyme or hormone synthesis without morphological lesions being apparent (84, 118).

Fetal infection is also common after arenavirus exposure. The natural reservoir often transmits the virus to the fetus in utero (29), and in the clinical setting, all the human-pathogenic arenaviruses probably invade and damage the fetus with significant frequency.

Lymphocytic Choriomeningitis Virus

Human Disease Pathogenesis

The early phases of LCM are characterized by symptoms resembling the early stages of arenaviral HF, and in rare cases human LCMV infection has pursued a course similar to the one of arenaviral HF (143). Nonhuman primates infected with LCMV often have all the clinical manifestations of HF (34, 98, 112, 127, 143). In contrast, in humans the early febrile illness is relatively mild, although during this phase the virus may enter the CNS, leading to the later development of immunopathological meningitis. The role of the immune response is inferred from the sequence of CNS disease following the resolution of a bout of systemic viremia (49), the limited observations on immunosuppressed patients who do not develop CNS disease even in the presence of virus in the CNS (67), and the resemblance of human disease to the murine model.

Infection of the Mouse and Other Rodents with LCMV

The infection of laboratory mice with LCMV has provided an important model for many viral and immunologic phenomena (116, 117). Infection of the murine fetus in utero or of newborn mice leads to a persistent carrier state that is the basis for efficient intergenerational transfer of virus in nature. This prolonged carrier state is associated with the presence of immunosuppressive variants of LCMV in spleen as well as thymic epithelial cell infection.

Adult mice infected by a non-CNS route will develop an immune response and clear their viremia unless they are immunosuppressed, in which case they develop prolonged viremia similar to that found after newborn infection (132). Adult mice infected intracranially with LCMV provide the prototypic model for acute immunopathological encephalitis and also probably have a course similar to that of humans who develop aseptic meningitis after LCMV infection. After intracranial injection of laboratory mice, extensive virus growth follows, initially in the meninges, but no disease occurs unless an effective immune response occurs (132). Immune cells enter the meninges and result in an inflammatory state leading to convulsions and death; cytokine genes are activated in inflammatory cells but necrosis of host tissues is absent, emphasizing the functional changes induced which lead to abnormal brain physiology and barrier function. If terminal seizures are prevented by drugs, life is prolonged and ultrastructural degenerative changes in the choroid plexus become evident before death. The critical cells mediating the immunopathological encephalitis have been shown to be $CD8^+$ T lymphocytes. As few as 100 to 1,000 cloned LCMV-specific cells can mediate the response if injected directly into the infected nervous system (147).

In addition to mediating immunopathology in the intracranially infected mouse, the $CD8^+$ T-cell response is largely responsible for recovery. A similar dominant role of cellular immunity in humans is inferred from the late and inefficient virus-neutralizing antibody response in humans as well as mice (1, 7, 91). Passive transfer of virus-specific $CD8^+$ T cells can also clear the extensive infection found throughout the tissues of neonatally infected murine carriers. These immune cells result in the disappearance of virus from infected neurons. Although $CD8^+$ lymphocytes are potentially cytolytic, there is no necrosis of neurons because the lack of major histocompatibility complex (MHC) class I antigen expression on these cells precludes the necessary lethal interaction (75). Presumably cytokines can result in cellular "cure" from viral infection, as suggested for other viruses (153).

Another aspect of murine LCMV infection relates to the humoral arm of the immune system. Frank Dixon found immune complex glomerulonephritis in chronic LCMV carrier mice and established the presence of viral immune complexes in the basement membranes of the affected mice. Laboratory strains of mice neonatally infected with LCMV develop a chronic immune complex disease which is genetically specified by the MHC haplotype of the mouse, which determines the level of antibodies produced. The finding of a humoral immune response in chronically viremic, neonatally infected carriers demonstrates that this state is not one of true tolerance. Indeed, LCMV-specific cytolytic T-cell precursors also exist in these mice and can be activated if LCMV is eradicated.

The chronic immune complex disease seen in this model, based on selected laboratory strains of virus and inbred mice, has minimal relevance to the natural situation, in which there is little effect of the virus on the mouse's biological economy. In some circumstances, mouse colonies may undergo a transient decrease of fertility shortly after LCMV is introduced, suggesting the possibility of mutual genetic adaptation (119).

LCMV in animal models has a predilection for the ependyma (123), and this plus the inflammatory response may be reflected in the occasional case of acquired hydrocephalus seen in human infections. Several other models of ocular disease, cerebellar degeneration, behavorial change, and endocrinopathy have also been developed in mice and rats, but these are beyond the scope of this discussion (23).

Lassa Virus

The severe systemic impact of Lassa fever is accompanied by dysfunction in several organ systems, probably due to the combined effects of activation of soluble mediators and direct infection. Lassa virus-infected rhesus monkeys show extensive macrophage involvement, with limited infection of what appear to be endothelial cells, as determined by fluorescence microscopy (127). More or less extensive infection occurs in foci in several organs, but there is relatively little necrosis. The cytokines are thought to come from direct cellular infection, but the data on the cellular effects of Lassa virus are contradictory (9, 41, 101). There is activation of some inflammatory cytokines in patients, but this deserves further study (100).

Abnormal platelet aggregation in response to collagen or adenosine diphosphate occurs in Lassa fever (32, 52). Decreased platelet function is most marked in cases with hemorrhagic manifestations, suggesting that the functional defect may be responsible for the bleeding. There is no evidence for disseminated intravascular coagulation. Plasma from acute Lassa fever patients will induce a defect in aggregation, and this plasma also contains a substance(s) which inhibits the respiratory burst of neutrophils following f-Met-Leu-Phe.

Recovery from Lassa fever proceeds via cellular immunity. This is suggested in humans by the late appearance of protective or neutralizing antibodies in a pattern similar to that seen in LCMV infection (55). In strain 13 guinea pigs, spleen cell transfers establish the ability to adoptively immunize with immune lymphoid cells but not plasma at the time of recovery (127).

Viruses Causing South American HFs

The major differences between the pathogenesis of Lassa fever and that of the South American HFs are quantitative rather than qualitative. The two most notable are the frequent presence of neurologic involvement and bleeding in the South American diseases. Neurologic signs were found in virtually all of 120 Argentine HF cases but in only 40% of Lassa fever patients (103). This probably reflects the increased neuroinvasiveness of Junin virus in experimental animals and presumably humans as well.

Argentine HF patients have very high levels of alpha interferon, as well as elevated concentrations of tumor necrosis factor alpha; both are highest in the sickest patients (63, 93). Indeed, the serum interferon concentrations are among the highest measured and probably also contribute to the pathogenesis of the disease. Infusion of potent virus-neutralizing antibodies results in a prompt disappearance of viremia, improvement in clinical status, and also clearing of serum interferon. Among the toxic effects of interferon which may be reflected in Argentine HF patients are fever, chills, myalgia, backache, thrombocytopenia, leukopenia, and, later, hair loss.

Bleeding is much more common in Argentine HF and the other South American HFs than in Lassa fever. The coagulation defect has been studied in detail, and no definite conclusion has been reached; there are only modest abnormalities. Presumably hemorrhage is a reflection of vascular damage common to both Lassa and Junin virus infections and the low platelet counts routinely seen in Junin virus infection. In addition, Argentine HF patients have a plasma inhibitor of platelet aggregation that differs from that of Lassa fever in being heat stable. Examination of bone marrow from Junin virus patients shows globally decreased cellularity and maturation arrest of both megakaryocytes and erythroblasts, and platelet survival is commonly normal. There is no evidence of widespread complement activation or disseminated intravascular coagulation (35). However, these patients also are immunosuppressed as measured by a decrease in mitogen stimulation of peripheral blood lymphocytes and a decrease in circulating lymphocytes, particularly $CD4^+$ lymphocytes.

Clinical recovery in Junin virus-infected humans typically begins around days 10 to 12 of illness and corresponds to the appearance of antibodies (35). Similar findings are described for the guinea pig model, in which antibodies are highly effective in passive transfer and in which antibody-dependent cellular cytotoxicity is important in eradicating infected cells to bring about recovery (79, 127).

CLINICAL MANIFESTATIONS

Lymphocytic Choriomeningitis Virus

Subclinical infections are common, but their proportion of the total human exposure is unknown. Most symptomatic LCMV infections result in febrile disease which has been associated with several characteristic clinical and laboratory manifestations (Table 2) (49, 66, 131, 154). After an incubation period thought to last 1 to 2 weeks, fever, chills, myalgia, asthenia, and headache develop. Most patients have anorexia and often vomiting. Photophobia, dysesthesias, testicular or parotid pain, arthralgia or even arthritis, and pharyngitis are also found. Both orchitis and parotitis have also been described to occur during this acute phase (94, 154). Cough occurs but is an inconsistent finding. Several reports of infiltrates on chest radiographs suggest that an element of mild pulmonary involvement is not uncommon. Arthralgia and, rarely, true arthritis as well as rash have been reported but are uncommon. The clinical laboratory findings usually show leukopenia (sometimes less than 1,000), thrombocytopenia (typically moderate but as low as 38,000 reported), and mild elevations of liver enzymes. This phase of the illness may last 1 to 3 weeks.

CNS invasion occurs in a minority of LCMV infections (1, 12, 66, 105, 156). The onset of CNS involvement may continue directly from the febrile phase noted above, follow a brief defervesence, or, less often, begin without any prodrome. Patients are febrile, with signs of meningeal irritation, and most will have a clinical picture of simple aseptic meningitis with about 1 week's duration of illness. A minority will have a longer duration, and some will develop signs of diffuse viral encephalomyelitis. Presumably reflecting the ependymal infection seen in mice, an acute hydrocephalus may occur during the course of human illness and has even required shunting for temporary relief (66). Virtually all patients survive without sequelae, although asthenia, depression, and difficulty in mental concentration are complaints that may last weeks.

During the CNS phase the leukocyte count is usually normal or modestly elevated. Most other blood analyses are normal, with the exception of mild elevations of serum enzymes. CSF contains hundreds to a few thousand cells, and hypoglycorrachia is sometimes present and can be <20 mg%.

Rarely, other neurologic syndromes have been described in association with LCMV infection, including ascending paralysis, bulbar paralysis, transverse myelitis, encephalitis lethargica, acute Parkinson's disease, and some relapsing cases (1, 105). Myocarditis with serologic evidence of recent LCMV infection has also been reported. In general, these associations have not been pursued or confirmed, and many of the earlier reports suffer from imprecise diagnostic methods and cross-contamination of laboratory animals used in virus isolation (90).

A new syndrome associated with LCMV infection has been observed in transplant patients receiving organs from infected donors (5, 27a, 51, 120, 125). The immunosuppression leads to a fulminant systemic illness more resembling Lassa fever than classical LCM; this has been observed before in immunosuppressed tumor patients given LCMV in hopes of shrinking the tumor burden (67). The change in clinical syndrome is analogous to the sparing of mice from immunopathological CNS disease after direct brain inoculation (125). The onset of disease is typically 1 to 3 weeks after transplantation, with fever, systemic illness, CNS dysfunction, and multisystem failure. Patients are viremic and the antibody response is low or absent. Of the 13 patients receiving organs from 4 donors, 11 are known to have died, the outcome for 1 is unknown, and 1 survived. The survivor had a decrease in his immunosuppressive medications and administration of ribavirin.

Deafness has been reported in two cases. It seems likely that LCMV is responsible for eighth-nerve deafness occasionally, particularly given the findings with the related Lassa virus (see below).

LCM should be suspected in patients presenting with aseptic meningitis or encephalitis, but these cases can be correctly diagnosed only by laboratory tests. Additional features that suggest LCM include autumn or winter season of onset; several days' febrile prodrome, particularly with a brief remission of fever; high CSF lymphocyte count; and hypoglycorrachia. LCMV has been confused with partially treated bacterial meningitis and granulomatous meningitis. A history of exposure to wild mice may be elicited, but often the exposure was not noted by the patient, so such elements of the history as cleaning outbuildings, living in substandard urban housing, or residence near grain fields should also be sought. Pet hamsters or mice may also be a risk factor if the rodent was contaminated by wild mice or if the supplier's colony has LCMV circulation. The potential role of gerbils and other rodents as pet vectors is unknown.

LCMV was first implicated as a cause of fetal abnormalities by serologic studies in Lithuania (142) and subsequently confirmed elsewhere (11). The mother often has a history of a febrile disease during pregnancy and may have a history of rodent exposure. Hydrocephalus is often recognizable at birth and is usually severe, with an associated chorioretinitis. Increasing recognition of this entity suggests that a more agile surveillance and a more comprehensive evaluation of its importance are in order (17, 140, 158). The virus also may result in abortion and perinatal infection with fatal outcome (86).

Lassa Virus

After an incubation period of 5 to 16 days, this disease begins gradually, with fever, asthenia, malaise, and gastrointestinal symptoms leading to prostration (85, 103). Cough, chest pain, and sore throat are common, as are abdominal pain, diarrhea, nausea, and vomiting. Later in the course of illness, bleeding, conjunctival injection, facial edema, and rales are features. Pleural effusions are common, and pericardial effusions may occur later in illness, with one patient having a relapsing course culminating in constrictive pericarditis (31, 65). Diffuse mucosal bleeding is often present in severe cases, as is hypotension giving way to shock. The varied and nonspecific findings make the clinical diagnosis of Lassa fever difficult, but the many different findings as well as the severity of the disease contribute to the recognition of florid cases.

Neurologic findings in Lassa fever are less prominent than in Argentine HF but are nevertheless common. In addition to hearing loss, tremor, encephalopathy, encephalitis, and ataxic syndromes have been described (30, 146).

Deafness has been noted as a common and diagnostically useful complication that typically occurs during recovery from Lassa fever. About one-fifth of patients will develop significant sensorineural hearing impairment either unilaterally or bilaterally, and the loss of hearing is often permanent (33). This important accompaniment of Lassa fever is not related to disease severity. Notably, an increased prevalence of Lassa virus antibodies is present among deaf persons in areas of endemicity.

Hematocrit may be slightly elevated, and the white count is usually normal or modestly elevated. Platelet counts are usually normal or modestly increased, even in the face of bleeding. Proteinuria is common. The serum transaminase level is usually elevated and predicts the mortality rate in a proportional fashion. Aspartate aminotransferase AST levels of 150 or greater suggest the need for intravenous ribavirin therapy, and very severe cases may reach values of several hundred (74). This is not usually because of hepatitis per se but presumably reflects the extent of viral replication in the liver and elsewhere. Indeed, viremia presents a similar and perhaps more fundamental correlation (74).

The case fatality rate for hospitalized patients with Lassa fever is about 15% without ribavirin therapy. The occurrence of milder or subclinical cases is suspected based on longitudinal studies of fever patients in Sierra Leone villages, but the data are ambiguous because of the limitations of the fluorescent-antibody test (104). Both seroconversions and loss of antibody over time were found and suggest that supposedly seronegative individuals are not necessarily naïve; furthermore, titer increases are also reported to occur in persons with preexisting fluorescent antibodies, suggesting that reinfection might occur.

Lassa virus is highly invasive to the human fetus and results in fetal loss in more than 75% of infected pregnant women (130). In the third trimester, the maternal mortality rate is markedly increased (30%) and the fetal mortality rate is 92%. Uterine evacuation in these high-risk patients decreases the maternal mortality rate. High titers of virus and the presence of viral antigen in placentas (155; S. Zaki, unpublished observations) suggest that the placenta may serve as a continuing, overwhelming source of virus. Furthermore, the unusual down-regulation of both class I and class II MHC antigen expression on the placenta may well result in an escape from surveillance analogous to that hypothesized for neurons in LCMV infections.

Junin Virus

Argentine HF begins with the insidious onset of fever, myalgia, and malaise after an incubation period of typically 1 to 2 weeks (110, 133, 141). As the disease progresses, these symptoms intensify and are often accompanied by dizziness, headache, and gastrointestinal disturbances such as nausea, vomiting, meteorism, diarrhea, and constipation. During this period, there may be few physical signs, but flushing of the face and chest, conjunctival suffusion, mild hypotension, and tachycardia are often present. The full-blown disease includes prostration, hyperesthesia, confusion, cerebellar tremor of the hands and tongue, and early bleeding manifestations such as petechiae. Thrombocytopenia, leukopenia, and proteinuria are virtually always present at this stage. AST is normal or slightly elevated, and measures of renal function are proportional to circulatory compromise. In severe cases, bleeding gums and mucosal hemorrhages are common. Neurologic signs are common and include somnolence, hyporeflexia, hypotonia, palmomental reflex, and the presence of the Romberg sign.

In severe cases, hypotension proceeds to frank clinical shock, and there may be hemorrhage, neurologic disease, or both. Hemorrhage is usually mucosal and most often gastrointestinal or uterine, although renal, pulmonary, and other sites may be involved. Neurologic manifestations may accompany severe hemorrhagic disease, or coma, seizures, and shock may occur alone, with a particularly poor prognosis associated. Mild disease may last only a few days, but severe infections continue for up to 2 to 3 weeks. Typically, improvement occurs around days 10 to 14. There are no recognized permanent sequelae, but patients may suffer alopecia in convalescence and are often troubled for several weeks by symptoms such as fatigue, dizziness, and difficulty concentrating.

The mortality rate of untreated Argentine HF is about 15 to 30%. Occasionally, Junin virus antibodies are found in persons without a history of HF, suggesting that milder cases may occur; some strains of Junin virus are also thought to be naturally attenuated (134).

Pregnant women infected with Junin virus have an increased mortality rate and high fetal wastage, particularly in the third trimester (22).

Viruses Causing Other South American HFs

Bolivian HF is less well studied, but it resembles Argentine HF and has a mortality rate of about 25% (42, 73, 151). One hospital-based outbreak occurring at high altitude (2,700 m) was associated with a very high mortality rate and prominent jaundice (124). Sporadic cases continue to occur, some of which are diagnosed but some of which are not registered. A small epidemic in Magdalena, Bolivia, exemplifies the situation. It was only reported because of a very unusual dissemination of virus to five members of the family of the patient with the index case; a visiting team took samples and disseminated the information, allowing proper diagnosis and workup of the outbreak.

Venezuelan HF also is similar to Bolivian HF in clinical presentation (137, 138). In a study of 14 virologically confirmed patients, pharyngitis was more prominent, the mortality rate was 64%, and deafness occurred in convalescence in one of the 5 survivors. The mortality rate will probably decline as more experience is accumulated, and indeed, only 26 of the 104 clinically identified patients died.

Infection with Sabia virus was first detected in Brazil. The patient with the index case presented with a picture resembling other South American HFs, except that hepatic necrosis was severe. The only other untreated case observed was a laboratory infection that pursued a course resembling a moderately severe case of Argentine HF.

Other Arenaviruses

The pathogenic potential of most of the viruses listed in Table 1 is unknown. The arenaviruses known from North America are Bear Canyon, Tamiami, and Whitewater Arroyo viruses. There is suggestive evidence that severe natural infections with Whitewater Arroyo virus have occurred, but further experience is needed. Laboratory infections with Flexal or Tacaribe virus have resulted in febrile disease with prostration and metrorrhagia or with headache and suggestions of mild CNS involvement, respectively. Pichinde virus has caused a number of subclinical infections of laboratory workers. Although antibodies thought to be due to infection with some of the other viruses have been detected in human sera, there is no knowledge of whether they are pathogenic. The Old World arenaviruses Mopeia and Mobala viruses are innocuous for monkeys and strain 13 guinea pigs and are probably of reduced pathogenicity for humans (127).

Differential Diagnosis of the HFs

The HFs are suspected from a history of rural travel or residence in one of the known areas of endemicity (Table 2; Fig. 1 and 3) or, more rarely, from occupation in a virology laboratory. It seems likely that additional human-pathogenic arenaviruses will be discovered as well. The patient examined early in disease may show lower-than-normal blood pressure, with bradycardia or tachycardia and flushing of the face and thorax; the patient may seem more seriously ill than expected. Nondependent edema or petechiae may also be present. Enanthem and conjunctival injection are common but less specific. Proteinuria is a common laboratory finding, but serum creatinine will be abnormal only in patients with severe cardiovascular compromise. The South American HFs will usually have thrombocytopenia and leukopenia early in their course, but transaminases will be normal or only slightly elevated. The blood count in early Lassa fever is often normal; AST may be normal in mildly ill patients but will be elevated in severe cases. Lassa fever is often accompanied by sore throat, pharyngitis with or without exudate, and odynophagia, but the specificity of this finding is relatively low.

Rickettsial diseases, leptospirosis, malaria, and typhoid fever are readily confused with Lassa fever and must always be carefully excluded because they are common, potentially lethal, and treatable. In some situations, empirical treatment with tetracycline or an effective antimalarial may be indicated. Somewhat less commonly confused but important considerations include dysentery, relapsing fever, other HFs (depending on geography), sepsis, viral encephalitis, and some intoxications. The differential diagnosis may also include early stages of human immunodeficiency virus infection, measles, hepatitis, infectious mononucleosis, collagen vascular diseases, and early stages of nephritis.

LABORATORY DIAGNOSIS

Virus Isolation

Virus isolation can be made from blood during the initial febrile phase of LCM, but after the onset of CNS disease, attempts using CSF will be more fruitful. Viremia is present during the acute course of HF. Lassa virus has also been isolated from CSF when CNS involvement was present.

The most general approach to arenavirus isolation is inoculation of Vero cells with serum or CSF. Viral antigen can be demonstrated by staining with direct or indirect fluorescent-antibody methods because cytopathic effect may be mild or absent. Antigen may be detectable within 3 days but may not appear for 2 weeks in low-titer samples. Although serum has been widely used, blood is believed by some to be slightly more sensitive, and in the case of Argentine HF, cocultivation of peripheral blood mononuclear cells can be positive after routine blood inoculation of Vero cells or suckling mice is negative (3). Animal inoculation intracranially with whole blood has been used widely in the past and in some cases may be marginally more sensitive than use of Vero cells, but it carries a greater biohazard and the possibility of cross-contamination. Suckling mice may be used for Junin virus (3), suckling hamsters for Machupo virus (73), adult mice for LCMV (24, 40, 90), and adult mice for Lassa virus (24). Inoculation of suckling mice with LCMV will only produce a carrier state (132), and similar results may occur with Lassa virus, depending on the mouse strain (129). Blind passage has been used for primary isolation of some virus strains.

In fatal cases, the spleen is the optimum source of virus, although isolations have been made from the lymph nodes, liver, kidneys, and other organs. The brain has been a poor source of virus, but isolation should be attempted, particularly in atypical cases.

Antigen Detection ELISA

Antigen detection enzyme-linked immunosorbent assay (ELISA) has been used with acute-phase sera from patients with HF and is quite promising. In Lassa fever an initial evaluation has yielded a diagnosis in virtually all cases if combined with immunoglobulin (IgM) antibody ELISA (13, 70). Junin and Machupo virus antigens are readily detected in patient sera using Junin virus reagents (T. G. Ksiazek and colleagues, unpublished observations).

RNA Detection

Very sensitive reverse transcription-PCR RT-PCR has been applied to several arenavirus systems, but there are no large patient evaluations that take into account the ample genetic diversity present in one arenavirus species. RT-PCR has the marked advantage that samples can be inactivated as RNA is extracted, and thus it provides a safe diagnostic procedure that can be used in many laboratories that do not have extensive containment. Primers have been designed and used for LCMV (14, 121). The technology has been proposed for Lassa virus and has been useful in limited geographic settings but requires generalization (19) and field experience (39, 43, 99, 115). Junin virus RT-PCR is also promising but requires further work to define the sensitivity (96). Consensus primers for other New World arenaviruses are available, and additional PCR-based diagnostic approaches are anticipated (18, 97).

Pathological Examination

Histology alone may be characteristic but is unlikely to be diagnostic, and particles are not plentiful by electron microscopy. Immunohistochemistry has been useful in Lassa fever and Bolivian HF.

Serology

Serologic relatedness among arenaviruses is seen in cross-reactive tests such as the indirect fluorescent antibody test using clinical sera or hyperimmune hamster and mouse sera (128). Neutralization tests are used to distinguish individual viruses. The serologic patterns of arenavirus infections have important differences according to the virus considered. Infection of humans or experimental animals with some of the viruses, such as Junin, Machupo, Tacaribe, and Amapari viruses, results in neutralizing antibodies readily detectable by standard techniques using 50 to 100 PFU of virus and differing serum dilutions; others, such as LCMV and Lassa, Pichinde, and Latino viruses, require a constant-serum, varying virus format with the addition of complement yielding a log neutralization index (LNI) according to the reduction of the virus titer (49, 69, 71, 90, 91). People or experimental animals infected with viruses that elicit brisk serum dilution neutralization titers usually develop antibodies around the time of recovery or slightly afterwards, but with Lassa virus or LCMV, the LNI may require several additional weeks to become positive and is very complement dependent. The serum dilution plaque reduction neutralization test is useful for distinguishing different arenavirus species, and titers are predictive of protection by passive antibody transfer for viruses such as Junin or Machupo virus (46). The LNI has also been useful for the same ends in experimental animals, but there is little experience with humans (69, 127).

Indirect fluorescent-antibody tests are widely used for arenavirus diagnosis and for detecting cross-reactions when assessing new virus isolates (128, 159). The antibody pattern with this test is found to be somewhat different when Lassa virus is compared to Junin and Machupo viruses. Lassa fever patients may develop detectable IgG or IgM antibodies as early as the first week of illness, and the appearance of antibodies does not necessarily correspond to clinical improvement (74). Argentine and Bolivian HF patients develop fluorescent antibodies around the time of clinical improvement or afterwards (35, 128). In LCM, fluorescent antibodies are usually present by the time of CNS involvement. If highly specific conjugates are available, IgM antibodies are useful in diagnosis and may be found in CSF (36, 95).

ELISA antibody tests are becoming the standard approach to serodiagnosis or seroepidemiology of arenavirus infections. IgM capture assays become positive early in convalesence (or, in the case of Lassa fever, during the disease course) and are more reliable than IgM fluorescent-antibody tests (13, 58; Ksiazek and colleagues, unpublished observations). Recombinant antigens are possible to avoid the infectious hazard from reagents, but the sera may be infectious in acutely ill patients (136). The IgG tests are positive for years after acute infections, a time when the fluorescent-antibody tests are negative or the antibodies have fallen to titers that are difficult to interpret; their virus specificity appears to be greater than that of the fluorescent-antibody test.

Laboratory Facilities

All arenaviruses with which there is experience are aerosol infectious, and therefore all members of the family should be treated with appropriate respect in the laboratory. High-nervous-system-passage LCMV strains such as today's Armstrong strain are highly attenuated (60) and are classified as requiring biosafety level 2 (BSL-2), but most other strains, including recent human isolates, are handled at BSL-3. Those that cause HF are all classified as BSL-4 agents in the United States. Inactivation of viruses with gamma irradiation provides a safe method for preparing sera for antigen or antibody tests and many other assays (102, 108). Diagnostic sera from patients with acute HF are best sent to qualified laboratories for testing. In the United States, diagnostic testing is available at the Centers for Disease Control and Prevention, which can be contacted at (404) 639-1115 or (404) 639-2888.

PREVENTION

Lymphocytic Choriomeningitis Virus

The epidemiology of LCMV in the United States is not well studied, but there are clearly active foci of virus transmission. Exclusion of wild mice from urban and rural dwellings is particularly important for the protection of pregnant women. Since LCMV is highly pathogenic for many nonhuman primate species (112, 127), they should also be protected from wild mice and substandard sources of laboratory mice. Breeding of rodents for pets, reptile food, or laboratory use or for pet sales should be done only by those willing to ensure rodent-proof facilities and to maintain surveillance of their operation for viral intrusion. Most large commercial breeders of laboratory animals maintain a regular survey of their rodents for LCMV and other viruses, and their animals are safe. However, there is no legal control for them or for pet rodent breeders, who are less cognizant of the risks. The serious consequences of LCMV in pregnant women and the immunosuppressed suggest a need for regulation to ensure a safe product (5, 17, 51). LCMV causes inapparent infections not only of rodents, but also of transplanted tumors and cell cultures, and thus concern for these sources of infection is also indicated.

Lassa Virus

Lassa virus is spread by one of the most ubiquitous and prolific rodents in Africa (Fig. 1). Control of the rodent inside or outside houses is unlikely to be highly effective or sustainable in that setting. Vaccination of humans seems to be the only approach likely to be useful. The potential for a Lassa virus vaccine has been convincingly demonstrated by using recombinant vaccinia viruses expressing Lassa virus glycoprotein genes which are protective in nonhuman primates and guinea pigs. Recombinants expressing the nucleoprotein gene have sometimes been effective in guinea pigs. Vesicular stomatitis virus containing the Lassa virus glycoprotein gene in place of the vesicular stomatitis virus glycoprotein gene has also proven to be highly attenuated in mice, guinea pigs, and monkeys, but this platform has never been used in humans (59). Another promising approach has incorporated the Lassa virus glycoprotein gene within the yellow fever virus 17D vaccine genome, yielding an attenuated and immunogenic construct in experimental animals which conferred immunity to both Lassa fever and yellow fever (20). Development of a vectored vaccine against Lassa virus is a tempting strategy, since the same vector might be expected to provide protection against the large number of South American arenaviruses if their genes were replaced.

Cross-protection against Lassa virus infection of macaques and guinea pigs has been demonstrated with Mopeia and Mobala viruses, and LCMV (127). Although some strains of these viruses are highly attenuated for nonhuman primates and guinea pigs, their development as Lassa virus immunogens is not practical.

Patients with convalescent Lassa fever may excrete virus in urine or semen. The duration of shedding is not well characterized, but virus can be isolated from urine at least 32 days after onset (24). Patients should be cautioned to use disinfectant in the toilet bowl before urination and practice safe sex until they are virus negative.

Junin Virus

Argentine HF (Fig. 3) is an inevitable occupational risk for the agricultural worker in the affected areas of the pampas and should be prevented by the use of a live attenuated vaccine, Candid #1. Lower attack rates in rural towns and less heavily exposed persons should eventually lead to targeting of these populations for vaccine prevention.

The vaccine was developed by serial passage of Junin virus in mice and then in cell culture. Cloning resulted in a virus that is attenuated, nonneuroinvasive, and nonneurovirulent in laboratory models such as the macaque and the strain 13 inbred guinea pig (47). The genetic basis for attenuation is not known, but the virus is more readily neutralized in vitro, is sensitive to complement inactivation, and is of markedly decreased pathogenicity even in immature laboratory hosts (47, 82). It was protective against parenteral and aerosol challenge in the same experimental hosts. Safety testing was successful, and although the antibody response was less than that following natural infection, the cellular immune response was strongly induced. Tests in the area of endemicity have found the vaccine to be more than 95% protective, and safety has been confirmed in adults, with additional safety data accumulating for pregnant women and children. More than 250,000 high-risk adults in the area of endemicity have been vaccinated without incident, and the annual number of cases has been reduced to fewer than 100 (D. Enria, unpublished data).

Recovering patients should be counseled about the possibility of virus excretion in semen, and precautions should be taken for the period of infectivity. The duration of infectiousness is presently unknown, but 4 to 6 weeks or until negative laboratory tests are obtained would be reasonable. Indeed, these precautions could be applicable to other arenavirus HFs.

Machupo Virus

Bolivian HF may be acquired by rural residents who come into contact with virus-infected rodents in savannas or, particularly, cultivated fields in the area of endemicity (Fig. 3). Attack rates are currently low, but if transmission increases, there is the possibility of using the Junin virus vaccine. In experimental animals, this vaccine protects against virulent Machupo virus challenge (P. B. Jahrling, G. A. Eddy, and C. J. Peters, unpublished observations). Currently, rodent control programs in towns and villages protect against severe epidemics like those seen in the 1960s.

Guanarito Virus

Venezuelan HF (Fig. 3) has not been sufficiently studied to examine preventive strategies aimed at rodents, and the Junin virus vaccine is not cross-protective in experimental animals.

Nosocomial and Laboratory Precautions

The role of nosocomial transmission and the precautions that are needed for patient care are controversial. In the zones of endemicity, mask, gown, and glove precautions are all that are used, and few episodes of spread to medical staff have been noted (64). However, occasional hospital or family epidemics have occurred with Lassa fever, Argentine HF, and Bolivian HF (124, 129). Analyses of the rare hospital epidemics, viral infectivity in experimental situations, and the limited human data on viral shedding suggest that the patient early in disease provides minimal risk, so expeditious evaluation of febrile travelers with only mask, gown, and glove precautions is feasible (126). Clinical laboratory samples should be minimized to those needed for diagnosis of an HF and the most important competing conditions; these samples should be handled cautiously, preferably within a laminar-flow hood, and waste should be properly disposed of (8). It is recommended that if the diagnosis of an arenaviral HF is made outside the area of endemicity, additional attention should be paid to the isolation of the patient, protection of medical staff, and minimization of environmental contamination (27).

TREATMENT

Lymphocytic Choriomeningitis Virus

There is no established therapy for LCMV other than support. The virus is sensitive to the antiviral drug ribavirin in vitro, but there is no clinical experience and no obvious scenario for its successful clinical use. In transplant patients or patients in other immunosuppressive situations, withdrawal of immunosuppression combined with ribavirin is worthwhile (51, 125).

Viruses Causing Arenaviral HFs

The arenaviral HFs require intensive supportive therapy. Movement should be atraumatic and minimized. Intramuscular injections and drugs such as aspirin that may interfere with coagulation or platelet function are contraindicated. Hydration should be cautious because of the propensity for pulmonary edema, the clinical manifestation of mild edema and interstitial pneumonitis seen pathologically. Bacterial superinfections are common and should be watched for and treated appropriately. Blood transfusions or clotting factor replacement is not required in most cases, but platelet transfusions should be used in the South American HFs as clinically indicated. Because much of the pathogenesis of these diseases is believed to result from release of cytokines and other soluble mediators (123), blocking agents may be developed as adjuncts to therapy in the future.

Lassa Virus

Ribavirin has been used in severe Lassa fever, with success in reducing the mortality rate compared to that for retrospective controls stratified for severity using serum AST or viremia (74). Patients with AST levels over 150 U/ml should be treated with intravenous drug in a dosage of 32 mg/kg of body weight given by slow intravenous infusion (53) followed by 16 mg/kg four times a day for 4 days and 8 mg/kg three times a day for 7 additional days. The expected side effects include reversible suppression of erythropoiesis, mild hemolysis, and mild direct hyperbilirubinemia.

Passive antibody has been successful in experimental models, but large amounts of carefully selected material are needed (127). The possibility of developing monoclonal antibodies with activity could eliminate the need for selected convalescent-phase plasma. This could provide a useful adjunct in Lassa fever therapy, since some patients with high AST or late presentation for therapy still have a high mortality rate. Antibody has been shown to enhance ribavirin therapy in macaques with experimental Lassa fever (72).

The value of oral or intravenous ribavirin in prophylaxis of exposures to Lassa virus and other arenaviruses is uncertain, in part as neither the dose nor the duration for humans is established. In experimental arenavirus infections, treatment for periods of 7 to 10 days has resulted only in delay of onset, and longer drug administration has not prevented the emergence of CNS disease in Junin virus-infected guinea pigs (78). Given the low risk of disease after exposure, it is preferable to closely observe contacts and initiate ribavirin only after the onset of fever and a presumptive diagnosis of an arenaviral HF. If prophylaxis is to be given, an oral dosage of 2 g daily for at least 14 to 21 days should be used.

Viruses Causing South American HFs

Argentine HF can be treated successfully with convalescent-phase plasma given within the first 8 days of disease onset (48). Two units were used during a randomized, double-blind trial to establish efficacy, and later dose seeking defined the actual amount of plasma needed based on the neutralizing-antibody titer and the recipient's weight. Although this approach has reduced the mortality rate from 15 to 30% to <1% within the area of endemicity, the economic burden of obtaining plasma and the possibility of blood-borne diseases remain. Patients who receive passive antibody therapy have lower antibody responses than do vaccine recipients, further complicating the logistics of this therapy.

About 10% of those receiving plasma therapy develop a late neurologic syndrome. These patients, after a symptom-free interval of 4 to 6 weeks, experience the gradual onset of fever, headache, and dizziness which last several days before the patients generally have a complete recovery. Cerebellar signs and oculomotor palsies may be present. Modestly increased mononuclear cells and protein are found in the CSF; Junin virus antibodies are present, but virus has never been isolated. The syndrome may be due to residual Junin virus in the CNS finally being eradicated by the immune system; antibody titers rise later and to higher levels in patients with neurologic involvement.

In the guinea pig model, murine monoclonal antibodies are effective in treating Junin virus infection (R. H. Kenyon and C. J. Peters, unpublished observations), and one of these has been converted to a human framework with retention of similar in vitro activity (A. Schmaljohn, unpublished observations), but further development is not being pursued.

Ribavirin studies with guinea pigs and nonhuman primates have shown a positive effect on the course of visceral disease, but ribavirin has not prevented CNS involvement (78, 127). In humans, intravenous ribavirin has been used with a favorable trend on viremia and survival and no untoward effects except anemia (48). Until controlled trials are conducted, the drug would be a reasonable substitute in treating patients outside the zone of endemicity if passive antibody is not available.

Experimental Bolivian HF has been treated successfully both with passive antibody and with ribavirin (149). There is no controlled experience with either modality in humans, although intravenous ribavirin has shown promise in recent clinical experience (83) and would be a reasonable choice to treat Machupo virus infections.

There is no experience in the therapy of other human arenaviral HFs except a single observation made on a scientist infected with Sabia virus in the laboratory. He was treated early in the course of disease with intravenous ribavirin; within 24 h of initiation of therapy he was afebrile and clinically much improved, and virus could no longer be isolated from his blood (10).

Several additional candidate drugs with activity against arenavirus have been identified by in vitro screening, and others are being discovered through the intensive interest generated by biodefense programs. An immunomodulator and one of the inhibitory compounds, selenazofurin, have been tested in animals, without significant activity (144). It seems unlikely that any of these drugs will be developed for clinical use in arenavirus diseases, but if they are brought into use for other agents, they may have some utility against arenaviruses. Small interfering RNA has been effective in vitro against Lassa virus, and this may eventually be developed with a proper in vivo delivery system (113).

REFERENCES

1. **Adair, C. V., R. L. Gauld, and J. E. Smadel.** 1953. Aseptic meningitis, a disease of diverse etiology: clinical and etiologic studies on 854 cases. *Ann. Intern. Med.* **39:**675–704.
2. **Ahmed, R., and M. B. Oldstone.** 1988. Organ-specific selection of viral variants during chronic infection. *J. Exp. Med.* **167:**1719–1724.
3. **Ambrosio, A. M., D. A. Enria, and J. I. Maiztegui.** 1986. Junin virus isolation from lympho-mononuclear cells of patients with Argentine hemorrhagic fever. *Intervirology* **25:**97–102.
4. **Ambrosio, A. M., M. R. Feuillade, G. S. Gamboa, and J. I. Maiztegui.** 1994. Prevalence of lymphocytic choriomeningitis virus infection in a human population of Argentina. *Am. J. Trop. Med. Hyg.* **50:**381–386.
5. **Amman, B. R., B. I. Pavlin, C. G. Albariño, J. A. Comer, B. R. Erickson, J. B. Oliver, T. K. Sealy, M. J. Vincent, S. T. Nichol, C. D. Paddock, A. J. Tumpey, K. D. Wagoner, R. D. Glauer, K. A. Smith, K. A. Winpisinger, M. S. Parsely, P. Wyrick, C. H. Hannafin, U. Bandy, S. Zaki, P. E. Rollin, and T. G. Ksiazek.** 2007. Pet rodents and fatal lymphocytic choriomeningitis in transplant patients. *Emerg. Infect. Dis.* **13:**719–725.
6. **Andrews, B. S., A. N. Theofilopoulos, C. J. Peters, D. J. Loskutoff, W. E. Brandt, and F. J. Dixon.** 1978. Replication of dengue and Junin viruses in cultured rabbit and human endothelial cells. *Infect. Immun.* **20:**776–781.
7. **Armstrong, C., and R. D. Lillie.** 1934. Experimental lymphocytic choriomeningitis of monkeys and mice produced by a virus encountered in studies of the 1933 St. Louis encephalitis epidemic. *Public Health Rep.* **49:**1027.
8. **Armstrong, L. R., L. M. Dembry, P. M. Rainey, M. B. Russi, A. S. Khan, S. H. Fischer, S. C. Edberg, T. G. Ksiazek, P. E. Rollin, and C. J. Peters.** 1999. Management of a Sabia virus-infected patient in a US hospital. *Infect. Control Hosp. Epidemiol.* **20:**176–182.

9. **Baize, S., J. Kaplon, C. Faure, D. Pannetier, M. C. Georges-Courbot, and V. Deubel.** 2004. Lassa virus infection of human dendritic cells and macrophages is productive but fails to activate cells. *J. Immunol.* **172:**2861–2869.
10. **Barry, M., M. Russi, L. Armstrong, D. Geller, R. Tesh, L. Dembry, J. P. Gonzalez, A. S. Khan, and C. J. Peters.** 1995. Brief report: treatment of a laboratory-acquired Sabia virus infection. *N. Engl. J. Med.* **333:**294–296.
11. **Barton, L. L., S. C. Budd, W. S. Morfitt, C. J. Peters, T. G. Ksiazek, R. F. Schindler, and M. T. Yoshino.** 1993. Congenital lymphocytic choriomeningitis virus infection in twins. *Pediatr. Infect. Dis. J.* **12:**942–946.
12. **Baum, S. G., A. M. Lewis, Jr., W. P. Rowe, and R. J. Huebner.** 1966. Epidemic nonmeningitic lymphocytic-choriomeningitis-virus infection. An outbreak in a population of laboratory personnel. *N. Engl. J. Med.* **274:** 934–936.
13. **Bausch, D. G., P. E. Rollin, A. H. Demby, M. Coulibaly, J. Kanu, A. S. Conteh, K. D. Wagoner, L. K. McMullan, M. D. Bowen, C. J. Peters, and T. G. Ksiazek.** 2000. Diagnosis and clinical virology of Lassa fever as evaluated by enzyme-linked immunosorbent assay, indirect fluorescent-antibody test, and virus isolation. *J. Clin. Microbiol.* **38:**2670–2677.
14. **Besselsen, D. G., A. M. Wagner, and J. K. Loganbill.** 2003. Detection of lymphocytic choriomeningitis virus by use of fluorogenic nuclease reverse transcriptase-polymerase chain reaction analysis. *Comp. Med.* **53:**65–69.
15. **Blumenthal, W., R. Ackermann, and W. Scheid.** 1968. Distribution of the lymphocytic choriomeningitis virus in an endemic area. *Dtsch. Med. Wochenschr.* **93:**944–948. (In German.)
16. **Bonner, P. C., W. P. Schmidt, S. R. Belmain, B. Oshin, D. Baglole, and M. Borchert.** 2007. Poor housing quality increases risk of rodent infestation and Lassa fever in refugee camps of Sierra Leone. *Am. J. Trop. Med. Hyg.* **77:** 169–175.
17. **Bonthius, D. J., R. Wright, B. Tseng, L. Barton, E. Marco, B. Karacay, and P. D. Larsen.** 2007. Congenital lymphocytic choriomeningitis virus infection: spectrum of disease. *Ann. Neurol.* **62:**347–355.
18. **Bowen, M. D., C. J. Peters, and S. T. Nichol.** 1997. Phylogenetic analysis of the Arenaviridae: patterns of virus evolution and evidence for cospeciation between arenaviruses and their rodent hosts. *Mol. Phylogenet. Evol.* **8:**301–316.
19. **Bowen, M. D., P. E. Rollin, T. G. Ksiazek, H. L. Hustad, D. G. Bausch, A. H. Demby, M. D. Bajani, C. J. Peters, and S. T. Nichol.** 2000. Genetic diversity among Lassa virus strains. *J. Virol.* **74:**6992–7004.
20. **Bredenbeek, P. J., R. Molenkamp, W. J. Spaan, V. Deubel, P. Marianneau, M. S. Salvato, D. Moshkoff, J. Zapata, I. Tikhonov, J. Patterson, R. Carrion, A. Ticer, K. Brasky, and I. S. Lukashevich.** 2006. A recombinant Yellow Fever 17D vaccine expressing Lassa virus glycoproteins. *Virology* **345:**299–304.
21. **Briggiler, A. M., D. Enria, M. R. Feuillade, and J. I. Maiztegui.** 1987. Contagio interhumano e infeccion inaparente por virus Junin en matrimonios del area endemica de fiebre hemorragica argentina. *Medicina* (Buenos Aires) **47:**565.
22. **Briggiler, A. M., S. Levis, D. Enria, A. M. Ambrosio, and J. I. Maiztegui.** 1990. Argentine hemorrhagic fever in pregnant women. *Medicina* (Buenos Aires) **50:**443.
23. **Buchmeier, M., J.-C. de la Torre, and C. Peters.** 2007. *Arenaviridae:* the viruses and their replication, p. 1791–1827. *In:* D. M. Knipe, P. M. Howley, D. E. Griffin, R. A. Lamb, M. A. Martin, B. Roizman, and S. E. Straus (ed.), *Fields Virology*, 5th ed. Lippincott Williams & Wilkins, Philadelphia, PA.
24. **Buckley, S. M., and J. Casals.** 1970. Lassa fever, a new virus disease of man from West Africa. 3. Isolation and characterization of the virus. *Am. J. Trop. Med. Hyg.* **19:** 680–691.
25. **Capul, A. A., M. Perez, E. Burke, S. Kunz, M. J. Buchmeier, and J. C. de la Torre.** 2007. Arenavirus Z-glycoprotein association requires Z myristoylation but not functional RING or late domains. *J. Virol.* **81:**9451–9460.
26. **Carey, D. E., G. E. Kemp, H. A. White, L. Pinneo, R. F. Addy, A. L. Fom, G. Stroh, J. Casals, and B. E. Henderson.** 1972. Lassa fever. Epidemiological aspects of the 1970 epidemic, Jos, Nigeria. *Trans. R. Soc. Trop. Med. Hyg.* **66:**402–408.
27. **Centers for Disease Control and Prevention.** 1995. Update: management of patients with suspected viral hemorrhagic fever—United States. *JAMA* **274:**374–375.
27a. **Centers for Disease Control and Prevention.** 2008. Brief report: lymphocytic choriomeningitis virus transmitted through solid organ transplantation—Massachusetts, 2008. *Morb. Mortal. Wkly. Rep.* **57:**799–801.
28. **Childs, J., and C. Peters.** 1993. Ecology and epidemiology of arenaviruses and their hosts, p. 331–373. *In* M. S. Salvato (ed.), *The Arenaviridae*. Plenum Press, New York, NY.
29. **Childs, J. E., G. E. Glass, G. W. Korch, T. G. Ksiazek, and J. W. Leduc.** 1992. Lymphocytic choriomeningitis virus infection and house mouse (Mus musculus) distribution in urban Baltimore. *Am. J. Trop. Med. Hyg.* **47:**27–34.
30. **Cummins, D., D. Bennett, S. P. Fisher-Hoch, B. Farrar, S. J. Machin, and J. B. McCormick.** 1992. Lassa fever encephalopathy: clinical and laboratory findings. *J. Trop. Med. Hyg.* **95:**197–201.
31. **Cummins, D., D. Bennett, S. P. Fisher-Hoch, B. Farrar, and J. B. McCormick.** 1989. Electrocardiographic abnormalities in patients with Lassa fever. *J. Trop. Med. Hyg.* **92:**350–355.
32. **Cummins, D., S. P. Fisher-Hoch, K. J. Walshe, I. J. Mackie, J. B. McCormick, D. Bennett, G. Perez, B. Farrar, and S. J. Machin.** 1989. A plasma inhibitor of platelet aggregation in patients with Lassa fever. *Br. J. Haematol.* **72:**543–548.
33. **Cummins, D., J. B. McCormick, D. Bennett, J. A. Samba, B. Farrar, S. J. Machin, and S. P. Fisher-Hoch.** 1990. Acute sensorineural deafness in Lassa fever. *JAMA* **264:**2093–2096.
34. **Danes, L., R. Benda, and M. Fuchsova.** 1963. Experimental inhalation infection with the lymphocytic choriomeningitis virus (WE strain) of the monkeys of the *Macacus cynomolgus* and *Macacus rhesus* species. *Bratisl. Lek. Listy* **43:**21–34.
35. **deBracco, M. M., M. T. Rimoldi, P. M. Cossio, A. Rabinovich, J. I. Maiztegui, G. Carballal, and R. M. Arana.** 1978. Argentine hemorrhagic fever. Alterations of the complement system and anti-Junin-virus humoral response. *N. Engl. J. Med.* **299:**216–221.
36. **Deibel, R., and G. D. Schryver.** 1976. Viral antibody in the cerebrospinal fluid of patients with acute central nervous system infections. *J. Clin. Microbiol.* **3:**397–401.
37. **Deibel, R., J. P. Woodall, W. J. Decher, and G. D. Schryver.** 1975. Lymphocytic choriomeningitis virus in man. Serologic evidence of association with pet hamsters. *JAMA* **232:**501–504.
38. **Delgado, S., B. R. Erickson, R. Agudo, P. J. Blair, E. Vallejo, C. G. Albarino, J. Vargas, J. A. Comer, P. E. Rollin, T. G. Ksiazek, J. G. Olson, and S. T. Nichol.**

2008. Chapare virus, a newly discovered arenavirus isolated from a fatal hemorrhagic fever case in Bolivia. *PloS Pathog.* **4:**e1000047.

39. **Demby, A. H., J. Chamberlain, D. W. Brown, and C. S. Clegg.** 1994. Early diagnosis of Lassa fever by reverse transcription-PCR. *J. Clin. Microbiol.* **32:**2898–2903.
40. **deSouza, M., and A. L. Smith.** 1989. Comparison of isolation in cell culture with conventional and modified mouse antibody production tests for detection of murine viruses. *J. Clin. Microbiol.* **27:**185–187.
41. **Djavani, M. M., O. R. Crasta, J. C. Zapata, Z. Fei, O. Folkerts, B. Sobral, M. Swindells, J. Bryant, H. Davis, C. D. Pauza, I. S. Lukashevich, R. Hammamieh, M. Jett, and M. S. Salvato.** 2007. Early blood profiles of virus infection in a monkey model for Lassa fever. *J. Virol.* **81:** 7960–7973.
42. **Douglas, R., N. Wiebenga, and R. B. Couch.** 1965. Bolivian hemorrhagic fever probably transmitted by personal contact. *Am. J. Epidemiol.* **82:**8591.
43. **Drosten, C., S. Gottig, S. Schilling, M. Asper, M. Panning, H. Schmitz, and S. Gunther.** 2002. Rapid detection and quantification of RNA of Ebola and Marburg viruses, Lassa virus, Crimean-Congo hemorrhagic fever virus, Rift Valley fever virus, dengue virus, and yellow fever virus by real-time reverse transcription-PCR. *J. Clin. Microbiol.* **40:**2323–2330.
44. **Dykewicz, C. A., V. M. Dato, S. P. Fisher-Hoch, M. V. Howarth, G. I. Perez-Oronoz, S. M. Ostroff, H. Gary, Jr., L. B. Schonberger, and J. B. McCormick.** 1992. Lymphocytic choriomeningitis outbreak associated with nude mice in a research institute. *JAMA* **267:**1349–1353. (Erratum, **268:**874.)
45. **Eichler, R., T. Strecker, L. Kolesnikova, J. ter Meulen, W. Weissenhorn, S. Becker, H. D. Klenk, W. Garten, and O. Lenz.** 2004. Characterization of the Lassa virus matrix protein Z: electron microscopic study of virus-like particles and interaction with the nucleoprotein (NP). *Virus Res.* **100:**249–255.
46. **Enria, D., S. G. Franco, A. Ambrosio, D. Vallejos, S. Levis, and J. Maiztegui.** 1986. Current status of the treatment of Argentine hemorrhagic fever. *Med. Microbiol. Immunol.* **175:**173–176.
47. **Enria, D. A., and J. G. Barrera Oro.** 2002. Junin virus vaccines. *Curr. Top. Microbiol. Immunol.* **263:**239–261.
48. **Enria, D. A., and J. I. Maiztegui.** 1994. Antiviral treatment of Argentine hemorrhagic fever. *Antivir. Res.* **23:** 23–31.
49. **Farmer, T. W., and C. A. Janeway.** 1942. Infections with the virus of lymphocytic choriomeningitis. *Medicine* **21:** 1–64.
50. **Fichet-Calvet, E., E. Lecompte, L. Koivogui, B. Soropogui, A. Doré, F. Kourouma, O. Sylla, S. Daffis, K. Koulémou, and J. ter Meulen.** 2007. Fluctuation of abundance and Lassa virus prevalence in Mastomys natalensis in Guinea, West Africa. *Vector Borne Zoonot. Dis.* **7:**119–128.
51. **Fischer, S. A., M. B. Graham, M. J. Kuehnert, C. N. Kotton, A. Srinivasan, F. M. Marty, J. A. Comer, J. Guarner, C. D. Paddock, D. L. DeMeo, W.-J. Shieh, B. R. Erikson, U. Bandy, A. DeMaria, Jr., J. P. Davis, F. L. Delmonico, B. Pavlin, A. Likos, M. J. Vincent, T. K. Sealy, C. S. Goldsmith, D. B. Jernigan, P. E. Rollin, M. M. Packard, M. Patel, C. Rowland, R. F. Helfand, S. T. Nichol, J. A. Fishman, T. Ksiazek, S. R. Zaki, and the LCMV in Transplant Recipients Investigation Team.** 2006. Transmission of lymphocytic choriomeningitis virus via organ transplantation. *N. Engl. J. Med.* **354:**2235–2249.
52. **Fisher-Hoch, S., J. B. McCormick, D. Sasso, and R. B. Craven.** 1988. Hematologic dysfunction in Lassa fever. *J. Med. Virol.* **26:**127–135.
53. **Fisher-Hoch, S. P., S. Gborie, L. Parker, and J. Huggins.** 1992. Unexpected adverse reactions during a clinical trial in rural west Africa. *Antivir. Res.* **19:**139–147.
54. **Frame, J. D., J. M. Baldwin, Jr., D. J. Gocke, and J. M. Troup.** 1970. Lassa fever, a new virus disease of man from West Africa. I. Clinical description and pathological findings. *Am. J. Trop. Med. Hyg.* **19:**670–676.
55. **Frame, J. D., P. B. Jahrling, J. E. Yalley-Ogunro, and M. H. Monson.** 1984. Endemic Lassa fever in Liberia. II. Serological and virological findings in hospital patients. *Trans. R. Soc. Trop. Med. Hyg.* **78:**656–660.
56. **Fulhorst, C. F., M. D. Bowen, R. A. Salas, G. Duno, A. Utrera, T. G. Ksiazek, N. M. De Manzione, E. De Miller, C. Vasquez, C. J. Peters, and R. B. Tesh.** 1999. Natural rodent host associations of Guanarito and Pirital viruses (Family Arenaviridae) in central Venezuela. *Am. J. Trop. Med. Hyg.* **61:**325–330.
57. **Fulhorst, C. F., M. L. Milazzo, D. S. Carroll, R. N. Charrel, and R. D. Bradley.** 2002. Natural host relationships and genetic diversity of Whitewater Arroyo virus in southern Texas. *Am. J. Trop. Med. Hyg.* **67:**114–118.
58. **Garcia, F. S., A. M. Ambrosio, M. R. Feuillade, and J. I. Maiztegui.** 1988. Evaluation of an enzyme-linked immunosorbent assay for quantitation of antibodies to Junin virus in human sera. *J. Virol. Methods* **19:**299–305.
59. **Geisbert, T. W., S. Jones, E. A. Fritz, A. C. Shurtleff, J. B. Geisbert, R. Liebscher, A. Grolla, U. Ströher, L. Fernando, K. M. Daddario, M. C. Guttieri, B. R. Mothé, T. Larsen, L. E. Hensley, P. B. Jahrling, and H. Feldmann.** 2005. Development of a new vaccine for the prevention of Lassa fever. *PLoS Med.* **2:**e183.
60. **Genovesi, E. V., and C. J. Peters.** 1987. Immunosuppression-induced susceptibility of inbred hamsters (Mesocricetus auratus) to lethal-disease by lymphocytic choriomeningitis virus infection. *Arch. Virol.* **97:**61–76.
61. **Gonzalez, J. P., S. Emonet, X. de Lamballerie, and R. Charrel.** 2007. Arenaviruses. *Curr. Top. Microbiol. Immunol.* **315:**253–288.
62. **Gregg, M. B.** 1975. Recent outbreaks of lymphocytic choriomeningitis in the United States of America. *Bull. W. H. O.* **52:**549–553.
63. **Heller, M. V., M. C. Saavedra, R. Falcoff, J. I. Maiztegui, and F. C. Molinas.** 1992. Increased tumor necrosis factor-alpha levels in Argentine hemorrhagic fever. *J. Infect. Dis.* **166:**1203–1204.
64. **Helmick, C. G., P. A. Webb, C. L. Scribner, J. W. Krebs, and J. B. McCormick.** 1986. No evidence for increased risk of Lassa fever infection in hospital staff. *Lancet* **ii:**1202–1205.
65. **Hirabayashi, Y., S. Oka, H. Goto, K. Shimada, T. Kurata, S. P. Fisher-Hoch, and J. B. McCormick.** 1988. An imported case of Lassa fever with late appearance of polyserositis. *J. Infect. Dis.* **158:**872–875.
66. **Hirsch, M. S., R. C. Moellering, Jr., H. G. Pope, and D. C. Poskanzer.** 1974. Lymphocytic-choriomeningitis-virus infection traced to a pet hamster. *N. Engl. J. Med.* **291:**610–612.
67. **Horton, J., J. E. Hotchin, K. B. Olson, and J. N. Davies.** 1971. The effects of MP virus infection in lymphoma. *Cancer Res.* **31:**1066–1068.
68. Reference deleted.
69. **Jahrling, P. B.** 1983. Protection of Lassa virus-infected guinea pigs with Lassa-immune plasma of guinea pig, primate, and human origin. *J. Med. Virol.* **12:**93–102.
70. **Jahrling, P. B., B. S. Niklasson, and J. B. McCormick.** 1985. Early diagnosis of human Lassa fever by ELISA detection of antigen and antibody. *Lancet* **i:**250–252.

71. **Jahrling, P. B., and C. J. Peters.** 1986. Serology and virulence diversity among Old-World arenaviruses, and the relevance to vaccine development. *Med. Microbiol. Immunol.* **175:**165–167.
72. **Jahrling, P. B., C. J. Peters, and E. L. Stephen.** 1984. Enhanced treatment of Lassa fever by immune plasma combined with ribavirin in cynomolgus monkeys. *J. Infect. Dis.* **149:**420–427.
73. **Johnson, K. M., S. B. Halstead, and S. N. Cohen.** 1967. Hemorrhagic fevers of Southeast Asia and South America: a comparative appraisal. *Prog. Med. Virol.* **9:**105–158.
74. **Johnson, K. M., J. B. McCormick, P. A. Webb, E. S. Smith, L. H. Elliott, and I. J. King.** 1987. Clinical virology of Lassa fever in hospitalized patients. *J. Infect. Dis.* **155:**456–464.
75. **Joly, E., L. Mucke, and M. B. Oldstone.** 1991. Viral persistence in neurons explained by lack of major histocompatibility class I expression. *Science* **253:**1283–1285.
76. **Keenlyside, R. A., J. B. McCormick, P. A. Webb, E. Smith, L. Elliott, and K. M. Johnson.** 1983. Case-control study of Mastomys natalensis and humans in Lassa virus-infected households in Sierra Leone. *Am. J. Trop. Med. Hyg.* **32:**829–837.
77. **Kentsis, A., E. C. Dwyer, J. M. Perez, M. Sharma, A. Chen, Z. Q. Pan, and K. L. Borden.** 2001. The RING domains of the promyelocytic leukemia protein PML and the arenaviral protein Z repress translation by directly inhibiting translation initiation factor eIF4E. *J. Mol. Biol.* **312:**609–623.
78. **Kenyon, R. H., P. G. Canonico, D. E. Green, and C. J. Peters.** 1986. Effect of ribavirin and tributylribavirin on Argentine hemorrhagic fever (Junin virus) in guinea pigs. *Antimicrob. Agents Chemother.* **29:**521–523.
79. **Kenyon, R. H., R. M. Condie, P. B. Jahrling, and C. J. Peters.** 1990. Protection of guinea pigs against experimental Argentine hemorrhagic fever by purified human IgG: importance of elimination of infected cells. *Microb. Pathog.* **9:**219–226.
80. **Kenyon, R. H., D. E. Green, and C. J. Peters.** 1985. Effect of immunosuppression on experimental Argentine hemorrhagic fever in guinea pigs. *J. Virol.* **53:**75–80.
81. **Kenyon, R. H., K. T. McKee, Jr., P. M. Zack, M. K. Rippy, A. P. Vogel, C. York, J. Meegan, C. Crabbs, and C. J. Peters.** 1992. Aerosol infection of rhesus macaques with Junin virus. *Intervirology* **33:**23–31.
82. **Kenyon, R. H., and C. J. Peters.** 1989. Actions of complement on Junin virus. *Rev. Infect. Dis.* **11**(Suppl. 4)**:** S771–S776.
83. **Kilgore, P. E., T. G. Ksiazek, P. E. Rollin, J. N. Mills, M. R. Villagra, M. J. Montenegro, M. A. Costales, L. C. Paredes, and C. J. Peters.** 1997. Treatment of Bolivian hemorrhagic fever with intravenous ribavirin. *Clin. Infect. Dis.* **24:**718–722.
84. **Klavinskis, L. S., A. L. Notkins, and M. B. Oldstone.** 1988. Persistent viral infection of the thyroid gland: alteration of thyroid function in the absence of tissue injury. *Endocrinology* **122:**567–575.
85. **Knobloch, J., J. B. McCormick, P. A. Webb, M. Dietrich, H. H. Schumacher, and E. Dennis.** 1980. Clinical observations in 42 patients with Lassa fever. *Tropenmed. Parasitol.* **31:**389–398.
86. **Komrower, G. M., B. L. Williams, and P. B. Stones.** 1955. Lymphocytic choriomeningitis in the newborn; probable transplacental infection. *Lancet* **ii:**697–698.
87. **Kraft, V., and B. Meyer.** 1990. Seromonitoring in small laboratory animal colonies. A five year survey: 1984–1988. *Z. Verstierkd.* **33:**29–35.
88. **Lecompte, E., E. Fichet-Calvet, S. Daffis, K. Koulémou, O. Sylla, F. Kourouma, A. Doré, B. Soropogui, V. Aniskin, B. Allali, S. Kouassi Kan, A. Lalis, L. Koivogui, S. Günther, C. Denys, and J. ter Meulen.** 2006. Mastomys natalensis and Lassa fever, West Africa. *Emerg. Infect. Dis.* **12:**1971–1974.
89. **Lecompte, E., J. ter Meulen, S. Emonet, S. Daffis, and R. N. Charrel.** 2007. Genetic identification of Kodoko virus, a novel arenavirus of the African pigmy mouse (Mus Nannomys minutoides) in West Africa. *Virology* **364:**178–183.
90. **Lehmann-Grube, F.** 1971. *Lymphocytic Choriomeningitis Virus*. Springer-Verlag, New York, NY.
91. **Lehmann-Grube, F., M. Kallay, B. Ibscher, and R. Schwartz.** 1979. Serologic diagnosis of human infections with lymphocytic choriomeningitis virus: comparative evaluation of seven methods. *J. Med. Virol.* **4:**125–136.
92. **Lenz, O., J. ter Meulen, H. Feldmann, H. D. Klenk, and W. Garten.** 2000. Identification of a novel consensus sequence at the cleavage site of the Lassa virus glycoprotein. *J. Virol.* **74:**11418–11421.
93. **Levis, S. C., M. C. Saavedra, C. Ceccoli, M. R. Feuillade, D. A. Enria, J. I. Maiztegui, and R. Falcoff.** 1985. Correlation between endogenous interferon and the clinical evolution of patients with Argentine hemorrhagic fever. *J. Interferon Res.* **5:**383–389.
94. **Lewis, J. M., and J. P. Utz.** 1961. Orchitis, parotitis and meningoencephalitis due to lymphocytic-choriomeningitis virus. *N. Engl. J. Med.* **265:**776–780.
95. **Lewis, V. J., P. D. Walter, W. L. Thacker, and W. G. Winkler.** 1975. Comparison of three tests for the serological diagnosis of lymphocytic choriomeningitis virus infection. *J. Clin. Microbiol.* **2:**193–197.
96. **Lozano, M. E., D. Enria, J. I. Maiztegui, O. Grau, and V. Romanowski.** 1995. Rapid diagnosis of Argentine hemorrhagic fever by reverse transcriptase PCR-based assay. *J. Clin. Microbiol.* **33:**1327–1332. (Erratum, *J. Clin. Microbiol.* **34:**1351, 1996.)
97. **Lozano, M. E., D. M. Posik, C. G. Albarino, G. Schujman, P. D. Ghiringhelli, G. Calderon, M. Sabattini, and V. Romanowski.** 1997. Characterization of arenaviruses using a family-specific primer set for RT-PCR amplification and RFLP analysis. Its potential use for detection of uncharacterized arenaviruses. *Virus Res.* **49:** 79–89.
98. **Lukashevich, I. S., M. Djavani, J. D. Rodas, J. C. Zapata, A. Usborne, C. Emerson, J. Mitchen, P. B. Jahrling, and M. S. Salvato.** 2002. Hemorrhagic fever occurs after intravenous, but not after intragastric, inoculation of rhesus macaques with lymphocytic choriomeningitis virus. *J. Med. Virol.* **67:**171–186.
99. **Lunkenheimer, K., F. T. Hufert, and H. Schmitz.** 1990. Detection of Lassa virus RNA in specimens from patients with Lassa fever by using the polymerase chain reaction. *J. Clin. Microbiol.* **28:**2689–2692.
100. **Mahanty, S., D. G. Bausch, R. L. Thomas, A. Goba, A. Bah, C. J. Peters, and P. E. Rollin.** 2001. Low levels of interleukin-8 and interferon-inducible protein-10 in serum are associated with fatal infections in acute Lassa fever. *J. Infect. Dis.* **183:**1713–1721.
101. **Mahanty, S., K. Hutchinson, S. Agarwal, M. McRae, P. E. Rollin, and B. Pulendran.** 2003. Cutting edge: impairment of dendritic cells and adaptive immunity by Ebola and Lassa viruses. *J. Immunol.* **170:**2797–2801.
102. **Mahanty, S., R. Kalwar, and P. E. Rollin.** 1999. Cytokine measurement in biological samples after physicochemical treatment for inactivation of biosafety level 4 viral agents. *J. Med. Virol.* **59:**341–345.
103. **McCormick, J. B., I. J. King, P. A. Webb, K. M. Johnson, R. O'Sullivan, E. S. Smith, S. Trippel, and T. C. Tong.** 1987. A case-control study of the clinical diag-

nosis and course of Lassa fever. *J. Infect. Dis.* **155:**445–455.

104. **McCormick, J. B., P. A. Webb, J. W. Krebs, K. M. Johnson, and E. S. Smith.** 1987. A prospective study of the epidemiology and ecology of Lassa fever. *J. Infect. Dis.* **155:**437–444.
105. **Meyer, H. M., Jr., R. T. Johnson, I. P. Crawford, H. E. Dascomb, and N. G. Rogers.** 1960. Central nervous system syndromes of "vital" etiology. A study of 713 cases. *Am. J. Med.* **29:**334–347.
106. **Mills, J. N., B. A. Ellis, J. E. Childs, K. T. McKee, Jr., J. I. Maiztegui, C. J. Peters, T. G. Ksiazek, and P. B. Jahrling.** 1994. Prevalence of infection with Junin virus in rodent populations in the epidemic area of Argentine hemorrhagic fever. *Am. J. Trop. Med. Hyg.* **51:**554–562.
107. **Mills, J. N., B. A. Ellis, K. T. McKee, Jr., T. G. Ksiazek, J. G. Oro, J. I. Maiztegui, G. E. Calderon, C. J. Peters, and J. E. Childs.** 1991. Junin virus activity in rodents from endemic and nonendemic loci in central Argentina. *Am. J. Trop. Med. Hyg.* **44:**589–597.
108. **Mitchell, S. W., and J. B. McCormick.** 1984. Physicochemical inactivation of Lassa, Ebola, and Marburg viruses and effect on clinical laboratory analyses. *J. Clin. Microbiol.* **20:**486–489.
109. **Molteni, H. D., H. C. Guarinos, C. O. Petrillo, and F. Jaschek.** 1961. Clinico-statistical study of 338 patients with epidemic hemorrhagic fever in the northwest of the province of Buenos Aires. *Sem. Med.* **118:**839–855. (In Spanish.)
110. **Monson, M. H., A. K. Cole, J. D. Frame, J. R. Serwint, S. Alexander, and P. B. Jahrling.** 1987. Pediatric Lassa fever: a review of 33 Liberian cases. *Am. J. Trop. Med. Hyg.* **36:**408–415.
111. **Monson, M. H., J. D. Frame, P. B. Jahrling, and K. Alexander.** 1984. Endemic Lassa fever in Liberia. I. Clinical and epidemiological aspects at Curran Lutheran Hospital, Zorzor, Liberia. *Trans. R. Soc. Trop. Med. Hyg.* **78:**549–553.
112. **Montali, R. J., B. M. Connolly, D. L. Armstrong, C. A. Scanga, and K. V. Holmes.** 1995. Pathology and immunohistochemistry of callitrichid hepatitis, an emerging disease of captive New World primates caused by lymphocytic choriomeningitis virus. *Am. J. Pathol.* **147:**1441–1449.
113. **Müller, S., and S. Günther.** 2007. Broad-spectrum antiviral activity of small interfering RNA targeting the conserved RNA termini of Lassa virus. *Antimicrob. Agents Chemother.* **51:**2215–2218.
114. **Nicklas, W., V. Kraft, and B. Meyer.** 1993. Contamination of transplantable tumors, cell lines, and monoclonal antibodies with rodent viruses. *Lab. Anim. Sci.* **43:**296–300.
115. **Niedrig, M., H. Schmitz, S. Becker, S. Günther, J. ter Meulen, H. Meyer, H. Ellerbrok, A. Nitsche, H. R. Gelderblom, and C. Drosten.** 2004. First international quality assurance study on the rapid detection of viral agents of bioterrorism. *J. Clin. Microbiol.* **42:**1753–1755.
116. **Oldstone, M. B.** 2002. Arenaviruses. I. The epidemiology molecular and cell biology of arenaviruses. Introduction. *Curr. Top. Microbiol. Immunol.* **262:**V–XII.
117. **Oldstone, M. B.** 2002. Arenaviruses. II. The molecular pathogenesis of arenavirus infections. Introduction. *Curr. Top. Microbiol. Immunol.* **263:**V–XII.
118. **Oldstone, M. B., R. Ahmed, M. J. Buchmeier, P. Blount, and A. Tishon.** 1985. Perturbation of differentiated functions during viral infection in vivo. I. Relationship of lymphocytic choriomeningitis virus and host strains to growth hormone deficiency. *Virology* **142:**158–174.
119. **Oldstone, M. B., A. Tishon, and M. J. Buchmeier.** 1983. Virus-induced immune complex disease: genetic control of C1q binding complexes in the circulation of mice persistently infected with lymphocytic choriomeningitis virus. *J. Immunol.* **130:**912–918.
120. **Palacios, G., J. Druce, L. Du, T. Tran, C. Birch, T. Briese, S. Conlan, P. L. Quan, J. Hui, J. Marshall, J. F. Simons, M. Egholm, C. D. Paddock, W. J. Shieh, C. S. Goldsmith, S. R. Zaki, M. Catton, and W. I. Lipkin.** 2008. A new arenavirus in a cluster of fatal transplant-associated diseases. *N. Engl. J. Med.* **358:**991–998.
121. **Park, J. Y., C. J. Peters, P. E. Rollin, T. G. Ksiazek, B. Gray, K. B. Waites, and C. B. Stephensen.** 1997. Development of a reverse transcription-polymerase chain reaction assay for diagnosis of lymphocytic choriomeningitis virus infection and its use in a prospective surveillance study. *J. Med. Virol.* **51:**107–114.
122. **Park, J. Y., C. J. Peters, P. E. Rollin, T. G. Ksiazek, C. R. Katholi, K. B. Waites, B. Gray, H. M. Maetz, and C. B. Stephensen.** 1997. Age distribution of lymphocytic choriomeningitis virus serum antibody in Birmingham, Alabama: evidence of a decreased risk of infection. *Am. J. Trop. Med. Hyg.* **57:**37–41.
123. **Peters, C. J.** 1996. Pathogenesis of viral hemorrhagic fevers, p. 779–799. *In* N. Nathanson, R. Ahmed, F. Gonzales-Scarano, D. Griffin, K. V. Holmes, F. A. Murphy, and H. L. Robinson (ed.), *Viral Pathogenesis*. Lippincott-Raven, Philadelphia, PA.
124. **Peters, C. J., R. W. Kuehne, R. R. Mercado, R. H. Le Bow, R. O. Spertzel, and P. A. Webb.** 1974. Hemorrhagic fever in Cochabamba, Bolivia, 1971. *Am. J. Epidemiol.* **99:**425–433.
125. **Peters, C. J.** 2006. Lymphocytic choriomeningitis virus—an old enemy up to new tricks. *N. Engl. J. Med.* **354:**2208–2211.
126. **Peters, C. J., P. B. Jahrling, and A. S. Khan.** 1996. Patients infected with high-hazard viruses: scientific basis for infection control. *Arch. Virol. Suppl.* **11:**141–168.
127. **Peters, C. J., P. B. Jahrling, C. T. Liu, R. H. Kenyon, K. T. McKee, Jr., and J. G. Barrera Oro.** 1987. Experimental studies of arenaviral hemorrhagic fevers. *Curr. Top. Microbiol. Immunol.* **134:**5–68.
128. **Peters, C. J., P. A. Webb, and K. M. Johnson.** 1973. Measurement of antibodies to Machupo virus by the indirect fluorescent technique. *Proc. Soc. Exp. Biol. Med.* **142:**526–531.
129. **Peters, C. J.** 1991. Arenaviruses, p. 541–570. *In* R. Belshe (ed.), *Textbook of Human Virology*, 2nd ed. Mosby Year Book, St. Louis, MO.
130. **Price, M. E., S. P. Fisher-Hoch, R. B. Craven, and J. B. McCormick.** 1988. A prospective study of maternal and fetal outcome in acute Lassa fever infection during pregnancy. *BMJ* **297:**584–587.
131. **Rousseau, M. C., M. F. Saron, P. Brouqui, and A. Bourgeade.** 1997. Lymphocytic choriomeningitis virus in southern France: four case reports and a review of the literature. *Eur. J. Epidemiol.* **13:**817–823.
132. **Rowe, W. P.** 1954. Studies on pathogenesis and immunity in lymphocytic choriomeningitis infection of the mouse. Naval Medical Research Institute, National Naval Medical Center. *Res. Rep.* **12:**167–220.
133. **Ruggiero, H. R., H. Ruggiero, C. Gonzales-Cambaceres, F. A. Cintora, F. Maglio, C. C. Magnoni, L. N. Astarloa, G. J. Squassi, A. Giacosa, and D. Fernandez.** 1964. Argentine hemorrhagic fever. II. Clinical studies. *Rev. Asoc. Med. Argent.* **78:**281–294.
134. **Sabattini, M. S., and M. S. Contigiani.** 1982. Ecological and biological factors influencing the maintenance of arenaviruses in nature, with special reference to the agent

of Argentinean haemorrhagic fever, p. 251–262. *In International Symposium on Tropical Arboviruses and Haemorrhagic Fevers*. Academia Brasileira de Ciencias, Rio de Janeiro, Brazil.

135. **Sabattini, M. S., L. E. Gonzalez de Rios, G. Diaz, and V. R. Vega.** 1977. Enfeccion natural y experimental de roedores con virus Junin. *Medicina* (Buenos Aires) **37:** 149–161.
136. **Saijo, M., M. C. Georges-Courbot, P. Marianneau, V. Romanowski, S. Fukushi, T. Mizutani, A. J. Georges, T. Kurata, I. Kurane, and S. Morikawa.** 2007. Development of recombinant nucleoprotein-based diagnostic systems for Lassa fever. *Clin. Vaccine Immunol.* **14:**1182–1189.
137. **Salas, R., N. de Manzione, R. B. Tesh, R. Rico-Hesse, R. E. Shope, A. Betancourt, O. Godoy, R. Bruzual, M. E. Pacheco, and B. Ramos.** 1991. Venezuelan haemorrhagic fever. *Lancet* **338:**1033–1036.
138. **Salas, R. A., N. de Manzione, and R. Tesh.** 1998. Venezuelan hemorrhagic fever: eight years of observation. *Acta Cient. Venez.* **49**(Suppl. 1)**:**46–51. (In Spanish.)
139. **Salazar-Bravo, J., L. A. Ruedas, and T. L. Yates.** 2002. Mammalian reservoirs of arenaviruses. *Curr. Top. Microbiol. Immunol.* **262:**25–63.
140. **Schulte, D. J., J. A. Comer, B. R. Erickson, P. E. Rollin, S. T. Nichol, T. G. Ksiazek, and D. Lehman.** 2006. Congenital lymphocytic choriomeningitis virus: an underdiagnosed cause of neonatal hydrocephalus. *Pediatr. Infect. Dis. J.* **25:**560–562.
141. **Schwarz, E. R., O. G. Mando, J. I. Maiztegui, and A. M. Vilches.** 1970. Sintomas y signos iniciales de mayor valor diagnostico en la fiebre hemorragica argentina. *Medicina* (Buenos Aires) **30**(Suppl. 1)**:**8–14.
142. **Sheinbergas, M. M., R. S. Ptashekas, R. L. Pikelite, I. Tuliavichene, and I. Sverdlov.** 1977. Clinical and pathomorphologic findings in hydrocephalus caused by prenatal infection with lymphocytic choriomeningitis virus. *Zh. Nevropatol. Psikhiatr. Im. S. S. Korsakova* **77:**1004–1007. (In Russian.)
143. **Smadel, J. E., R. H. Green, R. F. Paltauf, and T. A. Gonzales.** 1942. Lymphocytic choriomeningitis; two human fatalities following an unusual febrile illness. *Proc. Soc. Exp. Biol.* **49:**683–686.
144. **Smee, D. F., J. Gilbert, J. A. Leonhardt, B. B. Barnett, J. H. Huggins, and R. W. Sidwell.** 1993. Treatment of lethal Pichinde virus infections in weanling LVG/Lak hamsters with ribavirin, ribamidine, selenazofurin, and ampligen. *Antivir. Res.* **20:**57–70.
145. **Smith, A. L., F. X. Paturzo, E. P. Gardner, S. Morgenstern, G. Cameron, and H. Wadley.** 1984. Two epizootics of lymphocytic choriomeningitis virus occurring in laboratory mice despite intensive monitoring programs. *Can. J. Comp. Med.* **48:**335–337.
146. **Solbrig, M. V.** 1993. Lassa virus and central nervous system diseases, p. 331–373. *In* M. S. Salvato (ed.), *The Arenaviridae*. Plenum Press, New York, NY.
147. **Southern, P.** 1996. *Arenaviridae:* the viruses and their replication, p. 1505–1551. *In* B. N. Fields, D. M. Knipe, and P. M. Howley (ed.), *Fields Virology*, 3rd ed. Lippincott-Raven Publishers, Philadelphia, PA.
148. **Spiropoulou, C. F., S. Kunz, P. E. Rollin, K. P. Campbell, and M. B. A. Oldstone.** 2002. New World arenavirus clade C, but not clade A and B viruses, utilizes α-dystroglycan as its major receptor. *J. Virol.* **76:**5140–5146.
149. **Stephen, E. L., S. K. Scott, G. A. Eddy, and H. B. Levy.** 1977. Effect of interferon on togavirus and arenavirus infections of animals. *Tex. Rep. Biol. Med.* **35:**449–454.
150. **Stephenson, E. H., E. W. Larson, and J. W. Dominik.** 1984. Effect of environmental factors on aerosol-induced Lassa virus infection. *J. Med. Virol.* **14:**295–303.
151. **Stinebaugh, B. J., F. X. Schloeder, K. M. Johnson, R. B. Mackenzie, G. Entwisle, and E. De Alba.** 1966. Bolivian hemorrhagic fever. A report of four cases. *Am. J. Med.* **40:**217–230.
152. **Strecker, T., A. Maisa, S. Daffis, R. Eichler, O. Lenz, and W. Garten.** 2006. The role of myristoylation in the membrane association of the Lassa virus matrix protein *Z. Virol. J.* **3:**93.
153. **Uprichard, S. L., S. F. Wieland, A. Althage, and F. V. Chisari.** 2003. Transcriptional and posttranscriptional control of hepatitis B virus gene expression. *Proc. Natl. Acad. Sci. USA* **100:**1310–1315.
154. **Vanzee, B. E., R. G. Douglas, R. F. Betts, A. W. Bauman, D. W. Fraser, and A. R. Hinman.** 1975. Lymphocytic choriomeningitis in university hospital personnel. Clinical features. *Am. J. Med.* **58:**803–809.
155. **Walker, D. H., J. B. McCormick, K. M. Johnson, P. A. Webb, G. Komba-Kono, L. H. Elliott, and J. J. Gardner.** 1982. Pathologic and virologic study of fatal Lassa fever in man. *Am. J. Pathol.* **107:**349–356.
156. **Warkel, R. L., C. F. Rinaldi, W. H. Bancroft, R. D. Cardiff, G. E. Holmes, and R. E. Wilsnack.** 1973. Fatal acute meningoencephalitis due to lymphocytic choriomeningitis virus. *Neurology* **23:**198–203.
157. **Weaver, S. C., R. A. Salas, N. de Manzione, C. F. Fulhorst, G. Duno, A. Utrera, J. N. Mills, T. G. Ksiazek, D. Tovar, and R. B. Tesh.** 2000. Guanarito virus (Arenaviridae) isolates from endemic and outlying localities in Venezuela: sequence comparisons among and within strains isolated from Venezuelan hemorrhagic fever patients and rodents. *Virology* **266:**189–195.
158. **Wright, R., D. Johnson, M. Neumann, T. G. Ksiazek, P. Rollin, R. V. Keech, D. J. Bonthius, P. Hitchon, C. F. Grose, W. E. Bell, and J. F. Bale, Jr.** 1997. Congenital lymphocytic choriomeningitis virus syndrome: a disease that mimics congenital toxoplasmosis or cytomegalovirus infection. *Pediatrics* **100:**E9.
159. **Wulff, H., and K. M. Johnson.** 1979. Immunoglobulin M and G responses measured by immunofluorescence in patients with Lassa or Marburg virus infections. *Bull. W. H. O.* **57:**631–635.
160. **Zinkernagel, R. M.** 2002. Lymphocytic choriomeningitis virus and immunology. *Curr. Top. Microbiol. Immunol.* **263:**1–5.

Enteroviruses

JOSÉ R. ROMERO

45

VIROLOGY

Taxonomy

The genus *Enterovirus* was so designated because its members replicate in the human gastrointestinal (GI) tract. The original taxonomic classification of the enteroviruses (EVs) recognized 64 prototype serotypes within the family *Picornaviridae* ("pico" meaning small, "rna" for RNA genome) (Table 1) (191, 203). Additional serotypes continue to be discovered, and members of the genus currently exceed 90 confirmed or potential serotypes (123, 180, 181, 185, 186, 244). The "traditional" species designation within the genus includes the polioviruses, coxsackieviruses A and B, echoviruses, and the "numbered" EVs (Table 1). This original subclassification of the EVs was based on the ability of individual serotypes to grow in various cell cultures and produce disease in animal systems (191).

A century ago, the polioviruses were the first of the EVs identified as a result of their pathogenicity for humans (144). In animal models, they could produce flaccid paralysis in monkeys but failed to induce disease in murine systems. With the advent of tissue culture, they were found to replicate prolifically in cells of human and simian origin. The coxsackieviruses followed as the next species within the genus to be identified. The type A coxsackievirus serotypes characteristically are capable of replication in suckling mice which results in a diffuse myositis and flaccid paralysis. In cell culture they did not readily replicate in simian- or human-derived cells. In contrast, type B coxsackieviruses grow readily in tissue cultures of both simian and human origin as well as in suckling mice. Their pathology in suckling mice differed from that of type A serotypes in that the myositis was more focal, and direct infection of brain, myocardium, pancreas, and liver also occurred. Neither type A nor type B coxsackieviruses were pathogenic for monkeys. The echoviruses (enteric cytopathic human orphan viruses), so designated because of their initial apparent lack of association with human disease, were defined by their ability to grow well in simian-derived tissue culture cells but not at all in suckling mice or monkeys. The original distinctions based on cell culture and animal systems became significantly blurred as new strains were identified and by use of new cell lines that have resulted in crossover patterns of EV growth. For that reason, serotypes reported from 1974 to date have been designated "numbered" EVs (EVs 68, 69, etc.) (161).

Assignment of new serotypes within each of the EV species was based on generation of antisera against the new serotype and reciprocal cross-neutralization testing using a complete panel of prototype strains and antisera (51). Even using such an approach, misclassification occurred which required reclassification of several of the original EV serotypes. Coxsackievirus A23 and echovirus 8 were found to be identical to echoviruses 9 and 1, respectively. Echoviruses 10 and 28 have been reclassified as reovirus 1 and human rhinovirus 1A, respectively.

The advent of molecular virology opened the way for further refinement of definition of the genus *Enterovirus* and its species and constituent serotypes. Hepatitis A virus (EV 72) was moved into a new genus, *Hepatovirus*. Sequence analysis of echoviruses 22 and 23 has demonstrated them to be genotypically distinct from other members of the genus (110) and led to their reclassification into a genus unto themselves called *Parechovirus*. Phylogenetic analysis using the complete coding sequence of VP1, the major EV capsid protein, has been found to be extremely useful in defining EV taxonomy at the species and serotype levels (183, 184, 244). Using this approach, it was recognized that several EVs originally accepted as individual serotypes were, in fact, strains of one another (coxsackieviruses A11 [prototype strain Belgium-1], A15 [prototype strain G-9], A13 [prototype strain Flores], and A18 [prototype strain G-13]) (183).

A redefinition of the criteria for species demarcation within the genus *Enterovirus*, based on molecular and biological characteristics, has been issued by the International Committee on Taxonomy of Viruses (244). Criteria currently in use for species demarcation of the EVs require that members of an EV species share greater than 70% amino acid identity in the viral capsid P1 coding region and the nonstructural proteins 2C and 3CD; share a limited range of natural hosts and host receptors; possess a genome base composition of guanine and cytosine that varies by no more than 2.5%; and share a significant degree of compatibility in proteolytic processing, replication, encapsidation, and genetic recombination. Based on these criteria, the human EVs are now classified into five species: *Poliovirus* and *Human enterovirus* A through *Human enter-*

TABLE 1 The human EVs[a]

Traditional classification	Revised classification
Poliovirus (3 serotypes) Polioviruses 1–3	Poliovirus Polioviruses 1–3
Coxsackievirus Group A (23 serotypes) Coxsackievirus A1–A22, A24[b] Group B (6 serotypes) Coxsackieviruses B1–B6	Human EV A Coxsackieviruses A2–A8, 10, 12, 14, 16 EVs 71, 76, 89, 90[c] Human EV B Coxsackievirus A9 Coxsackieviruses B1–B6
Echovirus (28 serotypes) Echoviruses 1–7, 9, 11–21, 24–27, 29–33[b]	Echoviruses 1–7, 9, 11–21, 24–27, 29–33
Numbered EVs (4 serotypes) EVs 68–71[b]	EVs 69, 73–75, 77, 78, *79–88, 100, 101*[c] Human EV C Coxsackieviruses A1, A11, A13, A17, A19–A22, A24 Human EV D EVs 68, 70

[a] See references 37, 43, and 244.
[b] Coxsackievirus A23, echoviruses 8, 10, 22, 23, and 28, and enterovirus 72 have been reclassified.
[c] Serotypes in italics are not yet recognized by the International Committee on Taxonomy of Viruses.

ovirus D. This has resulted in a redistribution of the original EVs into new groupings (Table 1).

Recombination between the vaccine strains of poliovirus (Sabin strains) and the nonpoliovirus EVs occurs in nature and can give rise to vaccine-derived polioviruses (VDPVs). These recombinant events generally occur between the C species EVs and Sabin strains of poliovirus (131). VDPVs are 1 to 15% divergent with their parental Sabin strains. Further characterization is based on epidemiological or clinical characteristics. Circulating VDPVs (cVDPVs) emerge in areas with inadequate oral poliovirus vaccine coverage. Strains isolated from individuals with primary immunodeficiencies who have had prolonged infections with VDPV as a result of exposure to one of the Sabin strains of poliovirus, usually as a result of vaccination, are designated immunodeficiency-associated VDPVs. VDPV strains isolated from individuals without an immunodeficiency or isolates from the environment of persons for whom the ultimate source was not identified are designated ambiguous VDPVs.

Viral Structure

Like other members of the family *Picornaviridae*, the EVs are small (30 nm in diameter), consisting of a nonenveloped protein capsid and a single strand of positive (message)-sense RNA (203). The encapsulated RNA of the human EVs constitutes approximately 30% of the virion mass. The buoyant density of the EVs in CsCl is 1.30 to 1.34 g/cm^3 (203, 244). Because of their lack of a lipid envelope, EVs are insensitive to organic solvents. They are insensitive to nonionic detergents. EVs are stable at an acid pH of 3.0 or lower, a characteristic that allows them to traverse the stomach and gain access to the intestine, where they replicate. The EVs are inactivated by heat (>56°C), UV light, chlorination, and formaldehyde. These physical and chemical characteristics confer environmental stability on the EVs, permitting them to survive for days to weeks in water and sewage.

The capsid is comprised of four proteins: VP1, VP2, VP3, and VP4. The amino acid chains that comprise proteins VP1, VP2, and VP3 arrange themselves to form eight stranded antiparallel β-sheet structures in what has been playfully designated a "β-barrel jelly roll" (96) (Fig. 1). The amino acids that connect the β-strands and that make up the N- and C-terminal sequences extending from the β-barrel domain provide each EV serotype with its surface topography and unique antigenicity. The four capsid proteins assemble to yield a protomer with proteins VP1, VP2, and VP3 exposed on the surface of the virion and VP4 beneath them, lacking a surface exposure (Fig. 1). Five protomeric units assemble to form a pentamer. In turn, 12 pentamers assemble to form the mature virion. Thus, each virion is comprised of 60 repeating protomeric units consisting of equimolar amounts of each capsid. For all poliovirus serotypes, neutralization sites are most densely clustered on VP1, the largest and most surface exposed of the capsid proteins (165).

The atomic structures of several EVs have been resolved and reveal multiple common structural motifs (93, 96, 173). The apex of each pentameric unit (i.e., fivefold axis of symmetry) forms a "star-shaped" promontory or "plateau" surrounded by a deep cleft or "canyon" (Fig. 1). The canyon serves as the viral receptor binding site. At the floor of the canyon is a hydrophobic "pocket" that tunnels toward the fivefold axis. At the threefold axis of symmetry, the surface topography of the EV resembles that of a "propeller."

Viral Genome

The RNA genome of the EVs is approximately 7.4 kb in length (Fig. 2) (203). At the 5′ end of the genome is a virally encoded, covalently linked polypeptide, VPg (3B). A long 5′ noncoding region (NCR) of approximately 1/10 the length of the total genome precedes a single open reading frame (ORF) which spans from approximately nucleotide (nt) 740 to nt 7370. The ORF is followed by a short 3′ NCR and a terminal polyadenylated tail.

The 5′ NCR possesses regions of high nucleotide identity in which nucleotide sequences with absolute (or near absolute) conservation exist among the EVs (214, 216). These regions have been exploited for the design of primers and probes used for the detection of EVs through nucleic acid amplification techniques (e.g., reverse transcription-PCR [RT-PCR] and nucleic acid sequence-based amplification [NASBA]) (215). Additionally, internal RNA-RNA interactions within this region result in higher-order structures that have essential functions in replication and translation (5, 91, 196, 246) of the EV genome.

The EV ORF is subdivided into three regions, designated P1 to P3 (203). The P1 region codes for the four structural proteins (VP1 to VP4) that form the viral capsid. The capsid protein coding sequences are contiguous to one another and are organized 5′ to 3′ as VP4 (1A), VP2 (1B), VP3 (1C), and VP1 (1D), without intervening stop codons (Fig. 2). The largest and most surface exposed of the capsid proteins is VP1. It contains type-specific epitopes correlating with serotype (164, 183, 208, 244). For all poliovirus serotypes, neutralization sites are most densely clustered on VP1. Additional major neutralizing epitopes have been identified on VP2 and VP3. It is probable that immuno-

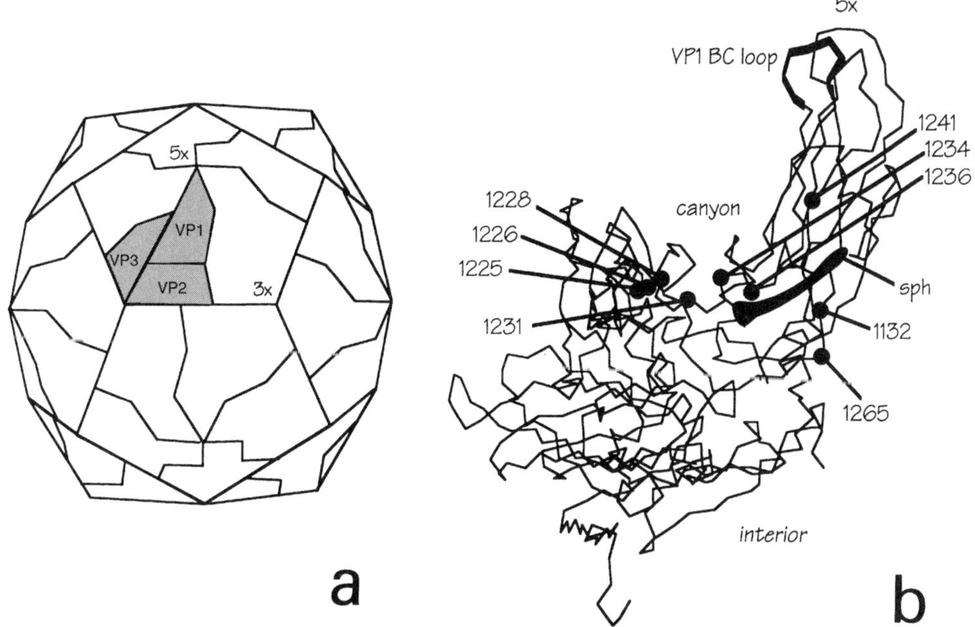

FIGURE 1 (a) Schematic representation of the icosahedral viral capsid structure of the EV. The fivefold (5x) and threefold (3x) axes of symmetry are indicated, as is the position of one of the 60 repeating protomeric units, each comprised of VP1, VP2, and VP3 surface proteins. (b) Line drawing of the VP1 and VP2 proteins in their tertiary configuration. The canyon structure, into which the cellular receptor for the EVs fits, is illustrated with its sphingosine (sph) hydrocarbon-binding pocket. (Reprinted from reference 202 with permission.)

dominant epitopes also exist on the VP1 proteins of other EVs. VP1 coding sequences serve as the target for "molecular serotyping" of the EVs (184). Destabilization of VP4, as a result of viral binding to its receptor, results in virus uncoating (15).

The P2 and P3 regions code for seven nonstructural proteins (5′-2A, 2B, 2C, 3A, 3B, 3C, and 3D-3′) and intermediates required for the viral life cycle (Fig. 2) (203). The EV genome codes for two proteases: $2A^{pro}$ and $3C^{pro}$. An intermediate protein product, $3CD^{pro}$, also possesses proteolytic activity. $2A^{pro}$ may also play a role in viral replication. The 2B protein plays a not yet clearly elucidated role in viral RNA synthesis which may include proliferation of membrane vesicles, the site of RNA replication. Protein 2C may have two functions, one as an NTPase and the other directing replication complexes to the cell membranes. Protein 3AB is believed to anchor VPg (3B) to membranes for priming of RNA synthesis. Enteroviruses encode a viral RNA-dependent RNA polymerase designated $3D^{pol}$.

Viral Replication

The viral life cycle begins with attachment of EV to its cellular receptor. Multiple cell surface molecules have been identified that serve as receptors or coreceptors for EV (202, 203). For the polioviruses, a single protein, CD155 or PVr (poliovirus receptor), is sufficient for cell entry (162). The poliovirus receptor maps to chromosome 19. CD155 is an adhesion molecule and a member of the immunoglobulin superfamily that helps to form adherens junctions and is a recognition molecule for natural killer cells. The polioviruses interact with CD155 via the canyon that surrounds the fivefold axis of symmetry of the virion, where domain 1 of the receptor inserts itself.

In the case of other EVs (i.e., coxsackieviruses B3 and A21), interaction with two cell surface proteins may be required for access to the cell cytoplasm. For coxsackievirus B3 interaction with CD55, decay-accelerating factor (a protein of the complement cascade) is required in order to transport the virus from the apical surface of the cell to the tight junction of the cell (52), where it can interact with its primary receptor, coxsackievirus and adenovirus receptor (18). Coxsackievirus A21 binds to CD55 but requires intracellular cell adhesion molecule 1 (ICAM-1) for infection (178). For both coxsackieviruses B3 and A21, interaction with the primary cellular receptor also occurs at the level of the canyon (278). Coreceptors are believed to be required for several group B coxsackieviruses and echoviruses (203).

Lastly, coxsackievirus A9 interaction with its cellular receptor occurs at a 3-amino-acid stretch (Arg-Gly-Asp) located in a 17-amino-acid extension of the C terminus of the capsid protein VP1 (212). However, altering the Arg-Gly-Asp motif does not completely nullify viral infection of cells, indicating that a secondary receptor may be used by coxsackievirus A9 (107).

The effect of binding of the cellular receptor to the EV canyon has been extensively studied for poliovirus and has led to several models for creation of a transmembrane pore that could be used for translocation of the viral RNA across the cell membrane into the cellular cytoplasm (15, 28). Receptor binding to the canyon results in shifts of the capsid proteins VP1, VP2, and VP3 that would allow for extrusion of VP4 and the hydrophobic N terminus of VP1.

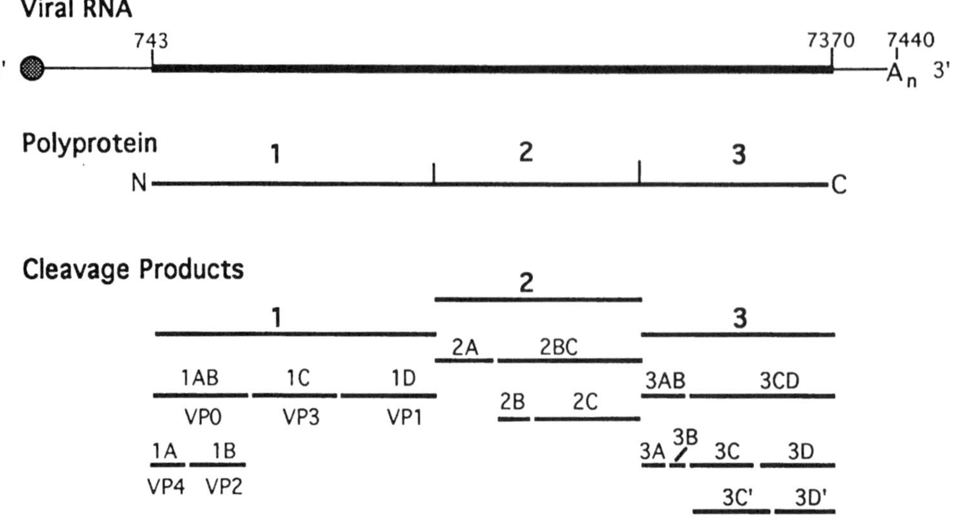

FIGURE 2 Genomic organization and translation products of the EVs, as represented by poliovirus. The cross-hatched circle indicates the covalently attached VPg molecule at the 5′ end of the RNA. The coding region (nt 743 to 7370 on this map) is shown as a thick line. The poly(A) tail at the 3′ end of the RNA is indicated by "A_n." The polyprotein coded for by the single ORF is then posttranslationally modified by viral proteases to form the viral protein cleavage products. (Reprinted from reference 121a with permission.)

Depending on the model, (i) the hydrophobic N termini of VP1 form a pore traversing the cell membrane; (ii) the hydrophobic N termini of VP1 serve as a membrane anchor, while VP4 plays a major role in forming a transmembrane pore; or (iii) the hydrophobic N termini of VP1 act together with VP4 to form a transmembrane pore.

Upon entry into the cell, the VPg protein covalently linked to the 5′ end of the viral genome is removed by a cellular protein. The EV 5′ and 3′ NCRs play critical roles in viral regulatory activities such as translation and replication (203). EVs subvert host cell protein synthesis by inhibiting the formation of the cap binding complex (eIF4F) essential for translation of the majority of cellular mRNAs. The EV protease $2A^{pro}$ cleaves eIF4G so that it cannot interact with the cap-binding protein eIF4E and serves to recruit the eIF3-40S ribosomal complex to the mRNA. Within as little as 2 h after infection, all host cell protein synthesis has been shut down by the EV.

Translation of the viral genome is carried out in a noncanonical cap-independent manner and is mediated by an approximately 500-nt-long discontinuous region of the 5′ NCR designated the internal ribosome entry site (IRES) (196). This highly structured region promotes binding of the 40S ribosomal subunit, which then scans to the initiation codon located at approximately nt 740. The model for 40S ribosomal subunit binding to the IRES proposes that EV protease-cleaved eIF4G binds to the IRES. The C-terminal domain of eIF4G interacts with the eIF3-40S ribosomal complex, recruiting it to the IRES (203). Additional cellular proteins [La, polypyrimidine tract-binding protein, unr, and poly r(C)-binding protein] have been shown to be important for IRES function (246).

Translation of the EV genome results in the generation of a single, large polyprotein (Fig. 2) that is immediately posttranslationally processed by three virally encoded proteases: $2A^{pro}$, $3C^{pro}$, and $3CD^{pro}$. $2A^{pro}$ and $3C^{pro}$ are active in the polyprotein and release themselves for it autocatalytically. $3CD^{pro}$ also self-releases from the polyprotein. The primary cleavage between the P1 and P2 regions is carried out by $2A^{pro}$. In addition, it cleaves cellular proteins eIF4GI, eIF4GII, poly(A)-binding protein 1, and dystrophin. $3C^{pro}$ is responsible for the cleave between 2C and 3A. $3CD^{pro}$ is more efficient than $3C^{pro}$ in the cleavage of the capsid proteins contained in the P1 precursor.

Genomic RNA replicates itself thousands of times within each infected cell via the virally encoded RNA-dependent RNA polymerase $3D^{pol}$ (Fig. 2). Synthesis of viral RNA is asymmetric, resulting in a 30- to 70-fold excess of positive-sense RNA (203). Viral proteins $2A^{pro}$, 2BC, 2B, 2C, 3AB, and 3B (VPg) (Fig. 2) are also involved in RNA replication. EV infection of a host cell results in cytoplasmic accumulation of smooth membrane vesicles, the surfaces of which serve as a platform for viral RNA replication. Several models have been proposed for the actual molecular mechanism of viral RNA synthesis, all of which include a replicative intermediate entity consisting of both positive- and negative-sense RNA.

In one model (203), a ribonucleoprotein complex formed by the binding of poly r(C)-binding protein and $3CD^{pro}$ to a cloverleaf domain located at the extreme upstream portion of the 5′ NCR interacts with poly(A)-binding protein 1 bound to the terminal polyadenylate tail of the viral genome. This results in circularization of the viral genome template. Binding of $3D^{pol}$, $3CD^{pro}$, and VPg to a specific viral genomic element within the 2C protein coding (cre element) results in uridylylation of VPg (i.e., VPg-pUpU). $3D^{pol}$ then uses VPg-pUpU bound to the poly(A) tail as a protein primer for negative-strand synthesis.

Assembly of the virion begins with cleavage of capsid precursor protein P1 from P2 by $2A^{pro}$. The protein $3CD^{pro}$ further cleaves P1 to yield capsid proteins VP0, VP3, and VP1. These proteins self-assemble into a protomer. Five protomers, in turn, self-assemble to yield a pentamer.

Twelve pentamers assemble to form the 80S empty capsid. One model proposes that positive-sense viral RNA threads itself into the 80S capsid to yield a 150S provirion. Final maturation of the virion occurs with cleavage of VP0 to VP2 and VP4, resulting in an infectious 160S virion. In another model, the pentamers assemble around the RNA to yield the 150S provirion. Maturation of the provirion occurs with cleavage of VP0. In this scenario, the empty 80S capsid serves merely as a depot for pentamers.

Infectious virions are released by cell lysis. The cytopathic effect of EVs in tissue culture cells has been well described (102) and remains an important diagnostic tool. Light microscopy reveals a characteristic rounding of cells and ultimately detachment from the tissue culture dish (Fig. 3). By electron microscopy, a series of changes occurs, beginning with alteration of nucleus morphology and margination of the chromatin (236). Ribosomes aggregate in the cytoplasm, and many clusters of membranous vesicles form; ultimately, the rounded and detached cells lyse.

EPIDEMIOLOGY

Humans are the only natural reservoir for the EVs. The nonpoliovirus EVs are estimated to cause between 10 million and 15 million symptomatic infections in the United States each year (248); however, the EVs are worldwide in their distribution (6, 8, 37, 85, 248, 256, 258). While the polioviruses have been largely controlled in developed countries with the introduction of vaccines, underdeveloped parts of the world continue to experience significant morbidity and mortality from those pathogens. In temperate climates, EV infections appear with a marked summer/fall seasonality (37); a high year-round incidence occurs in tropical and subtropical areas, with a higher incidence during the rainy season (157).

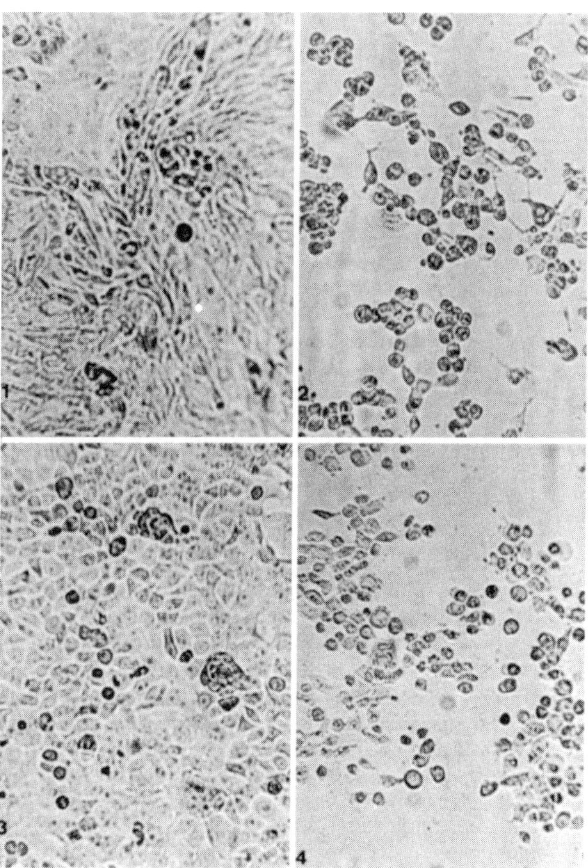

FIGURE 3 Cytopathic effect of poliovirus type 1 infection of tissue culture cells. (panel 1) Uninfected rhesus monkey kidney cells. (panel 2) Poliovirus-infected rhesus monkey kidney cells 24 h after infection. (panel 3) Uninfected HEp-2 cells. (panel 4) Poliovirus-infected HEp-2 cells 24 h after infection. (Reprinted from reference 102 with permission.)

The fecal-oral spread of these agents appears to be facilitated, particularly among children, during periods of warm weather and sparse clothing. In addition to transmission by direct person-to-person contact, EVs may be recovered from houseflies, wastewater, and sewage (17, 128, 167, 230, 263), but their role in outbreaks has not been established. In contrast, water-associated outbreaks of EVs have been demonstrated (92, 156).

Wild-type polioviruses, once major contributors to the epidemiological profile of the EVs in the United States, are no longer causes of acute flaccid paralysis (33). However, occasional imported cases of VDPV infections and vaccine-associated paralytic poliomyelitis continue to occur (34, 35), stressing the need for maintaining continued immunization against the polioviruses. Although efforts toward the global eradication of poliovirus infections resulted in the elimination of wild-type infections from the western hemisphere in 1991, polio continued to be a problem elsewhere in the world (64).

In developing countries, the prevalence of paralytic disease remained high (2 to 11 cases/1,000 population) throughout the 1970s. In 1988, the World Health Assembly resolved to eradicate poliomyelitis worldwide (39). In 1988, poliovirus was endemic to 125 countries (36), and in the early 1990s, as many as 15,000 cases of paralytic disease were estimated to occur worldwide annually. Significant progress toward worldwide eradication of poliovirus continued into the new millennium. Transmission of wild-type 2 poliovirus has not been detected anywhere in the world since October 1999 (32). By 2001, the number of countries in which polio was endemic had fallen to 10 and the annual number of cases of paralytic poliomyelitis had plummeted to 483 (276). Despite setbacks, progress toward total elimination of poliovirus transmission worldwide continues. In 2006, although the reported number of cases was four times higher than in 2001 (the result of importation of polio to countries previously polio free), the number of countries with endemic poliovirus transmission decreased to four (India, Nigeria, Pakistan, and Afganistan) (38, 276). However, importation of polio from these countries to surrounding and distant countries continues to be an ongoing problem. That same year, 13 countries reported reintroduction of polivirus, 5 of which had not reported cases in the preceding 5 years (38, 276).

A novel, unforeseen issue encountered as a result of vaccination efforts directed toward global interruption of poliovirus transmission is the appearance of VDPVs (131). The first reported outbreak of poliomyelitis secondary to these agents occurred in 2000 on the island of Hispaniola (130). VDPV-related paralytic disease or isolates have been reported in Haiti, the Dominican Republic, Madagascar, Egypt, the Philippines, Indonesia, Cambodia, and the United States (35, 39, 130). Factors favoring their development include low oral polio vaccine coverage and dense populations (130).

For the nonpoliovirus EVs, each EV season, in each part of the world, is dominated by only a few serotypes (6, 8, 37, 85, 256, 258), and in any given year, multiple EV serotypes may circulate within a community or geographic region (6, 8, 37, 85, 139, 256, 258). During the years 1970 to 2005, the predominant nonpoliovirus EV isolates identified in the United States, listed in descending order, were echoviruses 9, 11, and 30; coxsackievirus B5; echovirus 6; coxsackievirus B2; coxsackievirus A9; echovirus 4; coxsackievirus B3; echovirus 7; coxsackievirus B4; echovirus 18; coxsackievirus B1; and echoviruses 3 and 5 (37). These 15 serotypes account for approximately 80% of all EVs reported during that period.

The annual determination of predominant serotypes may be biased by reporting bias and the inability to readily grow numerous serotypes in tissue culture, particularly the group A coxsackieviruses, as well as by a skew toward those serotypes causing more serious disease (and, hence, prompting more laboratory investigation). The predominant serotypes cycle with various periodicities (37), a reflection of the availability of new susceptible host populations, especially children, within a community. Children are, indeed, the primary victims of EV infections. Data are derived from a number of sources, including the ambitious virus watch programs of the 1960s and 1970s, in which the overall incidences of infections with coxsackieviruses and echoviruses were highest among children (37, 76, 85, 139).

Because central nervous system (CNS) infections generate the most medical attention among the many manifestations of the EVs, much of the age-related incidence data come from surveys of meningitis and encephalitis. In a large Finnish cohort (206), an annual incidence of viral meningitis of 219/100,000 children less than 1 year of age was noted, versus 19/100,000 in children between the ages of 1 and 4 years. The incidence dropped even further with increased age. The vast majority of identified viral pathogens were EVs. Other surveys of meningitis and encephalitis have revealed a similar skew toward young infants (20, 85, 249); an incidence peak among young school-age children, 5 to 10 years of age, has also been reported in several studies (60, 207, 279); occasional outbreaks of EV CNS infections occur predominantly among adults (31, 137, 172).

A possible explanation for these seemingly conflicting age incidence findings may lie in the recent history of particular serotypes in the geographic area studied. Serotypes with "endemic" patterns, i.e., occurring with significant incidence every year, are most likely to affect only the youngest children (37). They are the most susceptible to these serotypes for the same reason they are most susceptible to many common infections—the absence of previous exposure and immunity. Older children and adults are more likely to predominate in an outbreak of a serotype which has not been present in a community for several years, creating a reservoir of susceptible individuals among children born since the last appearance of that serotype. Although EVs are the most common cause of aseptic meningitis among adults as well, the lower incidence and the greater ease of physical assessment in adults, compared with young infants, reduce the vigor with which a specific viral etiology is sought. When a serotype is introduced into a community which has many susceptible adults, perhaps because it has been many years since that serotype last appeared or because an antigenic variant of a common serotype has emerged, the large number of affected adults will spark renewed interest in and increased efforts toward a specific diagnosis (31, 85, 112, 137, 146). EV infections other than meningitis and encephalitis are also more commonly identified in children than adults (85, 112, 146), but because of the benign nature of many of these infections, investigations of these other diseases are less commonly performed.

While infection incidence is higher in children, the severity of infection as a function of age varies from disease to disease and sometimes from serotype to serotype. Traditional teaching has been that adults suffer the most severe infections with the polioviruses, manifesting paralytic disease much more commonly than children, in whom asymptomatic infection, aseptic meningitis, and abortive infection are the more common presentations (194, 268). A reexamination of the epidemiology of poliomyelitis, however, finds that the apparent increase in paralytic case/infection ratios with age may actually be the result of increasing immunity within a population following initial introduction of the viruses (177). In poliovirus-naïve populations in which poliomyelitis had never appeared, the highest rate of paralysis occurred in the youngest infants (177). Only subsequent to the introduction of polioviruses, as immunity and hygiene increase in parallel, does the incidence of paralysis appear to increase with increasing age, probably because the actual incidence of susceptible individuals increases with increasing age (177). Similarly, neonates are more likely to suffer severe complications of infections with the echoviruses and coxsackieviruses than are older children or adults (2, 125, 169). Comparison of case series of adults versus children with aseptic meningitis due to the EVs suggests a more severe disease in adults (3, 65); the same is true for pleurodynia (85), an illness usually due to coxsackie B viruses. Myocarditis is most common and most severe in infants less than 6 months of age and in young adults; patients from 10 to 19 years of age account for 10% of cases, while patients between the ages of 20 and 39 years constitute 52% of cases; the incidence then decreases so that patients over 60 years of age comprise only 5% of all cases of EV myocarditis (154).

Host factors which predispose to, or increase the severity of, EV infections, other than age and immunodeficiency, have been difficult to identify. Tonsillectomy and adenoidectomy around the time of poliovirus infection predispose to bulbar poliomyelitis. Perhaps by the same mechanism, physical exercise is an established risk factor for paralytic poliomyelitis (98, 228, 229) and a hypothesized one for enteroviral myocarditis (80). A male-to-female incidence ratio for EV infections of 1.4:1 is seen in individuals <20 years of age (132). The male predominance in cases is not observed in older individuals and may be a reflection of more female caregivers being exposed to the EV. Rates of infection with the nonpoliovirus EVs are higher among persons of lower socioeconomic status and in areas of crowding (171). In contrast, poliomyelitis incidence transiently increases with improved societal hygiene as the time of first poliovirus infection is shifted to an older age group. Pregnancy may increase the severity of poliovirus infection and myocarditis (154).

PATHOGENESIS

Patterns of Virus Replication

The pathogenesis of EV infections has been studied at molecular, cellular, and organ system levels (87, 191, 203,

204), and while much has been learned, much more remains unexplained. The majority of what is known about the pathogenesis of EV infections in humans has been based on the study of the polioviruses, the prototypic members of the genus, in experimental infections using chimpanzees more than four decades ago and, most recently, from transgenic mice expressing the poliovirus receptor CD155 (22, 23, 204). Observations in humans have supplemented these findings.

The EVs are transmitted by the fecal-oral route and, less commonly, by respiratory droplets and transplacentally. The virus may be shed for up to 2 weeks from the nasopharynx and for several weeks to months in the feces. While some replication occurs in the nasopharynx, with spread to upper respiratory tract lymphatics (poliovirus can be isolated from the tonsillar tissue in infected humans), most of the virus inoculum is swallowed (231). The characteristic stability of EVs at acid pH allows them to traverse the stomach en route to the site of primary infection in the lower GI tract. In human infection, poliovirus has been identified within the ileal wall and mesenteric nodes (231). It is believed that the EVs infect enterocytes or M cells in the lower GI tract. Supporting this is the fact that CD155 protein has been identified on the surface of intestinal epithelium and M cells and in the germinal centers of Peyer's patches (114). Additionally, M cells have been shown to bind and endocytose polioviruses, suggesting a similar role in in vivo infection (241).

A minor (primary) viremia follows replication in the lower GI tract and possibly the nasopharynx, seeding numerous organ systems, including the CNS, liver, lungs, and heart. More significant replication at these sites results in a major (secondary) viremia associated with the signs and symptoms of viral infection. If the CNS has not been seeded with the initial viremic episode, spread there may occur with the major viremia. The exact route by which polioviruses and other EVs gain entry to the CNS is still unclear, but two routes have been proposed and supported by observational and experimental data.

Viremia has been shown to be essential for development of paralytic disease in chimpanzees and supports this route as a mode of entry to the CNS (22). Further support for this mode of access to the CNS comes from studies comparing poliovirus accumulation in the CNS of CD155 transgenic mice and nontransgenic mice (280). Pharmacokinetic analysis of poliovirus injected into these two mouse strains indicates that poliovirus is delivered to the brain in significantly greater amounts than would be expected from the vascular concentration. The mechanism by which EVs leave the blood and enter the CNS is unknown. Endothelial cells may express EV receptors that may influence tissue susceptibility (105) and facilitate virus entry into the CNS and other organs. During clinical infections, EVs have been recovered from both the cellular and plasma fractions of the blood (200), and the more important of the blood compartments for establishing specific organ system infection is not known. Differences in susceptibility of mononuclear cells to various EV serotypes have been demonstrated (58, 70) and may impact patterns of neurotropism if cell-associated transport is important.

Evidence for access to the CNS via a neural route is available from simian, murine, and human studies. Sciatic-nerve inoculation of poliovirus in monkeys results in spread of virus along the nerve and the spinal cord (108). In monkeys and CD155 transgenic mice, the initial limb to develop paralysis following inoculation of poliovirus is the one injected (175, 190, 209). Freezing or transsection of the sciatic nerve prevents the development of paralysis of the limb of monkeys or CD155 transgenic mice inoculated intramuscularly with poliovirus (108, 209). Historically, among children inadvertently inoculated with an incompletely inactivated polio vaccine, a significant number developed initial paralysis in the limb receiving the vaccine (176). Trauma to a limb is associated with paralysis of that limb following poliovirus infection. This so-called "provocation poliomyelitis" is well described to occur following intramuscular injections into the leg or arm of a patient incubating wild-type polioviruses or those that receive live attenuated poliovirus vaccines (247, 251). Using the CD155 transgenic mouse model, it was discovered that the mechanism of provocation poliomyelitis appears to be the induction of retrograde axonal transport (88). Poliovirus may gain access to neurons at the level of the neuromuscular junction, which had been shown to have CD155 protein (145). Experimental evidence indicates that intact poliovirus virions (160S) are transported in endocytic vesicles along the axon by fast retrograde transport (190). Upon arrival at the neuronal body, viral RNA is released and replication ensues (204).

The ability of EVs to replicate in different tissues is not determined solely by the presence of a viral receptor on the cell surface. In humans and CD155 transgenic mice, CD155 expression has been documented to occur in tissues that are not sites of poliovirus replication (78, 162, 209). Although it was initially suggested that the IRES was a determinant of cell tropism for polioviruses, subsequent experiments failed to support this hypothesis (204). However, the same may not hold true for all the EVs. A chimera containing the 5′ NCR of echovirus 12 (Travis strain) in the background of a full-length infectious clone of coxsackievirus B3 failed to replicate in murine cells that normally supported the replication of coxsackievirus B3 (26). Because the chimera contained the capsid of coxsackievirus B3 and its nonstructural proteins, viral entry was eliminated as a replication-limiting factor. This was supported by the finding that the chimera replicated with an efficiency equal to that of coxsackievirus B3 in HeLa cells. Using reverse genetics, the block to replication in murine cells was localized to a specific stem-loop structure within the 5′ NCR, indicating that for the nonpoliovirus EVs, the 5′ NCR may be a determinant of tissue tropism.

Experimental evidence indicates that for the polioviruses, the alpha/beta interferon (IFN-α/β) response may determine cell tropism (111). Infection of CD155 transgenic mice lacking the IFN-α/β receptor with poliovirus resulted in viral replication in the liver, spleen, pancreas, and CNS; all of these organs expressed CD155. Infection of CD155 transgenic mice expressing the IFN-α/β receptor yielded viral replication in the brain and spinal cord only. In the latter mice, poliovirus infection of extraneural tissues led to rapid and robust production of IFN-stimulated genes that limited viral replication in those tissues. In both groups of mice, IFN-stimulated gene expression in neural tissue was low in the noninfected state, and a robust response after infection was not observed. Thus, IFN-α/β may function as a determinant of cell tropism in CD155 transgenic mice. Further support for this hypothesis was found by documenting that poliovirus-susceptible monkey and mouse kidney cells in culture as well as primate cell lines failed to provide a rapid IFN response upon infection (282).

The finding that IFN-α/β is a determinant of poliovirus tissue tropism may provide a long-sought-after explanation for the relatively rare occurrence of paralytic disease as a result of poliovirus infection (204). In the majority of individuals infected with poliovirus, the IFN-α/β response limits the replication of poliovirus in extraneural tissues, thereby preventing extension of infection into the CNS. In the <1% of individuals infected with poliovirus who develop paralytic disease, the IFN-α/β response may be defective, allowing for significant replication of poliovirus in extraneural tissues that permits CNS infection.

Molecular determinants of pathogenesis are being investigated to understand the clinical phenotypes of specific EV serotypes and subgroups. While all three serotypes of wild-type polioviruses are known to be neurotropic and neurovirulent, specific tissue tropisms and virulence patterns vary widely among the nonpoliovirus EVs, with certain serotypes consistently reported as causes of specific organ system disease and others only rarely so. The echoviruses and coxsackie B viruses are the principal causes of EV meningitis (20, 37, 57). The EV serotypes most frequently associated with meningitis, in descending order of frequency, are echoviruses 9, 11, and 30; coxsackievirus B5; echovirus 6; coxsackieviruses B2 and A9; echovirus 4; coxsackievirus B4; and echoviruses 7, 18, and 5 (37). Coxsackie B viruses are the most frequent EVs implicated in heart infection (154). Echovirus 11 and several other echovirus and coxsackie B virus serotypes are the most important pathogens of neonatal EV sepsis (2, 132); echovirus 11 is also the most common serotype causing chronic meningoencephalitis in antibody-deficient patients (155). Confounding the analysis of genotype-phenotype correlation is the observation that while certain serotypes are more commonly associated with certain diseases, virtually every EV serotype has been associated with virtually every EV disease manifestation.

The determinants of neurotropism and neurovirulence have been investigated extensively for the polioviruses. Following vaccination with attenuated strains, reversion to virulence has been observed in fecally shed virions recovered from healthy children (165). The viral RNAs of both wild-type and attenuated (vaccine) strains have been sequenced, and only a few differences exist between them. Comparison of wild-type, vaccine, and revertant poliovirus strains has been extremely useful in identifying neuroattenuating regions of the poliovirus genomes. For the polioviruses, the 5′ NCR has been documented to be a major determinant of virulence phenotype (i.e., the ability to cause paralysis) (163). For all three poliovirus Sabin strains, the major neurovirulence attenuating sites are clustered within a 10-nt region of the 5′ NCR (nt 472 to 484 relative to type 3 Sabin strain of poliovirus). Additional determinants of virulence are also found in the amino acids encoded in the P1 and P3 coding regions. Neurovirulence-determining genomic regions have yet to be identified for the nonpoliovirus EVs.

The search for determinants of virulence in other EVs has been less conclusive. Coxsackievirus B4 strains with murine pancreatic tropism and virulence are distinguished from avirulent coxsackievirus B4 strains by a single amino acid residue in the VP1 capsid protein (29). The extension of this finding to humans has yet to be established. Genotypic determinants of myocarditis remain to be conclusively identified. One mechanism of coxsackievirus B-induced cardiomyopathy may involve the ability of that virus' 2A protease molecule to cleave dystrophin, a cytoskeletal protein found in the heart (10). Using a series of intratypic capsid and 5′ NCR chimeras derived from laboratory and clinical strains of coxsackievirus B3 with cardiovirulent and noncardiovirulent phenotypes in mice, a genomic determinant was mapped to the 5′ NCR (69). Subsequent evaluation revealed that a higher-order RNA structure with the 5′ portion (stem loop II) of the 5′ NCR was a major determinant of cardiovirulence in mice (68).

Immune Responses

As with other viral infections, the host immune response to EV infection has both humoral and cell-mediated components (reviewed in reference 257); our knowledge to date suggests that the humoral response is the more important of the two in human EV disease. Anti-EV immunoglobulin M (IgM) antibodies are rapidly produced and persist for up to 6 months; IgA and IgG antibodies to the EVs may be detectable for many years following infection. Poliovirus vaccination has demonstrated the protective benefits of humoral immunity (see below), as has the observation that repeat infections with the same nonpoliovirus EV serotype rarely, if ever, occur. The importance of antibody formation in clearance of and recovery from EV infections is most compellingly illustrated by the severity and chronicity of EV infections in agammaglobulinemic individuals (155); intravenous immunoglobulin is used with some success for the prevention and treatment of EV infections in antibody-deficient patients. Similarly, the severity and timing of neonatal EV infections likely reflect antibody deficiency. There are four primary antigenic sites on the polioviruses to which neutralizing antibodies attach (203), and all but one of them are combinatorial. Chimeric viruses derived from polioviruses and coxsackievirus B serotypes have been used to show that the BC loop of VP1 (Fig. 1) is an important neutralizing epitope of poliovirus 1 and coxsackievirus B4 (208). Other epitopes for the nonpoliovirus EVs remain to be determined.

The study of cell-mediated immune responses to EVs has been much more limited, and the importance of the cellular response in preventing or clearing infection is still unclear (257). T-cell epitopes have been identified on the capsid, near previously discussed B-cell antigens, as well as on nonstructural proteins of coxsackieviruses and polioviruses. These studies have largely been descriptive and conducted in murine models; the relevance of T-cell epitopes and lymphocyte responses to human EV infections is still debated. Similarly, EVs and the T-cell responses to them have been implicated in the actual pathogenesis of chronic diseases. Myocarditis, for example, appears to represent an intricate interplay between virus and host genetics and/or immunity in which direct viral injury (e.g., by dystrophin injury, as noted above) and innocent-bystander damage due to the immune response both probably affect the ultimate outcome of disease (10, 154, 257). Similar interactions between EVs and host response have been implicated in the pathogenesis of chronic dilated cardiomyopathy (154), juvenile-onset diabetes mellitus (210), and inflammatory muscle diseases (61).

Histopathology

The benign nature of most EV infections has made human pathological data somewhat sparse. In patients dying of acute poliomyelitis, mixed inflammatory infiltrates (lymphocytes and neutrophils) and neuronal necrosis are found within the gray matter of the spinal cord's anterior horn and motor nuclei of the hindbrain (21). Small hemorrhages and edema are associated with the inflammation. Involvement of the cerebellum, cerebrum, and midbrain may also be found.

Only occasional pathological descriptions of nonpoliovirus EV meningitis have been reported. A patient who died of coxsackievirus B5 myocarditis with comcomitant meningitis (201) was noted to have inflammation of the choroid plexus of the lateral and fourth ventricles, fibrosis of the vascular walls with focal destruction of the ependymal lining, and fibrotic basal leptomeninges. Parenchymal findings were limited to moderate, symmetric dilation of the ventricles and an increase in number and size of subependymal astrocytes. The inflammatory reaction at the choroid plexus supports the concept of viremic spread to the CNS. An adolescent presenting with a similar constellation of findings died of systemic coxsackievirus B3 infection (250). The dura was grossly distended, with swelling also of the pia, arachnoid, and brain parenchyma. Microscopically, round cell infiltrates were noted in the meninges overlying the cerebellum; the brain parenchyma was congested with increased numbers of oligodendrocytes. Lymphocytic infiltration was most prominent around blood vessels in the cerebral white matter and in the basal ganglia, again suggesting viremic access to the CNS; focal areas of necrosis and hemorrhage were also seen. An immunosuppressed adult with coxsackievirus B4 meningoencephalitis who succumbed to myocarditis was found to have necrosis of the substantia nigra, with nearly complete loss of pigmented neurons and numerous macrophages, some containing melanin (54). Basophilic spicules, consistent with mineralized material, were scattered throughout the lesions. Similar, smaller lesions were symmetrically located in the lateral and superior aspects of the tegmentum. The thalamus, inferior olivary and dentate nuclei, and cerebellar cortex had sparse microglial nodules. The dentate nucleus of the cerebellum was hypercellular, with astrocytosis and neuronal loss. The macrophages and microglia were accompanied by a few scattered lymphocytes.

The pathological findings in EV myocarditis, as with myocarditis due to other etiologies, are classified according to parameters established in 1984 and known as the Dallas criteria (7). Inflammation with mononuclear cells, usually in the interstitium (Fig. 4), is associated with widespread myocardial necrosis. With resolution, fibrosis may replace most inflammatory changes. Findings may be quite focal, with a wide spectrum of severity in the inflammatory response and resultant myocardial damage.

CLINICAL MANIFESTATIONS

Neurologic Illnesses

Poliomyelitis

A total of 90 to 95% of wild-type poliovirus infections are asymptomatic. Only 1 to 2% of poliovirus infections during epidemics and <0.1% of infections under nonepidemic conditions result in paralysis. The remaining 4 to 8% of infections result in a flu-like illness termed "abortive poliomyelitis" or "minor illness" (43, 97). In these patients, fever, fatigue, headache, anorexia, myalgias, and sore throat may last 2 to 3 days, followed by complete recovery. Symptoms suggestive of an upper respiratory tract infection (fever and sore throat) are more commonly reported to occur in children (268). Older adolescents and adults may report a "grippe"-like prodrome characterized by fever and generalized aching (268).

The onset of the major illness (i.e., CNS involvement) may be more abrupt in children than in adults (97) and may follow, rather than accompany, the flu-like minor illness. Particularly in young infants and children, the illness may take on a biphasic appearance, with minor illness preceding "major illness" (97, 268). A biphasic or "dromedary" pattern of fever may occur and is commonly seen in approximately one-third of children. The onset of major illness in adults is more gradual and may occur up to 2 weeks from the onset of nonspecific signs and symptoms. Approximately one-third of patients with CNS involvement develop aseptic meningitis ("nonparalytic poliomyelitis") which is indistinguishable from that due to the nonpoliovirus EVs.

Paralysis is often preceded by severe myalgias, more so in adults (268). The pain is most commonly localized to the lower back and the involved limb(s). Hyperesthesias and paresthesias may be observed in the same affected muscle groups. Soreness and stiffness of the neck and back may be prominent. Exercise relieves the muscle aches, resulting in anxious movement by affected patients. Loss of superficial and deep tendon reflex precedes the development of weakness or paralysis. Paresis or paralysis typically appears within 1 to 2 days of onset of myalgias. The risk of onset of paralysis or of its progression continues until the fever subsides.

The paralytic manifestations of poliovirus infection reflect the regions of the CNS most severely affected (9, 97, 151, 268). The distribution of the paralysis is characteristically asymmetric, with proximal muscles more affected than distal muscles and legs more than arms. Single-limb involvement is most common, but quadriplegia may occur. Paralysis of the muscles of the diaphragm may also occur and result in respiratory failure. Paralysis of the bladder and intestinal atony are common.

Cranial nerve involvement may result in so-called "bulbar paralysis," with resultant difficulties in any or all of speech, swallowing, breathing, eye movement, and facial muscle movements. Medullary centers controlling respiration and vasomotor function can become involved, with potentially fatal outcome (9). Similarly, involvement of the cranial nerves IX, X, and XII can result in paralysis of the tongue, pharynx, and larynx, resulting in airway obstruction.

The natural history of the illness is highly variable, ranging from transient paresis with complete resolution to rapid progression with complete and permanent paralysis. The short-term outcome, i.e., resolution or paralysis, is evident within several days. The long-term outcome of paralytic poliomyelitis appears to be determined during the first 6 months after onset; absence of improvement during that time period usually suggests permanent paralysis with concomitant limb atrophy and deformity. If improvement occurs, the greatest strength gains occur during the first 6 months (264) and may continue for up to 9 months. The overall mortality of spinal poliomyelitis is approximately 5%. Bulbar and medullary poliomyelitis had high mortality rates (50% or greater) during the epidemic years in the

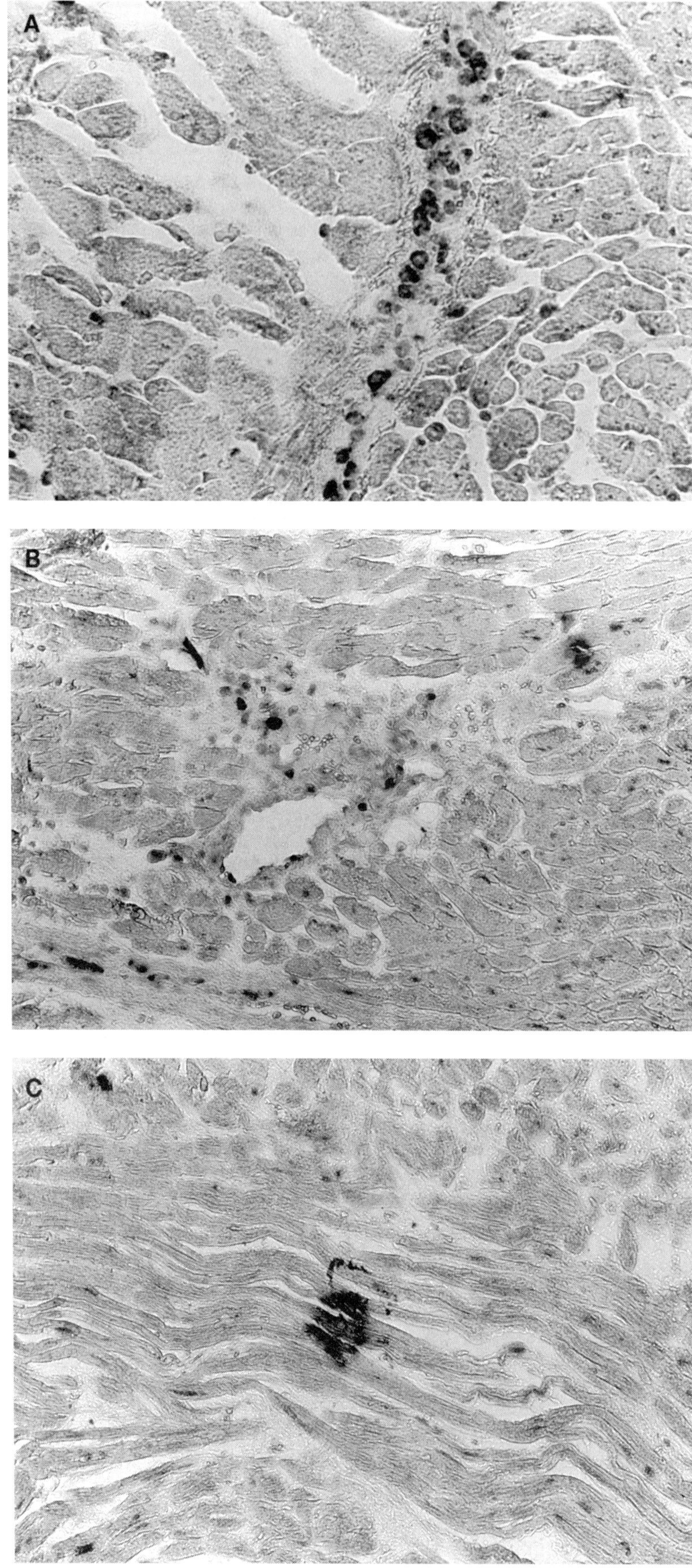
A
B
C

United States when modern respiratory support techniques were not available (9).

As many as 25% of individuals who recover from paralytic disease may develop the syndrome of postpoliomyelitis muscular atrophy (63). Characterized by recurrent weakness, pain, and atrophy 25 to 30 years after the initial acute infection, the clinical course of this manifestation is usually a gradual one that seldom results in total disability of the affected areas. While ongoing viral infection or reactivation has been postulated, and some laboratory evidence has been found to corroborate that mechanism (62, 174, 240), most believe that the postpoliomyelitis syndrome is a result, at least in part, of aging and neuronal dropout in already compromised neuromuscular connections (62).

Aseptic Meningitis and Encephalitis

The clinical disease observed during EV meningitis varies with the host's age and immune status. Neonates are at risk for severe systemic illness, of which meningitis or meningoencephalitis is commonly a part (2, 4, 125, 169). Group B coxsackieviruses were associated with aseptic meningitis in 62% of infants less than 3 months of age in one study (125). Echoviruses identified in infants <2 weeks of age were associated with meningitis or meningoencephalitis in 27% of cases (169). In a prospective study of neonates (<2 weeks of age) with proved EV infection, 75% had clinical or laboratory evidence of meningitis (4).

EV meningitis outside of the immediate (<2 weeks of age) neonatal period is rarely associated with severe disease or poor outcome. The natural history of typical EV meningitis is shown in Fig. 5 (99). Onset is usually sudden, and fever of 38 to 40°C is the most consistent clinical finding, occurring in 76 to 100% of patients (125, 195, 218, 223, 242, 243, 272). The fever pattern may be biphasic (99, 125), appearing first with nonspecific constitutional symptoms, followed by resolution and reappearance with the onset of meningeal signs. Nuchal rigidity is found in more than half of the patients, particularly in children older than 1 to 2 years of age (65, 195, 223, 272), but may be less common in infants (218). Headache is nearly always present in adults and children old enough to report it, and photophobia is also common. Nonspecific and constitutional signs and symptoms of viral infection, in decreasing order of occurrence, include vomiting, anorexia, rash, diarrhea, cough and upper respiratory findings (particularly pharyngitis), diarrhea, and myalgias (99, 125, 146, 195, 223, 272). Symptoms other than fever may also be biphasic, a presentation observed more often in adults than children.

Aseptic meningitis with certain EV serotypes is associated with particular clinical stigmata; e.g., hand-foot-and-mouth syndrome frequently occurs with EV 71 meningitis (95, 103), and nonspecific rashes are especially common with echovirus 9 meningitis (243), although both incidental findings can occur with numerous other serotypes as well (43).

Neurologic abnormalities are unusual; the literature on EV meningitis rarely includes more than 10% of patients with abnormal neurologic examinations. Febrile seizures are among those neurologic "abnormalities" which may complicate aseptic meningitis in children without implicating parenchymal brain involvement. The syndrome of inappropriate antidiuretic hormone was reported in 9 of 102 cases of EV meningitis in one study (42). Additional complications of meningitis include seizures, coma, and increased intracranial pressure (42, 218).

Cytochemical examination of the cerebrospinal fluid (CSF) of patients with EV meningitis usually reveals a modest monocytic pleocytosis (100 to 1,000 cells/mm^3) with normal or slightly depressed glucose levels and normal to slightly increased protein. Importantly, however, wide variations in these findings have been reported (reviewed in reference 220), with cell counts ranging from zero to several thousand, marked hypoglycorrhachia, and markedly elevated CSF protein amounts. Neutrophils may be the predominant cell type in early EV meningitis, with a shift to monocyte predominance within 24 to 48 h (220). Interestingly, CSF eosinophilia has been reported with meningitis due to coxsackievirus B4 (45).

A history of concomitant family illness is often obtained, including rashes and upper respiratory or GI symptoms and, occasionally, meningitis (75). The duration of illness due to EV meningitis is usually less than 1 week, with many patients feeling better immediately after the lumbar puncture (115), presumably due to the transient reduction of intracranial pressure with fluid removal. Adult patients often have symptoms that persist for several weeks (223), an observation not frequently made in children. Comparison of case series of adult EV meningitis (137, 172, 223) with similar series in children (20, 60, 249, 272, 279) suggests that the disease is more severe in adults. Difficulties in eliciting symptoms from young infants may contribute to this impression, in contrast to the case with adults, who readily attest to prolonged headaches, dizziness, photophobia, etc.

The short-term prognosis for young children with EV meningitis early in life appears to be good; however, there has been some controversy as to possible later sequelae. Uncontrolled studies found numerous subtle long-term behavioral and neurologic abnormalities (136). Neurologic, cognitive, and developmental and/or language abnormalities have been reported in controlled studies of long-term outcome in children with EV meningitis during infancy (11, 19, 74, 119, 237, 273). In the largest and most meticulously controlled study, however, no differences between patients and controls in any of the neurodevelopmental parameters studied could be demonstrated (217). Less well studied are the ultimate outcomes of aseptic meningitis cases in older children and adolescents; preliminary data suggest possible learning difficulties, but control patients were not studied (71).

Encephalitis due to the EVs is well known but is thought to be an unusual complication (219, 270). Improved diagnostic methods such as PCR may result in increased recognition of the EVs in cases of encephalitis (225).

In contrast to the typical focal disease seen with herpes simplex virus encephalitis, EVs have been more commonly

FIGURE 4 In situ hybridization study of an adult patient with EV myocarditis. Darkly staining cells indicate the presence of EV RNA. Infection is seen within the inflammatory infiltrate (A and B) as well as in nearby myocardial muscle cells (C). (Reprinted from reference 99.)

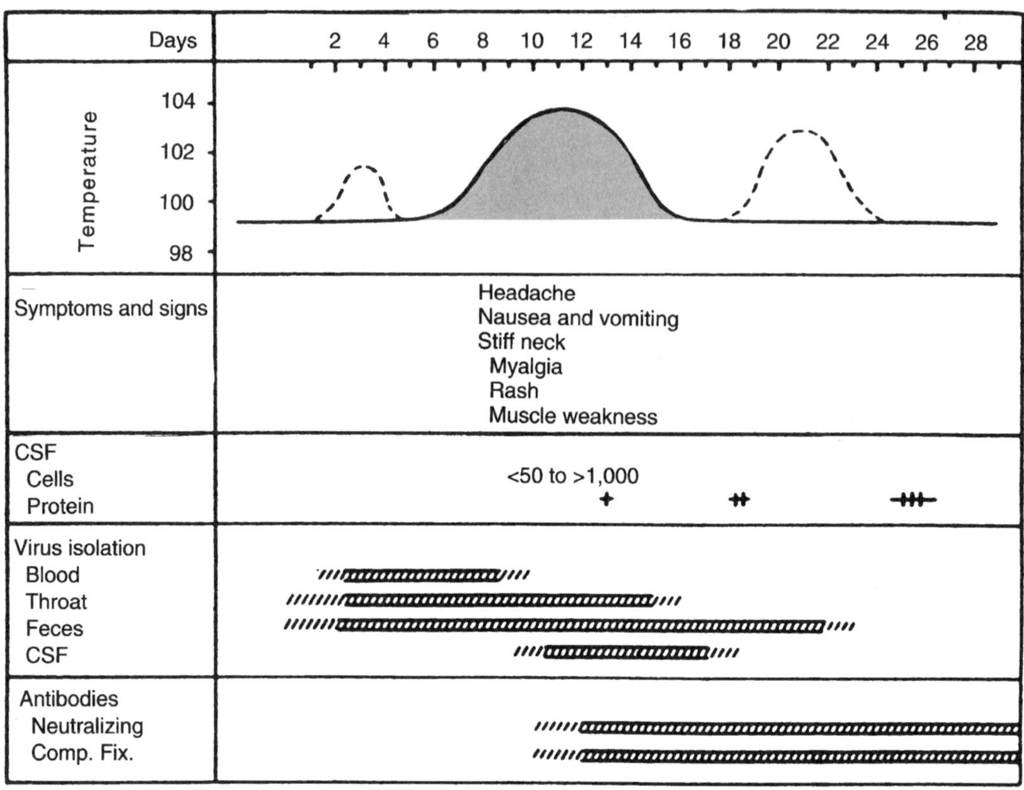

FIGURE 5 Natural history of EV aseptic meningitis. Comp. Fix., complement fixation. (Reprinted from reference 58 with permission.)

associated with global encephalitis and generalized neurologic depression (60, 101, 223, 255). The illness usually begins like aseptic meningitis, with a prodrome of fever, myalgias, and upper respiratory symptoms. Onset of CNS signs and symptoms is often abrupt, with confusion, weakness, lethargy, drowsiness, or irritability. Progression to coma or generalized seizures may occur. When meningeal signs and CSF pleocytosis accompany these findings, meningoencephalitis is the appropriate term. Unusual, but occasional, findings in EV encephalitis include blurred optic disks and other signs of increased intracranial pressure, multifocal encephalomyelopathy, apnea, truncal ataxia, abnormalities of cranial nerves, and paralysis; the last sign is usually a manifestation of spinal cord involvement and, when accompanying central signs and symptoms, is appropriately termed encephalomyelitis.

Focal EV encephalitis is less commonly reported than global disease, but it may be underappreciated. EVs are demonstrable by brain biopsy in 13% of patients suspected of having herpes simplex virus encephalitis, the most commonly identified cause of focal encephalitis (270, 271). Modlin et al. reported four cases of focal EV encephalitis and reviewed an additional three from the literature (168). A variety of focal neurologic findings were seen, as well as abnormalities by imaging studies. Cultures from the CSF of only two of the reported patients grew EVs; the remaining five individuals were confirmed to have EV infection by serologic methods. Hence, EVs must be included in the differential diagnosis of both generalized and focal encephalitis.

An EV 71-associated rhombencephalitis merits special mention (103). The onset of encephalitis may follow a biphasic course, during which the onset of the principal neurologic manifestation, myoclonus, is preceded by either hand-foot-and-mouth disease or herpangina. Myoclonus associated with tremor and/or ataxia (grade I rhombencephalitis) comprises the majority of cases. Either grade II rhombencephalitis, myoclonus plus cranial nerve involvement which may include ocular disturbances, or grade III rhombencephalitis, rapidly progressive cardiopulmonary failure occurring after a brief period of myoclonus, may occur in the remainder of cases.

Unlike aseptic meningitis, encephalitis due to EVs may have profound acute disease and long-term sequelae. For children with EV 71 infections, CNS involvement and brain stem involvement were associated with neurologic sequelae, delayed neurodevelopment, and reduced cognitive functioning (40, 104). However, those with CNS involvement without cardiopulmonary failure did well on neurodevelopment tests.

The unique situation of a child or adult with absent or deficient humoral immunity illustrates an important "experiment of nature" with regard to EV infections of the CNS. Unlike other viruses, which are largely controlled by cellular immune mechanisms, the EVs are cleared from the host by antibody-mediated mechanisms. Agammaglobulinemic individuals infected with EVs may develop chronic meningitis or meningoencephalitis lasting many years, often with fatal outcome (155); although this syndrome can occur in patients with mixed humoral and cellular immunodeficiencies, normal cell-mediated immune function can be documented for most affected patients. Although CSF culture-negative periods occur, more consistent evidence of persistent virus has been obtained using the PCR (225). Approximately 50% of these infected patients also develop a rheumatologic syndrome, most often dermatomyositis, which is also thought to be a direct result of EV infection of the affected tissues (155). Treatment with antibody preparations intravenously and intrathecally or intraventricularly has resulted in stabilization of some of these patients; however, virus persistence during therapy has been documented (155, 225). With the availability of intravenous preparations of immune globulin and the early recognition of this illness, fewer patients appear to be progressing to the classic description of this disease, and atypical neurologic presentations have appeared, including emotional lability, dementia, ataxia, paresthesias, deafness, memory loss, and dysarthria (223, 266). The expanded clinical spectrum of chronic EV meningoencephalitis has been revealed by PCR studies of CSF from patients with these atypical manifestations (266).

Other Neurologic Syndromes Associated with EV Infections

Although acute flaccid paralysis has been traditionally linked to the polioviruses, several nonpoliovirus EVs can also cause this syndrome. In regions of the world where the polioviruses have been eradicated, the nonpoliovirus EVs and circulating VDPVs are now the principal causes of EV acute flaccid paralysis. Several nonpoliovirus EVs have been associated with outbreaks of acute flaccid paralysis, including coxsackievirus A7 (86), EV 70 (262), and EV 71 (103). Sporadic cases of paralysis have been reported in association with isolation of an EV from the CNS or stool. In the latter situation, causality is difficult to establish due to the known prolonged fecal shedding period of the EVs. Reported nonpoliovirus EV serotypes associated with acute flaccid paralysis include coxsackieviruses A4, A7, A21, A24, B2, B3, and B5; echoviruses 3, 7, 9, 18, 19, and 33; and EVs 68 and 71 (37, 66, 81, 84–86, 152). Acute flaccid paralysis due to the nonpoliovirus EVs tends to be milder than that observed with poliovirus infection. It lacks fever at the time of onset of paralysis, affects the upper extremities and face more frequently, is associated with a more rapid recovery, and is less likely to be associated with atrophy. Interestingly, acute flaccid paralysis due to the nonpoliovirus EVs tends to be more severe in infants (66).

Febrile seizures in association with RT-PCR detection of the EV genome in CSF have been reported (100). Cerebellar ataxia has occasionally been associated with EV infections, as have Guillain-Barré syndrome and transverse myelitis (43). All such associations suffer from the same difficulty in distinguishing pathogenicity of a throat or stool isolate from coincidental shedding.

Infections of the Neonate and Young Infant

Neonatal EV Infection and Sepsis

The infected neonate appears to be at the greatest risk for severe morbidity and mortality when signs and symptoms develop in the first days of life, consistent with either intrapartum or perinatal acquisition (2, 4, 125, 169) (Fig. 6). The timing of maternal infection versus delivery of the infant appears to be critical: when enough time for antibody formation in the mother has elapsed, passive protection of the baby occurs. If, however, delivery occurs during maximal viremia and prior to adequate maternal antibody formation, the prognosis for the neonate is worse (2, 4, 169). An additional risk factor for disease severity may be EV serotype. A 20-year evaluation of the epidemiology of neonatal EV infections identified case fatality rates that ranged from approximately 17 to 20% for infants <1 month of age infected with echoviruses 6, 11, 20, and 30 and coxsackievirus B4 (132). However, only coxsackievirus B4 was associated with a higher risk of death than other EVs (odds ratio, 6.5; 95% confidence interval, 2.4 to 17.7).

The onset of clinical illness within the first 2 weeks of life is associated with a greater risk of development of severe disease than in older neonates and infants (4, 169). A history of maternal illness in the form of fever, abdominal pain, or a respiratory syndrome has been reported for 59 to 68% of infected neonates (2, 4, 125, 169). Even in the youngest patients, fever is generally present. In some, hypothermia or temperature instability may occur. Nonspecific signs such as irritability, lethargy, anorexia, emesis, abdominal distention, and jaundice are common (4, 125, 141). An exanthem may be present and has been variously described as macular, maculopapular, and, on occasion, papulovesicular, nodular, or bullous (Color Plate 53) (2). Upper respiratory findings may be present and consist of apnea, tachypnea, grunting, retractions, cough, and wheezing (4, 113, 125, 141). Diarrhea, sometimes associated with blood, may occur but is not a major finding (141). The illness may be biphasic in some infants (125).

In the majority of neonates, the infection is benign and self-limited, with fever resolving in an average of 3 days and other signs and symptoms resolving in about a week (4, 125, 141). In some, a biphasic course may occur with a mild nonspecific febrile illness preceding the onset of more severe disease. As the neonatal disease progresses, major systemic manifestations such as hepatic necrosis, myocarditis, and meningoencephalitis may develop (2). Severe neonatal EV disease is a multisystem organ syndrome comprised of multiple combinations of hepatitis, meningoencephalitis, myocarditis, coagulopathy, sepsis, and pneumonia. Two major clinical presentations are generally encountered: encephalomyocarditis syndrome (severe myocarditis in association with heart failure and meningoencephalitis) and hepatitis-hemorrhage syndrome (severe hepatitis with hepatic failure and disseminated intravascular coagulopathy) (132). The former syndrome is predominantly associated with infections due to the group B coxsackieviruses, while the latter is often associated with echovirus 11 infection (125, 169). Neurologic involvement may or may not be associated with signs of meningeal inflammation, including nuchal rigidity and bulging anterior fontanelle. CNS disease may progress to a more encephalitic picture with lethargy, seizures, and focal neurologic findings suggestive of herpes simplex virus. Cardiomegaly, hepatomegaly, poor perfusion, cyanosis, congestive heart failure, and arrhythmias are indicative of myocarditis. The severe nature of the hepatitis is evidenced by hepatomegaly, jaundice, increased transaminases, and hyperbilirubinemia. Disseminated intravascular coagulation and other findings of "sepsis" result in a patient with illness which may be indistinguishable from that due to overwhelming bacterial infection. The pneumonia may require mechanical ventilation. Renal failure, intracranial hemorrhage, adrenal hemorrhage, necrotizing enterocolitis, and

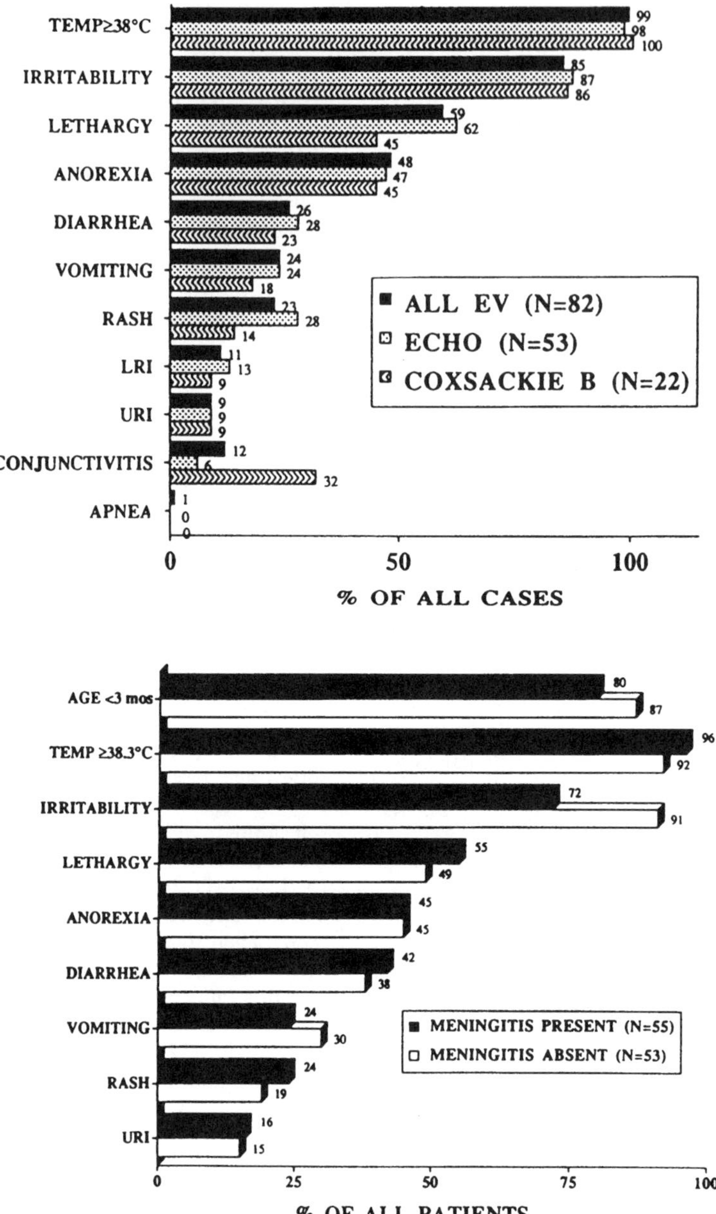

FIGURE 6 Clinical features of young infants with EV infections and the relationship of those features to the infecting serotype (echoviruses [ECHO] versus coxsackieviruses [COXSACKIE B], top panel) and to the presence or absence of meningitis (bottom panel). LRI, lower respiratory infection; URI, upper respiratory infection. (Reprinted from reference 56 with permission.)

inappropriate secretion of antidiuretic hormone have been reported (2).

The reported incidences of morbidity and mortality due to perinatal EV infections are not precisely known, but they may be as high as 80 and 10%, respectively (4, 120, 125, 141, 169). Although a more recent report indicated that the incidence of fatal outcome among EV-infected neonates was found to be 3.3%, neonates had a higher risk of death than persons ≥1 month of age (11.5%, versus 2.5%) infected with EV (132). When death occurs, it is typically due to hepatic failure with echoviruses or myocarditis with coxsackieviruses.

Nonspecific Febrile Illnesses of Infancy

It is estimated that between 10 million and 15 million people in the United States annually develop minor EV infections characterized by fever and nonspecific symptoms, with or without rashes (170, 248). These illnesses are of significance mainly for other diseases that they mimic, including bacterial sepsis, other viral exanthematous diseases, and herpes simplex virus infections; also, their age distribution makes them of great practical concern to the clinician. Most affected patients are young infants (<1 year of age), in whom differentiation of viral illness from the more alarming causes of nonspecific fevers and rashes is extremely difficult. In a prospective study of newborn infants in Rochester, NY, as many as 13% of infants born in the summer months were infected with EVs during the first month of life; 21% of the infected babies were admitted to the hospital with suspected bacterial sepsis and received unnecessary antibiotics or antiviral therapy (120). It was calculated that during the months of seasonal prevalence, about 7 infants per 1,000 live births require hospitalization for neonatal EV infection. Indeed, EVs have been shown by many investigators to be the major cause of hospitalization of young infants for suspected sepsis during the summer and fall months (226). Clinical manifestations include abrupt onset of fever, usually >39°C, with accompanying irritability; the fever may be biphasic (56). Additional symptoms, in order of decreasing frequency, include lethargy, anorexia, diarrhea, vomiting, rash (23% of patients), and respiratory symptoms. Signs and symptoms do not differ in this age group between the echoviruses and coxsackieviruses (56) (Fig. 6). Aseptic meningitis may accompany the nonspecific symptoms of EV infection in infants, and there are no clinical features that distinguish between EV-infected babies with and without meningitis (56). The systemic, global nature of this illness results in hospitalization of many of these infants to rule out bacterial sepsis. The duration of symptomatic illness in young infants beyond the neonatal period is usually 4 to 5 days.

Respiratory Illnesses

Many EV infections are accompanied by nonspecific respiratory signs and symptoms which are usually mild in nature. Summer cold, pharyngitis, tonsillitis, and laryngotracheobronchitis (croup) have been frequently reported (56). Bronchiolitis, pneumonia, and influenza-like syndromes are less commonly seen (24, 56). Most EV respiratory illnesses are benign, but symptoms may persist for many days and the resultant disruption in school days and workdays may be substantial. The EVs are responsible for approximately 15% of upper respiratory infections (URIs) for which an etiology is identified (46); conversely, respiratory illness is the major manifestation reported in 15 to 20% of EV infections (85, 170). In a 10-year review of EV-associated respiratory illnesses, 46% of patients presented with URIs, 13% presented with respiratory distress/apnea, 13% presented with pneumonia, 12% presented with otitis media, and fewer presented with bronchiolitis, croup, and pharyngotonsillitis (46). In two recent studies using RT-PCR detection, EVs were identified in 18% of children with lower respiratory infections and 25% with acute wheezing (49, 117). Many EV serotypes are identified in respiratory infections, approximately equally divided among the major subgroups (85, 170). The clinical manifestations of EV-associated URIs, otitis media, wheezing, and pharyngotonsillitis are indistinguishable from those due to other respiratory viruses. Pneumonia due to the EVs has been associated with numerous serotypes in infants and children (43). The clinical manifestations caused by these agents include fever, hyperpnea, and cyanosis. The laboratory findings usually include a normal leukocyte count, although extreme leukocytosis is occasionally encountered. Chest X ray may reveal perihilar infiltrates. Fatalities have occurred among infants and young children. Histopathological study of the lungs reveals thickening and infiltration of the alveolar septa but no necrosis or giant cells. In adults, bronchopneumonia has been associated with coxsackievirus B3 and echovirus 9 (43, 46).

Herpangina

Group A coxsackieviruses are the most common causes of herpangina, but the syndrome has been reported with the coxsackie B viruses, echoviruses, and numbered EVs as well (44, 95). The highest incidence is among children 1 to 7 years old (199), but infection has also been described to occur in neonates and adults. There is usually an abrupt onset of high fever associated with sore throat, dysphagia, sialorrhea, and malaise. One-fourth of patients may have vomiting and abdominal pain. Early in the illness the enanthem appears as grayish white vesicles measuring 1 to 4 mm in diameter. The lesions are located primarily on anterior pillars of the tonsillar fauces but may involve the posterior portion of the palate, uvula, and occasionally the oropharynx (Fig. 7). The vesicles are discrete, surrounded by erythema, and usually number fewer than 20. Over 2 to 3 days the vesicles usually rupture, leaving punched-out ulcers that may enlarge slightly, while new vesicles may appear. There may also be mild cervical adenopathy, headache, myalgia, arthralgia, and, rarely, parotitis or aseptic meningitis. Clinical laboratory studies are usually normal. The fever lasts 1 to 4 days, local and systemic symptoms begin to improve in 4 to 5 days, and recovery is usually complete within 7 to 10 days of onset (44, 192, 199).

Hand-Foot-and-Mouth Disease

Although hand-foot-and-mouth disease is one of the more common and unique syndromes typically associated with coxsackievirus A16, other coxsackievirus and EV serotypes (in particular EV 71) may be isolated (45, 95). In outbreaks, the highest attack rates are among children younger than 4 years of age, but adults are also frequently affected. The disease is usually mild, and the onset is associated with a sore throat with or without a low-grade fever. Scattered vesicular lesions occur randomly on the oral structures, the pharynx, and the lips; these ulcerate readily, leaving shallow lesions with red areolae. Approximately 85% of patients also develop sparse grayish vesicles (3 to 5 mm in diameter, surrounded by erythematous areolae) on the dorsum of the fingers, particularly in periungal areas, and on the margins of heels (Fig. 8). Occasionally, palmar, plantar, and groin lesions may appear, particularly in young children (43). Resolution is usually complete within 1 week. Certain outbreaks, particularly those due to EV 71, have been associated with diffuse systemic and neurologic disease (95).

Hemorrhagic Conjunctivitis

Acute hemorrhagic conjunctivitis (AHC) is associated with EV 70 and coxsackievirus A 24 variant (CA24v), and both of these viruses have been associated with pandemics of AHC (171). Epidemics and pandemics of EV 70 AHC first arose in 1969. Molecular fingerprinting has indicated that the common origin for all EV 70 strains was west Africa approximately 2 to 3 years prior to the first known pandemic. EV 70 was responsible for an outbreak in Florida (193).

Outbreaks of CA24v have also been widespread (171). Although originally confined to Southeast Asia and the Indian subcontinent, in 1985 it spread to Japan, Taiwan, Oceania, South America, and Africa. Phylogenetic analysis of CA24v isolates from outbreaks in Japan, Taiwan, and

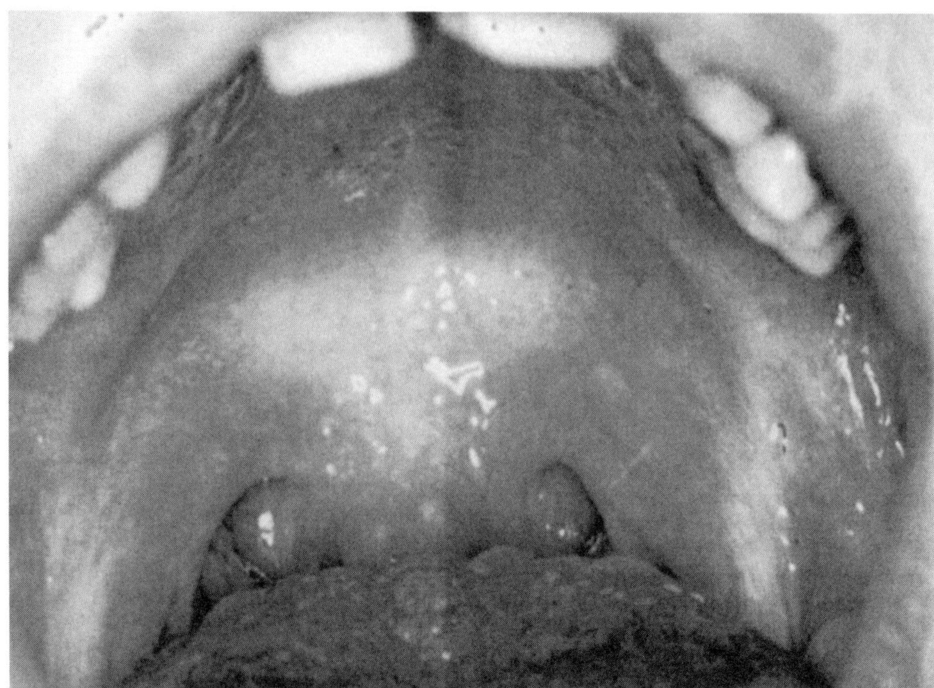

FIGURE 7 Herpangina due to coxsackie A viruses. Small, discrete vesicles surrounded by erythema are seen on the palate and uvula and elsewhere in the posterior oropharynx.

China indicate that the AHC outbreaks in these countries were the result of three successive waves of genetically distinct CA24v strains.

The illnesses caused by the two serotypes are indistinguishable from each other, although CA24v-associated AHC cases may be more commonly accompanied by upper respiratory and systemic symptoms and may have less severe conjunctival hemorrhage (232). After an incubation period of about 1 to 2 days, rapid onset of swelling of the eyelids, with congestion, lacrimation, and severe ocular pain, occurs (94). Photophobia and blurring of vision are common. Subconjunctival hemorrhages vary from petechiae to large blotches. Epithelial keratitis is common, transient, and seldom followed by subepithelial opacities. Fever is an uncommon accompaniment. Preauricular adenopathy is frequent. Occasionally, a mucopurulent discharge from the eyes is found. The illness is generally nonsystemic, although transient lumbar radiculomyelopathy and a poliomyelitis-like illness were described in some cases (261, 262). Recovery is usually complete within 1 to 2 weeks of onset. High secondary-attack rates within households are common.

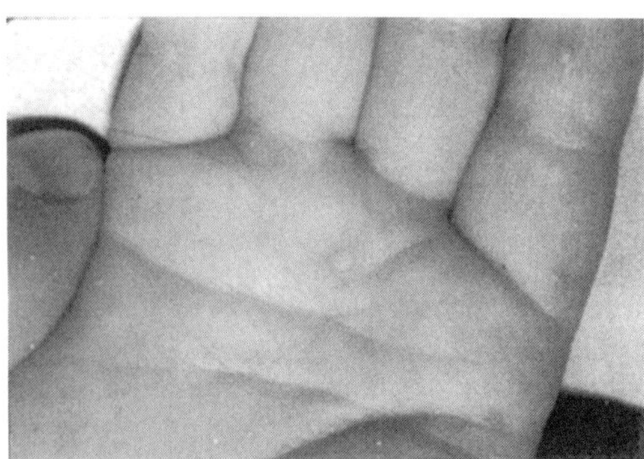

FIGURE 8 Characteristic lesions of EV hand-foot-and-mouth syndrome involving the dorsum of the hand and fingers.

Other EV serotypes have been known to cause outbreaks of acute conjunctivitis or keratoconjunctivitis, usually without hemorrhagic manifestations (43).

Muscular Syndromes

Pleurodynia

Pleurodynia is in reality a misnomer for a clinical condition which is, in actuality, primarily a disease of muscle with clinical manifestations that suggest a pleuritic origin. The disease was fully characterized in 1934 by Sylvest, who also provided its common geographically linked name: Bornholm disease (252). It is variably known by other descriptive designations: epidemic myalgia, devil's grip, etc. Various members of the group B coxsackieviruses are the usual causes of sporadic and epidemic pleurodynia. However, like all other EV-associated illnesses, it may also be caused by other EV serotypes (43).

An incubation period of approximately 4 days precedes the onset of illness, which is abrupt in about three-fourths of patients; the remainder first develop prodromal symptoms of headache, malaise, anorexia, and vague myalgia lasting 1 to 10 days. The major symptom is severe paroxysmal pain referred to the lower ribs or the sternum (85, 106, 124). Deep breathing, coughing, sneezing, or other movement accentuates the pain, which is described as knife-like stabbing, smothering, or catching; it may radiate to the shoulders, neck, or scapulae and is characteristically absent between paroxysms. Abdominal pain occurs concomitantly in about half of patients, but it may occur alone. Abdominal pain may be more commonly seen in children. Other symptoms include fever, headache, cough, anorexia, nausea, vomiting, and diarrhea. Fever is usually about 38°C but ranges to 40°C and may be biphasic. The mean duration of the illness is 3.5 days, varying from 1 to 14 days. Muscle tenderness is ordinarily not prominent, nor is frank myositis or muscle swelling, but some patients experience marked cutaneous hyperesthesia over the affected areas. A pleural friction rub may be heard in 25% of patients. There may be splinting and tenderness on abdominal examination, especially in the upper quadrants and periumbilical area. The chest X ray is typically normal.

Inflammatory Myositis

It is known that EVs can cause inflammatory r-muscle disease, because about 50% of agammaglobulinemia patients with chronic CNS EV infections also develop myositis (155). In these patients, cultivable virus is recovered from muscle tissue. An occasional patient with myositis and normal immunoglobulin concentrations has responded to gamma globulin therapy, with improvement or resolution of the disease.

In much the same way that diabetes is thought to be an autoimmune response to a triggering EV infection, there is also evidence for such a mechanism in polymyositis and dermatomyositis. The evidence for associating these rheumatologic diseases with EVs, as with diabetes, includes serologic studies (259). In addition, EV-like particles have been seen by electron microscopy in muscle biopsy specimens from these patients (48). Certain in situ, dot blot hybridization, and PCR studies of muscle tissue suggest the presence of EV RNA (25, 67). Other investigators, using the similar molecular techniques, failed to find evidence of the EV genome in affected muscles from myositis patients.

Cardiovascular Illnesses

Acute Myocarditis

The EVs are among the most commonly identified etiologies of myocarditis, although most cases of that disease may be undiagnosed (presenting as sudden death without autopsy) or, if diagnosed, have no identifiable cause. EVs may cause between 25 and 35% of cases of myocarditis for which a cause is found based on serologic, nucleic acid hybridization, or PCR-based studies of endomyocardial biopsies and autopsy specimens (89, 154). Conversely, it is estimated that only 1 to 2% of all symptomatic EV infections have associated signs or symptoms of myocardial involvement (85), with the latter more common during coxsackie B virus infections than with other serotypes. Bias in the estimation of frequency of myocarditis during EV infection is possible in both directions: the subclinical nature of some cardiac involvement may result in an underestimate of the true cardiopathogenicity of the EVs, but the study of patients presenting to physicians and hospitals with EV infections probably selects for the sickest patients and may overestimate the cardiac impact of EVs.

Neonates and young infants (<6 months of age) are particularly susceptible to coxsackie B virus-associated myocarditis accompanying systemic infection with those serotypes (125). Most cases occur in adults between the ages of 20 and 39 years. Males are affected more frequently than females (male/female ratio, approximately 1.5:1). Rigorous exercise is anecdotally reported as a precedent to many cases of myocarditis; in animal models, exercise increases the incidence and severity of myocardial involvement during EV infections (80).

Clinical manifestations reflect the regions and extent of cardiac involvement. Symptoms include palpitations and chest pain, often with accompanying fever or a history of recent viral respiratory illness. Arrhythmias and sudden death reflect a prominent involvement of the conducting system which may be of very recent onset; congestive heart failure or myocardial infarction-like presentation suggests more significant necrosis of myocytes and likely longer-standing disease. Pericardial friction rub indicates myopericarditis. Electrocardiographic findings include an evolution from early-stage S-T segment elevation and T-wave inversion to intermediate-stage normalization to late-stage recurrence of T-wave inversion (154). Myocardial enzyme elevations are detected in the blood. Magnetic resonance imaging and nuclear imaging may be of ancillary help in establishing a diagnosis of myocarditis, but endomyocardial biopsy remains the "gold standard" technique for confirming the histopathological diagnosis of myocarditis (see above) (154).

While most patients recover uneventfully from clinically apparent myocarditis, many have residual electrocardiographic or echocardiographic abnormalities for months to years. Smaller percentages of patients develop congestive heart failure, chronic myocarditis, or dilated cardiomyopathy.

Chronic Dilated Cardiomyopathy

There is a growing body of evidence to suggest that some cases of acute myocarditis progress to chronic dilated cardiomyopathy. The latter syndrome is characterized by dilation and dysfunction of the cardiac ventricles. The incidence of this chronic illness is estimated at between 1 and 10/100,000 population, and the contribution of preceding EV myocarditis to those figures is highly disputed. Some serologic, nucleic acid hybridization, and PCR studies suggest ongoing EV involvement in 15 to 30% of cases, less than that in acute myocarditis but still substantial (154). Other investigators consistently fail to find evidence of persistent EVs in patients with chronic cardiomyopathy (55, 127, 147, 153).

Like acute myocarditis, heart failure, chest pain, or arrhythmias may herald the onset of recognizable disease in patients with dilated cardiomyopathy. Ventricular dilation and its concomitant physical findings of mitral insufficiency, cardiomegaly, and congestive heart failure dominate the physical examination, electrocardiographic, and echocardiographic findings. Active myocarditis may be found concomitantly with chronic changes by endomyocardial biopsy, reinforcing the relationship between these processes in some patients.

GI Illnesses

EVs derive their name from their site of replication and shedding in the GI tract; however, enteric illness (vomiting and diarrhea) is usually a minor manifestation of EV infection (43). Neither coxsackieviruses nor echoviruses have been epidemiologically implicated as important primary causes of acute gastroenteritis. Isolation of an EV from the feces of a patient with gastroenteritis must be interpreted with caution because it may represent asymptomatic carriage in a patient made ill by a noncultivable agent. Coxsackie B viruses have been rarely associated with acute abdominal pain and mesenteric adenitis syndromes, which may mimic acute appendicitis. In addition to the occurrence of hepatitis as one aspect of general disease in the newborn, coxsackieviruses B2, B3, and A9 have been associated with hepatitis in older children (43). In adults, coxsackieviruses B3 and B5 have been associated with hepatitis on rare occasions.

Possible EV-Associated Diseases

Juvenile-Onset Diabetes Mellitus

Many serologic studies have found higher titers of antibodies to coxsackievirus B in children with diabetes than in controls (13, 14, 210). An occasional patient dying of ketoacidosis as the initial presentation of diabetes has had coxsackievirus isolated from the pancreas and elsewhere at autopsy (281). EV RNA has been purportedly identified by PCR in the serum of children with newly onset diabetes mellitus (50). Maternal EV infections during pregnancy appear to be correlated with later development of diabetes in offspring (59). Occasional patients have developed anti-islet cell antibodies in close proximity to acute EV infection (150). Diabetes occurs with an inverse seasonality to EV infections (i.e., trough incidence during EV season and peak incidence in the winter), consistent with a postinfectious autoimmune disease mechanism (79). However, a nested matched case control study of incident cases of beta-cell autoimmunity within two prospective cohorts of genetically high-risk children found no evidence that EV infection was a risk factor for the development of autoimmunity to beta cells (83). Numerous animal models have been developed that prove the diabetogenic potential of EVs in mice and rats. The most widely accepted model for encompassing epidemiological, immunologic, and genetic observations from studies of diabetes is that an EV infection in a genetically susceptible host results in an exaggerated autoimmune response and destruction of pancreatic islet cells (210).

LABORATORY DIAGNOSIS

Virus Isolation

John Enders and colleagues received the Nobel Prize in 1954 for successfully propagating poliovirus in a cell culture system (73). Isolation of EVs in cell culture remains the manner by which the majority of clinical laboratories attempt detection of EVs. The commercial availability of increasing numbers and types of continuous cell lines has provided numerous options for routine EV culture (215). The susceptibilities of commonly used cell lines for the EVs are summarized in Table 2. Monkey kidney cell lines have good sensitivity for the polioviruses, coxsackie B viruses, and echoviruses, whereas human diploid fibroblasts like WI-38 and human embryonic lung fibroblasts (HELF) have higher yields for coxsackie A viruses. RD cells, derived from a human rhabdomyosarcoma, are the most sensitive for detection of coxsackie A viruses (149) but fail with most coxsackie B viruses. Even with the addition of newer cell lines, such as Caco-2, A549, and NCI-H292 as well as genetically engineered cell lines expressing the poliovirus receptor or decay-accelerating factor, no single cell line is optimal for all EV serotypes (215). Most laboratories use a combination of a primary monkey kidney cell line, such as CMK (cynomolgus monkey kidney), with a human diploid fibroblast line (such as WI-38, MRC-5, or HELF). Studies have shown improved yield and speed of EV detection with the addition of BGMK (buffalo green monkey kidney) and RD cells. Commercially available mixtures of cell lines may be useful in attempting to achieve maximum sensitivity (215).

Isolation of EVs in cell culture and recognition of cytopathic effect require a high level of expertise and may be quite labor-intensive. Some EV serotypes, particularly within the coxsackievirus A group, do not grow at all in cell culture (102, 149, 191, 215, 269, 274). Of greater significance, 25 to 35% of specimens from patients with characteristic EV infections of any serotype will be negative by cell culture (47) because of antibody neutralization in situ; because of inadequate collection, handling, and processing of the samples; or because of intrinsic insensitivity to the cell lines used. EVs which do grow in cell culture may do so slowly. Reported mean times for EV isolation from CSF range from 3.7 to 8.2 days (224); EVs from other sites, where viral titers are higher, often grow more rapidly (47, 118, 166, 274). Shell vial culture may shorten detection time to 2 to 3 days.

TABLE 2 Commonly used cell lines for isolation of EVs and their susceptibilities

Cell line	Susceptibility[a] of cell line to:			
	Polioviruses	Coxsackieviruses		Echoviruses
		Type A	Type B	
Monkey kidney				
Rhesus	+++	+	+++	+++
Cynomolgus	++++	+	+++	+++
Buffalo green monkey	+++	+	++++	++
Human				
HeLa	+++	+	+++	+
Kidney (HK)	+++	+	++	+++
WI-38	++	++	+	+++
Embryonic lung (HELF)	+++	++	+	+++
MRC-5	+++	+	+	+++
Rhabdomyosarcoma (RD)	+++	+++	+	+++
HEp-2	+++	+	+++	+
A549	+++		+++	+++

[a] Relative susceptibilities: +, minimally susceptible; ++++, maximally susceptible.

Although it is the most sensitive method for laboratory diagnosis of some coxsackievirus A infections, isolation of EVs in suckling mice is rarely performed any longer because of the difficulties of the technique and of animal maintenance.

Nucleic Acid Amplification

The most significant development in rapid, direct detection of the EVs has been the application of nucleic acid amplification technology in the forms of RT-PCR and NASBA (215, 216). Nucleic acid amplification detection of EVs is rapidly becoming the standard for clinically useful methodologies for the detection of EVs. With the recent licensure of an FDA-approved RT-PCR assay, it is possible that this approach to diagnosis will extend beyond academic centers and reference laboratories (140).

Three strategies have been employed for the detection of EVs using traditional RT-PCR: "genus-specific," or universal, detection of all EV serotypes (reviewed in reference 215); detection of a limited number of serotypes, or "species-specific" detection (187); and "strain-specific" detection within a single serotype (215). For general diagnostic purposes, genus-specific detection of EVs is the most useful. Species- and strain-specific approaches to RT-PCR diagnosis may be useful for the screening of uncharacterized EV isolates (187), discrimination of wild-type polioviruses from nonpoliovirus EV isolates (135) or from vaccine strains (134), and the detection of specific serotypes, such as EV 71 (27).

The first reports of sets of primers and probes for universal amplification of the EVs appeared between 1989 and 1990; all sets were broadly reactive among many EV serotypes and had high specificity for the EVs (41, 109, 221). All are directed at highly conserved regions of the EV 5′ NCR. Many additional reports followed (215, 216). RT-PCR has provided a sensitive, specific, rapid, versatile, and clinically useful (205, 214, 253) method for the detection of EVs. In turn, species-specific primers designed to detect members of the human EVs A to D have been targeted to the EV 3′ NCR or VP1 (135, 187).

In the research setting, RT-PCR detection of EV has been demonstrated to be exquisitely sensitive: capable of detecting as few as 1 to 100 molecules of the EV genome, 0.001 to 1 PFU, or 0.003 to 0.1 50% tissue infective dose (reviewed in reference 215). However, it should be borne in mind that the robustness of RT-PCR assays for EV detection in the clinical setting may be significantly lower. The sensitivity and specificity of RT-PCR for the detection of the EVs in CSF compared to the traditional criterion standard of cell culture have been shown to range from 86 to 100% and from 92 to 100%, respectively (215, 238). The sensitivity and specificity of EV detection using RT-PCR in serum appear to be similarly high, ranging from 81 to 92% and 98 to 100%, respectively.

No cross-amplification has been found with a myriad of nonrelated viruses, bacteria, fungi, and yeasts (214). This being said, some primer pairings may amplify a limited number of rhinoviruses (129), a finding that is not surprising given that the rhinoviruses are members of the same viral family and share 5′ NCR sequence motifs. This should be of minor importance when samples such as CSF, serum, or nonrespiratory tract tissues are being tested but would be significant when testing throat or nasal specimens.

In the clinical setting, RT-PCR has been demonstrated to be extremely sensitive for the detection of EV in CSF specimens (222, 233). Paired analysis (i.e., viral culture and RT-PCR testing) of RT-PCR detection of EV from CSF specimens demonstrated it to be consistently and substantially more sensitive than cell culture (215). Using RT-PCR, it is possible to detect EV CNS infection in agammaglobulinemic patients with associated meningoencephalitis or encephalopathy in the absence of cell culture recovery of viruses (225, 266). RT-PCR results can usually be available in less than a day, a substantial time savings compared to the 4 to 8 days required for detection of positivity by cell culture. This reduction in time to positive detection of EVs has been documented to shorten hospital stay, reduce antibiotic use, and impact patient management (205, 245, 253).

In addition to "traditional" RT-PCR methodologies, real-time RT-PCR is also being applied for the clinical diagnosis of EV infections (reviewed in reference 215). Real-time RT-PCR offers the advantages of simultaneous detection of the amplicon, using DNA-binding fluorophores or fluorophore-labeled oligonucleotide probes, during amplification. An additional advantage is the shorter amplification times than with traditional RT-PCR. The assay can generally be completed in ≤4 h, including the time required for extraction of the viral RNA. Optimization of the assay is crucial, because reports indicate that some single-tube protocols may be less sensitive than traditional RT-PCR. Well-designed real-time RT-PCR assays for EV detection appear to be at least as sensitive as traditional in-house assays (215).

NASBA-based assays for detection of EVs in clinical specimens have been reported (reviewed in reference 215). The lower limits of detection have ranged from 10 to 10^2 RNA copies per reaction. As with RT-PCR, NASBA-based systems are more sensitive than cell culture for detection of EVs from clinical specimens (82, 142). In one study, a NASBA-based assay was found to be as sensitive as a commercially available RT-PCR assay for detection of EVs in clinical specimens (143). A problem encountered in the development of a commercially available NASBA assay has been the frequency of invalid results as a result of inhibition of the NASBA reaction (30, 82, 142). This appears to occur more frequently with the use of stool, rectal, throat, and nasopharyngeal samples than with CSF (30, 142, 143). In one study, CSF samples that yielded an indeterminate NASBA result all had significant amounts of blood contaminating the sample (82).

Serologic Assays

Serologic testing using immunoassays has had a limited role in EV diagnosis because of the great diversity of EV serotypes and the failure to identify a single common EV antigen, lack of sensitivity, and cross-reaction with non-EV members of the *Picornaviridae* family (reviewed in reference 215). The sensitivities of hetero- and homotypic immunoassays for the diagnosis of EV infections pale in comparison to that of RT-PCR, ranging from 34 to 75% for patients with RT-PCR-confirmed EV meningitis and 46% for patients for whom EV was detected in stool by RT-PCR (53, 254).

If the specific serotype of an infecting EV is known or suspected, e.g., in community-wide outbreaks, confirmatory homotypic serology can be performed for individual patients to document a rise in antibody titer from the acute to the convalescent phase of infection, thus providing useful epidemiological information. In a situation in which an EV is recovered from the feces or throat of a patient with unusual clinical manifestations, the etiologic role of the EV may be more firmly established by documenting a fourfold rise in titer of antibody to that serotype in paired acute- and convalescent-phase sera. In the usual scenario in which a patient presents with meningitis or other acute manifestations of illness and an EV is suspected, serology is not a practical option.

Specific Identification of EVs

The traditional criterion standard for determination of EV serotype is the use of intersecting pools of equine antisera, as established by Lim and Benyesh-Melnick (LBM pools) (148, 159, 160). Two sets of antibody pools are available: eight pools (A to H) of antisera that identify 42 EVs and seven pools (J to P) of antisera that identify 19 strains of group A coxsackieviruses. A checkerboard analysis localizes the isolate to a single serotype designation on the basis of the pattern of neutralization with the intersecting serum pools. The LBM pools are available in limited supplies from the World Health Organization.

While generally useful, several limitations exist with this methodology (16, 182). LBM pools identify only 40 of the 64 originally described EV serotypes and fail to identify the newly identified EVs. Because the LBM pools were developed over 30 years ago, genetic drift has given rise to antigenic variants of the prototypic strains, which may be difficult to conclusively serotype. Lastly, viral aggregation may negatively impact the performance of the pools, the procedure is labor-intensive and time-consuming, and the supply of LBM pools available from the World Health Organization is limited.

Broadly reactive and serotype-specific EV monoclonal antibodies have been developed and applied to cell culture confirmation by immunofluorescence. However, a review would appear to indicate that monoclonal antibodies for EV identification should best be used as a preliminary screen for species or serotype identification. They lack sensitivity, and reports of cross-reactivity with the rhinoviruses exist (138). The concordance of results of species identification of clinical EV isolates using monoclonal blends versus neutralization assay has demonstrated the latter to be significantly superior for identification of EVs (211). Multiple studies have documented the lack of reactivity of monoclonal blends in detecting EV 71 (260).

The use of bioinformatics in combination with nucleic acid amplification technology has resulted in the ability to "molecularly type" EVs, a powerful method for specific identification of EVs (183, 184, 189). This approach relies on amplification of sequences with the VP1 coding region of EVs. The amplicons generated are rapidly sequenced using PCR and computationally compared to a database of known EV VP1 sequences to establish identity. This method greatly reduces the time required for identification of EVs from weeks to days. Molecular typing has been extremely useful in identification of isolates previously classified as nontypeable EVs because they failed to be neutralized by the traditional LBM pools (182). This approach has led to the identification of multiple new EV serotypes (180–182, 186, 188). It is currently possible to perform species identification directly from clinical specimens (179).

The determination of the specific serotype of an infecting EV is often unnecessary because the diseases caused by the EVs are not serotype specific. Further identification of an EV to the level of specific serotype may be useful under certain circumstances. Epidemiological studies of patterns of EV infections require knowledge of specific serotypes, as do descriptions of unusual or novel clinical manifestations, such as flaccid paralysis due to nonpoliovirus EVs or cVDPVs and incursions of previously rarely encountered serotypes. In most circumstances, therefore, it is adequate and useful for the diagnostic laboratory to report the presence of "an EV" without further detail. The most common exception to this principle is in pediatrics, in which distinguishing between vaccine strain polioviruses and nonpolioviruses is critical to interpretation of viral culture results. In regions of the world where live attenuated poliovirus vaccines continue to be used, most children less than 2 years of age are repeatedly immunized with trivalent oral polio vaccine (Sabin strains), which, like all EVs, may be shed from the throat for 1 to 2 weeks and in the feces for several weeks to months. Hence, isolates from those two sites must be identified as either nonpoliovirus or poliovirus serotypes, with the latter presumed to be of vaccine origin unless unusual clinical circumstances suggest wild-type infection. Vaccine poliovirus has only rarely been recovered from CSF or blood (90, 158); thus, further characterization of EV isolates from those sites is less important, unless the clinical picture warrants (i.e., acute flaccid paralysis).

The standard method for distinguishing between polioviruses and nonpoliovirus EVs employs neutralization of the isolate with a pool of antisera directed against the three poliovirus serotypes. Molecular typing of wild-type poliovirus, vaccine poliovirus, and cVDPV is now possible and extremely useful (133, 134).

Interpretation of Results

The body site from which EVs are isolated is critical to the interpretation of EV detection assays and to the differentiation between EV "colonization" and actual EV-associated disease. The nasopharynx and GI tract are permissive sites of infection; i.e., EVs have ready access to these sites and may remain as "colonizers" for weeks to months. Detection of EVs by virus isolation or PCR at these sites must be interpreted cautiously because their presence alone does not establish causality of the illness in question (121). Indeed, virtually 100% of patients with EV aseptic meningitis will have detectable EV in feces (166), but most persons shedding EV in the feces at any particular time are asymptomatic; feces are thus the most sensitive and least specific site for detecting true EV-associated illness. Since the shedding period in the nasopharynx after EV infection is shorter than in the feces, the specificity of an EV isolate from the nasopharynx for true causation of current symptoms is better than with feces, but such shedding falls far short of a definitive association.

In contrast, the CNS, bloodstream, and genitourinary tract are not usually colonized with EVs; i.e., detection of virus in specimens from these sites implies true invasive infection and a high likelihood of association with current illness. Reports of coinfections of the CSF by bacteria and EVs have appeared (12, 72, 277). In the affected patients, the bacterium-associated clinical sequelae usually dominate. In the much more common situation, in which the clinical presentation is typical of viral meningitis, coinfection with a clinically "silent" bacterium would be extraordinarily unlikely. Hence, identification of an EV from a site not ordinarily colonized in a patient with a clinically compatible illness is usually sufficient evidence for establishing EV causality.

PREVENTION

Vaccines are available only for the polioviruses, and those provide no protection against the nonpoliovirus EV serotypes. In an attempt to eliminate the few remaining vaccine-associated cases of poliomyelitis that occurred annually in the United States, the use of live attenuated oral poliovirus vaccines was abandoned nearly a decade ago. Today, only inactivated poliovirus vaccines are used for immunization of children in this country. Elsewhere in the world, however, the majority of countries continue to use live attenuated oral poliovirus vaccines as a part of their vaccination regimens.

TREATMENT

As with other viral pathogens, there are several steps in the replication cycle of the picornaviruses that are potential targets in antiviral therapy. Cell susceptibility, viral attachment, viral uncoating, viral RNA replication, and viral protein synthesis have all been studied as targets of antipicornaviral compounds (Table 3).

Immunoglobulins

The primary mechanism of clearance of EVs by the host is via humoral immunity. As noted above, patients who lack antibody because of congenital or acquired immunodeficiencies are uniquely susceptible to infections with EVs (155). Similarly, healthy neonates are at high risk for severe EV disease because of a relative deficiency of EV antibodies (4). Antibodies act by binding to EVs and preventing attachment and binding to host cells, which correlates with "neutralization" of EVs observed in cell cultures treated with antibody.

Immune serum globulin has been used prophylactically and therapeutically against the EVs in two clinical settings: the neonate and the immunocompromised host. As noted above, neonates may develop an overwhelming sepsis syndrome from transplacental or peripartum acquisition of EV infection. The high mortality rate of this disease, coupled with the known association of severe EV disease with absolute or relative antibody deficiency states, has prompted numerous investigators to administer antibody preparations to neonates with EV sepsis. Anecdotal reports of clinical success with maternal serum or plasma (116) or commercial immunoglobulin preparations (122) against a variety of EV serotypes causing neonatal sepsis have been published; other reports describe progressive disease and death despite such therapy (275). A blinded, randomized controlled study was too small to demonstrate clinical benefit but did show a reduction in viral titer in babies receiving intravenous immunoglobulin preparations that were subsequently shown to contain high titers of antibody to the infecting serotype (4). Individuals with congenital or acquired antibody deficiencies are also at risk for severe EV infections (see above). Prior to the availability of intravenous immunoglobulin preparations, mixed results were reported with intramuscular and/or intrathecal administration of immunoglobulin preparations. As with neonatal sepsis, some antibody-deficient patients appeared to benefit by supplemental immunoglobulin; others progressed and died despite therapy (155, 266). Since known antibody-deficient patients have begun receiving maintenance supplementation with intravenous immunoglobulin, the incidence of chronic, progressive EV meningoencephalitis has fallen (demonstrating the prophylactic benefit of these preparations) and the clinical profile of patients developing such infections has been modified (155, 223). Therapeutic efficacy in established EV meningoencephalitis in antibody-deficient patients has only been anecdotally reported.

TABLE 3 Therapeutic strategies and candidate compounds for treatment of picornavirus infections

Target	Compound class
Cell susceptibility	Interferons
Virus attachment and binding to host cells	Antibodies, soluble ICAM
Viral uncoating and capsid function	Capsid function inhibitors
Viral replication	Enviromixime-like compounds
Viral protein synthesis	3C protease inhibitors

Capsid-Inhibiting Compounds

Capsid-inhibiting compounds block viral uncoating and/or viral attachment to host cell receptors. As noted above, the resolved three-dimensional structure of the EVs reveals a canyon formed by the junctions of VP1 and VP3. Beneath the canyon lies a pore which leads to a hydrophobic pocket into which a variety of diverse hydrophobic compounds can integrate (Table 3; Fig. 1). Although the compounds integrate into a virus capsid via a number of noncovalent, hydrophobic-type interactions, the affinity is high, with constants ranging from 2.0×10^{-8} to 2.9×10^{-7} M (77). Several hypotheses have been proposed for the mechanism of picornavirus inhibition by compounds that affect the function of the virus capsid. Filling the hydrophobic pocket results in increased stability of the virus, making the virus more resistant to uncoating. The increased stability of the virus-compound complex is evidenced by the resistance to thermal inactivation (213). It is also possible that a degree of capsid flexibility may be required for uncoating, and activity of these compounds within the hydrophobic pocket may reduce this necessary flexibility, inducing a more rigid structure. Alternatively, changes in the conformation of the canyon floor as a result of drug activity within the underlying pocket may affect attachment of the virus to the host cell receptor (197). It has been shown, however, that such perturbations in the canyon floor do not absolutely correlate with antiviral potency (283).

Pleconaril (3-[3,5-dimethyl-4[[3-(3-methyl-5-isoxazolyl) propyl]olyl]phenyl]-5-(trifluoromethyl)-1,2,4-oxadiazole) is the first of a new generation of metabolically stable capsid function inhibitors. This compound has demonstrated broad-spectrum and potent anti-EV and anti-rhinovirus activity and is highly orally bioavailable (1, 198, 265). In a mouse model of multiorgan system infection following subcutaneous and intraperitoneal inoculation of EVs, pleconaril has been shown to reduce viral titers in all affected organs and to prevent death of the animals (198). High levels of pleconaril are achieved in the CNS and in the nasal epithelial tract (M. McKinlay, personal communication). Pharmacokinetic studies of pleconaril have been undertaken in adults, children, and neonates (126, 265). In adults, the pharmacokinetics of pleconaril is best characterized as a one-compartment open model with first-order absorption (1). Concentrations of pleconaril 12 h after a single oral dose remain 2.5-fold greater than required to inhibit 95% of EVs in vitro. The pharmacokinetic profiles in neonates and older children are similar. Oral bioavailability in animals and humans approaches 70%.

Several abstracts indicating a potential efficacy of pleconaril for the treatment of meningitis have been published. In a placebo-controlled study involving 39 adults with laboratory-confirmed EV meningitis, the treatment group received either 200 or 400 mg of pleconaril three times daily for 7 days (267). The treatment groups exhibited a 45% reduction in disease duration (5 days, versus 11.5 days), a 50% reduction in time to complete resolution of headache (7 days, versus 14.2 days), and a 50% reduction in analgesic use (6 days, versus 12 days).

A multicenter, double-blind, placebo-controlled trial evaluated pleconaril at 200 or 400 mg three times daily for the treatment of EV meningitis in adolescents and adults aged 14 to 65 years (239). Patients receiving pleconaril at 200 mg three times daily experienced a 2-day reduction in the duration of headache and returned to work or school 2 days sooner than the placebo group. A 2-day reduction in meningitis symptoms other than headache was noted in treated patients.

In another study of pleconaril for the treatment of EV meningitis in children, 221 subjects, aged 4 to 14 years, were randomized to receive placebo, pleconaril at 2.5 mg/kg of body weight three times daily, or pleconaril at 5 mg/kg three times daily for 7 days (234). The duration of illness was determined using time to absence of headache and systemic symptoms as assessed by a global assessment score (GAS) and total morbidity score (TMS). Subjects receiving 2.5 mg/kg demonstrated sustained improvement in all parameters of assessment compared to those receiving placebo. Median reductions in GAS and TMS of 1 and 2 days, respectively, were seen in the treated groups. At days 4 and 8 of therapy, a reduction in viral shedding from the throat was observed in both pleconaril groups. While a statistically significant reduction in headache duration was observed in pleconaril-treated children >8 years of age, a similar significant reduction in children <8 years old was not seen. These findings may have been the result of the inability of the latter group to clearly identify this subjective symptom. Additionally, while patients receiving the high-dose pleconaril regimen initially demonstrated a reduction in headache, this was not sustained.

Peer-reviewed published reports of the therapeutic efficacy of pleconaril provide a mixed picture. In a randomized, double-blind, placebo-controlled challenge study, the efficacy of pleconaril in the reduction of viral shedding, relief of symptoms, and decrease in severity of clinical illness after infection with coxsackievirus A21 in nonimmune individuals was evaluated (235). Subjects received either placebo or 400 mg of pleconaril initially followed by 200 mg twice daily for 7 days. Fourteen hours after the initial dose of pleconaril or placebo, 100 PFU of coxsackievirus A21 was inoculated intranasally. Subjects receiving pleconaril demonstrated statistically significant lower viral titers in nasal secretions than controls on days 3, 4, and 7. The mean volume of nasal secretions in pleconaril-treated subjects was consistently less than in controls. Mean respiratory symptom scores in placebo-treated individuals were significantly higher than in the treated group.

A small clinical trial evaluating the use of pleconaril for the treatment of EV meningitis in infants has been conducted (3). Infants <12 months old were randomized to receive placebo or pleconaril at 5 mg/kg orally three times a day for 7 days. Pleconaril was tolerated; however, the treatment group had twice as many adverse events per patient. No significant differences were detected between the groups with regard to viral effect (EV detection by culture or PCR), duration of hospitalization, or symptoms. The authors concluded that the small numbers of patients, low yields of serial viral cultures, and the short, benign clinical course precluded the ability to demonstrate efficacy.

A post hoc subgroup analysis of two efficacy trials that failed to define clinical benefit for FDA registration of pleconaril indicated that it was beneficial in the acceleration of headache resolution (65). A combined analysis of two multicentered, randomized, placebo-controlled clinical trials of pleconaril for the treatment of EV meningitis in subjects greater than 14 years old documented a modest benefit in the time to complete resolution of headache. The analysis was restricted to subjects receiving pleconaril at 200 mg three times a day. A total of 607 patients were enrolled in both studies; 240 were confirmed to have EV meningitis. One hundred twenty-eight patients received pleconaril, and 112 received placebo. Although no statistically significant difference was observed between the pleconaril and placebo groups with regard to the median time to complete resolution of headache, subgroup analyses did reveal differences. Among patients presenting with moderate or severe nausea, the median time to resolution of headache was significantly shorter in the placebo-treated patients (7 days, versus 9.5 days). Patients with severe or very severe headache at baseline treated with pleconaril had shorter median times to complete resolution of headache (8 days, versus 9 days). Multivariate analysis documented that males had 50% faster resolution of headache than females.

Pleconaril has also been used in a compassionate-release protocol for the treatment of >90 patients with potentially life-threatening EV infections, 38 of whom have been monitored long enough to assess therapeutic responses (227). Among 16 antibody-deficient patients with chronic EV meningoencephalitis, 12 showed some clinical improvement and 3 others stabilized concurrently with therapy. Six of eight of these patients cleared the virus, and 8 of 9 had improvement in other laboratory parameters. Clinical responses were also seen in 3 of 4 patients with severe neonatal EV disease, 3 of 4 patients with myocarditis, 3 of 3 patients with chronic EV infection related to bone marrow transplantation, 2 of 3 patients with vaccine-associated or wild-type poliomyelitis, and 1 (of 1) patient with postpolio muscular atrophy syndrome.

A major setback for the licensure of pleconaril occurred after a 6-week prophylactic study for the prevention of picornaviral respiratory tract infection demonstrated an increase in menstrual irregularities in women receiving pleconaril (265). Further investigation revealed induction of cytochrome P450 3A activity by pleconaril and raised the possibility of the potential for drug interactions, in particular, interference with oral contraceptives and antiretroviral drugs (65). The FDA concluded that the risks of pleconaril use outweighed the modest benefits associated with its use and did not license pleconaril for treatment of the common cold (265).

Supportive care for the patient with EV meningitis is usually adequate to ensure complete recovery. Attention to fluid balance is necessary to avoid or ameliorate the syndrome of inappropriate antidiuretic hormone or brain edema. Electrolytes and, on occasion, urine and serum osmolality may require monitoring. Brain edema is a rare complication of EV meningitis but is readily managed with mannitol. Seizures may result from fever alone or may reflect direct viral or indirect inflammatory damage of brain parenchyma (in which case "encephalitis" is the more apt term). Phenytoin and phenobarbital are the preferred agents for managing this complication. Patients with EV 71 encephalitis may require respiratory support in the form of assisted mechanical ventilation.

Treatment for the neonate with sepsis or the child or adult with myocarditis is likewise symptomatic. Maintenance of blood pressure is, of course, paramount in each of those syndromes. Steroids have been widely debated in the therapy of myocarditis but are now thought to be contraindicated in most cases (154). No significant benefit has been reported for other immunosuppressive classes of drugs either, and some are clearly harmful in animal models.

Adequate hydration is the only indicated therapy for children with herpangina and hand-foot-and-mouth syndrome due to the EVs. Other respiratory manifestations of EV infections are managed symptomatically.

REFERENCES

1. **Abdel-Rahman, S. M., and G. L. Kearns.** 1999. Single oral dose escalation pharmacokinetics of pleconaril capsules in adults. *J. Clin. Pharmacol.* **39:**613–618.
2. **Abzug, M. J.** 2004. Presentation, diagnosis, and management of enterovirus infections in neonates. *Paediatr. Drugs* **6:**1–10.
3. **Abzug, M. J., G. Cloud, J. Bradley, P. J. Sánchez, J. Romero, D. Powell, M. Lepow, C. Mani, E. V. Capparelli, S. Blount, F. Lakeman, R. J. Whitley, and D. W. Kimberlin for the National Institute of Allergy and Infectious Diseases Collaborative Antiviral Study Group.** 2003. Double blind placebo-controlled trial of pleconaril in infants with enterovirus meningitis. *Pediatr. Infect. Dis. J.* **22:**335–341.
4. **Abzug, M. J., M. J. Levin, and H. A. Rotbart.** 1993. Profile of enterovirus disease in the first two weeks of life. *Pediatr. Infect. Dis. J.* **12:**820–824.
5. **Andino, R., G. E. Rieckhof, P. L. Achacoso, and D. Baltimore.** 1993. Poliovirus RNA synthesis utilizes an RNP complex formed around the 5′-end of viral RNA. *EMBO J.* **12:**3587–3598.
6. **Antona, D., N. Leveque, J. J. Chomel, S. Dubrou, D. Levy-Bruhl, and B. Lina.** 2007. Surveillance of enteroviruses in France, 2000–2004. *Eur. J. Clin. Microbiol. Infect. Dis.* **26:**403–412.
7. **Aretz, H. T.** 1987. Myocarditis: the Dallas criteria. *Hum. Pathol.* **18:**619–624.
8. **Ashwell, M. J., D. W. Smith, P. A. Phillips, and I. L. Rouse.** 1996. Viral meningitis due to echovirus types 6 and 9: epidemiological data from Western Australia. *Epidemiol. Infect.* **117:**507–512.
9. **Auld, P. A. M., S. V. Kevy, and R. C. Eley.** 1960. Poliomyelitis in children: experience with 956 cases in the 1955 Massachusetts epidemic. *N. Engl. J. Med.* **263:** 1093–1100.
10. **Badorff, C., G. H. Lee, B. J. Lamphear, M. E. Martone, K. P. Campbell, R. E. Rhoads, and K. U. Knowlton.** 1999. Enteroviral protease 2A cleaves dystrophin: evidence of a cytoskeletal disruption in an acquired cardiomyopathy. *Nat. Med.* **5:**320–326.
11. **Baker, R. C., A. W. Kummer, J. R. Schultz, H. Ho, and J. Gonzalez del Rey.** 1996. Neurodevelopmental outcome of infants with viral meningitis in the first three months of life. *Clin. Pediatr.* **35:**295–301.
12. **Balfour, H. H., Jr., G. L. Seifert, M. H. Seifert, Jr., P. G. Quie, C. K. Edelman, H. Bauer, and R. A. Siem.** 1973. Meningoencephalitis and laboratory evidence of triple infection with California encephalitis virus, echovirus 11 and mumps. *Pediatrics* **51:**680–684
13. **Banatvala, J. E.** 1987. Insulin-dependent (juvenile-onset, type 1) diabetes mellitus and coxsackie B viruses revisited. *Prog. Med. Virol.* **34:**33–54.
14. **Barrett-Connor, E.** 1985. Is insulin-dependent diabetes mellitus caused by coxsackie virus B infection? A review of the epidemiologic evidence. *Rev. Infect. Dis.* **7:**207–215.
15. **Belnap, D. M., D. J. Filman, B. L. Trus, N. Cheng, F. P. Booy, J. F. Conway, S. Curry, C. N. Hiremath, S. K. Tsang, A. C. Steven, and J. M. Hogle.** 2000. Molecular tectonic model of virus structural transitions: the putative cell entry states of poliovirus. *J. Virol.* **74:**1342–1354.
16. **Bendig, J., and P. Earl.** 2005. The Lim Benyesh-Melnick antiserum pools for serotyping human enterovirus cell culture isolates—still useful, but may fail to identify current strains of echovirus 18. *J. Virol. Methods* **127:**96–99.
17. **Bendinelli, M., and A. Ruschi.** 1969. Isolation of human enterovirus from mussels. *Appl. Microbiol.* **18:**531–532.
18. **Bergelson, J. M., J. A. Cunningham, G. Droguett, E. A. Kurt-Jones, A. Krithivas, J. S. Hong, M. S. Horwitz, R. L. Crowell, and R. W. Finberg.** 1997. Isolation of a common receptor for coxsackie B viruses and adenoviruses 2 and 5. *Science* **275:**1320–1323.
19. **Bergman, I., M. J. Painter, E. R. Wald, D. Chiponis, A. L. Holland, and H. G. Taylor.** 1987. Outcome in children with enteroviral meningitis during the first year of life. *J. Pediatr.* **110:**705–709.
20. **Berlin, L. E., M. L Rorabaugh, F. Heidrich, K. Roberts, T. Doran, and J. F. Modlin.** 1993. Aseptic meningitis in infants <2 years of age: diagnosis and etiology. *J. Infect. Dis.* **168:**888–892.
21. **Bodian, D.** 1949. Histopathologic basis of the clinical findings in poliomyelitis. *Am. J. Med.* **6:**563.
22. **Bodian, D.** 1952. Pathogenesis of poliomyelitis. *Am. J. Public Health* **42:**1388–1402.
23. **Bodian, D.** 1955. Emerging concept of poliomyelitis infection. *Science* **122:**105–108.
24. **Boivin, G., A. D. Osterhaus, A. Gaudreau, H. C. Jackson, J. Groen, and P. Ward.** 2002. Role of picornaviruses in flu-like illnesses of adults enrolled in an oseltamivir treatment study who had no evidence of influenza virus infection. *J. Clin. Microbiol.* **40:**330–334.
25. **Bowles, N. E., T. A. Bayston, H. Y. Zhang, D. Doyle, R. J. Lane, L. Cunningham, and L. C. Archard.** 1993. Persistence of enterovirus RNA in muscle biopsy samples suggests that some cases of chronic fatigue syndrome result from a previous, inflammatory viral myopathy. *J. Med.* **24:** 145–160.
26. **Bradrick, S. S., E. A. Lieben, B. M. Carden, and J. R. Romero.** 2001. A predicted secondary structural domain within the internal ribosome entry site of echovirus 12 mediates a cell-type-specific block to viral replication. *J. Virol.* **75:**6472–6481.

27. **Brown, B. A., D. R. Kilpatrick, M. S. Oberste, and M. A. Pallansch.** 2000. Serotype-specific identification of enterovirus 71 by PCR. *J. Clin. Virol.* **16:**107–112.
28. **Bubeck, D. D., J. Filman, N. Cheng, A. C. Steven, J. M. Hogle, and D. M. Belnap.** 2005. The structure of the poliovirus 135S cell entry intermediate at 10-angstrom resolution reveals the location of an externalized polypeptide that binds to membranes. *J. Virol.* **79:**7745–7755.
29. **Caggana, M., P. Chan, and A. Ramsingh.** 1993. Identification of a single amino acid residue in the capsid protein VP1 of coxsackievirus B4 that determines the virulent phenotype. *J. Virol.* **67:**4797–4803.
30. **Capaul, S. E., and M. Gorgievski-Hrisoho.** 2005. Detection of enterovirus RNA in cerebrospinal fluid (CSF) using NucliSens EasyQ Enterovirus assay. *J. Clin. Virol.* **32:** 236–240.
31. **Carrol, E. D., M. B. Beadsworth, N. Jenkins, L. Ratcliffe, I. Ashton, B. Crowley, F. J. Nye, and N. J. Beeching.** 2006. Clinical and diagnostic findings of an echovirus meningitis outbreak in the northwest of England. *Postgrad. Med. J.* **82:**60–64.
32. **Centers for Disease Control and Prevention.** 2001. Apparent global interruption of wild poliovirus type 2 transmission. *Morb. Mortal. Wkly. Rep.* **50:**222.
33. **Centers for Disease Control and Prevention.** 2005. Summary of notifiable diseases—United States. *Morb. Mortal. Wkly. Rep.* **54:**1–92.
34. **Centers for Disease Control and Prevention.** 2005. Poliovirus infections in four unvaccinated children—Minnesota, August–October. *Morb. Mortal. Wkly. Rep.* **54:**1053–1055.
35. **Centers for Disease Control and Prevention.** 2006. Imported vaccine-associated paralytic poliomyelitis—United States. *Morb. Mortal. Wkly. Rep.* **55:**97–99.
36. **Centers for Disease Control and Prevention.** 2006. Progress toward interruption of wild poliovirus transmission—worldwide, January 2005–March 2006. *Morb. Mortal. Wkly. Rep.* **55:**458–462.
37. **Centers for Disease Control and Prevention.** 2006. Enterovirus surveillance—United States, 1970–2005. *Morb. Mortal. Wkly. Rep.* **55:**1–20.
38. **Centers for Disease Control and Prevention.** 2007. Progress toward interruption of wild poliovirus transmission—worldwide, January 2006–May 2007. *Morb. Mortal. Wkly. Rep.* **56:**682–685.
39. **Centers for Disease Control and Prevention.** 2007. Update on vaccine-derived polioviruses—worldwide, January 2006–August 2007. *Morb. Mortal. Wkly. Rep.* **56:**996–1001.
40. **Chang, L. Y., L. M. Huang, S. S. Gau, Y. Y. Wu, S. H. Hsia, T. Y. Fan, K. L. Lin, Y. C. Huang, C. Y. Lu, and T. Y. Lin.** 2007. Neurodevelopment and cognition in children after enterovirus 71 infection. *N. Engl. J. Med.* **356:**1226–1234.
41. **Chapman, N. M., S. Tracy, C. J. Gauntt, and U. Fortmueller.** 1990. Molecular detection and identification of enteroviruses using enzymatic amplification and nucleic acid hybridization. *J. Clin. Microbiol.* **28:**843–850.
42. **Chemtob, S., E. R. Reece, and E. L. Mills.** 1985. Syndrome of inappropriate secretion of antidiuretic hormone in enteroviral meningitis. *Am. J. Dis. Child.* **139:**292–294.
43. **Cherry, J. D.** 2004. Enteroviruses and parechoviruses, p. 1984–2041. *In* R. D. Feigin, J. D. Cherry, G. J. Demmler, and S. L. Kaplan (ed.), *Textbook of Pediatric Infectious Diseases*, 5th ed. W. B. Saunders, Philadelphia, PA.
44. **Cherry, J. D., and C. L. Jahn.** 1965. Herpangina: the etiologic spectrum. *Pediatrics* **36:**632–634.
45. **Chesney, J. C., G. E. Hoganson, and M. H. Wilson.** 1980. CSF eosinophilia during an acute coxsackie B4 viral meningitis. *Am. J. Dis. Child.* **134:**703.
46. **Chonmaitree, T., and L. Mann.** 1995. Respiratory infections, p. 255–270. *In* H. A. Rotbart (ed.), *Human Enterovirus Infections*. ASM Press, Washington, DC.
47. **Chonmaitree, T., M. A. Menegus, and K. R. Powell.** 1982. The clinical relevance of CSF viral culture. A two-year experience with aseptic meningitis in Rochester, New York. *JAMA* **247:**1843–1847.
48. **Chou, S. M., and L. Gutmann.** 1970. Picornavirus-like crystals in subacute polymyositis. *Neurology* **20:**205–213.
49. **Chung, J. Y., T. H. Han, S. W. Kim, and E. S. Hwang.** 2007. Respiratory picornavirus infections in Korean children with lower respiratory tract infections. *Scand. J. Infect. Dis.* **39:**250–254.
50. **Clements, G. B., D. N. Galbraith, and K. W. Taylor.** 1995. Coxsackie B virus infection and onset of childhood diabetes. *Lancet* **346:**221–223.
51. **Committee on the Enteroviruses.** 1962. The enteroviruses. *Virology* **16:**501–504.
52. **Coyne, C. B., and J. M. Bergelson.** 2006. Virus-induced Abl and Fyn kinase signals permit coxsackievirus entry through epithelial tight junctions. *Cell* **124:**119–131.
53. **Craig, M. E., P. Robertson, N. J. Howard, M. Silink, and W. D. Rawlinson.** 2003. Diagnosis of enterovirus infection by genus-specific PCR and enzyme-linked immunosorbent assays. *J. Clin. Microbiol.* **41:**841–844.
54. **Cree, B. C., G. L. Bernardini, A. P. Hays, and G. Lowe.** 2003. A fatal case of coxsackievirus B4 meningoencephalitis. *Arch. Neurol.* **60:**107–112.
55. **Crespo-Leiro, M. G., M. Hermida-Prieto, F. Peña, F. Portela, J. Muñiz, L. F. Hermida, A. Juffe-Stein, and A. Castro-Beiras.** 2000. Absence of enteroviral RNA in hearts explanted from patients with dilated cardiomyopathy. *J. Heart Lung Transplant.* **19:**134–138.
56. **Dagan, R., and M. A. Menegus.** 1995. Nonpolic enteroviruses and the febrile infant, p. 239–254. *In* H. A. Rotbart (ed.), *Human Enterovirus Infections*. ASM Press, Washington, DC.
57. **Dagan, R., J. A. Jenista, and M. A. Menegus.** 1988. Association of clinical presentation, laboratory findings, and virus serotypes with the presence of meningitis in hospitalized infants with enterovirus infections. *J. Pediatr.* **113:** 975–978.
58. **Dagan, R., and M. A. Menegus.** 1992. Replication of enteroviruses in human mononuclear cells. *Isr. J. Med. Sci.* **28:**369–372.
59. **Dahlquist, G. G., S. Ivarsson, B. Lindberg, and M. Forsgren.** 1995. Maternal enteroviral infection during pregnancy as a risk factor for childhood IDDM. A population-based control study. *Diabetes* **44:**408–413.
60. **Dai-Ming, W., Z. Guo-Chang, and Z. Shi-Mei.** 1993. An epidemic of encephalitis and meningoencephalitis in children caused by echovirus type 30 in Shanghai. *Chin. Med. J.* **106:**767–769.
61. **Dalakas, M. C.** 1995. Enteroviruses and human neuromuscular diseases, p. 387–398. *In* H. A. Rotbart (ed.), *Human Enterovirus Infections*. ASM Press, Washington, DC.
62. **Dalakas, M. C., H. Bartfield, and T. Kurland (ed.).** 1995. *Annals of the New York Academy of Sciences*, vol. 753. *The Post-Polio Syndrome: Advances in the Pathogenesis and Treatment*. New York Academy of Sciences, New York, NY.
63. **Dalakas, M. C., J. L. Sever, D. L. Madden, N. M. Papadopoulos, I. C. Shekarchi, P. Albrecht, and A. Krezlewicz.** 1984. Late post-poliomyelitis muscular atrophy:

clinical, virological, and immunological studies. *Rev. Infect. Dis.* **6:**5562–5567.
64. **de Quadros, C. A., J. K. Andrus, J. M. Olive, C. Guerra de Macedo, and D. A. Henderson.** 1992. Polio eradication from the Western Hemisphere. *Annu. Rev. Public Health* **13:**239–252.
65. **Desmond, R. A., N. A. Accortt, L. Talley, S. A. Villano, S. J. Soong, and R. J. Whitley.** 2006. Enteroviral meningitis: natural history and outcome of pleconaril therapy. *Antimicrob. Agents Chemother.* **50:**2409–2414.
66. **Dietz, V., J. Andrus, J. M. Olive, S. Cochi, and C. de Quadros.** 1995. Epidemiology and clinical characteristics of acute flaccid paralysis associated with non-polio enterovirus isolation: the experience in the Americas. *Bull. W. H. O.* **73:**597–603.
67. **Douche-Aourik, F., W. Berlier, L. Féasson, T. Bourlet, R. Harrath, S. Omar, F. Grattard, C. Denis, and B. Pozzetto.** 2003. Detection of enterovirus in human skeletal muscle from patients with chronic inflammatory muscle disease or fibromyalgia and healthy subjects. *J. Med. Virol.* **71:**540–547.
68. **Dunn, J. J., S. S. Bradrick, N. M. Chapman, S. M. Tracy, and J. R. Romero.** 2003. The stem loop II within the 5′ nontranslated region of clinical coxsackievirus B3 genomes determines cardiovirulence phenotype in a murine model. *J. Infect. Dis.* **187:**1552–1561.
69. **Dunn, J. J., N. M. Chapman, S. Tracy, and J. R. Romero.** 2000. Genomic determinants of cardiovirulence in coxsackievirus B3 clinical isolates: localization to the 5′ nontranslated region. *J. Virol.* **74:**4787–4794.
70. **Eberle, K. E., V. T. Nguyen, and M. S. Freistadt.** 1995. Low levels of poliovirus replication in primary human monocytes: possible interactions with lymphocytes. *Arch. Virol.* **140:**2135–2150.
71. **Efter, C. G., J. Wedgwood, and U. B. Schaad.** 1991. Aseptische Meningitiden in der Padiatrie. *Schweiz. Med. Wochenschr.* **121:**1120–1126.
72. **Eglin, R. P., R. A. Swann, D. Isaacs, and E. R. Moxon.** 1984. Simultaneous bacterial and viral meningitis. *Lancet* **ii:**984.
73. **Enders, J. F., T. H. Weller, and F. C. Robbins.** 1949. Cultivation of the Lansing strain of poliomyelitis virus in culture of various human embryonic tissues. *Science* **109:** 85–99.
74. **Farmer, K., G. A. MacArthur, and M. M. Clay.** 1975. A follow-up study of 15 cases of neonatal meningoencephalitis due to coxsackie virus B5. *J. Pediatr.* **87:**568–571.
75. **Faulkner, R. S., A. J. MacLeod, and C. E. Van Rooyen.** 1957. Virus meningitis—seven cases in one family. *Can. Med. Assoc. J.* **77:**439–444.
76. **Fox, J. P., C. E. Hall, M. K. Cooney, R. E. Luce, and R. A. Kronmal.** 1972. The Seattle virus watch. II. Objectives, study population and its observation, data processing and summary of illnesses. *Am. J. Epidemiol.* **98:** 270–285.
77. **Fox, M. P., M. A. McKinlay, G. D. Diana, and F. J. Dutko.** 1991. Binding affinities of structurally related human rhinovirus capsid-binding compounds are related to their activities against human rhinovirus type 14. *Antimicrob. Agents Chemother.* **35:**1040–1047.
78. **Freistadt, M. S., G. Kaplan, and V. R. Racaniello.** 1990. Heterogeneous expression of poliovirus receptor-related proteins in human cells and tissues. *Mol. Cell. Biol.* **10:** 5700–5706.
79. **Gamble, D. R., and K. W. Taylor.** 1969. Seasonal incidence of diabetes mellitus. *Br. Med. J.* **3:**631–633.
80. **Gatmaitan, B. G., J. L. Chason, and A. M. Lerner.** 1970. Augmentation of the virulence of murine coxsackievirus B-3 myocardiopathy by exercise. *J. Exp. Med.* **131:**1121–1136.
81. **Gear, J. H.** 1984. Nonpolio causes of polio-like paralytic syndromes. *Rev. Infect. Dis.* **6**(Suppl. 2)**:**S379–S384.
82. **Ginocchio, C. C.** 2005. Development, technical performance, and clinical evaluation of a NucliSens basic kit application for detection of enterovirus RNA in cerebrospinal fluid. *J. Clin. Microbiol.* **43:**2616–2623.
83. **Graves, P. M., H. A. Rotbart, W. A. Nix, M. A. Pallansch, H. A. Erlich, J. M. Norris, M. Hoffman, G. S. Eisenbarth, and M. Rewers.** 2003. Prospective study of enteroviral infections and development of beta-cell autoimmunity. Diabetes autoimmunity study in the young (DAISY). *Diabetes Res. Clin. Pract.* **59:**51–61.
84. **Grimwood, K., Q. S. Huang, L. G. Sadleir, W. A. Nix, D. R. Kilpatrick, M. S. Oberste, and M. A. Pallansch.** 2003. Acute flaccid paralysis from echovirus type 33 infection. *J. Clin. Microbiol.* **41:**2230–2232.
85. **Grist, N. R., E. J. Bell, and F. Assaad.** 1978. Enteroviruses in human disease. *Prog. Med. Virol.* **24:**114–157.
86. **Grist, N. R., and E. J. Bell.** 1984. Paralytic poliomyelitis and nonpolio enteroviruses: studies in Scotland. *Rev. Infect. Dis.* **6**(Suppl. 2)**:**S385–S386.
87. **Gromeier, M., and A. Nomoto.** 2002. Determinants of poliovirus pathogenesis, p. 367–379. *In* B. L. Semler and E. Wimmer (ed.), *Molecular Biology of Picornaviruses.* ASM Press, Washington, DC.
88. **Gromeier, M., and E. Wimmer.** 1998. Mechanism of injury-provoked poliomyelitis. *J. Virol.* **72:**5056–5060.
89. **Guarner, J., J. Bhatnagar, W. J. Shieh, K. B. Nolte, D. Klein, M. S. Gookin, S. Peñaranda, M. S. Oberste, T. Jones, C. Smith, M. A. Pallansch, and S. R. Zaki.** 2007. Histopathologic, immunohistochemical, and polymerase chain reaction assays in the study of cases with fatal sporadic myocarditis. *Hum. Pathol.* **38:**1412.
90. **Gutierrez, K. M., and M. J. Abzug.** 1990. Vaccine-associated poliovirus meningitis in children with ventriculoperitoneal shunts. *J. Pediatr.* **117:**424–427.
91. **Haller, A. A., and B. L. Semler.** 1995. Translation and host cell shutoff, p. 113–133. *In* H. A. Rotbart (ed.), *Human Enterovirus Infections.* ASM Press, Washington, DC.
92. **Hawley, H. B., D. P. Morin, M. E. Geraghty, J. Tomkow, and C. A. Phillips.** 1973. Coxsackievirus B epidemic at a boy's summer camp. Isolation of virus from swimming water. *JAMA* **226:**33–36.
93. **Hendry, E., H. Hatanaka, E. Fry, M. Smyth, J. Tate, G. Stanway, J. Santti, M. Maaronen, T. Hyypiä, and D. Stuart.** 1999. The crystal structure of coxsackievirus A9: new insights into the uncoating mechanisms of enteroviruses. *Structure* **7:**1527–1538.
94. **Hierholzer, J. C., K. A. Hilliard, and J. J. Esposito.** 1975. Serosurvey for "acute hemorrhagic conjunctivitis" virus (enterovirus 70) antibodies in the southeastern United States, with review of the literature and some epidemiologic implications. *Am. J. Epidemiol.* **102:**533–544.
95. **Ho, M., E. R. Chen, K. H. Hsu, S. J. Twu, K. T. Chen, S. F. Tsai, J. R. Wang, and S. R. Shih.** 1999. An epidemic of enterovirus 71 infection in Taiwan. *N. Engl. J. Med.* **341:**929–935.
96. **Hogle, J. M., M. Chow, and D. J. Filman.** 1985. Three-dimensional structure of poliovirus at 2.9A resolution. *Science* **229:**1358–1365.
97. **Horstmann, D. M.** 1949. Clinical aspects of acute poliomyelitis. *Am. J. Med.* **6:**592.
98. **Horstmann, D. M.** 1950. Acute poliomyelitis: relation of physical activity at the time of onset to the course of the disease. *JAMA* **142:**236–241.
99. **Horstmann, D. M., and N. Yamada.** 1968. Enterovirus infections of the central nervous system. *Res. Publ. Assoc. Nerv. Ment. Dis.* **44:**236–253.

100. **Hosoya, M., M. Sato, K. Honzumi, M. Katayose, Y. Kawasaki, H. Sakuma, K. Kato, Y. Shimada, H. Ishiko, and H. Suzuki.** 2001. Association of nonpolio enteroviral infection in the central nervous system of children with febrile seizures. *Pediatrics* **107:**E12.
101. **Howden, C. W., W. R. Lang, and J. Laws.** 1966. An epidemic of ECHO 9 virus meningitis in Auckland. *N. Z. Med. J.* **65:**763–765.
102. **Hsiung, G. O.** 1995. Enteroviruses. *In* G. D. Hsiung (ed.), *Diagnostic Virology*. Yale University Press, New Haven, CT.
103. **Huang, C. C., C. C. Liu, Y. C. Chang, C. Y. Chen, S. T. Wang, and T. F. Yeh.** 1999. Neurologic complications in children with enterovirus 71 infections. *N. Engl. J. Med.* **341:**936–942.
104. **Huang, M. C., S. M. Wang, Y. W. Hsu, H. C. Lin, C. Y. Chi, and C. C. Liu.** 2006. Long-term cognitive and motor deficits after enterovirus 71 brainstem encephalitis in children. *Pediatrics* **118:**e1785–e1788.
105. **Huber, S. A., C. Haisch, and P. A. Lodge.** 1990. Functional diversity in vascular endothelial cells—role in coxsackievirus tropism. *J. Virol.* **64:**4516–4522.
106. **Huebner, R. J., J. A. Risser, J. A. Bell, E. A. Beeman, P. M. Beigelman, and J. C. Strong.** 1953. Epidemic pleurodynia in Texas; a study of 22 cases. *N. Engl. J. Med.* **248:**267–274.
107. **Hughes, P. J., C. Horsnell, T. Hyypiä, and G. Stanway.** 1991. RGD-dependent entry of coxsackievirus A9 into host cells and its bypass after cleavage of VP1 protein by intestinal proteases. *J. Virol.* **65:**4735–4740.
108. **Hurst, E. W.** 1936. The newer knowledge of virus diseases of the nervous system: a review and an interpretation. *Brain* **59:**1–34.
109. **Hyypia, T., P. Auvinen, and M. Maaronen.** 1989. Polymerase chain reaction for human picornaviruses. *J. Gen. Virol.* **70:**3261–3268.
110. **Hyypia, T., C. Horsnell, M. Maaronen, M. Khan, N. Kalkkinen, P. Auvinen, L. Kinnunen, and G. Stanway.** 1992. A distinct picornavirus group identified by sequence analysis. *Proc. Natl. Acad. Sci. USA* **89:**8847–8851.
111. **Ida-Hosonuma, M., T. Iwasaki, T. Yoshikawa, N. Nagata, Y. Sato, T. Sata, M. Yoneyama, T. Fujita, C. Taya, H. Yonekawa, and S. Koike.** 2005. The alpha/beta interferon response controls tissue tropism and pathogenicity of poliovirus. *J. Virol.* **79:**4460–4469.
112. **Irvine, D. H., A. B. H. Irvine, and P. S. Gardner.** 1967. Outbreak of ECHO virus type 30 in a general practice. *Br. Med. J.* **4:**774–776.
113. **Isacsohn, M., A. L. Eidelman, M. Kaplan, A. Goren, B. Rudensky, R. Handsher, and Y. Barak.** 1994. Neonatal coxsackievirus group B infections: experience of a single department of neonatology. *Isr. J. Med. Sci.* **30:**371–374.
114. **Iwasaki, A., R. Welker, S. Mueller, M. Linehan, A. Nomoto, and E. Wimmer.** 2002. Immunofluorescence analysis of poliovirus receptor expression in Peyer's patches of humans, primates, and CD155 transgenic mice: implications for poliovirus infection. *J. Infect. Dis.* **186:**585–592.
115. **Jaffe, M., I. Srugo, E. Tirosh, A. A. Colin, and Y. Tal.** 1989. The ameliorating effect of lumbar puncture in viral meningitis. *Am. J. Dis. Child.* **143:**682–685.
116. **Jantausch, B. A., N. L. C. Luban, L. Duffy, and W. J. Rodriquez.** 1995. Maternal plasma transfusion in the treatment of disseminated neonatal echovirus 11 infection. *Pediatr. Infect. Dis. J.* **14:**154–155.
117. **Jartti, T., P. Lehtinen, and T. Vuorinen.** 2004. Respiratory picornaviruses and respiratory syncytial virus as causative agents of acute expiratory wheezing in children. *Emerg. Infect. Dis.* **10:**1095–1101.
118. **Jarvis, W. R., and G. Tucker.** 1981. Echovirus type 7 meningitis in young children. *Am. J. Dis. Child.* **135:**1009–1012.
119. **Jenista, J. A., L. E. Daizell, P. W. Davidson, and M. A. Menegus.** 1984. Outcome studies of neonatal enterovirus infection. *Pediatr. Res.* **18:**230A.
120. **Jenista, J. A., K. R. Powell, and M. A. Menegus.** 1984. Epidemiology of neonatal enterovirus infection. *J. Pediatr.* **104:**685–690.
121. **Johnson, G. M., G. A. McAbee, E. D. Seaton, and S. M. Lipson.** 1992. Suspect value of non-CSF viral cultures in the diagnosis of enteroviral CNS infection in young infants. *Dev. Med. Child Neurol.* **34:**876–884.
121a. **Johnson, K. L., and P. Sarnow.** 1995. Viral RNA synthesis, p. 95–112. *In* H. A. Rotbart (ed.), *Human Enterovirus Infections*. ASM Press, Washington, DC.
122. **Johnston, J. M., and J. C. Overall, Jr.** 1989. Intravenous immunoglobulin in disseminated neonatal echovirus 11 infection. *Pediatr. Infect. Dis. J.* **8:**254–256.
123. **Junttila, N., N. Lévêque, J. P. Kabue, G. Cartet, F. Mushiya, J. J. Muyembe-Tamfum, A. Trompette, B. Lina, L. O. Magnius, J. J. Chomel, and H. Norder.** 2007. New enteroviruses, EV-93 and EV-94, associated with acute flaccid paralysis in the Democratic Republic of the Congo. *J. Med. Virol.* **79:**393–400.
124. **Kantor, F. S., and G. D. Hsiung.** 1962. Pleurodynia associated with echo virus type 8. *N. Engl. J. Med.* **266:**661–663.
125. **Kaplan, M. H., S. W. Klein, J. McPhee, and R. G. Harper.** 1983. Group B coxsackievirus infections in infants younger than three months of age: a serious childhood illness. *Rev. Infect. Dis.* **5:**1019–1032.
126. **Kearns, G. L., S. M. Abdel-Rahman, L. P. James, D. L. Blowey, J. D. Marshall, T. G. Wells, and R. F. Jacobs.** 1999. Single-dose pharmacokinetics of a pleconaril (VP63843) oral solution in children and adolescents. *Antimicrob. Agents Chemother.* **43:**634–638.
127. **Keeling, P., J. Jeffrey, S. Caforio, R. Taylor, G. F. Bottazzo, M. J. Davies, and W. J. McKenna.** 1992. Similar prevalence of enteroviral genome within the myocardium from patients with idiopathic dilated cardiomyopathy and controls by the polymerase chain reaction. *Br. Heart J.* **68:**554–559.
128. **Kelly, S., W. Winkelstein, Jr., and J. Winsser.** 1957. Poliomyelitis and other enteric viruses in sewage. *Am. J. Public Health Nations Health* **47:**72–77.
129. **Kessler, H. H., B. Santner, H. Rabenau, A. Berger, A. Vince, C. Lewinski, B. Weber, K. Pierer, D. Stuenzner, E. Marth, and H. W. Doerr.** 1997. Rapid diagnosis of enterovirus infection by a new one-step reverse transcription-PCR assay. *J. Clin. Microbiol.* **35:**976–977.
130. **Kew, O., V. Morris-Glasgow, M. Landaverde, C. Burns, J. Shaw, Z. Garib, J. André, E. Blackman, C. J. Freeman, J. Jorba, R. Sutter, G. Tambini, L. Venczel, C. Pedreira, F. Laender, H. Shimizu, T. Yoneyama, T. Miyamura, H. van Der Avoort, M. S. Oberste, D. Kilpatrick, S. Cochi, M. Pallansch, and C. de Quadros.** 2002. Outbreak of poliomyelitis in Hispaniola associated with circulating type 1 vaccine-derived poliovirus. *Science* **296:**356–359.
131. **Kew, O. M., R. W. Sutter, E. M. de Gourville, W. R. Dowdle, and M. A. Pallansch.** 2005. Vaccine-derived polioviruses and the endgame strategy for global polio eradication. *Annu. Rev. Microbiol.* **59:**587–635.
132. **Khetsuriani, N., A. Lamonte, M. S. Oberste, and M. Pallansch.** 2006. Neonatal enterovirus infections reported to the national enterovirus surveillance system in

the United States, 1983–2003. *Pediatr. Infect. Dis. J.* **25:** 889–893.

133. **Kilpatrick, D. R., K. Ching, J. Iber, R. Campagnoli, C. J. Freeman, N. Mishrik, H. M. Liu, M. A. Pallansch, and O. M. Kew.** 2004. Multiplex PCR method for identifying recombinant vaccine-related polioviruses. *J. Clin. Microbiol.* **42:**4313–4315.

134. **Kilpatrick, D. R., B. Nottay, C. F. Yang, S. J. Yang, E. Da Silva, S. Penaranda, M. Pallansch, and O. Kew.** 1998. Serotype-specific identification of polioviruses by PCR using primers containing mixed-base or deoxyinosine residues at positions of codon degeneracy. *J. Clin. Microbiol.* **36:**352–357.

135. **Kilpatrick, D. R., B. Nottay, C.-F. Yang, S.-J. Yang, M. N. Mulders, B. P. Holloway, M. A. Pallansch, and O. M. Kew.** 1996. Group-specific identification of polioviruses by PCR using primers containing mixed-base or deoxyinosine residues at positions of codon degeneracy. *J. Clin. Microbiol.* **34:**2990–2996.

136. **King, D. L., and D. T. Karzon.** 1975. An epidemic of aseptic meningitis syndrome due to echo virus type 6. *Pediatrics* **53:**432–437.

137. **Kinnunen, E., Hovi, T. Stenvik, O. Hellström, J. Porras, M. Kleemola, and M. L. Kantanen.** 1987. Localized outbreak of enteroviral meningitis in adults. *Acta Neurol. Scand.* **74:**346–351.

138. **Klespies, S. L., D. E. Cebula, C. L. Kelley, D. Galehouse, and C. C. Maurer.** 1996. Detection of enteroviruses from clinical specimens by spin amplification shell vial culture and monoclonal antibody assay. *J. Clin. Microbiol.* **34:**1465–1467.

139. **Kogon, A., I. Spigland, T. E. Frothingham, L. Elveback, C. Williams, C. E. Hall, and J. P. Fox.** 1969. The virus watch program: a continuing surveillance of viral infections in metropolitan New York families. VII. Observations on viral excretion, seroimmunity, intrafamilial spread and illness association in coxsackie and echovirus infections. *Am. J. Epidemiol.* **89:**51–61.

140. **Kost, C. B., B. Rogers, M. S. Oberste, C. Robinson, B. L. Eaves, K. Leos, S. Danielson, M. Satya, F. Weir, and F. S. Nolte.** 2007. Multicenter beta trial of the GeneXpert enterovirus assay. *J. Clin. Microbiol.* **45:** 1081–1086.

141. **Lake, A. M., B. A. Lauer, J. C. Clark, R. L. Wesenberg, and K. McIntosh.** 1976. Enterovirus infections in neonates. *J. Pediatr.* **89:**787–791.

142. **Landry, M. L., R. Garner, and D. Ferguson.** 2003. Rapid enterovirus RNA detection in clinical specimens by using nucleic acid sequence-based application. *J. Clin. Microbiol.* **41:**346–350.

143. **Landry, M. L., R. Garner, and D. Ferguson.** 2003. Comparison of the NucliSens Basic kit (nucleic acid sequence-based amplification) and the Argene Biosoft Enterovirus Consensus reverse transcription-PCR assays for rapid detection of enterovirus RNA in clinical specimens. *J. Clin. Microbiol.* **41:**5006–5010.

144. **Landsteiner, K., and E. Popper.** 1909. Uebertragung der Poliomyelitis acuta auf Affen. *Z. Immunitaetsforsch.* **2:** 377–390.

145. **Leon-Monzon, M. E., I. Illa, and M. C. Dalakas.** 1995. Expression of poliovirus receptor in human spinal cord and muscle. *Ann. N. Y. Acad. Sci.* **753:**48–57.

146. **Lerner, A. M., J. O. Klein, J. D. Cherry, and M. Finland.** 1963. New viral exanthems. *N. Engl. J. Med.* **269:** 678–685.

147. **Liljeqvist, J. A., T. Bergström, S. Holmström, A. Samuelson, G. E. Yousef, F. Waagstein, and S. Jeansson.** 1993. Failure to demonstrate enterovirus aetiology in Swedish patients with dilated cardiomyopathy. *J. Med. Virol.* **36:**6–10.

148. **Lim, K. A., and M. Benyesh-Melnick.** 1960. Typing of viruses by combinations of antisera pools. Application to typing of enteroviruses (coxsackie and echo). *J. Immunol.* **84:**309–317.

149. **Lipson, S. M., R. Waiderman, P. Costello, and K. Szabo.** 1988. Sensitivity of rhabdomyosarcoma and guinea pig embryo cell cultures to field isolates of difficult-to-cultivate group A coxsackieviruses. *J. Clin. Microbiol.* **26:**1298–1303.

150. **Lönnrot, M., M. Knip, M. Roivaninen, P. Koskela, H. K. Akerblom, and H. Hyöty.** 1998. Onset of type 1 diabetes mellitus in infancy after enterovirus infections. *Diabet. Med.* **15:**431–434.

151. **Lucchesi, P. F.** 1934. Poliomyelitis: a study of 410 patients at the Philadelphia Hospital for Contagious Diseases. *Am. J. Med. Sci.* **4:**515–523.

152. **Magoffin, R. L., and E. H. Lennette.** 1962. Nonpolioviruses and paralytic disease. *Calif. Med.* **97:**1–7.

153. **Mahon, N. G., B. Zal, G. Arno, P. Risley, J. Pinto-Basto, W. J. McKenna, M. J. Davies, and C. Baboonian.** 2001. Absence of viral nucleic acids in early and late dilated cardiomyopathy. *Heart* **86:**687–692.

154. **Martino, T. A., P. Liu, M. Petric, and M. J. Sole.** 1995. Enteroviral myocarditis and dilated cardiomyopathy: a review of clinical and experimental studies, p. 291–351. *In* H. A. Rotbart (ed.), *Human Enterovirus Infections*. ASM Press, Washington, DC.

155. **McKinney, R. E., Jr., S. L. Katz, and C. M. Wilfert.** 1987. Chronic enteroviral meningoencephalitis in agammaglobulinemic patients. *Rev. Infect. Dis.* **9:**334–356.

156. **McLaughlin, J. B., B. D. Gessner, T. V. Lynn, E. A. Funk, and J. P. Middaugh.** 2004. Association of regulatory issues with an echovirus 18 meningitis outbreak at a children's summer camp in Alaska. *Pediatr. Infect. Dis. J.* **23:**875–877.

157. **Melnick, J. L.** 1989. Enteroviruses, p. 191–263. *In* A. S. Evans (ed.), *Viral Infections of Humans, Epidemiology and Control*, 3rd ed. Plenum, New York, NY.

158. **Melnick, J. L., R. O. Proctor, A. R. Ocampo, A. R. Diwan, and E. Ben-Porath.** 1966. Free and bound virus in serum after administration of oral poliovirus vaccine. *Am. J. Epidemiol.* **84:**329–342.

159. **Melnick, J. L., V. Rennick, B. Hampil, N. J. Schmidt, and H. H. Ho.** 1973. Lyophilized combination pools of enterovirus equine antisera: preparation and test procedures for the identification of field strains of 42 enteroviruses. *Bull. W. H. O.* **48:**263–268.

160. **Melnick, J. L., N. J. Schmidt, B. Hampil, and H. H. Ho.** 1977. Lyophilized combination pools of enterovirus equine antisera: preparation and test procedures for the identification of field strains of 19 group A coxsackievirus serotypes. *Intervirology* **8:**172–181.

161. **Melnick, J. L., I. Tagaya, and H. Von Magnus.** 1974. Enteroviruses 69, 70, and 71. *Intervirology* **4:**369–370.

162. **Mendelsohn, C. L., E. Wimmer, and V. R. Racaniello.** 1989. Cellular receptor for poliovirus: molecular cloning, nucleotide sequence and expression of a new member of the immunoglobulin superfamily. *Cell* **56:**855–865.

163. **Minor, P. D.** 1992. The molecular biology of poliovaccines. *J. Gen. Virol.* **73:**3065–3077.

164. **Minor, P. D., M. Ferguson, D. M. Evans, J. W. Almond, and J. P. Icenogle.** 1986. Antigenic structure of polioviruses of serotypes 1, 2 and 3. *J. Gen. Virol.* **67:** 1283–1291.

165. **Minor, P. D., A. John, M. Ferguson, and J. P. Icenogle.** 1986. Antigenic and molecular evolution of the vaccine

strain of type 3 poliovirus during the period of excretion by a primary vaccinee. *J. Gen. Virol.* **67:**693–706.

166. **Mintz, L., and W. L. Drew.** 1980. Relation of culture site to the recovery of nonpolio enteroviruses. *Am. J. Clin. Pathol.* **74:**324–326.
167. **Mitchell, J. R., M. W. Presnell, E. W. Akin, J. M. Cummins, and O. C. Liu.** 1966. Accumulation and elimination of poliovirus by the eastern oyster. *Am. J. Epidemiol.* **84:**40–50.
168. **Modlin, J. F., R. Dagan, L. E. Berlin, D. M. Virshup, R. H. Yolken, and M. Menegus.** 1991. Focal encephalitis with enterovirus infections. *Pediatrics* **88:**841–845.
169. **Modlin, J. F.** 1986. Perinatal echovirus infection: insights from a literature review of 61 cases of serious infection and 16 outbreaks in nurseries. *Rev. Infect. Dis.* **8:**918–926.
170. **Moore, M.** 1982. Enteroviral disease in the United States, 1970–1979. *J. Infect. Dis.* **146:**103–108.
171. **Morens, D. M., and M. A. Pallansch.** 1995. Epidemiology, p. 3–23. *In* H. A. Rotbart (ed.), *Human Enterovirus Infections*. ASM Press. Washington, DC.
172. **Moses, E. B., A. G. Dean, M. H. Hatch, and A. L. Barron.** 1977. An outbreak of aseptic meningitis in the area of Fort Smith, Arkansas, 1975, due to echovirus type 4. *J. Ark. Med. Soc.* **74:**121–125.
173. **Muckelbauer, J. K., M. Kremer, I. Minor, G. Diana, F. J. Dutko, J. Groarke, D. C. Pevear, and M. G. Rossmann.** 1995. The structure of coxsackievirus B3 at 3.5 A resolution. *Structure* **3:**653–667.
174. **Muir, P., F. Nicholson, M. K. Sharief, E. J. Thompson, N. J. Cairns, P. Lantos, G. T. Spencer, H. J. Kaminski, and J. E. Banatvala.** 1995. Evidence for persistent enterovirus infection of the central nervous system in patients with previous paralytic poliomyelitis. *Ann. N. Y. Acad. Sci.* **753:**219–232.
175. **Nathanson, N., and D. Bodian.** 1961. Experimental poliomyelitis following intramuscular virus injection. 1. The effect of neural block on a neurotropic and a pantropic strain. *Bull. Johns Hopkins Hosp.* **108:**308–319.
176. **Nathanson, N., and A. Langmuir.** 1963. The Cutter incident: poliomyelitis following formaldehyde-inactivated poliovirus vaccination in the United States during the spring of 1955. III. Comparison of the clinical character of vaccinated and contact cases occurring after use of high rate lots of Cutter vaccine. *Am. J. Hyg.* **78:** 61–81.
177. **Nathanson, N., and J. R. Martin.** 1979. The epidemiology of poliomyelitis—enigmas surrounding its appearance, epidemicity, and disappearance. *Am. J. Epidemiol.* **110:**672–692.
178. **Newcombe, N. G., L. G. Beagley, D. Christiansen, B. E. Loveland, E. S. Johansson, K. W. Beagley, R. D. Barry, and D. R. Shafren.** 2004. Novel role for decay-accelerating factor in coxsackievirus A21-mediated cell infectivity. *J. Virol.* **78:**12677–12682.
179. **Nix, W. A., M. S. Oberste, and M. A. J. Pallansch.** 2006. Sensitive, seminested PCR amplification of VP1 sequences for direct identification of all enterovirus serotypes from original clinical specimens. *Clin. Microbiol.* **44:**2698–2704.
180. **Norder, H., L. Bjerregaard, L. Magnius, B. Lina, M. Aymard, and J. J. Chomel.** 2003. Sequencing of 'untypable' enteroviruses reveals two new types, EV-77 and EV-78, within human enterovirus type B and substitutions in the BC loop of the VP1 protein for known types. *J. Gen. Virol.* **84:**827–836.
181. **Oberste, M. S.** 2001. Molecular identification of new picornaviruses and characterization of a proposed enterovirus 73 serotype. *J. Gen. Virol.* **82:**409–416.
182. **Oberste, M. S., K. Maher, M. R. Flemister, G. Marchetti, D. R. Kilpatrick, and M. A. Pallansch.** 2000. Comparison of classic and molecular approaches for the identification of untypeable enteroviruses. *J. Clin. Microbiol.* **38:**1170–1174.
183. **Oberste, M. S., K. Maher, D. R. Kilpatrick, and M. A. Pallansch.** 1999. Molecular evolution of the human enteroviruses: correlation of serotype with VP1 sequence and application to picornavirus classification. *J. Virol.* **73:**1941–1948.
184. **Oberste, M. S., K. Maher, D. R. Kilpatrick, M. R. Flemister, B. A. Brown, and M. A. Pallansch.** 1999. Typing of human enteroviruses by partial sequencing of VP1. *J. Clin. Microbiol.* **37:**1288–1293.
185. **Oberste, M. S., K. Maher, S. M. Michele, G. Belliot, M. Uddin, and M. A. Pallansch.** 2005. Enteroviruses 76, 89, 90 and 91 represent a novel group within the species Human enterovirus A. *J. Gen. Virol.* **86:**445–451.
186. **Oberste, M. S., K. Maher, W. A. Nix, S. M. Michele, M. Uddin, D. Schnurr, S. al-Busaidy, C. Akoua-Koffi, and M. A. Pallansch.** 2007. Molecular identification of 13 new enterovirus types, EV79-88, EV97, and EV100-101, members of the species Human Enterovirus B. *Virus Res.* **128:**34–42.
187. **Oberste, M. S., K. Maher, A. J. Williams, N. Dybdahl-Sissoko, B. A. Brown, M. S. Gookin, S. Peñaranda, N. Mishrik, M. Uddin, and M. A. Pallansch.** 2006. Species-specific RT-PCR amplification of human enteroviruses: a tool for rapid species identification of uncharacterized enteroviruses. *J. Gen. Virol.* **87:**119–128.
188. **Oberste, M. S., S. M. Michele, K. Maher, D. Schnurr, D. Cisterna, N. Junttila, M. Uddin, J. J. Chomel, C. S. Lau, W. Ridha, S. al-Busaidy, H. Norder, L. O. Magnius, and M. A. Pallansch.** 2004. Molecular identification and characterization of two proposed new enterovirus serotypes, EV74 and EV75. *J. Gen. Virol.* **85:** 3205–3212.
189. **Oberste, M. S., W. A. Nix, K. Maher, and M. A. Pallansch.** 2003. Improved molecular identification of enteroviruses by RT-PCR and amplicon sequencing. *J. Clin. Virol.* **26:**375–377.
190. **Ohka, S., W. X. Yang, E. Terada, K. Iwasaki, and A. Nomoto.** 1998. Retrograde transport of intact poliovirus through the axon via the fast transport system. *Virology* **250:**67–75.
191. **Pallansch, M. A., and R. P. Roos.** 2007. Enteroviruses: polioviruses, coxsackieviruses, echoviruses, and newer enteroviruses, p. 839–893. *In* D. M. Knipe, P. M. Howley, D. E. Griffin, R. A. Lamb, M. A. Martin, B. Roizman, and S. E. Straus (ed.), *Fields Virology*, 5th ed. Lippincott Williams & Wilkins, Philadelphia, PA.
192. **Parrott, R. H., S. Ross, F. G. Burke, and E. C. Rice.** 1951. Herpangina: clinical studies of a specific infectious disease. *N. Engl. J. Med.* **245:**275–280.
193. **Patriarca, P. A., I. M. Onorato, V. E. F. Sklar, L. B. Schonberger, R. M. Kaminski, M. H. Hatch, D. M. Morens, and R. K. Forster.** 1983. Acute hemorrhagic conjunctivitis. Investigation of a large-scale community outbreak in Dade County, Florida. *JAMA* **249:**1283–1289.
194. **Paul, J. R., and D. M. Horstmann.** 1955. A survey of poliomyelitis virus antibodies in French Morocco. *Am. J. Trop. Med. Hyg.* **4:**512–524.
195. **Peigue-Lafeuille, H., N. Croquez, H. Laurichesse, P. Clavelou, O. Aumaître, J. Schmidt, M. Maillet-Vioud, C. Henquell, C. Archimbaud, J. L. Bailly, and M. Chambon.** 2002. Enterovirus meningitis in adults in

1999–2000 and evaluation of clinical management. *J. Med. Virol.* **67:**47–53.

196. **Pelletier, J., and N. Sonenberg.** 1988. Internal initiation of translation of eukaryotic mRNA directed by a sequence derived from poliovirus RNA. *Nature* **334:**320–325.

197. **Pevear, D. C., M. J. Fancher, P. J. Felock, M. G. Rossmann, M. S. Miller, G. D. Diana, A. M. Treasurywala, M. A. McKinlay, and F. J. Dutko.** 1989. Conformational change in the floor of the human rhinovirus canyon blocks adsorption to HeLa cell receptors. *J. Virol.* **63:**2002–2007.

198. **Pevear, D. C., T. M. Tull, M. E. Seipel, and J. M. Groarke.** 1999. Activity of pleconaril against enteroviruses. *Antimicrob. Agents Chemother.* **43:**2109–2115.

199. **Pichichero, M. E., S. McLinn, H. A. Rotbart, M. A. Menegus, M. Cascino, and B. E. Reidenberg.** 1998. Clinical and economic impact of enterovirus illness in private pediatric practice. *Pediatrics* **102:**1126–1134.

200. **Prather, S. L., R. Dagan, J. A. Jenista, and M. A. Menegus.** 1984. The isolation of enteroviruses from blood: a comparison of four processing methods. *J. Med. Virol.* **14:**221–227.

201. **Price, R. A., J. H. Garcia, and W. A. Rightsel.** 1970. Choriomeningitis and myocarditis in an adolescent with isolation of coxsackie B-5 virus. *Am. J. Clin. Pathol.* **53:** 825–831.

202. **Racaniello, V. R.** 1995. Early events in infection: receptor binding and cell entry, p. 73–93. *In* H. A. Rotbart (ed.), *Human Enterovirus Infections*. ASM Press, Washington, DC.

203. **Racaniello, V. R.** 2007. Picornaviridae: the viruses and their replication, p. 795–838. *In* D. M. Knipe, P. M. Howley, D. E. Griffin, R. A. Lamb, M. A. Martin, B. Roizman, and S. E. Straus (ed.), *Fields Virology*, 5th ed. Lippincott Williams & Wilkins, Philadelphia, PA.

204. **Racaniello, V. R.** 2006. One hundred years of poliovirus pathogenesis. *Virology* **344:**9–16.

205. **Ramers, C., G. Billman, M. Hartin, S. Ho, and M. H. Sawyer.** 2000. Impact of a diagnostic cerebrospinal fluid enterovirus polymerase chain reaction test on patient management. *JAMA* **283:**2680–2685.

206. **Rantakallio, P., M. Leskinen, and L. von Wendt.** 1986. Incidence and prognosis of central nervous system infections in a birth cohort of 12,000 children. *Scand. J. Infect. Dis.* **18:**287–294.

207. **Ray, C. G., R. H. McCollough, I. L. Doto, J. C. Todd, W. P. Glezen, and T. D. Chin.** 1966. Echo 4 illness. Epidemiological, clinical and laboratory studies of an outbreak in a rural community. *Am. J. Epidemiol.* **84:** 253–267.

208. **Reimann, B., R. Zell, and R. Kandolf.** 1991. Mapping of a neutralizing antigenic site of coxsackievirus B4 by construction of an antigenic chimera. *J. Virol.* **65:**3475–3480.

209. **Ren, R., and V. Racaniello.** 1992. Human poliovirus receptor gene expression and poliovirus tissue tropism in transgenic mice. *J. Virol.* **66:**296–304.

210. **Rewers, M., and M. Atkinson.** 1995. The possible role of enteroviruses in diabetes mellitus, p. 353–395. *In* H. A. Rotbart (ed.), *Human Enterovirus Infections*. ASM Press, Washington, DC.

211. **Rigonan, A. S., L. Mann, and T. Chonmaitree.** 1998. Use of monoclonal antibodies to identify serotypes of enterovirus isolates. *J. Clin. Microbiol.* **36:**1877–1881.

212. **Roivainen, M., T. Hyypiä, L. Piirainen, N. Kalkkinen, G. Stanway, and T. Hovi.** 1995. The coxsackievirus A9 RGD motif is not essential for virus viability. *J. Virol.* **69:**8035–8040.

213. **Rombaut, B., R. Vrijsen, and A. Boeye.** 1985. Comparison of arildone and 3-methylquercetin as stabilizers of poliovirus. *Antivir. Res.* **1985**(Suppl. 1)**:**67–73.

214. **Romero, J. R.** 1999. Reverse-transcription-polymerase chain reaction detection of the enteroviruses: overview and clinical utility in pediatric enteroviral infections. *Arch. Pathol. Lab. Med.* **123:**1161–1169.

215. **Romero, J. R.** 2006. Enteroviruses and parechoviruses, p. 1392–1404. *In* P. R. Murray, E. J. Baron, J. H. Jorgensen, M. L. Landry, and M. A. Pfaller (ed.), *Manual of Clinical Microbiology*, 9th ed. ASM Press, Washington, DC.

216. **Romero, J. R., and H. A. Rotbart.** 1994. PCR-based strategies for the detection of human enteroviruses, p. 341–374. *In* G. D. Ehrlich, and S. Greenberg (ed.), *PCR-Based Diagnostics in Infectious Disease*. Blackwell Scientific Publications, Boston, MA.

217. **Rorabaugh, M. L., L. E. Berlin, L. Rosenberg, and J. Modlin.** 1992. Absence of neurodevelopmental sequelae from aseptic meningitis. *Pediatr. Res.* **30:**177A.

218. **Rorabaugh, M. L., L. E. Berlin, F. Heldrich, K. Roberts, L. A. Rosenberg, T. Doran, and J. F. Modlin.** 1993. Aseptic meningitis in infants younger than 2 years of age: acute illness and neurologic complications. *Pediatrics* **92:**206–211.

219. **Rotbart, H. A.** 1995. Meningitis and encephalitis, p. 271–289. *In* H. A. Rotbart (ed.), *Human Enterovirus Infections*. ASM Press, Washington, DC.

220. **Rotbart, H. A.** 1997. Viral meningitis and the aseptic meningitis syndrome, p. 23–47. *In* W. M. Scheld, R. J. Whitley, and D. T. Durack (ed.), *Infections of the Central Nervous System*, 2nd ed. Lippincott-Raven, Philadelphia, PA.

221. **Rotbart, H. A.** 1990. Enzymatic RNA amplification of the enteroviruses. *J. Clin. Microbiol.* **28:**438–442.

222. **Rotbart, H. A.** 1990. Diagnosis of enteroviral meningitis with the polymerase chain reaction. *J. Pediatr.* **117:**85–89.

223. **Rotbart, H. A., P. J. Brennan, K. H. Fife, J. R. Romero, J. A. Griffin, M. A. McKinlay, and F. G. Hayden.** 1998. Enterovirus meningitis in adults. *Clin. Infect. Dis.* **27:**896–898.

224. **Rotbart, H. A.** 1999. Enteroviruses, p. 990–998. *In* P. R. Murray, E. J. Baron, M. A. Pfaller, F. C. Tenover, and R. H. Yolken (ed.), *Manual of Clinical Microbiology*, 7th ed. ASM Press, Washington, DC.

225. **Rotbart, H. A., J. P. Kinsella, and R. L. Wasserman.** 1990. Persistent enterovirus infection in culture-negative meningoencephalitis—demonstration by enzymatic RNA amplification. *J. Infect. Dis.* **161:**787–791.

226. **Rotbart, H. A., G. H. McCracken, R. J. Whitley, J. F. Modlin, M. Cascino, S. Shah, and D. Blum.** 1999. Clinical significance of enteroviruses in serious summer febrile illnesses of children. *Pediatr. Infect. Dis. J.* **18:** 869–874.

227. **Rotbart, H. A., A. D. B. Webster, and Pleconaril Treatment Registry Group.** 2001. Treatment of potentially life-threatening enterovirus infections with pleconaril. *Clin. Infect. Dis.* **32:**228–235.

228. **Russell, W. R.** 1947. Poliomyelitis; pre-paralytic stage and effect of physical activity on severity of paralysis. *Br. Med. J.* **2:**1023.

229. **Russell, W. R.** 1949. Paralytic poliomyelitis. The early symptoms and the effect of physical activity on the course of disease. *Br. Med. J.* **1:**465–471.

230. **Sabin, A. B., and R. Ward.** 1941. Flies as carriers of poliomyelitis virus in urban epidemics. *Science* **94:**590–591.

231. **Sabin, A. B., and R. Ward.** 1941. The natural history of human poliomyelitis. I. Distribution of virus in nervous and non-nervous tissues. *J. Exp. Med.* **73:**771–793.
232. **Sawyer, L. A., R. C. Hershow, M. A. Pallansch, D. B. Fishbein, P. F. Pinsky, S. F. Broerman, B. B. Grimm, L. J. Anderson, D. B. Hall, and L. B. Schonberger.** 1989. An epidemic of acute hemorrhagic conjunctivitis in American Samoa caused by coxsackievirus A24 variant. *Am. J. Epidemiol.* **130:**1187–1198.
233. **Sawyer, M. H., D. Holland, N. Aintablian, J. D. Connor, E. F. Keyser, and N. J. Waecker, Jr.** 1994. Diagnosis of enteroviral central nervous system infection by polymerase chain reaction during a large community outbreak. *Pediatr. Infect. Dis. J.* **13:**177–182.
234. **Sawyer, M. H., X. Saez-Llorenz, C. L. Aviles, M. O'Ryan, and J. Romero.** 1999. Oral pleconaril reduces the duration and severity of enteroviral meningitis in children. *Pediatr. Res.* **45**(Part 2)**:**173A.
235. **Schiff, G., and J. Sherwood.** 2000. Clinical activity of pleconaril in an experimentally induced coxsackievirus A21 respiratory infection. *J. Infect. Dis.* **181:**20–26.
236. **Schlegel, A., and K. Kirkegaard.** 1995. Cell biology of enterovirus infection, p. 135–154. *In* H. A. Rotbart (ed.), *Human Enterovirus Infections*. ASM Press, Washington, DC.
237. **Sells, C. J., R. L. Carpenter, and C. G. Ray.** 1975. Sequelae of central-nervous-system enterovirus infections. *N. Engl. J. Med.* **293:**1–4.
238. **Seme, K., T. Mocilnik, K. F. Komlos, A. Doplihar, D. H. Persing, and M. Poljak.** 2008. GeneXpert enterovirus assay: one-year experience in a routine laboratory setting and evaluation on three proficiency panels. *J. Clin. Microbiol.* **46:**1510–1513.
239. **Shafran, S. D., W. Halota, D. Gilbert, J. Bernstein, H. Meislin, and M. Reiss.** 1999. Pleconaril is effective for enteroviral meningitis in adolescents and adults: a randomized placebo-controlled multicenter trial, abstr. 1904. *Abstr. 39th Intersci. Conf. Antimicrob. Agents Chemother.* American Society for Microbiology, Washington, DC.
240. **Sharief, M. K., R. Hentges, and M. Ciardi.** 1991. Intrathecal immune response in patients with the post-polio syndrome. *N. Engl. J. Med.* **325:**749–755.
241. **Sicinski, P., J. Rowinski, J. B. Warchok, Z. Jarzabek, W. Gur, B. Szczygiel, K. Bielechi, and G. Koch.** 1990. Poliovirus type 1 enters the human host through intestinal M cells. *Gastroenterology* **98:**56–58.
242. **Singer, J. I., P. R. Maur, J. P. Riley, and P. B. Smith.** 1980. Management of central nervous system infections during an epidemic of enteroviral aseptic meningitis. *J. Pediatr.* **96:**559–563.
243. **Solomon, P., L. Weinstein, and T. W. Chang.** 1959. Epidemiologic, clinical and laboratory features of an epidemic of type 9 Echo virus meningitis. *J. Pediatr.* **55:** 609–619.
244. **Stanway, G., F. Brown, P. Christian, T. Hovi, T. Hyypiä, A. M. Q. King, N. J. Knowles, S. M. Lemon, P. D. Minor, M. A. Pallansch, A. C. Palmenberg, and T. Skern.** 2005. Family *Picornaviridae*, p. 757–778. *In* C. M. Fauquet, M. A. Mayo, J. Maniloff, U. Desselberger, and L. A. Ball (ed.), *Virus Taxonomy. Eighth Report of the International Committee on Taxonomy of Viruses*. Elsevier/Academic Press, San Diego, CA.
245. **Stellrecht, K. A., I. Harding, A. M. Woron, M. L. Lepow, and R. A. Venezia.** 2002. The impact of an enteroviral RT-PCR assay on the diagnosis of aseptic meningitis and patient management. *J. Clin. Virol.* **1:** S19–S26.
246. **Stewart, S., and B. Semler.** 1997. RNA determinants of picornavirus cap independent translation initiation. *Semin. Virol.* **8:**242–255.
247. **Strebel, P. M., N. Ion-Nedelcu, A. L. Baughman, R. W. Sutter, and S. L. Cochi.** 1995. Intramuscular injections within 30 days of immunization with oral poliovirus vaccine—a risk factor for vaccine-associated paralytic poliomyelitis. *N. Engl. J. Med.* **332:**500–506.
248. **Strikas, R. A., L. J. Anderson, and A. Parker.** 1986. Temporal and geographic patterns of isolates of nonpolio enterovirus in the United States, 1970–1983. *J. Infect. Dis.* **153:**346–351.
249. **Sumaya, C. V., and L. I. Corman.** 1982. Enteroviral meningitis in early infancy: significance in community outbreaks. *Pediatr. Infect. Dis.* **3:**151–154.
250. **Sutinen, S., J. L. Kalliomaki, R. Pohjonen, and R. Vastamaki.** 1971. Fatal generalized coxsackie B3 virus infection in an adolescent with successful isolation of the virus from pericardial fluid. *Ann. Clin. Res.* **3:**241–246.
251. **Sutter, R. W., P. A. Patriarca, A. J. Suleiman, S. Brogan, P. G. Malankar, S. L. Cochi, A. A. Al-Ghassani, and M. S. el-Bualy.** 1992. Attributable risk of DTP (diphtheria and tetanus toxoids and pertussis vaccine) injection in provoking paralytic poliomyelitis during a large outbreak in Oman. *J. Infect. Dis.* **165:**444–449.
252. **Sylvest, E.** 1934. *Epidemic Myalgia: Bornholm Disease*. Oxford University Press, London, England. (Translated by H. Andersen.)
253. **Tattevin, P., S. Minjolle, C. Arvieux, V. Clayessen, R. Colimon, J. Bouget, and C. Michelet.** 2002. Benefits of management strategy adjustments during an outbreak of enterovirus meningitis in adults. *Scand. J. Infect. Dis.* **34:**359–361.
254. **Terletskaia-Ladwig, E., C. Metzger, G. Schalasta, and G. Enders.** 2000. Evaluation of enterovirus serological tests IgM-EIA and complement fixation in patients with meningitis, confirmed by detection of enteroviral RNA by RT-PCR in cerebrospinal fluid. *J. Med. Virol.* **61:**221–227.
255. **Thivierge, B., and G. Delage.** 1982. Infections du systeme nerveux central a enterovirus: 223 cas vus a un hopital pediatrique entre 1973 et 1981. *Can. Med. Assoc. J.* **127:**1097–1102.
256. **Thoelen, I., P. Lemey, I. Van Der Donck, K. Beuselinck, A. M. Lindberg, and M. Van Ranst.** 2003. Molecular typing and epidemiology of enteroviruses identified from an outbreak of aseptic meningitis in Belgium during the summer of 2000. *J. Med. Virol.* **70:**420–429.
257. **Tracy, S., N. M. Chapman, R. J. Rubocki, and M. A. Beck.** 1995. Host immune responses to enterovirus infections, p. 175–191. *In* H. A. Rotbart (ed.), *Human Enterovirus Infections*. ASM Press, Washington, DC.
258. **Trallero, G., I. Casas, A. Tenorio, J. E. Echevarria, A. Castellanos, A. Lozano, and P. P. Brena.** 2000. Enteroviruses in Spain: virological and epidemiological studies over 10 years (1988–97). *Epidemiol. Infect.* **124:**497–506.
259. **Travers, R. L., G. R. V. Hughes, G. Cambridge, and J. R. Sewell.** 1977. Coxsackie B neutralisation titres in polymyositis/dermatomyositis. *Lancet* **i:**268.
260. **Van Doornum, G. J., and J. C. De Jong.** 1998. Rapid shell vial culture technique for detection of enteroviruses and adenoviruses in fecal specimens: comparison with conventional virus isolation method. *J. Clin. Microbiol.* **36:**2865–2868.
261. **Wadia, N. H., S. M. Katrak, V. P. Misra, K. Miyamura, K. Hashimoto, T. Ogino, T. Hikiji, and R. Kono.** 1983. Polio-like motor paralysis associated with acute hemor-

rhagic conjunctivitis in an outbreak in 1981 in Bombay, India: clinical and serologic studies. *J. Infect. Dis.* **147:** 660–668.

262. **Wadia, N. H., P. N. Wadia, S. M. Katrak, and V. P. Misra.** 1983. A study of the neurological disorder associated with acute haemorrhagic conjunctivitis due to enterovirus 70. *J. Neurol. Neurosurg. Psychiatry* **46:**599–610.
263. **Ward, R., J. L. Melnick, and D. M. Horstmann.** 1945. Poliomyelitis virus in fly-contaminated food collected at an epidemic. *Science* **101:**491–493.
264. **Watkins, A.** 1949. *Poliomyelitis: Papers and Discussions Presented at the First International Poliomyelitis Conference*, p. 142–143. J. B. Lippincott, Philadelphia, PA.
265. **Webster, A. D. B.** 2005. Pleconaril—an advance in the treatment of enteroviral infection in immunocompromised patients. *J. Clin. Virol.* **32:**1–6
266. **Webster, A. D. B., H. A. Rotbart, T. Warner, P. Rudge, and N. Hyman.** 1993. Diagnosis of enterovirus brain disease in hypogammaglobulinemic patients by polymerase chain reaction. *Clin. Infect. Dis.* **17:**657–661.
267. **Weiner, L. B., H. A. Rotbart, D. L. Gilbert, F. G. Hayden, J. H. Mynhardt, D. E. Dwyer, H. Trocha, J. M. Rogers, and M. A. McKinlay.** 1997. Treatment of enterovirus meningitis with pleconaril (VP 63843), an antipicornaviral agent, abstr. LB-27, p. 14. *Abstr. 37th Intersci. Conf. Antimicrob. Agents Chemother.* American Society for Microbiology, Washington, DC.
268. **Weinstein, L., A. Shelokov, and R. Seltser.** 1952. A comparison of the clinical features of poliomyelitis in adults and children. *N. Engl. J. Med.* **246:**296.
269. **Wenner, H. A., and M. F. Lenahan.** 1961. Propagation of group A coxsackie viruses in tissue cultures. *Yale J. Biol. Med.* **34:**421–438.
270. **Whitley, R. J., C. G. Cobbs, C. A. Alford, Jr., S. J. Soong, M. S. Hirsch, J. D. Connor, L. Corey, D. F. Hanley, M. Levin, and D. A. Powell.** 1989. Diseases that mimic herpes simplex encephalitis. *JAMA* **262:** 234–239.
271. **Whitley, R. J., S. J. Soong, M. S. Hirsch, A. W. Karchmer, R. Dolin, G. Galasso, J. K. Dunnick, and C. A. Alford.** 1981. Herpes simplex encephalitis. *N. Engl. J. Med.* **304:**313–318.
272. **Wilfert, C. M., S. N. Lehrman, and S. L. Katz.** 1983. Enteroviruses and meningitis. *Pediatr. Infect. Dis.* **2:**333–341.
273. **Wilfert, C. M., R. J. Thompson, T. R. Sunder, A. O'Quinn, J. Zeller, and J. Blacharsh.** 1981. Longitudinal assessment of children with enteroviral meningitis during the first three months of life. *Pediatrics* **67:**811–815.
274. **Wilfert, C. M., and J. Zeller.** 1985. Enterovirus diagnosis, p. 85–107. *In* L. M. de la Maza and E. M. Peterson (ed.), *Medical Virology IV.* Lawrence Erlbaum Associates, Publishers, Hillsdale, NJ.
275. **Wong, S. N., A. Y. Tam, T. H. Ng, W. F. Ng, C. Y. Tong, and T. S. Tang.** 1989. Fatal coxsackie B1 virus infection in neonates. *Pediatr. Infect. Dis. J.* **8:**638–641.
276. **World Health Organization.** 30 January 2008. *Wild Poliovirus Weekly Update.* http://www.polioeradication.org/casecount.asp.
277. **Wright, H. T., R. M. McAllister, and R. Ward.** 1962. "Mixed" meningitis: reports of a case with isolation of Haemophilus influenzae type b and echovirus type 9 from the cerebrospinal fluid. *N. Engl. J. Med.* **267:**142–144.
278. **Xiao, C., C. M. Bator, V. D. Bowman, E. Rieder, Y. He, B. Hébert, J. Bella, T. S. Baker, E. Wimmer, R. J. Kuhn, and M. G. Rossmann.** 2001. Interaction of coxsackievirus A21 with its cellular receptor, ICAM-1. *J. Virol.* **75:**2444–2451.
279. **Yamashita, K., K. Miyamura, S. Yamadera, N. Kato, M. Akatsuka, S. Inouye, and S. Yamazaki.** 1992. Enteroviral aseptic meningitis in Japan, 1981–1991. *Jpn. J. Med. Sci. Biol.* **45:**151–161.
280. **Yang, W. X., T. Terasaki, K. Shiroki, S. Ohka, J. Aoki, S. Tanabe, T. Nomura, E. Terada, Y. Sugiyama, and A. Nomoto.** 1997. Efficient delivery of circulating poliovirus to the central nervous system independently of poliovirus receptor. *Virology* **229:**421–428.
281. **Yoon, J. W., M. Austin, T. Onodera, and A. Notkins.** 1979. Virus-induced diabetes mellitus: isolation of a virus from the pancreas of a child with diabetic ketoacidosis. *N. Engl. J. Med.* **300:**1173–1179.
282. **Yoshikawa, T., T. Iwasaki, M. Ida-Hosonuma, M. Yoneyama, T. Fujita, H. Horie, M. Miyazawa, S. Abe, B. Simizu, and S. Koike.** 2006. Role of the alpha/beta interferon response in the acquisition of susceptibility to poliovirus by kidney cells in culture. *J. Virol.* **80:**4313–4325.
283. **Zhang, A., R. G. Nanni, D. A. Oren, E. J. Rozhon, and E. Arnold.** 1992. Three-dimensional structure-activity relationships for antiviral agents that interact with picornavirus capsids. *Semin. Virol.* **3:**453–471.

Rhinovirus

RONALD B. TURNER AND WAI-MING LEE

46

Human rhinoviruses (HRVs) constitute the largest genus in the *Picornaviridae* family (24). The name "rhinovirus" stems from the virus's special adaptation to growth in the nasal passages. Rhinoviruses have been implicated in 30 to 50% of all cases of acute respiratory disease and represent the single most important causative agent of common colds. It was already known in 1930 that "colds" were easily transmitted from human to human and to higher apes and that the responsible agent was probably a virus (19, 63), but it was not until the adaptation of cell culture to viral isolation in 1956 that the first rhinovirus was discovered (83, 85). Isolation and classification of the HRVs were facilitated by the use of human embryonic lung cell cultures (60) and the discovery of the low temperature optimum (32 to 35°C) for replication (103). Since the 1960s, at least 100 distinct serotypes have been described (39, 57, 58). In addition, rapid progress has been made in understanding the clinical characteristics and epidemiology of the rhinoviruses (34, 35). The first complete genome sequence was determined for HRV14 in 1984 (96), a reverse-genetics system was developed in 1985 (69), and the X-ray crystallographic structures of the viral capsids of five serotypes (1A, 2, 3, 14, and 16) were solved soon afterward (37, 61, 76, 90, 105, 112). Thus, remarkable progress in rhinovirus research, from initial virus identification to characterization at the atomic level, has been made in the last few decades.

VIROLOGY

Classification

The family *Picornaviridae* consists of nine genera. Four of these—*Rhinovirus*, *Enterovirus*, *Parechovirus*, and *Hepatovirus*—cause human infections. The parechoviruses and hepatovirus were formerly classified as enteroviruses. One of the defining characteristics of the HRVs is their acid lability (i.e., their infectivity is reduced at least 10-fold when they are incubated at pH 4 for 1 h at 37°C in 0.1 M sodium citrate). In contrast, most human enteroviruses are stable under these conditions. All HRVs so far examined exhibit higher buoyant density (1.38 to 1.42 g/ml) in cesium chloride solution than do enteroviruses, which characteristically band at 1.34. This property is due mainly, if not entirely, to replacement of potassium ions bound to the RNA genome of rhinoviruses by heavier cesium ions. Cesium-potassium exchange does not occur in enteroviruses because the protein shell is impermeable to the cesium ion.

Serotypes

Rhinovirus infectivity is neutralized by specific antisera. The absence of cross-reactivity with antisera specific for known serotypes would indicate the existence of a new serotype. A total of 101 serotypes (1A to 100 and 1B) were identified by 1987 (39). HRV-Hanks, a strain that has been used frequently in experimental rhinovirus studies, has been typed as HRV21 (64). By cross-neutralization tests with rabbit antisera prepared for 90 serotypes (1A, 1B, and 2 through 89), serologic relationships have been identified among 16 clusters encompassing 50 serotypes: (1A,1B), (2,49), (3,6,14,79), (9,32,67), (11,15,40,74,76), (12,78), (13,41), (22,61), (5,17,19,21,29,30,42,43,44,70), (18,36,50,58,89), (38,60), (39,54), (48,55), (56,57), (59,63,85), and (66,77), leading to the proposal that rhinoviruses are divided into antigenic subgroups (11). More-

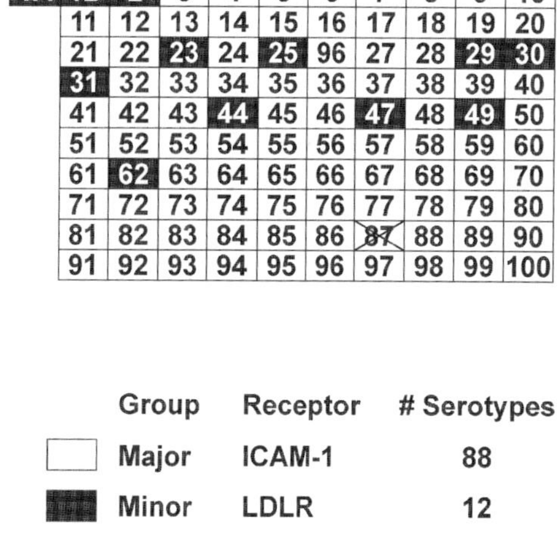

1A	1B	2	3	4	5	6	7	8	9	10
	11	12	13	14	15	16	17	18	19	20
	21	22	23	24	25	96	27	28	29	30
	31	32	33	34	35	36	37	38	39	40
	41	42	43	44	45	46	47	48	49	50
	51	52	53	54	55	56	57	58	59	60
	61	62	63	64	65	66	67	68	69	70
	71	72	73	74	75	76	77	78	79	80
	81	82	83	84	85	86	~~87~~	88	89	90
	91	92	93	94	95	96	97	98	99	100

Group	Receptor	# Serotypes
Major	ICAM-1	88
Minor	LDLR	12

FIGURE 1 Classification of human rhinovirus serotypes into two receptor groups. HRV87 has been reclassified as an enterovirus.

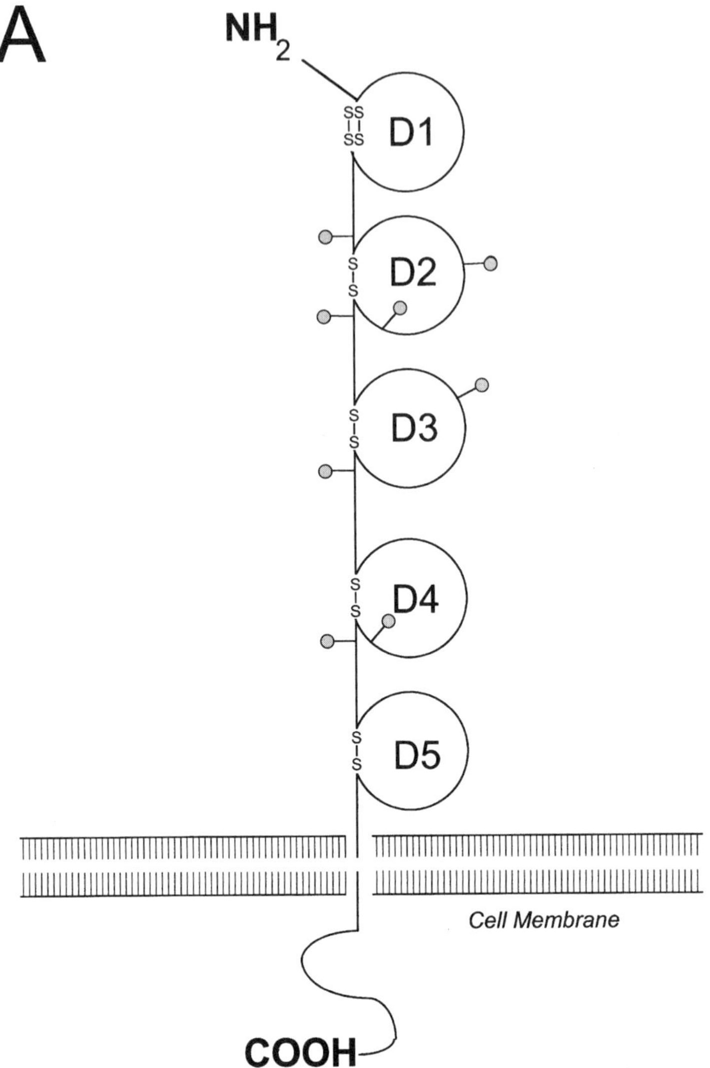

FIGURE 2 *(Continued on following page)*

over, certain serotypes, such as type 17, appear to be prone to antigenic hypervariation (81).

Phylogenetic Groups

Nucleotide sequences have been determined for the 5′ untranslated regions (UTR) and the VP4, VP2, and VP1 genes of all serotypes (64, 65, 92). Complete genome sequences have been determined for 46 serotypes (62, 97). Phylogenetic analysis of these sequences showed that 100 rhinovirus serotypes are divided into two genetic groups or species (A and B) (24, 48, 64, 92) and that HRV87 is an enterovirus (enterovirus 68). (75). HRV group A (HRVA) consists of 75 serotypes, and HRVB consists of 25 serotypes. In addition, the results of direct sequencing of rhinoviruses in original clinical specimens indicate the existence of many previously unrecognized rhinovirus strains and additional new genetic groups (62, 63a, 65, 68a). These new strains escaped detection in the past probably because they could not be cultured in traditional cell lines for rhinovirus isolation (65).

Receptor Types

Rhinovirus serotypes are also divided into two groups on the basis of receptor specificity (Fig. 1). The "major" receptor group, containing 88 serotypes, utilizes intercellular adhesion molecule 1 (ICAM-1 [Fig. 2A]) as a receptor for infecting host cells (30). This receptor is a member of the immunoglobulin superfamily and maps to human chromosome 19 (30). The major group of rhinoviruses is highly specific and does not recognize ICAM-1 from species other than humans, with the probable exception of chimpanzees (4). Twelve serotypes, constituting the "minor" receptor group, utilize the low-density lipoprotein receptor (LDLR) and related proteins as receptors (88, 106). All members of the minor receptor group are in HRVA, while the major receptor group consists of viruses in both HRVA and HRVB.

Composition

The virion has no lipid envelope and is composed of a single-stranded RNA genome tightly packed into the cen-

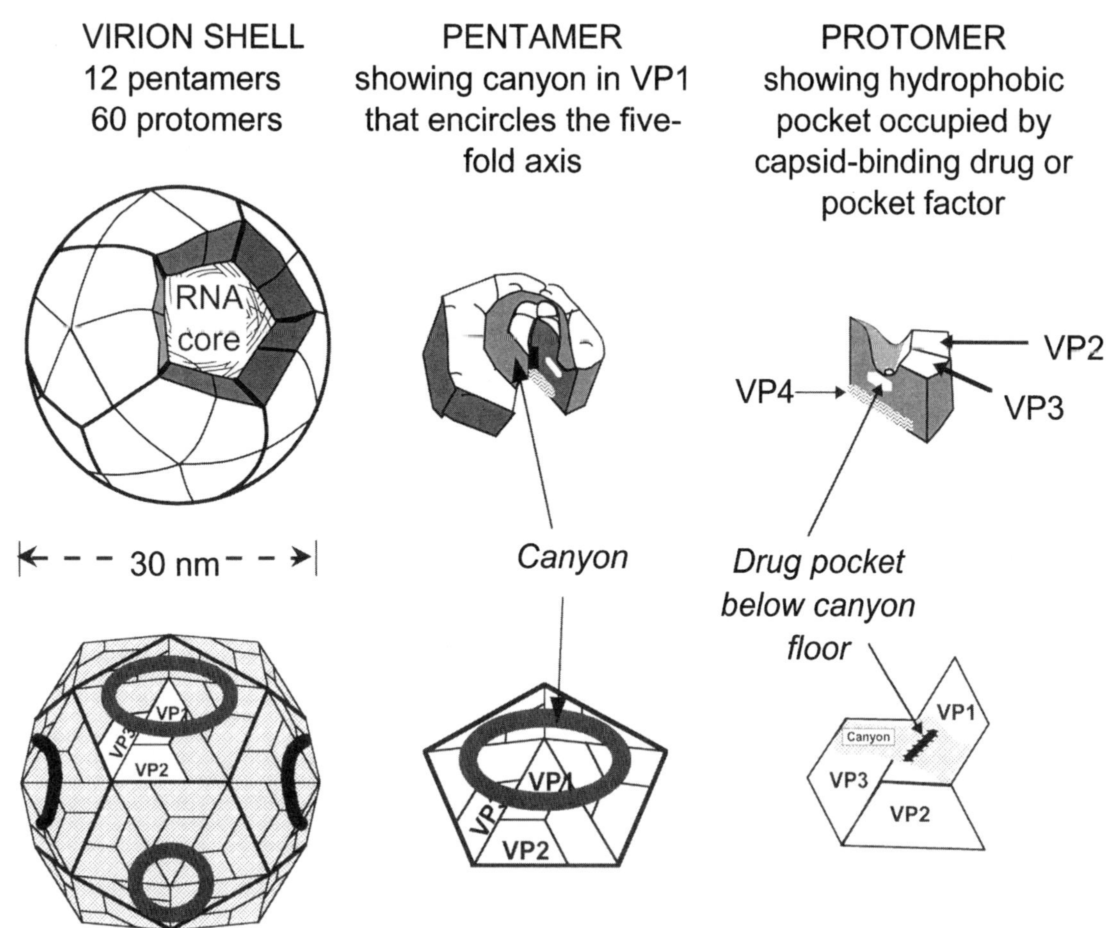

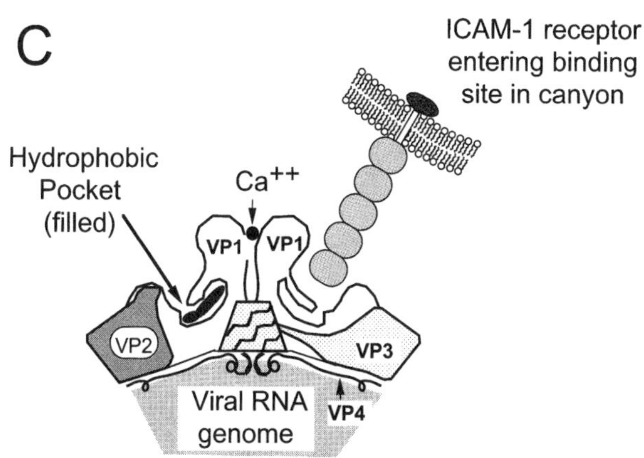

FIGURE 2 (A) Schematic drawing of ICAM-1, the receptor used by the major group of rhinoviruses. S-S represents disulfide bridges, and small circles represent sites of glycosylation. (B) Key features of the structure of a human rhinovirus. The virion shell consists of 12 pentamers, 1 of which has been removed to show the approximate location of the RNA packed tightly into a central cavity. Each pentamer, in turn, consists of five wedge-shaped protomer subunits. The canyon (shaded) is shown encircling the fivefold axis of the pentamer; the hydrophobic (drug-binding) pocket is indicated below the floor of the canyon in VP1. (C) Side view of the pentamer showing the spatial relationship between the receptor-binding site and the hydrophobic pocket. An ion, located at each pentamer center in serotypes 1A, 14, and 16, is tentatively identified as calcium.

ter of a protein shell known as the capsid (Fig. 2B). The concentration of purified virions can be measured spectrophotometrically with a conversion factor of 9.4×10^{12} virions per unit of optical density at 260 nm (91). Water is an important part of the virion structure. In its fully hydrated state (observed during conventional X-ray crystallography or by cryoelectron microscopy), the particle is about 30 nm in diameter. When dried (e.g., during preparation for conventional electron microscopy), the virion shrinks about 30% and loses infectivity. The protein shell, about 5 nm thick, is composed of 60 copies of each of four viral proteins, termed VP1 to VP4. Protein subunits called protomers, consisting of one copy of each of the four viral proteins, are organized into 12 pentamers. Each of the 12 pentamers contains a prominent depression or "canyon" in VP1 running moat-like around a central plateau (i.e., around the fivefold axis of symmetry).

Amino acid residues at the canyon base are more conserved than residues at exposed viral surfaces. Evidence indicates that the canyon region contains the binding site for the ICAM-1 receptor (10, 77). For example, it has been shown by cryoelectron microscopy (using purified fragments consisting of the distal two domains of ICAM-1) that the canyon (Fig. 2C) is the site at which the receptor binds to HRV16 and that purified virions can bind up to 60 such receptor fragments (77). Initially, it was hypothesized that a 20-Å-deep canyon was used to hide the viral receptor attachment site on a viral surface from immune surveillance (89). However, the X-ray structure of the HRV14-Fab complex showed that the antibody molecule penetrated deep into the canyon space (94). While the canyon may not conceal the receptor-binding site, the canyon plays a critical role in steps following attachment by providing a flexible region for the conformational change in the viral capsid. The binding of multiple receptors per virus particle (receptor "recruiting") appears to trigger a major rearrangement of the protein, accompanied by a 20% expansion of the shell, thus inducing conformational changes critical to allowing the eventual release of RNA.

At the base of the canyon lies a hydrophobic "pocket," which in HRV14 is empty but which in many other rhinoviruses (e.g., HRV16) is filled with a still-uncharacterized molecule called "pocket factor." Pocket factor may play a role in the replication cycle of rhinoviruses (59, 67, 91). This pocket is the binding site for several classes of picornavirus capsid-binding antivirals. In general, capsid-binding antivirals inhibit growth of picornaviruses by blocking virus-receptor interactions and uncoating of attached virus.

The rhinoviral genome is a single strand of positive-sense RNA of approximately 7,200 bases. Sequence analysis indicates a genome organization similar to that of poliovirus, the prototype enterovirus (Fig. 3A). Both viruses contain poly(A) tracts which are required for infectivity of the RNA, and both are covalently linked through the 5′-terminal uridylic acid to a small viral protein (VPg) which can be removed from the RNA without reducing its infectivity. The single large polyprotein, containing nearly

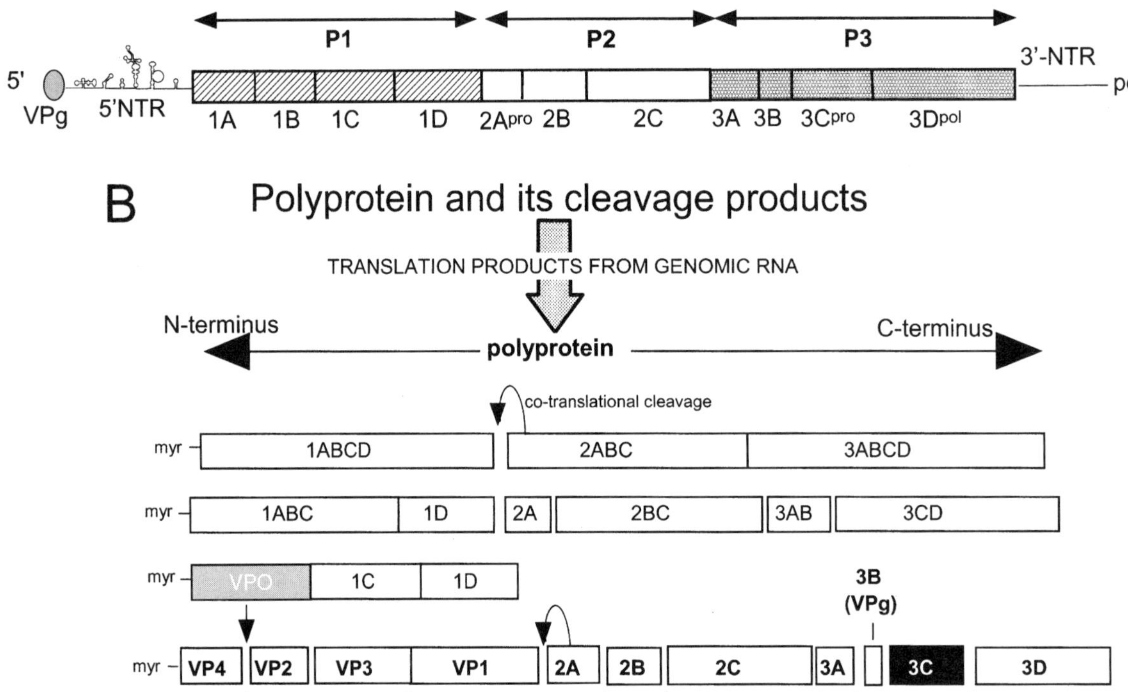

FIGURE 3 (A) RNA genome of an HRV. P1, P2, and P3 are precursor proteins which are subsequently processed to produce 11 end products. (B) Cleavage of the polyprotein is accomplished by two viral proteases, 2A and 3C. The 2A protease cotranslationally releases the coat precursor, P1, from nascent polyprotein, whereas the 3C (or precursor 3CD) protease cleaves all the remaining precursors and intermediates except for VP0. Cleavage of VP0 to VP4 and VP2 (maturation cleavage) occurs only after the RNA has been packaged in the protein shell. The VP0 cleavage site lies buried inside the shell near the RNA; the active site for this cleavage is not yet precisely known and might include bases in the RNA genome. The amino termini of coat proteins P1 and 1A are blocked by a myristoyl group. *cis* cleavage of the N terminus of 2A is shown by an arrow; black triangles indicate 3C cleavage sites.

2,200 amino acids, represents about 91% of the total genome. Both polio- and rhinoviruses have unusually long UTR (600 to 750 bases) at the 5′ ends with distinctive secondary and tertiary structures that enable ribosomes to initiate translation internally (i.e., without the need of the "cap" used by most cellular mRNAs). Internal ribosomal entry sites (IRES) are widely used by positive-stranded RNA viruses; some eukaryotic genes also employ this strategy. The rhinovirus genome also includes a relatively short 3′ UTR that is required for efficient viral replication (5).

The organization of the polyprotein of rhinoviruses is also very similar to that of poliovirus (Fig. 3B), though much less is known of the details of rhinoviral processing and assembly because of the less vigorous translation of rhinoviral RNA in cultured cells and its feebler shutoff of host protein synthesis (67). The rhinovirus genome, like that of polio virus, is organized into three major regions based on proteolytic processing: *P1*, *P2*, and *P3*, representing genes for precursor proteins. These precursors are subsequently cleaved into four, three, and four end products, respectively. Protein P1 is a precursor for the four coat proteins. P2 and P3 are precursors for proteases 2A and 3C and for proteins required for replication of the viral RNA.

Before assembly, the coat precursor protein, P1, is cleaved twice to form immature protomers (VP0, VP1, and VP3), which then package RNA to form noninfectious provirions containing 60 subunits (Fig. 4) (66, 67). The maturation cleavage of VP0, producing VP4 and VP2, occurs only after the RNA has been packaged in the protein shell (67). The VP0 cleavage site lies buried inside the shell near the RNA. The proteolytic process responsible for this cleavage is thus thought to be an element of the coat protein and may actually use bases in the RNA genome as part of its active site (90). The *P1* region is released by a *cis* cleavage at the N terminus of the 2A protease. All remaining cleavages are carried out by the 3C protease or its precursor form, 3CD. A molecule of myristic acid, which appears to play a role during virus assembly and disassembly, is covalently linked to the amino termini of VP4 and its precursor forms.

Biology

Replication Strategy

Rhinovirus replication follows the model developed from poliovirus research and takes place entirely in the cytoplasm. The initial event in infection is attachment of the virion to specific receptor units embedded in the plasma membrane (Fig. 5, step 1). Receptors then bring the virion close to the membrane. Recruitment of additional receptors (step 2) eventually triggers the uncoating of the virion, which involves extrusion of VP4 and delivery of the viral RNA genome across the membrane and into the cytosol (step 3), where translation can begin. The study of the uncoating pathway of rhinoviruses has been difficult because the interpretation of biochemical data is clouded by the fact that only 1% or fewer input virions initiate a successful infection. One major reason for the low infection efficiency is elution of noninfectious 135S and 80S subparticles. More than 50% of attached particles are typically lost to this abortive event. The role of endocytosis in uncoating of rhinoviruses is still not well defined. The site of uncoating, whether the cell surface plasma membrane or endocytic vesicle, may be determined by the stability of the virus-receptor complexes. For some serotypes whose receptor complexes are labile at neutral pH (47), binding of the virus to the receptors on the cell surface is sufficient to trigger uncoating. For the serotypes whose complexes are stable at neutral pH (47), some additional stimulus such as low pH is required, so uncoating is delayed until they are transported by normal trafficking of receptors into the endosomes (91).

Translation (step 4) is the crucial first step of viral replication because synthesis of new viral RNA cannot begin until the virus has successfully manufactured the necessary viral proteins. By using the IRES to confiscate ribosomes and other protein synthesizing machinery from the host cell, the incoming RNA strand directs synthesis of a polyprotein that is progressively cleaved into the final products described above.

The initial step in synthesis of new viral RNA is copying of the incoming genomic RNA to form complementary minus-stranded RNA (step 5), which then serves as a template for synthesis of new positive strands (step 6). Synthesis of positive-stranded RNA, which occurs in virus-induced membranous vesicles derived from the endoplasmic reticulum, is initiated so rapidly (20 to 50 times faster than for minus strands) that it generates multistranded replicative intermediates consisting of one minus-stranded template and many nascent positive-stranded copies. The initiation of minus-strand synthesis is apparently down-regulated by the presence of translating ribosomes on the positive strands (3). A molecule of VPg is covalently linked to all RNAs involved in transcription. The role of VPg in the initiation of minus-stranded RNA transcription has been elucidated for poliovirus. Following uridylylation by the 3D polymerase, VPg primes the transcription of poly(A) RNA to produce VPg-linked poly(U). The primary template for the uridylylation reaction exists as a small RNA hairpin within the coding region of protein 2C (82). This hairpin is recognized as an essential *cis*-acting replication element (CRE) for poliovirus. The CRE hairpin structure is also present in rhinovirus. Unlike polioviruses, the CRE hairpin structure locates within the 2A sequence and the VP1 sequence of HRVA and HRVB viruses, respectively (62, 68b).

During the early steps of replication, newly synthesized positive-stranded RNA molecules are recycled to form additional replication centers (step 7) until, with an ever-expanding pool of positive-stranded RNA, an increasing fraction of the positive-stranded RNA in the replication complex is packaged into virions. The replication machinery interacts directly with the capsid proteins so that only newly synthesized RNAs are packaged (74).

Virion assembly (steps 8 to 10) is controlled by a number of events. Before assembly can begin, coat precursor protein P1 must be cleaved to form immature protomers composed of three tightly aggregated proteins (VP0, VP3, and VP1). Early in the infection cycle this cleavage is likely very slow because of the low concentrations of P1 and its protease. Later, with increasing protease activity, the rising concentration of immature (5S) protomers triggers assembly into pentamers that then package the positive-stranded VPg-RNA to form provirions. Formation of infectious 150S to 160S particles results from the final maturation cleavage (66). Completed virus particles are ultimately released by infection-mediated disintegration of the host cell (step 11).

Throughout the replication cycle, virus associates intimately with cellular factors and organelles. Rhinovirus

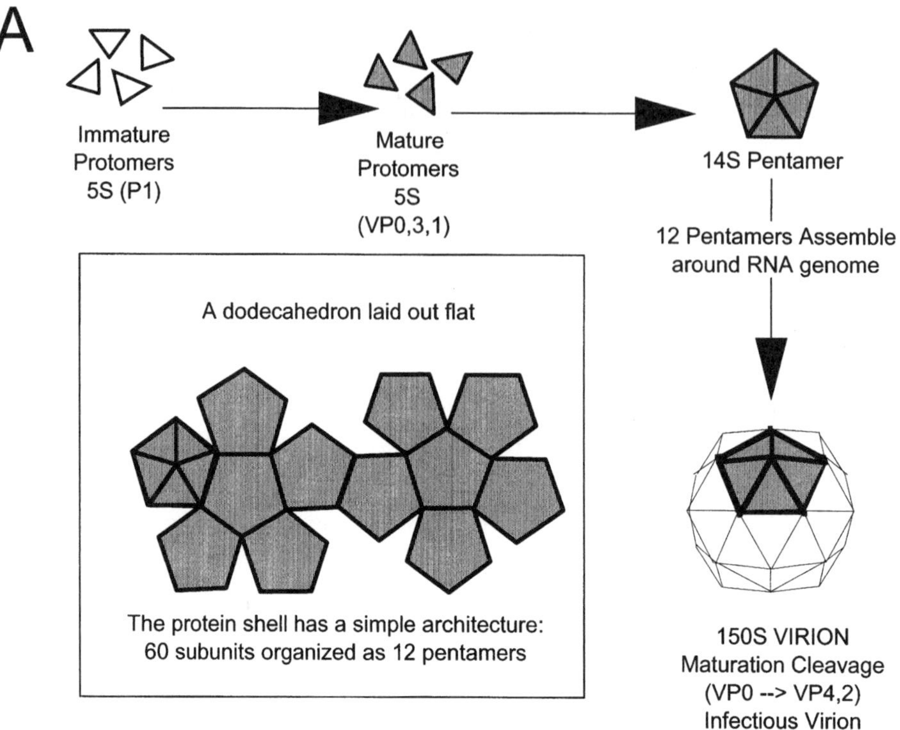

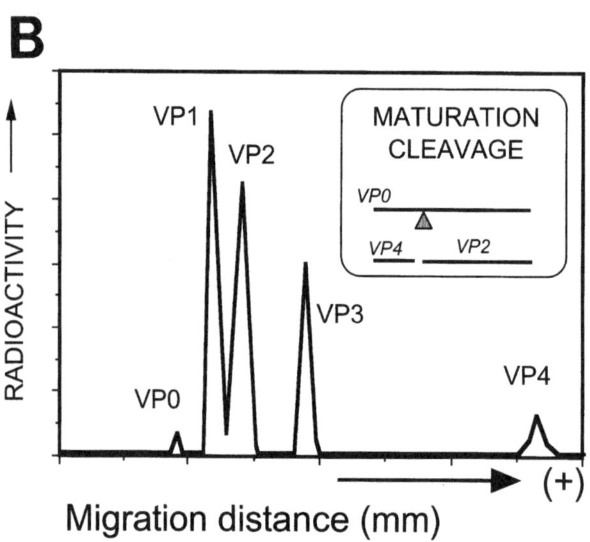

FIGURE 4 (A) Diagram representing virion architecture and assembly. (B) The mature virion contains four major proteins (VP1, -2, -3, and -4) plus traces of VP0, representing residual precursor following the maturation cleavage required for acquisition of infectivity. SDS, sodium dodecyl sulfate.

translation has been shown to require the direct participation of various cellular proteins, including most of the canonical translation initiation factors, with the exception of the cap-binding protein eIF4E (eukaryotic translation initiation factor 4E), and three additional cellular proteins, PTB (polypyrimidine tract-binding protein), PCBP2 [poly(rC)-binding protein 2], and Unr (upstream of N-ras). In addition, rhinovirus replication specifically shuts down host-cell translation via the cleavage of the eIF4G subunit of the cap-binding protein complex by the 2A protease and, by analogy with poliovirus, shuts off transcription of host RNA polymerases I, II, and III via the cleavage of multiple cellular transcription factors by the 3C protease.

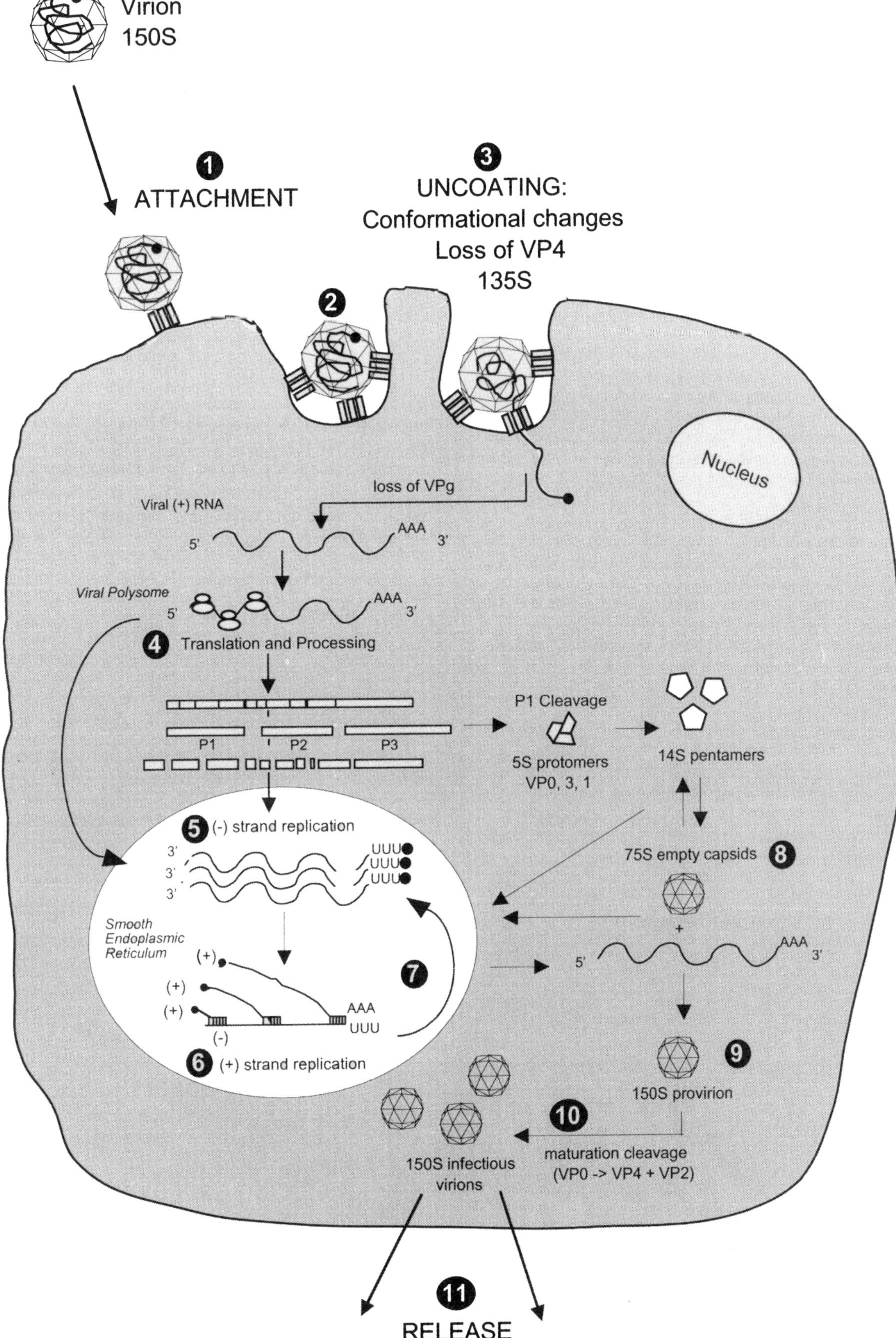

FIGURE 5 Overview of the rhinovirus infection cycle.

Host Range

Rhinoviruses have a high degree of species specificity. First, major group viruses (88 serotypes) do not recognize ICAM-1 from species other than humans, with the probable exception of chimpanzees (4). Although minor group viruses can utilize murine LDLR, mouse cells are nonpermissive for their intracellular replication, with the exception of HRV1A and HRV1B (88, 102a). Rhinoviruses can be adapted to replicate in mouse cells through multiple passages in culture (41).

Experimental studies on pathogenesis, prevention, and cure of HRV infection are hampered by the fact that their host range is restricted to humans and higher primates. Chimpanzees exposed intranasally to HRV14 and HRV43 (500 to 10,000 tissue culture infective doses [$TCID_{50}$]) did not have clinically detectable illness, although they did shed virus for several days, produced specific neutralizing antibody, and were apparently not infected when rechallenged with the same virus. Recently, transgenic mice expressing human ICAM-1 have been bred (22). This may be the first step to create an animal model of major group rhinovirus infection.

Growth in Cell Culture

Strains of human diploid embryonic lung cells (e.g., WI-38 and MRC-5) and H1 HeLa cells are the most commonly used cell lines for studies of rhinovirus growth in cell culture (Fig. 6). Human embryonic lung cells are useful for isolating HRV from clinical samples and producing virus inocula for human studies but have a finite passage life, about 50 cell divisions, and require a solid substrate for growth. H1 HeLa cells (66) can be grown in suspension and passaged indefinitely in culture. H1 HeLa cells have been used widely for studying the molecular biology of rhinoviruses, including producing the large quantity of virus required for X-ray crystallography studies (90). However, these cells have the disadvantage that they are derived from a human cervical carcinoma and are therefore unsuitable for preparing virus inocula for human use. In cultured H1 HeLa cells, the time required for a replication cycle of HRV16, from infection to completion of virus assembly, is about 6 h at 35°C, with a yield of about 300 PFU per cell (67). However, timing of the growth cycle and virus yield varies widely with variables such as pH, temperature, virus serotype, host cell and its nutritional vigor, and number of particles used to infect the cell (91). Details of the rhinovirus growth curve must therefore be determined empirically for any specific virus-cell system.

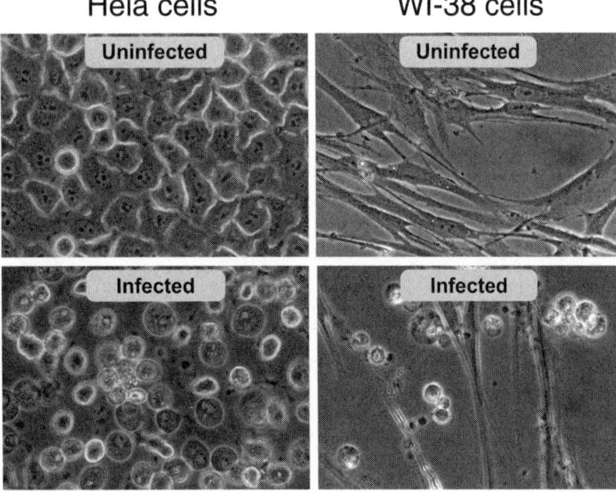

FIGURE 6 Cytopathic effect of HRV16 on H1 HeLa cells (ATCC CRL 1958) and WI-38 human diploid embryonic lung cells (ATCC CCL75). Cells were exposed to 100 PFU per cell and incubated at 35°C. Cytopathic effect in HeLa cells was apparent by 12 h but required about 48 h in WI-38 cells.

Recently, in vitro-differentiated tracheobronchial epithelial cultures have been exploited as a model for studying rhinovirus infection of the native airway (6). These cultures were developed by differentiating primary airway epithelial cells, isolated from human tracheobronchial tissues, in air-liquid interface cultures to form polarized mucociliary epithelium with structural characteristics similar to those of native airway tissues (111).

Inactivation by Physical and Chemical Agents

When subjected to any of a variety of treatments, including gentle heating, UV light, high pH, mercurials, phenol, and desiccation, rhinovirus virions lose their infectivity and their native antigenicity and acquire a new set of surface determinants called the coreless or heated antigens. Rhinoviruses are characteristically sensitive to acidic pH less than about 5 or to alkaline pH exceeding 9. Increasing ionic strength generally increases thermostability. Capsid-binding inhibitors that inhibit virus uncoating, such as chalcones, 4′,6-dicyanoflavan, R61837, and WIN compounds, also markedly stabilize rhinoviruses against heat and acid inactivation (72). This stabilizing effect has been attributed to either increasing rigidity of the coat proteins or increasing compressibility of the capsid.

Sodium dodecyl sulfate, particularly in the presence of organic acids such as malate and citrate, inactivates rhinoviruses rapidly even at room temperature. Infectivity of aqueous suspensions of rhinovirus survives extraction with diethyl ether, a treatment commonly used for the selective killing of bacterial and fungal contaminants and as a preliminary test to distinguish lipid enveloped viruses from nonenveloped ones. Infectivity is less refractory to extraction with more polar organic solvents such as chloroform, possibly because of the removal of the hydrophobic pocket factor, partial solvent denaturation of the protein shell, or oxidation due to contamination of the solvent by phosgene. Chemicals that alter the nucleic acid include nitrous acid, which deaminates purine and pyrimidine bases, and alkaline reagents such as ammonia, which cleaves RNA within the virus particle. Halogens (chlorine, bromine, and iodine), hydrogen peroxide, and ozone are also commonly used disinfectants.

Neutralization by Immunoglobulins

Several mechanisms for antibody-mediated neutralization of rhinoviruses have been proposed, including aggregation, virion stabilization, induction of conformational changes, and abrogation of cellular attachment (71, 93). Available evidence suggests that neutralization of rhinovirus in vitro results from steric blockage of the interaction between the virus and its receptors due to the binding of the antibody molecules on the virion surface (93). Rhinovirus virions can also be neutralized by saturation with excess soluble ICAM-1.

EPIDEMIOLOGY

Geographic Distribution

Rhinovirus is distributed worldwide, and antibody to rhinovirus is detected in serum specimens collected from many different parts of the world. Of particular interest has been the detection of rhinovirus antibody in serum specimens collected from members of an isolated Amazon Indian tribe shortly after their initial contact with civilization (98). Infection in this group was presumably acquired through intermittent contact with semicivilized tribes in the same region.

Incidence and Prevalence of Infection

In adults in the United States, the incidence of rhinovirus infection, based on virus isolation, is approximately 0.75 infection per person year. In children, the incidence is higher, with rates of 1.2 infections per year. Recent studies using reverse transcriptase PCR (RT-PCR) for the detection have reported similar incidence rates in young children, although systematic studies of incidence using this more sensitive diagnostic technique have not been done.

Approximately one-quarter of rhinovirus infections are asymptomatic. In studies of naturally acquired infection, 12 to 37% of infections detected by virus isolation and 12 to 22% of infections detected by RT-PCR have been asymptomatic (33, 54, 73, 104, 109, 110). Similarly, 20 to 30% of infections in subjects experimentally infected by intranasal inoculation of rhinovirus are asymptomatic.

Rhinovirus infection is a universal experience, and risk of infection with a new serotype is primarily a function of exposure to the virus. The prevalence of rhinovirus antibody in serum indicates that infection with the various serotypes begins in early childhood and continues throughout life (33). The peak prevalence of rhinovirus antibody is found in young adults, probably reflecting exposure to young children in the home, and the subsequent decline in rhinovirus antibody prevalence is probably related to less frequent exposure to the virus in older adults. Type-specific neutralizing antibody provides serotype-specific protection, but this is associated with little reduction in overall infection risk due to the large number of rhinovirus serotypes.

Seasonality

Frost and Gover (25), based on epidemiological observations made between 1923 and 1925, suggested that the respiratory disease season is composed of "successions of epidemics" due to different infectious agents. This ingenious observation was confirmed with the subsequent detection of the several families of respiratory viruses. In temperate areas of the northern hemisphere, a distinct peak of colds is observed in September (18, 25). This early-fall peak of colds begins the respiratory disease season and is strongly associated with rhinovirus infections, a finding confirmed by studies using culture or RT-PCR. In young adults in Charlottesville, VA, the rhinovirus infection rate reaches its highest annual point (3.5 illnesses/1,000 persons/day) during this period (35). Thereafter, rhinovirus prevalence declines, usually remaining low throughout the late fall, winter, and early spring (109). A second period of increased rhinovirus activity occurs in late spring, April and May. Although the overall incidence of colds is low during the summer months, rhinovirus accounts for up to 50% of the illnesses which occur during this season (35, 109). In the temperate areas of the southern hemisphere, the seasonal incidence of infection mirrors that in the northern hemisphere. In tropical climates, rhinovirus activity is detected throughout the year, with a peak incidence in the autumn months (95).

The cause of the seasonality of colds has been the subject of much speculation but remains largely unexplained. However, at least two factors influence this phenomenon: the effect of relative humidity on virus survival and the herding of children during the school term (32). Rhinovirus and other nonenveloped viruses survive best in conditions of high relative humidity. In contrast, enveloped viruses such as influenza virus survive best when humidity is low. Based on these observations, Hemmes et al. (44) suggested in 1960 that the relative humidity indoors is an important factor controlling the seasonal fluctuations of the different virus families.

Observations on the seasonal occurrence of rhinovirus colds support the above hypothesis. In a 15-year longitudinal study in Charlottesville, the occurrence of rhinovirus colds was greatest from April to October, which is the period when indoor relative humidity tends to remain above 45% (32). In 9 of 13 years, frontal systems with marked falls in maximum daily temperature, heavy cloud cover, and precipitation occurred 5 to 11 days before common cold rates reached defined peak levels. In 2 years, no frontal systems came through the area and no illness peaks occurred. School openings were also correlated with the fluctuating incidence of colds. In 8 of 14 years, the interval between the date of school opening and the date on which cold rates reached the defined peak was 11 to 14 days.

These observations suggest that climate has both biological and behavioral consequences which influence the incidence of rhinovirus infection. The rhinovirus season begins in April, when indoor relative humidity rises above 45%. This period corresponds to the late-spring peak of rhinovirus colds. With the beginning of summer, common-cold rates decline because children, the major reservoir of the virus, disperse during vacation. School openings in September reassemble this rhinovirus reservoir. The school openings, especially when coupled with rainy days keeping children indoors, enhance virus transmission, leading to an increase in the infection rate and the characteristic early-fall rhinovirus peak. When relative indoor humidity falls below the 45% threshold for optimal rhinovirus survival, the period of high rhinovirus prevalence ends until relative humidity rises again in the late spring.

Transmission

Rhinovirus infection is readily initiated by inoculation of virus onto the nasal mucosa. In those lacking serotype-specific neutralizing antibody, the 50% human infectious dose (HID_{50}) has ranged from 0.1 to 6 $TCID_{50}$ after intranasal inoculation. In contrast, experimental inoculation of rhinovirus into the mouth or exposure to infected volunteers by prolonged kissing is an inefficient method of initiating infection (14). A similar difference in susceptibility is observed between the upper and lower respiratory tracts. The HID_{50} for antibody-free volunteers given rhinovirus type 15 by nasal drops corresponded to 0.032 $TCID_{50}$, compared to 0.68 $TCID_{50}$ when the virus was given by small-particle aerosol (13). This 20-fold disparity in infectious dose between nose drops and inhaled particles suggests that the lower respiratory tract is less susceptible to rhinovirus infection than is the nasopharynx. In addition, interferon applied intranasally by drops or coarse spray is very effective in preventing natural rhinovirus infection (20, 42). Since application of interferon by this method would not be expected to prevent infection in the lower airway, this also points to the upper airway as the usual portal of entry for rhinovirus.

Delivery of rhinovirus to the nasal mucosa can occur either by droplets or by direct contact. Sneezes and coughs generate both large- and small-particle aerosols, but the amount of rhinovirus in respiratory secretions produced by coughs and sneezes is usually small. Although the rhinovirus genome may be present in small-particle aerosols, such aerosols do not appear to be an important mechanism of spread. Large-particle aerosols produced by coughs and sneezes and deposited onto the nasal or conjunctival mucosa may contribute to transmission (17).

Direct contact appears to be the most efficient mechanism of transmission of rhinovirus. Studies done under experimental conditions have demonstrated that rhinovirus is recovered from the fingers of approximately 65% of infected volunteers after finger-to-nose contact and that the contaminating virus survives for several hours on skin (45, 87). Contact with the contaminated fingers reliably transfers virus to the skin of a recipient individual. Once the fingertips of the recipient are contaminated, infection is readily induced by self-inoculation of the nasal mucosa by rubbing the nose or the eyes. The role of fomites in the transmission of virus is less clear. The virus contaminating the hands is readily transferred to objects in the environment. When fingertips have been experimentally contaminated with nasal mucus containing known amounts of rhinovirus, 13% of the starting virus titer was transferred to inanimate objects after brief contact, although transfer was less efficient if the virus inoculum was allowed to dry (45, 87). Virus on nonporous environmental surfaces may survive for up to 3 to 4 days and can be transmitted to the skin by contact. Although these various steps in fomite transmission have been demonstrated, there is a substantial loss of infectious virus at each step. An attempt to document transmission of infection from fomites under experimental conditions that would favor transmission was unsuccessful, suggesting that this mechanism may not be efficient for the spread of rhinovirus infections (51).

Studies in the natural setting have confirmed many of these steps in virus transmission. Virus is recovered from the skin of the hands of approximately 40% of individuals with natural rhinovirus colds and from 6 to 15% of objects in their environment (45, 87). Individuals in the natural setting routinely make finger-to-eye or finger-to-nose contact in a manner that would transfer virus to the nasal mucosa. In spite of these suggestive data, the mechanism of transmission of virus under natural conditions can be determined only by blocking transmission in the natural setting using an intervention which is specific for a particular route. In one trial using a 2% aqueous iodine as a virucidal treatment for the hands (45), regular applications to the fingers by mothers who had been exposed to a child with a fresh cold in the home reduced colds by 67% compared to placebo. None of 11 mothers using iodine became infected with the same rhinovirus recovered from the index case, compared to 31% of mothers using placebo. Another study of the hand contact route of cold transmission in asthmatic children (12) found that a group of children trained to avoid finger-to-nose contact had better outcomes than untrained controls. During several months of observation, the trained group had significantly less self-inoculatory behavior, fewer viral respiratory infections, and fewer attacks of asthma. These findings also support the finger-to-nose and finger-to-eye self-inoculation routes of cold transmission. Thus, direct evidence is available that supports the hypothesis that rhinovirus colds are transmitted by accidental self-inoculation of the nose following inadvertent contamination of the fingers with virus.

The duration of infectiousness for rhinovirus colds parallels the period of maximum virus shedding in nasal secretions. Rhinovirus concentrations in nasal secretions are highest during the second and third days after viral challenge. Deliberate infection of one member of a dually susceptible (i.e., antibody-free) married couple (15) determined that the features of the donors that were associated with transmission included a concentration of >1,000 $TCID_{50}$ of virus in nasal washings, virus on the hands and anterior nares, and symptoms of at least a moderately severe cold. In most instances, these conditions occurred only on the second and third days after virus inoculation. In households, secondary cases are seen after 1 to 3 days of exposure to an index case.

PATHOGENESIS IN HUMANS

Incubation Period

In experimentally infected volunteers, rhinovirus is first recovered in nasal washes from 8 to 18 h after inoculation, and the median period to virus recovery is 10 h. Respiratory symptoms occur surprisingly early, with the throat becoming sore and/or scratchy between 10 and 12 h after virus inoculation as newly produced virus appears (40). Nasal symptoms also appear early, although serial nasal washes are a confounder. Recent studies suggest that rhinovirus may be detected by RT-PCR 1 to 2 weeks prior to the onset of symptoms in some individuals, but these reports are at odds with the consistently short incubation period in experimental infections (50, 109). It seems more likely that these reports represent sequential infections rather than a prolonged incubation. The availability of convenient methods for genotyping virus detected in these natural colds will resolve this issue.

Patterns of Virus Replication

Virus replicates in ciliated and nonciliated epithelial cells in the nasopharynx and nasal passages of the human airway and is shed into respiratory secretions. Rhinovirus concentrations are highest in nasal secretions, with viral titers of approximately 300 $TCID_{50}$/ml, compared to 30 and 10 $TCID_{50}$/ml in oropharyngeal secretions and saliva, respectively. Most rhinovirus replication occurs in the nasopharynx and nasal passages. It has been difficult to determine whether growth occurs in the trachea and large bronchi because of the problem of obtaining lower-airway secretions which are not contaminated with nasopharyngeal secretions. Recently, in situ hybridization for rhinovirus RNA detection demonstrated that rhinovirus replication was present in bronchial biopsy samples of volunteers with experimental infection (78). Factors controlling sites of replication are not well understood but are thought to include temperature and the availability of viral receptors. Rhinovirus grows best around 33°C, the temperature of the upper airway, trachea, and large bronchi, and growth is inhibited at the core body temperature of 37°C. While the rhinovirus receptor (ICAM-1) has been identified in many tissues of the body, in the normal, nonstimulated epithelium of the nasopharynx and nasal passages, ICAM-1 has been identified primarily on nonciliated cells and not on ciliated epithelium. However, rhinovirus does infect ciliated cells in the epithelium during colds, perhaps as a result of up-regulation of ICAM-1 expression in the presence of rhinovirus (1, 80).

Following experimental infections, rhinovirus shedding usually reaches a peak 48 to 72 h after viral challenge and then rapidly declines. Less commonly, virus shedding may have a delayed onset and lower peak titers. These "late-low" shedders tend to have milder symptoms. Rhinovirus is usually no longer recoverable after 3 weeks, and the infection is presumed to be completely cleared. Prolonged or persistent infection of the lower airway may occur in immunocompromised hosts (56).

Factors in Disease Expression

An impressive feature of rhinovirus pathogenesis is that the nonspecific defense mechanisms of the nose are unable to prevent infection in the nonimmune individual and may, in fact, contribute to the pathogenesis of rhinovirus-associated illness. Following intranasal rhinovirus challenge, infection rates of more than 90% are routinely achieved in nonimmune volunteers, irrespective of the season of the year or of the allergic status, smoking history, physical condition, or stress level of the subject (33). Following infection, symptomatic individuals shed higher titers of virus in nasal secretions than do asymptomatic individuals.

Infection with rhinovirus produces no detectable histopathological change in the respiratory epithelium. Nucleic acid hybridization studies demonstrate small foci of infection interspersed among large areas of uninfected cells (16), and examination of nasal secretions with labeled rhinovirus antibody demonstrates occasional antigen-positive epithelial cells that have been shed from the nasal mucosa (102). These studies suggest that rhinovirus infection involves sparse and scattered areas of the nasal epithelium and that infected cells are shed from the epithelium, with rapid repair of the involved areas.

Despite the absence of overt histopathological damage to the nasal mucosa, inflammatory responses occur in the nasal epithelium and increased numbers of nasal epithelial cells are shed in secretions. Polymorphonuclear leukocytes (PMN) infiltrate the nasal epithelium early after infection, and PMN concentrations increase in the nasal secretions and peripheral blood. Of interest, this inflammatory response is seen only in symptomatic individuals. The correlation between the lymphocytic response to rhinovirus infection and symptomatic illness is less clearly characterized. There are conflicting data about the effect of rhinovirus infection on the peripheral lymphocyte count, but modest increases in T-lymphocyte concentrations have been reported both for the nasal mucosa and for nasal secretions during rhinovirus infection. Few B lymphocytes are noted in the nasal mucosa.

The evidence summarized above suggests that nonspecific host inflammatory responses may play a role in symptom expression (Fig. 7). A number of inflammatory mediators are increased in nasal secretions and/or the serum during rhinovirus colds, including bradykinin, interleukin 1b (IL-1b), IL-6, IL-8, interferon-inducible protein 10, and tumor necrosis factor alpha. The concentrations of IL-6 and IL-8 in nasal secretions have a modest correlation with symptom severity, and intranasal instillation of IL-8 in healthy volunteers produces symptoms that are similar to the common cold. Inhalation of bradykinin by healthy volunteers produces nasal obstruction, rhinorrhea, and sore throat. The detection of these mediators in association with illness, however, does not provide definitive evidence of a role in rhinovirus-associated illness. The role of kinins, in particular, is unclear in light of a study demonstrating that inhibition of the kinins with corticosteroids had no effect on cold symptoms (31).

Neurogenic mechanisms also appear to play a role in the expression of illness during rhinovirus infections (Fig. 7). The parasympathetic nervous system controls the se-

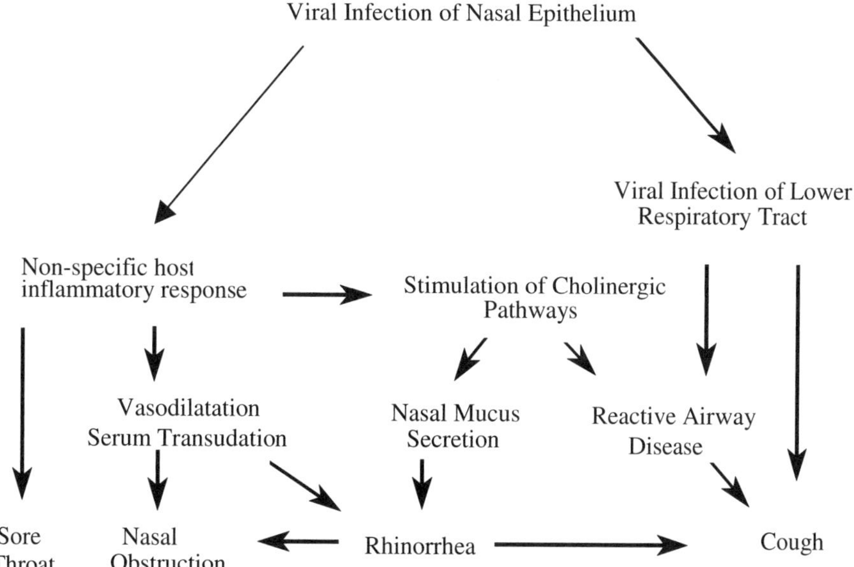

FIGURE 7 Proposed pathogenesis of symptoms associated with rhinovirus infection.

cretory activity of nasal seromucous glands. These glands, in association with plasma transudation, provide most of the nasal fluid produced during a rhinovirus cold. Drugs with anticholinergic activity, such as atropine methonitrate and ipratropium bromide, given intranasally and first-generation antihistamines given orally reduce mean nasal fluid volumes by approximately 30% in volunteers with experimental rhinovirus colds. These findings support the role of the parasympathetic nervous system in rhinovirus pathogenesis.

The mechanisms by which these mediators and neurogenic reflexes are stimulated by rhinovirus remain unknown. In addition to the obvious interaction between rhinovirus and the known cellular receptors ICAM-1 and LDLR, other nonspecific interactions may play a role in pathogenesis. Toll-like receptor 3, which recognizes double-stranded RNA, appears to mediate some cellular responses to rhinovirus (27). Rhinovirus also interacts with ceramide-enriched cell membrane platforms that may play a role in stimulating relevant signaling pathways (29). A number of secondary signaling pathways have been implicated in the elaboration of inflammatory mediators in vitro, but the relevance of these studies to the in vivo elaboration of mediators remains to be determined.

Another factor is the possible role of the host psychological state in promoting infection or illness. Available studies suggest that stress is not a factor in the acquisition of infection but that chronic stress in particular is associated with the development of more severe symptoms (9). Other studies suggest that personality type may also impact symptom severity. Introverted individuals are reported to have more severe illness (7). In contrast, a positive emotional style, associated with vigor and a feeling of well-being, is associated with a reduction in symptom severity (8).

Immune Response

Individuals who develop symptomatic rhinovirus illness have a prompt inflammatory response, with elaboration of inflammatory mediators and PMN infiltration. However, these inflammatory responses appear to play no role in control of the infection. There is less viral shedding in asymptomatic individuals, who also have a decreased inflammatory response, and the times to final viral clearance are comparable in symptomatic and asymptomatic individuals. Peak virus shedding occurs at approximately the same time as the peak of symptoms, and virus concentrations in secretions fall coincidently with the resolution of symptoms. Low levels of virus shedding continue for 2 to 3 weeks, however, and the termination of viral shedding and protection from subsequent infection are most closely correlated with the appearance of neutralizing antibody. Serum neutralizing antibody titers rise in 40 to 80% of persons following natural or experimental rhinovirus infection, depending on the serotype involved (33). The reason for the differences in antigenicity of the various rhinovirus serotypes is unknown. Studies using serial specimens collected from the same individuals have shown that serum neutralizing antibody persists for years (33). Serum neutralizing antibody levels of ≥8 are associated with good protection following natural exposure in the home, and levels of ≥16 are generally associated with solid immunity (33). However, artificial challenge with high concentrations (10,000 $TCID_{50}$) of rhinovirus has resulted in the infection of persons with antibody titers of up to 128.

The relative importance of serum versus nasal neutralizing antibody for protection has been difficult to determine, because serum antibody is found in close association with nasal antibody (101). The ratio of nasal to serum antibody following recent infection is in the range of 1:2. Over time the ratio falls to the range of 1:16, apparently because nasal antibody concentrations decline more rapidly than in the serum.

The dynamics and the role of neutralizing antibody during acute illness vary depending on the antibody status of the host. During the acute phase of rhinovirus colds, there is considerable transudation of serum proteins into nasal secretions (101). In individuals with preexisting serum neutralizing antibody, transudation of this antibody may modify the severity of the illness. In seronegative persons, rhinovirus neutralizing antibody appears in serum and nasal secretions approximately 2 weeks after onset of infection. The neutralizing activity is present in the immunoglobulin A (IgA) and IgG antibody classes, as well as in IgM in early infection. Neutralizing titers rapidly increase during the third and fourth weeks, at which time viral shedding in nasal secretions is no longer detectable (108).

While it appears that neutralizing antibody is important in elimination of rhinovirus shedding from nasal secretions, recovery from illness and the initial reduction in the viral load in nasal secretions occur before specific antibody appears. The mechanism of this early response to infection is not known. Alpha interferon may play a role in some individuals but is detected in the nasal secretions during only one-third of infections. Preinfection gamma interferon concentrations are inversely correlated with both severity of illness and duration of virus shedding during experimental colds (28). It is likely that other, as-yet-undetermined mechanisms are involved in the resolution of symptoms associated with rhinovirus infections.

CLINICAL MANIFESTATIONS

The major clinical syndrome associated with rhinovirus infection is rhinosinusitis, which is traditionally characterized as "the common cold." Rhinovirus colds frequently begin as a sore or scratchy throat that is followed closely by development of nasal obstruction and rhinorrhea. Over the course of the illness, the signs and symptoms of rhinovirus colds typically include various combinations of sneezing, rhinorrhea, nasal obstruction, facial pressure, sore and/or scratchy throat, hoarseness, cough, headache, malaise, chilliness, and feverishness. Cough occurs in approximately 30% of colds; it frequently appears after the onset of nasal symptoms and often persists longer. The clinical features of rhinovirus colds are similar in adults and older children. Infants and young children may at times only display mucus discharge from the nose.

Rhinovirus illness is quite variable; natural rhinovirus colds have shown durations ranging from 1 to 33 days in prospective epidemiological studies (34). The median length of these colds was 7 days, with approximately one-fourth lasting 2 weeks. Resolution of the most severe symptoms occurs quite rapidly in most cases, and lingering minor symptoms generally account for the prolonged duration of illness reported by some individuals.

Acute Sinusitis and Otologic Changes

Rhinovirus has been recovered from sinus aspirates of patients with acute community-acquired sinusitis, and rhinovirus RNA has also been detected in brushings from the sinus cavities of similar patients. Sinus imaging studies show that sinus involvement is an inherent feature of colds; thus, a rhinovirus cold is a viral rhinosinusitis. In young adults with early self-diagnosed common colds, sinus cavity abnormalities have been observed on computed tomography in up to 87% of patients (36). These individuals recover from their illness without intervention.

Rhinovirus infection also results in abnormalities of the eustachian tube and middle ear (23, 68). Abnormalities in middle ear pressures are seen in 40 to 75% of volunteers with experimental rhinovirus colds and 72 to 76% of patients with natural rhinovirus colds, sometimes in association with middle ear effusions. Rhinovirus has been recovered alone and in combination with bacteria in middle ear fluids from 24% of patients with otitis media (84). It is unclear whether viral invasion of the middle ear is required for the development of the eustachian tube and middle ear abnormalities.

Laboratory Abnormalities

Routine laboratory tests are not useful in the clinical evaluation of patients with suspected rhinovirus colds. During experimental rhinovirus infection, there is a modest increase in blood neutrophils, and a moderate elevation of the erythrocyte sedimentation rate in some volunteers (33). A predominance of PMN in the nasal secretions is characteristic of uncomplicated colds and does not aid in the diagnosis of bacterial superinfection. Nasal resistance has been shown to be increased and nasal mucus transport times have been shown to be mildly decreased in patients with natural and experimental rhinovirus colds. Also, sinus and nasal cavity computed tomography scans show abnormalities (36). None of the latter tests are appropriate or useful in the clinical management of patients with rhinovirus colds.

Complications

Acute Bacterial Sinusitis

The incidence of secondary acute bacterial sinusitis is difficult to ascertain given the changes that occur in the sinuses in uncomplicated rhinovirus colds. Various reports have estimated that 0.5 to 8% of viral colds are complicated by bacterial sinusitis. The factors leading to secondary bacterial invasion of the sinus cavity during colds are incompletely understood. Nose blowing propels nasal secretions into the sinuses, and occlusion of the ethmoid infundibulum in many patients with colds may trap nasopharyngeal bacteria in the sinus cavity, thus leading to secondary bacterial infection.

Acute Bacterial Otitis Media

Acute bacterial otitis media complicates an estimated 2% of colds in adults and up to 30% of colds in children. A high incidence of eustachian tube dysfunction during the common cold has been reported, and bacteria presumably reach the middle ear by a mechanism similar to that described above for sinusitis.

Exacerbations of Chronic Bronchitis

Up to 40% of exacerbations of chronic bronchitis have been associated with rhinovirus infections (33). The episodes are characterized by fever, increased purulence of the sputum, and worsening of ventilation. One longitudinal study of patients with chronic obstructive pulmonary disease documented viral infections in 23% of hospitalizations; rhinovirus was the most frequently identified agent. Treatment with antimicrobial drugs is beneficial in the prevention and treatment of these exacerbations, which suggests that bacterial infection also plays a role in the condition. Transient decreases in pulmonary function have occurred in patients with chronic obstructive pulmonary disease experiencing natural rhinovirus colds. The pathogenesis of these abnormalities is unknown but could involve direct viral invasion of the large airways or reflex mechanisms from upper respiratory tract disease.

Asthma

Rhinovirus is the principal virus implicated in precipitating asthma attacks in older children and adults and is associated with 60 to 70% of the asthma exacerbations in school-age children (53, 86). Both a fall peak of asthma exacerbation and the fall increase in the incidence of rhinovirus infection have been reported in association with the start of the school year (32, 52). Rhinovirus is particularly important in precipitating episodes of asthma in children over 2 years of age, in whom the infection is often associated with allergen-specific IgE (21), and the timing of the asthma peak may be due to a convergence of rhinovirus infection spread among schoolchildren and seasonal allergen exposure. The mechanisms by which rhinovirus infection induces wheezing are not well understood (26).

Other Lower Respiratory Syndromes

Rhinoviruses can be isolated from a small fraction of children admitted to hospitals with a diagnosis of bronchiolitis or pneumonia. Higher proportions of rhinovirus infections have been reported in studies that have used RT-PCR techniques for detection of rhinovirus. Rhinovirus was the only pathogen detected in 10% of children under 1 year of age with acute bronchiolitis in one recent study (79). Another study of bronchiolitis in children under 3 years of age found rhinovirus in 21% of patients, but it was isolated as the sole pathogen from only 4 (2%) of 192 patients (49). Rhinovirus has also been detected in the upper respiratory tract of patients with pneumonia. One study reported that 24% of children with pneumonia had rhinovirus detected in the upper respiratory tract by RT-PCR (55), although over one-half of these patients had evidence of a concurrent bacterial infection. These data demonstrate an association between rhinovirus and lower respiratory tract disease in immunocompetent children, but the frequency of rhinovirus infection in the general population makes assessment of a causal role for rhinovirus in the lower respiratory tract disease difficult.

Infections in Immunocompromised Patients

Rhinovirus has been isolated from the lower respiratory tract of a small number of immunocompromised patients. The significance of these isolates has been questioned given the prevalence of rhinovirus in the general population, the potential for contamination of the lower airway specimens by upper respiratory secretions, and the fact that most of the rhinovirus isolates were associated with concurrent isolation of more typical lower respiratory pathogens. A recent study, however, has provided definitive evidence for active and persistent infection of the lower respiratory tract in patients following lung transplantation (56). This observation adds to the growing body of evidence that rhinovirus does infect the lower respiratory tract and is consistent with a conclusion that rhinovirus is a real, although uncommon, cause of lower respiratory disease in this patient population.

CLINICAL DIAGNOSIS

Colds are familiar to everyone, and the illness is usually self-diagnosed before the patient seeks medical attention. The physical findings in the common cold are limited to the upper respiratory tract. Increased nasal secretion is frequently obvious, and a change in the color or consistency of the secretions is common during the course of the illness and is not an indication of sinusitis or bacterial superinfection. Examination of the nasal cavity may reveal swollen, erythematous nasal turbinates; however, this finding is nonspecific and of limited diagnostic usefulness.

Colds are different from episodes of allergic rhinitis; persistent sneezing, thin nasal discharge, watery eyes, and sensation of mucosal itch are more common in the latter. Also, other symptoms of colds such as sore throat, cough, malaise, and headache are less common with allergic or vasomotor rhinitis. When viral culture and nasal smear eosinophilia were used as criteria for diagnosis, adults were able to reliably distinguish colds from allergic rhinitis.

The clinical features of rhinovirus infection do not allow reliable differentiation from respiratory infections caused by other viral pathogens. Knowing the seasonal prevalence of the different respiratory viruses helps in suspecting the specific viral etiology of a cold, but a firm diagnosis depends on viral culture or serology, which is usually not practical or necessary for routine patient care.

Distinguishing the rhinosinusitis of a rhinovirus cold from a secondary acute bacterial sinusitis is often difficult. Two clinical presentations of acute bacterial sinusitis can be recognized. First, the classical features of acute bacterial sinusitis include fever and facial pain, swelling, or tenderness. There may also be maxillary toothache, if the infection is of dental origin. The features of this presentation, while specific, are often not present and thus lack sensitivity. The second and more common presentation of acute bacterial sinusitis is that of an acute respiratory illness which begins as a cold or "flu" but lasts longer than expected. Most natural rhinovirus colds have ended by 12 to 14 days, and almost all colds have improved by a week (34, 107). Therefore, in acute respiratory illnesses which have not improved or are worse after 10 days, the diagnosis of secondary bacterial sinusitis should be suspected. Radiographic imaging for diagnosis of bacterial sinusitis is of limited utility (36), and the imaging abnormalities seen with viral and bacterial sinusitis are often indistinguishable. An exception is the presence of a classical air fluid level showing thin fluid in the sinus cavity. This finding was associated with an 89% rate of bacterial recovery from sinus aspirates from patients who presented with suspected acute community-acquired sinusitis (38). However, a classic air fluid level was present in only 37% of the abnormal X rays for these patients. For this reason, the finding is not sensitive enough to justify the routine use of sinus imaging to distinguish viral from bacterial sinusitis.

LABORATORY DIAGNOSIS

Virus Isolation

Rhinovirus is found primarily in respiratory secretions from the upper airway, with the highest concentration in nasal fluids. Specimens used for viral culture have been primarily deep nasal swabs, aspirates, or nasal washes. Specimens of respiratory secretions intended for rhinovirus culture should be placed in a viral collection broth that contains proteins to "stabilize" the virus.

Cell culture is the standard method for rhinovirus isolation and propagation. Most work has been done in human embryonic lung cells (see above). Diploid fetal tonsil cells and heteroploid cell lines such as HeLa have also been used. Different lots of these cells may vary 100-fold or more in their sensitivity to rhinovirus for unknown reasons. Therefore, cell cultures should be monitored for sensitivity when used for growing rhinovirus.

Rhinovirus grows best at temperatures of 33 to 34°C under conditions of motion (e.g., roller drum). Cytopathic effect of rhinoviruses is readily apparent in sensitive cells (Fig. 6). The HID_{50} and the $TCID_{50}$ (in sensitive cells) are essentially the same for rhinovirus in limited testing (33). However, some rhinoviruses that did not grow initially in cell culture have been recovered in tracheal organ culture (46). Comparison of organ culture to cell culture has failed to show clear superiority for either, and the use of both systems is necessary for optimal viral recovery (46). Experimental infection with human rhinovirus has been produced in chimpanzees and gibbons, but native rhinovirus does not grow in lower animal species.

Antigen Detection

Fluorescent-antibody and immunoperoxidase methods for detecting rhinovirus antigen have been used in experimental studies. However, these techniques are generally serotype specific. Because of the relative difficulty of growing rhinovirus in cell culture and the low concentration of rhinovirus in respiratory secretions, these methods have not been adapted for clinical use. Commercially available assays for rhinovirus antigen are not available.

Nucleic Acid Detection

RT-PCR has become the standard diagnostic tool for the detection of rhinoviruses in clinical specimens, because it is more sensitive and faster and easier to perform than traditional virus isolation and antigen detection methods. The 5′ UTR of the rhinoviral genomic RNA has several short stretches of sequence that are almost completely conserved among all 100 serotypes (65). The RT-PCR primers based on these conserved sequences have been used for sensitive and specific detection of all rhinoviruses as a group. Recently, a molecular typing assay was developed for rapid identification of individual rhinovirus serotypes or strains in original clinical samples. This new assay uses sensitive pan-HRV primers and seminested PCR to amplify a 260-bp variable region in the 5′ UTR of the rhinoviral genome for sequence determination. The serotype or strain is then determined by phylogenetic comparisons of the resulting sequence to homologous reference sequences of 100 known serotypes (65). In situ hybridization using rhinovirus-specific probes has been used to locate the anatomic sites and cell types which support viral replication in the airways of infected subjects (1, 83a), making it useful to study pathogenesis.

Serologic Assays

Viral neutralization assay is the standard serologic method for rhinoviruses (33). Complement fixation and hemagglutination tests have not proven useful. The neutralization assay is used to identify specific viral serotypes and to measure antibody in human serum and nasal secretions. Viral shedding is a more sensitive indicator of infection than serologic response with experimental rhinovirus infections (33). In natural infections, either procedure alone has identified about two-thirds of the total diagnosed infections, and in family studies, 20 to 40% of infections were detected only by serologic assays.

A major problem with using the neutralization assay for diagnosis is the existence of at least 100 distinct rhinovirus serotypes (39). Thus, serologic diagnosis is practical only when the serotype of the infecting virus is known or suspected, such as in experimental virus challenge studies or in family studies where a rhinovirus has been recovered from a family member. Epidemiological studies based on viral culture and serologic assay have indicated that most rhinovirus serotypes circulating in the United States have been identified and that new types are not emerging at a rapid rate (70).

Hyperimmune rhinovirus antisera for neutralization testing have been produced in several animal species (33). The traditional method for identification of a rhinovirus serotype is neutralization of a virus inoculum containing 10 to 300 $TCID_{50}$ of virus by an antiserum concentration containing 20 U of antibody (33). Identification of rhinovirus serotypes in epidemiological studies has been done using antiserum pooled by a combinatorial method which has been adapted to a microtitration system. In order to measure rhinovirus neutralizing antibody in human serum and nasal washes, a small inoculum (3 to 30 $TCID_{50}$) of virus should be used in the neutralization assay to provide sufficient sensitivity to detect the relatively low concentration of antibody in these specimens.

PREVENTION

Hope for the development of a common-cold vaccine was considerably reduced when the large number of common-cold viruses was discovered in the 1950s and 1960s. Also, an attempt to achieve enhanced and broadened antigenicity through the use of polyvalent rhinovirus vaccines was disappointing (101). At present, work on rhinovirus vaccines is not being pursued.

Antiviral chemoprophylaxis for rhinovirus colds may have practical value, but no commercial product of proven efficacy is available. Alpha interferon applied topically in the nose is effective in reducing the incidence of colds in persons who are exposed to a family member with a fresh cold (20, 42). This approach reduces the overall risk of colds by 40% and almost eliminates proven rhinovirus colds in contacts. In spite of this substantial benefit, alpha interferon has not been developed as prophylaxis for rhinovirus infection because of the substantial incidence of nasal side effects associated with prolonged use of this agent. Other antiviral agents (capsid-binding compounds [e.g., pirodavir and R61837] and receptor-blocking antibody) have prophylactic activity in experimentally induced infections but have not been studied in the natural setting.

The only source of rhinovirus is the human airway and possibly sites in the environment contaminated with virus-containing nasal secretions. Thus, it may be possible to lower the risk of infection by avoiding exposure through a modification of personal behavior (see above) and by selected environmental measures. When possible, contact with cold sufferers should be avoided or reduced, especially when they are in the first 3 days of the illness. Hand washing after contact with an infected individual or with objects he or she may have touched is recommended, as is keeping fingers out of the eyes or nose during periods of exposure. Hand washing by infected persons will also limit the amount of infectious virus on their hands. Eradication of virus contaminating the hands by use of virucidal agents is an attractive approach to prevention of rhinovirus infection. A 2% aqueous iodine hand treatment appeared to be useful as prophylaxis against rhinovirus infection (45) (see above), but the cosmetic properties of the iodine solution prevent its practical use as a virucidal finger treatment. Commonly used hand sanitizers containing 62% ethanol are effective for removing rhinovirus from the hands. More recently, cosmetically acceptable hand treatments containing organic acids have been shown in experimental studies to have potent virucidal activity that persists for several hours after application (100). Whether these agents are effective for prevention of rhinovirus infection in the natural setting has not been determined.

TREATMENT

Symptomatic Therapies

The current treatment of rhinovirus-associated illness relies on remedies directed at specific symptoms. For common colds the efficacy of treatments for nasal obstruction, rhinorrhea, and the pain symptoms (i.e., sore throat and headache) has been demonstrated in studies done with adults (99). Attempts to demonstrate beneficial effects of these agents in children have failed, although it is not clear whether this failure is due to a lack of effect in children or simply due to the difficulty in assessing subjective symptoms in this population.

Adrenergic agents used either by topical intranasal administration or by oral administration have demonstrable effects on nasal obstruction. Topical administration of phenylephrine, oxymetazoline, or xylometazoline produces a prompt and marked reduction in nasal obstruction, with a gradual return to the baseline over a period of several hours. The use of these agents may be associated with nasal irritation, and prolonged use may be associated with rebound nasal obstruction. Although there has been no systematic comparison of the effect of topical and oral adrenergic agents on the nasal obstruction associated with the common cold, it appears that the oral agents produce about a 20% reduction in obstruction severity, compared to about 80% with the topical agents. The oral agents may also be associated with systemic side effects, including irritability and insomnia.

Rhinorrhea can also be treated topically or systemically. The first-generation antihistamines are the most commonly used treatment for runny nose and reduce rhinorrhea severity by approximately 25%. The effect on rhinorrhea appears to be related to the anticholinergic effects of the first-generation antihistamines, since the second-generation (nonsedating) antihistamines that have reduced anticholinergic side effects have no effect on the common cold. Sedation is a major side effect of the first-generation antihistamines and can be incapacitating for some individuals. Ipratropium bromide is a topical anticholinergic agent that is marketed for treatment of rhinorrhea and has effects comparable to those of the first-generation antihistamines. Nasal irritation and occasional bloody nasal mucus are side effects.

Cough associated with the common cold is frequently bothersome, but there are no satisfactory treatments for this symptom. Treatment with the antitussives codeine and dextromethorphan has not been shown to have a clinically significant effect on cough in colds. Treatment with a sedating-type antihistamine or antihistamine-decongestant combination may modestly benefit cough. This effect is presumed to be a result of drying of secretions in individuals with cough due to postnasal drip, but the treatment effect is small and not well defined. Some patients with cough during a cold may have reactive airway disease and might benefit from bronchodilator therapy; however, this intervention has not been subjected to careful study.

Although these symptomatic treatments appear to have beneficial effects on common-cold symptoms, there is no evidence that the use of these treatments will have an impact on the otitis media, sinusitis, or exacerbations of asthma that complicate this otherwise benign illness. The use of symptomatic therapies in children must take into account the inability to demonstrate beneficial effects in this population as well as the potential side effects associated with their use. Recent reports highlighting deaths in young children associated with errors in administration of common-cold treatments suggest that the use of these agents in young children should be discouraged.

Other Remedies

The lack of specific therapies, concern about the relative risk of symptomatic treatments, and the relatively benign nature of the common cold have produced significant interest in the use of alternative medicines for treatment of this illness. Many different nonconventional remedies have been promoted, but few have been subjected to rigorous scientific evaluation.

A potential role for zinc as a treatment for the common cold was first suggested by the observation that zinc is an inhibitor of 3C protease, an enzyme essential for rhinovirus replication. Although zinc has never been shown to have a significant antiviral effect in vivo, this observation produced numerous clinical trials to evaluate the effectiveness of zinc as a common-cold therapy. The results of these studies range from dramatic reductions in common-cold severity to no detectable effect. The studies that found no effect of zinc have been criticized as having small sample sizes or for using inadequate doses of zinc or formulations of zinc that might inactivate the zinc salts. The studies reporting a significant effect of zinc have been criticized for inadequate blinding either by the use of poorly matched placebos or because the active preparation was associated with a high incidence of adverse effects. Studies in the experimental rhinovirus cold model have consistently shown either no or relatively modest treatment effects of zinc preparations on common cold illness. The uncertain treatment effects of zinc must also be viewed in light of the side effects of this treatment. Oral zinc lozenges may be associated with sore mouth and occasional nausea. Intranasal zinc may cause nasal irritation and has been anecdotally linked to anosmia.

Echinacea is a traditional remedy for the common cold, with the use of this herb for treatment of respiratory symptoms dating to the late 1800s. There are three species of echinacea with different phytochemical characteristics that are used for medicinal purposes. The phytochemical composition of echinacea preparations may also vary due to differences in the part of the plant used, the type of extraction, and even the geographic location and time of year the plant is harvested. In spite of the differences in the echinacea preparations, only recently have there been attempts to standardize and characterize the material used in clinical trials. Many studies of echinacea prevention or treatment of the common cold have been reported, but the lack of characterization of the product and inattention to careful study design limit the interpretation and generalizability of the results (2). Although early studies suggested that echinacea may have beneficial treatment effects, recent more rigorous studies have failed to find any effect of echinacea on common-cold symptoms. Given the variation in echinacea products, the possibility that echinacea preparations with different phytochemical profiles might be beneficial cannot be excluded. The accumulating evidence, however, suggests that it is prudent to assume that echinacea has no beneficial effect until positive evidence of a treatment effect is produced.

Antiviral Treatment

A variety of antiviral approaches to prevention or treatment of rhinovirus infections have been studied, but no antiviral therapies are currently approved for the treatment of rhinovirus infections in the United States. The failure of this effort to produce useful antiviral therapies is due, in part, to the fact that rhinovirus colds are self-limited and usually benign and of short duration. As a result, treatments for the common cold must be rapidly effective, inexpensive, and virtually without toxicity or side effects.

Interferons, given as either prophylaxis or treatment for rhinovirus infections, have been studied extensively. Recombinant alpha interferon given intranasally either as seasonal prophylaxis or as contact prophylaxis was effective for prevention of rhinovirus colds, but interferon was not effective when given as treatment after onset of symptoms. Capsid-binding agents that bind in a pocket below the "canyon" region of the virion act by altering the conformation of the canyon to prevent receptor binding and/or by stabilizing the capsid and preventing uncoating. Compounds exhibiting this mechanism of action include a variety of isoxazole derivatives, flavonoids, pyridazines, and others. Pleconaril was the most extensively studied of these compounds. In large phase III clinical trials, an oral formulation of this drug reduced the total duration of colds by about 1 day and reduced symptom severity by about 19% (43). This drug was not approved for use as a common-cold treatment by the U.S. Food and Drug Administration because of safety concerns related to induction of cytochrome P450 3A isoenzymes. Decoy soluble ICAM-1, antibody to ICAM-1, 3C protease inhibitors, interferon inducers, and the benzimidazole derivative enviroxime have all been studied as common-cold treatments, but none of these has been developed into an effective product for prevention or treatment of the rhinovirus infection. Small interfering RNA technology may provide a new avenue for development of effective antirhinovirus treatments.

REFERENCES

1. **Arruda, E., T. R. Boyle, B. Winther, D. C. Pevear, J. M. Gwaltney, Jr., and F. G. Hayden.** 1995. Localization of human rhinovirus replication in the upper respiratory tract by in situ hybridization. *J. Infect. Dis.* **171:**1329–1333.

2. **Barrett, B.** 2003. Medicinal properties of Echinacea: a critical review. *Phytomedicine* **10:**66–86.
3. **Barton, D. J., B. J. Morasco, and J. B. Flanegan.** 1999. Translating ribosomes inhibit poliovirus negative-strand RNA synthesis. *J. Virol.* **73:**10104–10112.
4. **Bella, J., and M. G. Rossmann.** 1999. Review: rhinoviruses and their ICAM receptors. *J. Struct. Biol.* **128:**69–74.
5. **Brown, D. M., C. T. Cornell, G. P. Tran, J. H. Nguyen, and B. L. Semler.** 2005. An authentic 3′ noncoding region is necessary for efficient poliovirus replication. *J. Virol.* **79:**11962–11973.
6. **Chen, Y., E. Hamati, P. K. Lee, W. M. Lee, S. Wachi, D. Schnurr, S. Yagi, G. Dolganov, H. Boushey, P. Avila, and R. Wu.** 2006. Rhinovirus induces airway epithelial gene expression through double-stranded RNA and IFN-dependent pathways. *Am. J. Respir. Cell. Mol. Biol.* **34:**192–203.
7. **Cohen, S., W. J. Doyle, R. Turner, C. M. Alper, and D. P. Skoner.** 2003. Sociability and susceptibility to the common cold. *Psychol. Sci.* **14:**389–395.
8. **Cohen, S., W. J. Doyle, R. B. Turner, C. M. Alper, and D. P. Skoner.** 2003. Emotional style and susceptibility to the common cold. *Psychosom. Med.* **65:**652–657.
9. **Cohen, S., E. Frank, W. J. Doyle, D. P. Skoner, B. S. Rabin, and J. M. Gwaltney, Jr.** 1998. Types of stressors that increase susceptibility to the common cold in healthy adults. *Health Psychol.* **17:**214–223.
10. **Colonno, R. J., J. H. Condra, S. Mizutani, P. L. Callahan, M. E. Davies, and M. A. Murcko.** 1988. Evidence for the direct involvement of the rhinovirus canyon in receptor binding. *Proc. Natl. Acad. Sci. USA* **85:**5449–5453.
11. **Cooney, M. K., J. P. Fox, and G. E. Kenny.** 1982. Antigenic groupings of 90 rhinovirus serotypes. *Infect. Immun.* **37:**642–647.
12. **Corley, D. L., R. Gevirtz, R. Nideffer, and L. Cummins.** 1987. Prevention of post-infectious asthma in children by reducing self-inoculatory behavior. *J. Pediatr. Psychol.* **12:**519–531.
13. **Couch, R. B., T. R. Cate, R. G. Douglas, Jr., P. J. Gerone, and V. Knight.** 1966. Effect of route of inoculation on experimental respiratory viral disease in volunteers and evidence for airborne transmission. *Bacteriol. Rev.* **30:**517–529.
14. **D'Alessio, D. J., C. K. Meschievitz, J. A. Peterson, C. R. Dick, and E. C. Dick.** 1984. Short-duration exposure and the transmission of rhinoviral colds. *J. Infect. Dis.* **150:**189–194.
15. **D'Alessio, D. J., J. A. Peterson, C. R. Dick, and E. C. Dick.** 1976. Transmission of experimental rhinovirus colds in volunteer married couples. *J. Infect. Dis.* **133:**28–36.
16. **de Arruda, E., III, T. E. Mifflin, J. M. Gwaltney, Jr., B. Winther, and F. G. Hayden.** 1991. Localization of rhinovirus replication in vitro with in situ hybridization. *J. Med. Virol.* **34:**38–44.
17. **Dick, E. C., L. C. Jennings, K. A. Mink, C. D. Wartgow, and S. L. Inhorn.** 1987. Aerosol transmission of rhinovirus colds. *J. Infect. Dis.* **156:**442–448.
18. **Dingle, J. H., G. F. Badger, and W. S. Jordan, Jr.** 1964. *Illness in the Home: a Study of 25,000 Illnesses in a Group of Cleveland Families.* Case Western Reserve University Press, Cleveland, OH.
19. **Dochez, A. R., G. S. Shibley, and K. C. Mills.** 1930. Studies on the common cold. IV. Experimental transmission of the common cold to anthropoid apes and human beings by means of a filtrable agent. *J. Exp. Med.* **52:**701–716.
20. **Douglas, R. M., B. W. Moore, H. B. Miles, L. M. Davies, N. M. Graham, P. Ryan, D. A. Worswick, and J. K. Albrecht.** 1986. Prophylactic efficacy of intranasal alpha 2-interferon against rhinovirus infections in the family setting. *N. Engl. J. Med.* **314:**65–70.
21. **Duff, A. L., E. S. Pomeranz, L. E. Gelber, G. W. Price, H. Farris, F. G. Hayden, T. A. Platts-Mills, and P. W. Heymann.** 1993. Risk factors for acute wheezing in infants and children: viruses, passive smoke, and IgE antibodies to inhalant allergens. *Pediatrics* **92:**535–540.
22. **Dufresne, A. T., and M. Gromeier.** 2004. A nonpolio enterovirus with respiratory tropism causes poliomyelitis in intercellular adhesion molecule 1 transgenic mice. *Proc. Natl. Acad. Sci. USA* **101:**13636–13641.
23. **Elkhatieb, A., G. Hipskind, D. Woerner, and F. G. Hayden.** 1993. Middle ear abnormalities during natural rhinovirus colds in adults. *J. Infect. Dis.* **168:**618–621.
24. **Fauquet, C. M., M. A. Mayo, J. Maniloff, U. Desselberger, and L. A. Ball.** 2005 Picornaviridae, p. 757–778. *In* C. M. Fauquet, M. A. Mayo, J. Maniloff, U. Desselberger, and L. A. Ball (ed.), *Virus Taxonomy: Eighth Report of the International Committee on Taxonomy of Viruses.* Elsevier Academic Press. San Diego, CA.
25. **Frost, W. H., and M. Gover.** 1941. The incidence and time distribution of common colds in several groups kept under continuous observation, p. 359. *In* K. F. Maxcy (ed.), *Papers of Wade Hampton Frost.* The Commonwealth Fund, New York, NY.
26. **Gern, J. E., and W. W. Busse.** 1999. Association of rhinovirus infections with asthma. *Clin. Microbiol. Rev.* **12:**9–18.
27. **Gern, J. E., D. A. French, K. A. Grindle, R. A. Brockman-Schneider, S. Konno, and W. W. Busse.** 2003. Double-stranded RNA induces the synthesis of specific chemokines by bronchial epithelial cells. *Am. J. Respir. Cell. Mol. Biol.* **28:**731–737.
28. **Gern, J. E., R. Vrtis, K. A. Grindle, C. Swenson, and W. W. Busse.** 2000. Relationship of upper and lower airway cytokines to outcome of experimental rhinovirus infection. *Am. J. Respir. Crit. Care Med.* **162:**2226–2231.
29. **Grassme, H., A. Riehle, B. Wilker, and E. Gulbins.** 2005. Rhinoviruses infect human epithelial cells via ceramide-enriched membrane platforms. *J. Biol. Chem.* **280:**26256–26262.
30. **Greve, J. M., G. Davis, A. M. Meyer, C. P. Forte, S. C. Yost, C. W. Marlor, M. E. Kamarck, and A. McClelland.** 1989. The major human rhinovirus receptor is ICAM-1. *Cell* **56:**839–847.
31. **Gustafson, M., D. Proud, J. O. Hendley, F. G. Hayden, and J. M. Gwaltney, Jr.** 1996. Oral prednisone therapy in experimental rhinovirus infections. *J. Allergy Clin. Immunol.* **97:**1009–1014.
32. **Gwaltney, J. M., Jr.** 1984. The Jeremiah Metzger lecture. Climatology and the common cold. *Trans. Am. Clin. Climatol. Assoc.* **96:**159–175.
33. **Gwaltney, J. M., Jr.** 1997. Rhinoviruses, p. 815–838. *In* A. S. Evans (ed.), *Viral Infection of Humans: Epidemiology and Control*, 4th ed. Plenum Press, New York, NY.
34. **Gwaltney, J. M., Jr., J. O. Hendley, G. Simon, and W. S. Jordan, Jr.** 1967. Rhinovirus infections in an industrial population. II. Characteristics of illness and antibody response. *JAMA* **202:**494–500.
35. **Gwaltney, J. M., Jr., J. O. Hendley, G. Simon, and W. S. Jordan, Jr.** 1966. Rhinovirus infections in an industrial population. I. The occurrence of illness. *N. Engl. J. Med.* **275:**1261–1268.
36. **Gwaltney, J. M., Jr., C. D. Phillips, R. D. Miller, and D. K. Riker.** 1994. Computed tomographic study of the common cold. *N. Engl. J. Med.* **330:**25–30.

37. **Hadfield, A. T., W. Lee, R. Zhao, M. A. Oliveira, I. Minor, R. R. Rueckert, and M. G. Rossmann.** 1997. The refined structure of human rhinovirus 16 at 2.15 A resolution: implications for the viral life cycle. *Structure* **5:** 427–441.
38. **Hamory, B. H., M. A. Sande, A. Sydnor, Jr., D. L. Seale, and J. M. Gwaltney, Jr.** 1979. Etiology and antimicrobial therapy of acute maxillary sinusitis. *J. Infect. Dis.* **139:**197–202.
39. **Hamparian, V. V., R. J. Colonno, M. K. Cooney, E. C. Dick, J. M. Gwaltney, Jr., J. H. Hughes, W. S. Jordan, Jr., A. Z. Kapikian, W. J. Mogabgab, A. Monto, C. A. Phillips, R. R. Rueckert, J. H. Schieble, E. J. Stott, and D. A. J. Tyrrell.** 1987. A collaborative report: rhinoviruses—extension of the numbering system from 89 to 100. *Virology* **159:**191–192.
40. **Harris, J. M., II, and J. M. Gwaltney, Jr.** 1996. Incubation periods of experimental rhinovirus infection and illness. *Clin. Infect. Dis.* **23:**1287–1290.
41. **Harris, J. R., and V. R. Racaniello.** 2005. Amino acid changes in proteins 2B and 3A mediate rhinovirus type 39 growth in mouse cells. *J. Virol.* **79:**5363–5373.
42. **Hayden, F. G., J. K. Albrecht, D. L. Kaiser, and J. M. Gwaltney, Jr.** 1986. Prevention of natural colds by contact prophylaxis with intranasal alpha2-interferon. *N. Engl. J. Med.* **314:**71–75.
43. **Hayden, F. G., D. T. Herrington, T. L. Coats, K. Kim, E. C. Cooper, S. A. Villano, S. Liu, S. Hudson, D. C. Pevear, M. Collett, M. McKinlay, and the Pleconaril Respiratory Infection Study Group.** 2003. Efficacy and safety of oral pleconaril for treatment of colds due to picornaviruses in adults: results of 2 double-blind, randomized, placebo-controlled trials. *Clin. Infect. Dis.* **36:**1523–1532.
44. **Hemmes, J. H., K. C. Winkler, and S. M. Kool.** 1960. Virus survival as a seasonal factor in influenza and poliomyelitis. *Nature* **188:**430–437.
45. **Hendley, J. O., and J. M. Gwaltney, Jr.** 1988. Mechanisms of transmission of rhinovirus infections. *Epidemiol. Rev.* **10:**243–258.
46. **Higgins, P. G., E. M. Ellis, and D. A. Woolley.** 1969. A comparative study of standard methods and organ culture for the isolation of respiratory viruses. *J. Med. Microbiol.* **2:**109–115.
47. **Hoover-Litty, H., and J. M. Greve.** 1993. Formation of rhinovirus-soluble ICAM-1 complexes and conformational changes in the virion. *J. Virol.* **67:**390–397.
48. **Horsnell, C., R. E. Gama, P. J. Hughes, and G. Stanway.** 1995. Molecular relationships between 21 human rhinovirus serotypes. *J. Gen. Virol.* **76**(Pt. 10):2549–2555.
49. **Jacques, J., M. Bouscambert-Duchamp, H. Moret, J. Carquin, V. Brodard, B. Lina, J. Motte, and L. Andreoletti.** 2006. Association of respiratory picornaviruses with acute bronchiolitis in French infants. *J. Clin. Virol.* **35:** 463–466.
50. **Jartti, T., P. Lehtinen, T. Vuorinen, M. Koskenvuo, and O. Ruuskanen.** 2004. Persistence of rhinovirus and enterovirus RNA after acute respiratory illness in children. *J. Med. Virol.* **72:**695–699.
51. **Jennings, L. C., E. C. Dick, K. A. Mink, C. D. Wartgow, and S. L. Inhorn.** 1988. Near disappearance of rhinovirus along a fomite transmission chain. *J. Infect. Dis.* **158:**888–892.
52. **Johnston, N. W., S. L. Johnston, G. R. Norman, J. Dai, and M. R. Sears.** 2006. The September epidemic of asthma hospitalization: school children as disease vectors. *J. Allergy Clin. Immunol.* **117:**557–562.
53. **Johnston, S. L., P. K. Pattemore, G. Sanderson, S. Smith, F. Lampe, L. Josephs, P. Symington, S. O'Toole, S. H. Myint, D. A. J. Tyrrell, and S. T. Holgate.** 1995. Community study of role of viral infections in exacerbations of asthma in 9–11 year old children. *Br. Med. J.* **310:**1225–1229.
54. **Johnston, S. L., G. Sanderson, P. K. Pattemore, S. Smith, P. G. Bardin, C. B. Bruce, P. R. Lambden, D. A. Tyrrell, and S. T. Holgate.** 1993. Use of polymerase chain reaction for diagnosis of picornavirus infection in subjects with and without respiratory symptoms. *J. Clin. Microbiol.* **31:**111–117.
55. **Juven, T., J. Mertsola, M. Waris, M. Leinonen, O. Meurman, M. Roivainen, J. Eskola, P. Saikku, and O. Ruuskanen.** 2000. Etiology of community-acquired pneumonia in 254 hospitalized children. *Pediatr. Infect. Dis. J.* **19:**293–298.
56. **Kaiser, L., J. D. Aubert, J. C. Pache, C. Deffernez, T. Rochat, J. Garbino, W. Wunderli, P. Meylan, S. Yerly, L. Perrin, I. Letovanec, L. Nicod, C. Tapparel, and P. M. Soccal.** 2006. Chronic rhinoviral infection in lung transplant recipients. *Am. J. Respir. Crit. Care Med.* **174:** 1392–1399.
57. **Kapikian, A. Z., R. M. Conant, V. V. Hamparian, R. M. Chanock, P. J. Chapple, E. C. Dick, J. D. Fenters, J. M. Gwaltney, Jr., D. Hamre, J. C. Holper, W. S. Jordan, Jr., E. H. Lennette, J. L. Melnick, W. J. Mogabgab, M. A. Mufson, C. A. Phillips, J. H. Scheible, and D. A. J. Tyrrell.** 1967. Rhinoviruses: a numbering system. *Nature* **213:**761–762.
58. **Kapikian, A. Z., R. M. Conant, V. V. Hamparian, R. M. Chanock, E. C. Dick, J. M. Gwaltney, Jr., D. Hamre, W. S. Jordan, Jr., G. E. Kenny, E. H. Lennette, J. L. Melnick, W. J. Mogabgab, C. A. Phillips, J. H. Scheible, E. J. Stott, and D. A. J. Tyrrell.** 1971. A collaborative report: rhinoviruses—extension of the numbering system. *Virology* **43:**524–526.
59. **Katpally, U., and T. J. Smith.** 2007. Pocket factors are unlikely to play a major role in the life cycle of human rhinovirus. *J. Virol.* **81:**6307–6315.
60. **Ketler, A., V. V. Hamparian, and M. R. Hilleman.** 1962. Characterization and classification of ECHO 28-rhinovirus-coryzavirus agents. *Proc. Soc. Exp. Biol. Med.* **110:**821–831.
61. **Kim, S. S., T. J. Smith, M. S. Chapman, M. C. Rossmann, D. C. Pevear, F. J. Dutko, P. J. Felock, G. D. Diana, and M. A. McKinlay.** 1989. Crystal structure of human rhinovirus serotype 1A (HRV1A). *J. Mol. Biol.* **210:**91–111.
62. **Kistler, A. L., D. R. Webster, S. Rouskin, V. Magrini, J. J. Credle, D. P. Schnurr, H. A. Boushey, E. R. Mardis, H. Li, and J. L. DeRisi.** 2007. Genome-wide diversity and selective pressure in the human rhinovirus. *Virol. J.* **4:**40.
63. **Kruse, W.** 1914. Die Errger van Husten and Schupfen. *Muench. Med. Wochenschr.* **61:**1547–1552.
63a. **Lamson, D., N. Renwick, V. Kapoor, Z. Liu, G. Palacios, J. Ju, A. Dean, K. St. George, T. Briese, and W. I. Lipkin.** 2006. MassTag polymerase-chain-reaction detection of respiratory pathogens, including a new rhinovirus genotype, that caused influenza-like illness in New York State during 2004–2005. *J. Infect. Dis.* **194:** 1398–1402.
64. **Ledford, R. M., N. R. Patel, T. M. Demenczuk, A. Watanyar, T. Herbertz, M. S. Collett, and D. C. Pevear.** 2004. VP1 sequencing of all human rhinovirus serotypes: insights into genus phylogeny and susceptibility to antiviral capsid-binding compounds. *J. Virol.* **78:**3663–3674.

65. **Lee, W. M., K. Grindle, T. Pappas, D. J. Marshall, M. J. Moser, E. L. Beaty, P. A. Shult, J. R. Prudent, and J. E. Gern.** 2007. High-throughput, sensitive, and accurate multiplex PCR-microsphere flow cytometry system for large-scale comprehensive detection of respiratory viruses. *J. Clin. Microbiol.* **45:**2626–2634.
66. **Lee, W. M., S. S. Monroe, and R. R. Rueckert.** 1993. Role of maturation cleavage in infectivity of picornaviruses: activation of an infectosome. *J. Virol.* **67:**2110–2122.
67. **Lee, W. M., and W. Wang.** 2003. Human rhinovirus type 16: mutant V1210A requires capsid-binding drug for assembly of pentamers to form virions during morphogenesis. *J. Virol.* **77:**6235–6244.
68. **McBride, T. P., W. J. Doyle, F. G. Hayden, and J. M. Gwaltney, Jr.** 1989. Alterations of the eustachian tube, middle ear, and nose in rhinovirus infection. *Arch. Otolaryngol. Head Neck Surg.* **115:**1054–1059.
68a. **McErlean, P., L. A. Shackelton, S. B. Lambert, M. D. Nissen, T. P. Sloots, and I. M. Mackay.** 2007. Characterisation of a newly identified human rhinovirus, HRV-QPM, discovered in infants with bronchiolitis. *J. Clin. Virol.* **39:**67–75.
68b. **McKnight, K. L.** 2003. The human rhinovirus internal cis-acting replication element (cre) exhibits disparate properties among serotypes. *Arch. Virol.* **148:**2397–2418.
69. **Mizutani, S., and R. J. Colonno.** 1985. In vitro synthesis of an infectious RNA from cDNA clones of human rhinovirus type 14. *J. Virol.* **56:**628–632.
70. **Monto, A. S., E. R. Bryan, and S. Ohmit.** 1987. Rhinovirus infections in Tecumseh, Michigan: frequency of illness and number of serotypes. *J. Infect. Dis.* **156:**43–49.
71. **Mosser, A. G., D. M. Leippe, and R. R. Rueckert.** 1989. Neutralization of picornaviruses: support for the pentamer bridging hypothesis, p. 155. *In* B. Semler, and E. Ehrenfeld (ed.), *Molecular Aspects of Picornavirus Infection and Detection*. American Society for Microbiology, Washington, DC.
72. **Mosser, A. G., and R. R. Rueckert.** 1996. Picornavirus capsid binding agents, p. 114. *In* D. D. Richman (ed.), *Antiviral Drug Resistance*. John Wiley & Sons, Ltd., New York, NY.
73. **Nokso-Koivisto, J., T. J. Kinnari, P. Lindahl, T. Hovi, and A. Pitkaranta.** 2002. Human picornavirus and coronavirus RNA in nasopharynx of children without concurrent respiratory symptoms. *J. Med. Virol.* **66:**417–420.
74. **Nugent, C. I., K. L. Johnson, P. Sarnow, and K. Kirkegaard.** 1999. Functional coupling between replication and packaging of poliovirus replicon RNA. *J. Virol.* **73:**427–435.
75. **Oberste, M. S., K. Maher, D. Schnurr, M. R. Flemister, J. C. Lovchik, H. Peters, W. Sessions, C. Kirk, N. Chatterjee, S. Fuller, J. M. Hanauer, and M. A. Pallansch.** 2004. Enterovirus 68 is associated with respiratory illness and shares biological features with both the enteroviruses and the rhinoviruses. *J. Gen. Virol.* **85:**2577–2584.
76. **Oliveira, M. A., R. Zhao, W. M. Lee, M. J. Kremer, I. Minor, R. R. Rueckert, G. D. Diana, D. C. Pevear, F. J. Dutko, M. A. McKinlay, and M. C. Rossmann.** 1993. The structure of human rhinovirus 16. *Structure* **1:**51–68.
77. **Olson, N. H., P. R. Kolatkar, M. A. Oliveira, R. H. Cheng, J. M. Greve, A. McClelland, T. S. Baker, and M. G. Rossmann.** 1993. Structure of a human rhinovirus complexed with its receptor molecule. *Proc. Natl. Acad. Sci. USA* **90:**507–511.
78. **Papadopoulos, N. G., P. J. Bates, P. G. Bardin, A. Papi, S. H. Leir, D. J. Fraenkel, J. Meyer, P. M. Lackie, G. Sanderson, S. T. Holgate, and S. L. Johnston.** 2000. Rhinoviruses infect the lower airways. *J. Infect. Dis.* **181:**1875–1884.
79. **Papadopoulos, N. G., M. Moustaki, M. Tsolia, A. Bossios, E. Astra, A. Prezerakou, D. Gourgiotis, and D. Kafetzis.** 2002. Association of rhinovirus infection with increased disease severity in acute bronchiolitis. *Am. J. Respir. Crit. Care Med.* **165:**1285–1289.
80. **Papi, A., and S. L. Johnston.** 1999. Rhinovirus infection induces expression of its own receptor intercellular adhesion molecule 1 (ICAM-1) via increased NF-kappaB-mediated transcription. *J. Biol. Chem.* **274:**9707–9720.
81. **Patterson, L. J., and V. V. Hamparian.** 1997. Hyper-antigenic variation occurs with human rhinovirus type 17. *J. Virol.* **71:**1370–1374.
82. **Paul, A. V., E. Rieder, D. W. Kim, J. H. van Boom, and E. Wimmer.** 2000. Identification of an RNA hairpin in poliovirus RNA that serves as the primary template in the in vitro uridylylation of VPg. *J. Virol.* **74:**10359–10370.
83. **Pelon, W., W. J. Mogabgab, I. A. Phillips, and W. E. Pierce.** 1957. A cytopathogenic agent isolated from naval recruits with mild respiratory illnesses. *Proc. Soc. Exp. Biol. Med.* **94:**262–267.
83a. **Pitkaranta, A., T. Puhakka, M. J. Makela, O. Ruuskanen, O. Carpen, and A. Vaheri.** 2003. Detection of rhinovirus RNA in middle turbinate of patients with common colds by in situ hybridization. *J. Med. Virol.* **70:**319–323.
84. **Pitkaranta, A., A. Virolainen, J. Jero, E. Arruda, and F. G. Hayden.** 1998. Detection of rhinovirus, respiratory syncytial virus, and coronavirus infections in acute otitis media by reverse transcriptase polymerase chain reaction. *Pediatrics* **102:**291–295.
85. **Price, W. H.** 1956. The isolation of a new virus associated with respiratory clinical disease in humans. *Proc. Natl. Acad. Sci. USA* **42:**892–896.
86. **Rakes, G. P., E. Arruda, J. M. Ingram, G. E. Hoover, J. C. Zambrano, F. G. Hayden, T. A. Platts-Mills, and P. W. Heymann.** 1999. Rhinovirus and respiratory syncytial virus in wheezing children requiring emergency care. IgE and eosinophil analyses. *Am. J. Respir. Crit. Care Med.* **159:**785–790.
87. **Reed, S. E.** 1975. An investigation of the possible transmission of rhinovirus colds through indirect contact. *J. Hyg.* **75:**249–258.
88. **Reithmayer, M., A. Reischl, L. Snyers, and D. Blaas.** 2002. Species-specific receptor recognition by a minor-group human rhinovirus (HRV): HRV serotype 1A distinguishes between the murine and the human low-density lipoprotein receptor. *J. Virol.* **76:**6957–6965.
89. **Rossmann, M. G.** 1989. The canyon hypothesis. Hiding the host cell receptor attachment site on a viral surface from immune surveillance. *J. Biol. Chem.* **264:**14587–14590.
90. **Rossmann, M. G., E. Arnold, J. W. Erickson, E. A. Frankenberger, J. P. Griffith, H.-J. Hecht, J. E. Johnson, G. Kamer, M. Luo, A. G. Mosser, R. Rueckert, B. Sherry, and G. Vriend.** 1985. The structure of a human common cold virus (rhinovirus 14) and its functional relations to other picornaviruses. *Nature* **317:**145–153.
91. **Rueckert, R.** 1996. Picornaviridae: the viruses and their replication, p. 609–654. *In* B. N. Fields, D. M. Knipe, P. M. Howley, et al. (ed.), *Fields Virology*, 3rd ed. Lippincott-Raven Publishers, Philadelphia, PA.
92. **Savolainen, C., S. Blomqvist, M. N. Mulders, and T. Hovi.** 2002. Genetic clustering of all 102 human rhinovirus prototype strains: serotype 87 is close to human enterovirus 70. *J. Gen. Virol.* **83:**333–340.

93. **Smith, T. J., and T. Baker.** 1999. Picornaviruses: epitopes, canyons, and pockets. *Adv. Virus Res.* **52:**1–23.
94. **Smith, T. J., E. S. Chase, T. J. Schmidt, N. H. Olson, and T. S. Baker.** 1996. Neutralizing antibody to human rhinovirus 14 penetrates the receptor-binding canyon. *Nature* **383:**350–354.
95. **Souza, L. S., E. A. Ramos, F. M. Carvalho, V. M. Guedes, L. S. Souza, C. M. Rocha, A. B. Soares, F. Velloso Lde, I. S. Macedo, F. E. Moura, M. Siqueira, S. Fortes, C. C. de Jesus, C. M. Santiago, A. M. Carvalho, and E. Arruda.** 2003. Viral respiratory infections in young children attending day care in urban Northeast Brazil. *Pediatr. Pulmonol.* **35:**184–191.
96. **Stanway, G., P. J. Hughes, R. C. Mountford, P. D. Minor, and J. W. Almond.** 1984. The complete nucleotide sequence of a common cold virus: human rhinovirus 14. *Nucleic Acids Res.* **12:**7859–7875.
97. **Tapparel, C., T. Junier, D. Gerlach, S. Cordey, S. Van Belle, L. Perrin, E. M. Zdobnov, and L. Kaiser.** 2007. New complete genome sequences of human rhinoviruses shed light on their phylogeny and genomic features. *BMC Genomics* **8:**224.
98. **Thwing, C. J., E. Arruda, J. P. B. V. Filho, A. C. Filho, and J. M. Gwaltney, Jr.** 1993. Rhinovirus antibodies in an isolated Amazon Indian tribe. *Am. J. Trop. Med. Hyg.* **48:**771–775.
99. **Turner, R. B.** 2001. The treatment of rhinovirus infections: progress and potential. *Antiviral Res.* **49:**1–14.
100. **Turner, R. B., K. A. Biedermann, J. M. Morgan, B. Keswick, K. D. Ertel, and M. F. Barker.** 2004. Efficacy of organic acids in hand cleansers for prevention of rhinovirus infections. *Antimicrob. Agents Chemother.* **48:** 2595–2598.
101. **Turner, R. B., and R. B. Couch.** 2007. Rhinoviruses, p. 895–909. *In* D. M. Knipe, P. M. Howley, D. E. Griffin, R. A. Lamb, M. A. Martin, B. Roizman, and S. E. Straus (ed.), *Fields Virology*, 5th ed. Lippincott Williams and Wilkins. Philadelphia, PA.
102. **Turner, R. B., J. O. Hendley, and J. M. Gwaltney, Jr.** 1982. Shedding of infected ciliated epithelial cells in rhinovirus colds. *J. Infect. Dis.* **145:**849–853.
102a. **Tuthill, T. J., N. G. Papadopoulos, P. Jourdan, L. J. Challinor, N. A. Sharp, C. Plumpton, K. Shah, S. Barnard, L. Dash, J. Burnet, R. A. Killington, D. J. Rowlands, N. J. Clarke, E. D. Blair, and S. L. Johnston.** 2003. Mouse respiratory epithelial cells support efficient replication of human rhinovirus. *J. Gen. Virol.* **84:**2829–2836.
103. **Tyrrell, D. A., and R. Parsons.** 1960. Some virus isolations from common colds. III. Cytopathic effects in tissue cultures. *Lancet* **i:**239–242.
104. **van Benten, I., L. Koopman, B. Niesters, W. Hop, B. van Middelkoop, L. de Waal, K. van Drunen, A. Osterhaus, H. Neijens, and W. Fokkens.** 2003. Predominance of rhinovirus in the nose of symptomatic and asymptomatic infants. *Pediatr. Allergy Immunol.* **14:**363–370.
105. **Verdaguer, N., D. Blaas, and I. Fita.** 2000. Structure of human rhinovirus serotype 2 (HRV2). *J. Mol. Biol.* **300:** 1179–1194.
106. **Vlasak, M., M. Roivainen, M. Reithmayer, I. Goesler, P. Laine, L. Snyers, T. Hovi, and D. Blaas.** 2005. The minor receptor group of human rhinovirus (HRV) includes HRV23 and HRV25, but the presence of a lysine in the VP1 HI loop is not sufficient for receptor binding. *J. Virol.* **79:**7389–7395.
107. **Wald, E. R., N. Guerra, and C. Byers.** 1991. Upper respiratory tract infections in young children: duration of and frequency of complications. *Pediatrics* **87:**129–133.
108. **Winther, B., J. M. Gwaltney, Jr., N. Mygind, R. B. Turner, and J. O. Hendley.** 1986. Sites of rhinovirus recovery after point inoculation of the upper airway. *JAMA* **256:**1763–1767.
109. **Winther, B., F. G. Hayden, and J. O. Hendley.** 2006. Picornavirus infections in children diagnosed by RT-PCR during longitudinal surveillance with weekly sampling: association with symptomatic illness and effect of season. *J. Med. Virol.* **78:**644–650.
110. **Wright, P. F., A. M. Deatly, R. A. Karron, R. B. Belshe, J. R. Shi, W. C. Gruber, Y. Zhu, and V. B. Randolph.** 2007. Comparison of results of detection of rhinovirus by PCR and viral culture in human nasal wash specimens from subjects with and without clinical symptoms of respiratory illness. *J. Clin. Microbiol.* **45:** 2126–2129.
111. **Wu, R., Y. H. Zhao, and M. M. Chang.** 1997. Growth and differentiation of conducting airway epithelial cells in culture. *Eur. Respir. J.* **10:**2398–2403.
112. **Zhao, R., D. C. Pevear, M. J. Kremer, V. L. Giranda, J. A. Kofron, R. J. Kuhn, and M. G. Rossmann.** 1996. Human rhinovirus 3 at 3.0 A resolution. *Structure* **4:** 1205–1220.

Hepatitis A Virus

PHILIP R. SPRADLING, ANNETTE MARTIN, AND STEPHEN M. FEINSTONE

47

Hepatitis A is an acute, self-limiting infection of the liver by an enterically transmitted picornavirus, hepatitis A virus (HAV). Hepatitis A may occasionally result in fulminant hepatitis and death, but chronic hepatitis A is unknown.

Reports of icteric disease in early Chinese literature and the writings of Hippocrates may represent hepatitis A but cannot be distinguished from jaundice due to other causes (177). The earliest documented outbreaks of probable hepatitis A occurred in soldiers in Europe in the 17th and 18th centuries. Since then, hepatitis has been recognized as a camp follower, and many of the earliest terms used to describe the disease, like "kriegsikterus" and "jaunisse des camps," reflect its close association with the military.

During World War II, studies of epidemics of hepatitis among troops and civilians clearly established the existence of two forms of the disease, known as hepatitis A and hepatitis B (77). Experimental transmission studies rapidly defined the major features of hepatitis A, including a relatively short incubation period (15 to 49 days), its fecal-oral mode of transmission (77), and long-lasting immunity that could be passively transferred. An animal model of HAV infection using tamarin monkeys was established in 1968 (51). In 1973, HAV was visualized by immunoelectron microscopy, a finding that also resulted in a crude but sensitive test for antibody to HAV (anti-HAV). Virus-like particles approximately 27 nm in diameter were first identified in the stools of volunteers experimentally infected several years earlier with the MS-1 strain of HAV (59). These particles were specifically aggregated by convalescent-phase but not by preinfection serum (Fig. 1). The identification of HAV and the demonstration that infection could be transmitted to tamarins and later to seronegative chimpanzees ushered in a new era of research on hepatitis A which culminated in the propagation of the virus in cell culture, molecular cloning and sequencing of the viral genome, and, subsequently, the development and licensure of safe, effective vaccines (5, 44, 128, 156). In countries where vaccine programs have been instituted, the incidence of new hepatitis A cases has dropped significantly. In contrast, in countries in which hepatitis A endemicity is relatively high but sanitation is improving, epidemiological shift is resulting in an increase in susceptible young adults and a potential for large outbreaks.

VIROLOGY

Classification and Diversity

Classification

HAV is a positive-strand RNA virus classified within the family *Picornaviridae*, which includes many other medically and veterinary important pathogens subclassified into nine genera. HAV shares a similar genomic organization with members of this family, particularly those in the genus *Aphthovirus* (foot-and-mouth disease virus) and the genus *Cardiovirus* (e.g., encephalomyocarditis virus). However, limited nucleotide homology (44) and a number of attributes of the virus (107) distinguish it from other picornaviruses. Hence, HAV has been classified as the type species of a separate genus, *Hepatovirus*. One other distinct species of picornavirus, avian encephalomyelitis virus, has been tentatively classified within the *Hepatovirus* genus on the basis of a remarkably close phylogenetic relationship to HAV (146).

Genetic and Antigenic Diversity

The genetic diversity of HAV has been investigated by determining the partial genomic nucleotide sequences of numerous human HAV strains recovered from various human or simian sources and geographic areas (94, 131). Circulating human strains of HAV are relatively closely related genetically, especially compared to the genetic diversity evident among other picornaviruses. Two major human HAV genotypes (genotypes I and III) and two minor genotypes (II and VII) have been documented, the sequences of which differ from each other by 15 to 25% of base positions in the genomic region studied (VP1-2A junction). Three other genotypes (genotypes IV, V, and VI) each include a single simian HAV strain (131). A few HAV strains have been entirely sequenced (42, 44, 117, 122) and further used as laboratory strains that can be propagated in cell culture (24, 128, 140).

Comparisons of the nucleotide sequences of HAV strains demonstrated high amino acid conservation (greater than 70%) in the sequences of the viral capsid proteins. Viruses belonging to distinct genotypes elicit antibodies with substantial cross-neutralizing activity, suggesting that there is only one recognized HAV serotype (94, 147). Although some monoclonal antibodies are ca-

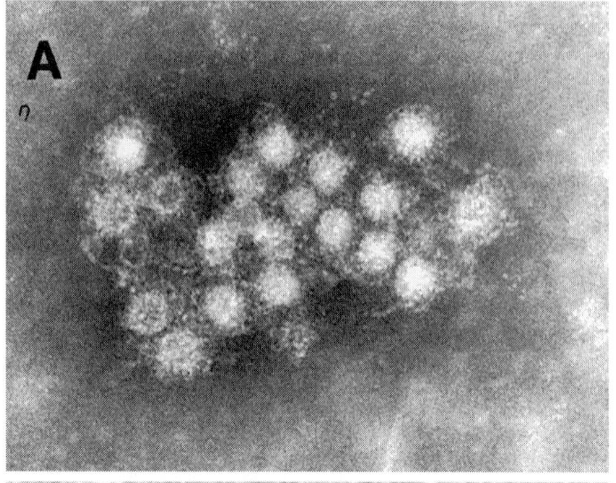

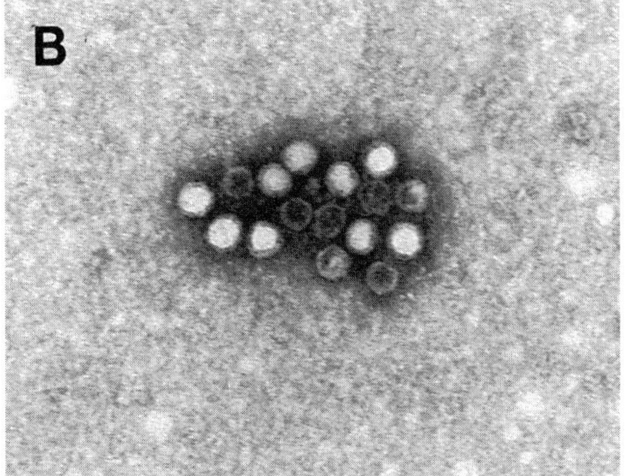

FIGURE 1 Electron micrographs of HAV. (A) Immunoelectron micrograph of HAV particles from human stool reacted with convalescent-phase serum. The particles are heavily coated with and aggregated by antibody. Both "full" and "empty" particles can be seen. (B) Immunoelectron micrograph showing particles from human stool reacted with a preinfection serum. The 27- to 28-nm particles are nearly devoid of antibody, and some fine structure can be seen.

pable of distinguishing unique epitopes that are variably present in strains of HAV isolated from humans or from naturally infected cynomolgus and African green monkeys (115, 158), even simian and human strains of HAV demonstrate substantial antigenic cross-reactivity.

Composition of the Virus

Virion Structure

HAV is a nonenveloped, 27- to 28-nm spherical virus, as determined by immunoelectron microscopy and negative staining (Fig. 1) (59). Mature HAV virions purified from feces collected from infected humans or chimpanzees band at 1.32 to 1.34 g/cm^3 in cesium chloride (CsCl) and sediment at approximately 160 S. Particles with lower density that band at about 1.27 g/cm^3 in CsCl and sediment at 70 to 80 S can often be detected in HAV preparations (Fig. 1) and may represent empty capsids devoid of genomic RNA (95, 141).

Attempts to determine the atomic structure of HAV by X-ray crystallography have not been successful, although such studies have provided high-resolution images of virus particles from each of the other major picornaviral genera. Medium-resolution images of the HAV particle by cryoelectron microscopy (Fig. 2) suggest that the HAV protein shell has an icosahedral structure similar to that of other picornaviruses, except for the apparent absence of depressions on the surface of the particle.

The HAV capsid encloses the viral genome, which is a single-stranded 35S RNA molecule of positive polarity approximately 7.5 kb in length, possessing structured 5′ and 3′ termini and a 3′ poly(A) tail (42). The viral genome encodes a single polyprotein that is subsequently cleaved essentially by the unique virus-encoded protease to generate four capsid proteins (VP1 to VP4) at its N terminus and the nonstructural proteins involved in genome replication at its C terminus (Fig. 3).

Antigenic Structure

Although a variety of genotypes of HAV have been identified, there appears to be only one serotype of HAV worldwide (94). This has important implications for the development of effective vaccines. Neutralizing murine monoclonal antibodies do not recognize denatured capsid proteins. Antisera raised to proteins expressed from recombinant DNAs show only weak reactivity with native capsids and have very limited virus neutralization activity (79), complicating the development of a vaccine based on recombinant DNA technology.

Antigenic variants of HAV that resist neutralization by neutralizing monoclonal antibodies have been selected in cell culture by continued passage of cell culture-adapted virus in the presence of these antibodies. Competition studies with these mutants suggest the existence of a single immunodominant site (149), and sequencing of the genomic regions encoding their capsid proteins indicated the presence of closely spaced neutralization epitopes in polypeptide loops within VP3 and VP1 (125). The critical neutralization epitopes of HAV are thus conformationally

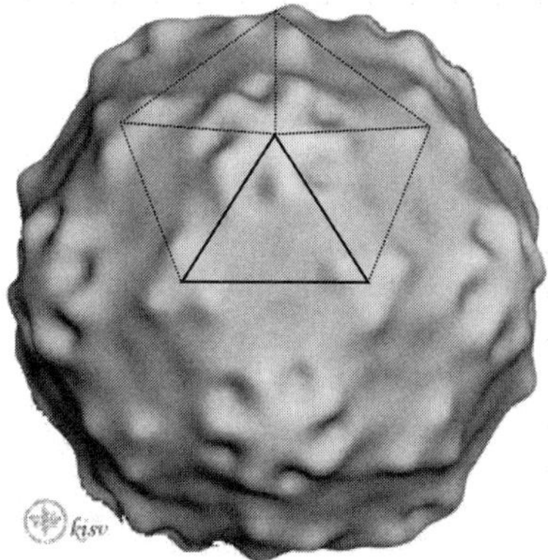

FIGURE 2 Medium-resolution image of the structure of the HAV particle as revealed by cryoelectron microscopy. The top of the solid triangle defines a fivefold axis of symmetry of the particle. Five such triangles, centered around the fivefold axis of symmetry, delineate a pentamer assembly subunit (dashed footprint). The mature particle contains 12 pentamers. Image reconstructions show significant surface features but suggest that there is no marked canyon around the fivefold axis of symmetry like that found in other picornaviruses. This unique image of the HAV particle was kindly provided in advance of publication by Holland Cheng, University of California at Davis.

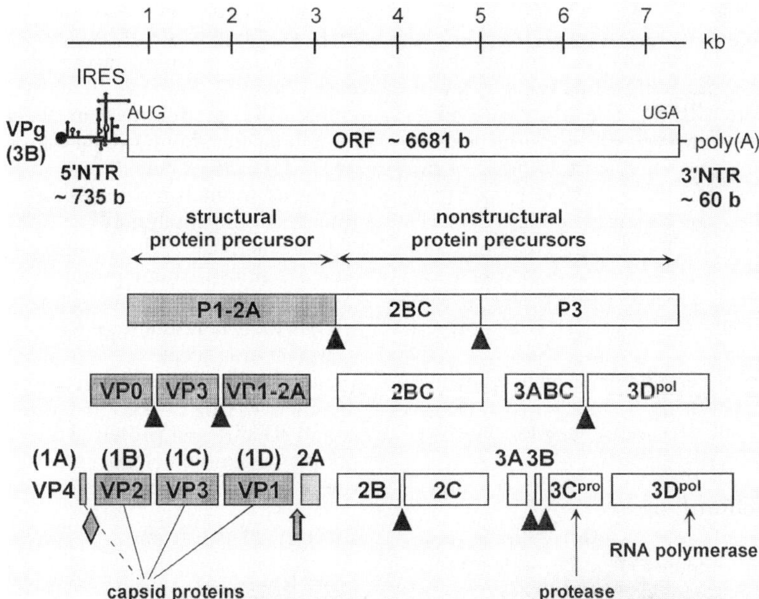

FIGURE 3 HAV genome organization and polyprotein processing. The positive-strand RNA genome, approximately 7.5 kb in length, contains a single open reading frame (ORF) and 5′ and 3′ NTRs of the indicated lengths (bases [b]). The initiator AUG and terminator UGA codons are indicated. The 5′ NTR is covalently linked to the genome-encoded protein 3B (otherwise termed VPg) and contains a structured IRES that determines the cap-independent mechanism of RNA translation initiation. The ORF encodes a polyprotein that is co- and posttranslationally cleaved by the viral protease $3C^{pro}$ (at sites indicated by black triangles), a yet-to-be-identified cellular protease (at the site indicated by a gray arrow), or an unknown proteolytic activity (at the site indicated by a gray diamond) to release the mature structural (dark gray boxes) and nonstructural (white boxes) proteins, as well as intermediate precursors (see also Table 1).

derived structures rather than linear epitopes and involve residues of VP1 and VP3 that are likely to be closely positioned on the surface of the HAV particle. Analogous residues within the poliovirus capsid do not lie in close proximity to each other, as demonstrated by the atomic-level resolution structural models. This feature distinguishes HAV from prototype picornaviruses.

HAV Resistance to Physical and Chemical Agents

In common with the enteroviruses, HAV is stable at low pH (pH less than 3.0) (138). However, the thermal stability of HAV is considerably greater than that of other picornaviruses (142). Incubation of the virus for 4 weeks at room temperature results in only a 100-fold decrease in infectivity. Significant loss of infectivity starts to occur with exposure at 60°C for short periods, and infectivity is destroyed almost instantaneously by heating above 90°C (121). However, outbreaks of hepatitis A have been reported following ingestion of partially cooked shellfish, suggesting that even steaming may be insufficient to destroy the virus. In addition, HAV infectivity is highly resistant to drying, and infectious virus has been recovered from acetone-fixed cell sheets. It is also highly resistant to detergents, surviving a 1% concentration of sodium dodecyl sulfate, as well as to organic solvents like diethyl ether, chloroform, and trichlorotrifluoroethane (124, 142). Solvent-detergent inactivation procedures thus do not reduce the infectivity of HAV, explaining why hepatitis A transmission has occasionally been associated with the administration of high-purity clotting factor concentrates (93). These properties of the virus are likely to contribute significantly to its ability to be spread through the environment and to cause common-source outbreaks of hepatitis.

HAV can be reliably inactivated by autoclaving (121°C for 30 min) and exposure to hypochlorite (chlorine bleach) in concentrations of 1.5 to 2.5 mg/liter for 15 min (124). Although chlorine is most commonly used to avoid HAV contamination in water, environmental surfaces can also be decontaminated by quaternary ammonium formulations containing 23% HCl (toilet bowl cleaner). Glutaraldehyde (2%), iodine (3 mg/liter for 5 min), and potassium permanganate (30 mg/liter for 5 min) are probably also effective. HAV is also inactivated by short incubation (5 min at 25°C) in 3% formalin or in diluted formalin for 3 days at 37°C and by UV irradiation (110).

Genome Structure

The single-stranded RNA genome of HAV (Fig. 3) does not have a cap structure at its 5′ end but, instead, has a small, covalently bound, virus-encoded protein termed VPg (3B), like other picornaviruses (168). The nucleotide sequence of the HAV genome begins at the 5′ end with two uridyl residues, typical of picornaviruses, followed by a relatively lengthy 5′ nontranslated region (5′ NTR), ~734 to 747 bases long. The 5′ NTR has a high level of secondary RNA structure comprising several complex stem-loop structures (25). The RNA secondary structure within this segment of the genome has been established by a combination of phylogenetic comparative sequence analyses, functional genetic studies, and direct biophysical and nuclease mapping techniques (25). The 5′ NTR RNA sequences contain both RNA replication elements and a highly structured RNA segment that functions as an internal ribosome entry site (IRES). The IRES determines the initiation of viral translation in a 5′-cap-independent fashion. Initiation of translation may start at either of two AUG codons at positions 735 to 737 and 741 to 743 (42), although the second of these codons is preferred (153). The AUG codon begins a single large open reading frame encoding a polyprotein of ~2,227 amino acid residues in length that is proteolytically processed into both structural (P1-2A) and nonstructural (2BC and P3) viral polypeptides (Fig. 3).

Following a translation terminator sequence, the genome ends with a 3′ NTR of 63 nucleotides that is followed by a poly(A) tail of various lengths typical of picornavirus genomes.

Structural and Replication Proteins

The primary cleavage of the polyprotein occurs between the P1-2A and 2BC-P3 segments (Fig. 3), under the direction of the only protease encoded by the virus, the 3C protein (83, 106).

The P1-2A segment comprises four structural polypeptides: 1A to 1D or, in order, VP4, VP2, VP3, and VP1, named according to their homologs in the poliovirus capsid based on relative molecular masses, with VP1 being the largest (Fig. 3). These proteins are approximately 23, 222, 246, and 273 amino acids in length, respectively (42, 74, 105). VP1 (1D), however, has a heterogeneous carboxy terminus (74), reflecting a unique maturation mechanism. While VP2 (1B), VP3 (1C), and VP1 comprise the viral capsid, VP4 (1A) is substantially smaller than its homologs in other picornaviruses and has never been experimentally determined to be part of the HAV capsid (Table 1). The 2A protein of HAV lacks homology with any other picornaviral 2A proteins and does not possess the *cis*-active protease activity found in the 2A proteins of other picornaviruses. 2A functions in viral assembly as a fusion precursor with 1D (VP1) and remains attached to some otherwise fully formed virions (4).

Nonstructural proteins derived from the 2BC-P3 segment of the polyprotein probably all contribute directly to the assembly of the membrane-bound viral replicase complex (Table 1). Proteins 2B and 2C (probably also the precursor 2BC) are involved in directing the rearrangements of cellular membranes required for replicase assembly (71, 155). The 2B protein is very hydrophobic and has been suggested to anchor the replicase complexes to altered intracellular membranes (71). 2C, on the other hand, has NTPase activity and contains a helicase sequence motif. The P3 nonstructural proteins include a putative RNA-dependent RNA polymerase (3D) and a cysteine protease (3C) which is responsible for most cleavages in the viral polyprotein (except for VP4/VP2 and VP1/2A cleavages) (2, 82a). P3 also generates protein 3B (VPg), which is attached to the 5′ end of both positive- and negative-strand RNAs, and protein 3A, which comprises a hydrophobic 21-amino-acid stretch that is believed to anchor the 3AB precursor of VPg to cellular membranes.

Biology of the Virus

Host Range

HAV infects humans and nonhuman primates. Serologic and experimental infectivity studies in nonhuman primates have revealed that HAV may infect chimpanzees and other Old World primates, like vervet, rhesus, and cynomolgus monkeys, as well as several species of New World primates, like tamarins *(Saguinus)*, marmosets *(Callithrix)*, squirrel monkeys, *(Saimiri)*, and owl monkeys *(Aotus)* (9). Chimpanzees, tamarins, and marmosets have been most extensively used as animal models of HAV infection. There are several reports of isolation of HAV-related viruses from monkeys in the wild, several of which have significant sequence variation and minor antigenic differences from human HAV (26).

Growth in Cell Culture

HAV was first isolated ex vivo in marmoset liver explant cultures and was subsequently propagated in continuous fetal rhesus monkey kidney cells (128). HAV can be propagated in a variety of mammalian cells, including cells of

TABLE 1 HAV structural and regulatory proteins

Viral protein	Function	Properties
1A (VP4)	Structural protein?	Found as VP4-VP2 precursor in immature viral particles but may be absent from mature particles
1B (VP2)	Structural protein	
1C (VP3)	Structural protein	
1D (VP1)	Structural protein	Also found as VP1-2A fusion precursor in immature particles
2A	Involved in capsid assembly	
2B	Drives cellular membrane rearrangements, allowing replicase complex assembly	Also found as a functional 2BC precursor
2C	NTPase, helicase	
3A	Membrane anchor for 3B?	
3B (VPg)	Initiation of RNA replication?	Covalently linked to the 5′ end of the genome
3C	Cysteine protease	Cleaves all protein junctions except for VP1/2A and VP4/VP2. Precursor 3ABC cleaves MAVS, an essential cellular signaling protein involved in protective cellular interferon responses
3D	RNA-dependent RNA polymerase	

primate origin like BS-C-1, FRhK-4, and MRC-5 cells (47, 63). However, wild-type viral strains collected from infected patients usually replicate very slowly and to relatively low titers in cultured cells, requiring weeks or even months to reach maximal titers. With continued in vitro passage, the virus becomes progressively adapted to growth in cell culture, replicating more rapidly and achieving higher titers (43, 47). Cells of guinea pig, porcine, or dolphin origin can also support HAV growth (55), and experimental infection in guinea pigs results in virus replication, but without any sign of clinical disease (78).

In contrast to the invariably transient nature of HAV infections in infected humans, infection of cultured cells is typically not associated with any dramatic cellular injury and commonly leads to long-term persistence of the virus in cells. These observations are consistent with the fact that HAV replication does not induce the shutdown of cellular protein or nucleic acid synthesis as observed with poliovirus. Highly adapted variants of HAV that replicate rapidly and cause cytopathic effects in cultured cells have been described (23, 92). Cellular injury appears to arise from the induction of apoptotic pathways leading to programmed cell death (23, 70). Continuous passage of the virus in cell culture frequently results in a reduction in the ability of the virus to replicate and cause disease in primates (127). Adaptive mutations that permit HAV to replicate efficiently in cell culture include those within the IRES that enhance cap-independent viral translation in a cell-type-specific fashion and within 2B that promote viral RNA replication in multiple cell types (49, 56, 73, 175).

Recently, a subpopulation of human hepatoma Huh7 cells that support efficient growth of wild-type HAV strains without requiring further genetic adaptation has been selected. These cells may prove useful to characterize wild-type HAV strains isolated from patients and environmental samples (88).

As with other positive-strand viruses, purified genomic RNA, whether extracted from virions or produced synthetically from cloned cDNA, is replication competent when transfected into permissive cultured cells (43). However, the recovery of virus from synthetic wild-type RNA is very difficult in transfected cell cultures and usually requires inoculation into the liver of susceptible primates (57). Using infectious cDNA in cell culture and findings from other picornaviruses, it has been possible to elucidate a number of features of the HAV replication strategy.

Replication Strategy (Fig. 4)

Attachment and Entry

Mature virus particles attach to cultured cells and undergo relatively slow uncoating, with release of viral RNA into the cytoplasm by about 4 h postinfection (17). A candidate cellular receptor (HAVcr1), a mucin-like glycoprotein, was first identified in cultured monkey kidney cells, and a human homolog was also shown to interact with the virus particle (58, 85). The binding of HAV to the cysteine-rich, globular C-terminal extracellular domain of HAVcr1 leads to particle alteration and uncoating (143). HAVcr1 is widely distributed in different tissues and is an important atopy susceptibility protein (TIM1) in humans within the T-cell immunoglobulin mucin (TIM) family (111). Interestingly, immunoglobulin A11 (IgA1λ) has been shown to be a specific ligand of HAVcr1/TIM1. This receptor-ligand association enhances interaction of HAV with HAVcr1/TIM1, a feature that may be important to promote in vivo infection by HAV under conditions where HAVcr1/TIM1 is present in limiting levels (151). However, the tropism of HAV for the liver cannot be determined by virus interaction with this ubiquitous molecule, and the hepatocellular asialoglycoprotein receptor may play a role in viral entry by mediating the uptake of IgA-virus complexes (54).

RNA Translation and Replication

HAV RNA translation and replication seem to take place in association with a tubular-vesicular membranous network rearranged from cytosolic membranes in HAV-infected cells (71, 155), as is the case for other picornaviruses. The uncoated RNA is translated via an IRES-dependent mechanism that uniquely requires intact cellular initiation factor eIF4G to function, unlike other picornavirus IRESs, which utilize a cleavage fragment of this factor (21). The HAV IRES appears to be highly stimulated by several cellular proteins, including polypyrimidine tract-binding protein (70). Within the membrane-bound replicase complex (71), the virion RNA serves as a template for negative-strand RNA synthesis by the RNA-dependent RNA polymerase 3D. This negative-strand intermediate then acts as a template for the synthesis of several positive-strand RNA molecules, which can be translated into proteins, replicated, or packaged into new virions. In poliovirus, 3B (VPg), the small genome-linked protein, functions as a protein primer for viral RNA synthesis in these reactions, which are templated by an internal *cis*-acting RNA element *(cre)*, forming a stem-loop structure (123). Similar RNA structures have further been identified in the genomes of other picornaviruses but have yet to be recognized in HAV.

Like for many other RNA viruses, HAV RNA replication generates double-stranded RNA molecules that trigger the cellular antiviral interferon responses. HAV has evolved a strategy to counteract these protective host innate immune responses (60). The 3ABC polypeptide, a stable and proteolytically active 3C protease precursor, is able to cleave the adaptor molecule (MAVS) of the RIG-I-mediated signaling pathway, thus inactivating this interferon signaling pathway (173).

Particle Assembly and Release

The mechanisms of HAV particle assembly appear to differ significantly from those of other picornaviruses. The presence of the N-terminal part of nonstructural protein 2A as a C-terminal extension of P1 appears to be essential for proper folding of the capsid protein precursor P1-2A, required for efficient 3C-mediated processing and assembly of pentamers containing five copies each of the VP4-VP2, VP3, and VP1-2A polypeptides (45, 126). These pentamers subsequently assemble into complete capsids, after which cleavage at the VP1-2A junction releases the mature VP1 protein. This cleavage appears to be mediated by a cellular rather than viral protease, resulting in a heterogeneous VP1 C terminus (74, 105). The VP4 proteins of other picornaviruses are considerably larger than the VP4 sequence encoded by the HAV genome. They also are myristylated at their N termini, a feature that plays an essential role in the capsid assembly process during replication of these viruses (38). The VP4 molecule of HAV is not myristylated, despite the presence of an internal consensus myristylation signal (154). The VP4 polypeptide is incorporated into nascent particles in the form of a VP4-VP2 precursor, VP0 (1AB), which is cleaved into its two con-

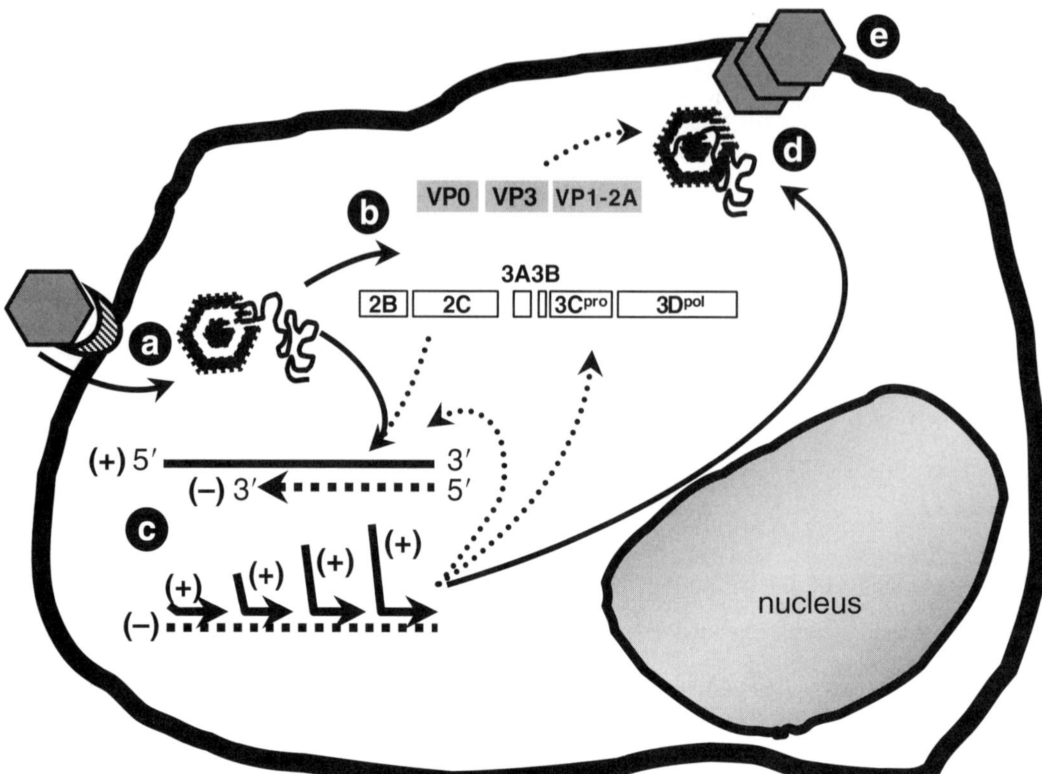

FIGURE 4 HAV replication cycle. (a) The viral particle interacts with a cellular receptor (possibly HAVcr1/TIM1) at the hepatocyte surface and is internalized, and the viral genome is uncoated; (b) the positive-strand RNA genome released in the cell cytoplasm is translated through an IRES-dependent mechanism. The resulting polyprotein is proteolytically processed to generate nonstructural proteins involved in genome replication (2B, 2C, 3AB, and $3D^{pol}$) and the protease ($3C^{pro}$), as well as capsid proteins. Translation is likely to occur in close proximity to the membranous web induced by 2BC proteins, where RNA replication takes place. (c) Nonstructural proteins assemble into a membrane-bound replicase complex that initiates the synthesis of a minus-strand RNA intermediate, which is then used as a template to generate multiple copies of positive-strand RNA by $3D^{pol}$. These newly synthesized RNAs can be reengaged into either translation or replication processes or (d) encapsidated to generate viral progeny. (e) Newly assembled particles are released from the infected cells by an as-yet-unidentified mechanism.

stituent polypeptides following assembly of the virus particle and packaging of the viral RNA, by an as-yet-undetermined mechanism. Although a large proportion of the newly synthesized particles remain cell associated, there is extensive release of progeny virus into cell culture supernatant fluids by an as-yet-unknown mechanism. In polarized human colonic epithelial cell (Caco-2) cultures, virus is released almost exclusively into apical supernatant fluids, mimicking the secretion of HAV across the apical canalicular membrane of the hepatocyte into the biliary system (18). Interestingly, this process is largely blocked by an inhibitor of the cellular secretory pathway (brefeldin A), suggesting that virus release may involve vectorial cellular vesicular transport mechanisms.

EPIDEMIOLOGY

Distribution and Geography

HAV is a common cause of hepatitis worldwide and is a classic example of an infectious disease for which the degree of endemicity is clearly attributable to the level of economic development and associated living conditions. Worldwide, three principal patterns of HAV infection can be described based on age-specific prevalence of antibodies to HAV (anti-HAV) (Fig. 5). In areas of high endemicity in Asia, Africa, Latin America, and the Middle East, the prevalence of anti-HAV reaches 90% in adults, and most children have been infected by 10 years of age. In areas of intermediate endemicity in some countries in Asia and Europe, only 50 to 60% of adults and 20 to 30% of 10-year-old children have been infected. In areas of low endemicity like North America and northern Europe, only 30% of adults have anti-HAV (11).

In addition to the three classic patterns, a fourth major pattern of worldwide HAV infection has recently been defined. Because the level of hepatitis A endemicity is closely related to the level of development, like improvements in sanitation and access to clean water, overall improvement in socioeconomic status results in an epidemiological shift manifested by a decline in the age-specific prevalence of immunity to HAV and an increase in the number of

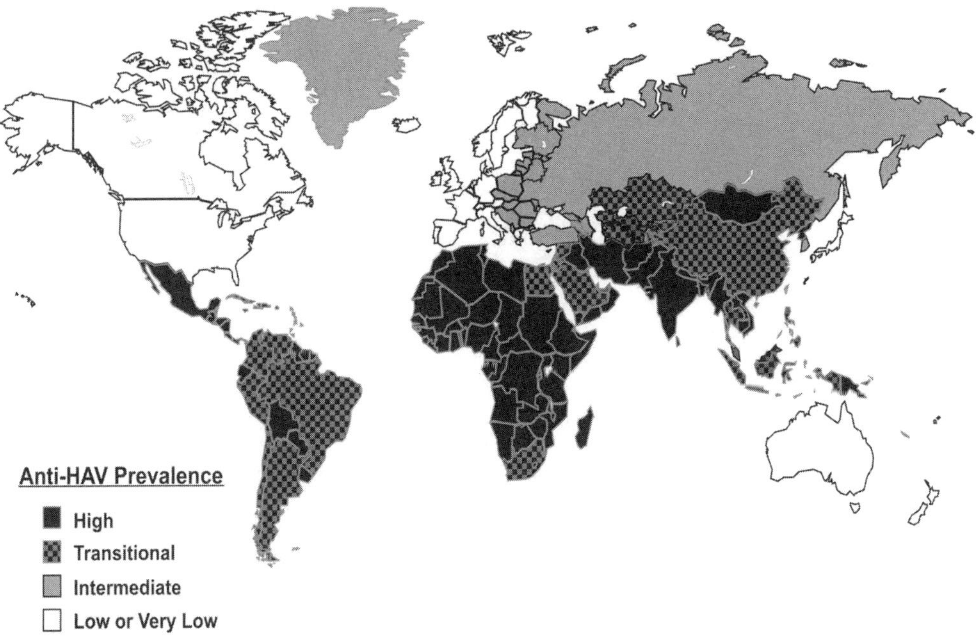

FIGURE 5 World map indicating patterns of endemicity of HAV infection (generalized from available data). (Source: CDC.)

susceptible older children, adolescents, and adults (11). Regions of transitional endemicity include China and countries in South America, central and Southeast Asia, and the Middle East.

The transition from high to intermediate endemicity can be expected to result in disease patterns characterized by increased morbidity, as cohorts of susceptible older children, adolescents, and adults become infected, and by a potential for outbreaks, as the susceptible population grows but relatively high levels of circulating virus persist. The most spectacular of these occurred in Shanghai, China, in 1988, in which the outbreak, caused by the ingestion of raw clams contaminated with HAV, resulted in nearly 300,000 cases (174). More recently, large outbreaks occurred in central Asia in 1995 to 1997, with peak incidence rates of more than 1,000 per 100,000 (11).

Incidence and Prevalence of Infection in the United States

Prevaccine Era

Before licensure of an effective vaccine in 1995, hepatitis A incidence in the United States was primarily cyclical, with peaks occurring every 10 to 15 years. During the 1980s and 1990s, an average of 26,000 hepatitis A cases was reported annually to public health agencies. The outcome of one incidence model, however, predicted an average of 271,000 infections per year between 1980 and 1999, thereby suggesting that only 1 in 10 cases of acute hepatitis A was reported. More than one-half of these infections, according to the model, occurred in children less than the age of 10 years and would have been clinically unrecognizable as hepatitis (6).

During the prevaccine era, approximately one-third of reported cases occurred among children aged less than 15 years, with the overall highest incidence involving children aged 5 to 14 years (35). In this period before hepatitis A vaccination, age, ethnicity, and birthplace were the most important determinants of HAV infection in the United States. Large serosurveys conducted from 1988 to 1994 found that the overall prevalence of anti-HAV was 31.3% and increased markedly with age, ranging from 9.4% among persons aged 6 to 11 years to 74.6% among persons ≥70 years of age. The age-adjusted prevalence was significantly higher among foreign-born than among U.S.-born participants and was highest among Mexican-Americans and lowest among non-Hispanic whites. In multivariate analysis, only Mexican-American ethnicity and income below the poverty level were associated with HAV infection among U.S.-born children (12).

Vaccine Era

The marked effectiveness of universal early childhood vaccination has been described in settings where the prevaccine-era hepatitis A incidence was moderately high. Since the licensure of hepatitis A vaccine and the implementation of a national childhood immunization strategy, hepatitis A rates in the United States have fallen dramatically (Fig. 6 to 8). Historically, however, epidemics of hepatitis A have occurred in the United States every 6 to 18 years, followed by declines in incidence. The most recent nationwide epidemic of hepatitis A occurred between 1994 and 1996, a period that preceded the Advisory Committee on Immunization Practices (ACIP) recommendations of 1996 and 1999 (see below). Because of the natural cyclic variation in hepatitis A incidence, it was problematic to discern to what degree the decline in incidence was attributable—if any—to vaccination. Allowing for herd immunity, one mathematical model estimated that 98,000 hepatitis A cases were prevented due to vaccination during 1995 through 2001; assuming no herd immunity, an estimated 32,000 cases were prevented (136). An estimated 50% of hepatitis A cases were averted by vaccination among children 2 to 18 years old despite low

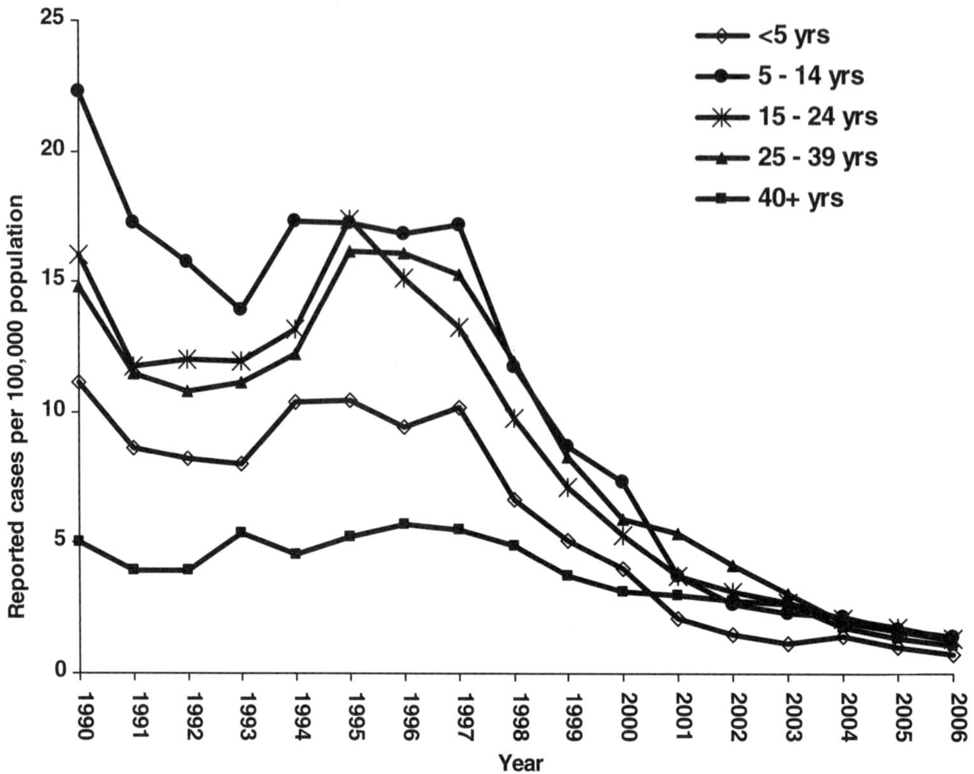

FIGURE 6 Rate of reported hepatitis A, by age group and year, United States, 1990 to 2006. (Source: National Notifiable Disease Surveillance System.)

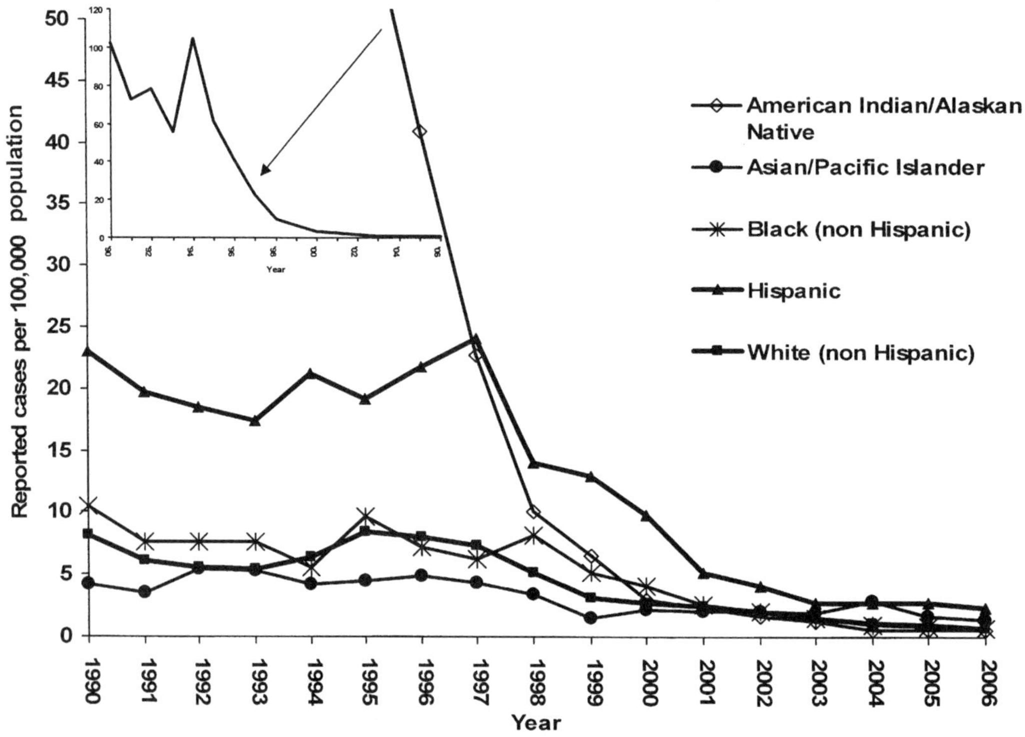

FIGURE 7 Rate of reported hepatitis A, by race/ethnicity, United States, 1990 to 2006. (Source: National Notifiable Disease Surveillance System.)

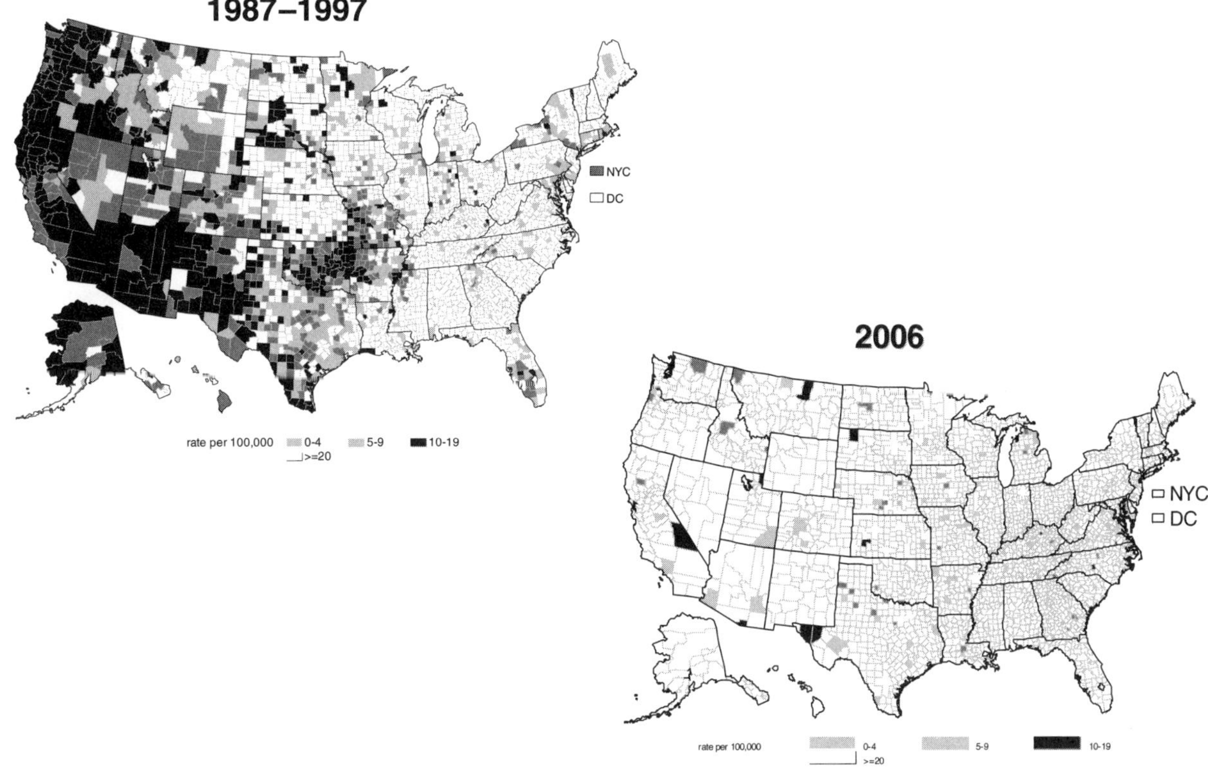

FIGURE 8 Rate of hepatitis A by county, United States, 1987 to 1997 and 2006. (Source: National Notifiable Disease Surveillance System.)

vaccination coverage (10%), demonstrating the strong effect of herd immunity. Another mathematical model predicted that nationwide routine hepatitis A vaccination at 1 year of age with 70% coverage would prevent 60% of additional cases during the period from 1995 to 2029, compared with the regional strategy recommended by ACIP in 1999, further highlighting the importance of herd immunity induced by early childhood vaccination (161).

Between the period from 1990 to 1997 and 2003, the hepatitis A rate in vaccinating states declined 88%, compared with 53% elsewhere, and whereas vaccinating states accounted for 65% of cases from 1990 to 1997, they accounted for 33% of cases in 2003 (166) (Fig. 8). In 2005, the incidence of reported hepatitis A in the United States was 1.5 per 100,000 population, an 88% decline from 1995 and the lowest rate ever recorded (35). In 2005, hepatitis A rates in the United States were highest among men aged 20 to 24 years (2.2 per 100,000 population), and the most predominant risk characteristic was international travel (15% of cases).

Concurrent with the overall decline in hepatitis A incidence in the United States in the vaccine era has been the narrowing of historic differences in rates among racial/ethnic populations and geographic locations (Fig. 7). Among Native Americans and Alaska Natives, rates indicate a 99% decline compared with the prevaccine era and are now approximately the same as or less than those of other racial/ethnic populations (15). Rates among Hispanic-Americans have fallen almost 90% during the same period, although they remain higher than those for non-Hispanics (35).

Transmission and Risk Factors

The most important means of transmission is undoubtedly from person to person via the fecal-oral route. During the prevaccine era, nearly one-half of hepatitis A cases in the United States involved no identifiable source of infection (13). Of those cases with an identifiable source, the majority resulted from person-to-person spread of HAV during community-wide outbreaks (13). Cyclic outbreaks, however, occurred among users of illicit drugs and among men who had sex with other men (MSM) (28). Overall, these data suggested that nationwide reductions in incidence were more likely to result from routine childhood vaccination than from targeted vaccination of high-risk groups, because children often have unrecognized or asymptomatic infection and play a major role in perpetuating HAV transmission during outbreaks.

In 2005, the most frequently identified risk factor for hepatitis A was international travel (15% of cases overall and 25% of cases among children aged <15 years). Most travel-related cases involved travel to Mexico and Central or South America (81%). Sexual contact and household contact with another person with hepatitis A have traditionally been among the most frequently identified risk factors, but in 2005 these were reported for only 12% of cases. In 2005, MSM accounted for 3% of all reported cases (5% of cases that occurred among males). From 1997 to 2004, the proportion of persons who reported injection of street drugs ranged from 6 to 10%; in 2005, the proportion reported was 5% (35).

Groups at Increased Risk for Hepatitis A

Travelers

Hepatitis A remains one of the most common vaccine-preventable diseases acquired during international travel. Persons from developed (low-endemicity) countries who travel to developing (medium- or high-endemicity) countries are at significant risk for acquiring hepatitis A (150) (Fig. 5). The risk will be higher among travelers visiting areas with poor sanitation and limited access to clean water, although it occurs in travelers who report observing strict protective measures and stay in more developed cities or upscale hotels (CDC, unpublished data, 2005). Hepatitis A among Hispanic children who live along the United States-Mexico border has been associated with cross-border travel to Mexico and food-borne exposures during travel (167).

MSM

Numerous outbreaks of hepatitis A have been reported among MSM in the United States, Canada, Europe, and Australia, sometimes occurring in the setting of a larger community-wide outbreak (13, 28, 114, 164). However, surveys of anti-HAV prevalence among MSM have not consistently demonstrated a greater propensity for infection compared with a similarly aged population, nor have specific sex practices been consistently identified (164).

Users of Illicit Drugs

Outbreaks among drug users, injecting and noninjecting, have been reported frequently in the United States and other developed countries since the 1980s (13). In the United States, many outbreaks have involved the use of methamphetamine, where case control studies have identified both percutaneous and fecal-oral transmission (81). Injection drug users appear to have a higher prevalence of anti-HAV than does the general U.S. population (164).

Persons with Clotting Factor Disorders

Because of its structure, HAV is resistant to solvent-detergent treatment used to inactivate enveloped viruses in plasma derivatives. Before improvements in viral inactivation procedures, widespread hepatitis A vaccination coverage, and improved donor screening methods, rare outbreaks of hepatitis A among persons with clotting factor disorders and hemophilia were reported in Europe and the United States (102, 145). However, an analysis of 140 hemophilia treatment centers from 1998 to 2002 identified no cases of hepatitis A attributed to administration of blood products (32).

Risk of Hepatitis A in Particular Settings

Food Service Establishments

Food-borne hepatitis A outbreaks are recognized relatively infrequently in the United States. Annually, only 2 to 3% of cases are identified through routine surveillance report association with common-source outbreaks of disease transmitted by food or water. Some hepatitis A transmission attributed to personal contact or another risk factor, however, is likely to have been food borne (61). The proportion of sporadic cases that might be from food sources is unknown but could be considerable, as approximately 50% of reported cases of hepatitis A still do not have an identified source of infection. HAV contamination of food can occur at any point during cultivation, harvesting, processing, distribution, or preparation. Recognizing food-borne outbreaks using routine surveillance may be difficult because (i) of problems of recall of food consumption, (ii) of gradual accrual of cases, (iii) of focal contamination, (iv) of unrecognized HAV infection, (v) of preexisting immunity, and (vi) cases may be geographically scattered after food consumption (61).

A single HAV-infected food handler can transmit HAV to dozens or even hundreds of persons. Common themes of large food-borne outbreaks have included (i) an HAV-infected food handler who worked while potentially infectious (2 weeks before to 1 week after symptom onset) and had contact with uncooked food or food after it had been cooked, (ii) secondary cases among other food handlers who ate food contaminated by the person with the index case, and (iii) relatively low attack rates among patrons (61). However, food handlers are not at a higher risk of hepatitis A because of their occupation, and most food handlers do not transmit HAV to consumers or restaurant patrons.

Molecular epidemiological techniques comparing RNA sequences of HAV allow for identification of previously unrecognized links between cases. In an outbreak in 1997, schoolchildren in Maine and Michigan with hepatitis A were linked with others in Wisconsin, Arizona, and Louisiana who had eaten strawberries from the same vendor; all outbreak cases shared identical viral sequences, and these were different from viral sequences obtained from non-outbreak-related cases (80). More recently, this approach confirmed the presence of an identical hepatitis A sequence obtained from both the implicated food product and 39 case patients infected by consumption of oysters (14).

Child Care Centers

The frequency of outbreaks among children attending day care centers and persons employed at these centers has decreased substantially as overall hepatitis A incidence among children has declined over the last decade (27). Because infection among children is typically mild or asymptomatic, outbreaks are often not identified until adult contacts become ill (76).

Health Care Institutions

Nosocomial transmission of HAV is rare, and persons with typical cases of hepatitis A are not routinely admitted to hospitals. In the past, outbreaks have occurred from adult patients because of fecal incontinence, but because most patients are hospitalized after the onset of jaundice, the period of peak infectivity has passed, and therefore, the probability of transmission is low (69). Rarely, outbreaks have been described to occur in neonatal intensive care units as the result of infants acquiring infection from blood products and subsequently transmitting hepatitis A to staff and other infants (118, 134).

Schools

In the United States, the appearance of cases of hepatitis A in schools is ordinarily a reflection of disease acquisition and transmission in the community. Secondary transmission to other students is uncommon; however, if multiple cases occur among students, a common source of infection is possible and should be investigated (34).

Workers Exposed to Sewage

No work-related instances of HAV transmission have been reported among wastewater workers in the United States, and serologic surveys have shown no substantial or consistent increase in the prevalence of anti-HAV among wastewater workers (157). Surveys performed in other countries indicate a possible elevated risk for HAV infection among workers exposed to sewage; however, these analyses did not control for other factors, like socioeconomic status (99).

PATHOGENESIS

As mentioned above, while HAV shares many virologic characteristics with enteroviruses, it has several unique in vitro properties that are probably reflected in the replication and pathogenic characteristics of HAV in the natural host.

Incubation Period

The incubation period for HAV infection ranges from 2 to 7 weeks, with a mean duration of about 28 days (90, 174). In experimentally infected tamarins, the duration of the incubation period (as measured to the onset of elevated liver enzymes) is inversely correlated to the inoculum dose, increasing approximately 5 days for each $\log_{10}$ reduction in dose of the inoculum (Fig. 9) (129). Clinically, the onset of symptoms may be abrupt, but early symptoms of hepatitis are often vague and nonspecific. Therefore, jaundice, usually first recognized by the patient as the appearance of dark urine, is more typically identified as the point of onset that defines the incubation period. The mean incubation period has been reported to be shorter in persons parenterally infected from contaminated blood products.

Viral Replication

Because the virus is acid resistant, it can survive passage through the stomach and may replicate initially somewhere lower in the intestine. Evidence of viral replication in humans in tissues other than the liver is sparse. Nevertheless, some cells of the gastrointestinal tract are probably susceptible to HAV, since the fecal-oral route is the most important mode of transmission. HAV has been identified by immunofluorescence in the epithelial cells of the intestinal crypts of both the jejunum and ileum of experimentally infected monkeys (7). Evidence of replication in the oropharynx has been obtained in orally inoculated chimpanzees, and this could also be an initial site of entry (41). While there may be extrahepatic sites of replication of HAV, the major recognized pathology is restricted to the liver. HAV, like many other picornaviruses, is very organ specific, perhaps because of specific hepatocyte receptors or intracellular replication factors. Virus is shed from infected liver cells into the bile canaliculi and passes into the intestine, after which it is excreted in the feces.

In infected persons, HAV replicates in the liver, is excreted in bile, and is shed in stool. Peak infectivity of infected persons occurs during the 2-week period before onset of jaundice or elevation of liver enzymes, when the concentration of virus in stool is highest (152) (Fig. 10). The concentration of virus in stool declines after jaundice appears. Children can shed HAV for longer periods than do adults, up to 10 weeks after onset of clinical illness; infants infected as neonates in one nosocomial outbreak shed HAV for up to 6 months (132, 134). Chronic shedding of HAV in feces does not occur; however, recurrent shedding occurs during relapses among persons who have relapsing illness (144). Viremia occurs soon after infection and persists through the period of liver enzyme elevation, but at concentrations several orders of magnitude lower than in stool (22, 97).

Because viremia occurs early, before the appearance of symptoms, blood-related transmission is possible. In addition, HAV is not inactivated by many of the techniques used to remove viruses from plasma products, like the solvent-detergent system. Cases of transfusion-associated hepatitis A and one outbreak of disease associated with factor VIII concentrate have been recognized (102). The disease following intravenous transmission appears to be no different than orally acquired infections.

Liver biopsy samples are generally not obtained for acute hepatitis. However, when biopsies have been performed, the morphological changes observed are similar to

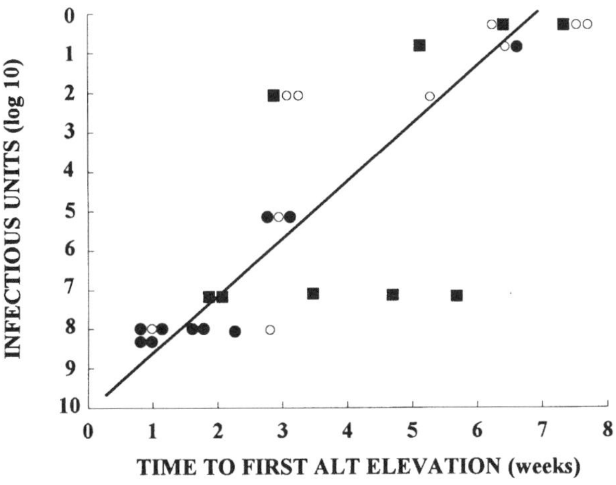

FIGURE 9 Experimental inoculation of marmosets (closed markers) and chimpanzees (open markers) with two strains of HAV, HM175 (circles) and MS-1 (squares), showing the inverse relationship between dose and incubation period. (From reference 129 with permission.)

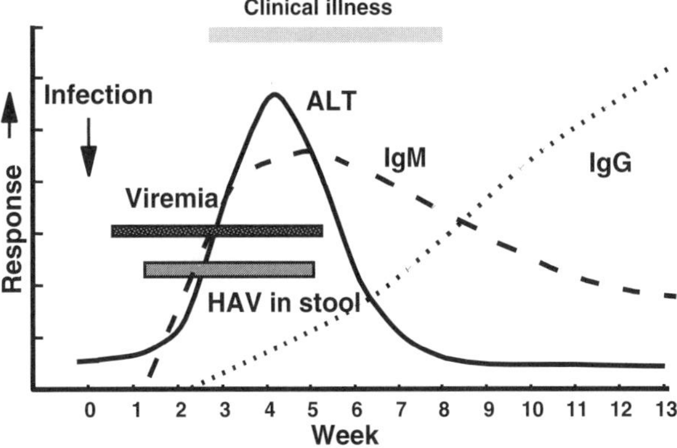

FIGURE 10 Clinical, virologic, and serologic events after HAV infection. (Source: http://www.cdc.gov/ncidod/diseases/hepatitis/slideset/hep_a/slide_1.htm.)

those seen in other forms of acute hepatitis (120). Hepatocytes are generally swollen and have distinct plasma membranes, enlarged nuclei, and ballooning degeneration. Cells might become shriveled and eosinophilic, and there is a diffuse accumulation of mononuclear cells throughout the lobules. The portal tracts are enlarged by edema and inflammatory cells (Fig. 11). In general, regeneration occurs rapidly and the liver returns to normal within 8 to 12 weeks. HAV antigen and HAV particles can be detected in the cytoplasm of infected cells by immunofluorescence, immunoperoxidase staining, or thin-section electron microscopy (Fig. 12) (109, 139).

Virus replication precedes the appearance of clinical and laboratory evidence of hepatitis by at least 2 weeks. HAV is not thought to be directly cytopathic, and the histopathology does not suggest widespread necrosis or apoptosis of hepatocytes. The presence of large quantities of virus in hepatocytes before the onset of hepatitis also argues against a major direct cytopathic effect of HAV. Clinical hepatitis coincides with the appearance of cellular and humoral immune responses, and the pathology of HAV infection appears to be largely the result of cell-mediated immune responses to the infection (159).

In tamarins inoculated with a large dose of HAV intravenously, HAV antigen in hepatocytes and mildly abnormal liver function were detectable within 1 week, possibly suggesting that there is a small, direct pathological effect of the replicating virus. After the initial mild elevation, liver enzyme levels stabilized or even declined until the third week after inoculation, when a second, higher peak was observed coincident with the appearance of serum antibodies and histopathological changes in the liver, suggesting an immunologic origin for the acute hepatitis (Fig. 13). Human studies revealed that lymphocytes recovered from the livers of patients with acute hepatitis A contained HAV-specific $CD8^+$ cytotoxic T cells, while during convalescence, there were more $CD4^+$ T cells, consistent with the hypothesis that $CD8^+$ T lymphocytes mediate liver cell damage (64). Furthermore, natural killer cells have been demonstrated to be capable of lysing HAV-infected tissue culture cells (8). Although liver damage occurs at the time that circulating antibodies become detectable, antibody-dependent cytotoxicity has not been demonstrated in

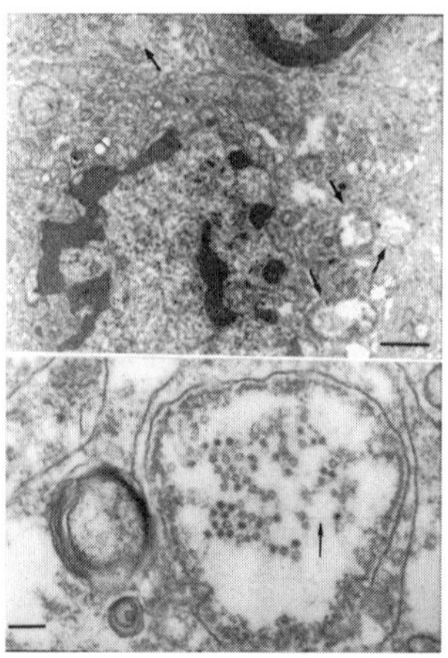

FIGURE 12 Electron micrographs of a marmoset hepatocyte during acute hepatitis A. The arrows in the upper panel point to cytoplasmic vesicles containing HAV. The lower panel is a higher-power view of one of the vesicles clearly showing the HAV particles. Bars, 500 nm in the upper panel and 100 nm in the lower. (Reprinted from reference 139 with permission.)

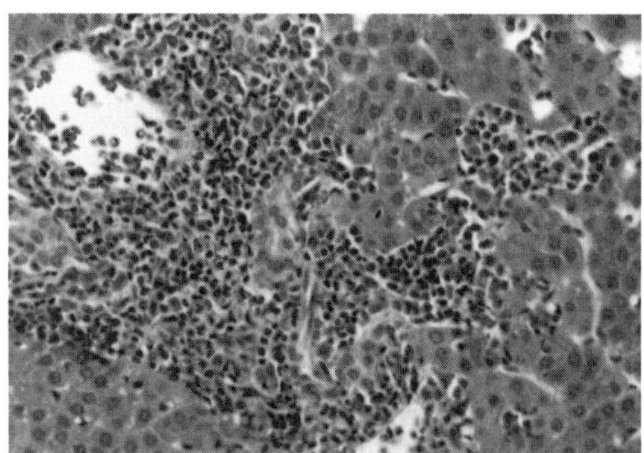

FIGURE 11 Photomicrograph of a liver biopsy sample taken from an aotus monkey during acute hepatitis A. There is a portal tract infiltration of mononuclear cell, primarily lymphocytes. Some of the inflammatory cells disrupt the limiting plate and extend into the lobule. Magnification, ×193. (Courtesy of Ludmila Asher, Walter Reed Army Institute of Research.)

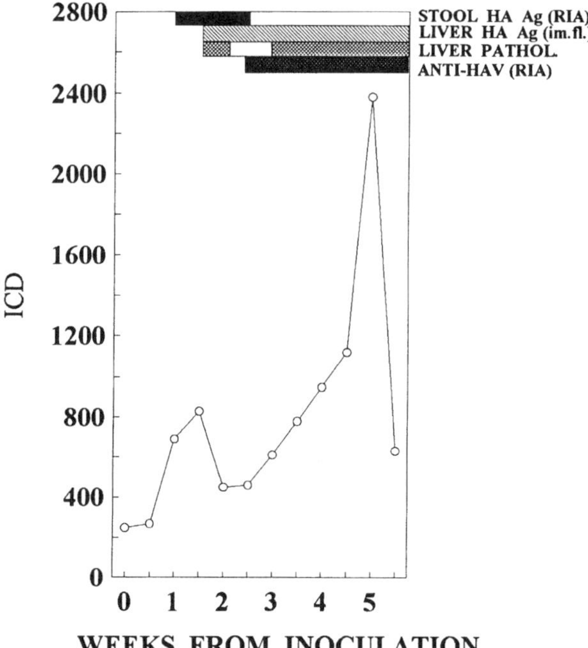

FIGURE 13 Biphasic enzyme elevation in a tamarin inoculated with 10^8 infectious units of HAV. There is mild pathology at the time of the first enzyme elevation. The second enzyme elevation begins at about the time of the appearance of serum antibody, and the liver pathology (PATHOL.) is more pronounced than during the first elevation. ICD, isocitric dehydrogenase; HA Ag, HAV antigen (measured by radioimmunoassay [RIA]); im.fl., immunofluorescence.

hepatitis A (65). While circulating immune complexes containing HAV and HAV-specific antibodies (primarily IgM) have been found during infection, immunoglobulin and complement deposits were not found at the sites of liver cell damage, and resolution of disease occurred at a time when antibody levels were rising and HAV antigen could still be easily detected in the liver (104).

Immunity

As second infections with HAV are unknown, immunity to HAV persists for life following natural infection. In some areas of endemicity where exposure to the virus is common, the mean antibody levels in the population decline in older age groups, suggesting that reexposure to HAV does not result in reinfection and boosting of the immune response.

The antibody response following HAV infection is vigorous and long lasting. Passive immunization with immune globulin (IG) resulting in relatively low levels of circulating antibody can provide complete protection against infection, indicating that serum antibody alone is sufficient to prevent infection. It has been difficult to judge the effect of mucosal immunity because antibodies in saliva or feces either are not detected or are present at very low levels (148). T-cell responses to HAV infections may be important for recovery and pathogenesis (see above). However, the role of cell-mediated immunity in protection is not known.

HAVcr1/TIM1 has been identified as a functional receptor for HAV. Members of the TIM gene family encode cell surface receptors that are important in T-cell regulation. TIM1 stimulates T-cell expansion and cytokine production and is associated with atopic disease. An inverse relationship between asthma and childhood exposure to HAV has been suggested (111). One hypothesis is that activation of T cells through TIM1 by HAV or by its natural ligand may affect T-cell differentiation and the development of Th2-driven allergic inflammatory responses, such that the reductions in childhood HAV infections may be associated with the observed increasing incidence of atopic diseases (111). However, other epidemiological studies have failed to confirm this finding. The presence of HAV antibodies may simply be an indicator of exposure to a number of infectious agents that may relate to a reduced risk of atopic disease.

CLINICAL FEATURES

Hepatitis A is an acute infection of the liver which may result in an icteric or anicteric clinical illness. The likelihood of having symptoms with HAV infection is related to age. In children aged <6 years, 70% of infections are asymptomatic. If illness does occur, it is typically not accompanied by jaundice (76). Among older children and adults, infection typically is symptomatic, with jaundice occurring in >70% of patients (91). The ratio of anicteric to icteric cases has been reported to vary from 12:1 to 1:3.5 in different outbreaks and largely depends on the age of the patients (91).

Mortality

The overall case fatality ratio among cases reported through the National Notifiable Diseases Surveillance System is approximately 0.3 to 0.6% but reaches 1.8% among adults aged >50 years. Host factors reportedly associated with an increased risk of fulminant hepatitis include old age and underlying chronic liver disease (1, 10, 97). In the 1988 Shanghai epidemic, which primarily involved adolescents and young adults, there were 47 deaths (0.015%) recorded among 310,746 cases (174). Of the 47 deaths, 25 were due to fulminant hepatitis, 15 were associated with underlying liver disease, and 7 were not directly hepatitis related (174).

Clinical Course (Fig. 10)

Infection with HAV, as evidenced by detection of anti-HAV IgM in serum, may produce a wide spectrum of outcomes ranging from inapparent (asymptomatic, without elevation of serum aminotransferase levels) to subclinical (asymptomatic, with elevation of serum aminotransferase levels) to clinically evident (with symptoms).

The clinical symptoms of acute hepatitis A are indistinguishable from those caused by other forms of hepatitis. The onset of the prodromal period, particularly in older children and adults, can be quite abrupt and is characterized by increasing fatigue, malaise, anorexia, fever, myalgias, abdominal pain, nausea, and vomiting. Younger children may have diarrhea or, less commonly, respiratory symptoms. If present, typical symptoms of hepatitis, beginning with darkening of the urine and followed by jaundice and pale or clay-colored stools, will appear after a period of several days to a week.

In the largest recorded series, the Shanghai epidemic, the prodromal symptoms included anorexia (82%), malaise (80%), fever (76%), nausea (69%), and vomiting (47%) among hospitalized patients; 91% had elevated bilirubin levels and 84% were overtly jaundiced (174). Itching, often a sign of cholestasis, occurs in less than 5% of symptomatic patients but may be severe enough to require antipruritics and corticosteroid therapy. In addition to jaundice and scleral icterus, physical findings may include hepatomegaly and tenderness. During the Shanghai outbreak, hepatomegaly was observed in 87% of the hospitalized patients and splenomegaly was found in 9%. Skin rashes were rarely seen (174). Spider nevi may appear on the trunk and usually disappear during convalescence. The return of color to the stools occurs within 2 or 3 weeks after the onset of illness and is a good sign of resolution of the disease.

Liver function tests, especially levels of alanine aminotransferase (ALT) and aspartate aminotransferase (AST) in serum, are sensitive, but they are nonspecific measures of parenchymal liver damage. ALT elevations, usually more than AST, may be found even during the prodromal stage. During icteric infections, the serum ALT levels, which are usually less than 2,000 IU/liter, may exceed 20,000 IU/liter. While high ALT levels occur in patients with severe hepatitis, the elevation of ALT is not necessarily correlated with the severity of the illness. Alkaline phosphatase levels are usually only mildly elevated in hepatitis A except when the illness is complicated by cholestasis. Biochemical abnormalities may persist for 2 to 3 weeks in children and, rarely, longer than 4 weeks in young adults (53).

The duration of illness varies. In many patients the appearance of jaundice is associated with a rapid resolution of the prodromal symptoms of nausea and fever. After 3 to 4 weeks, most patients feel better, have lost their hepatomegaly, and have normal or near-normal levels of ALT and bilirubin in serum. Prolonged jaundice or a relapsing pattern may also occur, but ultimate resolution in these cases is universal. Infection with HAV does not become chronic. Hepatitis A is not more severe in pregnant women. It is not passed to the fetus, nor is there an effect on fetal health or survival (176).

Complications

Prolonged jaundice in hepatitis A, often associated with fever and pruritus, is an indication of cholestatic hepatitis. Peak serum bilirubin levels may reach 12 to 29 mg/dl, and jaundice may continue for up to 18 weeks. In such cases, peak ALT levels are below 500 IU/liter during the icteric phase but alkaline phosphatase levels are elevated (137). Liver biopsies reveal centrilobular cholestasis and portal inflammation.

Relapsing disease has been reported to occur in some patients with hepatitis A (40, 144). One study reported that 12.5% of 297 adult patients had polyphasic courses and one-fifth had more than one relapse. HAV can be found in the stools of some patients during relapse. While the mechanism of relapse has not been elucidated, it is important to recognize that all reported cases resolved without any chronic sequelae (144).

Other atypical clinical features and complications, including immunologic, neurologic, hematologic, and renal extrahepatic manifestations, are rare (137). Although these are possibly manifestations of immune complex disease, the relationship of these syndromes to HAV infection is not established.

Fulminant hepatitis, characterized by rapid onset of liver failure and coma, is rarely associated with HAV infection. The initial clinical presentation in fulminant HAV infection is not significantly different from other cases of symptomatic acute HAV infection (67). However, encephalopathy and coagulopathy generally begin within 1 to 2 weeks after onset of symptoms, although death has been reported as early as 3 days after the onset of jaundice. Fulminant disease is more common in older age groups, and recovery from severe disease is less common in patients over 50 years of age. Serious and even fatal hepatitis A does occur in children (50). Severe disease also occurs more commonly in patients with underlying chronic liver disease, especially chronic hepatitis B or hepatitis C (67). Laboratory (decrease in clotting factors) and clinical (deepening coma) evidence of deteriorating liver function correlates with a histologic picture of virtually complete destruction of the hepatic parenchyma, with only a reticulin framework and portal tracts remaining. Occasionally, small groups of surviving hepatocytes can be seen close to portal tracts, which may be evidence of regeneration. Paradoxically, there may be limited or no evidence of an inflammatory response (108). Rates of spontaneous recovery from fulminant hepatitis A range between 30 and 60%, and survivors regain complete liver function. Prognosis is influenced by age, clotting factor levels, stage of coma, and presence of kidney disease. Recovery from fulminant hepatitis is difficult to predict, and the only effective treatment at this time is liver transplantation. Therefore, the decision on when to transplant requires careful consideration of all the clinical information.

LABORATORY DIAGNOSIS

The diagnosis of acute hepatitis A is most commonly confirmed by detection of specific antibody to HAV of the IgM class (primarily antibodies against capsid antigens), which indicates current or recent infection (Fig. 10). A number of methods have been used to detect IgM anti-HAV, including radioimmunoassay, immunochemical staining, enzyme-linked immunosorbent assay, immunoblotting, and dot blot immunogold filtration. IgM anti-HAV enzyme immunoassays are available commercially. Although the commercial assays are reportedly configured not to detect the low levels of IgM that may persist in patients more than 6 months after acute HAV infection, these assays may detect IgM anti-HAV in persons recently administered hepatitis A vaccine (171).

Persons who are unlikely to have acute viral hepatitis should not be tested for IgM anti-HAV, and the use of IgM anti-HAV as a screening tool or as part of testing panels used in the workup of nonacute liver function abnormalities should be discouraged. Testing of persons with no clinical symptoms of acute viral hepatitis, and among populations with a low prevalence of acute HAV infection, lowers the predictive value of the IgM anti-HAV test. Use of diagnostic tests for viral hepatitis among persons without symptoms of hepatitis A can lead to IgM anti-HAV test results that are falsely positive for acute HAV infection or of no clinical importance. This might be occurring with use of laboratory test panels that include routine testing for IgM anti-HAV without requiring a specific order for the test (i.e., "reflex testing" or use of a "hepatitis panel") among persons who are not being evaluated for possible acute hepatitis (e.g., persons with liver function test abnormalities or persons being screened for hepatitis C) (33).

Detection of IgG anti-HAV in the absence of IgM indicates previous or resolved HAV infection. Commercially available assays, however, detect total anti-HAV (both IgG and IgM antibodies). Still, the presence of total anti-HAV and the absence of IgM anti-HAV can be used to differentiate past and current infections.

Conversely, the absence of anti-HAV in a sample collected during the acute phase of illness or early convalescence is strong evidence against a diagnosis of HAV infection. If the clinical or epidemiological situation strongly suggests HAV infection and the patient has a negative serologic test, it may be worthwhile to repeat the test a few days to a week or more after the initial test.

Liver biopsy is rarely indicated to establish a diagnosis of acute hepatitis. This procedure is associated with discomfort to the patient and a small but finite risk, and the tissue morphology is usually not diagnostic.

Detection of virus or viral antigen in the stools of patients is a useful research tool but has no place in routine clinical diagnosis. Since HAV clinical isolates usually replicate very slowly and to very low titers in cell culture, virus isolation is insensitive, unreliable, and expensive, so it is not used for diagnosis or environmental studies.

Nucleic acid detection techniques are more sensitive than immunoassays for viral antigen to detect HAV in samples of different origins (e.g., clinical specimens, environmental samples, or food). Amplification of viral RNA by reverse transcription-PCR (RT-PCR) is currently the most sensitive and widely used method for detection of HAV RNA (116). Real-time PCR has revolutionized nucleic acid detection because it is rapid, sensitive, reproducible, and quantitative and reduces the risk of false positives due to contamination.

Nucleic acid sequencing is performed on PCR products to confirm their specificity and provide the ultimate means to identify and characterize the organism (116). Sequencing of selected genomic regions of HAV is used to determine the genetic relatedness of isolates for epidemiological investigations (114, 131). Real-time PCR permits rapid analysis of specimens in outbreak situations, with less than 36 h required from amplification to nucleic acid sequence results (116).

Today, PCR may be used for HAV detection in environmental samples (52, 75). The same characteristics that facilitate the likelihood of transmission of HAV by contaminated food and water—the stability of HAV in the environment, especially when associated with organic matter, and its resistance to low pH and heating—also improve the likelihood of detection in environmental samples. HAV detection in food has not been included traditionally as a part of outbreak investigations because of the long disease incubation period and the fact that the implicated foods usually have been consumed or discarded by the time the outbreak is recognized (89); unless there is ongoing contamination, the same holds true for waterborne outbreaks.

TREATMENT

Treatment of typical hepatitis A is supportive, as there are no antiviral agents approved that are effective against HAV. Hospitalization is rarely required, and while nosocomial spread of hepatitis A is rare, enteric isolation procedures are indicated for hospitalized patients. The course and symptomatology of cholestatic hepatitis may be reduced by a short course of corticosteroids (137).

Many agents have been studied for the treatment of fulminant hepatitis (e.g., corticosteroids, prostaglandin E, interferon, ribavirin, and amantadine), with inconclusive results. Liver transplantation is successful for some persons, although the criteria for choosing patients for liver transplantation are difficult to establish. Some transplant centers use the presence of severe coagulopathy and older age as criteria for transplantation, and others include hyperbilirubinemia and prolonged jaundice. The survival rate is moderately high even for patients with coma (approximately 66%), and no single factor is predictive of a poor outcome. The survival rate is 55 to 75% among patients undergoing transplantation (119).

PREVENTION

General

The prevention of hepatitis A is primarily a political, social, economic, and engineering concern. The provision of clean water, the availability of proper waste disposal, and general improvement in the overall living conditions rapidly reduce the incidence of hepatitis A within a population. A paradoxical consequence of socioeconomic development and of declining hepatitis A seroprevalence is the possibility that hepatitis A might become a greater public health problem because of the reciprocal increase in the number of persons susceptible to infection and symptomatic illness. General hygienic measures are most important in limiting person-to-person transmission in the home, school, or work setting. While nosocomial transmission is rare and hospitalized patients require only enteric precautions and private rooms (66), gloves should be worn when handling anything that is potentially contaminated with feces. Frequent hand washing should be emphasized and enforced.

Passive Immunization

Before the licensure of effective hepatitis A vaccines in 1995 to 1996, IG was the sole means of prevention of hepatitis A for people who either were likely to become infected or had been recently exposed. IG is a sterile preparation of concentrated antibodies (immunoglobulins) made from pooled human plasma processed by cold ethanol fractionation (46). In the United States, only plasma that has tested negative for HBV surface antigen, antibody to human immunodeficiency virus (HIV), and antibody to HCV is used to produce IG. Since 1995, the Food and Drug Administration (FDA) has required that the process used to make IG include a specific virus inactivation step or that final products test negative for HCV RNA by PCR (34). Despite concern that the decline in the prevalence of anti-HAV in the population might reduce the effectiveness of IG, there is no standard for anti-HAV levels in IG preparations, and there is at present no evidence of reduced efficacy of IG (147).

IG provides protection against hepatitis A through passive transfer of antibody. No transmission of HBV, HCV, HIV, or other viruses from intramuscular (i.m.) IG injection has been reported. When administered for preexposure prophylaxis, one dose of 0.02 ml/kg of body weight i.m. confers protection for no more than 3 months, and one dose of 0.06 ml/kg i.m. confers protection for 3 to 5 months (Table 2). When administered within 2 weeks after an exposure to HAV (0.02 ml/kg i.m.), IG is 80 to 90% effective in preventing hepatitis A (100, 113). Efficacy is greatest when IG is administered early in the incubation period. When administered later in the incubation period, IG might only attenuate the clinical manifestations of HAV infection (172).

The level of anti-HAV detected in persons 1 week after the administration of a single i.m. 5-ml dose of IG (see Table 2 for IG dosing) is typically in the range of 100 mIU/ml. By comparison, the titer of anti-HAV detected after recent infection often exceeds 15,000 mIU/ml, and following active immunization with three doses of HAV vaccine, it is approximately 3,500 mIU/ml. While measurable antibody following IG may disappear rapidly, neutralizing antibody and its associated protection are retained for several months (147).

Serious adverse events from IG are rare. Because anaphylaxis has been reported after repeated administration to persons with IgA deficiency, these persons should not receive IG. Pregnancy or lactation is not a contraindication to receipt of IG. A thimerosal-free preparation of IG is available and is preferable for use in infants and pregnant women (34).

TABLE 2 Recommended doses of IG for hepatitis A preexposure and postexposure prophylaxis[a]

Setting	Duration of coverage	Dose (ml/kg)[b]
Preexposure	Short term (1–2 mo)	0.02
	Long term (3–5 mo)	0.06[c]
Postexposure		0.02

[a] Source: reference 34.

[b] IG should be administered by i.m. injection into either the deltoid or gluteal muscle. For children aged <24 months, IG can be administered in the anterolateral thigh muscle.

[c] Repeat every 5 months if continued exposure to HAV virus occurs.

IG does not interfere with the immune response to live, attenuated poliovirus vaccine or yellow fever vaccine or, in general, to inactivated vaccines. However, IG can interfere with the response to other live attenuated vaccines (e.g., measles, mumps, and rubella [MMR] vaccine and varicella vaccine) when given as either individual or combination vaccines. Administration of MMR vaccine should be delayed for at least 3 months and varicella vaccine for at least 5 months after administration of IG for hepatitis A prophylaxis. IG should not be administered less than 2 weeks after administration of MMR vaccine or less than 3 weeks after administration of varicella vaccine unless the benefits of IG exceed the benefits of vaccination (31). If IG is administered less than 2 weeks after administration of MMR vaccine or less than 3 weeks after varicella vaccine, the person should be revaccinated, but not sooner than 3 months after IG administration for MMR or 5 months for varicella vaccine (31).

Active Immunization

Existing Vaccines

Inactivated and attenuated hepatitis A vaccines have been developed and evaluated in nonhuman primate models of HAV infection and in human clinical trials. For the most part, vaccines made from inactivated HAV have been evaluated for efficacy in controlled clinical trials (82, 170). However, a live attenuated HAV vaccine was developed in and has been used extensively in the People's Republic of China since 1992, reportedly with effective results (103).

The vaccines containing HAV antigen that are currently licensed in the United States are the single-antigen vaccines HAVRIX (GlaxoSmithKline, Rixensart, Belgium) and VAQTA (Merck & Co., Inc., Whitehouse Station, NJ) and the combination vaccine TWINRIX (containing both HAV and HBV antigens; GlaxoSmithKline). All are inactivated vaccines.

Inactivated hepatitis A vaccines are prepared by propagation of cell culture-adapted virus in human fibroblasts, purification by ultrafiltration and gel chromatography or other methods, formalin inactivation, and, in distinction from inactivated polio vaccine, adsorption to an aluminum hydroxide adjuvant; HAVRIX, TWINRIX, and VAQTA are formulated without a preservative. For HAVRIX and TWINRIX, the antigen content is determined by reactivity in a quantitative immunoassay for HAV antigen, and final vaccine potency (per dose) is expressed as enzyme-linked immunosorbent assay units (EL.U.). For VAQTA, the antigen content is expressed as units of HAV antigen (34).

The vaccine should be administered i.m. into the deltoid muscle. A needle length appropriate for the person's age and size should be used. VAQTA is licensed in two formulations which differ according to the person's age. Persons aged 12 months to 18 years should receive 25 U per dose in a two-dose schedule; persons aged >18 years should receive 50 U per dose in a two-dose schedule (Table 3). HAVRIX is available in two formulations which differ according to the person's age. Persons aged 12 months to 18 years should receive 720 EL.U. per dose in a two-dose schedule; persons aged >18 years should receive 1,440 EL.U. per dose in a two-dose schedule (Table 3). TWINRIX is licensed for use in persons aged >18 years. TWINRIX is a combined hepatitis A and hepatitis B vaccine containing 720 EL.U. of HAV antigen (half of the HAVRIX adult dose) and 20 μg of recombinant HBV surface antigen (the same as the ENGERIX-B adult dose). Primary immunization consists of three doses according to the same schedule as that commonly used for single-antigen hepatitis B vaccine (0, 1, and 6 months) (Table 3). TWINRIX contains aluminum phosphate and aluminum hydroxide as the adjuvant. After three doses of TWINRIX, antibody responses to both antigens are equivalent to responses seen after the single-antigen vaccines are administered separately on standard schedules (87). Clinicians may choose to use an accelerated schedule for TWINRIX (i.e., doses at days 0, 7, and 21). The FDA has approved the accelerated schedule for TWINRIX but not for the monovalent hepatitis B vaccine. Persons who receive a vaccination on an accelerated schedule should also receive a booster dose at 1 year after the start of the series to promote long-term immunity (19). Table 4 shows the minimum intervals between doses for HAVRIX, VAQTA, and TWINRIX.

TABLE 3 Recommended schedule for vaccines to prevent hepatitis A[a,b]

Vaccine[c]	Age (yr)	No. of doses	Schedule[d]
HAVRIX (pediatric formulation)	1	2	0, 6–12 mo
VAQTA (pediatric formulation)	1	2	0, 6–18 mo
TWINRIX (adult formulation)	18	3	0, 1, 6 mo

[a] Source: CDC (http://www.cdc.gov/vaccines/programs/vfc/downloads/resolutions/0607-1hepa.pdf).

[b] All children should receive hepatitis A vaccine at 1 year of age (i.e., 12 to 23 months). Vaccination should be completed according to the licensed schedules and integrated into the routine childhood vaccination schedule. Children who are not vaccinated by 2 years of age can be vaccinated subsequently. States, counties, and communities with existing hepatitis A vaccination programs for children 2 to 18 years are encouraged to maintain these programs. In these areas, new efforts focused on routine vaccination of 1-year-old children should enhance, not replace, ongoing programs directed at a broader population of children. In areas without existing hepatitis A vaccination programs, catch-up vaccination of unvaccinated children aged 2 to 18 years can be considered. Such programs might especially be warranted in the context of rising incidence or ongoing outbreaks among children or adolescents. Clinicians may choose to use an accelerated schedule for TWINRIX (i.e., doses at days 0, 7, and 21). The FDA has approved the accelerated schedule for TWINRIX, but not for the monovalent hepatitis B vaccine. Persons who receive a vaccination on an accelerated schedule should also receive a booster dose at 1 year after the start of the series to promote long-term immunity (19).

[c] Use of brand names is not meant to preclude the use of other hepatitis A vaccines where appropriate.

[d] 0 months represents timing of the initial dose; subsequent numbers represent months after the initial dose.

Vaccine Efficacy

Before widespread use of vaccine in the United States, the highest hepatitis A rates and majority of cases were concentrated in a limited number of states and counties in the western and southwestern parts of the country (166). From 1987 to 1997, one-half of all United States cases occurred among residents in 11 states that together constituted 22% of the total U.S. population and where the average annual incidence was over 20 cases per 100,000 population, twice the national average of 10 cases per 100,000 (34).

With the licensure of inactivated hepatitis A vaccines by the FDA during the period from 1995 to 1996, hepatitis A became the most frequently reported vaccine-preventable disease in the United States. In 1996, the

TABLE 4 Dosage intervals[a,b]

Vaccine	Minimum age (dose 1)	Minimum interval between doses (mo.)		
		Dose 1 to 2	Dose 2 to 3	Dose 1 to 3
HAVRIX (pediatric formulation)	12 mo	6	NA[c]	NA
VAQTA (pediatric formulation)	12 mo	6	NA	NA
TWINRIX (adult formulation)	18 yr	1	5	6

[a] Source: CDC (http://www.cdc.gov/vaccines/programs/vfc/downloads/resolutions/0607-1hepa.pdf).
[b] See Table 3, footnote b.
[c] NA, not applicable.

ACIP recommended targeted hepatitis A vaccination of high-risk populations, like MSM, users of illicit drugs, and travelers to countries where hepatitis A is endemic (29). Routine vaccination was recommended for children living in communities with the highest hepatitis A rates (e.g., Native American communities). The recommendations for vaccination were expanded by the ACIP in 1999 to include routine vaccination of children living in states and communities in which the average hepatitis A rate during the baseline period of 1987 to 1997 was ≥20 cases per 100,000 population, approximately twice the national average, and for consideration of vaccination of children in those states and communities in which the average rate during the baseline period was at least the national average (30). Further broadening of recommendations by the ACIP occurred in 2006, that all children should receive hepatitis A vaccine at the age of 1 year (i.e., 12 to 23 months) in accord with the licensed schedules and as part of the routine childhood vaccination schedule. Children not already vaccinated by age 2 could be vaccinated subsequently. States, counties, and communities were suggested to either continue ongoing or consider catch-up programs for vaccination of children aged 2 to 18 years (34).

Although it is expected that the 2005 licensure of the hepatitis A vaccine for use in younger children (aged ≥12 months) and the 2006 ACIP guideline for routine hepatitis A vaccination of all children aged ≥12 months should result in improved vaccination coverage and further reductions in disease incidence, results from the National Immunization Survey for coverage in the period from 2004 to 2005 among children aged 24 to 35 months demonstrate the need for improvement. Even in states where hepatitis A vaccination was recommended, coverage remained below levels observed for other vaccinations that were recommended during a comparable period. For example, one-dose vaccination coverage of varicella vaccine, which has been routinely recommended for children aged 12 to 18 months since 1996, was 76.3% in 2001 and 80.6% in 2002 for children aged 19 to 35 months. Coverage with one dose of MMR vaccine, which became available in 1971, was 93.0% in 2004 (36).

For hepatitis A vaccination, a statistically significant increase was observed in estimated national one-dose coverage, from 17.6% in 2004 to 21.3% in 2005. Coverage was greater in states where vaccination was recommended by the ACIP than in states where vaccination was to be considered or where no specific recommendation was in effect. In the 11 states where vaccination was recommended, one-dose coverage was 54.4% (range, 8.6 to 74.4%) in 2004 and 56.5% (range, 12.9 to 71.0%) in 2005. In the six states where vaccination was to be considered, one-dose coverage was 26.8% (range, 1.4 to 34.7%) in 2004 and 43.2% (range, 1.9 to 57.5%) in 2005. In the District of Columbia and the 33 states where no specific recommendation for vaccination was in effect, coverage was 1.5% (range, 0 to 10.3%) in 2004 and 2.9% (range, 0 to 8.4%) in 2005 (36).

Levels of antibody achieved following administration of vaccine are 10- to 100-fold lower than those produced after natural infection. To measure lower concentrations of antibody, more sensitive immunoassays were developed for immunogenicity studies that correlate more closely with neutralizing-antibody assays (96). Anti-HAV concentrations are measured in comparison with a WHO reference reagent and are expressed as milli-international units per milliliter. The lower limits of detection have typically been approximately 100 mIU/ml by commercial assays and 10 mIU/ml by more sensitive assays (34). A positive anti-HAV result by a standard assay indicates protection. However, after vaccination, persons who are anti-HAV negative by standard assays might nevertheless be protected, as the absolute lower limit of anti-HAV required to prevent HAV infection has not been defined. To define a protective antibody response, clinical studies conducted with HAVRIX have used levels of >20 mIU/ml, or >33 mIU/ml in more recent studies, and studies conducted with VAQTA have used levels of >10 mIU/ml (39).

Data thus far indicate that vaccines currently on the market provide long-term protection against hepatitis A. All 31 adults who received three doses of HAVRIX (720 EL.U. per dose at 0-, 1-, and 6-month intervals) had anti-HAV levels of >15 mIU/ml 12 years after the initial dose (162). Ten years after vaccination, more than 300 adults administered two doses of 1,440 EL.U. of HAVRIX had anti-HAV levels of >20 mIU/ml (162). Protective levels of anti-HAV were still observed in 544 (99%) of 549 children evaluated 5 to 6 years after receiving VAQTA (169). Antibody persistence derived from models of antibody decline predicts that protective levels of anti-HAV could be present for more than 25 years in adults and for at least 14 to 20 years in children (160). Whether other mechanisms (e.g., cellular memory) also contribute to long-term protection is unknown, but it is clear from passive-immunization studies that antibody alone is sufficient to protect against HAV infection.

Diminished vaccine response has been observed in infants with passively acquired antibody as the result of previous maternal HAV infection (34), which is why hepatitis A vaccination is deferred until 12 months of age. In the majority of studies, all infants subsequently had protective levels of antibody, but the final levels were substantially lower than those of infants born to anti-HAV-negative mothers and vaccinated according to the same schedule. Despite lower antibody levels after the primary series, the majority of infants with passively acquired antibody respond to a booster dose 1 to 6 years later (34, 62, 101).

Passively acquired antibody declines to undetectable levels in the majority of infants by the age of 1 year. After 1 year of age, hepatitis A vaccine is highly immunogenic, regardless of maternal anti-HAV status (34).

Hepatitis A vaccine using a standard dose and schedule is immunogenic for children and adults with HIV infection who are not immunocompromised (CD4 count of >200 cells/mm^3). Protective levels of antibody developed after vaccination in 61 to 87% of HIV-infected adults (86, 165) and in 100% of 32 HIV-infected children (72). Immunologic reconstitution with highly active antiretroviral therapy is likely to restore the ability to respond to the vaccine, because a low CD4 cell count at the time of vaccination (not the nadir) is associated with a lack of response (130).

In adults, simultaneous administration of hepatitis A vaccine with diphtheria, poliovirus (oral and inactivated), tetanus, typhoid (both oral and i.m.), cholera, Japanese encephalitis, rabies, or yellow fever vaccine does not appear to decrease the immune response to either vaccine or increase the frequency of reported adverse events (16). Studies indicating that hepatitis B vaccine can be administered simultaneously with hepatitis A vaccine without affecting either vaccine's immunogenicity or increasing the frequency of adverse events led to the licensure of TWINRIX (3). Among infants and children aged <18 months, simultaneous administration of hepatitis A vaccine with diphtheria-tetanus-acellular pertussis, *Haemophilus influenzae* type b, hepatitis B, MMR, or inactivated poliovirus vaccine does not affect the immunogenicity or reactogenicity of these vaccines (48).

Side Effects and Adverse Events

Approximately 50,000 persons were administered HAVRIX in prelicensure clinical studies (68). No serious adverse events were attributed definitively to hepatitis A vaccine. Among adults, the most frequently reported side effects occurring <3 days after the 1,440-EL.U. dose were soreness at the injection site (56%), headache (14%), and malaise (7%). In clinical studies among children, the most frequently reported side effects were soreness at the injection site (15%), feeding problems (8%), headache (4%), and injection site induration (4%). The frequency of side effects after administration of TWINRIX was similar to those reported when the two single-antigen vaccines were administered (84, 87). Approximately 10,000 persons were administered VAQTA in prelicensure clinical studies, and no serious adverse events were reported among participants (112). Among adults and children, the most frequent side effects that occurred <5 days after vaccination included tenderness, pain, and warmth at the injection site and headache.

An estimated 1.3 million persons in Europe and Asia were vaccinated with HAVRIX before the vaccine's licensure in the United States in 1995. Reports of serious adverse events were not higher than would be expected for an unvaccinated population (CDC, unpublished data, 1995). In a postlicensure study of 11,417 children and 25,023 adults who were administered VAQTA, no serious adverse events occurred that were considered to be associated with administration of the vaccine (Merck & Co., Inc., unpublished data, 2005). Since its licensure in 1995, approximately 188 million doses of VAQTA have been sold worldwide, including 50 million doses in the United States (GlaxoSmithKline, unpublished data, 2005; Merck & Co., Inc., unpublished).

Vaccination of a person who is immune because of previous infection does not increase the risk of adverse events. In populations that have expected high rates of previous HAV infection, prevaccination testing may be considered to reduce costs by not vaccinating persons who are already immune. Testing of children is not indicated because of their expected low prevalence of infection. For adults, the decision to test should be based on (i) the expected prevalence of immunity, (ii) the cost of vaccination compared with the cost of serologic testing (including the cost of an additional visit), and (iii) the likelihood that testing will not interfere with initiation of vaccination. For example, if the cost of screening (including laboratory and office visits) is one-third the cost of the vaccine series, then screening potential recipients in populations for which the prevalence of infection is likely to be >33% should be cost-effective (27).

Postvaccination testing is not indicated because of the high rate of vaccine response among adults and children. Furthermore, not all testing methods approved for routine diagnostic use in the United States have the sensitivity to detect low anti-HAV concentrations after vaccination.

Use of Hepatitis A Vaccine for Preexposure Protection against HAV Infection

The recommendations for hepatitis A vaccination are intended to further reduce hepatitis A morbidity and mortality rates in the United States and make possible consideration of eventual elimination of HAV transmission. Hepatitis A vaccination is recommended routinely for children, for persons who are at increased risk of infection, and for any person wishing to obtain immunity.

All children should receive hepatitis A vaccine at the age of 1 year (i.e., 12 to 23 months). Vaccination should be completed according to the licensed schedules (Table 3) and integrated into the routine childhood vaccination schedule. Children who are not vaccinated by age 2 can be vaccinated subsequently. States, counties, and communities with existing hepatitis A vaccination programs for children aged 2 to 18 years are encouraged to maintain these programs. In these areas, new efforts focused on routine vaccination of children aged 1 year should enhance, not replace, ongoing programs directed at a broader population of children. In areas without existing hepatitis A vaccination programs, catch-up vaccination of unvaccinated children aged 2 to 18 years can be considered. Such programs might especially be warranted in the context of increasing incidence or ongoing outbreaks among children or adolescents (34).

Vaccination of Persons at Increased Risk of HAV Infection

Vaccination is also recommended for MSM. Prevaccination testing generally is not indicated but might be warranted for older adults, in whom the probability of previous infection is substantial. Health care providers in primary-care and specialty medical settings in which MSM receive care should offer hepatitis A vaccine to patients at risk. Strategies to overcome barriers and increase coverage (e.g., use of standing orders) should be considered (34).

Vaccination is recommended for users of injection and noninjection illicit drugs. Prevaccination testing generally is not indicated but might be warranted for older adults. Providers should obtain a thorough history to identify patients who use or are at risk of using illicit drugs and might benefit from hepatitis A vaccination. Strategies to overcome barriers and increase coverage (e.g., use of standing orders) should be considered (34).

Persons who work with nonhuman primates (98) or with HAV in a research laboratory setting should be vaccinated. No other populations have been demonstrated to be at increased risk of HAV infection because of occupational exposure (34).

Although changes in clotting factor preparation practices and donor screening have greatly reduced the risk of hepatitis A for recipients of clotting factors, susceptible persons who are administered clotting factor concentrates should receive hepatitis A vaccine (34).

Vaccination of Persons with Chronic Liver Disease

Because persons with chronic liver disease may be predisposed to the development of fulminant hepatitis A, susceptible persons with chronic liver disease should be vaccinated. Susceptible persons who either are awaiting or have received liver transplants should be vaccinated (34).

Efficacy of Vaccine or IG for Postexposure Prophylaxis of Hepatitis A

Hepatitis A vaccine can prevent HAV infection if administered shortly after exposure in chimpanzees (133). Because the incubation period of hepatitis A can be 50 days, the fact that no cases of hepatitis A occurred in recipients after 17 days postvaccination during a clinical efficacy trial also suggested a possible postexposure effect (170). In a limited randomized trial, vaccine was 79% efficacious in preventing IgM anti-HAV positivity after household exposure to hepatitis A compared with no treatment, but confidence intervals were extremely wide (7 to 95%) and no comparison group received IG (135). Subsequently, hepatitis A vaccine was adopted for use for postexposure prophylaxis in Italy and other European countries.

The adoption of use of hepatitis A vaccine for postexposure prophylaxis in the United States by the ACIP in 2007 was based on results of a randomized trial comparing the efficacy of hepatitis A vaccine with that of IG in Almaty, Kazakhstan, among more than 4,500 contacts of patients with hepatitis A. Symptomatic HAV infection occurring between 15 and 56 days after exposure occurred was laboratory confirmed in 25 contacts who received vaccine (4.4%) and in 17 contacts who received IG (3.3%) (relative risk, 1.35; 95% confidence interval, 0.70 to 2.67), proving that hepatitis A vaccine and IG each provide good protection (163). The experiences of other countries (e.g., Canada and the United Kingdom) where hepatitis A vaccine has been recommended for postexposure use for >5 years supported these findings and led to the change in policy (37) (Table 5).

Persons who recently have been exposed to HAV and who have not received hepatitis A vaccine should be administered a single dose of single-antigen vaccine or IG (0.02 ml/kg) as soon as possible. No data are available about the relative efficacy of vaccine compared to IG postexposure in persons with underlying medical conditions. Therefore, decisions to use vaccine or IG should take into account the potential for severe manifestations of hepatitis A, including patient age and the presence of chronic liver disease (37).

Selected Special Categories for Exclusive Use of IG

IG should be used in healthy children younger than 12 months of age, immunocompromised persons, persons with chronic liver disease, and persons for whom vaccine is contraindicated. For healthy children aged 12 months through 18 years, hepatitis A vaccine at the age-appropriate dose is preferred to IG because of its long-term protection and ease of administration. Persons administered IG for whom hepatitis A vaccine is also recommended should receive a dose of vaccine simultaneously with IG. For persons who receive vaccine, the second dose should be administered according to the licensed schedule to complete the series. The efficacy of IG or vaccine when administered more than 2 weeks after exposure has not been established (37, 163).

Because hepatitis A cannot be reliably diagnosed on clinical presentation alone, serologic confirmation of HAV infection in index patients by IgM anti-HAV testing is recommended before postexposure treatment of contacts. Screening of contacts for immunity before administering postexposure prophylaxis is not recommended because screening would result in delay.

All previously unvaccinated household and sexual contacts of persons with serologically confirmed hepatitis A should be administered postexposure prophylaxis. In addition, persons who have shared illicit drugs with a person who has serologically confirmed hepatitis A should receive postexposure prophylaxis (34).

Postexposure prophylaxis should be administered to all previously unvaccinated staff and attendees of child care centers if one or more cases of hepatitis A are recognized

TABLE 5 Summary of updated recommendations for prevention of hepatitis A after exposure to HAV and in departing international travelers

Indication	Hepatitis A vaccine	IG
Postexposure prophylaxis	1. Healthy persons aged 12 mo to 40 yr at the age-appropriate dose 2. Healthy persons aged >40 yr if vaccine cannot be obtained	1. Persons aged >40 yr 2. Children aged <12 mo 3. Immunocompromised persons and persons with chronic liver disease, or for whom vaccine is contraindicated
International travel[a]	For most healthy persons, one dose of single antigen before travel	Persons who elect not to receive vaccine, are aged <12 mo, or are allergic to a vaccine component
	Older adults, immunocompromised persons, and persons with chronic liver disease or other chronic medical conditions planning to depart to an area ≤2 weeks should receive the initial dose of vaccine and also simultaneously can be administered IG at a separate anatomic site	

[a] To countries with high or intermediate hepatitis A endemicity.

in children or employees or cases are recognized in two or more households of center attendees. In centers that do not provide care to children who wear diapers, postexposure prophylaxis need be administered only to classroom contacts of an index patient. When an outbreak occurs (i.e., hepatitis A cases in three or more families), postexposure prophylaxis also should be considered for members of households that have children (center attendees) in diapers (34).

If a food handler is diagnosed with hepatitis A, postexposure prophylaxis should be administered to other food handlers at the same establishment. Because common-source transmission to patrons is unlikely, postexposure prophylaxis administration to patrons is usually not necessary but may be considered if the food handler both directly handled uncooked foods or foods after cooking and had diarrhea or poor hygienic practices while likely to be infectious and patrons can be identified and treated within 2 weeks of the exposure. Stronger consideration of postexposure prophylaxis use might be warranted for settings in which repeated exposures to HAV might have occurred (34).

Prevention of Hepatitis A before International Travel

Hepatitis A vaccination is recommended to prevent hepatitis A among travelers to countries with high or intermediate hepatitis A endemicity. In June 2007, the ACIP concluded that if hepatitis A vaccine alone can be recommended for prophylaxis after exposure to HAV, vaccine also should be recommended for healthy international travelers aged <40 years regardless of their scheduled dates for departure. For certain international travelers (e.g., older adults or those with underlying medical conditions), the performance of vaccine alone is unknown and clinical manifestations of hepatitis A tend to be more severe. Hence, under the updated recommendations for international travelers, for optimal protection, IG can be considered in addition to vaccine for older adults, immunocompromised persons, and persons with chronic liver disease or other chronic medical conditions who are traveling to an area of endemicity within 2 weeks (37).

Recommendations for Preexposure Protection against Hepatitis A for Travelers (Table 5)

All susceptible persons traveling to or working in countries that have high or intermediate hepatitis A endemicity are at increased risk of HAV infection and should be vaccinated or receive IG before departure. Hepatitis A vaccination at the age-appropriate dose is preferred to IG. Data are not available regarding the risk of hepatitis A for persons traveling to certain areas of the Caribbean, although prophylaxis should be considered if travel to areas with questionable sanitation is anticipated. Travelers to Australia, Canada, Western Europe, Japan, or New Zealand (i.e., countries in which endemicity is low) are at no greater risk of infection than persons living or traveling in the United States (37).

The first dose of hepatitis A vaccine should be administered as soon as travel is considered. Based on limited data indicating equivalent postexposure efficacies of IG and vaccine among healthy persons aged <40 years, one dose of single-antigen hepatitis A vaccine administered at any time before departure can provide adequate protection for most healthy persons. However, no data are available for other populations or other hepatitis A vaccine formulations (e.g., TWINRIX). For optimal protection, older adults, immunocompromised persons, and persons with chronic liver disease or other chronic medical conditions planning to depart to an area of endemicity in <2 weeks should receive the initial dose of vaccine and also can be simultaneously administered IG (0.02 ml/kg) at a separate anatomic injection site. Completion of the vaccine series according to the licensed schedule is necessary for long-term protection (37).

Travelers who elect not to receive vaccine, are aged <12 months, or are allergic to a vaccine component should receive a single dose of IG (0.02 ml/kg), which provides effective protection against hepatitis A for up to 3 months. Such travelers whose travel period is expected to be >2 months should be administered IG at 0.06 ml/kg; administration must be repeated if the travel period is >5 months (34).

REFERENCES

1. **Akriviadis, E. A., and A. G. Redeker.** 1989. Fulminant hepatitis A in intravenous drug users with chronic liver disease. *Ann. Intern. Med.* **110:**838–839.
2. **Allaire, M., M. M. Chernaia, B. A. Malcolm, and M. N. James.** 1994. Picornaviral 3C cysteine proteinases have a fold similar to chymotrypsin-like serine proteinases. *Nature* **369:**72–76.
3. **Ambrosch, F., F. E. André, A. Delem, E. D'Hondt, S. Jonas, C. Kunz, A. Safary, and G. Wiedermann.** 1992. Simultaneous vaccination against hepatitis A and B: results of a controlled study. *Vaccine* **10**(Suppl. 1)**:**S142–S145.
4. **Anderson, D. A., and B. C. Ross.** 1990. Morphogenesis of hepatitis A virus: isolation and characterization of subviral particles. *J. Virol.* **64:**5284–5289.
5. **Andre, F. E.** 1995. Approaches to a vaccine against hepatitis A: development and manufacture of an inactivated vaccine. *J. Infect. Dis.* **171**(Suppl. 1)**:**S33–S39.
6. **Armstrong, G. L., and B. P. Bell.** 2002. Hepatitis A virus infections in the United States: model-based estimates and implications for childhood immunization. *Pediatrics* **109:**839–845.
7. **Asher, L. V., L. N. Binn, T. L. Mensing, R. H. Marchwicki, R. A. Vassell, and G. D. Young.** 1995. Pathogenesis of hepatitis A in orally inoculated owl monkeys (Aotus trivirgatus). *J. Med. Virol.* **47:**260–268.
8. **Baba, M., H. Hasegawa, M. Nakayabu, K. Fukai, and S. Suzuki.** 1993. Cytolytic activity of natural killer cells and lymphokine activated killer cells against hepatitis A virus infected fibroblasts. *J. Clin. Lab. Immunol.* **40:**47–60.
9. **Balayan, M. S.** 1992. Natural hosts of hepatitis A virus. *Vaccine* **10:**S27–S31.
10. **Bell, B. P.** 2000. Hepatitis A and hepatitis B vaccination of patients with chronic liver disease. *Acta Gastro-Enterol. Belg.* **63:**359–365.
11. **Bell, B. P.** 2002. Global epidemiology of hepatitis A: implications for control strategies, p. 9–14. *In* H. S. Margolis, M. J. Alter, J. Liang, and J. Dienstag (ed.), *Viral Hepatitis and Liver Disease.* International Medical Press, Atlanta, GA.
12. **Bell, B. P., D. Kruszon-Moran, C. N. Shapiro, S. B. Lambert, G. M. McQuillan, and H. S. Margolis.** 2005. Hepatitis A virus infection in the United States: serologic results from the Third National Health and Nutrition Examination Survey. *Vaccine* **23:**5798–5806.
13. **Bell, B. P., C. N. Shapiro, M. J. Alter, L. A. Moyer, F. N. Judson, K. Mottram, M. Fleenor, P. L. Ryder, and H. S. Margolis.** 1998. The diverse patterns of hepatitis A

epidemiology in the United States—implications for vaccination strategies. *J. Infect. Dis.* **178:**1579–1584.

14. **Bialek, S. R., P. A. George, G. Xia, M. B. Glatzer, M. L. Motes, J. E. Veazey, R. M. Hammond, T. Jones, Y. C. Shieh, J. Wamnes, G. Vaughn, Y. Khudyakov, and A. E. Fiore.** 2007. Use of molecular epidemiology to confirm a multistate outbreak of hepatitis A caused by consumption of oysters. *Clin. Infect. Dis.* **44:**838–840.
15. **Bialek, S. R., D. A. Thoroughman, D. Hu, E. P. Simard, J. Chattin, J. Cheek, and B. P. Bell.** 2004. Hepatitis A incidence and hepatitis A vaccination among American Indians and Alaska Natives, 1990–2001. *Am. J. Public Health* **94:**996–1001.
16. **Bienzle, U., H. L. Bock, J. Kruppenbacher, F. Hofmann, G. E. Vogel, and R. Clemens.** 1996. Immunogenicity of an inactivated hepatitis A vaccine administered according to two different schedules and the interference of other "travelers" vaccines with the immune response. *Vaccine* **14:**501–505.
17. **Bishop, N. E., and D. A. Anderson.** 2000. Uncoating kinetics of hepatitis A virus virions and provirions. *J. Virol.* **74:**3423–3426.
18. **Blank, C. A., D. A. Anderson, M. Beard, and S. M. Lemon.** 2000. Infection of polarized cultures of human intestinal epithelial cells with hepatitis A virus: vectorial release of progeny virions through apical cellular membranes. *J. Virol.* **74:**6476–6484.
19. **Bock, H. L., T. Loscher, N. Scheiermann, R. Baumgarten, M. Wiese, W. Dutz, R. Sänger, and R. Clemens.** 1995. Accelerated schedule for hepatitis B immunization. *J. Travel Med.* **2:**213–217.
20. Reference deleted.
21. **Borman, A. M., and K. M. Kean.** 1997. Intact eukaryotic initiation factor 4G is required for hepatitis A virus internal initiation of translation. *Virology* **237:**129–136.
22. **Bower, W. A., O. V. Nainan, X. Han, and H. S. Margolis.** 2000. Duration of viremia in hepatitis A virus infection. *J. Infect. Dis.* **182:**12–17.
23. **Brack, K., W. Frings, A. Dotzauer, and A. Vallbracht.** 1998. A cytopathogenic, apoptosis-inducing variant of hepatitis A virus. *J. Virol.* **72:**3370–3376.
24. **Bradley, D. W., C. A. Schable, K. A. McCaustland, E. H. Cook, B. L. Murphy, H. A. Fields, J. W. Ebert, C. Wheeler, and J. E. Maynard.** 1984. Hepatitis A virus: growth characteristics of in vivo and in vitro propagated wild and attenuated virus strains. *J. Med. Virol.* **14:**373–386.
25. **Brown, E. A., S. P. Day, R. W. Jansen, and S. M. Lemon.** 1991. The 5′ nontranslated region of hepatitis A virus RNA: secondary structure and elements required for translation in vitro. *J. Virol.* **65:** 5828–5838.
26. **Brown, E. A., R. W. Jansen, and S. M. Lemon.** 1989. Characterization of a simian hepatitis A virus (HAV): antigenic and genetic comparison with human HAV. *J. Virol.* **63:**4932–4937.
27. **Bryan, J. P., and M. Nelson.** 1994. Testing for antibody to hepatitis A to decrease the cost of hepatitis A prophylaxis with immune globulin or hepatitis A vaccines. *Arch. Intern. Med.* **154:**663–668.
28. **Centers for Disease Control.** 1992. Hepatitis A among homosexual men—United States, Canada, and Australia. *Morb. Mortal. Wkly. Rep.* **41:**155, 161–164.
29. **Centers for Disease Control and Prevention.** 1996. Prevention of hepatitis A through active or passive immunization: recommendations of the Advisory Committee on Immunization Practices (ACIP). *Morb. Mortal. Wkly. Rep.* **45**(RR-15)**:**1–30.
30. **Centers for Disease Control and Prevention.** 1999. Prevention of hepatitis A through active or passive immunization: recommendations of the Advisory Committee on Immunization Practices (ACIP). *Morb. Mortal. Wkly. Rep.* **48**(RR-12)**:**1–37.
31. **Centers for Disease Control and Prevention.** 2002. General recommendations on immunization; recommendations of the Advisory Committee on Immunization Practices (ACIP) and the American Academy of Family Physicians (AAFP). *Morb. Mortal. Wkly. Rep.* **51**(RR-2)**:** 1–36.
32. **Centers for Disease Control and Prevention.** 2003. Blood safety monitoring among persons with bleeding disorders—United States, May 1998–June 2002. *Morb. Mortal. Wkly. Rep.* **51:**1152–1154.
33. **Centers for Disease Control and Prevention.** 2005. Positive test results for acute hepatitis A virus infection among persons with no recent history of acute hepatitis—United States, 2002–2004. *Morb. Mortal. Wkly. Rep.* **54:** 453–456.
34. **Centers for Disease Control and Prevention.** 2006. Prevention of hepatitis A through active or passive immunization. Recommendations of the Advisory Committee on Immunization Practices (ACIP). *Morb. Mortal. Wkly. Rep.* **55**(RR-7)**:**1–23.
35. **Centers for Disease Control and Prevention.** 2007. Surveillance for acute viral hepatitis—United States, 2005. *Morb. Mortal. Wkly. Rep.* **56**(SS-3)**:**1–24.
36. **Centers for Disease Control and Prevention.** 2007. Hepatitis A vaccination coverage among children aged 24—35 months—United States, 2004–2005. *Morb. Mortal. Wkly. Rep.* **56:**678–681.
37. **Centers for Disease Control and Prevention.** 2007. Update: Prevention of hepatitis A after exposure to hepatitis A virus and in international travelers. Updated recommendations of the Advisory Committee on Immunization Practices (ACIP). *Morb. Mortal. Wkly. Rep.* **56:**1080–1084.
38. **Chow, M., J. F. Newman, D. Filman, J. M. Hogle, D. J. Rowlands, and F. Brown.** 1987. Myristylation of picornavirus capsid protein VP4 and its structural significance. *Nature* **327:**482–486.
39. **Clemens, R., A. Safary, A. Hepburn, C. Roche, W. J. Stanbury, and F. E. André.** 1995. Clinical experience with an inactivated hepatitis A vaccine. *J. Infect. Dis.* **171**(Suppl. 1)**:**S44–S49.
40. **Cobden, I., and O. F. James.** 1986. A biphasic illness associated with acute hepatitis A virus infection. *J. Hepatol.* **2:**19–23.
41. **Cohen, J. I., S. Feinstone, and R. H. Purcell.** 1989. Hepatitis A virus infection in a chimpanzee: duration of viremia and detection of virus in saliva and throat swabs. *J. Infect. Dis.* **160:**887–890.
42. **Cohen, J. I., B. Rosenblum, J. R. Ticehurst, R. J. Daemer, S. M. Feinstone, and R. H. Purcell.** 1987. Complete nucleotide sequence of an attenuated hepatitis A virus: comparison with wild-type virus. *Proc. Natl. Acad. Sci. USA* **84:**2497–2501.
43. **Cohen, J. I., J. R. Ticehurst, S. M. Feinstone, B. Rosenblum, and R. H. Purcell.** 1987. Hepatitis A virus cDNA and its RNA transcripts are infectious in cell culture. *J. Virol.* **61:**3035–3039.
44. **Cohen, J. I., J. R. Ticehurst, R. H. Purcell, A. Buckler-White, and B. M. Baroudy.** 1987. Complete nucleotide sequence of wild-type hepatitis A virus: comparison with different strains of hepatitis A virus and other picornaviruses. *J. Virol.* **61:**50–59.
45. **Cohen, L., D. Benichou, and A. Martin.** 2002. Analysis of deletion mutants indicates that the 2A polypeptide of hepatitis A virus participates in virion morphogenesis. *J. Virol.* **76:**7495–7505.

46. **Cohn, E. J., J. L. Oncley, L. E. Strong, W. L. Hughes, Jr., and S. H. Armstrong.** 1944. Chemical, clinical, and immunological studies on the products of human plasma fractionation. I. The characterization of the protein fractions of human plasma. *J. Clin. Investig.* **23:**417–432.
47. **Daemer, R. J., S. M. Feinstone, I. D. Gust, and R. H. Purcell.** 1981. Propagation of human hepatitis A virus in African green monkey kidney cell culture: primary isolation and serial passage. *Infect. Immun.* **32:**388–393.
48. **Dagan, R., J. Amir, A. Mijalovsky, I. Kalmanovitch, A. Bar-Yochai, S. Thoelen, A. Safary, and S. Ashkenazi.** 2000. Immunization against hepatitis A in the first year of life: priming despite the presence of maternal antibody. *Pediatr. Infect. Dis. J.* **19:**1045–1052.
49. **Day, S. P., P. Murphy, E. A. Brown, and S. M. Lemon.** 1992. Mutations within the 5′ nontranslated region of hepatitis A virus RNA which enhance replication in BS-C-1 cells. *J. Virol.* **66:**6533–6540.
50. **Debray, D., P. Cullufi, D. Devictor, M. Fabre, and O. Bernard.** 1997. Liver failure in children with hepatitis A. *Hepatology* **26:**1018–1022.
51. **Deinhardt, F., D. Peterson, G. Cross, L. Wolfe, and A. W. Holmes.** 1975. Hepatitis in marmosets. *Am. J. Med. Sci.* **270:**73–80.
52. **Deng, M. Y., S. P. Day, and D. O. Cliver.** 1994. Detection of hepatitis A virus in environmental samples by antigen-capture PCR. *Appl. Environ. Microbiol.* **60:**1927–1933.
53. **Dienstag, J. L.** 1980. Hepatitis viruses: characterization and diagnostic techniques. *Yale J. Biol. Med.* **53:**61–69.
54. **Dotzauer, A., M. Brenner, U. Gebhardt, and A. Vallbracht.** 2005. IgA-coated particles of hepatitis A virus are translocalized antivectorially from the apical to the basolateral site of polarized epithelial cells via the polymeric immunoglobulin receptor. *J. Gen. Virol.* **86:**2747–2751.
55. **Dotzauer, A., S. M. Feinstone, and G. Kaplan.** 1994. Susceptibility of nonprimate cell lines to hepatitis A virus infection *J. Virol.* **68:**6064–6068. (Erratum, **68:**6829.)
56. **Emerson, S. U., Y. K. Huang, and R. H. Purcell.** 1993. 2B and 2C mutations are essential but mutations throughout the genome of HAV contribute to adaptation to cell culture. *Virology* **194:**475–480.
57. **Emerson, S. U., M. Lewis, S. Govindarajan, M. Shapiro, T. Moskal, and R. H. Purcell.** 1992. cDNA clone of hepatitis A virus encoding a virulent virus: induction of viral hepatitis by direct nucleic acid transfection of marmosets. *J. Virol.* **66:**6649–6654.
58. **Feigelstock, D., P. Thompson, P. Mattoo, Y. Zhang, and G. G. Kaplan.** 1998. The human homolog of HAVcr-1 codes for a hepatitis A virus cellular receptor. *J. Virol.* **72:**6621–6628.
59. **Feinstone, S. M., A. Z. Kapikian, and R. H. Purcell.** 1973. Hepatitis A: detection by immune electron microscopy of a viruslike antigen associated with acute illness. *Science* **182:**1026–1028.
60. **Fensterl, V., D. Grotheer, I. Berk, S. Schlemminger, A. Vallbracht, and A. Dotzauer.** 2005. Hepatitis A virus suppresses RIG-I-mediated IRF-3 activation to block induction of beta interferon. *J. Virol.* **79:**10968–10977.
61. **Fiore, A. E.** 2004. Hepatitis A transmitted by food. *Clin. Infect. Dis.* **38:**705–715.
62. **Fiore, A. E., C. N. Shapiro, K. Sabin, K. Labonte, K. Darling, D. Culver, B. P. Bell, and H. S. Margolis.** 2003. Hepatitis A vaccination of infants: effect of maternal antibody status on antibody persistence and response to a booster dose. *Pediatr. Infect. Dis. J.* **22:**354–359.
63. **Flehmig, B.** 1980. Hepatitis A-virus in cell culture. I. Propagation of different hepatitis A-virus isolates in a fetal rhesus monkey kidney cell line (Frhk-4). *Med. Microbiol. Immunol.* **168:**239–248.
64. **Fleischer, B., S. Fleischer, K. Maier, K. H. Wiedmann, M. Sacher, H. Thaler, and A. Vallbracht.** 1990. Clonal analysis of infiltrating T lymphocytes in liver tissue in viral hepatitis A. *Immunology* **9:**14–19.
65. **Gabriel, P., A. Vallbracht, and B. Flehmig.** 1986. Lack of complement-dependent cytolytic antibodies in hepatitis A virus infection. *J. Med. Virol.* **20:**23–31.
66. **Garner, J. S., and the Hospital Infection Control Practices Advisory Committee.** 1996. Guidelines for isolation precautions in hospitals. *Infect. Control Hosp. Epidemiol.* **17:**53–80.
67. **Gimson, A. E., Y. S. White, A. L. Eddleston, and R. Williams.** 1983. Clinical and prognostic differences in fulminant hepatitis type A, B, and non-A, non-B. *Gut* **24:**1194–1198.
68. **GlaxoSmithKline Biologicals.** 2005. HAVRIX®. Package insert. GlaxoSmithKline Biologicals, Rixensart, Belgium.
69. **Goodman, R. A.** 1985. Nosocomial hepatitis A. *Ann. Intern. Med.* **103:**452–454.
70. **Gosert, R., K. H. Chang, R. Rijnbrand, M. Yi, D. V. Sangar, and S. M. Lemon.** 2000. Transient expression of cellular polypyrimidine-tract binding protein stimulates cap-independent translation directed by both picornaviral and flaviviral internal ribosome entry sites in vivo. *Mol. Cell. Biol.* **20:**1583–1595.
71. **Gosert, R., D. Egger, and K. Bienz.** 2000. A cytopathic and a cell culture adapted hepatitis A virus strain differ in cell killing but not in intracellular membrane rearrangements. *Virology* **266:**157–169.
72. **Gouvea, A. F., M. I. De Moraes-Pinto, E. Ono, M. I. Dinelli, D. M. Machado, L. Y. Weckx, and R. C. Succi.** 2005. Immunogenicity and tolerability of hepatitis A vaccine in HIV-infected children. *Clin. Infect. Dis.* **41:**544–548.
73. **Graff, J., and S. U. Emerson.** 2003. Importance of amino acid 216 in nonstructural protein 2B for replication of hepatitis A virus in cell culture and in vivo. *J. Med. Virol.* **71:**7–17.
74. **Graff, J., O. C. Richards, K. M. Swiderek, M. T. Davis, F. Rusnak, S. A. Harmon, X. Y. Jia, D. F. Summers, and E. Ehrenfeld.** 1999. Hepatitis A virus capsid protein VP1 has a heterogeneous C terminus. *J. Virol.* **73:**6015–6023.
75. **Graff, J., J. Ticehurst, and B. Flehmig.** 1993. Detection of hepatitis A virus in sewage sludge by antigen capture polymerase chain reaction. *Appl. Environ. Microbiol.* **59:**3165–3170.
76. **Hadler, S. C., H. M. Webster, J. J. Erben, J. E. Swanson, and J. E. Maynard.** 1980. Hepatitis A in day-care centers: a community-wide assessment. *N. Engl. J. Med.* **302:**1222–1227.
77. **Havens, W. P. J.** 1947. The etiology of infectious hepatitis. *JAMA* **134:**653–655.
78. **Hornei, B., R. Kammerer, P. Moubayed, W. Frings, V. Gauss-Muller, and A. Dotzauer.** 2001. Experimental hepatitis A virus infection in guinea pigs. *J. Med. Virol.* **64:**402–409.
79. **Hughes, J. V., and L. W. Stanton.** 1985. Isolation and immunizations with hepatitis A viral structural proteins: induction of antiprotein, antiviral, and neutralizing responses. *J. Virol.* **55:** 395–401.
80. **Hutin, Y. J. F., V. Pool, E. H. Cramer, O. V. Nainan, J. Weth, I. T. Williams, S. T. Goldstein, K. F. Gensheimer, B. P. Bell, C. N. Shapiro, M. J. Alter, and H. S. Margolis for the National Hepatitis A Investigation Team.** 1999. A multistate, foodborne outbreak of hepatitis A. *N. Engl. J. Med.* **340:**595–602.

81. **Hutin, Y. J. F., K. M. Sabin, L. C. Hutwanger, L. Schaben, G. M. Shipp, D. M. Lord, J. S. Conner, M. P. Quinlisk, C. N. Shapiro, and B. P. Bell.** 2000. Multiple modes of hepatitis A virus transmission among methamphetamine users. *Am. J. Epidemiol.* **152:**186–192.

82. **Innis, B. L., R. Snitbhan, P. Kunasol, T. Laorakpongse, W. Poopatanakool, C. A. Kozik, S. Suntayakorn, T. Suknuntapong, A. Safary, and D. B. Tang.** 1994. Protection against hepatitis A by an inactivated vaccine. *JAMA* **271:**1328–1334.

82a. **Jia, X. Y., E. Ehrenfeld, and D. F. Summers.** 1991. Proteolytic activity of hepatitis A virus 3C protein. *J. Virol.* **65:**2595–2600.

83. **Jia, X. Y., D. F. Summers, and E. Ehrenfeld.** 1993. Primary cleavage of the HAV capsid protein precursor in the middle of the proposed 2A coding region. *Virology* **193:** 515–519.

84. **Joines, R. W., M. Blatter, B. Abraham, F. Xie, N. De Clercq, Y. Baine, K. S. Reisinger, A. Kuhnen, and D. L. Parenti.** 2001. A prospective, randomized, comparative US trial of a combination hepatitis A and B vaccine (Twinrix®) with corresponding monovalent vaccines (Havrix® and Engerix-B®) in adults. *Vaccine* **19:**4710–4719.

85. **Kaplan, G., A. Totsuka, P. Thompson, T. Akatsuka, Y. Moritsugu, and S. M. Feinstone.** 1996. Identification of a surface glycoprotein on African green monkey kidney cells as a receptor for hepatitis A virus. *EMBO J.* **15:** 4282–4296.

86. **Kemper, C. A., R. Haubrich, I. Frank, G. Dubin, C. Buscarino, J. A. McCutchan, and S. C. Deresinski for the California Collaborative Treatment Group.** 2003. Safety and immunogenicity of hepatitis A vaccine in human immunodeficiency virus-infected patients: a double-blind, randomized, placebo-controlled trial. *J. Infect. Dis.* **187:**1327–1331.

87. **Knöll, A., B. Hottenträger, J. Kainz, B. Bratschneider, and W. Jilg.** 2000. Immunogenicity of a combined hepatitis A and B vaccine in healthy young adults. *Vaccine* **18:**2029–2032.

88. **Konduru, K., and G. G. Kaplan.** 2006. Stable growth of wild-type hepatitis A virus in cell culture. *J. Virol.* **80:** 1352–1360.

89. **Koopmans, M., C. H. von Bonsdorff, J. Vinje, D. de Medici, and S. Monroe.** 2002. Foodborne viruses. *FEMS Microbiol. Rev.* **26:**187–205.

90. **Krugman, S., J. P. Giles, and J. Hammond.** 1967. Infectious hepatitis: evidence for two distinctive clinical, epidemiological, and immunological types of infection. *JAMA* **200:**365–373.

91. **Lednar, W. M., S. M. Lemon, J. W. Kirkpatrick, R. R. Redfield, M. L. Fields, and P. W. Kelley.** 1985. Frequency of illness associated with epidemic hepatitis A virus infection in adults. *Am. J. Epidemiol.* **122:**226–233.

92. **Lemon, S. M., P. C. Murphy, P. A. Shields, L. H. Ping, S. M. Feinstone, T. Cromeans, and R. W. Jansen.** 1991. Antigenic and genetic variation in cytopathic hepatitis A virus variants arising during persistent infection: evidence for genetic recombination. *J. Virol.* **65:**2056–2065.

93. **Lemon, S. M., P. C. Murphy, A. Smith, J. Zou, J. Hammon, S. Robinson, and B. Horowitz.** 1994. Removal/neutralization of hepatitis A virus during manufacture of high purity, solvent/detergent factor VIII concentrate. *J. Med. Virol.* **43:**44–49.

94. **Lemon, S. M., R. W. Jansen, and E. A. Brown.** 1992. Genetic, antigenic and biological differences between strains of hepatitis A virus. *Vaccine* **10:**S40–S44.

95. **Lemon, S. M., R. W. Jansen, and J. E. Newbold.** 1985. Infectious hepatitis A virus particles produced in cell culture consist of three distinct types with different buoyant densities in CsCl. *J. Virol.* **54:**78–85.

96. **Lemon, S. M., P. C. Murphy, P. J. Provost, I. Chalikonda, J. P. Davide, T. L. Schofield, D. R. Nalin, and J. A. Lewis.** 1997. Immunoprecipitation and virus neutralization assays demonstrate qualitative differences between protective antibody responses to inactivated hepatitis A vaccine and passive immunization with immune globulin. *J. Infect. Dis.* **176:**9–19.

97. **Lemon, S. M., and C. N. Shapiro.** 1994. The value of immunization against hepatitis A. *Infect. Agents Dis.* **3:** 38–49.

98. **Lemon, S. M., and D. L. Thomas.** 1997. Vaccines to prevent viral hepatitis. *N. Engl. J. Med.* **336:**196–204.

99. **Lerman, Y., G. Chodick, H. Aloni, J. Ribak, and S. Ashkenazi.** 1999. Occupations at increased risk of hepatitis A: a 2-year nationwide historical prospective study. *Am. J. Epidemiol.* **150:**312–320.

100. **Lerman, Y., T. Shohat, S. Ashkenazi, R. Almog, S. L. Heering, and J. Shemer.** 1993. Efficacy of different doses of immune serum globulin in the prevention of hepatitis A: a three-year prospective study. *Clin. Infect. Dis.* **17:** 411–414.

101. **Letson, G. W., C. N. Shapiro, D. Kuehn, C. Gardea, T. K. Welty, D. S. Krause, S. B. Lambert, and H. S. Margolis.** 2004. Effect of maternal antibody on immunogenicity of hepatitis A vaccine in infants. *J. Pediatr.* **144:**327–332.

102. **Mannucci, P. M., S. Gdovin, A. Gringeri, M. Colombo, A. Mele, N. Schinaia, N. Ciavarella, S. U. Emerson, R. H. Purcell, and the Italian Collaborative Group.** 1994. Transmission of hepatitis A to patients with hemophilia by factor VIII concentrates treated with organic solvent and detergent to inactivate viruses. *Ann. Intern. Med.* **120:**1–7.

103. **Mao, J. S., S. A. Chai, R. Y. Xie, N. L. Chen, Q. Jiang, X. Z. Zhu, S. Y. Zhang, H. Y. Huang, H. W. Mao, X. N. Bao, and C. J. Liu.** 1997. Further evaluation of the safety and protective efficacy of live attenuated hepatitis A vaccine (H2-strain) in humans. *Vaccine* **15:**944–947.

104. **Margolis, H. S., and Nainan, O. V.** 1990. Identification of virus components in circulating immune complexes isolated during hepatitis A virus infection. *Hepatology* **11:**31–37.

105. **Martin, A., D. Bénichou, S. F. Chao, L. M. Cohen, and S. M. Lemon.** 1999. Maturation of the hepatitis A virus capsid protein VP1 is not dependent on processing by the $3C^{pro}$ proteinase. *J. Virol.* **73:**6220–6227.

106. **Martin, A., N. Escriou, S. F. Chao, M. Girard, S. M. Lemon, and C. Wychowski.** 1995. Identification and site-directed mutagenesis of the primary (2A/2B) cleavage site of the hepatitis A virus polyprotein: functional impact on the infectivity of HAV RNA transcripts. *Virology* **213:**213–222.

107. **Martin, A., and S. M. Lemon.** 2002. The molecular biology of hepatitis A virus, p. 23–50. *In* J.-H. Ou (ed.), *Hepatitis Viruses.* Kluwer Academic Publishers, Norwell, MA.

108. **Masada, C. T., B. W. Shaw, Jr., R. K. Zetterman, S. S. Kaufman, and R. S. Markin.** 1993. Fulminant hepatic failure with massive necrosis as a result of hepatitis A infection. *J. Clin. Gastroenterol.* **17:**158–162.

109. **Mathiesen, L. R., J. Drucker, D. Lorenz, J. A. Wagner, R. J. Gerety, and R. H. Purcell.** 1978. Localization of hepatitis A antigen in marmoset organs during acute in-

fection with hepatitis A virus. *J. Infect. Dis.* **138:**369–377.

110. **Mbithi, J. N., V. S. Springthorpe, and S. A. Sattar.** 1990. Chemical disinfection of hepatitis A virus on environmental surfaces. *Appl. Environ. Microbiol.* **56:**3601–3604.
111. **McIntire, J. J., D. T. Umetsu, and R. H. DeKruyff.** 2004. TIM-1, a novel allergy and asthma susceptibility gene. *Springer Semin. Immunopathol.* **25:**335–348.
112. **Merck & Co., Inc.** 2001. VAQTA®. Package insert. Merck & Co., Inc., Whitehouse Station, NJ.
113. **Mosley, J. W., D. M. Reisler, D. Brachott, D. Roth, and J. Weiser.** 1968. Comparison of two lots of immune serum globulin for prophylaxis of infectious hepatitis. *Am. J. Epidemiol.* **87:**539–550.
114. **Nainan, O. V., G. L. Armstrong, X. H. Han, I. Williams, B. P. Bell, and H. S. Margolis.** 2005. Hepatitis A molecular epidemiology in the United States, 1996–1997: sources of infection and implications of vaccination policy. *J. Infect. Dis.* **191:**957–963.
115. **Nainan, O. V., H. S. Margolis, B. H. Robertson, M. Balayan, and M. A. Brinton.** 1991. Sequence analysis of a new hepatitis A virus naturally infecting cynomolgus macaques (Macaca fascicularis). *J. Gen. Virol.* **72:**1685–1689.
116. **Nainan, O. V., G. Xia, G. Vaughn, and H. S. Margolis.** 2006. Diagnosis of hepatitis A virus: a molecular approach. *Clin. Microbiol. Rev.* **19:**63–79.
117. **Najarian, R., D. Caput, W. Gee, S. J. Potter, A. Renard, J. Merryweather, G. Van Nest, and D. Dina.** 1985. Primary structure and gene organization of human hepatitis A virus. *Proc. Natl. Acad. Sci. USA* **82:**2627–2631.
118. **Noble, R. C., M. A. Kane, S. A. Reeves, and I. Roeckel.** 1984. Posttransfusion hepatitis A in a neonatal intensive care unit. *JAMA* **252:**2711–2715.
119. **O'Grady, J.** 1992. Management of acute and fulminant hepatitis A. *Vaccine* **10**(Suppl. 1):S21.
120. **Okuno,T., A. Sano, T. Deguchi, Y. Katsuma, T. Ogasawara, T. Okanoue, and T. Takino.** 1984. Pathology of acute hepatitis A in humans. Comparison with acute hepatitis B. *Am. J. Clin. Pathol.* **81:**162–169.
121. **Parry, J. V., and P. P. Mortimer.** 1984. The heat sensitivity of hepatitis A virus determined by a simple tissue culture method. *J. Med. Virol.* **14:**277–283.
122. **Paul, A. V., H. Tada, K. von der Helm, T. Wissel, R. Kiehn, E. Wimmer, and F. Deinhardt.** 1987. The entire nucleotide sequence of the genome of human hepatitis A virus (isolate MBB). *Virus Res.* **8:**153–171.
123. **Paul, A. V., J. H. van Boom, D. Filippov, and E. Wimmer.** 1998. Protein-primed RNA synthesis by purified poliovirus RNA polymerase. *Nature* **393:**280–284.
124. **Peterson, D. A., T. R. Hurley, J. C. Hoff, and L. G. Wolfe.** 1983. Effect of chlorine treatment on infectivity of hepatitis A virus. *Appl. Environ. Microbiol.* **45:**223–227.
125. **Ping, L. H., and S. M. Lemon.** 1992. Antigenic structure of human hepatitis A virus defined by analysis of escape mutants selected against murine monoclonal antibodies. *J. Virol.* **66:**2208–2216.
126. **Probst, C., M. Jecht, and V. Gauss-Muller.** 1999. Intrinsic signals for the assembly of hepatitis A virus particles. Role of structural proteins VP4 and 2A. *J. Biol. Chem.* **274:**4527–4531.
127. **Provost, P. J., F. S. Banker, P. A. Giesa, W. J. McAleer, E. B. Buynak, and M. R. Hilleman.** 1982. Progress toward a live, attenuated human hepatitis A vaccine. *Proc. Soc. Exp. Biol. Med.* **170:**8–14.
128. **Provost, P. J., and M. R. Hilleman.** 1979. Propagation of human hepatitis A virus in cell culture in vitro. *Proc. Soc. Exp. Biol. Med.* **160:**213–221.
129. **Purcell, R. H., S. M. Feinstone, J. R. Ticehurst, R. J. Daemer, and B. M. Baroudy.** 1984. Hepatitis A virus, p. 9–22. *In* G. N. Vyas, J. L. Dienstag, and J. H. Hoofnagle (ed.), *Viral Hepatitis and Liver Disease*. Grune & Stratton, Inc., Orlando, FL.
130. **Rimland, D., and J. L. Guest.** 2005. Response to hepatitis A vaccine in HIV patients in the HAART era. *AIDS* **19:**1702–1704.
131. **Robertson, B. H., R. W. Jansen, B. Khanna, A. Totsuka, O. V. Nainan, G. Siegl, A. Widell, H. Margolis, S. Isomura, K. Ito, T. Ishizu, Y. Moritsugu, and S. M. Lemon.** 1992. Genetic relatedness of hepatitis A virus strains recovered from different geographical regions. *J. Gen. Virol.* **73:**1365–1377.
132. **Robertson, B. H., F. Averhoff, T. L. Cromeans, X. Han, B. Khoprasert, O. V. Nainan, J. Rosenberg, L. Paikoff, E. DeBess, C. N. Shapiro, and H. S. Margolis.** 2000. Genetic relatedness of hepatitis A virus isolates during a community-wide outbreak. *J. Med. Virol.* **62:**144–150.
133. **Robertson, B. H., E. H. D'Hondt, J. Spelbring, H. Tian, K. Krawczynski, and H. S. Margolis.** 1994. Effect of postexposure vaccination in a chimpanzee model of hepatitis A virus infection. *J. Med. Virol.* **43:**249–251.
134. **Rosenblum, L. S., M. E. Villarino, O. V. Nainan, M. E. Melish, S. C. Hadler, P. P. Pinsky, W. R. Jarvis, C. E. Ott, and H. S. Margolis.** 1991. Hepatitis A outbreak in a neonatal intensive care unit: risk factors for transmission and evidence of prolonged viral excretion among preterm infants. *J. Infect. Dis.* **164:**476–482.
135. **Sagliocca, L., P. Amoroso, T. Stroffolini, B. Adamo, M. E. Tosti, G. Lettieri, C. Esposito, S. Buonocore, P. Pierri, and A. Mele.** 1999. Efficacy of hepatitis A vaccine in prevention of secondary hepatitis A infection: a randomized trial. *Lancet* **353:**1136–1139.
136. **Samandari, T., B. P. Bell, and G. L. Armstrong.** 2004. Quantifying the impact of hepatitis A immunization in the United States, 1995–2001. *Vaccine* **22:**4342–4350.
137. **Schiff, E. R.** 1992. Atypical clinical manifestations of hepatitis A. *Vaccine* **10**(Suppl. 1):S18–S20.
138. **Scholz, E., U. Heinricy, and B. Flehmig.** 1989. Acid stability of hepatitis A virus. *J. Gen. Virol.* **70**(Pt. 9)**:**2481–2485.
139. **Shimizu, Y. K., L. R. Mathiesen, D. Lorenz, J. Drucker, S. M. Feinstone, J. A. Wagner, and R. H. Purcell.** 1978. Localization of hepatitis A antigen in liver tissue by peroxidase-conjugated antibody method: light and electron microscopic studies. *J. Immunol.* **121:**1671–1679.
140. **Siegl, G., J. deChastonay, and G. Kronauer.** 1984. Propagation and assay of hepatitis A virus in vitro. *J. Virol. Methods* **9:**53–67.
141. **Siegl, G., G. G. Frosner, V. Gauss-Muller, J. D. Tratschin, and F. Deinhardt.** 1981. The physicochemical properties of infectious hepatitis A virions. *J. Gen. Virol.* **57:**331–341.
142. **Siegl, G., M. Weitz, and G. Kronauer.** 1984. Stability of hepatitis A virus. *Intervirology* **22:**218–226.
143. **Silberstein, E., L. Xing, W. van de Beek, J. Lu, H. Cheng, and G. G. Kaplan.** 2003. Alteration of hepatitis A virus (HAV) particles by a soluble form of HAV cellular receptor 1 containing the immunoglobin- and mucin-like regions. *J. Virol.* **77:**8765–8774.
144. **Sjogren, M. H., H. Tanno, O. Fay, S. Sileoni, B. D. Cohen, D. S. Burke, and R. J. Feighny.** 1987. Hepatitis

A virus in stool during clinical relapse. *Ann. Intern. Med.* **106:**221–226.

145. **Soucie, J. M., B. H. Robertson, B. P. Bell, K. A. McCaustland, and B. L. Evatt.** 1998. Hepatitis A virus infections associated with clotting factor concentrate in the United States. *Transfusion* **38:**573–579.
146. **Stanway, G., F. Brown, P. Christian, T. Hovi, T. Hyypiä, A. M. Q. King, N. J. Knowles, S. M. Lemon, P. D. Minor, M. A. Pallansch, A. C. Palmenberg, and T. Skern.** 2005. Family *Picornaviridae*, p. 757–778. *In* C. M. Fauquet, M. A. Mayo, J. Maniloff, U. Desselberger, and L. A. Ball (ed.), *Virus Taxonomy. Eighth Report of the International Committee on Taxonomy of Viruses*. Elsevier /Academic Press, San Diego, CA.
147. **Stapleton, J. T., R. Jansen, and S. M. Lemon.** 1985. Neutralizing antibody to hepatitis A virus in immune serum globulin and in the sera of human recipients of immune serum globulin. *Gastroenterology* **89:** 637–642.
148. **Stapleton, J. T., D. K. Lange, J. W. LeDuc, L. N. Binn, R. W. Jansen, and S. M. Lemon.** 1991. The role of secretory immunity in hepatitis A virus infection. *J. Infect. Dis.* **163:**7–11.
149. **Stapleton, J. T., and S. M. Lemon.** 1987. Neutralization escape mutants define a dominant immunogenic neutralization site on hepatitis A virus. *J. Virol.* **61:** 491–498.
150. **Steffen, R., M. A. Kane, C. N. Shapiro, N. Billo, K. J. Schoellhorn, and P. van Damme.** 1994. Epidemiology and prevention of hepatitis A in travelers. *JAMA* **272:** 885–889.
151. **Tami, C., E. Silberstein, M. Manangeeswaran, G. J. Freeman, S. E. Umetsu, R. H. DeKruyff, D. T. Umetsu, and G. G. Kaplan.** 2007. Immunoglobulin A (IgA) is a natural ligand of hepatitis A virus cellular receptor 1 (HAVCR1), and the association of IgA with HAVCR1 enhances virus-receptor interactions. *J. Virol.* **81:**3437–3446.
152. **Tassopoulos, N. C., G. J. Papaevangelou, J. R. Ticehurst, and R. H. Purcell.** 1986. Fecal excretion of Greek strains of hepatitis A virus in patients with hepatitis A and in experimentally infected chimpanzees. *J. Infect. Dis.* **154:**231–237.
153. **Tesar, M., S. A. Harmon, D. F. Summers, and E. Ehrenfeld.** 1992. Hepatitis A virus polyprotein synthesis initiates from two alternative AUG codons. *Virology* **186:**609–618.
154. **Tesar, M., X. Y. Jia, D. F. Summers, and E. Ehrenfeld.** 1993. Analysis of a potential myristoylation site in hepatitis A virus capsid protein VP4. *Virology* **194:**616–626.
155. **Teterina, N. L., K. Bienz, D. Egger, A. E. Gorbalenya, and E. Ehrenfeld.** 1997. Induction of intracellular membrane rearrangements by HAV proteins 2C and 2BC. *Virology* **237:**66–77.
156. **Ticehurst, J. R., V. R. Racaniello, B. M. Baroudy, D. Baltimore, R. H. Purcell, and S. M. Feinstone.** 1983. Molecular cloning and characterization of hepatitis A virus cDNA. *Proc. Natl. Acad. Sci. USA* **80:** 5885–5889.
157. **Trout, D., C. Mueller, L. Venczel, and A. Krake.** 2000. Evaluation of occupational transmission of hepatitis A virus among wastewater workers. *J. Occup. Environ. Med.* **42:**83–88.
158. **Tsarev, S. A., S. U. Emerson, M. S. Balayan, J. Ticehurst, and R. H. Purcell.** 1991. Simian hepatitis A virus (HAV) strain AGM-27: comparison of genome structure and growth in cell culture with other HAV strains. *J. Gen. Virol.* **72:**1677–1683.
159. **Vallbracht, A., and B. Fleischer.** 1992. Immune pathogenesis of hepatitis A. *Arch. Virol. Suppl.* **4:**3–4.
160. **Van Damme, P., J. Banatvala, O. Fay, S. Iwarson, B. McMahon, K. Van Herck, D. Shouval, P. Bonanni, B. Connor, G. Cooksley, G. Leroux-Roels, F. Von Sonnenburg, and the International Consensus Group on Hepatitis A Virus Immunity.** 2003. Hepatitis A booster vaccination: is there a need? *Lancet* **362:**1065–1071.
161. **Van Effelterre, T. P., T. K. Zink, B. J. Hoet, W. P. Hausdorff, and P. Rosenthal.** 2006. A mathematical model of hepatitis A transmission in the United States indicates value of universal childhood immunization. *Clin. Infect. Dis.* **43:**158–164.
162. **Van Herck, K., P. Van Damme, I. Dieussaert, and M. Stoffel.** 2004. Antibody persistence 10 years after immunization with a two-dose inactivated hepatitis A vaccine. *Int. J. Infect. Dis.* 8(Suppl. 1):S225 (Abstract.)
163. **Victor, J. C., A. S. Monto, T. Y. Surdina, S. Z. Suleimenova, G. Vaughan, O. V. Nainan, M. O. Favorov, H. S. Margolis, and B. P. Bell.** 2007. Hepatitis A vaccine versus immune globulin for postexposure prophylaxis. *N. Engl. J. Med.* **357:**1685–1694.
164. **Villano, S. A., K. E. Nelson, D. Vlahov, R. H. Purcell, A. J. Saah, and D. L. Thomas.** 1997. Hepatitis A among homosexual men and injection drug users: more evidence for vaccination. *Clin. Infect. Dis.* **25:**726–728.
165. **Wallace, M. R., C. J. Brandt, K. C. Earhart, B. J. Kuter, A. D. Grosso, H. Lakkis, and S. A. Tasker.** 2004. Safety and immunogenicity of an inactivated hepatitis A vaccine among HIV-infected subjects. *Clin. Infect. Dis.* **39:**1207–1213.
166. **Wasley, A., T. Samandari, and B. P. Bell.** 2005. Incidence of hepatitis A in the United States in the era of vaccination. *JAMA* **294:**194–201.
167. **Weinberg, M., J. Hopkins, L. Farrington, L. Gresham, M. Ginsberg, and B. P. Bell.** 2004. Hepatitis A in Hispanic children who live along the United States-Mexico border: the role of international travel and food-borne exposures. *Pediatrics* **114:**68–73.
168. **Weitz, M., B. M. Baroudy, W. L. Maloy, J. R. Ticehurst, and R. H. Purcell.** 1986. Detection of a genome-linked protein (VPg) of hepatitis A virus and its comparison with other picornaviral VPgs. *J. Virol.* **60:** 124–130.
169. **Werzberger, A., B. Kuter, and D. Nalin.** 1998. Six years' follow-up after hepatitis A vaccination. *N. Engl. J. Med.* **338:**1160. (Letter.)
170. **Werzberger, A., B. Mensch, B. Kuter, L. Brown, J. Lewis, R. Sitrin, W. Miller, D. Shouval, B. Wiens, and G. Calandra.** 1992. A controlled trial of a formalin-inactivated hepatitis A vaccine in healthy children. *N. Engl. J. Med.* **327:**453–457.
171. **Wiedmann, M., S. Boehm, W. Schumacher, C. Swysen, and M. Zauke.** 2003. Evaluation of three commercial assays for detection of hepatitis A virus. *Eur. J. Clin. Microbiol. Infect. Dis.* **22:**129–130.
172. **Winokur, P. L., and J. T. Stapleton.** 1992. Immunoglobulin prophylaxis for hepatitis A. *Clin. Infect. Dis.* **14:**580–586.
173. **Yang, Y., Y. Liang, L. Qu, Z. Chen, M. Yi, K. Li, and S. M. Lemon.** 2007. Disruption of innate immunity due to mitochondrial targeting of a picornaviral protease precursor. *Proc. Natl. Acad. Sci. USA* **104:**7253–7258.
174. **Yao, G.** 1991. Clinical spectrum and natural history of viral hepatitis A in a 1988 Shanghai epidemic, p. 76–78. *In* F. B. Hollinger, S. M. Lemon, and H. S. Margolis

(ed.), *Viral Hepatitis and Liver Disease*. Williams and Wilkins, Baltimore, MD.

175. **Yi, M., and S. M. Lemon.** 2002. Replication of subgenomic hepatitis A virus RNAs expressing firefly luciferase is enhanced by mutations associated with adaptation of virus to growth in cultured cells. *J. Virol.* **76:**1171–1180.

176. **Zhang, R. L., J. S. Zeng, and H. Z. Zhang.** 1990. Survey of 34 pregnant women with hepatitis A and their neonates. *Chin. Med. J. (Engl. Ed.)* **103:**552–555.

177. **Zuckerman, A. J.** 1983. The history of viral hepatitis from antiquity to the present, p. 3–32. *In* F. Deinhardt and J. Deinhardt (ed.), *Viral Hepatitis: Laboratory and Clinical Science*. Marcel Dekker, New York, NY.

Human Caliciviruses

ROBERT L. ATMAR AND MARY K. ESTES

48

Norwalk virus (NV) was first recognized from an outbreak of epidemic gastroenteritis in an elementary school in Norwalk, Ohio, in 1968, in which 50% of the students and teachers became ill and secondary cases occurred in 32% of family contacts (1). Subsequently, NV was visualized using immunoelectron microscopy (IEM) and described as a 27-nm filterable agent (57). This provided definitive proof that viruses cause diarrhea, an idea initially proposed during the 1940s and 1950s when a filterable infectious agent (although not cultured in cell culture) was passaged serially in volunteers. The first clear description of the basic virologic, clinical, and immunologic responses to nonbacterial infections came from studies in volunteers administered a bacterium-free fecal filtrate of NV (20) (see below). The history of these early investigations leading to visualization of the agent by IEM provides an excellent example of how major scientific advances often require and parallel new technological opportunities (33). The subsequent application of IEM to other diarrheal stool samples ultimately led to the discovery of other viral agents of gastroenteritis (see chapters 4, 26, 35, and 50).

VIROLOGY

Classification

Although the first report of the visualization of NV was in 1972, NV was not classified until 1990. Classification required the successful cloning of the viral genome because, even today, NV and related agents remain noncultivatable in cell culture. Molecular cloning and characterization of the NV genome allowed this virus to be classified as a member of the family *Caliciviridae* (48). Caliciviruses are nonenveloped, icosahedral particles containing a single-stranded RNA of positive polarity, approximately 7.7 kb in size. The name calicivirus, from the Latin *calyx* meaning "cup" or "goblet," describes the cup-shaped depressions observed by electron microscopy (EM) (Fig. 1). Although structural studies confirm that NV contains cup-shaped depressions, these depressions are often clearer in other strains of animal caliciviruses and human caliciviruses (HuCVs) (Fig. 1).

There are four genera currently recognized within the *Caliciviridae* family (67). Two of these genera (*Norovirus* and *Sapovirus*) contain human and a few animal strains, while the other two genera, *Vesivirus* (e.g., vesicular exanthem virus of swine, feline calicivirus, and San Miguel sea lion virus) and *Lagovirus* (e.g., rabbit hemorrhagic disease virus and European brown hare syndrome virus), contain only animal strains. The bovine enteric calicivirus, strain NB, belongs to a possible fifth, currently unassigned, genus. Classification of NV as a calicivirus based on its genomic characteristics replaces a previous interim classification in which these and other small fecal viruses were classified morphologically according to whether they contained visible structural features. In this morphological system, two groups of human viruses that contain members of the *Caliciviridae* family were recognized: the classical (or morphologically typical) caliciviruses and the small round structured viruses (SRSVs). NV was the prototype SRSV strain. Although most morphologically typical caliciviruses have been found to be sapoviruses (SaVs) and most SRSVs have been identified as noroviruses (NoVs), a few morphologically typical caliciviruses have been found to be NoVs. Thus, correct classification requires obtaining sequence information. Although electron microscopists in diagnostic laboratories may continue to use the morphological appearance as a tentative classification system, other rapid diagnostic assays to detect HuCVs are available (see below).

Serotypes and Antigenicity

NoV and SaV serotypes are not yet defined due to the lack of any cultivation systems. However, based on cross-challenge studies in volunteers and some comparisons of different prototype particles by IEM and enzyme-linked immunosorbent assay (ELISA), an initial proposal (before classification into genera) identified at least five serotypes, represented by NV, Hawaii agent (HV), Snow Mountain agent (SMA), the Taunton agent, and Sapporo virus (SV). Subsequently, additional antigenic groups were proposed based on IEM studies. These serotype designations assume that antibody reactivity by IEM reflects reactivity of antibody with neutralization epitopes on the surfaces of particles. However, some polyclonal and monoclonal antibodies that bind virus do not block virus binding to cells (129). The antigenic relationships between a subset of these viruses have been evaluated in ELISAs using hyperimmune antisera generated against recombinant virus-like particles (VLPs). Although only limited comparisons

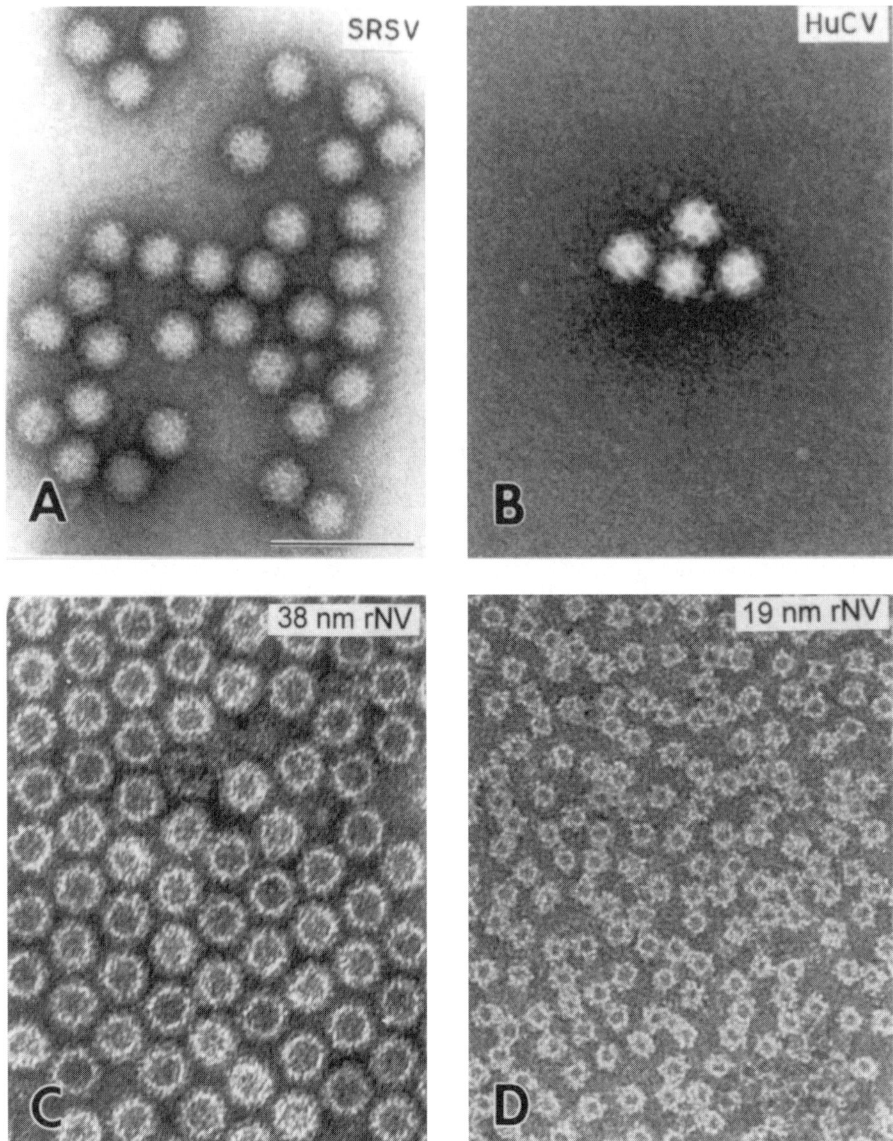

FIGURE 1 Electron micrographs of caliciviruses. Negative-stain electron micrographs of an NoV (previously called SRSV) from the stool of a volunteer given NoV/NV/8fIIa (A); an SaV with the classical calicivirus morphological features, including distinct cup-like indentations in the surface of the particles, taken from the stool of a child and containing SaV/Sapporo (B); 38-nm rNV particles produced and purified from insect cells infected with a baculovirus recombinant that expresses NV ORF2 (C); and 19-nm particles produced and purified from insect cells infected with a baculovirus recombinant that expresses NV ORF2 (D). Bar, 50 nm. (Panel D kindly provided by L. White.)

have been performed to date, viruses belonging to distinct genotypes (see below) are antigenically distinct from strains belonging to other genotypes for both NoVs (77) and SaVs (40).

Genogroups and Genotypes

The availability of the first NoV nucleotide sequence opened a new era in the characterization of HuCVs, including the agents previously characterized as SRSVs. Primers were designed to amplify viral sequences from clinical samples, and numerous different strains were identified (127). Eventually, the complete sequences of several HuCV strains were reported, and phylogenetic analyses of these and other virus strains allowed the classification of a virus strain into the genus *Norovirus* or *Sapovirus* (33).

Strains within a genus can be further subdivided based upon phylogenetic analysis of the polymerase region, the capsid region, or the third open reading frame (ORF3). Such analyses have allowed the subdivision of NoVs and SaVs into five genogroups each and virus strains in both genera into different genotypes (Table 1). Criteria for the separation of NoVs into genogroups and further into genotypes have been proposed based upon the complete amino acid sequence of the major structural protein, VP1 (134).

TABLE 1 Prototype strains of *Norovirus* and *Sapovirus* by genogroups and genotypes[a]

Norovirus genogroup and genotype	Prototype strain	*Sapovirus* genogroup and genotype	Prototype strain
I.1	Hu/NoV/Norwalk/1968/US	I.1	Hu/SaV/Sapporo/1982/JP
I.2	Hu/NoV/Southampton/1991/UK	I.2	Hu/SaV/Parkville/1994/US
I.3	Hu/NoV/Desert Shield 395/1990/SA	I.3	Hu/SaV/Stockholm 318/1997/SE
I.4	Hu/NoV/Chiba 407/1987/JP		
I.5	Hu/NoV/Musgrove/1989/UK	II.1	Hu/SaV/London/1992/UK
I.6	Hu/NoV/Hesse/1997/DE	II.2	Hu/SaV/Mex340/1990/MX
I.7	Hu/NoV/Winchester/1994/UK	II.3	Hu/SaV/Cruise ship/2000/US
I.8	Hu/NoV/Boxer/2001/US		
		III.1	Sw/SaV/PEC-Cowden/1980/US
II.1	Hu/NoV/Hawaii/1971/US		
II.2	Hu/NoV/Melksham/1994/UK	IV.1	Hu/SaV/Hou7-1181/1990/US
II.3	Hu/NoV/Toronto 24/1991/CA		
II.4	Hu/NoV/Bristol/1993/UK	V.1	Hu/SaV/Arg39/AR
II.5	Hu/NoV/Hillingdon/1990/UK		
II.6	Hu/NoV/Seacroft/1990/UK		
II.7	Hu/NoV/Leeds/1990/UK		
II.8	Hu/NoV/Amsterdam/1998/NL		
II.9	Hu/NoV/VA97207/1997/US		
II.10	Hu/NoV/Erfurt 546/2000/DE		
II.11	Sw/NoV/Sw918/1997/JP		
II.12	Hu/NoV/Wortley/1990/UK		
II.13	Hu/NoV/Fayetteville/1998/US		
II.14	Hu/NoV/M7/1999/US		
II.15	Hu/NoV/J23/1999/US		
II.16	Hu/NoV/Tiffin/1999/US		
II.17	Hu/NoV/CS-E1/2002/US		
II.18	Sw/NoV/OH-QW101/2003/US		
II.19	Sw/NoV/OH-QW170/2003/US		
III.1	Bo/NoV/Jena/1980/DE		
III.2	Bo/NoV/CH126/1998/NL		
IV.1	Hu/NoV/Alphatron/1998/NL		
IV.2	Lion/NoV/387/2006/IT		
V.1	Mu/NoV/MNV-1/2003/US		

[a] See references 84, 128, and 134.

Strains within a genotype and within a genogroup would have <15 and <45% pairwise differences, respectively, in the complete VP1 amino acid sequences analyzed by the uncorrected-distance method. A similar method has been used for SaVs, although the degree of genetic diversity is lower (28). In general, similar phylogenetic relationships have been obtained when either the polymerase or capsid region of the genome was analyzed (124). Discordant results are being noted increasingly within a genogroup due to recombination occurring between two NoV strains (7). Recombination occurs among both NoVs and SaVs, most commonly near the start of the VP1 gene, and is likely a common mechanism by which new strains are generated (5, 7, 41).

Recombinant VLPs have been used to characterize serologic immune responses of individuals involved in outbreaks of NoV infection (96). The likelihood of detecting a serologic response is greater when the antigen used is derived from a virus in the same genotype, but there are not enough data available at this time to determine the significance (in terms of biological or type differences) of a genotype. For example, patients infected with genogroup I viruses from genotypes distinct from NV (GI.1) show seroresponses to NV VLPs similar to those seen when the infecting strain is from the NV genotype. In contrast, patients infected with genogroup II viruses have such "homologous" responses to Toronto virus (GII.3) and HV (GII.1) VLPs only when the infecting strain is in the genotype from which the test antigen strain was derived (96).

Viruses with similar antigenic reactivities have been identified at different times and geographic locations. Viruses antigenically similar to the prototype viruses are still circulating, and these strains show relatively good conservation of amino acid sequences over long periods (127). Analysis of the amino acid sequences of the major capsid proteins of GII.4 strains identified over a 15-year period found that changes preferentially accumulated in the outer portion of the capsid protein (the P domain; see below) (117). Phylogenetic analysis of these viral sequences found a chronological pattern in the emergence of new viral strains, and combined with the observed patterns of epidemic disease raised the possibility that immunity in the human population drives genetic drift and the evolution of noroviruses (116, 117).

Composition

Virion Morphology, Structure, and Size

NV originally was described as a 27-nm particle based on analysis of particles obtained from stools that were aggregated with antibody (57). Structural analysis of particles from stool is limited by the necessity to perform IEM due to the low numbers of particles present in most samples. Based on such micrographs, NV appeared to have a feathery outer edge that lacked a definitive surface substructure (Fig. 1A); in certain orientations, NV has minor surface indentations.

A more precise description of the structure of NV is now available based on the analysis of recombinant NV (rNV) particles produced in insect cells infected with a baculovirus recombinant expressing the cDNA that encodes the capsid proteins (Fig. 1C and Color Plate 54) (53). The NV capsid is composed of 180 copies of a major polypeptide (VP1) that folds to produce the capsid structure and a few (<5) copies of another polypeptide (VP2) (30). By negative-stain EM, rNV particles have a morphology similar to that of the native NV (Fig. 1). The rNV particles have a distinct architecture and exhibit T=3 icosahedral symmetry (Color Plate 54) (106). The major capsid protein folds into 90 dimers that form a shell domain from which arch-like capsomers protrude (Color Plate 54b to d). The crystallographic structure of rNV particles shows that the major capsid protein is folded into two domains, a shell domain and a protruding domain. The shell domain has a classical eight-stranded beta sandwich motif found in many viral capsid structures, and the amino acid sequence of this domain is the most conserved region of the capsid protein sequence (105). The arches are made from the protruding domain and are arranged in such a way that there are large hollows at the icosahedral five- and threefold positions (Color Plate 54b) which appear as cup-like structures in classical caliciviruses. The three-dimensional structures of other caliciviruses are quite similar to that of NV (14). The S domain serves as an icosahedral scaffold (Color Plate 54d). The P2 domain is an insert into the P1 domain, and it has the greatest sequence and structural variability in the protein. The protruding domain of the classical calicivirus is longer than that for NV, and the shape of the top of the arch also differs in such a way that the NV would show a feathery appearance by negative-stain EM.

These three-dimensional structures provide independent evidence of the similarities of distinct morphological types of caliciviruses. They also are tantalizing in providing structural information on which to speculate about where antigenic epitopes and the cellular attachment site in the virus capsid might be located. The greatest sequence variation in the major capsid protein is in the top of the protruding arch region, a region that could contain determinants of strain specificity (105). It is possible that the virus binds to a cellular receptor either by recognition sites on the top of the protruding arches or by the receptor fitting into the hollow of the cup-like depressions on the virus surface. Although not yet proven to be cellular receptors for NoVs, the type A and B trisaccharides bind by extensive hydrogen bonding to the outer portion of the P2 domain of a GII.4 NoV (9).

Preparations of NoV (rNV and recombinant Mexico virus [GII.3]) particles also contain smaller particles (~19 nm) (Fig. 1d) (50). These particles probably represent an alternative assembly of the single capsid protein, and they possess binding and antigenic properties similar to those of the larger particles. Such smaller empty particles also have been observed in stools of children infected with these viruses, but it is not known if these smaller particles have any distinct biological properties.

Genome Organization and Virus-Specific Proteins

The first sequence of the NV genome was obtained from sequencing cloned DNA (cDNA) from virus partially purified from stools obtained from volunteers (48, 86). The full-length genomic sequence is known for more than 20 NoV strains and several SaV strains. Partial sequences of hundreds of other NoVs and SaVs have also been determined.

Comparison of the genome organization of the two genera of HuCVs with the other two genera in the *Caliciviridae* reveals both similarities and differences. The genome is a positive-sense, polyadenylated, single-stranded RNA approximately 7.4 to 8.3 kb in length, excluding the 3′ polyadenylated tail (67). After a short noncoding region at the 5′ sequence, the genome of the NoVs is predicted to contain three ORFs, as shown in Fig. 2. The first (ORF1) and second (ORF2) ORF sequences overlap by a short, variable (14 to 17) number of nucleotides. ORF3 is in a separate reading frame from ORF2, overlapping ORF2 by one (or a few) nucleotide(s). SaVs have only two ORFs, with the genes included in NoV ORF1 and ORF2 being in the same ORF (ORF1) of the SaVs (Fig. 2).

The longest NoV ORF, ORF1, encodes a polyprotein precursor of nonstructural proteins based on the identification of sequences similar to the picornavirus nonstructural proteins (Table 2). In vitro translation of the ORF1 from Southampton virus (a GI.2 NoV) yields a polyprotein that is cotranslationally cleaved to give three major products: a 48-kDa N–terminal protein (NS1-2), a 41-kDa protein NTPase (NS3), and a 113-kDa protein that is homologous to the 3ABCD region of picornaviruses. The 113-kDa protein can be cleaved further into a 22-kDa protein (NS4), a 16-kDa protein (NS5, VPg), a 19-kDa protein (NS6, the 3C protease), and a 57-kDa protein (NS7, the RNA-dependent RNA polymerase). Similar findings have been noted when the ORF1 of a GII NoV (NoV/Camberwell 101922/1994/AU) virus) was expressed in COS cells using a simian virus 40-based expression vector (115). The structures of a GI.1 NoV protease and of a GII.4 polymerase have been solved and could serve as targets in future development of antiviral drugs (94, 133).

Proteins expressed from ORF1 are immunoreactive based on detection by human immune sera of a fusion protein expressed in a λgt11 library and immunoprecipitation of a 57-kDa protein expressed from ORF1 in insect cells (54, 86). These results indicate that infected individuals make antibodies to proteins other than the capsid protein, an observation that should be considered when interpreting early data on the antigenic relatedness of these viruses determined by radioimmunoassay (RIA) or ELISA using stool extracts as antigen and sera from adult volunteers.

The second ORF of NV encodes a protein of 530 amino acids (aa) with a calculated molecular weight of 56,571, similar in size to the viral capsid protein (Fig. 2). The NV ORF2 contains a conserved amino acid motif of PPG that also is found in the picornavirus capsid protein VP3 (86). Expression of ORF2 and ORF3 in insect cells infected with a baculovirus recombinant containing this gene and the expression of ORF2 alone in cell-free translation systems produce products similar in size to that observed for the

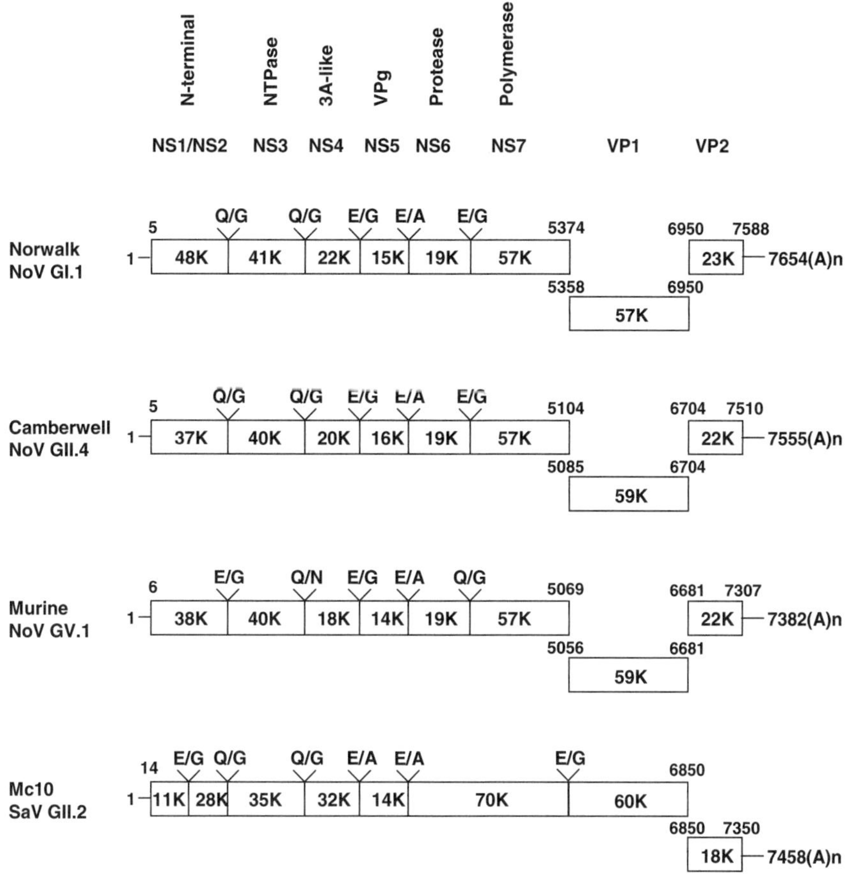

FIGURE 2 Genomic organization of NoVs and SaVs. Schematic of the genomic organization of two human genogroup I and II NoVs, the murine genogroup V NoV, and a human genogroup II SaV. The NoVs have three predicted ORFs: ORF1, which encodes a polyprotein that contains the nonstructural proteins NS1 to NS7; ORF2, which encodes the major capsid protein (VP1); and ORF3, which encodes a minor capsid protein (VP2). For SaVs, ORF1 is longer and contains VP1 (see text for details). Nucleotide numbers denoting ORFs are indicated for each of the viruses. Molecular weights of each of the viral proteins are also indicated. Among the NoVs, NS1 and NS2 form a single protein, and for the SaV strain indicated, NS6 and NS7 form a single protein. This information is compiled from GenBank sequences M87661 (NV), AF145896 (Camberwell), AY228235 (murine), and AY237420 (Mc10) and references 42, 97, 98, 115, and 118.

TABLE 2 HuCV structural and nonstructural proteins

Protein	Size (kDa)	ORF	Function	Comments
N-terminal (NS1/NS2)	37–41	ORF1	Unknown	NS1/NS2 is cleaved into two peptides in some NoV and SaV strains
NTPase (NS3)	40–41	ORF1	NTPase	Has sequence homology to RNA helicases
3A-like (NS4)	19–32	ORF1	Unknown	Location in ORF1 analogous to that of picornavirus 3A protein
VPg (NS5)	14–16	ORF1	VPg	Binds cellular initiation factors involved in protein synthesis
Protease (NS6)	13–19	ORF1	Cysteine protease	Mediates cleavage of ORF1-encoded polyprotein
Polymerase (NS7)	57	ORF1	RNA-dependent RNA polymerase	May also have protease and polymerase function as uncleaved precursor protein (NS6/NS7)
VP1	58–60	ORF2 (NoV) ORF1 (SaV)	Major structural protein	180 copies per virion, part of ORF1 in SaVs
VP2	12–29	ORF3 (NoV) ORF2 (SaV)	Minor structural protein	A few copies per virion of this basic protein

capsid protein of native NV particles, confirming that ORF2 encodes the capsid protein that self-assembles into VLPs (Fig. 1C).

A soluble viral antigen with a molecular weight of approximately 30,000 is excreted in the stools of volunteers infected with NV (86), and this antigen has been shown to result from the specific cleavage of the capsid protein (43). The amino terminus of the soluble protein detected in the stools of volunteers given NV is the same as that obtained following trypsin treatment of preparations of rNV particles (43). However, this cleavage product is made not from intact capsid protein but from soluble capsid protein, suggesting that the cleavage site is buried within intact particles. As predicted, the high-resolution structure shows that the cleavage site is buried in the hinge region between the protruding domain and shell domain. This indicates that this specific cleavage may not be important in activation of infectivity; it remains unknown if it affects the immunogenicity or pathogenicity of these viruses.

ORF3 is at the 3′ end of the genome. For NV, it encodes a small protein (212 aa) with a molecular mass of 22.5 kDa and a very basic charge (isoelectric point of 10.99). Sequences of ORF3 of other NoVs indicate that the protein encoded by this gene ranges from 211 to 268 aa. The NV ORF3 protein is a minor structural protein, being present in both native virions and VLPs expressed from a baculovirus recombinant containing both ORF2 and ORF3 (30). In native virions, the apparent molecular mass of the ORF3 protein was found to be 35 kDa. The higher molecular mass apparently results from phosphorylation of the ORF3 protein, based on the observation that the 35-kDa protein is lost following phosphatase treatment of baculovirus-expressed ORF3 recombinants (30). The role of the ORF3 protein is still unknown, although it may be involved in nucleic acid binding and encapsidation of the viral RNA (30).

The overall genomic organization of SaVs differs from that of NoVs, more closely resembling that of the animal calicivirus rabbit hemorrhagic disease virus. As noted earlier, the VP1 gene lies at the 3′ end of ORF1. In vitro translation experiments show that ORF1 of SaV/Mc10/2000/Thailand is cleaved into the same proteins as were described for NoVs, with the exception that the N-terminal protein is cleaved into two peptides, NS1 (11 kDa) and NS2 (28 kDa), and no cleavage of the protease and polymerase (NS6–7) occurs (97, 98). ORF2 is in frame −1 relative to ORF1 at the 3′ end of the genome, and it could encode a basic, hydrophilic protein that contains no cysteine residues and is analogous to ORF3 of the NoVs.

Biology

Norovirus Replication Strategy

Many human noroviruses bind to carbohydrate histo-blood group antigens (HBGAs) present on the surface of epithelial cells (82). There are strain-specific differences in NoV recognition of HBGAs, and for some NoVs, no HBGA to which the virus binds has been identified (45). The specific HBGA to which a NoV strain binds has been proposed to be a potential viral receptor based upon the lack of susceptibility to infection of persons who have genetic mutations that prevent the expression of the HBGA on the surface of the cell (46, 74, 121). So far, HBGAs have not been found to play a role in the binding of SaVs to epithelial cells (41).

The mechanism by which the virus enters the cell is not known. However, after entry, the NoV genomic RNA serves as an mRNA template from which the nonstructural proteins are produced. A subgenomic RNA containing ORF2 and ORF3 is produced during viral replication and serves as a template for production of the structural proteins, VP1 and VP2 (3). Besides the genomic RNA, a major species of subgenomic RNA (over 2 kb) has also been observed in stools of a volunteer infected with NV (54). The recent development of in vitro replication models (3, 59), and the availability of a murine NoV cell culture system (131), should lead to improved understanding of the replication strategies of these viruses.

Host Range and Animal Infection

Natural infections with HuCVs suggest that these viruses are species specific. Attempts to experimentally transmit NV and other HuCVs to a wide range of animals (chickens, mice, guinea pigs, rabbits, kittens, puppies, piglets, calves, baboons, and various monkey species) have largely been unsuccessful. Some rhesus monkeys and rabbits have seroconverted when fed HuCV, and a chimpanzee fed NV shed soluble antigen and responded serologically. More recently, replication of a human GII NoV strain has been successfully demonstrated in gnotobiotic piglets (13). Nevertheless, available data suggest that the host range specificity for HuCVs is narrow. Animal (porcine, bovine, and lion) strains have been noted in both the *Norovirus* and *Sapovirus* genera (33, 37, 75, 84), but it is not known whether these strains can be transmitted to humans. To date, no virus strain identified in a human has had the sequence of an animal NoV. The factors responsible for host restriction are not known at this time. Animal caliciviruses (vesiviruses and lagoviruses) have been noted to cause extraintestinal disease and to have a broad host range, being able to infect more than one species of animal. Additional human illnesses and cross-transmission between species may be discovered as the HuCVs become better characterized.

Growth in Cell Culture

The HuCVs have been refractory to cultivation in cell culture and in animal models. The propagation of NoVs has also been reported to occur in suspensions containing three-dimensional aggregates of human embryonic small intestinal cells (INT-407) (119), although earlier attempts to propagate NoVs in monolayers of this cell line failed (25). Confirmatory studies of this finding are still needed. A variety of cell lines (including human and animal cells) bind rNV particles, suggesting that host range specificity does not occur at the level of cell binding (129). In addition, NV RNA transfected into several of the mammalian cells that bind virus is infectious, producing viral particles (36). In a feline calicivirus infection model, both infection-permissive cells and nonpermissive cells can bind feline calicivirus, but infection-permissive cells bind the virus more efficiently than nonpermissive cells (68). The block to virus replication in the feline calicivirus-nonpermissive cell lines and for NV appears to be at a step in binding, internalization, or uncoating.

Inactivation by Physical and Chemical Agents

Studies of the stability of the HuCVs have been done by experimental infection of humans. Consistent with the fact that these agents are the most important cause of foodborne and waterborne disease, NV is resistant to inactivation following treatment with chlorine concentrations usually present in drinking water, and NV is more resistant to inactivation by chlorine than poliovirus 1, human rotavirus (Wa), simian rotavirus (SA11), or f2 bacteriophage (61). NV retains infectivity for volunteers following (i) exposure to pH 2.7 for 3 h at room temperature, (ii) treatment with 20% ether at 4°C for 24 h, or (iii) incubation at 60°C for 30 min (19). NoVs also have retained infectivity after freezing. Feline calicivirus, used as a surrogate calicivirus to study virus inactivation by different disinfectants, retains infectivity following exposure to ethanol, a detergent, or quarternary ammonium but is inactivated by glutaraldehyde, by an iodine-based disinfectant, and by 1,000 ppm of freshly reconstituted granular hypochlorite (22, 23). NoV-contaminated surfaces can be disinfected effectively using a combination of detergent and sodium hypochlorite (6).

EPIDEMIOLOGY

The cloning and expression of the NV genome resulted in the development of new assays and reagents that permit large-scale epidemiological studies. Epidemiological studies indicate that infection with NoVs is much more widespread than previously recognized (5, 27).

Geographic and Temporal Distribution

NoVs are the major causes of epidemic gastroenteritis in both developed and developing countries (5, 27). Epidemic viral gastroenteritis usually occurs in family- or community-wide outbreaks, affecting adults, school-age children, family contacts, and young children. Epidemic viral gastroenteritis is usually mild and self-limited, generally distinguishing it from infantile gastroenteritis caused by rotaviruses, which is generally a severe (often life-threatening) diarrheal illness in infants and young children. Infections by NoVs have been detected on all continents, and these viruses appear to have a worldwide distribution. Infections with NoVs occur year-round, although a distinct increase in occurrence of disease has been noted during cold-weather months (91).

Incidence and Prevalence of Infection

Specific incidence data for illness associated with NoVs and SaVs are not available for the United States. However, observations regarding the incidence of enteric illnesses of undefined etiology in family studies indicate that, on average, each family member experiences more than one such illness per year (89). In The Netherlands, NoVs were the most common cause of gastroenteritis in one population-based study, while they were seen with a frequency similar to that of rotavirus in subjects ill enough to present to a physician's office for care (17, 18). In the physician-based study, rotavirus infection was more common in patients less than 5 years of age, while NoVs were the most frequently detected virus in persons over 5 years of age. In Finland, NoVs were detected in 21% of the episodes of gastroenteritis in children under 2 years of age, making these viruses the second most commonly identified agent after rotavirus (100). NoVs also have been detected in patients with gastroenteritis in the developing world and are a common cause of traveler's diarrhea (5, 11, 64).

NV antibody seroprevalence was examined in relatively large studies performed in the 1970s using reagents from volunteers and an RIA or immune adherence hemagglutination assay (4). These studies indicated antibody to NV is acquired gradually, beginning slowly in childhood and accelerating in adult years, so that >50% of adults possess antibody to NV by age 50. Similar observations have been made in the United Kingdom, Japan, and Sweden using rNV capsid antigens, although a greater percentage of adults (89 to 98%) possessed antibody to NV. The higher detection rate for antibody likely reflects the greater sensitivity of the rNV antibody test (35). Other recombinant NoV and SaV capsid antigens have been used in seroprevalence studies in both developed and developing countries (4, 101). From these studies, several new observations have been made. NoV-specific antibody is transferred transplacentally, with up to 90% or more of newborns having measurable serum antibody (101). Antibody seroprevalence declines during the first 6 months of life, and then it rises progressively thereafter. Infection with NoVs can occur at a younger age (less than 1 year) than previously recognized.

A number of different NoV strains circulate in a community at any given time. During the epidemic period, strain diversity is greatest at the beginning of the season and declines as the season progresses (29). GI NoVs have been identified more commonly as causes of traveler's diarrhea and are also more commonly associated with shellfish-associated disease, while GII strains are most commonly associated with sporadic infection and outbreaks of gastroenteritis (5, 11, 64, 70). The reason for the observed differences between genogroups is not known, although NV (a GI NoV) has been shown to specifically bind to oyster tissues (69, 122). GI and GII NoVs may exhibit different stabilities under different environmental conditions.

Importance of NoVs and SaVs in Outbreaks of Gastroenteritis

Much of our understanding of the epidemiology of NoVs has come from studying the cause of outbreaks of water-borne and food-borne gastroenteritis. NoVs are now recognized as the most common cause of outbreaks of nonbacterial gastroenteritis in the United States, Europe, and Japan, with 60 to >90% of these outbreaks being associated with NoV infection (5). Outbreaks have occurred in recreational camps, cruise ships, communities, hospitals, schools (elementary or college), the military, nursing homes, and families. They have been associated with contaminated drinking water, swimming water, and consumption of uncooked or poorly cooked shellfish, ice, bakery products (frosting), various types of salads (potato, fruit, and tossed), and cold foods (celery, melon, vermicelli, consommé, sandwiches, and cold cooked ham) (113). Outbreaks can occur year-round and affect primarily school-aged children and adults.

Infections with SaVs were first detected among young children with gastroenteritis (81), although infections of adults and the elderly also occur. They have been associated with outbreaks in orphanages, day care centers, schools, and hospital wards (41). SaVs also have been associated with food-borne outbreaks, but much less frequently than NoVs (5).

Nosocomial infection with HuCVs may be quite common (110). Asymptomatic infections can occur (31, 85), and affected persons may be the source of some outbreaks. NoV infections occur in immunocompromised hosts, and prolonged (>1 year) symptomatic shedding has been described (95). A high rate of nosocomial infection has been associated with immunocompromised children (72). While

NoVs have been found in the stools of human immunodeficiency virus (HIV)-positive patients, its role in the etiology of gastroenteritis or infection in this group has not been reported to be greater than in non-HIV-infected controls (15, 109). Outbreaks have been associated with military personnel during field or shipboard maneuvers and with the elderly, often in nursing homes or hospital settings (34, 88, 110). These infections can be devastating because of high secondary attack rates leading to sustained chains of transmission, and such outbreaks can last several months. Repeated outbreaks on cruise ships have also occurred (47). Reinfections with the same agent can occur, as clearly demonstrated by the susceptibility of volunteers to infection and symptomatic or asymptomatic illness following multiple challenges with infectious virus (55, 103).

Since the mid-1990s, the GII.4 genotype has been the predominant cause of NoV outbreaks worldwide (79, 96). Symptomatic infection with these strains has been positively associated with secretor status (expression of the fucosyl transferase 2 [FUT2] gene) (62). Novel GII.4 variants emerged over the decade and caused epidemic disease (79, 117). Although the reason for the emergence of the new variants has not been determined, it is possible that the development of immunity in the population may drive the evolution of these viruses (116, 117).

Transmission

NV is highly infectious, and infections spread rapidly. In semiclosed communities or in volunteer studies, attack rates are high (>50% to as high as 90%) and patients present with explosive diarrhea and vomiting. There often is substantial spread to secondary contacts (>50% attack rate), and these characteristics may necessitate the closure and disinfection of hospital wards, cruise ships, or hotels (5, 12). Transmission occurs largely by the fecal-oral route, and exposure risks decrease as sanitary conditions improve and population density decreases. However, transmission by the fecal-oral route alone does not fully explain the rapid spread of these infections. Increasing evidence suggests that some outbreaks have been due to airborne or fomite transmission (12, 83). Proximity to persons suffering from projectile vomiting has been identified as a risk factor, and virus has been detected in vomitus.

An unresolved question related to transmission is the duration that an affected individual is infectious. The duration of symptomatic illness is 48 to 72 h. Monitoring of virus excretion by early IEM studies indicated that peak virus shedding occurs within 72 h, and shedding occurs in <50% of ill persons and does not persist beyond 100 h after the initial infection (120). Recent studies using more sensitive antigen detection and reverse transcriptase PCR (RT-PCR) assays have shown that NV excretion occurs in >90% of ill volunteers, shedding is detected in asymptomatic individuals, and antigen shedding starts earlier (15 h after infection and before symptomatic illness) and is more prolonged than previously thought, being detectable several weeks after infection (31, 92, 99). Correspondingly, epidemiological studies have identified transmission of NoVs in association with presymptomatic (76) and postsymptomatic (104) infection.

PATHOGENESIS

In volunteer studies with NV and SMA, the incubation periods ranged from 10 to 51 h and 19 to 41 h, respectively (21, 132). Illness usually lasted 24 to 48 h. The pathogenesis of NV illness has been examined in volunteer studies in adults from whom proximal intestinal biopsy samples were taken (2, 130). Histologic changes were seen in jejunal biopsy samples from ill volunteers (Fig. 3). Symptomatic illness was correlated with a broadening and blunting of the intestinal villi, crypt cell hyperplasia, cytoplasmic vacuolization, and infiltration of polymorphonuclear and mononuclear cells into the lamina propria, but the mucosa itself remained intact. Histologic changes were not seen in the gastric fundus, antrum, or colonic mucosa (130) or in convalescent-phase biopsy samples. The extent of small intestinal involvement remains unknown because studies have examined only the proximal small intestine, and the site of virus replication has not been determined. Clinical studies also showed that small intestinal brush border enzymatic activities (alkaline phosphatase, sucrase, and trehalase) were decreased, resulting in mild steatorrhea and transient carbohydrate malabsorption (2). Jejunal adenylate cyclase activity was not elevated (71), and gastric secretion of HCl, pepsin, and intrinsic factor was associated with these histologic changes. In contrast, gastric emptying was delayed (90). It has been suggested that reduced gastric motility may be responsible for the nausea and vomiting associated with this gastroenteritis.

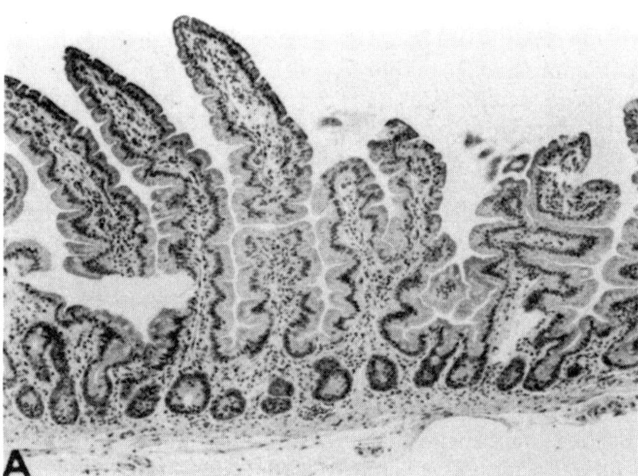

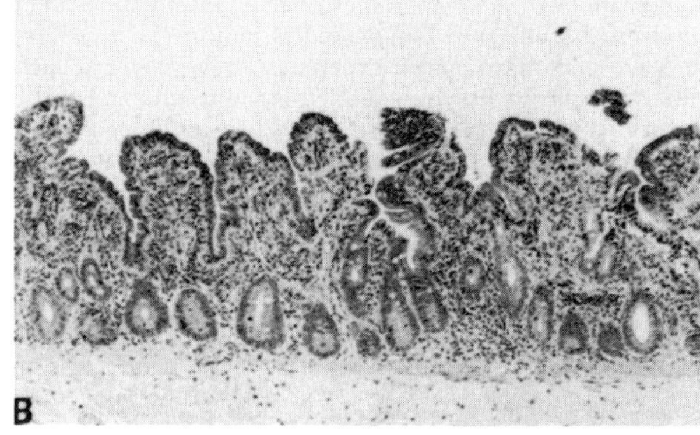

FIGURE 3 Histologic alterations observed in a volunteer after challenge with NV. Jejunal tissues from biopsy samples of a volunteer prior to challenge (A) and after challenge (B) with NV are shown. The villi are broadened and flattened during NV gastroenteritis illness. Hematoxylin and eosin stain; magnification × 62. (Reproduced from reference 2 with permission.)

Immune Responses

Limited studies of immunity have evaluated clinical resistance to infection or illness based upon the preinfection antibody status of volunteers administered NV (GI.1), SMA (GII.2), or HV (GII.1) and of individuals involved in outbreaks (19, 103, 132). These studies characterized the seroresponses of individuals who had various clinical outcomes following exposure to virus. The assays used for most analyses of immunity have been the first-generation tests such as IEM, RIAs, and ELISAs that used human reagents due to the inability to cultivate the NoVs. In vitro neutralization assays are not available. Therefore, analysis of immunity in volunteers is complicated by several factors, including the following: (i) the preinfection status of exposure to any of the NoV agents of the adult volunteer is not known, and (ii) neutralization assays with well-characterized cultivated viruses are not available. Due to these limitations, the results of available assays may reflect responses to common or shared nonneutralizing epitopes.

At least 50% of adult volunteers become ill following administration of NV, HV, or SMA. Short-term homologous immunity develops, based upon the results of early challenge studies in which volunteers who became ill following an initial NV challenge failed to become ill on rechallenge with the same agent 6 to 14 weeks later (103). In several volunteer studies, elevated preexisting levels of serum or intestinal antibody to NV did not correlate with resistance to illness; instead, higher antibody levels were associated with increased susceptibility to illness (55, 103). In contrast, short-term resistance to infection induced by prior homologous infection was correlated with antibody levels in other studies, and a correlation between the level of serum antibody and protection was observed in epidemiological studies (55, 112, 132).

Few studies have examined immunity to SaV infection in young children. One study that measured immunity to SaV/Sapporo/82 using an RIA with hyperimmune antiserum that measured type-specific antibodies found that the presence of serum antibody was clearly correlated with resistance to illness but not to infection (93).

Analysis of volunteers given NV using the new molecular assays has confirmed that ~50% of volunteers are susceptible to illness, but a larger number (82%) of volunteers are infected, often asymptomatically (31). Uninfected individuals are more likely to have lower preexisting serum and intestinal antibody titers than are all infected subjects (31, 99). At least some of these subjects have lower antibody levels because they have a nonfunctional FUT2 gene and are genetically resistant to infection with NV (due to lack of expression of an HBGA to which the virus can bind) (46, 74). Even so, among those with a functional FUT2 gene, those who were infected were significantly more likely to have measurable preexisting serum antibody than those not infected (74).

Taken together, these results suggest that our knowledge about immunity to NoV infections remains incomplete, and the conflicting data may be clarified once assays that measure responses to neutralizing epitopes become available. Genetic resistance appears to be due to lack of expression of certain HBGAs in the gastrointestinal epithelium (46, 74, 82); however, a number of HBGA binding patterns exist for the different NoV strains such that most, if not all, persons have the potential to be susceptible to at least some NoV strains (45). Short-term resistance to illness appears to be induced by infection, and this immunity may correlate with the level of serum antibody. On the other hand, long-term resistance to illness appears to be more complicated and may be influenced by additional factors (74).

CLINICAL MANIFESTATIONS

The hallmark of infection with NV and other HuCVs is the acute onset of vomiting or diarrhea or both. No prodrome is seen, and the spectrum of illness may vary widely in individual patients. For example, in adults infected with the same experimental inoculum, one volunteer vomited 20 times and required parenteral fluid therapy, whereas a second volunteer had no vomiting but eight diarrheal stools (20). The relative frequencies of these and other symptoms were described in a study of 50 volunteers challenged with NV (31) (Table 3) and are similar to those seen in natural outbreaks and in infection with related viruses (132). Of 50 volunteers orally administered NV, 41

TABLE 3 Responses of 50 adult volunteers (19 to 39 years old) given NV[a]

Response	% of infected volunteers (n = 41)[b]	% of uninfected volunteers (n = 9)
Seroconversion	98	0
Antigen excretion	88	0
Infection	100	0
Asymptomatic	32	0
Symptomatic	68	0
Symptoms with clinical illness (n = 28)		
Diarrhea	86	0
Vomiting	57	0
Nausea	96	10
Abdominal cramps	96	0
Headache/bodyache	96	40
Chills	36	0
Fever (>37.8°C)	32	0

[a] Data from reference 31.
[b] Infection determined by antigen shedding and/or antibody response.

(82%) became infected; of these infections, 68% were symptomatic and 32% were asymptomatic. The most common symptoms with clinical illness are nausea, malaise, and abdominal cramps. Diarrhea, which is usually watery and without mucus, blood, or leukocytes, occurs in most patients, and vomiting is seen in most. Subjective or documented fever and chills occur in a minority of patients. Figure 4 shows the clinical course of two volunteers infected with NV after oral challenge. The illness is generally mild and self-limited, with symptoms lasting 12 to 48 h, and illnesses caused by the different NoVs are clinically indistinguishable.

More severe disease can be seen in certain populations. Symptomatic illness lasts longer in children <1 year of age and in hospitalized patients (5, 80, 108). Volume depletion with renal insufficiency and hypokalemia are more common in the elderly and in persons with underlying disease (e.g., those with cardiovascular disease and the immunocompromised) (87). Disseminated intravascular coagulation developed as a complication of NoV infection in a group of previously healthy soldiers exposed to severe environmental stress (10). Chronic diarrhea lasting months to years can be seen in immunocompromised patients (60, 95). Most complications are associated with volume depletion or aspiration of vomitus and can include death, especially in the elderly.

A provisional diagnosis of infection during outbreaks of gastroenteritis is possible if the following criteria are met: (i) absence of bacterial or parasitic pathogens, (ii) vomiting in more than 50% of cases, (iii) mean (or median) duration of illness ranging from 12 to 60 h, and (iv) an incubation period of 24 to 48 h. These criteria were met in 81 to 100% of ill individuals in 38 NV outbreaks and have been used successfully in several epidemiological studies (58). A definitive diagnosis, desirable for both clinical and epidemiological studies, requires the use of a detection method for antigen, the viral genome, or antibody responses.

LABORATORY DIAGNOSIS

Because HuCVs cannot be grown in cell culture, and particle-positive stools are not readily available, initial assays for viral diagnosis were developed using reagents (pre- and postinfection serum and stool) from volunteer studies (reviewed in reference 4). The first immunologic test de-

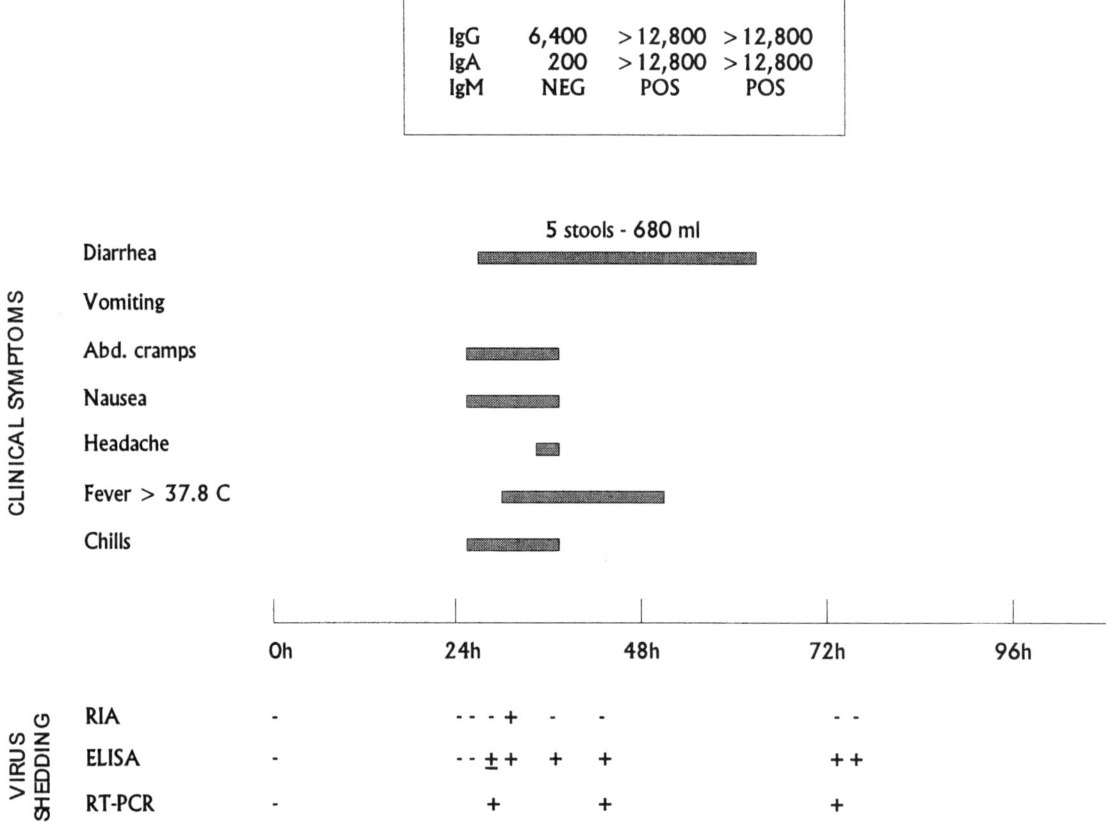

FIGURE 4 Clinical outcome of infection with NV in two volunteers. The clinical course of two volunteers who became ill after challenge with 8fIIa NV inoculum (at 0 h) is depicted. Both volunteers were considered to have severe disease. Volunteer 503 was a 29-year-old man, while volunteer 516 was a 23-year-old woman (31). NEG, negative; POS, positive; Ab, antibody; Abd, abdominal; −, negative; +, positive; ±, equivocal.

VOLUNTEER
516

SERUM ELISA Ab TITERS

Isotype	Day 0	Day 9	Day 16
IgG	400	3,200	>12,800
IgA	400	800	3,200
IgM	NEG	POS	POS

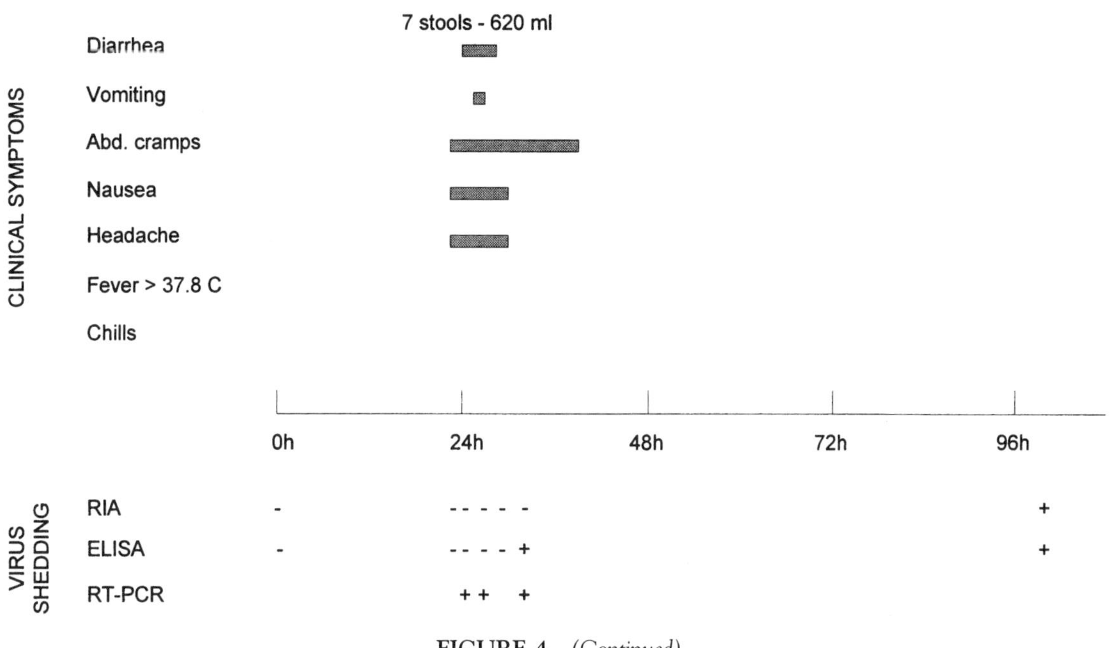

FIGURE 4 *(Continued)*

veloped for NV diagnosis was IEM (57), and this method has remained widely used for the examination of fecal samples for the presence of NV and other HuCVs in diagnostic laboratories worldwide. Although EM is still used, laboratory diagnosis of HuCV infections has changed over the last several years based on the cloning and sequencing of NV and subsequent expression of the NV capsid protein (Table 4). Recombinant VLPs have been produced for several NoVs and SaVs and have been used to develop new diagnostic assays, described below. However, the use of many of these assays remains restricted to research laboratories.

Antigen Detection

The first immunologic assays developed to detect antigen and amenable to large-scale use were RIAs and, subsequently, enzyme immunoassays (EIAs) (4). All the solid-phase assays for NoVs initially used human volunteer preinfection and convalescent-phase serum antibodies as capture and detector antibodies. These reagents have now been replaced with hyperimmune antisera made to rVLPs. Hyperimmune antiserum to rNV VLPs produced in guinea pigs, mice, and rabbits reacts with high titer of antibody to the immunogen and to native NV in stool (31, 35, 53), showing that the previous lack of success of producing high-titered antiserum was not due to any inherent poor antigenicity of NV, but rather to the paucity of pure immunogen. Hyperimmune antisera have been used to develop an antigen EIA that has been shown to be highly sensitive and specific for NV antigen (31, 51). The test sensitivity of the standard antigen EIA was determined to be ~0.025 ng of capsid protein (1.4×10^6 virions), and antigen was detected in the stools of volunteers at dilutions as high as 1:10,000 (31). The rNV antigen EIA can detect both virus particles and soluble protein.

Additional antigen detection EIAs were developed using other NoV and SaV rVLPs as antigens for production of hyperimmune antisera (4, 39). Each of these types of rEIAs has been found to be both sensitive and type specific (4, 39, 51). Initially, the type specificity of the antigen rEIAs was a surprise because antigen EIAs using volunteer convalescent-phase antisera often were more broadly cross-reactive. Apparently, the cross-reactive antibodies in convalescent-phase sera represent past exposure to multiple HuCV types and the cross-reactive epitopes of the rVLPs are not immunodominant. Cross-reactive epitopes that are shared within an NoV genogroup or across genogroups have now been identified, and monoclonal antibodies that detect GI-specific or GII-specific epitopes have been used to produce more broadly reactive antigen rEIAs (8, 63, 102, 107). These assays have been made commercially available outside of the United States, but improvements in sensitivity and specificity are needed before they are useful as a diagnostic for individual patients (8, 16, 107).

TABLE 4 Comparison of methods to detect HuCVs

Feature detected	Method	Comment	Specificity	Sensitivity	Reference(s)
Viral antigen	IEM	Detects particles	Depends on antiserum used	10^5–10^6 pp/ml[a]	57
	SPIEM[b]	Detects particles	Depends on antiserum used	10^5–10^6 pp/ml	73
	rEIA	Detects particles and soluble antigen	Type-specific with polyclonal hyperimmune anti-rVLP sera	Particulate and soluble antigen 0.025 ng of protein	4, 8, 39, 51, 63, 102, 107
Genomic RNA	Hybridization	Detects genome	Probes determine specificity	~10^4 genomes, if no inhibitors are present	52, 65
	RT-PCR	Need several primer sets and probes to detect all HuCVs	Primers and probes determine specificity	10–40 genomic copies, if no inhibitors are present	4, 41, 56, 66, 78, 97, 125, 126
Seroresponses	IEM	Labor-intensive	Type specificity depends on antigen used	Not known, but less sensitive than EIAs using rVLPs	35
	EIA	Broadly reactive using VLPs as antigen	Type specificity depends on antigen used		4, 32, 53, 96, 101

[a] pp/ml, physical particles per milliliter.
[b] SPIEM, solid-phase IEM.

Nucleic Acid Detection

Nucleic acid hybridization and RT-PCR assays have been developed to detect NoVs and SaVs in stool samples and other clinical and environmental samples. Hybridization assays for NV and SaV have been able to detect ~10^4 to 10^5 viral particles per ml of stool sample, which is similar to the detection limits of antigen detection EIAs. On the other hand, RT-PCR assays can generally detect lower quantities of virus, with as few as 10 to 40 genomic copies being identified (114). Because of the high specificity of the antigen rEIAs, RT-PCR assays have become the favored method for the diagnosis of NoV and SaV infection.

Several factors can affect the sensitivity and specificity of RT-PCR assays (4). Clinical samples and environmental samples may contain inhibitory substances that prevent amplification of viral RNA. A variety of methods have been developed to purify viral nucleic acids from these samples, and these methods vary in the ability to remove inhibitors successfully. A strategy for detection of the presence of inhibitors is the use of an internal standard RNA that is amplified only in the absence of significant amounts of inhibitor (114).

A number of different primer pairs and different RT-PCR conditions have been described for the detection of NoVs and SaVs (4, 41, 56, 66, 78, 97, 125, 126). No single primer pair will detect all NoVs or SaVs, and no assay has been universally accepted as a standard (126). Several different conserved regions of the genome have been targets for nucleic acid amplification (VP1, capsid specific, and NTPase), but recognition that the ORF1-ORF2 junction is highly conserved in NoVs has made this a prime target for amplification (56, 66, 78). Because no single primer pair detects all NoVs or SaVs, two or more primer pairs must be used to have a reasonable likelihood of virus detection. Following amplification, the results must then be interpreted using an additional test because of the nonspecific bands on gels of products amplified from stools, food, or environmental samples. The most commonly used confirmatory tests are hybridization assays with virus-specific probes and direct sequencing of the amplicons. As with the selection of primers, the selection of probes is complicated by the genetic diversity of these viruses. The generation of sequence data can be useful in linking clinical cases in epidemiological studies. Sensitive real-time RT-PCR assays are also available for both NoVs and SaVs (56, 78, 97).

RT-PCR assays are most commonly used to detect virus in stool samples, but they also have been used to detect virus in vomitus and throat swabs (4). RT-PCR assays are being used increasingly to detect NoVs in foods (primarily shellfish), water samples, sewage, and other environmental samples (e.g., swabs collected from areas potentially contaminated by ill persons) associated with outbreaks of viral gastroenteritis (4, 113). The potential utility of these methods for food and water safety is under evaluation.

Serologic Assays

EIAs to detect antibody responses have been developed using rVLPs as the antigen (4, 31, 53, 96). The assays were first performed by coating microtiter plates with rVLPs, followed by incubation steps with the human sera being tested, an anti-human immunoglobulin antiserum conjugate, and its substrate. Total or class- or subclass-specific serum antibodies are detected depending on the reagents used to detect the bound human antibody (32, 53, 123). The assay can be modified to detect virus-specific immunoglobulin A (IgA) in fecal samples or to detect virus-specific IgM using an antibody capture EIA format (4, 99).

The first assay to be developed used rNV VLPs as the antigen, and subsequently other recombinant antigens have been used (4, 32, 53, 96, 101). The rNV antibody EIA is as specific and efficient as previously described methods for detecting NV infection, and often it is more sensitive (31, 53). The increased test sensitivity is attributed to the very low assay background, which enables sera lacking antibody or containing very low levels of antibody to be detected, and the specificity of test results can be documented by use of the rNV antigen for antibody adsorption (31). Higher antibody titers are obtained with the rNV antibody EIA than with older antibody assays that relied on human reagents (35). In a volunteer study, detection of ≥4-fold rises in serum antibody titers was the most sensitive indicator of infection, although RNA detection methods were not evaluated (31). Significant rises in virus-specific IgA and IgG titers can be detected as early as 8 to 11 days after infection (32). Virus-specific IgM antibody also can be detected within 2 weeks of infection.

Heterologous antibody responses can often be detected in subjects following infection (e.g., antibody rise to SMA following infection with NV) (38, 96, 123). A heterologous response appears to occur only if a homologous antibody response also has occurred, and the heterologous response is of a lower magnitude than that of the homologous response (e.g., a 4-fold rise in antibody titer versus a 16-fold rise) (123). Heterologous responses involving IgM or IgA antibody occur infrequently (38, 123).

Antibody that blocks binding of VLPs to HBGAs has been proposed as a surrogate for NoV neutralizing antibody, since culture systems have not been available for these viruses (44). Although increases in HBGA-blocking antibody occur after infection, the sensitivity and specificity of these assays have not yet been determined.

Comparative Status of Tests

Each of the approaches described above can be useful for the detection of NoV and SaV infection (4). Because of the relative simplicity of performing EIAs, these should be the assays of choice for virus detection. The relatively poor sensitivity of currently licensed antigen EIAs has limited the utility of these assays for diagnosis of NoV infection in individual patients; however, these assays can be useful for identification of an NoV outbreak when multiple samples are available for testing (24, 107).

RT-PCR assays are the most widely used assays at present. These assays should be positive during acute illness if the appropriate primers and probes are selected, and they can even detect virus in stool samples 1 to 2 weeks following illness. The principal limitation of the RT-PCR assays is the lack of a universal set of primers for detection of all HuCVs.

Serologic assays are used to determine the presence of virus-specific IgM in individual sera or rising total antibody levels in paired (acute- and convalescent-phase) sera. The greatest value of IgM assays may be when only a single serum sample is available or when the initial serum is collected more than 10 days after the onset of illness. The selection of one or more of these diagnostic assays ultimately depends upon the availability of the clinical samples to be tested (serum and stool) and the availability of the reagents to perform the assay. The recombinant antigens and hyperimmune antisera are not widely available, so most laboratories depend upon EM and RT-PCR for the diagnosis of HuCV infection.

PREVENTION

No specific methods are available for the prevention of HuCV infection or illness. Because these agents are highly infectious, hand washing and disposal or disinfection of contaminated material may decrease transmission within a family or institution. Special care must also be given to the hygienic processing of food in view of the frequent occurrence of food-borne outbreaks of NoV infection. Ill food handlers should not prepare food for a minimum of 3 days after their illness, and plastic gloves should be worn to prepare foods. Consumption of raw shellfish is a risk, since outbreaks have occurred from the consumption of shellfish that meet current microbial (bacterial) sanitary standards. Human breast milk from women with a functional FUT2 gene contains fucosylated mucins that block binding of some NoV strains to HBGAs expressed on epithelial cells and may play a role in protecting infants from NoV infection (49, 111).

Immunoprophylaxis

Because our understanding of protective immunity to NV and other HuCVs is incomplete, it is unclear whether vaccination strategies will be able to prevent such illnesses. Vaccines could prove effective, based on short-term immunity to reinfection with NV following repeated experimental challenge (55, 103), or the apparent widespread and broad immunity to the SaVs after childhood, and on the observations in less well-developed countries of the correlation of the presence of serum antibodies to NV with resistance to infection (112). It is possible that repeated immunization will be required to induce long-lasting immunity; the availability of large amounts of stable recombinant VLPs makes this feasible. The rNV particles are safe and immunogenic when given to volunteers as a solution of VLPs or in a food matrix (expressed in transgenic potatoes). It is likely that evaluation of the immune response to these particles will help us understand immunity to these enteric infections (26).

Management of Outbreaks

Outbreaks can result in significant morbidity and economic loss because of frequent secondary transmission of diseases. Outbreaks are a particular concern in closed environments such as hospitals, nursing homes, and ships because all personnel can rapidly become disabled. Virus can persist in the environment and lead to recurrent outbreaks (47). Ill persons should be isolated, and hand washing and disposal or disinfection of contaminated material should be put into effect immediately. Control measures for outbreaks of viral gastroenteritis should focus on the removal of an ongoing common source of infection (e.g., an ill food handler or the contamination of a water supply), adequate disinfection of contaminated areas, and interruption of person-to-person transmission, which can perpetuate an outbreak in a population after the common source has been removed.

The facts that asymptomatic infection occurs more frequently than previously realized and that antigen may be shed for 2 to 3 weeks after exposure need to be recognized in managing such outbreaks. This is particularly important in instituting and overseeing the hygienic processing of food for and care of the elderly. The potential for contaminated water sources must be eliminated. Methods for outbreak management will probably improve as new tests are used in epidemiological studies of virus transmission in various settings. For example, if asymptomatic food handlers or hospital staff can be identified, they may be furloughed until they are no longer excreting virus and potentially infectious. Because improvements in environmental hygiene may not be accompanied by reductions of endemic diarrhea caused by viruses, immunization may play an important role in future control.

TREATMENT

As discussed above, the illnesses caused by these viruses are generally mild and self-limited, and resolution occurs without sequelae (5). Hospitalization or rehydration is rarely required for adults, and the major impact of this disease has been morbidity and loss of time from work and school. Treatment involves symptomatic therapy, with oral rehydration generally being sufficient. In rare cases, parenteral administration of intravenous fluids is required. Deaths from NV gastroenteritis have been reported for the elderly and from HuCV infections in immunocompromised children, although some of these have been attributable to other primary causes. The use of human milk or oral immunoglobulin therapy anecdotally has not had any therapeutic efficacy in an immunocompromised patient (95). Currently no antiviral drugs exist to treat the caliciviruses, but this may change once these viruses are successfully propagated or with the recent availability of high-resolution structures of several of the viral proteins that have enzymatic activities.

We gratefully acknowledge support for our research on NV and HuCVs provided by the FDA, EPA, Thrasher Research Fund, NOAA, and NIH.

REFERENCES

1. **Adler, J. L., and R. Zickl.** 1969. Winter vomiting disease. *J. Infect. Dis.* **119:**668–673.
2. **Agus, S. G., R. Dolin, R. G. Wyatt, A. J. Tousimis, and R. S. Northrup.** 1973. Acute infectious nonbacterial gastroenteritis: intestinal histopathology. Histologic and enzymatic alterations during illness produced by the Norwalk agent in man. *Ann. Intern. Med.* **79:**18–25.
3. **Asanaka, M., R. L. Atmar, V. Ruvolo, S. E. Crawford, F. H. Neill, and M. K. Estes.** 2005. Replication and packaging of Norwalk virus RNA in cultured mammalian cells. *Proc. Natl. Acad. Sci. USA* **102:**10327–10332.
4. **Atmar, R. L., and M. K. Estes.** 2001. Diagnosis of noncultivatable gastroenteritis viruses, the human caliciviruses. *Clin. Microbiol. Rev.* **14:**15–37.
5. **Atmar, R. L., and M. K. Estes.** 2006. The epidemiologic and clinical importance of norovirus infection. *Gastroenterol. Clin. N. Am.* **35:**275–290.
6. **Barker, J., I. B. Vipond, and S. F. Bloomfield.** 2004. Effects of cleaning and disinfection in reducing the spread of norovirus contamination via environmental surfaces. *J. Hosp. Infect.* **58:**42–49.
7. **Bull, R. A., G. S. Hansman, L. E. Clancy, M. M. Tanaka, W. D. Rawlinson, and P. A. White.** 2005. Norovirus recombination in ORF1/ORF2 overlap. *Emerg. Infect. Dis.* **11:**1079–1085.
8. **Burton-MacLeod, J. A., E. M. Kane, R. S. Beard, L. A. Hadley, R. I. Glass, and T. Ando.** 2004. Evaluation and comparison of two commercial enzyme-linked immunosorbent assay kits for detection of antigenically diverse human noroviruses in stool samples. *J. Clin. Microbiol.* **42:**2587–2595.
9. **Cao, S., Z. Lou, M. Tan, Y. Chen, Y. Liu, Z. Zhang, X. C. Zhang, X. Jiang, X. Li, and Z. Rao.** 2007. Structural basis for the recognition of blood group trisaccharides by norovirus. *J. Virol.* **81:**5949–5957.
10. **Centers for Disease Control and Prevention.** 2002. Outbreak of acute gastroenteritis associated with Norwalk-like viruses among British military personnel—Afghanistan, May 2002. *Morb. Mortal. Wkly. Rep.* **51:**477–479.
11. **Chapin, A. R., C. M. Carpenter, W. C. Dudley, L. C. Gibson, R. Pratdesaba, O. Torres, D. Sanchez, J. Belkind-Gerson, I. Nyquist, A. Karnell, B. Gustafsson, J. L. Halpern, A. L. Bourgeois, and K. J. Schwab.** 2005. Prevalence of norovirus among visitors from the United States to Mexico and Guatemala who experience traveler's diarrhea. *J. Clin. Microbiol.* **43:**1112–1117.
12. **Cheesbrough, J. S., J. Green, C. I. Gallimore, P. A. Wright, and D. W. Brown.** 2000. Widespread environmental contamination with Norwalk-like viruses (NLV) detected in a prolonged hotel outbreak of gastroenteritis. *Epidemiol. Infect.* **125:**93–98.
13. **Cheetham, S., M. Souza, T. Meulia, S. Grimes, M. G. Han, and L. J. Saif.** 2006. Pathogenesis of a genogroup II human norovirus in gnotobiotic pigs. *J. Virol.* **80:** 10372–10381.
14. **Chen, R., J. D. Neill, J. S. Noel, A. M. Hutson, R. I. Glass, M. K. Estes, and B. V. Prasad.** 2004. Inter- and intragenus structural variations in caliciviruses and their functional implications. *J. Virol.* **78:**6469–6479.
15. **Cunningham, A. L., G. S. Grohman, J. Harkness, C. Law, D. Marriott, B. Tindall, and D. A. Cooper.** 1988. Gastrointestinal viral infections in homosexual men who were symptomatic and seropositive for human immunodeficiency virus. *J. Infect. Dis.* **158:**386–391.
16. **De Bruin, E., E. Duizer, H. Vennema, and M. P. Koopmans.** 2006. Diagnosis of norovirus outbreaks by commercial ELISA or RT-PCR. *J. Virol. Methods* **137:**259–264.
17. **de Wit, M. A., M. P. Koopmans, L. M. Kortbeek, N. J. van Leeuwen, A. I. Bartelds, and Y. T. van Duynhoven.** 2001. Gastroenteritis in sentinel general practices, The Netherlands. *Emerg. Infect. Dis.* **7:**82–91.
18. **de Wit, M. A., M. P. Koopmans, L. M. Kortbeek, W. J. Wannet, J. Vinje, F. van Leusden, A. I. Bartelds, and Y. T. van Duynhoven.** 2001. Sensor, a population-based cohort study on gastroenteritis in the Netherlands: incidence and etiology. *Am. J. Epidemiol.* **154:**666–674.
19. **Dolin, R., N. R. Blacklow, H. DuPont, R. F. Buscho, R. G. Wyatt, J. A. Kasel, R. Hornick, and R. M. Chanock.** 1972. Biological properties of Norwalk agent of acute infectious nonbacterial gastroenteritis. *Proc. Soc. Exp. Biol. Med.* **140:**578–583.
20. **Dolin, R., N. R. Blacklow, H. DuPont, S. Formal, R. F. Buscho, J. A. Kasel, R. P. Chames, R. Hornick, and R. M. Chanock.** 1971. Transmission of acute infectious nonbacterial gastroenteritis to volunteers by oral administration of stool filtrates. *J. Infect. Dis.* **123:**307–312.
21. **Dolin, R., R. C. Reichman, K. D. Roessner, T. S. Tralka, R. T. Schooley, W. Gary, and D. Morens.** 1982. Detection by immune electron microscopy of the Snow Mountain agent of acute viral gastroenteritis. *J. Infect. Dis.* **146:**184–189.
22. **Doultree, J. C., J. D. Druce, C. J. Birch, D. S. Bowden, and J. A. Marshall.** 1999. Inactivation of feline calicivirus, a Norwalk virus surrogate. *J. Hosp. Infect.* **41:**51–57.
23. **Duizer, E., P. Bijkerk, B. Rockx, A. De Groot, F. Twisk, and M. Koopmans.** 2004. Inactivation of caliciviruses. *Appl. Environ. Microbiol.* **70:**4538–4543.
24. **Duizer, E., A. Pielaat, H. Vennema, A. Kroneman, and M. Koopmans.** 2007. Probabilities in norovirus outbreak diagnosis. *J. Clin. Virol.* **40:**38–42.
25. **Duizer, E., K. J. Schwab, F. H. Neill, R. L. Atmar, M. P. Koopmans, and M. K. Estes.** 2004. Laboratory efforts to cultivate noroviruses. *J. Gen. Virol.* **85:**79–87.
26. **Estes, M. K., J. M. Ball, R. A. Guerrero, A. R. Opekun, M. A. Gilger, S. S. Pacheco, and D. Y. Graham.** 2000.

Norwalk virus vaccines: challenges and progress. *J. Infect. Dis.* **181:**S367–S373.
27. **Estes, M. K., B. V. Prasad, and R. L. Atmar.** 2006. Noroviruses everywhere: has something changed? *Curr. Opin. Infect. Dis.* **19:**467–474.
28. **Farkas, T., W. M. Zhong, Y. Jing, P. W. Huang, S. M. Espinosa, N. Martinez, A. L. Morrow, G. M. Ruiz-Palacios, L. K. Pickering, and X. Jiang.** 2004. Genetic diversity among sapoviruses. *Arch. Virol.* **149:**1309–1323.
29. **Gallimore, C. I., M. Iturriza-Gomara, J. Xerry, J. Adigwe, and J. J. Gray.** 2007. Inter-seasonal diversity of norovirus genotypes: emergence and selection of virus variants. *Arch. Virol.* **152:**1295–1303.
30. **Glass, P. J., C. Q. Zeng, and M. K. Estes.** 2003. Two nonoverlapping domains on the Norwalk virus open reading frame 3 (ORF3) protein are involved in the formation of the phosphorylated 35K protein and in ORF3-capsid protein interactions. *J. Virol.* **77:**3569–3577.
31. **Graham, D. Y., X. Jiang, T. Tanaka, A. R. Opekun, H. P. Madore, and M. K. Estes.** 1994. Norwalk virus infection of volunteers: new insights based on improved assays. *J. Infect. Dis.* **170:**34–43.
32. **Gray, J. J., C. Cunliffe, J. Ball, D. Y. Graham, U. Desselberger, and M. K. Estes.** 1994. Detection of immunoglobulin M (IgM), IgA, and IgG Norwalk virus-specific antibodies by indirect enzyme-linked immunosorbent assay with baculovirus-expressed Norwalk virus capsid antigen in adult volunteers challenged with Norwalk virus. *J. Clin. Microbiol.* **32:**3059–3063.
33. **Green, K. Y.** 2007. *Caliciviridae:* the noroviruses, p. 949–979. *In* D. M. Knipe, P. M. Howley, D. E. Griffin, R. A. Lamb, M. A. Martin, B. Roizman, and S. E. Straus (ed.), *Fields Virology*, 5th ed. Lippincott Williams & Wilkins, Philadelphia, PA.
34. **Green, K. Y., G. Belliot, J. L. Taylor, J. Valdesuso, J. F. Lew, A. Z. Kapikian, and F. Y. Lin.** 2002. A predominant role for Norwalk-like viruses as agents of epidemic gastroenteritis in Maryland nursing homes for the elderly. *J. Infect. Dis.* **185:**133–146.
35. **Green, K. Y., J. F. Lew, X. Jiang, A. Z. Kapikian, and M. K. Estes.** 1993. Comparison of the reactivities of baculovirus-expressed recombinant Norwalk virus capsid antigen with those of the native Norwalk virus antigen in serologic assays and some epidemiologic observations. *J. Clin. Microbiol.* **31:**2185–2191.
36. **Guix, S., M. Asanaka, K. Katayama, S. E. Crawford, F. H. Neill, R. L. Atmar, and M. K. Estes.** 2007. Norwalk virus RNA is infectious in mammalian cells. *J. Virol.* **81:**12238–12248.
37. **Guo, M., K. O. Chang, M. E. Hardy, Q. Zhang, A. V. Parwani, and L. J. Saif.** 1999. Molecular characterization of a porcine enteric calicivirus genetically related to Sapporo-like human caliciviruses. *J. Virol.* **73:**9625–9631.
38. **Hale, A. D., D. C. Lewis, X. Jiang, and D. W. Brown.** 1998. Homotypic and heterotypic IgG and IgM antibody responses in adults infected with small round structured viruses. *J. Med. Virol.* **54:**305–312.
39. **Hansman, G. S., R. Guntapong, Y. Pongsuwanna, K. Natori, K. Katayama, and N. Takeda.** 2006. Development of an antigen ELISA to detect sapovirus in clinical stool specimens. *Arch. Virol.* **151:**551–561.
40. **Hansman, G. S., K. Natori, T. Oka, S. Ogawa, K. Tanaka, N. Nagata, H. Ushijima, N. Takeda, and K. Katayama.** 2005. Cross-reactivity among sapovirus recombinant capsid proteins. *Arch. Virol.* **150:**21–36.
41. **Hansman, G. S., T. Oka, K. Katayama, and N. Takeda.** 2007. Human sapoviruses: genetic diversity, recombination, and classification. *Rev. Med. Virol.* **17:**133–141.
42. **Hardy, M. E., T. J. Crone, J. E. Brower, and K. Ettayebi.** 2002. Substrate specificity of the Norwalk virus 3C-like proteinase. *Virus Res.* **89:**29–39.
43. **Hardy, M. E., L. J. White, J. M. Ball, and M. K. Estes.** 1995. Specific proteolytic cleavage of recombinant Norwalk virus capsid protein. *J. Virol.* **69:**1693–1698.
44. **Harrington, P. R., L. Lindesmith, B. Yount, C. L. Moe, and R. S. Baric.** 2002. Binding of Norwalk virus-like particles to ABH histo-blood group antigens is blocked by antisera from infected human volunteers or experimentally vaccinated mice. *J. Virol.* **76:**12335–12343.
45. **Huang, P., T. Farkas, W. Zhong, M. Tan, S. Thornton, A. L. Morrow, and X. Jiang.** 2005. Norovirus and histo-blood group antigens: demonstration of a wide spectrum of strain specificities and classification of two major binding groups among multiple binding patterns. *J. Virol.* **79:**6714–6722.
46. **Hutson, A. M., F. Airaud, J. LePendu, M. K. Estes, and R. L. Atmar.** 2005. Norwalk virus infection associates with secretor status genotyped from sera. *J. Med. Virol.* **77:**116–120.
47. **Isakbaeva, E. T., M. A. Widdowson, R. S. Beard, S. N. Bulens, J. Mullins, S. S. Monroe, J. Bresee, P. Sassano, E. H. Cramer, and R. I. Glass.** 2005. Norovirus transmission on cruise ship. *Emerg. Infect. Dis.* **11:**154–158.
48. **Jiang, X., D. Y. Graham, K. N. Wang, and M. K. Estes.** 1990. Norwalk virus genome cloning and characterization. *Science* **250:**1580–1583.
49. **Jiang, X., P. Huang, W. Zhong, M. Tan, T. Farkas, A. L. Morrow, D. S. Newburg, G. M. Ruiz-Palacios, and L. K. Pickering.** 2004. Human milk contains elements that block binding of noroviruses to human histo-blood group antigens in saliva. *J. Infect. Dis.* **190:**1850–1859.
50. **Jiang, X., D. O. Matson, F. R. Velazquez, J. J. Calva, W. M. Zhong, J. Hu, G. M. Ruiz-Palacios, and L. K. Pickering.** 1995. Study of Norwalk-related viruses in Mexican children. *J. Med. Virol.* **47:**309–316.
51. **Jiang, X., J. Wang, and M. K. Estes.** 1995. Characterization of SRSVs using RT-PCR and a new antigen ELISA. *Arch. Virol.* **140:**363–374.
52. **Jiang, X., J. Wang, D. Y. Graham, and M. K. Estes.** 1992. Detection of Norwalk virus in stool by polymerase chain reaction. *J. Clin. Microbiol.* **30:**2529–2534.
53. **Jiang, X., M. Wang, D. Y. Graham, and M. K. Estes.** 1992. Expression, self-assembly, and antigenicity of the Norwalk virus capsid protein. *J. Virol.* **66:**6527–6532.
54. **Jiang, X., M. Wang, K. Wang, and M. K. Estes.** 1993. Sequence and genomic organization of Norwalk virus. *Virology* **195:**51–61.
55. **Johnson, P. C., J. J. Mathewson, H. L. Dupont, and H. B. Greenberg.** 1990. Multiple-challenge study of host susceptibility to Norwalk gastroenteritis in US adults. *J. Infect. Dis.* **161:**18–21.
56. **Kageyama, T., M. Shinohara, K. Uchida, S. Fukushi, F. B. Hoshino, S. Kojima, R. Takai, T. Oka, N. Takeda, and K. Katayama.** 2004. Coexistence of multiple genotypes, including newly identified genotypes, in outbreaks of gastroenteritis due to norovirus in Japan. *J. Clin. Microbiol.* **42:**2988–2995.
57. **Kapikian, A. Z., R. G. Wyatt, R. Dolin, T. S. Thornhill, A. R. Kalica, and R. M. Chanock.** 1972. Visualization by immune electron microscopy of a 27-nm particle associated with acute infectious nonbacterial gastroenteritis. *J. Virol.* **10:**1075–1081.
58. **Kaplan, J. E., R. Feldman, D. S. Campbell, C. Lookabaugh, and G. W. Gary.** 1982. The frequency of a Norwalk-like pattern of illness in outbreaks of acute gastroenteritis. *Am. J. Public Health* **72:**1329–1332.

59. **Katayama, K., G. S. Hansman, T. Oka, S. Ogawa, and N. Takeda.** 2006. Investigation of norovirus replication in a human cell line. *Arch. Virol.* **151:**1291–1308.

60. **Kaufman, S. S., N. K. Chatterjee, M. E. Fuschino, D. L. Morse, R. A. Morotti, M. S. Magid, G. E. Gondolesi, S. S. Florman, and T. M. Fishbein.** 2005. Characteristics of human calicivirus enteritis in intestinal transplant recipients. *J. Pediatr. Gastroenterol. Nutr.* **40:**328–333.

61. **Keswick, B. H., T. K. Satterwhite, P. C. Johnson, H. L. Dupont, S. L. Secor, J. A. Bitsura, G. W. Gary, and J. C. Hoff.** 1985. Inactivation of Norwalk virus in drinking water by chlorine. *Appl. Environ. Microbiol.* **50:**261–264.

62. **Kindberg, E., B. Akerlind, C. Johnsen, J. D. Knudsen, O. Heltberg, G. Larson, B. Bottiger, and L. Svensson.** 2007. Host genetic resistance to symptomatic norovirus (GGII.4) infections in Denmark. *J. Clin. Microbiol.* **45:** 2720–2722.

63. **Kitamoto, N., T. Tanaka, K. Natori, N. Takeda, S. Nakata, X. Jiang, and M. K. Estes.** 2002. Cross-reactivity among several recombinant calicivirus virus-like particles (VLPs) with monoclonal antibodies obtained from mice immunized orally with one type of VLP. *J. Clin. Microbiol.* **40:**2459–2465.

64. **Ko, G., C. Garcia, Z. D. Jiang, P. C. Okhuysen, J. Belkind-Gerson, R. I. Glass, and H. L. Dupont.** 2005. Noroviruses as a cause of traveler's diarrhea among students from the United States visiting Mexico. *J. Clin. Microbiol.* **43:**6126–6129.

65. **Kogawa, K., S. Nakata, S. Ukae, N. Adachi, K. Numata, D. O. Matson, M. K. Estes, and S. Chiba.** 1996. Dot blot hybridization with a cDNA probe derived from the human calicivirus Sapporo 1982 strain. *Arch. Virol.* **141:**1949–1959.

66. **Kojima, S., T. Kageyama, S. Fukushi, F. B. Hoshino, M. Shinohara, K. Uchida, K. Natori, N. Takeda, and K. Katayama.** 2002. Genogroup-specific PCR primers for detection of Norwalk-like viruses. *J. Virol. Methods* **100:** 107–114.

67. **Koopmans, M. P., K. Y. Green, T. Ando, I. N. Clarke, M. K. Estes, D. O. Matson, S. Nakata, J. D. Neill, A. W. Smith, M. J. Studdert, and H. J. Thiel.** 2005. *Caliciviridae*, p. 843–851. *In* C. M. Fauquet, M. A. Mayo, J. Maniloff, U. Desselberger, and L. A. Ball (ed.), *Virus Taxonomy: Classification and Nomenclature of Viruses. Eighth Report of the International Committee on Taxonomy of Viruses.* Elsevier Academic Press, San Diego, CA.

68. **Kreutz, L. C., B. S. Seal, and W. L. Mengeling.** 1994. Early interaction of feline calicivirus with cells in culture. *Arch. Virol.* **136:**19–34.

69. **Le Guyader, F., F. Loisy, R. L. Atmar, A. M. Hutson, M. K. Estes, N. Ruvoen-Clouet, M. Pommepuy, and J. Le Pendu.** 2006. Norwalk virus-specific binding to oyster digestive tissues. *Emerg. Infect. Dis.* **12:**931–936.

70. **Le Guyader, F. S., and R. L. Atmar.** 2007. Viruses in shellfish, p. 207–229. *In* A. Bosch (ed.), *Human Viruses in Water.* Elsevier B.V., Boston, MA.

71. **Levy, A. G., L. Widerlite, C. J. Schwartz, R. Dolin, N. R. Blacklow, J. D. Gardner, D. V. Kimberg, and J. S. Trier.** 1976. Jejunal adenylate cyclase activity in human subjects during viral gastroenteritis. *Gastroenterology* **70:** 321–325.

72. **Lew, J. F., M. Petric, A. Z. Kapikian, X. Jiang, M. K. Estes, and K. Y. Green.** 1994. Identification of minireovirus as a Norwalk-like virus in pediatric patients with gastroenteritis. *J. Virol.* **68:**3391–3396.

73. **Lewis, D. C.** 1990. Three serotypes of Norwalk-like virus demonstrated by solid-phase immune electron microscopy. *J. Med. Virol.* **30:**77–81.

74. **Lindesmith, L., C. Moe, S. Marionneau, N. Ruvoen, X. Jiang, L. Lindblad, P. Stewart, J. LePendu, and R. Baric.** 2003. Human susceptibility and resistance to Norwalk virus infection. *Nat. Med.* **9:**548–553.

75. **Liu, B. L., P. R. Lambden, H. Gunther, P. Otto, M. Elschner, and I. N. Clarke.** 1999. Molecular characterization of a bovine enteric calicivirus: relationship to the Norwalk-like viruses. *J. Virol.* **73:**819–825.

76. **Lo, S. V., A. M. Connolly, S. R. Palmer, D. Wright, P. D. Thomas, and D. Joynson.** 1994. The role of the pre-symptomatic food handler in a common source outbreak of food-borne SRSV gastroenteritis in a group of hospitals. *Epidemiol. Infect.* **113:**513–521.

77. **Lobue, A. D., L. Lindesmith, B. Yount, P. R. Harrington, J. M. Thompson, R. E. Johnston, C. L. Moe, and R. S. Baric.** 2006. Multivalent norovirus vaccines induce strong mucosal and systemic blocking antibodies against multiple strains. *Vaccine* **24:**5220–5234.

78. **Loisy, F., R. L. Atmar, P. Guillon, P. Le Cann, M. Pommepuy, and F. S. Le Guyader.** 2005. Real-time RT-PCR for norovirus screening in shellfish. *J. Virol. Methods* **123:** 1–7.

79. **Lopman, B., H. Vennema, E. Kohli, P. Pothier, A. Sanchez, A. Negredo, J. Buesa, E. Schreier, M. Reacher, D. Brown, J. Gray, M. Iturriza, C. Gallimore, B. Bottiger, K. O. Hedlund, M. Torven, C. H. von Bonsdorff, L. Maunula, M. Poljsak-Prijatelj, J. Zimsek, G. Reuter, G. Szucs, B. Melegh, L. Svennson, Y. van Duijnhoven, and M. Koopmans.** 2004. Increase in viral gastroenteritis outbreaks in Europe and epidemic spread of new norovirus variant. *Lancet* **363:**682–688.

80. **Lopman, B. A., M. H. Reacher, I. B. Vipond, J. Sarangi, and D. W. Brown.** 2004. Clinical manifestation of norovirus gastroenteritis in health care settings. *Clin. Infect. Dis.* **39:**318–324.

81. **Madeley, C. R., and B. P. Cosgrove.** 1976. Letter: caliciviruses in man. *Lancet* **i:**199–200.

82. **Marionneau, S., N. Ruvoen, B. Moullac-Vaidye, M. Clement, A. Cailleau-Thomas, G. Ruiz-Palacois, P. Huang, X. Jiang, and J. Le Pendu.** 2002. Norwalk virus binds to histo-blood group antigens present on gastroduodenal epithelial cells of secretor individuals. *Gastroenterology* **122:**1967–1977.

83. **Marks, P. J., I. B. Vipond, F. M. Regan, K. Wedgwood, R. E. Fey, and E. O. Caul.** 2003. A school outbreak of Norwalk-like virus: evidence for airborne transmission. *Epidemiol. Infect.* **131:**727–736.

84. **Martella, V., M. Campolo, E. Lorusso, P. Cavicchio, M. Camero, A. L. Bellacicco, N. Decaro, G. Elia, G. Greco, M. Corrente, C. Desario, S. Arista, K. Banyai, M. Koopmans, and C. Buonavoglia.** 2007. Norovirus in captive lion cub *(Panthera leo)*. *Emerg. Infect. Dis.* **13:**1071–1073.

85. **Matson, D. O., M. K. Estes, T. Tanaka, A. V. Bartlett, and L. K. Pickering.** 1990. Asymptomatic human calicivirus infection in a day care center. *Pediatr. Infect. Dis. J.* **9:**190–196.

86. **Matsui, S. M., J. P. Kim, H. B. Greenberg, W. Su, Q. Sun, P. C. Johnson, H. L. Dupont, L. S. Oshiro, and G. R. Reyes.** 1991. The isolation and characterization of a Norwalk virus-specific cDNA. *J. Clin. Investig.* **87:** 1456–1461.

87. **Mattner, F., D. Sohr, A. Heim, P. Gastmeier, H. Vennema, and M. Koopmans.** 2006. Risk groups for clinical complications of norovirus infections: an outbreak investigation. *Clin. Microbiol. Infect.* **12:**69–74.

88. **McCarthy, M., M. K. Estes, and K. C. Hyams.** 2000. Norwalk-like virus infection in military forces: epidemic potential, sporadic disease, and the future direction of pre-

vention and control efforts. *J. Infect. Dis.* **181:**S387–S391.

89. **Mead, P. S., L. Slutsker, V. Dietz, L. F. Mccaig, J. S. Bresee, C. Shapiro, P. M. Griffin, and R. V. Tauxe.** 1999. Food-related illness and death in the United States. *Emerg. Infect. Dis.* **5:**607–625.
90. **Meeroff, J. C., D. S. Schreiber, J. S. Trier, and N. R. Blacklow.** 1980. Abnormal gastric motor function in viral gastroenteritis. *Ann. Intern. Med.* **92:**370–373.
91. **Mounts, A. W., T. Ando, M. Koopmans, J. S. Bresee, J. Noel, and R. I. Glass.** 2000. Cold weather seasonality of gastroenteritis associated with Norwalk-like viruses. *J. Infect. Dis.* **181:**S284–S287.
92. **Murata, T., N. Katsushima, K. Mizuta, Y. Muraki, S. Hongo, and Y. Matsuzaki.** 2007. Prolonged norovirus shedding in infants <=6 months of age with gastroenteritis. *Pediatr. Infect. Dis. J.* **26:**46–49.
93. **Nakata, S., S. Chiba, H. Terashima, T. Yokoyama, and T. Nakao.** 1985. Humoral immunity in infants with gastroenteritis caused by human calicivirus. *J. Infect. Dis.* **152:**274–279.
94. **Ng, K. K., N. Pendas-Franco, J. Rojo, J. A. Boga, A. Machin, J. M. Alonso, and F. Parra.** 2004. Crystal structure of Norwalk virus polymerase reveals the carboxyl terminus in the active site cleft. *J. Biol. Chem.* **279:** 16638–16645.
95. **Nilsson, M., K. O. Hedlund, M. Thorhagen, G. Larson, K. Johansen, A. Ekspong, and L. Svensson.** 2003. Evolution of human calicivirus RNA in vivo: accumulation of mutations in the protruding P2 domain of the capsid leads to structural changes and possibly a new phenotype. *J. Virol.* **77:**13117–13124.
96. **Noel, J. S., T. Ando, J. P. Leite, K. Y. Green, K. E. Dingle, M. K. Estes, Y. Seto, S. S. Monroe, and R. I. Glass.** 1997. Correlation of patient immune responses with genetically characterized small round-structured viruses involved in outbreaks of nonbacterial acute gastroenteritis in the United States, 1990 to 1995. *J. Med. Virol.* **53:**372–383.
97. **Oka, T., K. Katayama, G. S. Hansman, T. Kageyama, S. Ogawa, F. T. Wu, P. A. White, and N. Takeda.** 2006. Detection of human sapovirus by real-time reverse transcription-polymerase chain reaction. *J. Med. Virol.* **78:**1347–1353.
98. **Oka, T., M. Yamamoto, K. Katayama, G. S. Hansman, S. Ogawa, T. Miyamura, and N. Takeda.** 2006. Identification of the cleavage sites of sapovirus open reading frame 1 polyprotein. *J. Gen. Virol.* **87:**3329–3338.
99. **Okhuysen, P. C., X. Jiang, L. Ye, P. C. Johnson, and M. K. Estes.** 1995. Viral shedding and fecal IgA response after Norwalk virus infection. *J. Infect. Dis.* **171:** 566–569.
100. **Pang, X. L., J. Joensuu, and T. Vesikari.** 1999. Human calicivirus-associated sporadic gastroenteritis in Finnish children less than two years of age followed prospectively during a rotavirus vaccine trial. *Pediatr. Infect. Dis. J.* **18:** 420–426.
101. **Parker, S. P., W. D. Cubitt, and X. Jiang.** 1995. Enzyme immunoassay using baculovirus-expressed human calicivirus (Mexico) for the measurement of IgG responses and determining its seroprevalence in London, UK. *J. Med. Virol.* **46:**194–200.
102. **Parker, T. D., N. Kitamoto, T. Tanaka, A. M. Hutson, and M. K. Estes.** 2005. Identification of genogroup I and genogroup II broadly reactive epitopes on the norovirus capsid. *J. Virol.* **79:**7402–7409.
103. **Parrino, T. A., D. S. Schreiber, J. S. Trier, A. Z. Kapikian, and N. R. Blacklow.** 1977. Clinical immunity in acute gastroenteritis caused by Norwalk agent. *N. Engl. J. Med.* **297:**86–89.
104. **Patterson, T., P. Hutchings, and S. Palmer.** 1993. Outbreak of SRSV gastroenteritis at an international conference traced to food handled by a post-symptomatic caterer. *Epidemiol. Infect.* **111:**157–162.
105. **Prasad, B. V. V., M. E. Hardy, T. Dokland, J. Bella, M. G. Rossmann, and M. K. Estes.** 1999. X-ray crystallographic structure of the Norwalk virus capsid. *Science* **286:**287–290.

105a. **Prasad, B. V. V., M. E. Hardy, and M. K. Estes.** 2000. Structural studies of recombinant Norwalk capsids. *J. Infect. Dis.* **181:**S317–S321.

106. **Prasad, B. V. V., R. Rothnagel, X. Jiang, and M. K. Estes.** 1994. Three-dimensional structure of baculovirus-expressed Norwalk virus capsids. *J. Virol.* **68:**5117–5125.
107. **Richards, A. F., B. Lopman, A. Gunn, A. Curry, D. Ellis, H. Cotterill, S. Ratcliffe, M. Jenkins, H. Appleton, C. I. Gallimore, J. J. Gray, and D. W. Brown.** 2003. Evaluation of a commercial ELISA for detecting Norwalk-like virus antigen in faeces. *J. Clin. Virol.* **26:** 109–115.
108. **Rockx, B., M. De Wit, H. Vennema, J. Vinje, E. De Bruin, Y. Van Duynhoven, and M. Koopmans.** 2002. Natural history of human calicivirus infection: a prospective cohort study. *Clin. Infect. Dis.* **35:**246–253.
109. **Rodriguez-Guillen, L., E. Vizzi, A. C. Alcala, F. H. Pujol, F. Liprandi, and J. E. Ludert.** 2005. Calicivirus infection in human immunodeficiency virus seropositive children and adults. *J. Clin. Virol.* **33:**104–109.
110. **Russo, P. L., D. W. Spelman, G. A. Harrington, A. W. Jenney, I. C. Gunesekere, P. J. Wright, J. C. Doultree, and J. A. Marshall.** 1997. Hospital outbreak of Norwalk-like virus. *Infect. Control Hosp. Epidemiol.* **18:**576–579.
111. **Ruvoen-Clouet, N., E. Mas, S. Marionneau, P. Guillon, D. Lombardo, and J. Le Pendu.** 2006. Bile-salt-stimulated lipase and mucins from milk of 'secretor' mothers inhibit the binding of Norwalk virus capsids to their carbohydrate ligands. *Biochem. J.* **393:**627–634.
112. **Ryder, R. W., N. Singh, W. C. Reeves, A. Z. Kapikian, H. B. Greenberg, and R. B. Sack.** 1985. Evidence of immunity induced by naturally acquired rotavirus and Norwalk virus infection on two remote Panamanian islands. *J. Infect. Dis.* **151:**99–105.
113. **Schwab, K. J., M. K. Estes, and R. L. Atmar.** 2000. Norwalk and other human caliciviruses: molecular characterization, epidemiology, and pathogenesis, p. 460–493. *In* J. W. Cary, J. E. Linz, and D. Bhatnagar (ed.), *Microbial Foodborne Diseases: Mechanisms of Pathogenicity and Toxin Synthesis*. Technomic Publishing Co., Inc., Lancaster, PA.
114. **Schwab, K. J., M. K. Estes, F. H. Neill, and R. L. Atmar.** 1997. Use of heat release and an internal RNA standard control in reverse transcription-PCR detection of Norwalk virus from stool samples. *J. Clin. Microbiol.* **35:**511–514.
115. **Seah, E. L., J. A. Marshall, and P. J. Wright.** 1999. Open reading frame 1 of the Norwalk-like virus Camberwell: completion of sequence and expression in mammalian cells. *J. Virol.* **73:**10531–10535.
116. **Siebenga, J. J., H. Vennema, E. Duizer, and M. P. Koopmans.** 2007. Gastroenteritis caused by norovirus GGII.4, The Netherlands, 1994–2005. *Emerg. Infect. Dis.* **13:**144–146.
117. **Siebenga, J. J., H. Vennema, B. Renckens, E. de Bruin, B. van der Veer, R. J. Siezen, and M. Koopmans.** 2007. Epochal evolution of GGII.4 norovirus capsid proteins from 1995 to 2006. *J. Virol.* **81:**9932–9941.

118. **Sosnovtsev, S. V., G. Belliot, K. O. Chang, V. G. Prikhodko, L. B. Thackray, C. E. Wobus, S. M. Karst, H. W. Virgin, and K. Y. Green.** 2006. Cleavage map and proteolytic processing of the murine norovirus nonstructural polyprotein in infected cells. *J. Virol.* **80:** 7816–7831.
119. **Straub, T. M., K. Höner zu Bentrup, P. Orosz-Coghlan, A. Dohnalkova, B. K. Mayer, R. A. Bartholomew, C. O. Valdez, C. J. Bruckner-Lea, C. P. Gerba, M. Abbaszadegan, and C. A. Nickerson.** 2007. In vitro cell culture infectivity assay for human noroviruses. *Emerg. Infect. Dis.* **13:**396–403.
120. **Thornhill, T. S., A. R. Kalica, R. G. Wyatt, A. Z. Kapikian, and R. M. Chanock.** 1975. Pattern of shedding of the Norwalk particle in stools during experimentally induced gastroenteritis in volunteers as determined by immune electron microscopy. *J. Infect. Dis.* **132:**28–34.
121. **Thorven, M., A. Grahn, K. O. Hedlund, H. Johansson, C. Wahlfrid, G. Larson, and L. Svensson.** 2005. A homozygous nonsense mutation (428G→A) in the human secretor (FUT2) gene provides resistance to symptomatic norovirus (GGII) infections. *J. Virol.* **79:** 15351–15355.
122. **Tian, P., A. H. Bates, H. M. Jensen, and R. E. Mandrell.** 2006. Norovirus binds to blood group A-like antigens in oyster gastrointestinal cells. *Lett. Appl. Microbiol.* **43:**645–651.
123. **Treanor, J. J., X. Jiang, H. P. Madore, and M. K. Estes.** 1993. Subclass-specific serum antibody responses to recombinant Norwalk virus capsid antigen (rNV) in adults infected with Norwalk, Snow Mountain, or Hawaii virus. *J. Clin. Microbiol.* **31:**1630–1634.
124. **Vinje, J., J. Green, D. C. Lewis, C. I. Gallimore, D. W. Brown, and M. P. Koopmans.** 2000. Genetic polymorphism across regions of the three open reading frames of "Norwalk-like viruses." *Arch. Virol.* **145:**223–241.
125. **Vinje, J., R. A. Hamidjaja, and M. D. Sobsey.** 2004. Development and application of a capsid VP1 (region D) based reverse transcription PCR assay for genotyping of genogroup I and II noroviruses. *J. Virol. Methods* **116:** 109–117.
126. **Vinje, J., H. Vennema, L. Maunula, C. H. von Bonsdorff, M. Hoehne, E. Schreier, A. Richards, J. Green, D. Brown, S. S. Beard, S. S. Monroe, E. De Bruin, L. Svensson, and M. P. Koopmans.** 2003. International collaborative study to compare reverse transcriptase PCR assays for detection and genotyping of noroviruses. *J. Clin. Microbiol.* **41:**1423–1433.
127. **Wang, J., X. Jiang, H. P. Madore, J. Gray, U. Desselberger, T. Ando, Y. Seto, I. Oishi, J. F. Lew, and K. Y. Green.** 1994. Sequence diversity of small, round-structured viruses in the Norwalk virus group. *J. Virol.* **68:**5982–5990.
128. **Wang, Q. H., M. G. Han, S. Cheetham, M. Souza, J. A. Funk, and L. J. Saif.** 2005. Porcine noroviruses related to human noroviruses. *Emerg. Infect. Dis.* **11:** 1874–1881.
129. **White, L. J., J. M. Ball, M. E. Hardy, T. N. Tanaka, N. Kitamoto, and M. K. Estes.** 1996. Attachment and entry of recombinant Norwalk virus capsids to cultured human and animal cell lines. *J. Virol.* **70:**6589–6597.
130. **Widerlite, L., J. S. Trier, N. R. Blacklow, and D. S. Schreiber.** 1975. Structure of the gastric mucosa in acute infectious bacterial gastroenteritis. *Gastroenterology* **68:** 425–430.
131. **Wobus, C. E., S. M. Karst, L. B. Thackray, K. O. Chang, S. V. Sosnovtsev, G. Belliot, A. Krug, J. M. Mackenzie, K. Y. Green, and H. W. Virgin.** 2004. Replication of norovirus in cell culture reveals a tropism for dendritic cells and macrophages. *PLoS Biol.* **2:**e432.
132. **Wyatt, R. G., R. Dolin, N. R. Blacklow, H. L. Dupont, R. F. Buscho, T. S. Thornhill, A. Z. Kapikian, and R. M. Chanock.** 1974. Comparison of three agents of acute infectious nonbacterial gastroenteritis by cross-challenge in volunteers. *J. Infect. Dis.* **129:**709–714.
133. **Zeitler, C. E., M. K. Estes, and B. V. V. Prasad.** 2006. X-ray crystallographic structure of the Norwalk virus protease at 1.5-Å resolution. *J. Virol.* **80:**5050–5058.
134. **Zheng, D. P., T. Ando, R. L. Fankhauser, R. S. Beard, R. I. Glass, and S. S. Monroe.** 2006. Norovirus classification and proposed strain nomenclature. *Virology* **346:** 312–323.

Hepatitis E Virus

DAVID A. ANDERSON AND ISWAR L. SHRESTHA

49

Hepatitis E virus (HEV) is the causative agent of hepatitis E, known as enterically transmitted non-A, non-B hepatitis prior to the molecular cloning of HEV by Reyes and colleagues in 1990 (89). Hepatitis E is an acute and generally self-limiting infection of the liver, but HEV is unique among the hepatitis viruses in causing a high mortality rate during pregnancy. Clinical hepatitis E is of most importance in developing countries, where it is a major disease burden. Practical and accurate diagnostic assays are available, and an effective vaccine has been developed but is not yet available commercially. It is well established that animal strains of HEV are common throughout the world, with at least some potential for zoonotic infection and a low level of locally acquired disease in developed countries, in addition to that seen in travelers returned from regions where human infection is endemic. Wider use of the improved diagnostic assays that are now available should help to define the true incidence of HEV infection and disease in both developed and developing countries. The recent establishment of practical cell culture systems together with infectious cDNA clones of the virus is leading to a rapid expansion of our knowledge of HEV.

VIROLOGY

Classification

HEV was tentatively assigned to the *Caliciviridae* family for some years on the basis of its particle structure and overall genome organization; however, detailed analysis of the viral genome (41) together with more extensive studies of many human and animal caliciviruses provided the impetus for the reassignment of HEV to the new genus *Hepevirus*, family *Hepeviridae* (26). A related virus of chickens (avian HEV) (43, 48, 49) is the only other family member known at this time.

Serotypes and Antigenicity

There is insufficient evidence to support the division of HEV isolates into serotypes; however, antigenic variation in a number of epitopes has an impact on the sensitivities of some serologic tests. Type specificity of many epitopes was first recognized (127) in comparisons of the Burmese (89, 101) and Mexican (47) strains of HEV. In addition, some viral antigens appear to elicit highly variable antibody responses in different individuals. For example, many experimentally infected animals (and some patients) fail to develop antibodies to the ORF3 protein (65, 66).

Conversely, all isolates of mammalian HEV share some important cross-reactive antigens, and there is evidence for some limited antigenic cross-reactivity between "mammalian" HEV strains and avian HEV (43). Immunization of macaques with recombinant PORF2 proteins of 55 kDa (soluble; 112 to 607 amino acids [aa]) or 62 kDa (virus-like particles [VLPs]; 112 to 636 aa) expressed using a baculovirus system confers immunity to both homologous and heterologous virus challenge (87, 113, 114, 126), suggesting that major protective epitopes are common among HEV genotypes. One immunodominant, conformational epitope has also been identified in the HEV capsid (90). This ORF2.1 epitope is highly conserved between HEV strains and represents as much as 60% of the total convalescent-phase antibody repertoire (90). The ORF2.1 epitope appears to be distinct from the major neutralizing epitope, however (132).

Genotypes

Initial studies of the prototype Burmese strain of HEV (89, 101) and a highly divergent Mexican strain (47) demonstrated wide genetic variation, and the recent reports of many equally divergent HEV strains provide a basis for classification of strains into genotypes, with around 75% nucleotide identities between genotypes. Wang and colleagues (121) have suggested the following classifications: the Burmese (89, 101) and related strains (including most Chinese strains) as genotype 1, the Mexican strain (47) as genotype 2, the swine HEV strain discovered in the United States (77) and closely related strains isolated from patients infected in the United States (92) as genotype 3, and distinct isolates from patients in China (T1 strain) (121) and both patients and swine in Taiwan (45, 46) as genotype 4. Genotype 2 (Mexico) has also been detected in Africa (15, 71), apparently cocirculating with genotype 1 (120). The strong relationship between swine and human HEV isolates in the United States (77, 92), Taiwan (45, 46), Korea (2), and Japan (75, 99) demonstrates the importance of viral genotypes in helping to understand the epidemiology of HEV infection, especially in countries where it is not endemic. Avian HEV shares only around 50% nucleotide sequence identity with human and swine strains (49), and it is unclear whether this virus should be a member of the same genus or, rather, a separate genus as in the case of the mammalian and avian hepatitis B viruses (HBVs) (*Orthohepadnavirus* and *Avihepadnavirus* genera, respectively).

Composition of Virus

Virion Morphology, Structure, and Size

Virions of HEV isolated from the bile or feces are nonenveloped, icosahedral particles around 32 nm in diameter, without any obvious distinguishing morphology (Fig. 1). Because HEV is not present in large amounts in clinical material and yields from cell culture are extremely low, there has been very little characterization of authentic viral particles. However, the expression of truncated PORF2 (aa 112 to 636) in the baculovirus system leads to the formation of HEV VLPs (68, 125, 126). At around 27 nm, these VLPs are smaller than the intact virus particle, but cryoelectron microscopy (4, 67, 124) suggests that HEV VLPs are assembled as a T=1, icosahedral particle containing 30 dimeric subunits of 50-kDa PORF2, with the potential to form an intact virion of the correct size with a T=3 arrangement of 90 dimeric subunits (124). PORF2 dimerization appears to be due to noncovalent interactions in the C-terminal part of the protein and may contribute to the assembly of the immunodominant ORF2.1 epitope (4, 6). It is not known whether the PORF2 protein is truncated in viral particles (as it is in VLPs), and further characterization of infectious viral particles will be required to enhance our understanding of HEV structure.

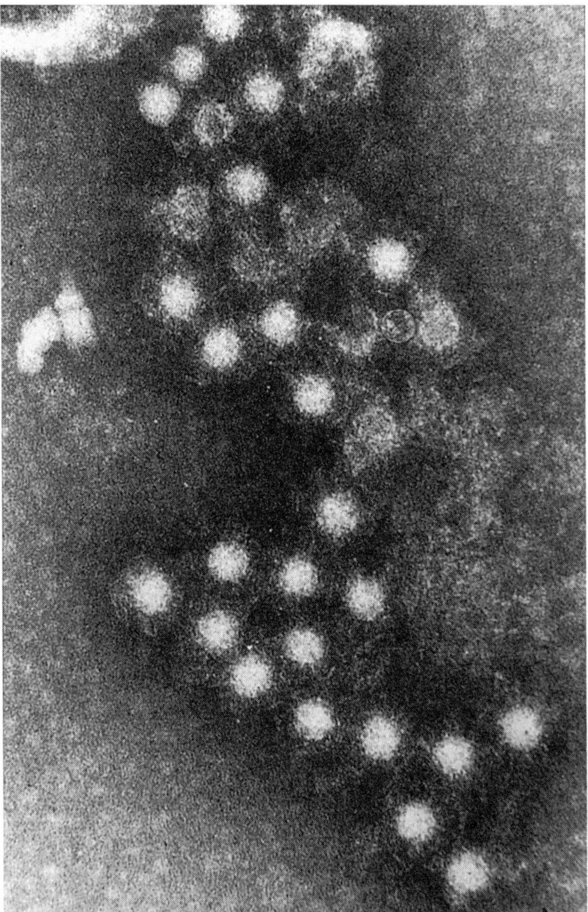

FIGURE 1 Particles of HEV from the stools of an experimentally infected macaque, complexed with acute-phase patient serum. (Courtesy of Zhuang Hui, Beijing Medical University.)

Genome Length and Composition

HEV has a single-stranded RNA genome of positive polarity. The prototype infectious cDNA clone of the SAR55 strain is 7,204 nucleotides [nt] (30). "Full-length" HEV sequences deposited in GenBank range in size up to 7,251 nt plus the poly(A) tail.

The 5′ end of the genome has a 7-methylguanosine cap (55) that is essential for infectivity (30). The viral RNA has short, highly conserved 5′ and 3′ untranslated regions of 35 and 68 to 75 nt, respectively, which are likely to have roles in RNA replication and encapsidation. The HEV genome contains three open reading frames (ORFs), organized as 5′-ORF1-ORF3-ORF2-3′ (Fig. 2), with ORF3 and ORF2 largely overlapping.

Early studies described the presence of subgenomic viral RNAs in the liver of infected macaques (101). However, the development of functional "replicons" of HEV RNA has recently allowed the identification of a single subgenomic RNA that functions as a bicistronic mRNA for translation of both ORF2 and ORF3 proteins (38).

Structural and Regulatory Proteins

The HEV genome encodes three proteins; PORF1 (replicative polyprotein), PORF3 (required for replication in vivo but dispensable in cell culture), and PORF2 (capsid protein).

Translation of ORF1 is expected to yield a polyprotein (PORF1) of approximately 186 kDa containing sequence motifs of methyltransferase, papain-like protease, RNA helicase, and RNA-dependent RNA polymerase (RDRP) activities (101). Expression of PORF1 alone in HepG2 cells or in an in vitro translation system failed to demonstrate any proteolytic processing into mature products (7), suggesting that other cofactors may be required for correct processing.

PORF3 is a very basic protein (pI ≈ 12.5) and is the most variable protein among HEV strains. PORF3 appears to be initiated from the third in-frame AUG codon (50), with a mass of around 11 to 13 kDa. PORF3 is associated with the cytoskeleton and is phosphorylated at serine 80 by mitogen-activated protein kinase (128); a number of host cell protein interactions occur with PORF3 (58, 61, 83, 119), suggesting a regulatory role for PORF3 in viral replication.

The role and importance of PORF3 in viral replication were unclear for many years but were greatly clarified by the identification of a *cis*-reactive element in the ORF for PORF3 that is essential for replication, such that many site-directed mutations were having primary effects on RNA structure rather than the protein (37). The ORF3 protein itself proved to be dispensable for replication in cell culture (29) but essential for infectivity in nonhuman primates (37) and pigs (50), consistent with a putative role in pathogenesis rather than replication. Phosphorylation does not appear to be essential for these functions (37).

The capsid protein (PORF2) is translated as a 660-aa protein, and a large proportion of the nascent protein is modified by N glycosylation following heterologous ex-

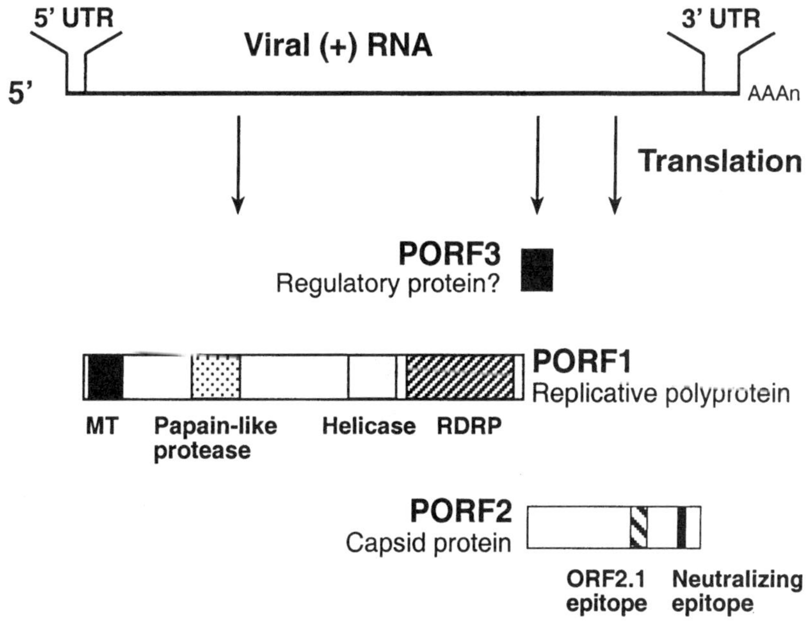

FIGURE 2 Genome organization and major antigenic domains of HEV. The genome, of around 7,200 nt, contains a 5′ 7-methylguanosine cap and highly conserved 5′ and 3′ untranslated regions (UTRs) of 35 and 68 to 75 nt, respectively. Three ORFs, organized as 5′-ORF1-ORF3-ORF2-3′, encode the viral proteins, which may be translated from a set of subgenomic mRNA molecules, but it is not known which mRNA species may encode each protein. The PORF1 polyprotein contains protein domains consistent with replicative proteins (methyltransferase, protease, helicase, and RDRP), and PORF2 is the major capsid protein. The function of PORF3 is unknown; this protein is dispensable for replication in cell culture but essential in vivo. Linear antigenic domains have been identified by peptide scanning throughout each of the three proteins, while within PORF2 a conformational, immunodominant epitope (the ORF2.1 epitope) is found between aa 394 and 457, while a conformational, neutralizing epitope is found between aa 578 and 607.

pression in mammalian cells (53, 112). However, this glycosylated form of the protein is highly unstable (111), and it is not clear whether the authentic viral particle contains glycosylated capsid proteins. A protein the size of full-length, nonglycosylated PORF2 has been detected in HEV replicon cell lines (107), but this may not represent mature virus particles. When PORF2 is expressed in insect cells, it is cleaved at a predominant site between aa 111 and 112 and at various sites within the C terminus of the protein. At least some of these truncated forms of PORF2 have the ability to self-assemble into VLPs or subviral particles (68, 76, 91, 115, 131).

Biology

Replication Strategy

The in vitro propagation of HEV was first demonstrated in primary macaque hepatocytes (102, 103), but this system did not permit any detailed studies. More recently, a reproducible cell culture system for HEV has been established in a subclone of liver-derived HepG2 cells (28). The combination of this system with both infectious cDNA clones and subgenomic replicons has begun to provide significant advances in our understanding of HEV replication (28, 29, 36–38), including the role of PORF3 in viral replication and identification of a bicistronic mRNA for PORF2 and PORF3 as outlined above.

Unfortunately, the yield of HEV in cell culture remains very low, precluding studies of many aspects of replication. It is reasonable to expect that the virus will now progressively adapt to cell culture as seen for hepatitis A virus (HAV), and it may further be hoped that some animal strains of HEV (either swine or avian) may prove less refractory to cell culture, noting the important role that duck HBV has played in defining the replication cycle of the HBV family. At present, however, the general outline of HEV replication can only be inferred (Fig. 3).

Following ingestion of HEV, the virus may be absorbed directly through the gastrointestinal mucosa into the circulation to reach the liver, or following one or more rounds of amplification in enterocytes. However, no evidence has been obtained for replication of HEV at this site, in contrast to the case with HAV, for which replication in enterocyte-derived Caco-2 cells is well established (11). HEV presumably interacts with one or more specific receptors or coreceptors, leading to penetration and uncoating of the virus, and the input viral RNA then serves as mRNA for PORF1. The PORF1 polyprotein is then cleaved by viral (and perhaps cellular) proteases to yield the mature replicative proteins. The RDRP then copies the input viral genome to yield negative-strand RNA, which in turn serves as a template for the transcription of further positive-strand RNA molecules, including new genomes.

Studies in cell culture have detected only a single subgenomic mRNA, suggesting that PORF1 is translated

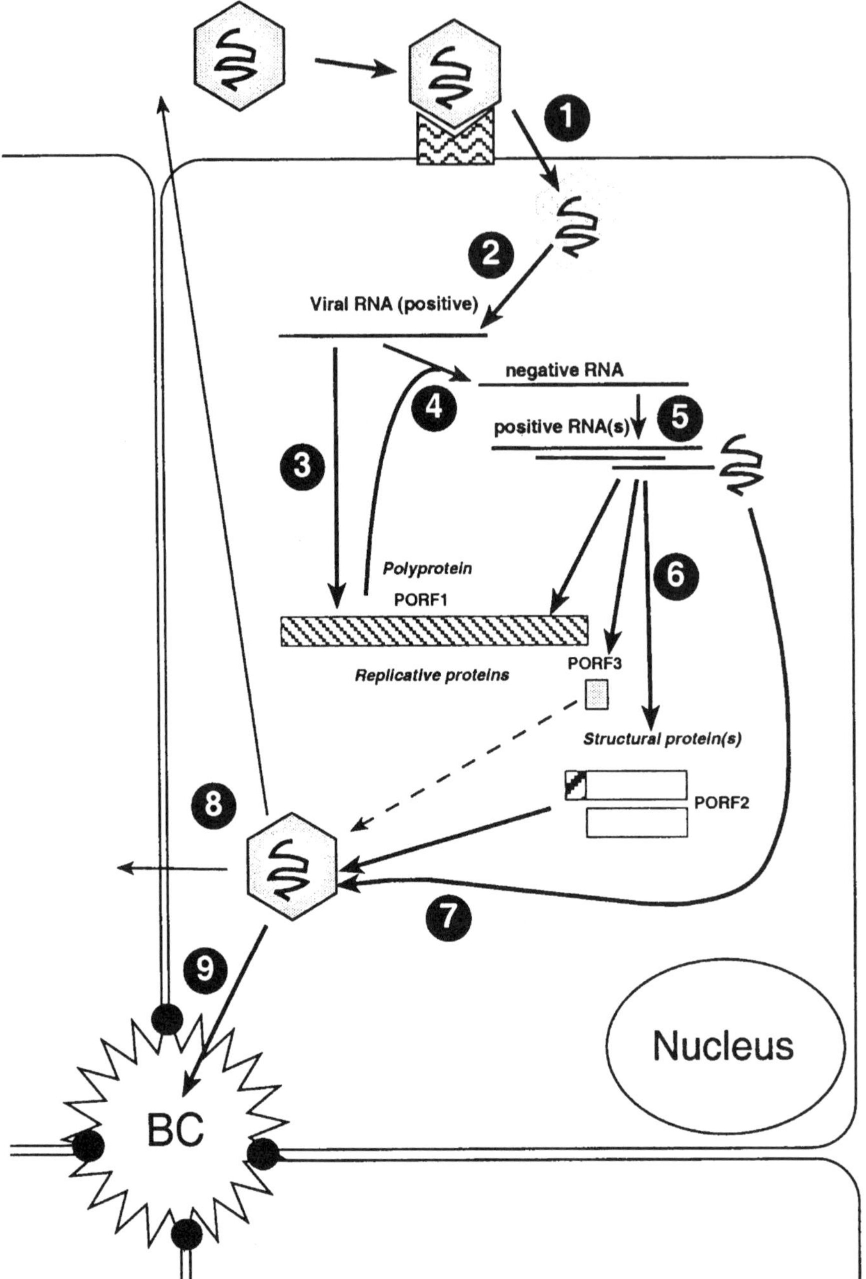

FIGURE 3 Putative replication cycle of HEV. After oral ingestion, HEV particles reach the liver, where they attach to an unidentified receptor on the basolateral domain of hepatocytes, leading to virus penetration (step 1) and uncoating of the genome (step 2) within the cell. Translation of the input genome (step 3) yields the PORF1 polyprotein, which is cleaved at unknown sites to yield the replicative proteins, which copy the input genome to yield full-length negative-strand RNAs (step 4), followed by subgenomic positive-strand mRNAs and full-length positive-strand RNAs (new viral genomes) (step 5). These subgenomic RNAs are translated to yield further molecules of PORF1, PORF2 (capsid), and PORF3 (regulatory) proteins (step 6). PORF2 and new viral genomes assemble into virions (step 7); it is not known whether virions contain full-length or truncated PORF2 products, and the role of membranes in assembly is unclear. Release of progeny virus through basolateral domains of the infected cell (step 8) may result in viremia and infection of distal hepatocytes, and/or infection of neighboring hepatocytes, but transmission to new hosts through the environment is achieved via release of progeny through the apical domain (step 9) to the bile canaliculi (BC) and ultimately the feces.

from the full-length genomic strand, while the subgenomic mRNA is bicistronic, encoding both PORF2 and PORF3 (38). However, we do not know whether the subgenomic mRNA is transcribed from a full-length negative strand or, conversely, from multiple subgenomic negative strands.

The site of HEV assembly in the cell and the role of proteins other than the capsid protein (PORF2) in assembly are also unknown.

A small amount of HEV is found in plasma during infection, consistent with release of progeny virus through the basolateral domains of hepatocytes leading to spread through the liver, but the majority of virus appears to be excreted through the biliary system to complete the replication cycle, consistent with release of virus through the apical domain of hepatocytes.

Host Range

Human strains of HEV can readily infect and cause disease in many nonhuman primates, with cynomolgus macaques *(Macaca fascicularis)* and rhesus macaques *(Macaca mulatta)* being widely used for experimental purposes. Swine HEV was first detected in pigs in the United States (77) and subsequently shown to be endemic in swine worldwide, as well as in wild deer in Japan (73, 82, 99, 100, 106). Swine HEV has been transmitted to macaques, and human HEV has been transmitted to swine (78, 81). Swine do not appear to develop clinical or biochemical disease following infection with either swine or human isolates of HEV (41).

Growth in Cell Culture

Propagation of HEV was first demonstrated in macaque hepatocytes (102, 103), but this system is not widely available or practicable. A more robust cell culture system uses a subclone of hepatocyte-derived HepG2 cells. Virus yields in this system remain very low, but it has allowed some key questions of virus replication to be addressed (28, 29, 36–38), as well as providing a system for the study of virus neutralization (27). It is likely that the virus will be able to adapt to cell culture over time to give yields sufficient for studies of other replicative events. Growth and serial passage of HEV have been described with PLC/PRF/5 cells (105).

Inactivation by Physical and Chemical Agents

Because HEV is transmitted via the fecal-oral route, it must withstand exposure to bile salts during excretion and low pH during ingestion, but it is generally considered more labile than the extremely stable HAV. HEV is inactivated at temperatures higher than 70°C but withstands incubation at 56°C for 30 min (105). Available cell culture systems for HEV are not sufficiently quantitative to allow precise measurement of inactivation kinetics under different conditions.

In areas of endemicity, boiling is the most reliable treatment for water (44), as chlorination may be ineffective in the presence of large amounts of organic matter (for example, contamination of water with feces) and indeed was shown to be inadequate during an outbreak in the Darfur region of Sudan (40). However, boiling is likely to be impractical in many of the settings where HEV is endemic or epidemic, such as refugee camps.

EPIDEMIOLOGY

There is a wide divergence in the sensitivity, specificity, and concordance of serologic assays for HEV in use around the world (72), and hence in the resulting estimates for prevalence of HEV infection. In general, there is broad agreement regarding the epidemiology of HEV infection in developing countries where clinical HEV infection is common; however, the situation in developed countries is less clear.

Distribution

Contamination of water sources with human feces is the most common risk factor for epidemic HEV infection, as for hepatitis A. Consequently, the major disease burden of HEV is in developing countries, with the Indian subcontinent, Egypt, and parts of China being recognized as areas of high endemicity. HEV is the most common cause of acute hepatitis in these countries. HEV infection appears to be less common in the developing countries of South America, although this conclusion may be biased by the small numbers of studies undertaken there using the more advanced diagnostic tests, as studies in Cuba have shown quite high prevalence of clinical HEV infection (63, 88). In many developing countries, the incidence and prevalence of HEV infection have not been examined, and it should be assumed that countries with poor sanitation have a high risk for endemic HEV infection and disease.

However, the distribution of HEV within countries where it is endemic is also highly variable, providing ideal conditions for epidemics in conditions of population displacement when combined with poor sanitary conditions. This is typically the case for refugee camps but is also likely to be a factor in the high attack rate of HEV that is commonly seen in army recruits in developing countries. In rural Tibet, very wide variations exist in HEV seroprevalence among individual villages (110). Because of limited internal migration between these villages and the majority transmission of HEV via water, the prevalence of HEV immunoglobulin G (IgG) was found to provide a marker for predicting historical water quality in each village, correlating in many cases with engineering surveys but identifying other villages where HEV prevalence was very high without obvious sources of contamination. Such studies may allow more targeted efforts in upgrading of water supplies in countries where HEV is endemic.

Clinical HEV infection in developed countries where HEV is not endemic will frequently be associated with recent travel to areas of endemicity. However, swine HEV strains have a worldwide distribution (2, 16, 19, 45, 79, 82, 99, 123), and in view of the close relationship between swine HEV and strains isolated from some patients in the United States (77, 92), Taiwan (45, 46), Korea (2), and Japan (75, 99), HEV infection should be considered a possibility in acute hepatitis patients who do not have a relevant travel history or markers of other hepatitis viruses.

The true rate of HEV infection in developed countries remains controversial. Serologic assays based on truncated PORF2 protein (aa 112 to 660) expressed using the baculovirus system have yielded seroprevalence rates of over 20% in blood donors from Baltimore, MD (108), whereas rates of less than 2% were found in Australian blood donors using the ORF2.1 protein (aa 394 to 660) expressed in *Escherichia coli* (5, 96), yet the two assays appear to be equally sensitive when applied to samples from countries where HEV is endemic. Somewhat higher HEV IgG prevalence rates, of between 3.7 and 6.7% in Japan (34, 104) and 11.9% in Korea (2), have been reported.

Avian HEV appears to share some antigenic cross-reactivity with human HEV strains (39, 43), and rats have also been implicated as a potential reservoir of HEV (54). It appears unlikely that these HEV-like viruses cause disease in humans (unlike the case for swine HEV), but exposure and cross-reactive antibody may contribute to the high estimates of seroprevalence obtained using some assays.

Incidence and Prevalence of Infection

Subclinical Infection Rate

In countries where HEV is endemic and clinical HEV infection is common, the majority of HEV infections appear to be subclinical, with a clinical/subclinical ratio of between 1:2.6 and 1:7 reported (70). In countries where HEV is not endemic, the rate of clinical HEV infection is clearly much lower, but it is impossible to estimate the subclinical attack rate because of the limited use of specific diagnostic tests in possible acute hepatitis E and the very wide divergence in seroprevalence rates obtained using different assays (see above). Factors that may influence the clinical attack rate in developed countries include the possibility that swine strains of HEV may be attenuated for humans (41, 80, 81) and the tendency of low-dose infections to produce mild or no disease, as observed in experimentally infected animals. Such low-dose exposure might be expected in developed countries, where massive fecal contamination of water supplies is rare.

Epidemic Patterns

In countries where HEV is endemic, sporadic HEV infection is often the most common form of viral hepatitis on an annual basis, accounting for around 70% of cases in Kathmandu, Nepal (3, 21), but above this background major epidemics also occur with a period of around 7 to 10 years. For example, HEV was responsible for 16 of 17 epidemics of enterically transmitted hepatitis in India (8), but HEV is also responsible for at least 25% of sporadic hepatitis cases between epidemics (56). In general, epidemics are associated with the wet season (summer in most countries where HEV is endemic). Large outbreaks of HEV were seen after flooding that coincided with the conflict and displacement of 1.8 million civilians in the Darfur region of Sudan (12, 40). From July to December 2004, 2,621 hepatitis E cases were recorded in the Mornay refugee camp of 78,800 inhabitants (an attack rate of 3.3%), with an overall case fatality rate of 1.7%. Epidemics of HEV have not been reported in developed countries.

Age-Specific Attack Rates

Clinical HEV infection in countries where HEV is endemic is most common in adolescents and young adults, but it occurs to a lesser extent from childhood (52) to late ages. There appear to be considerable differences in exposure rates between countries where HEV is considered endemic: in Egypt, around 60% of children were exposed to HEV by the age of 10, and this rate did not increase further with age (24, 33), whereas in Nepal, only 16% of 12-year-olds had evidence of exposure to HEV; exposure peaked at 31% later in life (21). It is likely that the risk of clinical disease increases with age, as for hepatitis A, but while clinical HAV infection is uncommon in many developing countries because of high exposure rates in children (for example, 100% HAV seropositive by the age of 1 to 3 years in one study in Egypt [24]), HEV exposure rates are never as high as for HAV, and a large proportion of the population remains susceptible.

Risk Factors and High-Risk Groups

For residents of developed countries, travel to countries where HEV is endemic remains the greatest risk factor for clinical HEV infection, but sporadic cases do occur in the absence of travel. Risk factors for these rare sporadic cases have not been clearly identified, but they may be different than for hepatitis A, as the prevalence of anti-HEV does not correspond with risk groups for HAV exposure (108). There is some evidence for increased seroprevalence in groups with occupational exposure to swine (57).

In developing countries, exposure to water contaminated with human waste is a clear risk factor, and close contact with domestic animals (including pigs) may also be a risk.

Reinfections

Levels of HEV-specific antibody decline rapidly in the first year after infection and may become negative by some assays, but antibodies to some parts of the PORF2 protein probably remain stable for many years thereafter. The presence of antibody to HEV appears to be protective for individuals in epidemics (14), but antibody may not persist at protective levels for life. Although it is not clear whether seropositive individuals have sterilizing immunity, clinical HEV infection appears to be limited to individuals who are seronegative at the time of exposure (14).

Seasonality

Peak rates of HEV infection occur in the wet season in some countries where HEV is endemic (for example Nepal, China, and India), associated with fecal contamination of water supplies. However, in some regions there appears to be no seasonal variation (23), and at least one study has shown an increased rate of infection associated with a period of unusually low rainfall, presumably by concentrating human wastes in a riverine ecology (22).

Analysis of serologic results from sporadic hepatitis patients in Kathmandu, Nepal, shows an interesting seasonal relationship for both the rate of infections and the level of anti-HEV IgM reactivity in patients during a nonepidemic year (Fig. 4). HEV-specific IgM was detectable in almost 60% of acute hepatitis cases seen at the Siddhi Polyclinic in 1997 (using a prototype version of the commercial ORF2.1 IgM ELISA [18]), but the levels of reactivity for positive sera may suggest different epidemiological patterns for infections giving high reactivity (for example, human HEV strains and/or high infectious doses spread via contaminated water, with a peak in the wet season) versus low reactivity (for example, zoonotic HEV strains spread via close contact or low infectious doses, at a constant rate through the year). Further studies are required to clarify the transmission patterns of HEV in different settings.

Transmission

Routes and Risk Factors

Hepatitis E is transmitted via the fecal-oral route. Consumption of contaminated water is by far the most common route of transmission for clinical cases of HEV in countries where HEV is endemic.

Most human isolates of HEV detected in countries where HEV is not considered endemic are more closely

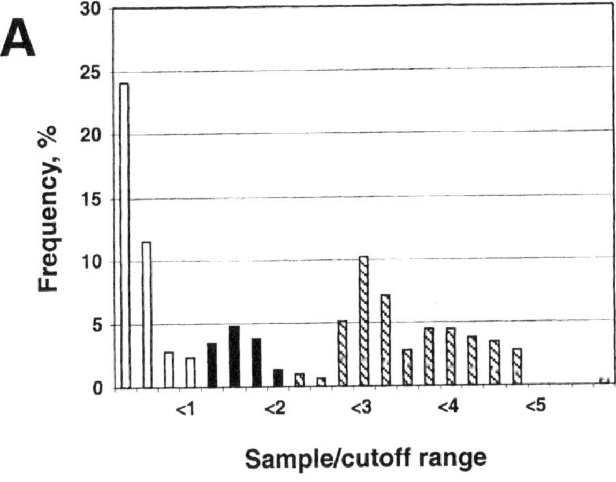

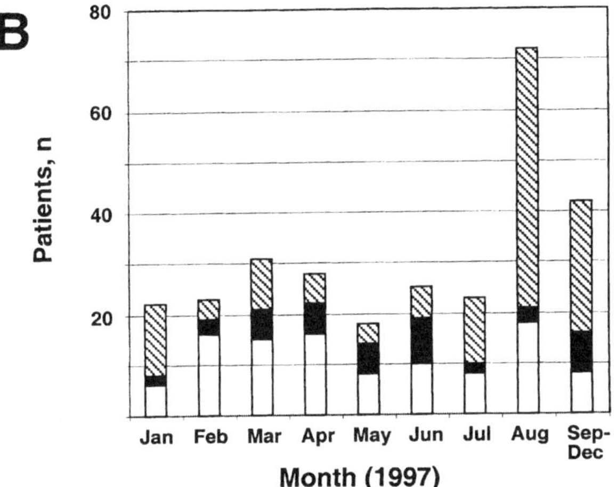

FIGURE 4 HEV-specific IgM levels in patients with acute, sporadic hepatitis in Kathmandu, Nepal. All patients seen at the Siddhi Polyclinic with symptoms and biochemical markers consistent with acute hepatitis during 1997 were tested using a prototype IgM ELISA based on the ORF2.1 antigen, and the results are shown as a frequency histogram of the ratio of sample to cutoff for patient samples (A). Almost 60% of patients tested positive in the HEV IgM ELISA, but with two distinct patterns of reactivity (low positive [■] and high positive [▧]). White bars indicate patients who tested negative. (B) The level of IgM reactivity did not correlate with patient age, sex, or levels of biochemical markers, but patients with highly positive results were more likely to present during the peak (wet) season. (Data from our laboratories.)

related to swine HEV strains, and there have been clearly defined cases of zoonotic HEV infection in Japan associated with consumption of HEV-infected pig or deer meat, and swine HEV has been detected in both wild pigs and deer in Japan (73, 82, 99, 100, 106). However, in most countries where HEV is not endemic, the true rate of zoonotic infection remains unclear due to limited testing (see reference 78 for a review of zoonotic HEV infection).

Risk of Transmission after Specific Exposures

Hepatitis E is not commonly transmitted by person-to-person contact (in contrast to hepatitis A), and household transmission is therefore not a significant risk factor. However, common-source exposure within homes or schools and other institutions via contaminated water should certainly be considered, especially in countries where HEV is endemic.

Nosocomial Infection

Nosocomial infections with HEV are probably very rare, but transfusion-associated HEV has been reported in Japan (74) and is likely to be more common in countries where HEV is highly endemic.

Duration of Infectiousness

Excretion of HEV in feces is the only significant risk for person-to-person infection. Although detection of virus in feces by reverse transcription-PCR (RT-PCR) is technically difficult, HEV RNA is detectable in 50% of patients 2 weeks after onset (20) and, in one case, has been detected at 52 days after onset (86).

PATHOGENESIS

Incubation Period

The incubation period for hepatitis E is reduced, and the likelihood of clinical disease is increased, with increasing doses of virus (117). The incubation period for hepatitis E is most commonly 5 to 6 weeks (range, 3 to 8 weeks), but in experimental infections of macaques with intravenous challenge and high doses of virus, disease can be evident as early as 2 weeks after exposure (66, 117).

Patterns of Virus Replication

HEV replication has not been observed in tissues other than liver, but it seems likely that a low level of replication may occur in enteric epithelium before infection of the liver, as for HAV (9). Small amounts of HEV can be detected in serum during the late incubation period and for 2 to 6 weeks after the onset of illness. HEV is excreted in feces; virus has not been reported to be found in other excretions.

The generalized course of infection and serologic responses to HEV are shown in Fig. 5. Infection is presumed to be initiated via cells lining the alimentary tract. Virus then spreads via the bloodstream to the liver, eventually infecting a large proportion of the hepatocyte population but without causing direct cytolytic damage. After an incubation period of 5 to 6 weeks, liver damage results and is thought to be mediated by the cellular immune response to the virus. As for HAV, infections in young children more often follow a benign course, but disease is possible at any age.

Characteristic Histopathological Changes

Histopathological studies of liver specimens obtained from patients involved in epidemics have demonstrated that infection with HEV can produce morphological changes in the liver comprising both cholestatic and classical acute hepatitis (13, 62, 122, 133), but these features are not unique or diagnostic in hepatitis E. Typical histopathological changes include lobular disarray with enlargement of portal tracts, Kupffer cell proliferation, focal hepatocyte necrosis and bridging necrosis, ballooning of hepatocytes, and acidophilic degeneration of hepatocytes as well as mononuclear cell infiltration. Within hepatocytes there is dilatation of the cisternae of the endoplasmic reticulum with an increase in the number and size of lysosomes

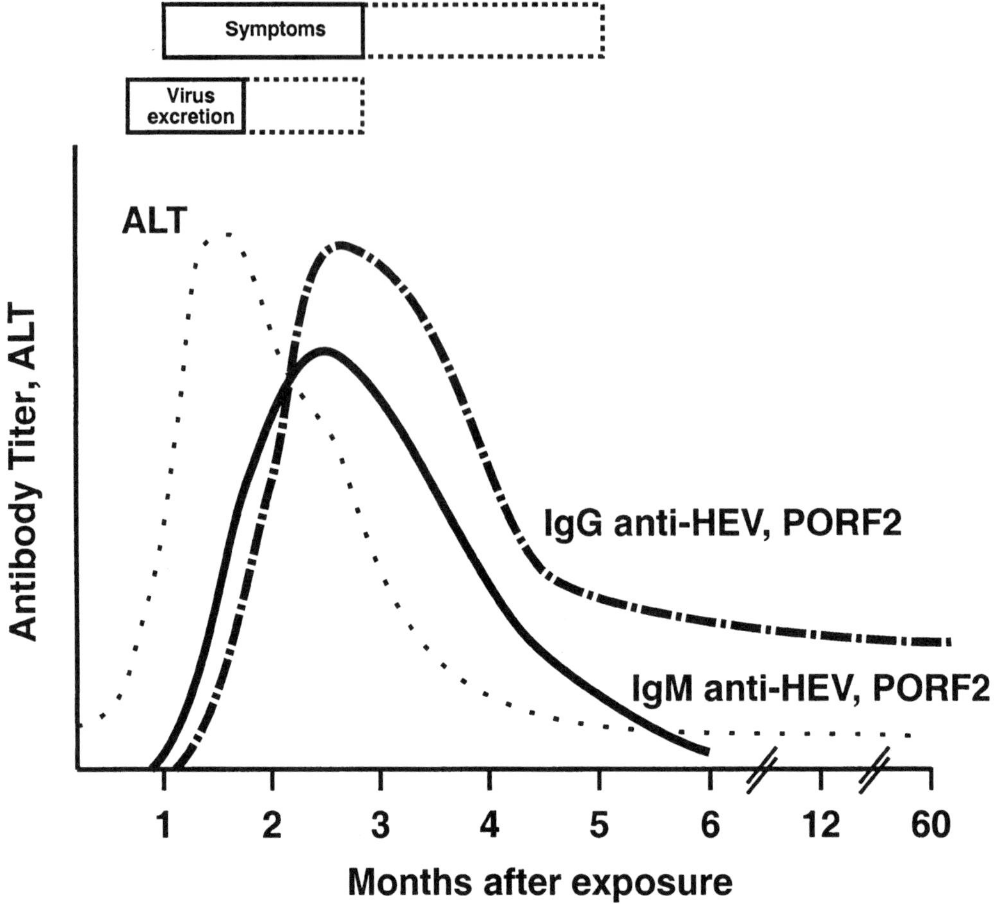

FIGURE 5 Course of HEV infection and characteristic humoral immune responses. After reaching high levels during the acute phase, HEV PORF2-specific IgG declines rapidly over 6 to 12 months and might not persist at protective levels for life. The serologic responses to the PORF2 protein as shown are those which probably occur in most patients, but the detection of these responses varies widely among different assays. Conversely, the responses to PORF3 appear to be highly variable (not illustrated), with a proportion of patients mounting no detectable response to the antigen, while others maintain reactivity to PORF3 for many years. (Modified from reference 3 with permission.)

within the cytoplasm. Condensation of the matrix within mitochondria together with dilatation of the outer mitochondrial membrane has also been reported.

Cholestatic hepatitis of hepatitis E is characterized by bile stasis in canaliculi and gland-like transformation of hepatocytes, degeneration of hepatocytes, and intralobular and portal tract infiltrates of lymphocytes and polymorphonuclear leukocytes. A prominent feature is the presence of cholestasis and glandular transformation of the liver cell plates, with the cholestatic changes persisting until clinical recovery occurs. These histopathological changes gradually resolve over a period of 3 to 6 months.

Patients with fulminant HEV infection demonstrate necrosis of parenchyma with collapse of liver lobules; swelling of hepatocytes, which have a foamy appearance; arrangement of hepatocytes into an acinar pattern; proliferation of small bile ductules; phlebitis of portal and central veins; and portal inflammation with lymphocytic and polymorphonuclear leukocyte infiltration (10, 42, 62).

Immune Responses

Nonspecific (Cytokines and Inflammatory Mediators)

Cytokine responses during HEV infection have not been studied.

Specific (Humoral, Cell-Mediated, and Mucosal Immunity)

The typical patterns of IgG and IgM class antibody responses during HEV infection are shown in Fig. 5. However, it should be noted that antibody responses to individual viral antigens are highly variable, due to both strain-specific differences in some epitopes and differences in responses to single antigens among individual patients (see "Serotypes and antigenicity" above). For example, PORF3 varies greatly among strains, but even in macaques challenged with a common-source inoculum, as few as one in three individuals will mount a detectable IgG response to PORF3, and this response is transient (66). In contrast, the 55- to 63-kDa antigens expressed with a baculovirus system, and the ORF2.1 protein expressed in *E. coli*, detect specific IgG and IgM responses in the great majority of patients. Typically, both IgG and IgM antibodies are detectable at the onset of disease, with IgM declining to undetectable levels over a period of 2 to 6 months, while an approximately 10-fold decline in IgG levels is seen over this period but levels then stabilize.

IgA responses to HEV (as a correlate of mucosal immunity) have been detected in around 50% of patients (17), but these antibodies rapidly declined to undetectable levels. The role of IgA in immunity to HEV infection is unknown, but as passive immunization with IgG appears to be sufficient for protection (114), it is likely that IgA is not essential.

Cellular immune responses during HEV infection have not been extensively studied. T-cell responses (proliferation) in HEV patients to peptide libraries derived from the PORF2 and PORF3 proteins are observed with peptide pools (but not individual peptides) derived from PORF2, but not PORF3 (1).

Correlates of Immune Protection

Antibody is sufficient for protection, as shown by successful passive immunization of macaques (114). Subsequent preclinical (87) and clinical (98) development of the truncated PORF2 (aa 112 to 607) vaccine produced using the baculovirus system has firmly established the ability of this vaccine to produce protective antibody responses.

However, a clearer understanding of antigenic structure and correlates of immune protection will be important in fully utilizing HEV vaccines, particularly with respect to the duration of protection beyond the scope of clinical trials. The development and implementation of effective vaccines for hepatitis A and B over the past 20 years have been aided by serologic assays in which the level of reactivity (dominated by only a few epitopes) is highly predictive of immunity, by virtue of the correlation between the immunodominant epitopes and protection. This correlation does not appear to be true for HEV. Within the 660-aa PORF2, the conformational ORF2.1 epitope appears to be immunodominant, with very long-lasting antibody (64–66, 90), but its role in protection is unclear. Other, less dominant epitopes appear to be responsible for protection via neutralizing antibody (94, 95, 130).

CLINICAL MANIFESTATIONS

Major Clinical Syndromes

Prodrome

Hepatitis E is clinically indistinguishable from other forms of acute viral hepatitis. The clinical presentation of acute viral hepatitis commonly begins with nonspecific, "flu-like" prodromal symptoms lasting from 1 to 10 days, consisting of fatigue, malaise, anorexia, nausea, vomiting, and some alteration in taste and smell. A low-grade fever, between 38° and 39°C, is common.

The first distinctive signs of hepatitis are often dark urine and pale clay-colored stools followed by onset of clinical jaundice. With the appearance of clinical jaundice, the prodromal symptoms usually subside; however, some patients may not show visible signs of jaundice despite severe symptoms. Abdominal examination may reveal an enlarged and tender liver associated with pain and discomfort in the right upper quadrant. The spleen may be enlarged in 10 to 15% of patients. Occasionally, patients may present with cholestasis, which is more common in pregnant women.

Resolution of HEV is accompanied by normalization of biochemical markers (serum alanine aminotransferase [ALT] levels and bilirubin) over a period of 6 weeks in most patients, whereas histologic changes may persist for up to 6 months without overt disease. Small numbers of patients appear to have a protracted course of disease, with resolution taking many months.

HEV infection during pregnancy is associated with a high mortality rate due to fulminant hepatitis, around 25% in the third trimester (42, 51, 118). Interestingly, a marked difference in the clinical progression of HEV was also observed between African citizens and French soldiers who acquired their infections in Africa, with none of 27 French soldiers having fulminant hepatitis but with a mean time to recovery of over 8 weeks, whereas 7 of 44 adult male Africans had fulminant hepatitis, with 6 deaths, yet a reduced time to recovery in the other patients (mean of around 3 weeks) (109).

The reason for the differing clinical courses between the French soldiers and male African citizens is unexplained. Similarly, the basis of the high mortality rate during pregnancy is not understood; studies of pregnant macaques have not demonstrated any increase in disease severity (116). While hormonal factors may contribute to pathogenesis during pregnancy, other factors may also be important, such as the underlying general health status or chronic infection with HBV or hepatitis C virus in patients at the time of HEV infection. No specific pathogenic factors have yet been identified.

Vertical transmission of HEV with severe hepatitis in the infant has been demonstrated (59), but it is unclear whether anything can be done to prevent this once the mother is infected. HEV has not been associated with congenital abnormalities.

Laboratory Abnormalities

Liver function tests are an important adjunct to diagnosis. The serum aminotransferases ALT and aspartate aminotransferase show variable increases during the prodromal phase. The ALT level peaks at the onset of symptoms before the serum bilirubin begins to increase. Peak levels of ALT vary from 1,000 to 2,000 U/liter at onset. ALT progressively diminishes during the recovery phase. The level of ALT, however, does not correlate with the degree of liver cell damage. Some patients presenting with anicteric acute HEV infection have only raised ALT, which is helpful in the early diagnosis of clinically suspected cases, along with the presence of anti-HEV IgM in the serum.

Jaundice is visible in sclera or skin when the serum total bilirubin level exceeds 2.5 mg/dl, usually following the peak levels of ALT. Peak serum total bilirubin levels range from 5 to 25 mg/dl; both conjugated and unconjugated fractions are increased. In cholestatic HEV infection (around 10% of patients), serum bilirubin may remain elevated for prolonged periods.

Prothrombin time and international normalized ratio may be increased in acute viral hepatitis, especially in fulminant hepatitis, indicating extensive hepatocellular necrosis and a worse prognosis. Similarly, a reduction in the serum albumin level may occur. Reduced blood glucose levels leading to hypoglycemia may be observed in patients with prolonged nausea, vomiting, and inadequate carbohydrate intake. Neutropenia, lymphopenia, and atypical lymphocytes may occasionally be observed during the acute phase of viral hepatitis.

Age-Related Differences

The risk and severity of clinical HEV disease increase with age at exposure, as with hepatitis A. Fever as the presenting sign of hepatitis E may be more common in the young (109). There is evidence that HEV infection contributes to fetal death and other complications when the mother has symptomatic hepatitis E (42, 118), but the situation with subclinical infections is unclear.

Disease in Immunocompromised Patients

The course of HEV disease in immunocompromised patients has not been studied. As the mechanism of liver damage is likely to be immune mediated, there may be no increased disease risk in the immunocompromised. However, there is no adequate explanation for the high case fatality rate in pregnant women, and it is conceivable that this could be related to their immunologic status.

Complications

The major complications of HEV infection are fulminant hepatitis, observed in less than 1% of patients from the general population but in up to 30% during the third trimester of pregnancy, with a high death rate in most studies. Cholestatic hepatitis is seen in around 10 to 25% of patients (60), with a prolonged period of cholestasis observed in some studies.

Clinical Diagnosis, Including Differential Diagnosis

Acute hepatitis E has no distinguishing clinical characteristics that allow a differential diagnosis from other forms of acute viral hepatitis. In many cases, the nonspecific symptoms found in the prodromal phase (fatigue, anorexia, abdominal pain, nausea and vomiting, and fever) may not lead to a suspicion of acute viral hepatitis unless the patient becomes jaundiced or has a relevant history, such as travel to an area of endemicity. Due to their identical clinical presentations and predominant modes of transmission, hepatitis E may be suspected in the same circumstances as hepatitis A, but it must be noted that HAV infection is far more common than HEV infection in developed countries. Conversely, in countries where HEV is endemic, it is often the most common cause of acute hepatitis.

LABORATORY DIAGNOSIS

Specific diagnosis of HEV infection remains problematic. A variety of nucleic acid and serologic assays are used in research laboratories, but routine (commercial) diagnostic assays vary widely in their sensitivities and specificities.

Virus Isolation

Virus isolation is not appropriate for HEV; like other hepatitis viruses, HEV is refractory to routine isolation in cell culture.

Antigen Detection

Detection of viral particles in feces by immunoelectron microscopy provides a specific diagnostic marker but is no longer in use due to the technical demands and very poor sensitivity of the technique. Other antigen detection methods have not been adopted.

Nucleic Acid Detection

Detection of HEV RNA in serum by RT-PCR provides the "gold standard" in specificity for diagnosis of acute hepatitis E but is not suitable for routine use. RT-PCR has been very useful in research situations for the detection of divergent HEV strains with which the serologic responses may not have been detected by some assays (46, 71, 93, 120, 121). RT-PCR remains an important research level confirmatory assay for positive HEV IgM tests in countries where HEV is not endemic, but its sensitivity is constrained by the duration and level of viremia and the stability of HEV RNA in samples.

Serologic Assays

A number of research and commercial immunoassays are available in various countries but showed major differences in their sensitivities and specificities (72, 84). More recently developed commercial assays appear to have improved on this performance through the use of better recombinant antigens and assay formats (detailed below), but first- and second-generation tests are still commercially available in most parts of the world. The appropriate use and interpretation of serologic assays for HEV infection must take into account the quality of different tests, together with the pattern of serologic responses (IgG and IgM) to various antigens and the widely varying prevalence of clinical HEV infection worldwide (3).

Diagnosis of HEV Infection in Areas of Low or Intermediate Prevalence

In areas with a low incidence of clinical HEV infection, such as the United States, Australia, and western Europe, or intermediate prevalence, such as Japan, Korea, and Taiwan, assay specificity will have a very large impact on the predictive value of HEV serologic tests. Diagnostic assays for the detection of HEV-specific IgG (manufactured by MP Biomedicals Asia Pacific, Singapore [formerly Genelabs Diagnostics], and Abbott Diagnostics, Chicago, IL) have considerable value for the diagnosis of acute hepatitis in travelers returned from areas of endemicity (25), among whom the incidence may be higher than the background rate of reactivity—around 2% in the healthy population. However, with the recognition that HEV should be considered in the diagnosis of sporadic acute hepatitis without a history of travel to recognized regions of endemicity (92, 93), the need for more specific tests becomes evident. For example, if the incidence of HEV infection among acute hepatitis patients in the United States is 0.2%, then only 1 in 10 patients whose samples are reactive in a test for HEV-specific IgG would be true positives, leading to an unacceptable positive predictive value.

The detection of HEV-specific IgM should therefore become the method of choice for diagnosis of acute HEV infection in areas of low prevalence. Until recently, a single HEV IgM assay was commercially available in most countries (MP Biomedicals Asia Pacific) based on the same recombinant HEV antigens as the widely available IgG tests. This assay had a reported false-positivity rate in U.S. blood donors of 26 of 856 (3%) (1998 technical bulletin, Genelabs), which would make it no more suitable than HEV IgG tests for diagnosis in areas of nonendemicity.

Published studies have also demonstrated that the recombinant antigens used in this assay may fail to detect antibody in around 40% of patients with acute HEV infection (125).

Enzyme-linked immunosorbent assays (ELISAs) with improved reactivity are in use in research laboratories; these assays are based on recombinant antigens derived from baculovirus-based (68, 91, 97, 125, 132) or *E. coli*-based (5, 32) expression systems but have not been widely adopted for commercially available assays. However, the ORF2.1 antigen, representing aa 394 to 660 derived from a Chinese strain of HEV expressed in *E. coli* (5, 65, 66), has been shown to represent immunodominant and highly conserved epitopes of HEV (90) and forms the basis of the recently developed commercial HEV IgM ELISA and ASSURE rapid, point-of-care (RPOC) tests produced by MP Biomedicals Asia Pacific. In the first published study, the IgM ELISA demonstrated a sensitivity of 99.3% (150 of 151 HEV-infected patients) and a specificity of 97.6% (203 of 208 controls), while the RPOC test demonstrated a slightly reduced sensitivity (96.7%; 146 of 151) and a slightly higher specificity (98.6%; 205 of 208) on the same samples (18). In a separate study of the HEV IgM RPOC test, where the comparator assay was an in-house quantitative IgM ELISA based on baculovirus-expressed HEV antigen (97), the RPOC assay was also found to have a high sensitivity (93%; 186 of 200) and specificity (99.7%; 320 of 321) (85). The RPOC test takes around 5 min in total and requires minimal training and no specialized equipment; representative assay results with the ASSURE HEV IgM test are shown in Fig. 6. The sensitivity of the commercially available ORF2.1-based ELISA and RPOC tests is clearly adequate for diagnosis of acute HEV infection, but the likely false-positivity rate of between 0.3 and 2.4% is around the same as that of previous assays, and caution must still be exercised in interpreting positive results from patients without a history of travel outside areas of low endemicity.

Substantial numbers of HEV cases have been reported from Taiwan (45, 46), Korea (2), and Japan (75, 99). Serologic diagnosis using HEV IgM tests is likely to have a higher positive predictive value in these populations than in the United States and other countries of lowest endemicity.

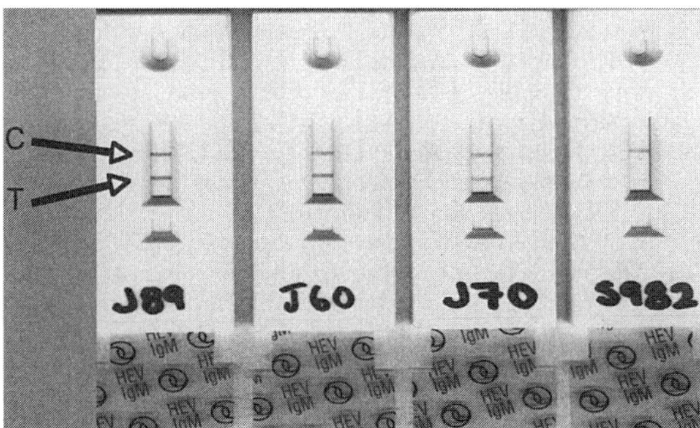

FIGURE 6 Representative test results obtained with the ASSURE HEV IgM RPOC test. A sample with no detectable HEV-specific IgM (S982) shows a single line (control [C]), while samples with HEV-specific IgM (J89, J60, and J70) show both control and test (T) lines. (Data from our laboratories.)

Diagnosis of HEV Infection in Areas of High Prevalence

Although the titer of HEV-specific IgG tends to decline markedly in the first year after infection, this relationship is not reliable enough to form the basis of differential diagnosis (5, 35). The detection of HEV-specific IgG is therefore of little use for diagnosis of acute infection in developing countries where HEV is endemic and large numbers of patients will have antibody from past infections. Detection of HEV-specific IgM must therefore be the method of choice in areas of endemicity.

In settings of endemicity, assay sensitivity is of primary concern. This includes the robustness of assays, in order that assays can be processed and interpreted manually, where equipment such as ELISA washers and readers is not available. In this context, the ASSURE HEV IgM RPOC test (Fig. 6) appears especially suitable for use in areas where HEV is endemic, with a sensitivity and specificity substantially equivalent to those of both the commercial ELISA based on the same antigen (18) and a quantitative research ELISA (85). While these studies have been performed with pedigreed sera and plasma samples, the test is designed for use with fresh whole blood, which further enhances its utility for resource-poor and emergency settings.

Although the HEV IgM RPOC test can offer performance equivalent to that of ELISAs, many laboratories will have a preference for the more traditional format of tests. The MP Biomedicals HEV IgM ELISA based on ORF2.1 antigen shows greatly improved sensitivity over the former Genelabs Diagnostics/MP Biomedicals HEV IgM ELISA (18) and is progressively replacing that test in most countries, although it is not currently available in the United States. Commercially available ELISA-based HEV IgM kits manufactured by ADALTIS (Bologna, Italy) and BIOKIT (Barcelona, Spain) are available in many countries, but to date there have been no published evaluations of assay performance for these tests.

As HEV accounts for as much as 70% of the cases of acute sporadic hepatitis in countries where HEV is endemic, the specificity of assays is less critical in these settings. For example, if the false-positivity rate of an assay is 2%, then only 1 in 35 hepatitis patients in areas of endemicity might be misdiagnosed as having acute HEV. Higher specificity would of course be favorable, and at least one HEV IgM assay in research use has been reported with a false-positivity rate of only 0.1% (69), while the ASSURE HEV IgM RPOC test has a false-positivity rate between 0.3 and 1.4% (18, 85).

PREVENTION

General

Environmental

The most significant influence on HEV infection is protection of water supplies from contamination with human fecal waste. Many epidemics in developing countries have occurred due to leakage of sewerage pipes into municipal water supply pipes laid in the same or adjacent trenches. A barrier between these two supplies is essential for long-term prevention. Chlorination and filtration systems are generally inadequate if the source water is contaminated.

Personal and Behavioral

Travelers to regions of endemicity must take precautions against the consumption of contaminated water. Only boiled or bottled water should be used. Although infection via food appears to be much less common for hepatitis E than for hepatitis A, it is important that travelers maintain vigilance about the risks of contaminated water, ice, and food. This is especially true for individuals who have been vaccinated against hepatitis A and B and may have a false sense of security with respect to all forms of hepatitis. Women should avoid unnecessary travel to areas of endemicity during pregnancy.

Isolation of Infected Persons

Isolation does not appear to be justified, due to the very low rates of person-to-person transmission; however, infected individuals should not be involved in food preparation or handling until symptoms have fully resolved.

Passive Immunoprophylaxis

Passive immunization has the potential to protect against disease (114), but gamma globulin prepared in countries where HEV is not endemic is ineffective, and even pools prepared in countries where it is endemic may offer little or no protective efficacy. Protective epitopes have now been characterized (27, 94, 95), and the development of an ELISA specific for the protective epitopes (132) may allow identification of suitable high-titer plasma pools in the future.

Active Immunization

Prospects for active immunization are very promising. Vaccines based on the PORF2 protein (aa 112 to 607 or 660) expressed in insect cells are clearly protective in animal studies (76, 87, 113, 126, 129). The recombinant 53-kDa vaccine represents aa 112 to 607, and a clinical trial in Nepalese army recruits demonstrated that the vaccine was highly effective in this population (98). A total of 1,794 healthy HEV-seronegative adults received three doses of either the 53-kDa vaccine or placebo at months 0, 1, and 6 and were monitored for a median of 804 days. Hepatitis E developed in 66 of 896 placebo recipients, versus 3 of 898 vaccine recipients, with an efficacy of 95.5% (98). It is hoped that the vaccine will eventually be available for use in countries where HEV is endemic and the impact of disease is greatest, rather than only as a "boutique" vaccine for the protection of travelers and military personnel from developed countries. The duration of vaccine protection will be an important consideration for use in endemic populations, and the recent development of an ELISA that appears to be specific for the major neutralizing antibody species in HEV, based on peptide 458-607 (minimum neutralization site), is likely to provide an important tool for such studies (132).

Management of Outbreaks

Outbreaks are most often associated with massive contamination of water supplies, commonly due to weather conditions. This is especially problematic in refugee or other emergency settings. The Darfur outbreaks of 2004 were explosive, with the first cases occurring in July and reaching a peak only 6 weeks later (12, 40), which offers little opportunity for active immunization in control of outbreaks once they have commenced. The recommended procedures for chlorination of water supplies appeared to be inadequate to control HEV in this outbreak, although no bacteria were present in the chlorinated water samples tested (40). Boiling of water is unlikely to be practical in such settings, but special efforts should be taken to supply pregnant women with safe water during outbreaks even if this is not possible for the whole population. These studies highlight the need for timely detection of acute HEV in such settings. Notably, diagnosis of HEV in the Darfur outbreak relied on ELISA and RT-PCR testing of sera transported to a reference laboratory in Cairo, Egypt, but the RPOC HEV IgM test became available toward the end of the outbreak and appeared to perform well in the field (G. Armstrong, CDC, personal communication).

TREATMENT

Symptomatic and Anti-Inflammatory Treatment

No specific symptomatic or anti-inflammatory treatments can be advised for hepatitis E. Bed rest where possible and attention to diet (avoiding fatty foods) may minimize symptoms and speed recovery; alcohol intake should be minimized. Pruritus is a feature of cholestatic hepatitis A which may justify the cautious use of corticosteroids (31); this may also be true in hepatitis E, in which cholestasis is quite common, but controlled studies have not been performed.

Role of End-Organ Support in Severe Disease

There is no specific treatment for acute liver failure, and management strategies for severe hepatitis E are not well established, but it appears that intensive supportive medical care, as for acute liver failure due to other causes, may be able to reduce the high mortality rate seen in regions of endemicity for fulminant hepatitis E during pregnancy. Two pregnant HEV patients have been described who acquired infection in countries where HEV is endemic but presented in the United Kingdom (51). One recovered without specific interventions; the other required ventilation and a bolus of mannitol, which may have aided full recovery.

Antiviral Treatment

Antivirals are not available for hepatitis E.

REFERENCES

1. **Aggarwal, R., R. Shukla, S. Jameel, S. Agrawal, P. Puri, V. K. Gupta, A. P. Patil, and S. Naik.** 2007. T-cell epitope mapping of ORF2 and ORF3 proteins of human hepatitis E virus. *J. Viral Hepat.* **14:**283–292.
2. **Ahn, J. M., S. G. Kang, D. Y. Lee, S. J. Shin, and H. S. Yoo.** 2005. Identification of novel human hepatitis E virus (HEV) isolates and determination of the seroprevalence of HEV in Korea. *J. Clin. Microbiol.* **43:**3042–3048.
3. **Anderson, D. A.** 2000. Waterborne hepatitis, p. 295–305. *In* S. C. Specter, R. L. Hodinka, and S. A. Young (ed.), *Clinical Virology Manual.* ASM Press, Washington, DC.
4. **Anderson, D. A., and R. H. Cheng.** 2005. Hepatitis E: structure and molecular virology, p. 603–610. *In* H. C. Thomas, S. Lemon, and A. J. Zuckerman (ed.), *Viral Hepatitis,* 3rd ed. Blackwell Publishing, Malden, MA.
5. **Anderson, D. A., F. Li, M. A. Riddell, T. Howard, H.-F. Seow, J. Torresi, G. Perry, D. Sumarsidi, S. M. Shrestha, and I. L. Shrestha.** 1999. ELISA for IgG-class antibody to hepatitis E virus based on a highly conserved,

conformational epitope expressed in *Eschericia coli*. *J. Virol. Methods* **81:**131–142.

6. **Anderson, D. A., M. A. Riddell, J. D. Chandler, and F. Li.** 2002. Molecular biology of hepatitis E virus, p. 82–89. *In* H. S. Margolis, M. J. Alter, T. J. Liang, and J. L. Dienstag (ed.), *Viral Hepatitis and Liver Disease*. International Medical Press, London, England.
7. **Ansari, I. H., S. K. Nanda, H. Durgapal, S. Agrawal, S. K. Mohanty, D. Gupta, S. Jameel, and S. K. Panda.** 2000. Cloning, sequencing, and expression of the hepatitis E virus (HEV) nonstructural open reading frame 1 (ORF1). *J. Med. Virol.* **60:**275–283.
8. **Arankalle, V. A., M. S. Chadha, S. A. Tsarev, S. U. Emerson, A. R. Risbud, K. Banerjee, and R. H. Purcell.** 1994. Seroepidemiology of water-borne hepatitis in India and evidence for a third enterically-transmitted hepatitis agent. *Proc. Natl. Acad. Sci. USA* **91:**3428–3432.
9. **Asher, L. V., L. N. Binn, T. L. Mensing, R. H. Marchwicki, R. A. Vassell, and G. D. Young.** 1995. Pathogenesis of hepatitis A in orally inoculated owl monkeys (Aotus trivirgatus). *J. Med. Virol.* **47:**260–268.
10. **Asher, L. V., B. L. Innis, M. P. Shrestha, J. Ticehurst, and W. B. Baze.** 1990. Virus-like particles in the liver of a patient with fulminant hepatitis and antibody to hepatitis E virus. *J. Med. Virol.* **31:**229–233.
11. **Blank, C. A., D. A. Anderson, M. Beard, and S. M. Lemon.** 2000. Infection of polarized cultures of human intestinal epithelial cells with hepatitis A virus: vectorial release of progeny virions through apical cellular membranes. *J. Virol.* **74:**6476–6484.
12. **Boccia, D., J. P. Guthmann, H. Klovstad, N. Hamid, M. Tatay, I. Ciglenecki, J. Y. Nizou, E. Nicand, and P. J. Guerin.** 2006. High mortality associated with an outbreak of hepatitis E among displaced persons in Darfur, Sudan. *Clin. Infect. Dis.* **42:**1679–1684.
13. **Bradley, D. W.** 1992. Hepatitis E: epidemiology, aetiology and molecular biology. *Rev. Med. Virol.* **2:**19–28.
14. **Bryan, J. P., S. A. Tsarev, M. Iqbal, J. Ticehurst, S. Emerson, A. Ahmed, J. Duncan, A. R. Rafiqui, I. A. Malik, R. H. Purcell, and L. J. Legters.** 1994. Epidemic hepatitis E in Pakistan: patterns of serologic response and evidence that antibody to hepatitis E virus protects against disease. *J. Infect. Dis.* **170:**517–521.
15. **Buisson, Y., M. Grandadam, E. Nicand, P. Cheval, H. van Cuyck-Gandre, B. Innis, P. Rehel, P. Coursaget, R. Teyssou, and S. Tsarev.** 2000. Identification of a novel hepatitis E virus in Nigeria. *J. Gen. Virol.* **81:**903–909.
16. **Chandler, J. D., M. A. Riddell, F. Li, R. J. Love, and D. A. Anderson.** 1999. Serological evidence for swine hepatitis E virus infection in Australian pig herds. *Vet. Microbiol.* **68:**95–105.
17. **Chau, K. H., G. J. Dawson, K. M. Bile, L. O. Magnius, M. H. Sjogren, and I. K. Mushahwar.** 1993. Detection of IgA class antibody to hepatitis E virus in serum samples from patients with hepatitis E virus infection. *J. Med. Virol.* **40:**334–338.
18. **Chen, H. Y., Y. Lu, T. Howard, D. Anderson, P. Y. Fong, W. P. Hu, C. P. Chia, and M. Guan.** 2005. Comparison of a new immunochromatographic test to enzyme-linked immunosorbent assay for rapid detection of immunoglobulin M antibodies to hepatitis E virus in human sera. *Clin. Diagn. Lab. Immunol.* **12:**593–598.
19. **Clayson, E. T., B. L. Innis, K. S. Myint, S. Narupiti, D. W. Vaughn, S. Giri, P. Ranabhat, and M. P. Shrestha.** 1995. Detection of hepatitis E virus infections among domestic swine in the Kathmandu Valley of Nepal. *Am. J. Trop. Med. Hyg.* **53:**228–232.
20. **Clayson, E. T., K. S. Myint, R. Snitbhan, D. W. Vaughn, B. L. Innis, L. Chan, P. Cheung, and M. P. Shrestha.** 1995. Viremia, fecal shedding, and IgM and IgG responses in patients with hepatitis E. *J. Infect. Dis.* **172:**927–933.
21. **Clayson, E. T., M. P. Shrestha, D. W. Vaughn, R. Snitbhan, K. B. Shrestha, C. F. Longer, and B. L. Innis.** 1997. Rates of hepatitis E virus infection and disease among adolescents and adults in Kathmandu, Nepal. *J. Infect. Dis.* **176:**763–766.
22. **Corwin, A., K. Jarot, I. Lubis, K. Nasution, S. Suparmawo, A. Sumardiati, S. Widodo, S. Nazir, G. Orndorff, Y. Choi, R. Tan, A. Sie, S. Wignall, R. Graham, and K. Hyams.** 1995. Two years' investigation of epidemic hepatitis E virus transmission in West Kalimantan (Borneo), Indonesia. *Trans. R. Soc. Trop. Med. Hyg.* **89:**262–265.
23. **Corwin, A. L., T. C. Dai, D. D. Duc, P. I. Suu, N. T. Van, L. D. Ha, M. Janick, L. Kanti, A. Sie, R. Soderquist, R. Graham, S. F. Wignall, and K. C. Hyams.** 1996. Acute viral hepatitis in Hanoi, Viet Nam. *Trans. R. Soc. Trop. Med. Hyg.* **90:**647–648.
24. **Darwish, M. A., R. Faris, J. D. Clemens, M. R. Rao, and R. Edelman.** 1996. High seroprevalence of hepatitis A, B, C, and E viruses in residents in an Egyptian village in the Nile Delta: a pilot study. *Am. J. Trop. Med. Hyg.* **54:**554–558.
25. **Dawson, G. J., I. K. Mushahwar, K. H. Chau, and G. L. Gitnick.** 1992. Detection of long-lasting antibody to hepatitis E virus in a US traveller to Pakistan. *Lancet* **340:**426–427.
26. **Emerson, S. U., D. Anderson, A. Arankalle, X. J. Meng, M. Purdy, and G. G. Schlauder.** 2005. Hepevirus, p. 851–855. *In* C. M. Fauquet, M. A. Mayo, J. Maniloff, U. Desselberger, and L. A. Ball (ed.), *Virus Taxonomy: Eighth Report of the International Committee on Taxonomy of Viruses*. Elsevier Academic Press, San Diego, CA.
27. **Emerson, S. U., P. Clemente-Casares, N. Moiduddin, V. A. Arankalle, U. Torian, and R. H. Purcell.** 2006. Putative neutralization epitopes and broad cross-genotype neutralization of hepatitis E virus confirmed by a quantitative cell-culture assay. *J. Gen. Virol.* **87:**697–704.
28. **Emerson, S. U., H. Nguyen, J. Graff, D. A. Stephany, A. Brockington, and R. H. Purcell.** 2004. In vitro replication of hepatitis E virus (HEV) genomes and of an HEV replicon expressing green fluorescent protein. *J. Virol.* **78:**4838–4846.
29. **Emerson, S. U., H. Nguyen, U. Torian, and R. H. Purcell.** 2006. ORF3 protein of hepatitis E virus is not required for replication, virion assembly, or infection of hepatoma cells in vitro. *J. Virol.* **80:**10457–10464.
30. **Emerson, S. U., M. Zhang, X. J. Meng, H. Nguyen, M. St. Claire, S. Govindarajan, Y. K. Huang, and R. H. Purcell.** 2001. Recombinant hepatitis E virus genomes infectious for primates: importance of capping and discovery of a cis-reactive element. *Proc. Natl. Acad. Sci. USA* **98:**15270–15275.
31. **Fagan, E. A., and T. J. Harrison.** 2000. *Viral Hepatitis*. BIOS, Oxford, England.
32. **Favorov, M. O., Y. E. Khudyakov, E. E. Mast, T. L. Yashina, C. N. Shapiro, N. S. Khudyakova, D. L. Jue, G. G. Onischenko, H. S. Margolis, and H. A. Fields.** 1996. IgM and IgG antibodies to hepatitis E virus (HEV) detected by an enzyme immunoassay based on an HEV-specific artificial recombinant mosaic protein. *J. Med. Virol.* **50:**50–58.
33. **Fix, A. D., M. Abdel-Hamid, R. H. Purcell, M. H. Shehata, F. Abdel-Aziz, N. Mikhail, H. el Sebai, M. Nafeh, M. Habib, R. R. Arthur, S. U. Emerson, and G. T. Strickland.** 2000. Prevalence of antibodies to hepatitis E in two rural Egyptian communities. *Am. J. Trop. Med. Hyg.* **62:**519–523.

34. **Fukuda, S., J. Sunaga, N. Saito, K. Fujimura, Y. Itoh, M. Sasaki, F. Tsuda, M. Takahashi, T. Nishizawa, and H. Okamoto.** 2004. Prevalence of antibodies to hepatitis E virus among Japanese blood donors: identification of three blood donors infected with a genotype 3 hepatitis E virus. *J. Med. Virol.* **73:**554–561.
35. **Ghabrah, T. M., S. Tsarev, P. O. Yarbough, S. U. Emerson, G. T. Strickland, and R. H. Purcell.** 1998. Comparison of tests for antibody to hepatitis E virus. *J. Med. Virol.* **55:**134–137.
36. **Graff, J., H. Nguyen, C. Kasorndorkbua, P. G. Halbur, M. St. Claire, R. H. Purcell, and S. U. Emerson.** 2005. In vitro and in vivo mutational analysis of the 3′-terminal regions of hepatitis E virus genomes and replicons. *J. Virol.* **79:**1017–1026.
37. **Graff, J., H. Nguyen, C. Yu, W. R. Elkins, M. St. Claire, R. H. Purcell, and S. U. Emerson.** 2005. The open reading frame 3 gene of hepatitis E virus contains a *cis*-reactive element and encodes a protein required for infection of macaques. *J. Virol.* **79:**6680–6689.
38. **Graff, J., U. Torian, H. Nguyen, and S. U. Emerson.** 2006. A bicistronic subgenomic mRNA encodes both the ORF2 and ORF3 proteins of hepatitis E virus. *J. Virol.* **80:**5919–5926.
39. **Guo, H., E. M. Zhou, Z. F. Sun, X. J. Meng, and P. G. Halbur.** 2006. Identification of B-cell epitopes in the capsid protein of avian hepatitis E virus (avian HEV) that are common to human and swine HEVs or unique to avian HEV. *J. Gen. Virol.* **87:**217–223.
40. **Guthmann, J. P., H. Klovstad, D. Boccia, N. Hamid, L. Pinoges, J. Y. Nizou, M. Tatay, F. Diaz, A. Moren, R. F. Grais, I. Ciglenecki, E. Nicand, and P. J. Guerin.** 2006. A large outbreak of hepatitis E among a displaced population in Darfur, Sudan, 2004: the role of water treatment methods. *Clin. Infect. Dis.* **42:**1685–1691.
41. **Halbur, P. G., C. Kasorndorkbua, C. Gilbert, D. Guenette, M. B. Potters, R. H. Purcell, S. U. Emerson, T. E. Toth, and X. J. Meng.** 2001. Comparative pathogenesis of infection of pigs with hepatitis E viruses recovered from a pig and a human. *J. Clin. Microbiol.* **39:**918–923.
42. **Hamid, S. S., S. M. Jafri, H. Khan, H. Shah, Z. Abbas, and H. Fields.** 1996. Fulminant hepatic failure in pregnant women: acute fatty liver or acute viral hepatitis? *J. Hepatol.* **25:**20–27.
43. **Haqshenas, G., F. F. Huang, M. Fenaux, D. K. Guenette, F. W. Pierson, C. T. Larsen, H. L. Shivaprasad, T. E. Toth, and X. J. Meng.** 2002. The putative capsid protein of the newly identified avian hepatitis E virus shares antigenic epitopes with that of swine and human hepatitis E viruses and chicken big liver and spleen disease virus. *J. Gen. Virol.* **83:**2201–2209.
44. **Hau, C. H., T. T. Hien, N. T. Tien, H. B. Khiem, P. K. Sac, V. T. Nhung, R. P. Larasati, K. Laras, M. P. Putri, R. Doss, K. C. Hyams, and A. L. Corwin.** 1999. Prevalence of enteric hepatitis A and E viruses in the Mekong River delta region of Vietnam. *Am. J. Trop. Med. Hyg.* **60:**277–280.
45. **Hsieh, S. Y., X. J. Meng, Y. H. Wu, S. T. Liu, A. W. Tam, D. Y. Lin, and Y. F. Liaw.** 1999. Identity of a novel swine hepatitis E virus in Taiwan forming a monophyletic group with Taiwan isolates of human hepatitis E virus. *J. Clin. Microbiol.* **37:**3828–3834.
46. **Hsieh, S. Y., P. Y. Yang, Y. P. Ho, C. M. Chu, and Y. F. Liaw.** 1998. Identification of a novel strain of hepatitis E virus responsible for sporadic acute hepatitis in Taiwan. *J. Med. Virol.* **55:**300–304.
47. **Huang, C. C., D. Nguyen, J. Fernandez, K. Y. Yun, K. E. Fry, D. W. Bradley, A. W. Tam, and G. R. Reyes.** 1992. Molecular cloning and sequencing of the Mexico isolate of hepatitis E virus (HEV). *Virology* **191:**550–558.
48. **Huang, F. F., G. Haqshenas, H. L. Shivaprasad, D. K. Guenette, P. R. Woolcock, C. T. Larsen, F. W. Pierson, F. Elvinger, T. E. Toth, and X. J. Meng.** 2002. Heterogeneity and seroprevalence of a newly identified avian hepatitis E virus from chickens in the United States. *J. Clin. Microbiol.* **40:**4197–4202.
49. **Huang, F. F., Z. F. Sun, S. U. Emerson, R. H. Purcell, H. L. Shivaprasad, F. W. Pierson, T. E. Toth, and X. J. Meng.** 2004. Determination and analysis of the complete genomic sequence of avian hepatitis E virus (avian HEV) and attempts to infect rhesus monkeys with avian HEV. *J. Gen. Virol.* **85:**1609–1618.
50. **Huang, Y. W., T. Opriessnig, P. G. Halbur, and X. J. Meng.** 2007. Initiation at the third in-frame AUG codon of open reading frame 3 of the hepatitis E virus is essential for viral infectivity in vivo. *J. Virol.* **81:**3018–3026.
51. **Hussaini, S. H., S. J. Skidmore, P. Richardson, L. M. Sherratt, B. T. Cooper, and J. G. O'Grady.** 1997. Severe hepatitis E infection during pregnancy. *J. Viral Hepat.* **4:**51–54.
52. **Hyams, K. C., M. C. McCarthy, M. Kaur, M. A. Purdy, D. W. Bradley, M. M. Mansour, S. Gray, D. M. Watts, and M. Carl.** 1992. Acute sporadic hepatitis E in children living in Cairo, Egypt. *J. Med. Virol.* **37:**274–277.
53. **Jameel, S., M. Zafrullah, M. H. Ozdener, and S. K. Panda.** 1996. Expression in animal cells and characterization of the hepatitis E virus structural proteins. *J. Virol.* **70:**207–216.
54. **Kabrane-Lazizi, Y., J. B. Fine, J. Elm, G. E. Glass, H. Higa, A. Diwan, C. J. Gibbs, Jr., X. J. Meng, S. U. Emerson, and R. H. Purcell.** 1999. Evidence for widespread infection of wild rats with hepatitis E virus in the United States. *Am. J. Trop. Med. Hyg.* **61:**331–335.
55. **Kabrane-Lazizi, Y., X. J. Meng, R. H. Purcell, and S. U. Emerson.** 1999. Evidence that the genomic RNA of hepatitis E virus is capped. *J. Virol.* **73:**8848–8850.
56. **Kar, P., S. Budhiraja, A. Narang, and A. Chakravarthy.** 1997. Etiology of sporadic acute and fulminant non-A, non-B viral hepatitis in north India. *Indian J. Gastroenterol.* **16:**43–45.
57. **Karetnyi, Y. V., M. J. Gilchrist, and S. J. Naides.** 1999. Hepatitis E virus infection prevalence among selected populations in Iowa. *J. Clin. Virol.* **14:**51–55.
58. **Kar-Roy, A., H. Korkaya, R. Oberoi, S. K. Lal, and S. Jameel.** 2004. The hepatitis E virus open reading frame 3 protein activates ERK through binding and inhibition of the MAPK phosphatase. *J. Biol. Chem.* **279:**28345–28357.
59. **Khuroo, M. S., S. Kamili, and S. Jameel.** 1995. Vertical transmission of hepatitis E virus. *Lancet* **345:**1025–1026.
60. **Khuroo, M. S., V. K. Rustgi, G. J. Dawson, I. K. Mushahwar, G. N. Yattoo, S. Kamili, and B. A. Khan.** 1994. Spectrum of hepatitis E virus infection in India. *J. Med. Virol.* **43:**281–286.
61. **Korkaya, H., S. Jameel, D. Gupta, S. Tyagi, R. Kumar, M. Zafrullah, M. Mazumdar, S. K. Lal, L. Xiaofang, D. Sehgal, S. R. Das, and D. Sahal.** 2001. The ORF3 protein of hepatitis E virus binds to Src homology 3 domains and activates MAPK. *J. Biol. Chem.* **276:**42389–42400.
62. **Krawczynski, K.** 1993. Hepatitis E. *Hepatology* **17:**932–941.
63. **Lemos, G., S. Jameel, S. Panda, L. Rivera, L. Rodriguez, and J. V. Gavilondo.** 2000. Hepatitis E virus in Cuba. *J. Clin. Virol.* **16:**71–75.
64. **Li, F., M. A. Riddell, H. F. Seow, N. Takeda, T. Miyamura, and D. A. Anderson.** 2000. Recombinant subunit ORF2.1 antigen and induction of antibody against im-

munodominant epitopes in the hepatitis E virus capsid protein. *J. Med. Virol.* **60:**379–386.
65. **Li, F., J. Torresi, S. A. Locarnini, H. Zhuang, W. Zhu, X. Guo, and D. A. Anderson.** 1997. Amino-terminal epitopes are exposed when full-length open reading frame 2 of hepatitis E virus is expressed in Escherichia coli, but carboxy-terminal epitopes are masked. *J. Med. Virol.* **52:** 289–300.
66. **Li, F., H. Zhuang, S. Kolivas, S. A. Locarnini, and D. A. Anderson.** 1994. Persistent and transient antibody responses to hepatitis E virus detected by Western immunoblot using open reading frame 2 and 3 and glutathione S-transferase fusion proteins. *J. Clin. Microbiol.* **32:**2060–2066.
67. **Li, T. C., N. Takeda, T. Miyamura, Y. Matsuura, J. C. Wang, H. Engvall, L. Hammar, L. Xing, and R. H. Cheng.** 2005. Essential elements of the capsid protein for self-assembly into empty virus-like particles of hepatitis E virus. *J. Virol.* **79:**12999–13006.
68. **Li, T. C., Y. Yamakawa, K. Suzuki, M. Tatsumi, M. A. Razak, T. Uchida, N. Takeda, and T. Miyamura.** 1997. Expression and self-assembly of empty virus-like particles of hepatitis E virus. *J. Virol.* **71:**7207–7213.
69. **Li, T. C., J. Zhang, H. Shinzawa, M. Ishibashi, M. Sata, E. E. Mast, K. Kim, T. Miyamura, and N. Takeda.** 2000. Empty virus-like particle-based enzyme-linked immunosorbent assay for antibodies to hepatitis E virus. *J. Med. Virol.* **62:**327–333.
70. **Longer, C. F., J. E. Elliot, J. D. Caudill, L. B. Binn, J. P. Bryan, M. Iqbal, B. L. Innis, E. T. Clayson, M. P. Shrestha, S. A. Tsarev, H. Y. Zhang, and J. Ticehurst.** 1996. Observations on subclinical hepatitis E virus (HEV) infection and protection against reinfection, p. 362–372. *In* Y. Buisson, P. Coursaget, and M. Kane (ed.), *Enterically-Transmitted Hepatitis Viruses.* La Simarre, Joue-les-Tours, France.
71. **Maila, H. T., S. M. Bowyer, and R. Swanepoel.** 2004. Identification of a new strain of hepatitis E virus from an outbreak in Namibia in 1995. *J. Gen. Virol.* **85:**89–95.
72. **Mast, E. E., M. J. Alter, P. V. Holland, and R. H. Purcell for the Hepatitis E Virus Antibody Serum Panel Evaluation Group.** 1998. Evaluation of assays for antibody to hepatitis E virus by a serum panel. *Hepatology* **27:** 857–861.
73. **Masuda, J., K. Yano, Y. Tamada, Y. Takii, M. Ito, K. Omagari, and S. Kohno.** 2005. Acute hepatitis E of a man who consumed wild boar meat prior to the onset of illness in Nagasaki, Japan. *Hepatol. Res.* **31:**178–183.
74. **Matsubayashi, K., Y. Nagaoka, H. Sakata, S. Sato, K. Fukai, T. Kato, K. Takahashi, S. Mishiro, M. Imai, N. Takeda, and H. Ikeda.** 2004. Transfusion-transmitted hepatitis E caused by apparently indigenous hepatitis E virus strain in Hokkaido, Japan. *Transfusion* **44:**934–940.
75. **Matsuda, H., K. Okada, K. Takahashi, and S. Mishiro.** 2003. Severe hepatitis E virus infection after ingestion of uncooked liver from a wild boar. *J. Infect. Dis.* **188:**944.
76. **McAtee, C. P., Y. Zhang, P. O. Yarbough, T. R. Fuerst, K. L. Stone, S. Samander, and K. R. Williams.** 1996. Purification and characterization of a recombinant hepatitis E protein vaccine candidate by liquid chromatography-mass spectrometry. *J. Chromatogr. B* **685:** 91–104.
77. **Meng, X.-J., R. H. Purcell, P. G. Halbur, J. R. Lehman, D. M. Webb, T. S. Tsareva, J. S. Haynes, B. J. Thacker, and S. U. Emerson.** 1997. A novel virus in swine is closely related to the human hepatitis E virus. *Proc. Natl. Acad. Sci. USA* **94:**9860–9865.
78. **Meng, X. J.** 2003. Swine hepatitis E virus: cross-species infection and risk in xenotransplantation. *Curr. Top. Microbiol. Immunol.* **278:**185–216.
79. **Meng, X. J., S. Dea, R. E. Engle, R. Friendship, Y. S. Lyoo, T. Sirinarumitr, K. Urairong, D. Wang, D. Wong, D. Yoo, Y. Zhang, R. H. Purcell, and S. U. Emerson.** 1999. Prevalence of antibodies to the hepatitis E virus in pigs from countries where hepatitis E is common or is rare in the human population. *J. Med. Virol.* **59:**297–302.
80. **Meng, X. J., P. G. Halbur, J. S. Haynes, T. S. Tsareva, J. D. Bruna, R. L. Royer, R. H. Purcell, and S. U. Emerson.** 1998. Experimental infection of pigs with the newly identified swine hepatitis E virus (swine HEV), but not with human strains of HEV. *Arch. Virol.* **143:**1405–1415.
81. **Meng, X. J., P. G. Halbur, M. S. Shapiro, S. Govindarajan, J. D. Bruna, I. K. Mushahwar, R. H. Purcell, and S. U. Emerson.** 1998. Genetic and experimental evidence for cross-species infection by swine hepatitis E virus. *J. Virol.* **72:**9714–9721.
82. **Michitaka, K., K. Takahashi, S. Furukawa, G. Inoue, Y. Hiasa, N. Horiike, M. Onji, N. Abe, and S. Mishiro.** 2007. Prevalence of hepatitis E virus among wild boar in the Ehime area of western Japan. *Hepatol. Res.* **37:**214–220.
83. **Moin, S. M., M. Panteva, and S. Jameel.** 2007. The hepatitis E virus Orf3 protein protects cells from mitochondrial depolarization and death. *J. Biol. Chem.* **282:**21124–21133.
84. **Myint, K. S., T. P. Endy, R. V. Gibbons, K. Laras, M. P. Mammen, Jr., E. R. Sedyaningsih, J. Seriwatana, J. S. Glass, S. Narupiti, and A. L. Corwin.** 2006. Evaluation of diagnostic assays for hepatitis E virus in outbreak settings. *J. Clin. Microbiol.* **44:**1581–1583.
85. **Myint, K. S., M. Guan, H. Y. Chen, Y. Lu, D. Anderson, T. Howard, H. Noedl, and M. P. Mammen, Jr.** 2005. Evaluation of a new rapid immunochromatographic assay for serodiagnosis of acute hepatitis E infection. *Am. J. Trop. Med. Hyg.* **73:**942–946.
86. **Nanda, S. K., I. H. Ansari, S. K. Acharya, S. Jameel, and S. K. Panda.** 1995. Protracted viremia during acute sporadic hepatitis E virus infection. *Gastroenterology* **108:** 225–230.
87. **Purcell, R. H., H. Nguyen, M. Shapiro, R. E. Engle, S. Govindarajan, W. C. Blackwelder, D. C. Wong, J. P. Prieels, and S. U. Emerson.** 2003. Preclinical immunogenicity and efficacy trial of a recombinant hepatitis E vaccine. *Vaccine* **21:**2607–2615.
88. **Quintana, A., L. Sanchez, O. Larralde, and D. Anderson.** 2005. Prevalence of antibodies to hepatitis E virus in residents of a district in Havana, Cuba. *J. Med. Virol.* **76:**69–70.
89. **Reyes, G. R., M. A. Purdy, J. P. Kim, K. C. Luk, L. M. Young, K. E. Fry, and D. W. Bradley.** 1990. Isolation of a cDNA from the virus responsible for enterically transmitted non-A, non-B hepatitis. *Science* **247:**1335–1339.
90. **Riddell, M. A., F. Li, and D. A. Anderson.** 2000. Identification of immunodominant and conformational epitopes in the capsid protein of hepatitis E virus by using monoclonal antibodies. *J. Virol.* **74:**8011–8017.
91. **Robinson, R. A., W. H. Burgess, S. U. Emerson, R. S. Leibowitz, S. A. Sosnovtseva, S. Tsarev, and R. H. Purcell.** 1998. Structural characterization of recombinant hepatitis E virus ORF2 proteins in baculovirus-infected insect cells. *Protein Expr. Purif.* **12:**75–84.
92. **Schlauder, G. G., G. J. Dawson, J. C. Erker, P. Y. Kwo, M. F. Knigge, D. L. Smalley, J. E. Rosenblatt, S. M. Desai, and I. K. Mushahwar.** 1998. The sequence and phylogenetic analysis of a novel hepatitis E virus isolated from a patient with acute hepatitis reported in the United States. *J. Gen. Virol.* **79:**447–456.

93. **Schlauder, G. G., S. M. Desai, A. R. Zanetti, N. C. Tassopoulos, and I. K. Mushahwar.** 1999. Novel hepatitis E virus (HEV) isolates from Europe: evidence for additional genotypes of HEV. *J. Med. Virol.* **57:**243–251.
94. **Schofield, D. J., J. Glamann, S. U. Emerson, and R. H. Purcell.** 2000. Identification by phage display and characterization of two neutralizing chimpanzee monoclonal antibodies to the hepatitis E virus capsid protein. *J. Virol.* **74:**5548–5555.
95. **Schofield, D. J., R. H. Purcell, H. T. Nguyen, and S. U. Emerson.** 2003. Monoclonal antibodies that neutralize HEV recognize an antigenic site at the carboxy-terminus of an ORF2 protein vaccine. *Vaccine* **22:**257–267.
96. **Seow, H.-F., N. M. B. Mahomed, J.-W. Mak, M. A. Riddell, F. Li, and D. A. Anderson.** 1999. Seroprevalence of antibodies to hepatitis E virus in the normal blood donor population and two aboriginal communities in Malaysia. *J. Med. Virol.* **59:**164–168.
97. **Seriwatana, J., M. P. Shrestha, R. M. Scott, S. A. Tsarev, D. W. Vaughn, K. S. Myint, and B. L. Innis.** 2002. Clinical and epidemiological relevance of quantitating hepatitis E virus-specific immunoglobulin M. *Clin. Diagn. Lab. Immunol.* **9:**1072–1078.
98. **Shrestha, M. P., R. M. Scott, D. M. Joshi, M. P. Mammen, Jr., G. B. Thapa, N. Thapa, K. S. Myint, M. Fourneau, R. A. Kuschner, S. K. Shrestha, M. P. David, J. Seriwatana, D. W. Vaughn, A. Safary, T. P. Endy, and B. L. Innis.** 2007. Safety and efficacy of a recombinant hepatitis E vaccine. *N. Engl. J. Med.* **356:**895–903.
99. **Sonoda, H., M. Abe, T. Sugimoto, Y. Sato, M. Bando, E. Fukui, H. Mizuo, M. Takahashi, T. Nishizawa, and H. Okamoto.** 2004. Prevalence of hepatitis E virus (HEV) infection in wild boars and deer and genetic identification of a genotype 3 HEV from a boar in Japan. *J. Clin. Microbiol.* **42:**5371–5374.
100. **Takahashi, K., N. Kitajima, N. Abe, and S. Mishiro.** 2004. Complete or near-complete nucleotide sequences of hepatitis E virus genome recovered from a wild boar, a deer, and four patients who ate the deer. *Virology* **330:**501–505.
101. **Tam, A. W., M. M. Smith, M. E. Guerra, C. C. Huang, D. W. Bradley, K. E. Fry, and G. R. Reyes.** 1991. Hepatitis E virus (HEV): molecular cloning and sequencing of the full-length viral genome. *Virology* **185:**120–131.
102. **Tam, A. W., R. White, E. Reed, M. Short, Y. Zhang, T. R. Fuerst, and R. E. Lanford.** 1996. In vitro propagation and production of hepatitis E virus from in vivo-infected primary macaque hepatocytes. *Virology* **215:**1–9.
103. **Tam, A. W., R. White, P. O. Yarbough, B. J. Murphy, C. P. McAtee, R. E. Lanford, and T. R. Fuerst.** 1997. In vitro infection and replication of hepatitis E virus in primary cynomolgus macaque hepatocytes. *Virology* **238:**94–102.
104. **Tanaka, E., N. Takeda, L. Tian-Chen, K. Orii, T. Ichijo, A. Matsumoto, K. Yoshizawa, T. Iijima, T. Takayama, T. Miyamura, and K. Kiyosawa.** 2001. Seroepidemiological study of hepatitis E virus infection in Japan using a newly developed antibody assay. *J. Gastroenterol.* **36:**317–321.
105. **Tanaka, T., M. Takahashi, E. Kusano, and H. Okamoto.** 2007. Development and evaluation of an efficient cell-culture system for hepatitis E virus. *J. Gen. Virol.* **88:**903–911.
106. **Tei, S., N. Kitajima, K. Takahashi, and S. Mishiro.** 2003. Zoonotic transmission of hepatitis E virus from deer to human beings. *Lancet* **362:**371–373.
107. **Thakral, D., B. Nayak, S. Rehman, H. Durgapal, and S. K. Panda.** 2005. Replication of a recombinant hepatitis E virus genome tagged with reporter genes and generation of a short-term cell line producing viral RNA and proteins. *J. Gen. Virol.* **86:**1189–1200.
108. **Thomas, D. L., P. O. Yarbough, D. Vlahov, S. A. Tsarev, K. E. Nelson, A. J. Saah, and R. H. Purcell.** 1997. Seroreactivity to hepatitis E virus in areas where the disease is not endemic. *J. Clin. Microbiol.* **35:**1244–1247.
109. **Tong, M. J., R. Roue, M. Nahor N'Gawara, J. Desrame, Y. Buisson, and P. Coursaget.** 1996. Clinical aspects of hepatitis E and hepatitis A: a comparison, p. 1–10. *In* Y. Buisson, P. Coursaget, and M. Kane (ed.), *Enterically-Transmitted Hepatitis Viruses*. La Simarre, Joue-les-Tours, France.
110. **Toole, M. J., F. Claridge, D. A. Anderson, H. Zhuang, C. Morgan, B. Otto, and T. Stewart.** 2006. Hepatitis E virus infection as a marker for contaminated community drinking water sources in Tibetan villages. *Am. J. Trop. Med. Hyg.* **74:**250–254.
111. **Torresi, J., F. Li, S. A. Locarnini, and D. A. Anderson.** 1999. Only the non-glycosylated fraction of hepatitis E virus capsid (open reading frame 2) protein is stable in mammalian cells. *J. Gen. Virol.* **80:**1185–1188.
112. **Torresi, J., J. Meanger, P. Lambert, F. Li, S. A. Locarnini, and D. A. Anderson.** 1997. High level expression of the capsid protein of hepatitis E virus in diverse eukaryotic cells using the Semliki Forest virus replicon. *J. Virol. Methods* **69:**81–91.
113. **Tsarev, S. A., T. S. Tsareva, S. U. Emerson, S. Govindarajan, M. Shapiro, J. L. Gerin, and R. H. Purcell.** 1997. Recombinant vaccine against hepatitis E: dose response and protection against heterologous challenge. *Vaccine* **15:**1834–1838.
114. **Tsarev, S. A., T. S. Tsareva, S. U. Emerson, S. Govindarajan, M. Shapiro, J. L. Gerin, and R. H. Purcell.** 1994. Successful passive and active immunization of cynomolgus monkeys against hepatitis E. *Proc. Natl. Acad. Sci. USA* **91:**10198–10202.
115. **Tsarev, S. A., T. S. Tsareva, S. U. Emerson, A. Z. Kapikian, J. Ticehurst, W. London, and R. H. Purcell.** 1993. ELISA for antibody to hepatitis E virus (HEV) based on complete open-reading frame-2 protein expressed in insect cells: identification of HEV infection in primates. *J. Infect. Dis.* **168:**369–378.
116. **Tsarev, S. A., T. S. Tsareva, S. U. Emerson, M. K. Rippy, P. Zack, M. Shapiro, and R. H. Purcell.** 1995. Experimental hepatitis E in pregnant rhesus monkeys: failure to transmit hepatitis E virus (HEV) to offspring and evidence of naturally acquired antibodies to HEV. *J. Infect. Dis.* **172:**31–37.
117. **Tsarev, S. A., T. S. Tsareva, S. U. Emerson, P. O. Yarbough, L. J. Legters, T. Moskal, and R. H. Purcell.** 1994. Infectivity titration of a prototype strain of hepatitis E virus in cynomolgus monkeys. *J. Med. Virol.* **43:**135–142.
118. **Tsega, E., K. Krawczynski, B. G. Hansson, and E. Nordenfelt.** 1993. Hepatitis E virus infection in pregnancy in Ethiopia. *Ethiop. Med. J.* **31:**173–181.
119. **Tyagi, S., M. Surjit, A. K. Roy, S. Jameel, and S. K. Lal.** 2004. The ORF3 protein of hepatitis E virus interacts with liver-specific alpha1-microglobulin and its precursor alpha1-microglobulin/bikunin precursor (AMBP) and expedites their export from the hepatocyte. *J. Biol. Chem.* **279:**29308–29319.
120. **van Cuyck, H., F. Juge, and P. Roques.** 2003. Phylogenetic analysis of the first complete hepatitis E virus

(HEV) genome from Africa. *FEMS Immunol. Med. Microbiol.* **39:**133–139.

121. **Wang, Y., R. Ling, J. C. Erker, H. Zhang, H. Li, S. Desai, I. K. Mushahwar, and T. J. Harrison.** 1999. A divergent genotype of hepatitis E virus in Chinese patients with acute hepatitis. *J. Gen. Virol.* **80:**169–177.
122. **Wong, D. C., R. H. Purcell, M. A. Sreenivasan, S. R. Prasad, and K. M. Pavri.** 1980. Epidemic and endemic hepatitis in India: evidence for a non-A, non-B hepatitis virus aetiology. *Lancet* **ii:**876–879.
123. **Wu, J. C., C. M. Chen, T. Y. Chiang, I. J. Sheen, J. Y. Chen, W. H. Tsai, Y. H. Huang, and S. D. Lee.** 2000. Clinical and epidemiological implications of swine hepatitis E virus infection. *J. Med. Virol.* **60:**166–171.
124. **Xing, L., K. Kato, T. Li, N. Takeda, T. Miyamura, L. Hammar, and R. H. Cheng.** 1999. Recombinant hepatitis E capsid protein self-assembles into a dual-domain T = 1 particle presenting native virus epitopes. *Virology* **265:**35–45.
125. **Yarbough, P. O., E. Garza, A. W. Tam, Y. Zhang, P. McAtee, and T. R. Fuerst.** 1996. Assay development of diagnostic tests for IgM and IgG antibody to hepatitis E virus, p. 294–296. *In* Y. Buisson, P. Coursaget, and M. Kane (ed.), *Enterically-Transmitted Hepatitis Viruses*. La Simarre, Joue-les-Tours, France.
126. **Yarbough, P. O., K. Krawczynski, A. W. Tam, C. P. McAtee, K. A. McCaustland, Y. Zhang, N. Garcon, J. Spellbring, D. Carson, F. Myriam, J. D. Lifson, M. Slaoui, J. P. Prieels, H. Margolis, and T. R. Fuerst.** 1997. Prevention of hepatitis E using r62K ORF 2 subunit vaccine: full protection against heterologous HEV challenge in cynomolgus macaques, p. 650–655. *In* M. Rizzetto, R. H. Purcell, J. L. Gerin, and G. Verme (ed.), *Viral Hepatitis and Liver Disease*. Edizioni Minervi Medica, Turin, Italy.
127. **Yarbough, P. O., A. W. Tam, K. E. Fry, K. Krawczynski, K. A. McCaustland, D. W. Bradley, and G. R. Reyes.** 1991. Hepatitis E virus: identification of type-common epitopes. *J. Virol.* **65:**5790–5797.
128. **Zafrullah, M., M. H. Ozdener, S. K. Panda, and S. Jameel.** 1997. The ORF3 protein of hepatitis E virus is a phosphoprotein that associates with the cytoskeleton. *J. Virol.* **71:**9045–9053.
129. **Zhang, M., S. U. Emerson, H. Nguyen, R. Engle, S. Govindarajan, W. C. Blackwelder, J. Gerin, and R. H. Purcell.** 2002. Recombinant vaccine against hepatitis E: duration of protective immunity in rhesus macaques. *Vaccine* **20:**3285–3291.
130. **Zhang, M., S. U. Emerson, H. Nguyen, R. E. Engle, S. Govindarajan, J. L. Gerin, and R. H. Purcell.** 2001. Immunogenicity and protective efficacy of a vaccine prepared from 53 kDa truncated hepatitis E virus capsid protein expressed in insect cells. *Vaccine* **20:**853–857.
131. **Zhang, Y., P. McAtee, P. O. Yarbough, A. W. Tam, and T. Fuerst.** 1997. Expression, characterization, and immunoreactivities of a soluble hepatitis E virus putative capsid protein species expressed in insect cells. *Clin. Diagn. Lab. Immunol.* **4:**423–428.
132. **Zhou, Y. H., R. H. Purcell, and S. U. Emerson.** 2004. An ELISA for putative neutralizing antibodies to hepatitis E virus detects antibodies to genotypes 1, 2, 3, and 4. *Vaccine* **22:**2578–2585.
133. **Zhuang, H.** 1992. Hepatitis E and strategies for its control. *Monogr. Virol.* **19:**126–139.

Astrovirus

ERNESTO MÉNDEZ AND CARLOS F. ARIAS

50

VIROLOGY

Astroviruses are present in a wide variety of animal species, including mammals and birds. In many species, including humans, these viruses are associated with gastrointestinal diseases. Human astroviruses (HAstV) were first identified in fecal samples of children with diarrhea by electron microscopy (EM) as small particles with a star-like morphology, a feature that Madeley and Cosgrove (42) used in 1975 to name this group of viruses (*astron* = star in Greek). This morphology, however, is observed in only a small proportion of the particles present in stool samples, and expertise in EM is required for their identification. Development of more sensitive and specific diagnostic methods, such as enzyme immunoassays (EIA) and reverse transcription coupled with PCR (RT-PCR), has revealed that HAstV represent serious gastrointestinal pathogens that affect distinct groups in the population. Adaptation of HAstV to tissue cultures and the molecular characterization of human as well as of animal viruses have contributed to the recent advances in the knowledge of their molecular biology; however, an in vivo system to study HAstV pathogenesis is still required.

Classification

The *Astroviridae* family includes icosahedral nonenveloped viruses with characteristic features that distinguish them from other naked viruses with a monopartite RNA genome, like those in the *Caliciviridae* and *Picornaviridae* families. Members of the family *Astroviridae* contain a single-stranded RNA genome of positive polarity organized in three open reading frames (ORFs). The virions are formed by three proteins that result from the proteolytic processing of a precursor polypeptide (8, 48). During infection with astroviruses a viral subgenomic RNA (sgRNA) is used as a template for the synthesis of the structural proteins (57). Additional features used to distinguish this family are the lack of RNA helicase and methyltransferase domains in the nonstructural proteins, and the use of a ribosomal frameshifting mechanism to translate the viral RNA-dependent RNA polymerase (RdRp) (31).

Astroviruses have been found in several species of mammals and birds, a distinguishing feature used to classify them into two genera: *Mamastrovirus* and *Avastrovirus*. The genus *Mamastrovirus* includes viruses found in humans, lambs, calves, deer, piglets, kittens, mice, dogs, and mink, while avastroviruses have been isolated from turkeys, chickens, ducks, and guinea fowls. Based on their reactivities in neutralization assays, HAstV have been classified into eight serotypes (HAstV-1 to HAstV-8) (27, 36, 69). This classification correlates with the virus genotype determined by the nucleotide sequence of the 3′ end of ORF2 (see below), although it does not correlate with genotypes defined by comparing other regions of the genome. In animals, more than one serotype has been found in viruses isolated from calves (76), chickens (6), and turkeys (34).

Composition of Virus

Astroviruses have been described as 28- to 30-nm particles with small projections from the surface, and occasional star-like structures have been observed in viruses from fecal samples and in infected cell cultures (42) (Fig. 1A). The images of HAstV obtained by cryo-EM and image processing analysis show a smoothly rippled, solid capsid shell with a diameter of 33 nm and 30 dimeric spikes centered at the twofold axis of symmetry that extend about 5 nm from the surface (45).

The astrovirus genome varies from 6.8 to 7.3 kb in length, depending on the species of origin (47). The genome of HAstV is around 6.8 kb, is polyadenylated, and contains three ORFs (Fig. 2), each encoding a polyprotein that is proteolytically processed into smaller products during the virus replication cycle. The two ORFs located towards the 5′ end of the genome, designated ORF1a and ORF1b, code for nonstructural proteins that are involved in replication and transcription of the genomic RNA, as well as in other functions relevant for virus replication, like the proteolytic processing of the precursor viral polypeptides (31). ORF2, localized at the 3′ end, encodes the structural polyprotein (Fig. 2). As a positive single-stranded RNA virus, the RNA extracted from virions is able to initiate productive infection. Infectious RNA has also been transcribed from a full-length cDNA clone derived from the genome of a HAstV-1 strain (19). Three proteins in the range of 24 to 35 kDa are present in fully infectious particles (48, 65) (see below). One hundred eighty copies of one protein of 70 or 90 kDa are predicted to form the virions (37).

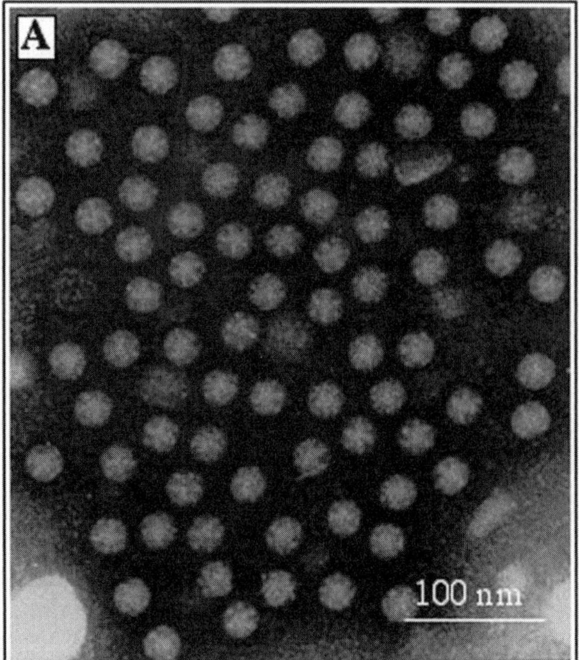

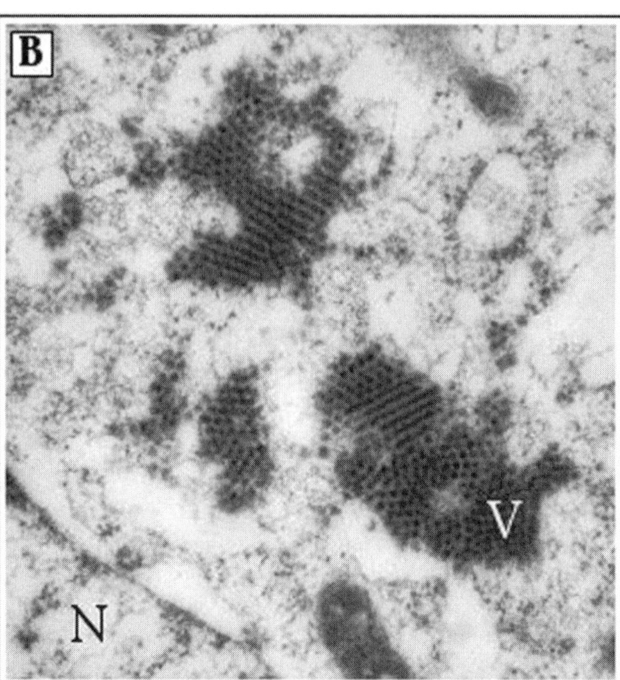

FIGURE 1 (A) The six- and five-point star-like morphology of astrovirus can be observed in fecal samples by negative staining and EM. (B) Paracrystalline arrays of human astrovirus particles observed by transmission EM in infected Caco-2 cells; virus clusters (V) are usually localized at the periphery of nuclei (N).

The protein product of ORF1a, called nsp1a, is around 920 amino acid residues in length, while ORF1b encodes a polypeptide of 515 to 528 amino acids. nsp1a is predicted to have five to six helical transmembrane motifs followed by a serine protease motif and a nuclear localization signal (NLS) (31) that overlaps a putative VPg protein that shows similarity to the VPg protein of calicivirus (3). The calicivirus VPg protein is covalently linked to its RNA 5′ end and is important for the translation, as well as for the replication of the genomic RNA (gRNA) (21). The putative VPg protein of astrovirus, however, has not been identified, and its existence is questionable. In addition, the biological relevance of the astrovirus NLS is uncertain, since nonstructural proteins have rarely been detected in the nuclei of infected cells. One specific region of nsp1a downstream of the NLS in which insertions or deletions are found has been suggested to have a role in RNA replication, since strains with differences in that region synthesize distinct amounts of viral RNA (26). In addition, a phosphorylated protein derived from the carboxy-terminal end of nsp1a has also been implicated in RNA replication (26) (Fig. 2).

The viral RdRp, encoded in ORF1b, is synthesized as part of a long polyprotein, called nsp1ab, that results from translation of ORF1a and ORF1b as a single polypeptide, through a ribosomal frameshift mechanism directed by highly conserved *cis*-acting sequences (the heptanucleotide AAAAAAC and one pseudoknot) localized in the overlap region between ORF1a and ORF1b (40) (Fig. 2). nsp1a and nsp1ab are processed at their amino termini by a cellular protease, probably a signalase, to release a 20 kDa protein (18, 50). Most of the downstream cleavage events are thought to be carried out by the viral serine protease, although the exact cleavage sites have not been defined (18) (Fig. 2).

The structural proteins encoded in ORF2 are translated from an sgRNA as a polyprotein precursor of 87 to 90 kDa. Two domains can be clearly distinguished in this protein: the first 415 amino acid residues form the highly conserved amino-terminal domain (more than 80% identical among human strains) with two small variable regions, while the second domain includes the hypervariable region downstream of amino acid residue 416, whose homology among different HAstVs can be as low as 36% (52, 74). This domain has been suggested to form the spikes of the particles and to be involved in the first interactions of the virus with the host cell (37) (Fig. 3).

The ORF2 primary translation product is processed to yield three final proteins that are present in fully infectious virions. The processing pathway of this precursor protein has been described in detail for a serotype 8 human isolate (Yuc8 strain) (48, 49). In this case, the primary protein product, of 90 kDa (VP90), is assembled into particles and is then processed by intracellular proteases at its carboxy-terminal region to yield a protein of 70 kDa (VP70) (49). This processing is carried out by caspases, cellular proteases activated during virus infection that are involved in cell death by apoptosis; the caspase cleavages correlate with, and are apparently required for, the release of virions from the cells. The released virions formed by VP70 are poorly infectious, and full activation of their infectivity requires that VP70 be cleaved by extracellular trypsin. Processing of the VP70-containing particles by this enzyme is sequential, producing final protein products of 34, 27, and 25

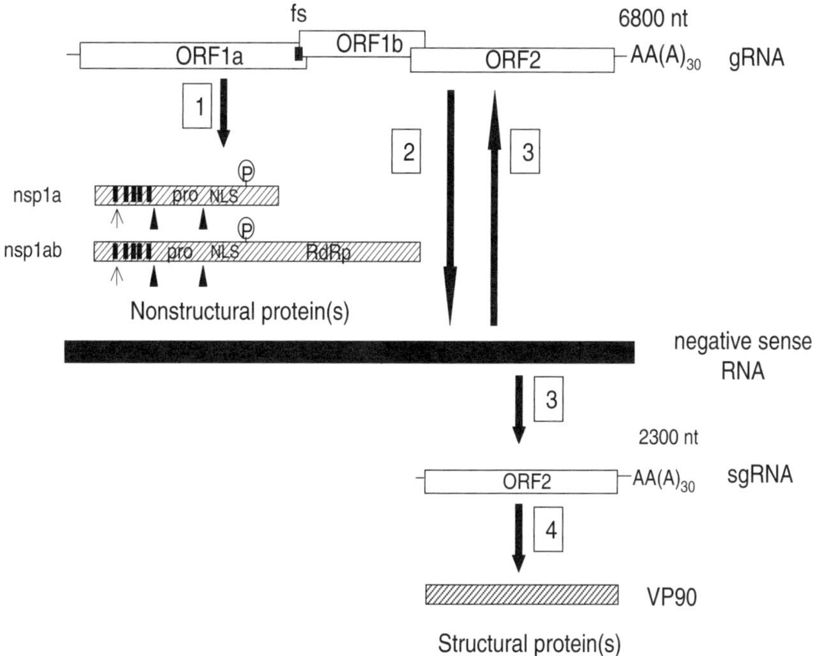

FIGURE 2 The gRNA of HAstV is organized into three ORFs (ORF1a, ORF1b, and ORF2), with 5′ and 3′ untranslated regions of 80 nucleotides, approximately, and a poly(A) tail. This RNA is used as a template for the synthesis of the nsp1a and nsp1ab nonstructural proteins. nsp1ab is produced by a translational frameshift mechanism using the signal (fs). nsp1a and nsp1ab participate in the synthesis of the three species of viral RNA. The negative-sense RNA is used as a template to produce more gRNA and the sgRNA, which codes for the structural protein. Motifs identified in the nonstructural proteins include hydrophobic small regions (black boxes), a serine protease (pro), an NLS, and an RdRp. A phosphorylation site (P) has been identified in nsp1a. The numbers in the squares represent the hypothetical order of the genome replication steps.

kDa, through at least eight intermediary polypeptides (48) (Fig. 3). Thus, the intracellular particles of HAstVs are constituted by polyprotein VP90, while extracellular virions are formed by either VP70 or its final cleavage products VP34, VP27, and VP25. Proteins in the size ranges of 32 to 35, 26 to 29, and 24 to 26 kDa have been found as final cleavage products of the structural polyproteins of different HAstV strains, suggesting that trypsin processing of the precursor capsid polypeptide is similar in other HAstVs (4, 8, 65). Neutralizing antibodies recognize epitopes on the 24- to 29-kDa proteins, which are derived from the hypervariable region of the precursor polypeptide (5, 65).

Biology

Two positive-sense viral RNAs are produced during infection: the gRNA (approximately 6.8 kb) and an sgRNA (approximately 2.4 kb), which are colinear at their 3′ ends (58). The first, besides being encapsidated, serves as a template for the synthesis of the nonstructural proteins nsp1a and nsp1ab. The sgRNA directs the synthesis of the structural 90-kDa polyprotein. Given the similarities of the genome structure of astroviruses with that of caliciviruses and alphaviruses, presumably both positive-sense astrovirus RNAs are produced from a negative-sense full-length antigenomic RNA (Fig. 2); however, this RNA has not yet been identified in astrovirus-infected cells. Conserved sequences at the 5′ end of the genome, and the sequence just upstream of the transcription initiation site of the sgRNA, suggest that the sgRNA is synthesized from an internal promoter in the negative-sense RNA (Fig. 3) (32).

In general, particular astroviruses demonstrate a limited host range (71); however, recent studies have suggested that interspecies transmission in birds could occur (12). Mammalian astroviruses have been associated primarily with gastrointestinal illness, although asymptomatic infections have been observed in calves (77). On the other hand, members of the *Avastrovirus* genus are associated with different diseases depending on the species. Astroviruses isolated from ducks are associated with liver disease (22); isolates from chickens are associated with renal and gastrointestinal diseases (29). Turkey astrovirus causes not only enteritis but also immunopathology leading to a disease called high-mortality syndrome (35).

HAstV were originally isolated in primary human embryonic kidney cells and subsequently adapted to grow in a continuous monkey kidney epithelial cell line (LLC-MK2), although these cells could not be infected directly with astrovirus extracted from fecal specimens. Recent studies revealed that HAstV infect a wide variety of cell lines, mainly of human and monkey origin, although with different efficiencies (10). Human cell lines of intestinal (like Caco-2, T84, and HT-29) and hepatoma (PLC/PRF/5) origin efficiently allow growth of different serotypes of HAstV of different serotypes. Baby hamster kidney (BHK) cells, and probably others, support efficient replication

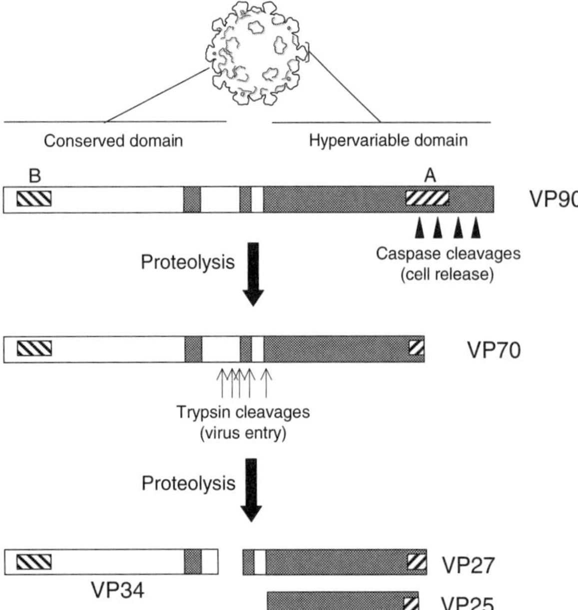

FIGURE 3 Scheme of a viral particle and the structural proteins of HAstV. Comparative sequence analysis of VP90 with structural proteins of other viruses suggests that the hypervariable region of VP90 (shaded box) forms the spikes of the particle, while the conserved domain (white box) forms the structured core (37). The structural protein contains basic (B) and acidic (A) regions that are highly conserved among astroviruses. Assembled virus particles containing VP90 are intracellularly processed by caspases (arrowheads) to yield particles formed by VP70 that are released from the cell. These particles are then cleaved by trypsin at specific sites (arrows) to yield fully infectious viruses containing proteins of 34, 27, and 25 kDa (VP34, VP27, and VP25). These data are based on studies carried out with a HAstV-8 strain (Yuc8) (48, 49). The drawing of the astrovirus particle at the top is based on images obtained by cryo-EM (45).

when transfected with authentic astrovirus RNA or with in vitro-transcribed full-length astrovirus RNA, although they are not easily infected, suggesting that barriers at the entry level could determine the susceptibility of some cells to virus infection (19). Limited studies indicate that HAstV enter cells by endocytosis through a clathrin-dependent mechanism (15).

Stability and Inactivation

Astrovirus particles are stable at a wide pH range (3 to 10) (63) and tolerate exposure to detergents, such as octylglucoside (65), and lipid solvents. HAstV infectivity is slightly affected when the virus is incubated at 4°C for 45 days in drinking water, although the titer drops by about 2 logs when the virus is maintained at 20°C (1). Temperatures of 60°C for more than 5 min drastically reduce infectivity. At −70 to −85°C, virus infectivity is retained for several years, although with repeated freezing and thawing, infectivity declines. Cesium chloride, frequently used to purify virus particles, destabilizes the integrity of HAstV if exposure exceeds 12 h (E. Mendez et al., unpublished data).

EPIDEMIOLOGY

Distribution, Incidence, and Prevalence of Infection

HAstV have been isolated from fecal samples of patients with gastrointestinal disease from all around the world. HAstV infections are recognized mainly in young children, elderly people, and immunocompromised patients, although infections in healthy adults can occasionally occur. An outbreak among the children of a single family has also been reported (68). From several epidemiological outpatient studies it has been determined that HAstV are an important cause of viral gastroenteritis in young children (mostly under 5 years of age), second only to rotavirus. About 75% of children older than 10 years have antibodies to astrovirus. With the use of more sensitive molecular methods for diagnosis, the incidence of astrovirus infections has been estimated at between 5 and 10% in children with gastroenteritis (41, 56), compared to less than 2% in healthy children. These rates were previously underestimated, mainly due to the less sensitive methods employed. Isolated studies have reported prevalences of HAstV as high as 26% in children with gastroenteritis (43).

HAstV have been associated with outbreaks in day care centers for children (54) and adults (44). Some of the largest outbreaks were observed in Japan, where more than 4,700 primary and junior high school students and staff were affected in a single outbreak (61). Outbreaks in aged care centers showed attack rates between 12 and 100%, with serotype 1 strains being the most common (44). Although caliciviruses are also important intestinal pathogens and cause severe infections in children, these viruses are most related to epidemic gastroenteritis that involves patients of all ages, not only children, and they have been responsible for 5 to 66% of the outbreaks in particular regions (13).

In immunodeficient patients, the frequency of astroviruses reported as a cause of gastroenteritis is variable. Some studies report HAstV as the principal viral cause of diarrhea in human immunodeficiency virus-positive patients (12% with diarrhea, versus 2% without) (24, 64), yet other studies suggest other viruses as the main cause (17). HAstV can establish persistent infections in the immunocompromised host (66).

Serotype Prevalence

As noted above, eight HAstV serotypes have been reported based on neutralization assays with polyclonal antisera. Since the sequence of the hypervariable carboxy terminus of the structural protein correlates with serotypes, serotypes are now commonly inferred from genotypes, determined by sequencing DNA fragments obtained by RT-PCR. Studies from different countries have shown that HAstV strains of serotype 1 are the most frequently found (in about 50% of the astrovirus-positive samples) (56), although other serotypes, like serotype 2, have also been found as the most common in some studies (73). Strains of serotype 7 have rarely been found (56).

Seasonality

In most temperate regions HAstV infections are more frequent in the winter, while in tropical regions astroviruses are more frequently detected during the rainy season (72). Also, high water flow in areas where poor water quality or sewage contamination exists is one of the causes of fecal contamination (62) and, therefore, of transmission of astrovirus and other enteropathogens.

Transmission

Contaminated food or water is the most frequent source of astrovirus infections. Large outbreaks of gastroenteritis in different countries (70), and sequence analysis of the astrovirus strains present in water supplies and in fecal samples from hospitalized patients in South Africa, have confirmed that food and water are important sources for virus infection (59). HAstV was found in 43% of raw sewage samples collected in an 8-month period in Hungary, indicating a high potential for transmission of this virus through this source (46). HAstV is able to survive on inert materials for long periods, and it has been suggested that it can also be transmitted through fomites in nosocomial infections (2).

PATHOGENESIS AND IMMUNE RESPONSE

Pathogenesis

HAstV has a specific tropism for epithelial cells of the small intestine. However, there is limited information on the pathogenesis of HAstV infection. Histopathological studies of biopsy samples from an immunodeficient patient showed that astrovirus infections are limited mainly to epithelial cells in the small intestine, particularly the jejunum, although the duodenum can also be affected (Fig. 4) (66). Studies with this patient, as well as with turkeys in-

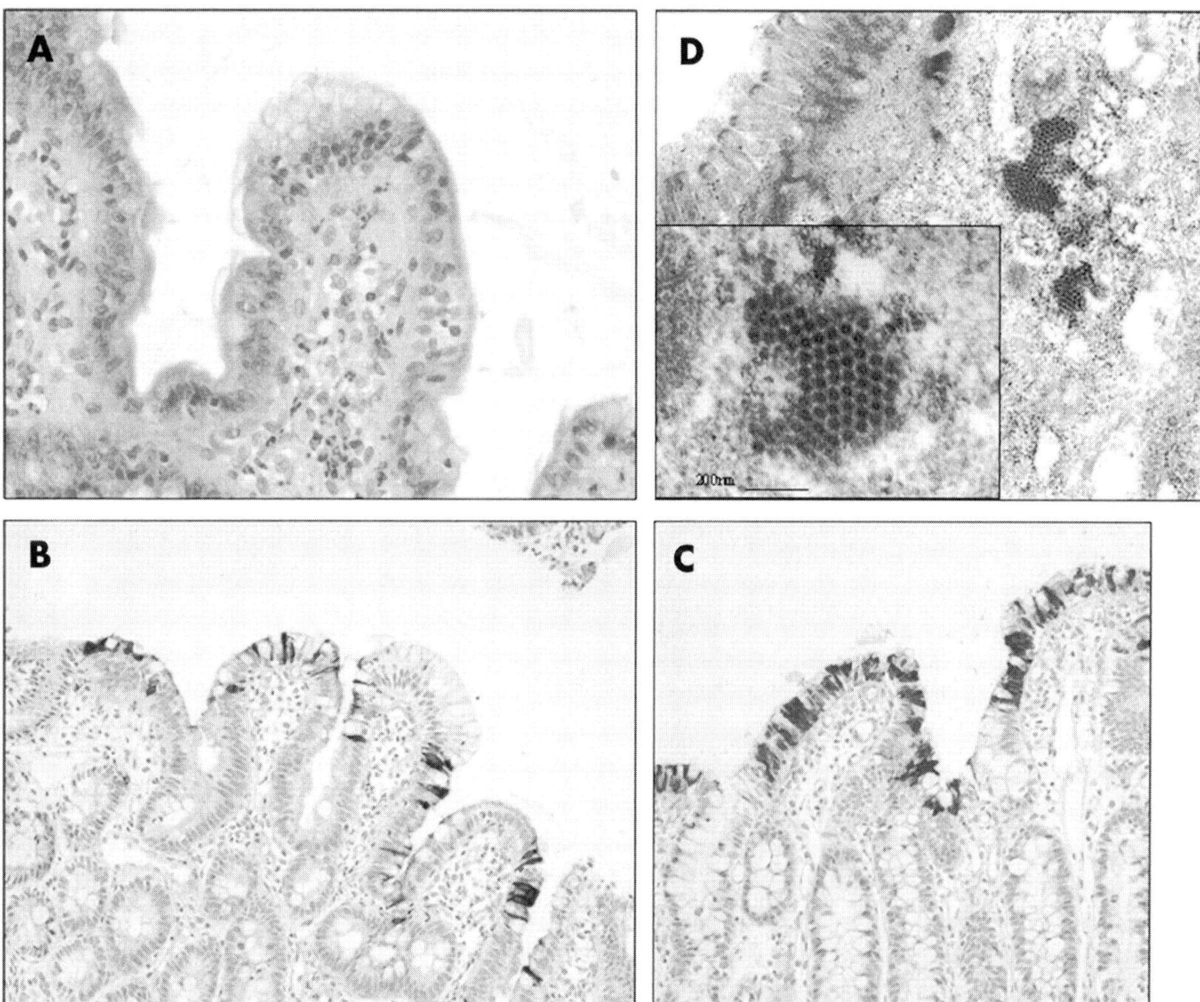

FIGURE 4 (A) Photomicrograph of a jejunal biopsy specimen from a bone marrow transplant recipient with astrovirus infection demonstrating villus blunting, nonspecific alterations in surface epithelial cells, and a mixed lamina propria inflammatory infiltrate, but without the presence of viral inclusion bodies (original magnification, ×100). Also shown are photomicrographs of duodenal (B) and jejunal (C) biopsy samples from a bone marrow transplant recipient with astrovirus infection immunostained with antiastrovirus antibody and demonstrating progressively extensive staining of surface epithelial cells, most commonly near the villus tips (original magnifications, ×40 and ×100, respectively). (D) Electron micrographs of a jejunal enterocyte demonstrating cytoplasmic paracrystalline viral arrays of astrovirus (original magnifications, ×32,000 and ×100,000 [inset]). (Adapted from reference 66 with permission.)

fected with a homologous astrovirus (33), indicate that inflammation is not central to illness pathogenesis. The fact that astrovirus induces cell death by apoptosis in cultured cells of human origin (25, 49) suggests that this programmed cell death, frequently associated with a very low inflammation response, could play a role in disease pathogenesis. In turkey astrovirus infections, virus can be recovered from different organs, although the small intestine seems to be the only organ where astrovirus replicates (7). Histologic studies with tissues from mammals infected with astrovirus, which are probably more similar to human infections, indicate that the virus is localized in the epithelial cells as well as in subepithelial macrophages of the small intestine. Intestinal epithelial cells are the primary site of astrovirus replication in humans, reflecting that high quantities of virus particles are present in fecal samples. Up to 10^{10} astrovirus particles may be shed per milliliter of stool (26), although many samples may contain much smaller amounts of virus. Virus can be present in fecal samples of infected children up to 2 weeks after symptoms disappear, but this period frequently is much longer in immunodeficient patients with chronic infections (72). Infection of gnotobiotic lambs with ovine viruses revealed that the incubation period of the disease is less than 2 days, with diarrhea that ends 4 days postinoculation (67). In this animal model infection occurred primarily in the dome of epithelial cells overlying jejunal and ileal Peyer's patches, and virus secretion occurred between days 2 and 9 postinoculation.

Immune Response

The existence of several HAstV serotypes suggests that neutralizing antibodies exert an immune selection pressure on the virus. In adult volunteers, HAstV seroconversion occurred after inoculation, and in some cases the antibodies recognized serotypes additional to the one contained in the inoculum, indicating that cross-neutralizing antibodies can be elicited upon infection (39, 53). The role of antibodies in controlling a natural infection is not clear, and it is not known if primary infections in childhood provide heterotypic protection for subsequent infection, although symptomatic infections in elderly patients suggest that antibodies acquired early in life (38) do not provide protection from illness at a late age.

The mucosal immune system could be important in protecting individuals from repeated astrovirus infections. T cells that recognize astrovirus antigens in a human leukocyte antigen (HLA)-restricted manner were found to reside in the intestinal lamina propria of healthy adults (55). These HAstV-specific $CD4^+$ T cells produced helper T-cell subtype 1 cytokines, interferon gamma, and tumor necrosis factor when activated.

CLINICAL MANIFESTATIONS

The incubation period is 3 to 4 days in adult human volunteers (39, 53). A typical astrovirus infection in humans is characterized by acute gastroenteritis, consisting of watery diarrhea for 2 to 3 days that may be accompanied by vomiting, fever, anorexia, abdominal pain, and a variety of constitutional symptoms that last no more than 4 days (72). Symptoms are similar to those caused by other gastrointestinal viruses, like rotavirus and calicivirus, but are usually not severe enough to require hospitalization. Cases of severe astrovirus infections have been reported during infections with serotype 6 (16) and 3 (11) strains; however, it is not clear if the severity was due to the particular virulence of the infecting strains, rather than being a general feature of the strains belonging to those serotypes. Recently, a case of intussusception in a 28-month-old child was associated with astrovirus infection (30). The severity of an astrovirus infection can be associated with the immune status of the patient, since immunodeficient patients have shown persistent infections with an extended course of infection and viral shedding (24). Illness due to astrovirus may also be more severe in elderly people, given the likelihood of general debility and serious medical conditions in this group of patients (44). Death associated with astrovirus infection is extremely rare.

LABORATORY DIAGNOSIS

Virus Isolation

Caco-2 is the cell line of choice for virus isolation from human fecal samples (10, 75). Trypsin treatment of the sample is necessary to successfully adapt HAstV to cells. Since the cytopathic effect caused by an astrovirus infection is difficult to observe in most cases, especially in the first passages in Caco-2 cells, this technique should be complemented with additional methods to enhance specificity and sensitivity (see below). Immunofluorescence staining of infected cells with group-specific antibodies is frequently necessary to confirm astrovirus isolation. EM of infected cells can also be used to confirm the isolation of astrovirus in culture, since characteristic paracrystalline structures around the nucleus formed by multiple particles can be observed (Fig. 1B). As mentioned earlier, T84 and PLC/PRF/5 hepatoma cells may also be used for isolation of HAstV directly from fecal specimens. Other cell lines, like HEK-293, HT-29, MA104, and LLC-MK2, that have been used to grow cell culture-adapted astrovirus strains are not easily infected with the virus present in fecal samples.

Electron Microscopy

EM has been used to distinguish this virus from other viruses of similar size; however, this technique requires qualified personnel to obtain reliable results, since a low percentage of particles in fecal samples show the star-like morphology. A total of 10^6 to 10^7 particles per g of stool are required for detection by this method (20). The sensitivity of EM can be improved by treating the sample with astrovirus-specific antibodies in order to agglutinate viral particles, facilitating detection.

Antigen Detection

EIA have been developed to detect HAstV antigens in fecal samples. Variations of this assay have used monoclonal antibodies that recognize a group antigen, as well as serotype-specific polyclonal antibodies. The most widely used EIA is a commercial assay (IDEIA Astrovirus; DAKO Corporation, Carpenteria, CA) based on a monoclonal antibody (28) that recognizes all human serotypes known so far. EIA is useful to detect astroviruses in a large number of samples, showing specificities in the range of 90 to 98%. It has been estimated that a positive EIA requires at least 10^5 and 10^6 viral particles per g of stool (20).

Nucleic Acid Detection

Astrovirus nucleic acid can be detected in fecal samples by RT-PCR. The most useful oligonucleotide primers to detect serologically distinct strains of HAstV were selected from highly conserved regions, such as the 5′-terminal region of ORF2, the 3′ end of the genome, and the RdRp gene (60). However, oligonucleotide primers from the hypervariable region of ORF2 have also been used to genotype human isolates, since the amino acid sequence of this region correlates with the serotype (51). The sensitivity of RT-PCR (approximately 10 to 100 particles per g of stool) (20) is higher than the sensitivity of EIA, although it can depend on several other factors such as the primers used, the protocol to obtain the viral RNA, and the reaction conditions. The sensitivity of RT-PCR for detection of HAstV may be enhanced when it is combined with cell culture. This combined method has been successfully used to detect HAstV in water samples (23). Sequencing of the amplified DNA fragment by RT-PCR from a fecal sample can be useful to confirm the presence of astrovirus in that sample and to distinguish genotypes or serotypes.

RT-PCR assays have also been used to confirm the presence of astrovirus in animal samples. However, the design of primers applicable for all animal astroviruses, especially avian, has been difficult because of the low identity among these strains (34).

PREVENTION

Prophylactic measures to avoid astrovirus spread in the population are important but may be difficult to achieve. Sanitation is particularly important in institutions such as day care centers, aged care centers, and hospitals with children and with immunocompromised patients, where outbreaks can emerge. Since astroviruses are resistant to a number of chemical treatments, appropriate disinfectants should be used. Soapy water and ethanol wipes were shown to reduce diarrhea due to astrovirus in a medical unit attending children with immune disorders (14). Standard water chlorination, although not totally effective, can help to diminish astrovirus viability (1). Universal hygienic procedures must be used to prepare the food.

TREATMENT

As mentioned above, the gastroenteritis caused by astrovirus is not as severe as that caused by other viruses, and it is self-limiting. Generally, astrovirus infections do not require a specific therapy, other than rehydration. However, in immunodeficient patients with persistent infections, intravenous immunoglobulin administration has been used. Immunoglobulin therapy of immunocompromised patients with persistent astrovirus infection has resulted in virus clearance and resolution of diarrhea (9), but this treatment did not work for bone marrow transplant patients with chronic diarrhea, even though this preparation was demonstrated to have antibodies to the homologous infecting astrovirus serotype (14). In this group, virus excretion was reduced in two patients when a T-cell response started to be detected after transplantation, suggesting that CD4^{+} T cells could be important to control virus replication, either directly or through activation of B cells to produce antibodies (14, 55). No antiviral agents have been developed with activity against astrovirus infections.

REFERENCES

1. **Abad, F. X., R. M. Pinto, C. Villena, R. Gajardo, and A. Bosch.** 1997. Astrovirus survival in drinking water. *Appl. Environ. Microbiol.* **63:**3119–3122.
2. **Abad, F. X., C. Villena, S. Guix, S. Caballero, R. M. Pinto, and A. Bosch.** 2001. Potential role of fomites in the vehicular transmission of human astroviruses. *Appl. Environ. Microbiol.* **67:**3904–3907.
3. **Al-Mutairy, B., J. E. Walter, A. Pothen, and D. K. Mitchell.** 2005. Genome prediction of putative genome-linked viral protein (VPg) of astroviruses. *Virus Genes* **31:** 21–30.
4. **Bass, D. M., and S. Qiu.** 2000. Proteolytic processing of the astrovirus capsid. *J. Virol.* **74:**1810–1814.
5. **Bass, D. M., and U. Upadhyayula.** 1997. Characterization of human serotype 1 astrovirus-neutralizing epitopes. *J. Virol.* **71:**8666–8671.
6. **Baxendale, W., and T. Mebatsion.** 2004. The isolation and characterisation of astroviruses from chickens. *Avian Pathol.* **33:**364–370.
7. **Behling-Kelly, E., S. Schultz-Cherry, M. Koci, L. Kelley, D. Larsen, and C. Brown.** 2002. Localization of astrovirus in experimentally infected turkeys as determined by in situ hybridization. *Vet. Pathol.* **39:**595–598.
8. **Belliot, G., H. Laveran, and S. S. Monroe.** 1997. Capsid protein composition of reference strains and wild isolates of human astroviruses. *Virus Res.* **49:**49–57.
9. **Bjorkholm, M., F. Celsing, G. Runarsson, and J. Waldenstrom.** 1995. Successful intravenous immunoglobulin therapy for severe and persistent astrovirus gastroenteritis after fludarabine treatment in a patient with Waldenstrom's macroglobulinemia. *Int. J. Hematol.* **62:**117–120.
10. **Brinker, J. P., N. R. Blacklow, and J. E. Herrmann.** 2000. Human astrovirus isolation and propagation in multiple cell lines. *Arch. Virol.* **145:**1847–1856.
11. **Caballero, S., S. Guix, W. M. El-Senousy, I. Calico, R. M. Pinto, and A. Bosch.** 2003. Persistent gastroenteritis in children infected with astrovirus: association with serotype-3 strains. *J. Med. Virol.* **71:**245–250.
12. **Cattoli, G., C. De Battisti, A. Toffan, A. Salviato, A. Lavazza, M. Cerioli, and I. Capua.** 2007. Co-circulation of distinct genetic lineages of astroviruses in turkeys and guinea fowl. *Arch. Virol.* **152:**595–602.
13. **Centers for Disease Control and Prevention.** 2007. Norovirus activity—United States, 2006–2007. *Morb. Mortal. Wkly. Rep.* **56:**842–846.
14. **Cubitt, W. D., D. K. Mitchell, M. J. Carter, M. M. Willcocks, and H. Holzel.** 1999. Application of electron microscopy, enzyme immunoassay, and RT-PCR to monitor an outbreak of astrovirus type 1 in a paediatric bone marrow transplant unit. *J. Med. Virol.* **57:**313–321.
15. **Donelli, G., F. Superti, A. Tinari, and M. L. Marziano.** 1992. Mechanism of astrovirus entry into Graham 293 cells. *J. Med. Virol.* **38:**271–277.
16. **Gabbay, Y. B., A. C. Linhares, E. L. Cavalcante-Pepino, L. S. Nakamura, D. S. Oliveira, L. D. da Silva, J. D. Mascarenhas, C. S. Oliveira, T. A. Monteiro, and J. P. Leite.** 2007. Prevalence of human astrovirus genotypes associated with acute gastroenteritis among children in Belem, Brazil. *J. Med. Virol.* **79:**530–538.
17. **Gallimore, C. I., D. W. Cubitt, A. F. Richards, and J. J. Gray.** 2004. Diversity of enteric viruses detected in patients with gastroenteritis in a tertiary referral paediatric hospital. *J. Med. Virol.* **73:**443–449.
18. **Geigenmuller, U., T. Chew, N. Ginzton, and S. M. Matsui.** 2002. Processing of nonstructural protein 1a of human astrovirus. *J. Virol.* **76:**2003–2008.

19. **Geigenmuller, U., N. H. Ginzton, and S. M. Matsui.** 1997. Construction of a genome-length cDNA clone for human astrovirus serotype 1 and synthesis of infectious RNA transcripts. *J. Virol.* **71:**1713–1717.
20. **Glass, R. I., J. Noel, D. Mitchell, J. E. Herrmann, N. R. Blacklow, L. K. Pickering, P. Dennehy, G. Ruiz-Palacios, M. L. de Guerrero, and S. S. Monroe.** 1996. The changing epidemiology of astrovirus-associated gastroenteritis: a review. *Arch. Virol. Suppl.* **12:**287–300.
21. **Goodfellow, I., Y. Chaudhry, I. Gioldasi, A. Gerondopoulos, A. Natoni, L. Labrie, J. F. Laliberte, and L. Roberts.** 2005. Calicivirus translation initiation requires an interaction between VPg and eIF 4 E. *EMBO Rep.* **6:** 968–972.
22. **Gough, R. E., M. S. Collins, E. Borland, and L. F. Keymer.** 1984. Astrovirus-like particles associated with hepatitis in ducklings. *Vet. Rec.* **114:**279.
23. **Grimm, A. C., J. L. Cashdollar, F. P. Williams, and G. S. Fout.** 2004. Development of an astrovirus RT-PCR detection assay for use with conventional, real-time, and integrated cell culture/RT-PCR. *Can. J. Microbiol.* **50:** 269–278.
24. **Grohmann, G. S., R. I. Glass, H. G. Pereira, S. S. Monroe, A. W. Hightower, R. Weber, and R. T. Bryan for the Enteric Opportunistic Infections Working Group.** 1993. Enteric viruses and diarrhea in HIV-infected patients. *N. Engl. J. Med.* **329:**14–20.
25. **Guix, S., A. Bosch, E. Ribes, L. Dora Martínez, and R. M. Pintó.** 2004. Apoptosis in astrovirus-infected CaCo-2 cells. *Virology* **319:**249–261.
26. **Guix, S., S. Caballero, A. Bosch, and R. M. Pinto.** 2005. Human astrovirus C-terminal nsP1a protein is involved in RNA replication. *Virology* **333:**124–131.
27. **Herrmann, J. E., R. W. Hudson, D. M. Perron-Henry, J. B. Kurtz, and N. R. Blacklow.** 1988. Antigenic characterization of cell-cultivated astrovirus serotypes and development of astrovirus-specific monoclonal antibodies. *J. Infect. Dis.* **158:**182–185.
28. **Herrmann, J. E., N. A. Nowak, D. M. Perron-Henry, R. W. Hudson, W. D. Cubitt, and N. R. Blacklow.** 1990. Diagnosis of astrovirus gastroenteritis by antigen detection with monoclonal antibodies. *J. Infect. Dis.* **161:**226–229.
29. **Imada, T., S. Yamaguchi, M. Mase, K. Tsukamoto, M. Kubo, and A. Morooka.** 2000. Avian nephritis virus (ANV) as a new member of the family *Astroviridae* and construction of infectious ANV cDNA. *J. Virol.* **74:** 8487–8493.
30. **Jakab, F., J. Peterfai, T. Verebely, E. Meleg, K. Banyai, D. K. Mitchell, and G. Szucs.** 2007. Human astrovirus infection associated with childhood intussusception. *Pediatr. Int.* **49:**103–105.
31. **Jiang, B., S. S. Monroe, E. V. Koonin, S. E. Stine, and R. I. Glass.** 1993. RNA sequence of astrovirus: distinctive genomic organization and a putative retrovirus-like ribosomal frameshifting signal that directs the viral replicase synthesis. *Proc. Natl. Acad. Sci. USA* **90:**10539–10543.
32. **Jonassen, C. M., T. T. Jonassen, T. M. Sveen, and B. Grinde.** 2003. Complete genomic sequences of astroviruses from sheep and turkey: comparison with related viruses. *Virus Res.* **91:**195–201.
33. **Koci, M. D., L. A. Moser, L. A. Kelley, D. Larsen, C. C. Brown, and S. Schultz-Cherry.** 2003. Astrovirus induces diarrhea in the absence of inflammation and cell death. *J. Virol.* **77:**11798–11808.
34. **Koci, M. D., and S. Schultz-Cherry.** 2002. Avian astroviruses. *Avian Pathol.* **31:**213–227.
35. **Koci, M. D., B. S. Seal, and S. Schultz-Cherry.** 2000. Molecular characterization of an avian astrovirus. *J. Virol.* **74:**6173–6177.
36. **Koopmans, M. P., M. H. Bijen, S. S. Monroe, and J. Vinje.** 1998. Age-stratified seroprevalence of neutralizing antibodies to astrovirus types 1 to 7 in humans in The Netherlands. *Clin. Diagn. Lab. Immunol.* **5:**33–37.
37. **Krishna, N. K.** 2005. Identification of structural domains involved in astrovirus capsid biology. *Viral Immunol.* **18:** 17–26.
38. **Kurtz, J., and T. Lee.** 1978. Astrovirus gastroenteritis age distribution of antibody. *Med. Microbiol. Immunol.* **166:** 227–230.
39. **Kurtz, J. B., T. W. Lee, J. W. Craig, and S. E. Reed.** 1979. Astrovirus infection in volunteers. *J. Med. Virol.* **3:** 221–230.
40. **Lewis, T. L., and S. M. Matsui.** 1997. Studies of the astrovirus signal that induces (−1) ribosomal frameshifting. *Adv. Exp. Med. Biol.* **412:**323–330.
41. **Liu, M. Q., B. F. Yang, J. S. Peng, D. J. Zhou, L. Tang, B. Wang, Y. Liu, S. H. Sun, and W. Z. Ho.** 2007. Molecular epidemiology of astrovirus infection in infants in Wuhan, China. *J. Clin. Microbiol.* **45:**1308–1309.
42. **Madeley, C. R., and B. P. Cosgrove.** 1975. Letter: 28 nm particles in faeces in infantile gastroenteritis. *Lancet* **ii:** 451–452.
43. **Maldonado, Y., M. Cantwell, M. Old, D. Hill, M. L. Sanchez, L. Logan, F. Millan-Velasco, J. L. Valdespino, J. Sepulveda, and S. Matsui.** 1998. Population-based prevalence of symptomatic and asymptomatic astrovirus infection in rural Mayan infants. *J. Infect. Dis.* **178:**334–339.
44. **Marshall, J. A., L. D. Bruggink, K. Sturge, N. Subasinghe, A. Tan, and G. G. Hogg.** 2007. Molecular features of astrovirus associated with a gastroenteritis outbreak in an aged-care centre. *Eur. J. Clin. Microbiol. Infect. Dis.* **26:**67–71.
45. **Matsui, S. M., D. Kiang, N. Ginzton, T. Chew, and U. Geigenmuller-Gnirke.** 2001. Molecular biology of astroviruses: selected highlights. *Novartis Found. Symp.* **238:** 219–233.
46. **Meleg, E., F. Jakab, B. Kocsis, K. Banyai, B. Melegh, and G. Szucs.** 2006. Human astroviruses in raw sewage samples in Hungary. *J. Appl. Microbiol.* **101:**1123–1129.
47. **Mendez, E., and C. F. Arias.** 2007. Astroviruses, p. 981–1000. *In* D. M. Knipe, P. M. Howley, D. E. Griffin, R. A. Lamb, M. A. Martin, B. Roizman, and S. E. Straus (ed.), *Fields Virology*, 5th ed., vol. 1. Lippincott Williams & Willkins, Philadelphia, PA.
48. **Méndez, E., T. Fernández-Luna, S. López, M. Méndez-Toss, and C. F. Arias.** 2002. Proteolytic processing of a serotype 8 human astrovirus ORF2 polyprotein. *J. Virol.* **76:**7996–8002.
49. **Mendez, E., E. Salas-Ocampo, and C. F. Arias.** 2004. Caspases mediate processing of the capsid precursor and cell release of human astroviruses. *J. Virol.* **78:**8601–8608.
50. **Mendez, E., M. P. Salas-Ocampo, M. E. Munguia, and C. F. Arias.** 2003. Protein products of the open reading frames encoding nonstructural proteins of human astrovirus serotype 8. *J. Virol.* **77:**11378–11384.
51. **Mendez-Toss, M., D. D. Griffin, J. Calva, J. F. Contreras, F. I. Puerto, F. Mota, H. Guiscafre, R. Cedillo, O. Munoz, I. Herrera, S. Lopez, and C. F. Arias.** 2004. Prevalence and genetic diversity of human astroviruses in Mexican children with symptomatic and asymptomatic infections. *J. Clin. Microbiol.* **42:**151–157.
52. **Mendez-Toss, M., P. Romero-Guido, M. E. Munguia, E. Mendez, and C. F. Arias.** 2000. Molecular analysis of a serotype 8 human astrovirus genome. *J. Gen. Virol.* **81:** 2891–2897.
53. **Midthun, K., H. B. Greenberg, J. B. Kurtz, G. W. Gary, F. Y. Lin, and A. Z. Kapikian.** 1993. Characterization

and seroepidemiology of a type 5 astrovirus associated with an outbreak of gastroenteritis in Marin County, California. *J. Clin. Microbiol.* **31:**955–962.

54. **Mitchell, D. K., D. O. Matson, X. Jiang, T. Berke, S. S. Monroe, M. J. Carter, M. M. Willcocks, and L. K. Pickering.** 1999. Molecular epidemiology of childhood astrovirus infection in child care centers. *J. Infect. Dis.* **180:** 514–517.
55. **Molberg, O., E. M. Nilsen, L. M. Sollid, H. Scott, P. Brandtzaeg, E. Thorsby, and K. E. Lundin.** 1998. $CD4^+$ T cells with specific reactivity against astrovirus isolated from normal human small intestine. *Gastroenterology* **114:** 115–122.
56. **Monroe, S. S.** 2003. Molecular epidemiology of human astroviruses, p. 607–616. *In* U. Desselberger and J. J. Gray (ed.), *Perspectives in Medical Virology*, vol. 9. *Viral Gastroenteritis*. Elsevier, Amsterdam, The Netherlands.
57. **Monroe, S. S., B. Jiang, S. E. Stine, M. Koopmans, and R. I. Glass.** 1993. Subgenomic RNA sequence of human astrovirus supports classification of *Astroviridae* as a new family of RNA viruses. *J. Virol.* **67:**3611–3614.
58. **Monroe, S. S., S. E. Stine, L. Gorelkin, J. E. Herrmann, N. R. Blacklow, and R. I. Glass.** 1991. Temporal synthesis of proteins and RNAs during human astrovirus infection of cultured cells. *J. Virol.* **65:**641–648.
59. **Nadan, S., J. E. Walter, W. O. Grabow, D. K. Mitchell, and M. B. Taylor.** 2003. Molecular characterization of astroviruses by reverse transcriptase PCR and sequence analysis: comparison of clinical and environmental isolates from South Africa. *Appl. Environ. Microbiol.* **69:** 747–753.
60. **Noel, J. S., T. W. Lee, J. B. Kurtz, R. I. Glass, and S. S. Monroe.** 1995. Typing of human astroviruses from clinical isolates by enzyme immunoassay and nucleotide sequencing. *J. Clin. Microbiol.* **33:**797–801.
61. **Oishi, I., K. Yamazaki, T. Kimoto, Y. Minekawa, E. Utagawa, S. Yamazaki, S. Inouye, G. S. Grohmann, S. S. Monroe, S. E. Stine, et al.** 1994. A large outbreak of acute gastroenteritis associated with astrovirus among students and teachers in Osaka, Japan. *J. Infect. Dis.* **170:** 439–443.
62. **Riou, P., J. C. Le Saux, F. Dumas, M. P. Caprais, S. F. Le Guyader, and M. Pommepuy.** 2007. Microbial impact of small tributaries on water and shellfish quality in shallow coastal areas. *Water Res.* **41:**2774–2786.
63. **Risco, C., J. L. Carrascosa, A. M. Pedregosa, C. D. Humphrey, and A. Sanchez-Fauquier.** 1995. Ultrastructure of human astrovirus serotype 2. *J. Gen. Virol.* **76**(Pt. 8):2075–2080.
64. **Rossit, A. R., M. T. de Almeida, C. A. Nogueira, J. G. da Costa Oliveira, D. M. Barbosa, A. C. Moscardini, J. D. Mascarenhas, Y. B. Gabbay, F. R. Marques, L. V. Cardoso, C. E. Cavasini, and R. L. Machado.** 2007. Bacterial, yeast, parasitic, and viral enteropathogens in HIV-infected children from Sao Paulo State, Southeastern Brazil. *Diagn. Microbiol. Infect. Dis.* **57:**59–66.
65. **Sanchez-Fauquier, A., A. L. Carrascosa, J. L. Carrascosa, A. Otero, R. I. Glass, J. A. Lopez, C. San Martin, and J. A. Melero.** 1994. Characterization of a human astrovirus serotype 2 structural protein (VP26) that contains an epitope involved in virus neutralization. *Virology* **201:**312–320.
66. **Sebire, N. J., M. Malone, N. Shah, G. Anderson, H. B. Gaspar, and W. D. Cubitt.** 2004. Pathology of astrovirus associated diarrhoea in a paediatric bone marrow transplant recipient. *J. Clin. Pathol.* **57:**1001–1003.
67. **Snodgrass, D. R., K. W. Angus, E. W. Gray, J. D. Menzies, and G. Paul.** 1979. Pathogenesis of diarrhoea caused by astrovirus infections in lambs. *Arch. Virol.* **60:**217–226.
68. **Tanaka, H., J. J. Kisielius, M. Ueda, R. I. Glass, and P. P. Joazeiro.** 1994. Intrafamilial outbreak of astrovirus gastroenteritis in Sao Paulo, Brazil. *J. Diarrhoeal Dis. Res.* **12:**219–221.
69. **Taylor, M. B., J. Walter, T. Berke, W. D. Cubitt, D. K. Mitchell, and D. O. Matson.** 2001. Characterisation of a South African human astrovirus as type 8 by antigenic and genetic analyses. *J. Med. Virol.* **64:**256–261.
70. **Utagawa, E. T., S. Nishizawa, S. Sekine, Y. Hayashi, Y. Ishihara, I. Oishi, A. Iwasaki, I. Yamashita, K. Miyamura, and S. Yamazaki.** 1994. Astrovirus as a cause of gastroenteritis in Japan. *J. Clin. Microbiol.* **32:**1841–1845.
71. **van Hemert, F. J., B. Berkhout, and V. V. Lukashov.** 2007. Host-related nucleotide composition and codon usage as driving forces in the recent evolution of the Astroviridae. *Virology* **361:**447–454.
72. **Walter, J. E., and D. K. Mitchell.** 2003. Astrovirus infection in children. *Curr. Opin. Infect. Dis.* **16:**247–253.
73. **Walter, J. E., D. K. Mitchell, M. L. Guerrero, T. Berke, D. O. Matson, S. S. Monroe, L. K. Pickering, and G. Ruiz-Palacios.** 2001. Molecular epidemiology of human astrovirus diarrhea among children from a periurban community of Mexico City. *J. Infect. Dis.* **183:**681–686.
74. **Wang, Q. H., J. Kakizawa, L. Y. Wen, M. Shimizu, O. Nishio, Z. Y. Fang, and H. Ushijima.** 2001. Genetic analysis of the capsid region of astroviruses. *J. Med. Virol.* **64:**245–255.
75. **Willcocks, M. M., M. J. Carter, F. R. Laidler, and C. R. Madeley.** 1990. Growth and characterisation of human faecal astrovirus in a continuous cell line. *Arch. Virol.* **113:**73–81.
76. **Woode, G. N., N. E. Gourley, J. F. Pohlenz, E. M. Liebler, S. L. Mathews, and M. P. Hutchinson.** 1985. Serotypes of bovine astrovirus. *J. Clin. Microbiol.* **22:**668–670.
77. **Woode, G. N., J. F. Pohlenz, N. E. Gourley, and J. A. Fagerland.** 1984. Astrovirus and Breda virus infections of dome cell epithelium of bovine ileum. *J. Clin. Microbiol.* **19:**623–630.

Coronaviruses

KENNETH McINTOSH AND J. S. M. PEIRIS

51

The first coronavirus to be recovered was infectious bronchitis virus (IBV) from chickens with respiratory disease, reported by Beaudette and Hudson in 1937 (7). Another group of animal coronaviruses, the murine hepatitis viruses (MHV), was first recognized by Cheever et al. (19) at the Rockefeller Institute in 1949 and independently by Gledhill and Andrewes (37) in London, England, in 1951. Transmissible gastroenteritis in swine was first recognized in 1946 (24). These three important animal diseases were, however, considered unrelated until after the human coronaviruses (HCoVs) were discovered in the 1960s and the *Coronavirus* genus was defined.

Tyrrell and Bynoe (128) described the first HCoV, B814, recovered from a schoolboy with a cold and passaged in organ cultures of human embryonic trachea. The virus, when examined by electron microscopy (EM) (3), was found to resemble avian IBV. At about the same time, Hamre and Procknow (44) recovered five virus strains in tissue culture from medical students with colds. The prototype strain HCoV 229E was examined by Almeida and Tyrrell (3), and its morphology was found to be identical to that of B814 and IBV. The organ culture technique was subsequently used to recover six further strains, including the prototype strain HCoV OC43, and three strains considered antigenically unrelated to either OC43 or 229E (84).

In the winter of 2002–2003 an unusual and often lethal form of pneumonia appeared in Guangdong Province of China (150), a disease subsequently labeled severe acute respiratory syndrome (SARS). Within days of this disease spreading to Hong Kong in late February, international air travel spread the virus far and wide, seeding outbreaks in Vietnam; Singapore; Toronto, Canada; and elsewhere. By the end of this brief but global epidemic in July 2003, 8,096 cases had been recorded, 744 of them fatal, in 29 countries across 5 continents. Spread within health care settings was a notable feature, accounting for 21% of all cases. The virus, termed the SARS coronavirus (SARS-CoV), initially emerged from an animal reservoir from live-animal markets in Guangdong, where diverse animal species are held and traded to serve the restaurant trade and the demand for exotic food. Within these markets, small mammals such as civet cats were found to harbor viruses closely related to SARS-CoV (39), and these markets are the likely source for the initial interspecies transmission to humans. However, civet cats in the wild do not harbor these viruses (104) and thus were unlikely to be the natural reservoir of the virus. Recently, the precursor virus has been found in species of *Rhinolophus* bats (65, 70, 125).

VIROLOGY

Classification

Coronaviruses have been classified as members of the order *Nidovirales*, positive-sense RNA viruses that replicate using a nested ("nido") set of mRNAs. The family *Coronaviridae* contains two genera, *Torovirus* and *Coronavirus*. The original basis for classification of the coronaviruses into a separate genus lay in the distinct morphology of the members (2) (Fig. 1). This classification has been clearly justified by the unique chemical structure and strategy of replication. The *Coronavirus* genus is a large one, with representative viruses infecting multiple species, including chickens, turkeys, ducks, geese, other birds, mice, cats, dogs, rabbits, cattle, bats, and humans. Many of the animal coronaviruses are of great economic importance. On the basis of antigenic relationships and genetic homologies, the coronaviruses were divided into three groups (Table 1). The first contains HCoV 229E and several animal strains; the second contains OC43, MHV, and several other animal strains; and the third contains IBV and several other avian coronaviruses.

Several coronavirus species cause gastroenteritis in newborn or young animals, and it was therefore not surprising when coronavirus-like particles (CVLPs) were found by EM in human feces. The identity of CVLPs in human intestinal contents and their role in disease are, however, still matters of some controversy. All but a few strains have been detected only by EM of negatively stained preparations of feces (18, 73, 80, 133). Their morphology is sometimes different from that of other coronaviruses (74). On the other hand, several strains have been propagated in intestinal organ cultures (16, 106), and both antigenic and biophysical studies have been performed on several isolates (34, 106). Certain strains have been found to be related both to calf diarrhea virus and to OC43 (34, 149). One strain, recovered from infants with outbreak-associated diarrhea and originally isolated in fetal intestinal organ cul-

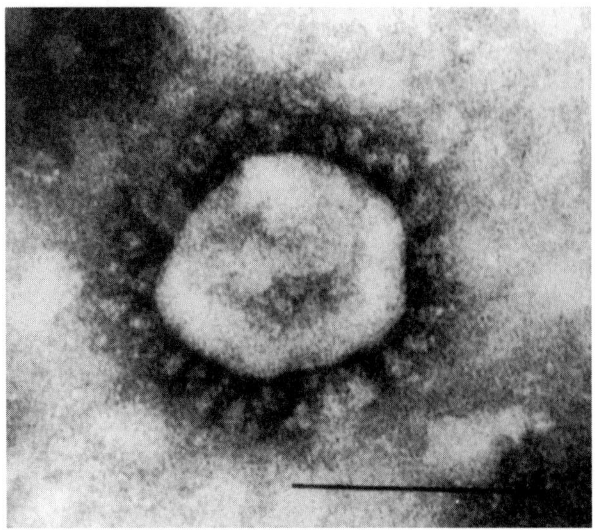

FIGURE 1 Coronavirus OC16, viewed by EM and negatively stained. The characteristic round, or oval, shape is seen, along with the petal-shaped peplomers. Bar, 100 nm. (Reprinted from reference 84 with permission.)

ture, has been adapted to growth in a mouse macrophage line and a mosquito cell line and appears not to be related to other HCoVs or animal coronaviruses (72). Further study of this strain may yield important information about the role of enteric coronaviruses in human intestinal disease.

Some of the confusion about the role of enteric coronaviruses as causes of diarrhea may be related to the similar appearance of toroviruses by EM of negatively stained stool specimens. Toroviruses are well-characterized causes of diarrhea in calves and horses. Human toroviruses, partially purified from stool samples, have been shown to be serologically related to both equine and bovine toroviruses (6, 56) and to contain sequences at the 3′ end almost identical to those of equine torovirus (26). With the help of this serologic specificity, microscopic identification and differentiation from coronaviruses are possible (26), and it appears likely that the distinct roles of toroviruses and enteric coronaviruses will be clarified in the future.

A novel coronavirus was isolated by several laboratories from SARS patients using African green monkey (Vero E6) or fetal rhesus monkey cells (25, 58, 99). The viral RNA sequence showed that the virus was only distantly related to previously characterized coronaviruses (25, 58, 77, 99, 111).

TABLE 1 Classification of coronaviruses[a]

Group	Virus(es)	Host(s)	Respiratory infection	Enteric infection	Hepatitis	Neurologic infection	Other[b]
1	HCoV 229E	Human	X			?	
	HCoV NL63	Human	X				
	Transmissible gastroenteritis virus, porcine epidemic diarrhea virus	Pig	X	X			X
	Porcine respiratory coronavirus	Pig	X				
	Canine coronavirus	Dog		X			
	Feline enteric coronavirus	Cat		X			
	Feline infectious peritonitis virus	Cat	X	X	X	X	X
	Rabbit coronavirus	Rabbit		X			X
	Bat coronavirus HKU2[c]	Bat					
2	HCoV OC43	Human	X	?		?	
	HCoV HKU1	Human	X				
	SARS-CoV	Civet, human[d]	X	X		X	X
	Hemagglutinating encephalomyelitis virus	Pig	X	X		X	
	MHV	Mouse	X	X	X	X	
	Sialodacryoadenitis virus	Rat					X
	Bovine coronavirus	Cow		X			
	Bat coronavirus HKU1[c]	Bat					
3	IBV	Chicken	X		X		X
	Turkey coronavirus	Turkey	X	X			

[a] Modified from reference 62, with permission.

[b] Other diseases caused by coronaviruses include immunologic disorders (leukopenia, lymphopenia, and autoimmune disorders), peritonitis, runting, nephritis, pancreatitis, parotitis, myocarditis, and sialodacryoadenitis.

[c] The pathogenicity of coronaviruses in bats is not clear.

[d] The natural host of SARS-CoV is not known.

In the wake of the SARS epidemic, two more HCoVs have been discovered: NL63, a group 1 virus isolated first from a child with bronchiolitis (130) and subsequently found to have worldwide distribution (5, 9, 22, 27, 29, 45, 55, 88), and HKU1, a group 2 virus first isolated from an adult with chronic pulmonary disease (142) and subsequently found also worldwide (35, 61, 66, 120, 129, 143). Both of these new coronaviruses are genetically and clinically closer to the traditional respiratory coronaviruses 229E and OC43 than to SARS-CoV.

The search for the animal reservoir of SARS-CoV has led to the recognition of a number of novel coronaviruses in bats (104, 125). These bat viruses fall within both group 1 and 2 coronaviruses (Fig. 2). Phylogenetic analysis of currently known coronaviruses has shown that bat coronaviruses appear to be in evolutionary stasis and well adapted to this host species, leading to the hypothesis that all animal coronaviruses and HCoVs derive from bat viruses and to the proposal that the taxonomic grouping of coronaviruses be revised in light of the current understanding (134).

Composition of Virus

Virion Morphology, Structure, and Size

Coronavirus virions are round, membrane-bound, moderately pleomorphic, medium-sized particles measuring 100 to 150 nm in diameter and covered with a distinctive fringe of widely spaced, club-shaped surface projections (Fig. 1) (81). The projections are about 20 nm in length. They represent the spike (S) protein, which aggregates in trimers to form the characteristic peplomers of the virus. Some members of group 2 coronaviruses, including OC43, also contain a shorter S protein, named hemagglutinin-esterase (HE). Also exposed on the surface is the amino-terminal end of the membrane (M) protein, the most abundant protein in the virus particle.

In thin sections of infected cells, the particles have a diameter of 85 nm and have a typical bilayer external membrane and a coiled nucleic acid core which is, in cross-section, 9 to 11 nm in diameter. These particles have been observed to bud from the membranes of the Golgi apparatus or endoplasmic reticulum (ER) and to accumulate in

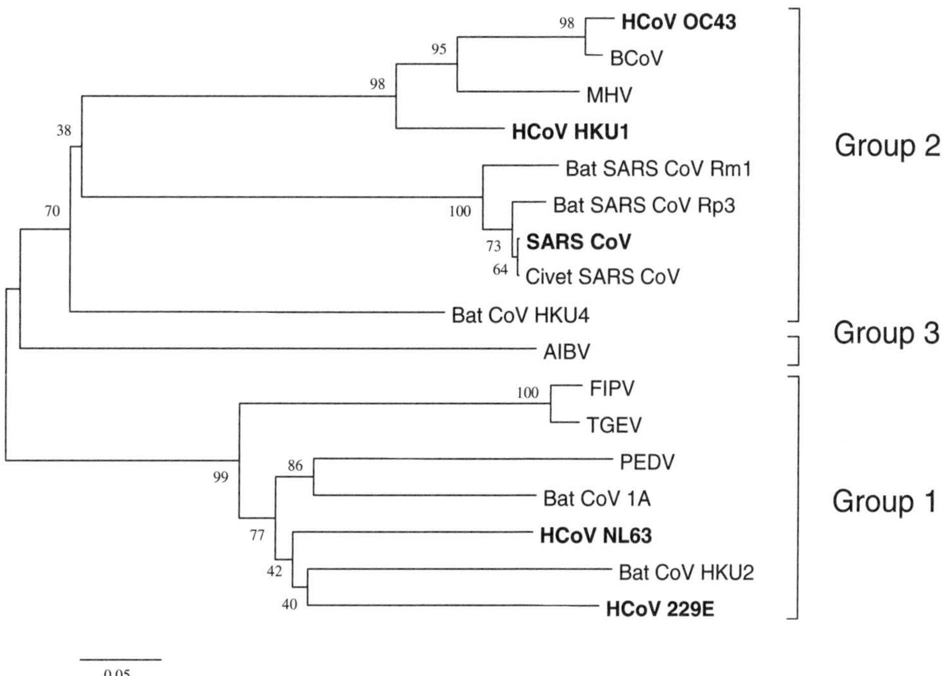

FIGURE 2 Phylogenetic analysis of RNA sequences coding for the RNA-dependent RNA polymerase (ORF1b) (partial sequence, 1,176 bp). The phylogenetic tree was constructed by the neighbor-joining method, and bootstrap values were determined with 1,000 replicates. The virus sequences used were HCoV OC43 (GenBank accession no. AY585229), bovine coronavirus (BCoV) (GenBank accession no. AF391541), MHV A59 (GenBank accession no. NC_001846), HCoV HKU1 (GenBank accession no. NC_006577), bat SARS-CoV Rm1/2004 (Rm1) (GenBank accession no. NC_009696), bat SARS-CoV Rp3/2004 (Rp3) (GenBank accession no. NC_009693), SARS-CoV (GenBank accession no. AY278491), civet SARS-CoV SZ3 (GenBank accession no. AY304486), bat coronavirus (CoV) HKU4 (GenBank accession no. NC_009019), avian IBV (AIBV) (GenBank accession no. AY319651), feline infectious peritonitis virus (GenBank accession no. AY994055), transmissible gastroenteritis virus (TGEV) (GenBank accession NC_002306), porcine epidemic diarrhea virus (PEDV) (GenBank accession no. NC_003436), bat CoV 1A (unpublished data), HCoV NL63 (GenBank accession no. NC_005831), bat CoV HKU2 (GenBank accession no. DQ249235), and HCoV 229E (GenBank accession no. NC_002645).

cytoplasmic vesicles (8) (Fig. 3). Infected cells often have virus particles on the cell surface which likely represent virus disgorged from cytoplasmic vesicles rather than budding of virus at the plasma membrane.

Genome Length and Composition

The genome of coronaviruses is the largest known RNA virus genome, 27 to 32 kb in size. It is single stranded, positive sense, capped, and adenylated. The order of genes is shown in Fig. 4 and is roughly identical throughout all coronavirus species, namely, 5′-replicase-S-envelope-M-nucleocapsid (N)-3′. In those species containing the HE gene, this is found between the replicase gene and the S protein gene. Many species have additional genes that code for accessory proteins.

Major Structural and Regulatory Proteins

The large surface glycoprotein, the S protein, is oriented with its amino terminus facing outward, is N glycosylated, and forms the club-shaped surface projections. It is this protein that is responsible for the stimulation of neutralizing antibody. The S protein is also involved in interaction with cellular receptors and thereby probably determines the tissue specificity of the virus. In group 1 and 3 coronaviruses it is cleaved into S1 (the portion involved in interaction with receptors) and S2 (the portion involved in fusion of the viral and cellular membranes).

There is a shorter HE glycoprotein also found on the surface of the virion on some group 2 coronaviruses, including strains OC43 and HKU1. The HE glycoprotein is, curiously, genetically related to a similar protein in influenza C virus. The esterase function may have a role in the release of virus from infected cells. Embedded in the membrane of the virus particle is the M protein, a 20- to 35-kDa glycosylated protein which penetrates the membrane three times and has a key role in viral assembly and probably interacts with the RNA-nucleoprotein complex of the virus during the maturation of the particle. Also present in the membrane is a sparsely represented protein, the envelope (E) protein. The nucleoprotein itself is a 50- to 60-kDa phosphoprotein which binds to and presumably stabilizes the positive-strand RNA of the virus. Open reading frame 1a/b (ORF1a/b) of the coronavirus genome encodes a huge polyprotein that is cleaved by cellular and viral proteases into some 16 proteins, including an RNA-dependent RNA polymerase, several RNases, several proteases, and several other essential proteins. For details of the viral structure and biology, readers are referred to the review by Masters (79).

The proteins of enteric HCoVs have not been well characterized, although it appears that their size and number are similar to those of other coronaviruses (106).

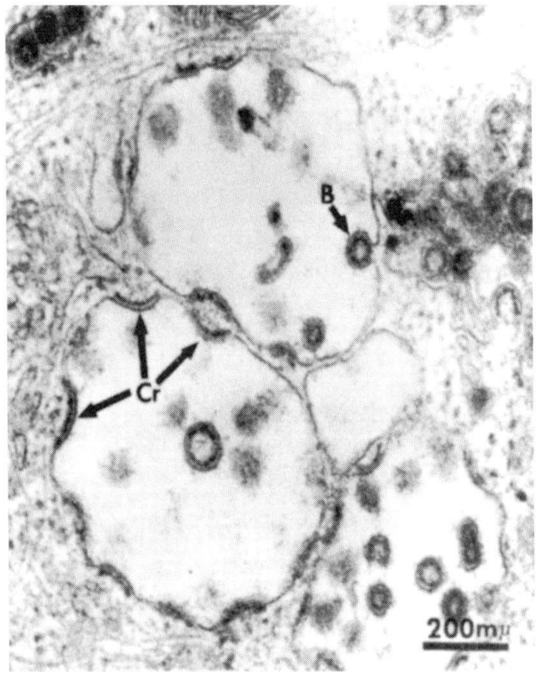

FIGURE 3 Coronavirus 229E in WI38 cells. Characteristic crescents (Cr) of budding particles (B) are seen, as well as particles which are free in cytoplasmic vesicles. (Reprinted from reference 8 with permission.)

Biology

Replication Strategy

The biology of coronaviruses has been reviewed (62, 79). Coronaviruses bind to cells through receptors which are probably quite specific, although the details are not presently known for all members of the genus. Coronavirus 229E, a group 1 virus, binds specifically the metalloprotease human aminopeptidase N (145). The other group 1 HCoV, NL63, binds specifically to another metalloprotease, angiotensin-converting enzyme 2 (ACE2) (47). Group 2 viruses use both S protein and (if present) HE to bind to 9-O-acetylated neuraminic acid molecules on many biological membranes, although the specificity of this binding is in question. MHV has another more specific receptor which belongs to the carcinoembryonic antigen family (141), but analogous receptors for OC43 and HKU1 have not been found. SARS-CoV was the first coronavirus shown to use ACE2 as a receptor (69).

Viral entry is accomplished through fusion of the plasma membrane with the viral membrane or by receptor-mediated endocytosis. The fusion activity is mediated by the S2 portion of the S protein. Once in the cytoplasm, the genomic viral RNA is translated by host machinery to produce a polyprotein from gene 1 that is then cleaved by a papain-like protease and the main protease to produce (among other proteins) an RNA-dependent RNA polymerase. This enzyme then is used to make a minus-sense copy of the full-length genome and also a nested set of minus-strand RNAs from the genomic RNA which serve as a template for mRNA synthesis. Each of the nested-set mRNAs begins with a leader sequence, identical to the leader sequence found at the 5′ end of the full-length genomic RNA, then an intergenic sequence, then the translated ORF, and then all bases through to the 3′ polyadenylated end. Thus, all of the mRNAs except the smallest, that coding for the N protein, are polycistronic, containing sequences coding for more than one protein, although only the first cistron in line is actually translated during protein synthesis (79).

The various viral proteins are synthesized, processed, and transported by cellular cytoplasmic machinery. Coronaviruses can replicate in enucleated cells. The S protein and HE are cotranslationally N glycosylated in the ER and processed in the Golgi apparatus, where the S protein is oligomerized into a trimer. The S protein of OC43 (but

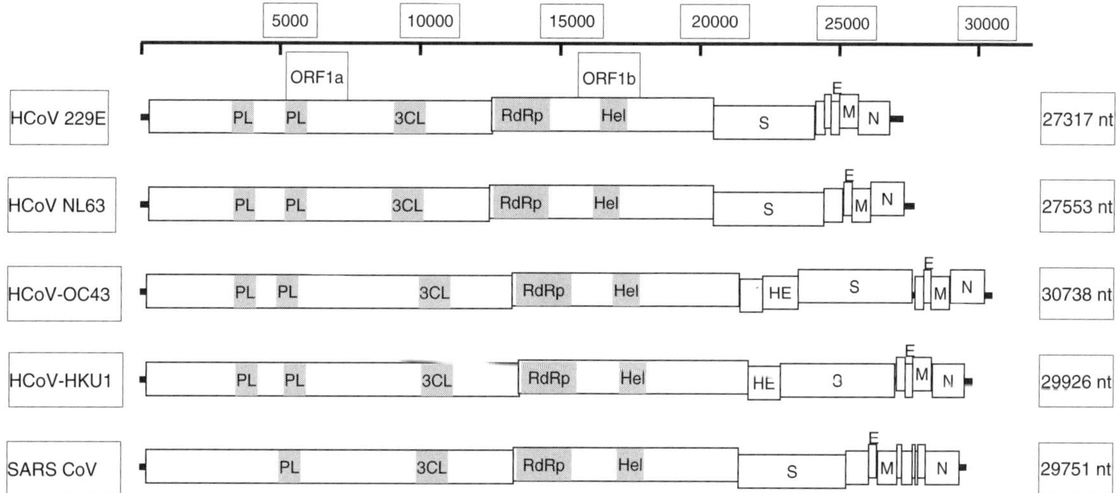

FIGURE 4 Genomic organization of HCoVs. Strains 229E and NL63 belong to group 1, OC43 and HKU1 belong to group 2a, and SARS-CoV belongs to group 2b. ORF1 comprises ORF1a and ORF1b, which overlap. Translation of ORF1b depends on a ribosomal frameshift. ORF1 and ORF2 are translated into polyproteins that are cleaved into 16 nonstructural proteins, nsp1 to nsp16, by papain-like proteases (PL) encoded by ORF1a and a chymotrypsin-like protease (3CL). ORF1b encodes the viral RNA-dependent RNA polymerase (RdRp) and a multifunctional helicase (Hel) which has NTPase, dNTPase, and 5′-triphosphatase activities in addition to its helicase function. The main structural proteins present in all coronaviruses are the S, envelope (E), M, and N proteins. Some coronaviruses have an additional HE glycoprotein. Recently the ORF3a product has also been reported to be a structural protein in SARS-CoV. These genes are interspersed with ORFs encoding nonstructural proteins which differ markedly in their number and gene order between different coronavirus groups. nt, nucleotides.

not 229E) undergoes proteolytic cleavage either intra- or extracellularly. The M protein is inserted into the ER shortly after synthesis and accumulates in the Golgi apparatus.

Assembly takes place when the N protein binds to genomic RNA and probably recognizes signals on the M protein in the ER or the Golgi apparatus. The S protein and HE are incorporated into the ER and Golgi membranes at the time of budding, and viruses accumulate in large numbers in smooth-walled cytoplasmic vesicles. These probably fuse with the plasma membrane and virus is released. After release, the virus particles collect in large numbers along the outer surface of the plasma membrane of the cell.

Host Range

Although multiple animal strains of coronaviruses exist, it is not clear whether any of the HCoVs (with the exception of SARS-CoV) naturally infects any species other than humans. Two strains, OC38 and OC43, which are antigenically identical and related to MHV, were adapted from human tracheal organ culture to growth in suckling-mouse brain (82). SARS-CoV has been reported to replicate in multiple species after experimental infection, including rhesus and cynomolgus macaques, ferrets, hamsters, guinea pigs, mice, rats, cats, and pigs (137). Neither 229E, NL63, nor HKU1 has been adapted to growth in animals. Growth of human strains in embryonated eggs has not been described.

Growth in Cell Culture

None of the HCoVs grows easily in cell culture without extensive adaptation by passage. Strains related to 229E can be grown in primary or secondary human embryonic kidney cell lines, in many diploid human fibroblast lines, and in a few heteroploid lines (12, 52). The most sensitive cell line for isolation of 229E from clinical specimens appears to be the diploid intestinal cell line MA-177 (52). NL63 grows and produces cytopathic effect (CPE) in LLC-MK2 and Vero B4 cells, but the CPE is somewhat nonspecific (113). Although in the first report of its identification, HKU1 was not reported to grow in any of a wide variety of cell culture systems (142), a subsequent report indicated that it consistently grew from clinical samples and produced CPE in HUH7 cells (129). Clinical strains of both OC43 and 229E have also been shown to grow in HUH7 cells (30, 33).

The highest titers of both 229E and OC43 have been obtained by growth in human rhabdomyosarcoma cells (114). Plaque assays for HCoV-229E can be performed in human diploid fibroblasts (43), and those for both 229E and OC43 can be performed in rhabdomyosarcoma and fetal tonsil diploid cells (114).

Although a number of isolates of SARS-CoV are available, primary isolation, especially from extrarespiratory sites, proved to be a challenge. SARS-CoV was isolated first in Vero E6 or fetal rhesus kidney cell lines with production of CPE (25, 58, 99). Vero E6 cells are now routinely used for its growth and also for plaque assays of infectivity (124). In addition, the virus has been adapted to growth in a number of other cell lines which express the ACE2 receptor.

Enteric coronaviruses have been very difficult to propagate in vitro. Success has been achieved in human embryonic intestinal organ cultures, where several strains have been passaged, with consistent production of characteristic particles and antigens (16, 106). There is a report of the growth of virus from a child with diarrhea in human rectal tumor cells (HRT-18), with resultant syncytial CPE. The virus, designated HECV-4408, was both antigenically and genetically almost identical to bovine coronavirus, however, suggesting the possibility of either an interspecies infection or laboratory contamination (149). The growth of another strain in mouse macrophages and a mosquito cell line (72) was described above.

Inactivation by Physical and Chemical Agents

The HCoVs were found early to be sensitive to ether and chloroform, but it was only after the appearance of SARS and the recognition of its nosocomial potential that it became critical to know about the survival and inactivation of HCoVs in various body fluids and on various surfaces. SARS-CoV was found to survive with loss of as little as 0.5 or 1.0 $\log_{10}$ infectious titer for 1 day on surfaces at room temperature, and for much longer at 4°C (63). This stability of the virus may have in part contributed to the explosive outbreaks in health care facilities. On the other hand, treatment with household bleach and simple detergent rapidly inactivated all viral infectivity in 5 min or less.

EPIDEMIOLOGY

Geographic Distribution

Surveys of human serum collections have demonstrated antibody to OC43 and 229E in essentially all areas of the world. In England in 1976, 100 and 94% of healthy adults were found by this method to have antibody to OC43 and 229E, respectively. Antibody to both OC43 and 229E appears in early childhood and increases in prevalence rapidly with age (86). Recent surveys that have searched for 229E, OC43, NL63, and HKU1 by PCR have also found these viruses in all corners of the world.

Given its emergence from a zoonotic reservoir, SARS was unusual in its geographic distribution. The outbreak that lasted from November 2002 until July 2003 emerged in Guangdong Province in China and spread to involve 29 countries across 5 continents (98). However, with the interruption of human-to-human transmission, that outbreak was aborted, and presently this human-adapted SARS-CoV exists only in freezers within virology laboratories. Three laboratory outbreaks have been reported in Singapore, Taiwan, and Beijing, the last leading to some limited community transmission which was again aborted by the use of public health measures. Another four instances of zoonotic transmission occurred in December 2003 to January 2004. These most likely also arose from the live-animal markets, caused mild disease, and did not result in detectable human-to-human transmission (121). SARS was unusual among respiratory viruses in that asymptomatic infection was uncommon (67). Thus, antibody to SARS-CoV is found only in those who have had clinical SARS, a small number of contacts who have been asymptomatically infected, and a fraction of individuals who work in these live-animal markets and have presumably been exposed to the precursor SARS-CoV-like virus (39).

The geographic distribution of the gastrointestinal coronaviruses is less clearly delineated. CVLPs have been found in the stools of adults and children in many parts of the developed and developing world. It has been common to find them in equal frequencies in both healthy and sick persons.

Incidence and Prevalence of Infection

The rate of coronavirus infection among adults with upper respiratory illness varies between respiratory seasons. In one of the first surveys, a 6-year study of 229E infection among medical students, infections were detected by rises in neutralizing antibody. By this method, only 1% of acute respiratory illnesses in the period from 1964 to 1965 could be attributed to 229E, but from 1966 to 1967 the proportion was 35% (42). The average rate of infection was 15%. The proportion of coronavirus-associated minor respiratory illnesses in a general population in Tecumseh, MI, during the same peak year was 34% (90), and a rate of 24% was found in Bethesda, MD (52).

Serosurveys of OC43 infection in adults have shown quite similar proportions. During peak seasons, 25% (90) to 29% (86) of colds could be associated with OC43 infection; overall, 17% of individuals developed antibody rises each year. In a serologic survey of OC43 infection in high-risk adult populations in Houston, TX, 8 to 9% of acute respiratory episodes in outpatient adults with underlying chronic obstructive pulmonary disease or asthma were attributable to OC43 infection (36). The vast majority of infections occurred between November and February. In England a study of asthmatic adults with acute respiratory symptoms from 1990 to 1992 showed infection with OC43 and 229E in 16% (95). Among Finnish adults surveyed by serologic techniques over a 10-month period, 8.5% of colds were associated with infection with either 229E- or OC43-related strains. In the same period, rhinoviruses were found in 52.5% by PCR (76).

Two community studies of acute respiratory illness using PCR for detection of 229E and OC43 have been performed in patients cared for by general practitioners in The Netherlands (38, 132). Both studies are among the very few that include equal numbers of control patients sampled during asymptomatic periods. The first study was of adults 60 years or older, covered a single respiratory season, and demonstrated that these two coronaviruses were found in 17% of 107 elderly subjects during acute respiratory disease, in contrast to only 2% of controls. In the same cohort, 32% of episodes were associated with rhinovirus infection (2% of controls), and 7% were associated with influenza infection (0% of controls) (38). In the second study, subjects of all ages were sampled over 3 years. The mean age of the sampled population was 35 years. In contrast to the findings in the exclusively elderly, in this population coronavirus infection was not significantly associated with illness, being found in 6 of 166 influenza-like illnesses (3.6%), 29 of 376 other respiratory illness (7.7%), and 21 of 541 controls (3.9%) (132). There have been no systematic, adequately controlled studies of either NL63 or HKU1 in adults or children with outpatient respiratory illness.

A number of recent surveys of hospitalized patients have looked for HCoVs using PCR as the detection method, examining patients of all ages with acute respiratory illnesses. Very few of these studies have, however, included asymptomatic controls. A study spanning two respiratory seasons in Pavia, Italy, looked at 823 patients admitted to a hospital with acute respiratory disease, most of whom were infants and children (501 under 5 years).

Among the older subjects, more than half were immunocompromised (33). HCoV strains 229E, OC43, and NL63 were specifically sought by PCR. A total of 47 infections were found (5.7%), 25 with OC43 (occurring in both respiratory seasons), 10 with 229E (occurring only in the first year), and 9 with NL63 (occurring only in the second year). Three HCoVs were found that could not be characterized further. Most patients had lower-tract involvement. All infected adults (5 total) were immunocompromised. Another study covering one respiratory season (2004–2005) in Hong Kong examined 4,181 patients admitted with acute respiratory disease (mean age, 22 years) to two hospitals and looked for all four HCoV strains. HCoVs were found in 87 patients (2.1%): OC43 was found in 53, NL63 in 17, HKU1 in 13, and 229E in 4 (66). A 20-month survey covering all four HCoV types in Lausanne, Switzerland, in 540 bronchoalveolar lavage samples from 279 hospitalized adults identified HCoVs in 29 (5.4%) samples, one-third of all respiratory viruses detected. Two-thirds of the HCoVs detected were OC43 or 229E. More than half the patients sampled and 12 of 29 with HCoVs were lung transplant patients, and many of the remainder were immunosuppressed. Most carried a diagnosis of pneumonia (32). Another recent study of hospitalized patients with acute respiratory disease, two-thirds of whom were children, looked for all four of the HCoV strains by PCR and immunofluorescence during a single respiratory season and found infections in 48 of 426 (11.3%). All but a few of the adults were immunocompromised, and coinfections with other viruses were frequent (about half) (35). None of these studies included control, asymptomatic patients.

Infection rates in children seen in hospitals with acute lower respiratory tract disease have been studied more extensively. Six such surveys are shown in Table 2, where coronavirus detection rates are compared with the rates of detection of multiple other respiratory viruses. Only two of the surveys looked for all four known HCoV strains by PCR (61, 66). None of these studies included control, asymptomatic children. A prospective, controlled study of all acute respiratory illnesses in the first year of life in 263 children at high risk for asthma in Perth, Australia, indicated that HCoV infections (strains 229E and OC43, detected by PCR) occurred in 5.5% of respiratory episodes and 4.4% of asymptomatic controls (60). A similar study in 82 unselected, healthy infants, not including controls but testing for NL63 as well and performed in Berne, Switzerland, identified HCoVs in 13 episodes (16%) of lower-tract disease in the first year of life (51).

Several recent studies have looked specifically for one or another of the newer HCoV strains. NL63 has been found in hospitalized children in Europe, North America, Japan, and Australia, with rates ranging from 1.2 to 9.3% (5, 9, 27, 55, 88). In only one of these studies were control children sampled, and in that case the rates of identification of NL63 were 3.0% in ill subjects and 1.7% in asymptomatic subjects ($P = 0.6$). A survey of 418 patients with mean age of 49 years admitted to four hospitals with community-acquired pneumonia in Hong Kong over a 1-year period (2003 to 2004) yielded HKU1 in 10 (2.4%), 9 of them adults (143).

Coronaviruses, along with rhinoviruses, influenza virus, and respiratory syncytial virus (RSV), are commonly associated with acute respiratory disease in the elderly. When increases in antibody to both 229E and OC43 are measured, the frequency of infection appears to be about half that of rhinovirus infection and the same as, or somewhat greater than, that of influenza virus and RSV (94, 136). The character and severity of illness are very similar to those of rhinovirus infections and somewhat less severe than those of influenza virus and RSV, rarely leading to hospitalization (38, 94, 136).

Enteric coronaviruses or CVLPs have been most frequently associated with gastrointestinal disease in neonates and infants less than 12 months of age. Particles have been found in the stools of adults with AIDS, in some studies more frequently in the presence of diarrhea than in its absence (116). Asymptomatic shedding is common, and particles are apparently shed for prolonged periods (54, 78, 91, 133). SARS-CoV was detected frequently and for prolonged periods by PCR in stool during infection, and more recent studies of HKU1 have identified virus in stool samples as well as respiratory samples from children hospitalized because of severe diarrhea and dehydration (129).

A discussion of the incidence and prevalence of SARS-CoV is not relevant in this context since there is no human-to-human transmission of this virus at present.

Seasonality

Both OC43 and 229E are epidemic, with peak incidence in the winter or early spring and well-defined outbreaks. In the 1960s and 1970s, 229E-like strains appeared to cause nationwide outbreaks in the United States at roughly 2-year intervals, whereas OC43-like outbreaks occur at less regular intervals and may be quite localized (89). Surveys of NL63 have clearly shown that it is predominantly seen in the winter in temperate countries and that its epidemic behavior varies widely in given locations from year to year (9, 55). While similar longitudinal studies of HKU1 have not been published, there is no reason to believe that its variability from year to year will be any different.

On the basis of the limited data currently available, enteric coronaviruses appear to have little or no seasonality (96).

Transmission

Both 229E and OC43, as well as several less well-characterized strains of coronaviruses (B814, LP, EVS, OC16, OC37, OC38, OC44, and OC48), were transmitted by intranasal inoculation to adult volunteers in the Common Cold Research Unit, and all produced clinical upper respiratory illness (11). Presumably, the respiratory route is the primary mode of infection with these viruses, although the details of their spread have not been studied.

After infection of adult volunteers, virus is shed beginning 48 h after inoculation, at about the time symptoms begin, and shedding continues for 5 days (92). Presumably, infected subjects are themselves infectious during this time.

As with other respiratory viruses, nosocomial transmission of coronaviruses does occur. An outbreak of respiratory coronaviruses in a neonatal intensive care unit has been described involving 10 infections among 40 premature infants monitored prospectively (119). All infections were associated with symptoms of generalized acute illness in this population. A report of NL63 infection in hospitalized children in New Haven, CT, also included an outbreak in a neonatal intensive care unit (27). However, the most dramatic examples of nosocomial transmission of coronaviruses occurred with SARS; 21% of cases were in health care workers, and the consequence of such transmission was severe. The virus spread readily in the hospital

TABLE 2 Published surveys of respiratory coronavirus infection in various pediatric populations and in relation to other respiratory viruses

Parameter	Description in reference[a]:					
	83	49	9	21	22	61
Population sampled	Inpatients	Inpatients	Inpatients	Inpatients	Inpatients	Inpatients and emergency room patients
Location	Chicago, IL	Christchurch, New Zealand	Quebec City, Canada	Hong Kong	Seoul, South Korea	Seattle, WA
Type of respiratory disease	Bronchiolitis or pneumonia	Any	Any	Any	Any	Any
No. of patients	380	75	396	587	515	1,061
No. of respiratory seasons	4	1	2	1	5	1
Method for HCoV detection	Serology	RT-PCR	RT-PCR	RT-PCR	RT-PCR	RT-PCR
Coronavirus(es) sought	229E, OC43	229E, OC43	NL63	229E, OC43, NL63	229E, OC43, NL63	229E, OC43, NL63, HKU1
All respiratory viruses (% positive)	55.0	87	NR	36.3	60.6	NR
RSV (%)	27.9	48	50.2	7.0	23.7	23
Rhinovirus (%)	NT	15	NT	NT	5.8	NT
Influenza viruses (%)	4.0	13	12.7	8.0	6.4	12
Parainfluenza viruses (%)	27.5	9	NT	4.3	8.0	9
Human metapneumovirus (%)	NT	5	5.5	4.9	4.7	7
Coronaviruses (%)	7.9	5	3.0	4.3	1.7	6.3
Adenovirus (%)	6.8	13	NT	5.5	6.8	13
Enteroviruses (%)	NT	7	NT	NT	NT	NT
Human bocavirus (%)	NT	NT	NT	NT	11.3	NT
Noncoronavirus coinfection rate (%)	NR	22.7	NR	2.2	11.5	NT
Coronavirus coinfection rate (%)	NR	75	60	20	NR	NT

[a] NR, not reported; NT, not tested.

environment, particularly early in the epidemic of 2002–2003, when the recognition of the disease was poor, confirmatory diagnosis was lacking, and appropriate precautions were not being taken (107). Barrier methods (wearing of personal protective gear and isolation of exposed or symptomatic persons) were the major weapons for combating what threatened to be a devastating epidemic. Retrospective studies in hospitals indicated that the enforcement of droplet and contact precautions was strongly associated with protection (118). However, in some instances when aerosol-generating procedures were used (e.g., nebulizers, intubation, and high-flow oxygen therapy), transmission also occurred via small-particle aerosols. In Hong Kong, approximately half of the health care workers who were infected had a history of taking part in such procedures. The unusual stability of the virus also likely predisposed it to spread via direct or indirect contact. SARS-CoV was merciless in exploiting the occasional lapse in infection control measures.

While the majority of cases did not transmit infection at all, a few were responsible for explosive outbreaks, the so-called "super spreading incidents" (112). In a number of these instances, it is the overall epidemiological context rather than the nature of the individual index patient that was crucial to such superspreading events. The risk factors associated with SARS outbreaks in hospital wards were narrow space between beds, lack of availability of washing or changing facilities for staff, performance of resuscitation in the ward, and the use of oxygen therapy or bilevel positive-airway-pressure ventilation (148).

There has been much speculation on why SARS did not, in fact, continue to spread globally, given that it was clearly contagious by the respiratory route and the world population had no preexisting immunity. The number of secondary cases produced by a single case was estimated to be 2.2 to 3.7, not much different from that now estimated for pandemic influenza (71). A physiological explanation for the success of public health measures in interrupting transmission is that unlike with many other respiratory viral infections, transmission predominantly took place later in the illness, after day 5 of symptoms. This correlated with low viral load in the upper respiratory tract early in the illness and provided a window of opportunity for case detection and isolation prior to maximal transmissibility, allowing public health measures to interrupt transmission in the community (97, 108). In addition, there was extraordinary cooperation and communication among nations and public health workers, contributing significantly to control of spread. It is interesting to speculate whether SARS-CoV might have become an endemic respiratory infection if not for the determined international global public health efforts implemented in 2003.

PATHOGENESIS IN HUMANS

Incubation Period

The incubation period of respiratory coronavirus infection in adult volunteers is, on average, 2 days, 1 day longer than that of rhinovirus infection and somewhat shorter than the incubation period of RSV or parainfluenza virus infection in the same host (127). The peak of respiratory symptoms is not reached until 3 or 4 days after inoculation.

The incubation period for SARS-CoV has been estimated to average 4 to 6 days, with a range of 1 to 14 days (71, 108).

Patterns of Virus Replication

Presumably the pattern of virus replication of coronaviruses is at least in part determined by cell tropism, and this, in turn, is determined by virus-receptor interaction. The cell surface tissue distributions of aminopeptidase N and ACE2 are very wide (69, 145), including several organs in which strains 229E and NL63 do not normally produce disease. It seems likely either that secondary receptors play a role in infection or that other factors are critical. In acute respiratory HCoV infections (other than with SARS-CoV), viral replication appears to be confined to the respiratory epithelium.

There is also some evidence for the presence of respiratory coronavirus genomes in the central nervous system in conjunction with chronic neurologic syndromes, particularly multiple sclerosis and acute demyelinating encephalomyelitis (4, 13, 122, 146). It appears clear that human "respiratory" coronaviruses are capable of entering the central nervous system. Assignment of a pathogenic role in demyelinating diseases of humans, so well demonstrated in the murine model, must, however, await further studies.

Factors in Disease Production

A histopathological study describes the nasal mucosa of a young girl with chronic rhinitis and bronchitis who showed the typical EM changes of a coronavirus infection (1). Brush biopsy specimens showed morphologically typical coronavirus particles in large numbers in cytoplasmic vesicles and the Golgi apparatus of ciliated epithelial cells (and not in goblet cells). Interestingly, the infected cells appeared not to show signs of cell death and to have intact synthetic activity. On the other hand, degenerative changes affecting the cilia and loss of cilia were seen. Presumably, ciliary function would have been affected in this child. It is interesting that EM of SARS-CoV infection of the human gastrointestinal tract seems to reveal a similar pattern, with viral infection occurring with minimal CPE (23, 68).

The pathogenesis of SARS has been widely studied in human subjects. SARS-CoV infects the alveolar epithelium, leading to diffuse alveolar damage, desquamation of pneumocytes, hyaline membrane formation, and clinically acute respiratory distress syndrome. Although the virus spreads to other organs (e.g., the gastrointestinal tract), the severity of the disease and fatal outcome are due to the pathology in the respiratory tract. The primary mechanism of pathology appears to be infection of type 1 and type 2 pneumocytes, which are key target cells for the virus (93, 98). Whether immunopathology contributes to the disease process is still unresolved (100). Proinflammatory cytokines (interleukin 1 [IL-1], IL-6, and IL-12) and chemokines (IL-8, CCL-2, and CXCL10) have been found to be elevated in patients with SARS, but it is not clear whether they drive pathogenesis or are a reflection of virus-induced cell pathology. There is also controversy over whether SARS-CoV evades activating type 1 interferon responses. In vitro studies appear to suggest that there is both poor interferon induction and signaling (31, 138), while some studies with peripheral blood leukocytes from SARS-CoV-infected patients suggest otherwise (15). The availability of an infectious clone of SARS-CoV now allows a detailed analysis of the virulence determinants of the virus (147). STAT1-deficient mice have increased susceptibility to SARS (48).

While a number of animal models for SARS have been investigated and are useful for vaccine efficacy studies, they fail to realistically reproduce the human disease (110). Intriguingly, young BALB/c mice infected with SARS-CoV replicate the virus with minimal lung pathology, while old mice manifest significant pathology, reminiscent of the age-related severity of human SARS (109).

Immune Responses

Serum antibody to the major structural antigens of the virus (primarily to the S protein but also to the M and N proteins) is made in adult volunteers in response to inoculation and infection with coronaviruses (115). Antibody titers, as measured by enzyme-linked immunosorbent assay, rise significantly in essentially all volunteers who shed virus (57). Adults and children often carry some measurable antibody in preinfection serum, and this reflects the experience of other investigators examining natural infection in adults and children (17, 53).

From volunteer studies with 229E and 229E-like strains, it appears that reinfection after a period of 1 year is possible, with production of symptoms. It is not clear, however, whether this is due to waning immunity or to slight differences in the antigenicities of different virus strains (105). Sequencing of several variants of 229E has revealed somewhat contradictory data regarding the antigenic stability of the S protein over time and space, but with consensus regarding the lack of evidence for recombination events (20). The S protein of OC43 has been shown to vary in the same community from year to year, but it is not clear that such variation is adequate to explain reinfection (135).

The mechanism by which recovery from respiratory coronavirus infection occurs has not been studied. As mentioned above, infections in immunocompromised subjects are very common and are associated with hospitalization, although the role of the coronavirus infection in illness is not clear. As with other respiratory viruses, prolonged shedding of virus (for 38 days) was recently documented to occur in a 3-year-old child who underwent stem cell transplantation (35). Severe but self-limited pneumonia was described to occur in an adult following autologous bone marrow transplantation, with diagnosis by EM (28), and another report describes two immunocompromised adults with 229E-related pneumonia, one of whom died as a result of the illness (101). An autopsy was not performed, so there is no anatomic information to elucidate the role of virus in the pneumonia.

Aspects of the immune responses to SARS have been reviewed in detail elsewhere (100). Neutralizing immune responses appear in the second week of the illness, peak at around 30 days, and remain detectable for years. The S protein is the predominant target of neutralizing immunity, and the major antibody neutralizing epitopes are in the region from residues 441 to 700 of the S protein.

CLINICAL MANIFESTATIONS

Major Clinical Syndromes

Human Respiratory Coronaviruses

Most of the human respiratory coronaviruses that were isolated in the 1960s were originally recovered during upper respiratory illness. The evidence for their pathogenicity comes from volunteer studies in which all strains tested caused illness in volunteers (10, 11, 64, 105). Bradburne et al. (10) and Tyrrell et al. (127) have summarized the characteristics of the respiratory symptoms produced by coronaviruses in volunteers. While the incubation period of coronavirus colds averages a day longer than that for rhinovirus, the course of illness is clinically indistinguishable. For coronavirus-infected volunteers, low-grade fever was present in about one in five, and malaise was frequent.

Volunteer studies have not been done with the newer respiratory coronaviruses. Particularly in young children, coronaviruses are frequently found by PCR of respiratory samples from both asymptomatic individuals (60, 132) and hospitalized patients without acute respiratory symptoms (9). Thus, although volunteer studies prove a level of pathogenicity for several of the respiratory coronaviruses (all those tested), it is very difficult in an individual case to attribute illness, particularly illness that is unlike that produced in the volunteers, to infection.

Despite such reservations, however, more serious lower respiratory tract illness is probably also caused by coronavirus infection. Early serologic surveys of infections in hospitalized pediatric patients with bronchiolitis and pneumonia found evidence of infection in about 8% of these children (83, 86, 87). Viruses antigenically identical to 229E were recovered from two infants with acute pneumonia in the absence of other detectable pathogens (83), and since the advent of PCR diagnosis, virus has been detected widely in such patients. But coinfection with other viruses is very common in such children, and when suitable controls are surveyed, virus is found also in asymptomatic subjects. One of the respiratory coronaviruses, NL63, has been found preferentially in children hospitalized with croup (22, 45, 131), and this stands as corroborative evidence for causality in this particular syndrome.

In young children with asthma, acute exacerbations were seen during infection by OC43 and 229E (85), although recent studies using PCR for detection of rhinoviruses have shown that this virus genus is by far the most important cause of acute wheezing in children with underlying asthma (50). Coronavirus infection of marine recruits has been associated with pneumonia and pleural reaction in about 33% (140). In adults with chronic pulmonary disease or asthma, several serologic studies have shown significant association between coronavirus infection and acute exacerbations of respiratory symptoms (14, 36, 38, 40, 95). Infection in the elderly, particularly in those with underlying cardiopulmonary disease, is commonly associated with lower respiratory tract symptoms, although these rarely lead either to hospitalization or to death (94, 136). Finally, a study of acute lower tract viral infections in patients after lung transplantation found respiratory viruses in 66%, with coronaviruses (OC43, 229E, and NL63) being present in rank order right behind rhinoviruses and ahead of others, and a highly significant association of viral infection with a decline in one-second forced expiratory volume (FEV-1), acute rejection, and likely development of bronchiolitis obliterans syndrome (59).

The role of respiratory coronaviruses in otitis media has been elucidated in studies which used PCR to detect viral nucleic acid in both nasal secretions and middle ear fluids. Among 92 children with acute otitis media, coronavirus sequences were found in 16 children (17%), with 14 children harboring the virus in the nasopharynx and 7 harboring it in the middle ear fluid (103). This incidence was lower than for both RSV (28%) and rhinovirus (35%).

Coronaviruses were less frequently found in middle ear effusions at the time of tube placement (3 of 100) (102).

SARS

SARS began with fever and myalgia and then progressed to cough (often with minimal upper respiratory symptoms), followed by dyspnea. Individuals seen at this stage often had scattered ground-glass peripheral lung infiltrates, and over the course of the next several days they either improved gradually or worsened, with increasing oxygen requirement and then, in severe cases, development of a full-blown acute respiratory distress syndrome. Overall mortality was between 9 and 12%, with the highest rates being in those over 60 years and those with underlying disease. Interestingly, children had milder illness. Laboratory abnormalities included leukopenia (with a particularly striking panlymphopenia in severe cases) and a transaminitis. Detailed clinical features are described elsewhere (97–99).

Enteric Coronaviruses

The clinical features of possible enteric infections with coronaviruses have not been clearly described. CVLPs have been detected in stools from healthy subjects as frequently as in stools from those with enteritis (80). On the other hand, studies of disease in neonates and infants in the first year of life have found statistically significant associations between CVLPs and illness, either mild and self-limited (34, 133) or severe and, in some neonates, requiring surgical intervention (18). Another study drew attention to differences between rotavirus diarrhea and CVLP-associated diarrhea. Fever and vomiting were of similar incidences, but stools from children excreting CVLPs were more often occult blood positive (18 versus 0%), less often watery (66 versus 92%) and more often mucoid (32 versus 8%) (91).

Complications

The major complications of respiratory coronavirus infections have been seen in children or adults with underlying cardiopulmonary disease. They have been, on the whole, of moderate severity and confined to wheezing or exacerbations of chronic obstructive disease.

LABORATORY DIAGNOSIS

Respiratory coronaviruses are difficult to grow in tissue culture. Subpassage is frequently required, as well as the use of special cell lines (52). The hepatoma line HUH7 has been recently used with success for isolation of HKU1, OC43, and 229E from clinical samples (30, 129). LLC-MK2 and Vero B4 cells have been helpful in isolation of NL63. Organ cultures of human embryonic trachea, while a sensitive culture system, are not practical for diagnostic laboratories. Although two strains have been adapted to growth in suckling mice (82), direct isolation in mice from respiratory tract specimens has not been reported.

Reverse transcriptase PCR (RT-PCR), either conventional or real-time, has become the diagnostic method of choice for detection of all HCoV strains. Although there have been attempts to develop a set of "pancoronavirus" primers and probes (27, 88), and such systems have been used with success (59), type-specific systems appear to be of greater sensitivity. In SARS, the small amount of virus present in all clinical samples obtained in the early phase of the illness proved to be a diagnostic challenge even with sensitive RT-PCR methods. The use of multiple specimens (including stool and blood) increased diagnostic yield in the first few days of SARS illness.

Coronaviruses can be detected by immunofluorescence of cells shed from the respiratory tract using commercially available reagents (119) or polyclonal (87) or monoclonal (35) reagents developed in individual laboratories. An enzyme-linked immunosorbent assay for coronavirus antigen in nasal swabs or secretions has been reported (75), but this test has limited usefulness.

The diagnosis of enteric coronavirus infection depends on finding the characteristic particles in stool samples examined by EM. At this writing, no culture, antigen detection, or nucleic acid amplification system exists for these viruses.

PREVENTION

While we lack detailed information on the mode of spread of respiratory HCoV infections (that is, the importance of small versus large droplets and aerosols versus fomites or direct transmission of infected secretions), it is reasonable to believe that barrier methods used to contain the spread of other respiratory viruses would prevent transmission. Interest in prevention of SARS was intense from the very beginning of the epidemic. As mentioned above, early case detection and barrier methods (personal protective devices and quarantine) were the major modes of prevention that ultimately resulted in the waning and finally disappearance of the outbreak. This subject has been recently reviewed (117).

SARS-CoV vaccine development is ongoing. Antibodies to the S protein are neutralizing, the critical epitopes being those in the receptor-binding domain. Subunit vaccines, whole-virus inactivated vaccines, vaccines that use various live-virus vectors, and DNA vaccines have been tested in various animal model systems, and many of these modalities have shown promise. Tests in human subjects have been much more limited but also show antigenicity. Antigenic diversity and lack of cross-neutralization between the human SARS-CoV used for vaccine development and precursor SARS-CoV-like viruses found in small mammals in live-game markets (e.g., civets) and bats, both of which are likely sources of any new SARS outbreak, pose a problem for vaccine development (144). However, some monoclonal antibodies appear to cross-neutralize and cross-protect against both human and animal (palm civet) coronaviruses but perhaps not those from bats (151). Vaccines for coronaviruses carry the risk that paradoxical disease enhancement may occur, as has been seen with vaccines for feline peritonitis virus (139). There is little evidence of this being a problem with SARS vaccines so far, but caution is clearly warranted for future coronavirus vaccines.

Animal studies on vaccine-induced protection, on adoptive transfer, and on T-cell depletion suggest that antibody is necessary and sufficient to confer protection. Since the precursor SARS-CoVs from animals (civets and bats) are still not culturable, and the virus isolates from the earliest stages of the SARS outbreak are not available, lentiviral pseudotypes incorporating SARS-CoV S protein have been used to explore the extent of cross-neutralization between these related viruses. While pseudotypes bearing the S protein of prototype SARS-CoV

(Urbani) are neutralized by antisera to both homologous antisera and those raised to animal-like SARS-CoV, e.g., GD03, the GD03-like pseudotype was refractory to neutralization with antiserum raised to either virus. This has worrying implications for the potential efficacy of a vaccine based on SARS-CoV prototypes against a SARS-CoV-like animal virus that may cause a future outbreak (144).

The only published information on chemoprophylaxis of respiratory HCoV infections describes the use of intranasal alpha interferon (4 million units three times a day) from 1 day before inoculation of virus until 2 days after (46). Under these conditions, the severity of symptoms and signs and virus replication were all beneficially affected to a significant extent.

TREATMENT

Because of its clinical severity, treatment of SARS was attempted immediately, with little or no information based on clinical trials or animal studies. During the outbreak of 2002–2003, most patients were treated with intravenous or oral ribavirin and those with severe disease also received corticosteroids. Later it was shown that various protease inhibitors, in particular, lopinavir-ritonavir, had activity against SARS-CoV in vitro. Pegylated interferons had therapeutic efficacy in macaques, and alpha interferon may have had some beneficial effect in a preliminary clinical study in humans (41). Because of a lack of controlled trials, it has been very difficult to evaluate the effectiveness of these treatments. A recent review of a very large published clinical experience concludes that none of the treatments used, including ribavirin, corticosteroids, interferon, antibody in various forms, or lopinavir-ritonavir, were conclusively demonstrated to have any beneficial effect (123).

Passive immunotherapy has shown some promise in animal models of SARS (126).

We acknowledge the kind assistance of Daniel K. W. Chu for the preparation of Fig. 2 and 4. K McIntosh also acknowledges support from the Bruce R. and Jolene M. McCaw Fund.

REFERENCES

1. **Afzelius, B. A.** 1994. Ultrastructure of human nasal epithelium during an episode of coronavirus infection. *Virchows Arch.* **424:**295–300.
2. **Almeida, J. D., D. M. Berry, C. H. Cunningham, K. McIntosh, and D. A. J. Tyrrell.** 1968. Coronaviruses. *Nature* **220:**650.
3. **Almeida, J. D., and D. A. J. Tyrrell.** 1967. The morphology of three previously uncharacterized human respiratory viruses that grow in organ culture. *J. Gen. Virol.* **1:**175–178.
4. **Arbour, N., R. Day, J. Newcombe, and P. J. Talbot.** 2000. Neuroinvasion by human respiratory coronaviruses. *J. Virol.* **74:**8913–8921.
5. **Bastien, N., J. L. Robinson, A. Tse, B. E. Lee, L. Hart, and Y. Li.** 2005. Human coronavirus NL-63 infections in children: a 1-year study. *J. Clin. Microbiol.* **43:**4567–4573.
6. **Beards, G. M., D. W. Brown, J. Green, and T. H. Flewett.** 1986. Preliminary characterisation of torovirus-like particles of humans: comparison with Berne virus of horses and Breda virus of calves. *J. Med. Virol.* **20:**67–78.
7. **Beaudette, F. R., and C. B. Hudson.** 1937. Cultivation of the virus of infectious bronchitis. *J. Am. Vet. Med. Assoc.* **90:**51–60.
8. **Becker, W. B., K. McIntosh, J. H. Dees, and R. M. Chanock.** 1967. Morphogenesis of avian infectious bronchitis virus and a related human virus (strain 229E). *J. Virol.* **1:**1019–1027.
9. **Boivin, G., M. Baz, S. Cote, R. Gilca, C. Deffrasnes, E. Leblanc, M. G. Bergeron, P. Dery, and G. De Serres.** 2005. Infections by human coronavirus-NL in hospitalized children. *Pediatr. Infect. Dis. J.* **24:**1045–1048.
10. **Bradburne, A. F., M. L. Bynoe, and D. A. Tyrrell.** 1967. Effects of a "new" human respiratory virus in volunteers. *Br. Med. J.* **3:**767–769.
11. **Bradburne, A. F., and B. A. Somerset.** 1972. Coronavirus antibody titres in sera of healthy adults and experimentally infected volunteers. *J. Hyg.* **70:**235–244.
12. **Bradburne, A. F., and D. A. J. Tyrrell.** 1971. Coronaviruses of man. *Prog. Med. Virol.* **13:**373–403.
13. **Burks, J. S., B. L. DeVald, L. D. Jankovsky, and J. C. Gerdes.** 1980. Two coronaviruses isolated from central nervous system tissue of two multiple sclerosis patients. *Science* **209:**933–934.
14. **Buscho, R. O., D. Saxtan, P. S. Shultz, E. Finch, and M. A. Mufson.** 1978. Infections with viruses and Mycoplasma pneumoniae during exacerbations of chronic bronchitis. *J. Infect. Dis.* **137:**377–383.
15. **Cameron, M. J., L. Ran, L. Xu, A. Danesh, J. F. Bermejo-Martin, C. M. Cameron, M. P. Muller, W. L. Gold, S. E. Richardson, S. M. Poutanen, B. M. Willey, M. E. DeVries, Y. Fang, C. Seneviratne, S. E. Bosinger, D. Persad, P. Wilkinson, L. D. Greller, R. Somogyi, A. Humar, S. Keshavjee, M. Louie, M. B. Loeb, J. Brunton, A. J. McGeer, and D. J. Kelvin.** 2007. Interferon-mediated immunopathological events are associated with atypical innate and adaptive immune responses in patients with severe acute respiratory syndrome. *J. Virol.* **81:**8692–8706.
16. **Caul, E. O., and S. I. Egglestone.** 1977. Further studies on human enteric coronaviruses. *Arch. Virol.* **54:**107–117.
17. **Cavallaro, J. J., and A. S. Monto.** 1970. Community-wide outbreak of infection with a 229E-like coronavirus in Tecumseh, Michigan. *J. Infect. Dis.* **122:**272–279.
18. **Chany, C., O. Moscovici, P. Lebon, and S. Rousset.** 1982. Association of coronavirus infection with neonatal necrotizing enterocolitis. *Pediatrics* **69:**209–214.
19. **Cheever, F. S., J. B. Daniels, A. M. Pappenheimer, and O. T. Bailey.** 1949. A murine virus (JHM) causing disseminated encephalomyelitis with extensive destruction of myelin. I. Isolation and biologic properties of the virus. *J. Exp. Med.* **89:**181–194.
20. **Chibo, D., and C. Birch.** 2006. Analysis of human coronavirus 229E spike and nucleoprotein genes demonstrates genetic drift between chronologically distinct strains. *J. Gen. Virol.* **87:**1203–1208.
21. **Chiu, S. S., K. H. Chan, K. W. Chu, S. W. Kwan, Y. Guan, L. L. Poon, and J. S. Peiris.** 2005. Human coronavirus NL63 infection and other coronavirus infections in children hospitalized with acute respiratory disease in Hong Kong, China. *Clin. Infect. Dis.* **40:**1721–1729.
22. **Choi, E. H., H. J. Lee, S. J. Kim, B. W. Eun, N. H. Kim, J. A. Lee, J. H. Lee, E. K. Song, S. H. Kim, J. Y. Park, and J. Y. Sung.** 2006. The association of newly identified respiratory viruses with lower respiratory tract infections in Korean children, 2000–2005. *Clin. Infect. Dis.* **43:**585–592.
23. **Cinatl, J., Jr., G. Hoever, B. Morgenstern, W. Preiser, J. U. Vogel, W. K. Hofmann, G. Bauer, M. Michaelis, H. F. Rabenau, and H. W. Doerr.** 2004. Infection of cultured intestinal epithelial cells with severe acute respira-

tory syndrome coronavirus. *Cell. Mol. Life Sci.* **61:**2100–2112.

24. **Doyle, L. P., and L. M. Hutchings.** 1946. A transmissible gastroenteritis in pigs. *J. Am. Vet. Assoc.* **108:**257–259.
25. **Drosten, C., S. Gunther, W. Preiser, S. van der Werf, H. R. Brodt, S. Becker, H. Rabenau, M. Panning, L. Kolesnikova, R. A. Fouchier, A. Berger, A. M. Burguiere, J. Cinatl, M. Eickmann, N. Escriou, K. Grywna, S. Kramme, J. C. Manuguerra, S. Muller, V. Rickerts, M. Sturmer, S. Vieth, H. D. Klenk, A. D. Osterhaus, H. Schmitz, and H. W. Doerr.** 2003. Identification of a novel coronavirus in patients with severe acute respiratory syndrome. *N. Engl. J. Med.* **348:**1967–1976.
26. **Duckmanton, L., B. Luan, J. Devenish, R. Tellier, and M. Petric.** 1997. Characterization of torovirus from human fecal specimens. *Virology* **239:**158–168.
27. **Esper, F., C. Weibel, D. Ferguson, M. L. Landry, and J. S. Kahn.** 2005. Evidence of a novel human coronavirus that is associated with respiratory tract disease in infants and young children. *J. Infect. Dis.* **191:**492–498.
28. **Folz, R. J., and M. A. Elkordy.** 1999. Coronavirus pneumonia following autologous bone marrow transplantation for breast cancer. *Chest* **115:**901–905.
29. **Fouchier, R. A., N. G. Hartwig, T. M. Bestebroer, B. Niemeyer, J. C. de Jong, J. H. Simon, and A. D. Osterhaus.** 2004. A previously undescribed coronavirus associated with respiratory disease in humans. *Proc. Natl. Acad. Sci. USA* **101:**6212–6216.
30. **Freymuth, F., A. Vabret, F. Rozenberg, J. Dina, J. Petitjean, S. Gouarin, L. Legrand, S. Corbet, J. Brouard, and P. Lebon.** 2005. Replication of respiratory viruses, particularly influenza virus, rhinovirus, and coronavirus in HuH7 hepatocarcinoma cell line. *J. Med. Virol.* **77:**295–301.
31. **Frieman, M., M. Heise, and R. Baric.** 20 April 2007. SARS coronavirus and innate immunity. *Virus Res.* doi: 10.1016/j.virusres.2007.03.015.
32. **Garbino, J., S. Crespo, J. D. Aubert, T. Rochat, B. Ninet, C. Deffernez, W. Wunderli, J. C. Pache, P. M. Soccal, and L. Kaiser.** 2006. A prospective hospital-based study of the clinical impact of non-severe acute respiratory syndrome (non-SARS)-related human coronavirus infection. *Clin. Infect. Dis.* **43:**1009–1015.
33. **Gerna, G., G. Campanini, F. Rovida, E. Percivalle, A. Sarasini, A. Marchi, and F. Baldanti.** 2006. Genetic variability of human coronavirus OC43-, 229E-, and NL63-like strains and their association with lower respiratory tract infections of hospitalized infants and immunocompromised patients. *J. Med. Virol.* **78:**938–949.
34. **Gerna, G., N. Passarani, M. Battaglia, and E. G. Rondanelli.** 1985. Human enteric coronaviruses: antigenic relatedness to human coronavirus OC43 and possible etiologic role in viral gastroenteritis. *J. Infect. Dis.* **151:**796–803.
35. **Gerna, G., E. Percivalle, A. Sarasini, G. Campanini, A. Piralla, F. Rovida, E. Genini, A. Marchi, and F. Baldanti.** 2007. Human respiratory coronavirus HKU1 versus other coronavirus infections in Italian hospitalised patients. *J. Clin. Virol.* **38:**244–250.
36. **Gill, E. P., E. A. Dominguez, S. B. Greenberg, R. L. Atmar, B. G. Hogue, B. D. Baxter, and R. B. Couch.** 1994. Development and application of an enzyme immunoassay for coronavirus OC43 antibody in acute respiratory illness. *J. Clin. Microbiol.* **32:**2372–2376.
37. **Gledhill, A. W., and C. H. Andrewes.** 1951. A hepatitis virus of mice. *Br. J. Exp. Pathol.* **32:**559–568.
38. **Graat, J. M., E. G. Schouten, M. L. Heijnen, F. J. Kok, E. G. Pallast, S. C. de Greeff, and J. W. Dorigo-Zetsma.** 2003. A prospective, community-based study on virologic assessment among elderly people with and without symptoms of acute respiratory infection. *J. Clin. Epidemiol.* **56:**1218–1223.
39. **Guan, Y., B. J. Zheng, Y. Q. He, X. L. Liu, Z. X. Zhuang, C. L. Cheung, S. W. Luo, P. H. Li, L. J. Zhang, Y. J. Guan, K. M. Butt, K. L. Wong, K. W. Chan, W. Lim, K. F. Shortridge, K. Y. Yuen, J. S. Peiris, and L. L. Poon.** 2003. Isolation and characterization of viruses related to the SARS coronavirus from animals in southern China. *Science* **302:**276–278.
40. **Gump, D. W., C. A. Phillips, B. R. Forsyth, K. McIntosh, K. R. Lamborn, and W. H. Stouch.** 1976. Role of infection in chronic bronchitis. *Am. Rev. Respir. Dis.* **113:**465–474.
41. **Haagmans, B. L., and A. D. Osterhaus.** 2006. Coronaviruses and their therapy. *Antivir. Res.* **71:**397–403.
42. **Hamre, D., and M. Beem.** 1972. Virologic studies of acute respiratory disease in young adults. V. Coronavirus 229E infections during six years of surveillance. *Am. J. Epidemiol.* **96:**94–106.
43. **Hamre, D., D. A. Kindig, and J. Mann.** 1967. Growth and intracellular development of a new respiratory virus. *J. Virol.* **1:**810–816.
44. **Hamre, D., and J. J. Procknow.** 1966. A new virus isolated from the human respiratory tract. *Proc. Soc. Exp. Biol. Med.* **121:**190–193.
45. **Han, T. H., J. Y. Chung, S. W. Kim, and E. S. Hwang.** 2007. Human coronavirus-NL63 infections in Korean children, 2004–2006. *J. Clin. Virol.* **38:**27–31.
46. **Higgins, P. G., R. J. Phillpotts, G. M. Scott, J. Wallace, L. L. Bernhardt, and D. A. Tyrrell.** 1983. Intranasal interferon as protection against experimental respiratory coronavirus infection in volunteers. *Antimicrob. Agents Chemother.* **24:**713–715.
47. **Hofmann, H., K. Pyrc, L. van der Hoek, M. Geier, B. Berkhout, and S. Pohlmann.** 2005. Human coronavirus NL63 employs the severe acute respiratory syndrome coronavirus receptor for cellular entry. *Proc. Natl. Acad. Sci. USA* **102:**7988–7993.
48. **Hogan, R. J., G. Gao, T. Rowe, P. Bell, D. Flieder, J. Paragas, G. P. Kobinger, N. A. Wivel, R. G. Crystal, J. Boyer, H. Feldmann, T. G. Voss, and J. M. Wilson.** 2004. Resolution of primary severe acute respiratory syndrome-associated coronavirus infection requires Stat1. *J. Virol.* **78:**11416–11421.
49. **Jennings, L. C., T. P. Anderson, A. M. Werno, K. A. Beynon, and D. R. Murdoch.** 2004. Viral etiology of acute respiratory tract infections in children presenting to hospital: role of polymerase chain reaction and demonstration of multiple infections. *Pediatr. Infect. Dis. J.* **23:**1003–1007.
50. **Johnston, S. L., P. K. Pattemore, G. Sanderson, S. Smith, F. Lampe, L. Josephs, P. Symington, S. O'Toole, S. H. Myint, D. A. Tyrrell, and S. T. Holgate.** 1995. Community study of role of viral infections in exacerbations of asthma in 9–11 year old children. *BMJ* **310:**1225–1229.
51. **Kaiser, L., N. Regamey, H. Roiha, C. Deffernez, and U. Frey.** 2005. Human coronavirus NL63 associated with lower respiratory tract symptoms in early life. *Pediatr. Infect. Dis. J.* **24:**1015–1017.
52. **Kapikian, A. Z., H. D. James, S. J. Kelly, J. H. Dees, H. C. Turner, K. McIntosh, H. W. Kim, R. H. Parrott, M. M. Vincent, and R. M. Chanock.** 1969. Isolation from man of "avian infectious bronchitis virus-like" viruses (coronaviruses) similar to 229E virus, with some epidemiological observations. *J. Infect. Dis.* **119:**282–290.
53. **Kaye, H. S., H. B. Marsh, and W. R. Dowdle.** 1971. Seroepidemiologic survey of coronavirus (strain OC 43)

related infections in a children's population. *Am. J. Epidemiol.* **94:**43–49.

54. **Kern, P., G. Muller, H. Schmitz, P. Racz, W. Meigel, G. Riethmuller, and M. Dietrich.** 1985. Detection of coronavirus-like particles in homosexual men with acquired immunodeficiency and related lymphadenopathy syndrome. *Klin. Wochenschr.* **63:**68–72.
55. **Koetz, A., P. Nilsson, M. Linden, L. van der Hoek, and T. Ripa.** 2006. Detection of human coronavirus NL63, human metapneumovirus and respiratory syncytial virus in children with respiratory tract infections in south-west Sweden. *Clin. Microbiol. Infect.* **12:**1089–1096.
56. **Koopmans, M., M. Petric, R. I. Glass, and S. S. Monroe.** 1993. Enzyme-linked immunosorbent assay reactivity of torovirus-like particles in fecal specimens from humans with diarrhea. *J. Clin. Microbiol.* **31:**2738–2744.
57. **Kraaijeveld, C. A., S. E. Reed, and M. R. Macnaughton.** 1980. Enzyme-linked immunosorbent assay for detection of antibody in volunteers experimentally infected with human coronavirus strain 229E. *J. Clin. Microbiol.* **12:** 493–497.
58. **Ksiazek, T. G., D. Erdman, C. S. Goldsmith, S. R. Zaki, T. Peret, S. Emery, S. Tong, C. Urbani, J. A. Comer, W. Lim, P. E. Rollin, S. F. Dowell, A. E. Ling, C. D. Humphrey, W. J. Shieh, J. Guarner, C. D. Paddock, P. Rota, B. Fields, J. DeRisi, J. Y. Yang, N. Cox, J. M. Hughes, J. W. LeDuc, W. J. Bellini, and L. J. Anderson.** 2003. A novel coronavirus associated with severe acute respiratory syndrome. *N. Engl. J. Med.* **348:**1953–1966.
59. **Kumar, D., D. Erdman, S. Keshavjee, T. Peret, R. Tellier, D. Hadjiliadis, G. Johnson, M. Ayers, D. Siegal, and A. Humar.** 2005. Clinical impact of community-acquired respiratory viruses on bronchiolitis obliterans after lung transplant. *Am. J. Transplant.* **5:**2031–2036.
60. **Kusel, M. M., N. H. de Klerk, P. G. Holt, T. Kebadze, S. L. Johnston, and P. D. Sly.** 2006. Role of respiratory viruses in acute upper and lower respiratory tract illness in the first year of life: a birth cohort study. *Pediatr. Infect. Dis. J.* **25:**680–686.
61. **Kuypers, J., E. T. Martin, J. Heugel, N. Wright, R. Morrow, and J. A. Englund.** 2007. Clinical disease in children associated with newly described coronavirus subtypes. *Pediatrics* **119:**e70–e76.
62. **Lai, M. M., and K. V. Holmes.** 2007. Coronaviridae: The viruses and their replication, p. 1305–1335. *In* D. M. Knipe, P. M. Howley, D. E. Griffin, R. A. Lamb, M. A. Martin, B. Roizman, and S.E. Straus (ed.), *Fields Virology*, 5th ed. Lippincott Williams & Wilkins, Philadelphia, PA.
63. **Lai, M. Y., P. K. Cheng, and W. W. Lim.** 2005. Survival of severe acute respiratory syndrome coronavirus. *Clin. Infect. Dis.* **41:**e67–e71.
64. **Larson, H. E., S. E. Reed, and D. A. Tyrrell.** 1980. Isolation of rhinoviruses and coronaviruses from 38 colds in adults. *J. Med. Virol.* **5:**221–229.
65. **Lau, S. K., P. C. Woo, K. S. Li, Y. Huang, H. W. Tsoi, B. H. Wong, S. S. Wong, S. Y. Leung, K. H. Chan, and K. Y. Yuen.** 2005. Severe acute respiratory syndrome coronavirus-like virus in Chinese horseshoe bats. *Proc. Natl. Acad. Sci. USA* **102:**14040–14045.
66. **Lau, S. K., P. C. Woo, C. C. Yip, H. Tse, H. W. Tsoi, V. C. Cheng, P. Lee, B. S. Tang, C. H. Cheung, R. A. Lee, L. Y. So, Y. L. Lau, K. H. Chan, and K. Y. Yuen.** 2006. Coronavirus HKU1 and other coronavirus infections in Hong Kong. *J. Clin. Microbiol.* **44:**2063–2071.
67. **Leung, G. M., W. W. Lim, L. M. Ho, T. H. Lam, A. C. Ghani, C. A. Donnelly, C. Fraser, S. Riley, N. M. Ferguson, R. M. Anderson, and A. J. Hedley.** 2006. Seroprevalence of IgG antibodies to SARS-coronavirus in asymptomatic or subclinical population groups. *Epidemiol. Infect.* **134:**211–221.
68. **Leung, W. K., K. F. To, P. K. Chan, H. L. Chan, A. K. Wu, N. Lee, K. Y. Yuen, and J. J. Sung.** 2003. Enteric involvement of severe acute respiratory syndrome-associated coronavirus infection. *Gastroenterology* **125:** 1011–1017.
69. **Li, W., M. J. Moore, N. Vasilieva, J. Sui, S. K. Wong, M. A. Berne, M. Somasundaran, J. L. Sullivan, K. Luzuriaga, T. C. Greenough, H. Choe, and M. Farzan.** 2003. Angiotensin-converting enzyme 2 is a functional receptor for the SARS coronavirus. *Nature* **426:**450–454.
70. **Li, W., Z. Shi, M. Yu, W. Ren, C. Smith, J. H. Epstein, H. Wang, G. Crameri, Z. Hu, H. Zhang, J. Zhang, J. McEachern, H. Field, P. Daszak, B. T. Eaton, S. Zhang, and L. F. Wang.** 2005. Bats are natural reservoirs of SARS-like coronaviruses. *Science* **310:**676–679.
71. **Lipsitch, M., T. Cohen, B. Cooper, J. M. Robins, S. Ma, L. James, G. Gopalakrishna, S. K. Chew, C. C. Tan, M. H. Samore, D. Fisman, and M. Murray.** 2003. Transmission dynamics and control of severe acute respiratory syndrome. *Science* **300:**1966–1970.
72. **Luby, J. P., R. Clinton, and S. Kurtz.** 1999. Adaptation of human enteric coronavirus to growth in cell lines. *J. Clin. Virol.* **12:**43–51.
73. **Maass, G., H. G. Baumeister, and N. Freitag.** 1977. Viruses as causal agents of gastroenteritis in infants and young children. *Muench. Med. Wochenschr.* **119:**1029–1034. (In German; author's translation.)
74. **Macnaughton, M. R., and H. A. Davies.** 1981. Human enteric coronaviruses. Brief review. *Arch. Virol.* **70:**301–313.
75. **Macnaughton, M. R., D. Flowers, and D. Isaacs.** 1983. Diagnosis of human coronavirus infections in children using enzyme-linked immunosorbent assay. *J. Med. Virol.* **11:**319–325.
76. **Makela, M. J., T. Puhakka, O. Ruuskanen, M. Leinonen, P. Saikku, M. Kimpimaki, S. Blomqvist, T. Hyypia, and P. Arstila.** 1998. Viruses and bacteria in the etiology of the common cold. *J. Clin. Microbiol.* **36:**539–542.
77. **Marra, M. A., S. J. Jones, C. R. Astell, R. A. Holt, A. Brooks-Wilson, Y. S. Butterfield, J. Khattra, J. K. Asano, S. A. Barber, S. Y. Chan, A. Cloutier, S. M. Coughlin, D. Freeman, N. Girn, O. L. Griffith, S. R. Leach, M. Mayo, H. McDonald, S. B. Montgomery, P. K. Pandoh, A. S. Petrescu, A. G. Robertson, J. E. Schein, A. Siddiqui, D. E. Smailus, J. M. Stott, G. S. Yang, F. Plummer, A. Andonov, H. Artsob, N. Bastien, K. Bernard, T. F. Booth, D. Bowness, M. Czub, M. Drebot, L. Fernando, R. Flick, M. Garbutt, M. Gray, A. Grolla, S. Jones, H. Feldmann, A. Meyers, A. Kabani, Y. Li, S. Normand, U. Stroher, G. A. Tipples, S. Tyler, R. Vogrig, D. Ward, B. Watson, R. C. Brunham, M. Krajden, M. Petric, D. M. Skowronski, C. Upton, and R. L. Roper.** 2003. The genome sequence of the SARS-associated coronavirus. *Science* **300:**1399–1404.
78. **Marshall, J. A., W. L. Thompson, and I. D. Gust.** 1989. Coronavirus-like particles in adults in Melbourne, Australia. *J. Med. Virol.* **29:**238–243.
79. **Masters, P. S.** 2006. The molecular biology of coronaviruses. *Adv. Virus Res.* **66:**193–292.
80. **Mathan, M., V. I. Mathan, S. P. Swaminathan, and S. Yesudoss.** 1975. Pleomorphic virus-like particles in human faeces. *Lancet* **i:**1068–1069.
81. **McIntosh, K.** 1974. Coronaviruses: a comparative review. *Curr. Top. Microbiol. Immunol.* **63:**83–129.
82. **McIntosh, K., W. B. Becker, and R. M. Chanock.** 1967. Growth in suckling-mouse brain of "IBV-like" viruses

from patients with upper respiratory tract disease. *Proc. Natl. Acad. Sci. USA* **58:**2268–2273.

83. **McIntosh, K., R. K. Chao, H. E. Krause, R. Wasil, H. E. Mocega, and M. A. Mufson.** 1974. Coronavirus infection in acute lower respiratory tract disease of infants. *J. Infect. Dis.* **130:**502–507.
84. **McIntosh, K., J. H. Dees, W. B. Becker, A. Z. Kapikian, and R. M. Chanock.** 1967. Recovery in tracheal organ cultures of novel viruses from patients with respiratory disease. *Proc. Natl. Acad. Sci. USA* **57:**933–940.
85. **McIntosh, K., E. F. Ellis, L. S. Hoffman, T. G. Lybass, J. J. Eller, and V. A. Fulginiti.** 1973. The association of viral and bacterial respiratory infections with exacerbations of wheezing in young asthmatic children. *J. Pediatr.* **82:**578–590.
86. **McIntosh, K., A. Z. Kapikian, H. C. Turner, J. W. Hartley, R. H. Parrott, and R. M. Chanock.** 1970. Seroepidemiologic studies of coronavirus infection in adults and children. *Am. J. Epidemiol.* **91:**585–592.
87. **McIntosh, K., J. McQuillin, S. E. Reed, and P. S. Gardner.** 1978. Diagnosis of human coronavirus infection by immunofluorescence: method and application to respiratory disease in hospitalized children. *J. Med. Virol.* **2:**341–346.
88. **Moes, E., L. Vijgen, E. Keyaerts, K. Zlateva, S. Li, P. Maes, K. Pyrc, B. Berkhout, L. van der Hoek, and M. Van Ranst.** 2005. A novel pancoronavirus RT-PCR assay: frequent detection of human coronavirus NL63 in children hospitalized with respiratory tract infections in Belgium. *BMC Infect. Dis.* **5:**6.
89. **Monto, A. S.** 1974. Medical reviews. Coronaviruses. *Yale J. Biol. Med.* **47:**234–251.
90. **Monto, A. S., and S. K. Lim.** 1974. The Tecumseh study of respiratory illness. VI. Frequency of and relationship between outbreaks of coronavirus infection. *J. Infect. Dis.* **129:**271–276.
91. **Mortensen, M. L., C. G. Ray, C. M. Payne, A. D. Friedman, L. L. Minnich, and C. Rousseau.** 1985. Coronaviruslike particles in human gastrointestinal disease. Epidemiologic, clinical, and laboratory observations. *Am. J. Dis. Child.* **139:**928–934.
92. **Myint, S., D. Harmsen, T. Raabe, and S. G. Siddell.** 1990. Characterization of a nucleic acid probe for the diagnosis of human coronavirus 229E infections. *J. Med. Virol.* **31:**165–172.
93. **Nicholls, J. M., J. Butany, L. L. Poon, K. H. Chan, S. L. Beh, S. Poutanen, J. S. Peiris, and M. Wong.** 2006. Time course and cellular localization of SARS-CoV nucleoprotein and RNA in lungs from fatal cases of SARS. *PLoS Med.* **3:**e27.
94. **Nicholson, K. G., J. Kent, V. Hammersley, and E. Cancio.** 1997. Acute viral infections of upper respiratory tract in elderly people living in the community: comparative, prospective, population based study of disease burden. *BMJ* **315:**1060–1064.
95. **Nicholson, K. G., J. Kent, and D. C. Ireland.** 1993. Respiratory viruses and exacerbations of asthma in adults. *BMJ* **307:**982–986.
96. **Payne, C. M., C. G. Ray, V. Borduin, L. L. Minnich, and M. D. Lebowitz.** 1986. An eight-year study of the viral agents of acute gastroenteritis in humans: ultrastructural observations and seasonal distribution with a major emphasis on coronavirus-like particles. *Diagn. Microbiol. Infect. Dis.* **5:**39–54.
97. **Peiris, J. S., C. M. Chu, V. C. Cheng, K. S. Chan, I. F. Hung, L. L. Poon, K. I. Law, B. S. Tang, T. Y. Hon, C. S. Chan, K. H. Chan, J. S. Ng, B. J. Zheng, W. L. Ng, R. W. Lai, Y. Guan, and K. Y. Yuen.** 2003. Clinical progression and viral load in a community outbreak of coronavirus-associated SARS pneumonia: a prospective study. *Lancet* **361:**1767–1772.
98. **Peiris, J. S., Y. Guan, and K. Y. Yuen.** 2004. Severe acute respiratory syndrome. *Nat. Med.* **10:**S88–S97.
99. **Peiris, J. S., S. T. Lai, L. L. Poon, Y. Guan, L. Y. Yam, W. Lim, J. Nicholls, W. K. Yee, W. W. Yan, M. T. Cheung, V. C. Cheng, K. H. Chan, D. N. Tsang, R. W. Yung, T. K. Ng, and K. Y. Yuen.** 2003. Coronavirus as a possible cause of severe acute respiratory syndrome. *Lancet* **361:**1319–1325.
100. **Peiris, J. S. M., Y. Guan, L. L. M. Poon, V. C. C. Cheng, J. M. Nicholls, and K. Y. Yuen.** 2006. Severe acute respiratory syndrome (SARS), p. 23–50. *In* W. M. Scheld, D. C. Hooper, and J. M. Hughes (ed.), *Emerging Infections 7*. ASM Press, Washington, DC.
101. **Pene, F., A. Merlat, A. Vabret, F. Rozenberg, A. Buzyn, F. Dreyfus, A. Cariou, F. Freymuth, and P. Lebon.** 2003. Coronavirus 229E–related pneumonia in immunocompromised patients. *Clin. Infect. Dis.* **37:**929–932.
102. **Pitkaranta, A., J. Jero, E. Arruda, A. Virolainen, and F. G. Hayden.** 1998. Polymerase chain reaction-based detection of rhinovirus, respiratory syncytial virus, and coronavirus in otitis media with effusion. *J. Pediatr.* **133:** 390–394.
103. **Pitkaranta, A., A. Virolainen, J. Jero, E. Arruda, and F. G. Hayden.** 1998. Detection of rhinovirus, respiratory syncytial virus, and coronavirus infections in acute otitis media by reverse transcriptase polymerase chain reaction. *Pediatrics* **102:**291–295.
104. **Poon, L. L., D. K. Chu, K. H. Chan, O. K. Wong, T. M. Ellis, Y. H. Leung, S. K. Lau, P. C. Woo, K. Y. Suen, K. Y. Yuen, Y. Guan, and J. S. Peiris.** 2005. Identification of a novel coronavirus in bats. *J. Virol.* **79:** 2001–2009.
105. **Reed, S. E.** 1984. The behaviour of recent isolates of human respiratory coronavirus in vitro and in volunteers: evidence of heterogeneity among 229E-related strains. *J. Med. Virol.* **13:**179–192.
106. **Resta, S., J. P. Luby, C. R. Rosenfeld, and J. D. Siegel.** 1985. Isolation and propagation of a human enteric coronavirus. *Science* **229:**978–981.
107. **Reynolds, M. G., B. H. Anh, V. H. Thu, J. M. Montgomery, D. G. Bausch, J. J. Shah, S. Maloney, K. C. Leitmeyer, V. Q. Huy, P. Horby, A. Y. Plant, and T. M. Uyeki.** 2006. Factors associated with nosocomial SARS-CoV transmission among healthcare workers in Hanoi, Vietnam, 2003. *BMC Public Health* **6:**207.
108. **Riley, S., C. Fraser, C. A. Donnelly, A. C. Ghani, L. J. Abu-Raddad, A. J. Hedley, G. M. Leung, L. M. Ho, T. H. Lam, T. Q. Thach, P. Chau, K. P. Chan, S. V. Lo, P. Y. Leung, T. Tsang, W. Ho, K. H. Lee, E. M. Lau, N. M. Ferguson, and R. M. Anderson.** 2003. Transmission dynamics of the etiological agent of SARS in Hong Kong: impact of public health interventions. *Science* **300:**1961–1966.
109. **Roberts, A., C. Paddock, L. Vogel, E. Butler, S. Zaki, and K. Subbarao.** 2005. Aged BALB/c mice as a model for increased severity of severe acute respiratory syndrome in elderly humans. *J. Virol.* **79:**5833–5838.
110. **Roberts, A., and K. Subbarao.** 2006. Animal models for SARS. *Adv. Exp. Med. Biol.* **581:**463–471.
111. **Rota, P. A., M. S. Oberste, S. S. Monroe, W. A. Nix, R. Campagnoli, J. P. Icenogle, S. Penaranda, B. Bankamp, K. Maher, M. H. Chen, S. Tong, A. Tamin, L. Lowe, M. Frace, J. L. DeRisi, Q. Chen, D. Wang, D. D. Erdman, T. C. Peret, C. Burns, T. G. Ksiazek, P. E. Rollin, A. Sanchez, S. Liffick, B. Holloway, J. Limor, K. McCaustland, M. Olsen-Rasmussen, R. Fouchier, S. Gunther, A. D. Osterhaus, C. Drosten, M. A.**

Pallansch, L. J. Anderson, and W. J. Bellini. 2003. Characterization of a novel coronavirus associated with severe acute respiratory syndrome. *Science* **300:**1394–1399.

112. **SARS Investigation Team from DMERI and SGH.** 2005. Strategies adopted and lessons learnt during the severe acute respiratory syndrome crisis in Singapore. *Rev. Med. Virol.* **15:**57–70.
113. **Schildgen, O., M. F. Jebbink, M. de Vries, K. Pyrc, R. Dijkman, A. Simon, A. Muller, B. Kupfer, and L. van der Hoek.** 2006. Identification of cell lines permissive for human coronavirus NL63. *J. Virol. Methods* **138:** 207–210.
114. **Schmidt, O. W., M. K. Cooney, and G. E. Kenny.** 1979. Plaque assay and improved yield of human coronaviruses in a human rhabdomyosarcoma cell line. *J. Clin. Microbiol.* **9:**722–728.
115. **Schmidt, O. W., and G. E. Kenny.** 1981. Immunogenicity and antigenicity of human coronaviruses 229E and OC43. *Infect. Immun.* **32:**1000–1006.
116. **Schmidt, W., T. Schneider, W. Heise, T. Weinke, H. J. Epple, M. Stöffler-Meilicke, O. Liesenfeld, R. Ignatius, M. Zeitz, E. O. Riecken, and R. Ullrich for the Berlin Diarrhea/Wasting Syndrome Study Group.** 1996. Stool viruses, coinfections, and diarrhea in HIV-infected patients. *J. Acquir. Immune Defic. Syndr. Hum. Retrovirol.* **13:**33–38.
117. **Seto, W. H., P. T. Y. Ching, and P. L. Ho.** 2006. Understanding and ensuring that infection control of SARS is achievable in the hospital, p. 161–177. *In* J. C. K. Chan and V. C. W. TaAm. Wong (ed.), *Challenges of Severe Acute Respiratory Syndrome.* Elsevier, New York, NY.
118. **Seto, W. H., D. Tsang, R. W. Yung, T. Y. Ching, T. K. Ng, M. Ho, L. M. Ho, and J. S. Peiris.** 2003. Effectiveness of precautions against droplets and contact in prevention of nosocomial transmission of severe acute respiratory syndrome (SARS). *Lancet* **361:**1519–1520.
119. **Sizun, J., D. Soupre, M. C. Legrand, J. D. Giroux, S. Rubio, J. M. Cauvin, C. Chastel, D. Alix, and L. de Parscau.** 1995. Neonatal nosocomial respiratory infection with coronavirus: a prospective study in a neonatal intensive care unit. *Acta Paediatr.* **84:**617–620.
120. **Sloots, T. P., P. McErlean, D. J. Speicher, K. E. Arden, M. D. Nissen, and I. M. Mackay.** 2006. Evidence of human coronavirus HKU1 and human bocavirus in Australian children. *J. Clin. Virol.* **35:**99–102.
121. **Song, H. D., C. C. Tu, G. W. Zhang, S. Y. Wang, K. Zheng, L. C. Lei, Q. X. Chen, Y. W. Gao, H. Q. Zhou, H. Xiang, H. J. Zheng, S. W. Chern, F. Cheng, C. M. Pan, H. Xuan, S. J. Chen, H. M. Luo, D. H. Zhou, Y. F. Liu, J. F. He, P. Z. Qin, L. H. Li, Y. Q. Ren, W. J. Liang, Y. D. Yu, L. Anderson, M. Wang, R. H. Xu, X. W. Wu, H. Y. Zheng, J. D. Chen, G. Liang, Y. Gao, M. Liao, L. Fang, L. Y. Jiang, H. Li, F. Chen, B. Di, L. J. He, J. Y. Lin, S. Tong, X. Kong, L. Du, P. Hao, H. Tang, A. Bernini, X. J. Yu, O. Spiga, Z. M. Guo, H. Y. Pan, W. Z. He, J. C. Manuguerra, A. Fontanet, A. Danchin, N. Niccolai, Y. X. Li, C. I. Wu, and G. P. Zhao.** 2005. Cross-host evolution of severe acute respiratory syndrome coronavirus in palm civet and human. *Proc. Natl. Acad. Sci. USA* **102:**2430–2435.
122. **Stewart, J. N., S. Mounir, and P. J. Talbot.** 1992. Human coronavirus gene expression in the brains of multiple sclerosis patients. *Virology* **191:**502–505.
123. **Stockman, L. J., R. Bellamy, and P. Garner.** 2006. SARS: systematic review of treatment effects. *PLoS Med.* **3:**e343.
124. **Stroher, U., A. DiCaro, Y. Li, J. E. Strong, F. Aoki, F. Plummer, S. M. Jones, and H. Feldmann.** 2004. Severe acute respiratory syndrome-related coronavirus is inhibited by interferon-alpha. *J. Infect. Dis.* **189:**1164–1167.
125. **Tang, X. C., J. X. Zhang, S. Y. Zhang, P. Wang, X. H. Fan, L. F. Li, G. Li, B. Q. Dong, W. Liu, C. L. Cheung, K. M. Xu, W. J. Song, D. Vijaykrishna, L. L. Poon, J. S. Peiris, G. J. Smith, H. Chen, and Y. Guan.** 2006. Prevalence and genetic diversity of coronaviruses in bats from China. *J. Virol.* **80:**7481–7490.
126. **ter Meulen, J., A. B. Bakker, E. N. van den Brink, G. J. Weverling, B. E. Martina, B. L. Haagmans, T. Kuiken, J. de Kruif, W. Preiser, W. Spaan, H. R. Gelderblom, J. Goudsmit, and A. D. Osterhaus.** 2004. Human monoclonal antibody as prophylaxis for SARS coronavirus infection in ferrets. *Lancet* **363:**2139–2141.
127. **Tyrrell, D. A., S. Cohen, and J. E. Schlarb.** 1993. Signs and symptoms in common colds. *Epidemiol. Infect.* **111:** 143–156.
128. **Tyrrell, D. A. J., and M. L. Bynoe.** 1965. Cultivation of a novel type of common-cold virus in organ cultures. *Br. Med. J.* **1:**1467–1470.
129. **Vabret, A., J. Dina, S. Gouarin, J. Petitjean, S. Corbet, and F. Freymuth.** 2006. Detection of the new human coronavirus HKU1: a report of 6 cases. *Clin. Infect. Dis.* **42:**634–639.
130. **van der Hoek, L., K. Pyrc, M. F. Jebbink, W. Vermeulen-Oost, R. J. Berkhout, K. C. Wolthers, P. M. Wertheim-van Dillen, J. Kaandorp, J. Spaargaren, and B. Berkhout.** 2004. Identification of a new human coronavirus. *Nat. Med.* **10:**368–373.
131. **van der Hoek, L., K. Sure, G. Ihorst, A. Stang, K. Pyrc, M. F. Jebbink, G. Petersen, J. Forster, B. Berkhout, and K. Uberla.** 2005. Croup is associated with the novel coronavirus NL63. *PLoS Med.* **2:**e240.
132. **van Gageldonk-Lafeber, A. B., M. L. Heijnen, A. I. Bartelds, M. F. Peters, S. M. van der Plas, and B. Wilbrink.** 2005. A case-control study of acute respiratory tract infection in general practice patients in The Netherlands. *Clin. Infect. Dis.* **41:**490–497.
133. **Vaucher, Y. E., C. G. Ray, L. L. Minnich, C. M. Payne, D. Beck, and P. Lowe.** 1982. Pleomorphic, enveloped, virus-like particles associated with gastrointestinal illness in neonates. *J. Infect. Dis.* **145:**27–36.
134. **Vijaykrishna, D., G. J. Smith, J. X. Zhang, J. S. Peiris, H. Chen, and Y. Guan.** 2007. Evolutionary insights into the ecology of coronaviruses. *J. Virol.* **81:**4012–4020.
135. **Vijgen, L., E. Keyaerts, P. Lemey, E. Moes, S. Li, A. M. Vandamme, and M. Van Ranst.** 2005. Circulation of genetically distinct contemporary human coronavirus OC43 strains. *Virology* **337:**85–92.
136. **Walsh, E. E., A. R. Falsey, and P. A. Hennessey.** 1999. Respiratory syncytial and other virus infections in persons with chronic cardiopulmonary disease. *Am. J. Respir. Crit. Care Med.* **160:**791–795.
137. **Wang, L. F., Z. Shi, S. Zhang, H. Field, P. Daszak, and B. T. Eaton.** 2006. Review of bats and SARS. *Emerg. Infect. Dis.* **12:**1834–1840.
138. **Wathelet, M. G., M. Orr, M. B. Frieman, and R. S. Baric.** 2007. Severe acute respiratory syndrome coronavirus evades antiviral signaling: role of nsp1 and rational design of an attenuated strain. *J. Virol.* **81:**11620–11633.
139. **Weiss, R. C., and F. W. Scott.** 1981. Antibody-mediated enhancement of disease in feline infectious peritonitis: comparisons with dengue hemorrhagic fever. *Comp. Immunol. Microbiol. Infect. Dis.* **4:**175–189.
140. **Wenzel, R. P., J. O. Hendley, J. A. Davies, and J. M. Gwaltney.** 1974. Coronavirus infections in military re-

cruits. Three–year study with coronavirus strains OC43 and 229E. *Am. Rev. Respir. Dis.* **109:**621–624.

141. **Williams, R. K., G. S. Jiang, and K. V. Holmes.** 1991. Receptor for mouse hepatitis virus is a member of the carcinoembryonic antigen family of glycoproteins. *Proc. Natl. Acad. Sci. USA* **88:**5533–5536.

142. **Woo, P. C., S. K. Lau, C. M. Chu, K. H. Chan, H. W. Tsoi, Y. Huang, B. H. Wong, R. W. Poon, J. J. Cai, W. K. Luk, L. L. Poon, S. S. Wong, Y. Guan, J. S. Peiris, and K. Y. Yuen.** 2005. Characterization and complete genome sequence of a novel coronavirus, coronavirus HKU1, from patients with pneumonia. *J. Virol.* **79:** 884–895.

143. **Woo, P. C., S. K. Lau, H. W. Tsoi, Y. Huang, R. W. Poon, C. M. Chu, R. A. Lee, W. K. Luk, G. K. Wong, B. H. Wong, V. C. Cheng, B. S. Tang, A. K. Wu, R. W. Yung, H. Chen, Y. Guan, K. H. Chan, and K. Y. Yuen.** 2005. Clinical and molecular epidemiological features of coronavirus HKU1-associated community-acquired pneumonia. *J. Infect. Dis.* **192:**1898–1907.

144. **Yang, Z. Y., H. C. Werner, W. P. Kong, K. Leung, E. Traggiai, A. Lanzavecchia, and G. J. Nabel.** 2005. Evasion of antibody neutralization in emerging severe acute respiratory syndrome coronaviruses. *Proc. Natl. Acad. Sci. USA* **102:**797–801.

145. **Yeager, C. L., R. A. Ashmun, R. K. Williams, C. B. Cardellichio, L. H. Shapiro, A. T. Look, and K. V. Holmes.** 1992. Human aminopeptidase N is a receptor for human coronavirus 229E. *Nature* **357:**420–422.

146. **Yeh, E. A., A. Collins, M. E. Cohen, P. K. Duffner, and H. Faden.** 2004. Detection of coronavirus in the central nervous system of a child with acute disseminated encephalomyelitis. *Pediatrics* **113:**e73–e76.

147. **Yount, B., K. M. Curtis, E. A. Fritz, L. E. Hensley, P. B. Jahrling, E. Prentice, M. R. Denison, T. W. Geisbert, and R. S. Baric.** 2003. Reverse genetics with a full-length infectious cDNA of severe acute respiratory syndrome coronavirus. *Proc. Natl. Acad. Sci. USA* **100:** 12995–13000.

148. **Yu, I. T., Z. H. Xie, K. K. Tsoi, Y. L. Chiu, S. W. Lok, X. P. Tang, D. S. Hui, N. Lee, Y. M. Li, Z. T. Huang, T. Liu, T. W. Wong, N. S. Zhong, and J. J. Sung.** 2007. Why did outbreaks of severe acute respiratory syndrome occur in some hospital wards but not in others? *Clin. Infect. Dis.* **44:**1017–1025.

149. **Zhang, X. M., W. Herbst, K. G. Kousoulas, and J. Storz.** 1994. Biological and genetic characterization of a hemagglutinating coronavirus isolated from a diarrhoeic child. *J. Med. Virol.* **44:**152–161.

150. **Zhao, Z., F. Zhang, M. Xu, K. Huang, W. Zhong, W. Cai, Z. Yin, S. Huang, Z. Deng, M. Wei, J. Xiong, and P. M. Hawkey.** 2003. Description and clinical treatment of an early outbreak of severe acute respiratory syndrome (SARS) in Guangzhou, PR China. *J. Med. Microbiol.* **52:**715–720.

151. **Zhu, Z., S. Chakraborti, Y. He, A. Roberts, T. Sheahan, X. Xiao, L. E. Hensley, P. Prabakaran, B. Rockx, I. A. Sidorov, D. Corti, L. Vogel, Y. Feng, J. O. Kim, L. F. Wang, R. Baric, A. Lanzavecchia, K. M. Curtis, G. J. Nabel, K. Subbarao, S. Jiang, and D. S. Dimitrov.** 2007. Potent cross-reactive neutralization of SARS coronavirus isolates by human monoclonal antibodies. *Proc. Natl. Acad. Sci. USA* **104:**12123–12128.

Arthropod-Borne Flaviviruses

LYLE R. PETERSEN AND ALAN D. T. BARRETT

52

The prototype flavivirus disease, yellow fever, was the first human illness shown to be caused by a filterable virus (in 1901) and the first member of the virus family to be isolated (in 1927). The *Flaviviridae* derive their name from yellow (*flavus*, Latin) fever. From the medical perspective, the flaviviruses are the most important group of arthropod-borne viruses (arboviruses). Dengue fever and dengue hemorrhagic fever (DHF) are major causes of human morbidity worldwide. Yellow fever remains an epidemic threat in Africa and South America. Since its introduction into North America, West Nile virus (WNV) has caused annual outbreaks of encephalitis and febrile illness in North America, and Japanese encephalitis (JE) remains a major cause of viral encephalitis in Asia.

VIROLOGY

Classification

The *Flaviviridae* constitute a structurally unique virus family of positive-sense, single-stranded RNA viruses, divided into the genera *Flavivirus*, *Pestivirus*, and *Hepacivirus*. There are over 70 distinct agents in the *Flavivirus* genus, most of which are transmitted by arthropods (mosquitoes or ticks); more than half are associated with human disease (Table 1). Classification of viruses within the *Flavivirus* genus has been based traditionally on antigenic distinctions. Using the neutralization test, flaviviruses have been classified into at least eight antigenic complexes, of which six contain human pathogens (13). More recently, nucleotide sequencing has taken a prominent role in determining relationships among viruses and identifying which are termed species. Twelve virus groups have been identified, plus an additional group of viruses that are found only in insects. Tamana bat and Ngoye viruses, isolated from a bat and tick, respectively, are tentative species in the genus *Flavivirus* but appear to be only distantly related to other members in the genus. The classification of the tick-borne flaviviruses is still being debated (50).

The viruses within the tick-borne encephalitis virus (TBEV), dengue virus, and JE virus serocomplexes are most closely related to each other, sharing up to 77% amino acid sequence homology, whereas homology across the serocomplexes is only 40 to 45%. Immunologic cross-protection between viruses is not observed for agents with <70% sequence homology, but incomplete or partial cross-protection may be present across closely related viruses within a serocomplex having sequence homologies of >70%.

Flaviviruses have evolved principally by mutational change. The high rate of mutation of these RNA viruses, which exist as quasispecies containing multiple genetic variants, is tempered by the requirement to maintain sufficient genetic stability to ensure infectivity for hosts and vectors belonging to different phyla. Intramolecular recombinational events within species contribute to strain variation of hyperendemic viruses (such as dengue virus) that have high rates of coinfection of hosts and vectors (67). An analysis of phylogenetic change by comparisons of virion complete envelope (E) glycoprotein gene sequences showed that the mosquito-borne flaviviruses (like dengue virus) have undergone explosive genetic diversification within the last 200 years, whereas the more primitive tick-borne viruses evolved slowly (176), probably due in part to the different ecologies of the viruses. The recent evolution of dengue viruses is associated with the expanding size and dispersal of human host and vector populations, while the tick-borne agents are transmitted in stable environments between small terrestrial mammal hosts and vectors with a long reproductive cycle.

Composition

Flavivirus particles are approximately 50 nm in diameter and have a spherical nucleocapsid surrounded by a lipid bilayer envelope with small surface projections, representing E glycoprotein dimers anchored to the virus membrane. Lipases, organic solvents, and detergents disrupt the virus envelope and inactivate flaviviruses.

The flavivirus genome is a single strand of RNA containing approximately 11,000 nucleotides (24) and is composed of a short 5′ noncoding region, a single long open reading frame containing more than 10,000 nucleotides, and a 3′ noncoding region that is usually devoid of poly(A) tracts. The long open reading frame encodes three structural proteins at the 5′ end, which are the capsid, premembrane (prM), and E proteins. These are followed downstream by seven nonstructural (NS) proteins in the sequence NS1-NS2A-NS2B-NS3-NS4A-NS4B-NS5 (Table 2). The structural proteins are included in the mature virion, whereas the NS proteins play various roles in virus

TABLE 1 List of members and tentative members of genus *Flavivirus*[a]

Vector	Group	Species or strain	Subtype	Comments	Genomic sequence
Tick	Mammalian tick borne	*Gadgets Gully virus*			+
		Kadam virus			+
		Karshi *virus*			+
		Kyasanur Forest disease virus			+
			Alkhumra	Genetic variant of Kyasanur Forest disease virus	+
		Langat virus			+
		Louping ill virus	British		+
			Irish		+
			Greek		+
			Spanish		+
			Turkish		+
		Omsk hemorrhagic fever virus			+
		Powassan virus			+
			Deer tick	Genetic variant of Powassan virus	+
		Royal Farm virus			+
		Tick-borne encephalitis virus	Central European		+
			Far Eastern		+
			Siberian		+
Tick	Seabird tick borne	*Meaban virus*			+
		Saumarez Reef virus			+
		Tyuleniy virus			+
Mosquito	Aroa	*Aroa virus*			
		Bussuquara			+
		Iguape			+
		Naranjal			
Mosquito	Dengue	Dengue virus 1			+
		Dengue virus 2			+
		Dengue virus 3			+
		Dengue virus 4			+
Mosquito		*Kedougou virus*			+
Mosquito	JE	Alfuy virus			+
		Cacipacore virus			
		Koutango virus			
		Japanese encephalitis virus			+
		Murray Valley encephalitis virus			+
		St. Louis encephalitis virus			+
		Usutu virus			+
		West Nile virus			+
			Kunjin		+
		Yaounde virus			
Mosquito	Kokobera	*Kokobera virus*			+
		New Mapoon		Tentative species	
		Stratford			

(Continued on next page)

TABLE 1 *(Continued)*

Vector	Group	Species or strain	Subtype	Comments	Genomic sequence
Mosquito	Ntaya	*Bagaza virus*			+
		Ilheus virus			+
		Israel turkey meningoencephalomyelitis virus			
		Ntaya virus			
		Rocio virus			+
		Tembusu virus			
Mosquito	Spondweni	Spondweni virus			
		Zika virus			+
Mosquito	Yellow fever	*Banzi virus*			
		Bouboui virus			
		Edge Hill virus			
		Jugra virus			
		Saboya virus			
			Potiskum		
		Sepik virus			+
		Uganda S virus			
		Wesselsbron virus			
		Yellow fever virus			+
No known vector	Entebbe bat	*Entebbe bat virus*		Genetically, the Entebbe bat group is in the yellow fever group.	+
			Sokoluk		
		Yokose virus			+
No known vector	Modoc	*Apoi virus*			+
		Cowbone Ridge virus			
		Jutiapa virus			
		Modoc virus			+
		Sal Vieja virus			
		San Perlita virus			
No known vector	Rio Bravo	*Bukalasa bat virus*			
		Carey Island virus			
		Dakar bat virus			
			Batu Cave		
		Montana myotis leukoencephalitis virus			+
		Phnom Penh bat virus			
		Rio Bravo virus			+
Insect	?	Cell fusing agent virus		Mosquito	+
		Culex flavivirus		Mosquito	+
		Kamiti River virus		Mosquito	+
		Ngoye virus		Tentative species isolated from a tick	
		Tamana bat virus		Tentative species isolated from a bat	+

[a] "Vector" refers to whether mosquitoes or ticks transmit the virus to vertebrate hosts. "Insect" refers to viruses that are found only in insects and do not appear to infect vertebrates. "Tentative species" refers to viruses for which there is insufficient information at present to determine if they are a species in the genus. For genome sequence, a plus sign indicates availability of the genome sequence in GenBank.

TABLE 2 Flavivirus proteins and their known or suspected functions

Protein	Location	Mol mass (kDa)	Function	
			Replication	Immunity
C	Capsid	9–12	Associates with RNA in nucleocapsid	T-cell epitopes
prM	Premembrane (immature virion)	18–19	Chaperone for E protein; proper folding and stabilization during virus maturation and exocytosis	Protective immunity (minor role, induces low-titer neutralizing antibody)
M	Membrane (mature virion)	7–9	Control of fusion events (with E)	T-helper epitope?, induces low-titer neutralizing antibody
E	Envelope	55–60	Receptor binding; mediation of membrane fusion in endosome and virus internalization; dissociation of nucleocapsids	Neutralizing (protective) antibody, CTL epitope(s), T-helper epitopes, immune enhancement, HI antibody
NS1	Nonstructural	42–50	Involved in RNA replication and virion maturation	Antibody, complement-dependent cell lysis; CTL epitopes
NS2A		18–22	Processing of NS2	?CTL epitope; interferon antagonist for WNV
NS2B		13–15	Central domain associated with functional NS3 protease	
NS3		67–70	Serine protease (posttranslational processing of viral proteins), helicase, nucleoside triphosphatase, RNA capping	Nonneutralizing antibody; CTL epitopes
NS4A		16	Integral membrane protein; part of replication complex	?CTL epitope
NS4B		27–28	Integral membrane protein; part of replication complex	?CTL epitope; interferon antagonist for WNV and dengue 2 virus, and others?
NS5		104–106	RNA-dependent RNA polymerase, methyltransferase, RNA capping	Nonneutralizing antibody; CTL epitope; interferon antagonist for Langat and JE viruses; induction of IL-8

replication and polypeptide processing. The polyprotein is co- and posttranslationally cleaved to yield the individual proteins. Translation occurs at the rough endoplasmic reticulum (ER), so that the prM, E, and NS1 proteins are translocated, whereas the others remain on the cytoplasmic side of the host cell membrane. Cell-associated virions within the ER are morphologically identical to extracellular particles.

The capsid protein interacts with RNA to form the virion nucleocapsid. The prM glycoprotein forms an intracellular heterodimer, stabilizing the E polypeptide during exocytosis. The prM protein is cleaved before virus release from the cell, leaving a small M structural protein anchored in the virus envelope and releasing the larger 18- to 19-kDa "pr" glycopeptide segment into the extracellular medium.

The E glycoprotein contains antigenic determinants for hemagglutination and neutralization. Antibodies directed at E determinants also mediate the phenomenon of antibody-dependent enhancement of infection in the pathogenesis of DHF. This protein is also involved in attachment to cells and fusion of the viral and host cell membrane during virus entry into the cell and thus is a major factor in virus virulence.

The three-dimensional crystallographic structure of the E glycoprotein reveals a head-to-tail dimer composed of a 170-Å-long rod anchored to the membrane at its basal end, with its long axis parallel to the virion surface (145), and is typical of a class II fusion protein characteristic of alphaviruses and flaviviruses. The C terminus resembles an immunoglobulin constant domain and is connected by a hinge region to a central portion of the molecule (domain I) with up-and-down topology consisting of eight antiparallel strands and containing the N terminus. Two long loops (domain II) extend outward from this part of the protein and play a role in dimerization of the molecule. A conserved stretch of 14 amino acids at the end of one of the domain II loops is responsible for fusion of the viral envelope and the membrane of the host cell (30). The fusion event is acid dependent and occurs within endosomal vesicles, releasing the uncoated nucleocapsids into the cytoplasm of the infected cell. The fusion process also results in an irreversible rearrangement of the E protein into a trimeric form. Domain III contains a ligand(s) involved in binding cell receptors. An Arg-Gly-Asp (RGD) peptide sequence in domain III is involved in attachment to glycosaminoglycan receptors (e.g., heparan sulfate) on cell membranes, but other ligand-receptor interactions probably also occur. Discontinuous (conformational) neutralization determinants are scattered across all three structural domains but tend to be located on the accessible surface of the E protein, with critical determinants located on domain III. In addition to infectious virions, several noninfectious subvirus structures are present on or are released from infected cells.

The NS1 protein is both released extracellularly and also associated with the plasma membrane of infected cells in the form of a dimeric structure anchored to glycosylphosphotidylinositol (75). The secreted form is antigenic ("soluble complement fixing" antigen) and contains both virus-specific and cross-reactive epitopes. Antibodies to NS1 do not react with the virion and exhibit no neutralizing activity. Protective immunity is mediated by antibody- and complement-mediated lysis of cells bearing NS1 targets (154).

NS3 functions as a serine protease involved in posttranslational cleavage of the virus polyprotein and also has RNA helicase and RNA triphosphatase activities. The protein is present in cell membranes, stimulates virus-specific T-cell responses, and is a target for attack by cytotoxic T cells, containing multiple dominant epitopes for $CD4^+$ and $CD8^+$ T lymphocytes in both mice and humans (106). Like NS3, the NS5 protein is also highly conserved. It functions both as the RNA-dependent RNA polymerase in virus replication and as a methyltransferase in 5′ cap methylation. The functions of the other NS proteins in replication are poorly defined. NS4B has been shown to be an interferon antagonist for WNV and dengue 2 virus, while NS5 has been shown to have the same activity for Langat and JE viruses.

Flavivirus NS proteins are processed in a major histocompatibility complex class I (MHC-I)-dependent fashion, resulting in serotype-specific and cross-reactive T-cell clones. Cytotoxic T cells recognizing NS proteins in infected cells are involved in postinfection virus clearance. The structural proteins, particularly E and prM, as well as NS1, stimulate MHC-II-restricted responses and generate antibodies protective against subsequent infection. However, the E and NS1 proteins also play a role in the generation of cytotoxic T lymphocytes (CTLs).

Replication Strategy

Flaviviruses enter cells by attachment to heparan sulfate or other, as-yet-undefined receptors, followed by endocytosis in clathrin-coated vesicles. The nucleocapsids are released from lysosomes into the cytoplasm after an acid-mediated change in the configuration of domain II of the E glycoprotein, which results in fusion with lysosomal membrane. The uncoated genomic mRNA is used for translation of the polyprotein, which includes the polymerase, protease, and helicase enzymes (NS5 and NS3) required for continued replication. They also form the template for synthesis of complementary minus RNA strands, which serve, in turn, as templates for full-length plus strands. The progeny genomic mRNA synthesizes further negative strands and NS and structural viral proteins required for continued replication and virion assembly. Assembly of virus particles occurs in close association with ER. Virus particles are transported through the ER to the plasma membrane, where they are exocytosed.

Growth in Cell Culture

Many cell cultures derived from human, monkey, rodent, swine, and avian tissues are useful for the replication and assay of flaviviruses (Table 3). Monkey kidney (Vero and LLC-MK2), hamster kidney (BHK-21), porcine kidney (PS), human adrenal carcinoma (SW-13), and primary chicken and duck embryo cells have been widely used. Virus titers of 10^6 to 10^8 tissue culture infective doses ($TCID_{50}$) or PFU per milliliter are readily achievable for most viruses in the genus. Both cytopathic effects (CPE) and plaque formation are observed in these cells, but these vary considerably with the specific virus and host cell (see below). Flavivirus replication in cultured cells may also be measured by detection of antigen or nucleic acid in the cytoplasm of cells by immunocytochemistry or in supernatant fluids by enzyme-linked immunosorbent assay (ELISA), complement fixation (CF), or reverse transcriptase PCR (RT-PCR).

Mosquito cell cultures, including C6/36 *Aedes albopictus* cells, are widely used for virus isolation or assay. CPE (syncytium formation) and plaque formation occur after infection with some viruses, but others are noncytopathic. Tick-borne flaviviruses replicate in tick cell cultures without causing CPE. The mosquito-borne viruses replicate well in mosquito but not tick cell cultures; the converse is true for the tick-borne viruses (92). The no-vector group does not replicate in either tick or mosquito cell cultures, while all flavivirures replicate in vertebrate cell cultures (92). Some mosquito- and tick-borne viruses can replicate to some extent in tick and mosquito cell cultures, respectively, which correlates with occasional field observations of some flaviviruses being isolated from both mosquitoes and ticks.

Multiplication in cell culture consists of a rapid absorption phase, followed by an eclipse phase of approximately 10 to 12 h, after which infectious virus first appears and enters a log phase of replication lasting 18 to 24 h. Peak titers in fluid phase cultures may appear after 24 h at high multiplicities of infection, but multiplication of many flaviviruses is considerably slower. Persistent infection without cytopathology has been demonstrated in a variety of arthropod and vertebrate cell lines. Progeny virus from such cultures may have altered antigenic properties, reduced virulence, or temperature sensitivity.

Inactivation by Physical and Chemical Agents

Flaviviruses are rapidly inactivated by ionic and nonionic detergents, trypsin, UV light, gamma irradiation, formaldehyde, β-propriolactone, ethyleneimine, and most disinfectants, including chlorine, iodine, phenol, and alcohol. The viruses are optimally stable at temperatures below −70°C, and they are rapidly inactivated in blood or other liquids within 30 min at 56°C. Flaviviruses are optimally stable at pH 8.4 to 8.8 and are rapidly degraded at low pH. Sensitivity to acid, bile, lipases, and proteases in the gastrointestinal tract generally precludes infection by the oral route, although TBEV may be acquired by ingestion of milk.

BIOLOGY

Host Range and Route of Infection

The host range of specific flaviviruses varies considerably by individual agent. In general, laboratory rodents (mice and hamsters) are susceptible to infection and develop lethal encephalitis after intracerebral inoculation (Table 3). Flaviviruses enter and infect their natural vertebrate hosts via the bite of blood-feeding arthropods. Several mosquito-borne viruses in the JE complex cause central nervous system (CNS) disease in both humans and domesticated livestock, particularly horses. Viruses in this group also infect wild birds, which serve as intermediary hosts in transmission cycles. In a balanced virus ecosystem, wild birds

TABLE 3 Host range and cell culture systems most useful for isolation and assay of flaviviruses, and vectors demonstrating infection and transmission in the laboratory[a]

Virus	Laboratory host (lethal infection)	Economically important animal	Nonhuman primate	Cell culture	Arthropod vectors
CEE virus	SM (i.c., i.p.), WM (i.c.), WH (i.c.), CE	Goat, sheep (encephalitis, i.c.)	Rhesus, cynomolgus (encephalitis, i.c.)	Vero, CE, BHK, HeLa, PS	*Ixodes* ticks
DEN virus	SM (i.c.),[b] WM (i.p.)[c]		Rhesus (s.c., viremia)	Vero, LLC-MK2, BHK, PMK, C6/36	*Aedes* and *Toxorhynchites* mosquitoes
JE virus	SM (i.c., i.p.), WM (i.c.), CE	Horse (encephalitis, i.c., i.n.), pig (viremia, s.c.)		Vero, LLC-MK2, CE, C6/36	*Culex* and *Aedes* mosquitoes
KFD virus	SM (i.c., i.p.), SH (i.c.), WM (i.c., i.p.)		Rhesus (viremia, i.c., s.c.)	BHK, PMK, LLC-MK2, Vero, HeLa, CE	*Haemaphysalis* ticks
OHF virus	SM (i.c., i.p.), WM (i.c., i.p.), WH (i.c.), GP (i.c.)	Muskrat (hemorrhagic disease)	Rhesus (encephalitis, i.c.)	BHK, PS, HeLa, CE	*Dermacentor* ticks and *Culex* and *Aedes* mosquitoes
MVE virus	CE, SM (i.c., i.p.), WM (i.c., i.p.), WH (i.c., i.p.)	Sheep (encephalitis, i.c.)		CE, PS, BHK, Vero, LLC-MK2	
POW virus	SM (i.c., i.p.), WM (i.c., i.p.)		Rhesus (encephalitis, i.c.)	BHK, LLC-MK2, Vero, PS	*Ixodes* ticks
ROC virus	SM (i.c., i.p.), WM (i.c., i.p.), SH (i.c., i.p.), WH (i.c., i.p.)			DE, Vero, PS, BHK, MA104	*Aedes* mosquitoes
SLE virus	SM (i.c., i.p.), SM (i.c., i.p.); WH (i.c.), WH (i.c.)		Rhesus (encephalitis, i.c.)	DE, CE, Vero, LLC-MK2, PS, BHK, SW-13	*Culex* mosquitoes
WNV	SM (i.c., i.p.), WM (i.c., i.p.), chick (i.c., s.c.), WH (i.c.)	Horse (viremia)	Rhesus (encephalitis, i.c.)	CE, BHK, Vero, LLC-MK2, PS, C6/36	*Culex*, *Aedes*, and *Anopheles* mosquitoes
YF virus	SM (i.c., i.p.), WM (i.c.), WH (i.c.), WH (i.p.)[d]		Rhesus, cynomolgus (encephalitis, i.c.; hepatitis, s.c.)	AP-61, Vero, LLC-MK2, BHK, SW-13, C6/36	*Aedes* and *Toxorhynchites* mosquitoes

[a] DEN, dengue; KFD, Kyasanur Forest disease; OHF, Omsk hemorrhagic fever; POW, Powassan; ROC, Rocio; YF, yellow fever; SM, suckling mouse; WM, weaned mouse; WH, weaned hamster; CE, primary chicken embryo; SH, suckling hamster; GP, guinea pig; i.c., intracerebral route; i.p., intraperitoneal route; i.n., intranasal route; s.c., subcutaneous route; BHK, baby hamster kidney; PMK, primary monkey kidney; PS, porcine kidney; DE, primary duck embryo. Vero, LLC-MK2, and MA104 are monkey kidney cells. C6/36 is a line of *A. albopictus* cells, SW-13 is a human adrenal carcinoma line, and AP-61 is a line of *A. pseudoscutellaris* cells.

[b] Often requires adaption by brain serial passage.

[c] AG129 and nude mice.

[d] Often requires adaption by liver serial passage.

infected with flaviviruses typically do not suffer overt illness. Rodents, insectivores, and birds are involved in transmission of TBE complex viruses, typically without causing disease in these hosts. Tick-borne flaviviruses also infect and cause disease in humans and domestic livestock. Kyasanur Forest disease virus (a member of the TBE complex) causes fatal illness in nonhuman primates, and Omsk hemorrhagic fever causes illness and death in an exotic rodent species (muskrats) introduced from North America to Russia. Yellow fever and dengue viruses are principally human pathogens but also infect certain nonhuman primates and, in the case of yellow fever, produce a similar illness (hepatitis) in certain neotropical monkey species.

Arthropod-borne flaviviruses are infectious for mosquito and tick vectors by the oral route and replicate to high titers in arthropod tissues. Of the approximately 70 flaviviruses, 16 have no known arthropod vector and are presumably transmitted directly between specific vertebrate reservoir host species, including rodents and bats. Contact infection of these hosts may be transmitted by the respiratory or oral route or by bites. Only isolated cases of human illness caused by a rodent-borne virus (Modoc virus) or bat-borne virus (Dakar bat virus) have been reported, but this observation may reflect lack of exposure rather than host range restriction.

Arthropod Infection

Medically important flaviviruses are transmitted by the bite of infected mosquitoes or ticks, which are true biological (as opposed to mechanical) vectors. After ingestion of a blood meal containing virus, replication occurs in midgut epithelial cells, and virus is released into the hemolymph, whence it invades the salivary gland; ultimately virus is secreted in saliva during refeeding on a susceptible vertebrate host. The interval between the ingestion of virus-containing blood and the salivary secretion of virus (extrinsic incubation period) is critical to transmission, as this interval must not exceed the life span of the arthropod. Increased temperature shortens the extrinsic incubation period and may thus increase the rate of virus transmission in nature. In general, flaviviruses do not induce pathological changes in the arthropod vector.

Mosquito-borne flaviviruses are amplified in nature by sequential passage through vectors and vertebrate hosts. Because of the small volume of blood ingested by the vector, the threshold concentration of virus in vertebrate blood required to infect 1% of vectors is quite high (~3 to 5 $\log_{10}$ infectious units/ml). Hosts that do not circulate virus at high titers are excluded from transmission cycles and are thus called "dead-end hosts." This is true for human beings for most flaviviruses, notable exceptions being dengue and yellow fever. Ticks imbibe much larger volumes of blood over a long period. This adaptation requires down-regulation of the host's coagulation, inflammatory, and immunologic responses by proteins contained in tick saliva (124). TBEVs are transmitted efficiently from infected to uninfected ticks via tick saliva shared during simultaneous feeding on a vertebrate host. WNV can be transmitted from infected to uninfected mosquitoes simultaneously feeding on birds.

Vertical transmission in arthropods is an important mechanism for overwinter survival of some flaviviruses. Flaviviruses infect the genital tract of male and female mosquitoes, and virus enters the ovum at the time of fertilization. Venereal transmission of flaviviruses from male to female mosquitoes also occurs. The mechanism of transovarial transmission of tick-borne flaviviruses remains to be elucidated.

PATHOGENESIS

Virus-Host Interactions

Human disease caused by flaviviruses may be classified as either (i) CNS infection, (ii) hemorrhagic fever, or (iii) fever-arthralgia with or without rash. By contrast, mice develop encephalitis after infection with all flaviviruses and have been widely used as a model for study of pathogenesis. After subcutaneous inoculation, flaviviruses replicate in subcutaneous tissues, with subsequent spread to regional lymph nodes, whence they are transported via lymphatics to the thoracic duct and then to the bloodstream. Langerhans dendritic cells appear to be important for transport of virus to lymphoid tissues (46, 79). After inoculation of virus in mosquito saliva, replication in local tissues may occur for several hours before vascular dissemination. Components of mosquito or tick saliva appear to facilitate flavivirus transmission by interfering with aspects of both innate and adaptive immunity (23, 155). After dissemination to and replication in extraneural tissues, high-titer viremia develops. Viremia is terminated around 1 week after infection by both innate and adaptive immune responses. Depending on the specific agent, extraneural cells and tissues involved in flavivirus replication include macrophages and other lymphoid cells, skeletal muscle and myocardium, smooth muscle, and endocrine and exocrine glands. Although no comprehensive analysis of flavivirus-cell interactions in vivo is possible, the special interactions of dengue viruses with dendritic cells and monocytes/macrophages, of dengue and yellow fever viruses with hepatocytes, and of the encephalitis viruses with neural cells underlie pathogenesis.

Invasion of the CNS appears to be closely linked to virus replication in extraneural sites and to the level of viremia. Factors that impair the blood-brain barrier, including immaturity, traumatic disruption of the barrier, or concurrent infection of the brain with unrelated agents, potentiate neuroinvasion and encephalitis. The mechanism by which flavivirus particles enter the CNS during natural infection remains uncertain. Postulated mechanisms include entry via leukocytes, direct entry across the blood-brain barrier, and entry by retrograde axonal transport via the peripheral nervous system (82). In the mouse, WNV RNA could be detected in the brain stem and spinal cord within the first 2 days of infection and viral antigen was observed in the cortex, hippocampus, and choroid plexus by the third day, suggesting multiple routes of CNS invasion (72). Although neuroinvasive flaviviruses can be identified from most regions of the CNS, a predilection for involvement of the anterior horn cells of the spinal cord as well as the thalamus, substantia nigra, pons, and cerebellum accounts for the acute flaccid paralysis and movement disorders clinically observed following infection in monkeys and humans.

Persistence of immunoglobulin M (IgM) antibody following acute infection has been noted for some flaviviruses, raising the question of persistent infection (91). Several animal models have demonstrated viral persistence, and chronic infections sometimes associated with progressive neuropathology have been observed (91). In humans, persistent infection with recurrent neurologic disease has been reported for patients following JE and TBE.

Age-related resistance in mice develops around 1 to 2 weeks of age with maturity of the blood-brain barrier, at which time parenteral injection of virus elicits inapparent infection, whereas intracerebral inoculation still causes lethal encephalitis. In humans, some flaviviruses (e.g., St. Louis encephalitis [SLE] virus and WNV) cause severe disease principally in the elderly, whereas others have a bimodal distribution, with an excess of cases at both age extremes (e.g., JE and Murray Valley encephalitis [MVE] viruses).

The genetic background of the host plays an important role in susceptibility to infection. In the mouse, presence of a truncated form of the 2′,5′-oligoadenylate synthetase gene located on chromosome 5 increases susceptibility to flavivirus encephalitis (135). Although a similar mutation has not been observed in humans, an increased frequency of a 2′,5′-oligoadenylate synthetase allele that contained a splice enhancer site was observed in patients hospitalized with WNV infection (174). It is possible that humans with a deletion in the CCR5 gene may be at higher risk for poor outcome following WNV infection (38, 49).

Immune Responses

Innate immune responses, including natural killer (NK) cells, alpha interferon (IFN-α) and other cytokines, and nitric oxide production by macrophages, are the first line of defense and also modulate virus-specific immune responses that rapidly follow infection (153). Abortive (subclinical) infections with WNV, which are the norm, are the presumed result of robust innate and acquired immune responses that outpace virus-mediated cell damage, as well as virus-induced apoptotic cell death that limits the progression of infection in the host.

Antibodies appear to play the primary role in protection against reinfection, while both antibodies and cellular immune responses are responsible for clearance of virus-infected cells and recovery from active infection. Neutralizing antibodies directed against determinants on the E glycoprotein provide long-lived, virus-specific protection against reinfection. Thus, infection by one virus gives lifelong immunity to that particular virus but not other flaviviruses. Infection also elicits antibody responses against the NS1 protein that decorates the surface of infected cells, and anti-NS1 antibodies may protect against reinfection and play a role in recovery from infection.

Pathological events in vivo are principally the result of direct virus injury. The extent to which the host's immunologic response to infection plays a role in pathogenesis in human infection is uncertain, except in the case of DHF (see below). In flavivirus encephalitis, neuroinvasion and rapid accumulation of viral antigen in the critical target tissues occur late in the course of infection and may elicit inflammatory responses that enhance lesions and accelerate death. NK cells and CTLs lyse infected neurons, and CTLs interact with infected astrocytes (99). Infection of these cells in the brain appears to result in an enhanced expression of MHC-I, with increased CTL recognition of infected cells. The increase in MHC-I molecules on infected cell surfaces may be induced by interferon or may be a result of flavivirus peptide transport to the ER. In addition to cell-mediated clearance, antibodies can be shown to cause early death in mice infected with yellow fever and MVE viruses. This effect is attributed to complement-mediated cytolysis of infected cells. Infiltration of neutrophils into perivascular areas of the infected brain in response to tumor necrosis factor alpha (TNF-α) and neutrophil chemotactic factor results in the expression of inducible nitric oxide synthase activity, which appears to increase damage (2), possibly by inducing apoptosis. An additional possible immunopathological mechanism includes antibody binding to glucosylphosphatidylinositol-anchored NS1, followed by signal transduction, activation of superoxide anions, and apoptosis (75). The relevance of experimental observations to human disease remains uncertain. Further study is needed on the effects of active and passive immunization against heterologous flaviviruses on the course and outcome of neurologic infection. It should be emphasized that there is evidence for cross-protection between flaviviruses in humans, whereas immunopathological responses have not been clearly defined except in the case of dengue disease.

The most important example of immunopathological response in humans is antibody-dependent enhancement of flavivirus replication in Fcγ receptor-bearing peripheral blood monocytes (62). This phenomenon is thought to determine the severity of dengue (see section on DHF below). However, recent studies have postulated a role for excessive cytokine production in severe dengue disease (130). Antibody attack against molecular mimics has also been postulated to play a role in dengue disease pathogenesis. The dengue virus E protein contains a 20-amino-acid region of homology with plasminogen, the mediator of fibrinolysis. It is speculated that anti-E antibodies may interfere with fibrinolysis and contribute to disseminated intravascular coagulopathy (70).

Virus-Specific Factors in Virulence

Differences have often been noted in the expression of disease caused by the same flavivirus among individual patients, among geographic regions, or between the early and late phases of an epidemic. These variations may be due in part to strain-specific differences in virulence genes. Virulence is multigenic, including altered by mutations in the E gene affecting attachment and uncoating, or in NS genes affecting the replication rate. Live, attenuated vaccines have been developed by serial passage in tissues or cell cultures, with fixation of specific mutations. Neurovirulence determinants in the E protein genes of yellow fever virus, JE virus, and TBEV have been partially mapped by comparing virulent strains and attenuated vaccines derived therefrom, or by sequencing attenuated neutralization escape mutants and mutants unable to bind brain membrane receptors (109, 172). E gene virulence determinants include (i) amino acid residues at the interface of domains I and II involved in reconfiguration of the E protein and trimer formation under acidic conditions in the endosome, (ii) residues (E98 to E120) in the fusion domain at the end of domain II, (iii) residues (E305 to E315) in the upper lateral surface of domain III involved in virus-cell attachment (172), and (iv) residues in the C-terminal stem anchor region involved in E protein conformational changes during fusion. Other studies have identified mutations in NS genes NS1, NS3, NS4B, and NS5 and in the 5′ and 3′ untranslated region that result in decreased virulence by down-regulating the rate of virus replication.

FEATURES OF SPECIFIC FLAVIVIRUSES

Viruses Causing CNS Infection

SLE Virus

Biology

SLE virus is a member of the JE antigenic complex, and antigenic cross-reactivities between SLE virus and other members of the complex are demonstrable with polyclonal and monoclonal antibodies. All SLE virus strains belong to a single serotype defined by neutralization, but strain variation is detectable at the molecular level. The nucleotide sequence of the SLE virus E protein varies by <10% among strains spanning a >60-year interval (88), suggesting that the virus is adapted to a highly constrained system of virus maintenance in vectors and vertebrate hosts. SLE virus strains from North America and from Central and South America can be assigned to seven lineages, which are predominantly, but not strictly, geographically distinct (88).

Among commonly used laboratory animals, hamsters are most susceptible to lethal infection, followed by mice (Table 3). Young animals are most susceptible to lethal encephalitis. Neurovirulence is greater with epidemic than with endemic strains. SLE virus is lethal for chicken embryos or after intracerebral inoculation of young hatchling birds, but birds infected naturally develop asymptomatic viremic infections. Birds are the principal virus-amplifying hosts in the transmission cycle. The absence of overt disease associated with SLE virus infection of birds is due to a long coevolution of virus strains with their hosts in the Americas. Although various wild and domestic mammals can be infected with SLE virus, these infections are also usually asymptomatic. Antibodies have been found in a wide array of wild mammals in North and South America.

Epidemiology

Distribution and geography. SLE virus is widely distributed in the United States, Canada, Mexico, and Central and South America. Outbreaks or sporadic cases have been reported from nearly all U.S. states (Fig. 1). The geography of SLE in the United States can be best understood in terms of its three enzootic transmission cycles sustained by *Culex pipiens* and *Culex quinquefasciatus* in the Ohio and Mississippi River basin states and areas farther east, *Culex nigripalpus* in Florida, and *Culex tarsalis* in the central and western states (Fig. 2). In the east, SLE is transmitted periodically in localized and sometimes regional outbreaks occurring at intervals of years and even decades apart and without significant enzootic or endemic transmission in intervening years. In Florida, the disease is absent in some years and in others causes sporadic human cases or focal or widespread outbreaks. In the west, SLE is transmitted perennially and at a low level in the enzootic transmission cycle, resulting in sporadic endemically acquired infections, a higher level of naturally acquired immunity, and, occasionally, outbreaks that are usually smaller than those occurring in the east.

Incidence and prevalence. More than 10,000 SLE cases have been reported in the United States over the last five decades. Most cases have occurred in sporadic outbreaks, and the annual reported incidence has fluctuated from 0.003 to 0.752 per 100,000, with a median number of about 35 reported cases per year (Fig. 3). In 1975, the largest SLE outbreak ever reported led to 1,967 cases in 31 states. Most cases occur in states in the Ohio and Mississippi River basins and on the Gulf Coast. It remains unknown whether WNV, a related JE serogroup flavivirus utilizing the same mosquito vectors and avian hosts as SLE virus, will replace SLE virus in its ecological niche and decrease SLE incidence.

Seroprevalence rates vary locally but are generally low. In locations with recent outbreaks, seroprevalence has ranged from 3 to 15%. Surveys have shown that only 1 of approximately 300 infections is clinically apparent. Although infections are uniform across the age spectrum, clinical attack rates rise steeply with age, resulting in inapparent/apparent infection ratios ranging from 800:1 in children under 10 years to 85:1 in adults. The biological basis for this increased susceptibility has not been defined.

In rural areas of the western United States, human infections occur sporadically, incidental to the enzootic transmission cycle involving mosquitoes and birds (Fig. 2). Hyperendemic transmission appears in years in which heavy snowpack and flooding have expanded the *C. tarsalis* larval habitat, whereas no more than a few sporadic cases are reported in most years.

SLE in eastern states follows an unpredictable pattern of localized outbreaks, usually in urban areas (117). The principal vectors, *C. pipiens* and *C. quinquefasciatus*, are typically found in peridomestic habitats. Outbreaks often have occurred in small towns or in older lower-socioeconomic-status sections of cities. Older construction featuring open foundations, porches, lack of air-conditioning, and poor screens contributes to an increased risk of exposure. Local or regional outbreaks occur infrequently, sometimes separated by decades when for unknown reasons virus transmission in the enzootic cycle becomes sufficiently intense to create substantial human infection risk. The overwintering mechanism for SLE virus remains unclear.

SLE transmission in Florida has followed a pattern of periodic outbreaks. Drought conditions might concentrate *C. nigripalpus* mosquitoes in relatively moist, densely vegetated "hammock" habitats at a time when nesting birds also make use of the hammocks (34). This forcing of birds and mosquitoes together fosters epizootic SLE amplification. During subsequent wet periods, infected birds and mosquitoes disperse and carry the virus from the hammocks.

Risk factors associated with human disease. Risk of exposure and risk of infection are independent of age; however, neuroinvasive disease incidence and case fatality rates are approximately 10-fold higher in persons older than 70 years than in young adults and children. Hypertension, arteriosclerosis, and other chronic diseases have been noted in fatal cases. Although such associations with symptomatic illness have not been controlled for age, they suggest that virus neuroinvasion might be facilitated through compromised vascular endothelia. Human immunodeficiency virus (HIV) infection has been associated with increased risk of acquiring SLE in recent outbreaks, but a confounding effect of homelessness or other exposure-related risk factors has been difficult to assess. Reduced risk of acquiring SLE in Florida was associated with flavivirus immunity

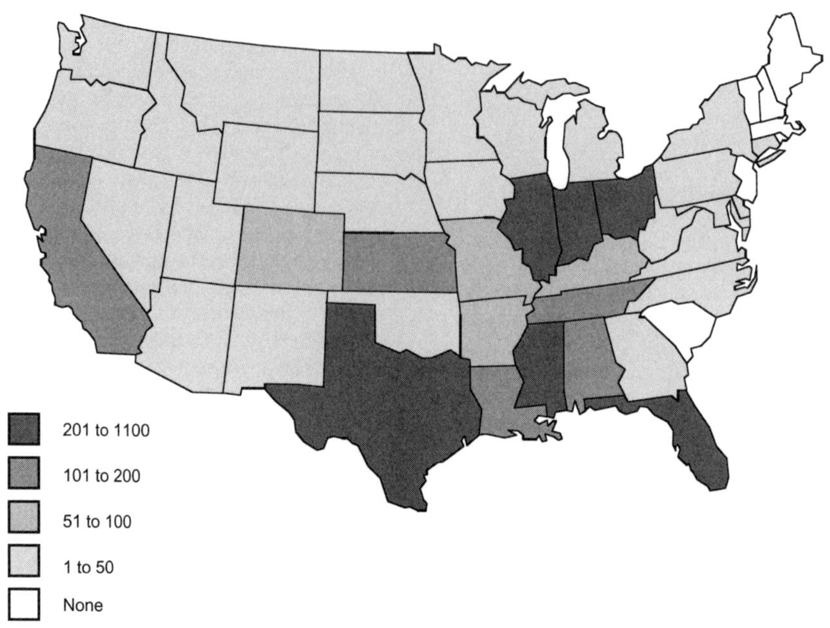

FIGURE 1 Reported SLE incidence per 100,000, by state, 1964 to 2005.

acquired during the last dengue disease outbreak in Florida in 1934.

The principal risk factor for C. *tarsalis*-borne SLE is residence in, or outdoor occupational or avocational exposure to, rural areas where the enzootic cycle is maintained. Risk is greatest in persons who are outdoors in the evening, when C. *tarsalis* is most active. In Florida, a similar pattern holds because C. *nigripalpus* also has exophilic crepuscular biting habits. In some C. *tarsalis*-borne outbreaks, risk has been higher in males, possibly reflecting occupational or avocational exposures to open areas with grassy swales used as mosquito breeding sites. The peridomestic habits of SLE vectors (C. *quinquefasciatus* and C. *pipiens)* elsewhere in the eastern states have been associated with higher incidence in females in some outbreaks, although this pattern is not consistent. Risk factors such as lack of air-conditioning, poor screens, and sitting on an unscreened porch suggest that exposure occurs indoors or near residences. In recent urban outbreaks, a large proportion of cases have occurred in homeless people.

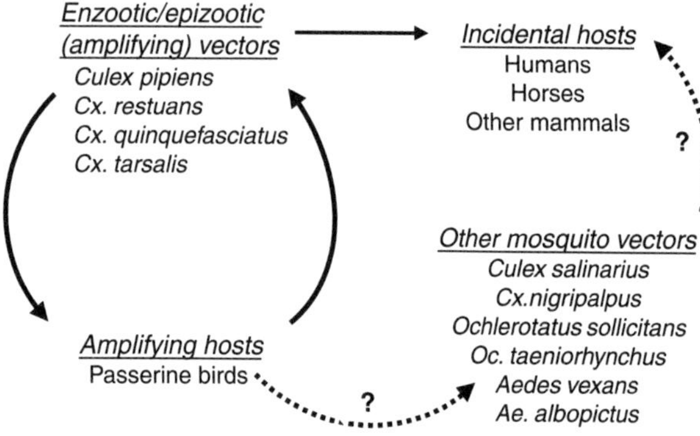

FIGURE 2 Transmission cycle of SLE virus and WNV. Both viruses are transmitted in a cycle between birds and *Culex* mosquitoes. C. *pipiens* is an important vector in the northern United States and Canada. *Culex quinquefasciatus* is important in the southern United States, whereas C. *tarsalis* is important in the western United States. In addition, C. *nigripalpus* is a vector in Florida. Other mosquito species may be "bridge" vectors to horses, humans, and other dead-end hosts, which typically do not develop high-level viremia and do not participate in the transmission cycle. However, bridge vectors likely have a minor role compared to enzootic vectors in viral transmission to dead-end hosts.

SLE cases are usually noted no earlier than June and peak in August and September. Transmission may extend to as late as December/January in Florida and in parts of southern California. Elevated temperatures enhance multiplication of SLE virus in C. *tarsalis*. Rainfall patterns also markedly influence SLE virus transmission. Years of high spring and summer rainfall or excessive runoff from snowmelt favor vector density and virus amplification in areas where C. *nigripalpus* and C. *tarsalis* are responsible for transmission. In contrast, midsummer drought conditions

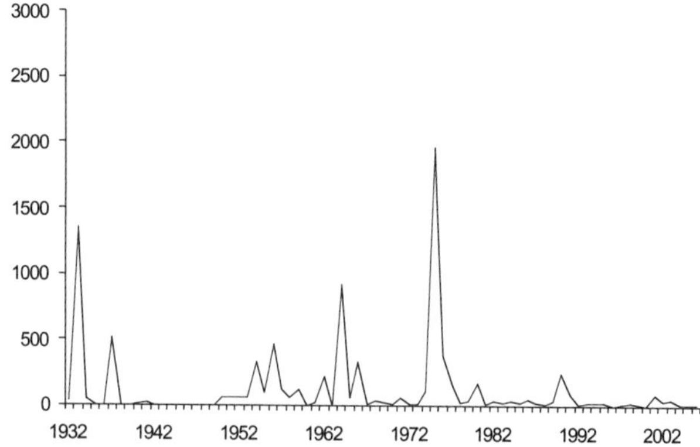

FIGURE 3 Number of reported cases of SLE, 1932 to 2006.

appear to favor amplification in the *C. pipiens-C. quinquefasciatus* transmission cycle, since these vectors breed in stagnant water pools susceptible to being flushed and cleaned by rainfall.

Transmission. Natural infections are transmitted by mosquito bites. Laboratory infection has occurred by mucous membrane or respiratory exposure. SLE virus antigen has been recovered from nasal secretions of infected mice, and hamsters can be experimentally infected by intranasal inoculation, suggesting the potential for infection by the olfactory apparatus. No nosocomial cases or instances of congenital infection have been reported. One possible transmission via breast milk has been reported.

Pathogenesis

Pathological changes in humans have been reported only for the CNS; however, SLE virus has been isolated from the vitreous humor, lungs, liver, spleen, and kidneys. In fatal cases, the brain and meninges appear to be congested, but cerebral edema is unusual. Pathological changes are widely distributed in the brain and spinal cord but are most pronounced in the substantia nigra, thalamus, hypothalamus, cerebellar and cerebral cortices, basal ganglia, and the brain stem and cervical spinal cord. Changes are most prevalent in gray matter nuclei, but lesions also are found in the subcortical and deep cerebral white matter and long tracts of the brain stem and spinal cord. Microscopic changes consist of diffuse parenchymal inflammation and substantial perivascular infiltrates with destruction of vessels and extensive microgliosis. The inflammatory infiltrate is a mixture of small lymphocytes, histiocytes, plasma cells, and rare neutrophils. Degenerating neurons may be surrounded by microglial nodules. Axonal destruction and demyelination are not usually present. SLE virus virions have been identified by electron microscopy in postmortem brain samples.

Clinical Manifestations

The incubation period has been estimated to be 4 to 21 days. Illness begins with nonspecific symptoms of malaise, fever, headache, and myalgias, sometimes accompanied by cough, sore throat, abdominal pain, vomiting, or diarrhea. Dysuria, urgency, and incontinence are early symptoms in some patients. The illness may evolve quickly, with development of meningismus, increased headache, tremulousness, ataxia, and mental clouding. Other patients have a more insidious progression of nonspecific symptoms, especially myalgias, backache, headache, photophobia, and gastrointestinal complaints, followed days later by neurologic symptoms.

Neurologic involvement most frequently results in an altered state of consciousness, which may be clinically subtle, manifested by only mild confusion or decreased cognitive facility. Deep coma occurs in about 15% of cases. Most patients exhibit tremors involving the eyelids, tongue, lips, and extremities. Cranial nerve palsies are present in about 25% of patients and are often asymmetrical or unilateral. Cerebellar signs are also common; ambulatory patients may exhibit an ataxic gait. Involuntary movements such as myoclonic jerking, nystagmus, and, rarely, opsoclonus may be present. Convulsions are unusual, occurring mainly in children and in severe cases in adults, and signal a poor prognosis. Nuchal rigidity is variable and may be more common in children. Presentation with focal weakness or paralysis is unusual. Occasional cases have presented with Guillain-Barré syndrome.

The peripheral white cell count is usually normal or slightly elevated. Proteinuria, microscopic hematuria, and pyuria are found in some patients. More than one-third of cases have hyponatremia due to inappropriate antidiuretic hormone (ADH) secretion. Liver enzymes may be slightly elevated. Lumbar puncture discloses an elevated opening pressure in the range of 200 to 250 mm Hg in about one-third of cases and cerebrospinal fluid (CSF) protein elevated above 45 mg/dl in more than two-thirds of cases. A moderate CSF pleocytosis of five to several hundred cells is typical, with the proportion of mononuclear cells increasing from 50 to 100% during the first week of illness. Electroencephalograms (EEGs) show diffuse generalized slowing and delta wave activity. Focal discharges and spike activity have been observed occasionally.

Defervescence and neurologic improvement are seen over several days, with a rapid reversal of altered sensorium. Overall, 17% of cases are fatal; deaths generally occur within the first or second week of illness. A prolonged convalescence is typical, characterized principally by emotional lability but also by asthenia, forgetfulness, headache, tremor, dizziness, and unsteadiness; such manifestations may persist for months to years after initial recovery. Muscle tremors, asymmetric deep tendon reflexes, and visual disturbances are present in about one-third of patients several months after the acute illness. One patient had postinfectious encephalomyelitis; otherwise, chronic, persistent, or relapsing infections have not been reported.

Diagnosis

SLE should be considered in patients with onset of acute encephalitis in summer or early fall and with exposure to an endemic or epidemic focus. Clinical features may overlap those of other virus infections, especially WNV, enteroviruses, western and eastern equine encephalitis, and herpesvirus. Mycoplasmal, bacterial, and fungal meningitis, especially partially treated bacterial meningitis, leptospirosis, cat scratch encephalopathy, and listeria encephalitis, may cause a CNS syndrome similar to SLE.

The limited viremia preceding onset of neurologic symptoms precludes virus isolation in most cases with clinical encephalitis. Virus isolation from CSF is generally unsuccessful, but virus can be recovered from brain and other postmortem tissues. Viral antigen can be detected by immunofluorescence (IF) or immunocytochemical staining in brain tissue, but the sensitivity of this technique is low because of the sparse distribution of infected cells. Antigen detection ELISAs and RT-PCR developed to identify infected mosquitoes have not been evaluated on clinical samples, but they are likely to be less sensitive than serology.

The principal serologic tests in use are IgM capture ELISA and IF. When both CSF and serum samples are examined, sensitivity of the former test approaches 100% by the 10th day after onset. The sensitivity of indirect IF is lower, especially when CSF is examined or if only acute-phase serum is examined. When both IgG and IgM are measured by indirect IF or ELISA in paired serum samples, sensitivity approaches 100%. Cross-reactive antibodies in patients who have had previous flavivirus infections, especially dengue virus and WNV, limit the specificity of serologic tests. More specific serologic tests (e.g., neutralization) are needed to sort out such reactions.

Prevention

Efforts to prevent SLE epidemics are based on mosquito and bird or sentinel chicken surveillance that measures enzootic virus activity in the spring and summer. Early, increased transmission in the enzootic cycle signals the possibility of spillover to humans and should trigger emergency mosquito control with insecticides and public health warnings to avoid mosquito exposure. Reduction of larval habitat by improving drainage is a long-term approach to reduce risk. Repairing screens, avoiding outdoor exposure in the evening, and applying mosquito repellents may reduce mosquito exposure. No vaccine is currently available.

Treatment

No specific antiviral therapy is currently available. As with other flaviviruses, ribavirin is active in vitro at relatively high concentrations. Although SLE virus is sensitive to IFN-α, treatment after onset of clinical signs has no benefit.

JE Virus

Biology

JE virus is the prototype of an antigenic complex that includes SLE and MVE viruses, WNV, and several other flaviviruses of lesser medical importance (Table 1). Although JE virus represents a single antigenic serotype (166), fine distinctions of no recognized clinical importance exist between JE virus strains serologically, genetically, and by biological assays such as cross-protection in mice and neurovirulence. Overall, two major immunotypes have been differentiated: Nakayama and Beijing-1/JaGAr-01. Nucleotide sequencing of portions of the genome has identified four genotypes (genetic clusters) of JE virus. Genotype I includes isolates from Cambodia and northern Thailand; genotype II includes isolates from Indonesia, southern Thailand, and Malaysia; genotype III includes isolates from temperate regions of Asia (Japan, China, Taiwan, India, Nepal, Sri Lanka, and the Philippines); and genotype IV includes certain isolates from Indonesia. During the past 25 years, genotype I has been replacing genotype III in China, Japan, Korea, and Vietnam. Phylogenetic studies suggest that JE virus originated in Indonesia/Malaysia, with genotype IV being ancestral to the other genotypes. At least five antigenic groups exist, and their relationship to the four genotypes is not clear at present.

Complete nucleotide sequences of several JE virus strains have been reported, including those of three attenuated vaccine strains derived from the wild-type SA14 strain. Although mutations in the NS genes may contribute to attenuation, it is clear that mutations in the E gene play a role, since a chimeric yellow fever 17D virus containing the E gene of wild-type JE virus is neurovirulent, while a chimera with the E gene of JE vaccine strain SA14-14-2 vaccine is not (25). Site-directed mutagenesis has identified amino acids E107 (fusion peptide at the tip of domain II) and E176/E177, E138, and E279 at the interface of domains I and II as important virulence determinants. The wild-type E138 Glu residue is changed to Lys in the SA14-14-2 vaccine strain and also plays an important role in neurovirulence.

Epidemiology

Distribution and geography. JE is transmitted in nearly every country of Asia from the far east of Russia to areas of Pakistan in west Asia (Fig. 4). Approximately 50,000 cases are reported annually, principally from China, Southeast Asia, and India. In most areas, transmission is endemic, with annual fluctuations in the number of cases depending on environmental factors. Within a single country, transmission may be localized to certain regions where appropriate ecological conditions prevail (in general, in rural areas where rice is grown). In developed countries such as Japan, Korea, and Taiwan, the few reported cases reflect high immunization rates despite the persistence of enzootic virus transmission.

JE appeared in Oceania in outbreaks in 1947 and on Guam and the Northern Mariana Islands in 1990. In 1995 and 1998, outbreaks affected residents in Badu and other islands in the Torres Straits, which separate Papua New Guinea and Australia. In 1998, a human JE case and evidence for infection of feral pigs were detected in a localized area at the mouth of the Mitchell River, Queensland, Australia. Subsequent surveillance failed to identify enzootic JE virus transmission in Australia until 2004, when seroconverting pigs and a positive *Culex sitiens* mosquito pool were identified.

Incidence and prevalence. Estimates of the subclinical/clinical infection ratio usually center around 300:1, although values range from 25:1 to 1,000:1 (167). Exposure to JE virus occurs in childhood, and antibody prevalence approaches 80% by early adulthood. Annual incidence rates in locations of endemicity typically range from 1 to 10 cases/100,000, and epidemic attack rates may exceed 100/100,000. With immunization, the incidence in Thailand dropped from 4 to 6 cases/100,000 in the early 1980s to less than 1/100,000 since 1996. In China, vaccination reduced JE morbidity from 2.5/100,000 in 1990 to 0.5/100,000. In Japan and other developed Asian countries, JE risk is highest in the elderly, reflecting high vaccine coverage of children and undefined biological risk factors associated with aging. In most areas, a slight (1.5:1) excess of cases in boys has been observed. In areas with overlapping religious and cultural affiliations (e.g., Malaysia and Indonesia), Muslims who eschew pork and do not keep pigs are at lower risk; conversely, Hindu Bali and principally Buddhist Chinese Sarawak have the highest reported JE activity in their respective countries. Household crowding, low socioeconomic status, and lack of air-conditioning appear to be risk factors for acquiring JE.

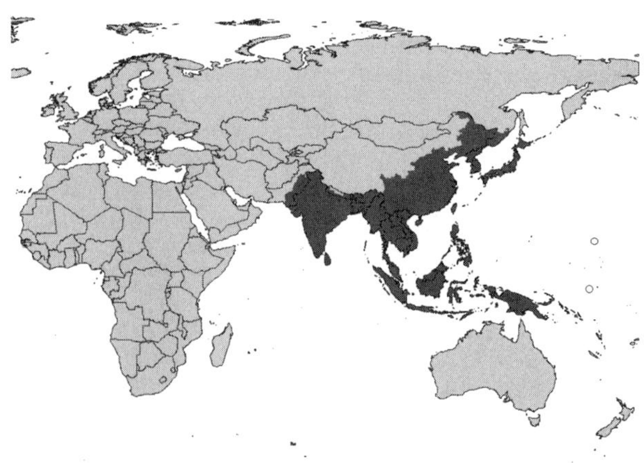

FIGURE 4 Geographic distribution of JE.

In countries where JE is endemic, JE is mostly a disease of children and young adults due to the fact that most adults are already immune. Increased incidence in the elderly in Japan and Korea, who presumably had been previously immune from early exposure to the virus, may indicate waning immunity. Prior antiflavivirus antibodies do not appear to protect against infection with JE virus but may decrease morbidity (54). Repeated clinical infections have not been reported, but subclinical reinfections are common in areas of endemicity and probably provide natural immunity and boosters to immunization.

Transmission. With the rare exception of laboratory-acquired cases, infection is transmitted only by bites of infected mosquitoes. In temperate regions, JE virus is transmitted in the late summer and early fall after the virus has been amplified by vector mosquitoes and pigs and, in some areas, by a preceding phase of amplification in birds (Fig. 5). Pigs play a central role in virus amplification, because they develop high and sustained levels of viremia and because their high body temperature and large hairless body surface area attract thousands of mosquitoes nightly. The ubiquitous place of pigs as a backyard or even cohabiting livestock animal in rural Asia leads to high levels of human exposure in rural villages and often in household premises. In developed countries (like Japan), the centralization of pig rearing and modernized agricultural methods have been credited as factors leading to a decline in JE virus transmission. On the other hand, deforestation and agricultural development, especially the creation of irrigation schemes, have contributed to an increase in JE and other mosquito-borne diseases in other areas (e.g., central Sri Lanka and the Terai of Nepal).

The principal JE vectors are *Culex* mosquitoes that use ground pools and especially rice paddies for their larval stages. *Culex tritaeniorhynchus* is the principal vector in most areas of Asia; other important vectors include *Culex annulus* in Taiwan and Hong Kong; *Culex vishnui*, *Culex gelidus*, *Culex pseudovishnui*, *Culex fuscocephala*, *Culex bitaeniorhynchus*, and *Anopheles hyrcanus* in India and Nepal; *C. gelidus* in Indonesia; *Culex annulirostris* in the Pacific and Australia; and *Aedes togoi* in Russia. Most JE vectors are zoophilic, preferring animals to humans; are exophilic, biting outdoors; and crepuscular, most active in the evening and night.

The transmission season is well defined in temperate areas (e.g., northern China), with onset of cases in June, a September peak, and disappearance by October. Farther south, the transmission season begins earlier and ends later. More complex seasonal patterns are observed in tropical areas where mosquito densities are correlated with monsoons. Vector density and infection rates typically increase following the initiation of rice cultivation midyear. Mosquito infection rates are modulated by rising herd immunity in pigs, but high vector abundance in the wet-cool season (October-December) ensures a continued risk of human infection.

Pathogenesis

The vast majority of infections are cleared before neuroinvasion occurs and are subclinical or lead to mild illnesses without CNS signs. Circulating antibody plays a critical part, and heterologous flavivirus immunity (e.g., from prior dengue virus infection) may limit peripheral virus replication and neuroinvasion. Disruption of the blood-brain barrier may be a risk factor for neuroinvasion, since persons with fatal JE are more likely to have had concurrent neurocysticercosis than persons dying of other causes; dual infections with herpes virus or mumps virus also have been reported. Functional and structural changes due to hypertension, cerebrovascular disease, and head trauma have also been suggested as factors contributing to neuroinvasion.

At autopsy, inflammatory reactions are found in the myocardium, lungs, liver, spleen, lymph nodes, and kidneys. The brain appears swollen, and the ventricles may be narrowed by edema. Herniation of the cerebellar tonsils and hippocampal uncus may occur. The meninges are con-

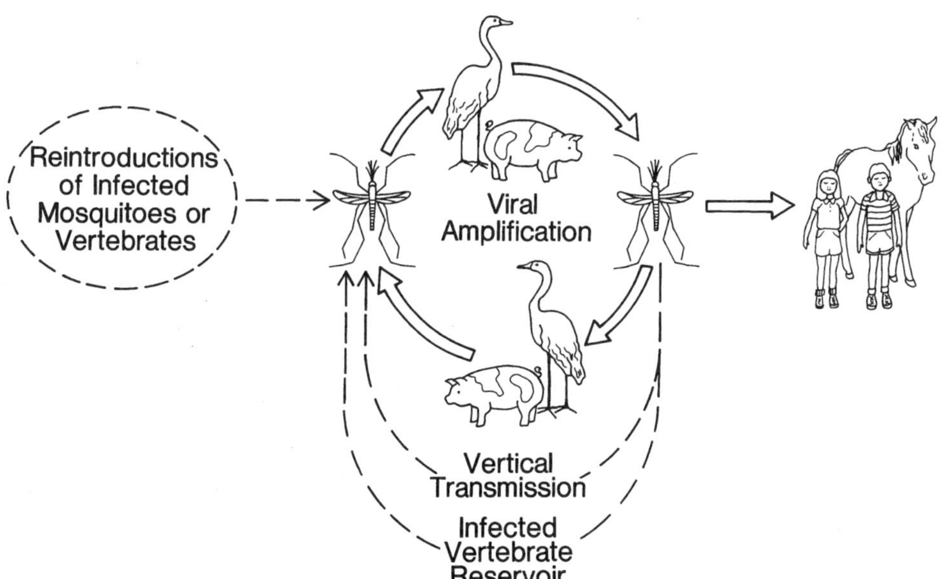

FIGURE 5 Transmission cycle of JE virus. Broken lines indicate speculative portions of the transmission cycle.

gested, and inflammatory changes are present. Pathological changes are distributed principally in the thalamus, substantia nigra, brain stem, hippocampus and temporal cortex, cerebellum, and spinal cord. Histopathological changes consist of focal neuronal degeneration, diffuse and focal microglial proliferation, and perivascular cuffing (78). Infected neurons contain antigen in their cell bodies, axons, and dendrites, suggesting that virus spreads from cell to cell within the brain. Antigen-containing neurons may have no associated microglial reaction until cell death has occurred. Small amounts of virus antigen may be present in vascular endothelia.

Infection elicits a broad inflammatory response of macrophages, T and B cells in perivascular cuffs, and predominantly T cells in the brain parenchyma. A greater proportion of $CD4^+$ T cells are seen in the CNS than in the blood. Degeneration of infected neurons, microglial proliferation, and neuronophagia lead to the formation of gliomesenchymal nodules. Intrathecal antibodies have been associated with a favorable outcome in some series, suggesting an important role for antibody-mediated virus neutralization in the brain. However, others suggest that specific antibodies cannot reach virus spreading directly from cell to cell and that neuronal damage occurs by an immunopathological mechanism. This view is supported by observations of intrathecal neurofilament protein antibodies and/or myelin basic protein antibodies in 49% of cases and their association with fatal outcome (36). Immune complexes, found in the CSF of 17% of patients, also were associated with death (35). Limited studies of the cellular immune response to infection have shown that immune $CD4^+$ and $CD8^+$ T cells proliferate in response to JE virus or infected cell lysates. Cellular proliferative and humoral responses are not correlated, and no association between cellular proliferative response and outcome has been found (35). In vivo models indicate that activation of microglial cells may produce proinflammatory mediators instrumental in inducing neuronal cell death (48).

Clinical Manifestations

After a mosquito bite, 4 to 14 days elapse before the onset of symptoms. A prodromal illness of fever, headache, lethargy, nausea, and vomiting lasting several days precedes the onset of CNS signs. Neurologic signs reflect damage to the brain stem, thalamus, cerebral cortex, and spinal cord. The central feature is an altered state of consciousness, ranging from mild mental clouding to drowsiness and stupor, or agitation and delirium (144). Some children exhibit personality changes, slurred speech, and mutism. Early-onset seizures occur in at least half of hospitalized children and a quarter of adults. Seizures are usually generalized tonic-clonic but may also be partial motor, or with more subtle clinical manifestations, such as twitching of a digit or eyebrow, or nystagmus. Patients with subtle seizures are usually in status epilepticus. Extrapyramidal features include dull, expressionless facies, generalized hypertonia, and cogwheel rigidity.

Significant stupor or coma is usual, tremor and involuntary movements are common, and signs of meningeal irritation may be present. Disconjugate gaze and facial and other cranial nerve palsies are found in one-third of cases. Papilledema is seen in fewer than 10% of cases. The muscular tone is usually increased, and hyperreflexia and pathological reflexes may be elicited. Weakness or paralysis may be generalized or asymmetric in distribution and spastic or flaccid in character. Autonomic disturbances, especially hyperpnea, may occur.

A modest peripheral leukocytosis may be present in the first week of illness. The serum sodium often is depressed due to inappropriate ADH secretion. The CSF typically is clear and under normal pressure, with normal or mildly elevated protein and normal glucose concentrations. A pleocytosis of 10 to several hundred white cells is typical in the first week of illness, and the cell count may remain elevated until the third week. EEG tracings show generalized delta wave slowing, consistent with a thalamic involvement. Computed tomography (CT) scans show diffuse white matter edema and nonenhancing low-density lesions mainly in the thalamus, basal ganglia, and pons. Unilateral or bilateral thalamic hemorrhages are common. Magnetic resonance imaging (MRI) discloses a similar pattern of high-signal-intensity lesions in the thalamus, basal ganglia, cerebellum, pons, midbrain, and spinal cord.

Defervescence occurs during the second week of illness; choreoathetosis and extrapyramidal signs may appear as other neurologic manifestations improve. The substantia nigra is a site of predominant injury in some patients, as detected by MRI and clinical presentation, with cogwheel rigidity and opsoclonus during the acute phase and emergence of typical Parkinsonism during convalescence, from which patients generally recover (142). Convalescence is slow; consciousness and motor functions are slowly regained. Illness is fatal in 10 to 35% of cases, most often within the first week of illness, and fatality rates have been decreasing with improved clinical management. Children less than 10 years old are more likely to die and to have serious neurologic sequelae, such as motor weakness and paralysis, abnormal muscular tone, seizures, blindness, ataxia, and extrapyramidal movement disorders (150). One-third to one-half of patients surviving the acute illness have such major neurologic sequelae 1 year later, and EEG abnormalities may be present in 50% of recovered children. At 5 years after recovery, 75% have behavioral disorders and subnormal performance on age-standardized psychological tests.

JE acquired during the first and second trimesters of pregnancy has led to fetal death and abortion, with recovery of virus isolates from products of conception (27). It is unknown whether congenital infection causes fetal malformations, as occurs in pigs. The few reported cases of JE in the third trimester have been associated with a normal fetal outcome.

The most common complications are bacterial infections, especially pneumonia, and stasis ulcers. In a few cases, clinical relapse occurred several months after recovery from the acute illness. JE virus-infected peripheral blood mononuclear cells were demonstrated in these and other asymptomatic recovered patients, implying the persistence of infection. Evidence of subacute JE virus CNS infection has been demonstrated in 5% of cases by detecting JE virus or antigen in CSF 3 weeks after recovery or intrathecal IgM at 50 to 180 days. The clinical significance of these findings is unclear.

Diagnosis

In Asia, the most important diagnostic considerations in children with signs of acute CNS infection are bacterial meningitis, tuberculosis, malaria, typhoid fever with associated tremors and ataxia, dengue disease with encephalopathy or encephalitis, WNV encephalitis, MVE (in

Australia and Papua New Guinea), Nipah virus encephalitis, and enterovirus (particularly enterovirus 71) infection. Other disorders that overlap the clinical presentation of JE are hyperthermia and scrub typhus. JE occasionally may present as Guillain-Barré syndrome or acute psychosis. In Asia, the percentage of children presenting with acute encephalitic illness who had JE ranged from 23 to 67%. Central hyperpneic breathing and extrapyramidal signs were the best clinical predictors that such an illness was JE, with a sensitivity of 41% and specificity of 81% (90).

JE virus rarely can be isolated from blood early in the illness, usually no later than 6 to 7 days after onset. Virus is seldom recovered from the CSF except in cases with a poor outcome. RT-PCR of CSF specimens is not a more sensitive technique. IF staining of CSF mononuclear cells provides laboratory confirmation most rapidly but has a reported sensitivity of only 60%.

The standard laboratory diagnostic method is serology by IgM capture ELISA, which has a sensitivity approaching 100% when both CSF and serum samples are tested and samples from 1 to 2 weeks after onset are used. An evaluation of three commercially available IgM capture ELISA kits demonstrated sensitivities of at least 89%; however, specificities ranged from 56 to 99% (76). Specificities were at least 96% when dengue virus IgM-positive samples were excluded. Samples taken too early in the illness may be negative. Anti-JE virus IgM was detected in nearly all serum samples collected at least 9 days after symptom onset and in all CSF samples collected at least 7 days after symptom onset (26). This and all serologic tests are limited by the potential for cross-reactions with cocirculating flaviviruses, principally dengue virus and WNV. Representative flavivirus antigens relevant to the patient's site of exposure should be included in serologic tests. Some laboratories have established diagnostic IgM ELISA absorbance ratios based on comparative reactivities to the respective antigens. Fourfold changes in IF, hemagglutination-inhibiting (HI), CF, and neutralizing antibodies (in order of increasing specificity) may provide a clear diagnosis in patients with their first flavivirus infection, but cross-reactions may be uninterpretable for patients with multiple previous flavivirus infections or immunization with JE and yellow fever vaccines.

Prevention

Formalin-inactivated, mouse brain-derived vaccine is produced in several countries, but manufacture is being phased out in place of Vero cell culture-derived inactivated vaccines. In the United States, mouse brain-derived vaccine manufactured by BIKEN (Osaka, Japan) is licensed as JE-VAX. The vaccine has a protective efficacy of 91% and is nearly 100% immunogenic after three doses (given either on days 0, 7, and 14 or on days 0, 7, and 30) (66). Immunity persists for at least 3 years, after which a booster may be given. The vaccine elicits antibodies that are cross-reactive against JE virus strains. The mouse brain-derived vaccine has several major limitations—high cost, three-dose vaccination schedule, and safety concerns. Several cases of acute disseminated encephalomyelitis temporally associated with JE vaccination have suggested a possible etiologic relationship. The principal vaccine-associated adverse event of concern is hypersensitivity, consisting of generalized urticaria and angioedema, appearing 1 to 3 days after immunization. Delayed reactions (occurring 2 to 3 days after vaccination), particularly after the second dose, have been reported. Hypersensitivity reactions have occurred in 18 to 64/10,000 persons immunized in the West for travel and have generally required oral or parenteral steroid therapy; several reactors have developed respiratory distress necessitating resuscitation and hospitalization. Systemic hypersensitivity reactions have been less frequently reported in Japan and Korea. Individuals with a history of urticaria, allergic rhinitis, or other allergic reactions appear to be at higher risk. Because of these potentially serious adverse events and the vaccine's high cost, vaccination is recommended only for expatriates, for persons with a high risk of exposure (e.g., in rural areas during the transmission season), and for persons with longer itineraries in areas of endemicity, arbitrarily greater than 30 days. JE vaccine may be safely administered to HIV-infected persons but is significantly less immunogenic, with respect to both the seroconversion rate and the level of neutralizing antibodies.

A live, attenuated vaccine (SA14-14-2) produced in primary hamster kidney cell culture was licensed in China in 1988, and over 200 million doses have been administered. Optimal dosing for the SA14-14-2 vaccine has not been established, but a single dose of the SA14-14-2 vaccine was shown to be 96% effective in Nepalese children 5 years after immunization (162). Investigational vaccines include formalin-inactivated vaccines produced in Vero cells; a live, attenuated chimeric yellow fever-JE vaccine; a live, attenuated chimeric dengue virus-JE vaccine; and DNA vaccines.

Exposure to JE mosquito vectors can be reduced by avoiding rural areas and outdoor activity during the evening; staying in air-conditioned or well-screened quarters; using repellents; and wearing long-sleeved clothing and long pants. Specific public health interventions to control vector mosquitoes are implemented in a few locations. These include the addition of larvicides and predatory fish to irrigated fields and periodically changing their water level to interfere with the vectors' aquatic stages. In epidemic emergencies, adulticide applications provide short-term reductions of vector mosquito populations.

Treatment

No specific antiviral therapy is currently available. In a double-blind, placebo-controlled trial, IFN-α2a did not improve the outcome of patients with JE (160). The introduction of intensive-care equipment and training has reduced the mortality rate from more than 30 to 5%. Acute coma, seizures, and respiratory failure necessitate rapid anticonvulsive therapy, ventilator support, and intensive monitoring of fluid and electrolyte balance. Osmotic agents to reduce intracranial pressure may be needed in some cases; a controlled study of early dexamethasone therapy found no clinical benefit (or harm) with its routine use. Hyponatremia due to inappropriate ADH secretion is a frequent complication usually responsive to free water restriction alone.

MVE Virus

Biology

MVE virus is a member of the JE antigenic complex and has a close genetic relationship to JE virus. Australian MVE virus strains share a high degree of sequence homogeneity, whereas strains from Papua New Guinea differ, indicating that this area may represent a separate focus of virus activity. The host range of MVE virus and susceptibility of cell cultures are shown in Table 3. Alfuy virus, also found in Australia, is a distinct species from MVE virus (107).

Epidemiology

Distribution and incidence. MVE virus occurs in Australia, Papua New Guinea, and probably islands in the eastern part of the Indonesian archipelago (101). Localized seasonal outbreaks or sporadic cases have been reported intermittently from southeastern Australia, the Kimberley region in Western Australia, and the Northern Territory. Although the disease is clinically severe, the incidence is low. Approximately 100 confirmed human cases occurred between 1951 and 1984, principally in the setting of small outbreaks. Some of these cases may have been due to the closely related Kunjin virus (a variant of WNV). An outbreak in 1974 extended over a wide geographic area involving Queensland, the Northern Territory, South Australia, the Ord River Basin of Western Australia, and Papua New Guinea. The virus appears to be endemic in the tropical Kimberley area of Western Australia.

MVE primarily strikes the young and the elderly, with approximately 50% of the cases in infants and children under 10 years old and 25% in persons over 50 years old. An excess of cases among males has been observed in several outbreaks. The case fatality rate is 30 to 40%. Subclinical infections are frequent, and only 1 in 1,000 to 2,000 infections appears to result in illness. Serologic surveys conducted after epidemics have revealed evidence of recent infection in 4.5 to 36% of the residents.

Virus activity is seasonal, occurring during the summer months (January to May), and is associated with periods of abnormally high rainfall over two consecutive years. Ecological factors influencing vector density, such as the development of irrigation projects, have been linked to the emergence of MVE epidemics.

Transmission. The primary summertime transmission cycle involves wild avian hosts and *Culex annulirostris* mosquitoes, a species that breeds in temporary pools. Aquatic birds, such as herons, egrets, and pelicans, serve as the major viremic hosts, but mammals (especially rabbits and possibly kangaroos) may also play a role in transmission. *Culex annulirostris* has been implicated in tangential transmission of MVE virus to humans, which are dead-end hosts and do not perpetuate the cycle. No human-to-human spread is recognized. The overwintering mechanism and the factors responsible for emergence of intermittent epidemics are unknown.

Pathogenesis

Like other members of the JE virus complex, MVE virus is highly neurotropic. The virus has been recovered from brain tissue obtained postmortem from human cases. Pathological findings are similar to those in JE (149) and are limited to the CNS. The major features include perivascular lymphocytic inflammation affecting gray matter of the cerebral cortex and spinal cord and, to a lesser extent, white matter and meninges; patchy infiltrates in deeper areas of the brain; neuronal degeneration and neuronophagia; destruction of cerebellar Purkinje cells; focal areas of demyelination; and capillary hemorrhages.

HI and neutralizing antibodies appear during the first week after onset. IgM antibodies appear early and may persist for weeks. Immunity to reinfection is believed to be lifelong. The presence of closely related flaviviruses in Australia, including Kunjin virus (WNV) and JE, dengue, and Kokobera viruses, complicates serodiagnosis.

Clinical Manifestations

The incubation period has not been established. A 2- to 5-day nonspecific illness precedes CNS involvement, with sudden onset of fever, headache, myalgia, generalized malaise, anorexia, and nausea. This is followed by the onset of nuchal rigidity and neurologic signs. In infants the disease progresses rapidly, and coma and death may occur within 24 h of onset of neurologic signs, often with clinical signs of involvement of the brain stem and spinal cord. The clinical features are classified by illness severity (11): (i) mild cases with altered levels of consciousness and variable neurologic abnormalities, but without coma or respiratory depression, and stabilization of neurologic signs within 5 to 10 days; (ii) severe cases with seizures, coma, and paralysis, often requiring respiratory assistance; and (iii) fatal cases with spastic quadriplegia and progressive CNS damage or severe disease with superimposed bacterial infection. Seizures and flaccid paralysis are rare in adult patients. The CSF shows pleocytosis, which shifts from polymorphonuclear to mononuclear predominance after a few days of onset; normal or mildly elevated protein; and normal glucose concentration. Neurologic sequelae occur in up to 40% of the mild cases and in all of the severe cases from which patients recover. Abnormalities include cerebral atrophy, paraplegia, impaired gait and motor coordination, and intellectual deterioration. Subclinical infections are common. Attempts to associate MVE virus with mild febrile illnesses without neurologic signs have not been successful.

Recovery or death generally occurs within 2 weeks of onset. Respiratory failure, intercurrent bacterial infections, and the residual neuropsychiatric deficits represent the most important complications of MVE.

Diagnosis

Viremia is present early in infection, but virus isolation from blood (or CSF) has not generally been successful, although RT-PCR on serum provided an early diagnosis in one case. Serologic diagnosis is based on ELISA or HI, CF, or neutralization tests. IgM antibodies appear to be quite specific and useful for early diagnosis, the test becoming positive around 7 days after onset. Cross-reactions with Kunjin virus and other flaviviruses may confuse interpretation. An epitope-blocking ELISA with MVE virus monoclonal antibodies distinguished MVE virus infections from those with other flaviviruses. Postmortem diagnosis is possible by examination of brain tissue by virus culture, direct detection of the virus genome by RT-PCR, or detection of virus antigen by immunohistochemistry.

Prevention and Treatment

No vaccine is available. Mice immunized with JE vaccine and challenged with MVE virus were not protected and in fact had accelerated deaths, consistent with an immunopathological process. In areas prone to recurrent epidemics (e.g., the Murray-Darling River basin), reduction of *Culex annulirostris* breeding by use of larvicides is practiced. Treatment of MVE is symptomatic.

WNV

WNV was first isolated from the blood of a patient with fever in Uganda in 1937. It is one of the most widely distributed of all arboviruses but had not been identified in the New World before its discovery in 1999 in the area of New York, NY (122).

Biology

WNV is a member of the JE antigenic complex and is represented by a single serotype. Antigenic analyses differentiate strains of WNV from Africa, Europe, and the Middle East from strains isolated in India and the Far East (63). Two major genetic lineages exist (97). Within lineage 1 are strains from Europe, the Middle East, West Africa, and Central Africa and distinguishable clades representing strains from India and Australia (Kunjin virus). Lineage 2 represents strains from various regions of Africa. The close genetic relationship between viral isolates identified in New York in 1999 and from a goose from Israel in 1998 suggests that the virus in the United States originated from the Middle East. Following its introduction into the United States, WNV has undergone microevolution, with the "New York" clade being replaced in 2002 by the "North America" clade as the virus spread across the country (33). Although the North America clade viruses appear to be as virulent as the New York clade viruses, the former viruses appear to disseminate faster in mosquitoes (77).

The virus is maintained in an enzootic cycle between birds and *Culex* mosquitoes (Fig. 2). Wild birds develop prolonged high levels of viremia and serve as amplifying hosts (86). Passerine birds develop high levels of viremia, are abundant, and become infected in high numbers during epizootics, suggesting that they may be the principal reservoir hosts for WNV. The major mosquito vector in Africa and the Middle East is *Culex univittatus*, with *Culex poicilipes*, *Culex neavei*, *Culex decens*, *Aedes albocephalus*, or *Mimomyia* spp. important in some areas (71, 158). In Europe, *C. pipiens*, *Culex modestus*, and *Coquillettidia richiardii* are important. In Asia, *C. tritaeniorhynchus*, *C. vishnui*, and *C. quinquefasciatus* predominate.

In the United States, more than 60 mosquito species have been infected with WNV. WNV and SLE virus appear to share the same maintenance vectors: *C. pipiens* and *Culex restuans* in the northeastern United States and Canada, *C. quinquefasciatus* in the southern United States, and *C. tarsalis* in the western United States and Canada. *C. nigripalpus* may be important in Florida. *Culex salinarius* was implicated in the epidemic on Staten Island in 2000 and might be an important bridge vector.

Culex mosquitoes are important for their role in overwintering the virus in temperate climates, where they hibernate as adults (121). The amplification cycle begins when infected overwintering mosquitoes emerge in the spring and infect birds. Amplification within the bird-mosquito-bird cycle continues until late summer and fall, when *Culex* mosquitoes begin diapause and rarely blood feed. The importance of vertical transmission in maintaining the virus is unknown, but it may be an important mechanism of infection of mosquitoes entering diapause.

In the Old World, naturally acquired disease in wild birds is uncommon, suggesting a balanced relationship between virus and hosts. A notable exception was mortality in domestic geese (5) and migrating storks (104) in Israel resulting from infection by a strain similar to the "New York" strain. This strain and its North American descendants have caused lethal infection in more than 320 resident and exotic avian species (21) and marked declines in populations of highly susceptible species, such as American crows, in the United States (95). Experimental inoculation of American crows demonstrated markedly higher mortality from the "New York" strain than from two other lineage 1 WNV strains (KUN and a strain isolated in Kenya) (8). A single nucleotide change in the NS3 gene was responsible for the increased mortality in American crows (7).

WNV grows and produces CPE or plaques in primary chicken embryo cells and in continuous cells of human, primate, swine, and mosquito origin. Mice and hamsters are susceptible to lethal infection by the intracerebral and intraperitoneal routes. Equine encephalitis outbreaks have occurred in many countries. In the United States, incidence peaked in 2002 and subsequently decreased after an equine WNV vaccine became available. Approximately 10% of experimentally infected horses develop clinical illness (10). Clinical series indicate a 20 to 40% mortality rate among ill horses. Age, vaccination status, inability to rise, and female gender are associated with the risk of death (152). Viremia in horses is low and of short duration; thus, horses are unlikely to serve as important amplifying hosts for WNV in nature (10).

Epidemiology

Distribution and geography. WNV is present throughout Africa, the Middle East, continental Europe, India, Indonesia, and Australia (14, 138). Notably, the virus has rarely been identified from areas where JE is endemic. In the New World, its distribution has expanded from its discovery site in New York City in 1999 to Argentina in 2006 (118) (Fig. 6).

Before 1995, human infection with WNV was mainly associated with little or no disease. Serologic data for the Nile Delta of Egypt showing 6% seroprevalence in schoolchildren and 40% seroprevalence in young adults suggest that infection is very common (31). In 1974, Cape Province, South Africa, experienced an outbreak with a 55% incidence of infection with thousands of clinical cases, yet

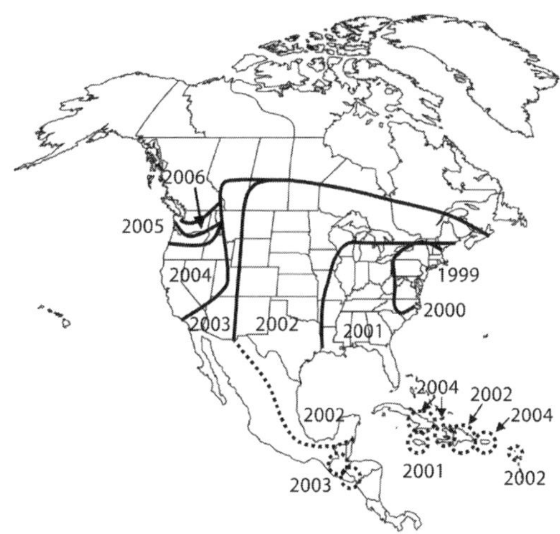

FIGURE 6 Expansion of WNV in North America, Central America, and the Caribbean, 1999 to 2006. Areas demarcated by solid lines are confirmed by virologic means in mosquitoes or vertebrates. Areas demarcated by dashed lines are those with serologic evidence in vertebrates only. Serologic evidence of WNV was found in Colombia and Venezuela in 2004, and WNV caused an equine outbreak in Argentina in 2006.

illness was mild and without encephalitis. Outside of Africa, small outbreaks or sporadic cases of CNS infection have been reported from Israel, India, and European countries (71). A marked upswing in WNV activity began in the mid-1990s coincident with the emergence of a group of genetically similar lineage I viruses of apparent increased pathogenicity (8, 96). Outbreaks associated with a high incidence of severe neuroinvasive disease occurred in Algeria (1994), Romania (1996), Tunisia (1997), Russia (1999 to 2001), the United States (1999), Israel (2000), and Sudan (2002) (102).

Subsequent to the 1999 outbreak in New York City, a national surveillance system that monitors WNV illness in humans, birds, and horses and other animals and infection in mosquitoes and sentinel chickens was established first in the United States and then in Canada. Because avian mortality proved a very sensitive measure of incursion of the virus into an area, surveillance could effectively monitor the virus's rapid dispersion across North America (Fig. 6).

Surveillance south of the U.S. border has been complicated by an unexplained lack of significant morbidity and mortality in birds, humans, and horses and by serologic cross-reactivity of other circulating flaviviruses, such as dengue virus. WNV was first detected south of the U.S. border in 2001, when a resident of the Cayman Islands developed WNV encephalitis. Serologic studies in birds and horses suggested that WNV has circulated in the Dominican Republic, Jamaica, Guadeloupe, El Salvador, Colombia, Cuba, Puerto Rico, and Argentina and widely in Mexico (85). The first outbreak of equine neuroinvasive disease was documented in Argentina in 2005 (39). WNV activity in Canada parallels that occurring in the northern United States.

Incidence and prevalence. The initial outbreak in New York City caused 62 cases and 7 deaths in Queens and surrounding areas (122). Despite the extensive spread of WNV in nature from 1999 through 2001, human disease was infrequent until 2002, when a multistate outbreak throughout the Midwest resulted in more than 4,000 reported cases (127). In 2003, another outbreak of similar magnitude occurred, followed by outbreaks of at least 1,100 cases of neuroinvasive disease from 2004 through 2007. The case fatality rate among persons with neuroinvasive disease is approximately 10%.

Serologic surveys indicate that even in areas experiencing outbreaks, less than 10% of the population has been exposed to the virus. Approximately 1.5 million persons are estimated to have been infected with WNV in the United States through 2006 (136). Human WNV infection incidence increases in early summer and peaks in August or early September. However, an outbreak in Phoenix, AZ, in 2004 began in May and peaked in late June and early July. In the United States, within large regional WNV epidemics, the incidence of human disease varies markedly from county to county, suggesting the importance of local ecological conditions. Males and persons living in a rural area were approximately 1.4 and 3.4 times, respectively, more likely than females or persons living in suburban or urban locations to have WNV infection. Farming, increased environmental temperatures from April through October, vegetation abundance in an urban area, and living in an inner suburb have been linked to increased WNV incidence.

Risk factors associated with human disease. Serologic surveys in Romania (165) and New York City (120) as well as blood donor screening data (84) indicate that WNV infection incidence is constant across all age groups during outbreaks. Age is the most important host risk factor for development of neuroinvasive disease after infection. The incidence of neuroinvasive disease increases approximately 1.5-fold for each decade of life, resulting in a risk approximately 30 times greater for a person 80 to 90 years old than for a child younger than 10 years old (127).

Immunosuppression substantially increases the likelihood of neuroinvasive disease following infection. One outpatient transplant clinic study found that the risk of neuroinvasive disease following infection was 40% (89). WNV neuroinvasive disease has occurred in recipients of kidney, kidney/pancreas, liver, lung, heart, bone marrow, and stem cell transplants. Neuroinvasive disease has been reported for patients with other immunocompromising conditions, including acute myelogenous leukemia, common variable immunodeficiency, and HIV infection. However, it is impossible to determine whether these conditions were predisposing factors. In human experimental studies of WNV as a cancer treatment, the risk of adverse outcomes was related to underlying severity of illness, particularly among patients with hematologic malignancies (161). A case control study showed that cancer and chemotherapy increased at least sixfold the risk of developing meningitis or encephalitis (131).

Older age, alcohol abuse, diabetes, hypertension, heart disease, kidney disease, and chemotherapy have been associated with WNV encephalitis. Persons homozygous for a deletion in the CCR5 gene (CCR5Δ32) were shown to be at increased risk for symptomatic infection and death from WNV (49).

Transmission. Nearly all human infections of WNV are due to mosquito bites (Fig. 2). Transmission has also been described to occur via transfused blood (133), transplanted organs (19, 74), transplacental transmission (17), occupational transmission via percutaneous exposure and laboratory exposure via inhalation, and conjunctival exposure and in a dialysis center by unidentified means. Transmission via breast milk is also likely, although this mode of transmission appears to be uncommon (65). An outbreak of WNV infection occurred among turkey farm workers; however, the means of transmission in that setting was unknown (18).

WNV transmission via transfused red blood cells, platelets, and fresh frozen plasma was documented in 2002 (133). Since 2003, the United States and Canadian blood supplies have been screened for WNV using nucleic acid amplification tests (NAT). Through 2006, screening identified approximately 1,800 potentially viremic blood donors, with as many as 1 in 150 donors being viremic in some outbreak areas. However, not all donations from NAT-positive blood donors are capable of transmitting WNV. All 32 documented transmissions through 2006 were from donations that were WNV IgM antibody negative (22, 133), suggesting that NAT-positive donations with IgM antibody are not infectious. Blood centers conduct NAT on minipools of 6 to 16 specimens, depending on the test kit manufacturer. Minipool NAT screening has reduced sensitivity for identification of donations with very low virus levels, which has resulted in nine "breakthrough" transmissions through 2006. To reduce this risk, blood centers now switch to individual donation testing in areas experiencing outbreaks (22).

Transmission via donated organs was first documented in 2002 (74). The organ donor was viremic on the day the organs were harvested, and all four recipients of organs from this patient developed febrile illnesses and three had encephalitis. In 2005, transmission via donated organs occurred from a donor whose serum from the day of organ harvest was positive for WNV-specific IgG and IgM antibodies but was negative for WNV RNA (19). Two organ recipients developed encephalitis, one had WNV nucleic acid and IgG antibodies in serum but remained asymptomatic, and another remained asymptomatic without serologic evidence of WNV infection.

A causal relationship between WNV and fetal abnormalities has not been proven. One woman with WNV encephalitis during the 27th week of pregnancy subsequently delivered a term infant with chorioretinitis and laboratory evidence of congenitally acquired WNV infection (17). Four percent of cord blood samples obtained after a community-wide epidemic tested positive for WNV-specific IgG antibodies, but none were positive for IgM antibodies (129). There were no significant differences between infants of seropositive and seronegative mothers with respect to birth outcomes. Of 72 live infants born to women infected with WNV during pregnancy, none had proven congenital WNV infection (126). Three infants born to women who had developed symptomatic WNV infection within 3 weeks of delivery had symptomatic WNV disease at or shortly after delivery (126), so intrauterine infection or infection at the time of delivery was possible.

Pathogenesis

WNV has been isolated from the lungs, heart, skeletal muscle, skin, lymph nodes, liver, small intestine, kidneys, thyroid, spinal cord, pons, basal ganglia, cerebellum, and cerebrum in patients dying within 1 month of receiving WNV for treatment of cancer during the 1950s (161). In fatal WNV encephalomyelitis cases, glial nodules with variable loss of neurons and perivascular cuffing by mononuclear cells are observed (55). Mononuclear inflammation and loss of neurons are most prominent in the gray matter of the medulla, pons, and midbrain. Inflammation of the spinal cord is universally present, particularly in the anterior horns. Immunohistochemical assays show viral antigens in the cytoplasm of neurons and neuronal processes. Experimental infection of monkeys demonstrated viral persistence of at least 5 months, mainly in the cerebellum, cerebral subcortical ganglia, lymph nodes, and kidneys (139). A decrease in neurovirulence was noted according to the duration of persistence.

Clinical Manifestations

Most persons infected with WNV are asymptomatic, and symptoms are seen in only about 20%. The typical incubation period for infection ranges from 2 to 14 days, although longer incubation periods have been observed among immunosuppressed hosts (133). The usual presentation is a self-limited febrile illness, called West Nile fever, which is indistinguishable from dengue fever and other viral infections. West Nile fever is characterized by fever, headache, malaise, back pain, myalgias, and anorexia persisting for 3 to 6 days. Eye pain, pharyngitis, nausea, vomiting, diarrhea, and abdominal pain can also occur. Rash appears in approximately one-half of patients with West Nile fever and is less frequent in patients with neuroinvasive disease. The rash is typically maculopapular; involves the chest, back, and arms; generally lasts for less than 1 week; and is sometimes accompanied by complaints of dysesthesia and pruritus. Generalized lymphadenopathy is rare in contemporary outbreaks.

Although West Nile fever was initially considered a mild, febrile illness, recent studies indicate that many patients experience a more severe and prolonged course. In a follow-up study of patients with West Nile fever, the frequency and median duration of symptoms were as follows: fatigue, 96% and 36 days; fever, 81% and 5 days; headache, 71% and 10 days; muscle weakness, 61% and 28 days; and difficulty concentrating, 53% and 14 days (168). Hospitalization was required for 30 patients for a median of 5 days, and 79% missed work or school for a median of 10 days. At 30 days, 63% were symptomatic. In another follow-up study of patients with West Nile fever, 53% reported symptoms of at least 30 days in duration and 79% reported missing work for a median of 16 days (131).

Neuroinvasive disease, which occurs in approximately 1 in 140 infected persons, can present as encephalitis, meningitis, or flaccid paralysis or a mixed pattern of disease. Encephalitis that is associated with muscle weakness and flaccid paralysis is particularly suggestive of WNV infection. Fever is present in at least 90%, with weakness, nausea, vomiting, and headache in approximately one-half of patients. Other neurologic manifestations include tremor, myoclonus, and Parkinsonian features such as rigidity, postural instability, and bradykinesia (134, 157).

WNV infection also causes an acute flaccid paralysis syndrome. Paralysis from WNV poliomyelitis is asymmetric and can occur without overt meningitis or encephalitis (156). Although Guillain-Barré syndrome can occur, most paralysis results from an anterior horn cell process suggestive of poliomyelitis. Cranial nerve palsies can occur, resulting in facial weakness, vertigo, dysarthria, and dysphagia. Facial paralysis appears to have a favorable prognosis. Dysarthria and dysphagia accompanied by acute flaccid paralysis indicate a high risk of impending respiratory failure (156). WNV infection infrequently causes other forms of weakness, including brachial plexopathy, radiculopathy, and a predominantly demyelinating peripheral neuropathy similar to Guillain-Barré syndrome. Other neurologic complications with WNV include seizures, cerebellar ataxia, optic neuritis, and hearing loss.

Ocular manifestations, including chorioretinitis and vitreitis, are commonly reported. The chorioretinal lesions are multifocal, with a "target-like" appearance. A prospective study of patients presenting to a hospital with WNV infection in Tunisia found that 80% had multifocal chorioretinitis with a mild vitreous inflammatory reaction (1). Most patients were asymptomatic and symptoms were self-limited. Other reported ocular findings include iridocyclitis, occlusive vasculitis, and uveitis. WNV infection has been associated with many other infrequently reported complications, including rhabdomyolysis; myocarditis, which has been seen pathologically, but clinical correlation with cardiac dysfunction in humans has not been conclusively demonstrated; hepatitis; pancreatitis; central diabetes insipidus; stiff person syndrome; and hemorrhagic manifestations.

CT of the brain typically shows no evidence of acute disease. MRI shows abnormalities in 20 to 70% of patients.

Hyperintensity on T2-weighed MR images may be seen in regions such as the basal ganglia, thalami, caudate nuclei, brain stem, and spinal cord. EEG for patients with meningitis or encephalitis typically shows generalized, continuous slowing, which is more prominent in the frontal or temporal regions. Patients with acute flaccid paralysis have electrodiagnostic studies showing normal sensory nerve action potentials with compound motor action potentials varying between normal and markedly decreased, depending on the degree of paralysis.

Diagnosis

WNV should be considered in patients who have unexplained febrile illness, encephalitis, meningitis, or acute flaccid paralysis during mosquito season. Evidence of WNV enzootic activity or other human cases, either locally or in a region where the patient has traveled, should raise the index of suspicion.

Total leukocyte counts in peripheral blood are mostly normal or elevated. In cases with signs of CNS involvement, the CSF usually demonstrates a pleocytosis often with a predominance of lymphocytes as well as an elevated protein concentration. A few patients with meningitis or encephalitis have normal (<5 per mm^3) CSF cell counts (3 and 5%, respectively). Over 90% of patients have elevated CSF protein levels.

Viremic blood donors develop IgM antibody in plasma within 9 days after donation (143). Serum or CSF can be tested with the IgM antibody capture ELISA. Nearly all patients with meningitis or encephalitis have a positive IgM antibody capture ELISA result at clinical presentation; however, limited data suggest that many patients with West Nile fever lack demonstrable antibody in serum obtained within 8 days of clinical onset and can be documented to have WNV infection only after NAT or convalescent-phase samples demonstrate antibody (164). IgM antibody to WNV may persist for 6 months or longer. False-positive ELISA results can occur due to recent immunization with yellow fever or JE vaccines or due to infections with other related flaviviruses, such as SLE and dengue viruses.

WNV can be isolated or viral antigen or nucleic acid detected in CSF, tissue, or other body fluids, although the low sensitivities of these methods preclude their routine clinical diagnostic use. NAT such as real-time PCR has been positive for up to 55% of CSF samples. NAT of plasma from blood donors indicates that viremia is of a low titer and detectable for a median of 6.9 days (12). Among patients with neuroinvasive disease, NAT of serum or plasma has a sensitivity less than 15%. However, patients with West Nile fever have been diagnosed by NAT, serology, and a combined approach of these two methods in 45, 58, and 94% of cases, respectively (164). NAT in serum or CSF may be valuable for severely immunocompromised patients, who may have prolonged viremia and lack IgM antibody.

Treatment

Treatment is supportive. Controlled studies to evaluate specific therapies for WNV infection have not been completed. IFN-α has efficacy against WNV in vitro and in animal models. Anecdotal use of standard IFN-α2b within 72 h of encephalitis presentation has been reported; however, two patients receiving IFN-α2b and ribavirin for hepatitis C virus infection developed West Nile fever after mosquito exposure (68).

Ribavirin has in vitro activity against WNV, but its use increased the mortality rate in Syrian golden hamsters when administered 2 days after inoculation (119). Uncontrolled data from Israel suggested that ribavirin use in some patients with WNV neuroinvasive disease appeared to be ineffective and possibly detrimental (28). Polyclonal antisera, monoclonal antibodies directed against the WNV E glycoprotein, and high-titer human intravenous immunoglobulin can protect mice against neuroinvasive disease, although efficacy diminishes rapidly after CNS invasion occurs.

Prevention

No licensed human vaccine exists. A formalin-inactivated, virus-infected whole-cell lysate equine vaccine was introduced in 2003. Equine neuroinvasive disease cases decreased from 14,539 in 2002 to 5,135 in 2003 and continue to decrease, suggesting that the vaccine has had considerable veterinary public health impact. Two additional equine WNV vaccines have since been licensed and marketed: a canarypox virus-based recombinant virus expressing the prM and E genes of WNV (111) and a chimeric virus vaccine in which the gene segments containing the prM and E genes of the 17D yellow fever virus vaccine strain were replaced by the corresponding gene segments of WNV (116). In addition, an equine WNV DNA vaccine was licensed by the U.S. Department of Agriculture in 2006, the first DNA vaccine to be licensed in any country (32). The equine DNA vaccine also has proven effective in birds and likely saved the highly susceptible, endangered California condor *(Gymnogyps californianus)* from extinction. A phase I human clinical trial of the WNV DNA vaccine produced neutralizing antibodies at levels shown to be protective in horses and produced significant T-cell responses against peptides derived from the M and E proteins. Similarly, phase I clinical trials of a modified version of the chimeric yellow fever-WNV vaccine described above were successful.

CEE and RSSE (TBEV)

Russian spring-summer encephalitis (RSSE) virus was isolated from human brain tissue in the far east of the former Soviet Union in 1937. A similar disease was first described in Czechoslovakia in 1948, and the causative virus (Central European encephalitis [CEE] virus) was shown to be serologically related to RSSE virus. These agents, transmitted by the bite of small ixodid ticks, cause severe neurologic infections and represent an important health threat over large areas of Europe and Asia.

Biology

Originally, the TBEV complex contained 14 antigenically related agents, 8 of which were human pathogens (Table 1). Genetic studies have resulted in the TBEV complex being divided into two complexes: the mammalian tick-borne virus group and the seabird tick-borne virus group. Within the mammalian tick-borne virus group are nine distinct species: Gadgets Gully, Kadam, Kyasanur Forest disease, Langat, louping ill, Omsk hemorrhagic fever, Powassan, and Royal Farm viruses and TBEV (50). TBEV has three subtypes: CEE virus (also called western subtype), RSSE virus (also called far eastern subtype), and Siberian (also called Vasilchenko virus) (41, 51). Louping ill virus has at least five subtypes (British, Greek, Irish, Spanish, and Turkish), and Kyasanur Forest disease virus has Alkhumra virus as a subtype. These viruses' close antigenic and genetic relationships create difficulty in identifying individual virus species. Nonetheless, immunity to CEE and RSSE is cross-protective. Within a subtype, strains are homogeneous, varying by a maximum of 2.2%, while a maximum difference between subtypes is 5.6%. It is proposed that the TBEVs evolved approximately 2,000 years ago. Evolution of this group of viruses is characterized by the emergence of a small number of stable lineages, reflecting the low rate of transmission of these agents and restricted movements of vectors and terrestrial (rodent) hosts.

The host range and cell culture susceptibility of tick-borne flaviviruses are shown in Table 3. Within a subtype, strains may vary considerably in virulence (140). Single amino acid changes in the E protein have been shown to alter the virulence of CEE virus (145). Most domestic livestock (cows, goats, and sheep) develop viremia and secrete virus in their milk but do not develop clinical illness. Dogs are susceptible to encephalitis acquired by tick bite.

Epidemiology

Distribution and incidence. TBE occurs in an endemic pattern over a wide area of Russia and the independent states of the former Soviet Union, Central and Eastern Europe, and Scandinavia, Switzerland, Germany, Italy, Greece, Albania, China, and Japan (Fig. 7). Austria, the Czech Republic, Slovakia, Slovenia, and Hungary experience the highest incidences, with several hundred cases each year and morbidity rates between 1 and 20 per 100,000. In the former Soviet Union, 3,000 to 6,000 cases occur annually. In Japan, sporadic cases of RSSE occur in Hokkaido. The highest incidence is in western Siberia, with morbidity rates of 5 to 10 per 100,000. Among American military personnel and travelers in Germany, the risk of infection was found to be approximately 1 per 1,000 person-months of exposure (110).

TBE has relatively constant distribution coinciding with ecological habitats favorable for tick activity. The rate of transmission and number of human cases vary in relation to fluctuating populations of the rodent hosts for immature ixodid ticks. The risk of human exposure to ticks largely depends on outdoor activities. Occupations (forestry and farming), mushroom and berry picking, and recreational activities in forested and scrub areas are risk factors for infection. Approximately two-thirds of the cases occur in young adults (20 to 40 years of age), and males are at slightly higher risk than females. Serologic surveys indicate that subclinical infections are common, and the illness-to-infection ratio is between 1:25 and 1:200. Antibody prevalence varies widely with region but ranges from 10 to 30% in adults living in areas of endemicity in Eastern Europe.

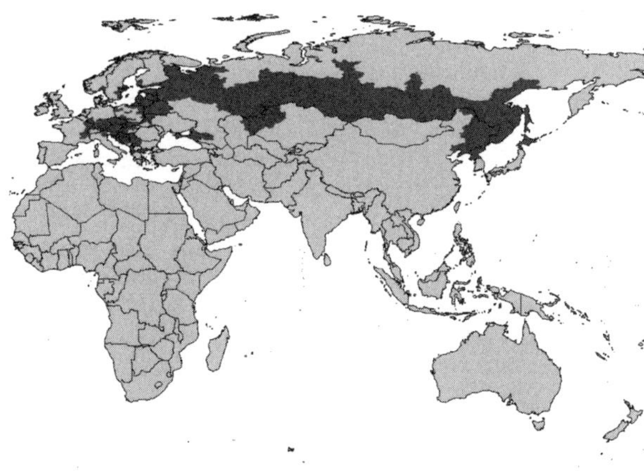

FIGURE 7 Geographic distribution of TBE.

Transmission. RSSE occurs from May to August, whereas CEE cases occur from May to October. The natural transmission cycle involves larval and nymphal ixodid ticks and wild rodents and insectivores (52). *Ixodes ricinus* (the species also responsible for Lyme disease transmission in Europe) and *Ixodes persulcatus* are responsible for transmission in Europe and Russia, respectively (Fig. 8). *Ixodes ovatus* is the vector in Hokkaido. In nature, ixodid vectors may reach high population densities (100 to 500/m^2), with up to 20% of the ticks infected with virus. The active transmission cycle is initiated in the spring, when adult and nymphal ticks emerge from hibernation. Adult ticks feed on large mammals, including domestic livestock, and lay eggs that produce larvae, a small proportion of which are transovarially infected. Goats, sheep, cows, and other large mammals provide a source of blood for adult ticks and are critical to maintaining the vector population, but these hosts are not or are rarely involved in virus transmission. Infected overwintering nymphal ticks feed together with larval ticks on small rodents and insectivores. Rodents may develop viremia and infect attached ticks, but direct transmission apparently also occurs between infected and uninfected ticks cofeeding on small mammals in the absence of detectable viremia (94). These mechanisms for passage from nymphal to larval ticks ensure amplification of the virus. CEE and RSSE viruses are passed from larva to nymph and from nymph to adult during tick molting. Human infection occurs on exposure to adult ticks that were infected during the previous or current season.

Infected sheep and goats secrete virus, with concentrations as high as 10^5 PFU/ml in milk, and human outbreaks with RSSE or CEE viruses have followed ingestion of unpasteurized sheep or goat's milk or cheese. Since flaviviruses are inactivated by gastric acid and intestinal bile, it is likely that virus entry occurs in the oropharynx, presumably via tonsillar lymphoid tissue. Laboratory infections with RSSE and CEE viruses occurred frequently before the use of biological containment procedures and vaccines and were often acquired by the aerosol route. Regardless of the route of infection, the patient is not contagious and does not perpetuate transmission by ticks or interhuman contact.

Pathogenesis

Pathological findings are limited to the CNS and are generally similar to those in other flavivirus encephalitides, with a predilection for damage to brain stem structures. Lymphocytic infiltration of the meninges and perivascular inflammation, neuronal degeneration and necrosis, neuronophagia, and glial nodule formation around necrotic neurons are widely scattered throughout the cerebral and cerebellar cortices, brain stem, basal ganglia, and spinal cord. The anterior horn cells of the cervical cord are especially affected in RSSE, which explains the lower motor neuron paralysis of the upper extremities, a hallmark of the disease. Indeed, the pathological picture and clinical manifestations (flaccid paralysis) may lead to confusion with

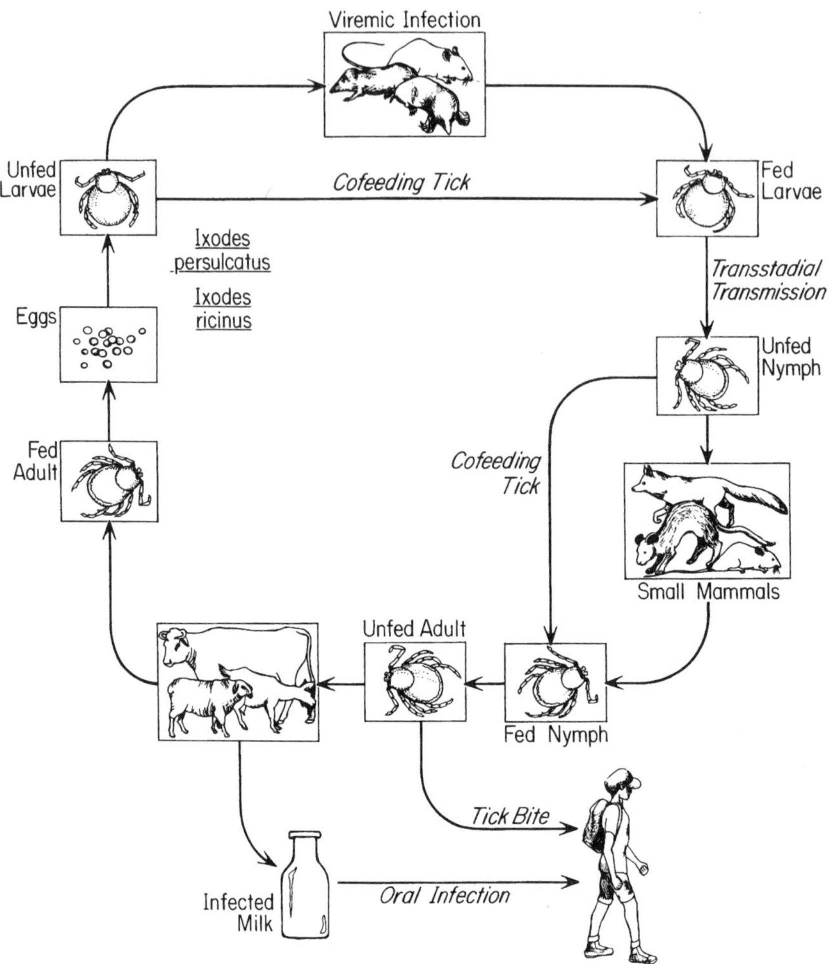

FIGURE 8 Transmission cycle of TBE. (Reprinted from reference 115a with permission of Lippincott Williams & Wilkins.)

poliomyelitis, but in TBE, the cerebral cortex is more heavily involved. Apoptosis has been proposed as one mechanism of cell death in TBE (73). An interesting feature of members of the TBEV complex is their propensity to cause persistent infections in experimentally infected monkeys, hamsters, and, possibly, humans. Chronic infection in animals is characterized by mutations in the virus (possibly related to evasion of the immune response) and destructive changes to neurons and other cell types in the brain in the absence of significant inflammation. Chronic progressive human encephalitis and seizure disorders in humans (including "Kozhevnikov epilepsy," a form of epilepsia partialis continua) have been associated with RSSE virus (125), and virus has been isolated from the CSF of a patient with a disease clinically resembling amyotrophic lateral sclerosis. However, chronic active infection appears to be rare.

Severity of disease has been correlated with high CSF cell counts and low serum neutralizing antibody levels, suggesting that these patients had a delayed immune response.

Clinical Manifestations

Up to two-thirds of patients give a history of tick bite. CEE virus has long been considered less virulent than RSSE virus. The incubation period is 3 to 7 days. CEE usually has a biphasic course, with an initial systemic illness lasting about a week and characterized by fever of 38 to 39°C, chills, malaise, headache, arthralgia, myalgia, and vomiting. This is followed by remission with fatigue but no other symptoms, lasting up to a week. Most patients experience an abortive infection and recover fully without further symptoms. However, up to one-third of patients develop a second phase of the disease which takes the form of aseptic meningitis in 10 to 50% and encephalitis, myelitis, or radiculitis in the remainder (52). Encephalitic signs include alteration of consciousness, ataxia, paresis or paralysis, and cranial nerve abnormalities. The case fatality rate is 1 to 3%, and death usually occurs within 1 week of onset of neurologic signs. The disease is less severe in children than in adults. Adult patients have higher levels of albumin and specific IgG in the CSF, indicating increased virus replication, and they more often require treatment for brain swelling than children. Adults aged at least 60 years have more severe initial illness and less favorable outcome than younger adults (100). The CSF changes in TBE are similar to those in other virus encephalitides. Other clinical laboratory abnormalities include leukocytosis and elevated erythrocyte sedimentation rate. Abnormalities in the EEG and MRI are seen for most patients with encephalitis signs.

About 10 to 30% of patients with acute involvement of brain parenchyma have neuropsychiatric sequelae (52). Postencephalitic signs and symptoms correlate with severity of the acute disease, and patients with coma or a requirement for assisted ventilation have increased sequelae. Objective neurologic sequelae (radicular signs and paresis) generally resolve over several months, but inability to work, chronic fatigue, memory and concentration deficits, and other cognitive changes may persist for years.

In RSSE, illness onset is more often gradual than acute, with a prodromal phase including fever, headache, anorexia, nausea, vomiting, and photophobia. These symptoms are followed by stiff neck, sensorial changes, visual disturbances, and neurologic dysfunction. The neurologic features are highly variable and include predominantly cerebrocortical forms with obtundation, convulsions, paresis or paralysis, and hyperkinesia; predominant involvement of the brain stem with respiratory depression, cardiac arrhythmia, oculomotor deficits, and paralysis of the shoulder girdle and upper extremities; and myelitic forms with lower motor neuron paralysis and little alteration of consciousness. Kozhevnikov epilepsy may occur in the acute stage or become part of a chronic postencephalitic syndrome. In fatal cases, death occurs within the first week after onset. Case fatality rates as high as 20% for RSSE have been reported, but such rates may be overestimates. The case fatality rate of the Siberian subtype appears to be similar to that of CEE. Neurologic sequelae, including residual flaccid paralyses of the shoulder girdle and arms, resembling the sequelae of poliomyelitis, occur in as many as 30 to 60% of survivors of RSSE.

Diagnosis

Diagnosis is most often made by serologic tests, especially the detection of serum and CSF IgM antibodies by ELISA. IgM antibodies in serum may be detectable for up to 10 months after disease onset. The virus (or viral antigen) may be isolated from the blood during the first phase of illness and from brain tissue of patients dying during the early phase of the disease, but the success rate is less than 10%. RT-PCR on brain tissue may be useful in postmortem diagnosis.

Prevention

Vaccination is warranted in persons living in areas of endemicity, persons working under high-risk conditions, or travelers engaged in high-risk activities. In Europe, two equivalent, safe, and effective inactivated TBE vaccines are available in adult and pediatric formulations: FSME-IMMUN (Baxter Vaccine AG, Vienna, Austria) and Encepur (Novartis Vaccines, Marburg, Germany). Two inactivated TBE vaccines are available in Russia. A two-dose primary series, followed by a booster at 1 year and subsequent booster doses at 3- to 5-year intervals, is practiced. For travelers, an accelerated dosing schedule at 0, 7, and 21 days, followed by a booster dose at 12 to 18 months, is available. Vaccine efficacy for both products is estimated at more than 95%.

The use of repellents or protective clothing may reduce the risk of tick bite. Permethrin-impregnated clothing is effective in repelling ticks during outdoor exposure (whereas *N,N*-diethyl-*m*-toluamide [DEET] is less effective).

Other Flavivirus Encephalitis Viruses

Flaviviruses associated with rare and sporadic cases of human disease are shown in Table 4. Selected agents of interest are described below.

Rocio Virus

In 1975 a new agent named Rocio virus was isolated from fatal human cases during an epidemic of encephalitis on the south coast of São Paulo State, Brazil (37). Epidemics in coastal São Paulo State in 1975 and 1976 resulted in 971 cases, with attack rates of up to 38 per 1,000 inhabitants. Young adult males with outdoor exposure (e.g., during fishing) were primarily affected. The disease appears to have virtually disappeared, with only rare subsequent suspect cases in the area originally affected and serologic evidence for circulation in Bahia State. The clinical features resembled those of SLE. The case fatality rate in hospitalized patients was 4%. Neurologic sequelae occurred in 20% of survivors. Virus is not recoverable from blood, but postmortem diagnosis may be made by virus isolation from brain tissue. Diagnosis in nonfatal cases is by serology (IgM ELISA).

Louping Ill Virus

Louping ill virus causes encephalitis in sheep in the British Isles and is a member of the TBEV complex, closely related to CEE virus. Minor differences in the genome distinguish strains from Scotland, Wales, and Ireland. Furthermore, there is evidence of closely related viruses that are considered to be subtypes of louping ill virus—British, Greek, Irish, Spanish, and Turkish—but whether or not they are subtypes of louping ill virus is still subject to debate. Infected sheep develop a biphasic illness with fever and prolonged viremia, followed by cerebellar ataxia, tremors, and paralyses. The transmission cycle of louping ill virus involves *Ixodes ricinus* ticks and both sheep and grouse. Approximately 43 human cases have been reported, of which 26 resulted from laboratory exposure and 17 resulted from tick bites or direct exposure of abattoir workers, butchers, and veterinarians to blood and tissues of sheep. The incubation period (4 to 7 days) closely resembles that of CEE virus, and clinical expression in humans is biphasic and closely resembles CEE. No deaths have been reported. Hemorrhagic disease may occur. Laboratory diagnosis is by virus isolation from blood or CSF during the early phase of illness, or by standard serologic tests. Treatment is symptomatic.

Powassan Virus

Powassan virus, a member of the TBE antigenic complex, was isolated in 1958 from a patient with fatal encephalitis in Ontario, Canada. Cases have been recognized subsequently in Russia, Canada, and the northeastern United States, and virus isolations from ticks or mammals and antibodies indicate a wide distribution including the western United States, Canada, and northern Mexico. Viruses isolated in North America are separable by nucleotide sequencing into two genotypic variants.

Thirty-two cases of Powassan encephalitis have been reported, most involving persons less than 20 years old, and males, probably reflecting increased outdoor activity and exposure to ticks (16). The seroprevalence in the United States and Canada is 0.5 to 4%. The virus is transmitted in a cycle involving small mammals (principally woodchucks) and *Ixodes* ticks, principally *Ixodes cookei*.

TABLE 4 Flaviviruses causing sporadic human disease[a]

Virus	Human disease			Veterinary disease species affected	Geographic distribution	Transmission cycle
	No. of cases	Clinical features	Severity			
Banzi virus	<10	Nonspecific febrile illness	Self-limited	None known	Southern and East Africa	Mosquitoes (*Culex*)-rodents
Bussuquara virus	1	Fever, arthralgia	Self-limited	None known	Brazil, Colombia, Panama	Mosquitoes (*Culex*)-rodents
Edge Hill virus	1	Fever, myalgia, arthralgia	Self-limited	None known	Australia	Mosquitoes (*Aedes*)-wallabies
Ilheus virus	6	Fever, myalgia, encephalitis[b]	Potentially severe (no deaths)	None known	Brazil, Colombia, Panama, Trinidad	Mosquitoes (*Psorophora*)-birds
Kokobera virus	3	Fever, rash, arthralgia	Self-limited	None known	Australia, Papua New Guinea	Mosquitoes (*Culex*)-?
Koutango virus	1[c]	Fever, rash, arthralgia	Self-limited	None known	West Central Africa	Ticks (several genera)-rodents
Kunjin virus	<20	Fever, rash, encephalitis	Potentially severe (no deaths)	Horses (rare)[e]	Australia, Sarawak, Thailand	Mosquitoes (*Culex*)-birds
Langat virus	<10	Fever, encephalitis[b]	Potentially severe (no deaths)	None known	Malaysia, Thailand, USSR	Ticks (*Ixodes*)-rodents
Louping ill virus	39[d]	Similar to CEE[f]	Potentially severe (no deaths)	Sheep[g]	United Kingdom, Ireland	Ticks (*Ixodes*)-sheep, grouse
Modoc virus	1	Aseptic meningitis	Self-limited	None known	Western United States, Canada	Rodent-rodent[h]
Negishi virus	>3[i]	Encephalitis	Potentially fatal	None known	Japan, China	Ticks-?
Rio Bravo virus	6 (11)	Febrile illness, meningitis, orchitis	Self-limited	None known	Western United States, Mexico	Bat-bat
Sepik virus	1	Febrile illness, (hospitalized)	Self-limited	None known	New Guinea	Mosquitoes (*Mansonia*)-?
Spondweni virus	3	Fever, arthralgia, rash	Self-limited	None known	South and West Africa	Mosquitoes (*Aedes*)-?
Usutu virus	1	Fever, rash	Self-limited	None known	South and Central Africa, Central Europe	Mosquitoes (*Culex*)-birds
Wesselsbron virus	<20	Fever, arthralgia, rash, encephalitis	Potentially severe (no deaths)	Sheep[h]	Sub-Saharan Africa, Thailand	Mosquitoes (*Aedes*)-?
Zika virus	>14	Fever, rash, arthralgia	Self-limited	None known	West, East, and Central Africa, Indonesia	Mosquitoes (*Aedes*)-monkeys

[a] The recognition of these diseases has often occurred in the setting of general virus investigations and surveillance projects. Infection (disease) may be more common than indicated, and the clinical spectrum may differ from that delineated by the few recognized cases.
[b] Includes cancer patients intentionally infected who developed encephalitis.
[c] Laboratory infection.
[d] Twenty-six cases were laboratory infections.
[e] Encephalomyelitis.
[f] In one case a hemorrhagic diathesis was described.
[g] Encephalitis (cerebellar syndrome). Sporadic disease has also been described for dogs, horses, cows, goats, pigs, and deer.
[h] Virus without known intermediate arthropod vector; transmission by contact or aerosol.
[i] Includes a laboratory infection.

The virus has also been isolated from *Ixodes marxi*, *Ixodes spinipalpis*, *Ixodes scapularis*, and *Dermacentor andersoni* ticks. Powassan virus has been isolated from both ticks and mosquitoes in Russia, but there is no evidence for mosquito transmission in North America.

The disease is characterized by a prodrome of fever and nonspecific symptoms (including rash in several cases), followed by neurologic signs of meningeal irritation and encephalitis, which are often severe. Serious neurologic sequelae have occurred in 35% of the reported cases; in one, clinical illness resembled RSSE with shoulder girdle involvement, and in another, it resembled herpes encephalitis with temporal lobe involvement. In Russia, prominent cerebellar signs differentiated the disease from RSSE. Case fatality rates are 10 to 15% (47). Laboratory diagnosis is by serology or virus isolation from brain tissues of patients who died from the disease.

Flaviviruses Associated Primarily with Febrile Syndromes with Rash

Dengue Viruses

Dengue disease was first described in the 18th century, but the causative agent was not isolated until 1944. Between 1944 and 1956 it was shown that four distinct viruses, designated dengue virus types 1 to 4, were responsible for the same clinical syndrome. In 1956, a severe form of the disease, DHF/dengue shock syndrome (DHF/DSS), was described for the first time, although in retrospect, earlier isolated outbreaks probably occurred in Australia and South Africa. DHF/DSS is described in the section on hemorrhagic fevers below.

Biology

Dengue virus fever is caused by four antigenically and genetically related but distinct viruses (dengue virus types 1 to 4) distinguished by neutralization tests. Infection with an individual dengue virus serotype confers lifelong protection to that serotype; however, sequential infections with different serotypes occur because cross-protection between serotypes in vivo is absent or of short duration. At the genomic level, strains of dengue virus belonging to the same serotype are >90% homologous, whereas homology across serotypes is approximately 65% (61). Distinct E gene genotypes have evolved in different geographic regions. In many areas of the world, two or more genotypes cocirculate, reflecting either the evolution of autochthonous variants over time or the introduction and spread of a distinct genotype from another region. In addition to mutational events, intertypic recombination appears to play a role in the evolution of variants within dengue virus serotypes (67) but not between serotypes.

The structure and replication strategy of dengue viruses are similar to those of other flaviviruses, but their host range and growth characteristics in vitro are distinctive. Unadapted isolates of dengue virus often do not cause CPE in cell culture and are not pathogenic for infant mice. Neuroadaptation by sequential passage is required to produce consistent pathogenicity. In general, cells of monkey (Vero and LLC-MK2) and mosquito (*A. albopictus* C6/36) origin are most useful for virus isolation and propagation in vitro (Table 3). Syncytium formation occurs in mosquito cells. Dengue viruses replicate to high titers in mosquitoes after intrathoracic inoculation.

Epidemiology

Distribution and incidence. Dengue viruses occur worldwide in tropical regions; their distribution is determined by the presence of the principal mosquito vector (*Aedes aegypti*) (Fig. 9). In tropical areas where the vector is active year-round, dengue virus infection occurs throughout the year, with increased transmission during the rainy season. This is due to higher mean temperatures and attendant shorter extrinsic incubation periods in the vector and to higher humidity and enhanced survival of adult mosquitoes. In temperate zones, transmission is limited to the summer months. Dengue fever epidemics occasionally struck temperate parts of North America, Europe, South Africa, and Argentina up to the early part of the 20th century. Dengue fever is an important travel-associated infection, and about 100 to 200 imported cases of dengue fever are reported each year for travelers returning to the United States, Europe, and Australia.

It is estimated that over 2.5 billion people inhabit tropical areas at risk of infection (56). Since World War II, dengue fever has expanded in incidence and geography, due principally to urbanization and the attendant increase

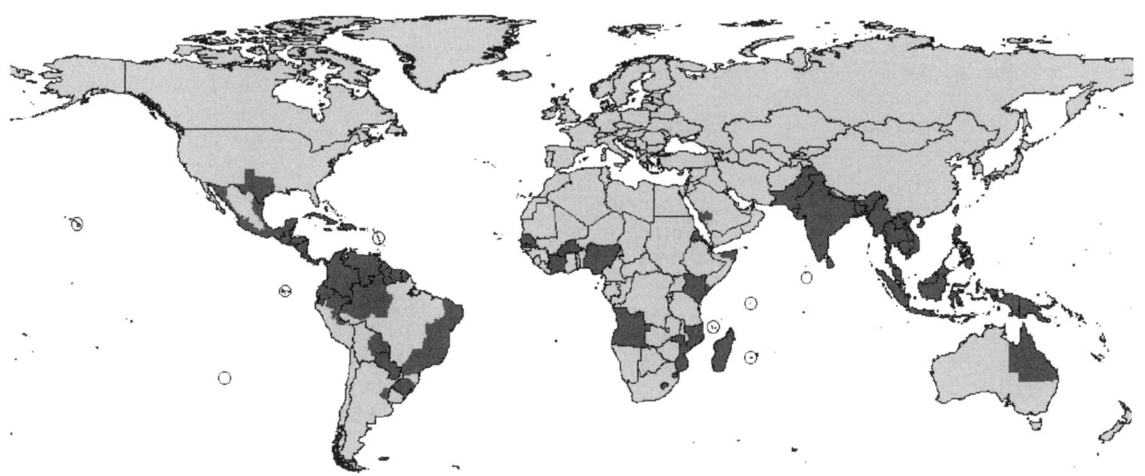

FIGURE 9 Geographic distribution of dengue fever.

in domestic *A. aegypti* populations, and to the increased movement of infected people by airplanes (56). Dengue virus infections are most prevalent in Southeast Asia, where all four serotypes are continuously present. In recent years, the Indian subcontinent, southern China, and Taiwan have experienced epidemics. Among island nations in Oceania, all four serotypes have been introduced episodically, but the island outbreaks have generally been caused by a single serotype. Intermittent transmission of dengue virus has occurred in Queensland, Australia. All four serotypes have been isolated in tropical Africa, but their medical impact remains unclear due to poor surveillance.

Control programs in the mid-20th century effectively eliminated the *A. aegypti* mosquito from much of the Americas, and dengue virus activity was reduced to sporadic activity in the Caribbean (137). However, discontinuation of the control program in the 1970s resulted in reinfestation of *A. aegypti* to its former range by the mid-1990s. Subsequently, reported dengue fever cases increased from 66,000 in 1980 to 300,000 to 700,000 cases from 1995 to 2003, which have occurred over a widening geographic range (59, 137). In addition to the increased incidence of classical dengue fever, large outbreaks of DHF began in 1981 with the introduction of a dengue virus type 2 variant from Southeast Asia (see below). All four dengue virus serotypes are now endemic in the Americas.

Dengue fever epidemics have occurred occasionally in the continental United States since the end of World War II (Louisiana in 1945 and Texas in 1980, 1986, 1995, 2000, and 2005). The Texas outbreaks resulted from amplified transmission in northern Mexico and included both imported cases and cases derived from secondary spread (20). Following a 56-year hiatus, an outbreak vectored by the *A. albopictus* mosquito occurred in Hawaii from 2001 to 2002 (43).

It is estimated that over 100 million cases of dengue fever occur annually throughout the world, but reports underestimate the true incidence. In areas of hyperendemicity of Southeast Asia, the annual incidence of infection is 10 to 20%, and most children have experienced at least one dengue virus infection by the age of 7 years. In these areas, dengue fever is a childhood disease, and adults are protected by cumulative immunity. In island communities or in naïve populations undergoing virgin soil epidemics, the incidence of dengue fever has been 70% or higher, with similar attack rates across all age groups. In some outbreaks, a higher incidence of dengue fever has been found in females, possibly indicating risk of infection around the home by the domestic, daytime-biting vector, *A. aegypti*. The ratio of inapparent to apparent infections is probably highly variable due to age, other host factors, and virus strain variation. Field studies have found inapparent-to-apparent infection ratios of between 6:1 and 15:1 for primary infection (57), but experimental infections of adults produce illness in nearly all subjects (151). The risk of dengue fever following primary infection increases with age (44).

Immunity acquired after infection with one serotype confers full (probably lifelong) protection against reinfection with that serotype but predisposes individuals to more severe disease (DHF) on sequential infection with another dengue virus serotype. The ratio of inapparent to apparent infections is significantly lower in secondary infection.

Transmission. Mosquitoes transmit dengue virus, and humans are the intermediate host. The period of viremia during which humans are infectious for blood-feeding adult female vectors is 3 to 5 days (123). The threshold viremia level for infection of mosquitoes is not known, but humans may sustain high-titer viremias, up to 8.3 $\log_{10}$/ml (57). After blood feeding, an extrinsic incubation period of 10 to 14 days must elapse before *A. aegypti* can transmit the virus upon refeeding (123). *A. aegypti* is a domestic species that breeds in artificial containers and bites in and around human habitation. Peak biting activity occurs in the early morning and late afternoon. In tropical areas where storage of drinking water is practiced, 10 to 20 female *A. aegypti* mosquitoes may be found per room, of which 5 to 10% may be infected with dengue virus. However, outbreaks with vector densities of fewer than 1 female mosquito per house have also been recorded. *A. aegypti* is a furtive mosquito and may probe several persons before completing a blood meal, enhancing the rate of virus transmission. The vector population threshold for dengue virus transmission has not been established. In rural areas in some parts of the world, *A. albopictus* plays a secondary role in interhuman transmission of dengue virus. *A. albopictus* spread from Asia to the New World in the 1980s, and in 1995 it was implicated in dengue virus transmission for the first time, in Mexico.

The maintenance of dengue viruses between epidemics has not been clearly defined, especially in rural areas with relatively sparse human populations. Vertical transmission of dengue virus in *A. aegypti* and in sylvatic *Aedes* spp. has been documented and probably contributes to virus maintenance. In Southeast Asia and West Africa, a sylvatic cycle of transmission occurs, involving nonhuman primates and tree hole-breeding *Aedes* spp., similar to the cycle for yellow fever (Fig. 10). However, in Africa, virus strains involved in the sylvatic cycle are distinct from strains associated with human disease outbreaks (146).

Dengue virus infections have occurred by needlestick, bone marrow transplantion, and blood transfusion.

Pathogenesis

The primary cell subset infected after inoculation in mosquito saliva is probably dendritic cells in the skin (173), which subsequently migrate to draining lymph nodes (79). After initial replication in skin and draining lymph nodes, virus is present in blood during the acute febrile phase, generally for 3 to 5 days, and may be recovered from serum and from peripheral blood mononuclear cells (83). Blood-derived dendritic cells are highly permissive to infection; one study found that the principal subset of peripheral blood mononuclear cells infected were $CD20^+$ B cells (81). The genesis of systemic symptoms in dengue fever is uncertain, but the release of cytokines and chemokines as a result of virus injury to dendritic cells may play an important role. In uncomplicated dengue fever, elevated levels of soluble interleukin 2 (IL-2) receptor, IL-2, soluble CD4, and IFN-γ in plasma or blood (174), and other cytokines like TNF-α, IL-1β, and platelet-activating factor in plasma or blood, are present. High levels of IFN-α have been documented for a week or more after illness onset. Leukopenia due to transient bone marrow suppression is a feature of dengue fever and also may be due to cytokine effects.

Because classic dengue fever is a self-limited disease, there are few reports of pathological changes. Biopsy specimens of rash lesions from human patients have shown

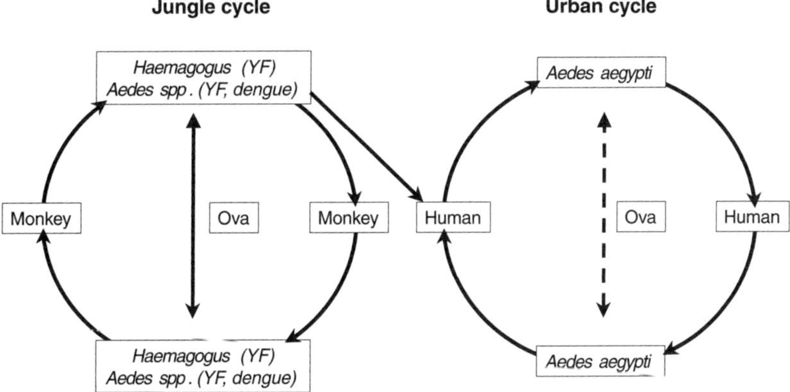

FIGURE 10 Simplified transmission cycle of dengue and yellow fever viruses. Both viruses have a jungle cycle involving tree hole mosquitoes. In the Americas, *Haemagogus* transmits yellow fever, but no jungle cycle for dengue fever has been discovered. In Africa, both viruses are transmitted in jungle cycles involving *Aedes* spp. Yellow fever does not exist in Asia, but in Malaysia, Sri Lanka, and probably elsewhere, dengue virus is transmitted in a jungle cycle involving *Aedes* spp. The relationship between the jungle cycle of dengue fever and human infections is not clear. However, the jungle cycle of yellow fever is a source of human infections in the Americas and Africa. Dengue fever transmission occurs principally in urban environments, where domestic *A. aegypti* serves as the vector and humans serve as the viremic hosts. A similar cycle of yellow fever transmission occurs commonly in West Africa. No urban outbreaks of yellow fever have occurred in the Americas since 1964, except possibly for a very limited outbreak in Bolivia in 1997 to 1998.

swelling of endothelial cells of small vessels, perivascular edema, and infiltration of mononuclear cells.

The viremic period is terminated coincident with the appearance of serum antibodies. In most patients, humoral and cellular responses result in recovery from infection and long-lasting protection against reinfection with the homologous serotype. Serotype-specific neutralizing antibodies directed against the E protein and serotype-specific $CD4^+$ and $CD8^+$ cytotoxic lymphocytes directed against structural and NS virus targets on infected cells are responsible for protection and recovery. Cross-protection against other dengue virus serotypes is short-lived, and in a subset of individuals experiencing secondary infection with a heterologous serotype, a severe immunopathological disease (DHF/DSS) occurs and is mediated by the interaction of antibodies and T cells (see the discussion of DHF below).

Clinical Manifestations

The incubation period is 2 to 7 days. Dengue fever begins abruptly with high fever, chilliness, headache, retrobulbar pain, lumbosacral aching pain, conjunctival congestion, puffiness of the eyelids, and facial flushing. Fever may be sustained for up to 6 to 7 days or may have a biphasic (saddleback) course. Fever is accompanied by generalized malaise, prostration, anorexia, and nausea. The pulse rate is slow in relation to the fever. Myalgia, arthralgia, and deep bone pain ("breakbone fever") are characteristic features of the disease. Respiratory symptoms (cough, sore throat, and rhinitis) are not uncommon, especially in children. A transient, generalized macular or mottled rash may appear on the first or second day. Coincident with defervescence on the third to fifth day, a maculopapular or morbilliform rash appears on the trunk and then on the face and limbs, sparing palms and soles. The rash is nonpruritic, lasts 1 to 5 days, and may result in desquamation on healing. Other signs and symptoms may include generalized lymphadenopathy, cutaneous hyperesthesia, and altered (metallic) taste sensation. Minor hemorrhagic signs are noted in some patients (petechiae and epistaxis).

Leukopenia with an absolute neutropenia is typical, and the platelet count may fall to less than 100×10^9/liter. Reactive lymphocytes are seen in the peripheral blood smear. Elevations in serum lactate dehydrogenase, aspartate aminotransferase, and alanine aminotransferase occur in more than half of cases. Myocarditis and various neurologic disorders have been associated with dengue fever. Myocarditis is self-limited and does not result in progressive heart failure. Neurologic manifestations include encephalitis (active infection and injury of the brain), encephalopathy (without evidence of brain infection), transverse myelitis, peripheral mononeuropathy, polyneuritis, Guillain-Barré syndrome, Bell's palsy, and Reye syndrome. Neurologic complications are likely caused by both nonspecific causes (the result of cerebral edema and systemic physiological alterations during the acute disease) and actual encephalitis due to viral neuroinvasion in individual cases (112, 159). Ocular disturbances are rare but include decreased visual acuity accompanied by retinal hemorrhage, cotton wool exudates, and macular lesions. Convalescence may be prolonged, lasting several weeks, with generalized weakness, psychological depression, bradycardia, and ventricular extrasystoles. Persistent arthritis is not a feature of dengue fever, and there are no known permanent sequelae of classic dengue virus infection.

Maternal dengue virus infection generally results in a normal fetal outcome. Fetal deaths during acute dengue virus infection have been recorded; however, a causal relationship could not be determined. Fetal abnormalities have not been definitively linked to dengue virus infection. Maternal infection near the time of parturition has been reported to result in hemorrhagic complications, premature delivery (15), and transplacental infection and severe dengue disease in the neonatal period (29), but such events are rare.

Diagnosis

The disease may resemble influenza, rubella, rubeola, malaria, scrub typhus, leptospirosis, and a variety of other arbovirus infections, especially WNV and chikungunya, O'nyong nyong, Sindbis, Mayaro, Edge Hill, Kokobera, Spondweni, Barmah Forest, Zika, and Ross River virus diseases. Serologic cross-reactions complicate the clinical and laboratory differentiation of dengue virus from other flaviviruses causing similar illnesses.

Diagnosis may be made by RT-PCR or by viral isolation from blood during the first 3 to 5 days of illness. *Toxorhynchites* mosquitoes inoculated by intrathoracic injection are very sensitive hosts for virus isolation, but virus can be identified by IF only after 10 to 14 days. *Toxorhynchites amboinensis* (TRA-284), *A. albopictus* (C6/36), and *Aedes pseudoscutellaris* (AP-61) cell cultures are highly susceptible to dengue virus infection, and virus antigen is detected by IF within a few days, depending upon the titer of virus in the sample. Monoclonal antibody IF staining and RT-PCR with type-specific primers are useful for serotype-specific diagnosis. Multiplex RT-PCR can provide a method for detection and typing multiple dengue viruses in clinical samples or cell culture fluids.

Serologic diagnosis depends on the demonstration of a ≥4-fold rise (or fall) in antibody titers. The IgM antibody capture ELISA is a useful diagnostic test, and a positive result on a single serum sample provides a presumptive diagnosis. IgM antibodies appear shortly after defervescence (on days 4 to 6 after onset) and wane after 1 to 2 months. IgM antibodies are found following both primary and secondary infections. The HI, CF, and neutralization tests may also be employed for serodiagnosis. Preferably an acute-phase sample is obtained as early as possible (in the febrile phase), and a second specimen is obtained 2 to 3 weeks later. A negative IgM test before the sixth day after onset is not definitive, whereas a negative result after that day is indicative of another etiology of the illness; however, a small proportion of cases of secondary infection will have no detectable IgM response. Serotype-specific diagnosis by a ≥4-fold rise in antibody titer is relatively simple in the case of primary infections, but considerable difficulties arise in serotype-specific diagnosis in cases of secondary infections because of broad cross-reactions. The plaque reduction neutralization test, which is more specific than other tests, or epitope-blocking ELISA employing monoclonal antibodies may help to distinguish specific from cross-reactive antibody responses. In the case of sequential dengue virus infections, the antibody response to the initial infecting virus type may exceed that to the current infecting type ("original antigenic sin"). Secondary dengue virus infections are characterized by the presence of HI antibodies at titers greater than 20 in the acute-phase sample and by high titers (>1,280) in convalescent-phase sera. The ratio of IgM and IgG antibodies determined by ELISA has been used to distinguish primary from secondary infections; in primary infections the IgM/IgG ratio in acute-phase sera or convalescent-phase sera obtained during the first month after onset generally exceeds 1.5, whereas secondary infections are characterized by an excess of IgG (93). Several commercialized ELISA kits for measuring dengue virus antibody are available, and they have variable sensitivities and specificities (53).

Simple and quick modifications of ELISA have been developed and marketed, including a dipstick enzyme immunoassays, dot blot assays, and immunochromatographic methods. These tests have high specificities and reasonably high sensitivities (53). The IgG ELISA can be used to distinguish primary from secondary dengue virus infections. Dengue virus antibodies can be measured in saliva and CSF using the commercial kits. Sensitivity is reported to be >90%. Screening of Puerto Rican, Brazilian, and Honduran blood donors with an investigational NAT based on the WNV blood donor screening NAT found prevalences of dengue virus RNA of approximately 1:1,000 during epidemics.

Prevention

Prevention of dengue virus transmission by control or eradication of *A. aegypti* depends on elimination of breeding sites. This approach has been successful in only a few locales (e.g., Singapore and Cuba) where intensive efforts have been sustainable. However, even in Singapore, dengue fever has resurged in recent years as a result of lowered herd immunity, virus transmission outside the home, an increase in the age of infection, and adoption of a case-reactive approach to vector control (128). One model used to estimate the *A. aegypti* density (expressed as the standing crop of pupae per human inhabitant) representing the threshold for virus transmission (45) found that the levels ranged, under different assumptions of immunity in the human population and environmental conditions, between 0.5 and 1.5, thus illustrating the extreme difficulty in dengue fever prevention by means of vector source reduction. Unfortunately, epidemic control by use of aerial or ground applications of mosquito adulticides has not been highly successful, in part because *A. aegypti* resting places are not reached by aerosols.

The long-term solution to the control of dengue virus infection is the development and wide-scale use of safe, effective, and inexpensive vaccines against all four dengue virus serotypes. Because of the possibility that vaccine immunity might predispose individuals to immunopathological events associated with DHF, it is necessary to simultaneously immunize against all four serotypes. Many approaches to dengue virus vaccines are currently under investigation (170). Development of live, attenuated vaccines has been delayed by problems with viral interference between serotypes and difficulties in achieving an appropriate level of attenuation. Nevertheless, a live, attenuated, tetravalent dengue virus vaccine developed by the Walter Reed Army Institute of Research and GlaxoSmithKline and produced by serial passage in primary dog kidney (PDK) cells is in phase II testing.

Two live, attenuated chimeric vaccines have progressed to clinical trials. Reverse genetics was used to introduce an attenuating 30-nucleotide (Δ30) deletion mutation into the 3′ untranslated region of cDNA clones of each dengue virus serotype (40). Clinical trials in humans and monkeys showed that the recombinant dengue virus serotype 1 and 4 vaccine candidates produced low viremia, were strongly immunogenic, and were minimally reactogenic. Subsequently, chimeric vaccine candidates for serotypes 1 to 3 were produced by replacing the respective M and E structural proteins of the wild-type viruses in the recombinant serotype 4 Δ30 vaccine candidate backbone (6). These candidate vaccines are currently in monovalent phase II clinical trials. Another strategy using Acambis's (Cambridge, MA) ChimeriVax technology replaces the M and E structural proteins of the licensed 17D yellow fever vaccine virus with the comparable proteins from the four dengue viruses (58). The tetravalent ChimeriVax vaccine against the four dengue virus serotypes was well tolerated in volunteers vaccinated at 0 and 6 months (42), and a phase III trial is scheduled to begin in 2008. Both of these live, attenuated chimeric vaccines have limited replication in mosquitoes.

Another vaccine under development is a live, attenuated chimeric vaccine which utilizes the serotype 2 PDK-53 vaccine strain (Mahidol University, Bangkok, Thailand), which is attenuated by three mutations in the NS genes (69). The tetravalent vaccine contains the serotype 2 PDK-53 vaccine strain plus three chimeras produced by the wild-type structural genes of the serotype 1, 3, and 4 viruses each incorporated into the serotype 2 PDK-53 backbone containing the attenuating mutations of the original vaccine strain. Whole-virus inactivated vaccines, recombinant subunit vaccines, DNA vaccines, recombinant vaccinia virus, and recombinant subunit vaccines are also under development.

Treatment

Treatment is supportive. Aspirin should be avoided due to the hemorrhagic diathesis and a possible relationship between dengue fever and Reye syndrome.

Other Flaviviruses Causing Febrile Illness

Flaviviruses associated with rare and sporadic human disease are listed in Table 4.

Viruses Causing the Hemorrhagic Fever Syndrome

Dengue Viruses

DHF and DSS are severe manifestations of dengue virus infection, first described in 1954 during an epidemic in the Philippines. In contrast to classic dengue fever, DHF is a life-threatening infection and a major cause of hospitalization. Nonetheless, severe forms of dengue fever can also result in hospitalization. The past several decades have seen the emergence of DHF as a major health threat in Southeast Asia and its geographic expansion into previously silent areas of the Americas, China, and the Middle East.

DHF/DSS is an acute immunopathological disease that occurs nearly exclusively in individuals sensitized by a prior infection and subsequently infected with a heterologous dengue virus serotype (60). The pathophysiological features include leakage of plasma from capillaries into the extravascular space manifested as hemoconcentration, pleural effusions, and hypotension; a hemorrhagic diathesis; and hepatic involvement (hepatomegaly, elevated transaminase, and focal pathological lesions) that resembles a less severe form of yellow fever. The case definition of DHF includes elevated hematocrit (>20% above normal), thrombocytopenia (<100,000/mm^3), and a positive tourniquet test. The case definition of DSS requires meeting the criteria for DHF plus a reduction in pulse pressure (<20 mm Hg) or in blood pressure. Grades of severity are recognized (Table 5).

TABLE 5 Classification of dengue fever, DHF, and DSS according to clinical and laboratory features

Disease	Grade	Clinical features	Hemorrhage	Hematocrit	Platelet count	Pulse pressure
Dengue fever		Fever, arthralgia, rash	None or minor[a]	Normal	Normal or >100,000	Normal
DHF	I	Fever, gastrointestinal and respiratory symptoms	None or minor[a]	Increased by 20%[b]	<100,000	Normal
	II	Fever, gastrointestinal and respiratory symptoms	Spontaneous hemorrhage	Increased by 20%[b]	<100,000	Normal
DSS	III	Same as above but with signs of hypotension[c]	None or spontaneous hemorrhage	Increased by 20%[b]	<100,000	≤20 mm Hg
	IV	Profound shock	None or spontaneous hemorrhage	Increased by 20%[c]	<100,000	≤20 mm Hg

[a] Often requires adaptation by brain serial passage.
[b] Over premorbid or convalescent-phase value.
[c] Other signs may include hepatomegaly, hypoalbuminemia, jaundice, and pleural effusion.

Biology

All four dengue virus serotypes cause DHF/DSS, but serotype 2 is the most important, followed by serotype 3. The sequence of infecting serotypes and strain differences in virulence appear to influence the occurrence of DHF. There is no animal model of DHF permitting study of these factors, as available dengue disease models in mice are characterized by encephalitis. Epidemiological studies and comparison of strains associated with different disease outcomes at the genome level have provided clues that virus-specified factors may contribute to the pathogenesis of DHF. In the Americas, two distinct genotypes of dengue serotype 2 virus have circulated since 1981, when a strain belonging to genotype I was introduced from Southeast Asia and superimposed on the endemic "American" genotype V (147). The Asian genotype has caused multiple epidemics of DHF/DSS in populations with prior immunity to serotype 1 (60), whereas the American genotype appears to be less pathogenic and has not caused outbreaks of severe disease in populations with a similar immunological background (169). Structural differences at critical determinants appear to be associated with the potential to cause DHF, specifically ones located at E390 (cell receptor interaction), a region of the 5′ noncoding region involved in the initiation of translation, and a region of the 3′ noncoding region believed to be important in the formation of replicative intermediates (98).

Epidemiology

Distribution and incidence. Dengue virus incidence has increased 30-fold in the last 50 years, and an average of 925,896 cases was reported annually from 2000 to 2005 to the WHO. A pandemic of unprecedented magnitude occurred in 1998, in which 1.2 million cases of dengue fever and DHF were reported from 56 countries worldwide. In Thailand, DHF ranks fifth as a cause of morbidity, third as a cause of death, and fifth as a cause of years of productive life lost. Case fatality rates elsewhere in Asia range from 1 to 5%, depending on availability and sophistication of hospital care. Outbreaks of DHF have occurred intermittently in the South Pacific and in southern China. In the American region, the first DHF epidemic occurred in Cuba in 1981 (10,000 cases and 158 deaths) (60). The incidence in the Americas has steadily increased; in 2001, the Americas alone reported over 652,212 cases of dengue fever, of which 15,500 were DHF.

The principal factor responsible for the increased incidence and geographic expansion of DHF is the cocirculation of multiple dengue virus serotypes. Human population growth, urbanization, the deterioration of sanitation favoring *A. aegypti* breeding and dengue virus transmission, and the rise in jet aircraft travel permitting dissemination of dengue viruses have contributed to the hyperendemicity of multiple dengue virus serotypes in Asia and in the Americas.

Risk factors associated with human disease. The principal risk factor for DHF/DSS is prior exposure to a heterologous dengue virus serotype. Approximately 90% of persons with DHF/DSS have secondary infections. The risk of DHF is estimated to be 15 times higher and that of DSS is estimated to be 50 to 100 times higher in secondary than in primary dengue virus infection (163).

Unlike classical dengue fever, DHF/DSS is principally a disease of childhood. Two peaks have been noted in age-specific incidence rates: incidence in children under 1 year old and incidence in children 3 to 5 years of age. The disease in infants is rare and is associated with primary infection in the presence of maternal antibody, whereas the vast majority of cases in older children are the result of secondary infections. In Thailand the highest incidence of DHF/DSS is in children 5 to 9 years of age. The 1981 DHF epidemic in Cuba illustrated the importance of age in DHF pathogenesis, since children had a higher incidence of severe disease than did adults with a similar immunologic predisposition (87). However, when dengue virus serotype 2 reinvaded in 1997, all individuals with prior exposure to serotype 1 had been infected at least 9 years before (serotype 1 struck Cuba in 1977 to 1978) and all patients hospitalized were >15 years old. The case fatality rate was higher in this outbreak than in 1981 (60).

The incidence of DHF (but not of dengue virus infection) is higher in females than males. It is hypothesized that females may have a more robust immune response to dengue virus infection or may be more susceptible to cytokine-mediated vascular injury. Malnutrition, which may reduce immune responsiveness, appears to spare children from DHF/DSS. Race influences disease severity; in Cuba, Caucasians and Asians had a significantly higher incidence of DHF/DSS than did Blacks (87). Underlying diseases (e.g., sickle cell disease, diabetes mellitus, and bronchial asthma) may increase the risk of developing severe disease. Peptic ulcer disease and menstruation may increase the risk of gastrointestinal hemorrhage and menorrhagia, respectively.

Pathogenesis

Human disease is characterized by diffuse capillary leakage and hemorrhage. Increased vascular permeability results in hemoconcentration, decreased effective blood volume, tissue hypoxia, lactic acidosis, and shock. These perturbations in homeostasis are mediated by cytokines, and there are consequently few pathological findings in fatal human cases. On autopsy, signs of capillary leak (pleural effusions and retroperitoneal edema) and of hemorrhage (petechiae, ecchymoses, and visceral hemorrhages) are evident. Histopathological examination reveals perivascular edema and hemorrhage, proliferation of lymphoid cells and plasmacytoid elements in spleen and lymph nodes, and necrosis of thymus-dependent areas of the spleen. Central or paracentral focal necrosis of hepatocytes, Councilman bodies, hypertrophy of Kupffer cells, and focal mononuclear cell infiltration may be evident in the liver. Bone marrow changes include maturational arrest of megakaryocytes. Focal dengue virus antigen has been demonstrated in skin, liver, and mononuclear leukocytes.

As with all pathogenic processes, there are multiple components that contribute to dengue virus pathogenesis, including virus and host genetic factors and the immune response induced by the viruses. The lack of suitable animal models has made dissection and understanding of the mechanism of dengue virus pathogenesis difficult. A direct role for virus in DHF seems unlikely, as plasma leakage takes place several days after viremia and supports a hypothesis for an immune-mediated mechanism for DHF.

Three immunopathological processes are associated with the genesis of DHF/DSS: (i) antibody-mediated enhancement of infection of monocytes/macrophages; (ii) activation of dengue virus-specific lymphocytes, with release of cytokines and activation of complement; and (iii) immune clearance of infected monocytes/macrophages, also with release of cytokines and activation of complement.

In the setting of a secondary dengue virus infection, preexisting nonneutralizing antibodies recognizing antigenic determinants on the E glycoprotein that are shared by the four dengue viruses (sometimes termed heterologous antibody) bind dengue virus and form infectious immune complexes. Dengue virus bound to IgG antibody gains access to the principal cell targets for replication (monocytes/macrophages) via Fcγ receptors, in particular FcRII. The number of infected cells in the host and the overall virus load are thus enhanced. This phenomenon of antibody-mediated enhancement of virus replication has been demonstrated in vitro but has been difficult to demonstrate in vivo. Indeed, many observations regarding the pathogenesis of DHF/DSS are based on extrapolations from in vitro studies, supported by measurements of cytokines in plasma samples. In addition to a role for the E protein, the NS1 protein may also play a role. NS1 is found in both cell-associated and secreted forms, with the latter associated with viremia in secondary infections. However, studies to date show no correlation between anti-NS1 antibodies and plasma leakage.

Primary infection also induces both serotype-specific and dengue virus cross-reactive CD4$^+$ and CD8$^+$ CTLs directed against cross-reactive structural and (especially) NS virion proteins expressed on the surface of infected monocytes. Activation of dengue virus-specific T lymphocytes interacting with infected monocytes/macrophages causes release of IFN-γ, IL-2, TNF-α, and TNF-β. Interestingly, CD4$^+$ T cells produce greater quantities of IFN-γ to the homologous virus causing the primary infection, while the ratio of TNF-α to IFN-γ is higher following stimulation with heterologous dengue viruses. It is hypothesized that low-avidity dengue virus cross-reactive T cells induced by the primary infecting dengue virus dominate during a secondary heterologous dengue virus infection. Furthermore, since plasma leakage is relatively short-lived, immune mediators, in particular proinflammatory mediators such as IL-6, IL-8, and TNF-α, likely play roles. Overall numbers of CD4$^+$ T cells, CD8$^+$ T cells, NK cells, and $\gamma\delta$ T cells have been found to be decreased in DHF patients compared to those with dengue fever.

Markers of T-cell activation include elevated levels of soluble CD4 and CD8, IL-2 receptor, and TNF receptors, and levels of these factors are higher in patients with DHF than in those with classical dengue fever. Activated CD4$^+$ and CD8$^+$ lymphocytes may themselves also be targets for dengue virus replication. Apoptosis or immune lysis of dengue virus-infected monocytes/macrophages by CD4$^+$ and CD8$^+$ CTLs results in the release of a variety of vasoactive mediators and procoagulants. IL-10 and secretory TNF-RII are significantly higher in DHF than in dengue fever patients, and IFN-γ peaks earlier in DHF patients, while IL-6, IL-1, and macrophage inhibitory factor were higher in fatal DHF cases. Higher levels of secreted viral NS1 occur in DHF patients, and complement activation (associated with the NS1 protein) appears to take place at the same time as plasma leakage.

Studies of dengue virus infection in cell culture indicate production of chemokines such as IL-8, RANTES, MIP-1α, and MIP-1β, which is consistent with studies in humans. IFN-γ up-regulates both the expression of Fcγ receptors on monocytes (augmenting the infection of these cells by infectious immune complexes) and the expression of MHC-I and -II molecules involved in recognition of these cells by cytotoxic T cells, thereby increasing the potential for enhanced dengue virus replication and release of cytokine mediators. Activation of complement by virus-antibody complexes or by cytokines released during immune clearance of infected cells is probably also involved in endothelial damage. Elevated levels of TNF-α, IL-6, C3a, C5a, and histamine have been described for DHF. TNF-α causes capillary endothelial permeability, and increased levels of this cytokine in particular in plasma have been associated with severe disease and shock. Dengue virus has been shown also to infect cells of the mast cell/basophil lineage in vitro, suggesting that release of histamine from mast cells contributes to capillary leakage.

A 43-kDa cytokine ("cytotoxic factor") produced by CD4$^+$ T cells has been demonstrated in sera from DHF patients. When administered to uninfected mice, cytotoxic factor induced vascular and blood-brain barrier permeability and lymphoid cell depletion, mimicking those seen in DHF. Immunization of mice with this cytokine prevented these effects. Although these observations strongly suggest that the disturbances in vascular permeability that account for DHF and DSS are mediated by cytokines, the precise mechanisms remain uncertain and are likely to be complex.

Another distinct mechanism postulated to play a role in the bleeding diathesis of DHF/DSS is the presence of cross-reactive antibodies against plasminogen in patients with dengue virus infections; the explanation for this phenomenon may be homology between a region of the dengue virus E protein and plasminogen. However, elucidation of the role of these antibodies in perturbation of fibrinolysis awaits further study.

Overall, there is strong evidence for dengue virus pathogenesis being immune mediated. However, the lack of an animal model and the complex interactions among components of the immune system have made it difficult to unravel the exact mechanism of pathogenesis of DHF. The prospects for therapeutic interventions in humans appear to be as problematic as or more problematic than for bacterial septic shock.

Clinical Manifestations

DHF is distinguished from dengue fever by the presence of fever, thrombocytopenia (platelet count, $<10^5$ per liter), and hemoconcentration (hematocrit increased by $>20\%$) (148). DSS is a more severe form of the disease, characterized by hypotension (pulse pressure, <20 mm Hg; cold, clammy extremities) or profound shock (171). The features distinguishing DHF and DSS are shown in Table 5.

The disease begins with a syndrome identical to classical dengue fever. However, on the second to fifth day the patient becomes increasingly ill, with prostration, restlessness, irritability, cold and clammy extremities, diaphoresis, circumoral and peripheral cyanosis, rapid respiration, rapid pulse, and hypotension. Hemorrhagic manifestations appear, including petechiae, ecchymoses, oozing from venipuncture sites, epistaxis, or intestinal hemorrhage. In 10 to 15% of cases, major hemorrhagic signs appear. Gastrointestinal hemorrhages or intracerebral bleeding may be life-threatening. Physical findings include skin hemorrhages, pleural effusions, hypotension, and hepatomegaly. Jaundice is a rare manifestation but can lead to confusion with yellow fever. Encephalopathy (stupor, coma, convulsions, and paresis) with normal CSF or (more rarely) true encephalitis occurs in a small proportion of cases. The hematocrit is elevated and serum albumin levels are reduced due to leakage of plasma from the intravascular space. Other laboratory abnormalities include neutropenia, relative lymphocytosis with atypical lymphocytes, thrombocytopenia, elevated serum transaminases, depletion of complement and fibrinogen, and the presence of fibrin split products in plasma. The chest X ray may reveal pleural effusions. Shock may be precipitous, and without specific intervention, death may occur in 25 to 50% of cases of DSS. However, early recognition and appropriate treatment have resulted in overall case fatality rates of 0.5 to 1.0%. Recovery is rapid and typically uneventful. Intercurrent bacterial infections, particularly bacterial sepsis from indwelling catheters, may contribute to morbidity and mortality. There are no known long-term sequelae of DHF/DSS.

The diagnosis of DHF is made on clinical and epidemiological grounds. In some areas, DHF overlaps with the distribution of other virus hemorrhagic fevers. Confusion in past outbreaks has occurred with yellow fever (in rare cases of DHF with jaundice), leptospirosis, and Venezuelan hemorrhagic fever (Guanarito virus). Other conditions to be differentiated in individual cases include severe malaria, bacterial sepsis, rickettsial infections, and typhoid fever. Clinical parameters highly predictive of DHF included (i) facial flushing and conjunctival injection without respiratory tract signs, (ii) enlargement and tenderness of the liver, and (iii) positive tourniquet test with or without leukopenia.

Techniques for virus isolation and RT-PCR from blood of acutely ill patients are discussed above. Serodiagnosis is possible, but identification of the infecting subtype is difficult because most cases of DHF occur in persons with prior dengue virus exposure who have secondary-type antibody responses. Antibodies to the NS proteins on Western blots, including NS1, NS3, and NS5, are more prominent in sera of patients with secondary than primary infections.

Treatment

The WHO has published guidelines for the management of cases (171). Triggers for hospitalization are the appearance of restlessness or lethargy, cold extremities or cyanosis, oliguria, rapid or weak pulse, hypotension, and hemoconcentration. Oxygen should be administered to all patients, and blood pressure, pulse pressure, urinary output, and vascular leak should be closely monitored by means of measurement of hematocrit and serum albumin. The key is careful fluid management during the period of capillary leakage, with the goal to maintain circulation without giving excess fluid and contributing to respiratory distress. Patients with grade I or II DHF should receive oral fluids but should be monitored closely. If signs of circulatory failure appear, such as a narrowing pulse pressure, intravenous fluids are required. Patients with shock (grade III or IV DSS) require more aggressive parenteral fluid therapy. Fluid therapy is discontinued as shock is controlled and the hematocrit comes into normal range, in order to avoid fluid overload and pulmonary edema. Those who do not respond and whose hematocrit is declining may have significant internal hemorrhage. Such patients or those with melena or other overt major blood loss are candidates for blood transfusion. Fresh whole blood should be given judiciously to avoid fluid overload. Electrolyte and acid-base balance should be carefully monitored; patients with metabolic acidosis who do not respond to fluid therapy should be treated with bicarbonate. Some patients with clear indications of disseminated intravascular coagulopathy and high levels of fibrin split products have been treated with heparin, with apparent clinical benefit. Salicylates and hepatotoxic drugs should be avoided. Corticosteroids are widely used; however, their effectiveness is unproved. The use of intravenous immunoglobulin has been advocated, based on the hypothesis that it may compete with dengue virus immune complexes for Fcγ receptors.

Specific antiviral therapy has not been extensively evaluated. An uncontrolled trial of human leukocyte interferon during the 1981 epidemic in Cuba suggested that deaths may have been averted, but this observation requires confirmation. Although ribavirin shows in vitro activity against dengue virus, concentrations required for in vivo efficacy are not achievable without toxicity. Future prospects include the development of virus protease inhibitors and antisense oligonucleotides. However, the rapidity of the disease process and the role of host cytokines in pathogenesis require that antiviral therapy be instituted before the full expression of disease.

Yellow Fever Virus

Yellow fever virus, the prototype member of the family *Flaviviridae*, causes a hemorrhagic fever syndrome characterized by high viremia; hepatic, renal, and myocardial injury; hemorrhage; and high lethality.

Biology

Yellow fever virus is a unique virus and has not been assigned to an antigenic complex or subgroup within the *Flavivirus* genus. Sequence analysis of the envelope gene revealed that yellow fever virus diverged earlier than other mosquito-borne viruses from the ancestral flaviviral lineage, approximately 3,000 years ago. Analyses of the yellow fever virus E gene sequence have distinguished at least seven genotypes: two in West Africa, with probable subdivisions between western (Senegal) and eastern (Nigeria) strains; one in Central and East Africa; one in East Africa; one in Angola; and two in South America. South American genotype I is present in Brazil, Colombia, and Ecuador, whereas genotype II is found in Peru and Bolivia. Genotype II exhibits a higher degree of microheterogeneity and a phylogenetic pattern suggesting independent evolution in localized geographic areas (9). Phylogenetic studies of the West African and South American genotype I strains show genetic relatedness, supporting the notion that yellow fever virus was introduced into the New World from West Africa during the slave trade. Homology across all yellow fever virus genotypes is >90%, suggesting that the virus is relatively resistant to mutational change, either because of gene flow within large geographic regions or because of restrictions on change based on the requirement for specific vectors and vertebrate hosts.

The host range of yellow fever virus is shown in Table 3. *Aedes pseudoscutellaris* (AP-61) mosquito cells are highly susceptible, with virus replication assessed by CPE, IF, or subpassage in mice or mammalian cells. Intrathoracic inoculation of mosquitoes (*Toxorhynchites* or *A. aegypti*) is also a sensitive method for isolation or assay of yellow fever virus. Asian (rhesus and cynomolgus) monkeys, as well as some New World monkeys, infected with yellow fever virus develop fatal hepatitis resembling the human disease, whereas African species with which the virus has coevolved are resistant to overt disease.

Epidemiology

Distribution and incidence. Yellow fever occurs only in tropical South America and sub-Saharan Africa (Fig. 11). Yellow fever virus has never invaded Asia. Possible explanations include (i) cross-protection afforded by dengue virus immunity, (ii) low vector competence of Asian strains of *A. aegypti* (there is experimental evidence to support both hypotheses), and (iii) occurrence of yellow fever in remote areas and exclusion of infected persons from routes of travel. Fifty to 300 cases are reported each year in South America and up to 5,000 cases are reported in Africa, but these reports may greatly underestimate the true impact. The highest number of cases reported to the WHO occurred from 1985 to 1994, largely due to a sustained series of epidemics in Nigeria. From 2000 through 2005, a total of 3,966 cases of yellow fever were reported to the WHO, of which 3,309 cases (83%) occurred in Africa. In South America, yellow fever occurs in the Amazon, Orinoco, and Araguaia River basins and contiguous areas, and intermittently on the island of Trinidad. From 2000 through 2005, a total of 659 cases were officially reported, particularly from Brazil, Colombia, and Peru. It should be emphasized that yellow fever is underreported and that the actual number of cases in Africa and South America may be as high as 200,000 per year. Ten fatal yellow fever virus infections occurred in travelers to countries in which yellow fever is endemic from 1996 to 2006; six of the patients had traveled to South America (3).

In South America the incidence of yellow fever is highest during months with peak rainfall, humidity, and temperature (January to March). In Africa, transmission peaks during the late rainy season and early dry season. In tropical America, jungle yellow fever principally affects young adult males exposed during forest-clearing activities to the vector (*Haemagogus* spp.), which inhabits the rain forest canopy. In Africa, a wider array of vectors is responsible for transmission, and they reach their highest densities in savanna habitats. Human infection is endemic, and the prevalence of immunity increases with age; therefore, children are at greater risk. There is little difference in incidence by gender.

During epidemics in Africa, the incidence of infection may be as high as 20% and the incidence of disease may be 3% (115). The infection/illness ratio ranges between 2:1 and 20:1. Immunity to certain heterologous flaviviruses ameliorates the disease and increases this ratio. The case fatality rate has varied widely in different epidemics, possibly reflecting virus strain variation in virulence and/or sensitivity of case detection. Rates higher than 50% are reported, but the lethality of yellow fever with jaundice usually approximates 20%.

Transmission. The virus is transmitted between wild nonhuman primates and diurnally active mosquitoes that breed in tree holes (*Haemagogus* spp. in the Americas and *Aedes africanus* in Africa) (4) (Fig. 10). Humans are infected when they are exposed to these vectors ("jungle yellow fever"), and epidemic spread from human to human can be maintained in rural areas by the same mosquitoes. Alternatively, *A. aegypti*, a domestic mosquito, may transmit yellow fever virus between humans as the sole viremic hosts in the cycle ("urban yellow fever"). In the moist savanna region of Africa, tree hole-breeding *Aedes* spp. (e.g., *Aedes furcifer* and *Aedes luteocephalus*) are implicated in endemic and epidemic transmission. The virus is maintained over the dry season by vertical transmission in mosquitoes.

Pathogenesis

Signs of specific organ dysfunction (hepatitis and renal injury) follow onset of illness by several days. The virus initially replicates in regional lymph nodes and then spreads via the bloodstream to other tissues, including the liver, spleen, bone marrow, and myocardium. In liver, Kupffer cells are infected first, followed by hepatocytes in the midzone (zone 2) of the liver lobule, which undergo coagulative necrosis, sparing cells bordering the central vein and portal tracts. The reason for this peculiar distribution of hepatic injury is unknown. However, midzonal necrosis has been described for low-flow hypoxia, due to ATP depletion and oxidative stress of marginally oxygenated cells at the border between anoxic and normoxic cells. A similar mechanism might operate in yellow fever virus infection.

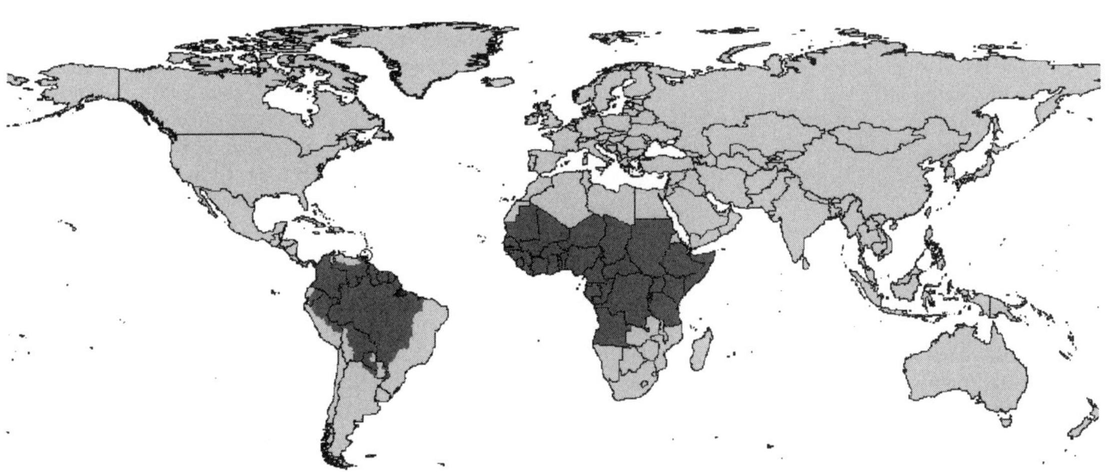

FIGURE 11 Geographic distribution of yellow fever.

Yellow fever virus antigen has been observed principally in hepatocytes in the midzone, suggesting a predilection of these cells for virus replication. Injury to hepatocytes is characterized by eosinophilic degeneration (Councilman bodies), rather than by ballooning and rarefaction necrosis typically seen in virus hepatitis. Several studies have shown that cytopathic changes (including Councilman bodies) are the result of programmed cell death (apoptosis), which, however, is induced too late to limit virus infection and prevent widespread tissue damage (105). Consistent with apoptotic cell death, only minimal mononuclear inflammation develops in yellow fever. Other hepatic pathological changes include microvesicular accumulation of fat, ceroid/lipofuchsin deposits, and intranuclear (Torres) bodies. The reticulin framework is preserved, and healing occurs without cirrhosis. Renal pathology is characterized principally by acute tubular necrosis and fatty change, which may represent late-stage injury following shock. Cerebral edema and petechial hemorrhages are common findings. Lymphocytic elements in the spleen and lymph nodes are depleted, and large mononuclear or histiocytic cells accumulate in the splenic follicles.

The disease is also characterized by hemorrhage and circulatory collapse. Decreased synthesis of vitamin K-dependent coagulation factors by the liver, disseminated intravascular coagulation, and altered platelet function contribute to the hemorrhagic diathesis (113). Direct virus injury to myocardial fibers, which show cloudy swelling and fatty changes, may contribute to shock. However, shock is undoubtedly mediated by cytokine dysregulation. TNF-α and inducible nitric oxide produced by infected and activated Kupffer cells and splenic macrophages might play a prominent role in cell injury, oxygen radical formation, microvascular damage and microthrombosis, tissue anoxia, and shock. Patients dying of yellow fever show cerebral edema at autopsy, probably the result of microvascular dysfunction.

Yellow fever virus infection is followed by a rapid immune response. Humoral, but not cellular, immune responses have been characterized. Neutralizing antibodies, cytolytic antibodies against viral proteins on the surface of infected cells, antibody-dependent cell-mediated cytotoxicity, and cytotoxic T cells are presumed to mediate the clearance of primary infection (114). Neutralizing antibodies appear toward the end of the first week after onset, and it is notable that antibody (and presumably cellular) responses occur coincident with the clinical crises. However, it is unclear whether immune mechanisms during the acute stage of disease contribute to pathogenesis. Neutralizing antibodies persist for life after yellow fever virus infection, and they provide complete protection against disease on reexposure to the virus.

Clinical Manifestations

The incubation period from the bite of an infected mosquito to onset of fever is 3 to 6 days. The clinical expression of disease varies from nonspecific febrile illness to life-threatening hemorrhagic fever (114). Onset is abrupt, with fever, chills, malaise, headache, lumbosacral pain, generalized myalgia, nausea, and dizziness. The patient appears toxic, with congestion of the conjunctivae and face; a furred tongue, with reddening of the edges; and a relative bradycardia in the face of fever (Faget sign). Leukopenia with a relative neutropenia is typically present. This "period of infection," during which the patient is viremic and may serve as a source of infection for blood-feeding mosquitoes, lasts up to several days. A distinct "period of remission" with abatement of fever and symptoms and lasting 2 to 24 h sometimes occurs, and the patient may simply recover. In other cases, the illness reappears, with fever, nausea, vomiting, epigastric pain, and the onset of jaundice, renal dysfunction, and a hemorrhagic diathesis. During this "period of intoxication," viremia is usually absent. Over the course of 3 to 5 days, jaundice and serum transaminase levels increase. The direct bilirubin reaches levels between 10 and 15 mg/dl. There is a marked increase in albuminuria, a reduction in urine output, and rising azotemia. Albumin levels in the urine range between 3 and 20 g/liter. Variable hemorrhagic phenomena occur, including coffee-grounds hematemesis, melena, metrorrhagia, petechiae, ecchymoses, epistaxis, oozing of blood from the gums, and excessive bleeding at needle puncture sites. Laboratory abnormalities include thrombocytopenia, prolonged clotting and prothrombin times, and reduced clotting factor levels, sometimes suggesting disseminated intravascular coagulation. Death occurs on the seventh to tenth day of illness. Preterminal events include hypothermia, agitated delirium, intractable hiccups, hypoglycemia, hyperkalemia, stupor, and coma. The electrocardiogram may show ST-T wave abnormalities. CSF is under increased pressure, with elevated albumin, but contains no increase in cells, findings consistent with cerebral edema.

Convalescence may be associated with weakness and fatigability lasting several weeks. Late deaths have occurred weeks after the illness and have been ascribed to cardiac arrhythmia. Elevations of serum transaminase levels have been documented to persist for at least 2 months after onset of yellow fever. As mentioned previously, the hepatitis resolves eventually without postnecrotic scarring.

Diagnosis

Diseases that must be differentiated clinically from yellow fever include viral hepatitis, leptospirosis, DHF, Rift Valley fever, Congo-Crimean hemorrhagic fever, severe malaria, Q fever, and typhoid fever. Other virus hemorrhagic fevers, including Lassa, Marburg, and Ebola virus diseases and Bolivian and Argentine hemorrhagic fevers, are not usually associated with jaundice. The high levels of protein in the urine help distinguish yellow fever from severe malaria (blackwater fever).

The virus is most readily recovered from blood during the first 4 days after onset. The virus may also be recovered from postmortem liver tissue. However, hepatic biopsy during the illness is contraindicated and has led to fatal hemorrhage in patients in whom this procedure was performed.

Virus is isolated by intracerebral inoculation of mice, intrathoracic inoculation of *Toxorhynchites* mosquitoes, or inoculation of mosquito cell cultures, particularly *A. pseudoscutellaris* cells, with detection of virus after 3 to 4 days by IF or RT-PCR. Viral antigen is detectable in serum by immunoassay in a high proportion of cases, and the test may detect noninfectious antigen in poorly handled specimens. RT-PCR may also be used for rapid detection of virus nucleic acid in blood. A definitive postmortem diagnosis is made by detection of yellow fever virus antigen in liver tissue sections by immunocytochemical staining or RT-PCR. There are no currently available commercial diagnostic tests; the assays described remain special procedures in research and reference laboratories. Although older methods for serologic diagnosis (HI, CF, indirect

IF, and neutralization tests) are useful procedures, they have largely been replaced by the ELISA, particularly the IgM capture immunoassay. The presence of IgM antibodies in a single sample provides a presumptive diagnosis, and confirmation is made by a rise in titer between paired acute- and convalescent-phase samples.

Prevention

The control of *A. aegypti* is discussed above for dengue virus. The control of yellow fever epidemics involving wild vector species is even more difficult. Aerial applications of ultralow-volume insecticides have been attempted in the past.

The risk of acquiring yellow fever illness among unvaccinated travelers to West Africa during the peak transmission season from July to October has been estimated at 50 per 100,000 for a 2-week stay. Measures to avoid mosquito bites are likely to provide incomplete protection, making immunization the best preventive strategy. A valid certificate of vaccination is required under the International Health Regulations for entry into countries where yellow fever is endemic and for travel from such countries to receptive (*A. aegypti*-infested) countries. Detailed information on these requirements can be obtained from the CDC website.

Yellow fever 17D is a highly effective and safe, live, attenuated vaccine. Protective immunity (conferred by neutralizing antibodies) occurs in >90% of vaccinees within 10 days and 99% in 30 days after vaccination, and vaccination probably provides lifelong protection after a single dose (141). The vaccine may be simultaneously administered with other vaccines used for childhood immunization (measles, polio, diphtheria-pertussis-tetanus, and hepatitis B) or travel (hepatitis A, oral cholera, and oral or parenteral typhoid). Severe or serious adverse reactions to 17D vaccine are extremely rare. The vaccine is thus not recommended for infants under 9 months of age (6 months during epidemic risk) and is contraindicated for infants up to 5 months old because of an elevated risk of encephalitis. Among older children and adults, encephalitis, acute disseminated encephalomyelitis, and Guillain-Barré syndrome occur at a rate of approximately 0.5 to 2 cases per million doses distributed (108). In 2001, a syndrome called acute viscerotropic disease (AVD) was described to occur among yellow fever vaccinees (64). AVD is characterized by nonspecific febrile illness that rapidly progresses to multisystem failure with thrombocytopenia. The mortality rate is approximately 50%. The vaccine strain can be found in high titers in blood and many organs, such as the kidneys, that are not usually associated with yellow fever. Genetic analysis of the implicated vaccines failed to find convincing evidence that the vaccine had reverted to a more virulent phenotype. Age greater than 60 years and history of thymus disease increase the risk of AVD; host genetic risk factors are postulated.

The vaccine is manufactured in embryonated chicken eggs and is contraindicated for persons with a history of egg allergy. An intradermal test can be administered to travelers who require immunization but have a history of egg allergy.

The safety of yellow fever vaccination during pregnancy has not been clearly established. In limited studies, congenital infection appears to occur at a low rate (probably 1 to 2%) but has not been clearly associated with fetal abnormalities. A case control study of vaccination in early pregnancy indicated a nonsignificant relative risk of spontaneous abortion of 2.3, and another study concluded that there was no medical rationale to interrupt pregnancy if inadvertent vaccination in pregnancy is performed. The immune response to yellow fever vaccination during pregnancy is impaired, and serologic evaluation to detect a protective immune response is advised. Other factors that may impair seroconversion in response to 17D vaccine include malnutrition, simultaneous administration of injected cholera vaccine, and HIV infection. Asymptomatic HIV-infected travelers with $CD4^+$ cell counts of $>200/mm^3$ who require the vaccine should be immunized, but it may be prudent to confirm that they have developed neutralizing antibodies. Adverse events do not appear more frequently in HIV-infected subjects, although one case of vaccine-associated neurologic disease occurring in an HIV-infected man with a low $CD4^+$ count ($108/mm^3$) has been reported.

Immunosuppressed persons who are unable to effectively resist viral infections should not be vaccinated. A history of thymus disease is a contraindication to yellow fever vaccination.

Treatment

Treatment of yellow fever is symptomatic. There is little experience in the management of patients in modern intensive-care settings. Salicylates should be avoided due to hemorrhagic diathesis. On theoretical grounds, severely ill patients should benefit from supplemental oxygen, fluid and electrolyte management, and circulatory support. In cases with severe hemorrhage, blood replacement may be indicated. ATP depletion of the liver might be countered by administration of glycolytic substrates (fructose). Heparin treatment to reverse disseminated intravascular coagulation has been proposed, but this should be considered only in cases that have been extensively evaluated and in which consumption of clotting factors and activation of fibrinolytic mechanisms appear to predominate over diminished production. Hemodialysis may be indicated in patients with severe renal impairment. No antiviral drug has proven effective in humans. Based on animal studies, interferon and immunoglobulin are not useful after onset of the disease. A novel inhibitor of viral RNA polymerase (T-1106) reduced mortality and viremia and improved clinical parameters when administered after yellow fever virus challenge (80). Liver transplantation has not been attempted.

Other Flaviviruses Associated with Hemorrhagic Fever

Kyasanur Forest Disease Virus

Kyasanur Forest virus, first isolated in Karnataka (then Mysore) State, India, in 1957, is a member of the TBEV antigenic complex that has been subsequently termed the mammalian tick-borne virus group. The virus occurs principally in a localized region of western India, but a closely related virus, Alkhumra virus, has been discovered in Saudi Arabia (175). Subsequent studies have shown that Alkhumra virus is a genetic variant of Kyasanur Forest disease virus.

Thousands of human cases of Kyasanur Forest disease have occurred in India, principally among persons working in the forest in Karnataka State. Several hundred cases occur annually, with higher rates during epidemic years. The case fatality rate is 3 to 5%. The transmission cycle involves ixodid ticks (*Haemaphysalis spinigera*) and wild rodents and insectivores. Wild and experimentally infected monkeys become infected and succumb to the disease. Domestic livestock are important as hosts sustaining tick populations, but their role in transmission is uncertain.

The clinical illness in humans is characterized by fever, headache, myalgia, cough, bradycardia, dehydration, gastrointestinal symptoms, leukopenia, and hemorrhagic manifestations with hypotension and shock (132). In some patients, a syndrome resembling CEE occurs, with a febrile illness lasting a week or more, followed by a remission, and then reappearance of fever and signs of meningoencephalitis. The cause of hemorrhage is unknown, but disseminated intravascular coagulation has been suspected. Diagnosis is by virus isolation from blood or serology. Virus is recoverable from blood during the first week of illness (and occasionally longer). A formalin-inactivated vaccine produced in chicken embryo fibroblasts is used in affected regions of India.

Alkhumra virus was first isolated in Jeddah, Saudi Arabia, in the 1990s from the blood of a butcher admitted to the hospital with a severe infectious syndrome. At least 24 cases have been recorded in the last 10 years; all were in Saudia Arabia and involved infection via affected goats, sheep, or camels. Clinical manifestations include fever, headache, retro-orbital pain, joint pain, generalized muscle pain, anorexia and vomiting associated with leukopenia, thrombocytopenia, and elevated levels of liver enzymes (103). Some patients have had clinical symptoms of hemorrhagic fever or encephalitis, and this has resulted in the virus sometimes been termed Alkhumra hemorrhagic fever virus. Overall, the case fatality rate is 25%.

Omsk Hemorrhagic Fever Virus

Omsk hemorrhagic fever virus was originally isolated in 1947 from a patient with hemorrhagic fever in Siberia. The virus is a member of the TBEV complex with a known distribution restricted to western Siberia. Approximately 1,500 cases were reported between 1945 and 1958, and the incidence in the late 1940s was high (500 to 1,400 per 100,000 population). Cases continue to occur but at considerably lower incidence. The transmission cycle involves ixodid ticks (principally *Dermacentor reticulatus*) and rodents, especially water voles (*Arvicola terrestris*). Muskrats develop epizootic illness. Sporadic cases acquired by tick bite occur in spring and summer. Muskrat hunters may become infected by contact with blood and tissues of infected animals, and such cases can occur during the winter months. The disease in humans closely resembles Kyasanur Forest disease except that sequelae (hearing loss, hair loss, and neuropsychiatric complaints) are relatively frequent. The case fatality rate is 0.5 to 3%. Laboratory diagnosis is by virus isolation from blood or by serology. No specific Omsk hemorrhagic fever vaccine has been developed, but TBE vaccines apparently provide cross-protective immunity and have been used in high-risk population groups.

REFERENCES

1. **Abroug, F., L. Ouanes-Besbes, M. Letaief, F. Ben Romdhane, M. Khairallah, H. Triki, and N. Bouzouiaia.** 2006. A cluster study of predictors of severe West Nile virus infection. *Mayo Clin. Proc.* **81:**12–16.
2. **Andrews, D. M., V. B. Matthews, L. M. Sammels, A. C. Carrello, and P. C. McMinn.** 1999. The severity of Murray Valley encephalitis in mice is linked to neutrophil infiltration and inducible nitric oxide synthase activity in the central nervous system. *J. Virol.* **73:**8781–8790.
3. **Barrett, A. D., and S. Higgs.** 2007. Yellow fever: a disease that has yet to be conquered. *Annu. Rev. Entomol.* **52:**209–229.
4. **Barrett, A. D., and T. P. Monath.** 2003. Epidemiology and ecology of yellow fever virus. *Adv. Virus Res.* **61:**291–315.
5. **Bin, H., Z. Grossman, S. Pokamunski, M. Malkinson, L. Weiss, P. Duvdevani, C. Banet, Y. Weisman, E. Annis, D. Gandaku, V. Yahalom, M. Hindyieh, L. Shulman, and E. Mendelson.** 2001. West Nile fever in Israel 1999–2000: from geese to humans. *Ann. N.Y. Acad. Sci.* **951:**127–142.
6. **Blaney, J. E., Jr., N. S. Sathe, C. T. Hanson, C. Y. Firestone, B. R. Murphy, and S. S. Whitehead.** 2007. Vaccine candidates for dengue virus type 1 (DEN1) generated by replacement of the structural genes of rDEN4 and rDEN4Delta30 with those of DEN1. *Virol. J.* **4:**23.
7. **Brault, A. C., C. Y. Huang, S. A. Langevin, R. M. Kinney, R. A. Bowen, W. N. Ramey, N. A. Panella, E. C. Holmes, A. M. Powers, and B. R. Miller.** 2007. A single positively selected West Nile viral mutation confers increased virogenesis in American crows. *Nat. Genet.* **39:**1162–1166.
8. **Brault, A. C., S. A. Langevin, R. A. Bowen, N. A. Panella, B. J. Biggerstaff, B. R. Miller, and N. Komar.** 2004. Differential virulence of West Nile strains for American crows. *Emerg. Infect. Dis.* **10:**2161–2168.
9. **Bryant, J., H. Wang, C. Cabezas, G. Ramirez, D. Watts, K. Russell, and A. Barrett.** 2003. Enzootic transmission of yellow fever virus in Peru. *Emerg. Infect. Dis.* **9:**926–933.
10. **Bunning, M. L., R. A. Bowen, C. B. Cropp, K. G. Sullivan, B. S. Davis, N. Komar, M. S. Godsey, D. Baker, D. L. Hettler, D. A. Holmes, B. J. Biggerstaff, and C. J. Mitchell.** 2002. Experimental infection of horses with West Nile virus. *Emerg. Infect. Dis.* **8:**380–386.
11. **Burrow, J. N., P. I. Whelan, C. J. Kilburn, D. A. Fisher, B. J. Currie, and D. W. Smith.** 1998. Australian encephalitis in the Northern Territory: clinical and epidemiological features, 1987–1996. *Aust. N.Z. J. Med.* **28:**590–596.
12. **Busch, M. P., S. Caglioti, E. F. Robertson, J. D. McAuley, L. H. Tobler, H. Kamel, J. M. Linnen, V. Shyamala, P. Tomasulo, and S. H. Kleinman.** 2005. Screening the blood supply for West Nile virus RNA by nucleic acid amplification testing. *N. Engl. J. Med.* **353:**460–467.
13. **Calisher, C. H., N. Karabatsos, J. M. Dalrymple, R. E. Shope, J. S. Porterfield, E. G. Westaway, and W. E. Brandt.** 1989. Antigenic relationships between flaviviruses as determined by cross-neutralization tests with polyclonal antisera. *J. Gen. Virol.* **70**(Pt. 1)**:**37–43.
14. **Campbell, G. L., A. A. Marfin, R. S. Lanciotti, and D. J. Gubler.** 2002. West Nile virus. *Lancet Infect. Dis.* **2:**519–529.
15. **Carles, G., A. Talarmin, C. Peneau, and M. Bertsch.** 2000. Dengue fever and pregnancy. A study of 38 cases in French Guiana. *J. Gynecol. Obstet. Biol. Reprod.* **29:**758–762.
16. **Centers for Disease Control and Prevention.** 2001. Outbreak of Powassan encephalitis—Maine and Vermont, 1999–2001. *Morb. Mortal. Wkly. Rep.* **50:**761–764.
17. **Centers for Disease Control and Prevention.** 2002. Intrauterine West Nile virus infection—New York, 2002. *Morb. Mortal. Wkly. Rep.* **51:**1135–1136.
18. **Centers for Disease Control and Prevention.** 2003. West Nile virus infection among turkey breeder farm workers—

Wisconsin, 2002. *Morb. Mortal. Wkly. Rep.* **52:**1017–1019.

19. **Centers for Disease Control and Prevention.** 2005. West Nile virus infections in organ transplant recipients—New York and Pennsylvania, August–September, 2005. *Morb. Mortal. Wkly. Rep.* **54:**1021–1023.
20. **Centers for Disease Control and Prevention.** 2007. Dengue hemorrhagic fever—U.S.-Mexico border, 2005. *Morb. Mortal. Wkly. Rep.* **56:**785–789.
21. **Centers for Disease Control and Prevention.** 2007. West Nile virus activity—United States, 2006. *Morb. Mortal. Wkly. Rep.* **56:**556–559.
22. **Centers for Disease Control and Prevention.** 2007. West Nile virus transmission through blood transfusion—South Dakota, 2006. *Morb. Mortal. Wkly. Rep.* **56:**76–79.
23. **Chambers, T. J., and M. S. Diamond.** 2003. Pathogenesis of flavivirus encephalitis. *Adv. Virus Res.* **60:**273–342.
24. **Chambers, T. J., C. S. Hahn, R. Galler, and C. M. Rice.** 1990. Flavivirus genome organization, expression, and replication. *Annu. Rev. Microbiol.* **44:**649–688.
25. **Chambers, T. J., A. Nestorowicz, P. W. Mason, and C. M. Rice.** 1999. Yellow fever/Japanese encephalitis chimeric viruses: construction and biological properties. *J. Virol.* **73:**3095–3101.
26. **Chanama, S., W. Sukprasert, A. Sa-ngasang, A. Anuegoonpipat, S. Sangkitporn, I. Kurane, and S. Anantapreecha.** 2005. Detection of Japanese encephalitis (JE) virus-specific IgM in cerebrospinal fluid and serum samples from JE patients. *Jpn. J. Infect. Dis.* **58:**294–296.
27. **Chaturvedi, U. C., A. Mathur, A. Chandra, S. K. Das, H. O. Tandon, and U. K. Singh.** 1980. Transplacental infection with Japanese encephalitis virus. *J. Infect. Dis.* **141:**712–715.
28. **Chowers, M. Y., R. Lang, F. Nassar, D. Ben-David, M. Giladi, E. Rubinshtein, A. Itzhaki, J. Mishal, Y. Siegman-Igra, R. Kitzes, N. Pick, Z. Landau, D. Wolf, H. Bin, E. Mendelson, S. D. Pitlik, and M. Weinberger.** 2001. Clinical characteristics of the West Nile fever outbreak, Israel, 2000. *Emerg. Infect. Dis.* **7:**675–678.
29. **Chye, J. K., C. T. Lim, K. B. Ng, J. M. Lim, R. George, and S. K. Lam.** 1997. Vertical transmission of dengue. *Clin. Infect. Dis.* **25:**1374–1377.
30. **Corver, J., A. Ortiz, S. L. Allison, J. Schalich, F. X. Heinz, and J. Wilschut.** 2000. Membrane fusion activity of tick-borne encephalitis virus and recombinant subviral particles in a liposomal model system. *Virology* **269:**37–46.
31. **Corwin, A., M. Habib, D. Watts, M. Darwish, J. Olson, B. Botros, R. Hibbs, M. Kleinosky, H. W. Lee, R. Shope, et al.** 1993. Community-based prevalence profile of arboviral, rickettsial, and Hantaan-like viral antibody in the Nile River Delta of Egypt. *Am. J. Trop. Med. Hyg.* **48:**776–783.
32. **Davis, B. S., G. J. Chang, B. Cropp, J. T. Roehrig, D. A. Martin, C. J. Mitchell, R. Bowen, and M. L. Bunning.** 2001. West Nile virus recombinant DNA vaccine protects mouse and horse from virus challenge and expresses in vitro a noninfectious recombinant antigen that can be used in enzyme-linked immunosorbent assays. *J. Virol.* **75:**4040–4047.
33. **Davis, C. T., G. D. Ebel, R. S. Lanciotti, A. C. Brault, H. Guzman, M. Siirin, A. Lambert, R. E. Parsons, D. W. Beasley, R. J. Novak, D. Elizondo-Quiroga, E. N. Green, D. S. Young, L. M. Stark, M. A. Drebot, H. Artsob, R. B. Tesh, L. D. Kramer, and A. D. Barrett.** 2005. Phylogenetic analysis of North American West Nile virus isolates, 2001–2004: evidence for the emergence of a dominant genotype. *Virology* **342:**252–265.
34. **Day, J. F., and G. A. Curtis.** 1999. Blood feeding and oviposition by Culex nigripalpus (Diptera: Culicidae) before, during, and after a widespread St. Louis encephalitis virus epidemic in Florida. *J. Med. Entomol.* **36:**176–181.
35. **Desai, A., V. Ravi, A. Chandramuki, and M. Gourie-Devi.** 1995. Proliferative response of human peripheral blood mononuclear cells to Japanese encephalitis virus. *Microbiol. Immunol.* **39:**269–273.
36. **Desai, A., V. Ravi, S. C. Guru, S. K. Shankar, V. G. Kaliaperumal, A. Chandramuki, and M. Gourie-Devi.** 1994. Detection of autoantibodies to neural antigens in the CSF of Japanese encephalitis patients and correlation of findings with the outcome. *J. Neurol. Sci.* **122:**109–116.
37. **de Souza Lopes, O., L. de Abreu Sacchetta, T. L. Coimbra, G. H. Pinto, and C. M. Glasser.** 1978. Emergence of a new arbovirus disease in Brazil. II. Epidemiologic studies on 1975 epidemic. *Am. J. Epidemiol.* **108:**394–401.
38. **Diamond, M. S., and R. S. Klein.** 2006. A genetic basis for human susceptibility to West Nile virus. *Trends Microbiol.* **14:**287–289.
39. **Diaz, L. A., V. Re, W. R. Almiron, A. Farias, A. Vazquez, M. P. Sanchez-Seco, J. Aguilar, L. Spinsanti, B. Konigheim, A. Visintin, J. Garcia, M. A. Morales, A. Tenorio, and M. Contigiani.** 2006. Genotype III Saint Louis encephalitis virus outbreak, Argentina, 2005. *Emerg. Infect. Dis.* **12:**1752–1754.
40. **Durbin, A. P., R. A. Karron, W. Sun, D. W. Vaughn, M. J. Reynolds, J. R. Perreault, B. Thumar, R. Men, C. J. Lai, W. R. Elkins, R. M. Chanock, B. R. Murphy, and S. S. Whitehead.** 2001. Attenuation and immunogenicity in humans of a live dengue virus type-4 vaccine candidate with a 30 nucleotide deletion in its 3′-untranslated region. *Am. J. Trop. Med. Hyg.* **65:**405–413.
41. **Ecker, M., S. L. Allison, T. Meixner, and F. X. Heinz.** 1999. Sequence analysis and genetic classification of tick-borne encephalitis viruses from Europe and Asia. *J. Gen. Virol.* **80**(Pt. 1)**:**179–185.
42. **Edelman, R.** 2007. Dengue vaccines approach the finish line. *Clin. Infect. Dis.* **45**(Suppl. 1)**:**S56–S60.
43. **Effler, P. V., L. Pang, P. Kitsutani, V. Vorndam, M. Nakata, T. Ayers, J. Elm, T. Tom, P. Reiter, J. G. Rigau-Perez, J. M. Hayes, K. Mills, M. Napier, G. G. Clark, and D. J. Gubler.** 2005. Dengue fever, Hawaii, 2001–2002. *Emerg. Infect. Dis.* **11:**742–749.
44. **Egger, J. R., and P. G. Coleman.** 2007. Age and clinical dengue illness. *Emerg. Infect. Dis.* **13:**924–925.
45. **Focks, D. A., R. J. Brenner, J. Hayes, and E. Daniels.** 2000. Transmission thresholds for dengue in terms of Aedes aegypti pupae per person with discussion of their utility in source reduction efforts. *Am. J. Trop. Med. Hyg.* **62:**11–18.
46. **Garcia-Tapia, D., D. E. Hassett, W. J. Mitchell, Jr., G. C. Johnson, and S. B. Kleiboeker.** 2007. West Nile virus encephalitis: sequential histopathological and immunological events in a murine model of infection. *J. Neurovirol.* **13:**130–138.
47. **Gholam, B. I., S. Puksa, and J. P. Provias.** 1999. Powassan encephalitis: a case report with neuropathology and literature review. *Can. Med. Assoc. J.* **161:**1419–1422.
48. **Ghoshal, A., S. Das, S. Ghosh, M. K. Mishra, V. Sharma, P. Koli, E. Sen, and A. Basu.** 2007. Proinflammatory mediators released by activated microglia induces neuronal death in Japanese encephalitis. *Glia* **55:**483–496.
49. **Glass, W. G., D. H. McDermott, J. K. Lim, S. Lekhong, S. F. Yu, W. A. Frank, J. Pape, R. C. Cheshier, and**

P. M. Murphy. 2006. CCR5 deficiency increases risk of symptomatic West Nile virus infection. *J. Exp. Med.* **203:** 35–40.

50. **Grard, G., G. Moureau, R. N. Charrel, J. J. Lemasson, J. P. Gonzalez, P. Gallian, T. S. Gritsun, E. C. Holmes, E. A. Gould, and X. de Lamballerie.** 2007. Genetic characterization of tick-borne flaviviruses: new insights into evolution, pathogenetic determinants and taxonomy. *Virology* **361:**80–92.
51. **Gritsun, T. S., T. V. Frolova, V. V. Pogodina, V. A. Lashkevich, K. Venugopal, and E. A. Gould.** 1993. Nucleotide and deduced amino acid sequence of the envelope gene of the Vasilchenko strain of TBE virus; comparison with other flaviviruses. *Virus Res.* **27:**201–209.
52. **Gritsun, T. S., V. A. Lashkevich, and E. A. Gould.** 2003. tick-borne encephalitis. *Antivir. Res.* **57:**129–146.
53. **Groen, J., P. Koraka, J. Velzing, C. Copra, and A. D. Osterhaus.** 2000. Evaluation of six immunoassays for detection of dengue virus-specific immunoglobulin M and G antibodies. *Clin. Diagn. Lab. Immunol.* **7:**867–871.
54. **Grossman, R. A., R. Edelman, P. Chiewanich, P. Voodhikul, and C. Siriwan.** 1973. Study of Japanese encephalitis virus in Chiangmai valley, Thailand. II. Human clinical infections. *Am. J. Epidemiol.* **98:**121–132.
55. **Guarner, J., W. J. Shieh, S. Hunter, C. D. Paddock, T. Morken, G. L. Campbell, A. A. Marfin, and S. R. Zaki.** 2004. Clinicopathologic study and laboratory diagnosis of 23 cases with West Nile virus encephalomyelitis. *Hum. Pathol.* **35:**983–990.
56. **Gubler, D. J.** 2002. Epidemic dengue/dengue hemorrhagic fever as a public health, social and economic problem in the 21st century. *Trends Microbiol.* **10:**100–103.
57. **Gubler, D. J., W. Suharyono, R. Tan, M. Abidin, and A. Sie.** 1981. Viraemia in patients with naturally acquired dengue infection. *Bull. W. H. O.* **59:**623–630.
58. **Guirakhoo, F., S. Kitchener, D. Morrison, R. Forrat, K. McCarthy, R. Nichols, S. Yoksan, X. Duan, T. H. Ermak, N. Kanesa-Thasan, P. Bedford, J. Lang, M. J. Quentin-Millet, and T. P. Monath.** 2006. Live attenuated chimeric yellow fever dengue type 2 (ChimeriVax-DEN2) vaccine: phase I clinical trial for safety and immunogenicity: effect of yellow fever pre-immunity in induction of cross neutralizing antibody responses to all 4 dengue serotypes. *Hum. Vaccines* **2:**60–67.
59. **Guzman, M. G., and G. Kouri.** 2003. Dengue and dengue hemorrhagic fever in the Americas: lessons and challenges. *J. Clin. Virol.* **27:**1–13.
60. **Guzman, M. G., G. Kouri, L. Valdes, J. Bravo, S. Vazquez, and S. B. Halstead.** 2002. Enhanced severity of secondary dengue-2 infections: death rates in 1981 and 1997 Cuban outbreaks. *Rev. Panam. Salud Publica* **11:** 223–227.
61. **Hahn, Y. S., R. Galler, T. Hunkapiller, J. M. Dalrymple, J. H. Strauss, and E. G. Strauss.** 1988. Nucleotide sequence of dengue 2 RNA and comparison of the encoded proteins with those of other flaviviruses. *Virology* **162:** 167–180.
62. **Halstead, S. B., and E. J. O'Rourke.** 1977. Dengue viruses and mononuclear phagocytes. I. Infection enhancement by non-neutralizing antibody. *J. Exp. Med.* **146:** 201–217.
63. **Hammam, H. M., and W. H. Price.** 1966. Further observations on geographic variation in the antigenic character of West Nile and Japanese B viruses. *Am. J. Epidemiol.* **83:**113–122.
64. **Hayes, E. B.** 2007. Acute viscerotropic disease following vaccination against yellow fever. *Trans. R. Soc. Trop. Med. Hyg.* **101:**967–971.
65. **Hinckley, A. F., D. R. O'Leary, and E. B. Hayes.** 2007. Transmission of West Nile virus through human breast milk seems to be rare. *Pediatrics* **119:**e666–e671.
66. **Hoke, C. H., A. Nisalak, N. Sangawhipa, S. Jatanasen, T. Laorakapongse, B. L. Innis, S. Kotchasenee, J. B. Gingrich, J. Latendresse, K. Fukai, et al.** 1988. Protection against Japanese encephalitis by inactivated vaccines. *N. Engl. J. Med.* **319:**608–614.
67. **Holmes, E. C., M. Worobey, and A. Rambaut.** 1999. Phylogenetic evidence for recombination in dengue virus. *Mol. Biol. Evol.* **16:**405–409.
68. **Hrnicek, M. J., and M. E. Mailliard.** 2004. Acute West Nile virus in two patients receiving interferon and ribavirin for chronic hepatitis C. *Am. J. Gastroenterol.* **99:** 957.
69. **Huang, C. Y.-M., S. Butrapet, K. R. Tsuchiya, N. Bhamarapravati, D. J. Gubler, and R. M. Kinney.** 2003. Dengue 2 PDK-53 virus as a chimeric carrier for tetravalent dengue vaccine development. *J. Virol.* **77:**11436–11447.
70. **Huang, Y. H., B. I. Chang, H. Y. Lei, H. S. Liu, C. C. Liu, H. L. Wu, and T. M. Yeh.** 1997. Antibodies against dengue virus E protein peptide bind to human plasminogen and inhibit plasmin activity. *Clin. Exp. Immunol.* **110:**35–40.
71. **Hubalek, Z., and J. Halouzka.** 1999. West Nile fever—a reemerging mosquito-borne viral disease in Europe. *Emerg. Infect. Dis.* **5:**643–650.
72. **Hunsperger, E. A., and J. T. Roehrig.** 2006. Temporal analyses of the neuropathogenesis of a West Nile virus infection in mice. *J. Neurovirol.* **12:**129–139.
73. **Isaeva, M. P., G. N. Leonova, V. B. Kozhemiako, V. G. Borisevich, O. S. Maistrovskaia, and V. A. Rasskazov.** 1998. Apoptosis as a mechanism for the cytopathic action of tick-borne encephalitis virus. *Vopr. Virusol.* **43:**182–186.
74. **Iwamoto, M., D. B. Jernigan, A. Guasch, M. J. Trepka, C. G. Blackmore, W. C. Hellinger, S. M. Pham, S. Zaki, R. S. Lanciotti, S. E. Lance-Parker, C. A. Diaz-Granados, A. G. Winquist, C. A. Perlino, S. Wiersma, K. L. Hillyer, J. L. Goodman, A. A. Marfin, M. E. Chamberland, and L. R. Petersen for the West Nile Virus in Transplant Recipients Investigation Team.** 2003. Transmission of West Nile virus from an organ donor to four transplant recipients. *N. Engl. J. Med.* **348:**2196–2203.
75. **Jacobs, M. G., P. J. Robinson, C. Bletchly, J. M. Mackenzie, and P. R. Young.** 2000. Dengue virus nonstructural protein 1 is expressed in a glycosylphosphatidylinositol-linked form that is capable of signal transduction. *FASEB J.* **14:**1603–1610.
76. **Jacobson, J. A., S. L. Hills, J. L. Winkler, M. Mammen, B. Thaisomboonsuk, A. A. Marfin, and R. V. Gibbons.** 2007. Evaluation of three immunoglobulin M antibody capture enzyme-linked immunosorbent assays for diagnosis of Japanese encephalitis. *Am. J. Trop. Med. Hyg.* **77:** 164–168.
77. **Jerzak, G., K. A. Bernard, L. D. Kramer, and G. D. Ebel.** 2005. Genetic variation in West Nile virus from naturally infected mosquitoes and birds suggests quasispecies structure and strong purifying selection. *J. Gen. Virol.* **86:**2175–2183.
78. **Johnson, R. T., D. S. Burke, M. Elwell, C. J. Leake, A. Nisalak, C. H. Hoke, and W. Lorsomrudee.** 1985. Japanese encephalitis: immunocytochemical studies of viral antigen and inflammatory cells in fatal cases. *Ann. Neurol.* **18:**567–573.
79. **Johnston, L. J., G. M. Halliday, and N. J. King.** 2000. Langerhans cells migrate to local lymph nodes following

cutaneous infection with an arbovirus. *J. Investig. Dermatol.* **114:**560–568.

80. **Julander, J. G., Y. Furuta, K. Shafer, and R. W. Sidwell.** 2007. Activity of T-1106 in a hamster model of yellow fever virus infection. *Antimicrob. Agents Chemother.* **51:** 1962–1966.
81. **King, A. D., A. Nisalak, S. Kalayanrooj, K. S. Myint, K. Pattanapanyasat, S. Nimmannitya, and B. L. Innis.** 1999. B cells are the principal circulating mononuclear cells infected by dengue virus. *Southeast Asian J. Trop. Med. Public Health* **30:**718–728.
82. **King, N. J., D. R. Getts, M. T. Getts, S. Rana, B. Shrestha, and A. M. Kesson.** 2007. Immunopathology of flavivirus infections. *Immunol. Cell Biol.* **85:**33–42.
83. **Kittigul, L., N. Meethien, D. Sujirarat, C. Kittigul, and S. Vasanavat.** 1997. Comparison of dengue virus antigens in sera and peripheral blood mononuclear cells from dengue infected patients. *Asian Pac. J. Allergy Immunol.* **15:**187–191.
84. **Kleinman, S., S. A. Glynn, M. Busch, D. Todd, L. Powell, L. Pietrelli, G. Nemo, G. Schreiber, C. Bianco, and L. Katz.** 2005. The 2003 West Nile virus United States epidemic: the America's Blood Centers experience. *Transfusion* **45:**469–479.
85. **Komar, N., and G. G. Clark.** 2006. West Nile virus activity in Latin America and the Caribbean. *Rev. Panam. Salud Publica* **19:**112–117.
86. **Komar, N., S. Langevin, S. Hinten, N. Nemeth, E. Edwards, D. Hettler, B. Davis, R. Bowen, and M. Bunning.** 2003. Experimental infection of North American birds with the New York 1999 strain of West Nile virus. *Emerg. Infect. Dis.* **9:**311–322.
87. **Kouri, G. P., M. G. Guzman, J. R. Bravo, and C. Triana.** 1989. Dengue haemorrhagic fever/dengue shock syndrome: lessons from the Cuban epidemic, 1981. *Bull. W. H. O.* **67:**375–380.
88. **Kramer, L. D., and L. J. Chandler.** 2001. Phylogenetic analysis of the envelope gene of St. Louis encephalitis virus. *Arch. Virol.* **146:**2341–2355.
89. **Kumar, D., M. A. Drebot, S. J. Wong, G. Lim, H. Artsob, P. Buck, and A. Humar.** 2004. A seroprevalence study of West Nile virus infection in solid organ transplant recipients. *Am. J. Transplant.* **4:**1883–1888.
90. **Kumar, R., A. S. Selvan, S. Sharma, A. Mathur, P. K. Misra, G. K. Singh, S. Kumar, and J. Arockiasamy.** 1994. Clinical predictors of Japanese encephalitis. *Neuroepidemiology* **13:**97–102.
91. **Kuno, G.** 2001. Persistence of arboviruses and antiviral antibodies in vertebrate hosts: its occurrence and impacts. *Rev. Med. Virol.* **11:**165–190.
92. **Kuno, G.** 2007. Host range specificity of flaviviruses: correlation with in vitro replication. *J. Med. Entomol.* **44:** 93–101.
93. **Kuno, G., I. Gomez, and D. J. Gubler.** 1991. An ELISA procedure for the diagnosis of dengue infections. *J. Virol. Methods* **33:**101–113.
94. **Labuda, M., and S. E. Randolph.** 1999. Survival strategy of tick-borne encephalitis virus: cellular basis and environmental determinants. *Zentbl. Bakteriol.* **289:**513–524.
95. **LaDeau, S. L., A. M. Kilpatrick, and P. P. Marra.** 2007. West Nile virus emergence and large-scale declines of North American bird populations. *Nature* **447:**710–713.
96. **Lanciotti, R. S., G. D. Ebel, V. Deubel, A. J. Kerst, S. Murri, R. Meyer, M. Bowen, N. McKinney, W. E. Morrill, M. B. Crabtree, L. D. Kramer, and J. T. Roehrig.** 2002. Complete genome sequences and phylogenetic analysis of West Nile virus strains isolated from the United States, Europe, and the Middle East. *Virology* **298:** 96–105.
97. **Lanciotti, R. S., J. T. Roehrig, V. Deubel, J. Smith, M. Parker, K. Steele, B. Crise, K. E. Volpe, M. B. Crabtree, J. H. Scherret, R. A. Hall, J. S. MacKenzie, C. B. Cropp, B. Panigrahy, E. Ostlund, B. Schmitt, M. Malkinson, C. Banet, J. Weissman, N. Komar, H. M. Savage, W. Stone, T. McNamara, and D. J. Gubler.** 1999. Origin of the West Nile virus responsible for an outbreak of encephalitis in the northeastern United States. *Science* **286:**2333–2337.
98. **Leitmeyer, K. C., D. W. Vaughn, D. M. Watts, R. Salas, I. Villalobos de Chacon, C. Ramos, and R. Rico-Hesse.** 1999. Dengue virus structural differences that correlate with pathogenesis. *J. Virol.* **73:**4738–4747.
99. **Liu, Y., N. King, A. Kesson, R. V. Blanden, and A. Mullbacher.** 1989. Flavivirus infection up-regulates the expression of class I and class II major histocompatibility antigens on and enhances T cell recognition of astrocytes in vitro. *J. Neuroimmunol.* **21:**157–168.
100. **Logar, M., P. Bogovic, D. Cerar, T. Avsic-Zupanc, and F. Strle.** 2006. Tick-borne encephalitis in Slovenia from 2000 to 2004: comparison of the course in adult and elderly patients. *Wien. Klin. Wochenschr.* **118:**702–707.
101. **Mackenzie, J. S., A. K. Broom, R. A. Hall, C. A. Johansen, M. D. Lindsay, D. A. Phillips, S. A. Ritchie, R. C. Russell, and D. W. Smith.** 1998. Arboviruses in the Australian region, 1990 to 1998. *Commun. Dis. Intell.* **22:**93–100.
102. **Mackenzie, J. S., D. J. Gubler, and L. R. Petersen.** 2004. Emerging flaviviruses: the spread and resurgence of Japanese encephalitis, West Nile and dengue viruses. *Nat. Med.* **10:**S98–S109.
103. **Madani, T. A.** 2005. Alkhumra virus infection, a new viral hemorrhagic fever in Saudi Arabia. *J. Infect.* **51:** 91–97.
104. **Malkinson, M., C. Banet, Y. Weisman, S. Pokamunski, R. King, M. T. Drouet, and V. Deubel.** 2002. Introduction of West Nile virus in the Middle East by migrating white storks. *Emerg. Infect. Dis.* **8:**392–397.
105. **Marianneau, P., A. M. Steffan, C. Royer, M. T. Drouet, A. Kirn, and V. Deubel.** 1998. Differing infection patterns of dengue and yellow fever viruses in a human hepatoma cell line. *J. Infect. Dis.* **178:**1270–1278.
106. **Mathew, A., I. Kurane, A. L. Rothman, L. L. Zeng, M. A. Brinton, and F. A. Ennis.** 1996. Dominant recognition by human CD8+ cytotoxic T lymphocytes of dengue virus nonstructural proteins NS3 and NS1.2a. *J. Clin. Investig.* **98:**1684–1691.
107. **May, F. J., M. Lobigs, E. Lee, D. J. Gendle, J. S. Mackenzie, A. K. Broom, J. V. Conlan, and R. A. Hall.** 2006. Biological, antigenic and phylogenetic characterization of the flavivirus Alfuy. *J. Gen. Virol.* **87:**329–337.
108. **McMahon, A. W., R. B. Eidex, A. A. Marfin, M. Russell, J. J. Sejvar, L. Markoff, E. B. Hayes, R. T. Chen, R. Ball, M. M. Braun, and M. Cetron.** 2007. Neurologic disease associated with 17D-204 yellow fever vaccination: a report of 15 cases. *Vaccine* **25:**1727–1734.
109. **McMinn, P. C.** 1997. The molecular basis of virulence of the encephalitogenic flaviviruses. *J. Gen. Virol.* **78**(Pt. 11)**:**2711–2722.
110. **McNeil, J. G., W. M. Lednar, S. K. Stansfield, R. E. Prier, and R. N. Miller.** 1985. Central European tick-borne encephalitis: assessment of risk for persons in the armed services and vacationers. *J. Infect. Dis.* **152:**650–651.
111. **Minke, J. M., L. Siger, K. Karaca, L. Austgen, P. Gordy, R. Bowen, R. W. Renshaw, S. Loosmore, J. C. Audonnet, and B. Nordgren.** 2004. Recombinant canarypoxvirus vaccine carrying the prM/E genes of West

Nile virus protects horses against a West Nile virus-mosquito challenge. *Arch. Virol. Suppl.* **18:**221–230.

112. **Misra, U. K., J. Kalita, U. K. Syam, and T. N. Dhole.** 2006. Neurological manifestations of dengue virus infection. *J. Neurol. Sci.* **244:**117–122.
113. **Monath, T. P.** 1987. Yellow fever: a medically neglected disease. Report on a seminar. *Rev. Infect. Dis.* **9:**165–175.
114. **Monath, T. P., and A. D. Barrett.** 2003. Pathogenesis and pathophysiology of yellow fever. *Adv. Virus Res.* **60:** 343–395.
115. **Monath, T. P., R. B. Craven, A. Adjukiewicz, M. Germain, D. B. Francy, L. Ferrara, E. M. Samba, H. N'Jie, K. Cham, S. A. Fitzgerald, P. H. Crippen, D. I. Simpson, E. T. Bowen, A. Fabiyi, and J. J. Salaun.** 1980. Yellow fever in the Gambia, 1978–1979: epidemiologic aspects with observations on the occurrence of Orungo virus infections. *Am. J. Trop. Med. Hyg.* **29:**912–928.

115a. **Monath, T. P., and F. X. Heinz.** 1996. Flaviviruses, p. 994. *In* B. N. Fields, D. M. Knipe, and P. M. Howley (ed.), *Fields Virology*, 3rd ed. Lippincott-Raven, Philadelphia, PA.

116. **Monath, T. P., J. Liu, N. Kanesa-Thasan, G. A. Myers, R. Nichols, A. Deary, K. McCarthy, C. Johnson, T. Ermak, S. Shin, J. Arroyo, F. Guirakhoo, J. S. Kennedy, F. A. Ennis, S. Green, and P. Bedford.** 2006. A live, attenuated recombinant West Nile virus vaccine. *Proc. Natl. Acad. Sci. USA* **103:**6694–6699.
117. **Monath, T. P., and T. F. Tsai.** 1987. St. Louis encephalitis: lessons from the last decade. *Am. J. Trop. Med. Hyg.* **37:**40S–59S.
118. **Morales, M. A., M. Barrandeguy, C. Fabbri, J. B. Garcia, A. Vissani, K. Trono, G. Gutierrez, S. Pigretti, H. Menchaca, N. Garrido, N. Taylor, F. Fernandez, S. Levis, and D. Enria.** 2006. West Nile virus isolation from equines in Argentina, 2006. *Emerg. Infect. Dis.* **12:** 1559–1561.
119. **Morrey, J. D., C. W. Day, J. G. Julander, L. M. Blatt, D. F. Smee, and R. W. Sidwell.** 2004. Effect of interferon-alpha and interferon-inducers on West Nile virus in mouse and hamster animal models. *Antivir. Chem. Chemother.* **15:**101–109.
120. **Mostashari, F., M. L. Bunning, P. T. Kitsutani, D. A. Singer, D. Nash, M. J. Cooper, N. Katz, K. A. Liljebjelke, B. J. Biggerstaff, A. D. Fine, M. C. Layton, S. M. Mullin, A. J. Johnson, D. A. Martin, E. B. Hayes, and G. L. Campbell.** 2001. Epidemic West Nile encephalitis, New York, 1999: results of a household-based seroepidemiological survey. *Lancet* **358:**261–264.
121. **Nasci, R. S., H. M. Savage, D. J. White, J. R. Miller, B. C. Cropp, M. S. Godsey, A. J. Kerst, P. Bennett, K. Gottfried, and R. S. Lanciotti.** 2001. West Nile virus in overwintering Culex mosquitoes, New York City, 2000. *Emerg. Infect. Dis.* **7:**742–744.
122. **Nash, D., F. Mostashari, A. Fine, J. Miller, D. O'Leary, K. Murray, A. Huang, A. Rosenberg, A. Greenberg, M. Sherman, S. Wong, and M. Layton.** 2001. The outbreak of West Nile virus infection in the New York City area in 1999. *N. Engl. J. Med.* **344:**1807–1814.
123. **Nishiura, H., and S. B. Halstead.** 2007. Natural history of dengue virus (DENV)-1 and DENV-4 infections: reanalysis of classic studies. *J. Infect. Dis.* **195:**1007–1013.
124. **Nuttall, P. A.** 1999. Pathogen-tick-host interactions: Borrelia burgdorferi and TBE virus. *Zentbl. Bakteriol.* **289:**492–505.
125. **Ogawa, M., H. Okubo, Y. Tsuji, N. Yasui, and K. Someda.** 1973. Chronic progressive encephalitis occurring 13 years after Russian spring-summer encephalitis. *J. Neurol. Sci.* **19:**363–373.
126. **O'Leary, D. R., S. Kuhn, K. L. Kniss, A. F. Hinckley, S. A. Rasmussen, W. J. Pape, L. K. Kightlinger, B. D. Beecham, T. K. Miller, D. F. Neitzel, S. R. Michaels, G. L. Campbell, R. S. Lanciotti, and E. B. Hayes.** 2006. Birth outcomes following West Nile virus infection of pregnant women in the United States: 2003–2004. *Pediatrics* **117:**e537–e545.
127. **O'Leary, D. R., A. A. Marfin, S. P. Montgomery, A. M. Kipp, J. A. Lehman, B. J. Biggerstaff, V. L. Elko, P. D. Collins, J. E. Jones, and G. L. Campbell.** 2004. The epidemic of West Nile virus in the United States, 2002. *Vector Borne Zoonot. Dis.* **4:**61–70.
128. **Ooi, E. E., K. T. Goh, and D. J. Gubler.** 2006. Dengue prevention and 35 years of vector control in Singapore. *Emerg. Infect. Dis.* **12:**887–893.
129. **Paisley, J. E., A. F. Hinckley, D. R. O'Leary, W. C. Kramer, R. S. Lanciotti, G. L. Campbell, and E. B. Hayes.** 2006. West Nile virus infection among pregnant women in a northern Colorado community, 2003 to 2004. *Pediatrics* **117:**814–820.
130. **Pang, T., M. J. Cardosa, and M. G. Guzman.** 2007. Of cascades and perfect storms: the immunopathogenesis of dengue haemorrhagic fever-dengue shock syndrome (DHF/DSS). *Immunol. Cell Biol.* **85:**43–45.
131. **Patnaik, J. L., H. Harmon, and R. L. Vogt.** 2006. Follow-up of 2003 human West Nile virus infections, Denver, Colorado. *Emerg. Infect. Dis.* **12:**1129–1131.
132. **Pavri, K.** 1989. Clinical, clinicopathologic, and hematologic features of Kyasanur Forest disease. *Rev. Infect. Dis.* **11**(Suppl. 4)**:**S854–S859.
133. **Pealer, L. N., A. A. Marfin, L. R. Petersen, R. S. Lanciotti, P. L. Page, S. L. Stramer, M. G. Stobierski, K. Signs, B. Newman, H. Kapoor, J. L. Goodman, and M. E. Chamberland.** 2003. Transmission of West Nile virus through blood transfusion in the United States in 2002. *N. Engl. J. Med.* **349:**1236–1245.
134. **Pepperell, C., N. Rau, S. Krajden, R. Kern, A. Humar, B. Mederski, A. Simor, D. E. Low, A. McGeer, T. Mazzulli, J. Burton, C. Jaigobin, M. Fearon, H. Artsob, M. A. Drebot, W. Halliday, and J. Brunton.** 2003. West Nile virus infection in 2002: morbidity and mortality among patients admitted to hospital in southcentral Ontario. *Can. Med. Assoc. J.* **168:**1399–1405.
135. **Perelygin, A. A., S. V. Scherbik, I. B. Zhulin, B. M. Stockman, Y. Li, and M. A. Brinton.** 2002. Positional cloning of the murine flavivirus resistance gene. *Proc. Natl. Acad. Sci. USA* **99:**9322–9327.
136. **Petersen, L. R., and E. B. Hayes.** 2004. Westward ho?—the spread of West Nile virus. *N. Engl. J. Med.* **351:**2257–2259.
137. **Petersen, L. R., and A. A. Marfin.** 2005. Shifting epidemiology of Flaviviridae. *J. Travel Med.* **12**(Suppl. 1)**:** S3–S11.
138. **Petersen, L. R., and J. T. Roehrig.** 2001. West Nile virus: a reemerging global pathogen. *Emerg. Infect. Dis.* **7:**611–614.
139. **Pogodina, V. V., M. P. Frolova, G. V. Malenko, G. I. Fokina, G. V. Koreshkova, L. L. Kiseleva, N. G. Bochkova, and N. M. Ralph.** 1983. Study on West Nile virus persistence in monkeys. *Arch. Virol.* **75:**71–86.
140. **Pogodina, V. V., and A. P. Savinov.** 1964. Variation in the pathogenicity of viruses of the tick-borne encephalitis complex for different animal species. I. Experimental infection of mice and hamsters. *Acta Virol.* **8:**424–434.
141. **Poland, J. D., C. H. Calisher, T. P. Monath, W. G. Downs, and K. Murphy.** 1981. Persistence of neutral-

izing antibody 30–35 years after immunization with 17D yellow fever vaccine. *Bull. W. H. O.* **59:**895–900.

142. **Pradhan, S., N. Pandey, S. Shashank, R. K. Gupta, and A. Mathur.** 1999. Parkinsonism due to predominant involvement of substantia nigra in Japanese encephalitis. *Neurology* **53:**1781–1786.
143. **Prince, H. E., L. H. Tobler, M. Lape-Nixon, G. A. Foster, S. L. Stramer, and M. P. Busch.** 2005. Development and persistence of West Nile virus-specific immunoglobulin M (IgM), IgA, and IgG in viremic blood donors. *J. Clin. Microbiol.* **43:**4316–4320.
144. **Rayamajhi, A., R. Singh, R. Prasad, B. Khanal, and S. Singhi.** 2006. Clinico-laboratory profile and outcome of Japanese encephalitis in Nepali children. *Ann. Trop. Paediatr.* **26:**293–301.
145. **Rey, F. A., F. X. Heinz, C. Mandl, C. Kunz, and S. C. Harrison.** 1995. The envelope glycoprotein from tick-borne encephalitis virus at 2 A resolution. *Nature* **375:** 291–298.
146. **Rico-Hesse, R.** 1990. Molecular evolution and distribution of dengue viruses type 1 and 2 in nature. *Virology* **174:**479–493.
147. **Rico-Hesse, R., L. M. Harrison, R. A. Salas, D. Tovar, A. Nisalak, C. Ramos, J. Boshell, M. T. de Mesa, R. M. Nogueira, and A. T. da Rosa.** 1997. Origins of dengue type 2 viruses associated with increased pathogenicity in the Americas. *Virology* **230:**244–251.
148. **Rigau-Perez, J. G.** 1997. Clinical manifestations of dengue hemorrhagic fever in Puerto Rico, 1990–1991. *Rev. Panam. Salud Publica* **1:**381–388.
149. **Robertson, E. G.** 1952. Murray Valley encephalitis; pathological aspects. *Med. J. Aust.* **1:**107–110.
150. **Sabchareon, A., and S. Yoksan.** 1998. Japanese encephalitis. *Ann. Trop. Paediatr.* **18**(Suppl.)**:**S67–S71.
151. **Sabin, A. B.** 1952. Research on dengue during World War II. *Am. J. Trop. Med. Hyg.* **1:**30–50.
152. **Salazar, P., J. L. Traub-Dargatz, P. S. Morley, D. D. Wilmot, D. J. Steffen, W. E. Cunningham, and M. D. Salman.** 2004. Outcome of equids with clinical signs of West Nile virus infection and factors associated with death. *J. Am. Vet. Med. Assoc.* **225:**267–274.
153. **Samuel, M. A., and M. S. Diamond.** 2006. Pathogenesis of West Nile virus infection: a balance between virulence, innate and adaptive immunity, and viral evasion. *J. Virol.* **80:**9349–9360.
154. **Schlesinger, J. J., M. W. Brandriss, J. R. Putnak, and E. E. Walsh.** 1990. Cell surface expression of yellow fever virus non-structural glycoprotein NS1: consequences of interaction with antibody. *J. Gen. Virol.* **71**(Pt. 3)**:** 593–599.
155. **Schneider, B. S., L. Soong, Y. A. Girard, G. Campbell, P. Mason, and S. Higgs.** 2006. Potentiation of West Nile encephalitis by mosquito feeding. *Viral Immunol.* **19:**74–82.
156. **Sejvar, J. J., A. V. Bode, A. A. Marfin, G. L. Campbell, D. Ewing, M. Mazowiecki, P. V. Pavot, J. Schmitt, J. Pape, B. J. Biggerstaff, and L. R. Petersen.** 2005. West Nile virus-associated flaccid paralysis. *Emerg. Infect. Dis.* **11:**1021–1027.
157. **Sejvar, J. J., M. B. Haddad, B. C. Tierney, G. L. Campbell, A. A. Marfin, J. A. Van Gerpen, A. Fleischauer, A. A. Leis, D. S. Stokic, and L. R. Petersen.** 2003. Neurologic manifestations and outcome of West Nile virus infection. *JAMA* **290:**511–515.
158. **Solomon, T.** 2004. Flavivirus encephalitis. *N. Engl. J. Med.* **351:**370–378.
159. **Solomon, T., N. M. Dung, D. W. Vaughn, R. Kneen, L. T. Thao, B. Raengsakulrach, H. T. Loan, N. P. Day, J. Farrar, K. S. Myint, M. J. Warrell, W. S. James, A. Nisalak, and N. J. White.** 2000. Neurological manifestations of dengue infection. *Lancet* **355:**1053–1059.
160. **Solomon, T., N. M. Dung, B. Wills, R. Kneen, M. Gainsborough, T. V. Diet, T. T. Thuy, H. T. Loan, V. C. Khanh, D. W. Vaughn, N. J. White, and J. J. Farrar.** 2003. Interferon alfa-2a in Japanese encephalitis: a randomised double-blind placebo-controlled trial. *Lancet* **361:**821–826.
161. **Southam, C. M., and A. E. Moore.** 1954. Induced virus infections in man by the Egypt isolates of West Nile virus. *Am. J. Trop. Med. Hyg.* **3:**19–50.
162. **Tandan, J. B., H. Ohrr, Y. M. Sohn, S. Yoksan, M. Ji, C. M. Nam, and S. B. Halstead.** 2007. Single dose of SA 14-14-2 vaccine provides long-term protection against Japanese encephalitis: a case-control study in Nepalese children 5 years after immunization. *Vaccine* **25:**5041–5045.
163. **Thein, S., M. M. Aung, T. N. Shwe, M. Aye, A. Zaw, K. Aye, K. M. Aye, and J. Aaskov.** 1997. Risk factors in dengue shock syndrome. *Am. J. Trop. Med. Hyg.* **56:** 566–572.
164. **Tilley, P. A., J. D. Fox, G. C. Jayaraman, and J. K. Preiksaitis.** 2006. Nucleic acid testing for West Nile virus RNA in plasma enhances rapid diagnosis of acute infection in symptomatic patients. *J. Infect. Dis.* **193:** 1361–1364.
165. **Tsai, T. F., F. Popovici, C. Cernescu, G. L. Campbell, and N. I. Nedelcu.** 1998. West Nile encephalitis epidemic in southeastern Romania. *Lancet* **352:**767–771.
166. **Tsarev, S. A., M. L. Sanders, D. W. Vaughn, and B. L. Innis.** 2000. Phylogenetic analysis suggests only one serotype of Japanese encephalitis virus. *Vaccine* **18**(Suppl. 2)**:**36–43.
167. **Vaughn, D. W., and C. H. Hoke, Jr.** 1992. The epidemiology of Japanese encephalitis: prospects for prevention. *Epidemiol. Rev.* **14:**197–221.
168. **Watson, J. T., P. E. Pertel, R. C. Jones, A. M. Siston, W. S. Paul, C. C. Austin, and S. I. Gerber.** 2004. Clinical characteristics and functional outcomes of West Nile fever. *Ann. Intern. Med.* **141:**360–365.
169. **Watts, D. M., K. R. Porter, P. Putvatana, B. Vasquez, C. Calampa, C. G. Hayes, and S. B. Halstead.** 1999. Failure of secondary infection with American genotype dengue 2 to cause dengue haemorrhagic fever. *Lancet* **354:**1431–1434.
170. **Whitehead, S. S., J. E. Blaney, A. P. Durbin, and B. R. Murphy.** 2007. Prospects for a dengue virus vaccine. *Nat. Rev. Microbiol.* **5:**518–528.
171. **World Health Organization.** 1997. *Dengue Haemorrhagic Fever: Diagnosis, Treatment, Prevention, and Control,* 2nd ed., p. 12–23. World Health Organization, Geneva, Switzerland.
172. **Wu, S. C., W. C. Lian, L. C. Hsu, and M. Y. Liau.** 1997. Japanese encephalitis virus antigenic variants with characteristic differences in neutralization resistance and mouse virulence. *Virus Res.* **51:**173–181.
173. **Wu, S. J., G. Grouard-Vogel, W. Sun, J. R. Mascola, E. Brachtel, R. Putvatana, M. K. Louder, L. Filgueira, M. A. Marovich, H. K. Wong, A. Blauvelt, G. S. Murphy, M. L. Robb, B. L. Innes, D. L. Birx, C. G. Hayes, and S. S. Frankel.** 2000. Human skin Langerhans cells are targets of dengue virus infection. *Nat. Med.* **6:**816–820.
174. **Yakub, I., K. M. Lillibridge, A. Moran, O. Y. Gonzalez, J. Belmont, R. A. Gibbs, and D. J. Tweardy.** 2005.

Single nucleotide polymorphisms in genes for 2′-5′-oligoadenylate synthetase and RNase L in patients hospitalized with West Nile virus infection. *J. Infect. Dis.* **192:**1741–1748.

175. **Zaki, A. M.** 1997. Isolation of a flavivirus related to the tick-borne encephalitis complex from human cases in Saudi Arabia. *Trans. R. Soc. Trop. Med. Hyg.* **91:**179–181.

176. **Zanotto, P. M., E. A. Gould, G. F. Gao, P. H. Harvey, and E. C. Holmes.** 1996. Population dynamics of flaviviruses revealed by molecular phylogenies. *Proc. Natl. Acad. Sci. USA* **93:**548–553.

Hepatitis C Virus

YARON ROTMAN AND T. JAKE LIANG

53

Hepatitis C virus (HCV), a member of the genus *Hepacivirus* in the *Flaviviridae* family, is a single-stranded RNA virus that infects humans and other higher primates and has a selective tropism to the liver. Following exposure, HCV is able to evade the host's immune system and establishes a chronic, often asymptomatic infection that may lead to liver failure, hepatocellular carcinoma, and death. Transmitted primarily through exposure to infected blood, but also through sexual and perinatal routes, the virus is estimated to infect 2% of the world's population. Originally termed non-A, non-B hepatitis, infection with HCV was a frequent cause of transfusion-related hepatitis until discovery of the virus in 1989 (31, 91) and the subsequent development of effective screening methods (see chapter 5 for a detailed discussion). Although great advances have been made in prevention and treatment of HCV infection, many patients still succumb to the disease, while many others remain undiagnosed.

VIROLOGY

Classification

Genotypes

Shortly after the identification of HCV, it became apparent that the virus is highly heterogeneous and that widely divergent genetic strains can be identified (27). The driving force for this variability is inherent to the replication strategy of the virus, which is mediated by an error-prone RNA-dependent RNA polymerase with a mutation rate of 10^{-4} to 10^{-5} per nucleotide (117), and a high replication level, with an estimated production rate of 10^{12} virions per day (113). This mutagenic tendency is balanced by viral and host constraints. The genetic variability can manifest at different levels, as genotypic, subgenotypic, or even quasispecies differences within the same host (103). These different levels of variability probably reflect different sources and selection pressures for heterogeneity. For instance, hypervariable region 1 (HVR-1) in the E2 gene has remarkable heterogeneity among different isolates, even within patients, probably as a consequence of its antigenicity and selective pressure by the host immune system. The genotypic variability, on the other hand, helps shed light on the evolutionary origin of the virus and its shared history with humankind. A suggested model, based on the genotype and subtype distribution, has been described for the endemic infection in sub-Saharan Africa and Southeast Asia, which has persisted for a considerable time. This infection then rapidly spread in the last century to the Western world and other countries with the advent of medical practices (blood transfusion and use of syringes) as well as with the epidemic of injection drug abuse (144).

On the basis of phylogenetic analysis, HCV can be classified into six distinct genotypes, differing from each other by 30 to 35% of their nucleotide sequences (Fig. 1). The genotypes themselves can be further subdivided into subtypes, with a genomic difference of 20 to 25% (144). The viral genotypes differ with respect to geographic origin and global distribution (Fig. 2) and respond differently to interferon-based treatment. In general, no specific genotype appears to be associated with disease severity, although genotype 3 is frequently associated with hepatic steatosis.

Serotypes and Antigenicity

Serotyping of HCV, although not commonly used in clinical practice, is possible. The nonstructural protein NS4 has an antigenic region that is highly variable among different viral types. This variability confers type-specific antibodies in infected patients. A commercial serotyping kit based on detection of antibodies with NS4-derived synthetic peptides has a reported sensitivity of 77% and a specificity of 94% (56). The low sensitivity, combined with the availability of more accurate nucleic acid-based methods, renders this assay less practical. In most clinical settings in the developed world, genotyping assays are preferred, although the serotyping method may be more practical for developing countries.

Composition of Virus

Virion Morphology, Structure, and Size

The lack of an efficient in vitro system for efficient replication and export has hampered the study of the physical properties of the HCV particle. However, even before the virus was successfully identified, inactivation by chloroform was demonstrated, suggesting a lipid membrane envelope (44), and filtration studies estimated the particle size at 30 to 60 nm. Electron microscopy studies identified HCV par-

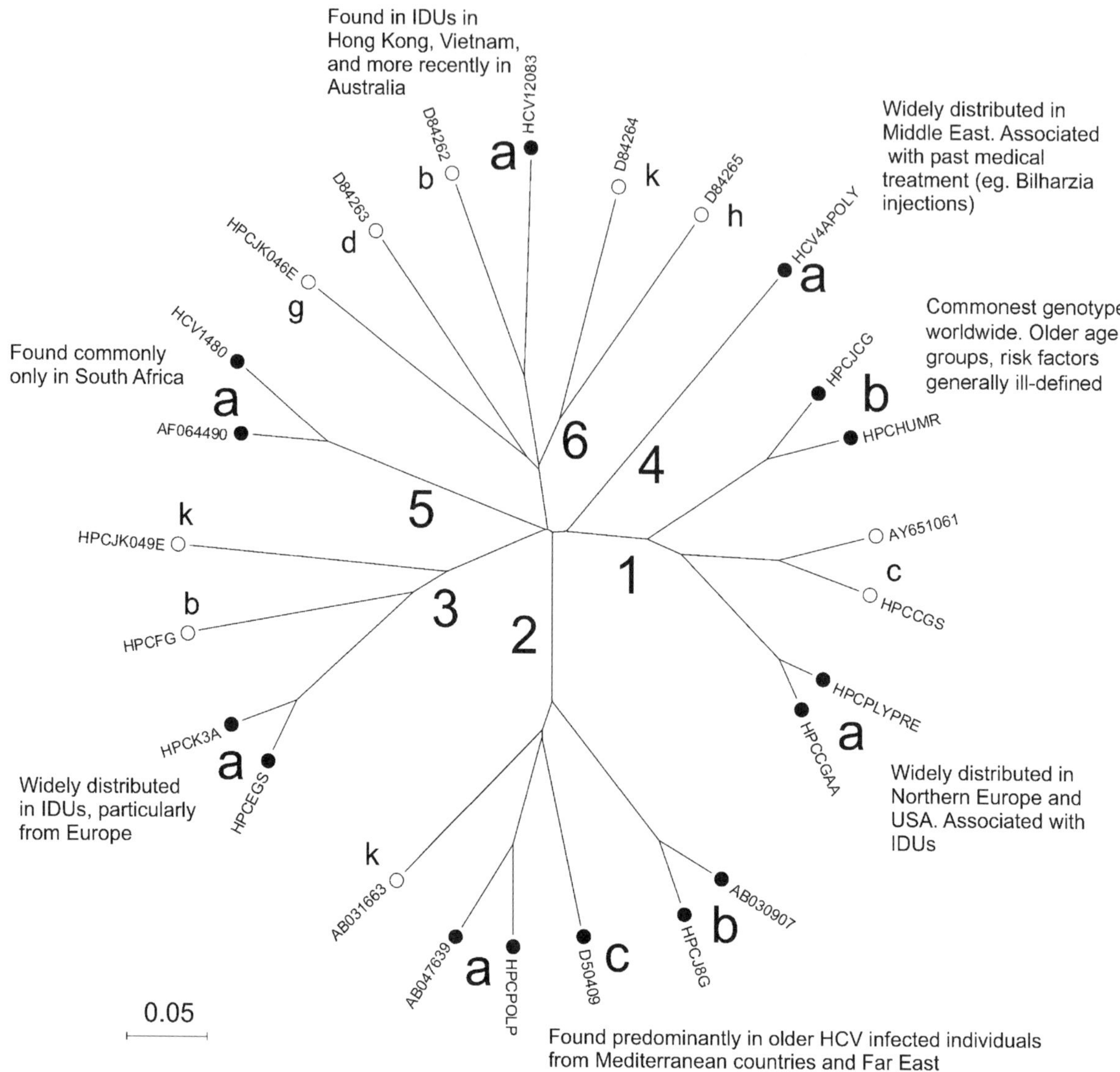
Found in IDUs in Hong Kong, Vietnam, and more recently in Australia
Widely distributed in Middle East. Associated with past medical treatment (eg. Bilharzia injections)
Commonest genotype worldwide. Older age groups, risk factors generally ill-defined
Found commonly only in South Africa
Widely distributed in Northern Europe and USA. Associated with IDUs
Widely distributed in IDUs, particularly from Europe
Found predominantly in older HCV infected individuals from Mediterranean countries and Far East
HCV12083
D84262
D84263
HPCJK046E
HCV1480
AF064490
HPCJK049E
HPCFG
HPCK3A
HPCEGS
AB031663
AB047639
HPCPOLP
D50409
HPCJ8G
AB030907
HPCCGAA
HPCPLYPRE
HPCCGS
AY651061
HPCHUMR
HPCJCG
HCV4APOLY
D84265
D84264
1
2
3
4
5
6
0.05

FIGURE 1 Phylogenetic analysis of complete open reading frame sequences demonstrating clustering to six genotypes and subgenotypes. The major epidemiological attributes of each genotype are noted. IDUs, injection drug users. (Reprinted from reference 144 with permission of Wiley-Liss, Inc., a subsidiary of John Wiley & Sons, Inc.)

ticles with sizes of 55 to 65 nm (83) (Fig. 3a). The reported density for virus particles has a wide range, <1.06 to 1.3 g/ml (8).

Although the HCV particle itself is difficult to demonstrate, by inferring from the virions of other *Flaviviridae*, the putative particle is composed of a nucleocapsid composed of the core protein and viral RNA, surrounded by a phospholipid membrane in which the viral envelope proteins are embedded. Apart from lipid-enveloped virions, naked nucleocapsids may also be circulating in the plasma, perhaps playing a role in the viral interaction with the immune system. Another form of viral particle circulating in the plasma is the lipo-viro-particle, which is rich in triglycerides and contains viral RNA, core protein, apolipoprotein B, and apolipoprotein E (8). Recent advances in a cell culture system provide a unique opportunity to visualize and study the structural features of HCV virions by electron microscopy (Fig. 3b).

Genome Organization and Composition

The HCV genome, like that of other members of the *Flaviviridae* family, is a single-stranded positive-sense RNA of about 9,600 nucleotides (nt). The genome contains a single large open reading frame, coding for a polyprotein of 3,300 amino acids, flanked by two highly conserved untranslated regions (UTRs) at the 5′ and 3′ ends (Fig. 4a).

The 5′ UTR (Fig. 4b) contains an internal ribosomal entry site (IRES) which interacts with the ribosomal machinery to facilitate cap-independent viral protein synthesis (50). The IRES has a conserved secondary structure comprising three domains that extend to the N-terminal core coding sequence and are essential for its function. Also contained in this region, upstream of the IRES, is a short sequence, conserved among all genotypes, that is recognized by a liver-specific microRNA (82). Mutations introduced into this conserved segment significantly reduce

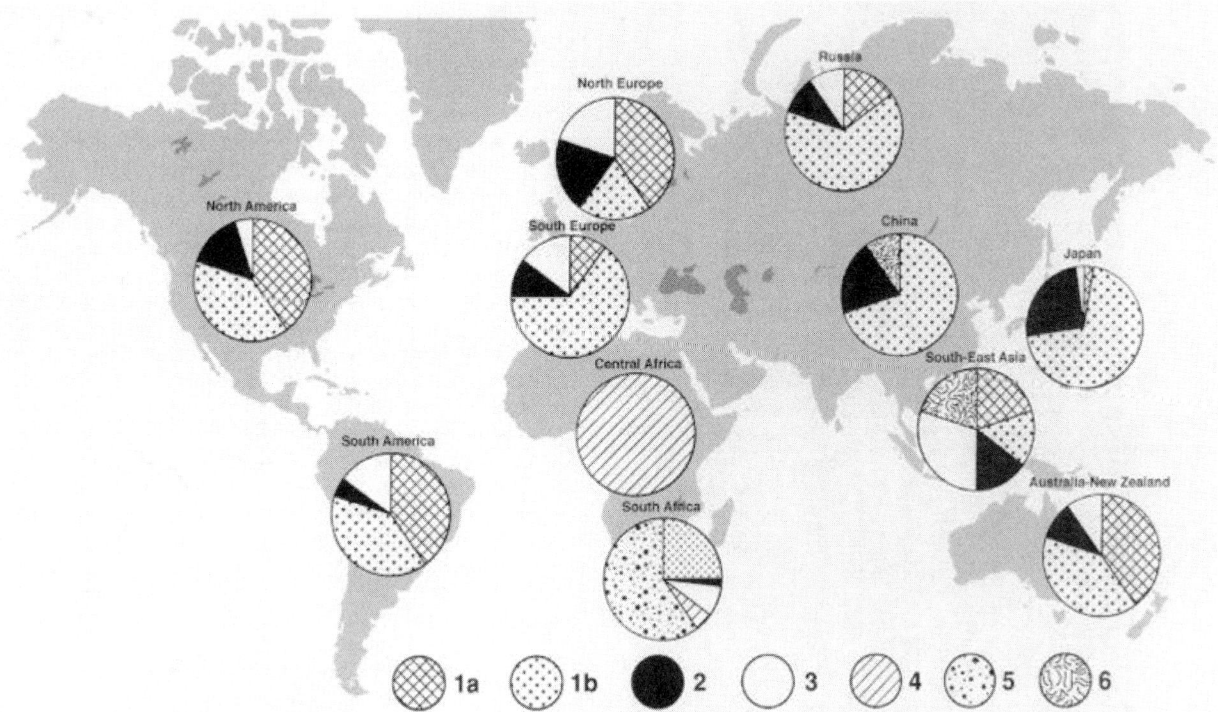

FIGURE 2 Geographic distribution of HCV genotypes. Genotype 1 is the most prevalent and can be seen worldwide. Genotype 3 is more common in south and Southeast Asia; genotype 4 is seen almost exclusively in patients from central Africa, Egypt, and Saudi Arabia; genotype 5 is mostly confined to South Africa; and genotype 6 is confined to Southeast Asia. (Reprinted from reference 47 with permission of Elsevier.)

viral replication in vitro, suggesting that this endogenous microRNA modulates the replication efficiency.

The UTR at the 3′ end of the HCV genome is required for replication. This region consists of three distinct domains: a highly variable 40-nt domain, a poly(U/C) tract of heterogeneous length, and a highly conserved, 98-nt-long "X" tail organized into three stem-loop structures (Fig. 4c). All of these domains are essential for effective replication (52, 164). The second stem-loop (stem-loop II) of the X segment is able to base-pair with another loop (stem-loop V) in the NS5B coding region, with the poly (U/C) tract probably serving as a flexible linker. As stem-loop V may be the binding site for the viral RNA polymerase, this closed-loop formation serves to bring the 3′ end of the positive-strand RNA into alignment with this site, to facilitate initiation of negative-strand synthesis.

Structural and Nonstructural Proteins

Translation of the open reading frame produces a single large polyprotein of about 3,300 amino acids. This polyprotein is then cleaved by host and viral proteases to produce three structural proteins (core, E1, and E2) and seven nonstructural proteins (p7 and NS2 to NS5) (Table 1).

The core protein is a basic, RNA-binding protein that together with the viral genome forms the viral nucleocapsid. After translation and cleavage of the first 191 amino acids of the viral polyprotein, it undergoes a series of posttranslational modifications before it becomes functional. The core protein is able to interact with multiple host proteins and induce gene expression. It has been implicated in the development of liver steatosis, carcinogenesis (112), apoptosis, and immunomodulation.

The two envelope proteins, E1 and E2, are type I transmembrane glycoproteins with an N-terminal ectodomain. After cleavage by signal peptidase, these proteins are associated with the endoplasmic reticulum (ER) membrane, where their ectodomain undergoes modification by N-linked glycosylation (154). They form noncovalent heterodimers that function as the building blocks for the assembly of the virion. Although both proteins are required for cell entry facilitation, E2 is probably the major viral protein to interact with host cell surface molecules and is thought to mediate viral entry.

p7 is a hydrophobic 63-amino-acid protein that is associated intracellularly with ER and mitochondrial membranes and is able to form a multimeric cation channel that can be blocked by amantadine (63). Its exact role in the viral life cycle is not clear; it is not required for in vitro replication but is essential for the formation of infectious virus (81). It is possible that the pore formed by p7 modulates intra-ER pH to protect viral glycoproteins during maturation and export.

NS2 is a 216-amino-acid protein that together with NS3 forms a cysteine protease (158) with an autocatalytic activity separating the two components from each other. The cleaved protein was also found to be essential for assembly of infectious virions, probably at an early morphogenesis stage (81).

The next nonstructural protein, NS3, has a chemotrypsin-like serine protease domain (11) followed by

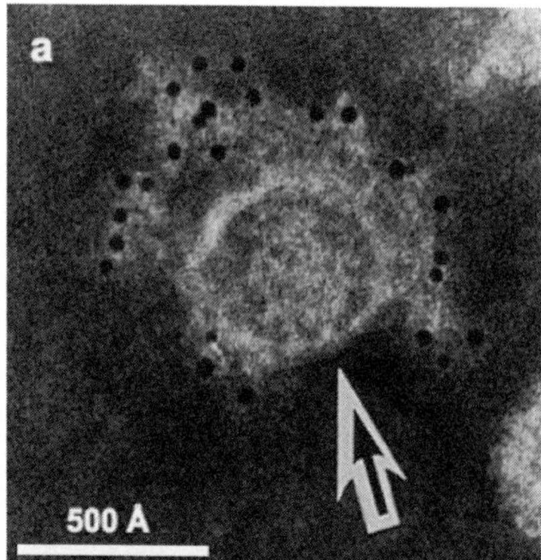

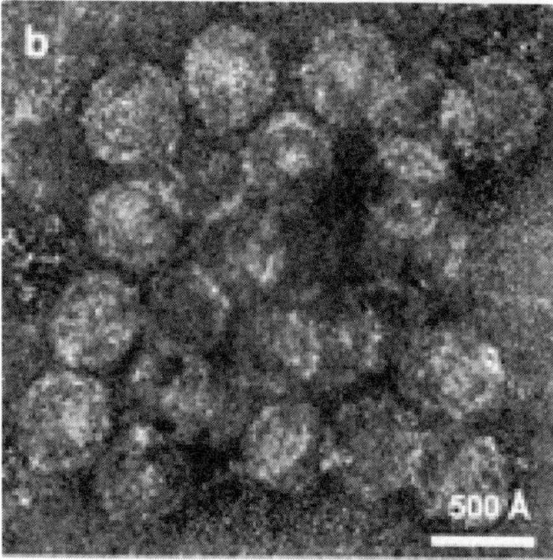

FIGURE 3 Electron microscopy of viral particles. (a) Immunogold electron microscopy of a viral particle from patient serum. The sample was incubated with anti-E1 polyclonal antibody and a secondary antibody conjugated to colloidal gold particles. An inner core (arrow) seems to be included within the particle. (Reprinted from reference 83 with permission.) (b) Negative-stain electron microscopy of HCV harvested from Huh7.5 cells infected in vitro with HCV strain JFH-1. Spherical particles of uniform size with inner cores can be seen.

an NTPase/RNA helicase (37). The serine protease activity requires NS4A as a cofactor, which anchors the complex to the ER membrane and changes the catalytic site conformation. This protease is responsible for cleavage of the downstream sites at the NS3/4A, NS4A/4B, NS4B/5A, and NS5A/5B junctions. The NS3/4A protease also targets several host cellular proteins, possibly playing a major role in other stages of the viral life cycle and the ability to evade the immune response (95, 109). The NS3 protease is an attractive target for antiviral therapy, and several specific NS3/4A protease inhibitors are being investigated as therapeutic agents (see below). The helicase domain acts as a molecular motor, unwinding double-stranded RNA in an ATP-dependent manner, and facilitates the activity of NS5B polymerase.

Not much is known about the role and structure of NS4B. This hydrophobic protein is an integral membrane protein in the ER membrane, is required for viral replication, and promotes the formation of unique membranous structures that serve as a scaffold for the formation of the membrane-associated replication complexes. NS4B also contains a GTP binding motif that is important for viral replication, although its function has not been defined. Sequence variations in the protein have a significant effect on the efficiency of viral replication (20).

The 447-amino-acid nonstructural protein NS5A is a hydrophilic, proline-rich protein, anchored to the ER membranes by its C terminus (77). Although its function has not been fully elucidated, this protein is probably a part of the replication complex. The protein is extensively phosphorylated by host kinases, and the degree of its phosphorylation is inversely related to the efficiency of viral replication in vitro. Adaptive mutations that reduce the degree of hyperphosphorylation are required for efficient replication of HCV replicons in tissue culture; however, the same mutations inhibit infectivity in vivo. This inverse relationship between in vivo infectivity and in vitro replication suggests that NS5A may act as a molecular switch, directing replication or assembly of virions according to the degree of its phosphorylation. Mutations in the interferon sensitivity-determining region within NS5A were initially thought to play a major role in the resistance to interferon of genotype 1 strains, but this was subsequently questioned by other studies (71). NS5A has been shown to interact with multiple host proteins and, like core and NS3/4A, is probably important for the ability of HCV to evade the host's interferon response.

The last protein encoded in the viral polyprotein is NS5B, the RNA-dependent RNA polymerase (9). This enzyme has the ability to initiate RNA synthesis de novo in the absence of a specific primer. Similar to other polymerases, the crystal structure of the catalytic domain demonstrates palm, finger, and thumb subdomains. A transmembrane C-terminal domain anchors the catalytic site to the membranous webs discussed below. This protein is responsible for the synthesis of the negative-strand intermediate and then the positive-strand viral genome. This essential role and the well-defined catalytic activity make this enzyme another attractive target for the development of specific inhibitors.

Translation from an alternative reading frame of the core-encoding region, with a +1 codon frameshift, yields a protein called F protein or ARFP (21). The reading frame for this protein does not start with the canonical AUG start codon, and translation is probably initiated by a programmed ribosomal frameshift. The evolutionary conservation of this frameshift product and the presence of antibodies to this protein in the sera of infected patients suggest that this protein is produced in vivo and probably has a role, yet to be elucidated, in the viral life cycle.

Biology

Replication Strategy

The complete replication cycle of HCV is not fully understood, although great advances have been made since the discovery of the virus. The replication cycle can be divided into stages: binding and entry into the cell; polyprotein translation and processing; RNA replication; and packaging, assembly, and release of the virion (Fig. 5).

Binding and Entry

The binding-and-entry stage has yet to be completely elucidated (12). The presence of E1 and E2 in a noncovalent heterodimer formation is essential for viral entry (14). Antibodies raised against E2 can efficiently inhibit binding and entry. Several cell surface molecules, mostly

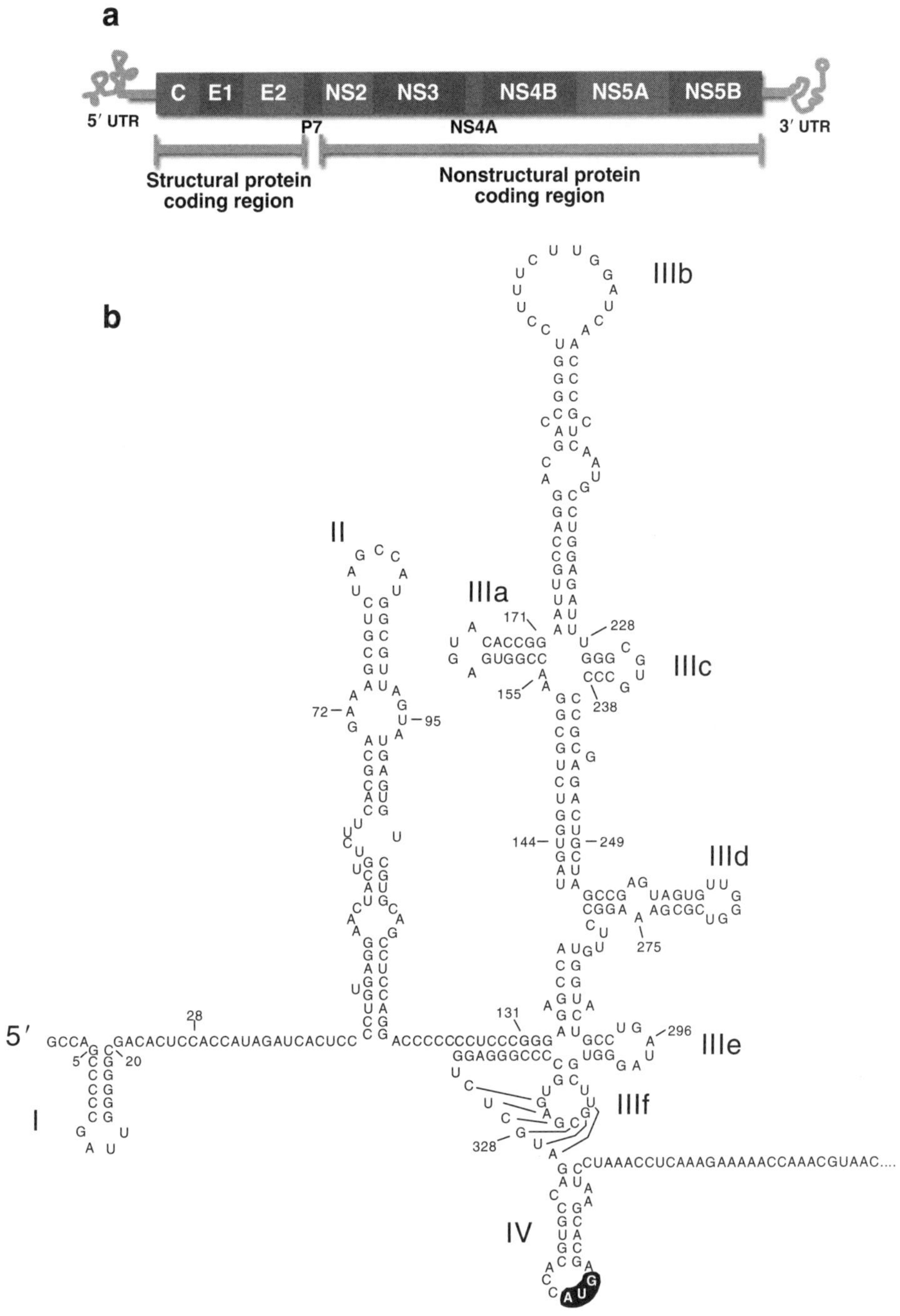

a

5′ UTR
C E1 E2 NS2 NS3 NS4B NS5A NS5B
P7 NS4A
3′ UTR
Structural protein coding region
Nonstructural protein coding region

b

5′ GCCA GACACUCCACCAUAGAUCACUCC ACCCCCCCUCCCGGG
GGAGGGCCC
CUAAACCUCAAAGAAAAACCAAACGUAAC....
I II IIIa IIIb IIIc IIId IIIe IIIf IV
5 20 28 72 95 131 144 155 171 228 238 249 275 296 328

c

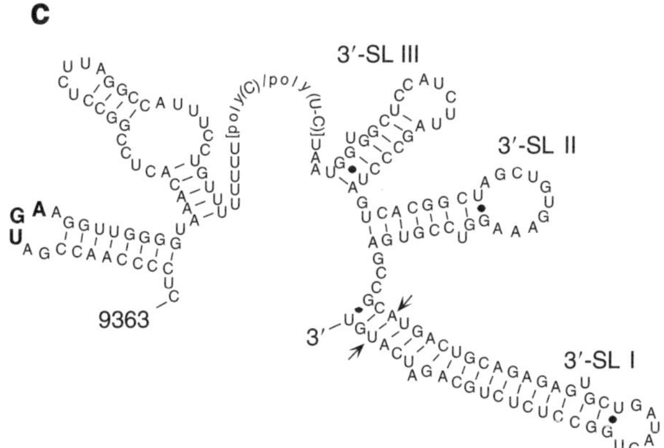

FIGURE 4 Genome structure of HCV. (a) The positive-sense single-stranded RNA genome of HCV has one long open reading frame containing genes for three structural and seven nonstructural proteins and flanked by two UTRs. (b) Sequence and secondary structure of the 5′ UTR. The AUG start codon for the open reading frame is highlighted in stem-loop IV. (c) Sequence and secondary structure of the 3′ UTR. Arrows indicate variable base pairs in the stem of stem-loop I, and the asterisk indicates the variable nucleotide in the loop of stem-loop I.

TABLE 1 Viral proteins and their function in the viral life cycle

Name	Size (amino acids)	Function	Intracellular location	Comment
Core	171	Viral capsid	ER membranes, membranous webs, lipid droplets	
E1	160	Viral envelope	RER[a] lumen (membrane anchored)	Glycoprotein
E2	334	Viral envelope	RER lumen (membrane anchored)	Glycoprotein, binds CD81
p7	63	Cation channel	RER membrane, mitochondrial membranes	Inhibited by amantadine and amiloride
NS2	216	Cysteine protease and viral assembly	RER membrane	Protease activity when joined with NS3
NS3	631	Serine protease, RNA helicase	Cytosol (anchored to ER membrane by NS4A)	Protease activity dependent on NS4A cofactor N-terminal protease and C-terminal helicase
NS4A	54	Protease cofactor	ER membrane	
NS4B	261	Scaffold for replication complex?	ER membrane	Induces membrane changes
NS5A	447	Regulating replication and assembly	ER membrane	
NS5B	591	RNA-dependent RNA polymerase	ER membrane	
F/ARFP		Unknown	Unknown	Product of an alternate reading frame of the core-encoding region

[a] RER, rough ER.

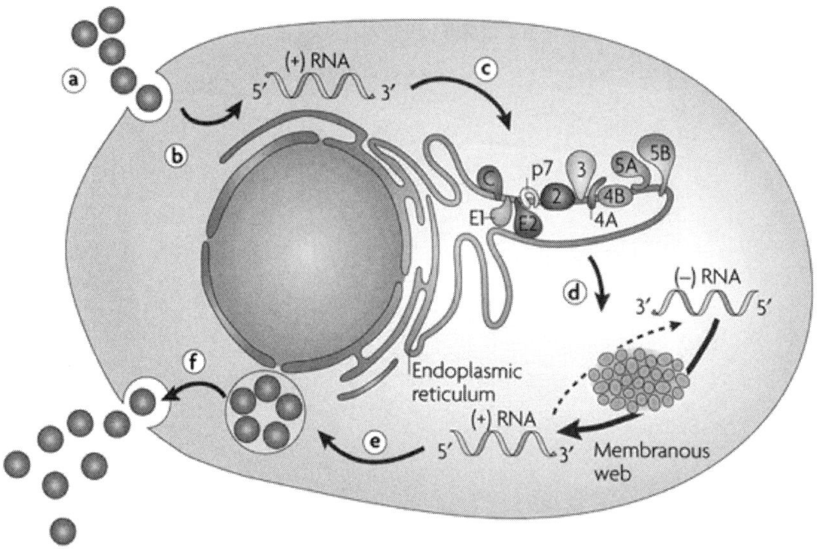

FIGURE 5 Viral replication cycle. Binding of the virus to the cell surface and internalization (a) are followed by release of the viral RNA (b), harnessing of the cellular ribosomes, and protein translation and processing (c). The viral proteins, associated with the ER membrane, promote the formation of replication complexes anchored to lipid membranous webs (d) in which the RNA-dependent polymerase NS5B creates copies of the viral RNA through a negative-strand RNA intermediate. HCV RNA is then packaged into membrane-covered viral particles (e) and exported from the cell, presumably through the exocytosis pathway (f). (Reprinted from reference 111 with permission of Macmillan Publishers Ltd.)

identified by screening for the ability to bind a soluble E2 protein, have been suggested as putative receptors that could facilitate virus-cell interaction and cell entry. The process is likely to involve several of these molecules, sequentially or in unison, as none alone was shown to be sufficient for entry. The 25-kDa tetraspanin CD81, a ubiquitous surface protein, is able to bind E2 (124) and is required for cell entry in a density-dependent manner. There is, however, evidence to suggest that CD81 is not required for binding but acts at a postbinding stage.

Another putative viral receptor is scavenger receptor class B type I (SR-BI), an 82-kDa, E2-binding (136) protein expressed on hepatocytes, dendritic cells, and steroidogenic tissue (adrenals and ovaries) and involved in binding of high-density lipoprotein (HDL), low-density lipoprotein (LDL), and oxidized LDL. The effect of SR-BI on HCV entry is enhanced by HDL cholesterol and inhibited by oxidized LDL. SR-BI and CD81 may interact with each other directly or indirectly, as HCV E2 is able to link the two molecules together, forming an E2-CD81-SR-BI complex (69).

A few other molecules have been suggested to be involved in this process. Highly sulfated heparan sulfate, a liver-specific form of heparan sulfate, was shown to bind E2 (13), and it may be the initial binding surface molecule. DC-SIGN and L-SIGN, two members of the C-type lectin family, were also shown to bind E2 and HCV particles. However, these proteins are expressed by dendritic cells and liver sinusoidal endothelial cells, respectively, but not by hepatocytes. Thus, they probably promote infection in trans by capturing virions and transporting them to the vicinity of hepatocytes (34). The LDL receptor was also found to be involved with HCV internalization (1), probably through association of viral particles with lipoproteins, because entry of naked HCV pseudoparticles is not mediated through this receptor (14). Most recently, claudin-1, a component of tight junctions that is highly expressed in the liver, was also found to be essential for viral entry into the cell (41).

Entry into the cell is clathrin and pH dependent, suggesting that after binding, the virus is endocytosed and that membrane fusion occurs in the endosome. In summary, although several surface molecules have been shown to bind viral proteins or particles and to facilitate cell entry, the process in vivo most likely involves several of these molecules interacting simultaneously or in sequence to bind, attach, endocytose, and internalize the virus.

Protein Translation and Processing

Following internalization and release of the viral RNA from the capsid, protein translation ensues. The IRES in the 5′ UTR is able to harness the 40S ribosomal subunit in the absence of other initiation factors (needed for cap-dependent translation) and direct it to the AUG start codon of the viral polyprotein. The eIF2–Met-tRNA–GTP ternary complex, eIF3, and the 60S subunit are then recruited to form the active 80S ribosome (50).

Following translation, the large polyprotein product is cleaved to the individual proteins by host and viral endogenous proteases. Four signal peptides are located in the polyprotein sequence—at the core protein and E1 junction, between E1 and E2, between E2 and p7, and at the p7 and NS2 junction. These signal peptides direct the elongating protein to the ER membrane and determine the location of the future cleavage products—cytosolic, ER membrane associated, or intraluminal. Cleavage at the site of the signal peptides is by the ER signal peptidase (161). The NS2/3 junction then undergoes autocatalytic cleavage following dimerization (158). Further downstream processing is dependent upon the NS3/4A protease, which cleaves the NS3/4A, NS4A/4B, NS4B/5A, and NS5A/5B junctions, with NS4A as a required cofactor (11).

RNA Replication

RNA replication occurs in a membrane-anchored complex of the viral nonstructural proteins and RNA, termed the replication complex or the replicase. Replication in vitro, and perhaps in vivo as well, occurs on unique membranous webs thought to be derived from the ER membranes by the action of NS4B (60). Host proteins such as cyclophilin B are also involved in regulating replication and may afford a potential target for antiviral treatment.

Packaging and Export

The process of packaging and export of HCV virions is assumed to involve budding of virions into the ER membrane and export through the secretory pathway. An interaction with the lipoprotein metabolism and export pathway may be involved. Aside from the structural proteins, p7 appears to be involved in this process, albeit with an unknown mechanism (81).

Host Range

In nature, HCV appears to infect only humans. A study in Gabon failed to detect HCV infection in 316 wild-born primates of different species (101). Chimpanzees can be experimentally infected with HCV, and this was actually shown even before HCV was identified. Although chimpanzees can develop a persistent infection like humans and develop similar inflammatory liver lesions, there are some important differences in disease behavior between the species. Persistent infection occurs after inoculation in only 30 to 40% of chimpanzees (as opposed to 85% in humans), and fibrosis and cirrhosis do not occur (93). The limited availability and the endangered status of chimpanzees, in addition to the financial cost, led to a search for other animal models. Tree shrews *(Tupaia belangeri chinensis)*, a species distantly related to primates, can be transiently infected with HCV (162).

The mechanism for the selective liver tropism is not clear but most likely involves selectivity of one or more of the cell surface molecules responsible for cell entry, although the specific molecule has not been identified. CD81 does not appear to be the tropism-conferring protein, as HCV E2 glycoprotein was shown to bind CD81 from tamarins (*Saguinus* sp.), which are not susceptible to HCV infection (106). Similarly, expression of CD81 from African green monkeys and rats in hepatoma cells confers susceptibility to HCV entry (46).

In an attempt to overcome viral selectivity and establish a small-animal model, several groups developed immunodeficient mouse strains harboring chimeric human-mouse livers (79, 107). HCV is able to replicate in the human-derived hepatocytes of these mice, but the absence of an effective immune response limits the value of this model in studying the pathogenesis of hepatitis C.

Cell Culture and In Vitro Model Systems

A robust cell culture system, capable of supporting efficient productive infection of HCV, has eluded researchers until recently. Various infectious culture systems have been reported, but none of them were subsequently shown to be sufficiently robust for practical application. Surrogate model systems, such as production of HCV-like particles and HCV retropseudoparticles, have been developed and provide valuable tools to study virus-cell interactions (12). The development of replicon systems was also instrumental in creating a system to study viral replication. These systems consist (98) of a bicistronic construct containing the nonstructural genome region (NS3-NS5B) downstream of the encephalomyocarditis virus (EMCV) IRES and a selectable marker driven by the HCV IRES (Table 2). Transfection of these subgenomic replicons to human hepatoma Huh7 cells resulted in viral replication. However, efficient viral replication depends on the appearance of adaptive mutations, especially in NS5A (123). This system is naturally limited by the absence of the structural proteins and hence is not amenable to study of the packaging and export process. Further modifications of the replicon system included the production of monocistronic subgenomic replicons and of a full-length replicon. None of these systems, however, produce potentially infectious virions. Moreover, the mutations required for adaptation to cell culture were found to inhibit replication and infectivity in vivo in chimpanzees (24).

Recently, Wakita et al. (156) transfected hepatoma cells with a full-length cDNA cloned from a patient with fulminant hepatitis C. This strain, termed JFH-1 and classified as genotype 2a, replicates efficiently in tissue culture without adaptive mutations and produces viral particles that are infectious to hepatoma cells in vitro and to chimpanzees in vivo. Since its description, studies utilizing this strain and chimeras derived from it have greatly enhanced our knowledge of the viral life cycle. However, the JFH-1 strain is unique, and information garnered from studying this strain may not be applicable to other more common strains, in particular genotype 1, the most frequent genotype in the world. Similar results have been obtained with a modified genotype 1 virus, but adaptive mutations were required to maintain in vitro replication and infectivity (165).

These approaches are all sequence dependent, and thus, results are not necessarily generalizable to other viral strains or genotypes. A sequence-independent system was recently described by Heller et al. (68) in which a viral cDNA is inserted between two self-splicing ribozymes and transfected into human hepatoma cells. This system can be applied to different HCV strains and genotypes to produce HCV particles capable of infecting chimpanzees (87). Finally, Lázaro et al. (94) were able to infect nontransformed human fetal hepatocytes in culture with HCV from genotypes 1, 2, and 3 from patient sera and demonstrated the release of infectious virions into the medium.

Inactivation by Physical and Chemical Agents

Although HCV played a major role in iatrogenic infection prior to its discovery and can be transmitted by invasive procedures, little data have been rigorously gathered on its survival in the environment and methods for inactivation. The lack of a robust cell culture system and the absence of a small-animal model hamper not only the ability to study the viral life cycle but also the development of methods to inactivate it. Some researchers focused on detection of (or the lack of) viral RNA by PCR as a surrogate for infectivity (29), while others examined the effects of various agents on binding of HCV to the Vero cell line (2). Many studies, however, are using the related pestivirus bovine viral diarrhea virus as a surrogate. The effectiveness of some agents is inferred from their effect on other lipid-enveloped viruses. Methodology also varies regarding the concentrations of various inactivating agents and times of exposure.

HCV is stable in stored serum and plasma samples at 4°C for at least 7 days (26). Even before the identification of HCV, treatment with heat, beta-propiolactone, UV radiation, and chloroform all were shown to prevent transmission of hepatitis to chimpanzees. Treatment of blood products by solvent-detergents, photochemical methods, or ultrafiltration seems to be sufficient to prevent transmission. The current recommendations for disinfecting reusable endoscopic equipment by mechanical washing with detergent and soaking in 2% glutaraldehyde were shown

TABLE 2 Tissue culture model systems

Model system	Method	Proteins expressed	Life cycle stage(s) studied	Infectivity in vivo	Comments
HCV-like particles (HCV-LP)	Assembly of envelope proteins in insect and mammalian cells	E1, E2	Binding and entry	–	
HCV pseudotype particles (HCVpp)	Envelope proteins assembled to a retroviral or lentiviral core particle	E1, E2	Binding and entry	–	
Subgenomic replicon	Expression driven by EMCV IRES	NS2–NS5B	Replication	–	Requires culture-adaptive mutations
Full genomic replicon	Expression driven by EMCV IRES	Entire genome	Replication	–	Requires culture-adaptive mutations
JFH-1 infectious strain (HCVcc)	A genotype 2a strain from a case of fulminant hepatitis	Entire genome	All	+++	Chimeras with other strains developed
DNA-ribozyme expression system	Transfection of viral cDNA between two ribozymes	Entire genome	All	++	Not sequence specific

to be sufficient to eliminate contamination with HCV (28). Alternative methods for cleaning medical instruments, such as the use of acidic electrolyte water or hydrogen peroxide, are also effective. The effectiveness of alcohol and diluted bleach was not formally tested against HCV, but the virus is most likely susceptible to these agents as well (135).

EPIDEMIOLOGY

Geographic Distribution

Infection with HCV is a global problem affecting up to 2% of the world's population (122). There is a great variability in seroprevalence rates among various countries and geographic regions (Fig. 6), reflecting differences in public health practices, transmission patterns, and population surveying schemes (140). In the developed world, injection drug use is currently the most common mode of infection and seroprevalence is generally low, ranging from 0.6% in Germany to 2.2 to 2.3% in Italy and Japan. The seroprevalence in the United States is reported at 1.6% (10). In the developing world, unsafe injections and contaminated medical instruments seem to be major risk factors. Egypt has the highest reported seroprevalence rate, 22%, attributable to mass public health campaigns of parenteral antischistosomal treatment (49). The WHO estimates that in the year 2000, 2 million people worldwide were iatrogenically infected by reused injection equipment (66). Blood transfusion is still a major risk factor for HCV transmission in the developing world, because of a lack of universal screening of blood donations as well as dependence on paid donors (140).

Transmission

Routes

The major route of HCV transmission is parenteral. In the past, transfusion of blood or blood products was the most common means of acquiring infection in the developed world. Posttransfusion hepatitis rates in patients undergoing open-heart surgery, for example, were as high as 33%. Products manufactured from pooled donor blood (such as anti-D globulin or coagulation factor concentrates) were implicated in large outbreaks of infection (88). However, changes in donor selection, including elimination of donor remuneration, exclusion of high-risk populations, screening donated blood for alanine aminotransferase (ALT) elevations, and the use of recombinant clotting factors, greatly reduced the risk of transmission even before HCV was actually identified (4) (Fig. 7). With the implementation of specific HCV tests, first serologic and then nucleic acid based, the risk of transfusion-associated HCV decreased further and is now estimated at 1:600,000 per unit.

With the elimination of blood transfusion as a risk factor, most of the parenteral exposure in the developed world is the result of injection drug use (18). Several practices, such as needle sharing, backloading, and sharing cotton, rinse water, and other paraphernalia, are associated with

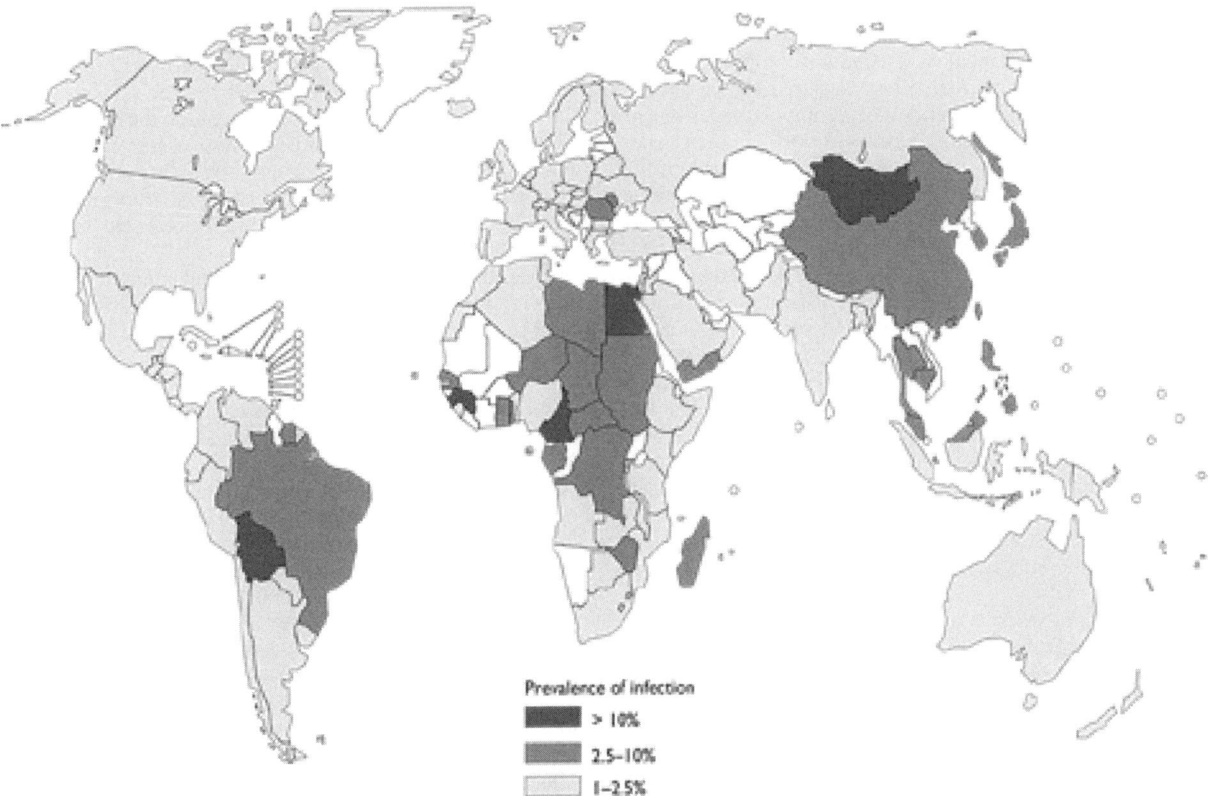

FIGURE 6 World distribution of HCV seroprevalence. The highest prevalence is in Egypt, 22%. Other countries with a high prevalence of infection include Mongolia, Bolivia, and several sub-Saharan nations. (Reprinted from *International Travel and Health* (160) with permission.)

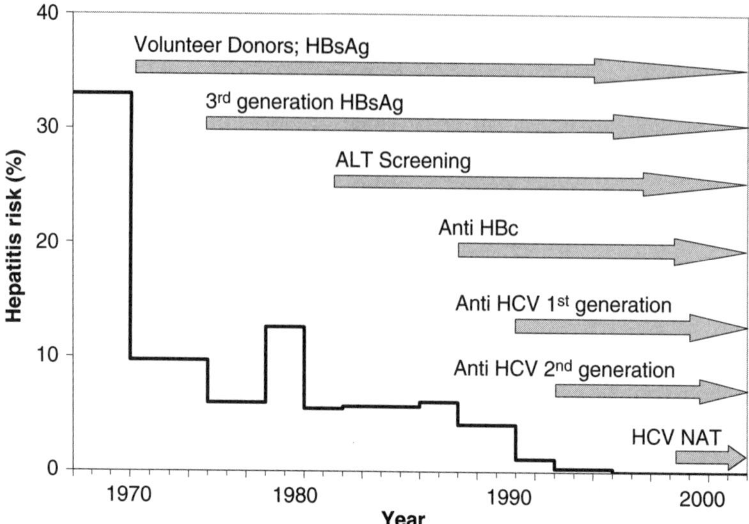

FIGURE 7 Evolution of screening methods for donated blood and the corresponding decrease in transfusion-related hepatitis. Data are shown for non-A, non-B hepatitis before the availability of anti-HCV testing and for HCV afterwards. HBsAg, hepatitis B virus surface antigen; anti-HBc, hepatitis B virus core antibodies; NAT, nucleic acid technology. (Adapted from reference 4.)

transmission. The seroprevalence of HCV antibodies increases with drug use duration, reaching a rate of 60 to 85% for persons using drugs for more than 6 years. Snorting cocaine has also been shown to be a risk factor for acquiring HCV, probably through contamination of shared snorting devices and nasal mucosal injury.

Iatrogenic transmission of hepatitis C has been associated with multiple medical procedures (134). Cases of transmission were reported to be associated with gastrointestinal and pulmonary endoscopy, ambulatory surgical procedures, chemotherapy, administration of anesthesia, radiological procedures, and, in general, any procedure involving parenteral access. Patients on hemodialysis are at an especially high risk for nosocomial infection (108), and a large number of outbreaks in dialysis units has been reported. The risk for dialysis patients can be decreased significantly by segregating patients to dedicated rooms and equipment based on HCV serology. In general, most cases of iatrogenic transmission in developed countries are associated with breaches of universal precautions and inadequate infection control practices, especially with the use of multidose vials. The source for most nosocomial outbreaks is a chronically infected patient, although transmission from an infected health care worker has been documented in rare cases. In the developing world, iatrogenic infection is associated with reuse of medical instruments, substandard hygienic practices, and treatment by nonprofessionals.

Health care workers are at risk for acquiring HCV infection through needlestick injuries. The risk is related to the size of the needle, the depth of the injury, use of intravenous or intra-arterial needles, higher viral load, and male gender (163). Overall, the risk of infection from a needlestick is usually quoted at 3% based on early reports, although a later analysis suggested that the risk is only 0.5% (80).

Hepatitis C can be transmitted vertically from mother to child. The risk of transmission is estimated at 2 to 5.5% (40, 104) in HCV-monoinfected mothers. The major risk factor for vertical transmission is coinfection with human immunodeficiency virus (HIV), which increases the transmission risk significantly (125). Other risk factors include maternal viral RNA and ALT level, prolonged labor (more than 6 h after rupture of the membranes), use of internal fetal monitoring devices during labor, and female gender of the newborn. The risk of transmission with vaginal delivery is not greater than with a cesarean section, and the latter should not be recommended routinely (105a). The timing of infection is either in utero or during delivery; whether postpartum transmission also occurs is not clear. Although HCV has been detected in breast milk from infected mothers, it does not seem to be transmissible by breast-feeding, and this should not be avoided by HCV-positive women (17).

Sexual transmission of HCV was documented in several case reports, but the actual risk of sexual transmission is hard to determine (150). Sexual exposure was found to be the only risk factor in 15% of acute hepatitis C cases (5), and hepatitis C is somewhat more common in populations at high risk for sexually transmitted diseases: HIV-infected persons, sex workers, men who have sex with men, persons with multiple sex partners, and those with other sexually transmitted diseases. However, studies of long-term monogamous heterosexual spouses of HCV-infected patients demonstrated a relatively low rate of infection, and those studies that utilized detailed analysis found that most infections were associated with other possible risk factors, such as drug abuse, sharing razors, high-risk sexual practices, etc. Moreover, when sequence analysis was used, only a small number of coinfected sexual partners were found to actually harbor the same strains. Two recent studies of low-risk monogamous couples (149, 152) found rates of HCV seropositivity of 2 to 3.8% in spouses of HCV-infected patients, although most infections were attributable to other risk factors. Prospective follow-up for up to 10 years did not identify any new case of interspousal transmission. Thus, sexual transmission is possible but appears to be very inefficient. This observation probably relates to a low titer of the virus in vaginal secretions, semen, and saliva; a lack of target cells in the genital system; and possibly other mechanisms as well.

The efficiency of sexual transmission during acute hepatitis C is less well defined. In a study of Egyptian health care workers with documented acute hepatitis C (84), 15% of spouses developed viremia, which spontaneously resolved in half of them. The breadth and magnitude of the polyclonal $CD4^+$ and $CD8^+$ T-cell response against HCV were greater in patients who eventually cleared viremia than in those who progressed to chronic infection. Interestingly, significant T-cell responses were also seen in some spouses of infected patients, although these spouses never developed viremia or seroconverted. This finding suggests that the host immune system plays a major role in the control of sexually transmitted HCV.

Currently the recommendation for a heterosexual, long-term, monogamous couple with one partner infected with HCV is to make no change to their sexual behavior. Couples may consider the use of barrier protection to reduce the already-low risk, or during higher-risk sexual practices, such as anal sex or intercourse during menses. The sharing of razors, toothbrushes, and nail clippers should be avoided. Persons who are in the high-risk groups mentioned above should use barrier protection to prevent HCV infection as well as other sexually transmitted diseases (150).

Risk Factors

Risk factors for infection with HCV stem directly from the routes of transmission discussed above. Thus, in the Western world, those at the highest risk for newly acquired infections are individuals who use intravenous drugs and share needles. Among non-drug users, transfusion of blood prior to 1992 or of clotting factors prior to 1987 constitutes a major risk. Patients on hemodialysis, past or present, are also a major risk group. Individuals incarcerated at correctional facilities are at a high risk of exposure to HCV, reflecting the prevalence of intravenous drug use and high-risk sexual behavior in this population. Estimates of HCV seroprevalence in incarcerated persons range from 16 to 41%, with chronic infection detected in 12 to 35% (157). Similarly, homeless persons with severe mental illnesses are also at a high risk of infection.

Promiscuity and high-risk sexual behavior were identified as risk factors for HCV seropositivity in cross-sectional studies (7). Although the prevalence is higher in female sex workers, it seems to be related more to drug abuse habits than to sexual transmission (92). Similarly, although epidemics of acute hepatitis C were recorded among men who have sex with men, this is mostly related to high-risk behavior and drug use (23).

Ethnicity and gender significantly modify the risk of HCV infection. In the United States, men are at a higher risk than women, with prevalence rates of 2.1 and 1.1%, respectively (10), and African-Americans have higher rates than Caucasian Americans. The highest rates were observed in non-Hispanic black males aged 40 to 49 years, for whom the prevalence is a striking 13.6%.

PATHOGENESIS IN HUMANS

Incubation Period

Since many acute infections with HCV are asymptomatic, it is difficult to define a precise incubation period. However, the relative kinetics of viral levels, liver enzymes, antibody appearance, and symptoms can be described based on observational studies of humans and experimental infection of chimpanzees. Typically in chimpanzees after HCV inoculation, HCV RNA is detectable rather quickly in the blood, usually within 2 weeks (100). The viral level then quickly rises until onset of hepatitis and activation of the host immune response, when the viral level can decrease, fluctuate, or become intermittently positive until either complete viral clearance is achieved or the animal progresses to chronic infection. Once chronicity is established, the viral levels remain relatively stable. Similar patterns are seen in human HCV infection, although viral levels may have much wider fluctuations. Some studies suggest that following HCV exposure, patients may have intermittently low-level viremia for a period that may last as long as 2 months but usually lasts about 2 weeks (58). This is followed by a ramp phase lasting 8 to 10 days in which viral levels increase rapidly in an exponential manner, with a doubling time of 11 h. Viral levels then reach a high-titer plateau for about 40 to 60 days. Serum ALT levels, marking liver injury, increase during the plateau phase, typically reaching a peak 7 to 8 weeks after infection. Symptoms and jaundice may appear at that time, although commonly these elevations are asymptomatic and thus often missed. Antibodies against HCV appear shortly after ALT starts to increase, and their appearance coincides with a decrease in viremia and either resolution or development of chronicity.

Patterns of Virus Replication

Organ Specificity

The selective infection of human hepatocytes by HCV is probably attributable to viral interaction with cell surface molecules specifically expressed on liver cells. Viral replication in extrahepatic sites, on the other hand, has been inconsistently demonstrated (19). In peripheral blood mononuclear cells (PBMCs), negative-strand RNA has been detected (albeit in a minority of cells) in dendritic cells and B lymphocytes. It has also been suggested that HCV is able to replicate in the central nervous system, possibly in microglia (48).

Quasispecies distribution and, perhaps, subgenotypic distribution (133) appear to differ between the hepatic, serum, and the extrahepatic compartments. PBMC-specific mutations and amino acid changes occur in the E1–HVR-1 region (19) and the IRES region in the 5′ UTR (133). Similar findings were reported for clones detected in the central nervous system (48). This may reflect strains with tropism for different compartments or emergence of tissue-specific adaptive mutations. The clinical significance of these observations is not clear. The detection of HCV RNA in PBMCs of patients who were treated successfully and are free of viremia and liver disease for a long period, as well as the absence of PBMC-specific strains in the serum of the same patients, suggests that even if extrahepatic replication occurs in PBMCs, it is associated with low viral replication and perhaps failure to mature or export the virus.

Factors in Disease Production

Histopathology

The basic histopathological findings in chronic hepatitis C (CHC) are similar to those of other chronic viral hepatitides (detailed in chapter 5) and can be separated into inflammatory and fibrotic components, thought to reflect the disease activity ("grade") and cumulative damage ("stage"), respectively (90). The characteristic inflammatory component consists of a chronic, predominantly monocytic, cellular infiltration of the portal tracts, which can extend into the limiting plate of hepatocytes bordering the tract ("piecemeal necrosis") and can be accompanied by various degrees of necroinflammatory changes in the lobules (see Fig. 2 in chapter 5). Not all components are seen in every biopsy, and these findings probably represent various degrees of severity. Fibrosis begins by accumulation of extracellular matrix and expansion of the portal tracts. This is followed by formation of septae, which are fibrotic bridges connecting vascular tracts and are mostly porto-portal but also porto-central. Progressive accumulation of these fibrotic bands distorts the liver architecture, and when coupled with regeneration and formation of nodules, is defined as cirrhosis, the end point of most chronic liver diseases (see Fig. 3 in chapter 5). Various scales have been developed to semiquantitatively describe those changes. Some histopathological characteristics more common in CHC than other chronic viral hepatitides include the presence of lymphoid aggregates or follicles in the portal tracts (Fig. 8a), inflammatory damage to small bile ducts with reactive changes, mild iron overload, and, occasionally, histologic findings similar to those with autoimmune hepatitis with a predominantly plasma cell infiltrate.

Steatosis, the accumulation of fat in the hepatocytes, is commonly observed in CHC (Fig. 8b), particularly in cases of infection with genotype 3. In non-genotype 3 cases, steatosis mostly reflects the presence of the metabolic syndrome or its components ("metabolic" steatosis), while for genotype 3, steatosis is probably a direct consequence of the viral infection ("viral" steatosis) (70) and appropriately disappears following successful viral eradication (128). In vitro data suggest that the core protein is responsible for the development of steatosis, possibly through inhibition of microsomal triglyceride transfer protein (a critical factor in maturation of very-low-density lipoprotein particles) or a genotype-specific effect on fatty acid synthase. The presence of steatosis is associated with accelerated fibrosis and possibly with reduced responsiveness to antiviral therapy.

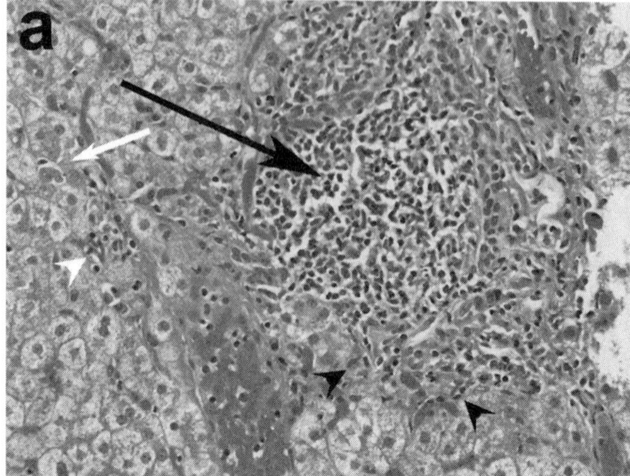

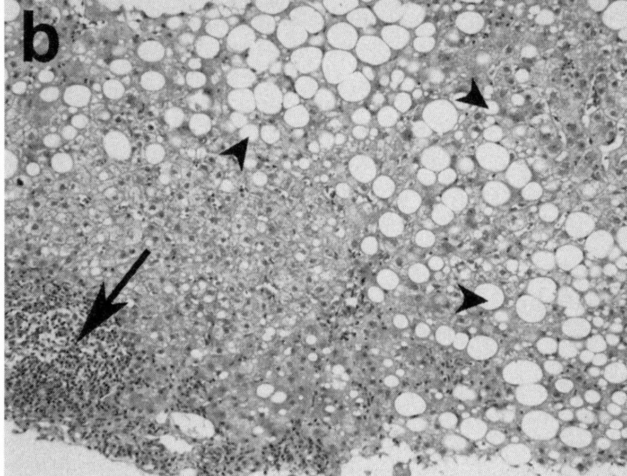

FIGURE 8 Histopathological findings in CHC. (a) Moderate inflammatory activity. The portal area is expanded by an inflammatory infiltrate and a lymphoid follicle (black arrow). The infiltrate disrupts the limiting plate between portal area and hepatic parenchyma ("interface hepatitis," black arrowheads). Foci of lobular inflammation can also be seen (white arrowhead) as well as an acidophil body (white arrow). Hematoxylin and eosin stain; magnification, ×400. (b) HCV-associated steatosis. The inflammatory infiltrate (arrow) is accompanied by fat droplets in hepatocytes (arrowheads). Hematoxylin and eosin stain; magnification, ×138. (Images provided by David Kleiner, National Cancer Institute, Bethesda, MD.)

Immune Responses

HCV, capable of causing chronic infection in most infected individuals, has multiple mechanisms of evading the immune system. Thus, the discussion of the host's immune response is coupled here to a discussion of viral evasion mechanisms (Fig. 9).

Nonspecific Immune Responses—Cytokines, Inflammatory Mediators, and the Innate Immune System

The single-stranded RNA genome of HCV contains numerous secondary-structure components. Upon infection of hepatocytes, these secondary structures are detected by Toll-like receptor 3 and retinoic acid-inducible gene I (RIG-I), the intracellular detectors of double-stranded RNA. This initiates a cascade of kinase activation that results in induction of beta interferon expression and its secretion to the surrounding milieu. Beta interferon then acts in an autocrine and paracrine manner, and through dimerization of the type I interferon receptor and activation of Jak1/Tyk2 and of the STAT system, induces the transcription of multiple interferon-stimulated genes (ISGs) that confer an antiviral state. HCV has developed several strategies of evading this pathway at multiple levels (54). The afferent arm of the host response, upstream of interferon induction, is effectively blocked by the NS3/4A serine protease, which cleaves and inactivates CARDIF (109) and TRIF (95), the downstream mediators of RIG-I and Toll-like receptor 3, respectively. The interferon signaling pathway is inhibited by induction of the inhibitory proteins SOCS1 and SOCS3 and by hypomethylation of STAT1, which attenuates its function. Finally, PKR, an interferon-stimulated protein that promotes an antiviral state, is inhibited by the NS5A and E2 viral proteins.

Interestingly, an increased pretreatment hepatic expression of several ISGs was found in patients for whom subsequent interferon-based treatment failed (30). Similarly,

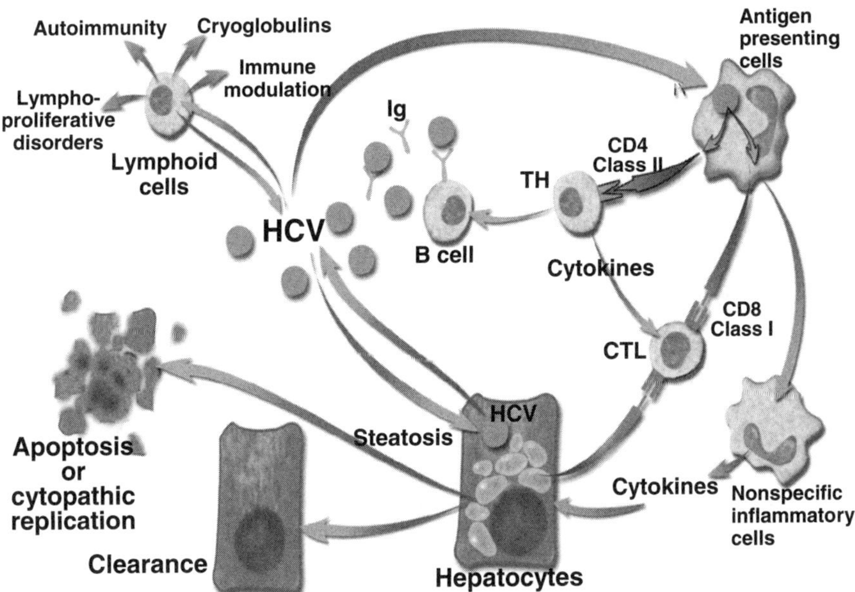

FIGURE 9 Immune response to HCV infection. HCV infection induces innate and adaptive immune responses. Induction of HCV-specific cytotoxic T cells by antigen-presenting cells is crucial in viral clearance and prevention of chronic infection, through both cytopathic and non-cytopathic mechanisms. Antibodies against HCV, secreted by B cells, appear late and do not seem to have an important role in viral control. Activation of nonspecific inflammatory cells causes liver injury. Chronic stimulation of lymphoid cells can induce autoimmunity and lymphoproliferative disorders, including cryoglobulinemia and lymphoma. TH, T helper; Ig, immunoglobulin; CTL, cytotoxic T lymphocyte.

levels of IP-10 (CXCL10), another ISG, in plasma were higher in patients with a slow response to interferon treatment (132). This observation suggests a maximal, but ineffective, activation of the type I interferon pathway in response to HCV infection in some patients.

Natural killer (NK) cells, the cellular effector arm of the innate immune system, are also important in HCV clearance, chronicity, and pathogenesis of liver damage. NK cells are held under a constant inhibitory influence by interaction of self major histocompatibility complex class I ligands with killer cell immunoglobulin-like receptors (KIRs) on their surface. A specific HLA-C–KIR genotype combination, which has a weaker inhibitory effect on NK cells, was shown to increase the rates of clearance of acute HCV infection in patients infected with a small inoculum (89). This suggests an important role for NK cells in prevention of chronicity. The interaction of NK and dendritic cells is important for dendritic cell maturation and efficient antigen presentation, crucial for recruitment of the adaptive cellular response. The E2 protein of HCV seems to be able to inhibit NK cell activity directly by cross-linking of CD81 receptors on the NK cell surface, and this may be a crucial link in the development of the defective adaptive response discussed below (59).

HCV-Specific Humoral and Cellular Immune Responses

The adaptive immune response against HCV tends to be weak and slow in onset compared to that against other viral infections (130). Upon acute infection, a specific cellular response appears after 4 to 12 weeks and is correlated with an increase in liver enzymes, marking the cellular immune response as the cause of hepatocyte injury, as opposed to viral cytopathicity per se. In general, patients who are able to mount a broad and vigorous $CD4^+$ $CD8^+$ response tend to recover spontaneously, while patients who become chronically infected have a late, transient, or narrowly focused and weak response. This defect in cellular immunity is HCV specific and is not associated with a wider immunodeficiency. Moreover, the virus-specific T cells seem to lose, over time, their ability to proliferate and produce cytokines in chronic infection (129).

Several mechanisms have been proposed to explain the attenuated cellular response. First, inhibition of NK cells and impaired dendritic cell maturation can lead to ineffective antigen presentation to the T cells. Second, continuous exposure to the persistent viral antigenemia may be the cause of the observed $CD8^+$ cell functional exhaustion. Third, direct viral inhibition of T cells may occur; the viral core protein binds to C1qR on these cells, thereby reducing their function and cytokine secretion. Fourth, escape mutations can develop as a result of the $CD8^+$ T-cell selective pressure (155). And finally, increased HCV-specific regulatory T cells in the liver of patients with CHC may be responsible for down-regulation of the T-cell response. Irrespective of the mechanism, it seems that the inability to mount and sustain an efficient $CD4^+$ cell response is the hallmark of progression to chronic infection.

HCV-specific antibodies also appear late during the course of acute infection, typically more than 4 weeks after initial infection. Although antibodies against epitopes in the envelope proteins have been demonstrated to protect against infection in a chimpanzee model, these "neutralizing" antibodies are not protective in humans (130). In fact, the titer of these antibodies is highest in patients with CHC, and such antibodies are often absent in patients who resolve infection, probably reflecting the rapid emergence of viral escape mutants during active replication (155). In general, anti-HCV antibodies do not seem to play a major role in the pathogenesis, clearance, and chronicity of hepatitis C.

Correlates of Immune Protection and Disease Resolution

The presence of cellular and humoral immune responses against HCV does not render full protection from reinfection upon recurrent exposure. Chimpanzees that recovered from HCV infection can be experimentally reinfected, although the recurrent disease seems to be attenuated in severity. This attenuation is dependent on the presence of both memory CD8$^+$ (143) and CD4$^+$ T cells (61). Reinfection has been reported for human patients in high-risk groups, such as active drug users or multitransfused children with thalassemia. Reinfection is possible after spontaneous recovery, after successful antiviral treatment, and even during treatment. Intravenous-drug users who spontaneously cleared viremia are less likely to be infected again upon reexposure and have lower rates of persistence to chronicity than do previously nonexposed controls, as long as they are HIV negative, again suggesting some degree of protection from acquired cellular immunity (62).

Patients who recover from HCV infection have persistent serum antibodies against HCV for a long duration, possibly for life, although a waning titer and sometimes disappearance have been documented after many years. Specific T-cell responses against HCV epitopes also seem to persist for life after spontaneous recovery from acute HCV infection.

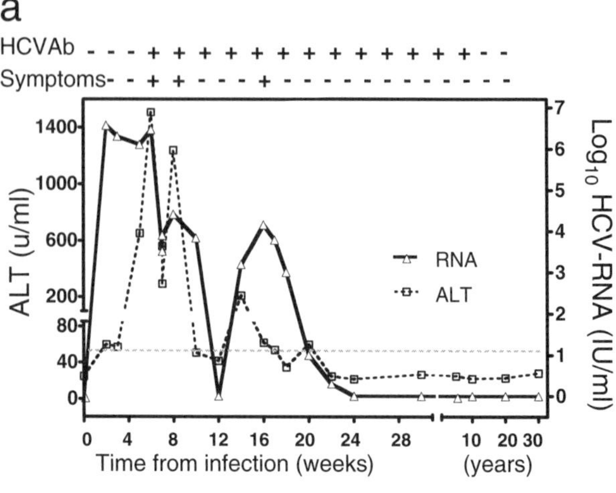

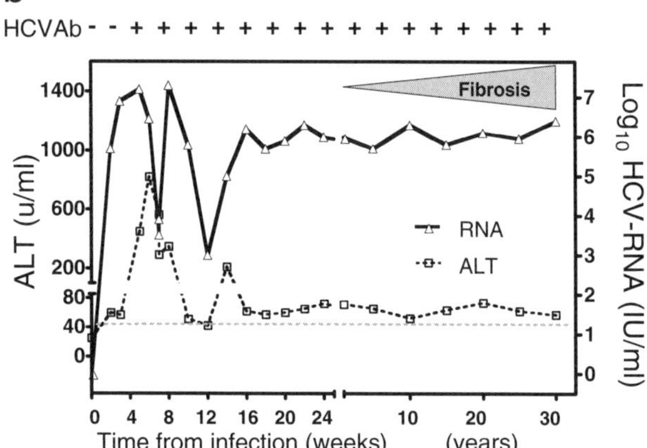

FIGURE 10 Clinical course and natural history of HCV infection. (a) Acute, spontaneously resolving hepatitis C. The liver enzyme elevation, symptoms, and appearance of antibodies usually lag behind viremia. Seropositivity persists for years after recovery but may decline after decades. (b) Acute infection progressing to CHC. Viral levels and enzyme elevations are relatively stable in the chronic phase. Accumulation of fibrosis occurs gradually, over many years. The gray dashed line represents the upper limit of the norm for ALT. HCVAb, anti-HCV antibodies.

CLINICAL MANIFESTATIONS

Major Clinical Syndromes

Acute Hepatitis C

Following infection with HCV, most patients develop intermittent viremia and elevated aminotransferases. Symptoms, however, are usually absent or very mild, and thus, most cases do not come to medical attention (67). Some patients do develop symptoms of hepatitis, which may include nausea, loss of appetite, or jaundice. It is estimated that only 20 to 25% of patients with acute hepatitis C will experience resolution of the infection, usually within 4 to 6 months, while for most cases, the disease will evolve to chronic infection (Fig. 10). The percentage of resolving cases is a rough estimate, at best, as many cases of acute asymptomatic disease go unnoticed, and is mostly based on serologic cross-sectional studies (72). Young age, female gender, African-American race, and presence of symptoms seem to be associated with resolution, and so are the vigor and breadth of the immune response. Conversely, immunosuppression is associated with higher rates of chronicity.

CHC

CHC is usually associated with mild, vague symptoms, if any. The most common symptom reported is fatigue, which is experienced by 50 to 75% of patients and is associated with age, female gender, and advanced disease (127). A vague, right upper quadrant pain is sometimes associated with CHC. Other associated symptoms may include arthralgia (23%), paresthesia (17%), myalgia (15%), pruritus (15%), and sicca syndrome (11%). Some patients present only with symptoms of advanced liver disease, such as jaundice, ascites, or gastrointestinal hemorrhage. Physical findings are usually absent unless cirrhosis is present, in which case jaundice, splenomegaly, spider angiomas, and other cirrhosis-associated manifestations may be seen.

Mild elevation of aminotransferases is commonly observed, predominantly of ALT, although up to one-third of asymptomatic patients have persistently normal enzymes (33). Antibodies against HCV, as well as relatively stable levels of serum HCV RNA, are universally present.

As discussed above, liver histology in CHC generally consists of inflammatory infiltrate and some degree of fibrosis, ranging from minimal expansion of portal tracts to cirrhosis. The fibrotic process, driven by the liver inflammation, can progress over time, although patients differ greatly in rates of progression. In some patients (nonprogressors), no increase in fibrosis is seen over decades of follow-up, while in others, it may progress rapidly to cirrhosis within a few years (126). Since the hepatic complications of CHC are generally limited to cirrhotic patients, defining predictive factors that affect the rate of progression, and thus prognosis, is of utmost importance (45). The most important predictors of rapid progression are immunosuppression, alcohol consumption, male gender, older age at infection, obesity, and degree of histologic activity. Estimates of the percentage of patients who progress to cirrhosis range from 4 to 22% at 20 years of infection, depending on methodology and patient population (51).

Acute Liver Failure

Few cases of acute liver failure attributable to HCV have been reported (42). Acute hepatitis C causing liver failure appears to be very rare; for example, none of the 308 cases observed by the U.S. Acute Liver Failure Study Group (116) were caused by HCV. A few cases were reported for patients with CHC developing fulminant liver failure upon withdrawal of immunosuppressive or chemotherapeutic treatment for other disorders. Fulminant liver failure can also be seen in patients chronically infected with HCV who suffer an acute infection with hepatitis A virus (153) or hepatitis B virus (32), although the association with acute hepatitis A has been debated.

Extrahepatic Manifestations

Although hepatitis C is mostly hepatotrophic, extrahepatic manifestations are not uncommon, presenting clinically or solely as laboratory abnormalities. Some are immunologic phenomena, while others may reflect actual viral presence in the affected organ. In a large, cross-sectional study (25), 39% of HCV-infected patients had at least one extrahepatic manifestation, most notably, various skin disorders, arthralgias, sicca syndrome, and peripheral neuropathy. Autoantibodies, mostly antinuclear antibodies or rheumatic factor, can be detected in 70% of tested sera. Antithyroid antibodies are often detected in HCV patients and can be associated with autoimmune thyroid disease. A common extrahepatic manifestation is HCV-associated mixed cryoglobulinemia (MC; previously termed essential MC or type II MC). The hallmark of this immunologic disorder is the presence in the serum of a cryoprecipitating monoclonal immunoglobulin M (IgM) directed against a polyclonal IgG. High concentrations of HCV can be detected within the cryoprecipitate. Low levels of cryoglobulins can be detected in up to 59% of infected patients (3), mostly without clinical manifestations. However, 10% of the patients develop small and medium-sized vessel leukocytoclastic vasculitis manifesting as palpable purpura, arthralgias or arthritis, peripheral neuropathy, glomerulonephritis, and, occasionally, involvement of other organs. The pathogenesis of HCV-associated MC is assumed to be chronic inflammatory stimulation of B cells with the subsequent formation of a clonal lymphoproliferative disorder and, at times, frank non-Hodgkin's lymphoma. Interferon therapy reduces cryoglobulin levels and decreases symptoms during treatment. This response is durable only if a sustained virologic response is achieved.

Apart from MC-related purpura, other skin manifestations of chronic hepatitis are pruritus, porphyria cutanea tarda, and lichen planus (3). Autoimmune thyroid disease is also commonly seen. Membranoproliferative glomerulonephritis, with or without cryoglobulins, is the most common renal manifestation of HCV infection. Sjögren-like lymphocytic sialoadenitis is histologically present in three-quarters of patients with hepatitis C, although only a minority have symptoms of the sicca syndrome. Diabetes mellitus type 2 is more frequent in patients with CHC than in control patients or patients with chronic hepatitis B. This may be related to the impaired glucose tolerance seen with cirrhosis, as well as to insulin resistance promoted directly by HCV.

Disease in Children

HCV infection in children is usually acquired vertically, although transfusion-associated disease used to account for many cases of HCV infection, especially in children with inherited coagulation disorders. During the first two decades of life, the disease seems to be mild and asymptomatic, although cirrhosis and complications have been reported (38). Spontaneous clearance of infection in vertically infected children can be seen in 20 to 25% of patients and can occur as late as age 3 years and, occasionally, even later. For the remaining 80%, noninvasive studies suggest mild asymptomatic disease in 50% and active disease in 30% (40). However, liver biopsies, although usually demonstrating mild disease, can also demonstrate progression of fibrosis with prolonged disease duration (64). Thus, although symptomatic disease is not commonly seen in children, it is not clear whether this reflects a true difference in disease behavior from the adult population or is just reflective of the shorter duration of disease.

Disease in Immunocompromised Hosts

Immunosuppression has a significant effect on HCV natural history. Coinfection with HIV is common, and it is estimated that 30% of HIV-infected patients in the United States and Europe are coinfected with HCV, with even higher rates in hemophiliacs and intravenous-drug abusers (131). Rates of coinfection in Africa appear to be much lower (110), perhaps because the dominant route of transmission for HIV is sexual in these regions. Since the advent of highly active antiretroviral therapy, with prolonged survival of HIV-infected patients, liver disease has emerged as a leading cause of mortality, ranking second only to AIDS-related death and surpassing cardiovascular causes (148). Coinfection is associated with higher serum HCV RNA levels, worse histopathological findings, and accelerated rates of fibrosis. Cirrhosis, hepatocellular carcinoma (HCC), and death from liver disease tend to appear after a shorter duration of infection in coinfected patients. Highly active antiretroviral therapy can slow the progression of liver fibrosis, although the rates of drug hepatotoxicity are increased in coinfected patients. Anti-HCV treatment is also associated with lower success rates in coinfected patients, and treatment results are directly related to $CD4^+$ cell counts (142).

Organ transplantation, and its associated prolonged immune suppression, can also affect the progression of hepatitis C. Patients in need of an organ transplant tend to have higher rates of HCV infection, probably because of the need for blood products and for multiple, invasive therapeutic and diagnostic interventions. This is especially true for kidney transplant recipients, for whom hemodialysis is a major risk factor and for whom more data are available. Serum HCV levels increase after kidney transplantation, and this was found to be particularly prominent after a course of antilymphocyte antibodies. HCV infection portends a worse outcome after kidney transplantation, with decreased rates of graft and patient survival, although most deaths are not due to liver disease (159). The limited data on progression of the liver disease in HCV-infected kidney transplant recipients suggest more advanced fibrosis in these patients (121). In hematopoietic-stem-cell transplant recipients, hepatitis C seems to progress more rapidly to cirrhosis than in patients who have not received transplants (120), and preexisting hepatitis C with elevated enzymes increases the risk for severe veno-occlusive disease, a serious hepatic complication of stem cell transplantation (147). Curiously, cancer chemotherapy and its associated profound immunosuppression may be associated with minor liver enzyme elevations but rarely with serious flares of hepatitis C.

Liver transplantation for hepatitis C is unique, since the infected organ itself is removed and is replaced by an uninfected organ. Universal reinfection of the graft is the rule and is associated with recurrence of hepatitis and cirrhosis in a significant number of patients, resulting in lower rates of graft and patient survival than for patients who had a liver transplantation for indications other than hepatitis C (151). A significant factor affecting survival is the need for immunosuppressive treatment of acute rejection episodes with bolus steroids, lymphocyte-depleting agents, or anti-interleukin 2 receptor antibodies. In fact, maintaining a stable immunosuppressive dose and avoiding rapid changes were shown to improve outcome significantly (15).

Complications

When liver cirrhosis is established as a result of CHC, decompensation and complications may occur. These complications are not unique to infection with HCV and can be seen with other etiologies of cirrhosis. The complications include hypersplenism, bleeding from esophageal varices or portal hypertensive gastropathy, hepatic encephalopathy, ascites, spontaneous bacterial peritonitis, renal failure, and death. Not all cirrhotic individuals are symptomatic or present with complications. Decompensation occurs at an estimated rate of about 4% per year (43, 76).

Hepatocellular carcinoma (HCC) can develop as a complication of cirrhosis, irrespective of the etiology, although some etiologies are associated with a much higher likelihood of HCC. The yearly incidence of HCC in patients with cirrhosis due to HCV infection is estimated at 2 to 8% (22). The risk for noncirrhotic patients appears to be much lower, although underestimation of the severity of the underlying liver disease may lead to false assurance in these patients. As discussed below, successful eradication of hepatitis C with antiviral treatment significantly reduces, but does not eliminate completely, the risk of HCC.

Differential Diagnosis

Diagnosis of CHC is straightforward when the appropriate laboratory tests are available. The differential diagnosis of elevated liver enzymes is vast; other causes of infectious hepatitis are discussed in chapter 5. However, a positive serum HCV antibody is almost always a marker of exposure to HCV, and a positive serum HCV RNA test is diagnostic for the disease. These tests should be performed for all patients with elevated aminotransferases and can be used to screen high-risk patients and blood or organ donors.

LABORATORY DIAGNOSIS

Virus Detection

Nucleic acid testing is the "gold standard" for detecting active HCV replication. Detection of viral genome sequence in the plasma, quantitatively or qualitatively, is now possible using automated assays with sensitivity and specificity nearing 100% (138). Qualitative assays to detect the presence of HCV most commonly utilize the PCR method and have a lower detection limit, 50 IU/ml. Assays based on the transcription-mediated amplification method are even more sensitive, with a lower threshold of 5 IU/ml. In most clinical scenarios, a qualitative result is sufficient for the diagnosis and monitoring of patients with chronic and acute hepatitis C. Quantitative measurement of HCV viral load is required before and during treatment of patients to assess their response and can be performed using quantitative PCR, branched-DNA assays, and real-time PCR, which recently became available for this purpose. The quantitative PCR has a limited dynamic range and a lower limit of detection, 600 IU/ml. However, the newer assays based on real-time PCR methodology have a sensitivity comparable to those of the earlier qualitative tests and a wider range of linearity, spanning from 10^1 to 10^8 IU/ml. Comparison of results from different quantitative assays is difficult, as tests differ with respect to the units used. To facilitate standardization, the World Health Organization developed a panel of standard calibration samples and promoted the use of the arbitrary international units.

An assay for detection of an HCV core protein antigen has been developed (139). An immune complex dissociation step (to diminish interference from naturally occurring anticore antibodies) is followed by an enzyme immunoassay (EIA) step. The assay has a detection threshold of 20,000 IU/ml, with a specificity of more than 99%. Despite the excellent performance of the assay, it is still inferior to nucleic acid detection assays, which become positive earlier, during the window period.

Serologic Assays

Serologic assays for detecting HCV infection were rapidly developed and improved following the initial discovery of the virus because of the urgent need to screen blood donors and prevent transmission. The first-generation EIA contained a single recombinant antigen derived from the NS4 protein and was limited in both sensitivity and specificity. Development of a second-generation test, with additional antigens from the core and NS3 proteins, and a third-generation test, with reconfigured core- and NS3-based antigens as well as an antigen from NS5, markedly improved the test performance and shortened the window period between infection and seroconversion. The currently available third-generation assays, especially those utilized in the Western world, provide sensitivity of 100% and specificity of nearly 100% when tested against standardized panels. As opposed to their use in diagnosing CHC in a clinically suspected case, the positive predictive value of the EIAs is lower when they are used for screening of a low-prevalence population, such as blood donors, and often requires a confirmatory test. A recombinant immunoblot assay can be used to confirm a positive EIA in this setting, although the nucleic acid tests discussed above are superior. With the current sensitivity and specificity of the EIA assays, a confirmatory test may no longer be necessary in the context of screening a low-risk population (118).

PREVENTION

General

Persons infected with HCV should be advised to avoid sharing toothbrushes, razors, nail clippers, and other personal-care articles that may become contaminated with blood (6). Patients in a long-term monogamous relationship need not alter their sexual practices, although testing the partner for exposure and counseling on the potential risk are advised. Patients involved in high-risk sexual behavior (persons with multiple partners, persons who engage in violent sex, sex workers, etc.) should be advised to use barrier protection to prevent HCV transmission and infection with other sexually transmitted diseases (150). Drug users should be counseled to avoid sharing of needles, syringes, and other injection and snorting paraphernalia. Needle exchange programs have been shown to reduce HCV seroprevalence.

Since alcohol consumption is associated with acceleration of liver injury and fibrosis, minimizing alcohol intake should be recommended for all patients. Routine vaccination against hepatitis A and B viruses should be done to reduce the risk of superinfection and potential liver failure.

Passive Immunoprophylaxis

Passive immunoprophylaxis against hepatitis C has been attempted in the context of liver transplantation, in light of the success in the use of hepatitis B immunoglobulin to prevent hepatitis B virus reinfection of the graft. Anti-HCV-enriched human immunoglobulin preparation failed to prevent reinfection in HCV patients after liver transplantation (35). The use of a monoclonal anti-E2 antibody in this setting in a phase II, randomized, controlled trial had only a transient effect on viral levels (137). The same antibody demonstrated short-term (less than 48 h) reduction of viral levels when administered to patients with CHC who had not undergone transplantation (55).

Active Immunization

An extensive effort is under way to develop an effective and safe HCV vaccine. Several strategies are being pursued (75). In the chimpanzee model, an adjuvant E1/E2-based vaccine that elicits antibody production and a CD4$^+$ response did not offer complete protection against acute infection but prevented development of chronicity. The use of HCV-like particles containing structural proteins was also shown recently to induce cellular and humoral responses and to prevent progression to chronicity in chimpanzees (39). The approach of priming with a DNA vaccine followed by a booster viral-vector vaccine is being pursued and showed promise in animal studies. No efficacy results for active prophylactic immunization in humans have been reported so far. One study examined the use of an E1 therapeutic vaccine in patients with CHC (114) and suggested that fibrosis was decreased in treated patients, although the mechanism is not clear, as viral levels were not reduced.

Antiviral Chemoprophylaxis

As discussed below, in documented cases of acute HCV infection, antiviral treatment is withheld for 8 to 16 weeks to allow the patients a chance to clear the virus on their own. Because interferon and ribavirin are expensive and fraught with side effects, chemoprophylaxis after exposure or in high-risk populations is not advised.

Management of Outbreaks

Outbreaks of hepatitis C associated with a single source of transmission are often detected late, as most cases of acute infection are asymptomatic and go unnoticed. When such an outbreak is detected, screening of all potentially affected patients, reviewing of potential breaches of standard care, and offering treatment to infected individuals should be undertaken.

Prevention of Perinatal and Congenital Infection

Although HCV can be transmitted vertically, there is no effective method to prevent transmission. Cesarean section was not proven to prevent infection of the newborn and should not be recommended routinely for HIV-negative mothers (105a). Invasive fetal monitoring during pregnancy was reported to be associated with increased risk of transmission (104). Thus, it is prudent to avoid invasive monitoring if possible, without compromising maternal or fetal safety

TREATMENT

Indication

In general, antiviral treatment is indicated for any adult patient with CHC who is viremic and has elevated aminotransferases or histologic evidence of progressive liver disease, i.e., fibrosis extending beyond the portal tracts (74). Normal aminotransferase levels should not exclude patients from therapy, as up to one-third of patients may be found to have advanced disease on histopathology. A liver biopsy is helpful in determining the degree of disease severity and can provide prognostic information. However, a biopsy is not an absolute requirement prior to treatment. In patients with genotype 2 or 3 infection, because of the high likelihood of response to a shorter course, treatment can be generally recommended irrespective of the histologic findings in suitable patients. Various noninvasive markers of advanced fibrosis that could potentially replace a liver biopsy have been tested to predict fibrosis. The current models, based on combinations of blood tests or sonographic measurement of liver stiffness, have reasonable accuracy in diagnosing advanced disease (cirrhosis) or very mild disease; for borderline cases, these models are less accurate.

Contraindications for antiviral treatment include pregnancy, breast-feeding, and allergy to the medications. Comorbidities that would increase the potential for complications, such as cardiac disease (which could worsen with ribavirin-induced anemia), depression (which may deteriorate with interferon treatment), seizure disorder, or advanced, decompensated liver disease, should be considered as relative contraindications. Caution should be exercised when treating patients with preexisting hematologic cytopenia and patients with renal failure, for whom the ribavirin dose should be decreased and the potential for adverse effects of treatment is high.

Interferon-Based Therapy

The mainstay of treatment of HCV infection is alpha interferon and its derivatives. Even before the virus was identified, treatment with interferon was shown to be efficacious (73), although at a low rate. Interferon induces a multitude of genes that promote an antiviral state. With the addition of ribavirin and pegylation of interferon, which attaches a polyethylene glycol (PEG) molecule to interferon and prolongs its half-life, a marked improvement in sustained virologic responses can be achieved (Fig. 11). Currently, the standard treatment of CHC consists of pegylated interferon and ribavirin (53, 102).

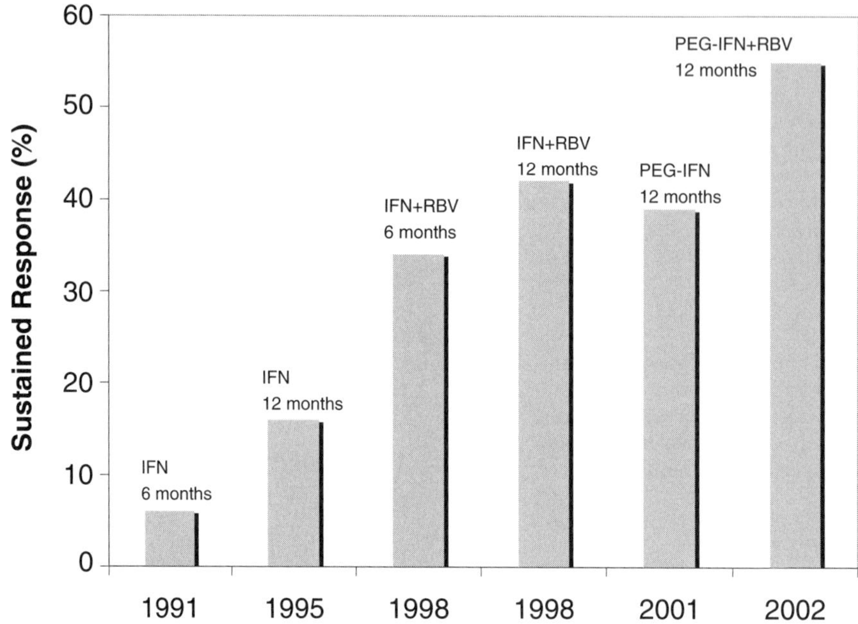

FIGURE 11 Evolution of treatment regimens for CHC and corresponding rates of sustained virologic response. IFN, alfa interferon; PEG-IFN, pegylated alfa interferon; RBV, ribavirin.

Two pegylated interferon formulations are currently available, pegylated alfa-2a interferon (Pegasys [Roche Pharmaceuticals]) and pegylated alfa-2b interferon (Pegintron [Schering-Plough]), differing in their active ingredient, PEG moiety, and pharmacological, pharmacodynamic, and pharmacokinetic properties (detailed in chapter 12). The treatment results for the two agents seem to be comparable, although no large head-to-head comparison study has been published to date.

Ribavirin (Copegus [Roche Pharmaceuticals] and Rebetol [Schering-Plough]) is a synthetic oral guanosine nucleoside analog. It is not effective against hepatitis C as monotherapy (36), although aminotransferase levels may decrease on treatment. However, in combination with interferon or pegylated interferon, ribavirin significantly enhances rates of viral eradication by decreasing rates of relapse. The mechanism of action of ribavirin has not been fully elucidated (99). The medication is administered orally twice daily, dosed according to weight and genotype (see below).

Treatment duration and the dose of ribavirin are determined by the infecting genotype (65) (Table 3). In general, patients with genotype 1 infection are treated for 48 weeks with a higher dose of ribavirin, while for patients with genotype 2 or 3, a 24-week course and a lower ribavirin dose are sufficient. Genotype 4 seems to require a treatment course similar to that of genotype 1, while data are lacking for genotypes 5 and 6 (115). Response to treatment is assessed by using a sensitive nucleic acid test in the serum, usually by PCR. An end-of-treatment response with current standard treatment is achieved in 69% of genotype 1 patients and 94% of genotype 2 or 3 patients. A sustained virologic response (SVR), defined as a negative HCV RNA test 24 weeks after the end of treatment, is achieved in 52% of patients with genotype 1; for genotypes 2 and 3 the response rate is 84% (65). Although the infecting genotype is the most important prognostic factor predicting response, several other pretreatment factors affect the rates of response to treatment. Among them, a high viral load, African-American race, obesity, and advanced fibrosis are the unfavorable factors.

Using frequently sampled viral level measurements from patients treated with interferon, Neumann et al. (113) demonstrated a biphasic response, with a rapid decline over the first 2 days and a slower, second-phase decline lasting at least up to day 14 of treatment. Mathematical

TABLE 3 Treatment of CHC

Genotypes	Type and dose of pegylated interferon	Ribavirin dosage	Duration	SVR rates[a]
1 and 4	Alfa-2a, 180 μg/w, alfa-2b, 1.5 μg/kg/wk	For persons >75 kg, 600 mg twice daily For persons <75 kg, 500 mg twice daily	48 wks	52% (genotype 1) and 82% (genotype 4)
2 and 3	Alfa-2a, 180 μg/w, alfa-2b, 1.5 μg/kg/wk	400 mg twice daily	24 wks	84%

[a] See reference 65.

modeling applied to these data suggests that the first phase represents rapid clearance of the virus from the serum on the basis of inhibition of replication and of new virion production by interferon. The second phase corresponds to the death and clearance of infected cells in addition to inhibition of viral replication. The parameters of viral kinetics are predictive of treatment result and have been applied as early predictors of nonresponse. Failure to achieve an early virologic response, defined as negativity or more than a 2-log decrease in viral load by week 12, or failure to become HCV RNA negative by week 24 of treatment (74), has a very high (>95%) negative predictive value for response and allows clinicians to terminate the treatment course early for some patients.

The treatment indications and regimen for acute hepatitis C are less standardized, with fewer, smaller studies available, mainly because this disease is frequently asymptomatic and likely to be missed. In general, treatment should be deferred for 8 to 16 weeks from the time of infection, to allow for possible spontaneous clearance to occur, especially in symptomatic patients. Treatment using standard or pegylated interferon monotherapy can be offered. Treatment for genotype 1 infection should probably last 24 weeks, while for genotype 2, 3 or 4, a course of 8 to 12 weeks of treatment seems to be sufficient (86). A high likelihood of treatment success, with SVR rates above 90%, was reported in several series, suggesting that at least for genotype 1 infection, treatment before chronicity develops should be attempted whenever possible (85).

Achievement of an SVR, inherently a virologic outcome, is a valid surrogate marker for beneficial clinical outcomes. Patients who become persistently HCV RNA negative are less likely to progress to decompensated liver disease, to die from hepatic causes, or to develop HCC, even if they already have established cirrhosis (78). In general, the likelihood of relapse later than 6 months after treatment (the currently accepted time point for SVR determination) is very low. HCV RNA sequences can occasionally be detected by PCR or transcription-mediated amplification in PBMCs or liver tissue (see above) but have not been shown to be associated with enzyme elevation or histologic worsening of liver disease. The significance of these findings remains unknown.

TABLE 4 Specifically targeted antiviral therapeutic agents against hepatitis C in clinical trials

Life cycle and target	Name(s)	Manufacturer(s)	Current status
Cell entry			
Polyclonal immunoglobulin	Civacir	NABI Biopharmaceuticals	Phase II[a] (liver transplant patients)
Monoclonal antibodies	HCV-AB 68, HCV-AB 65	XTL Biopharmaceuticals	Phase Ib
RNA translation			
Antisense oligonucleotide to 5′ UTR	ISI-14803	ISIS Pharmaceuticals	Phase II[b]
	AVI-4065	AVI Biopharma	Phase II[a]
HCV IRES	VGX-410C (mifepristone)	VGX Pharmaceuticals	Phase II[a]
Protein processing			
NS3/4A protease inhibition	BILN-2061	Boehringer-Ingelheim	Phase I[b]
	Telaprevir (VX-950)	Vertex Pharmaceuticals	Phase II
	SCH 503034	Schering-Plough	Phase II[a]
	ACH-806/GS-9132	Achillion Pharmaceuticals, Gilead Sciences	Phase I[b]
Viral replication			
NS5B polymerase inhibitor	Valopicitabine (NM283)	Idenix Pharmaceuticals, Novartis	Phase II[b]
	R1626	Roche Pharmaceuticals	Phase II
	HCV-796	ViroPharma, Wyeth	Phase II[a]
	GSK625433	GlaxoSmithKline	Phase I[a]
Cyclophilin B inhibitor	DEBIO-025	DebioPharm	Phase I
	NIM 811	Novartis	Phase I
NS3 helicase inhibitor	Molixan (NOV-205)	Novelos Therapeutics	Phase I[a]
Assembly and release			
α-Glucosidase inhibitor	Celgosivir (MX-3253)	Migenix	Phase II[a]
Therapeutic vaccines			
Saccharomyces cerevisiae-based vaccine	GI-5005	GlobeImmune	Phase I[a]
Virosome expressing HCV proteins	PeviTER, PeviPRO	Pevion Biotech	Phase I[a]

[a] Actively recruiting as of July 2007 (http://clinicaltrials.gov, accessed 27 July, 2007).
[b] Medication withdrawn.

Side Effects

Current treatment regimens are frequently accompanied by side effects (53, 102), detailed in chapter 12. Of interferon's side effects, the hematologic toxicity (especially neutropenia [146] and thrombocytopenia) is the one that most commonly necessitates dose reduction or interruption, in up to 20% of patients. Interestingly, psychiatric side effects of interferon, especially depression, are more common in HCV patients than in patients with chronic hepatitis B treated with the same doses. Ribavirin-induced hemolysis also frequently limits dosing. Side effects of the medications can be managed by dose modification, although this approach is undesirable, as it is associated with decreased rates of response to treatment (105), especially if dose adjustments are made early into the treatment course. Alternatively, supportive care can be given using, for example, acetaminophen for fever and pain or antidepressants for psychiatric disturbances. Hematopoietic growth factors such as granulocyte colony-stimulating factor and erythropoietin are often used to avoid dose reductions due to neutropenia and anemia, respectively, although this practice has yet to be shown to improve SVR rates.

Modified and New Therapies

The less-than-optimal rate of response to standard therapy, especially for genotype 1 patients, and the frequency of side effects have prompted the search for different therapeutic strategies. Modifications of dosage of pegylated interferon and ribavirin and of treatment duration have been studied in various situations (16, 96, 97, 141), but there has been no consensus regarding these issues. Modifications of interferon other than pegylation can potentially increase the response to treatment. Interferon alfacon-1 (Infergen; Intermune) is a synthetic recombinant interferon generated as a consensus sequence of naturally occurring alpha interferon subtypes. In combination with ribavirin, it seems to provide efficacy comparable to that of pegylated interferon, although the dosing regimen needs to be optimized (145). As mentioned above, ribavirin treatment is accompanied by hemolytic anemia in most cases, limiting its maximal dose and its applicability to patients who are not able to tolerate anemia, such as patients with atherosclerotic disease. Ribavirin analogs with decreased hematologic toxicity such as viramidine and taribavirin (57) are being explored. At least for viramidine, the results are currently disappointing.

In the past 5 years, several antiviral compounds which specifically target the HCV life cycle have been developed (119) (Table 4). Several agents targeted against the NS3/NS4A serine protease have reached advanced clinical trials. In general, these medications demonstrate rapid and significant inhibition of viral replication and in combination with pegylated interferon can achieve rapid viral clearance. Long-term results and safety data are yet to be reported for these agents, and resistant mutants have been detected during and after treatment. An alternative target for specific antiviral treatment is the NS5B polymerase. Specific inhibitors of this enzyme, both nucleoside analogs and nonnucleosides, have also reached advanced clinical trials. Medications in these groups have shown potent inhibition of viral replication, especially in combination with pegylated interferon, although achieving an effective dose may be limited for some of these agents because of dose-dependent side effects. Again, long-term efficacy data are not yet available, and concerns of safety, selection of resistant mutants, and possible interaction of nucleoside analogs with ribavirin need to be addressed.

When antiviral therapy fails to eradicate infection, an alternative approach is to attempt to halt, or even reverse, the ongoing liver damage and accumulation of fibrosis. One option is long-term treatment with low-dose interferon. Three large randomized trials were conducted to determine the efficacy of maintenance pegylated interferon in preventing decompensation of liver disease. The results have not been published so far. Another option is the use of an antifibrotic agent; limited data are currently available.

REFERENCES

1. **Agnello, V., G. Abel, M. Elfahal, G. B. Knight, and Q. X. Zhang.** 1999. Hepatitis C virus and other Flaviviridae viruses enter cells via low density lipoprotein receptor. *Proc. Natl. Acad. Sci. USA* **96:**12766–12771.
2. **Agolini, G., A. Russo, and M. Clementi.** 1999. Effect of phenolic and chlorine disinfectants on hepatitis C virus binding and infectivity. *Am. J. Infect. Control* **27:**236–239.
3. **Ali, A., and N. N. Zein.** 2005. Hepatitis C infection: a systemic disease with extrahepatic manifestations. *Clevel. Clin. J. Med.* **72:**1005–1019.
4. **Alter, H. J., and M. Houghton.** 2000. Clinical Medical Research Award. Hepatitis C virus and eliminating post-transfusion hepatitis. *Nat. Med.* **6:**1082–1086.
5. **Alter, M. J.** 1997. Epidemiology of hepatitis C. *Hepatology* **26:**62S–65S.
6. **Alter, M. J.** 2002. Prevention of spread of hepatitis C. *Hepatology* **36:**S93–S98.
7. **Alter, M. J., D. Kruszon-Moran, O. V. Nainan, G. M. McQuillan, F. Gao, L. A. Moyer, R. A. Kaslow, and H. S. Margolis.** 1999. The prevalence of hepatitis C virus infection in the United States, 1988 through 1994. *N. Engl. J. Med.* **341:**556–562.
8. **Andre, P., G. Perlemuter, A. Budkowska, C. Brechot, and V. Lotteau.** 2005. Hepatitis C virus particles and lipoprotein metabolism. *Semin. Liver Dis.* **25:**93–104.
9. **Appel, N., T. Schaller, F. Penin, and R. Bartenschlager.** 2006. From structure to function: new insights into hepatitis C virus RNA replication. *J. Biol. Chem.* **281:**9833–9836.
10. **Armstrong, G. L., A. Wasley, E. P. Simard, G. M. McQuillan, W. L. Kuhnert, and M. J. Alter.** 2006. The prevalence of hepatitis C virus infection in the United States, 1999 through 2002. *Ann. Intern. Med.* **144:**705–714.
11. **Bartenschlager, R.** 1999. The NS3/4A proteinase of the hepatitis C virus: unravelling structure and function of an unusual enzyme and a prime target for antiviral therapy. *J. Viral Hepat.* **6:**165–181.
12. **Barth, H., T. J. Liang, and T. F. Baumert.** 2006. Hepatitis C virus entry: molecular biology and clinical implications. *Hepatology* **44:**527–535.
13. **Barth, H., C. Schafer, M. I. Adah, F. Zhang, R. J. Linhardt, H. Toyoda, A. Kinoshita-Toyoda, T. Toida, T. H. Van Kuppevelt, E. Depla, F. Von Weizsacker, H. E. Blum, and T. F. Baumert.** 2003. Cellular binding of hepatitis C virus envelope glycoprotein E2 requires cell surface heparan sulfate. *J. Biol. Chem.* **278:**41003–41012.
14. **Bartosch, B., J. Dubuisson, and F. L. Cosset.** 2003. Infectious hepatitis C virus pseudo-particles containing functional E1-E2 envelope protein complexes. *J. Exp. Med.* **197:**633–642.

15. **Berenguer, M., V. Aguilera, M. Prieto, F. San Juan, J. M. Rayon, S. Benlloch, and J. Berenguer.** 2006. Significant improvement in the outcome of HCV-infected transplant recipients by avoiding rapid steroid tapering and potent induction immunosuppression. *J. Hepatol.* **44:** 717–722.
16. **Berg, T., M. von Wagner, S. Nasser, C. Sarrazin, T. Heintges, T. Gerlach, P. Buggisch, T. Goeser, J. Rasenack, G. R. Pape, W. E. Schmidt, B. Kallinowski, H. Klinker, U. Spengler, P. Martus, U. Alshuth, and S. Zeuzem.** 2006. Extended treatment duration for hepatitis C virus type 1: comparing 48 versus 72 weeks of peginterferon-alfa-2a plus ribavirin. *Gastroenterology* **130:** 1086–1097.
17. **Bhola, K., and W. McGuire.** 2007. Does avoidance of breast feeding reduce mother-to-infant transmission of hepatitis C virus infection? *Arch. Dis. Child.* **92:**365–366.
18. **Bialek, S. R., and N. A. Terrault.** 2006. The changing epidemiology and natural history of hepatitis C virus infection. *Clin. Liver Dis.* **10:**697–715.
19. **Blackard, J. T., N. Kemmer, and K. E. Sherman.** 2006. Extrahepatic replication of HCV: insights into clinical manifestations and biological consequences. *Hepatology* **44:**15–22.
20. **Blight, K. J.** 2007. Allelic variation in the hepatitis C virus NS4B protein dramatically influences RNA replication. *J. Virol.* **81:**5724–5736.
21. **Branch, A. D., D. D. Stump, J. A. Gutierrez, F. Eng, and J. L. Walewski.** 2005. The hepatitis C virus alternate reading frame (ARF) and its family of novel products: the alternate reading frame protein/F-protein, the double-frameshift protein, and others. *Semin. Liver Dis.* **25:**105–117.
22. **Bruix, J., and M. Sherman.** 2005. Management of hepatocellular carcinoma. *Hepatology* **42:**1208–1236.
23. **Buffington, J., P. J. Murray, K. Schlanger, L. Shih, T. Badsgard, R. R. Hennessy, R. Wood, I. B. Weisfuse, and R. A. Gunn.** 2007. Low prevalence of hepatitis C virus antibody in men who have sex with men who do not inject drugs. *Public Health Rep.* **122**(Suppl. 2)**:**63–67.
24. **Bukh, J., T. Pietschmann, V. Lohmann, N. Krieger, K. Faulk, R. E. Engle, S. Govindarajan, M. Shapiro, M. St Claire, and R. Bartenschlager.** 2002. Mutations that permit efficient replication of hepatitis C virus RNA in Huh-7 cells prevent productive replication in chimpanzees. *Proc. Natl. Acad. Sci. USA* **99:**14416–14421.
25. **Cacoub, P., C. Renou, E. Rosenthal, P. Cohen, I. Loury, V. Loustaud-Ratti, A.-M. Yamamoto, A.-C. Camproux, P. Hausfater, L. Musset, P. Veyssier, G. Raguin, and J.-C. Piette for the GERMIVIC (Groupe d'Etude et de Recherche en Medecine Interne et Maladies Infectieuses sur le Virus de l'Hepatite C).** 2000. Extrahepatic manifestations associated with hepatitis C virus infection: a prospective multicenter study of 321 patients. *Medicine* (Baltimore) **79:**47–56.
26. **Cardoso, M. S., K. Koerner, W. Hinz, C. Lenz, A. Schwandt, and B. Kubanek.** 1999. Hepatitis C virus stability: the issue! *Vox Sang.* **76:**124–127.
27. **Cha, T., E. Beall, B. Irvine, J. Kolberg, D. Chien, and M. S. Urdea.** 1992. At least five related, but distinct, hepatitis C viral genotypes exist. *Proc. Natl. Acad. Sci. USA* **89:**7144–7148.
28. **Chanzy, B., D. L. Duc-Bin, B. Rousset, P. Morand, C. Morel-Baccard, B. Marchetti, J. Fauconnier, M. R. Mallaret, J. Calop, J. P. Zarski, and J. M. Seigneurin.** 1999. Effectiveness of a manual disinfection procedure in eliminating hepatitis C virus from experimentally contaminated endoscopes. *Gastrointest. Endosc.* **50:**147–151.
29. **Charrel, R. N., R. de Chesse, A. Decaudin, P. De Micco, and X. de Lamballerie.** 2001. Evaluation of disinfectant efficacy against hepatitis C virus using a RT-PCR-based method. *J. Hosp. Infect.* **49:**129–134.
30. **Chen, L., I. Borozan, J. Feld, J. Sun, L. L. Tannis, C. Coltescu, J. Heathcote, A. M. Edwards, and I. D. McGilvray.** 2005. Hepatic gene expression discriminates responders and nonresponders in treatment of chronic hepatitis C viral infection. *Gastroenterology* **128:**1437–1444.
31. **Choo, Q. L., G. Kuo, A. J. Weiner, L. R. Overby, D. W. Bradley, and M. Houghton.** 1989. Isolation of a cDNA clone derived from a blood-borne non-A, non-B viral hepatitis genome. *Science* **244:**359–362.
32. **Chu, C. M., C. T. Yeh, and Y. F. Liaw.** 1999. Fulminant hepatic failure in acute hepatitis C: increased risk in chronic carriers of hepatitis B virus. *Gut* **45:**613–617.
33. **Conry-Cantilena, C., M. VanRaden, J. Gibble, J. Melpolder, A. O. Shakil, L. Viladomiu, L. Cheung, A. DiBisceglie, J. Hoofnagle, J. W. Shih, et al.** 1996. Routes of infection, viremia, and liver disease in blood donors found to have hepatitis C virus infection. *N. Engl. J. Med.* **334:**1691–1696.
34. **Cormier, E. G., R. J. Durso, F. Tsamis, L. Boussemart, C. Manix, W. C. Olson, J. P. Gardner, and T. Dragic.** 2004. L-SIGN (CD209L) and DC-SIGN (CD209) mediate transinfection of liver cells by hepatitis C virus. *Proc. Natl. Acad. Sci. USA* **101:**14067–14072.
35. **Davis, G. L., D. R. Nelson, N. Terrault, T. L. Pruett, T. D. Schiano, C. V. Fletcher, C. V. Sapan, L. N. Riser, Y. Li, R. J. Whitley, and J. W. Gnann, Jr., for the Collaborative Antiviral Study Group.** 2005. A randomized, open-label study to evaluate the safety and pharmacokinetics of human hepatitis C immune globulin (Civacir) in liver transplant recipients. *Liver Transplant.* **11:**941–949.
36. **Di Bisceglie, A. M., H. S. Conjeevaram, M. W. Fried, R. Sallie, Y. Park, C. Yurdaydin, M. Swain, D. E. Kleiner, K. Mahaney, and J. H. Hoofnagle.** 1995. Ribavirin as therapy for chronic hepatitis C. A randomized, double-blind, placebo-controlled trial. *Ann. Intern. Med.* **123:** 897–903.
37. **Dumont, S., W. Cheng, V. Serebrov, R. K. Beran, I. Tinoco, Jr., A. M. Pyle, and C. Bustamante.** 2006. RNA translocation and unwinding mechanism of HCV NS3 helicase and its coordination by ATP. *Nature* **439:**105–108.
38. **Elisofon, S. A., and M. M. Jonas.** 2006. Hepatitis B and C in children: current treatment and future strategies. *Clin. Liver Dis.* **10:**133–148, vii.
39. **Elmowalid, G. A., M. Qiao, S. H. Jeong, B. B. Borg, T. F. Baumert, R. K. Sapp, Z. Hu, K. Murthy, and T. J. Liang.** 2007. Immunization with hepatitis C virus-like particles results in control of hepatitis C virus infection in chimpanzees. *Proc. Natl. Acad. Sci. USA* **104:**8427–8432.
40. **European Paediatric Hepatitis C Virus Network.** 2005. A significant sex—but not elective cesarean section—effect on mother-to-child transmission of hepatitis C virus infection. *J. Infect. Dis.* **192:**1872–1879.
41. **Evans, M. J., T. von Hahn, D. M. Tscherne, A. J. Syder, M. Panis, B. Wolk, T. Hatziioannou, J. A. McKeating, P. D. Bieniasz, and C. M. Rice.** 2007. Claudin-1 is a hepatitis C virus co-receptor required for a late step in entry. *Nature* **446:**801–805.
42. **Farci, P., H. J. Alter, A. Shimoda, S. Govindarajan, L. C. Cheung, J. C. Melpolder, R. A. Sacher, J. W. Shih, and R. H. Purcell.** 1996. Hepatitis C virus-associated fulminant hepatic failure. *N. Engl. J. Med.* **335:**631–634.

43. **Fattovich, G., G. Giustina, F. Degos, F. Tremolada, G. Diodati, P. Almasio, F. Nevens, A. Solinas, D. Mura, J. T. Brouwer, H. Thomas, C. Njapoum, C. Casarin, P. Bonetti, P. Fuschi, J. Basho, A. Tocco, A. Bhalla, R. Galassini, F. Noventa, S. W. Schalm, and G. Realdi.** 1997. Morbidity and mortality in compensated cirrhosis type C: a retrospective follow-up study of 384 patients. *Gastroenterology* **112:**463–472.
44. **Feinstone, S. M., K. B. Mihalik, T. Kamimura, H. J. Alter, W. T. London, and R. H. Purcell.** 1983. Inactivation of hepatitis B virus and non-A, non-B hepatitis by chloroform. *Infect. Immun.* **41:**816–821.
45. **Feld, J. J., and T. J. Liang.** 2006. Hepatitis C—identifying patients with progressive liver injury. *Hepatology* **43:**S194–S206.
46. **Flint, M., T. von Hahn, J. Zhang, M. Farquhar, C. T. Jones, P. Balfe, C. M. Rice, and J. A. McKeating.** 2006. Diverse CD81 proteins support hepatitis C virus infection. *J. Virol.* **80:**11331–11342.
47. **Forns, X., and J. Bukh.** 1999. The molecular biology of hepatitis C virus. Genotypes and quasispecies. *Clin. Liver Dis.* **3:**693–716, vii.
48. **Forton, D. M., P. Karayiannis, N. Mahmud, S. D. Taylor-Robinson, and H. C. Thomas.** 2004. Identification of unique hepatitis C virus quasispecies in the central nervous system and comparative analysis of internal translational efficiency of brain, liver, and serum variants. *J. Virol.* **78:**5170–5183.
49. **Frank, C., M. K. Mohamed, G. T. Strickland, D. Lavanchy, R. R. Arthur, L. S. Magder, T. El Khoby, Y. Abdel-Wahab, E. S. Aly Ohn, W. Anwar, and I. Sallam.** 2000. The role of parenteral antischistosomal therapy in the spread of hepatitis C virus in Egypt. *Lancet* **355:**887–891.
50. **Fraser, C. S., and J. A. Doudna.** 2007. Structural and mechanistic insights into hepatitis C viral translation initiation. *Nat. Rev. Microbiol.* **5:**29–38.
51. **Freeman, A. J., G. J. Dore, M. G. Law, M. Thorpe, J. Von Overbeck, A. R. Lloyd, G. Marinos, and J. M. Kaldor.** 2001. Estimating progression to cirrhosis in chronic hepatitis C virus infection. *Hepatology* **34:**809–816.
52. **Friebe, P., and R. Bartenschlager.** 2002. Genetic analysis of sequences in the 3′ nontranslated region of hepatitis C virus that are important for RNA replication. *J. Virol.* **76:**5326–5338.
53. **Fried, M. W., M. L. Shiffman, K. R. Reddy, C. Smith, G. Marinos, F. L. Goncales, Jr., D. Haussinger, M. Diago, G. Carosi, D. Dhumeaux, A. Craxi, A. Lin, J. Hoffman, and J. Yu.** 2002. Peginterferon alfa-2a plus ribavirin for chronic hepatitis C virus infection. *N. Engl. J. Med.* **347:**975–982.
54. **Gale, M., Jr., and E. M. Foy.** 2005. Evasion of intracellular host defence by hepatitis C virus. *Nature* **436:**939–945.
55. **Galun, E., N. A. Terrault, R. Eren, A. Zauberman, O. Nussbaum, D. Terkieltaub, M. Zohar, R. Buchnik, Z. Ackerman, R. Safadi, Y. Ashur, S. Misrachi, Y. Liberman, L. Rivkin, and S. Dagan.** 2007. Clinical evaluation (Phase I) of a human monoclonal antibody against hepatitis C virus: safety and antiviral activity. *J. Hepatol.* **46:**37–44.
56. **Gault, E., P. Soussan, Y. Morice, L. Sanders, A. Berrada, B. Rogers, and P. Deny.** 2003. Evaluation of a new serotyping assay for detection of anti-hepatitis C virus type-specific antibodies in serum samples. *J. Clin. Microbiol.* **41:**2084–2087.
57. **Gish, R. G., S. Arora, K. Rajender Reddy, D. R. Nelson, C. O'Brien, Y. Xu, and B. Murphy.** 2007. Virological response and safety outcomes in therapy-naïve patients treated for chronic hepatitis C with taribavirin or ribavirin in combination with pegylated interferon alfa-2a: a randomized, phase 2 study. *J. Hepatol.* **47:**51–59.
58. **Glynn, S. A., D. J. Wright, S. H. Kleinman, D. Hirschkorn, Y. Tu, C. Heldebrant, R. Smith, C. Giachetti, J. Gallarda, and M. P. Busch.** 2005. Dynamics of viremia in early hepatitis C virus infection. *Transfusion* (Paris) **45:**994–1002.
59. **Golden-Mason, L., and H. R. Rosen.** 2006. Natural killer cells: primary target for hepatitis C virus immune evasion strategies? *Liver Transplant.* **12:**363–372.
60. **Gosert, R., D. Egger, V. Lohmann, R. Bartenschlager, H. E. Blum, K. Bienz, and D. Moradpour.** 2003. Identification of the hepatitis C virus RNA replication complex in Huh-7 cells harboring subgenomic replicons. *J. Virol.* **77:**5487–5492.
61. **Grakoui, A., N. H. Shoukry, D. J. Woollard, J. H. Han, H. L. Hanson, J. Ghrayeb, K. K. Murthy, C. M. Rice, and C. M. Walker.** 2003. HCV persistence and immune evasion in the absence of memory T cell help. *Science* **302:**659–662.
62. **Grebely, J., B. Conway, J. D. Raffa, C. Lai, M. Krajden, and M. W. Tyndall.** 2006. Hepatitis C virus reinfection in injection drug users. *Hepatology* **44:**1139–1145.
63. **Griffin, S., D. Clarke, C. McCormick, D. Rowlands, and M. Harris.** 2005. Signal peptide cleavage and internal targeting signals direct the hepatitis C virus p7 protein to distinct intracellular membranes. *J. Virol.* **79:**15525–15536.
64. **Guido, M., F. Bortolotti, G. Leandro, P. Jara, L. Hierro, J. Larrauri, C. Barbera, R. Giacchino, L. Zancan, F. Balli, C. Crivellaro, E. Cristina, A. Pucci, and M. Rugge.** 2003. Fibrosis in chronic hepatitis C acquired in infancy: is it only a matter of time? *Am. J. Gastroenterol.* **98:**660–663.
65. **Hadziyannis, S. J., H. Sette, Jr., T. R. Morgan, V. Balan, M. Diago, P. Marcellin, G. Ramadori, H. Bodenheimer, Jr., D. Bernstein, M. Rizzetto, S. Zeuzem, P. J. Pockros, A. Lin, and A. M. Ackrill.** 2004. Peginterferon-alpha2a and ribavirin combination therapy in chronic hepatitis C: a randomized study of treatment duration and ribavirin dose. *Ann. Intern. Med.* **140:**346–355.
66. **Hauri, A. M., G. L. Armstrong, and Y. J. Hutin.** 2004. The global burden of disease attributable to contaminated injections given in health care settings. *Int. J. STD AIDS* **15:**7–16.
67. **Heller, T., and B. Rehermann.** 2005. Acute hepatitis C: a multifaceted disease. *Semin. Liver Dis.* **25:**7–17.
68. **Heller, T., S. Saito, J. Auerbach, T. Williams, T. R. Moreen, A. Jazwinski, B. Cruz, N. Jeurkar, R. Sapp, G. Luo, and T. J. Liang.** 2005. An in vitro model of hepatitis C virion production. *Proc. Natl. Acad. Sci. USA* **102:**2579–2583.
69. **Heo, T. H., S. M. Lee, B. Bartosch, F. L. Cosset, and C. Y. Kang.** 2006. Hepatitis C virus E2 links soluble human CD81 and SR-B1 protein. *Virus Res.* **121:**58–64.
70. **Hezode, C., F. Roudot-Thoraval, E. S. Zafrani, D. Dhumeaux, and J. M. Pawlotsky.** 2004. Different mechanisms of steatosis in hepatitis C virus genotypes 1 and 3 infections. *J. Viral Hepat.* **11:**455–458.
71. **Hofmann, W. P., S. Zeuzem, and C. Sarrazin.** 2005. Hepatitis C virus-related resistance mechanisms to interferon alpha-based antiviral therapy. *J. Clin. Virol.* **32:**86–91.
72. **Hoofnagle, J. H.** 2002. Course and outcome of hepatitis C. *Hepatology* **36:**S21–S29.
73. **Hoofnagle, J. H., K. D. Mullen, D. B. Jones, V. Rustgi, A. Di Bisceglie, M. Peters, J. G. Waggoner, Y. Park, and E. A. Jones.** 1986. Treatment of chronic non-A, non-

B hepatitis with recombinant human alpha interferon. A preliminary report. *N. Engl. J. Med.* **315:**1575–1578.
74. **Hoofnagle, J. H., and L. B. Seeff.** 2006. Peginterferon and ribavirin for chronic hepatitis C. *N. Engl. J. Med.* **355:**2444–2451.
75. **Houghton, M., and S. Abrignani.** 2005. Prospects for a vaccine against the hepatitis C virus. *Nature* **436:**961–966.
76. **Hu, K. Q., and M. J. Tong.** 1999. The long-term outcomes of patients with compensated hepatitis C virus-related cirrhosis and history of parenteral exposure in the United States. *Hepatology* **29:**1311–1316.
77. **Huang, Y., K. Staschke, R. De Francesco, and S. L. Tan.** 2007. Phosphorylation of hepatitis C virus NS5A nonstructural protein: a new paradigm for phosphorylation-dependent viral RNA replication? *Virology* **364:**1–9.
78. **Iacobellis, A., M. Siciliano, F. Perri, B. E. Annicchiarico, G. Leandro, N. Caruso, L. Accadia, G. Bombardieri, and A. Andriulli.** 2007. Peginterferon alfa-2b and ribavirin in patients with hepatitis C virus and decompensated cirrhosis: a controlled study. *J. Hepatol.* **46:**206–212.
79. **Ilan, E., J. Arazi, O. Nussbaum, A. Zauberman, R. Eren, I. Lubin, L. Neville, O. Ben-Moshe, A. Kischitzky, A. Litchi, I. Margalit, J. Gopher, S. Mounir, W. Cai, N. Daudi, A. Eid, O. Jurim, A. Czerniak, E. Galun, and S. Dagan.** 2002. The hepatitis C virus (HCV)-Trimera mouse: a model for evaluation of agents against HCV. *J. Infect. Dis.* **185:**153–161.
80. **Jagger, J., V. Puro, and G. De Carli.** 2002. Occupational transmission of hepatitis C virus. *JAMA* **288:**1469.
81. **Jones, C. T., C. L. Murray, D. K. Eastman, J. Tassello, and C. M. Rice.** 2007. Hepatitis C virus p7 and NS2 proteins are essential for production of infectious virus. *J. Virol.* **81:**8374–8383.
82. **Jopling, C. L., M. Yi, A. M. Lancaster, S. M. Lemon, and P. Sarnow.** 2005. Modulation of hepatitis C virus RNA abundance by a liver-specific microRNA. *Science* **309:**1577–1581.
83. **Kaito, M., S. Watanabe, K. Tsukiyama-Kohara, K. Yamaguchi, Y. Kobayashi, M. Konishi, M. Yokoi, S. Ishida, S. Suzuki, and M. Kohara.** 1994. Hepatitis C virus particle detected by immunoelectron microscopic study. *J. Gen. Virol.* **75**(Pt. 7)**:**1755–1760.
84. **Kamal, S. M., A. Amin, M. Madwar, C. S. Graham, Q. He, A. Al Tawil, J. Rasenack, T. Nakano, B. Robertson, A. Ismail, and M. J. Koziel.** 2004. Cellular immune responses in seronegative sexual contacts of acute hepatitis C patients. *J. Virol.* **78:**12252–12258.
85. **Kamal, S. M., A. E. Fouly, R. R. Kamel, B. Hockenjos, A. Al Tawil, K. E. Khalifa, Q. He, M. J. Koziel, K. M. El Naggar, J. Rasenack, and N. H. Afdhal.** 2006. Peginterferon alfa-2b therapy in acute hepatitis C: impact of onset of therapy on sustained virologic response. *Gastroenterology* **130:**632–638.
86. **Kamal, S. M., K. N. Moustafa, J. Chen, J. Fehr, A. Abdel Moneim, K. E. Khalifa, L. A. El Gohary, A. H. Ramy, M. A. Madwar, J. Rasenack, and N. H. Afdhal.** 2006. Duration of peginterferon therapy in acute hepatitis C: a randomized trial. *Hepatology* **43:**923–931.
87. **Kato, T., T. Matsumura, T. Heller, S. Saito, R. K. Sapp, K. Murthy, T. Wakita, and T. J. Liang.** 2007. Production of infectious hepatitis C virus of various genotypes in cell cultures. *J. Virol.* **81:**4405–4411.
88. **Kenny-Walsh, E., for The Irish Hepatology Research Group.** 1999. Clinical outcomes after hepatitis C infection from contaminated anti-D immune globulin. *N. Engl. J. Med.* **340:**1228–1233.
89. **Khakoo, S. I., C. L. Thio, M. P. Martin, C. R. Brooks, X. Gao, J. Astemborski, J. Cheng, J. J. Goedert, D. Vlahov, M. Hilgartner, S. Cox, A. M. Little, G. J. Alexander, M. E. Cramp, S. J. O'Brien, W. M. Rosenberg, D. L. Thomas, and M. Carrington.** 2004. HLA and NK cell inhibitory receptor genes in resolving hepatitis C virus infection. *Science* **305:**872–874.
90. **Kleiner, D. E.** 2005. The liver biopsy in chronic hepatitis C: a view from the other side of the microscope. *Semin. Liver Dis.* **25:**52–64.
91. **Kuo, G., Q. L. Choo, H. J. Alter, G. L. Gitnick, A. G. Redeker, R. H. Purcell, T. Miyamura, J. L. Dienstag, M. J. Alter, C. E. Stevens, et al.** 1989. An assay for circulating antibodies to a major etiologic virus of human non-A, non-B hepatitis. *Science* **244:**362–364.
92. **Kweon, S. S., M. H. Shin, H. J. Song, D. Y. Jeon, and J. S. Choi.** 2006. Seroprevalence and risk factors for hepatitis C virus infection among female commercial sex workers in South Korea who are not intravenous drug users. *Am. J. Trop. Med. Hyg.* **74:**1117–1121.
93. **Lanford, R. E., C. Bigger, S. Bassett, and G. Klimpel.** 2001. The chimpanzee model of hepatitis C virus infections. *ILAR J.* **42:**117–126.
94. **Lázaro, C. A., M. Chang, W. Tang, J. Campbell, D. G. Sullivan, D. R. Gretch, L. Corey, R. W. Coombs, and N. Fausto.** 2007. Hepatitis C virus replication in transfected and serum-infected cultured human fetal hepatocytes. *Am. J. Pathol.* **170:**478–489.
95. **Li, K., E. Foy, J. C. Ferreon, M. Nakamura, A. C. Ferreon, M. Ikeda, S. C. Ray, M. Gale, Jr., and S. M. Lemon.** 2005. Immune evasion by hepatitis C virus NS3/4A protease-mediated cleavage of the Toll-like receptor 3 adaptor protein TRIF. *Proc. Natl. Acad. Sci. USA* **102:**2992–2997.
96. **Liang, T. J.** 2007. Shortened therapy for hepatitis C virus genotype 2 or 3—is less more? *N. Engl. J. Med.* **357:** 176–178.
97. **Lindahl, K., L. Stahle, A. Bruchfeld, and R. Schvarcz.** 2005. High-dose ribavirin in combination with standard dose peginterferon for treatment of patients with chronic hepatitis C. *Hepatology* **41:**275–279.
98. **Lohmann, V., F. Korner, J. Koch, U. Herian, L. Theilmann, and R. Bartenschlager.** 1999. Replication of subgenomic hepatitis C virus RNAs in a hepatoma cell line. *Science* **285:**110–113.
99. **Lutchman, G., S. Danehower, B. C. Song, T. J. Liang, J. H. Hoofnagle, M. Thomson, and M. G. Ghany.** 2007. Mutation rate of the hepatitis C virus NS5B in patients undergoing treatment with ribavirin monotherapy. *Gastroenterology* **132:**1757–1766.
100. **Major, M. E., H. Dahari, K. Mihalik, M. Puig, C. M. Rice, A. U. Neumann, and S. M. Feinstone.** 2004. Hepatitis C virus kinetics and host responses associated with disease and outcome of infection in chimpanzees. *Hepatology* **39:**1709–1720.
101. **Makuwa, M., S. Souquiere, P. Telfer, E. Leroy, O. Bourry, P. Rouquet, S. Clifford, E. J. Wickings, P. Roques, and F. Simon.** 2003. Occurrence of hepatitis viruses in wild-born non-human primates: a 3 year (1998–2001) epidemiological survey in Gabon. *J. Med. Primatol.* **32:**307–314.
102. **Manns, M. P., J. G. McHutchison, S. C. Gordon, V. K. Rustgi, M. Shiffman, R. Reindollar, Z. D. Goodman, K. Koury, M. Ling, and J. K. Albrecht.** 2001. Peginterferon alfa-2b plus ribavirin compared with interferon alfa-2b plus ribavirin for initial treatment of chronic hepatitis C: a randomised trial. *Lancet* **358:**958–965.
103. **Martell, M., J. I. Esteban, J. Quer, J. Genesca, A. Weiner, R. Esteban, J. Guardia, and J. Gomez.** 1992.

Hepatitis C virus (HCV) circulates as a population of different but closely related genomes: quasispecies nature of HCV genome distribution. *J. Virol.* **66:**3225–3229.

104. **Mast, E. E., L. Y. Hwang, D. S. Seto, F. S. Nolte, O. V. Nainan, H. Wurtzel, and M. J. Alter.** 2005. Risk factors for perinatal transmission of hepatitis C virus (HCV) and the natural history of HCV infection acquired in infancy. *J. Infect. Dis.* **192:**1880–1889.

105. **McHutchison, J. G., M. Manns, K. Patel, T. Poynard, K. L. Lindsay, C. Trepo, J. Dienstag, W. M. Lee, C. Mak, J. J. Garaud, and J. K. Albrecht.** 2002. Adherence to combination therapy enhances sustained response in genotype-1-infected patients with chronic hepatitis C. *Gastroenterology* **123:**1061–1069.

105a. **McIntyre, P. G., K. Tosh, and W. McGuire.** 2006. Caesaren section versus vaginal delivery for preventing mother to infant hepatitis C virus transmission. *Cochrane Database of Systematic Reviews,* issue 4.

106. **Meola, A., A. Sbardellati, B. Bruni Ercole, M. Cerretani, M. Pezzanera, A. Ceccacci, A. Vitelli, S. Levy, A. Nicosia, C. Traboni, J. McKeating, and E. Scarselli.** 2000. Binding of hepatitis C virus E2 glycoprotein to CD81 does not correlate with species permissiveness to infection. *J. Virol.* **74:**5933–5938.

107. **Mercer, D. F., D. E. Schiller, J. F. Elliott, D. N. Douglas, C. Hao, A. Rinfret, W. R. Addison, K. P. Fischer, T. A. Churchill, J. R. Lakey, D. L. Tyrrell, and N. M. Kneteman.** 2001. Hepatitis C virus replication in mice with chimeric human livers. *Nat. Med.* **7:**927–933.

108. **Meyers, C. M., L. B. Seeff, C. O. Stehman-Breen, and J. H. Hoofnagle.** 2003. Hepatitis C and renal disease: an update. *Am. J. Kidney Dis.* **42:**631–657.

109. **Meylan, E., J. Curran, K. Hofmann, D. Moradpour, M. Binder, R. Bartenschlager, and J. Tschopp.** 2005. Cardif is an adaptor protein in the RIG-I antiviral pathway and is targeted by hepatitis C virus. *Nature* **437:** 1167–1172.

110. **Modi, A. A., and J. J. Feld.** 2007. Viral hepatitis and HIV in Africa. *AIDS Rev.* **9:**25–39.

111. **Moradpour, D., F. Penin, and C. M. Rice.** 2007. Replication of hepatitis C virus. *Nat. Rev. Microbiol.* **5:**453–463.

112. **Moriya, K., H. Fujie, Y. Shintani, H. Yotsuyanagi, T. Tsutsumi, K. Ishibashi, Y. Matsuura, S. Kimura, T. Miyamura, and K. Koike.** 1998. The core protein of hepatitis C virus induces hepatocellular carcinoma in transgenic mice. *Nat. Med.* **4:**1065–1067.

113. **Neumann, A. U., N. P. Lam, H. Dahari, D. R. Gretch, T. E. Wiley, T. J. Layden, and A. S. Perelson.** 1998. Hepatitis C viral dynamics in vivo and the antiviral efficacy of interferon-alpha therapy. *Science* **282:**103–107.

114. **Nevens, F., T. Roskams, H. Van Vlierberghe, Y. Horsmans, D. Sprengers, A. Elewaut, V. Desmet, G. Leroux-Roels, E. Quinaux, E. Depla, S. Dincq, C. Vander Stichele, G. Maertens, and F. Hulstaert.** 2003. A pilot study of therapeutic vaccination with envelope protein E1 in 35 patients with chronic hepatitis C. *Hepatology* **38:**1289–1296.

115. **Nguyen, M. H., and E. B. Keeffe.** 2005. Prevalence and treatment of hepatitis C virus genotypes 4, 5, and 6. *Clin. Gastroenterol. Hepatol.* **3:**S97–S101.

116. **Ostapowicz, G., R. J. Fontana, F. V. Schiødt, A. Larson, T. J. Davern, S. H. B. Han, T. M. McCashland, A. O. Shakil, J. E. Hay, L. Hynan, J. S. Crippin, A. T. Blei, G. Samuel, J. Reisch, W. M. Lee, and the U.S. Acute Liver Failure Study Group.** 2002. Results of a prospective study of acute liver failure at 17 tertiary care centers in the United States. *Ann. Intern. Med.* **137:** 947–954.

117. **Pawlotsky, J. M.** 2003. Hepatitis C virus genetic variability: pathogenic and clinical implications. *Clin. Liver Dis.* **7:**45–66.

118. **Pawlotsky, J. M.** 2002. Use and interpretation of virological tests for hepatitis C. *Hepatology* **36:**S65–S73.

119. **Pawlotsky, J. M., S. Chevaliez, and J. G. McHutchison.** 2007. The hepatitis C virus life cycle as a target for new antiviral therapies. *Gastroenterology* **132:** 1979–1998.

120. **Peffault de Latour, R., V. Levy, T. Asselah, P. Marcellin, C. Scieux, L. Ades, R. Traineau, A. Devergie, P. Ribaud, H. Esperou, E. Gluckman, D. Valla, and G. Socie.** 2004. Long-term outcome of hepatitis C infection after bone marrow transplantation. *Blood* **103:**1618–1624.

121. **Perez, R. M., A. S. Ferreira, J. O. Medina-Pestana, M. Cendoroglo-Neto, V. P. Lanzoni, A. E. Silva, and M. L. Ferraz.** 2006. Is hepatitis C more aggressive in renal transplant patients than in patients with end-stage renal disease? *J. Clin. Gastroenterol.* **40:**444–448.

122. **Perz, J. F., L. A. Farrington, C. Pecoraro, Y. J. Hutin, and G. L. Armstrong.** 2004. Estimated global prevalence of hepatitis C virus infection. Annual meeting of the Infectious Diseases Society of America, Boston, MA.

123. **Pietschmann, T., and R. Bartenschlager.** 2003. Tissue culture and animal models for hepatitis C virus. *Clin. Liver Dis.* **7:**23–43.

124. **Pileri, P., Y. Uematsu, S. Campagnoli, G. Galli, F. Falugi, R. Petracca, A. J. Weiner, M. Houghton, D. Rosa, G. Grandi, and S. Abrignani.** 1998. Binding of hepatitis C virus to CD81. *Science* **282:**938–941.

125. **Polis, C. B., S. N. Shah, K. E. Johnson, and A. Gupta.** 2007. Impact of maternal HIV coinfection on the vertical transmission of hepatitis C virus: a meta-analysis. *Clin. Infect. Dis.* **44:**1123–1131.

126. **Poynard, T., P. Bedossa, and P. Opolon for the OBSVIRC, METAVIR, CLINIVIR, and DOSVIRC Groups.** 1997. Natural history of liver fibrosis progression in patients with chronic hepatitis C. *Lancet* **349:** 825–832.

127. **Poynard, T., P. Cacoub, V. Ratziu, R. P. Myers, M. H. Dezailles, A. Mercadier, P. Ghillani, F. Charlotte, J. C. Piette, and J. Moussalli.** 2002. Fatigue in patients with chronic hepatitis C. *J. Viral Hepat.* **9:**295–303.

128. **Poynard, T., V. Ratziu, J. McHutchison, M. Manns, Z. Goodman, S. Zeuzem, Z. Younossi, and J. Albrecht.** 2003. Effect of treatment with peginterferon or interferon alfa-2b and ribavirin on steatosis in patients infected with hepatitis C. *Hepatology* **38:**75–85.

129. **Rehermann, B.** 2007. Chronic infections with hepatotropic viruses: mechanisms of impairment of cellular immune responses. *Semin. Liver Dis.* **27:**152–160.

130. **Rehermann, B., and M. Nascimbeni.** 2005. Immunology of hepatitis B virus and hepatitis C virus infection. *Nat. Rev. Immunol.* **5:**215–229.

131. **Rockstroh, J. K., and U. Spengler.** 2004. HIV and hepatitis C virus co-infection. *Lancet Infect. Dis.* **4:**437–444.

132. **Romero, A. I., M. Lagging, J. Westin, A. P. Dhillon, L. B. Dustin, J. M. Pawlotsky, A. U. Neumann, C. Ferrari, G. Missale, B. L. Haagmans, S. W. Schalm, S. Zeuzem, F. Negro, E. Verheij-Hart, and K. Hellstrand.** 2006. Interferon (IFN)-gamma-inducible protein-10: association with histological results, viral kinetics, and outcome during treatment with pegylated IFN-alpha 2a and ribavirin for chronic hepatitis C virus infection. *J. Infect. Dis.* **194:**895–903.

133. **Roque-Afonso, A. M., D. Ducoulombier, G. Di Liberto, R. Kara, M. Gigou, E. Dussaix, D. Samuel, and C. Feray.** 2005. Compartmentalization of hepatitis C virus genotypes between plasma and peripheral blood mononuclear cells. *J. Virol.* **79:**6349–6357.
134. **Rotman, Y., and R. Tur-Kaspa.** 2001. Transmission of hepatitis B and C viruses—update. *Isr. Med. Assoc. J.* **3:** 357–359.
135. **Sattar, S. A., J. Tetro, V. S. Springthorpe, and A. Giulivi.** 2001. Preventing the spread of hepatitis B and C viruses: where are germicides relevant? *Am. J. Infect. Control* **29:**187–197.
136. **Scarselli, E., H. Ansuini, R. Cerino, R. M. Roccasecca, S. Acali, G. Filocamo, C. Traboni, A. Nicosia, R. Cortese, and A. Vitelli.** 2002. The human scavenger receptor class B type I is a novel candidate receptor for the hepatitis C virus. *EMBO J.* **21:**5017–5025.
137. **Schiano, T. D., M. Charlton, Z. Younossi, E. Galun, T. Pruett, R. Tur-Kaspa, R. Eren, S. Dagan, N. Graham, P. V. Williams, and J. Andrews.** 2006. Monoclonal antibody HCV-AbXTL68 in patients undergoing liver transplantation for HCV: results of a phase 2 randomized study. *Liver Transplant.* **12:**1381–1389.
138. **Scott, J. D., and D. R. Gretch.** 2007. Molecular diagnostics of hepatitis C virus infection: a systematic review. *JAMA* **297:**724–732.
139. **Seme, K., M. Poljak, D. Z. Babic, T. Mocilnik, and A. Vince.** 2005. The role of core antigen detection in management of hepatitis C: a critical review. *J. Clin. Virol.* **32:**92–101.
140. **Shepard, C. W., L. Finelli, and M. J. Alter.** 2005. Global epidemiology of hepatitis C virus infection. *Lancet Infect. Dis.* **5:**558–567.
141. **Shiffman, M. L., F. Suter, B. R. Bacon, D. Nelson, H. Harley, R. Sola, S. D. Shafran, K. Barange, A. Lin, A. Soman, and S. Zeuzem.** 2007. Peginterferon alfa-2a and ribavirin for 16 or 24 weeks in HCV genotype 2 or 3. *N. Engl. J. Med.* **357:**124–134.
142. **Shire, N. J., J. A. Welge, and K. E. Sherman.** 2007. Response rates to pegylated interferon and ribavirin in HCV/HIV coinfection: a research synthesis. *J. Viral Hepat.* **14:**239–248.
143. **Shoukry, N. H., A. Grakoui, M. Houghton, D. Y. Chien, J. Ghrayeb, K. A. Reimann, and C. M. Walker.** 2003. Memory CD8+ T cells are required for protection from persistent hepatitis C virus infection. *J. Exp. Med.* **197:**1645–1655.
144. **Simmonds, P., J. Bukh, C. Combet, G. Deleage, N. Enomoto, S. Feinstone, P. Halfon, G. Inchauspe, C. Kuiken, G. Maertens, M. Mizokami, D. G. Murphy, H. Okamoto, J. M. Pawlotsky, F. Penin, E. Sablon, I. T. Shin, L. J. Stuyver, H. J. Thiel, S. Viazov, A. J. Weiner, and A. Widell.** 2005. Consensus proposals for a unified system of nomenclature of hepatitis C virus genotypes. *Hepatology* **42:**962–973.
145. **Sjogren, M. H., R. Sjogren, Jr., M. F. Lyons, M. Ryan, J. Santoro, C. Smith, K. R. Reddy, H. Bonkovsky, B. Huntley, and S. Faris-Young.** 2007. Antiviral response of HCV genotype 1 to consensus interferon and ribavirin versus pegylated interferon and ribavirin. *Dig. Dis. Sci.* **52:**1540–1547.
146. **Soza, A., J. E. Everhart, M. G. Ghany, E. Doo, T. Heller, K. Promrat, Y. Park, T. J. Liang, and J. H. Hoofnagle.** 2002. Neutropenia during combination therapy of interferon alfa and ribavirin for chronic hepatitis C. *Hepatology* **36:**1273–1279.
147. **Strasser, S. I., D. Myerson, C. L. Spurgeon, K. M. Sullivan, B. Storer, H. G. Schoch, S. Kim, M. E. Flowers, and G. B. McDonald.** 1999. Hepatitis C virus infection and bone marrow transplantation: a cohort study with 10-year follow-up. *Hepatology* **29:**1893–1899.
148. **Sulkowski, M. S., and Y. Benhamou.** 2007. Therapeutic issues in HIV/HCV-coinfected patients. *J. Viral Hepat.* **14:**371–386.
149. **Tahan, V., C. Karaca, B. Yildirim, A. Bozbas, R. Ozaras, K. Demir, E. Avsar, A. Mert, F. Besisik, S. Kaymakoglu, H. Senturk, Y. Cakaloglu, C. Kalayci, A. Okten, and N. Tozun.** 2005. Sexual transmission of HCV between spouses. *Am. J. Gastroenterol.* **100:**821–824.
150. **Terrault, N. A.** 2002. Sexual activity as a risk factor for hepatitis C. *Hepatology* **36:**S99–S105.
151. **Thuluvath, P. J., K. L. Krok, D. L. Segev, and H. Y. Yoo.** 2007. Trends in post-liver transplant survival in patients with hepatitis C between 1991 and 2001 in the United States. *Liver Transplant.* **13:**719–724.
152. **Vandelli, C., F. Renzo, L. Romano, S. Tisminetzky, M. De Palma, T. Stroffolini, E. Ventura, and A. Zanetti.** 2004. Lack of evidence of sexual transmission of hepatitis C among monogamous couples: results of a 10-year prospective follow-up study. *Am. J. Gastroenterol.* **99:** 855–859.
153. **Vento, S., T. Garofano, C. Renzini, F. Cainelli, F. Casali, G. Ghironzi, T. Ferraro, and E. Concia.** 1998. Fulminant hepatitis associated with hepatitis A virus superinfection in patients with chronic hepatitis C. *N. Engl. J. Med.* **338:**286–290.
154. **Voisset, C., and J. Dubuisson.** 2004. Functional hepatitis C virus envelope glycoproteins. *Biol. Cell* **96:**413–420.
155. **von Hahn, T., J. C. Yoon, H. Alter, C. M. Rice, B. Rehermann, P. Balfe, and J. A. McKeating.** 2007. Hepatitis C virus continuously escapes from neutralizing antibody and T-cell responses during chronic infection in vivo. *Gastroenterology* **132:**667–678.
156. **Wakita, T., T. Pietschmann, T. Kato, T. Date, M. Miyamoto, Z. Zhao, K. Murthy, A. Habermann, H. G. Krausslich, M. Mizokami, R. Bartenschlager, and T. J. Liang.** 2005. Production of infectious hepatitis C virus in tissue culture from a cloned viral genome. *Nat. Med.* **11:**791–796.
157. **Weinbaum, C. M., K. M. Sabin, and S. S. Santibanez.** 2005. Hepatitis B, hepatitis C, and HIV in correctional populations: a review of epidemiology and prevention. *AIDS* **19**(Suppl. 3)**:**S41–S46.
158. **Welbourn, S., and A. Pause.** 2007. The hepatitis C virus NS2/3 protease. *Curr. Issues Mol. Biol.* **9:**63–69.
159. **Wells, J. T., M. R. Lucey, and A. Said.** 2006. Hepatitis C in transplant recipients of solid organs, other than liver. *Clin. Liver Dis.* **10:**901–917.
160. **World Health Organization.** 2007. *International Travel and Health.* World Health Organization, Geneva, Switzerland.
161. **Wu, J. Z.** 2001. Internally located signal peptides direct hepatitis C virus polyprotein processing in the ER membrane. *IUBMB Life* **51:**19–23.
162. **Xie, Z. C., J. I. Riezu-Boj, J. J. Lasarte, J. Guillen, J. H. Su, M. P. Civeira, and J. Prieto.** 1998. Transmission of hepatitis C virus infection to tree shrews. *Virology* **244:**513–520.
163. **Yazdanpanah, Y., G. De Carli, B. Migueres, F. Lot, M. Campins, C. Colombo, T. Thomas, S. Deuffic-Burban, M. H. Prevot, M. Domart, A. Tarantola, D. Abiteboul, P. Deny, S. Pol, J. C. Desenclos, V. Puro, and E. Bouvet.** 2005. Risk factors for hepatitis C virus transmission to health care workers after occupational exposure: a

European case-control study. *Clin. Infect. Dis.* **41:**1423–1430.

164. **Yi, M., and S. M. Lemon.** 2003. 3′ nontranslated RNA signals required for replication of hepatitis C virus RNA. *J. Virol.* **77:**3557–3568.

165. **Yi, M., R. A. Villanueva, D. L. Thomas, T. Wakita, and S. M. Lemon.** 2006. Production of infectious genotype 1a hepatitis C virus (Hutchinson strain) in cultured human hepatoma cells. *Proc. Natl. Acad. Sci. USA* **103:**2310–2315.

Alphaviruses

DAVID W. SMITH, JOHN S. MACKENZIE, AND SCOTT C. WEAVER

54

Alphavirus infections occur throughout the world, causing predominantly encephalitis in the Americas and polyarthralgic illness elsewhere. Disease due to the New World alphaviruses was first recognized when outbreaks of equine encephalitis occurred in Massachusetts in the early 19th century, followed by other outbreaks in the United States and South America (17). Western equine encephalitis virus (WEEV) was the first alphavirus successfully cultured, in 1930; eastern equine encephalitis virus (EEEV) and Venezuelan equine encephalitis virus (VEEV) were also isolated from horses later that decade. The earliest descriptions of human disease due to Old World alphaviruses were epidemics of likely chikungunya virus (CHIKV) illness occurring in India and Southeast Asia for over 200 years. Outbreaks of polyarthritis, probably due to Ross River virus (RRV), were described in eastern Australia and New Guinea in the late 19th and early 20th centuries. CHIKV, RRV, and Sindbis virus (SINV) were subsequently isolated from mosquitoes and patients in the 1950s and 1960s.

Alphavirus encephalitis has remained a rare, and declining, clinical disease in animals and humans, though the threat remains while these viruses continue to circulate. In contrast, the alphaviruses causing arthritis continue to cause human illness worldwide with regular epidemics, including massive CHIKV outbreaks.

The alphaviruses are principally mosquito-borne, positive-strand RNA viruses in the family *Togaviridae* that exhibit a broad range of pathogenicity in humans and animals (130, 142). Members of the genus are distributed worldwide in diverse ecological niches, where they are usually maintained in cycles between mosquitoes and birds or mammals. While human infections generally are incidental to the transmission cycles, in some instances human-mosquito-human cycles can maintain transmission and lead to large outbreaks and epidemics. Among the 24 alphaviruses listed in Table 1, 16 have been associated with human illness. Clinically, these manifest most commonly as polyarthralgia, often accompanied by fever and/or rash, or as central nervous system (CNS) infections.

VIROLOGY

Classification

The alphaviruses form a genus within the *Togaviridae*. Genetic studies have shown similarities in genomic organization to rubella virus (genus *Rubivirus* in the *Togaviridae*) and to two fish viruses and have suggested an evolutionary origin from a plant virus. The alphaviruses are classified into at least seven antigenic complexes (Table 1); this classification is generally supported by analyses of available genomic sequences (Fig. 1) (130, 142). The phylogenetic division into complexes of viruses related to EEEV, VEEV, SINV, and Semliki Forest virus (SFV) diverges from the antigenic classification in the placements of Middelburg virus (MIDV) and WEEV. Although WEEV is antigenically related to SINV, genetically it is a recombinant of an EEEV-like virus and an ancestral, perhaps extinct, SINV-like virus (145).

Genotypes

Alphaviruses are estimated to have evolved at a rate on the order of 10^{-4} substitutions/nucleotide/year, approximately 10- to 100-fold lower than that of most non-arthropod-borne RNA viruses, presumably reflecting constraints imposed by alternating host (vertebrate and arthropod) replication cycles (144). Molecular taxonomic studies have been instructive in tracing the movements of alphaviruses between continents, indicating the recent divergence of several medically important alphaviruses. The geographic origin of the alphaviruses is unclear, but phylogenetic analyses suggest that the modern alphaviruses have resulted from a combination of movement of viruses between the Old World and the New World 2,000 to 3,000 years ago and of evolution within the hemispheres. Later movements between the hemispheres and further recombinations between Old and New World viruses have contributed to the diversity (130, 142). For example, a later recombination between ancestral EEEV-like and SINV-like viruses, presumably in the New World, generated an intermediary that subsequently diverged into WEEV and related Fort Morgan (FMV) and Highlands J (HJV) viruses (145).

EEEV has four antigenic subtypes. Three of these occur exclusively in Latin America and are associated with equine but not human disease. The other subtype occurs in eastern North America, the Caribbean, and Mexico, where it is associated with human and equine disease (13). The North American lineage is highly conserved both genetically and antigenically, while the South and Central American lineages are more diverse. The lack of virulence

TABLE 1 Selected characteristics of alphaviruses[a]

Antigenic complex	Virus	Subtype(s)/variety	Clinical syndrome	Transmission cycle	Geographic distribution
EEE	**EEEV**	**North America**[b]	Encephalitis	Mosquito-bird	United States, Canada, Caribbean, Central and South America
		South America		Mosquito-mammal/bird	
VEE	**VEEV**	**IAB, IC, IE** (epizootic/ epidemic)	Febrile illness, encephalitis	Mosquito/equine	Central America, Mexico, Trinidad, Colombia, Venezuela, Peru, Ecuador
		ID, IE, IF (sylvatic)	Febrile illness, encephalitis	Mosquito-rodent/bird	Mexico, Central America, Brazil, Colombia, Peru, Venezuela
	EVERV	**II**	Encephalitis	Mosquito-rodent	Florida
	Mucambo virus	**IIIA**	Febrile illness, encephalitis	Mosquito-rodent/marsupial	Trinidad, Brazil, French Guiana, Surinam
	Tonate/Bijou Bridge virus	**IIIB**	Febrile illness, encephalitis	Mosquito-rodent/swallow bug-bird	French Guiana, Surinam, United States
	71D-1252 virus	IIIC		Unknown	Peru
	Pixuna virus	IV		Unknown	Brazil
	Cabassou virus	**V**	Febrile illness	Unknown	French Guiana
	AG80-663	**VI**	Febrile illness	Unknown	Argentina
WEE	**WEEV**[c]		Encephalitis	Mosquito-bird/hare	North America, Argentina, Brazil, Uruguay
		AG80-646		Mosquito-?	Argentina
	SINV[b]		Febrile illness, rash, arthritis	Mosquito-bird	Europe, Asia, Australia, Africa
		Ockelbo	Febrile illness, rash, arthritis	Mosquito-bird	Europe
		Kyzlagach		Mosquito?-bird	Azerbaijan
	Fort Morgan virus			Swallow bug-bird	Western United States
	HJV			Mosquito-bird	Eastern United States
	Aura virus			Mosquito-mammal	Brazil, Argentina
	Whataroa virus			Mosquito-bird	Australia, New Zealand, Oceania

Semliki Forest	**SFV**		Febrile illness, encephalitis	Mosquito-mammal/bird	Africa, Asia
	Me Tri		Encephalitis	Unknown	Vietnam
	CHIKV		Febrile illness, rash, arthritis	Mosquito-primate/other mammal; mosquito-human	Africa, Asia
	ONNV		Febrile illness, rash, arthritis	Mosquito-human epidemic cycle	Africa
		Igbo-Ora	Febrile illness, rash, arthritis	Mosquito-?	Africa
	MAYV		Febrile illness, rash, arthritis	Mosquito-primate, other mammal/marsupial/bird	Central and South America, Caribbean
		Una			Central and South America, Caribbean
	RRV		Febrile illness, rash, arthritis	Mosquito-mammal; mosquito-human (epidemic)	Australia, Oceania
		Sagiyama		Mosquito-?	Japan
	Getah virus			Mosquito-pig/other mammals	Asia
	Bebaru virus			Mosquito-?	Malaysia
Barmah Forest	**BFV**		Febrile illness, rash, arthritis	Mosquito-mammal	Australia
Middelburg[d]				Unknown	Africa
Ndumu				Unknown	Africa

[a] Viruses in bold type are human pathogens. Individual viruses are distinguished by standard serologic procedures; strains that exhibit slight differences (e.g., unidirectional fourfold difference in cross-neutralization tests) are regarded as subtypes, and lesser but consistent antigenic differences define viral varieties.
[b] Additonal antigenic subtypes or varieties are recognized.
[c] WEEV is a genetic recombinant of EEE-like and ancestral Sindbis-like viruses but is antigenically related to Sindbis complex viruses.
[d] Middelburg virus is antigenically distinct from viruses in other alphavirus complexes but is related genetically to SFV.

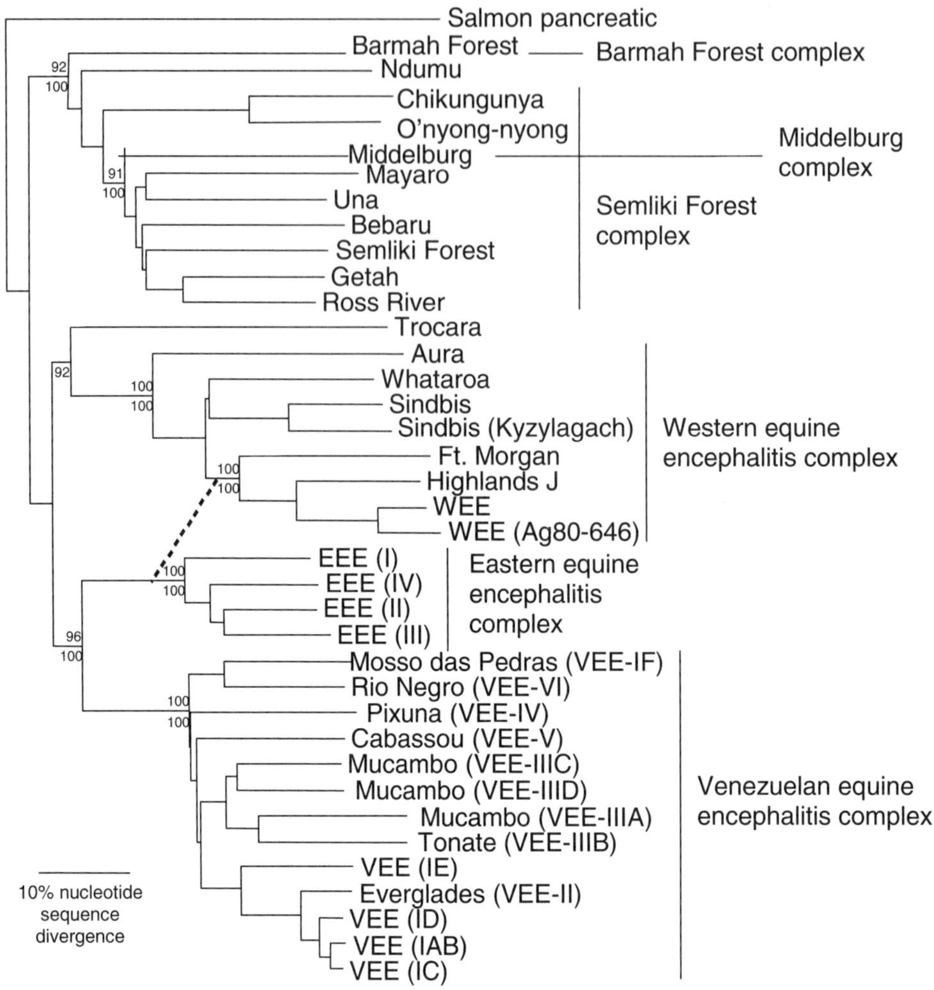

FIGURE 1 Genetic relationship of alphavirus species and some major subtypes (shown in parentheses) based on partial sequences of E1 glycoprotein gene. The main antigenic complexes are indicated on the right. The dotted line represents the recombination event between SINV and EEEV. Numbers on the lines indicate bootstrap values for clades to the right using the neighbor-joining (numbers above branches) or Bayesian (numbers below line) method. (Reprinted from reference 49 with permission.)

of the Latin American subtypes in humans may be related to their greater sensitivity to human type I interferons (1).

The VEEV antigenic complex, a sister group to EEEV, is even more diverse, with at least 10 different subtypes and varieties. These viruses are distributed in a mostly non-overlapping pattern in the Central and South American tropics and subtropics. The greater diversity of the VEEV complex may be explained by the low mobility of their rodent hosts compared to the avian hosts of EEEV. However, WEEV, which also cycles among birds, exhibits highly conserved lineages spanning North and South America (139, 143).

Composition

The alphaviruses are small icosahedral viruses with a lipid bilayer envelope closely enshrouding a nucleocapsid with a diameter of 40 nm (Fig. 2) (142). Eighty glycoprotein spikes extend from the virion surface in a T=4 lattice, giving the virion a total diameter of 69 nm. The flower-like spikes, heterotrimers comprised of an E1 protein and an E2 dimer, are anchored in and span the envelope to form 1:1 associations with nucleocapsid monomers via paired helical transmembrane segments. Nucleocapsids also are arranged in icosahedral T=4 symmetry, in pentamer and hexamer capsid protein clusters linked by N-terminal arms that also define interactive sites with the glycoprotein spikes. The positively charged outer rim of the capsomers is oriented toward the membrane, and the highly charged N-terminal domain binds the viral RNA.

The viral genome is a single strand of positive-sense RNA, 11 to 12 kb in length, with a poly(A) tail and a 5′-terminal cap (Fig. 3). The genome consists of regions encoding nonstructural protein replicases located at the 5′ two-thirds of the genome and the three structural proteins at the 3′ one-third (130). The nonstructural proteins are translated as a polyprotein that subsequently is cleaved into a number of functional intermediates and ultimately to four nonstructural proteins. The structural proteins are

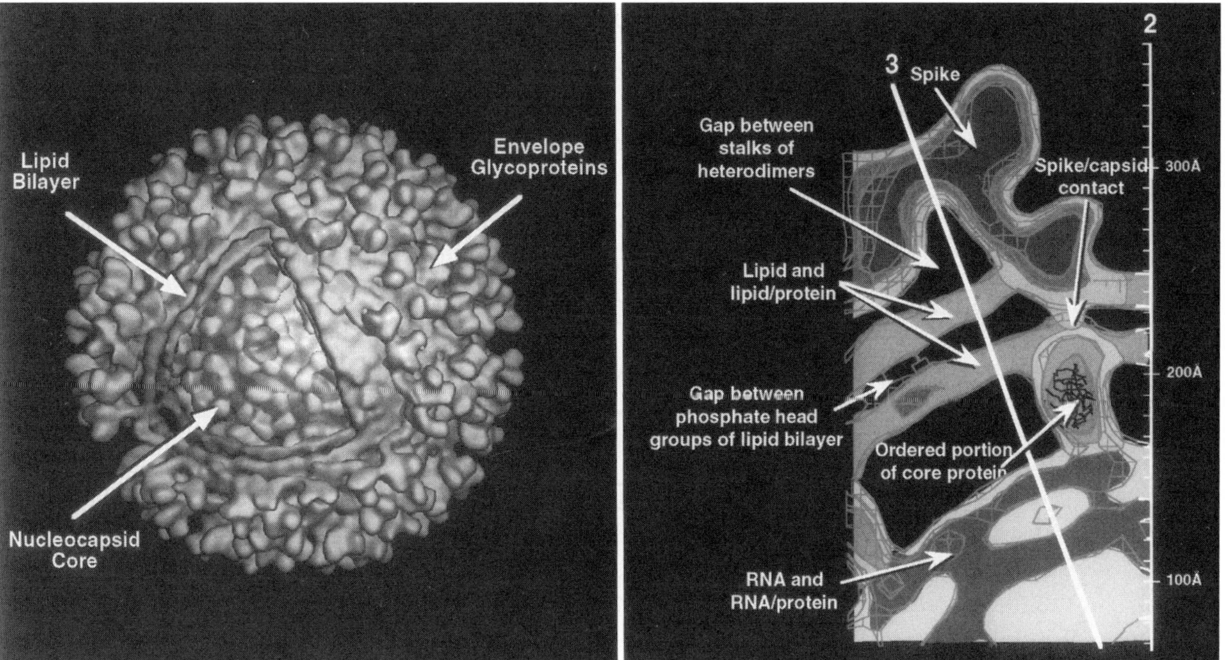

FIGURE 2 RRV. (Left) Cryoelectron microscopic image reconstruction of RRV showing the flower-like envelope protein spikes, virion membrane, and nucleocapsid core. (Right) Relationships of spike and capsid proteins and virion RNA. (Courtesy of R. J. Kuhn.)

translated from a 26S subgenomic mRNA (ca. 4.1 kb) and cleaved from a polyprotein into two envelope proteins, the capsid protein, and 6K and E3 polypeptides. Conserved sequences in the junction between nonstructural and structural domains and in 5′- and 3′-terminal nontranslated regions serve as promoters.

Characteristics of structural and nonstructural proteins are summarized in Table 2. Two domains on the E2 protein are principally associated with antibody-mediated viral neutralization, of which the most important is a small linear sequence of two antigenic sites between amino acids 180 to 216 for SINV and VEEV and in a corresponding position for RRV; a second domain is discontinuous and conformationally dependent. The former lies in spatial proximity to an E1 neutralizing domain and may define a virus receptor binding site on the E1-E2 spike. The E1 glycoprotein contains the viral hemagglutinin, fusion properties, and cross-reactive neutralizing epitopes. Epitopes that elicit protective nonneutralizing antibodies have been identified.

Other important viral phenotypic characteristics, including neurovirulence, have been linked to specific E1 and E2 amino acid substitutions. Among them is a Q55-H mutation in the SINV E2 protein that increases neurovirulence, growth in neuronal and nonneuronal cells, and resistance to the protective effects of *bcl-2* gene expression on virus-induced apoptosis (50, 52). Additional attenuating loci have been identified at other E2 loci, in the 5′ noncoding region, and in nsP1 of SFV, VEEV, and SINV. Importantly, natural viral determinants of equine virulence associated with epizootic VEEV emergence and viral capacity to replicate and disseminate in mosquito vectors also have been identified in the E2 protein (139).

BIOLOGY

Replication

Several different cellular protein receptors in vertebrate and mosquito cells have been identified for alphaviruses. The high-affinity laminin receptor serves as a mammalian and mosquito cell (in vitro) receptor for SINV, while other protein receptors for SINV have been identified in mouse neural and chicken cells. Other less conserved protein receptors or accessory factors may be involved in infection of the mosquito midgut. After binding to the cell membrane, virions are taken up in endocytic vesicles (Fig. 4). Virion spikes, especially through the E1 fusion-promoting protein, induce bridging of virion and vesicle membranes with release of the nucleocapsid. Acidic conditions in the vesicle lead to shrinkage of the capsid, exposure of a ribosomal binding domain, and uncoating, with release of RNA from the capsid matrix. In the cytoplasm, the positive-sense viral genome functions as mRNA. Nonstructural proteins are translated as polyproteins, principally as a P123 moiety when translation is terminated by an opal (UAG) codon between nsP3 and nsP4 or, when replaced by a sense codon, as a P1234 polyprotein. Replicase activities are associated with the polyprotein intermediates and individual nonstructural proteins, as well as host factors (130).

The replication complexes of alphaviruses are associated with cytoplasmic membranes, and the main determinant of membrane attachment seems to be nsP1, which is hydrophobically modified by palmitoylation of cysteine residues. RNA is replicated with the production of negative-sense RNA templates which are transcribed either to full-length genomic positive-sense RNA or, when initiated

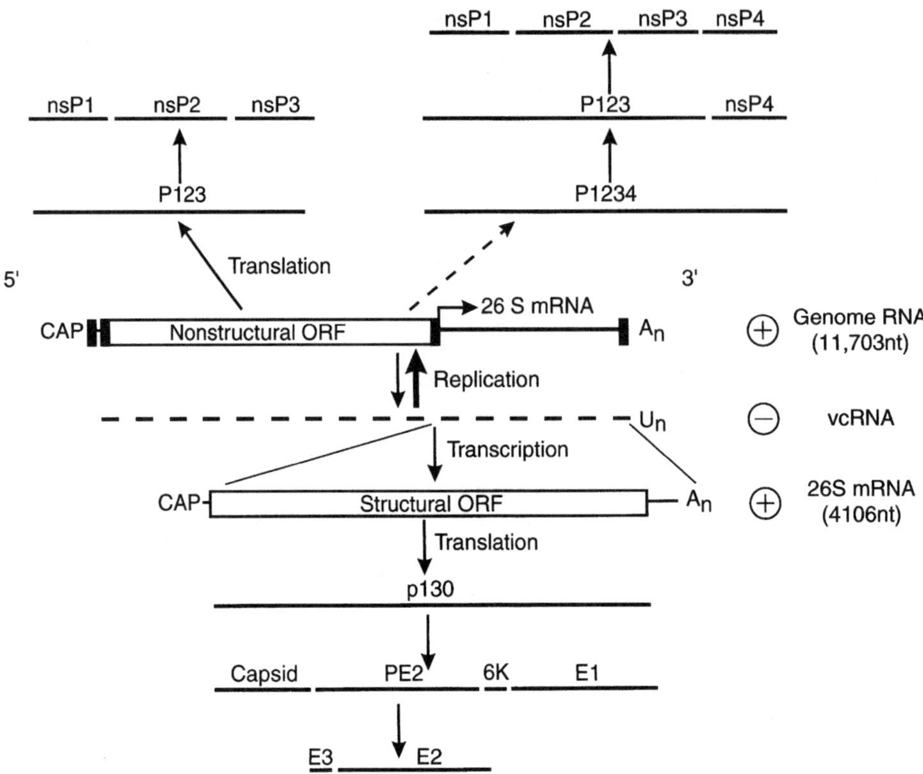

FIGURE 3 Schematic diagram of alphavirus genome [positive (⊕) sense RNA with poly(A) (A_n) tail and 5′ terminal cap (CAP); viral complementary RNA (vcRNA) of negative (⊖) sense; and subgenomic mRNA of positive sense]. Viral nonstructural proteins are translated from the 5′ two-thirds region of the genome, yielding polyprotein intermediates and nonstructural proteins nsP1 to nsP4. RNA is replicated into negative-sense RNA templates and transcribed into 26S subgenomic RNA. Cotranslational processing of the subgenomic mRNA yields the three principal structural proteins: capsid and envelope glycoproteins (E1 and E2). ORF, open reading frame; nt, nucleotide.

TABLE 2 Alphavirus proteins

Protein	Length (amino acids)[a]	Characteristics and function
Structural		
Capsid	264	30-kDa monomers organized as 12 pentamers and 30 hexamers; multiple copies bind to viral RNA genome, ribosome, and cytoplasmic domain of transmembrane spike
E1	439	52-kDa glycosylated transmembrane (spike) protein; fusion domain for viral membrane penetration; hemagglutination, neutralization, and protection
E2	423	49-kDa glycosylated transmembrane (spike) protein; epitopes for viral neutralization, neurovirulence, hemagglutination, viral receptor interactions
E3	64	10-kDa glycoprotein cleaved with E2 from PE2 intermediate; associated with virion spike in SFV
Nonstructural		
nsP1	540	Initiation of RNA minus-strand synthesis; guanyltransferase function, modulation of nsP2 activity
nsP2	807	N-terminal domain—RNA helicase, NTP binding, initiation of 26 mRNA transcription; C-terminal domain—nonstructural proteinase; 50% of SFV activity in nucleus (function unknown)
nsP3	556	N-terminal domain conserved in length and sequence; C-terminal domain variable in length and sequence; functions unclear
nsP4	610	RNA polymerase; unstable and rapidly degraded

[a] Length in SINV.

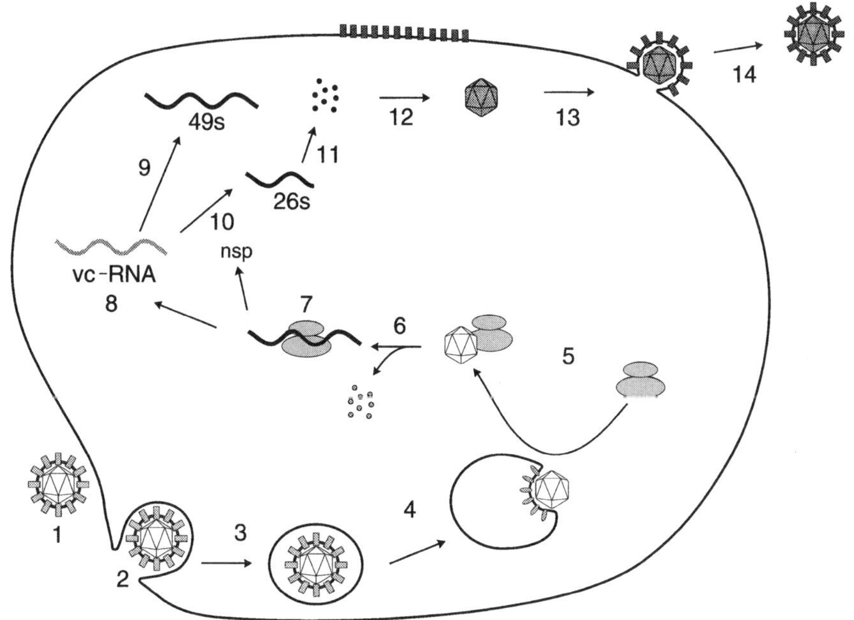

FIGURE 4 After binding to the cell membrane (step 1), virions are taken up in endocytic vesicles (steps 2 and 3). The virion and vesicular membranes fuse, releasing the nucleocapsid (step 4). The viral nucleocapsid binds to a ribosome (step 5) and is uncoated, freeing viral RNA (step 6) from the individual capsid (gray dots). Positive-sense viral RNA (heavy line) is replicated (step 7), producing complementary negative-sense RNA (gray line) (step 8), which in turn is transcribed to full-length genomic positive-sense RNA (step 9) or subgenomic RNA (step 10). Nonstructural proteins (nsp) are translated from genomic RNA. Subgenomic RNA is translated to produce capsid proteins (black dots) and envelope proteins, which are modified before insertion into the cell membrane (gray bars) (step 11). Genomic RNA is packaged with capsid proteins into nucleocapsid cores (step 12); capsid and E2 proteins associate (step 13) prior to viral budding (step 14).

at the internal junction site, to 26S subgenomic RNA. The 5′ ends of both are capped and methylated. Genomic RNA can bind to replicases, producing more negative-strand templates; to ribosomes, where translation leads to additional nonstructural proteins; or, after they become available, to capsid proteins for arrangement into nucleocapsids. Subgenomic RNA is cotranslationally processed, with rapid autoproteolytic release of the capsid protein, the first protein encoded from the 5′ terminus. This cleavage exposes an N-terminal signal sequence that facilitates transport and insertion of the PE2 polyprotein (containing E2) into the endoplasmic reticulum (ER) membrane. Subsequent signals on PE2 lead to insertion of the 6K protein and translocation and cleavage of E1. The envelope proteins are modified in the ER lumen by addition of carbohydrate chains and fatty acids and are further modified during transport through the Golgi apparatus. PE2-E1 dimers are formed in the ER; during transport through the Golgi apparatus, PE2 is cleaved to form E2 and E3. The envelope spikes are transported to the cell plasma membrane, where the E2 cytoplasmic domain associates with the nucleocapsid C-terminal domain prior to viral budding.

The highly productive and rapid alphavirus replication cycle has been exploited in a novel approach to produce nonreplicating particles (replicons) as immunogens. Foreign genes from a variety of viruses, including human immunodeficiency virus, Ebola virus, and Marburg virus, have been introduced in place of VEEV or SINV structural protein genes, with helper systems providing the alphavirus structural proteins that allow packaging of recombinant particles that cannot replicate, while allowing high-level expression of the desired antigen.

Host Range in Animals

Alphaviruses are transmitted to vertebrate hosts principally by mosquitoes but in some instances by ticks, mites, or other arthropods. The capacity of specific mosquito vectors to transmit infection requires competency to support viral replication in their midgut cells, followed by dissemination within the mosquito and infection of salivary glands (extrinsic incubation period). Salivary gland infection and the resultant capacity to transmit infection with subsequent blood feedings often persist for the life of the mosquito. Barriers to midgut and salivary gland infection have been identified in some species; e.g., a midgut barrier to CHIKV infection in *Aedes aegypti* has been linked to eye color at a chromosome 3 locus. Recently, a point mutation in CHIKV has been identified that appears to confer increased ability to disseminate from the midgut to the salivary glands in *Aedes albopictus* (136). Transovarial transmission of RRV in mosquitoes has been demonstrated experimentally and confirmed in Australian field studies.

Natural alphavirus infections are observed in a broad range of animal species, including birds, mammals, reptiles, and amphibians. Only animals that develop a higher-titer viremia (ca. $\geq 10^{3.5}$/ml) for a sustained period of several days contribute to further virus transmission. Many alphaviruses cause clinically silent infections of birds and rodents. Individual alphaviruses produce symptomatic infections in various animal species as described below. However, horses are unusually susceptible to a number of alphaviruses, e.g., EEEV, WEEV, VEEV, SFV, Getah virus, the Una strain of Mayaro virus (MAYV), RRV, and Middelburg virus, while EEEV is virulent for an extensive range of avian and mammalian species.

Alphaviruses produce lethal infections in wet chicks and embryonated eggs. Mice exhibit an age-dependent susceptibility; 2- to 3-day-old suckling mice develop fatal encephalitis when inoculated intracerebrally, while weanling and older mice are variably susceptible after intracerebral and peripheral inoculation. Differential ratios of fatal infection after inoculation by these routes have been linked to neuroinvasiveness and virulence of specific viral strains. Strains of o'nyong-nyong virus (ONNV) may kill suckling mice only after adaptation by serial passage. Other laboratory animals, such as hamsters, guinea pigs, rats, rabbits, and nonhuman primates, develop encephalitis after intracerebral inoculation with encephalitogenic alphaviruses.

Growth in Cell Culture

Alphaviruses can be propagated in a variety of cell cultures but generally grow best in mosquito cell lines such as C6/36, AP-61, and TRA-284. As may be expected with viruses that replicate in insects at ambient temperatures, they often grow better at low temperatures. However, the cytopathic effect (CPE) is minimal or absent in mosquito cells, so blind passage to another cell line is required. They rapidly produce destructive CPE in primary duck and chicken embryo cells and in most mammalian cell lines, including BHK-21, Vero, and HeLa cells. EEEV and VEEV produce cell rounding, degeneration, and lysis within 18 to 24 h and complete destruction of cell monolayers by 48 to 72 h; WEEV-induced CPE appears 24 to 48 h later. Viral yields usually range on the order of 10^7 to 10^{10} PFU/ml. These viruses are adapted to mosquitoes and to birds, whose body temperatures can exceed 40°C, and viral replication in vitro occurs over a broad range of temperatures, from 25 to 41°C. In mosquito cell cultures, after an initial phase that may produce some degree of CPE, a persistent infection without visible cytopathology can be maintained indefinitely. Numerous differences in viral nucleotide use, maturation, and replication have been demonstrated in mammalian and insect cells (144).

Inactivation by Physical and Chemical Agents

As enveloped RNA viruses, alphaviruses are labile in the environment and are inactivated by lipid solvents like ether and chloroform, by deoxycholate, and by common laboratory disinfectants such as hypochlorite, 70% alcohol, phenol, paraformaldehyde, and formaldehyde. Commercial procedures to eliminate potential viral contaminants of human biologics are effective in removing alphaviruses, e.g., ethanol fractionation and polyethylene glycol precipitation, virucidal treatments with tri(*n*-butyl) phosphate in combination with sodium cholate or Tween, and pasteurization at 60°C for 1 h (137).

PATHOGENESIS

Natural infection of vertebrates is initiated when mosquitoes deposit infected saliva in extravascular tissues while blood feeding. Most alphaviruses replicate initially in skeletal muscle cells in mouse models (56), although VEEV is taken up into Langerhans cells. The latter may be important in natural human infections, with virus then travelling within leukocytes to draining lymph nodes and eventually spreading to target tissues in the nervous system, joints, or skin.

For the neurotropic alphaviruses, local replication results in a brief viremia, followed by CNS invasion through the cerebral vascular endothelium or olfactory epithelium. Unlike EEEV and WEEV, which are principally neurotropic in humans, VEEV also produces a systemic illness with pathological changes in the lung and lymphoid tissue of the gastrointestinal tract, spleen, and peripheral nodes. CNS pathology in VEEV infection reflects both viral and immunopathological processes, in which the induction of cytokines, interferons, tumor necrosis factor alpha, and NO appear to be important in the balance of viral clearance and immune-mediated damage.

Variants of VEEV produced by site-directed mutagenesis have elucidated patterns of viral spread in mice after peripheral inoculation; specific changes in the E2 protein have been associated with delayed and sporadic infection of local lymph nodes, limitation of viral spread beyond the lymph nodes, and infection of local lymph nodes and other lymphatic tissue without significant viremia or neuroinvasion. In comparing the neurotropic wild-type VEEV Trinidad donkey IAB strain with its attenuated (vaccine) derivative, TC-83, attenuation appears to involve a combination of alterations in the E2 glycoprotein, perhaps affecting viral attachment and cell entry and, in the 5′ nontranslated region, affecting viral RNA synthesis. A mutation at amino acid position 120 in E2 corresponds to a locus associated with attenuation of SINV strains exhibiting rapid cellular penetration. The attenuated strain is more rapidly cleared from blood, reducing opportunities for neuroinvasion (faster cell penetration expedites peripheral viral clearance). The mutation in the 5′ noncoding region may reduce viral replication in infected CNS cells, leading to decreased necrosis, inflammation, and CNS spread. The vaccine's limited neurovirulence has been shown by direct intracerebral inoculation of horses, which results in a minimal inflammatory reaction. Thus, attenuation is speculated to be a combined effect of reduced neuroinvasion and neurovirulence.

In a murine model of alphavirus encephalitis, cellular genes that regulate the cell death pathway can modulate the outcome of SINV infection. Cellular *bax* and *bak* genes, which accelerate cell death, also accelerate SINV-induced apoptosis, while apoptotic inhibitors, like *bcl-2*, suppress alphavirus-induced apoptosis and can facilitate a persistent infection (52). During SFV-induced murine encephalitis, infiltrating leukocytes and neural precursor cells undergo apoptosis, while productively infected neurons undergo necrosis.

In humans, an age-dependent susceptibility of infants and the elderly to CNS infection has been observed epidemiologically, although its pathogenesis has not been elucidated. Immature mouse neurons infected with SINV or SFV die of caspase-dependent apoptosis, while mature neurons survive by producing factors inhibiting virus-induced apoptosis (50). Apoptosis is induced at the time of alphavirus fusion with the cell membrane, and virus replication is not required. Virus fusion apparently initiates the apoptotic cascade by inducing sphingomyelin degradation and ceramide release. In mature mice, antibody clears replicating virus from the infected cells, though viral RNA has been shown to persist in neurons and can protect the animal from fatal infection (51), and may act as a source of reactivation if there is interruption of continued antibody production. In contrast, T cells are not protective, although $CD8^+$ cells may act indirectly, possibly via cytokines, to assist in the clearance of viral RNA from neurons. In the special circumstance of airborne infection, induction of local respiratory tract immunity, including specific immunoglobulin G (IgG) as well as IgA, correlates with protection against VEEV challenge. Protection apparently is mediated by a Th1 mechanism, with elaboration of IgG2a subclass antibodies and gamma interferon in the absence of changes in interleukin 4.

The mechanism of antibody-mediated protection is only partially understood. Clearance of SINV from the murine nervous system in nonfatal infections relies on antibodies to the E2 glycoprotein and does not kill infected neurons. Release of budding virus is prevented and viral replication is inhibited through unknown antiviral mechanisms not requiring an interferon response; however, this nonlytic mechanism that controls viral infection results in viral RNA persistence (51). Alpha/beta interferon protects adult mice from SINV infection by rapidly conferring an antiviral state on otherwise permissive cell types, both locally and systemically. Persistence of alphavirus infections in humans has not been proven, but there is evidence that it may be involved in chronic illness following RRV infection (117, 131).

In alphavirus infections characterized by rash and polyarthritis, infection of skin structures has been demonstrated by viral isolation and direct detection by PCR for SINV, and by immunohistochemical staining of RRV antigen in basal epidermal and eccrine duct epithelial cells (43, 60). Skin biopsy samples from RRV patients show a perivascular mononuclear cell infiltrate of predominantly cytotoxic T cells which, in the rare cases of purpuric rash, also lead to capillary damage and extravasation of blood (43). In experimentally infected mice, viral infection of and extensive necrotic changes in muscles, tendons, connective tissue, and periosteum offer a possible explanation for the musculoskeletal symptoms in humans (58, 78), though these may also be immune mediated.

In mice, macrophages have been directly implicated as the primary mediators of muscle damage (78). RRV infects macrophages both via a natural virus receptor and by Fc receptor-mediated antibody-dependent enhancement. Infection interferes with transcription of the interferon regulatory factor 1 and NF-κB genes and translation of tumor necrosis factor and inducible nitric oxide synthase.

Joint fluids from the acute and chronic phases of RRV disease contain an exudate comprised almost entirely of mononuclear cells that exhibit vacuolation, mitotic figures, and other signs of activation. Synovium shows an extensive mononuclear cell infiltrate, predominantly cytotoxic T cells, with areas of necrosis and fibrin deposition (24, 131). Viral antigen and RNA, but not infectious virus, have been detected in joint synovium and macrophages for as long as 5 weeks after onset of symptoms (24, 128). RRV, Barmah Forest virus (BFV), CHIKV, and SINV infect synovial monocytes/macrophages in animal models and some in vitro systems, while RRV can also be found in synovial cells (131). Complement activation and immune complexes have not generally been detected in serum or joint fluid and, even when found, as in SINV disease, were not correlated with disease activity (64); however, gamma interferon has been found in joint fluid of RRV-infected humans. Natural killer cells obtained from an affected joint killed uninfected autologous synovial cells. In both the joints and skin, lymphocytes are principally CD8 T cells. A combination of release of inflammatory mediators from the infected monocytes/macrophages and the cytotoxic T-cell responses to viral antigens is the likely explanation for the synovial swelling, effusion, and joint pain experienced in acute alphavirus infection.

Genetic susceptibility to RRV polyarthritis has been linked to Gm phenotype and HLA-DR7 haplotype, which may have a role in reducing the cytotoxic T-cell response and delaying viral clearance (42, 131).

Joint symptoms persist for months or years in a substantial proportion of patients with alphavirus polyarthritis. RRV RNA has been shown by PCR to persist within synovial tissue, and the virus can also persist in macrophages in vitro, even in the presence of neutralizing antibodies (117, 131). Alphaviruses may be able to establish a persistent, nonreplicative infection in joints and provoke an ongoing immune response to viral antigens.

The pathogenesis of the hemorrhagic diathesis in some cases of chikungunya is uncertain. Experimental studies with a passaged African strain showed that the virus bound to platelets; however, platelet function was not studied (74).

EASTERN EQUINE ENCEPHALITIS VIRUS

Virology

Classification and Composition

The virus was first isolated in 1933 after an equine epizootic in New Jersey and Virginia, though outbreaks had been occurring in horses for over a century prior to that, and then was identified as a cause of human encephalitis in 1938. Two antigenic varieties, of North and South American origin, are recognized (13, 142). The respective strains exhibit important biological differences in their transmission cycles and virulence, but serologically, they can be distinguished only by special assays such as plaque reduction neutralization, kinetic hemagglutination inhibition (HI), and reactivity with monoclonal antibodies. Genetically, the North American strains are relatively homogeneous and stable, whereas South American strains are antigenically and genetically heterogeneous. Enzootic foci within North America are segregated to a degree; however, viral movement within the continent and selective pressures over a longer time frame have maintained the virus in one or two phylogenetic groups over the entire >50-year period during which strains have been available for study (Fig. 1).

Biology

Severe, often lethal, CNS infection occurs in humans, horses, and pheasants. In contrast, whooping cranes, turkeys, and emus develop rapidly fatal viscerotropic infection, with necrotic lesions variously in spleen, liver, pancreas, intestines, kidneys, adrenals, and lungs, without CNS lesions. Other patterns of organ tropism have been described for various avian and mammalian species.

Devastating outbreaks have occurred in commercial pheasant, partridge, turkey, and emu flocks. Infection is rapidly spread among pheasants by pecking and probably

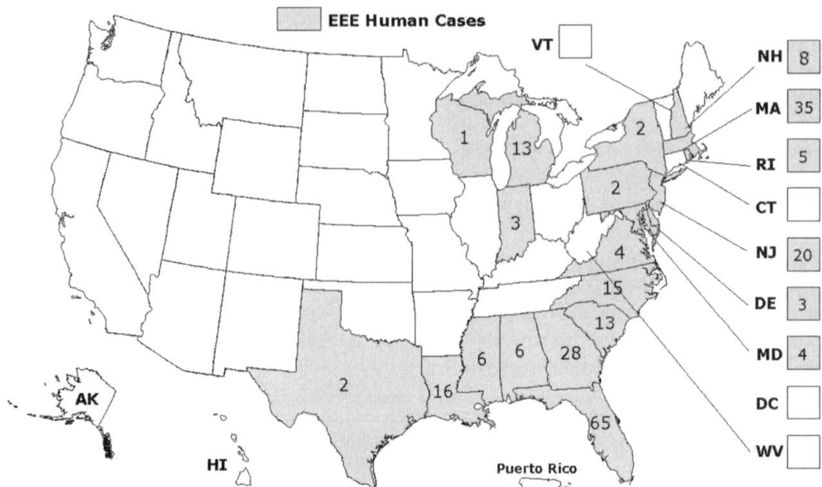

FIGURE 5 Reported cases of EEE among humans in the United States, 1964 to 2006. The reported incidence is highest in Florida, where equine cases are reported perennially from the northeastern coast and throughout the peninsula. Relatively constant inland foci of transmission have been identified in upstate New York, southwestern Michigan, northeastern Indiana, and southcentral Georgia. In Massachusetts, human cases have been reported almost entirely from the eastern counties and in New Jersey from the southern counties. (Reprinted from the Centers for Disease Control and Prevention at http://www.cdc.gov/ncidod/dvbid/arbor/arbocase.htm.)

by preening as well, since virus can be isolated from quills for up to 6 days after experimental inoculation and the birds can be infected orally. An outbreak in precious captive whooping cranes had nearly disastrous consequences, killing 7 of 39 of the endangered birds. The episode was an exception to the rule that native birds generally are resistant to infection, while exotic (introduced) species such as sparrows, pheasants, and emus develop lethal infections. The copious bloody diarrhea in ill whooping cranes and emus probably contributes to direct bird-to-bird transmission.

Horses have been considered dead-end hosts because viremia levels usually are too low to infect mosquitoes, though occasional horses may achieve circulating virus in the range of $10^{3.5}$ to $10^{5.5}$ PFU/ml and experimental horse-to-horse transmission by *Aedes sollicitans* mosquitoes has been shown.

Epidemiology

Distribution

The virus is transmitted only in the western hemisphere, where disease in horses or humans has been reported as far north as the Ontario and Quebec provinces in Canada, as far west as Wisconsin and eastern Texas, in the Caribbean, and in areas of South America as far south as central Argentina (13, 30, 48, 135). Outbreaks in the Caribbean and Mexico were caused by North American varieties of the virus. In the United States, transmission is concentrated in coastal areas on the Atlantic seaboard and Gulf Coast, but certain relatively constant inland foci of transmission also have been recognized (21) (Fig. 5).

The potential for viral transmission generally corresponds to the freshwater woodland swamp distribution of *Culiseta melanura* mosquitoes, the principal enzootic vector, with passerine birds as the major vertebrate hosts (48, 69). Its larval stages breed in depressions of mucky peat soils principally associated with upland red maples; a coastal biotype, where Atlantic white cedar swamps drain into salt marshes, and in the South, with loblolly bay vegetation.

In Central and South America, horse cases and enzootic viral transmission have been reported from many countries, and outbreaks of human disease have been reported from Jamaica, Trinidad, and the Dominican Republic (57). The enzootic vectors appear to be *Culex taeniopus* in the Caribbean and *Culex (melanoconion)* spp. in Central and South America. A wide range of species that feed on birds, mammals, and humans act as bridging vectors for epidemics.

Incidence and Prevalence of Human Infection

In the United States, infections have been steadily declining (17): they are rare and sporadic, with a median of five reported cases annually over the last four decades (Fig. 6).

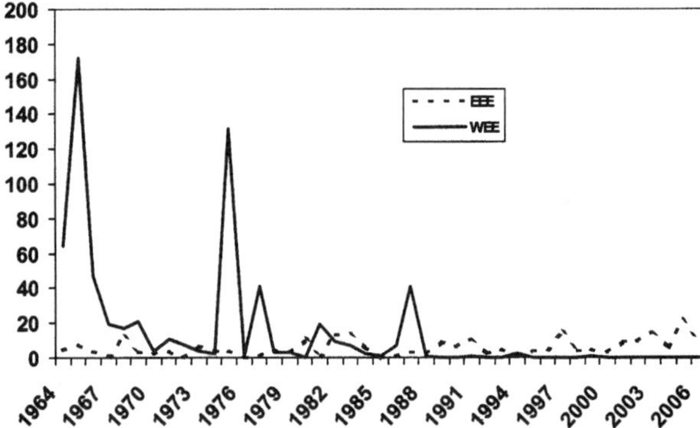

FIGURE 6 Reported cases of EEE (broken line) and WEE (solid line), United States, 1964 to 2006. (Reprinted from the Centers for Disease Control and Prevention at http://www.cdc.gov/ncidod/dvbid/arbor/arbocase.htm.)

Subclinical infections typically have been found in only 0.05 to 0.17% of persons surveyed in epidemic areas, so levels of immunity in human populations remain low (47). In Canada, equine outbreaks have occurred without associated human cases. Rare human cases have been reported from South America, and antibody prevalence rates have been highly variable, from 0 to 19%, depending on location (30).

Epidemic Patterns

Few outbreaks have been reported, and outbreaks are typically preceded by an epizootic in horses. An early Massachusetts outbreak led to 34 cases and, typical of EEE epidemics, was preceded by an epizootic of 300 equine cases in the state and simultaneous epizootics among horses in Rhode Island and Connecticut and an epornitic among pheasants the same summer (45). The last outbreak of note occurred in New Jersey in 1959, when 32 cases (22 fatal) were reported, yielding an epidemic attack rate of 101/100,000 (47).

In North America, the virus is transmitted in a freshwater swamp enzootic cycle among birds and strictly ornithophilic *Culiseta melanura* mosquitoes (Fig. 7). Viral transmission is concentrated at the edge of and within the swamp interior. Other mosquito vectors that feed on both birds and mammals are required to bridge the enzootic cycle, carrying the virus to locations where humans, horses, and other susceptible dead-end hosts are exposed. Several species have been identified as bridge or epizootic vectors (Fig. 7). The virus also has been isolated from *A. albopictus*, an Asian mosquito introduced into the southeastern United States; however, its role in transmitting infections to horses or humans has not been shown.

Viral amplification through the summer initially is manifested by rising viral infection rates in *Culiseta melanura*, followed by an increasing population of infected epizootic vectors (48). Infections in *Culiseta melanura* with HJV, a benign WEEV-related virus transmitted in the same enzootic cycle, often foreshadows other indicators of EEEV transmission. Human infections are usually preceded by cases in horses. Immunization has lessened the predictive value of equine deaths, but pheasant, partridge, pig, and goat deaths also may signal a risk for human cases.

The permanence of EEEV foci has suggested a local overwintering reservoir, but attempts to demonstrate vertical transmission in *Culiseta melanura* have not been convincing. Observations in enzootic coastal foci in New Jersey suggest that persistently infected permanent resident birds might carry the virus through the winter, with the intervention of an unknown amplification mechanism preceding transmission in the *Culiseta melanura* cycle. The maintenance of temperate overwintering foci also is supported by genetic analyses of viral strains from disparate locations. Viral transmission in South America occurs in forests among *Culex (melanoconion)* spp., especially *Culex taeniopus*, and rodents, marsupials, and, to a lesser degree, birds. Sporadic equine epizootics, often in conjunction with VEEV, have been reported. A wide range of bridging vectors is probably involved in transmission to humans and other mammals. Studies at an enzootic focus of EEEV in Peru suggest that people are regularly exposed but rarely seroconvert, presumably because the South

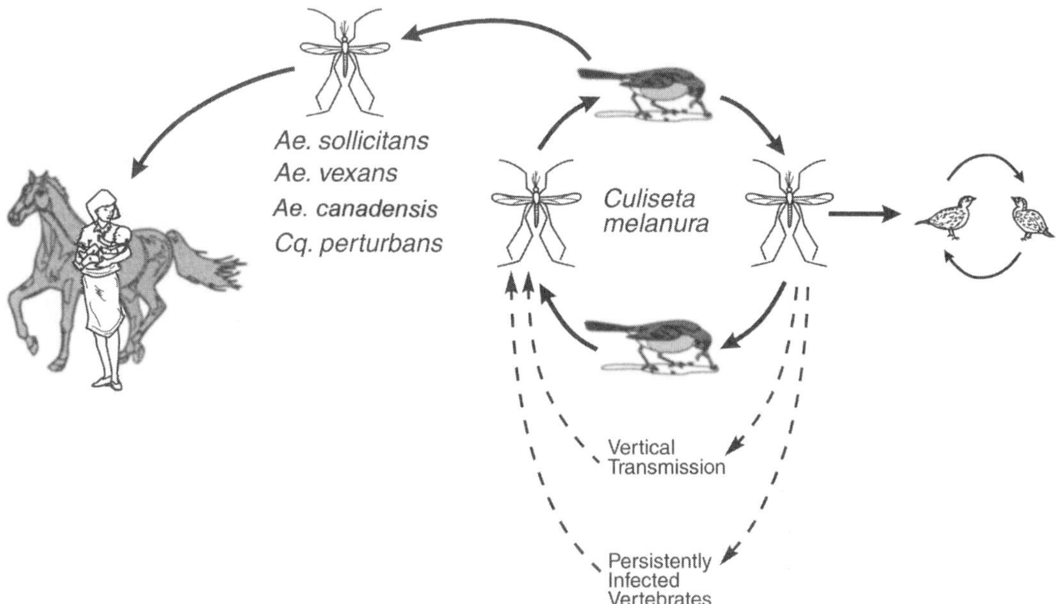

FIGURE 7 Schematic diagram of the EEE transmission cycle; solid lines show known portions, and broken lines show speculative portions. The principal enzootic mosquito vector, *Culiseta melanura*, transmits the virus among birds and occasionally initiates an outbreak among pheasants or other captive birds. Various other species bridge the enzootic cycle to infect humans and horses, which are dead-end hosts; the principal species include *Aedes sollicitans*, found in salt marsh coastal habitat; *Aedes vexans*, associated with open meadows and flooded ground pools; *Aedes canadensis*, associated with woodland pools; and *Coquillettidia perturbans*, found in open freshwater swamps with emerging vegetation. The viral overwintering mechanism is unknown but potentially includes vertically infected mosquitoes, persistently infected birds, and other vertebrates.

American strains that circulate there are poorly infectious for humans (2).

Risk Factors

Young children and the elderly are most likely to develop illness (47, 77). In the 1959 New Jersey outbreak, infections occurred equally in all age groups, but clinical attack rates were higher in children <4 years old and in adults >55 years old. Respective inapparent-to-apparent case ratios were 8:1 and 16:1, while at intermediate ages the ratio was 29:1 (47). Factors underlying increased biological susceptibility at the extremes of age have not been defined.

Many patients had a history of residence near or, exposure to, tidal or freshwater swampy locations where epizootic vectors might be prevalent. However, the movements of birds and vectors from these habitats into adjoining suburban residential areas place people over a much wider area at potential risk. Horse ownership and occupational exposure to infected pheasants have not been associated with increased risk of acquiring illness or infection. However, emu owners and veterinarians may be infected when exposed to highly infectious bloody discharges or organs while nursing or handling ill or dead animals. Brains of horses that die of acute EEE also may contain high viral titers, placing veterinarians at potential risk. Four laboratory-acquired infections, two by aerosol exposure, have been reported (138).

Seasonality

In Florida, equine and human cases are reported throughout the year, although 76% of human cases have had onset between June and August (Fig. 8) (9). In mid-Atlantic and New England states, human cases usually occur no earlier than July and can appear through the end of October or until the intervention of cold weather (77). Heavy rainfall in the preceding year and heavy late summer precipitation have been associated with increased risk of EEEV infection (48). Increased rainfall, creating a high water table, augments the breeding habitat of *Culiseta melanura*, and late summer rains expand the population of bridging vectors at an opportune stage for epizootic viral transmission.

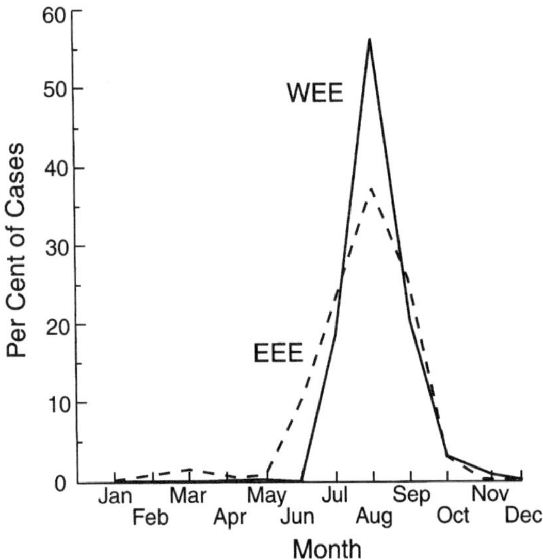

FIGURE 8 Reported cases of EEE and WEE by month, United States, 1972 to 1989. (Data from the Centers for Disease Control and Prevention at http://www.cdc.gov/ncidod/dvbid/arbor/arbocase.htm.)

Pathology

Visceral and pulmonary congestion or pneumonia may be present. The brain appears swollen, with flattened convolutions and narrowed sulci, while the meninges are congested (5, 44, 63). Inflammatory infiltrates of lymphocytes, histiocytes, and neutrophils are present in a perivascular distribution and in the parenchyma of the cerebral cortex, lentiform nuclei, thalamus, and brain stem, particularly in gray matter regions. The spinal cord may be affected at all levels, with lesions principally in the gray matter, but this is unusual. There is a mild to moderate loss of neurons, with neuronophagia, microglial reaction, and loss of oligodendrocytes with demyelinated lesions. Infection occurs preferentially in neurons, with occasional involvement of perivascular macrophages (44). Demyelinating lesions are more prevalent in patients dying after a longer period of illness.

Clinical Manifestations

The diagnosis should be considered in the summer or early fall in persons with a history of exposure to an enzootic focus, particularly in the context of recent mosquito exposure. Public health surveillance data can shed light on current transmission levels (48).

The incubation period has not been defined but is likely to be in the range of 3 to 10 days. The initial descriptions of cases, principally in infants, emphasized the dramatic onset and rapid evolution of neurologic symptoms leading to coma and death in 30 to 75% of cases (9, 148). However, in many cases in children and adults, a prodromal illness of fever, chills, malaise, and myalgia has been described, evolving over 1 to 2 weeks, after which patients may recover or progress to more severe illness requiring hospitalization (57, 111, 148). Early symptoms may also include headache, photophobia, and dysethesias. Those who deteriorate develop worsening headache, dizziness, vomiting, lethargy, and, later, neck stiffness, confusion, and convulsions. These events are compressed in infants, in whom illness begins with a rapid elevation of temperature, irritability, vomiting, and diarrhea, followed quickly by reducing conscious state or intermittent convulsions, leading to coma in 24 to 48 h.

High fever, often above 39°C, is common, and the conscious state varies from mildly depressed to comatose. Meningismus is common. The initial cranial nerve and motor examination may be normal, but more frequently, abnormalities such as nystagmus, gaze deviation, or sluggish pupils are present and alterations in tone, flaccid or spastic paralysis, and abnormal reflexes are present or evolve over several days. Some patients exhibit unilateral seizures, hemiparesis or hemiplegia, emotional lability, or aphasia reflecting focal damage. Clinical signs and radiological evidence of cerebral edema have been reported frequently, and brain swelling and uncal or subtentorial herniation have been described pathologically. Hyponatremia is common and can be severe due to inappropriate antidiuretic hormone secretion.

Patients with a prodrome of more than 4 days preceding the onset of neurologic symptoms have a better outcome than those with a more rapid clinical course, suggesting that the early systemic immune response may modulate neuroinvasion and neurologic disease (23, 57, 111, 148). This is supported by one unusual case in which a patient with preexisting MAYV antibodies had only a systemic febrile illness without headache or neurologic signs (23), suggesting partial cross-protection.

A mild case with limb dysesthesia and weakness, but no disturbances of consciousness suggesting encephalitis, indicated the possibility of myelitis without brain infection (23). In one case, severe encephalitis and coma during the third trimester of pregnancy did not interfere with a good outcome of the pregnancy (29).

Laboratory Abnormalities

The peripheral leukocyte (WBC) count may be normal but more often ranges from 15×10^9 to 35×10^9/liter, with a neutrophil predominance and left shift (29, 57, 111, 148). The cerebrospinal fluid (CSF) may be xanthochromic and show increased pressure. The CSF WBC count is greatly elevated (10×10^6 to $2{,}000 \times 10^6$/liter), with a predominance of polymorphonuclear cells early in infection, followed by a mononuclear cell predominance. The ratio of mononuclear cells increases over several days, but in individual cases, a neutrophil pleocytosis has persisted into the second week of illness. Red blood cells are usually present, the protein content may be elevated, and the ratio of CSF to serum glucose is reduced to below 50% in half of cases. Results of imaging studies have varied according to the stage of illness. In about three-quarters of reported cases, computed tomography scans have shown only diffuse cerebral edema, but focal abnormalities are sometimes seen in the frontal region and areas of low attenuation with mass effect are seen in the thalami, midbrain, and lentiform nucleus (95). These are seen more frequently by magnetic resonance imaging. Abnormalities generally improve over several weeks (29). Electroencephalogram (EEG) tracings show background slowing, with focal slowing in 50% of cases. Burst suppression patterns, disorganized background activity, and high-voltage delta wave slowing have been associated with reduced survival rates and poor outcome (111).

Outcomes

Progressive neurologic deterioration leads to death in up to 75% of encephalitis cases, usually within 10 days. Fatality rates are highest in the elderly, intermediate in children, and lowest in middle-aged adults (47, 77, 111). Although children are more likely to survive the illness than adults, infants are most likely to have residual neurologic abnormalities and to suffer permanent sequelae of motor weakness, paralysis, aphasia, mental retardation, and continued seizures. In one series, nearly half of children <9 years old who survived the infection had residual sequelae (9). In general, patients with a short prodromal illness (e.g., <4 days) before onset of neurologic symptoms have a higher likelihood of fatal outcome, regardless of age (111, 148).

Differential Diagnosis

The principal considerations in the differential diagnosis are bacterial cerebritis/cerebral abscess, herpes simplex encephalitis, or other viral encephalitides.

Laboratory Diagnosis

The virus has been isolated from serum 2 days after onset of illness in at least one case, but that is unusual (23). Virus often has been recovered from brain specimens of patients with fatal illness, and viral antigen has been demonstrated by immunohistochemical staining in brain biopsy and autopsy specimens. PCR assays are more sensitive than cell culture and should increase diagnostic sensitivity (72). Detection of EEEV IgM in serum is suggestive of recent infection, especially if accompanied by IgG seroconversion or a rise in titer. Detection of specific IgM in CSF is highly suggestive of encephalitis.

Prevention

Although in most years, at most one EEE case will occur in any single state, even the threat of a case can cause great concern in the general population. Public anxiety about EEE has led to reduced tourism in seaside resorts and to concern among owners of valuable racehorses. Thus, surveillance and preventive mosquito control programs are maintained in many areas with enzootic transmission. Personal protective measures are advisable when entering marshy and woodland areas where the enzootic cycle is maintained, bearing in mind that important epizootic vectors bite during the day as well as in the evening. Infants are less able to defend themselves against mosquitoes and should be kept under screened bassinets when outdoors.

An inactivated vaccine is available on an investigational basis for laboratory workers and others at high risk. Commercial, inactivated equine vaccine formulated with WEEV and VEEV offers a high degree of protection for horses, but annual boosters are required to maintain immunity.

Treatment

No specific antiviral therapy is currently available. The reduction of the EEE mortality rate nationally, from 50% between 1955 and 1971 to 33% between 1972 and 1989, most likely reflects the lifesaving effects of intensive supportive care (77). Anticonvulsants may be needed acutely to treat seizures and also are important to prevent increased pressure arising from convulsions. Respiratory support, reduction of cerebral edema, prevention and management of hyponatremia, support of vital functions, and treatment of secondary bacterial infections are all important parts of patient management.

WESTERN EQUINE ENCEPHALITIS VIRUS

Virology

Classification and Composition

WEEV was identified in 1930 as a cause of equine encephalitis in California. It was isolated in 1938 from the brain of an encephalitic child. It is a member of the SINV complex, which includes HJV, FMV, and Aura virus in the New World and several viruses in the Old World, including SINV. Only WEEV and SINV cause human infections (Table 1). Several antigenic subtypes or varieties have been recognized, including an enzootic WEEV strain transmitted in subtropical Argentina (AG80-646), which differs in mouse pathogenicity and other biological characteristics (8). Genetic similarities of North and South American strains in the principal WEEV lineages indicate that the virus has moved between the continents.

Amino acid and nucleotide sequences of the viral capsid and envelope proteins are most similar to those of EEEV and SINV, respectively, indicating that WEEV is a recombinant of EEEV and an ancestral New World Sindbis-like virus (145). The recombinant event is speculated to have occurred thousands of years ago, before the divergence of EEEV strains into North and South American varieties, and presumably occurred within the avian-mosquito transmission cycle shared by all three viruses.

Host Range

Humans, horses, and emus develop clinical symptoms after natural infection. In the eastern United States, HJV, transmitted in the same enzootic cycle as EEEV, is a rare cause of equine encephalitis but has produced outbreaks of fatal illness among pheasants, turkeys, and chukar partridges. There is one report of encephalitis in four humans, though all were also infected with St. Louis encephalitis virus (SLEV) (91). Captive exotic emus die of a fulminant viscerotropic infection, similar to that caused by EEEV. Experimental infection produces antibody without illness or viremia in cattle, illness without encephalitis in burros, and neurologic infections in a small proportion of ponies. Fatal illnesses are produced in certain wild rodents. The Argentine enzootic strain is avirulent in horses and exhibits minimal neurovirulence in mice (8).

Epidemiology

Distribution

WEEV activity has been reported from the western United States and Canadian provinces, Mexico, Guyana, Brazil, Argentina, and Uruguay (Fig. 9) (20, 34, 75, 90). Small equine outbreaks without human disease have occurred in Brazil and Guyana. In the temperate provinces of Argentina, intermittent epizootics have occurred in an area between latitudes 28° and 40°S, and from the Andes to the Atlantic coast, spilling over to adjacent areas of Uruguay. The enzootic WEEV subtype is transmitted in the subtropical Chaco province (8).

Incidence and Prevalence

Subclinical infections are common among residents of rural areas where the viral transmission cycle is maintained. Estimates of the ratios of apparent to inapparent cases have ranged from 1:1 for children <1 year old to 1:58 for children 1 to 4 years old to 1:1,150 for adults (17). In an outbreak where seroconversions were monitored, the overall ratio of reported cases to infections was 1:160.

Epidemic Patterns

WEEV now occurs as a very rare sporadic infection in the western United States and Canada, with only five cases reported since 1988. However, past outbreaks have resulted in thousands of cases, and the epidemic potential of the virus should not be overlooked. In the largest recorded outbreak, in 1941, 3,400 human and hundreds of thousands of equine cases were reported from Minnesota, North and South Dakota, Nebraska, Montana, Alberta, Manitoba, and Saskatchewan, with an estimated incidence of 167/100,000 in North Dakota (34). Between 1945 and 1958, more than 600 cases were reported from California, 375 in 1952 alone, with an incidence rate of 340/100,000 in rural Kern County, and in 1975, a regional outbreak produced 145 cases in Manitoba and 132 cases in the Red River Valley of North Dakota, with an estimated attack rate of 11/100,000 residents (75, 90). The last major outbreak, in 1987, led to 41 cases in the great plains and mountain states and 30 cases in Colorado. Active case finding in the state found an incidence of 1.6/100,000 in affected counties (20). Incidence rates consistently are highest in rural areas where the viral transmission cycle is maintained, with a lower risk in town and urban residents.

Previously, seroprevalence rates of 20% were common in areas of the western United States. However, a decline in the rural population and changes in land use patterns and lifestyles have reduced the risk of acquiring infection, such that current antibody levels in some areas of endemicity are in the range of 1%. Few human cases have been reported from South America, despite active surveillance in areas experiencing epizootics in horses. The epizootic strains appear to be virulent variants of enzootic strains (8). Clusters of human cases were reported in 1972–1973 and again in 1982–1983; a total of seven cases with one

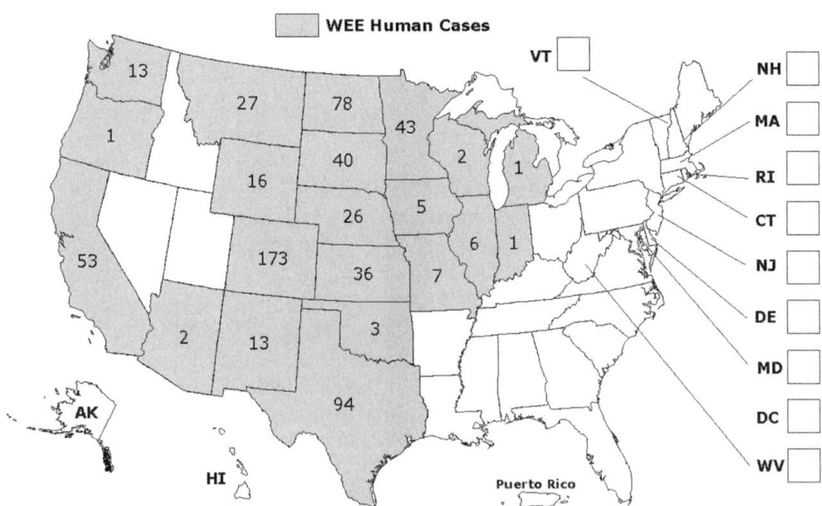

FIGURE 9 Reported cases of WEE among humans in the United States, 1964 to 2006. (Reprinted from the Centers for Disease Control and Prevention at http://www.cdc.gov/ncidod/dvbid/arbor/arbocase.htm.)

death were recognized, for an estimated attack rate of 3/1,000 inhabitants.

Transmission

In the western United States, the virus is transmitted between *Culex tarsalis* mosquitoes and passerine birds, principally sparrows and house finches. *Culex tarsalis* is adapted to naturally flooded ground pools and irrigated pastures, found mainly in rural and agricultural areas where most human and equine cases are acquired. Viral amplification and epidemic risk are increased by heavy winter snowpack, spring precipitation, and flooding, which expand vector larval habitat. Another cycle involving *Aedes melanimon* and the blacktail jackrabbit has also been identified (17). Concurrent outbreaks of WEEV and SLEV, transmitted in the same enzootic cycle in the western United States, have been reported frequently. However, extrinsic incubation of SLEV in vector mosquitoes is slower and requires higher temperatures, delaying transmission, often after WEEV activity has subsided.

Risk Factors

A bimodal age distribution of risk has been observed, with a sharp increase in risk with advanced age and a secondary peak in infants (20). Residence in rural areas is a principal risk factor; however, the long flight range of the mosquito vector allows it to infiltrate towns and suburban areas, and often, more cases are reported from these populated locations, while incidence rates are higher in thinly populated rural areas (90). In semiarid locations, WEEV incidence is highest in irrigated areas along the major river basins. Incidence rates in the United States and Argentina have been higher in males, probably reflecting greater outdoor exposure in ranch and farming activities. Cases occasionally are reported among persons engaged in outdoor leisure activities. Seven laboratory-acquired cases, including two deaths, have been reported through 1980, among them a well-documented case resulting from conjunctival or respiratory infection (39, 46).

Pathology

The brain appears normal or exhibits a moderate degree of vascular congestion (26, 75, 99, 116). There is a mild patchy, sometimes extensive, infiltration of the meninges and prominent vascular congestion. Inflammatory infiltrates of lymphocytes, plasma cells, and neutrophils are found in a perivascular distribution, with invasion of the vessel wall and vascular necrosis in some instances. Parenchymal lesions are typified by widely scattered, discrete foci of tissue necrosis with microglial proliferation and inflammatory cell infiltration. Neurons are found in various stages of degeneration. Lesions are distributed mainly in the subcortical white matter, the internal capsule, thalami, basal ganglia, substantia nigra, dentate nucleus, and molecular layer of the cerebellum and gray matter of the brain stem and spinal cord. Widely scattered focal areas of demyelination are seen. Infections acquired in infancy have led to significant disturbances in brain development resulting in cerebral atrophy and demyelination, with the formation of multiple glia-lined cysts and vascular calcification (26, 99).

Clinical Manifestations

The reported incubation period has been as short as 2 days in one case and, in a fatal laboratory-acquired infection, no longer than 10 days. In another laboratory-acquired case, illness began 4 days after an infectious fluid was splashed onto the face and eyes (39, 46). Illness typically begins with the sudden onset of headache, usually followed by dizziness, chills, fever, myalgias, and malaise (34, 39, 46, 75). These progressively worsen over a few days and may be followed by dizziness, tremor, irritability, photophobia, and neck stiffness. Patients typically appear to be drowsy or may be restless, with a moderately elevated temperature. Meningismus is present in about 50% of cases. Neurologic abnormalities are usually limited to weakness and generalized tremulousness, especially of the hands, lips, and tongue. A minority of patients (<5%) exhibit cranial nerve palsy, motor weakness, spasticity, or convulsions. Hemiplegia, quadriplegia, and focal weakness or seizures are unusual (~3% of cases). Stupor or coma develops in <10% of cases, with respiratory failure in some cases. Hyponatremia occurs occasionally but less frequently than with EEE. General improvement begins several days after the resolution of fever, typically within a week to 10 days after the onset. Cases of mild illness have been described in which fever, headache, and afternoon fatigue persist for several days to a week, without more serious manifestations.

In infants, the initial presentation and clinical progression are more rapid, evolving from a nonspecific illness of fever, irritability, and diarrhea to convulsions and coma (26, 99, 104, 126). Infants frequently present with a tense fontanel, spasticity, and sometimes in opisthotonus. Seizures usually are generalized but may have a focal component. Increased muscular tone, often to a point of generalized rigidity, is typical. Rapid fatal outcome or significant residual brain damage was common among cases reported from the 1940s to 1950s.

Outcomes

The overall mortality rate is 4% and is highest among persons >75 years old. However, serious sequelae are more prevalent in recovered infants and children, with the most serious outcomes in the youngest infants (25). Among infants <3 months old at the onset of illness, 44% have had extensive brain damage resulting in serious neurologic sequelae, and >25% have had mental retardation necessitating institutionalization. Other sequelae included lesser degrees of developmental delay, convulsions, spasticity, and extrapyramidal movement disorders. Sequelae have been less severe and more likely to improve in older infants and children.

Signs of parkinsonism were reported on follow-up in at least 11 cases (46, 96, 116). However, a case control study in Kansas, where WEEV is considered to be endemic, found no association between Parkinson's disease and previous WEEV infection.

Five cases of perinatal illness following late-trimester or postpartum maternal infection have been reported in which vertical transmission of infection was surmised. The neonates became ill 3 to 6 days after delivery, while maternal illness began on the same postpartum day in two cases and in the others had occurred 3 or 10 days prepartum (25, 125).

Laboratory Abnormalities

The peripheral WBC count is usually normal or elevated to 15×10^9 to 25×10^9/liter (34, 75). The CSF rarely is xanthochromic; the WBC count is usually elevated to 110×10^6 to $1,500 \times 10^6$/liter, with an early neutrophil and later mononuclear cell predominance. CSF protein is moderately elevated in about 50% of cases; glucose is usually normal. When recorded, CSF pressure was elevated in about two-thirds of cases.

Brain scans, cerebral angiography, and contrast-enhanced computed tomography findings have been unremarkable in the few cases in which they have been reported (3, 7, 75, 124, 129). One neonatal case showed diffuse low-attenuation lesions in the white matter, accompanied by multifocal EEG epileptiform discharges. Follow-up studies 4 months later showed severe diffuse seizure activity and enlarged ventricles, encephalomalacia, and numerous intracranial calcifications in the insular cortex and thalamus bilaterally. In several cases mimicking the focal presentation of herpes encephalitis, EEGs showed diffuse slowing with focal delta activity in the temporal region (3, 7, 124, 129).

Differential Diagnosis

Due to its overlapping geographic, seasonal, and transmission patterns, as well as its similar clinical features, SLEV infection is the principal alternative diagnosis. Even with the epidemiological clues of occurrence during a recognized outbreak, clinical differentiation of WEEV from other causes of acute CNS infection is difficult. Other clinical diagnoses that were later proved to be due to WEEV or SLEV are shown in Table 3 (68).

Laboratory Diagnosis

Viremia is generally considered to have cleared before the onset of CNS signs, and virus is rarely recovered from blood. Virus was isolated from the CSF of only 2 of 21 patients in one series of attempts and, in two cases, from brain biopsy samples that were obtained to rule out herpes encephalitis (125). PCR-based tests appear to be more sensitive than culture (72). Detection of virus-specific IgM in CSF or serum provides the most rapid laboratory confirmation. Serologic cross-reactions with other alphaviruses have not been a major concern in the western United States and Canada.

TABLE 3 Initial diagnosis of diseases ultimately proven by laboratory test to be either WEE or St. Louis encephalitis[a]

Infectious causes
Polioencephalomyelitis
Bacterial meningitis
Brain abscess
Tuberculous meningitis
Mumps encephalitis
Coccidioidal infection
Lymphocytic choriomeningitis
CNS syphilis
Coxsackie encephalitis
Pneumonia
Otitis media
Subacute bacterial endocarditis
Sydenham's chorea
Noninfectious causes
Brain trauma
Cerebrovascular accident
Intracranial hemorrhage
Intracranial neoplasm
Convulsive disorder
Cardiac failure

[a] Data from reference 68.

Prevention and Treatment

Where WEE has occurred in epidemics and epizootics, public health programs have been established to survey viral activity in mosquitoes and birds and to preemptively control vector mosquitoes. An experimental inactivated vaccine is available on an investigational basis to laboratory workers and other persons at high risk of exposure. Horses in enzootic areas should be immunized on an annual basis.

No specific therapy is available. Equine immune serum given on the third day of illness after a laboratory exposure was followed by a clinical course with coma and recovery with complications of acute parkinsonism. Supportive care consists mainly of anticonvulsant therapy and airway protection in patients with a reduced level of consciousness.

VENEZUELAN EQUINE ENCEPHALITIS VIRUS

Virology

Classification and Composition

VEEV was first detected in an outbreak of equine encephalitis in Colombia and Venezuela in 1936 and only later was found in human encephalitis cases occurring during a period of epizootic activity. Several subtypes of VEEV comprise a complex of six antigenically related but epidemiologically and ecologically disparate viruses. Only type I (VEEV) and type II (Everglades virus [EVEV]) are known to cause human disease. VEEV is further subdivided into IAB, IC, ID, IE, and IF strains. Epizootic viruses (IAB, IC, and IE) emerge at unpredictable intervals of years or decades, producing extensive outbreaks in equines and humans. By contrast, the sylvatic VEEV subtypes (ID, IE, and IF) are transmitted continuously in forest or swamp foci, causing sporadic human infections but, in general, no equine disease. Subtypes can be distinguished by special serologic procedures and by monoclonal antibodies; in addition, they differ biologically in characteristics such as plaque size, viremia levels, rapidity of clearance from blood, and host range (32, 150). In one Venezuelan focus, the close genetic relationships of sylvatic ID and epizootic IC viruses (<1% nucleotide substitutions in their entire genomes) suggested that the epizootic strain may have arisen by mutation from continuously circulating sylvatic viruses, and recent epizootic strains of IE have arisen from enzootic strains (139, 146). In contrast to spontaneous epizootics due to IC viruses, certain IAB virus outbreaks are speculated to have arisen from improperly inactivated equine vaccine, as the IAB strains isolated during many later epizootics were virtually identical to the Trinidad donkey and other early strains of IAB virus used to produce inactivated equine vaccine (143).

After the divergence of VEEV and EEEV, the VEEV lineage diverged into several enzootic lineages that generally occupy nonoverlapping distributions in the tropical and subtropical areas. Of these enzootic lineages, one genotype of subtype ID virus evidently generated the epizootic strains implicated in outbreaks dating to the 1920s (subtypes IAB and IC) (Fig. 1) (110, 113). Geographically isolated sylvatic viruses such as subtypes II (EVEV-Florida) and IIIB (Bijou Bridge-Colorado) may have become established through introductions by migratory birds, with their subsequent adaptations to local enzootic cycles. The latter, presumably an introduction of Tonate virus from South America, is believed to have been a contemporary event, occurring only ~40 years ago.

Host Range

Illnesses and encephalitis in horses and burros have been fatal in 20 to 40% of animals, without apparent age-related susceptibility (32, 101). Goat deaths have been reported in outbreaks, and dogs occasionally die with evidence of CNS pathology. Experimental infections have produced high mortality rates in species of North American rodents, dogs, and coyotes. Beef cattle, pigs, some bats, rodents, and birds (especially herons) develop sufficient viremia to participate in viral amplification.

Horses experimentally infected with sylvatic viral strains develop fever, mild leukopenia, and an insignificant viremia, while epizootic strains produce an illness with high fever, severe leukopenia, depressed hematocrit, high viremia, and encephalitis (32). Equine virulence patterns generally are mirrored in experimentally infected English shorthaired guinea pigs, except for some enzootic subtype ID strains (139). Rhesus monkeys experimentally infected with epizootic strains develop febrile illness with elevated hepatic transaminases, while enzootic strains produce no symptoms or fever (93).

Epidemiology

Distribution

Sylvatic viruses are transmitted in tropical and subtropical swamp and forested foci in North, Central, and South America. Epizootics have occurred principally in northern South America in Colombia, Venezuela, Trinidad, Peru, and Ecuador, but a series of outbreaks between 1969 and 1972 extended from Guatemala through all the countries of Central America, except Panama, and invaded Mexico and Texas (Fig. 10) (53).

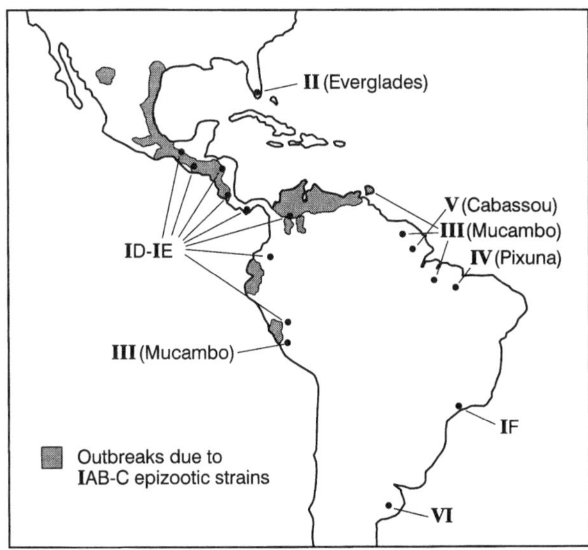

FIGURE 10 Geographic distribution of VEE epizootics and sylvatic viral subtypes.

Incidence and Prevalence

A low ratio of apparent to inapparent infections, 1:10, is typical; however, airborne transmission has resulted in illness in >75% of laboratory-infected persons (70).

Epidemic Patterns

Sylvatic viruses are transmitted in swampy and forested locations principally by *Culex melanoconion* mosquitoes among small mammals and aquatic birds (Fig. 11A). Sylvatic VEEV infections occur among persons living near or entering enzootic foci, e.g., among soldiers on jungle bivouacs (31, 102, 120, 141). In certain locations, endemic transmission to local residents leads to age-dependent seroprevalence rates of >50%.

Epidemic VEE occurs in conjunction with epizootic transmission among horses, leading to combined outbreaks of tens of thousands of human cases and hundreds of thousands of equine cases (Fig. 11B) (12, 14, 53, 113). In the 1995 outbreak in Venezuela and Colombia, >85,000 human cases were estimated, 3,000 with neurologic symptoms (4%) and 300 fatal ones (113, 146). A serosurvey found that 36% of the resident population had been infected and up to 8% of the state's equines had died. Similar statistics have been reported from previous outbreaks.

A susceptible equine population is essential for epizootic emergence and spread. Horses are potent amplifying hosts, their high viremia facilitating rapid animal-to-animal transmission by a variety of mosquito vectors, including floodwater *Aedes taeniorhychus*, *Psorophora confinnis*, *Mansonia* spp., and *Deinocerites* spp. Other biting insects may transmit the virus mechanically. Outbreaks frequently occur in normally dry locations when heavy rainfall and flooding have expanded mosquito breeding habitats and mosquito and rodent populations. In areas with susceptible horses, outbreaks spread at rates of several kilometers per day, followed by associated human cases several weeks later (53, 113). Transmission continues inexorably until susceptible horses have been depleted by natural infection or immunization or until the onset of dry weather and diminishing mosquito numbers. Transmission sometimes has resumed with the return of the rainy season. The intensity of transmission and high attack rates among horses and humans create a high level of immunity that may contribute to the periodicity of outbreaks every 10 to 20 years.

Age-Specific Attack Rates

Exposure during previous epidemics creates an age cohort effect in susceptibility. In the 1962 Zulia state outbreak, attack rates were 183.5/1,000/month in children <15 years old and 72.9 in persons >15 years old, reflecting immunity acquired during a series of outbreaks from 1942 to 1949. Six years later, in 1968, VEE recurred, and attack rates were highest in children <6 years of age. Infants <1 year old may be protected by maternal immunity. In the immunologically naïve Texas population, age-specific immunity rates after the 1971 outbreak were highest (21/100,000) in the 20- to 39-year age group, presumably reflecting outdoor exposure in occupational and leisure activities (12).

Risk Factors

Outbreaks occur principally in rural areas where horses and burros still are commonly used as transportation. Native Indians have been at greater risk because of residence

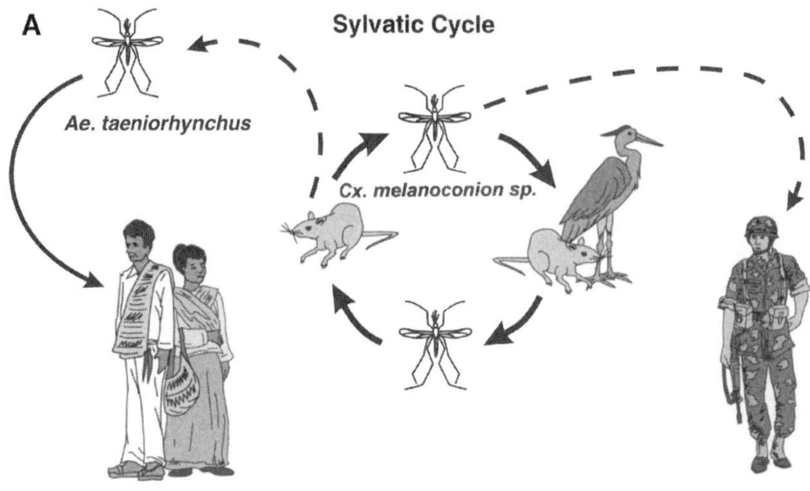

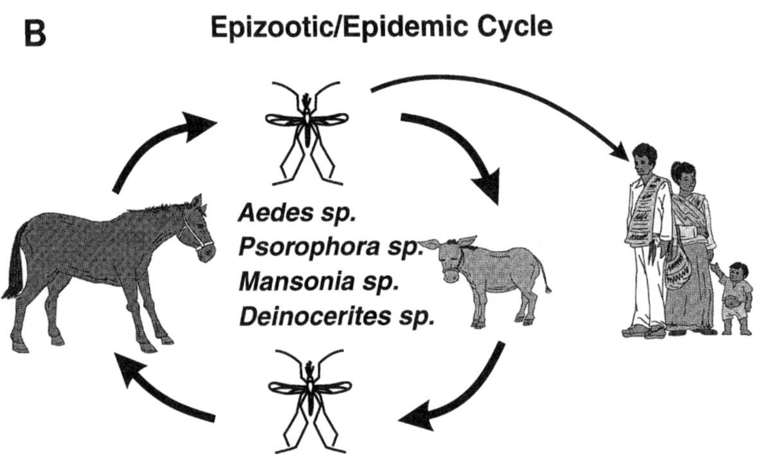

FIGURE 11 (A) Sylvatic VEEVs circulate continuously in silent tropical and subtropical foci among *Culex melaconion* mosquitoes and small mammals or aquatic birds. Humans (e.g., soldiers on jungle bivouacs) are infected when they chance upon transmission foci. Bridging vectors (e.g., *Aedes taeniorhychus*) that feed on viremic vertebrates in a sylvatic focus can carry the virus to nearby areas of human activity. (B) In contrast to the continuous cycling of sylvatic VEEV subtypes, until recently, epizootic VEEV had never been isolated except during periodic outbreaks. Once introduced, epizootic viruses are rapidly amplified among equines (horses and burros). Equines develop high viremia levels, so various mosquito species can function as biological vectors (only some important species are shown) and other biting insects, such as blackflies, can spread the virus mechanically. Humans develop illness with high viremia levels but probably have an insignificant role, if any, in viral amplification. Transmission declines as susceptible equines are exhausted by natural infection or immunization. It is speculated that epizootic IC viruses arise by mutation from sylvatic ID viruses; the subpopulation circulates in a sylvatic cycle and under appropriate conditions is amplified, leading to epizootic and epidemic spread.

in rural rancherias and other factors related to increased mosquito exposure or horse ownership (113).

Seasonality

Outbreaks occur during the rainy season, the monthly distribution of cases varying with local and secular changes in rainfall patterns. Outbreaks in northwestern Venezuela often have started in April, peaked in June or July, and subsided by December. Sylvatic viral strains are transmitted continuously in their tropical and subtropical foci.

Transmission

In outbreaks where few equine deaths were noted, the possibility of supplemental viral amplification in humans was considered. The viremia in humans is sufficiently high to infect mosquitoes, and peridomestic *A. aegypti* mosquitoes are potential vectors. In addition, direct person-to-person spread seems possible because virus can be isolated from the pharynx in 6 to 40% of acutely ill patients, sometimes on successive days (11). However, no clinical or serologic evidence of household clustering or intrafamilial spread is recognized, suggesting a minor role, if any, for person-to-person spread or for the importance of humans as amplifying hosts (11, 113).

Numerous laboratory outbreaks have been traced to airborne infection, with a total of 150 cases and one death reported through 1980 (70, 141). Very brief exposures in persons not working directly with the virus (e.g., walking through a laboratory) have been sufficient for infection to occur.

Pathology

Histopathological lesions have consistently been found in the CNS, lungs, heart, spleen, lymph nodes, liver, and gastrointestinal tract and, less often, in the kidneys and adrenal glands (27). The respiratory and intestinal mucosa appears hyperemic, with microscopic evidence of vascular congestion, hemorrhage, and vascular injury. Inflammatory reactions are most prominent in the lungs, with diffuse or patchy alveolar septal infiltrates, intra-alveolar edema, and, rarely, hemorrhage. Myocarditis and centrilobular hepatic necrosis may be seen. The brain appears swollen and hyperemic. Diffuse cellular infiltrates involve the meninges, and, in one-third of cases, the brain and spinal cord. Encephalomyelitis is characterized by perivascular inflammatory infiltrates, hemorrhages, foci of neuronal degeneration, and glial proliferation. Lesions are distributed in the cerebral gray and white matter, especially in the substantia nigra. The lymph nodes and spleen exhibit extensive follicular necrosis, germinal center lymphoid depletion, neutrophil infiltration, lymphophagocytosis, and vasculitis.

Spontaneous abortions after VEE-like infections have been associated with massive cerebral necrosis and typical acute lesions in the aborted fetuses, including cerebral calcifications similar to those associated with toxoplasmosis in one case (147). Congenital VEEV infection has been confirmed virologically by recovery of the virus from aborted fetuses (148). Infections acquired early in pregnancy have been associated with fetal hydranencephaly, porencephaly, and cerebral dysgenesis, a pattern of lesions reproduced in experimentally infected fetal rhesus monkeys.

Clinical Manifestations

The incubation period has been characterized from laboratory and other outbreaks as <1 to 5 days, usually 2 to 3 days (70). Well-documented cases have had onset 12 h after laboratory exposure.

The onset of illness is abrupt and rapidly incapacitating, with sudden chills, headache, fever, body aches, and prostration (12, 31, 70, 120). Headache is nearly unbearable and may be exacerbated by even the smallest movements of the eyes or neck and is worsened by bright light. Asthenia, dizziness, and acute discomfort are incapacitating. Nausea and vomiting are common. The temperature is moderately elevated, and the face appears flushed, with injected or suffused conjunctivae. Pharyngeal pain and inflammation are accompanied by cervical and other lymphadenitis. There may be mild subcostal abdominal tenderness. Symptoms settle over several days with defervescence, but a dull headache and weakness may persist several days longer. Occasionally, fever and symptoms recrudesce after an initial remission.

Despite the disease name, severe neurologic symptoms and encephalitis occur in only 4 to 14% of cases overall, principally in children and the elderly; however, tremulousness and somnolence suggesting milder neurologic involvement are not uncommon in a larger proportion of cases (14, 53, 113, 148). Among patients hospitalized with neurologic symptoms, up to 85% are children <10 years old, 15% are adults >50 years old, and only 1% are young adults. The risk for neurologic infection in children compared to adults has been estimated to be 10-fold greater (4% of all symptomatic cases versus 0.4%). Neurologic symptoms often appear late in the illness, sometimes after defervescence. Seizures are common and have a focal component in 40% of cases (92, 113). Cranial nerve palsy, motor weakness, paralysis, and specific signs of cerebellitis are present in 5 to 10% of hospitalized patients, while stupor and coma occur less frequently. More than half of hospitalized patients may exhibit clinical signs of elevated intracranial pressure. Meningismus is found in the majority of childhood cases.

Outcomes

The case fatality rate among encephalitis cases is 10 to 25%, with higher mortality rates in children <4 years old. Overall, between 0.2 and 1% of all symptomatic cases are fatal, nearly all in children. The outcome of recovered cases has not been well characterized; however, forgetfulness, nervousness, asthenia, and headache are not uncommon, at least through the first year. Recurrent seizures, motor impairment, psychomotor retardation, and behavioral disorders are sequelae in children (76).

When attenuated VEEV vaccine was given as an experimental palliative to eight patients with lymphoreticular tumors, the patients had typical self-limited illnesses without encephalitis; clinical and radiological regression was seen in four. Virus was recovered from one patient's bone marrow on multiple occasions from the 2nd to the 18th day after vaccination.

Sylvatic viruses generally produce a self-limited febrile illness; however, in one case, death evidently followed secondary infection and lymphoreticular involvement rather than encephalitis, as occurs in experimentally infected guinea pigs (141). Fatal encephalitis occurred after Tonate virus (IIIB subtype) infection in one study (59). All three recognized cases of subtype II (EVEV) infection produced encephalitis and coma without sequelae.

Laboratory Abnormalities

Leukopenia is characteristic, resulting from an early lymphopenia that rebounds over a week, while the absolute neutrophil count moves in the opposite direction, declining to 0.5×10^9 to 2×10^9/liter after 5 to 7 days. The net result is a declining total WBC count in the range of 2×10^9 to 6×10^9/liter (12). CSF contains a variable pleocytosis, usually with a lymphocytic predominance. Elevated CSF glucose has been reported; CSF protein typically is normal and rarely is elevated. About one-third of patients have had moderately elevated serum liver transaminases. Volunteers receiving live attenuated vaccine have exhibited transient attenuated or depressed T waves on electrocardiograms.

Differential Diagnosis

Sylvatic infections are indistinguishable from many ordinary or tropical viral infections, such as Oropouche virus and other bunyavirus fevers, while the absence of a rash and joint symptoms helps to rule out MAYV disease. The neurologic syndrome cannot be differentiated from that due to EEEV, SLEV, or other pathogens that occur in the same locations. Even in the context of an epidemic, the clinical diagnosis based on symptoms of acute febrile illness has been accurate in only about two-thirds of cases. The absence of rash and hemorrhagic phenomena aids in excluding epidemic dengue. An ongoing equine epizootic is the most helpful clue to the diagnosis.

Laboratory Diagnosis

Virus can be recovered from blood most easily in the first 3 days of illness, with declining sensitivity up to the eighth day (11, 141). Viral titers remain in the range of $10^{3.8}$ to $10^{5.7}$ PFU/ml through at least the fourth day of illness. In addition, virus can be recovered from the pharynx in 7 to 40% of cases in the same time frame (11, 14). PCR appears to be highly sensitive in detecting virus in acute-phase serum samples (80). Viral isolations also have been made from decidua of abortions and from bone marrow but have been inconsistent from brain (144). The subtype of viral isolates should be rapidly identified to inform public health decisions on control measures.

Detection of virus-specific IgM in acute-phase serum provides a rapid presumptive diagnosis in both horses and humans (115, 141). No cross-reactions with WEEV or EEEV antibodies are detected using available IgM and IgG enzyme-linked immunosorbent assay kits using IAB viral antigen. Antibodies to epizootic viruses can be differentiated from those to enzootic viruses by using an epitope-blocking enzyme immunoassay (EIA) (140). Neutralization (NT) titers may also provide subtype specificity of the antibodies. Specific IgM has persisted for several months after immunization with TC-83 vaccine, but its longevity after natural infection is unknown.

Prevention and Treatment

Systematic equine immunization should dampen epizootic transmission and, in principle, can prevent the emergence of outbreaks. Only the live attenuated TC-83 vaccine should be used, to avoid risk of inadequate inactivation and iatrogenic transmission. Attenuated equine vaccine is no longer produced in the United States, but production and distribution are maintained in support of public veterinary vaccination programs in several Latin American countries.

TC-83 strain and killed (TC-84) experimental human vaccines have been used extensively to protect laboratory workers and others at high risk of exposure (107). Direct studies of the former's efficacy are lacking; however, effectiveness can be inferred from the reduction of laboratory-acquired cases with its use and from experimental-challenge experiments in which vaccinated animals have been protected against airborne challenge infection. A single dose produces a neutralizing antibody response in 82% of vaccinees and induction of specific IgA, with 56% retaining a neutralizing antibody titer of >1:20 for 10 years (36). The strain is only partially attenuated, and self-limited influenza-like illness or aseptic meningitis similar to those of natural infection occurs in 23% of vaccinees. Virus has been recovered from blood and pharyngeal swabs as in the natural infection; therefore, immunosuppressive conditions or pregnancy in either the intended vaccinee or his or her household contacts is a reason for exclusion.

Among the 18% who fail to respond serologically, 76% seroconvert after reimmunization with the killed TC-84 vaccine. Preexisting antibodies from prior alphavirus vaccinations may interfere with a proper immune response, and other vaccinees show a persistent failure to respond to the live vaccine (88, 107). Although vaccination with inactivated TC-84 vaccine is recommended in live-vaccine nonresponders, inactivated vaccine may not protect against infection by the respiratory route, the principal concern in laboratories. In addition, titers of TC-84-induced antibody to enzootic ID and IE subtypes are lower, and these infections have occurred in vaccinees. Because of the limitations of available vaccine, all laboratory manipulations should be undertaken in biosafety level 3 (BSL-3) facilities. Other vaccines are under development.

Nonreplicating VEEV replicon particles have shown promise as a vehicle for delivery of chimeric vaccines for a range of other infectious agents.

Personal protection is based on avoiding foci of enzootic and epidemic transmission, using mosquito repellents, and wearing protective clothing. Treatment is symptomatic, with analgesics and bed rest in mild cases and supportive therapy in more severe cases. Fatality rates in children with neurologic symptoms remain high, in part because outbreaks occur in relatively undeveloped rural areas. Pneumonia is the principal nonneurologic illness, with evidence of secondary infection in some cases. In addition, significant lymphoid depletion could predispose to bacterial infection through the gastrointestinal tract. Appropriate early antibacterial therapy is important in acutely ill patients.

CHIKUNGUNYA VIRUS

Virology

Classification and Composition

The name of CHIKV derives from a Kimakonde root verb, *kungunyala*, meaning "to dry up or become contorted," specifically modified in early times to describe the bent posture of patients with painful joints (82). The disease occurs over a wide geographic area from west Africa, where genetic studies suggest the virus may have originated, to the Philippine archipelago in Asia, where it was transported a few hundred years ago (109). The west African strains form one major genetic lineage, while the other major lineage has spread widely and is divided into east African and Asian sublineages, which also show phenotypic and antigenic differences (10). Individual epidemics may be caused by specific genetic variants (123). The different lineages and sublineages do not have clear pathogenic differences, though strains causing hemorrhagic disease in humans do show increased pathogenicity in mice.

Host Range

Disease has not been observed in naturally infected animals. Monkeys and baboons, the principal vertebrate hosts in the viral transmission cycle, develop a viremia after infection but remain asymptomatic. Viremia of a sufficient level to potentially support viral transmission has been experimentally produced in some species of rodents and bats.

Epidemiology

Distribution

Viral transmission has been reported within a vast area of Asia and sub-Saharan Africa (Fig. 12); serologic evidence of infection also has been found in Pakistan, Saudi Arabia, and Iraq. Historical accounts and the known clinical differences between dengue and chikungunya suggest that

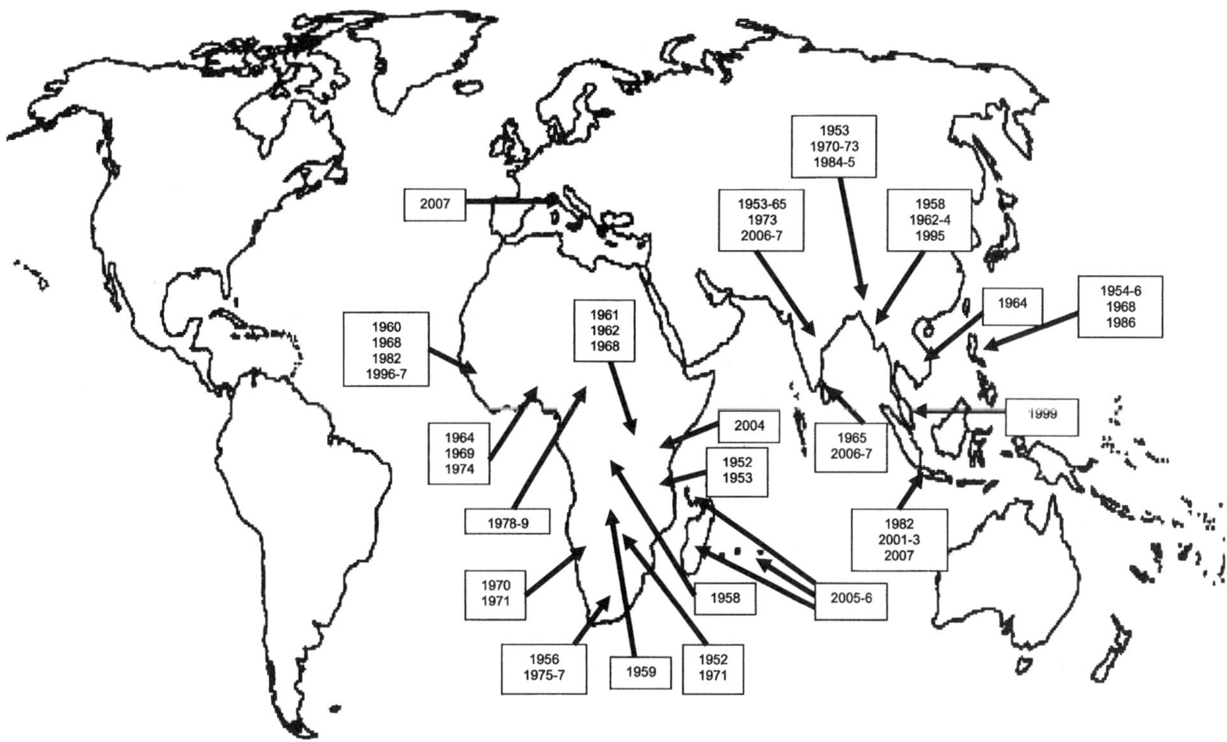

FIGURE 12 Reported chikungunya epidemics by year.

CHIKV also may have been transferred to the western hemisphere with the slave trade, as was yellow fever virus. However, the involvement of other viruses (e.g., MAYV) causing a similar clinical syndrome cannot be excluded. The virus is transmitted from human to human predominantly by *A. aegypti* mosquitoes, but *A. albopictus* and other *Aedes* species play a role in Asia and the Indian Ocean region. *A. albopictus* appears to have been the important vector in the recent epidemic in the Indian Ocean region (105) and in Italy in 2007 (112).

Incidence and Prevalence

Extensive epidemics were reported between 1952 and 1977 in eastern and southern Africa, with polyarthritis attack rates of 50% and village-to-village spread occurring in 2- to 3-week intervals. A high rate of milder or inapparent infection occurs within Africa, as seroprevalence rates of 30 to 100% have been found. Epidemics have been infrequent in Africa, the most recent occurring in Kinshasa in 1999–2000. Sporadic human infections occur with exposure to the forest or savanna transmission cycle in occupational activities or from nearby villages. Transmission occurs mainly in the rainy season, when mosquito numbers increase.

In Asia, explosive *A. aegypti*-borne outbreaks have occurred mainly in urban locations where peridomestic breeding sites in discarded containers and water storage reservoirs are prevalent. An estimated 400,000 cases occurred during an outbreak in Madras, India, in 1964, and in Bangkok, Thailand, 40,000 to 70,000 outpatient pediatric cases were seen in 1962 (55). However, by 1988 the disease had disappeared from the city. In a sudden reversal, scattered outbreaks in Thailand reemerged without warning in 1995. A similar disappearance from Calcutta, India, was demonstrated in a 1994 serosurvey that showed a 12% antibody prevalence in persons >50 years old but no evidence of infection in children or young adults. Malaysia experienced spread of the virus in 1998–1999, and CHIKV outbreaks also occurred in Indonesia in 1982 and again in 2001 to 2003. The most recent epidemic of over a million cases began in Kenya in late 2004, spread to the Comoros in early 2005, and spread to the Seychelles, Réunion, Mayotte, Mauritius, and in 2006 to India, predominantly the western coastal provinces, and Sri Lanka (105). Attack rates have approached or exceeded 50% of the population in many areas. It also spread to Italy in 2007 and was the first entry of CHIKV into Europe. Transmission has been predominantly due to *A. albopictus* in the Indian Ocean and Italy (105, 112, 136), possibly due to a point mutation in the E1 protein of that strain that increases its fitness for transmission by *A. albopictus* (136). Therefore, there is concern that this strain may spread internationally, including in Europe and North America, due to the wide distribution of *A. albopictus*.

In Africa, reduction of human infections in areas of previous activity parallels the natural transmission cycle of infections among forest monkeys and sylvatic *Aedes* mosquitoes, in which the virus circulates locally in 5- to 7-year cycles determined by the availability of susceptible animals. The virus is maintained by the continuous movement of epizootics over large regions, refreshed by the birth of new cohorts of susceptible animals. *A. aegypti*-borne outbreaks also have occurred in Africa (including the Tanganyika outbreak that led to the initial recognition of the disease) fueled by the prevalence of peridomestic mosquito breeding sites and, in arid areas, by receptacles of stored water.

Little is known about transmission cycles in Asia, although seropositive monkeys have been found, indicating the possibility of a similar forest primate-mosquito cycle. *A. albopictus* and *Aedes vittatus* are capable of transmitting the virus and are prevalent in areas where outbreaks have occurred, and the former has been shown to be important in the Indian Ocean and European outbreaks (105, 112, 136).

Cases have been reported for travellers and expatriates in tropical locations (35, 127). CHIKV is highly contagious in the laboratory. At least 39 cases due to percutaneous and nonpercutaneous exposures have been reported. Laboratory manipulations of live virus should be confined to BSL-3 facilities (138).

Clinical Manifestations

The incubation period is estimated to be 2 to 10 days. The onset of malaise, fever, and joint pains is sudden and typically without prodromal symptoms and is rapidly incapacitating (28, 61, 94, 114). Arthralgia is usually symmetrical, involving the knees, elbows, fingers, feet, ankles, and, less often, the shoulders and hips (66, 131). Backache and headache are common. Inflammation of the fascia of the sole of the foot and the wrist is often reported, and pressure on nerves due to swelling of the fascia may cause tingling in the extremities.

Patients appear to be distressed, holding their extremities motionless. In children, high fevers (>40°C) are typical, but fever may be entirely absent in adults (61). The conjunctivae are suffused, and the pharynx may be mildly inflamed. Rarely, the ear pinnae may be painful and inflamed (61, 134). Lymph nodes may be slightly enlarged and tender. Affected joints are warm and painful to palpation and exhibit periarticular fullness; however, definite effusions are present in about 10% of cases. Stiffness and intense pain accompany movement. Rash occurs in up to 50% of cases, appearing either with the onset of symptoms or several days later with the decline of fever. It is a faint irritating or pruritic maculopapular rash initially on the trunk and face and spreading to the extremities, including the palms and soles. Those with hemorrhagic disease may develop fine petechiae, and occasional purpura may appear on the trunk and limbs, especially on the legs and feet, with or without gingival bleeding. The liver may be slightly enlarged, although not as prominently as in dengue hemorrhagic fever.

After 2 to 4 days of illness, improvement is rapid, while joint pain and stiffness resolve more slowly and can persist for months or years in some cases (see below). Arthritic symptoms consist of morning stiffness, pain, and swelling of the joints, impairing function. Fever may be biphasic in children. The rash also may reappear in 3 to 7 days, with as many as three successive eruptions. Hemorrhagic phenomena are relatively uncommon and usually are limited to petechiae, but gum bleeding, epistaxis, hematemesis, melena, and rare cases of fatal shock have been reported (98, 122, 134). CNS involvement, consisting of meningismus, nuchal rigidity, ophthalmoplegia, slurred speech, and limb weakness, has been described in individual cases, and persistent convulsions associated with neurologic sequelae have been reported for infants (22, 61). Acute polyneuropathy and paralysis were described in a laboratory-confirmed case (18, 134).

Laboratory Abnormalities

The peripheral WBC count usually is normal or slightly depressed, while children may present with a neutrophilia followed by a relative lymphocytosis (18, 28, 61, 134). Markedly depressed platelet counts, $<50 \times 10^9$/liter, have been observed in patients with hemorrhagic manifestations. Prothrombin and bleeding times have been normal in a few reported cases. The erythrocyte sedimentation rate (ESR) may be increased to 20 to 50 mm/h, with elevated C-reactive protein. Various joint fluid abnormalities have been described in cases with persistent arthritic symptoms (see below).

In infants and children with convulsions and in anecdotal cases with various neurologic abnormalities, CSF has been uniformly normal except for an elevated protein in one case (18, 61). Routine electrocardiographs have disclosed changes suggestive of myocarditis in three cases (134).

Complications

Severe and fatal cases of CHIKV infection have been reported mainly for infants and children, particularly in a form associated with high fever, prolonged convulsions, and neurologic deficits suggesting primary encephalitis (18, 61, 134). During the 2005 Indian Ocean outbreak of CHIKV infection, there was a much higher incidence of serious disease than had previously been described (105). However, it is also believed that many of these cases involved other underlying illnesses that contributed to the poor outcomes. During that outbreak there was also a high rate of transmission to neonates from mothers who were symptomatic at delivery, with severe disease in the neonates. Ocular involvement, including uveitis and optic neuritis, was described in Indian cases.

Children and young adults typically have mild transitory joint pains, while arthritic symptoms are substantially more severe and persistent in older people. Morning stiffness and other symptoms typically persist for several weeks or months and, in a small percentage of cases, continue for years. A 3- to 5-year follow-up of 107 patients found that one-third had fully recovered within several weeks; one-third had a slower resolution, over about a year; and in 14%, recovery took 2 to 3 years (16). Fully recovered patients were younger, with a mean age of 37 years. Residual symptoms ranged from mild discomfort and stiffness to persistent pain with effusions or synovial thickening but no destructive changes or muscular atrophy. Joint fluids in three cases showed an elevated WBC count (2×10^9 to 5×10^9/liter) and, in one case, reduced complement levels (40). Low titers of rheumatoid factor (mean, 1:2), indicative of low-grade inflammation, and elevated ESRs (15 to 25 mm/h) have been reported for patients with persistent arthritic symptoms. Radiographs have shown mainly soft tissue swelling, but small erosions were noted in a metacarpophalangeal joint of one patient (40).

Differential Diagnosis

Dengue is the principal consideration in the differential diagnosis because of its overlapping geographic distribution, vectors, and transmission season and its similar clinical presentation, with acute fever and musculoskeletal pain. CHIKV produces a more severe and immediately debilitating illness, with prominent polyarthralgia and more rapid recovery. Dengue is characterized by more severe constitutional symptoms, retro-orbital headache, and eye pain and is less likely to produce a clinically apparent rash, and if it does, the rash differs from the maculopapular rash seen with CHIKV infection. Thrombocytopenia is relatively common in dengue compared with chikungunya. The illnesses are less easily differentiated in children, who have milder joint symptoms than do adults with CHIKV infection. ONNV illness is very similar, but with more prominent cervical lymphadenitis and conjunctivitis. SINV disease also occurs in southern Africa and causes polyarthralgia and rash, though with a milder illness and less fever than that due to CHIKV. In addition, rheumatic symptoms may be associated with various parasitic infections endemic in Africa or Asia. The differential diagnosis also should include cosmopolitan infections due to viruses producing acute polyarthritis, including hepatitis B and C viruses, human immunodeficiency virus, parvovirus B19, rubella virus, mumps virus, enteroviruses, and Epstein-Barr virus, and post- and parainfectious arthritis due to acute rheumatic fever, bacterial and parasitic enteric infections, Reiter's syndrome, and disseminated gonococcal infection. Serum sickness and Henoch-Schönlein purpura also should be considered in the diagnosis. Cases with acute arthritis involving small joints of the hands, wrists, knees, and elbows can mimic acute rheumatoid arthritis, and the chronicity of symptoms in some cases adds to the difficulty of making the appropriate diagnosis.

Laboratory Diagnosis

High and relatively persistent levels of viremia have been observed ($>10^{8.0}$ PFU/ml), with mean mouse 50% lethal doses of $10^{5.0}$ PFU/ml in the first 2 days of illness, declining to approximately $10^{1.0}$ PFU/ml by the fifth day (18). Viral RNA can often be detected in blood within 1 week of onset (105). Virus has not been recovered in the few CSF samples that have been tested (18). Joint fluids of acutely ill patients have not been examined virologically; in a few patients with persistent symptoms and high serum antibody titers, virus could not be isolated from joint fluid or blood.

Most diagnoses are serologic, using HI, immunofluorescence (IF), or, most commonly, EIA. Indirect and isotype capture EIAs for virus-specific IgM are positive within the first few days of illness and generally indicate recent infection. However, IgM persists for several weeks or months and may indicate recent past infection. A $\geq$4-fold rise in IgG titer or IgG seroconversion supports recent infection. Cross-reacting antibodies are uncommon but may occur due to ONNV, and where potential exposure to both viruses has occurred, then tests should be carried out for both. If this fails to distinguish between them, then NT tests are required.

Prevention

Outbreaks of *A. aegypti*-borne disease are best prevented by destroying or removing containers holding water that serve as breeding sites, following the approaches described for dengue control. Control measures for *A. albopictus* should be used where that is implicated as a vector. Personal protective measures against mosquito bites are indicated to prevent exposure in sylvatic settings.

A formalin-inactivated vaccine and a live CHIKV 181/clone 25 vaccine, attenuated by serial passage of an Asian strain in MRC-5 cells, have produced neutralizing antibodies in humans, but their efficacies have not been studied.

Treatment

Symptomatic treatment with nonsteroidal anti-inflammatory drugs provides relief from joint stiffness and pain in many patients, though individuals respond variably to the different drugs. Rest, heat, and gentle exercise may assist, but vigorous exercise should be avoided. There are no specific antiviral agents for any of the alphaviruses. Chloroquine was reported as being effective in a pilot study in southern Africa, but that has not yet been confirmed in controlled trials (15). Corticosteroids generally should be avoided, though short-term use may provide temporary relief in severe cases.

O'NYONG-NYONG VIRUS

The name of ONNV derives from the Acholi term meaning "very painful and weak," which was given to describe the illness in the first recorded outbreak (149). The epidemic, resulting in an estimated two million cases, emerged in 1959 in Uganda and spread rapidly in east Africa, south to Mozambique, and west to Zaire, and to Senegal in west Africa before dying out 3 years later. Another outbreak occurred in the Ivory Coast in the mid-1980s, but the virus did not reappear in east Africa until another major epidemic erupted in 1996–1997, leading to an extensive outbreak in southern Uganda (67, 121). In retrospect, the virus had been circulating locally at a low level as early as 1994–1995, as shown in a study of febrile patients presenting to hospitals in nearby areas. Virus recovered from those patients and the 1996 and 1959 strains proved to be similar genetically (73; R. Swanepoel, E. Sanders, and T. Tsai, unpublished data). Most recently the virus has been found in Chad (6).

As previous field studies indicated, *Anopheles funestus* was implicated as the principal mosquito vector in outbreaks. Adaptation of the virus to peridomestic *Anopheles* mosquitoes, a trait unique among alphaviruses, undoubtedly contributes to the explosive nature of its epidemic transmission (109). Other aspects of the viral transmission cycle have not been elucidated, but the presence of an unidentified nonhuman mammalian host may account for the maintenance of the virus between epidemics.

Clinically, the illness resembles that due to CHIKV and is characterized by fever, constitutional symptoms, joint pain, rash, and lymphadenitis, the full syndrome appearing in 40% of cases. Differentiation may be difficult; however, lymphadenopathy, occurring in 50% of cases, seems to be more marked in ONNV disease (67).

Virus can be recovered from acute-phase blood samples taken within the first 6 days after onset, and virus recovery may be successful in afebrile patients (67, 121). Laboratory diagnosis is usually done by serology, as discussed for CHIKV.

Personal protective measures against malaria should also be effective against acquiring ONNV, i.e., using mosquito nets impregnated with permethrin and avoiding unprotected evening and nighttime exposure.

Igbo-Ora virus, which can be distinguished antigenically from CHIKV and ONNV only by cross-complement fixation tests, has been shown to be a genetic variant of ONNV (73, 103). The virus was isolated in 1966 from blood samples of febrile patients in Igbo-Ora and Ibadan, Nigeria, and cases subsequently were reported from the Central African Republic and the Ivory Coast. The clinical illness, described in only one case, consisted of fever, polyarthritis, and pharyngitis.

SINDBIS VIRUS

SINV, named after the northern Egyptian district where the virus was first isolated, is transmitted in Europe, Africa,

Asia, and Australia. Strains are separated into Europe/Africa and Asia/Australia lineages, the close genetic relationship of Swedish and South African strains suggesting a recent introduction from South Africa to Scandinavia by migratory birds (100, 119). A third lineage has been identified in the southwest of Western Australia (119). Within these lineages there is evidence of both geographic and temporal evolution.

Epidemiology

In Africa, sporadic cases and occasional outbreaks numbering in hundreds or thousands of cases have been reported since 1954 to 1956, principally from areas of South Africa during the summer from December to April (65, 89). SINV antibodies have been detected in travellers returning from Africa, but SINV is very uncommon compared to other arboviruses such as CHIKV (35).

Novel outbreaks occurring in 1981 in Sweden, Finland, and the adjacent Karelia area of Russia were given local names: Ockelbo, Pogosta, and Karelian fevers, respectively. Subsequently, endemic transmission was recognized in those locales and in Norway. In Sweden, 600 to 1,200 cases are estimated annually (37, 83), while Pogosta disease recurs in a 7-year cycle. Transmission is localized to a zone between latitude 60° and 63°N, with declining incidence and seroprevalence north and south of this zone. Most cases occur from July to September, during the season of most active viral transmission among middle-aged adults with woodland exposure (e.g., while picking berries or gathering mushrooms).

In contrast, SINV rarely causes human disease in Asia or Australia, despite the fact that serologic studies in Australia have shown evidence of regular human infections. This suggests that there may be pathogenicity differences between the different lineages (84).

The maintenance cycle for SINV is thought to be a mosquito-bird cycle. Humans are dead-end hosts infected by the bite of ornithophilic mosquito species or by bridging mosquito vectors with broader feeding habits. These include *Aedes*, *Culex*, *Culiseta*, and *Mansonia* spp.

Clinical Manifestations

The incubation period for Ockelbo and Pogosta fevers is up to 1 week. The principal clinical features are arthralgia and rash (37, 65, 83, 89). Symptoms may be preceded by a short prodrome of fever, headache, and malaise followed by progressive musculoskeletal pain. All the joints may be symmetrically involved, although the ankles, wrists, knees, fingers, and toes are most frequently affected, followed by the hips, shoulders, elbows, and, occasionally, the neck and back. Joints are swollen due to synovial and periarticular edema, and some patients are unable to walk. Tendons may be inflamed as well. Pharyngitis and lymphadenopathy may be present. Discrete macules on the trunk and limbs, including the palms and soles, evolve to small (3-mm-diameter) papules generally sparing the face and head (Fig. 13). Lesions may occasionally vesiculate. The ESR may be elevated during the acute illness, occasionally to >25 mm/h. Other laboratory examinations have been unremarkable.

Joint symptoms usually resolve over a period of weeks, but residual symptoms persist for several years in one-third of cases (97). Convalescence is characterized by asthenia and fatigue.

The principal consideration in the differential diagnosis is West Nile virus infection, which is transmitted in the same season, enzootic cycle, and in an overlapping geographic distribution in Africa and Asia. However, West Nile virus causes less prominent joint pains, rash is less common, and lymphadenopathy may be more prominent. Other conditions to be differentiated are described in the section on CHIKV above (85).

Laboratory Diagnosis

Virus has been recovered from both blood and skin lesions of a minority of infected individuals, but this has limited diagnostic value (71). Serologic tests are preferred for routine diagnosis. Specific IgM generally appears within a week after onset, and IgG appears a few days later (71). IgM declines slowly, over a period of years (97). Cross-reacting antibody has not been described as a problem, but it should be considered where exposure to other alphaviruses may have occurred.

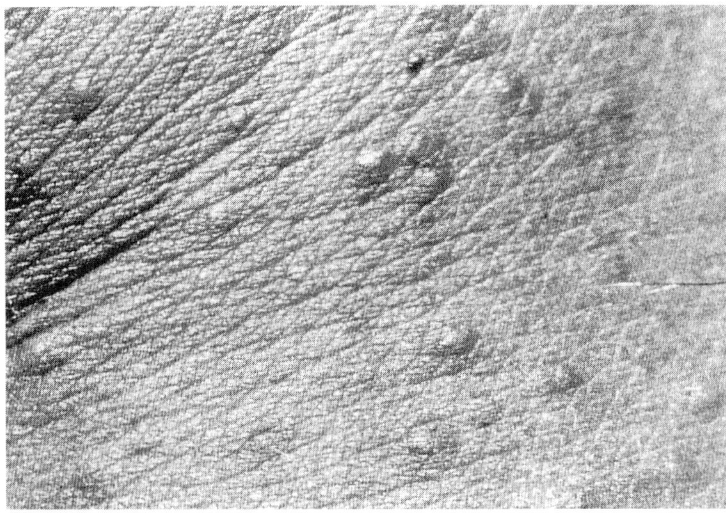

FIGURE 13 Small papular lesions seen in Sindbis (Ockelbo) fever. (Courtesy of B. Niklasson.)

Prevention and Treatment

Individuals planning excursions to known enzootic areas during the transmission season should use precautions against mosquito bites. No specific therapy is available. Symptomatic treatment with nonsteroidal anti-inflammatory drugs may provide relief from joint symptoms.

MAYARO VIRUS

MAYV is the principal New World representative of alphaviruses within the SFV complex. Viral activity is widely distributed in forested locations in Central America and the northern parts of South America, resulting in a high level of endemic transmission and seroprevalence rates of >50% in some areas. The virus was isolated in 1954 from febrile humans in scattered areas of Trinidad and named after the island's Mayaro district (4). Subsequently, four outbreaks were reported from Bolivia, Brazil, and Surinam among forestry and agricultural workers and soldiers (19, 106). In the Belterra epidemic in Brazil, serosurveys estimated infection in 20% of the town's population of 4,000 (106). The outbreaks were typified by forest exposure; high attack rates, often with higher risk among males of working age; and occurrence in the rainy season. The epidemiological pattern is explained by the forest cycle of viral transmission, probably between *Hemagogus* mosquitoes and wild vertebrates, including monkeys and marmosets, analogous to the sylvatic cycle of yellow fever.

The incubation period is <6 to 12 days (19, 62, 106). Onset of illness is sudden, with severe headache, vertigo, chills, myalgias, malaise, and fever, up to 40°C. Movement of the eyes, head, and neck is painful, and the conjunctivae may be injected. Joint pain and swelling are the principal features of the illness, affecting (in decreasing frequency) the fingers, wrists, ankles, toes, elbows, and knees. The hands may be so swollen that they cannot be closed. In the Belterra outbreak, incapacitated persons were seen hobbling around the village. Joint pains sometimes precede the onset of fever and range in severity from mild to incapacitating. In two-thirds of cases, a morbilliform rash appears late in the illness, often with the resolution of fever. The eruption consists of fine, blanching, often coalescent papules, principally on the trunk and extremities, mostly sparing the face. Rash occurs more often in children than in adults. Inguinal lymphadenopathy is present in about half the cases. Slight liver enlargement and mild jaundice have been reported. Fever remits after 1 to 6 days, and patients with mild symptoms are able to resume work in 2 to 3 days. Others remain incapacitated with fatigue and joint stiffness for several weeks. Polyuria and transient pneumonitis have been reported; however, their connection with other concurrent infections could not be ruled out. Hemorrhagic disease has been described, but no fatalities have been attributed to the illness.

Leukopenia with a relative lymphocytosis is a constant finding in the first week, returning to normal in the second week. Moderate albuminuria and slight elevations of liver transaminases and direct bilirubin have been reported for a few patients (62, 106).

Clinically the illness may be mistaken for dengue. An epidemiological history of forest exposure suggests the diagnosis, and other considerations are discussed in the section on CHIKV above (85).

The virus can be readily isolated from blood obtained within the first 3 or 4 days of illness (4, 106, 132). Detection of specific IgM and detection of a ≥4-fold or greater rise in IgG titer provides a serologic diagnosis of recent infection, but reciprocal testing with antigens against other local alphaviruses may be needed (132).

Infection is best prevented by avoiding forested areas, particularly during the day, when *Hemagogus* mosquitoes are active. Live attenuated CHIKV vaccine provided cross-protection in experimental monkey studies.

The Una subtype produces a febrile illness with arthritis in horses but is not known to cause human disease.

ROSS RIVER VIRUS

Virology

RRV is the most common arbovirus to cause infection in Australia. Outbreaks of "epidemic polyarthritis" infection were recognized in 1886 and 1928 and during World War II before the virus was isolated from *A. vigilax* mosquitoes collected along the Ross River in Queensland. The virus exhibits a high degree of conservation, with strains from the known region of viral transmission spanning a 30-year period showing only a 3.3% divergence in the nucleotide sequences of the E2 and E3 genes. Strains separate into three genotypes: genotype 1 was present in northern Queensland until the mid-1970s, when it was replaced by genotype 2, which also caused the outbreaks in the Pacific Islands. Genotype 3 is restricted to the southwestern corner of Western Australia but was largely replaced by genotype 2 in 1996, and that is now the dominant strain throughout Australia (84, 118). Complete genome sequences are available for genotype 1 (T48) and genotype 2 (NB5092) strains, and a full-length cDNA clone of the T48 strain has been constructed.

Epidemiology

Cases have been reported from all states of Australia, Papua New Guinea, New Caledonia, the Solomon Islands, and, in a single extensive outbreak in 1979–1980, from Fiji, American Samoa, Tonga, and the Cook Islands in the South Pacific (84). Several thousand cases of RRV disease are reported each year in Australia, the majority occurring in the heavily populated areas of southeastern Queensland, coastal New South Wales, and the southwest of Western Australia (118), though the highest attack rates actually occur in the sparsely populated northern tropical areas (Fig. 14) (81). In the tropical areas, human infections occur mainly in the December-to-May wet season and, in the central arid regions, they occur following irregular heavy rainfall and flooding. In the southerly temperate climates, infection is highest in the late spring, early summer, and autumn, when it is warm and wet. A low level of viral transmission may occur throughout the year, even in temperate southern Australia. Epidemics in these temperate areas generally occur every 2 to 4 years, likely related to the climatic conditions resulting in increases in vector numbers and to the availability of susceptible amplifying marsupial hosts.

The principal vectors are salt marsh *Aedes* species, especially *A. vigilax* in coastal areas and *Culex annulirostris* and other freshwater species in the interior (84, 118). Natural infections occur in a broad range of animals, including birds, marsupials, and placental mammals. The principal viral transmission cycle in Australia involves kangaroos, wallabies, and other macropods as vertebrate hosts, with

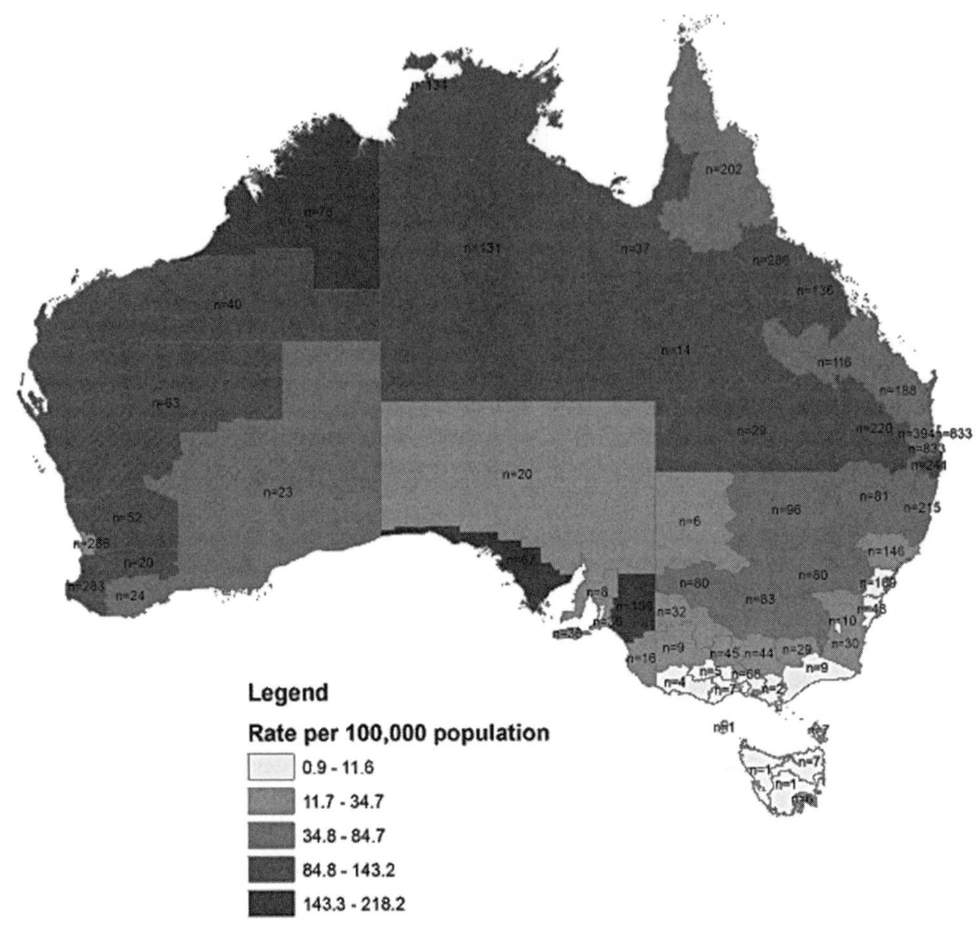

FIGURE 14 Notifications and notification rates of RRV infections, Australia, 2005–2006, by Statistical Division of residence. (Reprinted from reference 81 with permission.)

humans as incidental hosts. Short cycles of human-mosquito-human transmission have occurred during major epidemics (84) but are not sustained and do not significantly contribute to maintenance of the virus.

Epidemics typically have been preceded by increased rainfall and increased tidal inundation of coastal swamps, leading to expanded vector mosquito populations. Risk is associated with outdoor exposure during the periods of greatest mosquito activity, during the day and at night for *A. vigilax* and in the period before and after dusk and dawn for *C. annulirostris*. Cases in travellers are not unusual, and outbreaks have occurred among expatriate groups engaged in field activities, such as the military.

Clinical Manifestations

The estimates of clinical illness following RRV infection have varied widely, with case-to-infection ratios between 1:80 and 3:1 or higher (42, 56, 131). The incubation period is 3 to 21 days, usually 7 to 9 days (42). The acute illness consists of malaise, fatigue, muscle pains, joint pains, and, in only one-half of cases, low-grade fever (38, 84). Some patients have diarrhea, headache, neck stiffness, or sore throat. Within a few days, a maculopapular erythematous rash appears in 50 to 60% of cases, initially on the trunk and limbs and sometimes spreading to the palms, soles, and face. It may appear as early as 11 days before or up to 15 days after onset. Occasionally the rash is predominantly papular and, rarely, vesicular. Enanthems of the oral mucosa are uncommon. The rash generally fades or desquamates within 10 days, although lesions may recur. Painful joints are almost universal, and in 80 to 90% there is joint pain, tiredness, stiffness, and swelling. This is usually symmetric and typically involves the wrists, knees, ankles, and small joints of the hands and fingers. The elbows, shoulders, feet, back, and jaw may also be involved and, less frequently, the hips and costochondral junctions. Inflammation may extend to wrist and ankle tendons and the plantar fascia, causing nerve compression and paresthesias.

Most patients recover within a month, with joint pain, lethargy, and muscle pains being the slowest to resolve (56). The majority of infections with the arthritogenic alphaviruses are benign but temporarily debilitating. Fever and rash, if present, usually last less than a week; many recover fully within 4 weeks, and most return to full physical activity within 3 to 6 months. Joint pains, muscle pains, and lethargy are the slowest to resolve. One study in Western Australia found that at 12 months after onset, 90% of patients still had joint pain, 80% had tiredness, 75% had joint stiffness, and 50% had muscle or tendon pain (N. Prow, A. J. Plant, D. W. Smith, and A. K. Broom, unpublished data).

Glomerulonephritis and associated loin pain have been noted in several cases (56). Vertical infections have been demonstrated in experimentally infected mice and may occur rarely in humans, but there is no evidence of any associated fetal disease in humans. While headache is relatively common, there is no convincing evidence of more serious neurologic disease due to RRV.

The blood count is nearly always normal, and the C-reactive protein is rarely elevated. Rheumatoid factor and other autoantibodies are absent. Cases with glomerulonephritis may have hematuria with the presence of glomerular red cells, pyuria, and proteinuria. The ESR may be moderately elevated during the first week of illness and usually declines to normal despite the persistence of symptoms. Joints, even if swollen, often have very little excess synovial fluid, though amounts up to 70 ml have been reported. The joint fluid is clear, opalescent, and free of clots and exhibits a mononuclear pleocytosis of 1×10^9 to 60×10^9 cells/liter. Radiographs show no erosive changes or deformities.

The differential diagnosis includes other arboviruses found in Australia that cause acute arthritis, e.g., BFV, Kokobera virus, Kunjin virus, and, rarely, SINV (38, 84). Other considerations in the differential diagnosis are mentioned in the section on CHIKV above (85).

Laboratory Diagnosis

Humans have a transient viremia, so virus is only occasionally isolated from acute-phase blood. Culture is usually done in C6/36 cells, though blind passage to indicator cells, such as Vero, BHK, or chicken embryo cells, is needed to see a CPE. Intrathoracic injection of *Toxorhynchites* mosquitoes or inoculation of mice is less common. Detection of viral RNA is more sensitive but is also usually negative by the time patients present to a medical practitioner, and it is not used routinely.

Laboratory diagnosis is usually made serologically. Confirmed recent infection is indicated either by IgG seroconversion by EIA or NT or by a fourfold rise in IgG titer by HI or NT. Virus-specific IgM antibodies can be detected by EIA or IF and appear within 1 week of onset of illness. False-positive reactions can occur, and IgM commonly persists for several months. Detection of IgM alone is therefore only presumptive evidence of recent infection. Cross-reactions between RRV and BFV antibodies are very uncommon and usually occur with EIA IgM tests; they can be resolved with paired IgG tests or retesting using a different assay.

Prevention and Treatment

Mosquito control measures can be undertaken to control breeding in areas near human populations. Personal protective measures are recommended for people either living in or visiting areas of RRV activity. There are no vaccines available.

Rest during the acute period of illness is prudent, followed by gentle exercise. Heat assists some patients. Nonsteroidal anti-inflammatory drugs provide rapid relief of symptoms and hasten resumption of activities in most patients (42). Steroids have been used and provide temporary relief, but they are not recommended due to a lack of data on benefits.

BARMAH FOREST VIRUS

BFV, named after the site in northern Victoria where it was first isolated from *Culex annulirostris* mosquitoes, is antigenically distinct from other alphaviruses, including RRV and SINV, that are also found in Australia (33, 79, 84). The diseases are clinically indistinguishable, although arthritis and arthralgias are more severe, occur more frequently, and persist longer in RRV disease. Rash is more prominent in BFV disease (38). Their seasonality and transmission cycles have overlapping features, but independent outbreaks have occurred. Overall, the notification rates in Australia are usually 5 to 10% of those for RRV disease (Fig. 15) (81). The increase in notifications in recent years may reflect an increase in testing for this infection. Patient management is the same as for RRV.

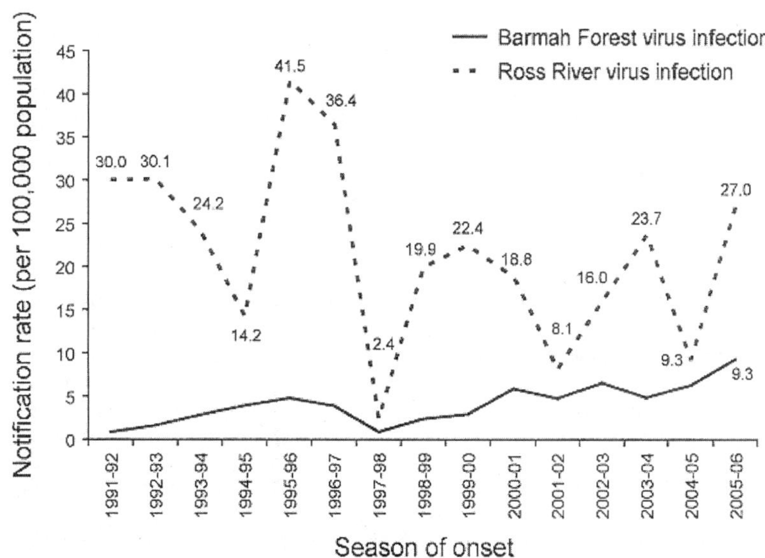

FIGURE 15 Crude annual rate of BFV and RRV infection notifications, Australia, 1 July 1991 to 30 June 2006, by season of onset. (Reprinted from reference 81 with permission.)

MISCELLANEOUS ALPHAVIRUSES

Semliki Forest Virus

In Central Africa, SFV is transmitted in a sylvatic cycle analogous to that of yellow fever virus (87). While human infections are common, disease is rare, with one case of febrile illness with severe persistent headache in humans following natural infection in Africa and one laboratory-acquired case of fatal encephalitis in Germany.

Me Tri Virus

Me Tri virus was isolated from *Culex tritaeniorhynchus* and has been associated with sporadic encephalitis cases in children in Vietnam (54). Genetic studies indicate that Me Tri virus is a variant of SFV (108).

Getah Virus

Getah virus is distributed widely in Asia and Oceania. It causes disease in horses and abortion in pigs and is a rare cause of febrile illness in humans.

LABORATORY DIAGNOSIS

Viral Detection

Most alphaviruses are assigned to BSL-2. However, in laboratories working routinely with EEEV and WEEV, vaccination of staff with the respective experimental inactivated vaccines is recommended. VEEV, CHIKV, MAYV, SFV, and others are highly transmissible in the laboratory or have caused serious laboratory infection (e.g., fatal SFV encephalitis), and work with these viruses should be confined to BSL-3 laboratories (138). Where appropriate, staff should be immunized with VEEV and CHIKV vaccines.

The viruses can be isolated from blood, CSF, pharyngeal secretions, skin, and other tissue specimens, the most appropriate sources varying individually for each of the viruses. Most are readily isolated in a variety of cell lines found in diagnostic laboratories, including Vero, A549, and MRC-5 cells. Reference laboratories often employ mosquito cell lines and occasionally intrathoracic inoculation of mosquitoes. Spin amplification has been shown to improve recovery of EEEV.

Antigen detection and PCR assays to detect viral products in blood, CSF, joint fluid, and skin have been described for several alphavirus infections, but few have been extensively evaluated. Reverse transcription-PCR assays have shown promise for rapid detection of virus in human blood and mosquito pools and for the detection of virus in the CSF in encephalitis cases.

Serology

The most sensitive serologic assays detect virus-specific IgM by capture EIA or indirect IF methods (86, 97, 115, 133). Specific IgM can be detected in serum within the first 7 to 10 days of illness in nearly all cases of alphavirus infection and in the CSF in encephalitis cases. However, serum IgM can persist for several months after acute infection and is not necessarily indicative of recent infection. Detection of specific IgM in the CSF is considered diagnostic of recent encephalitis. IgM testing for alphaviruses is relatively specific, with cross-reactions occurring only among viruses within the same antigenic complex, e.g., among viruses related to SINV.

A ≥4-fold rise in antibodies by HI, indirect IF, EIA, complement fixation (CF), or NT in paired serum samples confirms a recent infection. Elevated antibody titers in a single serum specimen provide a presumptive diagnosis (e.g., HI ≥ 160; CF ≥ 32; IF ≥ 160; NT ≥ 80), especially if accompanied by detection of IgM. Cross-reactions are uncommon for all of these assays but are most likely with IF, EIA, and HI, while CF antibodies are relatively specific and NT is highly specific. HI, IF, EIA, and NT antibodies rise in the first week after onset of illness, with a ≥4-fold change usually noted by the second week. HI and NT antibodies decline minimally after 30 months and may persist for years. CF antibodies rise more slowly and may not be detected until 2 to 3 weeks after illness onset. The half-life of CF antibodies is 2 to 3 years, and they remain detectable in only 15% of patients after 5 years, providing an alternate approach to identify recent past infections.

PREVENTION

General

Alphaviruses principally are maintained in zoonotic transmission cycles in natural habitats. Consequently, little can be done in an ecologically acceptable manner to control levels of virus circulation, and eradication is not feasible. Prevention is based on individual protection and public health measures to reduce vector numbers. Approaches to vector control are tailored to specific viral transmission cycles and habits of individual vector species. In general, these can be divided into steps to eliminate sources of mosquito vectors by environmental modifications, to minimize the emergent vector mosquito population by applications of larvicides, and to reduce adult mosquitoes by the emergency application of adulticides using backpack sprayers, trucks, or planes.

Examples of source reduction strategies include community projects to eliminate *A. aegypti* breeding sites in peridomestic containers to control CHIKV and environmental modifications, such as draining swamps and improving groundwater runoff, to control EEEV, WEEV, and RRV. Large-scale environmental modifications may be prohibitively expensive or conflict with other environmental priorities. Nevertheless, environmental modifications can achieve some reduction in vectors, especially when combined with systematic applications of larvicides to breeding sites.

Emergency vector control with adulticides can temporarily reduce vector mosquitoes that pose an immediate human risk. Typically, the decision to implement a large-scale adulticide program is stimulated by surveillance indicating large vector populations, high vector infection rates, seroconversions in sentinel animals, or cases in indicator animals, such as horses. These interventions are immediately effective in reducing adult mosquitoes on the wing, but infiltration of mosquitoes from surrounding untreated areas and their continued emergence necessitate repeated applications. The effectiveness of emergency vector control in preventing human disease has been difficult to prove because of inherent difficulties in conducting controlled evaluations under natural conditions. Large-scale insecticide applications are expensive and sometimes are met with local opposition because of concerns about pesticide toxicity for humans, birds, fish, and commercial bees. Nevertheless, adulticide use combined with public health advisories to avoid activities associated with exposure to vectors is the only available intervention to prevent epidemic transmission, and its expense, compared with the potential costs of even a single human EEE case, has been shown to be justified.

Personal Protection

Avoidance of mosquito exposure is the principal means of personal protection. This is most clear for diseases due to viruses such as MAYV and VEEV, in which infections occur in individuals or groups who chance upon enzootic viral foci. Specific advice to minimize exposure should be tailored to individual vector mosquito habits. For example, *Culex tarsalis*, a vector of WEEV, is found outdoors and is mainly active around sunset. In contrast, certain vectors of EEEV and VEEV are diurnal and feed during the day. *Culex tarsalis* is most prevalent in rural areas, whereas *A. aegypti*, the major epidemic vector of CHIKV, is associated with human dwellings and the disease is transmitted in urban locations.

Permethrin, a repellent and insecticide, should be applied to clothing, shoes (to prevent tick attachment), and camping gear, including bed nets. It is highly effective in preventing mosquito bites and when used by a group can temporarily achieve a local reduction of mosquitoes. Permethrin is approved for single applications as a scabicide (5% cream) and as a pediculicidal shampoo; however, no formulations are approved for repeated application to the skin as a repellent. Diethyl-*m*-toluamide (DEET) is the most effective repellent that is approved for use on skin. It also can be used on clothing, but permethrin is recommended (41). As a rule of thumb, each 10% of DEET in a formulation provides 1 h of protection. Although preparations containing up to 100% DEET are available, concentrations of 30 to 50% are recommended for adults and children over 2 months of age. In intertriginous areas, 50 to 75% DEET has produced deep skin ulcerations, and at lower concentrations, local and generalized hypersensitivity reactions have been reported. However, the most serious side effects are neurologic. Ingestion is associated with potentially fatal seizures, hepatitis, and encephalopathy, but dermal absorption and inhalation have also been associated with encephalopathy and seizures, principally in children. More than half of a topically applied dose penetrates the skin, and 17% is absorbed systemically. Severe or fatal encephalopathy has been reported in several cases, and DEET toxicity should be included in the differential diagnosis of neurologic infections in patients exposed to arboviruses. Irritability, sleeplessness, memory loss, and other psychological disturbances have been reported during chronic use in adults. To minimize toxicity, microcapsulated formulations that produce less absorption and confer a longer degree of protection at reduced concentrations are best. Repellents should be washed off after they are no longer needed, and for infants and children, they should not be applied to hands and the face, to reduce ingestion.

Picaridin, available at 7 and 15% concentrations, can be used but requires more frequent application and is slightly less effective than DEET.

For children under 2 months old, physical measures should be used to protect them from insect exposure. Specific recommendations for safe and effective use of repellents are summarized in Table 4.

Our thanks go to Theodore F. Tsai and Thomas P. Monath for allowing us to use text, figures, and tables from the previous edition of this chapter as a basis for this revision.

TABLE 4 Precautions to minimize exposure to mosquitoes and ticks[a]

Use an insect repellent on exposed skin to repel mosquitoes, ticks, fleas, and other arthropods. EPA-registered repellents include products containing DEET and picaridin. DEET concentrations of 30–50% are effective for several hours. Picaridin, available at 7 and 15% concentrations, needs more frequent application.
DEET formulations as high as 50% are recommended for both adults and children over 2 mo of age. Protect infants less than 2 mo of age by using a carrier draped with mosquito netting with an elastic edge for a tight fit.
When using sunscreen, apply sunscreen first and then repellent. Repellent should be washed off at the end of the day before going to bed.
Wear long-sleeved shirts (which should be tucked in), long pants, and hats to cover exposed skin. When you visit areas with ticks and fleas, wear boots, not sandals, and tuck pants into socks.
Inspect your body and clothing for ticks during outdoor activity and at the end of the day. Wear light-colored or white clothing so ticks can be more easily seen. Removing ticks right away can prevent some infections.
Apply permethrin-containing or other insect repellents to clothing, shoes, tents, mosquito nets, and other gear for greater protection. Permethrin is not labeled for use directly on skin. Most repellent is generally removed from clothing and gear by a single washing, but permethrin-treated clothing is effective for up to five washings.
Be aware that mosquitoes that transmit malaria are most active during twilight periods (dawn and dusk or in the evening).
Stay in air-conditioned or well-screened housing, and/or sleep under an insecticide-treated bed net. Bed nets should be tucked under mattresses and can be sprayed with a repellent if not already treated with an insecticide.
Daytime biters include mosquitoes that transmit dengue virus and CHIKV and sand flies that transmit leishmaniasis.

[a] Adapted from the Centers for Disease Control and Prevention recommendations (http://wwwn.cdc.gov/travel/contentMosquitoTick.aspx).

REFERENCES

1. **Aguilar, P. V., S. Paessler, A. S. Carrara, S. Baron, J. Poast, E. Wang, A. C. Moncayo, M. Anishchenko, D. Watts, R. B. Tesh, and S. C. Weaver.** 2005. Variation in interferon sensitivity and induction among strains of eastern equine encephalitis virus. *J. Virol.* **79:**11300–11310.
2. **Aguilar, P. V., R. M. Robich, M. J. Turell, M. L. O'Guinn, T. A. Klein, A. Huaman, C. Guevara, Z. Rios, R. B. Tesh, D. M. Watts, J. Olson, and S. C. Weaver.** 2007. Endemic eastern equine encephalitis in the Amazon region of Peru. *Am. J. Trop. Med. Hyg.* **76:** 293–298.
3. **Anderson, B. A.** 1984. Focal neurologic signs in western equine encephalitis. *Can. Med. Assoc. J.* **130:**1019–1021.
4. **Anderson, C. R., W. G. Downs, G. H. Wattley, N. W. Ahin, and A. A. Reese.** 1957. Mayaro virus: a new human disease agent. II. Isolation from blood of patients in Trinidad, B.W.I. *Am. J. Trop. Med. Hyg.* **6:**1012–1016.
5. **Bastian, F. O., R. D. Wende, D. B. Singer, and R. S. Zeller.** 1975. Eastern equine encephalomyelitis. Histopathologic and ultrastructural changes with isolation of the virus in a human case. *Am. J. Clin. Pathol.* **64:**10–13.

6. **Bessaud, M., C. N. Peyrefitte, B. A. Pastorino, P. Gravier, F. Tock, F. Boete, H. J. Tolou, and M. Grandadam.** 2006. O'nyong-nyong virus, Chad. *Emerg. Infect. Dis.* **12:** 1248–1250.
7. **Bia, F. J., G. F. Thornton, A. J. Main, C. K. Fong, and G. D. Hsiung.** 1980. Western equine encephalitis mimicking herpes simplex encephalitis. *JAMA* **244:**367–369.
8. **Bianchi, T. I., G. Aviles, T. P. Monath, and M. S. Sabattini.** 1993. Western equine encephalomyelitis: virulence markers and their epidemiological significance. *Am. J. Trop. Med. Hyg.* **49:**322–328.
9. **Bigler, W. J., E. B. Lassing, E. E. Buff, E. C. Prather, E. C. Beck, and G. L. Hoff.** 1976. Endemic eastern equine encephalomyelitis in Florida: a twenty-year analysis, 1955–1974. *Am. J. Trop. Med. Hyg.* **25:**884–890.
10. **Blackburn, N. K., T. G. Besselaar, and G. Gibson.** 1995. Antigenic relationship between chikungunya virus strains and o'nyong nyong virus using monoclonal antibodies. *Res. Virol.* **146:**69–73.
11. **Bowen, G. S., and C. H. Calisher.** 1976. Virological and serological studies of Venezuelan equine encephalomyelitis in humans. *J. Clin. Microbiol.* **4:**22–27.
12. **Bowen, G. S., T. R. Fashinell, P. B. Dean, and M. B. Gregg.** 1976. Clinical aspects of human Venezuelan equine encephalitis in Texas. *Bull. Pan. Am. Health Organ.* **10:**46–57.
13. **Brault, A. C., A. M. Powers, C. L. Chavez, R. N. Lopez, M. F. Cachon, L. F. Gutierrez, W. Kang, R. B. Tesh, R. E. Shope, and S. C. Weaver.** 1999. Genetic and antigenic diversity among eastern equine encephalitis viruses from North, Central and South America. *Am. J. Trop. Med. Hyg.* **61:**579–586.
14. **Briceno Rossi, A. L.** 1967. Rural epidemic encephalitis in Venezuela caused by a group A arbovirus (VEE). *Prog. Med. Virol.* **9:**176–203.
15. **Brighton, S. W.** 1984. Chloroquine phosphate treatment of chronic chikungunya arthritis. An open pilot study. *S. Afr. Med. J.* **66:**217–218.
16. **Brighton, S. W., O. W. Prozesky, and A. L. de la Harpe.** 1983. Chikungunya virus infection. A retrospective study of 107 cases. *S. Afr. Med. J.* **63:**313–315.
17. **Calisher, C. H.** 1994. Medically important arboviruses of the United Sates and Canada. *Clin. Microbiol. Rev.* **7:**89–116.
18. **Carey, D. E., R. M. Myers, C. M. DeRanitz, M. Jadhav, and R. Reuben.** 1969. The 1964 chikungunya epidemic at Vellore, South India, including observations on concurrent dengue. *Trans. R. Soc. Trop. Med. Hyg.* **63:**434–445.
19. **Causey, O. R., and O. M. Maroja.** 1957. Mayaro virus: a new human disease agent. III. Investigation of an epidemic of acute febrile illness on the River Guana in Para, Brazil and isolation of Mayaro virus as causative agent. *Am. J. Trop. Med. Hyg.* **6:**1017–1023.
20. **Centers for Disease Control.** 1988. Arboviral infections of the central nervous system—United States, 1987. *Morb. Mortal. Wkly. Rep.* **37:**506–515.
21. **Centers for Disease Control and Prevention.** 2006. Eastern equine encephalitis—New Hampshire and Massachusetts, August–September 2005. *Morb. Mortal. Wkly. Rep.* **55:**697–700.
22. **Chatterjee, S. N., S. K. Chakravarti, A. C. Mitra, and J. K. Sarkar.** 1965. Virological investigation of cases with neurological complications during the outbreak of haemorrhagic fever in Calcutta. *J. Indian Med. Assoc.* **45:** 314–316.
23. **Clarke, D. H.** 1961. Two nonfatal human infections with the virus of eastern equine encephalitis. *Am. J. Trop. Med. Hyg.* **10:**67–70.
24. **Clarris, B. J., R. L. Doherty, J. R. Fraser, E. L. French, and K. D. Muirden.** 1975. Epidemic polyarthritis: a cytological, virological and immunochemical study. *Aust. N. Z. J. Med.* **5:**450–457.
25. **Copps, S. C., and L. E. Giddings.** 1959. Transplacental transmission of western equine encephalitis. *Pediatrics* **24:** 31–33.
26. **Davis, J. H.** 1940. Equine encephalomyelitis (western type) in children: report of cases with residual atrophy of the brain. *J. Pediatr.* **16:**591–595.
27. **de la Monte, S., F. Castro, N. J. Bonilla, A. Gaskin de Urdaneta, and G. M. Hutchins.** 1985. The systemic pathology of Venezuelan equine encephalitis virus infection in humans. *Am. J. Trop. Med. Hyg.* **34:**194–202.
28. **Deller, J. J., and P. K. Russell.** 1968. Chikungunya disease. *Am. J. Trop. Med. Hyg.* **17:**107–111.
29. **Deresiewicz, R. L., S. J. Thaler, L. Hsu, and A. A. Zamari.** 1997. Clinical and neuroradiographic manifestations of eastern equine encephalitis. *N. Engl. J. Med.* **336:**1867–1874.
30. **Dickerman, R. W., F. P. Pinheiro, O. F. Oliva, J. F. Travassos da Rosa, and C. H. Calisher.** 1980. Eastern encephalitis virus from virgin forests of Northern Brazil. *Bull. Pan. Am. Health Organ.* **14:**15–21.
31. **Dietz, W. H., Jr., P. H. Peralta, and K. M. Johnson.** 1979. Ten clinical cases of human infection with Venezuelan equine encephalomyelitis virus, subtype I-D. *Am. J. Trop. Med. Hyg.* **28:**329–334.
32. **Dietz, W. H., Jr., O. Alvarez, Jr., D. H. Martin, T. E. Walton, L. J. Ackerman, and K. M. Johnson.** 1978. Enzootic and epizootic Venezuelan equine encephalomyelitis virus in horses infected by peripheral and intrathecal routes. *J. Infect. Dis.* **137:**227–237.
33. **Doggett, S. L., R. C. Russell, J. Clancy, J. Haniotis, and M. J. Cloonan.** 1999. Barmah Forest virus epidemic on the south coast of New South Wales, Australia, 1994–5: viruses, vectors, human cases and environmental factors. *J. Med. Entomol.* **36:** 861–868.
34. **Ecklund, C. M.** 1946. Human encephalitis of the western equine encephalitis type in Minnesota in 1941: clinical and epidemiological study of serologically positive cases. *Am. J. Hyg.* **43:**171–193.
35. **Eisenhut, M., T. F. Schwarz, and B. Hegenscheid.** 1999. Seroprevalence of dengue, chikungunya and Sindbis virus infections in German aid workers. *Infection* **27:**82–85.
36. **Engler, R. J., J. A. Mangiafico, P. Jahrling, T. G. Ksiazek, M. Pedrotti-Krueger, and C. J. Peters.** 1992. Venezuelan equine encephalitis-specific immunoglobulin responses: live attenuated TC-83 versus inactivated C-84 vaccine. *J. Med. Virol.* **38:**305–310.
37. **Espmark, A., and B. Niklasson.** 1984. Ockelbo disease in Sweden: epidemiological, clinical, and virological data from the 1982 outbreak. *Am. J. Trop. Med. Hyg.* **33:** 1203–1211.
38. **Flexman, J. P., D. W. Smith, J. S. Mackenzie, J. R. Fraser, S. P. Bass, L. Hueston, M. D. Lindsay, and A. L. Cunningham.** 1998. A comparison of the diseases caused by Ross River virus and Barmah Forest virus. *Med. J. Aust.* **169:**159–163.
39. **Fothergill, L. D., M. Holden, and R. W. G. Wyckoff.** 1939. Western equine encephalomyelitis in a laboratory worker. *JAMA* **113:**206–207.
40. **Fourie, E. D., and J. G. Morrison.** 1979. Rheumatoid arthritic syndrome after chikungunya fever. *S. Afr. Med. J.* **56:**130–132.
41. **Fradin, M. S.** 1998. Mosquitoes and mosquito repellents: a clinician's guide. *Ann. Intern. Med.* **128:**931–940.
42. **Fraser, J. R.** 1986. Epidemic polyarthritis and Ross River virus disease. *Clin. Rheum. Dis.* **12:**369–388.

43. **Fraser, J. R., V. M. Ratnamohan, J. P. Dowling, G. J. Becker, and G. A. Varigos.** 1983. The exanthem of Ross River virus infection. Histology, location of virus antigen and nature of inflammatory infiltrate. *J. Clin. Pathol.* **36:** 1256–1263.
44. **Garen, P. D., T. F. Tsai, and J. M. Powers.** 1999. Human eastern equine encephalitis: immunohistochemistry and ultrastructure. *Mod. Pathol.* **12:**646–652.
45. **Getting, V. A.** 1941. Equine encephalomyelitis in Massachusetts. *N. Engl. J. Med.* **224:**999–1006.
46. **Gold, H., and B. Hampil.** 1942. Equine encephalomyelitis in a laboratory technician with recovery. *Ann. Intern. Med.* **16:**556–559.
47. **Goldfield, M., J. N. Welsh, and B. F. Taylor.** 1968. The 1959 outbreak of Eastern encephalitis in New Jersey. 5. The inapparent infection:disease ratio. *Am. J. Epidemiol.* **87:**32–33.
48. **Grady, G. F., H. K. Maxfield, S. W. Hildreth, R. J. Timperi, Jr., R. F. Gilfillan, B. J. Rosenau, D. B. Francy, C. H. Calisher, L. C. Marcus, and M. A. Madoff.** 1978. Eastern equine encephalitis in Massachusetts, 1957–1976. A prospective study centered upon analyses of mosquitoes. *Am. J. Epidemiol.* **107:**170–178.
49. **Griffin, D. E.** 2007. Alphaviruses, p. 1023–1067. *In* D. M. Knipe, P. M. Howley, D. E. Griffin, R. A. Lamb, M. A. Martin, B. Roizman, and S. E. Straus (ed.), *Fields Virology*, 5th ed. Lippincott Williams & Wilkins, Philadelphia, PA.
50. **Griffin, D. E., B. Levine, S. Ubol, and J. M. Hardwick.** 1994. The effects of alphavirus infection on neurons. *Ann. Neurol.* **35:**S23-S27.
51. **Griffin, D., B. Levine, W. Tyor, S. Ubol, and P. Desprès.** 1997. The role of antibody in recovery from alphavirus encephalitis. *Immunol. Rev.* **159:**155–161.
52. **Griffin, D. E., and J. M. Hardwick.** 1997. Regulators of apoptosis on the road to persistent alphavirus infection. *Annu. Rev. Microbiol.* **51:**565–592.
53. **Gutierrez, V. E., T. P. Monath, A. A. Alava, B. D. Uriguen, R. M. Arzube, and R. W. Chamberlain.** 1975. Epidemiologic investigations of the 1969 epidemic of Venezuelan encephalitis in Ecuador. *Am. J. Epidemiol.* **102:**400–413.
54. **Ha, D. Q., C. H. Calisher, P. H. Tien, N. Karabatsos, and D. J. Gubler.** 1995. Isolation of a newly recognized alphavirus from mosquitoes in Vietnam and evidence for human infection and disease. *Am. J. Trop. Med. Hyg.* **53:** 100–104.
55. **Halstead, S. B., J. E. Scanlon, P. Umpaivit, and S. Udomsakdi.** 1969. Dengue and chikungunya virus infection in man in Thailand, 1962–1964. IV. Epidemiologic studies in the Bangkok metropolitan area. *Am. J. Trop. Med. Hyg.* **18:**997–1021.
56. **Harley, D., A. Sleigh, and S. Ritchie.** 2001. Ross River virus transmission, infection and disease: a cross-disciplinary review. *Rev. Clin. Microbiol.* **14:**909–932.
57. **Hart, K. L., D. Keen, and E. A. Belle.** 1964. An outbreak of eastern equine encephalomyelitis in Jamaica, West Indies. I. Description of human cases. *Am. J. Trop. Med. Hyg.* **13:**331–334.
58. **Heise, M. T., D. A. Simpson, and R. E. Johnston.** 2000. Sindbis-group alphavirus replication in periosteum and endosteum of long bones in adult mice. *J. Virol.* **74:**9294–9299.
59. **Hommel, D., J. M. Heraud, A. Hulin, and A. Talarmin.** 2000. Association of Tonate virus (subtype IIIB of the Venezuelan equine encephalitis complex) with encephalitis in a human. *Clin. Infect. Dis.* **30:**188–190.
60. **Hörling, J., S. Vene, C. Franzén, and B. Niklasson.** 1993. Detection of Ockelbo virus RNA in skin biopsies by polymerase chain reaction. *J. Clin. Microbiol.* **31:**2004–2009.
61. **Jadhav, M., M. Namboodripad, R. H. Carman, D. E. Carey, and R. M. Myers.** 1965. Chikungunya disease in infants and children in Vellore: a report of clinical and haematological features of virologically proved cases. *Indian J. Med. Res.* **53:**764–776.
62. **Jonkers, A. H., L. Spence, and J. Karbaat.** 1968. Arbovirus infections in Dutch military personnel stationed in Surinam. Further studies. *Trop. Geogr. Med.* **20:**251–256.
63. **Jordan, R. A., J. A. Wagner, and F. R. McCrumb.** 1965. Eastern equine encephalitis: report of a case with autopsy. *Am. J. Trop. Med. Hyg.* **14:**470–474.
64. **Julkunen, I., M. Brummer-Korvenkontio, A. Hautanen, P. Kuusisto, P. Lindstrom, O. Wager, and K. Penttinen.** 1986. Elevated serum immune complex levels in Pogosta disease, an acute alphavirus infection with rash and arthritis. *J. Clin. Lab. Immunol.* **21:**77–82.
65. **Jupp, P. G., N. K. Blackburn, D. L. Thompson, and G. M. Meenehan.** 1986. Sindbis and West Nile virus infections in the Witwatersrand-Pretoria region. *S. Afr. Med. J.* **70:**218–220.
66. **Kennedy, A. C., J. Fleming, and L. Solomon.** 1980. Chikungunya viral arthropathy: a clinical description. *J. Rheumatol.* **7:**231–236.
67. **Kiwanuka, N., E. J. Sanders, E. B. Rwaguma, J. Kawamata, F. P. Ssengooba, R. Najjemba, W. A. Were, M. Lamunu, G. Bagambisa, T. R. Burkot, L. Dunster, J. J. Lutwama, D. A. Martin, C. B. Cropp, N. Karabatsos, R. S. Lanciotti, T. F. Tsai, and G. L. Campbell.** 1999. O'nyong-nyong fever in south-central Uganda, 1996–1997: clinical features and validation of a clinical case definition for surveillance purposes. *Clin. Infect. Dis.* **29:** 1243–1250.
68. **Kokernot, R. H., H. R. Shinefield, and W. A. Longshore, Jr.** 1953. The 1952 outbreak of encephalitis in California. Differential diagnosis. *Calif. Med.* **79:**73–77.
69. **Komar, N., and A. Spielman.** 1994. Emergence of eastern encephalitis in Massachusetts. *Ann. N. Y. Acad. Sci.* **740:** 157–168.
70. **Koprowski, H., and H. R. Cox.** 1947. Human laboratory infection with Venezuelan equine encephalomyelitis virus. *N. Engl. J. Med.* **236:**647–654.
71. **Kurkela, S., T. Manni, J. Myllynen, A. Vaheri, and O. Vapalahti.** 2005. Clinical and laboratory manifestations of Sindbis virus infection: prospective study, Finland, 2002–2003. *J. Infect. Dis.* **191:**1820–1829.
72. **Lambert, A. J., D. A. Martin, and R. S. Lanciotti.** 2003. Detection of North American eastern and western equine encephalitis viruses by nucleic acid amplification assays. *J. Clin. Microbiol.* **41:**379–385.
73. **Lanciotti, R. S., M. L. Ludwig, E. B. Rwaguma, J. J. Lutwama, T. M. Cram, N. Karabatsos, B. C. Cropp, and B. R. Miller.** 1998. Emergence of epidemic O'nyong-nyong fever in Uganda after a 35 year absence: genetic characterization of the virus. *Virology* **252:**258–268.
74. **Larke, R. P., and E. F. Wheelock.** 1970. Stabilization of chikungunya virus infectivity by human blood platelets. *J. Infect. Dis.* **122:**523–531.
75. **Leech, R. W., J. C. Harris, and R. M. Johnson.** 1981. 1975 encephalitis epidemic in North Dakota and western Minnesota. An epidemiologic, clinical, and neuropathologic study. *Minn. Med.* **64:**545–548.
76. **Leon, C. A.** 1975. Sequelae of Venezuelan equine encephalitis in humans: a four year follow-up. *Int. J. Epidemiol.* **4:**131–140.
77. **Letson, G. W., R. E. Bailey, J. Pearson, and T. F. Tsai.** 1993. Eastern equine encephalitis (EEE): a description of the 1989 outbreak, recent epidemiologic trends, and the

association of rainfall with EEE occurrence. *Am. J. Trop. Med. Hyg.* **49:**677–685.

78. **Lidbury, B. A., C. Simeonovic, G. E. Maxwell, I. D. Marshall, and A. J. Hapel.** 2000. Macrophage-induced muscle pathology results in morbidity and mortality for Ross River virus-infected mice. *J. Infect. Dis.* **181:**27–34.
79. **Lindsay, M. D., C. A. Johansen, D. W. Smith, M. J. Wallace, and J. S. Mackenzie.** 1995. An outbreak of Barmah Forest virus disease in the south-west of Western Australia. *Med. J. Aust.* **162:**291–294.
80. **Linssen, B., R. M. Kinney, P. Aguilar, K. L. Russell, D. M. Watts, O. R. Kaaden, and M. Pfeffer.** 2000. Development of reverse transcription-PCR assays specific for detection of equine encephalitis viruses. *J. Clin. Microbiol.* **38:**1527–1535.
81. **Liu, C., C. Johansen, N. Kurucz, and P. Whelan.** 2006. Communicable Diseases Network Australia National Arbovirus and Malaria Advisory Committee annual report, 2005–06. *Commun. Dis. Intell.* **30:**411–429.
82. **Lumsden, W. H. R.** 1955. An epidemic of virus disease in Southern Province, Tanganyika Territory, in 1952–53. *Trans. R. Soc. Trop. Med. Hyg.* **49:**33–57.
83. **Lundström, J. O., S. Vene, A. Espmark, M. Engvall, and B. Niklasson.** 1991. Geographical and temporal distribution of Ockelbo disease in Sweden. *Epidemiol. Infect.* **106:**567–574.
84. **Mackenzie, J. S., M. D. Lindsay, R. J. Coelen, A. K. Broom, R. A. Hall, and D. W. Smith.** 1994. Arboviruses causing human disease in the Australasian zoogeographic region. *Arch. Virol.* **136:**447–467.
85. **Mangi, R. J.** 1994. Viral arthritis—the great masquerader. *Bull. Rheum. Dis.* **43:**5–6.
86. **Martin, D. A., D. A. Muth, T. Brown, A. J. Johnson, N. Karabatsos, and J. T. Roehrig.** 2000. Standardization of immunoglobulin M capture enzyme-linked immunosorbent assays for routine diagnosis of arboviral infections. *J. Clin. Microbiol.* **38:**1823–1826.
87. **Mathiot, C. C., G. Grimaud, P. Garry, J. C. Bouquety, A. Mada, A. M. Daguisy, and A. J. Georges.** 1990. An outbreak of human Semliki Forest virus infections in Central African Republic. *Am. J. Trop. Med. Hyg.* **42:**386–393.
88. **McClain, D. J., P. R. Pittman, H. H. Ramsburg, G. O. Nelson, C. A. Rossi, J. A. Mangiafico, A. L. Schmaljohn, and F. J. Malinoski.** 1998. Immunologic interference from sequential administration of live attenuated alphavirus vaccines. *J. Infect. Dis.* **177:**634–641.
89. **McIntosh, B. M., G. M. McGillivray, D. B. Dickinson, and H. Malherbe.** 1964. Illness caused by Sindbis and West Nile viruses in South Africa. *S. Afr. Med. J.* **38:** 291–294.
90. **Medovy, H.** 1976. The history of western encephalomyelitis in Manitoba. *Can. J. Public Health* **67**(Suppl. 1)**:** S13–S14.
91. **Meehan, P. J., D. L. Wells, W. Paul, E. Buff, A. Lewis, D. Muth, R. Hopkins, N. Karabatsos, and T. F. Tsai.** 2000. Epidemiological features of and public health response to a St. Louis encephalitis epidemic in Florida, 1990–1. *Epidemiol. Infect.* **125:**181–188.
92. **Molina, O. M., M. C. Morales, I. D. Soto, J. A. Pena, R. S. Haack, D. P. Cardozo, and J. J. Cardozo.** 1999. Venezuelan equine encephalitis. 1995 outbreak: clinical profile of the case with neurologic involvement. *Rev. Neurol.* **29:**296–298.
93. **Monath, T. P., C. H. Calisher, M. Davis, G. S. Bowen, and J. White.** 1974. Experimental studies of rhesus monkeys infected with epizootic and enzootic subtypes of Venezuelan equine encephalitis virus. *J. Infect. Dis.* **129:** 194–200.
94. **Moore, D. L., S. Reddy, F. M. Akinkugbe, V. H. Lee, T. S. David-West, O. R. Causey, and D. E. Carey.** 1974. An epidemic of chikungunya fever at Ibadan, Nigeria, 1969. *Ann. Trop. Med. Parasitol.* **68:**59–68.
95. **Morse, R. P., M. L. Bennish, and B. T. Darras.** 1992. Eastern equine encephalitis presenting with a focal brain lesion. *Pediatr. Neurol.* **8:**473–475.
96. **Mulder, D. W., M. Parrott, and M. Thaler.** 1951. Sequelae of western equine encephalitis. *Neurology* **1:**318–327.
97. **Niklasson, B. A., A. Espmark, and J. Lundström.** 1988. Occurrence of arthralgia and specific IgM antibodies three to four years after Ockelbo disease. *J. Infect. Dis.* **157:**832–835.
98. **Nimmannitya, S., S. B. Halstead, S. N. Cohen, and M. R. Margiotta.** 1969. Dengue and chikungunya virus infection in man in Thailand, 1962–1964. I. Observations on hospitalized patients with hemorrhagic fever. *Am. J. Trop. Med. Hyg.* 18:954–971.
99. **Noran, H. H., and A. B. Bake.** 1943. Sequels of equine encephalomyelitis. *Arch. Neurol. Psychiatry* 49:398–413.
100. **Norder, H., J. O. Lundström, O. Kozuch, and L. O. Magnius.** 1996. Genetic relatedness of Sindbis virus strains from Europe, Middle East, and Africa. *Virology* **222:**440–445.
101. **Oberste, M. S., M. Fraire, R. Navarro, C. Zepeda, M. L. Zarate, G. V. Ludwig, J. F. Konig, S. C. Weaver, J. F. Smith, and R. Rico-Hesse.** 1998. Association of Venezuelan equine encephalitis virus subtype IE with two equine epizootics in Mexico. *Am. J. Trop. Med. Hyg.* **59:**100–107.
102. **Oberste, M. S., S. C. Weaver, D. M. Watts, and J. F. Smith.** 1998. Identification and genetic analysis of Panama-genotype Venezuelan equine encephalitis virus subtype ID in Peru. *Am. J. Trop. Med. Hyg.* **58:**41–46.
103. **Olaleye, O. D., S. A. Omilabu, and A. H. Fagbami.** 1988. Igbo-Ora virus (an alphavirus isolated in Nigeria): a serological survey for haemagglutination inhibiting antibody in humans and domestic animals. *Trans. R. Soc. Trop. Med. Hyg.* **82:**905–906.
104. **Palmer, R. J., and K. H. Finley.** 1956. Sequelae of encephalitis: report of a study after the California epidemic. *Calif. Med.* **84:**98–100.
105. **Pialoux, G., B-A. Gaüzère, S. Jauréguiberry, and M. Strobel.** 2007. Chikungunya, an epidemic arbovirosis. *Lancet Infect. Dis.* **7:**319–327.
106. **Pinheiro, F. P., R. B. Freitas, J. F. Travassos da Rosa, Y. B. Gabbay, W. A. Mello, and J. W. LeDuc.** 1981. An outbreak of Mayaro virus disease in Belterra, Brazil. I. Clinical and virological findings. *Am. J. Trop. Med. Hyg.* **30:**674–681.
107. **Pittman, P. R., R. S. Makuch, J. A. Mangiafico, T. L. Cannon, P. H. Gibbs, and C. J. Peters.** 1996. Long-term duration of detectable neutralizing antibodies after administration of live-attenuated VEE vaccine and following booster vaccination with inactivated VEE vaccine. *Vaccine* **14:**337–343.
108. **Powers, A. M., A. C. Brault, Y. Shirako, E. G. Strauss, W. Kang, J. H. Strauss, and S. C. Weaver.** 2001. Evolutionary relationships and systematics of the alphaviruses. *J. Virol.* **75:**10118–10131.
109. **Powers, A. M., A. C. Brault, R. B. Tesh, and S. C. Weaver.** 2000. Re-emergence of chikungunya and o'nyong-nyong viruses: evidence for distinct geographical lineages and distant evolutionary relationships. *J. Gen. Virol.* **81:**471–479.
110. **Powers, A. M., M. S. Oberste, A. C. Brault, R. Rico-Hesse, S. M. Schmura, J. F. Smith, W. Kang, W. P. Sweeney, and S. C. Weaver.** 1997. Repeated emergence of epidemic/epizootic Venezuelan equine encephalitis

from a single genotype of enzootic subtype ID virus. *J. Virol.* **71:**6697–6705.

111. **Przelomski, M. M., E. O'Rourke, G. F. Grady, V. P. Berardi, and H. G. Markley.** 1988. Eastern equine encephalitis in Massachusetts: a report of 16 cases, 1970–1984. *Neurology* **38:**736–739.

112. **Rezza, G., L. Nicoletti, R. Angelini, R. Romi, A. C. Finarelli, M. Panning, P. Cordioli, C. Fortuna, S. Boros, F. Magurano, G. Silvi, P. Angelini, M. Dottori, M. G. Ciufolini, G. C. Majori, and A. Cassone for the CHIKV Study Group.** 2007. Infection with chikungunya virus in Italy: an outbreak in a temperate region. *Lancet* **370:**1840–1846.

113. **Rivas, F., L. A. Diaz, V. M. Cardenas, E. Daza, L. Bruzon, A. Alcala, O. De la Hoz, F. M. Caceres, G. Aristizabal, J. W. Martinez, D. Revelo, F. De la Hoz, J. Boshell, T. Camacho, L. Calderon, V. A. Olano, L. I. Villarreal, D. Roselli, G. Alvarez, G. Ludwig, and T. Tsai.** 1997. Epidemic Venezuelan equine encephalitis in La Guajira, Colombia, 1995. *J. Infect. Dis.* **175:**828–832.

114. **Robinson, M. C.** 1955. An epidemic of virus disease in Southern Province, Tanganyika Territory, in 1952–53. *Trans. R. Soc. Trop. Med. Hyg.* **49:**28–32.

115. **Rosato, R. R., F. F. Macasaet, and P. B. Jahrling.** 1988. Enzyme-linked immunosorbent assay detection of immunoglobulins G and M to Venezuelan equine encephalomyelitis virus in vaccinated and naturally infected humans. *J. Clin. Microbiol.* **26:**421–425.

116. **Rozdilsky, B., H. E. Robertson, and J. Chorney.** 1968. Western encephalitis: report of eight fatal cases, Saskatchewan epidemic, 1965. *Can. Med. Assoc. J.* **98:**79–86.

117. **Rulli, N. E., J. Melton, A. Wilmes, G. Ewart, and S. Mahalingam.** 2007. The molecular and cellular aspects of arthritis due to alphavirus infections. *Ann. N. Y. Acad. Sci.* **1102:**96–108.

118. **Russell, R.** 2002. Ross River virus: ecology and distribution. *Annu. Rev. Entomol.* **47:**1–31.

119. **Sammels, L. M., M. D. Lindsay, M. Poidinger, R. J. Coelen, and J. S. Mackenzie.** 1999. Geographic distribution and evolution of Sindbis virus in Australia. *J. Gen. Virol.* **80:**739–748.

120. **Sanchez, J. L., E. T. Takafuji, W. M. Lednar, J. W. LeDuc, F. F. Macasaet, J. A. Mangiafico, R. R. Rosato, D. P. Driggers, and J. C. Haecker.** 1984. Venezuelan equine encephalomyelitis: report of an outbreak associated with jungle exposure. *Mil. Med.* **149:**618–621.

121. **Sanders, E. J., E. B. Rwaguma, J. Kawamata, N. Kiwanuka, J. J. Lutwama, F. P. Ssengooba, M. Lamunu, R. Najjemba, W. A. Were, G. Bagambisa, and G. L. Campbell.** 1999. O'nyong-nyong fever in south-central Uganda, 1996–97: description of the epidemic and results of a household-based seroprevalence survey. *J. Infect. Dis.* **180:**1436–1443.

122. **Sarkar, J. K., S. N. Chatterjee, S. K. Chakravarti, and A. C. Mitra.** 1965. Chikungunya virus infection with haemorrhagic manifestations. *Indian J. Med. Res.* **53:**921–925.

123. **Schuffenecker, I., I. Iteman, A. Michault, S. Murri, L. Frangeul, M. C. Vaney, R. Lavenir, N. Pardigon, J. M. Reynes, F. Petinelli, L. Biscornet, L. Diancourt, S. Michel, S. Duquerroy, G. Guigon, M. P. Frenkiel, A. C. Bréhin, N. Cubito, P. Desprès, F. Kunst, F. A. Rey, H. Zeller, and S. Brisse.** 2006. Genome microevolution of chikungunya viruses causing the Indian Ocean outbreak. *PLoS Med.* **3:**e263.

124. **Schultz, D. R., J. S. Barthal, and G. Garrett.** 1977. Western equine encephalitis with rapid onset of parkinsonism. *Neurology* **27:**1095–1096.

125. **Sciple, G. W., G. Ray, L. C. LaMotte, P. Holden, P. Gardner, G. Crane, and M. D. Bublis.** 1967. Western encephalitis with recovery of virus from cerebrospinal fluid. *Neurology* **17:**169–171.

126. **Shinefield, H. R., and T. E. Townsend.** 1953. Transplacental transmission of western equine encephalomyelitis. *J. Pediatr.* **43:**21–25.

127. **Simon, F., P. Parola, M. Grandadam, S. Fourcade, M. Oliver, P. Brouqui, P. Hance, P. Kraemer, A. Ali Mohamed, X. de Lamballerie, R. Charrel, and H. Tolou.** 2007. Chikungunya infection: an emerging rheumatism among travelers returned from Indian Ocean islands. Report of 47 cases. *Medicine* (Baltimore) **86:**123–137.

128. **Soden, M., H. Vasudevan, B. Roberts, R. J. Coelen, G. Hamlin, S. Vasudevan, and J. La Brooy.** 2000. Detection of viral ribonucleic acid and histologic analysis of inflamed synovium in Ross River virus infection. *Arthritis Rheum.* **43:**365–369.

129. **Somekh, E., M. P. Glode, T. T. Reiley, and T. F. Tsai.** 1991. Multiple intracranial calcifications after western equine encephalitis. *Pediatr. Infect. Dis. J.* **10:**408–409.

130. **Strauss, J. H., and E. G. Strauss.** 1994. The alphaviruses: gene expression, replication, and evolution. *Microbiol. Rev.* **58:**491–562.

131. **Suhrbier, A., and M. La Linn.** 2004. Clinical and pathological aspects of arthritis due to Ross River virus and other alphaviruses. *Curr. Opin. Rheumatol.* **16:**374–379.

132. **Tesh, R. B., D. M. Watts, K. L. Russell, C. Damodaran, C. Calampa, C. Cabezas, G. Ramirez, B. Vasquez, C. G. Hayes, C. A. Rossi, A. M. Powers, C. L. Hice, L. J. Chandler, B. C. Cropp, N. Karabatsos, J. T. Roehrig, and D. J. Gubler.** 1999. Mayaro virus disease: an emerging mosquito-borne zoonosis in tropical South America. *Clin. Infect. Dis.* **28:**67–73.

133. **Thein, S., M. La Linn, J. Aaskov, M. M. Aung, M. Aye, A. Zaw, and A. Myint.** 1992. Development of a simple indirect enzyme-linked immunosorbent assay for the detection of immunoglobulin M antibody in serum from patients following an outbreak of chikungunya virus infection in Yangon, Myanmar. *Trans. R. Soc. Trop. Med. Hyg.* **86:**438–442.

134. **Thiruvengadam, K. V., V. Kalyanasundaram, and J. Rajgopal.** 1965. Clinical and pathological studies on chikungunya fever in Madras city. *Indian J. Med. Res.* **53:**729–744.

135. **Tikasingh, E. S., P. Ardoin, C. O. Everard, and J. B. Davies.** 1973. Eastern equine encephalitis in Trinidad. Epidemiological investigations following two human cases of South American strain in Santa Cruz. *Trop. Geogr. Med.* **25:**355–361.

136. **Tsetsarkin, K. A., D. L. Vanlandingham, C. E. McGee, and S. Higgs.** 2007. A single mutation in chikungunya virus affects vector specificity and epidemic potential. *PLoS Pathog.* **3:**e201.

137. **Uemura, Y., J. H. Yang, C. M. Heldebrant, K. Takechi, and K. Yokoyama.** 1994. Inactivation and elimination of viruses during preparation of human intravenous immunoglobulin. *Vox Sang.* **67:**246–254.

138. **U.S. Department of Health and Human Services, Centers for Disease Control and Prevention, and National Institutes of Health.** 1999. *Biosafety in Microbiological and Biomedical Laboratories (BMBL)*, 4th ed. U.S. Government Printing Office, Washington, DC. http://www.cdc.gov/OD/ohs/biosfty/bmbl4/bmbl4toc.htm.

139. **Wang, E., R. Barrera, J. Boshell, C. Ferro, J. E. Freier, J. C. Navarro, R. Salas, C. Vasquez, and S. C. Weaver.** 1999. Genetic and phenotypic changes accompanying the emergence of epizootic subtype IC Venezuelan

equine encephalitis viruses from an enzootic subtype ID progenitor. *J. Virol.* **73:**4266–4271.

140. **Wang, E., S. Paesslar, P. V. Aguilar, D. R. Smith, L. L. Coffey, W. Kang, M. Pfeffer, J. Olsen, P. J. Blair, C. Guevara, J. Estrada-Franco, and S. C. Weaver.** 2005. A novel, rapid assay for detection and differentiation of serotype-specific antibodies to Venezuelan equine encephalitis complex alphaviruses. *Am. J. Trop. Med. Hyg.* **72:**805–810.
141. **Watts, D. M., J. Callahan, C. Rossi, M. S. Oberste, J. T. Roehrig, M. T. Wooster, J. F. Smith, C. B. Cropp, E. M. Gentrau, N. Karabatsos, D. Gübler, and C. G. Hayes.** 1998. Venezuelan equine encephalitis febrile cases among humans in the Peruvian Amazon River region. *Am. J. Trop. Med. Hyg.* **58:**35–40.
142. **Weaver. S. C., T. K. Frey, H. V. Huang, R. M. Kinney, C. M. Rice, J. T. Roehrig, R. E. Shope, and E. G. Strauss.** 2005. Family *Togaviridae*, p. 999–1008. *In* C. M. Fauquet, M. A. Mayo, J. Maniloff, U. Desselberger, and L. A. Ball (ed.), *Virus Taxonomy: Classification and Nomenclature of Viruses. Eighth Report of the International Committee on Taxonomy of Viruses*. Academic Press, San Diego, CA.
143. **Weaver, S. C., M. Pfeffer, K. Marriott, W. Kang, and R. M. Kinney.** 1999. Genetic evidence for the origins of Venezuelan equine encephalitis virus subtype IAB outbreaks. *Am. J. Trop. Med. Hyg.* **60:**441–448.
144. **Weaver, S. C., A. C. Brault, W. Kang, and J. J. Holland.** 1999. Genetic and fitness changes accompanying adaptation of an arbovirus to vertebrate and invertebrate cells. *J. Virol.* **73:**4316–4326.
145. **Weaver, S. C., W. Kang, Y. Shirako, T. Rumenapf, E. G. Strauss, and J. H. Strauss.** 1997. Recombinational history and molecular evolution of western equine encephalomyelitis complex alphaviruses. *J. Virol.* **71:** 613–623.
146. **Weaver, S. C., R. Salas, R. Rico-Hesse, G. V. Ludwig, M. S. Oberste, J. Boshell, and R. B. Tesh.** 1996. Reemergence of epidemic Venezuelan equine encephalomyelitis in South America. *Lancet* **348:**436–440.
147. **Wenger, F.** 1977. Venezuelan equine encephalitis. *Teratology* **16:**359–362.
148. **Wesselhoeft, C., E. C. Smith, and C. F. Branch.** 1938. Human encephalitis: eight fatal cases with four due to virus of equine encephalomyelitis. *JAMA* **111:**1735–1741.
149. **Williams, M. C., J. P. Woodall, and J. D. Gillett.** 1965. O'nyong-nyong fever: an epidemic virus disease in east Africa. VII. Virus isolations from man and serological studies up to July 1961. *Trans. R. Soc. Trop. Med. Hyg.* **59:**186–197.
150. **Young, N. A., and K. M. Johnson.** 1969. Antigenic variants of Venezuelan equine encephalitis virus: their geographic distribution and epidemiologic significance. *Am. J. Epidemiol.* **89:**286–307.

Rubella Virus

DAVID W. KIMBERLIN

55

Rubella was known to early Arabian physicians by the name *al-hamikah,* but it was initially considered to be a form of measles (20). In 1752 and 1758, the German physicians de Bergen and Orlow first described rubella as a unique clinical entity (38, 147). Rubella subsequently was reported in England (82, 147, 151) and the United States (65, 147). In 1866, Henry Veale introduced the name rubella, believing that the name of a disease "should be short for the sake of convenience in writing, and euphonious for ease in pronunciation" (140). At the International Congress of Medicine in London, England, in 1881, these developments culminated in the consensus that rubella was a distinct disease (43, 136). Rubella is commonly called German measles, and it is the third of the six viral exanthems of childhood, with measles and scarlet fever being first and second, respectively (125).

Rubella was thought to be a benign disease until 1941, when the Australian ophthalmologist Norman McAlister Gregg first described the congenital defects of infants of mothers who had developed rubella early in pregnancy (46, 54). Although initially met with skepticism by the worldwide medical community, Gregg's keen observations were quickly confirmed in Australia (41, 129, 130), the United States (40), and the United Kingdom (80). By 1947, 521 cases of congenital rubella had been reported in the medical literature (148).

In 1938, Hiro and Tasaka (62) established the viral etiology and transmissibility of rubella by subcutaneously inoculating 16 nonimmune children with filtered nasopharyngeal saline washings collected from patients in the eruptive stage of rubella. Habel (56) used similar nasal washings obtained within 24 h of the appearance of the rash to infect *Macaca mulatta* monkeys. Rubella was successfully cultivated in tissue culture in 1962 by Weller and Neva (146) in Boston and by Parkman et al. (97) in Washington, DC. The methodology of Parkman and colleagues for the isolation of the noncytopathic rubella virus exploited its interference with the growth of enteroviruses in African green monkey kidney (AGMK) cell culture, and this soon became the standard method for rubella virus isolation.

The increasing recognition of congenital rubella syndrome during and after the pandemic of 1962 to 1965 emphasized the need for the development of an efficacious vaccine. Between 1965 and 1967, several attenuated rubella virus strains were developed and evaluated in clinical trials (86, 108, 112). Results of these investigations culminated in the convening of the International Conference on Rubella Immunization in February 1969 (78). During the same year, three strains of live attenuated rubella vaccines were licensed in various countries: HPV-77, grown in duck embryos for five passages (DE-5) or dog kidney cells for 12 passages (DK-12); Cendehill, grown in primary rabbit cells; and RA27/3, grown in human diploid fibroblast culture (85, 87, 108, 112). Since 1979, the RA27/3 vaccine has been used exclusively in the United States (103, 106). More than 170 million doses of rubella vaccine have been administered in the United States since licensure in 1969 (25). Due to the overwhelming success of the rubella immunization program, endemic transmission of rubella has been eliminated in the United States (15), and cases of rubella and of congenital rubella syndrome in the United States have declined 99.9 and 99.3%, respectively, compared to the prevaccine era (116).

VIROLOGY

Classification

Rubella virus is the sole member of the *Rubivirus* genus of the *Togaviridae* family. The other genus in the family of *Togaviridae* is *Alphavirus*. In contrast to the alphaviruses, which replicate in arthropods and in vertebrates, rubella virus has no invertebrate hosts. The only known host for rubella virus is humans.

Only one immunologically distinct serotype of rubella virus exists, and rubella virus is serologically unrelated to other known viruses. At least two genotypes can be distinguished by E1 gene sequences. Rubella genotype I isolates, predominant in Europe, Japan, and the western hemisphere, segregated into discrete subgenotypes. Rubella genotype II viruses are limited to Asia and Europe, demonstrate greater genetic diversity, and may consist of multiple genotypes (156). However, these biological variations are not the consequence of antigenic differences, as determined by protein composition or serologic analysis (6, 17).

Viral Composition

The spherical particles of rubella virus measure 50 to 70 nm in diameter (1, 5). An individual virion is composed of a 30-nm core structure surrounded by a single-layered envelope measuring 10 nm in thickness. The envelope is acquired during budding through the host nuclear or plasma membrane (5, 64). Glycoprotein projections measuring 5 to 6 nm in length are located on the viral surface (64, 104).

The viral core contains the single-stranded, positive-sense 40S RNA genome, composed of approximately 10,000 nucleotides, with a molecular weight of about 3.8×10^6 (121, 153). The structural protein known as protein C (or capsid protein) is one of three structural proteins of rubella virus and is associated with the 40S RNA. Protein C is nonglycosylated and has a molecular mass of 33 kDa (104). The other two major structural proteins, E1 and E2, are envelope glycoproteins that together comprise the viral surface projections described above. The molecular masses of E1 and E2 are 58 and 42 to 47 kDa, respectively. E1 is the viral hemagglutinin, and the exact function of E2 is unclear. A 42-kDa E2 molecule (designated E2a) and a 47-kDa E2 molecule (designated E2b) have been recognized (104).

Biology

Viral genomic and subgenomic RNA species are detectable in tissue culture 12 h postinfection, with peak RNA synthesis occurring by 26 h following initial infection (59). In comparison, viral protein production can be initially detected by immunofluorescence at 12 h postinfection, and peak structural protein synthesis occurs by 16 h after initial infection (59).

Propagation of rubella virus in tissue culture does not produce a reliable or distinctive cytopathic effect (CPE) by light microscopy. In general, growth of rubella virus in continuous cell lines (hamster, rabbit, simian, and human) produces a variable CPE which depends upon adaptation of the viral isolate to the cell line and on the passage history of the cell line, among other factors (153). Of the continuous cell lines, the kidney cell lines from the rabbit (RK-13), African green monkey (Vero), and baby hamster (BHK-21) are used most frequently for the detection of CPE.

Detection of rubella virus in primary cell culture (human, simian, bovine, rabbit, canine, or duck) is accomplished by means of an interference assay. Although infection with rubella virus in primary cell cultures does not produce CPE, superinfection by many additional viruses is blocked. AGMK cells have proven superior for isolation of virus from human specimens by the interference technique: infection in AGMK tissue culture by rubella virus is suggested by the failure of the typical enteroviral CPE to occur after challenge with echovirus 11 or other enteroviruses. The presence of rubella virus is then confirmed by an additional technique, such as neutralization or fluorescence with specific antirubella serum.

Although natural rubella virus infection occurs only in humans, infection in experimental animals can be achieved. The complete spectrum of acquired or congenital disease is not manifested in any of these animal models, however. Following intranasal, intramuscular, or intravenous administration, rhesus monkeys develop viremia and shed virus in nasopharyngeal secretions (99). Other species of monkeys can also be infected with rubella virus (67). Attempts at mimicking congenital rubella have resulted in recovery of virus from the amnion and placenta of monkeys, although the embryos are not consistently infected (100, 123). The ferret also has proven to be a very useful animal model in the study of rubella disease following both subcutaneous and intracerebral inoculation of virus (25). Additional animals that have been experimentally infected with rubella virus include rabbits, hamsters, guinea pigs, rats, and suckling mice.

Rubella virus is heat labile. Rapid inactivation occurs at 56°C, and a slower decrease in activity is noted at 37°C (98). In the presence of protein, the virus remains viable at 4°C for a week or more. However, infectivity is rapidly lost at temperatures of −10 to −20°C (98). Specimens can be stored indefinitely at −60°C. The addition of $MgSO_4$ stabilizes the virus with respect to heat inactivation, allowing for safe transport on ice (144). Extremes of pH (less than 6.8 or greater than 8.1), UV light, and chemicals such as ether, acetone, chloroform, deoxycholate, formalin, β-propiolactone, ethylene oxide, free chlorine, and 70% alcohol all inactivate rubella virus (16, 107).

EPIDEMIOLOGY

Geographic Distribution

Rubella has a worldwide distribution, although clinically recognized disease occurs less frequently in tropical regions than in temperate zones (21). Because humans are the only known natural host for rubella virus, the virus must circulate continuously within populations of people between periods of epidemics. Such endemic spread of rubella virus occurs in most areas of the globe, although small islands that are geographically isolated can lack endemicity (20, 61). Rubella epidemics have occurred as well on several large islands without the establishment of subsequent endemic spread of the virus among the island populations (48, 51, 153).

Incidence and Prevalence of Infection

Reporting of rubella was not required in the United States until 1966. Since widespread vaccination programs were initiated only 3 years later, there is a paucity of thorough data on the incidence and prevalence of rubella in the prevaccination era. The majority of cases of rubella prior to 1969 occurred in children 5 to 9 years of age (13). In comparison, rubella outbreaks in recent years have predominantly occurred in adolescents and young adults, with 49 to 63% of cases in 1992 and 1993 occurring in persons at least 20 years of age (14).

Before 1969, epidemics of rubella occurred in 6- to 9-year intervals, with worldwide pandemics ensuing every 10 to 30 years (25). An individual epidemic usually lasted 3 to 4 years, with cases peaking at the middle of the cycle (68). The widespread use of rubella vaccine has interrupted this epidemic pattern in those countries with effective vaccination programs. The last epidemic of rubella in the United States occurred in 1964 as part of the worldwide pandemic of 1962 to 1965. During that epidemic, 12.5 million cases of rubella were reported in the United States (69), with some 20,000 cases of congenital rubella syndrome (153).

Rubella is a highly contagious disease, and the incidence of rubella virus infection during an epidemic cycle approaches 100% of susceptible hosts in closed populations (e.g., military recruits) (70, 71, 111). Virtually all susceptible household contacts are infected during such outbreaks (48). The overall incidence of disease among susceptible hosts at the community level during an epidemic ranges from 50 to 90% (20). Clinically apparent cases of rubella occur with equal frequencies in boys and girls; however, rubella is more commonly diagnosed in women than men in adult populations, possibly due to heightened awareness of the risk of congenital rubella among women of child-bearing age (123).

At least half of all serologically confirmed childhood primary rubella virus infections result in clinically inapparent illness (71, 153). Reinfection with rubella virus can occur following natural infection, but it is usually asymptomatic (70). Viremia is rarely documented, although systemic symptoms such as arthritis and rash may occur (150). Reinfection following vaccination occurs more commonly than following natural infection, but it is also usually asymptomatic and not associated with viremia (33, 149). Up to 80% of persons previously vaccinated against rubella will be reinfected during an epidemic (33, 70). Reinfections are more likely to occur in persons with lower rubella antibody titers (33, 70, 149). Rubella virus reinfection during pregnancy can result in congenital rubella syndrome, although this is a very rare event (32, 47).

The success of the rubella control program is illustrated in the 40 years following licensure of the rubella vaccine in the United States (Fig. 1). By 2005, endemic transmission of rubella had been eliminated in the United States (15), and cases of rubella and of congenital rubella syndrome in the United States in 2007 were 99.9 and 99.3% lower, respectively, than in the prevaccine era (116). Since 2001, fewer than 25 rubella cases have been reported each year in the United States, and vaccination coverage is at least 95% among school-age children (15). An estimated 91% of the U.S. population is immune to rubella (15). The remarkable success in decreasing the incidence of rubella in this country and others has led scientists and international organizations to consider the goal of rubella eradication (42, 83, 105, 109, 145). According to a survey of the member countries in the World Health Organization, the number of countries that have incorporated rubella-containing vaccine into their routine national immunization programs increased from 65 (33%) in 1996 to 110 (57%) in 2003 (15). However, rubella continues to be endemic in many parts of the world, with the number of infants with congenital rubella syndrome born each year worldwide estimated in 1999 to be 110,000 (30).

Seasonality

In the temperate climates such as North America and Europe, rubella is most prevalent in March, April, and May (152). This seasonal pattern occurs both in years with high rates of infection and in years with low rates of infection (20).

Transmission

Rubella virus is transmitted primarily by virus-laden droplets from the respiratory secretions of infected persons. In studies conducted with volunteers, rubella virus can be detected in nasopharyngeal secretions from 7 days prior to 14 days following the onset of the rash (53, 58), with maximal shedding of virus occurring from 5 days before to 6 days after the appearance of the exanthem (20). The incubation period of rubella is usually 16 to 18 days, but can

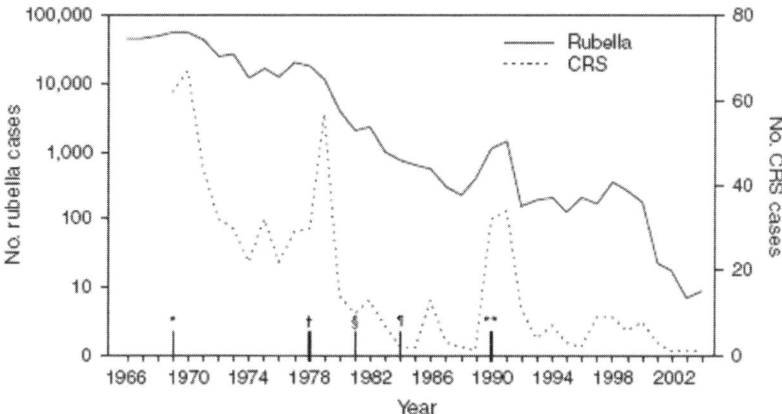

FIGURE 1 Number of reported cases of rubella and congenital rubella syndrome (CRS), by year, and chronology of rubella vaccination recommendations by the Advisory Committee on Immunization Practices, United States, 1966 to 2004. *, 1969—first official recommendations are published for the use of rubella vaccine. Vaccination is recommended for children aged 1 year to puberty. †, 1978—recommendations for vaccination are expanded to include adolescents and certain adults, particularly females. Vaccination is recommended for adolescent or adult females and males in populations in colleges, certain places of employment (e.g., hospitals), and military bases. §, 1981—recommendations place increased emphasis on vaccination of susceptible persons in training and educational settings (e.g., universities or colleges) and military settings and vaccination of workers in health care settings. ¶, 1984—recommendations are published for vaccination of workers in day care centers, schools, colleges, companies, government offices, and industrial sites. Providers are encouraged to conduct prenatal testing and postpartum vaccination of susceptible women. Recommendations for vaccination are expanded to include susceptible persons who travel abroad. **, 1990—recommendations include implementation of a new two-dose schedule for MMR vaccine. (Modified from reference 15.)

range from 14 to 23 days (2). Persons with subclinical cases of rubella are contagious and can transmit infection to others. Recipients of the rubella vaccine do not transmit rubella, however, even though the virus can be isolated from the pharynx.

Infants with congenital rubella syndrome are capable of transmission of virus to susceptible persons (118). At 1 year of age, between 10 and 20% of infants with congenital rubella syndrome continue to shed virus in the nasopharynx (114). Viral shedding occurs for as long as 20 months after birth in up to 3% of congenitally infected infants (23), a finding which can be of particular concern in hospital environments (52).

Individuals vary in their ability to transmit rubella. A minority of patients who have a high likelihood of transmitting virus to susceptible contacts have been identified during rubella epidemics ("spreaders") (57). In contrast, most individuals transmit rubella virus less efficiently ("nonspreaders"). Genetic factors may correlate with the ability to transmit rubella virus, with persons bearing the major histocompatibility complex antigens HLA-A1 and HLA-A8 being more likely to spread rubella during infection (20, 66).

Congenital Rubella

Fetal infection can occur throughout pregnancy, with the risk of infection being greatest during the first trimester, decreasing during the second trimester, and then rising again as the fetus approaches term. In one study, the risk of fetal infection in infants whose mothers had rubella during the first trimester was determined to be 81% (Fig. 2) (89). The infection rate following second-trimester exposure was 39%, and the infection rate was 53% after exposure during the third trimester (89). In a second study, the risk of fetal infection following maternal rubella during the second trimester was 32%; the risk following third-trimester maternal infection was 24% overall, but when maternal infection occurred near term, that rate rose to 58% (27).

The risk of congenital anomalies in live-born children following fetal infection also varies according to the month of pregnancy in which maternal infection occurs. One study reported that 85% of infants born to women infected with rubella virus during the first 8 weeks of pregnancy had anomalies detected during the first 4 years of life (102). Detectable defects occurred in 52% of infants born to mothers infected at 9 to 12 weeks' gestation, in 16% of infants born to women infected at 13 to 20 weeks' gestation, and in no infants born to mothers infected beyond 20 weeks' gestation (102). In another investigation that monitored infected infants until 2 years of age, 100% (9 of 9) of infants infected within the first 11 weeks of gestation had detectable congenital defects (89). In addition, 50% (2 of 4) of infants infected from 11 to 12 weeks' gestation demonstrated congenital anomalies; thus, 85% (11 of 13) infants infected during the first trimester had detectable defects in this study (Fig. 2) (89). A study of congenital rubella syndrome among children born to Amish women during the rubella outbreak of 1990 to 1991 reported a similar rate of defects (80%) among congenitally infected infants whose mothers had first-trimester infections (84).

For counseling purposes, determination of the risk of congenital defects after confirmed maternal infection can be calculated by multiplying the rates of fetal infections by the rates of defects in infected infants. Accordingly, the risks are 90% for maternal infection before the 11th week of gestation, 33% for infection occurring during weeks 11 and 12, 11% for infection from weeks 13 to 14, and 24% for infection between weeks 15 and 16 (25).

PATHOGENESIS IN HUMANS

Virus Replication

Following initial infection of cells of the nasopharyngeal respiratory epithelium, rubella virus spreads rapidly to the regional lymph nodes by means of the lymphatics and possibly by transient viremia. Viral replication continues in localized areas of the nasopharynx and regional lymph nodes for another 7 to 9 days, followed by viremic spread to multiple sites throughout the body (25). Maximal vi-

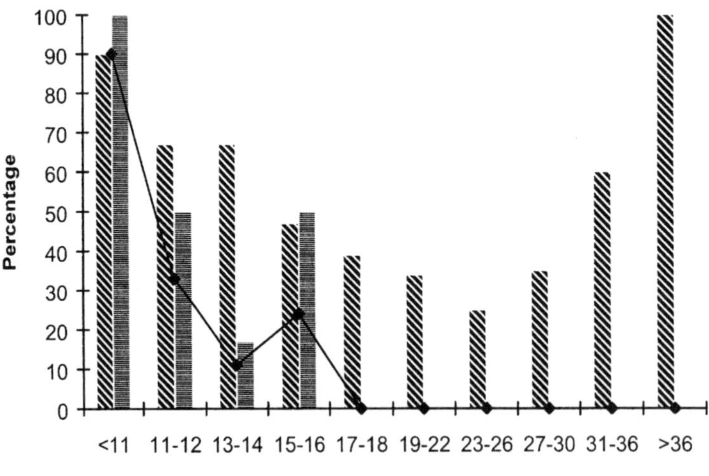

FIGURE 2 Likelihood and outcome of congenital rubella syndrome as a function of time of acquisition of maternal rubella virus infection. Hatched bars, rate of fetal infection; striped bars, rate of defects in infected persons; diamonds, overall risk of defects after maternal infection. (Adapted from reference 89 with permission.)

remia and viruria occur 10 to 17 days after infection, and heavy viral shedding from the nasopharynx continues from 10 to 24 days postexposure (20).

Rash develops 16 to 18 days after infection. At the same time, antibody begins to be detected, in association with clearance of viremia (25). Virus in tissues also clears rapidly as antibody becomes detectable. While virus can usually be cultured from nasopharyngeal secretions from 7 days before to 14 days after the onset of the rash, maximal viral transmission occurs during the period from 5 days prior to 6 days after the appearance of the rash (25). Other sites from which rubella virus has been cultured include lymph nodes, urine, cerebrospinal fluid (CSF), the conjunctival sac, breast milk, synovial fluid, lung tissue, and skin (at sites both with and without rash) (20).

Histopathology

Postnatal Rubella

Rubella acquired in the postnatal period is typically a mild disease, and death as a consequence of postnatally acquired rubella is exceedingly uncommon. From 1966 to 1975, 0.05% of reported cases of rubella in the United States resulted in death (12). As a result, a paucity of information exists on the tissue pathology that results from postnatally acquired rubella. Reported morphological changes in lymphoreticular tissues, central nervous system specimens, and synovial tissue have been nonspecific (20). Follicular hyperplasia and edema in lymph nodes and splenic tissue have been documented. In addition, minimal meningeal and perivascular exudate has been noted in neural tissue from a fatal case, as has diffuse swelling and nonspecific degeneration of brain (20). Lymphocytic infiltration, increased vascularity, and synovial cell hyperplasia are seen on synovial biopsy specimens from patients with rubella arthritis.

Congenital Rubella

While direct cellular destruction by rubella virus accounts for some of the tissue damage seen in congenital rubella syndrome, vascular injury and resulting insufficiency are more important in the pathogenesis of congenital defects (25, 37, 134). The amount of inflammation produced in target organs is much less than that seen with other congenital viral infections. In addition, rubella virus infection in vitro disrupts actin microfilaments (9), and mitotic arrest has been demonstrated in vivo (94). Such disruption and arrest may account for the decreased numbers of cells in many organs of congenitally infected infants, resulting in their generalized intrauterine growth restriction.

The pathological findings of the placenta include extensive perivasculitis, endovasculitis, and perivascular fibrosis (37, 134). Edema, fibrosis, and necrosis of the chorionic villi also occur, resulting in a small placenta. Cellular necrosis and other evidence of cytolysis are also present but are less widespread than the vascular lesions.

Numerous organs are involved in congenital rubella syndrome. In general, affected organs are hypoplastic, in part due to the reduction in the total numbers of cells. The necrotizing angiopathy of small blood vessels is characteristically seen in affected organs, including the placenta. Cellular and tissue necrosis can also be demonstrated in affected organs, although much less frequently than the vascular findings. As would be expected with a chronic infection, new and old lesions frequently can be seen in a single tissue specimen (37, 134).

Immune Responses to Rubella Virus Infection

Postnatal Rubella

Humoral Immune Response

Rubella-specific immunoglobulin M (IgM) antibodies can be detected by hemagglutination inhibition assay (HAI), immunofluorescence assay (IFA), radioimmunoassay, or enzyme-linked immunosorbent assay (ELISA) (25, 28). IgM antibodies can usually be detected within a few days of the onset of the rubella rash (Fig. 3). After a rapid peak, however, the IgM component of the host antibody response rapidly declines, becoming undetectable by 8 weeks following initial infection. Rarely, patients can have persistence of rubella-specific IgM for prolonged periods

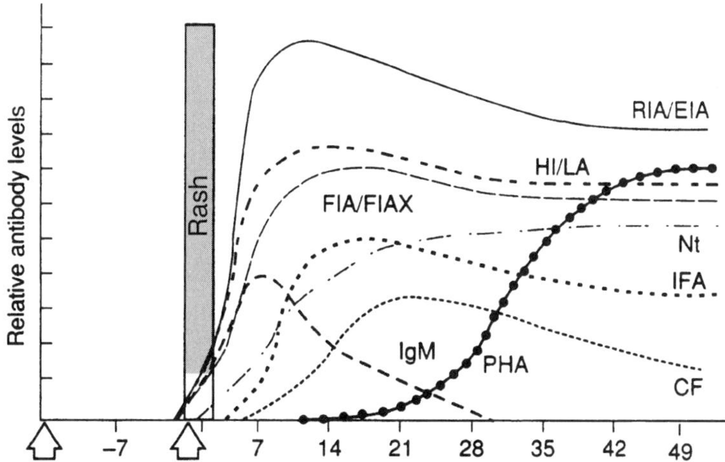

FIGURE 3 Schematic of the immune response in acute rubella virus infection. Values on the x axis indicate number of days. RIA, radioimmunoassay; EIA, enzyme immunoassay; HI, hemagglutination inhibition; LA, latex agglutination; FIA/FIAX and IFA, immunofluorescence; Nt, neutralization; PHA, passive agglutination. (Reprinted from reference 25 with permission of Elsevier.)

(101). IgM is usually not seen with reinfection. When IgM is present, reinfection can be distinguished from primary rubella by testing of the avidity of the IgG produced, which is higher in reinfection (8, 55).

Neutralizing and HAI IgG antibodies are first detectable in serum 14 to 18 days following infection, at the time of the rash (53). The quantity of HAI antibodies peaks around 2 weeks later and then gradually declines over the following year and persists thereafter for life. IgG antibodies measured by latex agglutination, neutralization, IFA, single radial hemolysis, RIA, and ELISA generally parallel this HAI pattern of IgG antibody kinetics (Fig. 3) (25). Passive hemagglutination IgG antibodies become detectable somewhat later, at 3 to 4 weeks following onset of rash (20). These antibodies then slowly rise to peak levels over the ensuing weeks and probably persist for life (25). Complement fixation (CF) IgG antibodies are first detectable 7 to 10 days after the onset of the rash, peaking at 1 to 3 months. CF antibodies subsequently diminish to the point of being undetectable over several years in the majority of patients.

The principal IgG subclass detected by the above assays is IgG1 (39). In addition, IgA mucosal HAI and neutralizing antibodies are usually produced following postnatally acquired rubella infection. Roughly half of patients who receive the rubella vaccine RA27/3 subcutaneously will produce detectable amounts of rubella-specific nasal IgA antibody (20).

Cellular Immune Response

Cell-mediated immune responses following postnatal rubella infection can be detected by lymphocyte transformation response, secretion of interferon or macrophage migration inhibitory factor, induction of delayed hypersensitivity to skin testing, and release of lymphokines by cultured lymphocytes (25). Cell-mediated responses can usually be demonstrated 1 week prior to the initiation of humoral immunity, peaking about 2 weeks after the onset of rash and then persisting for years (25). Transient suppression of lymphocyte function can occur initially, thus explaining the suppressed response to purified protein derivative within the month following acute rubella virus infection (91).

Congenital Rubella

Humoral Immune Response

Following maternal rubella infection, the transplacental transfer of maternal IgG is minimal during the first half of pregnancy but increases considerably beginning around 16 to 20 weeks' gestation. As a consequence, until the middle of the second trimester the amount of maternal rubella-specific IgG present in the fetal circulation is only 5 to 10% of that present in the maternal circulation (25). At roughly the same time that transplacental transport of rubella-specific IgG is increasing at midgestation, the fetal humoral system is beginning to produce detectable quantities of fetal immunoglobulin. The predominant class of fetal antibody produced in the latter half of pregnancy is IgM, although fetal IgG and IgA are also made (Fig. 4) (50). Nevertheless, rubella-specific IgG is more abundant overall, due to the combined amounts of both maternal and fetal antibody of this class. As the concentrations of maternal IgG decline following birth, rubella-specific IgM will predominate for a period of several months before declining to levels that are less than those of the increasing neonatal IgG. Virtually all congenitally infected infants have detectable IgM during the first 3 months of life; IgM

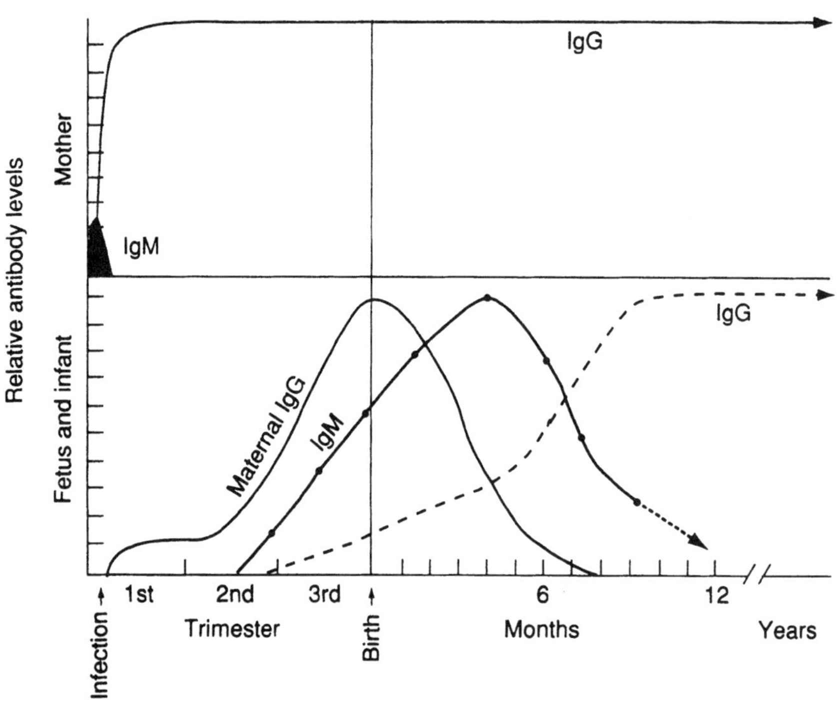

FIGURE 4 Schematic of the immune response in the mother, fetus, and infant after maternal and fetal rubella virus infections in the first trimester of pregnancy. (Reprinted from reference 25 with permission of Elsevier.)

is detectable in about half of such infants between 3 and 6 months of age, and about one-third have detectable IgM from 6 months to 2 years of age (26). Over the first several years of life, the amounts of rubella-specific IgG can decrease markedly, and some children can lose detectable amounts of such IgG altogether (24, 138). Low-avidity IgG can persist even after the disappearance of rubella-specific IgM (60).

Cellular Immune Response

Rubella-specific cell-mediated immune responses (lymphocyte-mediated cytotoxicity, lymphocyte transformation, lymphocyte interferon production, and leukocyte migration inhibition factor production) in infants with congenital rubella are diminished compared to those of children following postnatally acquired disease (11, 20). Additionally, abnormal delayed-hypersensitivity skin reactions can occur in congenitally infected persons (25). The degree of cellular immune dysfunction is greater in children exposed to rubella virus earlier in gestation, with the greatest impairment noted in infants whose mothers were infected during the first 8 weeks of pregnancy (11).

CLINICAL MANIFESTATIONS

Postnatal Rubella

In children who acquire rubella postnatally, a distinct prodromal period is rare. Adolescents and adults, on the other hand, usually will have prodromal symptoms from 1 to 5 days prior to the development of the rash. Symptoms include some combination of lymphadenopathy, low-grade fever, ophthalmalgia, mild conjunctivitis, headache, malaise, anorexia, aches, chills, cough, coryza, and sore throat. Lymph nodes that are characteristically involved include the suboccipital, posterior auricular, and posterior cervical chains. Such nodes are usually painful in adults. In volunteer studies with young adults, it was found that the lymph node enlargement usually lasts from 5 to 8 days (119), although resolution may take several weeks. While frequently occurring together in older patients with rubella, the combination of suboccipital lymphadenopathy and rash is not pathognomonic for rubella virus infection.

At least half of all serologically confirmed childhood primary rubella virus infections result in subclinical illness (71, 153). In those patients who do develop symptoms, the rash usually appears after an incubation period of 16 to 18 days. The exanthem initially appears on the face and then spreads rapidly to the trunk and distal extremities. The erythematous, maculopapular rash usually does not coalesce, and it typically spreads to the entire body within 24 h. During the second day of the exanthem, the rash begins to fade on the face, and by the end of the third day it has resolved across the entire body (hence the term "three-day measles"). The rash is frequently pruritic, especially in adults. Desquamation can occur during the convalescent stage of disease. If the patient had been febrile during the prodromal period, defervescence usually occurs within 1 day of the appearance of the rash.

Roughly 100 years ago, Forcheimer (44) described an exanthem of rubella consisting of small "rose red spots" on the soft palate and uvula that fade within 24 h, "sometimes leaving a yellowish brown pigmentation." In another article, however, Forcheimer refers to the exanthem as "small, discrete, dark red, but not dusky papules which disappear in a short time, leaving no trace behind" (147). Regardless of the type of exanthem noted, neither is pathognomonic for rubella, in contrast to the Koplik spots of measles.

Patients with postnatally acquired rubella frequently have leukopenia at the time of onset of rash. Studies with adult volunteers documented leukopenia beginning 1 day before the onset of rash and persisting for 4 to 5 days (119). Elevation of the erythrocyte sedimentation rate can develop during the first week of illness (20).

Recently, rubella virus has been associated with Fuchs heterochromic iridocyclitis (34, 126).

Complications

Arthritis and Arthralgias

Joint manifestations occur commonly following natural rubella virus infections in adults. Acute polyarticular arthritis occurs in 33 to 52% of women with natural rubella disease, while only 9 to 10% of men experience acute arthritis following rubella virus infection (132). Symptoms range from joint pain alone to frank arthritis, with swelling, joint effusions, decreased articular mobility, and local warmth and erythema. Joint complaints begin 1 to 6 days after the onset of the rash and can take several weeks to resolve completely (20). Chronic arthritis can develop, although this occurs infrequently. Arthritis and arthralgias can also occur following rubella immunization, although at a lower frequency than following infection with wild-type virus (132).

The pathogenesis of rubella arthritis is not fully understood. Some studies have implicated circulating immune complexes in disease pathogenesis (142), while others have found no such direct role (127). Rubella virus has been cultured from the synovial fluid of patients with acute and recurrent rubella arthropathies (18, 19), as well as from peripheral blood mononuclear cells of patients with chronic arthritis (19). One patient with chronic polyarthritis had persistent synovial lymphocyte proliferative responses to rubella virus antigen for at least 7 years following disease onset, raising the possibility of ongoing rubella virus antigen production within the joint (18, 45). Persistent rubella virus infection has been achieved in cultured human joint tissue, suggesting the possibility that similar events may occur in vivo (29, 88).

Neurologic Involvement

Unlike the arthropathies described above, encephalitis and postinfectious encephalopathy are very rare complications of natural postnatal rubella virus infection. The rate of occurrence of such neurologic events ranges from 1 in 4,700 to 1 in 6,000 cases of rubella (79, 137). Neurologic symptoms appear abruptly 1 to 6 days after appearance of the rash, with headache, vomiting, lethargy, nuchal rigidity, and generalized seizures. CSF white blood cell counts range from 20 to 100 cells/mm^3, with a lymphocyte predominance; CSF protein concentrations are normal or slightly increased, and CSF glucose concentrations are normal (20). Electroencephalographic tracings are frequently abnormal (153).

Mortality rates due to the neurologic manifestations of rubella range from 20 to 50% (49). Survivors usually recover fully following disease resolution (153). The pathogenesis of such complications is unclear, with some reports suggesting a direct involvement of rubella virus and others reporting findings consistent with a postinfectious process.

Hemorrhagic Manifestations

While transient depression of the thrombocyte count occurs not infrequently in postnatal rubella, thrombocytopenic purpura is encountered in only 1 in 1,500 cases (137). The median interval between onset of the exanthem of rubella and development of purpura is about 4 days (20). Unlike the other complications of rubella discussed above, hemorrhagic manifestations of disease are more likely to occur in children than adults. The thrombocytopenia can last for weeks or months, but complete recovery eventually results in most cases.

Differential Diagnosis

The benign nature of rubella virus infection and its nonspecific symptoms contribute to the difficulty in diagnosing rubella on clinical grounds. In addition, the marked decrease in disease incidence has resulted in many physicians lacking personal experience in recognizing the disease. Consequently, rubella can be readily mistaken for such illnesses as scarlet fever, toxoplasmosis, infectious mononucleosis, measles, roseola, erythema infectiosum, and enteroviral infections (49). In adults, the pruritic component of the rubella exanthem can be confused with an allergic reaction.

Congenital Rubella

Unlike those of postnatal rubella disease, the clinical manifestations of congenitally acquired rubella are usually severe. The classic triad of congenital rubella consists of cataracts, cardiac abnormalities, and deafness. In addition, less frequent manifestations of congenital rubella syndrome were recognized during the large pandemic of 1962 to 1965 and are collectively referred to as the expanded congenital rubella syndrome, as detailed below.

The consequences of in utero rubella virus infection can be considered broadly as belonging to one of three categories: (i) signs and symptoms that are transiently apparent in affected infants, (ii) permanent manifestations that are noted within the first year of life, and (iii) manifestations of congenital rubella that are delayed in onset until later in life (2 years of age to adulthood) (25).

Transient Sequelae

Many of the transient clinical manifestations of congenital rubella were first recognized during the large pandemic of 1962 to 1965. As implied, these manifestations usually resolve over a period of weeks. They include dermal erythropoiesis ("blueberry muffin" rash), chronic rash, thrombocytopenic purpura, hemolytic anemia, generalized lymphadenopathy, interstitial pneumonitis, hepatitis, hepatosplenomegaly, nephritis, myositis, myocarditis, bone radiolucencies, and meningoencephalitis (20). Among the more common of these findings are rash (petechial or blueberry muffin rash), hepatosplenomegaly, jaundice, pulmonary involvement, meningoencephalitis, and radiographic abnormalities (Fig. 5) (20). The majority of such infants are intrauterine growth restricted at delivery (25).

Permanent Manifestations

Sensorineural hearing loss is the most common permanent manifestation of congenital rubella, with deafness occurring in 80% of congenitally infected patients (25). Additional permanent sequelae of congenital rubella include cardiovascular anomalies, ophthalmologic findings, and neurologic impairment.

Structural defects of the cardiovascular system occur in the majority of infants whose mothers acquired rubella during the first 2 months of gestation (20). Patent ductus ar-

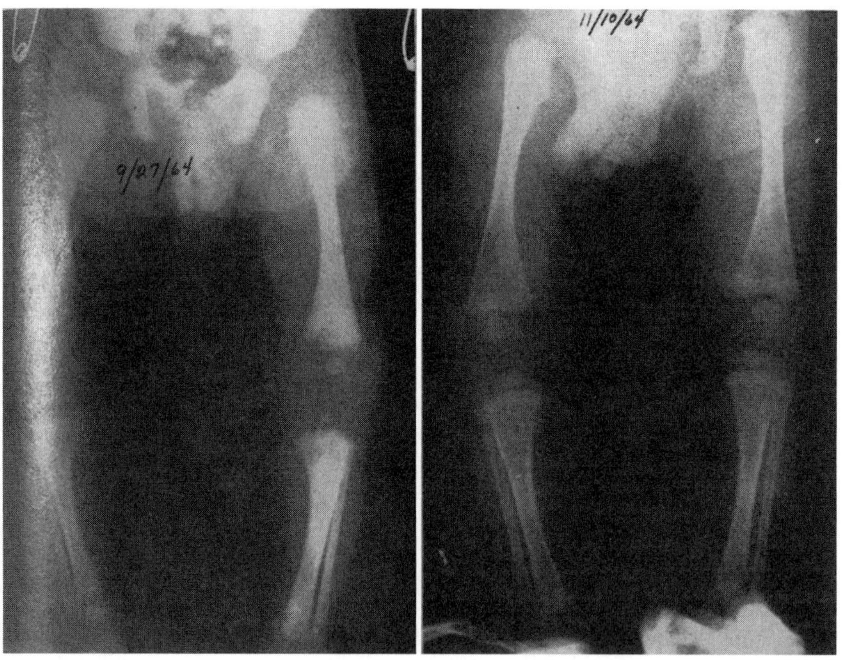

FIGURE 5 (Left) Provisional zones of calcification are poorly defined and irregular. Radiolucent defects are present in metaphyses of femora and tibiae and the parallel long axis of the bone. (Right) Lower extremities 2 months later show nearly complete disappearance of osseous abnormalities. (Reprinted from reference 117 with permission of the American Medical Association.)

teriosus is the most common of these cardiovascular sequelae, followed by pulmonary artery stenosis and pulmonary valvular stenosis. Two-thirds of patients with patent ductus arteriosus will have other cardiovascular lesions present (20).

Ophthalmologic findings include cataracts (bilateral or unilateral), retinopathy, and microphthalmia. The retinopathy results from pigmentary defects in the retina and usually does not interfere with vision. In contrast, a small number of patients have congenital glaucoma, which, if undetected, can result in visual impairment.

Permanent neurologic impairment can result from the active replication in the central nervous system of rubella virus both in utero and following delivery. Indeed, such neurologic sequelae as mental retardation and motor disabilities correlate with the severity and persistence of the acute meningoencephalitis that is present at delivery in 10 to 20% of infants with congenital rubella syndrome (20). Movement and behavioral disorders can also be seen in surviving patients.

Delayed Manifestations

Sequelae of congenital rubella that develop in childhood or adulthood but are not present in infancy include endocrinopathies, deafness, ocular damage, vascular effects, and progressive rubella panencephalitis (124, 135). Of these, the development of insulin-dependent diabetes mellitus occurs most frequently, with approximately 20% of patients being diagnosed with this form of diabetes by the time they reach adulthood (25). Autoimmune thyroid dysfunction can also be seen (22).

LABORATORY DIAGNOSIS

Rubella virus infection is definitively diagnosed by isolation of rubella virus in tissue culture, using one of several cell lines and primary cell strains. Viral interference in AGMK cells is one common culture technique by which the presence of rubella virus is demonstrated. When using such interference techniques, the presence of rubella virus is then confirmed by the specific detection of viral antigen by neutralization or immunofluorescence.

Virus can be readily isolated from throat swabs from patients with postnatal rubella virus infection for 6 days before and after the onset of rash (33, 153). Virus can be isolated from specimens from the nasopharynx, conjunctivae, urine, blood buffy coat, and CSF of patients with congenital rubella. In utero infection with rubella virus can be demonstrated by nucleic acid hybridization or by virus-specific antigen detection in specimens from the chorionic villus or fetus (73, 131). PCR assays have also been developed (155).

Despite the definitive results afforded by direct viral isolation in tissue culture, the majority of rubella cases are diagnosed serologically. A fourfold rise in rubella-specific IgG between acute- and convalescent-phase serum specimens confirms the diagnosis of postnatal rubella. Commercially available rubella virus IgG avidity assays are of variable sensitivity (92). Demonstration of the presence of rubella-specific IgM is also diagnostic for recent infection with rubella virus. Rarely, rubella-specific IgM can be detected with reinfection. Specific antigens of rubella virus can be identified by such serologic reactions as CF (122), HAI (128), precipitation (120), platelet aggregation (139), IFA (10), and ELISAs (141). Although the HAI remains the reference standard by which other tests are compared, simpler tests such as ELISAs have become the predominant assays used by commercial laboratories for the detection of rubella-specific IgG or IgM.

Serologic diagnosis of congenital rubella can be demonstrated by the presence of rubella-specific IgM in neonatal serum. Confirmation of the diagnosis based solely upon the presence of IgG is difficult. In such cases, it is necessary to test sequential sera from the infant for rubella-specific IgG. In most cases, the IgG titer will decrease over several months if it is solely of maternal origin, whereas it will rise if congenital infection has occurred and the infant is producing rubella-specific IgG.

PREVENTION

Hospitalized patients with postnatal rubella require contact isolation for 7 days after the onset of the rash. Postnatally infected children should be excluded from school or child care for the same period (2). In contrast, infants with congenital rubella should be considered contagious until their first birthday, unless nasopharyngeal and urine viral cultures obtained after 3 months of age are negative on several occasions.

Exposure to rubella virus during pregnancy can be especially anguishing (77). If a woman with such an exposure is known to be rubella immune from a previous pregnancy, she can be reassured with no further evaluation required. If, on the other hand, she is not immune to rubella or her rubella status is unknown, serologic testing should be performed immediately. If such testing performed around the time of the exposure demonstrates the presence of rubella antibody, it can be assumed that she is immune and thus not at risk. However, if no rubella-specific antibody is detected, she should have a second serum sample obtained 2 to 3 weeks after the exposure, and it should be tested for antibody simultaneously with the first specimen; seroconversion suggests that infection occurred with the exposure. If the second test is also negative, a final serologic analysis should be performed on a serum sample obtained 6 weeks following the initial exposure and also tested concurrently with the first specimen; a negative test result for both specimens indicates that infection has not occurred, and a positive result for the second but not the first (seroconversion) indicates recent infection (2).

Passive Immunoprophylaxis

Administration of immunoglobulin to susceptible persons experimentally exposed to rubella virus can prevent clinical rubella (81). However, there have also been many reports of the failure of immunoglobulin to prevent the anomalies of congenital rubella (36, 113). Therefore, the routine use of immunoglobulin for the prevention of rubella in an exposed pregnant patient cannot be recommended. Administration of immunoglobulin should be considered only if termination of the pregnancy is not an option. Limited data indicate that intramuscular immunoglobulin in a dose of 0.55 ml/kg of body weight may decrease clinically apparent infection in an exposed susceptible person from 87 to 18% compared with placebo (2). However, the absence of clinical signs in a woman who has received intramuscular immunoglobulin does not guarantee that fetal infection has been prevented (2).

Active Immunization

Since 1979, the RA27/3 rubella vaccine has been used exclusively in the United States (103, 106). Vaccination results in IgG antibody production in more than 98% of vaccine recipients, and a single dose confers long-term (probably lifelong) immunity against clinical and asymptomatic infection in more than 90% of vaccinees (2). Recent data suggest that cellular and humoral immune responses to rubella vaccination may be influenced by the HLA alleles of the vaccine recipient (95, 96). Subcutaneous administration of vaccine induces production of IgM antibodies that peak at 1 month postvaccination (26). Additionally, the generation of secretory IgA following subcutaneous vaccine administration may provide protection against reinfection by wild-type virus by blocking mucosal replication of virus.

Rubella vaccine given after exposure to wild-type rubella virus theoretically can prevent illness if administered within 3 days of exposure (2). Immunization of exposed nonpregnant persons may be indicated because if the exposure did not result in infection, immunization will protect the person in the future.

Rubella vaccine is administered subcutaneously in combination with measles and mumps vaccine (MMR) or in combination with measles, mumps, and varicella vaccine (MMRV). In addition, monovalent rubella vaccine and a combined rubella-measles vaccine are also available. Current recommendations for rubella vaccination call for administration of the first MMR or MMRV vaccination at 12 to 15 months of age. Antibody responses following the first dose of a rubella-containing vaccine are similar for premature and term infants at 15 months of age (31). A second MMR or MMRV vaccination is then recommended at school entry at 4 to 6 years of age; those persons who have not received this dose at school entry should receive their second dose of a rubella containing vaccine as soon as possible but no later than 11 to 12 years of age.

Postpubertal females who are not known to be immune to rubella should be immunized. They should not receive the vaccine if they are pregnant, and they should be warned not to get pregnant within 3 months of vaccination. In addition, premarital serologic screening for rubella immunity will bolster attempts at identifying susceptible women of childbearing age. Finally, prenatal or antepartum serologic screening for rubella immunity should be routinely performed. Women who are found to be rubella susceptible should receive rubella vaccine in the immediate postpartum period prior to discharge. Breast-feeding is not a contraindication to such immunization.

Adverse Reactions

From 5 to 15% of children receiving rubella vaccine develop rash, fever, or lymphadenopathy between 5 and 12 days after vaccination. Approximately 0.5% of children and 25% of susceptible postpubertal female vaccinees develop arthralgias beginning 7 to 21 days after vaccination. Such symptoms usually involve small peripheral joints. The incidence of joint manifestations after vaccination is lower than that following natural infection at the corresponding age (2). MMR vaccination rarely can cause idiopathic thrombocytopenic purpura, with cases occurring in approximately 1 in 22,000 doses; children with a history of idiopathic thrombocytopenic purpura do not have relapses following receipt of MMR (90).

A possible relationship between rubella vaccination and chronic arthritis in adult women is controversial. Following a 20-month review, the Institute of Medicine (IOM) in 1991 found that the evidence is consistent with a causal relation between the RA27/3 rubella vaccine strain and chronic arthritis in adult women, although the evidence is limited in scope (74). In a subsequent special report, the IOM stated that "proving that rubella vaccination can cause chronic arthritis will require an understanding of pathogenetic mechanisms and additional well-designed studies" (75). One such large retrospective cohort study was published in 1997 and found no evidence of any increased risk of new-onset chronic arthropathies or neurologic conditions in women receiving the RA27/3 rubella vaccine (115). Other reports also have not demonstrated a definitive association between rubella vaccine and persistent or recurrent joint manifestations, although additional investigations are needed to definitively disprove such a relationship (7, 133).

In 1998, a possible link between MMR vaccine and inflammatory bowel disease was published by Wakefield et al. (143). Over the ensuing years, their results could not be reproduced by others, and in 2004 it came to light that Wakefield's work had actually been funded by lawyers in Britain who were filing class action lawsuits regarding such claims. In 2004, 10 of the 12 coauthors of the original paper published a retraction (93), and the editors of *The Lancet* detailed these misgivings and others in an editorial (72).

Another allegation of the initial Wakefield paper from 1998 was that MMR was also associated with autism. Again, numerous studies subsequently found no such association, leading to an Immunization Safety Review Committee of the IOM review of the epidemiological and other evidence on MMR vaccine and risk for autism spectrum disorders. The conclusion of the IOM was that the evidence favors rejection of a causal relationship (76). Despite the unequivocal conclusions of the scientific community, confusion and doubt remain within the general population (35), illustrating the dangers of recklessly raising safety concerns for vaccines which have had such a positive impact on human health worldwide.

Contraindications

Rubella vaccine is contraindicated in pregnancy. Based upon data from the Centers for Disease Control and Prevention, the maximal theoretical risk for the occurrence of congenital rubella syndrome following administration of the RA27/3 vaccine during the first trimester of pregnancy is 1.6% (2). While asymptomatic rubella virus infection has been reported for 2% of such infants, no cases of congenital rubella syndrome resulting from live-virus vaccination of the mother have been reported (2). Persistence of fetal infection following inadvertent rubella vaccination during early pregnancy has been documented, but with no apparent adverse clinical sequelae (63).

Patients with altered immunity should not receive the rubella vaccine. These include patients with immunodeficiency diseases (except human immunodeficiency virus infection), patients receiving immunosuppressive therapy, and patients receiving large systemic doses of corticosteroids, alkylating agents, antimetabolites, or radiation. Immunocompetent children with minor illnesses with or without fever may be vaccinated. Rubella vaccine should not be given in the 2 weeks prior to or the 3 months following the administration of immunoglobulin or blood products.

TREATMENT

Postnatal rubella virus infection is usually either subclinical or so mild that no therapy is warranted. Complications of rubella virus infection can be treated symptomatically. Management of rubella arthritis in adults may require bed rest and administration of aspirin or nonsteroidal anti-inflammatory agents. Likewise, postinfectious encephalopathy and encephalitis are managed with supportive care, as are the thrombocytopenic and hemorrhagic manifestations of rubella.

Patients with congenital rubella require supportive care not only in the neonatal period but throughout life for such permanent impairments as deafness and heart defects. Prompt identification of such afflictions is of the utmost importance.

Interferon and amantadine have been used in individual cases of congenital rubella syndrome (4, 110). Results have been equivocal, however, and no controlled trials have been performed. Interferon has also been used in the treatment of chronic arthritis secondary to postnatal rubella virus infection, again with indeterminate results (3). Isoprinosine has been administered to patients with progressive rubella panencephalitis, without apparent therapeutic benefit (154).

REFERENCES

1. **Alain, R., F. Nadon, C. Seguin, P. Payment, and M. Trudel.** 1987. Rapid virus subunit visualization by direct sedimentation of samples on electron microscope grids. *J. Virol. Methods* **16:**209–216.
2. **American Academy of Pediatrics.** 2006. Rubella, p. 574–579. *In* L. K. Pickering (ed.), *2006 Red Book: Report of the Committee on Infectious Diseases*, 26th ed. American Academy of Pediatrics, Elk Grove Village, IL.
3. **Armstrong, R. D., A. Sinclair, G. O'Keeffe, and R. Grahame.** 1985. Interferon treatment of chronic rubella associated arthritis. *Clin. Exp. Rheumatol.* **3:**93–94.
4. **Arvin, A. M., N. J. Schmidt, K. Cantell, and T. C. Merigan.** 1982. Alpha interferon administration to infants with congenital rubella. *Antimicrob. Agents Chemother.* **21:**259–261.
5. **Bardeletti, G., N. Kessler, and M. Aymard-Henry.** 1975. Morphology, biochemical analysis and neuraminidase activity of rubella virus. *Arch. Virol.* **49:**175–186.
6. **Best, J. M., and J. E. Banatvala.** 1970. Studies on rubella virus strain variation by kinetic haemagglutination-inhibition tests. *J. Gen. Virol.* **9:**215–223.
7. **Bosma, T. J., J. Etherington, S. O'Shea, K. Corbett, F. Cottam, L. Holt, J. E. Banatvala, and J. M. Best.** 1998. Rubella virus and chronic joint disease: is there an association? *J. Clin. Microbiol.* **36:**3524–3526.
8. **Bottiger, B., and I. P. Jensen.** 1997. Maturation of rubella IgG avidity over time after acute rubella infection. *Clin. Diagn. Virol.* **8:**105–111.
9. **Bowden, D. S., J. S. Pedersen, B. H. Toh, and E. G. Westaway.** 1987. Distribution by immunofluorescence of viral products and actin-containing cytoskeletal filaments in rubella virus-infected cells. *Arch. Virol.* **92:**211–219.
10. **Brown, G. C., H. F. Maassab, J. A. Veronelli, and T. J. Francis, Jr.** 1964. Rubella antibodies in human serum: detection by the indirect fluorescent antibody technic. *Science* **145:**943–945.
11. **Buimovici-Klein, E., P. B. Lang, P. R. Ziring, and L. Z. Cooper.** 1979. Impaired cell-mediated immune response in patients with congenital rubella: correlation with gestational age at time of infection. *Pediatrics* **64:**620–626.
12. **Center for Disease Control.** 1976. Reported morbidity and mortality for the United States, 1975. *Morb. Mortal. Wkly. Rep.* **24:**2.
13. **Centers for Disease Control.** 1989. Rubella and congenital rubella syndrome—United States, 1985–1988. *Morb. Mortal. Wkly. Rep.* **38:**173–178.
14. **Centers for Disease Control and Prevention.** 1994. Rubella and congenital rubella syndrome—United States, January 1, 1991–May 7, 1994. *Morb. Mortal. Wkly. Rep.* **43:**391, 397–401.
15. **Centers for Disease Control and Prevention.** 2005. Elimination of rubella and congenital rubella syndrome—United States, 1969–2004. *Morb. Mortal. Wkly. Rep.* **54:**279–282.
16. **Chagnon, A., and P. Laflamme.** 1964. Effect of acidity on rubella virus. *Can. J. Microbiol.* **10:**501–502.
17. **Chantler, J. K.** 1979. Rubella virus: intracellular polypeptide synthesis. *Virology* **98:**275–278.
18. **Chantler, J. K., D. M. da Roza, M. E. Bonnie, G. D. Reid, and D. K. Ford.** 1985. Sequential studies on synovial lymphocyte stimulation by rubella antigen, and rubella virus isolation in an adult with persistent arthritis. *Ann. Rheum. Dis.* **44:**564–568.
19. **Chantler, J. K., A. J. Tingle, and R. E. Petty.** 1985. Persistent rubella virus infection associated with chronic arthritis in children. *N. Engl. J. Med.* **313:**1117–1123.
20. **Cherry, J. D.** 1992. Rubella, p. 1792–1817. *In* R. D. Feigin and J. D. Cherry (ed.), *Textbook of Pediatric Infectious Diseases*, 3rd ed. The W. B. Saunders Co., Philadelphia, PA.
21. **Clarke, M., G. C. Schild, J. Boustred, I. A. McGregor, and K. Williams.** 1980. Epidemiological studies of rubella virus in a tropical African community. *Bull. W.H.O.* **58:**931–935.
22. **Clarke, W. L., K. A. Shaver, G. M. Bright, A. D. Rogol, and W. E. Nance.** 1984. Autoimmunity in congenital rubella syndrome. *J. Pediatr.* **104:**370–373.
23. **Cooper, L. Z.** 1968. Rubella: a preventable cause of birth defects, p. 23. *In* D. Bergman (ed.), *Intrauterine Infections.* The National Foundation, New York, NY.
24. **Cooper, L. Z., A. L. Florman, P. R. Ziring, and S. Krugman.** 1971. Loss of rubella hemagglutination inhibition antibody in congenital rubella. Failure of seronegative children with congenital rubella to respond to HPV-77 rubella vaccine. *Am. J. Dis. Child.* **122:**397–403.
25. **Cooper, L. Z., S. R. Preblud, and C. A. Alford, Jr.** 1995. Rubella, p. 268–311. *In* J. S. Remington and J. O. Klein (ed.), *Infectious Diseases of the Fetus and Newborn Infant*, 4th ed. The W. B. Saunders Co., Philadelphia, PA.
26. **Cradock-Watson, J. E., and M. K. Ridehalgh.** 1976. Specific immunoglobulins in infants with the congenital rubella syndrome. *J. Hyg.* **76:**109–123.
27. **Cradock-Watson, J. E., M. K. Ridehalgh, M. J. Anderson, J. R. Pattison, and H. O. Kangro.** 1980. Fetal infection resulting from maternal rubella after the first trimester of pregnancy. *J. Hyg.* **85:**381–391.
28. **Cubie, H., and E. Edmond.** 1985. Comparison of five different methods of rubella IgM antibody testing. *J. Clin. Pathol.* **38:**203–207.
29. **Cunningham, A. L., and J. R. Fraser.** 1985. Persistent rubella virus infection of human synovial cells cultured in vitro. *J. Infect. Dis.* **151:**638–645.
30. **Cutts, F. T., and E. Vynnycky.** 1999. Modelling the incidence of congenital rubella syndrome in developing countries. *Int. J. Epidemiol.* **28:**1176–1184.

31. **D'Angio, C. T., P. A. Boohene, A. Mowrer, S. Audet, M. A. Menegus, D. S. Schmid, and J. A. Beeler.** 2007. Measles-mumps-rubella and varicella vaccine responses in extremely preterm infants. *Pediatrics* **119:**e574–e579.
32. **Das, B. D., P. Lakhani, J. B. Kurtz, N. Hunter, B. E. Watson, K. A. Cartwright, E. O. Caul, and A. P. Roome.** 1990. Congenital rubella after previous maternal immunity. *Arch. Dis. Child.* **65:**545–546.
33. **Davis, W. J., H. E. Larson, J. P. Simsarian, P. D. Parkman, and H. M. Meyer, Jr.** 1971. A study of rubella immunity and resistance to infection. *JAMA* **215:**600–608.
34. **de Groot-Mijnes, J. D., L. de Visser, A. Rothova, M. Schuller, A. M. van Loon, and A. J. Weersink.** 2006. Rubella virus is associated with Fuchs heterochromic iridocyclitis. *Am. J. Ophthalmol.* **141:**212–214.
35. **DeStefano, F.** 2007. Vaccines and autism: evidence does not support a causal association. *Clin. Pharmacol. Ther.* **82:**756–759.
36. **Doege, T. C., and K. S. Kim.** 1967. Studies of rubella and its prevention with immune globulin. *JAMA* **200:** 584–590.
37. **Driscoll, S. G.** 1969. Histopathology of gestational rubella. *Am. J. Dis. Child.* **118:**49–53.
38. **Emminghaus, H.** 1870. Über Rubeolen. *Jahrb. Kinder* **4:** 47–59.
39. **Enders, G., and F. Knotek.** 1989. Rubella IgG total antibody avidity and IgG subclass-specific antibody avidity assay and their role in the differentiation between primary rubella and rubella reinfection. *Infection* **17:**218–226.
40. **Erickson, C. A.** 1944. Rubella early in pregnancy causing congenital malformations of eyes and heart. *J. Pediatr.* **25:** 281–283.
41. **Evans, M. W.** 1944. Congenital dental defects in infants subsequent to maternal rubella during pregnancy. *Med. J. Aust.* **2:**225–228.
42. **Fenner, F.** 1998. Candidate viral diseases for elimination or eradication. *Bull. W.H.O.* **76**(Suppl. 2)**:**68–70.
43. **Forbes, J. A.** 1969. Rubella: historical aspects. *Am. J. Dis. Child.* **118:**5–11.
44. **Forcheimer, F.** 1898. The enanthem of German measles. *Trans. Am. Pediatr. Soc.* **10:**118–128.
45. **Ford, D. K., G. D. Reid, A. J. Tingle, L. A. Mitchell, and M. Schulzer.** 1992. Sequential follow up observations of a patient with rubella associated persistent arthritis. *Ann. Rheum. Dis.* **51:**407–410.
46. **Forrest, J. M., F. M. Turnbull, G. F. Sholler, R. E. Hawker, F. J. Martin, T. T. Doran, and M. A. Burgess.** 2002. Gregg's congenital rubella patients 60 years later. *Med. J. Aust.* **177:**664–667.
47. **Forsgren, M., and L. Soren.** 1985. Subclinical rubella reinfection in vaccinated women with rubella-specific IgM response during pregnancy and transmission of virus to the fetus. *Scand. J. Infect. Dis.* **17:**337–341.
48. **Gale, J. L., R. Detels, K. S. Kim, R. P. Beasley, K. P. Chen, and J. T. Grayston.** 1972. The epidemiology of rubella on Taiwan. 3. Family studies in cities of high and low attack rates. *Int. J. Epidemiol.* **1:**261–265.
49. **Gershon, A. A.** 1995. Rubella virus (German measles), p. 1459–1465. *In* G. L. Mandell, J. E. Bennett, and R. Dolin (ed.), *Principles and Practice of Infectious Diseases*, 4th ed. Churchill Livingstone, New York, NY.
50. **Grangeot-Keros, L., J. Pillot, F. Daffos, and F. Forestier.** 1988. Prenatal and postnatal production of IgM and IgA antibodies to rubella virus studied by antibody capture immunoassay. *J. Infect. Dis.* **158:**138–143.
51. **Grayston, J. T., J. L. Gale, and R. H. Watten.** 1972. The epidemiology of rubella on Taiwan. I. Introduction and description of the 1957–1958 epidemic. *Int. J. Epidemiol.* **1:**245–252.
52. **Greaves, W. L., W. A. Orenstein, H. C. Stetler, S. R. Preblud, A. R. Hinman, and K. J. Bart.** 1982. Prevention of rubella transmission in medical facilities. *JAMA* **248:**861–864.
53. **Green, R. H., M. R. Balsamo, J. P. Giles, S. Krugman, and G. S. Mirick.** 1965. Studies of the natural history and prevention of rubella. *Am. J. Dis. Child.* **110:**348–365.
54. **Gregg, N. M.** 1941. Congenital cataract following German measles in the mother. *Trans. Ophthalmol. Soc. Aust.* **3:**35–46.
55. **Gutierrez, J., M. J. Rodriguez, F. De Ory, G. Piedrola, and M. C. Maroto.** 1999. Reliability of low-avidity IgG and of IgA in the diagnosis of primary infection by rubella virus with adaptation of a commercial test. *J. Clin. Lab. Anal.* **13:**1–4.
56. **Habel, K.** 1942. Transmission of rubella to Macacus mulatta monkeys. *Public Health Rep.* **57:**1126–1139.
57. **Hattis, R. P., S. B. Halstead, K. L. Herrmann, and J. J. Witte.** 1973. Rubella in an immunized island population. *JAMA* **223:**1019–1021.
58. **Heggie, A. D., and F. C. Robbins.** 1969. Natural rubella acquired after birth. Clinical features and complications. *Am. J. Dis. Child.* **118:**12–17.
59. **Hemphill, M. L., R. Y. Forng, E. S. Abernathy, and T. K. Frey.** 1988. Time course of virus-specific macromolecular synthesis during rubella virus infection in Vero cells. *Virology* **162:**65–75.
60. **Herne, V., K. Hedman, and P. Reedik.** 1997. Immunoglobulin G avidity in the serodiagnosis of congenital rubella syndrome. *Eur. J. Clin. Microbiol. Infect. Dis.* **16:** 763–766.
61. **Hillenbrand, F. K.** 1956. Rubella in a remote community. *Lancet* **271:**64–66.
62. **Hiro, Y., and S. Tasaka.** 1938. Die Roteln sind eine Viruskrankheit. *Monatsschr. Kinderheilkd.* **76:**328–332.
63. **Hofmann, J., M. Kortung, B. Pustowoit, R. Faber, U. Piskazeck, and U. G. Liebert.** 2000. Persistent fetal rubella vaccine virus infection following inadvertent vaccination during early pregnancy. *J. Med. Virol.* **61:**155–158.
64. **Holmes, I. H., M. C. Wark, and M. F. Warburton.** 1969. Is rubella an arbovirus? II. Ultrastructural morphology and development. *Virology* **37:**15–25.
65. **Homans, J.** 1848. Roetheln, p. 370. *Boston Society for Medical Improvement, Records of Meetings* (manuscript). Boston Medical Library. Boston Society for Medical Improvements, Boston, MA.
66. **Honeyman, M. C., D. C. Dorman, M. A. Menser, J. M. Forrest, J. J. Guinan, and P. Clark.** 1975. HL-A antigens in congenital rubella and the role of antigens 1 and 8 in the epidemiology of natural rubella. *Tissue Antigens* **5:**12–18.
67. **Horstmann, D. M.** 1969. Discussion paper: the use of primates in experimental viral infections—rubella and the rubella syndrome. *Ann. N. Y. Acad. Sci.* **162:**594–597.
68. **Horstmann, D. M.** 1990. Rubella, p. 617. *In* A. S. Evans (ed.), *Viral Infections of Humans: Epidemiology and Control*, 3rd ed. Plenum Medical Book Company, New York, NY.
69. **Horstmann, D. M.** 1971. Rubella: the challenge of its control. *J. Infect. Dis.* **123:**640–654.
70. **Horstmann, D. M., H. Liebhaber, G. L. Le Bouvier, D. A. Rosenberg, and S. B. Halstead.** 1970. Rubella: reinfection of vaccinated and naturally immune persons exposed in an epidemic. *N. Engl. J. Med.* **283:**771–778.
71. **Horstmann, D. M., J. T. Riordan, M. Ohtawara, and J. C. Niederman.** 1965. A natural epidemic of rubella in a closed population: virological and epidemiological observations. *Arch. Gesamte Virusforsch.* **16:**483–487.

72. **Horton, R.** 2004. A statement by the editors of The Lancet. *Lancet* **363:**820–821.
73. **HoTerry, L., G. M. Terry, P. Londesborough, K. R. Rees, F. Wielaard, and A. Denissen.** 1988. Diagnosis of fetal rubella infection by nucleic acid hybridization. *J. Med. Virol.* **24:**175–182.
74. **Howe, C. J., and C. P. Howson.** 1991. Adverse effects of pertussis and rubella vaccines. *In* C. J. Howe, C. P. Howson, and H. V. Fineberg (ed.), *Adverse Effects of Pertussis and Rubella Vaccines*. National Academy Press, Washington, DC.
75. **Howson, C. P., M. Katz, R. B. Johnston, Jr., and H. V. Fineberg.** 1992. Chronic arthritis after rubella vaccination. *Clin. Infect. Dis.* **15:**307–312.
76. **Immunization Safety Review Committee.** 2004. Immunization Safety Review. *In* Institute of Medicine (ed.), *Vaccines and Autism Board of Health Promotion and Disease Prevention*. National Academy Press, Washington, DC.
77. **Kimberlin, D. W.** 1997. Rubella immunization. *Pediatr. Ann.* **26:**366–370.
78. **Krugman, S. E.** 1969. International Conference on Rubella Immunization. *Am. J. Dis. Child.* **118:**2–410.
79. **Margolis, F. J., J. L. Wilson, and F. H. Top.** 1943. Postrubella encephalomyelitis. Report of cases in Detroit and review of the literature. *J. Pediatr.* **23:**158–165.
80. **Martin, S. M.** 1945. Congenital defects and rubella. *Br. Med. J.* **1:**855.
81. **Martin du Pan, R., B. Koechli, and A. Douath.** 1972. Protection of nonimmune volunteers against rubella by intravenous administration of normal human gamma globulin. *J. Infect. Dis.* **126:**341–344.
82. **Maton, W. G.** 1815. Some account of rash, liable to be mistaken for scarlatina. *Med. Trans. R. Coll. Physicians* **5:** 149–165.
83. **Meissner, H. C., S. E. Reef, and S. Cochi.** 2006. Elimination of rubella from the United States: a milestone on the road to global elimination. *Pediatrics* **117:**933–935.
84. **Mellinger, A. K., J. D. Cragan, W. L. Atkinson, W. W. Williams, B. Kleger, R. G. Kimber, and D. Tavris.** 1995. High incidence of congenital rubella syndrome after a rubella outbreak. *Pediatr. Infect. Dis. J.* **14:**573–578.
85. **Meyer, H. M., Jr., H. E. Hopps, P. D. Parkman, and F. A. Ennis.** 1978. Control of measles and rubella through use of attenuated vaccines. *Am. J. Clin. Pathol.* **70:**128–135.
86. **Meyer, H. M., Jr., P. D. Parkman, T. E. Hobbins, H. E. Larson, W. J. Davis, J. P. Simsarian, and H. E. Hopps.** 1969. Attenuated rubella viruses. Laboratory and clinical characteristics. *Am. J. Dis. Child.* **118:**155–165.
87. **Meyer, H. M., Jr., P. D. Parkman, and T. C. Panos.** 1966. Attenuated rubella virus. II. Production of an experimental live-virus vaccine and clinical trial. *N. Engl. J. Med.* **275:**575–580.
88. **Miki, N. P., and J. K. Chantler.** 1992. Differential ability of wild-type and vaccine strains of rubella virus to replicate and persist in human joint tissue. *Clin. Exp. Rheumatol.* **10:**3–12.
89. **Miller, E., J. E. Cradock-Watson, and T. M. Pollock.** 1982. Consequences of confirmed maternal rubella at successive stages of pregnancy. *Lancet* **ii:**781–784.
90. **Miller, E., P. Waight, C. P. Farrington, N. Andrews, J. Stowe, and B. Taylor.** 2001. Idiopathic thrombocytopenic purpura and MMR vaccine. *Arch. Dis. Child.* **84:**227–229.
91. **Mori, T., and K. Shiozawa.** 1985. Suppression of tuberculin hypersensitivity caused by rubella infection. *Am. Rev. Respir. Dis.* **131:**886–888.
92. **Mubareka, S., H. Richards, M. Gray, and G. A. Tipples.** 2007. Evaluation of commercial rubella immunoglobulin G avidity assays. *J. Clin. Microbiol.* **45:**231–233.
93. **Murch, S. H., A. Anthony, D. H. Casson, M. Malik, M. Berelowitz, A. P. Dhillon, M. A. Thomson, A. Valentine, S. E. Davies, and J. A. Walker-Smith.** 2004. Retraction of an interpretation. *Lancet* **363:**750.
94. **Naeye, R. L., and W. Blanc.** 1965. Pathogenesis of congenital rubella. *JAMA* **194:**1277–1283.
95. **Ovsyannikova, I. G., R. M. Jacobson, J. E. Ryan, N. Dhiman, R. A. Vierkant, and G. A. Poland.** 2007. Relationship between HLA polymorphisms and gamma interferon and interleukin-10 cytokine production in healthy individuals after rubella vaccination. *Clin. Vaccine Immunol.* **14:**115–122.
96. **Ovsyannikova, I. G., R. M. Jacobson, R. A. Vierkant, V. S. Pankratz, and G. A. Poland.** 2007. HLA supertypes and immune responses to measles-mumps-rubella viral vaccine: findings and implications for vaccine design. *Vaccine* **25:**3090–3100.
97. **Parkman, P. D., E. L. Buescher, and M. S. Artenstein.** 1962. Recovery of rubella virus from army recruits. *Proc. Soc. Exp. Biol. Med.* **111:**225–230.
98. **Parkman, P. D., E. L. Buescher, M. S. Artenstein, J. M. McCown, F. K. Mundon, and A. D. Druzd.** 1964. Studies of rubella. I. Properties of the virus. *J. Immunol.* **93:**595–607.
99. **Parkman, P. D., P. E. Phillips, R. L. Kirschstein, and H. M. Meyer, Jr.** 1965. Experimental rubella virus infection in the rhesus monkey. *J. Immunol.* **95:**743–752.
100. **Parkman, P. D., P. E. Phillips, and H. M. Meyer, Jr.** 1965. Experimental rubella virus infection in pregnant monkeys. *Am. J. Dis. Child.* **110:**390–394.
101. **Pattison, J. R.** 1975. Persistence of specific IgM after natural infection with rubella virus. *Lancet* **i:**185–187.
102. **Peckham, C. S.** 1972. Clinical and laboratory study of children exposed in utero to maternal rubella. *Arch. Dis. Child.* **47:**571–577.
103. **Perkins, F. T.** 1985. Licensed vaccines. *Rev. Infect. Dis.* **7**(Suppl. 1)**:**S73–S76.
104. **Pettersson, R. F., C. Oker-Blom, N. Kalkkinen, A. Kallio, I. Ulmanen, L. Kaariainen, P. Partanen, and A. Vaheri.** 1985. Molecular and antigenic characteristics and synthesis of rubella virus structural proteins. *Rev. Infect. Dis.* **7**(Suppl. 1)**:**S140–S149.
105. **Plotkin, S. A.** 2006. The history of rubella and rubella vaccination leading to elimination. *Clin. Infect. Dis.* **43**(Suppl. 3)**:**S164–S168.
106. **Plotkin, S. A.** 1988. Rubella vaccine, p. 235–262. *In* S. A. Plotkin and E. A. Mortimer, Jr. (ed.), *Vaccines*. The W. B. Saunders Co., Philadelphia, PA.
107. **Plotkin, S. A.** 1969. Rubella virus, p. 364. *In* E. H. Lennette and N. J. Schmidt (ed.), *Diagnostic Procedures for Viral and Rickettsial Infections*. American Public Health Association, New York, NY.
108. **Plotkin, S. A., J. D. Farquhar, M. Katz, and F. Buser.** 1969. Attenuation of RA 27-3 rubella virus in WI-38 human diploid cells. *Am. J. Dis. Child.* **118:**178–185.
109. **Plotkin, S. A., M. Katz, and J. F. Cordero.** 1999. The eradication of rubella. *JAMA* **281:**561–562.
110. **Plotkin, S. A., R. M. Klaus, and J. P. Whitely.** 1966. Hypogammaglobulinemia in an infant with congenital rubella syndrome; failure of 1-adamantane to stop virus excretion. *J. Pediatr.* **69:**1085–1091.
111. **Pollard, R. B., and E. A. Edwards.** 1975. Epidemiologic survey of rubella in a military recruit population. *Am. J. Epidemiol.* **101:**431–437.
112. **Prinzie, A., C. Huygelen, J. Gold, J. Farquhar, and J. McKee.** 1969. Experimental live attenuated rubella virus vaccine. Clinical evaluation of Cendehill strain. *Am. J. Dis. Child.* **118:**172–177.

113. **Public Health Laboratory Service Working Party on Rubella.** 1970. Studies of the effect of immunoglobulin on rubella in pregnancy. Report of the Public Health Laboratory Service Working Party on Rubella. *Br. Med. J.* **2:**497–500.
114. **Rawls, W. E., A. Phillips, J. L. Melnick, and M. M. Desmond.** 1967. Persistent virus infection in congenital rubella. *Arch. Ophthalmol.* **77:**430–433.
115. **Ray, P., S. Black, H. Shinefield, A. Dillon, J. Schwalbe, S. Holmes, S. Hadler, R. Chen, S. Cochi, and S. Wassilak for the Vaccine Safety Datalink Team.** 1997. Risk of chronic arthropathy among women after rubella vaccination. *JAMA* **278:**551–556.
116. **Roush, S. W., T. V. Murphy, and the Vaccine-Preventable Disease Working Group.** 2007. Historical comparisons of morbidity and mortality for vaccine-preventable diseases in the United States. *JAMA* **298:** 2155–2163.
117. **Rudolph, A. J., E. B. Singleton, H. S. Rosenberg, D. B. Singer, and C. A. Phillips.** 1965. Osseous manifestations of the congenital rubella syndrome. *Am. J. Dis. Child.* **110:**428–433.
118. **Schiff, G. M., and M. S. Dine.** 1965. Transmission of rubella from newborns. A controlled study among young adult women and report of an unusual case. *Am. J. Dis. Child.* **110:**447–451.
119. **Schiff, G. M., J. L. Sever, and R. J. Huebner.** 1965. Experimental rubella. Clinical and laboratory findings. *Arch. Intern. Med.* **116:**537–543.
120. **Schmidt, N. J., and B. Styk.** 1968. Immunodiffusion reactions with rubella antigens. *J. Immunol.* **101:**210–216.
121. **Sedwick, W. D., and F. Sokol.** 1970. Nucleic acid of rubella virus and its replication in hamster kidney cells. *J. Virol.* **5:**478–489.
122. **Sever, J. L., R. J. Huebner, G. A. Castellano, P. S. Sarma, A. Fabiyi, G. M. Schiff, and C. L. Cusumano.** 1965. Rubella complement fixation test. *Science* **148:** 385–387.
123. **Sever, J. L., G. W. Meier, W. F. Windle, G. M. Schiff, G. R. Monif, and A. Fabiyi.** 1966. Experimental rubella in pregnant rhesus monkeys. *J. Infect. Dis.* **116:**21–26.
124. **Sever, J. L., M. A. South, and K. A. Shaver.** 1985. Delayed manifestations of congenital rubella. *Rev. Infect. Dis.* **7**(Suppl. 1):S164–S169.
125. **Shapiro, L.** 1965. The numbered diseases: first through sixth. *JAMA* **194:**680.
126. **Siemerink, M. J., K. M. Sijssens, J. D. de Groot-Mijnes, and J. H. de Boer.** 2007. Rubella virus-associated uveitis in a nonvaccinated child. *Am. J. Ophthalmol.* **143:**899–900.
127. **Singh, V. K., A. J. Tingle, and M. Schulzer.** 1986. Rubella-associated arthritis. II. Relationship between circulating immune complex levels and joint manifestations. *Ann. Rheum. Dis.* **45:**115–119.
128. **Stewart, G. L., P. D. Parkman, H. E. Hopps, R. D. Douglas, J. P. Hamilton, and H. M. Meyer, Jr.** 1967. Rubella-virus hemagglutination-inhibition test. *N. Engl. J. Med.* **276:**554–557.
129. **Swan, C., A. L. Tostevin, H. Mayo, et al.** 1944. Further observations on congenital defects in infants following infectious diseases during pregnancy, with special reference to rubella. *Med. J. Aust.* **1:**409–413.
130. **Swan, C., A. L. Tostevin, B. Moore, et al.** 1943. Congenital defects in infants following infectious diseases during pregnancy. With special reference to the relationship between German measles and cataract, deaf-mutism, heart disease and microcephaly, and to the period of pregnancy in which the occurrence of rubella is followed by congenital abnormalities. *Med. J. Aust.* **2:** 201–210.
131. **Terry, G. M., L. Ho-Terry, R. C. Warren, C. H. Rodeck, A. Cohen, and K. R. Rees.** 1986. First trimester prenatal diagnosis of congenital rubella: a laboratory investigation. *Br. Med. J. (Clin. Res. Ed.)* **292:**930–933.
132. **Tingle, A. J., M. Allen, R. E. Petty, G. D. Kettyls, and J. K. Chantler.** 1986. Rubella-associated arthritis. I. Comparative study of joint manifestations associated with natural rubella infection and RA 27/3 rubella immunisation. *Ann. Rheum. Dis.* **45:**110–114.
133. **Tingle, A. J., L. A. Mitchell, M. Grace, P. Middleton, R. Mathias, L. MacWilliam, and A. Chalmers.** 1997. Randomised double-blind placebo-controlled study on adverse effects of rubella immunisation in seronegative women. *Lancet* **349:**1277–1281.
134. **Tondury, G., and D. W. Smith.** 1966. Fetal rubella pathology. *J. Pediatr.* **68:**867–879.
135. **Townsend, J. J., J. R. Baringer, J. S. Wolinsky, N. Malamud, J. P. Mednick, H. S. Panitch, R. A. Scott, L. Oshiro, and N. E. Cremer.** 1975. Progressive rubella panencephalitis. Late onset after congenital rubella. *N. Engl. J. Med.* **292:**990–993.
136. **Transactions of the International Congress of Medicine.** 1881. *Trans. Intl. Congr. Med.* **4:**14–34.
137. **Ueda, K., F. Sasaki, K. Tokugawa, K. Segawa, and H. Fujii.** 1984. The 1976–1977 rubella epidemic in Fukuoka city in southern Japan: epidemiology and incidences of complications among 80,000 persons who were school children at 28 primary schools and their family members. *Biken J.* **27:**161–168.
138. **Ueda, K., K. Tokugawa, J. Fukushige, H. Yoshikawa, and S. Nonaka.** 1987. Hemagglutination inhibition antibodies in congenital rubella syndrome. A 17-year follow-up in the Ryukyu Islands. *Am. J. Dis. Child.* **141:** 211–212.
139. **Vaheri, A., and T. Vesikari.** 1971. Small size rubella virus antigens and soluble immune complexes: analysis by the platelet aggregation technique. *Arch. Gesamte Virusforsch.* **35:**10–24.
140. **Veale, H.** 1866. History of epidemic of Rotheln, with observations on its pathology. *Edinb. Med. J.* **12:**404–414.
141. **Vejtorp, M.** 1978. Enzyme-linked immunosorbent assay for determination of rubella IgG antibodies. *Acta Pathol. Microbiol. Scand. Sect. B* **86B:**387–392.
142. **Vergani, D., P. Morgan-Capner, E. T. Davies, A. W. Anderson, D. E. Tee, and J. R. Pattison.** 1980. Joint symptoms, immune complexes, and rubella. *Lancet* **ii:** 321–322.
143. **Wakefield, A. J., S. H. Murch, A. Anthony, J. Linnell, D. M. Casson, M. Malik, M. Berelowitz, A. P. Dhillon, M. A. Thomson, P. Harvey, A. Valentine, S. E. Davies, and J. A. Walker-Smith.** 1998. Ileal-lymphoid-nodular hyperplasia, non-specific colitis, and pervasive developmental disorder in children. *Lancet* **351:**637–641.
144. **Wallis, C., J. L. Melnick, and F. Rapp.** 1965. Different effects of MgC12 and MgSO4 on the thermostability of viruses. *Virology* **26:**694–699.
145. **Watson, J. C., S. C. Hadler, C. A. Dykewicz, S. Reef, and L. Phillips.** 1998. Measles, mumps, and rubella—vaccine use and strategies for elimination of measles, rubella, and congenital rubella syndrome and control of mumps: recommendations of the Advisory Committee on Immunization Practices (ACIP). *Morb. Mortal. Wkly. Rep. Recomm. Rep.* **47:**1–57.
146. **Weller, T. H., and F. A. Neva.** 1962. Propagation in tissue culture of cytopathic agents from patients with

rubella-like illness. *Proc. Soc. Exp. Biol. Med.* **111:**215–225.

147. **Wesselhoeft, C.** 1947. Rubella (German measles). *N. Engl. J. Med.* **236:**943–950.
148. **Wesselhoeft, C.** 1947. Rubella (German measles) (concluded). *N. Engl. J. Med.* **236:**978–988.
149. **Wilkins, J., J. M. Leedom, B. Portnoy, and M. A. Salvatore.** 1969. Reinfection with rubella virus despite live vaccine induced immunity. Trials of HPV-77 and HPV-80 live rubella virus vaccines and subsequent artificial and natural challenge studies. *Am. J. Dis. Child.* **118:** 275–294.
150. **Wilkins, J., J. M. Leedom, M. A. Salvatore, and B. Portnoy.** 1972. Clinical rubella with arthritis resulting from reinfection. *Ann. Intern. Med.* **77:**930–932.
151. **Willan (cited by G. Gregory).** 1843. *Lectures on the Eruptive Fevers*, p. 102. Henry Renshaw, London, United Kingdom.
152. **Witte, J. J., A. W. Karchmer, G. Case, K. L. Herrmann, E. Abrutyn, I. Kassanoff, and J. S. Neill.** 1969. Epidemiology of rubella. *Am. J. Dis. Child.* **118:**107–111.
153. **Wolinsky, J. S.** 1990. Rubella, p. 815–838. *In* B. N. Fields, D. M. Knipe, R. M. Chanock, M. S. Hirsch, J. L. Melnick, T. P. Monath, and B. Roizman (ed.), *Virology*, 2nd ed. Raven Press, New York, NY.
154. **Wolinsky, J. S., P. C. Dau, E. Buimovici-Klein, J. Mednick, B. O. Berg, P. B. Lang, and L. Z. Cooper.** 1979. Progressive rubella panencephalitis: immunovirological studies and results of isoprinosine therapy. *Clin. Exp. Immunol.* **35:**397–404.
155. **Zhao, L. H., Y. Y. Ma, H. Wang, S. P. Zhao, W. M. Zhao, H. Li, and L. Y. Wang.** 2006. Establishment and application of a TaqMan real-time quantitative reverse transcription-polymerase chain reaction assay for rubella virus RNA. *Acta Biochim. Biophys. Sin.* **38:**731–736.
156. **Zheng, D. P., T. K. Frey, J. Icenogle, S. Katow, E. S. Abernathy, K. J. Song, W. B. Xu, V. Yarulin, R. G. Desjatskova, Y. Aboudy, G. Enders, and M. Croxson.** 2003. Global distribution of rubella virus genotypes. *Emerg. Infect. Dis.* **9:**1523–1530.

Hepatitis D Virus

ANTONINA SMEDILE, ALESSIA CIANCIO, AND MARIO RIZZETTO

56

Hepatitis delta virus (HDV) is a defective minus-strand RNA virus that accelerates disease progression upon superinfection of hepatitis B carriers. This virus was recognized in the late 1970s as a new cause of hepatitis. The cloning and sequencing of the viral genome in 1986 established the peculiar features that make HDV unique among animal viruses. The biological features resemble those of plant RNA viruses such as the viroids and satellite RNAs.

VIROLOGY

HDV is the only member of the family *Deltaviridae*, genus *Deltavirus* (52). To establish infection in vivo, HDV depends on helper functions provided by hepatitis B virus (HBV). The HDV virion is a chimera composed of the HDV RNA genome and an antigen (HDAg), both enveloped by the surface antigen of HBV (HBsAg) (Fig. 1). Several genotypes of HDV with different geographic and demographic distributions and clinical pathogenicity (121) (Table 1) have been identified by comparative phylogenetic analysis. HDV exhibits 81 to 89% homology in nucleotide sequences within the same genotype. There is 27 to 34% divergence in nucleotide sequences between different genotypes (21). A lesser degree of heterogeneity was revealed in a novel genotype (II b) closely related to genotype II and in mixed HDV genotypes (I-II) reported in Taiwan, Japan, and Russia (48, 136). Recently, studies of HDV genome variability in highly divergent groups (African origin) suggest an ancient African lineage of *Deltavirus* among at least seven major clades or genotypes (98). Two serotypes of HDV have been identified (124).

Genome Structure

The genome consists of a circular, rod-shaped, single minus-strand RNA (Fig. 2) (39). The biological features conform to those of plant RNA viruses such as the viroids and satellite RNAs (125). The HDV particle isolated from sera of humans, chimpanzees, and woodchucks is 35 to 41 nm in diameter. Similar to plant virus RNAs, it is self-complementary and folds into an unbranched rod structure in which about 70% of the nucleotides are base paired (123). Three major RNA species have been found in infected cells and humans. The first is the 1.7-kb genomic RNA of negative polarity, which is predominant in the virions; the second is the complementary antigenomic RNA of positive polarity, which is present in greater amounts in the liver; and the third is a polyadenylated mRNA that is shorter than full-length genome RNA (0.8 kb) and is present in lesser amounts in the liver (126).

Like subviral agents of plants, HDV replicates through a rolling-circle mechanism. HDV RNA has two unique features that are crucial to this type of replication. The first is transcription by a host RNA polymerase II, and the second is the presence of a ribozyme conferring autocatalytic capacity (self-cleavage and self-ligation) for both the genomic and antigenomic strands (31). This type of replication produces linear multimers of both genomic and antigenomic RNAs, whose self-cleaving activity processes the RNAs to unit length. The autocatalytic RNA segments have been isolated and studied in vitro (63). Peculiar to the HDV ribozyme is its sensitivity to denaturants and lack of requirement for specific metal ions (20). It is the fastest naturally occurring self-cleaving RNA required for viability in a human pathogen. It is different from the hammerhead ribozymes described in plant viruses, suggesting that the catalytic domain of HDV RNA represents a new and different ribozyme motif (87). Mutagenesis and biochemical analyses support the concept that it has a pseudoknot structure (46).

The recent crystallization of the HDV ribozyme has provided a three-dimensional scaffold for understanding the mode of action of the RNA catalyst. The HDV RNA molecule is made by a compact catalytic core that comprises five helical segments connected in an intricate nested double pseudoknot (86). Despite the modest size of the HDV ribozyme, a complex three-dimensional architecture is generated; the cleft in the active site, produced by the juxtaposition of the helices and strand crossover with the surrounding biochemical backbone and base functional groups, is reminiscent of protein enzymes. The finding that the HDV ribozyme is capable of a process called base catalysis during self-cleavage sheds new light not only on the mechanism of RNA catalysis but also on the chemical evolution of RNA in a hypothetical probiotic RNA world (111). The features of the genomic ribozyme are illustrated in Fig. 3. The absences of the capping loop L4 and the helical crossover J1/2, which tightly interlace the two helical stacks of the ribozyme, significantly and independently impact the catalytic activity of the HDV ribozyme (128).

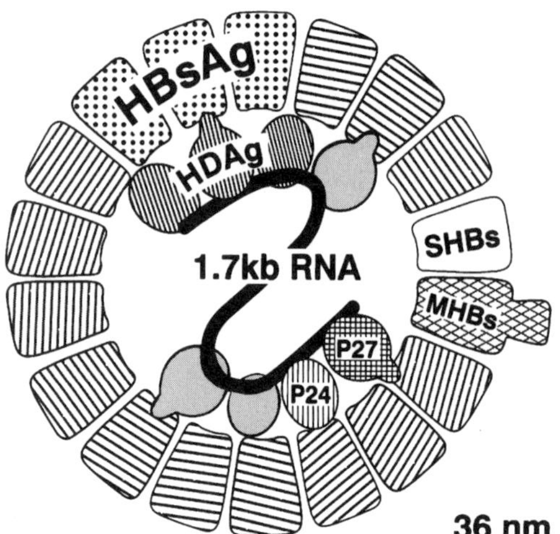

FIGURE 1 Schematic representation of HDV.

A U-turn motif (U-1) confers fast site-specific catalysis, which is also critical for double-rolling-circle replication of the virus (112). Further studies using a mutant with a mutation of the C-41 motif provide insight into the positioning and thermodynamic linkage of two metal ions (Mg^{2+} and H^+) and protons involved and influencing the self-cleavage activity of the ribozyme (75). Both the genomic and antigenomic ribozymes of HDV cleave faster in the presence of divalent metal ions than in monovalent cations, with the genomic form cleaving moderately faster in the presence of Mg^{2+} than of Ca^{2+} while the reverse is true for the antigenomic ribozyme. The metal ion reactivity preference correlates with a single U in the genomic sequence and a C in the antigenomic sequence (88). The HDV ribozyme carries out general acid-base catalysis by using the C-75 base and a divalent metal ion (89, 107) (Fig. 3).

Proteins and Transcription

HDV encodes a single protein, the HDAg, which is translated from a 0.8-kb mRNA transcribed from the genomic RNA. Transcription produces two isoforms of the HDV protein (large [L-HDAg] and small [S-HDAg]) that are identical in sequence except that the large isoform contains 19 additional amino acids at its carboxyl terminus (Fig. 4) (69). The HDV proteins contain several functional domains that are essential for viral replication, assembly, propagation, and spread of the virus in the liver: (i) a coiled-coil-rich domain that mediates formation of HDAg dimers, (ii) arginine-rich motifs that are necessary for RNA binding activity, (iii) an isoprenylation signal sequence at the C terminus, and (iv) a nuclear localization signal required for HDV RNA to be transported to the nucleus for RNA replication after HDV infection. The nuclear import of HDAg-HDV RNA complex is mediated by kariopherin (or importin) α-2B (74). The two forms of HDAg, HDAg-p24 and HDAg-p27, are derived from the same open reading frame during the replication cycle of HDV through a specific posttranscriptional RNA editing process that changes the coding capacity of the viral genome (92). HDV RNA is modified such that the amber stop codon (UAG) for S-HDAg is converted to a tryptophan codon (UGG). This modification occurs at an adenosine at position 1012 in the antigenomic RNA. HDV RNA editing was documented initially in transfected cells but also occurs in infected humans, chimpanzees, and woodchucks (25). A host double-stranded RNA adenosine deaminase that acts on RNA (ADARs) is responsible for the editing in the antigenomic strand (91). Of the two host genes (ADAR1 and ADAR2) responsible for RNA editing via deamination of adenosines in double-stranded RNAs, ADAR1a is primarily responsible for editing HDV genotypes I, II, and III (61). Mammalian cells express two forms of ADAR1, a large form (ADAR1-L) that localizes mainly to the cytoplasm and a small form (ADAR1-S) that resides in the nucleus. Using vectors that overexpress either form and specific ADAR1 small interfering RNAs, it was shown that ADAR1-S edits HDV RNA during replication and that editing occurs in the nucleus (62); overexpression of ADARs inhibits HDV RNA replication and compromises viral viability (134).

The efficiency of the editing process is variable in different genotypes and isolates, as shown by the variable levels of virion RNA in serum, which range from 10 to 35% over the course of replication (24). The editing at position 1012, referred to as the amber/W site, requires a highly conserved base-paired structure within the unbranched rod

TABLE 1 Genotypes of HDV

Genotype	Subgroup	Region(s) where detected	Yr detected	Reference
I	IA	United States, Europe, Middle East	1993	21
	IB	Northern and southern Italy	1995	Niro et al.[a]
II	IIA	Japan and Taiwan	1991	59
	IIB	Japan and Taiwan	1995	137
III		Colombia, Venezuela, Peru (northern region of South America)	1995	26
IV		Africa	2004	98
V		Africa	2004	98
VI		Africa	2004	98

[a] G. Niro, A. Smedile, A. Andriulli, M. Rizzetto, J. L. Gerin, and J. L. Casey, The predominance of hepatitis delta virus genotype I among chronically infected Italian patients, *Hepatology* **25:**728–734, 1997.

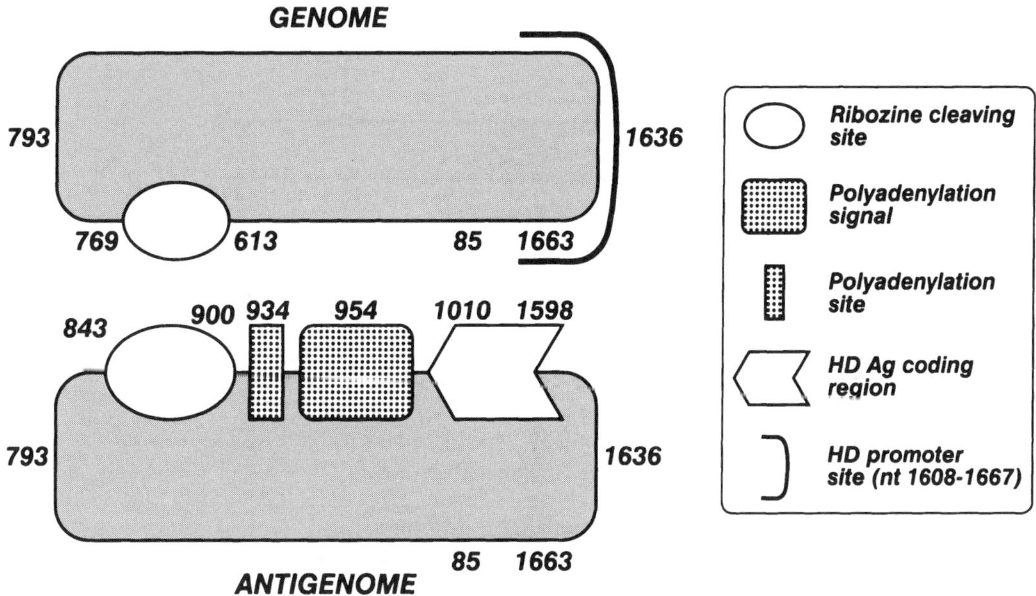

FIGURE 2 HDV RNA genome structure.

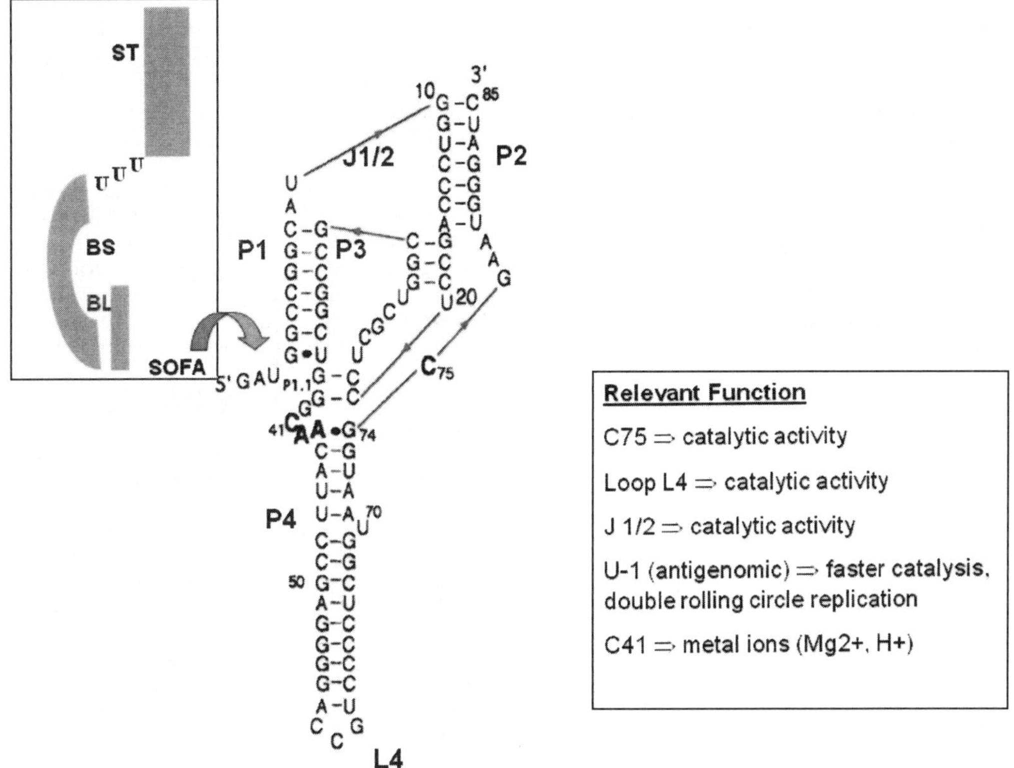

FIGURE 3 Sequence and secondary structure of the HDV genomic ribozyme. In the left box the specific on/off adaptor (SOFA) delta ribozyme module is shown. BL, blocker; BS, biosensor; ST, stabilizer. A search for ribozymes in the human genome map showed that a ribozyme segment structurally and biochemically related to the HDV ribozyme is contained in a conserved mammalian sequence residing in an intron of the CPEB3 gene, which belongs to a family of genes regulating mRNA polyadenylation (107). On the basis of these observations, it is thought that HDV ribozymes and the CPEB3 ribozyme are evolutionarily related and that HDV may have arisen from the human transcriptome.

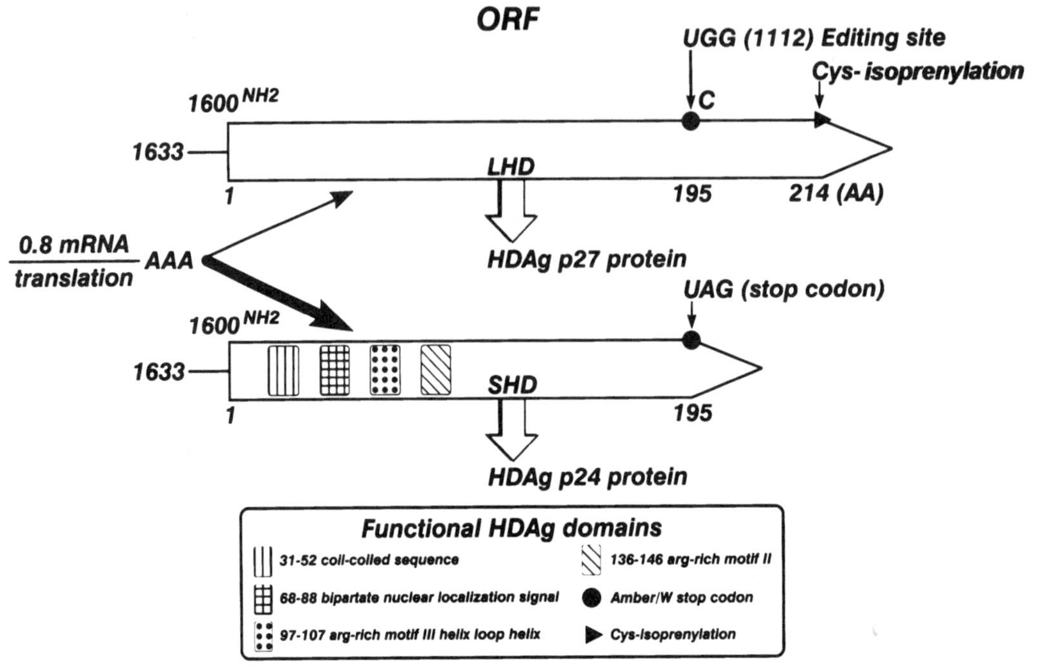

FIGURE 4 HDAg gene and protein domains. ORF, open reading frame.

structure of HDV RNA. HDAg-p24 promotes HDV replication and is produced by infectious RNA. HDAg-p27 inhibits replication and is required for virion assembly. The specificity of HDV editing in transfected cells expressing HDV RNAs does not require either virus replication or HDAg. However, HDAg is able to suppress the editing that occurs at the amber/W site and thus could play a role in regulating the efficiency of HDV replication (40). Transcription studies in vitro have demonstrated that a 199-nucleotide genomic-sense RNA molecule containing a region that represents one end of the HDV rod, upstream of the HDAg gene, has promoter activity in vitro (70).

A computer-generated analysis of the secondary structure of HDV promoter has revealed a highly ordered RNA secondary structure with an internal and external bulge region and a stem-loop conserved region between group I and II HDV isolates.

In the case of HDV genotype III, the highly conserved base pairing within the context of the unbranched rod structure is disrupted. This may affect the editing process, causing a significant difference in editing in genotypes I and III, with functional as well as pathogenic implications (19). Genotype II HDV has low RNA-editing efficiency, resulting in lower serum HDV RNA levels compared to genotype I HDV, and secretes fewer viral particles than genotype I; this, in turn, may reduce the extent of infection of hepatocytes (33a).

BIOLOGY

Virus Replication

Since the HDV virion is coated with the envelope proteins of the helper HBV, it is likely that HBV and HDV share a common receptor on the hepatocyte membrane recognized by the pre-S1 domain of the L-HBsAg. Inside the cytoplasm, HDV is transported to the nucleus, where replication occurs. The nuclear localization signal domain identified in the HDAg gene seems to mediate the initial step. The viral genome is then replicated by host DNA-dependent RNA polymerase II, interacting with the specific 199-nucleotide region of the RNA that contains the RNA promoter, allowing the transcription of the only open reading frame of HDAg. In this model, circular genomic RNA is transcribed by polymerase II to yield multimeric linear transcripts of antigenomic sense that undergo autocatalytic cleavage and ligation to produce circular monomeric antigenomic RNA. The antigenomic RNA then serves as a template for replication of circular genomic RNA by similar transcription and processing. Meanwhile, the extent of the editing process regulates the production of the L-HDAg (57). The large form acts as a dominant negative inhibitor of genome replication and is also needed for packaging of HDV RNA into the virus particles. Recent studies suggest that not only RNA polymerase II but also polymerase I or closely related nucleolus-associated polymerase I are involved (66).

Both the L-HBsAg and small HBsAg proteins are required for the encapsidation of HDV. This takes place by budding into the endoplasmic reticulum of the Golgi apparatus of the hepatocyte. Mutants generated by point mutations, small insertions, or deletions at the top of the rod structure may affect HDV replication by reducing its efficiency 100- to 1,000-fold compared to the wild type. The C terminus of the L-HDAg, where most of the genotype-specific sequence divergence is found, is involved in virion formation and inhibition of replication. Substantial variations between the structures of the RNA editing sites of the different genotypes suggest possible effects on the efficiency or mechanisms of editing. These observations suggest the possibility of subtle variations in the strategy of virus replication to accommodate different strains of HBV (26).

Hepatitis delta antigen binds to the clamp of RNA polymerase II and affects its structure and conformation. A recent hypothesis suggested that by loosening the clamp, HDAg may increase the rate of transcriptional elongation and affect transcriptional fidelity in vitro. By binding to the clamp, HDAg has been speculated to affect not only the decision of which nucleotide is incorporated but also the recognition of templates by polymerase II (139).

Infection in Experimental Animals

The host range of HDV infection includes humans, chimpanzees, woodchucks, and ducks carrying HBV-related hepadnaviruses (HBV, woodchuck hepatitis virus [WHV], and duck hepatitis virus (93, 95, 101). Infections in animals have reproduced the modes of HDV infection, coinfection, and superinfection that occur in humans. Infection has also been initiated by direct injection in the liver of HDV cDNA clones capable of generating virions. In transgenic mice not susceptible to HBV infection, direct infection of liver cells with HDV RNA in the absence of helper HBV results in the production of replicative intermediates of HDV and HDAg in the liver (79). A common feature of experimental HDV infection is the inhibition of HBV, shown by a decrease in the levels of HBsAg and HBV DNA in the serum and liver. Serial passage of HDV in chimpanzees and woodchucks has resulted in a shortening of the period of incubation and an increased severity of hepatitis D (96). In chimpanzees, the end-point titer of HDV infectivity may be as low as 10^{11} genomes (101). Studies of woodchucks have addressed whether genetic variations in the HDV genome could be relevant to the course of HDV infection (28),

Growth in Cell Culture

HDV has not been propagated in cell cultures (127). Primary hepatocyte cultures from woodchucks and chimpanzees infected with HDV have yielded a single cycle of replication in a small proportion of cells. A novel cell culture system maintaining a low level of continuous HDV genome replication has been described (32). With this model it was shown that the length of the RNA genome was maintained throughout 1 year of replication, except for some single-nucleotide deletions and insertions. Only single-nucleotide substitutions, with a prevalence of base transitions rather than transversions, were observed. These genetic changes did not affect the ability of HDV genome to replicate (33). Sequence stability was likewise observed in patients with chronic HDV infection who were monitored for decades (personal observation).

EPIDEMIOLOGY

Transmission

The parenteral route is the most efficient for HDV transmission; this explains the high rates of infection in drug addicts and hemophiliacs (84). The screening of blood for HBV infection has led to the virtual elimination of the risk of posttransfusion hepatitis D infection. The risk of HDV infection in medical personnel, hemodialysis units, and institutionalized patients has varied depending on the standards of HBV control. With improvement in HBV prophylaxis in developed countries, HDV infection in these settings has become rare (77). Infection has also declined in injection drug users.

Transmission of HDV in areas of endemic infection in the developing world occurs through inapparent parenteral routes; poor hygiene and overcrowding favor the spread of the virus. Sexual transmission has been documented in prostitutes and sexual partners of HDV-infected carriers (68). In southern Italy, cohabitation with an HDV carrier was identified as a major risk for HDV transmission (9). Body piercing and tattooing may represent modes of transmission (34, 71).

Geographic Distribution and Risk Factors

HDV infection is present worldwide (102). Prevalence rates in patients with chronic HBsAg-positive liver diseases have varied from less than 1% in temperate and cold climates to more than 30% in several tropical and subtropical countries. A major determinant of the prevalence of hepatitis D is the prevalence of HBV infection. In Europe, the improved control of HBV achieved in recent years has led to a marked decline of HDV infection. Public health measures to control the AIDS epidemic have also had an impact on the transmission of both HBV and HDV, which are transmitted through the same routes as human immunodeficiency virus (HIV). Among clinical categories, the highest prevalence of HDV infection is found in patients with advanced liver diseases (cirrhosis) and older patients (the highest prevalence is in patients older than 50 years). One Italian study (51) found that the prevalence of anti-HDV antibodies in chronic HBsAg carriers was 8.3% in 1997 compared to 14% in 1992 and 23% in 1987; however, another survey of chronic HBV carriers in Italy in 2007 found an 8 to 10% prevalence of HDV infection. The recent wave of immigrants from Eastern European and North African countries where HBV is still endemic may account for this finding; an impact of immigration on resurgence of HDV infection also has been noted in other European countries (132). More accurate testing for HDV as a consequence of the screening for HBV markers in patients undergoing nucleoside analogue therapy has also led to an increased recognition of HDV infection (55).

Risk factors associated with HDV infection included cohabitation with an anti-HDV-positive subject, intravenous drug abuse, residence in southern Italy, and cirrhosis.

New HDV infections have been reported recently in regions experiencing economic growth, such as Turkey, India, Russia, Egypt, and China. In these countries, HDV infection is present in 10 to 20% of infected HBV chronic carriers due to the rapid spread of drug addiction and other high-risk behavior (2, 122, 140). In Mongolia a high prevalence of HDV infection was also reported among apparently healthy adults (60), and despite a moderate endemicity for HBV infection, high rates of HDV coinfection were observed in Bangladesh (141).

Foci of infection have been identified in St. Petersburg, Russia (49); the island of Okinawa in Japan (106); and villages in China (6), northern India (115), and Albania (36). Another emerging hot spot for HDV infection is Samara (formerly Kuibyshev), a city in eastern European Russia; over 30% of patients with acute HBV infection are also coinfected with HDV (49). Regions of northern South America (Peru, Colombia, Ecuador, and Venezuela, in particular the subtropical area close to the jungle), as well as areas of northern India (115), remain an important reservoir for epidemics of HDV infection (26). Injection drug abusers remain at high risk of HDV infection in metropolitan areas, as shown by the recent outbreak reported in Washington, DC, during which 3 of 12 patients with acute hepatitis B plus HDV coinfection had a fulminant course and died (8).

HDV infection remains the second most common recognized cause of fulminant viral hepatitis worldwide (110). Severe outbreaks of hepatitis D have been reported in the Yupca Indians of South America, where HDV continues to be highly endemic despite efforts to implement HBV vaccination. In this setting, hepatitis D is acquired predominantly through superinfection (116).

Analysis of HDV RNA sequences reveals three major genotypes with different geographic and demographic distributions (85). Genotype I is predominant in the United States, Europe, and the Middle East; genotype II has been isolated in Japan and Taiwan; and genotype III is the only genotype isolated in the northern region of South America, where genotype F of HBV predominates (76). In Taiwan, a new genotype (genotype IV or a subtype of genotype II) has been identified (106). A recent sequence analysis of HDV isolated from sera of African origin and a comparison of the sequence with already available HDV sequences indicated the presence of additional genotypes, leading to subgrouping of HDV sequences into seven genotypes.

PATHOGENESIS

Virus Factors

The pattern of disease associated with chronic HDV infections may vary in different epidemiological settings. Relatively benign forms of liver disease and asymptomatic carriage of HDV have been reported to occur in some areas where HDV is endemic. However, in the areas of most heavily endemic infection, like South America (Venezuela, Colombia, Peru, and Ecuador), the course of HDV disease is often severe; a subfulminant or fulminant course has been observed in aboriginal communities and military personnel stationed in the Amazon jungles. The outcome is also severe in areas where HDV is not endemic (northern Europe and North America) and most of the patients are intravenous drug abusers. Interest in explaining the different patterns of infection has focused on geographic genetic diversity and virus interactions. Genotype III seems to correlate with the severe and fulminant acute hepatitis D among the Yupca Indians in Venezuela (56). Likewise, virologic analysis of HDV and HBV strains responsible for an outbreak that occurred in 1992 and 1993 among troops stationed at four jungle outposts in Peru demonstrated that the HDV isolate was exclusively of genotype III and the HBV isolate was of genotype F (27, 97).

Genotype II HDV, isolated in the Irabu islands of Okinawa, Japan, seems to cause only a mild form of HDV infection. In this area of endemic HBV-HDV infection, 210 (9.5%) of 2,207 subjects tested were HBsAg positive and 47 (22.4%) of them were positive for anti-HDV. Of 43 subjects with anti-HDV, 21 were positive for HDV RNA by PCR assay. Subjects with anti-HDV from this population rarely exhibited biochemical alterations or histologic lesions in the liver. The HDV isolates obtained from these patients were phylogenetically identified as a new genotypic subgroup within HDV genotype II and classified as II b; all had a T-to-C nucleotide change at position 1014. This mutation is also seen in HDV genotype I isolated from Nauru and in Greek isolates. The finding of genotype I isolates with the 1014 C mutation is also associated with less severe liver disease.

Genotype I, prevalent in Italy and North America, is heterogeneous. Phylogenetic analysis of 46 HDV samples from Italian carriers of HDV has shown that this genotype segregates into two major subgroups (IA and IB), although no clear correlation with disease severity was found. This type of phylogenetic analysis may help to track the transmission of HDV among drug addicts and their families (80, 137).

Pathology and Pathological Mechanisms

The liver histologic pattern of hepatitis D is nonspecific and is similar to other types of viral hepatitis (see chapter 5). In outbreaks in South America, HDV superinfection induced peculiar histologic features, characterized by extensive small-droplet steatosis in hepatocytes with necrosis as well as portal lymphocytic infiltration. The intralobular inflammatory cells were mainly macrophages containing periodic acid-Schiff-positive nonglycogenic granules. These cells, called morula cells, were first described during the outbreak of Labrea fever in the Amazon River and were shown to contain HDAg (37). HDV-associated microsteatosis has also been described in other cases of hepatitis D and in experimentally infected woodchucks that died after acute HDV hepatitis (F. Callea and A. Ponzetto, personal observation). The mechanism underlying this cytopathology is not understood. Possibly the overload of cellular organelles with virus gene products (about 300,000 copies of HDV RNA per cell) results in the storage of fat or phospholipids typical for this type of cell damage. Clusters of shrunken apoptotic hepatocytes with deeply acidophilic cytoplasm, in which the nucleus is absent or undergoing pyknosis, are often seen in hepatitis D. These cells have irregular outlines and sometimes assume irregular or rhomboid shapes (129).

The role of the immune system in HDV disease is incompletely understood. T-cell responses, responsible for cytotoxic effects in the liver, have been suggested (78), and HDV elicits humoral immune responses of the immunoglobulin M (IgM) and IgG classes. Resolved HDV infection induces immunity from early reinfection. Chronic HBV carrier chimpanzees reinfected with HDV 6 months after recovering from a previous HDV infection exhibited no hepatitis after the rechallenge whereas animals rechallenged 4 to 5 years after the primary HDV infection developed a mild and transient HDV infection, indicating that specific immunity might wane with time (94). On the other hand, T-cell responsiveness to HDAg in peripheral blood mononuclear cells isolated from individuals chronically infected with HDV has been correlated with reduced active disease. Chronic HDV infection in experimentally infected woodchucks correlated with clustered genetic variations that may provide escape from host immune pressure (59). Changes in the HDAg immunogenic domains may occur in patients chronically infected with HDV, with the production of HDV genetic diversity (138).

Vaccine consisting of the adjuvanted small nucleoprotein, sHDAg (p24), was used to study humoral and T-cell-mediated responses to HDAg in woodchucks chronically infected with WHV. Vaccination with HDAg induced humoral and cellular responses (Th-1 and Th-2 inducer), with a favorable outcome. The use of this vaccine in the woodchuck model has shown a potential to clear the virus from the liver (41). Vaccination with HDV DNA vaccine was also tested in woodchucks. Although immunized animals were not protected from HDV superinfection, the course of infection was milder, HDV viremia occurred later, fluctuations of HDV RNA levels were absent, and

HDV antibodies were not detectable (47). Following DNA vaccination, HDV antibody levels increased. The immune responses generated by L-HDAg- and S-HDAg-encoding DNA vaccines are different. DNA vaccine generated in mice with L-HDAg demonstrated a low humoral immunogenicity. HDV antibody levels were not improved by different dosage, gene gun immunization, or in vivo electroporation (114). The isoprenylation motif can mask the epitope at residues 174 to 195 of HDAg but does not interfere with cellular immunity following DNA-based immunization (58). The capacity to mount a strong $CD8^+$ T-cell response to DNA-based immunization with L-HDAg in different mouse haplotypes was demonstrated. The cytotoxic T-lymphocyte response to HDV antigens also appeared to protect against tumor formation and growth in mice (73).

CLINICAL MANIFESTATIONS

Acute Infection

Coinfection and Superinfection

No clinical feature differentiates acute hepatitis D from other types of acute viral hepatitis. The clinical presentation of acute HDV infection acquired through coinfection with HBV varies from simple enzymatic alterations to fulminant disease. Serologic profiles vary with the severity of clinical disease (Fig. 5). With subclinical and mild hepatitis, viremia is not detectable and coinfection by HDV is recognized only from the delayed rise in the titers of the IgM and IgG antibodies to HDV. In severe disease there is early viremia (HDAg and HDV RNA in serum) followed by seroconversion first to IgM and then to IgG antibody to HDV. IgM responses wane in a few weeks and IgG responses wane after a few months, usually leaving no serologic evidence of prior HDV infection (4, 118). Of note, the majority of patients with acute hepatitis D in Italy in recent years have required hospitalization, suggesting that the overall course is more severe than that of acute hepatitis B alone (105). Acute coinfection resolves in over 95% of cases.

Primary HDV disease acquired after superinfection is usually severe and is accompanied by jaundice and liver dysfunction; it has a worse prognosis than the form acquired by coinfection (110). Subclinical liver disease due to HBV can suddenly decompensate due to the superimposed acute hepatitis type D. In such patients early HDV viremia is a frequent finding, followed by brisk rises in IgM and IgG antibody levels. Superinfection advances to chronicity in over 70% of cases (Fig. 6). In superinfection that resolves, the IgM antibody level wanes in a few weeks and the IgG antibody level persists for 1 to 2 years. In superinfections that progress to chronicity, levels of both antibodies rise to high titers and persist (44).

The IgM antibody in patients with chronic infections is composed mainly of monomeric 7S IgM molecules, in contrast to the predominance of 19S pentameric molecules in those with acute infections (12).

Serum HDAg in patients with chronic infections is not detectable by ordinary immunologic assays because the antigen is masked in immune complexes (104).

Chronic Infection

No specific clinical feature marks the progression of hepatitis D from acute to chronic infection. Chronic infection is characterized by seroconversion to IgG anti-HDV antibody, the increase in the level of IgM anti-HDV antibody, and the persistence of HDV RNA in blood after the acute episode. Chronic HDV infection is rarely observed in healthy carriers of HBsAg. In areas where HDV is endemic, HDV infection is most frequent in cirrhotic patients and in patients with chronic active hepatitis (45). Chronic hepatitis D evolves to cirrhosis more rapidly than HBV infection alone, thus explaining the younger age-specific prevalence (by a decade) of patients with cirrhosis due to HBV-HDV compared with those with cirrhosis due to HBV alone (Tables 2 and 3). Although the progression to cirrhosis is usually rapid, when cirrhosis is established the disease course does not appear to differ from HBV cir-

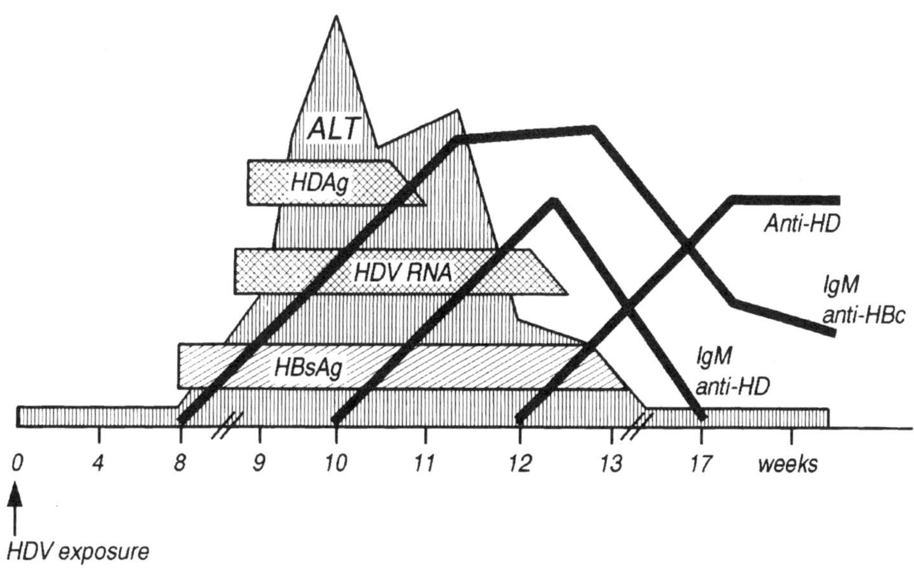

FIGURE 5 Serologic profile of HBV-HDV coinfection.

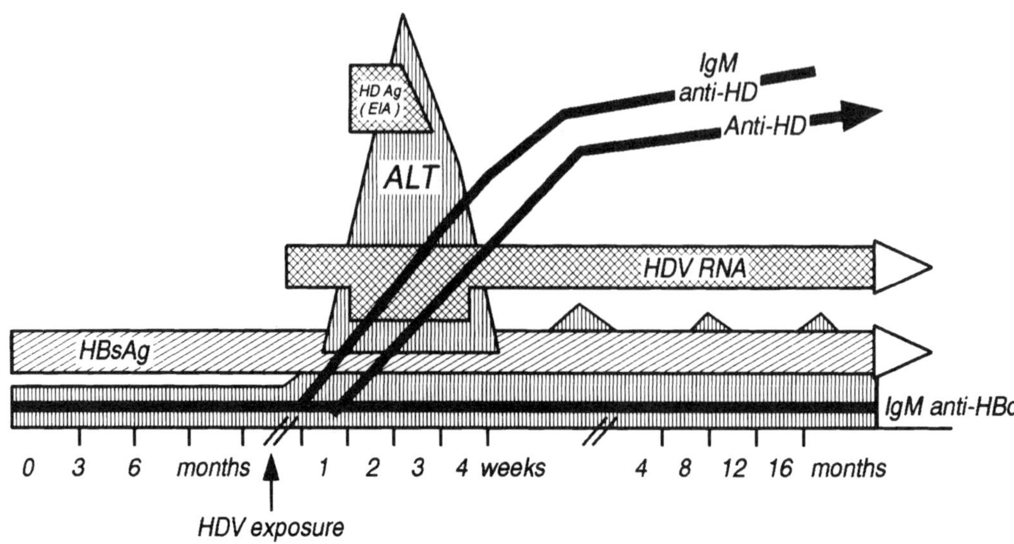

FIGURE 6 Serologic course of HDV superinfection evolving to chronicity.

rhosis. The estimated 5- and 10-year probabilities of survival without the need for liver transplantation in patients with chronic HDV infection compared to those with chronic HBV infection alone are as follows: 98 and 95%, respectively, for patients with chronic active hepatitis; 93 and 64%, respectively, for patients with histologically confirmed cirrhosis; and 49 and 29%, respectively, for patients with clinical cirrhosis. The estimated 93% 5-year survival is comparable to the 84 to 87% 5-year survival of patients with HBsAg-positive histologically confirmed cirrhosis. Natural history studies indicate that the course of HDV liver disease can also be slowly progressive and indolent for decades (38, 103; A. Gioustozi, E. K. Manesis, and S. Hadzyiannis, presented at the Fifth International Symposium of Hepatitis D Virus and Liver Disease, Gold Coast, Australia, 28 to 29 August 1995).

Three clinical phases of HDV liver disease have been proposed: an early stage with active HDV replication and suppression of HBV, a second stage characterized by moderate active disease with decreasing HDV and reactivating HBV levels, and a third late stage characterized either by the development of cirrhosis and hepatocellular carcinoma (HCC) or by remission of inflammation resulting from the reduction of replication of both viruses (67). The HBV status influences the final outcome of HDV disease; a rapid course to liver failure was reported in an Italian study of patients with HDV infection who had an active infection with both HBV and HDV. However, this outcome, typical in drug addicts, was in retrospect associated in some cases with coinfection with HCV (30, 119).

Disease in Children

HDV disease in children is acquired mainly by household contacts and only rarely by vertical transmission (142). The course of chronic HDV infection may be as severe as in adults. In two series from the early 1980s and at the beginning of the 1990s, the prevalence of HDV infection among children with chronic HBsAg-positive cirrhosis was, respectively, 34 and 30%; HDV is very rarely seen in pediatric carriers of HBsAg without liver disease (43). In Mediterranean countries HDV infection represents one of the most important causes of juvenile cirrhosis (13). In Moscow, where the prevalence of HBV infection is still high, HDV RNA was detected in 7 (4.7%) of 149 HBV DNA-positive children tested, 1 (2%) of 50 with acute hepatitis and 6 (8%) of 73 with chronic hepatitis (1).

Coinfections

Longitudinal evaluation of plasma HDV RNA levels in dually or multiply coinfected patients (HBV, HCV) has

TABLE 2 Progression from chronic HDV hepatitis to cirrhosis and liver dysfunction

Study	Yr of study	No. of patients with chronic hepatitis at baseline	Time of follow-up (yr) during study	No. (%) of patients with cirrhosis or liver dysfunction
Rizzetto et al. (102)	1983	75	4	31 (41%)
Buti et al. (15)	1995	66	6.5	14 (21%)
De Man et al. (38)	1995	9	4.8	4 (44%)
Rosina et al.[a]	1995	82	5.5	21 (25%)
Rosina et al. (103)	1999	159	6.8	73 (46%)
Fattovich et al. (45)	2000	39	6.6	12 (31%)

[a] F. Rosina, C. Pintus, and C. Meschievitz, A randomized controlled trial of a 12-month course of recombinant human interferon-alpha in chronic delta (type D) hepatitis: a multicenter Italian study, *Hepatology* **13**:1052–1056, 1991.

TABLE 3 Death (free of transplantation) from HDV cirrhosis

Study	Yr of study	No. of patients with cirrhosis at baseline	Time of follow-up (yr) during study	No. (%) of deaths	Concomitant HCV and/or HIV infection
Rizzetto et al. (102)	1983	26	4	8 (30%)	?
Buti et al. (15)	1995	16	6.5	12 (75%)	+ +
De Man et al. (38)	1995	18	4.8	9 (50%)	+ +
Rosina et al.[a]	1995	66	5.5	34 (51%)	+
Gioustozi et al.[b]	1995				
Archangelos		26	11.6	5 (19%)	–
Rest of Greece		37	5.4	12 (32%)	?
Rosina et al. (103)	1999	73	6.8	22 (30%)	–
Fattovich et al. (45)	2000	39	6.6	3 (15%)	–

[a] F. Rosina, C. Pintus, and C. Meschievitz, A randomized controlled trial of a 12-month course of recombinant human interferon-alpha in chronic delta (type D) hepatitis: a multicenter Italian study, *Hepatology* **13:**1052–1056, 1991.

[b] A. Gioustozi, E. K. Manesis, and S. Hadzyiannis, presented at Fifth International Symposium on Hepatitis D Virus and Liver Disease, Gold Coast, Australia, 28 to 29 August 1995.

shown a spectrum of virologic profiles changing over time. These viral coinfections present a dynamic and evolving profile of virus interactions, and monitoring of the viremic load for each coinfecting virus is essential to make a correct diagnosis and design the appropriate therapeutic regimen (99).

In HDV patients coinfected with both HBV and HCV, HCV viremia is usually suppressed. The inhibition of HCV replication may explain the less severe course of HCV posttransplantation hepatitis in patients multiply infected with HDV, HBV, and HCV compared with those infected with HCV alone (65). Injection drug users at high risk for HIV infection may exhibit triple coinfection with HIV, HBV, and HDV. In one study of 88 HBV-infected drug users in New York, HDV and HIV were present in 67 and 58%, respectively; HDV was associated with severe liver disease, but the severity was not further aggravated by concomitant HIV infection (84). In contrast, in an epidemic of HDV infection in drug users in Milan in the 1980s, patients coinfected with HIV, HBV, and HDV had a greater risk of developing chronic severe hepatitis than did those without HIV infection (16, 17). HDV infection does not affect the clinical, virologic, or immunologic response to highly active antiretroviral therapy but increases the risk of hepatitis flares, liver cirrhosis, hepatic decompensation, and death in patients with HBV-HIV coinfection (113).

Complications

HCC develops at approximately the same rate in chronic HDV carriers as in patients with HBV cirrhosis alone. HCC was the cause of death in 37% of HDV-infected cirrhotic patients monitored for a period of 5 to 10 years. Within 12 years of follow-up in Greece, 40% of HDV-infected subjects with cirrhosis developed HCC (Gioustozi et al., presented at the Fifth International Symposium on Hepatitis D Virus and Liver Disease). Like HCV, HDV can trigger autoimmune reactions. Patients with active HDV disease may develop autoantibodies against nuclear lamina (143), thymocytes, and autoantibodies reactive against the microsomal membranes of the liver and kidney (LKM antibodies) (3, 35, 133). The latter is called LKM3 to distinguish this virus-induced autoantibody from idiopathic LKM1 and LKM2 elicited in hepatitis induced by tienilic acid. LKM3 is directed against a 55-kDa microsomal band containing an antigen of the UDP glucoronyl transferase 1 gene family (UGT1) (90).

LABORATORY DIAGNOSIS

Serologic Diagnosis

HDV viremia can be diagnosed by the finding of HDV RNA or HDAg in serum (117). In coinfection the serologic profile is usually characterized by the presence of IgM antibodies to HBcAg and HBeAg (primary HBV infection) and IgM anti-HDV antibodies. In contrast, in superinfection the long-lasting HBV infection is marked by the presence of IgG anti-HBc and anti-HBe antibodies (chronic HBV infection) and the superimposed primary HDV infection is marked by the presence of the IgM antibody to HDAg (IgM anti-HDV), by the presence of HDV RNA, and by a rising titer of anti-IgG HD antibody. Recombinant HDAg is currently used as the standard antigen in the various assays. IgM anti-HDV antibody has been considered a marker of HDV-induced liver damage (44).

In drug addicts and among Amerindians in the western Brazilian Amazon, serum markers of HDV infection also could be detected without any HBV markers (50, 130).

Active infection may be diagnosed by the detection of HDAg in the liver (100, 101). Since the percentage of liver cells expressing HDAg diminishes as chronic hepatitis D progresses, immunohistologic analysis may give false-negative results for patients with advanced disease.

Genome Detection

Blot hybridization assays have detected the HDV RNA genome in 64% of patients with acute hepatitis D and 70% of patients with chronic hepatitis D (120). At present, the method of choice is reverse transcription-PCR (RT-PCR), which can detect 10 to 100 copies of the viral genome in serum. However, molecular assays are not commercially available and the choice of suitable primers for amplification of the viral genome is difficult because of the heterogeneity of different isolates. Amplification of the C-terminal segment of the HDAg coding region ensures the highest degree of efficiency. Assays have been developed using conserved primers from the C-terminal half of the HDAg-encoding region or using enzyme substrates to detect HDV amplicons (18). PCR techniques are more sensitive than other methods for the demonstration of virus in liver and serum. Detection of HDV RNA may help in the early diagnosis of acute infection during the seronegative period in immunosuppressed individuals and in the follow-up of treated patients who have very low initial or residual virus titers. HDV RNA is positive in 93% of patients with HBV-HDV coinfection and in 100% of those with superinfection, correlating with the intrahepatic expression of the HDAg.

Genotyping of HDV can be quickly performed by using restriction fragment length polymorphism (26). Quantification of HDV RNA by RT-PCR can be applied to direct analysis of HDV levels in patients with different forms of hepatitis and also in patients receiving antiviral therapy. Since the RT-PCR assay for HDV RNA is based on two steps, first PCR and then nested PCR (sensitivity, 10 to 100 genomes), the assay is qualitative. RT-PCR assays for HDV RNA quantification have been recently developed (64). The assay has been useful for monitoring HDV RNA levels during antiviral therapy (29). Direct in situ hybridization assays for the detection of HDV RNA in fixed liver tissue by nonradioactive procedures have been developed. These tests are limited to research laboratories.

Antigen Detection

HDAg is not detectable in serum by enzyme immunoassay or radioimmunoassay in immunocompetent patients with chronic hepatitis D, as these patients invariably have high titers of the homologous antibody that block the antigen in immune complexes. Polyacrylamide gel electrophoresis under denaturing conditions allows the separation of HDAg from anti-HDV antibody, permitting detection of the two isoforms of the viral antigen in patients with chronic hepatitis D. The test, however, is cumbersome and not practical (15).

PREVENTION

The main strategies for the prevention of HDV infection are (i) behavioral modifications to prevent disease transmission and (ii) active immunization against HBV. Changes in sexual practices in response to HIV infection have probably contributed to the declining incidence of HBV and HDV infection in the developed world and abroad, and improved methods for screening of blood products in blood banks have reduced the risk of transmission-associated hepatitis.

In animal models, passive immunoprophylaxis based on the administration of anti-HDV antibodies is not effective, probably due to lack of neutralizing activity of the antibodies. In HDV cirrhosis patients who have received transplants, passive immunoprophylaxis using hyperimmune anti-HBs immune globulin to prevent HBV reinfection has also been the best available strategy for the prevention of HDV reinfection (14).

By preventing infection with the helper virus HBV, active HBV vaccination constitutes effective prophylaxis against HDV infection. However, this mode of prevention is possible only for HBV-naïve individuals at risk of coinfection. Thus, universal immunization against HBV is the most effective measure for preventing HDV infection. Prophylaxis of HBV carriers from HDV superinfection remains an unresolved problem.

Management of Outbreaks

There is still a risk of major outbreaks of hepatitis D in poor countries in the tropical belt of South America and in new hot spots emerging in Europe, where the rate of HBV carriage remains high. Emergency measures previously adopted to manage the outbreak among the Yupca people of the Amazon included isolating the area at high risk of HDV superinfection and then starting a vaccine program against HBV in the local population of children and young adults. The widespread use of HBV vaccination of susceptible individuals has drastically reduced the number of new cases of HDV infection (116). Recent reports from the state of Acre in the western Amazon, however, have described severe hemorrhagic forms of hepatitis due to HBV (genotypes A and F) and HDV (genotype 3) among residents working on rubber plantations (130).

TREATMENT

Therapy with immunomodulators and antiviral agents such as steroids, thymosin, levamisole, and ribavarin has been disappointing (81).

Interferon

Standard alpha interferon (IFN) is the only approved drug for treatment of chronic hepatitis D. A proportion of patients respond initially with the normalization of alanine aminotransferase levels, but in the majority of responders infection and disease recur after cessation of therapy. When high doses of IFN are administered for a prolonged period (9 MU three times a week for 48 weeks), a consistent number of patients may have biochemical (71% normalization) and histologic responses while receiving therapy. In one study, histologic follow-up of the patients who responded to a protracted period of high-dose therapy showed a marked long-term histologic improvement with a significant reduction of the fibrotic score compared to that in nonresponders or controls.

Administration of pegylated IFN-α2b (pegIFN-α2b) for 12 months to 14 patients with chronic delta hepatitis resulted in a sustained biochemical response in 8 patients (57%) and a sustained virologic response in 6 patients (43%). Another study comparing pegIFN-α2b alone or combined with ribavarin, given for 18 months to 38 patients, found a sustained virologic response in only 21% of the patients. This study highlighted the potential efficacy of therapy in HDV-naïve individuals, the delayed clearance of HDV RNA from serum after discontinuation of therapy, and the lack of ribavirin efficacy. Unfortunately, tolerance of therapy was poor. The majority of patients originally had severe fibrosis or cirrhosis (82).

Nucleosides

By inhibiting the helper HBV, nucleoside analogs such as lamivudine (LAM), adefovir, and entecavir may indirectly provide a therapy for hepatitis D. HBV is spontaneously repressed by HDV infection; however, the initial experience with LAM and adefovir has been disappointing. In a controlled study in which LAM was given for 12 months to chronic HDV carriers with liver disease, no effect on HDV viremia was detected (83). Interestingly, however, an in vitro study has shown that LAM-resistant mutants corresponding to sW196L/S inhibit the secretion of HDV particles whereas mutants corresponding to sI195M do not affect secretion. These differences in HBsAg-encoding efficiency could affect the expression of HBsAg proteins of LAM-resistant HBV and might thus affect HDV secretion (131).

The nucleoside analog L-FMAU (clevudine) has significant antiviral activity against HBV in vitro in the duck and woodchuck models, with the unique property of inhibiting production of the surface antigen. L-FMAU has been tested in chronically HDV-infected woodchucks and has shown potent inhibition of HDV replication (22, 23). Studies of its effect on humans are lacking.

Other Approaches

Antisense oligonucleotides against functional domains of HDV are effective inhibitors of HDV replication in vitro. HBV antisense oligonucleotides were constructed to alter HBV functions that are considered essential for HDV replication (B. E. Korba, J. L. Casey, and J. L. Gerin, presented at Fifth International Symposium on Hepatitis Delta Virus and Liver Disease, Gold Coast, Australia, 28 Aug. to 3 Sept. 1995). A promising approach for the generation of a novel type of antiviral therapy is based on prenylation inhibition (53). Prenylation is a form of site-specific lipid modification of proteins. The large delta antigen of HDV was the first viral protein shown to undergo prenylation, and other viruses may also have prenylated proteins. The C-terminal 4 amino acids of L-HDAg are Cys-Arg-Pro-Gln, which is the motif for isoprenylation. The cysteine residue in the motif is readily isoprenylated (the addition of a 15-carbon farnesyl to the C terminus of a protein results in a substantial increase in hydrophobicity), and the isoprenyl group has a farnesyl rather than grenylgeranil group (54). Isoprenylation of the cysteine residue at the C terminus of the large HDAg appears to play a key role in the interaction with HBV surface proteins and leads to virion release. The abolition of L-HDAg prenylation by genetic mutation of the prenylation site prevents assembly of HDV virus-like particles, and prenylation inhibitors can pharmacologically abolish the assembly of HDV in a cell culture infection model (10, 11). This therapy has not been tested in humans.

The delta ribozyme may be an example of how to use ribozyme-based gene inactivation by using its property to act as a *cis*-acting RNA motif as well as *trans*-acting molecular scissors for the development of a gene inactivation system. This HDV ribozyme technology is unique; HDV is the only catalytic cleaving RNA motif described in humans which possesses a specific on/off adapter (SOFA) that switches the cleavage activity from off to on (riboswitch) solely in the presence of the appropriate substrate (5, 7). This property might be a target for ribozyme-based drugs.

Liver Transplantation

Although HDV disease is an uncommon indication for liver transplantation in the United States (135), it is still the reason for a sizable proportion of transplants in Italy and the rest of Europe (42). In Italy between 1985 and 1995, there were 154 transplants for HBV-associated cirrhosis; 59% of these patients were also anti-HDV positive. Prevention of recurrence of HBV by using passive immunoprophylaxis has also worked satisfactorily for the prevention of HDV reinfection. The reinfection rate after the introduction of standard HB immunoglobulin prophylaxis against HBV has dropped to 9 to 12% in two large series in Italy and France. The survival rate is excellent, with 98% of the HDV-positive transplant recipients surviving throughout a 7- to 10-year follow-up in France and in Italy (109). Prophylaxis with lamivudine pretransplantation and with lamivudine plus HB immunoglobulin posttransplantation has further diminished the residual rate of reinfection (72, 108). This combined prophylaxis is now also standard treatment for the prevention of HDV reinfection in transplant recipients.

REFERENCES

1. **Abe, K., E. Hayakawa, A. V. Sminov, A. L. Rossina, X. Ding, T. T. T. Huy, T. Sata, and V. F. Uchaikin.** 2004. Molecular epidemiology of hepatitis B, C, D and E viruses among children in Moscow, Russia. *J. Clin. Virol.* **30:**57–61.
2. **Altuglu, I., T. Ozacar, R. Sertoz, and S. Erensoy.** 2007. Hepatitis Delta virus (HDV) genotypes in patients with chronic hepatitis: molecular epidemiology of HDV in Turkey. *Int. J. Infect. Dis.* **11:**58–62.
3. **Amengual, M. J., M. Catalfamo, A. Pujol, C. Juarez, C. Gelpi, and J. L. Rodriguez.** 1989. Autoantibodies in chronic delta virus infection recognize a common protein of 46 KD in rat forestomach basal cell layer and stellate thymic epithelial cells. *Clin. Exp. Immunol.* **78:**80–84.
4. **Aragona, M., S. Macagno, F. Caredda, C. Lavarini, L. Bertolusso, P. Farci, and M. Rizzetto.** 1987. Serological response to the hepatitis delta virus in hepatitis D. *Lancet* **i:**478–480.
5. **Asif-Ullah, M., M. Lévesque, G. Robichaud, and J. P. Perreault.** 2007. Development of ribozyme-based gene inactivations: the example of the hepatitis delta virus ribozyme. *Curr. Gene Ther.* **7:**205–216.
6. **Bart, P. A., P. Jacquier, P. L. Zuber, D. Lavanchy, and P. C. Frei.** 1996. Seroprevalence of HBV (anti-HBc, HBsAg and anti-HBs) and HDV infections among 9006 women at delivery. *Liver* **16:**110–116.
7. **Bergeon, L., Jr., C. Reymond, and J. P. Perreault.** 2005. Functional characterization of the SOFA delta ribozyme. *RNA* **11:**1858–1868.
8. **Bialek, S. R., W. A. Bower, K. Mottram, D. Purchase, T. Nakano, O. Nainan, I. T. Williams, and B. P. Bell.** 2005. Risk factors for hepatitis B in an outbreak of hepatitis B and D among injection drug users. *J. Urban Health* **83:**468–478.
9. **Bonino, F., N. Caporaso, P. Dentico, G. Marinucci, L. Valeri, A. Craxi, A. Ascione, G. Raimondo, F. Piccinino, and G. Rocca.** 1985. Familiar clustering and spreading of delta infection. *J. Hepatol.* **1:**221–226.
10. **Bordier, B. B., H. B. Greenberg, K. Ohashi, M. A. Kay, and J. S. Glenn.** 2000. Prospects for prenylation inhibition-based anti-HDV therapy. *Antiviral Ther.* **5:**25.
11. **Bordier, B. B., J. Ohkanda, P. Liu, S. Y. Lee, F. H. Salazar, P. L. Marion, K. Ohashi, L. Meuse, M. A. Kay, J. L. Casey, A. M. Sebti, A. D. Hamilton, and J. S. Glenn.** 2003. In vivo antiviral efficacy of prenylation inhibitors against hepatitis delta virus. *J. Clin. Investig.* **112:**407–414.
12. **Borghesio, E., F. Rosina, A. Smedile, M. Lagget, M. G. Niro, G. Marinucci, and M. Rizzetto.** 1998. Serum IgM anti-HDV as a surrogate marker of hepatitis D in interferon-treated patients and in liver transplants. *Hepatology* **27:**873–876
13. **Bortolotti, F., V. Di Marco, P. Vajro, C. Crivellaro, L. Zancan, G. Nebbia, C. Barbera, M. Tedesco, A. Craxi, and M. Rizzetto.** 1993. Long-term evolution of chronic delta hepatitis in children. *J. Pediatr.* **122:**736.
14. **Burra, P., A. Smedile, A. Angelico, A. Ascione, and M. Rizzetto on behalf of the Study Group on Liver Transplantation of the Italian Association for the Study of**

the Liver (AISF). 2000. Liver transplantation in Italy: current status. *Dig. Liver Dis.* **32:**249–256.

15. **Buti, M., R. Esteban, and R. Jardi.** 1989. Chronic delta hepatitis: detection of hepatitis delta virus antigen in serum by immunoblot and correlation with other markers of delta viral replication. *Hepatology* **10:**907–910.
16. **Caredda, F., S. Antinori, C. Pastecchia, P. Coppin, A. Ponzetto, M. Rizzetto, and M. Moroni.** 1989. Presence and incidence of hepatitis delta virus infection in acute HBsAg-negative hepatitis. *J. Infect. Dis.* **159:**977–979.
17. **Caredda, F., L. Vag, F. Mainini, A. Di Marco, M. Nebuloni, and M. Moroni.** 1997. Strong association between hepatitis D virus (HDV) infection and liver cirrhosis in chronic carriers of HBsAg with AIDS, p. 906–910. *In* M. Rizzetto, R. H. Purcell, J. L. Gerin, and G. Verme (ed.), *Viral Hepatitis and Liver Disease*. Edizioni Minerva Medica, Turin, Italy.
18. **Cariani, E., A. Ravaggi, M. Puoti, G. Mantero, A. Alberti, and D. Primi.** 1992. Evaluation of hepatitis delta virus RNA levels during interferon therapy by analysis of polymerase chain reaction products with a non radioisotopic hybridization assay. *Hepatology* **15:**685–689.
19. **Casey, J. L.** 2002. RNA editing in hepatitis delta virus genotype III requires a branched double-hairpin RNA structure. *J. Virol.* **76:**7385–7397.
20. **Casey, J. L., K. F. Bergman, T. L. Brown, and J. L. Gerin.** 1992. Structural requirements for RNA editing in hepatitis delta virus: evidence for a uridine-to-cytidine editing mechanism. *Proc. Natl. Acad. Sci. USA* **89:**1749–1753.
21. **Casey, J. L., T. L. Brown, E. J. Colan, F. S. Wignall, and J. L. Gerin.** 1993. A genotype of hepatitis D virus that occurs in northern South America. *Proc. Natl. Acad. Sci. USA* **90:**9016–9020.
22. **Casey, J. L., P. J. Cote, C. K. Chung, B. C. Tennant, J. L. Gerin, and B. E. Korba.** 2000. Treatment of chronic hepatitis delta virus infection with L-FMAU strongly inhibits HDV viremia. *Antiviral Ther.* **5:**32.
23. **Casey, J. L., P. J. Cote, I. A. Toshkov, C. K. Chung, J. L. Gerin, W. E. Hornbuckle, B. C. Tennant, and B. E. Korba.** 2005. Clevudine inhibits hepatitis delta virus viremia: a pilot study of chronically infected woodchucks. *Antimicrob. Agents Chemother.* **49:**4396–4399.
24. **Casey, J. L., and J. L. Gerin.** 1995. Hepatitis delta virus RNA editing and genotype variations, p. 111–124. *In* G. Dinber-Gottlieb (ed.), *The Unique Hepatitis Delta Virus*. Springer-Verlag, New York, NY.
25. **Casey, J. L., and J. L. Gerin.** 1998. Genotype-specific complementation of hepatitis delta virus RNA replication by hepatitis delta antigen. *J. Virol.* **72:**2806–2814.
26. **Casey, J. L., G. A. Niro, R. Engle, A. Vega, H. Gomez, M. McCarthy, D. M. Watts, K. C. Hyams, and J. L. Gerin.** 1996. Hepatitis B virus/hepatitis D virus coinfection in outbreaks of acute hepatitis in the Peruvian Amazon basin: the role of HDV genotype and HBV genotype F. *J. Infect. Dis.* **174:**920–926.
27. **Casey, J. L., A. G. Polson, B. L. Bass, and J. L. Gerin.** 1997. Molecular biology of HDV: analysis of RNA editing and genotype variation, p. 290–294. *In* M. Rizzetto, R. H. Purcell, J. L. Gerin, and G. Verme (ed.), *Viral Hepatitis and Liver Disease*. Edizioni: Minerva Medica, Turin, Italy.
28. **Casey, J. L., B. C. Tennant, and J. L. Gerin.** 2006. Genetic changes in hepatitis delta virus from acutely and chronically infected woodchucks. *J. Virol.* **80:**6469–6477.
29. **Castelnau, C., F. Le Gal, M. P. Ripault, E. Gordien, M. Martinot-Peignoux, N. Boyer, B. N. Pham, S. Maylin, P. Bedossa, P. Dény, P. Marcellin, and E. Gault.** 2006. Efficacy of peginterferon alpha 2b in chronic hepatitis delta: relevance of quantitative RT-PCR for follow up. *Hepatology* **44:**728–735.
30. **Castillo, I., J. Bartolome, A. Madejon, M. Melero, J. C. Porres, and V. Carreno.** 1991. Hepatitis delta virus RNA detection in chronic HBsAg carriers with and without HIV infection. *Digestion* **48:**149–156.
31. **Cech, T. R.** 1988. Ribozymes and their medical implications. *JAMA* **260:**3030–3034.
32. **Chang, J., S. O. Gudima, C. Tarn, X. Nie, and J. M. Taylor.** 2005. Development of a novel system to study hepatitis delta virus genome replication. *J. Virol.* **79:**8182–8188.
33. **Chang, J., S. O. Gudima, and J. M. Taylor.** 2005. Evolution of hepatitis delta virus RNA genome following long-term replication in cell culture. *J. Virol.* **79:**13310–13316.

33a. **Chou, H.-C., T.-Y. Hsieh, G.-T. Sheu, and M. C. Lai.** 1998. Hepatitis delta antigen mediates the nuclear import of hepatitis delta virus RNA. *J. Virol.* **72:**3684–3690.

34. **Coppola, R. C., G. Masia, P. Pradat, C. Trepò, G. Carboni, F. Argiolas, and M. Rizzetto.** 2000. Impact of hepatitis C virus infection on healthy subjects on an Italian island. *J. Viral Hepatitis* **7:**130–137.
35. **Crivelli, O., C. Lavarini, E. Chiaberge, A. Amoroso, P. Farci, F. Negro, and M. Rizzetto.** 1983. Microsomal autoantibodies in chronic infection with the HBsAg associated delta (d) agent. *Clin. Exp. Immunol.* **54:**232–238.
36. **Dalekos, G. N., E. Zervou, F. Karabini, and E. V. Tsianos.** 1995. Prevalence of viral markers among refugees from southern Albania: increased incidence of infection with hepatitis A, B and D viruses. *Eur. J. Gastroenterol.* **7:**553–558.
37. **de Fonseca, J. C. F., L. C. C. Gayotto, L. C. L. Ferreira, J. R. Araujo, W. D. Alecrim, R. T. Santos, J. P. Simonetti, and V. A. Alves.** 1985. Labrea hepatitis—hepatitis B and delta antigen expression in liver tissue: report of three autopsy cases. *Rev. Inst. Med. Trop. Sao Paulo* **27:**224.
38. **De Man, R. A., P. R. Sprey, H. G. M. Niesters, R. A. Heijtink, P. E. Zondervan, W. Hop, and S. W. Schalm.** 1995. Survival and complications in a cohort of patients with anti-delta positive liver disease presenting in a tertiary referral clinic. *J. Hepatol.* **23:**662–667.
39. **Denniston, K. J., B. H. Hoyer, A. Smedile, F. V. Wells, J. Nelson, and J. L. Gerin.** 1986. Cloned fragment of the hepatitis delta RNA genome sequence and diagnostic application. *Science* **232:**873–875.
40. **Dingle, K., V. Bichko, H. Zuccola, J. Hogle, and J. Taylor.** 1998. Initiation of hepatitis delta virus genome replication. *J. Virol.* **72:**4783–4788.
41. **D'Ugo, E., M. Paroli, G. Palmieri, R. Giuseppetti, C. Argentini, E. Tritarelli, R. Bruni, V. Barnaba, M. Houghton, and M. Rapicetta.** 2004. Immunization of woodchucks with adjuvanted sHDAg (p24): immune response and outcome following challenge. *Vaccine* **22:**457–466.
42. **Fagiouli, S., G. Leandro, A. Bellati, A. Gasbarrini, G. L. Rapaccini, M. Pompili, M. Rendina, S. De Notariis, A. Francavilla, G. Gasbarrini, G. Ideo, and R. Naccarato.** 1996. Liver transplantation in Italy: preliminary 10-year report. *Ital. J. Gastroenterol.* **28:**343–350.
43. **Farci, P., C. Barbera, C. Navone, F. Bortolotti, P. Vajro, N. Caporaso, A. Vegnente, N. Ansaldi, M. Rizzetto, and P. Tolentino.** 1985. Infection with delta agent in children. *Gut* **26:**4–7.
44. **Farci, P., J. L. Gerin, M. Aragona, I. Lindsey, O. Crivelli, A. Balestrieri, A. Smedile, H. C. Thomas, and M. Rizzetto.** 1986. Diagnostic and prognostic significance of

the IgM antibody to the hepatitis delta virus. *JAMA* **255:** 1443–1446.

45. **Fattovich, G., G. Giustina, E. Christensen, M. Pantalena, I. Zagni, G. Realdi, S. W. Schalm, and the European Concerted Action on Viral Hepatitis (EUROHEP).** 2000. Influence of hepatitis delta virus infection on morbidity and mortality in compensated cirrhosis type B. *Gut* **46:**420–426.
46. **Ferre-D'Amare, A. R., K. Zhou, and J. A. Doudna.** 1998. Crystal structure of a hepatitis delta virus ribozyme. *Nature* **395:**567–574.
47. **Fielder, M., M. Lu, F. Siegel, J. Whipple, and M. Roggendorf.** 2001. Immunization of woodchucks *(Marmotta monax)* with hepatitis delta virus DNA vaccine. *Vaccine* **19:**4618–4626.
48. **Flodgren, E., S. Bengtsson, M. Knutsson, E. A. Strebkova, H. A. Kidd, O. A. Alexeyev, and K. Kidd-Ljunggren.** 2000. Recent high incidence of fulminant hepatitis in Samara, Russia: molecular analysis of prevailing hepatitis B and D virus strains. *J. Clin. Microbiol.* **38:** 3311–3316.
49. **Flodgren, E., S. Bengtsson, O. Alexeyev, and K. Kidd-Ljunggren.** 2000. Samara, Russia—a previously isolated city facing a real hepatitis D virus challenge. *Antiviral Ther.* **5:**D3.
50. **Gaeta, G. B., D. F. Precone, A. Cozzi-Lepri, P. Cicconi, and A. D'Arminio Monforte.** 2006. Multiple viral infections. *J. Hepatol.* **44:**S108–S113.
51. **Gaeta, G. B., T. Stroffolini, M. Chiaramonte, T. Ascione, G. Stornaiuolo, S. Lobello, E. Sagnelli, M. R. Brunetto, and M. Rizzetto.** 2000. Chronic hepatitis D: a vanishing disease? A multicenter Italian study. *Hepatology* **32:**824–827.
52. **Gerin, J. L.** 1994 The taxonomy of hepatitis delta virus, p. 63–64. *In* K. Nishioka, H. Suzuki, S. Mishiro, and T. Oda (ed.), *Viral Hepatitis and Liver Disease*. Springer-Verlag, Tokyo, Japan.
53. **Glenn, J. S., J. A. Watson, C. M. Havel, and J. M. White.** 1992. Identification of a prevalent site in delta virus large antigen. *Science* **256:**1331–1333.
54. **Glenn, J. S., J. C. Marsters, and H. B. Greenberg.** 1998. Use of a prenylation inhibitor as a novel antiviral agent. *J. Virol.* **72:**9303–9306.
55. **Grattagliano, I., V. O. Palmieri, P. Portincasa, and G. Palasciano.** 2006. Adefovir dipivoxyl for the treatment of delta-related liver cirrhosis. *Ann. Pharmacother.* **40:**1681–1684.
56. **Hadler, S. C., M. de Monzon, A. Ponzetto, E. Anzola, D. Rivero, A. Mondolfi, A. Bracho, D. P. Francis, M. A. Gerber, and S. Thung.** 1984. Delta virus infection and severe hepatitis. An epidemic in Yupca Indians of Venezuela. *Ann. Intern. Med.* **100:**339–344.
57. **Hsu, S. C., W. J. Syu, I. J. Sheen, H. T. Liu, K. S. Jeng, and J. C. Wu.** 2002. Varied assembly and RNA efficiencies between genotype I and II hepatitis D virus and their implications. *Hepatology* **35:**665–672.
58. **Huang, Y. H., J. C. Wu, S. C. Hsu, and W. Syu, Jr.** 2003. Varied immunity generated in mice by DNA vaccines with large and small hepatitis Delta antigens. *J. Virol.* **77:**12980–12985.
59. **Imazeki, F., M. Omata, and M. Otho.** 1990. Heterogeneity and evolution rates of delta virus RNA sequences. *J. Virol.* **64:**5594.
60. **Inoue, J., M. Takahashi, T. Nishizawa, L. Narantuya, M. Sakuma, Y. Kagawa, T. Shimosegawa, and H. Okamoto.** 2005. High prevalence of hepatitis delta virus infection detectable by enzyme immunoassay among apparently healthy individuals in Mongolia. *J. Med. Virol.* **76:**333–340.
61. **Jayan, G. C., and J. L. Casey.** 2002. Increased RNA editing and inhibition of hepatitis delta virus replication by high-level expression of ADAR1 and ADAR2. *J. Virol.* **76:**3819–3827.
62. **Jayan, G. C., and J. L. Casey.** 2002. Inhibition of hepatitits delta virus RNA editing by short inhibitory RNA-mediated knockdown of ADAR1 but not ADAR2 expression. *J. Virol.* **76:**12399–12404
63. **Kuo, M. Y. P., M. Chao, and J. Taylor.** 1989. Initiation of replication of the human hepatitis delta virus genome from cloned DNA: role of delta antigen. *J. Virol.* **63:** 1945–1950.
64. **Le Gal, F., E. Gordien, D. Affolabi, T. Hanslik, C. Alloui, P. Dény, and E. Gault.** 2005. Quantification of hepatitis delta virus RNA in serum by consensus real-time PCR indicates different patterns of virological response to interferon therapy in chronically infected patients. *J. Clin. Microbiol.* **43:**2363–2369.
65. **Leone, N., B. Lavezzo, A. Smedile, M. Salizzoni, V. Ghisetti, and M. Rizzetto.** 2001. Clinical and virological course of multiple viral infections after liver transplantation. *Transplant. Proc.* **33:**2598–2599.
66. **Li, Y. J., T. Macnaughton, L. Gao, and M. M. C. Lai.** 2006. RNA-templated replication of hepatitis delta virus: genomic and antigenomic RNAs associate with different nuclear bodies. *J. Virol.* **80:**6478–6486.
67. **Liaw, Y. F.** 1995. Role of hepatitis C virus in dual and triple hepatitis virus infection. *Hepatology* **22:**1101–1108.
68. **Liaw, Y. F., K. W. Chin, C. M. Chen, I. S. Sheen, and M. J. Huang.** 1990. Heterosexual transmission of hepatitis delta virus in the general population of an area endemic for hepatitis B virus infection: a prospective study. *J. Infect. Dis.* **162:**1170–1172.
69. **Lin, J. H., M. F. Chang, S. C. Baker, S. Govindarajan, and M. M. C. Lai.** 1990. Characterization of hepatitis delta antigen: specific binding to hepatitis delta virus RNA. *J. Virol.* **64:**4051–4058.
70. **Macnaughton, T., M. Beard, M. Chao, E. Gowans, and M. Lai.** 1993. Endogenous promoters can direct the transcription of hepatitis delta virus RNA from a recircularized cDNA template. *Virology* **196:**629–636.
71. **Mariano, A., A. Mele, M. E. Tosti, A. Piolato, G. Gallo, P. Ragno, C. Zotti, P. Lopalco, M. G. Pompa, G. Graziani, and T. Stroffolini.** 2004. Role of beauty transmission on the spread of parenterally transmitted hepatitis viruses in Italy. *J. Med. Virol.* **74:**216–220.
72. **Marzano, A., S. Gaia, V. Ghisetti, S. Carenzi, A. Premoli, W. Debernardi-Venon, C. Alessandria, A. Franchello, M. Salizzoni, and M. Rizzetto.** 2005. Viral load at the time of liver transplantation and risk of hepatitis B virus recurrence. *Liver Transpl.* **11:**402–409.
73. **Mauch, C., C. Grimm, S. Meckel, J. R. Wands, H. E. Blum, M. Roggendorf, and M. Geissler.** 2001. Induction of cytotoxic T lymphocyte responses against hepatitis delta virus antigens which protect against tumor formation in mice. *Vaccine* **20:**170–180.
74. **Modahl, L. E., and M. M. C. Lai.** 2000. The large delta antigen of hepatitis delta virus potently inhibits genomic but not antigenomic RNA synthesis: a mechanism enabling initiation of viral replication. *J. Virol.* **74:**7375–7380.
75. **Nakano, S., and P. C. Bevilacqua.** 2007. Mechanism characterization of the HDV genomic ribozyme: a mutant of the C41 motif provides insight into the positioning and thermodynamic linkage of metal ions and protons. *Biochemistry* **46:**3001–3012.
76. **Nakano, T., C. N. Shapiro, S. Hadler, and J. L. Casey.** 2000. Characterization of hepatitis D virus among the

indigenous population in Venezuela. *Antiviral Ther.* 5(Suppl. 1):D3.

77. **Navascues, C. A., M. Rodriguez, N. G. Sotorrio, P. Sala, A. Linares, A. Suarez, and L. Rodrigo.** 1995. Epidemiology of hepatitis D virus infection: changes in the last 14 years. *Am. J. Gastroenterol.* **90:**1981–1984.
78. **Negro, F., and M. Rizzetto.** 1993. Pathobiology of hepatitis delta virus. *J. Hepatol.* **17:**S149–S153.
79. **Netter, H. J., K. Kajino, and J. M. Taylor.** 1993. Experimental transmission of human hepatitis delta virus to the laboratory mouse. *J. Virol.* **67:**3357–3362.
80. **Niro, G. A., J. L. Casey, E. Gravinese, M. Garubba, P. Conoscitore, E. Sagnelli, M. Durazzo, N. Caporaso, F. Perri, G. Leandro, D. Facciorusso, M. Rizzetto, and A. Andriulli.** 1999. Intrafamilial transmission of hepatitis delta virus: molecular evidence. *J. Hepatol.* **30:**564–569.
81. **Niro, G. A., F. Rosina, and M. Rizzetto.** 2005. Treatment of hepatitis D. *J. Viral Hepat.* **12:**2–9.
82. **Niro, G. A., A. Ciancio, G. B. Gaeta, A. Smedile, A. Marrone, A. Olivero, M. Stanzione, E. David, G. Brancaccio, R. Fontana, F. Perri, A. Andriulli, and M. Rizzetto.** 2006. Pegylated interferon alpha-2b as monotherapy or in combination with ribavirin in chronic hepatitis delta. *Hepatology* **44:**713–720.
83. **Niro, G. A., A. Ciancio, H. L. Tillman, M. Lagget, A. Olivero, F. Perri, R. Fontana, N. Little, F. Campbell, A. Smedile, M. P. Manns, A. Andriulli, and M. Rizzetto.** 2005. Lamivudine therapy in chronic delta hepatitis: a multicentre randomized-controlled pilot study. *Aliment. Pharmacol. Ther.* **22:**227–232.
84. **Novick, D. M., P. Farci, T. S. Croxson, M. B. Taylor, C. W. Schneebaum, M. E. Lai, N. Bach, R. T. Senie, A. M. Gelb, and M. J. Kreek.** 1988. Hepatitis D virus and human immunodeficiency virus antibodies in parenteral drug abusers who are hepatitis B surface antigen positive. *J. Infect. Dis.* **158:**795.
85. **Obaid Shakil, A., S. Hadziyannis, J. H. Hoofnagle, A. M. Di Bisceglie, J. L. Gerin, and J. L. Casey.** 1997. Geographic distribution and genetic variability of hepatitis delta virus genotype 1. *Virology* **234:**160–167.
86. **Perrotta, A. T., and M. D. Been.** 1991. A pseudoknot-like structure required for efficient self-cleavage of hepatitis delta virus RNA. *Nature* **350:**434–436.
87. **Perrotta, A. T., I.-H. Shih, and M. D. Been.** 1999. Imidazole rescue of a cytosine mutation in a self-cleaving ribozyme. *Science* **286:**3–6.
88. **Perotta, A. T., and M. D. Been.** 2007. A single nucleotide linked to a switch in metal ion reactivity preference in the HDV ribozymes. *Biochemistry* **46:**5124–5130.
89. **Perotta, A. T., T. S. Wadkins, and M. D. Been.** 2006. Chemical rescue, multiple ionizable groups, and general acid-base catalysis in the HDV genomic ribozyme. *RNA* **12:**1282–1291.
90. **Philipp, T., M. Durazzo, C. Trautwein, B. Alex, P. Straub, J. G. Lamb, E. F. Johnson, R. H. Tukey, and M. P. Manns.** 1994. Recognition of uridine diphosphate glucuronosyl transferases by LKM-3 autoantibodies in chronic hepatitis D. *Lancet* **344:**578–581.
91. **Polson, A., B. Bass, and J. Casey.** 1996. RNA editing of hepatitis delta virus antigenome by dsRNA-adenosine deaminase. *Nature* **380:**454–456.
92. **Polson, A. G., H. L. Ley III, B. L. Brass, and J. L. Casey.** 1998. Hepatitis delta virus RNA editing is highly specific for the Amber/W site and is suppressed by hepatitis delta antigen. *Mol. Cell. Biol.* **18:**1919–1926.
93. **Ponzetto, A., P. J. Cote, H. Popper, B. H. Hoyer, W. T. London, E. C. Ford, F. Bonino, R. H. Purcell, and J. L. Gerin.** 1984. Transmission of the hepatitis B-virus associated delta agent to the eastern woodchuck. *Proc. Natl. Acad. Sci. USA* **81:**2208–2212.
94. **Ponzetto, A., B. Forzani, I. Forzani, N. D'Urso, L. Avanzini, A. Smedile, and G. Verme.** 1989. Immunization with hepatitis delta antigen does not prevent superinfection with hepatitis delta virus in the woodchuck. *Gastroenterology* **96:**646.
95. **Ponzetto, A., B. Forzani, P. P. Parravicini, C. Hele, A. Zanetti, and M. Rizzetto.** 1985. Epidemiology of hepatitis delta virus infection. *Eur. J. Epidemiol.* **1:**257–263.
96. **Ponzetto, A., F. Negro, H. Popper, F. Bonino, R. Engle, M. Rizzetto, R. H. Purcell, and J. L. Gerin.** 1988. Serial passage of hepatitis delta virus in chronic hepatitis B virus carrier chimpanzees. *Hepatology* **8:**1655–1661.
97. **Popper, H., S. N. Thung, M. A. Gerber, S. C. Hadler, M. de Monzon, A. Ponzetto, E. Anzola, D. Rivera, A. Mondolfi, and A. Bracho.** 1983. Histologic studies of severe delta agent infection in Venezuelan Indians. *Hepatology* **3:**906–912.
98. **Radjef, N., E. Gordien, V. Ivaniushina, E. Gault, P. Anais, T. Drugan, J. C. Trinchet, D. Roulot, M. Tamby, M. C. Milinkovitch, and P. Dény.** 2004. Molecular phylogenetic analyses indicate a wide and ancient radiation of African hepatitis delta virus, suggesting a *Deltavirus* genus of at least seven major clades. *J. Virol.* **78:**2537–2544.
99. **Raimondo, G., M. R. Brunetto, P. Pontisso, A. Smedile, A. M. Maina, C. Saitta, G. Squadrito, N. Tono, and the AISF Cooperative Group.** 2006. Longitudinal evaluation reveals a complex spectrum of virological profiles in hepatitis B virus/hepatitis C virus-coinfected patients. *Hepatology* **43:**100–107.
100. **Rizzetto, M., M. G. Canese, S. Aricò, O. Crivelli, C. Trepò, F. Bonino, and G. Verme.** 1977. Immunofluorescence detection of a new antigen-antibody system (delta/anti delta) associated with hepatitis B virus in liver and in serum of HBsAg carriers. *Gut* **18:**997–1003.
101. **Rizzetto, M., M. G. Canese, J. L. Gerin, W. T. London, L. D. Sly, and R. H. Purcell.** 1980. Transmission of the hepatitis B virus-associated delta antigen to chimpanzees. *J. Infect. Dis.* **141:**590–602.
102. **Rizzetto, M., S. Hadziyannis, B. G. Hansson, A. Toukan, and I. Gust.** 1992. Hepatitis delta virus infection in the world, epidemiological patterns and clinical expression. *Gastroenterol. Int.* **5:**18–32.
103. **Rosina, F., P. Conoscitore, R. Cuppone, G. Rocca, A. Giuliani, R. Cozzolongo, G. Niro, A. Smedile, G. Saracco, A. Andriulli, O. G. Manghisi, and M. Rizzetto.** 1999. Changing pattern of chronic hepatitis D in Southern Europe. *Gastroenterology* **117:**161–166.
104. **Rosina, F., A. Fabiano, A. Garripoli, A. Smedile, A. Mattalia, M. R. Eckart, M. Houghton, and F. Bonino.** 1991. Rabbit-derived anti-HDV antibodies for HDVAg immunoblotting. *J. Hepatol.* **13**(Suppl. 4):S130–S133.
105. **Sagnelli, E., T. Stroffolini, A. Ascione, F. Bonino, M. Chiaramonte, M. Colombo, A. Craxi, G. Giusti, O. G. Manghisi, and G. Pastore.** 1992. The epidemiology of hepatitis delta infection in Italy. *J. Hepatol.* **15:**211–215.
106. **Sakugawa, H., H. Nakasone, T. Nakayoshi, Y. Kawakami, S. Miyazato, F. Kinjo, A. Saito, S. P. Ma, H. Hotta, and M. Kinoshita.** 1999. Hepatitis delta virus genotype II b predominates in an endemic area, Okinawa, Japan. *J. Med. Virol.* **58:**366–372.
107. **Salehi-Ashtiani, K., A. Luptak, A. Litovchick, and J. W. Szostak.** 2006. A genomewide search for ribozymes reveals an HDV-like sequence in the human CPEB3 gene. *Science* **313:**1788–1792.
108. **Salizzoni, M., E. Cerutti, R. Romagnoli, F. Lupo, A. Franchello, F. Zamboni, F. Gennari, P. Strignano, A.**

Ricchiuti, A. Brunati, M. M. Schellino, A. Ottobrelli, A. Marzano, B. Lavezzo, E. David, and M. Rizzetto. 2005. The first one thousand liver transplants in Turin: a single-center experience in Italy. *Transplant Int.* **18:** 1328–1335.

109. **Samuel, D., X. Forns, M. Berenguer, C. Trautwein, A. Burroughs, M. Rizzetto, and M. Trepò.** 2006. Report of the monothematic EASL conference on liver transplantation for viral hepatitis (Paris, France, January 12–14, 2006). *J. Hepatol.* **45:**127–143.

110. **Saracco, G., S. Maccagno, F. Caredda, S. Antinori, and M. Rizzetto.** 1988. Serologic markers with fulminant hepatitis in persons positive for hepatitis B surface antigen. A worldwide epidemiologic and clinical survey. *Ann. Intern. Med.* **106:**380–384.

111. **Scott, W. G., J. T. Finch, and A. Klung.** 1995. The crystal structure of an all-RNA hammerhead ribozyme: a proposed mechanism for RNA catalytic cleavage. *Cell* **81:**991–1002.

112. **Sefcikova, J., M. V. Krasovska, J. Sponer, and N. G. Walter.** 2007. The genomic HDV ribozyme utilizes a previously unnoticed U-turn motif to accomplish fast site-specific catalysis. *Nucleic Acids Res.* **35:**1933–1946.

113. **Sheng, W. H., C. C. Hung, J. H. Kao, S. Y. Chang, M. Y. Chen, S. M. Hsieh, P. J. Chen, and S. C. Chang.** 2007. Impact of hepatitis D virus infection on the long-term outcome of patients with hepatitis B virus and HIV coinfection in the era of highly active antiretroviral therapy: a matched cohort study. *Clin. Infect. Dis.* **44:** 988–995.

114. **Shiau, Y. T., Y. H. Huang, J. C. Wu, M. H. Tao, W. Syu, Jr., F. Y. Chang, and S. D. Lee.** 2006. Analysis of humoral immunity of hepatitis D virus DNA vaccine generated in mice by using different dosage, gene gun immunization and in vivo electroporation. *J. Chin. Med. Assoc.* **69:**7–13.

115. **Singh, V., M. K. Goenka, D. K. Bhasin, R. Kochahar, and K. Singh.** 1995. A study of delta virus infection in patients with acute and chronic liver disease from northern India. *J. Viral Hepat.* **2:**151–154.

116. **Sjogren, M. H., A. Colichon, H. Vildosola, R. Cantella, and J. Romero.** 1997. Initial and 8 years serologic follow-up of HBV and HDV in resident of a hyperendemic area in the Amazon basin, p. 119.A28. *In* M. Rizzetto, R. H. Purcell, J. L. Gerin, and G. Verme (ed.), *Viral Hepatitis and Liver Disease*. Edizioni Minerva Medica, Turin, Italy.

117. **Smedile, A., K. F. Bergmann, B. M. Baroudi, F. V. Wells, R. H. Purcell, F. Bonino, M. Rizzetto, and J. L. Gerin.** 1990. Riboprobe assay for HDV-RNA: a sensitive method for the detection of the HDV genome in clinical serum samples. *J. Med. Virol.* **30:**20–24.

118. **Smedile, A., C. Lavarini, O. Crivelli, G. Raimondo, M. Fassone, and M. Rizzetto.** 1982. Radioimmunoassay detection of IgM antibodies to the HBV-associated delta (d) antigen: clinical significance in delta infection. *J. Med. Virol.* **9:**131–138.

119. **Smedile, A., C. Lavarini, and P. Farci.** 1983. Epidemiologic patterns of infection with the hepatitis B virus-associated delta antigen in Italy. *Am. J. Epidemiol.* **117:** 223–229.

120. **Smedile, A., M. Rizzetto, K. Denniston, F. Bonino, F. Wells, G. Verme, F. Consolo, B. Hoyer, R. H. Purcell, and J. L. Gerin.** 1986. Type D hepatitis: the clinical significance of hepatitis D virus RNA in serum as detected by a hybridization based-assay. *Hepatology* **6:** 1297–1302.

121. **Smedile, A., M. Rizzetto, and J. L. Gerin.** 1994. Advances in hepatitis D virus biology and disease, p. 157–175. *In* J. L. Boyer, and R. K. Okner (ed.), *Progress in Liver Disease*, vol. XII. The W. B. Saunders Co, Philadelphia, PA.

122. **Su, C. W., Y. H. Huang, T. I. Huo, H. H. Shih, I. J. Sheen, S. W. Chen, P. C. Lee, D. S. Lee, and J. C. Wu.** 2006. Genotypes and viremia of hepatitis B and D viruses are associated with outcome of chronic hepatitis D patients. *Gastroenterology* **130:**1625–1635.

123. **Tanner, N. K., S. Schaff, G. Thill, E. Petit-Koskas, A. M. Crain-Denoyelle, and E. Westhof.** 1994. A three-dimensional model of hepatitis delta virus ribozyme based on biochemical and mutational analyses. *Curr. Biol.* **4:**488–498.

124. **Taylor, J. M.** 2006. Hepatitis delta virus. *Virology* **344:** 71–76.

125. **Taylor, J. M.** 1990. Structure and replication of hepatitis delta virus. *Semin. Virol.* **1:**135–141.

126. **Taylor, J. M.** 1990. Hepatitis delta virus: cis and trans functions required for replication. *Cell* **61:**371–373.

127. **Taylor, J. M., J. Mason, J. Summers, C. Goldenberg, L. Aldrich, J. Coates, J. L. Gerin, and E. Gowans.** 1987. Replication of human hepatitis delta virus in primary cultures of woodchuck hepatocytes. *J. Virol.* **61:** 2891–2895.

128. **Tinsley, R. A., and N. G. Walter.** 2007. Long-range impact of peripheral joining elements on structure and function of the hepatitis delta virus ribozyme. *Biol. Chem.* **388:**705–715.

129. **Verme, G., P. Amoroso, G. Lettieri, P. Pierri, E. David, F. Sessa, R. Rizzi, F. Bonino, S. Recchia, and M. Rizzetto.** 1986. A histologic study of hepatitis delta virus liver disease. *Hepatology* **6:**1303.

130. **Viana, S., R. Parana, R. C. Moreira, A. P. Compri, and V. Macedo.** 2005. High prevalence of hepatitis B and hepatitis D virus in the western Brazilian Amazon. *Am. J. Trop. Med. Hyg.* **73:**808–814.

131. **Vietheer, P. T. K., H. J. Netter, T. Sozzi, and A. Bartholomeusz.** 2005. Failure of the lamivudine-resistant rtM204I hepatitis B virus mutants to efficiently support hepatitis delta virus secretion. *J. Virol.* **79:**6570–6573.

132. **Wedemeyer, H., B. Heidrich, and T. Manns.** 2007. Hepatitis D virus infection—not a vanishing disease in Europe! *Hepatology* **45:**1331–1332.

133. **Wesierka-Gadek, J., E. Penner, E. R. Hitchaman, and G. Sauermann.** 1990. Antibodies to nuclear lamin C in chronic hepatitis delta virus infection. *Hepatology* **12:** 1129–1133.

134. **Wong, S. K., and D. W. Lazinski.** 2002. Replicating hepatitis Delta virus RNA is edited in the nucleus by the small form of ADAR1. *Proc. Natl. Acad. Sci. USA* **99:**15118–15123.

135. **Wright, T. L., and B. Pereira.** 1995. Liver transplantation for chronic viral hepatitis. *Liver Transplant Surg.* **1:** 30–42.

136. **Wu, J.-C., T.-Y. Chaing, and I. J. Sheen.** 1998. Characterization and phylogenetic analysis of a novel hepatitis D virus strain discovered by restriction fragment length polymorphism analysis. *J. Gen. Virol.* **79:**1105–1113.

137. **Wu, J. C., K. B. Choo, C. M. Chen, T. Z. Chen, T. I. Huo, and S. D. Lee.** 1995. Genotyping of hepatitis D virus by restriction fragment length polymorphism and relation to outcome of hepatitis D. *Lancet* **346:**939.

138. **Wu, J. C., S. Y. Wang, W. J. Syu, Y. S. Huang, C. C. Lin, and I. J. Sheen.** 2000. Replacement of dominant strains of hepatitis D virus in chronic hepatitis D: clustering of amino acid changes within immunogenic domains. *Antiviral Ther.* **5:**D4.

139. **Yamaguchi, Y., T. Mura, S. Chanarat, A. Okamoto, and H. Handa.** 2007. Hepatitis delta antigen binds to the clamp of RNA polymerase II and affects transcriptional fidelity. *Genes Cells* **12:**863–875.

140. **Zakaria, S., R. Fouad, O. Shaker, S. Zaki, A. Hashem, S. S. El-Kamary, G. Esmat, and S. Zakaria.** 2007. Changing patterns of acute viral hepatitis at a major urban referral center in Egypt. *Clin. Infect. Dis.* **44:**e30–e36.

141. **Zaki, H., G. L. Darmstadt, A. Baten, C. R. Ahsan, and S. K. Saha.** 2003. Seroepidemiology of hepatitis B and Delta virus infections in Bangladesh. *J. Trop. Pediatr.* **49:**371–374.

142. **Zanetti, A. R., P. Ferroni, E. M. Magliani, P. Pirovano, C. Lavarini, A. L. Massaro, R. Gavinelli, C. Fabris, and M. Rizzetto.** 1982. Perinatal transmission of hepatitis B virus associated delta agent from mothers to offspring in Northern Italy. *J. Med. Virol.* **9:**139–148.

143. **Zauli, D., C. Crespi, F. B. Bianchi, A. Craxi, and E. Pisi.** 1986. Autoimmunity in chronic liver disease caused by hepatitis delta virus. *J. Clin. Pathol.* **39:**897–899.

Transmissible Spongiform Encephalopathies

ADRIANO AGUZZI

57

Prion diseases, also termed transmissible spongiform encephalopathies (TSEs), are inevitably fatal neurodegenerative conditions which affect humans and a wide variety of animals (8). Although prion diseases may manifest certain morphological and pathophysiological features that parallel other progressive encephalopathies, such as Alzheimer's disease (AD) and Parkinson's disease (4, 10), they are unique in that they are transmissible. Homogenization of brain tissue from affected individuals and intracerebral inoculation into another individual of the same species will typically reproduce the disease. This important fact was recognized almost six decades ago in the case of scrapie (50), a prototypic prion disease that affects sheep and goats.

The agent that elicits TSEs was termed prion by Stanley B. Prusiner and was defined as "a small proteinaceous infectious particle which is resistant to inactivation by most procedures that modify nucleic acids" (148). However, within this chapter the term prion is used operationally to denote the infectious agent, without implying that it possesses particular chemical or structural characteristics.

Prions certainly differ from all other known infectious pathogens in several respects. First, prions do not appear to contain an informational nucleic acid genome longer than 50 bases that would code for their progeny. Second, the only known component of the prion is a modified protein that is encoded by a cellular gene. Third, the major, and possibly only, component of the prion is the scrapie isoform of the prion protein (PrP^{Sc} or PrP-res), which is a disease-associated conformer of the cellular isoform PrP^{C} (also termed PrP-sen).

A fundamental event in prion diseases is a conformational change which occurs during the conversion of PrP^{C} into PrP^{Sc} (Fig. 1). PrP^{C} has been identified in all mammals and birds examined to date, as well as in the frog *Xenopus laevis* (172) and in fish (133, 156). PrP^{C} is anchored to the external surface of cells by a glycolipid moiety (170). The function of PrP^{C} is unknown. All attempts to identify posttranslational chemical modifications that distinguish PrP^{Sc} from PrP^{C} have been unsuccessful to date (169). PrP^{C} contains ca. 45% α-helix and two very short stretches of β-sheet (154). Conversion to PrP^{Sc} creates a protein that contains ca. 30% α-helix and 45% β-sheet. The mechanism by which PrP^{C} is converted into PrP^{Sc} remains unknown, but PrP^{C} seems to bind to PrP^{Sc}, maybe along with ancillary proteins, to form an intermediate complex during the formation of nascent PrP^{Sc} (128). Studies with transgenic mice have provided genetic evidence that incoming prions in the inoculum interact preferentially with homotypic PrP^{C} during the propagation of prions (150, 160).

The human prion diseases are referred to as kuru, Creutzfeldt-Jakob disease (CJD), variant CJD (vCJD), Gerstmann-Sträussler-Scheinker (GSS) disease, and fatal familial insomnia (FFI). The most common prion diseases of animals are scrapie of sheep and goats; bovine spongiform encephalopathy (BSE), or mad cow disease; and chronic wasting disease of deer and elk. Kuru was the first of the human prion diseases to be transmitted to experimental animals, and it has often been suggested that kuru spread among the Fore people of Papua New Guinea by ritual cannibalism (64, 65). The experimental and presumed human-to-human transmission of kuru led to the belief that prion diseases are infectious disorders caused by unusual viruses similar to those causing scrapie in sheep and goats. Yet a paradox was presented by the occurrence of CJD in families, first reported almost 70 years ago (97, 127), which appeared to be a genetic disease. The significance of familial CJD remained largely unappreciated until mutations in the protein-coding region of the PrP gene on the short arm of chromosome 20 were discovered (88, 168). The earlier finding that brain extracts from patients who had died of familial prion diseases inoculated into experimental animals often transmit disease posed a conundrum that was resolved with the genetic linkage of these diseases to mutations of the *PRNP* gene, which encodes PrP^{C} (121, 147, 177). To date, all cases of familial prion disease have been shown to cosegregate with *PRNP* missense or, in one case, nonsense mutations.

The most common form of prion disease in humans is sporadic CJD (sCJD). Its cause is unknown. Many attempts to show that the sporadic prion diseases are caused by infection have been unsuccessful (32, 49, 76, 119). The discovery that inherited prion diseases are caused by germ line mutation of the PrP gene raised the possibility that sporadic forms of these diseases might result from a somatic mutation (147). Alternatively, since PrP^{Sc} is formed from the cellular isoform of the prion protein, PrP^{C}, by a posttranslational process (28), sporadic prion diseases may result from the spontaneous conversion of PrP^{C} into PrP^{Sc}.

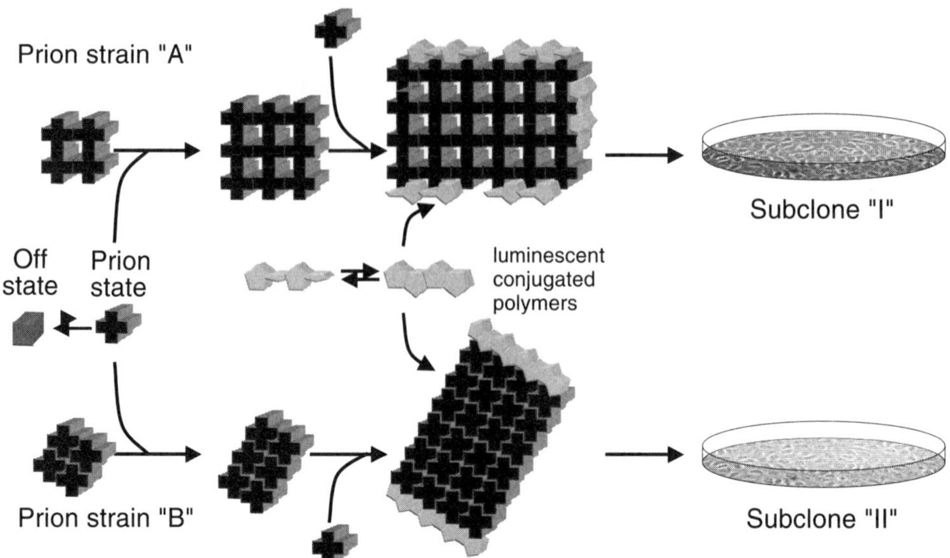

FIGURE 1 Model for prion strain propagation and detection. PrP^C (cube) exists in equilibrium with a misfolded monomeric isoform (cross). The latter can assemble into structurally heterogeneous yet highly ordered aggregated forms (upper versus lower assemblies) which replicate differentially in select cell lines. A panel of such lines, as provided by Mahal and colleagues, may form the basis for classifying prions. When stained with luminescent conjugated thiophene polymers, PrP^{Sc} aggregates stemming from distinct prion strains fluoresce in different colors.

CJD was reported to have a worldwide incidence of 1 case per 10^6 inhabitants annually (122). However, in countries that carry out active surveillance programs, reported CJD incidence is often higher (5), and in Switzerland it has reached $3.0/10^6$/year (70, 71), suggesting that many cases may go undetected. Less than 1% of CJD cases are infectious, and most of those seem to be iatrogenic. Between 10 and 15% of the cases of prion disease are inherited, while the remaining cases are sporadic. Kuru was once the most common cause of death among New Guinea women in the Fore region of the Highlands (63, 65, 66) but has virtually disappeared with the cessation of ritualistic cannibalism (16, 125). Most patients with CJD present primarily with dementia, but approximately 10% exhibit cerebellar dysfunction as the initial sign. People with either kuru or GSS disease usually present with ataxia, whereas those with FFI show insomnia and autonomic dysfunction (31, 89).

PrP^{CJD} has been found in the brains of most patients who died of prion disease. The term PrP^{CJD} is sometimes used when referring to the abnormal isoform of PrP in human brain. In this chapter, PrP^{Sc} is used interchangeably with PrP^{CJD}. PrP^{Sc} is always used after human CJD prions have been passaged into an experimental animal, because the nascent PrP^{Sc} molecules are produced from host PrP^C and the PrP^{CJD} in the inoculum serves only to initiate the process. In the brains of some patients with inherited prion diseases, as well as transgenic mice expressing mouse PrP with the human GSS point mutation (Pro→Leu), detection of PrP^{Sc} by Western blotting has been problematic despite clinical and neuropathological hallmarks of neurodegeneration (90, 91, 126), but histologic techniques such as histoblotting (176) have often revealed protease-resistant PrP.

Experimental transmission of neurodegeneration from the brains of patients with inherited prion diseases to inoculated rodents has been less frequent than with sporadic cases (177). Whether this distinction between transmissible and nontransmissible inherited prion diseases will persist is unclear. Transgenic mice expressing a chimeric human-mouse PrP gene are highly susceptible to human prions from sCJD and iatrogenic CJD (iCJD) cases (178), and—somewhat unexpectedly—transgenic mice expressing a full-length bovine *Prnp* transgene appear to be the best model for transmission of human prions to date (161). There is hope that suitable transgenic mice may eventually make the use of apes and monkeys for the study of human prion diseases unnecessary. To date, this is not yet possible for several reasons: (i) the molecular determinants of species barriers are not fully understood and may encompass species-specific host factors additional to PrP, and (ii) the peripheral pathophysiology of prion diseases may differ considerably between mice and humans.

Scrapie is the most common natural prion disease of animals. An investigation into the etiology of scrapie followed the vaccination of sheep for louping-ill virus with formalin-treated extracts of ovine lymphoid tissue unknowingly contaminated with scrapie prions (74). Two years later, more than 1,500 sheep developed scrapie from this vaccine. In the late 1990s a similar incident led to widespread scrapie infection of Italian sheep herds. Although the transmissibility of experimental scrapie became well established, the spread of natural scrapie within and among flocks of sheep remained puzzling. Parry argued that host genes were responsible for the development of scrapie in sheep. He was convinced that natural scrapie is a genetic disease which could be eradicated by proper breeding protocols (138, 139). He considered its transmission by inoculation to be of importance primarily for laboratory studies and communicable infection of little consequence in nature. Other investigators viewed natural scrapie as an infectious disease and argued that host genetics only modulates susceptibility to an endemic infectious agent (55).

Prion-infested offal is thought to be responsible for the epidemic of BSE (185). Prions in the offal from scrapie-infected sheep, or maybe from rare cows affected by hypothetical "sporadic BSE," seem to have survived the rendering process that produced meat and bone meal (MBM). Whether the "Ur-BSE prion" originated from sheep or was autochtonous to cows is a question that may not be solvable and is of mainly academic and legal significance.

The MBM was fed to cattle as a nutritional supplement. After BSE was recognized, MBM produced from domestic animal offal was banned from further use. Since 1986, when BSE was first recognized, >180,000 cattle have died of BSE. Over 130 persons have developed a "new variant" of CJD (43, 53, 186), which is likely to represent transmission of BSE to humans (35, 47, 81).

As we learn about the molecular and genetic characteristics of prion proteins, our understanding of prions and their place in biology will undoubtedly undergo considerable change. Indeed, the discovery of PrP, the identification of pathogenic *PRNP* gene mutations, and the differences in the structures of PrP^C and PrP^{Sc}, as well as studies of the process by which prions move from the site of infection to the brain, have already forced us to think about these diseases from viewpoints that had not been previously considered.

BASIC PRION BIOLOGY

The "Protein-Only" Hypothesis

The most widely accepted hypothesis on the nature of the infectious agent causing TSEs, which, as stated above, was termed prion by Stanley B. Prusiner (148), predicates that it consists essentially of a scrapie-like prion protein (PrP^{Sc}), an abnormally folded, protease-resistant, β-sheet-rich isoform of a normal cellular prion protein (PrP^C). According to this theory, the prion does not contain any informational nucleic acids, and its infective material propagates simply by recruitment and "autocatalytic" conformational conversion of cellular prion protein into disease-associated PrP^{Sc} (11).

A large body of experimental and epidemiological evidence is compatible with the protein-only hypothesis, and very stringently designed experiments have failed to disprove it. It would go well beyond the scope of this chapter to review all efforts that have been undertaken to this effect. Perhaps most impressively, knockout mice carrying a homozygous deletion of the murine *Prnp* gene, which encodes PrP^C (*Prnp*$^{0/0}$ mice), fail to develop disease upon inoculation with infectious brain homogenate (37), nor do their brains carry prion infectivity (159). Reintroduction of *Prnp* by transgenesis—even in a shortened, redacted form—restores infectibility and prion replication in *Prnp*$^{0/0}$ mice (57, 58, 163, 173). In addition, all familial cases of human TSEs are characterized by mutations in the human PrP^C gene (designated *PRNP*) (12, 151). Two recent studies go a long way toward settling the score as to the nature of the infectious agent by demonstrating that prions may be synthesized in cell-free systems (40, 108).

According to the protein-only hypothesis, the abnormal form of PrP^C, PrP^{Sc}, represents the infectious agent. Even if the protein-only hypothesis has not formally been proven, all studies agree that PrP^{Sc} represents an essential component of prion infectivity. The three-dimensional structure of PrP^C has been solved by nuclear magnetic resonance (NMR) spectroscopy; similar analyses have not been possible for PrP^{Sc} (86, 154). Studies employing Fourier transform infrared spectroscopy have demonstrated that PrP^{Sc} contains more β-sheets (about 40%) and fewer α-helical structures (about 30%) than PrP^C (135).

Whether prions multiply by template-directed refolding or by seeded nucleation, certain domains of PrP^C (or the entire protein) would need to rearrange such that the monomeric protein becomes capable of inducing the same change in further PrP^C monomers (Fig. 2A). This idea represents the core of the "template-directed refolding" hypothesis, which predicates an instructionist role for PrP^{Sc} onto PrP^C. The experimental evidence is compatible with this hypothesis, yet no positive evidence in its favor has been brought forward.

Alternatively, it has been proposed that PrP^{Sc} exists in a mass action equilibrium with PrP^C. Such equilibrium would be heavily shifted toward the side of PrP^C, so that only minute amounts of PrP^{Sc} would coexist with PrP^C. If that were the case, PrP^{Sc} could not possibly represent the infectious agent, since it would be ubiquitous. According to this "nucleation" hypothesis (92), however, the infectious agent would consist of a highly ordered aggregate of PrP^{Sc} molecules. The aggregated state would be an intrinsic property of infectivity: monomeric PrP^{Sc} would be harmless, but it might be prone to incorporation into nascent PrP^{Sc} aggregates (Fig. 2B).

Testing these hypotheses requires precise knowledge of the structural features of both PrP^C and PrP^{Sc}. To date, such knowledge has not progressed to a state which would allow for resolution of this issue. The structure of PrP^C has been studied extensively with high-resolution methods. Both crystallography (102) and NMR spectroscopy (154) have yielded detailed insights into the arrangement of PrP^C at the atomic level. PrP^{Sc}, however, has been amenable merely to low-resolution structural methods.

The NMR studies of recombinant PrP^C yielded a big surprise. The amino-proximal half of the molecule is not structured at all, whereas the carboxy-proximal half is globular and contains three α-helices (154, 155). This does not mean that the amino terminus must be randomly coiled in vivo: functional studies with transgenic mice imply that the domain comprising amino acids (aa) 32 to 121 carries out important physiological functions (163). Maybe the flexible tail of PrP^C acquires a defined structure once it reaches its natural habitat on rafts, which are specialized microdomains of the plasma membrane (131).

Why wasn't it yet possible to elucidate the structure of PrP^{Sc}? As discussed above, prion infective material can be recovered only from prion-infected mammalian organisms, or (in much lesser quantities) from infected cultured cells. In neither case is the purity of the recovered material satisfactory. Moreover, infectivity-associated PrP^{Sc} appears to consist obligatorily of aggregates: disaggregation sterilizes prions (149). But insoluble aggregates are resilient to most technologies for determination of protein structure; hence, all we know is that PrP^{Sc} consists mainly of a β-pleated sheet (42) and that PrP^{Sc} aggregates expose a remarkably ordered structure (187).

Neurotoxicity, Infectivity, and PrP^{Sc}

It is clear that prions exert their destructive effects predominantly, if not exclusively, within the central nervous

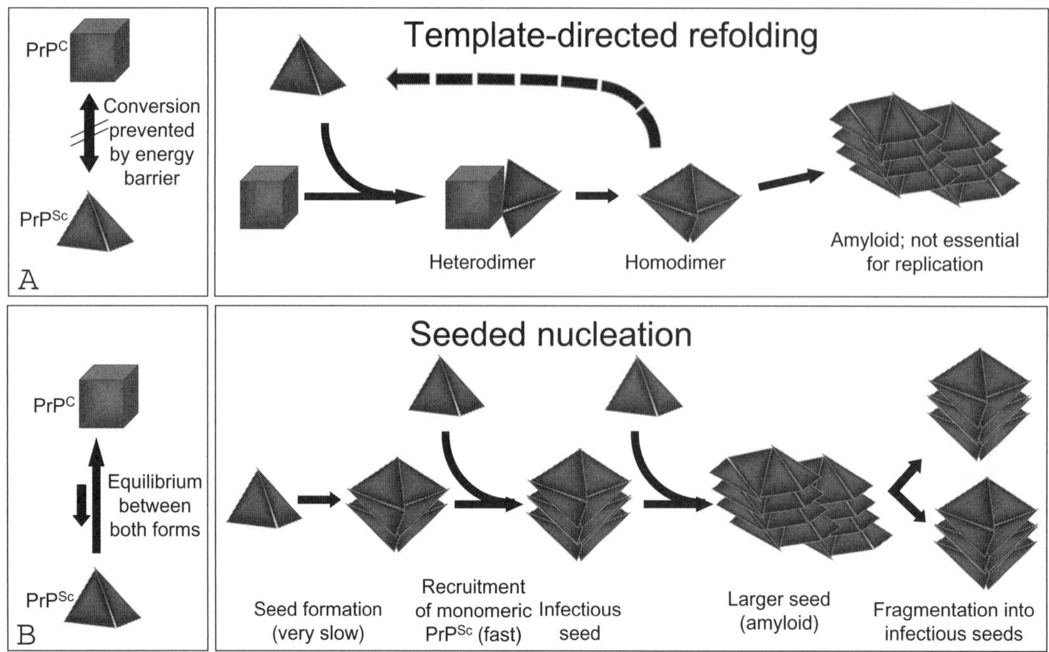

FIGURE 2 Models for the conformational conversion of PrP^C into PrP^{Sc}. (A) The "refolding" or template assistance model postulates an interaction between exogenously introduced PrP^{Sc} and endogenous PrP^C, which is induced to transform itself into further PrP^{Sc}. A high energy barrier may prevent spontaneous conversion of PrP^C into PrP^{Sc}. (B) The "seeding" or nucleation-polymerization model proposes that PrP^C and PrP^{Sc} are in a reversible thermodynamic equilibrium. Only if several monomeric PrP^{Sc} molecules are mounted into a highly ordered seed can further monomeric PrP^{Sc} be recruited and eventually aggregate to amyloid. Within such a crystal-like seed, PrP^{Sc} becomes stabilized. Fragmentation of PrP^{Sc} aggregates increases the number of nuclei, which can recruit further PrP^{Sc} and thus results in apparent replication of the agent.

system (CNS). However, the proximal cause of neurotoxicity remains unclear. PrP^C is required for prion replication, as mice devoid of PrP^C are resistant to prions (37). Dimeric PrP^C was found to efficaciously bind PrP^{Sc} (128), suggesting that its conversion is somehow instructed by the latter. The first evidence for PrP^C-mediated neurotoxicity was provided by grafting neural tissue overexpressing PrP^C into the brains of PrP-deficient mice (29). After intracerebral inoculation with scrapie prions, grafts accumulated high levels of PrP^{Sc} and infectivity development characteristic scrapie histopathology. It was then reported that depletion of endogenous neuronal PrP^C in mice with established prion infection reversed early spongiform changes and banned neuronal loss and progression to clinical disease (117).

PrP^C depletion during the conversion process is unlikely to cause pathology, since ablation of PrP^C does not result in scrapie-like symptoms (38). This is corroborated by postnatal PrP^C depletion which does not result in neurodegeneration (118). However, it could be possible that PrP^C function is altered upon conversion to PrP^{Sc}, leading to neurodegeneration (6, 9). Even though neurotoxic, quite surprisingly, high prion titers in lymphoid organs are not accompanied by significant histopathological changes (46, 54), even though murine scrapie infection was recently reported to cause an abnormal germinal-center reaction in the spleen (124).

Expression of a PrP variant targeted to the cytosol was found to be toxic to cultured cells and transgenic mice, and it was speculated that this feature might be common to diverse prion-related neurodegenerative disorders (111, 112). Mutant PrP^C, lacking a glycosylphosphatidylinositol (GPI) anchor and its signal peptide, retrogradely transported out of the endoplasmatic reticulum induced the generation of amorphous PrP aggregates that possessed partial proteinase K (PK) resistance in the cytosol (111). The disease was not reported to be transmissible—which is, after all, the crucial defining trait of a prion disease. Subsequent reports have argued against the contribution of a cytosolic neurotoxic PrP species to prion pathology (56), and therefore this issue should be considered unresolved at the present stage.

Transgenic mice expressing variants of PrP with N-terminal deletions were found to suffer from unexpected phenotypes, including cerebellar granular cell degeneration and leukoencephalopathy (153, 163). Deletions of aa 32 to 121 or 32 to 134 (collectively termed ΔPrP) confer strong neurotoxicity to PrP^C in vivo, a pathology that can be abrogated by reintroduction of wild-type, full-length PrP^C (163). The latter phenomenon suggests that ΔPrP is a functional antagonist of PrP^C. If so, suppression of ΔPrP toxicity may be used for probing the functional integrity of PrP mutants. This strategy has been extensively used, as it allows one to map functional domains within the *Prnp* gene—even if the function of PrP is still not understood.

PrP^C contains a highly hydrophobic stretch at the border between its flexible N-terminal part and its globular C-terminal part. This particular stretch is believed to play an important functional role, and its manipulation may provide significant functional insights: recent studies suggest that a small deletion within this hydrophobic stretch (aa 121 to 134) suffices to produce a highly neurotoxic molecule (22). Another neurotoxic type of PrP was reported by Hegde et al., who discovered that the hydrophobic domain acquires a transmembrane localization in a small fraction of PrP molecules, in contrast to abundantly GPI-anchored PrP molecules (77). Expression levels of transmembrane PrP (^{Ctm}PrP) are elevated in certain pathogenic PrP mutants, which are neurotoxic when expressed at high levels in transgenic animals (171). Surprisingly, when coexpressed with full-length PrP, ^{Ctm}PrP is even more neurotoxic. In this regard, it behaves very differently from N-terminally truncated PrP, whose toxicity is reduced or abolished by expression of full-length PrP.

Although the normal function of PrP is presumed to be beneficial, there is a growing list of malicious consequences that can be elicited by manipulating PrP—beyond eliciting prion diseases. No only do such consequences encompass the neurologic syndrome (called Shmerling's disease) elicited by ΔPrP family members, but also it was found that antibody-mediated cross-linking of PrP in vivo triggers neuronal apoptosis in the hippocampus and cerebellum (167). This effect was induced by dimerization of PrP^{C} through the intracranial stereotaxic delivery of bivalent immunoglobulins. None of the molecular mechanisms underlying these observations have been elucidated, but there has been much speculation that cross-linking may induce cytotoxic lethal signaling cascades. Recently, Chesebro et al. have generated an interesting *Prnp* transgene that lacks the signal peptide responsible for GPI anchoring (45). Consequently, transgenic mice expressed exclusively a secreted form of PrP^{C}. Even though GPI-negative transgenic mice did not develop clinical disease upon prion infection, their brains contained PrP^{Sc} plaques. Evidently, removal of the GPI anchor abolished the susceptibility to clinical disease while preserving the competence of the soluble PrP^{C} molecule to support prion replication (45). This observation fits with the growing body of evidence that PrP^{C} may function as a signaling molecule—just like other GPI-linked proteins (95).

Additionally, the brain, blood, and heart of GPI-negative transgenic mice contained both abnormal protease-resistant prion protein and prion infective material (181). Blood plasma of GPI-negative transgenic mice was found to be infectious (>7 log 50% lethal doses/ml) (181), mimicking a situation of blood-borne prion infectivity as known from sheep sick from scrapie (87), elk and deer with chronic wasting disease (123), and vCJD patients (110, 140). Interestingly, the hearts of these transgenic mice contained PrP^{Sc}-positive amyloid deposits leading to myocardial stiffness and cardiac disease (181).

Even though the exact composition of the infectious prion agent remains elusive, the size of the most infectious moiety was determined (166). The PK-resistant core of PrP^{Sc} was partially disaggregated, fractionated by size, and analyzed by light scattering and nondenaturing gel electrophoresis. Analyses revealed that nonfibrillar particles, with masses equivalent to 14 to 28 PrP molecules, are the most infectious particles. These very exciting data suggest that the "Ur-prion" is indeed an oligomeric seed, i.e., a small ordered aggregate which possesses the capability of growing by means of recruiting further monomeric PrP into itself.

David Harris and colleagues generated transgenic (PrP-EGFP) mice which express an enhanced green fluorescent protein (EGFP)-tagged version of the prion protein. This fusion protein behaves like endogenous PrP in terms of its posttranslational processing, subcellular localization, and functional activity—as measured by suppression of Shmerling's disease (19). Although not convertible to PrP^{Sc} when expressed by itself, the fusion protein was incorporated into scrapie fibrils in brains of prion-infected animals. Coexpression of the transgene and wild-type PrP resulted in progressive accumulation of fluorescent PrP-EGFP aggregates in neuropil, axons and the Golgi apparatus of neurons, upon prion inoculation. These results identified intracellular sites of PrP^{Sc} aggregation that had not been visualized thus far (20) and provide a novel and potentially extremely useful reagent for the study of PrP aggregation.

Prion Pathogenesis: Lessons from Mouse Models

PrP^{C} itself is involved in transporting prion infectivity from peripheral sites to the CNS. Adoptive transfer with wild-type bone marrow into *Prnp*$^{0/0}$ mice restores the capability of the spleen to accumulate high titers of prion infectivity, up to 300 dpi (27, 94). However, reconstitution experiments with wild-type bone marrow into *Prnp*$^{0/0}$ mice were insufficient to restore neuroinvasion. Therefore, hematopoietic cells (e.g., B and T cells, macrophages, and dendritic cells [DCs]) facilitate the transport of prions from peripheral entry sites to secondary lymphoid organs, in which prions accumulate and/or replicate, although the primary compartment for prion neuroinvasion appears to be nonhematopoietic, since it cannot be adopted by bone marrow reconstitution (27, 94, 98).

But how do prions reach the brain following a natural route of exposure, e.g., via ingestion? And which cellular and molecular preconditions enable efficient transport? These questions were intensively studied in vitro and in vivo: an in vitro study has shown that microfold cells (M cells), specialized intestinal epithelial cells which transfer antigens, including pathogens, through the epithelium, can transport infectious prions from the apical to the basolateral surface (79). Subsequently, prion neural entry and transit to the CNS may occur with direct prion uptake by nerve endings in the intestine (or spleen after an intraperitoneal exposure), and/or possibly following an amplification phase in the lymphoid tissue; Peyer's patches are required for prion disease development in the mouse (145). Many studies have shown disruption and delay in the development of prion disease upon interference with lymphoid prion accumulation (116, 130). Some of the lymphoid players crucial to peripheral prion accumulation have been revealed. Clearly, functional follicular dendritic cells (FDCs) are essential (114, 130)—but it is not entirely clear whether they are the only site of lymphoreticular prion replication or accumulation (27, 94). B lymphocytes are also necessary (98), as they provide maturation signals for FDCs. There is an ill-characterized bone marrow-derived cell population that clearly supports prion replication (27, 99), although this may not apply to all prion strains (30). In addition, morphological evidence based on time course studies indicates involvement of the vagus nerve and the sympathetic nervous system as routes of peripheral prion transport to the CNS (23). Glatzel et al. have shown that the sympathetic nervous system is essentially involved in neuroinvasion: mice with sympathectomy show a significantly prolonged incubation period, and transgenic mice overexpressing a nerve growth factor transgene that have sympathetic hyperinnervation of lymphoid organs show an accelerated incubation period after a peripheral prion exposure, illustrating the significance of these peripheral nerves in prion pathogenesis (69).

In the mouse scrapie model, some forms of immunodeficiency impair prion replication and delay disease development, illustrating the significant contribution of this early lymphoid phase. For example, severe combined immunodeficient (SCID) mice, RAG-$1^{-/-}$ mice, and μMT mice completely resist intraperitoneal prion infection (98). However, replacement of B-lymphocyte populations, whether they express PrP^{c} or not, restores prion infectibility, possibly due to the key role of mature B lymphocytes in FDC maturation by provision of tumor necrosis factor and lymphotoxins. PrP^{Sc} heavily decorates FDC membranes in secondary follicles of the spleen (93), lymph node, tonsils, and Peyer's patches in several prion diseases, including vCJD, scrapie, and chronic wasting disease.

The importance of FDCs in peripheral prion pathogenesis may be exploited for prion prevention strategies. Inhibiting the LTβR pathway in mice and nonhuman primates by treatment with LTβR-immunoglobulin fusion protein (LTβR-Ig) results in the disappearance of mature, functional FDCs (72, 73). Indeed, treatment with LTβR-Ig was found to impair peripheral prion pathogenesis (7, 114, 130).

The detection of PrP^{Sc} in spleens of sCJD patients (68) suggests that the interface between cells of the immune system and peripheral nerves might also be of relevance in sporadic prion diseases. Indeed, in mouse scrapie studies, there is no doubt that the microarchitecture of lymphoid organs crucially controls the efficacy of prion neuroinvasion: manipulation of the distance between FDCs and major splenic nerves affects the velocity of neuroinvasion (144). By ablation of the CXCR5 chemokine receptor, lymphocytes were directed toward specific microcompartments which reduced the distance between germinal center-associated FDCs and nerve endings (59). This resulted in an increased rate of prion entry into the CNS in CXCR$5^{-/-}$ mice, most likely due to repositioning of FDCs in juxtaposition with highly innervated, splenic arterioles. It remains to be determined whether the increased rate of neuroinvasion results from a passive diffusion of prions, such as from FDC-released exosomes (51, 52), or whether mobile cells such as DCs or B cells located in the germinal center are involved in an active process of transport. However, the cells involved in early transport remain unclear. Some evidence for the involvement of DCs has accrued (18). However, other mobile elements, including budding viruses, could also serve as vehicles of infectivity (107).

Since FDCs bind to opsonized antigens via the CD21 and CD35 complement receptors, is complement involved in prion pathogenesis? Indeed, mice that lack various complement factors, including C1q (100), or have been depleted of the C3 complement component (113) enjoy enhanced resistance to peripheral prion inoculation. C1q was shown to directly bind PrP in vitro (26). Human studies also point to a possible role for members of the classical complement cascade in prion pathogenesis (103); however, their precise role in prion disease is unknown.

As proinflammatory cytokines and immune cells are involved in lymphoid prion replication (30, 115, 130, 144), whether chronic inflammatory conditions within nonlymphoid organs could affect the dynamics of prion distribution was assessed. Indeed, inclusion body myositis, which is an inflammatory disease of muscle, was associated with large PrP^{Sc} deposits in muscle (104). Therefore, mice with nephritis, hepatitis, or pancreatitis were inoculated with mouse prions (RML strain) and were found to accumulate prions in these otherwise-prion-free organs. The presence of inflammatory foci consistently correlated with upregulation of LT and the ectopic induction of PrP^{C}-expressing FDCs (78).

These data raised concerns that analogous phenomena might occur in TSE-susceptible ruminants. Indeed, it was found that sheep with natural scrapie infections and concurrent mastitis harbored PrP^{Sc} in their mammary glands (109), indicating that inflammatory conditions induce accumulation of prions in organs previously believed to be prion free (Color Plate 55). PrP^{Sc} was identified in macrophages which end up being secreted in milk, which leads to the question of whether transmission of prions within flocks of sheep may occur via lactation (Color Plate 56). Therefore, inflammation might be indeed a "license" for prion replication in nonlymphoid peripheral organs (Color Plate 57), and other organized chronic inflammatory disorders could potentially be sites of prion accumulation and replication.

In addition, it was hypothesized that inflammatory conditions could result in the shedding of prions via excretory organs (e.g., the kidneys). To investigate this hypothesis, various transgenic and spontaneous mouse models of nephritis were analyzed to ascertain whether prions could be excreted via urine (162). Indeed, prion infectivity was observed in the urine of mice with both subclinical and terminal scrapie, and with inflammatory conditions of the kidney (162).

The genetic or environmental factors that enable horizontal prion spread between hosts have been perplexing. It is possible that the horizontal spread of prions is mediated by secreted body fluids (e.g., urine and milk) that are derived from potentially infectious secretory organs (e.g., mammary glands and kidneys). Placentas of infected ewes could provide a source of prion infectivity for horizontal transmission (182), but the set of data supporting the latter hypothesis is scant at best.

Public health considerations mandate that we increase our understanding of the altered prion tropism observed in ruminants (e.g., sheep, cattle, goats, elk, and deer) and the underlying mechanisms. Future experiments should include an analysis of the effects of other common chronic inflammatory disorders (e.g., granulomatous diseases) in prion-infected animals.

Does a chronic subclinical disease or a permanent carrier status occur in ruminants or in humans? Evidence that such a carrier status may be produced by the passage of the infectious agent across species was first reported by Race and Chesebro (13, 152) and has been confirmed by others (83)—at least for passage between hamsters and mice. Bruce Chesebro reported that hamster prions were inoculated into mice, which lived a long symptom-free life and did not accumulate detectable PrP^{Sc} (6). PrP^{Sc}-negative brains were then injected into other mice, which had no clinical disease for >650 days. The brains of these mice were then passaged into hamsters and resulted in rapid lethality. Therefore, the agent had silently replicated for several years in mice without inducing any clinical signs or histopathology but maintained full virulence for hamsters.

Immunodeficiency can also lead to a similar situation in which prions replicate silently in the body, even when there is no species barrier (62). So the problem of animal

TSEs could be more widespread than is assumed and may call for drastic prion surveillance measures in farm animals. Moreover, people carrying the infectious agent may transmit it horizontally (2), and the risks associated with this possibility can be met only if we know more about how the agent is transmitted and how prions reach the brain from peripheral sites.

Mechanistic Underpinnings of Prion Strains

The phenomenon of prion strains has intrigued scientists for decades. Prion strains are distinguishable by stable incubation periods and the pattern of histopathological lesions within the brains of members of the same host species. The propagation of different scrapie strains in mice homozygous with regard to their *Prnp* gene is the most difficult finding to be explained by the protein-only hypothesis (6, 9): it suggests that an incoming PrP^{Sc} strain can convert the same PrP precursor into a likeness of itself and that this alone can create distinct disease phenotypes, varying in clinical signs, organ tropism, and regions of prion accumulation in the brain.

It is challenging, but maybe not impossible, to reconcile these intriguing data with Prusiner's protein-only hypothesis: epigenetic, posttranslational strain characteristics of prions appear to dominate over the primary prion protein sequence of the infected host. The diversity of prion strains is largely believed to be due to the conformational flexibility of PrP^{Sc}. The host PrP^{Sc} structure is determined by both the PrP^{Sc} conformation in the donor inoculum and limitations imposed by the host primary PrP structure. Circumstantial evidence suggests that strain phenotypes may be encoded within different conformations of PrP^{Sc} with distinct properties, including stability against chaotropic salts and heat (158), the relative prevalence of the main glycosylated moieties, and the size of the PK-digested PrP^{Sc}. The strain-specific differences in the size of PK-digested PrP^{Sc} molecules are thought to result from individual conformations leading to exposure of distinct cleavage sites. This was first suggested by experiments with transmissible mink encephalopathy, indicating that prion diversity could indeed be conferred by a single protein with various three-dimensional structures (25). Although great strides have been made toward understanding the molecular origin of strains, the final proof that conformational variants of PrP^{Sc} represent the biological basis of prion strains is still lacking.

Recent in vivo evidence indicated that a similar phenomenon of conformational variants may occur in AD (129). Here the existence of $A\beta$ "strains" that can seed and accelerate aggregation and $A\beta$ pathology was posited. These intriguing observations support the hypothesis that the pathogenetic mechanisms operating in AD and in prion diseases have more in common than we often appreciate (4). Perhaps future studies will address whether different $A\beta$ strains with distinct biochemical or neuropathological characteristics occur in humans. Can multiple prion strains coexist and effect prion replication? Two subtypes of sCJD have been recently demonstrated to coexist in humans (143). Experimental studies have shown that when two strains infect the same host, one strain can impede the ability of the second strain to cause disease (120). Bartz and colleagues recently suggested that this might be caused by suppression of prion replication of the second strain (21). Strain features are useful for tracing prion infections between species. When transmitted to primates, BSE causes lesions strikingly similar to those of vCJD (14, 106). BSE is most likely transmissible to humans, too, and strong circumstantial evidence (1, 35, 81) suggests that BSE is the cause of vCJD, which has claimed more than 200 lives in the United Kingdom (85, 186) and a much smaller number in some other countries (43).

Analytical Differentiation of Prion Strains

Multiple TSE strains were historically distinguished by characteristic incubation periods in panels of differentially susceptible inbred mice (61). Different strains also differ in their capability of inducing morphologically diverse aggregates ranging from tiny deposits to huge amyloid plaques (164), and they can target distinct brain regions (34, 60). Combinations of these factors were used for establishing the uniqueness of the British BSE strain and its identity with the vCJD agent. However, strain determinations involving the inoculation of mice are unbearably slow and cumbersome and prohibitively expensive, and their reliability is merely based on correlative evidence (Table 1).

Meanwhile, a number of biochemical correlates for prion strains have been discovered. PrP^{Sc}s from distinct prion strains differ in electrophoretic mobility (24), immunoreactivity to amino-proximal antibodies after proteolysis (143), and relative glycoform prevalence (82). Also, the PrP^{Sc}-capturing efficacy of conformational antibodies (158) and the stability of PrP^{Sc} against heat and chaotropes

TABLE 1 Synopsis of currently used prion strain differentiation assays[a]

Assay principle	Test substrate	Speed	Cost
Incubation period in indicator mice (61)	Mice	Years	+++
Histologic lesion profile (176)	Mice	Years	+++
Histoblots (158)	Immunohistology	Days	++
Conformation-dependent immunoassay (141)	ELISA[b]	Days	+
Conformational-stability assay (25)	Western blot	Days	++
PK cleavage site (143)	Western blot	Days	+
Detection with N-terminal antibodies (82)	Western blot	Days	+
Glycosylation profile on Western blot (164)	Western blot	Days	+
Amyloid detection by thioflavin and Congo red stains (165)	Histochemistry	Hours	+
Luminescent conjugated polymers	Histochemistry	Hours	+
Cell panel assay	Cell culture	Weeks	++

[a] Most assays sport high discriminatory power among a few specific strains (e.g., glycosylation profiles for BSE and vCJD) but may perform poorly with other strains.

[b] ELISA, enzyme-linked immunosorbent assay.

(141) are to some extent strain dependent (Table 1). None of the above phenomena is conclusively discriminatory, yet they suggest that the structure of PrP^{Sc} aggregates might define prion strains (3). Alternative explanations have been put forward, including, e.g., differential binding to non-PrP^{Sc} components (184).

Yeasts carry self-propagating elements consisting of ordered protein aggregates that share traits with mammalian prions—including strains. The physical basis for yeast prion strains has been convincingly traced to the supramolecular assembly of the respective protein aggregates (179). By extension, the diversity of mammalian prion strains may plausibly reside within the conformational heterogeneity of PrP^{Sc}. Yet in the absence of definitive knowledge about its physical substrate, all strain differentiation methods—be they based on animal inoculations or on biochemical analyses—must be regarded as surrogate markers.

In this situation, any tool enabling strain discrimination from a new angle is welcome. The laboratory of Charles Weissmann described a panel of cell lines selectively permissive to distinct scrapie prion substrains. Mahal and colleagues have availed themselves of the previously described scrapie cell assay (101) to determine the efficiency with which four murine prion strains were propagated on four selected cell lines. Infectivity titers of the prion strain preparations, as measured by endpoint dilutions in susceptible animals, were almost identical, yet their "response index," the reciprocal of the dilution that results in a given proportion of infected cells under defined assay conditions, varied considerably among strains. As a consequence, the four strains could be clearly distinguished on the cell panel (Table 2).

Sibling subclones from a single cell line show surprisingly variable relative susceptibilities to individual strains. This provides a powerful tool for identifying factors controlling strain permissiveness. What could the identity of such factors be? Prion replication may be intrinsically controlled by the thermodynamics of aggregation, but it may also be modulated by cell-specific chaperones specifying the folding of PrP, or by putative "disaggregases" akin to Hsp104 of *Saccharomyces cerevisiae* (44) or the DnaK/ClpB system of bacteria (39).

If the strain-specific properties are enciphered by PrP^{Sc}, and the geometry of PrP^{Sc} amyloid affords sufficient degrees of freedom, cerebral PrP^{Sc} deposits of prion-infected individuals may exhibit subtle structural idiosyncrasies that are unique to distinct strains. This is confirmed by the observation that luminescent conjugated polymers (LCPs) fluoresce in distinct colors upon binding to PrP^{Sc} aggregates associated with various prion strains (165). The modulation of fluorescence is due to the rotational freedom bestowed by the single bonds between the thiophene building blocks of LCPs. Binding to PrP^{Sc} fixates the thiophenes in planar, orthogonal, or intermediate orientations, thereby altering their photophysical properties (Color Plate 57). Artificially assembled fibrils of pure, recombinant PrP also display conformation-dependent spectra, establishing that LCPs provide valid measurements of the supramolecular geometry of PrP^{Sc}.

TABLE 2 Response of the cell panel to four murine prion strains

Strain	Response[a] with cell line			
	CAD5	LD9	PK1	R33
22L	+	+	+	+
RML	+	+	+	−
Me7	+	+	−	−
301C	+	−	−	−

[a] Response is graded as efficient (+) or undetectable (−) prion replication, as measured by the scrapie cell assay on four cell lines.

Taken together, the studies discussed above add to the evidence that the host PrP^{Sc} structure is determined by both the PrP^{Sc} conformation within the inoculum and by constraints imposed by host factors. It is easy to imagine that important knowledge could be generated by combining Mahal's cell panel and LCP-based techniques.

Amyloid strains may be of broader significance than to prions. Strain-like amyloid conformational variants may occur in AD (129), suggesting that the pathogenetic mechanisms operating in AD and in prion diseases have more in common than typically appreciated (4). Ordered aggregation of proteins was also found to occur in most instances of type II diabetes, in chronic inflammatory conditions, and in many disorders of skeletal muscle. Therefore, a full understanding of the prion strain phenomenon may help in devising sensitive diagnostic procedures, and possibly also rational therapies, for many aggregation proteinopathies. Some of the latter diseases rank among the most prevalent chronic ailments of humankind.

EPIDEMIOLOGY

Human prion diseases manifest as sporadic, genetic, and acquired disorders. They are referred to as sCJD, familial or genetic CJD (gCJD), iCJD, and vCJD.

sCJD is a rapidly progressive dementia, usually leading to death within 6 months of disease onset (67). The cause of sCJD remains enigmatic. To date no obvious risk factors have been identified. Because of the short mean duration of this disease, incidence and mortality rates for sCJD are similar; thus, mortality rates are routinely used to describe the epidemiology of this disease. The overall annual mortality rate from sCJD in a panel of European and non-European countries, including Australia and Canada, is 1.39 cases per million for the period between 1999 and 2002 (105). Mortality rates are fairly constant, both over time and between countries, ranging from 0.41 case per million in 1994 in Spain to 2.63 cases per million in 2002 in Switzerland (70). Unlike other dementing diseases such as AD and Parkinson's disease, in which incidence rises with age, the peak incidence is between 55 and 65 years of age (70).

gCJD can be subdivided into three phenotypes: familial CJD, GSS disease, and FFI. The mode of inheritance in all of these diseases, which cosegregate with mutations in *PRNP*, is autosomal dominant (75). The overall annual mortality rate for gCJD in a panel of European and non-European countries, including Australia and Canada, is 0.17 case per million for the time period from 1999 to 2002. Between 1999 and 2002, mortality rates for gCJD were markedly different in various countries, ranging from 0.02 in The Netherlands to 1.07 in Slovakia (105).

iCJD is caused by prion exposure during neurosurgical procedures such as implantation of human dura mater, corneal graft implantation, or treatment with human cadaveric pituitary extracts (33). iCJD is rare, with fewer than 300 published cases. The majority of cases were caused by implantation of dura mater and injection of pituitary growth hormone (33). Recent epidemiological data confirm the observation that iCJD mainly affects individuals younger than 39 years (105).

vCJD, a relatively new member of the human prion disease family, was first reported in 1996 (186). Biochemical, neuropathological, and transmission studies have substantiated the concern that vCJD represents transmission of BSE prions to humans (1, 14, 35, 81). The incidence of vCJD in the United Kingdom rose each year from 1996 to 2001, evoking fears of a large upcoming epidemic. Since 2001, however, the incidence of vCJD in the United Kingdom appears to be stabilizing, and only a small number of other countries have seen isolated cases of vCJD. Although predictions on the future of the vCJD epidemic are still flawed with imprecision, there is growing evidence that the total number of vCJD victims will be limited (183). vCJD has a distinct clinicopathological profile, including age of onset. vCJD victims are much younger than sCJD patients (median age at death, 29 years) (105).

PATHOGENESIS IN HUMANS

CJD was, and fortunately continues to be, exceedingly rare: its incidence is typically $1/10^6$ inhabitants/year, but reaches $3/10^6$ inhabitants/year in Switzerland, which is currently reporting the highest number of cases (70, 71). Kuru, once decimating the population of Papua New Guinea, has almost disappeared. Iatrogenic transmission of CJD has principally occurred through improperly sterilized neurosurgical instruments, transplants of dura mater, and administration of pituitary hormones of cadaveric origin. While the last two routes of transmission no longer pose a major threat, a significant number of individuals may have been infected during a critical time window and may develop CJD in the coming years.

vCJD has caused some 140 deaths in the United Kingdom and a few cases in France, Italy, and Canada (http://www.gnn.gov.uk/environment/fullDetail.asp?ReleaseID=319104&NewsAreaID=2&NavigatedFromDepartment=False). Epidemiological, biochemical, and histologic evidence suggests that vCJD represents transmission of BSE prions to humans (1, 14, 35, 81). As stated above, the incidence of vCJD in the United Kingdom rose each year from 1996 to 2001; since the year 2001, however, the incidence of vCJD in the United Kingdom appears to be stabilizing (http://www.cjd.ed.ac.uk/vcjdq.htm). One may argue that it is too early to draw any far-reaching conclusions, but each year passing without any dramatic rise in the number of cases increases the hope that the total number of vCJD victims will be limited (183). Presently, there is reason to hope that the incidence of vCJD in the United Kingdom may already be subsiding (17).

vCJD prions accumulate prominently in lymphoreticular tissue, and the latter can be used for diagnostic purposes. Surprisingly, prions accumulate in lymphoid organs and muscle of sCJD patients (68).

Chronic Wasting Disease

There is uncertainty surrounding the danger of transmission to humans represented by chronic wasting disease. In fact, even transmissibility of BSE to humans relies on circumstantial evidence. Epidemiology and biochemistry favor the link between BSE and vCJD but are not ultimately conclusive. The Koch postulates (which would unambiguously assign an infectious agent to a disease) have never been fulfilled, and experimental inoculation of humans was—thankfully—never performed. Also, accidental exposure to BSE infectivity of a sizable collective at a precisely defined time point has never occurred or did not result in disease. Likewise, we do not know whether scrapie is just a veterinary problem that affects only sheep and goats or whether it can cross species barriers and affect humans. Finally, it is unknown whether BSE, upon transmission to sheep, remains as dangerous for humans as cow-derived BSE or whether it becomes attenuated and acquires the (allegedly) innocuous properties of bona fide sheep scrapie.

CLINICAL MANIFESTATIONS

Initial symptoms of sCJD include cognitive deficits, sleep disturbances, and behavioral abnormalities. As the disease progresses, other clinical features such as extrapyramidal and pyramidal symptoms, ataxia, and visual disturbances become obvious, and the patients usually develop myoclonus (67). Terminally affected sCJD patients typically develop a state of akinetic mutism prior to death. The disease course is usually short, the mean duration of the illness being 4 to 5 months (Table 3).

The clinical presentation of gCJD varies with the underlying mutation. Some mutants yield a clinical picture that is similar to that of sCJD. The age at onset tends to be younger and the disease duration longer than for sCJD. FFI and GSS disease represent exceptions. FFI has a unique clinical course which is characterized by profound disruption of the normal sleep-wake cycle, insomnia, and sympathetic overactivity (134), whereas GSS disease manifests as a progressive cerebellar ataxia.

In iCJD, the site of prion exposure seems to dictate the incubation time that intervenes between exposure and onset of prion disease-related symptoms. Direct intracerebral exposure to prions and implantation of prion-contaminated dura, for example, are associated with short incubation periods (16 to 28 months), whereas exposure to prions at sites outside the CNS results in long incubation times, ranging from 5 to 30 years (48). Furthermore, there is evidence that the route of prion exposure influences the clinical presentation. Dura mater- or growth hormone-related cases of iCJD are associated with a predominantly ataxic phenotype, whereas dementia was the initial symptom in cases in which prions were directly introduced into the CNS.

The fact that vCJD carries a distinct clinical profile has facilitated the formulation of diagnostic criteria. vCJD victims are much younger than sCJD patients (median age at death, 29 years). Furthermore, initial features and illness duration are relatively specific, with initial psychiatric symptoms and a median illness duration of 14 months (Table 3). It has been hard to estimate incubation times for vCJD due to the fact that the exact time points of prion exposure are not defined.

The diagnosis of human prion diseases is based on the appraisal of clinical signs and symptoms (described below) and a number of auxiliary examinations (48). Electroencephalography has historically been used to substantiate the diagnosis of a human prion disease. The usefulness of electroencephalography has been questioned due to its lim-

TABLE 3 Human prion diseases: clinical features

Human prion disease	Clinical features		
	Age at onset (yrs)	Mean disease duration (range)	Leading clinical symptoms
sCJD	60–70	6 m (1–35 m)	Progressive dementia and neurologic signs, e.g., myoclonus, cerebellar ataxia, visual problems, extrapyramidal symptoms
Inherited CJD			
gCJD	50–60	6 m (2–41 m)	Clinical symptoms similar to those of sCJD
GSS disease	50–60	5–6 yrs (3 m–13 yrs)	Cerebellar dysfunction (ataxia, nystagmus, dysarthria)
FFI	50 (20–63)	13–15 m (6–42 m)	Insomnia Autonomic dysfunction
Acquired CJD			
vCJD	26 (12–74)	14 m (6–24 m)	Early psychiatric symptoms (depression, anxiety, social withdrawal) dysesthesia, later neurologic deficits and cognitive decline
iCJD	—[a]	Similar to those of sCJD	Clinical symptoms similar to those of sCJD

[a] —, age at onset depends on iatrogenic exposure: incubation period, 1 to 30 years.

ited sensitivity (190). Recent advances in neuroimaging, and especially in magnetic resonance imaging (MRI), have revealed that different human prion diseases have specific patterns (180). For vCJD, the "pulvinar sign," a high T2 MRI signal in the posterior thalamus, seems to be relatively unique and is present in about 75% of patients with vCJD (189). For sCJD, fluid-attenuated inversion recovery and diffusion-weighted MRI sequences are associated with high sensitivity and specificity and may represent a relatively noninvasive method to corroborate the diagnosis of a human prion disease (157).

LABORATORY DIAGNOSIS

General Considerations

PrP^{Sc}, the form of the infectious agent that causes prion diseases, is present in an oligomeric or polymeric form. The tight association of PrP^{Sc} molecules in aggregates may be responsible for the extreme stability of PrP^{Sc}. Prion infectivity is thus resistant to a number of techniques customarily used for decontamination of conventional infectious agents. In clinical laboratories, personal protective clothing such as disposable gowns, gloves, and barrier protection for mucous membranes (eye protection or full-face visor) are recommended when working with potentially contaminated specimens. In addition, strict adherence to standard working procedures aimed at minimizing the chance of penetrating injuries is essential. Handling of potentially infectious material requires certain additional precautions as described below.

Collection of Samples

Whole blood may be used for isolation of DNA for genetic analysis (exclusion of gCJD and detection of the *PRNP* codon 129 status). Blood should be shipped in a chilled container. Currently, an approved blood-based screening test for human prion diseases is not available. Cerebrospinal fluid (CSF) is routinely used to monitor elevation of nonspecific neuronal injury markers. CSF should be shipped at 4°C. Tissue may be used for histopathology and biochemical examination. Brain biopsies can be recommended only in order to exclude the diagnosis of diseases for which therapeutic options are available. Nonneural tissues (lymphatic tissue or muscle) may be useful in order to confirm the suspicion of vCJD. Tissue should be fixed in formalin for histologic assessment as described above and snap-frozen for Western blotting. Formalin-fixed material may be shipped at room temperature, whereas snap-frozen material must be shipped on dry ice.

Transport of Samples

Shipping of infectious material via water, land (road or train), and air must comply with the "Recommendations of the United Nations Committee of Experts on the Transport of Dangerous Goods." In these guidelines, human prions are listed in category 6 (Toxic and Infectious Substances), division 2 (Infectious Substances). The code number UN 2900 applies for this type of pathogen. Certified shipping containers must be used.

Detection of the Agent by Microscopy

Whenever it is crucial to exclude any treatable nonprion entity as the cause of disease, histologic examination of CNS tissue can be diagnostically utilized premortem. Routine hematoxylin-eosin stains are used to interpret the vacuolization patterns, whereas immunohistochemical demonstration of PrP is necessary in order to determine PrP deposition patterns (Color Plate 58). Postmortem, defined regions within the CNS (cerebellum and thalamus) and nonneuronal tissues can be sampled to demonstrate distinct PrP deposition patterns (36). Histologically, prion diseases are characterized by spongiform changes, astrogliosis, and neuronal loss. These changes are most evident in the cerebral cortex and in the cerebellum. The prominent cerebellar involvement is typical for prion diseases and clearly separates this group of diseases from other dementing illnesses such as AD or diffuse Lewy body disease. White matter changes may be present in some cases and are thought to constitute secondary changes. In vCJD and in about 10 to 20% of sCJD patients, prion plaques are a prominent feature and may be demonstrated by Congo red staining or immunohistochemistry. Birefringence under polarized light, usually a characteristic feature of amyloid plaques, may be absent due to harsh pretreatment of fixed tissue.

Detection of PrP^{Sc} by Western Blotting

Western blotting is routinely performed on unfixed tissue originating from the CNS. Generally, this test is undertaken in a postmortem setting. In rare cases where a brain biopsy is justified, a biopsy specimen may be used for this test.

The basis of biochemical characterization of PrP^{Sc} resides in the relative resistance of PrP^{Sc} to proteolytic degradation. Whereas PrP^{C} is entirely digested by PK, identical treatment of PrP^{Sc} leads to removal of a variable number of N-terminal amino acids. Western blotting of digested PrP^{Sc} reveals three distinct bands, corresponding to di-, mono-, and unglycosylated forms (136). The molecular classification of PrP^{Sc} takes two parameters into account: the molecular weight of unglycosylated PrP^{Sc} and the relative amounts of PrP^{Sc} di-, mono-, and unglycosylated forms. The resulting information is then used to establish the "type" of PrP^{Sc} according to proposed provisional classification schemes (84, 137) (Fig. 3). Depending on the exact conditions under which the protease digestion and the Western blotting procedure are performed, between three and six different PrP^{Sc} types can be distinguished (84, 132). Distinct PrP^{Sc} types are thought to represent the molecular correlates of distinct prion strains. The fact that the PrP^{Sc} types found in vCJD patients and in BSE-diseased cattle are identical is one of the main arguments supporting the theory that BSE prions are responsible for the vCJD epidemic in humans (81). It is unknown how glycotype ratios can be faithfully maintained during prion replication; however, experiments with yeast prions indicate that this occurs in a synthetic prion replication system (96, 175). This phenomenon may be related to the quaternary structure of prion aggregates (3).

Genetic Investigations

For genetic testing, DNA is extracted from whole blood. The entire open reading frame may be amplified for sequencing using PCR (68). Sequencing of *PRNP* allows for the exclusion of gCJD (188). At least 29 disease-causing insertional or point mutations in *PRNP* have been identified to date (Table 4). In addition, there are several *PRNP* polymorphisms, one of which (codon 129M/V) may have a disease-modifying function. Homozygosity for methionine at codon 129 may constitute a risk factor for the development of prion disease (15): methionine homozygotes are clearly overrepresented among sCJD patients, and all individuals affected by vCJD are homozygous for methionine at codon 129. In addition, this polymorphism has a considerable effect on the clinical, biochemical, and neuropathological presentation of prion-diseased individuals (15).

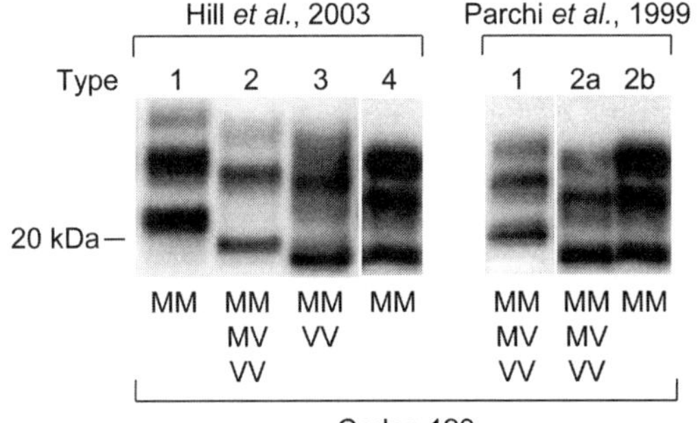

FIGURE 3 Western blot analysis of PrP^{Sc}. The currently most popular classification schemes for CJD (84, 137) reliably discriminate PrP^{Sc} types based on the mobility of the unglycosylated band of PrP^{Sc} and the signal intensity of di-, mono-, and unglycosylated forms of PrP^{Sc}. One scheme (84, 137) differentiates four principal PrP^{Sc} types (1 to 4) (84). Three principal PrP^{Sc} types (1, 2a, and 2b) are proposed in the second scheme (84). MM, homozygous methionine; MV, heterozygous methionine valine; VV, homozygous valine.

TABLE 4 Useful supplemental diagnostic tests and specimens for CJD[a]

Disorder	Supplemental diagnostic tests and specimens
sCJD	Histology, Western blotting, genetic testing for exclusion of gCJD, auxiliary tests such as determination of 14-3-3 or Tau protein in the CSF
gCJD	Genetic testing, histology, Western blotting, auxiliary tests such as determination of 14-3-3 or Tau protein in the CSF.
vCJD	Histology, Western blotting (lymphoid tissue and CNS tissue), genetic testing for exclusion of gCJD, auxiliary tests such as determination of 14-3-3 or Tau protein in the CSF.

[a] Clinical presentation is of primary diagnostic importance. Neuroimaging studies yield distinct results and can be useful.

Serologic Tests

To date there are neither serologic screening nor confirmatory tests for prion diseases. Instead, several studies had evaluated the usefulness of surrogate markers, such as 14-3-3 and Tau proteins that are found in CSF as a consequence of neuronal death. These proteins are ubiquitously expressed. 14-3-3 participates in protein kinase signaling and is involved in neuronal migration. Tau is a phosphoprotein that promotes the assembly and stability of neuronal axons by binding to microtubules. Elevation of these proteins is relatively nonspecific and can be seen in other conditions such as encephalitis, cerebral infarction, and paraneoplastic neurologic disorders.

The usefulness of current surrogate markers should not be overestimated. Satisfactory sensitivity and specificity (over 90%) can be achieved only in selected cohorts (190). Results from these tests, in combination with clinical data, may help at best to strengthen the diagnosis of a probable human prion disease. While 14-3-3 is routinely tested by Western blotting, Tau is often measured in a enzyme-linked immunosorbent assay format (190).

Evaluation, Reporting, and Interpretation of Results

The diagnosis of human prion disorders can be difficult to establish but is best approached through careful consideration of clinical presentation and other clinical studies such as neuroimaging. Brain biopsy and histologic assessment can be performed to rule out treatable disorders. Detection of spongiform changes and deposition of PrP^{Sc} in affected areas can help establish the diagnosis of prion disorders. The absence of these changes (for example, due to sampling bias) is not helpful in the exclusion of these disorders. Less invasive tests such as detection of surrogate markers (Tau and 14-3-3) in CSF can be helpful when considered in the context of available clinical neuroimaging information. Genetic testing can be performed to establish the diagnosis of genetic prion disorders. The constellation of tests that can be helpful in the diagnosis of each of these disorders is shown in Table 4. All testing other than neuropathology and sequencing of *PRNP* is usually performed on a research basis.

PREVENTION

Laboratory Handling of Potentially Contaminated Specimens

The highest titers of prion infective material can be found in CNS tissues (brain, spinal cord, and cranial nerves), but nonneural tissues such as lymphatic tissue or muscle may also contain infectious prions. Prions are not inactivated by formalin. A procedure recommended by the College of American Pathologists (http://www.cap.org) for safe handling of tissues is formalin fixation for at least 10 days, followed by formic acid treatment (50 to 100 ml of 95 to 100% [vol/vol]) for 1 h and formalin fixation for 2 days. Tissues can then be embedded. Formic acid inactivates formalin-treated prions but has minimal effect on the quality of histology. Disposable histologic equipment should be used whenever possible.

It is crucial for tissue preservation that formalin fixation be applied before formic acid inactivation. Reversing the order of the two reactions destroys the tissues to the extent of making them histologically uninterpretable.

Blood and bone marrow are presumed to contain low levels of infectivity (http://www.advisorybodies.doh.gov.uk/acdp/tseguidance/). These specimens can be handled safely under biosafety level 2 conditions by adhering to universal precautions for prevention of transmission of blood-borne pathogens. These specimens can be tested in automated analyzers found throughout clinical laboratories if instruments are enclosed and can contain spillage and if waste can be disposed of safely. Maintenance and emergency procedures that protect the user from exposure should be outlined in laboratory standard operating procedures and implemented. Manual processing (specimen decanting, for example) should be performed inside a negative-pressure laminar flow hood in a contained environment.

Prions can be substantially but not completely inactivated by physical exposure to steam or dry heat at high temperatures. Disposable laboratory equipment should be used whenever possible. Potentially contaminated laboratory waste should be autoclaved (134 to 137°C, 20 min) and then incinerated (http://www.advisorybodies.doh.gov.uk/acdp/tseguidance/). Chemical exposure to high concentrations of either sodium hypochlorite (>5.25% solution, freshly prepared) or sodium hydroxide (1 N solution) for 1 h is effective against prions and can be used to disinfect spills. Reusable laboratory material should be immersed in a freshly prepared >5.25% solution of sodium hypochlorite, or a 1 N solution of sodium hydroxide for 1 h, and then rinsed with water before being packaged for autoclave sterilization at 134°C for at least 20 min (http://www.advisorybodies.doh.gov.uk/acdp/tseguidance/).

TREATMENT

An impressive wealth of molecules has been proposed as potential antiprion compounds based on in vitro data (41, 142, 146, 174). Disappointingly, none of these compounds have been effective for actual therapy of prion disease in vivo. Transgenic expression of an immunoglobulin Fcγ domain fused to PrP^C drastically delays prion disease onset after peripheral and intracerebral prion challenge (128), raising the possibility that soluble prion protein mutants may be potential prionostatic compounds. Immunotherapy with anti-PrP antibodies has been shown to be effective in model systems (80) and may represent an alternative therapeutic approach.

REFERENCES

1. **Aguzzi, A.** 1996. Between cows and monkeys. *Nature* **381:**734.
2. **Aguzzi, A.** 2000. Prion diseases, blood and the immune system: concerns and reality. *Haematologica* **85:**3–10.
3. **Aguzzi, A.** 2004. Understanding the diversity of prions. *Nat. Cell. Biol.* **6:**290–292.
4. **Aguzzi, A., and C. Haass.** 2003. Games played by rogue proteins in prion disorders and Alzheimer's disease. *Science* **302:**814–818.
5. **Aguzzi, A., I. Hegyi, M. Peltola, and M. Glatzel.** 2000, posting date. Rapport des activitées 1996–1999. Hôpital universitaire de Zurich. Département de pathologie. Institut de neuropathologie. Centre nationale de référence pour les prionoses (NRPE).
6. **Aguzzi, A., and M. Heikenwalder.** 2003. Prion diseases: cannibals and garbage piles. *Nature* **423:**127–129.
7. **Aguzzi, A., and M. Heikenwalder.** 2005. Prions, cytokines, and chemokines: a meeting in lymphoid organs. *Immunity* **22:**145–154.
8. **Aguzzi, A., F. Montrasio, and P. S. Kaeser.** 2001. Prions: health scare and biological challenge. *Nat. Rev. Mol. Cell. Biol.* **2:**118–126.
9. **Aguzzi, A., and M. Polymenidou.** 2004. Mammalian prion biology. One century of evolving concepts. *Cell* **116:**313–327.
10. **Aguzzi, A., and A. J. Raeber.** 1998. Transgenic models of neurodegeneration. Neurodegeneration: of (transgenic) mice and men. *Brain Pathol.* **8:**695–697.
11. **Aguzzi, A., and C. Weissmann.** 1997. Prion research: the next frontiers. *Nature* **389:**795–798.
12. **Aguzzi, A., and C. Weissmann.** 1996. Sleepless in Bologna: transmission of fatal familial insomnia. *Trends Microbiol.* **4:**129–131.
13. **Aguzzi, A., and C. Weissmann.** 1998. Spongiform encephalopathies. The prion's perplexing persistence. *Nature* **392:**763–764.
14. **Aguzzi, A., and C. Weissmann.** 1996. Spongiform encephalopathies: a suspicious signature. *Nature* **383:**666–667.
15. **Alperovitch, A., I. Zerr, M. Pocchiari, E. Mitrova, J. de Pedro Cuesta, I. Hegyi, S. Collins, H. Kretzschmar, C. van Duijn, and R. G. Will.** 1999. Codon 129 prion protein genotype and sporadic Creutzfeldt-Jakob disease. *Lancet* **353:**1673–1674. (Letter.)
16. **Alpers, M.** 1988. Epidemiology and clinical aspects of kuru, p. 451–465. *In* S. B. Prusiner and M. P. McKinley (ed.), *Prions–Novel Infectious Pathogens Causing Scrapie and Creutzfeldt-Jakob Disease*. Academic Press, Orlando, FL.
17. **Andrews, N. J., C. P. Farrington, H. J. Ward, S. N. Cousens, P. G. Smith, A. M. Molesworth, R. S. Knight, J. W. Ironside, and R. G. Will.** 2003. Deaths from variant Creutzfeldt-Jakob disease in the UK. *Lancet* **361:** 751–752.
18. **Aucouturier, P., F. Geissmann, D. Damotte, G. P. Saborio, H. C. Meeker, R. Kascsak, R. I. Carp, and T. Wisniewski.** 2001. Infected splenic dendritic cells are suf-

ficient for prion transmission to the CNS in mouse scrapie. *J. Clin. Invest.* **108:**703–708.

19. **Barmada, S., P. Piccardo, K. Yamaguchi, B. Ghetti, and D. A. Harris.** 2004. GFP-tagged prion protein is correctly localized and functionally active in the brains of transgenic mice. *Neurobiol. Dis.* **16:**527–537.
20. **Barmada, S. J., and D. A. Harris.** 2005. Visualization of prion infection in transgenic mice expressing green fluorescent protein-tagged prion protein. *J. Neurosci.* **25:** 5824–5832.
21. **Bartz, J. C., M. L. Kramer, M. H. Sheehan, J. A. L. Hutter, J. I. Ayers, R. A. Bessen, and A. E. Kincaid.** 2007. Prion interference is due to a reduction in strain-specific PrP^{Sc} levels. *J. Virol.* **81:**689–697.
22. **Baumann, F., M. Tolnay, C. Brabeck, J. Pahnke, U. Kloz, H. H. Niemann, M. Heikenwalder, T. Rulicke, A. Burkle, and A. Aguzzi.** 2007. Lethal recessive myelin toxicity of prion protein lacking its central domain. *EMBO J.* **26:**538–547.
23. **Beekes, M., E. Baldauf, and H. Diringer.** 1996. Sequential appearance and accumulation of pathognomonic markers in the central nervous system of hamsters orally infected with scrapie. *J. Gen. Virol.* **77:**1925–1934.
24. **Bessen, R. A., and R. F. Marsh.** 1992. Biochemical and physical properties of the prion protein from two strains of the transmissible mink encephalopathy agent. *J. Virol.* **66:**2096–2101.
25. **Bessen, R. A., and R. F. Marsh.** 1994. Distinct PrP properties suggest the molecular basis of strain variation in transmissible mink encephalopathy. *J. Virol.* **68:**7859–7868.
26. **Blanquet-Grossard, F., N. M. Thielens, C. Vendrely, M. Jamin, and G. J. Arlaud.** 2005. Complement protein C1q recognizes a conformationally modified form of the prion protein. *Biochemistry* **44:**4349–4356.
27. **Blättler, T., S. Brandner, A. J. Raeber, M. A. Klein, T. Voigtländer, C. Weissmann, and A. Aguzzi.** 1997. PrP-expressing tissue required for transfer of scrapie infectivity from spleen to brain. *Nature* **389:**69–73.
28. **Borchelt, D. R., M. Scott, A. Taraboulos, N. Stahl, and S. B. Prusiner.** 1990. Scrapie and cellular prion proteins differ in their kinetics of synthesis and topology in cultured cells. *J. Cell. Biol.* **110:**743–752.
29. **Brandner, S., S. Isenmann, A. Raeber, M. Fischer, A. Sailer, Y. Kobayashi, S. Marino, C. Weissmann, and A. Aguzzi.** 1996. Normal host prion protein necessary for scrapie-induced neurotoxicity. *Nature* **379:**339–343.
30. **Brown, K. L., K. Stewart, D. L. Ritchie, N. A. Mabbott, A. Williams, H. Fraser, W. I. Morrison, and M. E. Bruce.** 1999. Scrapie replication in lymphoid tissues depends on prion protein-expressing follicular dendritic cells. *Nat. Med.* **5:**1308–1312.
31. **Brown, P.** 1992. The phenotypic expression of different mutations in transmissible human spongiform encephalopathy. *Rev. Neurol.* (Paris) **148:**317–327.
32. **Brown, P., F. Cathala, R. F. Raubertas, D. C. Gajdusek, and P. Castaigne.** 1987. The epidemiology of Creutzfeldt-Jakob disease: conclusion of a 15-year investigation in France and review of the world literature. *Neurology* **37:** 895–904.
33. **Brown, P., M. Preece, J. P. Brandel, T. Sato, L. McShane, I. Zerr, A. Fletcher, R. G. Will, M. Pocchiari, N. R. Cashman, J. H. d'Aignaux, L. Cervenakova, J. Fradkin, L. B. Schonberger, and S. J. Collins.** 2000. Iatrogenic Creutzfeldt-Jakob disease at the millennium. *Neurology* **55:**1075–1081.
34. **Bruce, M. E., P. A. McBride, and C. F. Farquhar.** 1989. Precise targeting of the pathology of the sialoglycoprotein, PrP, and vacuolar degeneration in mouse scrapie. *Neurosci. Lett.* **102:**1–6.
35. **Bruce, M. E., R. G. Will, J. W. Ironside, I. McConnell, D. Drummond, A. Suttie, L. McCardle, A. Chree, J. Hope, C. Birkett, S. Cousens, H. Fraser, and C. J. Bostock.** 1997. Transmissions to mice indicate that 'new variant' CJD is caused by the BSE agent. *Nature* **389:**498–501.
36. **Budka, H., A. Aguzzi, P. Brown, J. M. Brucher, O. Bugiani, F. Gullotta, M. Haltia, J. J. Hauw, J. W. Ironside, K. Jellinger, H. A. Kretzschmar, P. L. Lantos, C. Masullo, W. Schlote, J. Tateishi, and R. O. Weller.** 1995. Neuropathological diagnostic criteria for Creutzfeldt-Jakob disease (CJD) and other human spongiform encephalopathies (prion diseases). *Brain Pathol.* **5:**459–466.
37. **Büeler, H. R., A. Aguzzi, A. Sailer, R. A. Greiner, P. Autenried, M. Aguet, and C. Weissmann.** 1993. Mice devoid of PrP are resistant to scrapie. *Cell* **73:**1339–1347.
38. **Büeler, H. R., M. Fischer, Y. Lang, H. Bluethmann, H. P. Lipp, S. J. DeArmond, S. B. Prusiner, M. Aguet, and C. Weissmann.** 1992. Normal development and behaviour of mice lacking the neuronal cell-surface PrP protein. *Nature* **356:**577–582.
39. **Bukau, B., J. Weissman, and A. Horwich.** 2006. Molecular chaperones and protein quality control. *Cell* **125:** 443–451.
40. **Castilla, J., P. Saa, C. Hetz, and C. Soto.** 2005. In vitro generation of infectious scrapie prions. *Cell* **121:**195–206.
41. **Caughey, B., and R. E. Race.** 1992. Potent inhibition of scrapie-associated PrP accumulation by congo red. *J. Neurochem.* **59:**768–771.
42. **Caughey, B. W., A. Dong, K. S. Bhat, D. Ernst, S. F. Hayes, and W. S. Caughey.** 1991. Secondary structure analysis of the scrapie-associated protein PrP 27-30 in water by infrared spectroscopy. *Biochemistry* **30:**7672–7680.
43. **Chazot, G., E. Broussolle, C. Lapras, T. Blättler, A. Aguzzi, and N. Kopp.** 1996. New variant of Creutzfeldt-Jakob disease in a 26-year-old French man. *Lancet* **347:** 1181. (Letter.)
44. **Chernoff, Y. O., S. L. Lindquist, B. Ono, S. G. Inge-Vechtomov, and S. W. Liebman.** 1995. Role of the chaperone protein Hsp104 in propagation of the yeast prion-like factor [psi+]. *Science* **268:**880–884.
45. **Chesebro, B., M. Trifilo, R. Race, K. Meade-White, C. Teng, R. LaCasse, L. Raymond, C. Favara, G. Baron, S. Priola, B. Caughey, E. Masliah, and M. Oldstone.** 2005. Anchorless prion protein results in infectious amyloid disease without clinical scrapie. *Science* **308:**1435–1439.
46. **Clarke, M. C., and D. A. Haig.** 1971. Multiplication of scrapie agent in mouse spleen. *Res. Vet. Sci.* **12:**195–197.
47. **Collinge, J., K. C. Sidle, J. Meads, J. Ironside, and A. F. Hill.** 1996. Molecular analysis of prion strain variation and the aetiology of 'new variant' CJD. *Nature* **383:**685–690.
48. **Collins, P. S., V. A. Lawson, and P. C. Masters.** 2004. Transmissible spongiform encephalopathies. *Lancet* **363:** 51–61.
49. **Cousens, S. N., R. Harries Jones, R. Knight, R. G. Will, P. G. Smith, and W. B. Matthews.** 1990. Geographical distribution of cases of Creutzfeldt-Jakob disease in England and Wales 1970–84. *J. Neurol. Neurosurg. Psychiatry* **53:**459–465.
50. **Cuille, J., and P. L. Chelle.** 1939. Experimental transmission of trembling to the goat. *C. R. Seances Acad. Sci.* **208:**1058–1160.
51. **Denzer, K., M. J. Kleijmeer, H. F. Heijnen, W. Stoorvogel, and H. J. Geuze.** 2000. Exosome: from internal

vesicle of the multivesicular body to intercellular signaling device. *J. Cell Sci.* **113**(Pt. 19):3365–3374.

52. **Denzer, K., M. van Eijk, M. J. Kleijmeer, E. Jakobson, C. de Groot, and H. J. Geuze.** 2000. Follicular dendritic cells carry MHC class II-expressing microvesicles at their surface. *J. Immunol.* **165:**1259–1265.
53. **Department of Health.** 2007, posting date. Monthly Creutzfeldt-Jakob disease statistics. http://www.gnn.gov.uk/environment/fullDetail.asp?ReleaseID=319104&NewsAreaID=2&NavigatedFromDepartment=False.
54. **Dickinson, A. G., H. Fraser, V. M. Meikle, and G. W. Outram.** 1972. Competition between different scrapie agents in mice. *Nat. New Biol.* **237:**244–245.
55. **Dickinson, A. G., G. B. Young, J. T. Stamp, and C. C. Renwick.** 1965. An analysis of natural scrapie in Suffolk sheep. *Heredity Edinburgh* **20:**485–503.
56. **Drisaldi, B., R. S. Stewart, C. Adles, L. R. Stewart, E. Quaglio, E. Biasini, L. Fioriti, R. Chiesa, and D. A. Harris.** 2003. Mutant PrP is delayed in its exit from the endoplasmic reticulum, but neither wild-type nor mutant PrP undergoes retrotranslocation prior to proteasomal degradation. *J. Biol. Chem.* **278:**21732–21743.
57. **Fischer, M., T. Rülicke, A. Raeber, A. Sailer, M. Moser, B. Oesch, S. Brandner, A. Aguzzi, and C. Weissmann.** 1996. Prion protein (PrP) with amino-proximal deletions restoring susceptibility of PrP knockout mice to scrapie. *EMBO J.* **15:**1255–1264.
58. **Flechsig, E., D. Shmerling, I. Hegyi, A. J. Raeber, M. Fischer, A. Cozzio, C. von Mering, A. Aguzzi, and C. Weissmann.** 2000. Prion protein devoid of the octapeptide repeat region restores susceptibility to scrapie in PrP knockout mice. *Neuron* **27:**399–408.
59. **Forster, R., A. E. Mattis, E. Kremmer, E. Wolf, G. Brem, and M. Lipp.** 1996. A putative chemokine receptor, BLR1, directs B cell migration to defined lymphoid organs and specific anatomic compartments of the spleen. *Cell* **87:**1037–1047.
60. **Fraser, H., and A. G. Dickinson.** 1973. Scrapie in mice. Agent-strain differences in the distribution and intensity of grey matter vacuolation. *J. Comp. Pathol.* **83:**29–40.
61. **Fraser, H., and A. G. Dickinson.** 1968. The sequential development of the brain lesion of scrapie in three strains of mice. *J. Comp. Pathol.* **78:**301–311.
62. **Frigg, R., M. A. Klein, I. Hegyi, R. M. Zinkernagel, and A. Aguzzi.** 1999. Scrapie pathogenesis in subclinically infected B-cell-deficient mice. *J. Virol.* **73:**9584–9588.
63. **Gajdusek, D., and V. Zigas.** 1959. Clinical, pathological and epidemiological study of an acute progressive degenerative disease of the central nervous system among natives of the eastern highlands of New Guinea. *Am. J. Med.* **26:**442–469.
64. **Gajdusek, D. C.** 1977. Unconventional viruses and the origin and disappearance of kuru. *Science* **197:**943–960.
65. **Gajdusek, D. C., C. J. Gibbs, and M. Alpers.** 1966. Experimental transmission of a Kuru-like syndrome to chimpanzees. *Nature* **209:**794–796.
66. **Gajdusek, D. C., and V. Zigas.** 1957. Degenerative disease of the central nervous system in New Guinea—the endemic occurrence of 'kuru' in the native population. *N. Engl. J. Med.* **257:**974–978.
67. **Gambetti, P., Q. Kong, W. Zou, P. Parchi, and S. G. Chen.** 2003. Sporadic and familial CJD: classification and characterisation. *Br. Med. Bull.* **66:**213–239.
68. **Glatzel, M., E. Abela, M. Maissen, and A. Aguzzi.** 2003. Extraneural pathologic prion protein in sporadic Creutzfeldt-Jakob disease. *N. Engl. J. Med.* **349:**1812–1820.
69. **Glatzel, M., F. L. Heppner, K. M. Albers, and A. Aguzzi.** 2001. Sympathetic innervation of lymphoreticular organs is rate limiting for prion neuroinvasion. *Neuron* **31:**25–34.
70. **Glatzel, M., P. M. Ott, T. Lindner, J. O. Gebbers, A. Gmur, W. Wuest, G. Huber, H. Moch, M. Podvinec, B. Stamm, and A. Aguzzi.** 2003. Human prion diseases: epidemiology and integrated risk assessment. *Lancet Neurol.* **2:**757–763.
71. **Glatzel, M., C. Rogivue, A. Ghani, J. R. Streffer, L. Amsler, and A. Aguzzi.** 2002. Incidence of Creutzfeldt-Jakob disease in Switzerland. *Lancet* **360:**139–141.
72. **Gommerman, J. L., and J. L. Browning.** 2003. Lymphotoxin/light, lymphoid microenvironments and autoimmune disease. *Nat. Rev. Immunol.* **3:**642–655.
73. **Gommerman, J. L., F. Mackay, E. Donskoy, W. Meier, P. Martin, and J. L. Browning.** 2002. Manipulation of lymphoid microenvironments in nonhuman primates by an inhibitor of the lymphotoxin pathway. *J. Clin. Invest.* **110:**1359–1369.
74. **Gordon, W. S.** 1946. Advances in veterinary research. *Vet. Res.* **58:**516–520.
75. **Harder, A., K. Jendroska, F. Kreuz, T. Wirth, C. Schafranka, N. Karnatz, A. Theallier-Janko, J. Dreier, K. Lohan, D. Emmerich, J. Cervos-Navarro, O. Windl, H. A. Kretzschmar, P. Nurnberg, and R. Witkowski.** 1999. Novel twelve-generation kindred of fatal familial insomnia from Germany representing the entire spectrum of disease expression. *Am. J. Med. Genet.* **87:**311–316.
76. **Harries Jones, R., R. Knight, R. G. Will, S. Cousens, P. G. Smith, and W. B. Matthews.** 1988. Creutzfeldt-Jakob disease in England and Wales, 1980–1984: a case-control study of potential risk factors. *J. Neurol. Neurosurg. Psychiatry* **51:**1113–1119.
77. **Hegde, R. S., J. A. Mastrianni, M. R. Scott, K. A. DeFea, P. Tremblay, M. Torchia, S. J. DeArmond, S. B. Prusiner, and V. R. Lingappa.** 1998. A transmembrane form of the prion protein in neurodegenerative disease. *Science* **279:**827–834.
78. **Heikenwalder, M., N. Zeller, H. Seeger, M. Prinz, P. C. Klohn, P. Schwarz, N. H. Ruddle, C. Weissmann, and A. Aguzzi.** 2005. Chronic lymphocytic inflammation specifies the organ tropism of prions. *Science* **307:**1107–1110.
79. **Heppner, F. L., A. D. Christ, M. A. Klein, M. Prinz, M. Fried, J. P. Kraehenbuhl, and A. Aguzzi.** 2001. Transepithelial prion transport by M cells. *Nat. Med.* **7:**976–977.
80. **Heppner, F. L., C. Musahl, I. Arrighi, M. A. Klein, T. Rulicke, B. Oesch, R. M. Zinkernagel, U. Kalinke, and A. Aguzzi.** 2001. Prevention of scrapie pathogenesis by transgenic expression of anti-prion protein antibodies. *Science* **294:**178–182.
81. **Hill, A. F., M. Desbruslais, S. Joiner, K. C. Sidle, I. Gowland, J. Collinge, L. J. Doey, and P. Lantos.** 1997. The same prion strain causes vCJD and BSE. *Nature* **389:** 448–450. (Letter.)
82. **Hill, A. F., S. Joiner, J. A. Beck, T. A. Campbell, A. Dickinson, M. Poulter, J. D. Wadsworth, and J. Collinge.** 2006. Distinct glycoform ratios of protease resistant prion protein associated with PRNP point mutations. *Brain* **129:**676–685.
83. **Hill, A. F., S. Joiner, J. Linehan, M. Desbruslais, P. L. Lantos, and J. Collinge.** 2000. Species-barrier-independent prion replication in apparently resistant species. *Proc. Natl. Acad. Sci. USA* **29:**10248–10253.
84. **Hill, A. F., S. Joiner, J. D. Wadsworth, K. C. Sidle, J. E. Bell, H. Budka, J. W. Ironside, and J. Collinge.** 2003.

Molecular classification of sporadic Creutzfeldt-Jakob disease. *Brain* **126:**1333–1346.

85. **Hilton, D. A.** 2006. Pathogenesis and prevalence of variant Creutzfeldt-Jakob disease. *J. Pathol.* **208:**134–141.
86. **Hornemann, S., C. Korth, B. Oesch, R. Riek, G. Wider, K. Wuthrich, and R. Glockshuber.** 1997. Recombinant full-length murine prion protein, mPrP(23-231): purification and spectroscopic characterization. *FEBS Lett.* **413:**277–281.
87. **Houston, F., J. D. Foster, A. Chong, N. Hunter, and C. J. Bostock.** 2000. Transmission of BSE by blood transfusion in sheep. *Lancet* **356:**999–1000.
88. **Hsiao, K., H. F. Baker, T. J. Crow, M. Poulter, F. Owen, J. D. Terwilliger, D. Westaway, J. Ott, and S. B. Prusiner.** 1989. Linkage of a prion protein missense variant to Gerstmann-Sträussler syndrome. *Nature* **338:** 342–345.
89. **Hsiao, K., and S. B. Prusiner.** 1990. Inherited human prion diseases. *Neurology* **40:**1820–1827.
90. **Hsiao, K. K., D. Groth, M. Scott, S. L. Yang, H. Serban, D. Rapp, D. Foster, M. Torchia, S. J. DeArmond, and S. B. Prusiner.** 1994. Serial transmission in rodents of neurodegeneration from transgenic mice expressing mutant prion protein. *Proc. Natl. Acad. Sci. USA* **91:** 9126–9130.
91. **Hsiao, K. K., M. Scott, D. Foster, D. F. Groth, S. J. DeArmond, and S. B. Prusiner.** 1990. Spontaneous neurodegeneration in transgenic mice with mutant prion protein. *Science* **250:**1587–1590.
92. **Jarrett, J. T., and P. T. Lansbury, Jr.** 1993. Seeding "one-dimensional crystallization" of amyloid: a pathogenic mechanism in Alzheimer's disease and scrapie? *Cell* **73:**1055–1058.
93. **Jeffrey, M., G. McGovern, C. M. Goodsir, K. L. Brown, and M. E. Bruce.** 2000. Sites of prion protein accumulation in scrapie-infected mouse spleen revealed by immuno-electron microscopy. *J. Pathol.* **191:**323–332.
94. **Kaeser, P. S., M. A. Klein, P. Schwarz, and A. Aguzzi.** 2001. Efficient lymphoreticular prion propagation requires PrP^c in stromal and hematopoietic cells. *J. Virol.* **75:**7097–7106.
95. **Kimberley, F. C., B. Sivasankar, and B. Paul Morgan.** 2007. Alternative roles for CD59. *Mol. Immunol.* **44:**73–81.
96. **King, C. Y., and R. Diaz-Avalos.** 2004. Protein-only transmission of three yeast prion strains. *Nature* **428:** 319–323.
97. **Kirschbaum, W. R.** 1924. Zwei eigenartige Erkrankungen des Zentralnervensystems nach Art der spastischen Pseudosklerose (Jakob). *Z. Ges. Neurol. Psychiatr.* **92:** 175–220.
98. **Klein, M. A., R. Frigg, E. Flechsig, A. J. Raeber, U. Kalinke, H. Bluethmann, F. Bootz, M. Suter, R. M. Zinkernagel, and A. Aguzzi.** 1997. A crucial role for B cells in neuroinvasive scrapie. *Nature* **390:**687–690.
99. **Klein, M. A., R. Frigg, A. J. Raeber, E. Flechsig, I. Hegyi, R. M. Zinkernagel, C. Weissmann, and A. Aguzzi.** 1998. PrP expression in B lymphocytes is not required for prion neuroinvasion. *Nat. Med.* **4:**1429–1433.
100. **Klein, M. A., P. S. Kaeser, P. Schwarz, H. Weyd, I. Xenarios, R. M. Zinkernagel, M. C. Carroll, J. S. Verbeek, M. Botto, M. J. Walport, H. Molina, U. Kalinke, H. Acha-Orbea, and A. Aguzzi.** 2001. Complement facilitates early prion pathogenesis. *Nat. Med.* **7:**488–492.
101. **Klohn, P. C., L. Stoltze, E. Flechsig, M. Enari, and C. Weissmann.** 2003. A quantitative, highly sensitive cell-based infectivity assay for mouse scrapie prions. *Proc. Natl. Acad. Sci. USA* **100:**11666–11671.
102. **Knaus, K. J., M. Morillas, W. Swietnicki, M. Malone, W. K. Surewicz, and V. C. Yee.** 2001. Crystal structure of the human prion protein reveals a mechanism for oligomerization. *Nat. Struct. Biol.* **8:**770–774.
103. **Kovacs, G. G., P. Gasque, T. Strobel, E. Lindeck-Pozza, M. Strohschneider, J. W. Ironside, H. Budka, and M. Guentchev.** 2004. Complement activation in human prion disease. *Neurobiol. Dis.* **15:**21–28.
104. **Kovacs, G. G., E. Lindeck-Pozza, L. Chimelli, A. Q. Araújo, A. A. Gabbai, T. Ströbel, M. Glatzel, A. Aguzzi, and H. Budka.** 2004. Creutzfeldt-Jakob disease and inclusion body myositis: abundant disease-associated prion protein in muscle. *Ann. Neurol.* **55:**121–125.
105. **Ladogana, A., M. Puopolo, E. A. Croes, H. Budka, C. Jarius, S. Collins, G. M. Klug, T. Sutcliffe, A. Giulivi, A. Alperovitch, N. Delasnerie-Laupretre, J. P. Brandel, S. Poser, H. Kretzschmar, I. Rietveld, E. Mitrova, P. Cuesta Jde, P. Martinez-Martin, M. Glatzel, A. Aguzzi, R. Knight, H. Ward, M. Pocchiari, C. M. van Duijn, R. G. Will, and I. Zerr.** 2005. Mortality from Creutzfeldt-Jakob disease and related disorders in Europe, Australia, and Canada. *Neurology* **64:**1586–1591.
106. **Lasmezas, C. I., J. P. Deslys, R. Demaimay, K. T. Adjou, F. Lamoury, D. Dormont, O. Robain, J. Ironside, and J. J. Hauw.** 1996. BSE transmission to macaques. *Nature* **381:**743–744.
107. **Leblanc, P., S. Alais, I. Porto-Carreiro, S. Lehmann, J. Grassi, G. Raposo, and J. L. Darlix.** 2006. Retrovirus infection strongly enhances scrapie infectivity release in cell culture. *EMBO J.* **25:**2674–2685.
108. **Legname, G., I. V. Baskakov, H. O. Nguyen, D. Riesner, F. E. Cohen, S. J. DeArmond, and S. B. Prusiner.** 2004. Synthetic mammalian prions. *Science* **305:**673–676.
109. **Ligios, C., C. J. Sigurdson, C. Santucciu, G. Carcassola, G. Manco, M. Basagni, C. Maestrale, M. G. Cancedda, L. Madau, and A. Aguzzi.** 2005. PrP^{Sc} in mammary glands of sheep affected by scrapie and mastitis. *Nat. Med.* **11:**1137–1138.
110. **Llewelyn, C. A., P. E. Hewitt, R. S. Knight, K. Amar, S. Cousens, J. Mackenzie, and R. G. Will.** 2004. Possible transmission of variant Creutzfeldt-Jakob disease by blood transfusion. *Lancet* **363:**417–421.
111. **Ma, J., and S. Lindquist.** 2002. Conversion of PrP to a self-perpetuating PrPSc-like conformation in the cytosol. *Science* **298:**1785–1788.
112. **Ma, J., R. Wollmann, and S. Lindquist.** 2002. Neurotoxicity and neurodegeneration when PrP accumulates in the cytosol. *Science* **298:**1781–1785.
113. **Mabbott, N. A., M. E. Bruce, M. Botto, M. J. Walport, and M. B. Pepys.** 2001. Temporary depletion of complement component C3 or genetic deficiency of C1q significantly delays onset of scrapie. *Nat. Med.* **7:**485–487.
114. **Mabbott, N. A., F. Mackay, F. Minns, and M. E. Bruce.** 2000. Temporary inactivation of follicular dendritic cells delays neuroinvasion of scrapie. *Nat. Med.* **6:**719–720. (Letter.)
115. **Mabbott, N. A., G. McGovern, M. Jeffrey, and M. E. Bruce.** 2002. Temporary blockade of the tumor necrosis factor receptor signaling pathway impedes the spread of scrapie to the brain. *J. Virol.* **76:**5131–5139.
116. **Mabbott, N. A., J. Young, I. McConnell, and M. E. Bruce.** 2003. Follicular dendritic cell dedifferentiation by treatment with an inhibitor of the lymphotoxin pathway dramatically reduces scrapie susceptibility. *J. Virol.* **77:**6845–6854.

117. **Mallucci, G., A. Dickinson, J. Linehan, P. C. Klohn, S. Brandner, and J. Collinge.** 2003. Depleting neuronal PrP in prion infection prevents disease and reverses spongiosis. *Science* **302:**871–874.
118. **Mallucci, G. R., S. Ratte, E. A. Asante, J. Linehan, I. Gowland, J. G. Jefferys, and J. Collinge.** 2002. Postnatal knockout of prion protein alters hippocampal CA1 properties, but does not result in neurodegeneration. *EMBO J.* **21:**202–210.
119. **Malmgren, R., L. Kurland, B. Mokri, and J. Kurtzke.** 1979. The epidemiology of Creutzfeldt-Jakob disease, p. 93–112. *In* S. B. Prusiner and W. J. Hadlow (ed.), *Slow Transmissible Diseases of the Nervous System*, vol. 1. Academic Press, New York, NY.
120. **Manuelidis, L.** 1998. Vaccination with an attenuated Creutzfeldt-Jakob disease strain prevents expression of a virulent agent. *Proc. Natl. Acad. Sci. USA* **95:**2520–2525.
121. **Masters, C. L., D. C. Gajdusek, and C. J. Gibbs.** 1981. Creutzfeldt-Jakob disease virus isolations from the Gerstmann-Straussler syndrome with an analysis of the various forms of amyloid plaque deposition in the virus-induced spongiform encephalopathies. *Brain* **104:**559–588.
122. **Masters, C. L., and E. P. Richardson.** 1978. Subacute spongiform encephalopathy (Creutzfeldt-Jakob disease). The nature and progression of spongiform change. *Brain* **101:**333–344.
123. **Mathiason, C. K., J. G. Powers, S. J. Dahmes, D. A. Osborn, K. V. Miller, R. J. Warren, G. L. Mason, S. A. Hays, J. Hayes-Klug, D. M. Seelig, M. A. Wild, L. L. Wolfe, T. R. Spraker, M. W. Miller, C. J. Sigurdson, G. C. Telling, and E. A. Hoover.** 2006. Infectious prions in the saliva and blood of deer with chronic wasting disease. *Science* **314:**133–136.
124. **McGovern, G., K. L. Brown, M. E. Bruce, and M. Jeffrey.** 2004. Murine scrapie infection causes an abnormal germinal centre reaction in the spleen. *J. Comp. Pathol.* **130:**181–194.
125. **Mead, S., M. P. Stumpf, J. Whitfield, J. A. Beck, M. Poulter, T. Campbell, J. B. Uphill, D. Goldstein, M. Alpers, E. M. Fisher, and J. Collinge.** 2003. Balancing selection at the prion protein gene consistent with prehistoric kurulike epidemics. *Science* **300:**640–643.
126. **Medori, R., H. J. Tritschler, A. LeBlanc, F. Villare, V. Manetto, H. Y. Chen, R. Xue, S. Leal, P. Montagna, P. Cortelli, P. Tinuper, P. Avoni, M. Mochi, A. Baruzzi, J. J. Hauw, J. Ott, E. Lugaresi, L. A. Gambetti, and P. Gambetti.** 1992. Fatal familial insomnia, a prion disease with a mutation at codon 178 of the prion protein gene. *N. Engl. J. Med.* **326:**444–449.
127. **Meggendorfer, F.** 1930. Klinische und genealogische Beobachtungen bei einem Fall von spastischer Pseudosklerose Jakobs. *Z. Ges. Neurol. Psychiatr.* **128:**337–341.
128. **Meier, P., N. Genoud, M. Prinz, M. Maissen, T. Rulicke, A. Zurbriggen, A. J. Raeber, and A. Aguzzi.** 2003. Soluble dimeric prion protein binds PrP(Sc) in vivo and antagonizes prion disease. *Cell* **113:**49–60.
129. **Meyer-Luehmann, M., J. Coomaraswamy, T. Bolmont, S. Kaeser, C. Schaefer, E. Kilger, A. Neuenschwander, D. Abramowski, P. Frey, A. L. Jaton, J. M. Vigouret, P. Paganetti, D. M. Walsh, P. M. Mathews, J. Ghiso, M. Staufenbiel, L. C. Walker, and M. Jucker.** 2006. Exogenous induction of cerebral beta-amyloidogenesis is governed by agent and host. *Science* **313:**1781–1784.
130. **Montrasio, F., R. Frigg, M. Glatzel, M. A. Klein, F. Mackay, A. Aguzzi, and C. Weissmann.** 2000. Impaired prion replication in spleens of mice lacking functional follicular dendritic cells. *Science* **288:**1257–1259.
131. **Naslavsky, N., R. Stein, A. Yanai, G. Friedlander, and A. Taraboulos.** 1997. Characterization of detergent-insoluble complexes containing the cellular prion protein and its scrapie isoform. *J. Biol. Chem.* **272:**6324–6331.
132. **Notari, S., S. Capellari, A. Giese, I. Westner, A. Baruzzi, B. Ghetti, P. Gambetti, H. A. Kretzschmar, and P. Parchi.** 2004. Effects of different experimental conditions on the PrPSc core generated by protease digestion: implications for strain typing and molecular classification of CJD. *J. Biol. Chem.* **279:**16797–16804.
133. **Oidtmann, B., D. Simon, N. Holtkamp, R. Hoffmann, and M. Baier.** 2003. Identification of cDNAs from Japanese pufferfish (Fugu rubripes) and Atlantic salmon (Salmo salar) coding for homologues to tetrapod prion proteins. *FEBS Lett.* **538:**96–100.
134. **Padovani, A., M. D'Alessandro, P. Parchi, P. Cortelli, G. P. Anzola, P. Montagna, L. A. Vignolo, R. Petraroli, M. Pocchiari, E. Lugaresi, and P. Gambetti.** 1998. Fatal familial insomnia in a new Italian kindred. *Neurology* **51:**1491–1494.
135. **Pan, K.-M., M. Baldwin, J. Nguyen, M. Gasset, A. Serban, D. Groth, I. Mehlhorn, Z. Huang, R. J. Fletterick, F. E. Cohen, and S. B. Prusiner.** 1993. Conversion of alpha-helices into beta-sheets features in the formation of the scrapie prion proteins. *Proc. Natl. Acad. Sci. USA* **90:**10962–10966.
136. **Parchi, P., R. Castellani, S. Capellari, B. Ghetti, K. Young, S. G. Chen, M. Farlow, D. W. Dickson, A. A. F. Sima, J. Q. Trojanowski, R. B. Petersen, and P. Gambetti.** 1996. Molecular basis of phenotypic variability in sporadic Creutzfeldt-Jakob disease. *Ann. Neurol.* **39:**767–778.
137. **Parchi, P., A. Giese, S. Capellari, P. Brown, W. Schulz-Schaeffer, O. Windl, I. Zerr, H. Budka, N. Kopp, P. Piccardo, S. Poser, A. Rojiani, N. Streichemberger, J. Julien, C. Vital, B. Ghetti, P. Gambetti, and H. Kretzschmar.** 1999. Classification of sporadic Creutzfeldt-Jakob disease based on molecular and phenotypic analysis of 300 subjects. *Ann. Neurol.* **46:**224–233.
138. **Parry, H. B.** 1962. Scrapie: a transmissible and hereditary disease of sheep. *Heredity* **17:**75–105.
139. **Parry, H. B., and B. G. Livett.** 1973. A new hypothalamic pathway to the median eminence containing neurophysin and its hypertrophy in sheep with natural scrapie. *Nature* **242:**63–65.
140. **Peden, A. H., M. W. Head, D. L. Ritchie, J. E. Bell, and J. W. Ironside.** 2004. Preclinical vCJD after blood transfusion in a PRNP codon 129 heterozygous patient. *Lancet* **364:**527–529.
141. **Peretz, D., R. A. Williamson, G. Legname, Y. Matsunaga, J. Vergara, D. R. Burton, S. J. DeArmond, S. B. Prusiner, and M. R. Scott.** 2002. A change in the conformation of prions accompanies the emergence of a new prion strain. *Neuron* **34:**921–932.
142. **Pocchiari, M., S. Schmittinger, and C. Masullo.** 1987. Amphotericin B delays the incubation period of scrapie in intracerebrally inoculated hamsters. *J. Gen. Virol.* **68:** 219–223.
143. **Polymenidou, M., K. Stoeck, M. Glatzel, M. Vey, A. Bellon, and A. Aguzzi.** 2005. Coexistence of multiple PrPSc types in individuals with Creutzfeldt-Jakob disease. *Lancet Neurol.* **4:**805–814.
144. **Prinz, M., M. Heikenwalder, T. Junt, P. Schwarz, M. Glatzel, F. L. Heppner, Y. X. Fu, M. Lipp, and A. Aguzzi.** 2003. Positioning of follicular dendritic cells within the spleen controls prion neuroinvasion. *Nature* **425:**957–962.

145. **Prinz, M., G. Huber, A. J. Macpherson, F. L. Heppner, M. Glatzel, H. P. Eugster, N. Wagner, and A. Aguzzi.** 2003. Oral prion infection requires normal numbers of Peyer's patches but not of enteric lymphocytes. *Am. J. Pathol.* **162:**1103–1111.
146. **Priola, S. A., A. Raines, and W. S. Caughey.** 2000. Porphyrin and phthalocyanine antiscrapie compounds. *Science* **287:**1503–1506.
147. **Prusiner, S. B.** 1989. Creutzfeldt-Jakob disease and scrapie prions. *Alzheimer Dis. Assoc. Disord.* **3:**52–78.
148. **Prusiner, S. B.** 1982. Novel proteinaceous infectious particles cause scrapie. *Science* **216:**136–144.
149. **Prusiner, S. B., D. F. Groth, M. P. McKinley, S. P. Cochran, K. A. Bowman, and K. C. Kasper.** 1981. Thiocyanate and hydroxyl ions inactivate the scrapie agent. *Proc. Natl. Acad. Sci. USA* **78:**4606–4610.
150. **Prusiner, S. B., M. Scott, D. Foster, K. M. Pan, D. Groth, C. Mirenda, M. Torchia, S. L. Yang, D. Serban, G. A. Carlson, P. C. Hoppe, D. Westaway, and S. J. DeArmond.** 1990. Transgenetic studies implicate interactions between homologous PrP isoforms in scrapie prion replication. *Cell* **63:**673–686.
151. **Prusiner, S. B., M. R. Scott, S. J. DeArmond, and F. E. Cohen.** 1998. Prion protein biology. *Cell* **93:**337–348.
152. **Race, R., and B. Chesebro.** 1998. Scrapie infectivity found in resistant species. *Nature* **392:**770. (Letter.)
153. **Radovanovic, I., N. Braun, O. T. Giger, K. Mertz, G. Miele, M. Prinz, B. Navarro, and A. Aguzzi.** 2005. Truncated prion protein and Doppel are myelinotoxic in the absence of oligodendrocytic PrPC. *J. Neurosci.* **25:**4879–4888.
154. **Riek, R., S. Hornemann, G. Wider, M. Billeter, R. Glockshuber, and K. Wüthrich.** 1996. NMR structure of the mouse prion protein domain Prp(121-231). *Nature* **382:**180–182.
155. **Riek, R., S. Hornemann, G. Wider, R. Glockshuber, and K. Wüthrich.** 1997. NMR characterization of the full-length recombinant murine prion protein, mPrP(23-231). *FEBS Lett.* **413:**282–288.
156. **Rivera-Milla, E., C. A. Stuermer, and E. Malaga-Trillo.** 2003. An evolutionary basis for scrapie disease: identification of a fish prion mRNA. *Trends Genet.* **19:**72–75.
157. **Russmann, H., F. Vingerhoets, J. Miklossy, P. Maeder, M. Glatzel, A. Aguzzi, and J. Bogousslavsky.** 2005. Sporadic Creutzfeldt-Jakob disease: a comparison of pathological findings and diffusion weighted imaging. *J. Neurol.* **252:**338–342.
158. **Safar, J., H. Wille, V. Itri, D. Groth, H. Serban, M. Torchia, F. E. Cohen, and S. B. Prusiner.** 1998. Eight prion strains have PrP(Sc) molecules with different conformations. *Nat. Med.* **4:**1157–1165.
159. **Sailer, A., H. Büeler, M. Fischer, A. Aguzzi, and C. Weissmann.** 1994. No propagation of prions in mice devoid of PrP. *Cell* **77:**967–968.
160. **Scott, M., D. Groth, D. Foster, M. Torchia, S. L. Yang, S. J. DeArmond, and S. B. Prusiner.** 1993. Propagation of prions with artificial properties in transgenic mice expressing chimeric PrP genes. *Cell* **73:**979–988.
161. **Scott, M. R., R. Will, J. Ironside, H. O. Nguyen, P. Tremblay, S. J. DeArmond, and S. B. Prusiner.** 1999. Compelling transgenetic evidence for transmission of bovine spongiform encephalopathy prions to humans. *Proc. Natl. Acad. Sci. USA* **96:**15137–15142.
162. **Seeger, H., M. Heikenwalder, N. Zeller, J. Kranich, P. Schwarz, A. Gaspert, B. Seifert, G. Miele, and A. Aguzzi.** 2005. Coincident scrapie infection and nephritis lead to urinary prion excretion. *Science* **310:**324–326.
163. **Shmerling, D., I. Hegyi, M. Fischer, T. Blattler, S. Brandner, J. Gotz, T. Rulicke, E. Flechsig, A. Cozzio, C. von Mering, C. Hangartner, A. Aguzzi, and C. Weissmann.** 1998. Expression of amino-terminally truncated PrP in the mouse leading to ataxia and specific cerebellar lesions. *Cell* **93:**203–214.
164. **Sigurdson, C. J., G. Manco, P. Schwarz, P. Liberski, E. A. Hoover, S. Hornemann, M. Polymenidou, M. W. Miller, M. Glatzel, and A. Aguzzi.** 2006. Strain fidelity of chronic wasting disease upon murine adaptation. *J. Virol.* **80:**12303–12311.
165. **Sigurdson, C. J., K. P. R. Nilsson, S. Hornemann, G. Manco, M. Polymenidou, P. Schwarz, M. Leclerc, P. Hammarström, K. Wüthrich, and A. Aguzzi.** 18 November 2007. Prion strain discrimination using luminescent conjugated polymers. *Nat. Methods* doi:10.1038/nmeth1131.
166. **Silveira, J. R., G. J. Raymond, A. G. Hughson, R. E. Race, V. L. Sim, S. F. Hayes, and B. Caughey.** 2005. The most infectious prion protein particles. *Nature* **437:**257–261.
167. **Solforosi, L., J. R. Criado, D. B. McGavern, S. Wirz, M. Sanchez-Alavez, S. Sugama, L. A. DeGiorgio, B. T. Volpe, E. Wiseman, G. Abalos, E. Masliah, D. Gilden, M. B. Oldstone, B. Conti, and R. A. Williamson.** 2004. Cross-linking cellular prion protein triggers neuronal apoptosis in vivo. *Science* **303:**1514–1516.
168. **Sparkes, R. S., M. Simon, V. H. Cohn, R. E. K. Fournier, J. Lem, I. Klisak, C. Heinzmann, C. Blatt, M. Lucero, T. Mohandas, S. J. DeArmond, D. Westaway, S. B. Prusiner, and L. P. Weiner.** 1986. Assignment of the human and mouse prion protein genes to homologous chromosomes. *Proc. Natl. Acad. Sci. USA* **83:**7358–7362.
169. **Stahl, N., M. A. Baldwin, D. B. Teplow, L. Hood, B. W. Gibson, A. L. Burlingame, and S. B. Prusiner.** 1993. Structural studies of the scrapie prion protein using mass spectrometry and amino acid sequencing. *Biochemistry* **32:**1991–2002.
170. **Stahl, N., D. R. Borchelt, K. Hsiao, and S. B. Prusiner.** 1987. Scrapie prion protein contains a phosphatidylinositol glycolipid. *Cell* **51:**229–240.
171. **Stewart, R. S., P. Piccardo, B. Ghetti, and D. A. Harris.** 2005. Neurodegenerative illness in transgenic mice expressing a transmembrane form of the prion protein. *J. Neurosci.* **25:**3469–3477.
172. **Strumbo, B., S. Ronchi, L. C. Bolis, and T. Simonic.** 2001. Molecular cloning of the cDNA coding for Xenopus laevis prion protein. *FEBS Lett.* **508:**170–174.
173. **Supattapone, S., P. Bosque, T. Muramoto, H. Wille, C. Aagaard, D. Peretz, H. O. Nguyen, C. Heinrich, M. Torchia, J. Safar, F. E. Cohen, S. J. DeArmond, S. B. Prusiner, and M. Scott.** 1999. Prion protein of 106 residues creates an artificial transmission barrier for prion replication in transgenic mice. *Cell* **96:**869–878.
174. **Tagliavini, F., R. A. McArthur, B. Canciani, G. Giaccone, M. Porro, M. Bugiani, P. M. Lievens, O. Bugiani, E. Peri, P. Dall'Ara, M. Rocchi, G. Poli, G. Forloni, T. Bandiera, M. Varasi, A. Suarato, P. Cassutti, M. A. Cervini, J. Lansen, M. Salmona, and C. Post.** 1997. Effectiveness of anthracycline against experimental prion disease in Syrian hamsters. *Science* **276:**1119–1122.
175. **Tanaka, M., P. Chien, N. Naber, R. Cooke, and J. S. Weissman.** 2004. Conformational variations in an infectious protein determine prion strain differences. *Nature* **428:**323–328.
176. **Taraboulos, A., K. Jendroska, D. Serban, S. L. Yang, S. J. DeArmond, and S. B. Prusiner.** 1992. Regional mapping of prion proteins in brain. *Proc. Natl. Acad. Sci. USA* **89:**7620–7624.

177. **Tateishi, J., K. Doh-ura, T. Kitamoto, C. Tanchant, G. Steinmetz, J. M. Warter, and J. W. BoeMard.** 1992. Prion protein gene analysis and transmission studies of Creutzfeldt-Jakob disease, p. 129–138. *In* S. B. Prusiner, J. Collinge, J. Powell, and B. Anderton. (ed.), *Prion Diseases of Humans and Animals*. Ellis Horwood, London, United Kingdom.
178. **Telling, G. C., M. Scott, K. K. Hsiao, D. Foster, S. L. Yang, M. Torchia, K. C. Sidle, J. Collinge, S. J. DeArmond, and S. B. Prusiner.** 1994. Transmission of Creutzfeldt-Jakob disease from humans to transgenic mice expressing chimeric human-mouse prion protein. *Proc. Natl. Acad. Sci. USA* **91:**9936–9940.
179. **Toyama, B. H., M. J. Kelly, J. D. Gross, and J. S. Weissman.** 2007. The structural basis of yeast prion strain variants. *Nature* **449:**233–237.
180. **Tribl, G. G., G. Strasser, J. Zeitlhofer, S. Asenbaum, C. Jarius, P. Wessely, and D. Prayer.** 2002. Sequential MRI in a case of Creutzfeldt-Jakob disease. *Neuroradiology* **44:**223–226.
181. **Trifilo, M. J., T. Yajima, Y. Gu, N. Dalton, K. L. Peterson, R. E. Race, K. Meade-White, J. L. Portis, E. Masliah, K. U. Knowlton, B. Chesebro, and M. B. Oldstone.** 2006. Prion-induced amyloid heart disease with high blood infectivity in transgenic mice. *Science* **313:** 94–97.
182. **Tuo, W., D. Zhuang, D. P. Knowles, W. P. Cheevers, M. S. Sy, and K. I. O'Rourke.** 2001. Prp-c and Prp-Sc at the fetal-maternal interface. *J. Biol. Chem.* **276:** 18229–18234.
183. **Valleron, A. J., P. Y. Boelle, R. Will, and J. Y. Cesbron.** 2001. Estimation of epidemic size and incubation time based on age characteristics of vCJD in the United Kingdom. *Science* **294:**1726–1728.
184. **Weissmann, C.** 1991. A 'unified theory' of prion propagation. *Nature* **352:**679–683.
185. **Wilesmith, J. W., J. B. Ryan, W. D. Hueston, and L. J. Hoinville.** 1992. Bovine spongiform encephalopathy: epidemiological features 1985 to 1990. *Vet. Rec.* **130:** 90–94.
186. **Will, R. G., J. W. Ironside, M. Zeidler, S. N. Cousens, K. Estibeiro, A. Alperovitch, S. Poser, M. Pocchiari, A. Hofman, and P. G. Smith.** 1996. A new variant of Creutzfeldt-Jakob disease in the UK. *Lancet* **347:**921–925.
187. **Wille, H., M. D. Michelitsch, V. Guenebaut, S. Supattapone, A. Serban, F. E. Cohen, D. A. Agard, and S. B. Prusiner.** 2002. Structural studies of the scrapie prion protein by electron crystallography. *Proc. Natl. Acad. Sci. USA* **99:**3563–3568.
188. **Windl, O., M. Dempster, J. P. Estibeiro, R. Lathe, R. Desilva, T. Esmonde, R. Will, A. Springbett, T. A. Campbell, K. C. L. Sidle, M. S. Palmer, and J. Collinge.** 1996. Genetic basis of Creutzfeldt-Jakob disease in the United Kingdom—a systematic analysis of predisposing mutations and allelic variation in the Prnp gene. *Hum. Genet.* **98:**259–264.
189. **Zeidler, M., R. J. Sellar, D. A. Collie, R. Knight, G. Stewart, M. A. Macleod, J. W. Ironside, S. Cousens, A. C. Colchester, D. M. Hadley, R. G. Will, and A. F. Colchester.** 2000. The pulvinar sign on magnetic resonance imaging in variant Creutzfeldt-Jakob disease. *Lancet* **355:**1412–1418.
190. **Zerr, I., M. Pocchiari, S. Collins, J. P. Brandel, J. de Pedro Cuesta, R. S. Knight, H. Bernheimer, F. Cardone, N. Delasnerie-Laupretre, N. Cuadrado Corrales, A. Ladogana, M. Bodemer, A. Fletcher, T. Awan, A. Ruiz Bremon, H. Budka, J. L. Laplanche, R. G. Will, and S. Poser.** 2000. Analysis of EEG and CSF 14-3-3 proteins as aids to the diagnosis of Creutzfeldt-Jakob disease. *Neurology* **55:**811–815.

Index

Page numbers followed by f indicate figures; those followed by t indicate tables.